Preface to the Seventh Edition

In this edition, *Plumb's Veterinary Drug Handbook* continues with its mission to serve as a single volume reference to assist veterinarians, other health professionals, and animal caretakers in providing optimal drug therapy for veterinary patients. In addition to updating all the monographs, 20+ new systemic drug full monographs (see below) and several new ophthalmic and topical dermatologic drug monographs have been added. Additional information on compounding dosage forms has been added to many monographs.

Several monographs have been "retired" in this edition, primarily due to their withdrawal from the marketplace and/or being replaced in therapy with newer, ostensibly better, drug compounds. Two sections have been removed from the appendix. After consulting with several veterinary oncologists, I decided that listing chemotherapy drug protocols was not in the best interest of patient care. They change often and the drugs used have enough inherent safety issues that I believe "chemo" use in private practices must be carefully considered, in collaboration with oncologists and oncology-specific resources. The therapeutic diet tables have also been removed, again because they rapidly change and are outdated shortly after publication. Links to websites that provide this information are listed in the appendix.

New Systemic Monographs: Albumin, Alfaxalone, Butaphosphan (+Cyanocobalamin), Carbamazepine, Cefovecin, Cortisone Acetate, Desflurane, Fosfomycin, Immune Globulin, Fat Emulsion (IV), Lanthanum Carbonate, Mavacoxib, Metergoline, Metyrapone, Miltefosine, Pregabalin, Remifentanil, Robenacoxib, Rocuronium, Toceranib, Trazodone, and Trypan Blue.

"Retired" Systemic Monographs: Carbenicillin, Cefoperazone, Ethacrynic Acid, Ipecac Syrup, Methoxyflurane, Streptokinase, and Ticarcillin (alone).

Donald Plumb
March 2011

About the Author

Donald C. Plumb, PharmD., was formerly Director of Pharmacy Services and Hospital Director at the University of Minnesota's Veterinary Medical Center. Now retired from the University of Minnesota, he focuses full-time on providing veterinary drug information to veterinarians, other health professionals, and animal caretakers.

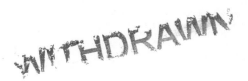

Notes and Cautions

Dosages and Extra-Label Use of Medications

Dosages for the various species for the drugs listed in this reference come from a variety of sources and are referenced to their source in the appendix. While a sincere effort has been made to assure that the dosages and information included in this book are accurate and reflect the original source's information, errors can occur; it is recommended that the reader refer to the original reference or the approved labeling information of the product for additional information and verification of all dosages.

Except for labeled dosages for veterinary-approved products (for a given species and indication,) dosages listed in this reference should be considered "extra-label" and are not necessarily endorsed by the manufacturer, the Food and Drug Administration (FDA) or this author. Veterinarians are responsible as per the Animal Medical Drug Use Clarification Act (AMDUCA) for the appropriate use of medications. The Animal Medicinal Drug Use Clarification Act of 1994 (AMDUCA) allows veterinarians to prescribe extralabel uses of certain approved animal drugs and approved human drugs for animals under certain conditions. Extralabel (or extra-label) use refers to the use of an approved drug in a manner that is not in accordance with the approved label directions. The key constraints of AMDUCA are that any extralabel use must be by or on the order of a veterinarian within the context of a veterinarian-client-patient relationship, must not result in violative residues in food-producing animals, and the use must be in conformance with the implementing regulations published at 21 CFR Part 530. A list of drugs specifically prohibited from extra-label use appears in the Code of Federal Regulations. For additional information go to the FDA-Center for Veterinary Medicine Website at: http://www.fda.gov/cvm/

Abbreviations: OTC & Rx

In addition to the abbreviations used in writing prescriptions (*e.g., tid*, q8h, etc.—see the abbreviation list in the appendix), the terms OTC or Rx are found in parentheses after a listed dosage form. If Rx, the drug is considered to be a prescription or legend product, and requires a prescription. OTC denotes that the item is available "over-the-counter" and does not legally require a prescription for purchase.

Trade and Proprietary Names

The notation used to signify trade names or proprietary names is an italicized, capitalized name followed by a ® (*e.g., Amoxi-Tabs®*). This notation may not accurately represent the drug's official registered copyright, trademark, or licensed status (*e.g.,* ™, etc.). For clarity, no use of ® or *italics* are used in the index.

Drug Interactions

Drug interaction identification and evaluation is in its infancy in veterinary medicine, as relatively little specific information is known on the subject for the variety of species treated. While drug interactions can be clinically significant and potentially life-threatening in veterinary patients, most of the interactions listed in the monographs are derived from human medicine (which is only slightly more informed than veterinary medicine on this topic) and are often included primarily to serve as cautions to the prescriber to be alert for unforeseen outcomes, or to enhance monitoring associated with the drug therapy. Additionally, it is likely there are potentially many other clinically significant interactions between drugs that are not listed; prescribers are reminded that the risk for adverse drug interactions occurring increases with the number of different drugs given to an individual patient.

Disclaimer

The author/publisher/distributor assume no responsibility for and make no warranty with respect to results that may be obtained from the uses, procedures, or dosages listed, and do not necessarily endorse such uses, procedures, or dosages. The author/publisher shall not be liable to any person whatsoever for any damages, or equivalencies, or by reason of any misstatement or error, negligent or otherwise obtained in this work. Should the purchaser not wish to be bound by the above, he/she may return the reference to the distributor for a full refund.

Contents

APPENDIX

Ophthalmic Products

ACARBOSE

(ay-**kar**-bose)   Precose®

ORAL ANTIDIABETIC

Prescriber Highlights

➤ Antihyperglycemic agent that reduces the rate & amount of glucose absorbed from the gut after a meal; may be useful for mild reductions in blood glucose in dogs or cats. Unlikely to be effective when used as sole therapy.

➤ Contraindications: Underweight animals, known hypersensitivity, diabetic ketoacidosis, inflammatory bowel disease, colonic ulceration, partial intestinal obstruction or predisposition to obstruction, chronic intestinal disease with marked disorders of digestion or absorption & when excessive gas formation would be detrimental.

➤ Dose–dependent loose stools, diarrhea & flatulence are the adverse effects most likely to be noted.

➤ Give with meals (preferably right before); drug is not very useful if feeding ad libitum.

➤ Expense may be an issue, but generics are now available.

Uses/Indications

May be useful for mild reductions in blood glucose concentrations (250–350 mg/dL range) in dogs and cats with non-insulin-dependent diabetes mellitus and as adjunctive treatment of insulin dependent diabetes mellitus. Acarbose is unlikely to give adequate glucose control when used alone and most recommend dietary therapy and other antihyperglycemic agents (e.g., insulin) instead.

Pharmacology/Actions

Acarbose competitively inhibits pancreatic alpha-amylase and alpha-glucosidases found in the small intestine. This delays the digestion of complex carbohydrates and disaccharides to glucose and other monosaccharides. Glucose is absorbed lower in the GI tract in lesser amounts than is normal thereby reducing insulin requirements during the postprandial hyperglycemic phase. Acarbose has no effect on lactase.

Pharmacokinetics

In dogs about 4% of an oral dose is absorbed; in humans only about 2% of an oral dose is absorbed from the gut that is then excreted by the kidneys. Practically all remaining drug in the gut is metabolized in the GI tract by intestinal bacteria. Patients with severe renal dysfunction attain serum levels approximately 5 times those of normal subjects.

Contraindications/Precautions/Warnings

Acarbose is contraindicated in patients with known hypersensitivity to the drug, diabetic ketoacidosis, inflammatory bowel disease, colonic ulceration, partial intestinal obstruction or predisposition to obstruction, chronic intestinal disease with marked disorders of digestion or absorption, and when excessive gas formation would be detrimental. Acarbose is not indicated in patients of low body weight (some say normal body weight as well) as it may have deleterious effects on nutrition status. Use caution in patients with renal dysfunction or severe liver disease.

Adverse Effects

Adverse effects reported in cats include flatulence, soft stools and diarrhea; in dogs, diarrhea and weight loss. Adverse effects are more likely at higher doses.

While acarbose alone does not cause hypoglycemia, it may contribute to it by reducing the rate and amount of glucose absorbed when the patient is receiving other hypoglycemic agents (insulin, oral hypoglycemics).

Reproductive/Nursing Safety

Safety in pregnancy has not been established; weigh any potential risks versus benefits in pregnant animals. In humans, the FDA categorizes this drug as category **B** for use during pregnancy (*Animal studies have not yet demonstrated risk to the fetus, but there are no adequate studies in pregnant women; or animal studies have shown an adverse effect, but adequate studies in pregnant women have not demonstrated a risk to the fetus in the first trimester of pregnancy, and there is no evidence of risk in later trimesters.*)

Overdosage/Acute Toxicity

Acute overdosages are likely to cause only diarrhea and flatulence. No treatment should be necessary. Should acute hypoglycemia occur secondary to other antihypoglycemics, parenteral glucose should be administered. If treating orally, use glucose (do not use sucrose).

Drug Interactions

The following drug interactions have either been reported or are theoretical in humans or animals receiving acarbose and may be of significance in veterinary patients:

■ **CHARCOAL:** Intestinal adsorbents may reduce the efficacy of acarbose

■ **DIGOXIN:** Acarbose may reduce digoxin blood concentrations

■ **HYPERGLYCEMIC AGENTS** (**corticosteroids, thiazides, estrogens, phenothiazines, thyroid hormones,** and **calcium channel blockers**): May negate the effects of acarbose

■ **PANCREATIN, PANCRELIPASE, OR AMYLASE:** Exogenous enzyme formulations may reduce the efficacy of acarbose

Laboratory Considerations

■ Increased **serum aminotransferase** levels have been noted in some humans taking high dosages for a long period

Doses

■ **DOGS:**

a) For dogs poorly controlled with insulin and dietary therapy when another reason for the poor control cannot be identified: Initially 12.5–25 mg total dose per dog PO with each meal. Give only at the time of feeding. May increase dose after two weeks to 50 mg per dog and then to 100 mg per dog (in large dogs, >25 kg) if response has been inadequate. There is a greater chance of diarrhea at the higher dosages. (Nelson 2005)

b) 12.5–20 mg (total dose) per meal PO (Daminet 2003)

■ **CATS:**

a) 12.5–25 mg (total dose) PO with meals. When acarbose is used with a low carbohydrate diet it may improve glycemic control and reduce insulin dependence. (Scherk 2005)

b) 12.5 mg per cat PO twice daily with meals. May be able to reduce insulin dosage and thereby reduce hypoglycemia occurrence. (Greco 2002)

c) 12.5–20 mg (total dose) per meal PO (Daminet 2003)

Monitoring

■ Serum glucose

■ Adverse effects (diarrhea)

Client Information

■ Give right before feeding for best results.

■ Diarrhea and/or gas most likely side effect(s); contact veterinarian if serious or continues.

■ Acarbose does not cause low blood sugar, but it may add to it if the animal is getting other drugs (including insulin) that lower blood sugar; watch for signs of low blood sugar: seizures (convulsions), collapse, rear leg weakness or paralysis, muscle twitching, unsteadiness, tiredness, or depression. If these occur call veterinarian immediately.

■ May take up to two weeks for the drug to work at its peak effect.

Chemistry/Synonyms

A complex oligosaccharide antihyperglycemic agent, acarbose occurs as white to off-white powder, is soluble in water and has a pKa of 5.1.

Acarbose may also be known as: Bay-g-5421, *Precose®, Asucrose®, Glicobase®, Glucobay®, Glucor®, Glumida®,* or *Prandase®.*

Storage/Stability

Do not store tablets above 25°C (77°F); protect from moisture.

Compatibility/Compounding Considerations

Tablets may be split or crushed and mixed with food just prior to administration.

Dosage Forms/Regulatory Status

VETERINARY-LABELED PRODUCTS: None

HUMAN-LABELED PRODUCTS:

Acarbose Oral Tablets: 25 mg, 50 mg & 100 mg; *Precose®* (Bayer), generic; (Rx)

References

Daminet, S (2003). Canine and Feline Diabetes Mellitus. Proceedings: World Small Animal Veterinary Assoc. World Congress. Accessed via: Veterinary Information Network. http://goo.gl/YRCPp

Greco, D (2002). Treatment of feline type 2 diabetes mellitus with oral hypoglycemic agents. Proceedings: Atlantic Coast Veterinary Conf. Accessed via: Veterinary Information Network. http://goo.gl/z0AuC

Nelson, R (2005). Diabetes Mellitus. *Textbook of Veterinary Internal Medicine: Diseases of the Dog and Cat 6th Ed.* S Ettinger and E Feldman Eds. Philadelphia, Elsevier. 2: 1563–1591.

Scherk, M (2005). Management of the Diabetic Cat. Proceedings: Western Veterinary Conference. Accessed via: Veterinary Information Network. http://goo.gl/dGiYr

ACEMANNAN

(ase-man-in)

NON-SPECIFIC IMMUNOSTIMULANT/ ANTIVIRAL

Prescriber Highlights

▶ Non-specific injectable immunostimulant that has been tried in FeLV-, FIV, or FIP-positive cats, & vaccine–induced fibrosarcomas (intralesional)

▶ Use is controversial; little, if any controlled study documentation supporting efficacy in veterinary medicine

▶ Adverse effects include: Possible hypersensitivity reactions, localized necrosis at injection sites; bolus IV administration can cause salivation, weakness, collapse, tachycardia, tachypnea; intralesional injection can cause prolonged pain at site; intraperitoneal injection can cause monocyte infiltrates on peritoneal surfaces, liver, & spleen with resultant abdominal pain, diarrhea and vomiting.

▶ Topical products available; potentially can reduce wound healing time

Uses/Indications

Veterinary acemannan injection is labeled for use in dogs or cats as an aid in the treatment (*i.e.,* surgery) and clinical management of fibrosarcoma. It has been tried as a treatment for FeLV, FIV, and FIP infections in cats, but clinical efficacy has not been adequately proven by controlled clinical studies.

Acemannan has been used in dogs as an intralesional injection for papillomatosis. It reportedly has been used in horses, but no specific information on this was located.

Pharmacology/Actions

Acemannan's immunostimulant activity is thought as a result of inducing increases in TNF-alpha, interferon, and IL-1. At injection sites, increased lymphocytic infiltration and accumulation have been noted. In tissue cultures, acemannan has suppressed HIV replication.

Pharmacokinetics

No information was located.

Contraindications/Precautions/Warnings

The manufacturer lists no contraindications to using acemannan, however, it should not be used in patients who have demonstrated past severe hypersensitivity reactions to it.

Adverse Effects

While the manufacturer does not list any specific adverse effects associated with use, hypersensitivity or localized injection reactions (*e.g.,* necrosis) are possible. Hyperactivity, lethargy, fever and hypotension have been reported with systemic use of the drug.

Bolus IV administration can cause salivation, weakness, collapse, hypotension, tachycardia and tachypnea. Intralesional injection can cause bleeding or prolonged pain at the injection site. Intraperitoneal injection can cause monocyte infiltrates on peritoneal surfaces, lung, liver, and spleen. Abdominal pain, vomiting and diarrhea have been reported with high dose, intraperitoneal injections.

Reproductive/Nursing Safety

No specific information was located on reproductive or nursing safety. The product label states, "The effects of this compound have not been studied in pregnant animals" and, also, ". . . the chemical nature of acemannan and the absence of significant toxicity in several animal species suggest the compound is not a teratogen."

Overdosage/Acute Toxicity

Single IP injections of 50 mg/kg in dogs resulted in no significant signs of toxicity. Acemannan fed orally to dogs at rates of up to 1.5 g/kg/day for 90 days showed no significant effects.

Drug Interactions

None were identified.

Laboratory Considerations

None were identified.

Doses

■ **DOGS/CATS:**

For labeled indications (aid in treatment and management of fibrosarcoma):

a) Prior to use, reconstitute with 10 mL sterile diluent. Five to 10 minutes may be necessary for complete dissolution. Shake well before using. Use within 4 hours after rehydration. Administer by concurrent intraperitoneal (IP) and intralesional injections weekly for a minimum of 6 treatments. Recommended IP dose is 1 mg/kg. Recommended intralesional dose is 2 mg injected deep into each tumor mass. When used as a prelude to surgery, give concurrent IP and intralesional injections weekly. Continue until delineation, necrosis or maximum tumor enlargement due to edema and immune cellular infiltration occur. Rapid necrosis, which accompanies this response, may happen within 2 to 4 weeks. Surgical excision is recommended immediately upon delineation, necrosis or maximum tumor enlargement. (Label Information; *Acemannan Immunostimulant*—VPL)

Monitoring

■ Clinical efficacy

■ Adverse effects (most likely local reactions)

Client Information

■ This compound is recommended for use by veterinary professionals only

■ Clients should be made aware of the "investigational" nature of using acemannan systemically; adverse effects are possible

Chemistry

Acemannan is a water soluble, complex carbohydrate polymer that is derived from Aloe vera. It is a long-chained polydispersed beta-(1,4)-acetylated polymannose with interspersed O-acetyl groups with a mannose:acetyl ratio of approximately 1:1.

Storage/Stability

Acemannan injection should be stored at temperatures less than 35°C (95°F); protect from extremes of heat or light.

Dosage Forms/Regulatory Status

VETERINARY-LABELED PRODUCTS:

Acemannan 10 mg vial with 10 mL vial of diluent (sterile saline) in kits of two vials (one of each) or eight vials (4 of each): *Acemannan Immunostimulant*® (VPL); OTC Biologic. Labeled for use in dogs or cats. **Note:** This product is a USDA-licensed biologic and is not an FDA-approved product.

Note: There are also topical products labeled for veterinary use that contain acemannan including a wound dressing and cleansing foam. Trade name is *CarraVet*® (VPL).

HUMAN-LABELED PRODUCTS: No systemic products located

ACEPROMAZINE MALEATE

(ase-*pro*-ma-zeen)   PromAce®, Aceproject®

PHENOTHIAZINE SEDATIVE/
TRANQUILIZER

Prescriber Highlights

▶ Negligible analgesic effects

▶ Dosage may need to be reduced in debilitated or geriatric animals, those with hepatic or cardiac disease, or when combined with other agents

▶ Inject IV slowly; do not inject into arteries

▶ Certain dog breeds (e.g., giant breeds, sight hounds) and dogs with the MDR1 mutation may be overly sensitive to effects and require dosage reduction

▶ May cause significant hypotension, cardiac rate abnormalities, hypo- or hyperthermia

▶ May cause penis protrusion in large animals (esp. horses)

Uses/Indications

Acepromazine is FDA-approved for use in dogs, cats, and horses. Labeled indications for dogs and cats include: ". . . as an aid in controlling intractable animals . . . alleviate itching as a result of skin irritation; as an antiemetic to control vomiting associated with motion sickness" and as a preanesthetic agent. The use of acepromazine as a sedative/tranquilizer in the treatment of adverse behaviors in dogs or cats has largely been supplanted by newer, effective agents that have fewer adverse effects. Its use for sedation during travel is controversial and many no longer recommend drug therapy for this purpose. In combination with analgesics (*e.g.*, opioids), acepromazine can potentiate their analgesic effect (neuroleptanalgesia).

In horses, acepromazine is labeled ". . . as an aid in controlling fractious animals," and in conjunction with local anesthesia for various procedures and treatments. It is also commonly used in horses as a pre-anesthetic agent at very small doses to help control behavior.

Although not FDA-approved, it is used as a tranquilizer (see doses) in other species such as swine, cattle, rabbits, sheep and goats. Acepromazine has also been shown to reduce the incidence of halothane-induced malignant hyperthermia in susceptible pigs.

Pharmacology/Actions

Acepromazine is a phenothiazine neuroleptic agent. While the exact mechanisms of action are not fully understood, the phenothiazines block post-synaptic dopamine receptors in the CNS and may also inhibit the release of, and increase the turnover rate of dopamine. They are thought to depress portions of the reticular activating system that assists in the control of body temperature, basal metabolic rate, emesis, vasomotor tone, hormonal balance, and alertness. Additionally, phenothiazines have varying degrees of anticholinergic, antihistaminic, antispasmodic, and alpha-adrenergic blocking effects.

The primary desired effect for the use of acepromazine in veterinary medicine is its tranquilizing action. Additional pharmacologic actions that acepromazine possess, include antiemetic, antispasmodic, and hypothermic actions. Some researchers have reported that acepromazine has anticonvulsant activity, but in veterinary medicine it is generally felt that phenothiazines should not be used in epileptic animals or those susceptible to seizures (*e.g.*, postmyelography) as it may precipitate seizures.

Acepromazine may decrease respiratory rates, but studies have demonstrated that little or no effect occurs with regard to the blood gas picture, pH or oxyhemoglobin saturation. A dose dependent decrease in hematocrit is seen within 30 minutes after dosing in horses and dogs. Hematocrit values in horses may decrease up to 50% of pre-dose values; this is probably due to increased splenic sequestration of red cells.

Besides lowering arterial blood pressure in dogs, acepromazine causes increases in central venous pressure, a vagally induced bradycardic effect and transient sinoatrial arrest. The bradycardia may be negated by a reflex tachycardic effect secondary to decreases in blood pressure. Acepromazine also has antidysrhythmic effects. Acepromazine has been demonstrated to inhibit the arrhythmias induced by ultra-short acting barbiturates, and protect against the ventricular fibrillatory actions of halothane and epinephrine. Other pharmacologic actions are discussed in the adverse effects section below.

Pharmacokinetics

The pharmacokinetics of acepromazine has been studied in the horse (Ballard et al. 1982). The drug has a fairly high volume of distribution (6.6 L/kg), and is more than 99% protein bound. The onset of action is fairly slow, requiring up to 15 minutes following IV administration, with peak effects seen in 30–60 minutes. The elimination half-life in horses is approximately 3 hours.

Acepromazine is metabolized in the liver with both conjugated and unconjugated metabolites eliminated in the urine. Metabolites may be found in equine urine up to 96 hours after dosing.

Contraindications/Precautions/Warnings

Animals may require lower dosages of general anesthetics following acepromazine. Use cautiously and in smaller doses in animals with hepatic dysfunction, mild cardiac disease, or general debilitation. Because of its hypotensive effects, acepromazine is relatively contraindicated in patients with significant cardiac disease, hypovolemia, hypotension or shock. Acepromazine has been said to decrease platelet aggregation and its use avoided in patients with coagulopathies or thrombocytopenia, but a study in 6 healthy dogs showed no platelet inhibition (Conner *et al.* 2009). Phenothiazines are relatively contraindicated in patients with tetanus or strychnine intoxication due to effects on the extrapyramidal system.

Intravenous injections should be made slowly. Do not administer intra-arterially in horses since it may cause severe CNS excitement/depression, seizures and death. Because of its effects on thermoregulation, use cautiously in very young or debilitated animals.

Two retrospective studies in dogs (McConnell *et al.* 2007), (Tobias & Marioni-Henry 2006) did not show any increase in seizure activity after administration of acepromazine.

When used alone, acepromazine has no analgesic effects; treat animals with appropriate analgesics to control pain. The tranquilization effects of acepromazine can be overridden and it cannot always be counted upon when used as a restraining agent. Do not administer to racing animals within 4 days of a race.

In dogs, acepromazine's effects may be individually variable and breed dependent. Dogs with MDR1 mutations (many Collies, Australian shepherds, etc.) may develop a more pronounced sedation that persists longer than normal. The Veterinary Clinical Pharmacology Lab at Washington State recommends reducing the dose by 25% in dogs heterozygous for the MDR1 mutation (mutant/normal) and by 30–50% in dogs homozygous for the MDR1 mutation (mutant/mutant). (WSU-VetClinPharmLab 2009)

Acepromazine should be used very cautiously as a restraining agent in aggressive dogs as it may make the animal more prone to startle and react to noises or other sensory inputs. In geriatric patients, very low doses have been associated with prolonged effects of the drug. Giant breeds and greyhounds may be extremely sensitive to the drug while terrier breeds are somewhat resistant to its effects. Atropine may be used with acepromazine to help negate its bradycardic effects.

In addition to the legal aspects (not FDA-approved) of using acepromazine in cattle, the drug may cause regurgitation of ruminal contents when inducing general anesthesia.

Adverse Effects

Acepromazine's effect on blood pressure (hypotension) is well described and an important consideration in therapy. This effect is thought to be mediated by both central mechanisms and through the alpha-adrenergic actions of the drug. Cardiovascular collapse (secondary to bra-

dycardia and hypotension) has been described in all major species. Dogs may be more sensitive to these effects than other animals.

Acepromazine has been shown to decrease tear production in cats (Ghaffari *et al.* 2010).

In male large animals acepromazine may cause protrusion of the penis; in horses, this effect may last 2 hours. Stallions should be given acepromazine with caution as injury to the penis can occur with resultant swelling and permanent paralysis of the penis retractor muscle. Other clinical signs that have been reported in horses include excitement, restlessness, sweating, trembling, tachypnea, tachycardia and, rarely, seizures and recumbency.

Acepromazine's effects of causing penis extension in horses and prolapse of the membrana nictitans in horses and dogs, may make its use unsuitable for show animals. There are also ethical considerations regarding the use of tranquilizers prior to showing an animal or having the animal examined before sale.

Occasionally an animal may develop the contradictory clinical signs of aggressiveness and generalized CNS stimulation after receiving acepromazine. IM injections may cause transient pain at the injection site.

Reproductive/Nursing Safety

In humans, the FDA categorizes phenothiazines as category **C** for use during pregnancy (*Animal studies have shown an adverse effect on the fetus, but there are no adequate studies in humans; or there are no animal reproduction studies and no adequate studies in humans.*) In a separate system evaluating the safety of drugs in canine and feline pregnancy (Papich 1989), this drug is categorized as in class: **B** (*Safe for use if used cautiously. Studies in laboratory animals may have uncovered some risk, but these drugs appear to be safe in dogs and cats or these drugs are safe if they are not administered when the animal is near term.*)

Overdosage/Acute Toxicity

The LD_{50} in mice is 61 mg/kg after IV dosage and 257 mg/kg after oral dose. While a toxicity study in dogs reported no adverse effects in dogs receiving 20–40 mg/kg over 6 weeks, since 2004 the ASPCA Animal Poison center has documented adverse effects in dogs receiving single doses between 20–42 mg/kg. Dogs have survived oral dosages up to 220 mg/kg, but overdoses can cause serious hypotension, CNS depression, pulmonary edema and hyperemia.

There were 70 exposures to acepromazine maleate reported to the ASPCA Animal Poison Control Center (APCC) during 2008–2009. In these cases 49 were dogs with 37 showing clinical signs and the remaining 21 reported cases were cats with 17 cats showing clinical signs. Common findings in dogs recorded in decreasing frequency included ataxia, sedation, lethargy, depression, and protrusion of the third eyelid, somnolence, bradycardia, and recumbency. Common findings in cats recorded in decreasing frequency included sedation, ataxia, lethargy, protrusion of the third eyelid, and depression.

Because of the apparent relatively low toxicity of acepromazine, most overdoses can be handled by monitoring the animal and treating clinical signs as they occur; massive oral overdoses should definitely be treated by emptying the gut if possible. Hypotension should not be treated initially with fluids; alpha-adrenergic pressor agents (epinephrine, phenylephrine) can be considered if fluids do not maintain adequate blood pressure. Seizures may be controlled with barbiturates or diazepam. Doxapram has been suggested as an antagonist to the CNS depressant effects of acepromazine.

Drug Interactions
The following drug interactions have either been reported or are theoretical in humans or animals receiving acepromazine or other phenothiazines and may be of significance in veterinary patients:

- **ACETAMINOPHEN:** Possible increased risk for hypothermia
- **ANTACIDS:** May cause reduced GI absorption of oral phenothiazines
- **ANTIDIARRHEAL MIXTURES** (*e.g.*, **Kaolin/pectin, bismuth subsalicylate mixtures**): May cause reduced GI absorption of oral phenothiazines
- **CNS DEPRESSANT AGENTS** (**barbiturates, narcotics, anesthetics,** etc.): May cause additive CNS depression if used with acepromazine
- **DOPAMINE:** Acepromazine may impair the vasopressive action of dopamine.
- **EMETICS:** Acepromazine may reduce the effectiveness of emetics
- **EPINEPHRINE, EPHEDRINE:** Phenothiazines block alpha-adrenergic receptors; concomitant use of epinephrine or ephedrine can lead to unopposed beta-activity causing vasodilation and increased cardiac rate
- **METOCLOPRAMIDE:** May increase risks for extrapyramidal adverse effects
- **OPIATES:** May enhance the hypotensive effects of acepromazine; dosages of acepromazine are generally reduced when used with an opiate
- **ORGANOPHOSPHATE AGENTS:** Acepromazine should not be given within one month of worming with these agents as their effects may be potentiated
- **PHENYTOIN:** Metabolism may be decreased if given concurrently with phenothiazines
- **PROCAINE:** Activity may be enhanced by phenothiazines
- **PROPRANOLOL:** Increased blood levels of both drugs may result if administered with phenothiazines

- **QUINIDINE:** With phenothiazines may cause additive cardiac depression

Doses
Note: The manufacturer's dose of 0.5–2.2 mg/kg for dogs and cats is considered by many clinicians to be 10 times greater than is necessary for most indications. Give IV doses slowly; allow at least 15 minutes for onset of action.

- **DOGS:**
  a) 0.55–2.2 mg/kg PO or 0.55–1.1 mg/kg IV, IM or SC (Package Insert; *PromAce®* —Fort Dodge)
  b) Restraint/sedation: 0.025–0.2 mg/kg IV; maximum of 3 mg or 0.1–0.25 mg/kg IM; Preanesthetic: 0.1–0.2 mg/kg IV or IM; maximum of 3 mg; 0.05–1 mg/kg IV, IM or SC (Morgan 1988)
  c) To reduce anxiety in the painful patient (not a substitute for analgesia): 0.05 mg/kg IM, IV or SC; do not exceed 1 mg total dose (Carroll 1999)
  d) Premedication: 0.03–0.05 mg/kg IM or 1–3 mg/kg PO at least one hour prior to surgery (not as reliable) (Hall & Clarke 1983)
  e) As a premedicant with morphine: acepromazine 0.05 mg/kg IM; morphine 0.5 mg/kg IM (Pablo 2003)

- **CATS:**
  a) 1.1–2.2 mg/kg PO, IV, IM or SC (Package Insert; *PromAce®* —Fort Dodge)
  b) To reduce anxiety in the painful patient (not a substitute for analgesia): 0.05 mg/kg IM, IV or SC; do not exceed 1 mg total dose (Carroll 1999)
  c) Restraint/sedation: 0.05–0.1 mg/kg IV, maximum of 1 mg (Morgan 1988)
  d) 0.11 mg/kg with atropine (0.045–0.067 mg/kg) 15–20 minutes prior to ketamine (22 mg/kg IM). (Booth 1988)

- **FERRETS:**
  a) As a tranquilizer: 0.25–0.75 mg/kg IM or SC; has been used safely in pregnant jills; use with caution in dehydrated animals. (Finkler 1999)
  b) 0.1–0.25 mg/kg IM or SC; may cause hypotension/hypothermia (Williams 2000)

- **RABBITS/RODENTS/SMALL MAMMALS:**
  a) Rabbits: As a tranquilizer: 1 mg/kg IM, effect should begin in 10 minutes and last for 1–2 hours (Booth 1988)
  b) Rabbits: As a premed: 0.1–0.5 mg/kg SC; 0.25–2 mg/kg IV, IM, SC 15 minutes prior to induction. No analgesia; may cause hypotension/hypothermia. (Ivey & Morrisey 2000)
  c) Mice, Rats, Hamsters, Guinea pigs, Chinchillas: 0.5 mg/kg IM. Do *not* use in Gerbils. (Adamcak & Otten 2000)

■ **CATTLE:**

a) Sedation: 0.01–0.02 mg/kg IV or 0.03–0.1 mg/kg IM (Booth 1988)

b) 0.05–0.1 mg/kg IV, IM or SC (Howard 1986)

c) Sedative one hour prior to local anesthesia: 0.1 mg/kg IM (Hall & Clarke 1983)

■ **HORSES:** (**Note**: ARCI UCGFS Class 3 Drug)

a) 0.044–0.088 mg/kg (2–4 mg/100 lbs. body weight) IV, IM or SC (Package Insert; *PromAce®*—Fort Dodge)

b) For mild sedation: 0.01–0.05 mg/kg IV or IM. Onset of action is about 15 minutes for IV; 30 minutes for IM (Taylor, P. 1999)

c) 0.02–0.05 mg/kg IM or IV as a preanesthetic (Booth 1988)

d) Neuroleptanalgesia: 0.02 mg/kg given with buprenorphine (0.004 mg/kg IV) or xylazine (0.6 mg/kg IV) (Thurmon & Benson 1987)

e) For adjunctive treatment of laminitis (developmental phase): 0.066–0.1 mg/kg 4–6 times per day (Brumbaugh *et al.* 1999)

■ **SWINE:**

a) 0.1–0.2 mg/kg IV, IM, or SC (Howard 1986)

b) 0.03–0.1 mg/kg (Hall & Clarke 1983)

c) For brief periods of immobilization: acepromazine 0.5 mg/kg IM followed in 30 minutes by ketamine 15 mg/kg IM. Atropine (0.044 mg/kg IM) will reduce salivation and bronchial secretions. (Lumb & Jones 1984)

■ **SHEEP & GOATS:**

a) 0.05–0.1 mg/kg IM (Hall & Clarke 1983)

■ **ZOO, EXOTIC, WILDLIFE SPECIES:**

For use of acepromazine in zoo, exotic and wildlife medicine refer to specific references, including:

a) *Zoo Animal and Wildlife Immobilization and Anesthesia.* West, G, Heard, D, Caulkett, N. (eds.). Blackwell Publishing, 2007.

b) *Handbook of Wildlife Chemical Immobilization, 3rd Ed.* Kreeger, T.J. and J.M. Arnemo. 2007.

c) *Restraint and Handling of Wild and Domestic Animals.* Fowler, M (ed.), Iowa State University Press, 1995

d) *Exotic Animal Formulary, 3rd Ed.* Carpenter, J.W., Saunders. 2005

e) The 2009 American Association of Zoo Veterinarian Proceedings by D. K. Fontenot also has several dosages listed for restraint, anesthesia, and analgesia for a variety of drugs for carnivores and primates. VIN members can access them at: http://goo.gl/BHRih or http://goo.gl/9UJse

Monitoring

■ Cardiac rate/rhythm/blood pressure if indicated and possible to measure

■ Degree of tranquilization

■ Male horses should be checked to make sure penis retracts and is not injured

■ Body temperature (especially if ambient temperature is very hot or cold)

Client Information

■ May discolor the urine to a pink or red-brown color; this is not abnormal

■ Acepromazine is FDA-approved for use in dogs, cats, and horses not intended for food

Chemistry/Synonyms

Acepromazine maleate (formerly acetylpromazine) is a phenothiazine derivative that occurs as a yellow, odorless, bitter tasting powder. One gram is soluble in 27 mL of water, 13 mL of alcohol, and 3 mL of chloroform.

Acepromazine Maleate may also be known as: acetylpromazine maleate, "ACE", ACP, *Aceproject®*, *Aceprotabs®*, *PromAce®*, *Plegicil®*, *Notensil®*, and *Atravet®*.

Storage/Stability

Store protected from light. Tablets should be stored in tight containers. Acepromazine injection should be kept from freezing.

Although controlled studies have not documented the compatibility of these combinations, acepromazine has been mixed with atropine, buprenorphine, chloral hydrate, ketamine, meperidine, oxymorphone, and xylazine. Both glycopyrrolate and diazepam have been reported to be physically **incompatible** with phenothiazines, however, glycopyrrolate has been demonstrated to be **compatible** with promazine HCl for injection.

Compatibility/Compounding Considerations

A study (Taylor, B.J. *et al.* 2009) evaluating the stability, sterility, pH, particulate formation and efficacy in laboratory rodents of compounded ketamine, acepromazine and xylazine (KAX) supported the finding that the drugs are stable and efficacious for at least 180 days after mixing if stored at room temperature in the dark.

Combinations of acepromazine mixed with atropine, buprenorphine, chloral hydrate, meperidine, and oxymorphone have been commonly used, but studies documenting their compatibility and stability were not located. Both glycopyrrolate and diazepam have been reported to be physically **incompatible** with phenothiazines, however glycopyrrolate has been demonstrated to be **compatible** with promazine HCl for injection.

Dosage Forms/Regulatory Status

VETERINARY-LABELED PRODUCTS:

Acepromazine Maleate for Injection: 10 mg/mL

for injection in 50 mL vials; *PromAce®* (Fort Dodge); generic; (Rx). FDA-approved forms available for use in dogs, cats and horses not intended for food.

Acepromazine Maleate Tablets: 5 mg, 10 mg & 25 mg in bottles of 100 and 500 tablets; *PromAce®* (Fort Dodge); generic; (Rx). FDA-approved forms available for use in dogs, cats and horses not intended for food.

When used in an extra-label manner in food animals, it is recommended to use the withdrawal periods used in Canada: Meat: 7 days; Milk: 48 hours. Contact FARAD (see appendix) for further guidance.

The ARCI (Racing Commissioners International) has designated this drug as a class 3 substance. See the appendix for more information.

HUMAN-LABELED PRODUCTS: None

References

Adamcak, A & B Otten (2000). Rodent Therapeutics. *Vet Clin NA: Exotic Anim Pract* **3:**1(Jan): 221–240.

Booth, NH (1988). Drugs Acting on the Central Nervous System. *Veterinary Pharmacology and Therapeutics – 6th Ed.* NH Booth and LE McDonald Eds. Ames, Iowa State University Press: 153–408.

Brumbaugh, G, H Lopez, et al. (1999). The pharmacologic basis for the treatment of laminitis. *The Veterinary Clinics of North America: Equine Practice* **15:**2(August).

Carroll, G (1999). Common Premedications for pain management: Pain management made simple. Proceedings: The North American Veterinary Conference, Orlando.

Conner, B, R Hanel, et al. (2009). The effects of acepromazine upon adenosine diphosphate– and arachidonic acid– mediated platelet activation in healthy dogs. Proceedings: IVECCS. Accessed via: Veterinary Information Network. http://goo.gl/qKFbT

Finkler, M (1999). Anesthesia in Ferrets. Proceedings: Central Veterinary Conference, Kansas City.

Ghaffari, MS, A Malmasi, et al. (2010). Effect of acepromazine or xylazine on tear production as measured by Schirmer tear test in normal cats. *Veterinary Ophthalmology* **13**(1): 1–3.

Hall, LW & KW Clarke (1983). *Veterinary Anesthesia 8th Ed.* London, Bailliere Tindall.

Howard, JL, Ed. (1986). *Current Veterinary Therapy 2, Food Animal Practice.* Philadelphia, W.B. Saunders.

Ivey, E & J Morrisey (2000). Therapeutics for Rabbits. *Vet Clin NA: Exotic Anim Pract* **3:**1(Jan): 183–216.

Lumb, WV & EW Jones (1984). *Veterinary Anesthesia, 2nd Ed.* Philadelphia, Lea & Febiger.

McConnell, J, R Kirby, et al. (2007). Administration of acepromazine maleate to 31 dogs with a history of seizures. *Journal of Veterinary Emergency and Critical Care* **17**(3): 262–267.

Morgan, RV, Ed. (1988). *Handbook of Small Animal Practice.* New York, Churchill Livingstone.

Pablo, L (2003). Total IV anesthesia in small animals. Proceedings: World Small Animal Veterinary Assoc World Congress. Accessed via: Veterinary Information Network. http://goo.gl/e1v31

Taylor, BJ, SA Orr, et al. (2009). Beyond–Use Dating of Extemporaneously Compounded Ketamine, Acepromazine, and Xylazine: Safety, Stability, and Efficacy over Time. *Journal of the American Association for Laboratory Animal Science* **48**(6): 718–726.

Taylor, P (1999). Tranquilizers in the horse – Choosing the right one. Proceedings: The North American Veterinary Conference, Orlando.

Thurmon, JC & GJ Benson (1987). Injectable anesthetics and anesthetic adjuncts. *Vet Clin North Am (Equine Practice)* **3**(1): 15–36.

Tobias, KM & K Marioni–Henry (2006). A retrospective study on the use of acepromazine maleate in dogs with seizures. *Journal of the American Animal Hospital Association* **42**(4): 283–289.

Williams, B (2000). Therapeutics in Ferrets. *Vet Clin NA: Exotic Anim Pract* **3:**1(Jan): 131–153.

WSU–VetClinPharmLab (2009). "Problem Drugs." http://goo.gl/aIGlM.

ACETAMINOPHEN

(ah-seet-a-*min*-a-fen)
Tylenol®, APAP, Paracetamol

ORAL ANALGESIC, ANTIPYRETIC

Prescriber Highlights

▶ Contraindicated in cats at any dosage; ferrets may be as sensitive to acetaminophen as cats

▶ At recommended dosages, not overly toxic to dogs, rodents, or rabbits. Dogs are more susceptible to red blood cell toxicity than are humans, so dose carefully.

▶ Often used in combined dosage forms with codeine; see codeine monograph for more information

Uses/Indications

Acetaminophen is occasionally used as an oral analgesic in dogs and small mammals. It may be particularly beneficial in dogs with renal dysfunction for the treatment of chronic pain conditions. In situations where moderate pain occurs, it may be used in combination products containing codeine, hydrocodone, or tramadol. See the codeine, hydrocodone and tramadol monographs for more information on the use of acetaminophen combination preparations.

Pharmacology/Actions

Acetaminophen's exact mechanism of actions are not completely understood; it produces analgesia and antipyresis via a weak, reversible, isoform-nonspecific inhibition of cyclooxygenase (COX-3; Cox-1–v1). Unlike aspirin, it does not possess significant antiinflammatory activity nor inhibit platelet function when given at clinically recommended dosages.

Pharmacokinetics

Specific pharmacokinetic information in domestic animals was not located. In humans, acetaminophen is rapidly and nearly completely absorbed from the gut and is rapidly distributed into most tissues. Approximately 25% is plasma protein bound. Dogs apparently exhibit dose dependent metabolism (saturable).

Contraindications/Precautions/Warnings

Acetaminophen is contraindicated in cats at any dosage. Severe methemoglobinemia, hematuria, and icterus can be seen. Cats are unable to significantly glucuronidate acetaminophen leading to toxic metabolites being formed and resultant toxicity. Acetaminophen should not be used in ferrets as they may be as sensitive to acetaminophen as are cats. At this time, acetaminophen should not be used in Sugar Gliders or Hedgehogs as its safety has not been determined.

Dogs do not metabolize acetaminophen as well as humans and its use must be judicious. While dogs are not as sensitive to acetaminophen as cats, they may also be susceptible to methemoglobinemia when given high dosages. In dogs, it is generally not recommended to use acetaminophen during the immediate post-operative phase (first 24 hours) due to an increased risk of hepatotoxicity.

Adverse Effects
Because acetaminophen is not routinely used in veterinary medicine, experience on its adverse effect profile is limited. At suggested dosages in dogs, there is some potential for renal, hepatic, GI, and hematologic effects occurring.

Reproductive/Nursing Safety
Absolute reproductive safety has not been established, but acetaminophen is apparently relatively safe for occasional use in pregnancy (no documented problems in humans). Animal data was not located. In humans, the FDA categorizes this drug as category *B* for use during pregnancy (*Animal studies have not yet demonstrated risk to the fetus, but there are no adequate studies in pregnant women; or animal studies have shown an adverse effect, but adequate studies in pregnant women have not demonstrated a risk to the fetus in the first trimester of pregnancy, and there is no evidence of risk in later trimesters.*) In a separate system evaluating the safety of drugs in canine and feline pregnancy (Papich 1989), this drug is categorized as in class: *C* (*These drugs may have potential risks. Studies in people or laboratory animals have uncovered risks, and these drugs should be used cautiously as a last resort when the benefit of therapy clearly outweighs the risks.*)

Acetaminophen is excreted in milk in low concentrations with reported milk:plasma ratios of 0.91 to 1.42 at 1 and 12 hours, respectively. In nursing human infants, no adverse effects have been reported.

Overdosage/Acute Toxicity
Because of the potentially severe toxicity associated with acetaminophen, consultation with an animal poison control center is highly recommended (see appendix). Effects can include methemoglobinemia, liver necrosis, renal effects, facial and paw swelling, and keratoconjunctivitis sicca (KCS). Liver effects are more common in dogs; facial and paw swelling and methemoglobinemia are more common in cats.

There were 1192 exposures to acetaminophen reported to the ASPCA Animal Poison Control Center (APCC) during 2008–2009. In these cases, 1083 were dogs with 187 showing clinical signs, 99 were cats with 47 showing clinical signs, 6 were birds with 1 showing clinical signs, 1 was a pig that showed clinical signs. The remaining 3 cases involved 2 ferrets and 1 lagomorph that showed no clinical signs. Common findings in dogs recorded in decreasing frequency included vomiting, lethargy, methemoglobinemia, edema of the face, elevated ALT, chemosis (conjunctival swelling/edema), and trembling. Common findings in cats recorded in decreasing frequency included methemoglobinemia, cyanosis, lethargy, vomiting, hypothermia, and anorexia.

For overdosage in dogs or cats, standard gut emptying techniques and supportive care should be administered when applicable. Further treatment with acetylcysteine, s-adenosyl methionine (SAMe), oxygen, and blood transfusions may be warranted (Richardson 2000), (Aronson & Drobatz 1996), (Mariani & Fulton 2001), (Steenbergen 2003).

Drug Interactions
The following drug interactions have either been reported or are theoretical in humans or animals receiving acetaminophen and may be of significance in veterinary patients:

■ **OTHER ANALGESICS:** Chronic use with acetaminophen may lead to renal pathologies

■ **BARBITURATES:** Increased conversion of acetaminophen to hepatotoxic metabolites; potentially increased risk for hepatotoxicity

■ **DOXORUBICIN:** May deplete hepatic glutathione, thereby leading to increased hepatic toxicity

■ **HALOTHANE:** Acetaminophen is not recommended for use for post-operative analgesia in animals that received halothane anesthesia

■ **ISONIAZID:** Possible increased risk of hepatotoxicity

■ **PHENOTHIAZINES:** Possible increased risk for hypothermia

■ **PROPYLENE GLYCOL:** Foods containing propylene glycol (often found in wet cat foods) may increase the severity of acetaminophen-induced methemoglobinemia or Heinz body formation.

■ **WARFARIN:** While acetaminophen is relatively safe to use, large doses may potentiate anticoagulant effects

Laboratory Considerations
■ False positive results may occur for urinary **5-hydroxyindoleacetic acid**

Doses
Note: For dosages of acetaminophen/codeine, and acetaminophen/hydrocodone combination products refer to the codeine and hydrocodone monographs.

■ **DOGS:**

As an analgesic:
a) 15 mg/kg PO q8h (Dodman 1992), (McLaughlin 2000)
b) 10 mg/kg PO q12h (Kelly 1995)

c) 10–15 mg/kg PO q12h for 5 days (Gaynor 2008)

d) In the treatment of degenerative myelopathy (in German Shepherds): 5 mg/kg PO (not to exceed 20 mg/kg per day) (Clemmons 1991)

■ **RABBITS/RODENTS/SMALL MAMMALS:**

As an analgesic:

a) Using Children's *Tylenol®*: 1–2 mg/mL in drinking water. Effective for controlling low-grade nociception. (Huerkamp 2000)

b) Mice, Rats, Gerbils, Hamsters, Guinea pigs, Chinchillas: 1–2 mg/mL in drinking water (Adamcak & Otten 2000)

Monitoring

■ When used at recommended doses for pain control in otherwise healthy animals, little monitoring should be necessary. However, with chronic therapy, occasional liver, renal and hematologic monitoring may be warranted, particularly when clinical signs occur.

Client Information

■ Follow directions carefully; do not exceed dosage or increase dosing frequency. Do not administer to cats or ferrets for any reason. Keep out of reach of children.

Chemistry/Synonyms

A synthetic non-opiate analgesic, acetaminophen (also known as paracetamol) occurs as a crystalline, white powder with a slightly bitter taste. It is soluble in boiling water and freely soluble in alcohol. Acetaminophen is known in the U.K. as paracetamol.

Acetaminophen may also be known as: paracetamol, MAPAP or APAP; many trade names are available.

Storage/Stability

Acetaminophen products should be stored at temperatures less than 40°C. Do not freeze oral solution or suspension.

Dosage Forms/Regulatory Status

VETERINARY-LABELED PRODUCTS: None

The ARCI (Racing Commissioners International) has designated this drug as a class 4 substance. See the appendix for more information.

HUMAN-LABELED PRODUCTS:

There are many different trade names and products of acetaminophen available. The most commonly known trade name is *Tylenol®*. Acetaminophen is commonly available in 325 mg, 500 mg, 650 mg tablets; 80 mg chewable tablets; 650 mg extended release tablets; 160 mg, 500 mg, & 650 mg caplets; 500 mg gelcaps; 325 mg, & 500 mg capsules, 80 mg and 160 mg sprinkle capsules; 80 mg/0.8 mL drops; 80 mg/2.5 mL, 80 mg/5 mL, 120 mg/5 mL, & 160 mg/5 mL elixirs; 160 mg/5 mL, 500 mg/15 mL, and 100 mg/mL liquids and solutions; 80 mg, 120 mg, 125 mg, 300 mg, 325 mg and 650 mg suppositories. Combinations with other analgesics (aspirin, codeine phosphate, hydrocodone, tramadol, oxycodone or propoxyphene) are also available.

References

Adamcak, A & B Otten (2000). Rodent Therapeutics. *Vet Clin NA: Exotic Anim Pract* 3:1(Jan): 221–240.

Aronson, L & KJ Drobatz (1996). Acetaminophen Toxicosis in 17 Cats. *Vet Emerg Crit Care* 6: 65–69.

Clemmons, R (1991). Therapeutic considerations for degenerative myelopathy of German Shepherds. Proceedings of the Ninth Annual Veterinary Medical Forum, New Orleans, American College of Veterinary Internal Medicine.

Dodman, N (1992). Advantages and guidelines for using antiprostaglandins. *The Veterinary Clinics of North America; Small Animal Practice* 22(2: March): 367–369.

Gaynor, JS (2008). Control of Cancer Pain in Veterinary Patients. *Veterinary Clinics of North America–Small Animal Practice* 38(6): 1429–+.

Huerkamp, M (2000). The use of analgesics in rodents and rabbits. Emory University, Division of Animal Resources.

Kelly, M (1995). Pain. *Textbook of Veterinary Internal Medicine: Diseases of the Dog and Cat*. S Ettinger and E Feldman Eds. Philadelphia, WB Saunders: 21–25.

Mariani, C & R Fulton (2001). Atypical Reaction to Acetaminophen Intoxication in a Dog. *Vet Emerg Crit Care* 10: 123–126.

McLaughlin, R (2000). Management of Osteoarthritic Pain. *Vet ClinNA: Small Anim Pract* 30:4(July): 933–947.

Richardson, J (2000). Management of Acetaminophen and Ibuprofen Toxicosis in Dogs and Cats. *Vet Emerg Crit Care* 10: 285–291.

Steenbergen, V (2003). Acetaminophen and Cats A Dangerous Combination. *Vet Tech*: 43–45.

ACETAZOLAMIDE
ACETAZOLAMIDE SODIUM

(ah-seet-a-*zole*-a-mide)
Diamox®, Dazamide®

CARBONIC ANHYDRASE INHIBITOR DIURETIC; ANTIGLAUCOMA AGENT

Prescriber Highlights

▶ Used sometimes for metabolic alkalosis or glaucoma in small animals; HYPP in horses

▶ Contraindicated in patients with significant hepatic, renal, pulmonary or adrenocortical insufficiency, hyponatremia, hypokalemia, hyperchloremic acidosis or electrolyte imbalance

▶ Give oral doses with food if GI upset occurs

▶ Electrolytes & acid/base status should be monitored with chronic or high dose therapy

▶ Monitor with tonometry if using for glaucoma

Uses/Indications

Acetazolamide has been used principally in veterinary medicine for its effects on aqueous humor production in the treatment of glaucoma, metabolic alkalosis, and for its diuretic action. It may be useful as an adjunctive treatment for syringomyelia in dogs. Acetazolamide's use in small animals is complicated by a relatively high occurrence of adverse effects.

In horses, acetazolamide is used as an adjunctive treatment for hyperkalemic periodic paralysis (HYPP).

In humans, the drug has been used as adjunctive therapy for epilepsy and for acute high-altitude sickness.

Pharmacology/Actions

The carbonic anhydrase inhibitors act by a noncompetitive, reversible inhibition of the enzyme carbonic anhydrase. This reduces the formation of hydrogen and bicarbonate ions from carbon dioxide thereby reducing the availability of these ions for active transport into body secretions.

Pharmacologic effects of the carbonic anhydrase inhibitors include: decreased formation of aqueous humor, thus reducing intraocular pressure, increased renal tubular secretion of sodium and potassium and, to a greater extent, bicarbonate, leading to increased urine alkalinity and volume. Acetazolamide has some anticonvulsant activity, which is independent of its diuretic effects (mechanism is not fully understood, but may be due to carbonic anhydrase or a metabolic acidosis effect).

In anesthetized cats, methazolamide did not, but acetazolamide did reduce the hypoxic ventilatory response. The authors believe this not as a result of carbonic anhydrase inhibition, but due to acetazolamide's effects on carotid bodies or type I cells (Teppema *et al.* 2006).

Pharmacokinetics

The pharmacokinetics of this agent have apparently not been studied in domestic animals. One report (Roberts 1985) states that after a dose of 22 mg/kg, the onset of action is 30 minutes; maximal effects occur in 2–4 hours; duration of action is about 4–6 hours in small animals.

In humans, the drug is well absorbed after oral administration with peak levels occurring within 1–3 hours. It is distributed throughout the body with highest levels found in the kidneys, plasma and erythrocytes. Acetazolamide has been detected in the milk of lactating dogs and it crosses the placenta (in unknown quantities). Within 24 hours of administration, an average of 90% of the drug is excreted unchanged into the urine by tubular secretion and passive reabsorption processes.

Contraindications/Precautions/Warnings

Carbonic anhydrase inhibitors are contraindicated in patients with significant hepatic disease (may precipitate hepatic coma), renal or adrenocortical insufficiency, hyponatremia, hypo-

kalemia, hyperchloremic acidosis, or electrolyte imbalance. They should not be used in patients with severe pulmonary obstruction that are unable to increase alveolar ventilation or in those who are hypersensitive to them. Long-term use of carbonic anhydrase inhibitors is contraindicated in patients with chronic, noncongestive, angle-closure glaucoma as angle closure may occur and the drug may mask the condition by lowering intraocular pressures.

Acetazolamide should be used with caution in patients with severe respiratory acidosis or having preexisting hematologic abnormalities. Cross sensitivity between acetazolamide and antibacterial sulfonamides may occur.

Adverse Effects

Potential adverse effects that may be encountered include: GI disturbances, CNS effects (sedation, depression, weakness, excitement, etc.), hematologic effects (bone marrow depression), renal effects (crystalluria, dysuria, renal colic, polyuria), hypokalemia, hyperglycemia, hyponatremia, hyperuricemia, hepatic insufficiency, dermatologic effects (rash, etc.), and hypersensitivity reactions.

At the dosages used for HYPP in horses adverse effects are reportedly uncommon.

Reproductive/Nursing Safety

Acetazolamide has been implicated in fetal abnormalities in mice and rats when used at high (10X) dosages and fetal toxicity has been noted when the drug has been used in pregnant humans. In humans, the FDA categorizes this drug as category *C* for use during pregnancy *(Animal studies have shown an adverse effect on the fetus, but there are no adequate studies in humans; or there are no animal reproduction studies and no adequate studies in humans.)*

In humans, the manufacturer states that either nursing or the drug must be discontinued if the mother is receiving acetazolamide. Veterinary significance is not clear.

Overdosage/Acute Toxicity

Information regarding overdosage of this drug was not located. In the event of an overdose, it is recommended to contact an animal poison control center. Monitor serum electrolytes, blood gases, volume status, and CNS status during an acute overdose; treat symptomatically and supportively.

Drug Interactions

The following drug interactions have either been reported or are theoretical in humans or animals receiving acetazolamide and may be of significance in veterinary patients:

■ **ALKALINE URINE:** Drugs where acetazolamide-caused alkaline urine may affect their excretion rate: Decreased urinary excretion of **quinidine, procainamide, tricyclic antidepressants;** Increased urinary excretion of **salicylates, phenobarbital**

■ **ASPIRIN** (or **other salicylates**): Increased

risk of acetazolamide accumulation and toxicity; increased risk for metabolic acidosis

■ **DIGOXIN:** As acetazolamide may cause hypokalemia, increased risk for toxicity

■ **INSULIN:** Rarely, carbonic anhydrase inhibitors interfere with the hypoglycemic effects of insulin

■ **METHENAMINE COMPOUNDS:** Acetazolamide may negate methenamine effects in the urine

■ **DRUGS AFFECTING POTASSIUM (corticosteroids, amphotericin B, corticotropin, or other diuretics):** Concomitant use may exacerbate potassium depletion

■ **PRIMIDONE:** Decreased primidone concentrations

Laboratory Considerations

■ By alkalinizing the urine, carbonic anhydrase inhibitors may cause false positive results in determining **urine protein** when using bromphenol blue reagent (*Albustix®, Albutest®, Labstix®*), sulfosalicylic acid (*Bumintest®, Exton's Test Reagent®*), nitric acid ring test, or heat and acetic acid test methods

■ Carbonic anhydrase inhibitors may **decrease iodine uptake** by the thyroid gland in hyperthyroid or euthyroid patients

Doses

Directions for reconstitution of injection: Reconstitute 500 mg vial with at least 5 mL of Sterile Water for Injection; use within 24 hours after reconstitution.

■ **DOGS:**

For adjunctive treatment of metabolic alkalosis:

a) 10 mg/kg four times daily (may aggravate volume contraction and hypokalemia) (Hardy and Robinson 1986)

For adjunctive therapy of glaucoma:

a) 10–25 mg/kg divided 2–3 times daily (Brooks 2002)

b) 50–75 mg/kg PO 2–3 times a day (Bedford 2003)

c) 50 mg/kg IV one time; 7 mg/kg, PO three times daily (Vestre 1985)

For adjunctive therapy of hydrocephalus in pediatric patients:

a) 0.1 mg/kg PO q8h (Coates 2002)

■ **CATS:**

For adjunctive therapy of glaucoma:

a) 50 mg/kg IV once; 7 mg/kg, PO three times daily (Vestre 1985)

■ **HORSES:** (**Note:** ARCI UCGFS Class 4 Drug)

For adjunctive therapy of hyperkalemic periodic paralysis (HYPP):

a) 2.2–4.4 mg/kg PO twice daily (Schott II 2004)

b) 0.5–2.2 mg/kg PO twice daily (Mayhew 2005)

c) 2–3 mg/kg PO q8-12h when diet adjustment does not control episodes. (Valberg 2008)

■ **RUMINANTS:**

a) 6–8 mg/kg IV, IM, or SC (Howard 1986)

■ **SWINE:**

a) 6–8 mg/kg IV, IM, or SC (Howard 1986)

Monitoring

■ Intraocular pressure tonometry (if used for glaucoma)

■ Blood gases if used for alkalosis

■ Serum electrolytes

■ Baseline CBC with differential and periodic retests if using chronically

■ Other adverse effects

Client Information

■ Give with food if using oral preparation and GI upset occurs

■ Notify veterinarian if abnormal bleeding or bruising occurs or if animal develops tremors or a rash

Chemistry/Synonyms

A carbonic anhydrase inhibitor, acetazolamide occurs as a white to faintly yellowish-white, odorless, crystalline powder with pK_as of 7.4 and 9.1. It is very slightly soluble in water, sparingly soluble in hot water (90–100°C) and alcohol. Acetazolamide sodium occurs as a white lyophilized solid and is freely soluble in water. The injection has a pH of 9.2 after reconstitution with Sterile Water for Injection.

Acetazolamide may also known as: acetazolam, acetazolamidum, or sodium acetazolamide; many trade names are available.

Storage/Stability

Acetazolamide products should be stored at room temperature.

To prepare parenteral solution: reconstitute with at least 5 mL of Sterile Water for Injection. After reconstitution, the injection is stable for one week when refrigerated, but as it contains no preservatives, it should be used within 24-hours.

Compatibility/Compounding Considerations

Acetazolamide sodium for injection is reportedly physically **compatible** with all commonly used IV solutions and cimetidine HCl for injection.

COMPOUNDED PREPARATION STABILITY: Acetazolamide oral suspension compounded from commercially available tablets has been published (Allen, 1996). Triturating twelve (12) 250 mg tablets with 60 mL of *Ora-Plus®* and *qs ad* to 120 mL with *Ora-Sweet®* (or *Ora-Sweet® SF*) yields a 25 mg/mL suspension that retains >90% potency for 60 days stored at both 5°C and 25°C. The stability of acetazolamide aqueous liquids decreases at pH values above 9. The optimal stability is reported to be between 3 and 5. Compounded preparations of acetazolamide should be protected from light.

Dosage Forms/Regulatory Status

VETERINARY-LABELED PRODUCTS: None

The ARCI (Racing Commissioners International) has designated this drug as a class 4 substance. See the appendix for more information.

HUMAN-LABELED PRODUCTS:

Acetazolamide Oral Tablets: 125 mg, 250 mg; generic; (Rx)

Acetazolamide Extended-Release Oral Capsules: 500 mg; *Diamox Sequels*® (Barr); generic (Rx)

Acetazolamide Injection (lyophilized powder for solution): 500 mg; generic; (Rx)

References

Allen, L.V. & M.A. Erickson (1996). Stability of acetazolamide, allopurinol, azathioprine, clonazepam, and flucytosine in extemporaneously compounded oral liquids. *Am J Health Syst Pharm* 53(16): 1944–1949.

Bedford, P (2003). Glaucoma–Is effective treatment a reality. Proceedings: World Small Animal Veterinary Association World Congress. Accessed via: Veterinary Information Network. http://goo.gl/93MTL

Brooks, DE (2002). Glaucoma–Medical and Surgical Treatment. Proceedings: Western Veterinary Conference. Proceedings: Veterinary Information Network. http://goo.gl/LwKdh

Coates, J (2002). Seizures in the pediatric dog and cat. Proceedings: ACVIM Forum. Accessed via: Veterinary Information Network. http://goo.gl/9iCR0

Howard, JL, Ed. (1986). *Current Veterinary Therapy 2, Food Animal Practice*. Philadelphia, W.B. Saunders.

Mayhew, J (2005). Differential Diagnosis for Botulism. Proceedings: ACVIM2005. Accessed via: Veterinary Information Network. http://goo.gl/GIADB

Roberts, SE (1985). Assessment and management of the ophthalmic emergency. *Comp CE* 7(9): 739–752.

Schott II, H (2004). Drugs action on the urinary system. *Equine Clinical Pharmacology*. J Bertone and L Horspool Eds., Elsevier: 155–175.

Teppema, LJ, H Bijl, et al. (2006). The carbonic anhydrase inhibitors methazolamide and acetazolamide have different effects on the hypoxic ventilatory response in the anaesthetized cat. *Journal of Physiology–London* 574(2): 565–572.

Valberg, S (2008). Muscle Tremors in Horses. Proceedings: Western Veterinary Conference. Accessed via: Veterinary Information Network. http://goo.gl/xNHsO

Vestre, WA (1985). Ophthalmic Diseases. *Handbook of Small Animal Therapeutics*. LE Davis Ed. New York, Chirchill Livingstone: 549–575.

ACETIC ACID

(ah-*see*-tick *ass*-id)   Vinegar

GI ACIDIFIER

Prescriber Highlights

▶ Used primarily for treatment of non-protein nitrogen-induced ammonia toxicosis (secondary to urea poisoning, etc.) in ruminants or enterolith prevention in horses

▶ Contraindicated if potential lactic acidosis (grain overload, rumen acidosis) is possible

▶ Given via stomach tube

Uses/Indications

Acetic acid is used via its acidifying qualities in ruminants to treat non-protein nitrogen-induced (*e.g.*, urea poisoning) ammonia toxicosis. It is also used as a potential treatment to prevent enterolith formation in horses by reducing colonic pH.

Pharmacology/Actions

Acetic acid in the rumen lowers pH due to shifting ammonia to ammonium ions and reducing absorption. It may also slow the hydrolysis of urea.

Pharmacokinetics

No information was noted.

Contraindications/Precautions/Warnings

Should not be administered to ruminants until potential lactic acidosis (grain overload, rumen acidosis) is ruled out.

Adverse Effects

Because of the unpleasant taste and potential for causing mucous membrane irritation, acetic acid is generally recommended for administration via stomach tube.

Overdosage/Acute Toxicity

When used for appropriate indications there is little likelihood of serious toxicity occurring after minor overdoses. Due to its potential corrosiveness, the greatest concern would occur if a concentrated form of acetic acid was mistakenly used. However, one human patient who had glacial acetic acid used instead of 5% acetic acid during colposcopy (cervix) demonstrated no detectable harm.

Drug Interactions

There are no documented drug interactions with oral acetic acid, but because of its acidic qualities it could, potentially, affect the degradation of several drugs in the gut.

Doses

■ **CATTLE/RUMINANTS:**

For cattle with putrefaction of rumen associated with a high rumen pH:

a) 4–10 liters of vinegar (Constable 1993)

For treatment of urea poisoning:

a) Using 5% acetic acid (vinegar) infuse 2–6 liters (for cattle) into rumen; may be repeated as necessary if clinical signs reoccur. Recovery ranges from 8–24 hours. A post-recovery pro-biotic rumen inoculation may enhance the gain and productivity of urea poisoned animals. (Hall 2006)

■ **HORSES:**

For enterolith prevention:

a) Using vinegar: 250 mL/450 kg body weight PO once daily (Robinson 1992)

Chemistry/Synonyms

Glacial acetic acid is $C_2H_4O_2$. Acetic acid has a distinctive odor and a sharp acid taste. It is miscible with water, alcohol or glycerin. Much confusion can occur with the percentages of $C_2H_4O_2$ contained in various acetic acid solutions. Acetic Acid USP is defined as having a concentration of 36–37% $C_2H_4O_2$. Diluted Acetic Acid NF contains 5.7–6.3% w/v of $C_2H_4O_2$. Solutions containing approximately 3–5% w/v of $C_2H_4O_2$ are commonly known as vinegar. Be certain of the concentration of the product you are using and your dilutions.

Acetic acid may also be known as: E260, eisessig (glacial acetic acid), essigsaure, etanoico, or ethanoic acid.

Storage/Stability
Acetic acid solutions should be stored in airtight containers.

Compatibility/Compounding Considerations
If diluting more concentrated forms of acetic acid to concentrations equivalent to vinegar (3-5%), use safety precautions to protect eyes and skin. It is strongly recommended to have someone check your calculations to prevent potentially serious consequences.

Dosage Forms/Regulatory Status
VETERINARY-LABELED PRODUCTS: None

HUMAN-LABELED PRODUCTS: None
There are no systemic products commercially available. Acetic acid (in various concentrations) may be purchased from chemical supply houses. Distilled white vinegar is available in gallon sizes from grocery stores.

References
Hall, J (2006). Urea and Nitrate Poisoning of Ruminants. Proceedings: Western Veterinary Conference. Accessed via: Veterinary Information Network. http://goo.gl/7CdEa

ACETOHYDROXAMIC ACID

(ah-seet-oh-*hy*-drox-am-ik) Lithostat®, AHA

UREASE INHIBITOR

Prescriber Highlights

▶ Used occasionally in dogs for persistent struvite uroliths & persistent urease-producing bacteriuria

▶ Contraindicated in patients with renal impairment & during pregnancy; do not use in cats

▶ Adverse effects are common & can include GI effects (anorexia, vomiting, mouth/esophageal ulcers), hemolytic anemia, hyperbilirubinemia & bilirubinuria

▶ Monitor renal function (incl. urinalysis), CBC's, & bilirubin levels

Uses/Indications
Acetohydroxamic acid can be used in dogs as adjunctive therapy in some cases of recurrent urolithiasis or in the treatment of persistent urinary tract infections caused by the following bacteria: *E. coli, Klebsiella, Morganella morganii, Staphylococci* spp., and *Pseudomonas aeruginosa.* Adverse effects limit its usefulness.

Pharmacology/Actions
AHA inhibits urease thereby reducing production of urea and subsequent urinary concentrations of ammonia, bicarbonate and carbonate. While the drug does not directly reduce urine pH, by reducing ammonia and bicarbonate production by urease-producing bacteria, it prevents increases in urine pH. The drug may act synergistically with several antimicrobial agents (*e.g.,* carbenicillin, gentamicin, clindamycin, trimethoprim-sulfa or chloramphenicol) in treating some urinary tract infections. The drug's effects on urinary pH and infection also indirectly inhibit the formation of urinary calculi (struvite, carbonate-apatite).

Pharmacokinetics
No canine specific data was located. In humans, the drug is rapidly absorbed after PO administration. Absolute bioavailability "in animals" is reported to be 50–60%. AHA is well distributed throughout body fluids. It is partially metabolized to acetamide, which is active; 36–65% of a dose is excreted in the urine unchanged, and 9–14% excreted in the urine as acetamide. The remainder is reportedly excreted as CO_2 via the respiratory tract.

Contraindications/Precautions/Warnings
AHA is contraindicated in patients with poor renal function (*e.g.,* serum creatinine >2.5 mg/dL) or when it is not specifically indicated (see Indications).

Acetohydroxamic acid is reportedly very toxic in cats and should not be used in felines.

Adverse Effects
In dogs, GI effects (anorexia, vomiting, mouth/esophageal ulcers), hemolytic anemia, hyperbilirubinemia and bilirubinuria have been reported. Other potential adverse effects include: CNS disturbances (anxiety, depression, tremulousness), hematologic effects (reticulocytosis, bone marrow depression), phlebitis, and skin rashes/alopecia. Effects on bilirubin metabolism have also been reported.

Reproductive/Nursing Safety
AHA use is considered contraindicated during pregnancy. In pregnant beagles, doses of 25 mg/kg/day caused cardiac, coccygeal, and abdominal wall abnormalities in puppies. At high doses (>750 mg/kg) leg deformities have been noted in test animals. Higher doses (1500 mg/kg) caused significant encephalopathologies. In humans, the FDA categorizes this drug as category **X** for use during pregnancy (*Studies in animals or humans demonstrate fetal abnormalities or*

adverse reaction; reports indicate evidence of fetal risk. The risk of use in pregnant women clearly outweighs any possible benefit.)

Overdosage/Acute Toxicity
In humans, mild overdoses have resulted in hemolysis after several weeks of treatment, particularly in patients with reduced renal function. Acute overdoses are expected to cause clinical signs such as anorexia, tremors, lethargy, vomiting and anxiety. Increased reticulocyte counts and a severe hemolytic reaction are laboratory findings that would be expected. Treatment for an acute overdose may include intensive hematologic monitoring with adjunctive supportive therapy, including possible transfusions.

Drug Interactions
The following drug interactions have either been reported or are theoretical in humans or animals receiving acetohydroxamic acid (AHA) and may be of significance in veterinary patients:
- **IRON:** AHA may chelate iron salts in the gut if given concomitantly
- **METHENAMINE:** AHA may have a synergistic effect with methenamine in inhibiting the urine pH increases caused by urease-producing *Proteus* spp.; AHA may also potentiate the antibacterial effect of methenamine against these bacteria
- **ALCOHOL:** In humans, AHA with alcohol has resulted in rashes

Laboratory Considerations
- Although AHA is a true urease inhibitor, it apparently does not interfere with urea nitrogen determination using one of the following: urease-Berthelot, urease-glutamate dehydrogenase or diacetyl monoxime methods.

Doses
- **DOGS:**
  For adjunctive therapy of persistent struvite uroliths and persistent urease-producing bacteria after treating with antibiotics and calculolytic diets:
  a) 12.5 mg/kg twice daily PO (Osborne *et al.* 1993), (Lulich *et al.* 2000)

Monitoring
- CBC
- Renal/Hepatic (bilirubin) function
- Efficacy

Client Information
- This medication can cause several adverse effects in dogs; contact veterinarian if dog develops persistent or severe vomiting, has a lack of appetite, a change in urine color, develops yellowing of the whites of the eyes, or has decreased energy/activity.

Chemistry/Synonyms
An inhibitor of urease, acetohydroxamic acid occurs as a white crystal having a pKa of 9.32–9.4 and a pH of about 9.4. 850 mg are soluble in one mL of water, and 400 mg are soluble in one mL of alcohol.

Acetohydroxamic acid may also be known as: AHA, Acetic acid oxime, N-Acetylhydroxylamine, N-Hydroxyacetamide, *Lithostat®* or *Uronefrex®*.

Storage/Stability
Tablets should be stored in tight containers.

Dosage Forms/Regulatory Status
VETERINARY-LABELED PRODUCTS: None

HUMAN-LABELED PRODUCTS: Acetohydroxamic Acid Oral Tablets: 250 mg; *Lithostat®* (Mission); (Rx)

References
Lulich, J, C Osborne, et al. (2000). Canine Lower Urinary Tract Disorders. *Textbook of Veterinary Internal Medicine: Diseases of the Dog and Cat.* S Ettinger and E Feldman Eds. Philadelphia, WB Saunders. 2: 1747–1781.

Osborne, C, J Lulich, et al. (1993). Canine and feline urolithiasis: Relationship and etiopathogenesis with treatment and prevention. *Disease mechanisms in small animal surgery.* M Bojrab Ed. Philadelphia, Lea & Febiger: 464–511.

ACETYLCYSTEINE
(assah-teel-*sis*-tay-een)
N-acetylcysteine, Mucomyst®, NAC

ANTIDOTE; MUCOLYTIC

Prescriber Highlights

▶ Used primarily as a treatment for acetaminophen toxicity or other hepatotoxic conditions where glutathione synthesis is inhibited or oxidative stress occurs.

▶ Also has been used as an inhaled solution for its mucolytic effect and, anecdotally for treating degenerative myelopathy

▶ Acetylcysteine is used as a topical ophthalmic (see the Topical Ophthalmic section in the appendix)

▶ Has caused hypersensitivity & bronchospasm when used in pulmonary tree

▶ Administer via gastric- or duodenal tube for acetaminophen poisoning in animals on an empty stomach

Uses/Indications
Acetylcysteine is used in veterinary medicine as both a mucolytic agent in the pulmonary tree and as a treatment for acetaminophen, xylitol, or phenol toxicity in small animals. Acetylcysteine is used investigatively as an antiinflammatory for chronic upper respiratory disease in cats, as an adjunct in heavy metal removal, and topically in the eye to halt the melting effect of collagenases and proteinases on the cornea.

It has been used anecdotally with aminocaproic acid to treat degenerative myelopathy in dogs, but data is lacking showing efficacy.

In horses with strangles, acetylcysteine instilled into the gutteral pouch has been used to help break up chondroids and avoid the need for surgical removal. Acetylcysteine enemas have been used in neonatal foals to break up meconium refractory to repeated enemas.

Pharmacology/Actions

When administered into the pulmonary tree, acetylcysteine reduces the viscosity of both purulent and nonpurulent secretions and expedites the removal of these secretions via coughing, suction, or postural drainage. The free sulfhydryl group on the drug is believed to reduce disulfide linkages in mucoproteins; this effect is most pronounced at a pH from 7–9. The drug has no effect on living tissue or fibrin.

Acetylcysteine can reduce the extent of liver injury or methemoglobinemia after ingestion of acetaminophen or phenol, by providing an alternate substrate for conjugation with the reactive metabolite of acetaminophen, thus maintaining or restoring glutathione levels.

Pharmacokinetics

When given orally, acetylcysteine is absorbed from the GI tract. When administered via nebulization or intratracheally into the pulmonary tract, most of the drug is involved in the sulfhydryl-disulfide reaction and the remainder is absorbed. Absorbed drug is converted (deacetylated) into cysteine in the liver and then further metabolized.

Contraindications/Precautions/Warnings

Acetylcysteine is contraindicated (for pulmonary indications) in animals hypersensitive to it. There are no contraindications for its use as an antidote.

Because acetylcysteine may cause bronchospasm in some patients when used in the pulmonary system, animals with bronchospastic diseases should be monitored carefully when using this agent.

Adverse Effects

When given orally for acetaminophen toxicity, acetylcysteine can cause GI effects (nausea, vomiting) and rarely, urticaria. Because the taste of the solution is very bad, taste-masking agents (*e.g.*, colas, juices) have been used. Since oral dosing of these drugs may be very difficult in animals, gastric or duodenal tubes may be necessary.

Intravenous administration appears to be very well tolerated in veterinary patients. IV boluses in humans have caused changes in blood pressure (hyper-, hypo-tension), GI effects and allergic reactions.

Rare adverse effects reported when acetylcysteine is administered into the pulmonary tract, include: hypersensitivity, chest tightness, bronchoconstriction, and bronchial or tracheal irritation.

Reproductive/Nursing Safety

Reproduction studies in rabbits and rats have not demonstrated any evidence of teratogenic or embryotoxic effects when used in doses up to 17 times normal. In humans, the FDA categorizes this drug as category *B* for use during pregnancy (*Animal studies have not yet demonstrated risk to the fetus, but there are no adequate studies in pregnant women; or animal studies have shown an adverse effect, but adequate studies in pregnant women have not demonstrated a risk to the fetus in the first trimester of pregnancy, and there is no evidence of risk in later trimesters.*)

It is unknown if acetylcysteine enters milk. Use caution when administering to a nursing dam.

Overdosage/Acute Toxicity

The LD_{50} of acetylcysteine in dogs is 1 g/kg (PO) and 700 mg/kg (IV). It is believed that acetylcysteine is quite safe (with the exception of the adverse effects listed above) in most overdose situations.

Drug Interactions

■ **ACTIVATED CHARCOAL:** The use of activated charcoal as a gut adsorbent of acetaminophen is controversial, as charcoal may also adsorb acetylcysteine. Because cats can develop methemoglobinemia very rapidly after ingestion of acetaminophen, do not delay acetylcysteine treatment and preferably give the first dose intravenously. If using the solution (not labeled for injectable use), it is preferable to use a 0.2 micron in-line filter.

Doses

■ **DOGS:**

For acetaminophen toxicity:

a) A 2–3 hour wait between activated charcoal and PO administration of acetylcysteine (NAC) is necessary. Give NAC as an initial oral loading dose of 140 mg/kg (dilute to 5% in dextrose or sterile water), followed by 70 mg/kg PO four times daily (q6h) for 7 treatments. With ingestion of massive quantities, some authors suggest using a 280 mg/kg loading dose and continuing treatment for 12–17 doses. May also be given IV after diluting to 5% and given via slow IV over 15–20 minutes. Additional therapy may include IV fluids, blood or *Oxyglobin®*, ascorbic acid and SAMe. (Wismer 2006)

b) 150 mg/kg PO or IV initially, then 50 mg/kg q4h for 17 additional doses (Bailey 1986)

c) Loading dose of 140 mg/kg PO, then 70 mg/kg PO every 6 hours for 7 treatments (Grauer & Hjelle 1988)

For phenol toxicity:

a) 140 mg/kg PO or IV initially, then 50 mg/kg q4h for 3 days. May be partially effective to reduce hepatic and renal injury. Resultant methemoglobinemia should be treated with ascorbic acid or methylene blue. (Dorman & Dye 2005)

For hepatotoxicity secondary to xylitol poisoning:

a) Acetylcysteine at 140–280 mg/kg loading dose IV, PO; followed by 70 mg/kg four times daily; vitamin K (phytonadione) at 1.25–2.5 mg/kg PO twice daily; plasma, SAMe at 20 mg/kg/day PO; vitamin E at 100–400 Units twice daily PO; and silymarin 20–50 mg/kg/day PO. (Talcott 2008)

For degenerative myelopathy:

a) 25 mg/kg PO q8h for 2 weeks, then q8h every other day. The 20% solution should be diluted to 5% with chicken broth or suitable diluent. Used in conjunction with aminocaproic acid (500 mg per dog PO q8h indefinitely). Other treatments may include prednisone (0.25–0.5 mg/kg PO daily for 10 days then every other day), Vitamin C (1000 mg PO q12h) and Vitamin E (1000 Units PO q12h). **Note:** No treatment has been shown to be effective in published trials. (Shell 2003)

■ **CATS:**

For acetaminophen toxicity:

a) A 2–3 hour wait between activated charcoal and PO administration of acetylcysteine (NAC) is necessary. Give NAC as an initial oral loading dose of 140 mg/kg (dilute to 5% in dextrose or sterile water), followed by 70 mg/kg PO four times daily (q6h) for 7 treatments. With ingestion of massive quantities, some authors suggest using a 280 mg/kg loading dose and continuing treatment for 12–17 doses. May also be given IV after diluting to 5% and given via slow IV over 15–20 minutes. Additional therapy may include IV fluids, blood or Oxyglobin®, ascorbic acid and SAMe. (Wismer 2006)

For phenol toxicity:

a) 140 mg/kg PO or IV initially, then 50 mg/kg q4h for 3 days. May be partially effective to reduce hepatic and renal injury. Resultant methemoglobinemia should be treated with ascorbic acid or methylene blue. (Dorman & Dye 2005)

For adjunctive treatment of hepatic lipidosis (see also Carnitine):

a) Identify underlying cause of anorexia and provide a protein replete feline diet, give acetylcysteine (NAC) at 140 mg/kg IV over 20 minutes, then 70 mg/kg IV q12h; dilute 10% NAC with saline 1:4 and ad-

minister IV using a 0.25 micron filter; correct hypokalemia and hypophosphatemia, beware of electrolyte changes with re-feeding phenomenon (Center 2006)

■ **HORSES:**

To help break up chondroids in the gutteral pouch:

a) Instill 20% solution (Foreman 1999)

In neonatal foals to break up meconium refractory to repeated enemas:

a) 8 grams in 20 g sodium bicarbonate in 200 mL water (pH of 7.6), give as enema as needed to effect (Freeman 1999)

b) With foal in lateral recumbency, insert a 30 french foley catheter with a 30 cc bulb for a retention enema. Using gravity flow, infuse slowly 100–200 mL of 4% acetylcysteine solution and retain for 30–45 minutes. IV fluids and pain medication should be considered. Monitor for possible bladder distention. (Pusterla *et al.* 2003)

Monitoring

When used for acetaminophen poisoning:

■ Hepatic enzymes (particularly in dogs)

■ Acetaminophen level, if available (particularly in dogs)

■ Hemogram, with methemoglobin value (particularly in cats)

■ Serum electrolytes, hydration status

Client Information

■ This agent should be used in a clinically supervised setting only

Chemistry/Synonyms

The N-acetyl derivative of L-cysteine, acetylcysteine occurs as a white, crystalline powder with a slight acetic odor. It is freely soluble in water or alcohol.

Acetylcysteine may also be known as: N-acetylcysteine or N-acetyl-L-cysteine, NAC, 5052 acetylcysteinum, NSC-111180, *Acetadote®*, *Mucomyst®* or *ACC®*.

Storage/Stability

When unopened, vials of sodium acetylcysteine should be stored at room temperature (15–30°C). After opening, vials should be kept refrigerated and used within 96 hours. The product labeled for IV use states to use within 24 hours.

Compatibility/Compounding Considerations

Acetylcysteine is **incompatible** with oxidizing agents; solutions can become discolored and liberate hydrogen sulfide when exposed to rubber, copper, iron, and during autoclaving. It does not react to aluminum, stainless steel, glass or plastic. If the solution becomes light purple in color, potency is not appreciably affected, but it is best to use non-reactive materials when giving the drug via nebulization. Acetylcysteine solutions are **incompatible** with amphotericin B, ampicillin sodium, erythromycin lactobionate, tetracycline, oxytetracycline, iodized oil, hydrogen peroxide and trypsin.

Dosage Forms/Regulatory Status

VETERINARY-LABELED PRODUCTS: None

HUMAN-LABELED PRODUCTS:

Acetylcysteine injection: 20% (200 mg/mL) in 30 mL single-dose vials, preservative free; *Acetadote®* (Cumberland); (Rx)

Acetylcysteine Oral Solution: 10% & 20% (as sodium) in 4 mL, 10 mL, & 30 mL vials; *Mucomyst®* (Sandoz); generic; (Rx)

Acetylcysteine Inhalation Solution: 10% & 20% (as sodium) in 4 mL, 10 mL, 30 mL vials & 100 mL vials (20% only); *Mucomyst®* (Apothecon); generic (Rx) **Note:** If using this product for dilution and then intravenous dosing, it is preferable to use a 0.2 micron in-line filter.

Acetylcysteine is also available in the USA as an oral OTC nutritional product. It is usually labeled as NAC N-Acetylcysteine and is commonly found as 600 mg capsules.

References

Bailey, EM (1986). Emergency and general treatment of poisonings. *Current Veterinary Therapy (CVT) IX Small Animal Practice*. RW Kirk Ed. Philadelphia, W.B. Saunders: 135–144.

Center, S (2006). Treatment for Severe Feline Hepatic Lipidosis. Proceedings: WSAVA. Accessed via: Veterinary Information Network. http://goo.gl/N7g14

Dorman, D & J Dye (2005). Chemical Toxicities. *Textbook of Veterinary Internal Medicine: Diseases of the Dog and Cat, 6th Ed*. S Ettinger and E Feldman Eds. Philadelphia, Elsevier: 256–261.

Foreman, J (1999). Equine respiratory pharmacology. *The Veterinary Clinics of North America: Equine Practice* 15:3(December): 665–686.

Freeman, D (1999). Gastrointestinal Pharmacology. *The Veterinary Clinics of North America: Equine Practice* 15:3(December): 535–559.

Grauer, GF & JJ Hjelle (1988). Household Drugs. *Handbook of Small Animal Practice*. RV Morgan Ed. New York, Churchill Livingstone: 1115–1118.

Pusterla, N, K Magdesian, et al. (2003). Evaluation and use of acetylcysteine retention enemas in the treatment of meconium impaction in foals. Proceedings: ACVIM Forum. Accessed via: Veterinary Information Network. http://goo.gl/PMYXr

Shell, L (2003). "Degenerative Myelopathy (Degenerative Radiculomyelopathy)." *Associates Database*.

Talcott, P (2008). New and Used Topics in Toxicology. Proceedings: Western Veterinary Conference. Accessed via: Veterinary Information Network. http://goo.gl/g6SuY

Wismer, T (2006). Hepatic Toxins and the Emergent Patient. Proceedings: IVECC Symposium. Accessed via: Veterinary Information Network. http://goo.gl/SbjSx

Acetylsalicylic Acid—See Aspirin

ACITRETIN

(ase-a-*tre*-tin)   Soriatane®

RETINOID

Note: Originally etretinate was used for certain dermatologic indications in small animals (primarily dogs). It has been withdrawn from the market and replaced with acitretin, an active metabolite of etretinate with the same indications, but a much shorter half-life. Much of the information below is extrapolated from etretinate data.

Prescriber Highlights

▶ Retinoid that may be useful for certain dermatologic conditions in small animals

▶ Contraindications: Pregnancy; Caution: Cardiovascular disease, hypertriglyceridemia or sensitivity to retinoids

▶ Adverse Effects: Limited experience; appears to be fairly well tolerated in small animals Potentially: anorexia/vomiting or diarrhea, cracking of foot pads, pruritus, ventral abdominal erythema, polydipsia, lassitude, joint pain/stiffness, eyelid abnormalities & conjunctivitis (KCS), swollen tongue, & behavioral changes

▶ Known teratogen; do not use in households with pregnant women present (Plumb's recommendation)

▶ May be very expensive; may need to compound smaller capsules for small dogs or cats

▶ Drug-drug; drug-lab interactions

Uses/Indications

Acitretin may be useful in the treatment of canine lamellar ichthyosis, solar-induced precancerous lesions in Dalmatians or bull Terriers, actinic keratoses, squamous cell carcinomas, and intracutaneous cornifying epitheliomas (multiple keratoacanthomas).

While the drug has provided effective treatment of idiopathic seborrhea (particularly in cocker spaniels), it is not effective in treating the ceruminous otitis that may also be present. Results have been disappointing in treating idiopathic seborrhea seen in basset hounds and West Highland terriers.

Acitretin's usage in cats is very limited, but etretinate has shown some usefulness in treating paraneoplastic actinic keratosis, solar-induced squamous cell carcinoma and Bowen's Disease in this species.

Pharmacology/Actions

Acitretin is a synthetic retinoid agent potentially useful in the treatment of several disorders related to abnormal keratinization and/or sebaceous gland abnormalities in small animals. The drug has some antiinflammatory activity, but its exact mechanism of action is not known.

Pharmacokinetics

Acitretin absorption is enhanced by food in the gut and is highly bound to plasma proteins. The drug is metabolized to conjugate forms that are excreted in the bile and urine. Terminal half-life averages 50 hours in humans.

Contraindications/Precautions/Warnings

Acitretin use should not be considered when the following conditions exist: cardiovascular disease, hypertriglyceridemia or known sensitivity to acitretin. Use with caution in patients with renal or hepatic failure.

Adverse Effects

Veterinary experience with this medication is limited, but the incidence of adverse effects appears to be less in companion animals than in people. Most animals treated (thus far) do not exhibit adverse effects. Potential adverse effects include: anorexia/vomiting/diarrhea, cracking of foot pads, pruritus, ventral abdominal erythema, polydipsia, lassitude, joint pain/stiffness, eyelid abnormalities and conjunctivitis (KCS), swollen tongue, and behavioral changes.

The most common adverse effect seen in cats is anorexia with resultant weight loss. If cats develop adverse effects, the time between doses may be prolonged (*e.g.*, Every other week give every other day) to reduce the total dose given.

Reproductive/Nursing Safety

Acitretin is a known teratogen. Major anomalies have been reported in children of women receiving acitretin. It should not be handled by pregnant women nor used in a household where women are pregnant or planning to become pregnant. It should be considered absolutely contraindicated in pregnant veterinary patients. In humans, the FDA categorizes this drug as category *X* for use during pregnancy (*Studies in animals or humans demonstrate fetal abnormalities or adverse reaction; reports indicate evidence of fetal risk. The risk of use in pregnant women clearly outweighs any possible benefit.*)

Acitretin is excreted in rat milk. At this time, it cannot be recommended for use in nursing dams.

Overdosage/Acute Toxicity

Information on overdoses with this agent remains limited. One oral overdose (525 mg) in a human patient resulted only in vomiting. The oral LD50 in rats and mice is >4 grams/kg.

Drug Interactions

The following drug interactions have either been reported or are theoretical in humans or animals receiving acitretin and may be of significance in veterinary patients:

■ **ALCOHOL:** Acitretin can form etretinate in the presence of alcohol; etretinate is a teratogen with an extremely long terminal half-life and (can persist in adipose tissue for years)

■ **HEPATOTOXIC DRUGS** (especially **methotrexate** and potentially **anabolic steroids, androgens, asparaginase, erythromycins, estrogens, fluconazole, halothane, ketoconazole, sulfonamides** or **valproic acid**): May be increased potential for hepatotoxicity

■ **OTHER RETINOIDS** (**isotretinoin, tretinoin,** or **vitamin A**): May cause additive toxic effects.

■ **TETRACYCLINES:** Acitretin with tetracyclines may increase the potential for the occurrence of pseudotumor cerebri (cerebral edema and increased CSF pressure)

Laboratory Considerations

■ In humans, acitretin may cause significant increases in **plasma triglycerides, serum cholesterol, serum ALT (SGPT), serum AST (SGOT), and serum LDH concentrations. Serum HDL** (high density lipoprotein) concentrations may be decreased. Veterinary significance of these effects is unclear.

Doses

■ **DOGS:**

For dermatologic conditions where retinoids may be useful:

a) 0.5−1 mg/kg PO once daily (Kwochka 2003)

b) 0.5−2 mg/kg PO once daily (Merchant 2000)

c) For sebaceous adenitis: 0.5−1 mg/kg once daily PO (Bloom 2006)

■ **CATS:**

For actinic keratosis/solar-induced squamous cell carcinoma; or Bowen's Disease:

a) 10 mg per cat once daily PO. (Power & Ihrke 1995) **Note:** This dose is for etretinate, but as the smallest capsule is 10 mg, this dose may need to suffice as well for cats.

b) For Bowen's Disease: 3 mg/kg/day (Guaguere *et al.* 1999), (Hnilica 2003)

Monitoring

■ Efficacy

■ Liver function tests (baseline and if clinical signs appear)

■ Schirmer tear tests (monthly—especially in older dogs)

Client Information

■ Acitretin should not be handled by pregnant women in the household; veterinarians must take responsibility to educate clients of the potential risk of ingestion by pregnant females

■ Food will increase the absorption of acitretin. To reduce variability of absorption, either have clients consistently give with meals or when fasted

■ Long-term therapy can be quite expensive

Chemistry/Synonyms
Acitretin, a synthetic retinoid occurs as a yellow to greenish-yellow powder.

Acitretin may also be known as: acitretinum, etretin, Ro-10-1670, Ro-10-1670/000, *Soriatane®, Acetrizoic Acid®,* or *Iodophil Viscous®.*

Storage/Stability
Store at room temperature and protected from light. After bottle is opened, protect from high temperature and humidity.

Dosage Forms/Regulatory Status
VETERINARY-LABELED PRODUCTS: None

HUMAN-LABELED PRODUCTS:

Acitretin Capsules: 10 mg, 17.5 mg, 22.5 mg & 25 mg; *Soriatane®* (Connetics); (Rx)

References
Bloom, P (2006). Nonpruritic alopecia in the dog. Proceedings: Western Vet Conf 2006. Accessed via: Veterinary Information Network. http://goo.gl/Qh57f
Guaguere, E, T Olivry, et al. (1999). Demodex cati infestation in association with feline cutaneous squamous cell carcinoma in situ: a report of five cases. *Veterinary Dermatology* 10(1): 61–67.
Hnilica, K (2003). "New" Feline Skin Diseases. Proceedings: Western Veterinary Conf. Accessed via: Veterinary Information Network. http://goo.gl/ONKxx
Kwochka, K (2003). Treatment of scaling disorders in dogs. Proceedings: Atlantic Coast Veterinary Conference. Accessed via: Veterinary Information Network. http://goo.gl/CnVgl
Merchant, S (2000). New Therapies in Veterinary Dermatology. Proceedings: American Animal Hospital Association 67th Annual Meeting, Toronto.
Power, H & P Ihrke (1995). The use of synthetic retinoids in veterinary medicine. *Kirk's Current Veterinary Therapy:XII.* J Bonagura Ed. Philadelphia, W.B. Saunders: 585–590.

ACTH—See Corticotropin
Activated Charcoal—See Charcoal, Activated

ACYCLOVIR
(ay-sye-kloe-vir)   Zovirax®
ANTIVIRAL (HERPES)

Prescriber Highlights
▶ Used primarily in birds for Pacheco's disease; may be useful in cats for Herpes infection
▶ If given rapidly IV, may be nephrotoxic
▶ Oral use may cause GI distress
▶ Reduce dosage with renal insufficiency
▶ May be fetotoxic at high dosages

Uses/Indications
Acyclovir may be useful in treating herpes infections in a variety of avian species and in cats with corneal or conjunctival herpes infections. Its use in veterinary medicine is not well es-tablished, however, and it should be used with caution. Acyclovir has relatively mild activity against *Feline Herpesvirus-1* when compared to some of the newer antiviral agents (*e.g.,* ganciclovir, cidofovir, or penciclovir).

Acyclovir is being investigated as a treatment for equine herpes virus type-1 myeloencephalopathy in horses, but clinical efficacy has not yet been proven and the drug's poor oral bioavailability is problematic. There continues to be interest in finding a dosing regimen that can achieve therapeutic levels and be economically viable, particularly since the drug's use during a recent outbreak appeared to have some efficacy in reducing morbidity and mortality (not statistically proven). Also, intravenous acyclovir may be economically feasible to treat some neonatal foals.

Pharmacology/Actions
Acyclovir has antiviral activity against a variety of viruses including herpes simplex (types I and II), cytomegalovirus, *Epstein-Barr,* and *varicella-Zoster.* It is preferentially taken up by these viruses, and converted into the active triphosphate form where it inhibits viral DNA replication.

Pharmacokinetics
In dogs, acyclovir bioavailability varies with the dose. At doses of 20 mg/kg and below, bioavailability is about 80%, but declines to about 50% at 50 mg/kg.

Bioavailability in horses after oral administration is very low (<4%) and oral doses of up to 20 mg/kg may not yield sufficient levels to treat equine herpes virus. Elimination half-lives in dogs, cats and horses are approximately 3 hours, 2.6 hours, and 10 hours, respectively.

In humans, acyclovir is poorly absorbed after oral administration (approx. 20%) and absorption is not significantly affected by the presence of food. It is widely distributed throughout body tissues and fluids including the brain, semen, and CSF. It has low protein binding and crosses the placenta. Acyclovir is primarily hepatically metabolized and has a half-life of about 3 hours in humans. Renal disease does not significantly alter half-life unless anuria is present.

Contraindications/Precautions/Warnings
Acyclovir is potentially contraindicated (assess risk vs. benefit) during dehydrated states, pre-existing renal function impairment, hypersensitivity to it or other related antivirals, neurologic deficits, or previous neurologic reactions to other cytotoxic drugs.

Adverse Effects
With parenteral therapy potential adverse effects include thrombophlebitis, acute renal failure, and ecephalopathologic changes (rare). GI disturbances may occur with either oral or parenteral therapy.

Preliminary effects noted in cats, include leukopenia and anemias, which are apparently reversible with discontinuation of therapy.

Reproductive/Nursing Safety

Acyclovir crosses the placenta, but rodent studies have not demonstrated any teratogenic effects thus far. Acyclovir crosses into maternal milk but associated adverse effects have not been noted. In humans, the FDA categorizes this drug as category *C* for use during pregnancy (*Animal studies have shown an adverse effect on the fetus, but there are no adequate studies in humans; or there are no animal reproduction studies and no adequate studies in humans.*)

Acyclovir concentrations in milk of women following oral administration have ranged from 0.6 to 4.1 times those found in plasma. These concentrations would potentially expose the breastfeeding infant to a dose of acyclovir up to 0.3 mg/kg/day. Data for animals was not located. Use caution when administering to a nursing patient.

Overdosage/Acute Toxicity

Acute oral overdosage is unlikely to cause significant toxicity. GI signs predominate although renal failure is possible with higher doses. Crystalluria and elevated renal values occurred at 188.7 mg/kg in a dog. There were 85 exposures to acyclovir reported to the ASPCA Animal Poison Control Center (APCC) during 2008–2009. In these cases 75 were dogs with 9 showing clinical signs. The remaining 10 cases were cats with 4 showing clinical signs. Common findings in dogs recorded in decreasing frequency included vomiting, diarrhea, and lethargy. Common findings in cats include vomiting.

Consider decontamination at 150 mg/kg or higher. Below 150 mg/kg, GI signs will likely predominate.

Drug Interactions

The following drug interactions have either been reported or are theoretical in humans or animals receiving acyclovir and may be of significance in veterinary patients:

■ **NEPHROTOXIC MEDICATIONS:** Concomitant administration of IV acyclovir with nephrotoxic medications may increase the potential for nephrotoxicity occurring. Amphotericin B may potentiate the antiviral effects of acyclovir but it also increases chances for development of nephrotoxicity.

■ **ZIDOVUDINE:** Concomitant use with zidovudine may cause additional CNS depression.

Doses

■ **BIRDS:**

For treatment of Pacheco's Disease:

a) 80 mg/kg PO q8h or 40 mg/kg q8h IM (do not use parenterally for more than 72 hours as it can cause tissue necrosis at site of injection) (Oglesbee & Bishop 1994)

b) 80 mg/kg in oral suspension once daily PO; mix suspension with peanut butter or add to drinking water 50 mg in 4 oz of water for 7–14 days) (Jenkins 1993)

c) When birds are being individually treated: 80 mg/kg PO or IM twice daily (Speer 1999)

d) For prophylaxis: Exposed birds are given 25 mg/kg IM once (give IM with caution as it is very irritating), and then acyclovir is added to drinking water at 1 mg/mL and to the food at 400 mg/quart of seed for a minimum of 7 days. Quaker parrots have been treated with a gavage of acyclovir at 80 mg/kg q8h for 7 days. (Johnson-Delaney 2005)

■ **CATS:**

For Herpesvirus-1 infections:

a) 10–25 mg/kg PO twice daily. Never begin therapy until diagnostic evaluation is completed. May be toxic in cats; monitor CBC every 2–3 weeks. (Lappin 2003)

■ **HORSES:**

a) Although efficacy is undetermined, anecdotal use of acyclovir orally at 10 mg/kg PO 5 times daily or 20 mg/kg PO q8h may have had some efficacy in preventing or treating horses during EHV-1 outbreaks. *However, the drug's very low oral bioavailability suggests that oral dosing is unlikely to be of much benefit. Additional studies may further clarify the usefulness of such dosing regimens—Plumb 2010;* based upon (Wilkins 2004) & (Henninger *et al.* 2007)

Monitoring

■ Renal function tests (BUN, Serum Cr) with prolonged or IV therapy

■ Cats: CBC

Chemistry/Synonyms

An antiviral agent, acyclovir (also known as ACV or acycloguanosine), occurs as a white, crystalline powder. 1.3 mg are soluble in one mL of water. Acyclovir sodium has a solubility of greater than 100 mg/mL in water. However, at a pH of 7.4 at 37°C it is practically all unionized and has a solubility of only 2.5 mg/mL in water. There is 4.2 mEq of sodium in each gram of acyclovir sodium.

Acyclovir may be known as: aciclovirum, acycloguanosine, acyclovir, BW-248U, *Zovirax®*, *Acic®*, *Aciclobene®*, *Aciclotyrol®*, *Acivir®*, *Acyrax®*, *Cicloviral®*, *Geavir®*, *Geavir®*, *Herpotern®*, *Isavir®*, *Nycovir®*, *Supraviran®*, *Viclovir®*, *Virherpes®*, *Viroxy®*, *Xorox®*, or *Zovirax®*.

Storage/Stability

Acyclovir capsules and tablets should be stored in tight, light resistant containers at room temperature. Acyclovir suspension and sodium sterile powder should be stored at room temperature.

Compatibility/Compounding Considerations

When reconstituting acyclovir sodium do not use bacteriostatic water with parabens as precipitation may occur. The manufacturer does not recommend using bacteriostatic water for injection with benzyl alcohol because of the potential toxicity in neonates. After reconstitution with 50–100 mL of a standard electrolyte or dextrose solution, the resulting solution is stable at 25°C for 24 hours. Acyclovir is reportedly **incompatible** with biologic or colloidial products (*e.g.*, blood products or protein containing solutions). It is also **incompatible** with dopamine HCl, dobutamine, fludarabine phosphate, foscarnet sodium, meperidine and morphine sulfate. Many other drugs have been shown to be **compatible** in specific situations. Compatibility is dependent upon factors such as pH, concentration, temperature and diluent used; consult specialized references or a hospital pharmacist for more specific information.

Dosage Forms/Regulatory Status

VETERINARY-LABELED PRODUCTS: None

HUMAN-LABELED PRODUCTS:

Acyclovir Oral Tablets: 400 mg & 800 mg; *Zovirax®* (GlaxoSmithKline); generic; (Rx)

Acyclovir Oral Capsules: 200 mg; *Zovirax®* (GlaxoSmithKline); generic; (Rx)

Acyclovir Oral Suspension: 200 mg/5 mL in 473 mL; *Zovirax®* (GlaxoSmithKline); generic; (Rx)

Acyclovir Sodium Injection (for IV infusion only): 50 mg/mL (as sodium); generic; (Rx)

Acyclovir Powder for Injection: 500 mg/vial (as sodium) in 10 mL vials; 1000 mg/vial (as sodium) in 20 mL vials; generic; (Rx)

Acyclovir Ointment: 5% (50 mg/g) in 15 g; *Zovirax®* (Biovail); (Rx)

Acyclovir Cream: 5% (50 mg/g) in 2g tubes; *Zovirax®* (Biovail); (Rx)

References

Henninger, R, S Reed, et al. (2007). Outbreak of neurologic disease caused by Equine Herpesvirus–1 at a university equestrian center. *J Vet Intern Med* 21(157–165).

Jenkins, T (1993, Last Update). "Personal Communication."

Johnson–Delaney, C (2005). Avian Viral Diseases. Proceedings: Atlantic Coast Veterinary Conference. Accessed via: Veterinary Information Network. http://goo.gl/Phux8

Lappin, M (2003). Infectious upper respiratory diseases I and II. Proceedings: Western Veterinary Conference. Accessed via: Veterinary Information Network. http://goo.gl/qsOaI

Oglesbee, B & C Bishop (1994). *Saunders Manual of Small Animal Practice.* S Birchard and R Sherding Eds. Philadelphia, W.B. Saunders Company: 1257–1270.

Speer, B (1999). The Big "P" diseases. Proceedings: Central Veterinary Conference, Kansas City.

Wilkins, P (2004). Acyclovir in the treatment of EHV–1 Myeloencephalopathy. Proceedings: ACVIM Forum. Accessed via: Veterinary Information Network. http://goo.gl/E8Icj

AGLEPRISTONE

(a-gle-*pris*-tone)   Alizin®, Alizine®

INJECTABLE PROGESTERONE BLOCKER

Prescriber Highlights

▶ Injectable progesterone blocker indicated for pregnancy termination in bitches; may also be of benefit in inducing parturition or in treating pyometra complex in dogs & progesterone-dependent mammary hyperplasia in cats

▶ Not currently available in USA; marketed for use in dogs in Europe, South America, etc.

▶ Localized injection site reactions are most commonly noted adverse effect; other adverse effects reported in >5% of patients include: anorexia (25%), excitation (23%), depression (21%), & diarrhea (13%)

Uses/Indications

Aglepristone is labeled (in the U.K. and elsewhere) for pregnancy termination in bitches up to 45 days after mating.

In dogs, aglepristone may prove useful in inducing parturition or treating pyometra complex (often in combination with a prostaglandin F analog such as cloprostenol).

In cats, it may be of benefit for pregnancy termination (one study documented 87% efficacy when administered at the recommended dog dose at day 25) or in treating mammary hyperplasias or pyometras.

Pharmacology/Actions

Aglepristone is a synthetic steroid that binds to the progesterone (P4) receptors thereby preventing biological effects from progesterone. In dogs, it has an affinity for uterine progesterone receptors approximately three times that of progesterone. In queens, affinity is approximately nine times greater than the endogenous hormone. As progesterone is necessary for maintaining pregnancy, pregnancy can be terminated or parturition induced. Abortion occurs within 7 days of administration.

Benign feline mammary hyperplasias (fibroadenomatous hyperplasia; FAHs) are usually under the influence of progesterone and aglepristone can be used to medically treat this condition.

When used for treating pyometra in dogs, aglepristone can cause opening of the cervix and resumption of miometral contractility.

Within 24 hours of administration, aglepristone does not appreciably affect circulating plasma levels of progesterone, cortisol, prostaglandins or oxytocin. Plasma levels of prolactin are increased within 12 hours when used in dogs during mid-pregnancy which is probably the cause of mammary gland congestion often seen in these dogs.

Aglepristone also binds to glucocorticoid receptors but has no glucocorticoid activity; it can prevent endogenous or exogenously administered glucocorticoids from binding and acting at these sites.

Pharmacokinetics

In dogs, after injecting two doses of 10mg/kg 24 hours apart, peak serum levels occur about 2.5 days later and mean residence time is about 6 days. The majority (90%) of the drug is excreted via the feces.

Contraindications/Precautions/Warnings

Aglepristone is contraindicated in patients who have documented hypersensitivity to it and during pregnancy, unless used for pregnancy termination or inducing parturition.

When being considered for use in treating pyometra in bitches, peritonitis must be ruled out before using.

Because of its antagonistic effects on glucocorticoid receptors, the drug should not be used in patients with hypoadrenocorticism or in dogs with a genetic predisposition to hypoadrenocorticism.

The manufacturer does not recommend using the product in patients in poor health, with diabetes, or with impaired hepatic or renal function as there is no data documenting its safety with these conditions.

Adverse Effects

As the product is in an oil-alcohol base, localized pain and inflammatory reactions (edema, skin thickening, ulceration, and localized lymph node enlargement) can be noted at the injection site. Resolution of pain generally occurs shortly after injection; other injection site reactions usually resolve within 2–4 weeks. The manufacturer recommends light massage of the injection site after administration. Larger dogs should not receive more than 5 mL at any one subcutaneous injection site. One source states that severe injection reactions can be avoided if the drug is administered into the scruff of the neck.

Systemic adverse effects reported from field trials include: anorexia (25%), excitation (23%), depression (21%), vomiting (2%), diarrhea (13%) and uterine infections (3.4%). Transient changes in hematologic (RBC, WBC indices) or biochemical (BUN, creatinine, chloride, potassium, sodium, liver enzymes) laboratory parameters were seen in <5% of dogs treated.

When used for pregnancy termination, a brown mucoid vaginal discharge can be seen approximately 24 hours before fetal expulsion. This discharge can persist for an additional 3–5 days. If used in bitches after the 20th day of gestation, abortion may be accompanied with other signs associated with parturition (e.g., inappetence, restlessness, mammary congestion).

Bitches may return to estrus in as little as 45 days after pregnancy termination.

Reproductive/Nursing Safety

Unless used for pregnancy termination or at term to induce parturition, aglepristone is contraindicated during pregnancy.

One study (Baan et al. 2005) using aglepristone to induce parturition (day 58) demonstrated no significant differences in weight gain between those puppies in the treatment group versus the control group suggesting that aglepristone did not have effect on milk production of treated bitches.

Overdosage/Acute Toxicity

When administered at 3X (30mg/kg) recommended doses, bitches demonstrated no untoward systemic effects. Localized reactions were noted at the injection site, presumably due to the larger volumes injected.

Drug Interactions

No documented drug interactions were noted. Theoretically, the following interactions may occur with aglepristone:

- ◾ **PROGESTINS** (**natural** or **synthetic**): Could reduce the efficacy of aglepristone
- ◾ **GLUCOCORTICOIDS:** Aglepristone could reduce the efficacy of glucocorticoid treatment
- ◾ **KETOCONAZOLE, ITRACONAZOLE, ERYTHROMYCIN:** The manufacturer states that although there is no data, these drugs may interact with aglepristone

Laboratory Considerations

None were noted

Doses

WARNING: As accidental injection of this product can induce abortion; it should not be administered or handled by pregnant women. Accidental injection can also cause severe pain, intense swelling and ischemic necrosis that can lead to serious sequelae, including loss of a digit. In cases of accidental injection, prompt medical attention must be sought.

- ◾ **DOGS:**

   To terminate pregnancy (up to day 45):
   a) 10 mg/kg (0.33 mL/kg) subcutaneous injection only. Repeat one time, 24 hours after the first injection. A maximum of 5 mL should be injected at any one site. Light massage of the injection site is recommended after administration. (Label information; *Alizin*®—Virbac U.K.)

   To induce parturition:
   a) At day 60 (post-estimated LH surge): 15 mg/kg SC and another dose 24 hours later. Subsequently, give oxytocin 0.15 Units/kg SC at hourly intervals until last pup is delivered. Additional studies confirming efficacy and safety are warranted before routine clinical application

can be recommended. (Fieni, F. & Gogny 2009)

b) On or after day 58 of pregnancy: 15 mg/kg subcutaneously; repeat in 9 hours. In treated group, expulsion of first pup occurred between 32 and 56 hours after treatment. Use standard protocols to assist with birth (including oxytocin to assist in pup expulsion if necessary) or to intervene if parturition does not proceed. (Baan *et al.* 2005)

As an adjunct to treating pyometra/metritis:

a) When attempting to preserve fertility (mating should occur in the first or second estrus post-treatment) in bitches up to 5 years old with a lack of detectable ovarian cysts: Treatment begun at week 2-4 of diestrus with a single SC injection of aglepristone at 10 mg/kg. Doses are repeated at days 2, 7, and 14. During first 7 days, daily injections of amoxicillin/clavulanic acid were also given. (Jurka *et al.* 2010)

b) For closed cervix: 6 mg/kg twice daily on the first day followed by the same dose once daily on days 2, 3, and 4. Some prefer using larger doses (10mg/kg) once daily on days 1, 3, and 8, then follow up also on days 15 and 28 depending on the bitch's condition. (Romagnoli 2003)

c) For metritis: 10 mg/kg subcutaneously once daily on days 1, 2 and 8.

For open or closed pyometra: aglepristone 10 mg/kg subcutaneously once daily on days 1, 2 and 8 and cloprostenol 1 microgram/kg subcutaneously on days 3 to 7. Bitches with closed pyometra or with elevated temperature or dehydration should also receive intravenous fluids and antibiotics (*e.g.,* amoxicillin/clavulanate at 24 mg/kg/day on days 1–5). If pyometra has not resolved, additional aglepristone doses should be given on days 14 and 28. (Fieni, F 2006)

d) 10 mg/kg SC on days 1, 2, 8, 15, & 29. Give misoprostol 10 micrograms/kg PO twice daily on days 3 through 12. Approximately 75% of cases show significant clinical improvement without developing the adverse effects associated with the prostaglandins (F2alpha, cloprostenol). (Fontbonne 2007)

■ **CATS:**

For treating mammary fibroadenomatous hyperplasia:

a) 20 mg/kg aglepristone subcutaneously once weekly until resolution of signs. Cats who present with heart rates greater than 200 BPM should receive atenolol at 6.25 mg (total dose) until heart rate is less than 200 BPM with regression in size of

the mammary glands. (Gorlinger *et al.* 2002)

b) 10 mg/kg SC on two consecutive days, once weekly. Complete mammary regression occurs on average 3-4 weeks once treatment begun. Relapses can occur, particularly in cats that have been treated with a long acting progestin (medroxyprogesterone acetate). These cats should be treated with aglepristone for 5 weeks. (Jurka & Max 2009)

To terminate pregnancy (up to day 45):

a) 15 mg/kg SC twice 24 hours apart. Efficacy is 95% if administered before implantation, 85% if after implantation. Termination occurs within 3 days in 50% of queens. (Fontbonne 2007)

Monitoring

■ Clinical efficacy

■ For pregnancy termination: ultrasound 10 days after treatment and at least 30 days after mating

■ Adverse effects (see above)

Client Information

■ Only veterinary professionals should handle and administer this product

■ When used for pregnancy termination in the bitch, clients should understand that aglepristone might only be 95% effective in terminating pregnancy when used between days 26–45

■ A brown mucoid vaginal discharge can be seen approximately 24 hours before fetal expulsion

■ Bitch may exhibit the following after treatment: lack of appetite, excitement, restlessness or depression, vomiting, or diarrhea

■ Clients should be instructed to contact veterinarian if bitch exhibits a purulent or hemorrhagic discharge after treatment or if vaginal discharge persists 3 weeks after treatment

■ When used for pyometra, there is a substantial risk of treatment failure and ovario-hysterectomy may be required

Chemistry/Synonyms

Aglepristone is a synthetic steroid. The manufactured injectable dosage form is in a clear, yellow, oily, non-aqueous vehicle that contains arachis oil and ethanol. No additional antimicrobial agent is added to the injection.

Aglepristone may also be known as RU-534, *Alizine®*, or *Alizin®*.

Storage/Stability

Aglepristone injection should be stored below 25°C and protected from light. The manufacturer recommends using the product within 28 days of withdrawing the first dose.

Compatibility/Compounding Considerations

Although no incompatibilities have been reported, due to the product's oil/alcohol vehicle formulation it should not be mixed with any other medication.

Dosage Forms/Regulatory Status

VETERINARY-LABELED PRODUCTS:

Note: Not presently available or approved for use in the USA. In several countries:

Aglepristone 30 mg/mL in 5 mL & 10 mL vials; *Alizine®* or *Alizin®* (Virbac); (Rx)

The FDA may allow legal importation of this medication for compassionate use in animals; for more information, see the *Instructions for Legally Importing Drugs for Compassionate Use in the USA* found in the appendix.

HUMAN-LABELED PRODUCTS: None

References

Baan, M, M Taverne, et al. (2005). Induction of parturition in the bitch with the progesterone–receptor blocker aglepristone. *Theriogenology* 63(17): 1958–1972.

Fieni, F (2006). Clinical evaluation of the use of aglepristone, with or without cloprostenol, to treat cystic endometrial hyperplasia–pyometra complex. *Theriogenology* 66(6–7): 1550–1556.

Fieni, F & A Gogny (2009). Clinical Evaluation of the Use of Aglepristone Associated with Oxytocin to Induce Parturition in Bitch. *Reproduction in Domestic Animals* 44: 167–169.

Fontbonne, A (2007). Anti–Progestins Compounds in Reproduction. Proceedings: World Small Animal Veterinary Association Congress. Accessed via: Veterinary Information Network. http://goo.gl/vbjmP

Gorlinger, S, H Kooistra, et al. (2002). Treatment of fibroadenomatous hyperplasia in cats with aglepristone. *J Vet Intern Med* 16: 710–713.

Jurka, P & A Max (2009). Treatment of fibroadenomatosis in 14 cats with aglepristone—changes in blood parameters and follow-up. *Veterinary Record* 165(22): 657–660.

Jurka, P, A Max, et al. (2010). Age–Related Pregnancy Results and Further Examination of Bitches after Aglepristone Treatment of Pyometra. *Reproduction in Domestic Animals* 45(3): 525–529.

Romagnoli, S (2003). Clinical Approach to Infertility in the Bitch. Proceedings: WSAVA 2003. Accessed via: Veterinary Information Network. http://goo.gl/xRScy

---

ALBENDAZOLE

(al-***ben***-da-zole)   Albenza®, Valbazen®

ANTIPARASITIC

Prescriber Highlights

▶ Broad spectrum against a variety of nematodes, cestodes & protozoa; labeled for cattle & sheep (suspension only)

▶ Contraindicated with hepatic failure, pregnancy, lactating dairy cattle

▶ May cause GI effects (including hepatic dysfunction) & rarely blood dyscrasias (aplastic anemia)

▶ Do not use in pigeons, doves or crias

Uses/Indications

Albendazole is labeled for the following endoparasites of cattle (not lactating): *Ostertagia ostertagi, Haemonchus* spp., *Trichostrongylus* spp., *Nematodius* spp., *Cooperia* spp., *Bunostomum phlebotomum, Oesphagostomum* spp., *Dictacaulus vivaparus* (adult and 4th stage larva), *Fasciola hepatica* (adults), and *Moniezia* spp.

In sheep, albendazole is FDA-approved for treating the following endoparasites: *Ostertagia circumcincta, Marshallagia marshalli, Haemonchus contortus, Trichostrongylus* spp., *Nematodius* spp., *Cooperia* spp., *Oesphagostomum* spp., *Chibertia ovina, Dictacaulus filaria, Fasciola hepatica, Fascioides magna, Moniezia expansa,* and *Thysanosoma actinoides.*

Albendazole is also used (extra-label) in small mammals, goats and swine for endoparasite control.

In cats, albendazole has been used to treat *Paragonimus kellicotti* infections. In dogs and cats, albendazole has been used to treat capillariasis. In dogs, albendazole has been used to treat Filaroides infections. It has been used for treating giardia infections in small animals, but concerns about bone marrow toxicity have diminished enthusiasm for the drug's use.

Pharmacology/Actions

Benzimidazole antiparasitic agents have a broad spectrum of activity against a variety of pathogenic internal parasites. In susceptible parasites, their mechanism of action is believed due to disrupting intracellular microtubular transport systems by binding selectively and damaging tubulin, preventing tubulin polymerization, and inhibiting microtubule formation. Benzimidazoles also act at higher concentrations to disrupt metabolic pathways within the helminth, and inhibit metabolic enzymes, including malate dehydrogenase and fumarate reductase.

Pharmacokinetics

Pharmacokinetic data for albendazole in cattle, dogs and cats was not located. The drug is thought better absorbed orally than other benzimidazoles. Approximately 47% of an oral dose was retrieved (as metabolites) in the urine over a 9-day period.

After oral dosing in sheep, the parent compound was either not detectable or only transiently detectable in plasma due to a very rapid first-pass effect. The active metabolites, albendazole sulphoxide and albendazole sulfone, reached peak plasma concentrations 20 hours after dosing.

Contraindications/Precautions/Warnings

The drug is not FDA-approved for use in lactating dairy cattle. The manufacturer recommends not administering to female cattle during the first 45 days of pregnancy or for 45 days after removal of bulls. In sheep, it should not be administered to ewes during the first 30 days of pregnancy or for 30 days after removal of rams.

Pigeons and doves may be susceptible to albendazole and fenbendazole toxicity (intestinal crypt epithelial necrosis and bone marrow hypoplasia).

Nine alpaca crias receiving albendazole at dosages from 33–100 mg/kg/day once daily for 4 consecutive days developed neutropenia and severe watery diarrhea. All required treatment and 7 of 9 animals treated died or were euthanized secondary to sepsis or multiple organ failure. (Gruntman & Nolen-Walston 2006)

In humans, caution is recommended for use in patients with liver or hematologic diseases.

Albendazole was implicated as being an oncogen in 1984, but subsequent studies were unable to demonstrate any oncogenic or carcinogenic activity of the drug.

Adverse Effects

Albendazole is tolerated without significant adverse effects when dosed in cattle or sheep at recommended dosages.

Dogs treated at 50 mg/kg twice daily may develop anorexia. Cats may exhibit clinical signs of mild lethargy, depression, anorexia, and resistance to receiving the medication when albendazole is used to treat Paragonimus. Albendazole has been implicated in causing aplastic anemia in dogs, cats, and humans.

Reproductive/Nursing Safety

Albendazole has been associated with teratogenic and embryotoxic effects in rats, rabbits and sheep when given early in pregnancy. The manufacturer recommends not administering to female cattle during the first 45 days of pregnancy or for 45 days after removal of bulls. In sheep, it should not be administered to ewes during the first 30 days of pregnancy or for 30 days after removal of rams.

In humans, the FDA categorizes this drug as category *C* for use during pregnancy (*Animal studies have shown an adverse effect on the fetus, but there are no adequate studies in humans; or there are no animal reproduction studies and no adequate studies in humans.*)

Safety during nursing has not been established.

Overdosage/Toxicity

Doses of 300 mg/kg (30X recommended) and 200 mg/kg (20X) have caused death in cattle and sheep, respectively. Doses of 45 mg/kg (4.5X those recommended) did not cause any adverse effects in cattle tested. Cats receiving 100 mg/kg/day for 14–21 days showed signs of weight loss, neutropenia and mental dullness.

Drug Interactions

The following drug interactions have either been reported or are theoretical in humans or animals receiving albendazole and may be of significance in veterinary patients:

- **CIMETIDINE:** Increased albendazole levels in bile and cystic fluid
- **DEXAMETHASONE:** May increase albendazole serum levels
- **PRAZIQUANTEL:** May increase albendazole serum levels

Doses

- **DOGS:**

  For *Filaroides hirthi* infections:
  a) 50 mg/kg q12h PO for 5 days; repeat in 21 days. Clinical signs may suddenly worsen during therapy, presumably due to a reaction to worm death. (Hawkins *et al.* 1989)
  b) 25 mg/kg PO q12h for 5 days; may repeat in 2 weeks (also for *Oslerus osleri*) (Reinemeyer 1995)

  For *Filaroides osleri* (also known as *Oslerus osleri*) infections:
  a) 9.5 mg/kg for 55 days or 25 mg/kg PO twice daily for 5 days. Repeat therapy in 2 weeks. (Todd *et al.* 1985)

  For *Capillaria plica*:
  a) 50 mg/kg q12h for 10–14 days. May cause anorexia. (Brown & Barsanti 1989)

  For *Paragonimus kellicotti*:
  a) 25 mg/kg PO q12h for 14 days (Reinemeyer 1995)

  For Giardia:
  a) 25 mg/kg PO twice daily for 5 days (Barr & Bowman 1994)
  b) 25 mg/kg PO twice daily for 2–5 days (Lappin 2000)

  For Leishmaniasis:
  a) 10 mg/kg PO once daily for 30 days or 5 mg/kg PO q6h for 60 days (Greene and Watson 1998)

- **CATS:**

  For *Paragonimus kellicotti*:
  a) 25 mg/kg PO q12h for 14 days (Reinemeyer 1995)

  For Giardia:
  a) 25 mg/kg PO q12h for 3–5 days; may cause bone marrow suppression in dogs and cats. (Vasilopulos 2006)

  For treatment of liver flukes (Platynosum or Opisthorchiidae families):
  a) 50 mg/kg PO once daily until ova are gone (Taboada 1999)

- **RABBITS/RODENTS/SMALL MAMMALS:**
  a) **Rabbits:** For Encephalitozoon phacoclastic uveitis: 30 mg/kg PO once daily for 30 days, then 15 mg/kg PO once daily for 30 days (Ivey & Morrisey 2000)
  b) **Rabbits:** For *E. cuniculi*: 20 mg/kg PO once daily for 10 days. (Bryan 2009)
  c) **Chinchillas:** For Giardia: 50–100 mg/kg PO once a day for 3 days (Hayes 2000)

■ **CATTLE:**

For susceptible parasites:

a) 10 mg/kg PO (Labeled directions; *Valbazen®*—Pfizer)

b) 7.5 mg/kg PO; 15 mg/kg PO for adult liver flukes (Roberson 1988)

c) For adult liver flukes: 10 mg/kg PO; best used in fall when the majority are adults (little or no efficacy against immature forms). A second treatment in winter may be beneficial. (Herd 1986)

d) For gastrointestinal cestodes: 10 mg/kg PO (Herd 1986a)

■ **SWINE:**

For susceptible parasites:

a) 5–10 mg/kg PO (Roberson 1988)

■ **SHEEP & GOATS:**

For susceptible parasites:

a) 7.5 mg/kg PO (0.75 mL of the suspension per 25 lb. body weight). (Labeled directions; *Valbazen® Suspension*—Pfizer)

b) 7.5 mg/kg PO; 15 mg/kg PO for adult liver flukes (Roberson 1988)

c) For adult liver flukes in sheep: 7.6 mg/kg (Paul 1986)

d) For treatment of nematodes in sheep: 3 mL of suspension per 100 lbs of body weight PO (Bulgin 2003)

■ **BIRDS:**

a) Ratites: Using the suspension: 1 mL/22 kg of body weight twice daily for 3 days; repeat in 2 weeks. Has efficacy against flagellate parasites and tapeworms. (Jenson 1998)

Monitoring

■ Efficacy

■ Adverse effects if used in non-FDA-approved species or at dosages higher than recommended

■ Consider monitoring CBC's and liver enzymes (q4–6 weeks) if treating long-term (>1 month)

Client Information

■ Shake well before administering

■ Contact veterinarian if adverse effects occur (*e.g.*, vomiting, diarrhea, yellowish sclera/mucous membranes or skin)

Chemistry/Synonyms

A benzimidazole anthelmintic structurally related to mebendazole, albendazole has a molecular weight of 265. It is insoluble in water and soluble in alcohol.

Albendazole may also be known as albendazolum, SKF-62979, *Valbazen®* or *Albenza®*; many other trade names are available.

Storage/Stability

Albendazole suspension should be stored at room temperature (15–30°C); protect from freezing. Shake well before using. Albendazole paste should be stored at controlled room temperature (15–30°C); protect from freezing.

Dosage Forms/ Regulatory Status

VETERINARY-LABELED PRODUCTS:

Albendazole Suspension: 113.6 mg/mL (11.36%) in 500 mL, 1 liter, 5 liters; *Valbazen® Suspension* (Pfizer); (OTC). FDA-approved for use in cattle (not female cattle during first 45 days of pregnancy or for 45 days after removal of bulls, or of breeding age) and sheep (do not administer to ewes during the first 30 days of pregnancy or for 30 days after removal of rams). Slaughter withdrawal for cattle = 27 days at labeled doses. Slaughter withdrawal for sheep = 7 days at labeled dose. Since milk withdrawal time has not been established, do not use in female dairy cattle of breeding age. A milk withdrawal time of 7 milkings has been proposed for sheep (Athanasiou *et al.* 2009).

Albendazole Paste: 30% in 205 g (7.2 oz); *Valbazen®* (Pfizer); (OTC). FDA-approved for use in cattle (not female cattle during first 45 days of pregnancy or for 45 days after removal of bulls or of breeding age). Slaughter withdrawal = 27 days at labeled doses. Since withdrawal time in milk has not been established, do not use in female dairy cattle of breeding age.

HUMAN-LABELED PRODUCTS:

Albendazole Oral Tablets: 200 mg; *Albenza®* (GlaxoSmithKline); (Rx)

References

Athanasiou, LV, DC Orfanou, et al. (2009). Proposals for withdrawal period of sheep milk for some commonly used veterinary medicinal products: A review. *Small Ruminant Research* **86**(1–3): 2–5.

Barr, S & D Bowman (1994). Giardiasis in Dogs and Cats. *Comp CE* **16**(May): 603–610.

Brown, SA & JA Barsanti (1989). Diseases of the bladder and urethra. *Textbook of Veterinary Internal Medicine.* SJ Ettinger Ed. Philadelphia, WB Saunders. **2**: 2108–2141.

Bryan, J (2009). E. Cuniculi: Past, Present, and Future. Proceedings: Western Veterinary Conference. Accessed via: Veterinary Information Network. http://goo.gl/UEYVt

Bulgin, M (2003). Current drugs of choice for sheep and goats. Proceedings: Western Veterinary Conference. Accessed via: Veterinary Information Network. http://goo.gl/I5mz4

Gruntman, A & R Nolen–Walston (2006). Albendazole toxicity in nine alpaca crias. Proceedings: ACVIM Forum 2006. Accessed via: Veterinary Information Network. http://goo.gl/vbGVs

Hawkins, EC, SJ Ettinger, et al. (1989). Diseases of the lower respiratory tract (lung) and pulmonary edema. *Textbook of Veterinary Internal Medicine.* SJ Ettinger Ed. Philadelphia, WB Saunders. **1**: 816–866.

Hayes, P (2000). Diseases of Chinchillas. *Kirk's Current Veterinary Therapy: XIII Small Animal Practice.* J Bonagura Ed. Philadelphia, WB Saunders: 1152–1157.

Herd, R (1986). Trematode Infections—Cattle, Sheep, Goats. *Current Veterinary Therapy: Food Animal Practice 2.* JL Howard Ed. Philadelphia, W.B. Saunders: 756–759.

Ivey, E & J Morrisey (2000). Therapeutics for Rabbits. *Vet Clin NA: Exotic Anim Pract* **3**:1(Jan): 183–216.

Jenson, J (1998). Current ratite therapy. *The Veterinary Clinics of North America: Food Animal Practice* **16**:3(November).

Lappin, M (2000). Protozoal and Miscellaneous Infections. *Textbook of Veterinary Internal Medicine: Diseases of the Dog and Cat.* S Ettinger and E Feldman Eds. Philadelphia, WB Saunders. **1**: 408–417.

Paul, JW (1986). Anthelmintic Therapy. *Current Veterinary Therapy: Food Animal Practice 2.* JL Howard Ed. Philadelphia, W.B. Saunders: 39–44.

Reinemeyer, C (1995). Parasites of the respiratory system. *Kirk's Current Veterinary Therapy:XII.* J Bonagura Ed. Philadelphia, W.B. Saunders: 895–898.

Roberson, EL (1988). Anticestodal and antitrematodal drugs. *Veterinary Pharmacology and Therapeutics.* NH Booth and LE McDonald Eds. Ames, Iowa State University Press: 928–949.

Taboada, J (1999). Feline Liver Diseases. Proceedings: The North American Veterinary Conference, Orlando.

Todd, KS, AJ Paul, et al. (1985). Parasitic Diseases. *Handbook of Small Animal Therapeutics.* LE Davis Ed. New York, Churchill Livingstone: 89–126.

Vasilopulos, R (2006). Advances in diagnosis and treatment of feline protozoal diarrhea. Proceedings: ACVIM 2006. Accessed via: Veterinary Information Network. http://goo.gl/FYwOW

ALBUMIN, HUMAN
ALBUMIN, CANINE

(al-*byoo*-min)

NATURAL PROTEIN COLLOID

Prescriber Highlights

▶ Natural colloid that may be useful in increasing intravascular oncotic pressure and organ perfusion and decreasing edema secondary to crystalloid fluid replacement, particularly in critically ill animals with reversible diseases/conditions when hypoalbuminemia is present

▶ Significant concerns with adverse effects, especially immune-mediated reactions when using xeno-albumin products (*i.e.*, human albumin in dogs); "thoughtful consideration and extreme care" must be taken when deciding whether to use

▶ Canine albumin product (lyophilized) available commercially in USA, but little data available on its safety and efficacy

▶ Treatment can be relatively expensive, but may be cheaper than plasma and may reduce intensive care unit stays

Uses/Indications

Albumin (human or canine) may be useful as colloid fluid replacement therapy in critically ill small animals. Conditions where albumin therapy may be considered include times when the patient is severely hypoalbuminemic (albumin <2.0 g/dL), severely edematous, or has systemic inflammatory response syndrome/sepsis and increased vascular leak. Because of availability, human albumin is usually used in small animals, but this "xeno-albumin" use poses considerable risks. There is little information available on the use of human albumin in cats.

A retrospective study evaluating 25% albumin (human) in critically ill dogs and cats, found that it could be safely administered to critically ill animals, and increase albumin levels and systemic blood pressure (Mathews & Barry 2005). However, another retrospective study (Trow *et al.* 2008) evaluating albumin (human) use in 73 critically ill dogs, found that while albumin increased serum albumin, total protein, and colloid osmotic pressure, 23% of treated dogs developed at least one adverse effect that could potentially have been caused by albumin. The authors caution that given the risks for complications and uncertain positive influence, thoughtful consideration and extreme care must be taken when deciding whether to administer human albumin transfusions to critically ill dogs, and these concerns should be discussed with clients; frequent monitoring should always be used.

An Italian retrospective study evaluating 5% human albumin in 418 dogs and 170 cats with critical illnesses, severe hypersensitivity reactions such as anaphylaxis, angioedema, and urticaria were not noted in any patient record. In no case was it necessary to discontinue or interrupt the albumin infusion due to adverse effects. Diarrhea, hyperthermia, or tremors were noted in 43% of dogs and 36% of cats treated. A combination of these adverse reactions was seen in 32% of dogs and 34% of cats treated. Adverse reactions that developed one day or more after treatment were noted in 28% of dogs and 11% of cats treated. Reactions beyond Day 3 were not recorded. Perivascular inflammation at catheter sites following albumin were seen in 17% of dogs and 34% of cats. This study did not measure changes in total protein, colloid oncotic pressure or albumin.

All these studies were retrospective in nature, and prospective, controlled studies are necessary before albumin's true benefit and risk profiles are known.

Pharmacology/Actions

Albumin provides 75-80% of the oncotic pressure of plasma. When replacing endogenous albumin that has been lost, albumin helps prevent additional crystalloid fluids from leaking from capillaries by reducing hydrostatic pressure. This can allow using less volume of crystalloids and increase perfusion, with less risk for edema. Albumin (for a given species) also has other actions, including binding and transport of drugs, ions, hormones, lipids, and metals (including iron), maintenance of endothelial integrity and permeability control, antioxidant properties, metabolic and acid−base functions, decrease platelet aggregation, augment antithrombin and serving as a thiol-group. It is unknown what effect, if any, xeno-albumin has on these actions.

Pharmacokinetics

Endogenous circulating albumin represents 30-40% of total body albumin. Elimination of exogenously administered canine albumin is estimated to be between 20-24 days with a half-life of 8-10 days. The kinetics of human albumin in dogs or cats is not well described.

Contraindications/Precautions/Warnings
A history of hypersensitivity to albumin (human or canine) is a specific contraindication for use. Because of the risk for hypersensitivity, repeat administration of xeno-albumin is relatively contraindicated in otherwise healthy animals (volume depleted) albumin use should be avoided.

The label for the canine albumin products states: Dogs with a pre-existing condition resulting in volume overload should be monitored carefully during administration of hyperosmolar products like canine albumin. Dogs with anemia or extreme dehydration should not receive canine albumin unless concurrent red blood cell products or appropriate fluid therapy is first administered.

Adverse Effects
The incidence of adverse effects reported in retrospective studies in dogs and cats with human albumin vary widely, but they can be serious. Hypersensitivity, both immediate (anaphylactoid; anaphylactic) and delayed (type III hypersensitivity; serum sickness) is an issue when using human albumin in dogs. These effects can be serious and deaths have occurred. Immediate adverse effects reported include facial edema, vomiting, urticaria, hyperthermia, and shock. Should facial edema occur, diphenhydramine should be given at 1-2 mg/kg IM and repeated every 8 hours as required (Mathews 2008). Delayed adverse effects can include lethargy, lameness, edema, cutaneous lesions/vasculitis, vomiting, inappetence, renal failure and coagulopathies.

While the risk appears low, transmission of infectious agents from albumin products is possible.

The incidence of adverse effects in dogs associated with human albumin appears to be higher in healthy dogs than in critically ill dogs possibly due to the blunted immune response that can be seen in critically ill patients. In a study in 6 healthy dogs given 2 mL/kg of 25% human albumin during a 1-hour period an immediate hypersensitivity reaction (vomiting, facial edema) was seen in 1 dog and delayed adverse reactions were seen 5 to 13 days after albumin in all 6 dogs and included lethargy, lameness, peripheral edema, ecchymoses, vomiting, and anorexia. Delayed complications in 2 of these dogs resulted in death due to renal failure and coagulopathy and were suspected to have occurred because of serum sickness secondary to type III hypersensitivity reactions. Another dog had shock and sepsis secondary to a multi-drug resistant *E. coli* infection (Francis *et al.* 2007). Another study in 9 healthy dogs that were given one or two infusions of human albumin 25% at an initial infusion rate of 0.5 mL/kg/hour that

was increased incrementally to a maximum of 4 mL/kg/hour, adverse effects were seen after the first or second infusion in 3 dogs. Anaphylactoid reactions were observed in 1 of 9 dogs during the first infusion and in the 2 dogs that were administered a second infusion. Two dogs developed severe edema and urticaria 6 or 7 days after the initial infusion. All dogs developed anti-HSA antibodies (Cohn *et al.* 2007).

Rash, nausea, vomiting, tachycardia and hypotension have been reported in humans, but hypersensitivity reactions are very rare.

Reproductive/Nursing Safety
In humans, the FDA categorizes this drug as category *C* for use during pregnancy (*Animal studies have shown an adverse effect on the fetus, but there are no adequate studies in humans; or there are no animal reproduction studies and no adequate studies in humans.*) However, it is unlikely to pose much risk to the fetus, particularly when used appropriately. Albumin excretion into maternal milk is not known, but is unlikely to be harmful.

Overdosage/Acute Toxicity
To avoid the effects of hyperalbuminemia/hyperproteinemia, albumin levels should be followed. Most believe that serum albumin should not exceed 2.5 grams/dL (some say 2 grams/dL) when used clinically.

Drug Interactions
While the administration of exogenous albumin could bind drugs that are highly bound to plasma proteins and affect the amount of free drug circulating, this does not appear to be of significance when albumin is used clinically.

Laboratory Considerations
■ Exogenous administration of albumin may temporarily decrease serum concentrations of calcium

Doses
■ **DOGS/CATS**
a) Dogs: In a review of albumin (human) 25% (HSA) use in small animals the author describes when he considers using 25% human albumin: Patients with: **1**) refractory hypotension; **2**) Severe hypoalbuminemic patients [albumin <1.5 g/dL or (<1.8 g/dL during dehydration and hypovolemia) with ongoing losses (e.g., peritonitis, pleural effusion)]; **3**) Combined with FFP in hypoalbuminemic septic patients; **4**) Patients that have protein-losing enteropathy before surgical biopsy; **5**) Markedly hypoalbuminemic patients that continue to vomit (likely attributable to bowel edema); **6**) Refractory hypotension associated with gastric dilation-volvulus. The following is an edited dosage protocol (see the reference for more detailed information on use, etc.): When time permits

(non-emergent situation), a test dose of 0.25 mL/kg/h is given over 15 minutes while monitoring heart rate, respiratory rate, and temperature (baseline before transfusion and at end of test dose). Discontinue infusion if adverse signs (facial swelling, or other signs of anaphylaxis or anaphylactoid reaction) develop. The maximum volume administered to any dog by the author is 25 mL/kg (6.25 g/kg) administered continuously over 72 hours; the mean volume administered to any dog overall is 5 mL/kg (1.25 g/kg). The maximum volume given as a slow push or bolus to treat hypotension is 4 mL/kg (1 gram/kg), with a mean volume of 2 mL/kg (0.5 g/kg). The range for a continuous rate infusion (CRI) after a bolus administration is 0.1 to 1.7 mL/kg/h (0.025–0.425 g/kg) over 4 to 72 hours. Infusions are empirically selected to meet low normal values. The shorter infusion times are most commonly used for refractory hypotension. (Mathews 2008)

b) Dogs: The administration of 10% human albumin may be useful in dogs with reversible disease and clinically affected by marked hypoalbuminemia (serum albumin, <1.5 g/dL) and low colloid osmotic pressure (colloid osmotic pressure, <14 mm Hg), but given the risks for complications and uncertain positive influence, thoughtful consideration and extreme care must be taken when deciding whether to administer human albumin transfusions to critically ill dogs, and these concerns should be discussed with clients and frequent monitoring performed. Reasonable goals for human albumin administration may be to increase serum albumin to 2 to 2.5 g/dL and colloid osmotic pressure to 14 to 20 mm Hg. Dogs with surgical diseases and septic peritonitis should be especially considered because of the role of albumin in wound healing. The protocol most often used for calculating the dosage of human albumin in the study was: albumin deficit (g) = 10X (serum albumin desired–serum albumin of patient) X body weight (kg) X 0.3. Alternatively, some dogs received 0.5 to 1.25 g/kg. In the authors' institution, the calculated dosage of human albumin was aseptically diluted to a 10% solution with saline (0.9% NaCl) solution and administered over a 12-hour period with a transfusion filter. Because of the antigenicity of human albumin in dogs, no dog was eligible for receiving additional human albumin after 7 days following initial human albumin administration. (Trow *et al.* 2008)

c) Dogs: Using the canine albumin lyophilized product (5 gram) for the treatment of hypovolemic shock or hypoalbuminemia regardless of the etiology: Dilute to 16% (add 30 mL of diluent such as sterile normal saline, *Normasol®* or dextrose 5%; see Compatibility/Compounding below) and administer IV at a dosage rate of 1 mL/min. A total of 2.5–5 mL/kg body weight is recommended. Albumin may be diluted in 0.9% saline or Normosol for administration. (Product label; Canine Albumin 5gm lyophilized— Animal Blood Resources)

Monitoring

■ Pre and post serum albumin. Depending on the source, most suggest a target for serum albumin concentrations of 2–2.5 g/dL

■ Pre and post colloid osmotic pressure (if possible)

■ Adverse effects: body temperature, respiratory rate, blood pressure and heart rate

■ Signs of volume overload

■ Monitor for delayed reactions, which can occur weeks after administration

Client Information

■ The medication must be given in an inpatient setting.

■ Clients should understand and accept the risks, costs, and monitoring associated with albumin's use.

Chemistry/Synonyms

Human albumin is a highly soluble, globular protein with a molecular weight of 66,500. The 5% solution has a colloid osmotic pressure (COP) similar to that of normal plasma. Amino acid homology of human and canine albumin is about 79%, but the canine albumin molecule is 2 kDalton larger and has a different relative charge and isoelectric point.

Albumin (human) may also be known as Alb, albumine, HSA, or albuminum. "Salt-poor" albumin is a misnomer, but still occasionally used as a designation for 25% albumin. There are a variety of tradename products, including: *Albuminar®*, *Albutein®*, *Buminate®*, *Plasbumin®*, and *Flexbumin®*.

Storage/Stability

5% solution: Albumin (human) 5% solution is stable for 3 years, providing storage temperature does not exceed 30°C (89°F). Protect from freezing. 25% and 20% solutions: Store at room temperature not exceeding 30°C (86°F). Do not freeze. Do not use after expiration date.

Do not use solutions of they appear turbid or if sediment is noted. Solutions should not be used if more than 4 hours have passed since the container has been entered as it contains no preservatives. Do not use solutions that have been frozen.

The lyophilized canine albumin product should be stored at 4-6°C (refrigerated) until use. Product is stable for 15 months as labeled. After rehydration, it should not be stored longer than 24 hours. Refrigerated storage for rehydrated product is recommended.

Compatibility/Compounding Considerations

Albumin may be administered either in conjunction with or combined with other parenteral products such as whole blood, plasma, saline, glucose, or sodium lactate. It is reportedly **compatible** with usual carbohydrate or electrolyte solutions, diltiazem or midazolam at a Y-site.

Do not mix albumin with protein hydrolysates, amino acid solutions or solutions containing alcohol.

When preparing human albumin for administration use only 16-gauge needles or dispensing pins with 20 mL vial sizes and larger. Needles or dispensing pins should only be inserted within the stopper area delineated by the raised ring. The stopper should be penetrated perpendicular to the plane of the stopper within the ring.

Canine albumin 5 gram lyophilized, should be rehydrated by adding 30 mL of 0.9% sterile saline or *Normosol®* to make a 16% canine albumin solution. Dextrose 5% solution may also be used as a diluent. DO NOT use sterile water to rehydrate the product. After addition of the diluent, gently swirl the solution until all powder is rehydrated. Once diluent is added, the vial may be warmed in a 37°C water bath to speed rehydration. Add 49 mL of appropriate diluent to obtain a 10% albumin solution and 100 mL to obtain a 5% solution.

Dosage Forms/Regulatory Status

VETERINARY-LABELED PRODUCTS:

Albumin, Canine, 98% lyophilized 5 g, without preservatives or plasma byproducts. (Animal Blood Resources Intl.). Product labeled for intravenous use in dogs and only to be used by or on the order of licensed veterinarian.

HUMAN-LABELED PRODUCTS:

Albumin, Human 5% in 50 mL, 100 mL, 250 mL & 500 mL glass containers, and 25% in 20 mL, 50 mL & 100 mL vials or flex containers; *Albuminar®* (ZLB Behring), *Albutein®* (Grifols), *Albuminate®* (Baxter), *Flexbumin®* (flexible container; Baxter), *Plasbumin®* (Talecris), generic; (Rx)

References

Cohn, LA, ME Kerl, et al. (2007). Response of healthy dogs to infusions of human serum albumin. *American Journal of Veterinary Research* 68(6): 657–663.

Francis, AH, LG Martin, et al. (2007). Adverse reactions suggestive of type III hypersensitivity in six healthy dogs given human albumin. *Javma–Journal of the American Veterinary Medical Association* 230(6): 873–879.

Mathews, KA (2008). The therapeutic use of 25% human serum albumin in critically ill dogs and cats. *Veterinary Clinics of North America–Small Animal Practice* 38(3): 595–+.

Mathews, KA & M Barry (2005). The use of 25% human serum albumin: outcome and efficacy in raising serum albumin and systemic blood pressure in critically ill dogs and cats. *Journal of Veterinary Emergency and Critical Care* 15(2): 110–118.
Trow, AV, EA Rozanski, et al. (2008). Evaluation of use of human albumin in critically ill dogs: 73 cases (2003–2006). *Javma–Journal of the American Veterinary Medical Association* 233(4): 607–612.

ALBUTEROL SULFATE

(al-**byoo**-ter-ole)   Salbutamol, Proventil®, Ventolin®

BETA-ADRENERGIC AGONIST

Prescriber Highlights

▶ Used primarily as a bronchodilator after PO or inhaled dosing

▶ Use with caution in patients with cardiac dysrhythmias or dysfunction, seizure disorders, hypertension or hyperthyroidism

▶ May be teratogenic (high doses) or delay labor

Uses/Indications

Albuterol is used principally in dogs and cats for its effects on bronchial smooth muscle to alleviate bronchospasm or cough. It is also used in horses as a bronchodilator.

Pharmacology/Actions

Like other beta-agonists, albuterol is believed to act by stimulating production of cyclic AMP through activation of adenyl cyclase. Albuterol is considered to be predominantly a beta$_2$ agonist (relaxation of bronchial, uterine, and vascular smooth muscles). At usual doses, albuterol possesses minimal beta$_1$ agonist (heart) activity. Beta-adrenergics can promote a shift of potassium away from the serum and into the cell, perhaps via stimulation of Na$^+$-K$^+$-ATPase. Temporary decreases in either normal or high serum potassium levels are possible.

Pharmacokinetics

The specific pharmacokinetics of this agent have apparently not been thoroughly studied in domestic animals. In general, albuterol is absorbed rapidly and well after oral administration. Effects occur within 5 minutes after oral inhalation; 30 minutes after oral administration (*e.g.*, tablets). It does not cross the blood-brain barrier but does cross the placenta. Duration of effect generally persists for 3–6 hours after inhalation and up to 12 hours (depending on dosage form) after oral administration. The drug is extensively metabolized in the liver principally to the inactive metabolite, albuterol 4'-O-sulfate. After oral administration the serum half-life in humans has been reported as 2.7–5 hours.

Contraindications/Precautions/Warnings

Albuterol is contraindicated in patients hypersensitive to it. It should be used with caution in patients with diabetes, hyperthyroidism, hypertension, seizure disorders, or cardiac disease (especially with concurrent arrhythmias).

Use during the late stages of pregnancy may inhibit uterine contractions.

Adverse Effects

Most adverse effects are dose-related and those that would be expected with sympathomimetic agents including increased heart rate, tremors, CNS excitement (nervousness) and dizziness. These effects are generally transient and mild and usually do not require discontinuation of therapy. Decreased serum potassium values may be noted; rarely is potassium supplementation required.

The S-form of albuterol may potentially increase airway inflammation in cats. As "regular" albuterol is the racemic form (R,S-albuterol) it may also increase airway inflammation and its use in cats should probably be limited to acute, rescue treatment only and not for chronic treatment. (Reinero 2008), (Reinero 2009). Additionally, cats don't like the "hiss" occurring during actuation of the metered-dose inhaler or the taste of the drug/vehicle.

Reproductive/Nursing Safety

In very large doses, albuterol is teratogenic in rodents. It should be used (particularly the oral dosage forms) during pregnancy only when the potential benefits outweigh the risks. Like some other beta agonists, it may delay pre-term labor after oral administration. In humans, the FDA categorizes this drug as category **C** for use during pregnancy (*Animal studies have shown an adverse effect on the fetus, but there are no adequate studies in humans; or there are no animal reproduction studies and no adequate studies in humans.*)

Overdosage/Acute Toxicity

Clinical signs of significant overdose after systemic administration (including when dogs bite an aerosol canister) may include: arrhythmias (tachycardia and extrasystole), hypertension, fever, vomiting, mydriasis, tremors, and CNS stimulation. Hypokalemia and hypophosphatemia may occur. There were 658 exposures to Albuterol reported to the ASPCA Animal Poison Control Center (APCC) during 2008-2009. In these cases, 656 were dogs with 610 showing clinical signs, and 2 were cats with both showing clinical signs. Common findings in dogs recorded in decreasing frequency included tachycardia, lethargy, vomiting, hypokalemia, panting, agitation, trembling, and tachypnea. Common findings in cats included tachycardia.

If there is a recent ingestion of tablets, and if the animal does not have significant cardiac or CNS effects, it should be handled like other overdoses (empty gut, give activated charcoal and a cathartic). For inhalation exposure (when a dog bites an aerosol canister) decontamination is generally not effective. If cardiac arrhythmias require treatment a beta-blocking agent (*e.g.*, at-

enolol, metoprolol) can be used. Diazepam can be used for tremors. Potassium supplementation may be required. The oral LD 50 of albuterol in rats is reported to be greater than 2 g/kg. Contact an animal poison control center for further information.

Drug Interactions

The following drug interactions have either been reported or are theoretical in humans or animals receiving albuterol (primarily when albuterol is given orally and not via inhalation) and may be of significance in veterinary patients:

- ■ **BETA-ADRENERGIC BLOCKING AGENTS** (*e.g.*, **propranolol**): May antagonize the actions of albuterol

- ■ **DIGOXIN:** Albuterol may increase the risk of cardiac arrhythmias

- ■ **INHALATION ANESTHETICS** (*e.g.*, **halothane, isoflurane, methoxyflurane**): Albuterol may predispose the patient to ventricular arrhythmias, particularly in patients with pre-existing cardiac disease—use cautiously

- ■ **OTHER SYMPATHOMIMETIC AMINES:** Used with albuterol may increase the risk of developing adverse cardiovascular effects

- ■ **TRICYCLIC ANTIDEPRESSANTS OR MONO-AMINE OXIDASE INHIBITORS:** May potentiate the vascular effects of albuterol

Doses

- ■ **DOGS:**

  WARNING: There are several older references that state that the oral dose is 50 *mg*/kg q8h. **This is an obvious overdose and should not be followed.** A more reasonable dose orally in dogs is: 0.05 mg/kg (50 *micrograms*/kg) PO q8–12h.

  a) 0.05 mg/kg (50 *micrograms*/kg) PO q8h (Johnson 2000)

  b) 0.02 mg/kg PO q12h for 5 days; if no improvement and no adverse effects may increase to 0.05 mg/kg PO q8–12h. If patient responds, reduce to lowest effective dose. (Church 2003)

  c) For inhalation, based on a 60 lb dog: 0.5 mL of the 0.5% solution for nebulization in 4 mL of saline nebulized every 6 hours (McConnell & Hughey 1992)

- ■ **CATS:**

  a) For bronchodilation in feline asthma using the 90 micrograms/puff aerosol albuterol inhaler and an appropriate spacer and mask:

  > For mild symptoms give one puff albuterol as needed with one puff of 110 micrograms fluticasone twice daily.

  > Moderate symptoms may be treated with albuterol one puff as needed with a 5 day course of prednisone at 1 mg/kg PO daily, and 220 micrograms of fluticasone twice daily.

Severely affected cats should be treated on an emergency basis with oxygen, an intravenous dose of a glucocorticoid, 90 micrograms (one puff) albuterol every 30 minutes as needed.

Chronic therapy should include fluticasone 220 micrograms twice daily, 90 micrograms albuterol as needed and 1 mg/kg prednisone every other day. (Dowling 2003)

b) For intermittent (not daily) signs (*e.g.*, wheeze, increased cough or respiratory rate and effort at rest) of feline asthma: two puffs into an appropriate spacer (*e.g.*, *Aerokat®*) twice daily; cat should breathe through the mask and spacer for 7–10 seconds. Positive clinical effect should be seen within 5–10 minutes. Can be used every 1/2 hour for 2–4 hours in crisis. (Padrid 2006)

■ **HORSES: (**Note: ARCI UCGFS Class 3 Drug)
a) For rescue therapy in horses demonstrating respiratory difficulty at rest: 360 micrograms (4 puffs) inhaled; if severe airway obstruction, may give at 15 minute increments for up to 2 hours. Continue as needed every 4-6 hours. Beneficial effects may last approximately 1 hour in severely affected horses. Longer acting beta agonists may be necessary. Combination therapy with corticosteroids reduces tolerance that develops and enhances beta-adrenergic receptor protein expression.

For moderate to severe disease: 360 micrograms followed in 5 minutes with aerosolized corticosteroid (beclomethasone or fluticasone) therapy. (Davis & Rush 2002)

b) 2–3 micrograms/kg via inhalation using a specially designed mask and spacer (*Aeromask®* and *Aerovent®*) (Foreman 1999)

c) For heaves: 0.8–2 micrograms/kg in a metered dose inhaler (Lavoie 2003)

d) For short-acting bronchodilation: 450–900 micrograms (5–10 puffs) as needed, not to exceed 4 times per week unless in conjunction with a corticosteroid (Mazan 2003)

e) For heaves: 360 micrograms (4 puffs) inhaled as needed. Tolerance develops rapidly if used as a sole therapy. (Rush 2006)

Monitoring

■ Clinical symptom improvement; auscultation, blood gases (if indicated)

■ Cardiac rate, rhythm (if warranted)

■ Serum potassium, early in therapy if animal is susceptible to hypokalemia

Client Information

■ Contact veterinarian if animal's condition deteriorates or it becomes acutely ill.

■ If using the aerosol, shake well before using. Be certain how to appropriately administer the product to maximize effectiveness. Do not puncture or use near an open flame; do not allow exposure to temperatures greater than 120°F. Keep out of reach of children and pets.

Chemistry/Synonyms

A synthetic sympathomimetic amine, albuterol sulfate occurs as a white, almost tasteless crystalline powder. It is soluble in water and slightly soluble in alcohol. One mg of albuterol is equivalent to 1.2 mg of albuterol sulfate.

Albuterol sulfate may also be known as: salbutamol hemisulphate, salbutamol sulphate, or salbutamoli sulfas; many trade names are available.

Storage/Stability

Oral albuterol sulfate products should be stored at 2–30°C. The inhaled aerosol should be stored at room temperature; do not allow exposure to temperatures above 120°F or the canister may burst. The 0.5% nebs should be stored at room temperature; the 0.083% nebs should be stored in the refrigerator. Discard solutions if they become colored.

Dosage Forms/Regulatory Status

VETERINARY-LABELED PRODUCTS: None

The ARCI (Racing Commissioners International) has designated this drug as a class 3 substance. See the appendix for more information.

HUMAN-LABELED PRODUCTS:

Albuterol Oral Tablets: 2 mg & 4 mg; generic; (Rx)

Albuterol Extended Release Oral Tablets: 4 mg & 8 mg; *VoSpire® ER* (Dava); generic (Mylan); (Rx)

Albuterol Oral Syrup: 2 mg (as sulfate)/5 mL in 473 mL; generic; (Rx)

Albuterol Aerosol: Each actualization delivers 90 micrograms albuterol in 6.7g, 6.8g, 8.5g, 18g; *ProAir HFA®* (Teva); *Proventil HFA®* (Key); *Ventolin HFA®* (GlaxoSmithKline); generic; (Rx).

Albuterol Solution for Inhalation ("Nebs"): 0.083% (2.5 mg/3 mL) in 3 mL UD vials; 0.5% (5 mg/mL) in 0.5 mL vials & 20 mL with dropper; 0.021% preservative-free (0.63 mg/3mL) & 0.042% preservative-free (1.25 mg/3 mL), in 3 mL UD vials *Proventil®* (Schering); *AccuNeb®* (Dey); generic; (Rx)

Also available: 14.7 g aerosol metered dose inhaler containing 18 mcg ipratropium bromide (an inhaled anticholinergic) and 103 mcg albuterol sulfate per puff; *Combivent®* (B-I); (Rx) and 3 mL unit dose solution for inhalation (neb) containing 0.5 mg ipratropium bromide and 3 mg albuterol, *DuoNeb®* (Dey); (Rx)

References

Church, D (2003). Drugs used in the management of respiratory diseases. Proceedings: World Small Animal Veterinary Assoc. World Congress. Accessed via: Veterinary Information Network. http://goo.gl/f3mOr

Davis, E & BR Rush (2002). Equine recurrent airway obstruction: pathogenesis, diagnosis, and patient management. *Veterinary Clinics of North America–Equine Practice* 18(3): 453–+.

Dowling, P (2003). Inhalation therapy for coughing dogs and wheezing cats. Proceedings: Western Veterinary Conference. Accessed via: Veterinary Information Network. http://goo.gl/2aXnC

Foreman, J (1999). Equine respiratory pharmacology. *The Veterinary Clinics of North America: Equine Practice* 15:3(December): 665–686.

Johnson, L (2000). Diseases of the Bronchus. *Textbook of Veterinary Internal Medicine: Diseases of the Dog and Cat.* S Ettinger and E Feldman Eds. Philadelphia, WB Saunders. 2: 1055–1061.

Lavoie, J–P (2003). Heaves (recurrent airway obstruction): practical management of acute episodes and prevention of exacerbations. *Current Therapy in Equine Medicine 5.* N Robinson Ed., Saunders: 417–421.

Mazan, M (2003). Use of aerosolized bronchodilators and corticosteroids. *Current Therapy in Equine Medicine 5.* N Robinson Ed., Saunders: 440–445.

McConnell, VC & T Hughey (1992, Last Update). "Formulary 1989: Update, The University of Georgia, Veterinary Medical Teaching Hospital."

Padrid, P (2006). Diagnosis and therapy of feline asthma. Proceedings: ACVIM 2006. http://goo.gl/ovF3z

Reinero, CR (2008). The Beta–agonist Paradox: Is Albuterol Detrimental to Asthma? Proceedings: American College of Veterinary Internal Medicine. Accessed via: Veterinary Information Network. http://goo.gl/gxRsO

Reinero, CR (2009). Dispelling the myths about diagnosis and treatment of feline asthma. Proceedings: ACVIM. Accessed via: Veterinary Information Network. http://goo.gl/Xsqci

Rush, B (2006). Heaves and aerosol drug therapy. Proceedings: Western Vet Conf. Accessed via: Veterinary Information Network. http://goo.gl/7YYND

ALENDRONATE SODIUM

(a-*len*-droe-nate)   Fosamax®

ORAL BISPHOSPHONATE BONE RESORPTION INHIBITOR

Prescriber Highlights

▶ Orally dosed bisphosphonate that reduces osteoclastic bone resorption

▶ Potentially useful for refractory hypercalcemia, FORLs, osteosarcoma

▶ Very limited clinical experience with use of this drug in animals; adverse effect profile, dosages, etc. may significantly change with more experience & clinical research

▶ Potentially can cause esophageal erosions; risks are not clear for dogs or cats

▶ Accurate dosing may be difficult & bioavailability is adversely affected by food, etc.

▶ Cost may be an issue

Uses/Indications

Alendronate use in small animals has been limited, but it may prove useful for treating refractory hypercalcemia in dogs or cats, feline odontoclastic resorptive lesions (FORLs), and as an osteosarcoma treatment adjuvant.

Pharmacology/Actions

Alendronate, like other bisphosphonates, inhibits osteoclastic bone resorption by inhibiting osteoclast function after binding to bone hydroxyapatite. Secondary actions that may contribute to therapeutic usefulness in osteogenic neoplasms include promoting apoptosis and inhibiting osteoclastogenesis, angiogenesis and cancer cell proliferation.

Pharmacokinetics

Specific pharmacokinetic values are limited for dogs and apparently unavailable for cats. Oral bioavailability in all species studied is less than 2%. In humans, alendronate sodium has very low oral bioavailability (<1%) and the presence of food can reduce bioavailability further to negligible amounts. In women, taking the medication with coffee or orange juice reduced bioavailability by 60% when compared to plain water.

Absorbed drug is rapidly distributed to bone or excreted into the urine. The drug is reportedly not highly plasma protein bound in dogs, but it is in rats. Alendronate apparently accumulates on subgingival tooth surfaces and bordering alveolar bone. Plasma concentrations are virtually undetectable after therapeutic dosing.

Alendronate is not metabolized and drug taken up by bone is very slowly eliminated. It is estimated that the terminal elimination half-life in dogs is approximately 1000 days and, in humans, approximately 10 years, however once incorporated into bone, alendronate is no longer active.

Contraindications/Precautions/Warnings

Alendronate is contraindicated in human patients with esophageal abnormalities (*e.g.*, strictures, achalasia) that cause delayed esophageal emptying and those who cannot stand or sit upright for 30 minutes after administration. At present, it is not believed that small animal patients need to remain upright after administration. Because of a lack of experience, the drug is not recommended for use in human patients with severe renal dysfunction (CrCl <35 mL/min). Alendronate should not be used in patients who have demonstrated hypersensitivity reactions to it.

Alendronate use in small animals should be considered investigational at this point. Limited research and experience, dosing questions, risks of esophageal irritation or ulcers, and medication expense all are potential hindrances to its therapeutic usefulness.

Adverse Effects

Little information on the specific adverse effect profile for dogs or cats is published. In humans, alendronate can cause upper GI irritation and erosions. Anecdotal reports of GI upset, vomiting and inappetence have been reported in dogs receiving the drug. It has been suggested that after administration, walking or playing with the dog for 30 minutes may reduce the incidence of esophageal problems. In cats, buttering the lips after administration to induce salivation and reduce esophageal transit time has been suggested.

Other potential adverse effects of concern include jaw osteonecrosis and musculoskeletal pain.

Reproductive/Nursing Safety

Alendronate at dosages of 2 mg/kg in rats caused decreased post-implantation survival rates and at 1 mg/kg caused decreased weight gain in healthy pups. Higher dosages (10 mg/kg) caused incomplete fetal ossification of several bone types. In humans, the FDA categorizes alendronate as category *C* for use during pregnancy (*Animal studies have shown an adverse effect on the fetus, but there are no adequate studies in humans; or there are no animal reproduction studies and no adequate studies in humans.*)

While it is unknown if alendronate enters maternal milk, it would be unexpected that measurable quantities would be found in milk or enough would be absorbed in clinically significant amounts in nursing offspring.

Overdosage/Acute Toxicity

No lethality was observed in dogs receiving doses of up to 200 mg/kg. Lethality in mice and rats was seen at dosages starting at 966 mg/kg and 552 mg/kg, respectively. Observed adverse effects associated with overdoses included hypocalcemia, hypophosphatemia, and upper GI reactions.

A recently ingested overdose should be treated with orally administered antacids or milk to bind the drug and reduce absorption. Do not induce vomiting. Monitor serum calcium and phosphorus and treat supportively.

Drug Interactions

The following drug interactions have either been reported or are theoretical in humans or animals receiving alendronate and may be of significance in veterinary patients:

- **ASPIRIN:** Increased risk of upper GI adverse effects

- **CALCIUM-CONTAINING ORAL PRODUCTS or FOOD:** Likely to significantly decrease oral bioavailability of alendronate

- **RANITIDINE (IV):** increased oral alendronate bioavailability two-fold in a human study

- **NSAIDS:** Humans taking NSAIDs with alendronate had no higher rates of GI adverse reactions than when NSAIDs were used with placebo

Laboratory Considerations

- No specific laboratory concerns or interactions have been noted.

Doses

- **DOGS:**
  a) For refractory hypercalcemia: 0.5–1 mg/kg PO once daily (Davies 2005)
  b) For investigational treatment of histiocytic sarcoma complex: Loading dose of 70 mg/m^2 (NOT mg/kg) PO daily for 14 days, then every other day for 14 days, then once weekly. Monitor for esophageal problems (excessive salivation, regurgitation). (Kitchell 2008)

- **CATS:**
  a) For feline odontoclastic resorptive lesions (FORLs): 3 mg/kg PO q12h (Gores 2004) **Note:** Use for this indication in cats is at present very controversial. (Plumb 2006)
  b) For idiopathic hypercalcemia (after dietary change has been attempted): Initially 2 mg/kg PO once weekly. Most cats respond to 10 mg (total dose). Administer at least 6 mL of water after administration and butter the lips to increase salivation and increase transit. If efficacious, effects usually seen in 3–4 weeks. Monitor via serum ionized calcium. (Chew & Green 2006)

Monitoring

- Serum calcium (ionized)
- GI adverse effects. **Note:** Depending on diagnosis (*e.g.,* hypercalcemia, adjunctive treatment of osteogenic sarcomas, or FORLs) other monitoring of serum electrolytes (total calcium, phosphorus, potassium sodium) or disease-associated signs may be required

Client Information

- Inform clients of the "investigational" nature with using this drug in small animals
- Potentially can cause esophageal erosions; risks are not clear for dogs or cats. Be sure adequate liquid is consumed after dosage and, ideally, do not feed for at least 30 minutes after dosing. See Adverse Effects for suggestions to minimize risks in dogs and cats.

Chemistry/Synonyms

Alendronate sodium is a synthetic analog of pyrophosphonate with the chemical name: (4-amino-1-hydroxy-1-phosphono-butyl) phosphonic acid. One mg is soluble in one liter of water.

Alendronate may also be known as: Alendronic acid, *Acide Alendronique, Acido Alendronico, Acidum Alendronicum, Adronat®, Alendros®, Arendal®, Onclast®* or *Fosamax®.*

Storage/Stability

Alendronate tablets should be stored in well-closed containers at room temperature. The oral solution should be stored at room temperature; do not freeze.

Dosage Forms/Regulatory Status

VETERINARY PRODUCTS: None

HUMAN PRODUCTS:

Alendronate Sodium Oral Tablets: 5 mg, 10 mg, 35 mg, 40 mg, & 70 mg; *Fosamax®* (Merck); generic; (Rx)

Alendronate Oral Solution: 70 mg (as base) in 75 mL; raspberry flavor; *Fosamax®* (Merck); (Rx)

References

Chew, D & T Green (2006). "VIN/AAFP Rounds: Feline Idiopathic Hypercalcemia."

Davies, D (2005). Clinical Approach to Canine Blood Calcium Disorders. Proceedings: ACVSc2005. Accessed via: Veterinary Information Network. http://goo.gl/xEIC6

Gores, B (2004). Common Dental Disorders in Dogs and Cats. NEVC2004.

Kitchell, B (2008). Managing Histiocytic Diseases. Proceedings: WSAVA. Accessed via: Veterinary Information Network. http://goo.gl/q6XSW

ALFAXALONE

Al-*fax*-a-lone)   Alfaxan®

INTRAVENOUS ANESTHETIC

Prescriber Highlights

▶ Injectable anesthetic for small animals available in some countries (U.K. Australia, New Zealand)

▶ Negligible analgesic effects

▶ Respiratory depression/apnea can occur, particularly if administered rapidly IV

▶ Use with premeds allows lower dose (and cost)

Uses/Indications

Alfaxalone may be used in dogs or cats as an intravenous induction agent prior to inhalation anesthesia or as a sole anesthetic agent for the induction and maintenance of anesthesia for the performance of examination or surgical procedures. It can also be administered deep IM to cats as a deep sedative/light anesthetic.

Pharmacology/Actions

Alfaxalone is a neuroactive steroid molecule with properties of a general anesthetic. The primary mechanism for the anesthetic action of alfaxalone is the modulation of neuronal cell membrane chloride ion transport, induced by binding of alfaxalone to GABA cell surface receptors. Alfaxalone has negligible analgesic properties at clinical doses.

Pharmacokinetics

In dogs, alfaxalone's volume of distribution after a single injection of clinical doses (2 mg/kg) is approximately 2.5 L/kg. At this dose, clearance is about 54 mL/kg/minute and elimination terminal half-life around 27 minutes (Ferre *et al.* 2006). A study done in Greyhounds showed similar results when dogs were not premedicated; however, premedicated (acepromazine/morphine) Greyhounds had substantially longer (5X) anesthetic durations and elimination half-life was approximately 19% longer and clearance about 24% lower then when they were not premedicated (Pasloske *et al.* 2009).

In cats, the volume of distribution of alfaxalone is approximately 2 L/kg. Clearance is dosage dependent with doses of 5 mg/kg (clinical dose) averaging 25.1 mL/kg/minute and doses of 25 mg/kg (supraclinical dose) averaging 14.8 mL/kg/min. The elimination half-lives at these doses were 45.2 and 76.6 min respectively. Alfaxalone has nonlinear pharmacokinetics in the cat, but with multiple doses there was no clinically relevant accumulation. (Whittem *et al.* 2008)

Cat and dog hepatocyte (*in vitro*) studies show that alfaxalone undergoes both Phase I (cytochrome P450 dependent) and Phase II (conjugation dependent) metabolism in both species. Both cats and dogs form the same five Phase I metabolites. Phase II metabolites in cats are alfaxalone sulfate and alfaxalone glucuronide, while only alfaxalone glucuronide is found in dogs. Alfaxalone metabolites are likely to be eliminated from both the dog and cat by the hepatic/fecal and renal routes, similarly to other species studied.

At usual dosages, dogs or cats are expected to recover to sternal recumbency in 60-80 minutes.

Contraindications/Precautions/Warnings

Alfaxalone should not be used with other injectable general anesthetic agents. As post-induction apnea can occur, alfaxalone should only be used in circumstances where endotracheal (ET) intubation, positive pressure ventilation and oxygen support can be administered. Following induction, ET intubation with oxygen is recommended.

Use with caution in patients with significant hepatic dysfunction as they may require lower dosages or increased dosing intervals to maintain anesthesia. Use with caution in elderly, critically ill or debilitated animals.

Patients should be in appropriate facilities and under sufficient supervision during the post-anesthesia recovery period. During recovery, it is preferable that animals are not handled or disturbed as psychomotor excitement may occur. Premedication with only a benzodiazepine may increase this likelihood.

As alfaxalone does not provide analgesia, appropriate pain control should be provided.

Safety of alfaxalone has not been established in animals less than 12 weeks of age.

Adverse Effects

Respiratory depression and apnea are the biggest concerns with this agent. In clinical studies, 44% of dogs and 19% of cats experienced post-induction apnea (defined as the cessation of breathing for 30 seconds or more). The mean duration of apnea in these animals was 100 seconds in dogs and 60 seconds in cats. Giving the drug slowly IV with persistent monitoring should occur when using this agent. When sufficient anesthesia is induced, endotracheal intubation and oxygen supplementation should be done. Cardiac arrhythmias may occur, but are thought to occur primarily due to hypoxemia/hypercapnia; O_2 therapy is recommended as the primary treatment should these occur, followed by appropriate cardiotherapy if required.

Reproductive/Nursing Safety

The safety has not been established in pregnancy or during lactation. Studies in pregnant mice, rats and rabbits have not demonstrated deleterious effects on gestation of the treated animals or on the reproductive performance of their offspring. Alfaxalone's effects upon fertility have not been evaluated.

Overdosage/Acute Toxicity

Hypoventilation, apnea, and hypotension are the most likely consequences of overdoses up to 25 mg/kg. Cardiac arrhythmias are possible. Extended monitoring with appropriate cardiopulmonary support may be required.

Drug Interactions

The New Zealand label states that alfaxalone has been safely used in combination with the premeds acepromazine, atropine, methadone, butorphanol, diazepam and xylazine. The concomitant use with other CNS depressants is expected to potentiate the depressant effects of either drug, and appropriate dose adjustments should be made. A study evaluating the effects that medetomidine (4 microgram/kg) and/or butorphanol (0.1 mg/kg) had on the induction doses required for alfaxalone in dogs found that when either was used alone average induction dose was 1.2 mg/kg and when used together average alfaxalone induction dose was 0.8 mg/kg (Maddern *et al.* 2010).

Propofol, Thiopental: The label states that alfaxalone *should not* be used with **other injectable anesthetics.**

Laboratory Considerations

None noted.

Doses

■ **DOGS/CATS:**

a) **INDUCTION:**

Dogs: Premedicated: 3 mg/kg IV; Not premedicated 2 mg/kg IV.

Cats: Premedicated or not premedicated: 5 mg/kg IV.

The rate of administration should be that, if required, the total dose is given over the first 60 seconds. After that, if intubation is still not possible, one further similar dose may be administered to effect. Administration should continue until the clinician is satisfied that the depth of anesthesia is sufficient for endotrache-

al intubation or until the entire dose has been administered.

MAINTENANCE:

Following induction, the animal may be intubated and maintained on alfaxalone or an inhalation anesthetic agent. Maintenance doses of alfaxalone may be given as supplemental boluses or as constant-rate infusion. Alfaxalone has been used safely and effectively in both dogs and cats for procedures lasting up to one hour. The following doses suggested for maintenance of anesthesia are based on data taken from controlled laboratory and field studies and represent the average amount of drug required to provide maintenance anesthesia for a dog or cat; however, the actual dose will be based on the response of the individual patient.

	DOGS		CATS	
	Unpre-medicated	Pre-medicated	Unpre-medicated	Pre-medicated
Dose for constant rate infusion				
mg/kg/hour	8–9	6–7	10–11	7–8
mg/kg/minute	0.13–0.15	0.1–0.12	0.16–0.18	0.11–0.13
mL/kg/minute	0.013–0.015	0.01–0.012	0.016–0.018	0.011–0.013
Bolus dose for each 10 minutes maintenance				
mg/kg	1.3–1.5	1–1.2	1.6–1.8	1.1–1.3
mL/kg	0.13–0.15	0.1–0.12	0.16–0.18	0.11–0.13

Where maintenance of anesthesia is with alfaxalone for procedures lasting more than 5 to 10 minutes, a butterfly needle or catheter can be left in the vein, and small amounts of alfaxalone injected subsequently to maintain the required level and duration of anesthesia. In most cases the average duration of recovery when using alfaxalone for maintenance will be longer than if using an inhalant gas as a maintenance agent. (Adapted from label; *Alfaxan*®—Vetoquinol U.K.)

b) **INDUCTION:**

Dogs: 1–2 mg/kg IV slowly over 20–30 seconds while assessing the degree of anesthesia achieved.

Cats: 2–5 mg/kg IV slowly over 20–30 seconds while assessing the degree of anesthesia achieved.

MAINTENANCE:

Following induction, the animal may be maintained on alfaxalone or an inhalation anesthetic agent. Where maintenance of anesthesia is with alfaxalone for procedures lasting more than 5 to 10 minutes, a needle or catheter can be left in the vein, and small amounts of alfaxalone may be injected up to a total dose of 5–12 mg/kg (0.5–1.2 mL/kg). A total dose of 5–7 mg/kg (0.5–0.7 mL) would be expected to provide sufficient anesthesia for short surgical procedures such as castration. For longer procedures, a total dose of 8–12 mg/kg (0.8–1.2 mL/kg) may be required. Recovery is not prolonged significantly following incremental doses of alfaxalone.

As a deep sedative/light anesthetic in cats: 5–10 mg/kg IM (deep) (0.5–1 mL/kg). The suggested site of injection is the quadriceps muscle mass. A dose of 10 mg/kg IM is expected to induce deep sedation or light anesthesia sufficient to allow venepuncture or the practice of some minor surgical techniques such as the drainage of an abscess or the repair of small superficial wounds. (Adapted from label; *Alfaxan-CD RTU®*—Jurox N.Z.)

■ **SMALL MAMMALS:**
a) **Rabbits:** 6–9 mg/kg IV; 9 mg/kg IM. It is prudent to administer oxygen concurrently by facemask. Apnea can occur so the author recommends not using intravenous induction unless the operator is confident with intubation. Published doses of injectable agents are for surgical anesthesia in *healthy* rabbits without the concurrent use of a volatile agent and thus should be considered as the maximum dose, which may not be necessary in many cases. In practice, the combination of an injectable induction using lower doses of the agents than required for surgical anesthesia, followed by intubation and maintenance on isoflurane, is probably the most common approach.

Monitoring

■ Level of anesthesia/CNS effects

■ Respiratory depression

■ Cardiovascular status (cardiac rate/rhythm; blood pressure)

Chemistry/Synonyms

Alfaxalone is 3-alpha-hydroxy-5-alpha-pregnane-11,20-dione and has a molecular weight of 332.5. It occurs as a white to creamy white powder. It is practically insoluble in water or mineral spirits, soluble in alcohol, and freely soluble in chloroform.

The commercial injection occurs as a clear, colorless sterile solution without preservatives. It is a water-soluble formulation containing 2-hydroxypropyl-beta-cyclodextrin (HPCD) as the solubilizing agent. Another product containing alfaxalone, *Saffan®* was marketed in the 1970's as an intravenous anesthetic agent for cats, but contained a polyethoxylated castor oil as the solubilizing agent which caused significant histamine release via mast cell degranula-

tion. This product was subsequently removed from the market.

The UK labels states to discard any remaining solution in the vial after use, but the New Zealand label states that "Contents of broached vials should preferably be used within 24 hours, but may be stored if necessary at 4°C for up to 7 days provided contamination is avoided. Do not use broached vials if the solution is not clear, colorless and free from particulate matter."

Alfaxalone may also be known as alfaksaloni, alfaxalon, alfaxalona, alfaxalonum, alphaxalone, or GR-2/234. A common tradename is *Alfaxan®*.

Storage/Stability

Alfaxalone solution for injection should be stored at room temperature (<30°C) and protected from light. Do not freeze.

Dosage Forms/Regulatory Status

VETERINARY-LABELED PRODUCTS: None in the USA.

Alfaxalone is available in several other countries, including UK, New Zealand, and Australia as a 10 mg/mL injection and depending on the market, in 10 mL and 20 mL vials. Trade name is *Alfaxan®* (Vetoquinol, Jurox). It requires a veterinary prescription.

HUMAN-LABELED PRODUCTS: None

References

Ferre, PJ, K Pasloske, et al. (2006). Plasma pharmacokinetics of alfaxalone in dogs after an intravenous bolus of Alfaxan–CD RTU. *Veterinary Anaesthesia and Analgesia* 33(4): 229–236.

Maddern, K, VJ Adams, et al. (2010). Alfaxalone induction dose following administration of medetomidine and butorphanol in the dog. *Veterinary Anaesthesia and Analgesia* 37(1): 7–13.

Pasloske, K, B Sauer, et al. (2009). Plasma pharmacokinetics of alfaxalone in both premedicated and unpremedicated Greyhound dogs after single, intravenous administration of Alfaxan (R) at a clinical dose. *Journal of Veterinary Pharmacology and Therapeutics* 32(5): 510–513.

Whittem, T, KS Pasloske, et al. (2008). The pharmacokinetics and pharmacodynamics of alfaxalone in cats after single and multiple intravenous administration of Alfaxan((R)) at clinical and supraclinical doses. *Journal of Veterinary Pharmacology and Therapeutics* 31(6): 571–579.

ALFENTANIL HCL

(al-*fen*-ta-nil)   Alfenta®

OPIATE ANESTHETIC ADJUNCT

Prescriber Highlights

▶ Injectable, potent opiate that may be useful for adjunctive anesthesia, particularly in cats

▶ Marginal veterinary experience & little published data available to draw conclusions on appropriate usage in veterinary species

▶ Dose-related respiratory & CNS depression are the most likely adverse effects seen

▶ Dose may need adjustment in geriatric patients & those with liver disease

▶ Class-II controlled substance; relatively expensive

Uses/Indications

An opioid analgesic, alfentanil may be useful for anesthesia, analgesia, or sedation similar to fentanyl; fentanyl is generally preferred because of the additional experience with its use in veterinary patients and cost. Alfentanil may be particularly useful in cats as adjunctive therapy during anesthesia to reduce other anesthetic (*i.e.*, propofol or isoflurane) concentrations.

Pharmacology/Actions

Alfentanil is a potent *mu* opioid with the expected sedative, analgesic, and anesthetic properties. When comparing analgesic potencies after IM injection, 0.4–0.8 mg of alfentanil is equivalent to 0.1–0.2 mg of fentanyl and approximately 10 mg of morphine.

Pharmacokinetics

The pharmacokinetics of alfentanil have been studied in the dog. The drug's steady state volume of distribution is about 0.56 L/kg, clearance is approximately 30 mL/kg/minute, and the terminal half-life is approximately 20 minutes.

In humans, onset of anesthetic action occurs within 2 minutes after intravenous dosing, and within 5 minutes of intramuscular injection. Peak effects occur approximately 15 minutes after IM injection. The drug has a volume of distribution of 0.4–1 L/kg. About 90% of the drug is bound to plasma proteins. Alfentanil is primarily metabolized in the liver to inactive metabolites that are excreted by the kidneys into the urine; only about 1% of the drug is excreted unchanged into the urine. Total body clearance in humans ranges from 1.6–17.6 mL/minute/kg. Clearance is decreased by about 50% in patients with alcoholic cirrhosis or in those that are obese. Clearance is reduced by approximately 30% in geriatric patients. Elimination half-life in humans is about 100 minutes.

Contraindications/Precautions/Warnings

Alfentanil is contraindicated in patients hypersensitive to opioids. Because of the drug's potency and potential for significant adverse effects, it should only be used in situations where patient vital signs can be continuously monitored. Initial dosage reduction may be required in geriatric or debilitated patients, particularly those with diminished cardiopulmonary function.

Adverse Effects

Adverse effects are generally dose related and consistent with other opiate agonists. Respiratory depression, bradycardia, and CNS depression are most likely to be encountered. Bradycardia is usually responsive to anticholinergic agents. Dose-related skeletal muscle rigidity is not uncommon and neuromuscular blockers are routinely used. Alfentanil has rarely been associated with asystole, hypercarbia and hypersensitivity reactions.

Respiratory or CNS depression may be exacerbated if alfentanil is given with other drugs that cause those effects.

Reproductive/Nursing Safety

In humans, the FDA categorizes alfentanil as a category **C** drug for use during pregnancy (*Animal studies have shown an adverse effect on the fetus, but there are no adequate studies in humans; or there are no animal reproduction studies and no adequate studies in humans*). If alfentanil is administered systemically to the mother close to giving birth, offspring may show behavioral alterations (hypotonia, depression) associated with opioids. Although high dosages given for 10–30 days to laboratory animals have been associated with embryotoxicity, it is unclear if this is a result of direct effects of the drug or as a result of maternal toxicity secondary to reduced food and water intake.

The effects of alfentanil on lactation or its safety for nursing offspring is not well defined, but it is unlikely to cause significant effects when used during anesthetic procedures in the mother.

Overdosage/Acute Toxicity

Intravenous, severe overdosages may cause circulatory collapse, pulmonary edema, seizures, cardiac arrest and death. Less severe overdoses may cause CNS and respiratory depression, coma, hypotension, muscle flaccidity and miosis. Treatment is a combination of supportive therapy, as necessary, and the administration of an opiate antagonist such as naloxone. Although alfentanil has a relatively rapid half-life, multiple doses of naloxone may be necessary. Because of the drug's potency, the use of a tuberculin syringe to measure dosages less than 1 mL with a dosage calculation and measurement double-check system, are recommended.

Drug Interactions

The following drug interactions have either been reported or are theoretical in humans or animals

receiving alfentanil and may be of significance in veterinary patients:

- **DRUGS THAT INHIBIT HEPATIC ISOENZYME CYP3A4,** such as **erythromycin, cimetidine, ketoconazole, itraconazole, fluconazole or diltiazem:** May increase the half-life and decrease the clearance of alfentanil leading to prolonged effect and an increased risk of respiratory depression

- **DRUGS THAT DEPRESS CARDIAC FUNCTION OR REDUCE VAGAL TONE,** such as **beta-blockers** or **other anesthetic agents:** May produce bradycardia or hypotension if used concurrently with alfentanil

Laboratory Considerations

- Patients receiving opiates may have increased plasma levels of **amylase** or **lipase** secondary to increased biliary tract pressure. Values may be unreliable for 24 hours after administration of alfentanil.

Doses

(**Note:** in very obese patients, figure dosages based upon lean body weight.)

- **DOGS:**

    As a premed:
    a) 5 micrograms/kg alfentanil with 0.3–0.6 mg of atropine IV 30 seconds before injecting propofol can reduce the dose of propofol needed to induce anesthesia to 2 mg/kg, but apnea may still occur. (Hall *et al.* 2001b)

    As a constant rate infusion for pain:
    a) Loading dose of 0.5–1 micrograms/kg, then a CRI of 0.5–1 micrograms/kg per minute. (Grint 2008)

    As an analgesic supplement to anesthesia:
    a) 2–5 micrograms/kg IV q20 minutes. (Hall *et al.* 2001b), (Hall *et al.* 2001a)

    b) For intra-operative analgesia in patients with intracranial disease: 0.2 micrograms/kg/minute (Raisis 2005)

Monitoring

- Anesthetic and/or analgesic efficacy
- Cardiac and respiratory rate
- Pulse oximetry or other methods to measure blood oxygenation when used for anesthesia

Client Information

- Alfentanil is a potent opiate that should only be used by professionals in a setting where adequate patient monitoring is available

Chemistry/Synonyms

A phenylpiperidine opioid anesthetic-analgesic related to fentanyl, alfentanil HCl occurs as a white to almost white powder. It is freely soluble in alcohol, water, chloroform or methanol. The commercially available injection has a pH of 4–6 and contains sodium chloride for isotonicity. Alfentanil is more lipid soluble than morphine, but less so than fentanyl.

Alfentanil may also be known as: alfentanyl, *Alfenta®, Fanaxal®, Fentalim®, Limifen®,* or *Rapifen®.*

Storage/Stability

Alfentanil injection should be stored protected from light at room temperature.

Compatibility/Compounding Considerations

In concentrations of up to 80 micrograms/mL, alfentanil injection has been shown to be **compatible** with Normal Saline, D_5 in Normal Saline, D_5W, and Lactated Ringers.

Dosage Forms/Regulatory Status

VETERINARY-LABELED PRODUCTS: None

The ARCI (Racing Commissioners International) has designated this drug as a class 1 substance. See the appendix for more information.

HUMAN-LABELED PRODUCTS:

Alfentanil HCl for injection: 500 micrograms (as base)/mL in 2, 5 mL, 10 mL,& 20 mL amps; preservative-free; *Alfenta®* (Akorn); generic (Abbott); (Rx, C-II).

References

Grint, N (2008). Constant Rate Infusions (CRIS) in Pain Management. Proceedings: BSAVA. Accessed via: Veterinary Information Network. http://goo.gl/CIXUX

Hall, L, K Clarke, et al. (2001a). Anesthesia of the dog. *Veterinary Anesthesia, 10th Ed*London, Saunders: 385–440.

Hall, L, K Clarke, et al. (2001b). Principles of sedation, analgesia, and premedication. *Veterinary Anesthesia, 10th Ed*London, Saunders: 75–112.

Raisis, A (2005). Techniques for anesthetizing animals with intracranial disease. Proceedings: ACVSc2005. Accessed via: Veterinary Information Network. http://goo.gl/3lEQH

ALLOPURINOL

(al-oh-*pyoor*-i-nol)   Zyloprim®

XANTHINE OXIDASE INHIBITOR; PURINE ANALOG

Prescriber Highlights

▶ Used as a uric acid reducer in dogs, cats, reptiles & birds & as an alternative treatment Leishmaniasis & Trypanosomiasis in dogs

▶ Use with caution (dosage adjustment may be required) in patients with renal or hepatic dysfunction

▶ Contraindicated in red-tailed hawks & should be used with caution, if at all, in other raptors

▶ Diet may need to be adjusted to lower purine

▶ GI effects are most likely adverse effects, but hypersensitivity, hepatic & renal effects can occur

▶ Many potential drug interactions

Uses/Indications

The principle veterinary uses for allopurinol are for the prophylactic treatment of recurrent uric acid uroliths and hyperuricosuric calcium oxalate uroliths in dogs, particularly Dalmatians. It has also been used in an attempt to treat gout in pet birds and reptiles.

Allopurinol has been recommended as an alternative treatment for canine Leishmaniasis. Although it appears to have clinical efficacy, it must be used for many months of treatment and does not apparently clear the parasite in most dogs at usual dosages. Allopurinol may also be useful for American Trypanosomiasis.

Pharmacology/Actions

Allopurinol and its metabolite, oxypurinol, inhibit the enzyme xanthine oxidase. Xanthine oxidase is responsible for the conversion of oxypurines (*e.g.*, hypoxanthine, xanthine) to uric acid. Hepatic microsomal enzymes may also be inhibited by allopurinol. It does not increase the renal excretion of uric acid nor does it possess any antiinflammatory or analgesic activity.

Allopurinol is metabolized by *Leishmania* into an inactive form of inosine that is incorporated into the organism's RNA leading to faulty protein and RNA synthesis.

Allopurinol, by inhibiting xanthine oxidase, can inhibit the formation of superoxide anion radicals, thereby providing protection against hemorrhagic shock and myocardial ischemia in laboratory conditions. The clinical use of the drug for these indications requires further study.

Pharmacokinetics

In Dalmatians, absorption rates were variable between subjects. Peak levels occur within 1–3 hours after oral dosing. Elimination half-life is about 2.7 hours. In dogs (not necessarily Dalmatians), the serum half-life of allopurinol is approximately 2 hours and for oxipurinol, 4 hours. Food does not appear to alter the absorption of allopurinol in dogs.

In horses, oral bioavailability of allopurinol is low (approximately 15%). Allopurinol is rapidly converted to oxypurinol in the horse as the elimination half-life of allopurinol is approximately 5–6 minutes. Oxypurinol has an elimination half-life of about 1.1 hours in the horse.

In humans, allopurinol is approximately 90% absorbed from the GI tract after oral dosing. Peak levels after oral allopurinol administration occur 1.5 and 4.5 hours later, for allopurinol and oxypurinol, respectively.

Allopurinol is distributed in total body tissue water but levels in the CNS are only about 50% of those found elsewhere. Neither allopurinol nor oxypurinol are bound to plasma proteins, but both drugs are excreted into milk.

Xanthine oxidase metabolizes allopurinol to oxypurinol. In humans, the serum half-life for allopurinol is 1–3 hours and for oxypurinol, 18–30 hours. Half-lives are increased in patients with diminished renal function. Both allopurinol and oxypurinol are dialyzable.

Contraindications/Precautions/Warnings

Allopurinol is contraindicated in patients who are hypersensitive to it or have previously developed a severe reaction to it. It should be used cautiously and with intensified monitoring in patients with impaired hepatic or renal function. When used in patients with renal insufficiency, dosage reductions and increased monitoring are usually warranted.

Allopurinol does not appear to be effective in dissolving urate uroliths in dogs with portovascular anomalies.

Red-tailed hawks appear to be sensitive to the effects of allopurinol. Doses at 50 mg/kg PO once daily caused clinical signs of vomiting and hyperuricemia with renal dysfunction. Doses of 25 mg/kg PO once daily were safe but not effective in reducing plasma uric acid.

Adverse Effects

Adverse effects in dogs are apparently uncommon with allopurinol when fed low purine diets. There has been one report of a dog developing hemolytic anemia and trigeminal neuropathy while receiving allopurinol. Xanthine coatings have formed around ammonium urate uroliths in dogs that have been fed diets containing purine. If the drug is required for chronic therapy, reduction of purine precursors in the diet with dosage reduction should be considered.

Several adverse effects have been reported in humans including GI distress, bone marrow suppression, skin rashes, hepatitis, and vasculitis. Human patients with renal dysfunction are at risk for further decreases in renal function and other severe adverse effects unless dosages are reduced. Until further studies are performed in dogs with decreased renal function, the drug should be used with caution and at reduced dosages.

Reproductive/Nursing Safety

While the safe use of allopurinol during pregnancy has not been established, dosages of up to 20 times normal in rodents have not demonstrated decreases in fertility. Infertility in males (humans) has been reported with the drug, but a causal effect has not been firmly established. In humans, the FDA categorizes this drug as category **C** for use during pregnancy (*Animal studies have shown an adverse effect on the fetus, but there are no adequate studies in humans; or there are no animal reproduction studies and no adequate studies in humans.*)

Allopurinol and oxypurinol may be excreted into milk; use caution when allopurinol is administered to a nursing dam.

Overdosage/Acute Toxicity

Vomiting has been seen in dogs at doses >44 mg/kg per the APCC database. A human ingesting 22.5 grams did not develop serious toxicity. The oral LD 50 in mice is 78 mg/kg.

There were 52 exposures to allopurinol reported to the ASPCA Animal Poison Control Center (APCC) during 2008–2009. In these cases, 51 were dogs with 6 showing clinical signs. The remaining 1 reported case was a cat that showed no symptoms. Common findings recorded in decreasing frequency included vomiting and trembling.

Drug Interactions

The following drug interactions have either been reported or are theoretical in humans or animals receiving allopurinol and may be of significance in veterinary patients:

▪ **AMINOPHYLLINE** or **THEOPHYLLINE:** Large doses of allopurinol may decrease metabolism thereby increasing their serum levels

▪ **AMOXICILLIN** or **AMPICILLIN:** In humans, concomitant use with allopurinol has been implicated in increased occurrences of skin rashes; the veterinary significance of this interaction is unknown

▪ **AZATHIOPRINE** or **MERCAPTOPURINE:** Allopurinol may inhibit metabolism and increase toxicity; if concurrent use is necessary, dosages of the antineoplastic/immunosuppressive agent should be reduced initially to 25–33% of their usual dose and then adjusted, dependent upon patient's response

▪ **CHLORPROPAMIDE:** Allopurinol may increase risks for hypoglycemia and hepatorenal reactions

▪ **CYCLOPHOSPHAMIDE:** Increased bone marrow depression may occur in patients receiving both allopurinol and cyclophosphamide

▪ **CYCLOSPORINE:** Allopurinol may increase cyclosporine levels

▪ **DIURETICS (Furosemide, Thiazides, Diazoxide, and Alcohol):** Can increase uric acid levels

▪ **ORAL ANTICOAGULANTS (e.g., Warfarin):** Allopurinol may reduce the metabolism of warfarin thereby increasing effect

▪ **TRIMETHOPRIM/SULFAMETHOXAZOLE:** In a few human patients, thrombocytopenia has occurred when used with allopurinol

▪ **URICOSURIC AGENTS (e.g., Probenecid, Sulfinpyrazone):** May increase the renal excretion of oxypurinol and thereby reduce xanthine oxidase inhibition; in treating hyperuricemia the additive effects on blood uric acid may, in fact, be beneficial to the patient

▪ **URINARY ACIDIFIERS (e.g., Methionine, Ammonium Chloride)** May reduce the solubility of uric acid in the urine and induce urolithiasis

Doses

▪ **DOGS:**
For urate uroliths:
a) For dissolution: 15 mg/kg PO q12h; only in conjunction with low purine foods.

For prevention: 10–20 mg/kg/day; because prolonged high doses of allopurinol may result in xanthine uroliths, it may be preferable to minimize recurrence with dietary therapy, with the option of treating infrequent episodes of urate urolith formation with dissolution protocols. (Osborne *et al.* 2003)

b) 7–10 mg/kg PO three times daily for both dissolution and prevention. Goal is to reduce urine urate:creatinine ratio by 50%. (Senior 1989)

For Leishmaniasis:
a) First line treatment: Meglumine antimoniate (N-methylglucamine antimoniate) 75 - 100 mg/kg once daily for 4-8 weeks plus allopurinol 10 mg/kg PO twice daily for 6-12 months. Second line treatment: Miltofosine 2 mg/kg PO once daily for 4 weeks plus allopurinol 10 mg/kg PO twice daily for 6-12 months OR allopurinol alone at 10 mg/kg PO twice daily for 6-12 months. (Solano-Gallego *et al.* 2009)

b) Meglumine antimoniate (100 mg/kg/day SQ) until resolution, with allopurinol at 20 mg/kg PO q12h for 9 months.

An alternate protocol using allopurinol alone: allopurinol 10 mg/kg PO q8h or 10–20 mg/kg PO q12h for 1–4 months. (Brosey 2005)

c) If possible use with meglumine antimoniate, if not, use allopurinol alone at 10 mg/kg PO twice daily. If animal has renal insufficiency, use at 5 mg/kg PO twice daily. (Font 1999)

d) 15 mg/kg PO twice daily for months (Lappin 2000)

▪ **BIRDS:**
For gout:
a) In budgies and cockatiels: Crush one 100 mg tablet into 10 mL of water. Add 20 drops of this solution to one ounce of drinking water. (McDonald 1989)

b) For parakeets: Crush one 100 mg tablet into 10 mL of water. Add 20 drops of this solution to one ounce of drinking water or give 1 drop 4 times daily. (Clubb 1986)

▪ **REPTILES:**
a) For elevated uric acid levels in renal disease in lizards: 20 mg/kg PO once daily (de la Navarre 2003)

b) For gout: 20 mg/kg PO once daily. Suggested dosage based upon human data as dose is not established for reptiles. (Johnson-Delaney 2005)

c) For hyperuricemia in green iguanas: 25 mg/kg PO daily. (Hernandez-Divers *et al.* 2008)

Monitoring

■ Urine uric acid (for urolithiasis)

■ Adverse effects

■ Periodic CBC, liver and renal function tests (*e.g.*, BUN, Creatinine, liver enzymes); especially early in therapy

Client Information

■ Unless otherwise directed, administer after meals (usually 1 hour or so). Notify veterinarian if animal develops a rash, becomes lethargic or ill.

Chemistry/Synonyms

A xanthine oxidase inhibitor, allopurinol occurs as a tasteless, fluffy white to off-white powder with a slight odor. It melts above 300° with decomposition and has an apparent pK_a of 9.4. Oxypurinol (aka oxipurinol, alloxanthine), its active metabolite, has a pK_a of 7.7. Allopurinol is only very slightly soluble in both water and alcohol.

Allopurinol may also be known as: allopurinolum, BW-56-158, HPP, or NSC-1390; many trade names are available.

Storage/Stability

Allopurinol tablets should be stored at room temperature in well-closed containers. The drug is stated to be stable in both light and air. The powder for injection should be stored at 25°C; may be exposed to 15−30°C. Once diluted to a concentration ≤6 mg/mL, store at room temperature and use within 10 hours; do not refrigerate.

Compatibility/Compounding Considerations

When using the injection, compatible IV solutions include D5W and normal saline.

Compounded preparation stability: Allopurinol oral suspension compounded from commercially available tablets has been published (Allen, 1996). Triturating eight (8) 300 mg tablets with 60 mL of *Ora-Plus®* and *qs ad* to 120 mL with *Ora-Sweet®* (or *Ora-Sweet® SF*) yields a 20 mg/mL suspension that retains >95% potency for 60 days stored at both 5°C and 25°C. The optimal stability of allopurinol liquids is reported to be between 3.1 and 3.4. Compounded preparations of allopurinol should be protected from light.

Another extemporaneously prepared suspension containing 20 mg/mL allopurinol for oral use can be prepared from the commercially available tablets. Tablets are crushed and mixed with an amount of *Cologel®* suspending agent equal to 1/3 the final volume. A mixture of simple syrup and wild cherry syrup at a ratio of 2:1 is added to produce the final volume. This preparation has been reported to be stable for at least 14 days when stored in an amber bottle at either room temperature or when refrigerated.

Dosage Forms/Regulatory Status

VETERINARY-LABELED PRODUCTS: None

HUMAN-LABELED PRODUCTS:

Allopurinol Oral Tablets: 100 mg & 300 mg; Zyloprim® (Faro); generic; (Rx)

Allopurinol Powder for Injection, lyophilized: 500 mg preservative-free in 30 mL vials; *Aloprim®* (Nabi); generic (Bedford Labs); (Rx)

References

Allen, L.V. & M.A. Erickson (1996). Stability of acetazolamide, allopurinol, azathioprine, clonazepam, and flucytosine in extemporaneously compounded oral liquids. *Am J Health Syst Pharm* 53(16): 1944-1949.

Brosey, B (2005). Leishmaniasis. Proceedings: ACVIM 2005. Accessed via: Veterinary Information Network. http://goo.gl/qQ0Yr

Clubb, SL (1986). Therapeutics: Individual and Flock Treatment Regimens. *Clinical Avian Medicine and Surgery.* GJ Harrison and LR Harrison Eds. Philadelphia, W.B. Saunders: 327–355.

de la Navarre, B (2003). Acute and chronic renal disease (specifically in lizard species). Proceedings: Western Veterinary Conference. Accessed via: Veterinary Information Network.

Font, A (1999). Canine leishmaniasis. Proceedings: American College of Veterinary Internal Medicine: 17th Annual Veterinary Medical Forum, Chicago.

Hernandez−Divers, SJ, D Martinez−Jimenez, et al. (2008). Effects of allopurinol on plasma uric acid levels in normouricaemic and hyperuricaemic green iguanas (Iguana iguana). *Veterinary Record* 162(4): 112−+.

Johnson−Delaney, C (2005). Osteodystrophy and renal disease in reptiles. Proceedings: Atlantic Coast Veterinary Conference. Accessed via: Veterinary Information Network. http://goo.gl/iuvuG

Lappin, M (2000). Protozoal and Miscellaneous Infections. *Textbook of Veterinary Internal Medicine: Diseases of the Dog and Cat.* S Ettinger and E Feldman Eds. Philadelphia, WB Saunders. 1: 408–417.

McDonald, SE (1989). Summary of medications for use in psittacine birds. *JAAV* 3(5): 120–127.

Osborne, C, J Lulich, et al. (2003). The role of nutrition in management of lower urinary tract disorders. Proceedings: ACVIM Forum. Accessed via: Veterinary Information Network. http://goo.gl/d6iGa

Senior, DF (1989). Medical Management of Urate Uroliths. *Current Veterinary Therapy X: Small Animal Practice.* RW Kirk Ed. Philadelphia, WB Saunders: 1178–1181.

Solano−Gallego, L, A Koutinas, et al. (2009). Directions for the diagnosis, clinical staging, treatment and prevention of canine leishmaniosis. *Veterinary Parasitology* 165(1–2): 1–18.

ALPRAZOLAM

(al-*prah*-zoe-lam)   Xanax®

BENZODIAZEPINE SEDATIVE/
TRANQUILIZER

Prescriber Highlights

▶ Oral benzodiazepine that may be useful for unwanted behaviors in dogs or cats

▶ Contraindications: Aggressive animals (controversial), benzodiazepine hypersensitivity

▶ Caution: Hepatic or renal disease

▶ Adverse Effects: Sedation, behavior changes, & contradictory responses; physical dependence is a possibility; may impede training

▶ C-IV controlled substance

Uses/Indications

Alprazolam may be useful for adjunctive therapy in anxious, aggressive dogs or in those demonstrating panic reactions. (**Note:** Some clinicians believe that benzodiazepines are contraindicated in aggressive dogs as anxiety may actually restrain the animal from aggressive tendencies). It may be useful in cats to treat anxiety disorders.

Alprazolam may have less effect on motor function at low doses than does diazepam.

Pharmacology/Actions

Subcortical levels (primarily limbic, thalamic, and hypothalamic) of the CNS are depressed by alprazolam and other benzodiazepines thus producing the anxiolytic, sedative, skeletal muscle relaxant, and anticonvulsant effects seen. The exact mechanism of action is unknown, but postulated mechanisms include: antagonism of serotonin, increased release of and/or facilitation of gamma-aminobutyric acid (GABA) activity, and diminished release or turnover of acetylcholine in the CNS. Benzodiazepine specific receptors have been located in the mammalian brain, kidney, liver, lung, and heart. In all species studied, receptors are lacking in the white matter.

Pharmacokinetics

The pharmacokinetics of alprazolam have not been described for either dogs or cats. In humans, alprazolam is well absorbed and is characterized as having an intermediate onset of action. Peak plasma levels occur in 1–2 hours.

Alprazolam is highly lipid soluble and widely distributed throughout the body. It readily crosses the blood-brain barrier and is somewhat bound to plasma proteins (80%).

Alprazolam is metabolized in the liver to at least two metabolites, including alpha-hydroxy-alprazolam which is pharmacologically active. Elimination half-lives range from 6–27 hours in people.

Contraindications/Precautions/Warnings

Some clinicians believe that benzodiazepines are contraindicated in aggressive dogs as anxiety may actually restrain the animal from aggressive tendencies. This remains controversial. Alprazolam is contraindicated in patients with known hypersensitivity to the drug. Use cautiously in patients with hepatic or renal disease, narrow angle glaucoma and debilitated or geriatric patients. Benzodiazepines may impair the abilities of working animals.

Adverse Effects

Benzodiazepines can cause sedation, increased appetite, and transient ataxia. Cats may exhibit changes in behavior (irritability, increased affection, depression, aberrant demeanor) after receiving benzodiazepines.

Dogs may rarely exhibit a contradictory response (CNS excitement) following administration of benzodiazepines.

Chronic usage of benzodiazepines may induce physical dependence. Animals appear to be less likely than humans to develop physical dependence at doses normally administered.

Benzodiazepines may impede the ability of the animal to learn and may retard training.

Reproductive/Nursing Safety

Diazepam and other benzodiazepines have been implicated in causing congenital abnormalities in humans if administered during the first trimester of pregnancy. Infants born of mothers receiving large doses of benzodiazepines shortly before delivery have been reported to suffer from apnea, impaired metabolic response to cold stress, difficulty in feeding, hyperbilirubinemia, hypotonia, etc. Withdrawal symptoms have occurred in infants whose mothers chronically took benzodiazepines during pregnancy. The veterinary significance of these effects is unclear, but the use of these agents during the first trimester of pregnancy should only occur when the benefits clearly outweigh the risks associated with their use. In humans, the FDA categorizes this drug as category *D* for use during pregnancy (*There is evidence of human fetal risk, but the potential benefits from the use of the drug in pregnant women may be acceptable despite its potential risks.*)

Overdosage/Acute Toxicity

Alprazolam overdoses are generally limited to CNS signs. CNS depression can be seen and the severity is generally dose dependant. Hypotension, respiratory depression, and cardiac arrest have been reported in human patients, but apparently, are quite rare. The reported LD_{50} in rats for alprazolam is >330 mg/kg, but cardiac arrest occurred at doses as low as 195 mg/kg. Life threatening signs in small animals are rare. Some animals may present with a paradoxical type reaction (disorientation, vocalization, agitation, etc.). At times, those signs may be followed by CNS depression.

There were 695 exposures to alprazolam reported to the ASPCA Animal Poison Control Center (APCC) during 2008–2009. In these cases, 658 were dogs with 330 showing clinical signs, 34 were cats with 19 showing clinical signs, 2 were birds with 1 reported as having symptoms, and 1 case was a chinchilla reported as having symptoms. Common findings in dogs recorded in decreasing frequency included ataxia, hyperactivity, lethargy, agitation, disorientation, and vomiting. Common findings in cats recorded in decreasing frequency included ataxia, depression, hyperactivity, polyphagia, and vocalization.

Treatment of acute toxicity consists of standard protocols for decontamination. The decision to give activated charcoal should be weighed carefully, as in some cases the risk of activated charcoal may outweigh the benefit. Flumazenil (see separate monograph) may be used to reverse the sedative effects of benzodiazepines, but only if the CNS depression is significant, resulting in respiratory depression.

Drug Interactions

The following drug interactions have either been reported or are theoretical in humans or animals receiving alprazolam and may be of significance in veterinary patients:

■ **ANTACIDS:** May slow the rate, but not the extent of oral absorption of alprazolam; administer 2 hours apart to avoid this potential interaction

■ **CNS DEPRESSANT AGENTS (barbiturates, narcotics, anesthetics**, etc.): Additive effects may occur

■ **DIGOXIN:** Serum levels may be increased; monitor serum digoxin levels or clinical signs of toxicity

■ **FLUOXETINE, FLUVOXAMINE:** Increased alprazolam levels

■ **HEPATICALLY METABOLIZED DRUGS (e.g., Cimetidine, erythromycin, isoniazid, ketoconazole, itraconazole**): Metabolism of alprazolam may be decreased and excessive sedation may occur

■ **RIFAMPIN:** May induce hepatic microsomal enzymes and decrease the pharmacologic effects of benzodiazepines

■ **TRICYCLIC ANTIDEPRESSANTS (e.g., AMITRIPTYLINE, CLOMIPRAMINE, IMIPRAMINE**): Alprazolam may increase levels of these drugs; clinical significance is not known and some state that clomipramine and alprazolam together may improve efficacy for phobias (e.g., thunderstorm phobia)

Doses

■ **DOGS:**

a) For treatment of canine anxiety disorders: 0.01–0.1 mg/kg PO as needed for panic, not to exceed 4 mg/dog/day. Start with 1–2 mg (total dose) for a medium-sized dog. (Overall 1997)

b) For separation anxiety: 0.25 mg–2 mg (total dose) once daily to three times daily PO. (Hunthausen 2006)

c) For storm phobias: 0.02–0.4 mg/kg PO q4h as needed; helps to minimize impact of experiencing a severe storm (Crowell-Davis 2003a);

0.02 mg/kg PO as needed one hour before anticipated storm and every 4 hours as needed; used as an adjunct after behavior modification and prior clomipramine treatment (see clomipramine monograph for further information) (Crowell-Davis 2003b)

d) For phobias, night waking: 0.01–0.1 mg/kg or 0.25–2 mg (total dose) per dog PO q6–12h PO (Siebert 2003)

e) For acute anxiety: 0.05–0.1 mg/kg PO prn or three times a day. Administer 30–60 minutes prior to trigger event. (Neilson 2009)

■ **CATS:**

a) For treatment of feline anxiety disorders: 0.125–0.25 mg/kg PO q12h (Start at 0.125 mg/kg PO) (Overall 1997)

b) For refractory house soiling: 0.1 mg/kg or 0.125–0.25 mg (total dose) per cat PO q8–12h (Siebert 2003)

c) For urine marking: 0.05–0.2 mg/kg PO q12–24h (Virga 2002)

d) For fears/phobias/anxieties: 0.125–0.25 mg (total dose) PO once to three times a day. (Landsberg 2005)

e) For acute anxiety: 0.05 mg/kg PO prn or three times a day. Administer 30-60 minutes prior to trigger event. (Neilson 2009)

Monitoring

■ Efficacy

■ Adverse Effects

■ Consider monitoring hepatic enzymes particularly when treating cats chronically

Client Information

■ Try to dose approximately one hour in advance of storms or other anticipated stimuli that evokes negative responses

■ If difficulty with pilling the medication occurs, consider using the orally-disintegrating tablets; hands must be dry before handling

■ If excessive sedation or yellowing of the whites of eyes (especially in cats) occurs, contact veterinarian

Chemistry/Synonyms

A benzodiazepine, alprazolam occurs as a white to off-white, crystalline powder. It is soluble in alcohol and insoluble in water.

Alprazolam may also be known as D65 MT, U 31889, or alprazolamum; many trade names available internationally.

Storage/Stability

Alprazolam tablets should be stored at room temperature in tight, light-resistant containers. The orally disintegrating tablets should be stored at room temperature and protected from moisture.

Compatibility/Compounding Considerations

Compounded preparation stability: Alprazolam oral suspension compounded from commercially available tablets has been published (Allen, 1998). Triturating sixty (60) alprazolam 2 mg tablets with 60 mL of Ora-Plus® and qs ad to 120 mL with Ora-Sweet® (or Ora-Sweet® SF) yields a 1 mg/mL oral suspension that retains >90% potency for 60 days stored at both 5°C and 25°C. Compounded preparations of alprazolam should be protected from light.

Dosage Forms/Regulatory Status

VETERINARY-LABELED PRODUCTS: None

The ARCI (Racing Commissioners International) has designated this drug as a class 2 substance. See the appendix for more information.

HUMAN-LABELED PRODUCTS:

Alprazolam Oral Tablets: 0.25 mg, 0.5 mg, 1 mg & 2 mg; *Xanax®* (Pfizer); generic; (Rx; C-IV)

Alprazolam Extended-release Oral Tablets: 0.5 mg, 1 mg, 2 mg, & 3 mg; *Xanax XR®* (Pfizer); generic; (Rx; C-IV)

Alprazolam Orally Disintegrating Tablets: 0.25 mg, 0.5 mg, 1 mg, & 2 mg; *Niravam®* (Schwarz Pharma); (Rx; C-IV)

Alprazolam Oral Solution: 1 mg/mL in 30 mL; *Alprazolam Intensol®* (Roxane); (Rx; C-IV)

References

Allen, L.V. & M.A. Erickson (1998). Stability of alprazolam, chloroquine phosphate, cisapride, enalapril maleate, and hydralazine hydrochloride in extemporaneously compounded oral liquids. *Am J Health Syst Pharm* 55(18): 1915–1920.

Crowell–Davis, S (2003a). Treating storm phobias. Proceedings: Western Veterinary Conference. http://goo.gl/Iprm2

Crowell–Davis, S (2003b). Use of clomipramine, alprazolam and behavior modification for treatment of storm phobia in dogs. *JAVMA* 222: 744–748.

Hunthausen, W (2006). The dog who can't be left alone. Proceedings: Western Vet Conf 2006. Accessed via: Veterinary Information Network. http://goo.gl/nPhwx

Landsberg, G (2005). Fear, anxiety and phobias – diagnosis and treatment. Proceedings: Western Veterinary Conf. Accessed via: Veterinary Information Network.

Neilson, J (2009). Pharmacologic Interventions for Behavioral Problems. Proceedings: Western Veterinary Conference. Accessed via: Veterinary Information Network. http://goo.gl/HVVZL

Overall, K (1997). *Clinical behavioral medicine for small animals.* St Louis, Mosby.

Siebert, L (2003). Psychoactive drugs in behavioral medicine. Western Veterinary Conference.

Virga, V (2002). Which drugs and why: An update on psychopharmacology. Proceedings: Atlantic Coast Veterinary Conference. Accessed via: Veterinary Information Network. http://goo.gl/m8qr4

ALTRENOGEST

(al-*tre-noe*-jest)   Regu-Mate®, Matrix®

ORAL PROGESTIN

Prescriber Highlights

▶ Progestational drug used in horses to suppress estrus or maintain pregnancy when progestin deficient; used in swine to synchronize estrus

▶ May be used in dogs for luteal deficiency or as a treatment to prevent premature delivery

▶ Many "handling" warnings for humans (see below)

▶ Very sensitive to light

Uses/Indications

Altrenogest (*Regu-Mate®*) is indicated (labeled) to suppress estrus in mares to allow a more predictable occurrence of estrus following withdrawal of the drug. It is used clinically to assist mares to establish normal cycles during the transitional period from anestrus to the normal breeding season often in conjunction with an artificial photoperiod. It is more effective in assisting in pregnancy attainment later in the transition period. Some authors (Squires et al. 1983) suggest selecting mares with considerable follicular activity (mares with one or more follicles 20 mm or greater in size) for treatment during the transitional phase. Mares that have been in estrus for 10 days or more and have active ovaries are also considered excellent candidates for progestin treatment.

Altrenogest is effective in normally cycling mares for minimizing the necessity for estrus detection, for the synchronization of estrus, and permitting scheduled breeding. Estrus will ensue 2–5 days after treatment is completed and most mares ovulate between 8–15 days after withdrawal. Altrenogest is also effective in suppressing estrus expression in show mares or mares to be raced. Although the drug is labeled as contraindicated during pregnancy, it has been demonstrated to maintain pregnancy in oophorectomized mares and may be of benefit in mares that abort due to sub-therapeutic progestin levels.

The product *Matrix®* is labeled for synchronization of estrus in sexually mature gilts that have had at least one estrous cycle. Treatment with altrenogest results in estrus (standing heat) 4–9 days after completion of the 14-day treatment period.

Altrenogest has been used in dogs for luteal insufficiency and as a treatment to prevent premature delivery.

Pharmacology/Actions

Progestins are primarily produced endogenously by the corpus luteum. They transform proliferative endometrium to secretory endometrium, enhance myometrium hypertrophy and inhibit spontaneous uterine contraction. Progestins have a dose-dependent inhibitory effect on the secretion of pituitary gonadotropins and have some degree of estrogenic, anabolic and androgenic activity.

Pharmacokinetics

In horses, the pharmacokinetics of altrenogest have been studied (Machnik *et al.* 2007). After oral dosing of 44 mg/kg PO, peak levels usually occur within 15–30 minutes post-dose; 24 hours post-dose, levels were below the level of quantification. Elimination half-lives are approximately 2.5–4 hours. Altrenogest appears to be primarily eliminated in the urine. Peak urine levels occur 3–6 hours after oral dosing. Urine levels were detectable up to 12 days post-administration.

Contraindications/Precautions/Warnings

The manufacturer (*Regu-Mate®*—Intervet) lists pregnancy as a contraindication to the use of altrenogest, however it has been used clinically to maintain pregnancy in certain mares (see Dosages below). Altrenogest should also not be used in horses intended for food purposes.

Adverse Effects

Adverse effects of altrenogest appear to be minimal when used at labeled dosages. One study (Shideler et al. 1983) found negligible changes in hematologic and most "standard" laboratory tests after administering altrenogest to 4 groups of horses (3 dosages, 1 control) over 86 days. Occasionally, slight changes in Ca^{++}, K^+, alkaline phosphatase and AST were noted in the treatment group, but values were only slightly elevated and only noted sporadically. No pattern or definite changes could be attributed to altrenogest. No outward adverse effects were noted in the treatment group during the trial.

Use of progestational agents in mares with chronic uterine infections should be avoided as the infection process may be enhanced.

Overdosage/Acute Toxicity

The LD_{50} of altrenogest is 175–177 mg/kg in rats. No information was located regarding the effects of an accidental acute overdose in horses or other species.

Drug Interactions

The following drug interactions have either been reported or are theoretical in humans or animals receiving altrenogest and may be of significance in veterinary patients:

■ **RIFAMPIN:** May decrease progestin activity if administered concomitantly. This is presumably due to microsomal enzyme induction with resultant increase in progestin metabolism. The clinical significance of this potential interaction is unknown.

Laboratory Considerations

■ Unlike exogenously administered progesterone, altrenogest does not interfere or cross-react with progesterone assays

Doses

■ **DOGS:**

For luteal insufficiency:

a) Document luteal insufficiency and rule out infectious causes of pregnancy loss. Best to avoid during first trimester. Give equine product (*Regumate®*) at 2 mL per 100 lbs of body weight PO once daily. Monitor pregnancy with ultrasound. Remember that exogenous progesterone is the experimental model for pyometra in the bitch, so monitor carefully. (Purswell 1999)

b) For luteal insufficiency, pre-term labor: 0.1 mL per 10 lb body weight PO once daily. (Barber 2006)

c) To maintain pregnancy if tocolytics (*e.g.*, terbutaline) do not control myometrial contractility: 0.088 mg/kg once daily (q24h). Must be withdrawn 2–3 days prior to predicted whelp date. (Davidson 2006)

■ **HORSES:**

To suppress estrus for synchronization:

a) Administer 1 mL per 110 pounds body weight (0.044 mg/kg) PO once daily for 15 consecutive days. May administer directly on tongue using a dose syringe or on the usual grain ration. (Package insert; *Regu-Mate®*—Intervet)

For prevention of abortion/pregnancy loss:

a) 0.088 mg/kg PO once daily. (Dascanio 2009)

b) To maintain pregnancy in mares with deficient progesterone levels: 0.044 mg/kg PO once daily. Three options for treatment: 1) treatment until day 60 of pregnancy or greater AND measurement of endogenous progesterone level of >4 ng/mL; 2) treatment until day 120 of pregnancy; or 3) treatment until end of pregnancy. (McCue 2003)

c) To maintain pregnancy in mares with placentitis: 22–44 mg (total dose; 10–20 mL) PO daily. (Valla 2003)

To suppress estrus (long-term):

a) 0.044 mg/kg PO daily (Squires *et al.* 1983)

■ **SWINE:**

For synchronization of estrous in sexually mature gilts that have had at least one estrous cycle:

a) Follow label directions for safe use. Administer 6.8 mL (15 mg) per gilt for 14 consecutive days. Apply as a top-dressing on a portion of gilt's daily feed allowance. Estrous should occur 4–9 days after completing treatment. (Package insert; *Matrix®*—Intervet)

Client Information

■ The manufacturer (*Regu-Mate®, Matrix®*— Intervet) lists the following people as those who should not handle the product:

1. Women who are or suspect that they are pregnant
2. Anyone with thrombophlebitis or thromboembolic disorders or with a history of these events
3. Anyone having cerebrovascular or coronary artery disease
4. Women with known or suspected carcinoma of the breast
5. People with known or suspected estrogen-dependent neoplasias
6. Women with undiagnosed vaginal bleeding
7. People with benign or malignant tumor that developed during the use of oral contraceptives or other estrogen containing products

Altrenogest can be absorbed after skin contact and absorption can be enhanced if the drug is covered by occlusive materials (*e.g.*, under latex gloves, etc.). If exposed to the skin, wash off immediately with soap and water. If the eyes are exposed, flush with water for 15 minutes and get medical attention. If the product is swallowed, do not induce vomiting and contact a physician or poison control center.

This medication is prohibited from use in an extra-label manner to enhance food and/or fiber production in animals

Chemistry/Synonyms

An orally administered synthetic progestational agent, altrenogest has a chemical name of 17 alpha-Allyl-17beta-hydroxyestra-4,9,11-trien-3-one.

Altrenogest may also be known as: allyl trenbolone, A-35957, A-41300, RH-2267, or RU-2267, *Regu-Mate®,* or *Matrix®.*

Storage/Stability

Altrenogest oral solution should be stored at room temperature. Altrenogest is extremely sensitive to light; dispense in light-resistant containers.

Dosage Forms/Regulatory Status

VETERINARY-LABELED PRODUCTS:

Altrenogest 0.22% (2.2 mg/mL) in oil solution in 150 mL and 1000 mL bottles; *Regu-Mate®* (Intervet); (Rx). FDA-approved for use in horses not intended for food. This medication is banned in racing animals in some countries.

Altrenogest 0.22% (2.2 mg/mL) in 1000 mL bottles; *Matrix®* (Intervet); (OTC, but extralabel use prohibited). FDA-approved for use in sexually mature gilts that have had at least one estrous cycle. Gilts must not be slaughtered for

human consumption for 21 days after the last treatment. The FDA prohibits the extra-label use of this medication to enhance food and/or fiber production in animals.

HUMAN-LABELED PRODUCTS: None

References

Barber, J (2006). Whelping management in the bitch. Proceedings: Western Veterinary Conference. Accessed via: Veterinary Information Network. http://goo.gl/TtiVh

Dascanio, J (2009). Hormonal Control of Reproduction. Proceedings: ABVP. Accessed via: Veterinary Information Network. http://goo.gl/o2vHk

Davidson, A (2006). Myths in small animal reproduction. Proceedings: Canine Medicine Symposium. Accessed via: Veterinary Information Network. http://goo.gl/V9SnE

Machnik, M, I Hegger, et al. (2007). Pharmacokinetics of altrenogest in horses. *J Vet Phamacol Ther* **30**: 86–90.

McCue, P (2003). Ovarian problems in the non–pregnant mare. Proceedings: Western Veterinary Conference. Accessed via: Veterinary Information Network. http://goo.gl/MqNgK

Purswell, B (1999). Pharmaceuticals used in canine theriogenology – Part 1 & 2. Proceedings: Central Veterinary Conference, Kansas City.

Squires, EL, RK Shideler, et al. (1983). Clinical Applications of Progestins in Mares. *Comp CE* 5(1): S16–S22.

Valla, W (2003). Medical management of mares with complicated pregnancies. Proceedings: ACVIM Forum. Accessed via: Veterinary Information Network.

ALUMINUM HYDROXIDE

(ah-*loo*-min-um hye-*droks*-ide)   Amphogel®

ORAL ANTACID/PHOSPHATE BINDER

Prescriber Highlights

▶ Used to treat hyperphosphatemia in small animal patients & sometimes as a gastric antacid for ulcers

▶ Chronic use may lead to electrolyte abnormalities; possible aluminum toxicity

▶ Many potential drug interactions

▶ Bulk, dried powder available from several sources

Uses/Indications

Orally administered aluminum hydroxide is used to reduce hyperphosphatemia in patients with renal failure when dietary phosphorus restriction fails to maintain serum phosphorus concentrations in the normal range.

Pharmacology/Actions

Aluminum salts reduce the amount of phosphorus absorbed from the intestine by physically binding to dietary phosphorus.

Contraindications/Precautions/Warnings

Aluminum-containing antacids may inhibit gastric emptying; use cautiously in patients with gastric outlet obstruction.

Adverse Effects

In small animals, the most likely side effect of aluminum hydroxide is constipation. If the patient is receiving a low phosphate diet and the patient chronically receives aluminum antacids, hypophosphatemia can develop.

Potentially, aluminum toxicity could occur with prolonged use. While previously believed unlikely to occur in small animal patients, at least 2 dogs in renal failure have been documented to have developed aluminum toxicity after receiving aluminum-containing phosphate binders (Segev *et al.* 2008). Aluminum-containing and calcium-containing phosphate binders may be used in combination to reduce the dose of each to reduce the risk of aluminum toxicity or hypercalcemia.

Reproductive/Nursing Safety

In a system evaluating the safety of drugs in canine and feline pregnancy (Papich 1989), these drugs are categorized as in class: *A* (*Probably safe. Although specific studies may not have proved the safety of all drugs in dogs and cats, there are no reports of adverse effects in laboratory animals or women.*)

Overdosage/Acute Toxicity

Acute toxicity is unlikely with an oral overdose. If necessary, GI and electrolyte imbalances that occur with chronic or acute overdose should be treated symptomatically.

Drug Interactions

The following drug interactions have either been reported or are theoretical in humans or animals receiving oral aluminum salts and may be of significance in veterinary medicine:

Aluminum salts can **decrease** the amount absorbed or the pharmacologic effect of:

- ◼ **ALLOPURINOL**
- ◼ **CHLOROQUINE**
- ◼ **CORTICOSTEROIDS**
- ◼ **DIGOXIN**
- ◼ **ETHAMBUTOL**
- ◼ **FLUOROQUINOLONES**
- ◼ **H-2 ANTAGONISTS (RANITIDINE, FAMOTIDINE**, etc.)
- ◼ **IRON SALTS**
- ◼ **ISONIAZID**
- ◼ **PENICILLAMINE**
- ◼ **PHENOTHIAZINES**
- ◼ **TETRACYCLINES**
- ◼ **THYROID HORMONES**

Separate oral doses of aluminum hydroxide and these drugs by two hours to help reduce this interaction.

Doses

◼ **DOGS:**

For hyperphosphatemia:

a) Aluminum hydroxide: 30–100 mg/kg/day PO with meals. (Adams 2009)

b) Aluminum hydroxide gel, dried powder: 30–90 mg/kg/day PO prior to meals. The dried powder is virtually tasteless and accepted readily by most cats when mixed with canned food. (Wolf 2008)

c) 15–45 mg/kg PO q12h (Bartges 2002)

For adjunctive therapy for gastric ulcers:

a) Aluminum hydroxide suspension or aluminum hydroxide/magnesium hydroxide suspension: 2–10 mL PO q2–4h (Hall & Twedt 1989)

b) Aluminum hydroxide tablets: ½–1 tablet or strength PO q6h (Matz 1995)

◼ **CATS:**

For hyperphosphatemia:

a) Aluminum hydroxide: Initially at 30–90 mg/kg per day. Dosage must be individualized. Capsules or suspension are preferred as they are more easily mixed with food and dispersed throughout ingesta. Evaluate serum phosphate levels at 10–14 day intervals to determine optimum dosage. (Polzin & Osborne 1985)

b) 15–45 mg/kg PO q12h (Bartges 2002)

As an antacid:

a) Aluminum hydroxide tablets: ¼ tablet PO q6h (Matz 1995)

◼ **RABBITS/RODENTS/SMALL MAMMALS:**

a) Chinchillas: Aluminum hydroxide gel: 1 mL/animal PO as needed

Guinea pigs: 0.5–1 mL/animal PO as needed (Adamcak & Otten 2000)

◼ **CATTLE:**

As an antacid:

a) Aluminum hydroxide: 30 grams/animal (Jenkins 1988)

◼ **HORSES:**

For adjunctive gastroduodenal ulcer therapy in foals:

a) Aluminum/magnesium hydroxide suspension: 15 mL (total dose) 4 times a day (Clark and Becht 1987)

Monitoring

- ◼ Serum phosphorus (after a 12-hour fast), initially at 10–14 day intervals; once "stable", at 4–6 week intervals

- ◼ For aluminum toxicity: neuromuscular effects, progressive decreases in mean cell volume (MCV) and microcytosis

Client Information

- ◼ Oral aluminum hydroxide products are available without prescription (OTC), but should be used under the supervision of the veterinarian.

- ◼ Bulk, powder, tablets or capsules (may be compounded) are easier to administer than human liquids or suspensions

- ◼ Give either just before feeding or mixed in food

■ Report any unusual neuromuscular signs such as weakness, difficulty walking, or stumbling to veterinarian

Dosage Forms/Regulatory Status

VETERINARY-LABELED PRODUCTS: None

HUMAN-LABELED PRODUCTS:

Aluminum Hydroxide Oral Capsules: 500 mg, *Dialume®* (RPR): (OTC)

Aluminum Hydroxide Oral Tablets: 600 mg, *Amphojel®* (Wyeth-Ayerst); (OTC)

Aluminum Hydroxide Concentrated Gel Suspension/Liquid (Note: These products are usually flavored (mint) and not well accepted by dogs or cats.):

> 320 mg/5 mL in 360 & 480 mL, UD 15 & 30 mL; generic; (OTC)
>
> 450mg/5 mL in 500 mL and UD 30 mL; generic (Roxane); (OTC)
>
> 675 mg/5 mL in 180 and 500 mL, UD 20 and 30 mL; generic; (OTC)

Aluminum Hydroxide Concentrated Gel Liquid: 600 mg/5 mL in 30, 150, 180, 360 & 480 mL; *AlternaGEL®* (J & J-Merck); generic; (OTC)

Aluminum Hydroxide Gel, Dried Powder, USP; Bulk powder is available from a variety of sources including many compounding pharmacies. See: http://goo.gl/1lYJk for additional source information.

Note: There are also many products available that have aluminum hydroxide and a magnesium or calcium salt (*e.g., Maalox®*, etc.) that are used as antacids. All oral aluminum and magnesium hydroxide preparations are OTC.

References

Adamcak, A & B Otten (2000). Rodent Therapeutics. *Vet Clin NA: Exotic Anim Pract* **3:**1(Jan): 221–240.

Adams, L (2009). Updates in management of chronic kidney disease. Proceedings: Western Veterinary Conference. Accessed via: Veterinary Information Network. http://goo.gl/yZFlg

Bartges, J (2002). Rusty Plumbing: Chronic renal failure. Proceedings: Western Veterinary Conf. Accessed via: Veterinary Information Network. http://goo.gl/BR47c

Hall, JA & DC Twedt (1989). Diseases of the Stomach. *Handbook of Small Animal Practice.* RV Morgan Ed. New York, Churchill LIvingstone: 371–384.

Jenkins, WL (1988). Drugs affecting gastrointestinal functions. *Veterinary Pharmacology and Therapeutics 6th Ed.* NH Booth and LE McDonald Eds. Ames, Iowa Stae Univ. Press: 657–671.

Matz, M (1995). Gastrointestinal ulcer therapy. *Kirk's Current Veterinary Therapy:XII.* J Bonagura Ed. Philadelphia, W.B. Saunders: 706–710.

Polzin, DJ & CA Osborne (1985). Diseases of the Urinary Tract. *Handbook of Small Animal Therapeutics.* LE Davis Ed. New York, Churchill Livingstone: 333–395.

Segev, G, C Bandt, et al. (2008). Aluminum Toxicity Following Administration of Aluminum–based Phosphate Binders in 2 Dogs with Renal Failure. *J Vet Intern Med* **22**(6): 1432–1435.

Wolf, A (2008). Chronic progressive renal disease in the cat: Recognition and management. Proceedings: ACVC.

AMANTADINE HCL

(a-*man*-ta-deen)   Symmetrel®

ANTIVIRAL (INFLUENZA A); NMDA ANTAGONIST

Prescriber Highlights

▶ Antiviral drug with NMDA antagonist properties; may be useful in adjunctive therapy of chronic pain in small animals & treatment of equine influenza in horses

▶ Very limited clinical experience; dogs may exhibit agitation & GI effects, especially early in therapy

▶ Large interpatient variations of pharmacokinetics in horses limit its therapeutic usefulness

▶ Overdoses are potentially very serious; fairly narrow therapeutic index in dogs & cats; may need to be compounded

▶ Extra-label use prohibited (by FDA) in chickens, turkeys & ducks

Uses/Indications

While amantadine may have efficacy and clinical usefulness against some veterinary viral diseases, presently the greatest interest for its use in small animals is as a NMDA antagonist in the adjunctive treatment of chronic pain, often in those tolerant to opioids. It is generally used in combination with an NSAID, when the NSAID alone does not offer sufficient pain relief. It is also used as an adjunct drug for treating neuropathic pain. It has been suggested for use as an early intervention in the treatment of pain associated with osteosarcomas (Gaynor, J.S. 2008).

Amantadine has also been investigated for treatment of equine-2 influenza virus in the horse. However, because of expense, interpatient variability in oral absorption and other pharmacokinetic parameters, and the potential for causing seizures after intravenous dosing, it is not commonly used for treatment.

In humans, amantadine is used for treatment and prophylaxis of influenza A, parkinsonian syndrome, and drug-induced extrapyramidal effects. As in veterinary medicine, amantadine's effect on NMDA receptors in humans are of active interest, particularly its use as a co-analgesic with opiates and in the reduction of opiate tolerance development.

Pharmacology/Actions

Like ketamine, dextromethorphan and memantine, amantadine antagonizes the N-methyl-D-aspartate (NMDA) receptor. Within the central nervous system, chronic pain can be maintained or exacerbated when glutamate or aspartate bind to this receptor. It is believed that this receptor is particularly important in allodynia (sensation of pain resulting from a normally non-noxious stimulus). Amantadine alone is not a particularly good analgesic, but in combination with other analgesics (*e.g.*, opiates, NSAIDs), it is thought that it may help alleviate chronic pain.

Amantadine's antiviral activity is primarily limited to strains of influenza A. While its complete mechanism of action is unknown, it does inhibit viral replication by interfering with influenza A virus M2 protein.

Amantadine's antiparkinsonian activity is not well understood. The drug does appear to have potentiating effects on dopaminergic neurotransmission in the CNS and anticholinergic activity.

Pharmacokinetics

The pharmacokinetics of this drug have apparently not been described in dogs or cats. In horses, amantadine has a very wide interpatient variability of absorption after oral dosing; bioavailability ranges from 40–60%. The elimination half-life in horses is about 3.5 hours and the steady state volume of distribution is approximately 5 L/kg.

In humans, the drug is well absorbed after oral administration with peak plasma concentrations occurring about 3 hours after dosing. Volume of distribution is 3–8 L/kg. Amantadine is primarily eliminated via renal mechanisms. Oral clearance is approximately 0.28 L/hr/kg; half-life is around 17 hours.

Contraindications/Precautions/Warnings

In humans, amantadine is contraindicated in patients with known hypersensitivity to it or rimantadine, and in patients with untreated angle-closure glaucoma. It should be used with caution in patients with liver disease, renal disease (dosage adjustment may be required), congestive heart failure, active psychoses, eczematoid dermatitis or seizure disorders. In veterinary patients with similar conditions, it is advised to use the drug with caution until more information on its safety becomes available.

In 2006, the FDA banned the use of amantadine and other influenza antivirals in chickens, turkeys and ducks.

Adverse Effects

There is very limited experience in domestic animals with amantadine and its adverse effect profile is not well described. It has been reported that dogs given amantadine occasionally develop agitation, loose stools, flatulence or diarrhea, particularly early in therapy. Experience in cats is limited; an adverse effect profile has yet to be fully elucidated, but the safety margin appears to be narrow.

Reproductive/Nursing Safety

In humans, the FDA categorizes amantadine as a category *C* drug for use during pregnancy (*Animal studies have shown an adverse effect on the fetus, but there are no adequate studies in humans; or there are no animal reproduction studies and no adequate studies in humans*). High dosages in rats demonstrated some teratogenic effects.

Amantadine does enter maternal milk. The manufacturer does not recommend its use in women who are nursing. Veterinary significance is unclear.

Overdosage/Acute Toxicity

Toxic dose reported for cats is 30 mg/kg and behavioral effects may be noted at 15 mg/kg in dogs and cats.

In humans, overdoses as low as 2 grams have been associated with fatalities. Cardiac dysfunction (arrhythmias, hypertension, tachycardia), pulmonary edema, CNS toxicity (tremors, seizures, psychosis, agitation, coma), hyperthermia, renal dysfunction and respiratory distress syndrome have all been documented. There is no known specific antidote for amantadine overdose. Treatment should consist of gut emptying, if possible, intensive monitoring and supportive therapy. Forced urine acidifying diuresis may increase renal excretion of amantadine. Physostigmine has been suggested for cautious use in treating CNS effects.

Drug Interactions

The following drug interactions have either been reported or are theoretical in humans or animals receiving amantadine and may be of significance in veterinary patients:

■ **ANTICHOLINERGIC DRUGS:** May enhance the anticholinergic effects of amantadine

■ **CNS STIMULANTS** (including **selegiline**): Concomitant use with amantadine may increase the drug's CNS stimulatory effects

■ **TRIMETHOPRIM/SULFA, QUINIDINE, QUININE, THIAZIDE DIURETICS OR TRIAMTERENE:** May decrease the excretion of amantadine, yielding higher blood levels

■ **URINARY ACIDIFIERS** (**e.g., methionine, ammonium chloride, ascorbic acid**): May increase the excretion of amantadine

Laboratory Considerations

■ No laboratory interactions identified

Doses

■ **DOGS:**

As adjunctive therapy for chronic pain:

a) For osteoarthritis pain when NSAIDs alone are not effective: 3–5 mg/kg PO once daily in addition to an NSAID (meloxicam at approved doses used for this study) (Lascelles, B.D.X. *et al.* 2008)

b) 3–5 mg/kg PO once daily. (Gaynor, J. 2002), (Gaynor, J.S. 2008)

c) To decrease wind-up: 3–5 mg/kg PO once daily for one week. (Perkowski 2006)

■ **CATS:**

As adjunctive therapy for chronic pain:

a) 3 mg/kg PO once daily. May be useful addition to NSAIDs; not been evaluated for toxicity. May need to be compounded. (Lascelles, D. *et al.* 2003)

b) 3–5 mg/kg PO once daily. (Gaynor, J. 2002), (Gaynor, J.S. 2008)

c) 3 mg/kg PO once daily. (Hardie 2006)

■ **HORSES:**
For acute treatment of equine-2 influenza:
a) 5 mg/kg IV q4h (Rees *et al.* 1997)

Monitoring

■ Adverse effects (GI, agitation)
■ Efficacy

Client Information

■ When used in small animals, the drug must be given as prescribed to be effective and may take a week or so to show effect.

■ Gastrointestinal effects (loose stools, gas, diarrhea) or some agitation may occur, particularly early in treatment. Contact the veterinarian if these become serious or persist.

■ Overdoses with this medication can be serious; keep well out of reach of children and pets.

Chemistry/Synonyms

An adamantane-class antiviral agent with NMDA antagonist properties, amantadine HCl occurs as a white to practically white, bitter tasting, crystalline powder with a pKa of 9. Approximately 400 mg are soluble in 1 mL of water; 200 mg are soluble in 1 mL of alcohol.

Amantadine HCl may also be known as: adamantanamine HCl, *Adekin®*, *Amanta®*, *Amantagamma®*, *Amantan®*, *Amantrel®*, *Amixx®*, *Antadine®*, *Antiflu-DES®*, *Atarin®*, *Atenegine®*, *Cerebramed®*, *Endantadine®*, *Infectoflu®*, *Influ-A®*, *Lysovir®*, *Mantadine®*, *Mantadix®*, *Mantidan®*, *Padiken®*, *Symadine®*, *Symmetrel®*, *Viroifral®* and *Virucid®*.

Storage/Stability

Tablets, capsules and the oral solution should be stored in tight containers at room temperature. Limited exposures to temperatures as low as 15°C and as high as 30°C are permitted. Avoid freezing the liquid.

Dosage Forms/Regulatory Status

VETERINARY-LABELED PRODUCTS: None

HUMAN-LABELED PRODUCTS:

Amantadine HCl Oral Tablets & Capsules: 100 mg; *Symmetrel®* (Endo); generic; (Rx)

Amantadine HCl Oral Syrup: 10 mg/mL in 480 mL; *Symmetrel®* (Endo); generic; (Rx). Note: It is reported that the oral liquid has a very bad taste.

In 2006, the FDA banned the extra-label use of amantadine and other influenza antivirals in chickens, turkeys and ducks.

References

Gaynor, J (2002). Other drugs used to treat pain. *Handbook of Veterinary Pain Management.* J Gaynor and W Muir Eds., Mosby: 251–260.

Gaynor, JS (2008). Control of Cancer Pain in Veterinary Patients. *Veterinary Clinics of North America–Small Animal Practice* 38(6): 1429–+.

Hardie, E (2006). Managing intractable pain. Proceedings: Western Vet Conf 2006. Accessed via: Veterinary Information Network. http://goo.gl/sED8X

Lascelles, BDX, JS Gaynor, et al. (2008). Amantadine in a multimodal analgesic regimen for alleviation of refractory osteoarthritis pain in dogs. *Journal of Veterinary Internal Medicine* 22(1): 53–59.

Lascelles, D, S Robertson, et al. (2003). Can chronic pain in cats be managed? Yes! Proceedings: Pain Management 2003. Accessed via: Veterinary Information Network. http://goo.gl/2m6yx

Perkowski, S (2006). Alternatives for pain management for chronic pain. Proceedings: ACVIM 2006. Accessed via: Veterinary Information Network. http://goo.gl/MzVog

Rees, W, J Harkins, et al. (1997). Amantadine and equine influenza: pharmacology, pharmacokinetics and neurological effects in the horse. *Equine Vet Jnl* 29(2): 89–91.

AMIKACIN SULFATE

(am-i-**kay**-sin)   Amikin®, Amiglyde-V®

AMINOGLYCOSIDE ANTIBIOTIC

Prescriber Highlights

▶ Parenteral aminoglycoside antibiotic that has good activity against a variety of bacteria, predominantly gram-negative aerobic bacilli

▶ Adverse Effects: Nephrotoxicity, ototoxicity, neuromuscular blockade

▶ Cats may be more sensitive to toxic effects

▶ Risk factors for toxicity: Preexisting renal disease, age (both neonatal & geriatric), fever, sepsis & dehydration

▶ Now usually dosed once daily when used systemically

Uses/Indications

While parenteral use is only FDA-approved in dogs, amikacin is used clinically to treat serious gram-negative infections in most species. It is often used in settings where gentamicin-resistant bacteria are a clinical problem. The inherent toxicity of the aminoglycosides limit their systemic use to serious infections when there is either a documented lack of susceptibility to other, less toxic antibiotics or when the clinical situation dictates immediate treatment of a presumed gram-negative infection before culture and susceptibility results are reported.

Amikacin is also FDA-approved for intrauterine infusion in mares. It is used with intraarticular injection in foals to treat gram-negative septic arthritis.

Pharmacology/Actions

Amikacin, like the other aminoglycoside antibiotics, act on susceptible bacteria presumably by irreversibly binding to the 30S ribosomal subunit thereby inhibiting protein synthesis. It is considered a bactericidal concentration-dependent antibiotic.

Amikacin's spectrum of activity includes: coverage against many aerobic gram-negative and some aerobic gram-positive bacteria, including most species of *E. coli*, Klebsiella, Proteus, Pseudomonas, Salmonella, Enterobacter, Serratia, and Shigella, Mycoplasma, and Staphylococcus. Several strains of *Pseudomonas aeruginosa*, Proteus, and Serratia that are resistant to gentamicin will still be killed by amikacin.

Antimicrobial activity of the aminoglycosides is enhanced in an alkaline environment.

The aminoglycoside antibiotics are inactive against fungi, viruses and most anaerobic bacteria.

Pharmacokinetics

Amikacin, like the other aminoglycosides is not appreciably absorbed after oral or intrauterine administration, but is absorbed from topical administration (not from skin or the urinary bladder) when used in irrigations during surgical procedures. Patients receiving oral aminoglycosides with hemorrhagic or necrotic enteritises may absorb appreciable quantities of the drug. After IM administration to dogs and cats, peak levels occur from ½–1 hour later. Subcutaneous injection results in slightly delayed peak levels and with more variability than after IM injection. Bioavailability from extravascular injection (IM or SC) is greater than 90%.

After absorption, aminoglycosides are distributed primarily in the extracellular fluid. They are found in ascitic, pleural, pericardial, peritoneal, synovial and abscess fluids; high levels are found in sputum, bronchial secretions and bile. Aminoglycosides are minimally protein bound (<20%, streptomycin 35%) to plasma proteins. Aminoglycosides do not readily cross the blood-brain barrier nor penetrate ocular tissue. CSF levels are unpredictable and range from 0–50% of those found in the serum. Therapeutic levels are found in bone, heart, gallbladder and lung tissues after parenteral dosing. Aminoglycosides tend to accumulate in certain tissues such as the inner ear and kidneys, which may help explain their toxicity. Volumes of distribution have been reported to be 0.15–0.3 L/kg in adult cats and dogs, and 0.26–0.58 L/kg in horses. Volumes of distribution may be significantly larger in neonates and juvenile animals due to their higher extracellular fluid fractions. Aminoglycosides cross the placenta; fetal concentrations range from 15–50% of those found in maternal serum.

Elimination of aminoglycosides after parenteral administration occurs almost entirely by glomerular filtration. The approximate elimination half-lives for amikacin have been reported to be 5 hours in foals, 1.14–2.3 hours in adult horses, 2.2–2.7 hours in calves, 1–3 hours in cows, 1.5 hours in sheep, and 0.5–2 hours in dogs and cats. Patients with decreased renal function can have significantly prolonged half-lives. In humans with normal renal function, elimination rates can be highly variable with the aminoglycoside antibiotics.

Contraindications/Precautions/Warnings

Aminoglycosides are contraindicated in patients who are hypersensitive to them. Because these drugs are often the only effective agents in severe gram-negative infections, there are no other absolute contraindications to their use. However, they should be used with extreme caution in patients with preexisting renal disease with concomitant monitoring and dosage interval adjustments made. Other risk factors for the development of toxicity include age (both neonatal and geriatric patients), fever, sepsis and dehydration.

Because aminoglycosides can cause irreversible ototoxicity, they should be used with caution in "working" dogs (*e.g.*, "seeing-eye," herding, dogs for the hearing impaired, etc.).

Aminoglycosides should be used with caution in patients with neuromuscular disorders (*e.g.*, myasthenia gravis) due to their neuromuscular blocking activity.

Sighthound dogs may require reduced dosages of aminoglycosides as they have significantly smaller volumes of distribution.

Because aminoglycosides are eliminated primarily through renal mechanisms, they should be used cautiously, preferably with serum monitoring and dosage adjustment in neonatal or geriatric animals.

Aminoglycosides are generally considered contraindicated in rabbits/hares as they adversely affect the GI flora balance in these animals.

Adverse Effects

The aminoglycosides are infamous for their nephrotoxic and ototoxic effects. The nephrotoxic (tubular necrosis) mechanisms of these drugs are not completely understood, but are probably related to interference with phospholipid metabolism in the lysosomes of proximal renal tubular cells, resulting in leakage of proteolytic enzymes into the cytoplasm. Nephrotoxicity is usually manifested by: increases in BUN, creatinine, nonprotein nitrogen in the serum, and decreases in urine specific gravity and creatinine clearance. Proteinuria and cells or casts may be seen in the urine. Nephrotoxicity is usually reversible once the drug is discontinued. While gentamicin may be more nephrotoxic and amikacin less nephrotoxic than the other aminoglycosides, the incidences of nephrotoxicity with all of these agents require equal caution and monitoring.

Ototoxicity (8th cranial nerve toxicity) of the aminoglycosides can manifest by either auditory and/or vestibular clinical signs and may be irreversible. Vestibular clinical signs are more frequent with streptomycin, gentamicin, or tobramycin. Auditory clinical signs are more frequent with amikacin, neomycin, or kanamycin, but either form can occur with any of these drugs.

Cats are apparently very sensitive to the vestibular effects of the aminoglycosides.

The aminoglycosides can also cause neuromuscular blockade, facial edema, pain/inflammation at injection site, peripheral neuropathy and hypersensitivity reactions. Rarely, GI clinical signs, hematologic and hepatic effects have been reported.

Reproductive/Nursing Safety

Aminoglycosides can cross the placenta and while rare, may cause 8th cranial nerve toxicity or nephrotoxicity in fetuses. Because the drug should only be used in serious infections, the benefits of therapy may exceed the potential risks. In humans, the FDA categorizes this drug as category *C* for use during pregnancy (*Animal studies have shown an adverse effect on the fetus, but there are no adequate studies in humans; or there are no animal reproduction studies and no adequate studies in humans.*) In a separate system evaluating the safety of drugs in canine and feline pregnancy (Papich 1989), this drug is categorized as in class: *C* (*These drugs may have potential risks. Studies in people or laboratory animals have uncovered risks, and these drugs should be used cautiously as a last resort when the benefit of therapy clearly outweighs the risks.*)

Aminoglycosides are excreted in milk. While potentially, amikacin ingested with milk could alter GI flora and cause diarrhea, amikacin in milk is unlikely to be of significant concern after the first few days of life (colostrum period).

Overdosage/Acute Toxicity

Should an inadvertent overdosage be administered, three treatments have been recommended. Hemodialysis is very effective in reducing serum levels of the drug but is not a viable option for most veterinary patients. Peritoneal dialysis also will reduce serum levels but is much less efficacious. Complexation of drug with either carbenicillin or ticarcillin (12–20 g/day in humans) is reportedly nearly as effective as hemodialysis. Since amikacin is less affected by this effect than either tobramycin or gentamicin, it is assumed that reduction in serum levels will also be minimized using this procedure.

Drug Interactions

The following drug interactions have either been reported or are theoretical in humans or animals receiving amikacin and may be of significance in veterinary patients:

■ **BETA-LACTAM ANTIBIOTICS (penicillins, cephalosporins):** May have synergistic effects against some bacteria; some potential for physical inactivation of aminoglycosides *in vitro* (do not mix together) and *in vivo* (patients in renal failure)

■ **CEPHALOSPORINS:** The concurrent use of aminoglycosides with cephalosporins is somewhat controversial. Potentially, cephalosporins could cause additive nephrotoxicity when used with aminoglycosides, but this interaction has only been well documented with cephaloridine and cephalothin (both no longer marketed).

■ **DIURETICS, LOOP (e.g., furosemide, torsemide) or OSMOTIC (e.g., mannitol):** Concurrent use with loop or osmotic diuretics may increase the nephrotoxic or ototoxic potential of the aminoglycosides

■ **NSAIDS:** Because NSAIDs may cause nephrotoxic effects, some believe that concurrent use with aminoglycosides should be avoided.

■ **NEPHROTOXIC DRUGS, OTHER (e.g., cisplatin, amphotericin B, polymyxin B, or vancomycin):** Potential for increased risk for nephrotoxicity

■ **NEUROMUSCULAR BLOCKING AGENTS & ANESTHETICS, GENERAL:** Concomitant use with general anesthetics or neuromuscular blocking agents could potentiate neuromuscular blockade

Laboratory Considerations

■ Amikacin serum concentrations may be falsely decreased if the patient is also receiving **beta-lactam antibiotics** and the serum is stored prior to analysis. It is recommended that if assay is delayed, samples be frozen and, if possible, drawn at times when the beta-lactam antibiotic is at a trough.

Doses

Note: Most infectious disease clinicians now agree that aminoglycosides should be dosed once a day in most patients (mammals). This dosing regimen yields higher peak levels with resultant greater bacterial kill, and as aminoglycosides exhibit a "post-antibiotic effect", surviving susceptible bacteria generally do not replicate as rapidly even when antibiotic concentrations are below MIC. Periods where levels are low may also decrease the "adaptive resistance" (bacteria take up less drug in the presence of continuous exposure) that can occur. Once daily dosing may decrease the toxicity of aminoglycosides as lower urinary concentrations may mean less uptake into renal tubular cells. However, patients who are neutropenic (or otherwise immunosuppressed) may benefit from more frequent dosing (q8h). Patients with significantly diminished renal function who must receive aminoglycosides may need to be dosed at longer intervals than once daily. Clinical drug monitoring is strongly suggested for these patients.

■ **DOGS:**

For susceptible infections:

a) 15 mg/kg IV q24h or 20 mg/kg SC/IM q24h. In Greyhounds (and potentially other sighthounds) reduce dose to 10 mg/kg IV q24 or 15mg/kg SC/IM q24h. (KuKanich 2008)

b) 15 mg/kg (route not specified) once

daily (q24h). Neutropenic or immuno-compromised patients may still need to be dosed q8h (dose divided). (Trepanier 1999)

c) Sepsis: 20 mg/kg once daily IV (Hardie 2000)

d) For empiric therapy: 15–30 mg/kg *(route not specified, assume IV, IM or SC—Plumb)* (Autran de Morais 2009)

■ **CATS:**

For susceptible infections:

a) For empiric therapy: 10–15 mg/kg *(route not specified, assume IV, IM or SC—Plumb)* (Autran de Morais 2009)

b) 15 mg/kg (route not specified) once daily (q24h). Neutropenic or immuno-compromised patients may still need to be dosed q8h (dose divided). (Trepanier 1999)

c) Sepsis: 20 mg/kg once daily IV (Hardie 2000)

■ **FERRETS:**

For susceptible infections:

a) 8–16 mg/kg IM or IV once daily (Williams 2000)

b) 8–16 mg/kg/day SC, IM, IV divided q8–24h (Morrisey & Carpenter 2004)

■ **RABBITS/RODENTS/SMALL MAMMALS:**

a) **Rabbits:** 8–16 mg/kg daily dose (may divide into q8h–q24h) SC, IM or IV. Increased efficacy and decreased toxicity if given once daily. If given IV, dilute into 4 mL/kg of saline and give over 20 minutes. (Ivey & Morrisey 2000)

b) **Rabbits:** 5–10 mg/kg SC, IM, IV divided q8–24h

Guinea pigs: 10–15 mg/kg SC, IM, IV divided q8–24h

Chinchillas: 10–15 mg/kg SC, IM, IV divided q8–24h

Hamster, rats, mice: 10 mg/kg SC, IM q12h

Prairie Dogs: 5 mg/kg SC, IM q12h (Morrisey & Carpenter 2004)

c) **Chinchillas:** 2–5 mg/kg SC, IM q8–12h (Hayes 2000)

■ **CATTLE:**

For susceptible infections:

a) 10 mg/kg IM q8h or 25 mg/kg q12h (Beech 1987)

b) 22 mg/kg/day IM divided three times daily (Upson 1988)

■ **HORSES:**

For susceptible infections:

a) 21 mg/kg IV or IM once daily (q24h) (Moore 1999b); (Foreman 1999)

b) In neonatal foals: 21 mg/kg IV once daily (Magdesian *et al.* 2004)

c) In neonatal foals: Initial dose of 25 mg/kg

IV once daily; strongly recommend to in-dividualize dosage based upon therapeu-tic drug monitoring. (Bucki *et al.* 2004)

d) Adults: 10 mg/kg IM or IV once daily (q24h)

Foals (<30 days old): 20–25 mg/kg IV or IM once daily (q24h). (Geor & Papich 2003)

e) For treatment of septic joints: 20 mg/kg IV once daily. Usually used with a peni-cillin, at least until a definitive culture is obtained. (Moll 2009)

For uterine infusion:

a) 2 grams mixed with 200 mL sterile nor-mal saline (0.9% sodium chloride for injection) and aseptically infused into uterus daily for 3 consecutive days (Pack-age insert; *Amiglyde-V®*—Fort Dodge)

b) 1–2 grams intrauterine (Perkins 1999)

For intra-articular injection as adjunctive treatment of septic arthritis in foals:

a) If a single joint is involved, inject 250 mg daily or 500 mg every other day; fre-quency is dependent upon how often joint lavage is performed. Use cautiously in multiple joints as toxicity may result (particularly if systemic therapy is also given). (Moore 1999a)

For regional intravenous limb perfusion (RILP) administration in standing horses:

a) Usual dosages range from 500 mg–2 grams; dosage must be greater than 250 mg when a cephalic vein is used for perfusion and careful placement of tourniquets must be performed. (Parra-Sanchez *et al.* 2006)

■ **BIRDS:**

For susceptible infections:

a) For sunken eyes/sinusitis in macaws caused by susceptible bacteria: 40 mg/kg IM once or twice daily. Must also flush si-nuses with saline mixed with appropriate antibiotic (10–30 mL per nostril). May require 2 weeks of treatment. (Karpinski & Clubb 1986)

b) 15 mg/kg IM or SC q12h (Hoeffer 1995)

c) For gram-negative infections resistant to gentamicin: Dilute commercial so-lution and administer 15–20 mg/kg (0.015 mg/g) IM once a day or twice a day (Clubb 1986)

d) Ratites: 7.6–11 mg/kg IM twice daily; air cell: 10–25 mg/egg; egg dip: 2000 mg/gallon of distilled water pH of 6 (Jenson 1998)

■ **REPTILES:**

For susceptible infections:

a) For snakes: 5 mg/kg IM (forebody) load-ing dose, then 2.5 mg/kg q72h for 7–9 treatments. Commonly used in respiratory infections. Use a lower dose for Python curtus. (Gauvin 1993)

b) Study done in gopher snakes: 5 mg/kg IM loading dose, then 2.5 mg/kg q72h. House snakes at high end of their preferred optimum ambient temperature. (Mader *et al.* 1985)

c) For bacterial shell diseases in turtles: 10 mg/kg daily in water turtles, every other day in land turtles and tortoises for 7–10 days. Used commonly with a beta-lactam antibiotic. Recommended to begin therapy with 20 mL/kg fluid injection. Maintain hydration and monitor uric acid levels when possible. (Rosskopf 1986)

d) For Crocodilians: 2.25 mg/kg IM q 72–96h (Jacobson 2000) (Jacobson 2000)

e) For gram-negative respiratory disease: 3.5 mg/kg IM, SC or via lung catheter every 3–10 days for 30 days. (Klaphake 2005)

■ **FISH:**

For susceptible infections:

a) 5 mg/kg IM loading dose, then 2.5 mg/kg every 72 hours for 5 treatments. (Lewbart 2006)

Monitoring

■ Efficacy (cultures, clinical signs, WBC's and clinical signs associated with infection). Therapeutic drug monitoring is highly recommended when using this drug systemically. Attempt to draw samples at 1, 2, and 4 hours post dose. Peak level should be at least 40 micrograms/mL and the 4–hour sample less than 10 micrograms/mL.

■ Adverse effect monitoring is essential. Pretherapy renal function tests and urinalysis (repeated during therapy) are recommended. Casts in the urine are often the initial sign of impending nephrotoxicity.

■ Gross monitoring of vestibular or auditory toxicity is recommended.

Client Information

■ With appropriate training, owners may give subcutaneous injections at home, but routine monitoring of therapy for efficacy and toxicity must still be done

■ Clients should also understand that the potential exists for severe toxicity (nephrotoxicity, ototoxicity) developing from this medication

■ Use in food producing animals is controversial as drug residues may persist for long periods

Chemistry/Synonyms

A semi-synthetic aminoglycoside derived from kanamycin, amikacin occurs as a white, crystalline powder that is sparingly soluble in water. The sulfate salt is formed during the manufacturing process. 1.3 grams of amikacin sulfate is

equivalent to 1 gram of amikacin. Amikacin may also be expressed in terms of units. 50,600 Units are equal to 50.9 mg of base. The commercial injection is a clear to straw-colored solution and the pH is adjusted to 3.5–5.5 with sulfuric acid.

Amikacin sulfate may also be known as: amikacin sulphate, amikacini sulfas, or BB-K8; many trade names are available.

Storage/Stability

Amikacin sulfate for injection should be stored at room temperature (15–30°C); freezing or temperatures above 40°C should be avoided. Solutions may become very pale yellow with time but this does not indicate a loss of potency.

Amikacin is stable for at least 2 years at room temperature. Autoclaving commercially available solutions at 15 pounds of pressure at 120°C for 60 minutes did not result in any loss of potency.

Compatibility/Compounding Considerations

When given intravenously, amikacin should be diluted into suitable IV diluent *etc.* normal saline, D5W or LRS) and administered over at least 30 minutes.

Amikacin sulfate is reportedly **compatible** and stable in all commonly used intravenous solutions and with the following drugs: amobarbital sodium, ascorbic acid injection, bleomycin sulfate, calcium chloride/gluconate, cefoxitin sodium, chloramphenicol sodium succinate, chlorpheniramine maleate, cimetidine HCl, clindamycin phosphate, colistimethate sodium, dimenhydrinate, diphenhydramine HCl, epinephrine HCl, ergonovine maleate, hyaluronidase, hydrocortisone sodium phosphate/succinate, lincomycin HCl, metaraminol bitartrate, metronidazole (with or without sodium bicarbonate), norepinephrine bitartrate, pentobarbital sodium, phenobarbital sodium, phytonadione, polymyxin B sulfate, prochlorperazine edisylate, promethazine HCl, secobarbital sodium, sodium bicarbonate, succinylcholine chloride, vancomycin HCl and verapamil HCl.

The following drugs or solutions are reportedly **incompatible** or only **compatible in specific situations** with amikacin: aminophylline, amphotericin B, ampicillin sodium, carbenicillin disodium, cefazolin sodium, cephalothin sodium, cephapirin sodium, chlorothiazide sodium, dexamethasone sodium phosphate, erythromycin glucepate, heparin sodium, methicillin sodium, nitrofurantoin sodium, oxacillin sodium, oxytetracycline HCl, penicillin G potassium, phenytoin sodium, potassium chloride (in dextran 6% in sodium chloride 0.9%; stable with potassium chloride in "standard" solutions), tetracycline HCl, thiopental sodium, vitamin B-complex with C and warfarin sodium. Compatibility is dependent upon factors such as pH, concentration, temperature and diluent used; consult specialized references or a hospital pharmacist for more specific information.

In vitro inactivation of aminoglycoside antibiotics by beta-lactam antibiotics is well documented. While amikacin is less susceptible to this effect, it is usually recommended to avoid mixing these compounds together in the same syringe or IV bag unless administration occurs promptly. See also the information in the Drug Interaction and Drug/Lab Interaction sections.

Dosage Forms/Regulatory Status

VETERINARY-LABELED PRODUCTS:

Amikacin Sulfate Injection: 50 mg (of amikacin base) per mL in 50 mL vials; *Amiglyde-V®* (Fort Dodge), generic (Teva); (Rx). FDA-approved for use in dogs.

Amikacin Sulfate Intrauterine Solution: 250 mg (of amikacin base) per mL in 48 mL vials; *Amiglyde-V®* (Fort Dodge), generic (Teva); (Rx). FDA-approved for use in horses not intended for food.

Warning: Amikacin is not FDA-approved for use in cattle or other food-producing animals in the USA. Drug residues may persist for long periods, particularly in renal tissue. For guidance with determining use and withdrawal times, contact FARAD (see Phone Numbers & Websites in the appendix for contact information).

HUMAN-LABELED PRODUCTS:

Amikacin Injection: 50 mg/mL and 250 mg/mL in 2 mL & 4 mL vials and 2 mL syringes (250 mg/mL only); *Amikin®* (Apothecon); generic; (Rx)

References

Autran de Morais, H (2009). Empiric Antibiotic Therapy. Proceedings: WSAVA.

Beech, J (1987). Respiratory Tract—Horse, Cow. *The Bristol Handbook of Antimicrobial Therapy*. DE Johnston Ed. Evansville, Veterinary Learning Systems: 88–109.

Bucki, E, S Giguere, et al. (2004). Pharmacokinetics of once–daily amikacin in healthy foals and therapeutic drug monitoring in hospitalized equine neonates. *J Vet Intern Med* 18: 728–733.

Clubb, SL (1986). Therapeutics: Individual and Flock Treatment Regimens. *Clinical Avian Medicine and Surgery*. GJ Harrison and LR Harrison Eds. Philadelphia, W.B. Saunders: 327–355.

Foreman, J (1999). Equine respiratory pharmacology. *The Veterinary Clinics of North America: Equine Practice* 15:3(December): 665–686.

Gauvin, J (1993). Drug therapy in reptiles. *Seminars in Avian & Exotic Med* 2(1): 48–59.

Geor, R & M Papich (2003). Once–daily aminoglycoside dosing regimens. *Current Therapy in Equine Medicine: 5*. N Robinson Ed., Saunders: 850–853.

Hardie, E (2000). Therapeutic Mangement of Sepsis. *Kirk's Current Veterinary Therapy: XIII Small Animal Practice*. J Bonagura Ed. Philadelphia, WB Saunders: 272–275.

Hayes, P (2000). Diseases of Chinchillas. *Kirk's Current Veterinary Therapy: XIII Small Animal Practice*. J Bonagura Ed. Philadelphia, WB Saunders: 1152–1157.

Hoeffer, H (1995). Antimicrobials in pet birds. *Kirk's Current Veterinary Therapy:XII*. J Bonagura Ed. Philadelphia, W.B. Saunders: 1278–1283.

Ivey, E & J Morrisey (2000). Therapeutics for Rabbits. *Vet Clin NA: Exotic Anim Pract* 3:1(Jan): 183–216.

Jacobson, E (2000). Antibiotic Therapy for Reptiles. *Kirk's Current Veterinary Therapy: XIII Small Animal Practice*. J Bonagura Ed. Philadelphia, WB Saunders: 1168–1169.

Jenson, J (1998). Current ratite therapy. *The Veterinary Clinics of North America: Food Animal Practice* 16:3(November).

Karpinski, LG & SL Clubb (1986). Clinical aspects of ophthalmology in caged birds. *Current Veterinary Therapy IX: Small Animal Practice*. RW Kirk Ed. Philadelphia, W.B. Saunders: 616–621.

Klaphake, E (2005). Sneezing turtles and wheezing snakes. Proceedings: Western Vet Conf. Accessed via: Veterinary Information Network. http://goo.gl/ILwoc

KuKanich, B (2008). Canine breed specific differences in clinical pharmacology. Proceedings: WVC. Accessed via: Veterinary Information Network. http://goo.gl/GCUEn

Lewbart, G (2006). Medicating the pet fish patient. Proceedings: Western Vet Conf. Accessed via: Veterinary Information Network. http://goo.gl/Ia8b3

Mader, DR, GM Conzelman, et al. (1985). Effects of ambient temperature on the half–life and dosage regimen of amikacin in the gopher snake. *JAVMA* 187(11): 1134–1136.

Magdesian, K, W Wilson, et al. (2004). Pharmacokinetics of high dose amikacin administered at extended intervals to neonatal foals. *Am J Vet Res* 65: 473–479.

Moll, H (2009). Recognition and treatment of the septic joint. Proceedings: Western Veterinary Conference. Accessed via: Veterinary Information Network. http://goo.gl/pcos3

Moore, R (1999a). How I treat septic joints in foals. Proceedings: The North American Veterinary Conference, Orlando.

Moore, R (1999b). Medical treatment of abdominal pain in the horse: Enteric treatment and motility modifiers. Proceedings: The North American Veterinary Conference, Orlando.

Morrisey, J & J Carpenter (2004). Formulary. *Ferrets, Rabbits, and Rodents Clinical Medicine and Surgery 2nd ed.* K Quesenberry and J Carpenter Eds. St Louis, Saunders.

Parra–Sanchez, A, J Lugo, et al. (2006). Pharmacokinetics and pharmacodynamics of enrofloxacin and a low dose of amikacin administered via regional intravenous limb perfusion in standing horses. *AJVR* 67(10): 1687–1695.

Perkins, N (1999). Equine reproductive pharmacology. *The Veterinary Clinics of North America: Equine Practice* 15:3(December): 687–704.

Rosskopf, WJ (1986). Shell diseases in turtles and tortoises. *Current Veterinary Therapy (CVT) IX Small Animal Practice*. RW Kirk Ed. Philadelphia, WB Saunders: 751–759.

Trepanier, L (1999). Management of resistant infections in small animal patients. Proceedings: American Veterinary Medical Association: 16th Annual Convention, New Orleans.

Upson, DW (1988). *Handbook of Clinical Veterinary Pharmacology*. Manhattan, Dan Upson Enterprises.

Williams, B (2000). Therapeutics in Ferrets. *Vet Clin NA: Exotic Anim Pract* 3:1(Jan): 131–153.

AMINOCAPROIC ACID

(a-mee-noe-ka-*proe*-ik)   Amicar®

FIBRINOLYSIS INHIBITOR/ ANTIPROTEASE

Prescriber Highlights

▶ May be useful for treating degenerative myelopathies in dogs; efficacy questionable

▶ Treatment may be very expensive, especially with large dogs

▶ Contraindicated in DIC

▶ Infrequently causes GI distress

Uses/Indications

Aminocaproic acid has been used as a treatment to degenerative myelopathy (seen primarily in German shepherds), but no controlled studies documenting its efficacy were located. One study (Polizopoulou *et al.* 2008) in 12 dogs where aminocaproic acid was used with acetylcysteine and vitamins B, C, and E, no improvement was noted with treatment and all dogs' neurological signs worsened with time. There is some interest in evaluating aminocaproic acid for adjunctive treatment of thrombocytopenia in dogs, but efficacy and safety for this purpose remains to be investigated. In humans, it is primarily used for treating hyperfibrinolysis-induced hemorrhage.

Pharmacology/Actions

Aminocaproic acid inhibits fibrinolysis via its inhibitory effects on plasminogen activator substances and via some antiplasmin action.

Aminocaproic acid is thought to affect degenerative myelopathy by its antiprotease activity thereby reducing the activation of inflammatory enzymes that damage myelin.

Pharmacokinetics

No pharmacokinetic data was located for dogs.

In a study where 70 mg/kg doses were given IV to horses over 20 minutes, the drug was distributed rapidly and plasma levels remained above the proposed therapeutic level of 130 micrograms/mL for one hour after the end of the infusion. Elimination half-life was 2.3 hours. The authors proposed that a constant rate infusion of 15 mg/kg/hr after the original infusion would maintain more prolonged therapeutic levels (Ross *et al.* 2006).

In humans, the drug is rapidly and completely absorbed after oral administration. The drug is well distributed in both intravascular and extravascular compartments and penetrates cells (including red blood cells). It is unknown if the drug enters maternal milk. It does not bind to plasma proteins. Terminal half-life is about 2 hours in humans and the drug is primarily renally excreted as unchanged drug.

Contraindications/Precautions/Warnings

Aminocaproic acid is contraindicated in patients with active intravascular clotting. It should only be used when the benefits outweigh the risks in patients with preexisting cardiac, renal or hepatic disease.

Adverse Effects

In dogs treated, about 1% exhibit clinical signs of GI irritation. It potentially can cause hyperkalemia particularly in renal impaired patients.

Reproductive/Nursing Safety

Some, but not all, animal studies have demonstrated teratogenicity; use when risk to benefit ratio merits. In humans, the FDA categorizes this drug as category *C* for use during pregnancy (*Animal studies have shown an adverse effect on the fetus, but there are no adequate studies in humans; or there are no animal reproduction studies and no adequate studies in humans.*)

Overdosage/Acute Toxicity

There is very limited information on overdoses with aminocaproic acid. The IV lethal dose in dogs is reportedly 2.3 g/kg. At lower IV overdosages, tonic-clonic seizures were noted in some dogs. There is no known antidote, but the drug is dialyzable.

Drug Interactions

The following drug interactions have either been reported or are theoretical in humans or animals receiving aminocaproic acid and may be of significance in veterinary patients:

- ■ **ESTROGENS:** Hypercoagulation states may occur in patients receiving aminocaproic acid and estrogens

Laboratory Considerations

- ■ Serum **potassium** may be elevated by aminocaproic acid, especially in patients with preexisting renal failure

Doses

- ■ **DOGS:**

  For adjunctive treatment of degenerative myelopathy (seen primarily in German shepherds):

  a) Aminocaproic acid 500 mg/dog PO q8h indefinitely. Used in conjunction with acetylcysteine at 25 mg/kg PO q8h for 2 weeks, then q8h every other day. The 20% solution should be diluted to 5% with chicken broth or suitable diluent. Other treatments may include prednisone (0.25–0.5 mg/kg PO daily for 10 days then every other day), Vitamin C (1000 mg PO q12h) and Vitamin E (1000 Int. Units PO q12). **Note:** No treatment has been shown to be effective in published trials. (Shell 2003)

  As an antifibrinolytic:

  a) No published doses for dogs, but has been used anecdotally at 50–100 mg/kg IV or PO q6h. (Hopper 2006)

Client Information

- ■ Drug costs to treat a German shepherd-sized dog can be substantial
- ■ As no well controlled studies have documented that this drug is effective for treating degenerative myelopathy, its use should be considered investigational

Chemistry/Synonyms

An inhibitor of fibrinolysis, aminocaproic acid is a synthetic monamino carboxylic acid occurring as a fine, white crystalline powder. It is slightly soluble in alcohol and freely soluble in water and has pKa's of 4.43 and 10.75. The injectable product has its pH adjusted to approximately 6.8.

Aminocaproic acid may also be known as: acidum aminocaproicum, CL-10304 CY-116, EACA, epsilon aminocaproic acid, JD-177,

NSC-26154, *Amicar®, Capracid®, Capramol®, Caproamin®, Caprolisin®, Epsicaprom®, Hemocaprol®, Hemocid®, Hexalense®,* or *Ipsilon®.*

Storage/Stability

Products should be stored at room temperature. Avoid freezing liquid preparations. Discoloration will occur if aldehydes or aldehydic sugars are present.

Compatibility/Compounding Considerations

When given as an intravenous infusion, normal saline, D_5W and Ringer's Injection have been recommended for use as the infusion diluent.

Dosage Forms/Regulatory Status

VETERINARY-LABELED PRODUCTS: None

The ARCI (Racing Commissioners International) has designated this drug as a class 4 substance. See the appendix for more information.

HUMAN-LABELED PRODUCTS:

Aminocaproic Acid Oral Tablets: 500 mg & 1000 mg; *Amicar®* (Xanodyne); generic (VersaPharm); (Rx)

Aminocaproic Oral Solution: 250 mg/mL in 237 mL & 473 mL; Aminocaproic Acid (VersaPharm); *Amicar®* (Xanodyne); generic; (Rx)

Aminocaproic Acid Injection: 250 mg/mL in 20 mL vials; generic; (Rx)

References

Hopper, K (2006). Hemostatic agents. Proceedings: IVECC. Accessed via: Veterinary Information Network. http://goo.gl/K41Jk

Polizopoulou, ZS, AF Koutinas, et al. (2008). Evaluation of a proposed therapeutic protocol in 12 dogs with tentative degenerative myelopathy. *Acta Veterinaria Hungarica* 56(3): 293–301.

Ross, J, B Dallop, et al. (2006). Pharmacokinetics and pharmacodynamics of aminocaproic acid in horses. Proceedings: IVECC. Accessed via: Veterinary Information Network. http://goo.gl/ugtjW

Shell, L (2003). "Degenerative Myelopathy (Degenerative Radiculomyelopathy)." *Associates Database.*

AMINOPENTAMIDE HYDROGEN SULFATE

(a-mee-noe-*pent*-a-mide) Centrine®
ANTICHOLINERGIC/ANTISPASMODIC

Prescriber Highlights

▶ Anticholinergic/antispasmodic for GI indications in small animals

▶ Typical adverse effect profile ("dry, hot, red"); potentially could cause tachycardia

▶ Contraindicated in glaucoma; relatively contraindicated in tachycardias, heart disease, GI obstruction, etc.

Uses/Indications

The manufacturer states that the drug is indicated "in the treatment of acute abdominal visceral spasm, pylorospasm or hypertrophic gastritis and associated nausea, vomiting and/or diarrhea" for use in dogs and cats.

Pharmacology/Actions

Aminopentamide is an anticholinergic agent that when compared to atropine has been described as having a greater effect on reducing colonic contractions and less mydriatic and salivary effects. It reportedly may also reduce gastric acid secretion.

Pharmacokinetics

No information was located.

Contraindications/Precautions/Warnings

The manufacturer lists glaucoma as an absolute contraindication to therapy and to use the drug cautiously, if at all, in patients with pyloric obstruction. Additionally, aminopentamide should not be used if the patient has a history of hypersensitivity to anticholinergic drugs, tachycardias secondary to thyrotoxicosis or cardiac insufficiency, myocardial ischemia, unstable cardiac status during acute hemorrhage, GI obstructive disease, paralytic ileus, severe ulcerative colitis, obstructive uropathy or myasthenia gravis (unless used to reverse adverse muscarinic effects secondary to therapy).

Antimuscarinic agents should be avoided or used with extreme caution in patients with known or suspected GI infections (*e.g.,* parvovirus enteritis), or with autonomic neuropathy. Atropine or other antimuscarinic agents can decrease GI motility and prolong retention of the causative agent(s) or toxin(s) resulting in prolonged clinical signs.

Antimuscarinic agents should be used with caution in patients with hepatic disease, renal disease, hyperthyroidism, hypertension, CHF, tachyarrhythmias, prostatic hypertrophy, esophageal reflux, and in geriatric or pediatric patients.

Adverse Effects

Adverse effects resulting from aminopentamide therapy may include dry mouth, dry eyes, blurred vision, and urinary hesitancy. Urinary retention is a symptom of too high a dose and the drug should be withdrawn until resolved.

Overdosage/Acute Toxicity

No specific information was located regarding acute overdosage clinical signs or treatment for this agent. The following discussion is from the Atropine monograph that could be used as a guideline for treating overdoses:

If a recent oral ingestion, emptying of gut contents and administration of activated charcoal and saline cathartics may be warranted. Treat clinical signs supportively and symptomatically. Do not use phenothiazines as they may contribute to the anticholinergic effects. Fluid therapy and standard treatments for shock may be instituted.

The use of physostigmine is controversial and should probably be reserved for cases where the patient exhibits either extreme agitation and is at risk for injuring themselves or others, or for cases where supraventricular tachycardias and sinus tachycardias are severe or life threatening. The usual dose for physostigmine (human) is: 2 mg IV slowly (for average sized adult), if no response, may repeat every 20 minutes until reversal of toxic antimuscarinic effects or cholinergic effects takes place. The human pediatric dose is 0.02 mg/kg slow IV (repeat q10 minutes as above) and may be a reasonable choice for treatment of small animals. Physostigmine adverse effects (bronchoconstriction, bradycardia, seizures) may be treated with small doses of IV atropine.

Drug Interactions

No specific interactions were noted for this product. The following drug interactions have either been reported or are theoretical in humans or animals receiving atropine, a similar drug and may be of significance in veterinary patients:

- ◼ **ANTIHISTAMINES, PROCAINAMIDE, QUINIDINE, MEPERIDINE, BENZODIAZEPINES, PHENOTHIAZINES:** May enhance the activity of atropine and its derivatives

- ◼ **PRIMIDONE, DISOPYRAMIDE, NITRATES:** May potentiate the adverse effects of atropine and its derivatives

- ◼ **CORTICOSTEROIDS (long-term use):** May increase intraocular pressure

- ◼ **NITROFURANTOIN, THIAZIDE DIURETICS, SYMPATHOMIMETICS:** Atropine and its derivatives may enhance actions

- ◼ **METOCLOPRAMIDE:** Atropine and its derivatives may antagonize metoclopramide actions

Doses

- ◼ **DOGS:**
  a) May be administered every 8–12 hours via IM, SC or oral routes. If the desired effect is not attained, the dosage may be gradually increased up to 5 times those listed below: Animals weighing: 10 lbs or less: 0.1 mg; 11–20 lbs: 0.2 mg; 21–50 lbs: 0.3 mg; 51–100 lbs: 0.4 mg; over 100 lbs: 0.5 mg (Package Insert; *Centrine®*—Fort Dodge)

  b) To decrease tenesmus in malabsorption/maldigestion syndromes: 0.1–0.4 mg (total dose) SC, or IM twice daily–three times daily (Chiapella 1989)

- ◼ **CATS:**
  a) As in "a" above in dogs

  b) As second-line adjunctive therapy for refractory IBD: 0.1–0.4 mg/kg SC two to three times daily (Washabau 2000)

Monitoring

- ◼ Clinical efficacy
- ◼ Adverse effects (see above)

Client Information

- ◼ Contact veterinarian if animal has difficulty urinating or if animal is bothered by dry eyes or mouth

Chemistry/Synonyms

An antispasmodic, anticholinergic agent, aminopentamide hydrogen sulfate has a chemical name of 4-(dimethylamino)-2,2-diphenylvaleramide.

Aminopentamide hydrogen sulfate may also be known as dimevamid or *Centrine®*.

Storage/Stability

Store aminopentamide tablets and injection at controlled room temperature (15–30°C; 59–86°F).

Dosage Forms/Regulatory Status

VETERINARY-LABELED PRODUCTS:

Aminopentamide Hydrogen Sulfate Tablets: 0.2 mg; *Centrine®* (Pfizer); (Rx). FDA-approved for use in dogs and cats only.

Aminopentamide Hydrogen Sulfate Injection: 0.5 mg/mL in 10 mL vials; *Centrine®* (Pfizer); (Rx). FDA-approved for use in dogs and cats only.

HUMAN-LABELED PRODUCTS: None

References

Chiapella, AM (1989). Diseases of the Small Intestine. *Handbook of Small Animal Practice*. RV Morgan Ed. New York, Churchill Livingstone: 395–420.

Washabau, R (2000). Intestinal Diseases/IBD. Proceedings: American Association of Feline Practitioners.

AMINOPHYLLINE
THEOPHYLLINE

(am-in-*off*-i-lin); (thee-*off*-i-lin)

PHOSPHODIESTERASE INHIBITOR BRONCHODILATOR

Prescriber Highlights

- ▶ Bronchodilator drug with diuretic activity; used for bronchospasm & cardiogenic pulmonary edema

- ▶ Narrow therapeutic index in humans, but dogs appear to be less susceptible to toxic effects at higher plasma levels

- ▶ Therapeutic drug monitoring recommended

- ▶ Many drug interactions

Uses/Indications

The theophyllines are used primarily for their bronchodilatory effects, often in patients with myocardial failure and/or pulmonary edema. While they are still routinely used, the methylxanthines must be used cautiously due to their adverse effects and toxicity.

Pharmacology/Actions

The theophyllines competitively inhibit phosphodiesterase thereby increasing amounts of cyclic AMP that then increase the release of endogenous epinephrine. The elevated levels of cAMP may also inhibit the release of histamine and slow reacting substance of anaphylaxis (SRS-A). The myocardial and neuromuscular transmission effects that the theophyllines possess may be a result of translocating intracellular ionized calcium.

The theophyllines directly relax smooth muscles in the bronchi and pulmonary vasculature, induce diuresis, increase gastric acid secretion and inhibit uterine contractions. They have weak chronotropic and inotropic action, stimulate the CNS and can cause respiratory stimulation (centrally-mediated).

Pharmacokinetics

The pharmacokinetics of theophylline have been studied in several domestic species. After oral administration, the rate of absorption of the theophyllines is limited primarily by the dissolution of the dosage form in the gut. In studies in cats, dogs, and horses, bioavailabilities after oral administration are nearly 100% when non-sustained release products are used. One study in dogs that compared various sustained-release products (Koritz, Neff-Davis, and Munsiff 1986), found bioavailabilities ranging from approximately 30–76% depending on the product used.

Theophylline is distributed throughout the extracellular fluids and body tissues. It crosses the placenta and is distributed into milk (70% of serum levels). In dogs, at therapeutic serum levels only about 7–14% is bound to plasma proteins. The volume of distribution of theophylline for dogs has been reported to be 0.82 L/kg. The volume of distribution in cats is reported to be 0.46 L/kg, and in horses, 0.85–1.02 L/kg. Because of the low volumes of distribution and theophylline's low lipid solubility, obese patients should be dosed on a lean body weight basis.

Theophylline is metabolized primarily in the liver (in humans) to 3-methylxanthine which has weak bronchodilitory activity. Renal clearance contributes only about 10% to the overall plasma clearance of theophylline. The reported elimination half-lives (mean values) in various species are: dogs ≈ 5.7 hours; cats ≈ 7.8 hours, pigs ≈ 11 hours; and horses ≈ 11.9 to 17 hours. In humans, there are very wide interpatient variations in serum half-lives and resultant serum levels. It could be expected that similar variability exists in veterinary patients, particularly those with concurrent illnesses.

Contraindications/Precautions/Warnings

The theophyllines are contraindicated in patients who are hypersensitive to any of the xanthines, including theobromine or caffeine. Patients who are hypersensitive to ethylenediamine should not take aminophylline.

The theophyllines should be administered with caution in patients with severe cardiac disease, seizure disorders, gastric ulcers, hyperthy-roidism, renal or hepatic disease, severe hypoxia, or severe hypertension. Because it may cause or worsen preexisting arrhythmias, patients with cardiac arrhythmias should receive theophylline only with caution and enhanced monitoring. Neonatal and geriatric patients may have decreased clearances of theophylline and be more sensitive to its toxic effects. Patients with CHF may have prolonged serum half-lives of theophylline.

Adverse Effects

The theophyllines can produce CNS stimulation and gastrointestinal irritation after administration by any route. Most adverse effects are related to the serum level of the drug and may be symptomatic of toxic blood levels; dogs appear to tolerate levels that may be very toxic to humans. Some mild CNS excitement and GI disturbances are not uncommon when starting therapy and generally resolve with chronic administration in conjunction with monitoring and dosage adjustments.

Dogs and cats can exhibit clinical signs of nausea and vomiting, anorexia, increased gastric acid secretion, diarrhea, polyphagia, polydipsia, and polyuria. Side effects in horses are generally dose related and may include: nervousness, excitability (auditory, tactile, and visual), tremors, diaphoresis, tachycardia, and ataxia. Seizures or cardiac dysrhythmias may occur in severe intoxications.

Reproductive/Nursing Safety

In humans, the FDA categorizes this drug as category *C* for use during pregnancy (*Animal studies have shown an adverse effect on the fetus, but there are no adequate studies in humans; or there are no animal reproduction studies and no adequate studies in humans.*)

Overdosage/Acute Toxicity

Clinical signs of toxicity (see above) are usually associated with levels greater than 20 micrograms/mL in humans and become more severe as the serum level exceeds that value. Tachycardias, arrhythmias, and CNS effects (seizures, hyperthermia) are considered the most life-threatening aspects of toxicity. Dogs appear to tolerate serum levels higher than 20 micrograms/mL.

Treatment of theophylline toxicity is supportive. After an oral ingestion, the gut should be emptied, charcoal and a cathartic administered using the standardized methods and cautions associated with these practices. Patients suffering from seizures should have an adequate airway maintained and treated with IV diazepam. The patient should be constantly monitored for cardiac arrhythmias and tachycardia. Fluid and electrolytes should be monitored and corrected as necessary. Hyperthermia may be treated with phenothiazines and tachycardia treated with propranolol if either condition is considered life threatening.

Drug Interactions

The following drug interactions have either been reported or are theoretical in humans or animals receiving aminophylline or theophylline and may be of significance in veterinary patients:

The following drugs can *decrease* theophylline levels:

- **BARBITURATES (phenobarbital)**
- **CARBAMAZEPINE** (may increase or decrease levels)
- **CHARCOAL**
- **HYDANTOINS (phenytoin)**
- **ISONIAZID** (may increase or decrease levels)
- **KETOCONAZOLE**
- **LOOP DIURETICS (furosemide)**; (may increase or decrease levels)
- **RIFAMPIN**
- **SYMPATHOMIMETICS (beta-agonists)**

The following drugs can *increase* theophylline levels:

- **ALLOPURINOL**
- **BETA-BLOCKERS (non-selective such as propranolol)**
- **CALCIUM CHANNEL BLOCKERS (e.g., diltiazem, verapamil)**
- **CIMETIDINE**
- **CORTICOSTEROIDS**
- **FLUOROQUINOLONES (enrofloxacin, ciprofloxacin):** If adding either, consider reducing the dose of theophylline by 30%. Monitor for toxicity/efficacy. Marbofloxacin reduces clearance of theophylline in dogs, but not with clinical significance. In animals with renal impairment, marbofloxacin may interfere with theophylline metabolism in a clinically relevant manner.
- **MACROLIDES (e.g., erythromycin; clindamycin, lincomycin)**
- **THIABENDAZOLE**
- **THYROID HORMONES** (in hypothyroid patients)

Theophylline may decrease the effects of following drugs:

- **BENZODIAZEPINES**
- **LITHIUM**
- **PANCURONIUM**
- **PROPOFOL**
- **EPHEDRINE, ISOPROTERENOL:** Toxic synergism (arrhythmias) can occur if theophylline is used concurrently with sympathomimetics (especially ephedrine) or possibly isoproterenol
- **HALOTHANE:** Theophylline with halothane may cause increased incidence of cardiac dysrhythmias
- **KETAMINE:** Theophylline with ketamine can cause an increased incidence of seizures

Laboratory Considerations

- Theophylline can cause falsely elevated values of serum **uric acid** if measured by the Bittner or colorimetric methods. Values are not affected if using the uricase method.
- Theophylline serum levels can be falsely elevated by **furosemide, phenylbutazone, probenecid, theobromine, caffeine, sulfathiazole, chocolate, or acetaminophen** if using a spectrophotometric method of assay.

Doses

Note: Theophyllines have a relatively low therapeutic index; determine dosage carefully. Because of aminophylline/theophylline's pharmacokinetic characteristics, it should be dosed on a lean body weight basis in obese patients. Dosage conversions between aminophylline and theophylline can be easily performed using the information found in the Chemistry section below. Aminophylline causes intense local pain when administered IM and is rarely used or recommended via this route.

- **DOGS:**

a) Using *Theochron®* Extended-Release Tablets *or Theo-Cap®* Extended-Release Capsules: Give 10 mg/kg PO every 12 hours initially, if no adverse effects are observed and the desired clinical effect is not achieved, give 15 mg/kg PO q12h while monitoring for adverse effects. (Bach *et al.* 2004)

b) For adjunctive medical therapy for mild clinical signs associated with tracheal collapse (<50% collapse): aminophylline: 11 mg/kg PO, IM or IV three times daily. (Fossum 2005)

c) For adjunctive therapy of severe, acute pulmonary edema and bronchoconstriction: Aminophylline 4–8 mg/kg IV or IM, or 6–10 mg/kg PO every 8 hours. Long-term use is not recommended. (Ware 2003)

d) For cough: Aminophylline: 10 mg/kg PO, IV three times daily (Anderson-Westberg 2005)

e) As a bronchodilator for collapsing trachea: 11 mg/kg PO or IV q6–12h (Ettinger & Kantrowitz 2005)

- **CATS:**

a) Using *Theo-Dur®*: 20 mg/kg PO once daily in the PM; using *Slo-Bid®*: 25 mg/kg PO once daily in the PM (Johnson 2000) [**Note:** The products *Theo-Dur®* and *Slo-Bid®* mentioned in this reference are no longer available in the USA. Although hard data is not presently available to support their use in cats, a reasonable alternative would be to cautiously use the dog dose and products mentioned above in the reference by Bach et al—Plumb]

b) Using aminophylline tablets: 6.6. mg/kg PO twice daily; using sustained release tablets (*Theo-Dur®*): 25–50 mg (total dose) per cat PO in the evening (Noone 1999)

c) For adjunctive medical therapy for mild clinical signs associated with tracheal collapse (<50% collapse): aminophylline: 5 mg/kg PO, two times daily. (Fossom 2005)

d) For adjunctive therapy for bronchoconstriction associated with fulminant CHF: Aminophylline 4–8 mg/kg SC, IM, IV q8–12h. (Ware 2003)

e) For cough: Aminophylline: 5 mg/kg PO twice daily (Anderson-Westberg 2005)

■ **FERRETS:**

a) 4.25 mg/kg PO 2–3 times a day (Williams 2000)

■ **HORSES: (Note:** ARCI UCGFS Class 3 Drug) **Note:** Intravenous aminophylline should be diluted in at least 100 mL of D_5W or normal saline and administered slowly (not >25 mg/min).

For adjunctive treatment of pulmonary edema:

a) Aminophylline 2–7 mg/kg IV q6–12h; Theophylline 5–15 mg/kg PO q12h (Mogg 1999)

b) 11 mg/kg PO or IV q8–12h. To "load" may either double the initial dose or give both the oral and IV dose at the same time. IV infusion should be in approximately 1 liter of IV fluids and given over 20–60 minutes. Recommend monitoring serum levels. (Foreman 1999)

For adjunctive treatment for heaves (RAO):

a) Aminophylline: 5–10 mg/kg PO or IV twice daily. (Lavoie 2003)

b) Aminophylline: 4–6 mg/kg PO three times a day. (Ainsworth & Hackett 2004)

Monitoring

■ Therapeutic efficacy and clinical signs of toxicity

■ Serum levels at steady state. The therapeutic serum levels of theophylline in humans are generally described to be between 10–20 micrograms/mL. In small animals, one recommendation for monitoring serum levels is to measure trough concentration; level should be at least above 8–10 micrograms/mL (**Note:** Some recommend not exceeding 15 micrograms/mL in horses).

Client Information

■ Give dosage as prescribed by veterinarian to maximize the drug's benefit

Chemistry/Synonyms

Xanthine derivatives, aminophylline and theophylline are considered to be respiratory smooth muscle relaxants but, they also have other pharmacologic actions. Aminophylline differs from theophylline only by the addition of ethylenediamine to its structure and may have different amounts of molecules of water of hydration. 100 mg of aminophylline (hydrous) contains approximately 79 mg of theophylline (anhydrous);100 mg of aminophylline (anhydrous) contains approximately 86 mg theophylline (anhydrous). Conversely, 100 mg of theophylline (anhydrous) is equivalent to 116 mg of aminophylline (anhydrous) and 127 mg aminophylline (hydrous).

Aminophylline occurs as bitter-tasting, white or slightly yellow granules or powder with a slight ammoniacal odor and a pK_a of 5. Aminophylline is soluble in water and insoluble in alcohol.

Theophylline occurs as bitter-tasting, odorless, white, crystalline powder with a melting point between 270–274°C. It is sparingly soluble in alcohol and only slightly soluble in water at a pH of 7, but solubility increases with increasing pH.

Aminophylline may also be known as: aminofilina, aminophyllinum, euphyllinum, metaphyllin, theophyllaminum, theophylline and ethylenediamine, theophylline ethylenediamine compound, or theophyllinum ethylenediaminum; many trade names are available.

Theophylline may also be known as: anhydrous theophylline, teofillina, or theophyllinum; many trade names are available.

Storage/Stability

Unless otherwise specified by the manufacturer, store aminophylline and theophylline oral products in tight, light-resistant containers at room temperature. Do not crush or split sustained-release oral products unless label states it is permissible.

Aminophylline for injection should be stored in single-use containers in which carbon dioxide has been removed. It should also be stored at temperatures below 30°C and protected from freezing and light. Upon exposure to air (carbon dioxide), aminophylline will absorb carbon dioxide, lose ethylenediamine and liberate free theophylline that can precipitate out of solution. Do not inject aminophylline solutions that contain either a precipitate or visible crystals.

Compatibility/Compounding Considerations

Aminophylline for injection is reportedly **compatible** when mixed with all commonly used IV solutions, but may be **incompatible** with 10% fructose or invert sugar solutions.

Aminophylline is reportedly **compatible** when mixed with the following drugs: amobarbital sodium, bretylium tosylate, calcium gluconate, chloramphenicol sodium succinate, dexamethasone sodium phosphate, dopamine HCl, erythromycin lactobionate, heparin sodium, hydrocortisone sodium succinate, lidocaine HCl, mephentermine sulfate, methicillin sodium, methyldopa HCl, metronidazole with sodium bicarbonate, pentobarbital sodium, phenobarbital sodium, potassium chloride, secobarbital sodium, sodium bicarbonate, sodium iodide, terbutaline sulfate, thiopental sodium, and verapamil HCl.

Aminophylline is reportedly **incompatible** (or data conflicts) with the following drugs: amikacin sulfate, ascorbic acid injection, bleomycin sulfate, cephalothin sodium, cephapirin sodium, clindamycin phosphate, codeine phosphate, corticotropin, dimenhydrinate, dobutamine HCl, doxorubicin HCl, epinephrine HCl, erythromycin glucepate, hydralazine HCl, hydroxyzine HCl, insulin (regular), isoproterenol HCl, levorphanol bitartrate, meperidine HCl, methadone HCl, methylprednisolone sodium succinate, morphine sulfate, nafcillin sodium, norepinephrine bitartrate, oxytetracycline, penicillin G potassium, pentazocine lactate, procaine HCl, prochlorperazine edisylate or mesylate, promazine HCl, promethazine HCl, sulfisoxazole diolamine, tetracycline HCl, vancomycin HCl, and vitamin B complex with C. Compatibility is dependent upon factors such as pH, concentration, temperature, and diluent used and it is suggested to consult specialized references for more specific information.

Compounded preparation stability: Aminophylline oral suspension compounded from commercially available injectable solution has been published (Chong *et al.* 2000). Diluting 40 mL of aminophylline 25 mg/ml injection with 2.7 mL of *Ora-Plus®* and *qs ad* to 45.4 mL with *Ora-Sweet®* yields a 22 mg/mL oral suspension that retains >90% potency for 91 days stored at 25°C. Compounded preparations of aminophylline should be protected from light and should not be refrigerated due to development of crystalline precipitation and >20% loss of potency after 7 days.

Dosage Forms/Regulatory Status

VETERINARY-LABELED PRODUCTS: None
The ARCI (Racing Commissioners International) has designated this drug as a class 3 substance. See the appendix for more information.

HUMAN-LABELED PRODUCTS:
The listing below is a sampling of products and sizes available; consult specialized references for a more complete listing.

Aminophylline Tablets: 100 mg (79 mg theophylline) & 200 mg (158 mg theophylline); generic; (Rx)

Aminophylline Injection: 250 mg (equiv. to 197 mg theophylline) mL in 10 mL & 20 mL vials, amps and syringes; generic; (Rx)

Theophylline Time Released Capsules and Tablets: 100 mg, 125 mg 200 mg, 300 mg, 400 mg, 450 mg, & 600 mg. (**Note:** Different products have different claimed release rates which may or may not correspond to actual times in veterinary patients; Theophylline Extended-Release (Dey); *Theo-24®* (UCB Pharma); *Theophylline SR* (various); *Theochron®* (Forest, various); Theophylline (Able); *Theocron®* (Inwood); *Uniphyl®* (Purdue Frederick); generic; (Rx)

Theophylline Tablets and Capsules: 100 mg, 200 mg, & 300 mg; *Bronkodyl®* (Winthrop); *Elixophyllin®* (Forest); generic; (Rx)

Theophylline Elixir: 80 mg/15 mL (26.7 mg/5 mL) in pt, gal, UD 15 mL and 30 mL, *Asmalix®* (Century); *Elixophyllin®* (Forest); *Lanophyllin®* (Lannett); generic; (Rx)

Theophylline & Dextrose Injection: 200 mg/container in 50 mL (4 mg/mL) & 100 mL (2 mg/mL); 400 mg/container in 100 mL (4 mg/mL), 250 mL (1.6 mg/mL), 500 mL (0.8 mg/mL) & 1000 mL (0.4 mg/mL); 800 mg/container in 250 mL (3.2 mg/mL), 500 mL (1.6 mg/mL) & 1000 mL (0.8 mg/mL); Theophylline & 5% Dextrose (Abbott & Baxter); (Rx)

References

Ainsworth, D & R Hackett (2004). Disorders of the Respiratory System. *Equine Internal Medicine 2nd Ed.* M Reed, W Bayly and D Sellon Eds. Phila., Saunders: 289–354.

Anderson–Westberg, K (2005). Coughing. *Textbook of Veterinary Internal Medicine, 6th Ed.* S Ettinger and E Feldman Eds., Elsevier: 189–192.

Bach, J, B KuKanich, et al. (2004). Evaluation of the bioavailability and pharmacokinetics of two extended–release theophylline formulations in dogs. *JAVMA* 224: 1113–1119.

Chong, E, R Dumont, et al. (2000). Stability of aminophylline in extemporaneously prepared oral suspensions. *J Informed Pharmacother.* 2: 100–106.

Ettinger, S & B Kantrowitz (2005). Diseases of the trachea. *Textbook of Veterinary Internal Medicine, 6th Ed.* SJ Ettinger and E Feldman Eds. Philadelphia, Elsevier: 1217–1232.

Foreman, J (1999). Equine respiratory pharmacology. *The Veterinary Clinics of North America: Equine Practice* 15:3(December): 665–686.

Fossom, T (2005). Tracheal collapse: managing those difficult cases. Proceedings: ACVC. Accessed via: Veterinary Information Network. http://goo.gl/AxFfH

Johnson, L (2000). Diseases of the Bronchus. *Textbook of Veterinary Internal Medicine: Diseases of the Dog and Cat.* S Ettinger and E Feldman Eds. Philadelphia, WB Saunders. 2: 1055–1061.

Lavoie, J–P (2003). Heaves (recurrent airway obstruction): practical management of acute episodes and prevention of exacerbations. *Current Therapy in Equine Medicine 5.* N Robinson Ed., Saunders: 417–421.

Ware, W (2003). Cardiovascular system disorders. *Small Animal Internal Medicine, 3rd Ed.* R Nelson and C Couto Eds. St Louis, Mosby: 1–209.

Williams, B (2000). Therapeutics in Ferrets. *Vet Clin NA: Exotic Anim Pract* 3:1(Jan): 131–153.

AMIODARONE HCL

(a-mee-oh-*da*-rone) Cordarone®, Pacerone®

CLASS III ANTIARRHYTHMIC

Prescriber Highlights

▶ Antidysrhythmic agent that can be used in dogs for arrhythmias associated with left ventricular dysfunction or to convert atrial fib into sinus rhythm; very limited experience warrants cautious use

▶ May be useful in horses to convert atrial fib or V tach into sinus rhythm

▶ Contraindicated in 2nd, 3rd degree heart block, bradyarrhythmias

▶ In *Dogs*: GI disturbances (vomiting, anorexia) most likely adverse effect, but corneal deposits, neutropenia, thrombocytopenia, bradycardia, hepatotoxicity, positive Coombs' test reported

▶ In *Horses*: Limited use, accurate adverse effect profile to be determined; Hind limb weakness, increased bilirubin reported when used IV to convert atrial fib

▶ Many drug interactions

Uses/Indications

Because of its potential toxicity and lack of experience with use in canine and equine patients, amiodarone is usually used when other less toxic or commonly used drugs are ineffective. It may be useful in dogs and horses to convert atrial fib into sinus rhythm and in dogs for arrhythmias associated with left ventricular dysfunction. In horses, one horse with ventricular tachycardia was converted into sinus rhythm using amiodarone.

As the risk of sudden death is high in Doberman pinschers exhibiting rapid, wide-complex ventricular tachycardia or syncope with recurrent VPC's, amiodarone may be useful when other drug therapies are ineffective.

Pharmacology/Actions

Amiodarone's mechanism of action is not fully understood; it apparently is a potassium channel blocker that possesses unique pharmacology from other antiarrhythmic agents. It can be best classified a Class III antiarrhythmic agent that also blocks sodium and calcium channels, and beta-adrenergic receptors. Major properties include prolongation of myocardial cell action-potential duration and refractory period.

Pharmacokinetics

Amiodarone may be administered parenterally or orally. Amiodarone is widely distributed throughout the body and can accumulate in adipose tissue. Amiodarone is metabolized by the liver into the active metabolite desethylamiodarone. After oral administration of a single dose in normal dogs, amiodarone's plasma half-life averaged 7.5 hours, but repeated dosing increased its half-life from 11 hours to 3.2 days.

In horses, amiodarone has a low oral bioavailability (range from 6–34%) and peak levels of amiodarone and desethylamiodarone occur about 7–8 hours after an oral dose. After IV administration amiodarone is rapidly distributed with a high apparent volume of distribution of 31 L/kg. In horses, amiodarone is relatively highly bound to plasma proteins (96%). Clearance was 0.35 L/kg/hr and median elimination half-lives for amiodarone and desethylamiodarone were approximately 51 and 75 hours, respectively (De Clercq, Baert *et al.* 2006).

In humans, oral absorption is slow and variable, with bioavailabilities ranging from 22–86%. Elimination half-lives for amiodarone and desethylamiodarone range from 2.5–10 days after a single dose, but with chronic dosing, average 53 days and 60 days, respectively.

Contraindications/Precautions/Warnings

Amiodarone is considered contraindicated in patients (humans) hypersensitive to it, having severe sinus-node dysfunction with severe sinus bradycardia, 2nd or 3rd degree heart block, or bradycardial syncope.

Clinical experience in veterinary patients is limited. Consider use only when other less toxic and more commonly used drugs are ineffective.

Adverse Effects

Gastrointestinal effects (*e.g.*, anorexia, vomiting) are apparently the most likely adverse effects seen in the limited number of canine patients treated. Hepatopathy (bilirubinemia, increased hepatic enzymes) has been reported in dogs on amiodarone. Because hepatic effects can occur before clinical signs are noted, routine serial evaluation of liver enzymes and bilirubin is recommended. Other adverse effects reported in dogs include bradycardia, neutropenia, thrombocytopenia, or positive Coombs' test. During IV infusion, pain at injection site, and facial pruritus and hyperemia have been noted. Corneal deposits may be seen in dogs treated with amiodarone, but this affect apparently occurs less frequently in dogs than in humans.

Horses treated with IV amiodarone for 36 hours or longer have developed short-term hind limb weakness and diarrhea.

In human patients, adverse effects are very common while on amiodarone therapy. Those that most commonly cause discontinuation of the drug include: pulmonary infiltrates or pulmonary fibrosis (sometimes fatal), liver enzyme elevations, congestive heart failure, paroxysmal ventricular tachycardia, and thyroid dysfunction (hypo- or hyperthyroidism). An odd effect seen in some individuals is a bluish cast to their skin. Reversible corneal deposits are seen in a majority of humans treated with amiodarone.

Clinical experience in dogs is limited; the adverse effect profile of this drug in people warrants its use in veterinary patients only when other less toxic agents are ineffective and treatment is deemed necessary.

Reproductive/Nursing Safety
In laboratory animals, amiodarone has been embryotoxic at high doses and congenital thyroid abnormalities have been detected in offspring. Use during pregnancy only when the potential benefits outweigh the risks of the drug. In humans, the FDA categorizes this drug as category *D* for use during pregnancy (*There is evidence of human fetal risk, but the potential benefits from the use of the drug in pregnant women may be acceptable despite its potential risks.*)

Overdosage/Acute Toxicity
Clinical overdosage experience is limited; most likely adverse effects seen are hypotension, bradycardia, cardiogenic shock, AV block, and hepatotoxicity. Treatment is supportive. Bradycardia may be managed with a pacemaker or beta-1 agonists (*e.g.*, isoproterenol); hypotension managed with positive inotropic agents or vasopressors. Neither amiodarone nor its active metabolite are dialyzable.

Drug Interactions
Several potentially significant interactions may occur with amiodarone. The following is a partial list of interactions that have either been reported or are theoretical in humans or animals receiving amiodarone and may be of significance in veterinary patients:

Amiodarone may significantly **increase** the serum levels and/or pharmacologic or toxic effects of:

■ **ANTICOAGULANTS (warfarin)**

■ **DIGOXIN**

■ **CYCLOSPORINE**

■ **LIDOCAINE**

■ **METHOTREXATE (with prolonged amiodarone administration)**

■ **PHENYTOIN**

■ **PROCAINAMIDE**

■ **QUINIDINE**

Amiodarone may have **additive effects on QTc interval**; possible serious arrhythmias may result:

■ **AZOLE ANTIFUNGALS (ketoconazole, itraconazole, etc.)**

■ **CISAPRIDE**

■ **DISOPYRAMIDE**

■ **DOLASETRON**

■ **FLUOROQUINOLONE ANTIBIOTICS (some, such as moxifloxacin, not enrofloxacin, marbofloxacin, etc.)**

■ **MACROLIDE ANTIBIOTICS (e.g., erythromycin)**

■ **ONDANSETRON**

Other amiodarone drug interactions:

■ **ANESTHETICS, GENERAL:** Increased risks for hypotension or arrhythmias

■ **BETA-ADRENERGIC BLOCKERS:** Possible potentiation of bradycardia, AV block or sinus arrest

■ **CALCIUM-CHANNEL BLOCKERS (e.g., diltiazem, verapamil):** Possible potentiation of bradycardia, AV block or sinus arrest

■ **CIMETIDINE:** Increased amiodarone levels

■ **CYCLOSPORINE:** Increased cyclosporine levels; may increase creatinine

■ **FENTANYL:** Possible hypotension, bradycardia

■ **RIFAMPIN:** Decreased amiodarone levels

Laboratory Considerations
■ While most human patients remain euthyroid while receiving amiodarone, it may cause an increase in **serum T_4** and serum reverse T_3 levels, and a reduction in **serum T_3** levels

■ The human therapeutic serum concentrations of 1–2.5 micrograms/mL are believed to apply to dogs as well

■ Amiodarone may cause a **positive Coombs'** test result

Doses
Note: Some human references state that because of the potential for drug interactions with previous drug therapies, the life-threatening nature of the arrhythmias being treated, and the unpredictability of response from amiodarone, the drug should be initially given (loaded) over several days in an inpatient setting where adequate monitoring can occur.

■ **DOGS:**

a) For atrial fibrillation or ventricular arrhythmias primarily in ambulatory patients: 8–10 mg/kg PO every 12 hours. Use caution if patient has bradycardia, AV blocks, or thyroid disorders. (Mucha 2009)

b) For ventricular arrhythmias secondary to occult cardiomyopathy in Doberman pinschers: 10 mg/kg PO twice daily for one week and then 8 mg/kg PO once daily. After 6 months reduce to 5 mg/kg PO once daily. For severe V-Tach, mexiletine is added at 5–8 mg/kg three times daily for one week. Once efficacy confirmed, patient weaned off mexiletine. (Meurs 2005)

c) For ventricular tachycardia when other first line drugs (Class I antiarrhythmics ± beta-blockers) are ineffective: 10 mg/kg PO q12h for one week and then 5 mg/kg PO q12h for maintenance. (Smith 2009)

d) For SVTs or Vtach: 10–20 mg/kg PO

once daily (q24h) loading for 5-7 days; 5–10 mg/kg PO once daily thereafter. (Saunders, A. et al. 2006), (Saunders, A.B. 2008)

■ **HORSES:**

For conversion of atrial fibrillation or ventricular tachycardia:

a) 5 mg/kg/hr for one hour, followed by 0.83 mg/kg/hr for 23 hours and then 1.9 mg/kg/hour for the following 30 hours. In the study (A fib), infusion was discontinued when conversion occurred or when any side effects were noted. 4 of 6 horses converted from A fib; one horse from V tach. In order to increase success rate and decrease adverse effects, regimen should be further adapted based upon PK/PD studies in horses. (De Clercq, van Loon et al. 2006a), (De Clercq, van Loon et al. 2006b)

Monitoring

■ Efficacy (ECG)

■ Toxicity (GI effects; CBC, serial liver enzymes; thyroid function tests; blood pressure; pulmonary radiographs if clinical signs such as dyspnea/cough occur)

Client Information

■ Because relatively few canine/equine patients have received this agent and the drug's potential for toxicity, clients should give informed consent before the drug is prescribed or administered.

Chemistry/Synonyms

An iodinated benzofuran, amiodarone is unique structurally and pharmacologically from other antiarrhythmic agents. It occurs as a white to cream colored lipophilic powder having a pKa of approximately 6.6. Amiodarone 200 mg tablets each contain approximately 75 mg of iodine.

Amiodarone HCl may also be known as: amiodaroni hydrochloridum, L-3428, 51087N, or SKF-33134-A; many trade names are available.

Storage/Stability

Tablets should be stored in tight containers, at room temperature and protected from light. A 3-year expiration date is assigned from the date of manufacture.

Injection should be stored at room temperature and protected from light or excessive heat. While administering, light protection is not necessary.

Compatibility/Compounding Considerations

Use D5W as the IV diluent. Amiodarone is reportedly compatible with dobutamine, lidocaine, potassium chloride, procainamide, propafenone, and verapamil. Variable compatibility is reported with furosemide and quinidine gluconate.

Compounded preparation stability: Amiodarone oral suspension compounded from commercially available tablets has been published (Nahata, 1997). Triturating one (1) tablet of amiodarone 200 mg with 20 mL of *Ora-Plus®* and *qs ad* to 40 mL with *Ora-Sweet®* (or *Ora-Sweet®SF*) yields a 5 mg/mL oral suspension that retains >90% potency for 91 days stored at 5°C. Compounded preparations of amiodarone should be protected from light. Amiodarone suspensions may be stored at room temperature during short periods (such as travel).

Dosage Forms/Regulatory Status

VETERINARY-LABELED PRODUCTS: None

The ARCI (Racing Commissioners International) has designated this drug as a class 4 substance. See the appendix for more information.

HUMAN-LABELED PRODUCTS:

Amiodarone Oral Tablets: 100 mg, 200 mg & 400 mg; *Cordarone®* (Wyeth-Ayerst); *Pacerone®* (Upsher Smith); generic; (Rx)

Amiodarone Injection Solution: 50 mg/mL in 3 mL, 10 mL & 30 mL single-dose vials, 18 mL multiple-dose vials & 3 mL prefilled syringes; *Nexterone®* (Prism); generic; (Rx)

References

De Clercq, D, K Baert, et al. (2006). Evaluation of the pharmacokinetics and bioavailability of intravenously and orally administered amiodarone in horses. *Am J Vet Res* 67(3): 448–454.

De Clercq, D, G van Loon, et al. (2006a). Intravenous amiodarone treatment in horses with chronic atrial fibrillation. *Vet J* 172(1): 129–134.

De Clercq, D, G van Loon, et al. (2006b). Treatment with amiodarone of refractory ventricular tachycardia in a horse. *J Vet Intern Med* 21(4): 878–880.

Meurs, K (2005). Primary Myocardial Disease in the Dog. *Textbook of Veterinary Internal Medicine, 6th Ed.* S Ettinger and E Feldman Eds., Elsevier: 1077–1082.

Mucha, C (2009). Therapeutics in Heart Disease. Proceedings: WSAVA. Accessed via: Veterinary Information Network. http://goo.gl/ca6mX

Nahata, M.C. (1997). Stability of amiodarone in an oral suspension stored under refrigeration and at room temperature. *Ann Pharmacother* 31(7-8): 851–852.

Saunders, A, M Miller, et al. (2006). Oral amiodarone therapy in dogs with atrial fibrillation. *J Vet Intern Med* 20: 921–926.

Saunders, AB (2008). Current Antiarrhythmic Therapy. Proceedings: Western Veterinary Conference. Accessed via: Veterinary Information Network. http://goo.gl/8DTWt

Smith, F (2009). Update on Antiarrhythmic Therapy. Proceedings: Western Veterinary Conference. Accessed via: Veterinary Information Network. http://goo.gl/aiVDJ

Amitraz—See the Topical Dermatologic Agents section in the appendix

AMITRIPTYLINE HCL

(a-mih-*trip*-ti-leen)   Elavil®

TRICYCLIC BEHAVIOR MODIFIER;
ANTIPRURITIC; NEUROPATHIC PAIN
MODIFIER

Prescriber Highlights

▶ Tricyclic "antidepressant" used primarily for behavior disorders & neuropathic pain/pruritus in small animals

▶ May reduce seizure thresholds in epileptic animals

▶ Sedation & anticholinergic effects most likely adverse effects

▶ Overdoses can be very serious in both animals & humans

Uses/Indications

Amitriptyline has been used for behavioral conditions such as separation anxiety or generalized anxiety in dogs, and excessive grooming, spraying and anxiety in cats. Currently clomipramine is often chosen over amitriptyline for use in dogs when a tricyclic is to be tried for behavioral indications. Amitriptyline may be useful for adjunctive treatment of pruritus, or chronic pain of neuropathic origin in dogs and cats. In cats, it potentially could be useful for adjunctive treatment of lower urinary tract disease. Amitriptyline has been tried to reduce feather plucking in birds.

Pharmacology/Actions

Amitriptyline (and its active metabolite, nortriptyline) has a complicated pharmacologic profile. From a slightly oversimplified viewpoint, it has 3 main characteristics: blockage of the amine pump, thereby increasing neurotransmitter levels (principally serotonin, but also norepinephrine), sedation, and central and peripheral anticholinergic activity. Other pharmacologic effects include stabilizing mast cells via H-1 receptor antagonism, and antagonism of glutamate receptors and sodium channels. In animals, tricyclic antidepressants are similar to the actions of phenothiazines in altering avoidance behaviors.

Pharmacokinetics

Amitriptyline is rapidly absorbed from both the GI tract and from parenteral injection sites, but transdermal (PLO-gel based) absorption in cats is poor (Mealey *et al.* 2004). Peak levels occur in 1–2 hours after oral administration in cats and other species within 2–12 hours. Amitriptyline is highly bound to plasma proteins, enters the CNS, and enters maternal milk in levels at, or greater than those found in maternal serum. The drug is metabolized in the liver to several metabolites, including nortriptyline, which is active. In humans, the terminal half-life is approximately 30 hours. Half-life in dogs has been reported to be 6–8 hours.

Contraindications/Precautions/Warnings

These agents are contraindicated if prior sensitivity has been noted with any other tricyclic. Concomitant use with monoamine oxidase inhibitors is generally contraindicated. Use with extreme caution in patients with seizure disorders as tricyclic agents may reduce seizure thresholds. Use with caution in patients with thyroid disorders, hepatic disorders, KCS, glaucoma, cardiac rhythm disorders, diabetes, or adrenal tumors.

Adverse Effects

The most predominant adverse effects seen with the tricyclics are related to their sedating and anticholinergic (constipation, urinary retention) properties. Occasionally, dogs exhibit hyperexcitability and, rarely, develop seizures. However, adverse effects can run the entire gamut of systems, including cardiac (dysrhythmias), hematologic (bone marrow suppression), GI (diarrhea, vomiting), endocrine, etc. Cats may demonstrate the following adverse effects: sedation, hypersalivation, urinary retention, anorexia, thrombocytopenia, neutropenia, unkempt hair coat, vomiting, ataxia, disorientation and cardiac conductivity disturbances.

Reproductive/Nursing Safety

Isolated reports of limb reduction abnormalities have been noted; restrict use to pregnant animals only when the benefits clearly outweigh the risks. In humans, the FDA categorizes this drug as category *D* for use during pregnancy (*There is evidence of human fetal risk, but the potential benefits from the use of the drug in pregnant women may be acceptable despite its potential risks.*)

Overdosage/Acute Toxicity

Overdosage with tricyclics can be life-threatening (arrhythmias, cardiorespiratory collapse). Because the toxicities and therapies for treatment are complicated and controversial, it is recommended to contact an animal poison control center for further information in any potential overdose situation.

There were 178 exposures to amitriptyline reported to the ASPCA Animal Poison Control Center (APCC) during 2008-2009. In these cases, 113 were dogs with 21 showing clinical signs. The remaining 65 cases were cats with 39 showing clinical signs. Common findings in dogs recorded in decreasing frequency included lethargy and tachycardia. Common findings in cats recorded in decreased frequency included vocalization, ataxia, mydriasis, tachycardia, disorientation, lethargy, and agitation.

Drug Interactions

The following drug interactions have either been reported or are theoretical in humans or animals receiving amitriptyline and may be of significance in veterinary patients:

- **ANTICHOLINERGIC AGENTS:** Increased effects; hyperthermia and ileus possible

- **CIMETIDINE:** May inhibit tricyclic antidepressant metabolism and increase the risk of toxicity

- **CISAPRIDE:** May have additive effects on QTc interval; possible serious arrhythmias may result

- **CNS DEPRESSANTS:** Increased effects

- **DIAZEPAM:** Possible increased amitriptyline levels

- **MONOAMINE OXIDASE INHIBITORS** (including **selegiline, amitraz**): Potential life threatening serotonin syndrome; use together not recommended

- **QUINIDINE:** Increased risk for QTc interval prolongation and tricyclic adverse effects

- **SELECTIVE-SEROTONIN RE-UPTAKE INHIBITORS** (**SSRIs, fluoxetine**, etc.): Potential increased amitriptyline levels, increased risk for serotonin syndrome; **Note:** SSRI's and TCA's etc. amitriptyline are often used together in veterinary behavior medicine, but enhanced monitoring for adverse effects is suggested)

- **SYMPATHOMIMETIC AGENTS:** May increase the risk of cardiac effects (arrhythmias, hypertension, hyperpyrexia)

- **THYROID AGENTS:** Increased risk for arrhythmias; monitor

Laboratory Considerations

- Tricyclics can widen QRS complexes, prolong PR intervals and invert or flatten T-waves on **ECG**

- The response to **metapyrone** may be decreased by amitriptyline

- Tricyclics may alter (increase or decrease) **blood glucose** levels

Doses

- **DOGS:**
For adjunctive treatment of pruritus:
a) 1–2 mg/kg PO q12h (Paradis & Scott 1992)
b) For acral pruritic dermatitis: 2.2 mg/kg PO twice daily; only occasionally effective. A 2–4 week trial is recommended (Rosychuk 1991)

For behavior disorders amenable to tricyclics:
a) For separation anxiety or generalized anxiety: 1–2 mg/kg PO q12h; with behavior modification (Shanley & Overall 1992); (Line 2000); (Overall 2000)
b) 1–4 mg/kg PO q12h. Begin at 1–2 mg/kg PO q12h for 2 weeks, increase by 1 mg/kg up to maximum dosage (4 mg/kg) as necessary. If no clinical response, decrease by 1 mg/kg PO q12h for 2 weeks until at initial dosage. (Virga 2002)

c) 2.2–4.4 mg/kg PO q12h (Reisner & Houpt 2000)
d) 0.25–1.5 mg/kg PO every 12–24h (Crowell-Davis 1999)

For neuropathic pain:
a) 1–2 mg/kg PO q12–24h (Hardie 2000)
b) For adjunctive treatment of pain associated with appendicular osteosarcoma: 1–2 mg/kg PO q12–24h (Liptak & Ehrhart 2005)

- **CATS:**
For adjunctive treatment of behavior disorders amenable to tricyclics:
a) 5–10 mg per cat PO once daily (Miller 1989), (Marder 1991), (Reisner & Houpt 2000)
b) 0.5–2 mg/kg PO q12–24h; start at 0.5 mg/kg PO q12h (Overall 2000)
c) 0.5–1 mg/kg PO q12–24h (Crowell-Davis 1999)
d) 0.5–1 mg/kg PO q12–24h. Allow 3–4 weeks for initial trial. (Virga 2002)

For self-mutilation behaviors associated with anxiety:
a) 5–10 mg per cat PO once to twice daily; with behavior modification (Shanley & Overall 1992)
b) 1–2 mg/kg PO q12h (Line 2000)

For pruritus (after other more conventional therapies have failed):
a) 5–10 mg per cat PO once daily or 2.5–7.5 mg/cat once to twice daily. When discontinuing, taper dose over 1–3 weeks. (Messinger 2000)

For symptomatic therapy of idiopathic feline lower urinary tract disease (FLUTD):
a) 2.5–12.5 mg (total dose) PO once daily at night (Bartges 2006)
b) 5–10 mg (total dose) PO once daily at night; the drug is in popular use at present and further studies are needed (Senior 2006)
c) Reserved for cases with severe, recurrent signs; 2.5–12.5 mg (total dose) PO at the time the owner retires for the night. Dosage is adjusted to produce a barely perceptible calming effect on the cat. If no improvement is seen within 2 months, the medication may be gradually tapered and then stopped. (Buffington 2006)

For neuropathic pain:
a) 2.5–12.5 mg/cat PO once daily (Hardie 2000)
b) 0.5–2 mg/kg PO once daily; may be a useful addition to NSAIDs for chronic pain. (Lascelles et al. 2003)

- **BIRDS:**
For adjunctive treatment of feather plucking:
a) 1–2 mg/kg PO q12–24 hours. Anecdotal

reports indicate some usefulness. Barring side-effects, may be worth a more prolonged course of therapy to determine efficacy. (Lightfoot 2001)

Monitoring

■ Efficacy

■ Adverse effects; it is recommended to perform a cardiac evaluation, CBC and serum chemistry panel prior to therapy

■ For cats, some clinicians recommend that liver enzymes be measured prior to therapy, one month after initial therapy, and yearly, thereafter

Client Information

■ All tricyclics should be dispensed in child-resistant packaging and kept well away from children or pets.

■ Several weeks may be required before efficacy is noted and to continue dosing as prescribed. Do not abruptly stop giving medication without veterinarian's advice.

Chemistry/Synonyms

A tricyclic dibenzocycloheptene-derivative antidepressant, amitriptyline HCl occurs as a white or practically white, odorless or practically odorless crystalline powder that is freely soluble in water or alcohol. It has a bitter, burning taste and a pK_a of 9.4.

Amitriptyline may also be known as amitriptylini hydrochloridum; many trade names are available.

Storage/Stability

Amitriptyline tablets should be stored at room temperature. The injection should be kept from freezing and protected from light.

Dosage Forms/Regulatory Status

VETERINARY-LABELED PRODUCTS: None

The ARCI (Racing Commissioners International) has designated this drug as a class 2 substance. See the appendix for more information.

HUMAN-LABELED PRODUCTS:

Amitriptyline HCl Tablets: 10 mg, 25 mg, 50 mg, 75 mg, 100 mg, & 150 mg; generic; (Rx)

There are also fixed dose oral combination products containing amitriptyline and chlordiazepoxide, and amitriptyline and perphenazine.

References

Bartges, J (2006). What to do when there's nothing to do: Feline idiopathic cystitis. Proceedings: ACVC 2006. Accessed via: Veterinary Information Network. http://goo.gl/cvPKW

Buffington, C (2006). Treatment of feline idiopathic cystitis. Proceedings: ECVIM. Accessed via: Veterinary Information Network. http://goo.gl/GRZXn

Crowell–Davis, S (1999). Behavior Psychopharmacology Part 1: Principles, Antipsycotics, Antidepressants and CNS Stimulants. Proceedings: Central Veterinary Conference, Kansas City.

Hardie, E (2000). Pain: Management. *Textbook of Veterinary Internal Medicine: Diseases of the Dog and Cat.* S Ettinger and E Feldman Eds. Philadelphia, WB Saunders. 1: 23–25.

Lascelles, D, S Robertson, et al. (2003). Can chronic pain in cats be managed? Yes! Proceedings: Pain Management 2003. Accessed via: Veterinary Information Network. http://goo.gl/2m6yx

Lightfoot, T (2001). Feather "Plucking". Proceedings: Atlantic Coast Veterinary Conference. Accessed via: Veterinary Information Network. http://goo.gl/6qoTg

Line, S (2000). Sensory Mutilation and Related Behavior Syndromes. *Kirk's Current Veterinary Therapy: XIII Small Animal Practice.* J Bonagura Ed. Philadelphia, WB Saunders: 90–93.

Liptak, J & N Ehrhart (2005). Bone and joint tumors. *Textbook of Veterinary Internal Medicine, 6th Ed.* S Ettinger and E Feldman Eds., Elsevier: 760–773.

Mealey, KL, KE Peck, et al. (2004). Systemic absorption of amitriptyline and buspirone after oral and transdermal administration to healthy cats. *Journal of Veterinary Internal Medicine* 18(1): 43–46.

Messinger, L (2000). Pruritis Therapy in the Cat. *Kirk's Current Veterinary Therapy: XIII Small Animal Practice.* J Bonagura Ed. Philadelphia, WB Saunders: 542–545.

Overall, K (2000). Behavioral Pharmacology. Proceedings: American Animal Hospital Association 67th Annual Meeting, Toronto.

Paradis, M & D Scott (1992). Nonsteroidal therapy for canine and feline pruritis. *Current Veterinary Therapy XI: Small Animal Practice.* R Kirk and J Bonagura Eds. Philadelphia, W.B. Saunders Company: 563–566.

Reisner, I & K Houpt (2000). Behavioral Disorders. *Textbook of Veterinary Internal Medicine: Diseases of the Dog and Cat.* S Ettinger and E Feldman Eds. Philadelphia, WB Saunders. 1: 156–162.

Rosychuck, R (1991). Newer therapies in veterinary dermatology. Proceedings of the Ninth Annual Veterinary Medical Forum, New Orleans, American College of Veterinary Internal Medicine.

Senior, D (2006). Lower Urinary Tract Disease – Feline. Proceedings: WSAVA. Accessed via: Veterinary Information Network. http://goo.gl/2k6lt

Shanley, K & K Overall (1992). Psychogenic dermatoses. *Current Veterinary Therapy XI: Small Animal Practice.* R Kirk and J Bonagura Eds. Philadelphia, W.B. Saunders Company: 552–558.

Virga, V (2002). Which drug and why: An update on psychopharmacology. Proceedings: Atlantic Coast Veterinary Conference. Accessed via: Veterinary Information Network. http://goo.gl/m8qr4

AMLODIPINE BESYLATE

(am-loe-*di*-peen)   Norvasc®

CALCIUM CHANNEL BLOCKER

Prescriber Highlights

▶ Calcium channel blocker used most often for treating hypertension, especially in cats

▶ Slight negative inotrope; use with caution in patients with heart disease, hepatic dysfunction

▶ Potentially may cause anorexia & hypotension in cats early in therapy; gingival hyperplasia seen in some dogs

▶ Hypertension may rapidly reoccur if dosages are missed

Uses/Indications

Oral amlodipine appears to be a useful agent in the treatment of hypertension in cats and many consider it the drug of choice for this indication. In pharmacokinetic studies, amlodipine has decreased blood pressure in dogs with chronic renal disease, but its efficacy in treating hypertensive dogs has been disappointing. When used alone in healthy dogs in higher dosages, amlodipine has been shown to activate the renin-angiotensin-aldosterone system (RAAS). Use with an ACE inhibitor (enalapril) at least partially blocks this effect (Atkins *et al.* 2007).

Hypertension in cats is usually secondary to other diseases (often renal failure or cardiac causes such as thyrotoxic cardiomyopathy or primary hypertrophic cardiomyopathy, etc.) and is most often seen in middle-aged or geriatric cats. These animals often present with acute clinical signs such as blindness, seizures, collapse or paresis. A cat is generally considered hypertensive if systolic blood pressure is >160 mmHg. Early reports indicate that if antihypertensive therapy is begun acutely, some vision may be restored in about 50% of cases of blindness secondary to hypertension.

Pharmacology/Actions

Amlodipine inhibits calcium influx across cell membranes in both cardiac and vascular smooth muscle. It has a greater effect on vascular smooth muscle, thereby acting as a peripheral arteriolar vasodilator and reducing afterload. Amlodipine also depresses impulse formation (automaticity) and conduction velocity in cardiac muscle. After an initial dose in dogs, amlodipine has a mild diuretic action.

Pharmacokinetics

No feline-specific data on the drug's pharmacokinetics was located. In humans, amlodipine's bioavailability does not appear to be altered by the presence of food in the gut. The drug is slowly but almost completely absorbed after oral administration and is reported to be absorbed after rectal administration. In humans, peak plasma concentrations occur between 6–9 hours post-dose and effects on blood pressure are correspondingly delayed. In cats, effects on systemic blood pressure are usually seen within 4 hours of dosing and may persist for approximately 30 hours post dose (Brown 2009). The drug has very high plasma protein binding characteristics (approximately 93%). However, drug interactions associated with potential displacement from these sites have not been elucidated. Amlodipine is slowly, but extensively metabolized to inactive compounds in the liver. Terminal plasma half-life is approximately 30 hours in dogs and 35 hours in healthy humans, but is prolonged in the elderly and in those patients with hypertension or hepatic dysfunction.

Contraindications/Precautions/Warnings

Because amlodipine may have slight negative inotropic effects, it should be used cautiously in patients with heart failure or cardiogenic shock. It should also be used cautiously in patients with hepatic disease or at risk for developing hypotension. A relative contraindication for amlodipine exists for humans with advanced aortic stenosis.

There is concern that using amlodipine alone for treating hypertension in cats with renal disease may expose glomeruli to higher pressures secondary to efferent arteriolar constriction. This is caused by localized increases in renin-angiotensin-aldosterone (RAAS) axis activity thereby allowing progressive damage to glomeruli. It is postulated that using an ACE inhibitor with amlodipine may help prevent this occurrence (Stepien 2006). Whether routine use of ACE inhibitors with amlodipine is necessary and beneficial in animals with chronic kidney disease and hypertension is somewhat controversial, particularly in cats.

Adverse Effects

Because of amlodipine's relatively slow onset of action, hypotension and inappetence is usually absent in cats. Infrequently, cats may develop azotemia, lethargy, hypokalemia, reflex tachycardia and weight loss. In humans taking amlodipine, headache (7.3% incidence) is the most frequent problem reported.

In dogs, gingival hyperplasia has been reported when used long term (Thomason *et al.* 2009).

Reproductive/Nursing Safety

While no evidence of impaired fertility was noted in rats given 8X overdoses, amlodipine has been shown to be fetotoxic (intrauterine death rates increased 5 fold) in laboratory animals (rats, rabbits) at very high dosages. No evidence of teratogenicity or mutagenicity was observed in lab animal studies. In rats, amlodipine prolonged labor. It is unknown whether amlodipine enters maternal milk. In humans, the FDA categorizes this drug as category *C* for use during pregnancy (*Animal studies have shown an adverse effect on the fetus, but there are no adequate studies in humans; or there are no animal reproduction studies and no adequate studies in humans.*)

Overdosage/Acute Toxicity

Limited experience with other calcium channel blockers in humans has shown that profound hypotension and bradycardia may result. There were 35 exposures to amlodipine reported to the ASPCA Animal Poison Control Center (APCC) during 2006 - 2009. In these cases, 15 were dogs with 7 showing clinical signs and the remaining 20 cases were cats with 4 showing clinical signs. Common findings in dogs recorded in decreasing frequency included lethargy. Common findings in cats recorded in decreasing frequency included lethargy and vomiting.

Risk in animals with overdoses is for hypotension and reflex tachycardia (possible to see bradycardia). When possible, massive overdoses should be managed with gut emptying and supportive treatment. Beta-agonists, intravenous lipid therapy, and intravenous calcium may be beneficial.

Drug Interactions

The following drug interactions have either been reported or are theoretical in humans or animals receiving amlodipine and may be of significance in veterinary patients:

No clinically significant drug-drug interactions have been noted specifically with amlodipine at this time. However, concomitant use of **diuretics, beta-blockers**, other **vasodilators or other agents that may reduce blood pressure** (*e.g.*, **fentanyl**) may cause hypotension if used with amlodipine. **Grapefruit juice/powder** may alter bioavailability.

Laboratory Considerations

■ No specific concerns were noted

Doses

■ **CATS:**

For treatment of systemic hypertension:

a) As a first step drug when systolic BP >160 mmHg, diastolic >120 mmHg: **1)** amlodipine (0.625 mg per cat q24h, if cat greater then 6 kg, 1.25 mg/cat q24h), add ACE inhibitor if proteinuric; **2)** ACE inhibitor (benazepril/enalapril 0.5 mg/kg q12h); **3)** spironolactone (1–2 mg/kg twice daily); **4)** hydralazine 0.5 mg/kg PO twice daily. Each step added (except when increasing amlodipine dose) if after 1-2 weeks systolic BP > 160 mmHg. (Henik 2007)

b) 0.625–1.25 mg (total dose) PO once daily. Drug of choice; often successful as a single agent. Can be combined with an ACEI, beta-blocker or diuretic if needed. Maximum effect seen within 7 days of therapy. (Sparkes 2003)

■ **DOGS:**

For adjunctive therapy for refractory heart failure:

a) For treatment of advanced mitral valve degeneration as an afterload reducer after ACE inhibitor maintenance therapy has been established: 0.2–0.4 mg/kg PO twice daily. Initiate therapy at 0.1 mg/kg PO twice daily and up-titrate weekly while monitoring blood pressure. (Kraus 2003)

b) As an arterial vasodilator particularly in dogs moderately refractory, or recurrent CHF secondary to mitral regurgitation and maintained blood pressures: 0.1 mg/kg q12–24h initially; titrate up as needed to 0.25 mg/kg PO q12–24h; monitor blood pressure. (DeFrancesco 2006)

For treatment of systemic hypertension: in dogs with chronic renal disease:

a) In dogs with chronic renal disease: 0.1–0.5 mg/kg PO once daily (q24h), most often combined with an ACE inhibitor. Dogs may require weeks to months of therapy to achieve satisfactory blood pressure control. (Polzin 2009)

b) As a 2nd step drug for systolic hypertension >160 mmHg, diastolic >120 mmHg; after **1)** enalapril/benazepril (0.5 mg/kg q12h); **2)** amlodipine (0.1 mg/kg q24h); **3)** amlodipine (0.2 mg/kg q24h); **4)** spironolactone (1–2 mg/kg twice daily); **5)** hydralazine 0.5 mg/kg PO twice daily. Each step added (except when increasing amlodipine dose) if after 1-2 weeks systolic BP > 160 mmHg. (Henik 2007)

Monitoring

■ Blood pressure;
■ Ophthalmic exam
■ Adverse effects

Client Information

■ May give with food
■ Missing dosages can cause rapid redevelopment of symptoms and damage secondary to hypertension

Chemistry/Synonyms

Amlodipine besylate, a dihydropyridine calcium channel-blocking agent, occurs as a white crystalline powder that is slightly soluble in water and sparingly soluble in alcohol.

Amlodipine Besylate may also as: amlodipini besilas, UK-48340-26, or UK-48340-11 (amlodipine maleate); many trade names are available.

Storage/Stability

Store amlodipine tablets at room temperature, in tight, light resistant containers.

Compatibility/Compounding Considerations

Compounded preparation stability: Amlodipine oral suspension compounded from commercially available tablets has been published (Nahata et al. 1999). Triturating six (6) amlodipine 5 mg tablets with 15 mL of *Ora-Plus®* and *qs ad* to 30 mL with *Ora-Sweet®* yields a 1 mg/mL oral suspension that retains >90% potency for 91 days stored at both 5°C and 25°C. Compounded preparations of amlodipine should be protected from light.

Dosage Forms/Regulatory Status

VETERINARY-LABELED PRODUCTS: None

The ARCI (Racing Commissioners International) has designated this drug as a class 4 substance. See the appendix for more information.

HUMAN-LABELED PRODUCTS:

Amlodipine Oral Tablets: 2.5 mg, 5 mg, & 10 mg; *Norvasc®* (Pfizer); generic; (Rx)

Fixed-dose combination products with bena-zepril (*Lotrel®*) or atorvastatin (*Caduet®*) are available.

References

Atkins, CE, WP Rausch, et al. (2007). The effect of am-lodipine and the combination of amlodipine and enalapril on the renin–angiotensin–aldosterone system in the dog. *Journal of Veterinary Pharmacology and Therapeutics* **30**(5): 394–400.

Brown, S (2009). Amlodipine and Hypertensive Nephropathy in Cats. Proceedings: ECVIM. Accessed via: Veterinary Information Network. http://goo.gl/Jd3bk

DeFrancesco, T (2006). Refractory heart failure. Proceedings: IVECCS 2006. Accessed via: Veterinary Information Network. goo.gl/WObuJ

Henik, R (2007). Stepwise therapy of systemic hyperten-sion. Proceedings: IVECCS. Accessed via: Veterinary Information Network. http://goo.gl/nofKU

Kraus, M (2003). Syncope in small breed dogs. Proceedings: ACVIM Forum. Accessed via: Veterinary Information Network. http://goo.gl/u7CLL

Nahata, M.C., R.S. Morosco, et al. (1999). Stability of amlo-dipine besylate in two liquid dosage forms. *J Am Pharm Assoc* (Wash) **39**(3): 375–377.

Polzin, D (2009). Proteinuria and hypertension in chronic kidney disease. Proceedings: WSAVA. Accessed via: Veterinary Information Network. http://goo.gl/LLfMQ

Sparkes, A (2003). Feline systemic hypertension–A hidden killer. Proceedings: World Small Animal Veterinary Assoc. Accessed via: Veterinary Information Network. http://goo.gl/QgVkr

Stepien, R (2006). Diagnosis and treatment of systemic hy-pertension. Proceedings: ACVIM Forum.

Thomason, JD, TL Fallaw, et al. (2009). Gingival Hyperplasia Associated with the Administration of Amlodipine to Dogs with Degenerative Valvular Disease (2004–2008). *Journal of Veterinary Internal Medicine* **23**(1): 39–42.

AMMONIUM CHLORIDE

(ah-*moe*-nee-um)   Uroeze®

ACIDIFYING AGENT

Prescriber Highlights

▶ Urinary acidifier; treatment of meta-bolic alkalosis

▶ Contraindicated in patients with he-patic failure or uremia

▶ Potential adverse effects are primarily GI distress; IV use may lead to meta-bolic acidosis

▶ Very unpalatable; addition of sugar (not molasses) may improve palatabi-lity to goats and sheep

▶ May increase excretion of quinidine; decrease efficacy of erythromycin or aminoglycosides in urine

---

Uses/Indications

The veterinary indications for ammonium chlo-ride are as a urinary acidifying agent to help pre-vent and dissolve certain types of uroliths (*e.g.*, struvite), to enhance renal excretion of some types of toxins (*e.g.*, strontium, strychnine) or drugs (*e.g.*, quinidine), or to enhance the efficacy

of certain antimicrobials (*e.g.*, chlortetracycline, methenamine mandelate, nitrofurantoin, oxy-tetracycline, penicillin G or tetracycline) when treating urinary tract infections. Ammonium chloride has also been used intravenously for the rapid correction of metabolic alkalosis.

Because of changes in feline diets to restrict struvite and as struvite therapeutic diets (*e.g.*, s/d) cause aciduria, ammonium chloride is not commonly recommended for struvite uroliths in cats.

Ammonium chloride is still recommended to help prevent uroliths in small ruminants, but dietary changes can significantly affect its effi-cacy for this purpose.

Pharmacology/Actions

The acidification properties of ammonium chloride are caused by its dissociation into chlo-ride and ammonium ions *in vivo*. The ammoni-um cation is converted by the liver to urea with the release of a hydrogen ion. This ion combines with bicarbonate to form water and carbon di-oxide. In the extracellular fluid, chloride ions combine with fixed bases and decrease the alka-line reserves in the body. The net effects are de-creased serum bicarbonate levels and a decrease in blood and urine pH.

Excess chloride ions presented to the kidney are not completely reabsorbed by the tubules and are excreted with cations (principally so-dium) and water. This diuretic effect is usually compensated for in the kidneys after a few days of therapy.

Pharmacokinetics

No information was located on the pharmacoki-netics of this agent in veterinary species. In hu-mans, ammonium chloride is rapidly absorbed from the GI.

Contraindications/Precautions/Warnings

Ammonium chloride is contraindicated in pa-tients with severe hepatic disease as ammonia may accumulate and cause toxicity. In general, ammonium chloride should not be administered to uremic patients since it can intensify the metabolic acidosis already existing in some of these patients. As sodium depletion can occur, ammonium chloride should not be used alone in patients with severe renal insufficiency and metabolic alkalosis secondary to vomiting hy-drochloric acid. In these cases, sodium chloride repletion with or without ammonium chloride administration should be performed to correct both sodium and chloride deficits. Ammonium chloride is contraindicated in patients with urate calculi or respiratory acidosis and high total CO_2 and buffer base. Ammonium chlo-ride alone cannot correct hypochloremia with secondary metabolic alkalosis due to intracel-lular potassium chloride depletion; potassium chloride must be administered to these patients.

Do not administer subcutaneously, rectally or intraperitoneally.

Use ammonium chloride with caution in patients with pulmonary insufficiency or cardiac edema.

A high roughage/concentrate ratio diet can decrease the urine pH lowering effect of ammonium chloride in horses (Kienzle *et al.* 2006).

Adverse Effects

Development of metabolic acidosis (sometimes severe) can occur unless adequate monitoring is performed. When used intravenously, pain at the injection site can develop; slow administration lessens this effect. Gastric irritation, nausea and vomiting may be associated with oral dosing of the drug. Urinary acidification is associated with an increased risk for calcium oxalate urolith formation in cats.

Overdosage/Acute Toxicity

Clinical signs of overdosage may include: nausea, vomiting, excessive thirst, hyperventilation, bradycardias or other arrhythmias, and progressive CNS depression. Profound acidosis and hypokalemia may be noted on laboratory results.

Treatment should consist of correcting the acidosis by administering sodium bicarbonate or sodium acetate intravenously. Hypokalemia should be treated by using a suitable oral (if possible) potassium product. Intense acid-base and electrolyte monitoring should be performed on an ongoing basis until the patient is stable.

Reproductive/Nursing Safety

In humans, the FDA categorizes this drug as category *B* for use during pregnancy (*Animal studies have not yet demonstrated risk to the fetus, but there are no adequate studies in pregnant women; or animal studies have shown an adverse effect, but adequate studies in pregnant women have not demonstrated a risk to the fetus in the first trimester of pregnancy, and there is no evidence of risk in later trimesters.*) In a separate system evaluating the safety of drugs in canine and feline pregnancy (Papich 1989), this drug is categorized as in class: *B* (*Safe for use if used cautiously. Studies in laboratory animals may have uncovered some risk, but these drugs appear to be safe in dogs and cats or these drugs are safe if they are not administered when the animal is near term.*)

Drug Interactions

The following drug interactions have either been reported or are theoretical in humans or animals receiving ammonium chloride or other urinary acidifying agents and may be of significance in veterinary patients:

- ■ **AMINOGLYCOSIDES (e.g., gentamicin)** and **ERYTHROMYCIN**: Are more effective in an alkaline medium; urine acidification may diminish these drugs effectiveness in treating bacterial urinary tract infections
- ■ **QUINIDINE**: Urine acidification may increase renal excretion

Doses

■ **DOGS:**

For urine acidification:

a) As adjunctive therapy for struvite uroliths: 20 mg/kg PO three times daily (Labato 2002)

b) To enhance the renal elimination of certain toxins/drugs: 200 mg/kg/day divided four times daily (Grauer & Hjelle 1988)

c) To enhance elimination of strontium: 0.2–0.5 grams PO 3–4 times a day (used with calcium salts) (Bailey 1986)

For ATT (ammonia tolerance testing):

a) 2 mL/kg of a 5% solution of ammonium chloride deep in the rectum, blood sampled at 20 minutes and 40 minutes; or oral challenge with ammonium chloride 100 mg/kg (maximum dose = 3 grams) either in solution: dissolved in 20–50 mL warm water or in gelatin capsules, blood sampled at 30 and 60 minutes. Test may also be done by comparing fasting and 6–hour postprandial samples without giving exogenous ammonium chloride. (Center 2004)

■ **CATS:**

For urine acidification:

a) In struvite dissolution therapy if diet and antimicrobials do not result in acid urine or to help prevent idiopathic FUS in a non-obstructed cat: 20 mg/kg PO twice daily (Lage *et al.* 1988)

b) As adjunctive therapy for struvite uroliths: 20 mg/kg PO twice daily (Labato 2002)

■ **HORSES:**

a) 4–15 grams PO) (Swinyard 1975)

b) Ammonium chloride as a urinary acidifier: 60–520 mg/kg PO daily. Ammonium salts are unpalatable and will have to be dosed via stomach tube or dosing syringe. Alternatively, ammonium sulfate at 165 mg/kg PO per day is more palatable and may be accepted when mixed with grain or hay. (Jose-Cunilleras and Hinchcliff 1999)

c) As a urinary acidifier to enhance renal excretion of strychnine: 132 mg/kg PO (Schmitz 2004)

■ **CATTLE:**

For urolithiasis prevention:

a) 200 mg/kg PO (Howard 1986)

b) 15–30 grams PO (Swinyard 1975)

■ **SHEEP & GOATS:**

For urolithiasis prevention:

a) 300 mg/kg PO (Edmondson 2009)

b) 0.5–1% of the daily dry matter will acidify urine, but can be very unpalatable. Table sugar may improve palatability. (Snyder 2009), (Van Metre 2009).

Monitoring

■ Urine pH (Urine pH's of ≤6.5 are recommended as goals of therapy)

■ Blood pH if there are clinical signs of toxicity or treating metabolic alkalosis

■ Serum electrolytes, if using chronically or if treating metabolic acidosis

■ Prior to IV use, it is recommended that the carbon dioxide combining power of the patient's serum be measured to insure that serious acidosis is prevented

Client Information

■ Contact veterinarian if animal exhibits signs of nausea, vomiting, excessive thirst, hyperventilation or progressive lethargy

■ Powders may have a bitter taste and patients may not accept their food after mixing

Chemistry/Synonyms

An acid-forming salt, ammonium chloride occurs as colorless crystals or as white, fine or course, crystalline powder. It is somewhat hygroscopic, and has a cool, saline taste. When dissolved in water, the temperature of the solution is decreased. One gram is soluble in approximately 3 mL of water at room temperature; 1.4 mL at 100°C. One gram is soluble in approximately 100 mL of alcohol.

One gram of ammonium chloride contains 18.7 mEq of ammonium and chloride ions. The commercially available concentrate for injection (26.75%) contains 5 mEq of each ion per mL and contains disodium edetate as a stabilizing agent. The pH of the concentrate for injection is approximately 5.

Ammonium chloride may also be known as muriate of ammonia and sal ammoniac.

Storage/Stability

Ammonium chloride for injection should be stored at room temperature; avoid freezing. At low temperatures, crystallization may occur; it may be resolubolized by warming to room temperature in a water bath.

Compatibility/Compounding Considerations

Ammonium chloride should not be titrated with strong oxidizing agents (e.g., potassium chlorate) as explosive compounds may result.

Ammonium chloride is reported to be physically **compatible** with all commonly used IV replacement fluids and potassium chloride. It is **incompatible** with codeine phosphate, dimenhydrinate, methadone HCl, nitrofurantoin sodium, sulfisoxazole diolamine, and warfarin sodium. It is also reportedly **incompatible** with alkalis and their hydroxides.

Dosage Forms/Regulatory Status

VETERINARY-LABELED PRODUCTS:

Note: The following may not be FDA-approved products as they are not located in the "Green Book".

Ammonium Chloride Tablets: 200 mg, 400 mg; *UriKare® 200, 400 Tablets* (Neogen); (Rx). Labeled for use in cats and dogs.

Ammonium Chloride Granules: 200 mg per ¼ teaspoonful powder; *Uroeze® 200* (Virbac), *UriKare® 200* (Neogen); (Rx). Labeled for cats and dogs.

Ammonium Chloride Granules: 400 mg per ¼ teaspoonful powder; *Uroeze®* (Virbac), *UriKare® 400* (Neogen); (Rx). Labeled for cats and dogs.

Ammonium chloride is also found in some veterinary labeled cough preparations *e.g., Spect-Aid® Expectorant Granules* (7% guaifenesin, 75% ammonium chloride, potassium iodide 2%) and in some cough syrups (also containing guaifenesin, pyrilamine and phenylephrine).

When used in large animals, feed grade ammonium chloride can be obtained from feed mills.

HUMAN-LABELED PRODUCTS:

Ammonium Chloride Injection: 26.75% (5 mEq/mL) in 20 mL (100 mEq) vials; generic (Hospira); (Rx). Preparation of solution for IV administration: Dilute 1 or 2 vials (100–200 mEq) in either 500 or 1000 mL of sodium chloride 0.9% for injection. Do not administer at a rate greater than 5 mL/min (human adult).

References

Bailey, EM (1986). Emergency and general treatment of poisonings. *Current Veterinary Therapy (CVT) IX Small Animal Practice*. RW Kirk Ed. Philadelphia, W.B. Saunders: 135–144.

Center, S (2004). Current recommendations for liver function testing. Proceedings: ACVIM Forum. Accessed via: Veterinary Information Network. http://goo.gl/5U8Xb

Edmondson, M (2009). Urolithiasis in small ruminants. Proceedings: ABVP. Accessed via: Veterinary Information Network. http://goo.gl/Pmsfw

Grauer, GF & JJ Hjelle (1988). Household Toxins. *Handbook of Small Animal Practice*. RV Morgan Ed. New York, Churchill Livingstone: 1109–1114.

Howard, JL, Ed. (1986). *Current Veterinary Therapy 2, Food Animal Practice*. Philadelphia, W.B. Saunders.

Kienzle, E, K Sturmer, et al. (2006). A high roughage/concentrate ratio decreases the effect of ammonium chloride on acid–base balance in horses. *Journal of Nutrition* 136(7): 2048S–2049S.

Labato, M (2002). Those troublesome uroliths I and II. Proceedings: Tufts Animal Expo. Accessed via: Veterinary Information Network. http://goo.gl/Ffbhj

Lage, AL, D Polzin, et al. (1988). Diseases of the Bladder. *Handbook of Small Animal Practice*. RV Morgan Ed. New York, Churchill Livingstone: 605–620.

Schmitz, D (2004). Toxicologic problems. *Equine Internal Medicine 2nd Ed*. S Reed, W Bayly and D Sellon Eds. Philadelphia, Saunders: 1441–1512.

Snyder, J (2009). Small Ruminant Medicine & Surgery for Equine and Small Animal Practitioners I & II. Proceedings: WVC. Accessed via: Veterinary Information Network. http://goo.gl/hkoer

Swinyard, EA (1975). Diuretic Drugs. *Remington's Pharmaceutical Sciences*. A Osol Ed. Easton, Mack Publishing: 861–873.

Van Metre, D (2009). Urolithiasis in ruminants. Proceedings: Western Veterinary Conference. Accessed via: Veterinary Information Network. http://goo.gl/aHRWM

AMMONIUM MOLYBDATE

AMMONIUM TETRATHIO-MOLYBDATE

(ah-*moe*-nee-um moe-*lib*-date;
tet-ra-*thye*-oh-moe-*lib*-date)   Molypen®

COPPER POISONING TREATMENT

Prescriber Highlights

▶ Used primarily to treat copper poisoning in food animals (esp. sheep)

▶ Consider contacting FDA for guidance in treating food animals

Uses/Indications

Ammonium molybdate and ammonium tetrathiomolybdate (TTM) are used for the investigational or compassionate treatment of copper poisoning in food animals, primarily sheep.

Adverse Effects

After apparent successful treatment for copper poisoning with ammonium tetrathiomolybdate (TTM), a flock of sheep became infertile, progressively unthrifty, and died 2–3 years later. The authors concluded the TTM was retained in the CNS, pituitary and adrenal glands and caused a toxic endocrinopathy (Haywood *et al.* 2004).

Reproductive/Nursing Safety

In humans, the FDA categorizes this drug as category *C* for use during pregnancy (*Animal studies have shown an adverse effect on the fetus, but there are no adequate studies in humans; or there are no animal reproduction studies and no adequate studies in humans.*)

Doses

Note: In food animals, FARAD recommends a minimum 10 day preslaughter withdrawal time and a minimum 5 day milk withholding interval. (Haskell *et al.* 2005)

Ammonium tetrathiomolybdate does not go into solution readily and ammonium molybdate administered orally is often preferred.

■ **SHEEP:**

For treatment of copper poisoning:

a) Food animals: Ammonium molybdate: 200 mg per head PO once daily for 3 weeks. Ammonium tetrathiomolybdate: 1.7–3.4 mg per head IV or SC every other day for 3 treatments (Post & Keller 2000)

b) 100 mg with 1–gram sodium sulfate by mouth daily (Debuf 1991)

c) 200 mg ammonium or sodium molybdate plus 500 mg of sodium thiosulfate given daily PO for up to 3 weeks (Thompson & Buck 1993)

d) Ammonium tetrathiomolybdate: 1.7 mg/kg IV or 3.4 mg/kg SC every other day for 3 treatments. Alternatively, ammonium molybdate 50–500 mg PO once daily and sodium thiosulfate 300–1000 mg PO once daily for 3 weeks. (Plumlee 1996)

e) Ammonium tetrathiomolybdate: 2–15 mg/kg IV q24h (once daily) for 3-6 days. (Boileau 2009)

Dosage Forms/Regulatory Status/Synonyms

VETERINARY-LABELED PRODUCTS: None.

Note: Ammonium Molybdate or ammonium tetrathiomolybdate can be obtained from various chemical supply houses, but it is recommended to contact the FDA before treating for guidance when contemplating using molybdate.

HUMAN-LABELED PRODUCTS:

Ammonium Molybdate Injection: 25 micrograms/mL (as 46 micrograms/mL ammonium molybdate tetrahydrate) in 10 mL vial; *Molypen®* (American Pharmaceutical Partners); generic; (Rx)

Ammonium molybdate may also be known as: *Molybdene Injectable®*, or *Molypen®*. Ammonium tetrathiomolybdate may also be known as TTM.

References

Boileau, M (2009). Challenging cases in small ruminant medicine. Proceedings: ACVIM. Accessed via: Veterinary Information Network. http://goo.gl/ZEc1Z

Debuf, YM, Ed. (1991). *The Veterinary Formulary: Handbook of Medicines Used in Veterinary Practice.* London, The Pharmaceutical Press.

Haskell, S, M Payne, et al. (2005). Farad Digest: Antidotes in Food Animal Practice. *JAVMA* 226(6): 884–887.

Haywood, S, Z Dincer, et al. (2004). Molybdenum–associated pituitary endocrinopathy in sheep associated with ammonium tetrathiomolybdate. *J Comparative Path* 130(1): 21–31.

Plumlee, K (1996). Disorders caused by toxicants: Metals and other inorganic compounds. *Large Animal Internal Medicine 2nd Ed.* B Smith Ed., Mosby: 1902–1908.

Post, L & W Keller (2000). Current status of food animal antidotes. *The Veterinary Clinics of North America: Food Animal Practice* 16:3(November).

Thompson, JR & WB Buck (1993). Copper–Molybdenum Toxicosis. *Current Veterinary Therapy 3: Food Animal Practice.* JL Howard Ed. Philadelphia, W.B. Saunders: 396–398.

AMOXICILLIN

(a-mox-i-*sill*-in) Amoxil®, Amoxi-Tabs®

AMINOPENICILLIN

Prescriber Highlights

▶ Bactericidal aminopenicillin with same spectrum as ampicillin (ineffective against bacteria that produce beta-lactamase)

▶ Most likely adverse effects are GI-related, but hypersensitivity & other adverse effects rarely occur

▶ Available in oral & parenteral dosage forms in USA

Uses/Indications

The aminopenicillins have been used for a wide range of infections in various species. FDA-approved indications/species, as well as non-approved uses, are listed in the Dosages section below. According to one reference (Trepanier 2009), amoxicillin (alone) is a reasonable first choice for empiric treatment (before culture and susceptibility results are back) of abscesses in cats.

Pharmacology/Actions

Like other penicillins, amoxicillin is a time-dependent, bactericidal (usually) agent that acts by inhibiting cell wall synthesis. Although there may be some slight differences in activity against certain organisms, amoxicillin generally shares the same spectrum of activity and uses as ampicillin. Because it is better absorbed orally (in non-ruminants), higher serum levels may be attained than with ampicillin.

Penicillins are usually bactericidal against susceptible bacteria and act by inhibiting mucopeptide synthesis in the cell wall resulting in a defective barrier and an osmotically unstable spheroplast. The exact mechanism for this effect has not been definitively determined, but beta-lactam antibiotics have been shown to bind to several enzymes (carboxypeptidases, transpeptidases, endopeptidases) within the bacterial cytoplasmic membrane that are involved with cell wall synthesis. The different affinities that various beta-lactam antibiotics have for these enzymes (also known as penicillin-binding proteins; PBPs) help explain the differences in spectrums of activity the drugs have that are not explained by the influence of beta-lactamases. Like other beta-lactam antibiotics, penicillins are generally considered more effective against actively growing bacteria.

The aminopenicillins, also called the "broad-spectrum" or ampicillin penicillins, have increased activity against many strains of gram-negative aerobes not covered by either the natural penicillins or penicillinase-resistant penicillins, including some strains of *E. coli*, Klebsiella, and Haemophilus. Like the natural penicillins, they are susceptible to inactivation by beta-lactamase-producing bacteria (*e.g.*, *Staph aureus*). Although not as active as the natural penicillins, they do have activity against many anaerobic bacteria, including Clostridial organisms. Organisms that are generally not susceptible include *Pseudomonas aeruginosa*, Serratia, Indole-positive Proteus (*Proteus mirabilis* is susceptible), Enterobacter, Citrobacter, and Acinetobacter. The aminopenicillins also are inactive against Rickettsia, mycobacteria, fungi, Mycoplasma, and viruses.

In order to reduce the inactivation of penicillins by beta-lactamases, potassium clavulanate and sulbactam have been developed to inactivate these enzymes and thus extend the spectrum of those penicillins. When used with a penicillin, these combinations are often effective against many beta-lactamase-producing strains of otherwise resistant *E. coli, Pasturella* spp., *Staphylococcus* spp., Klebsiella, and Proteus. Type I beta-lactamases that are often associated with *E. coli*, Enterobacter, and Pseudomonas are not generally inhibited by clavulanic acid.

Pharmacokinetics

Amoxicillin trihydrate is relatively stable in the presence of gastric acid. After oral administration, it is about 74–92% absorbed in humans and monogastric animals. Food will decrease the rate, but not the extent of oral absorption and many clinicians suggest giving the drug with food, particularly if there is concomitant associated GI distress. Amoxicillin serum levels will generally be 1.5–3 times greater than those of ampicillin after equivalent oral doses.

After absorption, the volume of distribution for amoxicillin is approximately 0.3 L/kg in humans and 0.2 L/kg in dogs. The drug is widely distributed to many tissues, including liver, lungs, prostate (human), muscle, bile, and ascitic, pleural and synovial fluids. Amoxicillin will cross into the CSF when meninges are inflamed in concentrations that may range from 10–60% of those found in serum. Very low levels of the drug are found in the aqueous humor, and low levels found in tears, sweat and saliva. Amoxicillin crosses the placenta, but it is thought to be relatively safe to use during pregnancy. It is approximately 17–20% bound to human plasma proteins, primarily albumin. Protein binding in dogs is approximately 13%. Milk levels of amoxicillin are considered low.

Amoxicillin is eliminated primarily through renal mechanisms, principally by tubular secretion, but some of the drug is metabolized by hydrolysis to penicilloic acids (inactive) and then excreted in the urine. Elimination half-lives of amoxicillin have been reported as 45–90 minutes in dogs and cats, and 90 minutes in cattle. Clearance is reportedly 1.9 mL/kg/min in dogs.

Contraindications/Precautions/Warnings

Penicillins are contraindicated in patients with a history of hypersensitivity to them. Because there may be cross-reactivity, use penicillins cautiously in patients who are documented hypersensitive to other beta-lactam antibiotics (*e.g.*, cephalosporins, cefamycins, carbapenems).

Do not administer penicillins, cephalosporins, or macrolides to rabbits, guinea pigs, chinchillas, hamsters, etc. or serious enteritis and clostridial enterotoxemia may occur.

Do not administer systemic antibiotics orally in patients with septicemia, shock, or other grave illnesses as absorption of the medication from the GI tract may be significantly delayed or diminished. Parenteral (preferably IV) routes should be used for these cases.

Adverse Effects

Adverse effects with the penicillins are usually not serious and have a relatively low frequency of occurrence.

Hypersensitivity reactions unrelated to dose can occur with these agents and can manifest as rashes, fever, eosinophilia, neutropenia, agranulocytosis, thrombocytopenia, leukopenia, anemias, lymphadenopathy, or full-blown anaphylaxis.

When given orally, penicillins may cause GI effects (anorexia, vomiting, diarrhea). Because the penicillins may alter gut flora, antibiotic-associated diarrhea can occur and allow the proliferation of resistant bacteria in the colon (superinfections). Healthy dogs given oral amoxicillin had their gut flora altered with a shift in balance toward gram-negative bacteria that included resistant *Enterobacteriaceae* species (Gronvold *et al.* 2010).

High doses or very prolonged use have been associated with neurotoxicity (*e.g.*, ataxia in dogs). Although the penicillins are not considered hepatotoxic, elevated liver enzymes have been reported. Other effects reported in dogs include tachypnea, dyspnea, edema and tachycardia.

Reproductive/Nursing Safety

Penicillins have been shown to cross the placenta; safe use during pregnancy has not been firmly established, but neither have there been any documented teratogenic problems associated with these drugs. However, use only when the potential benefits outweigh the risks. In humans, the FDA categorizes this drug as category *B* for use during pregnancy (*Animal studies have not yet demonstrated risk to the fetus, but there are no adequate studies in pregnant women; or animal studies have shown an adverse effect, but adequate studies in pregnant women have not demonstrated a risk to the fetus in the first trimester of pregnancy, and there is no evidence of risk in later trimesters.*) In a separate system evaluating the safety of drugs in canine and feline pregnancy (Papich 1989), this drug is categorized as in class: *A* (*Probably safe. Although specific studies may not have proved the safety of all drugs in dogs and cats, there are no reports of adverse effects in laboratory animals or women.*)

Overdosage/Acute Toxicity

Acute oral penicillin overdoses are unlikely to cause significant problems other than GI distress but other effects are possible (see Adverse Effects). In humans, very high dosages of parenteral penicillins, especially in patients with renal disease, have induced CNS effects.

Drug Interactions

The following drug interactions have either been reported or are theoretical in humans or animals receiving amoxicillin and may be of significance in veterinary patients:

■ **BACTERIOSTATIC ANTIMICROBIALS (e.g., chloramphenicol, erythromycin and other macrolides, tetracyclines, sulfonamides, etc.):** Because there is evidence of *in vitro* antagonism between beta-lactam antibiotics and bacteriostatic antibiotics, use together has been generally not recommended in the past, but actual clinical importance is not clear and in doubt.

■ **METHOTREXATE:** Amoxicillin may decrease the renal excretion of MTX causing increased levels and potential toxic effects.

■ **PROBENECID:** Competitively blocks the tubular secretion of most penicillins, thereby increasing serum levels and serum half-lives.

Laboratory Considerations

■ Amoxicillin may cause false-positive **urine glucose determinations** when using cupric sulfate solution (Benedict's Solution, *Clinitest®*). Tests utilizing glucose oxidase (*Tes-Tape®, Clinistix®*) are not affected by amoxicillin.

■ As penicillins and other beta-lactams can inactivate **aminoglycosides** *in vitro* (and *in vivo* in patients in renal failure), serum concentrations of aminoglycosides may be falsely decreased if the patient is also receiving beta-lactam antibiotics and the serum is stored prior to analysis. It is recommended that if the assay is delayed, samples be frozen and, if possible, drawn at times when the beta-lactam antibiotic is at a trough.

Doses

■ **DOGS:**

For susceptible infections:

a) For Gram-positive infections: 10 mg/kg PO, IM, SC twice daily for at least 2 days after symptoms subside.

For Gram-negative infections: 20 mg/kg PO three times daily or IM, SC twice daily for at least 2 days after symptoms subside (Aucoin 2000)

b) For susceptible UTI's: 10–20 mg/kg PO q12h for 5–7 days.

For susceptible systemic infections (bacteremia/sepsis): 22–30 mg/kg IV, IM, SC q8h for 7 days.

For susceptible orthopedic infections: 22–30 mg/kg IV, IM, SC, or PO q6–8h for 7–10 days. (Greene *et al.* 2006)

c) For Lyme disease: 22 mg/kg PO q12h for 21–28 days (Appel & Jacobson 1995)

d) For susceptible urinary tract infections: 11 mg/kg PO q8h. For preventative therapy for repeated (>2 per 6 months) urinary tract Gram-positive bacterial infections: 20 mg/kg PO once daily before bedtime after the dog has urinated. Use only after effective treatment completed using full therapeutic doses. (Adams 2009)

■ **CATS:**

For susceptible infections:

a) For Gram-positive infections: 10 mg/kg PO, IM, SC twice daily for at least 2 days after symptoms subside.

For Gram-negative infections: 20 mg/kg PO three times daily or IM, SC twice daily for at least 2 days after symptoms subside) (Aucoin 2000)

b) For susceptible UTI's and soft tissue infections: 50 mg (total dose per cat) or 11–22 mg/kg PO once daily for 5–7 days.

For sepsis: 10–20 mg/kg IV, SC, or PO q12h for as long as necessary. **Note:** Duration of treatment are general guidelines, generally treat for at least 2 days after all signs of infection are gone. (Greene *et al.* 2006)

c) *C. perfringens*, bacterial overgrowth (GI): 22 mg/kg PO once daily for 5 days (Lappin 2000)

d) *C. perfringens* enterotoxicosis: 11–22 mg/kg PO two to three times daily for 7 days (Leib 2004)

e) For treating *H. pylori* infections using triple therapy: amoxicillin 20 mg/kg PO twice daily for 14 days; metronidazole 10–15 mg/kg PO twice daily; clarithromycin 7.5 mg/kg PO twice daily (Simpson 2003)

■ **FERRETS:**

For eliminating Helicobacter gastritis infections:

a) Using triple therapy: Metronidazole 22 mg/kg, amoxicillin 22 mg/kg and bismuth subsalicylate (original *Pepto-Bismol*®) 17.6 mg/kg PO. Give each 3 times daily for 3–4 weeks. (Hall & Simpson 2000)

b) Using triple therapy: Metronidazole 20 mg/kg PO q12h, amoxicillin 20 mg/kg PO q12h and bismuth subsalicylate 17.5 mg/kg PO q8h. Give 21 days. Sucralfate (25 mg/kg PO q8h) and famotidine (0.5 mg/kg PO once daily) are also

used. Fluids and assisted feeding should be continued while the primary cause of disease is investigated. (Johnson 2006)

For susceptible infections:

a) 10–35 mg/kg PO or SC twice daily (Williams 2000)

■ **RABBITS/RODENTS/SMALL MAMMALS:**

Note: See warning above in Contraindications

a) Hedgehogs: 15 mg/kg IM or PO q12h (Smith 2000)

■ **CATTLE:**

For susceptible infections:

a) 6–10 mg/kg SC or IM q24h (Withdrawal time = 30 days) (Jenkins 1986)

b) For respiratory infections: 11 mg/kg IM or SC q12h (Hjerpe 1986), (Beech 1987b)

c) Calves: Amoxicillin trihydrate: 7 mg/kg PO q8–12h (Baggot 1983)

■ **HORSES:**

For susceptible infections:

a) For respiratory infections: 20–30 mg/kg PO q6h (Beech 1987a)

b) Foals: Amoxicillin Sodium: 15–30 mg/kg IV or IM q6–8h; amoxicillin trihydrate suspension: 25–40 mg/kg PO q8h; amoxicillin/clavulanate 15–25 mg/kg IV q6–8h (Brumbaugh 1999)

■ **BIRDS:**

For susceptible infections:

a) 125 mg/kg q12h PO. Mix oral solution to double strength to a final concentration of 125 mg/mL. (Antinoff 2009)

b) 100 mg/kg q8h, IM, SC, PO (Hoeffer 1995)

c) Ratites: 15–22 mg/kg PO twice daily; in drinking water: 250 mg/gallon for 3–5 days (Jenson 1998)

■ **REPTILES:**

For susceptible infections:

a) For all species: 22 mg/kg PO q12–24h; not very useful unless used in combination with aminoglycosides (Gauvin 1993)

Monitoring

■ Because penicillins usually have minimal toxicity associated with their use, monitoring for efficacy is usually all that is required unless toxic signs develop. Serum levels and therapeutic drug monitoring are not routinely done with these agents.

Client Information

■ The oral suspension should preferably be refrigerated, but refrigeration is not absolutely necessary; any unused oral suspension should be discarded after 14 days

■ Amoxicillin may be administered orally without regard to feeding status

■ If the animal develops gastrointestinal symptoms (*e.g.*, vomiting, anorexia), giving with food may be of benefit

Chemistry/Synonyms

An aminopenicillin, amoxicillin is commercially available as the trihydrate. It occurs as a practically odorless, white, crystalline powder that is sparingly soluble in water. Amoxicillin differs structurally from ampicillin only by having an additional hydroxyl group on the phenyl ring.

Amoxicillin may also be known as: amoxycillin, p-hydroxyampicillin, or BRL 2333; many trade names are available.

Storage/Stability

Amoxicillin capsules, tablets, and powder for oral suspension should be stored at room temperature (15–30°C) in tight containers. After reconstitution, the oral suspension should preferably be refrigerated (refrigeration not absolutely necessary) and any unused product discarded after 14 days.

Dosage Forms/Regulatory Status/Withdrawal Times

VETERINARY-LABELED PRODUCTS:

Amoxicillin Oral Tablets: 50 mg, 100 mg, 150 mg, 200 mg, & 400 mg; *Amoxi-Tabs®* (Pfizer); (Rx). FDA-approved for use in dogs and cats.

Amoxicillin Powder for Oral Suspension 50 mg/mL (after reconstitution) in 15 mL or 30 mL bottles; *Amoxi-Drop®* (Pfizer); (Rx). FDA-approved for use in dogs and cats.

Amoxicillin Intramammary Infusion 62.5 mg/syringe in 10 mL syringes; *Amoxi-Mast®* (Schering-Plough); (Rx). FDA-approved for use in lactating dairy cattle. Slaughter withdrawal (when administered as labeled) = 12 days; Milk withdrawal (when administered as labeled) = 60 hours.

HUMAN-LABELED PRODUCTS:

Amoxicillin Oral Tablets (chewable): 125 mg, 200 mg, 250 mg, & 400 mg; *Amoxil®* (GlaxoSmithKline); generic; (Rx)

Amoxicillin Oral Tablets: 500 mg & 875 mg; *Amoxil®* (GlaxoSmithKline); generic; (Rx)

Amoxicillin Oral Capsules: 250 mg & 500 mg; *Amoxil®* (GlaxoSmithKline); generic; (Rx)

Amoxicillin Powder for Oral Suspension: 200 mg/5 mL in 50 mL, 75 mL & 100 mL; 250 mg/5 mL in 80 mL, 100 mL & 150 mL; 400 mg/5 mL in 50 mL, 75 mL & 100 mL; *Amoxil®* (GlaxoSmithKline); *Trimox®* (Sandoz); generic; (Rx)

Amoxicillin Oral Extended-Release Tablets: 775 mg in 30s & UD 10s; *Moxatag®* (Middlebrook) (Rx)

References

Adams, L (2009). Recurrent Urinary Tract Infections: Bad Bugs That Won't Go Away. Proceedings: WVC. Accessed via: Veterinary Information Network. http://goo.gl/eX3w6

Antinoff, N (2009). Avian Critical Care: What's Old, What's New. Proceedings: IVECCS. Accessed via: Veterinary Information Network. http://goo.gl/WVvLn

Appel, M & R Jacobson (1995). CVT Update: Canine Lyme Disease. *Kirk's Current Veterinary Therapy:XII.* J Bonagura Ed. Philadelphia, W.B. Saunders: 303–309.

Aucoin, D (2000). Antimicrobial Drug Formulary. *Target: The antimicrobial guide to effective treatment*Port Huron, MI, North American Compendiums Inc: 93–142.

Baggot, JD (1983). Systemic antimicrobial therapy in large animals. *Pharmacological Basis of Large Animal Medicine.* JA Bogan, P Lees and AT Yoxall Eds. Oxford, Blackwell Scientific Publications: 45–69.

Beech, J (1987a). Drug therapy of respiratory disorders. *Vet Clin North Am (Equine Practice)* 3(1): 59–80.

Beech, J (1987b). Respiratory Tract—Horse, Cow. *The Bristol Handbook of Antimicrobial Therapy.* DE Johnston Ed. Evansville, Veterinary Learning Systems: 88–109.

Brumbaugh, G (1999). Clinical Pharmacology and the Pediatric Patient. 45th Annual AAEP Convention, Albuquerque.

Gauvin, J (1993). Drug therapy in reptiles. *Seminars in Avian & Exotic Med* 2(1): 48–59.

Greene, C, K Hartmannn, et al. (2006). Appendix 8: Antimicrobial Drug Formulary. *Infectious Disease of the Dog and Cat.* C Greene Ed., Elsevier: 1186–1333.

Gronvold, AMR, TM L'Abee-Lund, et al. (2010). Changes in fecal microbiota of healthy dogs administered amoxicillin. *Fems Microbiology Ecology* 71(2): 313–326.

Hall, E & K Simpson (2000). Diseases of the Small Intestine. *Textbook of Veterinary Internal Medicine: Diseases of the Dog and Cat.* S Ettinger and E Feldman Eds. Philadelphia, WB Saunders. 2: 1182–1238.

Hjerpe, CA (1986). The bovine respiratory disease complex. *Current Veterinary Therapy: Food Animal Practice 2.* JL Howard Ed. Philadelphia, W.B. Saunders: 670–681.

Hoeffer, H (1995). Antimicrobials in pet birds. *Kirk's Current Veterinary Therapy:XII.* J Bonagura Ed. Philadelphia, W.B. Saunders: 1278–1283.

Jenkins, WL (1986). Antimicrobial Therapy. *Current Veterinary Therapy: Food Animal Practice 2.* JL Howard Ed. Philadelphia, W.B. Saunders: 8–23.

Jenson, J (1998). Current ratite therapy. *The Veterinary Clinics of North America: Food Animal Practice* 16:3(November).

Johnson, D (2006). Ferrets: the other companion animal. Proceedings: ACVC. Accessed via: Veterinary Information Network. http://goo.gl/bSeol

Lappin, M (2000). Infectious causes of feline diarrhea. The North American Veterinary Conference, Orlando.

Leib, M (2004). Chronic idiopathic large bowel diarrhea in dogs. Proceedings: ACVIM Forum. Accessed via: Veterinary Information Network. http://goo.gl/Nwoz8

Simpson, K (2003). Intragastric warfare in Helicobacter infected cats. Proceedings: ACVIM Forum. Accessed via: Veterinary Information Network. http://goo.gl/gSR3T

Smith, A (2000). General husbandry and medical care of hedgehogs. *Kirk's Current Veterinary Therapy: XIII Small Animal Practice.* J Bonagura Ed. Philadelphia, WB Saunders: 1128–1133.

Trepanier, L (2009). Appropriate empirical antimicrobial therapy: Making decisions without a culture. Proceedings: ACVIM. Accessed via: Veterinary Information Network. http://goo.gl/HWfc7

Williams, B (2000). Therapeutics in Ferrets. *Vet Clin NA: Exotic Anim Pract* 3:1(Jan): 131–153.

AMOXICILLIN/ CLAVULANATE POTASSIUM AMOXICILLIN/ CLAVULANIC ACID

(a-mox-i-*sill*-in clav-yue-*lan*-ate)

Clavamox®, Augmentin®

POTENTIATED AMINOPENICILLIN

Prescriber Highlights

▶ Bactericidal aminopenicillin with beta-lactamase inhibitor that expands its spectrum. Not effective against Pseudomonas or Enterobacter

▶ Most likely adverse effects are GI related, but hypersensitivity & other adverse effects rarely occur

Uses/Indications

Amoxicillin/potassium clavulanate tablets and oral suspension products are FDA-approved for use in dogs and cats for the treatment of urinary tract, skin and soft tissue infections caused by susceptible organisms. It is also indicated for canine periodontal disease due to susceptible strains of bacteria. According to one reference (Trepanier 2009), amoxicillin + clavulanate is a reasonable first choice for empiric treatment (before culture and susceptibility results are back) of bacterial cystitis in female dogs, and hepatobiliary infections (with a fluoroquinolone) in dogs or cats.

Pharmacology/Actions

For information on the pharmacology/actions of amoxicillin, refer that monograph.

Clavulanic acid has only weak antibacterial activity when used alone and presently it is only available in fixed-dose combinations with either amoxicillin (oral) or ticarcillin (parenteral). Clavulanic acid acts by competitively and irreversibly binding to beta-lactamases, including types II, III, IV, and V, and penicillinases produced by Staphylococcus. Staphylococci that are resistant to penicillinase-resistant penicillins (*e.g.*, oxacillin) are considered resistant to amoxicillin/potassium clavulanate, although susceptibility testing may indicate otherwise. Amoxicillin/potassium clavulanate is usually ineffective against type I cephalosporinases. These plasmid-mediated cephalosporinases are often produced by members of the family Enterobacteriaceae, particularly *Pseudomonas aeruginosa*. When combined with amoxicillin, there is little if any synergistic activity against organisms already susceptible to amoxicillin, but amoxicillin-resistant strains (due to beta-lactamase inactivation) may be covered.

When performing Kirby-Bauer susceptibility testing, the *Augmentin®* (human-product trade name) disk is often used. Because the amoxicillin:clavulanic acid ratio of 2:1 in the susceptibility tests may not correspond to *in vivo* drug levels, susceptibility testing may not always accurately predict efficacy for this combination.

Pharmacokinetics

The pharmacokinetics of amoxicillin are presented in that drug's monograph. There is no evidence to suggest that the addition of clavulanic acid significantly alters amoxicillin pharmacokinetics.

Clavulanate potassium is relatively stable in the presence of gastric acid and is readily absorbed. In dogs, the absorption half-life is reportedly 0.39 hours with peak levels occurring about 1 hour after dosing. Specific bioavailability data for dogs or cats was not located.

Clavulanic acid has an apparent volume of distribution of 0.32 L/kg in dogs and is distributed (with amoxicillin) into the lungs, pleural fluid and peritoneal fluid. Low concentrations of both drugs are found in the saliva, sputum and CSF (uninflamed meninges). Higher concentrations in the CSF are expected when meninges are inflamed, but it is questionable whether therapeutic levels are attainable. Clavulanic acid is 13% bound to proteins in dog serum. The drug readily crosses the placenta but is not believed to be teratogenic. Clavulanic acid and amoxicillin are both found in milk in low concentrations.

Clavulanic acid is apparently extensively metabolized in the dog (and rat) primarily to 1-amino-4-hydroxybutan-2-one. It is not known if this compound possesses any beta-lactamase inhibiting activity. The drug is also excreted unchanged in the urine via glomerular filtration. In dogs, 34–52% of a dose is excreted in the urine as unchanged drug and metabolites, 25–27% eliminated in the feces, and 16–33% into respired air. Urine levels of active drug are considered high, but may be only 1/5th of those of amoxicillin.

Contraindications/Precautions/Warnings

Penicillins are contraindicated in patients with a history of hypersensitivity to them. Because there may be cross-reactivity, use penicillins cautiously in patients who are documented hypersensitive to other beta-lactam antibiotics (*e.g.*, cephalosporins, cefamycins, carbapenems).

Do not administer systemic antibiotics orally in patients with septicemia, shock, or other grave illnesses as absorption of the medication from the GI tract may be significantly delayed or diminished.

Do not administer penicillins, cephalosporins, or macrolides to rabbits, guinea pigs, chinchillas, hamsters, etc. or serious enteritis and clostridial enterotoxemia may occur.

Adverse Effects

Adverse effects with the penicillins are usually not serious and have a relatively low frequency of occurrence.

Hypersensitivity reactions unrelated to dose can occur with these agents and can manifest as rashes, fever, eosinophilia, neutropenia, agranulocytosis, thrombocytopenia, leukopenia, anemias, lymphadenopathy, or full-blown anaphylaxis.

When given orally, penicillins may cause GI effects (anorexia, vomiting, diarrhea). Because the penicillins may alter gut flora, antibiotic-associated diarrhea can occur and allow the proliferation of resistant bacteria in the colon (superinfections).

Neurotoxicity (e.g., ataxia in dogs) has been associated with very high doses or very prolonged use. Although the penicillins are not considered hepatotoxic, elevated liver enzymes have been reported. Other effects reported in dogs include tachypnea; dyspnea, edema and tachycardia.

Reproductive/Nursing Safety

In humans, the FDA categorizes this drug as category *B* for use during pregnancy (*Animal studies have not yet demonstrated risk to the fetus, but there are no adequate studies in pregnant women; or animal studies have shown an adverse effect, but adequate studies in pregnant women have not demonstrated a risk to the fetus in the first trimester of pregnancy, and there is no evidence of risk in later trimesters.*) In a separate system evaluating the safety of drugs in canine and feline pregnancy (Papich 1989), this drug is categorized as in class: *A* (*Probably safe. Although specific studies may not have proved the safety of all drugs in dogs and cats, there are no reports of adverse effects in laboratory animals or women.*)

Overdosage/Acute Toxicity

Acute oral penicillin overdoses are unlikely to cause significant problems other than GI distress, but other effects are possible (see Adverse Effects). In humans, very high dosages of parenteral penicillins, especially in patients with renal disease, have induced CNS effects.

Drug Interactions

The following drug interactions have either been reported or are theoretical in humans or animals receiving amoxicillin-clavulanate and may be of significance in veterinary patients:

■ **BACTERIOSTATIC ANTIMICROBIALS (e.g., chloramphenicol, erythromycin and other macrolides, tetracyclines, sulfonamides, etc.):** Because there is evidence of *in vitro* antagonism between beta-lactam antibiotics and bacteriostatic antibiotics, use together has been generally not recommended in the past, but actual clinical importance is not clear and currently in doubt.

■ **METHOTREXATE:** Amoxicillin may decrease the renal excretion of MTX causing increased levels and potential toxic effects

■ **PROBENECID:** Competitively blocks the tubular secretion of most penicillins, thereby increasing serum levels and serum half-lives

Laboratory Considerations

■ Amoxicillin may cause false-positive **urine glucose determinations** when using cupric sulfate solution (Benedict's Solution, *Clinitest®*). Tests utilizing glucose oxidase (*Tes-Tape®, Clinistix®*) are not affected by amoxicillin.

■ As penicillins and other beta-lactams can inactivate **aminoglycosides** *in vitro* (and *in vivo* in patients in renal failure), serum concentrations of aminoglycosides may be falsely decreased if the patient is also receiving beta-lactam antibiotics and the serum is stored prior to analysis. It is recommended that if the assay is delayed, samples be frozen and, if possible, drawn at times when the beta-lactam antibiotic is at a trough.

Doses

Note: All doses are for combined quantities of both drugs (unless noted otherwise).

■ **DOGS:**

For susceptible infections:

a) 13.75 mg/kg PO twice daily; do not exceed 30 days of therapy (Package insert; *Clavamox®*—Pfizer)

b) For susceptible UTI's: 12.5 mg/kg PO q12h for 5−7 days

For susceptible skin, soft tissue infections: 12.5 mg/kg PO q12h for 5−7 days (may need to extend to 21 days; do not exceed past 30 days). Much higher doses have been recommended for resistant skin infections.

For susceptible deep pyodermas: 12.5 mg/kg PO q12h for 14−120 days

For systemic bacteremia: 22 mg/kg PO q8−12h for 7 days

Note: Duration of treatments are general guidelines; generally treat for at least 2 days after all signs of infection are gone. (Greene *et al.* 2006)

c) For Gram-positive infections: 10 mg/kg PO twice daily

For Gram-negative infections: 20 mg/kg PO three times daily (Aucoin 2000)

d) For non-superficial pyoderma: 10−25 mg/kg PO twice daily for 3−6 weeks. Maximum dose is 650 mg twice daily. Increase to three times daily if no response in 1 week. If no response by the 2nd week, discontinue. (Aucoin 2002)

e) For recurrent pyoderma: 13.75−22 mg/kg PO q8−12h (Hillier 2006)

f) For pyoderma: 22 mg/kg PO twice daily or 13.75 mg/kg PO q8h (Rosenkrantz 2009)

g) For susceptible urinary tract infections: 12.5 mg/kg PO q8h (Adams 2009)

■ **CATS:**

For susceptible infections:

a) 62.5 mg/cat PO twice daily; do not exceed 30 days of therapy (Package insert; *Clavamox®*—Pfizer)

b) For Gram-positive infections: 10 mg/kg PO twice daily;

For Gram-negative infections: 20 mg/kg PO three times daily (Aucoin 2000)

c) For susceptible UTI's: 62.5 mg/cat (total dose) PO q12h for 10–30 days;

For susceptible skin, soft tissue infections: 62.5 mg/cat (total dose) or 10–20 mg/kg PO q12h for 5–7 days;

For susceptible sepsis, pneumonia: 10–20 mg/kg PO q8h for 7–10 days

Note: Duration of treatment are general guidelines, generally treat for at least 2 days after all signs of infection are gone. (Greene *et al.* 2006)

■ **FERRETS:**

For susceptible infections:

a) 10–20 mg/kg PO 2–3 times daily (Williams 2000)

■ **BIRDS:**

For susceptible infections:

a) 50–100 mg/kg PO q6–8h (Hoeffer 1995)

b) Ratites: 10–15 mg/kg PO twice daily (Jenson 1998)

Client Information

■ The oral suspension should preferably be refrigerated, but refrigeration is not absolutely necessary; any unused oral suspension should be discarded after 10 days

■ Amoxicillin/clavulanate may be administered orally without regard to feeding status

■ If the animal develops gastrointestinal symptoms (*e.g.*, vomiting, anorexia), giving with food may be of benefit

Monitoring

■ Because penicillins usually have minimal toxicity associated with their use, monitoring for efficacy is usually all that is required unless toxic signs or symptoms develop. Serum levels and therapeutic drug monitoring are not routinely performed with these agents.

Chemistry/Synonyms

A beta-lactamase inhibitor, clavulanate potassium occurs as an off-white, crystalline powder that has a pK_a of 2.7 (as the acid) and is very soluble in water and slightly soluble in alcohol at room temperatures. Although available in commercially available preparations as the potassium salt, potency is expressed in terms of clavulanic acid.

Amoxicillin may also be known as: amoxycillin, p-hydroxyampicillin, or BRL 2333; many trade names are available. Clavulanate potassium may also be known as: clavulanic acid, BRL-14151K, or kalii clavulanas.

Storage/Stability

Clavulanate products should be stored at temperatures less than 24°C (75°F) in tight containers. Potassium clavulanate is reportedly very susceptible to moisture and should be protected from excessive humidity.

After reconstitution, oral suspensions are stable for 10 days when refrigerated. Unused portions should be discarded after that time. If kept at room temperature, suspensions are reportedly stable for 48 hours. The veterinary oral suspension should be reconstituted by adding 14 mL of water and shaking vigorously; refrigerate and discard any unused portion after 10 days.

Dosage Forms/Regulatory Status

VETERINARY-LABELED PRODUCTS:

Oral Tablets (4:1 ratio):

62.5 mg: Amoxicillin 50 mg/12.5 mg clavulanic acid (as the potassium salt)

125 mg: Amoxicillin 100 mg/25 mg clavulanic acid (as the potassium salt)

250 mg: Amoxicillin 200 mg/50 mg clavulanic acid (as the potassium salt)

375 mg: Amoxicillin 300 mg/75 mg clavulanic acid (as the potassium salt); *Clavamox Tablets®* (Pfizer); (Rx). FDA-approved for use in dogs and cats.

Powder for Oral Suspension:

Amoxicillin 50 mg/12.5 mg clavulanic acid (as the potassium salt) per mL in 15 mL dropper bottles; *Clavamox® Drops* (Pfizer); (Rx). FDA-approved for use in dogs and cats.

HUMAN-LABELED PRODUCTS:

Note: Human-labeled amoxicillin/clavulanate products have varying ratios of amoxicillin: clavulanate ranging from 2:1 to 7:1.

Amoxicillin (as trihydrate)/Clavulanic Acid (as potassium salt) Tablets: Amoxicillin 250 mg/125 mg clavulanic acid; Amoxicillin 500 mg/125 mg clavulanic acid; Amoxicillin 875 mg/125 mg clavulanic acid; *Augmentin®* (GlaxoSmithKline); generic (Rx)

Chewable Tablets: Amoxicillin 125 mg/31.25 mg clavulanic acid; Amoxicillin 200 mg/28.5 mg clavulanic acid; 250 mg/62.5 mg clavulanic acid & 400 mg/57 mg clavulanic acid; *Augmentin®* (GlaxoSmithKline); generic; (Rx)

Powder for Oral Suspension—Amoxicillin/Clavulanic Acid (as potassium salt) after reconstitution: Amoxicillin 125 mg/31.25 mg clavulanic acid per 5 mL in 75 mL, 100 mL & 150 mL; Amoxicillin 200 mg/28.5 mg clavulanic acid per 5 mL in 50 mL, 75 mL & 100 mL; Amoxicillin 250 mg/62.5 mg clavulanic acid per 5 mL in 75 mL, 100 mL & 150 mL; Amoxicillin 400 mg/57 mg clavulanic acid per 5 mL in 50 mL, 75 mL & 100 mL; 600 mg/42.9 mg clavulanic acid per 5 mL in 75 mL, 100 mL, 125 mL & 200 mL; *Augmentin®* & *Augmentin ES-600®* (GlaxoSmithKline); *Amoclan®* (West-ward); generic; (Rx)

References

Adams, L (2009). Recurrent Urinary Tract Infections: Bad Bugs That Won't Go Away. Proceedings: WVC. Accessed via: Veterinary Information Network. http://goo.gl/eX3w6

Aucoin, D (2000). Antimicrobial Drug Formulary. *Target: The antimicrobial guide to effective treatment*Port Huron, MI, North American Compendiums Inc: 93–142.

Aucoin, D (2002). Rational antimicrobial therapy in dermatitis (including Otitis Externa). Proceedings: Atlantic Coast Veterinary Conference. Accessed via: Veterinary Information Network.

Greene, C, K Hartmannn, et al. (2006). Appendix 8: Antimicrobial Drug Formulary. *Infectious Disease of the Dog and Cat*. C Greene Ed., Elsevier: 1186–1333.

Hillier, A (2006). Antibiotic therapy for pyoderma. Proceedings: ACVC. Accessed via: Veterinary Information Network. http://goo.gl/uLSKY

Hoeffer, H (1995). Antimicrobials in pet birds. *Kirk's Current Veterinary Therapy:XII*. J Bonagura Ed. Philadelphia, W.B. Saunders: 1278–1283.

Jenson, J (1998). Current ratite therapy. *The Veterinary Clinics of North America: Food Animal Practice* 16:3(November).

Rosenkrantz, W (2009). Pyoderma: Topical and Systemic Treatment. Proceedings: Western Veterinary Conference. Accessed via: Veterinary Information Network. http://goo.gl/Y2VCi

Trepanier, L (2009). Appropriate empirical antimicrobial therapy: Making decisions without a culture. Proceedings: ACVIM. Accessed via: Veterinary Information Network. http://goo.gl/HWfc7

Williams, B (2000). Therapeutics in Ferrets. *Vet Clin NA: Exotic Anim Pract* 3:1(Jan): 131–153.

AMPHOTERICIN B DESOXYCHOLATE AMPHOTERICIN B LIPID-BASED

(am-foe-*ter*-i-sin *bee*) Abelcet®, Fungizone®

ANTIFUNGAL

Prescriber Highlights

▶ Systemic antifungal used for serious mycotic infections

▶ Must be administered IV

▶ Nephrotoxicity is biggest concern (not in birds), particularly with the deoxycholate form; newer lipid based products are less nephrotoxic & penetrate into tissues better, but are more expensive

▶ Renal function monitoring essential

▶ Drug interactions

Uses/Indications

Because the potential exists for severe toxicity associated with this drug, it should only be used for progressive, potentially fatal fungal infections. Veterinary use of amphotericin has been primarily in dogs, but other species have been treated successfully. For further information on fungal diseases treated, see the Pharmacology and Dosage sections.

The liposomal form of amphotericin B can be used to treat Leishmaniasis.

Pharmacology/Actions

Amphotericin B is usually fungistatic, but can be fungicidal against some organisms depending on drug concentration. It acts by binding to sterols (primarily ergosterol) in the cell membrane and alters the permeability of the membrane allowing intracellular potassium and other cellular constituents to "leak out." Because bacteria and rickettsia do not contain sterols, amphotericin B has no activity against those organisms. Mammalian cell membranes do contain sterols (primarily cholesterol) and the drug's toxicity may be a result of a similar mechanism of action, although amphotericin binds less strongly to cholesterol than ergosterol.

Amphotericin B has *in vitro* activity against a variety of fungal organisms, including Blastomyces, Aspergillus, Paracoccidioides, Coccidioides, Histoplasma, Cryptococcus, Mucor, and Sporothrix. Zygomycetes is reportedly variable in its response to amphotericin. Aspergillosis in dogs and cats does not tend to respond satisfactorily to amphotericin therapy. Additionally, amphotericin B has *in vivo* activity against some protozoa species, including *Leishmania* spp. and *Naegleria* spp.

It has been reported that amphotericin B has immunoadjuvant properties but further work is necessary to confirm the clinical significance of this effect.

Pharmacokinetics

Pharmacokinetic data on veterinary species is apparently unavailable. In humans (and presumably animals), amphotericin B is poorly absorbed from the GI tract and must be given parenterally to achieve sufficient concentrations to treat systemic fungal infections. After intravenous injection, the drug reportedly penetrates well into most tissues but does not penetrate well into the pancreas, muscle, bone, aqueous humor, or pleural, pericardial, synovial, and peritoneal fluids. The drug does enter the pleural cavity and joints when inflamed. CSF levels are approximately 3% of those found in the serum. Approximately 90–95% of amphotericin in the vascular compartment is bound to serum proteins. The newer "lipid" forms of amphotericin B have higher penetration into the lungs, liver and spleen than the conventional form.

The metabolic pathways of amphotericin are not known, but it exhibits biphasic elimination. An initial serum half-life of 24–48 hours, and a longer terminal half-life of about 15 days have been described. Seven weeks after therapy has stopped, amphotericin can still be detected in the urine. Approximately 2–5% of the drug is recovered in the urine in unchanged (biologically active) form.

Contraindications/Precautions/Warnings

Amphotericin is contraindicated in patients who are hypersensitive to it, unless the infection is life-threatening and no other alternative therapies are available.

Because of the serious nature of the diseases treated with systemic amphotericin, it is not contraindicated in patients with renal disease, but it should be used cautiously with adequate monitoring.

Adverse Effects

Amphotericin B is notorious for its nephrotoxic effects; most canine patients will show some degree of renal toxicity after receiving the drug. The proposed mechanism of nephrotoxicity is via renal vasoconstriction with a subsequent reduction in glomerular filtration rate. The drug may directly act as a toxin to renal epithelial cells. Renal damage may be more common, irreversible and severe in patients who receive higher individual doses or have preexisting renal disease. Usually, renal function will return to normal after treatment is halted, but may require several months to do so.

Newer forms of lipid-complexed and liposome-encapsulated amphotericin B significantly reduce the nephrotoxic qualities of the drug. Because higher dosages may be used, these forms may also have enhanced effectiveness. A study in dogs showed that amphotericin B lipid complex was 8–10 times less nephrotoxic than the conventional form.

The patient's renal function should be aggressively monitored during therapy. A pretreatment serum creatinine, BUN (serum urea nitrogen/SUN), serum electrolytes (including magnesium if possible), total plasma protein (TPP), packed cell volume (PCV), body weight, and urinalysis should be done prior to starting therapy. BUN, creatinine, PCV, TPP, and body weight are rechecked before each dose is administered. Electrolytes and urinalysis should be monitored at least weekly during the course of treatment. Several different recommendations regarding the stoppage of therapy when a certain BUN is reached have been made. Most clinicians recommend stopping, at least temporarily, amphotericin treatment if the BUN reaches 30–40 mg/dL, serum creatinine >3 mg/dL or if other clinical signs of systemic toxicity develop such as serious depression or vomiting.

At least two regimens have been used in the attempt to reduce nephrotoxicity in dogs treated with amphotericin desoxycholate. Mannitol (12.5 grams or 0.5–1 g/kg) given concurrently with amphotericin B (slow IV infusion) to dogs may reduce nephrotoxicity, but may also reduce the efficacy of the therapy, particularly in blastomycosis. Mannitol treatment also increases the total cost of therapy. Sodium loading prior to treating has garnered considerable support in recent years. A tubuloglomerular feedback mechanism that induces vasoconstriction and decreased GFR has been postulated for amphotericin B toxicity; increased sodium load at the glomerulus may help prevent that feedback. One

clinician (Foil 1986), uses 5 mL/kg of normal saline given in two portions, before and after amphotericin B dosing and states that is has been ". . . helpful in averting renal insufficiency. . . ."

Cats are apparently more sensitive to the nephrotoxic aspects of amphotericin B, and many clinicians recommend using reduced dosages in this species (see Dosage section).

Adverse effects reported in horses include: tachycardia, tachypnea, lethargy, fever, restlessness, anorexia, anemia, phlebitis, polyuria and collapse.

Other adverse effects that have been reported in mammals with amphotericin B include: anorexia, vomiting, hypokalemia, distal renal tubular acidosis, hypomagnesemia, phlebitis, cardiac arrhythmias, non-regenerative anemia and fever (may be reduced with pretreatment with NSAIDs or a low dosage of steroids). Calcinosis cutis has been reported in dogs treated with amphotericin B. Amphotericin B can increase creatine kinase levels.

In birds, nephrotoxicity does not appear to be an issue with amphotericin B use. It has been postulated that the shorter half-life of the drug noted in birds may be responsible for the lack of nephrotoxicity.

Reproductive/Nursing Safety

The safety of amphotericin B during pregnancy has not been established, but there are apparently no reports of teratogenicity associated with the drug. The risks of therapy should be weighed against the potential benefits. In humans, the FDA categorizes this drug as category *B* for use during pregnancy (*Animal studies have not yet demonstrated risk to the fetus, but there are no adequate studies in pregnant women; or animal studies have shown an adverse effect, but adequate studies in pregnant women have not demonstrated a risk to the fetus in the first trimester of pregnancy, and there is no evidence of risk in later trimesters.*) In a separate system evaluating the safety of drugs in canine and feline pregnancy (Papich 1989), this drug is categorized as in class: *A* (*Probably safe. Although specific studies may not have proved the safety of all drugs in dogs and cats, there are no reports of adverse effects in laboratory animals or women.*)

Overdosage/Acute Toxicity

No case reports were located regarding acute intravenous overdose of amphotericin B. Because of the toxicity of the drug, dosage calculations and solution preparation procedures should be double-checked. If an accidental overdose is administered, renal toxicity may be minimized by administering fluids and mannitol as outlined above in the Adverse Effects section.

Drug Interactions

The following drug interactions have either been reported or are theoretical in humans or animals receiving amphotericin B and may be of significance in veterinary patients:

■ **CORTICOSTEROIDS:** May exacerbate the potassium-losing effects of amphotericin

■ **DIGOXIN:** Amphotericin B-induced hypokalemia may exacerbate digoxin toxicity

■ **FLUCYTOSINE:** Synergy (*in vitro*) between amphotericin and flucytosine may occur against strains of Cryptococcus and Candida, but increased flucytosine toxicity may also occur

■ **NEPHROTOXIC DRUGS (aminoglycosides, polymyxin B, colistin, cisplatin, cyclosporine, methoxyflurane or vancomycin):** Since the renal effects of other nephrotoxic drugs may be additive with amphotericin B, avoid, if possible the concurrent or sequential use of these AGENTS

■ **POTASSIUM-DEPLETING DRUGS (e.g., thiazide or loop diuretics)**

■ **SALINE SOLUTIONS OR WITH SOLUTIONS CONTAINING A PRESERVATIVE:** Reconstituting amphotericin B with these solutions may cause precipitation

■ **SKELETAL MUSCLE RELAXANTS (tubocurarine):** Amphotericin B-induced hypokalemia may enhance curariform effects

Doses

All dosages are for amphotericin B desoxycholate (regular amphotericin B) unless specifically noted for the lipid-based products.

Note: Some clinicians have recommended administering a 1 mg test dose (less in small dogs or cats) IV over anywhere from 20 minutes to 4 hours and monitoring pulse, respiration rates, temperature, and if possible, blood pressure. If a febrile reaction occurs some clinicians recommend adding a glucocorticoid to the IV infusion solution or using an antipyretic prior to treating, but these practices are controversial.

A published study (Rubin et al. 1989) demonstrated less renal impairment and systemic adverse effects in dogs who received amphotericin B IV slowly over 5 hours in 1 L of D_5W than in dogs who received the drug IV in 25 mL of D_5W over 3 minutes.

■ **DOGS:**

For treatment of susceptible systemic fungal infections:

a) Two regimens can be used; after diluting vial (as outlined below in preparation of solution section), either:

1) Rapid-Infusion Technique: Dilute quantity of stock solution to equal 0.25 mg/kg in 30 mL of 5% dextrose. Using butterfly catheter, flush with 10 mL of D_5W. Infuse amphotericin B solution IV over 5 minutes. Flush catheter with 10 mL of D_5W and remove catheter. Repeat above steps using 0.5 mg/kg 3 times a week until 9–12 mg/kg accumulated dosage is given.

2) Slow IV Infusion Technique: Dilute quantity of stock solution to equal 0.25 mg/kg in 250–500 mL of D5W. Place indwelling catheter in peripheral vein and give total volume over 4–6 hours. Flush catheter with 10 mL of D_5W and remove catheter. Repeat above steps using 0.5 mg/kg 3 times a week until 9–12 mg/kg accumulated dosage is given. (Noxon 1989)

b) In dehydrated, sodium-depleted animals, must rehydrate before administration. Dosage is 0.5 mg/kg diluted in D5W. In dogs with normal renal function, may dilute in 60–120 mL of D5W and give by slow IV over 15 minutes. In dogs with compromised renal function, dilute in 500 mL or 1 liter of D_5W and give over slowly IV over 3–6 hours. Re-administer every other day if BUN remains below 50 mg/dL. If BUN exceeds 50 mg/dL, discontinue until BUN decreases to at least 35 mg/dL. Cumulative dose of 8–10 mg/kg is required to cure blastomycosis or histoplasmosis. Coccidioidomycosis, aspergillosis and other fungal diseases require a greater cumulative dosage.) (Legendre, A. 1995)

c) For treating systemic mycoses using the lipid-based products: *AmBisome®*, *Amphocil®* or *Abelcet®*: Give test dose of 0.5 mg/kg; then 1–2.5 mg/kg IV q48h (or Monday, Wednesday, Friday) for 4 weeks or until the tested cumulative dose is reached. Use 1 mg/kg dose for susceptible yeast and dimorphic fungi until a cumulative dose of 12 mg/kg is reached; for more resistant filamentous fungal infections (*e.g.*, pythiosis) use the higher dose 2–2.5 mg/kg until a cumulative dose of 24–30 mg/kg is reached. (Greene, C. & Watson 1998)

d) For treating systemic mycoses using the amphotericin B lipid complex (ABLC; *Abelcet®*) product: 2–3 mg/kg IV three days per week for a total of 9–12 treatments (cumulative dose of 24–27 mg). Dilute to a concentration of 1 mg/mL in dextrose 5% (D5W) and infuse over 1–2 hours. (Grooters 1999)

e) For systemic mycoses using amphotericin B lipid complex (*Abelcet®*): Dilute in 5% dextrose to a final concentration of 1 mg/mL and administer at a dosage of 2–3 mg/kg three times per week for 9–12 treatments or a cumulative dosage of 24–27 mg/kg. (Schulman & Marks 2005)

For blastomycosis (see general dosage guidelines above):

a) Amphotericin B 0.5 mg/kg 3 times weekly until a total dose of 6 mg/kg is given, with ketoconazole at 10–20 mg/kg (30 mg/kg for CNS, bone or eye involvement) divided for 3–6 months. (Foil 1986)

b) Amphotericin B 0.15–0.5 mg/kg IV 3 times a week with ketoconazole 20 mg/day PO once daily or divided twice daily; 40 mg/kg divided twice daily for ocular or CNS involvement (for at least 2–3 months or until remission then start maintenance). When a total dose of amphotericin B reaches 4–6 mg/kg start maintenance dosage of amphotericin B at 0.15–0.25 mg/kg IV once a month or use ketoconazole at 10 mg/kg PO either once daily, divided twice daily or ketoconazole at 2.5–5 mg/kg PO once daily. If CNS/ocular involvement use ketoconazole at 20–40 mg/kg PO divided twice daily. (Greene, C.E. et al. 1984)

c) For severe cases, using amphotericin B lipid complex (*Abelcet*®): 1–2 mg/kg IV three times a week (or every other day) to a cumulative dose of 12–24 mg/kg. (Taboada 2000)

For cryptococcosis (see general dosage guidelines above):

a) Amphotericin B 0.5–0.8 mg/kg SC 2–3 times per week. Dose is diluted in 0.45% NaCl with 2.5% dextrose (400 mL for cats, 500 mL for dogs less than 20 kg and 1000 mL for dogs greater than 20 kg). Concentrations greater than 20 mg/L result in local irritation and sterile abscess formation. May combine with flucytosine or the azole antifungals. (Taboada 2000)

For histoplasmosis (see general dosage guidelines above):

a) Amphotericin B 0.15–0.5 mg/kg IV 3 times a week with ketoconazole 10–20 mg/day PO once daily or divided twice daily (for at least 2–3 months or until remission then start maintenance). When a total dose of amphotericin B reaches 2–4 mg/kg, start maintenance dosage of amphotericin B at 0.15–0.25 mg/kg IV once a month or use ketoconazole at 10 mg/kg PO either once daily, divided twice daily or at 2.5–5 mg/kg PO once daily. (Greene, C.E. et al. 1984)

b) As an alternative to ketoconazole treatment: 0.5 mg/kg IV given over 6–8 hours. If dose is tolerated, increase to 1 mg/kg given on alternate days until total dose of 7.5–8.5 mg/kg cumulative dose is achieved. (Macy 1987)

For Leishmaniasis:

a) Using the liposomal form of Amphotericin B: 3–3.3 mg/kg IV 3 times weekly for 3–5 treatments. (Lappin 2000)

b) Using *AmBisome*® (lipid-based product): Give initial test dose of 0.5 mg/kg, then 3–3.3 mg/kg IV every 72–96 hours until a cumulative dose of 15 mg/kg is reached.

May be possible to give the same cumulative dose with a lower level every 48 hours. (Greene, C. et al. 2006)

For gastrointestinal pythiosis:

a) Resect lesions that are surgically removable to obtain 5–6 cm margins. Follow-up medical therapy using the amphotericin B lipid complex (ABLC; *Abelcet*®) product: 1–2 mg/kg IV three times weekly for 4 weeks (cumulative dose 12–24 mg). May alternatively use itraconazole at 10 mg/kg PO once daily for 4–6 months. (Taboada 1999)

■ **CATS:**

For treatment of susceptible systemic fungal infections:

a) Rapid-Infusion Technique: After diluting vial (as outlined below in preparation of solution section), dilute quantity of stock solution to equal 0.25 mg/kg in 30 mL of 5% dextrose. Using butterfly catheter, flush with 10 mL of D_5W. Infuse amphotericin B solution IV over 5 minutes. Flush catheter with 10 mL of D_5W and remove catheter. Repeat above steps using 0.25 mg/kg 3 times a week until 9–12 mg/kg accumulated dosage is given. (Noxon 1989)

For cryptococcosis (see general dosage guidelines above):

a) As an alternative therapy to ketoconazole: Amphotericin B: 0.25 mg/kg in 30 mL D_5W IV over 15 minutes q48h with flucytosine at 200 mg/kg/day divided q6h PO. Continue therapy for 3–4 weeks after clinical signs have resolved or until BUN >50 mg/dL. (Legendre, A. 1995)

b) Amphotericin B 0.15–0.4 mg/kg IV 3 times a week with flucytosine 125–250 mg/day PO divided two to four times a day. When a total dose of amphotericin B reaches 4–6 mg/kg, start maintenance dosage of amphotericin B at 0.15–0.25 mg/kg IV once a month with flucytosine at dosage above or with ketoconazole at 10 mg/kg PO once daily or divided twice daily. (Greene, C.E. et al. 1984)

c) Amphotericin B 0.5–0.8 mg/kg SC 2–3 times per week. Dose is diluted in 0.45% NaCl with 2.5% dextrose (400 mL for cats, 500 mL for dogs less than 20 kg and 1000 mL for dogs greater than 20 kg). Concentrations greater than 20 mg/L result in local irritation and sterile abscess formation. May combine with flucytosine or the azole antifungals. (Taboada 2000)

d) For treating systemic mycoses using the amphotericin B lipid complex (ABLC; *Abelcet*®) product: 1 mg/kg IV three days per week for a total of 12 treatments (cumulative dose of 12 mg). Dilute to a concentration of 1 mg/mL in dextrose 5% (D5W) and infuse over 1–2 hours. (Grooters 1999)

For histoplasmosis (see general dosage guidelines above):

a) Amphotericin B: 0.25 mg/kg in 30 mL D₅W IV over 15 minutes q48h with ketoconazole at 10 mg/kg q12h PO. Continue therapy for 4–8 weeks or until BUN >50 mg/dL. If BUN increases greater than 50 mg/dL, continue ketoconazole alone. Ketoconazole is used long-term (at least 6 months of duration. (Legendre, A.M. 1989)

b) Amphotericin B 0.15–0.5 mg/kg IV 3 times a week with ketoconazole 10 mg/day PO once daily or divided twice daily (for at least 2–3 months or until remission, then start maintenance). When a total dose of amphotericin B reaches 2–4 mg/kg, start maintenance dosage of amphotericin B at 0.15–0.25 mg/kg IV once a month or use ketoconazole at 10 mg/kg PO either once daily, divided twice daily or at 2.5–5 mg/kg PO once daily. (Greene et al, 1984)

For blastomycosis (see general dosage guidelines above):

a) Amphotericin B: 0.25 mg/kg in 30 mL D₅W IV over 15 minutes q48h with ketoconazole: 10 mg/kg q12h PO (for at least 60 days). Continue amphotericin B therapy until a cumulative dose of 4 mg/kg is given or until BUN >50 mg/dL. If renal toxicity does not develop, may increase dose to 0.5 mg/kg of amphotericin B. (Legendre, 1989)

b) Amphotericin B 0.15–0.5 mg/kg IV 3 times a week with ketoconazole 10 mg/day PO once daily or divided twice daily (for at least 2–3 months or until remission then start maintenance). When a total dose of amphotericin B reaches 4–6 mg/kg start maintenance dosage of amphotericin B at 0.15–0.25 mg/kg IV once a month or use ketoconazole at 10 mg/kg PO either once daily, divided twice daily or ketoconazole at 2.5–5 mg/kg PO once daily. If CNS/ocular involvement, use ketoconazole at 20–40 mg/kg PO divided twice daily. (Greene, O'Neal, and Barsanti 1984)

■ **RABBITS/RODENTS/SMALL MAMMALS:**

a) **Rabbits:** 1 mg/kg/day IV (Ivey & Morrisey, 2000)

■ **HORSES:**

For treatment of susceptible systemic fungal infections:

a) For fungal pneumonia: Day 1: 0.3 mg/kg IV; Day 2: 0.4 mg/kg IV; Day 3:

0.6 mg/kg IV; days 4–7: no treatment; then every other day until a total cumulative dose of 6.75 mg/kg has been administered (Foreman 1999)

b) For phycomycoses and pulmonary mycoses: After reconstitution (see below) transfer appropriate amount of drug to 1L of D5W and administer using a 16 g needle IV at a rate of 1 L/hr. Dosage schedule follows: Day 1: 0.3 mg/kg IV; Day 2: 0.45 mg/kg IV; Day 3: 0.6 mg/kg IV; then every other day for 3 days per week (MWF or TThSa) until clinical signs of either improvement or toxicity occur. If toxicity occurs, a dose may be skipped, dosage reduced or dosage interval lengthened. Administration may extend from 10–80 days.) (Brumbaugh 1987)

c) For intrauterine infusion: 200–250 mg. Little science is available for recommending doses, volume infused, frequency, diluents, etc. Most intrauterine treatments are commonly performed every day or every other day for 3–7 days. (Perkins 1999)

■ **LLAMAS:**

For treatment of susceptible systemic fungal infections:

a) A single case report. Llama received 1 mg test dose, then initially at 0.3 mg/kg IV over 4 hours, followed by 3 L of LRS with 1.5 mL of B-Complex and 20 mEq of KCl added. Subsequent doses were increased by 10 mg and given every 48 hours until reaching 1 mg/kg q48h IV for 6 weeks. Animal tolerated therapy well, but treatment was ultimately unsuccessful (Coccidioidomycosis). (Fowler 1989)

■ **BIRDS:**

For treatment of susceptible systemic fungal infections:

a) For raptors and psittacines with aspergillosis: 1.5 mg/kg IV three times daily for 3 days with flucytosine or follow with flucytosine. May also use intratracheally at 1 mg/kg diluted in sterile water once to 3 times daily for 3 days in conjunction with flucytosine or nebulized (1 mg/mL of saline) for 15 minutes twice daily. Potentially nephrotoxic and may cause bone marrow suppression. (Clubb 1986)

b) 1.5 mg/kg IV q12h for 3–5 days; topically in the trachea at 1 mg/kg q12h; 0.3–1 mg/mL nebulized for 15 minutes 2–4 times daily. (Flammer 2003)

c) For treatment of Macrorhabdiasis (*Microrhabdus ornithogaster*): amphotericin B at 100–150 mg/kg *PO* q12h for 30 days; treatment failures are common especially with shorter durations of treatment. (Flammer 2008)

■ **REPTILES:**

For susceptible fungal respiratory infections:
a) For most species: 1 mg/kg diluted in saline and given intra-tracheally once daily for 14–28 treatments. (Gauvin 1993)

Monitoring

Also see Adverse Effects section

■ BUN and serum creatinine every other day while dosage is being increased, and at least weekly thereafter during therapy

■ Serum electrolytes (sodium, potassium and magnesium) weekly

■ Liver function tests weekly

■ CBC weekly

■ Urinalysis weekly

■ TPP at least weekly

■ Animal's weight

Client Information

■ Clients should be informed of the potential seriousness of toxic effects that can occur with amphotericin B therapy

■ The costs associated with therapy

Chemistry/Synonyms

A polyene macrolide antifungal agent produced by Streptomyces nodosus, amphotericin B occurs as a yellow to orange, odorless or practically odorless powder. It is insoluble in water and anhydrous alcohol. Amphotericin B is amphoteric and can form salts in acidic or basic media. These salts are more water soluble but possess less antifungal activity than the parent compound. Each mg of amphotericin B must contain not less than 750 micrograms of anhydrous drug. Amphotericin A may be found as a contaminant in concentrations not exceeding 5%. The commercially available powder for injection contains sodium desoxycholate as a solubilizing agent.

Newer lipid-based amphotericin B products are available that have less toxicity than the conventional desoxycholate form. These include amphotericin B cholesteryl sulfate complex (amphotericin B colloidal dispersion, ABCD, *Amphotec®*), amphotericin B lipid complex (ABLC, *Abelcet®*), and amphotericin B liposomal (ABL, L-AMB, *Ambisome®*).

Amphotericin B may also be known as: amphotericin; amphotericin B cholesteryl sulfate complex, amphotericin B lipid complex, amphotericin B liposome, amphotericin B phospholipid complex, amphotericin B-Sodium cholesteryl sulfate complex, anfotericina B, or liposomal amphotericin B; many trade names are available.

Storage/Stability

Vials of amphotericin B powder for injection should be stored in the refrigerator (2–8°C), protected from light and moisture. Reconstitution of the powder must be done with sterile water for injection (no preservatives—see directions for preparation in the Dosage Form section below).

After reconstitution, if protected from light, the solution is stable for 24 hours at room temperature and for 1 week if kept refrigerated. After diluting with D_5W (must have pH >4.3) for IV use, the manufacturer recommends continuing to protect the solution from light during administration. Additional studies however, have shown that potency remains largely unaffected if the solution is exposed to light for 8–24 hours.

One reference (Orosz 2000) states that for avian use, the conventional amphotericin B (amphotericin B deoxycholate) can be diluted with sterile water, divided into 10 ml aliquots using aseptic technique, and stored at -20°C for approximately 1 month. However, no published data was located documenting the stability of the drug for this practice.

Compatibility/Compounding Considerations

Amphotericin B deoxycholate is reportedly **compatible** with the following solutions and drugs: D_5W, D_5W in sodium chloride 0.2%, heparin sodium, heparin sodium with hydrocortisone sodium phosphate, hydrocortisone sodium phosphate/succinate and sodium bicarbonate.

Amphotericin B deoxycholate is reportedly **incompatible** with the following solutions and drugs: **normal saline, lactated Ringer's**, D_5-normal saline, D_5-lactated Ringer's, amino acids 4.25%–dextrose 25%, amikacin, calcium chloride/gluconate, carbenicillin disodium, chlorpromazine HCl, cimetidine HCl, diphenhydramine HCl, dopamine HCl, edetate calcium disodium (Ca EDTA), gentamicin sulfate, kanamycin sulfate, lidocaine HCl, metaraminol bitartrate, methyldopate HCl, nitrofurantoin sodium, oxytetracycline HCl, penicillin G potassium/sodium, polymyxin B sulfate, potassium chloride, prochlorperazine mesylate, streptomycin sulfate, tetracycline HCl, and verapamil HCl. Compatibility is dependent upon factors such as pH, concentration, temperature and diluent used; consult specialized references or a hospital pharmacist for more specific information.

Dosage Forms/Regulatory Status

VETERINARY-LABELED PRODUCTS: None

HUMAN-LABELED PRODUCTS:

Amphotericin B Desoxycholate Powder for Injection: 50 mg in vials; generic (Pharma-Tek); (Rx)

Directions for reconstitution/administration: Using strict aseptic technique and a 20 gauge or larger needle, rapidly inject 10 mL of sterile water for injection (without a bacteriostatic agent) directly into the lyophilized cake; immediately shake well until solution is clear. A 5 mg/mL colloidal solution results. Further dilute (1:50) for administration to a concentration of 0.1 mg/mL with 5%

dextrose in water (pH >4.2). An in-line filter may be used during administration, but must have a pore diameter >1 micron.

Amphotericin B Lipid-Based Suspension for Injection: 100 mg/20 mL (as lipid complex) in 10 mL & 20 mL vials with 5 micron filter needles: *Abelcet®* (Enzon); (Rx)

Amphotericin B Lipid-Based Powder for Injection: 50 mg (as cholesteryl) in 20 mL single-use vials; 100 mg (as cholesteryl) in 50 mL single-use vials; *Amphotec®* (Sequus Pharmaceuticals); 50 mg (as liposomal) in single-dose vials with 5-micron filter; *AmBisome®* (Astellas); (Rx)

Amphotericin B is also available in topical formulations: *Fungizone®* (Apothecon); (Rx)

References

Brumbaugh, GW (1987). Rational selection of antimicrobial drugs for treatment of infections in horses. *Vet Clin North Am (Equine Practice)* 3(1): 191–220.

Clubb, SL (1986). Therapeutics: Individual and Flock Treatment Regimens. *Clinical Avian Medicine and Surgery*. GJ Harrison and LR Harrison Eds. Philadelphia, W.B. Saunders: 327–355.

Flammer, K (2003). Antifungal therapy in avian medicine. Proceedings: Western Veterinary Conference. Accessed via: Veterinary Information Network. http://goo.gl/rgOfo

Flammer, K (2008). Avian Mycoses: Managing those difficult cases. Proceedings: AAV. Accessed via: Veterinary Information Network. http://goo.gl/iDsnR

Foil, CS (1986). Antifungal agents in dermatology. *Current Veterinary Therapy IX: Small Animal Practice*. RW Kirk Ed. Philadelphia, WB Saunders: 560–565.

Foreman, J (1999). Equine respiratory pharmacology. *The Veterinary Clinics of North America: Equine Practice* 15:3(December): 665–686.

Fowler, ME (1989). *Medicine and Surgery of South American Camelids*. Ames, Iowa State University Press.

Gauvin, J (1993). Drug therapy in reptiles. *Seminars in Avian & Exotic Med* 2(1): 48–59.

Greene, C, K Hartmannn, et al. (2006). Appendix 8: Antimicrobial Drug Formulary. *Infectious Disease of the Dog and Cat*. C Greene Ed., Elsevier: 1186–1333.

Greene, C & A Watson (1998). Antimicrobial Drug Formulary. *Infectious Diseases of the Dog and Cat*. C Greene Ed. Philadelphia, WB Saunders: 790–919.

Greene, CE, KG O'Neal, et al. (1984). Antimicrobial chemotherapy. *Clinical Microbiology and INfectious Diseases of the Dog and Cat*. CE Greene Ed. Philadelphia, WB Saunders: 144–188.

Grooters, A (1999). New directions in antifungal therapy. Proceedings: American College of Veterinary Internal Medicine: 17th Annual Veterinary Medical Forum, Chicago.

Ivey, E. & J. Morrisey (2000). Therapeutics for Rabbits. *Vet Clin NA: Exotic Anim Pract* 3:1(Jan): 183–216.

Lappin, M (2000). Protozoal and Miscellaneous Infections. *Textbook of Veterinary Internal Medicine: Diseases of the Dog and Cat*. S Ettinger and E Feldman Eds. Philadelphia, WB Saunders. 1: 408–417.

Legendre, A (1995). Antimycotic Drug Therapy. *Kirk's Current Veterinary Therapy:XII*. J Bonagura Ed. Philadelphia, W.B. Saunders: 327–331.

Legendre, AM (1989). Systemic mycotic infections. *The Cat: Diseases and Clinical Management*. RG Sherding Ed. New York, Churchill Livingstone. 1: 427–457.

Macy, DW (1987). Fungal Diseases—Dog, Cat. *The Bristol Handbook of Antimicrobial Therapy*. DE Johnston Ed. Evansville, Veterinary Learning Systems: 152–157.

Noxon, JO (1989). Systemic antifungal therapy. *Current Veterinary Therapy X: Small Animal Practice*. RW Kirk Ed. Philadelphia, WB Saunders: 1101–1108.

Orosz, SE (2000). Overview of aspergillosis: Pathogenesis and treatment options. *Seminars in Avian and Exotic Pet Medicine* 9(2): 59–65.

Perkins, N (1999). Equine reproductive pharmacology. *The Veterinary Clinics of North America: Equine Practice* 15:3(December): 687–704.

Schulman, R & S Marks (2005). Systemic Mycoses: Coast to Coast. Proceedings: ACVIM 2005. Accessed via: Veterinary Information Network. http://goo.gl/jvFUv

Taboada, J (1999). How I treat gastrointestinal pythiosis. Proceedings: The North American Veterinary Conference, Orlando.

Taboada, J (2000). Systemic Mycoses. *Textbook of Veterinary Internal Medicine: Diseases of the Dog and Cat*. S Ettinger and E Feldman Eds. Philadelphia, WB Saunders. 1: 453–476.

AMPICILLIN
AMPICILLIN SODIUM
AMPICILLIN TRIHYDRATE

(am-pi-*sill*-in; sul-*bak*-tam)   Polyflex®

AMINOPENICILLIN

Prescriber Highlights

▶ Bactericidal aminopenicillin with same spectrum as amoxicillin (ineffective against bacteria that produce beta-lactamase)

▶ Most likely adverse effects are GI-related, but hypersensitivity & other adverse effects rarely occur; may cause more GI effects than amoxicillin when used orally

▶ More susceptible than amoxicillin to food reducing oral absorption

▶ Available in both parenteral & oral forms

Uses/Indications

In dogs and cats, ampicillin is not as well absorbed after oral administration as amoxicillin and its oral use has largely been supplanted by amoxicillin. It is used commonly in parenteral dosage forms when an aminopenicillin is indicated in all species. Ampicillin at high dosages, is still an effective drug for treating penicillin-sensitive enterococci, particularly *E. faecium*. An aminoglycoside (*e.g.*, gentamicin) is often added to treat serious enterococcus infections caused by penicillin-sensitive organisms.

The aminopenicillins, also called the "broad-spectrum" or ampicillin penicillins, have increased activity against many strains of gram-negative aerobes not covered by either the natural penicillins or penicillinase-resistant penicillins, including some strains of *E. coli*, Klebsiella, and Haemophilus.

Pharmacology/Actions

Like other penicillins, ampicillin is a time-dependent, bactericidal (usually) agent that acts via inhibiting cell wall synthesis. Ampicillin and the other aminopenicillins have increased activity against many strains of gram-negative aerobes not covered by either the natural penicillins or penicillinase-resistant penicillins, including some strains of *E. coli,* Klebsiella and Haemophilus. Like the natural penicillins, they are susceptible to inactivation by beta-lactamase-producing bacteria (*e.g.,* Staph aureus). Although not as active as the natural penicillins, they do have activity against many anaerobic bacteria, including Clostridial organisms. Organisms that are generally not susceptible include *Pseudomonas aeruginosa,* Serratia, Indole-positive Proteus (*Proteus mirabilis* is susceptible), Enterobacter, Citrobacter, and Acinetobacter. The aminopenicillins also are inactive against Rickettsia, mycobacteria, fungi, Mycoplasma, and viruses.

In order to reduce the inactivation of penicillins by beta-lactamases, potassium clavulanate and sulbactam have been developed to inactivate these enzymes and extend the spectrum of those penicillins. See the ampicillin/sulbactam or amoxicillin/clavulanate monographs for more information.

Pharmacokinetics

Ampicillin anhydrous and trihydrate are relatively stable in the presence of gastric acid. After oral administration, ampicillin is about 30–55% absorbed in humans (empty stomach) and monogastric animals. Food will decrease the rate and extent of oral absorption.

When administered parenterally (IM, SC) the trihydrate salt will achieve serum levels of approximately 1/2 those of a comparable dose of the sodium salt. The trihydrate parenteral dosage form should not be used where higher MIC's are required for treating systemic infections.

After absorption, the volume of distribution for ampicillin is approximately 0.3 L/kg in humans and dogs, 0.167 L/kg in cats, and 0.16–0.5 L/kg in cattle. The drug is widely distributed to many tissues, including liver, lungs, prostate (human), muscle, bile, and ascitic, pleural and synovial fluids. Ampicillin will cross into the CSF when meninges are inflamed in concentrations that may range from 10–60% those found in serum. Very low levels of the drug are found in the aqueous humor; low levels are found in tears, sweat and saliva. Ampicillin crosses the placenta, but is thought to be relatively safe to use during pregnancy. Ampicillin is approximately 20% bound to plasma proteins, primarily albumin. Milk levels of ampicillin are considered low. In lactating dairy cattle, the milk to plasma ratio is about 0.3.

Ampicillin is eliminated primarily through renal mechanisms, principally by tubular secretion, but some of the drug is metabolized by hydrolysis to penicilloic acids (inactive) and then excreted in the urine. Elimination half-lives of ampicillin have been reported as 45–80 minutes in dogs and cats, and 60 minutes in swine.

Contraindications/Precautions/Warnings

Penicillins are contraindicated in patients with a history of hypersensitivity to them. Because there may be cross-reactivity, use penicillins cautiously in patients who are documented hypersensitive to other beta-lactam antibiotics (*e.g.,* cephalosporins, cefamycins, carbapenems).

Do not administer systemic antibiotics orally in patients with septicemia, shock, or other grave illnesses as absorption of the medication from the GI tract may be significantly delayed or diminished. Parenteral (preferably IV) routes should be used for these cases.

Do not administer penicillins, cephalosporins, or macrolides to rabbits, guinea pigs, chinchillas, hamsters, etc., or serious enteritis and clostridial enterotoxemia may occur.

Adverse Effects

Adverse effects with the penicillins are usually not serious and have a relatively low frequency of occurrence.

Hypersensitivity reactions unrelated to dose can occur with these agents and manifest as rashes, fever, eosinophilia, neutropenia, agranulocytosis, thrombocytopenia, leukopenia, anemias, lymphadenopathy, or full-blown anaphylaxis. In humans, it is estimated that up to 15% of patients hypersensitive to cephalosporins will also be hypersensitive to penicillins. The incidence of cross-reactivity in veterinary patients is unknown.

When given orally penicillins may cause GI effects (anorexia, vomiting, diarrhea). Because the penicillins may also alter gut flora, antibiotic-associated diarrhea can occur and allow the proliferation of resistant bacteria in the colon (superinfections).

Neurotoxicity (*e.g.,* ataxia in dogs) has been associated with very high doses or very prolonged use. Although the penicillins are not considered hepatotoxic, elevated liver enzymes have been reported. Other effects reported in dogs include tachypnea, dyspnea, edema and tachycardia.

Reproductive/Nursing Safety

Penicillins have been shown to cross the placenta; safe use during pregnancy has not been firmly established, but neither have there been any documented teratogenic problems associated with these drugs. However, use only when the potential benefits outweigh the risks. In humans, the FDA categorizes ampicillin as category *B* for use during pregnancy (*Animal studies have not yet demonstrated risk to the fetus, but there are no adequate studies in pregnant women; or animal studies have shown an adverse effect, but adequate studies in pregnant women have not demonstrated a risk to the fetus in the first trimester of pregnancy, and there is no evidence of risk in later trimesters.*) In a separate system evaluating the safety of drugs in canine and feline pregnancy (Papich 1989), this drug is categorized as in class: *A* (*Probably safe. Although specific studies may not have proved the safety of all drugs in dogs and cats, there are no reports of adverse effects in laboratory animals or women.*)

Overdosage/Acute Toxicity
Acute oral penicillin overdoses are unlikely to cause significant problems other than GI distress, but other effects are possible (see Adverse Effects). In humans, very high dosages of parenteral penicillins, particularly in patients with renal disease, have induced CNS effects.

Drug Interactions
The following drug interactions have either been reported or are theoretical in humans or animals receiving ampicillin and may be of significance in veterinary patients:

■ **BACTERIOSTATIC ANTIMICROBIALS (e.g., chloramphenicol, erythromycin and other macrolides, tetracyclines, sulfonamides, etc.):** Because there is evidence of *in vitro* antagonism between beta-lactam antibiotics and bacteriostatic antibiotics, use together has not been generally recommended in the past, but actual clinical importance is not clear and currently in doubt.

■ **METHOTREXATE:** Ampicillin may decrease the renal excretion of MTX causing increased levels and potential toxic effects

■ **PROBENECID:** Competitively blocks the tubular secretion of most penicillins thereby increasing serum levels and serum half-lives

Laboratory Considerations
■ Ampicillin may cause false-positive **urine glucose determinations** when using cupric sulfate solution (Benedict's Solution, *Clinitest*®). Tests utilizing glucose oxidase (*Tes-Tape*®, *Clinistix*®) are not affected by ampicillin.

■ As penicillins and other beta-lactams can inactivate **aminoglycosides** *in vitro* (and *in vivo* in patients in renal failure), serum concentrations of aminoglycosides may be falsely decreased if the patient is also receiving beta-lactam antibiotics and the serum is stored prior to analysis. It is recommended that if the assay is delayed, samples be frozen and, if possible, drawn at times when the beta-lactam antibiotic is at a trough.

Doses

■ **DOGS:**
For susceptible infections:
a) For Gram-positive infections: 10–20 mg/kg PO twice daily; 5 mg/kg IM, SC twice daily; 5 mg/kg IV three times daily.

For Gram-negative infections: 20–30 mg/kg PO three times daily; 10 mg/kg IM, SC three times daily;

10 mg/kg IV four times daily (Aucoin 2000)

b) For susceptible UTI's: 12.5 mg/kg PO q12h for 3–7 days, 6.6 mg/kg IM or SC q12h for 3–7 days;

For susceptible soft tissue infections: 10–20 mg/kg PO, IM or SC q8h for 7 days;

For pneumonia, systemic: 22 mg/kg PO, IV or SC q8h for 7–14 days;

For meningitis, orthopedic infections: 22 mg/kg PO, IV, IM, SC q6–8h as long as necessary;

For susceptible sepsis, bacteremia: 20–40 mg/kg IV, IM or SC q6–8h for as long as necessary;

For neonatal sepsis: 50 mg/ kg IV or intraosseous q4–6h as long as necessary;

For susceptible orthopedic infections or meningitis: 22 mg/kg IV, IM, SC, or PO q6–8h for as long as necessary (Greene *et al.* 2006)

c) For sepsis: 20–40 mg/kg IV q6–8h (Hardie 2000)

d) For susceptible UTI's: 25 mg/kg PO q8h (Polzin 2005)

e) To eliminate the leptospiremic phase of leptospirosis: 22 mg/kg q6–8h IV during the acute illness until patient is eating, then amoxicillin 22 mg/kg PO q8h (Lunn 2006)

■ **CATS:**
For susceptible infections:
a) For Gram-positive infections: 10–20 mg/kg PO twice daily; 5 mg/kg IM, SC twice daily; 5 mg/kg IV three times daily;

For Gram-negative infections: 20–30 mg/kg PO three times daily; 10 mg/kg IM, SC three times daily; 10 mg/kg IV four times daily (Aucoin 2000)

b) For susceptible UTI's: 20 mg/kg PO q8–12h for 7–14 days;

For soft tissue infections 20–40 mg/kg PO q8–12h for 14 days;

For systemic infections: 7–11 mg/kg IV, IM or SC q8–12h for as long as necessary; (Greene *et al.* 2006)

c) For sepsis: 20–40 mg/kg IV q6–8h (Hardie 2000)

■ **CATTLE:**
For susceptible infections:
a) For respiratory infections: Ampicillin trihydrate (*Polyflex*®): 22 mg/kg SC q12h (60 day slaughter withdrawal suggested) (Hjerpe 1986)

b) For respiratory infections: Ampicillin sodium 22 mg/kg SC q12h; Ampicillin trihydrate: 11 mg/kg IM q24h (Beech 1987b)

■ **HORSES:**

For susceptible infections:

a) Ampicillin sodium: 10–50 mg/kg IV or IM three times daily

Ampicillin trihydrate: 5–20 mg/kg IM twice daily (Robinson 1987)

Ampicillin sodium: 11–15 mg/kg IM or IV three to four times daily (Beech 1987a)

b) **Foals:** Ampicillin sodium 11 mg/kg q6h IM or IV (Furr 1999)

c) **Foals:** Ampicillin sodium 15–30 mg/kg IV or IM q 6–8h (Brumbaugh 1999)

d) For intrauterine infusion: 1–3 grams. Little science is available for recommending doses, volume infused, frequency diluents, etc. Most treatments are commonly performed every day or every other day for 3–7 days.) (Perkins 1999)

■ **FERRETS:**

For susceptible infections: 5–10 mg/kg IM, SC or IV twice daily (Williams 2000)

■ **RABBITS/RODENTS/SMALL MAMMALS:**

a) **Rabbits:** Not recommended as it can cause a fatal enteritis (Ivey & Morrisey 2000)

b) **Gerbils, Mice, Rats:** 20–100 mg/kg PO, SC, IM q8–12h

c) **Guinea pigs, Chinchillas, Hamsters:** Do NOT use as it may cause enterocolitis (Adamcak & Otten 2000)

d) **Hedgehogs:** 10 mg/kg IM or PO once daily (Smith 2000)

■ **SWINE:**

For susceptible infections:

a) Ampicillin sodium: 6–8 mg/kg SC or IM q8h (Baggot 1983)

■ **BIRDS:**

For susceptible infections:

a) Amazon parrots: 150–200 mg/kg PO twice daily–three times daily (poorly absorbed PO); 100 mg/kg IM (as the trihydrate/*Polyflex*®) q4h.

Pet birds: 250 mg capsule in 8 oz. of drinking water (poorly absorbed; rapidly excreted)

Chickens: 1.65 g/L drinking water (see above)

Most birds: 250 mg/kg via feed for 5–10 days. Sprinkle on favorite food, or add to mash or corn mix. (Clubb 1986)

b) 100 mg/kg IM or IM q8h (Hoeffer 1995)

c) **Ratites:** 11–15 mg/kg PO or IV 3 times daily; 15–20 mg/kg IM twice daily (Jenson 1998)

■ **REPTILES:**

For susceptible infections:

a) All species: 3–6 mg/kg PO, SC or IM every 12–24 hours for 2 weeks; not very useful unless used in combination with aminoglycosides (Gauvin 1993)

b) For Chelonians (turtles et al): 50 mg/kg IM q12h (Jacobson 2000)

Monitoring

■ Because penicillins usually have minimal toxicity associated with their use, monitoring for efficacy is usually all that is required unless toxic signs or symptoms develop. Serum levels and therapeutic drug monitoring are not routinely done with these agents.

Client Information

■ Unless otherwise instructed by the veterinarian, this drug should be given orally on an empty stomach, at least 1 hour before feeding or 2 hours after.

■ Keep oral suspension in the refrigerator and discard any unused suspension after 14 days. If stored at room temperature, discard unused suspension after 7 days.

Chemistry/Synonyms

A semi-synthetic aminopenicillin, ampicillin anhydrous and trihydrate occur as practically odorless, white, crystalline powders that are slightly soluble in water. At usual temperatures (<42°C), ampicillin anhydrous is more soluble in water than the trihydrate (13 mg/mL vs. 6 mg/mL at 20°C). Ampicillin anhydrous or trihydrate oral suspensions have a pH of 5–7.5 after reconstitution with water.

Ampicillin sodium occurs as an odorless or practically odorless, white to off-white, crystalline hygroscopic powder. It is very soluble in water or other aqueous solutions. After reconstitution, ampicillin sodium has a pH of 8–10 at a concentration of 10 mg/mL. Commercially available ampicillin sodium for injection has approximately 3 mEq of sodium per gram of ampicillin.

Potency of the ampicillin salts is expressed in terms of ampicillin anhydrous.

Ampicillin may also be known as: aminobenzylpenicillin, ampicillinum, ampicillin anhydricum, anhydrous ampicillin, AY-6108, BRL-1341, NSC-528986, or P-50; many trade names are available.

Storage/Stability

Ampicillin anhydrous or trihydrate capsules and powder for oral suspension should be stored at room temperature (15–30°C). After reconstitution, the oral suspension is stable for 14 days if refrigerated (2–8°C); 7 days when kept at room temperature.

Ampicillin trihydrate for injection (*Polyflex*®) was labeled as stable for 12 months when refrigerated (2–8°C and 3 months when kept at room temperature. Its new labeling states that it is stable for 3 months when refrigerated. It is not clear if this change is a result of more recent scientific stability studies.

Ampicillin sodium for injection is relatively unstable after reconstitution and should generally be used within 1 hour of reconstitution. As the concentration of the drug in solution increases, the stability of the drug decreases. Dextrose may also speed the destruction of the drug by acting as a catalyst in the hydrolysis of ampicillin.

While most sources recommend using solutions of ampicillin sodium immediately, studies have demonstrated that at concentrations of 30 mg/mL, ampicillin sodium solutions are stable up to 48 hours at 4°C in sterile water for injection or 0.9% sodium chloride (72 hours if concentrations are 20 mg/mL or less). Solutions with a concentration of 30 mg/mL or less have been shown to be stable up to 24 hours in solutions of lactated Ringer's solution if kept at 4°C. Solutions of 20 mg/mL or less are reportedly stable up to 4 hours in D5W if refrigerated.

Compatibility/Compounding Considerations

Ampicillin sodium is reportedly **compatible** with the following additives (see the above paragraph for more information): heparin sodium, chloramphenicol sodium succinate, procaine HCl and verapamil HCl.

Ampicillin sodium is reportedly **incompatible** with the following additives: amikacin sulfate, chlorpromazine HCl, dopamine HCl, erythromycin lactobionate, gentamicin HCl, hydralazine HCl, hydrocortisone sodium succinate, kanamycin sulfate, lincomycin HCl, oxytetracycline HCl, polymyxin B sulfate, prochlorperazine edisylate, sodium bicarbonate and tetracycline HCl. Compatibility is dependent upon factors such as pH, concentration, temperature and diluent used; consult specialized references or a hospital pharmacist for more specific information.

Dosage Forms/Regulatory Status

VETERINARY-LABELED PRODUCTS:

Ampicillin Trihydrate Injection Powder for Suspension: 10 g and 25 g (of ampicillin) vials; *Polyflex*® (Fort Dodge); (Rx). FDA-approved for use in dogs, cats, and cattle. Withdrawal times at labeled doses (cattle; do not treat for more than 7 days): Milk = 48 hours; Slaughter = 6 days (144 hours).

HUMAN-LABELED PRODUCTS:

Ampicillin Sodium Powder for Injection: 250 mg& 500 mg, 1 g & 2 g in vials; generic; (Rx)

Ampicillin Oral Capsules (as trihydrate): 250 mg & 500 mg; *Principen*® (Geneva); generic; (Rx)

Ampicillin (as trihydrate) Powder for Oral Suspension: 125 mg/5 mL (as trihydrate) when reconstituted in 100 mL, 150 mL & 200 mL;

250 mg/5 mL (as trihydrate) when reconstituted in 100 mL & 200 mL; *Principen*® (Geneva); (Rx)

References

Adamcak, A & B Otten (2000). Rodent Therapeutics. *Vet Clin NA: Exotic Anim Pract* 3:1(Jan): 221–240.

Aucoin, D (2000). Antimicrobial Drug Formulary. *Target: The antimicrobial guide to effective treatment*Port Huron, MI, North American Compendiums Inc: 93–142.

Baggot, JD (1983). Systemic antimicrobial therapy in large animals. *Pharmacological Basis of Large Animal Medicine*. JA Bogan, P Lees and AT Yoxall Eds. Oxford, Blackwell Scientific Publications: 45–69.

Beech, J (1987a). Drug therapy of respiratory disorders. *Vet Clin North Am (Equine Practice)* 3(1): 59–80.

Beech, J (1987b). Respiratory Tract—Horse, Cow. *The Bristol Handbook of Antimicrobial Therapy*. DE Johnston Ed. Evansville, Veterinary Learning Systems: 88–109.

Brumbaugh, G (1999). Clinical Pharmacology and the Pediatric Patient. 45th Annual AAEP Convention, Albuquerque.

Clubb, SL (1986). Therapeutics: Individual and Flock Treatment Regimens. *Clinical Avian Medicine and Surgery*. GJ Harrison and LR Harrison Eds. Philadelphia, W.B. Saunders: 327–355.

Furr, M (1999). Antimicrobial treatments for the septic foal. Proceedings: The North American Veterinary Conference, Orlando.

Gauvin, J (1993). Drug therapy in reptiles. *Seminars in Avian & Exotic Med* 2(1): 48–59.

Greene, C, K Hartmannn, et al. (2006). Appendix 8: Antimicrobial Drug Formulary. *Infectious Disease of the Dog and Cat*. C Greene Ed., Elsevier: 1186–1333.

Hardie, E (2000). Therapeutic Mangement of Sepsis. *Kirk's Current Veterinary Therapy: XIII Small Animal Practice*. J Bonagura Ed. Philadelphia, WB Saunders: 272–275.

Hjerpe, CA (1986). The bovine respiratory disease complex. *Current Veterinary Therapy: Food Animal Practice 2*. JL Howard Ed. Philadelphia, W.B. Saunders: 670–681.

Hoeffer, H (1995). Antimicrobials in pet birds. *Kirk's Current Veterinary Therapy:XII*. J Bonagura Ed. Philadelphia, W.B. Saunders: 1278–1283.

Ivey, E & J Morrisey (2000). Therapeutics for Rabbits. *Vet Clin NA: Exotic Anim Pract* 3:1(Jan): 183–216.

Jacobson, E (2000). Antibiotic Therapy for Reptiles. *Kirk's Current Veterinary Therapy: XIII Small Animal Practice*. J Bonagura Ed. Philadelphia, WB Saunders: 1168–1169.

Jenson, J (1998). Current ratite therapy. *The Veterinary Clinics of North America: Food Animal Practice* 16:3(November).

Lunn, K (2006). Update on Leptospiral Infections. Proceedings: BSAVC. Accessed via: Veterinary Information Network. http://goo.gl/Gs983

Perkins, N (1999). Equine reproductive pharmacology. *The Veterinary Clinics of North America: Equine Practice* 15:3(December): 687–704.

Polzin, D (2005). Urinary Tract Therapeutics—What, When & How. Proceedings: ACVC. Accessed via: Veterinary Information Network. http://goo.gl/jRZ0n

Robinson, NE (1987). Table of Common Drugs: Approximate Doses. *Current Therapy in Equine Medicine, 2*. NE Robinson Ed. Philadelphia, W.B. Saunders: 761.

Smith, A (2000). General husbandry and medical care of hedgehogs. *Kirk's Current Veterinary Therapy: XIII Small Animal Practice*. J Bonagura Ed. Philadelphia, WB Saunders: 1128–1133.

Williams, B (2000). Therapeutics in Ferrets. *Vet Clin NA: Exotic Anim Pract* 3:1(Jan): 131–153.

AMPICILLIN SODIUM + SULBACTAM SODIUM

(am-pi-*sill*-in; sul-*bak*-tam)   Unasyn®

INJECTABLE POTENTIATED
AMINOPENICILLIN

Prescriber Highlights

▶ Parenteral potentiated aminopenicillin that may be used for infections where amoxicillin/clavulanate would be appropriate but when an injectable antibiotic is required

▶ Hypersensitivity reactions possible; contraindicated in patients with documented severe hypersensitivity to penicillins

▶ Usually dosed IM or IV q6–8h

Uses/Indications

Ampicillin sodium/sulbactam sodium in a 2:1 ratio is effective when used parenterally for several types of infections caused by many beta-lactamase-producing bacterial strains of otherwise resistant *E. coli*, *Pasturella* spp., *Staphylococcus* spp., *Klebsiella*, and *Proteus*. Other aerobic bacteria commonly susceptible to this combination include *Streptococcus*, *Listeria monocytogenes*, *Bacillus anthracis*, *Salmonella*, *Pasturella*, and *Acinetobacter*. Anaerobic bacterial infections caused by *Clostridium*, *Bacteroides*, *Fusobacterium*, *Peptostreptococcus* or *Propionibacterium* may be effectively treated with ampicillin/ sulbactam.

Type I beta-lactamases that may be associated with *Citrobacter*, *Enterobacter*, *Serratia* and *Pseudomonas* are not generally inhibited by sulbactam or clavulanic acid. Ampicillin/sulbactam is ineffective against practically all strains of *Pseudomonas aeruginosa*.

In dogs and cats, ampicillin/sulbactam therapy may be considered when oral amoxicillin/clavulanate treatment is not viable (patient NPO, critically ill) or when large parenteral doses would be desirable (sepsis, pneumonia, other severe infections) for treating susceptible bacterial infections or prophylaxis.

Ampicillin/sulbactam has been used successfully to treat experimentally induced *Klebsiella* pneumonia in foals.

Pharmacology/Actions

When sulbactam is combined with ampicillin it extends its spectrum of activity to those bacteria that produce beta-lactamases of Richmond-Sykes types II-VI that would otherwise render ampicillin ineffective. Sulbactam binds to beta-lactamases thereby "protecting" the beta-lactam ring of ampicillin from hydrolysis.

Sulbactam has some intrinsic antibacterial activity against some bacteria (*Neisseria*, *Moraxella*, *Bacteroides*) at achievable levels. Sulbactam binding to certain penicillin-binding proteins (PBPs) may explain its activity. For most bacteria, sulbactam alone does not achieve levels sufficient to act alone as an antibacterial but when used in combination with ampicillin, synergistic effects may result.

On a mg for mg basis, clavulanic acid is a more potent beta-lactamase inhibitor than is sulbactam, but sulbactam has advantages of reduced likelihood of inducing chromosomal beta-lactamases, greater tissue penetration and greater stability.

For further information on the pharmacology of ampicillin, refer to that monograph.

Pharmacokinetics

As sulbactam sodium is not appreciably absorbed from the GI tract, this medication must be given parenterally. A covalently linked double ester form of ampicillin/sulbactam (sultamicillin) is orally absorbed, but this combination is not commercially available in the USA. When administered parenterally (IV/IM), sulbactam's pharmacokinetic profile closely mirrors that of ampicillin in most species studied. During the elimination phase in calves, plasma concentrations of sulbactam were consistently higher than those of ampicillin, leading the authors of the study to propose using a higher ratio (than 2:1 ampicillin/sulbactam) if the combination is used in calves.

Contraindications/Precautions/Warnings

Penicillins are contraindicated in patients with a history of severe hypersensitivity (*e.g.*, anaphylaxis) to them. Because there may be cross-reactivity, use penicillins cautiously in patients who are documented hypersensitive to other beta-lactam antibiotics (*e.g.*, cephalosporins, cefamycins, carbapenems).

Patients with severe renal dysfunction may require increased periods of time between doses.

Adverse Effects

Intramuscular injections may be painful. Intravenous injections may cause thrombophlebitis. Hypersensitivity reactions to penicillins occur infrequently in animals, but can be severe (anaphylaxis), particularly after IV administration.

High doses or very prolonged use of penicillins have been associated with neurotoxicity (*e.g.*, ataxia in dogs). Although the penicillins are not considered hepatotoxic, elevated liver enzymes have been reported. Other effects reported in dogs include tachypnea, dyspnea, edema and tachycardia.

Reproductive/Nursing Safety

Penicillins have been shown to cross the placenta and safe use during pregnancy has not been firmly established, but neither have there been any documented teratogenic problems associated with these drugs; however, use only when the potential benefits outweigh the risks. In humans, the FDA categorizes ampicillin as category *B* for use during pregnancy (*Animal studies have not yet demonstrated risk to the fetus, but there are no adequate studies in pregnant women; or animal studies have shown an adverse effect, but adequate studies in pregnant women have not demonstrated a risk to the fetus in the first trimester of pregnancy, and there is no evidence of risk in later trimesters.*) In a separate system evaluating the safety of drugs in canine and feline pregnancy (Papich 1989), ampicillin is categorized as in class: *A* (*Probably safe. Although specific studies may not have proved the safety of all drugs in dogs and cats, there are no reports of adverse effects in laboratory animals or women.*)

It is unknown if sulbactam crosses the placenta and safe use during pregnancy has not been established.

Both ampicillin and sulbactam are distributed into human breast milk in low concentrations. For humans, the World Health Organization (WHO) rates ampicillin as being **compatible** with breastfeeding and the American Academy of Pediatrics lists sulbactam as **compatible** with breastfeeding.

Overdosage/Acute Toxicity

Neurological effects (ataxia) have rarely been reported in dogs receiving very high dosages of penicillins; should these develop, weigh the risks of continued use versus those of dosage reduction or using a different antibiotic. In humans, very high dosages of parenteral penicillins, especially in those with renal disease, have induced CNS effects.

Drug Interactions

The following drug interactions have either been reported or are theoretical in humans or animals receiving ampicillin/sulbactam and may be of significance in veterinary patients:

■ **AMINOGLYCOSIDES (amikacin, gentamicin, tobramycin):** *In vitro* studies have demonstrated that penicillins can have synergistic or additive activity against certain bacteria when used with aminoglycosides. However, beta-lactam antibiotics can inactivate aminoglycosides *in vitro* and *in vivo* in patients in renal failure or when penicillins are used in massive dosages. Amikacin is considered the most resistant aminoglycoside to this inactivation.

■ **BACTERIOSTATIC ANTIMICROBIALS (e.g., chloramphenicol, erythromycin and other macrolides, tetracyclines, sulfonamides, etc.):** Because there is evidence of *in vitro* antagonism between beta-lactam antibiotics and bacteriostatic antibiotics, use together has been generally not recommended in the past, but actual clinical importance is not clear and in doubt.

■ **PROBENECID:** Can reduce the renal tubular secretion of both ampicillin and sulbactam, thereby maintaining higher systemic levels for a longer period of time. This potential "beneficial" interaction requires further investigation before dosing recommendations can be made for veterinary patients.

Laboratory Considerations

■ Ampicillin may cause false-positive **urine glucose** determinations when using cupric sulfate solution (Benedict's Solution, *Clinitest®*). Tests utilizing glucose oxidase (*Test-Tape®, Clinistix®*) are not affected by ampicillin.

■ As penicillins and other beta-lactams can inactivate **aminoglycosides** *in vitro* (and *in vivo* in patients in renal failure or when penicillins are used in massive dosages), serum concentrations of aminoglycosides may be falsely decreased particularly when the serum is stored prior to analysis. It is recommended that if the aminoglycoside assay is delayed, samples be frozen and, if possible, drawn at times when the beta-lactam antibiotic is at a trough.

Doses

■ **DOGS:**

For susceptible infections:

a) For respiratory infections: 50 mg/kg (combined) IV q8h (Hawkins 2003)

b) For respiratory infections: 20 mg/kg IV or IM q6–8h (Greene & Reinero 2006)

c) As adjunctive treatment of serious bite wounds: 30–50 mg/kg q8h IV (Bateman 2005)

d) For intra-abdominal infections: 20 mg/kg IV or IM q6–8h (Extrapolation of human dose with limited studies in dogs and cats) (Greene 2006)

■ **CATS:**

For susceptible infections:

a) For respiratory infections using ampicillin/sulbactam (*Unasyn®*): 50 mg/kg (combined) IV q8h (Hawkins 2003)

b) As adjunctive treatment of serious bite wounds: 30–50 mg/kg q8h IV (Bateman 2005)

c) For intra-abdominal infections: 20 mg/kg IV or IM q6–8h (Extrapolation of human dose with limited studies in dogs and cats) (Greene 2006)

Monitoring

■ Because penicillins usually have minimal toxicity associated with their use, monitoring for efficacy is usually all that is required unless toxic signs or symptoms develop

■ Serum levels and therapeutic drug monitoring are not routinely performed with these agents

Client Information

■ Because of the dosing intervals required this drug is best administered to inpatients only

Chemistry/Synonyms

Ampicillin sodium and sulbactam sodium for injection occurs as a white to off-white powder that is freely soluble in water or other aqueous solutions.

Ampicillin/Sulbactam may also be known as: Ampibactan®, Bacimex®, Begalin-P®, Bethacil®, Comabactan®, Galotam®, Loricin®, Sulam®, Sulperazon®, Synergistin®, Unacid®, Unacim®, Unasyn® or Unasyna®.

Storage/Stability

The unreconstituted powder should be stored at temperatures at, or below, 30°C.

Compatibility/Compounding Considerations

Diluents for reconstituting the powder for injection for IV use that are reported **compatible** with ampicillin/sulbactam include sterile water for injection, and 0.9% sodium chloride. If reconstituted to a concentration of 45 mg/mL (30/15), the resulting solution is stable for 8 hours at room temperature and for 48 hours at 4°C. If reconstituted to a concentration of 30 mg/mL (20/10), the resulting solution is stable for 72 hours at 4°C. After reconstitution and before administering, the solution should be further diluted into a 50 or 100 mL bag of 0.9% sodium chloride and administered IV over 15–30 minutes. Diluted solutions for IV administration are stable at room temperature for 8 hours.

When reconstituting for IM use, sterile water for injection or 0.5% or 2% lidocaine HCl injection may be used. 3.2 mL of diluent is added to the 1.5 g vial; 6.4 mL of diluent to the 3 g vial. After reconstituting, the solution should be administered within 1 hour.

Ampicillin/sulbactam injection is **not compatible** with aminoglycoside antibiotics (e.g., gentamicin, amikacin) and should not be mixed with these agents.

Ampicillin/sulbactam is **compatible** with vancomycin when mixed at concentrations of 50/25 mg/mL of ampicillin/sulbactam and 20 mg/mL or less of vancomycin.

Dosage Forms/Regulatory Status

VETERINARY-LABELED PRODUCTS: None
HUMAN-LABELED PRODUCTS:

Ampicillin Sodium/Sulbactam Sodium Powder (injection): 1.5 g (1 g ampicillin sodium/0.5 g sulbactam sodium), 3 g (2 g ampicillin sodium/1 g sulbactam sodium) in vials, piggyback bottles and ADD-Vantage vials, and 15 g (10 g ampicillin sodium/5 g sulbactam sodium) in bulk; Unasyn® (Roerig); generic; (Rx)

References

Bateman, S (2005). A tale of two teeth—Managing severe bite wounds. Proceedings: WVC2005. Accessed via: Veterinary Information Network. http://goo.gl/UINWY

Greene, C (2006). Gastrointestinal and Intraabdominal Infections. *Infectious Diseases of the Dog and Cat, 3rd Ed.* C Greene Ed., Elsevier: 883–912.

Greene, C & C Reinero (2006). Bacterial Respiratory Infections. *Infectious Diseases of the Dog and Cat, 3rd Ed.* C Greene Ed., Elsevier: 866–882.

Hawkins, E (2003). Respiratory system disorders. *Small Animal Internal Medicine, 3rd Ed.* R Nelson and C Couto Eds. St Louis, Mosby: 210–342.

AMPROLIUM HYDROCHLORIDE

(am-proe-lee-um) Amprovine®, Corid®

ANTICOCCIDIAL

Prescriber Highlights

➤ Thiamine analog antiprotozoal (coccidia)

➤ Prolonged high dosages may cause thiamine deficiency; treatment is usually no longer than 14 days

➤ Occasionally may cause GI or neurologic effects

➤ May be unpalatable

Uses/Indications

Amprolium has good activity against *Eimeria tenella* and *E. acervulina* in poultry and can be used as a therapeutic agent for these organisms. It only has marginal activity or weak activity against *E. maxima*, *E. mivati*, *E. necatrix*, or *E. brunetti*. It is often used in combination with other agents (e.g., ethopabate) to improve control against those organisms.

In cattle, amprolium has FDA-approval for the treatment and prevention of *E. bovis* and *E. zurnii* in cattle and calves.

Amprolium has been used in dogs, swine, sheep, and goats for the control of coccidiosis, although there are no FDA-approved products in the USA for these species.

Pharmacology/Actions

By mimicking its structure, amprolium competitively inhibits thiamine utilization by the parasite. Prolonged high dosages can cause thiamine deficiency in the host; excessive thiamine in the diet can reduce or reverse the anticoccidial activity of the drug.

Amprolium is thought to act primarily upon the first generation schizont in the cells of the intestinal wall, preventing differentiation of the metrozoites. It may suppress the sexual stages and sporulation of the oocysts.

Pharmacokinetics

No information was located for this agent.

Contraindications/Precautions/Warnings

Not recommended to be used for more than 12 days in puppies.

Adverse Effects

In dogs, neurologic disturbances, depression, anorexia, and diarrhea have been reported but are rare and are probably dose-related. See Overdosage section below for treatment recommendations. The undiluted liquid or pastes are reportedly unpalatable.

Overdosage/Acute Toxicity

Amprolium has induced polioencephalomalacia (PEM) in sheep when administered at 880 mg/kg PO for 4–6 weeks and at 1 gram/kg for 3–5 weeks. Erythrocyte production also ceased in lambs receiving these high dosages.

It is reported that overdoses of amprolium will produce neurologic clinical signs in dogs. Treatment should consist of stopping amprolium therapy and administering parenteral thiamine (1–10 mg/day IM or IV).

Drug Interactions

The following drug interactions have either been reported or are theoretical in animals receiving amprolium and may be of significance in veterinary patients:

- ◼ **THIAMINE:** Exogenously administered thiamine in high doses may reverse or reduce the efficacy of amprolium

Doses

- ◼ **DOGS:**

  For coccidiosis:
  a) Small Pups (< 10 kg adult weight): 100 mg (total dose) (using the 20% powder) in a gelatin capsule PO once daily for 7–12 days. Large pups (>10 kg adult weight): 200 mg (total dose) (using the 20% powder) in a gelatin capsule PO once daily for 7–12 days. *In food*, for pups or bitches: 250–300 mg total dose using the 20% powder on food once daily for 7–12 days. *In water*, for pups or bitches: 30 mL of the 9.6% solution in one gallon of water (no other water provided) for 7–10 days (Greene *et al.* 2006)

  b) Prophylaxis: 0.075% solution as drinking water (Matz 1995)

  c) 150 mg/kg of amprolium and 25 mg/kg of sulfadimethoxine for 14 days (Blagburn 2003)

  d) For control of coccidiosis: 1.5 tablespoonsful (22.5 mL) of the 9.6% solution per one gallon of water to be used as the sole drinking water source, not to exceed 10 days. Monitor water consumption both for treatment and hydration assurance; rarely some dogs may not drink the amprolium water due to its bitter taste. In situations where dogs are co-habitants, it is necessary to place enough water for all to have access. (Blagburn 2005), (Blagburn 2007)

- ◼ **CATS:**

  For coccidiosis:
  a) For *Cystoisospora* spp.: 60–100 mg total dose PO once daily for 7 days (Lappin 2000)

  b) *On food*: 300–400 mg/kg on food once daily for 5 days or 110–220 mg/kg on food once daily for 7–12 days. *In water*: 1.5 teaspoonsful (7.5 mL) of the 9.6% so-lution in one gallon of water per day for 10 days.

  In combination: amprolium at 150 mg/kg PO once daily with sulfadimethoxine (25 mg/kg PO once daily) for 14 days (Greene *et al.* 2006)

- ◼ **FERRETS:**

  For coccidiosis:
  a) 19 mg/kg PO once daily (Lennox 2006)

- ◼ **RABBITS/RODENTS/SMALL MAMMALS:**

  a) Rabbits for coccidiosis: Using 9.6% solu-tion: 1 mL/7 kg BW PO once daily for 5 days; in drinking water: 0.5 mL/500 mL for 10 days (Ivey & Morrisey 2000)

  b) Gerbils, Mice, Rats, Hamsters: 10–20 mg/kg total daily dose divided q8–24h SC or IM. Chinchillas: 10–15 mg/kg per day divided q8–24h SC, IM or IV (Adamcak & Otten 2000)

- ◼ **CATTLE:**

  For coccidiosis:
  a) Treatment: 10 mg/kg PO for 5 days; 5 mg/kg for 21 days for prophylaxis (Todd *et al.* 1986)

- ◼ **SWINE:**

  For coccidiosis:
  a) Treatment: 25–65 mg/kg PO once or twice daily for 3–4 days (Todd *et al.* 1986)

  b) 100 mg/kg/day in food or water (Howard 1986)

- ◼ **SHEEP & GOATS:**

  For coccidiosis:
  a) Lambs: 55 mg/kg daily PO for 19 days (Todd *et al.* 1986)

- ◼ **CAMELIDS (NEW WORLD):**

  For *Eimeria macusaniensis* (E.mac):
  a) 10 mg/kg PO once daily for 5 days (Wolff 2009)

  b) 10 mg/kg PO as a 1.5% solution PO once daily. Treat for 10-15 days and give thia-mine at 10 mg/kg SC once daily every 5 days during treatment. (Cebra *et al.* 2007)

- ◼ **BIRDS:**

  a) For coccidiosis in pet birds: 2 mL (us-ing the 9.6% solution)/gallon of water for 5 days or longer. Cages should be steam cleaned to prevent reinfection. Supplement diet with B vitamins. Some strains resistant in Toucans and Mynahs. (Clubb 1986)

  b) For chickens (broilers or layers), turkeys, and pheasants: Refer to individual prod-uct instructions.

Monitoring

- ◼ Clinical efficacy

Chemistry/Synonyms

A structural analogue of thiamine (vitamin B_1), amprolium hydrochloride occurs as a white or almost white, odorless or nearly odorless pow-der. One gram is soluble in 2 mL of water and is slightly soluble in alcohol.

Amprolium may also be known as amprocidi, *Amprol®*, *Corid®*, *Coxoid®*, *Coxiprol®* or *Nemapro®*.

Storage/Stability

Unless otherwise instructed by the manufacturer, amprolium products should be stored at room temperature (15–30°C).

Dosage Forms/Regulatory Status/Withdrawal Times

VETERINARY-LABELED PRODUCTS:

Amprolium 9.6% (96 mg/mL) Oral Solution in 1 gal jugs; *Amprovine®* or *Corid®* 9.6% *Oral Solution* (Huvepharma); (OTC). FDA-approved for use in calves (not veal calves). Slaughter withdrawal (when used as labeled) = 24 hours; a withdrawal period has not been established for pre-ruminating calves.

Amprolium 20% Soluble Powder; *Corid®* 20% *Soluble Powder* (Huvepharma); (OTC). FDA-approved for use in calves (not veal calves). Slaughter withdrawal (when used as labeled) = 24 hours. A withdrawal period has not been established for pre-ruminating calves.

There are also available medicated feeds (amprolium alone) and combination products (medicated feeds, feed additives) containing amprolium with other therapeutic agents. These products may be labeled for use in calves, chickens and/or turkeys.

HUMAN-LABELED PRODUCTS: None

References

Adamcak, A & B Otten (2000). Rodent Therapeutics. *Vet Clin NA: Exotic Anim Pract* 3:1(Jan): 221–240.

Blagburn, B (2003). Giardiasis and coccidiosis updates. Proceedings: Western Veterinary Conference. Accessed via: Veterinary Information Network. http://goo.gl/EZqfI

Blagburn, B (2005). Treatment and control of tick borne diseases and other important parasites of companion animals. Proceedings: ACVC2005. Accessed via: Veterinary Information Network. http://goo.gl/Pexfa

Blagburn, B (2007, Last Update). "Personal communication."

Cebra, CK, BA Valentine, et al. (2007). Eimeria macusaniensis infection in 15 llamas and 34 alpacas. *Javma– Journal of the American Veterinary Medical Association* **230**(1): 94–100.

Clubb, SL (1986). Therapeutics: Individual and Flock Treatment Regimens. *Clinical Avian Medicine and Surgery*. GJ Harrison and LR Harrison Eds. Philadelphia, W.B. Saunders: 327–355.

Greene, C, K Hartmannn, et al. (2006). Appendix 8: Antimicrobial Drug Formulary. *Infectious Disease of the Dog and Cat*. C Greene Ed., Elsevier: 1186–1333.

Howard, JL, Ed. (1986). *Current Veterinary Therapy 2, Food Animal Practice*. Philadelphia, W.B. Saunders.

Ivey, E & J Morrisey (2000). Therapeutics for Rabbits. *Vet Clin NA: Exotic Anim Pract* 3:1(Jan): 183–216.

Lappin, M (2000). Protozoal and Miscellaneous Infections. *Textbook of Veterinary Internal Medicine: Diseases of the Dog and Cat*. S Ettinger and E Feldman Eds. Philadelphia, WB Saunders. **1**: 408–417.

Lennox, A (2006). Working up gastrointestinal disease in the ferret. Proceedings: West Vet Conf. Accessed via: Veterinary Information Network. http://goo.gl/ijsym

Matz, M (1995). Gastrointestinal ulcer therapy. *Kirk's Current Veterinary Therapy:XII*. J Bonagura Ed. Philadelphia, W.B. Saunders: 706–710.

Todd, KS, JA Dipietro, et al. (1986). Coccidiosis. *Current*

Veterinary Therapy 2: Food Animal Practice. JL Howard Ed. Philadelphia, WB Saunders: 632–636.

Wolff, P (2009). Camelid Medicine. Proceedings: AAZV. Accessed via: Veterinary Information Network. http://goo.gl/4TEAy

Amrinone Lactate–See Inamrinone Lactate

Antacids, Oral–See Aluminum Hydroxide; or Magnesium Hydroxide

ANTIVENIN (CROTALIDAE) POLYVALENT (EQUINE ORIGIN) ANTIVENIN (CROTALIDAE) POLYVALENT IMMUNE FAB (OVINE ORIGIN)

(an-tie-*ven*-nin)

Pit Viper Antivenin; CroFab®

ANTIDOTE

Note: The location of antivenins for rare species and the telephone numbers for envenomation experts are available from the Arizona Poison and Drug Information Center (800-222-1222). The National Animal Poison Control Center (888-426-4435) is another source for up-to-date snakebite treatment recommendations.

Prescriber Highlights

▶ May cause hypersensitivity reactions

▶ Treatment can be very expensive

Uses/Indications

The equine-derived product is indicated for the treatment of envenomation from most venomous snake bites (pit vipers) in North America and those caused by several species found in Central and South America (fer-de-lance, Central and South American Rattlesnake). The ovine-derived product is indicated for North American Crotalid snake envenomation in humans, but has been used in dogs. There is a fair amount of controversy with regard to use of these products in domestic animals. The risks of administration (*e.g.*, anaphylaxis—see below) may outweigh their potential benefits in certain circumstances. However, these agents can be life saving when given early in select situations.

Many factors contribute to the potential for toxicity (victim's size and general health, bite site(s), number of bites, age, species and size of snake, etc.).

Pharmacology/Actions

Antivenins act by neutralizing the venoms (complex proteins) in patients via passive immunization of globulins obtained from horses immunized with the venom. Antivenin is very effective in reversing venom-related coagulation abnormalities, but Timber Rattlesnake venom-induced thrombocytopenia may be resistant to treatment.

Contraindications/Precautions/Warnings

Because there is a risk of anaphylaxis occurring secondary to equine-origin proteins, some recommend performing sensitivity testing before administration, but evaluation of results may be difficult and a test-dose is not provided with the veterinary-labeled product. Up to 50% of the veterinary-labeled product contains equine albumin and other equine proteins.

Adverse Effects

The most significant adverse effect associated with the use of the equine origin product is anaphylaxis secondary to its equine serum source; an incidence rate of less than 2% has been reported. A 1:10 dilution of the antivenin given intracutaneously at a dose of 0.02–0.03 mL has been suggested as a test for hypersensitivity. Wheal formation and erythema indicate a positive reaction and are generally seen within 30 minutes of administration. However, a negative response does not insure that anaphylaxis will be avoided and slow intravenous administration is usually sufficient to identify animals that will react to the product. A pre-treatment dose of diphenhydramine is often recommended before administering antivenin primarily to sedate the patient and, theoretically, reduce any possible allergic reactions to the antivenin. Should an anaphylactoid reaction be detected (nausea, pruritus, hyperemia of the inner pinna), stopping the infusion, giving an additional dose of diphenhydramine and restarting the infusion 5 minutes later at a slower rate may allow the dose to be administered without further problems.

One case of a dog developing antivenin-associated serum sickness has been reported after treatment using Crotilidae antivenin (Berdoulay *et al.* 2005).

Reproductive/Nursing Safety

In humans, the FDA categorizes this drug as category *C* for use during pregnancy (*Animal studies have shown an adverse effect on the fetus, but there are no adequate studies in humans; or there are no animal reproduction studies and no adequate studies in humans*).

Safety during nursing has not been established but it would unlikely pose much risk.

Drug Interactions

The following drug interactions have either been reported or are theoretical in humans or animals receiving antivenin and may be of significance in veterinary patients:

- ◼ **ANALGESICS/SEDATIVES:** Although reducing excessive movement and other supportive therapy are important parts of treating envenomation, drugs that can mask the clinical signs associated with the venom (*e.g.*, analgesics and sedatives) should initially be used with caution.

- ◼ **ANTIHISTAMINES:** It has been stated that antihistamines may potentiate the venom; however, documentation of this interaction was not located and diphenhydramine is routinely used by many clinicians treating snakebite in dogs.

- ◼ **BETA-BLOCKERS:** May mask the early signs associated with anaphylaxis

- ◼ **CORTICOSTEROID** use has fallen out of favor in the treatment of snakebite envenomation and is usually not employed, but controversy remains regarding their use. Corticosteroids may be useful to treat anaphylaxis, however.

- ◼ **HEPARIN:** Is reportedly not effective in treating the thrombin-like enzymes found in rattlesnake venom.

Doses

Note: The treatment of pit viper snakebite involves significant treatment (aggressive IV fluids, antibiotics) and monitoring beyond administration of antivenin. It is highly recommended to refer to specialized references *e.g.*, (Peterson 2006) or to contact an animal poison control center for guidance beyond what is listed below.

- ◼ **DOGS/CATS:**

  Crotilidae antivenin (equine origin):

  a) Dogs/Cats: Dose necessary is calculated relative to the amount of venom injected, body mass of patient and the bite site. Average dose required for dogs or cats is 1–2 vials of antivenin. The earlier the antivenin is administered the more effective it is. Intravascular bites or bites to the torso or tongue are serious and require prompt, aggressive antivenin administration. Smaller patients may require higher doses (as venom amount/kg body weight is higher), and multiple vials may be necessary. Initially, give one vial, by diluting to 100–250 mL of crystalloid fluids and initially administer by slow IV (if there are no problems, may increase rate and administer volume over 30 minutes). In smaller patients, adjust infusion volume to prevent fluid overload. (Peterson 2006)

  b) Dogs: Administer 1–5 rehydrated vials (10–50 mL) IV depending on severity of symptoms, duration of time after the bite, snake size, patient size (the smaller the victim, the larger the dose). Additional doses may be given every 2 hours as required. If unable to give IV, may administer IM as close to bite as practical. Give supportive therapy (*e.g.*, corticosteroids, antibiotics, fluid therapy, blood products, and tetanus prophylaxis) as required. (Package Insert; *Antivenin®*—Fort Dodge)

- ■ **HORSES:**
  a) Crotilidae Antivenin: Use only if necessary to treat systemic effects, otherwise avoid use. Administer 1–2 vials slowly IV diluted in 250–500 mL saline or lactated Ringer's. Administer antihistamines; corticosteroids are contraindicated. (Bailey & Garland 1992)

Monitoring
- ■ Signs associated with an allergic response to the antivenin (anaphylaxis, anaphylactoid-reactions, serum sickness)
- ■ CBC with platelets; coagulation parameters
- ■ Biochem profile; hydration status
- ■ ECG

Client Information
- ■ Clients must be made aware of the potential for anaphylaxis as well as the expenses associated with treatment, monitoring and hospitalization.

Chemistry
Antivenin products are concentrated serum globulins obtained from horses immunized with the venoms of several types of snakes. They are provided as refined, lyophilized product with a suitable diluent. Up to 50% of the proteins contained in the veterinary product may be equine-specific proteins.

Storage/Stability
Do not store above 98°F (37°C); avoid freezing and excessive heat. Reconstitute the vial with the diluent provided; gently swirl the vial (may require several minutes; do not shake) to prevent excessive foaming. Warming the vial to body temperature may speed up reconstitution. Once reconstituted the vial contents are often added to a crystalloid intravenous solution (D5W, normal saline often recommended) for infusion. Depending on dog size, one vial in 100–250 mL has been suggested for infusion (Peterson 2006).

The package insert for the veterinary-labeled product states that after rehydration the vial should be used immediately. One reference (anon 2007a) states that the human-labeled equine origin product can be used within 4 hours of reconstitution if refrigerated, but another (anon 2007b) states that it can be used within 48 hours after reconstitution and within 12 hours after further dilution into IV fluids.

The polyvalent immune fab (ovine) product should be stored in the refrigerator and used within 4 hours of reconstitution.

Dosage Forms/Regulatory Status
Note: The availability status of antivenins in the USA is in flux. It is highly recommended to contact a poison control center (see sample phone numbers at the top of this monograph) to get current recommendations on availability and treatment options.

VETERINARY-LABELED PRODUCTS:
Antivenin (Crotalidae) Polyvalent Equine Origin single dose vial lyophilized; 10 mL vials with diluent. *Antivenin®* (Fort Dodge); (Rx). Approved for use in dogs.

HUMAN-LABELED PRODUCTS:
Antivenin (Crotalidae) Polyvalent Powder for Injection (lyophilized): combo packs with 1 mL vial of normal horse serum (for testing) and 10 mL Bacteriostatic water for injection USP; *Antivenin (Crotalidae) Polyvalent®* (Wyeth); (Rx)

Antivenin (Crotalidae) Polyvalent Immune Fab (Ovine Origin) Powder for Injection (lyophilized); 1 g total protein per single use vial; *CroFab®* (Altana); (Rx)

References
anon (2007a). "Facts and Comparisons Online Edition."
anon (2007b). "USP DI® Drug Information for the Health Professional Online Edition."
Bailey, E & T Garland (1992). Management of Toxicoses. *Current Therapy in Equine Medicine 3.* N Robinson Ed. Philadelphia, W.B. Saunders Co.: 346–353.
Berdoulay, P, M Schaer, et al. (2005). Serum sickness in a dog associated with antivenin therapy for a snake bite caused by Crotalus adamanteus. *J Vet Emerg Crit Care* 15(3): 206–212.
Peterson, M (2006). Snake Bite: North American Pit Vipers. *Small Animal Toxicology, 2nd Ed.* M Peterson and P Talcott Eds., Elsevier: 1017–1038.

ANTIVENIN (MICRURUS FULVIAS) EASTERN AND TEXAS CORAL SNAKE

(an-tie-*ven*-nin)
North American Coral Snake Antivenin

ANTIDOTE

Note: The location of antivenins for rare species and the telephone numbers for envenomation experts are available from the Arizona Poison and Drug Information Center (800-222-1222). The National Animal Poison Control Center (888-426-4435) is another source for up-to-date snakebite treatment recommendations.

Prescriber Highlights
▶ May cause hypersensitivity reactions
▶ Treatment can be very expensive

Uses/Indications
This product is indicated for the treatment of envenomation from the Eastern coral snake

(*Micrurus fulvius fulvius*) and the Texas coral snake (*Micrurus fulvius tenere*). It will not neutralize the venom form the Sonoran or Arizona coral snake (*Micruroides euryxanthus*) or the Brazilian giant coral snake (*Micrurus frontalis*). Coral snake envenomation is quite rare in the United States and approximately 60% of coral snake bites do not result in envenomation. Unlike pit viper venom, coral snake venom primarily causes neurotoxicity and clinical signs may be delayed. It has been recommended that animals suspected of a coral snake envenomation be hospitalized with close observation for 24–48 hours post-bite.

Pharmacology/Actions

Antivenins act by neutralizing the venoms (complex proteins) in patients via passive immunization of globulins obtained from horses immunized with the venom. Each vial of antivenin will neutralize approximately 2 mg of *M. fulvius fulvius* venom.

Contraindications/Precautions/Warnings

The coral snake antivenin will not neutralize *M. euryxanthus* (Sonoran or Arizona Coral Snake) venom. Because there is a risk of anaphylaxis occurring secondary to the horse serum, many recommend performing sensitivity testing before administration.

Adverse Effects

The most significant adverse effect associated with the use of these products is anaphylaxis secondary to the equine serum source of this product. An incidence rate of less than 2% has been reported. A 1:10 dilution of the antivenin given intracutaneously at a dose of 0.02–0.03 mL may be useful as a test for hypersensitivity. Wheal formation and erythema indicate a positive reaction and are generally seen within 30 minutes of administration. A negative response does not insure that anaphylaxis will not occur, however. A pre-treatment dose of diphenhydramine is often recommended before administering antivenin. Should an anaphylactoid reaction be detected, stopping the infusion, giving an additional dose of diphenhydramine and restarting the infusion 5 minutes later at a slower rate may allow the dose to be administered without further problems.

Reproductive/Nursing Safety

In humans, the FDA categorizes this drug as category *C* for use during pregnancy (*Animal studies have shown an adverse effect on the fetus, but there are no adequate studies in humans; or there are no animal reproduction studies and no adequate studies in humans*).

Drug Interactions

The following drug interactions have either been reported or are theoretical in humans or animals receiving antivenin and may be of significance in veterinary patients:

- ■ **ANALGESICS/SEDATIVES:** Although reducing excessive movement and other support-

ive therapy are important parts of treating envenomation, drugs that can mask the clinical signs associated with the venom (*e.g.*, analgesics and sedatives) should initially be used with caution

- ■ **ANTIHISTAMINES:** It has been stated that antihistamines may potentiate the venom; however, documentation of this interaction was not located and diphenhydramine is routinely used by many clinicians treating snakebite in dogs.

- ■ **BETA-BLOCKERS:** May mask the early signs associated with anaphylaxis.

- ■ **CORTICOSTEROID** use has fallen out of favor in the treatment of snakebite envenomation and is usually considered contraindicated. Corticosteroids may be useful to treat anaphylaxis, however.

Doses

Note: The treatment of Coral snakebite involves significant treatment and monitoring beyond administration of antivenin. It is highly recommended to refer to specialized references *e.g.*, (Peterson 2006a) or to contact an animal poison control center for guidance beyond what is listed below.

- ■ **DOGS/CATS:**
  Coral Snake antivenin (not Sonoran or Arizona variety):
  a) Dogs: After testing for hypersensitivity give 1–2 vials initially, and more in 4–6 hours if necessary. Therapy is best started within 4 hours after envenomation. Supportive care includes broad-spectrum antibiotics, fluid therapy and mechanical ventilation if necessary. Corticosteroids are not recommended. (Marks, Mannella et al. 1990)

  b) Dogs/Cats: Dose necessary is calculated relative to the amount of venom injected and the body mass of patient. Average dose required for dogs or cats is 1–2 vials of antivenin. The earlier the antivenin is administered the more effective it is. Smaller patients may require higher doses (as venom amount/kg body weight is higher), and multiple vials may be necessary. Initially give one vial, by diluting to 100–250 mL of crystalloid fluids and initially administering by slow IV. In smaller patients, adjust infusion volume to prevent fluid overload. Give additional vials as indicated by the progression of the syndrome. (Peterson 2006b)

- ■ **HORSES:**
  Coral Snake Antivenin:
  a) Use only if necessary to treat systemic effects, otherwise avoid use. Administer 1–2 vials slowly IV diluted in 250–500 mL saline or lactated Ringer's. Administer antihistamines; corticosteroids are con-

traindicated. May be used with Crotilidae antivenin. (Bailey and Garland 1992)

Monitoring

- Signs associated with an allergic response to the antivenin (anaphylaxis, anaphylactoid-reactions, serum sickness)
- Cardiorespiratory monitoring; mechanical ventilation may be necessary
- Pulse oximetry

Client Information

- Clients must be made aware of the potential for anaphylaxis as well as the expenses associated with treatment, monitoring and hospitalization.

Chemistry

These products are concentrated serum globulins obtained from horses immunized with the venoms of several types of snakes. They are provided as refined, lyophilized product with a suitable diluent.

Storage/Stability

Product should be stored in the refrigerator. Avoid freezing and excessive heat. Reconstitute vial with 10 mL of the supplied diluent. Gentle agitation may be used to hasten dissolution of the lyophilized powder. Reconstituted vials should be used within 48 hours (keep refrigerated) and within 12 hours once added to IV solutions.

Dosage Forms/Regulatory Status

Note: The availability status of antivenins in the USA is in flux. It is highly recommended to contact a poison control center (see sample phone numbers at the top of this monograph) to get current recommendations on availability and treatment options.

VETERINARY-LABELED PRODUCTS: None

HUMAN-LABELED PRODUCTS:

Antivenin (*Micrurus fulvius*) Powder for Injection lyophilized: in single-use vials with 1 vial diluent (10 mL water for injection); *Antivenin (Micrurus fulvius)*; (Ayerst); (Rx). **Note:** The manufacturer has discontinued producing this product, but has enough antivenin on hand to satisfy demand for several years.

References

Peterson, M (2006a). Snake Bite: Coral Snakes. *Small Animal Toxicology, 2nd Ed.* M Peterson and P Talcott Eds., Elsevier: 1017–1038.

Peterson, M (2006b). Snake Bite: North American Pit Vipers. *Small Animal Toxicology, 2nd Ed.* M Peterson and P Talcott Eds., Elsevier: 1017–1038.

ANTIVENIN (LATRODECTUS MACTANS) BLACK WIDOW SPIDER

(an-tie-*ven*-nin)
Black Widow Spider Antivenin

ANTIDOTE

Note: The location of antivenins for rare species and the telephone numbers for envenomation experts are available from the Arizona Poison and Drug Information Center (800-222-1222). The National Animal Poison Control Center (888-426-4435) is another source for up-to-date envenomation treatment recommendations.

Prescriber Highlights

- ▶ May cause hypersensitivity reactions
- ▶ May be difficult for veterinarians to obtain

Uses/Indications

Black widow spider antivenin is used to treat envenomation caused by this spider. Cats, camels and horses are considered to be extremely sensitive to the venom. Primary toxic signs are due to neurotoxins in the venom.

Pharmacology/Actions

Antivenins act by neutralizing the venoms (complex proteins) in patients via passive immunization of globulins obtained from horses immunized with the venom. In humans, symptoms begin to subside in 1-2 hours after administration.

Contraindications/Precautions/Warnings

Because there is a risk of anaphylaxis occurring secondary to the horse serum, many recommend performing sensitivity testing before administration.

Adverse Effects

The most significant adverse effect associated with the use of the equine origin product is anaphylaxis secondary to its equine serum source; an incidence rate of less than 2% has been reported. A 1:10 dilution of the antivenin given intracutaneously at a dose of 0.02–0.03 mL has been suggested as a test for hypersensitivity. Wheal formation and erythema indicate a positive reaction and are generally seen within 30 minutes of administration. However, a negative response does not insure that anaphylaxis will be avoided and slow intravenous administration is usually sufficient to identify animals that will react to the product. A pre-treatment dose of diphenhydramine is often recommended before administering antivenin primarily to sedate the patient and, theoretically, to reduce any possible allergic reactions to the antivenin. Should an anaphylactoid reaction be detected (nausea, pruritus, hyperemia of the inner pinna), stopping the infusion, giving an additional dose of diphenhydramine and restarting the infusion 5 minutes later at a slower rate may allow the dose to be administered without further problems.

Reproductive/Nursing Safety

In humans, the FDA categorizes this drug as category *C* for use during pregnancy (*Animal studies have shown an adverse effect on the fetus, but there are no adequate studies in humans; or there are no animal reproduction studies and no adequate studies in humans*).

Drug Interactions

The following drug interactions have either been reported or are theoretical in humans or animals receiving black widow spider antivenin and may be of significance in veterinary patients:

- **BETA-BLOCKERS:** May mask the early signs associated with anaphylaxis

Doses

- **DOGS/CATS:**
  a) After reconstituting the antivenin, add to 100 mL of normal saline and administer via slow IV over 30 minutes. Pretreatment with 2–4 mg/kg of diphenhydramine SC may help calm the patient and may possibly protect against allergic reactions from the antivenin. Monitor inner pinna during infusion for signs of anaphylaxis (hyperemia). If hyperemia occurs, discontinue infusion and give a second dose of diphenhydramine. If allergic reactions abate, may restart infusion at a slower rate; if they recur, stop infusion and seek consultation. Use care with administration of IV fluids as envenomation can cause significant hypertension. Benzodiazepines may alleviate muscle cramping. (Peterson & McNalley 2006)
  b) Dissolve contents of one vial and add to 100–200 mL of warm 0.9% NaCl and infuse over 2–6 hours. Administer diphenhydramine at 0.5–1 mg/kg prior to infusion. (Atkins 2006)

Client Information

- Clients must be made aware of the potential for anaphylaxis as well as the expenses associated with treatment, monitoring and hospitalization.

Monitoring

- Signs associated with an allergic response to the antivenin (anaphylaxis, anaphylactoid-reactions, serum sickness)
- Respiratory/cardiac rate
- Blood pressure
- Serum chemistry (blood glucose mandatory)

- CBC
- Urine output; urinalysis

Chemistry

This product is concentrated serum globulins obtained from horses immunized with the venom of the black widow spider. It is provided as refined, lyophilized product with a suitable diluent.

Storage/Stability

Product should be stored in the refrigerator (2–8°C). It is reconstituted by adding 2.5 mL of the diluent provided; shake the vial to completely dissolve the contents. Do not freeze the reconstituted solution. For IV use, further dilute the solution in 10–100 mL of normal saline injection.

Dosage Forms/Regulatory Status

Note: The availability status of antivenins in the USA is in flux. It is highly recommended to contact a poison control center (see sample phone numbers at the top of this monograph) to get current recommendations on availability and treatment options.

VETERINARY-LABELED PRODUCTS: None

HUMAN-LABELED PRODUCTS:

Antivenin (*Latrodectus mactans*) Powder for Injection: greater than or equal to 6000 antivenin Units/vial in single-use vials with 1 vial diluent (2.5 mL vial of sterile water for injection) and 1 mL vial of normal horse serum (1:10 dilution) for sensitivity testing; Antivenin (Lactrodectus mactans); (Merck); (Rx)

References

Atkins, L (2006). Spiders and Snakes—Envenomation. Proceedings: IVECCS. Accessed via: Veterinary Information Network. http://goo.gl/djON1

Peterson, M & J McNalley (2006). Spider Envenomation: Black Widow. *Small Animal Toxicology, 2nd Ed.* M Peterson and P Talcott Eds., Elsevier: 1017–1038.

APOMORPHINE HCL

(a-poe-*mor*-feen)   Apokyn®

EMETIC

Prescriber Highlights

▶ Rapid acting, centrally-mediated emetic used in dogs & sometimes in cats

▶ Contraindicated in certain species (e.g., rodents, rabbits) & when vomiting may be deleterious (e.g., impending coma, aspiration)

▶ May cause protracted vomiting; naloxone should reverse CNS effects or cardio-respiratory depression, but not vomiting

▶ Availability & expense may be an issue

Uses/Indications

Apomorphine is used primarily as an emetic in dogs, and is considered the emetic of choice for dogs by many clinicians. It is sometimes used in cats, but its use in this species is somewhat controversial.

Pharmacology/Actions

Apomorphine stimulates dopamine receptors in the chemoreceptor trigger zone, thus inducing vomiting. It can cause both CNS depression and stimulation, but tends to cause more stimulatory effects. Medullary centers can be depressed with resultant respiratory depression.

Pharmacokinetics

Apomorphine is slowly absorbed after oral administration and has unpredictable efficacy when given by this route, therefore, it is usually administered parenterally or topically to the eye. When given intravenously in dogs, emesis occurs very rapidly; after IM use, vomiting occurs generally within 5 minutes but may be more prolonged. Topical administration to the conjunctival sac is usually effective but less so than either IV or IM administration.

Apomorphine is primarily conjugated in the liver and then excreted in the urine.

Contraindications/Precautions/Warnings

Emetics can be an important aspect in the treatment of orally ingested toxins, but must not be used injudiciously. Emetics should not be used in rodents or rabbits, because they are either unable to vomit or do not have stomach walls strong enough to tolerate the act of emesis. Emetics are also contraindicated in patients that are: hypoxic, dyspneic, in shock, lack normal pharyngeal reflexes, seizuring, comatose, severely CNS depressed or where CNS function is deteriorating, or extremely physically weak. Emetics should also be withheld in patients who have previously vomited repeatedly. Because of the risk for additional esophageal or gastric injury with emesis, emetics are contraindicated in patients who have ingested strong acids, alkalis, or other caustic agents. Because of the risks of aspiration, emetics are usually contraindicated after petroleum distillate ingestion, but may be employed when the risks of toxicity of the compound are greater than the risks of aspiration. Use of emetics after ingestion of strychnine or other CNS stimulants may precipitate seizures.

Emetics generally do not remove more than 80% of the material in the stomach (usually 40–60%) and successful induction of emesis does not signal the end of appropriate monitoring or therapy. In addition to the contraindications outlined in the general statement, apomorphine should not be used in cases of oral opiate or other CNS depressant (e.g., barbiturates) toxicity, or in patients hypersensitive to morphine.

The use of apomorphine in cats is controversial, and several clinicians state that it should not be used in this species as it is much less effective than either xylazine or ipecac syrup and possibly, less safe.

If vomiting does not occur within the expected time after apomorphine administration, repeated doses are unlikely to induce emesis and may cause clinical signs of toxicity.

Adverse Effects

At usual doses, the principal adverse effect that may be seen with apomorphine is protracted vomiting. Protracted vomiting after ophthalmic administration may be averted by washing the conjunctival sac with sterile saline or ophthalmic rinsing solution. Excitement, restlessness, CNS depression or respiratory depression are usually only associated with overdoses of the drug. Anecdotal reports of corneal ulcers have been noted after conjunctival administration.

Reproductive/Nursing Safety

The reproductive safety of this drug has not been established; weigh the risks of use versus the potential benefits.

Overdosage/Acute Toxicity

Excessive doses of apomorphine may result in respiratory and/or cardiac depression, CNS stimulation (excitement, seizures) or depression and protracted vomiting. Naloxone may reverse the CNS and respiratory effects of the drug but cannot be expected to halt the vomiting. Atropine has been suggested to treat severe bradycardias.

Drug Interactions

The following drug interactions have either been reported or are theoretical in humans or animals receiving apomorphine and may be of significance in veterinary patients:

- **ANTIDOPAMINERGIC DRUGS (e.g., phenothiazines)** may negate the emetic effects of apomorphine

- **ONDANSETRON:** A human patient that received ondansetron and apomorphine developed severe hypotension. In humans, use together is contraindicated.

- **OPIATES OR OTHER CNS OR RESPIRATORY DEPRESSANTS (e.g., barbiturates):** Additive CNS, or respiratory depression may occur when apomorphine is used with these agents

Doses

- **DOGS:**

For induction of emesis:

a) 0.03 mg/kg IV or 0.04 mg/kg IM (IV route preferred); alternatively a portion of tablet may be crushed in a syringe, dissolved with few drops of water and administered into the conjunctival sac. After sufficient vomiting occurs, rinse conjunctival sac free of unabsorbed apomorphine. (Beasley & Dorman 1990)

b) 0.04 mg/kg IV or 0.08 mg/kg IM or SC (Bailey 1989), (Riviere 1985), (Mount 1989)

c) 0.04 mg/kg IV, 0.07 mg/kg IM, or 0.25 mg/kg into the conjunctival sac (Jenkins 1988)

■ **CATS:**

Note: Use of apomorphine in cats is controversial and many recommend not using in this species.

a) For induction of emesis: 0.04 mg/kg IV or 0.08 mg/kg IM or SC (Bailey 1989), (Reid & Oehme 1989)

Monitoring

■ CNS, respiratory, and cardiac systems should be monitored

■ Vomitus should be quantified, examined for contents and saved for possible later analysis

Client Information

■ This agent must be used in a professionally supervised setting only

Chemistry/Synonyms

A centrally-acting emetic, apomorphine occurs as a white powder or minute, white or grayish-white crystals and is sparingly soluble in water or alcohol.

Apomorphine HCl may also be known as: apomorphini hydrochloridum, *APO-go®*, *APO-go Pen®*, *Apofin®*, *Apokinon®*, *Apokyn®*, *Apomine®*, *Britaject®*, *Ixense®*, *Taluvian®*, or *Uprima®*.

Storage/Stability

Apomorphine soluble tablets should be stored in tight containers at room temperature (15–30°C) and protected from light.

Upon exposure to light and air, apomorphine gradually darkens in color. Discolored tablets or discolored solutions (green to turquoise) should not be used. Apomorphine solutions are more stable in acidic than in alkaline solutions. A 0.3% solution of apomorphine has a pH of about 3–4.

Compatibility/Compounding Considerations

Solutions of apomorphine can be made by solubilizing tablets in at least 1–2 mL of either sterile water for injection or 0.9% sodium chloride for injection. After being sterilized by filtration, the solution is stable for 2 days if protected from light and air and stored in the refrigerator. Do not use solutions that are discolored or form a precipitate after filtering.

Compounded preparation stability: Apomorphine injectable solution compounded from the active pharmaceutical ingredient (API) has been published (Jaeger, 1976). Dissolving 10 mg apomorphine to a final volume of 10 mL with 0.1% sodium metabisulfite in sterile water and filtering through a 0.22micron sterilizing filter yields a 2.5 mg/mL sterile solution that retains potency for two months stored at 25°C. Compounded preparations of apomorphine should be protected from light. Solutions of apomorphine should be cold sterilized and not be autoclaved as autoclaving results in the development of a green color.

Dosage Forms/Regulatory Status

VETERINARY-LABELED PRODUCTS:

Pharmaceutical dosage forms of apomorphine have been occasionally difficult to obtain and compounding pharmacies may be required to obtain the drug.

The ARCI (Racing Commissioners International) has designated this drug as a class 1 substance. See the appendix for more information.

HUMAN-LABELED PRODUCTS:

Apomorphine HCl Injection: 10 mg/mL in 2 mL amps and 3 mL cartridges; *Apokyn®* (Vernalis); (Rx)

References

Bailey, EM (1989). Emergency and general treatment of poisonings. *Current Veterinary Therapy (CVT) X Small Animal Practice*. RW Kirk Ed. Philadelphia, W.B. Saunders: 116–125.

Beasley, VR & DC Dorman (1990). Management of Toxicoses. *Vet Clin of North America: Sm Anim Pract* 20(2): 307–337.

Jaeger, R.W. & F.J. de Castro (1976). Apomorphine: a stable solution. *Clin Toxicol* 9(2): 199–202.

Jenkins, WL (1988). Drugs affecting gastrointestinal functions. *Veterinary Pharmacology and Therapeutics 6th Ed.* NH Booth and LE McDonald Eds. Ames, Iowas Stae Univ. Press: 657–671.

Mount, ME (1989). Toxicology. *Textbook of Veterinary Internal Medicine.* SJ Ettinger Ed. Philadelphia, WB Saunders. 1: 456–483.

Reid, FM & FW Oehme (1989). Toxicoses. *The Cat: Diseases and Clinical Management.* RG Sherding Ed. New York, Churchill Livingstone. 1: 185–215.

Riviere, JE (1985). Clinical management of of toxicoses and adverse drug reactions. *Handbook of Small Animal Therapeutics.* LE Davis Ed. New York, Churchill Livingstone: 657–683.

APRAMYCIN SULFATE

(a-pra-*mye*-sin)   Apralan®

AMINOGLYCOSIDE ANTIBIOTIC

Prescriber Highlights

▶ Orally administered aminocyclitol antibiotic for porcine *E. coli* bacillosis in swine (sometimes used in calves—not FDA-approved)

▶ Products no longer available in USA

▶ May be partially absorbed in neonates; potentially nephro- & ototoxic if absorbed systemically

Uses/Indications

Apramycin is no longer commercially available in the USA, but it is used in some countries for the treatment of bacterial enteritis, colibacillosis, salmonellosis, etc. in pigs, calves and poultry.

Pharmacology/Actions

Apramycin is an aminoglycoside that is bactericidal against many gram-negative bacteria (*E. coli*, Pseudomonas, Salmonella, Klebsiella, Proteus, Pasturella, *Treponema hyodysenteriae*, *Bordetella bronchiseptica*), Staphylococcus and

Mycoplasma. It prevents protein synthesis by susceptible bacteria, presumably by binding to the 30S ribosomal subunit.

Pharmacokinetics

After oral administration, apramycin is partially absorbed, particularly in neonates. Absorption is dose related and decreases substantially with the age of the animal. Absorbed drug is eliminated via the kidneys unchanged.

Contraindications/Precautions/Warnings

Do not use in known cases of apramycin hypersensitivity. The drug apparently has a wide margin of safety when used orally and is safe to use in breeding swine. Apramycin is contraindicated in cats and in patients with myasthenia gravis.

Adverse Effects

When used as labeled, the manufacturer does not list any adverse reactions. Should substantial amounts of the drug be absorbed, both ototoxicity and nephrotoxicity are a distinct possibility.

Drug Interactions/Laboratory Considerations

None were noted. May have similar interaction potential as neomycin; refer to that monograph for more information.

Doses

■ **SWINE:**

For bacterial enteritis caused by susceptible organisms:

a) Treated pigs should consume enough water to receive 12.5 mg/kg body weight per day for 7 days. Add to drinking water at a rate of 375 mg per gallon. After adding to water, stir and allow to stand for 15 minutes, then stir again. (Label directions; *Apralan® Soluble Powder*—SKB)

b) 20–40 mg/kg PO daily in drinking water (Huber 1988)

c) Pigs: To be administered via the drinking water. Add 1 small measure (4.4 mL) or 1 sachet of soluble powder per 20 L of drinking water. (Label information; *Apralan Soluble Powder®*—Elanco U.K.)

■ **CATTLE:**

a) For bacterial enteritis caused by susceptible organisms: 20–40 mg/kg PO daily in drinking water (Huber 1988)

b) **Calves:** For the treatment of colibacillosis or salmonellosis: 1–2 sachets to be administered in the drinking water, milk, or milk replacer to provide 20–40 mg of apramycin activity per kg of bodyweight daily according to the severity of the disease. Continue treatment for 5 days. (Label information; *Apralan Soluble Powder®*—Elanco U.K.)

■ **POULTRY:**

a) For bacterial enteritis caused by susceptible organisms: To be administered via drinking water to provide 250–500 mg

of apramycin activity per liter for 5 days. This may be achieved by adding 50 g apramycin per 100–200 liters of water. (Label information; *Apralan Soluble Powder®*—Elanco U.K.)

Monitoring

■ Clinical efficacy

Chemistry/Synonyms

Apramycin is an aminocyclitol antibiotic produced from *Streptomyces tenebrarius*; it is soluble in water.

Apramycin may also be known as nebramycin factor 2, nebramycin II, apramycine, apramicina, AIDS166733, *Apralan®* or *Abylan®*.

Storage/Stability

Apramycin powder should be stored in a cool dry place, in tightly closed containers, protected from moisture. Store at temperatures less than 25°C. If exposed to rust, as in a rusty waterer, the drug can be inactivated. The manufacturer recommends preparing fresh water daily. Shelf life of the powder is 24 months.

Dosage Forms/Regulatory Status

VETERINARY-LABELED PRODUCTS:

None at present in the USA. A swine product: Apramycin Sulfate Soluble Powder 37.5 & 48 g (base) bottle; *Apralan®* (Elanco); (OTC), was formerly marketed in the USA and is still available in several countries.

In the UK: Apramycin Soluble Powder: 1 gram sachets and 50 g (apramycin activity) in 220 mL; *Apralan Soluble Powder®* (Elanco); (POM-V). In the UK when used as labeled: Slaughter withdrawal: Pigs = 14 days, Calves = 28 days, Poultry = 7 days. Not for use in laying hens where eggs are for human consumption.

HUMAN-LABELED PRODUCTS: None

References

Huber, WG (1988). Aminoglycosides, Macrolides, Lincosamides, Polymyxins, Chloramphenicol, and other Antibacterial Drugs. *Veterinary Pharmacology and Therapeutics*. NH Booth and LE McDonald Eds. Ames, Iowa State University Press: 822–848.

ASA–see Aspirin

ASCORBIC ACID
VITAMIN C

(a-*skor*-bik)

Prescriber Highlights

▶ Prevention/treatment of scurvy in Guinea pigs most accepted use

▶ At usual dosages, little downside to use; may exacerbate liver injury in copper toxicosis

▶ Some drug interactions, primarily due to its urinary acidification qualities

▶ May alter some lab results (urine glucose, occult blood in stool, serum bilirubin)

Uses/Indications

Ascorbic acid is used to prevent and treat scurvy in guinea pigs. It has been used as a urinary acidifier in small animals, but its efficacy is in question. Sodium ascorbate does not acidify the urine. In the past, it was used to treat copper-induced hepatopathy in dogs but this use has fallen into disfavor (see Contraindications below).

Pharmacology/Actions

Exogenously supplied ascorbic acid is a dietary requirement in some exotic species (including rainbow trout, Coho salmon), guinea pigs, and in primates. The other animal species are able to synthesize *in vivo* enough Vitamin C to meet their nutritional needs. Vitamin C is used for tissue repair and collagen formation. It may be involved with some oxidation-reduction reactions, and with the metabolism of many substances (iron, folic acid, norepinephrine, histamine, phenylalanine, tyrosine, some drug enzyme systems). Vitamin C is believed to play a role in protein, lipid and carnitine synthesis, maintaining blood vessel integrity and immune function.

Pharmacokinetics

Vitamin C is generally well absorbed in the jejunum (human data) after oral administration, but absorption may be reduced with high doses as an active process is involved with absorption. Ascorbic acid is widely distributed and only about 25% is bound to plasma proteins. Vitamin C is biotransformed in the liver. When the body is saturated with vitamin C and blood concentrations exceed the renal threshold, the drug is more readily excreted unchanged into the urine.

Contraindications/Precautions/Warnings

Vitamin C (high doses) should be used with caution in patients with diabetes mellitus due to the laboratory interactions (see below), or in patients susceptible to urolithiasis as it can promote hyperoxaluria.

Because there is some evidence that it may increase copper's oxidative damage to the liver, avoid vitamin C's use in animals with copper-associated hepatopathy.

Adverse Effects

At usual doses vitamin C has minimal adverse effects. Occasionally GI disturbances have been noted in humans. At higher dosages there is an increased potential for urate, oxalate or cystine stone formation, particularly in susceptible patients.

Reproductive/Nursing Safety

The reproductive safety of vitamin C has not been studied, but it is generally considered safe at moderate dosages. In humans, the FDA categorizes this drug as category *A* for use during pregnancy (*Adequate studies in pregnant women have not demonstrated a risk to the fetus in the first trimester of pregnancy, and there is no evidence of risk in later trimesters.*) But in dosages greater than the RDA, the FDA categorizes vitamin C as category *C* for use during pregnancy (*Animal studies have shown an adverse effect on the fetus, but there are no adequate studies in humans; or there are no animal reproduction studies and no adequate studies in humans.*)

Overdosage/Acute Toxicity

Very large doses may result in diarrhea and potentially urolithiasis. Generally, treatment should consist of monitoring and keeping the patient well hydrated.

Drug Interactions

The following drug interactions have either been reported or are theoretical in humans or animals receiving ascorbic acid (high dosages) and may be of significance in veterinary patients:

▪ **AMINOGLYCOSIDES:** (*e.g.,* **gentamicin**) and **ERYTHROMYCIN:** Are more effective in an alkaline medium; urine acidification may diminish these drugs' effectiveness in treating bacterial urinary tract infections

▪ **QUINIDINE:** Urine acidification may increase renal excretion

▪ **DEFEROXAMINE:** While vitamin C may be synergistic with deferoxamine in removing iron, it may lead to increased iron tissue toxicity, especially in cardiac muscle. It should be used with caution, particularly in patients with preexisting cardiac disease.

▪ **IRON SALTS:** Presence of vitamin C may enhance the oral absorption of iron salts

Laboratory Considerations

▪ **Urine Glucose:** Large doses of vitamin C may cause false-negative values

▪ **Stool occult blood:** False-negative results may occur if vitamin C is administered within 48–72 hours of an amine-dependent test

▪ **Bilirubin, serum:** Vitamin C may decrease concentrations

Doses

■ **CATS:**

a) For adjunctive treatment of FIP: 125 mg (total dose) PO q12h (Weiss 1994)

b) For adjunctive treatment of toxic (*e.g.,* acetaminophen) methemoglobinemia (with oxygen, acetylcysteine): 30 mg/kg PO q6h (Macintire 2006)

■ **RABBITS/RODENTS/SMALL MAMMALS:**

a) **Rabbits:** For soft stools (may reduce cecal absorption of clostridial endotoxins): 100 mg/kg PO q12h (Ivey & Morrisey 2000)

■ **GUINEA PIGS:**

For treatment of scurvy:

a) During pregnancy: 30 mg/kg either parenterally or PO (in feed or water) (Fish & Besch-Williford 1992)

b) 25–50 mg (total dose) parenterally once daily until improvement is noted, then give oral supplemental vitamin C (daily requirement is 15 mg/day) (Wilson 2005)

c) 10 mg/kg daily, by injection if necessary, plus supportive care. Recovery is relatively rapid, usually within a week. Prevention is adequate daily intake of vitamin C. (Burke 1999)

d) 50 mg/kg PO, IM or SC (Adamcak & Otten 2000)

For prevention of scurvy:

a) Add 200 mg vitamin C to one liter of dechlorinated water and add to water bottle. 10–30 mg/kg PO, SC or IM (Adamcak & Otten 2000)

■ **HORSES:**

a) For replacement therapy after stress (*e.g.,* strenuous exercise): 20 grams PO daily (Ferrante & Kronfeld 1992)

b) For adjunctive treatment of erythrocyte oxidative injury (*e.g.,* red maple toxicity): 10–20 grams PO once daily (Davis & Wilkerson 2003); 30–50 mg/kg IV twice daily diluted in 5–10 L of crystalloid fluids (Alward 2008).

c) As a urinary acidifier: 1–2 g/kg PO daily (Jose-Cunilleras & Hinchcliff 1999)

d) As adjunctive therapy for perinatal asphyxia syndrome in foals: 100 mg/kg per day IV (Slovis 2003)

■ **CATTLE:**

a) For vitamin C-responsive dermatitis in calves: 3 grams SC once or twice (Miller 1993)

Chemistry/Synonyms

A water-soluble vitamin, ascorbic acid occurs as white to slightly yellow crystal or powder. It is freely soluble in water and sparingly soluble in alcohol. The parenteral solution has a pH of 5.5–7.

Ascorbic acid may also be known as: acidum ascorbicum, L-ascorbic acid, cevitamic acid, E300, or vitamin C; many trade names are available.

Storage/Stability

Protect from air and light. Ascorbic acid will slowly darken upon light exposure; slight discoloration does not affect potency. Because with time ascorbic acid will decompose with the production of CO_2, open ampules and multidose vials carefully. To reduce the potential for excessive pressure within ampules, store in refrigerator and open while still cold.

Compatibility/Compounding Considerations

Ascorbic acid for injection is **compatible** with most commonly used IV solutions, but is **incompatible** with many drugs when mixed in syringes or IV bags. Compatibility is dependent upon factors such as pH, concentration, temperature and diluent used; consult specialized references or a hospital pharmacist for more specific information.

Dosage Forms/Regulatory Status

VETERINARY-LABELED PRODUCTS:

Parenteral Injection: 250 mg/mL (as sodium ascorbate) in 100 and 250 mL vials; generic; (Rx or OTC depending on labeling)

Ascorbic Acid Powder: 442.25 g/lb *Vita-Flex Pure C*® (Vita-Flex); 50 grams/lb *Mega-C Powder*® (AHC); 146 g/pack *Stabilized C*® (Alpharma); (OTC)

HUMAN-LABELED PRODUCTS:

As Ascorbic Acid Oral Tablets & Capsules: 250mg, 500 mg, 1000 mg & 1500 mg; *Cevi-Bid*® (Lee); generic; (OTC);

Ascorbic Acid Oral Extended-release Tablets: 500 mg & 1000 mg; generic; (OTC)

Ascorbic Acid Oral Crystals: 1000 mg per ¼ tsp. in 120 g and 1 lb; *Vita-C*® (Freeda); (OTC)

Ascorbic Acid Oral Powder: 1060 mg per ¼ tsp. in 120 g and 1 lb; 60 mg per ¼ tsp. in 454 g; *Dull-C*® (Freeda); Ascorbic Acid (Humco); (OTC)

Ascorbic Acid Oral Liquid/Solution: 100 mg/mL in 50 mL & 500 mg/5 mL in 120 mL & 480 mL; *Cecon*® (Abbott); generic; (OTC)

Ascorbic Acid Injection: 500 mg/mL in 50 mL vials; *Ascor L 500*® (McGuff) (0.025% EDTA, preservative-free); generic; (Rx)

References

Adamcak, A & B Otten (2000). Rodent Therapeutics. *Vet Clin NA: Exotic Anim Pract* 3:1(Jan): 221–240.

Alward, A (2008). Red Maple Leaf Toxicosis in Horses. Proceedings: ACVIM. Accessed via: Veterinary Information Network. http://goo.gl/lgdiO

Burke, T (1999). Husbandry and Medicine of Rodents and Lagomorphs. Proceedings: Central Veterinary Conference, Kansas City.

Davis, E & M Wilkerson (2003). Hemolytic anemia. *Current Therapy in Equine Medicine: 5.* N Robinson Ed., Saunders: 344–348.

Ferrante, P & D Kronfeld (1992). Ergogenic Diets and Nutrients. *Current Therapy in Equine Medicine 3.* N Robinson Ed. Philadelphia, W.B. Saunders Co.: 808–814.

Fish, R & C Besch–Williford (1992). Reproductive disorders in the rabbit and guinea pig. *Current Veterinary Therapy XI: Small Animal Practice*. R Kirk and J Bonagura Eds. Philadelphia, W.B. Saunders Company.

Ivey, E & J Morrisey (2000). Therapeutics for Rabbits. *Vet Clin NA: Exotic Anim Pract* 3:1(Jan): 183–216.

Jose–Cunilleras, E & K Hinchcliff (1999). Renal pharmacology. *The Veterinary Clinics of North America: Equine Practice* 15:3(December): 647–664.

Macintire, D (2006). Hematologic Emergencies. Proceedings: ACVC 2006. Accessed via: Veterinary Information Network. http://goo.gl/00dy9

Miller, W (1993). Nutritional, Endocrine, and Keratinization Abnormalities. *Current Veterinary Therapy 3: Food Animal Practice*. J Howard Ed. Philadelphia, W.B. Saunders Co.: 911–913.

Slovis, N (2003). Perinatal asphyxia syndrome (Hypoxic ischemic encephalopathy). Proceedings: ACVIM Forum. Accessed via: Veterinary Information Network. http://goo.gl/I6TgF

Weiss, R (1994). Feline infectious peritonitis virus: Advances in therapy and control. *Consultations in Feline Internal Medicine: 2*. J August Ed. Philadelphia, W.B. Saunders Company: 3–12.

Wilson, H (2005). Rodent emergencies and critical care. Proceedings: IVECCS. Accessed via: Veterinary Information Network. http://goo.gl/ZJduX

ASPARAGINASE

(a-*spar*-a-gin-ase)   L-Asparaginase, Elspar®

ANTINEOPLASTIC

Prescriber Highlights

▶ Antineoplastic useful in treating lymphomas and leukemias in dogs/cats

▶ Two primary adverse effects: hypersensitivity & effects on protein synthesis (usually manifested by: GI effects, hemorrhagic pancreatitis, hepatotoxicity or coagulation disorders);

▶ Bone marrow suppression is rare and it does not have significant GI mucosal toxicity

▶ Usually given IM or SC as IV administration may increase for anaphylaxis

Uses/Indications

Asparaginase has been useful in combination with other agents in the treatment of lymphoid malignancies. The drug is most useful in inducing remission of disease but is also used in maintenance or rescue protocols. It may also have benefit in treating leukemia, particularly ALL.

Use of asparaginase as part of an initial treatment lymphosarcoma protocol is now somewhat controversial, as one study (MacDonald *et al.* 2005) in dogs showed no statistical difference for response rates, remission or survival rate, remission or survival duration, or prevalence of toxicity and treatment delay in dogs treated with or without asparaginase as part of a standard CHOP protocol.

Pharmacology/Actions

Some malignant cells are unable to synthesize asparagine and are dependent on exogenous asparagine for DNA and protein synthesis.

Asparaginase catalyzes asparagine into ammonia and aspartic acid. The antineoplastic activity of asparaginase is greatest during the post mitotic (G_1) cell phase. While normal cells are able to synthesize asparagine intracellularly, some normal cells having a high rate of protein synthesis, require some exogenous asparagine and may be adversely affected by asparaginase.

Resistance to asparaginase can develop rapidly, but apparently, there is no cross-resistance between asparaginase and other antineoplastic agents.

Asparaginase possesses antiviral activity, but its toxicity prevents it from being clinically useful in this regard.

Pharmacokinetics

Asparaginase is not absorbed from the GI tract and must be given either IV or IM. After IM injection, serum levels of asparaginase are approximately 1/2 of those after IV injection. Because of its high molecular weight, asparaginase does not diffuse readily out of the capillaries and about 80% of the drug remains within the intravascular space.

In humans after IV dosing, serum levels of asparagine fall almost immediately to zero and remain that way as long as therapy continues. Once therapy is halted, serum levels of asparagine do not recover for at least 23 days.

The metabolic fate of asparaginase is not known. In humans, the plasma half-life is highly variable and ranges from 8–30 hours.

Contraindications/Precautions/Warnings

Asparaginase is contraindicated in patients who have exhibited anaphylaxis to it, or those with pancreatitis or a history of pancreatitis. Asparaginase should be used with caution in patients with preexisting hepatic, renal, hematologic, gastrointestinal, or CNS dysfunction.

No special precautions are required for handling asparaginase, but any inadvertent skin contact should be washed off, as the drug can be a contact irritant.

Adverse Effects

Asparaginase adverse reactions are classified in two main categories, hypersensitivity reactions and effects on protein synthesis. Hypersensitivity reactions can occur with clinical signs of vomiting, diarrhea, urticaria, pruritus, dyspnea, restlessness, hypotension and collapse. The likelihood of hypersensitivity reactions occurring increases with subsequent doses and intravenous administration. Some clinicians recommend giving a test dose before the full dose to test for local hypersensitivity. Most oncologists now recommend administering antihistamines (*e.g.*, diphenhydramine (at 2 mg/kg in dogs and 1 mg/kg in cats SC 30 minutes prior to administration) prior to dosing. If a hypersensitivity reaction occurs, diphenhydramine (0.2–0.5 mg/kg slow IV), dexamethasone sodium phosphate (1–2 mg/kg IV), intravenous fluids and, if severe, epinephrine (0.1–0.3 mL of a 1:1000 solution IV) have been suggested (O'Keefe & Harris 1990).

The other broad category of toxicity is associated with asparaginase's effects on protein synthesis. Hemorrhagic pancreatitis or other gastrointestinal disturbances, hepatotoxicity and coagulation defects may be noted. Large doses may be associated with hyperglycemia secondary to altered insulin synthesis. Bone marrow depression is an uncommon consequence of asparaginase therapy, but leukopenia has been reported.

Reproductive/Nursing Safety
In humans, the FDA categorizes this drug as category *C* for use during pregnancy (*Animal studies have shown an adverse effect on the fetus, but there are no adequate studies in humans; or there are no animal reproduction studies and no adequate studies in humans.*)

Overdosage/Acute Toxicity
Little information was located regarding overdosages with this agent. It would be expected that toxicity secondary to the protein synthesis altering effects of the drug would be encountered. In dogs, it has been reported that the maximally tolerated dose of asparaginase is 10,000 IU/kg and the lethal dose is 50,000 IU/kg.

It is recommended to treat supportively if an overdose occurs.

Drug Interactions
The following drug interactions have either been reported or are theoretical in humans or animals receiving asparaginase and may be of significance in veterinary patients:

■ **METHOTREXATE:** Asparaginase may reduce methotrexate effectiveness against tumor cells until serum asparagine levels return to normal

■ **PREDNISONE:** Use with asparaginase may increase risk for hyperglycemia; in humans, asparaginase is usually administered after prednisone

■ **VINCRISTINE:** In humans, increased toxicity (neuropathy and erythropoiesis disruption) may occur when asparaginase (IV) is given concurrently with or before vincristine. Myelosuppression reportedly occurs in a minority of dogs treated with vincristine/asparaginase; some veterinary oncologists separate the dosing by a few days to a week, but others do not feel this is beneficial.

Laboratory Considerations
■ **Serum ammonia and urea nitrogen:** levels may be increased by the action of the drug

■ **Thyroxine-binding globulin:** Asparaginase may cause rapid (within 2 days) and profound decreases in circulating TBG, which may alter interpretation of thyroid function studies; values may return to normal after approximately 4 weeks

Doses
Note: Because of the potential toxicity of this drug to patients, veterinary personnel and clients, and since chemotherapy indications, treatment protocols, monitoring and safety guidelines often change, the following dosages should be used only as a general guide. Consultation with a veterinary oncologist and referral to current veterinary oncology references [*e.g.*, (Henry & Higginbotham 2009); (Argyle *et al.* 2008); (Withrow & Vail 2007); (Villalobos 2007); (Ogilvie & Moore 2006); (Ogilvie & Moore 2001)] is *strongly recommended*.

■ **DOGS/CATS:**
The following is a usual dose or dose range for asparaginase and should be used only as a general guide: Asparaginase is usually dosed in dogs and cats at 400 Units/kg or 10,000 Units/m^2 (NOT Units/kg) IM or SC, with a maximum dose of 10,000 Units per patient. **Note:** Many oncologists recommend administering antihistamines such as diphenhydramine at 2 mg/kg for dogs and 1 mg/kg for cats SC 30 minutes prior to administration.

Monitoring
■ Animals should have hepatic, renal, pancreatic (blood glucose, amylase) and hematopoietic function determined prior to initiating therapy and regularly monitored during therapy.

Client Information
■ Clients must be briefed on the possibilities of severe toxicity developing from this drug, including drug-related mortality

■ Clients should contact the veterinarian if the patient exhibits any symptoms of profound depression, severe diarrhea, abnormal bleeding (including bloody diarrhea) and/or bruising

Chemistry/Synonyms
Asparaginase is an enzyme derived from *E. coli* and occurs as a white or almost white, slightly hygroscopic powder that is soluble in water. The commercially available product is a lyophilized powder that also contains mannitol that after reconstituting has a pH of about 7.4. Activity of asparaginase is expressed in terms of International Units (I.U.), or Units.

Asparaginase may also be known as: coloaspase, A-ase, ASN-ase, L-asparaginase, L-asparagine amidohydrolase, MK-965 NSC-109229, Re-82-TAD-15, *Crasnitin®*, *Crasnitine®*, *Elspar®*, *Erwinase®*, *Kidrolase®*, *L-Asp®*, *Laspar®*, *Leucogen®*, *Leunase®*, *Paronal®*, or *Serasa®*.

Storage/Stability
Asparaginase powder for injection should be stored at temperatures less than 8°C, but it is stable for at least 48 hours at room temperature. After reconstituting, the manufacturer states that the drug is stable when refrigerated for up

to 8 hours, but other sources state that it is stable for up to 14 days.

Solutions should be used only if clear; turbid solutions should be discarded. Upon standing, gelatinous fibers may be noted in the solution occasionally. These may be removed without loss of potency with a 5 micron filter. Some loss of potency may occur if a 0.2 micron filter is used.

The solution may be gently shaken while reconstituting, but vigorous shaking should be avoided as the solution may become foamy and difficult to withdraw from the vial and some loss of potency can occur. Recommended intravenous diluents for asparaginase include D_5W and sodium chloride 0.9%.

Dosage Forms/Regulatory Status

VETERINARY-LABELED PRODUCTS: None

HUMAN-LABELED PRODUCTS:

Asparaginase Powder for Injection, lyophilized: 10,000 Units in 10 mL vials (with 80 mg mannitol, preservative-free); Reconstitute vial with 5 mL Sodium Chloride Injection or Sterile Water for Injection for IV use. For IM use, add 2 mL Sodium Chloride Injection. See Storage/Stability section for more information. *Elspar®* (Merck); (Rx)

References

Argyle, D, M Brearly, et al. (2008). *Decision Making in Small Animal Oncology*, Wiley–Blackwell.

Henry, C & M Higginbotham (2009). *Cancer Management in Small Animal Practice*, Saunders.

MacDonald, V, D Thamm, et al. (2005). Does L–asparaginase influence efficacy or toxicity when added to a standard CHOP protocol for dogs with lymphoma? *J Vet Intern Med* 19: 732–736.

O'Keefe, DA & CL Harris (1990). Toxicology of Oncologic Drugs. *Vet Clinics of North America: Small Animal Pract* 20(2): 483–504.

Ogilvie, G & A Moore (2001). *Feline Oncology: A Comprehensive Guide to Compassionate Care*, Veterinary Learning Systems.

Ogilvie, G & A Moore (2006). *Managing the Canine Cancer Patient: A Practical Guide to Compassionate Care*, Veterinary Learning Systems.

Villalobos, A (2007). *Canine and Feline Geriatric Oncology*. Ames, Blackwell.

Withrow, S & D Vail (2007). *Withrow and MacEwen's Small Animal Clinical Oncology 4th Ed*. Philadelphia, Elsevier.

ASPIRIN

(ass-pir-in)   ASA, Acetylsalicylic Acid

ANALGESIC; ANTIPYRETIC; PLATELET AGGREGATION REDUCER; ANTIINFLAMMATORY

Prescriber Highlights

▶ NSAID used for analgesic, antiinflammatory & antiplatelet effects in a variety of species

▶ Contraindicated in patients hypersensitive to it or with active GI bleeds; Relatively contraindicated in patients with bleeding disorders, asthma, or renal insufficiency (but has been used to treat glomerular disease)

▶ Aspirin has a very long half life in cats (approx. 30 hours; dose carefully); dogs are relatively sensitive to GI effects (bleeding)

▶ Low grade teratogen & may delay labor; avoid use in pregnancy

▶ Many drug & lab interactions

Uses/Indications

Aspirin is used in all species for its analgesic and antipyretic effects. It is one of the few nonsteroidal antiinflammatory agents that is relatively safe to use in both dogs and cats, although it can cause significant GI bleeding in dogs. Besides its analgesic, antiinflammatory and antipyretic effects, aspirin is used therapeutically for its effects on platelet aggregation in the treatment of DIC and pulmonary artery disease secondary to heartworm infestation in dogs. It is also used in cats with cardiomyopathy. Aspirin (at low doses) may be of benefit in the adjunctive treatment of glomerular disease due to its antiplatelet and antiinflammatory activity.

Pharmacology/Actions

Aspirin inhibits cyclooxygenase (COX-1, prostaglandin synthetase) thereby reducing the synthesis of prostaglandins and thromboxanes (TXA2). These effects are thought to be how aspirin produces analgesia, antipyrexia, and reduces platelet aggregation and inflammation.

Most cells can synthesize new cyclooxygenase, but platelets cannot. Therefore, aspirin can cause an irreversible effect on platelet aggregation. A study in dogs investigating the platelet function effects of various aspirin doses, showed that doses less than 1 mg/kg/day or at 10 mg/kg/day PO did not have any statistically significant effect on platelet aggregation. Doses of 1 and 2 mg/kg/day inhibited platelet function and aggregation. (Shearer *et al.* 2009)

Aspirin has been shown to decrease the clinical signs of experimentally induced anaphylaxis in calves and ponies.

While aspirin does not directly inhibit COX-2, it can modify it to produce, with lipoxygenase

(LOX), a compound known as aspirin-triggered lipoxin (ATL), which appears to have gastric mucosal protective actions. This may explain why aspirin tends to have reduced gastric damaging effects when used over time.

Pharmacokinetics

Aspirin is rapidly absorbed from the stomach and proximal small intestine in monogastric animals. The rate of absorption is dependent upon factors as stomach content, gastric emptying times, tablet disintegration rates and gastric pH. Absorption is slow from the GI tract in cattle, but approximately 70% of an oral dose will be absorbed.

During absorption, aspirin is partially hydrolyzed to salicylic acid where it is distributed widely throughout the body. Highest levels may be found in the liver, heart, lungs, renal cortex, and plasma. The amount of plasma protein binding is variable depending on species, serum salicylate and albumin concentrations. At lower salicylate concentrations it is 90% protein bound, but only 70% protein bound at higher concentrations. Salicylate is excreted into milk but levels appear to be very low. Salicylate will cross the placenta and fetal levels may actually exceed those found in the mother.

Salicylate is metabolized in the liver primarily by conjugation with glycine and glucuronic acid via glucuronyl transferase. Because cats are deficient in this enzymatic pathway, they have prolonged half-lives (27-45 hours) and are susceptible to accumulating the drug. Minor metabolites formed include gentisic acid, 2,3-dihydroxybenzoic acid, and 2,3,5-trihydroxybenzoic acid. Gentisic acid appears to be the only active metabolite, but because of its low concentrations appears to play an insignificant role therapeutically. The rate of metabolism is determined by both first order kinetics and dose-dependent kinetics depending on the metabolic pathway. Serum half life in dogs is approximately 8 hours, while in humans it averages 1.5 hours. Generally, steady-state serum levels will increase to levels higher (proportionally) than expected with dosage increases. These effects have not been well studied in domestic animals, however.

Salicylate and its metabolites are rapidly excreted by the kidneys by both filtration and renal tubular secretion. Significant tubular reabsorption occurs which is highly pH dependent. Salicylate excretion can be significantly increased by raising urine pH to 5−8. Salicylate and metabolites may be removed using peritoneal dialysis or more rapidly using hemodialysis.

Contraindications/Precautions/Warnings

Aspirin is contraindicated in patients demonstrating previous hypersensitivity reactions to it or in patients with bleeding ulcers. It is relatively contraindicated in patients with hemorrhagic disorders, asthma, or renal insufficiency.

Because aspirin is highly protein bound to plasma albumin, patients with hypoalbuminemia may require lower dosages to prevent clinical signs of toxicity. Aspirin should be used cautiously with enhanced monitoring in patients with severe hepatic failure or diminished renal function. Because of its effects on platelets, aspirin therapy should be halted, if possible, one week prior to surgical procedures.

Aspirin must be used cautiously in cats because of their inability to rapidly metabolize and excrete salicylates. Clinical signs of toxicity may occur if dosed recklessly or without stringent monitoring. Aspirin should be used cautiously in neonatal animals; adult doses may lead to toxicity.

Adverse Effects

The most common adverse effect of aspirin at therapeutic doses is gastric (nausea, anorexia, vomiting) or intestinal irritation with varying degrees of occult GI blood loss occurring. The resultant irritation may result in vomiting and/or anorexia. Severe blood loss may result in a secondary anemia or hypoproteinemia. In dogs, plain uncoated aspirin may be more irritating to the gastric mucosa than either buffered aspirin or enteric-coated tablets. Hypersensitivity reactions have been reported in dogs although they are thought to occur rarely. Cats may develop acidosis from aspirin therapy.

Reproductive/Nursing Safety

Salicylates are possible teratogens and have been shown to delay parturition; their use should be avoided during pregnancy, particularly during the later stages. In humans, the FDA categorizes this drug as category **D** for use during pregnancy (*There is evidence of human fetal risk, but the potential benefits from the use of the drug in pregnant women may be acceptable despite its potential risks.*) In a separate system evaluating the safety of drugs in canine and feline pregnancy (Papich 1989), this drug is categorized as in class: **C** (*These drugs may have potential risks. Studies in people or laboratory animals have uncovered risks, and these drugs should be used cautiously as a last resort when the benefit of therapy clearly outweighs the risks.*)

Overdosage/Acute Toxicity

Clinical signs of acute overdosage in dogs and cats include: depression, vomiting (may be blood tinged), anorexia, hyperthermia, and increased respiratory rate. Initially, a respiratory alkalosis occurs with a compensatory hyperventilation response. A profound metabolic acidosis follows. If treatment is not provided, muscular weakness, pulmonary and cerebral edema, hypernatremia, hypokalemia, ataxia, and seizures may all develop with eventual coma and death.

There were 538 exposures to aspirin reported to the ASPCA Animal Poison Control Center (APCC) during 2008-2009. In these cases, 481 were dogs with 240 showing clinical signs and

54 cases were cats with 14 showing clinical signs. The remaining 3 cases were made up of 2 birds, and 1 lagomorph that showed no clinical signs. Common findings in dogs recorded in decreasing frequency included vomiting, lethargy, panting, hyperthermia, diarrhea, bloody vomitus, and polydipsia. Common findings in cats recorded in decreasing frequency included vomiting. Treatment of acute overdosage initially consists of emptying the gut if ingestion has occurred within 12 hours, giving activated charcoal and an oral cathartic, placing an intravenous line, beginning fluids and drawing appropriate lab work (*e.g.*, blood gases). Some clinicians suggest performing gastric lavage with a 3–5% solution of sodium bicarbonate to delay the absorption of aspirin. A reasonable choice for an intravenous solution to correct dehydration would be dextrose 5% in water. Acidosis treatment and forced alkaline diuresis with sodium bicarbonate should be performed for serious ingestions, but should only be attempted if acid-base status can be monitored. Diuresis may be enhanced by the administration of mannitol (1–2 grams/kg/hr). GI protectant medications should also be administered. Seizures may be controlled with IV diazepam. Treatment of hypoprothrombinemia may be attempted by using phytonadione (2.5 mg/kg divided q8–12h) and ascorbic acid (25 mg parenterally) but ascorbic acid may negate some of the urinary alkalinization effects of bicarbonate. Peritoneal dialysis or exchange transfusions may be attempted in very severe ingestions when heroic measures are desired.

Drug Interactions

The following drug interactions have either been reported or are theoretical in humans or animals receiving aspirin and may be of significance in veterinary patients:

- **DRUGS THAT ALKALINIZE THE URINE** (*e.g.*, **acetazolamide, sodium bicarbonate**) significantly increase the renal excretion of salicylates; because carbonic anhydrase inhibitors (*e.g.*, acetazolamide, dichlorphenamide) may cause systemic acidosis and increase CNS levels of salicylates, toxicity may occur.

- **AMINOGLYCOSIDES:** Some clinicians feel that aspirin should not be given concomitantly with aminoglycoside antibiotics because of an increased likelihood of nephrotoxicity developing. The actual clinical significance of this interaction is not clear, and the risk versus benefits should be weighed when contemplating therapy.

- **CORTICOSTEROIDS:** May increase the clearance of salicylates, decrease serum levels and increase the risks for GI bleeding. One dog study showed no significant difference in gastric mucosal injury when ultra-low dose (0.5 mg/kg/day) aspirin was added to prednisone therapy. Addition of aspirin did increase the incidence of mild, self-limiting diarrhea (Graham & Leib 2009).

- **DIGOXIN:** In dogs, aspirin has been demonstrated to increase plasma levels of digoxin by decreasing the clearance of the drug.

- **FUROSEMIDE:** May compete with the renal excretion of aspirin and delay its excretion; this may cause clinical signs of toxicity in animals receiving high aspirin doses.

- **HEPARIN or ORAL ANTICOAGULANTS:** Aspirin may increase the risks for bleeding.

- **METHOTREXATE:** Aspirin may displace MTX from plasma proteins increasing the risk for toxicity.

- **NSAIDS:** Increased chances of developing GI ulceration exist. Animals that have been on aspirin therapy that will be replaced with a COX-2 NSAID, should probably have a "wash out" period of 3–10 days between stopping aspirin and starting the NSAID (Bill 2008).

- **PHENOBARBITAL:** May increase the rate of metabolism of aspirin by inducing hepatic enzymes.

- **PROBENECID, SULFINPYRAZONE:** At usual doses, aspirin may antagonize the uricosuric effects of probenicid or sulfinpyrazone

- **SPIRONOLACTONE:** Aspirin may inhibit the diuretic activity of spironolactone

- **TETRACYCLINE:** The antacids in buffered aspirin may chelate tetracycline products if given simultaneously; space doses apart by at least one hour

- **URINARY ACIDIFYING DRUGS** (**methionine, ammonium chloride, ascorbic acid**): Can decrease the urinary excretion of salicylates

Laboratory Considerations

- At high doses, aspirin may cause false-positive results for **urinary glucose** if using the cupric sulfate method (*Clinitest®*, Benedict's solution) and false-negative results if using the glucose oxidase method (*Clinistix®* or *Tes-Tape®*).

- **Urinary ketones** measured by the ferric chloride method (Gerhardt) may be affected if salicylates are in the urine (reddish-color produced). **5-HIAA** determinations by fluorescent methods may be interfered by salicylates in the urine. Falsely elevated **VMA** (vanillylmandelic acid) may be seen with most methods used if salicylates are in the urine. Falsely lowered **VMA** levels may be seen if using the Pisano method.

- Urinary excretion of **xylose** may be decreased if aspirin is given concurrently. Falsely elevated **serum uric acid** values may be measured if using colorimetric methods.

- Aspirin can decrease serum concentrations of **total T4**.

Doses

■ **DOGS:**

Note: Recommend using buffered varieties of aspirin in dogs

a) For analgesia: 10 mg/kg PO q12h (Lascelles 2003)

b) As an antiinflammatory/antirheumatic: 25 mg/kg PO q8h (Holland & Chastain 1995)

c) For antipyrexia: 10 mg/kg PO twice daily (Holland & Chastain 1995)

d) Post-Adulticide therapy for heartworm disease: 7–10 mg/kg PO once a day (Calvert 1987)

To decrease platelet aggregation; as an antithrombotic:

a) For adjunctive therapy in IMHA: 0.5 mg/kg PO twice daily. At this low dose risk for gastric ulceration is low, but adding misoprostol (2–5 micrograms/kg PO three times) may reduce the risk. (Noonan 2009)

b) For adjunctive therapy of glomerular disease: 0.5 mg/kg PO q24h (DiBartola & Chew 2006)

c) For adjunctive therapy with azathioprine and glucocorticoids for immune-mediated hemolytic anemia: 0.5 mg/kg PO once daily (Weinkle *et al.* 2004)

As an analgesic/antiinflammatory prior to elective intraocular surgery:

a) 6.5 mg/kg two to three times daily (Wyman 1986)

■ **CATS:**

For analgesia/antipyrexia/antiinflammatory:

a) One "baby" aspirin (81 mg) PO every 2–3 days (Bill 2008)

b) 10 mg/kg PO every other day (Holland & Chastain, 1995)

c) 10 mg/kg PO q48–72h in food (Hardie, 2000)

As an antithrombotic agent:

a) For prophylaxis of arterial thromboembolism (ATE): 5 mg (total dose) per cat PO q72hours (every 3rd day) (Smith *et al.* 2003), (Smith 2009)

b) For prophylaxis of arterial thromboembolism: 81 mg (total dose; one "baby" aspirin) q72hours (every 3rd day). Likely a weaker, but less expensive option than clopidogrel/LMWH. Generally, aspirin therapy is recommended in all cats with atrial enlargement and cardiomyopathy. (Meurs 2006)

c) For prevention of thromboembolism: High dose: 40 mg per cat PO q72h, or Low dose: 5 mg per cat PO q72h. (Fuentes 2009)

■ **FERRETS:**

a) 10–20 mg/kg PO once daily (has short duration of activity) (Williams 2000)

■ **RABBITS/RODENTS/SMALL MAMMALS:**

a) **Rabbits:** 5–20 mg/kg PO once daily for low grade analgesia (Ivey & Morrisey 2000)

b) **Mice, Rats, Gerbils, Hamsters:** 100–150 mg/kg PO q4h. **Guinea pigs:** 87 mg/kg PO (Adamcak & Otten 2000)

■ **CATTLE:**

For analgesia/antipyrexia:

a) 100 mg/kg PO q12h (Walz 2006)

b) Mature Cattle: two to four 240 grain boluses PO; Calves: one to two 240 grain boluses, allow animals to drink water after administration (Label directions; Vedco Brand)

■ **HORSES:** (**Note:** ARCI UCGFS Class 4 Drug)

For analgesia:

a) Mature Horses: two to four 240 grain boluses PO; Foals: one to two 240 grain boluses; allow animals to drink water after administration (Label directions–Vedco Brand)

b) 25 mg/kg PO q12h initially, then 10 mg/kg once daily (Jenkins 1987)

c) 15–100 mg/kg PO once daily) (Robinson 1987)

For anti-platelet activity as an adjunctive treatment of laminitis:

a) 5–10 mg/kg PO q24–48 hours or 20 mg/kg PO every 4–5 days (Brumbaugh *et al.* 1999)

■ **SWINE:**

For analgesia:

a) 10 mg/kg q4h PO (Jenkins 1987), (Koritz 1986)

b) 10 mg/kg q6h PO (Davis 1979)

■ **AVIAN:**

a) 5 grams in 250 mL of water as sole water source (Clubb 1986) **Note:** Because of the significant hydrolysis that will occur, this solution should be freshly prepared every 12 hours if stored at room temperature or every 4 days if kept refrigerated at 5° C.

Monitoring

■ Analgesic effect &/or antipyretic effect

■ Bleeding times if indicated

■ PCV and stool guaiac tests if indicated

Client Information

■ Contact veterinarian if symptoms of GI bleeding or distress occur (black, tarry feces; anorexia or vomiting, etc.).

■ Because aspirin is a very old drug, formal approvals from the FDA for its use in animals have not been required. There is no listed meat or milk withdrawal times listed for food-producing animals but because there are salicylate-sensitive people, in the interest of public health, this author suggests a minimum of 1 day withdrawal time for either milk or meat.

Chemistry/Synonyms

Aspirin, sometimes known as acetylsalicylic acid or ASA, is the salicylate ester of acetic acid. The compound occurs as a white, crystalline powder or tabular or needle-like crystals. It is a weak acid with a pK_a of 3.5. Aspirin is slightly soluble in water and is freely soluble in alcohol. Each gram of aspirin contains approximately 760 mg of salicylate.

Aspirin may also be known as: ASA, acetylsal acid, acetylsalicylic acid, acidum acetylsalicylicum, polopiryna, or salicylic acid acetate; many trade names are available.

Storage/Stability

Aspirin tablets should be stored in tight, moisture resistant containers. Do not use products past the expiration date or if a strong vinegar-like odor is noted emitting from the bottle.

Aspirin is stable in dry air, but readily hydrolyzes to acetate and salicylate when exposed to water or moist air; it will then exude a strong vinegar-like odor. The addition of heat will speed the rate of hydrolysis. In aqueous solutions, aspirin is most stable at pH's of 2–3 and least stable at pH's below 2 or greater than 8. Should an aqueous solution be desirable as a dosage form, the commercial product Alka-Seltzer® will remain stable for 10 hours at room temperature in solution.

Compatibility/Compounding Considerations

Compounded preparation stability: Aspirin is hydrolyzed by water to degradative byproducts, acetic acid and salicylic acid.

Effervescent buffered aspirin tablets (Alka-Seltzer®) dissolved in water are demonstrated to be stable for 10 hours at room temperature and for 90 hours if refrigerated. Although pharmacists compound aspirin suspensions in fixed oils, the long term stability of these preparations has not been determined.

Dosage Forms/Regulatory Status
VETERINARY-LABELED PRODUCTS:

Note: Aspirin products may not be FDA-approved.

Aspirin Tablets (Enteric-Coated): 81 mg; (Hartz); (OTC). Labeled for use in dogs.

Aspirin Tablets (Buffered, Microencapsulated, Chewable for dogs): 150 mg & 450 mg; Canine Aspirin Chewable Tablets for Small & Medium (150 mg) or Large Dogs® (450 mg) (Pala-Tech); (OTC). Labeled for use in dogs.

Aspirin Tablets 60 grain (3.9 g): Aspirin 60 Grain (Butler); (OTC) and (Vedco); (Rx); Rx is labeled for use in horses, cattle, sheep and swine; not for use in horses intended for food or in lactating dairy animals.

Aspirin Boluses 240 grain (15.6 g): Labeled for use in horses, foals, cattle and calves; not for use in lactating animals. Aspirin 240 Grain Boluses, Aspirin Bolus (various); (OTC)

Aspirin Boluses 480 grain (31.2 g). Labeled for use in mature horses, & cattle. Aspirin 480 Grain Boluses (various); (OTC)

Oral Aspirin Gel: 250 mg/mL in 30 mL: Aspir-Flex® Aspirin Gel for Small and Medium Dogs (Durvet); 500 mg/1 mL in 30 mL: Aspir-Flex® Aspirin Gel for Large Dogs (Durvet); (OTC). Labeled for use in dogs.

Aspirin Powder: l lb. (various); (OTC); Aspirin Powder Molasses-Flavored 50% acetylsalicylic acid in base (Butler); Aspirin USP 204 g/lb (apple flavored) (Neogen); Acetylsalicylic acid; (OTC)

Aspirin Granules: 2.5 gram per 39 mL scoop (apple and molasses flavor); Arthri-Eze Aspirin Granules® (Durvet); (OTC); Labeled for use in horses

Aspirin Liquid Concentrate (equiv to 12% aspirin) for Dilution in Drinking Water in 32 oz btls. (AgriPharm, First Priority); (OTC). Labeled for addition to drinking water for swine, poultry, beef and dairy cattle

There are no listed meat or milk withdrawal times listed for food-producing animals, but because there are salicylate-sensitive people, in the interest of public health, this author suggests a minimum of 1 day withdrawal time for either milk or meat. For further guidance with determining use and withdrawal times, contact FARAD (see Phone Numbers & Websites in the appendix for contact information).

The ARCI (Racing Commissioners International) has designated this drug as a class 4 substance. See the appendix for more information.

HUMAN-LABELED PRODUCTS:

Note: Many dosage forms and brand names are commercially available; the following is an abbreviated list of some products that have been used for veterinary indications:

Aspirin, Chewable Tablets: 81 mg (1.25 grains); Bayer® Children's Aspirin (Bayer); St. Joseph® Adult Chewable Aspirin (Schering-Plough); (OTC)

Aspirin, Tablets; plain uncoated; 325 mg (5 grain), & 500 mg (7.8 grain); Genuine and Maximum Bayer® Aspirin Tablets and Caplets (Bayer); Empirin® (GlaxoWellcome); Arthritis Foundation® Pain Reliever (McNeil-CPC); Norwich® Regular Strength (Lee); Norwich Extra-Strength® (Procter & Gamble); generic; (OTC)

Aspirin Tablets, enteric coated: 81 mg, 165 mg, 325 mg, 500 mg, 650 mg, & 800 mg; Ecotrin® Adult Low Strength (GlaxoSmithKline Consumer Healthcare); Halfprin 81® and 1/2 Halfprin® (Kramer), Heartline® (BDI), Ecotrin® Tablets & Caplets and Ecotrin® Maximum Strength Caplets (SmithKline Beecham); Extra Strength Bayer® Enteric 500 Aspirin (Bayer); generic; (OTC)

Aspirin Extended-controlled Release Tablets: 81 mg, 650 mg, 800 mg & 975 mg; Extended Release Bayer® 8-hour Caplets (Bayer); (OTC),

ZORprin® (PAR); (Rx), *Bayer® Low Adult Strength* (Bayer); generic; (OTC)

Aspirin, Tablets; buffered uncoated; 325 mg (5 grain), with aluminum &/or magnesium salts; *Tri-Buffered Bufferin Tablets* and *Caplets®* (Bristol-Myers Squibb); *Bayer® Buffered Aspirin* (Bayer); *Asprimox®* and *Asprimox® Extra Protection for Arthritis* (Invamed); 500 mg with calcium carbonate, magnesium carbonate, & magnesium oxide; *Extra Strength Bayer® Plus Caplets* (Bayer); *Bufferin®* (Bristol-Myers); 500 mg with 237 mg calcium carbonate, 33 mg magnesium hydroxide, 33 mg aluminum hydroxide; *Ascriptin® Maximum Strength* (Novartis); 500 mg with 100 mg magnesium hydroxide and 27 mg aluminum hydroxide; *Arthritis Pain Formula®* (Whitehall); 325 mg with 75 mg aluminum hydroxide, 75 mg magnesium hydroxide and calcium carbonate; *Asprimox Extra Protection for Arthritis Pain®* (Invamed); generic; (OTC)

Aspirin Tablets: buffered coated: 325 mg & 500 mg. *Adprin-B®* (Pfeiffer); *Asprimox®* (Invamed); *Magnaprin®* and *Magnaprin® Arthritis Strength Captabs®* (Rugby); *Ascriptin®* and *Ascriptin® Extra Strength* (Rhone-Poulenc Rorer), *Bufferin®* (Bristol Myers); generic; (OTC)

Rectal suppositories, chewing gum and effervescent oral dosage forms are also available commercially for human use.

References

Adamcak, A & B Otten (2000). Rodent Therapeutics. *Vet Clin NA: Exotic Anim Pract* 3:1(Jan): 221–240.

Bill, R (2008). NSAIDs—Keeping up with all the changes. *Proceedings: ACVC*.

Brumbaugh, G, H Lopez, et al. (1999). The pharmacologic basis for the treatment of laminitis. *The Veterinary Clinics of North America: Equine Practice* 15:2(August).

Calvert, CA (1987). Indications for the use of aspirin and corticosteroid hormones in the treatment of canine heartworm disease. *Sem Vet Med Surg (Small Animal)* 2(1): 78–84.

Clubb, SL (1986). Therapeutics: Individual and Flock Treatment Regimens. *Clinical Avian Medicine and Surgery*. GJ Harrison and LR Harrison Eds. Philadelphia, W.B. Saunders: 327–355.

Davis, LE (1979). Fever. *JAVMA* 175: 1210.

DiBartola, S & D Chew (2006). Tips for managing protein–losing nephropathy. Proceedings: ACVIM. Accessed via: Veterinary Information Network. http://goo.gl/9QuRD

Fuentes, V (2009). Management of feline heart disease. Proceedings: WSAVA. Accessed via: Veterinary Information Network. http://goo.gl/EdvHu

Graham, AH & MS Leib (2009). Effects of Prednisone Alone or Prednisone with Ultralow–Dose Aspirin on the Gastroduodenal Mucosa of Healthy Dogs. *Journal of Veterinary Internal Medicine* 23(3): 482–487.

Holland, M & C Chastain (1995). Uses & misuses of aspirin. *Kirk's Current Veterinary Therapy:XII*. J Bonagura Ed. Philadelphia, W.B. Saunders: 70–73.

Ivey, E & J Morrisey (2000). Therapeutics for Rabbits. *Vet Clin NA: Exotic Anim Pract* 3:1(Jan): 183–216.

Jenkins, WL (1987). Pharmacologic aspects of analgesic drugs in animals: An overview. *JAVMA* 191(10): 1231–1240.

Koritz, GD (1986). Therapeutic management of inflammation. *Current Veterinary Therapy 2: Food Animal Practice*. JL Howard Ed. Phialdelphia, WB Saunders: 23–27.

Lascelles, B (2003). Case examples in the management of cancer pain in dogs and cats, and the future of cancer pain alleviation. Proceedings: American College of Veterinary Internal Medicine. Accessed via: Veterinary Information Network. http://goo.gl/Yxog0

Meurs, K (2006). Therapeutic management of feline cardiomyopathy. Proceedings: ACVIM. Accessed via: Veterinary Information Network. http://goo.gl/TNXxJ

Noonan, M (2009). Immune Mediated Hemolytic Anemia. Proceedings: IVECC. Accessed via: Veterinary Information Network. http://goo.gl/EaAXT

Robinson, NE (1987). Table of Common Drugs: Approximate Doses. *Current Therapy in Equine Medicine, 2*. NE Robinson Ed. Philadelphia, W.B. Saunders: 761.

Shearer, L, S Kruth, et al. (2009). Effects of aspirin and clopidogrel on platelet function in healthy dogs. Proceedings: ECVIM. Accessed via: Veterinary Information Network. http://goo.gl/PaCol

Smith, S (2009). Feline Arteriothromboembolism. Accessed via: Veterinary Information Network. http://goo.gl/YaGVk

Smith, S, A Tobias, et al. (2003). Arterial thromboembolism in cats: acute crisis in 127 cases (1992–2001) and long–term management with low–dose aspirin in 24 cases. *J Vet Intern Med* 17: 73–83.

Walz, P (2006). Practical management of pain in cattle. Proceedings: ABVP. Accessed via: Veterinary Information Network. http://goo.gl/hScVv

Weinkle, T, S Center, et al. (2004). Azathioprine and ultra–low–dose aspirin therapy for canine immune–mediated hemolytic anemia. Proceedings: ACVIM Forum. Accessed via: Veterinary Information Network. http://goo.gl/FLUuE

Williams, N (2000). Therapeutics in Ferrets. *Vet Clin NA: Exotic Anim Pract* 3:1(Jan): 131–153.

Wyman, M (1986). Contemporary ocular therapeutics. *Current Veterinary Therapy IX, Small Animal Practice*. RW Kirk Ed. Philadelphia, W.B. Saunders: 684–696.

ATENOLOL

(a-*ten*-oh-lol)   Tenormin®

BETA-ADRENERGIC BLOCKER

Prescriber Highlights

▶ Beta-blocker that is used primarily for hypertension & tachyarrhythmias in small animals

▶ Has minimal beta-2 activity at usual doses; comparatively safe to use in asthmatic patients

▶ Contraindicated in patients with bradycardic arrhythmias, or hypersensitivity to it

▶ Negative inotrope so must be used with caution in patients with CHF; use with caution in renal failure patients & those with sinus node dysfunction

▶ Higher dosages may mask clinical signs of hyperthyroidism or hypoglycemia; may cause hyper- or hypoglycemia—use with caution in brittle diabetics

▶ Primary adverse effects are lethargy, hypotension, or diarrhea

▶ If discontinuing, recommend withdrawing gradually

Uses/Indications

Atenolol may be useful in the treatment of supraventricular tachyarrhythmias, premature ventricular contractions (PVC's, VPC's), systemic hypertension and in treating cats with hypertrophic cardiomyopathy without accompanying pulmonary edema. Atenolol is relatively safe to use in animals with bronchospastic disease.

Pharmacology/Actions

Atenolol is a relatively specific Beta$_1$-blocker. At higher dosages, this specificity may be lost and Beta$_2$ blockade can occur. Atenolol does not possess any intrinsic sympathomimetic activity like pindolol nor does it possess membrane-stabilizing activity like pindolol or propranolol. Cardiovascular effects secondary to atenolol's negative inotropic and chronotropic actions include: decreased sinus heart rate, slowed AV conduction, diminished cardiac output at rest and during exercise, decreased myocardial oxygen demand, reduced blood pressure, and inhibition of isoproterenol-induced tachycardia.

Pharmacokinetics

Only about 50–60% of an oral dose is absorbed in humans, but is absorbed rapidly. In cats, it is reported to have a bioavailability of approximately 90%. The drug has very low protein binding characteristics (5–15%) and is distributed well into most tissues. Atenolol has low lipid solubility and unlike propranolol, only small amounts of atenolol are distributed into the CNS. Atenolol crosses the placenta and levels in milk are higher than those found in plasma. Atenolol is minimally biotransformed in the liver; 40–50% is excreted unchanged in the urine and the bulk of the remainder is excreted in the feces unchanged (unabsorbed drug). Reported half-lives: dogs = 3.2 hours; cats = 3.7 hours; humans = 6–7 hours. Duration of beta blockade effect in cats persists for about 12 hours.

Contraindications/Precautions/Warnings

Atenolol is contraindicated in patients with overt heart failure, hypersensitivity to this class of agents, greater than first-degree heart block, or sinus bradycardia. Non-specific beta-blockers are generally contraindicated in patients with CHF unless secondary to a tachyarrhythmia responsive to beta-blocker therapy. They are also relatively contraindicated in patients with bronchospastic lung disease. Atenolol may reduce survival or cause increased morbidity in cats with hypertrophic cardiomyopathy, particularly those with accompanying pulmonary edema.

Atenolol should be used cautiously in patients with significant renal insufficiency or sinus node dysfunction.

Atenolol (at high dosages) can mask the clinical signs associated with hypoglycemia. It can also cause hypoglycemia or hyperglycemia and, therefore, should be used cautiously in labile diabetic patients.

Atenolol can mask the clinical signs associated with thyrotoxicosis, however, it may be used clinically to treat the clinical signs associated with this condition.

Adverse Effects

It is reported that adverse effects most commonly occur in geriatric animals or those that have acute decompensating heart disease. Adverse effects considered clinically relevant include: bradycardia, inappetence, lethargy and depression, impaired AV conduction, CHF or worsening of heart failure, hypotension, hypoglycemia, and bronchoconstriction (less so with Beta$_1$ specific drugs like atenolol). Syncope and diarrhea have also been reported in canine patients with beta-blockers. Lethargy and hypotension may be noted within 1 hour of administration.

Exacerbation of symptoms has been reported following abrupt cessation of beta-blockers in humans. It is recommended to withdraw therapy gradually in patients who have been receiving the drug chronically.

Reproductive/Nursing Safety

In humans, the FDA categorizes this drug as category *C* for use during pregnancy (*Animal studies have shown an adverse effect on the fetus, but there are no adequate studies in humans; or there are no animal reproduction studies and no adequate studies in humans.*)

Overdosage/Acute Toxicity

There were 219 exposures to atenolol reported to the ASPCA Animal Poison Control Center (APCC) during 2008¢2009. In these cases, 159 were dogs with 19 showing clinical signs, and the remaining 60 cases were cats with 9 showing clinical signs. Common findings in dogs recorded in decreasing frequency included lethargy and vomiting. Common findings in cats recorded in decreasing frequency included lethargy and vomiting.

Humans have apparently survived dosages of up to 5 grams. The most predominant clinical signs expected would be extensions of the drug's pharmacologic effects: hypotension, bradycardia, bronchospasm, cardiac failure, hypoglycemia, and hyperkalemia.

If overdose is secondary to a recent oral ingestion, emptying the gut and charcoal administration may be considered. Monitor: ECG, blood glucose, potassium and, if possible, blood pressure. Treatment of the cardiovascular effects is symptomatic. Use fluids and pressor agents (dopamine or norepinephrine) to treat hypotension. Bradycardia may be treated with atropine. If atropine fails, isoproterenol given cautiously has been recommended. Insulin and dextrose may be needed for hyperkalemia and hypoglycemia. Use of a transvenous pacemaker may be necessary. Cardiac failure can be treated with a digitalis glycoside, diuretics and oxygen. Glucagon (5–10 mg IV; human dose) may increase heart rate and blood pressure and reduce the cardiodepressant effects of atenolol.

Drug Interactions

The following drug interactions have either been reported or are theoretical in humans or animals receiving atenolol and may be of significance in veterinary patients:

- **ANESTHETICS (myocardial depressant):** Additive myocardial depression may occur with the concurrent use of atenolol and myocardial depressant anesthetic agents

- **CALCIUM-CHANNEL BLOCKERS (_e.g._, diltiazem, verapamil, amlodipine):** Concurrent use of beta-blockers with calcium channel blockers (or other negative inotropics) should be done with caution, particularly in patients with preexisting cardiomyopathy or CHF

- **CLONIDINE:** Atenolol may exacerbate rebound hypertension after stopping clonidine therapy

- **FUROSEMIDE, HYDRALAZINE OR OTHER HYPOTENSIVE PRODUCING DRUGS:** May increase the hypotensive effects of atenolol

- **PHENOTHIAZINES:** With atenolol may exhibit enhanced hypotensive effects

- **RESERPINE:** Potential for additive effects (hypotension, bradycardia)

- **SYMPATHOMIMETICS (metaproterenol, terbutaline, beta-effects of epinephrine, phenylpropanolamine, etc.):** May have their actions blocked by atenolol and they may, in turn, reduce the efficacy of atenolol

Doses

- **DOGS:**
For indications where beta-blockade may be indicated (cardiac arrhythmias, obstructive heart disease, hypertension, myocardial infarction, etc.):
  a) 0.3–0.6 mg/kg PO q12h; for refractory VTach combine with mexiletine (5–8 mg/kg PO q8h) (Smith 2009)
  b) For moderate to severe sub-valvular aortic stenosis (SAS): 0.5–1 mg/kg PO twice a day (Meurs 2006)
  c) To attempt to decrease syncopal episodes associated with pulmonic stenosis: 0.25–1 mg/kg PO twice a day (Meurs 2006)
  d) For hypertension: 0.25–1 mg/kg PO q12h (Stepien 2006)

- **CATS:**
For treatment of hypertension or cardiac conditions (_e.g._, hypertrophic cardiomyopathy) where beta blockade may be indicated:
  a) 3 mg/kg PO q12h (or 6.25–12.5 mg total dose) PO q12h (Stepien 2006)
  b) 6.25–12.5 mg (total dose per cat) q12h (Kittleson 2009)
  c) 6.25–12.5 mg (total dose) PO q12–24h. Treatment of choice for hyperthyroid, hypertensive cats. Beta-blockers are rarely

sufficient alone to treat hypertension due to other causes. (Waddell 2005)

- **FERRETS:**
For hypertrophic cardiomyopathy:
  a) 6.25 mg (total dose) PO once daily (Williams 2000)
  b) 3.13–6.25 mg (total dose) PO once daily (Johnson-Delaney 2005)

Monitoring

- Cardiac function, pulse rate, ECG if necessary, BP if indicated
- Toxicity (see Adverse Effects/Overdosage)

Client Information

- To be effective, the animal must receive all doses as prescribed. Notify veterinarian if animal becomes lethargic or becomes exercise intolerant; develops shortness of breath or cough; or develops a change in behavior or attitude. Do not stop therapy without first conferring with veterinarian.

Chemistry/Synonyms

A beta$_1$-adrenergic blocking agent, atenolol occurs as a white, crystalline powder. At 37°C, 26.5 mg are soluble in 1 mL of water. The pH of the commercially available injection is adjusted to 5.5–6.5.

Atenolol may also be known as atenololum, or ICI-66082; many trade names are available.

Storage/Stability

Tablets should be stored at room temperature and protected from heat, light and moisture.

Compatibility/Compounding Considerations

Atenolol tablets may be crushed or split/cut into ¼ s or ½ s for appropriate dosing.

Compounded preparation stability: Atenolol oral suspensions should not be compounded with sugar-containing vehicles. Atenolol oral suspension compounded from either active pharmaceutical ingredient (API) or commercially available tablets has been published (Patel, 1997). Triturating an appropriate amount of API or tablets with equal volumes of _Ora-Plus®_ and _Ora-Sweet® SF_ yields a 2 mg/mL oral suspension that retains >90% potency for 90 days stored at both 5°C and 25°C. This investigation also reveals that the presence of sugars (_Ora-Sweet®_ and simple syrup) reduces the potency of compounded atenolol suspensions to <90% in 7–14 days after compounding. Atenolol preparations are most stable at pH 4. Atenolol should be stored protected from light as exposure to ultraviolet light results in drug decomposition at all pH ranges.

Dosage Forms/Regulatory Status

VETERINARY-LABELED PRODUCTS: None
The ARCI (Racing Commissioners International) has designated this drug as a class 3 substance. See the appendix for more information.

HUMAN-LABELED PRODUCTS:
Atenolol Oral Tablets: 25 mg, 50 mg, & 100 mg;
Tenormin® (AstraZeneca); generic; (Rx)

Also available in an oral fixed dose combination
product with chlorthalidone.

References

Johnson–Delaney, C (2005). Ferret Cardiology.
   Proceedings: Atlantic Coast Veterinary Conference.
   Accessed via: Veterinary Information Network. http://
   goo.gl/qiaGG
Kittleson, M (2009). Treatment of feline hypertrophic
   cardiomyopathy (HCM)—Lost Dreams. Proceedings:
   ACVIM. Accessed via: Veterinary Information
   Network. http://goo.gl/XvCZt
Meurs, K (2006). Therapeutic management of canine con-
   genital heart disease. Proceedings: ACVIM. Accessed
   via: Veterinary Information Network. http://goo.gl/
   VLcyn
Patel, D., D. Doshi, et al. (1997). Short-term stability of
   atenolol in oral liquid formulations. Int J Pharm
   Compound 1: 437-439.
Smith, F (2009). Update on antiarrhythmic thera-
   py. Proceedings: WVC. Accessed via: Veterinary
   Information Network. http://goo.gl/aiVDJ
Stepien, R (2006). Therapeutic management of systemic
   hypertension. Proceedings: ACVIM Forum. Accessed
   via: Veterinary Information Network. http://goo.gl/
   JFcdF
Waddell, L (2005). Feline Hypertension. Proceedings:
   IVECCS. Accessed via: Veterinary Information
   Network. http://goo.gl/BbBEi
Williams, B (2000). Therapeutics in Ferrets. *Vet Clin NA:
   Exotic Anim Pract* **3:**1(Jan): 131–153.

ATIPAMEZOLE HCL

(at-i-*pam*-a-zole)   Antisedan®

ALPHA-2 ADRENERGIC ANTAGONIST

Prescriber Highlights

▶ Alpha$_2$ adrenergic antagonist; antagonizes agonists such as medetomidine
   or xylazine

▶ No safety data on use in pregnant or
   lactating animals

▶ May reverse effects rapidly, including
   analgesia; animals should be observed
   & protected from self-harm or causing
   harm to others

▶ Adverse Effects may include vomiting,
   diarrhea, hypersalivation, tremors, or
   excitation

Uses/Indications

Atipamezole is labeled for use as a reversal agent
for medetomidine and dexmedetomidine. It
potentially could be useful for reversal of other
alpha$_2$-adrenergic agonists as well (*e.g.*, amitraz,
xylazine, clonidine, tizanidine, brimonidine).

Pharmacology/Actions

Atipamezole competitively inhibits alpha$_2$-
adrenergic receptors, thereby acting as a reversal agent for alpha$_2$-adrenergic agonists (*e.g.*,
medetomidine). Net pharmacologic effects are
to reduce sedation, decrease blood pressure,
increase heart and respiratory rates, and reduce
the analgesic effects of alpha$_2$-adrenergic ago-

nists. Atipamezole will antagonize the diuretic
action of xylazine in dogs (Talukder *et al.* 2009).

Pharmacokinetics

After IM administration in the dog, peak plasma
levels occur in about 10 minutes. Atipamezole
is apparently metabolized in the liver to compounds that are eliminated in the urine. The
drug has an average plasma elimination half-life
of about 2–3 hours.

Contraindications/Precautions/Warnings

While the manufacturer lists no absolute contraindications to the use of atipamezole, the drug is
not recommended in pregnant or lactating animals due to the lack of data establishing safety.
Caution should be used in administration of anesthetic agents to elderly or debilitated animals.

When used as a reversal agent (antidote) for
alpha$_2$-agonist toxicity, atipamezole's effects
may subside before non-toxic levels of the offending agent are reached; repeat dosing may be
necessary.

Do not give IV to reptiles as profound hypotension can occur.

Adverse Effects

Potential adverse effects include occasional
vomiting, diarrhea, hypersalivation, tremors,
and brief excitation or apprehensiveness.

Because reversal can occur rapidly, care
should be exercised as animals emerging from
sedation and analgesia may exhibit apprehen-
sive or aggressive behaviors. After reversal, animals
should be protected from falling. Additional analgesia (*e.g.*, butorphanol) should be considered,
particularly after painful procedures.

In reptiles, intravenous administration reportedly can cause profound hypotension.

Reproductive/Nursing Safety

The manufacturer states that the drug is not
recommended in pregnant or lactating animals,
or in animals intended for breeding due to lack
of data establishing safety in these animals. No
other data was noted.

Overdosage/Acute Toxicity

Dogs receiving up to 10X the listed dosage apparently tolerated the drug without major effects. When overdosed, dose related effects seen
included panting, excitement, trembling, vomiting, soft or liquid feces, vasodilatation of sclera
and some muscle injury at the IM injection site.
Specific overdose therapy should generally not
be necessary.

Drug Interactions

The manufacturer states that information on the
use of atipamezole with other drugs is lacking,
therefore, caution should be taken when using
with other drugs (other than medetomidine).
The following drug interactions have either been
reported or are theoretical in humans or animals
receiving atipamezole and may be of significance in veterinary patients:

■ **ALPHA₁-ADRENERGIC BLOCKERS (e.g., prazosin):** Atipamezole is a relatively specific alpha₂ blocker it can also partially block alpha₁ receptors and reduce the effects of prazosin

■ **ALPHA₂-ADRENERGICS AGONISTS (e.g., detomidine, clonidine, brimonidine, xylazine, amitraz, etc.):** Atipamezole can reduce the effects (toxic or therapeutic) of these agents

Doses

■ **DOGS:**

For reversal of medetomidine:

a) Give IM an equal volume of *Antisedan®* and *Domitor®* is administered (mL per mL). The actual concentration of *Antisedan®* will be 5X that of *Domitor®*, as *Antisedan®* is 5 mg/mL versus *Domitor®*'s 1 mg/mL. (Package Insert; *Antisedan®*—Pfizer)

b) As above, but may give IV as well as IM. If it has been at least 45 minutes since medetomidine was given, may give atipamezole at half the volume of medetomidine if administered IV. If after 10–15 minutes an IM dose of atipamezole has not seemed to reverse the effects of medetomidine, an additional dose of atipamezole at 1/2 the volume of the medetomidine dose may be given. (McGrath & Ko 1997)

For reversal of dexmedetomidine:

a) 0.2 mg/kg IM or IV (Teixereia Neto 2009)

For treatment of amitraz toxicity:

a) 50 micrograms/kg IM; doses may need to be repeated every 4-6 hours as the half life of amitraz is longer than atipamezole in dogs. (Hugnet, Buronrosse et al. 1996), (Papich 2009)

■ **CATS:**

a) For reversal of medetomidine as part of a medetomidine/butorphanol or buprenorphine/ketamine/carprofen or meloxicam anesthesia/analgesia injectable combination: Use an equal volume IM of atipamezole as medetomidine was used in the combination. (Ko 2005)

b) For reversal of dexmedetomidine: 0.2 mg/kg IM or IV (Teixereia Neto 2009)

■ **RABBITS/RODENTS/SMALL MAMMALS:**

a) **Rabbits:** For medetomidine reversal: 0.5 mg/kg IM or SC; 0.25 mg/kg IV (Vella 2009)

b) **Mice, Rats, Gerbils, Hamsters, Guinea pigs:** To reverse xylazine or medetomidine: 0.1–1 mg/kg IM, IP, IV or SC (Adamcak & Otten 2000)

■ **RUMINANTS:**

a) For reversal of alpha₂-adrenergic agonists in bovine, new world camelids, ovine and caprine species: 0.02–0.1 mg/kg IV to effect (Haskell 2005)

b) Small ruminants, camelids: 0.1–0.2 mg/kg slow IV or IM; as a rule of thumb, if induction included ketamine or Telazol do not reverse alpha₂ sooner than 30 and ideally 60 minutes after induction. This will allow enough of the ketamine or tiletamine to be metabolized. (Snyder 2009), (Wolff 2009)

■ **BIRDS:**

a) As a reversal agent for alpha₂-adrenergic agonists (e.g., xylazine, detomidine, etc.): 0.5 mg/kg IM (Clyde & Paul-Murphy 2000)

■ **REPTILES:**

a) Reversal of all dosages ketamine/medetomidine combination (see ketamine or medetomidine monographs) with atipamezole is 4–5 times the medetomidine dose (Heard 1999). Reversal may take longer (up to one hour) in reptiles than in other species; Do NOT give IV as profound hypotension can occur (Mehler 2009).

■ **ZOO, EXOTIC, WILDLIFE SPECIES:**

For use of atipamezole in zoo, exotic and wildlife medicine refer to specific references, including:

a) *Zoo Animal and Wildlife Immobilization and Anesthesia.* West, G, Heard, D, Caulkett, N. (eds.). Blackwell Publishing, 2007.

b) *Handbook of Wildlife Chemical Immobilization, 3rd Ed.* Kreeger, T.J. and J.M. Arnemo. 2007.

c) *Restraint and Handling of Wild and Domestic Animals.* Fowler, M (ed.), Iowa State University Press, 1995

d) *Exotic Animal Formulary, 3rd Ed.* Carpenter, J.W., Saunders. 2005

e) The 2009 American Association of Zoo Veterinarian Proceedings by D. K. Fontenot also has several dosages listed for restraint, anesthesia, and analgesia for a variety of drugs for carnivores and primates. VIN members can access them at: http://goo.gl/BHRih or http://goo.gl/9UJse

Monitoring

■ Level of sedation and analgesia

■ Heart rate

■ Body temperature

Client Information

■ Atipamezole should be administered by veterinary professionals only. Clients should be informed that occasionally vomiting, diarrhea, hypersalivation, excitation and tremors may be seen after atipamezole administration. Should these be severe or persist after leaving the clinic, clients should contact the veterinarian.

Chemistry/Synonyms

Atipamezole is an imidazole alpha$_2$-adrenergic antagonist. The injection is a clear, colorless solution.

Atipamezole HCl may also be known as MPV-1248 or *Antisedan®*.

Storage/Stability

Atipamezole HCl injection should be stored at room temperature (15°–30°C) and protected from light.

Dosage Forms/Regulatory Status

VETERINARY-LABELED PRODUCTS:

Atipamezole HCl for Injection: 5 mg/mL in 10 mL multidose vials; *Antisedan®* (Pfizer); (Rx). FDA-approved for use in dogs.

HUMAN-LABELED PRODUCTS: None

References

Adamcak, A & B Otten (2000). Rodent Therapeutics. *Vet Clin NA: Exotic Anim Pract* **3:**1(Jan): 221–240.

Clyde, V & J Paul–Murphy (2000). Avian Analgesia. *Kirk's Current Veterinary Therapy: XIII Small Animal Practice.* J Bonagura Ed. Philadelphia, WB Saunders: 1126–1128.

Haskell, R (2005). Development of a Small Ruminant Formulary. Proceedings: WVC. Accessed via: Veterinary Information Network. http://goo.gl/3tIK9

Heard, D (1999). Advances in Reptile Anesthesia. The North American Veterinary Conference, Orlando.

Ko, J (2005). New anesthesia–analgesia injectable combinations in dogs and cats. Proceedings: ACVC. Accessed via: Veterinary Information Network. http://goo.gl/Yklxx

McGrath, C & J Ko (1997). How to use the new alpha–2 antagonist, Atipamezole (Antisedan®) to reverse medetomidine (Domitor®) in the dog. *Virgina Veterinary Notes, Veterinary Teaching Hospital.*

Mehler, S (2009). Anaesthesia and care of the reptile. Proceedings: BSAVA. Accessed via: Veterinary Information Network. http://goo.gl/2QYZU

Papich, M (2009). Medication precautions for the neurologic patient. Proceedings: ACVIM. Accessed via: Veterinary Information Network. http://goo.gl/DZ1t2

Snyder, J (2009). Small Ruminant Medicine & Surgery for Equine and Small Animal Practitioners I & II. Proceedings: WVC. Accessed via: Veterinary Information Network. http://goo.gl/hkoer

Talukder, MH, Y Hikasa, et al. (2009). Antagonistic Effects of Atipamezole and Yohimbine on Xylazine–Induced Diuresis in Healthy Dogs. *Journal of Veterinary Medical Science* **71**(5): 539–548.

Teixeria Neto, F (2009). Dexmedetomidine: A new alpha–2 agonist for small animal practice. Proceedings: WSAVA. Accessed via: Veterinary Information Network. http://goo.gl/tcFmb

Vella, D (2009). Rabbit General Anesthesia. Proceedings: AAVAC–UEP. Accessed via: Veterinary Information Network. http://goo.gl/XKsCh

Wolff, P (2009). Camelid Medicine. Proceedings: AAZV. Accessed via: Veterinary Information Network. http://goo.gl/4TEAy

ATOVAQUONE

(ah-*toe*-va-kwone)   Mepron®
ORAL ANTIPROTOZOAL AGENT

Prescriber Highlights

▶ Atovaquone (with azithromycin) appears effective in treating dogs with Babesia gibsoni infections. Alone, it is a second-line agent (after trimethoprim/sulfa) for pneumocystosis in dogs.

▶ In combination with azithromycin, used to treat cytauxzoonosis in cats

▶ Limited use thus far; appears well-tolerated by dogs

▶ Treatment may be quite expensive

Uses/Indications

Atovaquone (with azithromycin) appears effective in treating dogs with *Babesia gibsoni* (Asian genotype) infections, particularly in dogs not immunosuppressed or splenectomized. Atovaquone may be of benefit for treating pneumocystosis in dogs, but it is considered second line therapy after potentiated sulfonamides.

Atovaquone (with azithromycin) may be of benefit in treating *Cytauxzoon felis* infections in cats.

Pharmacology/Actions

Atovaquone's antiprotozoal mechanism of action is not completely understood. It is believed that the hydroxynaphthoquinones, like atovaquone, selectively inhibit protozoan mitochondrial electron transport causing inhibition of *de novo* pyrimidine synthesis. Unlike mammalian cells, certain protozoa cannot salvage preformed pyrimidines.

Pharmacokinetics

Pharmacokinetic data for dogs or cats was not located. In humans after oral administration, bioavailability ranges from 23–47%. The presence of food, particularly high in fat, can increase bioavailability significantly (2+ fold over fasted administration). The drug is highly bound to human plasma proteins (99.9%) and levels in the CSF are approximately 1% of those found in plasma. Elimination half-life in people is about 70 hours presumably due to enterohepatic recycling. There may be limited hepatic metabolism, but the bulk of absorbed drug is eventually eliminated unchanged in the feces.

Contraindications/Precautions/Warnings

No absolute contraindications for using atovaquone in dogs or cats have been documented. Animals with malabsorption syndromes or that cannot take the drug with food should have alternate therapies considered.

The drug is contraindicated in human patients that develop or have a prior history of hypersensitivity reactions to the drug.

Reproductive/Nursing Safety

Studies in pregnant rats with atovaquone plasma levels approximately 2–3 times those found in humans receiving therapeutic dosages revealed no increase in teratogenicity. Similar studies in rabbits showed increased maternal and fetal toxicity (decreased fetal growth and increased early fetal resorption). In humans, the FDA categorizes atovaquone as category *C* for use during pregnancy (*Animal studies have shown an adverse effect on the fetus, but there are no adequate studies in humans; or there are no animal reproduction studies and no adequate studies in humans.*)

Little information is available on the safety of this drug during lactation. In rats, milk levels were approximately ⅓ those found in maternal plasma. It is unlikely atovaquone in milk poses much risk to nursing puppies.

Adverse Effects

Atovaquone use in dogs and cats has been limited and the adverse effect profile is not well known. One study (Birkenheuer, AJ *et al.* 2004) using atovaquone and azithromycin for treating *Babesia gibsoni* infections in 10 dogs reported that no adverse effects were noted. The combination product containing atovaquone and proguanil (*Malarone®*) reportedly causes severe gastrointestinal effects in dogs.

In humans treated with atovaquone, rashes (up to 39% of treated patients) and gastrointestinal effects (nausea, vomiting, diarrhea) are the most frequently reported adverse effects. Rashes or diarrhea may necessitate discontinuation of therapy. Other adverse effects reported in humans include hypersensitivity reactions, increased liver enzymes, CNS effects (headache, dizziness, insomnia), hyperglycemia, hyponatremia, fever, neutropenia, and anemia.

Overdosage/Acute Toxicity

Limited information is available for any species. Minimum toxic doses have not been established; laboratory animals have tolerated doses up to 31.5 grams. The current recommendation for treating overdoses is basically symptomatic and supportive.

Drug Interactions

The following drug interactions have either been reported or are theoretical in humans or animals receiving atovaquone and may be of significance in veterinary patients:

■ **METOCLOPRAMIDE:** Can decrease atovaquone plasma concentrations

■ **TETRACYCLINE:** Can decrease atovaquone plasma concentrations

■ **RIFAMPIN:** Can decrease atovaquone plasma concentrations

Laboratory Considerations

■ No specific issues; see Monitoring for recommendations for testing for efficacy

Doses

■ **DOGS:**

a) For *Babesia gibsoni* (Asian genotype) infections: Atovaquone 13.3 mg/kg PO q8h and Azithromycin 10 mg/kg PO once daily. Give both drugs for 10 days. Reserve immunosuppressive therapy for cases that are not rapidly responding (3–5 days) to anti-protozoal therapy. (Birkenheuer, AJ *et al.* 2004), (Birkenheuer, A 2006)

b) For Pneumocystosis: 15 mg/kg PO once daily for 3 weeks. (Greene *et al.* 2006)

■ **CATS:**

a) For Cytauxzoonosis (*Cytauxzoon felis*): Atovaquone 15 mg/kg PO q8h with azithromycin 10 mg/kg PO q24h. All cases were treated with IV fluids and most received heparin. (Birkenheuer, A *et al.* 2008)

Monitoring

■ Monitoring for therapy for *Babesia gibsoni* in dogs should include surveillance for potential adverse effects and signs for clinical efficacy, including monitoring serial CBCs

■ Severe cases may have elevated BUN or liver enzymes, and hypokalemia

■ Current recommendation for determining "clearing" of the organism (*B. gibsoni*) is to perform a PCR test at 60 days and 90 days post-therapy

Client Information

■ Store medication at room temperature and away from bright light

■ Before using, shake bottle gently

■ To increase the absorption from the GI tract, give with food high in fat (*e.g.*, ice cream, tuna oil, butter, meat fat)

■ Adverse effect profile in dogs and cats for this medication is not well known

■ Report any significant effects such as rash, or severe or persistent vomiting or diarrhea, to the veterinarian

Chemistry/Synonyms

Atovaquone is a synthetic, hydroxy-1,4-naphthoquinone antiprotozoal agent. It occurs as a yellow powder that is highly lipid soluble, insoluble in water and slightly soluble in alcohol.

Atovaquone may also be known as: BW-566C, Atovacuona, Atovakvon, Atovakvoni, Atovaquonnum, *Malanil®*, *Mepron®*, or *Wellvone®*.

Storage/Stability

The commercially available oral suspension should be stored at room temperature (15–25°C) in tight containers and protected from bright light; do not freeze.

Dosage Forms/Regulatory Status

VETERINARY-LABELED PRODUCTS: None

HUMAN-LABELED PRODUCTS:
Atovaquone Oral Suspension: 150 mg/mL in 210 mL bottles; citrus flavor; *Mepron®* (GlaxoWellcome); (Rx)

A tablet dosage form was previously available, but was discontinued when the oral suspension was approved by FDA; the suspension has much better oral bioavailability in humans. A combination tablet product containing atovaquone and proguanil HCl (*Malarone®*) is available that has labeled indications (human) for malaria prophylaxis and treatment. This combination has reportedly caused significant GI adverse effects in dogs.

References

Birkenheuer, A (2006). Infectious Hemolytic Anemias. ACVIM Proceedings. Accessed via: Veterinary Information Network. http://goo.gl/DPVKW

Birkenheuer, A, L Cohn, et al. (2008). Atovaquone and azithromycin for the treatment of Cytauxzoon felis. Proceedings: ACVIM. Accessed via: Veterinary Information Network. http://goo.gl/v8MfT

Birkenheuer, A, M Levy, et al. (2004). Efficacy of combined atovaquone and azithromycin for therapy of chronic Babesia gibsoni (Asian genotype) infections in dogs. *J Vet Intern Med* 18: 494–498.

Greene, C, F Chandler, et al. (2006). Pneumocystosis. *Infectious Diseases of the Dogs and Cat.* C Greene Ed., Elsevier: 651–658.

ATRACURIUM BESYLATE

(a-tra-*cure*-ee-um) Tracrium®

NONDEPOLARIZING NEUROMUSCULAR BLOCKER

Prescriber Highlights

▶ Non-depolarizing neuromuscular blocking agent; minimal cardiovascular effects; valuable in critically ill patients who cannot receive standard inhalant anesthesia concentrations

▶ Should never be given as a sole agent; has no sedative or analgesic effects

▶ More potent in horses than other species

▶ Relatively contraindicated in patients with myasthenia gravis, hypersensitivity to it

▶ Less incidence of histamine release than tubocurarine or metocurine

▶ Potential drug interactions

Uses/Indications

Atracurium is indicated as an adjunct to general anesthesia to produce muscle relaxation during surgical procedures or mechanical ventilation and also to facilitate endotracheal intubation. Atracurium can be used in patients with significant renal or hepatic disease. It is valuable to paralyze critically ill patients when very low settings, or no inhalant anesthesia can be used.

Pharmacology/Actions

Atracurium is a nondepolarizing neuromuscular blocking agent and acts by competitively binding at cholinergic receptor sites at the motor end-plate thereby inhibiting the effects of acetylcholine. Atracurium is considered ¼ to ⅓ as potent as pancuronium. In horses, atracurium is more potent than in other species tested and more potent than other nondepolarizing muscle relaxants studied.

Atracurium does not provide any analgesia or sedation.

Neuromuscular blockade (NMB) can be variably potentiated when used with different general anesthetics. A study in dogs, demonstrated that when compared with propofol, sevoflurane prolonged atracurium-induced NMB by about 15 minutes (Kastrup *et al.* 2005).

At usual doses, atracurium exhibits minimal cardiovascular effects, unlike most other nondepolarizing neuromuscular blockers. A related compound, cisatracurium (*Nimbex®*) has even less cardiovascular effects in cats than does atracurium. While atracurium can stimulate histamine release, it is considered to cause less histamine release than either tubocurarine or metocurine. In humans, less than one percent of patients receiving atracurium exhibit clinically significant adverse reactions or histamine release.

Pharmacokinetics

After IV injection, maximal neuromuscular blockade generally occurs within 3–5 minutes. The duration of maximal blockade increases as the dosage increases. Systemic alkalosis may diminish the degree and duration of blockade; acidosis potentiates it. In conjunction with balanced anesthesia, the duration of blockade generally persists for 20–35 minutes. Recovery times do not appreciably change after giving maintenance doses, so predictable blocking effects can be attained when the drug is administered at regular intervals.

Atracurium is metabolized by ester hydrolysis and Hofmann elimination that occur independently of renal or hepatic function. Physiologic pH and temperature can affect elimination of atracurium. Increased body temperature can enhance the elimination of the drug. Ester hydrolysis is enhanced by decreases in pH, while Hofmann elimination is reduced by decreases in pH.

Contraindications/Precautions/Warnings

Atracurium is contraindicated in patients who are hypersensitive to it. Because it may rarely cause significant release of histamine, it should be used with caution in patients where this would be hazardous (severe cardiovascular disease, asthma, etc.). Atracurium has minimal cardiac effects and will not counteract the bradycardia or vagal stimulation induced by other agents. Use of neuromuscular blocking agents must be done with extreme caution, or not at all, in patients suffering from myasthenia gravis. Atracurium has no analgesic or sedative/anesthetic actions. To provide amnesia in critically ill patients, when no inhalant anesthesia can be used, midazolam should be considered. Either intermittent boluses (0.1 mg/kg IV every 20–30 minutes) or a continuous IV infusion (0.1 mg/kg/hr) of midazolam has been recommended (Spelts 2009).

It is not known whether this drug is excreted in milk. Safety for use in the nursing mother has not been established.

Adverse Effects

Clinically significant adverse effects are apparently quite rare in patients (<1% in humans) receiving recommended doses of atracurium and usually are secondary to histamine release. They can include: allergic reactions, inadequate or prolonged block, hypotension vasodilatation, bradycardia, tachycardia, dyspnea, broncho-, laryngo-spasm, rash, urticaria, and a reaction at the injection site. Patients developing hypotension usually have preexisting severe cardiovascular disease.

Overdosage/Acute Toxicity

Overdosage possibilities can be minimized by monitoring muscle twitch responses to peripheral nerve stimulation. Increased risks of hypotension and histamine release occur with overdoses, as well as prolonged duration of muscle blockade.

Besides treating conservatively (mechanical ventilation, O_2, fluids, etc.), reversal of blockade may be accomplished by administering an anticholinesterase agent such as edrophonium (0.5 mg/kg IV), or neostigmine (0.02–0.04 mg/kg IV) with an anticholinergic (atropine or glycopyrrolate). Reversal is usually attempted (in humans) approximately 20–35 minutes after the initial dose, or 10–30 minutes after the last maintenance dose. Reversal is usually complete within 8–10 minutes. Because the duration of action of atracurium may be longer than the reversal agent, careful observation and monitoring is required. Readministration of the reversal agent may be necessary.

Drug Interactions

The following drug interactions have either been reported or are theoretical in humans or animals receiving atracurium and may be of significance in veterinary patients:

The following agents may enhance the neuromuscular blocking activity of atracurium:

■ **AMINOGLYCOSIDE ANTIBIOTICS (gentamicin,** etc.)

■ **ANESTHETICS, GENERAL (enflurane, isoflurane, halothane)**

■ **BACITRACIN, POLYMYXIN B (systemic)**

■ **PROCAINAMIDE**

■ **QUINIDINE**

■ **LITHIUM**

■ **MAGNESIUM SALTS**

■ **ANTICONVULSANTS (PHENYTOIN, CARBAMAZEPINE):** Have been reported to both decrease the effects and duration of neuromuscular blockade

■ **OTHER MUSCLE RELAXANT DRUGS:** May cause a synergistic or antagonistic effect

■ **SUCCINYLCHOLINE:** May speed the onset of action and enhance the neuromuscular blocking actions of atracurium. Do not give atracurium until succinylcholine effects have diminished.

Doses

■ **DOGS:**

a) For use in critically ill patients when low concentrations of, or no inhalant anesthesia can be used: 0.2 mg/kg IV initial dose; subsequent doses 0.1 mg/kg IV. Do not dose more frequently than every 20–30 minutes in critical patients unless a peripheral nerve stimulator is applied, or voluntary movement is observed. Positive pressure ventilation, preferably mechanical, is required. (Spelts 2009)

b) For neuromuscular blockade augmentation during corneal surgery: 0.15 mg/kg IV (Nasisse 2004)

c) As a muscle relaxant to facilitate intubation in patients with severe blunt trauma: IV started and acepromazine 0.01 mg/kg plus butorphanol 0.1 mg/kg plus ketamine 1 mg/kg is infused. If patient requires intubation, give atracurium at 0.25 mg/kg IV push. (Crowe 2004)

d) For induction of respiratory muscle paralysis during mechanical ventilation: Loading dose: 0.2–0.5 mg/kg IV, then a constant rate infusion 5 minutes later of 3–9 micrograms/kg/min. Use D5W or 0.9% sodium chloride for diluent; do not mix with other drugs. Respiratory and cardiovascular monitoring should be provided. (Dhupa 2005)

■ **CATS:**

a) Induction dose: 0.22 mg/kg IV, give 1/10th to 1/6th of this dose initially as a "priming" dose, followed 4–6 minutes later with the remainder and a sedative/hypnotic agent.

Intraoperative dose: 0.11 mg/kg IV (Mandsager 1988)

b) For induction of respiratory muscle paralysis during mechanical ventilation: Loading dose: 0.2–0.5 mg/kg IV, then a constant rate infusion 5 minutes later of 0.37 micrograms/kg/min. Use D5W or 0.9% sodium chloride for diluent; do not mix with other drugs. Respiratory and cardiovascular monitoring should be provided. (Dhupa 2005)

c) For use in critically ill patients when low concentrations of, or no inhalant anesthesia can be used: 0.2 mg/kg IV initial dose; subsequent doses 0.1 mg/kg IV. Do not dose more frequently than every 20–30 minutes in critical patients unless a peripheral nerve stimulator is applied, or voluntary movement is observed. Positive pressure ventilation, preferably mechanical, is required. (Spelts 2009)

◼ **RABBITS/RODENTS/SMALL MAMMALS:**

a) Rabbits: For paralysis for periophthalmic surgery: 0.1 mg/kg (Ivey & Morrisey 2000)

◼ **HORSES:** (**Note:** ARCI UCGFS Class 2 Drug)

a) Intraoperative dose: 0.055 mg/kg IV (Mandsager 1988)

Monitoring

◼ Level of neuromuscular blockade; recommend use of a peripheral nerve stimulator to evaluate "train of 4" twitches. If not available, watch for spontaneous ventilation and voluntary muscle movement.

◼ Cardiac rate

Client Information

◼ This drug should only be used by professionals familiar with its use.

Chemistry/Synonyms

A synthetic, non-depolarizing neuromuscular blocking agent, atracurium, is a bisquaternary, non-choline diester structurally similar to metocurine and tubocurarine. It occurs as white to pale yellow powder; 50 mg are soluble in 1 mL of water, 200 mg are soluble in 1 mL of alcohol, and 35 mg are soluble in 1 mL of normal saline.

Atracurium besylate may also be known as: 33A74, atracurium besilate, BW-33A, *Abbottracurium®*, *Atracur®*, *Faulcurium®*, *Ifacur®*, *Laurak®*, *Mycurium®*, *Relatrac®*, *Sitrac®*, *Trablok®*, *Tracrium®*, or *Tracur®*.

Storage/Stability

The commercially available injection occurs as clear, colorless solution and is a sterile solution of the drug in sterile water for injection. The pH of this solution is 3.25–3.65. Atracurium injection should be stored in the refrigerator and protected against freezing. At room temperature, approximately 5% potency loss occurs each month; when refrigerated, a 6% potency loss occurs over a year's time.

Compatibility/Compounding Considerations

Atracurium is **compatible** with the standard IV solutions, but while stable in lactated Ringer's for 8 hours, degradation occurs more rapidly. It should not be mixed in the same IV bag or syringe, or given through the same needle with alkaline drugs (*e.g.*, barbiturates) or solutions (sodium bicarbonate) as precipitation may occur. It is **incompatible** when mixed with propofol, diazepam, thiopental, aminophylline, cefazolin,

heparin, ranitidine, and sodium nitroprusside.

Dosage Forms/Regulatory Status

VETERINARY-LABELED PRODUCTS: None

The ARCI (Racing Commissioners International) has designated this drug as a class 2 substance. See the appendix for more information.

HUMAN-LABELED PRODUCTS:

Atracurium Besylate Injection: 10 mg/mL in 5 mL single-use & 10 mL multi-use vials; *Tracrium®* (GlaxoWellcome); generic (Bedford Labs); (Rx)

References

Crowe, D (2004). Severe blunt trauma: Surgical intervention into the unknown. Proceedings: IVECCS. Accessed via: Veterinary Information Network. http://goo.gl/x4pLR

Dhupa, N (2005). Constant rate infusions. *Textbook of Veterinary Internal Medicine, 6th Ed.* S Ettinger and E Feldman Eds., Elsevier: 544–550.

Ivey, E & J Morrisey (2000). Therapeutics for Rabbits. *Vet Clin NA: Exotic Anim Pract* 3:1(Jan): 183–216.

Kastrup, MR, F Marsico, et al. (2005). Neuromuscular blocking properties of atracurium during sevoflurane or propofol anaesthesia in dogs. *Veterinary Anaesthesia and Analgesia* 32(4): 222–227.

Mandsager, RE (1988, Last Update). "Personal Communication."

Nasisse, M (2004). Practical ophthalmic surgery. Proceedings: ACVC. Accessed via: Veterinary Information Network. http://goo.gl/JWvSY

Spelts, K (2009). Anesthesia for the critically ill patient. Proceedings: WVC.

ATROPINE SULFATE

(a-troe-peen)

ANTICHOLINERGIC

Prescriber Highlights

▶ Prototype antimuscarinic agent used for a variety of indications (bradycardia, premed, antidote, etc.)

▶ Contraindicated in conditions where anticholinergic effects would be detrimental (*e.g.*, narrow angle glaucoma, tachycardias, ileus, urinary obstruction, etc.)

▶ Adverse effects are dose related & anticholinergic in nature: 1) dry secretions, 2) initial bradycardia, then tachycardia, 3) slow gut & urinary tract, 4) mydriasis/cycloplegia

▶ Drug interactions

Uses/Indications

The principal veterinary indications for systemic atropine include:

◼ Preanesthetic to prevent or reduce secretions of the respiratory tract

◼ Treat sinus bradycardia, sinoatrial arrest, and incomplete AV block

◼ Differentiate vagally-mediated bradycardia for other causes

- As an antidote for overdoses of cholinergic agents (*e.g.*, physostigmine, etc.)
- As an antidote for organophosphate, carbamate, muscarinic mushroom, blue-green algae intoxication
- Hypersialism
- Treatment of bronchoconstrictive disease

Pharmacology/Actions

Atropine, like other antimuscarinic agents, competitively inhibits acetylcholine or other cholinergic stimulants at postganglionic parasympathetic neuroeffector sites. High doses may block nicotinic receptors at the autonomic ganglia and at the neuromuscular junction. Pharmacologic effects are dose related. At low doses salivation, bronchial secretions, and sweating (not horses) are inhibited. At moderate systemic doses, atropine dilates and inhibits accommodation of the pupil, and increases heart rate. High doses will decrease GI and urinary tract motility. Very high doses will inhibit gastric secretion.

Pharmacokinetics

Atropine sulfate is well absorbed after oral administration, IM injection, inhalation, or endotracheal administration. After IV administration peak effects in heart rates occur within 3–4 minutes.

Atropine is well distributed throughout the body and crosses into the CNS, across the placenta, and can distribute into the milk in small quantities.

Atropine is metabolized in the liver and excreted into the urine. Approximately 30–50% of a dose is excreted unchanged into the urine. The plasma half-life in humans has been reported to be between 2–3 hours.

Contraindications/Precautions/Warnings

Atropine is contraindicated in patients with narrow-angle glaucoma, synechiae (adhesions) between the iris and lens, hypersensitivity to anticholinergic drugs, tachycardias secondary to thyrotoxicosis or cardiac insufficiency, myocardial ischemia, unstable cardiac status during acute hemorrhage, GI obstructive disease, paralytic ileus, severe ulcerative colitis, obstructive uropathy, and myasthenia gravis (unless used to reverse adverse muscarinic effects secondary to therapy). Atropine may aggravate some signs seen with amitraz toxicity, leading to hypertension and further inhibition of peristalsis.

Antimuscarinic agents should be used with extreme caution in patients with known or suspected GI infections. Atropine or other antimuscarinic agents can decrease GI motility and prolong retention of the causative agent(s) or toxin(s) resulting in prolonged clinical signs. Antimuscarinic agents must also be used with extreme caution in patients with autonomic neuropathy.

Atropine reportedly is not effective in treating bradycardias in puppies before 14 days of age or kittens younger than 11 days old. It may also damage hypoxic myocardia in neonates (Trass 2009).

Glycopyrrolate is usually the anticholinergic of choice when treating rabbits as a large percentage (40%?) have endogenous atropinesterase present.

Antimuscarinic agents should be used with caution in patients with hepatic or renal disease, geriatric or pediatric patients, hyperthyroidism, hypertension, CHF, tachyarrhythmias, prostatic hypertrophy, or esophageal reflux. Systemic atropine should be used cautiously in horses as it may decrease gut motility and induce colic in susceptible animals. It may also reduce the arrhythmogenic doses of epinephrine. Use of atropine in cattle may result in inappetence and rumen stasis that may persist for several days.

When used in food animals at doses up to 0.2 mg/kg, FARAD recommends a 28 day meat and 6 day milk withdrawal time. (Haskell *et al.* 2005)

Adverse Effects

Adverse effects are basically extensions of the drug's pharmacologic effects and are generally dose related. At usual doses, effects tend to be mild in relatively healthy patients. The more severe effects listed tend to occur with high or toxic doses. GI effects can include dry mouth (xerostomia), dysphagia, constipation, vomiting, and thirst. GU effects may include urinary retention or hesitancy. CNS effects may include stimulation, drowsiness, ataxia, seizures, respiratory depression, etc. Ophthalmic effects include blurred vision, pupil dilation, cycloplegia, and photophobia. Cardiovascular effects include sinus tachycardia (at higher doses), bradycardia (initially or at very low doses), hypertension, hypotension, arrhythmias (ectopic complexes), and circulatory failure.

Reproductive/Nursing Safety

In humans, the FDA categorizes this drug as category *C* for use during pregnancy (*Animal studies have shown an adverse effect on the fetus, but there are no adequate studies in humans; or there are no animal reproduction studies and no adequate studies in humans.*) In a separate system evaluating the safety of drugs in canine and feline pregnancy (Papich 1989), this drug is categorized as in class: *B* (*Safe for use if used cautiously. Studies in laboratory animals may have uncovered some risk, but these drugs appear to be safe in dogs and cats or these drugs are safe if they are not administered when the animal is near term.*) Atropine use in pregnancy may cause fetal tachycardia.

Overdosage/Acute Toxicity

For signs and symptoms of atropine toxicity see adverse effects above. If a recent oral ingestion, emptying of gut contents and administration of activated charcoal and saline cathartics may be warranted. Treat clinical signs supportively and symptomatically. Do not use phenothiazines as they may contribute to the anticholinergic effects. Fluid therapy and standard treatments for shock may be instituted.

The use of physostigmine is controversial and should probably be reserved for cases where the patient exhibits either extreme agitation and is at risk for injuring themselves or others, or for cases where supraventricular tachycardias and sinus tachycardias are severe or life threatening. The usual dose for physostigmine (human) is: 2 mg IV slowly (for average sized adult). If no response, may repeat every 20 minutes until reversal of toxic antimuscarinic effects or cholinergic effects takes place. The human pediatric dose is 0.02 mg/kg slow IV (repeat q10 minutes as above) and may be a reasonable choice for initial treatment of small animals. Physostigmine adverse effects (bronchoconstriction, bradycardia, seizures) may be treated with small doses of IV atropine.

Drug Interactions

The following drug interactions have either been reported or are theoretical in humans or animals receiving atropine and may be of significance in veterinary patients:

The following drugs may enhance the activity or toxicity of atropine and its derivatives:

- ◼ **AMANTADINE**
- ◼ **ANTICHOLINERGIC AGENTS** (other)
- ◼ **ANTICHOLINERGIC MUSCLE RELAXANTS**
- ◼ **ANTIHISTAMINES** (e.g., diphenhydramine)
- ◼ **DISOPYRAMIDE**
- ◼ **MEPERIDINE**
- ◼ **PHENOTHIAZINES**
- ◼ **PROCAINAMIDE**
- ◼ **PRIMIDONE**
- ◼ **TRICYCLIC ANTIDEPRESSANTS** (e.g., amitriptyline, clomipramine)
- ◼ **ALPHA-2 AGONISTS** (e.g., dexmedetomidine, medetomidine): Use of atropine with alpha-2 blockers may significantly increase arterial blood pressure, heart rates and the incidence of arrhythmias (Congdon *et al.* 2009). Clinical use of atropine or glycopyrrolate to prevent or treat medetomidine- or dexmedetomidine-caused bradycardia is controversial and many discourage using together. This may be particularly important when using higher dosages of the alpha-2 agonist.
- ◼ **AMITRAZ:** Atropine may aggravate some signs seen with amitraz toxicity; leading to hypertension and further inhibition of peristalsis
- ◼ **ANTACIDS:** May decrease PO atropine absorption; give oral atropine at least 1 hour prior to oral antacids
- ◼ **CORTICOSTEROIDS** (long-term use): may increase intraocular pressure
- ◼ **DIGOXIN** (slow-dissolving): Atropine may

increase serum digoxin levels; use regular digoxin tablets or oral liquid

- ◼ **KETOCONAZOLE:** Increased gastric pH may decrease GI absorption; administer oral atropine 2 hours after ketoconazole
- ◼ **METOCLOPRAMIDE:** Atropine and its derivatives may antagonize the actions of metoclopramide

Doses

◼ **DOGS:**

As a preanesthetic adjuvant:

a) In geriatric patients: 0.01–0.02 mg/kg IM, IV; do not use anticholinergics indiscriminately in geriatric patients. (Carpenter *et al.* 2005)

b) 0.074 mg/kg IV, IM or SC (Package Insert; *Atropine Injectable*, S.A.—Fort Dodge)

c) 0.02–0.04 mg/kg SC, IM or IV (Morgan 1988)

For adjunctive treatment of bradycardias, Incomplete AV block, etc.

a) During cardiopulmonary cerebral resuscitation (CPCR) efforts: 0.04 mg/kg IV or IO; can repeat every 3–5 minutes for a maximum of 3 doses. For intra-tracheal (IT) administration: 0.08–0.1 mg/kg dilute in 5–10 mL of sterile water before administering (Plunkett & McMichael 2008).

b) 0.02–0.04 mg/kg IV or IM (Russell & Rush 1995)

To differentiate vagally-mediated bradyarrhythmias from non-vagal bradyarrhythmias (Atropine Response Test):

Rishniw Preference: **1)** Record ECG at baseline; **2)** Administer 0.04 mg/kg atropine IV; **3)** Wait 15 minutes; **4)** Record ECG for at least 2 minutes (use slow paper speed). If the response is incomplete, repeat steps 2–4. Persistent sinus tachycardia at >140 bpm is expected in most dogs with vagally-mediated bradycardia.

Kittleson Preference: **1)** Record ECG at baseline; **2)** Administer 0.04 mg/kg atropine SQ; **3)** Wait 30 minutes; **4)** Record ECG for at least 2 minutes (use slow paper speed). Persistent sinus tachycardia at >140 bpm is expected in most dogs with vagally-mediated bradycardia. (Rishniw & Kittleson 2007)

For treatment of cholinergic toxicity:

a) 0.2–0.5 mg/kg; 1/4 of the dose IV and the remainder IM or SC (Firth 2000)

For treatment of bronchoconstriction:

a) 0.02–0.04 mg/kg for a duration of effect of 1–1.5 hours (Papich 1986)

◼ **CATS:**

As a preanesthetic adjuvant:

a) In geriatric patients: 0.01–0.02 mg/kg IM, IV; do not use anticholinergics indiscriminately in geriatric patients. (Carpenter *et al.* 2005)

b) 0.074 mg/kg IV, IM or SC (Package Insert; *Atropine Injectable, S.A.*—Fort Dodge)

c) 0.02–0.04 mg/kg SC, IM or IV (Morgan 1988)

For treatment of bradycardias:

a) During cardiopulmonary cerebral resuscitation (CPCR) efforts: 0.04 mg/kg IV or IO; can repeat every 3–5 minutes for a maximum of 3 doses. For intra-tracheal (IT) administration: 0.08–0.1 mg/kg; dilute in 5–10 mL of sterile water before administering (Plunkett & McMichael 2008).

b) 0.02–0.04 mg/kg SC, IM or IV q4–6h (Miller 1985)

For treatment of cholinergic toxicity:

a) 0.2–2 mg/kg; give ¼th of the dose IV and the remainder SC or IM (Morgan 1988)

■ **FERRETS:**

a) As a premed: 0.05 mg/kg SC or IM (Williams 2000)

■ **RABBITS/RODENTS/SMALL MAMMALS:**

a) To treat organophosphate toxicity: 10 mg/kg SC q20 minutes (Ivey & Morrisey 2000)

■ **CATTLE:**

Note: When used in food animals at doses up to 0.2 mg/kg, FARAD recommends a 28 day meat and 6 day milk withdrawal time. (Haskell *et al.* 2005)

As a preanesthetic:

a) Because of a lack of extended efficacy and potential adverse reactions, atropine is not used routinely as a preoperative agent in ruminants. If it is desired for use, a dose of 0.06–0.12 mg/kg IM has been suggested.) (Thurmon & Benson 1986)

For adjunctive treatment of bovine hypersensitivity disease:

a) 1 gram per cow once daily followed by 0.5 gram/cow in 2–3 days (method of administration not specified) (Manning & Scheidt 1986)

For treatment of cholinergic toxicity (organophosphates):

a) 0.5 mg/kg (average dose); give ¼th of the dose IV and the remainder SC or IM; may repeat q3–4h for 1–2 days (Bailey 1986)

■ **HORSES:** (**Note:** ARCI UCGFS Class 3 Drug) For treatment of bradyarrhythmias due to increased parasympathetic tone:

a) 0.01–0.02 mg/kg IV (Mogg 1999)

b) 0.045 mg/kg parenterally (Hilwig 1987)

As a bronchodilator:

a) 5 mg IV for a 400–500 kg animal (Beech 1987)

b) 5–7 mg/kg IV for a 450 kg horse can serve as a rescue medication in cases with severe airway obstruction, but it has an abbreviated duration of action (0.5–2 hours) and adverse effects (ileus, CNS toxicity, tachycardia, increased mucus secretion, and impaired mucociliary clearance) limit its use to a single rescue dose. (Rush 2006)

For organophosphate poisoning:

a) Approximately 1 mg/kg given to effect, IV (use mydriasis and absence of salivation as therapy endpoints), may repeat every 1.5–2 hours as required subcutaneously (Oehme 1987)

b) 0.22 mg/kg, ¼th of the dose administered IV and the remainder SC or IM (Package Insert; *Atropine Injectable, L.A.*— Fort Dodge)

■ **SWINE:**

The equine dose (above) may be used to initially treat organophosphate toxicity in swine.

As an adjunctive preanesthetic agent:

a) 0.04 mg/kg IM (Thurmon & Benson 1986)

■ **SHEEP, GOATS:**

For treating organophosphate toxicity:

a) Use the dose for cattle (above).

■ **BIRDS:**

For organophosphate poisoning:

a) 0.2 mg/kg IM every 3–4 hours as needed; ¼th the initial dose is administered. Use with pralidoxime (not in raptors) at 10–20 mg/kg IM q8–12h as needed. Do not use pralidoxime in carbamate poisonings.

To assist in diagnosing organophosphate poisoning (with history, clinical signs, etc.) in birds presenting with bradycardia: May administer atropine at 0.02 mg/kg IV. If bradycardia does not reverse, may consider organophosphate toxicity. (LaBonde 2006)

As a preanesthetic:

a) 0.04–0.1 mg/kg IM or SC once (Clubb 1986)

■ **REPTILES:**

For organophosphate toxicity in most species:

a) 0.1–0.2 mg/kg SC or IM as needed. (Gauvin 1993)

For ptyalism in tortoises:

a) 0.05 mg/kg (50 micrograms/kg) SC or IM once daily (Gauvin 1993)

Monitoring

Dependent on dose and indication:

■ Heart rate and rhythm

■ Thirst/appetite; urination/defecation capability

■ Mouth/secretions dryness

Client Information

■ Parenteral atropine administration is best performed by professional staff and where adequate cardiac monitoring is available.

■ If animal is receiving atropine systemically, allow animal free access to water and encourage drinking if dry mouth is a problem.

Chemistry/Synonyms

The prototype tertiary amine antimuscarinic agent, atropine sulfate is derived from the naturally occurring atropine. It is a racemic mixture of d-hyoscyamine and l-hyoscyamine. The l-form of the drug is active, while the d- form has practically no antimuscarinic activity. Atropine sulfate occurs as colorless and odorless crystals, or white, crystalline powder. One gram of atropine sulfate is soluble in approximately 0.5 mL of water, 5 mL of alcohol, or 2.5 mL of glycerin. Aqueous solutions are practically neutral or only slightly acidic. Commercially available injections may have the pH adjusted to 3.0–6.5.

Atropine may also be known as dl-hyoscyamine. Atropine sulfate may also be known as: atrop. sulph., atropine sulphate, or atropini sulfas; many trade names are available.

Storage/Stability

Atropine sulfate tablets or soluble tablets should be stored in well-closed containers at room temperature (15-30°C). Atropine sulfate for injection should be stored at room temperature; avoid freezing.

Compatibility/Compounding Considerations

Atropine sulfate for injection is reportedly **compatible** with the following agents: benzquinamide HCl, butorphanol tartrate, chlorpromazine HCl, cimetidine HCl (not with pentobarbital), dimenhydrinate, diphenhydramine HCl, dobutamine HCl, droperidol, fentanyl citrate, glycopyrrolate, hydromorphone HCl, hydroxyzine HCl (also with meperidine), meperidine HCl, morphine sulfate, nalbuphine HCl, pentazocine lactate, pentobarbital sodium (OK for 5 minutes, not 24 hours), perphenazine, prochlorperazine edisylate, promazine HCl, promethazine HCl (also with meperidine), and scopolamine HBr.

Atropine sulfate is reported physically **incompatible** with norepinephrine bitartrate, metaraminol bitartrate, methohexital sodium, and sodium bicarbonate. Compatibility is dependent upon factors such as pH, concentration, temperature, and diluent used; consult specialized references for more specific information.

Dosage Forms/Regulatory Status

VETERINARY-LABELED PRODUCTS:

Atropine Sulfate for Injection: 0.54 mg/mL (1/120 grain); *Atroject®* (Vetus), *Atropine SA®* (Butler), generic, (various); (Rx)

Atropine Sulfate for Injection: 15 mg/mL (organophosphate treatment) 100 mL vial; *Atropine L.A.®* (Butler), (RXV); generic (various) (Rx)

Atropine is labeled for use in dogs, cats, horses, cattle, sheep, and swine in the USA. No withdrawal times are mandated when used in food animals in the USA, but FARAD recommends a 28 day meat and 6 day milk withdrawal time. (Haskell *et al.* 2005). In the UK, slaughter withdrawal for cattle, sheep, and pigs is 14 days when used as an antimuscarinic and 28 days when used as an antidote; milk withdrawal is 3 days when used as an antimuscarinic and 6 days when used as an antidote. For guidance with determining use associated withdrawal times, contact FARAD (see Phone Numbers & Websites in the appendix)

The ARCI (Racing Commissioners International) has designated this drug as a class 3 substance. See the appendix for more information.

HUMAN-LABELED PRODUCTS:

Atropine Sulfate for Injection:

0.05 mg/mL in 5 mL syringes; Atropine Sulfate (Hospira); (Rx)

0.1 mg/mL in 5 mL and 10 mL syringes; Atropine Sulfate (Hospira); (Rx)

0.3 mg/mL in 1 mL and 30 mL vials; generic; (Rx)

0.4 mg/mL in 1 mL amps and 1 mL, 20 mL, and 30 mL vials; generic; (Rx)

0.5mg/mL in 1mL and 30 mL vials & 5 mL syringes; generic; (Rx)

0.8 mg/mL in 0.5 mL and 1 mL amps and 0.5 mL syringes; generic; (Rx)

1 mg/mL in 1 mL amps and vials and 10 mL syringes; generic; (Rx)

0.5 mg, 1 mg & 2 mg pre-filled, auto-injectors; *AtroPen®* (Meridian Medical Technologies); (Rx)

Atropine Sulfate Tablets: 0.4 mg; *Sal-Tropine®* (Hope); (Rx)

See also the monograph for atropine sulfate for ophthalmic use in the appendix. Atropine sulfate ophthalmic drops have been used buccally to decrease excessive oral secretions in human patients.

References

Bailey, EM (1986). Management and treatment of toxicosis in cattle. *Current Veterinary Therapy 2: Food Animal Practice*. JL Howard Ed. Philadelphia, WB Saunders: 341–354.

Beech, J (1987). Drug therapy of respiratory disorders. *Vet Clin North Am (Equine Practice)* 3(1): 59–80.

Carpenter, RE, GR Pettifer, et al. (2005). Anesthesia for geriatric patients. *Veterinary Clinics of North America–Small Animal Practice* 35(3): 571–+.

Clubb, SL (1986). Therapeutics: Individual and Flock Treatment Regimens. *Clinical Avian Medicine and Surgery*. GJ Harrison and LR Harrison Eds. Philadelphia, W.B. Saunders: 327–355.

Congdon, J, M Marquez, et al. (2009). Cardiovascular and sedation paramerters during dexmedetomidine and atropine administration. Prtoceedings: IVECCS.

Firth, A (2000). Treatments used in small animal toxicoses. *Kirk's Current Veterinary Therapy: XIII Small Animal*

Practice. J Bonagura Ed. Philadelphia, WB Saunders: 207–211.

Gauvin, J (1993). Drug therapy in reptiles. *Seminars in Avian & Exotic Med* 2(1): 48–59.

Haskell, S, M Payne, et al. (2005). Farad Digest: Antidotes in Food Animal Practice. *JAVMA* 226(6): 884–887.

Hilwig, RW (1987). Cardiac arrhythmias. *Current Therapy in Equine Medicine.* NE Robinson Ed. Philadelphia, WB Saunders: 154–164.

Ivey, E & J Morrisey (2000). Therapeutics for Rabbits. *Vet Clin NA: Exotic Anim Pract* 3:1(Jan): 183–216.

LaBonde, J (2006). Avian Toxicology. Proceedings: AAV. Accessed via: Veterinary Information Network. http://goo.gl/ZH8fd

Manning, TO & VJ Scheidt (1986). Bovine hypersensitivity skin disease. *Current Veterinary Therapy 2 : Food Animal Practice.* JL Howard Ed. Philadelphia, WB Saunders: 934–936.

Miller, MS (1985). Treatment of cardiac arrhythmias and conduction disturbances. *Handbook of Small Animal Cardiology.* LP Tilley and JM Owens Eds. New York, Churchill Livingstone: 333–386.

Mogg, T (1999). Equine Cardiac Disease: Clinical pharmacology and therapeutics. *The Veterinary Clinics of North America: Equine Practice* 15:3(December).

Morgan, RV, Ed. (1988). *Handbook of Small Animal Practice.* New York, Churchill Livingstone.

Oehme, FW (1987). Insecticides. *Current Therapy in Equine Medicine.* NE Robinson Ed. Philadelphia, WB Saunders: 658–660.

Papich, MG (1986). Bronchdilator therapy. *Current Veterinary Therapy IX, Small Animal Practice.* RW Kirk Ed. Philadelphia, W.B. Saunders: 278–284.

Plunkett, SJ & M McMichael (2008). Cardiopulmonary resuscitation in small animal medicine: An update. *Journal of Veterinary Internal Medicine* 22(1): 9–25.

Rishniw, M & M Kittleson (2007). "Atropine Response Test."

Rush, B (2006). Use of inhalation therapy in management of recurrent airway obstruction. Proceedings: ACVIM. Accessed via: Veterinary Information Network. http://goo.gl/LhZJ8

Russell, L & J Rush (1995). Cardiac Arrhythmias in Systemic Disease. *Kirk's Current Veterinary Therapy:XII.* J Bonagura Ed. Philadelphia, W.B. Saunders: 161–166.

Thurmon, JC & GJ Benson (1986). Anesthesia in ruminants and swine. *Current Veterinary Therapy 2: Food Animal Practice.* JL Howard Ed. Philadelphia, WB Saunders: 51–71.

Trass, A (2009). Pediatric Emergencies. Proceedings: IVECCS.

Williams, B (2000). Therapeutics in Ferrets. *Vet Clin NA: Exotic Anim Pract* 3:1(Jan): 131–153.

AURANOFIN

(au-*rane*-oh-fin)   Ridaura®

ORAL GOLD IMMUNOSUPPRESSIVE

Prescriber Highlights

▶ Orally administered gold; used for pemphigus & idiopathic polyarthritis in dogs or cats

▶ Can be quite toxic & expensive, intensive ongoing monitoring required; dosages must be compounded from 3 mg capsules

▶ Probably less toxic, but also less efficacy than injectable gold

▶ Considered contraindicated in SLE (exacerbates)

▶ Known teratogen & maternotoxic

▶ Renal, hepatic & GI toxicity possible; dose dependent immune-mediated thrombocytopenia, hemolytic anemia or leukopenias have been seen

Uses/Indications

Auranofin has been used to treat idiopathic polyarthritis and pemphigus foliaceous in dogs and cats. Several clinicians report that while auranofin may be less toxic, it also less efficacious than injectable gold (aurothioglucose).

Pharmacology/Actions

Auranofin is an orally available gold salt. Gold has antiinflammatory, antirheumatic, immunomodulating, and antimicrobial (*in vitro*) effects. The exact mechanisms for these actions are not well understood. Gold is taken up by macrophages where it inhibits phagocytosis and may inhibit lysosomal enzyme activity. Gold also inhibits the release of histamine, and the production of prostaglandins. While gold does have antimicrobial effects *in vitro*, it is not clinically useful for this purpose. Auranofin suppresses helper T-cells, without affecting suppressor T-cell populations.

Pharmacokinetics

Unlike other available gold salts, auranofin is absorbed when given by mouth (20–25% of the gold) primarily in the small and large intestines. In contrast to the other gold salts, auranofin is only moderately bound to plasma proteins (the others are highly bound). Auranofin crosses the placenta and is distributed into maternal milk. Tissues with the highest levels of gold are kidneys, spleen, lungs, adrenals and liver. Accumulation of gold does not appear to occur, unlike the parenteral gold salts. About 15% of an administered dose (60% of the absorbed dose) is excreted by the kidneys, the remainder in the feces.

Contraindications/Precautions/Warnings

Auranofin should only be administered to animals where other less expensive and toxic therapies are ineffective and the veterinarian and owner are aware of the potential pitfalls of auranofin therapy and are willing to accept the associated risks and expenses. Gold salts are contraindicated in SLE as they may exacerbate the signs associated with this disease.

Adverse Effects

A dose dependent immune-mediated thrombocytopenia, hemolytic anemia or leukopenias have been noted in dogs. Discontinuation of the drug and administration of steroids has been recommended. Auranofin has a higher incidence of dose dependent GI disturbances (particularly diarrhea) in dogs than with the injectable products. Discontinuation of the drug or a lowered dose will generally resolve the problem. Renal toxicity manifested by proteinuria is possible as is hepatotoxicity (increased liver enzymes). These effects are less likely than either the GI or hematologic effects. Dermatosis and corneal ulcers have also been associated with auranofin therapy.

Reproductive/Nursing Safety

Auranofin has been demonstrated to be teratogenic and maternotoxic in laboratory animals; it should not be used during pregnancy unless the owner accepts the potential risks of use. In humans, the FDA categorizes this drug as category *C* for use during pregnancy (*Animal studies have shown an adverse effect on the fetus, but there are no adequate studies in humans; or there are no animal reproduction studies and no adequate studies in humans.*)

Following auranofin administration, gold is excreted in the milk of rodents. Trace amounts appear in the serum and red blood cells of nursing offspring. As this may cause adverse effects in nursing offspring, switching to milk replacer is recommended if auranofin is to be continued in the dam. Because gold is slowly excreted, persistence in milk will occur even after the drug is discontinued.

Overdosage/Acute Toxicity

Very limited data is available. The minimum lethal oral dose in rats is 30 mg/kg. It is recommended that gut-emptying protocols be employed after an acute overdose when applicable. Chelating agents (*e.g.*, penicillamine, dimercaprol) for severe toxicities have been used, but are controversial. One human patient who took an overdose over 10 days developed various neurologic sequelae, but eventually (after 3 months) recovered completely after discontinuation of the drug and chelation therapy.

Drug Interactions

The following drug interactions have either been reported or are theoretical in humans or animals receiving auranofin and may be of significance in veterinary patients:

■ **CYTOTOXIC AGENTS** (including **high dose corticosteroids**): Auranofin's safety when used with these agents has not been established; use with caution

■ **PENICILLAMINE or ANTIMALARIAL DRUGS:** Use with gold salts is not recommended due to the increased potential for hematologic or renal toxicity

Laboratory Considerations

■ In humans, response to **tuberculin skin tests** may be enhanced; veterinary significance is unclear

Doses

■ **DOGS:**

a) For immune-mediated arthropathies and dermatopathies: 0.05–0.2 mg/kg (up to 9 mg/day total dose) PO q12h (Vaden & Cohn 1994), (Kohn 2003)

b) For treatment of pemphigus complex (with corticosteroids): 0.12–0.2 mg/kg twice daily (White 2000)

■ **CATS:**

a) As a rescue drug for feline pemphigus and for idiopathic dermatoses and plasma cell pododermatitis/stomatitis: 0.2–0.3 mg/kg twice daily; must be reformulated for accurate dosing. (Morris 2004)

Monitoring

The following should be performed prior to therapy, then once monthly for 2–3 months, then every other month:

■ Hepatic and renal function tests (including urinalysis);

■ CBC, with platelet counts. **Note:** eosinophilia may denote impending reactions

Client Information

■ Clients must understand that several months may be required before a positive response may be seen.

■ Commitment to the twice daily dosing schedule, the costs associated with therapy, and the potential adverse effects should be discussed before initiating therapy.

Chemistry/Synonyms

An orally administered gold compound, auranofin occurs as a white, odorless, crystalline powder. It is very slightly soluble in water and soluble in alcohol. Auranofin contains 29% gold.

Auranofin may also be known as: SKF-39162, SKF-D-39162, *Crisinor®, Crisofin®, Goldar®, Ridaura®* or *Ridauran®*.

Storage/Stability

Store capsules in tight, light resistant containers at room temperature. After manufacture, expiration dates of 4 years are assigned to the capsules.

Dosage Forms/Regulatory Status

VETERINARY-LABELED PRODUCTS: None

HUMAN-LABELED PRODUCTS:

Auranofin Capsules: 3 mg; *Ridaura®* (SK-Beecham); (Rx)

References

Kohn, B (2003). Canine Immune–mediated Polyarthritis. Proceedings: World Small Animal Veterinary Association World Congress. Accessed via: Veterinary Information Network. http://goo.gl/9i1uX

Morris, D (2004). Immunomodulatory drugs in veterinary dermatology. Proceedings: Western Veterinary Conf 2004. Accessed via: Veterinary Information Network. http://goo.gl/PiK89

Vaden, S & L Cohn (1994). Immunosuppressive Drugs: Corticosteroids and Beyond. Proceedings of the Twelfth Annual Veterinary Medical Forum, San Francisco, American College of Veterinary Internal Medicine.

White, S (2000). Nonsteroidal Immunosuppressive Therapy. *Kirk's Current Veterinary Therapy: XIII Small Animal Practice.* J Bonagura Ed. Philadelphia, WB Saunders: 536–538.

Aurothioglucose—See Gold Salts, Injectable

AZAPERONE

(a-zap-*peer*-ohne)   Stresnil®

BUTYROPHENONE TRANQUILIZER

Prescriber Highlights

▶ A butyrophenone tranquilizer for swine; also used in wildlife

▶ Do not give IV, allow pigs to be undisturbed for 20 minutes after injecting

▶ No analgesic activity

▶ May cause transient piling, salivation & shivering

Uses/Indications

Azaperone is officially indicated for the "control of aggressiveness when mixing or regrouping weanling or feeder pigs weighing up to 36.4 kg" (Package Insert, *Stresnil®—P/M*; Mallinckrodt). It is also used clinically as a general tranquilizer for swine, to allow piglets to be accepted by aggressive sows, and as a preoperative agent prior to general anesthesia or cesarean section with local anesthesia.

Azaperone has been used as a neuroleptic in horses, but some horses develop adverse reactions (sweating, muscle tremors, panic reaction, CNS excitement) and IV administration has resulted in significant arterial hypotension. Because of these effects, most clinicians avoid the use of this drug in equines.

Azaperone, in combination with butorphanol and medetomidine (BAM), has been used as an immobilization combination in cervids, but it may not have additional benefit and may increase risk for hypoxia.

Pharmacology/Actions

The butyrophenones as a class cause tranquilization and sedation (sedation may be less than with the phenothiazines), anti-emetic activity, reduced motor activity, and inhibition of CNS catecholamines (dopamine, norepinephrine).

Azaperone appears to have minimal effects on respiration and may inhibit some of the respiratory depressant actions of general anesthetics. A slight reduction of arterial blood pressure has been measured in pigs after IM injections of azaperone, apparently due to slight alpha-adrenergic blockade. Azaperone has been demonstrated to prevent the development of halothane-induced malignant hyperthermia in susceptible pigs. Preliminary studies have suggested that the effects of butyrophenones may be antagonized by 4-aminopyridine.

Pharmacokinetics

Minimal information was located regarding actual pharmacokinetic parameters, but the drug is considered to have a fairly rapid onset of action following IM injections in pigs (5–10 minutes) with a peak effect at approximately 30 minutes post injection. It has a duration of action of 2–3 hours in young pigs and 3–4 hours in older swine. The drug is metabolized in the liver with 13% of it excreted in the feces. At 16 hours post-dose, practically all the drug is eliminated from the body; however in the UK a 10-day slaughter withdrawal has been assigned.

Contraindications/Precautions/Warnings

When used as directed, the manufacturer reports no contraindications (other than for slaughter withdrawal) for the drug. It should not be given IV as a significant excitatory phase may be seen in pigs. Avoid use in very cold conditions as cardiovascular collapse may occur secondary to peripheral vasodilation.

Do not exceed dosing recommendation in boars as the drug may cause the penis to be extruded.

Because Vietnamese Pot Bellied pigs may have delayed absorption due to sequestration of the drug in body fat, re-dose with extreme caution; deaths have resulted after repeat dosing.

Adverse Effects

Transient salivation, piling, panting and shivering have been reported in pigs. Pigs should be left undisturbed after injection (for approximately 20 minutes) until the drug's full effects have been expressed; disturbances during this period may trigger excitement.

Azaperone has minimal analgesic effects and is not a substitute for appropriate anesthesia or analgesia. Doses above 1 mg/kg may cause the penis to be extruded in boars.

In white-tailed deer, butorphanol, azaperone and medetomidine (BAM) caused greater hypoventilation and hypoxemia without significant reductions in immobilization times than butorphanol and medetomidine alone (Boesch *et al.* 2008).

Overdosage/Acute Toxicity

Azaperone overdoses can cause hypotension; doses >1 mg/kg in boars may cause penis extrusion leading to damage. There is no reversal agent for azaperone; treat supportively.

Drug Interactions

No specific drug interactions have been reported for azaperone. The following interactions have been reported for the closely related compounds, haloperidol or droperidol:

- ◼ **CNS DEPRESSANT AGENTS (barbiturates, narcotics, anesthetics**, etc.) may cause additive CNS depression if used with butyrophenones

Doses

- ◼ **SWINE:**

  For the approved indication of mixing feeder or weanling pigs:

  a) 2.2 mg/kg deeply IM (see client information below) (Package Insert; Stresnil®—P/M Mallinckrodt; **Note:** No longer on US market)

  For labeled indications (Stresnil®—Janssen U.K.):

  a) **Note:** all doses are to be given IM directly behind the ear using a long hypodermic needle and given as closely behind the ear as possible and perpendicular to the skin.

  Aggression (prevention and cure of fighting; including regrouping of piglets, porkers, fattening pigs): 2 mg/kg (1 mL/20 kg)

  Treatment of aggression in sows: 2 mg/kg (1 mL/20 kg)

  Stress (restlessness, anxiety, etc.): 1–2 mg/kg (0.5–1 mL/20 kg)

  Transport of boars: 1 mg/kg (0.5 mL/20 kg)

  Transport of weaners: 0.4–2 mg/kg (0.4–1 mL/20 kg)

  Obstetrics: 1 mg/kg (0.5 mL/20 kg)

  As a premed: 1–2 mg/kg (0.5–1 mL/20 kg)

Monitoring

- ◼ Level of sedation

Client Information

- ◼ Must be injected IM deeply, either behind the ear and perpendicular to the skin or in the back of the ham. All animals in groups to be mixed must be treated.

Chemistry/Synonyms

A butyrophenone neuroleptic, azaperone occurs as a white to yellowish-white macrocrystalline powder with a melting point between 90–95°C. It is practically insoluble in water; 1 gram is soluble in 29 mL of alcohol.

Azaperone may also be known as azaperonum, R-1929, Stresnil®, or Suicalm®.

Storage/Stability

Azaperone injection should be stored at controlled room temperature (15–25°C) and away from light. Do not store above 25°C. Once the vial is opened it should be used within 28 days.

Compatibility/Compounding Considerations

No published information was located regarding mixing azaperone with other compounds.

A compounded product that combines butorphanol, azaperone and medetomidine (BAM) is reportedly available.

Dosage Forms/Regulatory Status

VETERINARY-LABELED PRODUCTS: Note: No FDA-approved azaperone products are currently marketed in the USA. Compounded azaperone injection and a combination injection containing butorphanol, azaperone, and medetomidine (BAM) can be obtained from zoopharm.net

In the UK: Azaperone 40 mg/mL for Injection in 100 mL vials; Stresnil® (Janssen—UK); (POM-V) Pigs may be slaughtered for human consumption only after 10 days from the last treatment.

The ARCI (Racing Commissioners International) has designated this drug as a class 2 substance. See the appendix for more information.

HUMAN-LABELED PRODUCTS: None

References

Boesch, J, P Curtis, et al. (2008). Medetomidine–butorphanol with and without azaperone for immobilizing free–ranging North American White–tailed deer (Odocoileus virginianus). Proceedings: IVECCS.

AZATHIOPRINE
AZATHIOPRINE
SODIUM

(ay-za-**thye**-oh-preen)   Imuran®

IMMUNOSUPPRESSANT

Prescriber Highlights

- ▶ Purine antagonist immunosuppressive used for a variety of autoimmune diseases

- ▶ May take several weeks for immunosuppression to occur

- ▶ Often used in combination with corticosteroids to reduce doses and dosing frequency of each drug

- ▶ Known mutagen & teratogen; use with caution in patients with hepatic disease

- ▶ Bone marrow depression principal adverse effect; GI effects (including GI distress, anorexia, pancreatitis & hepatotoxicity) also seen

- ▶ Usually not used in cats as they are very sensitive to bone marrow effects

Uses/Indications

In veterinary medicine, azathioprine is used primarily as an immunosuppressive agent in the treatment of immune-mediated diseases in dogs. See Doses below for more information. For auto-agglutinizing immune mediated hemolytic anemia, azathioprine is generally recommended to start at the time of diagnosis. When used in combination with cyclosporine, azathioprine has been used to prevent rejection of MHC-matched renal allografts in dogs.

Azathioprine is often used in combination with corticosteroids, such as prednisolone, primarily to reduce the incidence of adverse effects of each drug by allowing dosage reductions and eventually, every other day dosing of each drug.

Although the drug can be very toxic to bone marrow in cats, it is sometimes used to treat feline autoimmune skin diseases.

Pharmacology/Actions

While the exact mechanism how azathioprine exerts its immunosuppressive action has not been determined, it is probably dependent on several factors. Azathioprine antagonizes purine metabolism thereby inhibiting RNA, DNA synthesis and mitosis. It may also cause chromosome breaks secondary to incorporation into nucleic acids and cellular metabolism may become disrupted by the drug's ability to inhibit coenzyme formation. Azathioprine has greater activity on delayed hypersensitivity and cellular immunity than on humoral antibody responses. Clinical response to azathioprine may require up to 6 weeks.

Pharmacokinetics

Azathioprine is poorly absorbed from the GI tract and is rapidly metabolized to mercaptopurine. Mercaptopurine is rapidly taken up by lymphocytes and erythrocytes. Mecaptopurine remaining in the plasma is then further metabolized to several other compounds that are excreted by the kidneys. Only minimal amounts of either azathioprine or mercaptopurine are excreted unchanged. Cats have low activity of thiopurine methyltransferase (TPMT), one of the routes used to metabolize azathioprine. Approximately 11% of humans have low thiopurine methyltransferase activity, and these individuals have a greater incidence of bone marrow suppression, but also greater azathioprine efficacy. Dogs have variable TMPT activity levels similar to that seen in humans, which may explain why some canine patients respond better and/or develop more myelotoxicity than others. However, one study (Rodriguez et al. 2004) in dogs did not show significant correlation between TMPT activity in red blood cells and drug toxicity.

Contraindications/Precautions/Warnings

Azathioprine is contraindicated in patients hypersensitive to it. The drug should be used cautiously in patients with hepatic dysfunction. Use of azathioprine in cats is controversial; they seem to be more susceptible to azathioprine's bone marrow suppressive effects.

Adverse Effects

The principal adverse effect associated with azathioprine is bone marrow suppression. Cats are more prone to develop these effects and the drug is generally not recommended for use in this species. Leukopenia is the most prevalent consequence, but anemias and thrombocytopenia may also be seen. GI upset/anorexia, poor hair growth, acute pancreatitis and hepatotoxicity have been associated with azathioprine therapy in dogs.

Because azathioprine depresses the immune system, animals may be susceptible to infections or neoplastic illnesses with long-term use.

In recovering dogs with immune-mediated hemolytic anemia, taper the withdrawal of the drug slowly over several months and monitor for early signs of relapse. Rapid withdrawal can lead to a rebound hyperimmune response.

Reproductive/Nursing Safety

Azathioprine is mutagenic and teratogenic in lab animals. In humans, the FDA categorizes this drug as category *D* for use during pregnancy (*There is evidence of human fetal risk, but the potential benefits from the use of the drug in pregnant women may be acceptable despite its potential risks.*) In a separate system evaluating the safety of drugs in canine and feline pregnancy (Papich 1989), this drug is categorized as in class: *C* (*These drugs may have potential risks. Studies in people or laboratory animals have uncovered risks, and these drugs should be used cautiously as a last resort when the benefit of therapy clearly outweighs the risks.*)

Azathioprine is distributed into milk; it is recommended to use milk replacer while the dam is receiving azathioprine.

Overdosage/Acute Toxicity

No specific information was located regarding acute overdose of azathioprine. It is suggested to use standard protocols to empty the GI tract if ingestion was recent and to treat supportively. Contact an animal poison control center for more information.

Drug Interactions

The following drug interactions have either been reported or are theoretical in humans or animals receiving azathioprine and may be of significance in veterinary patients:

- ■ **ACE INHIBITORS (benazepril, enalapril,** etc.): Increased potential for hematologic toxicity

- ■ **ALLOPURINOL:** The hepatic metabolism of azathioprine may be decreased by concomitant administration of allopurinol; in humans, it is recommended to reduce the azathioprine dose to ¼–⅓ usual if both drugs are to be used together

- ■ **AMINOSALICYLATES (sulfasalazine, mesalamine, olsalazine):** Increased risk for azathioprine toxicity

- ■ **NON-DEPOLARIZING MUSCLE RELAXANTS (e.g., pancuronium, tubocurarine):** The neuromuscular blocking activity of these drugs may be inhibited or reversed by azathioprine

- **CORTICOSTEROIDS:** Although azathioprine is often used with corticosteroids, there is greater potential risk for toxicity development
- **DRUGS AFFECTING MYELOPOIESIS (e.g., trimethoprim/sulfa, cyclophosphamide,** etc.): Increased potential for hematologic toxicity
- **WARFARIN:** Potential for reduced anticoagulant effect

Doses

- **DOGS:**

  As an immunosuppressive:

  a) For inflammatory bowel disease: Initially 2 mg/kg PO once daily for 2 weeks, then tapered to 2 mg/kg PO every other day for 2–4 weeks, then 1 mg/kg PO every other day. May take 2–6 weeks before beneficial effects are seen. (Moore 2004)

  b) For immune-mediated anemia, colitis, immune-mediated skin disease, and acquired myasthenia gravis: 2 mg/kg PO once daily (q24h); long-term therapy 0.5–1 mg/kg PO every other day, with prednisolone administered on the alternate days (Papich 2001)

  c) For adjunctive therapy in myasthenia gravis in non-responsive patients: Initially, 1 mg/kg PO once daily. CBC is evaluated every 1–2 weeks. If neutrophil and platelet counts are normal after 2 weeks, dose is increased to 2 mg/kg PO once daily. CBC is repeated every week for the first month and then monthly thereafter. Recommend to discontinue azathioprine if WBC falls below 4,000 cells/mcL or neutrophil count is less than 1,000 cells/mcL. Serum ACHR antibody concentrations reevaluated q4–6 weeks. Azathioprine dose is tapered to every other day when clinical remission occurs and serum ACHR antibody concentrations are normalized. (Coates 2000)

  d) For lymphoplasmacytic enteritis if clinical response to prednisolone is poor or the adverse effects (of prednisolone) predominate: azathioprine 2 mg/kg PO once daily for 5 days, then on alternate days to prednisolone (Simpson 2003)

  e) For severe cases (autoagglutination, hemolytic crisis with rapid decline of hematocrit, intravascular hemolysis, Cocker Spaniels) of immune-mediated hemolytic anemia: 2.2 mg/kg PO once daily (q24h) in addition to prednisone (initially at 2.2 mg/kg PO q12h until hematocrit reaches 25–30%; then dose is gradually tapered by approximately 25% q2–3 weeks until a dose of 0.5 mg/kg PO q48h is reached). (Macintire 2006)

  f) For use with glucocorticoids in acute immune-mediated hemolytic anemia (IMHA): Author starts all patients with IMHA with adjunctive immunosuppressants (usually azathioprine) at 1–2 mg/kg PO once daily. Often used for long-term maintenance as steroid side effects quickly become intolerable to many pet owners. Generally well tolerated in dogs but may cause bone marrow suppression and hepatotoxicity. (Noonan 2009)

  g) For severe and refractory inflammatory bowel disease: 2.2 mg/kg PO once daily; a lag time of 3–5 weeks is expected before clinical improvement is noted (Jergens & Willard 2000)

  h) For adjunctive treatment of ocular fibrous histiocytomas: 2 mg/kg PO daily for 2 weeks, reevaluate, and reduce to 1 mg/kg every other day for 2 weeks, then 1 mg/kg once weekly for 1 month (Riis 1986)

  i) In combination with cyclosporine, to prevent rejection of MHC-matched renal allografts in dogs: 1–5 mg/kg PO every other day (Gregory 2000)

  j) For perianal fistulas (anal furunculosis): In the study, initially 2 mg/kg PO once daily (q24h) until a reduction in the size, number or inflammation of the fistulas was seen or total WBC <5000 cells/mcL or neutrophil count was <3500 cells/mcL or platelet count <160,000 cells/mcL. Then reduce to 2 mg/kg PO every other day (q48h) and continued for 12 weeks as long as myelosuppression doesn't develop. After 12 weeks, reduce dose to 1 mg/kg PO every other day (q48h) with a planned therapy duration of 12 months. Prednisone was given at 2 mg/kg PO once daily for the first two weeks of therapy; then at 1 mg/kg PO once daily for another 2 weeks and then discontinued. All dogs were placed on a limited antigen diet. No correlation with efficacy and lymphocyte blastogenesis effect. Complete or partial remission in 64% of treated dogs, which is less than systemic cyclosporine or topical tacrolimus treatment, but azathioprine treatment is less expensive. (Harkin et al. 2007)

  k) For treatment of glomerulonephritis: 2 mg/kg PO once daily. Immunosuppressive treatment is controversial. (Labato 2006)

  l) To reduce inflammation in dogs with chronic hepatitis: 2.2 mg/kg PO once daily in combination with corticosteroids (Prednis(ol)one initially at 1–2 mg/kg/day PO; dose is gradually tapered with clinical improvement). Azathioprine dose is given every other day after 1–2 weeks. (Twedt 2010b), (Twedt 2010a)

- **CATS:**

  Note: Most do not recommend azathioprine for use in cats because of the potential for development of fatal toxicity and the difficulty in accurately dosing.

As an immunosuppressive:

a) For severe and refractory inflammatory bowel disease: Must be used with caution; myelotoxicity with severe neutropenia is possible. Azathioprine at 0.3 mg/kg PO once every other day; may take 3–5 weeks before any beneficial effects. Administration can be enhanced by crushing one 50 mg tablet and suspending it in 15 mL of syrup resulting in a concentration of 3.3 mg/mL. Must be shaken well before each use. If cat becomes ill, rectal temperature and WBC should be determined immediately. (Willard 2002)

■ **FERRETS:**

As an immunosuppressive:

a) For treating inflammatory bowel disease: Treatments include prednisone (1 mg/kg PO q12–24h), azathioprine (0.9 mg/kg PO q24–72h), and dietary management. (Johnson 2006)

■ **HORSES:**

As an immunosuppressive:

a) 3 mg/kg PO q24h. Although clinical experiences are still limited, azathioprine appears to be a relatively safe immunosuppressive treatment in the horse and its cost is relatively low. (Divers 2010)

b) For various autoimmune skin diseases (*e.g.*, pemphigus foliaceous): 1–3 mg/kg PO q24h for 1 month, then every other day (q48h). May cause thrombocytopenia. Azathioprine used as a steroid-sparing drug; used with corticosteroids in an attempt to eventually decrease the amount of steroid needed. (White 2006)

Monitoring

■ Hemograms (including platelets) should be monitored closely; initially every 1–2 weeks and every 1–2 months (some recommend q2 weeks) once on maintenance therapy. It is recommended by some clinicians that if the WBC count drops to between 5,000–7,000 cells/mm^3 the dose be reduced by 25%. If WBC count drops below 5,000 cells/mm^3 treatment should be discontinued until leukopenia resolves.

■ Liver function tests; serum amylase, if indicated

■ Efficacy

Client Information

■ There is the possibility of severe toxicity developing from this drug including drug-related neoplasms or mortality; routine testing to detect toxic effects are necessary

■ Contact veterinarian should the animal exhibit symptoms of abnormal bleeding, bruising, lack of appetite, vomiting or infection

■ Although, no special precautions are necessary with handling intact tablets, wash hands after administering the drug; if using a compounded formulation, wear protective gloves or wash hands immediately after administration

Chemistry/Synonyms

Related structurally to adenine, guanine and hypoxanthine, azathioprine is a purine antagonist antimetabolite that is used primarily for its immunosuppressive properties. Azathioprine occurs as an odorless, pale yellow powder that is insoluble in water and slightly soluble in alcohol. Azathioprine sodium powder for injection occurs as a bright yellow, amorphous mass. After reconstituting with sterile water for injection to a concentration of 10 mg/mL, it has an approximate pH of 9.6.

Azathioprine/Azathioprine sodium may also be known as: azathioprinum, BW-57322, or NSC-39084; many trade names are available.

Storage/Stability

Azathioprine tablets should be stored at room temperature in well-closed containers and protected from light.

The sodium powder for injection should be stored at room temperature and protected from light. It is reportedly stable at neutral or acidic pH, but will hydrolyze to mercaptopurine in alkaline solutions. This conversion is enhanced upon warming or in the presence of sulfhydryl-containing compounds (*e.g.*, cysteine). After reconstituting, the injection should be used within 24-hours as no preservative is present.

Compatibility/Compounding Considerations

Azathioprine sodium is reportedly **compatible** with the following intravenous solutions: dextrose 5% in water, and sodium chloride 0.45% or 0.9%. Compatibility is dependent upon factors such as pH, concentration, temperature and diluent used; consult specialized references or a hospital pharmacist for more specific information.

Compounded preparation stability: Azathioprine oral suspension compounded from commercially available tablets has been published (Allen, 1996). Triturating one-hundred twenty (120) azathioprine 50 mg tablets with 60 mL of *Ora-Plus®* and *qs ad* to 120 mL with *Ora-Sweet®* (or *Ora-Sweet® SF*) yields a 50 mg/mL suspension that retains >90% potency for 60 days stored at both 5°C and 25°C. The stability of azathioprine aqueous liquids decreases in the presence of alkaline pH. The optimal stability is reported to be between 5.5 and 6.5. Compounded preparations of azathioprine should be protected from light.

Dosage Forms/Regulatory Status

VETERINARY-LABELED PRODUCTS: None

HUMAN-LABELED PRODUCTS:

Azathioprine Tablets: 50 mg, 75 mg & 100 mg;

Azasan® (aaiPharma); *Imuran®* (Prometheus); generic (aaiPharma); (Rx)

Azathioprine Sodium Injection: 100 mg (as sodium)/vial in 20 mL vials; generic; (Rx)

References

Allen, L.V. & M.A. Erickson (1996). Stability of acetazolamide, allopurinol, azathioprine, clonazepam, and flucytosine in extemporaneously compounded oral liquids. *Am J Health Syst Pharm* 53(16): 1944-1949.

Coates, J (2000). Use of azathioprine in the myasthenia gravis patient. Proceedings: The North American Veterinary Conference, Orlando.

Divers, TJ (2010). Azathioprine – a useful treatment for immune–mediated disorders in the horse? *Equine Veterinary Education* 22(10): 501–502.

Gregory, C (2000). Immunosuppressive Agents. *Kirk's Current Veterinary Therapy: XIII Small Animal Practice.* J Bonagura Ed. Philadelphia, WB Saunders: 509–513.

Harkin, K, D Phillips, et al. (2007). Evaluation of azathioprine on lesion severity and lymphocyte blastogenesis in dogs with perianal fistulas. *J Am Anim Hosp Assoc* 43(21–26).

Jergens, A & M Willard (2000). Diseases of the large Intestine. *Textbook of Veterinary Internal Medicine: Diseases of the Dog and Cat.* S Ettinger and E Feldman Eds. Philadelphia, WB Saunders. 2: 1238–1256.

Johnson, D (2006). Ferrets: the other companion animal. Proceedings: ACVC. Accessed via: Veterinary Information Network. http://goo.gl/bSeol

Labato, M (2006). Improving survival for dogs with protein–losing nephropathies. Proceedings: ACVIM 2006. Accessed via: Veterinary Information Network. http://goo.gl/0jeng

Macintire, D (2006). New therapies for immune–mediated hemolytic anemia. Proceedings: ACVIM 2006. Accessed via: Veterinary Information Network. http://goo.gl/ILCPS

Moore, L (2004). Beyond corticosteroids for therapy of inflammatory bowel disease in dogs and cats. Proceedings: ACVIM Forum. Accessed via: Veterinary Information Network. http://goo.gl/MOJ1B

Noonan, M (2009). Immune Mediated Hemolytic Anemia. Proceedings: IVECC. Accessed via: Veterinary Information Network. http://goo.gl/EaAXT

Papich, M (2001). Immunosuppressive Drug Therapy. Proceedings: World Small Animal Veterinary Association World Congress. Accessed via: Veterinary Information Network. http://goo.gl/cbdMn

Riis, RC (1986). Tumors of the eye and adnexa. *Current Veterinary Therapy (CVT) IX Small Animal Practice.* RW Kirk Ed. Philadelphia, WB Saunders: 679–684.

Rodriguez, D, A Mackin, et al. (2004). Relationship between red blood cell thiopurine methyltransferase activity and myelotoxicity in dogs receiving azathioprine. *J Vet Intern Med* 18(3): 339–345.

Simpson, K (2003). Chronic enteropathies: How should I treat them. Proceedings: ACVIM Forum. Accessed via: Veterinary Information Network. http://goo.gl/nicNM

Twedt, D (2010a). How I treat chronic hepatitis. Proceedings: WSAVA.

Twedt, D (2010b). Medical therapy for hepatobiliary disease. Proceedings: WSAVA.

White, S (2006). Autoimmune diseases affection the skin. Proceedings: ACVIM. Accessed via: Veterinary Information Network. http://goo.gl/ippJr

Willard, M (2002). Stopping "unstoppable" diarrhea–How to stop the flood. Proceedings: Atlantic Coast Veterinary Conference. Accessed via: Veterinary Information Network. http://goo.gl/S7D3X

AZITHROMYCIN

(ay-zith-roe-*my*-sin)   Zithromax®

MACROLIDE ANTIBIOTIC

Prescriber Highlights

▶ Oral & parenteral human macrolide antibiotic; potentially useful for a variety of infections in veterinary patients; not effective for clearing Chlamydophila felis or Mycoplasma Haemofelis in cats.

▶ Very long tissue half-lives in dogs & cats

▶ Contraindications: Hypersensitivity to macrolides

▶ Caution: Hepatic disease

▶ Adverse Effects: Potentially GI distress, but less so than with erythromycin

▶ Relatively expensive, but prices are dropping secondary to the availability of generic products

Uses/Indications

Azithromycin with its relative broad spectrum and favorable pharmacokinetic profile may be useful for a variety of infections in veterinary species, including *Bordetella* pneumonias in dogs.

Azithromycin has been shown to be ineffective in the treatment of *Mycoplasma haemofelis* or eliminating *Chlamydophila felis* in cats.

Azithromycin may be potentially useful for treating Rhodococcus infections in foals.

Pharmacology/Actions

Like other macrolide antibiotics, azithromycin inhibits protein synthesis by penetrating the cell wall and binding to the 50S ribosomal subunits in susceptible bacteria. It is considered a bacteriostatic antibiotic.

Azithromycin has a relatively broad spectrum. It has *in vitro* activity (does not necessarily indicate clinical efficacy) against gram-positive organisms such as *Streptococcus pneumoniae*, *Staph aureus*; gram-negative organisms such as *Haemophilus influenzae*; *Bartonella* spp., *Bordetella* spp.; and *Mycoplasma pneumoniae*, *Borrelia burgdorferi* and *Toxoplasma* spp.

Pharmacokinetics

The pharmacokinetics of azithromycin have been described in cats and dogs. In dogs, the drug has excellent bioavailability after oral administration (97%). Tissue concentrations apparently do not mirror those in the serum after multiple doses and tissue half-lives in the dogs may be up to 90 hours. Greater than 50% of an oral dose is excreted unchanged in the bile. In cats, oral bioavailability is 58%. Tissue half-lives are less than in dogs, and range from 13 hours in adipose tissue to 72 hours in cardiac muscle.

As with dogs, cats excrete the majority of a given dose in the bile.

In foals, azithromycin is variably absorbed after oral administration with a mean systemic bioavailability ranging from 40–60%. It has a very high volume of distribution (11.6–18.6 L/kg). Elimination half-life is approximately 20–26 hours. The drug concentrates in bronchoalveolar cells and pulmonary epithelial fluid. Elimination half-life in PMN's is about 2 days. In adult horses, oral bioavailability is low (1–7%).

When compared to erythromycin, azithromycin has better absorption characteristics, longer tissue half-lives, and higher concentrations in tissues and white blood cells. Azithromycin achieves high concentrations in bronchial secretions and has excellent ocular penetration.

Goats have an elimination half-life of 32.5 hours (IV), 45 hours (IM), an apparent volume of distribution (steady-state) of 34.5 L/kg and a clearance of 0.85 L/kg/hr.

Rabbits have an elimination half-life of 24.1 hours (IV), and 25.1 hours (IM). IM injection has a high bioavailability, but causes some degree of muscle damage at the injection site.

Sheep have an elimination half-life average of 48 hours (IV), 61 hours (IM), an apparent volume of distribution (steady-state) of 34.5 L/kg and a clearance of 0.52 L/kg/hr.

Contraindications/Precautions/Warnings

Azithromycin is contraindicated in animals hypersensitive to any of the macrolides. It should be used with caution in patients with impaired hepatic function.

Adverse Effects

Azithromycin can cause vomiting in dogs if high doses are given, but compared to erythromycin, azithromycin has fewer GI adverse effects. Other adverse effects, particularly those associated with the liver, may become apparent in dogs and cats as more experience is attained. Local IV site reactions have occurred in patients receiving IV azithromycin. Foals may develop diarrhea while receiving the drug.

Reproductive/Nursing Safety

Safety during pregnancy has not been fully established; use only when clearly necessary. In humans, the FDA categorizes this drug as category **B** for use during pregnancy (*Animal studies have not yet demonstrated risk to the fetus, but there are no adequate studies in pregnant women; or animal studies have shown an adverse effect, but adequate studies in pregnant women have not demonstrated a risk to the fetus in the first trimester of pregnancy, and there is no evidence of risk in later trimesters.*)

Overdosage/Acute Toxicity

Acute oral overdoses are unlikely to cause significant morbidity other than vomiting, diarrhea and GI cramping.

Drug Interactions

The following drug interactions have either been reported or are theoretical in humans or animals receiving azithromycin and may be of significance in veterinary patients:

- ■ **ANTACIDS (oral; magnesium- and aluminum-containing):** May reduce the rate of absorption of azithromycin; suggest separating dosages by 2 hours

- ■ **CISAPRIDE:** No data on azithromycin, but other macrolides contraindicated with cisapride; use with caution

- ■ **CYCLOSPORINE:** Azithromycin may potentially increase cyclosporine blood levels; monitor carefully

- ■ **DIGOXIN:** No data on azithromycin, but other macrolides can increase digoxin levels; monitor carefully

- ■ **PIMOZIDE:** Azithromycin use is contraindicated in patients taking pimozide (unlikely to be used in vet med—used for Tourette's disorder in humans). Acute deaths have occurred.

Doses

■ **DOGS:**

For susceptible infections:

a) 5–10 mg/kg PO once daily for 3–5 days (Trepanier 1999), (Sykes 2003)

b) 5 mg/kg PO once daily for 2 days, then every 3–5 days for a total of 5 doses (Aucoin 2002)

c) For "Derm" infections: 5–10 mg/kg PO once daily for 5–7 days. For animals that are difficult to pill, a dose given every 5 days (after the initial 5–7 day course of therapy) may be effective if continued treatment is necessary. (Merchant 2000)

d) For canine pyoderma: 10 mg/kg PO once daily for 5–10 days (Ramadinha *et al.* 2002)

e) For *Babesia gibsoni* (Asian genotype) infections: Atovaquone 13.3 mg/kg PO q8h with a fatty meal and Azithromycin 10 mg/kg PO once daily. Give both drugs for 10 days. Reserve immunosuppressive therapy for cases that are not rapidly responding (3–5 days) to anti-protozoal therapy. (Birkenheuer, AJ *et al.* 2004), (Birkenheuer, A 2006)

f) For idiopathic lymphoplasmacytic (chronic) rhinitis: Long term administration of antibiotics having immunomodulatory effects combined with nonsteroidal antiinflammatory agents can be helpful in some dogs. Doxycycline 3–5 mg/kg PO q12h, or azithromycin 5 mg/kg PO q24h in combination with piroxicam 0.3 mg/kg PO q24h. (Kuehn 2010)

■ **CATS:**

For susceptible infections:

a) 5–10 mg/kg PO once daily for 3–5 days (Trepanier 1999), (Sykes 2003)

b) 5 mg/kg PO once daily for 2 days, then every 3–5 days for a total number of doses of 5 (Aucoin 2002)

c) For "Derm" infections: 7–15 mg/kg PO q12h daily for 5–7 days. For animals that are difficult to pill, a dose given every 5 days (after the initial 5–7 day course of therapy) may be effective if continued treatment is necessary. (Merchant 2000)

d) For susceptible upper respiratory infections: 5–10 mg/kg PO once daily for 5 days, then q72h (every 3rd day) long-term. If there is an initial positive response to the antibiotic, therapy should be continued for 6–8 weeks without changing the antibiotic. (Scherk 2006)

e) For Bartonellosis: 10 mg/kg PO once daily for 21 days. Response to therapy is rapid; most cats with anterior uveitis will show significant improvement in less than one week. Recurrence after 21 days of treatment, followed by good flea control, is low. Failure of Bartonella positive cats to respond indicates that Bartonella is part of a polymicrobial disease syndrome. (Ketring 2009)

■ **HORSES:**

For treatment of *R. equi* infections in foals:

a) 10 mg/kg PO once daily. Because of persistence of high levels in bronchoalveolar cells and pulmonary epithelial lining fluid, after 5 days of once daily treatment, every other day (q48h) dosing may be appropriate. (Jacks *et al.* 2001)

■ **RODENTS/SMALL MAMMALS:**

a) Rabbits: For Staphylococcus osteomyelitis: 50 mg/kg PO once daily with 40 mg/kg of rifampin q12h PO (Ivey & Morrisey 2000)

b) Rabbits: For jaw abscesses: 15–30 mg/kg PO once daily (q24h). Systemic antibiotic treatment is continued for 2–4 weeks post-operatively. Advise owners to discontinue treatment if anorexia or diarrhea occurs. (Johnson 2006b)

c) Guinea pigs: For Pneumonia: 15–30 mg/kg PO once daily (q24h). Advise owners to discontinue treatment if soft stools develop. (Johnson 2006a)

■ **BIRDS:**

a) For Chlamydiosis; study done in experimentally infected cockatiels: Azithromycin 40 mg/kg PO once every other day (q48h) for 21 days (as effective as a 21 or 45 day treatment with doxycycline). Birds were dosed via metallic feeding tube into crop using the commercially available (*Zithromax®*) human oral suspension. (Guzman *et al.* 2010)

Monitoring

■ Clinical efficacy

■ Adverse effects

Client Information

■ Give medication as prescribed. Do not refrigerate oral suspension and shake well before each use. If using the suspension, preferably give to an animal with an empty stomach. Discard any unused oral suspension after 14 days.

■ Contact veterinarian if animal develops severe diarrhea or vomiting, or if condition deteriorates after beginning therapy.

Chemistry/Synonyms

A semisynthetic azalide macrolide antibiotic, azithromycin dihydrate occurs as a white crystalline powder. In one mL of water at neutral pH and at 37° C, 39 mg are soluble. Although commercial preparations are available as the dihydrate, potency is noted as the anhydrous form.

Azithromycin may also be known as: azithromycinum, acitromicina, CP-62993, or XZ-450; many trade names are available.

Storage/Stability

The commercially available tablets should be stored at temperatures less than 30°C. Products for reconstitution for oral suspension should be stored between 5–30°C before reconstitution with water. After reconstitution the multiple dose product may be stored between 5–30°C for up to ten days and then discarded. The single dose packets should be given immediately after reconstitution.

The injectable product should be stored below 30°C. After reconstitution with sterile water for injection, solutions containing 100 mg/mL are stable for 24 hours if stored below 30°C.

Compatibility/Compounding Considerations

Azithromycin injection is physically and chemically **compatible** with several intravenous solutions, including: half-normal and normal saline, D5W, LRS, D5 with 0.3% or 0.45% sodium chloride, and D5 in LRS. When azithromycin injection is diluted into 250–500 mL of one of the above solutions, it remains physically and chemically stable for 24 hours at room temperature and up to 7 days if kept refrigerated at 5°C.

Dosage Forms/Regulatory Status

VETERINARY-LABELED PRODUCTS: None
Preparations compounded for dogs and cats may be available from compounding pharmacies.

HUMAN-LABELED PRODUCTS:

Azithromycin Oral Tablets: 250 mg, 500 mg & 600 mg (as dihydrate); *Zithromax®* (Pfizer); generic; (Rx)

Azithromycin Powder for Oral Suspension: After reconstitution: 100 mg/5 mL in 15 mL bottles; 200 mg/5 mL in 15, 22.5 & 30 mL bottles; 1 g/packet in single-dose packets of 3's & 10's; *Zithromax®* (Pfizer); generic; and extended-release powder for oral suspension in 2 g single-dose bottles *Zmax®* (Pfizer); (Rx)

Azithromycin Powder for Injection (lyophilized): 500 mg in 10 mL vials; *Zithromax®* (Pfizer); generic; (Rx)

References

Aucoin, D (2002). Rational approach to antimiocrobial therapy in companion animals. Proceedings: Atlantic Coast Veterinary Conference. Accessed via: Veterinary Information Network. http://goo.gl/5atZq

Birkenheuer, A (2006). Infectious Hemolytic Anemias. ACVIM Proceedings. Accessed via: Veterinary Information Network. http://goo.gl/DPVKW

Birkenheuer, A, M Levy, et al. (2004). Efficacy of combined atovaquone and azithromycin for therapy of chronic Babesia gibsoni (Asian genotype) infections in dogs. *J Vet Intern Med* **18**: 494–498.

Guzman, DSM, O Diaz–Figueroa, et al. (2010). Evaluating 21–day Doxycycline and Azithromycin Treatments for Experimental Chlamydophila psittaci Infection in Cockatiels (Nymphicus hollandicus). *Journal of Avian Medicine and Surgery* **24**(1): 35–45.

Ivey, E & J Morrisey (2000). Therapeutics for Rabbits. *Vet Clin NA: Exotic Anim Pract* **3:1**(Jan): 183–216.

Jacks, S, S Giguere, et al. (2001). Pharmacokinetics of azithromycin and concentration of body fluids and bronchoalveolar cells in foals. *Am J Vet Res* **62**: 1870–1875.

Johnson, D (2006a). Guinea Pig Medicine Primer. Proceedings: ACVC. Accessed via: Veterinary Information Network. http://goo.gl/WmWhU

Johnson, D (2006b). Treating jaw abscesses in rabbits. Proceedings: ACVC. Accessed via: Veterinary Information Network. http://goo.gl/DUfnQ

Ketring, K (2009). Feline Bartonellosis: The naysayers are wrong! It is the most under diagnosed feline ocular disease. Proceedings: WVC.

Kuehn, N (2010). CHRONIC NASAL DISEASE IN DOGS: DIAGNOSIS & TREATMENT. Proceedings: ACVIM.

Merchant, S (2000). New Therapies in Veterinary Dermatology. Proceedings: American Animal Hospital Association 67th Annual Meeting, Toronto.

Ramadinha, R, S Ribeiro, et al. (2002). Evaluation and efficiency of azithromycin (acitromicina) for treating bacterial pyodermas in dogs. Proceedings: World Small Animal Veterinary Association World Congress. Accessed via: Veterinary Information Network. http://goo.gl/U4UtB

Scherk, M (2006). Snots and Snuffles: Chronic Feline Upper Respiratory Syndrome. Proceedings: ACVIM. Accessed via: Veterinary Information Network. http://goo.gl/tWQ49

Sykes, J (2003). Azithromycin: What's all the fuss about? Proceedings: Australian College of Veterinary Scientists Science Week. Accessed via: Veterinary Information Network. http://goo.gl/e1rlF

Trepanier, L (1999). Management of resistant infections in small animal patients. Proceedings: American Veterinary Medical Association: 16th Annual Convention, New Orleans.

AZTREONAM

(az-**tree**-oh-nam)   Azactam®
INJECTABLE MONOBACTAM ANTIBACTERIAL

Prescriber Highlights

▶ Monobactam injectable antibiotic with good activity against a variety of gram-negative aerobic bacteria

▶ May be considered for use for treating serious infections, when aminoglycosides or fluoroquinolones are ineffective or relatively contraindicated

▶ Very limited information available regarding dosing & adverse effect profile

Uses/Indications

Aztreonam is a monobactam antibiotic that may be considered for use in small animals for treating serious infections caused by a wide variety of aerobic and facultative gram-negative bacteria, including strains of *Citrobacter, Enterobacter, E. coli, Klebsiella, Proteus, Pseudomonas* and *Serratia.* The drug exhibits good penetration into most tissues and low toxic potential and may be of benefit in treating infections when an aminoglycoside or a fluoroquinolone are either ineffective or are relatively contraindicated. Any consideration for using aztreonam must be tempered with the knowledge that little clinical experience or research findings have been published with regard to target species.

Aztreonam has also been used to treat pet fish (koi) infected with *Aeromonas salmonocida.*

Pharmacology/Actions

Aztreonam is a bactericidal antibiotic that binds to penicillin-binding protein-3 thereby inhibiting bacterial cell wall synthesis resulting in cell lyses and death of susceptible bacteria. Aztreonam is relatively stable to the effects of bacterial beta-lactamases and unlike many other beta-lactam antibiotics, it does not induce the activity of beta-lactamases.

Aztreonam has activity against many species and most strains of the following gram-negative bacteria: *Aeromonas, Citrobacter, Enterobacter, E. coli, Klebsiella, Pasturella, Proteus, Pseudomonas* and *Serratia.* It is not clinically efficacious against gram-positive or anaerobic bacteria.

Aztreonam can be synergistic against *Pseudomonas aeruginosa* and other gram-negative bacilli when used with aminoglycosides.

Pharmacokinetics

There is limited information published on the pharmacokinetic parameters of aztreonam in dogs and none was located for cats.

In dogs, after a 20 mg/kg dose was administered IM, peak plasma levels of approximately 40 micrograms/mL occurred in about 20 minutes. Serum protein binding is about 20–30%, compared to 65% in humans. High tissue levels are found in the kidney (approx. 2.5X that of plasma). Liver concentrations approximate those found in plasma and lower levels are found in the lung and spleen. The drug is primarily (80%) excreted unchanged in the dog. Elimination half-lives are approximately 0.7 hours after IV administration and 0.9 hours after IM administration. These values are approximately twice as short as those reported in humans (ages 1 yr to adult) with normal renal function.

Contraindications/Precaution/Warnings

Aztreonam should not be used in patients with documented severe hypersensitivity to the compound. Patients with serious renal dysfunction may need dosage adjustment. Use cautiously in patients with serious liver dysfunction.

Adverse Effects

Adverse effect profiles for aztreonam specific to target species were not located. Aztreonam's adverse effects in humans are similar to those of other beta-lactam antibiotics: hypersensitivity, gastrointestinal effects including GI bacterial overgrowth/Pseudomembranous colitis, pain and/or swelling after IM injection, and phlebitis after IV administration. Transient increases in liver enzymes, serum creatinine, and coagulation indices have been noted.

Reproductive/Nursing Safety

Aztreonam crosses that placenta and can be detected in fetal circulation. However, no evidence of teratogenicity or fetal toxicity have been reported after doses of up to 5 times normal were given to pregnant rats and rabbits. In humans, the FDA categorizes this drug as category *B* for use during pregnancy (*Animal studies have not yet demonstrated risk to the fetus, but there are no adequate studies in pregnant women; or animal studies have shown an adverse effect, but adequate studies in pregnant women have not demonstrated a risk to the fetus in the first trimester of pregnancy, and there is no evidence of risk in later trimesters.*)

Aztreonam has been detected in human breast milk at levels approximately 1% of those found in serum. As the drug is not absorbed orally, it is likely safe to use in nursing animals though antibiotic-associated diarrhea is possible.

Overdosage/Acute Toxicity

There is little reason for concern in patients with adequate renal function. The IV LD$_{50}$ for mice is 3.3 g/kg. Hemodialysis or peritoneal dialysis may be used to clear aztreonam from the circulation.

Drug Interactions

The following drug interactions have either been reported or are theoretical in humans or animals receiving aztreonam and may be of significance in veterinary patients:

■ **PROBENECID:** Can reduce the renal tubular secretion of aztreonam, thereby maintaining higher systemic levels for a longer period of time; this potential "beneficial" interaction requires further investigation before dosing recommendations can be made for veterinary patients

For *in vitro* interactions, see the Storage-Stability-Compatibility section.

Laboratory Considerations

■ Aztreonam may cause false-positive **urine glucose determinations** when using cupric sulfate solution (Benedict's Solution, *Clinitest®*). Tests utilizing glucose oxidase (*Tes-Tape®*, *Clinistix®*) are not affected by aztreonam.

Doses

■ **DOGS:**

Note: Dosages for this medication are not well established for use in veterinary pa-

tients. For dogs, an anecdotal dosing suggestion is to use the human pediatric dose of 30 mg/kg IM or IV q6–8h. When compared to humans, aztreonam has a shorter half-life, but is about half as bound to plasma proteins; the human pediatric dose may be a reasonable choice until more data becomes available.

■ **FISH:**

a) For treating *Aeromonas salmonicida* in koi: 100 mg/kg IM or ICe (intracoelemic) every 48 hours for 7 treatments. (Lewbart 2005)

Monitoring

■ Because monobactams usually have minimal toxicity associated with their use, monitoring for efficacy is usually all that is required unless toxic signs develop

■ Serum levels and therapeutic drug monitoring are not routinely performed with this agent

Client Information

■ Veterinary professionals only should administer this medication

■ Because of the dosing intervals required, this drug is best administered to inpatients only

Chemistry/Synonyms

Aztreonam is a synthetic monobactam antimicrobial. It occurs as a white, odorless crystalline powder.

Aztreonam may also be know as: Aztreonamum, Azthreonam, Attsreonaami, SQ-26776, *Monobac®*, *Azactam®*, *Aztreotic®*, *Azenam®*, *Primbactam®*, *Trezam®*, or *Urobactam®*.

Storage/Stability

Commercially available powder for reconstitution should be stored at room temperature (15°–30°C).

For IM use, add at least 3 mL of diluent (sterile water for injection, bacteriostatic sterile water for injection, NS, or bacteriostatic sodium chloride injection.) Solutions are stable for 48 hours at room temperature, 7 days if refrigerated.

For direct IV use, add 6–10 mL of sterile water for injection to each 15 or 30 mL vial. If the medication is to be given as an infusion, add at least 3 mL of sterile water for injection for each gram of aztreonam powder; then add the resulting solution to a suitable IV diluent (NS, LRS, D5W, etc.) so that the final concentration does not exceed 20 mg/mL. Inspect all solutions for visible particulate matter. Solutions may be colorless or a light, straw yellow color; upon standing, a light pink color may develop which does not affect the drug's potency. Intravenous solutions not exceeding concentrations of 20 mg/mL are stable for 48 hours at room temperature, 7 days if refrigerated. The package insert has specific directions for freezing solutions after dilution.

Compatibility/Compounding Considerations

Intravenous admixtures containing aztreonam are **compatible** with clindamycin, amikacin, gentamicin, tobramycin, ampicillin-sulbactam, imipenem-cilastatin, morphine, propofol, piperacillin-tazobactam, ticarcillin-clavulanate, ranitidine, sodium bicarbonate, potassium chloride, butorphanol, furosemide, hydromorphone, cefotaxime, cefuroxime, ceftriaxone and cefazolin. It is **not compatible** with metronidazole, nafcillin, amphotericin B, or vancomycin.

Dosage Forms/Regulatory Status

VETERINARY-LABELED PRODUCTS: None

HUMAN-LABELED PRODUCTS:

Aztreonam Injection (lyophilized cake or powder for solution): 500 mg. 1 g, 2 g single-dose vials; 1 g in single-dose vials, & single-dose 100 mL infusion bottles; & 2 g in single-dose vials, 30 mL single-dose vials and single-dose 100 mL infusion bottles; *Azactam*® (Squibb); generic (Rx)

Aztreonam Powder (lyophilized); for inhalation solution: 75 mg preservative free, arginine free (Lysine 46.7 mg) in 2 mL single-dose vials with 1 mL amp of sodium chloride 0.17% diluent; *Cayston*® (Gilead Sciences); (Rx)

Aztreonam is not commercially available in Canada.

References

Lewbart, G (2005). Antimicrobial and antifungal agents used in fish. *Exotic Animal Formulary 3rd Ed.* J Carpenter Ed., Elsevier; 5–12.

BACLOFEN

(**bak**-loe-fen)   Lioresal®

GABA DERIVATIVE MUSCLE RELAXANT

Prescriber Highlights

▶ Muscle relaxant that may be used for treating urinary retention in dogs

▶ Do not use in cats

▶ Adverse Effects: sedation, weakness, pruritus, & gastrointestinal distress

▶ Do not stop therapy abruptly

▶ Overdoses potentially serious

Uses/Indications

Baclofen may be useful to decrease urethral resistance in dogs to treat urinary retention. It is not recommended for cats.

Pharmacology/Actions

Considered a skeletal muscle relaxant, baclofen's mechanism of action is not well understood but it acts at the spinal cord level and decreases the frequency and amplitude of muscle spasm. It apparently decreases muscle spasticity by reducing gamma efferent neuronal activity. In the urethra, it reduces striated sphincter tone.

Pharmacokinetics

After oral administration, baclofen is rapidly and well absorbed but, at least in humans, there is wide interpatient variation. The drug is widely distributed with only a small percentage crossing the blood-brain barrier. Baclofen is eliminated primarily by the kidneys and less than 15% of a dose is metabolized by the liver. Elimination half-lives in humans range from 2.5–4 hours.

Baclofen crosses the placenta. It is unknown if it enters maternal milk in quantities sufficient to cause effects in offspring.

Contraindications/Precautions/Warnings

Baclofen is contraindicated in patients hypersensitive to it and is not recommended for use in cats. It should be used with caution in patients who have seizure disorders and working dogs that must be alert. Do not give the intrathecal medication by any other route.

Adverse Effects

Adverse effects reported in dogs include sedation, weakness, pruritus, salivation, and gastrointestinal distress (nausea, abdominal cramping).

Discontinue this medication gradually as hallucinations and seizures have been reported in human patients who have abruptly stopped the medication.

Reproductive/Nursing Safety

Very high doses caused fetal abnormalities in rodents. It is unknown if normal dosages affect fetuses; use during pregnancy with care. In humans, the FDA categorizes this drug as category C for use during pregnancy (*Animal studies have shown an adverse effect on the fetus, but there are no adequate studies in humans; or there are no animal reproduction studies and no adequate studies in humans.*)

Overdosage/Acute Toxicity

Deaths in dogs have been reported with baclofen doses as low as 8 mg/kg. Oral overdoses as low as 1.3 mg/kg may cause vomiting, depression, and vocalization. Other signs that may be noted include hypotonia or muscle twitching. Massive overdoses may cause respiratory depression, coma, or seizures. Onset of clinical signs after overdoses in dogs can occur from 15 minutes to 7 hours after ingestion and can persist for hours to days.

There were 288 exposures to baclofen reported to the ASPCA Animal Poison Control Center (APCC) during 2008-2009. In these cases, 272 were dogs with 233 showing clinical signs, and the remaining 16 cases were cats with 15 showing clinical signs. Common findings in dogs recorded in decreasing frequency included vocalization, vomiting, hypersalivation, ataxia, recumbency, hypothermia, and lethargy. Common findings in cats recorded in decreasing frequency included ataxia, vomiting, mydriasis, hypothermia, vocalization, and lethargy.

In alert patients, consider emptying the gut using standard techniques. Avoid the use of magnesium containing saline cathartics as they may compound CNS depression. Forced fluid diuresis may enhance baclofen excretion. Obtunded patients with respiratory depression may need to be mechanically ventilated. Monitor ECG and treat arrhythmias if needed. For patients who are vocalizing or disoriented, cyproheptadine (1.1 mg/kg orally or rectally) may be effective in alleviating the signs. Atropine has been suggested to improve ventilation, heart rate, BP, and body temperature. Diazepam may be useful for treating seizures. Intravenous lipids may potentially be useful as baclofen is lipid soluble. Contact an animal poison control center for further information and guidance.

Drug Interactions

The following drug interactions have either been reported or are theoretical in humans or animals receiving baclofen and may be of significance in veterinary patients:

- ■ **CNS DEPRESSANTS (other):** May cause additive CNS depression

Laboratory Considerations

- ■ Increased **AST, alkaline phosphate** and **blood glucose** have been reported in humans

Doses

- ■ **DOGS:**
  To treat urinary retention by decreasing urethral resistance:
  a) 1–2 mg/kg PO q8h (Coates 1999), (Labato 2005), (Lulich 2004)
  b) 5–10 mg (total dose) PO q8h (Senior 1999)

Monitoring

- ■ Efficacy
- ■ Adverse effects

Client Information

- ■ Do not stop therapy abruptly without veterinarian approval

Chemistry/Synonyms

A skeletal muscle relaxant that acts at the spinal cord level, baclofen occurs as white to off-white crystals. It is slightly soluble in water and has pKa values of 5.4 and 9.5.

Baclofen may also be known as: aminomethyl chlorohydrocinnamic acid, Ba-34647, baclofenum, *Baclo®*, *Baclohexal®*, *Baclon®*, *Baclopar®*, *Baclosal®*, *Baclospas®*, *Balgifen®*, *Clinispas®*, *Clofen®*, *Kemstro®*, *Lebic®*, *Lioresal®*, *Liotec®*, *Miorel®*, *Neurospas®*, *Nu-Baclo®*, *Pacifen®*, or *Vioridon®*.

Storage/Stability

Do not store tablets above 30°C (86°F). Intrathecal product should be stored at room temperature; do not freeze or heat sterilize.

Compatibility/Compounding Considerations

Compounded preparation stability: Baclofen oral suspension compounded from commercially available tablets has been published (Allen 1996). Triturating one-hundred twenty (120) baclofen 10 mg tablets with 60 mL of *Ora-Plus®* and *qs ad* to 120 mL with *Ora-Sweet®* (or *Ora-Sweet® SF*) yields a 10 mg/mL oral suspension that retains >90% potency for 60 days stored at both 5°C and 25°C. Compounded preparations of baclofen should be protected from light.

Another oral liquid compounding recipe has been described (Olin 2000): To prepare a 5 mg/mL liquid (35 day expiration date): Grind fifteen 20 mg tablets in a glass mortar to fine powder. Wet the powder with 10 mL of glycerin and form a fine paste. Slowly add 15 mL of simple syrup to the paste and transfer to a glass amber bottle. Rinse the mortar and pestle with another 15 mL of simple syrup and transfer to the bottle. Repeat until final volume is 60 mL. Shake well before each use and store in the refrigerator.

Dosage Forms/Regulatory Status

VETERINARY-LABELED PRODUCTS: None

The ARCI (Racing Commissioners International) has designated this drug as a class 4 substance. See the appendix for more information.

HUMAN-LABELED PRODUCTS:

Baclofen Tablets: 10 mg & 20 mg; *Lioresal®* (Novartis); generic; (Rx); 10 mg & 20 mg orally disintegrating tablets: *Kemstro®* (Schwarz); (Rx)

Baclofen Intrathecal Injection: 0.05 mg/mL (50 micrograms/mL) preservative-free in single-use amps, 10 mg per 20 mL (500 micrograms/mL) preservative-free in single-use amps (1 amp refill kit) & 10 mg/5 mL (2000 micrograms/mL) preservative-free in single-use amps (2 or 4 amp refill kits); *Lioresal® Intrathecal* (Medtronic); (Rx)

References

Allen, L.V. & M.A. Erickson (1996). Stability of baclofen, captopril, diltiazem hydrochloride, dipyridamole, and flecainide acetate in extemporaneously compounded oral liquids. *Am J Health Syst Pharm* 53(18): 2179–2184.

Coates, J (1999). Urethral dyssynergia in lumbosacral syndrome. Proceedings: 17th Annual Veterinary Medical Forum: ACVIM, Chicago.

Labato, M (2005). Micturition Disorders. *Textbook of Veterinary Internal Medicine, 6th Ed.* S Ettinger and E Feldman Eds., Elsevier: 105–109.

Lulich, J (2004). Managing functional urethral obstruction. Proceedings: ACVIM Forum. Accessed via: Veterinary Information Network. http://goo.gl/acf8d

Olin, B (2000). *Drug Facts and Comparisons: 2000.* St. Louis, Facts and Comparisons.

Senior, D (1999). Management of Micturition Disorders. American Animal Hospital Association Annual Meeting, Denver.

BAL in Oil — see Dimercaprol

BARBITURATE PHARMACOLOGY

(bar-*bich*-yoo-rate; bar-bi-*toor*-ate)

Also see the monographs for Methohexital, Phenobarbital, Pentobarbital, and Thiopental.

While barbiturates are generally considered CNS depressants, they can invoke all levels of CNS mood alteration from paradoxical excitement to deep coma and death. While the exact mechanisms for the CNS effects caused by barbiturates are unknown, they have been shown to inhibit the release of acetylcholine, norepinephrine, and glutamate. The barbiturates also have effects on GABA and pentobarbital has been shown to be GABA-mimetic. At high anesthetic doses, barbiturates have been demonstrated to inhibit the uptake of calcium at nerve endings.

The degree of depression produced is dependent on the dosage, route of administration, pharmacokinetics of the drug, and species treated. Additionally, effects may be altered by patient age, physical condition, or concurrent use of other drugs. The barbiturates depress the sensory cortex, lessen motor activity, and produce sedation at low dosages. In humans, it has been shown that barbiturates reduce the rapid-eye movement (REM) stage of sleep. Barbiturates have no true intrinsic analgesic activity.

In most species, barbiturates cause a dose-dependent respiratory depression, but, in some species, they can cause slight respiratory stimulation. At sedative/hypnotic doses, respiratory depression is similar to that during normal physiologic sleep. As doses increase, the medullary respiratory center is progressively depressed with resultant decreases in rate, depth, and volume. Respiratory arrest may occur at doses four times lower than those will cause cardiac arrest. These drugs must be used very cautiously in cats; they are particularly sensitive to the respiratory depressant effects of barbiturates.

Besides the cardiac arresting effects of the barbiturates at euthanatizing dosages, the barbiturates have other cardiovascular effects. In the dog, pentobarbital has been demonstrated to cause tachycardia, decreased myocardial contractility and stroke volume, and decreased mean arterial pressure and total peripheral resistance.

The barbiturates cause reduced tone and motility of the intestinal musculature, probably secondary to its central depressant action. The thiobarbiturates (thiamylal, thiopental) may, after initial depression, cause an increase in both tone and motility of the intestinal musculature; however, these effects do not appear to have much clinical significance. Administration of barbiturates reduces the sensitivity of the motor end-plate to acetylcholine thereby slightly relaxing skeletal muscle. Because the musculature is not completely relaxed, other skeletal muscle relaxants may be necessary for surgical procedures.

There is no direct effect on the kidney by the barbiturates, but severe renal impairment may occur secondary to hypotensive effects in overdose situations. Liver function is not directly affected when used acutely, but hepatic microsomal enzyme induction is well documented with extended barbiturate (especially phenobarbital) administration. Although barbiturates reduce oxygen consumption of all tissues, no change in metabolic rate is measurable when given at sedative dosages. Basal metabolic rates may be reduced with resultant decreases in body temperature when barbiturates are given at anesthetic doses.

BENAZEPRIL HCL

(ben-*a*-za-pril)   Fortekor®, Lotensin®

ANGIOTENSIN CONVERTING ENZYME (ACE) INHIBITOR

Prescriber Highlights

▶ ACE inhibitor that may be useful for treating heart failure, hypertension, chronic renal failure & protein-losing glomerulonephropathies in dogs & cats; particularly useful in patients with hypertension and proteinuria

▶ Caution in patients with hyponatremia, coronary or cerebrovascular insufficiency, SLE, hematologic disorders

▶ GI disturbances most likely adverse effects, but hypotension, renal dysfunction, hyperkalemia possible

▶ Mildly fetotoxic at high dosages

Uses/Indications

Benazepril may be useful as a vasodilator in the treatment of heart failure and as an antihypertensive agent, particularly in dogs. Reasonable evidence exists that ACE-inhibitors increase survival (when compared to placebo) in dogs with dilated cardiomyopathy and mitral valve disease. Benazepril may be of benefit in treating the clinical signs associated with valvular heart disease and left to right shunts. ACE inhibitors may also be of benefit in the adjunctive treatment of chronic renal failure and for protein losing nephropathies.

In cats, benazepril (or enalapril) can be used for treating hypertension, adjunctive treatment of hypertrophic cardiomyopathy, and reducing protein loss associated with chronic renal failure.

Pharmacology/Actions

Benazepril is a prodrug and has little pharmacologic activity of its own. After being hydrolyzed in the liver to benazeprilat, the drug inhibits the conversion of angiotensin-I to angiotensin-II by inhibiting angiotensin-converting enzyme (ACE). Angiotensin-II acts both as a vasoconstrictor and stimulates production of aldosterone in the adrenal cortex. By blocking angiotensin-II formation, ACE inhibitors generally reduce blood pressure in hypertensive patients and vascular resistance in patients with congestive heart failure. There is no evidence that ACE inhibitors reduce abnormal cardiac hypertrophy in cats.

When administered to dogs with heart failure at low dosages (0.1 mg/kg q12h), benazepril improved clinical signs, but did not significantly affect blood pressure (Wu & Juany 2006)

In cats with chronic renal failure, benazepril has been shown to reduce systemic arterial pressure and glomerular capillary pressure while increasing renal plasma flow and glomerular filtration rates. It may also help improve appetite.

ACE inhibitors' proteinuric reducing effects are most likely a result of reducing intraglomerular hypertension by a vasodilating effect on postglomerular arterioles.

Like enalapril and lisinopril, but not captopril, benazepril does not contain a sulfhydryl group. ACE inhibitors containing sulfhydryl groups (*e.g.*, captopril) may have a greater tendency of causing immune-mediated reactions.

Pharmacokinetics

After oral dosing in healthy dogs, benazepril is rapidly absorbed and converted into the active metabolite benazeprilat with peak levels of benazepril occurring approximately 75 minutes after dosing. The elimination half-life of benazeprilat is approximately 3.5 hours in healthy dogs. Unlike enalaprilat, which is approximately 95% cleared in dogs via renal mechanisms, benazeprilat is cleared via both renal (45%) and hepatic (55%) routes.

In cats, inhibition of ACE is long-lasting (half-life of 16–23 hours), despite relatively quick elimination of free benazeprilat, due to high affinity of benazeprilat to ACE. Because enalaprilat exhibits nonlinear binding of benazeprilat to ACE, doses greater than 0.25 mg/kg PO produced only small incremental increases in peak effect or duration of ACE inhibition. (King *et al.* 2003)

In humans, approximately 37% of an oral dose is absorbed after oral dosing and food apparently does not affect the extent of absorption. About 95% of the parent drug and active metabolite are bound to serum proteins. Benazepril and benazeprilat are primarily eliminated via the kidneys and mild to moderate renal dysfunction apparently does not significantly alter elimination as biliary clearance may compensate somewhat for reductions in renal clearances. Hepatic dysfunction or age does not appreciably alter benazeprilat levels.

Contraindications/Precautions/Warnings

Benazepril is contraindicated in patients who have demonstrated hypersensitivity to the ACE inhibitors.

ACE inhibitors should be used with caution in patients with hyponatremia or sodium depletion, coronary or cerebrovascular insufficiency, preexisting hematologic abnormalities or a collagen vascular disease (*e.g.*, SLE). Patients with severe CHF should be monitored very closely upon initiation of therapy.

Potentially, ACE inhibitors could worsen preexisting azotemia; using a lower dose and monitoring creatinine and BUN has been recommended (Bartges 2009).

Adverse Effects

Benazepril's adverse effect profile in dogs is not well described, but other ACE inhibitors effects in dogs usually center around GI distress (anorexia, vomiting, diarrhea). Potentially, hypotension, renal dysfunction and hyperkalemia could occur. Because it lacks a sulfhydryl group (unlike captopril), there is less likelihood that immune-mediated reactions will occur, but rashes, neutropenia and agranulocytosis have been reported in humans.

In healthy cats given mild overdoses (2 mg/kg PO once daily for 52 weeks), only increased food consumption and weight were noted.

Reproductive/Nursing Safety

Benazepril apparently crosses the placenta. High doses of ACE inhibitors in rodents have caused decreased fetal weights and increases in fetal and maternal death rates; no teratogenic effects have been reported to date, but use during pregnancy should occur only when the potential benefits of therapy outweigh the risks to the offspring. In humans, the FDA categorizes this drug as category *C* for use during the first trimester of pregnancy (*Animal studies have shown an adverse effect on the fetus, but there are no adequate studies in humans; or there are no animal reproduction studies and no adequate studies in humans.*) During the second and third trimesters, the FDA categorizes this drug as category *D* for use during pregnancy (*There is evidence of human fetal risk, but the potential benefits from the use of the drug in pregnant women may be acceptable despite its potential risks.*)

Benazepril is distributed into milk in very small amounts.

Overdosage/Acute Toxicity

In overdose situations, the primary concern is hypotension; supportive treatment with volume expansion with normal saline is recommended to correct blood pressure. Because of the drug's long duration of action, prolonged monitoring and treatment may be required. Recent massive overdoses should be managed using gut-emptying protocols as appropriate.

Drug Interactions

The following drug interactions have either been reported or are theoretical in humans or animals receiving benazepril and may be of significance in veterinary patients:

■ **ASPIRIN:** Aspirin may potentially negate the decrease in systemic vascular resistance induced by ACE inhibitors; however, one study in dogs using low-dose aspirin, the hemodynamic effects of enalaprilat (active metabolite of enalapril, a related drug) were not affected

■ **ANTIDIABETIC AGENTS (insulin, oral agents):** Possible increased risk for hypoglycemia; enhanced monitoring recommended

■ **DIURETICS (e.g., furosemide, hydrochlorothiazide):** Potential for increased hypotensive effects; some veterinary clinicians recommend reducing furosemide doses (by 25–50%) when adding enalapril or benazepril to therapy for heart failure

■ **DIURETICS, POTASSIUM-SPARING (e.g., spironolactone, triamterene):** Increased hyperkalemic effects, enhanced monitoring of serum potassium

■ **LITHIUM:** Increased serum lithium levels possible; increased monitoring required

■ **POTASSIUM SUPPLEMENTS:** Increased risk for hyperkalemia

Laboratory Considerations

■ When using **iodohippurate sodium I^{123}/I^{134} or Technetium Tc^{99} pententate renal imaging** in patients with renal artery stenosis, ACE inhibitors may cause a reversible decrease in localization and excretion of these agents in the affected kidney which may lead to confusion in test interpretation.

Doses

■ **DOGS:**

For adjunctive treatment of heart failure:

a) 0.25–0.5 mg/kg PO once daily (Miller & Tilley 1995); (Kittleson 2007)

b) 0.25–0.5 mg/kg PO once to twice daily (Ware 1997)

For adjunctive treatment of hypertension and/or proteinuria:

a) As a first step drug for systolic hypertension >160 mmHg, diastolic >120 mmHg; after **1)** enalapril/benazepril (0.5 mg/kg q12h); **2)** amlodipine (0.1 mg/kg q24h); **3)** amlodipine (0.2 mg/kg q24h); **4)** spironolactone (1–2 mg/kg twice daily); **5)** hydralazine 0.5 mg/kg PO twice daily. Each step added (except when increasing amlodipine dose) if after 1-2 weeks systolic BP > 160 mmHg. (Henik 2007)

b) 0.25–0.5 mg/kg q12–24h; Co-administration with a calcium channel antagonist may lower blood pressure when monotherapy is not sufficient. In diabetic

dogs, an ACE inhibitor may block adverse effects of calcium channel antagonists. (Brown 2003)

c) For hypertension associated with protein-losing renal disease: 0.5 mg/kg PO once daily (q24h) Response may be variable in dogs with hypertension secondary to other diseases; ACE inhibitors are usually well tolerated and can be tried in non-emergency hypertension. (Stepien 2006)

d) For proteinuria, hypertension: 0.25–1 mg/kg PO q12-24h. Potentially, ACE inhibitors could worsen preexisting azotemia; using a lower dose and monitoring creatinine and BUN is recommended (Bartges 2009).

■ **CATS:**

For adjunctive treatment of heart failure:

a) 0.25–0.5 mg/kg PO once daily (Kittleson 2007)

b) For CHF or hypertension: 0.25–0.5 mg/kg PO once to twice daily (Atkins 2003)

For adjunctive treatment of hypertension:

a) 0.5–1 mg/kg PO once daily (Sparkes 2003), (Adams 2009)

b) 0.25–1 mg/kg PO once to twice daily. Because of their antiproteinuric effects, ACE inhibitors are the drugs of first choice to treat hypertension in animals with proteinuria. (Langston 2003)

c) 0.25–0.5 mg/kg PO once daily (q24h) (Stepien 2006)

d) For proteinuria, hypertension associated with chronic kidney disease: 0.25–0.5 mg/kg PO once to twice daily (q12–24h); rarely higher (Polzin 2006)

e) For proteinuria, hypertension: 0.25–1 mg/kg PO q12-24h. Potentially, ACE inhibitors could worsen preexisting azotemia; using a lower dose and monitoring creatinine and BUN is recommended (Bartges 2009).

f) As a 2nd step drug when systolic BP >160 mmHg, diastolic >120 mmHg: **1)** amlodipine (0.625 mg per cat q24h, if cat greater then 6 kg, 1.25 mg/cat q24h), add ACE inhibitor if proteinuric; **2)** ACE inhibitor (benazepril/enalapril 0.5 mg/kg q12h); **3)** spironolactone (1–2 mg/kg twice daily); **4)** hydralazine 0.5 mg/kg PO twice daily. Each step added (except when increasing amlodipine dose) if after 1–2 weeks systolic BP > 160 mmHg. (Henik 2007)

Monitoring

■ Clinical signs of CHF

■ Serum electrolytes, creatinine, BUN, urine protein

■ Blood pressure (if treating hypertension or

clinical signs associated with hypotension arise)

Client Information
■ Do not abruptly stop or reduce therapy without veterinarian's approval. Contact veterinarian if vomiting or diarrhea persist or is severe or if animal's condition deteriorates.

Chemistry/Synonyms
Benazepril HCl, an angiotensin converting enzyme inhibitor, occurs as white to off-white crystalline powder. It is soluble in water and ethanol. Benazepril does not contain a sulfhydryl group in its structure.

Benazepril may also be known as: CGS-14824A (benazepril or benazepril hydrochloride), *Benace®, Boncordin®, Briem®, Cibace®, Cibacen®, Cibacen®, Cibacene®, Fortekor®, Labopal®, Lotensin®, Lotrel®, Tensanil®,* or *Zinadril®.*

Storage/Stability
Benazepril tablets (and combination products) should be stored at temperatures less than 86°F (30°C) and protected from moisture. They should be dispensed in tight containers.

Dosage Forms/Regulatory Status
VETERINARY-LABELED PRODUCTS: None in the USA

In the UK (and elsewhere): Benazepril Tablets: 2.5 mg, 5 mg, & 20 mg; *Fortekor®* (Novartis— UK); (POM-V) Labeled for use in cats for chronic renal insufficiency and for heart failure in dogs.

The ARCI (Racing Commissioners International) has designated this drug as a class 3 substance. See the appendix for more information.

HUMAN-LABELED PRODUCTS:

Benazepril HCl Oral Tablets: 5 mg, 10 mg, 20 mg, & 40 mg; *Lotensin®* (Novartis); generic; (Rx)

Also available in fixed dose combination products containing amlodipine (*Lotrel®*) or hydrochlorothiazide (*Lotensin HCT®*)

References

Adams, L (2009). Importance of proteinuria and hypertension in chronic kidney disease. Proceedings: WVC.

Atkins, C (2003). Therapeutic strategies in feline heart disease. Proceedings: ACVIM Forum. Accessed via: Veterinary Information Network. http://goo.gl/NSJtl

Bartges, J (2009). Update on management of proteinuria. Proceedings: WVC.

Brown, S (2003). Update on feline hypertension: diagnosis and treatment. Proceedings: World Small Animal Veterinary Association World Congress. Accessed via: Veterinary Information Network.

Henik, R (2007). Stepwise therapy of systemic hypertension. Proceedings: IVECCS. Accessed via: Veterinary Information Network. http://goo.gl/nofKU

King, J, M Maurer, et al. (2003). Pharmacokinetic/pharmacodynamic modeling of the disposition and effect of benazepril and benazeprilat in cats. *J Vet Phamacol Ther* 26: 213–224.

Kittleson, M (2007). Management of Heart Failure. *Small Animal Medicine Cardiology Textbook, 2nd Ed.,* Accessed Online via the Veterinary Drug Information Network.

Langston, C (2003). Management of chronic renal failure: The Pre–Transplant Period. Proceedings: Atlantic Coast Veterinary Conference. Accessed via: Veterinary Information Network. http://goo.gl/0oe3K

Miller, M & J Tilley (1995). *Manual of Canine and Feline Cardiology, 2nd Ed.*

Polzin, D (2006). Treating feline renal failure: an evidenced–based approach. Proceedings: WVC. Accessed via: Veterinary Information Network. http://goo.gl/C2JgZ

Sparkes, A (2003). Feline systemic hypertension–A hidden killer. Proceedings: World Small Animal Veterinary Assoc. Accessed via: Veterinary Information Network. http://goo.gl/QgVkr

Stepien, R (2006). Diagnosis and treatment of systemic hypertension. Proceedings: ACVIM Forum.

Ware, W (1997). Acquired Valvular Diseases. *Handbook of Small Animal Practice 3rd Ed.* R Morgan Ed. Philadelphia, WB Saunders: 91–97.

Wu, S & H Juany (2006). Effect of benazepril on systemic blood pressure in dogs with heart failure. Proceedings: WSAVA. Accessed via: Veterinary Information Network. http://goo.gl/sr9ZB

BETAMETHASONE
BETAMETHASONE ACETATE
BETAMETHASONE SODIUM PHOSPHATE

(bet-ta-*meth*-a-sone)   Celestone®

GLUCOCORTICOID

Note: For more information on the pharmacology of glucocorticoids refer to the monograph: Glucocorticoids, General information. For topical or otic use, see the Topical Dermatology & Otic sections in the appendix.

Prescriber Highlights

▶ Injectable (long-acting) & topical glucocorticoid

▶ Long acting; 25–40X more potent than hydrocortisone; no mineralocorticoid activity

▶ Goal is to use as much as is required & as little as possible for as short an amount of time as possible

▶ Primary adverse effects are "Cushingoid" in nature with sustained use

▶ Many potential drug & lab interactions when used systemically

Contraindications/Precautions/Warnings
For the product *Betasone®* (Schering), the manufacturer states that the drug is "contraindicated in animals with acute or chronic bacterial infections unless therapeutic doses of an effective antimicrobial agent are used." Systemic use of glucocorticoids is generally considered contraindicated in systemic fungal infections (un-

less used for replacement therapy in Addison's), when administered IM in patients with idiopathic thrombocytopenia and in patients hypersensitive to a particular compound. Use of sustained-release injectable glucocorticoids is contraindicated for chronic corticosteroid therapy of systemic diseases.

Animals that have received glucocorticoids systemically other than with "burst" therapy, should be tapered off the drugs. Patients who have received the drugs chronically should be tapered off slowly as endogenous ACTH and corticosteroid function may return slowly. Should the animal undergo a "stressor" (*e.g.*, surgery, trauma, illness, etc.) during the tapering process or until normal adrenal and pituitary function resume, additional glucocorticoids should be administered.

Corticosteroid therapy may induce parturition in large animal species during the latter stages of pregnancy.

Adverse Effects

Adverse effects are generally associated with long-term administration of these drugs, especially if given at high dosages or not on an alternate day regimen. Effects generally manifest as clinical signs of hyperadrenocorticism. When administered to young, growing animals, glucocorticoids can retard growth. Many of the potential effects, adverse and otherwise, are outlined in the Pharmacology section of the Glucocorticoids, General information monograph.

In dogs, polydipsia (PD), polyphagia (PP) and polyuria (PU), may all be seen with short-term "burst" therapy as well as with alternate-day maintenance therapy on days when given the drug. Adverse effects in dogs associated with long-term use can include: dull, dry haircoat, weight gain, panting, vomiting, diarrhea, elevated liver enzymes, pancreatitis, GI ulceration, lipidemias, activation or worsening of diabetes mellitus, muscle wasting and behavioral changes (depression, lethargy, viciousness). Discontinuation of the drug may be necessary; changing to an alternate steroid may also alleviate the problem. With the exception of PU/PD/PP, adverse effects associated with antiinflammatory therapy are relatively uncommon. Adverse effects associated with immunosuppressive doses are more common and potentially more severe.

Cats generally require higher dosages than dogs for clinical effect but tend to develop fewer adverse effects. Occasionally, polydipsia, polyuria, polyphagia with weight gain, diarrhea, or depression can be seen. Long-term, high dose therapy can lead to "Cushingoid" effects.

Reproductive/Nursing Safety

In addition to the contraindications, precautions and adverse effects outlined above, betamethasone has been demonstrated to cause decreased sperm output and semen volume and increased percentages of abnormal sperm in dogs.

Use with caution in nursing dams. Corticosteroids appear in milk and could suppress growth, interfere with endogenous corticosteroid production or cause other unwanted effects in the nursing offspring. However, in humans, several studies suggest that amounts excreted in breast milk are negligible when prednisone or prednisolone doses in the mother are less than or equal to 20 mg/day or methylprednisolone doses are less than or equal to 8 mg/day. Larger doses for short periods may not harm the infant.

Overdosage/Acute Toxicity

Glucocorticoids when given short-term are unlikely to cause harmful effects, even in massive dosages. One incidence of a dog developing acute CNS effects after accidental ingestion of glucocorticoids has been reported. Should clinical signs occur, use supportive treatment if required.

Chronic usage of glucocorticoids can lead to serious adverse effects. Refer to Adverse Effects above for more information.

Drug Interactions

The following drug interactions have either been reported or are theoretical in humans or animals receiving betamethasone systemically and may be of significance in veterinary patients:

- **AMPHOTERICIN B:** When administered concomitantly with glucocorticoids may cause hypokalemia

- **ANTICHOLINESTERASE AGENTS (e.g., pyridostigmine, neostigmine, etc.):** In patients with myasthenia gravis, concomitant glucocorticoid and anticholinesterase agent administration may lead to profound muscle weakness; if possible, discontinue anticholinesterase medication at least 24 hours prior to corticosteroid administration

- **ASPIRIN AND OTHER SALICYLATES:** Glucocorticoids may reduce salicylate blood levels

- **BARBITURATES:** May increase the metabolism of glucocorticoids

- **CYCLOPHOSPHAMIDE:** Glucocorticoids may inhibit the hepatic metabolism of cyclophosphamide; dosage adjustments may be required

- **CYCLOSPORINE:** Concomitant administration of glucocorticoids and cyclosporine may increase the blood levels of each by mutually inhibiting hepatic metabolism; clinical significance is not clear

- **DIGOXIN:** When glucocorticoids are used concurrently with digitalis glycosides, an increased chance of digitalis toxicity may occur should hypokalemia develop; diligent monitoring of potassium and digitalis glycoside levels is recommended.

■ **DIURETICS, POTASSIUM-DEPLETING (e.g., furosemide, thiazides):** When administered concomitantly with glucocorticoids may cause hypokalemia

■ **ESTROGENS:** May decrease corticosteroid clearance

■ **INSULIN:** Requirements may increase in patients receiving glucocorticoids

■ **ISONIAZID:** May have serum levels decreased by corticosteroids

■ **KETOCONAZOLE:** Corticosteroid clearance may be reduced and the AUC increased

■ **MITOTANE:** May alter the metabolism of steroids; higher than usual doses of steroids may be necessary to treat mitotane-induced adrenal insufficiency

■ **RIFAMPIN:** May increase the metabolism of glucocorticoids

■ **THEOPHYLLINES:** Alterations of pharmacologic effects of either drug can occur

■ **ULCEROGENIC DRUGS (e.g., NSAIDS):** Use with glucocorticoids may increase the risk of gastrointestinal ulceration

■ **VACCINES:** Patients receiving corticosteroids at immunosuppressive dosages should generally not receive live attenuated-virus vaccines as virus replication may be augmented; diminished immune response may occur after vaccine, toxoid, or bacterin administration in patients receiving glucocorticoids

Laboratory Considerations

■ Glucocorticoids may increase **serum cholesterol** and **urine glucose** levels

■ Glucocorticoids may decrease **serum potassium**

■ Glucocorticoids can suppress the release of thyroid stimulating hormone (TSH) and reduce T_3 & T_4 values; thyroid gland atrophy has been reported after chronic glucocorticoid administration

■ Uptake of I^{131} by the thyroid may be decreased by glucocorticoids

■ Reactions to **skin tests** may be suppressed by glucocorticoids

■ False-negative results of the **nitroblue tetrazolium test** for systemic bacterial infections may be induced by glucocorticoids

■ Betamethasone does not cross-react with the cortisol assay

Doses

■ **DOGS:**

For the control of pruritus:

a) *Betasone®* *Aqueous* *Suspension*: 0.25–0.5 mL per 20 pounds body weight IM. Dose dependent on severity of condition. May repeat when necessary. Relief averages 3 weeks in duration. Do not exceed more than 4 injections. (Package Insert; *Betasone®*—Schering) **Note:** Product no longer marketed in the USA.

■ **HORSES:** Source of product an issue. Alternative is triamcinolone (see that monograph for additional information). (**Note:** ARCI UCGFS Class 4 Drug)

As a relatively short-acting corticosteroid for intraarticular administration:

a) 6–15 mg per joint IA. Frequency of reinjection is limited to the minimum number needed to achieve soundness. (Frisbee 2003)

Monitoring

Monitoring of glucocorticoid therapy is dependent on its reason for use, dosage, agent used (amount of mineralocorticoid activity), dosage schedule (daily versus alternate day therapy), duration of therapy, and the animal's age and condition. The following list may not be appropriate or complete for all animals; use clinical assessment and judgment should adverse effects be noted:

■ Weight, appetite, signs of edema
■ Serum and/or urine electrolytes
■ Total plasma proteins, albumin
■ Blood glucose
■ Growth and development in young animals
■ ACTH stimulation test if necessary

Client Information

■ Clients should carefully follow the dosage instructions and should not discontinue the drug abruptly without consulting veterinarian beforehand

■ Clients should be briefed on the potential adverse effects that can be seen with these drugs and instructed to contact the veterinarian should these effects become severe or progress

Chemistry/Synonyms

A synthetic glucocorticoid, betamethasone is available as the base and as the dipropionate, acetate and sodium phosphate salts. The base is used for oral dosage forms. The sodium phosphate and acetate salts are used in injectable preparations. The dipropionate salt is used in topical formulations and in combination with the sodium phosphate salt in a veterinary-approved injectable preparation.

Betamethasone occurs as an odorless, white to practically white, crystalline powder. It is insoluble in water and practically insoluble in alcohol. The dipropionate salt occurs as a white or creamy-white, odorless powder. It is practically insoluble in water and sparingly soluble in alcohol. The sodium phosphate salt occurs as an odorless, white to practically white, hygroscopic powder. It is freely soluble in water and slightly soluble in alcohol.

Betamethasone may also be known as flubenisolone or *Celestone®*.

Storage/Stability

Betamethasone tablets should be stored in well-closed containers at 2–30°C. The oral solution should be stored in well-closed containers, protected from light and kept at temperatures less than 40°C. The sodium phosphate injection should be protected from light and stored at room temperature (15–30°C); protect from freezing. The combination veterinary injectable product (*Betasone®*) should be stored between 2–30°C and protected from light and freezing.

Compatibility/Compounding Considerations
When betamethasone sodium phosphate was mixed with heparin sodium, hydrocortisone sodium succinate, potassium chloride, vitamin B-complex with C, dextrose 5% in water (D₅W), D₅ in Ringer's, D₅ in lactated Ringer's, Ringer's lactate injection or normal saline, no physical incompatibility was noted immediately or after 4 hours.

Dosage Forms/Regulatory Status

VETERINARY-LABELED PRODUCTS:
The following product is apparently no longer marketed in the USA. Betamethasone Dipropionate Injection equivalent to 5 mg/mL of betamethasone and betamethasone sodium phosphate equivalent to 2 mg/mL betamethasone in 5 mL vials; *Betasone®* (Schering-Plough); (Rx). FDA-approved for use in dogs.

Betamethasone valerate is also found in *Gentocin® Otic, Gentocin® Topical Spray* and *Topagen® Ointment*, (Schering-Plough). There are several other otic and topical products containing betamethasone and gentamicin on the veterinary market. See the appendix for more information on these products.

The ARCI (Racing Commissioners International) has designated this drug as a class 4 substance. See the appendix for more information.

HUMAN-LABELED PRODUCTS:
Betamethasone Oral Solution: 0.6 mg/5 mL in 118 mL; *Celestone®* (Schering); (Rx)

Betamethasone Injection: betamethasone (as sodium phosphate) 3 mg/mL and betamethasone acetate 3 mg/mL suspension in 5 mL multi-dose vials; *Celestone Soluspan®* (Schering); (Rx)

References

Frisbee, D (2003). Intraarticular corticosteroids. *Current Therapy in Equine Medicine 5.* C Kawcak Ed. Philadelphia, Saunders: 551–554.

BETHANECHOL CHLORIDE

(beh-*than*-e-kole)   Urecholine®
CHOLINERGIC

Prescriber Highlights

▶ Cholinergic agent used primarily to increase bladder contractility; symptomatic treatment of dysautonomia

▶ Principle contraindications are GI or urinary tract obstructions or if bladder wall integrity is in question

▶ Adverse Effects: "SLUD" (salivation, lacrimation, urination, defecation)

▶ Cholinergic crisis possible if injecting IV or SC, have atropine at the ready

Uses/Indications

In veterinary medicine, bethanechol is used primarily to stimulate bladder contractions in small animals. It also can be used as an esophageal or general GI stimulant, although metoclopramide and/or neostigmine have largely supplanted it for these uses.

Pharmacology/Actions

Bethanechol directly stimulates cholinergic receptors. Its effects are principally muscarinic and at usual doses has negligible nicotinic activity. It is more resistant to hydrolysis than acetylcholine by cholinesterase and, therefore, has an increased duration of activity.

Pharmacologic effects include increased esophageal peristalsis and lower esophageal sphincter tone, increased tone and peristaltic activity of the stomach and intestines, increased gastric and pancreatic secretions, increased tone of the detrusor muscle of the bladder, and decreased bladder capacity. At high doses after parenteral administration, effects such as increased bronchial secretions and constriction, miosis, lacrimation, and salivation can be seen. When administered SC or orally, effects are predominantly on the GI and urinary tracts.

Pharmacokinetics

No information was located on the pharmacokinetics of this agent in veterinary species. In humans, bethanechol is poorly absorbed from the GI tract, and the onset of action is usually within 30–90 minutes after oral dosing. After subcutaneous administration, effects begin within 5–15 minutes and usually peak within 30 minutes. The duration of action after oral dosing may persist up to 6 hours after large doses and 2 hours after SC dosing. Subcutaneous administration yields a more enhanced effect on urinary tract stimulation than does oral administration.

Bethanechol does not enter the CNS after usual doses; other distribution aspects of the drug are not known. The metabolic or excretory fate of bethanechol has not been described.

Contraindications/Precautions/Warnings

Contraindications to bethanechol therapy include: bladder neck or other urinary outflow obstruction, when the integrity of the bladder wall is in question (*e.g.*, as after recent bladder surgery), hyperthyroidism, peptic ulcer disease or when other inflammatory GI lesions are present, recent GI surgery with resections/anastomoses, GI obstruction or peritonitis, hypersensitivity to the drug, epilepsy, asthma, coronary artery disease or occlusion, hypotension, severe bradycardia or vagotonia or vasomotor instability. If urinary outflow resistance is increased due to enhanced urethral tone (not mechanical obstruction!), bethanechol should only be used in conjunction with another agent that will sufficiently reduce outflow resistance [*e.g.*, diazepam, dantrolene (striated muscle) or phenoxybenzamine (smooth muscle).]

Adverse Effects

When administered orally to small animals, adverse effects are usually mild with vomiting, diarrhea, salivation, and anorexia being the most likely to occur. Cardiovascular (bradycardia, arrhythmias, hypotension) and respiratory effects (asthma, dyspnea) are most likely only seen after overdosage situations or with high dose SC therapy.

In horses, salivation, lacrimation and abdominal pain are potential adverse effects.

IM or IV use is not recommended except in emergencies when the IV route may be used. Severe cholinergic reactions are likely if given IV. If injecting the drug (SC or IV), it is recommended that atropine be immediately available.

Reproductive/Nursing Safety

In humans, the FDA categorizes this drug as category *C* for use during pregnancy (*Animal studies have shown an adverse effect on the fetus, but there are no adequate studies in humans; or there are no animal reproduction studies and no adequate studies in humans.*)

It is unknown if bethanechol is distributed into milk.

Overdosage/Acute Toxicity

Clinical signs of overdosage are basically cholinergic in nature. Muscarinic effects (salivation, urination, defecation, etc.) are usually seen with oral or SC administration. If given IM or IV, a full-blown cholinergic crisis can occur with circulatory collapse, bloody diarrhea, shock and cardiac arrest possible.

Treatment for bethanechol toxicity is atropine. Refer to the atropine monograph for more information on its use. Epinephrine may also be employed to treat clinical signs of bronchospasm.

Drug Interactions

The following drug interactions have either been reported or are theoretical in humans or animals receiving bethanechol and may be of significance in veterinary patients:

- ■ **ANTICHOLINERGIC DRUGS: (e.g., atropine, glycopyrrolate, propantheline)**: Can antagonize bethanechol's effects
- ■ **CHOLINERGIC DRUGS (e.g., neostigmine, physostigmine, pyridostigmine**: Because of additional cholinergic effects, bethanechol should generally not be used concomitantly with other cholinergic drugs
- ■ **GANGLIONIC BLOCKING DRUGS (e.g., mecamylamine)**: Can produce severe GI and hypotensive effects
- ■ **QUINIDINE, PROCAINAMIDE:** Can antagonize the effects of bethanechol

Doses

Note: The injectable product is no longer commercially marketed in the USA

- ■ **DOGS:**

  For urinary indications:
  a) To stimulate detrusor contractility: 5–25 mg (total dose) PO 2–3 times a day (Dickinson 2010)
  b) 5–15 mg (total dose) PO q8h (Lulich 2003)
  c) 5–25 mg (total dose) PO q8h (Bartges 2003)
  d) 2.5–25 mg (total dose) PO three times daily (Coates 2004)

  For increased esophageal sphincter tone:
  a) 0.5–1 mg/kg PO q8h (Jones 1985)

  For symptomatic treatment of dysautonomia:
  a) 2.5–7.5 mg (total dose) PO divided q8-12h; may improve gastrointestinal motility and bladder emptying (Sisson 2004)
  b) 1.25–5 mg (total dose) PO once daily (Willard 2003)
  c) 0.05 mg/kg SC q12h and slowly increase as necessary. While SC administration gives better results, can also use 1.25–5 mg (total dose) q12h PO. (O'Brien 2003)

- ■ **CATS:**

  To increase bladder contractility:
  a) 1.25–7.5 mg (total dose) PO two to three times daily (Lane 2003)
  b) 1.25–7.5 mg per cat PO q8h (Osborne *et al.* 2000), (Bartges 2003)

  For symptomatic treatment of dysautonomia:
  a) 2.5–7.5 mg (total dose) PO divided q8-12h; may improve gastrointestinal motility and bladder emptying (Sisson 2004)
  b) 1.25–5 mg (total dose) PO once daily (Willard 2003)

■ **HORSES:** (**Note:** ARCI UCGFS Class 4 Drug)
To stimulate detrusor muscle activity:

a) 0.025–0.075 mg/kg subcutaneously q8h.
Dosage is variable and should be adjusted for each patient. (Jose-Cunilleras & Hinchcliff 1999)

b) For post-surgery bladder atony in foals: 0.4 mg/kg PO 2–3 times a day in a tapering withdrawal may restore function. (McKenzie 2009)

c) If bladder is capable of weak contractions: 0.025–0.075 mg/kg SC 2–3 times; or 0.25–0.75 mg/kg PO 2–4 times a day. **Note:** Oral dose is 10X that of SC dose (Schott II & Carr 2003)

■ **CATTLE:**
For adjunctive medical therapy (with fluids, mineral oil, and NSAIDs if needed) of cecal dilation/dislocation (CDD):

a) Only if animal is "normal" or only slightly disturbed, defecation is present, and rectal exam does not reveal torsion or retroflexion. If these criteria are not met, or no improvement within 24 hours of medical therapy, surgical therapy is recommended. Bethanechol at 0.07 mg/kg SC three times daily for 2 days. Withhold feed for 24 hours and then gradually give increasing amounts of hay if defecation is present and CDD is resolved. (Meylan 2004)

Monitoring

■ Clinical efficacy

■ Urination frequency, amount voided, bladder palpation

■ Adverse effects (see above section)

Client Information

■ Give medication to animal with an empty stomach unless otherwise instructed by veterinarian

■ Contact veterinarian if salivation or GI (vomiting, diarrhea, or anorexia) effects are pronounced or persist

Chemistry/Synonyms

A synthetic cholinergic ester, bethanechol occurs as a slightly hygroscopic, white or colorless crystalline powder with a slight, amine-like or "fishy" odor. It exhibits polymorphism, with one form melting at 211° and the other form at 219°. One gram of the drug is soluble in approximately 1 mL of water or 10 mL of alcohol.

Bethanechol Chloride may also be known as: carbamylmethylcholine chloride, *Duvoid®, Miotonachol®, Muscaran®, Myo Hermes®, Myocholine®, Myotonine®, Ucholine®, Urecholine®, Urocarb®,* or *Urotonine®.*

Storage/Stability

Bethanechol tablets should be stored at room temperature in tight containers.

Compounded preparation stability: Beth-

anechol oral suspension compounded from commercially available tablets has been published (Allen, 1998). Triturating twelve (12) bethanechol 50 mg tablets with 60 mL of *Ora-Plus®* and *qs ad* to 120 mL with *Ora-Sweet®* (or *Ora-Sweet® SF*) yields a 5 mg/mL oral suspension that retains >90% potency for 60 days stored at both 5°C and 25°C. Compounded preparations of bethanechol should be protected from light.

Dosage Forms/Regulatory Status

VETERINARY-LABELED PRODUCTS: None
The ARCI (Racing Commissioners International) has designated this drug as a class 4 substance. See the appendix for more information.

HUMAN-LABELED PRODUCTS:

Bethanechol Chloride Oral Tablets: 5 mg, 10 mg, 25 mg & 50 mg; *Urecholine®* (Barr/Duramed); generic; (Rx)

An injectable product was formerly commercially available.

References

Allen, L.V. & M.A. Erickson (1998). Stability of bethanechol chloride, pyrazinamide, quinidine sulfate, rifampin, and tetracycline hydrochloride in extemporaneously compounded oral liquids. Am J Health Syst Pharm 55(17): 1804-1809.

Bartges, J (2003). Canine lower urinary tract cases. Proceedings: ACVIM Forum. Accessed via: Veterinary Information Network. http://goo.gl/HH41u

Coates, J (2004). Neurogenic micturition disorders. Proceedings: ACVIM Forum. Accessed via: Veterinary Information Network. http://goo.gl/260CO

Dickinson, P (2010). Disorders of micturition and continence. Proceedings: UCD Veterinary Neurology Symposium.

Jones, BD (1985). Gastrointestinal disorders. *Handbook of Small Animal Therapeutics.* LE Davis Ed. New York, Churchill Livingston: 397–462.

Jose–Cunilleras, E & K Hinchcliff (1999). Renal pharmacology. *The Veterinary Clinics of North America: Equine Practice* 15:3(December): 647–664.

Lane, I (2003). Incontinence and voiding disorders in cats. Proceedings: Western States Veterinary Conference. Accessed via: Veterinary Information Network. http://goo.gl/7jZKx

Lulich, J (2003). Urologic Logic: Challenging Cases I. Proceedings: Western Veterinary Conference. Accessed via: Veterinary Information Network. http://goo.gl/7ypV7

McKenzie, E (2009). Umbilical and urinary tract problems in foals. Proceedings: WVC.

Meylan, M (2004). Motility in the bovine large intestine and pathogenesis of cecal dilatation/dislocation. Proceedings: ACVIM Forum. Accessed via: Veterinary Information Network. http://goo.gl/KXraq

O'Brien, D (2003). Dysautonomia. Proceedings: ACVIM Forum. Accessed via: Veterinary Information Network. http://goo.gl/28rdr

Osborne, C, J Kruger, et al. (2000). Feline Lower Urinary Tract Diseases. *Textbook of Veterinary Internal Medicine: Diseases of the Dog and Cat.* S Ettinger and E Feldman Eds. Philadelphia, WB Saunders. 2: 1710–1747.

Schott II, H & E Carr (2003). Urinary incontinence in horses. Proceedings: ACVIM Forum. Accessed via: Veterinary Information Network. http://goo.gl/q7Uo2

Sisson, A (2004). Dysautonomia. *The 5–Minute Veterinary Consult: Canine and Feline 3rd Ed.* L Tilley and F Smith Eds., Lippincott Williams & Wilkins: 375.

Willard, M (2003). Digestive system disorders. *Small Animal Internal Medicine, 3rd Ed.* R Nelson and C Couto Eds. St Louis, Mosby: 343–471.

Bicarbonate — see Sodium Bicarbonate

BISACODYL

(bis-a-*koe*-dill)   Dulcolax®

ORAL/RECTAL LAXATIVE

Prescriber Highlights

▶ Stimulant laxative used in dogs & cats

▶ Contraindicated in GI obstruction

▶ GI cramping/diarrhea possible

▶ Don't give with milk products or antacids; do not crush or split tablets

Uses/Indications

Bisacodyl oral and rectal products are used as stimulant cathartics in dogs and cats.

Pharmacology/Actions

A stimulant laxative, bisacodyl's exact mechanism is unknown. It is thought to produce catharsis by increasing peristalsis by direct stimulation on the intramural nerve plexuses of intestinal smooth muscle. It has been shown to increase fluid and ion accumulation in the large intestine thereby enhancing catharsis.

Pharmacokinetics

Bisacodyl is minimally absorbed after either oral or rectal administration. Onset of action after oral administration is generally 6–10 hours and 15 minutes to an hour after rectal administration.

Contraindications/Precautions/Warnings

Stimulant cathartics are contraindicated in the following conditions: intestinal obstruction (not constipation), undiagnosed rectal bleeding, or when the patient is susceptible to intestinal perforation.

Bisacodyl should only be used short-term as chronic use can damage myenteric neurons.

Adverse Effects

Bisacodyl has relatively few side effects when used occasionally; cramping, nausea, or diarrhea may be noted after use.

Reproductive/Nursing Safety

In humans, the FDA categorizes this drug as category *B* for use during pregnancy (*Animal studies have not yet demonstrated risk to the fetus, but there are no adequate studies in pregnant women; or animal studies have shown an adverse effect, but adequate studies in pregnant women have not demonstrated a risk to the fetus in the first trimester of pregnancy, and there is no evidence of risk in later trimesters.*)

Bisacodyl may be distributed into milk but at quantities unlikely to cause any problems in nursing offspring.

Overdosage/Acute Toxicity

Overdoses may result in severe cramping, diarrhea, vomiting and potentially, fluid and electrolyte imbalances. Animals should be monitored and given replacement parenteral fluids and electrolytes as necessary.

Drug Interactions

The following drug interactions have either been reported or are theoretical in humans or animals receiving bisacodyl and may be of significance in veterinary patients:

■ **ANTACIDS/MILK:** Do not give milk or antacids within an hour of bisacodyl tablets as it may cause premature disintegration of the enteric coating.

■ **ORAL DRUGS:** Stimulant laxatives may potentially decrease GI transit time thereby affecting absorption of other oral drugs. Separate doses by two hours if possible.

Doses

Note: Bisacodyl enema products and pediatric suppositories are no longer available in the USA. Human pediatric suppositories were 5 mg; the 10 mg "adult" suppositories can be cut lengthwise to approximate one pediatric suppository.

■ **DOGS:**

As a cathartic:

a) One 5 mg tablet PO for small dogs; one to two 5 mg tablets (10–15 mg) for medium to large dogs. Do not break tablets. (Willard 2003)

b) 5–20 mg (1–4 tablets) PO once daily, or 1–3 pediatric suppositories (Sherding 1994)

■ **CATS:**

As a cathartic:

a) One 5 mg tablet PO; do not break tablets. (Willard 2003)

b) 5 mg (1 tablet) PO once daily, or 1–3 pediatric suppositories (Sherding 1994)

c) One 5 mg tablet PO q24h. May be given in combination with fiber supplementation. Avoid daily use if used chronically as it may damage myenteric neurons. (Washabau 2001)

Client Information

■ If using oral tablets, do not crush or allow animal to chew; intense cramping may occur.

■ Unless otherwise directed by veterinarian, bisacodyl should be used on an "occasional" basis only. Chronic use can damage the nerves in the colon and has lead to laxative dependence in humans.

Chemistry/Synonyms

A diphenylmethane laxative, bisacodyl occurs as white to off-white crystalline powder. It is practically insoluble in water and sparingly soluble in alcohol.

Bisacodyl may also be known as bisacodylum; many trade names are available.

Storage/Stability

Bisacodyl suppositories and enteric-coated tablets should be stored at temperatures less than 30°C.

Dosage Forms/Regulatory Status

VETERINARY-LABELED PRODUCTS: None

HUMAN-LABELED PRODUCTS:

Bisacodyl Enteric-coated Oral Tablets: 5 mg; *Alophen®* (Numark); *Bisa-Lax®* (Bergen Brunswig); *Dulcolax®* (Boehringer Ingelheim); *Ex-Lax Ultra®* (Novartis); *Fleet® Laxative* (Fleet); *Modane®* (Savage Labs); *Bisac-Evac®* (G & W Labs); *Caroid®* (Mentholatum Co); *Correctol®* (Schering-Plough); *Feen-a-mint®* (Schering-Plough); generic; (OTC)

Bisacodyl Rectal Suppositories: 10 mg; *Dulcolax®* (Boehringer Ingelheim); *Bisacodyl Uniserts®* (Upsher-Smith); *Bisa-Lax®* (Bergen Brunswig); *Bisac-Evac®* (G & W Labs), *Fleet® Laxative* (Fleet); generic; (OTC)

Bisacodyl enema products and pediatric suppositories are no longer available in the USA. Pediatric suppositories were 5 mg and the 10 mg "adult" suppositories can be cut lengthwise to approximate a pediatric suppository.

References
Sherding, R (1994). Anorectal diseases. *Saunders Manual of Small Animal Practice.* S Birchard and R Sherding Eds. Philadelphia, W.B. Saunders Company: 777–792.

Washabau, R (2001). Feline constipation, obstipation and megacolon: Prevention, diagnosis and treatment. Proceedings: World Small Animal Assoc. World Congress. Accessed via: Veterinary Information Network.

Willard, M (2003). Digestive system disorders. Small Animal Internal Medicine, 3rd Ed. R Nelson and C Couto Eds. St Louis, Mosby: 343–471.

BISMUTH SUBSALICYLATE

(*biz*-mith sub-sal-*iss*-ih-layt)
BSS, Pepto-Bismol®

ANTIDIARRHEAL

Prescriber Highlights

▶ Used to treat diarrhea & as a component of "triple therapy" for treating Helicobacter GI infections

▶ High doses may cause salicylism, use with caution in cats

▶ Constipation/impactions may occur

▶ Refrigeration may improve palatability

Uses/Indications

In veterinary medicine, bismuth subsalicylate products are used to treat diarrhea and as a component of "triple therapy" for treating Helicobacter GI infections. The drug is also used in humans for other GI symptoms (indigestion, cramps, gas pains) and in the treatment and prophylaxis of traveler's diarrhea.

Pharmacology/Actions

Bismuth subsalicylate is thought to possess protectant, anti-endotoxic and weak antibacterial properties. It is believed that the parent compound is cleaved in the small intestine into bismuth carbonate and salicylate. The protectant, anti-endotoxic and weak antibacterial properties are thought to be because of the bismuth. The salicylate component has antiprostaglandin activity that may contribute to its effectiveness and reduce clinical signs associated with secretory diarrheas.

Pharmacokinetics

No specific veterinary information was located. In humans, the amount of bismuth absorbed is negligible while the salicylate component is rapidly and completely absorbed. Salicylates are highly bound to plasma proteins and are metabolized in the liver to salicylic acid. Salicylic acid, conjugated salicylate metabolites and any absorbed bismuth are all excreted renally.

Contraindications/Precautions/Warnings

Salicylate absorption may occur; use with caution in patients with preexisting bleeding disorders. Because of the potential for adverse effects caused by the salicylate component, this drug should be used cautiously, if at all, in cats.

As bismuth is radiopaque, it may interfere with GI tract radiologic examinations.

Adverse Effects

Antidiarrheal products are not a substitute for adequate fluid and electrolyte therapy when required. May change stool color to a gray-black or greenish-black; do not confuse with melena. In human infants and debilitated individuals, use of this product may cause impactions to occur.

Reproductive/Nursing Safety

The FDA has not, apparently, given bismuth subsalicylate a pregnancy risk category. As it is a form of salicylate, refer to the aspirin monograph for further guidance. Use with caution in pregnant animals.

Use with caution in nursing dams.

Overdosage/Acute Toxicity

Bismuth subsalicylate liquid/suspension contains approximately 8.7 mg/mL salicylate. Two tablespoonsful (30 mL) is approximately equivalent to one 325 mg aspirin tablet. See the Aspirin monograph for more information.

Drug Interactions

The following drug interactions have either been reported or are theoretical in humans or animals

receiving bismuth subsalicylate and may be of significance in veterinary patients:

■ **TETRACYCLINE:** Bismuth containing products can decrease the absorption of orally administered tetracycline products. If both agents are to be used, separate drugs by at least 2 hours and administer tetracycline first.

■ **ASPIRIN:** Because bismuth subsalicylate contains salicylate, concomitant administration with aspirin may increase salicylate serum levels; monitor appropriately.

Laboratory Considerations

■ At high doses, salicylates may cause false-positive results for **urinary glucose** if using the cupric sulfate method (*Clinitest®*, Benedict's solution) and false-negative results if using the glucose oxidase method (*Clinistix®* or *Tes-Tape®*).

■ **Urinary ketones** measured by the ferric chloride method (Gerhardt) may be affected if salicylates are in the urine (reddish-color produced).

■ **5-HIAA** determinations by the fluorometric method may be interfered by salicylates in the urine.

■ Falsely elevated **VMA** (vanillylmandelic acid) may be seen with most methods used if salicylates are in the urine. Falsely lowered **VMA** levels may be seen if using the Pisano method.

■ Urinary excretion of **xylose** may be decreased if salicylates are given concurrently.

■ Falsely elevated **serum uric acid** values may be measured if using colorimetric methods.

Doses

Note: Doses of liquids below are for the 17.5 mg/mL (1.75%) liquids (veterinary suspensions; original *Pepto-Bismol®* liquid, etc.) unless otherwise specified.

■ **DOGS:**

For acute diarrhea:
a) 1 mL per 5 kg of body weight PO 3 times a day; should probably not exceed 5 days of therapy (Hall, E. & Simpson 2000)

b) *Pepto-Bismol®*: 0.25 mL/kg PO q4–6h, up to 2 mL/kg q 6–8h (Cote 2000)

For treating Helicobacter gastritis infections:
a) Using triple therapy: Metronidazole 15.4 mg/kg q8h, amoxicillin 11 mg/kg q8h and bismuth subsalicylate (original *Pepto-Bismol®*) 0.22 mL/kg PO q4–6h. Give each for 3 weeks (Hall, J. 2000)

b) Using triple therapy: Metronidazole 10 mg/kg PO q12h, amoxicillin 15 mg/kg q12h and bismuth subsalicylate 262 mg tablets given based upon body weight (<5kg = 0.25 tablet; 5-9.9 kg = 0.5 tablet; 10-24.9kg = 1 tablet; >25kg = 2 tablets) q12h. Give each for 2 weeks. (Leib *et al.* 2007)

As a gastroprotectant/coating agent in the adjunctive treatment of uremic gastritis:
a) 2 mL/kg PO q6–8h (Bartges 2006)

■ **CATS:**

For diarrhea:
a) *Pepto-Bismol®*: 0.25 mL/kg PO q4–6h; cats are sensitive to salicylates and probably should not receive frequent or high dosages (Cote 2000)

b) Using "*Pepto-Bismol® Regular*" or equivalent strength (17.5 mg/mL) liquid: 0.5–1 mL/kg PO q12h for 3 days. (Scherk 2005)

c) For diarrhea in kittens and young cats: 1–2 mL *Pepto-Bismol®* 3–4 times a day. Refrigeration may increase palatability. (Tams 1999)

For eliminating Helicobacter gastritis infections:
a) Using triple therapy: Metronidazole 15.4 mg/kg q8h, amoxicillin 11 mg/kg q8h and bismuth subsalicylate (original *Pepto-Bismol®*) 0.22 mL/kg PO q4–6h. Give each for 3 weeks. (Hall, J. 2000)

■ **FERRETS:**

For eliminating Helicobacter gastritis infections:
a) Using triple therapy: Metronidazole 20 mg/kg, amoxicillin 30 mg/kg and bismuth subsalicylate 7.5 mg/kg PO. Give each q8h for 3–4 weeks. (Johnson-Delaney 2009))

b) Using triple therapy: Metronidazole 20 mg/kg PO q12h, amoxicillin 20 mg/kg PO q12h and bismuth subsalicylate 17.5 mg/kg PO q8h; continue for 21 days. Used with famotidine (0.5 mg/kg PO once daily) and sucralfate (25 mg/kg PO q8h) (Johnson 2006)

■ **CATTLE:**

For diarrhea:
a) For calves: 60 mL two to four times a day for two days (Label Directions; *Corrective Mixture®*—Beecham).

b) 2–3 ounces PO 2–4 times a day (Braun 1986)

■ **HORSES:**

For diarrhea:
a) For foals: 3–4 ounces per 45 kg (100 lb.) body weight PO q6–8h (Madigan 2002)

b) For foals or adults: 1 ounce per 8 kg of body weight PO 3-4 times daily (Clark & Becht 1987)

c) For foals: 3–4 oz. PO q6–8h (Martens & Scrutchfield 1982)

d) For foals: 60 mL two to four times a day for two days (Label Directions; *Corrective Mixture®*—Beecham).

■ **SWINE:**

For diarrhea in baby pigs:

a) 2–5 mL PO two to four times a day for 2 days (Label Directions; *Corrective Mixture®*—Beecham)

Monitoring

■ Clinical efficacy

■ Fluid and electrolyte status in severe diarrhea

Client Information

■ Shake product well before using.

■ Refrigeration of the suspension may improve palatability. Do not mix with milk before administering.

■ If diarrhea persists, contact veterinarian.

■ May change stool color to a gray-black or greenish-black; contact veterinarian if stool becomes "tarry" black.

Chemistry/Synonyms

Bismuth subsalicylate occurs as white or nearly white, tasteless, odorless powder and contains about 58% bismuth. It is insoluble in water, glycerin and alcohol.

Bismuth subsalicylate may also be known as: BSS, basic bismuth salicylate, bismuth oxysalicylate, bismuth salicylate, bismuthi subsalicylas, *Bismu-kote®*, *Bismukote®*, *Bismupaste®*, *Bismatrol®*, *Bismed®*, *Bismusal®*, *Bismylate®*, *Bisval®*, *Equi-Phar®*, *Gastrocote®*, *Jatrox®*, *Kalbeten®*, *Kaopectate®*, *Katulcin-R®*, *PalaBIS®*, *Peptic Relief®*, *Pink Biscoat®*, *Pink Bismuth Rose®*, or *Ulcolind Wismut®*; many other human trade names are available.

Storage/Stability

Bismuth subsalicylate should be stored protected from light. Unless otherwise labeled store at room temperature; do not freeze.

Compatibility/Compounding Considerations

Bismuth subsalicylate is **incompatible** with mineral acids and iron salts. When exposed to alkali bicarbonates, bismuth subsalicylate decomposes with effervescence.

Dosage Forms/Regulatory Status

VETERINARY-LABELED PRODUCTS:

Bismuth Subsalicylate Paste:

5% (50 mg/mL) in 15 mL tubes; *Bismukote Paste for Small Dogs®* (Vedco), (OTC). Labeled for use in small dogs.

10% (100 mg/mL) in 15 mL & 30 mL tubes; *Bismukote Paste for Medium and Large Dogs®* (Vedco), *Bismupaste D®* (Butler); (OTC). Depending on product, labeled for use in small, medium and large dogs.

20% (200 mg/mL) in 60 mL tubes; *Bismupaste E®* (Butler), *Equi-Phar®* (Vedco), (OTC). Labeled for use in horses.

Bismuth Subsalicylate Oral Suspension:

Bismuth subsalicylate Oral Suspension 1.75% (17.5 mg/mL; 262 mg/15 mL). *Bismu-kote® Suspension* (Vedco), *Bismusal®* (Bimeda), *Bismusol® Suspension* (AgriPharm), *Bismusol®*

(First Priority), *Corrective Suspension®* (Phoenix), *Gastrocote®* (Butler); generic; (OTC). Available in gallons. Labeled for use in cattle, horses, calves, foals, dogs and cats. Each mL contains about 8.7 mg salicylate.

Bismuth Subsalicylate Tablets:

Bismuth Subsalicylate tablets (each tablet contains 262 mg of bismuth subsalicylate). Labeled for use in dogs. PalaBIS® (PharmX); (OTC). One tablet contains about 102 mg salicylate.

HUMAN-LABELED PRODUCTS:

Bismuth Subsalicylate (BSS) Liquid/Suspension: 87 mg/5 mL; 130 mg/15 mL; 262 mg/15 mL; 524 mg/15 mL; 525 mg/15 mL; in 120 mL, 236 mL, 237 mL, 240 mL, 355 mL, 360 mL, or 480 mL; *Kaopectate®* (Pfizer); *Kaopectate®*, *Kaopectate® Children's* & *Extra Strength* (Pharmacia); *Pink Bismuth* (various); *Kao-Tin®* (Major); *Peptic Relief®* (Rugby); *Pepto-Bismol®* & *Maximum Strength* (Procter & Gamble *Maalox® Total Stomach Relief Liquid* (Novartis); (OTC). **Note:** Regular strength (262 mg/mL) contains 8.7 mg salicylate per mL; Extra-Strength (525 mg/mL) contains 15.7 mg of salicylate per mL.

Bismuth Subsalicylate Tablets and Caplets: 262 mg (regular & chewable); *Kaopectate®* (Pfizer Consumer Health); *Bismatrol®* (Major); *Peptic Relief®* (Rugby); *Pepto-Bismol®* (Procter & Gamble)); (OTC). One tablet contains about 102 mg salicylate.

References

Bartges, J (2006). There's nothing cute about acute renal failure. Proceedings: ACVC 2006. Accessed via: Veterinary Information Network. http://goo.gl/1MekY

Braun, RK (1986). Dairy Calf Health Management. *Current Veterinary Therapy 2: Food Animal Practice.* JL Howard Ed. Philadelphia, WB Saunders: 126–135.

Clark, ES & JL Becht (1987). Clinical Pharmacology of the Gastrointestinal Tract. *Vet Clin North Am (Equine Practice)* 3(1): 101–122.

Cote, E (2000). Over–the–Counter Pharmaceuticals. *Textbook of Veterinary Internal Medicine: Diseases of the Dog and Cat.* S Ettinger and E Feldman Eds. Philadelphia, WB Saunders. 1: 318–320.

Hall, E & K Simpson (2000). Diseases of the Small Intestine. *Textbook of Veterinary Internal Medicine: Diseases of the Dog and Cat.* S Ettinger and E Feldman Eds. Philadelphia, WB Saunders. 2: 1182–1238.

Hall, J (2000). Diseases of the Stomach. *Textbook of Veterinary Internal Medicine: Diseases of the Dog and Cat.* S Ettinger and E Feldman Eds. Philadelphia, WB Saunders. 2: 1154–1182.

Johnson, D (2006). Ferrets: the other companion animal. Proceedings: ACVC. Accessed via: Veterinary Information Network. http://goo.gl/bSeol

Johnson–Delaney, C (2009). Gastrointestinal physiology and disease of carnivorous exotic companion animals. Proceedings: ABVP.

Leib, MS, RB Duncan, et al. (2007). Triple antimicrobial therapy and acid suppression in dogs with chronic vomiting and gastric Helicobacter spp. *Journal of Veterinary Internal Medicine* 21(6): 1185–1192.

Madigan, J (2002). Diarrhea. Proceedings: Western Veterinary Conf. Accessed via: Veterinary Information Network. http://goo.gl/tzBYZ

Martens, RJ & WL Scrutchfield (1982). Foal Diarrhea: Pathogenesis, Etiology, and Therapy. *Comp Cont Ed* 4(4): S175–S186.

Scherk, M (2005). The frustration of recurrent feline diarrhea. Proceedings: Western Veterinary Conference. Accessed via: Veterinary Information Network. http://goo.gl/mncY4

Tams, T (1999). Acute Diarrheal Diseases of the Dog and Cat. Proceedings: The North American Veterinary Conference, Orlando.

BLEOMYCIN SULFATE

(blee-oh-*mye*-sin)   Blenoxane®

ANTINEOPLASTIC

Prescriber Highlights

▶ Antibiotic antineoplastic agent infrequently used for a variety of neoplasms in dogs & cats; intralesional administration may have promise

▶ Two main toxicities: acute (fever, anorexia, vomiting, & allergic reactions) & delayed (dermatologic effects, stomatitis, pneumonitis & pulmonary fibrosis)

▶ Do not exceed total dosage recommendations

▶ Intensive adverse effect monitoring required when used systemically

Uses/Indications

Bleomycin has occasionally been used as adjunctive treatment of lymphomas, squamous cell carcinomas, teratomas, and nonfunctional thyroid tumors in both dogs and cats. Recent work has demonstrated that bleomycin may be promising for intralesional treatment for a variety of localized tumors with or without concomitant electropermeabilization.

Pharmacology/Actions

Bleomycin is an antibiotic that has activity against a variety of gram-negative and gram-positive bacteria as well as some fungi. While its cytotoxicity prevents it from being clinically useful as an antimicrobial, it can be useful against a variety of tumors in small animals.

Bleomycin has both a DNA binding site and a site that binds to the ferrous form of iron. By accepting an electron from ferrous ion to an oxygen atom in the DNA strand, DNA is cleaved.

Resistance to bleomycin therapy is via reduced cellular uptake of the drug, reduced ability to damage DNA and increased rates of DNA repair by the cell and, probably most importantly, via the enzyme bleomycin hydrolase.

Pharmacokinetics

Bleomycin is not appreciably absorbed from the gut and must be administered parenterally. It is mainly distributed to the lungs, kidneys, skin, lymphatics and peritoneum. In patients with normal renal function, terminal half-life is about 2 hours. In humans, 60–70% of a dose is excreted as active drug in the urine.

Contraindications/Precautions/Warnings

Because bleomycin is a toxic drug with a low therapeutic index, it should be used only by those having the facilities to actively monitor patients and handle potential complications. Bleomycin is contraindicated in patients with prior hypersensitivity reactions from the drug, preexisting pulmonary disease, or adverse pulmonary effects from prior therapy. The drug should be used very cautiously in patients with significant renal impairment and dosage reduction may be necessary. Bleomycin can be teratogenic; it should only be used in pregnant animals when the owners accept the associated risks.

Adverse Effects

Toxicity falls into two broad categories: acute and delayed. Acute toxicities include fever, anorexia, vomiting, and allergic reactions (including anaphylaxis). Delayed toxic effects include dermatologic effects (*e.g.*, alopecia, rashes, etc.), stomatitis, pneumonitis and pulmonary fibrosis. These latter two effects have been associated with drug-induced fatalities. Initial signs associated with pulmonary toxicity include pulmonary interstitial edema with alveolar hyaline membrane formation and hyperplasia of type II alveolar macrophages. Pulmonary toxicity is potentially reversible if treatment is stopped soon enough. Unlike many other antineoplastics, bleomycin does not usually cause bone marrow toxicity but thrombocytopenia, leukopenia and slight decreases in hemoglobin levels are possible. Renal toxicity and hepatotoxicity are potentially possible.

To reduce the likelihood of pulmonary toxicity developing, a total maximum dosage of 125–200 mg/m^2 should not be exceeded.

Reproductive/Nursing Safety

In humans, the FDA categorizes this drug as category *D* for use during pregnancy (*There is evidence of human fetal risk, but the potential benefits from the use of the drug in pregnant women may be acceptable despite its potential risks.*)

It is not known if bleomycin enters milk; it is not recommended to nurse while receiving the medication.

Overdosage/Acute Toxicity

No specific information was located. Because of the toxicity of the drug, it is important to determine dosages carefully.

Drug Interactions

The following drug interactions have either been reported or are theoretical in humans or animals receiving bleomycin and may be of significance in veterinary patients:

■ **ANESTHETICS, GENERAL:** Use of general anesthetics in patients treated previously with bleomycin should be exercised with caution. Bleomycin sensitizes lung tissue to oxygen (even to concentrations of inspired oxygen considered to be safe) and rapid deterioration of pulmonary function with post-operative pulmonary fibrosis can occur.

■ **PRIOR OR CONCOMITANT CHEMOTHERAPY WITH OTHER AGENTS OR RADIATION THERAPY:** Can lead to increased hematologic, mucosal and pulmonary toxicities with bleomycin therapy.

Doses

Note: Because of the potential toxicity of this drug to patients, veterinary personnel and clients, and since chemotherapy indications, treatment protocols, monitoring and safety guidelines often change, the following dosages should be used only as a general guide. Consultation with a veterinary oncologist and referral to current veterinary oncology references [*e.g.*, (Henry & Higginbotham 2009); (Argyle *et al.* 2008); (Withrow & Vail 2007); (Villalobos 2007); (Ogilvie & Moore 2006); (Ogilvie & Moore 2001)] is *strongly recommended*.

■ **SMALL ANIMALS:**
The following is a usual dosage or dose range for bleomycin and should be used only as a general guide: 10 Units mg/m^2 (NOT mg/kg) or 0.3–0.5 mg/kg (Note: 1 Unit = 1 mg). Some protocols use the drug once daily for a few days and then back off to once weekly; some give the drug once weekly at the start. To reduce the likelihood of pulmonary toxicity, a total maximum dosage of 125–200 mg/m^2 should not be exceeded.

Monitoring

■ Efficacy

■ Pulmonary Toxicity: Obtain chest films, (baseline and on a regular basis—in humans they are recommended q1–2 weeks); lung auscultation (dyspnea and fine rales may be early signs of toxicity); other initial signs associated with pulmonary toxicity include pulmonary interstitial edema with alveolar hyaline membrane formation and hyperplasia of type II alveolar macrophages

■ Blood chemistry (encompassing renal and hepatic function markers) and hematologic profiles (CBC) may be useful to monitor potential renal, hepatic and hematologic toxicities

■ Total dose accumulation

Client Information

■ Clients must be informed of the potential toxicities associated with therapy and urged to report any change in pulmonary function (*e.g.*, shortness of breath, wheezing) immediately

Chemistry/Synonyms

An antibiotic antineoplastic agent, bleomycin sulfate is obtained from *Streptomyces verticullis*. It occurs as a cream colored, amorphous powder that is very soluble in water and sparingly soluble in alcohol. After reconstitution, the pH

of the solution ranges from 4.5–6. Bleomycin is assayed microbiologically. One unit of bleomycin is equivalent to one mg of the reference Bleomycin A$_2$ standard.

Bleomycin sulfate may also be known as: bleomycin sulphate, bleomycini sulfas, *Bileco®, Blanoxan®, Blenamax®, Blenoxane®, Bleo®, Bleo-S®, Bleo-cell®, Bleocin®, Bleolem®, Blio®, Blocamicina®, Bonar®, Oil Bleo®,* or *Tecnomicina®.*

Storage/Stability

Powder for injection should be kept refrigerated. After reconstituting with sterile saline, water, or dextrose, the resulting solution is stable for 24 hours. Bleomycin is less stable in dextrose solutions than in saline. After reconstituting with normal saline, bleomycin is reportedly stable for at least two weeks at room temperature and for 4 weeks when refrigerated; however, since there are no preservatives in the resulting solution, the product is recommended for use within 24 hours.

Compatibility/Compounding Considerations

Bleomycin sulfate is reported to be **compatible** with the following drugs: amikacin sulfate, cisplatin, cyclophosphamide, dexamethasone sodium phosphate, diphenhydramine HCl, doxorubicin, heparin sodium, metoclopramide HCl, vinblastine sulfate, and vincristine sulfate. Compatibility is dependent upon factors such as pH, concentration, temperature and diluent used; consult specialized references or a hospital pharmacist for more specific information.

Dosage Forms/Regulatory Status

VETERINARY-LABELED PRODUCTS: None
HUMAN-LABELED PRODUCTS:
Bleomycin Sulfate Lyophilized Powder for Injection after reconstitution: 15 Units & 30 Units per vial; generic; (Rx)

References

Argyle, D, M Brearly, et al. (2008). *Decision Making in Small Animal Oncology*, Wiley–Blackwell.

Henry, C & M Higginbotham (2009). *Cancer Management in Small Animal Practice*, Saunders.

Ogilvie, G & A Moore (2001). *Feline Oncology: A Comprehensive Guide to Compassionate Care*, Veterinary Learning Systems.

Ogilvie, G & A Moore (2006). *Managing the Canine Cancer Patient: A Practical Guide to Compassionate Care*, Veterinary Learning Systems.

Villalobos, A (2007). *Canine and Feline Geriatric Oncology*. Ames, Blackwell.

Withrow, S & D Vail (2007). *Withrow and MacEwen's Small Animal Clinical Oncology 4th Ed.* Philadelphia, Elsevier.

BOLDENONE UNDECYLENATE

(bole-*di*-nohn un-de-sil-*en*-ate)
Equipoise®

ANABOLIC STEROID

Prescriber Highlights

▶ Long-acting anabolic steroid labeled for horses; possibly useful in cats to stimulate appetite

▶ Not recommended for use in stallions or pregnant mares

▶ May cause androgenic effects, including aggressiveness; potentially a hepatotoxin

▶ Potentially a drug of abuse by humans, watch for diversion scams

Uses/Indications

Boldenone is labeled for use as adjunctive therapy ". . . as an aid for treating debilitated horses when an improvement in weight, haircoat, or general physical condition is desired" (Package Insert; Equipoise®—Fort Dodge).

Boldenone may possibly be useful to stimulate appetite in cats.

Pharmacology/Actions

In the presence of adequate protein and calories, anabolic steroids promote body tissue building processes and can reverse catabolism. As these agents are either derived from or are closely related to testosterone, the anabolics have varying degrees of androgenic effects. Endogenous testosterone release may be suppressed by inhibiting luteinizing hormone (LH). Large doses can impede spermatogenesis by negative feedback inhibition of FSH.

Anabolic steroids can also stimulate erythropoiesis possibly by stimulation of erythropoietic stimulating factor. Anabolics can cause nitrogen, sodium, potassium and phosphorus retention and decrease the urinary excretion of calcium.

Pharmacokinetics

No specific information was located for this agent. It is considered a long-acting anabolic, with effects persisting up to 8 weeks. It is unknown if the anabolic agents cross into milk.

Contraindications/Precautions/Warnings

The manufacturer (Solvay) recommends not using the drug on stallions or pregnant mares. Other clinicians state that anabolic steroids should not be used in either stallions or nonpregnant mares intended for reproduction. Boldenone should not be administered to horses intended for food purposes.

In humans, anabolic agents are contraindicated in patients with hepatic dysfunction, hypercalcemia, patients with a history of myocardial infarction (can cause hypercholesterolemia), pituitary insufficiency, prostate carcinoma, in selected patients with breast carcinoma, benign prostatic hypertrophy and during the nephrotic stage of nephritis.

Adverse Effects

In the manufacturer's (Equipoise®—Solvay) package insert, only androgenic (over aggressiveness) effects are listed. However, in work reported in both stallions and mares (Squires and McKinnon 1987), boldenone caused a detrimental effect in testis size, and sperm production and quality in stallions. In mares, the drug caused fewer total and large follicles, smaller ovaries, increased clitoral size, shortened estrus duration, reduced pregnancy rates and severely altered sexual behavior.

Although not reported in horses, anabolic steroids have the potential to cause hepatic toxicity.

Reproductive/Nursing Safety

The anabolic agents are category **X** (*Risk of use outweighs any possible benefit*) agents for use in pregnancy and are contraindicated because of possible fetal masculinization.

Overdosage/Acute Toxicity

No information was located for this specific agent. In humans, sodium and water retention can occur after overdosage of anabolic steroids. It is suggested to treat supportively and monitor liver function should an inadvertent overdose be administered.

Drug Interactions

No drug interactions were located for boldenone specifically. The following drug interactions have either been reported or are theoretical in humans or animals receiving anabolic steroids and may be of significance in veterinary patients:

▪ **ANTICOAGULANTS** (**warfarin**): Anabolic agents as a class may potentiate the effects of anticoagulants; monitoring of INR and dosage adjustment of the anticoagulant (if necessary) are recommended

▪ **CORTICOSTEROIDS, ACTH:** Anabolics may enhance the edema that can be associated with ACTH or adrenal steroid therapy

▪ **INSULIN:** Diabetic patients receiving insulin may need dosage adjustments if anabolic therapy is added or discontinued; anabolics may decrease blood glucose and decrease insulin requirements

Laboratory Considerations

▪ Concentrations of **protein bound iodine** (**PBI**) can be decreased in patients receiving androgen/anabolic therapy, but the clinical significance of this is probably not important

▪ Androgen/anabolic agents can decrease amounts of **thyroxine-binding globulin** and decrease **total T$_4$** concentrations and increase **resin uptake of T$_3$ and T$_4$**; free thyroid hormones are unaltered and, clinically, there is no evidence of dysfunction.

- Both **creatinine** and **creatine excretion** can be decreased by anabolic steroids
- Anabolic steroids can increase the urinary excretion of **17-ketosteroids**
- Androgenic/anabolic steroids may alter **blood glucose** levels.
- Androgenic/anabolic steroids may suppress **clotting factors II, V, VII, and X**.
- Anabolic agents can affect **liver function tests** (BSP retention, SGOT, SGPT, bilirubin, and alkaline phosphatase)

Doses

- **HORSES:** (**Note:** ARCI UCGFS Class 4 Drug)
  a) 1.1 mg/kg IM; may repeat in 3 week intervals (most horses will respond with one or two treatments) (Package Insert; *Equipoise®*—Fort Dodge)
  b) 1 mg/kg IM; repeated at 3 week intervals (Robinson 1987)

- **CATS:**
  a) As an appetite stimulant: 5 mg (total dose) IM/SC every 7 days; anabolic steroids not as effective as many other appetite stimulants and may be associated with hepatotoxicity (Bartges 2003)

Monitoring

- Androgenic side effects
- Fluid and electrolyte status, if indicated
- Liver function tests if indicated
- Red blood cell count, indices, if indicated
- Weight, appetite

Client Information

- Because of the potential for abuse by humans, anabolic steroids are controlled drugs. Boldenone should be kept in a secure area and out of the reach of children.
- Contact veterinarian of patient develops yellowing of whites of the eyes, or develops a decreased appetite or lethargy.

Chemistry/Synonyms

An injectable anabolic steroid derived from testosterone, boldenone undecylenate has a chemical name of 17 beta-hydroxyandrosta-1,4-dien-3-one. The commercially available product is in a sesame oil vehicle.

Boldenone undecylenate may also be known as: Ba-29038, boldenone undecenoate, *Equipoise®*, or *Vebonol®*.

Storage/Stability

Boldenone injection should be stored at room temperature; avoid freezing.

Compatibility/Compounding Considerations

Because boldenone injection is in an oil vehicle, it should not be physically mixed with any other medications.

Dosage Forms/Regulatory Status

VETERINARY-LABELED PRODUCTS:

Boldenone Undecylenate for Injection: 25 mg/mL in 10 mL vials; 50 mg/mL in 10 mL & 50 mL vials; *Equipoise®* (Pfizer); (Rx, C-III). FDA-approved for use in horses not to be used for food.

The ARCI (Racing Commissioners International) has designated this drug as a class 4 substance. See the appendix for more information.

HUMAN-LABELED PRODUCTS: None

References

Bartges, J (2003). Enteral Nutrition. Proceedings: World Small Animal Veterinary Assoc. World Congress. Accessed via: Veterinary Information Network. http://goo.gl/IZLCY

Robinson, NE (1987). Table of Common Drugs: Approximate Doses. *Current Therapy in Equine Medicine, 2*. NE Robinson Ed. Philadelphia, W.B. Saunders: 761.

BROMIDES
POTASSIUM BROMIDE
SODIUM BROMIDE

(*broe*-mide)

ANTICONVULSANT

Prescriber Highlights

▶ Primary or adjunctive therapy for seizure disorders in dogs; 3rd line agent for cats (some say contraindicated in cats)

▶ Very long half-life, must give loading dose to see therapeutic levels within a month

▶ Most prevalent adverse effect in dogs is sedation, especially when used with phenobarbital. Polyphagia with resultant weight gain is also commonly noted, particularly in the first few months of therapy. Polydipsia and polyuria can also be seen.

▶ Cats may develop adverse respiratory effects

▶ Therapeutic levels in dogs approximately 1–3 mg/mL

▶ Do not feed salty snacks; keep chloride in diet stable

▶ Toxic effects include profound sedation to stupor, ataxia, tremors, hind limb paresis, or other CNS manifestations

▶ If using sodium bromide (vs. potassium bromide), dosage adjustments must be made

Uses/Indications

Bromides are used both as primary therapy and as adjunctive therapy to control seizures in dogs that are not adequately controlled by phenobarbital (or primidone) alone (when steady state trough phenobarbital levels are >30 micrograms/mL for at least one month). While historically bromides were only recommended for use alone in patients suffering from phenobarbital (or primidone) hepatotoxicity, they have frequently been used as a drug of first choice in recent years. However, as more experience is gained in veterinary medicine with newer human anticonvulsants (e.g., zonisamide, levetiracetem, gabapentin) and their transition to less expensive generically available products, bromide use in dogs may become less prevalent.

Although not frequently used, bromides are also considered suitable by some for use in cats with chronic seizure disorders, but cats may be more susceptible to the drug's adverse effects.

Pharmacology/Actions

Bromide's anti-seizure activity is thought to be the result of its generalized depressant effects on neuronal excitability and activity. Bromide ions compete with chloride transport across cell membranes resulting in membrane hyperpolarization, thereby raising seizure threshold and limiting the spread of epileptic discharges.

Pharmacokinetics

Bromides are well absorbed after oral administration, primarily in the small intestine. Bromides are also well absorbed after solutions are administered rectally in dogs (bioavailability of 60–100%). Bromide is distributed in the extracellular fluid and mimics the volume of distribution of chloride (0.2–0.4 L/Kg). It is not bound to plasma proteins and readily enters the CSF (in dogs: 87% of serum concentration; in humans: 37%). Bromides enter maternal milk (see Reproductive Safety below). Bromides are principally excreted by the kidneys. The half-life in dogs has been reported to be from 16–25 days; cats, 10 days; and humans, 12 days.

Contraindications/Precautions/Warnings

Older animals and those with additional diseases, may be prone to intolerance (see Adverse Effects below) at blood levels that are easily tolerable by younger, healthier dogs. Patients with renal dysfunction may need dosage adjustments.

Because bromides have been associated with sometimes serious pulmonary effects in cats, it should be used with extreme caution. Some state that the drug should not be used in cats.

Adverse Effects

A transient sedation (lasting up to 3 weeks) is commonly seen in dogs receiving bromides. Serum concentrations of bromide above 15 mMol/L (150 mg/dL) are considered "toxic" by some, but many dogs apparently tolerate levels of up to 30 mMol/L. Toxicity generally presents as profound sedation to stupor, ataxia, tremors, hind limb paresis, or other CNS manifestations. Pancreatitis has been reported in dogs receiving combination therapy of bromides with either primidone or phenobarbital; however, since this effect has been reported with both primidone and phenobarbital, its direct relationship with bromide is unknown. Additional potential adverse effects reported include: polyphagia with weight gain, polydipsia, polyuria, anorexia, vomiting, and constipation. Feeding a low calorie diet may help prevent weight gain. Pruritic dermatitis and paradoxical hyperactivity are rarely reported.

If administering an oral loading dose of potassium bromide, acute GI upset may occur if given too rapidly. Potentially, large loading doses could affect serum potassium levels in patients receiving potassium bromide.

If the patient cannot tolerate the gastrointestinal effects (vomiting) of potassium bromide and divided doses with food do not alleviate the problem, switching to sodium bromide may be tried.

Lower respiratory effects (cough, dyspnea) have been associated with bromide therapy in cats. Peribronchial infiltrates may be seen on radiographs and dyspnea may be serious or fatal. Signs appear to be reversible in most cats once bromides are discontinued. Other adverse effects in cats include polydipsia, sedation, and weight gain.

Reproductive/Nursing Safety

Reproductive safety has not been established. Human infants have suffered bromide intoxication and growth retardation after maternal ingestion of bromides during pregnancy. Bromide intoxication has also been reported in human infants breastfeeding from mothers taking bromides. Use with caution in pregnancy or lactation.

Overdosage/Acute Toxicity

Toxicity is more likely with chronic overdoses, but acute overdoses are a possibility. In addition to the adverse effects noted above, animals that have developed bromism (whether acute or chronic) may develop signs of muscle pain, conscious proprioceptive deficits, anisocoria, and hyporeflexia.

Standard gut removal techniques should be employed after a known acute overdose. Death after an acute oral ingestion is apparently rare as vomiting generally occurs spontaneously. Administration of parenteral (0.9% sodium chloride) or oral sodium chloride, parenteral glucose and diuretics (e.g., furosemide) may be helpful in reducing bromide loads in either acutely or chronically intoxicated individuals.

Drug Interactions

The following drug interactions have either been reported or are theoretical in humans or animals receiving bromides and may be of significance in veterinary patients:

■ **CNS SEDATING DRUGS:** Because bromides can cause sedation, other CNS sedating drugs may cause additive sedation

■ **DIURETICS (furosemide, thiazides):** May

enhance the excretion of bromides thereby affecting seizure control and dosage requirements

■ **LOW/HIGH SALT DIETS:** Bromide toxicity can occur if chloride ion ingestion is markedly reduced. Patients put on low salt diets may be at risk. Conversely, additional sodium chloride in the diet (including prescription diets high in chloride) could reduce serum bromide levels, affecting seizure control. Keep chloride content of diet relatively constant while bromides are being administered. If chloride content must be altered, monitor bromide levels more frequently.

■ **DRUGS THAT CAN LOWER SEIZURE THRESHOLD** (*e.g.*, **xylazine**): May potentially reduce efficacy of antiseizure medications

Laboratory Considerations

■ See drug interactions above regarding chloride. Bromide may interfere with **serum chloride** determinations yielding falsely high results.

■ Potassium bromide does not affect canine thyroid function test results

Doses

Note: Doses are listed for potassium bromide. If using sodium bromide reduce dose by approximately 15%.

■ **DOGS:**

Because of the extraordinarily long serum half-life in dogs, (it may take up to 4–5 months for blood levels to reach steady state concentrations), many dosing regimens include an initial oral bolus loading dose to reduce the period to attain therapeutic concentrations. An excellent review of treating idiopathic epilepsy in dogs and cats has been published (Thomas 2010). In this review, with respect to dosing bromides the author states: "Because of the variability in absorption, distribution, and speed of metabolism among patients, published dose recommendations serve as a general guide only. Because of sensitivity to side effects and lack of prior metabolic induction, most new patients are started at the lower end of the dose range. If necessary, the dose is slowly titrated upward until seizures are controlled or the maximum tolerated dose is reached. On the other hand, patients with frequent or severe seizures are often best managed by starting at the higher end of the dose range or using a loading dose. Once the seizures are controlled, the dose may need to be adjusted downward to minimize side effects."

a) Initially, potassium bromide: 20–30 mg/kg PO once daily, with food. If sodium bromide used, decrease dose by 15% (*i.e.*, 17–26 mg/kg). The dose is subsequently adjusted based on clinical effects and therapeutic monitoring (see Monitoring below).

A loading dose may be used to obtain target serum concentrations sooner, particularly in patients with frequent seizures or if phenobarbital must be rapidly withdrawn. Several protocols published; author's preference is: 400 mg/kg PO divided into 8 doses given over a 48-hour period (*i.e.*, 50 mg/kg every 6 hours for 2 days.) Giving entire loading dose at once will usually cause vomiting. Once loading dose given, start maintenance dose.

When bromide is added to phenobarbital to improve seizure control, the current phenobarbital dose is continued while maintenance dosing of bromide is started. After 3 months, if seizures well controlled and the serum concentration of bromide is at least 1.5 mg/mL, it may be possible to taper the phenobarbital, decreasing the dose in 25% increments every 2 to 4 weeks. If seizures become more frequent during phenobarb withdrawal, patient may require both drugs. If phenobarbital must be withdrawn quickly, a loading dose of bromide is administered and the phenobarbital is tapered over a 2-week period while maintenance doses of bromide are administered. (Thomas 2010)

b) For seizures: Loading dose: 400–600 mg/kg/day divided and given with food. May be given over 24 hours or more gradually over 5 days. Then go to initial maintenance dose: 20–30 mg/kg PO once daily (Munana 2004a)

c) A good starting dose is 35 mg/kg PO once daily, but the author often uses a loading dose: 125 mg/kg/day for 5 days PO divided q12h and then resume at 35 mg/kg PO once daily. For dogs where oral administration is not possible (*e.g.*, status epilepticus), may give rectally at 100 mg/kg body weight every 4 hours for 6 total doses. (Dewey 2005)

d) Using an intravenous *sodium bromide* loading dose to rapidly achieve minimum therapeutic concentration (1–1.5 mg/mL): Intravenous, 600–1200 mg/kg, diluted in a solution and administered over eight hours. If target serum bromide concentrations are not reached, additional intravenous sodium bromide may be administered. (USPC 2005) (**Note:** It has been anecdotally reported that a 3% solution of sodium bromide can be used intravenously. To prepare a 3% solution: add 30 grams of sodium bromide to 1000 mL of sterile water for injection; use an in-line IV filter. Use with caution—Plumb)

■ **CATS:**

a) As third choice (after phenobarbital and

diazepam) therapy of refractory seizures: 10–20 mg/kg/day PO. Follow same
guideline as dogs (Quesnel 2000)

b) As second line therapy for epilepsy:
30 mg/kg PO once daily (Munana 2004b)

Monitoring

■ Efficacy/Toxicity

■ Serum Levels. In dogs, therapeutic bromide
concentrations are generally agreed to be
1–3 mg/mL; lower range may be effective
for dogs on phenobarbital therapy and the
higher range for dogs on bromide alone.
Time of day (hours post-dose) for sampling
is not critical. Actual monitoring recommendations vary and depend on whether
the patient received a loading dose or not.
One recommendation (Boothe 2004) based
upon pharmacokinetic principles is: If no
load was given and maintenance dose was
used initially, monitor at 3–4 weeks and
then at steady-state (2.5–3 months). The
first sample indicates about 50% of what
will be achieved at steady-state and allows
adjustment of the dosage early. If a loading
dose was used, an immediate level after the
load (day 6 or 7 after a 5 day loading protocol), followed by a sample at 1 month
and then 3 months. The immediate sample
indicates what was achieved with loading;
the 1 month level indicates the success of
the maintenance dose, maintains what was
achieved with the loading dose and allows
dosage adjustment, if required; and the 3
month level establishes the new baseline.

Client Information

■ Clients must be committed to administering doses of anticonvulsant medications on
a regular basis. Lack of good compliance
with dosing regimens is a major cause of
therapeutic failures with anti-seizure medications. If a dose is missed, give it when remembered; a dose may be doubled the next
day, but should preferably be separated by
several hours to reduce the chance for gastrointestinal upset.

■ Clients should also understand and accept
that this treatment involves using a non-
approved (FDA) "drug."

■ Dose measurements of bromide solutions
should be done with a needle-less syringe or
other accurate measuring device. The dose
may either be sprinkled on the dog's food
(assuming he/she consumes it entirely) or
squirted in the side of the mouth.

■ Toxic effects (*e.g.*, profound sedation, ataxia,
stupor, GI effects) should be explained to
the owner and if they occur, they should be
reported to the veterinarian.

■ Dogs that cannot tolerate the gastrointestinal effects (vomiting) of potassium chloride
with single daily doses may better tolerate

doses divided through the day given with
food. Clients should not alter diet without
first consulting with veterinarian and to
avoid giving dogs salty treats (*e.g.*, pig ears).

Chemistry

Potassium bromide occurs as white, odorless, cubical crystals or crystalline powder. One
gram will dissolve in 1.5 mL of water. Potassium
bromide contains 67.2% bromide. Each gram
contains 8.4 mEq (mMol) of potassium and
bromide.

Sodium bromide occurs as white, odorless,
cubic crystals or granular powder. One gram will
dissolve in 1.2 mL of water. Sodium bromide
contains 77.7% bromide.

Because of the different molecular weights of
sodium and potassium, with respect to actual
bromide content, sodium bromide solutions of
250 mg/mL contain about 20% more bromide
than potassium bromide 250 mg/mL solution.
This is generally not clinically significant unless
changing from one salt to another for a given
patient.

Storage/Stability

Store in tight containers. Solutions may be
stored for up to one year in clear or brown,
glass or plastic containers at room temperature.
Refrigerating the solution may help reduce the
chance for microbial growth, but may cause
crystals or precipitants to form. Should precipitation occur, warming the solution should resolubolize the bromide.

Compatibility/Compounding Considerations

Bromides can precipitate out alkaloids in solution. Mixing with strong oxidizing agents can
liberate bromine. Metal salts can precipitate solutions containing bromides. Sodium bromide
is hygroscopic; potassium bromide is not.

At a concentration of 250 mg/mL, 25 grams
of potassium bromide are weighed and add a
sufficient amount of distilled water to a final
volume of 100 mL; potassium bromide dissolves
easily in water, sodium bromide may take longer
to dissolve. Flavoring agents are not usually necessary for patient acceptance.

Dosage Forms/Regulatory Status

At the time of writing, neither potassium or sodium bromide are available in FDA-approved
dosage forms in North America. Reagent grade
or USP grade may be obtained from various
chemical supply houses to compound an acceptable oral product. If purchasing a reagent grade,
specify American Chemical Society (ACS) grade.

References

Boothe, DM (2004). Bromide: The "old" new anticonvul-
sant. Proceedings: WSAVA. Accessed via: Veterinary
Information Network. http://goo.gl/F9Pvm
Dewey, C (2005). Managing the Seizure Patient.
Proceedings: IVECCS. Accessed via: Veterinary
Information Network. http://goo.gl/rmkrc
Munana, K (2004a). Managing the Epileptic Dog.
Proceedings: ACVIM Forum, Minneapolis. Accessed
via: Veterinary Information Network. http://goo.gl/
LcOO8

Munana, K (2004b). Seizures and cats. Proceedings: ACVIM Forum, Minneapolis. Accessed via: Veterinary Information Network. http://goo.gl/GwiPW

Quesnel, A (2000). Seizures. *Textbook of Veterinary Internal Medicine: Diseases of the Dog and Cat.* S Ettinger and E Feldman Eds. Philadelphia, WB Saunders. **1**: 148–152.

Thomas, W (2010). Idiopathic epilepsy in dogs and cats. *Vet Clin NA: Sm Anim Pract* **40**(1): 161–179.

USPC (2005). "Bromide (Veterinary–Systemic)." *USP Veterinary Pharmaceutical Information Monographs.* 2007.

BROMOCRIPTINE MESYLATE

(broe-moe-*krip*-teen)   Parlodel®

DOPAMINE AGONIST/PROLACTIN INHIBITOR

Prescriber Highlights

▶ Dopamine agonist & prolactin inhibitor occasionally used in dogs for pregnancy termination or pseudopregnancy; in horses for pituitary adenomas; in cats for acromegaly

▶ Many adverse effects possible; GI, CNS depression & hypotension are most likely; much more likely to cause emesis in dogs than cabergoline

▶ Interferes with lactation

Uses/Indications

Bromocriptine may potentially be of benefit in treating acromegaly/pituitary adenomas or pseudopregnancy in a variety of species. However, because of adverse effects, its potential value for treating hyperadrenocorticism in dogs is low. It has been used in dogs for pregnancy termination and pseudopregnancy.

Pharmacology/Actions

Bromocriptine exhibits multiple pharmacologic actions. It inhibits prolactin release from the anterior pituitary thereby reducing serum prolactin. The mechanism for this action is by a direct effect on the pituitary and/or stimulating postsynaptic dopamine receptors in the hypothalamus to cause release of prolactin-inhibitory factor. Bromocriptine also activates dopaminergic receptors in the neostriatum of the brain.

Pharmacokinetics

In humans, only about 28% of a bromocriptine dose is absorbed from the gut and, due to a high first-pass effect, only about 6% reaches the systemic circulation. Distribution characteristics are not well described but in humans, it is highly bound (90–96%) to serum albumin. Bromocriptine is metabolized by the liver to inactive and non-toxic metabolites. It has a biphasic half-life; the alpha phase is about 4 hours and the terminal phase is about 15 hours, but one source says 45–50 hours.

Contraindications/Precautions/Warnings

Bromocriptine is generally contraindicated in patients with hypertension. It should be used with caution in patients with hepatic disease as metabolism of the drug may be reduced.

Adverse Effects

Bromocriptine may cause a plethora of adverse effects that are usually dose related and minimized with dosage reduction. Some more likely possibilities include: gastrointestinal effects (nausea, vomiting), nervous system effects (sedation, fatigue, etc.), and hypotension (particularly with the first dose, but it may persist). At dosages used in dogs, more likely to cause emesis than cabergoline.

Reproductive/Nursing Safety

Usage during pregnancy is contraindicated in humans, although documented teratogenicity has not been established.

Because bromocriptine interferes with lactation, it should not be used in animals that are nursing.

Overdosage/Acute Toxicity

Overdosage may cause vomiting, severe nausea, and profound hypotension. There were 20 exposures to bromocriptine reported to the ASPCA Animal Poison Control Center (APCC) during 2008–2009. In these cases, all 20 were dogs with 18 showing clinical signs. Common findings in dogs recorded in decreasing frequency included vomiting, trembling, diarrhea, subdued, and tachycardia. Standardized gut removal techniques should be employed when applicable, but emesis often occurs spontaneously. Institute cardiovascular monitoring (blood pressure, heart rate) and support as needed.

Drug Interactions

The following drug interactions have either been reported or are theoretical in humans or animals receiving bromocriptine and may be of significance in veterinary patients:

◼ **ALCOHOL:** Use with alcohol may cause a disulfiram-type reaction

◼ **BUTYROPHENONES (e.g., haloperidol, azaperone), AMITRIPTYLINE, PHENOTHIAZINES, and RESERPINE:** May increase prolactin concentrations and bromocriptine doses may need to be increased

◼ **CYCLOSPORINE:** May elevate cyclosporine levels

◼ **ERYTHROMYCIN, CLARITHROMYCIN:** May increase bromocriptine levels

◼ **ESTROGENS or PROGESTINS:** May interfere with the effects of bromocriptine

◼ **ERGOT ALKALOIDS:** Use of bromocriptine and ergot alkaloids is not recommended; some human patients receiving both have developed severe hypertension and myocardial infarction

◼ **HYPOTENSIVE MEDICATIONS:** May cause additive hypotension if used with bromocriptine

◼ **MAO INHIBITORS** (including **amitraz,** and maybe **selegiline**): Avoid use of bromocriptine with these compounds

■ **METOCLOPRAMIDE:** May cause prolactin release in dogs, thereby negating the effects of bromocriptine for treating pseudopregnancy

■ **OCTREOTIDE:** May increase bromocriptine levels

■ **SYMPATHOMIMETICS** (*e.g.,* **phenylpropanolamine**): Enhanced bromocriptine effects have been reported in humans (rare), including ventricular tachycardia and cardiac dysfunction

Doses

■ **DOGS:**

For treatment of pseudocyesis (pseudopregnancy):

a) 10–100 micrograms/kg PO daily in divided doses until lactation ceases. Vomiting, depression and anorexia are common side effects, usually more problematic than the lactation. (Davidson & Feldman 2005)

b) 10–100 micrograms/kg PO twice daily for 10–14 days. Vomiting is very common; reducing dose and administering after meals may help. (Johnson 2003)

c) 10–50 micrograms/kg PO at least twice a day (Romagnoli 2009)

For pregnancy termination after mismating:

a) From day 35–45 after LH surge 50–100 micrograms/kg PO or IM twice daily for 4–7 days. Not uniformly effective and may cause vomiting at this dosage (a peripheral acting antiemetic 30 minutes before dose may be helpful) (Verstegen 2000)

b) As an abortifacient 25 days after LH surge: Cloprostenol at 1 microgram/kg SC q48 hours (every other day) plus bromocriptine at 30 micrograms/kg PO q24h (every day) (Johnson 2003)

■ **CATS:**

For adjunctive treatment of acromegaly:

a) Initial dose of 0.2 mg (total dose); may reduce insulin requirements (Jones 2004)

■ **HORSES: (Note:** ARCI UCGFS Class 2 Drug)

For treatment of pituitary adenoma:

a) 0.03–0.09 mg/kg (30–90 micrograms/kg) twice daily PO or SC, but its use is limited (Toribio 2004)

b) 5 mg (total dose) IM q12h. To prepare an injectable formulation for IM use from oral dosage forms: Bromocriptine mesylate 70 mg is added to 7 mL of a solution of 80% normal saline and 20% absolute alcohol (v/v). Final concentration is 1% (10 mg/mL) (Beck 1992)

Monitoring

■ Monitoring is dependent upon the reason for use to evaluate efficacy. However, blood pressures should be evaluated if patients have clinical signs associated with hypotension.

Client Information

■ Have client administer drug with food to attempt to reduce GI adverse effects.

Chemistry/Synonyms

A dopamine agonist and prolactin inhibitor, bromocriptine mesylate is a semisynthetic ergot alkaloid derivative. It occurs as a yellowish-white powder and is slightly soluble in water and sparingly soluble in alcohol.

Bromocriptine mesylate may also be known as: bromocryptine, brom-ergocryptine, 2-bromergocryptine, 2-bromocriptine methanesulphonate, bromocriptini mesilas, 2-bromo-alpha-ergocriptine mesylate, 2-bromoergocryptine monomethanesulfonate, or CB-154 (bromocriptine); many trade names are available.

Storage/Stability

Tablets and capsules should be protected from light and stored in tight containers at temperatures less than 25°C.

Dosage Forms/Regulatory Status

VETERINARY-LABELED PRODUCTS: None

The ARCI (Racing Commissioners International) has designated this drug as a class 2 substance. See the appendix for more information.

HUMAN-LABELED PRODUCTS:

Bromocriptine Mesylate Oral Capsules: 5 mg (as base); *Parlodel*® (Novartis); generic; (Rx)

Bromocriptine Mesylate Oral Tablets: 0.8 mg (as base); *Cycloset*® (Patheon); 2.5 mg; *Parlodel*® *SnapTabs* (Novartis); generic; (Rx)

References

Beck, D (1992). Effective long–term tratment of a suspected pituitary adenoma in a pony. *Equine Vet Educ* 4(3): 119–122.

Davidson, A & E Feldman (2005). Ovarian and Estrous Cycle Abnormalities. *Textbook of Veterinary Internal Medicine, 6th Ed.* S Ettinger and E Feldman Eds., Elsevier: 1649–1655.

Johnson, C (2003). Reproductive system disorders. *Small Animal Internal Medicine 3rd Ed.* R Nelson and C Couto Eds. Philadelphia, Mosby: 847–945.

Jones, B (2004). Less common feline endocrinopathies. Proceedings: WSAVA. Accessed via: Veterinary Information Network. http://goo.gl/Hsow1

Romagnoli, S (2009). An update on pseudopregnancy. Proceedings: WSAVA.

Toribio, R (2004). Pars intermedia dysfunction (Equine Cushing's Disease). *Equine Internal Medicine 2nd Edition.* M Reed, W Bayly and D Sellon Eds. Phila, Saunders: 1327–1340.

Verstegen, J (2000). Overview of mismating regimens for the bitch. *Kirk's Current Veterinary Therapy: XIII Small Animal Practice.* J Bonagura Ed. Philadelphia, WB Saunders: 947–954.

BUDESONIDE

(bue-*des*-oh-nide) Entocort EC®

GLUCOCORTICOID

Prescriber Highlights

▶ Orally administered glucocorticoid with limited systemic glucocorticoid effects; may be useful in treating IBD in small animals that are either refractory to, or intolerant of, systemic steroids

▶ Hyperadrenocorticism possible, but much less likely then with systemic steroids

▶ Limited veterinary experience

▶ Drug interactions (CYP3A inhibitors, antacids)

▶ Expense may be an issue; may need to be compounded to smaller dosage strengths

Uses/Indications

While there are inhalational forms of the medication for treating asthma or allergic rhinitis, most veterinary interest involves its potential oral use to treat inflammatory intestinal diseases in small animals that are either refractory to, or intolerant of, systemic steroids. In humans, oral budesonide is indicated for Crohn's disease.

Pharmacology/Actions

Budesonide is a potent glucocorticoid (15X more potent than prednisolone) with high topical activity. It has weak mineralocorticoid activity. By delaying dissolution until reaching the duodenum and subsequent controlled release of the drug, the drug can exert its topical antiinflammatory activity in the intestines. While the drug is absorbed from the gut into the portal circulation, it has a high first-pass metabolism effect through the liver that reduces systemic blood levels and resultant glucocorticoid effects of the drug. However, significant suppression of the HPA-axis does occur in patients taking the drug.

Pharmacokinetics

Budesonide's pharmacokinetics have been reported in dogs. The drug has a bioavailability of 10–20%. When dosed at 10 micrograms/kg, half-life is about 2 hours and clearance 2.2 L/hr/kg. At 100 micrograms/kg, half-life is slightly prolonged to 2–3 hours.

Upon oral administration of the commercially available product in humans, budesonide is nearly completely absorbed from the gut, but time to achieve peak concentrations are widely variable (30–600 minutes). The presence of food in the gut may delay absorption, but does not impact the amount of drug absorbed. Because of a high first-pass effect, only about 10% of a dose is systemically bioavailable in healthy adults. In patients with Crohn's disease, oral bioavailability may be twice that initially, but with further dosing, reduces to amounts similar to healthy subjects. Budesonide's mean volume of distribution in humans ranges from 2.2–3.9 L/kg. The drug is completely metabolized and these metabolites are excreted in the feces and urine. Budesonide's terminal half-life is about 4 hours.

Contraindications/Precautions/Warnings

Budesonide is contraindicated in patients hypersensitive to it. Because budesonide can cause systemic corticosteroid effects, it should be used with caution in any patient where glucocorticoid therapy may be problematic including those with GI ulcers, active infections, diabetes mellitus, or cataracts.

Adverse Effects

There are limited reports of the clinical use of budesonide in small animals and the determination of the drug's adverse effect profile is ongoing. Steroid hepatopathy is possible. In humans, oral budesonide is generally well tolerated and glucocorticoid adverse effects occur infrequently when the drug is used for courses of therapy of no more than 8 weeks duration. Patients with moderate to severe hepatic dysfunction may be more likely to develop signs associated with hypercorticism.

Because budesonide does suppress the HPA-axis, animals undergoing stressful procedures such as surgery, should be considered for exogenous steroid administration.

Reproductive/Nursing Safety

In humans, the FDA categorizes budesonide as a category *C* drug for use during pregnancy (*Animal studies have shown an adverse effect on the fetus, but there are no adequate studies in humans; or there are no animal reproduction studies and no adequate studies in humans*). Like other corticosteroids, budesonide has been demonstrated to be embryocidal and teratogenic in rats and rabbits.

Specific data on budesonide levels in maternal milk are not available and the manufacturer warns against use by nursing women; however, because of the drugs high first pass effect, the amounts are unlikely to be of clinical significance to nursing animal offspring.

Overdosage/Acute Toxicity

Acute, oral overdoses are unlikely to be of much concern although doses of 200 mg/kg were lethal in mice. Gut evacuation should be considered for massive overdoses.

Drug Interactions

The following drug interactions have either been reported or are theoretical in humans or animals receiving budesonide and may be of significance in veterinary patients:

■ **ERYTHROMYCIN, CIMETIDINE, KETOCONAZOLE, ITRACONAZOLE, FLUCONAZOLE, DILTIAZEM, GRAPEFRUIT JUICE POWDER,** etc: Because the hepatic enzyme CYP3A extensively metabolizes budesonide, drugs that inhibit this isoenzyme can significantly increase the amount of drug that enters the systemic circulation. Ketoconazole given with budesonide may increase the area under the curve (AUC) of budesonide by eight fold.

■ **ORAL ANTACIDS:** Because the dissolution of the drug's coating is pH dependent, oral antacids should not be given at the same time as the drug. Other drugs that potentially would increase gastric pH (*e.g.*, omeprazole, ranitidine, etc.) apparently do not significantly impact the oral pharmacokinetics of the drug.

Laboratory Considerations

■ While no specific laboratory interactions were located, budesonide could potentially alter laboratory test results similarly to other corticosteroids.

Doses

■ **DOGS**

For treatment of IBD:

a) 1 mg (total dose) PO once daily for small dogs and 2 mg (total dose) PO once daily for large dogs (Mackin 2002)

b) 3 mg/m^2 (NOT mg/kg) (0.5–3 mg per dog depending on body weight) PO once daily or every other day (Gaschen 2006)

■ **CATS:**

For treatment of IBD:

a) 1 mg (total dose) PO once daily (Mackin 2002)

b) 1 mg per cat PO once to twice daily. Main reason for use is in cats that respond to steroids, but cannot tolerate their systemic side effects. (Willard 2009)

Monitoring

■ Efficacy

■ Adverse effects

Client Information

■ Do not open the capsule unless your veterinarian instructs you to do so; do not crush or allow animal to chew capsules

■ This drug must be given as prescribed to be effective, do not stop therapy without contacting your veterinarian

■ If animal exhibits increased thirst or appetite or their coat changes, contact your veterinarian

Chemistry/Synonyms

Budesonide, a non-halogenated glucocorticoid, occurs as a white to off-white, odorless, tasteless powder. It is practically insoluble in water, freely soluble in chloroform and sparingly soluble in alcohol. The commercially available capsules contain a granulized micronized form of the drug that is coated to protect from dissolution in gastric juice, but will dissolve at pH >5.5. In humans, this pH usually corresponds with the drug reaching the duodenum.

Budesonide may also be known as S 1320, *Entocord®*, *Entocort EC®*, *Pulmicort®*, and *Rhinocort®*.

Storage/Stability

Budesonide oral capsules should be stored in tight containers at room temperature. Exposures to temperatures as low as 15°C (59°F) and as high as 30°C (86°F) are permitted.

Compatibility/Compounding Considerations

If reformulating into smaller capsules, do not alter (damage) the micronized enteric-coated sugar spheres inside of the capsules.

Dosage Forms/Regulatory Status

VETERINARY-LABELED PRODUCTS: None.

HUMAN-LABELED PRODUCTS:

Budesonide Capsules: 3 mg (micronized); *Entocort EC®* (Prometheus); (Rx)

Human budesonide capsules may need to be compounded into dosage strengths suitable for dogs or cats, but the enteric-coated sugar spheres found inside the capsule should not be altered or damaged.

There are also budesonide products (powder and suspension for oral inhalation, and nasal sprays) for the treatment of asthma or allergic rhinitis. Trade names for these products include *Pulmicort®* and *Rhinocort®*.

References

Gaschen, F (2006). Small Intestinal Diarrhea—Causes and Treatment. Proceedings: WSAVA. Accessed via: Veterinary Information Network. http://goo.gl/eKjft

Mackin, A (2002). Practical use of glucocorticoids. Proceedings: ACVIM. Accessed via: Veterinary Information Network. http://goo.gl/DBiRF

Willard, M (2009). Canine and Feline Diarrheas: Diagnosis/Management of Infiltrative Disorders. Proceedings: ACVIM.

BUPRENORPHINE HCL

(byoo-pre-*nor*-feen)   Buprenex®, Subutex®

OPIATE PARTIAL AGONIST

Prescriber Highlights

▶ Partial *mu* opiate agonist used primarily as an injectable & buccal analgesic in small animals, especially cats; has been used in horses also

▶ Often used, especially in cats, as a component of short-term immobilization "cocktails" in combination with an alpha-2 agonist (*e.g.*, dexmedetomidine) with a dissociative agent (*e.g.*, ketamine)

▶ Buccal administration in cats well tolerated & effective

▶ Rarely, may cause respiratory depression

▶ At standard doses, naloxone may not completely reverse respiratory depressant effects in overdoses

Uses/Indications

Buprenorphine is most often used as an analgesic for mild to moderate pain in small animals. In many species, it is not as an effective analgesic as pure *mu*-agonists (morphine, hydromorphone, etc.), but it generally causes fewer adverse effects. In cats, buccal (oral transmucosal) administration is often a practical, effective method for helping to control post-operative pain and it may provide better analgesia in cats than does parenteral morphine or oxymorphone. One study however, found that IV or IM buprenorphine provided better post-operative (OHE) analgesia than when the drug was administered SC or via the oral transmucosal route (Giordano *et al.* 2010). Combining opiates with short-term NSAIDs for post-op pain control is being used more commonly.

For acute pain control, buprenorphine may have the disadvantage of a longer onset of action than other opiates.

Buprenorphine has been used in horses, but its short duration of action and expense relative to other opiates limit its usefulness.

Pharmacology/Actions

Buprenorphine has partial agonist activity at the *mu*-receptor. This is in contrast to pentazocine that acts as an antagonist at the *mu*-receptor. Buprenorphine is considered 30 times as potent as morphine and exhibits many of the same actions as the opiate agonists. It produces a dose-related analgesia but at higher dosages analgesic effects may actually decrease. Buprenorphine appears to have a high affinity for *mu*-receptors in the CNS, which may explain its relatively long duration of action. Analgesia may persist for 12 hours, but usually a 6–8 hour duration of analgesic effect is typical.

The cardiovascular effects of buprenorphine may cause a decrease in both blood pressure and cardiac rate. Rarely, human patients may exhibit increases in blood pressure and cardiac rate. Respiratory depression is a possibility, and decreased respiratory rates have been noted in horses treated with buprenorphine. Gastrointestinal effects appear to be minimal in cats treated with buprenorphine.

Pharmacokinetics

Buprenorphine is rapidly absorbed following IM injection, with 40–90% absorbed systemically when tested in humans. The drug is also absorbed sublingually (bioavailability≈55%) in people. Oral doses appear to undergo a high first-pass effect with metabolism occurring in the GI mucosa and liver.

The distribution of the drug has not been well studied. Data from work done in rats reflects that buprenorphine concentrates in the liver, but is also found in the brain, GI tract, and placenta. It is highly bound (96%) to plasma proteins (not albumin), crosses the placenta, and it and its metabolites are found in maternal milk at concentrations equal to or greater than those found in plasma.

Buprenorphine is metabolized in the liver by N-dealkylation and glucuronidation. These metabolites are then eliminated by biliary excretion into the feces (≈70%) and urinary excretion (≈27%).

In cats, buprenorphine has a volume of distribution [Vd(ss)] of approximately 8 L/kg and a clearance of about 20 mL/kg/min. Elimination half-life is about 6–7 hours. When administered via oral mucosa (liquid placed into the side of cat's mouth), absorption was comparable to that seen with IM or IV administration. Subcutaneous administration may be less bioavailable and clinically effective than transmucosal administration. Human transdermal patch buprenorphine (*Transtac*®—Napp Pharm.; UK) applied to cats has demonstrated widely variable blood levels and without a loading dose does not appear to provide adequate analgesia.

In dogs, oral transmucosal administered buprenorphine is about 50% absorbed. The differences in oral mucosal bioavailability compared with cats may be a result of the pH differences in the oral cavity of each species; cats have a more alkaline oral pH.

In the horse, onset of action is approximately 15 minutes after IV dosing. The drug is very well absorbed after sublingual administration. The peak effect occurs in 30–45 minutes and the duration of action may last up to 8 hours. Elimination half-life after an IV dose is about 6 hours. Because acepromazine exhibits a similar onset and duration of action, many equine clinicians favor using this drug in combination with buprenorphine.

Contraindications/Precautions/Warnings

All opiates should be used with caution in patients with hypothyroidism, severe renal insufficiency, adrenocortical insufficiency (Addison's), and in geriatric or severely debilitated patients.

Rarely, patients may develop respiratory depression from buprenorphine; it, therefore, should be used cautiously in patients with compromised cardiopulmonary function. Like other opiates, buprenorphine must be used with extreme caution in patients with head trauma, increased CSF pressure or other CNS dysfunction (*e.g.*, coma).

Patients with severe hepatic dysfunction may eliminate the drug more slowly than normal patients. Buprenorphine may increase bile duct pressure and should be used cautiously in patients with biliary tract disease.

The drug is contraindicated in patients having known hypersensitivity to it.

Adverse Effects

Although rare, respiratory depression appears to be the major adverse effect to monitor for with buprenorphine; other adverse effects (sedation) may be noted. The primary side effect seen in humans is sedation with an incidence of approximately 66%. May cause urine retention or difficulty voiding, particularly with high IV doses or epidural administration.

In cats, buprenorphine is usually very well tolerated with GI effects (vomiting) only rarely been reported; hyperthermia does not appear to be a problem.

In horses, buprenorphine may cause some excitement and diminished gut sounds, but colic has not been a major concern.

Reproductive/Nursing Safety

Although no controlled studies have been performed in domestic animals or humans, the drug has exhibited no evidence of teratogenicity or causing impaired fertility in laboratory animals. In humans, the FDA categorizes this drug as category *C* for use during pregnancy (*Animal studies have shown an adverse effect on the fetus, but there are no adequate studies in humans; or there are no animal reproduction studies and no adequate studies in humans.*)

Overdosage/Acute Toxicity

The intraperitoneal LD_{50} of buprenorphine has been reported to be 243 mg/kg in rats. The ratio of lethal dose to effective dose is at least 1000:1 in rodents. Because of the apparent high index of safety, life-threatening acute overdoses should be a rare event in veterinary medicine, but most overdoses will cause signs. There were 55 exposures to buprenorphine reported to the ASPCA Animal Poison Control Center (APCC) during 2008-2009. In these cases, 34 were dogs with 25 showing clinical signs, and 20 were cats with 6 showing clinical signs. The 1 remaining case was a lagomorph that showed clinical signs. Common findings in dogs recorded in decreas-

ing frequency included vocalization, ataxia, hypersalivation, hypothermia, and lethargy.

Treatment with naloxone and doxapram have been suggested in cases of acute overdoses causing respiratory or cardiac effects. Secondary to buprenorphine's high affinity for the *mu* receptor, high doses of naloxone may be required to treat respiratory depression.

Drug Interactions

The following drug interactions have either been reported or are theoretical in humans or animals receiving buprenorphine and may be of significance in veterinary patients:

- **ANESTHETICS, LOCAL (mepivacaine, bupivacaine):** May be potentiated by concomitant use of buprenorphine

- **ANTICONVULSANTS (phenobarbital, phenytoin):** May decrease plasma buprenorphine levels

- **BENZODIAZEPINES:** Case reports of humans developing respiratory/cardiovascular/CNS depression; use with caution

- **CNS DEPRESSANTS (*e.g.*, anesthetic agents, antihistamines, phenothiazines, barbiturates, tranquilizers, alcohol, etc.):** May cause increased CNS or respiratory depression when used with buprenorphine

- **ERYTHROMYCIN:** Can increase plasma buprenorphine levels

- **FENTANYL** (and other **pure opiate agonists**): Buprenorphine may potentially antagonize some analgesic effects (**Note:** *This is controversial*), but may also reverse some of the sedative and respiratory depressant effects of pure agonists

- **HALOTHANE:** Potentially can increase buprenorphine effects

- **KETOCONAZOLE, ITRACONAZOLE, FLUCONAZOLE:** Can increase plasma buprenorphine levels

- **MONAMINE OXIDASE (MAO) INHIBITORS (*e.g.*, selegiline, amitraz):** Possible additive effects or increased CNS depression

- **NALOXONE:** May reduce analgesia associated with high dose buprenorphine

- **PANCURONIUM:** If used with buprenorphine may cause increased conjunctival changes

- **RIFAMPIN:** Potentially decrease plasma buprenorphine concentrations

Doses

- **DOGS:**

  For analgesia:
  a) 0.005–0.02 mg/kg IM, IV or SC q6–12h (Hendrix & Hansen 2000)

  b) As a continuous IV infusion: 2–4 micrograms/kg/hour (Hansen 2008)

  c) 0.005–0.03 mg/kg IV, IM, SC, epidural (Boothe 1999)

  d) 0.006–0.02 mg/kg IV, IM, SQ; duration of effect 6–12 hours and is a relatively effective analgesic, but may be difficult to reverse with naloxone if untoward effects are seen. (Perkowski 2006)

■ **CATS:**

For analgesia:

a) 0.01−0.03 mg/kg IM, IV, Buccal. Effects may last up to 6 hours. Buccal use is well accepted by cats. (Robertson & Lascelles 2003)

b) 0.01−0.03 mg/kg PO transmucosally (squirted directly into the mouth) q8h (Lichtenberger 2006)

c) 0.01−0.03 mg/kg IM, IV, SC q6−8h; 0.01−0.03 mg/kg PO q6−12h (Hansen 2003); As a continuous IV infusion: 1−3 micrograms/kg/hour (Hansen 2008)

d) In the emergent patient: Dose rates higher than 20 micrograms/kg (0.02 mg/kg) should be used. Higher doses produce better analgesia. SC administration of 20 micrograms/kg has limited effects and transmucosal, IV or IM routes preferred. (Leece 2009)

■ **FERRETS:**

a) 0.01−0.05 mg/kg SC or IM 2−3 times daily (Williams 2000)

■ **HORSES:** (**Note:** ARCI UCGFS Class 2 Drug)

For neuroleptanalgesia:

a) 0.004 mg/kg IV (given with acepromazine 0.02 mg/kg) (Thurmon & Benson 1987)

b) 0.006 mg/kg IV (given with xylazine 0.07 mg/kg) (Thurmon & Benson 1987)

■ **RABBITS/RODENTS/SMALL MAMMALS:**

As an analgesic (for control of acute or chronic visceral pain):

a) **Rabbits:** 0.01−0.05 mg/kg SC, IM or IV q6−12h; 0.5 mg/kg rectally q12h (Ivey & Morrisey 2000)

b) **Guinea pigs:** 0.05 mg/kg SC or IV q8−12h

Mice: 0.05−0.1 mg/kg SC q12h.

Rats: 0.01− 0.05 mg/kg SC or IV q8−12h or 0.1−0.25 mg/kg PO q8−12h. (Adamcak & Otten 2000)

As a premedication:

a) **Rabbits:** In compromised patients: 0.05−0.1 mg/kg SC alone. (Vella 2009)

b) **Rabbits:** In healthy animals before uncomplicated elective procedures: Buprenorphine 0.02−0.06 mg/kg with midazolam (0.25−0.5 mg/kg) IM within 20 minutes of procedure along with a local or line incisional block using lidocaine and bupivacaine. Protocols are modified for ill or unstable animals. (Lennox 2009)

■ **ZOO, EXOTIC, WILDLIFE SPECIES:**

For use of buprenorphine in zoo, exotic and wildlife medicine refer to specific references, including:

a) *Zoo Animal and Wildlife Immobilization and Anesthesia.* West, G, Heard, D, Caulkett, N. (eds.). Blackwell Publishing, 2007.

b) *Handbook of Wildlife Chemical Immobilization, 3rd Ed.* Kreeger, T.J. and J.M. Arnemo. 2007.

c) *Restraint and Handling of Wild and Domestic Animals.* Fowler, M (ed.), Iowa State University Press, 1995

d) *Exotic Animal Formulary, 3rd Ed.* Carpenter, J.W., Saunders. 2005

e) The 2009 American Association of Zoo Veterinarian Proceedings by D. K. Fontenot also has several dosages listed for restraint, anesthesia, and analgesia for a variety of drugs for carnivores and primates. VIN members can access them at: http://goo.gl/BHRih or http://goo.gl/9UJse

Monitoring

■ Analgesic efficacy
■ Respiratory status
■ Cardiac status

Client Information

■ This agent should be used parenterally in an inpatient setting or with direct professional supervision

■ Buccal/SL dosing may be performed at home, but pre-measuring dosages in syringes (if using the injection orally) should be considered

Chemistry/Synonyms

A thebaine derivative, buprenorphine is a synthetic partial opiate agonist. It occurs as a white, crystalline powder with a solubility of 17 mg/mL in water and 42 mg/mL in alcohol. The commercially available injectable product (*Buprenex®*—Norwich Eaton) has a pH of 3.5−5 and is a sterile solution of the drug dissolved in D_5W. Terms of potency are expressed in terms of buprenorphine. The commercial product contains 0.324 mg/mL of buprenorphine HCl, which is equivalent to 0.3 mg/mL of buprenorphine.

Buprenorphine HCl may also be known as: buprenorphini hydrochloridum, CL-112302, NIH-8805, UM-952; *Anorfin®, Buprenex®, Buprine®, Finibron®, Magnogen®, Nopan®, Norphin®, Pentorel®, Prefin®, Suboxone®, Subutex®, Temgesic®,* or *Temgesic-nX®.*

Storage/Stability

Buprenorphine should be stored at room temperature (15−30° C). Temperatures above 40° C or below freezing should be avoided. Buprenorphine products should be stored away from bright light. Autoclaving may considerably decrease drug potency. The drug is stable between a pH of 3.5−5.

Compatibility/Compounding Considerations

Buprenorphine is reported to be **compatible** with the following IV solutions and drugs:

acepromazine, atropine, diphenhydramine, D_5W, D_5W and normal saline, dexmedetomidine, droperidol, glycopyrrolate, hydroxyzine, lactated Ringer's, normal saline, scopolamine, and xylazine.

Although no published data could be located to support stability for this combination, buprenorphine injection has been mixed in syringes with dexmedetomidine and ketamine.

Buprenorphine is reportedly **incompatible** with diazepam and lorazepam.

Dosage Forms/Regulatory Status

VETERINARY-LABELED PRODUCTS: None
The ARCI (Racing Commissioners International) has designated this drug as a class 2 substance. See the appendix for more information.

A compounded sustained-release injectable (SC) product is reportedly available from zoopharm.net.

HUMAN-LABELED PRODUCTS:
Buprenorphine HCl for Injection: 0.324 mg/mL (equivalent to 0.3 mg/mL buprenorphine); 1 mL amps & *Carpuject*; *Buprenex*® (Reckitt Benkhiser); generic (Hospira); (Rx, C-III)

Buprenorphine HCl Sublingual Tablets: 2 & 8 mg (as base); *Subutex*® (Reckitt Benkhiser); generic (Roxane Labs); (Rx, C-III)

Buprenorphine HCl Transdermal System: *Butrans*® (Purdue); (Rx, C-III)

Buprenorphine HCl Combinations: Sublingual Tablets: 2 mg buprenorphine base/0.5 mg naloxone; 8 mg buprenorphine base/2 mg naloxone; *Suboxone*® (Reckitt Benkhiser); (C-III)

References

Adamcak, A & J Otten (2000). Rodent Therapeutics. *Vet Clin NA: Exotic Anim Pract* **3**:1(Jan): 221–240.

Boothe, DM (1999). What's new in drug therapy in small animals. Wild West Conference.

Giordano, T, PVM Steagall, et al. (2010). Postoperative analgesic effects of intravenous, intramuscular, subcutaneous or oral transmucosal buprenorphine administered to cats undergoing ovariohysterectomy. *Veterinary Anaesthesia and Analgesia* **37**(4): 357–366.

Hansen, B (2003). Opiate use in cardiovascular medicine. Proceedings: ACVIM Forum. Accessed via: Veterinary Information Network. http://goo.gl/Bxji6

Hansen, B (2008). Analgesia for the critically ill dog or cat: An update. *Vet Clin NA: Sm Anim Pract* **38**: 1353–1363.

Hendrix, P & B Hansen (2000). Acute Pain Management. *Kirk's Current Veterinary Therapy: XIII Small Animal Practice*. J Bonagura Ed. Philadelphia, WB Saunders: 57–61.

Ivey, E & J Morrisey (2000). Therapeutics for Rabbits. *Vet Clin NA: Exotic Anim Pract* **3**:1(Jan): 183–216.

Leece, E (2009). Soothing the pain 2 —Anaesthesia and analgesia in the ER. Proceedings: ESFM. Accessed via: Veterinary Information Network. http://goo.gl/r9euz

Lennox, A (2009). Anaesthesia and analgesia of the rabbit. Proceedings: BSAVA.

Lichtenberger, M (2006). Preop and surgical pain management protocols. Proceedings: Western Vet Conf. Accessed via: Veterinary Information Network. http://goo.gl/Oys8T

Perkowski, S (2006). Practicing pain management in the acute setting. Proceedings: ACVIM. Accessed via: Veterinary Information Network. http://goo.gl/TRPqy

Robertson, S & B Lascelles (2003). Safe and effective acute pain relief in cats. Proceedings: PAIN 2003. Accessed via: Veterinary Information Network. http://goo.gl/ORxDj

Thurmon, JC & GJ Benson (1987). Injectable anesthetics and anesthetic adjuncts. *Vet Clin North Am (Equine Practice)* **3**(1): 15–36.

Vella, D (2009). Rabbit General Anesthesia. Proceedings: AAVAC–UEP. Accessed via: Veterinary Information Network.

Williams, B (2000). Therapeutics in Ferrets. *Vet Clin NA: Exotic Anim Pract* **3**:1(Jan): 131–153.

BUSPIRONE HCL

(byoo-*spye*-rone)   BuSpar®

ANXIOLYTIC

Prescriber Highlights

▶ Non-benzodiazepine anxiolytic agent used in dogs & cats

▶ May take a week or more to be effective; not appropriate for acute treatment of situational anxieties

▶ Use with caution in patients with severe hepatic or renal disease

▶ Adverse Effects relatively uncommon; cats may exhibit behavior changes

▶ Human generic forms of medication relatively inexpensive

Uses/Indications

Buspirone may be effective in treating certain behavior disorders in dogs and cats, principally those that are fear/phobia related and especially those associated with social interactions. Buspirone may also be useful for urine spraying or treatment of motion sickness in cats. Approximately 50% of cats show improvement in urine marking when buspirone is given. Buspirone may be more effective in multi-cat households than in single cat households.

Pharmacology/Actions

Buspirone is an anxioselective agent. Unlike the benzodiazepines, buspirone does not possess any anticonvulsant or muscle relaxant activity and little sedative or psychomotor impairment activity. Buspirone does not share the same mechanisms as the benzodiazepines (does not have significant affinity for benzodiazepine receptors and does not affect GABA binding). It appears to act as a partial agonist at serotonin (5-HT1A) receptors and as an agonist/antagonist of dopamine (D2) receptors in the CNS. In neurons, buspirone slows the neuronal flow depletion of serotonin stores.

Pharmacokinetics

In humans, buspirone is rapidly and completely absorbed but a high first pass effect limits systemic bioavailability to approximately 5%. Binding to plasma proteins is very high (95%). In rats, highest tissue concentrations are found in the lungs, kidneys, and fat. Lower levels are found in the brain, heart, skeletal muscle, plasma and liver. Both buspirone and its metabolites are distributed into maternal milk. The elimination half-life (in humans) is about 2–4 hours. Buspirone is hepatically metabolized to several metabolites (including one that is active: 1-PP). These metabolites are excreted primarily in the urine.

In a limited study done in 6 cats (Mealey *et al.* 2004), oral administration of buspirone gave peak levels in about 1.4 hours, but oral bioavailability appeared to be significantly lower than in humans. Transdermal administration of buspirone (PLO-base) did not yield detectable levels (ELISA method).

Contraindications/Precautions/Warnings

Buspirone should be used with caution with either significant renal or hepatic disease. Because buspirone may reduce disinhibition, it should be used with caution in aggressive animals. While buspirone has far less sedating properties than many other anxiolytic drugs, it should be used with caution in working dogs.

Because buspirone often takes a week or more for effect, it should not be used as the sole therapy for situational anxieties.

Adverse Effects

Adverse effects are usually minimal in animals treated with buspirone and it is generally well tolerated. Bradycardia, GI disturbances and stereotypic behaviors are possible. Cats may demonstrate increased affection, which may be the desired effect. In multi-cat households, cats that have previously been extremely timid in the face of repeated aggression from other cats may, after receiving buspirone begin turning on their attacker.

The most likely adverse effect profile seen with buspirone in humans includes dizziness, headache, nausea/anorexia, and restlessness; other neurologic effects (including sedation) may be noted. Rarely, tachycardias and other cardiovascular clinical signs may be present.

Reproductive/Nursing Safety

While the drug has not been proven safe during pregnancy, doses of up to 30 times the labeled dosage in rabbits and rats demonstrated no teratogenic effects. In humans, the FDA categorizes this drug as category *B* for use during pregnancy (*Animal studies have not yet demonstrated risk to the fetus, but there are no adequate studies in pregnant women; or animal studies have shown an adverse effect, but adequate studies in pregnant women have not demonstrated a risk to the fetus in the first trimester of pregnancy, and there is no evidence of risk in later trimesters.*)

Buspirone and its metabolites have been detected in the milk of lactating rats; avoid use during nursing if possible.

Overdosage/Acute Toxicity

Limited information is available. The oral LD_{50} in dogs is 586 mg/kg. Oral overdoses may produce vomiting, dizziness, drowsiness, miosis and gastric distention. Standard overdose protocols should be followed after ingestion has been determined.

Drug Interactions

Buspirone may be used in combination with tricyclic or SSRI agents, but dosage reductions may be necessary to minimize adverse effects.

The following drug interactions have either been reported or are theoretical in humans or animals receiving buspirone and may be of significance in veterinary patients:

- **CNS DEPRESSANTS:** Potentially could cause increased CNS depression
- **DILTIAZEM:** May cause increased buspirone plasma levels and adverse effects
- **ERYTHROMYCIN:** May cause increased buspirone plasma levels and adverse effects
- **GRAPEFRUIT JUICE (powder):** May cause increased buspirone plasma levels and adverse effects
- **KETOCONAZOLE, ITRACONAZOLE:** May cause increased buspirone plasma levels and adverse effects
- **MONOAMINE OXIDASE INHIBITORS** (*e.g.,* **selegiline, amitraz**): Use with buspirone is not recommended because dangerous hypertension may occur
- **RIFAMPIN:** May cause decreased buspirone plasma levels
- **TRAZODONE:** Use with buspirone may cause increased ALT
- **VERAPAMIL:** May cause increased buspirone plasma levels

Doses

- **DOGS:**
  For low-grade anxieties and fears:
  a) 1 mg/kg PO q8–24h (mild anxiety); 2.5–10 mg (total dose) per dog PO q8–24h (mild anxiety); 10–15 mg per dog PO q8–12h (more severe anxiety, thunderstorm phobia) (Overall 2000)
  b) 1–2 mg/kg PO q12h; 5–15 mg (total dose) per dog PO q8–12h (Siebert 2003)
  c) 5–10 mg (total dose) PO q8–12h (Reisner & Houpt 2000)
  d) For global anxiety: 0.5–2 mg/kg PO q8–12h; may take 2–4 weeks until effect. (Horwitz 2006)
  e) 1 mg/kg PO q8–12h; most useful in social phobias; may also be useful for panic disorders (Virga 2005)

- **CATS:**
  For adjunctive treatment of low-grade anxieties/fears, spraying, overgrooming:
  a) 0.5–1 mg/kg PO q8–12h; 2.5–5 mg (total dose) per cat PO q8–12h for 6–8 weeks; some cats do well on once daily dosing (Overall 2000)

b) 2.5–5 mg (total dose) PO once a day to 3 times a day (Seksel 2003)

c) For urine marking: 2.5–7.5 mg (total dose) per cat PO q12h (Levine 2008)

d) 0.5–1 mg/kg PO q12h; 2.5–7.5 mg (total dose) per cat PO q12h (Siebert 2003)

e) 0.5–1 mg/kg PO q8–12h; most useful in social phobias; may also be useful for panic disorders (Virga 2005)

Monitoring
- Efficacy
- Adverse effect profiles

Chemistry/Synonyms
An arylpiperazine derivative anxiolytic agent, buspirone HCl differs structurally from the benzodiazepines. It occurs as a white, crystalline powder with solubilities at 25°C of 865 mg/mL in water and about 20 mg/mL in alcohol.

Buspirone HCl may also be known as MJ-9022; many trade names are available.

Storage/Stability
Buspirone HCl tablets should be stored in tight, light-resistant containers at room temperature. After manufacture, buspirone tablets have an expiration date of 36 months.

Dosage Forms/Regulatory Status

VETERINARY-LABELED PRODUCTS: None
The ARCI (Racing Commissioners International) has designated this drug as a class 2 substance. See the appendix for more information.

HUMAN-LABELED PRODUCTS:
Buspirone HCl Oral Tablets: 5 mg (4.6 mg as base), 7.5 mg (6.85 mg as base), 10 mg (9.1 mg as base), 15 mg (13.7 mg as base) and 30 mg (27.4 mg as base); BuSpar® (Bristol-Myers Squibb); generic; (Rx)

References

Horwitz, D (2006). Canine anxieties and phobias. Proceedings: Western Veterinary Conference. Accessed via: Veterinary Information Network. http://goo.gl/gfWHV

Levine, E (2008). Feline Fear and Anxiety. *Vet Clin NA: Sm Anim Pract* **38**: 1065–1079.

Mealey, KL, KE Peck, et al. (2004). Systemic absorption of amitriptyline and buspirone after oral and transdermal administration to healthy cats. *Journal of Veterinary Internal Medicine* **18**(1): 43–46.

Overall, K (2000). Behavioral Pharmacology. Proceedings: American Animal Hospital Association 67th Annual Meeting, Toronto.

Reisner, I & K Houpt (2000). Behavioral Disorders. *Textbook of Veterinary Internal Medicine: Diseases of the Dog and Cat.* S Ettinger and E Feldman Eds. Philadelphia, WB Saunders. **1**: 156–162.

Seksel, K (2003). When to use medication, What to use and why. Proceedings: World Small Animal Veterinary Association World Congress. Accessed via: Veterinary Information Network. http://goo.gl/sIRZn

Siebert, L (2003). Psychoactive drugs in behavioral medicine. Western Veterinary Conference.

Virga, V (2005). Psychopharmacology for anxiety disorders. Proceedings: Western Vet Cong 2005. Accessed via: Veterinary Information Network. http://goo.gl/4uZW3

BUSULFAN

(byoo-*sul*-fan)   Myleran®, Busulfex®

ANTINEOPLASTIC

Prescriber Highlights

- Antineoplastic sometimes used in treating chronic granulocytic leukemias in small animals
- Myelosuppression; may be severe
- May increase uric acid levels

Uses/Indications
Busulfan may be useful in the adjunctive therapy of chronic granulocytic leukemias or polycythemia vera in small animals. Not commonly used in veterinary medicine.

Pharmacology/Actions
Busulfan is a bifunctional alkylating agent antineoplastic and is cell cycle-phase nonspecific. The exact mechanism of action has not been determined but is thought to be due to its alkylating, cross-linking of strands of DNA and myelosuppressive properties. Busulfan's primary activity is against cells of the granulocytic series.

Pharmacokinetics
Busulfan is well absorbed after oral administration. Distribution characteristics are not well described but in humans, drug concentrations in the CSF are nearly equal to those found in plasma. It is unknown whether the drug enters maternal milk. Busulfan is rapidly, hepatically metabolized to at least 12 different metabolites that are slowly excreted into the urine. In humans, serum half-life of busulfan averages about 2.5 hours.

Contraindications/Precautions/Warnings
Busulfan is contraindicated in patients who have shown resistance to the drug in the past or are hypersensitive to it. Only veterinarians with the experience and resources to monitor the toxicity of this agent should administer this drug. The risk versus benefits of therapy must be carefully considered in patients with preexisting bone marrow depression or concurrent infections. Additive bone marrow depression may occur in patients undergoing concomitant radiation therapy.

Adverse Effects
The most commonly associated adverse effect seen with busulfan therapy is myelosuppression. In humans, anemia, leukopenia, and thrombocytopenia may be observed. Onset of leukopenia is generally 10–15 days after initiation of therapy and leukocyte nadirs occurring on average around 11–30 days. Severe bone marrow depression can result in pancytopenia that may take months to years for recovery. In humans, bronchopulmonary dysplasia with pulmonary fibrosis, uric acid nephropathy, and stomatitis

have been reported. These effects are uncommon and generally associated with chronic, higher dose therapy.

Reproductive/Nursing Safety

Busulfan's teratogenic potential has not been well documented, but it is mutagenic in mice and may potentially cause a variety of fetal abnormalities. It is generally recommended to avoid the drug during pregnancy, but because of the seriousness of the diseases treated with busulfan, the potential benefits to the mother must be considered. In humans, the FDA categorizes this drug as category *D* for use during pregnancy (*There is evidence of human fetal risk, but the potential benefits from the use of the drug in pregnant women may be acceptable despite its potential risks.*)

It is unknown if busulfan enters milk; avoid nursing if the dam is receiving the drug.

Overdosage/Acute Toxicity

There is limited experience with busulfan overdoses. The LD50 in mice is 120 mg/kg. Chronic overdosage is more likely to cause serious bone marrow suppression than is an acute overdose; however, any overdose, should be treated seriously with standard gut emptying protocols used when appropriate and supportive therapy initiated when required. There is no known specific antidote for busulfan intoxication.

Drug Interactions

The following drug interactions have either been reported or are theoretical in humans or animals receiving busulfan and may be of significance in veterinary patients:

■ **ACETAMINOPHEN:** Use within 72 hours prior to busulfan can reduce busulfan clearance by reducing glutathione concentrations in tissues and blood

■ **CYCLOPHOSPHAMIDE:** Can potentially reduce clearance of busulfan, probably by competing for available glutathione

■ **ITRACONAZOLE:** Potential decreased busulfan clearance

■ **MYELOSUPPRESSANT AGENTS:** Concurrent use with other bone marrow depressant medications may result in additive myelosuppression

■ **PHENYTOIN:** Possible increased clearance of busulfan

■ **THIOGUANINE:** Used concomitantly with busulfan may result in hepatotoxicity

Laboratory Considerations

■ Busulfan may raise serum **uric acid** levels. Drugs such as allopurinol may be required to control hyperuricemia.

Doses

Note: Because of the potential toxicity of this drug to patients, veterinary personnel and clients, and since chemotherapy indications, treatment protocols, monitoring and safety

guidelines often change, the following dosages should be used only as a general guide. Consultation with a veterinary oncologist and referral to current veterinary oncology references [*e.g.*, (Henry & Higginbotham 2009); (Argyle *et al.* 2008); (Withrow & Vail 2007); (Villalobos 2007); (Ogilvie & Moore 2006); (Ogilvie & Moore 2001)] is *strongly recommended*.

■ **SMALL ANIMALS:**
   a) Busulfan is rarely used in veterinary medicine, but when used it is usually dosed in a range of 2–4 mg/m^2 (NOT mg/kg) PO once daily.

Monitoring

■ CBC

■ Serum uric acid

■ Efficacy

Client Information

■ Clients must understand the importance of both administering busulfan as directed and reporting immediately any signs associated with toxicity (*e.g.*, abnormal bleeding, bruising, urination, depression, infection, shortness of breath, etc.).

Chemistry/Synonyms

An alkylsulfonate antineoplastic agent, busulfan occurs as white, crystalline powder. It is slightly soluble in alcohol and very slightly soluble in water.

Busulfan may also be known as: bussulfam, busulfanum, busulphan, CB-2041, GT-41, myelosan, NSC-750, WR-19508, *Bussulfam®*, *Busulfanum®*, *Busulivex®*, *Mielucin®*, *Misulban®*, or *Myleran®*.

Storage/Stability

Busulfan tablets should be stored in well-closed containers at room temperature.

Dosage Forms/Regulatory Status

VETERINARY-LABELED PRODUCTS: None
HUMAN-LABELED PRODUCTS:
Busulfan Oral Tablets: 2 mg; *Myleran®* (GlaxoSmithKline); (Rx)

Busulfan Injection Solution: 6 mg/mL in 10 mL single-use amps with syringe filters; *Busulfex®* (Otsuka America); (Rx)

References

Argyle, D, M Brearly, et al. (2008). *Decision Making in Small Animal Oncology*, Wiley–Blackwell.
Henry, C & M Higginbotham (2009). *Cancer Management in Small Animal Practice*, Saunders.
Ogilvie, G & A Moore (2001). *Feline Oncology: A Comprehensive Guide to Compassionate Care*, Veterinary Learning Systems.
Ogilvie, G & A Moore (2006). *Managing the Canine Cancer Patient: A Practical Guide to Compassionate Care*, Veterinary Learning Systems.
Villalobos, A (2007). *Canine and Feline Geriatric Oncology*. Ames, Blackwell.
Withrow, S & D Vail (2007). *Withrow and MacEwen's Small Animal Clinical Oncology 4th Ed.* Philadelphia, Elsevier.

BUTAPHOSPHAN WITH CYANOCOBALAMIN

(byoo-ta-*fos*-fan; sye-*an*-oh-koe-bal-ah-min)
Catosal®

INJECTABLE PHOSPHATE/VITAMIN B12

Prescriber Highlights

▶ An injectable organic phosphorous and vitamin B-12 product

▶ Not an FDA-approved drug

Because this product has not undergone FDA-approval process as a drug, there is a limited amount of information available; refer to the Cyanocobalamin and Phosphate monographs for more information

Uses/Indications

The combination product *Catosal®* contains butaphosphan with cyanocobalamin (Vitamin B-12). It is marketed in several countries for a variety of species (sheep, poultry, pigs, horses, goats, dogs, cattle, fur-bearing animals, and cats) when a parenteral source of phosphorous and vitamin B-12 is indicated. In the USA, the label states that it is a source of Vitamin B12 and phosphorus for prevention or treatment of deficiencies of these nutrients in cattle, swine, horses and poultry.

Pharmacology/Actions

For more detail on pharmacology/actions, see the *Cyanocobalamin* and *Phosphate* monographs. A study (Furll *et al.* 2010) done in dairy cattle where butaphosphan/cyanocobalamin was injected daily one to two weeks before parturition either 0, 3, or 6 times (0.1 mL/kg IV; 10 mg/kg butaphosphan and 5 micrograms/kg cyanocobalamin) showed that multiple daily IV injections before parturition increased serum cyanocobalamin levels, post-partum glucose availability, and decreased peripheral fat mobilization and ketone body formation. Puerperal infection rates in the first 5 days post-partum were decreased in the group receiving 6 injections versus the cows receiving placebo.

Another study done in dairy cattle to determine the effect of butaphosphan/cyanocobalamin on the prevalence of subclinical ketosis in dairy cattle in the early postpartum period has been published (Rollin *et al.* 2010). Cows received either placebo (25 mL sterile water SC) or butaphosphan/cyanocobalamin injection (25 mL SC) on the day of, and one day after, calving. Only mature cows (3 or more lactations) receiving the drug had a lower rate of hyperketonemia than the non-treated cattle. These mature cows also showed significantly lower increases in serum concentrations of beta-hydroxybutyrate (BHBA) when measured at 3 and 10 days post-calving.

Pharmacokinetics

No specific information located; refer to the phosphate and cyanocobalamin monographs for further information.

Contraindications/Precautions/Warnings

This product should *not* be used in patients with hyperphosphatemia. Use with caution in patients with chronic renal failure.

Use standard aseptic procedures during administration of injections. Volumes of more than 10 mL should be split and given at separate intramuscular or subcutaneous sites.

Adverse Effects

None noted.

Reproductive/Nursing Safety

No specific information located.

Overdosage/Acute Toxicity

No specific information located.

Drug Interactions

No specific information located. Refer to the phosphate monograph for more information.

Laboratory Considerations

No specific information located.

Doses

■ **HORSES:**

a) 1–2 mL per 100 lbs body weight SC, IM, or IV; repeat daily as needed. Use standard aseptic procedures during administration of injections. Volumes of more than 10 mL should be split and given at separate intramuscular or subcutaneous sites. (*Catosal®*; Bayer (USA) label information)

■ **CATTLE:**

a) 1–2 mL per 100 lbs body weight SC, IM, or IV; repeat daily as needed. Volumes of more than 10 mL should be split and given at separate intramuscular or subcutaneous sites. Calves: 2–4 mL per 100 lbs body weight; repeat daily as needed. (*Catosal®*; Bayer (USA) label information)

■ **SWINE:**

a) 2 - 5 mL per 100 lbs body weight SC, IM, or IV repeat daily as needed. Volumes of more than 10 mL should be split and given at separate intramuscular or subcutaneous sites. Piglets: 1–2.5 mL (total dose) per animal SC, IM, or IV; repeat daily as needed. (*Catosal®*; Bayer (USA) label information)

■ **BIRDS:**

a) Poultry (turkeys): 1–3 mL per liter of drinking water; repeat daily as needed. (*Catosal®*; Bayer (USA) label information)

Chemistry/Synonyms

Butaphosphan is 1-(n-Butylamino)-1-methylethyl phosphonous acid. One gram (10 mL of injection) provides 173 mg of phosphorous.

Storage/Stability

The injectable product should be stored at temperatures below 30°C (86°F); avoiding freezing.

Compatibility/Compounding Considerations

No specific information located. Consult the cyanocobalamin and Phosphate monographs for guidance.

Dosage Forms/Regulatory Status

VETERINARY-LABELED PRODUCTS:

Butaphosphan 100 mg/mL and Cyanocobalamin (Vitamin B-12) 0.05 mg/mL in 100 mL & 250 mL multidose (each mL contains 30 mg of n-Butyl alcohol as a preservative); *Catosal®* (Bayer). This is not an FDA-approved drug product (not listed in Green Book). The USA labeling for the product states that federal law (USA) restricts this drug to use by or on the order of a licensed veterinarian (Rx) and that there is a zero day withdrawal period for meat, milk, and eggs.

HUMAN-LABELED PRODUCTS: None

References

Furll, M, A Deniz, et al. (2010). Effect of multiple intravenous injections of butaphosphan and cyanocobalamin on the metabolism of periparturient dairy cows. *Journal of Dairy Science* 93(9): 4155–4164.

Rollin, E, RD Berghaus, et al. (2010). The effect of injectable butaphosphan and cyanocobalamin on postpartum serum beta–hydroxybutyrate, calcium, and phosphorus concentrations in dairy cattle. *Journal of Dairy Science* 93(3): 978–987.

BUTORPHANOL TARTRATE

(byoo-*tor*-fa-nol)

Stadol®, Torbutrol®, Torbugesic®

OPIATE PARTIAL AGONIST

Prescriber Highlights

▶ Partial opiate agonist/antagonist used in a variety of species as an analgesic, premed, antitussive, or antiemetic

▶ Not a good choice as an analgesic for moderate to severe pain in small animals, but a reasonably good analgesic for horses

▶ Contraindicated or caution in patients with liver disease, hypothyroidism, or renal insufficiency, Addison's, head trauma, increased CSF pressure or other CNS dysfunction (e.g., coma) & in geriatric or severely debilitated patients

▶ Reduce dose in dogs with MDR1 mutation

▶ Potential adverse effects in *Dogs/Cats:* Sedation, ataxia, anorexia or diarrhea (rarely)

▶ *Horses* (at usual doses): a transient ataxia & sedation, but CNS excitement possible

▶ Controlled substance (C-IV)

Uses/Indications

FDA-approved indication for dogs is "... for the relief of chronic non-productive cough associated with tracheobronchitis, tracheitis, tonsillitis, laryngitis and pharyngitis originating from inflammatory conditions of the upper respiratory tract" (Package Insert; *Torbutrol®*—Fort Dodge). It is also used in practice in both dogs and cats as a preanesthetic medication, analgesic, and as an antiemetic prior to cisplatin treatment (although not very effective in cats for this indication). Compared with other opiate analgesics, butorphanol is not very useful in small animals (particularly dogs) for treating pain and has to be dosed frequently. Butorphanol is a useful reversal agent for the CNS and respiratory depressant effects of *mu*-agonists. Due to its kappa effects, it can reverse CNS and respiratory depression without completely reversing the analgesic effect of the *mu* agonist drugs.

The FDA-approved indication for horses is "... for the relief of pain associated with colic in adult horses and yearlings" (Package Insert; *Torbugesic®*—Fort Dodge). It has also been used clinically as an analgesic in cattle.

Pharmacology/Actions

Butorphanol is considered to be, on a weight basis, 4–7 times as potent an analgesic as morphine, 15–30 times as pentazocine, and 30–50 times as meperidine; however a ceiling effect is reached at higher dosages, where analgesia is no longer enhanced and may be reduced. Its agonist activity is thought to occur primarily at the kappa and sigma receptors and the analgesic actions at sites in the limbic system (sub-cortical level and spinal levels). Its use as an analgesic in small animals has been disappointing, primarily because of its very short duration of action and ability to alleviate only mild to moderate pain.

The antagonist potency of butorphanol is considered to be approximately 30 times that of pentazocine and 1/40th that of naloxone and will antagonize the effect of true agonists (*e.g.*, morphine, meperidine, oxymorphone).

Besides the analgesic qualities of butorphanol, it possesses significant antitussive activity. In dogs, butorphanol has been shown to elevate CNS respiratory center threshold to CO_2 but, unlike opiate agonists, not depress respiratory center sensitivity. Butorphanol, unlike morphine, apparently does not cause histamine release in dogs. CNS depression may occur in dogs, while CNS excitation has been noted (usually at high doses) in horses and dogs.

Although possessing less cardiovascular effects than the classical opiate agonists, butorphanol can cause a decrease in cardiac rate secondary to increased parasympathetic tone and mild decreases in arterial blood pressures.

The risk of causing physical dependence seems to be minimal when butorphanol is used in veterinary patients.

Pharmacokinetics

Butorphanol is absorbed completely in the gut when administered orally but, because of a high first-pass effect, only about 1/6th of the administered dose reaches the systemic circulation. The drug has also been shown to be completely absorbed following IM administration.

Butorphanol is well distributed, with highest levels (of the parent compound and metabolites) found in the liver, kidneys, and intestine. Concentrations in the lungs, endocrine tissues, spleen, heart, fat tissue and blood cells are also higher than those found in plasma. Approximately 80% of the drug is bound to plasma proteins (human data). Butorphanol will cross the placenta and neonatal plasma levels have been roughly equivalent to maternal levels. The drug is also distributed into maternal milk.

Butorphanol is metabolized in the liver, primarily by hydroxylation. Other methods of metabolism include N-dealkylation and conjugation. The metabolites of butorphanol do not exhibit any analgesic activity. These metabolites and the parent compound are mainly excreted into the urine (only 5% is excreted unchanged), but 11–14% of a dose is excreted into the bile and eliminated with the feces.

Following IV doses in horses, the onset of action is approximately 3 minutes with a peak analgesic effect at 15–30 minutes. The duration of action in horses may be up to 4 hours after a single dose.

Contraindications/Precautions/Warnings

The drug is contraindicated in patients having known hypersensitivity to it. All opiates should be used with caution in patients with hypothyroidism, severe renal insufficiency, adrenocortical insufficiency (Addison's), and in geriatric or severely debilitated patients.

Like other opiates, butorphanol must be used with extreme caution in patients with head trauma, increased CSF pressure or other CNS dysfunction (e.g., coma).

Dogs with MDR1 mutations (many Collies, Australian shepherds, etc.) may develop a more pronounced sedation that persists longer than normal. The Washington State University Veterinary Clinical Pharmacology Lab recommends reducing the dose by 25% in dogs heterozygous for the MDR1 mutation and by 30-50% in dogs homozygous (mutant/mutant) for the mutation.

The manufacturer states that butorphanol "should not be used in dogs with a history of liver disease" and, because of its effects on suppressing cough, "it should not be used in conditions of the lower respiratory tract associated with copious mucous production." The drug should be used cautiously in dogs with heartworm disease, as safety for butorphanol has not been established in these cases.

Butorphanol may not be a very good analgesic and may cause respiratory depression in turtles or tortoises (Sladky *et al.* 2007).

Adverse Effects

Adverse effects reported in dogs/cats include sedation, excitement, respiratory depression, ataxia, anorexia or diarrhea (rarely). Adverse effects may be less severe than those seen with pure agonists.

Adverse effects seen in horses (at usual doses) may include a transient ataxia and sedation, but excitement has been noted as well (see below). Although reported to have minimal effects on the GI, butorphanol has the potential to decrease intestinal motility and ileus can occur. Horses may exhibit CNS excitement (tossing and jerking of head, increased ambulation, augmented avoidance response to auditory stimuli) if given high doses (0.2 mg/kg) IV rapidly. Very high doses IV (1–2 mg/kg) may lead to the development of nystagmus, salivation, seizures, hyperthermia and decreased GI motility. These effects are considered transitory in nature.

Reproductive/Nursing Safety

Although no controlled studies have been performed in domestic animals or humans, the drug has exhibited no evidence of teratogenicity or of causing impaired fertility in laboratory animals. The manufacturer, however, does not recommend its use in pregnant bitches, foals, weanlings (equine), and breeding horses. In humans, the FDA categorizes this drug as category *C* for use during pregnancy (*Animal studies have shown an adverse effect on the fetus, but there are no adequate studies in humans; or there are no animal reproduction studies and no adequate studies in humans.*) In a separate system evaluating the safety of drugs in canine and feline pregnancy (Papich 1989), this drug is categorized as in class: *B* (*Safe for use if used cautiously. Studies in laboratory animals may have uncovered some risk, but these drugs appear to be safe in dogs and cats; or these drugs are safe if they are not administered when the animal is near term.*)

Butorphanol can be distributed into milk, but not in amounts that would cause concern in nursing offspring.

Overdosage/Acute Toxicity

Acute life-threatening overdoses with butorphanol should be unlikely. The LD_{50} in dogs is reportedly 50 mg/kg. However, because butorphanol injection is available in two dosage strengths (0.5 mg/mL and 10 mg/mL) for veterinary use, the possibility exists that inadvertent overdoses may occur in small animals. It has been suggested that animals exhibiting clinical signs of overdose (CNS effects, cardiovascular changes, and respiratory depression) be treated immediately with intravenous naloxone. Additional supportive measures (e.g., fluids, O_2, vasopressor agents, and mechanical ventilation) may be required. Should seizures occur and persist, diazepam may be used for control.

Drug Interactions

The following drug interactions have either been reported or are theoretical in humans or animals receiving butorphanol and may be of significance in veterinary patients:

- **OTHER CNS DEPRESSANTS** (*e.g.,* **anesthetic agents, antihistamines, phenothiazines, barbiturates, tranquilizers, alcohol,** etc.): May cause increased CNS or respiratory depression when used with butorphanol; dosage may need to be decreased

- **ERYTHROMYCIN:** Could potentially decrease metabolism of butorphanol

- **FENTANYL** (and other **pure opiate agonists**): Butorphanol may potentially antagonize some analgesic effects (**Note:** this is controversial), but may also reverse some of the sedative and respiratory depressant effects of pure agonists

- **PANCURONIUM** If used with butorphanol may cause increased conjunctival changes

- **THEOPHYLLINE:** Could potentially decrease metabolism of butorphanol

Doses

Note: All doses are expressed in mg/kg of the *base* activity. If using the human product (*Stadol®*), 1 mg of tartrate salt = 0.68 mg base.

- **DOGS:**

  As an antitussive:
  a) 0.055–0.11 mg/kg SC q6–12h; treatment should not normally be required for longer than 7 days; or 0.55 mg/kg PO q6–12h; may increase dose to 1.1 mg/kg PO q6–12h (The oral doses correspond to one 5 mg tablet per 20 lbs. and 10 lbs. of body weight, respectively); treatment should not normally be required for longer than 7 days (Package Insert; *Torbutrol®*—Fort Dodge)

  b) 0.05–1 mg/kg PO q6–12h; goal is to suppress coughing without causing excessive sedation (Johnson, L 2000)

  c) 0.55–1.1 mg/kg PO as needed (Johnson, LR 2004)

  As an analgesic:
  a) 0.1–0.5 mg/kg IV, IM, SQ; provides only mild to moderate analgesia (good visceral analgesia); duration of sedative action 2–4 hours, but analgesic action may be 1 hour or less (Perkowski 2006)

  b) As a constant rate infusion: 0.1–0.4 mg/kg/hr; occasionally used for abdominal pain (Hellyer 2006)

  c) As an epidural analgesic: 0.25 mg/kg diluted with preservative-free saline (0.2 mL) or local anesthetic epidurally. Onset of action less than 30 minutes and duration is 2-4 hours. Has predominantly supraspinal effects. (Valverde 2008)

  In combination as an immobilizing agent:
  a) For difficult dogs and short procedures (nail trims, X-rays, etc): butorphanol 0.2 mg/kg; medetomidine 0.001–0.01 mg/kg; midazolam 0.05–0.2 mg/kg. All given IM.

  For dogs requiring more sedation: butorphanol 0.2 mg/kg; medetomidine 0.01–0.02 mg/kg; midazolam 0.05–0.2 mg/kg; all are given IM. Consider adding Telazol 1–2 mg/kg if insufficient sedation from above. For painful procedures consider adding buprenorphine at 0.02–0.04 mg/kg or substituting butorphanol or buprenorphine with either morphine 0.5–1 mg/kg or hydromorphone 0.1–0.2 mg/kg. More information available from www.vsag.org. (Moffat 2008)

  As reversal agent for the sedative and respiratory depressant effects of *mu*-agonist opiates:
  a) 0.05–0.1 mg/kg IV; the benefit of using butorphanol over naloxone is that it does not completely reverse analgesic effects. (Quandt 2009)

  As an anti-emetic prior to cisplatin treatment:
  a) 0.4 mg/kg IM 1/2 hour prior to cisplatin infusion (Klausner & Bell 1988)

- **CATS:**

  As an analgesic:
  a) 0.1–0.5 mg/kg IV, IM, SQ; provides only mild to moderate analgesia (good visceral analgesia); duration of sedative action 2–4 hours, but analgesic action may be 1 hour or less (Perkowski 2006)

  b) As a postoperative CRI (usually in combination with ketamine) for mild to moderate pain: Loading dose of 0.1–0.2 mg/kg IV, then a CRI of 0.1–0.2 mg/kg/hr; Ketamine is used at a loading dose of 0.1 mg/kg IV with a CRI of 0.4 mg/kg/hr. When used with an opioid CRI may allow reduction in dosage of both. (Lichtenberger 2006b)

  c) As an epidural analgesic: 0.25 mg/kg diluted with preservative-free saline (0.2 mL) or local anesthetic epidurally. Onset of action less than 30 minutes and duration is 2-4 hours. Has predominantly supraspinal effects. (Valverde 2008)

  As reversal agent for the sedative and respiratory depressant effects of *mu*-agonist opiates:
  a) 0.05–0.1 mg/kg IV; the benefit of using butorphanol over naloxone is that it does not completely reverse analgesic effects. (Quandt 2009)

  In combination as an immobilizing agent:
  a) For difficult cats and short procedures (nail trims, X-rays, etc): butorphanol 0.2 mg/kg; medetomidine

0.001–0.015 mg/kg; midazolam 0.05–0.2 mg/kg. All given IM.

For cats requiring more sedation: butorphanol 0.2 mg/kg; medetomidine 0.015–0.02 mg/kg; midazolam 0.05–0.2 mg/kg; add ketamine 1–5 mg/kg when insufficient sedation from opioid, higher doses of medetomidine, and midazolam; all are given IM. For painful procedures consider adding buprenorphine at 0.02–0.04 mg/kg or substituting butorphanol or buprenorphine with either morphine 0.5 mg/kg or hydromorphone 0.1 mg/kg. More information available from www.vsag.org. (Moffat 2008)

■ **FERRETS:**
a) As a sedative/analgesic:
Butorphanol alone 0.05–0.1 mg/kg IM, SC. Butorphanol/Xylazine: Butorphanol 0.2 mg/kg + Xylazine 2 mg/kg IM

For injectable anesthesia:
Butorphanol 0.1 mg/kg, Ketamine 5 mg/kg, medetomidine 80 micrograms/kg. Combine in one syringe and give IM. May need to supplement with isoflurane (0.5–1.5%) for abdominal surgery. (Finkler 1999)

b) Xylazine (2 mg/kg) plus butorphanol (0.2 mg/kg) IM;

Telazol (1.5 mg/kg) plus xylazine (1.5 mg/kg) plus butorphanol (0.2 mg/kg) IM; may reverse xylazine with yohimbine (0.05 mg/kg IM) (Williams 2000)

As an analgesic:
a) 0.05–0.5 mg/kg SC or IM q4h (Williams 2000)

b) For post-op analgesia: 0.1–0.2 mg/kg loading dose, then a constant rate infusion of 0.1–0.2 mg/kg/hr (Lichtenberger 2006a)

■ **RABBITS/RODENTS/SMALL MAMMALS:**
For chemical restraint in rabbits:
a) 0.1–0.5 mg/kg IV (Burke 1999); (Ivey & Morrisey 2000)

For analgesia:
a) For postsurgical analgesia in rabbits: 0.1–0.5 mg/kg IV or SC q2–4h; lower dosages may be more effective due to "ceiling effect" (Ivey & Morrisey 2000)

b) **Rabbits:** As an analgesic (post-operative pain): 0.4 mg/kg SC q4–6h; for surgical procedures (in combo with xylazine/ketamine): 0.1 mg/kg once IM or SC (Huerkamp 1995)

c) **Rabbits for post-op analgesia:** 0.1–0.2 mg/kg loading dose, then a constant rate infusion of 0.1–0.2 mg/kg/hr (Lichtenberger 2006a)

■ **BIRDS:**
As an analgesic:
a) As an analgesic, sedative, preanesthetic: 1–4 mg/kg IM, IV q2-3h (Lennox 2009)

b) 1–4 mg/kg q4h IM, IV, PO (Bays 2006)

■ **CATTLE:**
As an analgesic:
a) For surgery in adult cattle: 20–30 mg IV (jugular) (may wish to pretreat with 10 mg xylazine) (Powers 1985)

b) 0.02–0.25 mg/kg IV, SQ; 20–30 mg (total dose) IV for an adult animal. Duration of effect is 4 hours. An appropriate withdrawal period is 72 hours for milk, and 4 days for meat. (Walz 2006)

■ **HORSES:** (**Note:** ARCI UCGFS Class 3 Drug)
As an analgesic:
a) 0.1 mg/kg IV q3–4h; not to exceed 48 hours (Package Insert; *Torbugesic®*—Fort Dodge)

b) For moderate to marked abdominal pain: 0.01–0.02 mg/kg IV alone or in combination with xylazine (0.02–0.1 mg/kg IM) (Moore 1999)

c) For colic pain: 5–10 mg (total dose for a 450–500 kg horse) IV combined with 100–200 mg xylazine (total dose). Compared to IV bolus, a constant rate infusion of butorphanol at 23.7 micrograms/kg/hr induces fewer GI side effects while providing analgesia. (Zimmel 2003)

d) Foals: 0.1–0.2 mg/kg IV or IM (Robertson 2003)

e) Two studies have looked at butorphanol CRI in horses for post-op pain. **1)** Loading dose of 0.0178 mg/kg (17.8 micrograms/kg), then a constant rate infusion of 23.7 micrograms/kg/hr; **2)** Constant rate infusion of 13 micrograms/kg/hr (Mogg 2006)

As a preanesthetic, outpatient surgery, or chemical restraint:
a) 0.01–0.04 mg/kg IV (with xylazine 0.1–0.5 mg/kg IV) (Orsini 1988)

b) For field anesthesia: Sedate with xylazine (1 mg/kg IV; 2 mg/kg IM) given 5–10 minutes (longer for IM route) before induction of anesthesia with ketamine (2 mg/kg IV). Horse must be adequately sedated (head to the knees) before giving the ketamine (ketamine can cause muscle rigidity and seizures). If adequate sedation does not occur, either **1)** Redose xylazine: up to half the original dose, **2)** Add butorphanol (0.02–0.04 mg/kg IM). Butorphanol can be given with the original xylazine if you suspect that the horse will be difficult to tranquilize (*e.g.*, high-strung Thoroughbreds) or added before the ketamine. This combination will improve induction, increase analgesia and increase recumbency time by about 5–10 minutes. **3)** Diazepam (0.03 mg/kg IV). Mix the diazepam with the ketamine. This combination will improve induction when sedation is marginal, improve muscle relaxation during anesthesia and prolong anesthesia by about 5–10 minutes. **4)** Guaifenesin (5% solution administered IV to effect) can also be used to increase sedation and muscle relaxation. (Mathews 1999)

As an antitussive:

a) 0.02 mg/kg IM two to three times daily (Orsini 1988)

■ **CAMELIDS:** (llamas and alpacas):

a) As a sedative 0.1 mg/kg or 10 mg (total dose) IM.

As an anesthetic: butorphanol 0.07–0.1 mg/kg; ketamine 0.2–0.3 mg/kg; xylazine 0.2–0.3 mg/kg **IV** or butorphanol 0.05–0.1 mg/kg; ketamine 0.2–0.5 mg/kg; xylazine 0.2–0.5 mg/kg **IM** (Wolff 2009)

b) For procedural pain (*e.g.*, castrations) when recumbency (up to 30 minutes) is desired: Alpacas: butorphanol 0.046 mg/kg; xylazine 0.46 mg/kg; ketamine 4.6 mg/kg. Llamas: butorphanol 0.037 mg/kg; xylazine 0.37 mg/kg; ketamine 3.7 mg/kg. All drugs are combined in one syringe and given IM. May administer 50% of original dose of ketamine and xylazine during anesthesia to prolong effect up to 15 minutes.

If doing mass castrations on 3 or more animals, can make up bottle of the "cocktail." Add 10 mg (1 mL) of butorphanol and 100 mg (1 mL) xylazine to a 1 gram (10 ml vial) of ketamine. This mixture is dosed at 1 mL/40 lbs. (18 kg) for alpacas, and 1 ml per 50 lbs. (22 kg) for llamas. Handle quietly and allow plenty of time before starting procedure. Expect 20 minutes of surgical time; patient should stand 45 minutes to 1 hour after injection. (Miesner 2009)

c) For analgesia: 0.1 mg/kg IV, IM or SC q4-6h. (Miesner 2009)

■ **REPTILES/AMPHIBIANS:**

As an analgesic:

a) 0.05–1 mg/kg q12h IM, IV, PO, SC (up to 20 mg/kg in tortoises) (Bays 2006)

■ **ZOO, EXOTIC, WILDLIFE SPECIES:**

For use of butorphanol in zoo, exotic and wildlife medicine refer to specific references, including:

a) *Zoo Animal and Wildlife Immobilization and Anesthesia.* West, G, Heard, D, Caulkett, N. (eds.). Blackwell Publishing, 2007.

b) *Handbook of Wildlife Chemical Immobilization, 3rd Ed.* Kreeger, T.J. and J.M. Arnemo. 2007.

c) *Restraint and Handling of Wild and Domestic Animals.* Fowler, M (ed.), Iowa State University Press, 1995

d) *Exotic Animal Formulary, 3rd Ed.* Carpenter, J.W., Saunders. 2005

e) The 2009 American Association of Zoo Veterinarian Proceedings by D. K. Fontenot also has several dosages listed for restraint, anesthesia, and analgesia for a variety of drugs for carnivores and primates. VIN members can access them at: http://goo.gl/NNIWQ or http://goo.gl/9UJse

Monitoring

■ Analgesic and/or antitussive efficacy

■ Respiratory rate/depth

■ Appetite and bowel function

■ CNS effects

Client Information

■ Clients should report any significant changes in behavior, appetite, bowel or urinary function in their animals

Chemistry/Synonyms

A synthetic opiate partial agonist, butorphanol tartrate is related structurally to morphine but exhibits pharmacologic actions similar to other partial agonists such as pentazocine or nalbuphine. The compound occurs as a white, crystalline powder that is sparingly soluble in water and insoluble in alcohol. It has a bitter taste and a pK_a of 8.6. The commercial injection has a pH of 3–5.5. One mg of the tartrate is equivalent to 0.68 mg of butorphanol base.

Butorphanol tartrate may also be known as: levo-BC-2627 (butorphanol), *Dolorex®*, *Equanol®*, *Stadol®*, *Torbutrol®*, *Torbugesic®*, and *Verstadol®*.

Storage/Stability

The injectable product should be stored out of bright light and at room temperature; avoid freezing.

Compatibility/Compounding Considerations

The injectable product is reported to be **compatible** with the following IV fluids and drugs: acepromazine, atropine sulfate, chlorpromazine, diphenhydramine HCl, droperidol, fentanyl citrate, hydroxyzine HCl, meperidine, morphine sulfate, pentazocine lactate, perphenazine, prochlorperazine, promethazine HCl, scopolamine HBr, and xylazine.

The drug is reportedly **incompatible** with the following agents: dimenhydrinate, and pentobarbital sodium.

Dosage Forms/Regulatory Status

Note: Butorphanol is a class IV controlled substance. The veterinary products (*Torbutrol®*, *Torbugesic®*) strengths are listed as base activity. The human product (*Stadol®*) strength is labeled as the tartrate salt.

VETERINARY-LABELED PRODUCTS:

Butorphanol Tartrate Injection: 0.5 mg/mL (activity as base) in 10 mL vials; *Torbutrol®* (Fort-Dodge); (Rx, C-IV). FDA-approved for use in dogs.

Butorphanol Tartrate Injection: 2 mg/mL (activity as base) in 10 mL vials. *Torbugesic-SA®* (Fort Dodge); (Rx, C-IV). FDA-approved for use in cats.

Butorphanol Tartrate Injection: 10 mg/mL (activity as base) in 10 mL, 50 mL vials; *Torbugesic®* (Fort-Dodge), *Dolorex®* (Intervet), *Butorject®* (Phoenix), *Torphaject®* (Butler); *Equanol®* (Vedco) generic; (Rx, C-IV). FDA-approved for use in horses not intended for food.

Butorphanol Tartrate Tablets: 1 mg, 5 mg, and 10 mg (activity as base) tablets; bottles of 100; *Torbutrol®* (Fort-Dodge); (Rx, C-IV). FDA-approved for use in dogs.

The ARCI (Racing Commissioners International) has designated this drug as a class 3 substance. See the appendix for more information.

HUMAN-LABELED PRODUCTS:

Butorphanol Tartrate Injection: 1 mg/mL (as tartrate salt; equivalent to 0.68 mg base) in 1 & 2 mL vials; 2 mg/mL (as tartrate salt) in 1, 2 & 10 mL vials; *Stadol®* (Bristol-Myers Squibb); generic; (Rx, C-IV)

Butorphanol Nasal Spray: 10 mg/mL in 2.5 mL metered dose; generic; (Rx, C-IV)

References

Bays, T (2006). Recognizing and managing pain in exotic species. Proceedings: Western Vet Conf. Accessed via: Veterinary Information Network. http://goo.gl/C75Uv

Burke, T (1999). Husbandry and Medicine of Rodents and Lagomorphs. Proceedings: Central Veterinary Conference, Kansas City.

Finkler, M (1999). Anesthesia in Ferrets. Proceedings: Central Veterinary Conference, Kansas City.

Hellyer, P (2006). Pain assessment and multimodal analgesic therapy in dogs and cats. Proceedings: ABVP. Accessed via: Veterinary Information Network. http://goo.gl/LMXcX

Huerkamp, M (1995). Anesthesia and postoperative management of rabbits and pocket pets. *Kirk's Current Veterinary Therapy:XII.* J Bonagura Ed. Philadelphia, W.B. Saunders: 1322–1327.

Ivey, E & J Morrisey (2000). Therapeutics for Rabbits. *Vet Clin NA: Exotic Anim Pract* **3:1**(Jan): 183–216.

Johnson, L (2000). Diseases of the Bronchus. *Textbook of Veterinary Internal Medicine: Diseases of the Dog and Cat.* S Ettinger and E Feldman Eds. Philadelphia, WB Saunders. **2:** 1055–1061.

Johnson, L (2004). Canine airway collapse. Proceedings: ACVIM Forum. Accessed via: Veterinary Information Network. http://goo.gl/yKRzG

Klausner, JS & FW Bell (1988, Last Update). "Personal Communication."

Lennox, A (2009). Avian advanced anaesthesia, monitoring and critical care. Proceedings: BSAVA. Accessed via: Veterinary Information Network. http://goo.gl/er09t

Lichtenberger, M (2006a). Anesthesia Protocols and Pain Management for Exotic Animal Patients. Proceedings: Western Vet Conf. Accessed via: Veterinary Information Network. http://goo.gl/hB5Kt

Lichtenberger, M (2006b). Pain management protocols for the ICU patient. Proceedings: Western Vet Conf. Accessed via: Veterinary Information Network. http://goo.gl/duBz4

Mathews, N (1999). Anesthesia in large animals—Injectable (field) anesthesia: How to make it better. Proceedings: Central Veterinary Conference, Kansas City.

Miesner, M (2009). Field anesthesia techniques in camelids. Proceedings: WVC. Accessed via: Veterinary Information Network. http://goo.gl/aYHQB

Moffat, K (2008). Addressing canine and feline aggression in the veterinary clinic. *Vet Clin NA: Sm Anim Pract* **38**: 983–1003.

Mogg, T (2006). Pain management in horses. Proceedings: ACVIM. Accessed via: Veterinary Information Network. http://goo.gl/6YLPg

Moore, R (1999). Medical treatment of abdominal pain in the horse: Analgesics and IV fluids. Proceedings: The North American Veterinary Conference, Orlando.

Orsini, JA (1988). Butorphanol tartrate: Pharmacology and clinical indications. *Comp CE* **10**(7): 849–854.

Perkowski, S (2006). Practicing pain management in the acute setting. Proceedings: ACVIM. Accessed via: Veterinary Information Network. http://goo.gl/TRPqy

Powers, JF (1985). Butorphanol analgesia in the bovine. Proceedings: American Assoc. of Bovine Practitioners Conference, Buffalo.

Quandt, J (2009). Sedation and analgesia for the critically ill patient: Comprehensive review. Proceedings: ACVIM. Accessed via: Veterinary Information Network. http://goo.gl/wfkfQ

Robertson, S (2003). Sedation and general anesthesia of foals. *Current Therapy in Equine Medicine 5.* E Carr Ed. Philadelphia, Saunders: 115–120.

Sladky, KK, V Miletic, et al. (2007). Analgesic efficacy and respiratory effects of butorphanol and morphine in turtles. *Javma–Journal of the American Veterinary Medical Association* **230**(9): 1356–1362.

Valverde, A (2008). Epidural analgesia and anesthesia in dogs and cats. *Vet Clin NA: Sm Anim Pract* **38**: 1205–1230.

Walz, P (2006). Practical management of pain in cattle. Proceedings: ABVP. Accessed via: Veterinary Information Network. http://goo.gl/hScVv

Williams, B (2000). Therapeutics in Ferrets. *Vet Clin NA: Exotic Anim Pract* **3:1**(Jan): 131–153.

Wolff, P (2009). Camelid Medicine. Proceedings: AAZV. Accessed via: Veterinary Information Network. http://goo.gl/4TEAy

Zimmel, D (2003). Management of pain and dehydration in horses with colic. *Current Therapy in Equine Medicine 5.* A Blikslager Ed. Philadelphia, Saunders: 115–120.

n-Butylscopolammonium Bromide–See the monograph found in the "N's" before neomycin

CABERGOLINE

(ka-*ber*-go-leen)   Dostinex®, Galastop®

PROLACTIN INHIBITOR/DOPAMINE (D2) AGONIST

Prescriber Highlights

▶ Ergot derivative used for reducing prolactin levels in bitches and queens. Indications include: inducing/synchronizing estrus, inducing abortion, treating pseudopregnancy, mastitis, and pre-surgery for mammary tumors.

▶ Appears to be well tolerated in dogs & cats; vomiting has been infrequently reported, but adverse effects are much less than with bromocriptine.

▶ Potentially very expensive, particularly in large dogs, but generic tablets now available; usually must be compounded for accurate dosing.

Uses/Indications

For dogs and cats, cabergoline may be useful for inducing estrus, treatment of primary or secondary anestrus, mastitis, pseudopregnancy, as a treatment prior to mammary tumor surgery, and pregnancy termination in the second half of pregnancy. Cabergoline may be useful in treating some cases of pituitary-dependent hyperadrenocorticism (Cushing's).

Preliminary work has been done in psittacines (primarily Cockatiels) for adjunctive treatment of reproductive-related disorders, particularly persistent egg laying.

In humans, cabergoline is indicated for the treatment of disorders associated with hyperprolactenemia or the treatment of Parkinson's disease.

Pharmacology/Actions

Cabergoline has a high affinity for dopamine$_2$ (D$_2$) receptors and has a long duration of action. It exerts a direct inhibitory effect on the secretion of prolactin from the pituitary. When compared to bromocriptine it has greater D$_2$ specificity, a longer duration of action, and less tendency to cause vomiting.

Pharmacokinetics

The pharmacokinetics of cabergoline have apparently not been reported for dogs or cats. In humans, the drug is absorbed after oral dosing but its absolute bioavailability is not known. Food does not appear to significantly alter absorption. The drug is only moderately bound to plasma proteins ($\approx$50%). Cabergoline is extensively metabolized in the liver via hydrolysis; these metabolites and about 4% of unchanged drug are excreted into the urine. Half-life is estimated to be around 60 hours. Duration of pharmacologic action may persist for 48 hours or more. Renal dysfunction does not appear to significantly alter elimination characteristics of the drug.

Contraindications/Precautions/Warnings

Cabergoline is contraindicated in dogs and cats that are pregnant unless abortion is desired (see indications). Cabergoline should not be used in patients who are hypersensitive to ergot derivatives. Patients that do not tolerate bromocriptine may or may not tolerate cabergoline. In humans, cabergoline is contraindicated in patients who have uncontrolled hypertension.

Patients with significantly impaired liver function should receive the drug with caution, and if required, possibly at a lower dosage.

When using to induce estrus, it is recommended to wait at least 4 months after the prior cycle to allow the uterus to recover.

Adverse Effects

Cabergoline is usually well tolerated by animal patients. Vomiting has been reported, but may be alleviated by administering with food. Dogs receiving cabergoline for more than 14 days may exhibit changes in coat color.

Human patients have reported postural hypotension, dizziness, headache, nausea and vomiting while receiving cabergoline.

Reproductive/Nursing Safety

This drug can cause spontaneous abortion in pregnant dogs or cats. In pregnant humans, cabergoline is designated by the FDA as a category *B* drug (*Animal studies have not demonstrated risk to the fetus, but there are no adequate studies in pregnant women; or animal studies have shown an adverse effect, but adequate studies in pregnant women have not demonstrated a risk to the fetus during the first trimester of pregnancy, and there is no evidence of risk in later trimesters.*)

Because cabergoline suppresses prolactin, it should not be used in nursing mothers.

Overdosage/Acute Toxicity

Overdose information is not available for dogs or cats, and remains very limited for humans. It is postulated that cabergoline overdoses in people could cause hypotension, nasal congestion, syncope or hallucinations. Treatment is basically supportive and primarily focuses on supporting blood pressure.

Drug Interactions

The following drug interactions have either been reported or are theoretical in humans or animals receiving cabergoline and may be of significance in veterinary patients:

■ **HYPOTENSIVE DRUGS:** Because cabergoline may have hypotensive effects, concomitant use with other hypotensive drugs may cause additive hypotension

■ **METOCLOPRAMIDE:** Use with cabergoline may reduce the efficacy of both drugs and should be avoided

■ **PHENOTHIAZINES (e.g., acepromazine, chlorpromazine):** Use of cabergoline with dopamine (D$_2$) antagonists may reduce the efficacy of both drugs and should be avoided

Laboratory Considerations

■ No particular laboratory interactions or considerations were located for this drug.

Doses

Because of the dosage differences in animals versus human patients and the strength of the commercially available product, a compounding pharmacist must usually reformulate this medication.

■ **DOGS:**

For estrus induction:

a) 5 micrograms/kg PO once daily induces fertile proestrus in 4–25 days. (Davidson 2004)

b) 5 micrograms/kg PO once daily until an induced proestrus is pronounced for 2 days or until onset of estrus (Concannon 2005)

c) 0.6 micrograms/kg PO once daily. Make a 10 micrograms per mL solution by dissolving commercial tablets in warm distilled water (One 0.5 mg tablet (500 micrograms) per 50 mL of distilled water.) Give the appropriate dose for the patient within 15 minutes of preparation and discard the remaining solution. Continue until day 2 after the onset of the first signs of proestrus, or until day 42 without signs of proestrus. 81% (22 of 27) of dogs treated at this low dose showed proestrus between days 4 and 48. (Cirit *et al.* 2006)

To reduce milk production:

a) For pseudocyesis (pseudopregnancy): 5 micrograms/kg once a day PO for 5–10 days. (Gobello *et al.* 2001)

b) For pseudocyesis: 5 micrograms/kg once a day or every other day SC (likely needs to be compounded). (Davidson 2004)

c) For pseudocyesis: 5 micrograms/kg PO once daily for 4-5 days; occasional failures can be handled by repeating treatment and extending duration to 8-10 days. Additional protocols for treatment failures include combining cabergoline with metergoline (500 micrograms/kg PO twice daily), or cabergoline with bromocriptine (10–30 micrograms/kg PO twice daily). (Romagnoli 2009)

d) For adjunctive treatment of mastitis after puppies weaned: 5 micrograms/kg PO daily. (Traas & O'Conner 2009)

During the diestrous period to pre-treat mammary tumors prior to surgery:

a) 5 micrograms/kg PO 5–7 days before surgery. (Fontbonne 2007)

For pregnancy termination:

a) Administer after day 40: 5 micrograms/kg PO for 5 days; approximately 50% effective (Romagnoli 2006)

b) Between days 35–45: Cabergoline 5 micrograms/kg PO once daily for 7 days in food and cloprostenol at 1 microgram/kg SC (after a tenfold dilution with physiologic saline) on days 1 and 3 given at least 8 hours after food. If pregnancy not terminated by day 8, cabergoline continued (at same dose) until day 12. (Corrada *et al.* 2006)

For pituitary-dependent hyperadrenocorticism (Cushing's Disease):

a) 0.1 mg/kg PO every 3 days. Effective in 70% of dogs treated. Dogs with tumor sizes greater than 5 mm did not respond. (Castillo *et al.* 2005)

■ **CATS:**

For pregnancy termination:

a) At 30 days post-coitus, cabergoline at 5 micrograms/kg PO q24h and cloprostenol 5 micrograms/kg SC q48h in 7–13 days was used to induce abortion. (Davidson 2004)

To reduce prolactin production in queens:

a) 5 micrograms/kg PO once daily (Romagnoli 2009)

During the diestrous period to pre-treat mammary tumors prior to surgery:

a) 5 micrograms/kg PO 5–7 days before surgery. (Fontbonne 2007)

■ **BIRDS:**

For persistent egg laying in psittacines combination with removal of males, altered light cycle:

a) Initially 10–20 micrograms/kg PO daily; higher dosages were also used. Further work needed to determine the dose rate, etc. (Chitty *et al.* 2006)

Monitoring

■ Efficacy

■ Adverse effects

Client Information

■ Give this medication with food; contact veterinarian if vomiting persists

Chemistry/Synonyms

Cabergoline, a synthetic, ergot-derivative, dopamine agonist similar to bromocriptine, occurs as a white powder that is insoluble in water, and soluble in ethanol or chloroform. The commercially available tablets also contain the inactive ingredients, leucine and lactose.

Cabergoline may also be known as FCE-21336, cabergolina, *Cabasar®*, *Actualene®*, *Sostilar®*, *Dostinex®* or *Galastop®*.

Storage/Stability

The commercially available tablets should be stored at controlled room temperature (20°–25°C; 68°–77°F). The veterinary (Europe) oral liquid product *Galastop®* should be stored below

25°C and protected from light. Do not refrigerate. Once opened, it should be used within 28 days.

Compatibility/Compounding Considerations
It has been reported that the drug is unstable or degrades in aqueous suspensions and if compounded into a liquid that will not be used immediately, should be compounded into a lipid-based product. Preparing a fresh aqueous solution for immediate use should be stable (see estrus induction for dogs dose "c" above).

Dosage Forms/Regulatory Status

VETERINARY-LABELED PRODUCTS: None in USA.

Cabergoline is available in Europe as *Galastop®* (Ceva) 50 micrograms/mL oral liquid (miglyol base). An injectable product, *Galastop® Injectable* is available in some countries.

HUMAN-LABELED PRODUCTS:

Cabergoline Oral Tablets: 0.5 mg (500 micrograms); generic; (Rx)

References

Castillo, V, J Lalia, et al. (2005). Cushing's disease (pituitary dependent) in dogs: Its treatment with cabergoline. Proceedings: WSAVA. Accessed via: Veterinary Information Network. http://goo.gl/XBFZZ

Chitty, J, A Raftery, et al. (2006). Use of cabergoline in companion psittacine birds. Proceedings: AAV. Accessed via: Veterinary Information Network. http://goo.gl/xuaW6

Cirit, U, S Bacinoglu, et al. (2006). The effects of low dose cabergoline on induction of estrus and pregnancy rates in anestrus bitches. Anim Repro Sci **in press**.

Concannon, P (2005). Estrus induction in dogs: approaches, protocols and applications. Proceedings: WSAVA. Accessed via: Veterinary Information Network. http://goo.gl/IcPIK

Corrada, Y, R Rodriguez, et al. (2006). A combination of oral cabergoline and double cloprostenol injections to produce third–quarter gestation termination in the bitch. J Am Anim Hosp Assoc **42**(366–370).

Davidson, A (2004). Update: Therapeutics for reproductive disorders in small animal practice. Proceedings: ACVIM Forum. Accessed via: Veterinary Information Network. http://goo.gl/Fe4Gp

Fontbonne, A (2007). Hormones and antibiotics in canine and feline reproduction. Proceedings: WSAVA. Accessed via: Veterinary Information Network. http://goo.gl/JsqHc

Gobello, C, C Concannon, et al. (2001). Canine Pseudopregnancy: A Review. Recent Advances in Small Animal Reproduction. C Concannon, G England, J Verstegen and C Linde–Forsberg Eds. Ithaca, IVIS.

Romagnoli, S (2006). Control of reproduction in dogs and cats: Use and misuse of hormones. Proceedings: WSAVA World Congress. Accessed via: Veterinary Information Network. http://goo.gl/aGuBF

Romagnoli, S (2009). An update on pseudopregnancy. Proceedings: WSAVA. Accessed via: Veterinary Information Network. http://goo.gl/0FKV9

Traas, A & C O'Conner (2009). Postpartum Emergencies. Proceedings: IVECCS. Accessed via: Veterinary Information Network. http://goo.gl/KGCXC

CALCITONIN SALMON

(kal-si-*toe*-nin *sam*-in)
Miacalcin®, Calcimar®

OSTEOCLAST INHIBITING HORMONE

Prescriber Highlights

▶ Hormone used primarily to control hypercalcemia in dogs and hypercalcemia or nutritional secondary hyperparathyroidism in reptiles

▶ Hypersensitivity possible

▶ Young animals may be extremely sensitive to effects

▶ May cause GI effects

▶ Do not confuse with calcitriol

Uses/Indications

In small animals, calcitonin has been used as adjunctive therapy to control hypercalcemia. It potentially may be of use in the adjunctive treatment of pain, particularly when originating from bone. Calcitonin's use in veterinary medicine has been limited by expense, availability and resistance development to its effects after several days of treatment.

Pharmacology/Actions

Calcitonin has a multitude of physiologic effects. It principally acts on bone inhibiting osteoclastic bone resorption. By reducing tubular reabsorption of calcium, phosphate, sodium, magnesium, potassium and chloride, it promotes their renal excretion. Calcitonin also increases jejunal secretion of water, sodium, potassium and chloride (not calcium).

Pharmacokinetics

Calcitonin is destroyed in the gut after oral administration and therefore must be administered parenterally. In humans, the onset of effect after IV administration of calcitonin salmon is immediate. After IM or SC administration, onset occurs within 15 minutes with maximal effects occurring in about 4 hours. Duration of action is 8–14 hours after IM or SC injection. The drug is thought to be rapidly metabolized by the kidneys, in the blood and peripheral tissues.

Contraindications/Precautions/Warnings

Calcitonin is contraindicated in animals hypersensitive to it. Patients with a history of hypersensitivity to other proteins may be at risk. Young animals are reportedly up to 100 times more sensitive to calcitonin than are older animals (adults).

Adverse Effects

There is not a well-documented adverse effect profile for calcitonin in domestic animals. Anorexia and vomiting have been reported to occur in dogs. Overmedicating can lead to hypocalcemia. The following effects are documented in humans and potentially could be seen in animals: diarrhea, anorexia, vomiting, swelling and pain at injection site, redness and peripheral paresthesias. Rarely, allergic reactions may occur. Tachyphylaxis (resistance to drug therapy with time) may occur in some dogs treated.

Reproductive/Nursing Safety

There is little information on the reproductive safety of calcitonin; however, it does not cross the placenta. Very high doses have decreased birth weights in laboratory animals, presumably due to the metabolic effects of the drug. In humans, the FDA categorizes this drug as category *C* for use during pregnancy (*Animal studies have shown an adverse effect on the fetus, but there are no adequate studies in humans; or there are no animal reproduction studies and no adequate studies in humans.*)

Calcitonin has been shown to inhibit lactation. Safe use during nursing has not been established.

Overdosage/Acute Toxicity

Very limited data is available. Nausea and vomiting have been reported after accidental overdose injections. Chronic overdosing can lead to hypocalcemia.

Drug Interactions

The following drug interactions have either been reported or are theoretical in humans or animals receiving calcitonin and may be of significance in veterinary patients:

■ **VITAMIN D ANALOGS** or **CALCIUM** products: May interfere with the efficacy of calcitonin

Doses

■ **DOGS:**

For hypervitaminosis D (toxicity)/hypercalcemia:

a) 4–8 Units/kg SC two to three times a day. Effects are short-lived and multiple treatments are required. (Mooney 2008)

b) 4–6 Units/kg SC q2–3 hours until serum calcium levels are normalized (Firth 2000)

c) For adjunctive therapy if fluid deficit replacement, saline diuresis, furosemide and prednisone have failed to control calcium: 4 Units/kg IV, then 4–8 Units/kg SC q12–24h (Nelson & Elliott 2003)

d) 4–6 Units/kg SC q8–12h (Davies 2005)

■ **REPTILES:**

For hypercalcemia:

a) Green iguanas in combination with fluid therapy: 1.5 Units/kg SC q8h for several weeks if necessary (Gauvin 1993)

For nutritional secondary hyperparathyroidism (NSHP):

a) If reptile is not hypocalcemic: 50 Units/kg IM once weekly for 2–3 doses. (Hernandez-Divers 2005)

b) Correct husbandry problems and correct hypocalcemia with calcium and vitamin

D. Once calcium level is normal and patient is on oral calcium supplementation (usually about 7 days after starting therapy) give calcitonin at 50 Units/kg IM weekly for 2–3 doses. Supportive care can be tapered off once patient becomes stable. (Johnson 2004)

Monitoring

■ Serum Calcium

Chemistry/Synonyms

A polypeptide hormone, calcitonin is a 32-amino acid polypeptide having a molecular weight of about 3600. Calcitonin is available commercially as either calcitonin human or calcitonin salmon, both of which are synthetically prepared. Potency of calcitonin salmon is expressed in international units (IU), in this reference this is expressed as Units. Calcitonin salmon is approximately 50X more potent than calcitonin human on a per weight basis.

Calcitonin salmon may also be known as calcitonin-salmon, calcitoninum salmonis, salmon calcitonin, SCT-1, or *Calcimar*®; many other trade names are available internationally.

Storage/Stability

Calcitonin salmon for injection should be stored in the refrigerator (2–8°C). The nasal solution should be stored in the refrigerator but protected from freezing. Once in use it should be stored at room temperature in an upright position; use within 35 days.

Dosage Forms/Regulatory Status

VETERINARY-LABELED PRODUCTS: None

HUMAN-LABELED PRODUCTS:

Calcitonin Salmon for Injection: 200 IU/mL in 2 mL vials; *Miacalcin*® (Novartis); (Rx)

Calcitonin Salmon Intranasal Spray: 200 Units/activation (0.09 mL/dose) in 2 mL vials (*Miacalcin*®) and 3.7 mL metered-dose (*Fortical*®) glass bottle with pump; *Miacalcin*® (Novartis); *Fortical*® (Upsher-Smith)

References

Davies, D (2005). Clinical Approach to Canine Blood Calcium Disorders. Proceedings: ACVSc2005. Accessed via: Veterinary Information Network. http://goo.gl/xEIC6

Firth, A (2000). Treatments used in small animal toxicoses. Kirk's Current Veterinary Therapy: XIII Small Animal Practice. J Bonagura Ed. Philadelphia, WB Saunders: 207–211.

Gauvin, J (1993). Drug therapy in reptiles. Seminars in Avian & Exotic Med 2(1): 48–59.

Hernandez–Divers, S (2005). Reptile Non–Infectious Diseases. Proceedings: WSAVA World Congress. Accessed via: Veterinary Information Network. http://goo.gl/gHqcs

Johnson, D (2004). Metabolic bone disease in reptiles. Proceedings: ACVC. Accessed via: Veterinary Information Network. http://goo.gl/Lo63t

Mooney, C (2008). Hypercalcaemia—Distinguishing causes and preventing complications. Proceedings: WSAVA. Accessed via: Veterinary Information Network. http://goo.gl/HxLEc

Nelson, R & D Elliott (2003). Metabolic and electrolyte disorders. Small Animal Internal Medicine, 3rd Ed. R Nelson and C Couto Eds. St Louis, Mosby: 816–846.

CALCITRIOL

(kal-si-*trye*-ole)
Rocaltrol®, Calcijex®, Active Vitamin D3

VITAMIN D ANALOG

Prescriber Highlights

▶ Vitamin D analog may be useful in dogs (& possibly cats) for treatment of hypocalcemia, chronic renal disease or idiopathic seborrhea.

▶ Contraindications: Hypercalcemia, hyperphosphatemia, malabsorption syndromes

▶ Adverse Effects: Hypercalcemia, hypercalcuria or hyperphosphatemia greatest concerns

▶ May need to have oral dosage forms compounded

▶ Do not confuse with calcitonin

Uses/Indications

Calcitriol can be useful when combined with oral calcium therapy for the long-term treatment of hypocalcemia associated with hypoparathyroidism. It may be potentially beneficial in the adjunctive treatment of chronic renal disease in dogs and cats but its use is somewhat controversial, particularly the decision on how soon in the course of chronic renal insufficiency it should employed. It reportedly can improve cats' appetite and general well being. It may also be of benefit in treating some types of dermatopathies (primary idiopathic seborrhea).

Pharmacology/Actions

Calcitriol is a vitamin D analog. Vitamin D is considered a hormone and, in conjunction with parathormone (PTH) and calcitonin, regulates calcium homeostasis in the body. Active analogues (or metabolites) of vitamin D enhance calcium absorption from the GI tract, promote reabsorption of calcium by the renal tubules, and increase the rate of accretion and resorption of minerals in bone. Calcitriol has a rapid onset of action (approximately 1 day) and a short duration of action. Unlike other forms of vitamin D, calcitriol does not require renal activation for it to be effective.

Pharmacokinetics

If fat absorption is normal, vitamin D analogs are readily absorbed from the GI tract (small intestine). Bile is required for adequate absorption and patients with steatorrhea, liver or biliary disease will have diminished absorption. Calcitriol has a rapid onset of biologic action and has a short duration of action (<1 day to 2–3 days). Dogs and cats appear to require much smaller doses of calcitriol than do humans.

Contraindications/Precautions/Warnings

Calcitriol is contraindicated in patients with hypercalcemia, vitamin D toxicity, malabsorption syndrome, or abnormal sensitivity to the effects of vitamin D. It should be used with extreme caution in patients with hyperphosphatemia (many clinicians believe hyperphosphatemia or a combined calcium/phosphorous product of >70 is a contraindication to the use of vitamin D analogs). Using calcitriol in patients with hyperphosphatemia can increase risks for tissue mineralization with additional renal tissue damage and dysfunction. Generally, calcium and phosphorus levels should be in the low normal range before beginning treatment.

As calcitriol can promote hypercalciuria, it should be used with caution in animals susceptible to calcium oxalate uroliths.

Adverse Effects

While hypercalcemia is a definite concern, calcitriol administered in low dosages to dogs with chronic renal disease infrequently causes hypercalcemia, unless it is used with a calcium-containing phosphorus binder, particularly calcium carbonate. Signs of hypercalcemia include polydipsia, polyuria and anorexia. Hyperphosphatemia may also occur and patients' serum phosphate levels should be normalized before therapy is begun. Monitoring of serum calcium levels is mandatory while using this drug.

Reproductive/Nursing Safety

Calcitriol has proven to be teratogenic in laboratory animal when given at doses several times higher than those used therapeutically. In humans, the FDA categorizes this drug as category **C** for use during pregnancy (*Animal studies have shown an adverse effect on the fetus, but there are no adequate studies in humans; or there are no animal reproduction studies and no adequate studies in humans.*)

Safe use during lactation has not been established.

Overdosage/Acute Toxicity

Overdosage can cause hypercalcemia, hypercalciuria, and hyperphosphatemia. Intake of excessive calcium and phosphate may also cause the same effect. Acute ingestions should be managed using established protocols for removal or prevention of the drug being absorbed from the GI. Orally administered mineral oil may reduce absorption and enhance fecal elimination.

Hypercalcemia secondary to chronic dosing of the drug should be treated by first temporarily discontinuing (not dose reduction) calcitriol and exogenous calcium therapy. If the hypercalcemia is severe, furosemide, calcium-free IV fluids (*e.g.*, normal saline), urine acidification, and corticosteroids may be employed.

Drug Interactions

The following drug interactions have either been reported or are theoretical in humans or animals

receiving calcitriol and may be of significance in veterinary patients:

■ **CALCIUM-CONTAINING PHOSPHORUS BINDING AGENTS (e.g., calcium carbonate):** Use with calcitriol may induce hypercalcemia

■ **CORTICOSTEROIDS:** Can nullify the effects of vitamin D analogs

■ **DIGOXIN or VERAPAMIL:** Patients on verapamil or digoxin are sensitive to the effects of hypercalcemia; intensified monitoring is required

■ **PHENYTOIN, BARBITURATES or PRIMIDONE:** May induce hepatic enzyme systems and increase the metabolism of Vitamin D analogs thus decreasing their activity

■ **THIAZIDE DIURETICS:** May cause hypercalcemia when given in conjunction with Vitamin D analogs

Laboratory Considerations

■ **SERUM CHOLESTEROL** levels may be falsely elevated by vitamin D analogs when using the Zlatkis-Zak reaction for determination

Doses

■ **DOGS:**
To suppress secondary hyperparathyroidism in CRF:
a) Decision to use calcitriol must be made with caution because hypercalcemia is potentially a serious complication that if prolonged can result in a reduction (reversible or irreversible) of GFR. Hypercalcemia is an uncommon side effect (unless used with a calcium-containing phosphorus binding agent) if calcitriol is dosed at 2.5–3.5 nanograms/kg/day PO. (Polzin *et al.* 2005)

b) 2.5–3.5 nanograms/kg PO once daily. Dogs with refractory hyperparathyroidism may require up to 6 nanograms/kg/day. (Chew 2003)

c) **1)** Confirm the diagnosis of chronic renal failure (serum creatinine >2 mg/dL); **2)** Reduce hyperphosphatemia to <6 mg/dL; **3)** If serum creatinine between 2–3 mg/dL and serum phosphorus <6 mg/dL, start calcitriol at 2.5–3.5 nanograms/kg/day PO (so-called "preventative" dose); if serum creatinine >3 mg/dL and serum phosphorus <6 mg/dL, obtain a baseline PTH level and start calcitriol at 3.5 nanograms/kg/day.

Monitoring of preventative dose: assess serum calcium on days 7 and 14 after starting calcitriol and then every 6 months. Serum creatinine should be measured every 1–3 months. If hypercalcemia occurs, stop calcitriol for one week to determine if the drug is causing the hypercalcemia or if it's due to another cause (*e.g.*, too little calcitriol).

Monitoring patients with elevated PTH: monitor as above, but also determine PTH levels at 4–6 weeks after starting calcitriol. If still elevated increase dose by 1–2 nanograms/kg/day, but do not exceed 6.6 nanograms/kg/day unless monitoring ionized calcium. If higher daily doses are required (5–7 nanograms/kg/day), a pulsed-dosing strategy may be considered. This is usually about 20 nanograms/kg given twice weekly PO at bedtime on an empty stomach. (Nagode 2005)

For hypocalcemia:
a) For subacute and chronic maintenance treatment of hypocalcemia: Initially, 20–30 nanograms/kg/day PO divided twice a day for 3–4 days, then 5–15 nanograms/kg/day divided twice a day (Chew & Nagode 2000)

b) For long-term maintenance in animals with hypoparathyroidism: 0.03–0.06 micro-grams/kg/day. Maximal effect is in 1–4 days. Combine with oral calcium to reduce vitamin D dose requirements. Adjust dose by monitoring serum calcium. (Crystal 2007)

For primary idiopathic seborrhea (especially in spaniel breeds):
a) 10 nanograms/kg PO once daily. Give as far away from the main meal as possible. (Kwochka 1999)

■ **CATS:**
To suppress secondary hyperparathyroidism in CRF:
a) 1.5–3.5 nanograms/kg PO daily given separately from meals. Remove oil from capsule, dilute in corn oil, then give the appropriate volume. Store for up to 2 weeks. (Gunn-Moore 2008)

b) 2.5–3.5 nanograms/kg PO once daily (Chew 2003)

c) See the dog dose in "c" above (Nagode 2005)

For long-term maintenance in animals with hypoparathyroidism:
a) 0.03–0.06 micrograms/kg/day. Maximal effect is in 1-4 days. Combine with oral calcium to reduce vitamin D dose requirements. Adjust dose by monitoring serum calcium. (Crystal 2007)

Monitoring

■ Serum calcium, phosphate, creatinine. Baseline and at one week; then every 2–4 weeks thereafter

■ Serum PTH levels, especially in cats

■ Clinical efficacy (*e.g.*, improved appetite, activity level, slowed progression of disease)

Client Information

■ Clients should be briefed on the signs of hypercalcemia (polydipsia, polyuria, anorexia)

and hypocalcemia (muscle tremors, twitching, tetany, weakness, stiff gait, ataxia, behavioral changes, and seizures) and instructed to report these signs to the veterinarian

■ If using lower doses (<3.5 nanograms/kg/day) give with the morning meal; if using doses of >5 nanograms/kg/day; administer at bedtime on an empty stomach to reduce chance for hypercalcemia

Chemistry/Synonyms

Calcitriol, a vitamin D analog is synthesized for pharmaceutical use. It is a white crystalline compound and is insoluble in water.

Calcitriol may also be known as: calcitrolo, calcitriolum, 1,25-dihydroxycholecalciferol, 1-alpha,25 dihydrocholecalciferol, 1alpha, 25-Dihydroxyvitamin D_3 or 1,25-DHCC, 1,25-dihidroxyvitamin D_3, Ro 21-5535, U 49562, *Acuode®, Alpha D$_3$®, Bocatriol®, Calcijex®, Calcitriol KyraMed®, Calcitriol Purissimus®, Calcitriol-Nefro®, Calcitriolo®, Decostriol®, Dexiven®, Difix®, Hitrol®, Kalcytriol®, Kolkatriol®, Lotravel®, Osteotriol®, Renatriol®, Rexamat®, Rocaltrol®, Roical®, Rolsical®, Silkis®, Sitriol®,* or *Tirocal®.*

Storage/Stability

Protect from light. Store in tight, light resistant containers at room temperature. The injection does not contain preservatives and remaining drug should be discarded after opening ampule.

Dosage Forms/Regulatory Status

VETERINARY-LABELED PRODUCTS: None

HUMAN-LABELED PRODUCTS:

Note: Most doses are expressed in nanograms/kg (ng/kg); to convert micrograms to nanograms: 1 microgram = 1000 ng, 0.25 micrograms = 250 ng, etc. Reformulation by a compounding pharmacy is usually required to assure accurate dosing.

Calcitriol Oral Capsules: 0.25 micrograms & 0.5 micrograms; *Rocaltrol®* (Validus); Calcitriol (Teva); (Rx)

Calcitriol Oral Solution: 1 microgram/mL in 15 mL btls, *Rocaltrol®* (Roche); & single-use graduated oral dispensers; Calcitriol (Roxane); (Rx)

Calcitriol Injection: 1 microgram/mL & 2 micrograms/mL in 1 mL amps & vials; *Calcijex®* (Abbott); Calcitriol Injection (aaiPharma); (Rx)

Topical also available

References

Chew, D (2003). Chronic Renal Failure Treatment Updates. Proceedings: Western Veterinary Conf. Accessed via: Veterinary Information Network. http://goo.gl/qh2SQ

Chew, D & L Nagode (2000). Treatment of hypoparathyroidism. Kirk's Current Veterinary Therapy: XIII Small Animal Practice. J Bonagura Ed. Philadelphia, WB Saunders: 340–345.

Crystal, M (2007). Hypoparathyroidism. Backwell's 5-Minute Veterinary Consult: Canine & Feline. L Tilley and F Smith Eds., Blackwell: 720–721.

Gunn–Moore, D (2008). The diagnosis and treatment of renal insufficiency in cats. Proceedings: World Veterinary Congress. Accessed via: Veterinary Information Network. http://goo.gl/9dqhs

Kwochka, K (1999). The Cutting Edge of Dermatologic Therapy. Proceedings: North American Veterinary Conference, Orlando.

Nagode, L (2005). "Medical FAQ's: Protocol for calcitriol use in CRF dogs and cats." http://goo.gl/rJtvg.

Polzin, D, C Osborne, et al. (2005). Chronic Kidney Disease. Textbook of Veterinary Internal Medicine: Diseases of the Dog and Cat 6th Ed. S Ettinger and E Feldman Eds., Elsevier: 1756–1785.

CALCIUM ACETATE

(*kal*-see-um ass-a-*tate*)   PhosLo®
ORAL PHOSPHATE BINDER

Prescriber Highlights

▶ Oral phosphorus binding agent for use in treating hyperphosphatemia associated with chronic renal failure

▶ Must monitor serum phosphorus & calcium

Uses/Indications

Calcium acetate can be used for oral administration to treat hyperphosphatemia in patients with chronic renal failure. Secondary to its phosphorus binding efficiency and lower concentration of elemental calcium, calcium acetate is considered the most effective and having the lowest potential for causing hypercalcemia of the calcium-based phosphorus-binding agents. When compared to calcium carbonate, calcium acetate binds approximately twice as much phosphorus per gram of elemental calcium administered. Unlike calcium citrate, calcium acetate does not promote aluminum absorption.

Pharmacology/Actions

When calcium acetate is given with meals it binds to dietary phosphorus and forms calcium phosphate, an insoluble compound that is eliminated in the feces. Calcium acetate is soluble over a range of pH and, therefore, available for binding phosphorus in the stomach and proximal small intestine.

Pharmacokinetics

No information was located on the pharmacokinetics of calcium acetate in dogs and cats. In humans, approximately 30% is absorbed when given with food.

Contraindications/Precautions/Warnings

This agent should not be used when hypercalcemia is present. Because hypercalcemia can result from administering oral calcium products to animals with renal failure, adequate monitoring of serum ionized calcium and phosphorus is required.

Use calcium containing phosphate binders with caution in patients having a serum calcium and phosphorus product greater than 60.

Using calcium-based phosphate binders and

calcitriol together is controversial. Some authors state the combination is contraindicated, while others state that intensified monitoring for hypercalcemia is required.

Adverse Effects

Hypercalcemia is the primary concern associated with using high dosages of this agent; adequate monitoring is required.

In humans, GI intolerance (nausea) has been reported.

Reproductive/Nursing Safety

No reproductive safety studies were located and the human label states that it is not known whether the drug can cause fetal harm. However, it would be surprising if calcium acetate caused teratogenic effects. In humans, the FDA categorizes calcium acetate as category **C** for use during pregnancy (*Animal studies have shown an adverse effect on the fetus, but there are no adequate studies in humans; or there are no animal reproduction studies and no adequate studies in humans.*)

It would be expected that calcium acetate would be safe to administer during lactation.

Overdosage/Acute Toxicity

Potentially, acute overdoses could cause hypercalcemia. Patients should be monitored and treated symptomatically. If dosage was massive and recent, consider using standard protocols to empty the gut.

Drug Interactions

The following drug interactions have either been reported or are theoretical in humans or animals receiving calcium acetate and may be of significance in veterinary patients:

- ■ **CALCITRIOL:** If administered with calcium acetate, may lead to hypercalcemia; if calcitriol is used concomitantly, intensified monitoring for hypercalcemia is mandatory
- ■ **DIGOXIN:** Calcium acetate is not recommended for use in human patients that are on digoxin therapy, as hypercalcemia may cause serious arrhythmias
- ■ **FLUOROQUINOLONES, TETRACYCLINES:** Oral calcium-containing products can reduce absorption of fluoroquinolones; if both calcium acetate and one of these antibiotics are required, separate dosages by at least two hours

Laboratory Considerations

- ■ No specific concerns noted; see Monitoring

Doses

- ■ **DOGS/CATS:**
  For hyperphosphatemia associated with chronic renal failure:
  a) In conjunction with a low-phosphorus diet: Initial therapy at 60–90 mg/kg/day, with food or mixed with food, or just prior to each meal. Individualize dose to achieve desired serum phosphorus con-

centrations. Perform serial serum phosphorus evaluations at 2–4 week intervals. Decrease dose if serum calcium exceeds normal limits; additional aluminum-based phosphate binders should be used if hyperphosphatemia persists. (Polzin *et al.* 2005)

Monitoring

Initially at 10–14 day intervals; once "stable", at 4–6 week intervals:

- ■ Serum phosphorus (after a 12–hour fast)
- ■ Serum ionized calcium

Client Information

- ■ Give with meals; either just before or mixed into food
- ■ The veterinarian may prescribe additional doses to be administered between meals if additional calcium is required, give only with meals unless the veterinarian instructs to do so
- ■ Use of this medication will require ongoing laboratory monitoring

Chemistry/Synonyms

Calcium acetate is a white, odorless, hygroscopic powder that is freely soluble in water and slightly soluble in alcohol. Each gram contains approximately 254 mg of elemental calcium.

Calcium acetate may also be known as: calcii acetas, acetato de calcio, kalcio acetates, kalciumacetat, or kalciumasetaatti, *PhosLo®*.

Storage/Stability

The commercially available tablets, capsules and gelcaps should be stored at room temperature (25°C); excursions are permitted to 15–30°C.

Dosage Forms/Regulatory Status

VETERINARY-LABELED PRODUCTS: None

HUMAN-LABELED PRODUCTS:

Calcium Acetate Oral Tablets: 667 mg (169 mg elemental calcium); *Calphron®* (Nephro-Tech); *Eliphos®* (Hawthorn); (Rx)

Calcium Acetate Oral Capsules & Gelcaps: 667 mg (169 mg elemental calcium); *PhosLo®* (Fresenius); (Rx)

References

Polzin, D, C Osborne, et al. (2005). Chronic Kidney Disease. *Textbook of Veterinary Internal Medicine: Diseases of the Dog and Cat 6th Ed.* S Ettinger and E Feldman Eds., Elsevier: 1756–1785.

Calcium EDTA—see Edetate Calcium Disodium

CALCIUM SALTS
CALCIUM GLUCONATE
CALCIUM GLUCEPTATE
CALCIUM CHLORIDE
CALCIUM LACTATE

(kal-see-um)

ESSENTIAL CATION NUTRIENT

Prescriber Highlights

▶ Used to treat or prevent hypocalcemia; or as an oral antacid

▶ Contraindicated in V-fib or hypercalcemia

▶ Must NOT give IV too rapidly

▶ Must monitor therapy carefully depending on condition, etc.

▶ Drug interactions & incompatibilities prevalent

Uses/Indications

Calcium salts are used orally for the prevention of hypocalcemia or as a phoshorus binding agent. Parenteral calcium is used for; treatment of documented ionized hypocalcemia, calcium channel blocker toxicity, or hyperkalemia

Pharmacology/Actions

Calcium is an essential element that is required for many functions within the body, including proper nervous and musculoskeletal system function, cell membrane and capillary permeability, and activation of enzymatic reactions.

Pharmacokinetics

Calcium is absorbed in the small intestine in the ionized form only. Presence of vitamin D (in active form) and an acidic pH is necessary for oral absorption. Parathormone (parathyroid hormone) increases with resultant increased calcium absorption in calcium deficiency states and decreases as serum calcium levels rise. Dietary factors (high fiber, phytates, fatty acids), age, drugs (corticosteroids, tetracyclines), disease states (steatorrhea, uremia, renal osteodystrophy, achlorhydria), or decreased serum calcitonin levels may all cause reduced amounts of calcium to be absorbed.

After absorption, ionized calcium enters the extracellular fluid and then is rapidly incorporated into skeletal tissue. Calcium administration does not necessarily stimulate bone formation. Approximately 99% of total body calcium is found in bone. Of circulating calcium, approximately 50% is bound to serum proteins or complexed with anions and 50% is in the ionized form. Total serum calcium is dependent on serum protein concentrations. Total serum calcium changes by approximately 0.8 mg/dL for every 1.09 g/dL change in serum albumin. Calcium crosses the placenta and is distributed into milk.

Calcium is eliminated primarily in the feces, contributed by both unabsorbed calcium and calcium excreted into the bile and pancreatic juice. Only small amounts of the drug are excreted in the urine as most of the cation filtered by the glomeruli is reabsorbed by the tubules and ascending loop of Henle. Vitamin D, parathormone, and thiazide diuretics decrease the amount of calcium excreted by the kidneys. Loop diuretics (e.g., furosemide), calcitonin, and somatotropin increase calcium renal excretion.

Contraindications/Precautions/Warnings

Calcium is contraindicated in patients with ventricular fibrillation or hypercalcemia. Parenteral calcium should not be administered to patients with above normal serum calcium levels. Calcium should be used very cautiously in patients receiving digitalis glycosides, or having cardiac or renal disease. Calcium chloride, because it can be acidifying, should be used with caution in patients with respiratory failure, respiratory acidosis, or renal disease.

In dogs, calcium gluconate diluted 1:1 has been regarded as safe to administer subcutaneously for the treatment of primary hypoparathyroidism in the past, but there are now several case reports of severe tissue reactions (pyogranulomatous panniculitis, adipocyte mineralization, etc.) at the injection site; use with caution, particularly when using with calcitriol.

Adverse Effects

Hypercalcemia can be associated with calcium therapy, particularly in patients with cardiac or renal disease; animals should be adequately monitored. Other effects that may be seen include GI irritation and/or constipation after oral administration, mild to severe tissue reactions after IM or SC administration of calcium salts and venous irritation after IV administration. Calcium chloride may be more irritating than other parenteral salts and is more likely to cause hypotension. Too rapid intravenous injection of calcium can cause hypotension, cardiac arrhythmias and cardiac arrest.

Should calcium salts be infused perivascularly, stop the infusion; treatment then may include: infiltrating the affected area with normal saline, corticosteroids administered locally, applying heat and elevating the area, and infiltrating the affected area with 1% procaine and hyaluronidase.

Reproductive/Nursing Safety

Although parenteral calcium products have not been proven safe to use during pregnancy, they are often used before, during, and after parturition in cows, ewes, bitches, and queens to treat parturient paresis secondary to hypocalcemia. In humans, the FDA categorizes this drug as category *C* for use during pregnancy (*Animal studies have shown an adverse effect on the fetus, but there are no adequate studies in humans; or there are no animal reproduction studies and no adequate studies in humans.*)

Overdosage/Acute Toxicity

Unless other drugs are given concurrently that enhance the absorption of calcium, oral overdoses of calcium containing products are unlikely to cause hypercalcemia. Hypercalcemia can occur with parenteral therapy or oral therapy in combination with vitamin D or increased parathormone levels. Hypercalcemia should be treated by withholding calcium therapy and other calcium elevating drugs (*e.g.*, vitamin D analogs). Mild hypercalcemia generally will resolve without further intervention when renal function is adequate.

More serious hypercalcemia (>12 mg/dL) should generally be treated by hydrating with IV normal saline and administering a loop diuretic (*e.g.*, furosemide) to increase both sodium and calcium excretion. Potassium and magnesium must be monitored and replaced as necessary. ECG should also be monitored during treatment. Corticosteroids, and in humans calcitonin and hemodialysis, have also been employed in treating hypercalcemia.

Drug Interactions

The following drug interactions have either been reported or are theoretical in humans or animals receiving calcium and may be of significance in veterinary patients:

■ **CALCIUM CHANNEL BLOCKERS (e.g., diltiazem, verapamil, etc.):** Intravenous calcium may antagonize the effects of calcium-channel blocking agents

■ **DIGOXIN:** Patients on digitalis therapy are more apt to develop arrhythmias if receiving IV calcium—use with caution

■ **MAGNESIUM (oral):** With oral calcium may lead to increased serum magnesium and/or calcium, particularly in patients with renal failure.

■ **MAGNESIUM SULFATE:** Parenteral calcium can neutralize the effects of hypermagnesemia or magnesium toxicity secondary to parenteral magnesium sulfate

■ **NEUROMUSCULAR BLOCKERS** (*e.g.*, **tubocurarine, metubine, gallamine, pancuronium, atracurium, and vecuronium**): Parenteral calcium may reverse the effects of nondepolarizing neuromuscular blocking agents; calcium has been reported to prolong or enhance the effects of tubocurarine

■ **TETRACYCLINES, FLUOROQUINOLONES (oral):** Oral calcium can reduce the amount of tetracyclines or fluoroquinolones absorbed from the GI tract; separate dosages by two hours if possible

■ **POTASSIUM SUPPLEMENTS:** Patients receiving both parenteral calcium and potassium supplementation may have an increased chance of developing cardiac arrhythmias—use cautiously

■ **THIAZIDE DIURETICS:** Used in conjunction with large doses of calcium may cause hypercalcemia

■ **VITAMIN A:** Excessive intake of vitamin A may stimulate calcium loss from bone and cause hypercalcemia.

■ **VITAMIN D:** Concurrent use of large doses of vitamin D or its analogs may cause enhanced calcium absorption and induce hypercalcemia

Laboratory Considerations

■ **SERUM AND URINARY MAGNESIUM:** Parenteral calcium may cause false-negative results for serum and urinary magnesium when using the Titan yellow method of determination.

Doses

■ **DOGS**

For hypocalcemia:

a) Calcium gluconate injection: 94–140 mg/kg IV slowly to effect (intraperitoneal route may also be used). Monitor respirations and cardiac rate and rhythm during administration. (USPC 1990)

b) For acute hypocalcemia: Calcium gluconate 10% injection: Warm to body temperature and give IV at a rate of 50–150 mg/kg (0.5–1.5 mL/kg) over 20–30 minutes. If bradycardia develops, halt infusion. Following acute crisis, infuse 10–15 mL (of a 10% solution) per kg over a 24–hour period. Long-term therapy may be accomplished by increasing dietary calcium and using vitamin D. Calcium lactate may be given orally at a rate of 0.5–2 g/day. (Seeler & Thurmon 1985)

c) Calcium gluconate 10% 0.5–1.5 mL/kg or calcium chloride 10% 1.5–3.5 mL (total) IV slowly over 15 minutes; monitor heart rate or ECG during infusion. If ST segment elevation or Q-T interval shortening occur, temporarily discontinue infusion and reinstate at a slower rate when resolved. Maintenance therapy is dependent on cause of hypocalcemia. Hypoparathyroidism is treated with vitamin D analogs (refer to DHT monograph) with or without oral calcium supplementation. (Russo & Lees 1986)

d) For emergency treatment of tetany and seizures secondary to hypoparathyroidism: Calcium gluconate 10%: 0.5–1.5 mL/kg (up to 20 mL) over 15–30 minutes. May repeat at 6–8 hour intervals or give as continuous infusion at 10–15 mg/kg/hour. Monitor ECG and stop infusion if S-T segment elevates, Q-T interval shortens, or arrhythmias occur. For long-term therapy (with DHT—refer to that monograph), calcium supplementation may occasionally be useful. Calcium gluconate at 500–750 mg/kg/day divided three times daily, or calcium lactate at 400–600 mg/kg/day divided three times daily, or calcium carbonate 100–150 mg/kg/day divided twice daily. Monitor serum calcium and adjust as necessary. (Kay & Richter 1988)

e) For emergency treatment: Calcium gluconate 10% 5–15 mg/kg (0.5–1.5 mL/kg) slowly to effect over a ten minute period, or calcium chloride 10% (extremely caustic if administered extravascularly) 5–15 mg/kg (0.15–0.5 mL/kg); dose is the same but volume is 1/3 that of calcium gluconate; monitor heart rate or ECG (if possible) during infusion. If bradycardia or Q-T interval shortening occurs, temporarily discontinue infusion. Short-term treatment immediately after correction of tetany: Either give a constant rate infusion of calcium gluconate 10% at 60–90 mg/kg/day (6.5–9.75 mL/kg/day) added to the fluids or give the daily dosage SC in 3–4 divided doses per day after diluting with an equal volume of saline. (Crystal 2004)

For hyperkalemic cardiotoxicity:

a) Secondary to uremic crisis: Correct metabolic acidosis, if present, with sodium bicarbonate (bicarbonate may also be beneficial even if acidosis not present). Calcium gluconate (10%) indicated if serum K+ is >8 mEq/L. Give at an approximate dose of 0.5–1 mL/kg over 10–20 minutes; monitor ECG. Rapidly corrects arrhythmias but effects are very short (10–15 minutes). IV glucose (0.5–1 g/kg body weight with or without insulin) also beneficial in increasing intracellular K+ concentrations. (Polzin & Osborne 1985)

■ **CATS:**

For hypocalcemia:

a) Calcium gluconate injection: 94–140 mg/kg IV slowly to effect (intraperitoneal route may also be used). Monitor respirations and cardiac rate and rhythm during administration. (USPC 1990)

b) For acute hypocalcemia secondary to hypoparathyroidism: Using 10% calcium gluconate injection, give 1–1.5 mL/kg IV slowly over 10–20 minutes. Monitor ECG if possible. If bradycardia, or Q-T interval shortening occurs, slow rate or temporarily discontinue. Once life-threatening signs are controlled, add calcium to IV fluids and administer as a slow infusion at 60–90 mg/kg/day (of elemental calcium). This converts to 2.5 mL/kg every 6–8 hours of 10% cal-

cium gluconate. Carefully monitor serum calcium (once to twice daily) during this period and adjust dose as required. Begin oral calcium initially at 50–100 mg/kg/day divided 3–4 times daily of elemental calcium and dihydrotachysterol once animal can tolerate oral therapy. Give DHT initially at 0.125–0.25 mg PO per day for 2–3 days, then 0.08–0.125 mg per day for 2–3 days and finally 0.05 mg PO per day until further dosage adjustments are necessary. As cat's serum calcium is stabilized, intravenous calcium may be reduced and discontinued if tolerated. Stable serum calcium levels (8.5–9.5 mg/dL) are usually achieved in about a week. Continue to monitor and adjust dosages of DHT and calcium to lowest levels to maintain normocalcemia. (Peterson & Randolph 1989) (**Note:** refer to the DHT monograph for further information.)

c) For hypocalcemia secondary to phosphate enema toxicity or puerperal tetany: follow the guidelines for use of intravenous calcium in "b" above. (Peterson & Randolph 1989)

d) For emergency treatment: Calcium gluconate 10% 5–15 mg/kg (0.5–1.5 mL/kg) slowly to effect over a ten minute period, or calcium chloride 10% (extremely caustic if administered extravascularly) 5–15 mg/kg (0.15–0.5 mL/kg); dose is the same but volume is 1/3 that of calcium gluconate; monitor heart rate or ECG (if possible) during infusion. If bradycardia or Q-T interval shortening occurs, temporarily discontinue infusion. Short-term treatment immediately after correction of tetany: Either give a constant rate infusion of calcium gluconate 10% at 60–90 mg/kg/day (6.5–9.75 mL/kg/day) added to the fluids or give the daily dosage SC in 3–4 divided doses per day after diluting with an equal volume of saline. (Crystal 2004)

■ **CATTLE**

For hypocalcemia:

a) Calcium gluconate injection: 150–250 mg/kg IV slowly to effect (intraperitoneal route may also be used). Monitor respirations and cardiac rate and rhythm during administration. (USPC 1990)

b) Calcium gluconate 23% injection: 250–500 mL IV slowly, or IM or SC (divided and given in several locations, with massage at sites of injection) (Label directions; Calcium Gluc. Injection 23%—TechAmerica)

c) 8–12 grams of calcium IV infused over

a 5–10 minute period; use a product containing magnesium during the last month of pregnancy if subclinical hypomagnesemia is detected. (Allen & Sansom 1986)

■ **HORSES**

For hypocalcemia:

a) Calcium gluconate injection: 150–250 mg/kg IV slowly to effect (intraperitoneal route may also be used). Monitor respirations and cardiac rate and rhythm during administration. (USPC 1990)

b) Calcium gluconate 23% injection: 250–500 mL IV slowly, or IM or SC (divided and given in several locations, with massage at sites of injection) (Label directions; Calcium Gluconate Injection 23%—TechAmerica)

c) For lactation tetany: 250 mL per 450 kg body weight of a standard commercially available solution that also contains magnesium and phosphorous IV slowly while auscultating heart. If no improvement after 10 minutes, repeat. Intensity in heart sounds should be noted, with only an infrequent extrasystole. Stop infusion immediately if a pronounced change in rate or rhythm is detected. (Brewer 1987)

■ **SHEEP & GOATS:**

For hypocalcemia:

a) Sheep: Calcium gluconate injection: 150–250 mg/kg IV slowly to effect (intraperitoneal route may also be used). Monitor respirations and cardiac rate and rhythm during administration. (USPC 1990)

b) Sheep: Calcium gluconate 23% injection: 25–50 mL IV slowly, or IM or SC (divided and given in several locations, with massage at sites of injection) (Label directions; Calcium Gluconate Injection 23%—TechAmerica)

■ **SWINE:**

For hypocalcemia:

a) Calcium gluconate injection: 150–250 mg/kg IV slowly to effect (intraperitoneal route may also be used). Monitor respirations and cardiac rate and rhythm during administration. (USPC 1990)

b) Calcium gluconate 23% injection: 25–50 mL IV slowly, or IM or SC (divided and given in several locations, with massage at sites of injection) (Label directions; Calcium Gluconate Injection 23%—TechAmerica)

■ **BIRDS:**

For hypocalcemic tetany:

a) Calcium gluconate: 50–100 mg/kg IV slowly to effect; may be diluted and given

IM if a vein cannot be located (Clubb 1986)

For egg-bound birds:

a) Initially, calcium gluconate 1% solution 0.01–0.02 mL/g IM. Provide moist heat (80–85°F) and allow 24 hours for bird to pass egg. (Nye 1986)

■ **REPTILES:**

For egg binding in combination with oxytocin (oxytocin: 1–10 Units/kg IM):

a) Calcium glubionate: 10–50 mg/kg IM as needed until calcium levels back to normal or egg binding is resolved. Use care when giving multiple injections. Calcium/oxytocin is not as effective in lizards as in other species. (Gauvin 1993)

Monitoring

■ Serum calcium

■ Serum magnesium, phosphate, and potassium when indicated

■ Serum PTH (parathormone) if indicated

■ Renal function tests initially and as required

■ ECG during intravenous calcium therapy if possible

■ Urine calcium if hypercalcuria develops

Chemistry

Several different salts of calcium are available in various formulations. Calcium gluceptate and calcium chloride are freely soluble in water; calcium lactate is soluble in water; calcium gluconate and calcium glycerophosphate are sparingly soluble in water, and calcium phosphate and carbonate are insoluble in water. Calcium gluconate for injection has a pH of 6–8.2 and calcium chloride for injection has a pH of 5.5–7.5.

To determine calcium content per gram of various calcium salts:

Calcium Acetate: 253 mg (12.7 mEq)
Calcium Carbonate: 400 mg (20 mEq)
Calcium Chloride: 270 mg (13.5 mEq)
Calcium Citrate: 211 mg (10.6 mEq)
Calcium Gluceptate: 82 mg (4.1 mEq)
Calcium Gluconate: 90 mg (4.5 mEq)
Calcium Glycerophosphate: 191 mg (9.6 mEq)
Calcium Lactate: 130 mg (6.5 mEq)
Calcium Phosphate Dibasic
    Anhydrous: 290 mg (14.5 mEq)
    Dihydrate: 230 mg (11.5 mEq)
Calcium Phosphate Tribasic: 400 mg (20 mEq)

Storage/Stability

Calcium gluconate tablets should be stored in well-closed containers at room temperature. Calcium lactate tablets should be stored in tight containers at room temperature. Calcium gluconate injection, calcium gluceptate injection, and calcium chloride injection should be stored at room temperature and protected from freezing.

Compatibility/Compounding Considerations

Calcium chloride for injection is reportedly **compatible** with the following intravenous solutions and drugs: amikacin sulfate, ascorbic acid, bretylium tosylate, cephapirin sodium, chloramphenicol sodium succinate, dopamine HCl, hydrocortisone sodium succinate, isoproterenol HCl, lidocaine HCl, methicillin sodium, norepinephrine bitartrate, penicillin G potassium/sodium, pentobarbital sodium, phenobarbital sodium, sodium bicarbonate, verapamil HCl, and vitamin B-complex with C.

Calcium chloride for injection **compatibility information conflicts** or is dependent on diluent or concentration factors with the following drugs or solutions: fat emulsion 10%, dobutamine HCl, oxytetracycline HCl, and tetracycline HCl. Compatibility is dependent upon factors such as pH, concentration, temperature and diluent used.

Calcium chloride for injection is reportedly **incompatible** with the following solutions or drugs: amphotericin B, cephalothin sodium, and chlorpheniramine maleate.

Calcium gluconate for injection is reportedly **compatible** with the following intravenous solutions and drugs: sodium chloride for injection 0.9%, lactated Ringer's injection, dextrose 5%–20%, dextrose-lactated Ringer's injection, dextrose-saline combinations, amikacin sulfate, aminophylline, ascorbic acid injection, bretylium tosylate, cephapirin sodium, chloramphenicol sodium succinate, corticotropin, dimenhydrinate, erythromycin gluceptate, heparin sodium, hydrocortisone sodium succinate, lidocaine HCl, methicillin sodium, norepinephrine bitartrate, penicillin G potassium/sodium, phenobarbital sodium, potassium chloride, tobramycin sulfate, vancomycin HCl, verapamil and vitamin B-complex with C.

Calcium gluconate compatibility information conflicts or is dependent on diluent or concentration factors with the following drugs or solutions: phosphate salts, oxytetracycline HCl, prochlorperazine edisylate, and tetracycline HCl. Compatibility is dependent upon factors such as pH, concentration, temperature and diluent used.

Calcium gluconate is reportedly **incompatible** with the following solutions or drugs: intravenous fat emulsion, amphotericin B, cefamandole naftate, cephalothin sodium, dobutamine HCl, methylprednisolone sodium succinate, and metoclopramide HCl.

Consult specialized references or a hospital pharmacist for more specific information.

Dosage Forms/Regulatory Status

VETERINARY-LABELED PRODUCTS:

(Note: not necessarily a complete list; veterinary-labeled products are apparently not FDA-approved as they do not appear in the Green Book)

Parenteral Products:

Calcium Gluconate (as calcium borogluconate) 23% [230 mg/mL; 20.7 mg (1.06 mEq) calcium per mL]; in 500 mL bottles; *AmTech® Calcium Gluconate 23% Solution* (Phoenix Scientific); (OTC), *Calcium Gluconate 23%* (AgriPharm, AgriLabs, Aspen, Bimeda, Durvet, Phoenix Pharmaceutical, Vet Tek, Vetus); (OTC), *Cal-Nate 1069®* (Butler); (OTC). Depending on the product, labeled for use in cattle, horses, swine, sheep, cats, and dogs. No withdrawal times are required.

Calcium Gluconate oral 40 g–42 g calcium/300 mL tube. Supplement for use pre and post calving. *Cal Supreme Gel®* (Bimeda); (OTC)

Calcium Chloride 35% w/w or 47% w/v equivalent to 170 mg calcium/ mL (127 mg per g) in 300 mL (400 g) tube. *Clearcal 50®* (Vedco); (OTC)

Products are also available that include calcium, phosphorus, potassium and/or dextrose; refer to the individual product's labeling for specific dosage information. Trade names for these products include: *Norcalciphos®*—Pfizer, and *Cal-Dextro® Special, #2, C, and K*—Fort Dodge; (Rx).

Oral Products: No products containing only calcium (as a salt) are available commercially with veterinary labeling. There are several products (*e.g.*, *Pet-Cal®* and *Osteoform® Improved*) that contain calcium with phosphorous and vitamin D (plus other ingredients in some preparations).

HUMAN-APPROVED PRODUCTS: (not a complete list)

Parenteral Products:

Calcium Gluconate Injection 10% 100 mg/mL; equivalent to elemental calcium 0.465 mEq/mL (9.3 mg), preservative-free in 10 & 50 mL single-dose vials & 100 & 200 mL pharmacy bulk vials; generic; (Rx)

Calcium Chloride Injection 10% [100 mg/mL; 27.2 mg (1.36 mEq) calcium per mL] in 10 mL amps, vials, and syringes; generic; (Rx)

Oral Products:

Calcium Gluconate (9.3% calcium) Tablets: 500 mg (45 mg calcium), approx. 555.6 mg (50 mg calcium), 648 to 650 mg (58.5 to 60 mg calcium), 972 to 975 mg (87.75 to 90 mg calcium); generic; (OTC)

Calcium Gluconate Oral Powder: 1,040 mg/15 mL (346.7 mg/15 mL calcium, gluten free, sugar free) in 448 g; Calcium Gluconate (Freeda) (OTC)

Calcium Gluconate Capsules: 500 mg; Calcium Gluconate (Bio-Tech); 700 mg; *Cal-G®* (Key); (OTC)

Calcium Lactate (13% calcium) Tablets: 648 mg to 650 mg (84.5 mg calcium); 100 mg elemental calcium; generic (OTC); Capsules 500 mg (96 mg calcium), *Cal-Lac®* (Bio Tech); (OTC)

Also available are calcium carbonate tablets, suspension and capsules, calcium acetate tablets, calcium citrate tablets, and tricalcium phosphate tablets.

References

Allen, WM & BF Sansom (1986). Parturient paresis (milk fever) and hypocalcemia (cows, ewes, and goats). *Current Veterinary Therapy 2: Food Animal Practice*. JL Howard Ed. Philadelphia, WB Saunders: 311–317.

Brewer, BD (1987). Disorders of calcium metabolism. *Current Therapy in Equine Medicine*. NE Robinson Ed. Philadelphia, WB Saunders: 189–192.

Clubb, SL (1986). Therapeutics: Individual and Flock Treatment Regimens. *Clinical Avian Medicine and Surgery*. GJ Harrison and LR Harrison Eds. Philadelphia, W.B. Saunders: 327–355.

Crystal, M (2004). Hypocalcemia. *The 5–Minute Veterinary Consult: Canine and Feline 3rd Ed*. L Tilley and F Smith Eds., Lippincott Williams & Wilkins: 662–663.

Gauvin, J (1993). Drug therapy in reptiles. *Seminars in Avian & Exotic Med* 2(1): 48–59.

Kay, AD & KP Richter (1988). Diseases of the parathyroid glands. *Handbook of Small Animal Practice*. RV Morgan Ed. New York, Churchill Livingstone: 521–526.

Nye, RR (1986). Dealing with the Egg–bound Bird. *Current Veterinary Therapy (CVT) IX Small Animal Practice*. RW Kirk Ed. Philadelphia, W.B. Saunders: 746–747.

Peterson, ME & JF Randolph (1989). Endocrine Diseases. *The Cat: Diseases and Clinical Management*. RG Sherding Ed. New York, Churchill Livingstone. 2: 1095–1161.

Polzin, DJ & CA Osborne (1985). Diseases of the Urinary Tract. *Handbook of Small Animal Therapeutics*. LE Davis Ed. New York, Churchill Livingstone: 333–395.

Russo, EA & GE Lees (1986). Treatment of hypocalcemia. *Current Veterinary Therapy (CVT) IX Small Animal Practice*. RW Kirk Ed. Philadelphia, WB Saunders: 91–94.

Seeler, DC & JC Thurmon (1985). Fluid and Electrolyte Disorders. *Handbook of Small Animal Therapeutics*. LE Davis Ed. New York, Churchill Livingstone: 21–44.

USPC (1990). *Veterinary Information– Appendix III. Drug Information for the Health Professional* Rockville, United States Pharmacopeial Convention. 2: 2811–2860.

Camphorated Tincture of Opium — See Paregoric

CAPTOPRIL

(*kap*-toe-pril)   Capoten®

ANGIOTENSIN-CONVERTING ENZYME (ACE) INHIBITOR

Prescriber Highlights

▶ First available ACE inhibitor; use largely supplanted by enalapril & other newer ACE inhibitors

▶ Shorter duration of activity & more adverse effects than other newer ACE inhibitors

Uses/Indications

The principle uses of captopril in veterinary medicine, are as a vasodilator in the treatment of CHF and hypertension. Because of approval status and fewer adverse effects, enalapril and benazepril have largely supplanted the use of this drug in veterinary medicine.

Pharmacology/Actions

Captopril prevents the formation of angiotensin-II (a potent vasoconstrictor) by competing with angiotensin-I for the enzyme angiotensin-converting enzyme (ACE). ACE has a much higher affinity for captopril than for angiotensin-I. Because angiotensin-II concentrations are decreased, aldosterone secretion is reduced and plasma renin activity is increased.

The cardiovascular effects of captopril in patients with CHF include decreased total peripheral resistance, pulmonary vascular resistance, mean arterial and right atrial pressures; no change or decrease in heart rate; and increased cardiac index and output, stroke volume, and exercise tolerance. Renal blood flow can be increased with little change in hepatic blood flow.

Pharmacokinetics

In dogs, approximately 75% of an oral dose is absorbed but food in the GI tract reduces bioavailability by 30–40%. It is distributed to most tissues (not the CNS) and is 40% bound to plasma proteins in dogs. The half-life of captopril is about 2.8 hours in dogs and less than 2 hours in humans. Its duration of effect in dogs may only persist for 4 hours. The drug is metabolized and renally excreted. More than 95% of a dose is excreted renally, both as unchanged (45–50%) drug and as metabolites. Patients with significant renal dysfunction can have significantly prolonged half-lives.

Contraindications/Precautions/Warnings

Captopril is contraindicated in patients who have demonstrated hypersensitivity with ACE inhibitors. It should be used with caution and under close supervision in patients with renal insufficiency; doses may need to be reduced.

Captopril should also be used with caution in patients with hyponatremia or sodium depletion, coronary or cerebrovascular insufficiency, preexisting hematologic abnormalities or a collagen vascular disease (*e.g.*, SLE).

Patients with severe CHF should be monitored very closely upon initiation of therapy.

Adverse Effects

There have been some reports of hypotension, renal failure, hyperkalemia, vomiting and diarrhea developing in dogs after captopril administration. Captopril may have a higher incidence of gastrointestinal effects in dogs than other available ACE inhibitors. Although seen in people, skin rashes (4–7% incidence) and neutropenia/agranulocytosis (rare) have not been reported in dogs.

Reproductive/Nursing Safety

Captopril apparently crosses the placenta. High doses of ACE inhibitors in rodents have caused decreased fetal weights and increases in fetal and maternal death rates; no teratogenic effects have been reported to date, but use during pregnancy should occur only when the potential benefits of therapy outweigh the risks to the offspring. In humans, the FDA categorizes this drug as category *C* for use during the first trimester of pregnancy (*Animal studies have shown an adverse effect on the fetus, but there are no adequate studies in humans; or there are no animal reproduction studies and no adequate studies in humans.*) During the second and third trimesters, the FDA categorizes this drug as category *D* for use during pregnancy (*There is evidence of human fetal risk, but the potential benefits from the use of the drug in pregnant women may be acceptable despite its potential risks.*) In a separate system evaluating the safety of drugs in canine and feline pregnancy (Papich 1989), this drug is categorized as in class: *C* (*These drugs may have potential risks. Studies in people or laboratory animals have uncovered risks, and these drugs should be used cautiously as a last resort when the benefit of therapy clearly outweighs the risks.*)

Captopril enters milk in concentrations of about 1% of that found in maternal plasma.

Overdosage/Acute Toxicity

In overdose situations, the primary concern is hypotension; supportive treatment with volume expansion with normal saline is recommended to correct blood pressure. Dogs given 1.5 g/kg orally developed emesis and decreased blood pressure. Dogs receiving doses greater than 6.6 mg/kg q8h may develop renal failure.

Drug Interactions

The following drug interactions have either been reported or are theoretical in humans or animals receiving captopril and may be of significance in veterinary patients:

- **ANTACIDS:** Reduced oral absorption of captopril may occur if given concomitantly with antacids; it is suggested to separate dosing by at least two hours
- **CIMETIDINE:** Used concomitantly with captopril has caused neurologic dysfunction in two human patients
- **DIGOXIN:** Levels may increase 15–30% when captopril is added, automatic reduction in dosage is not recommended, but monitoring of serum digoxin levels should be performed
- **DIURETICS:** Concomitant diuretics may cause hypotension if used with captopril; titrate dosages carefully
- **NON-STEROIDAL ANTIINFLAMMATORY AGENTS (NSAIDS):** May reduce the clinical efficacy of captopril when it is being used as an antihypertensive agent
- **POTASSIUM or POTASSIUM SPARING DIURETICS (e.g., spironolactone):** Hyperkalemia may develop with captopril
- **PROBENECID:** Can decrease renal excretion of captopril and possibly enhance the clinical and toxic effects of the drug
- **VASODILATORS (e.g., prazosin, hydralazine, nitrates):** Concomitant vasodilators may cause hypotension if used with captopril; titrate dosages carefully

Laboratory Considerations

- Captopril may cause a false positive **urine acetone test** (sodium nitroprusside reagent).
- When using **iodohippurate sodium I^{123}/I^{134} or Technetium Tc^{99} pententate renal imaging** in patients with renal artery stenosis, ACE inhibitors may cause a reversible decrease in localization and excretion of these agents in the affected kidney which may lead confusion in test interpretation.

Doses

Note: Because of fewer adverse effects in dogs, longer duration of activity, and/or veterinary labeling/dosage forms, enalapril and other newer ACE inhibitors have largely supplanted the use of this drug in veterinary medicine.

- **DOGS:**
  a) 0.5–2 mg/kg PO three times daily (Atkins 2008)
  b) 0.5–2 mg/kg PO q8–12h (Bonagura & Muir 1986)
- **CATS:**
  a) ¼ to ½ of a 12.5 mg tablet PO q8–12h (Bonagura 1989)
  b) For dilative, restrictive or hypertrophic cardiomyopathy: 0.55–1.54 mg/kg PO q8–12h (Kittleson 2000))

Monitoring

- Clinical signs of CHF
- Serum electrolytes, creatinine, BUN, urine protein
- CBC with differential; periodic
- Blood pressure (if treating hypertension or signs associated with hypotension arise).

Client Information

- Give medication on an empty stomach unless otherwise instructed. Do not abruptly stop or reduce therapy without veterinarian's approval. Contact veterinarian if vomiting or diarrhea persist or are severe, or if animal's condition deteriorates.

Chemistry/Synonyms

Related to a peptide isolated from the venom of a South American pit viper, captopril occurs as a slightly sulfurous smelling, white to off-white, crystalline powder. It is freely soluble in water or alcohol.

Captopril may also be known as: captoprilum, or SQ-14225; many trade names are available.

Storage/Stability

Captopril tablets should be stored in tight containers at temperatures not greater than 30°C.

Compatibility/Compounding Considerations

Compounded preparation stability: Captopril oral suspension compounded from commercially available tablets has been published (Allen & Erickson 1996). Triturating one (1) captopril 100 mg tablet with 65 mL of *Ora-Plus*® and *qs ad* to 134 mL with *Ora-Sweet*® (or *Ora-Sweet*® SF) yields a 0.75 mg/mL oral suspension that retains >90% potency for 14 days stored at 5°C and for 7 days at 25°C. Compounded preparations of captopril should be protected from light.

Dosage Forms/Regulatory Status

VETERINARY-LABELED PRODUCTS: None

The ARCI (Racing Commissioners International) has designated this drug as a class 3 substance. See the appendix for more information.

HUMAN-LABELED PRODUCTS:

Captopril Oral Tablets: 12.5 mg, 25 mg, 50 mg, & 100 mg; *Capoten®* (Par); generic; (Rx)

Captopril and Hydrochlorothiazide Oral Tablets: 15 mg hydrochlorothiazide and 25 mg captopril; 15 mg hydrochlorothiazide and 50 mg captopril; 25 mg hydrochlorothiazide and 25 mg captopril; 25 mg hydrochlorothiazide and 50 mg captopril. *Capozide®*, (Par); generic; (Rx)

References

Allen, LV & MA Erickson (1996). Stability of baclofen, captopril, diltiazem hydrochloride, dipyridamole, and flecainide acetate in extemporaneously compounded oral liquids. *Am J Health Syst Pharm* 53(18): 2179–2184.

Atkins, C (2008). Therapeutic advances in the management of heart disease: An overview. Proceedings: World Veterinary Congress. Accessed via: Veterinary Information Network. http://goo.gl/NSs5x

Bonagura, JD (1989). Cardiovascular Diseases. *The Cat: Diseases and Clinical Management*. RG Sherding Ed. New York, Churchill Livingstone. 2: 649–686.

Bonagura, JD & W Muir (1986). Vasodilator therapy. *Current Veterinary Therapy (CVT) IX Small Animal Practice*. RW Kirk Ed. Philadelphia, WB Saunders: 329–334.

Kittleson, M (2000). Therapy of Heart Failure. *Textbook of Veterinary Internal Medicine: Diseases of the Dog and Cat*. S Ettinger and E Feldman Eds. Philadelphia, WB Saunders. 1: 713–737.

CARBAMAZEPINE

(Kar-*bam*-aye-zuh-peen)   Tegretol®

DIBENZAZEPINE ANTICONVULSANT, NEUROPATHIC PAIN & PSYCHOTHERAPEUTIC AGENT

Prescriber Highlights

▶ Potentially useful for behavior disorders (aggression), neuropathic pain states, or epilepsy in dogs and cats

▶ Very little information published on use, adverse effects, etc. for veterinary patients

▶ Pharmacokinetic profile in dogs a serious roadblock for clinical use

▶ Reportedly can be used successfully for photic head shaking in horses not responding to cyproheptadine

▶ Many potential drug interactions

Uses/Indications

Carbamazepine potentially could be useful for treating behavior disorders, neuropathic pain states, or epilepsy in dogs and cats, but its unfavorable pharmacokinetic profile in dogs is problematic, however. Despite this, there are sporadic case reports that it has had efficacy in dogs (aggression, psychomotor seizures) and it has been proposed that there may be an as of yet unidentified active metabolite in dogs that is more slowly eliminated. There is extremely scant information published on the use of this drug in cats, but it has been stated that it has had some efficacy in reducing aggression.

Until more information is available, carbamazepine should be considered as a 3rd-line agent for use in small animals, but if formulations can be developed to increase absorption and methods developed to reduce hepatic metabolism (*e.g.*, ketoconazole, grapefruit juice powder), its potential is intriguing.

In horses, with photic head shaking, cyproheptadine is generally the drug of first choice, but carbamazepine has been used.

Pharmacology/Actions

Carbamazepine has a variety of pharmacological effects similar to drugs such as phenytoin in the central nervous system, including modulation of ion channels (sodium and calcium) and receptor-mediated neurotransmission (GABA, glutamate, monoamines). Its antiseizure effects are due primarily to limiting seizure propagation by reduction of post-tetanic potentiation (PTP) of synaptic transmission. It also has antiarrhythmic, antidiuretic, anticholinergic, antidepressant, sedative, muscle relaxant, and neuromuscular transmission-inhibitory actions, but only mild analgesic effects.

Carbamazepine has been shown to reduce electrical- and chemical-induced seizures in rats and mice. It appears to act by reducing polysynaptic responses and blocking the post-tetanic potentiation. Carbamazepine has been shown in cats and rats to reduce or block pain induced by stimulation of the infraorbital nerve. Also in cats, it depresses thalamic potential and bulbar and polysynaptic reflexes, including the linguomandibular reflex.

The principal metabolite of carbamazepine, carbamazepine-10,11-epoxide, also has anticonvulsant activity.

Pharmacokinetics

When compared to humans, carbamazepine is eliminated much more rapidly in dogs. Humans may eliminate carbamazepine and its active metabolite, carbamazepine-10,11-epoxide, up to 25 times more slowly then dogs.

The pharmacokinetics of carbamazepine were reported in the dog in 1980 (Frey & Loscher 1980). Like the above study, the drug was better absorbed when given as liquid preparation than from tablets. Elimination half-life was 1.5 hours for carbamazepine and 2.2 hours for carbamazepine-10,11-epoxide. However after dosing for a week, plasma concentrations showed a pronounced and progressive decline from Day 2 and the authors concluded that carbamazepine was not a suitable drug for treating epilepsy in dogs.

A study evaluating the pharmacokinetics of carbamazepine in the dog using a 2-hydroxypropyl-beta-cyclodextrin-based formulation administered orally and intravenously compared with oral commercially available tablets and suspensions was published (Brewster *et al.* 1997). They found that the oral bioavailability of tablets was low in dogs (around 28%) and that oral suspensions or solutions increased bioavailability. After IV dosing, volume of distribution (steady-state) was 0.58 L/kg, and elimination half-life of carbamazepine was 38 minutes and 110 minutes for the epoxide metabolite. Renal clearance was only 12 mL/min or about 4% of total body clearance. Elimination half-life after tablet administration was 116 minutes. As this was a single-dose study (with a 2-week washout period between doses), no effect of hepatic enzyme induction could be measured.

A study comparing the oral bioavailability of carbamazepine in a beta-cyclodextrin complex with hydroxymethylcelluse matrix tablets (sustained-release; *Tegretol® CR 200*) in 4 Beagles found that the experimentally produced betacyclodextrin complexes had higher bioavailability then the commercial product. However, there was significant inter-subject variability. The dose given to these dogs was approximately 20 mg/kg of the commercial sustained release tablets. At this dosage, peak levels occurred at approximately 1 hour after dosing and averaged 0.5 micrograms/mL. Elimination half-life was 46 minutes. No determination of any metabolites was measured in this study.

Contraindications/Precautions/Warnings

There is extremely limited information for carbamazepine's safety in animals; the following pertains to humans and may apply to veterinary patients: Carbamazepine is **contraindicated** in patients with a history of bone marrow depression; concomitant use of an MAO-I, or use within 14 days of discontinuing an MAOI or hypersensitivity to carbamazepine or tricyclic compounds. Use with caution in patients with significant hepatic dysfunction.

Adverse Effects

There is extremely limited information for carbamazepine's adverse effect profile in animals. In humans, adverse effects (dizziness, drowsiness, nausea, and vomiting) are often seen when therapy is begun and the drug is usually started at a low dosage and then increased as the patient tolerates. Serious adverse effects reported in humans are usually associated with the cardiovascular (AV block, CHF) or hemopoietic system (aplastic anemia, agranulocytosis), skin (TEN, Stevens-Johnson Syndrome), and liver.

Reproductive/Nursing Safety

Carbamazepine can cause teratogenic effects. The drug crosses the placenta readily and has been implicated in increased rates of congenital malformations in humans. The FDA lists carbamazepine as a category *D* drug (*There is evidence of human fetal risk, but the potential benefits from the use of the drug in pregnant women may be acceptable despite its potential risks.*)

While carbamazepine is excreted into maternal milk and has the potential for some risks to nursing offspring, it is generally considered compatible with breast-feeding in humans.

Overdosage/Acute Toxicity

Reported oral median lethal dose (LD_{50}) in animals include: Mice: 1,100 to 3,750 mg/kg; Rats: 3,850 to 4,025 mg/kg: Rabbits: 1,500 to 2,680 mg/kg; and Guinea pigs: 920 mg/kg. Overdose treatment consists of using decontamination protocols when appropriate, and supportive care. In the event of an overdose in a veterinary species, contact a veterinary poison control center for further guidance.

Drug Interactions

The following drug interactions have either been reported or are theoretical in humans or animals receiving carbamazepine and may be of significance in veterinary patients:

The following drugs may *increase* the plasma levels or effects of carbamazepine:

- **ACETAZOLAMIDE**
- **AZOLE ANTIFUNGALS (e.g., KETACONAZOLE, ITRACONAZOLE)**
- **CALCIUM CHANNEL BLOCKERS, (e.g., DILTIAZEM, VERAPAMIL)**
- **CIMETIDINE**
- **DANAZOL**
- **GRAPEFRUIT JUICE**
- **ISONIAZID**
- **MACROLIDES (e.g., ERYTHROMYCIN, CLARITHROMYCIN)**
- **MAO INHIBITORS (including SELEGILINE)** Contraindicated in humans; discontinue MAOI at least 14 days prior to carbamazepine.
- **NIACIN**
- **SSRI ANTIDEPRESSANTS (FLUOXETINE, etc.)**
- **TRICYCLIC ANTIDEPRESSANTS (CLOMIPRAMINE, AMITRIPTYLINE, etc.)**
- **VALPROIC ACID**

The following drugs may *decrease* the plasma levels or effects of carbamazepine:

- **BARBITURATES (e.g., PHENOBARBITAL)**
- **CISPLATIN**
- **DOXORUBICIN**
- **FELBAMATE**
- **PHENYTOIN**
- **PRIMIDONE**

■ **RIFAMPIN**

■ **THEOPHYLLINE**

Carbamazepine may *increase* the plasma levels or effects of the following drugs:

■ **CLOMIPRAMINE**

■ **ISONIAZID**

Carbamazepine (particularly after chronic therapy) may *decrease* the effect of the following drugs/drug classes by lowering their serum concentrations or pharmacological effects:

■ **ACETAMINOPHEN**

■ **BENZODIAZEPINES**

■ **BUPROPION**

■ **BUSPRIONE**

■ **CALCIUM CHANNEL BLOCKERS**

■ **CYCLOSPORINE**

■ **DOXYCYCLINE**

■ **GLUCOCORTICOIDS**

■ **ITRACONAZOLE**

■ **LAMOTRIGINE**

■ **LEVOTHYROXINE**

■ **METHADONE**

■ **MIRTAZAPINE**

■ **NON-DEPOLARIZING   MUSCLE   BLOCKERS** (e.g., **ATRACURIUM**)

■ **PRAZIQUANTEL**

■ **TOPIRAMATE**

■ **TRAMADOL**

■ **ZONISAMIDE**

■ **TOPIRAMATE**

■ **TRAZODONE**

■ **TRICYCLIC ANTIDEPRESSANTS**

■ **VALPROIC ACID** (may also increase risk for phenobarbital toxicity)

■ **VERAPAMIL**

■ **WARFARIN**

Laboratory Considerations

■ In humans, thyroid function tests have been reported to show decreased values and interference with some pregnancy tests has been reported. Veterinary significance is unclear.

Doses

■ **DOGS:**

a) As a psychotherapeutic agent: 4–8 mg/kg PO q12h; not commonly used, but may have some utility in dogs that seem to have amygdalar hyperactivity; sometimes used in conjunction with SSRIs to control explosive aggression. (Haug 2008)

■ **HORSES:**

a) For photic head shaking: 10 mg/kg PO q6h or 29 mg/kg PO q12h. May be helpful in some horses that do not respond to cyproheptadine. (Brooks 2008)

Monitoring

■ Occasional CBC's and liver function tests are suggested

■ Clinical efficacy

Client Information

■ Clients should understand that this drug has been used very infrequently in animals and may not be safe or effective

■ This medication may need to be administered frequently if it is to be effective

■ Report any adverse effects noted to the veterinarian

Chemistry/Synonyms

Carbamazepine is a dibenzoazepine iminostilbene derivative and is chemically related to imipramine. It has the chemical name 5H-Dibenz[b,f]azepine-5-carboxamide and a molecular weight of 236.3. Carbamazepine is a white or off-white powder and is practically insoluble in water, but soluble in alcohol and in acetone.

Carbamazepine may also be known as G-32883, carbamazepine, carbamazepine, carbamazepinum, karbamatsepiini, karbamazepin, karbamazepinas, or karbamazepinum. Trade names include: *Tegretol®* and *Carbatrol®*.

Storage/Stability

Carbamazepine should be stored below 30°C (86°F) in airtight containers as humid conditions can reduce potency by up to one-third. Protect from light.

Compatibility/Compounding Considerations

Compounded preparation stability: Carbamazepine oral suspension compounded from commercially available tablets has been published (Burkart *et al.* 1981). Triturating one (1) carbamazepine 200 mg tablet with 5 mL simple syrup yields a 40 mg/mL oral suspension that retains >90% potency for 90 days stored at both 5°C and 25°C. Suspensions may separate over the 90 day storage period but can be resuspended when shaken vigorously. Compounded preparations of carbamazepine should be protected from light.

Dosage Forms/Regulatory Status

VETERINARY-LABELED PRODUCTS: None

HUMAN-LABELED PRODUCTS:

Carbamazepine Oral Tablets: 100 mg (regular and chewable), & 200 mg; *Tegretol®*, (Ciba-Geigy); *Epitol®* (Teva); generic; (Rx)

Carbamazepine Oral Tablets or Capsules Extended-Release (12-hour); *Tegretol® XR* (Ciba-Geigy); *Carbatrol®* (Rexar); *Equetro®* (Validus); generic; (Rx)

Carbamazepine Oral Suspension: *Tegretol®* (Ciba-Geigy), generic; (Rx)

References

Brewster, ME, WR Anderson, et al. (1997). Intravenous and oral pharmacokinetic evaluation of a 2–hydroxypropyl–beta–cyclodextrin–based formulation of carbamazepine in the dog: Comparison with commercially available tablets and suspensions. *Journal of Pharmaceutical Sciences* 86(3): 335–339.

Brooks, D (2008). Photic Head Shaking. *Blackwell's Five–Minute Veterinary Consult: Equine 2nd Edition.* J–P Lavoie and KW Hinchcliff Eds. Ames, IA, WIley–Blackwell: 590–591.

Burkart, G, R Hammond, et al. (1981). Stability of extemporaneous suspensions of carbamazepine. *Am J Hosp Pharm* 38: 1929.

Frey, HH & W Loscher (1980). PHARMACOKINETICS OF CARBAMAZEPINE IN THE DOG. *Archives Internationales De Pharmacodynamie Et De Therapie* 243(2): 180–191.

Haug, L (2008). Canine aggression toward unfamiliar people and dogs. *Vet Clin NA: Sm Anim Pract* 38: 1023–1041.

CARBIMAZOLE

(kar-*bi*-ma-zole)

Neo-Carbimazole®, Carbazole®

ANTI-THYROID

Note: This drug is not available in the USA, but is routinely used in Europe and elsewhere in place of methimazole

Prescriber Highlights

▶ Used outside of USA & Canada for medical treatment of feline hyperthyroidism

▶ Contraindications/Cautions: Hypersensitive to carbimazole; not recommended in cats intolerant to methimazole; history of or concurrent hematologic abnormalities, liver disease or autoimmune disease

▶ Adverse Effects: Most occur within first 3 months of treatment; vomiting, anorexia & depression most frequent. Eosinophilia, leukopenia, & lymphocytosis are usually transient. Rare, but serious: self-induced excoriations, bleeding, hepatopathy, thrombocytopenia, agranulocytosis, positive direct antiglobulin test, & acquired myasthenia gravis

▶ Dosing requirements may change with time

▶ Place kittens on milk replacer if mother receiving carbimazole

▶ Unlike methimazole, has no bitter taste

▶ Potentially efficacious when used transdermally in cats

Uses/Indications

Carbimazole (a pro-drug of methimazole) or methimazole are considered by most clinicians to be the agents of choice when using drugs to treat feline hyperthyroidism. Propylthiouracil has significantly higher incidences of adverse reactions when compared to methimazole.

Methimazole and therefore, carbimazole, may be useful for the prophylactic prevention of cisplatin-induced nephrotoxicity in dogs.

Pharmacology/Actions

Carbimazole is converted almost entirely to methimazole *in vivo*. Methimazole interferes with iodine incorporation into tyrosyl residues of thyroglobulin thereby inhibiting the synthesis of thyroid hormones. It also inhibits iodinated tyrosyl residues from coupling to form iodothyronine. Methimazole has no effect on the release or activity of thyroid hormones already formed or in the general circulation.

Pharmacokinetics

Carbimazole is rapidly absorbed from the GI tract and rapidly and nearly totally converted to methimazole. Because of differences in molar weight, to attain an equivalent serum level, carbimazole must be dosed approximately 2 times that of methimazole.

In cats, the volume of distribution of methimazole is variable (0.12–0.84 L/kg). Methimazole apparently concentrates in thyroid tissue and biologic effects persist beyond measurable blood levels. After oral dosing, plasma elimination half-life ranges from 2.3–10.2 hours. There is usually a 1–3 week lag time between starting the drug and significant reductions in serum T_4. Carbimazole may be amenable for use transdermally in cats to control hyperthyroidism.

In dogs, methimazole has a serum half-life of 8–9 hours.

Contraindications/Precautions/Warnings

Carbimazole is contraindicated in patients who are hypersensitive to it or methimazole. It should be used very cautiously in patients with a history of or concurrent hematologic abnormalities, liver disease or autoimmune disease.

Because carbimazole is a prodrug and is converted into methimazole, cats who have had prior serious reactions to methimazole should receive carbimazole with great caution.

Adverse Effects

Adverse effects are reported less often with carbimazole than methimazole. Whether they indeed occur less frequently is debatable. Most adverse effects associated with carbimazole or methimazole use in cats occur within the first three months of therapy with vomiting, anorexia and depression occurring most frequently. The GI effects may be related to the drug's bitter taste and are usually transient. Eosinophilia, leukopenia, and lymphocytosis may be noted in approximately 15% of cats treated within the first 8 weeks of therapy. These hematologic effects usually are also transient and generally do not require drug withdrawal. Other more serious but rare adverse effects include: self-induced excoriations (2.3%), bleeding (2.3%), hepatopathy (1.5%), thrombocytopenia (2.7%), agranulocytosis (1.5%), and positive direct antiglobulin test (1.9%). These effects generally require withdrawal of the drug and adjunctive therapy. Up to 50% of cats receiving methimazole chronically (>6 months), will develop a positive ANA, which requires dosage reduction. Rarely, cats will develop an acquired myasthenia gravis that requires either withdrawal or concomitant glucocorticoid therapy.

High levels of methimazole cross the placenta and may induce hypothyroidism in kittens born of queens receiving the drug. Levels higher than those found in plasma are found in human breast milk. It is suggested that kittens be placed on a milk replacer after receiving colostrum from mothers on methimazole.

Reproduction/Nursing Safety

Carbimazole, like methimazole (carbimazole is converted to methimazole), has been associated with teratogenic effects in humans (scalp defects). It may also affect offspring thyroid development or function. In humans, the FDA categorizes methimazole as category **D** for use during pregnancy (*There is evidence of human fetal risk, but the potential benefits from the use of the drug in pregnant women may be acceptable despite its potential risks.*)

As methimazole can enter milk and have deleterious effects on offspring, switch to milk replacer if carbimazole or methimazole are required for nursing dams.

Overdosage

Acute toxicity that may be seen with overdosage include those that are listed above under Adverse Effects. Agranulocytosis, hepatopathy, and thrombocytopenias are perhaps the most serious effects that may be seen. Treatment consists of following standard protocols in handling an oral ingestion (empty stomach if not contraindicated, administer charcoal, etc.) and to treat symptomatically and supportively.

Drug Interactions

The following drug interactions have either been reported or are theoretical in humans or animals receiving carbimazole and may be of significance in veterinary patients:

- **BUPROPION:** Potential for increased risk for hepatotoxicity; increased monitoring (LFT's) necessary
- **DIGOXIN:** Carbimazole may decrease digoxin efficacy
- **WARFARIN:** Potential for decreased anticoagulant efficacy if carbimazole added

Doses

See also Methimazole. Usually, carbimazole dosages are twice that of methimazole.

- **CATS:**
  For hyperthyroidism:
  a) 2.5–5 mg (total dose) per cat PO twice daily (Trepanier 2007)
  b) 10–15 mg total dose daily per cat in divided doses for 1–3 weeks will produce a euthyroid state for most patients. Then adjust dosage for the patient to the lowest effective dose. Most cats will need dosing at least once daily. (Debuf 1991)

c) Initially, give 5 mg (total dose) q8h for 2–3 weeks. Then adjust. May need to increase dose in approximately 10% of cats (be sure owner was compliant with previous dose). Most cats require 5 mg PO q12h to maintain euthyroidism. (Peterson 2000)

d) Using the sustained-release tablets (*Vidalta®*): 15 mg PO once daily at the same time each day. Do not break or crush tabs. Adjust dose upwards or downwards within a range of 10 mg–25 mg per day in 5 mg increments depending on clinical signs and TT4 (tablets cannot be split, so combinations of 10 mg and 15 mg tablets must be used). If cat requires doses less than 10 mg per day, use alternative treatment. (Adapted from label information; *Vidalta®*—Intervet UK)

Monitoring

During first 3 months of therapy (baseline values and every 2–3 weeks):

- CBC, platelet counts
- Serum T_4
- If indicated by clinical signs: liver function tests, ANA
- After stabilized (at least 3 months of therapy):
- T_4 at 3–6 month intervals
- Other diagnostic tests as dictated by adverse effects

Client Information

- It must be stressed to owners that this drug will decrease excessive thyroid hormones, but does not cure the condition
- Adherence with the treatment regimen is necessary for success

Chemistry/Synonyms

A thioimidazole-derivative antithyroid drug, carbimazole occurs as a white to creamy white powder having a characteristic odor. It is slightly soluble in water and soluble in alcohol.

Carbimazole may also be known as: carbimazolum, *Basolest®*, *Camazol®*, *Carbimazole®*, *Carbazole®*, *Carbistad®*, *Cazole®*, *Neo Tomizol®*, *Neo-Mercazole®*, *Neo-Thyreostat®*, *Thyrostat®*, *Tyrazol®*, or *Neo-morphazole®*.

Storage/Stability

Unless otherwise labeled, carbimazole tablets should be stored at room temperature in well-closed containers.

Dosage Forms/Regulatory Status

VETERINARY-LABELED PRODUCTS: None

HUMAN-LABELED PRODUCTS:

There are no FDA-approved products in the USA; elsewhere it may be available as:

Carbimazole Oral Tablets: 5 mg & 20 mg. Trade names include *Neo-Carbimazole®*, *Carbazole®*, *Neo Mercazole®*, etc.

Carbimazole Oral Sustained-Release Tablets: 10 mg & 15 mg; *Vidalta*® (Intervet-UK); POM-V

References

Debuf, YM, Ed. (1991). *The Veterinary Formulary: Handbook of Medicines Used in Veterinary Practice.* London, The Pharmaceutical Press.

Peterson, M (2000). Hyperthyroidism. *Textbook of Veterinary Internal Medicine: Diseases of the Dog and Cat.* S Ettinger and E Feldman Eds. Philadelphia, WB Saunders. **1**: 1400–1419.

Trepanier, L (2007). Pharmacologic management of feline hyperthyrodism. *Vet Clin NA: Sm Anim Pract* 37: 775–788.

CARBOPLATIN

(kar-boe-pla-tin)   Paraplatin®

ANTINEOPLASTIC

Prescriber Highlights

▶ Platinum antineoplastic agent used for a variety of carcinomas & sarcomas

▶ Unlike cisplatin, may be used in cats

▶ Contraindications: History of hypersensitivity to it or other platinum agents; severe bone marrow depression

▶ Caution: Hepatic/renal disease, hearing impairment, active infection

▶ Primary adverse effects: GI, Bone marrow depression. Nadir (neutrophils/platelets) in dogs about 14 days; in cats (neutrophils) about 17–21 days

▶ Fetotoxic

▶ Must be given IV in D5W

▶ May adversely affect vaccinations (safety/efficacy)

▶ Treatment may be very expensive

Uses/Indications

Like cisplatin, carboplatin may be useful in a variety of veterinary neoplastic diseases including squamous cell carcinomas, ovarian carcinomas, mediastinal carcinomas, pleural adenocarcinomas, nasal carcinomas and thyroid adenocarcinomas. Carboplatin's primary use currently in small animal medicine is in the adjunctive treatment (post amputation) of osteogenic sarcomas. Its effectiveness in treating transitional cell carcinoma of the bladder has been disappointing; however, intra-arterial administration with NSAID (*e.g.*, meloxicam) may prove to enhance efficacy. Intracavitary carboplatin for recurrent idiopathic or malignant pleural effusion after pericardectomy holds promise.

Carboplatin, unlike cisplatin, appears to be relatively safe to use in cats.

Carboplatin may be considered for intralesional use in conditions such as equine sarcoids or in treating adenocarcinoma in birds.

Whether carboplatin is more efficacious than cisplatin for certain cancers does not appear to be decided at this point, but the drug does ap-

pear to have fewer adverse effects (less renal toxicity and reduced vomiting) in dogs.

Pharmacology/Actions

Carboplatin's exact mechanism of action is not fully understood. Both carboplatin's and cisplatin's properties are analogous to those of bifunctional alkylating agents producing inter- and intrastrand crosslinks in DNA, thereby inhibiting DNA replication, RNA transcription, and protein synthesis. Carboplatin is cell-cycle nonspecific.

Pharmacokinetics

After IV administration, carboplatin is well distributed throughout the body; highest concentrations are found in the liver, kidney, skin and tumor tissue. The metabolic fate and elimination of carboplatin are complex and the discussion of this aspect of the drug's pharmacokinetics is beyond the scope of this reference. Suffice it to say, the parent drug degrades into platinum and platinum-complexed compounds that are primarily eliminated by kidneys. In dogs, almost one half of the dose is excreted in the urine within 24 hours and approximately 70% of the platinum administered is secreted in the urine after 72 hours.

Contraindications/Precautions/Warnings

Carboplatin is contraindicated in patients hypersensitive to it or other platinum-containing compounds. It is also contraindicated in patients with severe bone marrow suppression. Patients with severe carboplatin-induced myelosuppression should be allowed to recover their counts before additional therapy.

Caution is advised in patients with active infections, hearing impairment or preexisting renal or hepatic disease.

Do not give carboplatin IM or SC.

Adverse Effects

Established adverse effects in dogs include anorexia and/or vomiting that usually occur 2–4 days after a dose, and dose-related bone marrow suppression that is exhibited primarily as thrombocytopenia and/or neutropenia. The nadir of platelet and neutrophil counts generally occur about 14 days post treatment in dogs. Recovery is generally seen by day 21. In cats, thrombocytopenia occurs infrequently, but the neutrophil nadir occurs about 21 days post treatment. Recovery usually occurs by day 28 in cats.

Hepatotoxicity (increased serum bilirubin and liver enzymes) is seen in about 15% of human patients treated with carboplatin. Other potential adverse effects include: nephrotoxicity, neuropathies and ototoxicity. These effects occur with carboplatin therapy much less frequently than with cisplatin therapy. Anaphylactoid reactions have been reported rarely in humans that have received platinum-containing compounds (*e.g.*, cisplatin). Hyperuricemia may occur after therapy in a small percentage of patients.

Reproductive/Nursing Safety

Carboplatin is fetotoxic and embryotoxic in rats and the risks of its use during pregnancy should be weighed with its potential benefits. In humans, the FDA categorizes this drug as category **D** for use during pregnancy (*There is evidence of human fetal risk, but the potential benefits from the use of the drug in pregnant women may be acceptable despite its potential risks.*)

It is unknown whether carboplatin enters maternal milk. In humans, it is recommended to discontinue nursing if the mother is receiving the drug.

Overdosage/Acute Toxicity

There is limited information available. An overdose of carboplatin would be expected to cause aggravated effects associated with the drug's bone marrow nephro- and liver toxicity. Monitor for neurotoxicity, ototoxicity, hepatotoxicity and nephrotoxicity.

Treatment is basically supportive; no specific antidote is available. Plasmapheresis or hemodialysis could potentially be of benefit in removing the drug.

Drug Interactions

The following drug interactions have either been reported or are theoretical in humans or animals receiving carboplatin and may be of significance in veterinary patients:

- **AMINOGLYCOSIDES:** Potential for increased risk of nephrotoxicity or ototoxicity
- **CISPLATIN:** Human patients previously treated with cisplatin have an increased risk of developing neurotoxicity or ototoxicity after receiving carboplatin
- **MYLEOSUPPRESSIVE DRUGS:** The leukopenic or thrombocytopenic effects secondary to carboplatin may be enhanced by other myelosuppressive medications
- **RADIATION THERAPY:** Potential for increased hematologic toxicity
- **VACCINES:** Live or killed virus vaccines administered after carboplatin therapy may not be as effective as the immune response to these vaccines may be modified by carboplatin therapy; carboplatin may also potentiate live virus vaccines replication and increase the adverse effects associated with these vaccines

Doses

Note: Because of the potential toxicity of this drug to patients, veterinary personnel and clients, and since chemotherapy indications, treatment protocols, monitoring and safety guidelines often change, the following dosages should be used only as a general guide. Consultation with a veterinary oncologist and referral to current veterinary oncology references [*e.g.*, (Henry & Higginbotham 2009); (Argyle *et al.* 2008); (Withrow & Vail 2007); (Villalobos 2007); (Ogilvie & Moore 2006); (Ogilvie & Moore 2001)] is *strongly recommended.*

Do not confuse cisplatin and carboplatin dosages; cisplatin dosages are much lower.

The following is a usual dosage (dosage may need adjustment in patients with reduced renal function) or dose range for carboplatin and should be used only as a general guide:

Dogs: 300–350 mg/m^2 IV every 3 weeks.

Cats and Rabbits: 180–260 mg/m^2 IV every 3 weeks. It has also been administered intratumorally in cats for nasal planum carcinomas.

Monitoring

- CBC
- Serum electrolytes, uric acid
- Baseline renal and hepatic function tests

Client Information

- Clients should fully understand the potential toxicity of this agent and, ideally, should give informed consent for its use.
- As carboplatin (and any platinum containing metabolites) is principally excreted in the urine over several days after treatment, clients should be warned to avoid direct contact with patient's urine.

Chemistry/Synonyms

Carboplatin, like cisplatin, is a platinum-containing antineoplastic agent. It occurs as white to off-white crystalline powder having a solubility of 14 mg/mL in water and is insoluble in alcohol. The commercially available powder for injection contains equal parts of mannitol and carboplatin. After reconstitution with sterile water for injection, a resulting solution of 10 mg/mL of carboplatin has a pH of 5–7 and an osmolality of 94 mOsm/kg.

Carboplatin may also be known as: cis-Diammine-1,1-cyclobutanedicarboxylato-platinum, carboplatinum; CBDCA; JM-8; or NSC-241240; many trade names are available.

Storage/Stability

The powder for injection should kept stored at room temperature and protected from light.

After reconstitution, solutions containing 10 mg/mL are stable for at least 8 hours. Some sources say that the solution is stable for up to 24 hours and can be refrigerated, but because there are no preservatives in the solution, the manufacturer recommends discarding unused portions after 8 hours. Previous recommendations to avoid the use of solutions to dilute carboplatin containing sodium chloride are no longer warranted as only a minimal amount of carboplatin is converted to cisplatin in these solutions.

Because aluminum can displace platinum from carboplatin, the solution should not be prepared, stored or administered where aluminum-containing items can come into contact with the solution. Should carboplatin come into contact with aluminum, a black precipitate will form and the product should not be used.

Compatibility/Compounding Considerations

Directions for reconstitution for the 50 mg vial: Add 5 mL of either sterile water for injection, normal saline injection or D_5W that will provide a solution containing 10 mg/mL. May infuse directly (usually over 15 minutes) or further dilute. Visually inspect after reconstitution/dilution for discoloration or particulate matter.

Dosage Forms/Regulatory Status

VETERINARY-LABELED PRODUCTS: None

HUMAN-LABELED PRODUCTS:

Carboplatin lyophilized Powder for reconstitution and IV Injection: 50 mg, 150 mg , & 450 mg in single-dose vials (contains mannitol); generic (Baxter); (Rx)

Carboplatin Injection: 10 mg/mL in 5 mL, 15 mL & 45 mL single-use vials; generic; (Rx)

References

Argyle, D, M Brearly, et al. (2008). *Decision Making in Small Animal Oncology*, Wiley–Blackwell.

Henry, C & M Higginbotham (2009). *Cancer Management in Small Animal Practice*, Saunders.

Ogilvie, G & A Moore (2001). *Feline Oncology: A Comprehensive Guide to Compassionate Care*, Veterinary Learning Systems.

Ogilvie, G & A Moore (2006). *Managing the Canine Cancer Patient: A Practical Guide to Compassionate Care*, Veterinary Learning Systems.

Villalobos, A (2007). *Canine and Feline Geriatric Oncology*. Ames, Blackwell.

Withrow, S & D Vail (2007). *Withrow and MacEwen's Small Animal Clinical Oncology 4th Ed*. Philadelphia, Elsevier.

CARNITINE
LEVOCARNITINE
L-CARNITINE

(*kar*-ni-teen)   Carnitor®

NUTRIENT

Prescriber Highlights

▶ Nutrient required for normal fat utilization & energy metabolism

▶ May be useful in certain cardiomyopathies (including doxorubicin induced) in dogs

▶ Use only L (levo-) forms

▶ Preferably give with meals

Uses/Indications

Levocarnitine may be useful as adjunctive therapy of dilated cardiomyopathy in dogs. Up to 90% of dogs with dilated cardiomyopathy may have a carnitine deficiency. American Cocker spaniels, Boxers, dogs with cysteine or urate urolithiasis, and dilated cardiomyopathy may all especially benefit. Any breed with dilated cardiomyopathy may receive a trial of the drug as approximately 5% will respond.

Levocarnitine may also protect against doxorubicin-induced cardiomyopathy and reduce risks of myocardial infarction and it may be beneficial in the adjunctive treatment of valproic acid toxicity.

In cats, levocarnitine has been recommended as being useful as an adjunctive therapy in feline hepatic lipidosis by facilitating hepatic lipid metabolism. Its use for this indication is somewhat controversial.

Pharmacology/Actions

Levocarnitine is required for normal fat utilization and energy metabolism in mammalian species. It serves to facilitate entry of long-chain fatty acids into cellular mitochondria where they can be used during oxidation and energy production.

Severe chronic deficiency is generally a result of an inborn genetic defect where levocarnitine utilization is impaired and not the result of dietary insufficiency. Effects seen in levocarnitine deficiency may include hypoglycemia, progressive myasthenia, hepatomegaly, CHF, cardiomegaly, hepatic coma, neurologic disturbances, encephalopathy, hypotonia and lethargy.

Pharmacokinetics

In humans, levocarnitine is absorbed via the GI with a bioavailability of about 15%, but is absorbed rapidly in the intestine via passive and active mechanisms. Highest levels of levocarnitine are found in skeletal muscle. Levocarnitine is distributed in milk. Exogenously administered levocarnitine is eliminated by both renal and fecal routes. Plasma levocarnitine levels may be increased in patients with renal failure.

Contraindications/Precautions/Warnings

Levocarnitine may also be known as Vitamin B_T. Products labeled as such may have both D and L racemic forms. Use only Levo- (L-) forms as the D- form may competitively inhibit L- uptake with a resulting deficiency.

Adverse Effects

Adverse effect profile is minimal. Gastrointestinal upset is the most likely effect that may be noted and is usually associated with high dosages but is usually mild and limited to loose stools or possibly diarrhea; nausea and vomiting are possible. Human patients have reported increased body odor.

Reproductive/Nursing Safety

Studies done in rats and rabbits have demonstrated no teratogenic effects and it is generally believed that levocarnitine is safe to use in pregnancy though documented safety during pregnancy has not been established. In humans, the FDA categorizes this drug as category **B** for use during pregnancy (*Animal studies have not yet demonstrated risk to the fetus, but there are no adequate studies in pregnant women; or animal studies have shown an adverse effect, but adequate studies in pregnant women have not demonstrated a risk to the fetus in the first trimester of pregnancy, and there is no evidence of risk in later trimesters.*)

Overdosage/Acute Toxicity

Levocarnitine is a relatively safe drug. Minor overdoses need only to be monitored; with massive overdoses consider gut emptying. Refer to a poison control center for more information.

Drug Interactions

The following drug interactions have either been reported or are theoretical in humans or animals receiving levocarnitine and may be of significance in veterinary patients:

■ **VALPROIC ACID:** Patients receiving valproic acid may require higher dosages of levocarnitine

Doses

■ **DOGS:**

For myocardial carnitine deficiency associated with dilated cardiomyopathy:

a) As a trial for treating canine dilated cardiomyopathy: For a large or giant breed dog: 2 grams (approximately 1 teaspoonful of pure powder) PO q8–12h;

For adjunctive (with traditional pharmacotherapy) therapy of dilated cardiomyopathy in American Cocker spaniels: 1 gram (approximately 1/2 teaspoonful) PO q8–12h with taurine (Keene 2002)

b) For boxers with severe myocardial failure: Give 2–3 grams carnitine PO q12h for 2–4 months to determine if they respond (Kittleson 2006)

c) For adjunctive treatment of American cocker spaniels with dilated cardiomyopathy: Carnitine 1 g PO q12h with taurine 500 mg q12h PO (Kittleson 2006)

d) For cardiac indications (dilated cardiomyopathy) when carnitine supplementation may benefit:

American Cocker spaniels: 1 g PO q8h

Boxer dogs with dilated cardiomyopathy: 2 g PO q8h

Documented systemic carnitine deficiency: 50–100 mg/kg PO q8h.

Myocardial carnitine deficiency only: 200 mg/kg PO q8h (Smith 2009)

■ **CATS:**

a) As adjunctive dietary therapy in cats with severe hepatic lipidosis: 250 mg PO once daily (use *Carnitor*®); also supplement with taurine (250 mg once to twice daily), Vitamin E (10 Units/kg/day), water soluble vitamins and determine B12 status (treat while awaiting data at 1 mg/cat SC). See also Acetylcysteine. (Center 2006)

b) For supplementation in cats with liver disease: 250–500 mg/day (Zoran 2006)

Monitoring

■ Efficacy

■ Periodic blood chemistries have been rec-

ommended for human patients, their value in veterinary medicine is undetermined.

Client Information

■ Give with meals when possible to reduce likelihood of GI side effects.

■ The majority of dogs responding to carnitine therapy for dilated cardiomyopathy will require other medication to control clinical signs.

Chemistry/Synonyms

Levocarnitine (the L-isomer of carnitine) is an amino acid derivative, synthesized *in vivo* from methionine and lysine. It is required for energy metabolism and has a molecular weight of 161.

Carnitine may also be known as: vitamin B(T), L-carnitine, or levocarnitinum; many trade names are available.

Storage/Stability

Levocarnitine capsules, tablets and powder should be stored in well-closed containers at room temperature. The oral solution should be kept in tight containers at room temperature. The injection should be stored at room temperature in the original carton; discard any unused portion after opening, as the injection contains no preservative.

Dosage Forms/Regulatory Status

VETERINARY-LABELED PRODUCTS: None

HUMAN-LABELED PRODUCTS:

Levocarnitine Oral Tablets: 330 mg & 500 mg; *Carnitor*® (Sigma-Tau); L-Carnitine (Freeda Vitamins); Levocarnitine (Rising); (Rx & OTC)

Levocarnitine or L-Carnitine Oral Capsules: 250 mg; generic; (OTC—as a food supplement)

Levocarnitine Oral Solution: 100 mg/mL in 118 mL; *Carnitor*® (Sigma-Tau); Levocarnitine (Rising); (Rx)

Levocarnitine Injection: 200 mg/mL in single-dose vials & preservative-free in single-dose vials and amps; *Carnitor*® (Sigma-Tau); generic; (Rx)

Note: L-carnitine may also be available in bulk powder form from local health food stores

References

Center, S (2006). Treatment for Severe Feline Hepatic Lipidosis. Proceedings: WSAVA. Accessed via: Veterinary Information Network. *http://goo.gl/N7g14*

Keene, B (2002). Understanding the importance of carnitine, taurine and other nutraceuticals in the cardiology patient. Proceedings; ACVIM Forum. Accessed via: Veterinary Information Network. *http://goo.gl/wvp8P*

Kittleson, M (2006). "Chapt 10: Management of Heart Failure." *Small Animal Cardiology, 2nd Ed.*

Smith, F (2009). Alternative therapies for the cardiac diseases. Proceedings: WVC. Accessed via: Veterinary Information Network. *http://goo.gl/pGQPQ*

Zoran, D (2006). Inflammatory liver disease in cats. Proceedings: ABVP 2006. Accessed via: Veterinary Information Network. *http://goo.gl/lFyUT*

CARPROFEN

(kar-*pro*-fen)   Rimadyl®

NON-STEROIDAL ANTIINFLAMMATORY AGENT

Prescriber Highlights

▶ NSAID used in dogs & other small animals

▶ Contraindicated in dogs with bleeding disorders (e.g., Von Willebrand's), history of serious reactions to it or other propionic-class NSAIDs

▶ Caution: Geriatric patients or those with preexisting chronic diseases (e.g., inflammatory bowel disease, renal or hepatic insufficiency)

▶ GI adverse effects are less likely than with older NSAIDs but can occur

▶ Rarely may cause hepatic failure; monitor liver enzymes

Uses/Indications

Carprofen is labeled (in the USA) for the relief of pain and inflammation in dogs. It may also prove to be of benefit in other species as well, but data is scant to support its safety beyond very short-term use at this time. In Europe, carprofen is reportedly registered for single dose use in cats, but there have been reported problems (e.g., vomiting) with cats receiving more than a single dose.

Carprofen is being investigated for antineoplastic effects in dogs and may be a useful adjunctive treatment for some types of tumors with COX-2 overexpression.

Pharmacology/Actions

Like other NSAIDs, carprofen exhibits analgesic, antiinflammatory, and antipyretic activity probably through its inhibition of cyclooxygenase, phospholipase A_2 and inhibition of prostaglandin synthesis. Carprofen appears to be more sparing of COX-1 *in vitro* and in dogs appears to have fewer COX-1 effects (GI distress/ulceration, platelet inhibition, renal damage) when compared to older non-COX-2 specific agents. COX-2 specificity appears to be species, dose, and tissue dependent. Carprofen in horses or cats does not seem to be as COX-2 specific as it is in dogs.

Pharmacokinetics

When administered orally to dogs, carprofen is approximately 90% bioavailable. Peak serum levels occur between 1–3 hours post dosing. The drug is highly bound to plasma proteins (99%) and has a low volume of distribution (0.12–0.22 L/kg). Carprofen is extensively metabolized in the liver primarily via glucuronidation and oxidative processes. About 70–80% of a dose is eliminated in the feces; 10–20% eliminated in the urine. Some enterohepatic recycling of the drug occurs.

Elimination half-life of carprofen in the dog is approximately 8 hours with the S form having a longer half-life than the R form. The half-life of carprofen is reportedly 22 hours in horses and averages 20 hours in cats, but interindividual variability is very high in cats (9–49 hours). Half-life is not necessarily a good predictor of duration of effect, as the drug's high affinity for tissue proteins may act as a reservoir for the drug at inflamed tissue.

Contraindications/Precautions/Warnings

Carprofen is contraindicated in dogs with bleeding disorders (e.g., Von Willebrand's) or those that have had prior serious reactions to it or other propionic-class antiinflammatory agents. It should be used with caution in geriatric patients or those with preexisting chronic diseases (e.g., inflammatory bowel disease, renal or hepatic insufficiency).

Adverse Effects

Although adverse effects appear to be uncommon with carprofen use in dogs, they can occur. Mild gastrointestinal effects (vomiting, diarrhea, inappetence) or lethargy are the most likely to appear but incidence is low (<2%). Rarely, serious effects including hepatocellular damage and/or renal disease; hematologic and serious gastrointestinal effects (ulceration) have been reported. Increased risks for the development of renal toxicity include preexisting renal insufficiency, dehydration or sodium depletion.

Reported incidence of hepatopathy is approximately 0.05% or less in dogs. It has been postulated that this adverse effect could be caused by formation of reactive acyl glucuronide metabolites that bind to and form haptites on hepatocytes; an immunological reaction then occurs causing hepatotoxicity. Geriatric dogs or dogs with chronic diseases (e.g., inflammatory bowel disease, renal or hepatic insufficiency) may be at greater risk for developing hepatic toxicity while receiving this drug, but the effect may be idiosyncratic and unpredictable. Although not proven statistically significant, Labrador Retrievers have been associated with 1/4 of the initially reported cases associated with the reported hepatic syndrome; but it is not believed that this breed has any greater chance of developing this adverse effect than others. Before initiating therapy, pre-treatment patient evaluation and discussion with the owner regarding the potential risks versus benefits of therapy are advised.

Carprofen has been used in cats, but as cats have limited ability hepatically to glucuronidate there is a greater potential for drug accumulation with resultant adverse effects. In particular, cats appear to be more susceptible to developing renal adverse effects from NSAIDs. Prolonged administration of carprofen in cats has also caused gastrointestinal effects. Hepatotoxicity does not appear to be a significant concern with NSAID use in cats, perhaps since they do not form significant amounts of gulcuronidated metabolites.

Reproductive/Nursing Safety

The manufacturer states that the safe use of carprofen in dogs less than 6 weeks of age, pregnant dogs, dogs used for breeding purposes, or lactating bitches has not been established. Carprofen has been given to pregnant rats at dosages of up to 20 mg/kg during day 7–15 of gestation. While no teratogenic effects were noted in pups, the drug did delay parturition with an increased number of dead pups at birth.

Overdosage/Acute Toxicity

In dog toxicologic studies, repeated doses of up to 10X resulted in little adversity. Some dogs exhibited hypoalbuminemia, melena or slight increases in ALT. However, post-marketing surveillance suggests that there may be significant interpatient variability in response to acute or chronic overdoses. According to the APCC database, vomiting has been reported at doses as low as 5.3 mg/kg in dogs and 3.9 mg/kg in cats. The APCC level of concern for renal damage is 50 mg/kg in dogs and 8 mg/kg in cats.

There were 2235 exposures to carprofen reported to the ASPCA Animal Poison Control Center (APCC) during 2008-2009. In these cases, 1952 were dogs with 296 showing clinical signs and the remaining 283 cases were cats with 41 showing clinical signs. Common findings in dogs recorded in decreasing frequency included vomiting, lethargy, anorexia, diarrhea, azotemia, bloody vomitus, elevated BUN, elevated alkaline phosphatase, and elevated creatinine. Common findings in cats recorded in decreasing frequency included vomiting, anorexia, axotemia, hyperphosphatemia, and lethargy.

This medication is a NSAID. As with any NSAID, overdosage can lead to gastrointestinal and renal effects. Decontamination with emetics and/or activated charcoal is appropriate. For doses where GI effects are expected, the use of gastrointestinal protectants is warranted. If renal effects are also expected, fluid diuresis is warranted.

Drug Interactions

Note: Although the manufacturer does not list any specific drug interactions in the package insert, it does caution to avoid or closely monitor carprofen's use with other ulcerogenic drugs (*e.g.*, **corticosteroids** or other **NSAIDs**). While some advocate a multi-day washout period when switching from one NSAID to another (not aspirin—see below), there does not appear to be any credible evidence that this is required. Until so, consider starting the new NSAID when the next dose would be due for the old one.

The following drug interactions have either been reported or are theoretical in humans or animals receiving carprofen and may be of significance in veterinary patients:

- ■ **ACE INHIBITORS (e.g., benazepril, enalapril):** Because ACE inhibitors potentially can reduce renal blood flow, use with NSAIDs could increase the risk for renal injury. However, one study in dogs receiving tepoxalin did not show any adverse effect. It is unknown what effects, if any, occur if other NSAIDs and ACE inhibitors are used together in dogs.

- ■ **ASPIRIN:** When aspirin is used concurrently with carprofen, plasma levels of carprofen could decrease and an increased likelihood of GI adverse effects (blood loss) could occur. Concomitant administration of aspirin with carprofen cannot be recommended. Washout periods of several days is probably warranted when switching from an NSAID to aspirin therapy in dogs.

- ■ **CORTICOSTEROIDS:** Concomitant administration with NSAIDs may significantly increase the risks for GI adverse effects

- ■ **DIGOXIN:** Carprofen may increase serum levels of digoxin; use with caution in patients with severe cardiac failure

- ■ **FUROSEMIDE:** Carprofen may reduce the saluretic and diuretic effects of furosemide

- ■ **HIGHLY PROTEIN BOUND DRUGS (e.g., phenytoin, valproic acid, oral anticoagulants, other antiinflammatory agents, salicylates, sulfonamides, sulfonylurea antidiabetic agents):** Because carprofen is highly bound to plasma proteins (99%), it potentially could displace other highly bound drugs; increased serum levels and duration of actions may occur. Although these interactions are usually of little concern clinically, use together with caution.

- ■ **METHOTREXATE:** Serious toxicity has occurred when NSAIDs have been used concomitantly with methotrexate; use together with extreme caution

- ■ **PHENOBARBITAL, RIFAMPIN, or OTHER HEPATIC ENZYME INDUCING AGENTS:** As carprofen hepatotoxicity may be mediated by its hepatic metabolites, these drugs should be avoided if carprofen is required. One source states: Patients should not receive phenobarbital or other hepatic drug metabolizing enzyme inducers when receiving this drug (Boothe 2005).

- ■ **PROBENECID:** May cause a significant increase in serum levels and half-life of carprofen

Laboratory Considerations

- ■ In dogs, carprofen can have no effect or slightly lower **Free T$_4$**, **Total T$_4$** and **TSH** levels in dogs.

Doses

- ■ **DOGS:**
  As an antiinflammatory/analgesic:
  a) 4.4 mg/kg PO; may be given once daily or divided and given as 2.2. mg/kg twice

daily; round dose to nearest half caplet increment. For postoperative pain, administer approximately 2 hours before the procedure. Injectable is dosed as the oral products, but administered SC. (Package Insert; *Rimadyl®*—Pfizer)

b) Surgical pain: 4 mg/kg PO, IM, SC once. Pain/inflammation (non-surgical): 2.2 mg/kg PO q12–24h (Boothe 2005)

■ **CATS:**

As an antiinflammatory/analgesic: Extreme caution is advised, particularly with continued dosing.

a) For surgical pain: 1–4 mg/kg SC pre- or post-operatively. Analgesia may last 12–18 hours. Use of 1–2 mg/kg SC gives similar efficacy as the higher doses, but is safer (Robertson & Lascelles 2003)

b) 2 mg/kg PO q12h; limit to 2 days of therapy (Hardie 2000)

c) Less than 1 mg/kg PO once daily (q24h) for 2–3 treatments (Boothe 2005)

d) For surgical pain: 2 mg/kg or less (lean weight) SC once at induction (Mathews 2005)

■ **RABBITS/RODENTS/SMALL MAMMALS:**

a) **Rabbits:** For chronic joint pain: 2.2 mg/kg PO q12h (Ivey & Morrisey 2000)

b) **Rats:** 5 mg/kg SC or 5–10 mg/kg PO. Chinchillas: 4 mg/kg SC once daily (Adamcak & Otten 2000)

c) 1–4 mg/kg PO, SC q12–24h (Bays 2006)

■ **HORSES: (Note:** ARCI UCGFS Class 4 Drug)

a) As an antiinflammatory/analgesic: 0.7 mg/kg IV, one time (Clark & Clark 1999)

b) 0.7 mg/kg IV, one time; may follow with 0.7 mg/kg PO (granules, mixed with a little feed) for up to 4–9 days according to clinical response (Label information; *Rimadyl® Large Animal Solution, Rimadyl Granules®*—Pfizer U.K.)

■ **CATTLE:**

a) In young cattle (<12 months old) for adjunctive therapy of acute inflammation associated with respiratory disease: 1.4 mg/kg IV or SC once. Slaughter withdrawal = 21 days; not to be used in cows producing milk for human consumption. (Label information; *Rimadyl® Large Animal Solution*—Pfizer U.K.)

■ **BIRDS:**

As an antiinflammatory/analgesic:

a) 2 mg/kg PO q8–24 hours (Clyde & Paul-Murphy 2000)

b) 1 mg/kg SC. Study demonstrated increased walking ability in lame chickens. (Paul-Murphy 2003)

c) 1–4 mg/kg IM, IV, PO (Bays 2006)

■ **REPTILES:**

As an antiinflammatory/analgesic:

a) 1–4 mg/kg IV, IM, SC, PO q 24–72h (Bays 2006)

■ **ZOO, EXOTIC, WILDLIFE SPECIES:**

For use of carprofen in zoo, exotic and wildlife medicine refer to specific references, including:

a) *Exotic Animal Formulary, 3rd Ed.* Carpenter J. W. Saunders. 2005

b) The 2009 American Association of Zoo Veterinarian Proceedings by D. K. Fontenot also has several dosages listed for restraint, anesthesia, and analgesia for a variety of drugs for carnivores and primates. VIN members can access them at: http://goo.gl/BHRih or http://goo.gl/9UJse

Monitoring

■ Baseline (especially in geriatric dogs, dogs with chronic diseases, or when prolonged treatment is likely): physical exam, CBC, Serum chemistry panel (including liver and renal function tests), and UA. It is recommended to reassess the liver enzymes at one, two and 4 weeks of therapy and then at 3–6 month intervals. Should elevation occur, recommend discontinuing the drug.

■ Clinical efficacy

■ Signs of potential adverse reactions: inappetence, diarrhea, vomiting, melena, polyuria/polydipsia, anemia, jaundice, lethargy, behavior changes, ataxia or seizures

■ Chronic therapy: Consider repeating CBC, UA and serum chemistries on an ongoing basis

Client Information

■ Although rare, serious adverse effects have been reported with the use of this drug. Read and understand the client information sheet provided with this medication; contact the veterinarian with any questions or concerns.

■ Watch for signs of potential adverse effects including: decreased appetite, vomiting, diarrhea, dark or tarry stools, increased water consumption, increased urination, pale gums due to anemia, yellowing of gums, skin or white of the eye due to jaundice, incoordination, seizures, or behavioral changes. Should these signs present, clients should stop the drug immediately and contact their veterinarian.

■ Store the flavored chewable tablets out of reach of dogs to avoid the potential for overdose.

Chemistry/Synonyms

A propionic acid derivative non-steroidal antiinflammatory agent, carprofen occurs as a white crystalline compound. It is practically insoluble in water and freely soluble in ethanol at room temperature. Carprofen has both an S (+) enantiomer and R (-) enantiomer. The commercial product contains a racemic mixture of both. The S (+) enantiomer has greater antiinflammatory potency than the R (-) form.

Carprofen may also be known as: C-5720; Ro-20-5720/000, *Rimadyl®*, *Zinecarp®*, *Canidryl®*, *Novox®*, *Carprodyl®* or *Norocarp®*.

Storage/Stability

The commercially available caplets or chewable tablets should be stored at room temperature (15–30°C).

The commercially available (in the USA) injection should be stored in the refrigerator (2–8°C; 36–46°F). Once broached, the injection may be stored at temperatures of up to 25°C for 28 days.

Compatibility/Compounding Considerations

Compounded preparation stability: Carprofen oral suspension compounded from commercially available tablets has been published (Hawkins *et al.* 2006). Triturating one (1) carprofen 100 mg tablet with 10 mL of *Ora-Plus®* and *qs ad* to 20 mL with *Ora-Sweet®* yields a 5 mg/mL suspension that retains 90% potency for 21 days stored at both 5°C and 25°C. Compounded preparations of carprofen should be protected from light.

Dosage Forms/Regulatory Status

VETERINARY-LABELED PRODUCTS:

Carprofen Scored Caplets: 25 mg, 75 mg & 100 mg; *Rimadyl®* Caplets (Pfizer), *Novocox®* (Impax), *Vetprofen®* (Belcher), *Norocarp®* (Norbrook); (Rx). FDA-approved for use in dogs.

Carprofen Chewable Tablets: 25 mg, 75 mg & 100 mg; *Rimadyl®* Chewable Tablets (Pfizer); (Rx). FDA-approved for use in dogs.

Carprofen Sterile Injectable Solution: 50 mg/mL in 20 mL vials; *Rimadyl®* (Pfizer); (Rx). FDA-approved for use in dogs.

In the U.K., *Rimadyl®* Injection is labeled for use in dogs, cats, horses, ponies and cattle (less than 12 months old; slaughter withdrawal = 21 days; not to be used in cattle producing milk for human consumption). *Rimadyl®* Granules are labeled for use in horses and ponies. See Doses for more information.

The ARCI (Racing Commissioners International) has designated this drug as a class 4 substance. See the appendix for more information.

HUMAN-LABELED PRODUCTS: None

References

Adamcak, A & B Otten (2000). Rodent Therapeutics. *Vet Clin NA: Exotic Anim Pract* 3:1(Jan): 221–240.

Bays, T (2006). Recognizing and managing pain in exotic species. Proceedings: Western Vet Conf. Accessed via: Veterinary Information Network. *http://goo.gl/C75Uv*

Boothe, DM (2005). New information on nonsteroidal antiinflammatories: What every criticalist must know. Proceedings: IVECC. Accessed via: Veterinary Information Network. *http://goo.gl/xUukK*

Clark, J & T Clark (1999). Analgesia. *The Veterinary Clinics of North America: Equine Practice* 15:3(December): 705–723.

Clyde, V & J Paul–Murphy (2000). Avian Analgesia. *Kirk's Current Veterinary Therapy: XIII Small Animal Practice.* J Bonagura Ed. Philadelphia, WB Saunders: 1126–1128.

Hardie, E (2000). Pain: Management. *Textbook of Veterinary Internal Medicine: Diseases of the Dog and Cat.* S Ettinger and E Feldman Eds. Philadelphia, WB Saunders. **1**: 23–25.

Hawkins, MG, MJ Karriker, et al. (2006). Drug distribution and stability in extemporaneous preparations of meloxicam and carprofen after dilution and suspension at two storage temperatures. *J Am Vet Med Assoc* **229**(6): 968–974.

Ivey, E & J Morrisey (2000). Therapeutics for Rabbits. *Vet Clin NA: Exotic Anim Pract* 3:1(Jan): 183–216.

Mathews, K (2005). Nonsteroidal; Anti–Inflammatory Analgesics. *Textbook of Veterinary Internal Medicine, 6th Ed.* S Ettinger and E Feldman Eds., Elsevier: 518–521.

Paul–Murphy, J (2003). Managing pain in birds. Proceedings: Pain 2003. Accessed via: Veterinary Information Network. *http://goo.gl/dTYJA*

Robertson, S & B Lascelles (2003). Safe and effective acute pain relief in cats. Proceedings: PAIN 2003. Accessed via: Veterinary Information Network. *http://goo.gl/ORxDj*

CARVEDILOL

(kar-*vah*-da-lol)   Coreg®

BETA & ALPHA-1 ADRENERGIC BLOCKER

Prescriber Highlights

▶ Non-selective Beta-adrenergic blocker with selective alpha$_1$-adrenergic blocking activity that could be useful for treating heart failure in dogs; use is controversial

▶ Limited veterinary experience

▶ Negative inotrope that may prohibit its use in severely symptomatic patients; potentially could decompensate patient

▶ Additional adverse effects that may demonstrate intolerance include lassitude, inappetence, & hypotension

Uses/Indications

Carvedilol may be useful as adjunctive therapy in the treatment of heart failure (dilated cardiomyopathy) in dogs. There is a fair amount of controversy at present among veterinary cardiologists as to whether this drug will find a therapeutic niche. One study (Oyama & Prosek 2006) done in dogs with dilated cardiomyopathy showed that carvedilol dosed at 0.3 mg/kg PO q12h for 3 months did not produce any significant improvements in neurohormonal activation, heart size, or owner-perceived quality of life. The authors state that doses >0.3 mg/kg q12h are likely to be required to effect changes in ventricular remodeling and function.

Pharmacology/Actions

Carvedilol is a non-selective, beta-adrenergic blocker with selective alpha$_1$-adrenergic blocking activity. Despite their negative inotropic effects, chronic dosing of beta blockers in human patients with dilated cardiomyopathy can be useful in reducing both morbidity and mortality. Patients in heart failure, chronically activate their sympathetic nervous system, thereby leading to tachycardia, activation of the renin-angiotensin-aldosterone system, down-regulation of beta-receptors, induction of myocyte necrosis and myocyte energy substrate and calcium ion handling. By giving beta-blockers, these negative effects may be reversed or diminished. As carvedilol also inhibits alpha$_1$-adrenergic activity, it can cause vasodilation and reduce afterload. Carvedilol has free-radical scavenging and antidysrhythmic effects that could be beneficial in heart failure patients.

Pharmacokinetics

In dogs, a pilot study (Arsenault *et al.* 2003) showed carvedilol's bioavailability after oral dosing averaged about 23% in the 4 dogs studied, but in 3 of the 4, bioavailability ranged from 3−10%. Volume of distribution averaged about 1.4 L/kg; elimination half-life was about 100 minutes. At least 15 different metabolites of carvedilol have been identified after dosing in dogs. Hydroxylation of the carbazolyl ring and glucuronidation of the parent compound are the most predominant processes of metabolism in dogs.

In humans, carvedilol is rapidly and extensively absorbed but due to a high first-pass effect, bioavailability is about 30%. The drug is extensively bound to plasma proteins (98%). It is extensively metabolized and the R(+) enantiomer is metabolized 2−3 times greater than the S(-) form during the first pass. Both the R(+) and S(-) enantiomers have equal potency as non-specific beta- or alpha-adrenergic blockers. CYP2D6 and CYP2C9 are the P450 isoenzymes most responsible for hepatic metabolism. Some of these metabolites have pharmacologic activity. Metabolites are primarily excreted via the bile and feces. Elimination half-life of carvedilol in humans is about 8−9 hours.

Contraindications/Precautions/Warnings

In humans, carvedilol is contraindicated in class IV decompensated heart failure, bronchial asthma, 2nd or 3rd degree AV block, sick sinus syndrome (unless artificially paced), severe bradycardia, cardiogenic shock or hypersensitivity to the drug. Dogs with equivalent conditions should not receive the drug.

Adverse Effects

Veterinary experience is very limited and an accurate portrayal of adverse effects in dogs has yet to be elucidated. Too rapid beta blockade can cause decompensation in patients with heart failure; cautious dosage titration is mandatory. Dogs that do not tolerate the medication may show signs of inappetence, lassitude, or hypotension. Bronchospasm has been reported in humans.

Because the drug is extensively metabolized in the liver, patients with hepatic insufficiency should receive the drug with caution. In humans, carvedilol has on rare occasions, caused mild hepatocellular injury.

Reproductive/Nursing Safety

In humans, the FDA categorizes carvedilol as a category *C* drug for use during pregnancy (*Animal studies have shown an adverse effect on the fetus, but there are no adequate studies in humans; or there are no animal reproduction studies and no adequate studies in humans*). In rats and rabbits, carvedilol increased post-implantation loss.

It is unknown if carvedilol enters maternal milk in dogs, but it does enter milk in rats. Use with caution in nursing patients.

Overdosage/Acute Toxicity

The acute oral LD$_{50}$ in healthy rats and mice is greater than 8 grams/kg. Clinical signs associated with large overdoses include: severe hypotension, cardiac insufficiency, bradycardia, cardiogenic shock and death due to cardiac arrest. Gut emptying protocols should be considered if ingestion was recent. In humans, bradycardia is treated with atropine, and cardiovascular function supported with glucagon and sympathomimetics (*e.g.*, dobutamine, epinephrine, etc.). Contact an animal poison control center for specific information in the case of overdose.

Drug Interactions

The following drug interactions have either been reported or are theoretical in humans or animals receiving carvedilol and may be of significance in veterinary patients:

- **BETA-BLOCKERS (other):** Use with carvedilol may cause additive effects

- **CALCIUM CHANNEL BLOCKERS (e.g., diltiazem, verapamil):** Carvedilol may rarely cause hemodynamic compromise in patients taking diltiazem or verapamil

- **CIMETIDINE:** May decrease metabolism and increase AUC of carvedilol

- **CLONIDINE:** Carvedilol may potentiate the cardiovascular effects of clonidine

- **CYCLOSPORINE:** Carvedilol may increase cyclosporine levels

- **DIGOXIN:** Carvedilol can increase (in humans) digoxin plasma concentrations by approximately 15%

- **FLUOXETINE, PAROXETINE, QUINIDINE:** May increase R(+)-carvedilol concentrations and increase alpha-$_1$ blocking effects (vasodilation)

- **INSULIN; ORAL ANTIDIABETIC AGENTS:** Carvedilol may enhance the blood glucose lowering effects of insulin or other antidia-betic agents

◼ **RIFAMPIN:** Can decrease carvedilol plasma concentrations by as much as 70%

◼ **RESERPINE:** Drugs such as reserpine can cause increased bradycardia and hypotension in patients taking carvedilol

Laboratory Considerations
◼ No specific laboratory interactions or considerations noted

Doses

◼ **DOGS:**

a) Start at the low end of the dosing range and gradually titrate upward carefully watching to avoid negative inotropic effects. Usual starting dose: ¼−½ of a 3.125 mg tablet PO twice daily. (Kramer 2008)

b) Beta blockers are best employed in dogs that are minimally symptomatic with early/mild heart failure, or animals in later stages of CHF. Some cardiologists have used carvedilol at 0.2 mg/kg PO twice daily initially with slow titration upwards towards a dose of 0.8 mg/kg twice daily. Many dogs with CHF will not tolerate this upward titration. (Rush 2008)

c) A reasonable target plasma carvedilol concentration is 50−100 nanograms/mL. Based upon prior studies and the small series of dogs studied in this study, doses of 0.5 mg/kg PO twice daily should result in beta-blockade, but maximum beta-blockade may require doses of >0.7−0.9 mg/kg. Because of bioavailability variations, plasma monitoring, clinical trials and uptitration protocols may be beneficial. (Gordon *et al.* 2004)

Monitoring
◼ Clinical efficacy
◼ Adverse effects
◼ Plasma drug levels (see Doses above)

Client Information
◼ Give this medication exactly as veterinarian prescribes. Do not stop the medication without the approval and guidance of veterinarian

◼ Contact veterinarian if animal's condition worsens while receiving this medication, or if it shows signs of reduced appetite, fatigue or listlessness, and dizziness or unsteadiness

◼ Medication is best given with food

Chemistry/Synonyms
A non-selective beta-adrenergic blocker with selective alpha$_1$-adrenergic blocking activity, carvedilol occurs as a white to off-white crystalline powder that is practically insoluble in water, dilute acids, and gastric or intestinal fluids. It is sparingly soluble in ethanol. The compound exhibits polymorphism and contains both R(+) and S(-) enantiomers. It is a basic, lipophilic compound.

Carvedilol may also be known as: BM-14190, carvedilolum, *Cardilol®*, *Cardiol®*, *Carloc®*, *Carvil®*, *Carvipress®*, *Coreg®*, *Coritensil®*, *Coropres®*, *Dilatrend®*, *Dilbloc®*, *Dimitone®*, *Divelol®*, *Eucardic®*, *Hybridil®*, *Kredex®*, or *Querto®*.

Storage/Stability
Carvedilol tablets and extended release capsules should be stored below 30°C (86°F) and protected from moisture. They should be dispensed in tight, light-resistant containers.

Compatibility/Compounding Considerations
Compounded preparation stability: Carvedilol oral suspension compounded from commercially available tablets has been published (Yamreudeewong *et al.* 2006); however, HPLC analysis of drug samples in this study gave erratic and variable results indicating a loss of potency at refrigerated temperatures as compared to room temperature. Results of this study do not necessarily confirm that carvedilol is stable when prepared as an oral liquid.

Another published (Gordon *et al.* 2006) compounded oral suspension with documented 90 day stability to accurately dose dogs is to powder 25 mg tablets and add enough de-ionized water to make a paste, allowing the tablet coating to dissolve. Then suspend in a commercially available simple syrup to a concentration of either 2 mg/mL or 10 mg/mL. Store in amber bottles at temperatures not exceeding 25°C and protect from light for up to 90 days. Shake well before administering.

Dosage Forms/Regulatory Status

VETERINARY-LABELED PRODUCTS: None

The ARCI (Racing Commissioners International) has designated this drug as a class 3 substance. See the appendix for more information.

HUMAN-LABELED PRODUCTS:

Carvedilol Oral Tablets: 3.125 mg, 6.25 mg, 12.5 mg, & 25 mg; *Coreg®* (GlaxoSmithKline); generic; (Rx)

Carvedilol Extended-Release Oral Capsules: 10 mg, 20 mg, 40 mg & 80 mg (as phosphate); *Coreg CR®* (GlaxoSmithKline); (Rx)

References

Arsenault, W, D Boothe, et al. (2003). The pharmaco-kinetics of carvedilol in healthy dogs: A pilot study. Proceedings ACVIM Forum. Accessed via: Veterinary Information Network. *http://goo.gl/DgUQN*

Gordon, S, DM Boothe, et al. (2004). Plasma carvedilol levels in dogs with spontaneous cardiovascular disease receiving chronic oral carvedilol: A pilot study. Proceedings ACVIM Forum, Minneapolis. Accessed via: Veterinary Information Network. *http://goo.gl/h0jm8*

Gordon, S., D.M. Boothe, et al. (2006). Stability of carvedilol in an oral liquid preparation. Proceedings:

ACVIM. Accessed via: Veterinary Information Network. http://goo.gl/9SZwJ

Kramer, G (2008). New cardiac drugs. Proceedings: IVECCS. Accessed via: Veterinary Information Network. *http://goo.gl/XurmY*

Oyama, M & M Prosek (2006). Acute Conversion of atrial fibrillation in two dogs by intravenous amiodarone administration. *J Vet Intern Med* 20(5): 1224–1227.

Rush, J (2008). Heart failure in dogs and cats. Proceedings: IVECCS. Accessed via: Veterinary Information Network. *http://goo.gl/JSFRD*

Yamreudeewong, W., E. Dolence, et al. (2006). Stability of two extemporaneously prepared oral metoprolol and carvedilol liquids. Hosp Pharm 41: 254-259.

CASPOFUNGIN ACETATE

(kas-poe-*fun*-jin)   Cancidas®

PARENTERAL ANTIFUNGAL

Prescriber Highlights

▶ Parenteral antifungal that has potential for treating invasive aspergillosis or disseminated candidal infections in companion animals

▶ Very limited clinical experience in veterinary medicine

▶ Very Expensive

Uses/Indications

Caspofungin has potential for treating invasive aspergillosis or disseminated candidal infections in companion animals although little, if any, information on its use in dogs or cats is available.

Pharmacology/Actions

Caspofungin represents the echinocandins, a new class of antifungal agent. These drugs inhibit beta-glucan synthase, thereby blocking the synthesis of beta-(1,3)-D-glucan, a component found in cell walls of filamentous fungi. Caspofungin has activity against *Aspergillus* and *Candida* species and is effective in treating pneumonia caused by *Pneumocystis carinii*. Because it contains very little beta-glucan synthase, *Cryptococcus neoformans* infections are not effectively treated with caspofungin.

Pharmacokinetics

No information was located on the pharmacokinetics of caspofungin in dogs or cats.

In humans, the drug is not appreciably absorbed from the gut and must be administered IV. Protein binding (primarily to albumin) is high (97%) and the drug is distributed to tissues over a 36–48 hour period. Caspofungin is slowly metabolized via hydrolysis and N-acetylation. It also spontaneously degrades chemically. Caspofungin exhibits polyphasic elimination, but little drug is excreted or biotransformed during the first 30 hours post-administration. Elimination half-life for the primary phase is about 10 hours; the secondary phase between 40–50 hours. Excretion, consisting mostly as metabolites, is via the feces and urine. Only small amounts (1–2%) are excreted unchanged into the urine.

Contraindications/Precautions/Warnings

No specific information is available for veterinary patients. Caspofungin is contraindicated in human patients hypersensitive to it. Dosage adjustment is recommended in humans with moderate hepatic impairment. No information is available for use in patients with significant hepatic impairment; avoid use.

Reproductive/Nursing Safety

In humans, the FDA categorizes caspofungin as category C for use during pregnancy (*Animal studies have shown an adverse effect on the fetus, but there are no adequate studies in humans; or there are no animal reproduction studies and no adequate studies in humans.*) Studies with caspofungin performed in pregnant rats and rabbits demonstrated changes in fetal ossification. The drug should be avoided during the first trimester of pregnancy unless the benefits associated with treating outweigh the risks.

Although no data is available, because the drug is not appreciably absorbed from the gut, it would be expected that caspofungin would be safe to administer during lactation.

Adverse Effects

An adverse effect profile for animals has not been determined. In humans, caspofungin is generally well tolerated. Histamine-mediated signs have occurred (rash, facial swelling, pruritus) and anaphylaxis has been reported. Intravenous site reactions (pain, redness, phlebitis) have occurred. Hepatic dysfunction has been reported but frequency is unknown.

Overdosage/Acute Toxicity

Limited information is available. Dosages of 210 mg (about 3x) in humans were well tolerated. Some monkeys receiving 5–8 mg/kg (approx. 4–6X) over 5 weeks developed sites of microscopic subcapsular necrosis on their livers.

Drug Interactions

The following drug interactions have either been reported or are theoretical in humans or animals receiving caspofungin and may be of significance in veterinary patients:

■ **CARBAMAZEPINE:** Reduced caspofungin plasma levels

■ **CYCLOSPORINE:** Increased caspofungin plasma levels and increased risk of hepatic enzyme increases

■ **DEXAMETHASONE:** Reduced caspofungin plasma levels

■ **PHENYTOIN:** Reduced caspofungin plasma levels

■ **RIFAMPIN:** Reduced caspofungin plasma levels

Laboratory Considerations

■ No specific concerns noted; see Monitoring

Doses

■ **DOGS/CATS:**

No published doses for dogs or cats were located and the use of this medication in these patients must be considered highly investigational. Although not labeled for use in human pediatric patients, one study performed in immunocompromised human pediatric patients administered doses of 0.8–1.6 mg/kg in patients weighing less than 50 kg and 50–75 mg (total dose) in those weighing more than 50 kg. The drug was well tolerated in both groups.

Monitoring

■ Clinical efficacy

■ Periodic liver function tests, CBC, serum electrolytes

Client Information

■ This medication is appropriate for inpatient use only

■ Clients should understand the investigational nature and the associated expense of using this drug on veterinary patients

Chemistry/Synonyms

Caspofungin acetate is a semisynthetic echinocandin compound produced from a fermentation product of *Glarea lozoyensis*. It occurs as a white to off-white powder that is freely soluble in water and slightly soluble in ethanol. The commercially available lyophilized powder for injection also contains acetic acid, sodium hydroxide, mannitol and sucrose.

Caspofungin may also be known as: caspofungina, caspofungine, caspofungini, kaspofungiinia, kaspofungina, L-743873, MK-0991, or *Cancidas®*.

Storage/Stability

The commercially available product should be stored refrigerated (2–8°C). Refer to the package insert for very specific directions on preparing the solution for intravenous use.

Do not use if the solution is cloudy or has precipitated.

Compatibility/Compounding Considerations

It is recommended not to mix or infuse with any other medications and not to use with intravenous solutions containing dextrose.

Dosage Forms/Regulatory Status

VETERINARY-LABELED PRODUCTS: None

HUMAN-LABELED PRODUCTS:

Caspofungin Acetate Lyophilized Powder for Injection: 50 & 70 mg in single-use vials; *Cancidas®* (Merck); (Rx)

CEFACLOR

(**sef**-a-klor)   Ceclor®

ORAL 2ND GENERATION CEPHALOSPORIN

Prescriber Highlights

▶ Oral 2nd generation cephalosporin that is more active against some gram-negative bacteria then first generation (e.g., cephalexin) cephalosporins

▶ Potentially useful when an oral cephalosporin is desired to treat bacterial infections that are susceptible to cefaclor, but resistant to first generation cephalosporins

▶ Limited clinical experience in veterinary medicine

▶ Adverse effects most likely seen in small animals would be GI-related

Uses/Indications

Cefaclor may potentially be useful when an oral cephalosporin is desired to treat infections that are susceptible to it but resistant to first generation cephalosporins such as cephalexin or cefadroxil. Little information is available with regard to its clinical use in small animals, however.

Pharmacology/Actions

Cefaclor, like other cephalosporins, is bactericidal and acts via inhibiting cell wall synthesis. Its spectrum of activity is similar to that of cephalexin, but it is more active against gram-negative bacteria including strains of *E. coli*, *Klebsiella pneumoniae*, and *Proteus mirabilis*.

Pharmacokinetics

Limited information is available on the pharmacokinetics of cefaclor in dogs and none was located for cats. In dogs, about 75% of an oral dose is absorbed, but an apparent first-pass effect reduces bioavailability to about 60%. Cefaclor is distributed to many tissues, but levels are lower in interstitial fluid than those found in serum. Very high levels are excreted into the urine unchanged. Bile levels are higher than those found in serum. Dogs appear to metabolize a greater percentage of cefaclor than do rats, mice, or humans. Approximate elimination half-life is about 2 hours in dogs.

In humans, cefaclor is well absorbed after oral administration; food delays, but does not appreciably alter the amount absorbed. The drug is widely distributed, crosses the placenta and enters breast milk. Up to 85% of a dose is excreted unchanged into the urine; elimination half-life is less than 1 hour in patients with normal renal function.

Contraindications/Precautions/Warnings

No specific information is available for veterinary patients. Cefaclor is contraindicated in human patients hypersensitive to it and must be cautiously used in patients with penicillin-allergy. Dosage adjustment is recommended in humans with severe renal impairment.

Reproductive/Nursing Safety

In humans, the FDA categorizes cefaclor as category *B* for use during pregnancy (*Animal studies have not yet demonstrated risk to the fetus, but there are no adequate studies in pregnant women; or animal studies have shown an adverse effect, but adequate studies in pregnant women have not demonstrated a risk to the fetus in the first trimester of pregnancy, and there is no evidence of risk in later trimesters.*) Studies performed in pregnant rats (doses up 12X human dose) and ferrets (doses up to 3X human dose) demonstrated no overt fetal harm.

Cefaclor enters maternal milk in low concentrations. Although probably safe for nursing offspring the potential for adverse effects cannot be ruled out, particularly, alterations to gut flora with resultant diarrhea.

Adverse Effects

As usage of cefaclor in animals has been very limited, a comprehensive adverse effect profile has not been determined. In humans, cefaclor is generally well tolerated but commonly can cause gastrointestinal effects (nausea, diarrhea). Hypersensitivity reactions including anaphylaxis are possible; cefaclor appears to cause a higher incidence of serum-sickness-like reactions than other cephalosporins, particularly in children who have received multiple courses of treatment. Rare adverse effects reported include erythema multiforme, rash, increases in liver function tests, and transient increases in BUN and serum creatinine.

Overdosage/Acute Toxicity

Cefaclor appears quite safe in dogs. Dogs given daily PO doses of 200 mg/kg/day for 30 days developed soft stools and occasional emesis. Two dogs in this study group developed transient moderate decreases in hemoglobin. One dog in another study group that was given 400 mg/kg/day for one year developed a reversible thrombocytopenia.

Drug Interactions

The following drug interactions have either been reported or are theoretical in humans or animals receiving cefaclor and may be of significance in veterinary patients:

■ **ANTACIDS (magnesium- or aluminum-containing)**: Reduces extent of absorption of extended-release cefaclor tablets

■ **PROBENECID:** Reduced renal excretion of cefaclor

■ **WARFARIN:** Rare reports of increased anticoagulant effect

Laboratory Considerations

■ Except for cefotaxime, cephalosporins may cause false-positive **urine glucose determinations** when using the copper reduction method (Benedict's solution, Fehling's solution, *Clinitest*®); tests utilizing glucose oxidase (*Tes-Tape*®, *Clinistix*®) are not affected by cephalosporins

■ When using the Jaffe reaction to measure **serum or urine creatinine**, cephalosporins (not ceftazidime or cefotaxime) given in high dosages may cause falsely elevated values

■ In humans, particularly with azotemia, cephalosporins have caused a false-positive direct **Coombs' test**.

■ Cephalosporins may also cause falsely elevated **17-ketosteroid** values in urine

Doses

■ **DOGS/CATS:**

For susceptible infections:

a) For skin or soft tissue infections: 7 mg/kg PO q8h for 21–30 days.

For systemic, lower respiratory tract infections: 10–13 mg/kg PO q8h for 14 days. Maximum daily dose is 1 gram. (Greene *et al.* 2006)

Monitoring

■ Clinical efficacy

■ Patients with renal insufficiency should have renal function monitored

Client Information

■ Preferably should be administered to animal without food; however, if patient vomits or develops a lack of appetite while receiving medication it can be administered with food

■ Give as directed by the veterinarian; even if animal appears well, continue treating for the full duration prescribed

■ Contact veterinarian if animal develops severe vomiting/diarrhea or rash/itching

Chemistry/Synonyms

Cefaclor occurs as a white to off-white powder that is slightly soluble in water.

Cefaclor may also be known as: cefaclorum, cefaklor, cefkloras, kefakloori or compound 99638. There are many internationally registered trade names.

Storage/Stability

Capsules, tablets, and powder for suspension should be stored at room temperature (15–30°C). After reconstituting, the oral suspension should be stored in the refrigerator and discarded after 14 days.

Dosage Forms/Regulatory Status

VETERINARY-LABELED PRODUCTS: None

HUMAN-LABELED PRODUCTS:

Cefaclor Oral Capsules: 250 mg & 500 mg; *Ceclor*® *Pulvules* (Lilly), generic; (Rx)

Cefaclor Chewable Tablets: 125 mg, 187 mg, 250 mg, & 375 mg; *Raniclor*® (Ranbaxy); (Rx)

Cefaclor Extended-Release Oral Tablets: 375 mg & 500 mg; generic (Zenith Goldline); (Rx)

Cefaclor Powder for Oral Suspension: 125 mg/5 mL, 187 mg/5 mL, 250 mg/5 mL, & 375 mg/5 mL; *Ceclor®* (Eli Lilly); generic; (Rx)

References

Greene, C, K Hartmannn, et al. (2006). Appendix 8: Antimicrobial Drug Formulary. *Infectious Disease of the Dog and Cat.* C Greene Ed., Elsevier: 1186–1333.

CEFADROXIL

(sef-a-*drox*-ill)   Cefa-Drops®, Duricef®

1ST GENERATION CEPHALOSPORIN

Prescriber Highlights

▶ Oral 1st generation cephalosporin

▶ May be administered with food (especially if GI upset occurs)

▶ Most likely adverse effects are GI in nature

▶ May need to reduce dose in renal failure

▶ May be expensive when compared to generic cephalexin

Uses/Indications

Cefadroxil is FDA-approved for oral therapy in treating susceptible infections of the skin, soft tissue, and genitourinary tract in dogs and cats. The veterinary oral tablets have been discontinued (in the USA), but human-labeled oral capsules and tablets are still available.

Pharmacology/Actions

A first generation cephalosporin, cefadroxil exhibits activity against the bacteria usually covered by this class. First generation cephalosporins are usually bactericidal and act via inhibition of cell wall synthesis.

While there may be differences in MIC's for individual first generation cephalosporins, their spectrums of activity are quite similar. They generally possess excellent coverage against most gram-positive pathogens; variable to poor coverage against most gram-negative pathogens. These drugs are very active *in vitro* against groups A beta-hemolytic and B Streptococci, non-enterococcal group D Streptococci (S. bovis), *Staphylococcus intermedius* and *aureas, Proteus mirabilis* and some strains of *E. coli, Klebsiella* spp., Actinobacillus, Pasturella, *Haemophilus equigenitalis,* Shigella and Salmonella. With the exception of *Bacteroides fragilis,* most anaerobes are very susceptible to the first generation agents. Most species of Corynebacteria are susceptible, but *C. equi* (*Rhodococcus*) is usually resistant. Strains of *Staphylococcus epidermidis* are usually sensitive to the parenterally administered 1st generation drugs, but may have variable susceptibilities to the oral drugs. The following bacteria are regularly resistant to the 1st generation agents: Group D streptococci/enterococci (S. faecalis, S. faecium), Methicillin-resistant Staphylococci, *indole-positive Proteus* spp., *Pseudomonas* spp., *Enterobacter* spp., *Serratia* spp. and *Citrobacter* spp.

Pharmacokinetics

Cefadroxil is reportedly well absorbed after oral administration to dogs without regard to feeding state. After an oral dose of 22 mg/kg, peak serum levels of approximately 18.6 micrograms/mL occur within 1–2 hours of dosing. Only about 20% of the drug is bound to canine plasma proteins. The drug is excreted into the urine and has a half-life of about 2 hours. Over 50% of a dose can be recovered unchanged in the urine within 24 hours of dosing.

In cats, the serum half-life has been reported as approximately 3 hours.

Oral absorption of cefadroxil in adult horses after oral suspension was administered was characterized as poor and erratic. In a study done in foals (Duffee, Christensen, and Craig 1989), oral bioavailability ranged from 36–99.8% (mean=58.2%); mean elimination half-life was 3.75 hours after oral dosing.

Contraindications/Precautions/Warnings

Cephalosporins are contraindicated in patients with a history of hypersensitivity to them. Because there may be cross-reactivity, use cephalosporins cautiously in patients who are documented hypersensitive to other beta-lactam antibiotics (*e.g.,* penicillins, cefamycins, carbapenems).

Oral systemic antibiotics should not be administered in patients with septicemia, shock or other grave illnesses as absorption of the medication from the GI tract may be significantly delayed or diminished. Parenteral routes (preferably IV) should be used for these cases.

Adverse Effects

Adverse effects with the cephalosporins are usually not serious and have a relatively low frequency of occurrence.

Hypersensitivity reactions unrelated to dose can occur with these agents and can manifest as rashes, fever, eosinophilia, lymphadenopathy, or full-blown anaphylaxis. The use of cephalosporins in patients documented to be hypersensitive to penicillin-class antibiotics is controversial. In humans, it is estimated that up to 15% of patients hypersensitive to penicillins will also be hypersensitive to cephalosporins. The incidence of cross-reactivity in veterinary patients is unknown.

When given orally, cephalosporins may cause GI effects (anorexia, vomiting, diarrhea). Administering the drug with a small meal may help alleviate these effects. Because the cephalosporins may alter gut flora, antibiotic-associated diarrhea can occur and allow the proliferation of resistant bacteria in the colon (superinfections).

While cephalosporins (particularly cephalothin) have the potential for causing nephrotoxicity, at clinically used doses in patients with normal renal function, risks for the occurrence of this adverse effect appear minimal.

Cefadroxil or cephalexin may rarely cause tachypnea.

High doses or very prolonged use of cephalosporins have been associated with neurotoxicity, neutropenia, agranulocytosis, thrombocytopenia, hepatitis, positive Comb's test, interstitial nephritis, and tubular necrosis. Except for tubular necrosis and neurotoxicity, these effects have an immunologic component.

Reproductive/Nursing Safety

Cephalosporins have been shown to cross the placenta and safe use of them during pregnancy has not been firmly established, but neither have there been any documented teratogenic problems associated with these drugs. However, use only when the potential benefits outweigh the risks. In humans, the FDA categorizes this drug as category *B* for use during pregnancy (*Animal studies have not yet demonstrated risk to the fetus, but there are no adequate studies in pregnant women; or animal studies have shown an adverse effect, but adequate studies in pregnant women have not demonstrated a risk to the fetus in the first trimester of pregnancy, and there is no evidence of risk in later trimesters.*)

Cephalosporins can be distributed into milk, but are unlikely to pose much risk to nursing offspring; diarrhea is possible.

Overdosage/Acute Toxicity

Acute oral cephalosporin overdoses are unlikely to cause significant problems other than GI distress, but other effects are possible (see Adverse Effects section).

Drug Interactions

The following drug interactions have either been reported or are theoretical in humans or animals receiving cefadroxil and may be of significance in veterinary patients:

■ **PROBENECID:** Competitively blocks the tubular secretion of most cephalosporins thereby increasing serum levels and serum half-lives

Laboratory Considerations

■ Except for cefotaxime, cephalosporins may cause false-positive **urine glucose determinations** when using cupric sulfate solution (Benedict's Solution, *Clinitest*®). Tests utilizing glucose oxidase (*Tes-Tape*®, *Clinistix*®) are not affected by cephalosporins

■ When using the Jaffe reaction to measure **serum or urine creatinine**, cephalosporins (not ceftazidime or cefotaxime) in high dosages may falsely cause elevated values

■ In humans, particularly with azotemia, cephalosporins have caused a false-positive direct **Combs' test**

■ Cephalosporins may also cause falsely elevated **17-ketosteroid** values in urine

Doses

■ **DOGS:**

For susceptible infections:

a) 22 mg/kg PO twice daily. Treat skin and soft tissue infections for at least 3 days, and GU infections for at least 7 days. Treat for at least 48 hours after animal is afebrile and asymptomatic. Reevaluate therapy if no response after 3 days of treatment. Maximum therapy is 30 days. (Package Insert; *Cefa-Tabs*®—Fort-Dodge).

b) For susceptible Staph infections: 30 mg/kg PO q12h (may not be adequate dose for non-UTI's caused by *E. coli*) (Campbell & Rosin 1998)

c) For UTI: 11–22 mg/kg PO q12h for 7–30 days

For skin, pyoderma: 22–35 mg/kg PO q12h for 3–30 days

For systemic, orthopedic infections: 22 mg/kg PO q8–12h for 30 days (Greene & Watson 1998), (Greene *et al.* 2006)

d) 10 mg/kg q12h for susceptible gram-positive infections; 30 mg/kg q8h for susceptible gram-negative infections (Aucoin 2000)

e) For canine pyoderma/infectious otitis: 22 mg/kg PO q12h (Kwochka 2003); (Kwochka 2002)

f) For UTI: 10–20 mg/kg PO q8h. For acute urethrocystitis, treatment may be 7–10 days; for chronic urethrocystitis, up to 4 weeks of treatment may be necessary; for pyelonephritis, 4–8 weeks may be adequate (Brovida 2003)

g) For UTI: 30 mg/kg PO q8h (Dowling 2009)

h) For superficial and deep bacterial pyoderma: 22–33 mg/kg PO 2-3 times daily (Beale & Murphy 2006)

■ **CATS:**

For susceptible infections:

a) For UTI: 22 mg/kg PO once daily for 21 days or less

For skin, pyoderma: 22–35 mg/kg PO q12h for 3–30 days

For systemic, orthopedic infections: 22 mg/kg PO q8–12h for 30 days (Greene & Watson 1998)

b) 10 mg/kg q12h for susceptible gram-positive infections; 30 mg/kg q8h for susceptible gram-negative infections (Aucoin 2000)

c) 22 mg/kg PO q12h (Lappin 2002)

■ **FERRETS:**

For susceptible infections:

a) 15–20 mg/kg PO twice daily (Williams 2000)

Monitoring

■ Because cephalosporins usually have minimal toxicity associated with their use, monitoring for efficacy is usually all that is required.

■ Patients with diminished renal function may require intensified renal monitoring. Serum levels and therapeutic drug monitoring are not routinely performed with these agents.

Chemistry/Synonyms

A semisynthetic cephalosporin antibiotic, cefadroxil occurs as a white to yellowish-white, crystalline powder that is soluble in water and slightly soluble in alcohol. The commercially available product is available as the monohydrate.

Cefadroxil may also be known as: BL-S578; cefadroxilum, cephadroxil, or MJF-11567-3; many trade names are available.

Storage/Stability

Cefadroxil tablets, capsules and powder for oral suspension should be stored at room temperature (15–30°C) in tight containers. After reconstitution, the oral suspension is stable for 14 days when kept refrigerated (2–8°C).

Dosage Forms/Regulatory Status

VETERINARY-LABELED PRODUCTS:

Cefadroxil Powder for Oral Suspension: 50 mg/mL in 15 mL and 50 mL btls (orange-pineapple flavor); *Cefa-Drops®* (BIVI) (Rx). FDA-approved for use in dogs and cats.

HUMAN-LABELED PRODUCTS:

Cefadroxil Oral Tablets: 1 gram; generic; (Rx)

Cefadroxil Oral Capsules: 500 mg; generic; (Rx)

Cefadroxil Powder for Oral Suspension: 125 mg/5 mL, 250 mg/5 mL, & 500 mg/5 mL in 50, 75 (500 mg/5 mL only) & 100 mL; generic; (Rx)

References

Aucoin, D (2000). *Antimicrobial Drug Formulary. Target: The antimicrobial guide to effective treatment* Port Huron, MI, North American Compendiums Inc: 93–142.

Beale, K & M Murphy (2006). Selecting appropriate antimicrobial therapy for infections of the skin of the dog. Proceedings: Western Vet Conf. Accessed via: Veterinary Information Network. *http://goo.gl/aQoiv*

Brovida, C (2003). Urinary Tract Infection (UTI): How to diagnose correctly and treat. Proceedings: World Small Animal Veterinary Assoc World Congress. Accessed via: Veterinary Information Network. *http://goo.gl/F2zcU*

Campbell, B & E Rosin (1998). Effect on food on absorption of cefadroxil and cephalexin. *J Vet Pharmacol Therap* 21: 418–420.

Dowling, P (2009). Optimizing antimicrobial therapy of urinary tract infections. Proceedings: WVC.

Greene, C, K Hartmannn, et al. (2006). Appendix 8: Antimicrobial Drug Formulary. *Infectious Disease of the Dog and Cat.* C Greene Ed., Elsevier: 1186–1333.

Greene, C & A Watson (1998). Antimicrobial Drug Formulary. *Infectious Diseases of the Dog and Cat.* C Greene Ed. Philadelphia, WB Saunders: 790–919.

Kwochka, K (2002). Appropriate use of antimicrobials in dermatology and otology: Options for topical and systemic treatments. Proceedings: ACVIM Forum. Accessed via: Veterinary Information Network. *http://goo.gl/reiPh*

Kwochka, K (2003). Update on the use of systemic antibiotics for superficial and deep pyoderma. Proceedings: Atlantic Coast Veterinary Conference. Accessed via: Veterinary Information Network. *http://goo.gl/QrsXY*

Lappin, M (2002). Feline fevers of unknown origin I, II, III. Proceedings: Western Veterinary Conference. Accessed via: Veterinary Information Network. *http://goo.gl/JuGRY*

Williams, B (2000). Therapeutics in Ferrets. *Vet Clin NA: Exotic Anim Pract* 3:1(Jan): 131–153.

CEFAZOLIN SODIUM

(sef-a-**zoe**-lin)   Ancef®, Kefzol®, Zolicef®

1ST GENERATION CEPHALOSPORIN

Prescriber Highlights

▶ 1st generation parenteral cephalosporin

▶ Potentially could cause hypersensitivity reactions

▶ Can cause pain on IM injection; Give IV over 3–5 minutes (or more)

▶ May need to reduce dose in renal failure

Uses/Indications

In the United States, there are no cefazolin products FDA-approved for veterinary species but it has been used clinically in several species when an injectable, first generation cephalosporin is indicated. It is used for surgical prophylaxis, and for a variety of systemic infections (including orthopedic, soft tissue, sepsis) caused by susceptible bacteria. Most commonly given every 6–8 hours via parenteral routes, cefazolin constant rate intravenous infusion protocols are being developed as cefazolin is a time (above MIC)-dependent antibiotic, and serum/tissue concentrations can remain above MIC.

Pharmacology/Actions

A first generation cephalosporin, cefazolin exhibits activity against the bacteria usually covered by this class. First generation cephalosporins are usually bactericidal and act via inhibition of cell wall synthesis. They are considered time-dependent antibiotics.

While there may be differences in MIC's for individual first generation cephalosporins, their spectrums of activity are quite similar. They possess generally excellent coverage against most gram-positive pathogens; variable to poor coverage against most gram-negative pathogens. These drugs are very active *in vitro* against groups A beta-hemolytic and B Streptococci, non-enterococcal group D Streptococci (*S. bovis*), *Staphylococcus intermedius* and *aureus, Proteus mirabilis* and some strains of *E. coli, Klebsiella* spp., Actinobacillus, Pasturella, *Haemophilus equigenitalis*, Shigella and Salmonella. With the exception of *Bacteroides fragilis*, most anaerobes are very susceptible to the first generation agents. Most species of Corynebacteria are susceptible, but *C. equi*

(Rhodococcus) is usually resistant. Strains of *Staphylococcus epidermidis* are usually sensitive to the parenterally administered 1st generation drugs, but may have variable susceptibilities to the oral drugs. The following bacteria are regularly resistant to the 1st generation agents: Group D streptococci/enterococci (*S. faecalis, S. faecium*), Methicillin-resistant Staphylococci, *indole-positive Proteus* spp., *Pseudomonas* spp., *Enterobacter* spp., *Serratia* spp. and *Citrobacter* spp.

Pharmacokinetics

Cefazolin is not appreciably absorbed after oral administration and must be given parenterally to achieve therapeutic serum levels. Absorbed drug is excreted unchanged by the kidneys into the urine. Elimination half-lives may be significantly prolonged in patients with severely diminished renal function.

In dogs, peak levels occur in about 30 minutes after IM administration. The apparent volume of distribution at steady state is 700 mL/kg, total body clearance of 10.4 mL/min/kg with a serum elimination half-life of 48 minutes. Approximately 64% of the clearance can be attributed to renal tubular secretion. The drug is approximately 16–28% bound to plasma proteins in dogs.

In horses, the apparent volume of distribution at steady state is 190 mL/kg, total body clearance of 5.51 mL/min/kg with a serum elimination half-life of 38 minutes when given IV and 84 minutes after IM injection (gluteal muscles). Cefazolin is about 4–8% bound to equine plasma proteins. Because of the significant tubular secretion of the drug, it would be expected that probenecid administration would alter the kinetics of cefazolin. One study performed in horses (Donecker, Sams, and Ashcroft 1986), did not show any effect, but the authors concluded that the dosage of probenecid may have been sub-therapeutic in this species.

In calves, the volume of distribution is 165 mL/kg, and had a terminal elimination half-life of 49–99 minutes after IM administration.

Contraindications/Precautions/Warnings

Cephalosporins are contraindicated in patients with a history of hypersensitivity to them. Because there may be cross-reactivity, use cephalosporins cautiously in patients who are documented hypersensitive to other beta-lactam antibiotics (*e.g.*, penicillins, cefamycins, carbapenems).

Patients in renal failure may need dosage adjustments.

Adverse Effects

Adverse effects with the cephalosporins are usually not serious and have a relatively low frequency of occurrence.

Hypersensitivity reactions unrelated to dose can occur with these agents and can manifest as rashes, fever, eosinophilia, lymphadenopathy, or full-blown anaphylaxis. The use of cephalosporins in patients documented to be hypersensitive to penicillin-class antibiotics is controversial. In humans, it is estimated 1–15% of patients hypersensitive to penicillins will also be hypersensitive to cephalosporins. The incidence of cross-reactivity in veterinary patients is unknown.

Cephalosporins can cause pain at the injection site when administered intramuscularly, although this effect occurs less with cefazolin than with other agents. Sterile abscesses or other severe local tissue reactions are possible but are much less common. Thrombophlebitis is also possible after IV administration of these drugs.

While cephalosporins (particularly cephalothin) have the potential for causing nephrotoxicity at clinically used doses in patients with normal renal function, risks for the occurrence of this adverse effect appear minimal.

High doses or very prolonged use has been associated with neurotoxicity, neutropenia, agranulocytosis, thrombocytopenia, hepatitis, positive Comb's test, interstitial nephritis, and tubular necrosis. Except for tubular necrosis and neurotoxicity, these effects have an immunologic component. Cefazolin may be more likely than other cephalosporins to cause seizures at very high doses.

Reproductive/Nursing Safety

Cephalosporins have been shown to cross the placenta and safe use of them during pregnancy has not been firmly established, but neither have there been any documented teratogenic problems associated with these drugs. However, use only when the potential benefits outweigh the risks. In humans, the FDA categorizes this drug as category *B* for use during pregnancy (*Animal studies have not yet demonstrated risk to the fetus, but there are no adequate studies in pregnant women; or animal studies have shown an adverse effect, but adequate studies in pregnant women have not demonstrated a risk to the fetus in the first trimester of pregnancy, and there is no evidence of risk in later trimesters.*)

Cefazolin is distributed into milk and could potentially alter neonatal gut flora. Use with caution in nursing dams.

Overdosage/Acute Toxicity

Cephalosporin overdoses are unlikely to cause significant problems, but other effects are possible (see Adverse Effects section). Very high doses given IV rapidly could potentially cause seizures.

Drug Interactions

The following drug interactions have either been reported or are theoretical in humans or animals receiving cefazolin and may be of significance in veterinary patients:

■ **NEPHROTOXIC DRUGS:** The concurrent use of parenteral aminoglycosides or other nephrotoxic drugs (*e.g.*, amphotericin B) with cephalosporins is somewhat controversial. Potentially, cephalosporins could cause additive nephrotoxicity when used with these drugs, but this interaction has only been well documented with cephaloridine (no longer marketed). Nevertheless, use caution.

■ **PROBENECID:** Competitively blocks the tubular secretion of most cephalosporins thereby increasing serum levels and serum half-lives.

Laboratory Considerations

■ Except for cefotaxime, cephalosporins may cause false-positive **urine glucose determinations** when using cupric sulfate solution (Benedict's Solution, *Clinitest®*). Tests utilizing glucose oxidase (*Tes-Tape®*, *Clinistix®*) are not affected by cephalosporins.

■ When using the Jaffe reaction to measure **serum or urine creatinine**, cephalosporins (not ceftazidime or cefotaxime) in high dosages may falsely cause elevated values.

■ In humans, particularly with azotemia, cephalosporins have caused a false-positive direct **Coombs' test**.

■ Cephalosporins may also cause falsely elevated **17-ketosteroid** values in urine.

Doses

Note: If injecting IM, must be injected into a large muscle mass. IV injections should not be given faster than over 3–5 minutes.

■ **DOGS:**

For susceptible infections:

a) For surgical prophylaxis: Orthopedic procedures: 20 mg/kg IV at induction followed by 20 mg/kg IV every 90 minutes until wound closure; Soft tissue surgery: 20 mg/kg IV at time of surgery followed by a second dose of 20 mg/kg SC 6 hours later (Trepanier 2003)

b) Gram-positive infections: 10 mg/kg IV, or IM q8h; 10–30 mg/kg IV q8h
Gram-negative infections: 30 mg/kg IM or SC; 10–30 mg/kg IV q8h (Aucoin 2000)

c) For sepsis: 20–25 mg/kg IV q4–8h (Hardie 2000)

d) For surgical prophylaxis: 8 mg/kg IV just before and during surgery 1 hour apart or 20–22 mg/kg IV just before and during surgery 2 hours apart.
For systemic infections: 5–25 mg/kg IM or IV q6–8h as long as necessary.
For orthopedic infections: 22 mg/kg IV, IM or SC q6–8h for 7 days or less.
For sepsis, bacteremia: 15–25 mg/kg IV, IM or SC q4–8h for 7 days or less (Greene & Watson 1998)

e) For infections in neonates: 10–30 mg/kg IV or IO (intraosseous) q8h (Kampschmidt 2006)

■ **CATS:**

For susceptible infections:

a) Gram-positive infections: 10 mg/kg IV, or IM q8h; 10–30 mg/kg IV q8h
Gram-negative infections: 30 mg/kg IM or SC; 10–30 mg/kg IV q8h (Aucoin 2000)

b) For surgical prophylaxis: Orthopedic procedures: 20 mg/kg IV at induction followed by 20 mg/kg IV every 90 minutes until wound closure; Soft tissue surgery: 20 mg/kg IV at time of surgery followed by a second dose of 20 mg/kg SC 6 hours later (Trepanier 2003)

c) For sepsis: 20–25 mg/kg IV q4–8h (Hardie 2000)

d) For systemic infections: 33 mg/kg IV, or IM q8–12h as long as necessary (Greene & Watson 1998)

e) 20–25 mg/kg q8h IM or IV (Lappin 2002)

f) For infections in neonates: 10–30 mg/kg IV or IO (intraosseous) q8h (Kampschmidt 2006)

■ **HORSES:**

For susceptible infections:

a) 25 mg/kg IV, IM q6h (Bertone 2003)

b) 25 mg/kg IV, IM q6–8h (Papich 2003)

c) **Foals:** 20 mg/kg IV q8–12h (Caprile & Short 1987); (Brumbaugh 1999)

d) **Neonatal foals:** 15–20 mg/kg IV q8h (Magdesian 2003)

■ **REPTILES:**

For susceptible infections:

a) **Chelonians:** 22 mg/kg IM q24h (Johnson 2002)

Monitoring

■ Because cephalosporins usually have minimal toxicity associated with their use, monitoring for efficacy is usually all that is required.

■ Patients with diminished renal function may require intensified renal monitoring. Serum levels and therapeutic drug monitoring are not routinely done with these agents.

Chemistry/Synonyms

An injectable, semi-synthetic cephalosporin antibiotic, cefazolin sodium occurs as a practically odorless or having a faint odor, white to off-white, crystalline powder or lyophilized solid. It is freely soluble in water and very slightly soluble in alcohol. Each gram of the injection contains 2 mEq of sodium. After reconstitution, the solution for injection has a pH of 4.5–6 and has a light-yellow to yellow color.

Cefazolin sodium may also be known as: 46083, cefazolinum natricum, cephazolin sodium, or SKF-41558; many trade names are available.

Storage/Stability

Cefazolin sodium powder for injection and solutions for injection should be protected from light. The powder for injection should be stored at room temperature (15–30°C); avoid temperatures above 40°C. The frozen solution for injection should be stored at temperatures no higher than -20°C.

After reconstitution, the solution is stable for 24 hours when kept at room temperature; 96 hours if refrigerated. If after reconstitution, the solution is immediately frozen in the original container, the preparation is stable for at least 12 weeks when stored at -20°C.

Compatibility/Compounding Considerations

The following solutions are reportedly **compatible** with cefazolin: Amino acids 4.25%/dextrose 25%, D_5W in Ringer's, D_5W in Lactated Ringer's, D_5W in sodium chloride 0.2%–0.9%, D_5W, $D_{10}W$, Ringer's Injection, Lactated Ringer's Injection, and normal saline The following drugs are reportedly **compatible with cefazolin when given together at a Y-site:** amiodarone, atracurium, calcium gluconate, famotidine, cyclophosphamide, dexmedetomidine, diltiazem, doxorubicin liposome, heparin, hetastarch, insulin, lidocaine, magnesium sulfate, midazolam, metronidazole, morphine, propofol, ranitidine, vancomycin, vecuronium, verapamil HCl, and vitamin B-complex.

The following drugs or solutions are reportedly **incompatible** or only compatible in specific situations with cefazolin: amikacin sulfate, amobarbital sodium, ascorbic acid injection, bleomycin sulfate, calcium chloride/gluconate, cimetidine HCl, erythromycin gluceptate, kanamycin sulfate, lidocaine HCl, oxytetracycline HCl, pentobarbital sodium, polymyxin B sulfate, tetracycline HCl and vitamin B-complex with C injection.

Compatibility is dependent upon factors such as pH, concentration, temperature and diluent used; consult specialized references or a hospital pharmacist for more specific information.

Dosage Forms/Regulatory Status

VETERINARY-LABELED PRODUCTS: None

HUMAN-LABELED PRODUCTS:

Cefazolin Sodium Powder for Injection: 500 mg, 1 g, 5 g, 10 g, & 20 g in vials & piggyback vials; generic (Apothecon); (Rx)

Cefazolin Sodium for Injection (IV infusion): 1 g; in 50 mL plastic containers, or duplex bags; generic; (Rx)

References

Aucoin, D (2000). Antimicrobial Drug Formulary. *Target: The antimicrobial guide to effective treatment* Port Huron, MI, North American Compendiums Inc: 93–142.

Bertone, J (2003). Rational antibiotic choices. Proceedings: Western Veterinary Conf. Accessed via: Veterinary Information Network. *http://goo.gl/MxKfS*

Brumbaugh, G (1999). Clinical Pharmacology and the Pediatric Patient. 45th Annual AAEP Convention, Albuquerque.

Caprile, KA & CR Short (1987). Pharmacologic considerations in drug therapy in foals. *Vet Clin North Am (Equine Practice)* 3(1): 123–144.

Greene, C & A Watson (1998). Antimicrobial Drug Formulary. *Infectious Diseases of the Dog and Cat.* C Greene Ed. Philadelphia, WB Saunders: 790–919.

Hardie, E (2000). Therapeutic Mangement of Sepsis. *Kirk's Current Veterinary Therapy: XIII Small Animal Practice.* J Bonagura Ed. Philadelphia, WB Saunders: 272–275.

Johnson, J (2002). Medical management of ill chelonians. Proceedings; Western Veterinary Conference. Accessed via: Veterinary Information Network. *http://goo.gl/NTerN*

Kampschmidt, K (2006). Drug use in the neonatal pediatric small animal patient. Proceedings: Western Veterinary Conference. Accessed via: Veterinary Information Network. *http://goo.gl/hhAM5*

Lappin, M (2002). Feline fevers of unknown origin I, II, III. Proceedings: Western Veterinary Conference. Accessed via: Veterinary Information Network. *http://goo.gl/JuGRY*

Magdesian, K (2003). Neonatal pharmacology and therapeutics. *Current Therapy in Equine Medicine 5.* C Kollias–Baker Ed. Philadelphia, Saunders: 1–5.

Papich, M (2003). Antimicrobial therapy for horses. *Current Therapy in Equine Medicine 5.* C Kollias–Baker Ed. Philadelphia, Saunders: 6–11.

Trepanier, L (2003). Perioperative antimicrobial prophylaxis. Proceedings: International Veterinary Emergency and Critical Care Symposium. Accessed via: Veterinary Information Network. *http://goo.gl/Ixsc6*

CEFEPIME HCL

(sef-eh-*pim*)   Maxipime®

4TH GENERATION CEPHALOSPORIN

Prescriber Highlights

▶ Injectable 4th generation cephalosporin that is more active against some gram-negative & gram-positive bacteria than 3rd generation cephalosporins

▶ Potentially useful for treating neonatal foals & dogs with serious infections

▶ Limited clinical experience in veterinary medicine

▶ Adverse effects most likely seen in small animals or foals would be GI-related (diarrhea)

▶ Treatment may be very expensive

Uses/Indications

Cefepime is a semi-synthetic 4th generation cephalosporin with enhanced activity against many gram-negative and gram-positive pathogens. It potentially may be useful in treating serious infections in dogs or foals particularly when aminoglycosides, fluoroquinolones or other more commonly used beta-lactam drugs are ineffective or contraindicated.

Pharmacology/Actions

Cefepime, like other cephalosporins, is usually bactericidal and acts by inhibiting cell wall synthesis. It is classified as a 4th-generation cephalosporin, implying increased gram-negative activity (particularly against *Pseudomonas*) and better activity against many gram-positive bacteria than would be seen with the 3rd generation agents. It rapidly penetrates into gram-negative bacteria and targets penicillin-binding proteins (PBPs). Cefepime does not readily induce beta-lactamases and is highly resistant to hydrolysis by them.

Cefepime has activity against many gram-positive aerobes including many species and strains of Staphylococci and Streptococci. It is not clinically effective in treating infections caused by enterococci, *L. monocytogenes*, or methicillin-resistant staphylococci.

Cefepime has good activity against many gram-negative bacteria and has better activity than other cephalosporins against many Enterobacteriaceae including *Enterobacter* spp., *E. coli*, *Proteus* spp. and Klebsiella. Its activity against *Pseudomonas* is similar to, or slightly less than, that of ceftazidime.

Cefepime also has activity against certain atypicals like *Mycobacterium avium-intracellulare* complex.

Some anaerobes are sensitive to cefepime, but *Clostridia* and *Bacteroides* are not.

Pharmacokinetics

Cefepime is not absorbed from the GI tract and must be administered parenterally. In dogs, cefepime's volume of distribution at steady state is approximately 0.14 L/kg, elimination half-life about 1.1 hours and clearance 0.13 L/kg/hr.

In neonatal foals, cefepime's volume of distribution at steady state is approximately 0.18 L/kg, elimination half-life about 1.65 hours and clearance 0.08 L/kg/hr.

In humans, volume of distribution is about 18 L in adults; 20% of the drug is bound to plasma proteins. Elimination half-life is about 2 hours. Approximately 85% of a dose is excreted unchanged into the urine, less than 1% is metabolized.

Contraindications/Precautions/Warnings

No specific information is available for veterinary patients. Cefepime is contraindicated in human patients hypersensitive to it or other cephalosporins. Dosage adjustment is recommended in humans with severe renal impairment.

Adverse Effects

As usage of cefepime in animals has been very limited, a comprehensive adverse effect profile has not been determined.

There are some reports of dogs or foals developing loose stools or diarrhea after receiving cefepime. IM injections may be painful (alleviated by using 1% lidocaine as diluent).

Human patients generally tolerate cefepime well. Injection site inflammation and rashes occur in approximately 1% of treated patients. Gastrointestinal effects (dyspepsia, diarrhea) occur in less than 1% treated patients. Hypersensitivity reactions including anaphylaxis are possible. Rarely, patients with renal dysfunction who have received cefepime without any dosage adjustment will develop neurologic effects (see Overdosage).

Reproductive/Nursing Safety

Studies performed in pregnant mice, rats, and rabbits demonstrated no overt fetal harm. In humans, the FDA categorizes cefepime as category **B** for use during pregnancy (*Animal studies have not yet demonstrated risk to the fetus, but there are no adequate studies in pregnant women; or animal studies have shown an adverse effect, but adequate studies in pregnant women have not demonstrated a risk to the fetus in the first trimester of pregnancy, and there is no evidence of risk in later trimesters.*)

Cefepime enters maternal milk in very low concentrations. Although probably safe for nursing offspring, the potential for adverse effects cannot be ruled out, particularly alterations to gut flora with resultant diarrhea.

Overdosage/Acute Toxicity

No specific information was located for acute toxicity in veterinary patients.

Humans with impaired renal function receiving inadvertent overdoses have developed encephalopathy, seizures and neuromuscular excitability.

Drug Interactions

The following drug interactions have either been reported or are theoretical in humans or animals receiving cefepime and may be of significance in veterinary patients:

■ **AMINOGLYCOSIDES:** Potential for increased risk of nephrotoxicity—monitor renal function

Laboratory Considerations

■ Cefepime may cause false-positive **urine glucose determinations** when using the copper reduction method (Benedict's solution, Fehling's solution, *Clinitest®*); tests utilizing glucose oxidase (*Tes-Tape®*, *Clinistix®*) are not affected by cephalosporins

■ In humans, particularly with azotemia, cephalosporins have caused a false-positive direct **Coombs' test**

Doses

■ **DOGS:**

For susceptible infections:
a) 40 mg/kg IV q6h (Gardner & Papich 2001)

■ **HORSES:**

For susceptible infections in foals:
a) 11 mg/kg IV q8h; for gram-negative infections (Gardner & Papich 2001)
b) 11 mg/kg IV q8h; use has been limited primarily to neonates with poor aminoglycoside kinetics or documented multi-resistant infections (McKenzie 2005)

Monitoring

■ Clinical efficacy

■ Monitor renal function in patients with renal insufficiency

Client Information

■ Veterinary professionals only should administer this medication

■ Because of the dosing intervals required, this drug is best administered to inpatients only

Chemistry/Synonyms

Cefepime HCl occurs as a white to off-white, non-hygroscopic powder that is freely soluble in water.

Cefepime may also be known as: BMY-28142, cefepimi, or cefepima; internationally registered trade names include: *Axepime®, Biopime®, Cefepen®, Ceficad®, Cemax®, Cepim®, Cepimix®, Forpar®, Maxcef®, Maxipime®* or *Maxil®*.

Storage/Stability

The powder for injection should be stored between (2–25°C) and protected from light. Cefepime can be reconstituted and administered with a variety of diluents including normal saline and D5W. Generally, the solution is stable for up 24 hours at room temperature; up to 7 days if kept refrigerated.

Compatibility/Compounding Considerations

Drugs that may be admixed with cefepime include: amikacin (but not gentamicin or tobramycin), ampicillin, vancomycin, metronidazole and clindamycin. These admixtures have varying times that they remain stable. For more information on dosage preparation, stability and compatibility, refer to the package insert for *Maxipime®* or contact a hospital pharmacist.

Dosage Forms/Regulatory Status

VETERINARY-LABELED PRODUCTS: None
HUMAN-LABELED PRODUCTS:
Cefepime Powder for Injection: 500 mg, 1 gram & 2 gram in vials, 15 mL & 20 mL vials, ADD-Vantage vials, & 100 mL piggyback bottles; *Maxipime®* (Dura); generic (Apotex USA); (Rx)

Cefepime Injection Solution: 1g & 2 g in 50 mL & 100 mL (respectively) single-dose *Galaxy* containers; generic (Baxter); (Rx)

References

Gardner, S & M Papich (2001). Comparison of cefepime pharmacokinetics in neonatal foals and adult dogs. *J Vet Pharmacol Therap* 24: 187–192.

McKenzie, H (2005). Pathophysiology and treatment of pneumonia in foals. ACVIM 2005 Proceedings. Accessed via: Veterinary Information Network. *http://goo.gl/r2VHP*

CEFIXIME

(sef-*ix*-eem)   Suprax®

3RD GENERATION CEPHALOSPORIN

Prescriber Highlights

▶ Oral 3rd generation cephalosporin that may be useful in dogs; only available commercially (in the USA) as a pediatric oral suspension

▶ Contraindications: Hypersensitivity to it or other cephalosporins

▶ May need to adjust dose if patient has renal disease

▶ Adverse Effects: Primarily GI, but hypersensitivity possible

Uses/Indications

Uses for cefixime are limited in veterinary medicine. Its use should be reserved for those times when infections (systemic or urinary tract) are caused by susceptible gram-negative organisms where oral treatment is indicated or when FDA-approved fluoroquinolones or other 3rd generation cephalosporins (*e.g.*, cefpodoxime) are either contraindicated or ineffective.

Pharmacology/Actions

Like other cephalosporins, cefixime inhibits bacteria cell wall synthesis. It is considered bactericidal and relatively resistant to bacterial beta-lactamases.

Cefixime's main spectrum of activity is against gram-negative bacteria in the family Enterobacteriaceae (excluding Pseudomonas) including Escherichia, Proteus, and Klebsiella. It is efficacious against Streptococcus, Rhodococcus, and apparently, Borrelia. Efficacy for *E. coli* is rapidly decreasing as significant resistance has developed in recent years.

Cefixime is not efficacious against *Pseudomonas aeruginosa*, Enterococcus, Staphylococcus, Bordetella, Listeria, Enterobacter, Bacteroides, Actinomyces or Clostridium. For other than *Streptococcus* spp., it has limited efficacy against many gram-positive organisms or anaerobes.

Because sensitivity of various bacteria to the 3rd generation cephalosporin antibiotics is unique to a given agent, cefixime specific disks or dilutions must be used to determine susceptibility.

Pharmacokinetics

Cefixime is relatively rapidly absorbed after oral administration. Bioavailability in the dog is about 50%. Food may impede the rate, but not the extent, of absorption. The suspension may have a higher bioavailability than tablets. The drug is fairly highly bound to plasma proteins in the dog (about 90%). It is unknown if the drug penetrates into the CSF.

Elimination of cefixime is by both renal and non-renal means, but serum half-lives are prolonged in patients with decreased renal function. In dogs, elimination half-life is about 7 hours.

Contraindications/Precautions/Warnings

Cefixime is contraindicated in patients hypersensitive to it or other cephalosporins. Because cefixime is excreted by the kidneys dosages and/or dosage frequency may need to be adjusted in patients with significantly diminished renal function. Use with caution in patients with seizure disorders and patients allergic to penicillins.

Adverse Effects

Adverse effects in the dog may include GI distress (vomiting, etc.) and hypersensitivity reactions (urticaria and pruritus, possibly fever).

Reproductive/Nursing Safety

Cefixime has not been shown to be teratogenic, but should only be used during pregnancy when clearly indicated. In humans, the FDA categorizes this drug as category *B* for use during pregnancy (*Animal studies have not yet demonstrated risk to the fetus, but there are no adequate studies in pregnant women; or animal studies have shown an adverse effect, but adequate studies in pregnant women have not demonstrated a risk to the fetus in the first trimester of pregnancy, and there is no evidence of risk in later trimesters.*)

Overdosage/Acute Toxicity

Cephalosporin overdoses are unlikely to cause significant problems, but other effects are possible (see Adverse Effects section).

Drug Interactions

The following drug interactions have either been reported or are theoretical in humans or animals receiving cefixime and may be of significance in veterinary patients:

■ **PROBENECID:** Competitively blocks the tubular secretion of most cephalosporins thereby increasing serum levels and serum half-lives

■ **SALICYLATES:** May displace cefixime from plasma protein binding sites; clinical significance is unclear

Laboratory Considerations

■ Cefixime may cause false-positive **urine glucose determinations** when using cupric sulfate solution (Benedict's Solution, *Clinitest®*). Tests utilizing glucose oxidase (*Tes-Tape®, Clinistix®*) are not affected by cephalosporins.

■ If using the nitroprusside test for determining **urinary ketones,** cefixime may cause false-positive results.

Doses

■ **DOGS:**

For susceptible infections:
a) For infectious endocarditis when documented resistance against or other contraindications for fluoroquinolones and aminoglycosides: 10 mg/kg PO q12h (DeFrancesco 2000)

b) For UTI: 5 mg/kg PO once to twice daily for 7–14 days

For respiratory, systemic infections: 12.5 mg/kg PO q12h for 7–14 days. Duration of treatment dependent on chronicity of infection. (Greene & Watson 1998), (Greene *et al.* 2006)

c) 5 mg/kg PO once to twice a day (Boothe 1999)

■ **CATS:**

For susceptible infections:
a) 5–12.5 mg/kg PO q12h (Lappin 2002)

Monitoring

■ Efficacy

■ Adverse effects

Client Information

■ Can be given without regard to meals

■ Give as directed for as long as veterinarian recommends, even if patient appears well

Chemistry/Synonyms

An oral 3rd generation semisynthetic cephalosporin antibiotic, cefixime is available commercially as the trihydrate. Cefixime occurs as a white to slightly yellowish white crystalline powder with a characteristic odor and a pKa of 3.73. Solubility in water is pH dependent. At a pH of 3.2, 0.5 mg/mL is soluble and 18 mg/mL at pH 4.2. The oral suspension is strawberry flavored and after reconstitution has pH of 2.5–4.2.

Cefixime may also be known as: cefiximum, CL-284635, FK-027, FR-17027 and *Suprax®*; many internationally registered trade names are available.

Storage/Stability

Cefixime powder for suspension should be stored at room temperature in tight containers. After reconstitution of the oral suspension, refrigeration is not required, but it should be discarded after 14 days whether refrigerated or not.

Dosage Forms/Regulatory Status

VETERINARY-LABELED PRODUCTS: None

HUMAN-LABELED PRODUCTS:

Cefixime Powder for Oral Suspension: 100 mg/5 mL in 50 mL, 75 mL & 100 mL, 200 mg/5 mL in 25 mL, 37.5 mL, 50 mL, 75 mL & 100 mL; *Suprax®* (Lupin Pharma); (Rx)

References

Boothe, DM (1999). What's new in drug therapy in small animals. Wild West Conference.

DeFrancesco, T (2000). CVT Update: Infectious Endocarditis. *Kirk's Current Veterinary Therapy: XIII Small Animal Practice.* J Bonagura Ed. Philadelphia, WB Saunders: 768–772.

Greene, C, K Hartmannn, et al. (2006). Appendix 8: Antimicrobial Drug Formulary. *Infectious Disease of the Dog and Cat.* C Greene Ed., Elsevier: 1186–1333.

Greene, C & A Watson (1998). Antimicrobial Drug Formulary. *Infectious Diseases of the Dog and Cat.* C Greene Ed. Philadelphia, WB Saunders: 790–919.

Lappin, M (2002). Feline fevers of unknown origin I, II, III. Proceedings: Western Veterinary Conference. Accessed via: Veterinary Information Network. http://goo.gl/JuGRY

CEFOTAXIME SODIUM

(sef-oh-*taks*-eem)   Claforan®

3RD GENERATION CEPHALOSPORIN

Prescriber Highlights

▶ 3rd generation parenteral cephalosporin

▶ Potentially could cause hypersensitivity reactions, granulocytopenia, or diarrhea

▶ Causes pain on IM injection; give IV over 3–5 minutes (or more)

▶ May need to reduce dose in renal failure

Uses/Indications

In the United States, there are no cefotaxime products FDA-approved for veterinary species but it has been used clinically in several species when an injectable 3rd generation cephalosporin may be indicated.

Pharmacology/Actions

Cefotaxime is a third generation injectable cephalosporin agent and, like other cephalosporins, inhibits bacteria cell wall synthesis. It is usually bactericidal and it is a time-dependent antibiotic. Cefotaxime has a relatively wide spectrum of activity against both gram-positive and gram-negative bacteria. While less active against *Staphylococcus* spp. than the first generation agents, it still has significant activity against those and other gram-positive cocci. Cefotaxime, like the other 3rd generation agents, has extended coverage of gram-negative aerobes particularly in the family *Enterobacteriaceae*, including *Klebsiella* spp., *E. coli*, *Salmonella*, *Serratia marcescens*, *Proteus* spp., and *Enterobacter* spp. Cefotaxime's *in vitro* activity against *Pseudomonas aeruginosa* is variable and results are usually disappointing when the drug is used clinically against this organism. Many anaerobes are also susceptible to cefotaxime including strains of *Bacteroides fragilis*, *Clostridium* spp., *Fusobacterium* spp., *Peptococcus* spp., and *Peptostreptococcus* spp.

Because 3rd generation cephalosporins exhibit specific activities against bacteria, a 30 microgram cefotaxime disk should be used when performing Kirby-Bauer disk susceptibility tests for this antibiotic.

Pharmacokinetics

Cefotaxime is not appreciably absorbed after oral administration and must be given parenterally to attain therapeutic serum levels. After administration, the drug is widely distributed in body tissues including bone, prostatic fluid (human), aqueous humor, bile, ascitic and pleural fluids. Cefotaxime crosses the placenta and activity in amniotic fluid either equals or exceeds that in maternal serum. Cefotaxime distributes into milk in low concentrations. In humans, approximately 13–40% of the drug is bound to plasma proteins.

Unlike the first generation cephalosporins (and most 2nd generation agents), cefotaxime will enter the CSF in therapeutic levels (at high dosages) when the patient's meninges are inflamed.

Cefotaxime is partially metabolized by the liver to desacetylcefotaxime which exhibits some antibacterial activity. Desacetylcefotaxime is partially degraded to inactive metabolites by the liver. Cefotaxime and its metabolites are primarily excreted in the urine. Because tubular secretion is involved in the renal excretion of the drug, in several species probenecid has been demonstrated to prolong the serum half-life of cefotaxime.

Pharmacokinetic parameters in certain veterinary species follow: In dogs, the apparent volume of distribution at steady state is 480 mL/kg, and a total body clearance of 10.5 mL/min/kg after intravenous injection. Serum elimination half-lives of 45 minutes when given IV, 50 minutes after IM injection, and 103 minutes after SC injection have been noted. Bioavailability is about 87% after IM injection and approximately 100% after SC injection.

In cats, total body clearance is approximately 3 mL/min/kg after intravenous injection and the serum elimination half-life is about 1 hour. Bioavailability is about 93–98% after IM injection.

Contraindications/Precautions/Warnings

Cephalosporins are contraindicated in patients with a history of hypersensitivity to them. Because there may be cross-reactivity, use cephalosporins cautiously in patients who are documented hypersensitive to other beta-lactam antibiotics (*e.g.*, penicillins, cefamycins, carbapenems).

Patients in renal failure may need dosage adjustments.

Adverse Effects

Adverse effects with the cephalosporins are usually not serious and have a relatively low frequency of occurrence.

Hypersensitivity reactions unrelated to dose can occur with these agents and can manifest as rashes, fever, eosinophilia, lymphadenopathy, or full-blown anaphylaxis. The use of cephalosporins in patients documented to be hypersensitive to penicillin-class antibiotics is controversial. In humans, it is estimated 1–15% of patients hypersensitive to penicillins will also be hypersensitive to cephalosporins. The incidence of cross-reactivity in veterinary patients is unknown.

Cephalosporins can cause pain at the injection site when administered intramuscularly. Sterile abscesses or other severe local tissue reactions are also possible but are much less common. Thrombophlebitis is also possible after IV administration of these drugs.

Because the cephalosporins may also alter gut flora, antibiotic-associated diarrhea can occur and allow the proliferation of resistant bacteria in the colon (superinfections).

While cephalosporins (particularly cephalothin) have the potential for causing nephrotoxicity at clinically used doses in patients with normal renal function, risks for the occurrence of this adverse effect appear minimal.

High doses or very prolonged use has been associated with neurotoxicity, neutropenia, agranulocytosis, thrombocytopenia, hepatitis, positive Comb's test, interstitial nephritis, and tubular necrosis. Except for tubular necrosis and neurotoxicity, these effects have an immunologic component.

Reproductive/Nursing Safety

Cephalosporins have been shown to cross the placenta and safe use of them during pregnancy has not been firmly established, but neither have there been any documented teratogenic problems associated with these drugs. However, use only when the potential benefits outweigh the risks. In humans, the FDA categorizes this cefotaxime as category *B* for use during pregnancy (*Animal studies have not yet demonstrated risk to the fetus, but there are no adequate studies in pregnant women; or animal studies have shown an adverse effect, but adequate studies in pregnant women have not demonstrated a risk to the fetus in the first trimester of pregnancy, and there is no evidence of risk in later trimesters.*)

Most of these agents (cephalosporins) are excreted in milk in small quantities. Modification/alteration of bowel flora with resultant diarrhea is theoretically possible.

Overdosage/Acute Toxicity

Cephalosporin overdoses are unlikely to cause significant problems, but other effects are possible (see Adverse effects section).

Drug Interactions

The following drug interactions have either been reported or are theoretical in humans or animals receiving cefotaxime and may be of significance in veterinary patients:

■ **AMINOGLYCOSIDES/NEPHROTOXIC DRUGS:** The concurrent use of parenteral aminoglycosides or other nephrotoxic drugs (*e.g.*, amphotericin B) with cephalosporins is somewhat controversial. Potentially, cephalosporins could cause additive nephrotoxicity when used with these drugs, but this interaction has only been well documented with cephaloridine (no longer marketed). *In vitro* studies have demonstrated that cephalosporins can have synergistic or additive activity against certain bacteria when used

with aminoglycosides, but they should not be mixed together (administer separately).

■ **PROBENECID:** Competitively blocks the tubular secretion of most cephalosporins, thereby increasing serum levels and serum half-lives

Laboratory Considerations

■ In humans, particularly with azotemia, cephalosporins have caused a false-positive direct **Coombs' test.**

■ Cephalosporins may cause falsely elevated **17-ketosteroid** values in urine.

■ Cefotaxime like most other cephalosporins, may cause a **false-positive urine glucose determination** when using the cupric sulfate solution test (*e.g.*, *Clinitest®*), Benedict's solution or Fehling's solution.

Doses

■ **DOGS:**
For susceptible infections:
a) For soft tissue infections: 22 mg/kg IV, IM or SC q8h for 7 days or less or 50 mg/kg IV or IM q12h for 7 days or less.

  For orthopedic infections: 20–40 mg/kg IV, IM or SC q6–8h for 7 days or less.

  For severe bacteremia: 20–80 mg/kg IV q6h or 10–50 mg/kg IV q4–6h for as long as necessary (Greene & Watson 1998)

b) 25–50 mg/kg IV, IM or SC q8h (Riviere 1989); (Vaden & Papich 1995)

c) For sepsis: 20–80 mg/kg IV, IM q8h (Tello 2002)

d) For CNS infections (spinal cord): 25 mg–50 mg/kg IV, IM q8h (Dickinson 2003)

■ **CATS:**
For susceptible infections:
a) For severe bacteremia: 20–80 mg/kg IV or IM q6h as long as necessary (Greene & Watson 1998)

b) 25–50 mg/kg IV, IM or SC q8h (Vaden & Papich 1995), (Lappin 2002)

c) For sepsis: 20–80 mg/kg IV, IM q8h (Tello 2003)

  For CNS infections (spinal cord): 25 mg–50 mg/kg IV, IM q8h (Dickinson 2003)

d) To prevent bacterial colonization of pancreas in cats with severe pancreatitis, anorexia for long periods, or with systemic inflammatory response (SIRS): 50 mg/kg IM q8h (Zoran 2008)

■ **HORSES:**
For susceptible infections:
a) **Foals:** 40 mg/kg IV q6h (Giguere 2003)

b) For meningitis in foals: 40 mg/kg IV 3–4 times a day (Furr 1999)

c) Foals for systemic therapy: 20–30 mg/kg IV or IM q6-8h

Foals: As regional perfusion for adjunctive treatment of septic arthritis: 1 gram cefotaxime in 20 mL of saline. Tourniquet above and below joint. Inject antibiotic solution and leave tourniquet in place for 20 minutes. (Stewart 2008)

■ **BIRDS:**

For susceptible infections:

a) For most birds: 50–100 mg/kg IM three times a day; may be used with aminoglycosides, but nephrotoxicity may occur. Reconstituted vial good for 13 weeks if frozen. (Clubb 1986)

b) For bacterial infections, bacterial hepatitis: 75–100 mg/kg IM or IV q4–8h (Oglesbee 2009a), (Oglesbee 2009b)

c) Ratites (young birds): 25 mg/kg IM 3 times daily (Jenson 1998)

d) 75–100 mg/kg IM or IV q4–8h (Hess 2002)

e) 75 mg/kg IM q8h (Tully 2002)

■ **REPTILES:**

For susceptible infections:

a) 20–40 mg/kg IM once daily for 7–14 days (Gauvin 1993)

b) **Chelonians:** 20–40 mg/kg IM q24h (Johnson 2002)

c) Nebulized antibiotic therapy: 100 mg twice daily (Raiti 2003)

Monitoring

■ Because cephalosporins usually have minimal toxicity associated with their use, monitoring for efficacy is usually all that is required.

■ Patients with diminished renal function may require intensified renal monitoring.

Chemistry/Synonyms

A semisynthetic, 3rd generation, aminothiazolyl cephalosporin, cefotaxime sodium occurs as an odorless, white to off-white crystalline powder with a pK_a of 3.4. It is sparingly soluble in water and slightly soluble in alcohol. Potency of cefotaxime sodium is expressed in terms of cefotaxime. One gram of cefotaxime (sodium) contains 2.2 mEq of sodium.

Cefotaxime sodium may also be known as: cefotaximum natricum, CTX, HR-756, RU-24756 and *Claforan®*; many other trade names are available internationally.

Storage/Stability

Cefotaxime sodium sterile powder for injection should be stored at temperatures of less than 30°C; protected from light. The commercially available frozen injection should be stored at temperatures no greater than -20°C. Depending on storage conditions, the powder or solutions may darken which may indicate a loss in potency. Cefotaxime is not stable in solutions with pH >7.5 (sodium bicarbonate).

Compatibility/Compounding Considerations

All commonly used IV fluids and the following drugs are reportedly **compatible** with cefotaxime: clindamycin, metronidazole, and verapamil. Compatibility is dependent upon factors such as pH, concentration, temperature, and diluent used; consult specialized references or a hospital pharmacist for more specific information.

Dosage Forms/Regulatory Status

VETERINARY-LABELED PRODUCTS: None

HUMAN-LABELED PRODUCTS:

Cefotaxime Sodium Powder for Injection: 500 mg, 1 g, 2 g, & 10 g in vials, bottles, infusion bottles & *ADD-Vantage* system vials; *Claforan®* (Hoechst Marion Roussel); generic; (Rx)

Cefotaxime Sodium for Injection: 1 g & 2 g in infusion bottles, & premixed, frozen 50 mL; *Claforan®* (Hoechst Marion Roussel); generic (Cura); (Rx)

References

Clubb, SL (1986). Therapeutics: Individual and Flock Treatment Regimens. *Clinical Avian Medicine and Surgery*. GJ Harrison and LR Harrison Eds. Philadelphia, W.B. Saunders: 327–355.

Dickinson, P (2003). Infectious Diseases of the Spinal Cord. Proceedings: Western Veterinary Conference. Accessed via: Veterinary Information Network. http://goo.gl/DrnLg

Furr, M (1999). Antimicrobial treatments for the septic foal. Proceedings: The North American Veterinary Conference, Orlando.

Gauvin, J (1993). Drug therapy in reptiles. *Seminars in Avian & Exotic Med* 2(1): 48–59.

Giguere, S (2003). Antimicrobial therapy in foals. Proceedings: Western Veterinary Conference. Accessed via: Veterinary Information Network. http://goo.gl/pdKJZ

Greene, C & A Watson (1998). Antimicrobial Drug Formulary. *Infectious Diseases of the Dog and Cat*. C Greene Ed. Philadelphia, WB Saunders: 790–919.

Hess, L (2002). Practical emergency/critical care of pet birds. Proceedings: Atlantic Coast Veterinary Conference. Accessed via: Veterinary Information Network. http://goo.gl/GgVeM

Jenson, J (1998). Current ratite therapy. *The Veterinary Clinics of North America: Food Animal Practice* 16:3(November).

Johnson, J (2002). Medical management of ill chelonians. Proceedings; Western Veterinary Conference. Accessed via: Veterinary Information Network. http://goo.gl/NTerN

Lappin, M (2002). Feline fevers of unknown origin I, II, III. Proceedings: Western Veterinary Conference. Accessed via: Veterinary Information Network. http://goo.gl/JuGRY

Oglesbee, B (2009a). Liver disease in pet birds. Proceedings: WVC. Accessed via: Veterinary Information Network. http://goo.gl/eoO1Y

Oglesbee, B (2009b). Working up the pet bird with lower respiratory tract disorders. Proceedings: WVC. http://goo.gl/r0maj

Raiti, P (2003). Administration of aerosolized antibiotics to reptiles. Proceedings: Atlantic Coast Veterinary Conference. Accessed via: Veterinary Information Network. http://goo.gl/FYpIT

Stewart, A (2008). Equine Neonatal Sepsis. Proceedings: WVC. Accessed via: Veterinary Information Network. http://www.vin.com/Members/Proceedings/Proceedings.plx?CID=WVC2008&PID=PR19727&O=VIN

Tello, L (2002). Medical management of septic shock. Proceedings: World Small Animal Veterinary Assoc World Congress. Accessed via: Veterinary Information Network. http://goo.gl/iAbvR

Tello, L (2003). Septic patient: Approach and medical management. Proceedings: World Small Animal Veterinary Assoc World Congress. Accessed via: Veterinary Information Network. http://goo.gl/Tt7BL

Tully, T (2002). Avian Therapeutic Options. Proceedings: Western Veterinary Conference. Accessed via: Veterinary Information Network. http://goo.gl/7E5ce

Vaden, S & M Papich (1995). Empiric Antibiotic Therapy. Kirk's Current Veterinary Therapy:XII. J Bonagura Ed. Philadelphia, W.B. Saunders: 276–280.

Zoran, D (2008). Feline Pancreatitis. Proceedings: WVC. Accessed via: Veterinary Information Network. http://goo.gl/iiGcg

CEFOTETAN DISODIUM

(sef-oh-tee-tan)   Cefotan®

2ND GENERATION CEPHALOSPORIN (CEPHAMYCIN)

Prescriber Highlights

▶ 2nd to 3rd generation parenteral cephalosporin (cephamycin) similar to cefoxitin

▶ Pharmacokinetic profile better and may be more effective against E.coli in dogs than cefoxitin

▶ Contraindications: Hypersensitivity to it or cephalosporins

▶ Adverse Effects: Unlikely; potentially could cause bleeding

▶ If severe renal dysfunction, may need to increase time between doses

Uses/Indications

Cefotetan may be a reasonable choice for treating serious infections caused by susceptible bacteria, including E. coli or anaerobes. It appears to be well tolerated in small animals and may be given less frequently than cefoxitin.

Pharmacology/Actions

Often categorized as a 2nd or 3rd generation cephalosporin, cefotetan is usually bactericidal and acts by inhibiting mucopeptide synthesis in the bacterial cell wall.

Cefotetan's in vitro activity against aerobes include E.coli, Proteus, Klebsiella, Salmonella, Staphylococcus and most Streptococcus. It has efficacy against most strains of the following anaerobes: Actinomyces, Clostridium, Peptococcus, Peptostreptococcus and Propionibacterium. Many strains of Bacteroides are still sensitive to cefotetan.

Cefotetan is generally ineffective against Pseudomonas aeruginosa and Enterococci.

Because 2nd generation cephalosporins exhibit specific activities against bacteria, a 30-microgram cefoxitin disk should be used when performing Kirby-Bauer disk susceptibility tests for this antibiotic.

Pharmacokinetics

Cefotetan is not appreciably absorbed after oral administration and must be given parenterally to achieve therapeutic serum levels. The drug is well distributed into most tissues, but only has limited penetration into the CSF. Cefotetan is primarily excreted unchanged by the kidneys into the urine via both glomerular filtration (primarily) and tubular secretion. Elimination half-lives may be significantly prolonged in patients with severely diminished renal function.

Contraindications/Precautions/Warnings

Cephamycins are contraindicated in patients who have a history of hypersensitivity to them. Because there may be cross-reactivity, use cephalosporins cautiously in patients who are documented to be hypersensitive to other beta-lactam antibiotics (e.g., penicillins, cephalosporins, carbapenems).

Adverse Effects

There is little information on the adverse effect profile of this medication in veterinary species, but it appears to be well tolerated. In humans, less than 5% of patients report adverse effects. Because cefotetan contains an N-methylthiotetrazole side chain (like cefoperazone), it may have a greater tendency to cause hematologic effects (e.g. hypoprothrombinemia) or disulfiram-like reactions (vomiting, etc.) than other parenteral cephalosporins.

Hypersensitivity reactions unrelated to dose can occur with these agents and can manifest as rashes, fever, eosinophilia, lymphadenopathy, or full-blown anaphylaxis. The use of cephalosporins in patients documented to be hypersensitive to penicillin-class antibiotics is controversial. In humans, it is estimated 1–15% of patients hypersensitive to penicillins will also be hypersensitive to cephalosporins. The incidence of cross-reactivity in veterinary patients is unknown.

Cephalosporins can cause pain at the injection site when administered intramuscularly. Sterile abscesses or other severe local tissue reactions are also possible but are less common. Thrombophlebitis is also possible after IV administration of these drugs.

Even when administered parenterally, cephalosporins may alter gut flora and antibiotic-associated diarrhea or the proliferation of resistant bacteria in the colon (superinfections) can occur.

While cephalosporins (particularly cephalothin) have the potential for causing nephrotoxicity at clinically used doses in patients with normal renal function, risks for the occurrence of this adverse effect appear minimal. High doses or very prolonged use has been associated with neurotoxicity, neutropenia, agranulocytosis, thrombocytopenia, hepatitis, positive Comb's test, interstitial nephritis, and tubular necrosis. Except for tubular necrosis and neurotoxicity, these effects have an immunologic component.

Reproductive/Nursing Safety

Safe use during pregnancy has not been established; use only when justified. In humans, the

FDA categorizes this drug as category **B** for use during pregnancy (*Animal studies have not yet demonstrated risk to the fetus, but there are no adequate studies in pregnant women; or animal studies have shown an adverse effect, but adequate studies in pregnant women have not demonstrated a risk to the fetus in the first trimester of pregnancy, and there is no evidence of risk in later trimesters*)

Cefotetan enters maternal milk in small quantities. Alteration of bowel flora with resultant diarrhea is theoretically possible.

Overdosage/Acute Toxicity
Unlikely to cause adverse effects, unless massive or chronically overdosed; seizures possible. Treat symptomatically.

Drug Interactions
The following drug interactions have either been reported or are theoretical in humans or animals receiving cefotetan and may be of significance in veterinary patients:

- **ALCOHOL:** A disulfiram reaction is possible
- **AMINOGLYCOSIDES/NEPHROTOXIC DRUGS:** The concurrent use of parenteral aminoglycosides or other nephrotoxic drugs (*e.g.*, amphotericin B) with cephalosporins is somewhat controversial. Potentially, cephalosporins could cause additive nephrotoxicity when used with these drugs, but this interaction has only been well documented with cephaloridine (no longer marketed). *In vitro* studies have demonstrated that cephalosporins can have synergistic or additive activity against certain bacteria when used with aminoglycosides, but they should not be mixed together (administer separately).

Laboratory Considerations
- Except for cefotaxime, cephalosporins may cause false-positive **urine glucose determinations** when using cupric sulfate solution (Benedict's Solution, *Clinitest®*). Tests utilizing glucose oxidase (*Tes-Tape®, Clinistix®*) are not affected by cephalosporins.
- When using the Jaffe reaction to measure **serum or urine creatinine**, cephalosporins (not ceftazidime or cefotaxime) in high dosages may falsely cause elevated values.
- In humans, particularly with azotemia, cephalosporins have caused a false-positive direct **Coombs' test.**
- Cephalosporins may also cause falsely elevated **17-ketosteroid** values in urine.

Doses
- **DOGS:**
For susceptible infections:
a) 30 mg/kg SC q12h (Autran de Morais 2009)
b) For soft tissue infections: 30 mg/kg SC q12h for 7 days or less;
For bacteremia, sepsis: 30 mg/kg IV, SC q8h for as long as required. (Greene *et al.* 2006)

- **CATS:**
For susceptible infections:
a) For sepsis: 30 mg/kg q5-8h IV (Hardie 2000)

Monitoring
- Because cephalosporins usually have minimal toxicity associated with their use, monitoring for efficacy is usually all that is required.
- Patients with diminished renal function may require intensified renal monitoring. Serum levels and therapeutic drug monitoring are not routinely done with these agents.

Chemistry/Synonyms
A semisynthetic cephamycin similar to cefoxitin, cefotetan disodium occurs as a white to pale yellow, lyophilized powder. It is very soluble in water and alcohol. The injection contains approximately 3.5 mEq of sodium per gram of cefotetan and after reconstitution has a pH of 4–6.5.

Cefotetan Disodium may also be known as: ICI-156834, YM-09330, *Apacef®, Apatef®, Cefotan®, Ceftenon®, Cepan®, Darvilen®,* or *Yamatetan®.*

Storage/Stability
The sterile powder for injection should be stored below 22°C and protected from light. A darkening of the powder with time does not indicate lessened potency. After reconstituting with sterile water for injection, the resultant solution is stable for 24 hours if stored at room temperature, 96 hours if refrigerated, and at least one week if frozen at -20C.

Dosage Forms/Regulatory Status
VETERINARY-LABELED PRODUCTS: None

HUMAN-LABELED PRODUCTS:
Cefotetan Disodium Powder for Solution: 1 g, 2 g, & 10 g in 10 mL & 20 mL vials; generic; (Rx)

References
Autran de Morais, H (2009). Empiric Antibiotic Therapy. Proceedings: WSAVA. Accessed via: Veterinary Information Network. http://goo.gl/JSZKU

Greene, C, K Hartmannn, et al. (2006). Appendix 8: Antimicrobial Drug Formulary. *Infectious Disease of the Dog and Cat.* C Greene Ed., Elsevier: 1186–1333.

Hardie, E (2000). Therapeutic Mangement of Sepsis. *Kirk's Current Veterinary Therapy: XIII Small Animal Practice.* J Bonagura Ed. Philadelphia, WB Saunders: 272–275.

CEFOVECIN SODIUM

(sef-oh-**vee**-sin)   Convenia®

INJECTABLE LONG-ACTING
CEPHALOSPORIN

Prescriber Highlights

▶ Long-acting injectable cephalosporin
labeled for use in dogs and cats

▶ Primary benefit is for patients whose
owners have difficulty adhering to an
oral dosing regimen or when oral antibiotics are not tolerated or absorbed

Uses/Indications

In the USA, cefovecin is FDA-approved for dogs
to treat skin infections (secondary superficial
pyoderma, abscesses, and wounds) caused by
susceptible strains of *Staphylococcus intermedius*
and *Streptococcus canis* (Group G) and in cats
to treat skin infections (wounds and abscesses)
caused by susceptible strains of *Pasteurella
multocida*.

In the UK, cefovecin is also labeled for dogs
for skin and soft tissue infections caused by
E. coli and/or *Pasteurella multocida*, for the
treatment of urinary tract infections associated with *E. coli* and/or *Proteus* spp., and as
adjunctive treatment to mechanical or surgical
periodontal therapy of severe infections of the
gingival and periodontal tissues associated with
Porphyromonas spp. and *Prevotella* spp. Also in
the UK, cefovecin is labeled for use in cats for
skin infections caused by *Fusobacterium* spp.,
Bacteroides spp., *Prevotella* oralis, beta-hemolytic *Streptococci* and/or *Staphylococcus pseud-
intermedius*, and the treatment of urinary tract
infections associated with *E. coli*.

Cefovecin's long half-life in dogs and cats allows a single dose or extended dosing intervals
(determined by organism susceptibility and
MIC) for treating a variety of infections off-label
(in USA).

Pharmacology/Actions

Cefovecin is a cephalosporin antibiotic, one
source describes it as a 3rd-generation cephalosporin. Its mechanism of action in susceptible
bacteria, like other beta-lactams, is to bind to
and disrupt the actions of bacterial transpeptidase and carboxypeptidase thereby interfering
with bacterial cell wall synthesis.

Cefovecin is not active against *Pseudomonas*
spp. or enterococci and its high protein-binding
does not allow it (at labeled doses) to achieve effective serum levels to treat systemic (non-UTI)
E. coli infections.

Pharmacokinetics

After SC injection in dogs or cats, cefovecin is
completely absorbed. In dogs, peak levels occur about 6 hours after a dose, and in cats,
about 2 hours. The drug is highly bound to

plasma proteins (98.5% dogs; 99.8% cats)
that slowly dissociate giving the drug its long
elimination half-life. As cefovecin exhibits
non-linear kinetics, an increase in dosage does
not proportionally increase the plasma concentration. In the product label the following
additional pharmacokinetic values are listed: terminal elimination half-life: 133 ± 16 hours (dog),
166 ± 18 hours (cat), maximum plasma concentration: 121 ± 51 micrograms/mL (dog),
141 ± 12 micrograms/mL (cat); volume of distribution (steady-state): 0.122 ± 0.011 L/kg (dog),
0.09 ± 0.01 L/kg (cat); total body clearance:
0.76 ± 0.13 mL/hr/kg (dog), $0.350 \pm$
0.40 mL/kg/hr (cat).

Elimination of cefovecin is primarily via renal
mechanism and the majority of a dose is excreted unchanged in the urine, but a small amount
is excreted unchanged in the bile. Cefovecin is a
highly protein-bound molecule in dog plasma
(98.5%) and cat plasma (99.8%) and may compete with other highly protein-bound drugs
for plasma protein binding sites. Cefovecin
may persist in the body for up to 65 days.

Contraindications/Precautions/Warnings

Cefovecin is contraindicated in animals with a
known allergy to cefovecin or to other beta-lactam antibiotics. Anaphylaxis has been reported
with the use of this product. Because cefovecin
is primarily eliminated via renal mechanisms,
use with caution in animals with severe renal
dysfunction.

The UK labeling warns against using in small
herbivores (Guinea pigs, rabbits).

Safe use in dogs or cats less than 4 months of
age has not been established. The UK labeling
warns against using in dogs or cats less then 8
weeks old.

Adverse Effects

In dogs and cats, cefovecin appears to be well
tolerated. Pre-marketing (USA) studies in dogs
and cats found no significant increases in adverse effect types or rates when compared with
control. However, treated animals did have some
changes in laboratory values. Several dogs had
mild to moderate increases in liver enzymes
(GGT, ALT). In treated cats, 4/147 cats had increases (mild) in ALT concentrations, 24/147
had increases in BUN, and 6/147 had moderately elevated serum creatinine values.

In the FDA's Cumulative Veterinary Adverse
Drug Experience (ADE) Reports (through
November 2010), the most common adverse
effects listed (in decreasing order of frequency)
are: Dogs: depression/lethargy, anorexia, and
vomiting; Cats: anorexia, depression/lethargy,
and vomiting. As more experience is gained with
this agent, a clearer adverse drug reaction profile
is expected.

Hypersensitivity reactions, anaphylaxis and
death associated with this drug are possible
and have been reported. The manufacturer

also states: Occasionally, cephalosporins and NSAIDs have been associated with myelotoxicity, thereby creating a toxic neutropenia. Other hematological reactions seen with cephalosporins include neutropenia, anemia, hypoprothrombinemia, thrombocytopenia, prolonged prothrombin time (PT) and partial thromboplastin time (PTT), platelet dysfunction and transient increases in serum aminotransferases.

Because the drug can persist in the body for up to 65 days, adverse reactions may occur that require prolonged treatment.

Reproductive/Nursing Safety

The manufacturer states that safe use in breeding or lactating animals has not been determined. However, cephalosporins are generally considered safe to use during pregnancy and lactation and veterinarians and owners can weigh any risks of using the drug versus the benefits to the dam and offspring.

Overdosage/Acute Toxicity

Acute overdoses should be relatively safe. Dogs administered cefovecin SC up to 180 mg/kg (22.5X) showed only site irritation, vocalization, and edema. Edema resolved within 8–24 hours. Cats given the same dose (22.5X) injection showed the same signs but 10 days post had a lower mean white blood cell counts than controls, and one cat had a small amount of bilirubinuria on day 10.

Drug Interactions

As cefovecin is so highly bound to plasma proteins it potentially could displace (or be displaced) from plasma protein binding sties by other highly bound agents. The manufacturer reports that in an experimental *in vitro* system, cefovecin demonstrated that it could increase the free (active) concentrations of other highly protein-bound dugs such as **carprofen, furosemide, doxycycline,** and **ketoconazole.** They caution that concurrent use of these or other drugs that have a high degree of protein binding (*e.g.*, **NSAIDs, propofol, cardiac, anticonvulsant, and behavioral medications**) may compete with cefovecin-binding and cause adverse reactions; actual clinical significance has not been established, however.

Laboratory Considerations

- Cephalosporins may cause false-positive **urine glucose determinations** when using the copper reduction method (Benedict's solution, Fehling's solution, *Clinitest®*); tests utilizing glucose oxidase (*Tes-Tape®*, *Clinistix®*) are not affected by cephalosporins

- When using the Jaffe reaction to measure **serum or urine creatinine,** cephalosporins (not ceftazidime or cefotaxime) given in high dosages may cause falsely elevated values

- Cephalosporins may cause falsely lowered **albumin** levels when certain tests are used to measure albumin

- In humans, particularly with azotemia, cephalosporins have caused a false-positive direct **Coombs' test.**

- Cephalosporins may also cause falsely elevated **17-ketosteroid** values in urine

Doses

- **DOGS:**

  For labeled indications

  a) USA: Skin infections due to *S. intermedius* or *S. canis* (Group G)): Administer 8 mg/kg SC once. A second injection (same dose/route) may be administered if response to therapy is not complete 7 days later (for *S. intermedius* infections) and 14 days later for *S. canis* (Group G) infections. Maximum treatment should not exceed 2 injections. (Adapted from label information; *Convenia®*—Pfizer)

  b) UK (for indicated organisms see Uses above): Skin and soft tissue infections: 8 mg/kg SC once. If required, treatment may be repeated at 14 day intervals up to a further three times. In accordance with good veterinary practice, treatment of pyoderma should be extended beyond complete resolution of clinical signs.

  Severe infections of the gingival and periodontal tissues: 8 mg/kg SC once.

  UTI: 8 mg/kg SC once. (Adapted from label information; *Convenia®*—Pfizer UK)

- **CATS:**

  For labeled indications:

  a) USA: Skin infections (wounds and abscesses) caused by susceptible strains of *Pasteurella multocida*): 8 mg/kg SC as a single, one-time subcutaneous injection. Therapeutic concentrations are maintained for approximately 7 days for *Pasteurella multocida* infections. (Adapted from label information; *Convenia®*—Pfizer USA)

  b) UK (for indicated organisms see Uses above): Skin and soft tissue abscesses and wounds: 8 mg/kg SC once. If required, an additional dose may be administered 14 days after the first injection.

  UTI: 8 mg/kg SC once. (Adapted from label information; *Convenia®*—Pfizer UK)

Monitoring

- Efficacy
- Adverse effects

Client Information

- Clients should understand that this drug may persist in the body of a treated animal for approximately 2 months after injection and if any occur, report them to the veterinarian.

Chemistry/Synonyms

Cefovecin sodium is a 3rd-generation cephalosporin antibacterial agent with a molecular weight of 475.5. Each mL of reconstituted lyophilized powder contains cefovecin sodium equivalent to 80 mg of cefovecin; methylparaben 1.8 mg and propylparaben 0.2 mg are added as preservatives, and sodium citrate dihydrate 5.8 mg and citric acid monohydrate 0.1 mg, sodium hydroxide or hydrochloric acid are added to adjust pH.

Cefovecin sodium may also be known as UK-287074-02, cefovecina sodica, céfovécine sodique or natrii cefovecinum. A trade name is *Convenia®*.

Storage/Stability

Store the powder and the reconstituted product in the original carton, refrigerated at 2°–8°C (36°–46°F). Use the entire contents of the vial within 28 days of reconstitution. Cefovecin is light sensitive; protect from light. After each use return the unused portion back to the refrigerator in the original carton. Color of the solution may vary from clear to amber at reconstitution and may darken over time, but if stored as recommended, solution color does not adversely affect potency.

Compatibility/Compounding Considerations

To deliver the appropriate dose, aseptically reconstitute vial with 10 mL sterile water for injection. Shake and allow vial to sit until all material is visually dissolved. The resulting solution contains cefovecin sodium equivalent to 80 mg/mL of cefovecin.

Dosage Forms/Regulatory Status

VETERINARY-LABELED PRODUCTS:

Cefovecin Sodium (lyophilized) 800 mg (of cefovecin) per 10 mL multidose vial (80 mg/mL when reconstituted); *Convenia®* (Pfizer); (Rx). FDA-approved as labeled for use in dogs and cats.

HUMAN-LABELED PRODUCTS: None

CEFOXITIN SODIUM

(se-**fox**-i-tin)   Mefoxin®

2ND GENERATION CEPHALOSPORIN (CEPHAMYCIN)

Prescriber Highlights

▶ 2nd generation parenteral cephalosporin; effective against anaerobes, including Bacteroides

▶ Potentially could cause hypersensitivity reactions, thrombocytopenia, & diarrhea

▶ Causes pain on IM injection; Give IV over 3–5 minutes (or more)

▶ May need to reduce dose in renal failure

Uses/Indications

In the United States, there are no cefoxitin products FDA-approved for veterinary species, but it has been used clinically in several species when an injectable second generation cephalosporin may be indicated.

Pharmacology/Actions

Although not a true cephalosporin, cefoxitin is usually classified as a 2nd generation agent. Cefoxitin has activity against gram-positive cocci, but less so on a per weight basis than the 1st generation agents. Unlike the first generation agents, it has good activity against many strains of *E. coli*, Klebsiella and Proteus that may be resistant to the first generation agents. In human medicine, cefoxitin's activity against many strains of *Bacteroides fragilis* has placed it in a significant therapeutic role. While *Bacteroides fragilis* has been isolated from anaerobic infections in veterinary patients, it may not be as significant a pathogen in veterinary species as in humans.

Because 2nd generation cephalosporins exhibit specific activities against bacteria, a 30-microgram cefoxitin disk should be used when performing Kirby-Bauer disk susceptibility tests for this antibiotic.

Pharmacokinetics

Cefoxitin is not appreciably absorbed after oral administration and must be given parenterally to achieve therapeutic serum levels. The absorbed drug is primarily excreted unchanged by the kidneys into the urine via both tubular secretion and glomerular filtration. In humans, approximately 2% of a dose is metabolized to descarbamylcefoxitin, which is inactive. Elimination half-lives may be significantly prolonged in patients with severely diminished renal function.

In horses, the apparent volume of distribution at steady state is 110 mL/kg, total body clearance of 4.32 mL/min/kg with a serum elimination half-life of 49 minutes.

In calves, the volume of distribution is 318 mL/kg, and it has a terminal elimination half-life of 67 minutes after IV dosing, and 81 minutes after IM administration. Cefoxitin is approximately 50% bound to calf plasma proteins. Probenecid (40 mg/kg) has been demonstrated to significantly prolong elimination half-lives.

Contraindications/Precautions/Warnings

Cephalosporins are contraindicated in patients with a history of hypersensitivity to them. Because there may be cross-reactivity, use cephalosporins cautiously in patients who are documented hypersensitive to other beta-lactam antibiotics (*e.g.*, penicillins, cefamycins, carbapenems).

Patients in renal failure may need dosage adjustments.

Adverse Effects

Adverse effects with the cephalosporins are usually not serious and have a relatively low frequency of occurrence.

Hypersensitivity reactions unrelated to dose can occur with these agents and can manifest as rashes, fever, eosinophilia, lymphadenopathy, or full-blown anaphylaxis. The use of cephalosporins in patients documented to be hypersensitive to penicillin-class antibiotics is controversial. In humans, it is estimated 1–15% of patients hypersensitive to penicillins will also be hypersensitive to cephalosporins. The incidence of cross-reactivity in veterinary patients is unknown.

Cephalosporins can cause pain at the injection site when administered intramuscularly. Sterile abscesses or other severe local tissue reactions are also possible but are less common. Thrombophlebitis is also possible after IV administration of these drugs.

Even when administered parenterally, cephalosporins may alter gut flora and antibiotic-associated diarrhea or the proliferation of resistant bacteria in the colon (superinfections) can occur.

While cephalosporins (particularly cephalothin) have the potential for causing nephrotoxicity at clinically used doses in patients with normal renal function, risks for the occurrence of this adverse effect appear minimal. High doses or very prolonged use has been associated with neurotoxicity, neutropenia, agranulocytosis, thrombocytopenia, hepatitis, positive Comb's test, interstitial nephritis, and tubular necrosis. Except for tubular necrosis and neurotoxicity, these effects have an immunologic component.

Reproductive/Nursing Safety

Cephalosporins have been shown to cross the placenta and safe use of them during pregnancy has not been firmly established, but neither have there been any documented teratogenic problems associated with these drugs; however, use only when the potential benefits outweigh the risks. In humans, the FDA categorizes this drug as category *B* for use during pregnancy (*Animal studies have not yet demonstrated risk to the fetus, but there are no adequate studies in pregnant women; or animal studies have shown an adverse effect, but adequate studies in pregnant women have not demonstrated a risk to the fetus in the first trimester of pregnancy, and there is no evidence of risk in later trimesters.*)

Cefoxitin can be distributed into milk in low concentrations. It is unlikely to pose significant risk to nursing offspring.

Overdosage/Acute Toxicity

Acute oral cephalosporin overdoses are unlikely to cause significant problems other than GI distress, but other effects are possible (see Adverse Effects section).

Drug Interactions

The following drug interactions have either been reported or are theoretical in humans or animals receiving cefoxitin and may be of significance in veterinary patients:

■ **AMINOGLYCOSIDES/NEPHROTOXIC DRUGS:** The concurrent use of parenteral aminoglycosides or other nephrotoxic drugs (*e.g.*, amphotericin B) with cephalosporins is somewhat controversial. Potentially, cephalosporins could cause additive nephrotoxicity when used with these drugs, but this interaction has only been well documented with cephaloridine (no longer marketed). *In vitro* studies have demonstrated that cephalosporins can have synergistic or additive activity against certain bacteria when used with aminoglycosides, but they should not be mixed together (administer separately).

■ **PROBENECID:** Competitively blocks the tubular secretion of most cephalosporins thereby increasing serum levels and serum half-lives.

Laboratory Considerations

■ Except for cefotaxime, cephalosporins may cause false-positive **urine glucose determinations** when using cupric sulfate solution (Benedict's Solution, *Clinitest®*). Tests utilizing glucose oxidase (*Tes-Tape®, Clinistix®*) are not affected by cephalosporins.

■ When using the Jaffe reaction to measure **serum or urine creatinine**, cephalosporins (not ceftazidime or cefotaxime) in high dosages may falsely cause elevated values.

■ In humans, particularly with azotemia, cephalosporins have caused a false-positive direct **Coombs' test.**

■ Cephalosporins may also cause falsely elevated **17-KETOSTEROID** values in urine.

Doses

■ **DOGS:**
For susceptible infections:
a) For mixed infections (*e.g.*, aspiration pneumonia, bowel perforation): 30 mg/kg SC q8h; 30 mg/kg IV q4–6h (Trepanier 1999)

b) For sepsis: 30 mg/kg IV q5h (Hardie 2000)

c) For soft tissue infections: 30 mg/kg SC q8h or 30 mg/kg IV q5h
For bacteremia: 15–30 mg/kg IV, IM SC q6–8h
For orthopedic infections: 22 mg/kg IV, IM q6–8h
Use for all indications above as long as necessary to control initial infection, then switch to oral drugs for longer therapy. (Greene *et al.* 2006)

d) 30 mg/kg SC q8h (Autran de Morais 2009)

■ **CATS:**
For susceptible infections:
a) For systemic infections: 25–30 mg/kg IV or IM q8h; use for as long as necessary to control initial infection, then switch to oral drugs for longer therapy (Greene *et al.* 2006)

b) For sepsis: 30 mg/kg IV q5h (Hardie 2000)

c) 30 mg/kg IV q8h (Vaden & Papich 1995)

d) For second line treatment of non-tuberculosis mycobacteria (NTM): 30–40 mg/kg IV, IM or SC q6-8h (causes pain on injection with IM or SC) (Gunn-Moore 2008)

■ **HORSES:**

For susceptible infections:

a) **Foals:** 20 mg/kg IV q4–6h (Caprile and Short 1987); (Brumbaugh 1999)

Monitoring

■ Because cephalosporins usually have minimal toxicity associated with their use, monitoring for efficacy is usually all that is required.

■ Patients with diminished renal function may require intensified renal monitoring.

Chemistry/Synonyms

Actually a cephamycin, cefoxitin sodium is a semisynthetic antibiotic that is derived from cephamycin C that is produced by *Streptomyces lactamdurans*. It occurs as a white to off-white, somewhat hygroscopic powder or granules with a faint but characteristic odor. It is very soluble in water and only slightly soluble in alcohol. Each gram of cefoxitin sodium contains 2.3 mEq of sodium.

Cefoxitin may also be known as: MK-306, L-620-388, cefoxitinum, cefoxitina, cefoxitine, *Mefoxin®*, *Mefoxitin®*, *Cefociclin®*, or *Cefoxin®*.

Storage/Stability

Cefoxitin sodium powder for injection should be stored at temperatures less than 30°C and should not be exposed to temperatures greater than 50°C. The frozen solution for injection should be stored at temperatures no higher than -20°C.

After reconstitution, the solution is stable for 24 hours when kept at room temperature and from 48 hours to 1 week if refrigerated. If after reconstitution the solution is immediately frozen in the original container, the preparation is stable up to 30 weeks when stored at -20°C. Stability is dependent on the diluent used and the reader should refer to the package insert or other specialized references for more information. The powder or reconstituted solution may darken but this apparently does not affect the potency of the product.

Compatibility/Compounding Considerations

All commonly used IV fluids and the following drugs are reportedly **compatible** with cefoxitin: amikacin sulfate, cimetidine HCl, gentamicin sulfate, kanamycin sulfate, mannitol, metronidazole, multivitamin infusion concentrate, sodium bicarbonate, tobramycin sulfate and vitamin B-complex with C. Compatibility is dependent upon factors such as pH, concentration, temperature and diluent used; consult specialized references or a hospital pharmacist for more specific information.

Dosage Forms/Regulatory Status

VETERINARY-LABELED PRODUCTS: None

HUMAN-LABELED PRODUCTS:

Cefoxitin Sodium Powder for Injection: 1 g, 2 g, & 10 g in vials & infusion bottles; generic (American Pharmaceutical Partners); (Rx)

References

Autran de Morais, H (2009). Empiric Antibiotic Therapy. Proceedings: WSAVA. Accessed via: Veterinary Information Network. http://goo.gl/JSZKU

Brumbaugh, G (1999). Clinical Pharmacology and the Pediatric Patient. 45th Annual AAEP Convention, Albuquerque.

Greene, C, K Hartmannn, et al. (2006). Appendix 8: Antimicrobial Drug Formulary. *Infectious Disease of the Dog and Cat*. C Greene Ed., Elsevier: 1186–1333.

Gunn-Moore, D (2008). Feline Mycobacterial Infections. Proceedings: WSAVA. Accessed via: Veterinary Information Network. http://goo.gl/HSwHE

Hardie, E (2000). Therapeutic Mangement of Sepsis. *Kirk's Current Veterinary Therapy: XIII Small Animal Practice*. J Bonagura Ed. Philadelphia, WB Saunders: 272–275.

Trepanier, L (1999). Treating resistant infections in small animals. Proceedings: 17th Annual American College of Veterinary Internal Medicine Meeting, Chicago.

Vaden, S & M Papich (1995). Empiric Antibiotic Therapy. *Kirk's Current Veterinary Therapy:XII*. J Bonagura Ed. Philadelphia, W.B. Saunders: 276–280.

CEFPODOXIME PROXETIL

(sef-poe-*docks*-eem)   Simplicef®, Vantin®

3RD GENERATION CEPHALOSPORIN

Prescriber Highlights

▶ Oral 3rd generation cephalosporin that may be useful in dogs or cats

▶ Contraindications: Hypersensitivity to it or other cephalosporins

▶ May need to adjust dose if patient has renal disease

▶ Adverse Effects: Primarily GI, but hypersensitivity possible

Uses/Indications

In dogs, cefpodoxime is indicated for the treatment of skin infections caused by *Staphylococcus intermedius*, *Staphylococcus aureus*, *Streptococcus canis*, *E. coli*, *Proteus mirabilis*, and *Pasteurella multocida*. Although not currently FDA-approved for cats, it may also be useful as well.

Pharmacology/Actions

Like other cephalosporins, cefpodoxime inhibits bacterial cell wall synthesis. It is considered bactericidal and relatively resistant to bacterial beta-lactamases.

Cefpodoxime's main spectrum of activity is against gram-negative bacteria in the family *Enterobacteriaceae* (excluding Pseudomonas) including Escherichia, Proteus, and Klebsiella, and gram-positive streptococci (not enterococcus) and Staphylococci.

Cefpodoxime is not efficacious against

Pseudomonas aeruginosa, Enterococcus, anaerobes, and methicillin-resistant Staphylococcus strains.

Because sensitivity of various bacteria to the 3rd generation cephalosporin antibiotics is unique to a given agent, cefpodoxime specific disks or dilutions must be used to determine susceptibility.

Pharmacokinetics

Cefpodoxime proxetil is not active as an antibiotic. Cefpodoxime is active after the proxetil ester is cleaved *in vivo.* After single oral doses (10 mg/kg) to fasted dogs, bioavailability is approximately 63%; volume of distribution 10 mL/kg; peak concentrations about 16 mg/mL; time to peak was 2.2 hours; and terminal elimination half-life of approximately 5–6 hours.

In humans, cefpodoxime proxetil is about 40–50% absorbed from the GI tract. Food can alter the rate, but not the extent, of absorption. Cefpodoxime penetrates most tissues well; it is unknown if it penetrates into the CSF. The drug is eliminated in both the urine and feces. Serum half-life may be prolonged in patients with impaired renal function.

In foals after an oral dose (suspension) of 10 mg/kg, peak levels occur in about 100 minutes and peak at about 0.8 micrograms/mL. Elimination half-life is about 7 hours in foals. Levels in synovial and peritoneal fluids were similar to those found in the serum, but no drug was detected in the CSF.

Contraindications/Precautions/Warnings

Cefpodoxime is contraindicated in patients hypersensitive to it or other cephalosporins. Because cefpodoxime is excreted by the kidneys, dosages and/or dosage frequency may need to be adjusted in patients with significantly diminished renal function. Use with caution in patients with seizure disorders.

Adverse Effects

Although usage of this drug in veterinary patients remains limited to date, it appears to be tolerated very well. The most likely adverse effects seen with this medication have been inappetence, diarrhea, and vomiting. Hypersensitivity reactions are a possibility.

Cefpodoxime may occasionally induce a positive direct Coombs' test. Rarely, blood dyscrasias may be seen following high doses of cephalosporins.

Reproductive/Nursing Safety

Cefpodoxime has not shown to be teratogenic but should only be used during pregnancy when clearly indicated. The veterinary product is labeled: "The safety of cefpodoxime proxetil in dogs used for breeding, pregnant dogs, or lactating bitches has not been demonstrated." In humans, the FDA categorizes this drug as category **B** for use during pregnancy (*Animal studies have not yet demonstrated risk to the fetus, but there are no adequate studies in pregnant women; or animal studies have shown an adverse effect, but adequate studies in pregnant women have not demonstrated a risk to the fetus in the first trimester of pregnancy, and there is no evidence of risk in later trimesters.*)

The drug enters maternal milk in low concentrations. Modification/alteration of bowel flora with resultant diarrhea is theoretically possible.

Overdosage/Acute Toxicity

Cephalosporin overdoses are unlikely to cause significant problems but other effects are possible (see Adverse effects section).

Drug Interactions

The following drug interactions have either been reported or are theoretical in humans or animals receiving cefpodoxime and may be of significance in veterinary patients:

■ **AMINOGLYCOSIDES/NEPHROTOXIC DRUGS:** The concurrent use of parenteral aminoglycosides or other nephrotoxic drugs (*e.g.,* amphotericin B) with cephalosporins is somewhat controversial. Potentially, cephalosporins could cause additive nephrotoxicity when used with these drugs, but this interaction has only been well documented with cephaloridine (no longer marketed). *In vitro* studies have demonstrated that cephalosporins can have synergistic or additive activity against certain bacteria when used with aminoglycosides, but they should not be mixed together (administer separately).

■ **ANTACIDS:** Drugs that can increase stomach pH may decrease the absorption of the drug

■ **H-2 ANTAGONISTS (ranitidine, famotidine,** etc.): Drugs that can increase stomach pH may decrease the absorption of the drug

■ **PROBENECID:** Competitively blocks the tubular secretion of most cephalosporins thereby increasing serum levels and serum half-lives

■ **PROTON PUMP INHIBITORS** (*e.g.,* **omeprazole**): Drugs that can increase stomach pH may decrease the absorption of the drug

Laboratory Considerations

■ Cefpodoxime may cause false-positive **urine glucose determinations** when using cupric sulfate solution (Benedict's Solution, *Clinitest®*). Tests utilizing glucose oxidase (*Tes-Tape®, Clinistix®*) are not affected by cephalosporins.

■ If using the nitroprusside test for determining **urinary ketones**, cefpodoxime may cause false-positive results.

Doses

■ **DOGS:**

a) For susceptible skin infections: 5–10 mg/kg PO once daily. Should be administered for 5–7 days or 2–3 days beyond cessation of clinical signs, up to a maximum of 28 days. Treatment of acute infections should not be continued for more than 3–4 days if no response to therapy is seen. May be given with or without food. (Label information; *Simplicef®*—Pfizer)

■ **CATS:**

a) For susceptible skin and soft tissue infections: 5 mg/kg PO q12h or 10 mg/kg PO once daily (**Note:** Extrapolated from human dosage) (Greene & Watson 1998)

■ **HORSES:**

a) Foals (neonates) with bacterial infections: 10 mg/kg PO q6-12 hours. Additional studies required to confirm clinical efficacy and safety. (Carrillo *et al.* 2005)

Monitoring
■ Clinical efficacy

Client Information
■ Can be given without regard to meals (in humans presence of food enhances absorption).
■ Give as directed for as long as veterinarian recommends, even if patient appears well.

Chemistry/Synonyms
An orally administered semisynthetic 3rd generation cephalosporin, cefpodoxime proxetil is a prodrug that is hydrolyzed *in vivo* to cefpodoxime. The esterified form (proxetil) enhances lipid solubility and oral absorption.

Cefpodoxime proxetil may also be known as: CS-807; R-3763, U-76252, U-76253, *Banan®, Biocef®, Cefodox®, Cepodem®, Garia®, Instana®, Kelbium®, Orelox®, Otreon®, Podomexef®, Simplicef®,* or *Vantin®.*

Storage/Stability
Tablets and unreconstituted powder should be stored at 20–25°C in well-closed containers. After reconstitution, the oral suspension should be stored in the refrigerator and discarded after 14 days.

Dosage Forms/Regulatory Status

VETERINARY-LABELED PRODUCTS:
Cefpodoxime Proxetil Tablets: 100 mg & 200 mg; *Simplicef®* (Pfizer); (Rx). FDA-approved for use in dogs.

HUMAN-LABELED PRODUCTS:
Cefpodoxime Proxetil Oral Tablets: 100 mg & 200 mg; *Vantin®* (Pharmacia & Upjohn), generic (Aurobindo); (Rx)

Cefpodoxime Proxetil Granules for Suspension, Oral: 50 mg/5 mL & 100 mg/5 mL in 50 mL, 75 mL & 100 mL bottles; *Vantin®* (Pharmacia & Upjohn), generic (Aurobindo); (Rx)

References
Carrillo, NA, S Giguere, et al. (2005). Disposition of orally administered cefpodoxime proxetil in foals and adult horses and minimum inhibitory concentration of the drug against common bacterial pathogens of horses. *American Journal of Veterinary Research* 66(1): 30–35.
Greene, C & A Watson (1998). Antimicrobial Drug
Formulary. *Infectious Diseases of the Dog and Cat.* C Greene Ed. Philadelphia, WB Saunders: 790–919.

CEFTAZIDIME

(sef-*taz*-i-deem)   Ceptaz®, Fortaz®, Tazicef®

3RD GENERATION CEPHALOSPORIN

Prescriber Highlights

▶ 3rd generation cephalosporin used parenterally for gram-negative infections

▶ Particularly useful in reptiles

▶ Could cause hypersensitivity reactions, granulocytopenia, thrombocytopenia, diarrhea, mild azotemia

▶ May cause pain on IM injection; SC injection probably less painful

▶ May need to reduce dose in renal failure; use with caution

▶ Check drug-lab interactions

Uses/Indications
Ceftazidime is potentially useful in treating serious gram-negative bacterial infections particularly against susceptible Enterobacteriaceae including *Pseudomonas aeruginosa*, that are not susceptible to other, less-expensive agents, or when aminoglycosides are not indicated (due to their potential toxicity). It is of particular interest for treating gram-negative infections in reptiles due to a very long half-life.

Pharmacology/Actions
Ceftazidime is a third generation injectable cephalosporin agent. It is bactericidal and acts via its inhibition of enzymes responsible for bacterial cell wall synthesis. The third generation cephalosporins retain much of the gram-positive activity of the first and second generation agents, but, have much expanded gram-negative activity. As with the 2nd generation agents, enough variability exists with individual bacterial sensitivities that susceptibility testing is necessary for most bacteria. Ceftazidime is considered an anti-pseudomonal cephalosporin, but resistance development is an issue. A European study (Seol *et al.* 2002) looking at antibiotic susceptibility of *Pseudomonas aeruginosa* isolates obtained from dogs, demonstrated that 77% of strains tested were sensitive to ceftazidime.

Pharmacokinetics
Ceftazidime is not appreciably absorbed after oral administration. In dogs after SC injection, the terminal half-life of ceftazidime was 0.8 hours; a 30 mg/kg dose was above the MIC for *Pseudomonas aeruginosa* for 4.3 hours. When administered as a 4.1 mg/kg/hr constant rate infusion (after a loading dose of 4.4 mg/kg), mean serum concentration was above 165 micrograms/mL. The authors concluded that either dosage regimen would be appropriate treatment for infections in dogs caused by *Pseudomonas*

aeruginosa (Moore *et al.* 2000). Ceftazidime is widely distributed throughout the body, including into bone and CSF and is primarily excreted unchanged by the kidneys via glomerular filtration. As renal tubular excretion does not play a major role in the drug's excretion probenecid does not affect elimination kinetics.

Contraindications/Precautions/Warnings

Only prior allergic reaction to cephalosporins contraindicates ceftazidime's use. In humans documented hypersensitive to penicillin, up to 16% may also be allergic to cephalosporins; veterinary significance is unclear.

Because the drug is primarily excreted via the kidneys, accumulation may result in patients with significantly impaired renal function; use with caution and adjust dose as required.

Adverse Effects

Because veterinary usage of ceftazidime has been very limited, a full adverse effect profile has not been determined for veterinary patients. Gastrointestinal effects have been reported in dogs that have received the drug subcutaneously. When given IM, pain may be noted at the injection site; pain on injection could also occur after SC administration in animals.

Hypersensitivity reactions and gastrointestinal signs have been reported in humans and may or may not apply to veterinary patients. Pseudomembranous colitis (*C. difficile*) may occur with this antibiotic. Increased serum concentrations of liver enzymes have been described in 1–8% of human patients given ceftazidime.

Reproductive/Nursing Safety

In humans, the FDA categorizes this drug as category ***B*** for use during pregnancy (*Animal studies have not yet demonstrated risk to the fetus, but there are no adequate studies in pregnant women; or animal studies have shown an adverse effect, but adequate studies in pregnant women have not demonstrated a risk to the fetus in the first trimester of pregnancy, and there is no evidence of risk in later trimesters.*) No teratogenic effects were demonstrated in studies in pregnant mice and rats given up to 40X labeled doses of ceftazidime.

Because of the drug's low absorbability, it is unlikely to be harmful to nursing offspring, but alterations to GI flora of nursing animals could occur.

Overdosage/Acute Toxicity

An acute overdose in patients with normal renal function is unlikely to be of great concern; but in humans with renal failure, overdosage of ceftazidime has caused seizures, encephalopathy, coma, neuromuscular excitability, asterixis, and myoclonia. Treatment of signs associated with overdose is primarily symptomatic and supportive. Hemodialysis could be used to enhance elimination.

Drug Interactions

The following drug interactions have either been reported or are theoretical in humans or animals receiving ceftazidime and may be of significance in veterinary patients:

- **AMINOGLYCOSIDES/NEPHROTOXIC DRUGS:** The concurrent use of parenteral aminoglycosides or other nephrotoxic drugs (*e.g.*, amphotericin B) with cephalosporins is somewhat controversial. Potentially, cephalosporins could cause additive nephrotoxicity when used with these drugs, but this interaction has only been well documented with cephaloridine (no longer marketed). *In vitro* studies have demonstrated that cephalosporins can have synergistic or additive activity against certain bacteria when used with aminoglycosides, but they should not be mixed together (administer separately).

- **CHLORAMPHENICOL:** May be antagonistic to the ceftazidime's effects on gram-negative bacilli; concurrent use Is not recommended

Laboratory Considerations

- Ceftazidime, like most other cephalosporins, may cause a **false-positive urine glucose** determination when using the cupric sulfate solution test (*e.g.*, *Clinitest*®).

- In humans, ceftazidime rarely causes positive direct antiglobulin (**Coombs'**) tests and increased **prothrombin times**.

- When using Kirby-Bauer disk diffusion procedures for testing susceptibility, a specific 30 microgram ceftazidime disk should be used. An inhibition zone of 18 mm or more indicates susceptibility; 15–17 mm, intermediate; and 14 mm or less, resistant. When using a dilution susceptibility procedure, an organism with a MIC of 8 micrograms/mL or less is considered susceptible; 16 micrograms/mL intermediate; and 32 micrograms/mL or greater is resistant. With either method, infections caused by organisms with intermediate susceptibility may be effectively treated if the infection is limited to tissues where the drug concentrates, or when a higher than normal dose is used.

Doses

- **DOGS:**
  a) For initial antibiotic therapy of gram-negative infections: 25 mg/kg IM or SC q8–12h (Kruth 1998)
  b) For initial treatment of orthopedic infections: 25 mg/kg IV, IM q8–12h;

  For initial treatment of soft tissue infections: 30–50 mg/kg IV, IM q8–12h;

  For initial treatment of sepsis, bacteremia: 15–30 mg/kg IV, IM q6–8h. (Greene & Watson 1998)

■ **CATS:**

a) For initial treatment of systemic infections: 25–30 mg/kg IV, IM or intraosseous q8–12h (Greene & Watson 1998)

■ **REPTILES:**

a) For susceptible infections: 20 mg/kg IM or SC q72hours (every 3 days). (Lewbart 2001)

b) For bacterial infections in snakes, particularly when Enterobacteriaceae or Pseudomonas aeruginosa are confronted: 20 mg/kg IM q72h at 30°C. (Klingenberg 1996), (Johnson, R. 2008)

c) For chelonians: 50 mg/kg IM q24h (Johnson, J. 2002)

Monitoring

■ Efficacy

■ Baseline renal function

Client Information

■ Clients may be instructed to administer this drug SC for outpatient therapy. Be certain they understand the storage and stability issues before dispensing.

Chemistry/Synonyms

A semi-synthetic, third-generation cephalosporin antibiotic, ceftazidime occurs as a white to cream-colored crystalline powder that is slightly soluble in water (5 mg/mL) and insoluble in alcohol, chloroform and ether. The pH of a 0.5% solution in water is between 3 and 4.

Ceftazidime may also be known as ceftazidimum, GR-20263, or LY-139381, *Fortaz®*, *Ceptaz®*, *Tazicef®*, and *Tazidime®*; there are many international trade names.

Storage/Stability

Commercially available powders for injection should be stored at 15–30°C (59–86°F) and protected from light. The commercially available frozen ceftazidime for injection should be stored at temperatures no higher than −20°C (-4°F).

The commercial products containing the sodium carbonate (*Fortaz®*, *Tazicef®*, *Tazidime®*) all release carbon dioxide (effervesce) when reconstituted and are supplied in vials under negative pressure; do not allow pressure to normalize before adding diluent. The product containing arginine (*Ceptaz®*), does not effervesce.

Once reconstituted, the solution retains potency for 24 hours (18 hours for arginine formulation) at room temperature and 7 days when refrigerated. Solutions frozen in the original glass vial after reconstitution with sterile water are stable for 3 months when stored at −20°C (-4°F). While no stability data was located, veterinarians have anecdotally reported efficacy when individual dosages are frozen in plastic syringes. Once thawed, they should not be refrozen. Thawed solutions are stable for 8 hours at room temperature and 4 days when refrigerated.

Compatibility/Compounding Considerations

Ceftazidime is **compatible** with the following diluents when being prepared for IM (or SC) injection: sterile or bacteriostatic water for injection, 0.5% or 1% lidocaine. Once reconstituted it is **compatible** with the more commonly used IV fluids, including: D5W, normal saline or half-normal saline, Ringer's, or lactated Ringer's.

Do not use sodium bicarbonate solution for a diluent; it is not recommended to mix with aminoglycosides, vancomycin or metronidazole.

Dosage Forms/Regulatory Status

VETERINARY-LABELED PRODUCTS: None

HUMAN-LABELED PRODUCTS:

Ceftazidime Powder for Injection: 500 mg, 1 g, 2 g, & 6 g in 20 mL & 100 mL vials, infusion packs, *ADD-Vantage* vials & piggyback vials; *Fortaz®* & *Ceptaz®* (GlaxoWellcome); *Tazicef®* (Hospira); *Tazidime®* (Eli Lilly); (Rx)

Ceftazidime Injection: 1 g & 2 g premixed, frozen in 50 mL*Fortaz®* (GlaxoWellcome); 1 & 2 g in *Galaxy* containers; *Tazicef®* (Hospira); (Rx)

References

Greene, C & A Watson (1998). Antimicrobial Drug Formulary. *Infectious Diseases of the Dog and Cat.* C Greene Ed. Philadelphia, WB Saunders: 790–919.

Johnson, J (2002). Medical management of ill chelonians. Proceedings: Western Veterinary Conference. Accessed via: Veterinary Information Network. http://goo.gl/NTerN

Johnson, R (2008). Critical care of reptiles. Proccedings: AAVAC-UEP. Accessed via: Veterinary Information Network. http://goo.gl/ZeIou

Klingenberg, R (1996). Therapeutics. *Reptile Medicine and Surgery.* D Mader Ed. Philadelphia, Saunders: 299–321.

Kruth, S (1998). Gram–negative bacterial infections. *Infectious Diseases of the Dog and Cat.* C Greene Ed. Philadelphia, Saunders: 217–226.

Lewbart (2001). Reptile Formulary. Proceedings: Atlantic Coast Veterinary Conference. Accessed via: Veterinary Information Network. http://goo.gl/EEQmM

Moore, K, L Trepanier, et al. (2000). Pharmacokinetics of ceftazidime in dogs following subcutaneous administration and constant infusion and association with in vitro susceptibility of Pseudomonas aeruginosa. *Am J Vet Res* **61**(10): 1204–1208.

Seol, N, T Naglic, et al. (2002). In vitro antimicrobial susceptibility of 182 Pseudomonas aeruginosa strains isolated from dogs to selected antipseudomonal agents. *J Vet Med B Infect Dis Vet Public Health* **49**(4): 188–192.

CEFTIOFUR CRYSTALLINE FREE ACID

(sef-*tee*-oh-fur)   Excede®

3RD GENERATION CEPHALOSPORIN

Prescriber Highlights

▶ Veterinary-only 3rd generation cephalosporin labeled for use in cattle, horses & swine

▶ Potentially could cause hypersensitivity reactions, granulocytopenia, thrombocytopenia, or diarrhea

▶ Administered SC at the posterior aspect of ear in cattle; administered IM in swine

▶ Shake well prior to use

Uses/Indications

In beef, lactating and non-lactating cattle, ceftiofur crystalline free acid (CCFA) is labeled for the treatment of bovine respiratory disease (BRD, shipping fever, pneumonia) associated with *Mannheimia haemolytica, Pasteurella multocida, and Histophilus somni* and for the control of respiratory disease in cattle at high risk of developing BRD associated with *M. haemolytica, P. multocida, and H. somni.* It is also indicated for the treatment of foot rot (interdigital necrobacillosis) associated with *Fusobacterium necrophorum* and *Porphyromonas levii.*

In swine, ceftiofur CFAis labeled for the treatment of swine respiratory disease (SRD) associated with *Actinobacillus pleuropneumoniae, Pasteurella multocida, Haemophilus parasuis,* and *Streptococcus suis.*

In horses, ceftiofur CFA is FDA-approved for the treatment of lower respiratory tract infections caused by susceptible strains of *Streptococcus equi* ssp. *zooepidemicus.*

Pharmacology/Actions

Ceftiofur is a 3rd generation cephalosporin antibiotic active against a variety of gram-positive and gram-negative bacteria and like other cephalosporins, inhibits bacteria cell wall synthesis; it is usually bactericidal and is a time-dependent antibiotic.

After administration, the parent compound (ceftiofur) is rapidly cleaved into furoic acid and desfuroylceftiofur (active). Desfuroylceftiofur inhibits cell wall synthesis (at stage three) of susceptible multiplying bacteria and exhibits a spectrum of activity similar to that of cefotaxime. Parent ceftiofur and the primary metabolite are equally potent and assays to measure microbial sensitivity (plasma and tissue levels) are based on ceftiofur equivalents referred to as CE. The protein binding activity of ceftiofur creates a "reservoir effect" to maintain active levels at the site of infection.

In cattle, ceftiofur has a broad range of *in vitro* activity against a variety of pathogens including many species of Pasteurella, Streptococcus, Staphylococcus, Salmonella, and *E. coli.*

In Swine, ceftiofur CFA at a single IM dosage of 2.27 mg/lb (5 mg/kg) BW provides concentrations of ceftiofur and desfuroylceftiofur-related metabolites in plasma that are multiples above the MIC90 for an extended period of time for the swine respiratory disease (SRD) label pathogens *Actinobacillus pleuropneumoniae, Pasteurella multocida, Haemophilus parasuis* and *Streptococcus suis.*

Pharmacokinetics

In cattle, subcutaneous administration of ceftiofur CFA, in the middle third of the posterior aspect of the ear (middle third of the ear) of beef and non-lactating dairy cattle, or in the posterior aspect of the ear where it attaches to the head (base of the ear) of beef, non-lactating dairy, and lactating dairy cattle, provides therapeutic concentrations of ceftiofur and desfuroylceftiofur-related metabolites in plasma above the MIC90 for the bovine respiratory disease (BRD) label pathogens, *Pasteurella multocida, Mannheimia haemolytica* and *Histophilus somni* for generally not less than 150 hours after single administration.

Pharmacokinetic studies indicate that base of ear administrations (BOE) in dairy cattle are consistent with middle of ear (MOE) administration in beef cattle with blood levels at therapeutic threshold within 2 hours of administration at labeled doses.

The systemic safety of ceftiofur concentrations resulting from product administration at the base of the ear was established via a pharmacokinetic comparison of the two routes of administration (base of the ear versus middle third of the ear). Based upon the results of this relative bioavailability study, the two routes of administration are therapeutically equivalent.

In swine, therapeutic plasma levels for the parent compound and primary metabolite, desfuroylceftiofur, are reached within 1 hour of treatment. Plasma levels remained above the MIC for nearly 100% of target swine respiratory disease (SRD) pathogens for an average of 8 days.

In horses, ceftiofur CFA at 6.6 mg/kg IM is relatively slowly absorbed and eliminated. After the first dose the time to peak serum level is about 22 hours and after a second dose 96 hours apart from the first, time to peak was about 16 hours. When dosed at this regiment the drug and its active metabolites stay above the determined therapeutic concentration (0.2 micrograms/mL) for susceptible strains of *Streptococcus equi* spp. *zooepidemicus* for 10 days.

Contraindications/Precautions/Warnings

Cephalosporins are contraindicated in patients with a history of hypersensitivity to them. Because there may be cross-reactivity, use cephalosporins cautiously in patients who are documented hypersensitive to other beta-lactam antibiotics (e.g., penicillins, cefamycins, carbapenems).

Hypersensitivity reactions unrelated to dose can occur with these agents and can manifest as rashes, fever, eosinophilia, lymphadenopathy, or full-blown anaphylaxis. The use of cephalosporins in patients documented to be hypersensitive to penicillin-class antibiotics is controversial. In humans, it is estimated 1−15% of patients hypersensitive to penicillins will also be hypersensitive to cephalosporins. The incidence of cross-reactivity in veterinary patients is unknown.

Avoid direct contact of the product with the skin, eyes, mouth and clothing. Sensitization of the skin may be avoided by wearing latex gloves. Persons with a known hypersensitivity to penicillin or cephalosporins should avoid exposure to this product.

Administration of ceftiofur free acid into the ear arteries is likely to result in sudden death in cattle.

Following label use as a single treatment in cattle, slaughter withdrawal time = 13 days and zero day (no) milk discard time. Extra-label drug use may result in violative residues. A withdrawal period has not been established for this product in pre-ruminating calves; do not use in calves to be processed for veal.

In swine, slaughter withdrawal is 14 days. A maximum of 2 mL of formulation should be injected at each injection site. Injection volumes in excess of 2 mL may result in violative residues.

In horses, the manufacturer warns that if acute diarrhea is observed after dosing, additional doses should not be administered and appropriate therapy should be initiated. Use has not been evaluated in horses less than 4 months of age and inbreeding, pregnant, or lactating horses. The long-term effects on injection sites have not been evaluated. Additonally the manufacturer warns that due to the extended exposure in horses, based on the drug's pharmacokinetic properties, adverse reactions may require prolonged care. Approximately 17 days are needed to eliminate 97% of the dose from the body. Animals experiencing adverse reactions may need to be monitored for this duration of time.

Adverse Effects

Adverse effects with the cephalosporins are usually not serious and have a relatively low frequency of occurrence, but cephalosporins can cause allergic reactions in sensitized individuals. Topical exposures to such antimicrobials, including ceftiofur, may elicit mild to severe allergic reactions in some individuals. Repeated or prolonged exposure may lead to sensitization.

In cattle, administration of ceftiofur free acid into the ear arteries is likely to result in sudden death. Following SC injection in the middle third of the posterior aspect of the ear, thickening and swelling (characterized by aseptic cellular infiltrate) of the ear may occur. As with other parenteral injections, localized post-injection bacterial infections may result in abscess formation; attention to hygienic procedures can minimize occurrence. Following SC injections at the posterior aspect of the ear where it attaches to the head (base of the ear), areas of discoloration and signs of inflammation may persist at least 13 days post administration resulting in trim loss of edible tissue at slaughter. Injection of volumes greater than 20 mL in the middle third of the ear, may result in open draining lesions in a small percentage of cattle.

In horses, ceftiofur CFA may cause swelling at the injection site and diarrhea, soft or loose stools.

Reproductive/Nursing Safety

The manufacturer states that the effects of ceftiofur on bovine reproductive performance, pregnancy, and lactation have not been determined and the safety of ceftiofur has not been demonstrated for pregnant swine or swine intended for breeding. However, cephalosporins as a class are relatively safe to use during pregnancy, and teratogenic or embryotoxic effects would not be anticipated.

Target animal safety studies report administration of a single dose of ceftiofur free acid at the base of the ear to high-producing dairy cattle did not adversely affect milk production compared to untreated controls. Ceftiofur in maternal milk would unlikely pose significant risk to offspring.

Overdosage/Acute Toxicity

Cephalosporin overdoses are unlikely to cause significant problems other than GI distress, but other effects are possible (see Adverse Effects section). Use of dosages in excess of 6.6 mg ceftiofur equivalents (CE)/kg or administration by unapproved routes in cattle (subcutaneous injection in the neck or intramuscular injection) may cause violative residues. Dosages in excess of 5 mg ceftiofur equivalents (CE)/kg or administration by an unapproved route in swine may result in illegal residues in edible tissues. Contact FARAD (see appendix) for assistance in determining appropriate withdrawal times in circumstances where the drug has been used at higher than labeled dosages.

Drug Interactions

Although the manufacturer does not list any drug interactions on the label for ceftiofur, the following drug interactions have either been reported or are theoretical in humans or animals receiving injectable 3rd generation cephalosporins and may be of significance in veterinary patients receiving ceftiofur:

■ **AMINOGLYCOSIDES/NEPHROTOXIC DRUGS:** The concurrent use of parenteral aminoglycosides or other nephrotoxic drugs (*e.g.,* amphotericin B) with cephalosporins is somewhat controversial. Potentially, cephalosporins could cause additive nephrotoxicity when used with these drugs, but this interaction has only been well documented with cephaloridine (no longer marketed). *In vitro* studies have demonstrated that cephalosporins can have synergistic or additive activity against certain bacteria when used with aminoglycosides, but they should not be mixed together (administer separately).

■ **PROBENECID:** Competitively blocks the tubular secretion of most cephalosporins, thereby increasing serum levels and serum half-lives

Laboratory Considerations

Note: Ceftiofur is structurally similar to cefotaxime and it is not known if these interactions occur with ceftiofur.

■ Except for cefotaxime, cephalosporins may cause false-positive **urine glucose determinations** when using cupric sulfate solution (Benedict's Solution, *Clinitest®*). Tests utilizing glucose oxidase (*Tes-Tape®, Clinistix®*) are not affected by cephalosporins.

■ When using the Jaffe reaction to measure **serum or urine creatinine**, cephalosporins (not ceftazidime or cefotaxime) in high dosages may falsely cause elevated values.

■ In humans, particularly with azotemia, cephalosporins have caused a false-positive direct **Coombs' test**.

■ Cephalosporins may also cause falsely elevated **17-ketosteroid** values in urine.

Doses

■ **CATTLE:**

Beef and lactating cattle treatment dose: Administer as a single SC injection in the posterior aspect of the ear where it attaches to the head at the *base of the ear* to cattle at 3 mg per lb (6.6 mg ceftiofur equivalents per kg) body weight (1.5 mL sterile suspension per 100 lb body weight). The approved site of injection in lactating dairy cattle is at the base of the ear (BOE). (*Excede® Sterile Suspension*; Package Insert—Pfizer)

Beef and non-lactating dairy cattle treatment dose: Administer as a single SC injection in the *middle third* of the posterior aspect of the ear at a dosage of 6.6 mg ceftiofur equivalents/kg body weight (1.5 mL sterile suspension per 100 lb body weight).

Most animals will respond to treatment within 3–5 days. If no improvement is observed, the diagnosis should be reevaluated. Administration of ceftiofur free acid into the ear arteries is likely to result in sudden death in cattle.

Beef and non-lactating dairy cattle control dose: Administer as a SC injection either in the middle third of the posterior aspect of the ear or in the posterior aspect of the ear where it attaches to the head (base of the ear) to beef and non-lactating dairy cattle at a dosage of 6.6 mg ceftiofur equivalents (CE)/kg body weight (1.5 mL sterile suspension per 100 lb body weight). See package insert for graphics depicting locations of injection and anatomical landmarks to avoid. (*Excede® Sterile Suspension*; Package Insert—Pfizer)

■ **SWINE:**

Administer by IM injection in the post-auricular region of the neck as a single dosage of 2.27 mg ceftiofur equivalents (CE) per lb (5 mg CE/kg) body weight (BW). This is equivalent to 1 mL sterile suspension per 44 lb (20 kg) BW. No more than 2 mL should be injected in a single injection site

Injection volumes in excess of 2 mL may result in violative residues. Pigs heavier than 88 lb (40 kg) will require more than one injection.

Most animals will respond to treatment within 3–5 days. If no improvement is observed, the diagnosis should be reevaluated. (*Excede® For Swine*; Package Insert—Pfizer)

■ **HORSES:**

For lower respiratory tract infections caused by susceptible strains of *Streptococcus equi* ssp. *zooepidemicus*: 6.6 mg/kg IM; repeat in 4 days. A maximum of 20 mL per injection site may be administered. Shake well before using. (*Excede® Sterile Suspension*; Package Insert—Pfizer)

Monitoring

Because cephalosporins usually have minimal toxicity associated with their use, monitoring for efficacy is usually all that is required. Some clinicians recommend weekly CBC monitoring of small animals receiving ceftiofur. Patients with diminished renal function may require intensified renal monitoring. Serum levels and therapeutic drug monitoring are not routinely done with these agents.

Chemistry/Synonyms

Ceftiofur CFA has a molecular weight of 523.58.

Ceftiofur CFA may also be known as CM-31916, ceftiofuri, or *Excede®*.

Storage/Stability

Ceftiofur CFA cattle and swine products should be stored at controlled room temperature 20–25 °C (68–77°F). Shake well before using. Contents should be used within 12 weeks after the first dose is removed.

Dosage Forms/Regulatory Status

VETERINARY-LABELED PRODUCTS:

Ceftiofur Crystalline Free Acid equivalent to 200 mg/mL ceftiofur (in a *Miglyol®* cottonseed oil based suspension) in 100 mL vials; *Excede®* (Pfizer). FDA-approved for use in beef, lactating and non-lactating cattle. If used in an extralabel manner, contact FARAD (see appendix) for guidance in determining withdrawal times for milk or meat.

Ceftiofur Crystalline Free Acid equivalent to 100 mg/mL ceftiofur (in a *Miglyol®* cottonseed oil based suspension) in 100 mL vials; *Excede® for Swine* (Pfizer);

HUMAN-LABELED PRODUCTS: None

CEFTIOFUR HCL

(sef-*tee*-oh-fur)   Excenel®, Spectramast®

3RD GENERATION CEPHALOSPORIN

Prescriber Highlights

▶ A veterinary-only 3rd generation cephalosporin

▶ Potentially could cause hypersensitivity reactions, granulocytopenia, thrombocytopenia, or diarrhea

▶ Causes pain on IM injection to small animals

▶ May need to reduce dose in renal failure

Uses/Indications

In swine, ceftiofur HCl injection is labeled for the treatment and control of swine bacterial respiratory disease (swine bacterial pneumonia) associated with *Actinobacillus (Haemophilus) pleuropneumoniae, Pasteurella multocida, Salmonella choleraesuis* and *Streptococcus suis.*

In cattle, ceftiofur HCl is labeled for the treatment of the following bacterial diseases: Bovine respiratory disease (BRD, shipping fever, pneumonia) associated with *Mannheimia haemolytica, Pasteurella multocida,* and *Histophilus somni;* Acute bovine interdigital necrobacillosis (foot rot, pododermatitis) associated with *Fusobacterium necrophorum* and *Bacteroides melaninogenicus;* and acute metritis (0–14 days post-partum) associated with bacterial organisms susceptible to ceftiofur.

The intramammary syringe for dry dairy cattle (*Spectramast DC®*) is labeled for the treatment of subclinical mastitis in dairy cattle at the time of dry off associated with *Staphylococcus aureus, Streptococcus dysgalactiae,* and *Streptococcus uberis.* The intramammary syringe for lactating dairy cattle (*Spectramast LC®*) is labeled for the treatment of clinical mastitis in lactating dairy cattle associated with coagulase-negative staphylococci, *Streptococcus dysgalactiae,* and *Escherichia coli.*

Pharmacology

Ceftiofur is a 3rd generation cephalosporin antibiotic active against a variety of gram-positive and gram-negative bacteria and like other cephalosporins inhibits bacteria cell wall synthesis; it is usually bactericidal and is a time-dependent antibiotic.

After administration, the parent compound (ceftiofur) is rapidly cleaved into furoic acid and desfuroylceftiofur (active). Desfuroylceftiofur inhibits cell wall synthesis (at stage three) of susceptible multiplying bacteria and exhibits a spectrum of activity similar to that of cefotaxime. Parent ceftiofur and the primary metabolite are equally potent and assays to measure microbial sensitivity (plasma and tissue levels) are based on ceftiofur equivalents referred to as CE. The protein binding activity of ceftiofur creates a "reservoir effect" to maintain active levels at the site of infection.

In cattle, ceftiofur has a broad range of *in vitro* activity against a variety of pathogens, including many species of Pasturella, Streptococcus, Staphylococcus, Salmonella, and *E. coli.*

In swine, ceftiofur HCl has activity against the pathogens *Actinobacillus pleuropneumoniae, Pasteurella multocida, Haemophilus parasuis* and *Streptococcus suis* for an extended period of time.

Pharmacokinetics

In cattle and swine, ceftiofur is rapidly metabolized to desfuroylceftiofur, the primary metabolite. In cattle, ceftiofur sodium and HCl have practically equivalent pharmacokinetic parameters. The following pharmacokinetic values for cattle are for the active metabolite desfuroylceftiofur. The volume of distribution in cattle is about 0.3 L/kg. Peak levels are about 7 micrograms/mL after IM injection of ceftiofur sodium (*Naxcel®*), but areas under the curve are practically equal as well as elimination half-lives (approx. 8–12 hours).

The elimination kinetics of ceftiofur HCl in milk when used in an extralabel manner to treat coliform mastitis has been studied. Milk samples were tested after two, 300 mg doses (6 mL), administered 12 hours apart into the affected mammary quarters. The samples tested at less than the tolerance level for this drug set by FDA by 7 hours after the last intramammary administration. However, the authors noted considerable variability in the time required for samples from individual cows and mammary gland quarters to consistently show drug residues less than the tolerance level and reported that elimination rates of the drug may be related to milk production. Therefore, cows producing smaller volumes of milk many have prolonged withdrawal times. (Smith *et al.* 2004)

In lactating dairy cattle, active ceftiofur concentrations were measured after the administration of 1 mg/kg SC in healthy dairy cattle within 24 hours of calving. Drug concentrations were found to exceed MIC in uterine tissues and lochial fluid for common pathogens (Okker *et al.* 2002).

In swine, a study measuring tissue distribution following IM injection of varying doses revealed the highest concentration were detected in the kidneys, followed by lungs, liver and muscle tissue (Beconi-Barker *et al.* 1996). In swine, the intramuscular bioavailability of the ceftiofur sodium salt and the hydrochloride salt at doses of 3mg/kg or 5mg/kg were compared. The study reported similar therapeutic efficacy for both salt forms (Brown *et al.* 1999).

Contraindications/Precautions/Warnings

Cephalosporins are contraindicated in patients with a history of hypersensitivity to them. Because there may be cross-reactivity, use cephalosporins cautiously in patients who are documented hypersensitive to other beta-lactam antibiotics (*e.g.*, penicillins, cefamycins, carbapenems).

In swine, areas of discoloration associated with the injection site at time periods of 11 days or less may result in trim-out of edible tissues at slaughter.

In cattle, after intramuscular or subcutaneous administration in the neck, areas of discoloration at the site may persist beyond 11 days resulting in trim loss of edible tissues at slaughter. Following intramuscular administration in the rear leg, areas of discoloration at the injection site may persist beyond 28 days resulting in trim loss of edible tissues at slaughter.

Swine treated with ceftiofur HCl (*Excenel® RTU*) must not be slaughtered for 4 days following the last treatment.

Cattle treated with ceftiofur HCl (*Excenel® RTU*) must not be slaughtered for 3 days following the last treatment. There is no required milk discard time.

Cattle treated with *Spectramast DC®*, must not be slaughtered for 16 days following the last treatment. Milk taken from cows completing a 30 day dry cow period may be used with no milk discard. Following label use, no slaughter withdrawal period is required for neonatal calves born from treated cows regardless of colostrum consumption.

Cattle treated with *Spectramast LC®*, must not be slaughtered for 2 days following the last treatment. Milk taken from cows during treatment and for 72 hours after the last treatment must be discarded.

Patients in renal failure may need dosage adjustments.

Adverse Effects

Adverse effects with the cephalosporins are usually not serious and have a relatively low frequency of occurrence.

Hypersensitivity reactions unrelated to dose can occur with these agents and can manifest as rashes, fever, eosinophilia, lymphadenopathy, or full-blown anaphylaxis. The use of cephalosporins in patients documented to be hypersensitive to penicillin-class antibiotics is controversial. In humans, it is estimated 1–15% of patients hypersensitive to penicillins will also be hypersensitive to cephalosporins. The incidence of cross-reactivity in veterinary patients is unknown.

Swine safety data: results from a five-day tolerance study in normal feeder pigs indicated that ceftiofur sodium was well tolerated when administered at 125 mg ceftiofur equivalents/kg BW (more than 25 times the highest recommended daily dosage) for five consecutive days. Ceftiofur administered intramuscularly to pigs produced no overt adverse signs of toxicity.

Cattle safety data: results from a five-day tolerance study in feeder calves indicated that ceftiofur sodium was well tolerated at 55 mg ceftiofur equivalents/kg BW (25 times the highest recommended dose) for five consecutive days. Ceftiofur administered intramuscularly had no adverse systemic effects.

Reproductive/Nursing Safety

The effects of ceftiofur on cattle and swine reproductive performance, pregnancy, and lactation have not been determined. However, cephalosporins as a class are relatively safe to use during pregnancy, and teratogenic or embryotoxic effects would not be anticipated.

Overdosage/Acute Toxicity

Cephalosporin overdoses are unlikely to cause significant problems other than GI distress, but other effects are possible (see Adverse Effects section).

Cephalosporin overdoses are unlikely to cause significant problems other than GI distress, but other effects are possible (see Adverse Effects section). Use of dosages in excess of those labeled or by unapproved routes of administration may cause violative residues. Contact FARAD (see appendix) for assistance in determining appropriate withdrawal times in circumstances where the drug has been used at higher than labeled dosages.

Drug Interactions

Although the manufacturer does not list any drug interactions on the label for ceftiofur, the following drug interactions have either been reported or are theoretical in humans or animals receiving injectable 3rd generation cephalosporins and may be of significance in veterinary patients receiving injectable ceftiofur:

■ **AMINOGLYCOSIDES/NEPHROTOXIC DRUGS:** The concurrent use of parenteral aminoglycosides or other nephrotoxic drugs (*e.g.*, amphotericin B) with cephalosporins is somewhat controversial. Potentially, cephalosporins could cause additive nephrotoxicity when used with these drugs, but this interaction has only been well documented with cephaloridine (no longer marketed). *In vitro* studies have demonstrated that cephalosporins can have synergistic or additive activity against certain bacteria when used with aminoglycosides, but they should not be mixed together (administer separately).

■ **PROBENECID:** Competitively blocks the tubular secretion of most cephalosporins thereby increasing serum levels and serum half-lives

Laboratory Considerations

Note: Ceftiofur is structurally similar to cefotaxime and it is not known if these interactions occur with ceftiofur.

■ Except for cefotaxime, cephalosporins may cause false-positive **urine glucose determinations** when using cupric sulfate solution (Benedict's Solution, *Clinitest®*). Tests utilizing glucose oxidase (*Tes-Tape®, Clinistix®*) are not affected by cephalosporins.

■ When using the Jaffe reaction to measure **serum or urine creatinine**, cephalosporins (not ceftazidime or cefotaxime) in high dosages may falsely cause elevated values.

■ In humans, particularly with azotemia, cephalosporins have caused a false-positive direct **Coombs' test.**

■ Cephalosporins may also cause falsely elevated **17-ketosteroid** values in urine.

Doses

■ **SWINE:**

a) Administer IM at 3 to 5 mg/kg body weight (1 mL of sterile suspension per 22 to 37 lb body weight). Treatment should be repeated at 24–hour intervals for a total of three consecutive days. (*Excenel® RTU;* Package Insert—Pfizer)

■ **CATTLE:**

For bovine respiratory disease and acute bovine interdigital necrobacillosis:

a) Administer IM or SC at 1.1 to 2.2 mg/kg (1 to 2 mL sterile suspension per 100 lb) daily for a total of three consecutive days. Additional treatments may be administered on Days 4 and 5 for animals which do not show a satisfactory response. For or BRD only, administer IM or SC 2.2 mg/kg every other day on Days 1 and 3 (48h interval). Do not inject more than 15 mL per injection site. (*Excenel® RTU;* Package Insert—Pfizer)

For acute post-partum metritis:

a) Administer by IM or SC 2.2 mg/kg (2 mL sterile suspension per 100 lb) daily for five consecutive days. Do not inject more than 15 mL per injection site. (*Excenel® RTU;* Package Insert—Pfizer)

For neonatal salmonellosis:

a) Ceftiofur HCl 5 mg/kg IM once daily for 5 days (Fecteau *et al.* 2002)

For the treatment of subclinical mastitis in dairy cattle at time of dry off associated with *Staphylococcus aureus, Streptococcus dysgalactiae* or *Streptococcus uberis*:

a) Infuse one syringe of *Spectramast® DC* into each affected quarter at the time of dry off. (*Spectramast® DC*; Package Insert—Pfizer)

For the treatment of clinical mastitis in lactating dairy cattle associated with coagulase-negative staphylococci *Streptococcus dysgalactiae* or *E. coli*:

a) Infuse one syringe of *Spectramast® LC* into each affected quarter. Repeat this treatment in 24 hours. For extended duration therapy, once daily treatment may be repeated for up to 8 consecutive days. (*Spectramast® LC* Package Insert—Pfizer)

Monitoring

Because cephalosporins usually have minimal toxicity associated with their use, monitoring for efficacy is usually all that is required. Some clinicians recommend weekly CBC monitoring of small animals receiving ceftiofur. Patients with diminished renal function may require intensified renal monitoring. Serum levels and therapeutic drug monitoring are not routinely performed with these agents.

Chemistry/Synonyms

Ceftiofur HCl is a semisynthetic 3rd generation cephalosporin. Ceftiofur HCl is a weak acid and is acid stable and water-soluble with a molecular weight of 560. The injectable sterile suspension in a ready to use formulation that contains ceftiofur hydrochloride equivalent to 50 mg ceftiofur, 0.50 mg phospholipon, 1.5 mg sorbitan monooleate, 2.25 mg sterile water for injection, and cottonseed oil. Both *Spectramast®* products are sterile, oil based suspensions of ceftiofur HCl.

Ceftiofur HCl may also be known as U-64279A, ceftiofuri hydrochloridium or *Excenel RTU®*.

Storage/Stability

The ready-to-use injectable product should be stored at controlled room temperature 20 to 25 °C (68 to 77 °F). Shake well before using; protect from freezing.

The intramammary syringes should be stored at controlled room temperature 20 to 25 °C (68 to 77 °F). Protect from light. Store plastets in carton until used.

Dosage Forms/Regulatory Status

VETERINARY-LABELED PRODUCTS:

Ceftiofur HCL Sterile Suspension for injection, 50 mg/mL in 100 mL vials; *Excenel RTU®* (Pharmacia/Upjohn); (Rx). FDA-approved for use in cattle and swine. Slaughter withdrawal = 3 days in cattle, and 4 days in swine. There is no required milk discard time.

Ceftiofur HCl Sterile Suspension for Intramammary Infusion in Dry Cows 500 mg ceftiofur equivalents (as the HCl) per 10 mL syringe (plastets) in packages of 12 syringes with 70% isopropyl alcohol pads; *Spectramast® DC* (Pfizer); (Rx) Slaughter withdrawal for cattle = 16 days (no slaughter withdrawal required for neonatal calves born from treated cows)

Ceftiofur HCl Sterile Suspension for Intramammary Infusion in Lactating Cows 125 mg ceftiofur equivalents (as the HCl) per 10 mL syringe (plastets) in packages of 12 syringes with 70% isopropyl alcohol pads; *Spectramast® LC* (Pfizer); (Rx) Cattle slaughter withdrawal = 2 days; milk discard = 72 hours

HUMAN-LABELED PRODUCTS: None

References

Beconi–Barker, M, R Hornish, et al. (1996). Ceftiofur hydrochloride: plasma and tissue distribution in swine following intramuscular administration at various doses. *J Vet Phamacol Ther* 19(3): 192–199.

Brown, S, B Hanson, et al. (1999). Comparison of plasma pharmacokinetics and bioavailability of ceftiofur sodium and ceftiofur hydrochloride in pigs after a single intramuscular injection. *J Vet Phamacol Ther* 22: 35–40.

Fecteau, M–E, J House, et al. (2002). Efficacy of ceftiofur for treatment of bovine neonatal salmonellosis. Proceedings: ACVIM Forum. Accessed via: Veterinary Information Network. http://goo.gl/Ndw9q

Okker, H, SE J., et al. (2002). Pharmacokinetics of ceftiofur in plasma and uterine secretions and tissues after subcutaneous postpartum administration in lactating dairy cows. *J Vet Phamacol Ther* 25: 33–38.

Smith, G, R Gehring, et al. (2004). Elimination kinetics of ceftiofur hydrochloride after intramammary administration in lactating dairy cows. *JAVMA* 224(11).

CEFTIOFUR SODIUM

(sef-*tee*-oh-fur)   Naxcel®

3RD GENERATION CEPHALOSPORIN

Prescriber Highlights

▶ A veterinary-only 3rd generation cephalosporin

▶ Potentially could cause hypersensitivity reactions, granulocytopenia, thrombocytopenia, or diarrhea

▶ Causes pain on IM injection to small animals

▶ May need to reduce dose in patients with renal failure

Monograph by Elaine Lust, PharmD

Uses/Indications

Labeled indications for ceftiofur sodium:

In cattle for treatment of bovine respiratory disease (shipping fever, pneumonia) associated with *Mannheimia haemolytica*, *Pasteurella multocida* and *Histophilus somni*. It is also indicated for treatment of acute bovine interdigital necrobacillosis (foot rot, pododermatitis) associated with *Fusobacterium necrophorum* and *Bacteroides melaninogenicus*.

In swine for treatment/control of swine bacterial respiratory disease (swine bacterial pneumonia) associated with *Actinobacillus (Haemophilus) pleuropneumoniae*, *Pasteurella multocida*, *Salmonella choleraesuis* and *Streptococcus suis*.

In sheep/goats for treatment of sheep/caprine respiratory disease (sheep/goat pneumonia) associated with *Mannheimia haemolytica* and *Pasteurella multocida*.

In horses for treatment of respiratory infections in horses associated with *Streptococcus zooepidemicus*.

In dogs for the treatment of canine urinary tract infections associated with *E. coli* and *Proteus mirabilis*.

In day old chicks/poults for the control of early mortality, associated with *E. coli* organisms susceptible to ceftiofur.

Ceftiofur sodium has also been used in an extra-label manner in a variety of veterinary species (see Doses) to treat infections that likely to be susceptible to a 3rd generation cephalosporin.

Pharmacology/Actions

Ceftiofur is a 3rd generation cephalosporin antibiotic active against a variety of gram-positive and gram-negative bacteria and like other cephalosporins inhibits bacteria cell wall synthesis, is usually bactericidal and is a time-dependent antibiotic.

Ceftiofur is rapidly cleaved into furoic acid and desfuroylceftiofur, which is active. Desfuroylceftiofur inhibits cell wall synthesis (at stage three) of susceptible multiplying bacteria and exhibits a spectrum of activity similar to that of cefotaxime. It has a broad range of *in vitro* activity against a variety of pathogens, including many species of Pasteurella, Streptococcus, Staphylococcus, Salmonella, and *E. coli*.

Pharmacokinetics

In cattle, ceftiofur sodium and HCl have practically equivalent pharmacokinetic parameters. The following pharmacokinetic values for cattle are for the active metabolite desfuroylceftiofur. The volume of distribution in cattle is about 0.3 L/kg. Peak levels are about 7 micrograms/mL after IM injection of *Naxcel®*, but areas under the curve are practically equal as well as elimination half-lives (approx. 8–12 hours). Peak levels occur 30–45 minutes after IM dosing. Pharmacokinetic parameters of ceftiofur sodium are very similar for either SC or IM injection in cattle.

In dairy goats, dosing at 1.1 mg/kg or 2.2 mg/kg, administered IV or IM, demonstrated 100% bioavailability via the IM route. After 5 daily IM doses of the drug, serum concentrations were found to be dose-proportional (Courtin *et al.* 1997).

In horses, 2 grams of ceftiofur were administered via regional IV perfusion or systemic IV to determine radiocarpal joint synovial fluid and plasma concentrations. Mean synovial fluid concentrations were higher for the regional IV perfusion than systemic IV administration. The study concluded regional IV perfusion induced significantly higher intraarticular antibiotic concentrations in the radiocarpal joint compared to systemic IV administration. Additionally, synovial fluid drug concentrations remained above the MIC for common pathogens for more than 24 hours (Pille *et al.* 2005).

Contraindications/Precautions/Warnings

Cephalosporins are contraindicated in patients with a history of hypersensitivity to the drug. Because there may be cross-reactivity, use cephalosporins cautiously in patients who are documented hypersensitive to other beta-lactam antibiotics (*e.g.*, penicillins, cefamycins, carbapenems).

Hypersensitivity reactions unrelated to dose can occur with these agents and can manifest as rashes, fever, eosinophilia, lymphadenopathy, or full-blown anaphylaxis. The use of cephalosporins in patients documented to be hypersensitive to penicillin-class antibiotics is controversial. In humans, it is estimated 1−15% of patients hypersensitive to penicillins will also be hypersensitive to cephalosporins. The incidence of cross-reactivity in veterinary patients is unknown.

Withdrawal times: Cattle: 4-day slaughter withdrawal time is required. No milk discard time is required. Swine: A 4-day slaughter withdrawal time is required. Sheep/Goats: No slaughter withdrawal time or milk discard time is required. Not to be used in horses intended for human consumption.

Patients in renal failure may need dosage adjustments.

Adverse Effects

Adverse effects with the cephalosporins are usually not serious and have a relatively low frequency of occurrence. The use of ceftiofur may result in some signs of immediate and transient local pain to the animal. Following subcutaneous administration of ceftiofur sodium in the neck, small areas of discoloration at the site may persist beyond five days, potentially resulting in trim loss of edible tissues at slaughter. Localized post-injection bacterial infections may result in abscess formation in cattle. Attention to hygienic procedures can minimize their occurrence.

The administration of antimicrobials to horses under conditions of stress may be associated with acute diarrhea that could be fatal. If acute diarrhea is observed, discontinue use of this antimicrobial and initiate appropriate therapy. One report however, found that ceftiofur administered to horses (4 mg/kg IM) had minimal effects on fecal flora (Clark & Dowling 2005).

Hypersensitivity reactions unrelated to dose can occur with these agents and can manifest as rashes, fever, eosinophilia, lymphadenopathy, or full-blown anaphylaxis. The use of cephalosporins in patients documented to be hypersensitive to penicillin-class antibiotics is controversial. In humans, it is estimated 1−15% of patients hypersensitive to penicillins will also be hypersensitive to cephalosporins. The incidence of cross-reactivity in veterinary patients is unknown.

Reproductive/Nursing Safety

The effects of ceftiofur on the reproductive performance, pregnancy, and lactation of cattle, dogs, horses, swine, sheep, and goats have not been determined.

Cephalosporins have been shown to cross the placenta and safe use of them during pregnancy have not been firmly established, but neither have there been any documented teratogenic problems associated with these drugs. However, use only when the potential benefits outweigh the risks.

Most of these agents (cephalosporins) are excreted in milk in small quantities. Modification/alteration of bowel flora with resultant diarrhea is theoretically possible. When dosed as labeled, there are no milk withdrawal times necessary for ceftiofur products in dairy cattle.

Overdosage/Acute Toxicity

Cephalosporin overdoses are unlikely to cause significant problems other than GI distress, but other effects are possible (see Adverse Effects section). However, overdoses in food animals may result in significantly extended withdrawal times, contact FARAD (see appendix) for assistance.

Drug Interactions

Although the manufacturer does not list any drug interactions on the label for ceftiofur, the following drug interactions have either been reported or are theoretical in humans or animals receiving injectable 3rd generation cephalosporins and may be of significance in veterinary patients receiving ceftiofur:

■ **AMINOGLYCOSIDES/NEPHROTOXIC DRUGS:** The concurrent use of parenteral aminoglycosides or other nephrotoxic drugs (*e.g.*, amphotericin B) with cephalosporins is somewhat controversial. Potentially, cephalosporins could cause additive nephrotoxicity when used with these drugs, but this interaction has only been well documented with cephaloridine (no longer marketed). *In vitro* studies have demonstrated that cephalosporins can have synergistic or additive activity against certain bacteria when used with aminoglycosides, but they should not be mixed together (administer separately).

■ **PROBENECID:** Competitively blocks the tubular secretion of most cephalosporins thereby increasing serum levels and serum half-lives.

Laboratory Considerations

Note: Ceftiofur is structurally similar to cefotaxime and it is not known if these interactions occur with ceftiofur.

■ Except for cefotaxime, cephalosporins may cause false-positive **urine glucose determinations** when using cupric sulfate solution (Benedict's Solution, *Clinitest*®). Tests utilizing glucose oxidase (*Tes-Tape*®, *Clinistix*®) are not affected by cephalosporins..

■ When using the Jaffe reaction to measure **serum or urine creatinine**, cephalosporins (not ceftazidime or cefotaxime) in high dosages may falsely cause elevated values.

■ In humans, particularly with azotemia, cephalosporins have caused a false-positive direct **Coombs' test**.

■ Cephalosporins may also cause falsely elevated **17-ketosteroid** values in urine.

Doses

■ **CATTLE:**

a) Administer to cattle by IM or SC injection at 1.1 to 2.2 mg/kg of body weight (1–2 mL reconstituted sterile solution per 100 lbs body weight). Treatment should be repeated at 24-hour intervals for a total of three consecutive days. Additional treatments may be given on days four and five for animals which do not show a satisfactory response (not recovered) after the initial three treatments. (Package Insert; *Naxcel®*—Pfizer)

■ **SWINE:**

a) Administer to swine by IM injection at 3 to 5 mg/kg of body weight (1mL of reconstituted sterile solution per 22 to 37 lbs body weight). Treatment should be repeated at 24-hour intervals for a total of three consecutive days. (Package Insert; *Naxcel®*—Pfizer)

■ **SHEEP/GOATS:**

a) Administer to sheep/goats by IM injection at 1.1 to 2.2 mg/kg of body weight (1–2 mL reconstituted sterile solution per 100 lbs body weight). Treatment should be repeated at 24 hour intervals for a total of three consecutive days. Additional treatments may be given on days four and five for animals which do not show a satisfactory response (not recovered) after the initial three treatments. When used in lactating does, the high end of the dosage is recommended. (Package Insert; *Naxcel®*—Pfizer)

■ **HORSES:**

a) Administer to horses by IM injection at the dosage of 1 to 2 mg ceftiofur per pound (2.2 to 4.4 mg/kg) of body weight (2–4 mL reconstituted sterile solution per 100 lbs body weight). A maximum of 10 mL may be administered per injection site. Repeat treatment at 24-hour intervals, continued for 48 hours after symptoms have disappeared. Do not exceed 10 days of treatment. (Package Insert; *Naxcel®*—Pfizer)

b) 1–2 mg/kg IV or IM q12–24h (Bertone 2003)

c) For Lyme disease: 2.2–4.4 mg/kg IV q12 hours via a long-term catheter (Divers 1999)

d) Foals: 2.2–4.4 mg/kg IV or IM q12–24h (Brumbaugh 1999)

e) For strangles: Early in infection when only fever and depression are present: ceftiofur sodium 2.2 mg/kg IM q12–24h. If lymphadenopathy noted in otherwise healthy and alert horse do not treat. If lymphadenopathy present and horse is depressed, febrile, anorexic and especially if dyspneic, treat as above. (Foreman 1999)

f) For intrauterine infusion: 1 gram. Little science is available for recommending doses, volume infused, frequency, diluents, etc. Most treatments are commonly performed every day or every other day for 3–7 days. (Perkins 1999)

g) Foals: 2.2–5 mg/kg IM q12h (Giguere 2003)

■ **DOGS:**

a) For susceptible UTI's: 2.2 mg/kg SC once daily for 5–14 days Administer to dogs by subcutaneous injection at the dosage of 1 mg ceftiofur per pound (2.2 mg/kg) of body weight (0.1 mL reconstituted sterile solution per 5 lbs body weight). Treatment should be repeated at 24–hour intervals for 5–14 days. (Package Insert; *Naxcel®*—Pfizer)

b) 10 mg/kg once to twice daily (q12–24h) SC (Aucoin 2000)

c) For UTI: 2.2 mg/kg SC once daily for 5–14 days

   For systemic, soft tissue infections: 2.2 mg/kg q12h or 4.4 mg/kg q24h SC for 5–14 days

   For sepsis, bacteremia: 4.4 mg/kg q12h SC for 2–5 days (Greene & Watson 1998)

d) For neonatal septicemia: 2.5 mg/kg SC q12h for no longer than 5 days; presumptive therapy with vitamin K1 (0.01–1 mg per neonate SC) may be used in puppies and kittens less than 48 hours old (Davidson 2004), (Davidson 2009)

■ **CATS:**

a) For UTI: 2.2 mg/kg SC once daily for 5–14 days

   For systemic, soft tissue infections: 2.2 mg/kg q12h or 4.4 mg/kg q24h SC for 5–14 days

   For sepsis, bacteremia: 4.4 mg/kg q12h SC for 2–5 days (Greene & Watson 1998)

■ **BIRDS:**

a) Day-Old Turkey Poults: Administer by SC injection in the neck region of day-old turkey poults at the dosage of 0.17 to 0.5 mg ceftiofur/poult. One mL of the 50 mg/mL reconstituted solution will treat approximately 100 to 294 day-old poults.

Day Old Chicks: Administer by SC injection in the neck region of day-old chicks at the dosage of 0.08 to 0.20 mg ceftiofur per chick. One mL of the 50 mg/mL reconstituted solution will treat approximately 250 to 625 day-old chicks. A sterile 26 gauge needle and syringe or properly cleaned automatic injection machine should be used. (Package Insert; *Naxcel®*—Pfizer)

b) **Ratites:** 10–20 mg/kg IM twice daily (Jenson 1998)

■ **REPTILES:**

a) **Chelonians:** 4 mg/kg IM once daily for 2 weeks. Commonly used in respiratory infections. (Gauvin 1993)

b) **Green iguanas:** for microbes susceptible at > 2 μg/mL, 5 mg/kg, IM or SC, every 24 hours (Bensen *et al.* 2003)

c) For bacterial pneumonia: 2.2 mg/kg IM q24–48h; keep patient at upper end of ideal temperature range (Johnson 2004)

■ **EXOTICS/WILDLIFE:**

a) Captive Female Asian Elephants: 1.1 mg/kg IM given two to three times a day or, alternatively 1.1 mg/kg IV once daily, depending upon the MIC of the pathogen (Dumonceax *et al.* 2005)

Treatment Monitoring

Because cephalosporins usually have minimal toxicity associated with their use, monitoring for efficacy is usually all that is required. Some clinicians recommend weekly CBC monitoring of small animals receiving ceftiofur. Patients with diminished renal function may require intensified renal monitoring. Serum levels and therapeutic drug monitoring are not routinely done with these agents.

Chemistry/Synonyms

Ceftiofur sodium is a semisynthetic 3rd generation cephalosporin. Ceftiofur sodium is a weak acid and is acid stable and water-soluble.

Ceftiofur sodium may also be known as CM 31-916, U 64279E, ceftiofen sodium, *Excenel®* (not *Excenel® RTU*), *Naxcel®*, or *Accent®*.

Storage/Stability

Unreconstituted ceftiofur sodium powder for reconstitution should be stored at room temperature. Protect from light. Color of the cake may vary from off-white to tan, but this does not affect potency.

After reconstitution with bacteriostatic water for injection or sterile water for injection, the solution is stable up to 7 days when refrigerated and for 12 hours at room temperature (15–30°C). According to the manufacturer, if a precipitate should form while being stored refrigerated during this time, the product may be used if it goes back into solution after warming. If not, contact the manufacturer. Frozen reconstituted solutions are stable up to 8 weeks.

Thawing may be done at room temperature or by swirling the vial under running warm or hot water.

One-time salvage procedure for reconstituted product: At the end of the 7-day refrigeration or 12-hour room temperature storage period following reconstitution, any remaining reconstituted product may be frozen up to 8 weeks without loss in potency or other chemical properties. This is a one-time only salvage procedure for the remaining product. To use this salvaged product at any time during the 8-week storage period, hold the vial under warm running water, gently swirling the container to accelerate thawing, or allow the frozen material to thaw at room temperature. Rapid freezing or thawing may result in vial breakage. Any product not used immediately upon thawing should be discarded.

Dosage Forms/Regulatory Status

VETERINARY-LABELED PRODUCTS:

Ceftiofur Sodium Powder for Injection 50 mg ceftiofur/mL when reconstituted in 1 g & 4 g vials; *Naxcel®* (Pfizer), generic; (Rx). FDA-approved for various indications in cattle, swine, sheep, goats, horses, dogs, and day-old chicks or turkey poults. Withdrawal times: Cattle: 4-day slaughter withdrawal time is required. No milk discard time is required. Swine: A 4-day slaughter withdrawal time is required. Sheep/Goats: No slaughter withdrawal time or milk discard time is required. Not to be used in horses intended for human consumption.

HUMAN-LABELED PRODUCTS: None

References

Aucoin, D (2000). Antimicrobial Drug Formulary. *Target: The antimicrobial guide to effective treatment* Port Huron, MI, North American Compendiums Inc: 93–142.

Bensen, K, A Lee, et al. (2003). Pharmacokinetics of ceftiofur sodium after IM or SC administration in green iguanas (Iguana iguana). *Am J Vet Res* 64(10): 1278–1282.

Bertone, J (2003). Rational antibiotic choices. Western Veterinary Conf. Accessed via: Veterinary Information Network. http://goo.gl/MxKfS

Brumbaugh, G (1999). Clinical Pharmacology and the Pediatric Patient. 45th Annual AAEP Convention, Albuquerque.

Clark, C & P Dowling (2005). Antimicrobial–associated diarrhea in horses. Proceedings: ACVIM. Accessed via: Veterinary Information Network. http://goo.gl/3cDgv

Courtin, F, A Craigmill, et al. (1997). Pharmacokinetics of ceftiofur and metabolites after single intravenous and intramuscular administration and multiple intramuscular administration of ceftiofur sodium to dairy goats. *J Vet Pharmacol Ther* 20(5): 368–373.

Davidson, A (2004). Clinical neonatology in small animal practice. Proceedings: ACVIM Forum. Accessed via: Veterinary Information Network. http://goo.gl/OPzsW

Davidson, A (2009). Neonatal resuscitation: Techniques to improve outcome. Proceedings: WVC. Accessed via: Veterinary Information Network. http://goo.gl/ri9Os

Divers, T (1999). Lyme disease in horses – Diagnosis and treatment. Proceedings: The North American Veterinary Conference, Orlando.

Dumonceax, G, R Isaza, et al. (2005). Pharmacokinetics and IM bioavailability of ceftiofur in Asian elephants. *J Vet Pharmacol Ther* 28(5): 441–446.

Foreman, J (1999). Equine respiratory pharmacology. *The Veterinary Clinics of North America: Equine Practice* 15:3(December): 665–686.

Gauvin, J (1993). Drug therapy in reptiles. *Seminars in Avian & Exotic Med* 2(1): 48–59.

Giguere, S (2003). Antimicrobial therapy in foals. Proceedings: Western Veterinary Conference. Accessed via: Veterinary Information Network. http://goo.gl/pdKJZ

Greene, C & A Watson (1998). Antimicrobial Drug Formulary. *Infectious Diseases of the Dog and Cat.* C Greene Ed. Philadelphia, WB Saunders: 790–919.

Jenson, J (1998). Current ratite therapy. *The Veterinary Clinics of North America: Food Animal Practice* 16:3(November).

Johnson, D (2004). Reptile therapeutic protocols. Proceedings: ACVC. Accessed via: Veterinary Information Network. http://goo.gl/QcqNx

Perkins, N (1999). Equine reproductive pharmacology. *The Veterinary Clinics of North America: Equine Practice* 15:3(December): 687–704.

Pille, F, S De Baere, et al. (2005). Synovial fluid and plasma concentrations of ceftiofur after regional intravenous perfusion in the horse. *Veterinary Surgery* 34: 610–617.

CEFTRIAXONE SODIUM

(sef-try-*ax*-ohn)   Rocephin®

3RD GENERATION CEPHALOSPORIN

Prescriber Highlights

▶ 3rd generation cephalosporin; achieves high levels in CNS; long half life

▶ Potentially could cause hypersensitivity reactions, granulocytopenia/thrombocytopenia, diarrhea, mild azotemia, biliary "sludging"

▶ Causes pain on IM injection; Give IV over 30 minutes (or more)

▶ May need to reduce dose in renal failure; avoid with icterus

Uses/Indications

Ceftriaxone is used to treat serious infections, particularly against susceptible Enterobacteriaceae that are not susceptible to other less expensive agents or when aminoglycosides are not indicated (due to their potential toxicity). Its long half life, good CNS penetration, and activity against *Borrelia burgdorferi* also has made it a potential choice for treating Lyme's disease.

Pharmacology/Actions

Ceftriaxone is a third generation injectable cephalosporin agent. The third generation cephalosporins retain the gram-positive activity of the first and second-generation agents, but, have much expanded gram-negative activity. As with the 2nd generation agents, enough variability exists with individual bacterial sensitivities that susceptibility testing is necessary for most bacteria. Because of the excellent gram-negative coverage of these agents and when compared to the aminoglycosides and their significantly less toxic potential, they have been used on an increasing basis in veterinary medicine.

Pharmacokinetics

Ceftriaxone is not absorbed after oral administration and must be given parenterally. It is widely distributed throughout the body; CSF levels are higher when meninges are inflamed. Ceftriaxone crosses the placenta and enters maternal milk in low concentrations; no documented adverse effects to offspring have been noted. Ceftriaxone is excreted by both renal and non-renal mechanisms; in humans, elimination half-lives are approximately 6–11 hours.

In dogs, ceftriaxone bioavailability after IM or SC administration equal that of IV, but peak levels occur much faster after IM (approximately 30 minutes) than SC (80 minutes). Peak levels are higher with IM administration than SC, but total area under the curve is similar for both routes. Elimination half-life is longer after SC administration (1.73 hrs) than either IM (1.17 hrs) or IV administration (0.88 hrs). The authors of the study (Rebuelto *et al.* 2002) concluded that once or twice daily IM or SC injections of 50 mg/kg should be adequate to treat most susceptible infections in dogs.

Contraindications/Precautions/Warnings

Only prior allergic reaction to cephalosporins contraindicates ceftriaxone's use. In humans documented hypersensitive to penicillin, up to 16% may also be allergic to cephalosporins. The veterinary significance of this is unclear.

Although bleeding times have only been reported rarely in humans, ceftriaxone should be used with caution in patients with vitamin K utilization or synthesis abnormalities (*e.g.*, severe hepatic disease).

Patients in renal failure may need dosage adjustments; but are not generally required unless severely uremic, or with concomitant hepatic impairment.

Adverse Effects

Because veterinary usage of ceftriaxone is very limited, an accurate adverse effect profile has not been determined. The following adverse effects have been reported in humans and may or may not apply to veterinary patients: hematologic effects, including eosinophilia (6%), thrombocytosis (5%), leukopenia (2%) and, more rarely, anemia, neutropenia, lymphopenia and thrombocytopenia. Approximately 2–4% of humans get diarrhea. Very high dosages (100 mg/kg/day) in dogs have caused a "sludge" in bile. Hypersensitivity reactions (usually a rash) have been noted. Increased serum concentrations of liver enzymes, BUN, creatinine, and urine casts have been described in about 1–3% of patients. When given IM, pain may be noted at the injection site.

Reproductive/Nursing Safety

No teratogenic effects were demonstrated in studies in pregnant mice and rats given up to 20X labeled doses of ceftriaxone. In humans, the FDA categorizes this drug as category *B* for use during pregnancy (*Animal studies have not yet demonstrated risk to the fetus, but there are no adequate studies in pregnant women; or animal studies have shown an adverse effect, but adequate studies in pregnant women have not demonstrated a risk to the fetus in the first trimester of pregnancy, and there is no evidence of risk in later trimesters.*)

Ceftriaxone is distributed into milk in low concentrations and is unlikely to pose much risk to nursing offspring.

Overdosage/Acute Toxicity

Limited information available; overdoses should be monitored and treated symptomatically and supportively if required.

Drug Interactions

The following drug interactions have either been reported or are theoretical in humans or animals receiving ceftriaxone and may be of significance in veterinary patients:

■ **AMINOGLYCOSIDES/NEPHROTOXIC DRUGS:** The concurrent use of parenteral aminoglycosides or other nephrotoxic drugs (*e.g.,* amphotericin B) with cephalosporins is somewhat controversial. Potentially, cephalosporins could cause additive nephrotoxicity when used with these drugs, but this interaction has only been well documented with cephaloridine (no longer marketed). *In vitro* studies have demonstrated that cephalosporins can have synergistic or additive activity against certain bacteria when used with aminoglycosides.

■ **CALCIUM:** Concomitant use with calcium containing solutions have caused fatal calcium-ceftriaxone precipitates in lungs and kidneys of neonatal humans. Do not mix with calcium or administer calcium-containing solutions or products within 48 hours of ceftriaxone administration.

Laboratory Considerations

■ When using Kirby-Bauer disk diffusion procedures for testing susceptibility, a specific 30 micrograms ceftriaxone disk should be used. A cephalosporin-class disk containing cephalothin should not be used to test for ceftriaxone susceptibility. An inhibition zone of 18 mm or more indicates susceptibility; 14–17 mm, intermediate; and 13 mm or less, resistant.

■ When using a dilution susceptibility procedure, an organism with a MIC of 16 micrograms/mL or less is considered susceptible and 64 micrograms/mL or greater is considered resistant. With either method, infections caused by organisms with intermediate susceptibility may be effectively treated if the infection is limited to tissues where the drug is concentrated or if a higher than normal dose is used.

■ Ceftriaxone, like most other cephalosporins,

may cause a **false-positive urine glucose** determination when using the cupric sulfate solution test (*e.g., Clinitest®*).

■ Ceftriaxone in very high concentrations (50 micrograms/mL or greater) may cause falsely elevated **serum creatinine** levels when manual methods of testing are used. Automated methods do not appear to be affected.

Doses

■ **DOGS:**
  a) For meningitis/borreliosis: 15–50 mg/kg (maximum single dose in humans is 1 gram) IV or IM q12h for 4–14 days

     For preoperative/intraoperative use: 25 mg/kg (maximum single dose in humans is 1 gram) IM or IV one time

     For skin, genitourinary infections: 25 mg/kg IM once daily (q24h) for 7–14 days (Greene & Watson 1998)

  b) For infectious endocarditis and documented resistance against or other contraindications for fluoroquinolones and aminoglycosides in dogs: 20 mg/kg IV q12h (DeFrancesco 2000)

  c) 15–50 mg/kg (route not specified) once daily (Trepanier 1999)

■ **CATS:**
  For systemic infections:
  a) 25–50 mg/kg IV, IM or Intraosseous q12h as long as necessary (Greene & Watson 1998)

■ **HORSES:**
  For susceptible infections:
  a) 25–50 mg/kg q12h IV or IM.Excellent CSF and bone penetration; expensive. (Stewart 2008)

  b) 20 mg/kg IV q12h (Brumbaugh 1999)

Monitoring

■ Efficacy

■ If long-term therapy, occasional CBC, renal function (BUN, Serum Creatinine, urinalysis) and liver enzymes (AST, ALT) may be considered.

Chemistry/Synonyms

A third generation cephalosporin, ceftriaxone sodium occurs as a white to yellowish-orange crystalline powder. It is soluble in water (400 mg/mL at 25°C). Potencies of commercial products are expressed in terms of ceftriaxone. One gram of ceftriaxone sodium contains 3.6 mEq of sodium.

Ceftriaxone Sodium may also be known as: ceftriaxonum natricum, Ro-13-9904, or Ro-13-9904/000; many trade names are available.

Storage/Stability

The sterile powder for reconstitution should be stored at or below 25°C and protected from light.

After reconstituting with either 0.9% sodium chloride or D$_5$W, ceftriaxone solutions (at concentrations of approximately 100 mg/mL) are stable for 3 days at room temperature and for 10 days when refrigerated. Solutions of concentrations of 250 mg/mL are stable for 24 hours at room temperature and 3 days when refrigerated. At concentrations of 10–40 mg/mL solutions frozen at -20°C are stable for 26 weeks.

Compatibility/Compounding Considerations
The manufacturer does not recommend admixing any other anti-infective drugs with ceftriaxone sodium, but amikacin and metronidazole are reported **compatible**.

Do not mix with calcium or calcium-containing solutions, or administer calcium-containing solutions or products within 48 hours of ceftriaxone administration (see Drug Interactions).

Dosage Forms/Regulatory Status

VETERINARY-LABELED PRODUCTS: None
HUMAN-LABELED PRODUCTS:
Ceftriaxone Injection Powder for Solution: 250 mg & 500 mg, 1 g, 2 g, & 10 g, (as base) in vialssingle-use duplex containers and in bulk; *Rocephin*® (Roche); generic; (Rx)

References

Brumbaugh, G (1999). Clinical Pharmacology and the Pediatric Patient. 45th Annual AAEP Convention, Albuquerque.

DeFrancesco, T (2000). CVT Update: Infectious Endocarditis. *Kirk's Current Veterinary Therapy: XIII Small Animal Practice*. J Bonagura Ed. Philadelphia, WB Saunders: 768–772.

Greene, C & A Watson (1998). Antimicrobial Drug Formulary. *Infectious Diseases of the Dog and Cat*. C Greene Ed. Philadelphia, WB Saunders: 790–919.

Rebuelto, M, G Albarellos, et al. (2002). Pharmacokinetics of ceftriaxone administered by the intravenous, intramuscular and subcutaneous routes to dogs. *J Vet Phamacol Ther* 25: 73–76.

Stewart, A (2008). Equine Neonatal Sepsis. Proceedings: WVC. Accessed via: Veterinary Information Network. http://www.vin.com/Members/Proceedings/Proceedings.plx?CID=WVC2008&PID=PR19727&O=VIN

Trepanier, L (1999). Treating resistant infections in small animals. Proceedings: 17th Annual American College of Veterinary Internal Medicine Meeting, Chicago.

CEFUROXIME AXETIL
CEFUROXIME SODIUM
(sef-yoor-*oks*-eem)   Ceftin®, Zinacef®
2ND GENERATION CEPHALOSPORIN

Prescriber Highlights

▶ Oral & parenterally administered 2nd generation cephalosporin that is more active against some gram-negative bacteria than first generation (*e.g.*, cephalexin, cefazolin) cephalosporins

▶ Potentially useful in small animals when a cephalosporin is desired to treat bacterial infections susceptible to cefuroxime, but resistant to first generation cephalosporins, when enhanced gram-negative coverage is desired for surgery prophylaxis, or when high CNS levels are necessary

▶ Limited clinical experience in veterinary medicine

▶ Adverse effects most likely seen in small animals would be GI-related

Uses/Indications

Cefuroxime is a semi-synthetic 2nd generation cephalosporin with enhanced activity against some gram-negative pathogens when compared to the first generation agents. Cefuroxime is available in both oral and parenteral dosage forms. It potentially may be useful in small animals when a cephalosporin is desired to treat bacterial infections susceptible to cefuroxime, but resistant to first generation cephalosporins, when enhanced gram-negative coverage is desired for surgery prophylaxis, or when high CNS levels are necessary. Little information is available with regard to its clinical use in small animals, however.

Pharmacology/Actions

Cefuroxime, like other cephalosporins, is bactericidal and acts by inhibiting cell wall synthesis. Its spectrum of activity is similar to that of cephalexin, but it is more active against gram-negative bacteria including strains of *E. coli*, *Klebsiella pneumoniae*, Salmonella and Enterobacter. It is not effective against methicillin-resistant Staphylococcus, Pseudomonas, Serratia or Enterococcus.

Pharmacokinetics

No information was located for the pharmacokinetics of cefuroxime in dogs, cats or horses.

In humans, cefuroxime axetil is well absorbed after oral administration and is rapidly hydrolyzed in the intestinal mucosa and circulation to the parent compound. Bioavailability ranges on average from 37% (fasted) to 52% (with food). Peak serum levels occur in about 2–3 hours after oral dosing. When the sodium salt is administered IM, peak levels occur within 15 minutes to 1 hour. Cefuroxime is widely distributed after absorption, including to bone, aqueous humor and joint fluid. Therapeutic levels can be attained in the CSF if meninges are inflamed. Binding to human plasma proteins ranges from 35–50%. Cefuroxime is primarily excreted unchanged in the urine; elimination half-life in patients with normal renal function is between 1–2 hours.

Contraindications/Precautions/Warnings

No specific information is available for veterinary patients. In humans, cefuroxime is contraindicated in patients hypersensitive to it or other cephalosporins. Dosage adjustment is recommended in humans with severe renal impairment.

Adverse Effects

As usage of cefuroxime in animals has been limited, a comprehensive adverse effect profile has not been determined. A six-month toxicity study of oral cefuroxime axetil given at dosages ranging from 100 mg/kg/day to 1600 mg/kg day in Beagles demonstrated little adversity associated with cefuroxime. At the highest dosing levels (approximately 80X), some vomiting and slight suppression of body weight gain were noted. Minor reductions in neutrophils and red cells, with increases in prothrombin times were also seen.

When used clinically in dogs, gastrointestinal effects (inappetence, vomiting, diarrhea) would be the most likely expected adverse effects, but incidence rates are not known.

Cefuroxime is generally well tolerated in human patients. Injection site inflammation can occur when cefuroxime is used intravenously. Gastrointestinal effects (nausea, diarrhea) may occur, but are not frequently reported. Eosinophilia and hypersensitivity reactions (including anaphylaxis) are possible. Neurologic effects (hearing loss, seizures), pseudomembranous colitis, serious dermatologic reactions (TEN, Stevens-Johnson syndrome, etc.), hematologic effects (pancytopenia, thrombocytopenia), and interstitial nephritis have all been reported rarely in humans.

Reproductive/Nursing Safety

Studies performed in pregnant mice at dosages of up to 6400 mg/kg and rabbits at 400 mg/kg demonstrated no adverse fetal effects. In humans, the FDA categorizes cefuroxime as category *B* for use during pregnancy (*Animal studies have not yet demonstrated risk to the fetus, but there are no adequate studies in pregnant women; or animal studies have shown an adverse effect, but adequate studies in pregnant women have not demonstrated a risk to the fetus in the first trimester of pregnancy, and there is no evidence of risk in later trimesters.*)

Cefuroxime enters maternal milk in low concentrations. Although probably safe for nursing offspring the potential for adverse effects cannot be ruled out, particularly alterations to gut flora with resultant diarrhea.

Overdosage/Acute Toxicity

Beagles receiving daily dosages of up to 1600 mg/kg/day orally tolerated cefuroxime well (see Adverse Effects).

Cerebral irritation with seizures has been reported with large overdoses in humans. Plasma levels of cefuroxime can be reduced with hemodialysis or peritoneal dialysis.

Drug Interactions

The following drug interactions have either been reported or are theoretical in humans or animals receiving cefuroxime and may be of significance in veterinary patients:

■ **AMINOGLYCOSIDES:** Potential for increased risk of nephrotoxicity—monitor renal function; however, aminoglycosides and cephalosporins may have synergistic or additive actions against some gram-negative bacteria (Enterobacteriaceae)

■ **FUROSEMIDE, TORSEMIDE:** Possible increased risk of nephrotoxicity

■ **PROBENECID:** Reduced renal excretion of cefaclor

Laboratory Considerations

■ Cefuroxime may cause false-positive **urine glucose determinations** when using the copper reduction method (Benedict's solution, Fehling's solution, *Clinitest®*); tests utilizing glucose oxidase (*Tes-Tape®, Clinistix®*) are not affected by cephalosporins

■ In humans, particularly with azotemia, cephalosporins have caused a false-positive direct **Coombs' test**

Doses

■ **DOGS:**

For susceptible infections:

a) For soft tissue infections: 10 mg/kg PO q12h for 10 days. For systemic infections: 15 mg/kg IV q8h. For meningitis: 30 mg/kg IV q8h. **Note:** All dosages extrapolated from human dosages. (Greene *et al.* 2006)

For surgery prophylaxis:

a) 20 mg/kg IV 30 minutes prior to surgery and every 2 hours during surgery. (Greene *et al.* 2006)

Monitoring

■ Clinical efficacy

■ Monitor renal function in patients with renal insufficiency

Client Information

■ Give the oral tablets with food as it may enhance the absorption of the drug

■ Avoid crushing tablets; a strong, bitter taste results even if mixed into food; if tablets must be crushed, give with dairy products such as milk or chocolate milk to improve absorption and palatability

■ Give as directed by the veterinarian; even if animal appears well, continue treating for the full duration prescribed

■ Contact veterinarian if animal develops severe vomiting/diarrhea or rash/itching

Chemistry/Synonyms

Cefuroxime axetil occurs as a white or almost white, powder that is insoluble in water and slightly soluble in dehydrated alcohol.

Cefuroxime sodium occurs as a white or almost white, hygroscopic powder that is freely soluble in water.

Cefuroxime may also be known as: CCI-15641, cefuroxim, cefuroxima, cefuroximum, cefuroksiimi, or cefuroksimas; many internationally registered trade names are available.

Storage/Stability

Cefuroxime axetil tablets should be stored in tight containers at room temperature (15–30°C); protect from excessive moisture.

The powder for suspension should be stored at 2–30°C. Once reconstituted, it should be kept refrigerated (2–8°C) and any unused suspension discarded after 10 days.

The powder for injection of infusion should be stored at room temperature (15–30°C). The powder may darken, but this does not indicate any loss of potency. When reconstituted with sterile water to a concentration of 90 mg/mL, the resulting solution is stable for 24 hours at room temperature; 48 hours if refrigerated. If further diluted into a **compatible** IV solution such as D5W, normal saline or Ringer's, the resulting solution is stable for 24 hours at room temperature; up to 7 days if refrigerated.

Compatibility/Compounding Considerations

Drugs that are reportedly **compatible** when mixed with cefuroxime for IV use include, clindamycin, furosemide and metronidazole. Drugs that may be given at a Y-site with a cefuroxime infusion running include, morphine, hydromorphone, and propofol. Aminoglycosides, ciprofloxacin, or ranitidine should not be admixed with cefuroxime.

Dosage Forms/Regulatory Status

VETERINARY-LABELED PRODUCTS: None
HUMAN-LABELED PRODUCTS:

Cefuroxime Axetil Oral Tablets (film coated): 125 mg, 250 mg, & 500 mg; *Ceftin®* (GlaxoWellcome), generic (Ranbaxy); (Rx)

Cefuroxime Axetil Oral Suspension: 25 mg/mL & 50 mg/mL (125 mg/5 mL & 250 mg/5 mL; as base) when reconstituted in 50 &100 mL; generic, (Ranbaxy); (Rx)

Cefuroxime Sodium Powder for Injection: 750 mg, 1.5 g & 7.5 g (as sodium) in 10 mL & 20 mL vials, 100 mL piggyback vials, infusion packs, ADD-Vantage vials & bulk package; *Zinacef®* (GlaxoWellcome); generic; (Rx)

Cefuroxime Sodium Injection: 750 mg & 1.5 g (as sodium), premixed, frozen in 50 mL; *Zinacef®* (GlaxoWellcome); (Rx)

References

Greene, C, K Hartmannn, et al. (2006). Appendix 8: Antimicrobial Drug Formulary. *Infectious Disease of the Dog and Cat.* C Greene Ed., Elsevier: 1186–1333.

CEPHALEXIN

(sef-a-*lex*-in)   Keflex®

1ST GENERATION CEPHALOSPORIN

Prescriber Highlights

▶ 1st generation oral cephalosporin (available for injection in other countries)

▶ May be administered with food (especially if GI upset occurs)

▶ Most likely adverse effects are GI in nature; hypersensitivity reactions possible

▶ May need to reduce dose in patients with renal failure

Uses/Indications

There are no FDA-approved cephalexin products for veterinary use in the USA. However, it has been used clinically in dogs, cats, horses, rabbits, ferrets, and birds, particularly for susceptible Staphylococcal infections.

Pharmacology/Actions

A first generation cephalosporin, cephalexin exhibits activity against the bacteria usually covered by this class. Cephalosporins are bactericidal against susceptible bacteria and act by inhibiting mucopeptide synthesis in the cell wall resulting in a defective barrier and an osmotically unstable spheroplast. The exact mechanism for this effect has not been definitively determined, but beta-lactam antibiotics have been shown to bind to several enzymes (carboxypeptidases, transpeptidases, endopeptidases) within the bacterial cytoplasmic membrane that are involved with cell wall synthesis. The different affinities that various beta-lactam antibiotics have for these enzymes (also known as penicillin-binding proteins; PBPs) help explain the differences in spectrums of activity of these drugs that are not explained by the influence of beta-lactamases. Like other beta-lactam antibiotics, cephalosporins are generally considered to be more effective against actively growing bacteria.

While there may be differences in MIC's for individual first generation cephalosporins, their spectrums of activity are quite similar. They possess generally excellent coverage against most gram-positive pathogens and variable to poor coverage against most gram-negative pathogens. These drugs are very active *in vitro* against groups A beta-hemolytic and B Streptococci, non-enterococcal group D Streptococci (*S. bovis*), *Staphylococcus intermedius* and *aureas*, *Proteus mirabilis* and some strains of *E. coli*, *Klebsiella* spp., Actinobacillus, Pasturella, *Haemophilus equigenitalis*, Shigella and Salmonella. With the exception of *Bacteroides fragilis*, most anaerobes are very susceptible to the first generation agents. Most species of Corynebacteria are susceptible, but *C. equi* (Rhodococcus) is usually resistant. Strains of *Staphylococcus epidermidis* are usually sensitive to the parenterally administered 1st generation drugs, but may have variable susceptibilities to the oral drugs. The following bacteria are regularly resistant to the 1st generation agents: Group D streptococci/enterococci (*S. faecalis*, *S. faecium*), Methicillin-resistant Staphylococci, *indole-positive Proteus* spp., *Pseudomonas* spp., *Enterobacter* spp., *Serratia* spp. and *Citrobacter* spp.

Pharmacokinetics

After oral administration, cephalexin is rapidly and completely absorbed in humans. Cephalexin (base) must be converted to the HCl before absorption can occur and, therefore, absorption can be delayed. There is a form of cephalexin HCl commercially available for oral use that apparently is absorbed more rapidly, but the clinical significance of this is in question. Food apparently has little impact on absorption.

In a study done in dogs and cats (Silley et al. 1988), peak serum levels reached 18.6 micrograms/mL about 1.8 hours after a mean oral dose of 12.7 mg/kg in dogs, and 18.7 micrograms/mL, 2.6 hours after an oral dose of 22.9 mg/kg in cats. Elimination half-lives ranged from 1–2 hours in both species. Bioavailability was about 75% in both species after oral administration.

There may be temporal differences in pharmacokinetics depending on the time of day the drug is administered. Six beagles given cephalexin orally at 10:00 and 22:00 had significantly lower peak levels (77%) after the 22:00 dose versus the 10:00 dose. Additionally, the elimination half-life was approximately 50% longer with the evening dose versus the morning dose. Clinical significance is not clear as times above an MIC of 0.5 micrograms/mL were not different (Prados *et al.* 2007).

In horses, oral cephalexin has low bioavailability (approx. 5%) and a short plasma half-life (about 2 hours), but at doses of 30 mg/kg PO q8h sufficient plasma and interstitial levels were achieved to treat gram-positive bacteria (MIC ≤5 micrograms/mL) (Davis *et al.* 2005).

Outiside the USA, an oily suspension of the sodium salt (*Ceporex® Injection*—Glaxovet; Cefalexina Injection 20%—Labatorino Burnet) is available in several countries for IM or SC injection in animals. In calves, the sodium salt had a 74% bioavailability after IM injection and a serum half-life of about 90 minutes. When 7.5 mg/kg was injected either SC or IM in adult cattle, the 20% suspension had longer durations of time above MIC90 for common gram positive pathogens when injected SC versus IM (11–14 hours vs. 8-9 hours) (Dova *et al.* 2008).

Contraindications/Precautions/Warnings

Cephalosporins are contraindicated in patients with a history of hypersensitivity to them. Because there may be cross-reactivity, use cephalosporins cautiously in patients who are documented hypersensitive to other beta-lactam antibiotics (*e.g.*, penicillins, cefamycins, carbapenems).

Oral systemic antibiotics should not be administered in patients with septicemia, shock or other grave illnesses as absorption of the medication from the GI tract may be significantly delayed or diminished. Parenteral routes (preferably IV) should be used for these cases.

Adverse Effects

Adverse effects with the cephalosporins are usually not serious and have a relatively low frequency of occurrence.

In addition to the adverse effects listed below, cephalexin has reportedly caused salivation, tachypnea and excitability in dogs, and emesis and fever in cats. Nephrotoxicity occurs rarely during therapy with cephalexin, but patients with renal dysfunction, receiving other nephrotoxic drugs or that are geriatric may be more susceptible. Interstitial nephritis, a hypersensitivity reaction, has been reported with many of the cephalosporins including cephalexin. The incidence of these effects is not known.

Hypersensitivity reactions unrelated to dose can occur with these agents and can manifest as rashes, fever, eosinophilia, lymphadenopathy, or full-blown anaphylaxis. The use of cephalosporins in patients documented to be hypersensitive to penicillin-class antibiotics is controversial. In humans, it is estimated 1–15% of patients hypersensitive to penicillins will also be hypersensitive to cephalosporins. The incidence of cross-reactivity in veterinary patients is unknown.

When given orally, cephalosporins may cause GI effects (anorexia, vomiting, diarrhea). Administering the drug with a small meal may help alleviate these effects. Because the cephalosporins may also alter gut flora, antibiotic-associated diarrhea or proliferation of resistant bacteria in the colon can occur.

Rarely, cephalexin has been implicated in causing toxic epidermal necrolysis in cats.

While cephalosporins (particularly cephalothin) have the potential for causing nephrotoxicity at clinically used doses in patients with normal renal function, risks for the occurrence of this adverse effect appear minimal.

High doses or very prolonged use has been associated with neurotoxicity, neutropenia, agranulocytosis, thrombocytopenia, hepatitis, positive Coomb's test, interstitial nephritis, and tubular necrosis. Except for tubular necrosis and neurotoxicity, these effects have an immunologic component.

Reproductive/Nursing Safety

Cephalosporins have been shown to cross the placenta and safe use of them during pregnancy has not been firmly established, but neither have there been any documented teratogenic problems associated with these drugs. However, use only when the potential benefits outweigh the risks. In humans, the FDA categorizes cephalexin as category **B** for use during pregnancy (*Animal studies have not yet demonstrated risk to the fetus, but there are no adequate studies in pregnant women; or animal studies have shown an adverse effect, but adequate studies in pregnant women have not demonstrated a risk to the fetus in the first trimester of pregnancy, and there is no evidence of risk in later trimesters.*)

Small amounts of cephalexin may be distributed into maternal milk; it could potentially affect gut flora in neonates.

Overdosage/Acute Toxicity

Acute oral cephalosporin overdoses are unlikely to cause significant problems other than GI distress, but other effects are possible (see Adverse Effects section).

Drug Interactions

The following drug interactions have either been reported or are theoretical in humans or animals receiving cephalexin and may be of significance in veterinary patients:

■ **PROBENECID:** Competitively blocks the tubular secretion of most cephalosporins thereby increasing serum levels and serum half-lives

Laboratory Considerations

■ Except for cefotaxime, cephalosporins may cause false-positive **urine glucose determinations** when using cupric sulfate solution (Benedict's Solution, *Clinitest®*). Tests utilizing glucose oxidase (*Tes-Tape®*, *Clinistix®*) are not affected by cephalosporins.

■ When using the Jaffe reaction to measure **serum or urine creatinine**, cephalosporins (not ceftazidime or cefotaxime) in high dosages may falsely cause elevated values.

■ In humans, particularly with azotemia, cephalosporins have caused a false-positive direct **Coombs' test**. Cephalosporins may also cause falsely elevated **17-ketosteroid** values in urine.

Doses

■ **DOGS:**
For susceptible infections:

a) For superficial and deep pyoderma: 22–33 mg/kg PO two to three times daily (Beale & Murphy 2006)

b) For recurrent pyoderma: 22 mg/kg PO q12h (use at q8h for deep pyoderma) (Hillier 2006)

c) For superficial canine pyoderma: 30–40 mg/kg PO once daily (q24h) for 4 weeks. (Toma *et al.* 2008)

d) For pyoderma: 22–35 mg/kg PO q12h or 22 mg/kg PO q8h

For respiratory infections: 20–40 mg/kg PO q8h; For soft tissue infections: 30–50 mg/kg PO q12h

For systemic infections: 25–60 mg/kg PO q8h

For orthopedic infections: 22–30 mg/kg PO q6–8h for 28 days

For above doses, guideline for duration of therapy is treat for 5–7 days beyond resolution of clinical disease or preferably negative culture (Greene & Watson 1998)

e) For pyometra/metritis: 10–30 mg/kg PO q8–12h (Freshman 2002a)

f) For UTI: 30–40 mg/kg PO q8h. For acute urethrocystitis, treatment may be 7–10 days for chronic urethrocystitis, up to 4 weeks of treatment may be necessary; for pyelonephritis, 4–8 weeks may be adequate (Brovida 2003)

g) For neonates: 10–30 mg/kg PO (weak neonates should be given via stomach tube) twice daily–three times daily (Freshman 2002b)

h) For juvenile cellulitis in 3–16 week old puppies: 20 mg/kg PO three times daily (Macintire 2004)

i) For treating infectious otitis: 22 mg/kg PO q12h (Kwochka 2002)

■ **CATS:**
For susceptible infections:

a) For soft tissue infections: 30–50 mg/kg PO q12h

For systemic infections: 35 mg/kg PO q6–8h.

For above doses, guideline for duration of therapy is treat for 5–7 days beyond resolution of clinical disease or preferably negative culture (Greene & Watson 1998)

b) 22 mg/kg PO q8h; administer with food if GI upset occurs (Vaden & Papich 1995)

c) For Gram-positive infections: 22 mg/kg PO twice daily

d) For Gram-negative infections: 30 mg/kg PO three times daily (Aucoin 2000)

e) 20–40 mg/kg PO q8h (Lappin 2002)

■ **RABBITS/RODENTS/SMALL MAMMALS:**

a) **Rabbits:** 11–22 mg/kg PO q8h (Ivey & Morrisey 2000)

b) **Guinea pigs:** 50 mg/kg IM q24h (Adamcak & Otten 2000))

■ **FERRETS:**
For susceptible infections:

a) 15–25 mg/kg PO 2–3 times daily (Williams 2000)

■ **HORSES:**

For susceptible infections:

a) 30 mg/kg PO q8h (Davis *et al.* 2005)

b) 22–33 mg/kg PO q6h (Brumbaugh 1999)

■ **BIRDS:**

For susceptible infections:

a) 35–50 mg/kg PO four times daily (using suspension); most preps are well accepted (Clubb 1986)

b) 40–100 mg/kg q6h PO (Hoeffer 1995)

c) **Ratites:** 15–22 mg/kg PO three times daily; For megabacteriosis: 50 mg/kg PO 4 times daily for 5 days (Jenson 1998)

Monitoring

■ Because cephalosporins usually have minimal toxicity associated with their use, monitoring for efficacy is usually all that is required

■ Patients with diminished renal function may require intensified renal monitoring. Serum levels and therapeutic drug monitoring are not routinely done with these agents

Chemistry/Synonyms

A semi-synthetic oral cephalosporin, cephalexin (as the monohydrate) occurs as a white to off-white crystalline powder. It is slightly soluble in water and practically insoluble in alcohol.

Cephalexin may also be known as: cefalexin, 66873, or cefalexinum; many trade names are available.

Storage/Stability

Cephalexin tablets, capsules, and powder for oral suspension should be stored at room temperature (15–30°C) in tight containers. After reconstitution, the oral suspension is stable for 2 weeks.

Dosage Forms/Regulatory Status

VETERINARY-LABELED PRODUCTS: None

HUMAN-LABELED PRODUCTS:

Cephalexin Oral Capsules: 250 mg, 333 mg, 500 mg & 750 mg; Oral Tablets: 250 mg & 500 mg; *Keflex*® (Advancis); generic; (Rx)

Cephalexin Powder for Oral Suspension: 125 mg/5mL & 250 mg/5 mL (after reconstitution) in 100 mL & 200 mL; *Keflex*® (Advancis); generic; (Rx)

References

Adamcak, A & B Otten (2000). Rodent Therapeutics. *Vet Clin NA: Exotic Anim Pract* 3:1(Jan): 221–240.

Aucoin, D (2000). Antimicrobial Drug Formulary. *Target: The antimicrobial guide to effective treatment* Port Huron, MI, North American Compendiums Inc: 93–142.

Beale, K & M Murphy (2006). Selecting appropriate antimicrobial therapy for infections of the skin of the dog. Proceedings: Western Vet Conf. Accessed via: Veterinary Information Network. http://goo.gl/aQoiv

Brovida, C (2003). Urinary Tract Infection (UTI): How to diagnose correctly and treat. Proceedings: World Small Animal Veterinary Assoc World Congress. Accessed via: Veterinary Information Network. http://goo.gl/F2zcU

Brumbaugh, G (1999). Clinical Pharmacology and the Pediatric Patient. 45th Annual AAEP Convention, Albuquerque.

Clubb, SL (1986). Therapeutics: Individual and Flock Treatment Regimens. *Clinical Avian Medicine and Surgery.* GJ Harrison and LR Harrison Eds. Philadelphia, W.B. Saunders: 327–355.

Davis, J, J Salmon, et al. (2005). The pharmacokinetics and tissue distribution of cephalexin in the horse. Proceedings: ACVIM 2005. Accessed via: Veterinary Information Network. http://goo.gl/iSOGe

Dova, SW, G Albarellos, et al. (2008). Comparative pharmacokinetics of an injectable cephalexin suspension in beef cattle. *Research in Veterinary Science* 85(3): 570–574.

Freshman, J (2002a). Management of uterine infections in the bitch. Proceedings: Western Veterinary Conference. Accessed via: Veterinary Information Network. http://goo.gl/wFibP

Freshman, J (2002b). Puppy neonatology. Proceedings: Western Veterinary Conference. Accessed via: Veterinary Information Network. http://goo.gl/vE0Z7

Greene, C & A Watson (1998). Antimicrobial Drug Formulary. *Infectious Diseases of the Dog and Cat.* C Greene Ed. Philadelphia, WB Saunders: 790–919.

Hillier, A (2006). Antibiotic therapy for pyoderma. Proceedings: ACVC. Accessed via: Veterinary Information Network. http://goo.gl/uLSKY

Hoeffer, H (1995). Antimicrobials in pet birds. *Kirk's Current Veterinary Therapy:XII.* J Bonagura Ed. Philadelphia, W.B. Saunders: 1278–1283.

Ivey, E & J Morrisey (2000). Therapeutics for Rabbits. *Vet Clin NA: Exotic Anim Pract* 3:1(Jan): 183–216.

Jenson, J (1998). Current ratite therapy. *The Veterinary Clinics of North America: Food Animal Practice* 16:3(November).

Kwochka, K (2002). Appropriate use of antimicrobials in dermatology and otology: Options for topical and systemic treatments. Proceedings: ACVIM Forum. Accessed via: Veterinary Information Network. http://goo.gl/reiPh

Lappin, M (2002). Feline fevers of unknown origin I, II, III. Proceedings: Western Veterinary Conference. Accessed via: Veterinary Information Network. http://goo.gl/JuGRY

Macintire, D (2004). Pediatric Emergencies. Proceedings: ACVIM Forum. Accessed via: Veterinary Information Network. http://goo.gl/hIEyv

Prados, AP, L Arnbros, et al. (2007). Chronopharmacological study of cephalexin in dogs. *Chronobiology International* 24(1): 161–170.

Toma, S, S Colombo, et al. (2008). Efficacy and tolerability of once-daily cephalexin in canine superficial pyoderma: an open controlled study. *Journal of Small Animal Practice* 49(8): 384–391.

Vaden, S & M Papich (1995). Empiric Antibiotic Therapy. *Kirk's Current Veterinary Therapy:XII.* J Bonagura Ed. Philadelphia, W.B. Saunders: 276–280.

Williams, B (2000). Therapeutics in Ferrets. *Vet Clin NA: Exotic Anim Pract* 3:1(Jan): 131–153.

CEPHAPIRIN SODIUM
CEPHAPIRIN BENZATHINE

(sef-a-*pye*-rin)   Cefa-Lak®, Cefa-Dri®

1ST GENERATION CEPHALOSPORIN

Prescriber Highlights

▶ 1st generation intramammary cephalosporin; also used via intrauterine infusions for endometritis

▶ Potentially could cause hypersensitivity reactions

▶ Watch withdrawal times

Uses/Indications

In the USA, there are no longer parenterally administered cephapirin products available. A 500 mg intrauterine suspension (*Metricure®*) is available in many countries worldwide.

An intramammary cephapirin sodium product is FDA-approved in the USA for use in the treatment of mastitis in lactating dairy cows and cephapirin benzathine is FDA-approved in dry cows.

Pharmacology/Actions

A first generation cephalosporin, cephapirin exhibits activity against the bacteria usually covered by this class. A cephalothin disk is usually used to determine bacterial susceptibility to this antibiotic when using the Kirby-Bauer method. Cephalosporins are usually bactericidal against susceptible bacteria and act by inhibiting mucopeptide synthesis in the cell wall resulting in a defective barrier and an osmotically unstable spheroplast. The exact mechanism for this effect has not been definitively determined, but beta-lactam antibiotics have been shown to bind to several enzymes (carboxypeptidases, transpeptidases, endopeptidases) within the bacterial cytoplasmic membrane that are involved with cell wall synthesis. The different affinities that various beta-lactam antibiotics have for these enzymes (also known as penicillin-binding proteins; PBPs) help explain the differences in these drugs' spectrums of activity that are not explained by the influence of beta-lactamases. Like other beta-lactam antibiotics, cephalosporins are generally considered more effective against actively growing bacteria.

Pharmacokinetics

In cattle when used systemically, the apparent volume of distribution has been reported as 0.335–0.399 L/kg; total body clearance is 12.66 mL/min/kg and serum elimination half-life is about 64–70 minutes in cattle.

When cephapirin sodium (*Cefa-Lak®*) was administered to healthy (no mastitis) dairy cattle via intramammary infusion it was rapidly metabolized to the active metabolite desacetylcephaprin in milk. Times above MIC_{90} for common mastitis pathogens and time to reach FDA tolerance concentrations is similar whether the cow was milked two or three times daily. Additionally, giving the second dose 16 hours later (rather then 12 hours as labeled) to cows that are milked three times daily caused no significant effect on withdrawal times or times above MIC. Cows with low daily milk production (<25kg) appear to absorb more cephalothin systemically and had longer mean residence times than those with high milk production. The authors caution that extended withdrawal times would be prudent in cows with very low milk production and that more studies are required to determine the pharmacokinetics in animals with mastitis. (Stockler *et al.* 2009).

Contraindications/Precautions/Warnings

Cephalosporins are contraindicated in patients with a history of hypersensitivity to them. Because there may be cross-reactivity, use cephalosporins cautiously in patients who are documented hypersensitive to other beta-lactam antibiotics (*e.g.*, penicillins, cefamycins, carbapenems).

Adverse Effects

Adverse effects with the cephalosporins are usually not serious and have a relatively low frequency of occurrence.

Potentially, hypersensitivity reactions could occur with intramammary infusion. Hypersensitivity reactions unrelated to dose can occur with these agents and can manifest as rashes, fever, eosinophilia, lymphadenopathy, or full-blown anaphylaxis. The use of cephalosporins in patients documented to be hypersensitive to penicillin-class antibiotics is controversial. In humans, it is estimated 1–15% of patients hypersensitive to penicillins will also be hypersensitive to cephalosporins. The incidence of cross-reactivity in veterinary patients is unknown.

Reproductive/Nursing Safety

Cephalosporins have been shown to cross the placenta and safe use of them during pregnancy has not been firmly established, but neither have there been any documented teratogenic problems associated with these drugs. See label information for more information.

Overdosage/Acute Toxicity

No clinical effects would be expected but if used at doses or rates higher than labeled, withdrawal times may be prolonged.

Drug Interactions

No significant concerns when used via the intramammary or intrauterine routes.

Laboratory Considerations

■ No significant concerns when used via the intramammary route or intrauterine routes.

Doses

■ **CATTLE:**

For mastitis:
a) Lactating cow (*Cefa-Lak®*): After milking out udder, clean and dry teat area. Swab teat tip with alcohol wipe and allow to dry. Insert tip of syringe into teat canal; push plunger to instill entire contents. Massage quarter and do not milk out for 12 hours. May repeat dose q12h. (Label directions; *Cefa-Lak®*—BIVI)

b) Dry Cow (*Cefa-Dri®*): Same basic directions as above, but should be done at the time of drying off and not later than 30 days prior to calving. (Label directions; *Cefa-Dri®*—BIVI)

For subacute and chronic endometritis (at least 14 days after parturition) caused by cephapirin sensitive bacteria:
a) Using the Intrauterine suspension:

Contents of syringe (500 mg) instilled through the cervix into the lumen of the uterus; depending on response may retreat in 7-14 days if signs persist. May be used one day after insemination. If pyometra, pretreatment with a prostglandin recommended. (From label information; *Metricure®*—Intervet U.K.)

Monitoring

■ Because cephalosporins usually have minimal toxicity associated with their use, monitoring for efficacy is usually all that is required.

■ Patients with diminished renal function may require intensified renal monitoring. Serum levels and therapeutic drug monitoring are not routinely done with these agents.

Chemistry/Synonyms

A semi-synthetic cephalosporin antibiotic, cephapirin sodium occurs as a white to off-white, crystalline powder having a faint odor. It is very soluble in water and slightly soluble in alcohol. Each gram of the injection contains 2.36 mEq of sodium. After reconstitution, the solution for injection has a pH of 6.5–8.5.

Cephapirin sodium may also be known as: BL-P-1322, cefapirin, cefapirinum natricum, *Brisfirina®, Cefa-Dri®, Cefa-Lak®, Cefaloject®, Cefatrex®, Lopitrex®, Metricure®, Piricef®, ToDAY®* or *ToMORROW®*.

Storage/Stability

Cephapirin intramammary syringes should be stored at controlled room temperature (15–30°C); avoid excessive heat.

Dosage Forms/Regulatory Status

VETERINARY-LABELED PRODUCTS:

Cephapirin Sodium Mastitis Tube; 200 mg cephapirin per 10 mL tube; *ToDAY®* (BIVI), *Cefa-Lak®* (BIVI); (OTC). FDA-approved for use in lactating dairy cattle. Milk withdrawal = 96 hours; Slaughter withdrawal = 4 days.

Cephapirin Benzathine Mastitis Tube; 300 mg cephapirin per 10 mL tube; *ToMORROW®* (BIVI), *Cefa-Dri®* (BIVI); (OTC). FDA-approved for use in dry dairy cattle. Milk withdrawal = 72 hours after calving and must not be administered within 30 days of calving; Slaughter withdrawal = 42 days.

In many countries, including Canada, Australia and the UK, 500 mg cephapirin benzathine intrauterine infusion syringes are available for treating endometritis in dairy or beef cattle. *Metricure®* (Intervet); (Rx). Milk and meat withdrawal times may vary with each country; refer to the label, but usually: milk withdrawal = 0 hours and meat withdrawal = 48 hours.

HUMAN-LABELED PRODUCTS: None

References

Stockler, RM, DE Morin, et al. (2009). Effect of milking frequency and dosing interval on the pharmacokinetics of cephapirin after intramammary infusion in lactating dairy cows. *Journal of Dairy Science* 92(9): 4262–4275.

CETIRIZINE HCL

(she-*tih*-ra-zeen)   Zyrtec®

2ND GENERATION ANTIHISTAMINE

Prescriber Highlights

▶ Oral, relatively non-sedating antihistamine

▶ Limited clinical experience in veterinary medicine; recommended dosages for dogs & cats vary widely but the drug appears well tolerated

▶ Potentially may cause vomiting, hypersalivation, or somnolence in small animals

▶ Expensive when compared to 1st generation antihistamines; generic products becoming available

Uses/Indications

Cetirizine is a H1 receptor blocking antihistamine agent that may be useful for the adjunctive treatment of histamine-mediated pruritic conditions in dogs or cats. It may also find a role in treating horses.

Pharmacology/Actions

Cetirizine, a human metabolite of hydroxyzine, is a piperazine-class non-sedating (when compared to first generation drugs) antihistamine. It selectively inhibits peripheral H1 receptors. Also, cetirizine appears to decrease histamine release from basophils in some species, but in cats, cetirizine or cyproheptadine do not reduce eosinophilic airway inflammation (experimentally produced) (Schooley *et al.* 2007). Cetirizine does not possess significant anticholinergic or anti-serotonergic effects. Tolerance to its antihistaminic effects is thought not to occur.

Pharmacokinetics

No specific information was located for the pharmacokinetics of cetirizine in dogs. In a study performed in cats (Papich *et al.* 2006) after an oral dose of 5 mg, volume of distribution was 0.26 L/kg and clearance about 0.3 mL/L/minute. Terminal elimination half-life was approximately 11 hours. The mean plasma concentrations remained above 0.85 micrograms/mL (a concentration reported to be effective for humans) for 24 hours after dosing. In horses, the terminal elimination half-life is reported to be around 6 hours (Olsen *et al.* 2008). After oral administration to humans, cetirizine peak concentrations occur in about one hour. Food can delay, but not affect the extent of, absorption. It is 93% bound to human plasma proteins and brain levels are approximately 10% of those found in plasma. Approximately 80% is excreted in the urine, primarily as unchanged drug. Terminal elimination half-life is around 8 hours; antihistaminic effect generally persists for 24 hours after a dose.

Contraindications/Precautions/Warnings

No specific information is available for veterinary patients. In humans, cetirizine is contraindicated in patients hypersensitive to it or hydroxyzine. Dosage adjustment is recommended in humans with severe renal or hepatic impairment, or older than 76 years of age.

The combination product containing pseudoephedrine is not appropriate for use in dogs or cats.

Adverse Effects

Cetirizine appears well tolerated in dogs and cats. Vomiting or hypersalivation after dosing have been reported in some dogs. Drowsiness has been reported in small dogs at higher dosages.

A pharmacokinetic/pharmacodynamic study performed in a small number of horses yielded no visible adverse effects.

In humans, the primary adverse effects reported have been drowsiness (13%) and dry mouth (5%). Rarely, hypersensitivity reactions or hepatitis have been reported.

Reproductive/Nursing Safety

In pregnant mice, rats, and rabbits, dosages of approximately 40X, 180X, and 220X respectively, of the human dose when compared on mg/m^2 basis, caused no teratogenic effects. In humans, the FDA categorizes cetirizine as category *B* for use during pregnancy (*Animal studies have not yet demonstrated risk to the fetus, but there are no adequate studies in pregnant women; or animal studies have shown an adverse effect, but adequate studies in pregnant women have not demonstrated a risk to the fetus in the first trimester of pregnancy, and there is no evidence of risk in later trimesters.*)

In Beagles, approximately 3% of a dose was excreted into milk. Although probably safe for use in nursing veterinary patients, the manufacturer does not recommend using cetirizine in nursing women.

Overdosage/Acute Toxicity

Limited information is available. Reported minimum lethal oral doses for mice and rats are 237 mg/kg (95X human adult dose on a mg/m^2 basis) and 562 mg/kg (460X human adult dose on a mg/m^2 basis), respectively. Cetirizine may cross into the CNS in overdose situations and cause neurologic signs. Unlike the earlier non-sedating antihistamines, terfenadine and astemizole (both no longer available in the USA), cetirizine does not appreciably prolong the QT interval on ECG at high serum levels.

Overdoses of cetirizine products that also contain pseudoephedrine (*Zyrtec-D 12 Hour®*) may be serious. It is advised to contact an animal poison control center in this event.

Drug Interactions

The following drug interactions have either been reported or are theoretical in humans or animals receiving cetirizine and may be of significance in veterinary patients:

■ **CNS DEPRESSANTS:** Additive CNS depression if used with cetirizine

Laboratory Considerations

■ None noted, however discontinue medication well in advance of any **hypersensitivity skin testing**

Doses

■ **DOGS:**

a) For atopic dermatitis: 1 mg/kg PO once daily with or without food. Satisfactory control of pruritus in 18% of dogs evaluated in the study. (Cook *et al.* 2004)

b) For atopic dermatitis: 5–10 mg (total dose) PO once daily (Thomas 2005)

c) For allergic dermatitis: 1 mg/kg PO q12h (Hillier 2004)

d) For adjunctive treatment of pruritus: 0.5–1 mg/kg or 5–10 mg total dose once to twice daily. (MacDonald 2007)

■ **CATS:**

a) For adjunctive treatment of non-responsive chronic rhinosinusitis: 5 mg (total dose) PO q12h (Hawkins & Cohn 2006)

b) 5 mg (total dose) per cat PO once daily, no controlled studies evaluating effectiveness against other antihistamines. (Ashley 2009)

c) For adjunctive treatment of pruritus: 2.5–5 mg (total dose) per cat once daily. (MacDonald 2002), (MacDonald 2007)

■ **HORSES:**

a) Based on pharmacokinetic and pharmacodynamic data, cetirizine at 0.2–0.4 mg/kg PO q12h may be a useful antihistamine in horses. (Olsen *et al.* 2008)

Monitoring

■ Clinical efficacy

■ Adverse effects (vomiting, somnolence)

Client Information

■ Warn clients of the potential costs

■ Potential adverse effects include GI effects (vomiting, hypersalivation) and somnolence

■ May be given without regard to feeding status

Chemistry/Synonyms

Cetirizine HCl occurs as a white to almost white, crystalline powder that is freely soluble in water. A 5% solution has a pH of 1.2–1.8.

Cetirizine may also be known as: UCB-P071, P-071, cetirizina, cetirizini, cetirizin, ceterizino, or *Zyrtec®*; many internationally registered trade names are available.

Storage/Stability

Tablets should be stored at 20–25°C; excursions are permitted to 15–30°C. The oral syrup may be stored at room temperature or in the refrigerator.

Dosage Forms/Regulatory Status

VETERINARY-LABELED PRODUCTS: None

The ARCI (Racing Commissioners International) has designated this drug as a class 4 substance.

HUMAN-LABELED PRODUCTS:

Cetirizine HCl Oral Tablets (film-coated): 5 mg & 10 mg; *Zyrtec®* (McNeil Consumer), generic; (Rx)

Cetirizine HCl Chewable Tablets (grape flavor): 5 mg & 10 mg; *Zyrtec®* (McNeil Consumer); (Rx)

Cetirizine HCl Oral Syrup: 1 mg/mL (grape flavor) in 118 & 473 mL; *Zyrtec®* (McNeil Consumer); generic; (Rx)

Cetirizine HCl 5 mg with Pseudoephedrine HCl 120 mg Extended-Release Tablets; *Zyrtec-D 12 Hour®* (Pfizer); (Rx)

References

Ashley, P (2009). Thinking outside the box of DepoMedrol: Dermatology drug choices for cats. Proceedings: WVC. Accessed via: Veterinary Information Network. http://goo.gl/I1bRP

Cook, C, D Scott, et al. (2004). Treatment of canine atopic dermatitis with cetirizine, a second–generation antihistamine: a single–blinded, placebo–controlled study. *Can Vet J* 45: 414–417.

Hawkins, E & L Cohn (2006). Infectious rhinitis: What bugs? What drugs? Proceedings WVC2006. Accessed via: Veterinary Information Network. http://goo.gl/RNmIK

Hillier, A (2004). Practical symptomatic therapy for allergic dermatitis. Proceedings WVC2004. Accessed via: Veterinary Information Network. http://goo.gl/M9Zpr

MacDonald, J (2002). Current therapy for pruritus. Proceedings: Western Veterinary Conference. Accessed via: Veterinary Information Network. http://goo.gl/ErwOJ

MacDonald, J (2007). Treating the atopic dogs: Options to keep the pet owner happy. Proceedings: ACVC. Accessed via: Veterinary Information Network. http://goo.gl/bnR4Q

Olsen, L, U Bondesson, et al. (2008). Cetirizine in horses: Pharmacokinetics and pharmacodynamics following repeated oral administration. *Veterinary Journal* 177(2): 242–249.

Papich, M, E Schooley, et al. (2006). Cetirizine (Zyrtec®) pharmacokinetics in healthy cats. Proceedings: ACVIM 2006. Accessed via: Veterinary Information Network. http://goo.gl/T8BSW

Schooley, EK, JBM Turner, et al. (2007). Effects of cyproheptadine and cetirizine on eosinophilic airway inflammation in cats with experimentally induced asthma. *American Journal of Veterinary Research* 68(11): 1265–1271.

Thomas, R (2005). Canine atopic dermatitis II: Treatment. Proceedings: WVC2005. Accessed via: Veterinary Information Network. http://goo.gl/Zi2W7

CHARCOAL, ACTIVATED

(***char**-kole*)   Toxiban®

ORAL ADSORBENT

Prescriber Highlights

▶ Orally administered adsorbent for GI tract toxins/drug overdoses; recommend consulting with an animal poison control center before use

▶ Not effective for mineral acids/alkalis

▶ Too rapid administration may induce emesis/aspiration

▶ In small dogs & cats, monitor for hypernatremia

▶ Handle with care as charcoal stains clothing very easily; dry powder "floats"

Uses/Indications

Activated charcoal is administered orally to adsorb certain drugs or toxins to prevent or reduce their systemic absorption.

Pharmacology/Actions

Activated charcoal has a large surface area and adsorbs many chemicals and drugs via ion-ion, hydrogen bonding, dipole and Van der Walle forces in the upper GI tract thereby preventing or reducing their absorption. Efficiency of adsorption increases with the molecular size of the toxin and poorly water soluble organic substances are better adsorbed than small, polar, water-soluble organic compounds.

While activated charcoal also adsorbs various nutrients and enzymes from the gut, when used for acute poisonings, no clinical significance usually results. Activated charcoal reportedly is not effective in adsorbing cyanide, but this has been disputed in a recent study. It is not very effective in adsorbing alcohols, ferrous sulfate, lithium, caustic alkalies, nitrates, sodium chloride/chlorate, petroleum distillates or mineral acids. Activated charcoal slurries are more effective in adsorbing most toxins than are tablets.

Pharmacokinetics

Activated charcoal is not absorbed nor metabolized in the gut. As activated charcoal slurries can slow GI transit times, an osmotic cathartic is often given concurrently which can enhance expulsion of the toxin-charcoal moiety.

Contraindications/Precautions/Warnings

Charcoal should not be used for mineral acids or caustic alkalies as it is ineffective. Although not contraindicated for ethanol, methanol, or iron salts, activated charcoal is ineffective in adsorbing these products and may obscure GI lesions during endoscopy.

To enhance elimination of the charcoal-toxin moiety, an osmotic cathartic (*e.g.*, sorbitol) is often given with activated charcoal. If multiple doses of activated charcoal are administered, it has been recommended that only the first dose contain the cathartic to prevent diarrhea and dehydration (Jutkowitz & Schildt 2009).

Adverse Effects
Very rapid GI administration of charcoal can induce emesis. If aspiration occurs after activated charcoal is administered, pneumonitis/aspiration pneumonia may result. Charcoal can cause either constipation or diarrhea and feces will be black. Products containing sorbitol may cause loose stools and vomiting.

There have been reports of hypernatremia occurring in small dogs and cats after charcoal (with or without sorbitol) administration, presumably due an osmotic effect pulling water into the GI tract. Reduced sodium fluids (*e.g.*, D5W, 1/2 normal saline/D2.5W) with warm water enemas can be administered to alleviate the condition.

Charcoal powder is very staining and the dry powder tends to "float" covering wide areas.

Overdosage/Acute Toxicity
Potentially could cause electrolyte abnormalities; see Adverse Effects for more information.

Drug Interactions
The following drug interactions have either been reported or are theoretical in humans or animals receiving charcoal and may be of significance in veterinary patients:

■ **OTHER ORALLY ADMINISTERED THERAPEUTIC AGENTS:** Separate by at least 3 hours the administration of any other orally administered therapeutic agents from the charcoal dose

■ **DAIRY PRODUCTS:** May reduce the adsorptive capacity of activated charcoal

■ **MINERAL OIL:** May reduce the adsorptive capacity of activated charcoal

■ **POLYETHYLENE GLYCOL; ELECTROLYTE SOLUTIONS (*e.g., Go-Lytely®*):** May reduce the adsorptive capacity of activated charcoal

Doses

■ **DOGS & CATS:**
Note: Depending on the toxin exposure, recommendations for using activated charcoal can vary. It is highly recommended to contact an animal poison control center for specific guidance on using activated charcoal in veterinary patients.

Dogs and cats with no clinical signs may freely drink the charcoal suspension if administered via syringe. A small amount of food may be added to the solution to enhance palatability. In animals exhibiting clinical signs, administration of activated charcoal slurries/suspensions may be administered via an orogastric tube with a cuffed endotracheal tube in place to help prevent aspiration. Administration via a nasogastric tube may be useful, particularly in cats. (Jutkowitz & Schildt 2009)

As a gastrointestinal absorbent:
a) 10 mL of a 20% slurry (1 g of charcoal in 5 mL of water) per kg of body weight by stomach tube (Carson & Osweiler 2003)

For acute poisoning:
a) After decontamination of the GI tract give activated charcoal at 1–4 g/kg PO. Placement of a nasogastric tube can facilitate administration and reduce the incidence of aspiration in the sedated/fractious animal particularly when repeated administration is desired; repeat every 4–6 hours for toxins that are recirculated through the intestinal capillary network. (Rudloff 2006)

b) 1–4 g/kg in 50–200 mL of water. Concurrent with or within 30 minutes of giving charcoal, give an osmotic cathartic. Repeated doses of activated charcoal may also bind drugs that are enterohepatically recycled. (Beasley & Dorman 1990)

c) Administer in a bathtub or other easily cleanable area. Give activated charcoal at 1–5 g/kg PO (via stomach tube using either a funnel or large syringe) diluted in water at a concentration of 1 g charcoal/5 –10 mL of water. Follow in 30 minutes with sodium sulfate oral cathartic. (Bailey 1989)

■ **RUMINANTS:**
a) As a cathartic for plant intoxications: Activated charcoal (AC) slurry dosage range of 1–5 g/kg (~1 g of activated charcoal per 5 ml of water). Multi-dose activated charcoal is beneficial for a number of plant intoxications, including oleander. Administration of a cathartic mixed in the AC slurry helps to hasten elimination of contents from the gastrointestinal tract. Commonly used cathartics include sodium sulfate (Glauber's salts), magnesium sulfate (Epsom salts), and sorbitol. Sodium or magnesium sulfate can be administered at 250–500 mg/kg mixed in the AC slurry. Sorbitol (70%), also mixed in the AC slurry, can be administered at 3 ml/kg. There is little need to administer a cathartic if significant diarrhea is already present. (Puschner 2010)

■ **HORSES:**
a) **Foals:** 250 grams (minimum). Adult horses: up to 750 grams. Make a slurry by mixing with up to 4 L (depending on animal's size) of warm water and administer via stomach tube. Leave in stomach for 20–30 minutes and then give a laxative to hasten removal of toxicants. (Oehme 1987)

b) See the reference by Puschner in the Ruminants section above

Monitoring

■ Monitoring for efficacy of charcoal is usually dependent upon the toxin/drug that it is being used for and could include the drug/toxin's serum level, clinical signs, etc.

■ Serum sodium, particularly if patient develops neurologic signs associated with hypernatremia (tremors, ataxia, seizures)

Client Information

■ This agent should generally be used with professional supervision; if used on an outpatient basis patients must be observed for at least 4 hours after administration for signs associated with too much sodium in the blood (weakness, unsteadiness, tremors, convulsions). Should these occur, patients must immediately be seen by a veterinarian.

■ Charcoal can easily stain fabrics

Chemistry/Synonyms

Activated charcoal occurs as a fine, black, odorless, tasteless powder that is insoluble in water or alcohol. Commercially available activated charcoal products may differ in their adsorptive properties, but one gram must adsorb 100 mg of strychnine sulfate in 50 mL of water to meet USP standards.

Activated charcoal may also be known as: active carbon, activated carbon, carbo activatus, adsorbent charcoal, decolorizing carbon, or medicinal charcoal. There are many trade names available.

Storage/Stability

Store activated charcoal in well-closed glass or metal containers or in the manufacturer's supplied container.

Dosage Forms/Regulatory Status

VETERINARY-LABELED PRODUCTS:

In the USA, the following products are labeled for veterinary use, but there are no oral activated charcoal products listed as FDA-approved on the FDA's "Green Book" website.

Activated charcoal 47.5%, Kaolin 10% granules (free flowing and wettable) in 1 lb bottles, and 5 kg pails: *Toxiban® Granules* (Vet-A-Mix); (OTC). Labeled for use in both large and small animals.

Activated charcoal 10.4%, Kaolin 6.25% suspension in 240 mL bottles: *Toxiban® Suspension* (Vet-A-Mix); (OTC). Labeled for use in both large and small animals.

Activated charcoal 10%, Kaolin 6.25%, sorbitol 10% suspension in 240 mL bottles: *Toxiban® Suspension* with *Sorbitol* Vet-A-Mix); (OTC). Labeled for use in small animals.

Activated Charcoal 10%, Attapulgite 20%, sodium chloride 35 mg/mL, potassium chloride 35 mg/mL Gel/Paste in 80 mL & 300 mL: *D-Tox-Besc®* (AgriPharm); *Activated Charcoal Gel with Electrolytes®* & *DVM Formula®* (Bomac Plus Vet), *Activated Charcoal Paste®* (First Priority); (OTC). Labeled for use in small and large animals.

Activated Hardwood Charcoal and thermally activated attapulgite clay (concentrations not labeled) in an aqueous gel suspension in 8 fl oz bottle, 60 mL tube and 300 mL tube with easy dose syringe. *UAA® (Universal Animal Antidote) Gel* (Vedco); (OTC). Labeled for use in dogs, cats and grain overload in ruminants.

HUMAN-LABELED PRODUCTS:

Activated Charcoal Oral Powder: 15 g, 30 g, 40 g, 120 g, 240 g and UD 30 g; generic; (OTC)

Activated Charcoal Oral Liquid/Suspension with sorbitol: 15 g & 30 g in 150 mL & 50 g in 240 mL; *CharcoAid®* (Requa); 25 g in 120 mL & 50 g in 240 mL; *Actidose® with Sorbitol* (Paddock); (OTC)

Activated Charcoal Liquid/Suspension without sorbitol: 15 g & 50 g in 120 mL & 240 mL; *CharcoAid® 2000* (Requa); (OTC); 208 mg/mL — 12.5 g in 60 mL & 25 g in 120 mL; 12.5 g in 60 mL, 15 g in 75 mL, 25 g in 120 mL, 30 g in 120 mL, 50 g in 240 mL; *Actidose-Aqua®* (Paddock); generic; (OTC)

Activated Charcoal Oral Granules: 15 g in 120 mL; *CharcoAid® 2000* (Requa); (OTC)

References

Bailey, EM (1989). Emergency and general treatment of poisonings. *Current Veterinary Therapy (CVT) X Small Animal Practice.* RW Kirk Ed. Philadelphia, W.B. Saunders: 116–125.

Beasley, VR & DC Dorman (1990). Management of Toxicoses. *Vet Clin of North America: Sm Anim Pract* 20(2): 307–337.

Carson, T & G Osweiler (2003). Toxicology. *Handbook of Small Animal Practice.* R Morgan, R Bright and M Swartout Eds. Phil., Saunders: 1197–1244.

Jutkowitz, L & J Schildt (2009). Management of common household toxins. Proceedings: WVC. http://goo.gl/oiqBU

Oehme, FW (1987). General Principles in Treatment of Poisoning. *Current Therapy in Equine Medicine 2.* NE Robinson Ed. Philadelphia, W.B. Saunders.

Puschner, B (2010). Diagnostic and therapeutic approach to plant poisonings in large animals. Accessed via: Veterinary Information Network. http://www.vin.com/Members/Proceedings/Proceedings.plx?CID=AC VIM2010&PID=PR55815&O=VIN

Rudloff, E (2006). Poisonings and intoxications. Proceedings: Western Veterinary Conference. Accessed via: Veterinary Information Network. http://goo.gl/bFWOg

CHLORAMBUCIL

(klor-*am*-byoo-sil)   Leukeran®

IMMUNOSUPPRESSANT/
ANTINEOPLASTIC

Prescriber Highlights

▶ Nitrogen mustard derivative immunosuppressant & antineoplastic

▶ Used for severe autoimmune diseases
in cats (e.g., IBD, pemphigus, etc.) as it
is less toxic than cyclophosphamide or
azathioprine in cats

▶ Caution: Preexisting bone marrow
depression, infection

▶ Potential teratogen

▶ Adverse Effects primarily myelosuppression & GI toxicity

Uses/Indications

Chlorambucil may be useful in a variety of
neoplastic diseases, including lymphocytic
leukemia, multiple myeloma, polycythemia
vera, macroglobulinemia, and ovarian adenocarcinoma. It may also be useful as adjunctive
therapy for some immune-mediated conditions
(*e.g.*, glomerulonephritis, inflammatory bowel
disease, non-erosive arthritis, or immune-mediated skin disease). It has found favor as a routine
treatment for feline pemphigus foliaceous and
severe feline eosinophilic granuloma complex
due to the drug's relative lack of toxicity in cats
and efficacy.

Pharmacology/Actions

Chlorambucil is a cell-cycle nonspecific alkylating antineoplastic/immunosuppressive agent.
Its cytotoxic activity stems from cross-linking
with cellular DNA.

Pharmacokinetics

Chlorambucil is rapidly and nearly completely
absorbed after oral administration; peak levels
occur in about one hour. It is highly bound to
plasma proteins. While it is not known whether
it crosses the blood-brain barrier, neurological
side effects have been reported. Chlorambucil
crosses the placenta, but it is not known whether
it enters maternal milk. Chlorambucil is extensively metabolized in the liver, primarily
to phenylacetic acid mustard, which is active.
Phenylacetic acid mustard is further metabolized to other metabolites that are excreted in
the urine.

Contraindications/Precautions/Warnings

Chlorambucil is contraindicated in patients who
are hypersensitive to it or have demonstrated
resistance to its effects. It should be used with
caution in patients with preexisting bone marrow depression or infection, or are susceptible to
bone marrow depression or infection.

Adverse Effects

The most commonly associated major adverse
effects seen with chlorambucil therapy is myelosuppression manifested by anemia, leukopenia,
and thrombocytopenia and gastrointestinal
toxicity (vomiting, diarrhea). A greater likelihood of toxicity occurs with higher dosages.
This may occur gradually with nadirs occurring
usually within 7–14 days of the start of therapy.
Recovery generally takes from 7–14 days. Severe
bone marrow depression can result in pancytopenia that may take months to years for recovery. Alopecia and delayed regrowth of shaven
fur have been reported in dogs; Poodles or Kerry
blues are reportedly more likely to be affected
than other breeds. One case report of neurotoxicity (facial twitching, myoclonus, agitation,
seizures) after chlorambucil therapy in a cat has
been reported (Benitah *et al.* 2003).

In humans, bronchopulmonary dysplasia with
pulmonary fibrosis, neurotoxicity, and uric acid
nephropathy have been reported. These effects
are uncommon and generally associated with
chronic, higher dose therapy. Hepatotoxicity has
been reported rarely in humans.

Reproductive/Nursing Safety

Chlorambucil's teratogenic potential remains
poorly documented, but it may potentially
cause a variety of fetal abnormalities. It is generally recommended to avoid the drug during
pregnancy, but because of the seriousness of the
diseases treated with chlorambucil, the potential benefits to the mother must be considered.
Chlorambucil has been documented to cause
irreversible infertility in male humans, particularly when given during pre-puberty and puberty. In humans, the FDA categorizes this drug
as category *D* for use during pregnancy (*There
is evidence of human fetal risk, but the potential
benefits from the use of the drug in pregnant wom-
en may be acceptable despite its potential risks.*) In
a separate system evaluating the safety of drugs
in canine and feline pregnancy (Papich 1989),
this drug is categorized as in class: *C* (*These
drugs may have potential risks. Studies in people
or laboratory animals have uncovered risks, and
these drugs should be used cautiously as a last resort when the benefit of therapy clearly outweighs
the risks.*)

Overdosage/Acute Toxicity

The oral LD_{50} in mice is 123 mg/kg. There have
been limited experiences with acute overdoses
in humans. Doses of up to 5 mg/kg resulted in
neurologic (seizures) toxicity and pancytopenia (nadirs at 1–6 weeks post ingestion). All
patients recovered without long-term sequelae.
Treatment should consist of gut emptying when
appropriate (beware of rapidly changing neurologic status if inducing vomiting). Monitoring
of CBC's several times a week for several weeks
should be performed after overdoses and blood
component therapy may be necessary.

Drug Interactions

The following drug interactions have either been reported or are theoretical in humans or animals receiving chlorambucil and may be of significance in veterinary patients:

■ **MYELOSUPPRESSIVE DRUGS (e.g., other antineoplastics, chloramphenicol, flucytosine, amphotericin B, or colchicine):** Bone marrow depression may be additive

■ **IMMUNOSUPPRESSIVE DRUGS (e.g., azathioprine, cyclophosphamide, cyclosporine, corticosteroids):** Use with other immunosuppressant drugs may increase the risk of infection

Laboratory Considerations

■ Chlorambucil may raise serum **uric acid** levels. Drugs such as **allopurinol** may be required to control hyperuricemia in some patients.

Doses

For current specific dosing recommendations, indications, treatment protocols, monitoring and safety guidelines when chlorambucil is used as an antineoplastic agent, it is strongly recommended to work in collaboration with a veterinary oncologist and to refer to veterinary oncology references (Henry & Higginbotham 2009); (Argyle *et al.* 2008); (Withrow & Vail 2007); (Villalobos 2007); (Ogilvie & Moore 2006); (Ogilvie & Moore 2001).

■ **DOGS:**

For adjunctive therapy (as an immunosuppressant) in the treatment of glomerulonephritis:

a) 0.1–0.2 mg/kg PO once daily or every other day (Vaden & Grauer 1992)

For adjunctive therapy of lymphoreticular neoplasms, macroglobulinemia, and polycythemia vera:

a) For first level treatment of dogs of canine lymphoma where clients cannot afford, or will not accept combination chemotherapy due to risks of toxicity: Prednisone alone 40 mg/m^2 (NOT mg/kg) PO daily for 7 days then every other day) or in combination with chlorambucil at 6–8 mg/m^2 (NOT mg/kg) PO every other day. Perform a CBC every 2–3 weeks. (Ogilvie 2006)

b) For lymphoproliferative disease; macroglobulinemia: 2–4 mg/m^2 (NOT mg/kg) PO q24–48h (Gilson & Page 1994)

For treatment of pemphigus complex:

a) Prednisone 2–4 mg/kg PO divided q12h with chlorambucil 0.2 mg/kg q24–48h (Helton-Rhodes 1994)

b) Used in combination with corticosteroids. Chlorambucil 0.1–0.2 mg/kg once daily initially until marked improvement (or 75% improvement) of clinical signs (may require 4–8 weeks). Then alternate day dosing is begun and maintained for several weeks. If no exacerbation, alternately decrease chlorambucil and corticosteroids until lowest possible dose is attained. (White 2000)

For adjunctive treatment of inflammatory bowel disease:

a) 1.5 mg/m^2 (NOT mg/kg) PO every other day (Marks 2007)

■ **CATS:**

For adjunctive treatment of inflammatory bowel disease:

a) As a second choice (corticosteroids first choice) or refractory or severe IBD: Cats greater than 4 kg: 2 mg (total dose) PO q48 hours (every other day) for 2–4 weeks then tapered to the lowest effective dose (2 mg per cat q72–96 hours; every 3rd to 4th day). Cats less than 4 kg are started at 2 mg (total dose) q72 hours (every 3rd day). (Moore 2004)

b) 15 mg/m^2 (NOT mg/kg) PO once per day for 4 consecutive days, repeated every 3 weeks (in combination with prednisolone) appears highly effective in managing cats with severe IBD or intestinal lymphoma. Alternatively, may dose at 2 mg (total dose) per cat every 4 days indefinitely. (Marks 2007)

c) For lymphocytic-plasmacytic enteritis (LPE): Chlorambucil is sometimes useful for cats that do not respond to diet, prednisolone and metronidazole; limited experience, but seems it should be administered with prednisolone. Two methods for dosing: **1)** Initial dose is 2 mg/m^2 (NOT mg/kg) PO for 4–7 days, then decreased to 1 mg/m^2 (NOT mg/kg) for 7 days. If clinical signs are lessening, continue daily dosing but only every other week; it is common for patients to develop anemia. **2)** Large cats (>7 lb.) 2 mg PO twice weekly; smaller cats (<7 lb) 1 mg PO twice weekly. If a clinical response will occur, it should be seen in 4–6 weeks, after which the drug is slowly tapered to the lowest effective dose. Monitor CBC's anytime the cat seems to feel bad. (Willard 2006)

d) As an alternative (chlorambucil usually reserved for refractory cases) to prednisolone therapy: For cats < 2 kg: 2 mg (total dose) PO once weekly. For cats > 2 kg: 2 mg (total dose) PO once every 4 days. A good choice if no clear differentiation can be made between severe IBD and lymphoma. (Gruffyd-Jones 2009)

For adjunctive treatment of pemphigus complex or other immune-mediated dermatoses:

a) 2 mg (total dose per cat) every 48 hours.

May be used in combination with or as an alternative to steroids. (Ashley 2009)

b) For generalized pemphigus foliaceous: If cats have a poor response to prednisolone alone, may add chlorambucil at 0.1–0.2 mg/kg PO q24–48h; has slow onset of action and can cause bone marrow depression. (Hillier 2006)

c) For idiopathic dermatitis when nothing else works: 0.2 mg/kg PO q24–48h. Closely monitor during treatment. (Hnilica 2003)

For adjunctive treatment of FIP:

a) Prednisolone 4 mg/kg PO once daily with chlorambucil 20 mg/m^2 (NOT mg/kg) every 2–3 weeks (Weiss 1994)

For lymphocytic leukemia:

a) Chlorambucil 6 mg/m^2 (2 mg/5.3 kg cat) PO every other day and prednisolone 5 mg/cat/day. Supplemental cobalamin (1 mL SC q2–3 weeks) and folate/B-complex vitamins should also be given. (Simpson 2003)

■ **HORSES:**

For adjunctive therapy in treating lymphoma using the LAP protocol:

a) Cytosine arabinoside 200–300 mg/m^2 (NOT mg/kg) SC or IM once every 1–2 weeks; Chlorambucil 20 mg/m^2 (NOT mg/kg) PO every 2 weeks (alternating with cytosine arabinoside) and Prednisone 1.1–2.2 mg/kg PO every other day. If this protocol is not effective (no response seen in 2–4 weeks) add vincristine at 0.5 mg/m^2 (NOT mg/kg) IV once a week. Side effects are rare. (Couto 1994)

Monitoring

■ Efficacy

■ CBC, Platelets once weekly (or once stable every other week) during therapy; once stable, dogs may require only monthly monitoring. If neutrophils are <3,000/microL hold drug until recovered and reduce dose by 25% or increase dosing interval. Other references recommend CBCs at 0, 1, 2, 4, 8, & 12 weeks and then every 3-6 months (Mueller 2000) or in cats, CBCs at 2 to 3 weeks after starting therapy and every 3-6 months thereafter (Ashley 2009).

■ Uric acid, liver enzymes; if warranted

Client Information

■ Clients must understand the importance of both administering chlorambucil as directed and immediately reporting any signs associated with toxicity (*e.g.*, abnormal bleeding, bruising, urination, depression, infection, shortness of breath, etc.)

Chemistry/Synonyms

A nitrogen mustard derivative antineoplastic agent, chlorambucil occurs as an off-white, slightly granular powder. It is very slightly soluble in water.

Chlorambucil may also be known as: CB-1348, NSC-3088, WR-139013, chlorambucilun, chloraminophene, chlorbutinum, *Chloraminophene®*, *Leukeran®*, or *Linfolysin®*.

Storage/Stability

Chlorambucil tablets should be stored in light-resistant, well-closed containers under refrigeration (2–8°C; 36–46°F). Tablets can be stored at a maximum of 30°C (86°F) up to one week. An expiration date of one year after manufacture is assigned to the commercially available tablets.

Compatibility/Compounding Considerations

Compounded preparation stability: Chlorambucil oral suspension compounded from commercially available tablets has been published (Dressman & Poust 1983). Triturating six (6) chlorambucil 2 mg tablets with 2 mL *Cologel®* and *qs ad* to 6 mL with simple syrup yields a 2 mg/mL oral suspension that retains 90% potency for 7 days at 5°C. Suspensions of chlorambucil stored at room temperature rapidly decompose with losses >15% in one day. Chlorambucil is rapidly hydrolyzed independently of pH, but minimal hydrolysis occurs at pH 2. Refrigeration also slows hydrolysis.

Dosage Forms/Regulatory Status

VETERINARY-LABELED PRODUCTS: None

HUMAN-LABELED PRODUCTS:

Chlorambucil Oral Tablets (film-coated): 2 mg; *Leukeran®* (GlaxoSmithKline); (Rx)

References

Argyle, D, M Brearly, et al. (2008). *Decision Making in Small Animal Oncology*, Wiley–Blackwell.

Ashley, P (2009). Thinking outside the box of DepoMedrol: Dermatology drug choices for cats. Proceedings: WVC. Accessed via: Veterinary Information Network. http://goo.gl/I1bRP

Benitah, N, LP de Lorimier, et al. (2003). Chlorambucil–induced myoclonus in a cat with lymphoma. *Journal of the American Animal Hospital Association* 39(3): 283–287.

Couto, C (1994). Lymphoma in the Horse. Proceedings of the Twelfth Annual Veterinary Medical Forum, San Francisco, American College of Veterinary Internal Medicine.

Dressman, J & R Poust (1983). Stability of allopurinol and of five antineoplastics in suspension. *Am J Hosp Pharm* 40(4): 616–618.

Gilson, S & R Page (1994). Principles of Oncology. *Saunders Manual of Small Animal Practice*. S Birchard and R Sherding Eds. Philadelphia, W.B. Saunders Company: 185–192.

Gruffyd–Jones, T (2009). Feline Inflammatory Bowel Disease and Inflammatory LIver Disease. Proceedings: TuftsBG2009. Accessed via: Veterinary Information Network. http://goo.gl/cfGUw

Helton–Rhodes, K (1994). Immune–mediated dermatoses. *Saunders Manual of Small Animal Practice*. S Birchard and R Sherding Eds. Philadelphia, W.B. Saunders Company: 313–318.

Henry, C & M Higginbotham (2009). *Cancer Management in Small Animal Practice*, Saunders.

Hillier, A (2006). Update on autoimmune diseases. Proceedings: ACVC. Accessed via: Veterinary Information Network. http://goo.gl/ccGFb

Hnilica, K (2003). Managing Feline Pruritus. Proceedings: Western Veterinary Conference. Accessed via: Veterinary Information Network. http://goo.gl/U19xu

Marks, S (2007). Inflammatory Bowel Disease—More than a garbage can diagnosis. Proceedings: UCD Canine Medicine Symposium. Accessed via: Veterinary Information Network. http://goo.gl/ZGPg1

Moore, L (2004). Beyond corticosteroids for therapy of inflammatory bowel disease in dogs and cats. Proceedings: ACVIM Forum. Accessed via: Veterinary Information Network. http://goo.gl/MOJ1B

Mueller, R (2000). *Dermatology for the Small Animal Practitioner*, Teton New Media.

Ogilvie, G (2006). Canine Lymphoma. Proceedings WSAVA. Accessed via: Veterinary Information Network. http://goo.gl/yUtYJ

Ogilvie, G & A Moore (2001). *Feline Oncology: A Comprehensive Guide to Compassionate Care*, Veterinary Learning Systems.

Ogilvie, G & A Moore (2006). *Managing the Canine Cancer Patient: A Practical Guide to Compassionate Care*, Veterinary Learning Systems.

Simpson, K (2003). Chronic enteropathies: How should I treat them. Proceedings: ACVIM Forum. Accessed via: Veterinary Information Network. http://goo.gl/nicNM

Vaden, S & G Grauer (1992). Medical management of canine glomerulonephritis. *Current Veterinary Therapy XI: Small Animal Practice*. R Kirk and J Bonagura Eds. Philadelphia, W.B. Saunders Company: 861–864.

Villalobos, A (2007). *Canine and Feline Geriatric Oncology*. Ames, Blackwell.

Weiss, R (1994). Feline infectious peritonitis virus: Advances in therapy and control. *Consultations in Feline Internal Medicine: 2*. J August Ed. Philadelphia, W.B. Saunders Company: 3–12.

White, S (2000). Nonsteroidal Immunosuppressive Therapy. *Kirk's Current Veterinary Therapy: XIII Small Animal Practice*. J Bonagura Ed. Philadelphia, WB Saunders: 536–538.

Willard, M (2006). Chronic Diarrhea: Part 2. Proceedings: ACVC. Accessed via: Veterinary Information Network. http://goo.gl/LXXZ0

Withrow, S & D Vail (2007). *Withrow and MacEwen's Small Animal Clinical Oncology 4th Ed*. Philadelphia, Elsevier.

CHLORAMPHENICOL
CHLORAMPHENICOL SODIUM SUCCINATE

(klor-am-*fen*-i-kole)
Chloromycetin®, Duricol®, Viceton®
BROAD-SPECTRUM ANTIBACTERIAL

Prescriber Highlights

▶ Broad spectrum antibiotic

▶ Contraindications: Food animals (banned)

▶ Extreme caution/avoid use: Preexisting hematologic disorders, pregnancy, neonates, hepatic failure, renal failure (cats); IV use in patients with cardiac failure; use long-term (>14 days) in cats with caution

▶ May need to reduce dose in patients with hepatic or renal insufficiency

▶ Adverse Effects: GI; potentially myelo-suppressive, especially with high dose, long-term treatment

▶ Potentially toxic to humans; have dosage-giver avoid direct contact with medication

Uses/Indications

Chloramphenicol is used for a variety of infections in small animals and horses, particularly those caused by anaerobic bacteria. The FDA has prohibited the use of chloramphenicol in animals used for food production because of the human public health implications.

Pharmacology/Actions

Chloramphenicol usually acts as a bacterio-static antibiotic, but at higher concentrations or against some very susceptible organisms it can be bactericidal. Chloramphenicol acts by binding to the 50S ribosomal subunit of susceptible bacteria, thereby preventing bacterial protein synthesis. Erythromycin, clindamycin, lincomycin, tylosin, etc., also bind to the same site, but unlike these drugs, chloramphenicol appears to also have an affinity for mitochondrial ribosomes of rapidly proliferating mammalian cells (*e.g.*, bone marrow) that may result in reversible bone marrow suppression.

Chloramphenicol has a wide spectrum of activity against many gram-positive and gram-negative organisms. Gram-positive aerobic organisms that are generally susceptible to chloramphenicol include many streptococci and staphylococci. It is also effective against some gram-negative aerobes including Neisseira, Brucella, Salmonella, Shigella, and Haemophilus. Many anaerobic bacteria are sensitive to chloramphenicol including Clostridium, Bacteroides (including *B. fragilis*), Fusobacterium, and Veillonella. Chloramphenicol also has activity against Nocardia, Chlamydia, Mycoplasma, and Rickettsia.

Pharmacokinetics

Chloramphenicol is rapidly absorbed after oral administration with peak serum levels occurring approximately 30 minutes after dosing. The palmitate oral suspension produces significantly lower peak serum levels when administered to fasted cats. The sodium succinate salt is rapidly and well absorbed after IM or SC administration in animals and, contrary to some recommendations, need not be administered only intravenously. The palmitate and sodium succinate is hydrolyzed in the GI tract and liver to the base.

Chloramphenicol is widely distributed throughout the body. Highest levels are found in the liver and kidney, but the drug attains therapeutic levels in most tissues and fluids, including the aqueous and vitreous humor, and synovial fluid. CSF concentrations may be up to 50% of those in the serum when meninges are uninflamed and higher when meninges are inflamed. A 4–6 hour lag time before CSF peak levels occur may be seen. Chloramphenicol concentrations in the prostate are approximately 50% of those in the serum. Because only a small amount of the drug is excreted unchanged into the urine in dogs, chloramphenicol may not be the best choice for lower urinary tract infections in that species. The volume of distribution of chloramphenicol has been reported as 1.8 L/kg in the dog, 2.4 L/kg in the cat, and 1.41 L/kg in horses. Chloramphenicol is about 30–60% bound to plasma proteins, enters milk and crosses the placenta.

In most species, chloramphenicol is eliminated primarily by hepatic metabolism via glucuronidative mechanisms. Only about 5–15% of the drug is excreted unchanged in the urine. The cat, having little ability to glucuronidate drugs, excretes 25% or more of a dose as unchanged drug in the urine.

The elimination half-life has been reported as 1.1–5 hours in dogs, <1 hour in foals and ponies, and 4–8 hours in cats. The elimination half-life of chloramphenicol in birds is highly species variable, ranging from 26 minutes in pigeons to nearly 5 hours in bald eagles and peafowl.

The usual serum therapeutic range for chloramphenicol is 5–15 micrograms/mL.

Contraindications/Precautions/Warnings

Chloramphenicol is prohibited by the FDA for use in food animals.

Chloramphenicol is contraindicated in patients hypersensitive to it. Because of the potential for hematopoietic toxicity, the drug should be used with extreme caution, if at all, in patients with preexisting hematologic abnormalities, especially a preexisting non-regenerative anemia. The drug should only be used in patients in hepatic failure when no other effective antibiotics are available. Chloramphenicol should be used with caution in patients with impaired hepatic or renal function as drug accumulation may occur. Those patients may need dosing adjustment, and monitoring of blood levels should be considered.

Chloramphenicol should be used with caution in neonatal animals, particularly in young kittens. In neonates (humans), circulatory collapse (so-called "Gray-baby syndrome") has occurred with chloramphenicol, probably due to toxic levels accumulating secondary to an inability to conjugate the drug or excrete the conjugate effectively.

Adverse Effects

While the toxicity of chloramphenicol in humans has been much discussed, the drug is considered by most to have a low order of toxicity in adult companion animals when appropriately dosed.

The development of aplastic anemia reported in humans, does not appear to be a significant problem for veterinary patients; however, a dose-related bone marrow suppression (reversible) is seen in all species, primarily with long-term therapy. Early signs of bone marrow toxicity can include vacuolation of many of the early cells of the myeloid and erythroid series, lymphocytopenia, and neutropenia. Thrombocytopenia

associated with chloramphenicol use in cats has been reported.

Other effects that may be noted include anorexia, vomiting, diarrhea, and depression.

It has been said that cats tend to be more sensitive to developing adverse reactions to chloramphenicol than dogs, but this is probably more as a result of the drug's longer half-life in the cat. Cats dosed at 50 mg/kg q12h for 2–3 weeks do develop a high incidence of adverse effects and should be closely monitored when prolonged high-dose therapy is necessary.

Reproductive/Nursing Safety

Chloramphenicol has not been determined to be safe for use during pregnancy. The drug may decrease protein synthesis in the fetus, particularly in the bone marrow. It should only be used when the benefits of therapy clearly outweigh the risks. In humans, the FDA categorizes this drug as category *C* for use during pregnancy (*Animal studies have shown an adverse effect on the fetus, but there are no adequate studies in humans; or there are no animal reproduction studies and no adequate studies in humans.*) In a separate system evaluating the safety of drugs in canine and feline pregnancy (Papich 1989), this drug is categorized as in class: *C* (*These drugs may have potential risks. Studies in people or laboratory animals have uncovered risks, and these drugs should be used cautiously as a last resort when the benefit of therapy clearly outweighs the risks.*)

Because chloramphenicol is found in milk in humans at 50% of serum levels, the drug should be given with caution to nursing bitches or queens, particularly within the first week after giving birth.

Overdosage/Acute Toxicity

Because of the potential for serious bone marrow toxicity, large overdoses of chloramphenicol should be handled by emptying the gut using standard protocols. For more information on the toxicity of chloramphenicol, refer to the Adverse Effects section above.

Drug Interactions

The following drug interactions have either been reported or are theoretical in humans or animals receiving chloramphenicol and may be of significance in veterinary patients (**Note:** cats may be particularly susceptible to chloramphenicol's effects on the hepatic metabolism of other drugs):

■ **ANTI-ANEMIA DRUGS (Iron, Vitamin B12, folic acid):** Chloramphenicol may delay hematopoietic response

■ **BETA-LACTAM ANTIBIOTICS (penicillins, cephalosporins, aminoglycosides):** Potential for antagonism

■ **CIMETIDINE:** May reduce the metabolism of chloramphenicol increasing the risks for toxicity

■ **LIDOCAINE:** Chloramphenicol may delay hepatic metabolism

■ **MYELOSUPPRESSIVE DRUGS** (*e.g.*, **cyclophosphamide**): Potential for additive bone marrow depression

■ **PENTOBARBITAL:** Chloramphenicol has been demonstrated to prolong the duration of pentobarbital anesthesia by 120% in dogs, and 260% in cats

■ **PHENOBARBITAL:** Chloramphenicol may inhibit hepatic metabolism and phenobarbital may decrease chloramphenicol concentrations

■ **PRIMIDONE:** Anorexia and CNS effects may occur in dogs

■ **PROPOFOL:** Chloramphenicol may prolong anesthesia

■ **RIFAMPIN:** May decrease serum chloramphenicol levels

Laboratory Considerations

■ False-positive **glucosuria** has been reported, but the incidence is unknown.

Doses

■ **DOGS:**
For susceptible infections:
a) 45–60 mg/kg PO q8h; 45–60 mg/kg IM, SC or IV q6–8h (USPC 1990)
b) 40–50 mg/kg IV, IM, SC or PO q8h; avoid in young animals or in breeding or pregnant animals; avoid or reduce dosage in animals with severe liver failure. (Vaden & Papich 1995)
c) For urinary, rickettsial, localized soft tissue infections: 25–50 mg/kg PO q8h for 7 days.

For systemic infections: 50 mg/kg PO, IV, IM, SC q6–8h for 3–5 days

For severe bacteremia, sepsis: 50 mg/kg IV, IM or SC q4–6h for 3 days (Greene & Watson 1998)
d) For Rocky Mountain Spotted Fever: 15–20 mg/kg q8h PO, IM or IV for 14–21 days (Sellon & Breitschwerdt 1995)
e) For susceptible infectious otitis: 50 mg/kg PO q8h (Rosenkrantz 2006)

■ **CATS:**
For susceptible infections:
a) 25–50 mg/kg PO q12h; 12–30 mg/kg IM, SC or IV q12h (USPC 1990)
b) 50 mg (total dose) IV, IM, SC or PO q8h; avoid in young animals or in breeding or pregnant animals; avoid or reduce dosage in animals with severe liver failure (Vaden & Papich 1995)
c) For urinary, localized soft tissue infections: 50 mg per cat (total dose) PO q12h for 14 days.

For systemic infections: 25–50 mg/kg PO, IV, IM, SC q12h for 14 days or less

For severe bacteremia, sepsis: 50 mg per cat (total dose) PO, IV, IM or SC q6–

8h for 5 days or less. (Greene & Watson 1998)

■ **RABBITS/RODENTS/SMALL MAMMALS:**
a) **Rabbits:** 30–50 mg/kg PO, SC, IM, IV q8–24h (Ivey & Morrisey 2000)
b) **Hedgehogs:** 50 mg/kg PO q12h; 30–50 mg/kg SC, IM, IV or IO q12h (Smith 2000)
c) **Chinchillas:** 30–50 mg/kg PO, SC, IM q12h (Hayes 2000)
d) **Gerbils, Guinea Pigs, Hamsters, Mice, Rats:** 20–50 mg/kg (succinate salt) SC q6–12h (Adamcak & Otten 2000)
e) **Guinea pigs for pneumonia:** 30–50 mg/kg PO q12h (Johnson 2006b)

■ **FERRETS:**
For proliferative colitis:
a) 50 mg/kg q12h PO for 14–21 days (Johnson 2006a)

For susceptible infections:
a) 50 mg/kg PO twice daily (using palmitate salt—may be unavailable) or 50 mg/kg SC or IM twice daily (succinate salt) (Williams 2000)

■ **HORSES:**
For susceptible infections:
a) 45–60 mg/kg PO q8h; 45–60 mg/kg IM, SC or IV q6–8h (USPC 1990)
b) **Foals:** 20 mg/kg PO or IV q4h (Furr 1999)
c) **Foals:** Chloramphenicol sodium succinate: 25–50 mg/kg IV q4–8h; chloramphenicol base or palmitate: 40–50 mg/kg PO q6–8h (Brumbaugh 1999)

■ **BIRDS:**
For susceptible infections:
a) Chloramphenicol sodium succinate: 80 mg/kg IM two to three times daily, 50 mg/kg IV three to four times daily

Chloramphenicol palmitate suspension (30 mg/mL): 0.1 mL/30 grams of body weight three to four times daily. Do not use for initial therapy in life-threatening infections. Must use parenteral form if crop stasis occurs. (Clubb 1986)
b) Chloramphenicol palmitate suspension (30 mg/mL): 75 mg/kg three times a day; absorption is erratic, but well-tolerated and efficacious in baby birds with enteric infections being hand fed. Will settle out if added to drinking water. (McDonald 1989)
c) Succinate: 50 mg/kg IM or IV q8h; Palmitate: 75 mg/kg PO q8h (Hoeffer 1995)
d) Ratites (not to be used for food): 35–50 mg/kg PO, IM, IV or SC 3 times daily for 3 days (Jenson 1998)

■ **REPTILES:**
For susceptible infections:
a) For most species using the sodium succi-

nate salt: 20–50 mg/kg IM or SC for up to 3 weeks. Chloramphenicol is often a good initial choice until sensitivity results are available. (Gauvin 1993)

b) 30–50 mg/kg/day IV, or IM for 7–14 days (Lewbart 2001)

Monitoring
■ Clinical efficacy
■ Adverse effects; chronic therapy should be associated with routine CBC monitoring

Client Information
■ **MUST NOT** be used in any animal to be used for food production
■ There is evidence that humans exposed to chloramphenicol have an increased risk of developing fatal aplastic anemia. Products should be handled with care. Do not inhale powder and wash hands after handling tablets.
■ Crushed tablets or capsule contents are very bitter tasting and animals may not accept the drug if presented in this manner

Chemistry/Synonyms
Originally isolated from *Streptomyces venezuelae*, chloramphenicol is now produced synthetically. It occurs as fine, white to grayish, yellow white, elongated plates or needle-like crystals with a pK_a of 5.5. It is freely soluble in alcohol and about 2.5 mg are soluble in 1 mL of water at 25°C.

Chloramphenicol sodium succinate occurs as a white to light yellow powder. It is freely soluble in both water and alcohol. Commercially available chloramphenicol sodium succinate for injection contains 2.3 mEq of sodium per gram of chloramphenicol.

Chloramphenicol may also be known as: chloramphenicolum, chloranfenicol, cloranfenicol, kloramfenikol, or laevomycetinum; many trade names are available.

Storage/Stability
Chloramphenicol capsules and tablets should be stored in tight containers at room temperature (15–30°C). The palmitate oral suspension should be stored in tight containers at room temperature and protected from light or freezing.

The sodium succinate powder for injection should be stored at temperatures less than 40°, preferably between 15–30°C. After reconstituting the sodium succinate injection with sterile water, the solution is stable for 30 days at room temperature and 6 months if frozen. The solution should be discarded if it becomes cloudy.

Compatibility/Compounding Considerations
The following drugs and solutions are reportedly **compatible** with chloramphenicol sodium succinate injection: all commonly used intravenous fluids, amikacin sulfate, aminophylline, ampicillin sodium (in syringe for 1 hr.) ascorbic acid, calcium chloride/gluconate, cephalothin sodium, cephapirin sodium, colistimethate sodium, corticotropin, cyanocobalamin, dimenhydrinate, dopamine HCl, ephedrine sulfate, heparin sodium, hydrocortisone sodium succinate, hydroxyzine HCl, kanamycin sulfate, lidocaine HCl, magnesium sulfate, metaraminol bitartrate, methicillin sodium, methyldopate HCl, methylprednisolone sodium succinate, metronidazole with or without sodium bicarbonate, nafcillin sodium, oxacillin sodium, oxytocin, penicillin G potassium/sodium, pentobarbital sodium, phenylephrine HCl with or without sodium bicarbonate, phytonadione, plasma protein fraction, potassium chloride, promazine HCl, ranitidine HCl, sodium bicarbonate, thiopental sodium, verapamil HCl, and vitamin B-complex with C.

The following drugs and solutions are reportedly **incompatible** (or compatibility data conflicts) with chloramphenicol sodium succinate injection: chlorpromazine HCl, glycopyrrolate, metoclopramide HCl, oxytetracycline HCl, polymyxin B sulfate, prochlorperazine edislyate/mesylate, promethazine HCl, tetracycline HCl, and vancomycin HCl.

Compatibility is dependent upon factors such as pH, concentration, temperature and diluent used; consult specialized references or a hospital pharmacist for more specific information.

Dosage Forms/Regulatory Status
VETERINARY-LABELED PRODUCTS:
Chloramphenicol Oral Tablets and Capsules: 50 mg, 100 mg, 250 mg, 500 mg, & 1 g; FDA-approved for use in dogs only. *Trade names and manufacturers/sponsors vary* (Rx)

Chloramphenicol Injection: 100 mg/mL; (Rx). FDA-approved for use in dogs, but availability and marketing status unknown.

Chloramphenicol (as palmitate) Oral Suspension: 30 mg/mL, *Chloromycetin®* (BIVI); (Rx). FDA-approved for use in dogs, but availability and marketing status unknown.

Veterinary-labeled ophthalmic 1% ointments are also available.

HUMAN-LABELED PRODUCTS:
Chloramphenicol Powder for Injection: 1 gram (100 mg/mL (as sodium succinate when reconstituted); *Chloromycetin® Sodium Succinate* (Parke-Davis); generic; (Rx)

Ophthalmic preparations are also available.

References
Adamcak, A & B Otten (2000). Rodent Therapeutics. *Vet Clin NA: Exotic Anim Pract* 3:1(Jan): 221–240.
Brumbaugh, G (1999). Clinical Pharmacology and the Pediatric Patient. 45th Annual AAEP Convention, Albuquerque.
Clubb, SL (1986). Therapeutics: Individual and Flock Treatment Regimens. *Clinical Avian Medicine and Surgery*. GJ Harrison and LR Harrison Eds. Philadelphia, W.B. Saunders: 327–355.
Furr, M (1999). Antimicrobial treatments for the septic foal. Proceedings: The North American Veterinary Conference, Orlando.

Gauvin, J (1993). Drug therapy in reptiles. *Seminars in Avian & Exotic Med* 2(1): 48–59.

Greene, C & A Watson (1998). Antimicrobial Drug Formulary. *Infectious Diseases of the Dog and Cat.* C Greene Ed. Philadelphia, WB Saunders: 790–919.

Hayes, P (2000). Diseases of Chinchillas. *Kirk's Current Veterinary Therapy: XIII Small Animal Practice.* J Bonagura Ed. Philadelphia, WB Saunders: 1152–1157.

Hoeffer, H (1995). Antimicrobials in pet birds. *Kirk's Current Veterinary Therapy:XII.* J Bonagura Ed. Philadelphia, W.B. Saunders: 1278–1283.

Ivey, E & J Morrisey (2000). Therapeutics for Rabbits. *Vet Clin NA: Exotic Anim Pract* 3:1(Jan): 183–216.

Jenson, J (1998). Current ratite therapy. *The Veterinary Clinics of North America: Food Animal Practice* 16:3(November).

Johnson, D (2006a). Ferrets: the other companion animal. Proceedings: ACVC. Accessed via: Veterinary Information Network. http://goo.gl/bSeol

Johnson, D (2006b). Guinea Pig Medicine Primer. Proceedings: ACVC. Accessed via: Veterinary Information Network. http://goo.gl/WmWhU

Lewbart (2001). Reptile Formulary. Proceedings: Atlantic Coast Veterinary Conference. Accessed via: Veterinary Information Network. http://goo.gl/EEQmM

McDonald, SE (1989). Summary of medications for use in psittacine birds. *JAAV* 3(3): 120–127.

Rosenkrantz, W (2006). Systemic Therapy for Otitis Externa and Otitis Media. Proceedings: Western Vet Conf. Accessed via: Veterinary Information Network. http://goo.gl/QScyP

Sellon, R & E Breitschwerdt (1995). CVT Update: Rocky Mountain Spotted Fever. *Kirk's Current Veterinary Therapy:XII.* J Bonagura Ed. Philadelphia, W.B. Saunders: 293–297.

Smith, A (2000). General husbandry and medical care of hedgehogs. *Kirk's Current Veterinary Therapy: XIII Small Animal Practice.* J Bonagura Ed. Philadelphia, WB Saunders: 1128–1133.

USPC (1990). Veterinary Information– Appendix III. *Drug Information for the Health Professional* Rockville, United States Pharmacopeial Convention. 2: 2811–2860.

Vaden, S & M Papich (1995). Empiric Antibiotic Therapy. *Kirk's Current Veterinary Therapy:XII.* J Bonagura Ed. Philadelphia, W.B. Saunders: 276–280.

Williams, B (2000). Therapeutics in Ferrets. *Vet Clin NA: Exotic Anim Pract* 3:1(Jan): 131–153.

CHLORDIAZEPOXIDE ± CLIDINIUM BR

(klor-dye-az-e-*pox*-ide) ± (kli-*din*-ee-um)
Librium®, Librax®

BENZODIAZEPINE ± ANTIMUSCARINIC

Prescriber Highlights

▶ Benzodiazepine for behavior problems (phobias, etc.) & with an antimuscarinic (clidinium) for irritable bowel syndrome in dogs

▶ Not commonly used, so little has been published on adverse effects (similar to diazepam +/- atropine)

▶ Potentially teratogenic

Uses/Indications

Chlordiazepoxide alone may be a useful adjunct to treating certain behaviors where benzodiazepines may be useful including noise phobias in dogs; inter-cat aggression and urine spraying in cats. When combined with clidinium, it may be useful symptomatic therapy for dogs with irritable bowel syndrome.

Pharmacology/Actions

The subcortical levels (primarily limbic, thalamic, and hypothalamic) of the CNS are depressed by chlordiazepoxide and other benzodiazepines thus producing the anxiolytic, sedative, skeletal muscle relaxant and anticonvulsant effects seen. The exact mechanism of action is unknown but postulated mechanisms include: antagonism of serotonin, increased release of and/or facilitation of gamma-aminobutyric acid (GABA) activity, and diminished release or turnover of acetylcholine in the CNS. Benzodiazepine specific receptors have been located in the mammalian brain, kidney, liver, lung, and heart. In all species studied, receptors are lacking in the white matter.

Clidinium bromide is an antimuscarinic with its main action to reduce GI motility and secretion similarly to atropine. Clidinium is a quaternary ammonium compound and, unlike atropine, does not cross appreciably into the CNS or the eye and should not exhibit the same extent of CNS or ocular adverse effects that atropine possesses. For further information, refer to the atropine monograph.

Pharmacokinetics

Chlordiazepoxide is rapidly absorbed following oral administration. It is highly lipid soluble and is widely distributed throughout the body. It easily crosses the blood-brain barrier and is fairly highly bound to plasma proteins. Chlordiazepoxide is metabolized in the liver to several metabolites, including: desmethyldiazepam (nordiazepam), desmethylchlordiazepoxide and oxazepam, all of which are pharmacologically active and can have considerable half lives. These are eventually conjugated with glucuronide and eliminated primarily in the urine. Because of the active metabolites, serum values of chlordiazepoxide are not useful in predicting efficacy.

Little pharmacokinetic data for clidinium is available. The drug is incompletely absorbed from the gut (small intestine). Effects in humans are seen in about an hour; duration of effect is about 3 hours. As the compound is completely ionized *in vivo*, it does not enter the CNS or the eye and therefore unlike atropine does not have effects on those systems. The drug is metabolized principally in the liver, but is also excreted unchanged in the urine.

Contraindications/Precautions/Warnings

Use benzodiazepines cautiously in patients with hepatic or renal disease and in debilitated or geriatric patients. Chlordiazepoxide should only be administered very cautiously to patients in coma, shock or with significant respiratory depression. It is contraindicated in patients with known hypersensitivity to the drug.

Chlordiazepoxide should be used very cautiously, if at all, in aggressive patients as it may disinhibit the anxiety that may help prevent these animals from aggressive behavior. Benzodiazepines may impair the abilities of working animals. If administering the drug IV (rarely warranted), be prepared to administer cardiovascular or respiratory support. Give IV slowly.

Clidinium, like other antimuscarinic agents should not be used in patients with tachycardias secondary to thyrotoxicosis or cardiac insufficiency, myocardial ischemia, unstable cardiac status during acute hemorrhage, GI obstructive disease, paralytic ileus, severe ulcerative colitis, obstructive uropathy, or myasthenia gravis.

Antimuscarinic agents should be used with extreme caution in patients with known or suspected GI infections. Antimuscarinic agents can decrease GI motility and prolong retention of the causative agent(s) or toxin(s) resulting in prolonged effects of the toxin. Antimuscarinic agents must also be used with extreme caution in patients with autonomic neuropathy.

Antimuscarinic agents should be used with caution in patients with hepatic or renal disease, geriatric or pediatric patients, hyperthyroidism, hypertension, CHF, tachyarrhythmias, prostatic hypertrophy, or esophageal reflux. Systemic atropine should be used cautiously in horses as it can decrease gut motility and induce colic in susceptible animals. It may also reduce the arrhythmogenic doses of epinephrine. Use of atropine in cattle may result in inappetence and rumen stasis that may persist for several days.

Adverse Effects

Chlordiazepoxide's adverse effects are similar to other benzodiazepines, especially diazepam (they share several active metabolites). As there is much more information with respect to diazepam in dogs or cats than chlordiazepoxide, the following is extrapolated from diazepam information: Dogs could exhibit a contradictory response (CNS excitement) following administration of chlordiazepoxide. The effects with regard to sedation and tranquilization are extremely variable with each dog. Cats could exhibit changes in behavior (irritability, depression, aberrant demeanor) after receiving chlordiazepoxide. There have been reports of cats developing hepatic failure after receiving oral diazepam for several days. It is unknown if chlordiazepoxide also shares this effect. Clinical signs have been reported to occur 5–11 days after beginning oral therapy. Cats that receive diazepam should have baseline liver function tests. These should be repeated and the drug discontinued if emesis, lethargy, inappetence, or ataxia develops.

Clidinium's adverse effects are basically extensions of the drug's pharmacologic effects and are generally dose related. At usual doses effects tend to be mild in relatively healthy patients. More severe effects tend to occur with high or toxic doses. GI effects can include dry mouth (xerostomia), dysphagia, constipation, vomiting, and thirst. GU effects may include urinary retention or hesitancy. Cardiovascular effects include sinus tachycardia (at higher doses), bradycardia (initially or at very low doses), hypertension, hypotension, arrhythmias (ectopic complexes), and circulatory failure.

Reproductive/Nursing Safety

Benzodiazepines have been implicated in causing congenital abnormalities in humans if administered during the first trimester of pregnancy. Infants born of mothers receiving large doses of benzodiazepines shortly before delivery have been reported to suffer from apnea, impaired metabolic response to cold stress, difficulty in feeding, hyperbilirubinemia, hypotonia, etc. Withdrawal symptoms have occurred in infants whose mothers chronically took benzodiazepines during pregnancy. The veterinary significance of these effects is unclear, but the use of these agents during the first trimester of pregnancy should only occur when the benefits clearly outweigh the risks associated with their use. In humans, the FDA categorizes chlordiazepoxide as category *D* for use during pregnancy (*There is evidence of human fetal risk, but the potential benefits from the use of the drug in pregnant women may be acceptable despite its potential risks.*)

Benzodiazepines and their metabolites are distributed into milk and may cause CNS effects in nursing neonates.

Overdosage/Acute Toxicity

When administered alone, chlordiazepoxide overdoses are generally limited to significant CNS depression (confusion, coma, decreased reflexes, etc.). Hypotension, respiratory depression, and cardiac arrest have been reported in human patients but apparently are quite rare.

Treatment of acute toxicity consists of standard protocols for removing and/or binding the drug in the gut if taken orally, and supportive systemic measures. The use of analeptic agents (CNS stimulants such as caffeine) is generally not recommended. Flumazenil may be considered for adjunctive treatment of overdoses of benzodiazepines.

Drug Interactions

The following drug interactions have either been reported or are theoretical in humans or animals receiving chlordiazepoxide or other benzodiazepines and may be of significance in veterinary patients:

- ■ **DIGOXIN:** The pharmacologic effects of digoxin may be increased; monitor serum digoxin levels or signs of toxicity

- ■ **OTHER CNS DEPRESSANT DRUGS (e.g., barbiturates, opiates, anesthetics):** Additive effects may occur

- ■ **PROBENECID:** May interfere with benzodiazepine metabolism in the liver, causing increased or prolonged effects

■ **RIFAMPIN:** May induce hepatic microsomal enzymes and decrease the pharmacologic effects of benzodiazepines

The following drugs may decrease the metabolism of chlordiazepoxide and excessive sedation may occur:

■ **CIMETIDINE**

■ **ERYTHROMYCIN**

■ **FLUOXETINE**

■ **ISONIAZID**

■ **KETOCONAZOLE**

■ **METOPROLOL**

■ **PROPRANOLOL**

When using the product containing clidinium the following potential interactions noted with atropine may apply and the following drugs may enhance the activity or toxicity of clidinium:

■ **AMANTADINE**

■ **ANTICHOLINERGIC AGENTS (OTHER)**

■ **ANTICHOLINERGIC MUSCLE RELAXANTS**

■ **ANTIHISTAMINES** (*e.g.*, **diphenhydramine**)

■ **DISOPYRAMIDE**

■ **MEPERIDINE**

■ **PHENOTHIAZINES**

■ **PROCAINAMIDE**

■ **PRIMIDONE**

■ **TRICYCLIC ANTIDEPRESSANTS** (*e.g.*, **amitriptyline, clomipramine**)

■ **AMITRAZ:** Atropine may aggravate some signs seen with amitraz toxicity; leading to hypertension and further inhibition of peristalsis

■ **ANTACIDS:** May decrease PO atropine absorption; give oral atropine at least 1 hour prior to oral antacids

■ **CORTICOSTEROIDS (long-term use):** may increase intraocular pressure

■ **DIGOXIN (slow-dissolving):** Atropine may increase serum digoxin levels; use regular digoxin tablets or oral liquid

■ **KETOCONAZOLE:** Increased gastric pH may decrease GI absorption; administer atropine 2 hours after ketoconazole

■ **METOCLOPRAMIDE:** Atropine and its derivatives may antagonize the actions of metoclopramide

Laboratory Considerations

■ Chlordiazepoxide can cause interference with the Zimmerman reaction for **17-ketosteroids**, resulting in false results.

■ It can also cause a false-positive result in the *Gravindex®* **pregnancy** test.

Doses

■ **DOGS:**
Chlordiazepoxide alone:
For behavior indications (thunderstorm/noise phobias):

a) 2.2–6.6 mg/kg PO as needed (start low) (Overall 2000)

Chlordiazepoxide with clidinium:
For symptomatic treatment of irritable bowel syndrome:

a) Using the combination product (*e.g.*, *Librax®*), give 0.1–0.25 mg/kg of clidinium or 1–2 capsules PO two times to three times a day. Owner may give when abdominal pain or diarrhea first noticed or if stressful conditions are encountered. Drug can usually be discontinued in a few days. (Leib 2004)

b) Using the combination product (*e.g.*, *Librax®*), give 0.44–1.1 mg/kg of clidinium PO two to three times a day. Use at first signs of cramping or abdominal pain. Most dogs only require for a day to 2 weeks. Some require long-term treatment at 1–2 doses per day. (Tams 2000)

■ **CATS:**
As an anxiolytic:

a) Chlordiazepoxide: 0.5–1 mg/kg PO q12–24h (Virga 2002)

Monitoring

■ Clinical efficacy

■ Adverse effects

Client Information

■ Keep out of reach of children and in tightly closed containers

■ Notify veterinarian if animal's behavior worsens

Chemistry/Synonyms

A benzodiazepine, chlordiazepoxide HCl occurs as an odorless, white crystalline powder. It is soluble in water and alcohol, but is unstable in aqueous solutions.

A synthetic quaternary antimuscarinic agent similar to glycopyrrolate, clidinium bromide occurs as a white to nearly white, crystalline powder. It is soluble in alcohol and water.

Chlordiazepoxide HCl may also be known as: chlordiazepoxidi hydrochloridum, methaminodiazepoxide hydrochloride, NSC-115748, or Ro-5-0690; many trade names are available.

Storage/Stability

Chlordiazepoxide HCl capsules or tablets should be stored protected from light. The chlordiazepoxide HCl injection should be prepared immediately prior to use and any unused portions discarded. The diluent should be stored in the refrigerator before use.

Clidinium bromide and chlordiazepoxide capsules should be stored at room temperature in tight, light-resistant containers.

Dosage Forms/Regulatory Status

VETERINARY-LABELED PRODUCTS: None
The ARCI (Racing Commissioners International) has designated this drug as a class 2 substance. See the appendix for more information.

HUMAN-LABELED PRODUCTS:

Chlordiazepoxide HCl Oral Capsules: 5 mg, 10 mg & 25 mg; generic; (Rx, C-IV)

Chlordiazepoxide HCl 5 mg and Clidinium Br 2.5 mg Capsules; *Librax® Capsules* (Valeant); generic; (Rx, C-IV)

References

Leib, M (2004). Chronic idiopathic large bowel diarrhea in dogs. Proceedings: ACVIM Forum. Accessed via: Veterinary Information Network. http://goo.gl/Nwoz8

Overall, K (2000). Behavioral Pharmacology. Proceedings: American Animal Hospital Association 67th Annual Meeting, Toronto.

Tams, T (2000). Diagnosis and Management of Large Intestinal Disorders in Dogs. Proceedings: American Animal Hospital Association 67th Annual Meeting, Toronto.

Virga, V (2002). Which drug and why: An update on psychopharmacology. Proceedings: Atlantic Coast Veterinary Conference. Accessed via: Veterinary Information Network. http://goo.gl/m8qr4

CHLOROTHIAZIDE
CHLOROTHIAZIDE
SODIUM

(klor-oh-*thye*-a-zide)   Diuril®

THIAZIDE DIURETIC

Prescriber Highlights

▶ Thiazide diuretic used for nephrogenic diabetes insipidus & hypertension in dogs; udder edema in dairy cattle (cattle product now discontinued in USA)

▶ Contraindications: Hypersensitivity; pregnancy (relative contraindication)

▶ Extreme caution/avoid: Severe renal disease, preexisting electrolyte/water balance abnormalities, impaired hepatic function, hyperuricemia, SLE, diabetes mellitus

▶ Adverse Effects: Hypokalemia, hypochloremic alkalosis, other electrolyte imbalances, hyperuricemia, GI effects

▶ Many drug-drug & laboratory test interactions

Uses/Indications

In veterinary medicine, furosemide has largely supplanted the use of thiazides as a general diuretic (edema treatment). Thiazides are still used for the treatment of systemic hypertension, nephrogenic diabetes insipidus, and to help prevent the recurrence of calcium oxalate uroliths in dogs.

Chlorothiazide is FDA-approved for use in dairy cattle for the treatment of post parturient udder edema, but the veterinary labeled product has been discontinued in the USA.

Pharmacology/Actions

Thiazide diuretics act by interfering with the transport of sodium ions across renal tubular epithelium possibly by altering the metabolism of tubular cells. The principle site of action is at the cortical diluting segment of the nephron; enhanced excretion of sodium, chloride, and water results. Thiazides also increase the excretion of potassium, magnesium, phosphate, iodide, and bromide and decrease the glomerular filtration rate (GFR). Plasma renin and resulting aldosterone levels are increased which contributes to the hypokalemic effects of the thiazides. Bicarbonate excretion is increased, but effects on urine pH are usually minimal. Thiazides usually initially have a hypercalciuric effect but with continued therapy, calcium excretion is significantly decreased. But in dogs, hydrochlorothiazide, but not chlorothiazide, has been shown to decrease urinary calcium excretion. Uric acid excretion is also decreased by the thiazides. Thiazides can cause, or exacerbate, hyperglycemia in diabetic patients, or induce diabetes mellitus in prediabetic patients.

The antihypertensive effects of thiazides are well known, and these agents are used extensively in human medicine for treating essential hypertension. The exact mechanism of this effect has not been established.

Thiazides paradoxically reduce urine output in patients with diabetes insipidus (DI). They have been used as adjunctive therapy in patients with neurogenic DI and are the only drug therapy for nephrogenic DI.

Pharmacokinetics

The pharmacokinetics of the thiazides have apparently not been studied in domestic animals. In humans, chlorothiazide is only 10−21% absorbed after oral administration. The onset of diuretic activity occurs in 1−2 hours and peaks at about 4 hours. The serum half-life is approximately 1−2 hours and the duration of activity is from 6−12 hours. Like all thiazides, the antihypertensive effects of chlorothiazide can take several days to transpire.

Thiazides are found in the milk of lactating humans. Because of the chance of idiosyncratic or hypersensitive reactions, it is recommended that these drugs not be used in lactating females or nursing mothers.

Contraindications/Precautions/Warnings

Thiazides are contraindicated in patients hypersensitive to any one of these agents or to sulfonamides, and those with anuria. They are also contraindicated in pregnant females who are otherwise healthy and have only mild edema; newborn human infants have developed thrombocytopenia when their mothers received thiazides.

Thiazides should be used with extreme caution, if at all, in patients with severe renal disease or with preexisting electrolyte or water balance abnormalities, impaired hepatic function (may precipitate hepatic coma), hyperuricemia, lupus (SLE); or diabetes mellitus. Patients with conditions that may lead to electrolyte or water balance abnormalities (*e.g.*, vomiting, diarrhea, etc.) should be monitored carefully.

Adverse Effects

Hypokalemia is one of the most common adverse effects associated with the thiazides but rarely causes clinical signs or progresses further; however, monitoring of potassium is recommended with chronic therapy.

Hypochloremic alkalosis (with hypokalemia) may develop, especially if there are other causes of potassium and chloride loss (*e.g.*, vomiting, diarrhea, potassium-losing nephropathies, etc.) or if the patient has cirrhotic liver disease. Dilutional hyponatremia and hypomagnesemia may also occur. Hyperparathyroid-like effects of hypercalcemia and hypophosphatemia have been reported in humans, but have not led to effects such as nephrolithiasis, bone resorption, or peptic ulceration.

Hyperuricemia can occur but is usually asymptomatic.

Other possible adverse effects include GI reactions (vomiting, diarrhea, etc.), pancreatitis, hypersensitivity/dermatologic reactions, GU reactions (polyuria), hematologic toxicity, hyperglycemia, hyperlipidemias, and orthostatic hypotension.

Reproductive/Nursing Safety

In humans, the FDA categorizes this drug as category *B* for use during pregnancy (*Animal studies have not yet demonstrated risk to the fetus, but there are no adequate studies in pregnant women; or animal studies have shown an adverse effect, but adequate studies in pregnant women have not demonstrated a risk to the fetus in the first trimester of pregnancy, and there is no evidence of risk in later trimesters.*)

Chlorothiazide enters maternal milk and can reduce milk volume and suppress lactation. Generally, discontinuation of the drug or nursing is recommended in humans.

Overdosage

Acute overdosage may cause electrolyte and water balance problems, CNS effects (lethargy to coma and seizures), and GI effects (hypermotility, GI distress). Transient increases in BUN have also been reported.

Treatment consists of emptying the gut after recent oral ingestion using standard protocols. Avoid giving concomitant cathartics as they may exacerbate the fluid and electrolyte imbalances that may ensue. Monitor and treat electrolyte and water balance abnormalities supportively. Additionally, monitor respiratory, CNS and cardiovascular status; treat supportively and symptomatically, if required.

Drug Interactions

The following drug interactions have either been reported or are theoretical in humans or animals receiving chlorothiazide and may be of significance in veterinary patients:

■ **AMPHOTERICIN B:** Use with thiazides can lead to an increased risk for severe hypokalemia

■ **CORTICOSTEROIDS, CORTICOTROPIN:** Use with thiazides can lead to an increased risk for severe hypokalemia

■ **DIAZOXIDE:** Increased risk for hyperglycemia, hyperuricemia, and hypotension may occur

■ **DIGITALIS, DIGOXIN:** Thiazide-induced hypokalemia, hypo-magnesemia, and/or hypercalcemia may increase the likelihood of digitalis toxicity

■ **INSULIN:** Thiazides may increase insulin requirements

■ **LITHIUM:** Thiazides can increase serum lithium concentrations

■ **METHENAMINE:** Thiazides can alkalinize urine and reduce methenamine effectiveness

■ **NSAIDS:** Thiazides may increase risk for renal toxicity and NSAIDs may reduce diuretic actions of thiazides

■ **NEUROMUSCULAR BLOCKING AGENTS:** Tubocurarine or other nondepolarizing neuromuscular blocking agents response or duration may be increased in patients taking thiazide diuretics

■ **PROBENECID:** Blocks thiazide-induced uric acid retention (used to therapeutic advantage)

■ **QUINIDINE:** Half-life may be prolonged by thiazides (thiazides can alkalinize the urine)

■ **VITAMIN D OR CALCIUM SALTS:** Hypercalcemia may be exacerbated if thiazides are concurrently administered with Vitamin D or calcium salts

Laboratory Considerations

■ **AMYLASE:** Thiazides can increase serum amylase values in asymptomatic patients and those in the developmental stages of acute pancreatitis (humans)

■ **CORTISOL:** Thiazides can decrease the renal excretion of cortisol

■ **ESTROGEN, URINARY:** Hydrochlorothiazide may falsely decrease total urinary estrogen when using a spectrophotometric assay

■ **HISTAMINE:** Thiazides may cause false-negative results when testing for pheochromocytoma

■ **PARATHYROID-FUNCTION TESTS:** Thiazides may elevate serum calcium; recommend discontinuing thiazides prior to testing

■ **PHENOLSULFONPHTHALEIN (PSP):** Thiazides can compete for secretion at proximal renal tubules

■ **PHENTOLAMINE TEST:** Thiazides may give false-negative results

■ **PROTEIN-BOUND IODINE:** Thiazides may decrease values

■ **TRIIODOTHYRONINE RESIN UPTAKE TEST:** Thiazides may slightly reduce uptake

■ **TYRAMINE:** Thiazides can cause false-negative results.

Doses

■ **DOGS:**

For treatment of nephrogenic diabetes insipidus:

a) 20–40 mg/kg PO q12h (Polzin & Osborne 1985), (Nichols 1989), (Behrend 2003)

For treatment of systemic hypertension:

a) 20–40 mg/kg PO q12–24h with dietary salt restriction (Cowgill & Kallet 1986)

As a diuretic:

a) 20–40 mg/kg PO q12h (twice daily) (Mucha 2009)

■ **CATS:**

For treatment of diabetes insipidus:

a) 20–40 mg/kg PO q12h may be tried (Behrend 2003)

As a diuretic:

a) 20–40 mg/kg PO q12h (twice daily) (Mucha 2009)

■ **CATTLE:**

a) 4–8 mg/kg once or twice daily PO for adult cattle (Howard 1986)

b) 2 g PO once to twice daily (Swinyard 1975)

Monitoring

■ Serum electrolytes, BUN, creatinine, glucose

■ Hydration status

■ Blood pressure, if indicated

■ Hemograms, if indicated

Client Information

■ Clients should contact veterinarian if signs of water or electrolyte imbalance occur (*e.g.*, excessive thirst, lethargy, lassitude, restlessness, reduced urination, GI distress, or rapid heart rate)

Chemistry/Synonyms

Chlorothiazide is a thiazide diuretic and occurs as a white to practically white, odorless, crystalline powder having a slightly bitter taste. It is very slightly soluble in water and slightly soluble in alcohol.

Chlorothiazide may also be known as: chlorothiazidum, clorotiazida, *Azide®, Chlorzide®, Chlotride®, Diachlor®, Diuril®, Diurigen®, Pahtlisan®,* or *Saluric®.*

Storage/Stability

Tablets should be stored at room temperature. The oral suspension should be protected from freezing. The injectable preparation is stable for 24 hours after reconstitution. If the pH of the reconstituted solution is less than 7.4, precipitation will occur in less than 24 hours.

Compatibility/Compounding Considerations

Chlorothiazide sodium for injection is reportedly **compatible** with the following IV solutions: dextrose and/or saline products for IV infusion (with the exception of many Ionosol and Normosol products), Ringer's injection and Lactated Ringer's, 1/6 M sodium lactate, Dextran 6% with dextrose or sodium chloride, and fructose 10%. It is also reportedly **compatible** with the following drugs: cimetidine HCl, lidocaine HCl, nafcillin sodium, and sodium bicarbonate.

Chlorothiazide sodium is reportedly **incompatible** with the following drugs: amikacin sulfate, chlorpromazine HCl, codeine phosphate, hydralazine HCl, insulin (regular), morphine sulfate, norepinephrine bitartrate, polymyxin B sulfate, procaine HCl, prochlorperazine edisylate and mesylate, promazine HCl, promethazine HCl, streptomycin sulfate, tetracycline HCl, trifluopromazine HCl, and vancomycin HCl.

Dosage Forms/Regulatory Status

VETERINARY-LABELED PRODUCTS: None

The ARCI (Racing Commissioners International) has designated this drug as a class 4 substance. See the appendix for more information.

HUMAN-LABELED PRODUCTS:

Chlorothiazide Tablets: 250 mg & 500 mg; *Diuril®* (Merck); *Diurigen®* (Goldline); generic; (Rx)

Chlorothiazide Oral Suspension: 50 mg/mL in 237 mL; *Diuril®* (Merck); (Rx)

Chlorothiazide Sodium Powder for Injection (lyophilized): 500 mg (0.25 g mannitol) in 20 mL vials; *Diuril®* (Merck); (Rx)

References

Behrend, E (2003). Diabetes insipidus and other causes of polyuria/polydipsia. Proceedings: Western Veterinary Conference. Accessed via: Veterinary Information Network. http://goo.gl/pxzS4

Cowgill, LD & AJ Kallet (1986). Systemic Hypertension. *Current Veterinary Therapy IX, Small Animal Practice.* RW Kirk Ed. Philadelphia, WB. Saunders: 360–364.

Howard, JL, Ed. (1986). *Current Veterinary Therapy 2, Food Animal Practice.* Philadelphia, W.B. Saunders.

Mucha, C (2009). Therapeutics in Heart Disease. Proceedings: WSAVA. Accessed via: Veterinary Information Network. http://goo.gl/ca6mX

Nichols, R (1989). Diabetes Insipidus. *Current Veterinary Therapy X: Small Animal Practice.* RW Krik Ed. Philadeliphia, WB Saunders: 974–978.

Polzin, DJ & CA Osborne (1985). Diseases of the Urinary Tract. *Handbook of Small Animal Therapeutics.* LE Davis Ed. New York, Churchill Livingstone: 333–395.

Swinyard, EA (1975). Diuretic Drugs. *Remington's Pharmaceutical Sciences.* A Osol Ed. Easton, Mack Publishing: 861–873.

CHLORPHENIRAMINE MALEATE

(klor-fen-*ir*-a-meen)   Chlor-Trimetron®

ANTIHISTAMINE

Prescriber Highlights

▶ An alkylamine antihistamine used primarily for its antihistamine/antipruritic effects; occasionally used for CNS depressant (sedative) effects

▶ Contraindications: Hypersensitivity. Caution: narrow angle glaucoma, hypertension, GI or urinary obstruction, hypertension, hyperthyroidism, cardiovascular disease

▶ Adverse Effects: Sedation, anticholinergic effects, GI effects

Uses/Indications

Antihistamines are used in veterinary medicine to reduce or help prevent histamine mediated adverse effects. Chlorpheniramine is one of the more commonly used antihistamines in the cat for the treatment of pruritus. It may also be of benefit as a mild sedative in small animals due to its CNS depressant effects.

Pharmacology/Actions

Antihistamines (H_1-receptor antagonists) competitively inhibit histamine at H_1 receptor sites. They do not inactivate or prevent the release of histamine, but can prevent histamine's action on the cell. Besides their antihistaminic activity, these agents all have varying degrees of anticholinergic and CNS activity (sedation). Some antihistamines have antiemetic activity (*e.g.*, diphenhydramine) or antiserotonin activity (*e.g.*, cyproheptadine, azatadine).

Pharmacokinetics

Chlorpheniramine pharmacokinetics have not been described in domestic species. In humans, the drug is well absorbed after oral administration, but because of a relatively high degree of metabolism in the GI mucosa and the liver, only about 25–60% of the drug is available to the systemic circulation.

Chlorpheniramine is well distributed after IV injection; the highest distribution of the drug (in rabbits) occurs in the lungs, heart, kidneys, brain, small intestine, and spleen. In humans, the apparent steady-state volume of distribution is 2.5–3.2 L/kg and about 70% is bound to plasma proteins. It is unknown if chlorpheniramine is excreted into the milk.

Chlorpheniramine is metabolized in the liver and practically all the drug (as metabolites and unchanged drug) is excreted in the urine. In human patients with normal renal and hepatic function, the terminal serum half-life the drug ranges from 13.2–43 hours.

Contraindications/Precautions/Warnings

Chlorpheniramine is contraindicated in patients who are hypersensitive to it or other antihistamines in its class. Because of their anticholinergic activity, antihistamines should be used with caution in patients with angle closure glaucoma, prostatic hypertrophy, pyloroduodenal or bladder neck obstruction, and COPD if mucosal secretions are a problem. Additionally, they should be cautiously used in patients with hyperthyroidism, cardiovascular disease or hypertension.

Adverse Effects

Most commonly seen adverse effects are CNS depression (lethargy, somnolence) and GI effects (diarrhea, vomiting, anorexia). The sedative effects of antihistamines may diminish with time. Anticholinergic effects (dry mouth, urinary retention) are a possibility.

The sedative effects of antihistamines may adversely affect the performance of working dogs.

Chlorpheniramine may cause paradoxical excitement in cats. Palatability is also an issue with this drug and felines.

Reproductive/Nursing Safety

In humans, the FDA categorizes this drug as category *B* for use during pregnancy (*Animal studies have not yet demonstrated risk to the fetus, but there are no adequate studies in pregnant women; or animal studies have shown an adverse effect, but adequate studies in pregnant women have not demonstrated a risk to the fetus in the first trimester of pregnancy, and there is no evidence of risk in later trimesters.*)

It is unknown if chlorpheniramine is excreted into milk; use with caution in dams nursing neonates.

Overdosage/Acute Toxicity

Overdosage may cause CNS stimulation (excitement to seizures) or depression (lethargy to coma), anticholinergic effects, respiratory depression, and death. A 9-month-old dachshund ingesting 25 mg/kg showed signs of ataxia, tremors, bradycardia, coma, & cardiac arrest and died within 11 hours of ingestion (Murphy 2001).

Treatment consists of emptying the gut (if the ingestion was oral) using standard protocols. Induce emesis if the patient is alert and CNS status is stable. Administration of a saline cathartic and/or activated charcoal may be given after emesis or gastric lavage. Treatment of other clinical signs should be performed using symptomatic and supportive therapies. Phenytoin (IV) is recommended in the treatment of seizures caused by antihistamine overdoses in humans; barbiturates and diazepam should be avoided.

Drug Interactions

The following drug interactions have either been reported or are theoretical in humans or animals receiving chlorpheniramine and may be of significance in veterinary patients:

▪ **ANTICOAGULANTS (heparin, warfarin):** Antihistamines may partially counteract the anticoagulation effects of heparin or warfarin

■ **MAO INHIBITORS** (including **amitraz**, and possibly **selegiline**): May prolong and exacerbate anticholinergic effects

■ **OTHER CNS DEPRESSANT DRUGS:** Increased sedation can occur

Laboratory Considerations

■ Antihistamines can decrease the wheal and flare response to **antigen skin testing**. In humans, it is suggested that antihistamines be discontinued at least 4 days before testing.

Doses

Note: Contents of sustained-release capsules may be placed on food, but should not be allowed to dissolve before ingestion.

■ **DOGS:**

a) 4–8 mg (maximum of 0.5 mg/kg) PO q8–12h PO; many clinicians use as adjunctive treatment of chemotherapy of mast cell tumors (Papich 2000)

b) 4–12 mg (total dose) two to three times daily (MacDonald 2002)

c) 2–8 mg (total dose) per dog PO every 12 hours, not to exceed 0.5 mg/kg every 12 hours (Cote 2005)

For pruritus:

a) As a trial for pruritus in atopic dogs: 0.4–0.8 mg/kg two to three times daily (Rosychuk 2002)

b) 0.2–0.8 mg/kg PO 2-3 times a day (Marsella 2008)

As a mild sedative:

a) 0.22 mg/kg PO q8h; 4–20 mg (total dose per day) divided q8–12h (Overall 2000)

■ **CATS:**

a) 2 mg (total dose) per cat PO every 12 hours (Cote 2005)

b) 2–4 mg per cat q12–24h PO (Hnilica 2003), (Rosychuk 2002)

c) Most common dosage in cats is: 2 mg per cat two to three times daily (MacDonald 2002)

For pruritus:

a) 2–4 mg/cat twice daily; rarely may be maintained on once daily dosing. Palatability may be enhanced by dipping the split tablet into tuna fish "juice", butter or petrolatum; placing split tablets into empty gelatin capsules or sprinkling or mixing timed release beads (partial contents of an 8 mg capsule) with food. (Messinger 2000)

b) 0.5–2 mg (total dose; ¼ - ½ of a 4 mg tablet) PO 2-3 times per day (Marsella 2008)

As a mild sedative:

a) 1–2 mg per cat q12–24h (low dose), 2–4 mg per cat PO q12–24h (high dose) (Overall 2000)

■ **FERRETS:**

a) 1–2 mg/kg PO 2–3 times a day (Williams 2000)

■ **BIRDS:**

a) One 4 mg tablet in one cup (240 mL; 8 oz.) of bottled water to be used as drinking water; changed daily. (Clubb 2009)

Monitoring

■ Clinical efficacy

■ Adverse effects

Client Information

■ Chlorpheniramine is FDA-approved for use in humans; the oral dosage forms are either prescription or non-prescription agents, depending on the product's labeling

■ Most common adverse effects are drowsiness/sleepiness; cats may become excited

■ Do not crush or allow animal to chew sustained-release products

Chemistry/Synonyms

A propylamine (alkylamine) antihistaminic agent, chlorpheniramine maleate occurs as an odorless, white, crystalline powder with a melting point between 130–135° C and a pK_a of 9.2. One gram is soluble in about 4 mL of water or 10 mL of alcohol.

Chlorpheniramine maleate may also be known as chlorphenamini maleas; many trade names are available.

Storage/Stability

Chlorpheniramine tablets and sustained-release tablets should be stored in tight containers. The sustained-release capsules should be stored in well-closed containers. The oral solution should be stored in light-resistant containers; avoid freezing. All chlorpheniramine products should be stored at room temperature (15–30°C).

Dosage Forms/Regulatory Status

VETERINARY-LABELED PRODUCTS: None

The ARCI (Racing Commissioners International) has designated this drug as a class 4 substance. See the appendix for more information.

HUMAN-LABELED PRODUCTS:

Chlorpheniramine Maleate Oral Tablets: 2 mg (chewable), *Chlo-Amine*® (Hollister-Stier); (OTC); 4 mg tablets, *Aller-Chlor*® (Rugby); *Allergy*® (Major); *Allergy Relief*® (Zee Medical); generic; (OTC); Chlorpheniramine Maleate Extended-release Tablets & Capsules: 8 mg, 12 mg & 16 mg; *Chlor-Trimeton*® *Allergy 8* or *12 Hour* (Schering-Plough Healthcare); *Efidac*® *24* (Hogil); *QDALL AR*® (Atley); generic; (Rx & OTC)

Chlorpheniramine Caplets: 8 mg (as tannate); *ED-CHLOR-TAN*® (Edwards Pharmaceuticals); (Rx)

Chlorpheniramine Maleate Oral Syrup: 2 mg/5 mL in 118 mL; *Aller-Chlor*® (Rugby);

(OTC); Oral Suspension: 4 mg/5 mL in 118 mL; *Pediox-S®* (Atley); (Rx)

Many combination products are available that combine chlorpheniramine with decongestants, analgesics, and/or antitussives.

References

Clubb, S (2009). Feather damaging behavior. Proceedings; WVC.

Cote, E (2005). Over–the–counter human medications. *Textbook of Veterinary internal Medicine 6th Ed.* S Ettinger and E Feldman Eds., Elsevier: 509–511.

Hnilica, K (2003). Managing Feline Pruritus. Proceedings: Western Veterinary Conference. Accessed via: Veterinary Information Network. http://goo.gl/U19xu

MacDonald, J (2002). Current therapy for pruritus. Proceedings: Western Veterinary Conference. Accessed via: Veterinary Information Network. http://goo.gl/ErwOJ

Marsella, R (2008). Medical management of pruritus: Non–specific therapy for management of the pruritic dog or cat. Proceedings: ACVC.

Messinger, L (2000). Pruritis Therapy in the Cat. *Kirk's Current Veterinary Therapy: XIII Small Animal Practice.* J Bonagura Ed. Philadelphia, WB Saunders: 542–545.

Murphy, L (2001). Antihistamine Toxicosis. *Veterinary Medicine*(October 2001).

Overall, K (2000). Behavioral Pharmacology. Proceedings: American Animal Hospital Association 67th Annual Meeting, Toronto.

Papich, M (2000). Antihistamines: Current Therapeutic Use. *Kirk's Current Veterinary Therapy: XIII Small Animal Practice.* J Bonagura Ed. Philadelphia, WB Saunders: 49–53.

Rosychuk, R (2002). Newer therapies in dermatology: Part I. Proceedings: ACVIM Forum. Accessed via: Veterinary Information Network. http://goo.gl/hIqEj

Williams, B (2000). Therapeutics in Ferrets. *Vet Clin NA: Exotic Anim Pract* 3:1(Jan): 131–153.

CHLORPROMAZINE HCL

(klor-*proe*-ma-zeen)   Thorazine®

PHENOTHIAZINE SEDATIVE/
ANTIEMETIC

Prescriber Highlights

▶ Prototype phenothiazine used primarily as an antiemetic, may be particularly useful to treat motion sickness in cats

▶ Generally contraindicated in horses

▶ Negligible analgesic effects

▶ Dosage may need to be reduced in debilitated/geriatric animals, those with hepatic or cardiac disease or when combined with other agents

▶ Use with caution in dehydrated patients because phenothiazines can cause vasodilation & reduce perfusion; rehydrate before use

▶ Inject diluted solution IV slowly; do not inject into arteries; do not inject IM in rabbits

▶ May cause significant hypotension, cardiac rate abnormalities, hypo- or hyperthermia; may cause extrapyramidal effects at high doses in cats

Uses/Indications

The clinical use of chlorpromazine as a neuroleptic agent has diminished, but the drug is still used for its antiemetic effects in small animals and occasionally as a preoperative medication and tranquilizer. As an antiemetic, chlorpromazine will inhibit apomorphine-induced emesis in the dog but not the cat. It will also inhibit the emetic effects of morphine in the dog. It does not inhibit emesis caused by copper sulfate, or digitalis glycosides.

Once the principle phenothiazine used in veterinary medicine, chlorpromazine has been largely supplanted by acepromazine. It has similar pharmacologic activities as acepromazine, but is less potent and has a longer duration of action. For further information, refer to the acepromazine monograph.

Pharmacokinetics

Chlorpromazine is absorbed rapidly after oral administration, but undergoes extensive first pass metabolism in the liver. The drug is also well absorbed after IM injection, but onsets of action are slower than after IV administration.

Chlorpromazine is distributed throughout the body and brain concentrations are higher than those in plasma. Approximately 95% of chlorpromazine in plasma is bound to plasma proteins (primarily albumin).

The drug is extensively metabolized principally in the liver and kidneys, but little specific information is available regarding its excretion in dogs and cats.

Contraindications/Precautions/Warnings

Chlorpromazine causes severe muscle discomfort and swelling when injected IM into rabbits; use IV only in this species.

Animals may require lower dosages of general anesthetics following phenothiazines. Use cautiously and in smaller doses in animals with hepatic dysfunction, cardiac disease, or general debilitation. Because of its hypotensive effects, phenothiazines are relatively contraindicated in patients with hypovolemia or shock, and in patients with tetanus or strychnine intoxication due to effects on the extrapyramidal system.

Intravenous injections must be diluted with saline to concentrations of no more than 1 mg/mL and administered slowly. Chlorpromazine has no analgesic effects; treat animals with appropriate analgesics to control pain.

Dogs with MDR1 mutations (many Collies, Australian shepherds, etc.) may develop a more pronounced sedation that persists longer than normal with this agent. It may be prudent to reduce initial doses by 25% to determine the reaction of a patient identified or suspect of having this mutation.

Phenothiazines should be used very cautiously as restraining agents in aggressive dogs: it may make the animal more prone to startle and react to noises or other sensory inputs.

Adverse Effects

In addition to the possible effects listed in the acepromazine monograph (*e.g.*, hypotension, contradictory effects such as CNS stimulation, bradycardia), chlorpromazine may cause extrapyramidal signs in the cat when used at high dosages. These can include tremors, shivering, rigidity and loss of the righting reflexes. Lethargy, diarrhea, and loss of anal sphincter tone may also be seen.

Horses may develop an ataxic reaction with resultant excitation and violent consequences. These ataxic periods may cycle with periods of sedation. Because of this effect, chlorpromazine is rarely used in equine medicine today.

Reproductive/Nursing Safety

In humans, the FDA categorizes this drug as category *C* for use during pregnancy (*Animal studies have shown an adverse effect on the fetus, but there are no adequate studies in humans; or there are no animal reproduction studies and no adequate studies in humans.*)

Chlorpromazine is thought to be excreted into maternal milk and safety to nursing offspring cannot be assured.

Overdosage/Acute Toxicity

Most small overdoses cause only somnolence; larger overdoses can cause serious effects including coma, agitation/seizures, ECG changes/ arrhythmias, hypotension and extrapyramidal effects. Contact an animal poison control center in the event of a suspected large overdose or if multiple drugs are involved.

Most overdoses can be handled by monitoring the patient and treating signs as they occur; massive oral overdoses should definitely be treated by emptying the gut if possible. Hypotension should not be treated with epinephrine; use either phenylephrine or norepinephrine (levarterenol). Seizures may be controlled with barbiturates or diazepam.

Drug Interactions

The following drug interactions have either been reported or are theoretical in humans or animals receiving chlorpromazine or other phenothiazines and may be of significance in veterinary patients:

- **ACETAMINOPHEN:** Possible increased risk for hypothermia
- **ANTACIDS:** May cause reduced GI absorption of oral phenothiazines
- **ANTIDIARRHEAL MIXTURES (e.g., kaolin/ pectin, bismuth subsalicylate mixtures):** May cause reduced GI absorption of oral phenothiazines
- **CNS DEPRESSANT AGENTS (barbiturates, narcotics, anesthetics**, etc.**):** May cause additive CNS depression if used with phenothiazines
- **DIPYRONE:** May cause serious hypothermia
- **EPINEPHRINE:** Phenothiazines block alpha-adrenergic receptors and concomitant epinephrine can lead to unopposed beta-activity causing vasodilation and increased cardiac rate
- **OPIATES:** May enhance the hypotensive effects of the phenothiazines; dosages of chlorpromazine may need to be reduced when used with an opiate
- **ORGANOPHOSPHATE AGENTS:** Phenothiazines should not be given within one month of worming with these agents as their effects may be potentiated
- **PARAQUAT:** Toxicity may be increased by chlorpromazine
- **PHENYTOIN:** Metabolism may be decreased if given concurrently with phenothiazines
- **PHYSOSTIGMINE:** Toxicity may be enhanced by chlorpromazine
- **PROCAINE:** Activity may be enhanced by phenothiazines
- **PROPRANOLOL:** Increased blood levels of both drugs may result if administered with phenothiazines
- **QUINIDINE:** With phenothiazines may cause additive cardiac depression

Doses

- **DOGS:**
  As an antiemetic:
  a) 0.5 mg/kg IV, IM or SC three to four times daily (Dowling 2003)
  b) 0.2–0.4 mg/kg SC, IM q8h (Washabau 2006)
  c) 4–8 mg (total dose; do not exceed 0.5 mg/kg) per dog PO q12h (Marks 2008)

  As a muscle relaxant during tetanus:
  a) 2 mg/kg IM twice daily (Morgan 1988)

- **CATS:**
  As an antiemetic:
  a) 0.5 mg/kg IV, IM or SC three to four times daily (Dowling 2003)
  b) 2 mg (total dose) per cat PO q12h (Marks 2008)

  As a preanesthetic:
  a) up to 1.1 mg/kg IM 1–1.5 hours prior to surgery (Booth 1988)

- **CATTLE:**
  a) Premedication for cattle undergoing standing procedures: Up to 1 mg/kg IM (may cause regurgitation if animal undergoes general anesthesia) (Hall & Clarke 1983)

- **HORSES: (Note:** ARCI UCGFS Class 2 Drug)
  Note: Because of side effects (ataxia, panic reaction) this drug is not recommended for use in horses; use acepromazine or promazine if phenothiazine therapy is desired.

- **SWINE:**
  a) Premedication: 1 mg/kg IM (Hall & Clarke 1983)

b) 0.55–3.3 mg/kg IV; 2–4 mg/kg IM

c) Restraint: 1.1 mg/kg IM (effects are at peak in 45–60 minutes); Prior to barbiturate anesthesia: 2–4 mg/kg IM (Booth 1988)

■ **SHEEP & GOATS:**

a) 0.55–4.4 mg/kg IV, 2.2–6.6 mg/kg IM (Lumb & Jones 1984)

b) Goats: 2–3.5 mg/kg IV q5–6h (Booth 1988)

Monitoring

■ Cardiac rate/rhythm/blood pressure if indicated and possible to measure

■ Degree of tranquilization/anti-emetic activity if indicated

■ Body temperature (especially if ambient temperature is very hot or cold)

Client Information

■ Avoid getting solutions on hands or clothing; contact dermatitis may develop.

■ May discolor the urine to a pink or red-brown color; this is not abnormal.

Chemistry/Synonyms

A propylamino-phenothiazine derivative, chlorpromazine is the prototypic phenothiazine agent. It occurs as a white to slightly creamy white, odorless, bitter tasting, crystalline powder. One g is soluble in 1 mL of water and 1.5 mL of alcohol. The commercially available injection is a solution of chlorpromazine HCl in sterile water at a pH of 3–5.

Chlorpromazine HCl may also be known as aminazine, or chlorpromazini hydrochloridum; many trade names are available.

Storage/Stability

Protect from light and store at room temperature; avoid freezing the oral solution and injection. Dispense oral solution in amber bottles. Store oral tablets in tight containers. Do not store in plastic syringes or IV bags for prolonged periods as the drug may adsorb to plastic.

Chlorpromazine will darken upon prolonged exposure to light; do not use solutions that are darkly colored or if precipitates have formed. A slight yellowish color will not affect potency or efficacy.

Compatibility/Compounding Considerations

Alkaline solutions will cause the drug to oxidize.

The following products have been reported to be **compatible** when mixed with chlorpromazine HCl injection: all usual intravenous fluids, ascorbic acid, atropine sulfate, butorphanol tartrate, diphenhydramine, droperidol, fentanyl citrate, glycopyrrolate, heparin sodium, hydromorphone HCl, hydroxyzine HCl, lidocaine HCl, meperidine, metoclopramide, metaraminol bitartrate, morphine sulfate, pentazocine lactate, promazine HCl, promethazine, scopolamine HBr, and tetracycline HCl.

The following products have been reported as

being **incompatible** when mixed with chlorpromazine: aminophylline, amphotericin B, chloramphenicol sodium succinate, chlorothiazide sodium, dimenhydrinate, methicillin sodium, methohexital sodium, nafcillin sodium, penicillin g potassium, pentobarbital sodium, phenobarbital sodium, and thiopental sodium. Compatibility is dependent upon factors such as pH, concentration, temperature, and diluent used; consult specialized references or a hospital pharmacist for more specific information.

Dosage Forms/Regulatory Status

VETERINARY-LABELED PRODUCTS: None

The ARCI (Racing Commissioners International) has designated this drug as a class 2 substance. See the appendix for more information.

HUMAN-LABELED PRODUCTS:

Chlorpromazine Oral Tablets: 10 mg, 25 mg, 50 mg, 100 mg & 200 mg; generic; (Rx)

Chlorpromazine Injection: 25 mg/mL in 1 & 2 mL amps; generic; (Rx)

References

Booth, NH (1988). Drugs Acting on the Central Nervous System. *Veterinary Pharmacology and Therapeutics—6th Ed.* NH Booth and LE McDonald Eds. Ames, Iowa State University Press: 153–408.

Dowling, P (2003). GI Therapy: When what goes in won't stay down. Proceedings: Western Veterinary Conference. Accessed via: Veterinary Information Network. http://goo.gl/co8V8

Hall, LW & KW Clarke (1983). *Veterinary Anesthesia 8th Ed.* London, Bailliere Tindall.

Lumb, WV & EW Jones (1984). *Veterinary Anesthesia, 2nd Ed.* Philadelphia, Lea & Febiger.

Marks, S (2008). GI Therapeutics: Which Ones and When? Proceedings: IVECCS. Accessed via: Veterinary Information Network. http://goo.gl/RntHJ

Morgan, RV, Ed. (1988). *Handbook of Small Animal Practice.* New York, Churchill Livingstone.

Washabau, R (2006). Current anti-emetic therapy. Proceedings WVC 2006, Accessed via the Veterinary Information Network Jan 2007. Accessed via: Veterinary Information Network. http://goo.gl/LYKDB

CHLORPROPAMIDE

(klor-*proe*-pa-mide) Diabenese®

SULFONYLUREA ANTIDIABETIC

Prescriber Highlights

▶ Oral sulfonylurea antidiabetic agent sometimes used in dogs or cats for diabetes insipidus; potentially for diabetes mellitus

▶ Many contraindications/cautions

▶ Most likely adverse effects are hypoglycemia or GI distress

Uses/Indications

While chlorpropamide could potentially be of benefit in the adjunctive treatment of diabetes mellitus in small animals, its use has been primarily for adjunctive therapy in diabetes insipidus in dogs and cats.

Pharmacology/Actions

Sulfonylureas lower blood glucose concentrations in both diabetic and non-diabetic patients. The exact mechanism of action is not known, but these agents are thought to exert the effect primarily by stimulating the beta cells in the pancreas to secrete additional endogenous insulin. Ongoing use of the sulfonylureas appears to enhance peripheral sensitivity to insulin and reduce the production of hepatic basal glucose. The mechanisms causing these effects are yet to be fully explained. Chlorpropamide has antidiuretic activity, presumably by potentiating vasopressin's effects on the renal tubules. It may also stimulate secretion of vasopressin.

Pharmacokinetics

Chlorpropamide is absorbed well from the GI tract. Its distribution characteristics have not been well described, but it is highly bound to plasma proteins and is excreted into milk. Elimination half-lives have not been described in domestic animals, but in humans the elimination half-life is about 36 hours. The drug is both metabolized in the liver and excreted unchanged. Elimination of chlorpropamide is enhanced in alkaline urine; decreased in acidic urine.

Contraindications/Precautions/Warnings

Oral antidiabetic agents are considered contraindicated with the following conditions: severe burns, severe trauma, severe infection, diabetic coma or other hypoglycemic conditions, major surgery, ketosis, ketoacidosis, or other significant acidotic conditions. Chlorpropamide should only be used when its potential benefits outweigh its risks during untreated adrenal or pituitary insufficiency, thyroid, cardiac, renal or hepatic function impairment, prolonged vomiting, high fever, malnourishment or debilitated condition, or when fluid retention is present.

Adverse Effects

Hypoglycemia and GI disturbances are the most common adverse effects noted with this agent. Syndrome of inappropriate antidiuretic hormone (SIADH), anorexia, diarrhea, hepatotoxicity, skin eruptions, lassitude or other CNS effects, and hematologic toxicity are all potentially possible.

Reproductive/Nursing Safety

Safe use during pregnancy has not been established. In humans, the FDA categorizes this drug as category *C* for use during pregnancy (*Animal studies have shown an adverse effect on the fetus, but there are no adequate studies in humans; or there are no animal reproduction studies and no adequate studies in humans.*)

Chlorpropamide enters maternal milk; in humans it is not recommended for use during nursing.

Overdosage/Acute Toxicity

Profound hypoglycemia is the greatest concern after an overdose. Gut emptying protocols should be employed when warranted. Because of its long half-life, blood glucose monitoring and treatment with parenteral glucose may be required for several days. Overdoses may require additional monitoring (blood gases, serum electrolytes) and supportive therapy.

Drug Interactions

The following drug interactions have either been reported or are theoretical in humans or animals receiving chlorpropamide and may be of significance in veterinary patients:

- **ALCOHOL:** A disulfiram-like reaction (anorexia, nausea, vomiting) has been reported in humans who have ingested alcohol within 48–72 hours of receiving chlorpropamide
- **BARBITURATES:** Barbiturate duration of action may be prolonged

The following drugs may potentiate *hypoglycemia* if administered with chlorpropamide, or be displaced by chlorpropamide from plasma proteins thereby causing enhanced pharmacologic effects of the two drugs involved:

- **CHLORAMPHENICOL**
- **BETA-BLOCKERS,**
- **MAOI'S** (including **amitraz** and possibly, **selegiline**)
- **NSAIDS**
- **PROBENECID**
- **SALICYLATES**
- **SULFONAMIDES**
- **WARFARIN**

The following drugs may potentiate *hyperglycemia* if administered with chlorpropamide:

- **CALCIUM CHANNEL BLOCKERS (e.g., diltiazem, amlodipine)**
- **CORTICOSTEROIDS**
- **ESTROGENS**
- **ISONIAZID**
- **PHENOTHIAZINES**
- **PHENYTOIN**
- **THIAZIDES**
- **THYROID MEDICATIONS**

Laboratory Considerations

- Chlorpropamide may mildly increase values of **liver enzymes, BUN, or serum creatinine.**

Doses

For adjunctive therapy in diabetes insipidus in dogs and cats. Beneficial effects may be seen in less than 50% of animals treated. A trial period of at least one week of therapy should be given before assessing effect.

- **DOGS & CATS:**

  For adjunctive treatment of diabetes insipidus in animals with partial ADH deficiency:
  a) 10–40 mg/kg PO daily (Randolph and Peterson 1994), (Behrend 2003)

  b) Dogs: 50–250 mg (total dose) PO daily; Cats: 50 mg (total dose) PO daily (Hoskins 2005)

Monitoring

■ Serum electrolytes, plasma and urine osmolarity, urine output; if used for DI

■ Blood Glucose

Chemistry/Synonyms

An oral sulfonylurea antidiabetic agent, chlorpropamide occurs as a white, crystalline powder having a slight odor. It is practically insoluble in water.

Chlorpropamide may also be known as: chlorpropamidum, *Anti-D®, Chlomide®, Clordiabet®, Copamide®, Deavynfar®, Diabecontrol®, Diabeedol®, Diabemide®, Diabenese®, Diabet®, Diabexan®, Diabiclor®, Diabines®, Diabitex®, Dibecon®, Glicoben®, Gliconorm®, Glicorp®, Glycemin®, Glymese®, Hypomide®, Idle®, Insogen®, Normoglic®, Novo-Propamide®, Propamide®,* or *Trane®.*

Storage/Stability

Chlorpropamide tablets should be stored in well-closed containers at room temperature.

Dosage Forms/Regulatory Status

VETERINARY-LABELED PRODUCTS: None

HUMAN-LABELED PRODUCTS:

Chlorpropamide Oral Tablets: 100 mg & 250 mg; generic; (Rx)

References

Behrend, E (2003). Diabetes insipidus and other causes of polyuria/polydipsia. Proceedings: Western Veterinary Conference. Accessed via: Veterinary Information Network. http://goo.gl/pxzS4

Hoskins, J (2005). Geriatric medicine: Kidney diseases. Proceedings: ACVC 2006, Accessed from the Veterinary Information Network, Jan 2007. http://goo.gl/eLSHI

CHLORTETRACYCLINE

(klor-te-tra-sye-kleen)
Aureomycin®, Pennchlor®

TETRACYCLINE ANTIBIOTIC

Prescriber Highlights

▶ Tetracycline antibiotic used primarily in water or feed treatments or topically for ophthalmic use

▶ Many bacteria are now resistant; may still be very useful to treat mycoplasma, rickettsia, spirochetes, & Chlamydia

▶ Contraindications: Hypersensitivity. Extreme caution: Pregnancy. Caution: liver, renal insufficiency

▶ Adverse Effects: GI distress, staining of developing teeth & bones, superinfections, photosensitivity

▶ Drug-drug; drug-lab interactions

Uses/Indications

There are a variety of FDA-approved chlortetracycline products for use in food animals. It may also be useful in treating susceptible infections in dogs, cats, birds and small mammals (not Guinea pigs). For more information, refer to the Doses section below.

Pharmacology/Actions

Tetracyclines generally act as bacteriostatic antibiotics inhibiting protein synthesis by reversibly binding to 30S ribosomal subunits of susceptible organisms thereby preventing binding to those ribosomes of aminoacyl transfer-RNA. Tetracyclines are believed to reversibly bind to 50S ribosomes and additionally alter cytoplasmic membrane permeability in susceptible organisms. In high concentrations, tetracyclines can inhibit protein synthesis by mammalian cells.

As a class, the tetracyclines have activity against most mycoplasma, spirochetes (including the Lyme disease organism), Chlamydia, and Rickettsia. Against gram-positive bacteria, the tetracyclines have activity against some strains of staphylococcus and streptococci, but resistance of these organisms is increasing. Gram-positive bacteria that are usually covered by tetracyclines include: *Actinomyces* spp., *Bacillus anthracis, Clostridium perfringens* and *tetani, Listeria monocytogenes,* and Nocardia. Among gram-negative bacteria that tetracyclines usually have *in vitro* and *in vivo* activity include *Bordetella* spp., *Brucella,* Bartonella, *Haemophilus* spp., *Pasturella multocida,* Shigella, and *Yersinia pestis.* Many or most strains of *E. coli,* Klebsiella, Bacteroides, Enterobacter, Proteus and *Pseudomonas aeruginosa* are resistant to the tetracyclines. While most strains of *Pseudomonas aeruginosa* show *in vitro* resistance to tetracyclines, those compounds attaining high urine levels (*e.g.,* tetracycline, oxytetracycline) have been associated with clinical cures in dogs with UTI secondary to this organism.

Oxytetracycline, chlortetracycline, and tetracycline share nearly identical spectrums of activity and patterns of cross-resistance and a tetracycline susceptibility disk is usually used for *in vitro* testing for chlortetracycline susceptibility.

Pharmacokinetics

Refer to the oxytetracycline monograph for general information on the pharmacokinetics of tetracyclines.

Contraindications/Precautions/Warnings

Chlortetracycline is contraindicated in patients hypersensitive to it or other tetracyclines. Because tetracyclines can retard fetal skeletal development and discolor deciduous teeth, they should only be used in the last half of pregnancy when the benefits outweigh the fetal risks. Oxytetracycline, chlortetracycline and tetracycline are considered more likely to cause these abnormalities than either doxycycline or minocycline.

In patients with renal insufficiency or hepatic impairment, chlortetracycline must be used cautiously. Lower than normal dosages are recommended with enhanced monitoring of renal and hepatic function. Avoid concurrent administration of other nephrotoxic or hepatotoxic drugs.

Because it may cause clostridial enterotoxemia in guinea pigs, chlortetracycline should not be used this species.

Adverse Effects

Chlortetracycline given to young animals can cause discoloration of bones and teeth to a yellow, brown, or gray color. High dosages or chronic administration may delay bone growth and healing.

Tetracyclines in high levels can exert an antianabolic effect that can cause an increase in BUN and/or hepatotoxicity, particularly in patients with preexisting renal dysfunction. As renal function deteriorates secondary to drug accumulation, this effect may be exacerbated.

In ruminants, high oral doses can cause ruminal microflora depression and ruminoreticular stasis. Rapid intravenous injection of undiluted propylene glycol-based products can cause intravascular hemolysis with resultant hemoglobinuria. Propylene glycol based products have also caused cardiodepressant effects when administered to calves.

In small animals, tetracyclines can cause nausea, vomiting, anorexia, and diarrhea. Cats do not tolerate oral tetracycline or oxytetracycline very well; signs of colic, fever, hair loss, and depression may be seen. There are reports that long-term tetracycline use may cause urolith formation in dogs.

Horses that are stressed by surgery, anesthesia, trauma, etc., may break with severe diarrheas after receiving tetracyclines (especially with oral administration).

Tetracycline therapy (especially long-term) may result in overgrowth (superinfections) of non-susceptible bacteria or fungi.

Tetracyclines have been associated with photosensitivity reactions and, rarely, hepatotoxicity or blood dyscrasias.

Reproductive/Nursing Safety

In humans, the FDA categorizes this drug as category *D* (tetracyclines-general) for use during pregnancy (*There is evidence of human fetal risk, but the potential benefits from the use of the drug in pregnant women may be acceptable despite its potential risks.*)

Tetracyclines are excreted in milk, but because much of the drug will be bound to calcium in milk, it is unlikely to be of significant risk to nursing animals.

Overdosage/Acute Toxicity

Tetracyclines are generally well tolerated after acute overdoses. Dogs given more than 400 mg/kg/day orally or 100 mg/kg/day IM of oxytetracycline did not demonstrate any toxicity. Oral overdoses would most likely be associated with GI disturbances (vomiting, anorexia, and/or diarrhea). Should the patient develop severe emesis or diarrhea, fluids and electrolytes should be monitored and replaced if necessary. Chronic overdoses may lead to drug accumulation and nephrotoxicity.

High oral doses given to ruminants, can cause ruminal microflora depression and ruminoreticular stasis. Rapid intravenous injection of undiluted propylene glycol-based products can cause intravascular hemolysis with resultant hemoglobinuria.

Rapid intravenous injection of tetracyclines has induced transient collapse and cardiac arrhythmias in several species, presumably due to chelation with intravascular calcium ions. Overdose quantities of drug could exacerbate this effect if given too rapidly IV. If the drug must be given rapidly IV (less than 5 minutes), some clinicians recommend pre-treating the animal with intravenous calcium gluconate.

Drug Interactions

The following drug interactions have either been reported or are theoretical in humans or animals receiving chlortetracycline and may be of significance in veterinary patients:

■ **BETA-LACTAM OR AMINOGLYCOSIDE ANTIBIOTICS:** Bacteriostatic drugs, like the tetracyclines, may interfere with bactericidal activity of the penicillins, cephalosporins, and aminoglycosides; there is some controversy regarding the actual clinical significance of this interaction, however

■ **DIGOXIN:** Tetracyclines may increase the bioavailability of digoxin in a small percentage of patients (human) and lead to digoxin toxicity. These effects may persist for months after discontinuation of the tetracycline.

■ **DIVALENT OR TRIVALENT CATIONS (oral antacids, saline cathartics or other GI products containing aluminum, calcium, iron, magnesium, zinc, or bismuth cations):** When orally administered, tetracyclines can chelate divalent or trivalent cations that can decrease the absorption of the tetracycline or the other drug if it contains these cations; it is recommended that all oral tetracyclines be given at least 1–2 hours before or after the cation-containing products

■ **WARFARIN:** Tetracyclines may depress plasma prothrombin activity and patients on anticoagulant (*e.g.*, warfarin) therapy may need dosage adjustment.

Laboratory Considerations

■ Tetracyclines (not minocycline) may cause falsely elevated values of **urine catecholamines** when using fluorometric methods of determination.

■ Tetracyclines reportedly can cause false-positive **urine glucose** results if using the cupric sulfate method of determination (Benedict's reagent, *Clinitest®*), but this may be the result of ascorbic acid that is found in some parenteral formulations of tetracyclines. Tetracyclines have also reportedly caused false-negative results in determining urine glucose when using the glucose oxidase method (*Clinistix®*, *Tes-Tape®*).

Doses

■ **DOGS/CATS:**

For susceptible infections:

a) 25 mg/kg PO q6−8h (Papich 1992)

b) To prevent recurrence of mycoplasma or chlamydial conjunctivitis in large catteries where topical therapy is impractical: soluble chlortetracycline powder in food at a dose of 50 mg per day per cat for 1 month (Carro 1994)

■ **RABBITS/RODENTS/SMALL MAMMALS:**
Note: Not recommended for use in guinea pigs

a) **Rabbits:** 50 mg/kg PO q12−24h (Ivey & Morrisey 2000)

b) **Chinchillas:** 50 mg/kg PO q12h (Hayes 2000)

c) **Hamsters:** 20 mg/kg IM or SC q12h; Mice: 25 mg/kg SC or IM q12h; Rats: 6−10 mg/kg SC or IM q12h (Adamcak & Otten 2000)

■ **BIRDS:**

a) For the treatment of chlamydiosis: In small birds add chlortetracycline to food in a concentration of 0.05%; larger psittacines require 1% CTC. (Flammer 1992)

b) **Ratites:** 15−20 mg/kg PO three times daily (Jenson 1998)

c) **Pigeons:** 50 mg/kg PO q6−8h; or 1000−1500 mg/gallon drinking water; in warm weather mix fresh every 12 hours. Best used in combination with tylosin for ornithosis complex; calcium inhibits absorption therefore grit and layer pellets should be withheld during treatment. (Harlin 2006)

■ **CATTLE AND SWINE:**

For susceptible infections:

a) 6−10 mg/kg IV or IM; 10−20 mg/kg PO (**Note:** Although not specified in this reference, chlortetracycline is generally administered once daily.) (Howard 1993)

Chemistry/Synonyms

A tetracycline antibiotic, chlortetracycline occurs as yellow, odorless crystals. It is slightly soluble in water.

Chlortetracycline may also be known as clortetraciclina, A-377, NRRL-2209, SF-66, *Aureomycin®* or *CLTC® 100 MR*.

Storage/Stability

Chlortetracycline should be stored in tight containers and protected from light.

Dosage Forms/Regulatory Status

VETERINARY-LABELED PRODUCTS:
There are several feed additive/water mix preparations available containing chlortetracycline. Trade names include *Aureomycin®*; (BIVI), *CTC®* (AgriLabs) *CLTC® 100 MR* (Philbro); (AL Labs); *CLTC® 100 MR* (Pennfield/Durvet). There are also combination products containing chlortetracycline and sulfamethazine (*Aureomycin Sulmet®*, *Aureo S 700®*), chlortetracycline, sulfamethazine and penicillin (*Aureomix 500®*, *Pennclor SP 250 & 500®*), chlortetracycline, sulfathiazole, and penicillin (*Aureozol 500®*)

See individual labels for more information.

HUMAN-LABELED PRODUCTS: None

References

Adamcak, A & B Otten (2000). Rodent Therapeutics. *Vet Clin NA: Exotic Anim Pract* 3:1(Jan): 221−240.

Flammer, K (1992). An update on the diagnosis and treatment of avian chlamydiosis. *Current Veterinary Therapy XI: Small Animal Practice*. R Kirk and J Bonagura Eds. Philadelphia, W.B. Saunders Company: 1150−1153.

Harlin, R (2006). Practical pigeon medicine. Proceedings: AAV 2006. Accessed via: Veterinary Information Network. http://goo.gl/EW76N

Hayes, P (2000). Diseases of Chinchillas. *Kirk's Current Veterinary Therapy: XIII Small Animal Practice*. J Bonagura Ed. Philadelphia, WB Saunders: 1152−1157.

Howard, J (1993). Table of Common Drugs: Approximate Doses. *Current Veterinary Therapy 3: Food Animal Practice*. J Howard Ed. Philadelphia, W.B. Saunders Co.: 930−933.

Ivey, E & J Morrisey (2000). Therapeutics for Rabbits. *Vet Clin NA: Exotic Anim Pract* 3:1(Jan): 183−216.

Jenson, J (1998). Current ratite therapy. *The Veterinary Clinics of North America: Food Animal Practice* 16:3(November).

Chondroitin Sulfate–See Glucosamine/Chondroitin

CHORIONIC GONADOTROPIN (HCG)

(kor-ee-*on*-ic goe-*nad*-oh-troe-pin)
Chorulon®

REPRODUCTIVE HORMONE

Prescriber Highlights

▶ Human hormone that mimics luteinizing hormone & some FSH activity; used for a variety of theriogenology conditions in many species

▶ Only administered parenterally

▶ Contraindications: Androgen responsive neoplasias, hypersensitivity

▶ Adverse Effects: Antibodies/hypersensitivity, pain on injection

Uses/Indications

The veterinary product's labeled indication is for "parenteral use in cows for the treatment of nymphomania (frequent or constant heat) due to cystic ovaries." It has been used for other purposes in several species; refer to the Dosage section for more information.

Pharmacology/Actions

HCG mimics quite closely the effects of luteinizing hormone (LH) but also has some FSH-like activity. In males, HCG can stimulate the differentiation of, and androgen production by, testicular interstitial (Leydig) cells. It may also stimulate testicular descent when no anatomical abnormality is present.

In females, HCG will stimulate the corpus luteum to produce progesterone and can induce ovulation (possibly also in patients with cystic ovaries). In the bitch HCG will induce estrogen secretion.

Pharmacokinetics

HCG is destroyed in the GI tract after oral administration, so it must be given parenterally. After IM injection, peak plasma levels occur in about 6 hours.

HCG is distributed primarily to the ovaries in females and to the testes in males, but some may also be distributed to the proximal tubules in the renal cortex.

HCG is eliminated from the blood in biphasic manner. The initial elimination half-life is about 11 hours and the terminal half-life is approximately 23 hours.

Contraindications/Precautions/Warnings

In humans, HCG is contraindicated in patients with prostatic carcinoma or other androgen-dependent neoplasias, precocious puberty or having a previous hypersensitivity reaction to HCG. No labeled contraindications for veterinary patients were noted, but the above human contraindications should be used as guidelines.

Antibody production to this hormone has been reported after repetitive use, resulting in diminished effect.

Adverse Effects

Potentially, hypersensitivity reactions are possible with this agent. HCG may cause abortion in mares prior to the 35th day of pregnancy, perhaps due to increased estrogen levels. No other reported adverse reactions were noted for veterinary patients.

In humans, HCG has caused pain at the injection site, gynecomastia, headache, depression, irritability, and edema.

Reproductive/Nursing Safety

In humans, the FDA categorizes this drug as category *X* for use during pregnancy (*Studies in animals or humans demonstrate fetal abnormalities or adverse reaction; reports indicate evidence of fetal risk. The risk of use in pregnant women clearly outweighs any possible benefit.*)

It is unknown if HCG enters maternal milk.

Overdosage/Acute Toxicity

No overdosage cases have been reported with HCG.

Drug/Lab Interactions

No interactions have apparently been reported with HCG.

Doses

■ **DOGS:**

For cryptorchidism:

a) 500 Units injected twice weekly for 4–6 weeks (McDonald 1988)

For HCG Challenge test (to determine if testicular tissue remains in castrated male dogs; in females to diagnose sexual differentiation disorders or if functional ovarian tissue remains after ovariohysterectomy):

a) Male dogs or females with suspected sexual differentiation disorder: Take sample for resting testosterone level. Administer 44 micrograms/kg HCG IM and take a 4 hour post sample.

Female dogs: 100–1000 Units IM during apparent estrous episode. Measure progesterone level in 5–7 days. If above 1 ng/mL, this indicates functional ovarian tissue. (Shille & Olson 1989)

To produce luteinization of a persistent follicular cyst:

a) 500 Units IM; repeat in 48 hours. If effective, will convert from proestrus to estrus in 1–2 days and sexual behavior should stop within 2 weeks. (Barton & Wolf 1988)

For infertile bitches cycling normally with low progesterone due to lack of corpus luteum formation:

a) Next cycle, give 500 Units HCG SC on days 10–11 of heat cycle or when vaginal smear indicates breeding readiness. Breed 2 days after HCG administration. (Barton & Wolf 1988)

For male infertility secondary to low testosterone, LH and FSH:

a) HCG 500 Units SC twice weekly for 4 weeks. Add PMSG (Pregnant Mare Serum Gonadotropin) 20 Units/kg SC 3 times weekly. If PMSG is unavailable, use FSH-P at same dose (1 mg FSH = 10–14 IU). Continue for 3 months. Once spermatogenesis ensues, may continue with HCG only. (Barton & Wolf 1988)

■ **CATS:**

For HCG Challenge test (to determine if testicular tissue remains in castrated male cats; in females to diagnose sexual differentiation disorders or if functional ovarian tissue remains after ovariohysterectomy):

a) Male cats or females with suspected sexual differentiation disorder: Take sample for resting testosterone level. Administer 250 micrograms HCG IM and take a 4 hour post sample.

Queens: 50–100 Units IM during apparent estrous episode. Measure progesterone level in 5–7 days. If above 1 ng/mL, this indicates functional ovarian tissue. (Shille & Olson 1989)

For infertility, reduced libido, testis descent in male cats:

a) 50–100 Units repeated if necessary (Verstegen 2000)

For infertility in queens due to confirmed ovulation failure:

a) 100–500 Units IM (Barton & Wolf 1988)

To induce ovulation in anestrus queens:

a) Give FSH-P 2 mg IM daily (for up to 5 days) until estrus is observed. Give 250 micrograms HCG on first and second day of estrus (Kraemer & Bowen 1986)

After artificial insemination:

a) 50–75 Units IM immediately after insemination; repeat insemination and injection in 24 hours (Sojka 1986)

■ **FERRETS:**

a) 100 Units IM; repeat in 1 week as necessary. Most effective 14 days after onset of estrus. (Williams 2000)

■ **RABBITS/RODENTS/SMALL MAMMALS:**

a) **Guinea pigs:** For cystic ovaries: 1000 Units/animal IM, repeat in 7–10 days (Adamcak & Otten 2000)

■ **BIRDS:**

To reduce feather plucking (especially in female birds):

a) Dosage is empirical; 500–1,000 Units/kg IM. If no response in 3 days, repeat. If no response after second injection, unlikely to be of benefit at any dose. If reduces feather plucking, will need to repeat after 4–6 weeks. Major drawback is that with repeated usage, time between treatments is reduced. (Lightfoot 2001)

■ **CATTLE:**

For treatment of ovarian cysts:

a) 10,000 Units deep IM or 2500–5000 Units IV, may repeat in 14 days if animal's behavior or physical exam indicates a need for retreatment. Alternatively, 500–2500 Units injected directly into the follicle. (Package Insert; *Follutein®*—Solvay)

■ **HORSES:**

For cryptorchidism:

a) **Foals:** 1000 Units injected twice weekly for 4–6 weeks (McDonald 1988) (**Note:** Many clinicians believe that medical treatment is unwarranted and that surgery should be performed.)

To induce ovulation in early estrus when one, large, dominant follicle that is palpable with a diameter >35 mm is present:

a) HCG: 2000–3000 Units IV (preferable to treat mare 6 hours before mating) (Hopkins 1987)

For treatment of persistent follicles during the early transition period:

a) 1000–5000 Units (results are variable) (Van Camp 1986)

To hasten ovulation and reduce variability of estrus after prostaglandin synchronization:

a) HCG: 1500–3300 Units 5–6 days after the second prostaglandin treatment or on the first or second day of estrus (Bristol 1986)

Chemistry/Synonyms

A gonad-stimulating polypeptide secreted by the placenta, chorionic gonadotropin is obtained from the urine of pregnant women. It occurs as a white or practically white, amorphous, lyophilized powder. It is soluble in water and practically insoluble in alcohol. One International Unit (called Units in this reference) of HCG is equal to one USP unit. There are at least 1500 USP Units per mg.

Chorionic gonadotropin may also be known as: human chorionic gonadotropin, HCG, hCG, LH 500, CG, chorionic gonadotrophin, dynatropin, gonadotropine chorionique, gonadotrophinum chorionicum, choriogonadotrophin, chorionogonadotropin, pregnancy-urine hormone, or PU; there are many trade names internationally.

Storage/Stability

Chorionic gonadotropin powder for injection should be stored at room temperature (15–30°C) and protected from light. After reconstitution, the resultant solution is stable for 30–90 days (depending on the product) when stored at 2–15°C. The labels for the veterinary products, *Chorulon®* and *P.G. 600®* state to use the vial immediately after reconstituting with the supplied diluent.

Dosage Forms/Regulatory Status

VETERINARY-LABELED PRODUCTS:

Chorionic Gonadotropin (HCG) Injection: 10,000 Units per 10 mL double vial packs containing 10,000 USP Units per vial with bacteriostatic water for injection; single dose 10 mL vials of freeze-dried powder and five 10 mL vials of sterile diluent; *Chorulon®* (Intervet), *Chorionad®* (Vetcom); (Rx). FDA-approved for use in cows and finfish. No withdrawal time is required when used as labeled.

Chorionic Gonadotropin freeze-dried powder: Single dose 5 mL vials when reconstituted contains pregnant mare serum gonadotropin (PMSG) 400 Units and human chorionic gonadotropin (hCG) 200 Units; five dose 25 mL vials that when reconstituted contains pregnant mare serum gonadotropin (PMSG) 2,000 Units and human chorionic gonadotropin (hCG) 1,000 Units; *P.G. 600®* (Intervet); (OTC). FDA-approved for use in swine (prepubertal gilts and sows at weaning); no meat withdrawal time is required when used as labeled.

HUMAN-LABELED PRODUCTS:

Chorionic Gonadotropin Powder for Injection: 5,000 Units/vial with 10 mL diluent (to make 500 Units/mL); 10,000 Units/vial with 10 mL diluent (to make 1,000 Units/mL); 20,000 Units/vial with 10 mL diluent (to make 2,000 Units/mL) in 10 mL vials; *Profasi®* (Serono); *Choron 10®* (Forest); *Gonic®* (Hauck); *Novarel®* (Ferring); *Pregnyl®* (Organon); generic; (Rx)

References

Adamcak, A & B Otten (2000). Rodent Therapeutics. *Vet Clin NA: Exotic Anim Pract* 3:1(Jan): 221–240.

Barton, CL & AM Wolf (1988). Disorders of Reproduction. *Handbook of Small Animal Practice*. RV Morgan Ed. New York, Churchill Livingstone: 679–700.

Bristol, F (1986). Estrous synchronization in mares. *Current Therapy in Theriogenology 2: Diagnosis, Treatment and Prevention of Reproductive Diseases in Small and Large Animals*. DA Morrow Ed. Philadelphia, WB Saunders: 661–664.

Hopkins, SM (1987). Ovulation Management. *Current Therapy in Equine Medicine*. NE Robinson Ed. Philadelphia, WB Saunders: 498–500.

Kraemer, DC & MJ Bowen (1986). Embryo transfer in laboratory animals. *Current Therapy in Theriogenology 2: Diagnosis, Treatment and Prevention of Reproductive Diseases in Small and Large Animals*. DA Morrow Ed. Philadelphia, WB Saunders: 73–78.

Lightfoot, T (2001). Feather "Plucking". Proceedings: Atlantic Coast Veterinary Conference. Accessed via: Veterinary Information Network. http://goo.gl/6qoTg

McDonald, LE (1988). Hormones of the pituitary gland. *Veterinary Pharmacology and Therapeutics – 6th Ed.* NH Booth and LE McDonald Eds. Ames, Iowa State University Press: 581–592.

Shille, VM & PN Olson (1989). Dynamic testing in reproductive endocrinology. *Current Veterinary Therapy X: Small Animal Practice*. RW Kirk Ed. Philadelphia, WB Saunders: 1282–1291.

Sojka, NJ (1986). Management of artificial breeding in cats. *Current Therapy in Theriogenology 2: Diagnosis, Treatment and Prevention of Reproductive Diseases in Small and Large Animals*. DA Morrow Ed. Philadelphia, WB Saunders: 805–808.

Van Camp, SD (1986). Breeding soundness examination of the mare and common genital abnormalities encountered. *Current Therapy in Theriogenology 2: Diagnosis, Treatment and Prevention of Reproductive Diseases in Small and Large Animals*. DA Morrow Ed. Philadelphia, WB Saunders: 654–661.

Verstegen, J (2000). Feline Reproduction. *Textbook of Veterinary Internal Medicine: Diseases of the Dog and Cat*. S Ettinger and E Feldman Eds. Philadelphia, WB Saunders. 2: 1585–1598.

Williams, B (2000). Therapeutics in Ferrets. *Vet Clin NA: Exotic Anim Pract* 3:1(Jan): 131–153.

CHROMIUM
CHROMIUM PICOLINATE

(*kroe*-mee-um pik-oh-*lin*-ate)

TRANSITION TRACE METAL

Prescriber Highlights

▶ Trace metal "nutraceutical" that may be useful as an adjunctive treatment for diabetes mellitus & obesity in cats

▶ Efficacy in question, but probably safe

Uses/Indications

Chromium supplementation may be useful in the adjunctive treatment of diabetes mellitus or obesity, particularly in cats; there is controversy whether this treatment is beneficial. It does not appear to be useful in dogs with diabetes mellitus.

Pharmacology/Actions

Metallic chromium has no pharmacologic activity, but other valence states have activity. Chromium VI (hexavalent form) is used in the welding and chemical industries and is considered a carcinogen. Chromium III (trivalent) is the form used in supplements and found naturally in foods. Chromium is thought to play a role in insulin function. It is an active component of so-called glucose tolerance factor (GTF). GTF is a complex of molecules that includes glycine, glutamic acid, cystiene and nicotinic acid. Chromium's exact role in carbohydrate and nitrogen metabolism is not clear. It does not lower blood glucose levels in normal patients. In humans, chromium deficiency can cause impaired tolerance to glucose and insulin function, increased serum cholesterol and triglyceride levels, neuropathy, weight loss, impaired nitrogen metabolism, and decreased respiratory function.

Pharmacokinetics

Chromium is not absorbed very well from the GI tract and most of a dose is excreted in the feces. When given as a salt (picolinate, chloride, nicotinate), lipophilicity and solubility are increased and absorption is enhanced. Absorbed chromium is eliminated via the kidneys.

Contraindications/Precautions/Warnings

Chromium supplements could, potentially, exacerbate renal insufficiency; use with caution in these patients. Because the picolinate salt can potentially alter behavior, consider using chromium chloride, or chromium nicotinate in patients receiving SSRI's or other behavioral therapies.

Adverse Effects

Chromium supplements (Cr III) at usual dosages appear to be well tolerated. Some human patients have complained of cognitive, perceptual, and motor dysfunction after receiving the picolinate salt.

Reproductive/Nursing Safety

In humans, chromium (up to 8 micrograms/kg) is probably safe to use in pregnancy but information remains sketchy. Because cats may receive much higher dosages than the human dosages for treating diabetes, use cautiously in pregnant animals.

Chromium supplements are likely to be safe to use in lactating animals.

Overdosage/Acute Toxicity

Little information on acute overdoses was located. There are at least two case reports of women developing renal failure after taking excessive doses of chromium picolinate.

Drug Interactions

The following drug interactions have either been reported or are theoretical in humans or animals receiving chromium and may be of significance in veterinary patients:

■ **CORTICOSTEROIDS:** May increase the urinary excretion of chromium

■ **H₂ BLOCKERS (cimetidine, ranitidine, famotidine, etc.) or PROTON PUMP INHIBITORS (PPI's, omeprazole, etc.):** May decrease chromium levels by inhibiting their absorption; clinical significance is unclear

■ **NSAIDS:** May increase the absorption and retention of chromium; clinical significance is unlikely

■ **ZINC:** Theoretically, co-administration of zinc with chromium could decrease the oral absorption of both

Laboratory Considerations

■ No specific laboratory interactions or considerations noted

Doses

■ **CATS:**
For use as an oral hypoglycemic agent:
a) Chromium picolinate 200 micrograms (per cat) PO once a day. (Dowling 2000); (Greco 2002)
For adjunctive treatment of feline obesity:
a) Chromium picolinate 20 micrograms/kg PO every other a day (Flores 2004)

Monitoring

■ As there is no reliable way to measure chromium in the body, a clinical trial is the only way to determine whether chromium is effective in helping to control blood glucose. Standard methods of monitoring diabetes treatment efficacy should be followed (*e.g.,* fasting blood glucose, appetite, attitude, body condition/weight, PU/PD resolution and, perhaps, serum fructosamine and/or glycosylated hemoglobin levels).

Client Information

■ Clients should give the medication only as prescribed and not change brands without their veterinarian's approval.

Chemistry/Synonyms

A trace element (Cr; atomic number 24), oral chromium supplements are usually given as the picolinate salt (also known as chromium tripicolinate).

Storage/Stability

Chromium picolinate should be stored in tight containers. For storage recommendations, refer to the label for each product used.

Dosage Forms/Regulatory Status

VETERINARY-LABELED PRODUCTS: None
HUMAN-LABELED PRODUCTS:
No oral products FDA-approved as pharmaceuticals.

Injectable chromium: (as chromic chloride hexahydrate): 4 micrograms/mL (as 20.5 micrograms chromic chloride hexahydrate) and 20 micrograms/mL (as 102.5 micrograms chromic chloride hexahydrate) in 5 mL (20 micrograms/mL only), 10 mL & 30 mL (20 micrograms/mL only); *Chroma-Pak®* (Smith & Nephew SoloPak); generic; (Rx) Oral chromium products are considered to be nutritional supplements by the FDA. No standards have been accepted for potency, purity, safety or efficacy by regulatory bodies.

Supplements are available from a wide variety of sources. Most veterinary use in small animals is with chromium picolinate dosage forms. Common tablet sizes include 200 micrograms, 400 micrograms, 500 micrograms and 800 micrograms. Bioequivalence between products cannot be assumed.

References

Dowling, P (2000). Two transition metals show promise in treating diabetic cats. *Vet Med*(March): 190–192.

Flores, G (2004). Effect of chromium picolinate in the management of feline obesity. Proceedings: WSAVA. Accessed via: Veterinary Information Network. http://goo.gl/yKuo5

Greco, D (2002). Treatment of feline type 2 diabetes mellitus with oral hypoglycemic agents. Proceedings: Atlantic Coast Veterinary Conf. Accessed via: Veterinary Information Network. http://goo.gl/z0AuC

CIMETIDINE
CIMETIDINE HCL

(sye-***met***-i-deen)   Tagamet®

HISTAMINE2 BLOCKER

Prescriber Highlights

▶ Prototype histamine-2 (H₂) blocker used to reduce GI acid production

▶ Newer H₂ blockers (*e.g.,* ranitidine, famotidine) & other agents (*e.g.,* omeprazole) may be more effective, have longer duration of activity, & fewer drug interactions

▶ Caution: Geriatric patients, hepatic or renal insufficiency

▶ Compared with newer H₂ blockers, there are many drug interactions

Uses/Indications

In veterinary medicine, cimetidine has been used for the treatment and/or prophylaxis of gastric, abomasal and duodenal ulcers, uremic gastritis, stress-related or drug-induced erosive gastritis, esophagitis, duodenal gastric reflux, and esophageal reflux. It has also been employed to treat hypersecretory conditions associated with gastrinomas and systemic mastocytosis. Cimetidine has also been used investigationally as a immunomodulating agent (see doses) in dogs. Cimetidine has been used for the treatment of melanomas in horses, but the drug's poor bioavailability and subsequent high doses (48 mg/kg/day) in adult horses makes it a very expensive, unproven treatment. Its use in veterinary and human medicine has been largely supplanted by newer agents that compared to cimetidine are more effective, need less frequent dosing, and do not have as many drug interaction issues.

Pharmacology/Actions

At the H_2 receptors of the parietal cells, cimetidine competitively inhibits histamine thereby reducing gastric acid output both during basal conditions and when stimulated by food, pentagastrin, histamine, or insulin. Gastric emptying time, pancreatic or biliary secretion, and lower esophageal pressures are not altered by cimetidine. By decreasing the amount of gastric juice produced, cimetidine also decreases the amount of pepsin secreted.

Cimetidine has an apparent immunomodulating effect as it has been demonstrated to reverse suppressor T-cell-mediated immune suppression. It also possesses weak anti-androgenic activity.

Pharmacokinetics

In dogs, the oral bioavailability is reported to be approximately 95%, serum half-life is 1.3 hours and volume of distribution is 1.2 L/kg.

In horses, after intragastric administration oral bioavailability is only about 14%, steady-state volume of distribution 0.77 L/kg, median plasma clearance 8.2 mL/min/kg, and terminal elimination half-life is approximately 90 minutes.

In humans, cimetidine is rapidly and well absorbed after oral administration, but a small amount is metabolized in the liver before entering the systemic circulation (first-pass effect). The oral bioavailability is 70–80%. Food may delay absorption and slightly decrease the amount absorbed, but when given with food, peak levels occur when the stomach is not protected by the buffering capabilities of the ingesta.

Cimetidine is well distributed in body tissues and only 15–20% is bound to plasma proteins. The drug enters milk and crosses the placenta.

Cimetidine is both metabolized in the liver and excreted unchanged by the kidneys. More of the drug is excreted by the kidneys when administered parenterally (75%) than when given orally (48%). The average serum half-life is 2 hours in humans, but can be prolonged in elderly patients and those with renal or hepatic disease. Peritoneal dialysis does not appreciably enhance the removal of cimetidine from the body.

Contraindications/Precautions/Warnings

Cimetidine is contraindicated in patients with known hypersensitivity to the drug.

Cimetidine should be used cautiously in geriatric patients and in patients with significantly impaired hepatic or renal function. In humans meeting these criteria, increased risk of CNS effects (confusion) may occur; dosage reductions may be necessary.

Adverse Effects

Adverse effects appear to be very rare in animals at the dosages generally used. Potential adverse effects (documented in humans) that could be seen include mental confusion, headache (upon discontinuation of the drug), gynecomastia, and decreased libido. Rarely, agranulocytosis may develop and, if given rapidly IV, transient cardiac arrhythmias may be seen. Pain at the injection site may occur after IM administration.

Cimetidine does inhibit microsomal enzymes in the liver and may alter the metabolic rates of other drugs (see Drug Interactions below).

Reproductive/Nursing Safety

In humans, the FDA categorizes this drug as category *B* for use during pregnancy (*Animal studies have not yet demonstrated risk to the fetus, but there are no adequate studies in pregnant women; or animal studies have shown an adverse effect, but adequate studies in pregnant women have not demonstrated a risk to the fetus in the first trimester of pregnancy, and there is no evidence of risk in later trimesters.*) In a separate system evaluating the safety of drugs in canine and feline pregnancy (Papich 1989), this drug is categorized as in class: *B* (*Safe for use if used cautiously. Studies in laboratory animals may have uncovered some risk, but these drugs appear to be safe in dogs and cats or these drugs are safe if they are not administered when the animal is near term.*)

Cimetidine is distributed into milk; while safety during nursing is not assured, it is usually considered compatible with nursing in humans.

Overdosage/Acute Toxicity

Clinical experience with cimetidine overdosage is limited. In laboratory animals, very high dosages have been associated with tachycardia and respiratory failure; respiratory support and beta-adrenergic blockers have been suggested for use should these signs occur.

Drug Interactions

The following drug interactions have either been reported or are theoretical in humans or animals receiving cimetidine and may be of significance in veterinary patients:

Cimetidine may inhibit the hepatic microsomal enzyme system and thereby reduce the metabolism, prolong serum half-lives, and increase the serum levels of several drugs and/or reduce the hepatic blood flow and reduce the amount of hepatic extraction of drugs that have a high first-pass effect, including:

- ◼ **BENZODIAZEPINES (e.g., diazepam)**
- ◼ **BETA-BLOCKERS (e.g., propranolol)**
- ◼ **CALCIUM CHANNEL BLOCKERS (e.g., verapamil)**
- ◼ **CHLORAMPHENICOL**
- ◼ **LIDOCAINE**

- **METRONIDAZOLE**
- **PHENYTOIN**
- **PROCAINAMIDE**
- **THEOPHYLLINE**
- **TRIAMTERENE**
- **TRICYCLIC ANTIDEPRESSANTS**
- **WARFARIN**
- **ANTACIDS:** May decrease the absorption of cimetidine; stagger doses (separate by 2 hours if possible)
- **KETOCONAZOLE, ITRACONAZOLE,** etc: Cimetidine may decrease the absorption of these drugs; give these medications at least two hours before cimetidine
- **MYELOSUPPRESSIVE DRUGS:** Cimetidine may exacerbate leukopenias when used with myelosuppressive agents

Laboratory Considerations

- **Creatinine:** Cimetidine may cause small increases in plasma creatinine concentrations early in therapy; these increases are generally mild, non-progressive, and have disappeared when therapy is discontinued
- **Gastric Acid Secretion Tests:** Histamine$_2$ blockers may antagonize the effects of histamine and pentagastrin in the evaluation of gastric acid secretion; it is recommended that histamine$_2$ blockers be discontinued at least 24 hours before performing this test
- **Allergen Extract Skin Tests:** Histamine$_2$ antagonists may inhibit histamine responses; it is recommended that histamine$_2$ blockers be discontinued at least 24 hours before performing this test

Doses

- **DOGS:**
  For GI indications:
  a) 5–10 mg/kg PO four times daily may be given PO or via parenteral routes. (Leib 2008)

  As an immunomodulating agent (reverses suppressor T-cell-mediated immune suppression):
  a) 10–25 mg/kg PO twice daily (Desiderio & Rankin 1986)

- **CATS:**
  a) 5–10 mg/kg PO q6-8h or 10 mg/kg q6h as a slow (over 30 minutes) IV infusion (DeNovo 1986)

- **FERRETS:**
  For stress induced ulcers:
  a) 5–10 mg/kg PO, SC, IM or IV 3 times daily (Williams 2000)

- **RABBITS/RODENTS/SMALL MAMMALS:**
  a) **Rabbits:** For GI ulcers: 5–10 mg/kg PO, SC, IM or IV q8-12h (Ivey & Morrisey 2000)
  b) **Mice, Rats, Gerbils, Hamsters, Guinea pigs, Chinchillas:** 5–10 mg/kg PO, IM or

SC q6-12h (Adamcak & Otten 2000)

- **HORSES: (Note:** ARCI UCGFS Class 5 Drug)
  For foals:
  a) 1000 mg divided twice daily or three times daily PO, IV or IM (Robinson 1987)(
  b) 300–600 mg PO or IV 4 times a day (Clark & Becht 1987)

  For adjunctive treatment of melanomas:
  a) 48 mg/kg/day (*dosing interval not specified*) PO for 2–3 weeks following resolution of tumor growth; regression should be seen evident within 3 months of initiating treatment; if no improvement seen it will probably not be effective and should be discontinued. Some horses may require treatment their entire life. (Rashmir-Raven *et al.* 2006)

- **SWINE:**
  To treat gastric ulcers:
  a) 300 mg per animal twice daily (Wass *et al.* 1986)

- **REPTILES:**
  In most species:
  a) 4 mg/kg PO q8-12h (Gauvin 1993)

Monitoring

- Clinical efficacy (dependent on reason for use); monitored by decrease in symptomatology, endoscopic examination, blood in feces, etc.
- Adverse effects if noted

Client Information

- To maximize the benefit of this medication, it must be administered as prescribed by the veterinarian; signs may reoccur if dosages are missed.

Chemistry/Synonyms

An H$_2$- receptor antagonist, cimetidine occurs as a white to off-white, crystalline powder. It has what is described as an "unpleasant" odor and a pK$_a$ of 6.8. Cimetidine is sparingly soluble in water and soluble in alcohol. Cimetidine HCl occurs as white, crystalline powder and is very soluble in water and soluble in alcohol. It has a pK$_a$ of 7.11 and the commercial injection has a pH of 3.8–6.

Cimetidine may also be known as: cimetidinum, or SKF-92334; many trade names are available.

Storage/Stability

Cimetidine products should be stored protected from light and kept at room temperature. Do not refrigerate the injectable product as precipitation may occur. Oral dosage forms should be stored in tight containers.

Compatibility/Compounding Considerations

The cimetidine injectable product is **compatible** with the commonly used IV infusions solutions, including amino acid (TPN) solutions, but should be used within 48 hours of dilution.

Cimetidine is also reported to be **compatible** with the following drugs: acetazolamide sodium, amikacin sulfate, atropine sulfate, carbenicillin disodium, cefoxitin sodium, chlorothiazide sodium, clindamycin phosphate, colistimethate sodium, dexamethasone sodium phosphate, digoxin, epinephrine, erythromycin lactobionate, furosemide, gentamicin sulfate, heparin sodium, insulin (regular), isoproterenol HCl, lidocaine HCl, lincomycin HCl, methylprednisolone sodium succinate, nafcillin sodium, norepinephrine bitartrate, penicillin G potassium/sodium, phytonadione, polymyxin B sulfate, potassium chloride, protamine sulfate, quinidine gluconate, sodium nitroprusside, tetracycline HCl, vancomycin HCl, verapamil HCl, and vitamin B complex (with or without C).

The following drugs are reported to be either **incompatible** with cimetidine or data conflicts: amphotericin B, ampicillin sodium, cefamandole naftate, cefazolin sodium, cephalothin sodium, and pentobarbital sodium. Compatibility is dependent upon factors such as pH, concentration, temperature and diluent used; consult specialized references or a hospital pharmacist for more specific information.

Compounded preparation stability: Cimetidine oral suspension compounded from commercially available tablets has been published (Tortorici 1979). Triturating twenty-four (24) cimetidine 300 mg tablets with 10 mL of glycerin and *qs ad* to 120 mL with simple syrup yields a 60 mg/mL oral suspension that retains >90% potency for 17 days stored at 4°C.

Dosage Forms/Regulatory Status

VETERINARY-LABELED PRODUCTS: None
The ARCI (Racing Commissioners International) has designated this drug as a class 5 substance. See the appendix for more information.

HUMAN-LABELED PRODUCTS:
Cimetidine Oral Tablets: 200 mg, 300 mg, 400 mg, & 800 mg; *Tagamet®* & *Tagamet® HB 200* (GlaxoSmithKline & GSK Consumer); *Acid Reducer 200®* (Major); generic; (Rx, OTC)

Cimetidine HCl Oral Solution: 300 mg (as HCl)/5 mL in 240 mL, 480 mL & UD 5 mL; generic; (Rx)

Cimetidine HCl Injection: 150 mg/mL (as hydrochloride) in 2 mL vials single-dose & 8 mL multiple-dose vials; generic (Rx); Cimetidine in 0.9% Sodium Chloride Injection: 6 mg (as hydrochloride)/mL in premixed 50 mL single-dose container; generic (Hospira); (Rx)

References

Adamcak, A & B Otten (2000). Rodent Therapeutics. *Vet Clin NA: Exotic Anim Pract* 3:1(Jan): 221–240.

Clark, ES & JL Becht (1987). Clinical Pharmacology of the Gastrointestinal Tract. *Vet Clin North Am (Equine Practice)* 3(1): 101–122.

DeNovo, RC, Jr. (1986). Therapeutics of gastrointestinal diseases. *Current Veterinary Therapy (CVT) IX Small Animal Practice*. RW Kirk Ed. W.B. Saunders: 862–871.

Desiderio, JV & BM Rankin (1986). Immunomodulators. *Current Veterinary Therapy IX: Small Animal Practice*. RW Kirk Ed. Philadelphia, WB Saunders: 1091–1096.

Gauvin, J (1993). Drug therapy in reptiles. *Seminars in Avian & Exotic Med* 2(1): 48–59.

Ivey, E & J Morrisey (2000). Therapeutics for Rabbits. *Vet Clin NA: Exotic Anim Pract* 3:1(Jan): 183–216.

Leib, MS (2008). Drugs used to treat vomiting and upper GI diseases in dogs and cats. Proceedings: ACVC. Accessed via: Veterinary Information Network. http://goo.gl/MsdLP

Rashmir–Raven, A, J Foy, et al. (2006). Cutaneous Tumors in Horses. Proceedings: Western Vet Conference. Accessed via: Veterinary Information Network. http://goo.gl/XCmdJ

Robinson, NE (1987). Table of Common Drugs: Approximate Doses. *Current Therapy in Equine Medicine, 2*. NE Robinson Ed. Philadelphia, W.B. Saunders: 761.

Tortorici, M (1979). Formulation of a cimetidine oral suspension. *Am J Hosp Pharm* 36(1): 22.

Wass, WM, JR Thompson, et al. (1986). Gastric ulcer syndrome in swine. *Current Veterinary Therapy 2: Food Animal Practice*. JL Howard Ed. Philadelphia, WB Saunders: 723–724.

Williams, B (2000). Therapeutics in Ferrets. *Vet Clin NA: Exotic Anim Pract* 3:1(Jan): 131–153.

CIPROFLOXACIN

(sip-roe-*flox*-a-sin)   Cipro®

FLUOROQUINOLONE ANTIBIOTIC

Prescriber Highlights

▶ Human-label fluoroquinolone antibiotic

▶ In dogs, oral bioavailability lower than enrofloxacin

▶ Available as a true IV product

▶ Contraindications: Hypersensitivity. Relatively contraindicated for young, growing animals due to cartilage abnormalities

▶ Caution: Hepatic or renal insufficiency, dehydration

▶ Adverse Effects: GI distress, CNS stimulation, crystalluria, & hypersensitivity

▶ Administer PO preferably on an empty stomach

▶ Drug interactions

Uses/Indications

Because of its similar spectrum of activity, ciprofloxacin could be used as an alternative to enrofloxacin when a larger oral dosage form or intravenous product is desired. But the two compounds cannot be considered equivalent because of pharmacokinetic differences (see below).

Pharmacology/Actions

Ciprofloxacin is a bactericidal and a concentration dependent agent, with susceptible bacteria cell death occurring within 20–30 minutes of exposure. Ciprofloxacin has demonstrated a significant post-antibiotic effect for both gram-negative and gram-positive bacteria and is active in both stationary and growth phases of bacterial replication. Its mechanism of action is not thoroughly understood, but it is believed to act by inhibiting bacterial DNA-gyrase (a type-II topoisomerase), thereby preventing DNA super-coiling and DNA synthesis.

Both enrofloxacin and ciprofloxacin have similar spectrums of activity. These agents have good activity against many gram-negative bacilli and cocci, including most species and strains of P*seudomonas aeruginosa, Klebsiella* spp., *E. coli,* Enterobacter, Campylobacter, Shigella, Salmonella, Aeromonas, Haemophilus, Proteus, Yersinia, Serratia, and Vibrio species. Of the currently commercially available quinolones, ciprofloxacin and enrofloxacin have the lowest MIC values for the majority of these pathogens treated. Other organisms that are generally susceptible include *Brucella* spp. *Chlamydia trachomatis,* Staphylococci (including penicillinase-producing and methicillin-resistant strains), Mycoplasma, and *Mycobacterium* spp. (not the etiologic agent for Johne's disease). When combined with either ceftazidime or cefepime, fluorquinolones may have an additive or synergistic effect against certain bacteria.

The fluoroquinolones have variable activity against most Streptococci and are not usually recommended for use in treating these infections. These drugs have weak activity against most anaerobes and are ineffective in treating anaerobic infections.

Resistance does occur by mutation, particularly with *Pseudomonas aeruginosa, Klebsiella pneumonia,* Acinetobacter, and enterococci, but plasmid-mediated resistance does not seem to occur.

Pharmacokinetics

Both enrofloxacin and ciprofloxacin are well absorbed after oral administration in most species; in dogs however, enrofloxacin's bioavailability is at least twice that of ciprofloxacin after oral dosing. In humans, the oral bioavailability of ciprofloxacin has been reported to be between 50–85%. Studies of the oral bioavailability in ponies have shown that ciprofloxacin is poorly absorbed (2–12%) while enrofloxacin in foals apparently is well absorbed.

In humans, the volume of distribution in adults for ciprofloxacin is about 2–3.5 L/kg and it is approximately 20–40% bound to serum proteins.

Ciprofloxacin is one of the metabolites of enrofloxacin. Approximately 15–50% of the drugs are eliminated unchanged into the urine by both tubular secretion and glomerular filtration. Enrofloxacin/ciprofloxacin are metabolized to various metabolites that are less active than the parent compounds. Approximately 10–40% of circulating enrofloxacin is metabolized to ciprofloxacin in most species. These metabolites are eliminated in both the urine and feces. Because of the dual (renal and hepatic) means of elimination, patients with severely impaired renal

function may have slightly prolonged half-lives and higher serum levels but may not require dosage adjustment.

The pharmacokinetics of ciprofloxacin has been studied in dogs, calves, horses, and pigs. Oral bioavailability is approximately 50% in calves and 40% (only one pig studied) in pigs and it has an elimination half-life of about 2.5 hours in both species. Protein binding was significantly different for each species, with calves having about 70% of the drug bound and pigs only about 23% bound to plasma proteins. Elimination half-life is reported to be about 2.5 hours in dogs.

Contraindications/Precautions/Warnings

Ciprofloxacin, as is enrofloxacin, should be considered contraindicated in small and medium breed dogs from 2–8 months of age. Bubble-like changes in articular cartilage have been noted when the drug was given at 2–5 times recommended doses for 30 days, although clinical signs have only been seen at the 5X dose. To avoid cartilage damage, large and giant breed dogs may need to wait longer than the recommended 8 months since they may be in the rapid-growth phase past 8 months of age. Quinolones are also contraindicated in patients hypersensitive to them.

Because ciprofloxacin has occasionally been reported to cause crystalluria, animals should not be allowed to become dehydrated during therapy with either ciprofloxacin or enrofloxacin. In humans, ciprofloxacin has been associated with CNS stimulation and should be used with caution in patients with seizure disorders. Patients with severe renal or hepatic impairment may require dosage adjustments to prevent drug accumulation.

Use high dose ciprofloxacin in cats with caution. No reports of retinal toxicity (as can be seen with high dose enrofloxacin) secondary to ciprofloxacin in cats were located and retinal toxicity appears to be less likely since it is less lipophilic than enrofloxacin; however caution is advised.

Adverse Effects

With the exception of potential cartilage abnormalities in young animals (see Contraindications above), the adverse effect profile of fluoroquinolones appears to be minimal. GI distress (vomiting, anorexia) is the most frequently, yet uncommon, reported adverse effect. Although not reported thus far in animals, hypersensitivity reactions, crystalluria, and CNS effects (dizziness, stimulation) could potentially occur.

Reproductive/Nursing Safety

In humans, the FDA categorizes this drug as category *C* for use during pregnancy (*Animal studies have shown an adverse effect on the fetus, but there are no adequate studies in humans; or there are no animal reproduction studies and no adequate studies in humans.*)

Ciprofloxacin is distributed into milk, but oral absorption should be negligible. No adverse effects have been reported in nursing human infants of mothers receiving ciprofloxacin.

Overdosage

Little specific information is available. See the enrofloxacin monograph for more information.

Drug Interactions

The following drug interactions have either been reported or are theoretical in humans or animals receiving ciprofloxacin and may be of significance in veterinary patients:

- ◾ **ANTACIDS/DAIRY PRODUCTS** containing cations (Mg^{++}, Al^{+++}, Ca^{++}) may bind to ciprofloxacin and prevent its absorption; separate doses of these products by at least 2 hours from ciprofloxacin

- ◾ **ANTIBIOTICS, OTHER (aminoglycosides, 3rd-generation cephalosporins, penicillins— extended-spectrum):** Synergism may occur, but is not predictable, against some bacteria (particularly *Pseudomonas aeruginosa*) with these compounds. Although enrofloxacin/ ciprofloxacin has minimal activity against anaerobes, *in vitro* synergy has been reported when used with **clindamycin** against strains of Peptostreptococcus, Lactobacillus and *Bacteroides fragilis*.

- ◾ **CYCLOSPORINE:** Fluoroquinolones may exacerbate the nephrotoxicity, and reduce the metabolism of, cyclosporine (used systemically)

- ◾ **GLYBURIDE:** Severe hypoglycemia possible

- ◾ **IRON, ZINC (oral):** Decreased ciprofloxacin absorption; separate doses by at least two hours

- ◾ **METHOTREXATE:** Increased MTX levels possible with resultant toxicity

- ◾ **NITROFURANTOIN:** May antagonize the antimicrobial activity of the fluoroquinolones; concomitant use is not recommended

- ◾ **PHENYTOIN:** Ciprofloxacin may alter phenytoin levels

- ◾ **PROBENECID:** Blocks tubular secretion of ciprofloxacin and may increase its blood level and half-life

- ◾ **QUINIDINE:** Increased risk for cardiotoxicity

- ◾ **SUCRALFATE:** May inhibit absorption of ciprofloxacin; separate doses of these drugs by at least 2 hours

- ◾ **THEOPHYLLINE:** Ciprofloxacin may increase theophylline blood levels

- ◾ **WARFARIN:** Potential for increased warfarin effects

Laboratory Considerations

- ◾ In some human patients, the fluoroquinolones have caused increases in **liver enzymes, BUN,** and **creatinine** and decreases in **hematocrit**. The clinical relevance of these mild changes is not known at this time.

Doses

■ **DOGS:**

For susceptible infections:

a) 5–15 mg/kg PO q12h; Avoid or reduce dosage of these drugs in animals with severe renal failure; avoid in young animals or in pregnant or breeding animals. (Vaden & Papich 1995)

b) For UTI: 10 mg/kg PO once daily (q24h) for 7–14 days

For skin, soft tissue infections: 10–15 mg/kg PO once daily (q24h) for 7–14 days

For bone systemic infections, bacteremia and more resistant pathogens (*e.g.,* Enterobacter): 20 mg/kg PO once daily (q24h) for 7–14 days (Greene *et al.* 2006)

c) For pyoderma: 11 mg/kg PO q12h (Miller 2005)

■ **CATS:**

For susceptible infections:

a) Ciprofloxacin: 5–15 mg/kg PO q12h

Avoid or reduce dosage of these drugs in animals with severe renal failure; avoid in young animals or in pregnant or breeding animals. (Vaden & Papich 1995)

■ **FERRETS:**

For susceptible infections:

a) 5–15 mg/kg PO twice daily (Williams 2000)

■ **RABBITS/RODENTS/SMALL MAMMALS:**

a) **Rabbits:** 5–20 mg/kg PO q12h (Ivey & Morrisey 2000)

b) **Chinchillas, Gerbils, Guinea Pigs, Hamsters, Mice, Rats:** 7–20 mg/kg PO q12h (Adamcak & Otten 2000)

c) For treating pasteurellosis in rabbits: ciprofloxacin or enrofloxacin 15–20 mg/kg PO twice daily for a minimum of 14 days in mild cases and up to several months in chronic infections. (Antinoff 2008)

■ **BIRDS:**

For susceptible gram-negative infections:

a) Using ciprofloxacin 500 mg tablets: 20–40 mg/kg PO twice daily. Crushed tablet goes into suspension well, but must be shaken well before administering. (McDonald 1989)

b) Ciprofloxacin (using crushed tablets): 20 mg/kg PO q12h (Bauck & Hoefer 1993)

c) Ciprofloxacin (using crushed tablets or suspend) 10–15 mg/kg PO q12h (Hoeffer 1995)

d) **Ratites:** 3–6 mg/kg PO twice daily (Jenson 1998)

Monitoring

- ◾ Clinical efficacy
- ◾ Adverse effects

Chemistry/Synonyms

A fluoroquinolone antibiotic, ciprofloxacin HCl occurs as a faintly yellowish to yellow, crystalline powder. It is slightly soluble in water. Ciprofloxacin is related structurally to the veterinary-FDA-approved drug enrofloxacin (enrofloxacin has an additional ethyl group on the piperazinyl ring).

Ciprofloxacin may also be known as ciprofloxacine, ciprofloxacinum, ciprofloxacino, Bay-q-3939, or *Cipro®*.

Storage/Stability

Unless otherwise directed by the manufacturer, ciprofloxacin tablets should be stored in tight containers at temperatures less than 30°C. Protect from strong UV light. The injection should be stored at 5°–25°C and protected from light and freezing.

Compatibility/Compounding Considerations

The manufacturer recommends administering IV ciprofloxacin alone (temporarily discontinuing other solutions or drugs while ciprofloxacin running). However, other sources state that ciprofloxacin injection is reportedly **compatible** with the following IV solutions and drugs: Dextrose 5%, D5 and 1/4 or 1/2 NaCl, Ringer's, LRS, normal saline; **Y-site compatible with** amikacin sulfate, aztreonam, ceftazidime, cimetidine, cyclosporine, dexmedetomidine, dobutamine, dopamine, fluconazole, gentamicin, lidocaine, midazolam, KCl, ranitidine, tobramycin, and vitamin B complex.

Ciprofloxacin injection is reportedly **incompatible** with aminophylline, amphotericin B, azithromycin, cefuroxime, clindamycin, heparin sodium, sodium bicarbonate, and ticarcillin.

Compatibility is dependent upon factors such as pH, concentration, temperature and diluent used; consult specialized references or a hospital pharmacist for more specific information.

Dosage Forms/Regulatory Status

VETERINARY-LABELED PRODUCTS: None
HUMAN-LABELED PRODUCTS:

Ciprofloxacin Oral Tablets: 100 mg, 250 mg, 500 mg & 750 mg; *Cipro®* (Shering-Plough); generic; (Rx)

Ciprofloxacin Extended-Release Oral Tablets: 500 mg & 1000 mg; *Cipro XR®* (Shering-Plough); generic; (Rx)

Ciprofloxacin Microcapsules for Oral Suspension: 250 mg/5 mL (5%) & 500 mg/5 mL (10%) when reconstituted in 100 mL with diluent; *Cipro®* (Schering-Plough); (Rx)

Ciprofloxacin Solution for Injection: 200 mg & 400 mg in 100 mL &200 mL (respectively) in 5% dextrose flexible containers (0.2%); *Cipro®* I.V. (Schering-Plough); generic (Sandoz); (Rx)

References

Adamcak, A & B Otten (2000). Rodent Therapeutics. *Vet Clin NA: Exotic Anim Pract* 3:1(Jan): 221–240.

Antinoff, N (2008). Respiratory diseases of ferrets, rabbits, and rodents. Proceedings: IVECCS. Accessed via: Veterinary Information Network. http://goo.gl/bCQlM

Bauck, L & H Hoefer (1993). Avian antimicrobial therapy. *Seminars in Avian & Exotic Med* 2(1): 17–22.

Greene, C, K Hartmannn, et al. (2006). Appendix 8: Antimicrobial Drug Formulary. *Infectious Disease of the Dog and Cat*. C Greene Ed., Elsevier: 1186–1333.

Hoeffer, H (1995). Antimicrobials in pet birds. *Kirk's Current Veterinary Therapy:XII.* J Bonagura Ed. Philadelphia, W.B. Saunders: 1278–1283.

Ivey, E & J Morrisey (2000). Therapeutics for Rabbits. *Vet Clin NA: Exotic Anim Pract* 3:1(Jan): 183–216.

Jenson, J (1998). Current ratite therapy. *The Veterinary Clinics of North America: Food Animal Practice* 16:3(November).

McDonald, SE (1989). Summary of medications for use in psittacine birds. *JAAV* 3(3): 120–127.

Miller, W (2005). Pyoderma in 2005. Proceedings: ACVC. Accessed via: Veterinary Information Network. http://goo.gl/MX0g3

Vaden, S & M Papich (1995). Empiric Antibiotic Therapy. *Kirk's Current Veterinary Therapy:XII.* J Bonagura Ed. Philadelphia, W.B. Saunders: 276–280.

Williams, B (2000). Therapeutics in Ferrets. *Vet Clin NA: Exotic Anim Pract* 3:1(Jan): 131–153.

CISAPRIDE

(sis-a-pride)

PROMOTILITY AGENT

Prescriber Highlights

▶ Oral GI prokinetic agent, used in several species for GI stasis, reflux esophagitis, & constipation/megacolon (cats)

▶ No longer commercially available, must be obtained from a compounding pharmacy

▶ Contraindications: Hypersensitivity, GI perforation or obstruction, hemorrhage

▶ Caution: Pregnancy

▶ Adverse effects appear to be minimal in veterinary patients; vomiting, diarrhea, and abdominal discomfort can occur

▶ Drug interactions

Uses/Indications

Proposed uses for cisapride in small animals include esophageal reflux, esophagitis and treatment of primary gastric stasis disorders. Cisapride has been found to be useful in the treatment of constipation and megacolon in cats.

Pharmacology/Actions

Cisapride increases lower esophageal peristalsis and sphincter pressure and accelerates gastric emptying. The drug's proposed mechanism of action enhances the release of acetylcholine at the myenteric plexus, but does not induce nicotinic or muscarinic receptor stimulation. Acetylcholinesterase activity is not inhibited. Cisapride blocks dopaminergic receptors to a lesser extent than does metoclopramide and does not increase gastric acid secretion.

Pharmacokinetics

Human data: After oral administration, cisapride is rapidly absorbed with an absolute bioavailability of 35–40%. The drug is highly bound to plasma proteins and apparently extensively distributed throughout the body. Cisapride is extensively metabolized and its elimination half-life is about 8–10 hours.

Contraindications/Precautions/Warnings

Cisapride is contraindicated in patients in whom increased gastrointestinal motility could be harmful (*e.g.*, perforation, obstruction, GI hemorrhage) or those who are hypersensitive to the drug.

Adverse Effects

Cisapride appears to be safe in small animals at the dosages recommended. Occasionally vomiting, diarrhea, and abdominal discomfort may be noted. Although considered very rare in veterinary patients, prolonged QT intervals or other cardiac arrhythmias are possibilities.

In humans, the primary adverse effects are gastrointestinal related with diarrhea and abdominal pain most commonly reported, but the drug was removed from the market due to concerns with QT-interval prolongation.

Dosage may need to be decreased in patients with severe hepatic impairment.

Reproductive/Nursing Safety

Cisapride at high dosages (>40 mg/kg/day) caused fertility impairment in female rats. At doses 12 to 100 times the maximum recommended, cisapride caused embryotoxicity and fetotoxicity in rabbits and rats. Its use during pregnancy should occur only when the benefits outweigh the risks. Cisapride is excreted in maternal milk in low levels; use with caution in nursing mothers.

Overdosage/Acute Toxicity

LD_{50} doses in various lab animals range from 160 - 4000 mg/kg. The reported oral lethal dose in dogs is 640 mg/kg. In one reported human overdose of 540 mg, the patient developed GI distress and urinary frequency. There were 29 exposures to cisapride reported to the ASPCA Animal Poison Control Center (APCC) during 2008-2009. In these cases, 21 were cats with 6 showing clinical signs, and 8 were dogs with 5 showing clinical signs. Most common adverse effects seen in dogs and cats are diarrhea, lethargy, ataxia, hypersalivation, muscle fasciculations, agitation, abnormal behavior, hyperthermia, and possibly seizures (dogs) (APCC unpublished data).

Significant overdoses should be handled using standard gut emptying protocols when appropriate; supportive therapy should be initiated when required. Activated charcoal is effective in binding unabsorbed cisapride (Volmer 1996).

Drug Interactions

The following drug interactions have either been reported or are theoretical in humans or animals receiving cisapride and may be of significance in veterinary patients:

- **ANTICHOLINERGIC AGENTS:** Use of anticholinergic agents may diminish the effects of cisapride

- **BENZODIAZEPINES:** Cisapride may enhance the sedative effects of alcohol or benzodiazepines

- **WARFARIN:** Cisapride may enhance anticoagulant effects; additional monitoring and anticoagulant dosage adjustments may be required

- **ORAL DRUGS WITH A NARROW THERAPEUTIC INDEX:** May need serum levels monitored more closely when adding or discontinuing cisapride as cisapride can decrease GI transit times and potentially affect the absorption of other oral drugs

As cisapride is metabolized via cytochrome P450 (3A4 in humans), the following medications/foods that can inhibit this enzyme may lead to increased cisapride levels with an increased risk for cisapride cardiotoxicity:

- **AMIODARONE**
- **ANTIFUNGALS (ketoconazole, itraconazole, fluconazole)**
- **CHLORAMPHENICOL**
- **CIMETIDINE**
- **FLUVOXAMINE**
- **GRAPEFRUIT JUICE/POWDER**
- **MACROLIDE ANTIBIOTICS (except azithromycin) Note:** Erythromycin did not alter cisapride pharmacodynamics in one study in dogs

The following drugs may increase QT interval and use with cisapride may increase this risk:

- **AMIODARONE**
- **CLARITHROMYCIN**
- **MOXIFLOXACIN**
- **PROCAINAMIDE**
- **QUINIDINE**
- **SOTALOL**
- **TRICYCLIC ANTIDEPRESSANTS (amitriptyline, imipramine)**

Doses

- **DOGS:**

  As a promotility agent

  a) 0.1–0.5 mg/kg PO 2–3 times per day given 30 minutes before meals. Higher doses of 1 mg/kg may be required in some cases. (Twedt 2008)

  b) To reduce regurgitation associated with megaesophagus: 0.55 mg/kg PO once to three times daily. Practically: 2.5 mg per dose for dogs weighing between 5–10 lbs.; 5 mg per dose for dogs weighing between 11–40 lbs; and 10 mg per dose for dogs greater than 40 lbs. Administer no closer than 30 minutes before feeding. (Tams 1994)

c) For adjunctive treatment (with H-2 blockers or proton pump inhibitors such as omeprazole—preferred) for esophageal reflux: 0.1–0.5 mg/kg PO q8–24h (Willard 2006)

d) To reduce the risk for esophageal stricture formation in cases of esophagitis: 0.5–0.75 mg/kg PO three times daily. (Richter 2009)

To stimulate detrusor contraction for micturition disorders:

a) 0.5 mg/kg PO q8h (Coates 2004)

■ **CATS:**

As a promotility agent:

a) For chronic constipation (*e.g.*, megacolon): In combination with a stool softener (author recommends lactulose at a starting dose of 2–3 mL PO three times a day; then adjust as needed) and a bulk agent (*e.g.*, psyllium or pumpkin pie filling) cisapride is given initially at 2.5 mg (for cats up to 10 pounds) or 5 mg (for cats 11 pounds or heavier) three times daily, 30 minutes before food. Cats weighing greater than 16 pounds may require 7.5 mg. (Tams 1994)

b) For chronic constipation (*e.g.*, megacolon): Used adjunctively with conventional dietary therapeutics: 1.25–2.5 mg per cat two to three times a day; cats with hepatic insufficiency should be treated with half the usual dose; probably most effective when given 15 minutes before a meal. (Nixon 1994)

c) For chronic constipation (*e.g.*, megacolon): 2.5–5 mg per cat PO q8–12h (Carr 2009)

d) For chronic constipation (*e.g.*, megacolon): 5 mg per cat (total dose) PO q8–12h (Scherk 2003)

e) For gastric stasis: 0.1 mg/kg PO two to three times daily; cats tolerate 2.5 mg doses without problems (Twedt 2005)

f) To reduce the risk for esophageal stricture formation in cases of esophagitis: 0.5–0.75 mg/kg PO three times daily. (Richter 2009)

■ **RABBITS/RODENTS/SMALL MAMMALS:**

a) **Mice, Rats, Gerbils, Hamsters, Guinea pigs, Chinchillas:** 0.1–0.5 mg/kg PO q12h (Adamcak & Otten 2000)

b) Rabbits for GI stasis: 0.5 mg/kg PO q6–12h. With IV or SC fluids depending on amount of dehydration, feeding a high fiber slurry and with or without metoclopramide (0.2–1 mg PO, SC q6–8h). (Hess 2002)

c) For ileus if GI tract not obstructed in Guinea pigs, chinchillas: 0.5 mg/kg q8–12h (*Route not specified; assume PO*) (Orcutt 2005)

d) For gastric stasis in rabbits: Usually started at 0.5 mg/kg PO (via NG tube) q8h after first stools were produced or no intestinal obstruction appreciated. May be synergistic if used with ranitidine (0.5 mg/kg IV q24h). (Lichtenberger 2008)

■ **HORSES:**

As a promotility agent:

a) Foals with periparturient asphyxia: 10 mg (total dose) PO q6–8h. Adequate time for healing of damaged bowel before using prokinetic agents is essential. (Vaala 2003)

Monitoring

■ Efficacy

■ Adverse effects profile

Client Information

■ Inform client to watch carefully and report any adverse effects noted.

Chemistry/Synonyms

An oral GI prokinetic agent, cisapride is a substituted piperidinyl benzamide and is structurally, but not pharmacologically, related to procainamide. It is available commercially as a monohydrate, but potency is expressed in terms of the anhydrate.

Cisapride may also be known as: cisapridum, or R-51619; many trade names are registered.

Storage/Stability

Unless otherwise instructed by the manufacturer, store cisapride tablets in tight, light-resistant containers at room temperature.

Compatibility/Compounding Considerations

Compounded preparation stability: Cisapride oral suspension compounded from commercially available tablets has been published (Allen & Erickson 1998). Triturating twelve (12) cisapride 10 mg tablets with 60 mL of *Ora-Plus*® and qs ad to 120 mL with *Ora-Sweet*® with pH finally adjusted to 7 with sodium bicarbonate yields a 1 mg/mL oral suspension that retains >90% potency for 60 days stored at both 5°C and 25°C. Although cisapride tablets are no longer commercially available, the active pharmaceutical ingredient powder may be used to compound suitable oral suspensions of cisapride. Compounded preparations of cisapride should be protected from light.

Dosage Forms/Regulatory Status

VETERINARY-LABELED PRODUCTS: None

HUMAN-LABELED PRODUCTS: None

Because of adverse effects in humans, cisapride has been removed from the US market. It may be available from compounding pharmacies.

References

Adamcak, A & B Otten (2000). Rodent Therapeutics. *Vet Clin NA: Exotic Anim Pract* 3:1(Jan): 221–240.

Allen, LV & MA Erickson (1998). Stability of alprazolam, chloroquine phosphate, cisapride, enalapril maleate, and hydralazine hydrochloride in extemporaneously compounded oral liquids. *Am J Health Syst Pharm* 55(18): 1915–1920.

Carr, A (2009). Managing Constipation in Cats. Proceedings: ACVIM. Accessed via: Veterinary Information Network. http://goo.gl/13MBy

Coates, J (2004). Neurogenic micturition disorders. Proceedings: ACVIM Forum. Accessed via: Veterinary Information Network. http://goo.gl/260CO

Hess, L (2002). Practical Emergency/Critical Care of the Pet Rabbit. Proceedings: Atlantic Coast Veterinary Conference. Accessed via: Veterinary Information Network. http://goo.gl/4upFr

Lichtenberger, M (2008). What's new in small mammal critical care. Proceedings: AAV. http://goo.gl/f4wXv

Nixon, M (1994). Cisapride–The newest gastrointestinal prokinetic drug. *Academy of Feline Practioners Newsletter*: 6.

Orcutt, C (2005). Chinchilla and Guinea pig diseases. Proceedings: Western Veterinary Conf. Accessed via: Veterinary Information Network. http://goo.gl/mwRyI

Richter, K (2009). Esophageal Strictures—Update on Therapeutic Options. Proceedings: ACVIM. Accessed via: Veterinary Information Network. http://goo.gl/6RM8j

Scherk, M (2003). Feline megacolon. Proceedings: World Small Animal Veterinary Assoc World Congress. Accessed via: Veterinary Information Network. http://goo.gl/v69lu

Tams, T (1994). Cisapride: Clinical experience with the newest GI prokinetic drug. Proceedings: Twelfth Annual Veterinary Medical Forum, San Francisco, American College of Veterinary Internal Medicine.

Twedt, D (2005). The vomiting cat. Proceedings: ACVC. Accessed via: Veterinary Information Network. http://goo.gl/Ktzp4

Twedt, D (2008). Antiemetics, prokinetics & antacids. Proceedings: ACVIM. Accessed via: Veterinary Information Network. http://goo.gl/FCGyQ

Vaala, W (2003). Perinatal asphyxia syndrome in foals. *Current Therapy in Equine Medicine 5.* N Robinson and E Carr Eds. Phila., Saunders: 644–649.

Volmer, PA (1996). Cisapride toxicosis in dogs. *Veterinary and Human Toxicology* 38(2): 118–120.

Willard, M (2006). Rare esophageal problems that are not so rare. Proceedings: IVECCS. Accessed via: Veterinary Information Network. http://goo.gl/iVAyU

CISPLATIN

(*sis*-pla-tin)   Platinol-AQ®

ANTINEOPLASTIC

Prescriber Highlights

▶ Platinum antineoplastic agent used for a variety of carcinomas & sarcomas; palliative control of neoplastic pulmonary effusions with intracavitary administration; intralesional injection for skin tumors in horses

▶ Contraindications: Cats; preexisting significant renal impairment or myelosuppression

▶ Primary adverse effects: Vomiting (pretreat with antiemetic); nephrotoxicity (use forced saline diuresis); myelosuppression; many other adverse effects possible

▶ Drug related deaths possible

▶ Teratogenic, fetotoxic; may cause azoospermia

▶ Must be handled with care by dosage preparer/administerer

▶ Must be given as slow IV infusion; fast administration (<5 minutes) may increase toxicity

Uses/Indications

In veterinary medicine, the systemic use of cisplatin is presently limited to use in dogs. The drug has been, or may be, useful in a variety of neoplastic diseases including squamous cell carcinomas, transitional cell carcinomas, ovarian carcinomas, mediastinal carcinomas, osteosarcomas, pleural adenocarcinomas, nasal carcinomas, and thyroid adenocarcinomas.

Cisplatin may be useful for the palliative control of neoplastic pulmonary effusions after intracavitary administration.

In horses, cisplatin has been used for intralesional injection for skin tumors.

Pharmacology/Actions

While the exact mechanism of action of cisplatin has not been determined, its properties are analogous to those of bifunctional alkylating agents producing inter- and intrastrand crosslinks in DNA. Cisplatin is cell cycle nonspecific.

Pharmacokinetics

After administration, the drug concentrates in the liver, intestines and kidneys. Platinum will accumulate in the body and may be detected 6 months after a course of therapy has been completed. Cisplatin is highly bound (90%) to serum proteins.

In dogs, cisplatin exhibits a biphasic elimination profile. The initial plasma half-life is short (approximately 20–50 minutes), but the terminal phase is very long (about 60–80 hours). Approximately 80% of a dose can be recovered as free platinum in the urine within 48 hours of dosing in dogs.

Contraindications/Precautions/Warnings

The drug is contraindicated in cats because of severe dose-related primary pulmonary toxicoses (dyspnea, hydrothorax, pulmonary edema, mediastinal edema, and death). Cisplatin is also contraindicated in patients with preexisting significant renal impairment, myelosuppression, or a history of hypersensitivity to platinum-containing compounds. Because of the fluid loading required prior to dosing, it should be used with caution in patients with congestive heart failure.

When preparing the product for injection, wear gloves and protective clothing as local reactions may occur with skin or mucous membrane contact. Should accidental exposure occur, wash the area thoroughly with soap and water.

Adverse Effects

In dogs, the most frequent adverse effect seen after cisplatin treatment is vomiting, which usually occurs within 6 hours after dosing and persists for 1–6 hours. This is because of direct effects on the chemoreceptor trigger zone (CTZ). Maropitant, butorphanol, dexamethasone and metoclopramide have all been used successfully as antiemetics when given before cisplatin administration.

Nephrotoxicity may occur unless the animal is adequately diuresed with sodium chloride prior to, and after therapy; diuresis will generally significantly reduce the incidence and severity of nephrotoxicity in the majority of dogs. Intravenous methimazole (40 mg/kg) has been demonstrated to protect cisplatin-induced nephrotoxicity in dogs in experimental models.

Other adverse effects that have been reported include hematologic abnormalities (thrombocytopenia and/or granulocytopenia), ototoxicity (high-frequency hearing loss and tinnitus), anorexia, diarrhea (including hemorrhagic diarrhea), seizures, peripheral neuropathies, electrolyte abnormalities, hyperuricemia, increased hepatic enzymes, anaphylactoid reactions, and death.

Direct IV infusion over 1–5 minutes should be avoided as it may cause increased nephrotoxicity or ototoxicity.

Reproductive/Nursing Safety

Cisplatin's safe use in pregnancy has not been established. It is teratogenic and embryotoxic in mice. In human males, the drug may cause azoospermia and impaired spermatogenesis. In humans, the FDA categorizes this drug as category *D* for use during pregnancy (*There is evidence of human fetal risk, but the potential benefits from the use of the drug in pregnant women may be acceptable despite its potential risks.*) In a separate system evaluating the safety of drugs in canine and feline pregnancy (Papich 1989), this drug is categorized as in class: *C* (*These drugs may have potential risks. Studies in people or laboratory animals have uncovered risks, and these drugs should be used cautiously as a last resort when the benefit of therapy clearly outweighs the risks.*)

Overdosage/Acute Toxicity

The minimum lethal dose of cisplatin in dogs is reportedly 2.5 mg/kg ($\approx$80 mg/m^2). Because of the potential for serious toxicity associated with this agent, dosage calculations should be checked thoroughly to avoid overdosing. See Adverse Effects above for more information.

Drug Interactions

The following drug interactions have either been reported or are theoretical in humans or animals receiving cisplatin and may be of significance in veterinary patients:

- **AMINOGLYCOSIDES:** Potential for increased risk for nephrotoxicity and/or nephrotoxicity; if possible, delay aminoglycoside administration by at least two weeks after cisplatin

- **AMPHOTERICIN B:** Potential for increased risk for nephrotoxicity; if possible, delay amphotericin B administration by at least two weeks after cisplatin

- **FUROSEMIDE** (and other **loop diuretics**): Potential for increased ototoxicity

- **PHENYTOIN:** Cisplatin may reduce serum levels of phenytoin

Doses

Note: Because of the potential toxicity of this drug to patients, veterinary personnel and clients, and since chemotherapy indications, treatment protocols, monitoring and safety guidelines often change, the following dosages should be used only as a general guide. Consultation with a veterinary oncologist and referral to current veterinary oncology references [*e.g.*, (Henry & Higginbotham 2009); (Argyle *et al.* 2008); (Withrow & Vail 2007); (Villalobos 2007); (Ogilvie & Moore 2006); (Ogilvie & Moore 2001)] is *strongly recommended*.

- **DOGS:**
For potentially susceptible carcinomas and sarcomas:
a) The following is a usual dosage or dose range for cisplatin and should be used only as a general guide: Dogs: 30–70 mg/m^2 (NOT mg/kg) IV over 20 minutes to several hours every 3–5 weeks.

   Warning: Do not confuse cisplatin and carboplatin dosages; cisplatin dosages are much lower. Dogs must undergo saline diuresis before and after cisplatin therapy to reduce the potential for nephrotoxicity development. Some clinicians also recommend using either mannitol or furosemide with saline, but this is somewhat controversial.

Intracavitary administration for palliative control of neoplastic pulmonary effusions:

a) Give dog IV normal saline at 10 mL/kg/hr for 4 hours prior to treating. Dose cisplatin at 50 mg/m^2 (NOT mg/kg) (diluted in normal saline to a total volume of 250 mL/m^2). Warm solution to body temperature; place a 16-gauge over-the-needle catheter into the pleural space using sterile technique. Remove as much pleural fluid as possible and then slowly infuse cisplatin solution through same catheter. Once completed, remove catheter. May repeat every 3–4 weeks as needed to control effusion. If resolves completely, discontinue therapy after the 4th treatment. Reinstitute if effusion recurs. (Hawkins & Fossum 2000)

■ **HORSES:**

For intralesional injection of skin tumors:

a) Add 10 mg of cisplatin powder (if available) to 1 mL of water and 2 mL of medical-grade sesame oil. Resultant solution contains 3.3 mg of cisplatin per mL. Inject 1 mg per cm^3 of tumor/tumor bed intralesionally with a small gauge needle (22–25 gauge) attached to an extension set with Luer-lock connections. Inject in multiple planes no further than 0.6 to 1 cm apart. Because the volume of tumor is difficult to measure, the rule of thumb is to discontinue injection when fluid is extruded from the skin surface. Because recurrence at the periphery of the treated area is the primary cause of treatment failure, injection into 1–2 cm of normal tissue surrounding the tumor has been recommended. Intralesional injection is generally repeated at 2-week intervals for 4 total treatments. (Moll 2002)

Monitoring

Adapted primarily from the reference by Shapiro (Shapiro 1989).

■ Toxicity. Baseline laboratory data: urinalysis, hemogram, platelet count, serum biochemical and electrolyte determination. Repeat tests before each dose if animal is receiving high-dose therapy (≈monthly) or as needed if signs/symptoms of toxicity develop. Animals receiving frequent small doses should be monitored at least weekly. Not recommended to use cisplatin if WBC is <3200/mcl, platelets <100,000, creatinine clearance is <1.4 mL/min/kg, or uremia, electrolyte or acid-base imbalance is present. Reduce dose if rapid decreases occur with either WBC or platelets, changes in urine specific gravity or serum electrolytes, elevated serum creatinine or BUN, or if creatinine clearance is >1.4 but <2.9 mL/min/kg.

■ Efficacy. Tumor measurement and radiography at least monthly. In one study (Knapp et al. 1988), the authors state that dogs should be evaluated at 42 days into therapy. Dogs demonstrating complete or partial remission or stable disease should receive additional therapy. Dogs whose disease has progressed should have cisplatin therapy stopped and receive alternate therapies if warranted.

Client Information

■ Clients must be briefed on the possibilities of severe toxicity developing from this drug, including drug-related mortality.

Chemistry/Synonyms

An inorganic platinum-containing antineoplastic, cisplatin occurs as white powder. One mg is soluble in 1 mL of water or normal saline. The drug is available commercially as a solution for injection. Cisplatin injection (premixed solution) has a pH of 3.7–6.

Cisplatin may also be known as: cis-Platinum II, cis-DDP, CDDP, cis-diamminedichloroplatinum, cisplatina, cisplatinum, cis-platinum, DDP, NSC-119875, Peyrone's salt, or platinum diamminodichloride; many trade names are available.

Storage/Stability

The injection should be stored at room temperature and away from light; do not refrigerate as a precipitate may form. During use, the injection should be protected from direct bright sunlight, but does not need to be protected from normal room incandescent or fluorescent lights.

Do not use aluminum hub needles or aluminum containing IV sets as aluminum may displace platinum from the cisplatin molecule with the resulting formation of a black precipitate. Should a precipitate form from either cold temperatures or aluminum contact, discard the solution.

Compatibility/Compounding Considerations

Cisplatin is reportedly **compatible** with the following intravenous solutions and drugs: dextrose/saline combinations, sodium chloride 0.225%–0.9%, magnesium sulfate, and mannitol. It is also **compatible** in syringes or at Y-sites with: bleomycin sulfate, cyclophosphamide, doxorubicin HCl, droperidol, fluorouracil, furosemide, heparin sodium, leucovorin calcium, methotrexate, mitomycin, vinblastine sulfate, and vincristine sulfate.

Cisplatin **compatibility information conflicts** or is dependent on diluent or concentration factors with the following drugs or solutions: dextrose/saline combinations, dextrose 5% in water, and metoclopramide. Compatibility is dependent upon factors such as pH, concentration, temperature and diluent used; consult specialized references or a hospital pharmacist for more specific information.

Cisplatin is reportedly **incompatible** with the following solutions or drugs: sodium chloride 0.1% and sodium bicarbonate 5%.

Dosage Forms/Regulatory Status

VETERINARY-LABELED PRODUCTS: None

HUMAN-LABELED PRODUCTS:

Cisplatin Injection: 1 mg/mL in 50 mL, 100 mL & 200 mL multi-dose vials; generic; (Rx)

Cisplatin powder or compounded formulations appropriate for intralesional injection may be available from compounding pharmacies.

References

Argyle, D, M Brearly, et al. (2008). *Decision Making in Small Animal Oncology*, Wiley–Blackwell.

Hawkins, E & T Fossum (2000). Medical and Surgical Management of Pleural Effusion. *Kirk's Current Veterinary Therapy: XIII Small Animal Practice*. J Bonagura Ed. Philadelphia, WB Saunders: 819–825.

Henry, C & M Higginbotham (2009). *Cancer Management in Small Animal Practice*, Saunders.

Moll, H (2002). Skin tumor management. Proceedings: Western Veterinary Conference. Accessed via: Veterinary Information Network. http://goo.gl/xtUEh

Ogilvie, G & A Moore (2001). *Feline Oncology: A Comprehensive Guide to Compassionate Care*, Veterinary Learning Systems.

Ogilvie, G & A Moore (2006). *Managing the Canine Cancer Patient: A Practical Guide to Compassionate Care*, Veterinary Learning Systems.

Villalobos, A (2007). *Canine and Feline Geriatric Oncology*. Ames, Blackwell.

Withrow, S & D Vail (2007). *Withrow and MacEwen's Small Animal Clinical Oncology 4th Ed*. Philadelphia, Elsevier.

CITRATE SALTS
POTASSIUM CITRATE
SODIUM CITRATE AND
CITRIC ACID

(*sI*-trate)   Nutrived®, Urocit-K®

URINARY ALKALINIZER

Prescriber Highlights

▶ Oral administered precursor to bicarbonate; used for urinary alkalization & treatment of chronic metabolic acidosis; may be useful to prevent calcium oxalate urolith formation

▶ Many contraindications to therapy, including heart failure, severe renal impairment, UTI with calcium or struvite stones

▶ Contraindications for potassium citrate alone include hyperkalemia, ulcer disease; tablets in patients with delayed gastric emptying conditions, esophageal compression, or intestinal obstruction

▶ Most prevalent adverse effect is GI distress but, potentially, hyperkalemia, fluid retention & metabolic alkalosis possible

▶ Adequate lab monitoring mandatory

Uses/Indications

Citrate salts serve as source of bicarbonate; they are more pleasant tasting than bicarbonate preparations making them more palatable. They are used as urinary alkalinizers when an alkaline urine is desirable and in the management of chronic metabolic acidosis accompanied with conditions such as renal tubular acidosis or chronic renal insufficiency. Potassium citrate alone (*Uracit-K®*) has been used for the prevention of calcium oxalate uroliths. The citrate can complex with calcium thereby decreasing urinary concentrations of calcium oxalate. The urinary alkalinizing effects of the citrate also increase the solubility of calcium oxalate.

Pharmacology/Actions

Citrate salts are oxidized in the body to bicarbonate thereby acting as alkalinizing agents. The citric acid component of multi-component products is converted only to carbon dioxide and water and has only a temporary effect on systemic acid-base status.

Pharmacokinetics

Absorption and oxidation are nearly complete after oral administration; less than 5% of a dose is excreted unchanged.

Contraindications/Precautions/Warnings

Contraindications for products containing sodium citrate and/or potassium citrate: aluminum toxicity, heart failure, severe renal impairment (with azotemia or oliguria), UTI associated with calcium, or struvite stones. Additional contraindications for potassium citrate alone include hyperkalemia (or conditions that predispose to hyperkalemia such as adrenal insufficiency, acute dehydration, renal failure, uncontrolled diabetes mellitus), or peptic ulcer (particularly with the tablets). The potassium citrate tablets are contraindicated in patients with delayed gastric emptying conditions, esophageal compression, or intestinal obstruction or stricture. These products should be used with caution (weigh risks vs. benefit) in severe renal tubular acidosis or chronic diarrheal syndromes as they may be ineffective. Sodium citrate products should be used with caution in patients with congestive heart disease.

In dosages not resulting in hypernatremia, hyperkalemia or metabolic alkalosis, these products should not cause fetal harm.

Adverse Effects

The primary adverse effects noted with these agents are gastrointestinal in nature, however, most dogs receiving these products tolerate them well. Potassium citrate products have the potential of causing hyperkalemia, especially in susceptible patients. Sodium citrate products may lead to increased fluid retention in patients with cardiac disease. Rarely, metabolic alkalosis could occur.

Reproductive/Nursing Safety
In humans, the FDA categorizes potassium citrate as a category *C* drug for use during pregnancy (*Animal studies have shown an adverse effect on the fetus, but there are no adequate studies in humans; or there are no animal reproduction studies and no adequate studies in humans*).

No specific data is available on the safety of citrates during nursing, but no documented adverse effects have been reported.

Overdosage/Acute Toxicity
Overdosage and acute toxicity would generally fall into 4 categories: gastrointestinal distress and ulceration, metabolic alkalosis, hypernatremia (sodium citrate), or hyperkalemia (potassium citrate). Should an overdose occur and there are reasonable expectations of preventing absorption (especially with the tablets), gut-emptying protocols should be employed if not contraindicated. Otherwise, treat GI effects, if necessary, with intravenous fluids or other supportive care. Hyperkalemia, hypernatremia, and metabolic alkalosis should be treated if warranted. It is suggested to refer to an animal poison control center, an internal medicine text or other references for additional information for specific treatment modalities for these conditions.

Drug Interactions
The following drug interactions have either been reported or are theoretical in humans or animals receiving citrates and may be of significance in veterinary patients:

■ **AMPHETAMINES; PSEUDOEPHEDRINE; EPHEDRINE:** Alkalinized urine can decrease excretion

■ **ANTACIDS:** Citrate alkalinizers used with antacids (particularly those containing bicarbonate or aluminum salts) may cause systemic alkalosis, and aluminum toxicity (aluminum antacids only) particularly in patients with renal insufficiency. Sodium citrate combined with sodium bicarbonate may cause hypernatremia, and may cause the development of calcium stones in patients with preexisting uric acid stones.

■ **ASPIRIN:** Alkalinized urine can increase the excretion of salicylates

■ **FLUOROQUINOLONES:** The solubility of ciprofloxacin & enrofloxacin is decreased in an alkaline environment. Patients with alkaline urine should be monitored for signs of crystalluria.

■ **LITHIUM:** Alkalinized urine can decrease excretion

■ **METHENAMINE:** Concurrent use with methenamine is not recommended as it requires an acidic urine for efficacy.

■ **QUINIDINE:** Alkalinized urine can decrease excretion

■ **TETRACYCLINES:** Alkalinized urine can decrease excretion

With potassium citrate products, the following agents may lead to increases in serum potassium levels (including severe hyperkalemia), particularly in patients with renal insufficiency:

■ **ACE INHIBITORS (e.g., enalapril, lisinopril)**

■ **CYCLOSPORINE**

■ **DIGOXIN**

■ **HEPARIN**

■ **NONSTEROIDAL ANTIINFLAMMATORY DRUGS (NSAIDS)**

■ **POTASSIUM-CONTAINING DRUGS/FOODS**

■ **SPIRONOLACTONE; TRIAMTERENE**

Doses
■ **DOGS:**
For adjunctive therapy to inhibit calcium oxalate crystal formation in dogs with hypocitraturia:
a) Potassium citrate: 40–75 mg/kg PO q12h; avoid overzealous urinary alkalinization as calcium phosphate uroliths may form (Grauer 2003)
b) Potassium citrate: Initially 50 mg/kg PO q12h. Monitor urine pH; goal is to obtain values of 7–7.5 (Bartges, JW 2000)
c) To help decrease the possibility of calcium oxalate stone formation using *Nutrived® Potassium Citrate Granules*: 1 scoop mixed or sprinkled on food per 10 lb. body weight per day. (Label information; *Nutrived® Potassium Citrate Granules for Dogs & Cats*—Vedco)
d) If calcium oxalate crystalluria is persistent or calcium oxalate uroliths occur and dietary and hydrochlorothiazide (2 mg/kg PO q12h) therapy have been implemented, give potassium citrate to effect to achieve a urine pH of 6.5–7 using a starting dose of 50–75 mg/kg PO q12h. If urine pH already above 7–7.5, do not use potassium citrate. Monitor serum potassium levels monthly and reduce dose if hyperkalemia occurs. (Adams & Syme 2005)

For adjunctive therapy of chronic renal failure as a potassium supplement and alkalinizing agent:
a) Potassium citrate: Initially, 75 mg/kg PO q12h (Bartges, J 2002)

■ **CATS:**
For adjunctive therapy to inhibit calcium oxalate formation:
a) Potassium citrate: initially 50–100 mg kg PO q12h. Goal is to achieve a urine pH of approximately 7.5 (Bartges, J 2002)
b) To help decrease the possibility of calcium oxalate stone formation using *Nutrived® Potassium Citrate Granules*: 1 scoop mixed or sprinkled on food per day. (Label information; *Nutrived® Potassium Citrate Granules for Dogs & Cats*—Vedco)

c) Recommended dose is 100–150 mg/kg/day PO, but it is unclear whether this dose will actually increase urinary citrate in cats. (Westropp *et al.* 2005)

For adjunctive therapy of chronic renal failure as a potassium supplement and alkalinizing agent:

a) Potassium citrate: Initially, 75 mg/kg PO q12h (Bartges, J 2002)

b) If cat is significantly acidemic: 2.5 mEq (total dose) potassium or 15–30 mg/kg as potassium citrate PO q12h (Wolf 2006)

c) When cats with CRF are hypokalemic: 2–4 mEq (total dose) of potassium per day as potassium citrate or potassium gluconate. (DiBartola & Chew 2006)

Monitoring

Depending on patient's condition, product chosen and reason for use:

■ Serum potassium, sodium, bicarbonate, chloride

■ Acid/base status

■ Urine pH, Urinalysis

■ Serum creatinine, CBC, particularly in chronic renal failure

Chemistry/Synonyms

Generally used as alkalinizing agents, citric acid and citrate salts are available in several commercially available dosage forms. Citric acid occurs as an odorless or practically odorless, colorless, translucent crystal with a strong acidic taste. It is very soluble in water. Potassium citrate occurs as odorless, transparent crystals or a white, granular powder having a cooling, saline taste. It is freely soluble in water. 108 mg of potassium citrate contains approximately 1 mEq of potassium. Sodium citrate occurs as colorless crystals or a white, granular powder. The hydrous form is freely soluble in water.

Potassium citrate may also be known as citrate of potash, or citric acid tripotassium salt monohydrate. Sodium citrate and citric acid solutions may also be known as Shohl's solution.

Storage/Stability

Store solutions and potassium citrate tablets in tight containers at room temperature unless otherwise recommended by manufacturer.

Dosage Forms/Regulatory Status

VETERINARY-LABELED PRODUCTS:

Potassium Citrate and Fatty Acids Granules: each 5 g (one scoop) contains 300 mg potassium citrate (approximately 2.8 mEq of potassium) and 423 mg total fatty acids; also contains several amino acids—quantities not labeled; *Nutrived® Potassium Citrate Granules* for *Cats* and *Dogs* (Vedco); (OTC)

HUMAN-LABELED PRODUCTS:

Potassium Citrate Extended-Release Oral Tablets: 5 mEq (540 mg), 10 mEq (1080 mg) & 15 mEq; *Urocit-K®;* (Mission); generic (Rising) (Rx)

Potassium Citrate/Sodium Citrate Combinations:
Tablets: 50 mg potassium citrate and 950 mg sodium citrate. *Citrolith®* (Beach Pharm); (Rx)

Syrup: 550 mg potassium citrate, 500 mg sodium citrate, 334 mg citric acid/5 mL (1mEq K, 1 mEq Na per mL equivalent to 2 mEq bicarbonate); in 120 and 480 mL, *Polycitra®* (Willen); (Rx)

Solution: 550 mg K citrate, 500 mg sodium citrate, 334 mg citric acid/5 mL (1 mEq K, 1 mEq Na per mL; equiv to 2 mEq bicarbonate) in 120 and 480 mL. *Polycitra-LC®* (Willen); (Rx).

1100 mg potassium citrate, 334 mg citric acid/5 mL, (2 mEq K/mL; equiv. to 2 mEq bicarbonate) in 120 and 480. *Polycitra-K®* (Willen); (Rx)

Crystals for Reconstitution: 3300 mg K citrate, 1002 mg citric acid per UD packet (equiv. To 30 mEq bicarbonate) in single dose packets. *Polycitra-K®* (Willen); (Rx)

Citric Acid/Sodium Citrate Combinations:
Solutions: Sodium Citrate Dihydrate 490 mg sodium citrate and Citric Acid 640 mg per 5 mL (1 mEq sodium equiv to 1 mEq bicarbonate/mL) in 500 mL and UD 15 and 30 mL, *Oracit®*; (Carolina Medical); (Rx)

Sodium Citrate Dihydrate 500 mg sodium citrate and Citric 334 mg per 5 mL (1 mEq sodium equiv to 1 mEq bicarbonate/mL) in 120 and 473 mL and UD 15 and 30 mL; *Bicitra®;* (Alza Corp); (Rx)

Potassium Citrate, Sodium Citrate/Citric Acid Solutions:
550 mg potassium citrate monohydrate, 500 mg sodium citrate dihydrate, 334 mg citric acid monohydrate per 5 mL (1 mEq potassium and 1 mEq sodium per mL and is equivalent to 2 mEq bicarbonate in 60 oz bottles; *Cytra-LC®* (Cypress); (Rx)

1100 mg potassium citrate monohydrate and 334 mg citric acid monohydrate per 5 mL (2 mEq potassium per mL and is equivalent to 2 mEq bicarbonate) in 473 mL; *Cytra-K®* (Cypress); (Rx)

20 mEq potassium, 30 mEq citrate (20 g dextrose, 5 g fructose, 35 mEq chloride, 45 mEq sodium)/L in 1 liter; *Naturalyte® Oral Electrolyte Solution* (Unico); (OTC)

References

Adams, L & H Syme (2005). Canine lower urinary tract diseases. *Textbook of Veterinary Internal Medicine, 6th Ed.* S Ettinger and E Feldman Eds., Elsevier: 1850– 1874.

Bartges, J (2000). Calcium oxalate uroliths. The North American Veterinary Conference, Orlando.

Bartges, J (2002). Feline calcium oxalate uroliths. Proceedings: Western Veterinary Conference. Accessed via: Veterinary Information Network. http://goo.gl/c9X6V

DiBartola, S & D Chew (2006). Tips for managing chronic renal failure. Proceedings: ACVIM. Accessed via: Veterinary Information Network. http://goo.gl/hf5C4

Grauer, G (2003). Urinary Tract Disorders. *Small Animal Internal Medicine 3rd Edition*. R Nelson and C Couto Eds. Phila, Saunders: 568–659.

Westropp, J, C Buffington, et al. (2005). Feline lower urinary tract diseases. *Textbook of Veterinary Internal Medicine, 6th Ed.* S Ettinger and E Feldman Eds., Elsevier: 1828–1850.

Wolf, A (2006). Chronic progressive renal disease in the cat: Recognition and management. Proceedings: ABVP2006. Accessed via: Veterinary Information Network. http://goo.gl/1q5Bq

CLARITHROMYCIN

(klar-***ith***-ro-my-sin)   Biaxin®

MACROLIDE ANTIBIOTIC

Prescriber Highlights

▶ Macrolide antibiotic that may useful for treating atypical mycobacterial infections or treatment of *Helicobacter* spp. infections in dogs, cats, & ferrets; *Rhodococcus equi* infections in foals

▶ Appears to be well tolerated by domestic animals, but clinical experience is limited

▶ Many potential drug interactions

▶ Expense may be an issue, but generics now available

Uses/Indications

In small animal medicine, clarithromycin is primarily of interest in treating atypical mycobacterial infections or treatment of *Helicobacter* spp. infections in cats and ferrets. In equine medicine, clarithromycin may be useful in treating *Rhodococcus equi* infections in foals.

Pharmacology/Actions

Clarithromycin, like other macrolide antibiotics, penetrate susceptible bacterial cell walls and bind to the 50S ribosomal subunit inhibiting protein synthesis. The drug is usually bacteriostatic, but may be bactericidal at high concentrations in very susceptible organisms.

Clarithromycin's spectrum of activity is similar to that of erythromycin, but it also has activity against a variety of bacteria that are not easily treated with other antibiotics (*e.g.*, atypical mycobacteria). Activity against gram-positive aerobic cocci is similar to that of erythromycin, but lower concentrations are required to be effective against susceptible organisms. The drug is typically not effective against oxacillin-resistant Staph or coagulase-negative Staph. Clarithromycin also has activity against *Rhodococcus equi*. Activity against gram-negative aerobic bacteria includes *Haemophilus influenzae*, *Pasturella multocida*, *Legionella pneumophilia*, *Bordetella pertussis* and *Campylobacter* spp. Clarithromycin has inhibitory activity against a variety of atypical mycobacteria, including *M. avium complex* and *M. leprae*. Clarithromycin has good activity against *Mycoplasma pneu-*

moniae and *Ureaplasma ureatlyticum*. Other organisms where clarithromycin may have therapeutic usefulness include: *Nocardia* spp. *Toxoplasma gondii*, *Helicobacter pylori*, *Borrelia burgdorferi*, and *Cryptosporidium parvum*.

Pharmacokinetics

In horses (foals), the drug is apparently well absorbed after intragastric administration with peak serum concentrations occurring about 1.5 hours after dosing. Elimination half-life is about 4.8 hours.

In dogs, clarithromycin bioavailability ranges from 60–83% with the higher values obtained when given to fasted animals.

Contraindications/Precautions/Warnings

In humans, clarithromycin is contraindicated in patients hypersensitive to it or other macrolide antibiotics (*e.g.*, erythromycin, azithromycin).

Adverse Effects

The adverse effect profile for clarithromycin in domestic animals is not well described. With limited clinical experience, it appears to be well tolerated in dogs, cats, ferrets, and foals. Like all orally administered antibiotics, GI disturbances are possible. Pinnal or generalized erythema may be associated with this drug when used in cats.

Adverse effects in humans include gastrointestinal adverse effects (primarily nausea, vomiting, abdominal pain, abnormal taste, diarrhea) that, when compared with erythromycin, are milder and occur less frequently. Approximately 4% of treated humans develop transient, mildly elevated BUN levels. Rarely, prolonged QT interval (torsades de pointes), hepatotoxicity, thrombocytopenia, or hypersensitivity reactions have been reported. Pseudomembranous colitis secondary to *Clostridium difficile* has been reported after clarithromycin use.

Reproductive/Nursing Safety

In humans, the FDA categorizes clarithromycin as a category *C* drug for use during pregnancy (*Animal studies have shown an adverse effect on the fetus, but there are no adequate studies in humans; or there are no animal reproduction studies and no adequate studies in humans*). Teratogenic studies in rats and rabbits failed to document any teratogenic effects in some studies, but at high dosages (yielding plasma levels 2–17 times achieved in humans with maximum recommended dosages) in pregnant rats, rabbits and monkeys, some effects (cleft palate, cardiovascular abnormalities, fetal growth retardation) were noted.

Clarithromycin is excreted into milk of lactating animals and levels may be higher in milk than in the dam's plasma, but this is unlikely to be of clinical significance.

Overdosage/Acute Toxicity

Generally, overdoses of clarithromycin are usually not serious with only gastrointestinal effects seen. Patients ingesting large overdoses may be given activated charcoal/cathartic to remove any unabsorbed drug. Forced diuresis, peritoneal dialysis, or hemodialysis do not appear to be effective in removing the drug from the body.

Drug Interactions
The following drug interactions have either been reported or are theoretical in humans or animals receiving clarithromycin and may be of significance in veterinary patients:

■ **CISAPRIDE:** Clarithromycin can inhibit the metabolism of cisapride and the manufacturer states that use of these drugs together (in humans) is contraindicated

■ **FLUCONAZOLE:** Possible increased clarithromycin levels

■ **DIGOXIN:** Clarithromycin may increase the serum levels of digoxin

■ **OMEPRAZOLE:** Clarithromycin and omeprazole can increase the plasma levels of one another

■ **WARFARIN:** Clarithromycin may potentiate the effects of oral anticoagulant drugs

■ **ZIDOVUDINE:** Clarithromycin may decrease serum concentrations of zidovudine

Clarithromycin, like erythromycin, can inhibit the metabolism of other drugs that use the CYP3A subfamily of the cytochrome P450 enzyme system. Depending on the therapeutic index of the drug(s) involved, therapeutic drug monitoring and/or dosage reduction may be required if the drugs must be used together. These drugs include:

■ **ALFENTANIL**

■ **BROMOCRIPTINE**

■ **BUSPIRONE**

■ **CARBAMAZEPINE**

■ **DISOPYRAMIDE (also risk of increased QT interval)**

■ **METHYLPREDNISOLONE**

■ **MIDAZOLAM, ALPRAZOLAM, TRIAZOLAM**

■ **QUINIDINE** (also risk of increased QT interval)

■ **RIFABUTIN**

■ **TACROLIMUS (systemic)**

■ **THEOPHYLLINE**

Laboratory Considerations
■ No clarithromycin-related laboratory interactions noted.

Doses
■ **DOGS:**
For treatment of severe or refractory cases of canine leproid granuloma syndrome:
a) Using a combination of clarithromycin 15–25 mg/kg total daily dose PO given divided q8–12h; and rifampin 10–15 mg/kg PO once daily. Usually treatment should be continued for 4–8 weeks until lesions are at least substantially reduced in size and ideally have resolved completely. (Malik *et al.* 2001)

For susceptible infections:
a) 2.5–10 mg/kg PO twice daily (Boothe 1999)
b) 5–10 mg/kg PO q12h (Greene & Watson 1998)

■ **CATS:**
For treatment of feline leprosy:
a) Using a regimen of either two or three of the following drugs: clarithromycin: 62.5 mg per cat q12h; clofazimine: 25–50 mg once per day or 50 mg every other day; rifampin: 10–15 mg/kg once a day. (Malik *et al.* 2002)

For treatment of *Nocardia* (*N. nova*) infections:
a) Combination therapy with: amoxicillin 20 mg/kg PO twice daily with clarithromycin 62.5–125 mg (total dose per cat) PO twice daily and/or doxycycline 5 mg/kg or higher PO twice daily. (Malik 2006)

For treatment of *H. pylori* infections:
a) Combination therapy with: clarithromycin 7.5 mg/kg PO twice daily; metronidazole 10–15 mg/kg PO twice daily; amoxicillin 20 mg/kg PO twice daily for 14 days. (Simpson 2003)

For treatment of *M. tuberculosis-bovis* variant infections:
a) Using all three drugs: Clarithromycin 5–10 mg/kg PO q12h; rifampin 10–20 mg/kg PO once daily, enrofloxacin 5–10 mg/kg PO q12–24h. Treatment must continue for at least 2 months. Maintenance for additional 4 months using (at same dosages enrofloxacin and clarithromycin or rifampin and enrofloxacin). (Greene & Gunn-Moore 1998)

For susceptible infections:
a) 7.5 mg/kg PO q12h (Greene & Watson 1998)

■ **FERRETS:**
For treatment of *Helicobacter mustelae* infections:
a) Clarithromycin 12.5 mg/kg PO q12h with ranitidine bismuth citrate (**Note:** not currently available in the USA, but may be available from compounding pharmacies) 24 mg/kg PO q12h. Treat for 14 days. Same regimen, but given q8h is also published. (Johnson-Delaney 2009)
b) 12.5–50 mg/kg q8–24h with omeprazole at 0.7 mg/kg PO once daily (q24h) (Fisher 2005)

■ **HORSES:**
For treatment of *Rhodococcus equi* infection in foals:
a) 7.5 mg/kg PO q12h (Jacks *et al.* 2002), (Chaffin 2006)

b) 7.5 mg/kg PO q12h in combination with rifampin at 5 mg/kg PO q12h or 10 mg/kg PO q24h. (Giguere 2003)

Monitoring

■ Antibacterial efficacy

■ Adverse effects

Client Information

■ If using the oral suspension, do *not* refrigerate; keep at room temperature and discard 14 days after reconstituting

■ This drug may be given without regard to meals

■ Clarithromycin can interact with many other drugs; do not give any drugs to the animal without the veterinarian's knowledge

Chemistry/Synonyms

Clarithromycin is a semi-synthetic macrolide antibiotic related to erythromycin. It differs from erythromycin by the methylation of position 6 in the lactone ring. Clarithromycin occurs as a white to off-white crystalline powder. It is practically insoluble in water, slightly soluble in ethanol, and soluble in acetone. It is slightly soluble in a phosphate buffer at pH's of 2–5.

Clarithromycin may also be known as: 6-O-Methylerythromycin, TE-031, A-56268, *Adel®, Biaxin®, Biclar®, Bremon®, Clamicin®, Clamycin®, Claribid®, Clarimac®, Clarimax®, Claritab®, Cyllind®, Gervaken®, Heliclar®, Helicodid®, Karin®, Klacid®, Klaciped®, Klaricid®, Klaridex®, Kofron®, Lagur®, Mabicrol®, Macladin®, Maclar®, Mavid®, Monaxin®, Monocid®, Naxy®, Veclam®,* and *Zeclar®.*

Storage/Stability

The conventional 250 mg tablets should be protected from light and stored in well-closed containers at 15–30°C (59–86°F). The conventional or extended-release 500 mg tablets should be stored in well-closed containers at controlled room temperature (20–25°C; 68–77°F). The granules for reconstitution into an oral suspension should be stored in well-closed containers at 15–30°C. After reconstitution, it should be stored at room temperature (do not refrigerate) and any unused drug discarded after 14 days.

Dosage Forms/Regulatory Status

VETERINARY-LABELED PRODUCTS: None
HUMAN-LABELED PRODUCTS:

Clarithromycin Regular & Film-coated Oral Tablets: 250 mg & 500 mg; Extended-release Tablets: 500 mg; *Biaxin®* & *Biaxin® XL* (Abbott), generic; (Rx)

Clarithromycin Granules for Oral Suspension: 125 mg/5 mL & 250 mg/5 mL (after reconstitution) in 50 mL & 100 mL; *Biaxin®* (Abbott), generic; (Rx)

A pre-packaged combination containing lansoprazole, amoxicillin and clarithromycin for *H. pylori* is marketed as *Prevpak®* (TAP); (Rx)

References

Boothe, DM (1999). What's new in drug therapy in small animals. Wild West Conference.

Chaffin, M (2006). Treatment and chemoprophylaxis of Rhodococcus equi pneumonia in foals. Proceedings: ACVIM. Accessed via: Veterinary Information Network. http://goo.gl/wuP4O

Fisher, P (2005). Ferret Medicine I. Proceedings: Western Vet Conf. Accessed via: Veterinary Information Network. http://goo.gl/bSPRO

Giguere, S (2003). Rhodococcus equi infections. *Current Therapy in Equine Medicine 5.* C Kollias–Baker Ed. Philadelphia, Saunders.

Greene, C & D Gunn–Moore (1998). Mycobacterial Infections: Tuberculosis mycobacterial infections. *Infectious Diseases of the Dog and Cat.* C Greene Ed. Philadelphia, Saunders: 313–325.

Greene, C & A Watson (1998). Antimicrobial Drug Formulary. *Infectious Diseases of the Dog and Cat.* C Greene Ed. Philadelphia, WB Saunders: 790–919.

Jacks, S, S Giguere, et al. (2002). Disposition of oral clarithromycin in foals. *J Vet Phamacol Ther* 25(5): 359–362.

Johnson–Delaney, C (2009). Gastrointestinal physiology and disease of carnivorous exotic companion animals. Proceedings: ABVP. http://goo.gl/Nphb5

Malik, R (2006). Nocardia infections in cats. Proceedings Western Vet Conf. Accessed via: Veterinary Information Network. http://goo.gl/bY0lh

Malik, R, M Hughes, et al. (2002). Feline Leprosy – two different clinical syndromes. *J Feline Med Surg* 4(1): 43–59.

Malik, R, P Martin, et al. (2001). Treatment of canine leproid granuloma syndrome: preliminary findings in dogs. *Aust Vet J* 79(Jan): 30–36.

Simpson, K (2003). Intragastric warfare in Helicobacter infected cats. Proceedings: ACVIM Forum. Accessed via: Veterinary Information Network. http://goo.gl/gSR3T

Clavulanate/Amoxicillin — See Amoxicillin/Clavulanate

Clavulanate/Ticarcillin — See Ticarcillin /Clavulanate

CLEMASTINE FUMARATE

(*klem*-as-teen)   Tavist®

ANTIHISTAMINE

Prescriber Highlights

▶ Oral antihistamine with greater anticholinergic, but less sedative activity

▶ Poor pharmacokinetic profile for oral administration in dogs or horses

▶ Caution: Prostatic hypertrophy, bladder neck obstruction, severe cardiac failure, angle-closure glaucoma, or pyeloduodenal obstruction

▶ Most likely adverse effects: Dogs: Sedation, paradoxical hyperactivity & anticholinergic effects (dryness of mucous membranes, etc.); Cats: Diarrhea

Uses/Indications

Clemastine may be used for symptomatic relief of histamine$_1$-related allergic conditions.

Pharmacology/Actions

Like other H$_1$-receptor antihistamines, clemastine acts by competing with histamine for sites on H$_1$-receptor sites on effector cells. They do not block histamine release, but can antagonize its effects. Clemastine has greater anticholinergic activity, but less sedation than average.

Pharmacokinetics

In dogs, oral bioavailability is very low (3%). Clemastine has a high volume of distribution (13.4 L/kg; 98% protein bound) and clearance (2.1 L/hr/kg). After IV administration, elimination half-life is about 4 hours and completely inhibited wheal formation for 7 hours. Oral administration at 0.5 mg/kg only yielded minor inhibition of wheal formation. The authors of the study (Hansson *et al.* 2004) concluded that most oral dosage regimens in the literature are likely to give too low a systemic exposure of the drug to allow effective therapy.

In horses, clemastine has poor oral bioavailability (3–4%), a volume of distribution at steady-state of 3.8 L/kg, a clearance (TBC) of 0.79 L/hr/Kg and a terminal half-life of about 5.4 hours. The authors concluded that the drug is not appropriate for oral administration in the horse and must be dosed at least 3–4 times a day intravenously to maintain therapeutic plasma concentrations. (Torneke *et al.* 2003)

In humans, clemastine has a variable bioavailability (20–70%); its distribution is not well characterized, but does distribute into milk. Metabolic fate has not been clearly determined, but it appears to be extensively metabolized and those metabolites are eliminated in the urine. In humans, its duration of action is about 12 hours.

Contraindications/Precautions/Warnings

Clemastine is contraindicated in patients hypersensitive to it. It should be used with caution in patients with prostatic hypertrophy, bladder neck obstruction, severe cardiac failure, angle-closure glaucoma, or pyeloduodenal obstruction.

Adverse Effects

The most likely adverse effects seen in dogs receiving clemastine are sedation, paradoxical hyperactivity, and anticholinergic effects (dryness of mucous membranes, etc.). In cats, diarrhea has been noted most commonly; one cat reportedly developed a fixed drug reaction while on this medication.

Reproductive/Nursing Safety

Clemastine has been tested in pregnant lab animals in doses up to 312 times labeled without evidence of harm to fetuses. However, because safety has not been established in other species, its use during pregnancy should be weighed carefully. In humans, the FDA categorizes this drug as category **B** for use during pregnancy

(*Animal studies have not yet demonstrated risk to the fetus, but there are no adequate studies in pregnant women; or animal studies have shown an adverse effect, but adequate studies in pregnant women have not demonstrated a risk to the fetus in the first trimester of pregnancy, and there is no evidence of risk in later trimesters.*)

Clemastine enters maternal milk and may potentially cause adverse effects in offspring. Use with caution, especially with newborns.

Overdosage/Acute Toxicity

There are no specific antidotes available. Significant overdoses should be handled using standard gut emptying protocols, when appropriate, and supportive therapy initiated when required. The adverse effects seen with overdoses are an extension of the drug's side effects; principally CNS depression (although CNS stimulation may be seen), anticholinergic effects (severe drying of mucous membranes, tachycardia, urinary retention, hyperthermia, etc.), and possibly hypotension. Physostigmine may be considered to treat serious CNS anticholinergic effects and diazepam employed to treat seizures, if necessary.

Drug Interactions

The following drug interactions have either been reported or are theoretical in humans or animals receiving clemastine and may be of significance in veterinary patients:

■ **CNS DEPRESSANT MEDICATIONS:** Additive CNS depression may be seen if combining clemastine with other CNS depressant medications such as barbiturates, tranquilizers, etc.

■ **MONOAMINE OXIDASE INHIBITORS** (including **furazolidone, amitraz,** and possibly **selegiline**) may intensify the anticholinergic effects of clemastine

Laboratory Considerations

Because antihistamines can decrease the wheal and flair response to **skin allergen testing**, antihistamines should be discontinued 3–7 days (depending on the antihistamine used and the reference) before intradermal skin tests.

Doses

■ **DOGS:**

Note: Relatively recent published information (Hansson *et al.* 2004) on the pharmacokinetics of clemastine in dogs puts the efficacy of previously published doses for this drug in doubt, but some veterinary dermatologists still recommend its use. Usual doses published are approximately 0.05–0.1 mg/kg PO q12h; however oral bioavailability (see Pharmacokinetics above) in dogs is less than 5% versus approximately 20–70% in humans, and an oral dose of 0.5 mg/kg (10X most published doses) in dogs only inhibited histamine-induced wheal formation to a slight degree, while IV administration inhibited it for 7 hours. Further dosing studies must be performed before this drug can be recommended for therapeutic use in the dog.

■ **CATS:**

As an antihistamine:

a) 0.68 mg per cat PO twice daily (Miller 2005)

b) 0.34−0.68 mg per cat PO q12h (Messinger 2000)

c) For atopy: 0.15 mg/kg PO q 12 hrs. Efficacy may be increased by combining with omega 3 fatty acids. (Campbell 1999)

Monitoring

■ Efficacy

■ Adverse Effects, if any

Client Information

■ Clients should understand that antihistamines may be useful for symptomatic relief of allergic signs, but are not a cure for the underlying disease.

Chemistry/Synonyms

Also known as meclastine fumarate or mecloprodin fumarate, clemastine fumarate is an ethanolamine antihistamine. It occurs as an odorless, faintly yellow, crystalline powder. It is very slightly soluble in water and sparingly soluble in alcohol.

Tavist-D® contains clemastine fumarate in an immediate release outer shell and phenylpropanolamine HCl in a sustained release inner matrix.

Clemastine fumarate may also be known by the following synonyms and internationally registered trade names: clemastini fumaras, HS-592, meclastine fumarate, mecloprodine fumarate, *Agasten®, Aller-Eze®, Antihist-1®, Clamist®, Contac 12 Hour Allergy®, Dayhist-1®, Tavegil®, Tavegyl®* or *Tavist®.*

Storage/Stability

Oral tablets and solution should be stored in tight, light resistant containers at room temperature.

Dosage Forms/Regulatory Status

VETERINARY-LABELED PRODUCTS: None

The ARCI (Racing Commissioners International) has designated this drug as a class 3 substance. See the appendix for more information.

HUMAN-LABELED PRODUCTS:

Clemastine Fumarate Oral Tablets: 1.34 mg as fumarate (equivalent to 1 mg clemastine), 2.68 mg (equivalent to 2 mg clemastine); *Dayhist-1®* (Major); *Tavist® Allergy* (Novartis Consumer Health); generic; (Rx & OTC)

Clemastine Oral Syrup: 0.67 mg/5 mL (equivalent to 0.5 mg clemastine) in 118 & 120 mL; generic; (Rx)

References

Campbell, K (1999). New Drugs in Veterinary Dermatology. Proceedings: Central Veterinary Conference, Kansas City.

Hansson, H, U Bergvall, et al. (2004). Clinical pharmacology of clemastine in healthy dogs. *Vet Derm* 15: 152–158.

Messinger, L (2000). Pruritis Therapy in the Cat. *Kirk's Current Veterinary Therapy: XIII Small Animal Practice.* J Bonagura Ed. Philadelphia, WB Saunders: 542–545.

Miller, W (2005). Allergic Skin Diseases in 2005. Proceedings: ACVC. Accessed via: Veterinary Information Network. http://goo.gl/7Vxcs

Torneke, K, C Ingvast–Larsson, et al. (2003). Pharmacokinetics and pharmacodynamics of clemastine in healthy horses. *J Vet Phamacol Ther* 26(2): 151–157.

CLENBUTEROL HCL

(klen-*byoo*-ter-ol)   Ventipulmin®

Prescriber Highlights

▶ Beta-2-adrenergic agonist used in horses as a bronchodilator in the management of airway obstruction and for dystocia as a uterine relaxant

▶ Banned in food animals in USA and several other countries

▶ In pregnancy, antagonizes the effects of dinoprost (prostaglandin F2alpha) & oxytocin & can diminish normal uterine contractility

▶ Acute adverse effects include tachycardia, muscle tremors, sweating, restlessness, & urticaria

▶ Chronic administration can potentially cause deleterious effects on endocrine, immune and reproductive functions

Uses/Indications

Clenbuterol is FDA-approved for use in horses as a bronchodilator in the management of airway obstruction, such as recurrent airway obstruction (RAO; formerly COPD). It has been used both parenterally and orally as a uterine relaxant for the adjunctive treatment of dystocia.

It has been used as a partitioning agent in food producing animals, but its use for this purpose is banned in the USA as relay toxicity in humans has been documented.

Pharmacology/Actions

Like other beta-2 agonists, clenbuterol is believed to act by stimulating production of cyclic AMP through the activation of adenyl cyclase. By definition, beta-2 agonists have more smooth muscle relaxation activity (bronchial, vascular, and uterine smooth muscle) versus its cardiac effects (beta-1). Clenbuterol appears to have secondary modes of action in horses as it can inhibit the release from macrophages of proinflammatory cytokines such as interleukin−1(beta) and tumor necrosis factor (alpha), and increase ciliary beat frequency to enhance mucous clearance.

Compared to control, when clenbuterol was administered IV to healthy horses, aerobic capacity was not improved, insulin levels were increased, and treadmill velocities for defined heart rates were reduced (Ferraz *et al.* 2007).

Chronic administration of clenbuterol to horses can cause decreased aerobic performance, induce cardiac hypertrophy and infiltration of collagen in cardiac muscle, and suppress cortisol response to exercise. Chronic clenbuterol administration in combination with exercise training can alter immune function (reduced killer and CD8+ cells). In pregnant mares, clenbuterol can inhibit uterine tone and contractility, but these effects are not considered detrimental. In non-pregnant mares, clenbuterol's effects on uterine contractility may potentially increase risks for mating-induced endometritis. Some studies have shown that clenbuterol can impair reproductive funtion in males. (Kearns & McKeever 2009)

Pharmacokinetics

After oral administration to horses, peak plasma levels of clenbuterol occur 2 hours after administration and the average half-life is about 10–13 hours. The manufacturer states that the duration of effect varies from 6–8 hours. After multiple oral doses, the drug's volume of distribution is approximately 1.6 L/kg and clearance was 94 mL/kg/hr. Urinary concentrations of clenbuterol are approximately 100X those found in plasma and can persist at quantifiable levels for 288 hours (12 days) in urine after the last oral dose (Soma *et al.* 2004).

Contraindications/Precautions/Warnings

The drug is contraindicated in food producing animals (legal ramifications). The label states that the drug should not be used in horses suspected of having cardiovascular impairment as tachycardia may occur.

Adverse Effects

Muscle tremors, sweating, restlessness, urticaria, and tachycardia may be noted, particularly early in the course of therapy. Creatine kinase elevations have been noted in some horses and, rarely, ataxia can occur. Clenbuterol is reported to induce abortion in pregnant animals.

Clenbuterol has been touted in some body building circles as an alternative to anabolic steroids for muscle development and body fat reduction; however, its safe use for this purpose is in serious question. Be alert for scams to divert legitimately obtained clenbuterol for this purpose.

Reproductive/Nursing Safety

Clenbuterol's safety in breeding stallions and brood mares has not been established. Clenbuterol should not be used in pregnant mares near full-term as it antagonizes the effects of dinoprost (prostaglandin F2alpha) and oxytocin and can diminish normal uterine contractility.

Overdosage/Acute Toxicity

Some case reports of clenbuterol overdoses have been reported in various species. In recent years, clenbuterol has been used as an adulterant in illicit heroin. Depending on dosage and species, emptying gut may be appropriate, otherwise supportive therapy and administration of parenteral beta-blockers to control heart rate and rhythm and elevated blood pressure may be considered.

Drug Interactions

The following drug interactions have either been reported or are theoretical in humans or animals receiving clenbuterol and may be of significance in veterinary patients:

■ **ANESTHETICS, INHALANT:** Use with inhalation anesthetics (*e.g.*, **halothane, isoflurane, methoxyflurane**), may predispose the patient to ventricular arrhythmias, particularly in patients with preexisting cardiac disease—use cautiously

■ **BETA-BLOCKERS (*e.g.*, propranolol):** May antagonize clenbuterol's effects

■ **DIGOXIN:** Use with digitalis glycosides may increase the risk of cardiac arrhythmias

■ **DINOPROST:** Clenbuterol may antagonize the effects of dinoprost (prostaglandin F2alpha)

■ **OXYTOCIN:** Clenbuterol may antagonize the effects of oxytocin

■ **SYMPATHOMIMETIC AMINES, OTHER (*e.g.*, terbutaline, albuterol):** Concomitant administration with other sympathomimetic amines may enhance the adverse effects of clenbuterol

■ **TRICYCLIC ANTIDEPRESSANTS or MONOAMINE OXIDASE INHIBITORS:** May potentiate the vascular effects of clenbuterol

Doses

■ **HORSES: (Note:** ARCI UCGFS Class 3 Drug) As a bronchodilator:

a) Initially, 0.8 micrograms/kg (practically: 0.5 mL of the commercially available syrup/100 lb. BW) twice daily for 3 days; if no improvement increase to 1.6 micrograms/kg (practically: 1 mL of the commercially available syrup/100 lb. BW) twice daily for 3 days; if no improvement increase to 2.4 micrograms/kg (practically: 1.5 mL of the commercially available syrup/100 lb. BW) twice daily for 3 days; if no improvement increase to 3.2 micrograms/kg (practically: 2 mL of the commercially available syrup/100 lb. BW) twice daily for 3 days; if no improvement discontinue therapy. Recommended duration of therapy is 30 days; then withdraw therapy and reevaluate. If signs return, reinitiate therapy as above. (Package Insert; *Ventipulmin®*)

As adjunctive treatment for dystocia emergencies:

a) 300 micrograms per 500 kg mare IV slowly (Note: parenteral formulation not available commercially in the USA). The drug's fast onset of action when given IV allows veterinarian to decide quickly if uterine relaxation will correct the problem. Clenbuterol is particularly useful when repelling the equine fetus to allow manipulation of the head and limbs. May be used in combination with sedatives, analgesics and tranquilizers. Xyalazine and detomidine may potentiate uterine relaxant effects of clenbuterol. (Card 2002)

b) At the author's hospital: Upon arrival of a dystocia, on the clinician's orders the nurse administers 10 mls of clenbuterol syrup orally as the mare walks in the door. (McCafferty 2007)

Monitoring
- Clinical efficacy
- Adverse effects

Client Information
- Clients should be instructed on the restricted use requirements of this medication and to keep it secure from children or those who may "abuse" it.
- The drug may be prohibited from use by various equine associations (*e.g.*, racing or show).

Chemistry/Synonyms
A beta-2-adrenergic agonist, clenbuterol HCl's chemical name is 1-(4-Amino-3,5-dichlorophenyl)-2-tert-butyl aminoethanol HCl.

Clenbuterol HCl may also be known as: NAB-365, *Aeropulmin®*, *Broncodil®*, *Broncoterol®*, *Bronq-C®*, *Cesbron®*, *Clembumar®*, *Clenasma®*, *Clenbutol®*, *Contrasmina®*, *Contraspasmin®*, *Monores®*, *Novegam®*, *Oxibron®*, *Oxyflux®*, *Prontovent®*, *Spiropent®*, *Ventilan®*, *Ventipulmin®* or *Ventolase®*.

Storage/Stability
The commercially available syrup is colorless and should be stored at room temperature (avoid freezing). The manufacturer warns to replace the safety cap on the bottle when not in use.

Dosage Forms/Regulatory Status
VETERINARY-LABELED PRODUCTS:
Clenbuterol HCl Oral Syrup: 72.5 micrograms/mL in 100 mL, 330 mL, 460 mL bottles; *Ventipulmin® Syrup* (Boehringer Ingelheim); *Aeropulmin® Syrup* (Butler, Phoenix); (Rx). FDA-approved for use in horses not intended for use as food.

Extra-label clenbuterol use in food animals is prohibited by federal (USA) law.

The ARCI (Racing Commissioners International) has designated this drug as a class 3 substance. See the appendix for more information.

HUMAN-LABELED PRODUCTS: None

References
Card, C (2002). Dystocia in mares. *Large Animal Veterinary Rounds* 2(4).
Ferraz, GC, AR Teixeira–Neto, et al. (2007). Effect of acute administration of Clenbuterol on athletic performance in horses. *Journal of Equine Veterinary Science* 27(10): 446–449.
Kearns, CF & KH McKeever (2009). Clenbuterol and the horse revisited. *Veterinary Journal* 182(3): 384–391.
McCafferty, K (2007). Nursing's role in equine dystocia. Proceedings: IVECCS. Accessed via: Veterinary Information Network. http://goo.gl/FzsDz
Soma, L, C Uboh, et al. (2004). Pharmacokinetics and disposition of clenbuterol in the horse. *J Vet Phamacol Ther* 27: 71–77.

CLINDAMYCIN HCL
CLINDAMYCIN PALMITATE HCL
CLINDAMYCIN PHOSPHATE

(klin-da-*mye*-sin)   Antirobe®, Cleocin®

LINCOSAMIDE ANTIBIOTIC

Prescriber Highlights

▶ Lincosamide antibiotic, broad spectrum against many anaerobes, gram-positive aerobic cocci, Toxoplasma, etc.

▶ Contraindications: Horses, rodents, ruminants, lagomorphs; patients hypersensitive to lincosamides

▶ Caution: Liver or renal dysfunction; consider reducing dosage if severe

▶ Adverse Effects: gastroenteritis, esophageal injuries possible if "dry pilled," pain at injection site if given IM

Uses/Indications
Clindamycin products are FDA-approved for use in dogs and cats. The labeled indications for dogs include wounds, abscesses and osteomyelitis caused by *Staphylococcus aureus*. Because clindamycin has excellent activity against most pathogenic anaerobic organisms, it is also used extensively for those infections. Clindamycin is used for a variety of protozoal infections, including toxoplasmosis. For further information, refer to the Dosage or Pharmacology sections.

Pharmacology/Actions
The lincosamide antibiotics, lincomycin and clindamycin, share mechanisms of action and have similar spectrums of activity, although lincomycin is usually less active against susceptible organisms. Complete cross-resistance occurs between the two drugs; at least partial cross-resistance occurs between the lincosamides and

erythromycin. They may act as bacteriostatic or bactericidal agents, depending on the concentration of the drug at the infection site and the susceptibility of the organism. The lincosamides are believed to act by binding to the 50S ribosomal subunit of susceptible bacteria, thereby inhibiting peptide bond formation.

Most aerobic gram-positive cocci are susceptible to the lincosamides (*Strep. faecalis* is not) including Staphylococcus and Streptococci. Other organisms that are generally susceptible include: *Corynebacterium diphtheriae, Nocardia asteroides,* Erysepelothrix, Toxoplasma, and *Mycoplasma* spp. Anaerobic bacteria that are generally susceptible to the lincosamides include: *Clostridium perfringens, C. tetani* (not *C. difficile*), Bacteroides (including many strains of *B. fragilis*), Fusobacterium, Peptostreptococcus, Actinomyces, and Peptococcus.

Pharmacokinetics

In dogs, oral bioavailability is about 73%, elimination half-life is reportedly 2–5 hours after oral administration and 10–13 hours after subcutaneous administration. Volume of distribution is about 0.9 L/kg.

In humans, the drug is rapidly absorbed from the gut and about 90% of the total dose is absorbed. Food decreases the rate of absorption, but not the extent. Peak serum levels are attained about 45–60 minutes after oral dosing. IM administration gives peak levels about 1–3 hours post injection.

Clindamycin is distributed into most tissues. Therapeutic levels are achieved in bone, synovial fluid, bile, pleural fluid, peritoneal fluid, skin, and heart muscle. Clindamycin also penetrates well into abscesses, scar tissue, and white blood cells. CNS levels may reach 40% of those in the serum if meninges are inflamed. Clindamycin is about 93% bound to plasma proteins. The drug crosses the placenta and can be distributed into milk at concentrations equal to those in plasma.

Clindamycin is partially metabolized in the liver to both active and inactive metabolites. Unchanged drug and metabolites are excreted in the urine, feces, and bile. Half-lives can be prolonged in patients with severe renal or hepatic dysfunction.

Contraindications/Precautions/Warnings

Although there have been case reports of parenteral administration of lincosamides to horses, cattle, and sheep, the lincosamides are considered to be contraindicated for use in rabbits, hamsters, chinchillas, guinea pigs, horses, and ruminants because of serious gastrointestinal effects that may occur, including death. Clindamycin is contraindicated in patients with known hypersensitivity to it or lincomycin.

Clindamycin has been implicated in causing esophagitis and potentially, esophageal strictures in small animals. Avoid dry "pilling" when administering this drug.

Patients with very severe renal and/or hepatic disease should receive the drug with caution and the manufacturer suggests monitoring serum clindamycin levels during high-dose therapy; consider dosage reduction.

Clindamycin use is generally avoided in neonatal small animals.

Adverse Effects

Adverse effects after oral administration reported in dogs and cats include gastroenteritis (emesis, loose stools, and infrequently bloody diarrhea in dogs). There have been case reports of esophageal injuries (esophagitis, strictures) occurring in cats when solid dosage forms were given without food or a water bolus. Cats may occasional show hypersalivation or lip smacking after oral administration. IM injections reportedly cause pain at the injection site.

C. difficile–associated pseudomembranous colitis has been reported in some species, but does not appear to be a significant risk when clindamycin is used in dogs or cats.

Reproductive/Nursing Safety

Clindamycin crosses the placenta, and cord blood concentrations are approximately 46% of those found in maternal serum. Safe use during pregnancy has not been established, but neither has the drug been implicated in causing teratogenic effects. In humans, the FDA categorizes this drug as category *B* for use during pregnancy (*Animal studies have not yet demonstrated risk to the fetus, but there are no adequate studies in pregnant women; or animal studies have shown an adverse effect, but adequate studies in pregnant women have not demonstrated a risk to the fetus in the first trimester of pregnancy, and there is no evidence of risk in later trimesters.*) In a separate system evaluating the safety of drugs in canine and feline pregnancy (Papich 1989), this drug is categorized as in class: *A* (*Probably safe. Although specific studies may not have proved the safety of all drugs in dogs and cats, there are no reports of adverse effects in laboratory animals or women.*)

Because clindamycin is distributed into milk, nursing puppies or kittens of mothers receiving clindamycin may develop diarrhea. However, in humans, the American Academy of Pediatrics considers clindamycin compatible with breastfeeding.

Overdosage/Acute Toxicity

There is little information available regarding overdoses of this drug. In dogs, oral doses of up to 300 mg/kg/day for up to one year did not result in toxicity. Dogs receiving 600 mg/kg/day, developed anorexia, vomiting, and weight loss.

Drug Interactions

The following drug interactions have either been reported or are theoretical in humans or animals receiving clindamycin and may be of significance in veterinary patients:

- ■ **CYCLOSPORINE:** Clindamycin may reduce levels

- **ERYTHROMYCIN:** *in vitro* antagonism when used with clindamycin; concomitant use should probably be avoided

- **NEUROMUSCULAR BLOCKING AGENTS** (*e.g.,* **pancuronium**): Clindamycin possesses intrinsic neuromuscular blocking activity and should be used cautiously with other neuromuscular blocking agents

Laboratory Considerations

- Slight increases in **liver function tests** (AST, ALT, Alk. Phosph.) may occur. There is apparently not any clinical significance associated with these increases.

Doses

- **DOGS:**

  For susceptible bacterial infections:

  a) For infected wounds, abscesses and dental infections: 5.5–33 mg/kg PO q12h; for osteomyelitis: 11–33 mg/kg PO q12h. Treatment may continue for up to 28 days. If no response after 3–4 days, discontinue. (Package insert; *Antirobe®*—Pfizer)

  b) For staphylococcal pyoderma: 11 mg/kg PO once daily for 7–28 days

    For wounds, abscesses, dental infections, stomatitis: 5–11 mg/kg PO q12h for 7–28 days.

    For osteomyelitis: 11 mg/kg PO q12h for 28 days

    For systemic, bacteremia: 3–10 mg/kg IV, IM SC, PO q8h as long as needed (Greene & Watson 1998)

  c) 5–11 mg/kg IM, SC or PO q12h avoid or reduce dose in patients with severe liver failure (Vaden & Papich 1995)

  d) For sepsis: 11 mg/kg IV q12h (Hardie 2000)

  e) For recurrent superficial pyodermas: 11 mg/kg PO once daily to twice a day; resistance can develop quickly (Logas 2005)

  f) For actinomycosis: 5 mg/kg SC q12h (Edwards 2006)

  g) For susceptible hepatobiliary infections: 10–16 mg/kg SC once daily or 5–10 mg/kg PO q12h. In patients with liver function impairment: 5 mg/kg PO q12h or SC q24h (Center 2006)

  h) For anaerobic infections: 5–10 mg/kg PO, IV q12h (Greene & Jang 2006a)

  i) For intra-abdominal sepsis 5–11 mg/kg IV, SC, PO q8–12h for 5–7 days combined with gentamicin or a parenteral 3rd generation cephalosporin (such as cefotaxime) or enrofloxacin.

    For pancreatitis: 5–11 mg/kg IV, SC, PO q8–12h for 3–5 days. (Greene 2006)

  j) For susceptible respiratory infections: 10 mg/kg PO, SC q12h (Greene & Reinero 2006)

  k) For surgical prophylaxis for gram-positive aerobes and anaerobic coverage: 5–11 mg/kg PO 16–60 minutes preoperatively (Greene & Jang 2006b)

  For susceptible protozoal infections:

  a) For Toxoplasmosis: 12.5 mg/kg PO or IM q12h for 28 days

    For Neospora: 10 mg/kg q12h for 4 weeks. Used concurrently with trimethoprim/sulfa (15 mg/kg PO q12h for 4 weeks)

    For *Hepatozoon canis*: 10 mg/kg PO q8h for 2–4 weeks. Use concurrently with pyrimethamine (0.25 mg/kg PO once daily for 2–4 weeks) and trimethoprim/sulfa (15 mg/kg PO q12h for 2–4 weeks)

    For *Babesia* spp.: 12.5 mg/kg q12h PO for 2 weeks (Lappin 2000)

  b) For Babesia infections if specific antibabesial drugs (*e.g.,* diminazene, imidocarb, pentamidine) are not available: 25 mg/kg PO q12h for 7–21 days (Taboada & Lobetti 2006)

  c) For *Hepatozoon americanum* infections: 10 mg/kg PO q8h for 14 days. Use concurrently with trimethoprim/sulfa (15 mg/kg PO q12h 14 days) and pyrimethamine (0.25 mg/kg PO once daily for 14 days) and then follow with decoquinate (for 2 years) once clinical signs have resolved. (Macintire *et al.* 2006)

- **CATS:**

  For susceptible bacterial infections:

  a) 5–10 mg/kg PO q12h (Jenkins 1987b); (Trepanier 1999)

  b) For infected wounds, abscesses and dental infections: 11–33 mg/kg PO once a day (q24h). Do not treat acute infections for more than 3–4 days if no clinical response is seen. Maximum labeled treatment period = 14 days (Package insert; *Antirobe®*—Pfizer)

  c) For sepsis: 11 mg/kg IV q12h (Hardie 2000)

  d) For anaerobic infections: 5–10 mg/kg PO, IV q12h (Greene & Jang 2006a)

  e) For intra-abdominal sepsis 5–11 mg/kg IV, SC, PO q8–12h for 5–7 days combined with gentamicin or a parenteral 3rd generation cephalosporin (such as cefotaxime) or enrofloxacin.

    For pancreatitis: 5–11 mg/kg IV, SC, PO q8–12h for 3–5 days. (Greene 2006)

  f) For susceptible respiratory infections: 10–15 mg/kg PO, SC q12h (Greene & Reinero 2006)

  g) For surgical prophylaxis for gram-positive aerobes and anaerobic coverage: 5–11 mg/kg PO 16–60 minutes preoperatively (Greene & Jang 2006b)

For susceptible protozoal infections:

a) Toxoplasmosis:

To decrease zoonotic risk to susceptible humans by reducing shedding period in cats suspected of toxoplasmosis after fecal exam: 25–50 mg/kg PO daily; alternative medications include sulfonamides at 100 mg/kg PO daily, or pyrimethamine at 2 mg/kg daily PO.

For treatment of clinical toxoplasmosis: Clindamycin at 10 mg/kg PO q12h, trimethoprim-sulfonamide combination at 15 mg/kg PO q12h, and azithromycin at 10 mg/kg once daily for at least 28 days. Institute supportive care as needed. Patients with uveitis should receive topical, oral or parenteral glucocorticoids to reduce risk for secondary glaucoma and lens luxations. (Lappin 2004)

b) For enteroepithelial toxoplasmosis: 8–16 mg/kg PO or SC q8h for 14–28 days.

For systemic toxoplasmosis: 12.5–25 mg/kg PO or SC q12h for 14–28 days (Greene & Watson 1998)

■ **FERRETS:**

For susceptible infections:

a) 5–10 mg/kg PO twice daily (Williams 2000)

■ **BIRDS:**

For susceptible infections:

a) 25 mg/kg PO q8h (Tully 2002)

b) For mild spore-forming enteric bacterial infections: 50 mg/kg PO q12h for 5–10 days (Flammer 2006)

■ **REPTILES:**

For susceptible infections (anaerobes):

a) 5 mg/kg PO once daily (Lewbart 2001)

b) For respiratory infections (anaerobes, mycoplasma): 5 mg/kg PO once daily for 14 days (Klaphake 2005)

Monitoring

■ Clinical efficacy

■ Adverse effects; particularly severe diarrhea

■ Manufacturer recommends doing periodic liver and kidney function tests and blood counts if therapy persists for more than 30 days

Client Information

■ Clients should be instructed to report the incidence of severe, protracted, or bloody diarrhea to the veterinarian

■ If using oral tablets or capsules, especially in cats, give medication followed by at least 6 mL (a little more than a teaspoonful) of liquid

Chemistry/Synonyms

A semisynthetic derivative of lincomycin, clindamycin is available as the hydrochloride hydrate, phosphate ester, and palmitate hydrochloride. Potency of all three salts is expressed as milligrams of clindamycin. The hydrochloride occurs as a white to practically white, crystalline powder. The phosphate occurs as a white to off-white, hygroscopic crystalline powder. The palmitate HCl occurs as a white to off-white amorphous powder. All may have a faint characteristic odor and are freely soluble in water. With the phosphate, about 400 mg are soluble in one mL of water. Clindamycin has a pK_a of 7.45. The commercially available injection has a pH of 5.5–7.

Clindamycin HCl may also be known as: chlorodeoxylincomycin hydrochloride, (7S)-chloro-7-deoxy-lincomycin hydrochloride, clindamycini hydrochloridum, U-28508, or U-25179E; many trade names are available.

Storage/Stability

Clindamycin capsules and the palmitate powder for oral solution should be stored at room temperature (15–30°C). After reconstitution, the palmitate oral solution (human-product) should not be refrigerated or thickening may occur. It is stable for 2 weeks at room temperature. The veterinary oral solution should be stored at room temperature and has an extended shelf life.

Clindamycin phosphate injection should be stored at room temperature. If refrigerated or frozen, crystals may form which resolubolize upon warming.

Compatibility/Compounding Considerations

Clindamycin for injection is reportedly **compatible** for at least 24 hours in the following IV infusion solutions: D_5W, Dextrose combinations with Ringer's, lactated Ringer's, sodium chloride, $D_{10}W$, sodium chloride 0.9%, Ringer's injection, and lactated Ringer's injection. Clindamycin for injection is reportedly **compatible** with the following drugs: amikacin sulfate, ampicillin sodium, aztreonam, carbenicillin disodium, cefazolin sodium, cefonicid sodium, cefoperazone sodium, cefotaxime sodium, ceftazidime sodium, ceftizoxime sodium, cefuroxime sodium, cimetidine HCl, gentamicin sulfate, heparin sodium, hydrocortisone sodium succinate, kanamycin sulfate, methylprednisolone sodium succinate, magnesium sulfate, meperidine HCl, metoclopramide HCl, metronidazole, morphine sulfate, penicillin G potassium/sodium, piperacillin sodium, potassium chloride, sodium bicarbonate, tobramycin HCl (not in syringes), verapamil HCl, and vitamin B-complex with C.

Drugs that are reportedly **incompatible** with clindamycin include: aminophylline, ciprofloxacin, ranitidine HCl, and ceftriaxone sodium. Compatibility is dependent upon factors such as pH, concentration, temperature, and diluent used; consult specialized references or a hospital pharmacist for more specific information.

Dosage Forms/Regulatory Status

VETERINARY-LABELED PRODUCTS:

Clindamycin (as the HCl) Oral Capsules: 25 mg, 75 mg, 150 mg, 300 mg; *Antirobe® Capsules* (Pfizer) FDA-approved for use in dogs and cats. Generics also available in 25 mg, 75 mg, 150 mg, and 300 mg capsules; (Rx). FDA-approved for use in dogs.

Clindamycin (as the HCl) Oral Tablets: 25 mg, 75 mg, 150 mg; *Clintabs®* (Virbac); (Rx). FDA-approved for use in dogs.

Clindamycin (as the HCl) Oral Solution 25 mg/mL in 30 mL bottles. *Antirobe® Aquadrops* (Pfizer), *Clinsol®* (Virbac); generic; (Rx). FDA-approved for use in dogs and cats.

HUMAN-LABELED PRODUCTS:

Clindamycin (as the HCl) Oral Capsules: 75 mg, 150 mg, & 300 mg; *Cleocin®* (Pfizer); generic; (Rx)

Clindamycin (as the palmitate HCl) Granules for Oral Solution: 75 mg/5 mL in 100 mL; *Cleocin® Pediatric* (Pfizer); (Rx)

Clindamycin (as the Phosphate) Solution Concentrate for Injection: 150 mg/mL in 2 mL, 4 mL, 6 mL & 2 mL, 4 mL and 6 mL *ADD-Vantage* vials; *Cleocin® Phosphate* (Pharmacia & Upjohn); generic; (Rx)

Clindamycin (as the Phosphate) Injection: 300 mg, 600 mg & 900 mg in 50 mL *Galaxy* containers with dextrose 5%; *Cleocin Phosphate IV®*(Pharmacia & Upjohn) (Rx)

Clindamycin Phosphate Suppositories: 100 mg (as base) *Cleocin®* (Pfizer); (Rx)

Also available in topical and vaginal preparations.

References

Center, S (2006). Hepatobiliary infections. *Infectious Diseases of the Dog and Cat, 3rd Ed.* C Greene Ed., Elsevier: 912–935.

Edwards, D (2006). Actinomycosis and nocardiosis. *Infectious Diseases of the Dog and Cat, 3rd Ed.* C Greene Ed., Elsevier: 451–461.

Flammer, K (2006). Managing Avian Bacterial Diseases II. Proceedings: WVC2006. Accessed via: Veterinary Information Network. http://goo.gl/wPvdh

Greene, C (2006). Gastrointestinal and Intraabdominal Infections. *Infectious Diseases of the Dog and Cat, 3rd Ed.* C Greene Ed., Elsevier: 883–912.

Greene, C & S Jang (2006a). Anaerobic infections. *Infectious Diseases of the Dog and Cat, 3rd Ed.* C Greene Ed., Elsevier: 380–388.

Greene, C & S Jang (2006b). Surgical and traumatic wound infections. *Infectious Diseases of the Dog and Cat, 3rd Ed.* C Greene Ed., Elsevier: 524–531.

Greene, C & C Reinero (2006). Bacterial Respiratory Infections. *Infectious Diseases of the Dog and Cat, 3rd Ed.* C Greene Ed., Elsevier: 866–882.

Greene, C & A Watson (1998). Antimicrobial Drug Formulary. *Infectious Diseases of the Dog and Cat.* C Greene Ed. Philadelphia, WB Saunders: 790–919.

Hardie, E (2000). Therapeutic Mangement of Sepsis. *Kirk's Current Veterinary Therapy: XIII Small Animal Practice.* J Bonagura Ed. Philadelphia, WB Saunders: 272–275.

Klaphake, E (2005). Sneezing turtles and wheezing snakes. Proceedings: Western Vet Conf. Accessed via: Veterinary Information Network. http://goo.gl/ILwoc

Lappin, M (2000). Protozoal and Miscellaneous Infections.

Textbook of Veterinary Internal Medicine: Diseases of the Dog and Cat. S Ettinger and E Feldman Eds. Philadelphia, WB Saunders. 1: 408–417.

Lappin, M (2004). Toxoplasmosis. Proceedings: WSAVA World Congress. Accessed via: Veterinary Information Network. http://goo.gl/N54X3

Lewbart (2001). Reptile Formulary. Proceedings: Atlantic Coast Veterinary Conference. Accessed via: Veterinary Information Network. http://goo.gl/EEQmM

Logas, D (2005). Superficial and Deep Pyoderma. Proceedings: Western Veterinary Conf. Accessed via: Veterinary Information Network. http://goo.gl/qMbzy

Macintire, D, N Vincent–Johnson, et al. (2006). Hepatazooan americanum Infection. *Infectious Diseases of the Dog and Cat, 3rd Ed.* C Greene Ed., Elsevier: 705–711.

Taboada, J & R Lobetti (2006). Babesia. *Infectious Diseases of the Dog and Cat, 3rd Ed.* C Greene Ed., Elsevier: 722–736.

Trepanier, L (1999). Treating resistant infections in small animals. Proceedings: 17th Annual American College of Veterinary Internal Medicine Meeting, Chicago.

Tully, T (2002). Avian Therapeutic Options. Proceedings: Western Veterinary Conference. Accessed via: Veterinary Information Network. http://goo.gl/7E5ce

Vaden, S & M Papich (1995). Empiric Antibiotic Therapy. Kirk's Current *Veterinary Therapy:XII.* J Bonagura Ed. Philadelphia, W.B. Saunders: 276–280.

Williams, B (2000). Therapeutics in Ferrets. *Vet Clin NA: Exotic Anim Pract* 3:1(Jan): 131–153.

CLOFAZIMINE

(kloe-*fa*-zi-meen)   Lamprene®

ANTIMYCOBACTERIAL ANTIBIOTIC

Prescriber Highlights

▶ May be difficult for veterinarians to obtain & accurately dose

▶ Antimycobacterial antibiotic that may be used as part of multi-drug therapy for leprosy-like or M. avium-related diseases in small animals

▶ Very limited clinical experience & documentation supporting its use in veterinary patients

▶ Skin, eye, excretion staining noted & dose limiting gastrointestinal adverse effects

▶ Treatment usually must continue for weeks to months

Uses/Indications

In small animals, clofazimine is sometimes used as part of multi-drug therapy against mycobacterial diseases, primarily leprosy-like or *M. avium*-related disease states.

In humans, clofazimine is used primarily as part of a multi-drug regimen in the treatment of all forms of leprosy (with rifampin and dapsone), or the treatment of Mycobacterium avium complex (MAC) (with at least two of the following agents: clarithromycin or azithromycin, rifampin or rifabutin, and ethambutol). It has also been used in some treatment regimens for Crohn's disease, pyoderma gangrenosum, etc.

Pharmacology/Actions

Clofazimine binds to mycobacterial DNA and inhibits growth. It is considered to be slowly bactericidal against susceptible organisms. Clofazimine has activity against a variety of mycobacteria including: *M. leprae, M. tuberculosis, M. avium* complex (MAC), *M. bovis,* and *M. chelonei.* Resistance is thought to occur only rarely; cross-resistance with dapsone or rifampin apparently does not occur. Clofazimine may have some antileishmanial activity. Clofazimine has antiinflammatory and immunosuppressive effects, but the mechanisms of action for these effects are not understood.

Pharmacokinetics

Clofazimine's pharmacokinetics have apparently not been determined in domestic animals. In humans, the microcrystalline form of the drug is variably absorbed after oral administration; bioavailability ranges from 45–70%. Food enhances absorption but increasing the dosage decreases the percentage absorbed. Clofazimine is highly lipid soluble and is distributed primarily to lipid tissue and the reticuloendothelial system. Throughout the body macrophages take up clofazimine. The drug crosses the placenta and is distributed into milk, but does not apparently cross into the CNS or CSF. Clofazimine is retained in the body for a long period; its elimination half-life is at least 70 days long. Bile excretion may be responsible for the majority of the drug's excretion, but excretion in sputum, sebum, and sweat may also contribute.

Contraindications/Precautions/Warnings

It is suggested that clofazimine be used with caution in patients with pre-existing gastrointestinal conditions such as diarrhea or abdominal pain.

Adverse Effects

There is very limited clinical experience with this medication in domestic animals and its adverse effect profile is not well documented. Apparently, the skin, eye, and excretion discoloration (described below) also occurs in animals. Gastrointestinal effects have been reported. One case of a dog receiving clofazimine and rifampin to treat canine leproid granuloma resulted in hepatotoxicity. There is a report of one cat treated with clofazimine developing a photosensitization reaction (Bennett 2007).

In humans, clofazimine is usually well tolerated, particularly at dosages of 100 mg/day or less. The most troubling adverse effect in many patients is the dose-related skin, eye, and body fluid discoloration (pink to brownish-black) that occurs in most patients, as it may cause severe psychosocial effects; other drug regimens, not including clofazimine, are often chosen in patients with light skin color. This discoloration can persist for months to years after clofazimine has been discontinued. In dosages greater than 100 mg/day, gastrointestinal effects (pain, nau-sea, vomiting, diarrhea) become more likely and often limit the dosage that can be administered. Other adverse effects (CNS, increased liver enzymes, etc.) are reported in less than 1% of patients receiving the drug.

Reproductive/Nursing Safety

In humans, the FDA categorizes clofazimine as a category *C* drug for use during pregnancy (*Animal studies have shown an adverse effect on the fetus, but there are no adequate studies in humans; or there are no animal reproduction studies and no adequate studies in humans*). Very large doses (12–25X) demonstrated no teratogenic effects in rats or rabbits, but some effects were noted in mice. The World Health Organization (WHO) states that the drug is safe to use during pregnancy when used as part of one of their treatment protocols for leprosy.

Clofazimine does enter maternal milk and skin discoloration of nursing offspring can occur.

Overdosage/Acute Toxicity

Very limited data is available; the LD_{50} for rabbits is 3.3 g/kg and is greater than 5 g/kg in mice, rats, and guinea pigs. Treatment, if required, would include gut emptying and supportive care. Contact an animal poison control center for additional guidance.

Drug Interactions

The following drug interactions have either been reported or are theoretical in humans or animals receiving clofazimine and may be of significance in veterinary patients:

- **ISONIAZID:** May reduce the clofazimine levels in the skin and increase the amounts in plasma and urine; clinical significance unclear

- **DAPSONE:** There is sketchy evidence that suggests dapsone may reduce the antiinflammatory effects of clofazimine; clinical significance unclear

Laboratory Considerations

- No clofazimine-related laboratory interactions noted

Doses

- **DOGS:**

  For *Mycobacterium avium* complex (MAC) as part of a multi-drug regimen:
  a) 4 mg/kg PO once daily. Other drugs that may be used in combination include doxycycline, clarithromycin, and/or enrofloxacin. (Greene & Gunn-Moore 1998)

  For *M. avium intracellularae* complex infections, leprosy, or opportunistic mycobacteriosis:
  a) 4–8 mg/kg PO once a day for 4 weeks usually as part of a multi-drug protocol. (Greene & Watson 1998)

- **CATS:**

  For treatment of feline leprosy:

a) Using a regimen of either two or three of the following drugs: clarithromycin: 62.5 mg per cat q12h, clofazimine: 25-50 mg once per day or 50 mg every other day, Rifampin: 10-15 mg/kg once a day. (Malik *et al.* 2002)

For treatment of localized atypical mycobacterial infections:

a) Perform wide surgical excision of lesion if possible. Give long-term systemic antibacterial therapy, continued at least 4 weeks beyond complete clinical resolution. Base antibiotic selection on culture and susceptibility results, if available: Clofazimine 8 mg/kg PO once daily. Other doses listed in reference for marbofloxacin, doxycycline, minocycline, or clarithromycin. (Hnilica 2003)

For *M. avium intracellularae* complex infections, leprosy or opportunistic mycobacteriosis:

a) 4-8 mg/kg PO once a day for 4 weeks usually as part of a multi-drug protocol. (Greene & Watson 1998)

■ **BIRDS:**

For avian mycobacteriosis:

a) Treatment protocols include: **1**) rifampin 45 mg/kg, ethambutol 30 mg/kg and clofazimine 6 mg/kg PO once daily; or **2**) ethambutol 20 mg/kg, cycloserine 5 mg/kg, enrofloxacin 15 mg/kg q12h plus clofazimine 1.5 mg/kg PO q24h (recommended regime for raptors). Regular monitoring of fecal samples is needed; antifungal medication may be required. Surgery for discrete nodules may be curative. (Turner 2008)

Monitoring
■ Efficacy against mycobacterial disease
■ Adverse effects (primarily GI, but consider monitoring hepatic function in dogs)

Client Information
■ Unless otherwise instructed give this medication with food
■ This medication may cause your animal's skin to turn color (usually pink, but from red to orange to brown). It may also cause discoloring of tears, urine, feces, and other body fluids to a brownish-black color. This discoloration may persist for many months after therapy is concluded.

Chemistry/Synonyms
Clofazimine, a phenazine dye antimycobacterial agent, occurs as an odorless or nearly odorless, reddish-brown powder that is highly insoluble in water. In room temperature alcohol, clofazimine's solubility is 1 mg/mL.

Clofazimine may also be known as: B-663, G-30320, NSC-141046, Chlofazimine, *Clofozine®, Hansepran®, Lamcoin®, Lamprene®,* or *Lampren®.*

Storage/Stability
Clofazimine oral capsules should be stored in tight containers, protected from moisture at temperatures less than 30°C.

Compatibility/Compounding Considerations
The commercially available capsules are a micronized form of the drug in a wax matrix base; it may be difficult to obtain an accurate dosage for small animals. It is suggested to contact a compounding pharmacist for advice.

Dosage Forms/Regulatory Status

VETERINARY-LABELED PRODUCTS: None
HUMAN-LABELED PRODUCTS: None

In November 2004, clofazimine (*Lamprene®*) became available in the USA only on a limited basis. The FDA now restricts its use to physicians enrolled as investigators under an Investigational New Drug (IND) for treating Hansen's Disease (Leprosy) or multi-drug resistant tuberculosis. Its status for use in veterinary patients is uncertain at the time of writing; contact the FDA Center for Veterinary Medicine (see appendix) for more information.

References

Bennett, SL (2007). Photosensitisation induced by clofazimine in a cat. *Australian Veterinary Journal* 85(9): 375–380.

Greene, C & D Gunn–Moore (1998). Mycobacterial Infections: Tuberculosis mycobacterial infections. *Infectious Diseases of the Dog and Cat.* C Greene Ed. Philadelphia, Saunders: 313–325.

Greene, C & A Watson (1998). Antimicrobial Drug Formulary. *Infectious Diseases of the Dog and Cat.* C Greene Ed. Philadelphia, WB Saunders: 790–919.

Hnilica, K (2003). Atypical presentations in feline dermatology. Proceedings: Western Veterinary Conf. Accessed via: Veterinary Information Network. http://goo.gl/Brs6Q

Malik, R, M Hughes, et al. (2002). Feline Leprosy – two different clinical syndromes. *J Feline Med Surg* 4(1): 43–59.

Turner, K (2008). A review of avian mycobacteriosis. Proceedings: AAVAC–UEP. Accessed via: Veterinary Information Network. http://goo.gl/RVaNm

CLOMIPRAMINE HCL

(kloe-*mi*-pra-meen)
Clomicalm®, Anafranil®

TRICYCLIC ANTIDEPRESSANT

Prescriber Highlights

▶ Tricyclic antidepressant used in dogs & cats for obsessive compulsive disorders, but may be useful for other behavior disorders

▶ Used in birds to treat feather picking

▶ Caution: Seizure disorders, liver disease, cardiac rate/rhythm disorders, urinary retention or reduced GI motility

▶ Not a teratogen, but may affect testicular size/function

▶ Adverse Effects: Emesis, diarrhea, sedation, anticholinergic effects (dry mouth, tachycardia, etc.); cats may be more sensitive than dogs

Uses/Indications

In veterinary medicine, clomipramine is used primarily in dogs as a treatment for obsessive-compulsive disorders (ritualistic stereotypical behaviors) and may be useful for dominance aggression and anxiety (separation).

Clomipramine may also be useful in cats, particularly for behaviors such as urine spraying. One prospective, double-blinded controlled study in cats with psychogenic alopecia comparing clomipramine (0.5 mg/kg PO daily) versus placebo showed no statistic differences in study parameters (Mertens *et al.* 2006).

Clomipramine has been used to treat feather picking in birds.

Pharmacology/Actions

While the exact mechanism of action of tricyclic antidepressants is not completely understood, it is believed that their most significant effects result from their action in preventing the reuptake of norepinephrine and serotonin at the neuronal membrane. Clomipramine is predominantly an inhibitor of serotonin (5-HT) reuptake, but it also has effects on other neurotransmitters. Clomipramine's active metabolite, desmethylclomipramine has primarily noradrenergic activity and, at least in humans, may be responsible for the majority of the drug's adverse effects.

Pharmacokinetics

In dogs, after absorption, clomipramine is rapidly converted in the liver to its active metabolite desmethylclomipramine. Both the parent drug and the active metabolite are highly bound to plasma proteins (96%). Repeated oral dosing increases clomipramine concentrations but not desmethylclomipramine. The presence of food decreases the area under the curve for the parent compound by about 25% but not the metabo-lite. Giving without food probably is not necessary for efficacy. After a single dose in dogs, the elimination half-life of clomipramine averages 5 hours.

Cats appear to metabolize clomipramine more slowly than dogs and wide interpatient variability in pharmacokinetic parameters have been shown after single oral doses. Male cats may metabolize clomipramine more slowly than female cats. In a limited (6 subject) pharmacokinetic study, oral bioavailability averaged 90%.

In humans, the drug is well absorbed from the GI tract but a substantial first pass effect reduces its systemic bioavailability to approximately 50%. The presence of food in the gut apparently does not significantly alter its absorption.

Clomipramine is highly lipophilic and widely distributed throughout the body with an apparent volume of distribution of 17 L/kg. The drug crosses the placenta and into maternal milk. Plasma levels have been detected in nursing babies of mothers taking the drug. Both clomipramine and its active metabolite (desmethylclomipramine) cross the blood-brain barrier and significant levels are found in the brain. It should be noted that although therapeutic effects may take several weeks to be seen, adverse effects can occur early on in treatment.

Clomipramine is metabolized principally in the liver to several metabolites including desmethylclomipramine, which is active. About two-thirds of these metabolites are eliminated in the urine and the rest in the feces. After a single dose, the elimination half-life of clomipramine averages 32 hours and desmethylclomipramine averages 69 hours, but there remains wide interpatient variation.

Contraindications/Precautions/Warnings

These agents are contraindicated if prior sensitivity has been noted with any other tricyclic. Concomitant use with monoamine oxidase inhibitors is generally contraindicated. As aged cheeses can contain high levels of tyramine, avoid giving to animals receiving clomipramine.

In humans, these drugs (tricyclic antidepressants) may lower seizure threshold. Use with caution in animals with preexisting seizure disorders. Because of their anticholinergic effects, use with caution in patients with decreased GI motility, urinary retention, cardiac rhythm disturbances, or increased intraocular pressure. One study in dogs however, showed little effect on intra-ocular pressure or cardiac rhythm. In humans, tricyclic antidepressants have caused hepatic abnormalities. Baseline and annual monitoring of liver enzymes is suggested for animals receiving clomipramine long-term. Tricyclics should be used cautiously in patients with hyperthyroidism or those that are receiving thyroid supplementation as there may be an increased risk of cardiac rhythm abnormalities developing.

Adverse Effects

The primary adverse effects reported thus far with the use of clomipramine in dogs are anorexia, emesis, diarrhea, elevation of liver enzymes, and sedation/lethargy/depression. At therapeutic dosages dogs rarely develop anticholinergic (dry mouth, etc.) effects. Cardiac effects such as tachycardia secondary to the drugs anticholinergic activity may also result. One case of a dog developing pancreatitis after receiving clomipramine has been published (Kook *et al.* 2009).

Cats have been reported to be more susceptible to the adverse effects (anticholinergic effects, sedation) of clomipramine than dogs. This may be the result of slower elimination of the desmethyl metabolite in cats.

Adverse effects reported in birds include ataxia, drowsiness, and regurgitation.

Reproductive/Nursing Safety

No teratogenic effects were noted in mice and rats given clomipramine at dosages of up 20X usual maximum human dosage. Data in other domestic species appear to be lacking. The manufacturer warns not to use in breeding male dogs as high dose (12.5X) toxicity studies demonstrated testicular atrophy.

In humans, the FDA categorizes this drug as category *C* for use during pregnancy (*Animal studies have shown an adverse effect on the fetus, but there are no adequate studies in humans; or there are no animal reproduction studies and no adequate studies in humans.*)

Overdosage/Acute Toxicity

Clomipramine has a narrow margin of safety; significant clinical signs can be seen at or slightly above therapeutic range (at 2–3 mg/kg, APCC database). Overdosage with tricyclics can be life-threatening (arrhythmias, seizures, cardiorespiratory collapse). In dogs, lethal doses are approximately between 50 and 100 mg/kg/day PO (12.5–25X recommended dose).

There were 158 exposures to clomipramine reported to the ASPCA Animal Poison Control Center (APCC) during 2008-2009. In these cases, 112 were dogs with 40 showing clinical signs and the remaining 46 cases were cats with 22 showing clinical signs. Common findings in dogs recorded in decreasing frequency included lethargy, tachycardia, ataxia, depression, vocalization, and vomiting. Common findings in cats recorded in decreasing frequency included lethargy, mydriasis, tachypnea, ataxia, depression, and tachycardia. Because the toxicities and therapies for treatment are complicated and controversial, contact an animal poison control center for further information in any potential overdose situation.

Drug Interactions

The following drug interactions have either been reported or are theoretical in humans or animals receiving clomipramine and may be of significance in veterinary patients:

- **ANTICHOLINERGIC AGENTS:** Because of additive effects, use with clomipramine cautiously

- **BUTYREPHENONE ANTIPSYCHOTIC AGENTS (e.g., haloperidol):** There is a case report (Starkey *et al.* 2008) of a macaw developing extrapyramidal side effects after it had received a long acting haloperidol injection and then subsequently received clomipramine.

- **CIMETIDINE:** May inhibit tricyclic antidepressant metabolism and increase the risk of toxicity

- **CISAPRIDE:** Increased risk for prolonged QT interval

- **CLONIDINE:** May cause increased blood pressure

- **CNS DEPRESSANTS:** Because of additive effects, use with clomipramine cautiously

- **MEPERIDINE, PENTAZOCINE, DEXTROMETHORPHAN:** Increased risk for serotonin syndrome

- **QUINIDINE:** Increased risk for QTc interval prolongation and tricyclic adverse effects

- **RIFAMPIN:** May decrease tricyclic blood levels

- **SSRIs (*e.g.*, fluoxetine, paroxetine, sertraline, etc.):** Increased risk for serotonin syndrome

- **SYMPATHOMIMETIC AGENTS:** Use in combination with sympathomimetic agents may increase the risk of cardiac effects (arrhythmias, hypertension, hyperpyrexia)

- **MONOAMINE OXIDASE INHIBITORS** (including **amitraz** and possibly, **selegiline**): Concomitant use (within 14 days) with monoamine oxidase inhibitors is generally contraindicated (serotonin syndrome)

Laboratory Considerations

- **ECG:** Tricyclics can widen QRS complexes, prolong PR intervals and invert or flatten T-waves on ECG

- **METAPYRONE TEST:** The response to metapyrone may be decreased by clomipramine

- **GLUCOSE, BLOOD:** Tricyclics may alter (increase or decrease) blood glucose levels

- **THYROID TESTS:** Clomipramine may decrease T3, T4 and free T4 levels in dogs and cats

Doses

- **DOGS:**

  a) 2–4 mg/kg once daily or divided twice daily PO. (Label directions; *Clomicalm*®)

  b) 3 mg/kg q12h; start at a low dose (*e.g.*, 1 mg/kg for 2 weeks, then 2 mg/kg for 2 weeks, then 3 mg/kg) (Reisner & Houpt 2000)

  c) For treatment of male dimorphic behaviors (urine marking, mounting, roaming, inter-male aggression); fearful/fear aggression behaviors; noise phobias; obsessive/compulsive behaviors (self-mutilation, excessive grooming, stereotypies): 1 mg/kg PO every 12 hours for 2 weeks; then 2 mg/kg PO q12h for 2 weeks, then 3 mg/kg PO q12h for 4 weeks and maintain. May take 4–6 weeks to see apparent improvement. (Overall 1997)

d) For adjunctive treatment (with alprazolam and behavior modification) of storm phobia: Clomipramine 2 mg/kg PO q12h for 3 months, then 1 mg/kg PO q12h, then 0.5 mg/kg PO q12h for 2 weeks. Alprazolam 0.02 mg/kg PO as needed 1 hour before anticipated storms and q4h as needed (Crowell-Davis 2003)

■ **CATS:**

a) For urine marking/spraying; inter-cat aggression related to social hierarchy; redirected aggression; compulsive grooming/wool sucking: 0.5 mg/kg once daily PO (Overall 1997)

b) 0.3–0.5 mg/kg PO q24h (Landsberg 2008)

c) 0.5–1 mg/kg once daily (Reisner & Houpt 2000)

d) For urine marking: 0.3–0.5 mg/kg PO q24h (2.5–5 mg per cat q24h) (Levine 2008)

■ **BIRDS:**

a) For adjunctive treatment of feather picking: Reported dosages range from 0.5–9 mg/kg PO q12-24h (Siebert 2007)

Monitoring

■ Clinical efficacy

■ Adverse Effects: Baseline liver function tests; EKG

Client Information

■ Generally used in combination with behavior modification treatments

■ May take several weeks before beneficial effects are seen

■ May be given with or without food; if patient vomits from the medication, give with food

■ Do not stop therapy without veterinarian's guidance

■ Keep well out of reach of pets and children; overdoses can be very toxic

Chemistry/Synonyms

A dibenzazepine-derivative tricyclic antidepressant, clomipramine HCl occurs as a white to off-white crystalline powder and is freely soluble in water.

Clomipramine HCl may also be known as: chlorimipramine hydrochloride, clomipramini hydrochloridum, G-34586, monochlorimipramine hydrochloride, *Clofranil®*, *Clomicalm®*,

Clopram®, *Clopress®*, *Equinorm®*, *Hydiphen®*, *Maronil®*, *Novo-Clopamine®*, *Placil®*, *Tranquax®*, or *Zoiral®*.

Storage/Stability

The commercially available veterinary tablets should be stored in a dry place at controlled room temperature (15–30°C) in the original closed container. The (human label) capsules should be stored at temperatures less than 30°C in tight containers and protected from moisture. An expiration date of 3 years from the date of manufacture is assigned to the commercially available capsules.

Dosage Forms/Regulatory Status

VETERINARY-LABELED PRODUCTS:

Clomipramine HCl Oral Tablets: 5 mg, 20 mg, 40 mg, & 80 mg; FDA-approved for dogs. *Clomicalm®* (Novartis); (Rx)

The ARCI (Racing Commissioners International) has designated this drug as a class 2 substance. See the appendix for more information.

HUMAN-LABELED PRODUCTS:

Clomipramine Oral Capsules: 25 mg, 50 mg, & 75 mg; *Anafranil®* (Novartis); generic; (Rx)

References

Crowell-Davis, S (2003). Use of clomipramine, alprazolam and behavior modification for treatment of storm phobia in dogs. *JAVMA* 222: 744–748.

Kook, PH, A Kranjc, et al. (2009). Pancreatitis associated with clomipramine administration in a dog. *Journal of Small Animal Practice* 50(2): 95–98.

Landsberg, G (2008). Treating canine and feline anxiety: Drug therapy and pheromones. Proceedings: BSAVA. Accessed via: Veterinary Information Network. http://goo.gl/49u6s

Levine, E (2008). Feline fear and anxiety. *Veterinary Clinics Small Animal* 38: 1065–1079.

Mertens, P, S Torres, et al. (2006). The effects of clomipramine hydrochloride in cats with psychogenic alopecia: a prospective study. *J Am Anim Hosp Assoc* 42.

Overall, K (1997). *Clinical behavioral medicine for small animals*. St Louis, Mosby.

Reisner, I & K Houpt (2000). Behavioral Disorders. *Textbook of Veterinary Internal Medicine: Diseases of the Dog and Cat*. S Ettinger and E Feldman Eds. Philadelphia, WB Saunders. 1: 156–162.

Siebert, L (2007). Pharmacotherapy for behavioral disorders in pet birds. *Journal of Exotic Pet Medicine* 16(1): 30–37.

Starkey, SR, JK Morrisey, et al. (2008). Extrapyramidal Side Effects in a Blue and Gold Macaw (Ara ararauna) Treated With Haloperidol and Clomipramine. *Journal of Avian Medicine and Surgery* 22(3): 234–239.

CLONAZEPAM

(kloe-na-ze-pam)   Klonopin®

BENZODIAZEPINE

Prescriber Highlights

▶ Benzodiazepine anticonvulsant, used primarily as adjunctive therapy for short-term treatment of epilepsy in dogs & for longer-term adjunctive treatment of epilepsy in cats; may also be used as an anxiolytic

▶ Contraindications: Hypersensitivity to benzodiazepines, narrow angle glaucoma, significant liver disease

▶ May exacerbate myasthenia gravis

▶ If using for seizures, discontinue gradually

▶ Adverse Effects: Sedation & ataxia most prevalent; Cats: Possible hepatic necrosis, but thought less likely to occur than with diazepam

▶ Dogs: Tolerance to efficacy may occur (over a few weeks)

▶ Controlled substance (C-IV)

Uses/Indications

Clonazepam is used primarily as an short-term adjunctive anticonvulsant for the treatment of epilepsy in dogs. It has been considered as long-term adjunctive therapy in dogs not controlled with other, more standard therapies, but like diazepam, tolerance tends to develop in a few weeks of treatment. It can also be used as an anxiolytic agent.

Clonazepam has been used as an anxiolytic and in the treatment of epilepsy in cats.

Pharmacology/Actions

The subcortical levels (primarily limbic, thalamic, and hypothalamic) of the CNS are depressed by diazepam and other benzodiazepines thereby producing the anxiolytic, sedative, skeletal muscle relaxant, and anticonvulsant effects seen. The exact mechanism of action is unknown, but postulated mechanisms include: antagonism of serotonin, increased release of and/or facilitation of gamma-aminobutyric acid (GABA) activity, and diminished release or turnover of acetylcholine in the CNS. Benzodiazepine specific receptors have been located in the mammalian brain, kidney, liver, lung, and heart. In all species studied, receptors are lacking in the white matter.

Pharmacokinetics

In dogs, clonazepam's oral bioavailability is variable (20–60%) but absorption is rapid. Protein binding is about 82% and the drug rapidly crosses into the CNS. Clonazepam exhibits saturation kinetics in dogs as elimination rates are dose dependent.

In humans, the drug is well absorbed from the GI tract, crosses the blood-brain barrier and placenta and is metabolized in the liver to several metabolites that are excreted in the urine. Peak serum levels occur about 3 hours after oral dosing. Half-lives range from 19–40 hours.

Contraindications/Precautions/Warnings

Clonazepam is contraindicated in patients who are hypersensitive to it or other benzodiazepines, have significant liver dysfunction, or acute narrow angle glaucoma. Benzodiazepines have been reported to exacerbate myasthenia gravis.

Adverse Effects

There is very limited information on the adverse effect profile of this drug in domestic animals. Sedation (or excitement) and ataxia may occur. Clonazepam has been reported to cause a multitude of various adverse effects in humans. Some of the more significant effects include increased salivation, hypersecretion in upper respiratory passages, GI effects (vomiting, constipation, diarrhea, etc.), transient elevations of liver enzymes, and hematologic effects (anemia, leukopenia, thrombocytopenia, etc.). Tolerance (usually noted after several weeks) to the anticonvulsant effects has been reported in dogs.

In cats, clonazepam may cause sedation, ataxia and possibly, acute hepatic necrosis.

Patients discontinuing clonazepam, particularly those who have been on the drug chronically at high dosages, should be tapered off or status epilepticus may be precipitated. Vomiting and diarrhea may occur during this process.

Reproductive/Nursing Safety

Safe use during pregnancy has not been established; adverse teratogenic effects have been seen in rabbits and rats. In humans, the FDA categorizes this drug as category *D* for use during pregnancy (*There is evidence of human fetal risk, but the potential benefits from the use of the drug in pregnant women may be acceptable despite its potential risks.*)

It is not known if clonazepam drug is excreted into milk, but several other benzodiazepines have been documented to enter milk. Theoretically, accumulation of the drug and its metabolites to toxic levels are possible; use with caution in nursing dams.

Overdosage/Acute Toxicity

Overdoses commonly cause sedation, depression, and ataxia. Some animals will exhibit paradoxical signs, such as hyperactivity, disorientation, and vocalization. Emesis is generally not indicated. With mild to moderate overdoses, animals can often be monitored at home, as long as the animal is rousable and does not show paradoxical signs. Animals should be confined and stimulation kept to a minimum. Paradoxical excitation can be treated with a mild sedative, such as diphenhydramine.

There were 659 exposures to clonazepam reported to the ASPCA Animal Poison Control

Center (APCC) during 2008-2009. In these cases, 590 were dogs with 340 showing clinical signs, 66 were cats with 43 showing clinical signs, and 1 was a bird that showed clinical signs. The remaining 2 cases involved a rodent and a ferret that showed no clinical signs. Common findings in dogs recorded in decreasing frequency included ataxia, lethargy, hyperactivity, vomiting, disorientation, sedation, agitation, vocalization, and depression. Common findings in cats recorded in decreasing frequency included ataxia, sedation, lethargy, disorientation, agitation, and polyphagia.

Massive overdoses can lead to respiratory depression or hypotension. Flumazenil can be used to reverse respiratory depression or severe depression. The half-life of flumazenil is short and the animal may require multiple doses.

Drug Interactions

The following drug interactions have either been reported or are theoretical in humans or animals receiving clonazepam and may be of significance in veterinary patients:

- **ANTIFUNGALS, AZOLE (itraconazole, ketoconazole, etc.):** May increase clonazepam levels
- **CIMETIDINE:** May decrease metabolism of benzodiazepines
- **CNS DEPRESSANT DRUGS:** If clonazepam administered with other CNS depressant agents (barbiturates, narcotics, anesthetics, etc.) additive effects may occur
- **ERYTHROMYCIN:** May decrease the metabolism of benzodiazepines
- **PHENOBARBITAL:** May decrease clonazepam concentrations
- **PHENYTOIN:** May decrease clonazepam concentrations
- **PROPANTHELINE:** May decrease clonazepam concentrations
- **RIFAMPIN:** May induce hepatic microsomal enzymes and decrease the pharmacologic effects of benzodiazepines

Laboratory Considerations

- Benzodiazepines may decrease the thyroidal uptake of I^{123} or I^{131}.

Doses

- **DOGS:**
  As an adjunctive medication in the treatment of seizures:
  a) 1–2 mg/kg PO q12h (Dickinson 2010)
  b) 0.5 mg/kg PO two to three times a day; may need to lower phenobarbital dose by 10–20% (Neer 1994)
  As an anxiolytic:
  a) 0.05–0.25 mg/kg PO q12–24h (Virga 2005)
  b) 0.1–1 mg/kg PO two to three times a day (Landsberg 2005)

- **CATS:**
  As an anxiolytic:
  a) 0.05–0.25 mg/kg PO q12–24h (Virga 2005)
  b) 0.02–0.2 mg/kg PO once to two times a day (Landsberg 2005)
  c) 0.1–0.2 mg/kg PO as needed or up to two times a day. (Neilson 2009)
  As an adjunctive medication in the treatment of seizures:
  a) Starting dose is 0.5 mg (total dose) PO q12–24h (Podell 2006), (Podell 2008)
  b) 1/8th to 1/4 of a 0.5 mg tablet PO two to three times daily; anecdotally more effective for maintenance and to decrease cluster seizures; acute hepatic necrosis possible (Pearce 2006)

Monitoring

- Efficacy
- Adverse effects
- The therapeutic blood level has been reported as 0.015–0.07 micrograms/mL.
- Cats: Liver function tests

Client Information

- A major factor in anticonvulsant therapy failure is lack of compliance with the prescribed therapy; it is very important to give doses regularly
- Cats: If patient develops lack of appetite, vomits, or yellowish whites of eyes, contact veterinarian immediately
- Do not stop therapy abruptly without veterinarian's guidance

Chemistry/Synonyms

A benzodiazepine anticonvulsant, clonazepam occurs as an off-white to light yellow, crystalline powder having a faint odor. It is insoluble in water and slightly soluble in alcohol.

Clonazepam may also be known as: clonazepamum, Ro-5-4023, *Antelepsin®*, *Clonagin®*, *Clonapam®*, *Clonax®*, *Clonex®*, *Diocam®*, *Epitril®*, *Iktorivil®*, *Kenoket®*, *Klonopin®*, *Kriadex®*, *Neuryl®*, *Paxam®*, *Rivatril®*, *Rivotril®*, or *Solfidin®*.

Storage/Stability

Tablets should be stored in airtight, light resistant containers at room temperature. After manufacture, a 5-year expiration date is assigned.

Compatibility/Compounding Considerations

Compounded preparation stability: Clonazepam oral suspension compounded from commercially available tablets has been published (Allen & Erickson 1996). Triturating six (6) clonazepam 2 mg tablets with 60 mL of *Ora-Plus®* and *qs ad* to 120 mL with *Ora-Sweet®* (or *Ora-Sweet® SF*) yields a 0.1 mg/mL suspension that retains >90% potency for 60 days stored at both 5°C and 25°C. Compounded preparations of clonazepam should be protected from light.

Dosage Forms/Regulatory Status

VETERINARY-LABELED PRODUCTS: None
The ARCI (Racing Commissioners International) has designated this drug as a class 2 substance. See the appendix for more information.

HUMAN-LABELED PRODUCTS:

Clonazepam Oral Tablets: 0.5 mg, 1 mg, & 2 mg; *Klonopin*® (Roche); generic; (Rx, C-IV)

Clonazepam Orally Disintegrating Tablets: 0.125 mg, 0.25 mg, 0.5 mg, 1 mg & 2 mg (with mannitol); *Klonopin*® *Wafers* (Roche); generic (Barr); (Rx, C-IV)

References

Allen, LV & MA Erickson (1996). Stability of acetazolamide, allopurinol, azathioprine, clonazepam, and flucytosine in extemporaneously compounded oral liquids. *Am J Health Syst Pharm* 53(16): 1944–1949.

Dickinson, P (2010). Seizures: Why can't I get the seizures under control? Proceedings: UCD Veterinary Neurology Symposium. Accessed via: Veterinary Information Network. http://goo.gl/l78rr

Landsberg, G (2005). Fear, anxiety and phobias—Diagnosis and treatment. Proceedings: ACVC 2005. Accessed via: Veterinary Information Network. http://goo.gl/HXM4j

Neer, T (1994). Seizures (Part I & II). Proceedings of the Twelfth Annual Veterinary Medical Forum, San Francisco, American College of Veterinary Internal Medicine.

Neilson, J (2009). Pharmacologic Interventions for Behavioral Problems. Proceedings: Western Veterinary Conference. Accessed via: Veterinary Information Network. http://goo.gl/HVVZL

Pearce, L (2006). Seizures in cats; Why they are not little dogs. Proceedings: Western Vet Conf. Accessed via: Veterinary Information Network. http://goo.gl/dnvl3

Podell, M (2006). New Horizons in the treatment of epilepsy. Proceedings: ACVIM. Accessed via: Veterinary Information Network. http://goo.gl/PlHdG

Podell, M (2008). Novel approaches to feline epilepsy. Proceedings: ACVIM. Accessed via: Veterinary Information Network. http://goo.gl/0hc8Z

Virga, V (2005). How I use benzodiazepines for situational anxieties. Proceedings: Western Vet Conf. Accessed via: Veterinary Information Network. http://goo.gl/9rPs7

CLONIDINE

(kloe-ni-deen)   Duraclon®, Catapres®

CENTRAL ALPHA-2 AGONIST

Prescriber Highlights

▶ Centrally acting alpha-adrenergic agonist used as a diagnostic for growth hormone deficiency or pheochromocytoma in dogs, adjunctive treatment for IBD, &, potentially, epidurally as an adjunct for pain &/or anesthesia or a premed prior to surgery

▶ Limited experience in veterinary species for therapeutic purposes

▶ Potential adverse effects include: Transient hyperglycemia, dry mouth, constipation, sedation, aggressive behavior, hypotension, collapse, & bradycardia

Uses/Indications

Clonidine is of interest in veterinary medicine as a diagnostic agent to determine growth hormone deficiency or pheochromocytoma in dogs, and as an adjunctive treatment for refractory inflammatory bowel disease, particularly in cats. It is being investigated as a premed in dogs and in a variety of species as an epidural adjunct with or without opiates in the treatment of severe pain or for surgical procedures using epidural anesthesia.

Pharmacology/Actions

Clonidine acts centrally (brain stem), stimulating alpha-adrenoreceptors, thereby reducing sympathetic outflow from the CNS; decreased renal vascular resistance, peripheral resistance, cardiac rate, and blood pressure result. Renal blood flow and glomerular filtration rates are not affected. Clonidine stimulates growth hormone release by stimulating release of GHRH, but this effect does not persist with continued dosing. Clonidine possesses centrally acting analgesic effects probably at presynaptic and postjunctional alpha$_2$-adrenoreceptors in the spinal cord thereby blocking pain signal transmission to the brain. It may also increase seizure threshold but the clinical significance for this effect is unclear.

Pharmacokinetics

Limited information is available on the pharmacokinetics of clonidine in domestic animals. In cats, clonidine exhibits a two-compartment open model and penetrates into tissues rapidly.

In humans, the drug is well absorbed after oral administration. Peak plasma concentrations occur approximately 3–5 hours after oral administration. After epidural administration, maximal analgesia occurs within 30–60 minutes. Clonidine is apparently widely distributed into body tissues; tissue concentrations are higher than in plasma. Clonidine does enter into the CSF, but brain concentrations are low compared with other tissues. In humans with normal renal function, clonidine's half-life is 6–20 hours. Elimination may be prolonged with higher dosages (dose-dependent elimination kinetics) or in patients with renal dysfunction. Up to 60% of a dose is eliminated unchanged in the urine, but the remainder is metabolized in the liver; one active metabolite (p-hydroxyclonidine) has been identified.

Contraindications/Precautions/Warnings

Clonidine is contraindicated in patients known to be hypersensitive to it. It should be used with caution in patients with severe cardiovascular disease, including conduction disturbances or heart failure; it should be used very cautiously in patients with renal failure.

Adverse Effects

Reported adverse effects most likely to occur include: transient hyperglycemia, dry mouth, constipation, sedation, aggressive behavior, hypotension, collapse, and bradycardia (responsive to atropine). Tolerance to its therapeutic effects has been reported in humans.

Reproductive/Nursing Safety

At reasonable dosages no significant teratogenic effects have been described in laboratory animals, but at very high dosages some effects (increased perinatal mortality, growth retardation, cleft palates) have been seen. In humans, the FDA categorizes clonidine as a category *C* drug for use during pregnancy (*Animal studies have shown an adverse effect on the fetus, but there are no adequate studies in humans; or there are no animal reproduction studies and no adequate studies in humans*).

Clonidine does enter maternal milk at concentrations of about 20% of those found in plasma; clinical significance to nursing offspring is unknown, but clonidine was undetectable in plasma of an infant one hour after nursing from a mother taking clonidine.

Overdosage/Acute Toxicity

Clonidine has a narrow margin of safety. Common signs include hypotension, bradycardia, vomiting, weakness, and depression. Rarely, seizures or respiratory depression is seen. The LD_{50} values reported for oral clonidine in rats are 465 mg/kg and mice, 206 mg/kg.

There were 150 exposures to clonidine reported to the ASPCA Animal Poison Control Center (APCC) during 2008-2009. In these cases, 130 were dogs with 41 showing clinical signs and the remaining 20 cases were cats with 14 showing clinical signs. Common findings in dogs recorded in decreasing frequency included lethargy, tachycardia, ataxia, and hypertension. Common findings in cats recorded in decreasing frequency included lethargy.

Fluids and dopamine can be used to treat hypotension.

Treatment for large overdoses includes gut evacuation using standard protocols. Use of emetics should be carefully considered, as level of consciousness may deteriorate rapidly. Treatment of systemic effects is primarily symptomatic and supportive. Hypotensive effects may be treated, if necessary, using fluids or pressors (*e.g.*, dopamine); bradycardia may be treated with IV atropine, if required. Atipamezole or yohimbine may also be used to help reverse the cardiovascular effects, but multiple doses may be required, as signs can last up to 48 hours, depending on clonidine dosage.

Drug Interactions

The following drug interactions have either been reported or are theoretical in humans or animals receiving clonidine and may be of significance in veterinary patients:

■ **ANTIHYPERTENSIVE DRUGS, OTHER:** Possible additive hypotensive effects

■ **BETA-ADRENERGIC BLOCKING AGENTS (*i.e.*, propranolol)** may enhance bradycardia when given with clonidine. In patients receiving clonidine and beta-adrenergic blocking agents together: if clonidine is to be discontinued, the beta-blocker should be discontinued prior to clonidine and clonidine gradually discontinued, otherwise rebound hypertension may occur.

■ **CNS DEPRESSANT DRUGS (opiates, barbiturates, etc.):** Clonidine may exacerbate the actions of other CNS depressant drugs

■ **DIGOXIN:** Possible additive bradycardia

■ **PRAZOSIN:** May decrease the antihypertensive effects of clonidine

■ **TRICYCLIC ANTIDEPRESSANTS (e.g., amitriptyline):** May block the antihypertensive effects of clonidine

Laboratory Considerations

■ No specific laboratory interactions were noted for clonidine.

Doses

■ **DOGS:**

For diagnosing hyposomatotropism:

a) Dosage may be variable depending on the laboratory's protocol. Contact lab prior to test to determine protocol and sample handling instructions. Usual dose is 10 micrograms/kg IV. Obtain plasma for growth hormone (GH) levels, prior to clonidine dosing and at 15, 30, 45, 60, and 120 minutes. Larger dosages may cause a more pronounced and prolonged hyperglycemia and a higher incidence of other adverse reactions that may include sedation, aggressive behavior, hypotension, collapse, and bradycardia (responsive to atropine). Adverse effects may persist for 15−60 minutes post dose. Healthy dogs should demonstrate GH levels of 10 ng/mL after clonidine administration. (Feldman & Nelson 1996)

For adjunctive antidiarrheal therapy for refractory cases of inflammatory bowel disease:

a) 5−10 micrograms/kg PO or SC two to three times a day; can activate alpha$_2$-receptors in the CRT and cause vomiting. (Washabau 2009)

■ **CATS:**

For adjunctive antidiarrheal therapy for refractory cases of inflammatory bowel disease:

a) As fourth line therapy after prostaglandin synthetase inhibitors (*i.e.*, sulfasalazine, bismuth subsalicylate), opioid agonists (*i.e.*, loperamide), and 5-HT3 serotonergic antagonists (*i.e.*, ondansetron) are being used: clonidine 5−10 micrograms/kg two to three times a day, SC or PO. (Washabau 2000)

■ **CATTLE:**
For epidural analgesia/analgesia:
a) 2–3 micrograms/kg diluted to 8 mL with sterile normal saline epidurally; onset/ duration of analgesia = 19 minutes/192 minutes with 2 micrograms/kg dose and = 9 minutes/311 minutes with 3 micrograms/kg dose; peak effects from 60–180 minutes (De Rossi *et al.* 2003)

Monitoring
■ Dependent upon purpose for use. When used for determining GH levels, adverse effects (noted in dosage section) should be evaluated.

■ Blood pressure and cardiac rate are most likely to be affected, but effects usually only persist for an hour after dose.

■ When used for ongoing diarrhea treatment, evaluation of efficacy and adverse effect profile should be monitored.

Client Information
■ When used for chronic therapy, have clients report signs that may indicate adverse effects (weakness, lethargy, behavioral changes, etc.); caution not to alter or discontinue treatment without veterinarian's advice.

Chemistry/Synonyms
An imidazoline derivative centrally acting alpha-adrenergic agonist, clonidine HCl occurs as an odorless, bitter, white or almost white crystalline powder. It is soluble in water and alcohol. It is also considered highly lipid soluble. The commercially available injection for epidural use has its pH adjusted to between 5 to 7.

Clonidine may also be known as: ST-155, clonidini hydrochloridum, *Adesipress-TTS®, Arkamin®, Aruclonin®, Atensina®, Barclyd®, Cantanidin®, Caprysin®, Catanidin®, Catapresan®, Catapresan®, Catapres®, Catapressan®, Clonistada®, Clonnirit®, Dispaclonidin®, Dixarit®, Duraclon®, Epiclodina®, Glausine®, Haemiton®, Menograine®, Mirfat®, Normopresan®, Paracefan®,* or *Tenso-Timelets®.*

Storage/Stability
Clonidine tablets should be stored in tight, light-resistant containers at room temperature; excursions permitted to 15–30°C (59–86°F). The preservative-free injection for epidural use should be stored at controlled room temperature (25°C). Because it contains no preservative, unused portions of the injection should be discarded.

Dosage Forms/Regulatory Status

VETERINARY-LABELED PRODUCTS: None
The ARCI (Racing Commissioners International) has designated this drug as a class 3 substance. See the appendix for more information.

HUMAN-LABELED PRODUCTS:
Clonidine HCl Injection for epidural use:

100 micrograms/mL, & 500 micrograms/mL preservative-free in 10 mL vials; *Duraclon®* (aaiPharma); (Rx)

Clonidine HCl Oral Tablets: 0.1 mg, 0.2 mg & 0.3 mg; *Catapres®* (Boehringer Ingelheim); generic; (Rx)

Clonidine HCl Oral Modified-release Tablets: 0.1 mg (equivalent to 0.087 mg of base); *Jenloga®* (UPM Inc); (Rx)

Clonidine HCl Transdermal: 0.1 mg/24hrs (2.5 mg total clonidine content), 0.2 mg/24hrs (5 mg total clonidine content), & 0.3 mg/24hrs (7.5 mg total clonidine content); *Catapres-TTS-1®, 2®* or *3®* (Boehringer Ingelheim); (Rx)

References
De Rossi, R, G Bucker, et al. (2003). Perineal analgesic actions of epidural clonidine in cattle. *Vet Anaesth Analg* **30**: 63–70.
Feldman, E & R Nelson (1996). *Canine and Feline Endocrinology and Reproduction*. Philadelphia, Saunders.
Washabau, R (2000). Intestinal Diseases/IBD. Proceedings: American Association of Feline Practitioners.
Washabau, R (2009). Principles in the therapy of canine inflammatory bowel disease. Proceedings: WSAVA. Accessed via: Veterinary Information Network. http:// goo.gl/wvg8Y

CLOPIDOGREL BISULFATE
(kloe-***pid***-oh-grel)   Plavix®
PLATELET AGGREGATION INHIBITOR

Prescriber Highlights
▶ Oral, once-daily platelet aggregation inhibitor that may be useful in preventing thromboembolic disease in cats and in hypercoagulable states in dogs

▶ Limited clinical experience in feline medicine; but appears well tolerated

▶ Potentially may cause vomiting or bleeding

Uses/Indications
Clopidogrel, a platelet aggregation inhibitor, may be useful for preventing thrombi in susceptible cats. It may also improve pelvic limb circulation in cats after a cardiogenic embolic event via a vasomodulating effect secondary to inhibition of serotonin release from platelets. Research is ongoing. It may also prove to be of benefit in treating hypercoagulable states in dogs.

Pharmacology/Actions
Clopidogrel is metabolized to an active, highly unstable compound (not yet identified) that is responsible for its inhibitory platelet-aggregation (both primary and secondary aggregation) activity. This compound binds selectively to platelet surface low-affinity ADP-receptors and inhibits ADP binding to the site. This inhibits activation of the platelet glycoprotein Ib/IIIa

complex that is necessary for platelet-fibrinogen binding and inhibits the release from platelets other compounds that enhance platelet aggregation (*e.g.*, serotonin, calcium, fibrinogen, thrombospondin, ADP). Clopidogrel's active metabolite irreversibly alters the ADP receptor; the platelet is affected for its lifespan.

Clopidogrel's mechanism of action on platelet aggregation is different than aspirin's effects. Aspirin acetylates and inactivates COX-1 in platelets, thereby preventing formation of thromboxane A2.

Pharmacokinetics

No specific information was located for the pharmacokinetics of clopidogrel in cats. In a pharmacodynamic study in cats (Hogan *et al.* 2004), doses as low as 18.75 mg were as effective as higher dosages in reducing platelet aggregation; maximal effects were seen after 3 days of therapy and platelet function returned to normal 7 days after stopping treatment. While lower dosages may be effective in cats, they have not been evaluated and are not practical to administer with the presently available 75 mg human-labeled dosage form (tablets).

In humans, clopidogrel is rapidly absorbed with a bioavailability of about 50%. Food does not alter its absorption. Clopidogrel is highly bound to plasma proteins in humans and is rapidly hydrolyzed to a carboxylic acid derivative inactive metabolite that is excreted via the urine and feces. The 2% of drug that is covalently bound to platelets has an approximate elimination half-life of 11 days.

Contraindications/Precautions/Warnings

No specific information is available for cats. In humans, clopidogrel is contraindicated in patients with active pathologic bleeding or known hypersensitivity to the drug.

Adverse Effects

Clopidogrel appears well tolerated by cats, but numbers treated have been relatively few. Some cats may vomit or develop anorexia; giving the drug with food may alleviate these effects.

In humans, the primary adverse effects reported have been bleeding related. In a major pre-clinical study, major bleeding occurred in approximately 2% of patients treated. Use of aspirin with clopidogrel may increase this incidence. Rashes and gastrointestinal effects (diarrhea) have also been reported. Rarely, thrombotic thrombocytopenic purpura (TTP) has been noted; onset can occur after a short period of treatment (<2 weeks).

Reproductive/Nursing Safety

In pregnant rats and rabbits, dosages of approximately 65X and 78X respectively, of the human dose when compared on mg/m^2 basis, caused no teratogenic effects. In humans, the FDA categorizes clopidogrel as category *B* for use during pregnancy (*Animal studies have not yet demonstrated risk to the fetus, but there are no adequate studies in pregnant women; or animal studies have shown an adverse effect, but adequate studies in pregnant women have not demonstrated a risk to the fetus in the first trimester of pregnancy, and there is no evidence of risk in later trimesters.*)

In rats, clopidogrel or its metabolites are distributed into milk. Although probably safe to use in nursing veterinary patients, weigh the potential risks to nursing offspring before allowing patients receiving the drug to nurse their young, or use a milk replacer.

Overdosage/Acute Toxicity

Limited information is available. Reported lethal oral doses for mice and rats were 1500 mg/kg and 2000 mg/kg (460X human adult dose on a mg/m^2 basis), respectively. Acute toxic signs may include bleeding or vomiting. Platelet transfusions have been suggested if rapid reversal is required.

Drug Interactions

The following drug interactions have either been reported or are theoretical in humans or animals receiving clopidogrel and may be of significance in veterinary patients:

- **ASPIRIN:** Increased risk for bleeding, however many human patients take both medications

- **HEPARIN; LOW MOLECULAR WEIGHT HEPARINS:** Clopidogrel appears safe to use with heparin (both unfractionated and LMW)

- **NSAIDS:** Increased risk for bleeding; clopidogrel may interfere with metabolism

- **PHENYTOIN:** Clopidogrel may interfere with metabolism

- **PROTON PUMP INHIBITORS (e.g., omeprazole):** Proton pump inhibitors may decrease the efficacy of clopidogrel. The clinical significance of this interaction is unclear and being intensely debated in human medicine.

- **TORSEMIDE:** Clopidogrel may interfere with metabolism

- **WARFARIN:** Increased risk for bleeding; clopidogrel may interfere with metabolism

Laboratory Considerations

- None noted

Doses

- **DOGS:**

  As an anti-platelet agent:

  a) 1–3 mg/kg PO once daily; if used with aspirin give lower doses (0.5–1 mg/kg PO once daily) (Brainard 2008)

- **CATS:**

  To prevent thrombus formation:

  a) 18.75 mg (practically, 1/4 of a 75 mg tablet) PO once daily (Hogan 2006)

  b) 7 mg (total dose) PO once daily in combination with aspirin 40–81 mg (total dose) every 3 days. Clinical trials are needed to determine appropriate dosage and indications. (Moise 2007)

c) 1–3 mg/kg PO once daily; if used with aspirin give lower doses (0.5–1 mg/kg PO once daily) (Brainard 2008)

Monitoring

■ Clinical efficacy

■ Adverse effects (vomiting, bleeding)

Client Information

■ May be given without regard to feeding status

■ Potential adverse effects include vomiting, lack of appetite or bleeding

■ If vomiting occurs, give with food

■ Report any bleeding or black, tarry stools to veterinarian

Chemistry/Synonyms

Clopidogrel bisulfate, a thienopyridine, occurs as a white to off-white powder that is practically insoluble in water at a pH of 7, but freely soluble at a pH of 1.

Clopidogrel may also be known as: SR-259990C, PCR-4099, or clopedogreli. Internationally registered trade names for clopidogrel include: *Antiplaq, Clodian, Cloflow, Clopact, Clopivas, Clopod, Iscover, Iskimil, Nabratin, Noklot, Plavix®, Pleyar,* or *Troken*.

Storage/Stability

Clopidogrel tablets should be stored at 25°C; excursions are permitted to 15–30°C.

Compatibility/Compounding Considerations

Compounded preparation stability: Clopidogrel oral suspension compounded from commercially available tablets has been published (Skillman *et al.* 2010). Triturating four (4) clopidogrel 75 mg tablets with 30 mL of *Ora-Plus®* and *qs ad* to 60 mL with *Ora-Sweet®* (or *Ora-Sweet® SF*) yields a 5 mg/mL oral suspension that retains >90% potency for 60 days stored at both 5°C and 25°C. Compounded preparations of clopidogrel should be protected from light.

Dosage Forms/Regulatory Status

VETERINARY-LABELED PRODUCTS: None
HUMAN-LABELED PRODUCTS:

Clopidogrel Bisulfate Tablets: 75 mg & 300 mg; *Plavix®* (Bristol-Myers Squibb); (Rx)

References

Brainard, B (2008). Practical anticoagulation. Proceedings: IVECCS. Accessed via: Veterinary Information Network. http://goo.gl/Mge4p

Hogan, D (2006). Feline cardiogenic embolism: What do we know and where are going? Proceedings ACVIM2006. Accessed via: Veterinary Information Network. http://goo.gl/Hsdjv

Hogan, D, D Andrews, et al. (2004). Antiplatelet effects and pharmacodynamics of clopidogrel in cats. *JAVMA* 225(9): 1406–1411.

Moise, NS (2007). Presentation and management of thromboembolism in cats. *In Practice* 29(1): 2–8.

Skillman, KL, RL Caruthers, et al. (2010). Stability of an extemporaneously prepared clopidogrel oral suspension. *Am J Health Syst Pharm* 67(7): 559–561.

CLOPROSTENOL SODIUM

(kloe-***pros***-te-nol)   Estrumate®

PROSTAGLANDIN (F-CLASS)

Prescriber Highlights

▶ Synthetic F-class prostaglandin used in cattle to induce luteolysis, induce abortion, treat pyometra, endometritis, etc.

▶ Contraindications: Pregnancy (when abortion or induced parturition are not desired)

▶ Can cause cholinergic-like adverse effects in dogs

▶ Do not give IV

▶ Pregnant women should not handle; caution handling in humans with asthma & women of childbearing age

Uses/Indications

Cloprostenol is FDA-approved for use in beef or dairy cattle to induce luteolysis. It is recommended by the manufacturer for unobserved or undetected estrus in cows cycling normally, pyometra or chronic endometritis, expulsion of mummified fetus, luteal cysts, induced abortions after mismating, and to schedule estrus and ovulation for controlled breeding.

Cloprostenol has been used in dogs for pregnancy termination and treatment of open pyometra. The use of cloprostenol for pyometra is controversial as some believe dinoprost (PGF2alpha) is more effective and has fewer adverse effects than cloprostenol.

In horses, cloprostenol has been used for luteolysis, induce abortion, and stimulate uterine contractions.

Pharmacology/Actions

Prostaglandin F_{2alpha} and its analogues cloprostenol and fluprostenol are powerful luteolytic agents. They cause rapid regression of the corpus luteum and arrest its secretory activity. These prostaglandins also have direct stimulating effect on uterine smooth muscle causing contraction and a relaxant effect on the cervix.

In normally cycling animals, estrus will generally occur 2–5 days after treatment. In pregnant cattle treated between 10–150 days of gestation, abortion will usually occur 2–3 days after injection.

Pharmacokinetics

No information was located on the pharmacokinetics of cloprostenol. It is reported to have a longer duration of action than dinoprost tromethamine.

Contraindications/Precautions/Warnings

Should not be administered to pregnant animals when abortion is not desired.

Women of child-bearing age, persons with asthma or other respiratory diseases should use extreme caution when handling cloprostenol as the drug may induce abortion or acute broncho-constriction. Cloprostenol is readily absorbed through the skin and must be washed off imme-diately with soap and water.

Do not administer IV.

Adverse Effects

The manufacturer does not list any adverse ef-fects for this product when used as labeled. If used after the 5th month of gestation, increased risk of dystocia and decreased efficacy occur.

In dogs, cloprostenol can cause increased salivation, tachycardia, increased urination and defecation, gagging, vomiting, ataxia, and mild depression. Pretreatment with an anticholiner-gic drug (such as atropine) may reduce the se-verity of these effects.

At higher doses in horses, cloprostenol can cause sweating, cramping and loose stools, but incidence of adverse effects is less than with dinoprost tromethamine. In horses, uterine contractions are stimulated for approximately 5 hours post-dose.

Reproductive/Nursing Safety

Cloprostenol is contraindicated in pregnant animals when abortion or induced parturition is not desired.

Overdosage/Acute Toxicity

The manufacturer states that at doses of 50 and 100 times those recommended, cattle may show signs of uneasiness, slight frothing, and milk let-down.

Overdoses of cloprostenol or other synthetic prostaglandin F2alpha analogs in small animals reportedly can result in shock and death.

Drug Interactions

The following drug interactions have either been reported or are theoretical in humans or animals receiving cloprostenol and may be of signifi-cance in veterinary patients:

■ **OXYTOCIC AGENTS, OTHER:** Activity may be enhanced by cloprostenol

Doses

■ **DOGS:**

For adjunctive treatment of open cervix pyometra:

a) 1–5 micrograms/kg (0.001–0.005 mg/kg) (route not specified) once per day. May require up to 2–3 weeks of treatment. When starting treatment, start with one-half the normal dosage and gradu-ally achieve the full dose within 2–3 days. (Romagnoli 2002)

b) Cloprostenol at 1 microgram/kg SC (not during feeding) every 5 days for 15 days (if not cured earlier) with aglepristone at 10 mg/kg SC every 5 days until cured. Give *Clavamox®* (12.5 mg/kg PO twice daily and supportive hydration through-

out protocol, if indicated. (Threlfall 2006)

For pregnancy termination:

a) 1–2.5 micrograms/kg SC once daily for 4–7 days has been successful in terminat-ing pregnancy in dogs after 30 days gesta-tion (Davidson 2004)

b) 1–2.5 micrograms/kg SC every 48 hours for three doses. At higher dose (2.5 mg/kg); appears very effective start-ing at 30 days of pregnancy. Anticholin-ergic drug administration (*e.g.*, atropine) 15 minutes prior to dosing appears to lessen adverse effects. (Romagnoli 2006)

■ **CATTLE:**

For treatment of pyometra:

a) 500 micrograms IM (up to 97% efficacy) (McCormack 1986)

For pyometra or chronic endometritis, mummified fetus (manual assistance may be required to remove from vagina), luteal cysts:

a) 500 micrograms IM (Package Insert; *Es-trumate®*—Miles/Mobay)

For unobserved or undetected estrus in cows with continued ovarian cyclicity and a ma-ture corpus luteum:

a) 500 micrograms IM; estrus should com-mence in 2–5 days at which time the animal may be inseminated. If estrus detection is not possible or practical, ani-mal may be inseminated twice at 72 and 96 hours post injection. (Package Insert; *Estrumate®*—Miles/Mobay)

For abortion, from one week after mating to approximately the 150th day of gestation:

a) 500 micrograms IM; abortion gener-ally takes place in 4–5 days after injec-tion (Package Insert; *Estrumate®*—Miles/ Mobay)

For controlled breeding:

a) *Single injection method*: Use only animals with mature corpus luteum. Examine rectally to determine corpus luteum maturity, anatomic normality, and lack of pregnancy. Give 500 micrograms clo-prostenol IM. Estrus should occur in 2–5 days. Inseminate at usual time after detecting estrus, or inseminate once at 72 hours post injection, or twice at 72 and 96 hours post injection.

Double injection method: Examine rectal-ly to determine if animal is anatomically normal, not pregnant, and cycling nor-mally. Give 500 micrograms IM. Repeat dose 11 days later. Estrus should occur in 2–5 days after second injection. Insemi-nate at usual time after detecting estrus, or inseminate once at 72 hours post sec-ond injection, or twice at 72 and 96 hours post second injection.

Animals that come into estrus after first injection may be inseminated at the usual time after detecting estrus.

Any controlled breeding program should be completed by either observing animals and re-inseminating or hand mating after returning to estrus, or turning in clean-up bull(s) five to seven days after the last injection of cloprostenol to cover any animals returning to estrus. (Package Insert; *Estrumate®*—Miles/Mobay)

■ **HORSES:**

a) To cause abortion prior to the twelfth day of gestation: 100 micrograms IM, most effective day 7 or 8 post estrus. Mare will usually return to estrus within 5 days. (Lofstedt 1986)

b) For luteolysis and to stimulate uterine contractions: 250 micrograms (total dose) IM once. Research has shown that 1/10th of a dose can still cause luteolysis and if given on once or on two consecutive days can avoid side effects. (Dascanio 2009)

c) For luteolysis: 25–250 micrograms (0.1–1 mL) IM once. As an ecbolic: 250 micrograms (1 mL) IM q24h. Cloprostenol should not be used more than one day after ovulation because it can damage the corpus luteum and reduce progesterone. (Foss 2009)

■ **SWINE:**

To induce parturition in sows:

a) 175 micrograms IM; give 2 days or less before anticipated date of farrowing. Farrowing generally occurs in approximately 36 hours after injection. (Pugh 1982)

■ **SHEEP & GOATS:**

a) **Goats:** To induce parturition in does: 62.5–125 micrograms IM at 144 days of gestation in early morning. Deliveries will peak at 30–35 hours after injection. Maintain goat in usual surroundings and minimize outside disturbances. (Williams 1986)

b) **Goats:** To treat pseudopregnancy (hydrometra/mucometra): 125 micrograms IM once. (Tibary 2009)

■ **CAMELIDS:**

a) As a luteolytic: **Alpacas:** 100 micrograms IM once. **Llamas:** 250 micrograms IM once. Not to be given more than 4 days after ovulation. Luteolysis and abortion can be induced at any stage of pregnancy with 2-4 injections of cloprostenol. (Adams 2008)

Client Information

■ Cloprostenol should be used by individuals familiar with its use and precautions

■ Pregnant women, asthmatics or other persons with bronchial diseases should handle this product with extreme caution

■ Any accidental exposure to skin should be washed off immediately

Chemistry/Synonyms

A synthetic prostaglandin of the F class, cloprostenol sodium occurs as a white or almost white, amorphous, hygroscopic powder. It is freely soluble in water and alcohol. Potency of the commercially available product is expressed in terms of cloprostenol.

Cloprostenol sodium may also be known as ICI-80996, *Estrumate®,* or *estroPLAN®.*

Storage/Stability

Cloprostenol sodium should be stored at room temperature (15–30°C); protect from light.

Dosage Forms/Regulatory Status

VETERINARY-LABELED PRODUCTS:

Cloprostenol Sodium Injection equivalent to 250 micrograms/mL cloprostenol in 20 mL vials; *Estrumate®* (Schering-Plough); *estroPLAN® Injection* (Parnell); (Rx). FDA-approved for use in beef and dairy cattle. No preslaughter withdrawal or milk withdrawal is required; no specific tolerances for cloprostenol residues have been published.

HUMAN-LABELED PRODUCTS: None

References

Adams, G (2008). Breeding management of llamas and alpacas. Proceedings: WVC. Accessed via: Veterinary Information Network. http://goo.gl/f3oFl

Dascanio, J (2009). Hormonal Control of Reproduction. Proceedings: ABVP. Accessed via: Veterinary Information Network. http://goo.gl/o2vHk

Davidson, A (2004). Update: Therapeutics for reproductive disorders in small animal practice. Proceedings: ACVIM Forum. Accessed via: Veterinary Information Network. http://goo.gl/Fe4Gp

Foss, R (2009). Breeding the problem mare. Proceedings: WVC. Accessed via: Veterinary Information Network. http://goo.gl/ABWXx

Lofstedt, RM (1986). Termination of unwanted pregnancy in the mare. *Current Therapy in Theriogenology 2: Diagnosis, Treatment and Prevention of Reproductive Diseases in Small and Large Animals.* DA Morrow Ed. Philadelphia, WB Saunders: 715–718.

McCormack, J (1986). Pyometra in cattle. *Current Veterinary Therapy: Food Animal Practice 2.* JL Howard Ed. Philadelphia, W.B. Saunders: 777–778.

Pugh, DM (1982). The Hormones II: Control of reproductive function. *Veterinary Applied Pharmacology and Therapeutics* London, Baillière Tindall: 181–201.

Romagnoli, S (2002). Canine pyometra: Pathogenesis, therapy and clinical cases. Proceedings: World Small Animal Veterinary Association World Congress. Accessed via: Veterinary Information Network. http://goo.gl/aWLNz

Romagnoli, S (2006). Control of reproduction in dogs and cats: Use and misuse of hormones. Proceedings: WSAVA World Congress. Accessed via: Veterinary Information Network. http://goo.gl/aGuBF

Threlfall, W (2006). Hormonal Usage. Proceedings: ACVC. Accessed via: Veterinary Information Network. http://goo.gl/vg8nw

Tibary, A (2009). Infertility in goats: Individual & herd approach. Proceedings: WVC. Accessed via: Veterinary Information Network. http://goo.gl/1xjUF

Williams, CSF (1986). Practical management of induced parturition. *Current Therapy in Theriogenology 2: Diagnosis, Treatment and Prevention of Reproductive Diseases in Small and Large Animals.* DA Morrow Ed. Philadelphia, WB Saunders: 588–589.

CLORAZEPATE DIPOTASSIUM

(klor-*az*-e-pate)   Tranxene-SD®, Gen-Xene®

BENZODIAZEPINE

Prescriber Highlights

▶ Benzodiazepine anxiolytic, sedative-hypnotic, & anticonvulsant used in dogs & cats

▶ Contraindications: Hypersensitivity to benzodiazepines, narrow angle glaucoma, or significant liver disease

▶ Use extreme caution in aggressive animals (especially fear induced)

▶ May exacerbate myasthenia gravis

▶ Can interact with phenobarbital

▶ Adverse Effects: Sedation & ataxia most prevalent

Uses/Indications

Clorazepate has been used in dogs both as an adjunctive anticonvulsant (usually in conjunction with phenobarbital) and in the treatment of behavior disorders, primarily those that are anxiety or phobia-related. In dogs, clorazepate has been reported to develop tolerance to its anticonvulsant effects less rapidly than clonazepam.

Clorazepate may be useful as an anxiolytic agent in cats.

Pharmacology/Actions

The subcortical levels (primarily limbic, thalamic, and hypothalamic) of the CNS are depressed by clorazepate and other benzodiazepines thus producing the anxiolytic, sedative, skeletal muscle relaxant and anticonvulsant effects seen. The exact mechanism of action is unknown, but postulated mechanisms include: antagonism of serotonin, increased release of and/or facilitation of gamma-aminobutyric acid (GABA) activity and diminished release or turnover of acetylcholine in the CNS. Benzodiazepine specific receptors have been located in the mammalian brain, kidney, liver, lung and heart. In all species studied, receptors are lacking in the white matter.

Pharmacokinetics

In dogs, clorazepate peak serum levels generally occur within 1-2 hours. Volume of distribution is about 1.8 L/kg after multiple dosing. Clorazepate is metabolized to nordiazepam and other metabolites. Nordiazepam is active and has a very long half-life (in humans up to 100 hours). In dogs, the sustained release preparation apparently offers no pharmacokinetic advantage over the non-sustained preparations (Brown & Forrester 1989).

Contraindications/Precautions/Warnings

Clorazepate is contraindicated in patients who are hypersensitive to it or other benzodi-

azepines, have significant liver dysfunction or have acute narrow angle glaucoma. Clorazepate should be used very cautiously, if at all, in aggressive patients as it may disinhibit the anxiety that may help prevent these animals from aggressive behavior. Benzodiazepines have been reported to exacerbate myasthenia gravis.

Use with caution in dogs displaying fear-induced aggression; these drugs may actually provoke dogs to attack.

Adverse Effects

In dogs, the most likely adverse effects seen include sedation and ataxia. These effects apparently occur infrequently, are mild and usually transient. Physical dependence may occur and abrupt withdrawal of clorazepate may precipitate seizures.

In cats, clorazepate may cause sedation, ataxia and, potentially, acute hepatic necrosis.

Reproductive/Nursing Safety

Safe use during pregnancy has not been established; teratogenic effects of similar benzodiazepines have been noted in rabbits and rats. In humans, the FDA categorizes this drug as category **D** for use during pregnancy (*There is evidence of human fetal risk, but the potential benefits from the use of the drug in pregnant women may be acceptable despite its potential risks.*)

Nordiazepam is distributed into milk and may affect nursing neonates.

Overdosage/Acute Toxicity

When used alone, clorazepate overdoses are generally limited to significant CNS depression (confusion, coma, decreased reflexes, etc.). Treatment of significant oral overdoses consists of standard protocols for removing and/or binding the drug in the gut and supportive systemic measures. The use of analeptic agents (CNS stimulants such as caffeine, amphetamines, etc.) is generally not recommended. Flumazenil may be considered for very serious overdoses.

Drug Interactions

The following drug interactions have either been reported or are theoretical in humans or animals receiving clorazepate and may be of significance in veterinary patients:

▪ **ANTIFUNGALS, AZOLE (itraconazole, ketoconazole, etc.):** May increase levels

▪ **CIMETIDINE:** May decrease metabolism of benzodiazepines

▪ **CNS DEPRESSANT DRUGS:** If clorazepate is administered with other CNS depressant agents (**barbiturates, narcotics, anesthetics, etc.**) additive effects may occur

▪ **ERYTHROMYCIN:** May decrease the metabolism of benzodiazepines

▪ **PHENOBARBITAL:** While used together in the treatment of seizures in dogs, can interact with one another. Clorazepate (especially high serum concentrations), may increase the serum levels of phenobarbital, particularly if added to patients who received phenobarbital long-term. In time, clorazepate levels may decrease, leading to decreased phenobarbital levels.

■ **PHENYTOIN:** May decrease clorazepate concentrations

■ **RIFAMPIN:** May induce hepatic microsomal enzymes and decrease the pharmacologic effects of benzodiazepines

Laboratory Considerations

■ Benzodiazepines may decrease the thyroidal uptake of I^{123} or I^{131}.

■ Clorazepate may increase **serum alkaline phosphatase** and **serum cholesterol** levels; clinical significance is unclear.

Doses

■ **DOGS:**

As an adjunctive medication in the treatment of seizures:

a) In combination with phenobarbital: Clorazepate: 1–2 mg/kg PO q12h, but may need to divide q12h dose and give q8h to minimize adverse effects and maintain therapeutic levels (Boothe 1999)

b) In combination with phenobarbital: Clorazepate: 0.5–1 mg/kg PO q8h. No advantage gained with using sustained release products over regular caps or tabs. May affect phenobarb levels; monitor 2 and 4 weeks later. (Thomas 2000)

c) 1–2 mg/kg PO q12h (Podell 2006)

d) 2–4 mg/kg PO twice daily, some dogs may require three times daily (Dowling 2003)

e) As a third-line agent: 1–2 mg/kg PO q8–12h (Quesnel 2001)

f) For management of cluster seizures: Immediately after first seizure give clorazepate at 0.5–2 mg/kg two to three times daily for the next 48–96 hours and then stop clorazepate. It may be used in addition to the existing anticonvulsant maintenance therapy, but it is used only during the time of seizure activity and not as maintenance therapy. (Hoskins 2005)

As adjunctive therapy for the treatment of fears and phobias:

a) 11.25–22.5 mg per dog PO once to twice daily (recommends the sustained-delivery product (*Tranxene®-SD*). (Marder 1991)

b) Using the sustained delivery product (*Tranxene®-SD*), initially give 22.5 mg for large dogs, 11.25 mg for medium dogs and 5.6 mg for small dogs PO; adjust dosage according to dog's response (Shull-Selcer & Stagg 1991)

c) 0.55–2.2 mg/kg PO as needed up to q8h; titrate to clinical sedation—dose

may vary for individual dogs (Reisner & Houpt 2000), (Sherman & Mills 2008)

d) 0.2–1 mg/kg PO q12–24h (Virga 2002)

■ **CATS:**

a) As an anxiolytic or for compulsive behaviors: 0.2–0.5 mg/kg PO q12–24h (Virga 2002)

b) As an alternative drug to phenobarbital for seizures: 3.75–7.5 mg (total dose per cat) PO once to twice daily. Similar precautions are necessary as decribed for diazepam use in cats. (Podell 2008)

Monitoring

■ Efficacy

■ Adverse effects

Client Information

■ A major factor in anticonvulsant therapy failure is lack of compliance with the prescribed therapy; it is very important to give doses regularly

■ Do not stop giving this drug abruptly as convulsions may occur; contact veterinarian for guidance in stopping treatment

■ Cats: If patient develops lack of appetite, vomits, or yellowish whites of eyes, contact veterinarian immediately

Chemistry/Synonyms

A benzodiazepine anxiolytic, sedative-hypnotic, and anticonvulsant, clorazepate dipotassium occurs as a light yellow, fine powder that is very soluble in water and slightly soluble in alcohol.

Clorazepate dipotassium may also be known as Abbott-35616, AH-3232, 4306-CB, clorazepic acid, dipotassium clorazepate, dikalii clorazepas, or potassium clorazepate; many trade names are available.

Storage/Stability

Clorazepate dipotassium is unstable in the presence of water. It has been recommended to keep the dessicant packets in with the original container of the capsules and tablets and to consider adding a dessicant packet to the prescription vial when dispensing large quantities of tablets or capsules to the client.

Dosage Forms/Regulatory Status

VETERINARY-LABELED PRODUCTS: None
The ARCI (Racing Commissioners International) has designated this drug as a class 2 substance. See the appendix for more information.

HUMAN-LABELED PRODUCTS:
Clorazepate Dipotassium Tablets: 3.75 mg, 7.5 mg, & 15 mg; *Tranxene® T-tab* (Ovation); generic; (Rx, C-IV)

References

Boothe, D (1999). Anticonvulsant pharmacology: Improving management of refractory seizures. Proceedings: American College of Veterinary Internal Medicine: 17th Annual Veterinary Medical Forum, Chicago.

Brown, S & S Forrester (1989). Serum disposition of oral clorazepate from regular–release and sustained–release tablets in dogs. *J Vet Int Med* 3(2): 116.

Dowling, P (2003). Optimizing anticonvulsant therapy. Proceedings: Western Veterinary Conference. Accessed via: Veterinary Information Network. http://goo.gl/H9YKo

Hoskins, J (2005). Geriatric medicine: Nervous System. Proceedings: ACVC 2006. Accessed via: Veterinary Information Network. http://goo.gl/LHU4m

Marder, A (1991). Psychotropic drugs and behavioral therapy. *Veterinary Clinics of North America: Small Animal Practice* 21(2): 329–342.

Podell, M (2006). New Horizons in the treatment of epilepsy. Proceedings: ACVIM. Accessed via: Veterinary Information Network. http://goo.gl/PlHdG

Podell, M (2008). Novel approaches to feline epilepsy. Proceedings: ACVIM. Accessed via: Veterinary Information Network. http://goo.gl/0hc8Z

Quesnel, A (2001). Antiepileptic therapy in dogs and cats—an update, Proceedings: World Small Animal Veterinary Association World Congress. Accessed via: Veterinary Information Network. http://goo.gl/SAsJQ

Reisner, I & K Houpt (2000). Behavioral Disorders. *Textbook of Veterinary Internal Medicine: Diseases of the Dog and Cat.* S Ettinger and E Feldman Eds. Philadelphia, WB Saunders. **1**: 156–162.

Sherman, BL & DS Mills (2008). Canine anxieties and phobias: An update on separation anxiety and noise aversions. *Veterinary Clinics of North America–Small Animal Practice* 38(5): 1081–+.

Shull-Selcer, E & W Stagg (1991). Advances in the understanding and treatment of noise phobias. *Veterinary Clinics of North America: Small Animal Practice* 21(2): 353–367.

Thomas, W (2000). Idiopathic epilepsy in dogs. *Vet Clin NA: Small Anim Pract* 30:1(Jan): 183–206.

Virga, V (2002). Which drug and why: an update on psychopharmacology. Proceedings: Atlantic Coast Veterinary Conference. Accessed via: Veterinary Information Network. http://goo.gl/m8qr4

CLORSULON

(***klor**-su-lon*)   Curatrem®, Ivomec Plus®

ANTIPARASITIC (FLUKICIDE)

Prescriber Highlights

▶ Adult flukicide (*Fasciola hepatica*)

▶ Not for female dairy cattle

▶ Slaughter withdrawal 8 days at labeled doses for *Curatrem®*, 49 days for *Ivomec Plus®*

Uses/Indications

Clorsulon is FDA-approved for use in the treatment of immature and adult forms of *Fasciola hepatica* (Liver fluke) in cattle. It is not effective against immature flukes less than 8 weeks old. It also has activity against *Fasciola gigantica*. Although not FDA-approved, the drug has been used in practice in various other species (*e.g.*, sheep, llamas). It has activity against *F. magna* in sheep, but is not completely effective in eradicating the organism after a single dose, thus severely limiting its clinical usefulness against this parasite. Clorsulon is also not effective against the rumen fluke (Paramphistomum).

Pharmacology/Actions

In susceptible flukes, clorsulon inhibits the glycolytic enzymes 3-phosphoglycerate kinase and phosphoglyceromutase, thereby blocking the Emden-Myerhof glycolytic pathway; the fluke is deprived of its main metabolic energy source and dies. Clorsulon at 7 mg/kg is effective against migrating *F. hepatica* 8 weeks post-infection, but at 2 mg/kg is effective only against adult flukes (14 weeks post infection).

Pharmacokinetics

After oral administration to cattle, the drug is absorbed rapidly with peak levels occurring in about 4 hours. Approximately 75% of the circulating drug is found in plasma and 25% in erythrocytes. At 8–12 hours after administration, clorsulon levels peak in the fluke.

Contraindications/Precautions/Warnings

No milk withdrawal time has been determined, and the drug is labeled not for use in female dairy cattle of breeding age.

The combination injectable product (*Ivomec Plus®*) must be administered subcutaneously only; do not give IV or IM. The manufacturer warns to use in cattle only as severe reactions, including fatalities in dogs, may occur.

Adverse Effects

When used as directed adverse effects are unlikely to occur with the oral suspension (*Curatrem®*). Local swelling may occur at injection sites with *Ivomec Plus®*.

Reproductive/Nursing Safety

Clorsulon is considered safe to use in pregnant or breeding animals.

Overdosage/Acute Toxicity

Clorsulon is very safe when administered orally to cattle or sheep. Doses of up to 400 mg/kg have not produced toxicity in sheep. A dose that is toxic in cattle has also not been determined.

Drug Interactions/Laboratory Considerations

■ None identified

Doses

■ **CATTLE:**
  For *Fasciola hepatica* infections:
  a) 7 mg/kg PO; deposit suspension over the back of the tongue (Label directions; *Curatrem®*—Merial)

  For *Fasciola hepatica* infections, round worms, lungworms, cattle grubs, sucking lice, mange mites (see Ivermectin monograph or product label for more information on species covered):
  a) Inject 1mL per 110 lb. body weight SC behind the shoulder (Label directions; *Ivomec Plus®*—Merial)

■ **SHEEP:**
  For *Fasciola hepatica* infections:
  a) 7 mg/kg PO (Roberson 1988)

■ **LLAMAS:**
  For *Fasciola hepatica* infections:
  a) 7 mg/kg PO (Fowler 1989)

Monitoring

■ Clinical efficacy

Client Information

■ Shake well before using (*Curatrem®*)

■ Follow withdrawal times for slaughter (8 days for *Curatrem®*, 49 days for *Ivomec Plus®*)

■ Do not use in female dairy cattle of breeding age

Chemistry/Synonyms

A benzenesulfonamide, clorsulon has a chemical name of 4-amino-6-trichloroethenyl-1,3-benzenedisulfonamide.

Clorsulon may also be known as MK-401, *Curatrem®,* or *Ivomec®.*

Storage/Stability

Unless otherwise instructed by the manufacturer, clorsulon should be stored at room temperature (15–30°C).

Dosage Forms/Regulatory Status

VETERINARY APPROVED PRODUCTS:

Clorsulon 8.5% (85 mg/mL) Oral Drench in quarts or gallons; *Curatrem®* (Merial); (OTC). FDA-approved for use in cattle. Slaughter withdrawal = 8 days (when used as labeled); Because a withdrawal time in milk has not been established, do not use in female dairy cattle of breeding age.

Clorsulon 10% (100 mg/mL) and Ivermectin 1% (10 mg/mL) Injection in 50 mL, 200 mL, 500 mL, & 1000 mL. *Ivomec®* Plus (Merial); *Normectin®* Plus (Norbrook); (OTC). FDA-approved for subcutaneous injection use in cattle. Do not use within 49 days of slaughter; do not use in female dairy cattle of breeding age.

HUMAN APPROVED PRODUCTS: None

References

Fowler, ME (1989). *Medicine and Surgery of South American Camelids.* Ames, Iowa State University Press.

Roberson, EL (1988). Anticestodal and antitrematodal drugs. *Veterinary Pharmacology and Therapeutics.* NH Booth and LE McDonald Eds. Ames, Iowa State University Press: 928–949.

CLOXACILLIN SODIUM
CLOXACILLIN
BENZATHINE

(klox-a-*sill*-in)
Orbenin-DC®, Dry-Clox®, Dariclox®

ANTI-STAPHYLOCOCCAL PENICILLIN

Prescriber Highlights

▶ Intramammary isoxazolyl (anti-staph-ylococcal) penicillin

▶ Contraindicated: Hypersensitivity to penicillins

▶ Oral dosage forms (human) no longer marketed in USA

Uses/Indications

Cloxacillin is used via intramammary infusion in dry and lactating dairy cattle.

Pharmacology/Actions

Cloxacillin, dicloxacillin and oxacillin have nearly identical spectrums of activity and can be considered therapeutically equivalent when comparing *in vitro* activity. These penicillinase-resistant penicillins have a narrower spectrum of activity than the natural penicillins. Their antimicrobial efficacy is aimed directly against penicillinase-producing strains of gram-positive cocci, particularly Staphylococcal species. They are sometimes called anti-staphylococcal penicillins. There are documented strains of Staphylococci that are resistant to these drugs (so-called methicillin-resistant Staph), but these strains have not yet become a major problem in veterinary species. While this class of penicillins does have activity against some other gram-positive and gram-negative aerobes and anaerobes, other antibiotics (penicillins and otherwise) are usually better choices. The penicillinase-resistant penicillins are inactive against *Rickettsia*, mycobacteria, fungi, Mycoplasma, and viruses.

Pharmacokinetics

Cloxacillin is only available in intramammary dosage forms in the USA.

Contraindications/Precautions/Warnings

Penicillins are contraindicated in patients with a history of hypersensitivity to them. Because there may be cross-reactivity, use penicillins cautiously in patients who are documented hypersensitive to other beta-lactam antibiotics (*e.g.*, cephalosporins, cefamycins, carbapenems).

Adverse Effects

Adverse effects with the penicillins are usually not serious and have a relatively low frequency of occurrence.

Hypersensitivity reactions unrelated to dose can occur with these agents and can manifest as rashes, fever, eosinophilia, neutropenia, agranulocytosis, thrombocytopenia, leukopenia, anemias, lymphadenopathy, or full-blown anaphylaxis. In humans, it is estimated that 1–15% of patients hypersensitive to cephalosporins will also be hypersensitive to penicillins. The incidence of cross-reactivity in veterinary patients is unknown.

Reproductive/Nursing Safety

Penicillins have been shown to cross the placenta and safe use of them during pregnancy has not been firmly established, but neither have there been any documented teratogenic problems associated with these drugs. However, use only when the potential benefits outweigh the risks. In humans, the FDA categorizes this drug as category *B* for use during pregnancy (*Animal studies have not yet demonstrated risk to the fetus, but there are no adequate studies in pregnant women; or animal studies have shown an adverse effect, but adequate studies in pregnant women have not demonstrated a risk to the fetus in the first trimester of pregnancy, and there is no evidence of risk in later trimesters.*) In a separate system evaluating the safety of drugs in canine and feline pregnancy (Papich 1989), this drug is categorized as in class: *A (Probably safe. Although specific studies may not have proved the safety of all drugs in dogs and cats, there are no reports of adverse effects in laboratory animals or women.*)

Overdosage/Acute Toxicity

Overdosage of intramammary infusions is unlikely to pose much risk to the patient, but may prolong withdrawal times.

Drug Interactions

■ No significant interactions are likely when intramammary dosage forms are used as labeled.

Laboratory Considerations

■ No specific concerns noted

Doses

Note: Oral dosage forms are no longer available commercially in the USA—see Dicloxacillin for oral use

■ **DOGS:**

For susceptible infections:

a) 20–40 mg/kg PO q8h (Vaden & Papich 1995)

b) For Staph. pyoderma, diskospondylitis, osteoarthritis or skin infections: 10–15 mg/kg PO q6h for 14–84 days

c) For systemic infections, bacteremia: 10–40 mg/kg PO q6–8h for 7–14 days (Greene & Watson 1998)

■ **CATS:**

For susceptible infections:

a) 20–40 mg/kg PO or IM q6–8h (Papich 1988)

b) For Staph. pyoderma, diskospondylitis, osteoarthritis or skin infections: 10–15 mg/kg PO q6h for 14–84 days

c) For systemic infections, bacteremia: 10–40 mg/kg PO q6–8h for 7–14 days (Greene & Watson 1998)

■ **CATTLE:**

For mastitis (treatment or prophylaxis) caused by susceptible organisms:

a) Lactating cow (using lactating cow formula; *Dari-Clox®*): After milking out and disinfecting teat, instill contents of syringe; massage. Repeat q12h for 3 total doses.

Dry (non-lactating) cows (using dry cow formula; benzathine): After last milking (or early in the dry period), instill contents of syringe and massage into each quarter. (Package inserts; *Dari-Clox®*, *Orbenin-DC®*—Beecham; *Dri-Clox®*—Fort Dodge)

Monitoring

■ Because penicillins usually have minimal toxicity associated with their use, monitoring for efficacy is usually all that is required unless toxic signs develop. Serum levels and therapeutic drug monitoring are not routinely done with these agents.

Client Information

■ Dry cow products (benzathine; *Orbenin-DC®, Dry-Clox®*) slaughter withdrawal = 28–30 days (depending on product used)

■ Lactating cow product (*Dariclox®*) withdrawal times when used as labeled; milk withdrawal = 48 hours; slaughter withdrawal = 10 days

Chemistry/Synonyms

An isoxazolyl-penicillin, cloxacillin sodium is a semisynthetic, penicillinase-resistant penicillin. It is available commercially as the monohydrate sodium salt that occurs as an odorless, bitter-tasting, white, crystalline powder. It is freely soluble in water and soluble in alcohol and has a pK_a of 2.7. One mg of cloxacillin sodium contains not less than 825 micrograms of cloxacillin.

Cloxacillin benzathine occurs as white or almost white powder that is slightly soluble in water and alcohol. A 1% (10 mg/mL) suspension has a pH from 3–6.5.

Cloxacillin sodium may also be known as: BRL-1621, sodium cloxacillin, chlorphenyl-methyl isoxazolyl penicillin sodium, methyl-chlorophenyl isoxazolyl penicillin sodium, cloxacilina sodica, cloxacillinum natricum, or P-25; many trade names are available.

Storage/Stability

Unless otherwise instructed by the manufacturer, cloxacillin benzathine or cloxacillin sodium mastitis syringes should be stored at temperatures less than 25°C in tight containers.

Dosage Forms/Regulatory Status

VETERINARY-LABELED PRODUCTS:

Cloxacillin Benzathine 500 mg (of cloxacillin) in a peanut-oil gel; 10 mL syringe for intramammary infusion: *Orbenin-DC®* (Schering-Plough), *Dry-Clox®* (BIVI), *Boviclox®* (Norbrook); (Rx). FDA-approved for use in dairy cows during the dry period (immediately after last milking or early in the dry period). Do not use *Dry-Clox®* or *Boviclox®* within 30 days prior to calving; (28 days for *Orbenin-DC®*). Slaughter withdrawal for Dry-Clox® = 30 days; *Orbenin®-DC* = 28 days; *Boviclox®* = 72 hours for milk and meat. A tolerance of 0.01 ppm has been established for negligible residues in uncooked edible meat and milk from cattle.

Cloxacillin Sodium 200 mg (of cloxacillin) in vegetable oils; 10 mL syringe for intramammary infusion: *Dariclox®* (Schering-Plough); (Rx). FDA-approved for use in lactating dairy cows. When used as labeled, Milk withdrawal = 48 hours; Slaughter withdrawal = 10 days.

HUMAN-LABELED PRODUCTS: None

References

Greene, C & J A Watson (1998). Antimicrobial Drug Formulary. *Infectious Diseases of the Dog and Cat*. C Greene Ed. Philadelphia, WB Saunders: 790–919.

Papich, MG (1988). Therapy of gram–positive bacterial infections. *Vet Clin North America: Sm Animal Pract* 18(6): 1267–1285.

Vaden, S & M Papich (1995). Empiric Antibiotic Therapy. *Kirk's Current Veterinary Therapy:XII*. J Bonagura Ed. Philadelphia, W.B. Saunders: 276–280.

CODEINE PHOSPHATE CODEINE SULFATE

(koe-deen)

OPIATE

Prescriber Highlights

▶ Opiate used for analgesia, cough, & sometimes diarrhea in dogs & cats

▶ Contraindications: Hypersensitivity to narcotics, receiving MAOI's (amitraz, selegiline?), or diarrhea caused by a toxic ingestion until the toxin is eliminated

▶ Conditions where narcotics must be used with caution: Hypothyroidism, severe renal insufficiency, Addison's, head injuries or increased intracranial pressure, or acute abdominal conditions (e.g., colic) as it may obscure the diagnosis or clinical course of these conditions; in geriatric or severely debilitated patients; use extreme caution in patients with respiratory disease or acute respiratory dysfunction

▶ Adverse Effects most likely noted include: Sedation, constipation, high doses may cause respiratory depression. Cats may also show CNS stimulation.

▶ Controlled Substance (Class-II when used as a sole agent)

Uses/Indications

In small animal medicine, codeine is used principally as an oral analgesic when salicylates are not effective and parenteral opiates are not warranted. It may also be useful as an antitussive or an antidiarrheal.

Pharmacology/Actions

Codeine possesses activity similar to other opiate agonists. It is an effective antitussive and a mild analgesic. It produces similar respiratory depression, as does morphine at equianalgesic dosages. For further information on opiate pharmacology, refer to: Opiate Agonists, Pharmacology.

Pharmacokinetics

Very limited information is available for domestic animals. It has been stated that in dogs there is only limited evidence of oral absorption of codeine (Papich 2009). The following information is human data unless otherwise noted. After oral administration, codeine salts are rapidly absorbed. Codeine is about 2/3's as effective after oral administration when compared with parenteral administration. After oral dosing, onset of action is usually within 30 minutes and analgesic effects persist for 4–6 hours. Codeine is metabolized in the liver and then excreted into the urine.

Contraindications/Precautions/Warnings

All opiates should be used with caution in patients with hypothyroidism, severe renal insufficiency, adrenocortical insufficiency (Addison's disease), and in geriatric or severely debilitated patients. Codeine is contraindicated in cases where the patient is hypersensitive to narcotic analgesics, or in patients taking monamine oxidase inhibitors (MAOIs). It is also contraindicated in patients with diarrhea caused by a toxic ingestion (until the toxin is eliminated from the GI tract) or when used repeatedly in patients with severe inflammatory bowel disease.

Codeine should be used with caution in patients with head injuries or increased intracranial pressure, and in those with acute abdominal conditions (*e.g.*, colic) as it may obscure the diagnosis or clinical course of these conditions. Use with extreme caution in patients suffering from respiratory disease or from acute respiratory dysfunction (*e.g.*, pulmonary edema secondary to smoke inhalation).

Opiate analgesics are contraindicated in patients who have been stung by the scorpion species *Centruroides sculpturatus Ewing* and *C. gertschi Stahnke* as they may potentiate these venoms.

Do not use the combination product containing acetaminophen in cats.

Adverse Effects

Codeine generally is well tolerated, but adverse effects are possible, particularly at higher dosages or with repeated use. Sedation is the most likely effect seen. Potential gastrointestinal effects include anorexia, vomiting, constipation, ileus, and biliary and pancreatic duct spasms. Respiratory depression is generally not noted unless the patient receives high doses or is at risk (see contraindications above).

In cats, opiates may cause CNS stimulation with hyperexcitability, tremors, and seizures are possible.

Reproductive/Nursing Safety

Opiates cross the placenta. Very high doses in mice have caused delayed ossification. Use during pregnancy only when the benefits outweigh the risks, particularly with chronic use. In humans, the FDA categorizes this drug as category C for use during pregnancy (*Animal studies have shown an adverse effect on the fetus, but there are no adequate studies in humans; or there are no animal reproduction studies and no adequate studies in humans.*) In a separate system evaluating the safety of drugs in canine and feline pregnancy (Papich 1989), this drug is categorized as in class: **B** (*Safe for use if used cautiously. Studies in laboratory animals may have uncovered some risk, but these drugs appear to be safe in dogs and cats or these drugs are safe if they are not administered when the animal is near term.*)

Although codeine enters maternal milk, no documented problems have been associated with its use in nursing mothers.

Overdosage/Acute Toxicity

Opiate overdosage may produce profound respiratory and/or CNS depression in most species. Other effects can include cardiovascular collapse, hypothermia, and skeletal muscle hypotonia. Oral ingestions of codeine should be removed when possible using standard gut removal protocols. Because rapid changes in CNS status may occur, inducing vomiting should be attempted with caution. Naloxone is the agent of choice in treating respiratory depression. In massive overdoses, naloxone doses may need to be repeated and animals should be closely observed because naloxone's effects may diminish before subtoxic levels of codeine are attained. Mechanical respiratory support should also be considered in cases of severe respiratory depression. Serious overdoses involving any of the opiates should be closely monitored; it is suggested to contact an animal poison control center for further information.

Drug Interactions

The following drug interactions have either been reported or are theoretical in humans or animals receiving codeine and may be of significance in veterinary patients:

- ■ **ANTICHOLINERGIC DRUGS:** Use with codeine may increase the chances of constipation developing

- ■ **ANTIDEPRESSANTS (tricyclic/monoamine oxidase inhibitors):** May potentiate CNS depressant effects

- ■ **CNS DEPRESSANTS, OTHER (e.g., anesthetic agents, antihistamines, phenothiazines, barbiturates, tranquilizers, alcohol, etc.):** May cause increased CNS or respiratory depression when used with codeine

- ■ **QUINIDINE:** May inhibit the transformation of codeine to morphine in the liver thereby decreasing it efficacy

Laboratory Considerations

- ■ As they may increase biliary tract pressure, opiates can increase plasma amylase and lipase values up to 24 hours following their administration.

Doses

- ■ **DOGS:**

  As an antitussive:

  a) 1–2 mg/kg PO q6–12h (Fenner 1994)

b) Starting doses have been as low as 0.1–0.3 mg/kg PO q8–12h and as high as 1–2 mg/kg PO q6–12h. Whatever the starting point, the dose may need to be increased to achieve a satisfactory effective. (Church 2003)

As an analgesic:

a) For mild to moderate acute pain: 0.5–2 mg/kg PO titrated to effect q6–12h. May use for chronic pain at lowest effective dose (Mathews 2000)

b) In combination with acetaminophen: Using a 60 mg codeine and 300 mg acetaminophen fixed-dose tablet (*e.g.*, Tylenol® #4), give 1–2 mg/kg (of the codeine) PO q6–8h. Using codeine alone: 1–4 mg/kg PO q1– 6 hours (Hansen 1994); (Hardie 2000) **Note:** Do not use in cats.

c) 0.5–1 mg/kg PO q4-6h (Gaynor 2008)

As an antidiarrheal:

a) 0.25–0.5 mg/kg PO q6–8h (Sherding & Johnson 1994)

- ■ **CATS:**

Note: Do **NOT** use the combination product containing acetaminophen

As an analgesic:

a) For mild to moderate acute pain: 0.5–2 mg/kg PO titrated to effect q6–12h. May use for chronic pain at lowest effective dose (Mathews 2000)

b) 0.5–2 mg/kg PO q6–8h (Scherk 2003)

c) 0.5 mg/kg PO q6h (Gaynor 2008)

- ■ **RABBITS:**

Using acetaminophen and codeine elixir:

a) 1 mL in 10–20 mL of drinking water (add dextrose to enhance palatability) (Ivey & Morrisey 2000)

Monitoring

- ■ Efficacy
- ■ Adverse effects (see above)

Client Information

- ■ Keep out of reach of children
- ■ Do not use any product containing acetaminophen (*e.g.*, Tylenol #3) in cats
- ■ Report any significant changes in behavior or activity level, or GI effects (constipation, lack of appetite, vomiting) to veterinarian

Chemistry/Synonyms

A phenanthrene-derivative opiate agonist, codeine is available as the base and three separate salts. Codeine base is slightly soluble in water and freely soluble in alcohol. Codeine phosphate occurs as fine, white, needle-like crystals or white, crystalline powder. It is freely soluble in water. Codeine sulfate's appearance resembles codeine phosphate, but it is soluble in water.

Codeine phosphate may also be known as: codeine phosphate hemihydrate, codeini phos-

phas; codeini phosphas hemihydricus, or codei-
nii phosphas; many trade names are available.

Storage/Stability

Codeine phosphate and sulfate tablets should
be stored in light-resistant, well-closed containers at room temperature. Codeine phosphate
injection should be stored at room temperature
(avoid freezing) and protected from light. Do
not use the injection if it is discolored or contains a precipitate.

Compatibility/Compounding Considerations

Codeine phosphate injection is reportedly **compatible** with glycopyrrolate or hydroxyzine HCl.
It is reportedly **incompatible** with aminophylline, ammonium chloride, amobarbital sodium,
chlorothiazide sodium, heparin sodium, methicillin sodium, pentobarbital sodium, phenobarbital sodium, phenytoin sodium, secobarbital
sodium, sodium bicarbonate, sodium iodide,
and thiopental sodium.

Dosage Forms/Regulatory Status

VETERINARY-LABELED PRODUCTS: None.
The ARCI (Racing Commissioners International) has designated this drug as a class 1
substance. See the appendix for more information.

HUMAN-LABELED PRODUCTS:

There are many products available containing
codeine. The following is a partial listing:

Codeine Phosphate Solution: 15 mg/5 mL in
500 mL & UD 5 mL; Codeine Phosphate (Roxane); (Rx, C-II)

Codeine Sulfate Tablets: 15 mg, 30 mg & 60 mg;
generic; (Rx, C-II)

Codeine Phosphate Parenteral Injection:
15 mg/mL & 30 mg/mL in 2 mL *Carpuject* syringe; generic; (Rx, C-II)

Codeine Phosphate Antitussives with expectorants: 10 mg codeine phosphate and 200 mg
guaifenesin; 10 mg codeine phosphate and
100 mg guaifenesin; Many different trade
names available; (C-V; C-III; certain states may
restrict at a higher level; OTC or Rx)

Codeine Phosphate 7.5 mg (#1), 15 mg (#2),
30 mg (#3), 60 mg (#4) with Acetaminophen
300 mg tablets; *Tylenol® with Codeine #'s 1, 2,
3, 4* (McNeil); generic; (Rx, C-III) **Warning:** Do
not use in cats.

Codeine Phosphate 15 mg (#2), 30 mg (#3),
60 mg (#4) with Aspirin 320 mg tablets; *Empi-
rin® with Codeine #'s 2, 3, 4* (Glaxo Wellcome);
generic; (Rx, C-III)

Note: Codeine-only products are Class-II controlled substances. Combination products with
aspirin or acetaminophen are Class-III. Codeine containing cough syrups are either Class-
V or Class-III, depending on the state.

References

Church, D (2003). Drugs used in the management of re-
spiratory diseases. Proceedings: World Small Animal
Veterinary Assoc. World Congress. Accessed via:
Veterinary Information Network. http://goo.gl/f3mOr

Fenner, W (1994). Seizures, narcolepsy, and cataplexy.
Saunders Manual of Small Animal Practice. S Birchard
and R Sherding Eds. Philadelphia, W.B. Saunders
Company: 1147–1156.

Gaynor, JS (2008). Control of Cancer Pain in Veterinary
Patients. *Veterinary Clinics of North America–Small
Animal Practice* 38(6): 1429–+.

Ivey, E & J Morrisey (2000). Therapeutics for Rabbits. *Vet
Clin NA: Exotic Anim Pract* 3:1(Jan): 183–216.

Mathews, K (2000). Pain assessment and general approach to management. *Vet Clin NA: Small Anim Pract*
30:4(July): 729–756.

Papich, MG (2009). Analgesic drugs for small animals.
Proceedings: WVC.

Scherk, M (2003). Feline analgesia in 2003. Proceedings:
World Small Animal Veterinary Assoc World Congress.
Accessed via: Veterinary Information Network. http://
goo.gl/nXadm

Sherding, R & S Johnson (1994). Diseases of the intestines.
Saunders Manual of Small Animal Practice. S Birchard
and R Sherding Eds. Philadelphia, W.B. Saunders
Company: 687–714.

COLCHICINE

(*kol*-chi-seen)

ANTIINFLAMMATORY

Prescriber Highlights

▶ Unique antiinflammatory occasionally
used in dogs for hepatic cirrhosis/fibro-
sis; relatively experimental

▶ Contraindications: Serious renal, GI, or
cardiac dysfunction

▶ Caution: Geriatric or debilitated patients

▶ Teratogenic, reduces spermatogenesis

▶ Most likely adverse effects are GI distress (may be an early sign of toxicity),
but several serious effects are possible
including bone marrow suppression

Uses/Indications

In veterinary medicine, colchicine has been proposed as a treatment in small animals for amyloidosis. For colchicine to be effective, however,
it must be given early in the course of the disease
and it will be ineffective once renal failure has
occurred. At the time of writing, no conclusive
evidence exists for its efficacy for this indication
in dogs.

Colchicine has also been proposed for treating chronic hepatic fibrosis presumably by decreasing the formation and increasing the breakdown of collagen, but its efficacy is in question

A case report (Brown *et al.* 2008) using colchicine to treat endotracheal stent granulation
stenosis in a dog has been published and the
drug may find a place in therapy for this indication after further investigation.

Pharmacology/Actions

Colchicine inhibits cell division during metaphase by interfering with sol-gel formation and
the mitotic spindle. The mechanism for its anti-

fibrotic activity is believed secondary to collagenases activity stimulation.

Colchicine apparently blocks the synthesis and secretion of serum amyloid A (SAA; an acute-phase reactant protein) by hepatocytes thereby preventing the formation of amyloid-enhancing factor and preventing amyloid disposition.

Colchicine is best known in human medicine for its antigout activity. The mechanism for this effect is not fully understood, but it probably is related to the drug's ability to reduce the inflammatory response to the disposition of monosodium urate crystals.

Pharmacokinetics

No information was located specifically for domestic animals; the following information is human/lab animal data unless otherwise noted. After oral administration, colchicine is absorbed from the GI tract. Some of the absorbed drug is metabolized in the liver (first-pass effect). These metabolites and unchanged drug are re-secreted into the GI tract via biliary secretions where it is reabsorbed. This "recycling" phenomena may explain the intestinal manifestations noted with colchicine toxicity. Colchicine is distributed into several tissues, but is concentrated in leukocytes. Plasma half-life is about 20 minutes, but leukocyte half-life is approximately 60 hours. Colchicine is deacetylated in the liver and metabolized in other tissues. While most of a dose (as colchicine and metabolites) is excreted in the feces, some is excreted in the urine. More may be excreted in the urine in patients with hepatic disease. Patients with severe renal disease may have prolonged half-lives.

Contraindications/Precautions/Warnings

Colchicine is contraindicated in patients with serious renal, GI, or cardiac dysfunction and should be used with caution in patients in early stages of these disorders. It should also be used with caution in geriatric or debilitated patients.

Colchicine use in veterinary medicine is somewhat controversial as safety and efficacy have not been well documented.

Adverse Effects

There has been little experience with colchicine in domestic animals. There are reports that colchicine can cause nausea, vomiting, and diarrhea in dogs, but these are thought to occur infrequently at doses used. Neutropenia is a rare adverse effect.

In humans, GI effects have been noted (abdominal pain, anorexia, vomiting, diarrhea) and can be an early indication of toxicity; it is recommended to discontinue therapy (in humans) should these occur. Prolonged administration has caused bone marrow depression. Severe local irritation has been noted if extravasation occurs after intravenous administration; thrombophlebitis has also been reported.

Reproductive/Nursing Safety

Because colchicine has been demonstrated to be teratogenic in laboratory animals (mice and hamsters) it should be used during pregnancy only when its potential benefits outweigh its risks. Colchicine may decrease spermatogenesis. In humans, the FDA categorizes this drug as category *C* (ORAL) for use during pregnancy (*Animal studies have shown an adverse effect on the fetus, but there are no adequate studies in humans; or there are no animal reproduction studies and no adequate studies in humans.*) In humans, the FDA categorizes this drug as category *D* (PARENTERAL) for use during pregnancy (*There is evidence of human fetal risk, but the potential benefits from the use of the drug in pregnant women may be acceptable despite its potential risks.*)

It is unknown if colchicine enters maternal milk; use cautiously in nursing mothers.

Overdosage/Acute Toxicity

Colchicine can be a very toxic drug after relatively small overdoses. Deaths in humans have been reported with a single oral ingestion of as little as 7 mg, but 65 mg is considered the lethal dose in an adult human. GI manifestations are usually the presenting signs seen. These can range from anorexia and vomiting to bloody diarrhea or paralytic ileus. Renal failure, hepatotoxicity, pancytopenia, paralysis, shock, and vascular collapse may also occur.

There is no specific antidote to colchicine. Gut removal techniques should be employed when applicable. Because of the extensive GI "recycling" of the drug, repeated doses of activated charcoal and a saline cathartic may reduce systemic absorption. Other treatment is symptomatic and supportive. Dialysis (peritoneal) may be of benefit.

Drug Interactions

The following drug interactions have either been reported or are theoretical in humans or animals receiving colchicine and may be of significance in veterinary patients:

■ **BONE MARROW DEPRESSANT MEDICATIONS (e.g., antineoplastics, immunosuppressants, chloramphenicol, amphotericin B):** May cause additive myelosuppression when used with colchicine

Laboratory Considerations

■ Colchicine may cause false-positive results when testing for **erythrocytes or hemoglobin in urine.**

■ Colchicine may interfere with **17-hydroxy-corticosteroid** determinations in urine if using the Reddy, Jenkins, and Thorn procedure.

■ Colchicine may cause increased serum values of **alkaline phosphatase.**

Doses

Colchicine may have some efficacy in the treatment of amyloidosis, but veterinary dosages are apparently unavailable at this time.

■ **DOGS:**

For the adjunctive treatment of hepatic cirrhosis/fibrosis:

a) 0.03 mg/kg PO once daily (Leveille-Webster & Center 1995); (Twedt 1999); (Richter 2002); (Willard 2006)

b) 0.025–0.03 mg/kg PO once daily (probenecid-free drug). Not recommended for initial use with azathioprine, chlorambucil or methotrexate due to similar side effects (GI toxicity, bone marrow suppression). Used in many dogs and fewer cats without problems. (Center 2002), (Center 2006)

For amyloidosis:

a) For periodic fever syndrome in Shar Pei dogs: 0.03 mg/kg PO once daily. (Scherk & Center 2005)

b) To reduce the frequency and severity of fever and prevent the development of amyloidosis in dogs with Shar Pei Fever: 0.025–0.03 mg/kg PO q24h; no evidence supports use of colchicine once amyloidosis has resulted in renal failure (Vaden 2006)

■ **BIRDS:**

As an antifibrotic for the adjunctive treatment of hepatic fibrosis:

a) Psittacines: 0.2 mg/kg PO q12h. May potentiate gout in some cases. (Carpenter 2005), (Oglesbee 2009)

Monitoring

■ Efficacy

■ Adverse effects (see above)

■ CBC

Client Information

■ Clients should be informed of the "investigational" nature of colchicine use in dogs and should be informed of the potential adverse effects that may be seen

■ Report changes in appetite or other GI effects immediately to veterinarian

■ Keep well out of reach of children or pets

■ Pregnant women should avoid exposure to the drug or urine of animals being treated

Chemistry/Synonyms

An antigout drug possessing many other pharmacologic effects, colchicine occurs as a pale yellow, amorphous powder or scales. It is soluble in water and freely soluble in alcohol.

Colchicine may also be known as: colchicinum, *Artrex®*, *Colchily®*, *Colchicquim®*, *Colchis®*, *Colcine®*, *Colgout®*, *Goutichine®*, *Goutnil®*, *Reugor®*, *Ticolcin®*, or *Tolchicine®*.

Storage/Stability

Colchicine tablets should be stored in tight, light resistant containers. The injection should be diluted only in 0.9% sodium chloride for injection or sterile water for injection. Do not use D_5W or bacteriostatic sodium chloride for injection as precipitation may occur. Do not use solutions that have become turbid.

Dosage Forms/Regulatory Status

VETERINARY-LABELED PRODUCTS: None

The ARCI (Racing Commissioners International) has designated this drug as a class 4 substance. See the appendix for more information.

HUMAN-LABELED PRODUCTS:

Colchicine Oral Tablets: 0.6 mg (1/100 gr); *Colcrys®* (AR Scientific); generic; (Rx);

A combination oral product (tablets) containing colchicine 0.5 mg and probenecid 500 mg is also available (not likely to be useful in veterinary patients)

References
Brown, SA, JE Williams, et al. (2008). Endotracheal stent granulation stenosis resolution after colchicine therapy in a dog. *Journal of Veterinary Internal Medicine* 22(4): 1052–1055.

Carpenter, J (2005). *Exotic Animal Formulary, 3rd Ed.*, Elsevier.

Center, S (2002). Chronic hepatitis. Proceedings: Western Veterinary Conference. Accessed via: Veterinary Information Network. http://goo.gl/pvWQX

Center, S (2006). Chronic hepatitis. Proceedings; WSAVA World Congress. Accessed via: Veterinary Information Network. http://goo.gl/YANss

Leveille–Webster, C & S Center (1995). Chronic hepatitis: Therapeutic considerations. *Kirk's Current Veterinary Therapy:XII.* J Bonagura Ed. Philadelphia, W.B. Saunders: 749–756.

Oglesbee, B (2009). Liver disease in pet birds. Proceedings: WVC. Accessed via: Veterinary Information Network. http://goo.gl/eoO1Y

Richter, K (2002). Common canine hepatopathies. Proceedings: ACVIM Forum. Accessed via: Veterinary Information Network. http://goo.gl/pqRDc

Scherk, M & S Center (2005). Toxic, metabolic, infections, and neoplastic liver diseases. *Textbook of Veterinary Internal Medicine, 6th Ed.* S Ettinger and E Feldman Eds., Elsevier: 1464–1478.

Twedt, D (1999). Treatment of chronic hepatitis: Scientific research examines traditional therapies. Proceedings: American College of Veterinary interanl Medicine: 17th Annual Veterinary Medical Forum, Chicago.

Vaden, S (2006). Common familial renal diseases of dogs and cats. Proceedings: Western Vet Conf. Accessed via: Veterinary Information Network. http://goo.gl/PehVh

Willard, M (2006). General considerations in hepatic disease: part 2. Proceedings: ACVC. Accessed via: Veterinary Information Network. http://goo.gl/BITIz

Co-Trimoxazole; Co-trimazine — See Sulfa/Trimethoprim

CORTICOTROPIN (ACTH)

(kor-ti-koe-*troe*-pin) Acthar®

HORMONAL DIAGNOSTIC AGENT

Prescriber Highlights

▶ Stimulates cortisol release; used primarily to test for hyper- or hypoadrenocorticism (ACTH-stimulation test); use as a screening test for naturally occuring "Cushing's" is becoming less popular than in the past. Also used to test for iatrogenic Cushing's and to monitor therapy when treating with anti-adrenal drugs.

▶ Adverse Effects: Unlikely unless using chronically

▶ Do not administer gel form IV

▶ Issues include availability & expense; may need to obtain via a compounding pharmacy. Many have switched to using cosyntropine.

Uses/Indications

Availability of corticotropin in FDA-approved products is an issue as no commercially products were commercially available for veterinary use at the time writing and either cosyntropin (see monograph) or compounded ACTH products are required.

In veterinary medicine, an ACTH product (*Adrenomone®*—Summit Hill) was FDA-approved for use in dogs, cats, and beef or dairy cattle for stimulation of the adrenal cortex when there is a deficiency of ACTH and as a therapeutic agent in primary bovine ketosis, but apparently is no longer commercially available. In practice, ACTH tends to be used most often in the diagnosis of hypoadrenocorticism (ACTH-stimulation test), iatrogenic Cushing's syndrome, and to monitor the response to mitotane or trilostane therapy in Cushing's syndrome. It is less often recommended as a screening test for naturally occuring "Cushing's" syndrome in dogs as the test is relatively insensitive.

One reference (Behrend 2003) recommends using the ACTH stimulation test if the dog has non-adrenal illness, received any form of exogenous glucocorticoids (including topicals), or received phenobarbital. If the dog has no known non-adrenal illness and moderate to severe clinical signs of hyperadrenocorticism, use the low-dose dexamethasone suppression test. If using the ACTH-stim test, the author states that cosyntropin is the agent of choice (see that monograph). ACTH has been used for several purposes in human medicine for its corticosteroid stimulating properties, but as it must be injected, it is not commonly employed in veterinary patients.

Pharmacology/Actions

ACTH stimulates the adrenal cortex (principally the zona fasciculata) to stimulate the production and release of glucocorticoids (primarily cortisol in mammals and corticosterone in birds). ACTH release is controlled by corticotropin-releasing factor (CRF) activated in the central nervous system and via a negative feedback pathway, whereby either endogenous or exogenous glucocorticoids suppresses ACTH release.

Pharmacokinetics

Because it is rapidly degraded by proteolytic enzymes in the gut, ACTH cannot be administered PO. It is not effective if administered topically to the skin or eye.

After IM injection in humans, repository corticotropin injection is absorbed over 8–16 hours. The elimination half-life of circulating ACTH is about 15 minutes but because of the slow absorption after IM injection of the gel, effects may persist up to 24 hours.

Contraindications/Precautions/Warnings

When used for diagnostic purposes, it is unlikely that increases in serum cortisol levels induced by ACTH will have significant deleterious effects on conditions where increased cortisol levels are contraindicated (*e.g.*, systemic fungal infections, osteoporosis, peptic ulcer disease, etc.). ACTH gel should not be used in patients hypersensitive to porcine proteins.

Adverse Effects

Prolonged use may result in fluid and electrolyte disturbances and other adverse effects; if using on a chronic basis, refer to the human literature for an extensive listing of potential adverse reactions. The veterinary manufacturer suggests giving potassium supplementation with chronic therapy.

Do not administer the repository form (gel) IV.

Reproductive/Nursing Safety

ACTH should only be used during pregnancy when the potential benefits outweigh the risks. It may be embryocidal. Neonates born from mothers receiving ACTH should be observed for signs of adrenocortical insufficiency. In humans, the FDA categorizes this drug as category *C* for use during pregnancy (*Animal studies have shown an adverse effect on the fetus, but there are no adequate studies in humans; or there are no animal reproduction studies and no adequate studies in humans.*)

Overdosage/Acute Toxicity

When used for diagnostic purposes, acute inadvertent overdoses are unlikely to cause any significant adverse effects. Monitor as required and treat symptomatically if necessary.

Drug Interactions

The following drug interactions have either been reported or are theoretical in humans or animals receiving corticotropin for diagnostic purposes and may be of significance in veterinary patients:

■ **ANTICHOLINESTERASES (e.g., pyridostigmine):** ACTH may antagonize effects in patients with myasthenia gravis

■ **DIURETICS:** ACTH may increase electrolyte loss

Laboratory Considerations

■ Patients should not receive **hydrocortisone** or **cortisone** on test day

■ ACTH may decrease ^{131}I uptake by the thyroid gland

■ ACTH may suppress **skin test reactions**

■ ACTH may interfere with **urinary estrogen** determinations

■ Obtain specific information from the laboratory on sample handling and laboratory normals for cortisol when doing ACTH stimulation tests

Doses

Note: When using compounded ACTH products, it is recommended to get several post-ACTH samples, at a minimum one and two hours following injection. (Behrend 2005)

■ **DOGS:**

ACTH Stimulation Test:

a) Draw baseline blood sample for cortisol determination and administer 2.2 Units/kg of ACTH gel IM. Draw sample 120 minutes after injection. (Feldman & Peterson 1984), (Kemppainen & Zerbe 1989)

b) Draw baseline blood sample for cortisol determination and administer 0.5 Units/kg of ACTH gel IM. Draw sample 120 minutes after injection.

Normals: Pre-ACTH 1.1–8 micrograms/dL; Post-ACTH 6.2–16.8 micrograms/dL. Hyperadrenocorticism: Pre-ACTH 4–10.8 micrograms/dL; Post-ACTH 11.7–50 micrograms/dL.

Hypoadrenocorticism: Pre-ACTH and Post-ACTH: ≤ 1 microgram/dL (Morgan 1988)

■ **CATS:**

ACTH Stimulation Test:

a) Draw baseline blood sample for cortisol determination and administer 2.2 Units/kg of ACTH gel IM. Draw samples at 60 minutes and 120 minutes after injection. (Kemppainen & Zerbe 1989)

b) Draw baseline blood sample for cortisol determination and administer 0.5 Units/kg of ACTH gel IM. Draw sample 120 minutes after injection.

Normals: Pre-ACTH 0.33–2.6 micrograms/dL; Post-ACTH 4.8–7.6 micrograms/dL. Hyperadrenocorticism: Pre-ACTH 4–10.8 micrograms/dL; Post-ACTH 11.7–50 micrograms/dL.

Hypoadrenocorticism: Pre-ACTH and Post-ACTH: ≤ 1 microgram/dL (Morgan 1988)

■ **CATTLE:**

For ACTH deficiency or for primary bovine ketosis:

a) 200–600 Units initially followed by daily or semi-daily dose of 200–300 Units (Package Insert; *Adrenomone®*—Summit Hill)

■ **HORSES:**

ACTH Stimulation Test:

a) Draw baseline blood sample for cortisol determination and administer 1 Unit/kg IM of ACTH gel. Draw second sample 8 hours later. Normal stimulation will result in serum cortisol levels will increase 2–3 times. Horses with pituitary tumors will increase cortisol fourfold after ACTH. (Beech 1987)

b) Obtain pre-dose level. Administer 1 Unit/kg IM of ACTH gel between 8 and 10 AM; take post ACTH cortisol levels at 2 and 4 hours post dose. Horses with a functional adrenal gland should have a 2- to 3-fold increase in plasma cortisol when compared with baseline. (Toribio 2004)

■ **BIRDS:**

ACTH Stimulation Test:

a) Draw baseline blood sample for corticosterone (not cortisol) determination and administer 16–25 Units IM. Draw second sample 1–2 hours later. Normal baseline corticosterone levels vary with regard to species, but generally range from 1.5–7 ng/mL. After ACTH, corticosterone levels generally increase by 5–10 times those of baseline. Specific values are listed in the reference. (Lothrop & Harrison 1986)

Chemistry/Synonyms

A 39 amino acid polypeptide, corticotropin is secreted from the anterior pituitary. The first 24 amino acids (from the N-terminal end of the chain) define its biologic activity. While human, sheep, cattle and swine corticotropin have different structures, the first 24 amino acids are the same and, therefore, biologic activity is thought to be identical. Commercial sources of ACTH have generally been obtained from porcine pituitaries. One USP unit of corticotropin is equivalent to 1 mg of the international standard.

Corticotropin may also be known as: ACTH, adrenocorticotrophic hormone, adrenocorticotrophin, corticotrophin, corticotropinum, *Acethropan®, Acortan simplex®, Actharn®, Acthelea®, Acton prolongatum®, H.P. Acthar®* or *Cortrophin-Zinc®.*

Storage/Stability

Corticotropin in the past has been available commercially as corticotropin for injection, repository corticotropin for injection, and corticotropin zinc hydroxide suspension. Corticotropin is commonly called ACTH (abbreviated from adrenocorticotropic hormone). Repository corticotropin is often called ACTH gel and is the most commonly used ACTH product in veterinary medicine.

Corticotropin for injection (aqueous) can be stored at room temperature (15–30°C) before reconstitution. After reconstitution, it should be refrigerated and used within 24 hours. Repository corticotropin injection should be stored in the refrigerator (2–8°C). To allow ease in withdrawing the gel into a syringe, the vial may be warmed with warm water prior to use.

Dosage Forms/Regulatory Status

VETERINARY-LABELED PRODUCTS: None
Compounded ACTH products may be available from compounding pharmacies.

HUMAN-LABELED PRODUCTS:

Corticotropin Repository Injection: 80 Units/mL in 5 mL multi-dose vials; *H.P. Acthar® Gel* (Questcor); (Rx) **Note:** This product is only available through a specialty pharmacy distribution system and is not available via regular retail pharmacies or drug wholesalers.

References

Beech, J (1987). Respiratory Tract—Horse, Cow. *The Bristol Handbook of Antimicrobial Therapy*. DE Johnston Ed. Evansville, Veterinary Learning Systems: 88–109.

Behrend, E (2003). Common questions in endocrine diagnostic testing. Proceedings: Western Veterinary Conference. Accessed via: Veterinary Information Network. http://goo.gl/Z6mZ2

Behrend, E (2005). Use of compounded ACTH for adrenal function testing in dogs. Proceedings: ACVIM. Accessed via: Veterinary Information Network. http://goo.gl/FDMUK

Feldman, EC & ME Peterson (1984). Hypoadrenocorticism. *Vet Clin of North America: Small Anim Prac* 14(4): 751–766.

Kemppainen, RJ & CA Zerbe (1989). Common Endocrine Diagnostic Tests: Normal Values and Interpretation. *Current Veterinary Therapy X: Small Animal Practice*. RW Kirk Ed. Philadelphia, WB Saunders: 961–968.

Lothrop, CD & GJ Harrison (1986). Miscellaneous diagnostic tests. *Clinical Avian Medicine and Surgery*. GJ Harrison and LR Harrison Eds. Philadelphia, W.B. Saunders: 293–297.

Morgan, RV, Ed. (1988). *Handbook of Small Animal Practice*. New York, Churchill Livingstone.

Toribio, R (2004). The adrenal glands. *Equine Internal Medicine 2nd Edition*. M Reed, W Bayly and D Sellon Eds. Phila, Saunders: 1357–1361.

CORTISONE ACETATE

(kor-ti-*zone* ass-ah-tate)

ADRENAL CORTICOSTEROID

Prescriber Highlights

▶ Oral glucocorticoid with both glucocorticoid and mineralocorticoid effects; may be a lower drug cost way to manage Addison's by reducing dosage requirements for mineralocorticoid drugs

▶ Not commonly used in veterinary medicine; whether it has any clinically significant benefit in dogs over oral prednis(ol)one is controversial

▶ Typical cautions and adverse effects associated with other corticosteroid drugs if used at supra-physiologic replacement doses; otherwise should be very well tolerated

▶ Relatively inexpensive

Uses/Indications

Cortisone acetate potentially could be an alternative to predniso(lo)ne for the oral treatment of hypoadrenocorticism in dogs. *In vivo* it is rapidly converted to cortisol and thereby could serve as a total replacement for both glucocorticoid and mineralocorticoid effects. Whether cortisone acetate is any more effective then prednis(ol)one for long-term treatment in dogs is controversial as some believe that any benefit the increased mineralocorticoid activity cortisone acetate has is clinically insignificant.

Pharmacology/Actions

Cortisone/cortisol has effects on practically every body system. For a more complete description refer to the Hydrocortisone monograph.

Pharmacokinetics

Like other glucocorticoids, cortisone acetate's pharmacokinetics do not correlate with its pharmacodynamic activity. Cortisol acetate is absorbed and converted to cortisol *in vivo*. Oral bioavailability in humans ranges widely, but is approximately 50%.

Contraindications/Precautions/Warnings

When used for physiologic replacement in dogs with hypoadrenocorticism, cortisone acetate is contraindicated if the patient is hypersensitive to it. If used at supra-physiologic dosages, the typical contraindications and warnings for drugs like prednisone should be followed. See that monograph for more information.

Adverse Effects

When used for physiologic replacement in dogs with hypoadrenocorticism, cortisone acetate should be very well tolerated. Potentially, GI effects (vomiting, inappetence, diarrhea could occur and hypersensitivity reactions are theoretically possible. If used at supra-physiologic dosages, the typical adverse effect profile for drugs like prednisone is possible. See the prednisone monograph for more information.

Reproductive/Nursing Safety

Glucocorticoids are probably necessary for normal fetal development. They may be required for adequate surfactant production, myelin, retinal, pancreatic, and mammary development. However, excessive dosages early in pregnancy may lead to teratogenic effects. In humans, the FDA categorizes this drug as category *C* for use during pregnancy (*Animal studies have shown an adverse effect on the fetus, but there are no adequate studies in humans; or there are no animal reproduction studies and no adequate studies in humans.*)

Glucocorticoids unbound to plasma proteins will enter milk. High dosages or prolonged administration to mothers may potentially inhibit the growth of nursing newborns.

Overdosage/Acute Toxicity

Acute ingestion is rarely a clinical problem and clinical effects are unlikely with acute overdose. However, neuropsychiatric effects can occur; cardiac arrhythmias and anaphylaxis are possible, but very rare.

Drug Interactions

The following drug interactions have either been reported or are theoretical in humans or animals receiving hydrocortisone and may be of significance in veterinary patients:

■ **AMPHOTERICIN B:** Administered concomitantly with glucocorticoids may cause hypokalemia; in humans, there have been cases of CHF and cardiac enlargement reported after using hydrocortisone to treat Amphotericin B adverse effects

■ **ASPIRIN:** Glucocorticoids may reduce salicylate blood levels and increase risk for GI ulceration/bleeding

■ **DIURETICS, POTASSIUM-DEPLETING (e.g., spironolactone, triamterene):** Administered concomitantly with glucocorticoids may cause hypokalemia

■ **ESTROGENS:** The effects of hydrocortisone and, possibly other glucocorticoids, may be potentiated by concomitant administration with estrogens

■ **INSULIN; ANTIDIABETIC AGENTS:** Insulin requirements may increase in patients receiving glucocorticoids

■ **MITOTANE:** May alter the metabolism of steroids; higher than usual doses of steroids may be necessary to treat mitotane-induced adrenal insufficiency

■ **NSAIDS:** Administration of ulcerogenic drugs with glucocorticoids may increase the risk of gastrointestinal ulceration

■ **POTASSIUM-DEPLETING DRUGS (e.g., amphotericin B, furosemide, thiazides):** Adminis-

tered concomitantly with glucocorticoids may cause hypokalemia

■ **VACCINES:** Patients receiving corticosteroids at immunosuppressive dosages should generally not receive live attenuated-virus vaccines as virus replication may be augmented; a diminished immune response may occur after vaccine, toxoid, or bacterin administration in patients receiving glucocorticoids

■ **WARFARIN:** Hydrocortisone may affect INR's; monitor

Laboratory Considerations

■ Cortisone can cross react with cortisol in ACTH response test. This test must be performed before cortisone is administered. (**Note:** Dexamethasone does not cross react)

■ Glucocorticoids may increase **serum cholesterol**

■ Glucocorticoids may increase **urine glucose** levels

■ Glucocorticoids may decrease **serum potassium**

■ Glucocorticoids can suppress the release of **thyroid stimulating hormone** (TSH) and reduce T_3 & T_4 values. Thyroid gland atrophy has been reported after chronic glucocorticoid administration. Uptake of I^{131} by the thyroid may be decreased by glucocorticoids.

■ Reactions to **skin tests** may be suppressed by glucocorticoids

■ False-negative results of the **nitroblue tetrazolium** test for systemic bacterial infections may be induced by glucocorticoids

■ Glucocorticoids may cause **neutrophilia** within 4−8 hours after dosing and return to baseline within 24−48 hours after drug discontinuation

■ Glucocorticoids can cause **lymphopenia** which can persist for weeks after drug discontinuation in dogs

Doses

■ **DOGS:**

For long-term treatment of hypoadrenocorticism:

a) In the changeover period as animals recover from an acute crisis, start eating and drinking and are changed from parenteral to oral medication, traditionally a semi-selective mineralocorticoid (fludrocortisone) and a semi-selective glucocorticoid (cortisone acetate or prednisolone) are initially used together. The former is discontinued in a proportion of patients after one to two months. When using cortisone acetate most hypoadrenocorticoid dogs are started on a dose of 0.5−1 mg/kg PO q12-24h. Once stable, generally a dose of 0.5 mg/kg PO q12-24h provides adequate additional glucocorticoid supplementation. Some clinicians advocate prednisolone use as a glucocorticoid supplement in the long-term management of hypoadrenocorticism, but in the author's opinion cortisone acetate is a more effective alternative. (Church 2008), (Church 2009)

Client Information

■ Adherence to the prescribed dose and dosage schedule should be stressed and clients should not discontinue the drug abruptly without consulting with the veterinarian beforehand.

■ Clients should be briefed on the potential adverse effects that can be seen with this drug.

Monitoring

Monitoring of cortisone therapy is dependent on its reason for use, dosage, adjunctive mineralocorticoid therapy, dosage schedule (daily versus alternate day therapy), duration of therapy, and the animal's age and condition. The following list may not be appropriate or complete for all animals; use clinical assessment and judgment should adverse effects be noted:

■ Weight, appetite, signs of edema

■ Serum and/or urine electrolytes

■ Total plasma proteins, albumin

■ Blood glucose

■ Growth and development in young animals

■ ACTH stimulation test if necessary

Chemistry/Synonyms

Cortisone acetate is synthetic acetate ester of cortisone. It occurs as a white or practically white, odorless, crystalline powder. It is insoluble in water and slightly soluble in alcohol.

Cortisone acetate may also be known as acetato de cortisona, compound E acetate, acétate de cortisone, cortisoni acetas, or 11-dehydro-17-hydroxycorticosterone acetate.

Storage/Stability

Cortisone acetate tablets should be stored in well-closed containers at a temperature less than 40°C, preferably at 15-30°C.

Dosage Forms/Regulatory Status

VETERINARY-LABELED PRODUCTS: None

HUMAN-LABELED PRODUCTS:

Cortisone Acetate Oral Tablets; 25 mg; generic; (Rx)

References

Church, DB (2008). Addison's Disease: What's The Best Treatment? Proceedings: WSAVA. Accessed via: Veterinary Information Network. http://goo.gl/uXM7F

Church, DB (2009). Management of Hypoadrenocorticism. Proceedings: WSAVA. Accessed via: Veterinary Information Network. http://goo.gl/1YHrT

COSYNTROPIN

(koh-**sin**-troh-pin)   Cortrosyn®, Synacthen®

HORMONAL DIAGNOSTIC AGENT

Prescriber Highlights

▶ Alternative to ACTH for adrenal function tests

▶ Drug-lab interactions

▶ Availability & expense have been issues

Uses/Indications

Cosyntropin is used primarily as an alternative to ACTH to test for adrenocortical insufficiency (Addison's), or hyperadrenocorticism, particularly in animals who have reacted immunologically to corticotropin in the past or if ACTH gel is unavailable. In addition to its use to diagnose hypoadrenocorticism, the ACTH stimulation test is used to help diagnose iatrogenic Cushing's syndrome, and to monitor the response to mitotane or trilostane therapy in Cushing's syndrome. It is less often recommended as a screening test for naturally occurring "Cushing's" syndrome dogs as the test is relatively insensitive.

Pharmacology/Actions

Like endogenous corticotropin, cosyntropin stimulates the adrenal cortex (in normal patients) to secrete cortisol, corticosterone, etc. Because of its structure, corticotropin is not as immunogenic as endogenous corticotropin. Apparently, the bulk of immunogenicity resides in the C-terminal portion of corticotropin (22–39 amino acids) and cosyntropin ends after amino acid #24.

Pharmacokinetics

Cosyntropin must be given parenterally because it is inactivated by gut enzymes. It is rapidly absorbed after being given IM. After giving IM or rapid IV, plasma cortisol levels reach their peak within an hour. It is unknown how cosyntropin is inactivated or eliminated.

Contraindications/Precautions/Warnings

Contraindicated in patients with known hypersensitivity to cosyntropin. Use caution in patients who have shown hypersensitive reactions to ACTH in the past; there is a distinct possibility that cross-reactivity could occur.

Adverse Effects

When used short-term, the only real concern is hypersensitivity reactions.

Reproductive/Nursing Safety

In humans, the FDA categorizes this drug as category *C* for use during pregnancy (*Animal studies have shown an adverse effect on the fetus, but there are no adequate studies in humans; or there are no animal reproduction studies and no adequate studies in humans.*)

Overdosage/Acute Toxicity

Unlikely to be of clinical consequence if used one-time only.

Laboratory Considerations

- Patients should not receive **hydrocortisone** or **cortisone** on test day; dexamethasone sodium phosphate does not interfere with cortisol assays

- If using a fluorometric analysis: Falsely high values may be observed if the patient is taking **spironolactone**

- Falsely high values may be observed in patients with high **bilirubin** or if free plasma hemoglobin present

Doses

■ **DOGS:**

For testing (screening) adrenal function:

a) For tentative diagnosis of Addison's disease: **1)** Draw blood for hemogram, serum biochemistry and basal cortisol; **2)** Begin IV fluids and give 2–5 mg/kg dexamethasone sodium phosphate; **3)** Immediately give 0.25 mg (250 micrograms) of cosyntropin IV or IM; **4)** Draw a second blood sample for plasma cortisol 45–60 minutes later. Blood levels of <1 micrograms/dL are typical for hypoadrenocorticism, while those stimulating to only 2–3 micrograms/dL are also suggestive. (Schaer 2006)

b For ACTH Stimulation test: Two different protocols: 1 microgram/kg or 250 micrograms/dog IV or IM with serum cortisol measured before and 1 hour post injection. 80–85% of dogs with pituitary-dependent hyperadrenocorticism (PD) and 60% of dogs with adrenal tumor/hyperplasia (AT) will have an exaggerated response. Unfortunately, just about any other extra-adrenal illness can cause an exaggerated post-ACTH level. (Reine 2006)

c) Low dose ACTH stimulation test: 0.5 micrograms/kg IV; peak concentrations at 60 minutes after dose with a return to baseline at 240 minutes. (Martin *et al.* 2007)

■ **CATS:**

For testing (screening) adrenal function:

a) For tentative diagnosis of Addison's disease: **1)** Draw blood for hemogram, serum biochemistry and basal cortisol; **2)** Begin IV fluids and give 2–5 mg/kg dexamethasone sodium phosphate; **3)** Immediately give 0.125 mg of cosyntropin IV or IM; **4)** Draw a second blood sample for plasma cortisol 45–60 minutes later. Blood levels of <1 microgram/dL are typical for hypoadrenocorticism, while those stimulating to only 2–3 micrograms/dL are also suggestive. (Schaer 2006)

b) 0.125 mg (total dose—125 mcg) IM or IV. Begin test between 8–9 AM; obtain preinjection cortisol level and 30 minutes and 1 hour post. (Feldman 2000)

c) For diagnosis of hyperadrenocorticism in cats: 125 micrograms/cat IM or IV with cortisol measurements before and at 30 and 60 minutes post. (Reine 2006)

d) Low dose ACTH stimulation test: 5 micrograms/kg; cortisol concentrations peak at 60 minutes post-dose. (Martin *et al.* 2009)

■ **HORSES:**

For testing (screening) adrenal function:

a) For relative adrenal insufficiency (RIA) evaluation in critically ill horses: Draw blood for baseline cortisol and give cosyntropin at 0.1 micrograms/kg; cortisol will peak after 30 minutes. (Stewart, A 2006)

b) Obtain pre-dose level. Administer 1 mg IV of cosyntropin between 8 and 10 AM; take post ACTH cortisol levels at 2 hours post dose. Horses with a functional adrenal gland should have at least a two-fold increase in plasma cortisol when compared with baseline. (Toribio 2004)

c) **Foals:** 0.5 micrograms/kg IV. Peak cortisol levels occur at 30 minutes post dose. (Stewart, AJ *et al.* 2007)

Monitoring

■ See specific protocols for test procedures

Chemistry/Synonyms

A synthetic polypeptide that mimics the effects of corticotropin (ACTH), cosyntropin is commercially available as a lyophilized white to off-white powder containing mannitol. Cosyntropin's structure is identical to the first 24 (of 39) amino acids in natural corticotropin. 0.25 mg of cosyntropin is equivalent to 25 Units of corticotropin.

Cosyntropin may also be known as: tetracosactide, alpha(1–24)-corticotrophin, beta(1–24)-corticotrophin, tetracosactido, tetracosactidum, tetracosactrin, tetracosapeptide, *Cortrosina®, Cortrosyn®, Nuvacthen Depot®, Synacthen®, Synacthen Depot®, Synacthen Retard®,* or *Synacthene®.*

Storage/Stability

After reconstituting with sterile normal saline, the solution is stable for 24 hours at room temperature; 21 days if refrigerated. Do not add the drug to blood or plasma infusions. One study (Frank and Oliver 1998) showed that cosyntropin can be reconstituted and stored frozen (-20°C) in plastic syringes for up to 6 months and still show biologic activity in the dog. It is recommended to freeze in small aliquots as it is unknown what effect thawing and refreezing has on potency.

Dosage Forms/Regulatory Status

VETERINARY-LABELED PRODUCTS: None

HUMAN-LABELED PRODUCTS:

Cosyntropin Powder for Injection: 0.25 mg lyophilized (250 mcg) in single-dose vials with diluent; *Cortrosyn®* (Amphastar); (Rx)

Cosyntropin Solution for Injection: 0.25 mg/mL, preservative free in 1 mL single-dose vials; generic (Sandoz); (Rx)

References

Martin, LG, EN Behrend, et al. (2007). Effect of low doses of cosyntropin on serum cortisol concentrations in clinically normal dogs. *American Journal of Veterinary Research* 68(5): 555–560.

Martin, LG, A DeClue, et al. (2009). Effect of low doses of cosyntropin on cortisol concentrations in clinically healthy dogs. Proceedings: ACVIM.

Reine, N (2006). Understanding commonly used endocrine diagnostic tests. Proceedings: ACVIM. Accessed via: Veterinary Information Network. http://goo.gl/nX9Fa

Schaer, M (2006). Acute adrenocortical insufficiency. Proceedings: WSAVA World Congress. Accessed via: Veterinary Information Network. http://goo.gl/QpFSa

Stewart, A (2006). Endocrine monitoring in the ICU/NICU. Proceedings: IVECCS. Accessed via: Veterinary Information Network. http://goo.gl/PLK8a

Stewart, A, E Behrend, et al. (2007). Effect of low doses of cosyntropin on serum cortisol concentrations in clinically normal nenotal foals. Proceedings: IVECCS.

Toribio, R (2004). The adrenal glands. *Equine Internal Medicine 2nd Edition*. M Reed, W Bayly and D Sellon Eds. Phila, Saunders: 1357–1361.

CROMOLYN SODIUM (SYSTEMIC)

(***kroh***-mah-lin)
Disodium Cromoglycate, Sodium Cromoglicate, Intal®

MAST CELL STABILIZER

For ophthalmic use, see the monograph in the Ophthalmic Drug Appendix

Prescriber Highlights

▶ Inhaled mast cell stabilizer that may be useful adjunctive treatment in preventing airway hyper-reactivity in horses with type 2 (high mast cell count in BAL) IAD or with RAO (heaves)

▶ Not for treatment of acute bronchoconstriction; used as a preventative agent

▶ May take several days or weeks for efficacy

Uses/Indications

Cromolyn sodium is a mast cell stabilizer that may be useful in reducing airway hyper-reactivity in horses with type 2 (high mast cell count in bronchoalveolar lavage fluid; mast cells of >2% of the total cell count) inflammatory airway disease (IAD) or with recurrent airway obstruction (RAO; heaves). Use of this agent is somewhat controversial; studies have yielded conflicting efficacy results.

Pharmacology/Actions

Cromolyn inhibits the release of histamine and leukotrienes from sensitized mast cells found in lung mucosa, nasal mucosa and eyes. Its exact mechanism of activity is not understood, but it is thought to be a result from blocking indirect entry of calcium ions into cells. Other effects of cromolyn include inhibiting neuronal reflexes in the lung, inhibiting bronchospasm secondary to tachykins, inhibiting the movement of other inflammatory cells (neutrophils, monocytes, eosinophils), and preventing the down-regulation of beta-2 adrenergic receptors on lymphocytes. Cromolyn does not possess antihistaminic, anticholinergic, antiserotonin, corticosteroid-like, or antiinflammatory actions.

Pharmacokinetics

Limited information is available for horses. The amount of cromolyn reaching the distal airways is probably variable and dependent on the type of nebulizer used and the amount of concurrent bronchoconstriction present. Absorbed cromolyn is eliminated in the urine and via the bile into the feces.

In humans, less than 2% is absorbed from the GI tract after oral dosing. Approximately 8% is absorbed when inhaled into the lung. Absorbed drug is eliminated via the feces and urine as unchanged drug.

Contraindications/Precautions/Warnings

Do not use in patients with documented hypersensitivity to cromolyn.

Unlikely to be of benefit in treating horses with types 1 and 3 IAD. Cromolyn has no efficacy in treating acute bronchospasm.

Adverse Effects

Adverse effects associated with inhaled cromolyn use in horses are not well documented. Cough and treatment avoidance (secondary to bad taste?) have been reported. It has been proposed that pretreatment with albuterol may reduce the incidence of cough.

Humans can occasionally develop cough, throat irritation or complain of unpleasant taste. Rarely, bronchoconstriction and anaphylaxis (<0.0001%) have been reported.

Reproductive/Nursing Safety

Laboratory animal studies have shown no effect on fertility. Teratogenicity studies in mice, rats and rabbits have not demonstrated any teratogenic effects and it is likely safe to use during pregnancy. Extremely low (or undetectable) levels have been detected in milk; cromolyn is most likely safe to use during nursing.

Overdosage/Acute Toxicity

Because of the drug's low systemic bioavailability after inhalation or oral administration, acute overdoses are unlikely to cause significant morbidity.

Drug Interactions

No notable drug interactions have been reported.

Laboratory Considerations

No notable laboratory interactions or alterations have been reported.

Doses

- **HORSES:**
  a) For type 2 inflammatory airway disease: Using a jet nebulizer: 200 mg (total dose) q12 hours; using an ultrasonic nebulizer 80 mg once daily (q24h). (Couetil 2002)

  b) For RAO/IAD (either as long-term therapy or before exposure to allergens): Using the aerosol (800 micrograms/puff) and a suitable delivery system: 8–12 mg (10–15 puffs) once to twice daily. (Mazan 2003)

  c) If inflammatory airway disease is mast cell rich: Albuterol, fluticasone and cromolyn are used. Albuterol inhaler: 10 puffs twice daily for 2 weeks then once daily for 1 week. Albuterol is used 20 minutes before giving corticosteroid (fluticasone 250 micrograms: 10 puffs twice daily for for 2 weeks the once daily for 1 week.) Then give cromolyn: If using the *Intal®* 1 mg product: 10 puffs twice daily for 10 days then once daily for 10 days. If using the *Intal®* 5 mg product give 2 puffs twice daily for 10 days then once daily for 10 days. Instruct client to allow 20-30 seconds between each puff to maximize efficiency. (Lester & Secombe 2008)

Monitoring

- Clinical efficacy
- For horses with type 2 IAD, reductions in mast cell counts in bronchoalveolar lavage fluid could help confirm efficacy

Client Information

- This medication does not treat airway constriction but used to prevent airway constriction by reducing the release of substances from cells that can cause it; it should not be used to treat acute bronchoconstriction (difficulty breathing).
- This medicine the must be dosed once to twice daily and it may take several days or weeks before it can be determined if it is working.
- Proper use of the drug delivery device is very important; if any questions arise regarding proper use, contact the veterinarian.

Chemistry/Synonyms

Cromolyn sodium occurs as a white, odorless, hygroscopic, crystalline powder that is soluble in water and insoluble in alcohol.

Cromolyn sodium may also be known as cromoglicic acid, cromoglycic acid, sodium cromo-glicate, disodium cromoglycate, sodium cromo-glycate, DSCG, SCG, FPL–670, or DNSG; there are many international trade names.

Storage/Stability/Compatibility

Cromolyn sodium solution for inhalation should be stored below 40°C (104°F); preferably between 15–30°C. Protect from freezing, light and humidity. Store in foil pouch until ready for use. Do not use solution if it is cloudy or contains a precipitate. Solution remaining in nebulizers after use should be discarded.

Compatibility/Compounding Considerations

Cromolyn solution is reportedly **compatible** with acetylcysteine, albuterol, epinephrine, iso-etherine, isoproterenol, metaproterenol, or terbutaline solutions for up to 60 minutes. It is **not compatible** with bitolterol.

Dosage Forms/Regulatory Status

VETERINARY-LABELED PRODUCTS: None in the USA

HUMAN-LABELED PRODUCTS:

Cromolyn Sodium Solution for Inhalation: 20 mg/2 mL vials or amps; generic; (Rx)

Cromolyn Sodium Aerosol for Inhalation: 800 micrograms/actuation in 8.1 g (approx. 112 sprays) and 14.2 g (approx. 200 sprays); *Intal®* (Aventis); (Rx)

There is also an OTC nasal solution (*Nasal-crom®*), and an oral concentrate (*Gastrocrom®*) indicated for mastocystosis available, but these dosage forms are unlikely to be of use in veterinary medicine.

References

Couetil, L (2002). Aerosol medications for the management of inflammatory airway disease (IAD). Proceedings: ACVIM 2002. Accessed via: Veterinary Information Network. http://goo.gl/HHTnl

Lester, G & C Secombe (2008). Inflammatory airway disease. Proceedings: Australian Veterinary Association.

Mazan, M (2003). Use of aerosolized bronchodilators and corticosteroids. *Current Therapy in Equine Medicine 5.* N Robinson Ed., Saunders: 440–445.

CYANOCOBALAMIN (VITAMIN B12)

(sye-*an*-oh-koe-*bal*-ah-min)

VITAMIN/NUTRITIONAL

Prescriber Highlights

- ▶ Used for parenteral treatment of vitamin B12 deficiency
- ▶ Very safe

Uses/Indications

Cyanocobalamin is used for treating deficiencies of vitamin B12. Malabsorption of the nutrient secondary to gastrointestinal tract disease, or dietary chromium deficiencies (in ruminants) can be associated with dietary deficiencies of vitamin B12. As there appears to be a high percentage of cats with exocrine pancreatic insufficiency or gastrointestinal disease that are deficient in cobalamin, there is considerable interest in evaluating serum cobalamin (vitamin B12) in these patients. Giant schnauzers may have a genetic defect affecting the location of the cobalamin-intrinsic factor, causing cobalamin deficiency. Dogs with inflammatory bowel disease may also develop cobalamin deficiency.

Pharmacology/Actions

Vitamin B12 (cobalamin), a cobalt-containing water-soluble vitamin, serves as an important cofactor for many enzymatic reactions in mammals that are required for normal cell growth, function and reproduction, nucleoprotein and myelin synthesis, amino acid metabolism, and erythropoiesis. Cobalamin is required for folate utilization; B12 deficiency can cause functional folate deficiency. Unlike humans, macrocytic anemias do not appear to be a significant component to cobalamin deficiency in dogs or cats.

Clinical signs associated with cobalamin deficiency in cats may include weight loss, poor haircoat, vomiting, or diarrhea. Increases in serum methionine and methylmalonic acid, and decreased serum cystathionine and cysteine values may be noted. Homocysteine levels do not appear to be affected.

In dogs, cobalamin deficiency may cause or contribute to inappetence, diarrhea, weight loss, leukopenia, or methylmalonylaciduria.

In ruminants, vitamin B12 appears to be synthesized by rumen microflora and requires dietary cobalt to be present for its formation. Clinical signs seen with cobalamin deficiency states associated with cobalt deficiency in cattle and sheep include inappetence, lassitude, poor haircoat/fleece, poor milk production, weight loss, or failure to grow.

Pharmacokinetics

After food is consumed in monogastric mammals, cobalamin in food is bound to a protein (haptocorrin) in the stomach. Haptocorrin/cobalamin is degraded by pancreatic proteases in the duodenum, but cobalamin is then bound by Intrinsic factor (IF), a protein produced in the stomach and pancreas in dogs, in the pancreas (only) in cats, and in the stomach (only) in humans. The cobalamin-IF complex is absorbed in the small intestine where it binds to cubulin, which facilitates its entry into the portal circulation. A protein called transcobalamin 2 (TCII) then binds to cobalamin allowing its entry into target cells. Some cobalamin is rapidly excreted into the bile where entero-hepatic recirculation occurs. Dogs and cats, unlike humans, do not possess cobalamin-binding protein TC1. This means that dogs and cats with B12 dietary deficiency or malabsorption can rapidly deplete their stores of B12 in one to two months, whereas in humans it may require 1–2 years.

In normal cats, circulating half-life of cobalamin is approximately 13 days, but in two cats with inflammatory bowel disease, it was only 5 days (Simpson *et al.* 2001).

Contraindications/Precautions/Warnings

For injectable use, no contraindications are documented for domestic animals. In humans, cyanocobalamin is contraindicated in patients hypersensitive to it or hydroxocobalamin.

Adverse Effects

Cyanocobalamin appears very well tolerated when used parenterally in animals. In humans, anaphylaxis has been reported rarely after parenteral use. Some human patients complain of pain at the injection site, but this is uncommon.

Reproductive/Nursing Safety

Studies documenting safety during pregnancy have apparently not been done in humans or animals, but it is likely safe to use. Vitamin B12 deficiency states are thought to cause teratogenic effects.

While vitamin B12 can be excreted into milk, it is safe to use while nursing.

Overdosage/Acute Toxicity

No overdose information was located, but an inadvertent overdose of cyanocobalamin given via SC or IM injection is unlikely to cause significant morbidity.

Drug Interactions

No significant drug interactions have been identified when cyanocobalamin is administered parenterally.

Laboratory Considerations

- Serum samples to be analyzed for cobalamin and/or folate should be protected from bright light and excessive heat
- If a microbiologic method assay is used to determine cobalamin values, concurrent use of antibiotics can cause falsely low serum or red blood cell values

Doses

- **DOGS:**
    a) Cobalamin deficiency in dogs with severe GI disease (protein losing enteropathies, inflammatory bowel disease): Injectable cyanocobalamin at 25 micrograms/kg once per week for 4–6 weeks, then once monthly thereafter to maintain normal serum levels. May take as long as 3–4 weeks to see a response and lifelong therapy may be required. (Zoran 2008)
    b) Cobalamin deficiency associated with GI disease: Based on body size, 250–1200 micrograms (total dose) SC once weekly for 6 weeks, then every 14 days for 6 weeks, then one dose 30 days later. Recheck serum cobalamin concentration one month after that. If the

underlying disease process is resolved and cobalamin stores have been replenished, level should be supranormal. If levels are normal, continue treatment at least monthly. If subnormal, further workup is required and continue cobalamin treatment weekly or bi-weekly. (Steiner 2009)

c) Cobalamin deficiency associated with exocrine pancreatic insufficiency: 250–500 mcg (total dose) parenterally; repeat treatment based upon serum levels. (Westermarck *et al.* 2005)

■ **CATS:**

a) Cobalamin deficiency in cats with IBD: 250–500 micrograms (total dose per cat) SC once per week for 6 weeks, then every 1–2 months. (Marks 2003). For adjunctive treatment of idiopathic hepatic lipidosis: 250 micrograms (total dose) SC once per week for 6 weeks. Recheck serum B_{12} level in one to two weeks after cessation of treatment as some cats may need repeated administration. (Marks 2009)

b) Cobalamin deficiency associated with GI disease: Based on body size, 150–250 micrograms (total dose) SC once weekly for 6 weeks, then every 14 days for 6 weeks, then one dose 30 days later. Recheck serum cobalamin concentration one month after that. If the underlying disease process is resolved and cobalamin stores have been replenished, level should be supranormal. If levels are normal, continue treatment at least monthly. If subnormal, further workup is required and continue cobalamin treatment weekly or bi-weekly. (Steiner 2009)

c) Cobalamin deficiency associated with exocrine pancreatic insufficiency: 100–250 micrograms (total dose) SC once weekly; periodically assess cobalamin and folate levels. (Westermarck *et al.* 2005)

■ **HORSES:**

a) For vitamin B12 deficiency: 1–2 mL of a 1000 micrograms/mL injection (1000–2000 micrograms per horse) injected IM or SC; dosage may be repeated once or twice weekly, as indicated by condition or response. (Label information; Amtech Vitamin B12 1000 mcg—IVX)

■ **CATTLE, SHEEP:**

a) For treatment of vitamin B12 deficiency associated with cobalt deficiency: Lambs: 100 micrograms (total dose) injected once weekly. Adult sheep: 300 micrograms (total dose) injected once weekly. (Baxter 1986)

b) For treatment of vitamin B12 deficiency associated with cobalt deficiency: Cattle and sheep: 0.2–0.4 mL of a 5000 micro-

grams/mL injection (1000–2000 micrograms) injected IM or SC; dosage may be repeated in weekly intervals if necessary. (Label information; Vitamin B12 5000 micrograms—Butler)

■ **SWINE:**

a) For vitamin B12 deficiency: 0.1–0.4 mL of a 5000 micro-grams/mL injection (500–2000 micrograms) injected IM or SC; dosage may be repeated in weekly intervals if necessary. (Label information; Amtech Vitamin B12 5000 micrograms—IVX)

Monitoring

■ Cobalamin levels

■ In small animals: folate status; both before and after treatment with cyanocobalamin

■ Clinical signs associated with deficiency

■ CBC, baseline and ongoing if abnormal

Client Information

■ Several weeks after starting B12 therapy may be required before improvement is seen

■ Vitamin B12 deficiency in animals may require life-long treatment

■ As cyanocobalamin may be administered SC, clients can be instructed to administer at home, but the importance of ongoing follow-up with the veterinarian must be stressed

Chemistry/Synonyms

Cyanocobalamin occurs as dark red crystals or crystalline powder. It is sparingly soluble in water (1 in 80) and soluble in alcohol. When in the anhydrous form, it is very hygroscopic and can absorb substantial amounts of water from the air.

Vitamin B12 may also be known as cobalamins. Cyanocobalamin may also be known as: cyanocobalamine, cyanocobalaminum, cobamin, cianokobalaminas, cianocobalamina, or cycobemin; many internationally registered trade names.

Storage/Stability

Cyanocobalamin injection should be stored below 40°C; protect from light and freezing.

Compatibility/Compounding Considerations

Cyanocobalamin injection is reportedly **compatible** with all commonly used intravenous fluids.

Dosage Forms

VETERINARY-LABELED PRODUCTS:

Cyanocobalamin (Vitamin B12) Injection 1000, 3000 and 5000 micrograms/mL in 100 mL, 250 mL and 500 mL multi-dose vials depending on source; generic; (Rx). Products may be labeled as cyanocobalamin or vitamin B12, and be labeled for use in cattle, horses, dogs, cats, sheep, or swine.

There are many combination products, both oral and injectable, containing cyanocobalamin as one of the ingredients. These are not recommended for use when cobalamin deficiency states exist.

HUMAN-LABELED PRODUCTS:

Cyanocobalamin (crystalline, Vitamin B12) Injection 100 micrograms (0.1 mg) per mL and 1000 (1 mg) per mL, vial sizes range from 1 mL single-use to 10 mL and 30 mL multidose; generic; (Rx). Besides generically labeled products, there are several products available with a variety of trade names, including *Cyanoject®*, *Rubesol®*, *Crysti®*, or *Crystamine®*.

Oral tablet dosage forms are also available, but have not been shown to be appropriate for therapy of cobalamin deficient states in small animal medicine. A nasally administered product is marketed, but there is no information on its use in dogs or cats.

References

Baxter, J (1986). Deficiencies of mineral nutrients. *Current Veterinary Therapy: Food Animal Practice 2.* J Howard Ed., Sunders: 278–286.

Marks, S (2003). Advances in dietary management of gastrointestinal disease. Proceedings: IAMS2003. Accessed via: Veterinary Information Network. http://goo.gl/6C3cf

Marks, S (2009). How I treat feline hepatic lipidosis and feline cholangitis. Proceedings: WSAVA. Accessed via: Veterinary Information Network. http://goo.gl/Zme6I

Simpson, K, J Fyfe, et al. (2001). Subnormal concentrations of serum cobalamin (vitamin B12) in cats with gastrointestinal disease. *J Vet Intern Med* 15: 26–32.

Steiner, JM (2009). Cobalamin deficiency in dogs and cats: Why should you care? Proceedings: ACVIM.

Westermarck, E, M Wiberg, et al. (2005). Exocrine pancreatic insufficiency in dogs and cats. *Textbook of Veterinary internal Medicine 6th Ed.* S Ettinger and E Feldman Eds., Elsevier: 1492–1495.

Zoran, DL (2008). Protein losing enteropathies. World Veterinary Congress.

CYCLOPHOSPHAMIDE

(sye-kloe-*foss*-fa-mide)   Cytoxan®, Neosar®

IMMUNOSUPPRESSIVE/ ANTINEOPLASTIC

Prescriber Highlights

▶ Antineoplastic/immunosuppressive used in dogs & cats for a variety of conditions

▶ Low dose metronomic (continuous) therapy with piroxicam shows promise for preventing sarcoma recurrence in dogs with fewer adverse effects then high dose tx.

▶ Contraindications: Prior anaphylaxis; caution in patients with leukopenia, thrombocytopenia, previous radiotherapy, impaired hepatic or renal function, or in those for whom immunosuppression may be dangerous (e.g., infection)

▶ Potentially teratogenic, fetotoxic

▶ Primary adverse effects are myelosuppression, GI effects, alopecia (especially Poodles, Old English Sheepdogs, etc.), & hemorrhagic cystitis.

▶ Adequate monitoring essential

Uses/Indications

In veterinary medicine, cyclophosphamide is used primarily in small animals (dogs and cats) in combination with other agents both as an antineoplastic agent (lymphomas, leukemias, carcinomas, and sarcomas) and as an immunosuppressant (SLE, ITP, IMHA, pemphigus, rheumatoid arthritis, proliferative urethritis, etc.). Its use in treating acute immune-mediated hemolytic anemia is controversial; there is some evidence that it does not add beneficial effects when used with prednisone.

Cyclophosphamide has been used historically as a chemical shearing agent in sheep.

Pharmacology/Actions

While commonly categorized as an alkylating agent, the parent compound (cyclophosphamide) is a prodrug and cyclophosphamide's metabolites, such as phosphoramide mustard, act as alkylating agents interfering with DNA replication, RNA transcription and replication, and ultimately disrupting nucleic acid function. The cytotoxic properties of cyclophosphamide are also enhanced by the phosphorylating activity the drug possesses.

Cyclophosphamide has marked immunosuppressive activity and both white cells and antibody production are decreased, but the exact mechanisms for this activity have not been fully elucidated.

Pharmacokinetics

While the pharmacokinetics of cyclophosphamide apparently have not been detailed in dogs or cats, it is presumed that the drug is handled in a manner similar to humans. The drug is well absorbed after oral administration with peak levels occurring about 1 hour after dosing. Cyclophosphamide and its metabolites are distributed throughout the body, including the CSF (albeit in subtherapeutic levels). The drug is only minimally protein bound and is distributed into milk and presumed to cross the placenta.

Cyclophosphamide is metabolized in the liver to several metabolites. Which metabolites account for which portion of the cytotoxic properties of the drug is a source of controversy. After IV injection, the serum half-life of cyclophosphamide is approximately 4–12 hours, but drug/metabolites can be detected up to 72 hours after administration. The majority of the drug is excreted as metabolites and unchanged drug in the urine.

Contraindications/Precautions/Warnings

Cyclophosphamide should not be used in patients with prior anaphylactic reactions to the drug otherwise, there are no absolute contraindications to the use of cyclophosphamide. It must be used with caution, however in patients with leukopenia, thrombocytopenia, previous radiotherapy, impaired hepatic or renal function, or in those for whom immunosuppression may be dangerous (e.g., infected patients). Patients who develop myelosuppression should have subsequent doses delayed until adequate recovery occurs.

Because of the potential for development of serious adverse effects, cyclophosphamide should only be used in patients who can be adequately and regularly monitored.

Adverse Effects

Primary adverse effects in animals associated with cyclophosphamide are myelosuppression, gastroenterocolitis (anorexia, nausea, vomiting, diarrhea), alopecia (especially in breeds where haircoat continually grows, e.g., Poodles, Old English Sheepdogs), and hemorrhagic cystitis.

Cyclophosphamide's myelosuppressant effects primarily impact the white cells lines, but may also affect red cell and platelet production. The nadir for leukocytes generally occurs between 7–14 days after dosing and may require up to 4 weeks for recovery. When used with other drugs causing myelosuppression, toxic effects may be exacerbated.

Sterile hemorrhagic cystitis induced by cyclophosphamide is thought to be caused by the metabolite acrolein. Up to 30% of dogs receiving long-term (>2 months) cyclophosphamide can develop this problem. Furosemide administered with cyclophosphamide may reduce the occurrence of this adverse effect.

In cats, cyclophosphamide-induced-cystitis (CIC) is rare. Initial signs may present as hematuria and dysuria. Because bacterial cystitis is not uncommon in immunosuppressed patients, it must be ruled out by taking urine cultures. Diagnosis of CIC is made by a negative urine culture and inflammatory urine sediment found during urinalysis. Because bladder fibrosis and/or transitional cell carcinoma of the bladder is also associated with cyclophosphamide use, these may need to be ruled out by contrast radiography. It is believed that the incidence of CIC may be minimized by increasing urine production and frequent voiding. The drug should be given in the morning and animals should be encouraged to drink/urinate whenever possible. Recommendation for treatment of CIC includes discontinuing cyclophosphamide, furosemide, and corticosteroids. Refractory cases have been treated by surgical debridement, 1% formalin or 25% DMSO instillation in the bladder.

Other adverse effects that may be noted with CTX therapy include pulmonary infiltrates and fibrosis, depression, immune-suppression with hyponatremia, and leukemia.

In recovering dogs with immune-mediated hemolytic anemia, taper the withdrawal of the drug slowly over several months and monitor for early signs of relapse. Rapid withdrawal can lead to a rebound hyperimmune response.

Reproductive/Nursing Safety

Cyclophosphamide's safe use in pregnancy has not been established and it is potentially teratogenic and embryotoxic. Cyclophosphamide may induce sterility (may be temporary) in male animals. In humans, the FDA categorizes this drug as category *D* for use during pregnancy (*There is evidence of human fetal risk, but the potential benefits from the use of the drug in pregnant women may be acceptable despite its potential risks.*) In a separate system evaluating the safety of drugs in canine and feline pregnancy (Papich 1989), this drug is categorized as in class: *C* (*These drugs may have potential risks. Studies in people or laboratory animals have uncovered risks, and these drugs should be used cautiously as a last resort when the benefit of therapy clearly outweighs the risks.*)

Cyclophosphamide is distributed in milk and nursing is generally not recommended when dams are receiving the drug.

Overdosage/Acute Toxicity

There is only limited information on acute overdoses of this drug. The lethal dose in the dogs has been reported as 40 mg/kg IV. If an oral overdose occurs, gut emptying should proceed if indicated and the animal should be hospitalized for supportive care.

Drug Interactions

The following drug interactions have either been reported or are theoretical in humans or animals receiving cyclophosphamide and may be of significance in veterinary patients:

■ **ALLOPURINOL:** May increase the myelosuppression caused by cyclophosphamide

■ **CARDIOTOXIC DRUGS (e.g., doxorubicin):** Use caution when using cyclophosphamide with other cardiotoxic agents as potentiation of cardiotoxicity may occur

■ **CHLORAMPHENICOL:** May inhibit cyclophosphamide metabolism

■ **IMIPRAMINE:** May inhibit cyclophosphamide metabolism

■ **PHENOBARBITAL (or other barbiturates)** given chronically may increase the rate of metabolism of cyclophosphamide to active metabolites via microsomal enzyme induction and increase the likelihood of toxicity development

■ **PHENOTHIAZINES:** May inhibit cyclophosphamide metabolism

■ **POTASSIUM IODIDE:** May inhibit cyclophosphamide metabolism

■ **SUCCINYLCHOLINE:** Metabolism may be slowed with resulting prolongation of effects, as cyclophosphamide may decrease the levels of circulating pseudocholinesterases

■ **THIAZIDE DIURETICS:** May increase the myelosuppression caused by cyclophosphamide

■ **VITAMIN A:** May inhibit cyclophosphamide metabolism

Laboratory Considerations

■ **Uric acid** levels (blood and urine) may be increased after cyclophosphamide use.

■ The immunosuppressant properties of cyclophosphamide may cause false negative **antigenic skin test** results to a variety of antigens, including tuberculin, Candida, and Trichophyton.

Doses

Note: In oral tablets, the active ingredient is contained within an inner tablet surrounded by an inert flecked outer tablet. Accurate dosing may be difficult if splitting or crushing tablets. When dosing in cats or very small dogs, or if using low-dose therapy, compounding pharmacies may be able to compound oral dosage forms containing less than 25 mg. Another method has been suggested (Mackin 2009) to allow use of whole 25 mg tablets when used as an immunosuppressant: Convert daily (or every other day) doses into a weekly total dose and then administer whole tablets at a suitable interval to allow using whole tablets.

■ **DOGS:**

As an antineoplastic:

Note: Because of the potential toxicity of this drug to patients, veterinary personnel and clients, and since chemotherapy indications, treatment protocols, monitoring and safety guidelines often change, the following dosages should be used only as a general guide. Consultation with a veterinary oncologist and referral to current veterinary oncology references [e.g., (Henry & Higginbotham 2009); (Argyle *et al.* 2008); (Withrow & Vail 2007); (Villalobos 2007); (Ogilvie & Moore 2006); (Ogilvie & Moore 2001)] is *strongly recommended*.

a) To inhibit local recurrence in dogs with incompletely resected soft tissue sarcomas: 10 mg/m^2 (NOT mg/kg) PO once daily with piroxicam at 0.3 mg/kg PO once daily. If dog develops unacceptable adverse effects dosing interval increased to every other day. (Elmslie *et al.* 2008)

b) 50 mg/m^2 (NOT mg/kg) PO 4 days/week or a single dose of 250 mg/m^2 (NOT mg/kg) PO once every 3 weeks; IV doses range from 100–300 mg/m^2 (NOT mg/kg) weekly, depending on the protocol used (Kitchell 2005)

As an immunosuppressant:

a) For use with glucocorticoids in immune-mediated thrombocytopenia or acute immune-mediated hemolytic anemia (IMHA) in patients with marked anemia (PCV less than 10%), signs of marked clinical compromise (*e.g.*, weakness, stupor, collapse), disease severe enough to require transfusion, a strongly positive slide agglutination, or jaundice and/or hemoglobinemia or hemoglobinuria. Immunosuppressants may also be necessary within a few weeks of starting glucocorticoids therapy if patient fails to respond to steroids alone, or side effects (polydipsia, polyuria, polyphagia, tachypnea) become intolerable. May use azathioprine, cyclosporine or cyclophosphamide (personal choice as there is little concrete evidence to suggest one has clear benefits over the other two). If cyclophosphamide used: Start with 50 mg/m^2 (NOT mg/kg) PO every 2nd day; adjust dose to manage side effects. Because of adverse effects, prefer either cyclosporine or azathioprine for long-term therapy. (Mackin 2009)

b) For use with glucocorticoids in acute immune-mediated hemolytic anemia (IMHA): Author starts all patients with IMHA with adjunctive immunosuppressants (usually azathioprine); if using cyclophosphamide: 50 mg/m^2 (NOT mg/kg) PO daily for 4 days on, 3 days off, as a pulse therapy. Alternatively some clinicians use 50 mg/m^2 PO every other day or high dose IV therapy at 200 mg/m^2 at the outset (author rarely uses the high dose IV therapy unless patient is on IV fluid support as hemorrhagic cystitis is more more likely to occur. (Noonan 2009)

c) For polyarthritis: In most cases initial treatment is to attempt immunosuppression with high doses of corticosteroids (prednisolone at 2–4 mg/kg in a daily divided dose for 2 weeks and then gradually reduced over the next 4–8 weeks); maintain therapy to help prevent relapses. If relapses occur or the response to prednisolone is poor, add cyclophosphamide given PO daily at a dose of 1.5 mg/kg for dogs over 30 kg, 2 mg/kg for dogs 15–30 kg, and 2.5 mg/kg for dogs for dogs under 15 kg. Give cyclophosphamide doses on 4 consecutive days each week as close to the above dosing regimen as possible, allowing that tablets cannot be split. Oral prednisolone also given each day at 0.25–0.5 mg/kg. Continue treatment for 2–4 months, but do not treat with cyclophosphamide longer than 4 months because of bladder toxicity. Test urine weekly for blood, stop if overt blood detected. Monitor CBC q7–14 days; if white count falls below 6,000/mm3 or platelet count is <125,000/mm3 reduce dosage by 1/4th; if white count falls below 4,000/mm3 or platelet count is <100,000/mm3 stop drug for 2 weeks and the resume at 1/2 prior dose. If relapses occur or response still poor, may add levamisole (5–7 mg/kg PO every other day; max dose of 150 mg). Goal is to stop therapy in 3–6 months. (Bennett 2005)

d) As an alternative immunosuppressive agent for glomerulonephritis: 2.2 mg/kg PO q24h for 4 days, discontinue for 3 days and then repeat. (Labato 2006)

■ **CATS:**

As an antineoplastic: Cyclophosphamide has been used a sole agent and in a COP protocol to treat lymphomas in cats. Collaboration with a veterinary oncologist is highly recommended.

As an immunosuppressant:

a) For ITP or IMHA: Most cats respond to oral steroids alone (oral prednisolone starting dose 4 mg/kg/day) and other immunosuppressants are rarely needed. If cyclophosphamide is to be added, dose as in dogs (see Mackin dose above), but author prefers to use either cyclosporine or chlorambucil in cats. (Mackin 2009)

b) To slow progression of FIP: 2–4 mg/kg PO four times a week. (Foley 2005)

■ **HORSES:**

For neoplastic diseases; consultation with a veterinary oncologist is encouraged before use:

a) Usual doses used in horses are: 200 mg/m² (usually 1 gram per horse per dose) IV every 1-2 weeks. For generalized lymphoma the CAP protocol was used at

the time of publication by one of the authors. See the reference or the vincristine monograph for more information. (Mair & Couto 2006)

■ **RABBITS:**

As an antineoplastic (lymphoma) agent:

a) 50 mg/m² (NOT mg/kg) PO daily for 3 days each week or 100–200 mg/m² IV (cephalic or saphenous veins) every 7 days. Consider using a fully implantable vascular access device for multiple IV chemo administration. (Bryan 2009)

Monitoring

■ Efficacy; See the Protocol section or refer to the references from the Dosage section above for more information

■ Toxicity, see Adverse Effects above. Regular hemograms and urinalyses are mandatory.

Client Information

■ Clients must be briefed on the possibilities of severe toxicity developing from this drug, including drug-related mortality.

■ After dosing in dogs, frequent walks to encourage urination is suggested to attempt to lessen the risk for bladder toxicity.

■ Clients should contact veterinarian should the animal exhibit any signs of abnormal bleeding and/or bruising.

■ Although no special precautions are necessary when handling intact tablets, direct exposure should be avoided with crushed tablets, oral elixir, or the animal's urine or feces. Should exposure occur, wash the area thoroughly with soap and water.

Chemistry/Synonyms

A nitrogen-mustard derivative, cyclophosphamide occurs as a white, crystalline powder that is soluble in water and alcohol. The commercially available injection has pH of 3 to 7.5.

Cyclophosphamide may also be known as: CPM, CTX, CYT, B-518, ciclofosfamida, cyclophosphamidum, cyclophosphanum, NSC-26271, WR-138719, Alkyloxan®, Carloxan®, Ciclosmida®, Cicloxal®, Cyclan®, Cyclo-cell®, Cycloblastin®, Cycloblastine®, Cyclostin®, Cycloxan®, Cytophosphan®, Cytoxan®, Endoxan®, Endoxana®, Enduxan®, Fosfaseron®, Genoxal®, Genuxal®, Ledoxina®, Neosar®, Procytox®, or Sendoxan®.

Storage/Stability

Cyclophosphamide tablets and powder for injection should be stored at temperatures less than 25°C. They may be exposed to temperatures up to 30°C for brief periods, but should not be exposed to temperatures above 30°C. Tablets should be stored in tight containers. The commercially available tablets (Cytoxan®) are manufactured in a bi-level manner with a white tablet containing the cyclophosphamide found within a surrounding flecked outer tablet. Therefore, the person administering the drug need not protect their hands from cyclophosphamide exposure unless the tablets are crushed. Because of their construction, accurately splitting tablets is problematic and cannot be recommended.

Cyclophosphamide injection may be dissolved in aromatic elixir to be used as an oral solution. When refrigerated, it is stable for 14 days.

After reconstituting the powder for injection with either sterile water for injection or bacteriostatic water for injection, the product should be used within 24 hours if stored at room temperature; 6 days if refrigerated.

Compatibility/Compounding Considerations

Commercially available cyclophosphamide tablets may not have the active ingredient dispersed evenly throughout the tablet. To assure accurate oral dosing, it is recommended to obtain dosing forms from an experienced compounding pharmacist.

Cyclophosphamide is reportedly **compatible** with the following intravenous solutions and drugs: Amino acids 4.25%/dextrose 25%, D_5 in normal saline, D_5W, sodium chloride 0.9%. It is also **compatible** in syringes or at Y-sites for brief periods with the following: bleomycin sulfate, cefazolin, cisplatin, doxorubicin HCl, droperidol, fluorouracil, furosemide, heparin sodium, leucovorin calcium, methotrexate sodium, metoclopramide HCl, mitomycin, vinblastine sulfate, and vincristine sulfate. Compatibility is dependent upon factors such as pH, concentration, temperature and diluent used; consult specialized references or a hospital pharmacist for more specific information.

Dosage Forms/Regulatory Status

VETERINARY-LABELED PRODUCTS: None

HUMAN-LABELED PRODUCTS:

Cyclophosphamide Tablets: 25 mg & 50 mg; generic (Gensia Sicor); (Rx)

Cyclophosphamide Powder for Solution for Injection: 500 mg, 1 g and 2 g in vials; generic (Rx)

References

Argyle, D, M Brearly, et al. (2008). *Decision Making in Small Animal Oncology*, Wiley–Blackwell.

Bennett, D (2005). Immune–mediated and infective arthritis. Textbook of Veterinary Internal Medicine, 6th Ed. S Ettinger and E Feldman Eds., Elsevier: 1958–1965.

Bryan, J (2009). Neoplasia in rabbits: Therapy. Proceedings: WVC. Accessed via: Veterinary Information Network. http://goo.gl/b58mQ

Elmslie, RE, P Glawe, et al. (2008). Metronomic Therapy with Cyclophosphamide and Piroxicam Effectively Delays Tumor Recurrence in Dogs with Incompletely Resected Soft Tissue Sarcomas. *Journal of Veterinary Internal Medicine* 22(6): 1373–1379.

Foley, J (2005). Feline Infectious peritonitis and feline enteric coronavirus. Textbook of Veterinary Internal Medicine, 6th Ed. S Ettinger and E Feldman Eds., Elsevier: 663–666.

Henry, C & M Higginbotham (2009). *Cancer Management in Small Animal Practice*, Saunders.

Kitchell, B (2005). Practical Chemotherapy. Proceedings: AAFP Winter Meeting. Accessed via: Veterinary Information Network. http://goo.gl/NAhOF

Labato, M (2006). Improving survival for dogs with protein–losing nephropathies. Proceedings: ACVIM 2006. Accessed via: Veterinary Information Network. http://goo.gl/0jeng

Mackin, A (2009). Chronic managment of the immune–mediated blood disorders. Proceedings: World Veterinary Congress.

Mair, TS & CG Couto (2006). The use of cytotoxic drugs in equine practice. *Equine Veterinary Education* 18(3): 149–156.

Noonan, M (2009). Immune Mediated Hemolytic Anemia. Proceedings: IVECC. Accessed via: Veterinary Information Network. http://goo.gl/EaAXT

Ogilvie, G & A Moore (2001). *Feline Oncology: A Comprehensive Guide to Compassionate Care*, Veterinary Learning Systems.

Ogilvie, G & A Moore (2006). *Managing the Canine Cancer Patient: A Practical Guide to Compassionate Care*, Veterinary Learning Systems.

Villalobos, A (2007). *Canine and Feline Geriatric Oncology*. Ames, Blackwell.

Withrow, S & D Vail (2007). *Withrow and MacEwen's Small Animal Clinical Oncology 4th Ed*. Philadelphia, Elsevier.

CYCLOSPORINE (SYSTEMIC)

(sye-kloe-spor-een)
Atopica®, Neoral®, Sandimmune®

IMMUNOSUPPRESSIVE

Note: Cyclosporine topical ophthalmic information is found in the ophthalmology section in the appendix.

Prescriber Highlights

▶ Immunosuppressant (primarily cellular immunity)

▶ Adverse Effects: Primarily GI related, but uncommon at usual dosages

▶ If using human-labeled products, don't confuse Sandimmune® with Atopica®/Neoral®/Gengraf® dosages; they are not bioequivalent. When using generically labeled products, determine with which product they are bioequivalent & dose appropriately.

▶ Serum levels should be measured to assure efficacy & minimize adverse effect potential

▶ Cost may be an issue

▶ Drug-drug interactions

Uses/Indications

Cyclosporine may be useful as an immunosuppressant for immune-mediated diseases (see dosage section) and as part of a protocol to reduce the rejection of allografts in transplant medicine in dogs and cats. It has been postulated that cyclosporine may have beneficial effects in keratinization disorders.

Pharmacology/Actions

Cyclosporine is an immunosuppressant that focuses on cell-mediated immune responses (but it has some humoral immunosuppressive action). While cyclosporine's exact mechanism of action is not known, it is believed that it acts by a specific, reversible inhibition of immunocompetent lymphocytes in the G_0- or G_1-phase of the cell cycle. T-helper lymphocytes are the primary target, but T-suppressor cells are also affected. Lymphokine production and release (including interleukin-2, T-Cell Growth factor) are also inhibited by cyclosporine.

Pharmacokinetics

Cyclosporine is poorly absorbed after oral administration and bioavailability can vary widely between patients. The emulsion form oral product (*Neoral®*) reportedly achieves much higher blood levels in dogs and cats for a given dose and dosage recommendations change accordingly. Note: *Neoral®/Atopica®* and *Sandimmune®* are NOT bioequivalent.

In dogs, the veterinary-labeled oral product (*Atopica®*) is rapidly absorbed, but bioavailability is variable and can range from 23–45%. Food in the GI increases variability of bioavailability and reduces it by about 20%.

Cyclosporine is distributed in high levels into the liver, fat and blood cells (RBC's lymphocytes). It does not appreciably enter the CNS.

The drug is primarily metabolized in the liver via the cytochrome P450 system and excreted into the bile. Less than 1% of a dose is excreted unchanged into the urine. Elimination half-life in the dog is approximately 5–12 hours.

There is some controversy regarding dosing cyclosporine in overweight animals. It has been stated that since the drug is hydrophobic, it lends support to dosing based upon the patient's ideal weight rather than its actual weight (Diesel & Moriello 2008). However in humans, obesity does not significantly impact cyclosporine pharmacokinetics (Lindholm 1991) and no published studies were found for dogs comparing pharmacokinetics in non-obese and obese animals.

Contraindications/Precautions/Warnings

Cyclosporine is contraindicated in patients hypersensitive to it or any component (*e.g.*, polyoxyethylated castor oil) in the injectable micro-emulsion products. It is labeled as being contraindicated in dogs with a history of malignant neoplasia. Cyclosporine should be used with caution in patients with hepatic or renal disease.

Because of its immunosuppressant effects it has been recommended to check cats' FeLV and FIP status before using cyclosporine.

Cyclosporine is pumped by P-glycoprotein, but the Washington State University Clinical Pharmacology Lab reports that it has not seen any increased sensitivity to cyclosporine and does not recommend any dose reductions in dogs with MDR1 mutations. They do however, recommend therapeutic drug monitoring. (WSU-VetClinPharmLab 2009)

Adverse Effects

In dogs, vomiting, anorexia, and diarrhea are most commonly seen; gingival hyperplasia, hypertrichosis, excessive shedding, and papillomatosis have been reported. Quite commonly dogs will vomit when starting therapy, but this generally abates with time.

In order to reduce the incidence of vomiting in dogs when starting therapy, some clinicians will start at a low dose, give with food and gradually increase oral doses over the first week or so. One protocol (Bloom 2006) is: 1–2 mg/kg PO once daily for 2 days, 2–3 mg/kg PO once daily for 2 days, 3–4 mg/kg PO once daily for 3 days, and then 5 mg/kg PO once daily for 30 days. For the first 10 days metoclopramide is given 30 minutes prior to cyclosporine. For the first 14 days cyclosporine is given with a meal and after that, 2 hours prior to a meal.

Cats with high blood levels (1,000 ng/mL) may develop anorexia. Gastrointestinal upset may be seen in cats especially during the first month of therapy. Increased hair growth, gingival hyperplasia, flare of latent viral infections have also been noted in feline patients on cyclosporine. A case of a cat developing fatal systemic toxoplasmosis while on cyclosporin therapy has been reported.

While nephrotoxicity and hepatotoxicity are potentially an issue in dogs and cats, it appears that extremely high blood levels (>3,000 ng/mL) are necessary before this is a significant problem.

Animals who have levels greater than 1,000 ng/mL that persist for weeks or months may be more susceptible to bacterial or fungal infections. Long-term use, particularly in combination with other immunosuppressants (steroids), may predispose the patient to develop neoplastic diseases.

Because the drug has an unpleasant taste, it has been suggested that compounded dosages be placed in gelatin capsules or used with taste-masking flavoring agents.

Reproductive/Nursing Safety

Cyclosporine has been shown to be fetotoxic and embryotoxic in rats and rabbits at dosages 2–5 times normal. Use during pregnancy only when the risks outweigh the benefits. In humans, the FDA categorizes this drug as category *C* for use during pregnancy (*Animal studies have shown an adverse effect on the fetus, but there are no adequate studies in humans; or there are no animal reproduction studies and no adequate studies in humans.*)

Cyclosporine is distributed into milk and safety cannot be assured for nursing offspring. In humans, it is not recommended that women nurse while taking cyclosporine.

Overdosage/Acute Toxicity

Acute overdoses may cause transient renal- or hepato-toxicity. Overdoses may be treated with gut evacuation (emesis is apparently effective in humans if used within 2 hours of ingestion); otherwise, treat supportively and symptomatically.

Drug Interactions
The following drug interactions have either been reported or are theoretical in humans or animals receiving cyclosporine and may be of significance in veterinary patients:

The following drugs may **increase** cyclosporine blood levels and increase the risk for cyclosporine toxicity:

- **ACETAZOLAMIDE**
- **ALLOPURINOL**
- **AMIODARONE**
- **AMLODIPINE**
- **AZITHROMYCIN**
- **AZOLE ANTIFUNGALS** (*e.g.*, **ketoconazole, itraconazole, fluconazole**) Both ketoconazole and fluconazole have been used to therapeutic advantage to reduce the dose (and cost) required of cyclosporine in dogs.
- **BROMOCRIPTINE**
- **CALCIUM CHANNEL BLOCKERS** (*e.g.*, **verapamil, diltiazem**)
- **CARVEDILOL**
- **CIMETIDINE**
- **CHLORAMPHENICOL**
- **CIPROFLOXACIN/ENROFLOXACIN**
- **CISAPRIDE**
- **COLCHICINE** (colchicine levels may also increase)
- **CORTICOSTEROIDS**
- **DANAZOL**
- **DIGOXIN**
- **ESTROGENS**
- **FLUVOXAMINE**
- **GLIPIZIDE/GLYBURIDE**
- **GRAPEFRUIT JUICE/GRAPEFRUIT JUICE POWDER**
- **IMIPENEM**
- **LOSARTAN, VALSARTAN**
- **MACROLIDE ANTIBIOTICS** (*e.g.*, **erythromycin, clarithromycin**)
- **MEDROXYPROGESTERONE**
- **METOCLOPRAMIDE**
- **METRONIDAZOLE**
- **OMEPRAZOLE**
- **SERTRALINE**
- **TINIDAZOLE**
- The following drugs may **decrease** the blood levels of cyclosporine:
- **AZATHIOPRINE**
- **CARBAMAZEPINE**
- **CLINDAMYCIN** (may decrease cyclosporine bioavailability)
- **CYCLOPHOSPHAMIDE**
- **FAMOTIDINE**
- **GRISEOFULVIN**
- **NAFCILLIN**
- **OCTREOTIDE**
- **RIFAMPIN**
- **PHENOBARBITAL**
- **PHENYTOIN**
- **ST. JOHN'S WORT**
- **SULFADIAZINE/SULFAMETHOXAZOLE**
- **SULFASALAZINE**
- **TERBINAFINE**
- **TRIMETHOPRIM** (may also increase risk for nephrotoxicity)
- **WARFARIN** (may also reduce efficacy of warfarin)

Additional interactions/notes:

- **ACE INHIBITORS** (**benazepril, enalapril**, etc): Have been case reports in humans where renal function declined
- **DIGOXIN:** Cyclosporine can cause increased digoxin levels with possible toxicity
- **DOXORUBICIN:** Cyclosporine can increase doxorubicin and doxorubicinol (active metabolite) levels
- **KETOCONAZOLE** and other **azole antifungals:** Have been shown that they can substantially reduce the metabolism of cyclosporine in dogs or cats and many clinicians are using this interaction to reduce the dose and resultant cost of cyclosporine treatment. Attempt this with caution only, and with the realization that monitoring of cyclosporine levels may be required.
- **MELPHALAN:** Increased risk for renal failure
- **METHOTREXATE:** Cyclosporine may increase MTX levels
- **MYCOPHENOLATE:** Reduced levels of mycophenolate
- **NEPHROTOXIC DRUGS, OTHER** (*e.g.*, **acyclovir, amphotericin B, aminoglycosides, colchicine, vancomycin, NSAIDs, tacrolimus**): Possible additive nephrotoxicity
- **SPIRONOLACTONE** and other **potassium sparing diuretics:** Increased risk for hyperkalemia
- **VACCINATIONS:** May be less effective while patients are receiving cyclosporine; avoid the use of live attenuated vaccines

Doses
Note: Dosages are for *Sandimmune®* unless otherwise noted. *Atopica®* or *Neoral®* are not interchangeable with *Sandimmune®* dosages.

- **DOGS:**
For control of atopic dermatitis using *Atopica®* in dogs weighing at least 1.8 kg:
  a) 5 mg/kg (3.3–6.7 mg/kg) PO once daily for 30 days. Following this initial treatment period, dosage may be tapered to

every other day, and then 2 times per week, until a minimum frequency is reached that will maintain the desired therapeutic effect. Give at least one hour before, or two hours after meals. (Label information; *Atopica®*—Novartis)

b) 5–7 mg/kg/day or less. Ideally should be given on an empty stomach, but if causes GI upset, administration with food may help. In large dogs, administration of cyclosporine at 2.5 mg/kg/day with ketoconazole (5 mg/kg/day) may give good results and reduce expenses. (White 2007)

c) The standard dosage for atopic dermatitis is 5 mg/kg per day. Dosages of *Atopica®* of 2.5–3 mg/kg per day may be as effective as 5 mg/kg per day when given with generic ketoconazole at 5 mg/kg per day. After control of pruritus is achieved, the clinician may be able to reduce the daily dosage or switch to every second or third day therapy. (Ihrke 2009)

For inflammatory bowel disease using *Neoral®* or modified cyclosporine (*Atopica®*):

a) In dogs refractory to immunosuppressive doses of steroids: 5 mg/kg PO once daily. (Allenspach *et al.* 2006)

b) For inflammatory bowel disease refractory to azathioprine and prednisone: 5 mg/kg PO once daily (Marks 2007)

c) 2–5 mg/kg PO q12h; dose can be very individual, so it is recommended to monitor trough levels (aim for 500 ng/mL) (Moore 2004)

As an immunosuppressant (usually as part of an immunosuppressive protocol):

a) *Sandimmune®*: 10–25 mg/kg/day PO divided q12h. *Neoral®*: 5–10 mg/kg/day PO divided q12h. Trough level of approximately 500 ng/mL is goal (values are dependent on methodology used); may check level 24–48 hours after starting therapy. To reduce the cost of treatment in large dogs, may give ketoconazole at 10 mg/kg/day divided q12h with cyclosporine. (Gregory 2000)

b) For pemphigus: Using *Atopica®* or *Neoral®*: 5–10 mg/kg PO q24h with ketoconazole (5 mg/kg PO q24h). May be used as a sole agent or in combination with glucocorticoids. (Rosenkrantz 2004)

c) As an alternative immunosuppressive agent for refractory IMHA, especially those that are non-regenerative: 5–10 mg/kg PO divided twice daily to achieve plasma trough levels of >200 ng/mL (**Note:** *reference states >200 mg/mL, but it is believed this is a typo*). Large breed dogs can be dosed concurrently with ketoconazole (10 mg/kg/day) to allow reduction of cyclosporine dose. (Macintire 2006)

For perianal fistulas (anal furunculosis):

a) Induce remission of clinical signs by using cyclosporine alone (5 mg/kg orally twice daily) or combined with ketoconazole (cyclosporine: 5 mg/kg orally once daily; ketoconazole: 8 mg/kg orally once daily). Monitor the dog for signs of clinical improvement. Most dogs show some benefit within 2–4 weeks, but complete remission of clinical signs can take 16–20 weeks. Once clinical remission has been established, treat for an additional 4 weeks and then discontinue therapy. If a relapse occurs, repeat the above treatment protocol and then establish a maintenance dose that keeps the lesions in clinical remission. Some dogs have needed a dose as low as 25 mg daily or every other day. Univ. of Wisconsin School of Veterinary Medicine Protocol from: (Diesel & Moriello 2008)

b) Week 1: Tuesday: Hospitalization. Clip perineum to monitor healing and improve hygiene. Wednesday: Start treatment with: Cyclosporine (CyA) 10 mg/kg/day (*Neoral®*, 100 mg capsules) and Ketoconazole (KC) 5 mg/kg/day (*Nizoral®*, 200 mg tablets); Thursday: Maintain CyA dose; Friday: Check CyA plasma concentration, Maintain CyA dose; Saturday: Adjust CyA dose to obtain a trough plasma concentration of 240–400 ng/mL; Maintain KC dose during the entire period of treatment; Sunday: Maintain CyA dose

Week 2: Monday: Check CyA plasma concentration, Maintain CyA dose; Tuesday: Adjust CyA dose if needed; Wednesday: Maintain CyA dose; Thursday: Check CyA plasma concentration; Maintain CyA dose; Friday: Adjust CyA dose if needed; Discharge from hospital.

Week 3–Week 8: Check CyA plasma concentration every Tuesday. Check for possible side effects: Hair loss and hypertrichosis (CyA), pruritus (KC), gingival hyperplasia (CyA), vomiting (CyA, KC), diarrhea (CyA), kidney (CyA) and liver (CyA, KC) damage, cholestasis (KC), cutaneus papillomatosis (CyA), and viral and fungal infections (CyA).

CyA dose is adjusted if needed, KC dose is maintained.

Discontinue treatment after 8 weeks. Serious cases that are not healed but show substantial improvement may be treated for another 4 weeks. (van Sluijs 1999)

■ **CATS:**

As an immunosuppressant (usually as part of an immunosuppressive protocol):

a) *Sandimmune®*: 4–15 mg/kg/day PO divided q12h. *Neoral®*: 1–5 mg/kg/day PO divided q12h. Trough level of approximately 250–500 ng/mL is goal; may check level 24–48 hours after starting therapy. (Gregory 2000)

For feline asthma (in chronic severe cases where patients either require large doses of steroids or are steroid resistant):

a) *Sandimmune®*: Initial dose of 10 mg/kg PO q12h. Check blood levels at least weekly until a stable dose achieves trough blood levels of 500–1,000 ng/mL. (Padrid 2000)

For inflammatory bowel disease using *Neoral®* or modified cyclosporine (*Atopica®*):

a) 1–4 mg/kg PO q12–24h; dose can be very individual, so it is recommended to monitor trough levels (aim for 500 ng/mL). (Moore 2004)

b) As an alternative to prednisolone: 1–4 mg/kg PO twice a day (Gruffyd-Jones 2009)

For dermatologic conditions:

a) For atopic dermatitis 5 mg/kg PO q24h; (**Note:** Actual product used not identified in study; but drug was provided by Novartis-Pharma, makers of *Atopica®*) (Wisselink & Willemse 2009)

b) For atopic dermatitis or eosinophilc granuloma complex: 5–10 mg/kg PO daily (eosinophilic granuloma lesions may require up to 12.5 mg/day). When symptoms are controlled decrease frequency of administration. In cats difficult to dose orally, one colleague uses *Sandimmune®* at 2.5–5 mg/kg SC daily with decreased dosing frequency once controlled. (Ashley 2009)

Monitoring

■ Therapeutic efficacy

■ Adverse effects

■ Consider therapeutic drug monitoring, particularly when response is poor or adverse effects occur; ideally after 24–48 hours after starting therapy and then every 2–4 weeks; target trough levels (12 hours after last dose) have been suggested as 100–500 ng/mL in dogs and 250–1,000 ng/mL for cats (see dosage references) for immunosuppression. Because different methodologies may yield different results; contact the laboratory for recommendations on the evaluation of levels

■ CBC and biochem profile: baseline and then monthly to every 3 months has been suggested; others believe this is not warranted

Client Information

■ Clients should be briefed on the expense of this medication before prescribing.

■ Give to an animal with an empty stomach (one hour before or two hours after meals).

Importance of regular dosing must be stressed. If a dose is missed, the next dose should be administered (without doubling) as soon as possible, but dosing should be no more frequent than once daily.

■ There may be a lag time of up to 6 weeks before the drug demonstrates clinical benefit.

■ While the drug's label states that the dose may be tapered after 30 days of therapy, your veterinarian may wish to extend this time, as it has been shown that many animals benefit from getting the higher dosage for a longer period.

Chemistry/Synonyms

Also known as Cyclosporin A, cyclosporine is a naturally produced immunosuppressant agent. It is a non-polar, cyclic, polypeptide antibiotic consisting of 11 amino acids and occurs as a white, fine crystalline powder. It is relatively insoluble in water, but generally soluble in organic solvents and oils.

Commercially cyclosporine is available in several dosage forms, including an oral liquid, capsules, and a concentrate for injection. To increase oral absorption, a micro emulsion forming preparation (*Neoral®*) is also available in capsules and oral liquid. The veterinary product, *Atopica®*, is a micro-emulsion product equivalent to *Neoral®*.

Cyclosporine may also be known as: ciclosporin, 27-400, ciclosporinum, cyclosporine, cyclosporine A, OL-27-400, *Atopica®*, *Gengraf®*, *Neoral®*, *Sandimmune®*, or *Sigmasporin®*.

Storage/Stability

The veterinary product (*Atopica®*), should be stored and dispensed in the original unit-dose container at controlled room temperature (15–35°C; 59–77°F).

The oral liquid and oral capsules (*Sandimmune®*) should be stored in their original containers at temperatures less than 30°C; protect from freezing and do not refrigerate. After opening the oral liquid, use within 2 months.

The oral liquid and capsules for emulsion (*Neoral®*) should be stored in their original containers at 25°C. Temperatures below 20°C may cause the solution to gel or flocculate. Rewarming to 25° can reverse this process without harm.

The injection should be stored at temperatures less than 30°C and be protected from light. After diluting to a concentration of approximately 2 mg/mL, the resultant solution is stable for 24 hours in D5W or normal saline; if diluting with normal saline it would be wise to use the solution within 12 hours. It does not need to be protected from light after diluting.

Dosage Forms/Regulatory Status

VETERINARY-LABELED PRODUCTS:

Cyclosporine (Modified) Capsules: 10 mg, 25 mg, 50 mg, & 100 mg; *Atopica®* (Novartis); (Rx). FDA-approved for use in dogs.

See the appendix for more information on the topical ophthalmic preparation.

HUMAN-LABELED PRODUCTS:

Note: Determining bioequivalence between cyclosporine products is complicated; for the latest information see the FDA's Orange Book Website http://www.fda.gov/cder/ob/ and search on cyclosporine.

Cyclosporine Oral Capsules (Soft-gelatin): 25 mg, 50 mg & 100 mg; *Sandimmune®* (Novartis); generic; (Rx)

Cyclosporine (Microemulsion) Oral Capsules (Soft-gelatin): 25 mg, & 100 mg; *Neoral®* (Novartis); *Gengraf®* (Abbott); generic; (Eon Labs), (Pliva); (Rx)

Cyclosporine Oral Solution: 100 mg/mL in 50 mL btls with syringe; *Sandimmune®* (Novartis); (Rx)

Cyclosporine Oral Solution Microemulsion: 100 mg/mL in 50 mL btls; *Neoral®* (Novartis); generic, (Abbott; Pliva); (Rx)

Cyclosporine Concentrated Solution for Injection: 50 mg/mL in 5 mL single-use vials & amps; *Sandimmune®* (Novartis); generic (Bedford Labs); (Rx)

References

Allenspach, K, S Rufenacht, et al. (2006). Pharmacokinetics and clinical efficacy of cyclosporine treatment of dogs with steroid–refractory inflammatory bowel disease. *Journal of Veterinary Internal Medicine* 20(2): 239–244.

Ashley, P (2009). Thinking outside the box of DepoMedrol: Dermatology drug choices for cats. Proceedings: WVC. Accessed via: Veterinary Information Network. http://goo.gl/I1bRP

Bloom, P (2006). Cyclosporine and emesis. Proceedings: Western Vet Conf. Accessed via: Veterinary Information Network. http://goo.gl/C0qvb

Diesel, A & KA Moriello (2008). A busy clinician's review of CYCLOSPORINE. *Veterinary Medicine* 103(5): 266–+.

Gregory, C (2000). Immunosuppresive Agents. *Kirk's Current Veterinary Therapy: XIII Small Animal Practice.* J Bonagura Ed. Philadelphia, WB Saunders: 509–513.

Gruffyd–Jones, T (2009). Current thoughts on feline inflammatory bowel disease. Proceedings: WSAVA. Accessed via: Veterinary Information Network. http://goo.gl/joVX9

Ihrke, P (2009). The management of canine atopic dermatitis. Proceedings: Canine Medicine Symposium, UC–Davis. Accessed via: Veterinary Information Network. http://goo.gl/MCs7d

Lindholm, A (1991). Factors Iinfluencing the Pharmacokinetics of Cyclosporine in Man. *Therapeutic Drug Monitoring* 13(6): 465–477.

Macintire, D (2006). New therapies for immune–mediated hemolytic anemia. Proceedings: ACVIM 2006. Accessed via: Veterinary Information Network. http://goo.gl/ILCPS

Marks, S (2007). Inflammatory Bowel Disease—More than a garbage can diagnosis. Proceedings: UCD Canine Medicine Symposium. Accessed via: Veterinary Information Network. http://goo.gl/ZGPg1

Moore, L (2004). Beyond corticosteroids for therapy of inflammatory bowel disease in dogs and cats. Proceedings: ACVIM Forum. Accessed via: Veterinary Information Network. http://goo.gl/MOJ1B

Padrid, P (2000). Feline bronchial disease: Therapeutic recommendations for the 21st Century. Proceedings: The North American Veterinary Conference, Orlando.

Rosenkrantz, W (2004). Pemphigus: current therapy. *Vet Derm* 15: 90–98.

van Sluijs, F (1999). Treatment of Perianal Fistulas. Proceedings: North American Veterinary Conference, Orlando.

White, S (2007). Atopic dermatitis and its secondary infections. Proceedings: Canine Medicine Symposium. Accessed via: Veterinary Information Network. http://goo.gl/upBF7

Wisselink, MA & T Willemse (2009). The efficacy of cyclosporin A in cats with presumed atopic dermatitis: A double blind, randomised prednisolone–controlled study. *Veterinary Journal* 180(1): 55–59.

WSU–VetClinPharmLab (2009). "Problem Drugs." http://goo.gl/aIGlM.

CYPROHEPTADINE HCL

(sip-roe-*hep*-ta-deen)   Periactin®

ANTIHISTAMINE

Prescriber Highlights

▶ Serotonin antagonist antihistamine used as an appetite stimulant in cats & as an antipruritic/antihistamine in dogs & cats; used in horses for photic head shaking or treatment of equine Cushing's; may be useful for treating serotonin-syndrome in small animals

▶ Caution: Urinary or GI obstruction, severe CHF, narrow angle glaucoma

▶ Adverse Effects: Sedation (cats may demonstrate paradoxical hyperexcitability) & anticholinergic effects; some reports of hemolytic anemia in cats

Uses/Indications

Cyproheptadine may be useful in cats as an appetite stimulant. It potentially may be of benefit in the treatment of feline asthma or pruritus in cats, but clinical efficacy is marginal for these indications. Cyproheptadine use as monotherapy for eosinophilic airway inflammation in cats is not recommended (Schooley *et al.* 2007).

Cyproheptadine is an antihistamine but its efficacy is questionable for this indication in dogs. The drug may be useful as adjunctive therapy for Cushing's syndrome probably as result of its antiserotonin activity, however one study demonstrated efficacy in less than 10% of dogs treated for pituitary dependent hyperadrenocorticism.

Cyproheptadine may be useful as adjunctive treatment in dogs or cats with serotonin syndrome.

In horses, cyproheptadine has been used for treating photic head shaking and pituitary pars intermedia dysfunction (PPID, Equine Cushing's Disease). Pergolide is generally considered to be superior to cyproheptadine for treating PPID.

Pharmacology/Actions

Like other H_1-receptor antihistamines, cyproheptadine acts by competing with histamine for sites on H_1-receptor sites on effector cells.

Antihistamines do not block histamine release, but can antagonize its effects. Cyproheptadine also possesses potent antiserotonin activity and, reportedly, has calcium channel blocking action as well.

Pharmacokinetics

Limited data is available. Cyproheptadine is well absorbed after oral administration. Its distribution characteristics are not well described. Cyproheptadine is apparently nearly completely metabolized in the liver and these metabolites are then excreted in the urine; elimination is reduced in renal failure. Elimination half-life in cats averages about 13 hours, but there is wide interpatient variability.

Contraindications/Precautions/Warnings

Cyproheptadine is contraindicated in patients hypersensitive to it. It should be used with caution in patients with prostatic hypertrophy, bladder neck obstruction, severe cardiac failure, angle-closure glaucoma, or pyeloduodenal obstruction.

Adverse Effects

The most likely adverse effects seen with cyproheptadine are related to its CNS depressant (sedation) and anticholinergic effects (dryness of mucous membranes, etc.). Cats can develop a paradoxical agitated state that resolves upon dose reduction or discontinuation. There have been reports of cyproheptadine-induced hemolytic anemia in cats. Horses may show mild depression, anorexia, or lethargy.

At higher dosages, cyproheptadine has caused significant polyphagia in dogs.

Reproductive/Nursing Safety

Cyproheptadine has been tested in pregnant lab animals in doses up to 32X labeled dose without evidence of harm to fetuses. Nevertheless, because safety has not been established in other species, its use during pregnancy should be weighed carefully. In humans, the FDA categorizes this drug as category *B* for use during pregnancy (*Animal studies have not yet demonstrated risk to the fetus, but there are no adequate studies in pregnant women; or animal studies have shown an adverse effect, but adequate studies in pregnant women have not demonstrated a risk to the fetus in the first trimester of pregnancy, and there is no evidence of risk in later trimesters.*)

It is not known if cyproheptadine is distributed into milk.

Overdosage/Acute Toxicity

There are no specific antidotes available. Significant overdoses should be handled using standard gut emptying protocols when appropriate and supportive therapy when required. The adverse effects seen with overdoses are an extension of the drug's side effects, principally CNS depression (although CNS stimulation may be seen), anticholinergic effects (severe drying of mucous membranes, tachycardia, urinary retention, hyperthermia, etc.) and possibly hypotension. Physostigmine may be considered to treat serious CNS anticholinergic effects, and diazepam employed to treat seizures, if necessary.

Horses that have received doses 2 times greater than recommended apparently showed no untoward effects.

Drug Interactions

The following drug interactions have either been reported or are theoretical in humans or animals receiving cyproheptadine and may be of significance in veterinary patients:

■ **CNS DEPRESSANT MEDICATIONS:** Additive CNS depression may be seen if combining cyproheptadine with other CNS depressant medications, such as barbiturates, tranquilizers, etc.

■ **SSRIs (including sertraline, fluoxetine, paroxetine, etc.):** Cyproheptadine may decrease the efficacy of the SSRI

Laboratory Considerations

■ Because antihistamines can decrease the wheal and flair response to **skin allergen testing**, antihistamines should be discontinued from 3–7 days (depending on the antihistamine used and the reference) before intradermal skin tests.

■ Cyproheptadine may increase amylase and prolactin serum levels when administered with **thyrotropin-releasing hormone.**

Doses

■ **DOGS:**

As an antihistamine:

a) 0.3–2 mg/kg PO twice daily (Bevier 1990), (MacDonald 2002)

As an appetite stimulant:

a) 0.2 mg/kg PO q12h. May be dosed less frequently if inappetence is mild. (Moore 2005)

For adjunctive treatment of serotonin syndrome:

a) 1.1 mg/kg PO; doses may be repeated q4–6h as needed until signs have resolved. In cases where PO dosing not possible (severe vomiting), may crush tablets and mix with saline and give rectally. (Wismer 2006)

■ **CATS:**

As an appetite stimulant:

a) 2–4 mg per cat PO once or twice daily (Davenport 1994), (Ogilvie 2003)

b) 1–4 mg/cat PO, or 0.35–1 mg/kg PO once or twice a day (Frimberger 2000)

c) 2 mg per cat PO q12h (Smith 2003)

d) 0.35–1 mg/kg PO q12h. May be dosed less frequently if inappetence is mild. (Moore 2005)

e) In cats with renal insufficiency: 1 mg per cat PO q12h (Scherk 2008)

As an antihistamine/antipruritic:

a) 2 mg per cat PO q12h (Messinger 2000)

b) 2 mg per cat or 1.1 mg/kg PO q12h (Hnilica 2003)

c) For feline asthma (particularly when cats are maxed out on dosages of corticosteroids and terbutaline): 2 mg PO q12h. Therapeutic response may not be seen for 4–7 days, but CNS depression can occur in 24 hours. (Padrid 2000)

For adjunctive treatment of serotonin syndrome:

a) 2–4 mg (total dose) PO; doses may be repeated q4–6h as needed until signs have resolved. In cases where PO dosing not possible (severe vomiting), may crush tablets and mix with saline and give rectally. (Wismer 2006)

■ **HORSES:** (**Note:** ARCI UCGFS Class 4 Drug) For photic head shaking:

a) 0.3–0.6 mg/kg PO q12h (Dowling 1999)

b) 0.3 mg/kg PO twice daily (Mealey 2004)

For treatment of equine Cushing's:

a) 0.25 mg/kg PO once a day for 4–8 weeks; if no response (clinical signs and plasma ACTH), increase dosage frequency to twice daily. Approximately ⅓ of horses may benefit, non-responders should be switched to pergolide. (Toribio 2004)

b) 65–125 mg (total dose) PO once daily. Pergolide is the drug of choice as it is much more effective then cyproheptadine. (Young 2009)

c) If only a limited response to a pergolide dose of 0.006 mg/kg (3 mg a day for a 500 kg horse) and endocrinologic tests remain abnormal, typically add cyproheptadine at 0.5 mg/kg PO q12h. Clinical improvement may occur even if endocrinologic tests remain abnormal so continue to monitor blood glucose and endrinologic tests. (Schott II 2009)

Monitoring

■ Efficacy (weight if used for anorexia)

■ Adverse effects, if any

■ With long-term use, should occasionally monitor serum BUN in cats

Client Information

■ Possible side effects include sedation/lethargy and mucous membrane dryness

■ Cats may respond with agitation; contact veterinarian if this occurs; if cat becomes very lethargic, weak or develops pale mucous membranes contact veterinarian immediately

■ Horses may show mild depression, anorexia, or lethargy

Chemistry/Synonyms

An antihistamine that also possesses serotonin antagonist properties, cyproheptadine HCl occurs as a white to slightly yellow crystalline powder. Approximately 3.64 mg are soluble in one mL of water and 28.6 mg in one mL of alcohol.

Cyproheptadine HCl may also be known as: cyproheptadini hydrochloridum, *Ciplactin®*, *Cyheptine®*, *Cyprogin®*, *Cyprono®*, *Cyprosian®*, *Klarivitina®*, *Nuran®*, *Periactine®*, *Periactinol®*, *Periatin®*, *Peritol®*, *Polytab®*, *Practin®*, *Preptin®*, *Supersan®*, or *Trimetabol®*.

Storage/Stability

Cyproheptadine HCl tablets and oral solution should be stored at room temperature and freezing should be avoided.

Dosage Forms/Regulatory Status

VETERINARY-LABELED PRODUCTS: None

The ARCI (Racing Commissioners International) has designated this drug as a class 4 substance. See the appendix for more information.

HUMAN-LABELED PRODUCTS:

Cyproheptadine HCl Oral Tablets: 4 mg; generic; (Rx)

Cyproheptadine HCl Oral Syrup: 2 mg/5 mL in 473 mL; generic; (Rx)

References

Dowling, P (1999). Clinical pharmacology of nervous system diseases. *The Veterinary Clinics of North America: Equine Practice* 15:3(December): 575–588.

Frimberger, A (2000). Anticancer Drugs: New Drugs or Applications for Veterinary Medicines. *Kirk's Current Veterinary Therapy: XIII Small Animal Practice.* J Bonagura Ed. Philadelphia, WB Saunders: 474–478.

Hnilica, K (2003). Eosinophilic dermatopathies in cats. Proceedings: Western Veterinary Conf. Accessed via: Veterinary Information Network. http://goo.gl/IiCOD

MacDonald, J (2002). Current therapy for pruritus. Proceedings: Western Veterinary Conference. Accessed via: Veterinary Information Network. http://goo.gl/ErwOJ

Mealey, R (2004). Head shaking. *Equine Internal Medicine 2nd Edition.* M Reed, W Bayly and D Sellon Eds. Phila, Saunders: 657–659.

Messinger, L (2000). Pruritis Therapy in the Cat. *Kirk's Current Veterinary Therapy: XIII Small Animal Practice.* J Bonagura Ed. Philadelphia, WB Saunders: 542–545.

Moore, A (2005). Practical chemotherapy. *Textbook of Veterinary Internal Medicine, 6th Ed.* S Ettinger and E Feldman Eds., Elsevier: 713–720.

Ogilvie, G (2003). Nutrition and cancer: New keys for cure and control 2003! Proceedings; World Small Animal Veterinary Assoc. World Congress. Accessed via: Veterinary Information Network. http://goo.gl/s4u95

Padrid, P (2000). Feline bronchial disease: Therapeutic recommendations for the 21st Century. Proceedings: The North American Veterinary Conference, Orlando.

Scherk, M (2008). What's new pussycat? An update on feline renal insufficiency. Proceedings: WVC. Accessed via: Veterinary Information Network. http://goo.gl/fleYa

Schooley, EK, JBM Turner, et al. (2007). Effects of cyproheptadine and cetirizine on eosinophilic airway inflammation in cats with experimentally induced asthma. *American Journal of Veterinary Research* 68(11): 1265–1271.

Schott II, H (2009). Management of Pituitary Pars Intermedia Dysfunction. Proceedings: Western Vet Conf. Accessed via: Veterinary Information Network. http://goo.gl/2VC3p

Smith, A (2003). Special concerns in cat chemotherapy. Proceedings: ACVIM Forum. Accessed via: Veterinary Information Network. http://goo.gl/dnmJ3

Toribio, R (2004). Pars intermedia dysfunction (Equine Cushing's Disease). *Equine Internal Medicine 2nd Edition.* M Reed, W Bayly and D Sellon Eds. Phila, Saunders: 1327–1340.

Wismer, T (2006). Serotonin Syndrome. Proceedings: IVECC Symposium. Accessed via: Veterinary Information Network. http://goo.gl/ua96I

Young, J (2009). Equine laminitis causes and treatments. Proceedings: ACVIM. Accessed via: Veterinary Information Network. http://goo.gl/bK2iX

CYTARABINE

(sye-*tare*-a-bean)
Cytosine arabinoside, Cytosar-U®

ANTINEOPLASTIC

Prescriber Highlights

▶ Parenteral antineoplastic (lymphoreticular neoplasms, leukemias) for dogs & cats

▶ Contraindications: Hypersensitivity; potentially, embryotoxic & teratogenic

▶ Adverse Effects: Primarily myelosuppression, but GI & other toxicities can occur

▶ Adequate monitoring essential

Uses/Indications

In veterinary medicine, cytarabine is used primarily in small animals as an antineoplastic agent for lymphoreticular neoplasms, myeloproliferative disease (leukemias), and CNS lymphoma.

Pharmacology/Actions

Cytarabine is converted intracellularly into cytarabine triphosphate that apparently competes with deoxycytidine triphosphate, thereby inhibiting DNA polymerase with resulting inhibition of DNA synthesis. Cytarabine is cell phase specific, and acts principally during the S-phase (DNA synthesis). It may also, under certain conditions, block cells from the G_1 phase to the S phase.

Pharmacokinetics

Cytarabine has very poor systemic availability after oral administration and is only used parenterally. Following IM or SC injections, the drug peaks in plasma within 20–60 minutes, but levels attained are much lower than with an equivalent IV dose.

Cytarabine is distributed widely throughout the body, but crosses into the CNS in only a limited manner. If given via continuous IV infusion, CSF levels are higher than with IV bolus injection and can reach 20–60% of those levels found in plasma. Elimination half-life in the CSF is significantly longer than that of serum. In humans, cytarabine is only about 13% bound to plasma proteins. The drug apparently crosses the placenta, but it is not known if it enters milk.

Circulating cytarabine is rapidly metabolized by the enzyme cytidine deaminase, principally in the liver but also in the kidneys, intestinal mucosa, and granulocytes, to the inactive metabolite ara-U (uracil arabinoside). About 80% of a dose is excreted in the urine within 24 hours as both ara-U ($\approx$90%) and unchanged cytarabine ($\approx$10%).

Contraindications/Precautions/Warnings

Cytarabine is contraindicated in patients hypersensitive to it. Because of the potential for development of serious adverse reactions, cytarabine should only be used in patients who can be adequately and regularly monitored.

The person preparing or administering cytarabine for injection, need not observe any special handling precautions other than wearing gloves, however, should any contamination occur, thoroughly wash off the drug from skin or mucous membranes.

Adverse Effects

The principal adverse effect of cytarabine is myelosuppression (with leukopenia being most prevalent), but anemia and thrombocytopenia can also be seen. Myelosuppressive effects are more pronounced with IV administration and reach a nadir at 5–7 days, and generally recover at 7–14 days.

GI disturbances (anorexia, nausea, vomiting, diarrhea), conjunctivitis, oral ulceration, neurotoxicity, hepatotoxicity and fever may also be noted with cytarabine therapy, but occur rarely in veterinary patients. Anaphylaxis has been reported, but is believed to occur very rarely.

Cytarabine is a mutagenic and, potentially, carcinogenic agent.

Reproductive/Nursing Safety

Cytarabine's safe use in pregnancy has not been established and it is potentially teratogenic and embryotoxic. In humans, the FDA categorizes this drug as category *D* for use during pregnancy (*There is evidence of human fetal risk, but the potential benefits from the use of the drug in pregnant women may be acceptable despite its potential risks.*)

It is unknown if cytarabine enters milk; safe use during nursing cannot be assured.

Overdosage/Acute Toxicity

Cytarabine efficacy and toxicity (see Adverse Effects) are dependent not only on the dose, but also the rate the drug is given. In dogs, the IV LD_{50} is 384 mg/kg when given over 12 hours and 48 mg/kg when infused IV over 120 hours. Should an inadvertent overdose occur, supportive therapy should be instituted.

Drug Interactions

The following drug interactions have either been reported or are theoretical in humans or animals receiving cytarabine and may be of significance in veterinary patients:

◾ **DIGOXIN:** Presumably due to causing alterations in the intestinal mucosa, cytarabine may decrease the amount of digoxin (tablets only) absorbed after oral dosing; this effect may persist for several days after cytarabine has been discontinued

■ **FLUCYTOSINE (5-FC):** Limited studies have indicated that cytarabine may antagonize the anti-infective activity of fluorocytosine; monitor for decreased efficacy

■ **GENTAMICIN:** Limited studies have indicated that cytarabine may antagonize the anti-infective activity of gentamicin; monitor for decreased efficacy

Laboratory Considerations
■ None reported

Doses
Note: Because of the potential toxicity of this drug to patients, veterinary personnel and clients, and since chemotherapy indications, treatment protocols, monitoring and safety guidelines often change, the following dosages should be used only as a general guide. Consultation with a veterinary oncologist and referral to current veterinary oncology references [*e.g.*, (Henry & Higginbotham 2009); (Argyle *et al.* 2008); (Withrow & Vail 2007); (Villalobos 2007); (Ogilvie & Moore 2006); (Ogilvie & Moore 2001)] is *strongly recommended.*

■ **DOGS:**
For susceptible neoplastic diseases:
The following is a usual dosage or dose range for cytarabine in dogs and should be used only as a general guide: Usually, cytarabine is dosed at 100 mg/m^2 (NOT mg/kg) IV either as a continuous infusion over 2–3 days or divided and given IV or SC for 2–4 days.

■ **CATS:**
For susceptible neoplastic diseases:
The following is a usual dosage or dose range for cytarabine in cats and should be used only as a general guide: Usually, cytarabine is dosed at 100 mg/m^2 (NOT mg/kg) IV either as a continuous infusion over 2–3 days or divided and given IV or SC for 2–4 days. Cats are generally dosed similarly as dogs.

■ **HORSES:**
For neoplastic diseases; consultation with a veterinary oncologist is encouraged before use:
a) Usual doses used in horses are: 200–300 mg/m^2 (usually 1–1.5 grams per horse per dose) SC, IM or IV every 1–2 weeks. For generalized lymphoma the CAP protocol was used at the time of publication by one of the authors. See the reference or the vincristine monograph for more information. (Mair & Couto 2006)

Monitoring
■ Efficacy; see the Protocol section or refer to the references from the Dosage section above for more information

■ Toxicity; see Adverse Effects above. Regular hemograms are mandatory. Periodic liver and kidney function tests are suggested.

Client Information
■ Clients must be briefed on the possibilities of severe toxicity developing from this drug, including drug-related mortality

■ Clients should contact the veterinarian should the patient exhibit any signs of profound depression, abnormal bleeding and/or bruising

Chemistry/Synonyms
A synthetic pyrimidine nucleoside antimetabolite, cytarabine occurs as an odorless, white to off-white, crystalline powder with a pK$_a$ of 4.35. It is freely soluble in water and slightly soluble in alcohol.

Cytarabine may also be known as: 1-beta-D-arabinofuranosylcytosine, arabinosylcytosine, ara-C, cytarabine liposome, cytarabinum, cytosine arabinoside, liposomal cytarabine, NSC-63878, U-19920, U-19920A, WR-28453, ARA-cell®, *Alexan®, Arabine®, Aracytin®, Aracytine®, Citab®, Citagenin®, Citaloxan®, Cylocide Cytarbel®, Cytarine®, DepoCyt®, DepoCyte®, Erpalfa®, Ifarab®, Laracit®, Medsara®, Novutrax®, Serotabir®, Starasid®, Tabine®, Tarabine®* or *Udicil®.*

Storage/Stability
Cytarabine sterile powder for injection should be stored at room temperature (15–30°C). After reconstituting with bacteriostatic water for injection, solutions are stable for at least 48 hours when stored at room temperature. One study, however, demonstrated that the reconstituted solution retains 90% of its potency for up to 17 days when stored at room temperature. If the solution develops a slight haze, the drug should be discarded.

Compatibility/Compounding Considerations
Cytarabine is reportedly **compatible** with the following intravenous solutions and drugs: amino acids 4.25%/dextrose 25%, dextrose containing combinations, dextrose-saline combinations, dextrose-lactated Ringer's injection combinations, Ringer's injection, lactated Ringer's injection, sodium chloride 0.9%, sodium lactate 1/6 M, corticotropin, lincomycin HCl, methotrexate sodium, metoclopramide HCl, potassium chloride, prednisolone sodium phosphate, sodium bicarbonate, and vincristine sulfate.

Cytarabine **compatibility information conflicts** or is dependent on diluent or concentration factors with the following drugs or solutions: cephalothin sodium, gentamicin sulfate, hydrocortisone sodium succinate, and methylprednisolone sodium succinate. Compatibility is dependent upon factors such as pH, concentration, temperature and diluent used; consult specialized references or a hospital pharmacist for more specific information.

Cytarabine is reportedly **incompatible** with the following solutions or drugs: carbenicillin disodium, fluorouracil, regular insulin, nafcillin sodium, oxacillin sodium, and penicillin G sodium.

Dosage Forms/Regulatory Status

VETERINARY-LABELED PRODUCTS: None

HUMAN-LABELED PRODUCTS:

Cytarabine Powder for Injection: 100 mg, 500 mg, 1 g & 2 g in vials; generic; (Rx)

Cytarabine Injection: 10 mg/mL (liposomal) preservative free in 5 mL vials; *DepoCyt®* (Enzon); (Rx);

Cytarabine Injection: 20 mg/mL in 5 mL single- & multi-dose vials & preservative free 50 mL bulk package vials, & 100 mg/mL in 20 mL single-dose vials; *Tarabine®* PFS (Adria); generic (Mayne); (Rx)

References

Argyle, D, M Brearly, et al. (2008). *Decision Making in Small Animal Oncology*, Wiley–Blackwell.

Henry, C & M Higginbotham (2009). *Cancer Management in Small Animal Practice*, Saunders.

Mair, TS & CG Couto (2006). The use of cytotoxic drugs in equine practice. *Equine Veterinary Education* 18(3): 149–156.

Ogilvie, G & A Moore (2001). *Feline Oncology: A Comprehensive Guide to Compassionate Care*, Veterinary Learning Systems.

Ogilvie, G & A Moore (2006). *Managing the Canine Cancer Patient: A Practical Guide to Compassionate Care*, Veterinary Learning Systems.

Villalobos, A (2007). *Canine and Feline Geriatric Oncology*. Ames, Blackwell.

Withrow, S & D Vail (2007). *Withrow and MacEwen's Small Animal Clinical Oncology 4th Ed.* Philadelphia, Elsevier.

d-Panthenol —see Dexpanthenol

DACARBAZINE
DTIC

(da-*kar*-ba-zeen)

ANTINEOPLASTIC

Prescriber Highlights

- ▶ Parenteral antineoplastic used in dogs for relapsed lymphomas, soft tissue sarcomas, & melanoma
- ▶ Not recommended for use in cats
- ▶ Contraindications: Hypersensitivity; potentially teratogenic.
- ▶ Primary adverse effects are GI (can be severe & dose limiting) & bone marrow suppression; adequate monitoring essential
- ▶ Must give diluted IV; extravasation injuries can be serious

Uses/Indications

Dacarbazine has been used to treat relapsed canine lymphoma, soft tissue sarcomas and melanoma in dogs. In combination with doxorubicin, dacarbazine has been evaluated to treat dogs with relapsed lymphosarcoma. Ongoing studies evaluating various protocols are ongoing for this indication.

Pharmacology/Actions

The mechanism for dacarbazine's antineoplastic activity has not been precisely determined, but it is believed the drug acts as an alkylating agent through the formation of reactive carbonium ions. Dacarbazine also possesses antimetabolic activity by inhibiting DNA's of purine nucleoside. It possesses minimal immunosuppressant activity and is probably not a cell cycle-phase specific drug.

Pharmacokinetics

Dacarbazine (DTIC) is poorly absorbed from the GI tract and is administered intravenously. It is converted into an active form of the drug in the liver. The drug's distribution characteristics are not well known, but it is only slightly bound to plasma proteins and probably concentrates in the liver. Only limited amounts cross the blood-brain barrier; it probably crosses the placenta, but it is unknown if it is distributed into milk. Dacarbazine is extensively metabolized in the liver and is excreted in the urine via tubular secretion. Elimination half-life is about 5 hours.

Contraindications/Precautions/Warnings

Dacarbazine is not recommended for use in cats as it is unknown whether the feline liver can adequately metabolize it.

Dacarbazine (DTIC) is contraindicated in patients who are hypersensitive to it. DTIC can cause life-threatening toxicity. It should only be used where adequate monitoring and support can be administered. It should be used with caution in patients with preexisting bone marrow depression, hepatic or renal dysfunction, or infection.

Adverse Effects

Gastrointestinal toxicity (including vomiting, anorexia, diarrhea) can commonly be seen after administration and is dose limiting. Pretreatment with an antiemetic (*e.g.*, dolasetron, ondansetron) is used by some oncologists.

Bone marrow toxicity is usually asymptomatic with leukocyte and platelet nadirs seen several weeks after therapy. Occasionally severe hematopoietic toxicity can occur with fatal consequences. Other delayed toxic effects can include, alopecia, severe hepatotoxicity, renal impairment, and photosensitivity reactions. These delayed reactions appear rarely.

Because DTIC can cause extensive pain and tissue damage, avoid extravasation injuries. Venous spasm and phlebitis may occur during IV administration. Severe pain at the injection site can occur if giving the concentrated drug; dilution and administration by IV infusion is recommended. Pretreatment with dexamethasone and/or butorphanol has been suggested to reduce vasospasm, phlebitis and pain.

There is increasing evidence that chronic exposure by health care givers to antineoplastic drugs increases the mutagenic, teratogenic, and carcinogenic risks associated with these agents. Proper precautions in the handing, preparation, administration, and disposal of these drugs and supplies associated with their use are strongly recommended.

Reproductive/Nursing Safety

DTIC is teratogenic in rats at higher than clinically used dosages. It should be used during pregnancy only when the potential benefits outweigh its risks. In humans, the FDA categorizes this drug as category *C* for use during pregnancy (*Animal studies have shown an adverse effect on the fetus, but there are no adequate studies in humans; or there are no animal reproduction studies and no adequate studies in humans.*)

While it is unknown if DTIC enters milk, the potential carcinogenicity of the drug warrants using extreme caution in allowing the mother to continue nursing while receiving DTIC.

Overdosage/Acute Toxicity

Because of the toxic potential of this agent, iatrogenic overdoses must be avoided. Recheck dosage calculations. See Adverse Effects above for additional information on toxicity.

Drug Interactions

The following drug interactions have either been reported or are theoretical in humans or animals receiving dacarbazine and may be of significance in veterinary patients:

- ■ **MYELOSUPPRESSIVE DRUGS, OTHER** (*e.g.*, **other antineoplastics, immunosuppressives, chloramphenicol, flucytosine, colchicine,** etc.): May cause additive myelosuppression when used with DTIC
- ■ **RIFAMPIN:** May increase the metabolism of DTIC
- ■ **PHENOBARBITAL:** May increase the metabolism of DTIC
- ■ **PHENYTOIN:** May increase the metabolism of DTIC

Doses

Note: Because of the potential toxicity of this drug to patients, veterinary personnel and clients, and since chemotherapy indications, treatment protocols, monitoring and safety guidelines often change, the following dosages should be used only as a general guide. Consultation with a veterinary oncologist and referral to current veterinary oncology references [*e.g.*, (Henry & Higginbotham 2009); (Argyle *et al.* 2008); (Withrow & Vail 2007); (Villalobos 2007); (Ogilvie & Moore 2006); (Ogilvie & Moore 2001)] is **strongly recommended**.

■ **DOGS:**
Usual doses for DTIC in dogs (depending on the protocol used) are 800–1000 mg/m2 (NOT mg/kg) IV over 5–8 hours every 2–3 weeks.

Monitoring
- ■ Efficacy
- ■ Toxicity, including CBC with differential and platelets; renal and hepatic function tests

Client Information
- ■ Inform clients of the potential toxicities and risks associated with this therapy and report immediately any signs associated with serious toxicity (*e.g.*, bloody vomiting or diarrhea, abnormal bleeding, bruising, urination, depression, infection, shortness of breath, etc.).

Chemistry/Synonyms

An antineoplastic agent, dacarbazine occurs as a colorless to ivory colored crystalline solid. It is slightly soluble in water or alcohol. After reconstituting with sterile water, the injection has a pH of 3–4.

Dacarbazine may also be known as: dacarbazinum, DIC, DTIC, imidazole carboxamide, diemthyl triazeno imadazol carboxamide, NSC-45388, WR-139007, *Asercit®*, *DTI®*, *DTIC-Dome®*, *Dacarb®*, *Dacarbaziba®*, *Dacatic®*, *Deticene®*, *Detilem®*, *Detimedac®*, *Fauldetic®*, *Ifadac®*, or *Oncocarbil®*.

Storage/Stability

The powder for injection should be protected from light and kept refrigerated. If exposed to heat, the powder may change color from ivory to pink indicating some decomposition.

After reconstituting with sterile water for injection the resultant solution is stable for up to 72 hours if kept refrigerated; up to 8 hours at room temperature. If further diluted (up to 500 mL) with either D_5W or normal saline, the solution is stable for at least 24 hours when refrigerated; 8 hours at room temperature under normal room lighting.

Compatibility/Compounding Considerations

Drug additives that are reported to be **compatible** with dacarbazine include: bleomycin, cyclophosphamide, cytarabine, dactinomycin, doxorubicin, ondansetron and vinblastine. **Y-site compatibility** includes: doxorubicin liposome, granisetron, and ondansetron.

Compatibility is dependent upon factors such as pH, concentration, temperature and diluent used; consult specialized references or a hospital pharmacist for more specific information.

Dosage Forms/Regulatory Status

VETERINARY-LABELED PRODUCTS: None

HUMAN-LABELED PRODUCTS:

Dacarbazine Powder for Injection: 100 mg & 200 mg (may contain mannitol) vials; *DTIC-Dome®* (Bayer); generic; (Rx)

References

Argyle, D., M. Brearly, et al. (2008). *Decision Making in Small Animal Oncology*, Wiley–Blackwell.

Henry, C. & M. Higginbotham (2009). *Cancer Management in Small Animal Practice*, Saunders.

Ogilvie, G. & A. Moore (2001). *Feline Oncology: A Comprehensive Guide to Compassionate Care*, Veterinary Learning Systems.

Ogilvie, G. & A. Moore (2006). *Managing the Canine Cancer Patient: A Practical Guide to Compassionate Care*, Veterinary Learning Systems.

Villalobos, A. (2007). *Canine and Feline Geriatric Oncology*. Ames, Blackwell.

Withrow, S. & D. Vail (2007). *Withrow and MacEwen's Small Animal Clinical Oncology 4th Ed.* Philadelphia, Elsevier.

DACTINOMYCIN
ACTINOMYCIN D

(dak-ti-noe-*mye*-sin)   Cosmegen®

ANTINEOPLASTIC

Prescriber Highlights

▶ Parenteral antibiotic antineoplastic used in dogs & cats

▶ Contraindications: Hypersensitivity. Caution: Preexisting bone marrow depression, hepatic dysfunction, or infection

▶ Teratogenic

▶ Primary adverse effects are GI & bone marrow depression (may be life threatening); adequate monitoring essential

▶ Specific administration techniques required, avoid extravasation injuries

---

Uses/Indications

Dactinomycin has been used as adjunctive treatment of lymphoreticular neoplasms, bone and soft tissue sarcomas, and carcinomas in small animals. It appears to have low efficacy against most carcinomas and sarcomas. It is being investigated as a part of protocols for rescue therapy for canine lymphomas.

Pharmacology/Actions

Dactinomycin is an antibiotic antineoplastic. While it has activity against gram-positive bacteria, the drug's toxicity precludes its use for this purpose. Dactinomycin's exact mechanism of action for its antineoplastic activity has not been determined, but it apparently inhibits DNA-dependent RNA synthesis. Dactinomycin forms a complex with DNA and interferes with DNA's template activity. Dactinomycin also possesses immunosuppressing and some hypocalcemic activity.

Pharmacokinetics

Because dactinomycin is poorly absorbed it must be given IV. It is rapidly distributed and high concentrations may be found in bone marrow and nucleated cells. Dactinomycin crosses the placenta, but it is unknown whether it enters

maternal milk. The majority of the drug is excreted unchanged in the bile and urine.

Contraindications/Precautions/Warnings

Dactinomycin can cause life-threatening toxicity. It should only be used where adequate monitoring and support can be administered. Dactinomycin is contraindicated in patients who are hypersensitive to it. It should be used with caution in patients with preexisting bone marrow depression, hepatic dysfunction, or infection.

Dactinomycin is actively transported by the p-glycoprotein pump and certain breeds susceptible to MDR1-allele mutation (Collies, Australian Shepherds, Shelties, Long-haired Whippet) are at higher risk for toxicity. It is suggested to test susceptible breeds prior to treating (test available at Washington State Univ. Vet. School).

Adverse Effects

Adverse effects that may be seen more frequently include: anemia, leukopenia, thrombocytopenia (or other signs of bone marrow depression), diarrhea, and ulcerative stomatitis or other GI ulceration. Because dactinomycin may cause increased serum uric acid levels, allopurinol may be required to prevent urate stone formation in susceptible patients. Hepatotoxicity is potentially possible with this agent.

Because dactinomycin can cause extensive pain and tissue damage, avoid extravasation injuries. Dilution and administration by IV infusion is recommended or to administer slowly into a running IV line; use the "two-needle" technique.

There is increasing evidence that chronic exposure by health care givers to antineoplastic drugs increases the mutagenic, teratogenic and carcinogenic risks associated with these agents. Proper precautions in the handing, preparation, administration, and disposal of these drugs and supplies associated with their use are strongly recommended.

Reproductive/Nursing Safety

Dactinomycin has been demonstrated to be embryotoxic and teratogenic in rats, rabbits, and hamsters at higher than clinically used dosages. It should be used during pregnancy only when the potential benefits outweigh its risks. In humans, the FDA categorizes this drug as category *C* for use during pregnancy (*Animal studies have shown an adverse effect on the fetus, but there are no adequate studies in humans; or there are no animal reproduction studies and no adequate studies in humans.*)

While it is unknown if dactinomycin enters maternal milk, the potential mutagenicity and carcinogenicity of the drug warrants using extreme caution in allowing the mother to continue nursing while receiving dactinomycin.

Overdosage/Acute Toxicity

Because of the toxic potential of this agent, iatrogenic overdoses must be avoided; recheck dosage calculations. See Adverse Effects above for additional information on toxicity.

Drug Interactions

The following drug interactions have either been reported or are theoretical in humans or animals receiving dactinomycin and may be of significance in veterinary patients:

- **DOXORUBICIN:** Additive cardiotoxicity may occur if used concurrently or sequentially with doxorubicin
- **MYELOSUPPRESSIVE DRUGS, OTHER (e.g., other antineoplastics, chloramphenicol, flucytosine, colchicine, etc.):** May cause additive myelosuppression when used with dactinomycin
- **VITAMIN K:** Patients requiring vitamin K may require higher dosages when receiving dactinomycin

Laboratory Considerations

- Dactinomycin may interfere with determination of antibacterial **drug levels** if using bioassay techniques.

Doses

Note: Because of the potential toxicity of this drug to patients, veterinary personnel and clients, and since chemotherapy indications, treatment protocols, monitoring and safety guidelines often change, the following dosages should be used only as a general guide. Consultation with a veterinary oncologist and referral to current veterinary oncology references [e.g., (Henry & Higginbotham 2009); (Argyle *et al.* 2008); (Withrow & Vail 2007); (Villalobos 2007); (Ogilvie & Moore 2006); (Ogilvie & Moore 2001)] is *strongly recommended.*

- **DOGS:**
Depending on the protocol, usual doses for dactinomycin in dogs range from 0.5−1 mg/m^2 (NOT mg/kg) IV over 20 minutes; doses may be repeated (depending on the protocol) at 1−3 week intervals.

Monitoring

- Efficacy
- Toxicity: including CBC with differential and platelets; hepatic function tests; check inside patient's mouth for ulceration

Client Information

- Inform clients of the potential toxicities and risks associated with this therapy and to report immediately any signs associated with serious toxicity (*e.g.*, bloody vomiting or diarrhea, abnormal bleeding, bruising, urination, depression, infection, shortness of breath, etc.).

Chemistry/Synonyms

An antibiotic antineoplastic agent, dactinomycin (also known as actinomycin D) occurs as a bright red, crystalline powder. It is somewhat hygroscopic and soluble in water at 10°C and slightly soluble at 37°C. The commercially available preparation is a yellow lyophilized mixture of dactinomycin and mannitol.

Dactinomycin may also be known as: DTIC, ACT, actinomycin C(1), actinomycin D, meractinomycin, NSC-3053, *Ac-De®*, *Bioact-D®*, or *Dacmozen®*.

Storage/Stability

The commercially available powder should be stored at room temperature and protected from light. When reconstituting, sterile water for injection without preservatives must be used as preservatives may cause precipitation. After reconstituting, the manufacturer recommends using the solution immediately and discarding any unused portion (no preservatives). When stored in the refrigerator, reconstituted solution loses 2−3% potency over 6 hours. The reconstituted solution may be added to D$_5$W or normal saline IV infusions. IV fluid sterilizing filters (cellulose ester membrane) may partially remove dactinomycin.

Compatibility/Compounding Considerations

A precipitate may form when dactinomycin is added to sterile water that contains preservatives.

Drugs that reported to be **compatible with dactinomycin when injected at a Y-site** include: granisetron and ondansetron. Compatibility is dependent upon factors such as pH, concentration, temperature and diluent used; consult specialized references or a hospital pharmacist for more specific information

Dosage Forms/Regulatory Status

VETERINARY-LABELED PRODUCTS: None

HUMAN-LABELED PRODUCTS:

Dactinomycin Powder for Injection, lyophilized: 500 micrograms with mannitol 20 mg in vials; *Cosmegen®* (Merck); (Rx)

References

Argyle, D., M. Brearly, et al. (2008). *Decision Making in Small Animal Oncology*, Wiley–Blackwell.

Henry, C. & M. Higginbotham (2009). *Cancer Management in Small Animal Practice*, Saunders.

Ogilvie, G. & A. Moore (2001). *Feline Oncology: A Comprehensive Guide to Compassionate Care*, Veterinary Learning Systems.

Ogilvie, G. & A. Moore (2006). *Managing the Canine Cancer Patient: A Practical Guide to Compassionate Care*, Veterinary Learning Systems.

Villalobos, A. (2007). *Canine and Feline Geriatric Oncology*. Ames, Blackwell.

Withrow, S. & D. Vail (2007). *Withrow and MacEwen's Small Animal Clinical Oncology 4th Ed.* Philadelphia, Elsevier.

DALTEPARIN SODIUM

(*dahl*-tep-ah-rin)   Fragmin®

ANTICOAGULANT

Prescriber Highlights

▶ Low molecular weight (fractionated) heparin that may be useful for treatment or prophylaxis of thromboembolic disease

▶ Preferentially inhibits factor Xa & usually only minimally impacts thrombin & clotting time (TT or aPTT)

▶ Hemorrhage unlikely, but possible

▶ Must be given subcutaneously

▶ Cats & dogs may require very frequent dosing making outpatient administration impractical

▶ Expense may be an issue, particularly in large dogs/horses

Uses/Indications

Dalteparin may be useful for prophylaxis or treatment of deep vein thrombosis or pulmonary embolus. Recent pharmacokinetic work in dogs and cats, raises questions whether the drug can be effectively and practically administered long-term. In humans, it is also indicated for prevention of ischemic complications associated with unstable angina/non Q-wave MI.

Pharmacology/Actions

By binding to and accelerating antithrombin III, low molecular weight heparins (LMWHs) enhance the inhibition of factor Xa and thrombin. The potential advantage to using these products over standard (unfractionated) heparin is that they preferentially inhibit factor Xa and only minimally impact thrombin and clotting time (TT or aPTT).

Pharmacokinetics

In dogs, dalteparin is completely absorbed after SC injection. It has a volume of distribution of 50–70 mL/kg and a half-life of about 2 hours. Dalteparin half-life in dogs is shorter than in humans.

Cats appear to have a much shorter duration of activity (anti-Xa) associated with LMWHs than do humans and to maintain a therapeutic target of anti-XA activity of 0.5–1 IU/mL requires 150 Units/kg SC q4h dosing of dalteparin. (Alwood, A. *et al.* 2007)

In horses, dalteparin's pharmacokinetics are similar to humans.

In humans, after subcutaneous injection, dalteparin is absorbed rapidly with a bioavailability of about 87%; peak plasma levels (activity) occur in about 4 hours. Anti-factor Xa activity persists for up to 24 hours and doses are usually given once to twice a day. Dalteparin is excreted via the kidneys in the urine; elimina-

tion half-life is about 3–5 hours. Half-life may be prolonged in patients with renal dysfunction.

Contraindications/Precautions/Warnings

Dalteparin is contraindicated in patients who are hypersensitive to it, heparin, or pork products. It is also contraindicated in patients with major bleeding, or thrombocytopenia associated with positive *in vitro* tests for anti-platelet in the presence of dalteparin. Use dalteparin cautiously in patients with significant renal dysfunction as drug accumulation could result. It should be used with extreme caution in patients with heparin-induced thrombocytopenia or increased risk of hemorrhage.

Adverse Effects

In humans adverse effects do not routinely occur, but hemorrhage is a possibility. Injection site hematomas or pain, allergic reactions, and neurologic sequelae secondary to epidural or spinal hematomas have been reported.

Do not administer via IM or IV routes; dalteparin must be given via subcutaneous injection only. Dalteparin cannot be used interchangeably with other LMWHs or heparin sodium, as dosages differ for each.

Reproductive/Nursing Safety

In humans, dalteparin is designated by the FDA as a category *B* drug (*Animal studies have not demonstrated risk to the fetus, but there are no adequate studies in pregnant women; or animal studies have shown an adverse effect, but adequate studies in pregnant women have not demonstrated a risk to the fetus during the first trimester of pregnancy, and there is no evidence of risk in later trimesters.*)

Dalteparin is likely safe to use during nursing.

Overdosage/Acute Toxicity

Overdosage may lead to hemorrhagic complications. If treatment is necessary, protamine sulfate via slow IV may be administered. 1 mg of protamine sulfate can inhibit the effects of 100 units of administered anti-Xa dalteparin. Avoid overdoses of protamine.

Drug Interactions

The following drug interactions have either been reported or are theoretical in humans or animals receiving dalteparin and may be of significance in veterinary patients:

▪ **ANTICOAGULANTS, ORAL (Warfarin):** Increased risk for hemorrhage

▪ **PLATELET-AGGREGATION INHIBITORS (aspirin, clopidogrel):** Increased risk for hemorrhage

▪ **THROMBOLYTIC AGENTS:** Increased risk for hemorrhage

Laboratory Considerations

▪ Low molecular weight heparins may cause asymptomatic, fully-reversible increases in **AST** or **ALT**; **bilirubin** is only rarely increased in these patients, therefore, interpret these tests with caution, as increases do not necessarily indicate hepatic damage or dysfunction.

Doses

■ DOGS:

a) 150 Units/kg SC three times daily; twice daily dosing may be effective. Studies are ongoing to clarify efficacy and dosages. (Dunn 2006)

b) Initial dose 150 Units/kg SC q8h. (Alwood, A.J. 2008)

■ CATS:

a) Cats appear to have a much shorter duration of activity (anti-Xa) associated with LMWHs than do humans and to maintain a therapeutic target of anti-XA activity of 0.5–1 IU/mL requires 150 Units/kg SC q4h dosing of dalteparin. Current clinical dose recommendation is 180 Units/kg SC q4-6h (Alwood, A. *et al.* 2007), (Alwood, A.J. 2008)

■ HORSES:

a) For prophylaxis of coagulation disorders in colic patients: 50 Units/kg SC once daily (q24h) (Feige *et al.* 2003)

Monitoring

■ Baseline and ongoing during therapy CBC (with platelet count)

■ Urinalysis

■ Stool occult blood test

■ Routine coagulation tests (aPTT, PT) are usually insensitive measures of activity and normally not warranted

■ Factor Xa activity (available at Cornell Coagulation Laboratory) may be useful, particularly if bleeding occurs or patient has renal dysfunction. **Note:** To measure peak anti-Xa activity in cats, sample at 2 hours post-dose

Client Information

■ If this drug is to be used on an outpatient basis, clients must be instructed in proper injection technique for subcutaneous injection and to immediately report any signs associated with bleeding or pulmonary thrombosis. If not using the pre-filled syringes, use a very small gauge insulin or tuberculin syringe and needle (*e.g.*, 27 gauge).

■ Clients must understand that if they do not use the drug regularly (as prescribed), clots may form.

Chemistry/Synonyms

A low molecular weight heparin (LMWH), dalteparin sodium is obtained by nitrous acid depolymerization of heparin derived from pork intestinal mucosa. The average molecular weight is about 5000 and 90% ranges from 2000–9000 daltons (heparin sodium has a molecular weight around 12000). 1 mg of dalteparin is equivalent to not less than 110 Units and not more than 210 Units of anti-factor Xa.

Dalteparin sodium may also be known as: Daltaparinum natricum, Kabi-2165, *Boxol®, Fragmine®, Ligofragmin®,* or *Low Liquemine®.*

Storage/Stability

The manufacturer of the commercially available injection states the product should be stored at controlled room temperature (20–25°C, 68–77°F). Do not use if particulate matter or discoloration occur. Once the multi-dose vial is punctured, store at room temperature; discard any unused solution after 2 weeks.

A study showed that commercially available dalteparin solution was stable when drawn into syringes for up to 30 days when stored at room temperature or refrigerated. (Laposata & Johnson 2003)

Dosage Forms/Regulatory Status

VETERINARY-LABELED PRODUCTS: None

HUMAN-LABELED PRODUCTS:

Dalteparin Sodium Injection (Anti-factor Xa International Units): Available in a variety of preservative-free single dose syringes that range from 2500 Units (16 mg/0.2 mL) to 18,000 Units per 0.72 mL (115.2 mg/0.72 mL); these are less likely to be of clinical use in veterinary medicine. Multi-dose vials include: 95,000 Units per 9.5 mL (64 mg/mL), contains benzyl alcohol 14 mg/mL in 9.5 mL multidose vials; *Fragmin®* (Pfizer); (Rx)

References

Alwood, A., A. Downend, et al. (2007). Anticoagulant effects of low –molecular weight heparins in healthy cats. *J Vet Intern Med* 21(3): 378–387.

Alwood, A.J. (2008). Heparin Therapy in Critical Care— Should We Be Using Low Molecular Weight Heparins? Proceedings: IVECCS. Accessed via: Veterinary Information Network. http://goo.gl/LrRcQ

Dunn, M. (2006). Clinical experience with LMWH in dogs and cats. Proceedings: IVECCS. Accessed via: Veterinary Information Network. http://goo.gl/SaP1m

Feige, K., C. Schwarzwald, et al. (2003). Comparison of unfractionated and low molecular weight heparin for prophylaxis of coagulopathies in 52 horses with colic: a randomised double–blind clinical trial. *Equine Vet J* 35((5)): 506–513.

Laposata, M. & S. Johnson (2003). Assessment of the stability of dalteparin sodium in prepared syringes for up to thirty days: an in vitro study. *Clin Ther* 25(4): 1219–1225.

DANAZOL

(*da*-na-zole)   Danocrine®

ANDROGEN

Prescriber Highlights

▶ Synthetic androgen; suppresses the pituitary-ovarian axis. Used primarily for adjunctive treatment of autoimmune hemolytic anemia/thrombocytopenia in dogs & cats. Efficacy is unpredictable and slow.

▶ Caution: Severe cardiac, renal or hepatic function impairment, or undiagnosed abnormal vaginal bleeding

▶ Teratogenic

▶ Rare hepatotoxicity in dogs

▶ Expense may be an issue

Uses/Indications

Because of expense and unpredictable efficacy, danazol is not commonly used in veterinary medicine, but has been used as adjunctive therapy (with corticosteroids) in the treatment of canine immune-mediated thrombocytopenia and hemolytic anemia, particularly if the patient becomes refractory to glucocorticoids and other immunosuppressive therapy. There is apparently synergism when danazol is combined with corticosteroids for these indications. Once remission is attained, some dogs may have their dosage reduced or other medications may be eliminated and be controlled with danazol alone. In humans, danazol has been used for the treatment of endometriosis, fibrocystic breast disease, idiopathic thrombocytopenic purpura and a variety of other conditions.

Pharmacology/Actions

Danazol is a synthetic androgen with weak androgenic effects. It suppresses the pituitary-ovarian axis. Danazol probably directly inhibits the synthesis of sex steroids and binds to sex steroid receptors in tissues where it may express anabolic, weak androgenic, and antiestrogenic effects. Danazol appears to reduce affinity of antibody with the mononuclear phagocytic system Fc receptor. It also may compete with glucocorticoids on steroid-binding globulin, thereby allowing greater free glucocorticoid to act.

Pharmacokinetics

There is very limited data available. Danazol is absorbed from the GI tract, but appears to be a rate limited process as increasing the dosage does not yield a corresponding increase in serum level. Distribution information is practically nonexistent; the drug apparently crosses the placenta. Danazol is believed to be principally metabolized in the liver. In humans, half-lives average about 4–5 hours.

Contraindications/Precautions/Warnings

Danazol should be used in patients with severe cardiac, renal, or hepatic function impairment, or undiagnosed abnormal vaginal bleeding only when its benefits outweigh its risks.

Adverse Effects

Hepatotoxicity (incidence is rare) is the most significant of the adverse effects that have been reported thus far in dogs. Otherwise virilization in females is the most likely other effect that may be seen. Rarely, danazol may cause weight gain or lethargy. Human patients have developed vaginitis. Other potential adverse effects include edema, testicular atrophy, hirsutism, or alopecia.

Reproductive/Nursing Safety

Because of documented teratogenic effects, danazol is contraindicated during pregnancy. In humans, the FDA categorizes this drug as category X for use during pregnancy (*Studies in animals or humans demonstrate fetal abnormalities or adverse reaction; reports indicate evidence of fetal risk. The risk of use in pregnant women clearly outweighs any possible benefit.*)

While it is unknown if danazol enters milk, the potential adverse effects associated with androgens in young animals warrants caution. In humans, breastfeeding is contraindicated in patients taking danazol.

Overdosage/Acute Toxicity

No information was located. Significant overdoses should initially be handled by contacting an animal poison control center and initiate gut emptying protocols when applicable.

Drug Interactions

The following drug interactions have either been reported or are theoretical in humans or animals receiving danazol and may be of significance in veterinary patients:

■ **CYCLOSPORINE:** May significantly increase cyclosporine levels

■ **INSULIN:** By affecting carbohydrate metabolism, danazol may affect insulin requirements (doses may need to be increased) in diabetic patients

■ **WARFARIN:** Concomitant use of danazol with anticoagulants may enhance the anticoagulant effect as danazol may decrease the synthesis of procoagulant factors in the liver

Laboratory Considerations

■ Danazol may decrease **total serum thyroxine** (T4) and increase T3 uptake; because thyroid-binding globulin is decreased, free T4 and TSH remain normal.

■ **ALT** (SGPT) and **AST** (SGOT) may increase early in therapy but decrease towards baseline later in therapy. After discontinuation of danazol, levels usually return to baseline.

Doses

■ **DOGS:**

For adjunctive treatment of immune-mediated hemolytic anemia or thrombocytopenia:

a) As adjunctive therapy with glucocorticoids in non-regenerative forms of IMHA: 5 mg/kg PO three times daily. Used to reduce the dose of glucocorticoids needed for long-term therapy. (Chabanne 2006)

b) 5 mg/kg PO 2–3 times per day; rarely helpful. Costly and has limited effectiveness. (Noonan 2009)

c) Initially, (in addition to prednis(ol)one) danazol may be given at 10 mg/kg/day PO. Once anemia improves, corticosteroids may be slowly tapered and eventually DC'd. When remission maintained by danazol alone, may lower to 5 mg/kg/day. Slowly taper after 2–3 months of normal hemograms with frequent monitoring of hemograms. (Bucheler & Cotter 1995)

▪ **CATS:**

For adjunctive treatment of immune-mediated hemolytic anemia:

a) 5 mg/kg PO twice daily (Loar 1994)

Monitoring

For autoimmune hematologic disorders:

▪ Efficacy (CBC, platelets, etc.)

▪ Hepatic function, baseline and at regular intervals while on therapy

Client Information

▪ Clients should be informed that it may take several (2–3) months to see a positive response with this drug

▪ Clients should monitor for hepatotoxicity (jaundice) or changes in hematologic status (bleeding, tarry stools, etc.)

Chemistry/Synonyms

A synthetic derivative of ethisterone (ethinyl testosterone), danazol occurs as a white to pale yellow, crystalline powder. It is practically insoluble in water and sparingly soluble in alcohol.

Danazol may also be known as: Win-17757, *Anargil®, Azol®, Cyclomen®, D-Zol®, Danalem®, Danatrol®, Danazant®, Danogen®, Danocrine®, Danokrin®, Danol®, Ectopal®, Gonablok®, Kendazol®, Ladazol®, Ladogal®, Lisigon®, Mastodanatrol®, Norciden®, Vabon®, Winobanin®, Zendol®,* or *Zoldan-A®.*

Storage/Stability

Danazol capsules should be stored in well-closed containers at room temperature.

Dosage Forms/Regulatory Status

VETERINARY-LABELED PRODUCTS: None

The ARCI (Racing Commissioners International) has designated this drug as a class 4 substance. See the appendix for more information.

HUMAN-LABELED PRODUCTS:

Danazol Capsules: 50 mg, 100 mg, & 200 mg; generic; (Rx)

References

Bucheler, J. & S. Cotter (1995). Canine Immune–Mediated Hemolytic Anemia. *Kirk's Current Veterinary Therapy:XII.* J Bonagura Ed. Philadelphia, W.B. Saunders: 152–157.

Chabanne, L. (2006). Immune–Mediated Hemolytic Anemia In the Dog. Proceedings: WSAVA Congress. Accessed via: Veterinary Information Network. http://goo.gl/LICvo

Loar, A. (1994). Anemia: Diagnosis and treatment. *Consultations in Feline Internal Medicine: 2.* J August Ed. Philadelphia, W.B. Saunders Company: 469–487.

Noonan, M. (2009). Immune Mediated Hemolytic Anemia. Proceedings: IVECC. Accessed via: Veterinary Information Network. http://goo.gl/EaAXT

DANOFLOXACIN MESYLATE

(dan-oh-*floks*-a-sin)   A180®, Advocin®

INJECTABLE FLUOROQUINOLONE

Prescriber Highlights

▶ Parenteral fluoroquinolone antibiotic labeled for use in cattle (not dairy or veal) to treat BRD associated with *Mannheimia* (Pasturella) *hemolytica* & *P. multocida*; may also be of benefit in treating fluoroquinolone-susceptible infections in non-food producing species (horses, camelids, exotics)

▶ Labeled in cattle for two SC injections 48 hours apart

▶ FDA prohibits extra-label use in food animals

Uses/Indications

Danofloxacin mesylate injection is indicated for the treatment of Bovine Respiratory Disease (BRD) associated with *Mannheimia* (Pasturella) *hemolytica* and *P. multocida* in cattle (not dairy or veal). Because of the drug's spectrum of activity, it may also be of benefit in the treatment of infections caused by *Histophilus somni* (*Haemophilus somnus*) or *M. bovis*, but the drug is not labeled (at the time of writing) for treating these pathogens. In other countries, danofloxacin may be labeled for use in swine and chickens (non-laying), but in the USA it is illegal to use the drug in an extra-label manner in food-producing species.

Danofloxacin may be of benefit in treating susceptible infections in adult horses, camelids and other non-food producing species.

Pharmacology/Actions

Danofloxacin is a fluoroquinolone bactericidal antibiotic that inhibits bacterial DNA-gyrase, preventing DNA supercoiling and DNA synthesis. Fluoroquinolones have good activity against many gram-negative bacilli and some gram-positive cocci (*Staphylococcus aureus* and *Staphylococcus intermedius).* In general, fluoroquinolones have a dose or concentration dependant effect rather than a time-dependant bactericidal effect.

MIC90 values for *Mannheimia* (*Pasturella*) *hemolytica* and *Pasturella multocida* average 0.06 micrograms/mL and 0.015 micrograms/mL, respectively.

Pharmacokinetics

After subcutaneous injection in the neck in cattle, danofloxacin is reportedly rapidly absorbed with high bioavailability ($\approx$90%). Peak serum levels occur about 2–3 hours after dosing. Steady-state volume of distribution is approximately 2.7 L/kg; lung levels exceed those in plasma. Terminal elimination half-life ranges from 3–6 hours. In cattle, elimination is primarily unchanged drug into the urine. Other species may metabolize greater percentages of the drug into a desmethyl metabolite (desmethyldanofloxacin).

In horses, a research study on the pharmacokinetics of IM, IV and IG (intragastric) administration of danofloxacin at 1.25 mg/kg to healthy mature horses revealed favorable bioavailability with the IM route at 89% and poor bioavailability of the IG route at 22%. The authors reported good tolerability of the IG route (Fernandez-Varon *et al.* 2006).

In sheep, the drug quickly reaches high tissue concentrations. One hour after IM administration, the concentration peaks in lung tissue and interdigital skin. A study dosing sheep at 1.25 mg/kg IV and IM resulted in similar levels for serum, exudates and transudates (Aliabadi, Landoni *et al.* 2003).

In goats, a study of danofloxacin administered at 1.25 mg/kg IV or IM, revealed similar half-lives of 4.67 and 4.41 hours after IV and IM, respectively. Volume of distribution was high via either route with 100% bioavailability reported after IM administration. The drug's penetration into both exudates and transudates were slightly slower after IM administration (Aliabadi & Lees 2001). Another study found that goats challenged with *E. coli* endotoxin receiving danofloxacin at 1.25 mg/kg IV or IM had an altered clearance of the drug with significant increases in plasma concentrations and AUC (Ismail 2006).

In camels, IV administration of the drug at 1.25mg/kg results in a high volume of distribution, a half-life of 5.37 hours and rapid clearance. The IM administration of the drug at the same dose resulted in rapid and near complete absorption, with a half life of 5.71 hours (Aliabadi, Badrelin *et al.* 2003).

In pigs, the drug has been shown to reach a high concentration in lung tissue and gastrointestinal tissue, including mucosa. In the first 24-hours after an intramuscular dose of 2 mg/kg, 43% of the dose is eliminated in the urine. Elimination half-life in swine is about 7 hours.

Contraindications/Precautions/Warnings

The FDA prohibits extra-label usage of this drug in food animals. The manufacturer cautions use of danofloxacin in animals with known or suspected CNS disorders as quinolones have rarely caused CNS stimulation.

Adverse Effects

Hypersensitivity reactions and lameness have been reported after administration to calves at labeled dosages. Incidence rates are not known, but they are believed to occur uncommonly. In cattle, subcutaneous injections can cause a local tissue reaction that may result in trim loss.

Reproductive/Nursing Safety

Studies documenting safety during pregnancy in cattle are not available. In studies performed in rats (100 mg/kg/day), mice (50 mg/kg/day) and rabbits (15 mg/kg/day), no teratogenic effects were observed.

Danofloxacin safety during nursing is not known, but it is prohibited from use in lactating dairy cattle where the milk is for human consumption.

Overdosage/Acute Toxicity

Limited information is available for cattle. High dosages, 18–60 mg/kg for 3–6 days in feeder calves reportedly can cause arthropathies/lameness (consistent with other fluoroquinolones), CNS stimulation (ataxia, nystagmus, tremors), inappetence, recumbency, depression, and exophthalmos. Some (3/6) 21-day-old calves receiving 18 mg/kg twice 48 hours apart developed nasal pad erythema.

Studies performed in adult dogs given 2.4 mg/kg/day PO for 90 days developed no observable effects.

Drug Interactions

No specific interactions have been reported when danofloxacin is used in cattle. In humans:

- ■ **THEOPHYLLINE** (**aminophylline**): Some injectable fluoroquinolones (*e.g.*, ciprofloxacin) can potentially increase serum concentrations; increased monitoring of theophylline concentrations is recommended

Laboratory Considerations

- ■ No issues identified

Doses

- ■ **CATTLE:**
  For labeled indications:
  a) 6 mg/kg (1.5 mL per 100 lb body weight) SC. Repeat once in approximately 48 hours. Administered dosage volume should not exceed 15 mL. (Label directions; *A180*®—Pfizer)

Monitoring

- ■ Clinical efficacy

Client Information

■ If clients are to administer this product to food animals, they should be advised on proper injection technique and the importance of using the product per the label only

Chemistry/Synonyms

Danofloxacin mesylate is a synthetic fluoroquinolone that occurs as a white to off-white crystalline powder. Approximately 180 grams are soluble in 1 liter of water.

Danofloxacin may also be known by the following synonyms: CP-76136-27, danofloxacine or danofloxacino. Internationally registered trade names include: *Advocin®, Advocine®, Danocin®, Advocid®,* and *Advovet®.*

Storage/Stability

Danofloxacin mesylate for injection should be stored at or below 30° C and protected from light and freezing. The color of the injectable solution is yellow to amber and does not affect potency.

Danofloxacin injection for SC use should not be mixed with other medications or diluents. Fluoroquinolone injectable products can be very sensitive to pH changes or chelation with cationic substances (calcium, magnesium, zinc, etc.).

Dosage Forms/Regulatory Status

VETERINARY-LABELED PRODUCTS:

Danofloxacin Mesylate 180 mg/mL (of danofloxacin) in 100 mL & 250 mL multi-dose vials; *A180®* (Pfizer); (Rx). FDA-approved for use in cattle only. Not for use in cattle intended for dairy product or calves to be processed for veal. When administered per the label directions, slaughter withdrawal is 4 days from the time of the last treatment.

HUMAN-LABELED PRODUCTS: None

References

Aliabadi, F., H. Badrelin, et al. (2003). Pharmacokinetics and PH–PD modeling of danofloxacin in camel serum and tissue fluid cages. *Vet J* 165(2): 104–108.

Aliabadi, F., M. Landoni, et al. (2003). Pharmacokinetics (PK), pharmacodynamics (PD) and PK–PD integration of danofloxacin in sheep biological fluids. Antimicrob. Agents Chemother. Feb:47(2): 626–635. 2003. *Antimicrob. Agents Chemotherap.* 47(2): 626–635.

Aliabadi, F. & P. Lees (2001). Pharmacokinetics and pharmacodynamics of danofloxacin in serum and tissue fluids of goats following intravenous and intramuscular administration. *AJVR* 62(12): Dec 2001.

Fernandez–Varon, E., I. Ayala, et al. (2006). Pharmacokinetics of danofloxacin in horses after intravenous, intramuscular and intragastric administration. *Equine Vet J* 38(4): 342–346.

Ismail, M. (2006). A pharmacokinetic study of danofloxacin in febrile goats following repeated administration of endotoxin. *J Vet Phamacol Ther* 29: 313–316.

DANTROLENE SODIUM

(*dan*-troe-leen) Dantrium®

SKELETAL MUSCLE RELAXANT

Prescriber Highlights

▶ Direct acting muscle relaxant

▶ Primary indications: Horses: post-anesthesia myositis/acute rhabdomyolysis; *Dogs & Cats:* functional urethral obstruction, potentially rhabdomyolysis; *Swine:* malignant hyperthermia

▶ Extreme caution: Hepatic dysfunction

▶ Caution: Severe cardiac dysfunction or pulmonary disease

▶ Adverse Effects: Weakness, sedation, increased urinary frequency, GI effects; hepatotoxicity possible especially with chronic use.

▶ Injectable is very expensive

Uses/Indications

In humans, oral dantrolene is indicated primarily for the treatment associated with upper motor neuron disorders (*e.g.,* multiple sclerosis, cerebral palsy, spinal cord injuries, etc.). In veterinary medicine, its proposed indications include: the prevention and treatment of malignant hyperthermia syndrome in various species, the treatment of functional urethral obstruction due to increased external urethral tone in dogs and cats, the prevention and treatment of equine post-anesthetic myositis (PAM), and equine exertional rhabdomyolysis. It has also been recommended for use in the treatment of bites from Black Widow Spiders in small animals and the treatment of porcine stress syndrome.

Pharmacology/Actions

Dantrolene exhibits muscle relaxation activity by direct action on muscle. While the exact mechanism is not well understood, it probably acts on skeletal muscle by interfering with the release of calcium from the sarcoplasmic reticulum. It has no discernible effects on the respiratory or cardiovascular systems, but can cause drowsiness and dizziness. The reasons for these CNS effects are not known.

Pharmacokinetics

The bioavailability of dantrolene after oral administration in humans is only about 35% and after intragastric administration to horses, approximately 39%. The drug is fairly slowly absorbed, with peak levels occurring about 5 hours after oral administration (humans) and 1.5 hours in horses. The drug is substantially bound to plasma proteins (principally albumin), but many drugs may displace it from such (see Drug Interactions).

Dantrolene is rapidly eliminated from the horse (half-life≈130 minutes). The elimination half-life in humans is approximately 8 hours.

Dantrolene is metabolized in the liver and the metabolites are excreted in the urine. Only about 1% of the parent drug is excreted unchanged in the urine and bile.

In horses, oral dantrolene absorption is affected by food and must be given to fasted horse orally to achieve therapeutic levels.

Contraindications/Precautions/Warnings

Because dantrolene can cause hepatotoxicity, it should be used with extreme caution in patients with preexisting liver disease. It should be used with caution in patients with severe cardiac dysfunction or pulmonary disease.

Adverse Effects

The most significant adverse reaction with dantrolene therapy is hepatotoxicity. In humans, it is most commonly associated with high dose chronic therapy, but may also be seen after short high dose therapy. The incidence of this reaction is unknown in veterinary medicine, but monitor for its occurrence.

More common, but less significant are the CNS associated signs of weakness, sedation, dizziness, headache, and GI effects (nausea, vomiting, constipation). Also seen are increased urinary frequency and, possibly, hypotension.

Reproductive/Nursing Safety

The safe use of dantrolene during pregnancy has not been determined. In humans, the FDA categorizes this drug as category *C* for use during pregnancy (*Animal studies have shown an adverse effect on the fetus, but there are no adequate studies in humans; or there are no animal reproduction studies and no adequate studies in humans.*) In a separate system evaluating the safety of drugs in canine and feline pregnancy (Papich 1989), this drug is categorized as in class: *C* (*These drugs may have potential risks. Studies in people or laboratory animals have uncovered risks, and these drugs should be used cautiously as a last resort when the benefit of therapy clearly outweighs the risks.*)

Dantrolene is distributed into milk; safe use cannot be assured during nursing.

Overdosage/Acute Toxicity

There is no specific antidotal therapy to dantrolene overdoses, therefore, remove the drug from the gut if possible and treat supportively.

Drug Interactions

The following drug interactions have either been reported or are theoretical in humans or animals receiving dantrolene and may be of significance in veterinary patients:

- **BENZODIAZEPINES & OTHER CNS DEPRESSANTS:** Increased sedation may be seen if tranquilizing agents are used concomitantly with dantrolene

- **CALCIUM-CHANNEL BLOCKERS:** Rare reports of cardiovascular collapse in humans; concomitant use with dantrolene during malignant hyperthermia crises not recommended

- **ESTROGENS:** Increased risks of hepatotoxicity from dantrolene have been seen in women >35 years of age who are also receiving estrogen therapy; veterinary significance is unknown

- **WARFARIN:** Dantrolene may be displaced from plasma proteins by warfarin with increased effects or adverse reactions resulting

Doses

- **DOGS:**

For treatment of functional urethral obstruction due to increased external urethral tone:
a) 1–5 mg/kg PO q8–12h (Lane 2000), (Coates 2004)
b) 1 mg/kg PO q8h (Lulich 2004)

For canine stress syndrome (CSS)/Malignant Hyperthermia (MH):
a) To treat an acute attack: 0.2–3 mg/kg IV (Axlund 2004)
b) For MH-like syndrome associated with hops (*Humulus lupulus*) ingestion: 2–3 mg/kg IV or 3.5 mg/kg PO as soon as possible after ingestion. (Wismer 2004)

For adjunctive treatment of rhabdomyolysis:
a) 1.5 mg/kg PO q8h (from a case report; very intensive drug and supportive therapy used in this case). (Wells *et al.* 2009)

For adjunctive treatment of Black Widow Spider bite:
a) 1 mg/kg IV; followed by 1 mg/kg PO q4h (Bailey 1986)

- **CATS:**

For treatment of functional urethral obstruction due to increased external urethral tone:
a) 0.5–2 mg/kg PO q12h OR 0.5–1 mg/kg IV (IV product very expensive) (Gunn-Moore 2008)
b) 0.5–2 mg/kg PO three times daily (Coates 2004)
c) 2–10 mg (total dose) PO three times daily with either prazosin (0.5 mg/cat once to twice daily) or phenoxybenzamine (2.5–7.5 mg/cat once to twice daily) (Sparkes 2006)
d) 0.5–1 mg/kg PO q12h (Bartges 2009)

- **HORSES:**

For treatment of acute rhabdomyolysis:
a) 15–25 mg/kg slow IV four times daily (Robinson 1987)
b) 2–4 mg/kg PO via nasogastric tube once daily (Hanson 1999)

For prevention of rhabdomyolysis:
a) For prevention of recurrent exertional rhabdomyolysis in Thoroughbreds: 4 mg/kg PO in horses fasted (12-hour fast in study) prior to administration. (McKenzie *et al.* 2003)

b) Several dosage regimens have been recommended, but take care as use and efficacy are uncertain: 2 mg/kg PO once daily for 3–5 days and then every 3rd day for a month has been recommended. Drug is diluted in normal saline and given via stomach tube. Another dosage recommendation is 300 mg (total dose) PO once daily (may be preferable because the drug is hepatotoxic). Another recommendation is 500 mg (total dose) PO for 3–5 days and then 300 mg PO every third day. Monitor hepatic function and status. (MacLeay 2004)

c) 800 mg (total dose); within 30 minutes prior to administration contents of capsules mixed with 9 mL tap water to make a suspension and given PO one hour before exercise. (Edwards *et al.* 2003)

For prevention of post-anesthetic myositis (PAM):

a) To prevent muscle damage in horses undergoing hypotensive anesthesia: 6 mg/kg enterally (given via NG tube in study) 60 minutes prior to general anesthesia. Does not appear to prolong recovery time. (McKenzie & Mosley 2009)

b) 10 mg/kg PO (intragastric) 1.5 hours before surgery. This should give peak levels at the time surgery begins and maintain postulated therapeutic levels for an additional 2 hours. The intragastric preparation was made by dissolving/suspending the contents of oral capsules into 500 mL of normal saline. Should further doses be warranted, additional doses of 2.5 mg/kg PO (intragastric) q60 minutes can be given. Alternatively, IV doses of 1.9 mg/kg loading will give therapeutic levels but will only persist for about 20 minutes. An IV dose of 4 mg/kg will maintain therapeutic levels for about 2 hours, but peak levels will be quite high. (Court *et al.* 1987)

■ **SWINE:**

Prevention or treatment of malignant hyperthermia:

a) 3.5 mg/kg IV (Booth 1988)

Monitoring

Depending on the reason for use:

■ Baseline and periodic liver function tests (ALT, AST, Alk Phos, etc.) if projecting to be used chronically or using high dosages

■ Body temperature (malignant hyperthermia)

■ Urine volume, frequency, continence

Client Information

■ Dantrolene can cause GI upset (vomiting, lack of appetite), increased urinary frequency, and sedation (drowsiness)

■ Rarely, dantrolene can cause liver toxicity; contact veterinarian if patient develops persistent vomiting, lack of appetite, unexplained profound lethargy, or yellowish whites of eyes or mucous membranes

■ Intravenous use of this drug should only be used by professionals familiar with its use

Chemistry/Synonyms

A hydantoin derivative that is dissimilar structurally and pharmacologically from other skeletal muscle relaxant drugs, dantrolene sodium is a weak acid with a pK_a of 7.5. It occurs as an odorless, tasteless, orange, fine powder that is slightly soluble in water. It rapidly hydrolyzes in aqueous solutions to the free acid form that precipitates out of solution.

Dantrolene Sodium may also be known by the following synonyms and internationally registered trade names: F-440, F-368, *Danlene®*, *Dantamacrin®*, *Dantralen®*, or *Dantrolen®*.

Storage/Stability

Dantrolene capsules should be stored in well-closed containers at room temperature. Dantrolene powder for injection should be stored at temperatures less than 30°C and protected from prolonged exposure to light. After reconstitution, the powder for injection should be used within 6 hours when stored at room temperature and should be protected from direct light. It is **not compatible** with either normal saline or D_5W injection.

Compatibility/Compounding Considerations

To dose in small dogs or cats, it has been suggested to re-encapsulate ⅛th–¼th of the contents of a 25 mg capsule and place into a size 2 or 4 gelatin capsule (Gunn-Moore 2008).

Dosage Forms/Regulatory Status

VETERINARY-LABELED PRODUCTS: None

HUMAN-LABELED PRODUCTS:

Dantrolene Sodium Oral Capsules: 25 mg, 50 mg, & 100 mg; *Dantrium®* (JHP Pharm); generic; (Rx)

Dantrolene Sodium Powder for Injection Solution: 20 mg/vial (approx. 0.32 mg/mL dantrolene after reconstitution; with mannitol 3 g/vial) in 70 mL vials; *Dantrium® Intravenous* (JHP Pharm); (Rx*).* **Note:** Because of the expense, minimum order quantity, and non-returnable nature of the commercially available intravenous product, it may not be practical for veterinary use.

References

Axlund, T. (2004). Exercise induced collapse and hyperthermic myopathy: What every clinician should know. Proceedings: ACVC. Accessed via: Veterinary Information Network. http://goo.gl/UlcNw

Bailey, E.M. (1986). Emergency and general treatment of poisonings. *Current Veterinary Therapy (CVT) IX Small Animal Practice.* RW Kirk Ed. Philadelphia, W.B. Saunders: 135–144.

Bartges, J. (2009). Pipes are leaking: Urinary Incontinence.

Proceedings: WVC. Accessed via: Veterinary Information Network. http://goo.gl/X51gQ

Booth, N.H. (1988). Drugs Acting on the Central Nervous System. *Veterinary Pharmacology and Therapeutics – 6th Ed.* NH Booth and LE McDonald Eds. Ames, Iowa State University Press: 153–408.

Coates, J. (2004). Neurogenic micturition disorders. Proceedings: ACVIM Forum. Accessed via: Veterinary Information Network. http://goo.gl/260CO

Court, M.H., L.R. Engelking, et al. (1987). Pharmacokinetics of dantrolene sodium in horses. *J Vet Pharmacol Ther* 10(3): 218–226.

Edwards, J.G.T., J.R. Newton, et al. (2003). The efficacy of dantrolene sodium in controlling exertional rhabdomyolysis in the Thoroughbred racehorse. *Equine Veterinary Journal* 35(7): 707–711.

Gunn-Moore, D. (2008). Feline lower urinary tract disease (FLUTD)—Cystitis in cats. Proceedings: World Veterinary Congress. Accessed via: Veterinary Information Network. http://goo.gl/jBoEO

Hanson, R. (1999). Diagnosis and First Aid of Sporting Horse Injuries. Proceedings: Central Veterinary Conference, Kansas City.

Lane, I. (2000). Urinary Obstruction and Functional Urine Retention. *Textbook of Veterinary Internal Medicine: Diseases of the Dog and Cat.* S Ettinger and E Feldman Eds. Philadelphia, WB Saunders. 1: 93–96.

Lulich, J. (2004). Managing functional urethral obstruction. Proceedings: ACVIM Forum. Accessed via: Veterinary Information Network. http://goo.gl/acf8d

MacLeay, J. (2004). Diseases of the musculoskeletal system. *Equine Internal Medicine 2nd Ed.* S Reed, W Bayly and D Sellon Eds. Philadelphia, Saunders: 461–521.

McKenzie, E. & C. Mosley (2009). Dantrolene sodium prevents myopathy in horses undergoing hypotensive anesthesia. Proceedings: IVECCS. Accessed via: Veterinary Information Network. http://goo.gl/OH0GW

McKenzie, E., S. Valberg, et al. (2003). The effect of oral dantrolene sodium on post–exercise serum creatinine kinase activity in Thoroughbred horses with recurrent exertional rhabdomyolysis. Proceedings: ACVIM. Accessed via: Veterinary Information Network. http://goo.gl/MIS49

Robinson, N.E. (1987). Table of Common Drugs: Approximate Doses. *Current Therapy in Equine Medicine, 2.* NE Robinson Ed. Philadelphia, W.B. Saunders: 761.

Sparkes, A. (2006). Feline lower urinary tract disease. Proceedings: WSAVA Congress. Accessed via: Veterinary Information Network. http://goo.gl/PB0qs

Wells, R.J., C.D. Sedacca, et al. (2009). Successful management of a dog that had severe rhabdomyolysis with myocardial and respiratory failure. *Javma–Journal of the American Veterinary Medical Association* 234(8): 1049–1054.

Wismer, T. (2004). Newer antidotal therapies. Proceedings: IVECC Symposium. Accessed via: Veterinary Information Network. http://goo.gl/jNp8A

DAPSONE

(*dap*-sone)   DDS

ANTIMYCOBACTERIAL ANTIBIOTIC

Prescriber Highlights

▶ Potentially useful for treating mycobacterial & some protozoal (Pneumocystis) infections; may be used to treat Brown Recluse spider bites & cutaneous vasculitis

▶ Rarely used due to potential for severe adverse effects

▶ Relatively contraindicated in cats

▶ Adverse effects: hepatotoxicity, methemoglobinemia, anemia, thrombocytopenia, neutropenias, gastrointestinal effects, neuropathies, & cutaneous drug eruptions; photosensitivity reactions are possible

Uses/Indications

Dapsone may be useful as a second-line agent in the treatment of mycobacterial diseases in dogs and, possibly, cats. It potentially may be a useful treatment for *Pneumocystis jiroveci* (formerly *Pneumocystis carinii*) infections.

Because of its leukocyte inhibitory characteristics, dapsone may be useful for adjunctive treatment of Brown recluse spider (*Loxosceles rectusa recluse*) bites, or when an underlying etiology causing cutaneous vasculitis cannot be determined.

Pharmacology/Actions

The exact mechanism for dapsone's actions are not known. It probably has similar actions to that of the sulfonamides, primarily affecting folic acid synthesis in susceptible organisms. Dapsone also decreases neutrophil chemotaxis, complement activation, antibody production and lysosomal enzyme synthesis. The mechanisms for these actions are not well understood.

Pharmacokinetics

After oral administration to dogs, dapsone is rapidly and completely absorbed. Elimination half-life ranges from about 6–10 hours. In humans, the monoacetyl metabolite is almost completely bound to plasma proteins, but in dogs, it is only about 60% bound. Dapsone is primarily eliminated via the kidneys as conjugates and unidentified metabolites. Half-life in humans is widely variable and ranges from about 10–50 hours.

Contraindications/Precautions/Warnings

Because of increased incidences of neurotoxicity and hemolytic anemia, dapsone is generally not recommended for use in cats. Dapsone in contraindicated in patients hypersensitive to it or other sulfone drugs. It should not be used in patients with severe anemias or other preexisting blood dyscrasias. Because of its potential for causing hepatic toxicity, dapsone should be used with caution in animals with preexisting hepatic dysfunction.

Adverse Effects
Adverse effects include hepatotoxicity, dose-dependent methemoglobinemia, hemolytic anemia, thrombocytopenia, neutropenias, gastrointestinal effects, neuropathies, and cutaneous drug eruptions. Photosensitivity is possible. Dapsone is a potential carcinogen.

Reproductive/Nursing Safety
In pregnant animals, dapsone should be used with caution. In humans, the FDA categorizes dapsone as a category *C* drug for use during pregnancy (*Animal studies have shown an adverse effect on the fetus, but there are no adequate studies in humans; or there are no animal reproduction studies and no adequate studies in humans*). Animal studies have apparently not been performed with dapsone to determine its effects in pregnancy.

Dapsone is excreted into milk in concentrations equivalent to those found in plasma; and hemolytic reactions have been seen in human neonates. Consider switching to milk replacer if dapsone is required in a nursing dam.

Overdosage/Acute Toxicity
Because of its toxicity potential, specific species differences in sensitivity, and pharmacokinetics, it is recommended to contact an animal poison control center in cases of dapsone overdoses. In humans, dapsone overdoses generally cause nausea, vomiting, and hyperexcitability which can occur within minutes of an overdose. Methemoglobinemia with associated depression, seizures, and cyanosis can occur. Hemolysis may be delayed, occurring from 7–14 days after the overdose. Treatment in humans includes removal of drug from the gut, methylene blue for methemoglobinemia and, sometimes, hemodialysis to enhance removal of the drug and the monoacetyl metabolite.

Drug Interactions
The following drug interactions have either been reported or are theoretical in humans or animals receiving dapsone and may be of significance in veterinary patients:

- **PROBENECID:** May decrease the renal excretion of active metabolites of dapsone
- **PYRIMETHAMINE:** May increase risk of hematologic reactions occurring with dapsone
- **RIFAMPIN:** May decrease plasma dapsone concentrations (7–10 fold)
- **TRIMETHOPRIM:** May increase plasma dapsone concentrations (and vice versa) and potentially increase each other's toxicity

Laboratory Considerations
- No specific laboratory interactions or considerations noted

Doses
- **DOGS:**
  a) As an alternative treatment for pemphigus: Dapsone at 1 mg/kg PO q8h; with sulfasalazine at 10–40 mg/kg q8h. (Rosenkrantz 2004)
  b) For post-vaccination alopecia/vasculitis resistant to prednisone therapy: 1 mg/kg PO q8h (Lemarie 2003b)
  c) For treating mycobacteriosis: 1.1 mg/kg PO q6h until remission, then 0.3 mg/kg q8–12h after recovery (Greene & Watson 1998)
  d) For adjunctive therapy of vasculitis: 1 mg/kg PO q8h (Hillier 2006)
  e) For adjunctive treatment of Brown Recluse spider (*Loxosceles* spp.) bite: 1 mg/kg PO three times daily for 10 days (Peterson 2006)

- **CATS:**
  Caution: Dapsone can potentially cause serious side effects in cats (*e.g.*, blood dyscrasias, and hepatic or neuro toxicities); many consider its use relatively contraindicated in cats. If this drug is to be used, clients must accept the risks associated with its use; intensive monitoring for adverse effects must be performed.
  a) As an alternative to clofazimine for treating feline leprosy (see caution above): 1 mg/kg once daily PO. (Lemarie 2003a)
  b) For treating mycobacteriosis: 8 mg/kg PO once daily for 6 weeks (Greene & Watson 1998)
  c) For aural chondritis: 1 mg/kg PO q24h (Griffin 2006)

- **HORSES:**
  a) As an alternative treatment for *Pneumocystis carinii* pneumonia: 3 mg/kg PO once daily (q24h). **Note:** From one case report of treatment of a foal; treatment period was 56 days. (Clark-Price *et al.* 2004)

Monitoring
- CBC with platelets every 2–3 weeks during first 4 months of treatment and then every 3–4 months
- Liver function tests
- Other adverse effects (GI, drug eruptions, neurotoxicity, etc.)
- Efficacy

Client Information
- Clients should understand that limited experience has occurred with dapsone in domestic animals and that toxicity may occur.
- Because photosensitivity can occur, exposed skin should be protected from prolonged exposure to sunlight.

Chemistry/Synonyms

A sulfone antimycobacterial/antiprotozoan, dapsone occurs as a white or creamy-white, odorless, crystalline powder. It is very slightly soluble in water, freely soluble in alcohol, and insoluble in fixed or vegetable oils.

Dapsone may also be known as: DADPS, dapsonum, DDS, diaminodiphenylsulfone, NSC-6091, diaphenylsulfone, disulone, sulfonyldianiline, *Avlosulfone®*, *Daps®*, *Dapsoderm-X®*, *Dopsan®*, *Novasulfone®*, *Servidapsone®*, and *Sulfona®*.

Storage/Stability

Dapsone tablets should be stored protected from light at controlled room temperature (20–25°C, 68–77°F).

Compatibility/Compounding Considerations

Dapsone tablets may be compounded into a stable liquid dosage form. The simplest method is to use a 1:1 ratio of *Ora-Plus®:Ora-Sweet®* and use crushed tablets to make a concentration of 2 mg/mL. This preparation is stable either stored refrigerated or at room temperature for 90 days (Nahata *et al.* 2000).

Dosage Forms/Regulatory Status

VETERINARY-LABELED PRODUCTS: None

HUMAN-LABELED PRODUCTS:

Dapsone Oral Tablets: 25 mg & 100 mg (scored); generic (Jacobus); (Rx)

References

Clark–Price, S., J. Cox, et al. (2004). Use of dapsone on the treatment of Pneumocystis carinii pneumonia in a foal. *JAVMA* 224(3): 407–410.

Greene, C. & A. Watson (1998). Antimicrobial Drug Formulary. *Infectious Diseases of the Dog and Cat*. C Greene Ed. Philadelphia, WB Saunders: 790–919.

Griffin, C. (2006). Dermatologic diseases of the auricle. Proceedings: WSAVA Congress. Accessed via: Veterinary Information Network. http://goo.gl/Qllpg

Hillier, A. (2006). Life threatening skin diseases. Proceedings: ACVC. Accessed via: Veterinary Information Network. http://goo.gl/GkQ1e

Lemarie, S. (2003a). Cutaneous mycobacterium, nocardia and actinomyces. Proceedings Western Veterinary Conf. http://goo.gl/xhbNj

Lemarie, S. (2003b). Puppy skin diseases. Proceedings: Western Veterinary Conf. Accessed via: Veterinary Information Network. http://goo.gl/gCLCT

Nahata, M.C., R.S. Morosco, et al. (2000). Stability of dapsone in two oral liquid dosage forms. *Ann Pharmacother* 34(7–8): 848–850.

Peterson, M. (2006). Venomous arthropods. Proceedings: Western Vet Conf. Accessed via: Veterinary Information Network. http://goo.gl/QO8zX

Rosenkrantz, W. (2004). Pemphigus: current therapy. *Vet Derm* 15: 90–98.

DARBEPOETIN ALFA

(*dar*-beh-*poe*-eh-tin *al*-fah)   Aranesp®

ERYTHROPOIETIC AGENT

Prescriber Highlights

▶ Biosynthetic erythropoietic agent potentially useful for treating anemia of chronic kidney disease in dogs & cats

▶ May be less immunogenic (not proven) in dogs or cats than epoetin alfa (rHuEPO)

▶ Longer duration of effect, initially only dosed once per week

▶ Treatment expense may be formidable

Uses/Indications

Darbepoetin may potentially be useful in treating anemia of chronic kidney disease in dogs and cats. It may be less immunogenic than epoetin, but this is only theoretical and has not been documented. Another advantage is that doses may be administered less often to maintain PCV. Treatment costs may be higher than using epoetin, however.

Pharmacology/Actions

Darbepoetin is a recombinant DNA-produced protein related to erythropoietin. It stimulates erythropoiesis using the same mechanism as endogenous erythropoietin by interacting with progenitor stem cells to increase RBC production. Darbepoetin may be less immunogenic in animals than epoetin secondary to its formulation utilizing carbohydrates as part of its structure. Theoretically, carbohydrates may "shield" the sites on the drug of greatest antigenic potential from immune cell detection. Carbohydrates also increase the solubility and stability of the compound, causing less aggregate formation and, therefore, potentially less immunogenicity.

Pharmacokinetics

No information was located on the pharmacokinetics in dogs or cats. In humans with chronic renal failure after subcutaneous injection, bioavailability is about 37% and the drug is absorbed slowly with a distribution half-life of about 1.4 hours. It is extensively metabolized and terminal elimination half-life averages 21 hours. Terminal half-life is about 3 times greater than that of epoetin alfa.

Contraindications/Precautions/Warnings

Darbepoetin should not be used in dogs or cats with documented anti-rHuEPO antibodies. Antibody formation diagnosis is based upon high myeloid:erythroid ratio on bone marrow cytology and exclusion of other causes of anemia. In humans, darbepoetin is contraindicated in patients hypersensitive to it or excipients in the formulation and in those with uncontrolled hypertension.

Adverse Effects

The adverse effect profile for darbepoetin is unknown, but adverse effects reported with rHuEPO (epoetin) therapy in animals include: anti-rHuEPO antibody formation with resultant pure red blood cell aplasia (PRCA), hypertension, seizures, or iron deficiency.

Reproductive/Nursing Safety

Studies performed in pregnant rats and rabbits demonstrated no overt teratogenicity at IV dosages of up to 20 mg/kg/day. Decreased body weights were noted in some rat pups.

It is unknown if darbepoetin is distributed into milk, but it is unlikely to pose much risk to animals nursing.

Overdosage/Acute Toxicity

Little information is available. Humans have received therapeutic dosages of up to 8 micrograms/kg every week for 12 weeks. Polycythemia is possible and therapeutic phlebotomy may be required.

Drug Interactions

None have been identified. For epoetin (a related compound):

- **ANDROGENS:** May increase the sensitivity of erythroid progenitors and this interaction has been used for therapeutic effect

- **DESMOPRESSIN:** With EPO can decrease bleeding times

Laboratory Considerations

- No specific lab issues were identified; see Contraindications and Monitoring for more information.

Doses

- **DOGS/CATS:**

  Doses and dosing intervals for darbepoetin in dogs and cats have not been well established. Anecdotally it has been suggested to use the initial human dose of 0.45 micrograms/kg of darbepoetin in dogs and cats and adjust using clinical judgment and careful monitoring. Alternatively, animals that have received epoetin alfa (RHuEPO) can have their total weekly dosages converted using the following guidelines: Total weekly dose of epoetin in Units divided by 200 = once weekly dose in micrograms darbepoetin. Example: animal gets 400 Units of epoetin 3 times weekly = 1200 Units. Divide by 200 = 6 micrograms of darbepoetin once weekly.

Monitoring

- Before re-dosing check PCV each time
- Monitor patient's iron stores or supplement with iron
- Blood pressure

Client Information

- Clients must be committed to the expense and associated monitoring required for this treatment

- Therapeutic effects may not be noted for several weeks after starting treatment

Chemistry/Synonyms

Darbepoetin alfa is a 165-amino acid protein that is produced using recombinant DNA technology in Chinese hamster ovary cells. Two additional N-linked oligosaccharide chains are added to human erythropoietin yielding a glycoprotein with an approximate molecular weight of 37,000 daltons.

Darbepoetin may also be known by the following synonyms: NESP, novel erythropoiesis stimulating protein, darbepoetina or darbepoetinum. Internationally registered trade names include: *Aranesp*® and *Nespo*®.

Storage/Stability

The commercially available injection solutions (polysorbate or albumin-based) should be stored at 2−8°C and protected from light. Do not freeze or shake.

Dosage Forms/Regulatory Status

VETERINARY-LABELED PRODUCTS: None

The ARCI (Racing Commissioners International) has designated this drug as a class 2 substance. It is also prohibited on the premises of a racing facility.

HUMAN-LABELED PRODUCTS:

Darbepoetin Alfa Solution for Injection (preservative free); *Aranesp*® (Amgen); (Rx)

Each size is available in polysorbate or albumin-based solutions:

25 micrograms/0.42 mL preservative free in single-dose prefilled syringes

25 micrograms/mL preservative free, in single-dose vials

40 micrograms/0.4 mL preservative free in single-dose prefilled syringes

40 micrograms/mL preservative free in single-dose vials

60 micrograms/0.3 mL preservative free in single-dose prefilled syringes

60 micrograms/mL in single-dose vials

100 micrograms/0.5 mL preservative free in single-dose prefilled syringes

100 micrograms/mL in single-dose vials

150 micrograms/0.3 mL preservative free in single-dose prefilled syringes

150 micrograms/0.75 mL in single-dose vials

200 micrograms/0.4 mL preservative free in single-dose prefilled syringes

200 micrograms/mL in single-dose vials

300 micrograms/0.6 mL preservative free in single-dose prefilled syringes

300 micrograms/mL in single-dose vials

500 micrograms/mL preservative free in single-dose vials and prefilled syringes

DECOQUINATE

(de-koe-*kwin*-ate)   Deccox®

ANTIPROTOZOAL/COCCIDIOSTAT

Prescriber Highlights

▶ Coccidiostat

▶ Not FDA-approved for lactating dairy animals, laying chickens

▶ Not effective against adult coccidia; no effect on clinical coccidiosis; results in treating calves with cryptosporidiosis have been disappointing

Uses/Indications

Decoquinate is labeled for use in cattle for the prevention of coccidiosis in either ruminating or non-ruminating calves, cattle or young goats caused by the species *E. christenseni* or *E. ninakohlyakimoviae*. It is used for prevention of coccidiosis in broilers caused by *E. tenella*, *E. necatrix*, *E. acervulina*, *E. mivati*, *E. maxima* or *E. burnetti*.

It may be useful in dogs as prophylactic treatment for coccidiosis and hepatozoonosis relapse.

Pharmacology/Actions

Decoquinate is 4-hydroxy quinolone agent that has anticoccidial activity. Decoquinate acts on the sporozoite stage of the life cycle. The sporozoite apparently can still penetrate the host intestinal cell, but further development is prevented. The mechanism of action for decoquinate is to disrupt electron transport in the mitochondrial cytochrome system of coccidia.

Pharmacokinetics

No information was located.

Contraindications/Precautions/Warnings

Decoquinate is not effective for treating clinical coccidiosis and has no efficacy against adult coccidia. Decoquinate is not FDA-approved for use in animals producing milk for food or in laying chickens.

Adverse Effects

No adverse effects listed when given as directed.

Overdosage/Acute Toxicity

No specific information located. Decoquinate is considered to have a wide safety margin.

Drug Interactions/Laboratory Considerations

■ None noted

Doses

■ **DOGS:**

For coccidiosis prophylaxis:

a) 50 mg/kg PO once daily (Matz 1995)

For canine hepatozoonosis (*Hepatozoon americanum*): **Note:** When using decoquinate for this indication, obtain the decoquinate 6% (27.2 gram/lb.) powder. An approximate conversion is ¼ teaspoonful is

equivalent to approximately 45 mg decoquinate and 1 teaspoonful (5 mL) is equivalent to approximately 180 mg decoquinate.

a) For 14 days: Use TMP/Sulfa 15 mg/kg PO q12h; Clindamycin 10 mg/kg PO q8h; Pyrimethamine 0.25 mg/kg PO once daily);

Then to prevent relapse after TCP therapy: Decoquinate at 20 mg/kg PO q12h long-term. Recommend treating for 2 years and then performing muscle biopsy. If negative, may discontinue. When using the 27.2 gram/lb (6%) feed additive (*Deccox*®) the decoquinate powder can be administered at a rate of 1 teaspoon per 10 kg (22 lb) of body weight and fed twice daily. (Macintire *et al.* 2006), (Macintire 2007)

b) TMP/Sulfa 15 mg/kg PO daily for 14 days; Clindamycin 10 mg/kg PO q8h For 14 days; Pyrimethamine 0.25 mg/kg PO once daily For 14 days; then give Decoquinate: 10–20 mg/kg PO q12h for 24 months. (Blagburn 2005)

■ **CATTLE:**

a) For prophylaxis of coccidiosis: Using the 6% premix: 0.5 mg/kg per day in feed for at least 28 days (Penzhorn and Swan 1993) (McDougald & Roberson 1988)

■ **GOATS:**

For prophylaxis of coccidiosis:

a) 0.5 mg/kg per day in feed during periods of exposure (Bretzlaff 1993)

b) 0.5–1 mg/kg of body weight PO (de la Concha 2002)

■ **LLAMAS:**

a) For prophylaxis of coccidiosis: Using the 6% premix: 0.5 mg/kg per day in feed for at least 28 days (Johnson 1993)

Client Information

■ Decoquinate should be used for at least 4 weeks when used for preventing coccidiosis outbreaks

■ When used in dogs for Hepatozoonosis treatment may be for up to two years

■ Mix well into food

Chemistry/Synonyms

A coccidiostat, decoquinate occurs as a cream to buff-colored fine amorphous powder having a slight odor. It is insoluble in water.

Decoquinate may also be known as HC-1528, M&B-15497, or *Deccox*®.

Storage/Stability

Decoquinate is reportedly **incompatible** with strong bases or oxidizing material. Follow label storage directions; store in a cool, dry place, preferably in airtight containers.

Deccox® is labeled as being **compatible** (and cleared for use) with bacitracin zinc (with or without roxarsone), chlortetracycline, and lincomycin.

Dosage Forms/Regulatory Status

VETERINARY-LABELED PRODUCTS:

Decoquinate 6% (27.2 gram/lb.) Feed Additive (with corn meal, soybean oil, lecithin and silicon dioxide) in 50 lb bags; *Deccox®* (Alpharma); (OTC). FDA-approved for use in cattle, sheep, goats (**DO NOT** feed to cows, goats or sheep producing milk for food), and chickens (not laying chickens).

Decoquinate 0.5% (2.271 grams/lb) Feed Additive in 50 lb bags; *Doccox®-L* (Alpharma), (OTC). FDA-approved for use in ruminating and non-ruminating calves and cattle. **DO NOT** feed to cows producing milk for food.

Decoquinate 0.8% (3.632 grams/lb) in 5 lb and 50 lb bags. *Deccox®M* (Alpharma) (OTC). FDA-approved for use in ruminating and non-ruminating calves including veal calves.

Also available are calf milk replacers that contain 22.7 mg decoquinate per pound. For the prevention of coccidiosis in non-ruminating and calves and cattle. *Advance® Calvita® Supreme 20/21* (and *18/21*) *Medicated with Decoquinate* (MS Specialty Nutrition); (OTC)

HUMAN-LABELED PRODUCTS: None

References

Blagburn, B. (2005). Treatment and control of tick borne diseases and other important parasites of companion animals. Proceedings: ACVC2005. Accessed via: Veterinary Information Network. http://goo.gl/Pexfa

Bretzlaff, K. (1993). Production Medicine and Health Programs for Goats. *Current Veterinary Therapy 3: Food Animal Practice.* J Howard Ed. Philadelphia, W.B. Saunders Co.: 162–167.

de la Concha, A. (2002). Diseases of kids. Proceedings: Western Veterinary Conference. Accessed via: Veterinary Information Network. http://goo.gl/t2w7e

Johnson, L. (1993). Llama Herd health management. *Current Veterinary Therapy 3: Food Animal Practice.* J Howard Ed. Philadelphia, W.B. Saunders Co.: 172–177.

Macintire, D. (2007, Last Update). "Personal communication."

Macintire, D., N. Vincent–Johnson, et al. (2006). Hepatazooan americanum Infection. *Infectious Diseases of the Dog and Cat, 3rd Ed.* C Greene Ed., Elsevier: 705–711.

Matz, M. (1995). Gastrointestinal ulcer therapy. *Kirk's Current Veterinary Therapy:XII.* J Bonagura Ed. Philadelphia, W.B. Saunders: 706–710.

McDougald, L. & E. Roberson (1988). Antiprotazoan Drugs. *Veterinary Pharmacology and Therapeutics.* NH Booth and LE McDonald Eds. Ames, Iowa State University Press: 950–968.

DEFEROXAMINE MESYLATE

(de-fer-ox-a-meen)   Desferal®, DFO

Prescriber Highlights

▶ Parental iron chelating agent used primarily for treatment of iron or aluminum intoxication in dogs/cats; has been used as a ferric ion chelator in cardiac arrest/GDV

▶ Contraindications: Severe renal failure unless dialysis used

▶ Caution: Pregnancy

▶ Adverse Effects: Allergic reactions, auditory neurotoxicity, pain or swelling at injection sites, GI distress

▶ When used IV, must be given slowly

Uses/Indications

Deferoxamine is used for the treatment of either acute or chronic iron toxicity. It is being evaluated as an iron chelator for adjunctive treatment of acute cardiac ischemia and as a chelator for aluminum toxicity. Its efficacy in treating reperfusion injuries has been disappointing.

Pharmacology/Actions

Deferoxamine (DFO) binds ferric (Fe^{+++}) ions to its three hydroxamic groups forming ferrioxamine. This forms a stable, water-soluble compound that is readily excreted by the kidneys. DFO does not appear to chelate other trace metals (except aluminum) or electrolytes in clinically significant quantities.

Pharmacokinetics

DFO is poorly absorbed from the GI and is usually given parenterally. The drug is widely distributed in the body. DFO and ferrioxamine are excreted primarily in the urine. Ferrioxamine will give the urine a reddish color ("vin rosé") that indicates iron removal.

Contraindications/Precautions/Warnings

DFO is contraindicated in patients with severe renal failure, unless dialysis is used to remove ferrioxamine.

Adverse Effects

There is little veterinary experience with this drug. Potential adverse effects include, allergic reactions, auditory neurotoxicity (particularly with chronic, high-dose therapy), pain or swelling at injection sites, and GI distress. Too rapid IV injection may cause rapid heart rates, convulsions, hypotension, hives, and wheezing.

Oral administration of DFO is controversial. Some have recommended oral administration after oral iron ingestions, but DFO may actually increase the amount of iron absorbed from the gut. At present, oral sodium bicarbonate solution 5% given as a gastric lavage is probably a better treatment in reducing oral absorption of iron.

Reproductive/Nursing Safety

Because deferoxamine has caused skeletal abnormalities in animals at dosages just above those recommended for iron toxicity, it should be used during pregnancy only when its benefits outweigh its risks. In humans, the FDA categorizes this drug as category *C* for use during pregnancy (*Animal studies have shown an adverse effect on the fetus, but there are no adequate studies in humans; or there are no animal reproduction studies and no adequate studies in humans.*)

Overdosage/Acute Toxicity

See Adverse Effects above. Chronic high dose use may also lead to hypocalcemia and thrombocytopenia.

Drug Interactions

The following drug interactions have either been reported or are theoretical in humans or animals receiving deferoxamine and may be of significance in veterinary patients:

■ **PROCHLORPERAZINE:** Use with deferoxamine may cause temporary impairment of consciousness

■ **VITAMIN C:** May be synergistic with deferoxamine in removing iron, but could lead to increased tissue iron toxicity especially in cardiac muscle; it should be used with caution, particularly in patients with preexisting cardiac disease

Laboratory Considerations

■ DFO may interfere (falsely low values) with colorimetric **iron** assays

■ DFO may cause falsely high total iron binding capacity (**TIBC**) measurements

Doses

■ **DOGS & CATS:**

In dogs at risk for, or exhibiting signs of severe iron toxicosis; cat dosages not well established:

a) Most effective within the first 24 hours. Extrapolated animal dose is 40 mg/kg IM q4–8 hours. IM route is preferred as too rapid IV administration can cause hypotension and pulmonary edema. Efficacy can be increased by giving ascorbic acid **after** the gut has been cleared of iron. Deferoxamine-iron complex gives a salmon pink ("vin rose") color to urine. Continue to chelate until urine clears or serum iron levels return to normal. (Wismer 2004)

b) Initiate ASAP or at least within 12 hours of ingestion; give as a constant rate infusion at 15 mg/kg/hour. More rapid infusion may precipitate arrhythmias or aggravate hypotension. If constant rate infusion is not possible or are unable to monitor patient during infusion, give

40 mg/kg IM q4–8h, depending on clinical status. Continue therapy until serum iron levels are below 300 microliters/dL or decrease below the TIBC, whichever is lower. Chelation therapy may require 2–3 days of therapy. Following recovery, monitor for signs of GI obstruction, which may develop 4–6 weeks post-ingestion. (Greentree & Hall 1995)

c) 10 mg/kg IM or IV q8h for 24 hours (Firth 2000)

Experimentally, as a ferric ion chelator during treatment of cardiac arrest:

a) 5–15 mg/kg IV, IM or SC (Muir 1994)

b) 10 mg/kg IV, IM q2h twice, then three times daily for 24 hours (Hackett & Van pelt 1995)

Monitoring

For iron overload:

■ Efficacy (serum ferritin, serum iron, TIBC are recommended to monitor iron overload)

■ Treatment is continued until serum iron levels decrease below total iron-binding capacity or until urine loses its "vin rosé" color

■ Adverse effects (see above); additionally, if chronic iron overload: eye examinations (iron toxicity and its subsequent removal may adversely affect vision)

Chemistry/Synonyms

An iron-chelating agent, deferoxamine mesylate occurs as a white to off-white powder that is freely soluble in alcohol or water.

Deferoxamine mesylate may also be known as: desferoxamine mesylate, DFO, Ba-33112, Ba-29837, deferoxamini mesilas, desferrioxamine mesylate, desferrioxamine methanesulphonate, NSC-527604, *Desferal®* or *Desferin®*.

Storage/Stability

Store at room temperature. After aseptic reconstitution (2–5 mL for 500 mg vial; 8–20 mL for 2 gram vial) with sterile water for injection, the solution may be stored for up 24 hours at room temperature and protected from light. It is recommended not to mix this agent with other drugs; do not use if solution is turbid. Dilution in normal saline, lactated Ringer's or dextrose 5% has been recommended when administering as an intravenous infusion.

Dosage Forms/Regulatory Status

VETERINARY-LABELED PRODUCTS: None

HUMAN-LABELED PRODUCTS:

Deferoxamine Mesylate Powder for Injection (lyophilized): 500 mg & 2 g in vials; *Desferal®* (Novartis); generic; (Hospira); (Rx)

References

Firth, A. (2000). Treatments used in small animal toxicoses. *Kirk's Current Veterinary Therapy: XIII Small Animal Practice.* J Bonagura Ed. Philadelphia, WB Saunders: 207–211.

Greentree, W. & J. Hall (1995). Iron Toxicosis. *Kirk's*

Current Veterinary Therapy:XII. J Bonagura Ed. Philadelphia, W.B. Saunders: 240–242.

Hackett, T. & D. Van pelt (1995). Cardiopulmonary resuscitation. *Kirk's Current Veterinary Therapy:XII.* J Bonagura Ed. Philadelphia, W.B. Saunders: 167–175.

Muir, W. (1994). Cardiopulmonary cerebral resuscitation. *Saunders Manual of Small Animal Practice.* S Birchard and R Sherding Eds. Philadelphia, W.B. Saunders Company: 513–524.

Wismer, T. (2004). Newer antidotal therapies. Proceedings: IVECC Symposium. Accessed via: Veterinary Information Network. http://goo.gl/jNp8A

DERACOXIB

(*dare*-a-**cox**-ib)   Deramaxx®

NON-STEROIDAL ANTIINFLAMMATORY AGENT

Prescriber Highlights

▶ Coxib-class NSAID FDA-approved for use in dogs for treatment of post-operative pain (higher dose, 7 day maximum) & for treatment of pain & inflammation associated with osteoarthritis (lower dose, ongoing dosing)

▶ May be useful alternative to piroxicam in adjunctive treatment of transitional cell carcinoma of bladder

▶ At lower doses, appears to cause predominantly COX-2 inhibition

▶ Adverse effect profile still being fully determined, but GI & renal effects are possible

Uses/Indications

Deracoxib is indicated for the treatment of post-operative pain (higher dose, 7 day maximum), and for the treatment of pain and inflammation associated with osteoarthritis (lower dose, ongoing dosing) in dogs.

Like piroxicam, deracoxib is of interest in adjunctive treatment of transitional cell carcinoma of the bladder; investigations into this use are ongoing.

Pharmacology/Actions

Deracoxib is a coxib-class, nonsteroidal antiinflammatory drug (NSAID). It is believed to predominantly inhibit cyclooxygenase-2 (COX-2) and spare COX-1 at therapeutic dosages. This, theoretically, would inhibit production of the prostaglandins that contribute to pain and inflammation (COX-2) and spare those that maintain normal gastrointestinal and renal function (COX-1). However, COX-1 and COX-2 inhibition studies are done *in vitro* and do not necessarily correlate perfectly with clinical effects seen in actual patients.

Pharmacokinetics

After oral administration to dogs, bioavailability is greater than 90%; the time to peak serum concentration occurs at approximately 2 hours. The presence of food in the gut can enhance bioavailability. The drug has an apparent volume of distribution of 1.5 L/kg in dogs and is at least 90% bound to canine plasma proteins. Deracoxib is hepatically metabolized to four primary metabolites. These metabolites and unchanged drug are principally eliminated in the feces. Some excretion of metabolites occurs via renal mechanisms. Terminal elimination half-life in the dog is dependent upon dose. In dosages up to approximately 8 mg/kg, half-life is about 3 hours (clearance ≈ 5 mL/min/kg). Half-life at a dose of 20 mg/kg is approximately 19 hours (clearance ≈ 1.7 mL/min/kg). Drug accumulation can occur with higher dosages, leading to increased toxic effects as increased COX-1 inhibition can occur at higher concentrations. Serum half-life is not necessarily a good predictor of duration of efficacy, possibly due to the drug's high protein binding.

In cats, after 1 mg oral doses of deracoxib, peak levels (0.28 micrograms/mL) occurred about 3.6 hours after administration. Elimination half-life was about 8 hours (Gassel *et al.* 2006).

Contraindications/Precautions/Warnings

Deracoxib is contraindicated in patients known to be hypersensitive to it. It should be used with caution in patients with concurrent GI ulcerative diseases, renal or hepatic dysfunction, those in hypoproteinemic states, or with conditions that may predispose them to hypercoagulability.

Adverse Effects

In the majority of dogs treated, deracoxib appears to be well tolerated, particularly when dosed as labeled and not in conjunction with other NSAIDs or corticosteroids. However, like other NSAIDs used in dogs, many adverse effects associated with deracoxib have been reported and include: gastrointestinal (vomiting, anorexia/weight loss, diarrhea, melena, hematemesis, hematochezia, GI ulceration/perforation); urinary (azotemia, polydipsia, polyuria, UTI, hematuria, incontinence, renal failure); hematologic (anemia, thrombocytopenia); hepatic (increased hepatic enzymes, changes in total protein, etc.); neurologic (lethargy/weakness, seizures, etc.); cardiovascular/respiratory (tachypnea, bradycardia, cough); and dermatologic/immunologic (fever, facial/muzzle edema, urticaria, dermatitis). Rare occurrences of these effects are possible. As additional clinical experience is gained with this agent, relative instances of these effects and the potential risk for them to occur in a given patient population should be clarified.

Reproductive/Nursing Safety

No information on the drug's safety in pregnancy or in nursing pups was located. Use with caution in these animals.

Overdosage/Acute Toxicity

There is little data available regarding this drug's acute toxicity. A 14-day study in dogs demonstrated no clinically observable adverse effects in the dogs that received 10 mg/kg. Dogs who received 25 mg/kg, 50 mg/kg or 100 mg/kg per day for 10–11 days survived, but showed vomiting and melena; no hepatic or renal lesions were demonstrated in these dogs.

In safety studies performed by the drug manufacturer (Roberts *et al.* 2009), oral deracoxib was well tolerated by dogs when administered for up to six months at a variety of doses. Some dogs receiving ≥ 6 mg/kg/day (1.5–5X) showed signs of focal tubular degeneration/regeneration on histopathology. Focal tubular necrosis was seen in 4 dogs (of a total of 20) when dosed at 8 mg/kg/day (1 of 10 dogs) or 10 mg/kg/day (3 of 10 dogs) in the 6 month safety study.

There were 979 exposures to deracoxib reported to the ASPCA Animal Poison Control Center (APCC) during 2008-2009. In these cases 948 were dogs with 96 showing clinical signs and the remaining 31 cases were cats with 1 showing clinical signs. Common findings in dogs recorded in decreasing frequency included vomiting, diarrhea, lethargy, and elevated creatinine.

Because non-linear elimination occurs in dogs at dosages of 10 mg/kg and above, dogs acutely ingesting dosages above this amount should be observed for gastrointestinal erosion or ulceration and treated symptomatically for vomiting and GI bleeding.

This medication is a NSAID. As with any NSAID, overdosage can lead to gastrointestinal and renal effects. Decontamination with emetics and/or activated charcoal is appropriate. For doses where GI effects are expected, the use of gastrointestinal protectants is warranted. The ASPCA APCC recommends GI protectants at acute dosages of 15 mg/kg and above and IV fluid diuresis at dosages of 30 mg/kg and above in healthy dogs.

Drug Interactions

No specific drug interactions were noted, but the manufacturer warns that use in conjunction with other **NSAIDS** or **corticosteroids** be avoided, or monitored carefully. While some advocate a multi-day washout period when switching from one NSAID to another (not aspirin—see below), there does not appear to be any credible evidence that this is required. Until so, consider starting the new NSAID when the next dose would be due for the old one.

It is also possible deracoxib may cause increased renal dysfunction if used with other drugs that can cause or contribute to **renal dysfunction** (**e.g., diuretics, aminoglycosides**), but the clinical significance of this potential interaction is unclear.

The following drug interactions have either been reported or are theoretical in humans or animals receiving coxib-class NSAIDs and may be of significance in veterinary patients:

- **ACE INHIBITORS (e.g., enalapril, benazepril):** Some NSAIDs can reduce effects on blood pressure. Because ACE inhibitors potentially can reduce renal blood flow, use with NSAIDs could increase the risk for renal injury. However, one study in dogs receiving tepoxalin did not show any adverse effect. It is unknown what effects, if any, occur if other NSAIDs and ACE inhibitors are used together in dogs.

- **ASPIRIN:** May increase the risk of gastrointestinal toxicity (*e.g.*, ulceration, bleeding, vomiting, diarrhea). Washout periods several days long are probably warranted when switching from an NSAID to aspirin therapy in dogs.

- **CORTICOSTEROIDS (e.g., prednisone):** May increase the risk of gastrointestinal toxicity (*e.g.*, ulceration, bleeding, vomiting, diarrhea)

- **DIGOXIN:** NSAIDS may increase serum levels

- **FLUCONAZOLE:** Administration has increased plasma levels of celecoxib in humans and potentially could also affect deracoxib levels in dogs

- **FUROSEMIDE:** NSAIDs may reduce saluretic and diuretic effects

- **METHOTREXATE:** Serious toxicity has occurred when NSAIDs have been used concomitantly with methotrexate; use together with extreme caution

- **NEPHROTOXIC DRUGS (e.g., furosemide, aminoglycosides, amphotericin B, etc.):** May enhance the risk of nephrotoxicity development

- **NSAIDS, OTHER:** May increase the risk of gastrointestinal toxicity (*e.g.*, ulceration, bleeding, vomiting, diarrhea)

Laboratory Considerations

- No specific laboratory interactions were noted for deracoxib. Deracoxib does not appear to affect thyroid function tests in dogs.

Doses

- **DOGS:**
  a) For the control of pain and inflammation associated with osteoarthritis: 1–2 mg/kg PO once a day as needed.

  For treatment of post-operative pain: 3–4 mg/kg PO once a day as needed, not to exceed 7 days of therapy at this dosage. (Package insert; *Deramaxx*®)

Monitoring

- Baseline and periodic CBC and serum chemistry (including BUN/serum creatinine, and liver function assessment)

- Baseline history and physical

- Efficacy of therapy

- Adverse effect monitoring via client

Client Information

Note: The manufacturer provides a client information sheet they recommend be given with every prescription for this medication.

- Since dogs may find the chewable tablets' taste desirable, the drug should be stored out of reach of animals and children

- Owners should immediately report to the veterinarian if any of the following adverse effects occur: bloody stool/diarrhea or vomit, or allergic reaction (facial swelling face, hives, red, itchy skin)

- Owners should contact the veterinarian if any of the following adverse effects persist or are severe: loss of appetite, vomiting, change in bowel movements (*e.g.*, stool color), change in behavior, decrease in water consumption, or urination

- The manufacturer recommends that although the drug can be given on an empty stomach, it is preferable to be given with food; water should be available at all times to avoid dehydration

- Other drugs for pain or inflammation should not be used with this medication without the approval of the veterinarian

- Do not increase or alter the dose of this medication without the approval of the veterinarian.

Chemistry/Synonyms

Deracoxib is a diaryl-substituted pyrazole that is chemically related to other coxib-class NSAIDs such as celecoxib. Its molecular weight is 397.38.

Deracoxib's chemical name is: 4-[3-(difluoromethyl)-5-(3-fluoro-4-methoxyphenyl)-1H-pyrazole-1-yl] benzenesulfonamide.

Storage/Stability

The commercially available chewable tablets for dogs should be stored at room temperature between 15–30°C (59–86°F).

Dosage Forms/Regulatory Status

VETERINARY-LABELED PRODUCTS:

Deracoxib Chewable (scored) Tablets: 25 mg, 50 mg, 75 mg, & 100 mg in bottles of 7, 30 and 90 tablets; *Deramaxx®* (Novartis) (Rx). FDA-approved for use in dogs.

The ARCI (Racing Commissioners International) has designated this drug as a class 4 substance. See the appendix for more information.

HUMAN-LABELED PRODUCTS: None

References

Gassel, A.D., K.M. Tobias, et al. (2006). Disposition of deracoxib in cats after oral administration. *Journal of the American Animal Hospital Association* 42(3): 212–217.

Roberts, E.S., K.A. Van Lare, et al. (2009). Safety and tolerability of 3–week and 6–month dosing of Deramaxx((R)) (Deracoxib) chewable tablets in dogs. *Journal of Veterinary Pharmacology and Therapeutics* 32(4): 329–337.

Dermcaps® — see Fatty Acids

DES — see Diethylstilbestrol

DESFLURANE

(dez-*floor*-ane)   Suprane®

INHALANT ANESTHETIC

Prescriber Highlights

▶ Primary benefit is when very rapid recoveries are desired

▶ Similar effects on CNS, respiratory and cardiovascular systems as isoflurane

▶ Requires desflurane-specific vaporizer (electric, heated, pressurized, expensive)

Uses/Indications

Desflurane is a volatile anesthetic with a chemical structure identical to isoflurane except for substitution of a fluorine atom for chlorine at the alpha-ethyl carbon. Desflurane may be of particular use when rapid recoveries are desired.

Pharmacology/Actions

Desflurane is a halogenated inhalant anesthetic. It is structurally related to isoflurane (has a fluorine atom substituted for chlorine at the alpha-ethyl carbon). While the precise mechanism that inhalant anesthetics exert their general anesthetic effect is not precisely known, they may interfere with functioning of nerve cells in the brain by acting at the lipid matrix of the membrane. Like sevoflurane, desflurane has a very low blood/gas partition coefficient (0.42). Minimal Alveolar Concentration (MAC; %) in oxygen reported for desflurane: dogs = 7; cats = 9.8; horse = 7.23; rabbit = 8.9, alpacas/llamas = 7.8-8.

Some key pharmacologic effects noted with desflurane include: rapid inductions and recoveries; rapid recoveries may be a benefit, but could also be detrimental particularly if perioperative analgesics are not used. It is relatively resistant to biodegradation that may minimize risk for nephrotoxicity.

Like sevoflurane, desflurane does not potentiate catecholamine-induced arrhythmias, and like all the inhalant anesthetics it does decrease arterial blood pressure and depress ventilation in a dose-dependent manner. Unlike sevoflurane, it is a respiratory irritant, has a pungent odor and is not well suited for mask inductions.

Pharmacokinetics

Onset of action is very rapid after inhalation; some have described as "one breath" induction. At body temperature (37°C) desflurane has a blood/gas coefficient of 0.47, an oil/gas coefficient (indicates potency) of 19 and a brain/blood coefficient of 1.3.

Very little of desflurane is eliminated via hepatic routes as only 0.02% is recovered as metabolites. In humans, elimination half-life is 2.5 minutes (isoflurane about 9.5 minutes).

Contraindications/Precautions/Warnings

Desflurane is contraindicated in patients that are hypersensitive to it or other halogenated agents or that have a history or predilection towards malignant hyperthermia. It should be used with caution (benefits vs. risks) in patients with increased CSF pressure or head injury.

Because of its rapid action, use caution not to overdose during the induction phase. Because of the rapid recovery associated with desflurane, use caution (and appropriate analgesia and sedation during the recovery phase) particularly with large animals.

Geriatric or critically ill animals may require less inhalation anesthetic.

The National Institute for Occupational Safety and Health Administration has recommended that no worker should be exposed at ceiling concentrations greater than 2 ppm of any halogenated anesthetic agent over a sampling period not to exceed 1 hour.

Adverse Effects

Desflurane is usually very well tolerated. Hypotension and respiratory depression may occur and are considered dos-dependent. Like all halogenated anesthetics, desflurane can cause malignant hyperthermia in susceptible individuals (usually humans or pigs). Desflurane may have a lower incidence rate of this effect than other halogenated anesthetics.

When used for mask inductions, desflurane can cause respiratory irritation and cause salivation in dogs and cats. Rapid changes in desflurane concentrations may result in a sympathetic response and temporarily increase cardiac work.

Reproductive/Nursing Safety

Desflurane appears to be relatively safe to use during pregnancy, but data are limited. Because of its low solubility, desflurane may be one of the safest inhalant anesthetics for use during pregnancy. In rats and rabbits, no overt teratogenic effects were observed when exposed at 1 MAC-hour/day during organogenesis (10-13 days exposure). For humans, desflurane is categorized by the FDA as a category *B* drug (*Animal studies have not demonstrated risk to the fetus, but there are no adequate studies in pregnant women; or animal studies have shown an adverse effect, but adequate studies in pregnant women have not demonstrated a risk to the fetus during the first trimester of pregnancy, and there is no evidence of risk in later trimesters.*)

Desflurane is likely compatible with nursing as levels are low in milk and rapidly washout within 24 hours of use. However, safety during nursing has not been established.

Overdosage/Acute Toxicity

In the event of an overdosage, discontinue desflurane; maintain airway and support respiratory and cardiac function as necessary.

Drug Interactions

The following drug interactions have either been reported or are theoretical in humans or animals receiving desflurane and may be of significance in veterinary patients:

■ **ACE INHIBITORS OR OTHER HYPOTENSIVE AGENTS:** Concomitant use may increase risks for hypotension. Enalapril caused significant decreases in systolic blood pressure in cats and dogs undergoing isoflurane anesthesia (Ishikawa *et al.* 2007). Similar effects may be expected with desflurane.

■ **NON-DEPOLARIZING NEUROMUSCULAR BLOCKING AGENTS:** Additive neuromuscular blockade may occur

■ **SUCCINYLCHOLINE:** With inhalation anesthetics, may induce increased incidences of cardiac effects (bradycardia, arrhythmias, sinus arrest and apnea) and, in susceptible patients, malignant hyperthermia

Laboratory Considerations

■ Like other halogenated anesthetics, desflurane can cause transient increases in glucose and white blood cell count.

Doses

a) Clinically useful concentrations: Induction = 8–15%; Maintenance = 5–9% (Grubb 2004)

b) Approximate MAC for emergency patients: 6% (Gaynor 2010)

c) Following intravenous induction: the author usually starts with a vaporiser setting of about 8% (around MAC in most animals), increasing the concentration as required. (Clarke 2008)

Monitoring

■ Respiratory, ventilatory status
■ Cardiac rate/rhythm; blood pressure
■ Level of anesthesia
■ Body temperature,
■ Neuromuscular function

Chemistry/Synonyms

Desflurane has the chemical name: (±)-2-Difluoromethyl 1,2,2,2-tetrafluoroethyl ether and has molecular weight of 168. It is a clear, colorless, heavy liquid. It is non-flammable and non-explosive. At one atmosphere it has a boiling point of 22-23°C, a vapor pressure of 669mm Hg at 20°C, specific gravity is 1.465 at 20°C. Desflurane is practically insoluble in water, but miscible with anhydrous alcohol. Desflurane has a very low blood:gas solubility ratio of 0.42 (at 37°C).

Desflurane may also be known as I-653, desfluraani, desflurano, or desfluranum. A common trade name is *Suprane*®.

Storage/Stability

Desflurane solution should be stored in its original container at 15° to 30°C (59° to 86°F). Secure cap on bottle tightly after use. Protect from light.

Before opening, the contents of the bottle should be cooled to below 10°C (48°F). Desflurane is relatively stable in soda lime at room temperature, but can produce carbon monoxide and formaldehyde. At 80°C, rate of degradation per hour is 0.44%.

Dosage Forms/Regulatory Status

VETERINARY-LABELED PRODUCTS: None

HUMAN-LABELED PRODUCTS:

Desflurane Solution for Inhalation Anesthesia in 240 mL btls; *Suprane®* (Baxter); (Rx)

References

Clarke, K.W. (2008). Options for inhalation anaesthesia. *In Practice* 30(9): 513–518.

Gaynor, J.S. (2010). Critical Anesthesia: Not All Patients Are Created Equal. Proceedings: WVC. Accessed via: Veterinary Information Network. http://goo.gl/AHapL

Grubb, T. (2004). Gas Anesthetics: Where Are We Now? Proceedings: IVECCS. Accessed via: Veterinary Information Network. http://goo.gl/Ade69

Ishikawa, Y., M. Uechi, et al. (2007). Effect of Isoflurane Anesthesia on Hemodynamics Following Administration of an Angiotensin–Converting Enzyme Inhibitor in Cats. Proceedings: ACVIM. Accessed via: Veterinary Information Network. http://goo.gl/0ZZ3x

DESLORELIN ACETATE

(dess-*lor*-a-lin)   SucroMate®, Ovuplant®

HORMONAL AGENT

Prescriber Highlights

▶ Synthetic GnRH analog for estrual mares to induce & time ovulation; implants may also be effective to control reproduction in the bitch or as a contraceptive in male dogs

▶ No labeled contraindications

▶ Adverse Effects: May cause some local swelling, pain, etc; interovulatory period may be prolonged if implant not removed

Uses/Indications

Deslorelin is FDA-approved for inducing ovulation in estrual mares. There is also interest in developing dosages and dosage forms as a long-term, reversible contraceptive in a variety of animal species, as a treatment for prostatic disease in male dogs, and incontinence in ovariectomized dogs.

In humans, deslorelin has been investigated for treating children with precocious puberty, and in adults for prostate carcinoma, dysmenorrhea, fibroids, and endometriosis.

Pharmacology/Actions

Deslorelin increases the levels of endogenous luteinizing hormone (LH), thereby inducing ovulation. When developing follicles are greater than 30 mm in diameter, deslorelin induces ovulation in approximately 78% of mares within 48 hours of administration.

Pharmacokinetics

In horses after implantation of a 2.1 mg pellet, concentrations of LH and FSH peak about 12 hours after implant and return to pretreatment levels approximately 3–4 days after implantation. Oral dosing of 100 micrograms/kg to Beagles, demonstrated no increase in LF or FSH.

Contraindications/Precautions/Warnings

Deslorelin acetate is contraindicated in horses known to be hypersensitive to it. Do not use in horses intended for human consumption. Do not administer IV.

Adverse Effects

The IM gel can cause swelling at the site of injection. Swelling generally subsides with 5 days. With the implants, minor local swelling, sensitivity to touch, and elevated skin temperature at injection site may occur; these effects should resolve within 5 days of implantation.

There is some evidence that deslorelin implants can suppress pituitary FSH secretion and decrease follicular development in subsequent diestrus, leading to a prolonged interovulatory period. Some clinicians (see the dose recommendation by McCue 2003, below), recommend removing the implant to negate this possibility.

Reproductive/Nursing Safety

Abnormalities in foal viability or behavior related to the use of deslorelin have not been observed in foals born to treated mares.

Overdosage/Acute Toxicity

In 8 mares that received a single IM injection at 10X the recommended of 1.8 mg dose, one exhibited moderate tremors and hives 6 hours after injection. If inadvertent administration of additional implant is done, it should be removed upon detection if within 96 hours of implant.

Drug Interactions

■ No specific interactions noted

Laboratory Considerations

■ None noted

Doses

■ **DOGS:**

As a contraceptive in male dogs: Using the 4.7 mg implant (*Suprelorin-6®*—Virbac/Peptech): Implant SC every 6 months. Using the 9.4 mg implant (*Suprelorin-12®*-Peptech): Implant SC every 12 months. Implant in loose skin below lower neck and lumbar area; avoid implanting into fat. Pregnant women should not administer the implant. (Adapted from label information; see full label for further dosing instructions, precautions and adverse effects)

■ **HORSES:**

For induction of ovulation:

a) For inducing ovulation within 48 hours in cyclic estrous mares with an ovarian follicle between 30 and 40 mL in diameter: Shake vial well before drawing into syringe. Administer 1.8 mg (1 mL) by in-tramuscular injection in the neck. (Label Information—*SucroMate® Equine*)

b) If follicle is greater than 30 mm in diam-eter (as determined by rectal palpation or ultrasound), and breeding is to take place within 48 hours, place one implant subcutaneously in the neck. Implant site should be midway between head and shoulder over the muscle mass of the neck and away for subcutaneous nerves and vessels. Thoroughly disinfect site of implant. Insert the entire length of needle SC and fully depress the implanter plung-er. Slowly withdraw needle while pressing skin at injection site. Examine implanter to assure that implant has been admin-istered. Do not reuse implanter. Implant will be absorbed with time. (Package in-sert; *Ovuplant®*)

c) As above, but because interovulatory in-terval may be prolonged if implant is left in the mare, remove after approximately 48 hours.

Alternative dosing/removal method: Re-strain mare and briefly wash vulva with soap and water and then dry. One mL of lidocaine is infused into the edge of the vulva. The implant is inserted just beneath the epithelium in the blocked area. When the lidocaine is absorbed, the implant can be palpated. After ovulation, the implant can be gently "squeezed" out of the original opening created by the implant device. No treatment is required at the site after removal of the implant. (McCue 2003)

Monitoring
■ None required

Chemistry/Synonyms
Deslorelin acetate is a synthetic gonadotro-pin-releasing hormone (GnRH, gonadorelin) analog. It is a nonapeptide and has chemical modifications in the amino aide composition at positions 6 and 9/10.

Storage/Stability
Deslorelin implants or injectable suspension should be stored refrigerated (2–8°C, 36–46°F).

Dosage Forms/Regulatory Status
VETERINARY-LABELED PRODUCTS:
Deslorelin Suspension for Injection 1.8 mg/mL in 10 mL multi-dose vials; *SucroMate® Equine* (Thorn/Bioniche; NADA 141-319); (Rx). FDA-approved for horses (not intended for food).

Deslorelin 2.1 mg cylindrical implant with im-planter; 5 per box *Ovuplant®* (Peptech) (Rx). FDA-approved for ovulation induction in mares. Not for use in horses intended for food. This product is FDA-approved in the USA (per the FDA's Green Book), but it may not be cur-rently marketed.

In Australia, New Zealand (6 month only) and several EU countries: Deslorelin Implants 4.7 mg (6 month) and 9.4 mg (12 month) are available for contraceptive use in male dogs. Trade name is *Suprelorin®-6* or *Suprelorin®-12* (Peptech)

The FDA may allow legal importation of this medication for compassionate use in animals; for more information, see the *Instructions for Legally Importing Drugs for Compassionate Use in the USA* found in the appendix.

HUMAN-LABELED PRODUCTS: None

References
McCue, P. (2003). Hormone therapy: new aspects. Proceedings: Western Veterinary Conference. Accessed via: Veterinary Information Network. http://goo.gl/RfyuN

DESMOPRESSIN ACETATE

(des-moe-*press*-in)   Stimate®, DDAVP®

HORMONAL AGENT

Prescriber Highlights

▶ Synthetic vasopressin analogue used to treat diabetes insipidus & Von Wil-lebrand's disease (limited usefulness)

▶ Contraindications: Hypersensitivity to desmopressin, type IIB or platelet-type (pseudo) Von Willebrand's (German shorthair pointers?)

▶ Use caution in patients susceptible to thrombosis

▶ Adverse Effects: Eye irritation after conjunctival administration; hypersen-sitivity possible

▶ Overdoses can cause fluid retention/hyponatremia

Uses/Indications
Desmopressin has been found to be useful in the treatment of central diabetes insipidus in small animals. It may be useful in treating Von Willebrand's disease, but its short duration of activity (2–4 hours) in this condition, resistance development, and expense limit its usefulness for this disorder. Desmopressin may be useful perioperatively to reduce lymph node involve-ment and metastatic disease in canine mam-mary gland cancer.

Pharmacology/Actions
Desmopressin is related structurally to arginine vasopressin, but it has more antidiuretic activity and less vasopressor properties on a per weight basis. Desmopressin increases water reabsorp-tion by the collecting ducts in the kidneys, there-by increasing urine osmolality and decreasing net urine production. Therapeutic doses do not

directly affect either urinary sodium or potassium excretion.

Desmopressin causes a dose-dependent increase in plasma factor VIII and plasminogen factor and also causes smaller increases in factor VIII-related antigen and ristocetin cofactor activities.

Pharmacokinetics

Because desmopressin is destroyed in the GI tract, it usually is given parenterally or topically. Oral tablets have been used in those dogs that cannot tolerate ophthalmic administration, but bioavailability is very low. In humans, intranasal administration is commonly used, while in veterinary medicine topical administration to the conjunctiva is preferred. The onset of antidiuretic action in dogs usually occurs within one hour of administration, peaks in 2–8 hours, and may persist for up to 24 hours. Distribution characteristics of desmopressin are not well described, but it does enter maternal milk. The metabolic fate is also not well understood. Terminal half lives in humans after IV administration are from 0.4–4 hours.

Contraindications/Precautions/Warnings

Desmopressin is contraindicated in patients hypersensitive to it. It should not be used for treatment of type IIB or platelet-type (pseudo) Von Willebrand's disease as platelet-aggregation and thrombocytopenia may occur. German shorthair pointers apparently can have this type of vWD. Desmopressin should be used with caution in patients susceptible to thrombotic events.

When desmopressin is used to stimulate von Willebrand factor, with repeated administration tachyphylaxis (increasing lack of efficacy) will occur to a variable extent within 24 hours.

Adverse Effects

Side effects in small animals apparently are uncommon. Occasionally eye irritation may occur after conjunctival administration. Hypersensitivity reactions are possible. Humans using the drug have complained about increased headache frequency.

Reproductive/Nursing Safety

Safe use during pregnancy has not been established; however safe doses of up to 125 times the average human antidiuretic dose have been given to rats and rabbits without demonstration of fetal harm. In humans, the FDA categorizes this drug as category *B* for use during pregnancy (*Animal studies have not yet demonstrated risk to the fetus, but there are no adequate studies in pregnant women; or animal studies have shown an adverse effect, but adequate studies in pregnant women have not demonstrated a risk to the fetus in the first trimester of pregnancy, and there is no evidence of risk in later trimesters.*)

Desmopressin is likely safe to use during nursing.

Overdosage/Acute Toxicity

Oral doses of 0.2 mg/kg/day have been administered to dogs for 6 months without any significant drug-related toxicities reported. Dosages that are too high may lead to fluid retention and hyponatremia; dosage reduction and fluid restriction may be employed to treat. Adequate monitoring should be performed.

Drug Interactions

The following drug interactions have either been reported or are theoretical in humans or animals receiving desmopressin and may be of significance in veterinary patients:

■ **CHLORPROPAMIDE,   FLUORDROCORTISONE, UREA:** May enhance the antidiuretic effects of desmopressin

Laboratory Considerations

■ See Monitoring Parameters

Doses

Note: When doses listed below use "drops" of the nasal solution they are referencing the 0.1 mg/mL product and NOT the 1.5 mg/mL product (*Stimate®*). **Do not** confuse the two.

■ **DOGS:**

a) One drop placed twice daily in the conjunctival sac sufficiently controls polyuria in most dogs with central DI. Using one drop three times a day usually returns urine production to normal. (Rijnberk 2005)

b) For treatment of diabetes insipidus (central): 1–4 drops of the intranasal solution in the conjunctival sac once to twice daily; may use intranasal solution parenterally at 2–5 micrograms SC once to twice daily (Nichols 2000)

c) For treatment of complete and partial central diabetes insipidus: 1–4 drops of the intranasal solution in the conjunctival sac once a day to twice a day (Behrend 2003)

d) 1–2 drops into the conjunctival sac or 0.01–0.05 mL SC once a day to twice a day (Bruyette, D 2002)

e) As a trial in place of water deprivation test: one-half to one 0.1 or 0.2 mg DDAVP tablet PO q8h or 1–4 drops of nasal spray from an eye dropper into the conjunctival sac every 12 hours for 5–7 days. If central DI, owners should notice a decrease in PU/PD by the end of treatment period. Increase in urine specific gravity by 50% or more, compared with pre-treatment values, also support diagnosis of central DI. (Nelson 2002)

For treatment of Von Willebrand's disease:

a) For preoperative prophylaxis: 1 microgram/kg SC one-half hour before surgery. Close monitoring needed to determine extent and duration of response. Transfusion should be readily available. Desmopressin not effective for treatment or preoperative prophylaxis of severe Types 2 and 3 vWD. (Brooks 2003)

b) May be particularly useful to help prevent or control bleeding in association with surgery. Intranasal product is given subcutaneously at 1–4 micrograms/kg. Onset of activity occurs in 30 minutes and duration of effect is approximately 2 hours. (Carr & Panciera 2000)

■ **CATS:**

a) To help differentiate central diabetes insipidus from the nephrogenic form: 1 drop into the conjunctival sac twice daily for 2–3 days; a dramatic reduction in water intake or a 50% or greater increase in urine concentration gives strong evidence for a deficit in ADH production. For treatment of central DI: 1–2 drops into the conjunctival sac once or twice a day; duration of activity is 8–24 hours. (Bruyette, DS 1991)

b) For treatment of diabetes insipidus (central): 1– 4 drops of the intranasal solution in the conjunctival sac once to twice daily; may use intranasal solution parenterally at 2–5 micrograms SC once to twice daily (Nichols 2000)

c) For treatment of diabetes insipidus in cats whose owners find the intranasal or conjunctival application of desmopressin inconvenient: 25–50 micrograms (total dose; ¼th to ½ of a 100 microgram tablet) PO q12h. Dose and response may be variable. (Aroch *et al.* 2005)

■ **HORSES:**

For diagnosis of diabetes insipidus:

a) 20 micrograms IV (Barnes *et al.* 2002)

b) Dilute the nasal spray formulation (0.1 mg/ml) in sterile water and administer 0.05 micrograms/kg IV. Urine specific gravity (SG) should be measured every 2 hours. An increase in SG to 1.025 or greater within 2 to 7 hours is consistent with central DI. No change in urine SG is consistent with nephrogenic DI if medullary washout has been accounted for. (McKenzie 2009)

Monitoring

For Central DI:

■ Serum electrolytes

■ Urine osmolality and/or urine volume

■ For Von Willebrand's disease:

■ Bleeding times

Client Information

■ Keep solutions refrigerated whenever possible.

■ Instruct clients on the importance of compliance with administering this drug as di-

rected. It is a treatment, not a cure for the condition.

■ Clients should be counseled on the expense associated with using this drug long-term.

Chemistry/Synonyms

A synthetic polypeptide related to arginine vasopressin (antidiuretic hormone), desmopressin acetate occurs as a fluffy white powder with a bitter taste. The commercially available nasal solution has HCl added and the pH is approximately 4. This preparation also contains chlorobutanol 0.5% as a preservative.

Desmopressin Acetate may also be known as: 1-Deamino-8-D-Arginine Vasopressin, *DDAVP®*, *Concentraid®*, *D-Void®*, *Defirin®*, *Desmogalen®*, *Desmospray®*, *Desmotabs®*, *Emosint®*, *Minirin®*, *Minirin/DDAVP®*, *Minrin®*, *Minurin®*, *Nocutil®*, *Octim®*, *Octostim®*, *Presinex®*, or *Stimate®*.

Storage/Stability

The nasal solution should be refrigerated (2–8°C). It has an expiration date of one year after manufacture. While the nasal solution should be stored in the refrigerator, it is stable at room temperature for 3 weeks in the unopened bottle. The product for injection should be stored refrigerated (4°C); do not freeze.

Dosage Forms/Regulatory Status

VETERINARY-LABELED PRODUCTS: None

HUMAN-LABELED PRODUCTS:

Desmopressin Acetate Intranasal Spray Solution: 0.1 mg/mL (0.01%; 10 micrograms/spray) in 5 mL bottle or 2.5 mL rhinal tube delivery system; *DDAVP®* (Sanofi-Aventis); generic; (Rx)

Desmopressin Acetate Intranasal Spray Solution: 1.5 mg/mL (0.15%; 150 micrograms/spray) in 2.5 mL bottle; *Stimate®* (ZLB Behring); (Rx)

Desmopressin Acetate Injection Solution: 4 micrograms/mL in 1 mL single-dose amps & 10 mL multiple dose vials; *DDAVP®* (Sanofi-Aventis); generic; (Rx)

Desmopressin Acetate Oral Tablets: 0.1 mg & 0.2 mg; *DDAVP®* (Sanofi-Aventis); generic; (Rx)

References

Aroch, I., M. Mazaki–Tovi, et al. (2005). Central diabetes insipidus in five cats: clinical presentation, diagnosis and oral desmopressin therapy. *Journal of Feline Medicine and Surgery* 7(6): 333–339.

Barnes, D., H. Schott II, et al. (2002). Antidiuretic response to horses to DDAVP (desmopressin acetate). Proceedings ACVIM Forum. Accessed via: Veterinary Information Network. http://goo.gl/eTf6i

Behrend, E. (2003). Diabetes insipidus and other causes of polyuria/polydipsia. Proceedings: Western Veterinary Conference. Accessed via: Veterinary Information Network. http://goo.gl/pxzS4

Brooks, M. (2003). Transfusion therapy for hemostatic defects. Proceedings: ACVIM Forum. Accessed via: Veterinary Information Network. http://goo.gl/D1oX0

Bruyette, D. (1991). Polyuria and polydipsia. *Consultations in Feline Internal Medicine.* J August Ed. Philadelphia, W.B. Saunders Company: 227–235.

Bruyette, D. (2002). Diagnostic approach to polyuria and polydipsia. Proceedings: Atlantic Coast Veterinary Conference. Accessed via: Veterinary Information Network. http://goo.gl/fSN2L

Carr, A. & D. Panciera (2000). CVT Update: Diagnosis and Treatment of Immune–Mediated Hemolytic Anemia. *Kirk's Current Veterinary Therapy: XIII Small Animal Practice.* J Bonagura Ed. Philadelphia, WB Saunders: 434–438.

McKenzie, E. (2009). Polyuria/polydipsia in Horses. Proceedings: Western Veterinary Conference. Accessed via: Veterinary Information Network. http://goo.gl/fbeHt

Nelson, R. (2002). Polyuria, polydipsia, and diabetes insipidus. Proceedings: World Small Animal Veterinary Asssoc. World Congress. Accessed via: Veterinary Information Network. http://goo.gl/h6L1h

Nichols, R. (2000). Clinical use of DDAVP for the diagnosis and treatment of diabetes insipidus. *Kirk's Current Veterinary Therapy: XIII Small Animal Practice.* J Bonagura Ed. Philadelphia, WB Saunders: 325–326.

Rijnberk, A. (2005). Diabetes Insipidus. *Textbook of Veterinary Internal Medicine, 6th Ed.* S Ettinger and E Feldman Eds., Elsevier: 1503–1507.

DESOXYCORTICO-STERONE PIVALATE; DOCP

(de-sox-ee-kor-ti-*kost*-er-ohn *pih*-vah-late)
Percorten-V®

MINERALOCORTICOID

Prescriber Highlights

▶ Parenteral mineralocorticoid used to treat Addison's in dogs/cats

▶ Relative contraindications: congestive heart failure, severe renal disease, or edema; Caution: pregnancy

▶ Addison's patients must receive glucocorticoid supplementation in periods of high stress/illness

▶ May cause irritation at injection site

▶ Adjust dosage based upon monitoring parameters

Uses/Indications

DOCP is indicated for the parenteral treatment of adrenocortical insufficiency in dogs. It is also used in an extra-label manner in cats.

Pharmacology/Actions

Desoxycorticosterone pivalate (DOCP) is a long-acting mineralocorticoid agent. The site of action of mineralocorticoids is at the renal distal tubule where it increases the absorption of sodium. Mineralocorticoids also enhance potassium and hydrogen ion excretion. To be effective, mineralocorticoids require a functioning kidney.

Pharmacokinetics

Little information is available. It is injected IM (or subcutaneously) as a microcrystalline depot for slow dissolution into the circulation. DOCP usually has a duration of action in dogs for 21–30 days after injection.

Contraindications/Precautions/Warnings

The drug is contraindicated in dogs suffering from congestive heart failure, severe renal disease, or edema.

Because some animals may be more (or less) sensitive to the effects of the drug, "cookbook" dosing without ongoing monitoring is inappropriate. Some animals may require additional supplementation with a glucocorticoid agent on an ongoing basis that may cause polydipsia, polyuria, or polyphagia if doses are too high. All animals with hypoadrenocorticism should receive additional glucocorticoids (2–10 times basal) during periods of stress or acute illness.

Do not administer DOCP IV; acute collapse and shock may result. If given IV, treat immediately for shock with IV fluids and glucocorticoids.

Adverse Effects

Occasionally, irritation at the site of injection may occur. Adverse effects of DOCP are generally a result of excessive dosage (see Overdosage below).

Reproductive/Nursing Safety

The manufacturer states that the drug should not be used in pregnant dogs as safe use during pregnancy has not been established. Use in pregnant animals only when the potential benefits outweigh the risks.

DOCP should be safe for offspring when administered to nursing dams.

Overdosage/Acute Toxicity

Overdosage may cause polyuria, polydipsia, hypernatremia, hypertension, edema, and hypokalemia. Cardiac enlargement is possible with prolonged overdoses. Excessive weight gain may be indicative of fluid retention secondary to sodium retention. Electrolytes should be aggressively monitored and potassium may need to be supplemented. Discontinue the drug in patients until clinical signs associated with overdosage have resolved and then restart the drug at a lower dosage.

Drug Interactions

The following drug interactions have either been reported or are theoretical in humans or animals receiving DOCP and may be of significance in veterinary patients:

▪ **AMPHOTERICIN B:** Patients may develop hypokalemia if mineralocorticoids are administered concomitantly with amphotericin B

▪ **ASPIRIN:** DOCP may reduce salicylate levels

▪ **DIGOXIN:** Because DOCP may cause hypokalemia, it should be used with caution and increased monitoring when used in patients receiving digitalis glycosides

▪ **INSULIN:** Potentially, DOCP could increase the insulin requirements of diabetic patients

▪ **POTASSIUM-DEPLETING DIURETICS (e.g., fu-**

rosemide, thiazides): Patients may develop hypokalemia if mineralocorticoids are administered concomitantly with potassium-depleting diuretics; as diuretics can cause a loss of sodium, they may counteract the effects DOCP

Doses

■ **DOGS:**

Note: Dosage requirements are variable and should be individualized to the patient.

For hypoadrenocorticism:

a) 2.2 mg/kg IM every 25 days (Label information; *Percorten®-V*)

b) Initially, inject 2.2 mg/kg IM or SC every 25 days. Reevaluate at 12 and 25 days after initial injection. If hyponatremia and/or hyperkalemia are noted at 12 days, increase dose by 10%. If they are noted at 25 days (but not on day 12), shorten dosing interval by 2 days. (Reusch 2000)

c) 1.5–2.2 mg/kg IM q20–30 days (Lorenz & Melendez 2002)

d) Initially, 2.2 mg/kg IM q25 days. If electrolytes remain in normal range at 30 days, reduce dose by 10% a month. In our clinic, we have used a dose of DOCP as low as 1 mg/kg q30 days with good control of hypoadrenocorticism. (Scott-Moncrieff 2006)

■ **CATS:**

For maintenance therapy of hypoadrenocorticism:

a) 2.2 mg/kg IM every 25 days plus prednisolone (0.25–1 mg/cat PO twice daily; if daily oral dosing not feasible, may give 10 mg of methylprednisolone acetate once a month IM) (Reusch 2000)

b) 10–12.5 mg (total dose) IM per month. Adjust dose based-upon follow-up serum electrolyte concentrations monitored every 1–2 weeks during initial maintenance period. Normal electrolyte values 2 weeks following injection, suggests adequate dosing, but does not provide information regarding duration of action. Prednisone at 1.25 mg PO once a day or IM methylprednisolone acetate 10 mg once a month can provide long-term glucocorticoid supplementation. (Bruyette 2002)

Monitoring

■ Serum electrolytes, BUN, creatinine; initially every 1–2 weeks, then once stabilized, every 3–4 months

■ Weight, PE for edema

Client Information

■ Clients should be familiar with the symptoms associated with both hypoadrenocorticism (*e.g.*, weakness, depression, anorexia, vomiting, diarrhea, etc.) and DOCP overdosage (*e.g.*, edema) and report these to the veterinarian immediately.

■ If client is injecting the drug at home, instruct in proper technique for IM administration. Vial should be shaken vigorously to suspend the macrocrystals.

Chemistry/Synonyms

A mineralocorticoid, desoxycorticosterone pivalate (DOCP) occurs as a white or creamy white powder that is odorless and stable in air. It is practically insoluble in water, slightly soluble in alcohol and vegetable oils. The injectable product is a white aqueous suspension and has a pH between 5–8.5.

Desoxycorticosterone pivalate may also be known as: deoxycorticosterone pivalate, deoxycorticosterone trimethyl-acetate, deoxycortone pivalate, deoxycortone trimethylacetate, desoxycorticosterone pivalate, desoxycorticosterone trimethyl-acetate, *Cortiron®,* or *Percorten-V®.*

Storage/Stability

Store the injectable suspension at room temperature and protect from light or freezing. Do not mix with any other agent.

Dosage Forms/Regulatory Status

VETERINARY-LABELED PRODUCTS:

Desoxycorticosterone Pivalate Injectable Suspension: 25 mg/mL in 4 mL vials; *Percorten-V®* (Novartis); (Rx). FDA-approved for use in dogs.

The ARCI (Racing Commissioners International) has designated this drug as a class 4 substance. See the appendix for more information.

HUMAN-LABELED PRODUCTS: None

References

Bruyette, D. (2002). Feline adrenal disease. Proceedings: Atlantic Coast Veterinary Conference. Accessed via: Veterinary Information Network. http://goo.gl/1TBMB

Lorenz, M. & L. Melendez (2002). Hypoadrenocorticism. Proceedings: Western Veterinary Conference. Accessed via: Veterinary Information Network. http://goo.gl/6YGJd

Reusch, C. (2000). Hypoadrenocorticism. *Textbook of Veterinary Internal Medicine: Diseases of the Dog and Cat.* S Ettinger and E Feldman Eds. Philadelphia, WB Saunders. 2: 1488–1499.

Scott–Moncrieff, J. (2006). Canine hypoadrenocorticism: diagnosing and treating the difficult cases. Proceedings: ACVC. Accessed via: Veterinary Information Network. http://goo.gl/vLi0m

DETOMIDINE HCL

(de-*toe*-ma-deen)   Dormosedan®

Prescriber Highlights

▶ Alpha₂ sedative analgesic used primarily in horses

▶ Contraindications: Heart block, severe coronary, cerebrovascular, or respiratory disease, chronic renal failure

▶ Caution: Horses with endotoxic or traumatic shock or approaching shock, advanced hepatic or renal disease; stress due to temperature extremes, fatigue, or high altitude; patients treated for intestinal impactions; with suspected colic as it may mask abdominal pain or changes in respiratory & cardiac rates

▶ May respond (*i.e.*, kick) to external stimuli even after fully sedated; use caution, opioids may temper

▶ Adverse Effects: Initial blood pressure increase, then bradycardia/heart block, piloerection

Uses/Indications

At present, detomidine is only FDA-approved for use as a sedative analgesic in horses, but it has been used clinically in other species.

Pharmacology/Actions

Detomidine, like xylazine, is an alpha₂-adrenergic agonist that produces a dose-dependent sedative and analgesic effect, but it also has cardiac and respiratory effects. For more information, refer to the xylazine monograph or the adverse effects section below. Detomidine is approximately 50–100 times as potent as xylazine.

Pharmacokinetics

Detomidine is well absorbed after oral administration, but is used only parenterally currently. The drug is apparently rapidly distributed into tissues, including the brain after parenteral administration and is extensively metabolized and then excreted primarily into the urine. Peak sedative actions can range from 5–20 minutes post injection in horses.

Published mean or median pharmacokinetic values for detomidine in horses include: Volume of distribution: 0.47-0.59 L/kg (at rest), 1.3 L/kg (after exercise). Time to reach maximum blood level concentration: Approximately 2 minutes (IV), 77 minutes (IM). Clearance: 12-16 mL/min/kg. Elimination half-life: 24–26 minutes (IV, at rest), 46 minutes (IV, after exercise), 51 minutes (IM, at rest) (Hubbell, J.A.E. *et al.* 2009), (Mama *et al.* 2009). The oromucosal gel product (available in some countries) bioavailability is lower than IM (22% vs. 38%) (Kaukinen *et al.* 2009).

After exercise, the volume of distribution of detomidine is higher then at rest. Initial dose requirements may be higher and subsequent doses lower after exercise (Hubbell, J.A.E. *et al.* 2009).

Contraindications/Precautions/Warnings

Detomidine is contraindicated in horses with preexisting AV or SA heart block, severe coronary insufficiency, cerebrovascular disease, respiratory disease or chronic renal failure. Use cautiously in animals with endotoxic or traumatic shock or approaching shock, and advanced hepatic or renal disease. Horses who are stressed due to temperature extremes, fatigue, or high altitude should be given the drug carefully. Because this drug may inhibit gastrointestinal motility, use with prudence in patients treated for intestinal impactions. In horses with suspected colic, the use of detomidine analgesia should be used cautiously as it may mask abdominal pain and conceal changes in respiratory and cardiac rates, thereby making diagnosis more difficult.

Although animals may appear to be deeply sedated, some may respond (kick, etc.) to external stimuli; use appropriate caution. The addition of opioids (*e.g.*, butorphanol) may help temper this effect. The manufacturer recommends allowing the horse to stand quietly for 5 minutes prior to injection and for 10–15 minutes after injection to improve the effect of the drug. After administering detomidine, protect the animal from temperature extremes.

During times of ambient temperature extremes, especially summer heat, consider using dosages in the lower range to reduce chances for toxicity.

When using the gel, wear impermeable gloves during drug administration or doing procedures that require contact with the horse's mouth.

Adverse Effects

Detomidine can cause an initial rise in blood pressure that is then followed by bradycardia and heart block. Atropine at 0.02 mg/kg IV has been successfully used to prevent or correct the bradycardia that may be seen when the detomidine is used at labeled dosages. In addition, piloerection, sweating, ataxia, salivation, slight muscle tremors, and penile prolapse may all be noted after injection.

When compared to xylazine, detomidine causes more pronounced bradycardia and bradyarrhythmias. Because the sedative and muscle-relaxing effects of detomidine in horses can persist for up to 90 minutes, it may influence the quality of recovery and contribute to post-anesthesia ataxia.

Reproductive/Nursing Safety

The manufacturer states that "Information on the possible effects of detomidine HCl in breeding horses is limited to uncontrolled clinical reports; therefore, this drug is not recommended for use in breeding animals." No other information was located.

Overdosage/Acute Toxicity

The manufacturer states that detomidine is tolerated by horses at doses 5X (0.2 mg/kg) the high dose level (0.04 mg/kg). Doses of 0.4 mg/kg given daily for 3 consecutive days produced microscopic foci of myocardial necrosis in 1 of 8 horses tested. Doses of 10–40X recommended can cause severe respiratory and cardiovascular changes that can become irreversible and cause death. Yohimbine or atipamezole could be used to reverse some or all of the effects of the drug. Atipamezole, at a dose of 50–100 micrograms/kg has been successfully used to treat inadvertent overdoses of detomidine in horses.

Drug Interactions

The following drug interactions have either been reported or are theoretical in humans or animals receiving detomidine and may be of significance in veterinary patients:

■ **ALPHA-2 AGONISTS, OTHER (e.g., xylazine, medetomidine, romifidine, clonidine and including epinephrine):** Not recommended to be used together with detomidine as effects may be additive

■ **ANESTHETICS, OPIATES, SEDATIVE/HYPNOTICS:** Effects may be additive; dosage reduction of one or both agents may be required; potential for increased risk for arrhythmias when used in combination with thiopental, ketamine or halothane

■ **EPINEPHRINE:** As epinephrine possesses alpha agonist effects, do not use to treat cardiac effects caused by detomidine

■ **PHENOTHIAZINES (e.g., acepromazine):** Severe hypotension can result

■ **SEDATIVES OR ANALGESICS, OTHER:** The manufacturer warns to use with extreme caution in combination with other sedative or analgesic drugs

■ **SULFONAMIDES, POTENTIATED (e.g., trimethoprim/sulfa):** The manufacturer warns against using this agent with intravenous potentiated sulfonamides (e.g., trimethoprim/sulfa) as fatal dysrhythmias may occur

Doses

■ **HORSES: (Note:** ARCI UCGFS Class 3 Drug) For sedation/analgesia (**CAUTION:** Do not confuse micrograms/kg with mg/kg doses):

a) Injection: 20–40 micrograms/kg (0.02–0.04 mg/kg) IV or IM (IV only for analgesia). Effects generally occur within 2–5 minutes. Lower dose will generally provide 30–90 minutes of sedation and 30–45 minutes of analgesia. The higher dose will generally provide 90–120 minutes of sedation and 45–75 minutes of analgesia. Allow animal to rest quietly prior to and after injection.

Sublingual Gel: 0.04 mg/kg (0.018 mg/lb)

(0.040 mg/kg) placed beneath the tongue of the horse; not meant to be swallowed. The dosing syringe delivers the product in 0.25 mL increments. The package insert provides a dosing table to determine correct amount of gel to administer for the weight of the horse. (Package inserts; *Dormosedan®*; *Dormosedan Gel®*—Pfizer)

b) For horses with marked abdominal pain that are either not candidates for exploratory surgery or must be transported long distances for surgery: 0.01–0.02 mg/kg (10–20 micrograms/kg) IV or IM (Moore 1999)

c) Detomidine at 0.01–0.02 mg/kg IV or IM with or without butorphanol (0.02–0.03 mg/kg) (Taylor 1999)

d) For adjunctive treatment of moderate pain: 0.03–0.04 mg/kg IV;

For caudal epidural analgesia: 0.06 mg/kg, given between S4–S5; duration of analgesia is 2–3 hours *or* detomidine 0.03 mg/kg with morphine (0.2 mg mg/kg) given between S1–L6; duration of analgesia is >6 hours (Muir 2004)

e) For oral administration when horse is not amenable to injections: 0.06 mg/kg PO; profound sedation occurs in about 45 minutes (Hubbell, J. 2006)

f) As a CRI for standing chemical restraint and analgesia: Two protocols have been described:

1) Loading dose of 7.5 micrograms/kg IV bolus, followed by a CRI rate of 0.6 micrograms/kg/minute for the first 15 minutes; after this CRI rate is halved every 15 minutes. In many cases did not provide adequate analgesia alone and needed to be supplemented by local anesthetics, epidural analgesia, or supplemental detomidine and/or butorphanol. Average duration of procedures was 40 minutes.

2) Loading dose of 8.4 micrograms/kg IV bolus, then 0.5 micrograms/kg/minute for 15 minutes, then 0.3 micrograms/kg/minute for 15 minutes, then 0.15 micrograms/kg/minute thereafter. A butorphanol CRI was used if additional sedation and analgesia was required. (Mogg 2006)

■ **CATTLE:**

a) For sedation/analgesia: 30–60 micrograms/kg (0.03–0.06 mg/kg) IV or IM (Not FDA-approved) (Alitalo 1986)

b) For analgesia: 0.01 mg/kg IV; short (½ hour) duration of action. Appropriate withdrawal times are: Milk = 72 hours; Slaughter = 7 days. (Walz 2006)

- **SHEEP, GOATS:**
  a) For anesthesia: Detomidine at 0.01 mg/kg IM, followed by propofol at 3–5 mg/kg IV.

  For analgesia: 0.005–0.05 mg/kg IV or IM q3–6 hours (once) (Haskell 2005)

- **LLAMAS, ALPACAS:**
  a) For analgesia: 0.005–0.05 mg/kg IV or IM q3–6 hours (once) (Haskell 2005)

- **BIRDS:**
  a) For sedation/analgesia: 0.3 mg/kg IM; limited data available on duration of effect, adverse effects, etc. (Clyde & Paul-Murphy 2000)

Monitoring

- Level of sedation, analgesia
- Cardiac rate/rhythm; blood pressure if indicated

Client Information

- This drug should be used in a professionally supervised setting by individuals familiar with its properties.

Chemistry/Synonyms

An imidazoline derivative alpha$_2$-adrenergic agonist, detomidine HCl occurs as a white crystalline substance that is soluble in water.

Detomidine HCl may also be known as: demotidini hydrochloridum, MPV-253-AII, or *Dormosedan®*.

Storage/Stability

Detomidine HCl for injection should be stored at room temperature (59-85°F; 15–30°C) and protected from light.

Detomidine Gel for SL Administration should be stored at controlled room temperature (68-77°F; 20-25°C); excursions are permitted to 59-85°F (15–30°C).

Dosage Forms/Regulatory Status

VETERINARY-LABELED PRODUCTS:

Detomidine HCl for Injection: 10 mg/mL in 5 mL and 20 mL vials; *Dormosedan®* (Pfizer); (Rx). FDA-approved for use in mature horses and yearlings.

Detomidine HCL Oromucosal Gel for Sublingual Administration: 7.8 mg/mL in 3 mL graduated dosing syringes; *Dormosedan Gel®* (Pfizer); (Rx). FDA-approved for use in horses not intended for human consumption.

The ARCI (Racing Commissioners International) has designated this drug as a class 3 substance. See the appendix for more information.

HUMAN-LABELED PRODUCTS: None

References

Alitalo, I. (1986). Clinical Experiences with Domesedan® in Horses and Cattle: A Review. *Acta Vet Scand* 82: 193–196.

Clyde, V. & J. Paul–Murphy (2000). Avian Analgesia. *Kirk's Current Veterinary Therapy: XIII Small Animal Practice.* J Bonagura Ed. Philadelphia, WB Saunders: 1126–1128.

Haskell, R. (2005). Development of a Small Ruminant Formulary. Proceedings: WVC. Accessed via: Veterinary Information Network. http://goo.gl/3tIK9

Hubbell, J. (2006). Chemical Restraint of Standing Procedures in the Horse. Proceedings: NAVC.

Hubbell, J.A.E., R.A. Sams, et al. (2009). Pharmacokinetics of detomidine administered to horses at rest and after maximal exercise. *Equine Veterinary Journal* 41(5): 419–422.

Kaukinen, H., J. Aspegrén, et al. (2009). Bioavailability of Detomidine Administered to Horses as an Oromucosal (Sublingual) Gel and Comparison of Absorption of Detomidine by the Sublingual and Intramuscular Routes. Proceedings: ACVIM. Accessed via: Veterinary Information Network. http://goo.gl/dPZhP

Mama, K.R., K. Grimsrud, et al. (2009). Plasma concentrations, behavioural and physiological effects following intravenous and intramuscular detomidine in horses. *Equine Veterinary Journal* 41(8): 772–777.

Mogg, T. (2006). Pain management in horses. Proceedings: ACVIM. Accessed via: Veterinary Information Network. http://goo.gl/6YLPg

Moore, R. (1999). Medical treatment of abdominal pain in the horse: Analgesics and IV fluids. Proceedings: The North American Veterinary Conference, Orlando.

Muir, W. (2004). Recognizing and treating pain in horses. *Equine Internal Medicine, 2nd Ed.* S Reed, W Bayly and D Sellon Eds. Philadelphia, Saunders: 1529–1542.

Taylor, P. (1999). Tranquilizers in the horse – Choosing the right one. Proceedings: The North American Veterinary Conference, Orlando.

Walz, P. (2006). Practical management of pain in cattle. Proceedings: ABVP. Accessed via: Veterinary Information Network. http://goo.gl/hScVv

DEXAMETHASONE DEXAMETHASONE SODIUM PHOSPHATE

(dex-a-*meth*-a-zone)   Azium®, Dexasone®

GLUCOCORTICOID

Prescriber Highlights

- Injectable, oral & ophthalmic glucocorticoid
- Long acting; 30X more potent than hydrocortisone; no mineralocorticoid activity
- If using for therapy, goal is to use as much as is required & as little as possible for as short an amount of time as possible
- Primary adverse effects are "Cushingoid" in nature with sustained use, but acute effects (primarily GI, colon perforation in dogs after high doses) can be seen
- Many potential drug & lab interactions

Uses/Indications

Glucocorticoids have been used in an attempt to treat practically every malady that afflicts man or animal, but there are three broad uses and dosage ranges for use of these agents. 1) Replacement of glucocorticoid activity in patients with adrenal insufficiency, 2) as an antiinflammatory agent, and 3) as an immunosuppressive. Among some of the uses for glucocorticoids include treatment of: endocrine conditions (*e.g.*, adrenal insufficiency), rheumatic diseases (*e.g.*, rheumatoid arthritis), collagen diseases (*e.g.*, systemic lupus), allergic states, respiratory diseases (*e.g.*, asthma), dermatologic diseases (*e.g.*, pemphigus, allergic dermatoses), hematologic disorders (*e.g.*, thrombocytopenias, autoimmune hemolytic anemias), neoplasias, nervous system disorders (increased CSF pressure), GI diseases (*e.g.*, ulcerative colitis exacerbations), and renal diseases (*e.g.*, nephrotic syndrome). Some glucocorticoids are used topically in the eye and skin for various conditions or are injected intra-articularly or intra-lesionally. The above listing is certainly not complete. High dose fast-acting corticosteroids use for shock or CNS trauma is controversial; recent studies have not demonstrated significant benefit and it actually may cause increased deleterious effects.

Pharmacology/Actions

Glucocorticoids have effects on virtually every cell type and system in mammals. An overview of the effects of these agents follows:

Cardiovascular System: Glucocorticoids can reduce capillary permeability and enhance vasoconstriction. A relatively clinically insignificant positive inotropic effect can occur after glucocorticoid administration. Increased blood pressure can result from both the drugs' vasoconstrictive properties and increased blood volume that may be produced.

Cells: Glucocorticoids inhibit fibroblast proliferation, macrophage response to migration inhibiting factor, sensitization of lymphocytes and the cellular response to mediators of inflammation. Glucocorticoids stabilize lysosomal membranes.

CNS/Autonomic Nervous System: Glucocorticoids can lower seizure threshold, alter mood and behavior, diminish the response to pyrogens, stimulate appetite and maintain alpha rhythm. Glucocorticoids are necessary for normal adrenergic receptor sensitivity.

Endocrine System: When animals are not stressed, glucocorticoids will suppress the release of ACTH from the anterior pituitary, thereby reducing or preventing the release of endogenous corticosteroids. Stress factors (*e.g.*, renal disease, liver disease, diabetes) may sometimes nullify the suppressing aspects of exogenously administered steroids. Release of thyroid-stimulating hormone (TSH), follicle-stimulating hormone (FSH), prolactin, and luteinizing hormone (LH) may all be reduced when glucocorticoids are administered at pharmacological doses. Conversion of thyroxine (T_4) to triiodothyronine (T_3) may be reduced by glucocorticoids; plasma levels of parathyroid hormone increased. Glucocorticoids may inhibit osteoblast function. Vasopressin (ADH) activity is reduced at the renal tubules and diuresis may occur. Glucocorticoids inhibit insulin binding to insulin-receptors and the post-receptor effects of insulin.

Hematopoietic System: Glucocorticoids can increase the numbers of circulating platelets, neutrophils and red blood cells, but platelet aggregation is inhibited. Decreased amounts of lymphocytes (peripheral), monocytes and eosinophils are seen as glucocorticoids can sequester these cells into the lungs and spleen and prompt decreased release from the bone marrow. Removal of old red blood cells becomes diminished. Glucocorticoids can cause involution of lymphoid tissue.

GI Tract and Hepatic System: Glucocorticoids increase the secretion of gastric acid, pepsin, and trypsin. They alter the structure of mucin and decrease mucosal cell proliferation. Iron salts and calcium absorption are decreased while fat absorption is increased. Hepatic changes can include increased fat and glycogen deposits within hepatocytes, increased serum levels of alanine aminotransferase (ALT), and gamma-glutamyl transpeptidase (GGT). Significant increases can be seen in serum alkaline phosphatase levels. Glucocorticoids can cause minor increases in BSP (bromosulfophthalein) retention time.

Immune System (also see Cells and Hematopoietic System): Glucocorticoids can decrease circulating levels of T-lymphocytes; inhibit lymphokines; inhibit neutrophil, macrophage, and monocyte migration; reduce production of interferon; inhibit phagocytosis and chemotaxis; antigen processing; and diminish intracellular killing. Specific acquired immunity is affected less than nonspecific immune responses. Glucocorticoids can also antagonize the complement cascade and mask the clinical signs of infection. Mast cells are decreased in number and histamine synthesis is suppressed. Many of these effects only occur at high or very high doses and there are species differences in response.

Metabolic effects: Glucocorticoids stimulate gluconeogenesis. Lipogenesis is enhanced in certain areas of the body (*e.g.*, abdomen) and adipose tissue can be redistributed away from the extremities to the trunk. Fatty acids are mobilized from tissues and their oxidation is increased. Plasma levels of triglycerides, cholesterol, and glycerol are increased. Protein is mobilized from most areas of the body (not the liver).

Musculoskeletal: Glucocorticoids may cause muscular weakness (also caused if there is a lack of glucocorticoids), atrophy, and osteoporosis. Bone growth can be inhibited via growth hormone and somatomedin inhibition, increased calcium excretion and inhibition of vitamin D activation. Resorption of bone can be enhanced. Fibrocartilage growth is also inhibited.

Ophthalmic: Prolonged corticosteroid use

(both systemic or topically to the eye) can cause increased intraocular pressure and glaucoma, cataracts, and exophthalmos.

Renal, Fluid, & Electrolytes: Glucocorticoids can increase potassium and calcium excretion, sodium and chloride reabsorption, and extracellular fluid volume. Hypokalemia and/or hypocalcemia rarely occur. Diuresis may develop following glucocorticoid administration.

Skin: Thinning of dermal tissue and skin atrophy can be seen with glucocorticoid therapy. Hair follicles can become distended and alopecia may occur.

Pharmacokinetics

Pharmacokinetics of dexamethasone do not translate into pharmacologic effect. The half-life of dexamethasone in dogs is about 2–5 hours, but biologic activity can persist for 48 hours or more.

Contraindications/Precautions/Warnings

Because dexamethasone has negligible mineralocorticoid effect, it should generally not be used alone in the treatment of adrenal insufficiency.

Do not administer the propylene glycol base injectable product rapidly intravenously; hypotension, collapse, and hemolytic anemia can occur. Many clinicians only use dexamethasone sodium phosphate when giving the drug intravenously.

In dogs, dexamethasone can cause more gastrointestinal complications and bleeding than does prednisone, so careful attention to the minimum dosing necessary is required. There is a high incidence of gastrointestinal bleeding and colonic perforation in canine neurosurgical patients treated with dexamethasone (also seen with methylprednisolone sodium succinate); the dose and duration of therapy should be limited to as short a time as possible, and prednisone or prednisolone used when possible instead of dexamethasone (Wilson 2011).

Systemic use of glucocorticoids is generally considered contraindicated in systemic fungal infections (unless used for replacement therapy in Addison's), when administered IM in patients with idiopathic thrombocytopenia and in patients hypersensitive to a particular compound. Use of sustained-release injectable glucocorticoids is considered contraindicated for chronic corticosteroid therapy of systemic diseases.

Animals that have received glucocorticoids systemically other than with "burst" therapy, should be tapered off the drugs. Patients who have received the drugs chronically should be tapered off slowly as endogenous ACTH and corticosteroid function may return slowly. Should the animal undergo a "stressor" (e.g., surgery, trauma, illness, etc.) during the tapering process or until normal adrenal and pituitary function resume, additional glucocorticoids should be administered.

Animals, particularly cats, at risk for diabetes mellitus or with concurrent cardiovascular disease should receive glucocorticoids with caution due to these agents' potent hyperglycemic effect.

Adverse Effects

Adverse effects are generally associated with long-term administration of these drugs, especially if given at high dosages or not on an alternate day regimen. Effects generally are manifested as clinical signs of hyperadrenocorticism. Glucocorticoids can retard growth in young animals. Many of the potential effects, adverse and otherwise, are outlined above in the Pharmacology section.

In dogs, polydipsia (PD), polyphagia (PP) and polyuria (PU), may all be seen with short-term "burst" therapy as well as with alternate-day maintenance therapy on days when giving the drug. Very high doses in dogs with spinal chord injuries have caused fatal colon perforations. Other adverse effects in dogs can include: dull, dry haircoat, weight gain, panting, vomiting, diarrhea, elevated liver enzymes, pancreatitis, GI ulceration, lipidemias, activation or worsening of diabetes mellitus, muscle wasting, and behavioral changes (depression, lethargy, viciousness). Discontinuation of the drug may be necessary; changing to an alternate steroid may also alleviate the problem. With the exception of PU/PD/PP, adverse effects associated with antiinflammatory therapy are relatively uncommon. Adverse effects associated with immunosuppressive doses are more common and, potentially, more severe.

Cats generally require higher dosages than dogs for clinical effect, but tend to develop fewer adverse effects. Glucocorticoids appear to have a greater hyperglycemic effect in cats than other species. Occasionally, polydipsia, polyuria, polyphagia with weight gain, diarrhea, or depression can be seen. Long-term, high dose therapy can lead to "Cushingoid" effects, however.

Administration of dexamethasone or triamcinolone may play a role in the development of laminitis in horses.

Reproductive/Nursing Safety

Corticosteroid therapy may induce parturition in large animal species during the latter stages of pregnancy. In humans, the FDA categorizes this drug as category *C* for use during pregnancy (*Animal studies have shown an adverse effect on the fetus, but there are no adequate studies in humans; or there are no animal reproduction studies and no adequate studies in humans.*) In a separate system evaluating the safety of drugs in canine and feline pregnancy (Papich 1989), this drug is categorized as in class: *C* (*These drugs may have potential risks. Studies in people or laboratory animals have uncovered risks, and these drugs should be used cautiously as a last resort when the benefit of therapy clearly outweighs the risks.*)

Overdosage/Acute Toxicity

Glucocorticoids when given short-term are unlikely to cause significant harmful effects, even in massive dosages. One incidence of a dog developing acute CNS effects after accidental ingestion of glucocorticoids has been reported. Should clinical signs occur, use supportive treatment if required.

Chronic usage of glucocorticoids can lead to serious adverse effects. Refer to Adverse Effects above for more information.

Drug Interactions

The following drug interactions have either been reported or are theoretical in humans or animals receiving dexamethasone and may be of significance in veterinary patients:

■ **AMPHOTERICIN B:** Administered concomitantly with glucocorticoids may cause hypokalemia

■ **ANTICHOLINESTERASE AGENTS (e.g., pyridostigmine, neostigmine, etc.):** In patients with myasthenia gravis, concomitant glucocorticoid and anticholinesterase agent administration may lead to profound muscle weakness. If possible, discontinue anticholinesterase medication at least 24 hours prior to corticosteroid administration

■ **ASPIRIN:** Glucocorticoids may reduce salicylate blood levels

■ **BARBITURATES:** May increase the metabolism of glucocorticoids and decrease dexamethasone blood levels

■ **CYCLOPHOSPHAMIDE:** Glucocorticoids may also inhibit the hepatic metabolism of cyclophosphamide; dosage adjustments may be required

■ **CYCLOSPORINE:** Concomitant administration of glucocorticoids and cyclosporine may increase the blood levels of each, by mutually inhibiting the hepatic metabolism of each other; the clinical significance of this interaction is not clear

■ **DIAZEPAM:** Dexamethasone may decrease diazepam levels

■ **DIURETICS, POTASSIUM-DEPLETING (e.g., spironolactone, triamterene):** Administered concomitantly with glucocorticoids may cause hypokalemia

■ **EPHEDRINE:** May reduce dexamethasone blood levels and interfere with dexamethasone suppression tests

■ **INDOMETHACIN:** Can cause false negative test results in the dexamethasone suppression test

■ **INSULIN:** Insulin requirements may increase in patients receiving glucocorticoids

■ **KETOCONAZOLE AND OTHER AZOLE ANTIFUNGALS:** May decrease the metabolism of glucocorticoids and increase dexamethasone blood levels; ketoconazole may induce adrenal insufficiency when glucocorticoids are withdrawn by inhibiting adrenal corticosteroid synthesis

■ **MACROLIDE ANTIBIOTICS (erythromycin, clarithromycin):** May decrease the metabolism of glucocorticoids and increase dexamethasone blood levels

■ **MITOTANE:** May alter the metabolism of steroids; higher than usual doses of steroids may be necessary to treat mitotane-induced adrenal insufficiency

■ **NSAIDS:** Administration of ulcerogenic drugs with glucocorticoids may increase the risk of gastrointestinal ulceration

■ **PHENYTOIN:** May increase the metabolism of glucocorticoids and decrease dexamethasone blood levels

■ **RIFAMPIN:** May increase the metabolism of glucocorticoids and decrease dexamethasone blood levels

■ **DEXAMETHASONE:** In dogs, dexamethasone increased quinidine volume of distribution (49-78%) and elimination half-life (1.5-2.3X). (Zhang *et al.* 2006)

■ **VACCINES:** Patients receiving corticosteroids at immunosuppressive dosages should generally not receive live attenuated-virus vaccines as virus replication may be augmented; a diminished immune response may occur after vaccine, toxoid, or bacterin administration in patients receiving glucocorticoids

Laboratory Considerations

■ While dexamethasone does not interfere with the cortisol assay, over a few days it will suppress the HPA axis and suppress endogenous release of cortisol, so if using it to diagnose hypoadrenocorticism, **ACTH stimulation tests** should be performed as soon as possible.

■ Glucocorticoids may increase **serum cholesterol**

■ Glucocorticoids may increase **urine glucose** levels

■ Glucocorticoids may decrease **serum potassium**

■ Glucocorticoids can suppress the release of thyroid stimulating hormone (TSH) and reduce **T3 & T4** values. Thyroid gland atrophy has been reported after chronic glucocorticoid administration. Uptake of I^{131} by the thyroid may be decreased by glucocorticoids.

■ Reactions to **skin tests** may be suppressed by glucocorticoids

■ False-negative results of the **nitroblue tetrazolium** test for systemic bacterial infections may be induced by glucocorticoids

■ Glucocorticoids may cause **neutrophilia** within 4-8 hours after dosing and return to baseline within 24-48 hours after drug discontinuation

■ Glucocorticoids can cause **lymphopenia** in dogs which can persist for weeks after drug discontinuation

Doses

■ **DOGS:**

For labeled indications (antiinflammatory; glucocorticoid agent):

a) Injection: 0.5−1 mg IV or IM; may be repeated for 3−5 days; Tablets: 0.25−1.25 mg PO daily in single or two divided doses (Package Insert; *Azium*®— Schering)

As an antiinflammatory agent or immunosuppressive:

a) Generally, most veterinarians use prednisone or prednisolone when a glucocorticoid is administered orally to dogs. Despite a short circulating half-life, dexamethasone has a long biologic duration of effect (thought to be >48 hours, whereas the biologic duration of effect of prednisone is 12−36 hours). Thus, it is difficult to spare normal adrenal function, even when dexamethasone is given every other day. (Wilson 2011)

Replacement of glucocorticoid activity in patients with adrenal insufficiency (Note: Dexamethasone has no mineralocorticoid activity):

a) For Addisonian crises: give 0.1−0.2 mg/kg dexamethasone sodium phosphate IV as the initial dose. Dexamethasone is not measured on the cortisol assay, so the ACTH stimulation test will be valid after dexamethasone is used. If the dog is vomiting/inappetent, dexamethasone may be continued at a dose of 0.05−0.1 mg/kg q12h until able to switch to oral prednisone as the glucocorticoid replacement (see Prednisone monograph for more information) (Wilson 2011).

b) For Addisonian crisis: Dexamethasone sodium phosphate at 0.2−0.5 mg/kg IV once; maintenance therapy with prednisone. Dexamethasone, unlike prednisone will not interfere with cortisol assays. (Jutkowitz 2009)

c) For adjunctive acute treatment (including correction of hypotension/hypovolemia, electrolyte imbalances, acidosis, hypoglycemia, and hypercalcemia: Immediately place IV catheter in cephalic or jugular vein, and collect a blood sample for measurement of electrolytes and cortisol. Cosyntropin (synthetic ACTH) is then administered IV, and a second blood sample for measurement of cortisol collected 1 hour later. Fluid therapy (0.9% saline IV, 30−80 mL/kg/24 hours plus correction for dehydration) should be started immediately. After the second blood sample is collected, give prednisolone sodium succinate (4−20 mg/kg IV), or hydrocortisone hemisuccinate or hydrocortisone phosphate (2−4 mg/kg IV) or dexamethasone sodium phosphate at 0.5−2 mg/kg as an initial dose. Then add dexamethasone at a dose of 0.05−0.1 mg/kg q12 hours into fluids until able to switch to oral glucocorticoids. If animal is in shock, administration of steroids should be at shock doses and this should take precedence over establishing an immediate diagnosis. For dogs with hyperkalemia consider IV glucose and insulin to rapidly lower serum potassium, and calcium gluconate to protect the heart from the cardiosuppressive effects of hyperkalemia. (Scott-Moncrieff 2010)

For use a diagnostic agent:

Low-Dose Dexamethasone Suppression (LDDS) Test:

a) Obtain plasma samples for cortisol before and 4 and 8 hours after IV administration of 0.01 mg/kg dexamethasone. The 8-hour plasma cortisol is used as a screening test for hyperadrenocorticism, with concentrations >1.4 micrograms/dL being consistent with (not confirming) the diagnosis of Cushing's syndrome. Test is relatively sensitive and specific, but not perfect. Approximately 90% of dogs with Cushing's syndrome have an 8 hour post-dexamethasone plasma cortisol concentration >1.4 micrograms/dL and another 6 to 8% have values of 0.9-1.3 micrograms/dL. The results of a low dose test can also aid in discriminating pituitary-dependent hyperadrenocorticism (PDH) from adrenocortical tumor (ACT), using 3 criteria: **1)** an 8 hour plasma cortisol >1.4 micrograms/dL but <50% of the basal value; **2)** a 4 hour plasma cortisol concentration <1.0 micrograms/dl; and **3)** a 4 hour plasma cortisol concentration <50% of the basal value. If a dog has Cushing's and it meets any of these 3 criteria, it most likely has PDH. Approximately 65% of dogs with naturally occurring PDH demonstrate suppression, as defined by these 3 criteria. A dog with Cushing's that fails to meet any of these 3 criteria could have either PDH or ACT. However, if two relatively equal sized adrenals on abdominal ultrasonography, it most likely has PDH. (Feldman 2009)

High-Dose Dexamethasone Suppression (HDDS) Test:

a) Relatively easy to perform (plasma obtained before and 4 or 8 hours after IV administration of 0.1 mg/kg dexamethasone), readily available and inexpensive. If a dog has Cushing's syndrome and the plasma cortisol, 8 hours post-dexamethasone, is <50% of the basal value, the dog has pituitary-dependent hyperadrenocorticism (PDH). However, our experience with the LDDS and abdominal ultrasonography has limited the need and use of HDDS. Approximately 75% of dogs with PDH demonstrate suppression with the HDDS. Realizing that approximately 65% of PDH dogs demonstrate "suppression" consistent with PDH on the LDDS limits the value of this test by only identifying an additional 10% of afflicted dogs. (Feldman 2009)

■ **CATS:**

For labeled indications (antiinflammatory; glucocorticoid agent): Injection: 0.125–0.5 mg IV or IM; may be repeated for 3–5 days; Tablets: 0.125–0.5 mg daily in single or divided doses (Package Insert; *Azium®*— Schering)

As an antiinflammatory agent or immunosuppressive:

Generally, most veterinarians use prednisolone when a glucocorticoid is administered orally to cats. If using dexamethasone, figure the dose for prednisolone and administer 10-20% of that dose as dexamethasone. Approximately 0.75 mg of dexamethasone is equivalent to 5 mg prednisone.

Low-Dose Dexamethasone Suppression (LDDS) Test:

a) Test of choice for diagnosis of feline hyperadrenocorticism; uses a higher dose of dexamethasone (0.1 mg/kg IV) than in dogs. A base-line blood sample is collected, and additional samples are collected at 4 and 8 hours after dexamethasone administration. Cortisol concentration will be suppressed (<1.5 micrograms/dL) at 8 hours in normal cats but not in cats with hyperadrenocorticism. A few cats with HAC will suppress normally on the LDDS. If the index of suspicion for hyperadrenocorticism is high, a second test using the lower dose of dexamethasone (0.01 mg/kg) can be performed, but some normal cats will fail to suppress at this dose. (Scott-Moncrieff 2010)

■ **RABBITS/RODENTS/SMALL MAMMALS:**

a) **Mice, Rats, Gerbils, Hamsters, Guinea pigs, Chinchillas:** 0.6 mg/kg IM (as an antiinflammatory) (Adamcak & Otten 2000)

■ **CATTLE:**

For adjunctive therapy of insect bites or stings:

a) 2 mg/kg IM or IV q4h (use epinephrine if anaphylaxis develops) (Fowler 1993)

For primary bovine ketosis:

a) 5–20 mg IV or IM (Package Insert; *Azium®*— Schering)

■ **HORSES: (Note:** ARCI UCGFS Class 4 Drug)

For labeled indications (antiinflammatory; glucocorticoid agent):

a) Dexamethasone Injection: 2.5–5 mg IV or IM (Package Insert; *Azium®*— Schering)

Dexamethasone sodium phosphate injection: 2.5–5 mg IV (Package Insert; *Azium® SP*— Schering)

For recurrent airway obstruction (heaves):

a) For a 500 kg horse give 40 mg IM once every other day for 3 treatments, followed by 35 mg IM once every other day for 3 treatments, followed by 30 mg IM once every other day for 3 treatments, etc., until horse is weaned off dexamethasone. Corticosteroid use may be contraindicated in horses predisposed to laminitis or exhibiting endocrinopathies. (Ainsworth & Hackett 2004)

b) For short term treatment with environmental control: In the study, dexamethasone sodium phosphate was dosed at 0.1 mg/kg IM once daily for 4 days, 0.075 mg/kg IM once daily for 4 days, and 0.05 mg/kg IM for 4 days. Except for bronchoalveolar lavage cytology, oral prednisolone (1 mg/kg PO X 4d, 0.75 mg/kg PO x 4d, 0.5 mg/kg PO x 4d) was as effective as IM dexamethasone. (Courouce-Malblanc *et al.* 2008)

c) In this study, horses were under continuous antigen exposure: Dexamethasone was given at 0.05 mg/kg PO once daily for 7 days or prednisolone (2 mg/kg PO once daily for 7 days). Both were effective, but dexamethasone more so. (Leclere *et al.* 2010)

Dexamethasone suppression test:

a) 20 mg IM. Normal values: Cortisol levels decrease 50% in 2 hours, 70% in 4 hours, and 80% at 6 hours. At 24 hours, levels are still depressed about 30% of original value. (Beech 1987)

■ **SWINE:**

For glucocorticoid therapy:

a) 1–10 mg IV or IM (Howard 1986)

■ **LLAMAS:**

For adjunctive therapy of anaphylaxis:

a) 2 mg/kg IV (Smith 1989)

■ **BIRDS:**

For shock, trauma, gram-negative endotoxemia:

a) Dexamethasone 2 mg/mL injection: 2–4 mg/kg IM or IV once, twice or three times daily. Taper off drug when using long-term. (Clubb 1986)

■ **REPTILES:**

For septic shock in most species:

a) Using Dexamethasone Sodium Phosphate: 0.1–0.25 mg/kg IV or IM (Gauvin 1993)

Monitoring

Monitoring of glucocorticoid therapy is dependent on its reason for use, dosage, agent used (amount of mineralocorticoid activity), dosage schedule (daily versus alternate day therapy), duration of therapy, and the animal's age and condition. The following list may not be appropriate or complete for all animals; use clinical assessment and judgment should adverse effects be noted:

■ Weight, appetite, signs of edema

■ Serum and/or urine electrolytes

■ Total plasma proteins, albumin

■ Blood glucose

■ Growth and development in young animals

■ ACTH stimulation test if necessary

Client Information

■ Clients should carefully follow the dosage instructions and should not discontinue the drug abruptly without consulting with veterinarian beforehand.

■ Clients should be briefed on the potential adverse effects that can be seen with these drugs and instructed to contact the veterinarian should these effects become severe or progress.

Chemistry/Synonyms

A synthetic glucocorticoid, dexamethasone occurs as an odorless, white to practically white, crystalline powder that melts with some decomposition at about 250°C. It is practically insoluble in water and sparingly soluble in alcohol. Dexamethasone sodium phosphate occurs as an odorless or having a slight odor, white to slightly yellow, hygroscopic powder. One gram is soluble in about 2 mL of water; it is slightly soluble in alcohol

1.3 mg of dexamethasone sodium phosphate is equivalent to 1 mg of dexamethasone; 4 mg/mL of dexamethasone sodium phosphate injection is approximately equivalent to 3 mg/mL of dexamethasone.

Dexamethasone may also be known as: desamethasone, dexametasone, dexamethasonum, 9alpha-Fluoro-16alpha-methylprednisolone; hexadecadrol; many trade names are available.

Storage/Stability

Dexamethasone is heat labile and should be stored at room temperature (15–30°C) unless otherwise directed by the manufacturer. Dexamethasone sodium phosphate injection should be protected from light. Dexamethasone tablets should be stored in well-closed containers.

Compatibility/Compounding Considerations

Dexamethasone sodium phosphate for injection is reportedly **compatible** with the following drugs: amikacin sulfate, aminophylline, bleomy-

cin sulfate, cimetidine HCl, glycopyrrolate, lidocaine HCl, nafcillin sodium, netilmicin sulfate, prochlorperazine edisylate and verapamil.

Dexamethasone sodium phosphate is reportedly **incompatible** with: daunorubicin HCl, doxorubicin HCl, metaraminol bitartrate, and vancomycin. Compatibility is dependent upon factors such as pH, concentration, temperature and diluent used; consult specialized references or a hospital pharmacist for more specific information.

Dosage Forms/Regulatory Status

VETERINARY-LABELED PRODUCTS:

Dexamethasone Injection: 2 mg/mL; *Azium® Solution* (Schering-Plough), generic; (Rx). FDA-approved for use in dogs, cats, horses (those not intended for food) and cattle. There are no withdrawal times required when used in cattle. A withdrawal period has not been established for this product in preruminal calves; do not use in veal calves.

Dexamethasone Oral Powder: 10 mg crystalline in 10 mg packets. FDA-approved for use in cattle and horses (not horses intended for food). *Azium® Powder* (Schering-Plough); (Rx)

Dexamethasone Sodium Phosphate Injection: 4 mg/mL (equivalent to 3 mg/mL dexamethasone); generic; (Rx). FDA-approved for use in horses.

Dexamethasone 5 mg and trichlormethiazide 200 mg oral bolus: in boxes of 30 and 100 boluses; *Naquasone® Bolus* (Schering-Plough); (Rx). FDA-approved for use in cattle. Milk withdrawal = 72 hours.

The ARCI (Racing Commissioners International) has designated dexamethasone as a class 4 substance. See the appendix for more information.

HUMAN-LABELED PRODUCTS:

Dexamethasone Oral Tablets: 0.25 mg, 0.5 mg, 0.75 mg, 1 mg, 1.5 mg, 2 mg, 4 mg, & 6 mg; *Decadron®* (Merck); *DexPak® Day TaperPak* (ECR); *Zema-Pak® 10 & 13 Day* (Macoven); generic; (Rx)

Dexamethasone Oral Elixir/Solution: 0.5 mg/5 mL in 100 mL, 237 mL, 500 mL and UD 5 & UD 20 mL; 1 mg/mL (concentrate) in 30 mL with dropper; *Dexamethasone Intensol®* (Roxane); generic; (Rx)

Dexamethasone Sodium Phosphate Injection: 4 mg/mL (as sodium phosphate solution) in 1 mL, 5 mL, 10 mL & 30 mL vials, 1 mL syringe & 1 mL fill in 2 mL vials; generic; (Rx); 10 mg/mL (as sodium phosphate solution) in 1 mL and 10 mL vials & 1 mL syringes; generic; (Rx); 20 mg/mL (as sodium phosphate solution) in 5 mL vials (IV); *Hexadrol® Phosphate* (Organon), (Rx)

Dexamethasone is also available in topical ophthalmic (see ophthalmic products in the appendix) and inhaled aerosol dosage forms.

References

Adamcak, A. & B. Otten (2000). Rodent Therapeutics. *Vet Clin NA: Exotic Anim Pract* 3:1(Jan): 221–240.

Ainsworth, D. & R. Hackett (2004). Disorders of the Respiratory System. *Equine Internal Medicine 2nd Ed.* M Reed, W Bayly and D Sellon Eds. Phila., Saunders: 289–354.

Beech, J. (1987). Respiratory Tract—Horse, Cow. *The Bristol Handbook of Antimicrobial Therapy*. DE Johnston Ed. Evansville, Veterinary Learning Systems: 88–109.

Clubb, S.L. (1986). Therapeutics: Individual and Flock Treatment Regimens. *Clinical Avian Medicine and Surgery*. GJ Harrison and LR Harrison Eds. Philadelphia, W.B. Saunders: 327–355.

Courouce–Malblanc, A., G. Fortier, et al. (2008). Comparison of prednisolone and dexamethasone effects in the presence of environmental control in heaves–affected horses. *Veterinary Journal* 175(2): 227–233.

Feldman, E.C. (2009). Diagnosis & Treatment of Canine Cushing's I: Diagnosis of Hyperadrenocorticism (Cushing's Syndrome) in Dogs—Which Tests are Best? Proceedings: Western Veterinary Conference. Accessed via: Veterinary Information Network. http://goo.gl/n4XsM

Fowler, M.E. (1993). Zootoxins. *Current Veterinary Therapy: Food Animal Practice 3*. JL Howard Ed. Philadelphia, W.B. Saunders: 411–413.

Gauvin, J. (1993). Drug therapy in reptiles. *Seminars in Avian & Exotic Med* 2(1): 48–59.

Howard, J.L., Ed. (1986). *Current Veterinary Therapy 2, Food Animal Practice*. Philadelphia, W.B. Saunders.

Jutkowitz, L. (2009). Diagnosis and Management of the Addisonian Crisis. Proceedings: WVC. Accessed via: Veterinary information Network. http://goo.gl/WdDHS

Leclere, M., J. Lefebvre–Lavoie, et al. (2010). Efficacy of oral prednisolone and dexamethasone in horses with recurrent airway obstruction in the presence of continuous antigen exposure. *Equine Veterinary Journal* 42(4): 316–321.

Scott–Moncrieff, J.C. (2010). Hypoadrenocorticism in dogs and cats: Update on diagnosis & treatment. Proceedings: ACVIM Forum. Accessed via: Veterinary Information Network. http://goo.gl/DV3Xh

Smith, J.A. (1989). Noninfectious diseases, metabolic diseases, toxicities, and neoplastic diseases of South American camelids. *Vet Clin of North Amer: Food Anim Pract* 5(1): 101–143.

Wilson, S. (2011, Last Update). "Personal Communication."

Zhang, K.W., S. Kohno, et al. (2006). Clinical oral doses of dexamethasone decreases intrinsic clearance of quinidine, a cytochrome P450 3A substrate in dogs. *Journal of Veterinary Medical Science* 68(9): 903–907.

DEXMEDETOMIDINE

(deks-mee-deh-*toe*-mih-deen)
Dexdomitor®

ALPHA-2 ADRENERGIC AGONIST

Prescriber Highlights

▶ Alpha-2 agonist similar to medetomidine used as a sedation, analgesia in dogs & cats

▶ Contraindications: cardiac disease, liver or kidney diseases, shock, severe debilitation, or animals stressed due to heat, cold or fatigue; caution in very old or young animals, animals with seizure disorders, respiratory, renal or kidney disorders

▶ Adverse Effects: Bradycardia, occasional AV blocks, decreased respiration, hypothermia, urination, vomiting, hyperglycemia, & pain on injection (IM). Rarely: prolonged sedation, paradoxical excitation, hypersensitivity, apnea & death from circulatory failure

▶ Dosed in dogs based upon body surface area, not weight

▶ Effects may be reversed with atipamezole

Uses/Indications

In the USA, dexmedetomidine for dogs and cats is FDA-approved for use as a sedative and analgesic to facilitate clinical examinations, clinical procedures, minor surgical procedures, and minor dental procedures, and in dogs only as a preanesthetic to general anesthesia. In Europe, there is an additional indication in cats as a premed for use prior to ketamine general anesthesia.

Pharmacology/Actions

Dexmedetomidine is the dextrorotatory enantiomer of the alpha$_2$ adrenergic agonist, medetomidine. The other enantiomer, levomedetomidine is thought to be pharmacologically inactive so dexmedetomidine is about two times more potent than medetomidine.

Dexmedetomidine is much more specific than xylazine for alpha$_2$ receptors versus alpha$_1$ receptors. The pharmacologic effects of dexmedetomidine include: depression of CNS (sedation, anxiolysis), analgesia, GI (decreased secretions, varying affects on intestinal muscle tone) and endocrine functions, peripheral and cardiac vasoconstriction, bradycardia, respiratory depression, diuresis, hypothermia, analgesia (somatic and visceral), muscle relaxation (but not enough for intubation), and blanched or cyanotic mucous membranes. Effects on blood pressure are variable, but dexmedetomidine can cause hypertension longer than does xylazine.

Pharmacokinetics

In dogs after IM administration, dexmedetomidine is absorbed (bioavailability 60%) and reaches peak plasma levels in about 35 minutes. Volume of distribution is 0.9 L/kg and elimination half-life is approximately 40−50 minutes. The drug is primarily metabolized in the liver via glucuronidation and N-methylation. No metabolites are active and they are eliminated primarily in the urine and to lesser extent in the feces.

In cats after IM administration, dexmedetomidine is absorbed and reaches peak plasma levels of about 17 ng/mL occur in about 15 minutes. Oral transmucosal (OTM, buccal) administration of dexmedetomidine (40 micrograms/kg) appears to give similar levels (extrapolated from clinical effects) as IM administration in cats (Slingsby *et al.* 2009). But in comparing OTM versus IM dexmedetomidine (20 micrograms/kg combined with buprenorphine 20 micrograms/kg, another report found that cats in the IM group were more sedated than in the OTM group, but that OTM administration allowed placement of an IV catheter in 75% of the cats (Santos *et al.* 2009). Volume of distribution is 2.2 L/kg and elimination half-life is approximately 1 hour. Metabolites are eliminated primarily in the urine and to lesser extent in the feces.

In humans after IV administration, dexmedetomidine is rapidly distributed, undergoes almost complete biotransformation via both glucuronidation and CY-450 enzymes systems and has a terminal elimination half-life of about 2 hours. Metabolites are eliminated in the urine and feces.

Contraindications/Precautions/Warnings

The US labeling states not to use in dogs or cats with cardiovascular disease, respiratory disorders, liver or kidney diseases, or in conditions of shock, severe debilitation, or stress due to extreme heat, cold or fatigue. It is not recommended in cats with respiratory disease. Due to the pronounced cardiovascular effects of dexmedetomidine, only clinically healthy dogs and cats should be treated. While not contraindicated in pediatric or geriatric dogs or cats in the US label, it states that the drug has not been evaluated in dogs younger than 16 weeks of age or in cats younger than 12 weeks of age, or in geriatric dogs and cats.

The UK labeling states not to use in puppies less than 6 months old or in kittens less than 5 months old; in animals with cardiovascular disorders; in animals with severe systemic disease or that are moribund; or in animals known to be hypersensitive to the active substance or any of the excipients.

Use with caution in animals with, or prone to developing, seizures. Dexmedetomidine lowered the seizure threshold in cats undergoing anesthesia with enflurane.

Because blinking may be impaired in cats during sedation and dexmedetomidine/butorphanol has been shown to reduce tear production in dogs (Jalornaki & Eskelinen 2007), eye lubricants should be used when using dexmedetomidine.

Adverse Effects

The adverse effects reported with medetomidine or dexmedetomidine are essentially extensions of their pharmacologic effects including bradycardia, vasoconstriction, muscle tremors, transient hypertension, reduced tear production, occasional AV blocks, decreased respiration, hypothermia, urination, vomiting, hyperglycemia, and pain on injection (IM). Rare effects that have been reported include: prolonged sedation, paradoxical excitation, hypersensitivity, pulmonary edema, apnea, and death from circulatory failure.

Reproductive/Nursing Safety

The drug is not recommended for use in pregnant dogs or those used for breeding purposes because safety data for use during pregnancy is insufficient; therefore use only when the benefits clearly outweigh the drug's risks. However, no teratogenic effects were observed when rats were given up to 200 micrograms/kg SC from days 5−16 of gestation or when rabbits were given up 96 micrograms/kg IV from days 6−18 of gestation. In humans, the FDA categorizes this drug as category *C* for use during pregnancy (*Animal studies have shown an adverse effect on the fetus, but there are no adequate studies in humans; or there are no animal reproduction studies and no adequate studies in humans.*)

Dexmedetomidine is distributed into the milk of lactating rats; safe use during nursing has not been established.

Overdosage/Acute Toxicity

Single doses of up to 5X (IV) and 10X (IM) were tolerated in dogs, but adverse effects can occur (see above). Because of the potential of additional adverse effects occurring (heart block, PVC's, or tachycardia), treatment of dexmedetomidine-induced bradycardia with anticholinergic agents (atropine or glycopyrrolate) is usually not recommended. Atipamezole is probably a safer choice to treat any dexmedetomidine-induced effect.

Drug Interactions

Note: Before attempting combination therapy with dexmedetomidine, it is strongly advised to access references from veterinary anesthesiologists familiar with the use of this drug. The following drug interactions have either been reported or are theoretical in humans or animals receiving dexmedetomidine or medetomidine (a related compound) and may be of significance in veterinary patients:

- ◾ **ANESTHETICS, OPIATES, SEDATIVE/HYPNOT-ICS:** Effects may be additive; dosage reduction of one or both agents may be required. General anesthetic requirements may be reduced between 30-60%.

■ **ATROPINE, GLYCOPYRROLATE:** The use of atropine (or glycopyrrolate) with dexmedetomidine can significantly increase arterial blood pressure and heart rate; use together is not recommended in dogs (and probably other species) (Congdon *et al.* 2009).

■ **EPINEPHRINE:** As epinephrine possesses alpha agonist effects, do not use to treat cardiac effects caused by dexmedetomidine

■ **YOHIMBINE:** May reverse the effects of medetomidine; but atipamezole is preferred for clinical use to reverse the drug's effects

Laboratory Considerations
■ Medetomidine (and presumably dexmedetomidine) can inhibit ADP-induced **platelet aggregation** in cats.

Doses
■ **DOGS:**
a) For sedation and analgesia: 375 micrograms/m^2 body surface area (BSA) IV; 500 micrograms/m^2 BSA IM. The microgram/kg dosage decreases as body weight increases.

As a preanesthetic: Depending on duration and severity of the procedure and anesthetic regimen: 125−375 micrograms/m^2 IM. The microgram/kg dosage decreases as body weight increases. Accurate dosing is not possible with dogs weighing less than 2 kg. An extensive dosing table using patient weights is available in the package insert. It is recommended that patients are fasted for 12 hours prior to use. After injection allow animal to rest quietly for 15 minutes, sedation/analgesia occur within 5-15 minutes, with peak effects at 30 minutes post dose. (Label Information; *Dexdomitor*®—Pfizer)

b) For use in combination with an opioid and ketamine (so-called "doggie magic") to provide anesthesia and pain management (**Note:** reference has dosing tables for conversion of patient weight to various microgram/m^2 doses of dexmedetomidine; opioid concentrations used in the reference are: Butorphanol 10 mg/mL, Hydromorphone 2 mg/mL, Morphine 15 mg/mL, & Buprenorphine 0.3 mg/mL. Ketamine concentration is 100 mg/mL. As these drugs may be available in other concentrations, only use those products with the above concentrations if using this protocol.)

For geriatric dogs, dogs with renal or liver dysfunction as a premed prior to propofol or face mask induction, followed by maintenance on isoflurane or sevoflurane: dexmedetomidine at 62.5 micro-

grams/m^2. Combine with equal volumes of one of the opioids noted above and ketamine. May administer IM or IV.

For slightly heavier sedation in ASA class II or II dogs requiring sedation for radiographic procedures: Dexmedetomidine at 125 micrograms/m^2. Combine with equal volumes of one of the opioids noted above and ketamine. May administer IM or IV.

For dogs undergoing minor surgery, Penn hip or OFA-types of radiographic procedures that require significant muscle relaxation: Dexmedetomidine at 250 micrograms/m^2. Combine with equal volumes of one of the opioids noted above and ketamine. May administer IM or IV.

To induce a surgical plane of anesthesia for OHE, castration, or other abdominal surgery: Dexmedetomidine at 375 micrograms/m^2. Combine with equal volumes of one of the opioids noted above and ketamine. May administer IM or IV. Provides rapid immobilization; lateral recumbency in 5-8 minutes. Dogs can be intubated and maintained on oxygen. Supplemental low doses of isoflurane (0.5%) or sevoflurane (1%) can be used.

For immobilizing extremely fractious dogs and wolf-hybrid dogs: Dexmedetomidine at 500 micrograms/m^2. Combine with equal volumes of one of the opioids noted above and ketamine. Administer IM. This dose is rarely required.

To reverse above, atipamezole IM at the same volume as the dexmedetomidine. (Ko 2009)

c) As a constant rate infusion for postoperative pain management in critically ill dogs: After surgery a loading dose of 25 micrograms/m^2 IV, followed by a constant rate infusion for 24 hours at 25 micrograms/m^2/hr. In study, morphine at 0.2 mg/kg IV was used when rescue analgesia required (about half the dogs in the study). In this study, dexmedetomidine was as effective as morphine CRI (2.5 mg/m^2 load, and 2.5 mg/m^2/hr CRI). Authors concluded that CRI's of dexmedetomidine have potential to provide postoperative analgesia in critically ill patients, but additional studies required to determine appropriate doses and/or use with other analgesics to provide maximal and safe post-surgical analgesia. (Valtolina *et al.* 2009)

■ **CATS:**
a) For sedation and analgesia,: 40 micrograms/kg IM. A dosing table is available in the package insert. Recommended that patients be fasted for 12 hours prior to

use. Apply an eye lubricant. After injection allow animal to rest quietly for 15 minutes, sedation/analgesia occurs within 5-15 minutes, with peak effects at 30 minutes post dose. (Label Information; *Dexdomitor®*—Pfizer)

b) For use in combination with an opioid and ketamine (so-called "kitty magic", "DKT" or "Triple Combination") to provide sedation and analgesia (**Note:** Opioid concentrations used in the reference are: Butorphanol 10 mg/mL, Hydromorphone 2 mg/mL, Morphine 15 mg/mL, & Buprenorphine 0.3 mg/mL. Ketamine concentration is 100 mg/mL. Dexmedetomidine concentration is 0.5 mg/mL. As these drugs may be available in other concentrations, only use those products with the above concentrations if using this protocol.)

For the chart below: MILD = For sedation or as a premed prior to propofol or face mask induction; MODERATE = For castration or minor surgical procedures; PROFOUND = Invasive surgical procedures including OHE and declaws. Cats can be reversed immediately with an equal volume (of the dexmedetomidine dose) of atipamezole.

Cat Weight		Volume (of each) of: Dexmedetomidine-Opioid-Ketamine			IM Route
Lbs	Kg	MILD	MODERATE	PROFOUND	
4-7	2-3	0.025 mL	0.05 mL	0.1–0.15 mL	
7-9	3-4	0.05 mL	0.1 mL	0.2–0.25 mL	
9-13	4-6	0.1 mL	0.2 mL	0.3–0.35 mL	
14-15	6-7	0.2 mL	0.3 mL	0.4–0.45 mL	
15-18	7-8	0.3 mL	0.4 mL	0.5–0.55 mL	

(Ko 2009)

Monitoring
■ Level of sedation and analgesia; heart rate; body temperature
■ Heart rhythm, blood pressure, respiration rate, and pulse oximetry should be considered, particularly in higher risk patients

Client Information
■ This drug should be administered and monitored by veterinary professionals only
■ Clients should be made aware of the potential adverse effects associated with its use, particularly in dogs at risk (older, preexisting conditions)

Chemistry/Synonyms
Dexmedetomidine is the dextrorotatory enantiomer of medetomidine.

Dexmedetomidine HCl may also be known as (S)-medetomidine, (+)-medetomidine, MPV 1440, MPV 295, or MPV 785. Trade names include: *Precedex®* or *Dexdomitor®*.

Storage/Stability
Store the injection at room temperature (15–30°C); do not freeze.

Compatibility/Compounding Considerations
Information "on file" with the manufacturer states that dexmedetomidine 0.5 mg/mL solution for injection can be mixed with butorphanol 2 mg/mL or with ketamine 50 mg/mL solution, or with butorphanol 2 mg/mL solution and ketamine 50 mg/mL solution, in the same syringe and possesses no pharmacological risk. Anecdotal comments have been noted that buprenorphine, hydromorphone, morphine can also be mixed with dexmedetomidine.

Dosage Forms/Regulatory Status
VETERINARY-LABELED PRODUCTS:
Dexmedetomidine HCl 0.5 mg/mL (500 micrograms/mL) in 10 mL multidose vials; *Dexdomitor®* (Pfizer); (Rx).

HUMAN-LABELED PRODUCTS:
Dexmedetomidine HCl Concentrated Solution for Injection: 100 micrograms/mL (equiv. to dexmedetomidine hydrochloride 118 mcg), preservative free, sodium chloride 9 mg in 2 mL vials; *Precedex®* (Hospira); (Rx)

References
Congdon, J., M. Marquez, et al. (2009). Cardiovascular and sedation paramerters during dexmedetomidine and atropine administration. Prtoceedings: IVECCS.

Jalornaki, S. & E. Eskelinen (2007). Effect of dexmedetomidine–butorphanol combination on Schirmer 1 tear test (STT1) readings in dogs. Proceedings: ACVO. Accessed via: Veterinary Information Network. http://goo.gl/3erdT

Ko, J. (2009). Dexmedetomidine and its injectable anesthetic–pain management combinations. Proceedings: ACVC. Accessed via: Veterinary Information Network. http://goo.gl/8UTsp

Santos, L., J. Ludders, et al. (2009). Sedative and Cardiorespiratory Effects of Dexmedetomidine and Buprenorphine Administered to Cats via Oral Trans–Mucosal or Intramuscular Routes. Proceedings: IVECCS. http://goo.gl/q51PA

Slingsby, L., T. Monrow, et al. (2009). Thermal antinociception after dexmedetomidine administration in cats: a comparison between intramuscular and oral transmucosal administration. *Journal of Feline Medicine and Surgery* 11(829–834).

Valtolina, C., J.H. Robben, et al. (2009). Clinical evaluation of the efficacy and safety of a constant rate infusion of dexmedetomidine for postoperative pain management in dogs. *Veterinary Anaesthesia and Analgesia* 36(4): 369–383.

DEXPANTHENOL
D-PANTHENOL

(dex-*pan*-the-nole)   Ilopan®

Prescriber Highlights

▶ Precursor to Coenzyme A that ostensibly aids in production of acetylcholine

▶ Potentially may be useful in the prevention of post-surgical ileus, but efficacy is in doubt

▶ Contraindications: Ileus secondary to mechanical obstruction or in cases of colic caused by the treatment of cholinergic anthelmintics

Uses/Indications

Dexpanthenol has been suggested for use in intestinal atony or distension, postoperative retention of flatus and feces, prophylaxis and treatment of paralytic ileus after abdominal surgery or traumatic injuries, equine colic (not due to mechanical obstruction) and any other condition when there is an impairment of smooth muscle function. Controlled studies are lacking with regard to proving the efficacy of the drug for any of these indications.

Pharmacology/Actions

A precursor to pantothenic acid, dexpanthenol acts as a precursor to coenzyme A that is necessary for acetylation reactions to occur during gluconeogenesis and in the production of acetylcholine. It has been postulated that post-surgical ileus can be prevented by giving high doses of dexpanthenol, thereby assuring adequate levels of acetylcholine. However, one study in normal horses (Adams, Lamar, and Masty 1984) failed to demonstrate any effect of dexpanthenol on peristalsis.

Pharmacokinetics

Dexpanthenol is rapidly converted to pantothenic acid *in vivo*, which is widely distributed throughout the body, primarily as coenzyme A.

Contraindications/Precautions/Warnings

Dexpanthenol is contraindicated in ileus secondary to mechanical obstruction, or in cases of colic caused by the treatment of cholinergic anthelmintics. It is also contraindicated in humans with hemophilia as it may exacerbate bleeding.

Adverse Effects

Adverse reactions are reportedly rare. Hypersensitivity reactions have been reported in humans, but may have been due to the preservative agents found in the injectable product. Potentially, GI cramping and diarrhea are possible.

Reproductive/Nursing Safety

Safety in use during pregnancy has not been established. In humans, the FDA categorizes this drug as category *C* for use during pregnancy (*Animal studies have shown an adverse effect on the fetus, but there are no adequate studies in humans; or there are no animal reproduction studies and no adequate studies in humans.*)

Overdosage/Acute Toxicity

The drug is considered non-toxic even when administered in high doses.

Drug Interactions

The following drug interactions have either been reported or are theoretical in humans or animals receiving dexpanthenol and may be of significance in veterinary patients:

▪ **NEOSTIGMINE; SUCCINYLCHOLINE:** The manufacturers have recommended that dexpanthenol not be administered within 12 hours of neostigmine or other parasympathomimetic agents or within 1 hour of patients receiving succinylcholine. The clinical significance of these potential interactions has not been documented, however.

Doses

▪ **DOGS & CATS:**
a) 11 mg/kg IM; repeat if indicated at 4–6 hour intervals (Rossoff 1974)
b) 11 mg/kg IM; may be repeated in 2 hours after initial injection and followed every 6–8 hours until condition is alleviated. The time interval and duration of therapy will depend upon the degree of severity that the animal is exhibiting from the clinical standpoint. (Label Instructions; *d-Panthenol® Injectable*—Vedco)

▪ **HORSES:**
a) 2.5 grams IV or IM; repeat if indicated at 4–6 hour intervals (Rossoff 1974), (Label Instructions; *d-Panthenol® Injectable*—Vedco)

Monitoring

Clinical efficacy

Client Information

▪ Should be used in a professionally monitored situation where gastrointestinal motility can be monitored.

Chemistry/Synonyms

The alcohol of D-pantothenic acid, dexpanthenol occurs as a slightly bitter-tasting, clear, viscous, somewhat hygroscopic liquid. It is freely soluble in water or alcohol.

Dexpanthenol may also be known as: D-panthenol, dexpanthenolum, dextro-pantothenyl alcohol, pantothenol; many trade names are available.

Storage/Stability

Dexpanthenol should be protected from both freezing and excessive heat. It is incompatible with strong acids and alkalis.

Dosage Forms/Regulatory Status

VETERINARY-LABELED PRODUCTS:

Dexpanthenol Injection: 250 mg/mL in 100 mL vials; *D-Panthenol® Injectable* (Vedco), generic (Butler, Phoenix Pharmaceutical); (Rx). Labeled for use in dogs, cats, and horses.

HUMAN-LABELED PRODUCTS:

Dexpanthenol Injection: 250 mg/mL in 2 mL & 10 mL vials, UD *Stat-Pak* 2 mL disp syringes; *Ilopan®* (Adria); generic; (Rx)

References

Rossoff, I.S. (1974). *Handbook of Veterinary Drugs*. New York, Springer Publishing.

Dextrose—see the Tables of Parenteral Fluids in the Appendix

DEXRAZOXANE

(dex-ra-t-ane)   Zinecard®

ANTIDOTE

Prescriber Highlights

▶ May be useful in attenuating the cardiotoxic effects of doxorubicin in patients (dogs) showing signs of anthracycline cardiotoxicity, have cardiac disease, or are at maximum cumulative dosages of doxorubicin; also used to treat extravasation injuries associated with doxorubicin

▶ Potentially may reduce efficacy of doxorubicin & increase myelosuppression

▶ For extravasation treatment, must be administered within hours of injury

▶ Very expensive

Uses/Indications

Dexrazoxane may be useful to attenuate the cardiotoxic effects of doxorubicin in patients who are showing signs of anthracycline cardiotoxicity, have cardiac disease, or are at maximum cumulative dosages of doxorubicin. It is also used to treat extravasation injuries associated with doxorubicin.

While dexrazoxane has been shown to be cardioprotective when given at dosages of 10 times the doxorubicin dose, there is evidence that it may also partially protect the cancer cells being treated.

Pharmacology/Actions

Dexrazoxane is hydrolyzed to an active metabolite that chelates intracellular iron that is believed to prevent the formation of an anthracycline-iron complex thought to be the primary cause of anthracycline-induced cardiomyopathy.

Pharmacokinetics

In dogs, dexrazoxane's pharmacokinetics fit a two compartment open model. Steady-state volume of distribution is 0.67 L/kg, terminal half life is about 1.2 hours, and clearance about 11 mL/min/kg. Clearance was dose-independent and the drug showed low tissue and protein binding. Dexrazoxane is primarily excreted in the urine as unchanged drug and metabolites.

Contraindications/Precautions/Warnings

Dexrazoxane should not be used unless an anthracycline antineoplastic agent is being used.

Efficacy and safety for use in cats is not known.

Adverse Effects

Dexrazoxane may cause additive myelosuppression when used with other myelosuppressive agents. There is some evidence in humans, that dexrazoxane may reduce the efficacy of anthracycline antitumor agents. Clinical significance in veterinary patients is unknown.

Wear gloves when handling and use normal procedures for handling and disposal of anticancer medications. If unreconstituted powder contacts skin or mucous membranes, wash off thoroughly with soap and water.

Reproductive/Nursing Safety

Dexrazoxane has been shown to cause testicular atrophy in dogs when administered at usual doses for 13 weeks. In humans, the FDA categorizes dexrazoxane as a category *C* drug for use during pregnancy (*Animal studies have shown an adverse effect on the fetus, but there are no adequate studies in humans; or there are no animal reproduction studies and no adequate studies in humans*). In rats and rabbits, dexrazoxane was teratogenic at doses lower than those administered to humans.

It is unknown if dexrazoxane enters maternal milk; human mothers are advised to discontinue nursing if given the drug.

Overdosage/Acute Toxicity

Because of the method of administration and drug expense, overdoses are unlikely in veterinary medicine. As there is no known antidote, treatment would be supportive. Potentially, the drug could be removed via hemodialysis.

Drug Interactions

Dexrazoxane does not influence the pharmacokinetics of doxorubicin.

The following drug interactions have either been reported or are theoretical in humans or animals receiving dexrazoxane and may be of significance in veterinary patients:

■ **MYELOSUPPRESSIVE AGENTS, OTHER:** Additive myelo-suppression may occur when used with other myelosuppressive agents.

Laboratory Considerations

■ No specific laboratory interactions or considerations were noted.

Doses

■ **DOGS:**

For treatment of anthracycline (doxorubicin, epirubicin, etc.) extravasation:

a) Terminate doxorubicin infusion immediately, and infuse intravenously 1000 mg/m^2 of dexrazoxane in a separate infusion within 6 hours and again on day 2. Infuse 500 mg/m^2 on day 3. Acute surgical evaluation is performed. **Note:** Dosage recommendations are for human patients, but may apply to veterinary patients. (Langer *et al.* 2000)

b) Anecdotally; IV administration of dexrazoxane at 10 times the doxorubicin dose with 3 hours and again at 24 and 48 hours after extravasation significantly reduces local tissue injury. (Vail 2006)

For prevention of doxorubicin-induced cardiomyopathy:

a) Dexrazoxane to doxorubicin dose ratio is 10:1 (*e.g.,* 300 mg/m^2 of dexrazoxane to 30 mg/m^2 doxorubicin) given as slow IV bolus, starting 30 minutes of, and prior to the doxorubicin dose (as a short, IV bolus.) (Selting 2005)

b) Use can be considered in breeds at risk (Shelties, Collies, Australian Shepherds, etc.), dogs that are exceeding the usual cumulative dose cut-off, and in cases where there is preexisting cardiac disease and no effective chemo options exist: Dexrazoxane to doxorubicin dose ratio is 10:1 (*e.g.,* 300 mg/m^2 of dexrazoxane to 30 mg/m^2 doxorubicin) given as slow IV bolus, starting 30 minutes before doxorubicin is administered. (Vail 2006)

Monitoring

■ CBC

■ If used for cardioprotection: echocardiogram, ECG, etc.

Client Information

■ Clients should understand and accept the potential costs associated with this drug and that when used for extravasation injuries, may not be fully effective.

Chemistry/Synonyms

A derivative of EDTA, dexrazoxane occurs as a white crystalline powder that is soluble in water and slightly soluble in ethanol and practically insoluble in nonpolar organic solvents. It has a pKa of 2.1 and degrades rapidly at pH's above 7.

Dexrazoxane may also be known as: 2,6-Piperazinedione, ADR-529, ICRF-187, NSC-169780, *Zinecard®*, *Cardioxane®* or *Eucardion®*.

Storage/Stability

Unreconstituted dexrazoxane vials should be stored at 25°C (77°F); excursions permitted to 15–30°C (59–86°F). Once reconstituted with the supplied diluent, it is stable for 6 hours at room temperature or refrigerated. Unused solutions after that time should be discarded. After reconstitution, the resulting solution may be diluted with either 0.9% sodium chloride injection or D$_5$W in concentrations of 1.3–5 mg/mL. Inspect visually for particulate matter and discoloration prior to administering.

Compatibility/Compounding Considerations

The manufacturer states that dexrazoxane should not be mixed with any other drug.

Dosage Forms/Regulatory Status

VETERINARY-LABELED PRODUCTS: None

HUMAN-LABELED PRODUCTS:

Dexrazoxane Lyophilized Powder for Injection Solution: 250 mg in single-use vials with 25 mL vial of sodium lactate injection; and 500 mg regular & preservative free (equiv to dexrazoxane hydrochloride 589 mg) in single-use vials with 50 mL vial of sodium lactate injection; *Zinecard®* (Pfizer); *Totect®* (Topo Target); generic; (Rx)

References

Langer, S., M. Sehested, et al. (2000). Treatment of anthracycline extravasation with dexrazoxane. *Clin Cancer Res* 6(Sept): 3680–3686.

Selting, K. (2005). Cardiotoxicity: Getting to the heart of the matter. Proceedings: ACVIM. Accessed via: Veterinary Information Network. http://goo.gl/CPepk

Vail, D. (2006). New supportive therapies for cancer patients. Proceedings: ACVIM. Accessed via: Veterinary Information Network. http://goo.gl/r4oMT

DEXTRAN 70

(**dex**-tran)

PLASMA VOLUME EXPANDER

Note: *Dextran is also available as Dextran 40 and Dextran 75. As Dextran 70 is the most commonly used version in veterinary medicine, the following monograph is limited to it alone.*

Prescriber Highlights

▶ Branched polysaccharide plasma volume expander

▶ Contraindications: Preexisting coagulopathies

▶ Caution: Patients susceptible to circulatory overload (severe heart or renal failure), thrombocytopenia

▶ Adverse Effects: Quite rare in dogs. Increased bleeding times, acute renal failure & anaphylaxis possible (but very rare)

▶ Must monitor for fluid overload

Uses/Indications

Dextran 70 is a relatively low cost colloid for the adjunctive treatment of hypovolemic shock. Hetastarch is the more commonly employed synthetic colloid used today.

Pharmacology/Actions

Dextran 70 has osmotic effects similarly to albumin. Dextran's colloidal osmotic effect draws fluid into the vascular system from the interstitial spaces, resulting in increased circulating blood volume.

Pharmacokinetics

After IV infusion, circulating blood volume is increased maximally within one hour and effects can persist for 24 hours or more. Approximately 20-30% of a given dose remains in the intravascular compartment at 24 hours and it may be detected in the blood 4-6 weeks after dosing. Dextran 70 is slowly degraded to glucose by dextranase in the spleen and then metabolized to carbon dioxide and water. A small amount may be excreted directly into the gut and eliminated in the feces.

Contraindications/Precautions/Warnings

Patients overly susceptible to circulatory overload (severe heart or renal failure) should receive dextran 70 with great caution. Dextran 70 is contraindicated in patients with severe coagulopathies and should be used with caution in patients with thrombocytopenia as it can interfere with platelet function. Do not give dextran IM. Patients on strict sodium restriction should receive dextran cautiously as a 500 mL bag contains 77 mEq of sodium.

Adverse Effects

Dextran 70 may increase bleeding time and decrease von Willebrand's factor antigen and factor VIII activity. This does not usually cause clinical bleeding in dogs.

While anaphylactoid reactions are not rare in humans, they do occur rarely in dogs, but at a higher rate than with hetastarch. Unlike dextran 40, dextran 70 has rarely been associated with acute renal failure. In humans, GI effects (abdominal pain, nausea/vomiting) have been reported with use of dextran 70.

Reproductive/Nursing Safety

In humans, the FDA categorizes this drug as category **C** for use during pregnancy (*Animal studies have shown an adverse effect on the fetus, but there are no adequate studies in humans; or there are no animal reproduction studies and no adequate studies in humans.*)

Overdosage/Acute Toxicity

The drug should be dosed and monitored carefully as volume overload may result.

Drug Interactions

Dextran reportedly has no drug interactions that are clinically significant.

Laboratory Considerations

■ Dextran 70 may interfere with **blood cross-matching** as it can cross-link with red blood cells and appear as rouleaux formation. Isotonic saline may be used to negate this effect.

■ **Blood glucose** levels may be increased as dextran is degraded.

■ Falsely elevated **bilirubin** levels may be noted; reason unknown.

Doses

■ DOGS:

a) Small volume resuscitation techniques are recommended in any dog with closed cavity hemorrhage, head injury, pulmonary contusions or edema, cardiogenic shock, or oliguric renal failure. An initial dose of balanced isotonic crystalloids (10-15 mL/kg) for dogs is given. Either hetastarch or dextran-70 is then administered (5 mL/kg in dogs) over 1-5 minutes. The perfusion parameters are reassessed and the initial mL/kg bolus repeated as needed until the end-point of resuscitation is reached. (Kirby 2008)

b) 20 mL/kg/day; when acute resuscitation is required, may be given as a slow bolus over 30 minutes to an hour. May also be given as a constant rate infusion over a longer period to augment colloid oncotic pressure or decrease the volume of crystalloids infused, thereby reducing hemodilution. (Martin 2004)

■ CATS:

a) Small volume resuscitation techniques are recommended in the hypovolemic cat with closed cavity hemorrhage, head injury, pulmonary contusions or edema, cardiogenic shock, or oliguric renal failure. An initial dose of balanced isotonic crystalloids (5-10 mL/kg for cats) is given. Either hetastarch or dextran-70 is then administered (2-5 mL/kg in cats) over 1-5 minutes. The perfusion parameters are reassessed and the initial mL/kg bolus repeated as needed until the endpoint of resuscitation is reached. (Kirby 2008)

b) 10 mL/kg/day; when acute resuscitation is required. May be given as a slow bolus over 30 minutes to an hour. May also be given as a constant rate infusion over a longer period to augment colloid oncotic pressure or decrease the volume of crystalloids infused, thereby reducing hemodilution. (Martin 2004)

■ CATTLE:

a) For dehydrated (secondary to diarrhea) calves given as 6% Dextran 70 in 7.2% sodium chloride: To prepare solution, add 31.6 g sodium chloride into the barrel of a 60 mL syringe. Draw 60 mL of 6% dextran 70 in 0.9% NaCl from the bag/bottle to dilute the NaCl crystals. Re-inject the dissolved solution into the bag/bottle through a 0.22 micron filter giving a 6% dextran 70 in 7.2% NaCl solution. Resultant solution may be refrigerated for up to 3 months. Inject IV 4-5 mL/kg of this solution over 4–5 minutes, followed immediately by oral administration of isotonic electrolyte solution. Give dextran 70 solution one time only or hypernatremia may result and follow-up with isotonic fluids (oral or IV) are critical. (Sweeney 2003)

Monitoring

■ Other than the regular monitoring performed in patients that would require volume expansion therapy, there is no inordinate monitoring required specific to dextran therapy.

Chemistry/Synonyms

A branched polysaccharide used intravenously as a plasma volume expander, dextran 70 occurs as a white to light yellow amorphous powder. It is freely soluble in water and insoluble in alcohol. Dextran 70 contains (on average) molecules of 70,000 daltons. Each 500 mL of the commercially available 6% dextran 70 in normal saline provides 77 mEq of sodium. Dextran 70 in normal saline has a viscosity of 3.68 centipose (blood is 3 centipose) and a colloid osmotic pressure of 62 mmHg (canine plasma is approximately 20 mmHg).

Dextran 70 may also be known as: dextranum 70, polyglucin, *Dextran 70®*, *Fisiodex 70®*, *Gentran 70®*, *Hyskon®*, *Lomodex 70®*, *Longasteril 70®*, *Macrodex®*, *Macrohorm 70®*, *Neodextril 70®*, *Plander®*, *RescueFlow®*, or *Solplex 70®*.

Storage/Stability

Dextran 70 injection should be stored at room temperature; preferably in an area with little temperature variability. While only clear solutions should be used, dextran flakes can form but may be resolubolized by heating the solution in a boiling water bath until clear, or autoclaving at 110°C for 15 minutes.

Compatibility/Compounding Considerations

Dextran 70 is **compatible** with many other solutions and drugs; refer to specialized references or a hospital pharmacist for more information.

Dosage Forms/Regulatory Status

VETERINARY-LABELED PRODUCTS: None

HUMAN-LABELED PRODUCTS:

Dextran High Molecular Weight Injection: 6% dextran 70 in 0.9% sodium chloride in 500 mL; *Dextran 70®* (McGaw); (Rx), *Gentran70®* (Baxter); (Rx), *Macrodex®* (Medisan); (Rx)

Dextran High Molecular Weight Injection: 6% dextran 70 in 5% dextrose in 500 mL; *Macrodex®* (Medisan); (Rx)

References

Kirby, R. (2008). Shock and Resuscitation: Parts 1 & 2. "Be a Shock Buster . . . !". Proceedings: World Veterinary Congress. Accessed via: Veterinary Information Network. http://goo.gl/OGkk5

Martin, L. (2004). Plasma vs Synthetic Colloids: Do you know which to use? Proceedings: ACVIM Forum. Accessed via: Veterinary Information Network. http://goo.gl/rba5H

Sweeney, R. (2003). When salt water isn't enough: TPN, colloid, and blood product therapy in cattle. Proceedings: ACVIM Forum. Accessed via: Veterinary Information Network. http://goo.gl/Ew59P

DIAZEPAM

(dye-*az*-e-pam)   Valium®, Diastat®

BENZODIAZEPINE

Prescriber Highlights

▶ Benzodiazepine used for a variety of indications (anxiolytic, muscle relaxant, hypnotic, appetite stimulant, & anticonvulsant) in several species; use in cats is controversial

▶ In dogs, tolerance to anticonvulsant effects occurs with long-term use and make it less useful to treat status epilepticus

▶ Contraindications: Hypersensitivity to benzodiazepines, cats exposed to chlorpyrifos, significant liver disease (especially in cats)

▶ Caution: hepatic or renal disease, aggressive, debilitated or geriatric patients; patients in coma, shock or with significant respiratory depression

▶ Adverse Effects: Sedation & ataxia most prevalent. *Dogs:* CNS excitement, increased appetite; *Cats:* Hepatic failure or behavior changes; *Horses:* Muscle fasciculations

▶ Inject IV slowly

▶ May be teratogenic

▶ Drug interactions

▶ Controlled substance (C-IV)

Uses/Indications

Diazepam is used clinically for its anxiolytic, muscle relaxant, hypnotic, appetite stimulant, and anticonvulsant activities. It is also used in preanesthesia protocols for neuroleptanalgesia.

While diazepam is a drug of choice for treating status epilepticus and cluster seizures in dogs, it, and the other benzodiazepines are not very useful as maintenance anticonvulsants in dogs. They have short durations of action and long-term administration usually causes tolerance to their anticonvulsant effects. Additionally, long-term use in dogs may prevent effective use of diazepam for the emergency treatment of seizures. In cats, diazepam has a longer elimination half-life and tolerance does not appear to be a major concern, but many neurologists avoid its use in cats because of the risk for serious hepatotoxicity.

Pharmacology/Actions

The subcortical levels (primarily limbic, thalamic, and hypothalamic), of the CNS are depressed by diazepam and other benzodiazepines thus producing the anxiolytic, sedative, skeletal muscle relaxant, and anticonvulsant effects seen. The exact mechanism of action is unknown, but postulated mechanisms include: antagonism of serotonin, increased release of and/or facilitation of gamma-aminobutyric acid (GABA) activity, and diminished release or turnover of acetylcholine in the CNS. Benzodiazepine specific receptors have been located in the mammalian brain, kidney, liver, lung, and heart. In all species studied, receptors are lacking in the white matter.

Pharmacokinetics

Diazepam is rapidly absorbed following oral administration. Peak plasma levels occur within 30 minutes to 2 hours after oral dosing. The drug is slowly (slower than oral) and incompletely absorbed following IM administration. In dogs, rectally administered diazepam has a bioavailability of <10%, but when factoring in diazepam plus the active (20-50% of the anticonvulsant activity of diazepam) metabolites desmethyldiazepam and oxazepam, bioavailability is closer to 80%. When administered intranasally to dogs, bioavailability is about 80%.

Diazepam is highly lipid soluble and is widely distributed throughout the body. It readily crosses the blood-brain barrier and is fairly highly bound to plasma proteins. In the horse at a serum concentration of 75 ng/mL, 87% of the drug is bound to plasma proteins. In humans, this value has been reported to be 98–99%.

Diazepam is metabolized in the liver to several metabolites, including desmethyldiazepam (nordiazepam), temazepam, and oxazepam, all of which are pharmacologically active. These are eventually conjugated with glucuronide and eliminated primarily in the urine. Because of the active metabolites, serum values of diazepam are not useful in predicting efficacy. Serum half-lives (approximated) have been reported for diazepam and metabolites in dogs, cats, and horses:

	Dogs	Cats	Horses	Humans
Diazepam	2.5–3.2 hrs	5.5 hrs	7–22 hrs	20–50 hrs
Nordiazepam	3 hrs	21.3 hrs		30–200 hrs

Contraindications/Precautions/Warnings

Inject intravenously slowly. This is particularly true when using a small vein for access or in small animals; diazepam may cause significant thrombophlebitis. Rapid injection of intravenous diazepam in small animals or neonates may cause hypotension/cardiotoxicity secondary to the propylene glycol in the formulation. Intra-carotid artery injections must be avoided.

Use of diazepam in cats is controversial, primarily because of case reports of serious hepatotoxicity. Some are of the opinion that the drug should not be used chronically in cats.

Use cautiously in patients with hepatic or renal disease and in debilitated or geriatric patients. The drug should be administered to patients in coma, shock, or with significant respiratory depression very cautiously. It is contraindicated in patients with known hypersensitivity to the drug. Diazepam should be used very cautiously, if at all, in aggressive patients, as it may disinhibit the anxiety that may help prevent these animals from aggressive behavior. Benzodiazepines may impair the abilities of working animals. If administering the drug IV, be prepared to administer cardiovascular or respiratory support.

It is recommended not to use diazepam for seizure control in cats exposed to chlorpyrifos as organophosphate toxicity may be potentiated.

Animals who have toxicity from ingesting human sleep aids such as zolpidem (*Ambien*®) or eszopiclone (*Lunesta*®) should not receive benzodiazepines to treat paradoxical CNS stimulation as these drugs also increase GABA activity; IV phenothiazines such as acepromazine or chlorpromazine, or phenobarbital are recommended instead.

Rapid IV bolus administration can potentially cause hypotension; administer over 1–3 minutes depending on dose and patient size.

Adverse Effects

Rapid IV administration of diazepam can potentially cause hypotension; give IV slowly and flush IV catheter with fluids after administration to help prevent phlebitis.

Adverse effects reported in dogs include sedation, increased appetite, agitation, ataxia, and aggression. Additionally, dogs may exhibit a contradictory response (CNS excitement) following administration of diazepam. Doses of 0.8 mg/kg or higher are more likely to cause this effect. Diazepam's effects with regard to sedation and tranquilization in dogs can be variable and some feel that this makes it less than an ideal inpatient sedating agent, particularly when used alone.

Cats may exhibit changes in behavior (irritability, depression, aberrant demeanor) after receiving diazepam. There have been reports of cats developing hepatic failure after receiving oral diazepam (not dose dependent) for several days. Clinical signs (anorexia, lethargy, increased ALT/AST, hyperbilirubinemia) have been reported to occur 5–11 days after beginning oral therapy. Cats that receive diazepam should have baseline liver function tests. These should be repeated and the drug discontinued if emesis, lethargy, inappetence or ataxia develops.

In horses, diazepam may cause muscle fasciculations, weakness and ataxia at doses sufficient to cause sedation. Doses greater than 0.2 mg/kg may induce recumbency as a result of its muscle relaxant properties and general CNS depressant effects.

Reproductive/Nursing Safety

Diazepam has been implicated in causing congenital abnormalities in humans if administered during the first trimester of pregnancy. Infants born of mothers receiving large doses of benzodiazepines shortly before delivery have been reported to suffer from apnea, impaired metabolic response to cold stress, difficulty in feeding, hyperbilirubinemia, hypotonia, etc. Withdrawal symptoms have occurred in infants whose mothers chronically took benzodiazepines during pregnancy. The veterinary significance of these effects is unclear, but the use of these agents during the first trimester of pregnancy should only occur when the benefits clearly outweigh the risks associated with their use. In humans, the FDA categorizes this drug as category **D** for use during pregnancy (*There is evidence of human fetal risk, but the potential benefits from the use of the drug in pregnant women may be acceptable despite its potential risks.*) In a separate system evaluating the safety of drugs in canine and feline pregnancy (Papich 1989), this drug is categorized as in class: **C** (*These drugs may have potential risks. Studies in people or laboratory animals have uncovered risks, and these drugs should be used cautiously as a last resort when the benefit of therapy clearly outweighs the risks.*)

Benzodiazepines and their metabolites are distributed into milk and may cause CNS effects in nursing neonates.

Overdosage/Acute Toxicity

When administered alone, diazepam overdoses are generally limited to significant CNS depression (confusion, coma, decreased reflexes, etc.). Hypotension, respiratory depression, and cardiac arrest have been reported in human patients, but apparently are quite rare.

Treatment of acute toxicity consists of standard protocols for removing and/or binding the drug in the gut if taken orally, and supportive systemic measures. The use of analeptic agents (CNS stimulants such as caffeine) is generally not recommended. Flumazenil may be considered for adjunctive treatment of overdoses of benzodiazepines.

Drug Interactions

The following drug interactions have either been reported or are theoretical in humans or animals receiving diazepam and may be of significance in veterinary patients:

■ **AMITRIPTYLINE:** Diazepam may increase levels

■ **ANTACIDS:** May decrease oral diazepam absorption

■ **ANTIFUNGALS, AZOLE (itraconazole, ketoconazole, etc.):** May increase diazepam levels

■ **CIMETIDINE:** May decrease metabolism of benzodiazepines

■ **CNS DEPRESSANT DRUGS (barbiturates, narcotics, anesthetics, etc.):** If diazepam administered with other CNS depressant agents additive effects may occur

■ **DEXAMETHASONE:** May decrease diazepam levels

■ **DIGOXIN:** Diazepam may increase digoxin levels

■ **ERYTHROMYCIN:** May decrease the metabolism of benzodiazepines

■ **MINERAL OIL:** May decrease oral diazepam absorption

■ **OMEPRAZOLE:** May inhibit the metabolism of diazepam and increase levels

■ **PHENOBARBITAL:** May decrease diazepam concentrations

■ **PHENYTOIN:** May decrease diazepam concentrations

■ **QUINIDINE:** May increase diazepam levels

■ **RIFAMPIN:** May induce hepatic microsomal enzymes and decrease the pharmacologic effects of benzodiazepines

Laboratory Considerations

■ Patients receiving diazepam, may show false negative **urine glucose** results if using *Diastix®* or *Clinistix®* tests.

Doses

■ **DOGS:**

For treatment of seizures:

a) For cluster seizures or status epilepticus (for client treatment at home): 0.5 mg/kg rectally; if on phenobarbital, use diazepam at 2 mg/kg (using diazepam parenteral solution) per rectum. Administer at the onset of seizure and up to 3 times in a 24-hour period, but should not be given within 10 minutes of the prior dose. Owners should stay with dog for one hour after administration. (Podell 2000), (Podell 2006), (Podell 2009)

b) For cluster seizures (for client treatment at home): 1 mg/kg administered rectally at the onset of seizures; can be given up to 3 times over a 24 hour period. Dogs receiving phenobarbital should receive 2 mg/kg. Because diazepam is inactivated by light and adheres to plastic, it is best to dispense the drug in the original glass vial and instruct the owner to draw the required amount into a syringe when needed. A rubber catheter or teat cannula is then placed on the syringe for rectal administration. (Munana 2010)

c) For refractory status epilepticus using constant rate IV infusion: 0.1–0.5 mg/kg diluted in D5W. Rate administered per hour should be equal to the maintenance fluid requirement for the patient. Use with caution as diazepam can crystallize in solution and adsorb to PVC tubing.

For status or cluster seizure treatment at home: 0.5–2 mg/kg per rectum (Platt & McDonnell 2000)

d) For status epilepticus: Rule out hypoglycemia, electrolyte abnormalities as primary cause. Stop seizure with diazepam or midazolam 0.5–1 mg/kg IV, 1–2 mg/kg rectally or IV if patient on phenobarbital. Place IV catheter and initiate active cooling if necessary. If another seizure occurs, repeat IV diazepam or midazolam. Administer a long-acting anticonvulsant (e.g., phenobarbital at 5–8 mg/kg IV every 4–6h until seizures are under control regardless of additional therapy). If patient still has seizure activity, consider one or more of the following: **1)** continuous rate infusion of diazepam or midazolam, **2)** propofol or other means of anesthesia. (Knipe 2006), (Knipe 2009)

e) For status epilepticus: 0.5 mg/kg IV, intranasally or rectally. Dose may be repeated twice, if necessary. Anticonvulsant activity lasts only 15–30 minutes so a longer acting therapy is required if seizures stop. For at home therapy for cluster seizures, diazepam may be given rectally or intranasally at 0.5 mg/kg. Dogs who are on chronic phenobarbital therapy, may require higher doses (1–2 mg/kg). (Mariani 2010b)

Functional urethral obstruction/urethral sphincter hypertonus:

a) 2–10 mg q8h (Polzin and Osborne 1985); (Lane 2000)

b) 2–10 mg PO three times a day; 0.5 mg/kg IV (Chew et al. 1986)

c) 0.2 mg/kg PO q8h or 2–10 mg (total dose) PO q8h (Bartges 2003)

As a psychotherapeutic agent (e.g., situational anxiety):

a) 0.55–2.2 mg/kg PO q8-12h (Haug 2008)

b) 0.5–2.2 mg/kg prn for storms (Sherman & Mills 2008)

c) As a fast-acting anxiolytic: 0.5–2 mg/kg PO prn (Neilson 2009)

For adjunctive treatment of metronidazole toxicity (CNS):

a) Doses of diazepam averaged 0.43 mg/kg in the study and were given as an IV bolus once, and then PO q8h for 3 days. (Evans et al. 2002)

■ **CATS:**

As a psychotherapeutic agent:

a) Urine marking and anxiety: 0.2–0.4 mg/kg PO q12-24h (start at 0.2 mg/kg PO q12h) (Overall 2000)

b) For spraying: 1–2.5 mg per cat PO q8-12h; sedation and ataxia should abate within several days (Reisner & Houpt 2000)

c) As a fast-acting anxiolytic: 0.2–0.5 mg/kg PO prn (Neilson 2009)

For treatment of seizure disorders:

a) 0.25–0.5 mg/kg PO q8-12h. To halt an ongoing seizure, diazepam may be administered at 0.5–1 mg/kg IV. If cat has a history of receiving insulin, glucose may be more beneficial. Do not use if cat has been exposed to chlorpyrifos as organophosphate toxicity may be potentiated. (Shell 2000)

b) For maintenance therapy: 0.2–1 mg/kg PO q12h. Use with caution; associated with fatal hepatic necrosis. Phenobarbital is preferred as a maintenance drug in cats. (Mariani 2010a)

Functional urethral obstruction/urethral sphincter hypertonus:

a) 1–2.5 mg (total dose) PO q8h (Osborne et al. 2000)

b) 2.5–5 mg (total dose) PO q8h or as needed, or 0.5 mg/kg IV (Bartges 2003)

■ **FERRETS:**

For premedication/sedation:

a) 1–2 mg/kg IM; may be given with ketamine (10–20 mg/kg) (Morrisey & Carpenter 2004)

b) For sedation anesthesia: 0.5 mg/kg IM or IV (IV preferred); 0.2 mg/kg if using with ketamine (2–5 mg/kg) (Kaiser-Klingler 2009)

■ **RABBITS/RODENTS/SMALL MAMMALS:**

a) **Rabbits:** Pre-anesthetic: 2–10 mg/kg IM; 1–5 mg/kg IM or IV. Give IV to effect for seizures. (Ivey & Morrisey 2000)

b) **Rabbits:** For sedation: 0.5–2 mg/kg IV or IM (IV preferred).

For anesthesia: Diazepam 0.5–1 mg/kg with ketamine (20–35 mg/kg) IM or IV.

Hedgehogs: For long anesthesia: Diazepam at 0.5–2 mg/kg with ketamine at 5–20 mg/kg IM (Kaiser-Klingler 2009)

c) **Hamsters, Gerbils, Mice, Rats:** 3–5 mg/kg IM.

Guinea pigs: 0.5–3 mg/kg IM (Adamcak & Otten 2000)

■ **CATTLE:**

a) Sedative in calves: 0.4 mg/kg IV (Booth 1988)

b) As a tranquilizer: 0.55–1.1 mg/kg IM (Lumb & Jones 1984)

c) Treatment of CNS hyperactivity and seizures: 0.5–1.5 mg/kg IM or IV (Bailey 1986)

■ **HORSES: (Note:** ARCI UCGFS Class 2 Drug)
For field anesthesia:

a) Sedate with xylazine (1 mg/kg IV; 2 mg/kg IM) given 5–10 minutes (longer for IM route) before induction of anesthesia with ketamine (2 mg/kg IV). Horse must be adequately sedated (head to the knees) before giving the ketamine (ketamine can cause muscle rigidity and seizures).

If adequate sedation does not occur, either **1)** Redose xylazine: up to half the original dose; **2)** Add butorphanol (0.02–0.04 mg/kg IV). Butorphanol can be given with the original xylazine if you suspect that the horse will be difficult to tranquilize (*e.g.*, high-strung Thoroughbreds) or added before the ketamine. This combination will improve induction, increase analgesia and increase recumbency time by about 5–10 minutes; **3)** Diazepam (0.03 mg/kg IV). Mix the diazepam with the ketamine. This combination will improve induction when sedation is marginal, improve muscle relaxation during anesthesia and prolong anesthesia by about 5–10 minutes; **4)** Guaifenesin (5% solution administered IV to effect) can also be used to increase sedation and muscle relaxation. (Mathews 1999)

For seizures:

a) **Foals:** 0.05–0.4 mg/kg IV; repeat in 30 minutes if necessary

b) Adults: 25–50 mg IV; repeat in 30 minutes if necessary (Sweeney & Hansen 1987)

Treatment of seizures secondary to intra-arterial injection of xylazine or other similar agents:

a) 0.10–0.15 mg/kg IV (Thurmon & Benson 1987)

As an appetite stimulant:

a) 0.02 mg/kg IV; immediately after dosing, offer animal food. Keep loud noises and distractions to a minimum. If effective, usually only 2–3 treatments in a 24–48 hour period are required. (Ralston 1987)

■ **SWINE:**
For tranquilization:

a) 5.5 mg/kg IM (will develop posterior ataxia in 5 minutes and then recumbency within 10 minutes) (Booth 1988)

b) 0.55–1.1 mg/kg IM (Lumb & Jones 1984)

c) For sedation prior to pentobarbital anesthesia: 8.5 mg/kg IM (maximized at 30 minutes; reduces pentobarbital dose by 50%) (Booth 1988)

For treatment of CNS hyperactivity and seizures:

a) 0.5–1.5 mg/kg IM or IV (Howard 1986)

■ **SHEEP:**
As a tranquilizer:

a) 0.55–1.1 mg/kg IM (Lumb & Jones 1984)

■ **GOATS:**
For Bermuda grass induced toxicosis and tremors:

a) 0.8 mg/kg IV (Booth 1988)

To stimulate appetite:

a) 0.04 mg/kg IV; offer food immediately, duration of effect may last up to 45 minutes (Booth 1988)

■ **BIRDS:**

a) For adjunctive therapy of pain control (with analgesics): 0.5–2 mg/kg IV or IM (Clyde & Paul-Murphy 2000)

b) For sedation/induction: 0.5–2 mg/kg IV or IM. Doses apply to pet birds to the medium parrots. Adjustments would need to be made for large parrots or wild species such as raptors. (Kaiser-Klingler 2009)

■ **ZOO, EXOTIC, WILDLIFE SPECIES:**
For use of diazepam in zoo, exotic and wildlife medicine refer to specific references, including:

a) *Zoo Animal and Wildlife Immobilization and Anesthesia*. West, G, Heard, D, Caulkett, N. (eds.). Blackwell Publishing, 2007.

b) *Handbook of Wildlife Chemical Immobilization, 3rd Ed*. Kreeger, T.J. and J.M. Arnemo. 2007.

c) *Restraint and Handling of Wild and Domestic Animals*. Fowler, M (ed.), Iowa State University Press, 1995

d) *Exotic Animal Formulary, 3rd Ed*. Carpenter, J.W., Saunders. 2005

e) The 2009 American Association of Zoo Veterinarian Proceedings by D. K. Fontenot also has several dosages listed for restraint, anesthesia, and analgesia for a variety of drugs for carnivores and primates. VIN members can access them at: http://goo.gl/BHRih or http://goo.gl/9UJse

Monitoring

■ Horses should be observed carefully after receiving this drug.

■ Cats receiving diazepam should have baseline liver function tests. Repeat and discontinue drug if emesis, lethargy, inappetence, or ataxia develop. When used for seizure control in cats, one author (Quesnel 2000) recommends obtaining serum level 5 days after beginning therapy. Therapeutic serum concentration goals for seizure control in cats ranges from 2500–700 nmol/L (200–700 ng/mL), depending on the source.

Client Information

■ Keep out of reach of children and in tightly closed containers

■ Cats: If patient develops lack of appetite, vomits, or yellowish whites of eyes contact veterinarian immediately

Chemistry/Synonyms

A benzodiazepine, diazepam is a white to yellow, practically odorless crystalline powder with a melting point between 131°–135°C and pK$_a$ of 3.4. Diazepam is tasteless initially, but develops a bitter after-taste. One g is soluble in 333 mL of water, 25 mL of alcohol, and it is sparingly soluble in propylene glycol. The pH of the commercially prepared injectable solution is adjusted with benzoic acid/sodium benzoate to 6.2–6.9. It consists of a 5 mg/mL solution with 40% propylene glycol, 10% ethanol, 5% sodium benzoate/benzoic acid buffer, and 1.5% benzyl alcohol as a preservative.

Diazepam may also be known as: diazepamum, LA-III, NSC-77518, or Ro-5-2807; many trade names are available.

Storage/Stability

All diazepam products should be stored at room temperature (15°–30°C). The injection should be kept from freezing and protected from light. The oral dosage forms (tablets/capsules) should be stored in tight containers and protected from light.

Because diazepam may adsorb to plastic, it should not be stored drawn up into plastic syringes. The drug may also significantly adsorb to IV solution plastic (PVC) bags and to the infusion tubing. This adsorption appears to be dependent on several factors (temperature, concentration, flow rates, line length, etc.).

Compatibility/Compounding Considerations

The manufacturers of injectable diazepam do not recommend the drug be mixed with any other medication or IV diluent and diluting for infusion cannot be recommended. However, some studies have shown that dilution in some IV solutions at low concentrations do not exhibit visible precipitates; but microcrystal formation could not be ruled out

Mixing ketamine with diazepam in the same syringe or IV bag is not recommended as precipitation may occur. Although there are many anecdotal reports of mixing ketamine with diazepam in the same syringe just prior to injection there does not appear to be any published information documenting the stability of the drugs after mixing. Do not use if a visible precipitate forms.

Dosage Forms/Regulatory Status

VETERINARY-LABELED PRODUCTS: None

The ARCI (Racing Commissioners International) has designated this drug as a class 2 substance. See the appendix for more information.

HUMAN-LABELED PRODUCTS:

Diazepam Oral Tablets: 2 mg, 5 mg, & 10 mg; *Valium®* (Roche); generic; (Rx, C-IV)

Diazepam Oral Solution: 1 mg/mL in 500 mL, and 5 mg & 10 mg patient cups; generic (Roxane); (Rx, C-IV); Concentrated oral solution: 5 mg/mL in 30 mL with dropper; *Diazepam Intensol®* (Roxane); (Rx, C-IV)

Diazepam Injection: 5 mg/mL in 2 mL *Carpuject* cartridges; generic; (Rx, C-IV)

Diazepam Rectal Gel: 2.5 mg, 10 mg, & 20 mg; *Diastat®* (Xcel); (Rx, C-IV)

References

Adamcak, A. & B. Otten (2000). Rodent Therapeutics. *Vet Clin NA: Exotic Anim Pract* 3:1(Jan): 221–240.

Bailey, E.M. (1986). Management and treatment of toxicosis in cattle. *Current Veterinary Therapy 2: Food Animal Practice*. JL Howard Ed. Philadelphia, WB Saunders: 341–354.

Bartges, J. (2003). Canine lower urinary tract cases. Proceedings: ACVIM Forum. Accessed via: Veterinary Information Network. http://goo.gl/HH41u

Booth, N.H. (1988). Drugs Acting on the Central Nervous System. *Veterinary Pharmacology and Therapeutics – 6th Ed*. NH Booth and LE McDonald Eds. Ames, Iowa State University Press: 153–408.

Chew, D.J., S.P. DiBartola, et al. (1986). Pharmacologic Manipulation of Urination. *Current Veterinary Therapy IX: Small Animal Practice*. RV Kirk Ed. Philadelphia, W.B. Saunders: 1207–1212.

Clyde, V. & J. Paul–Murphy (2000). Avian Analgesia. *Kirk's Current Veterinary Therapy: XIII Small Animal Practice*. J Bonagura Ed. Philadelphia, WB Saunders: 1126–1128.

Evans, J., D. Levesque, et al. (2002). The use of diazepam in the treatment of metronidazole toxicosis in the dog. Proceedings: ACVIM Forum. Accessed via: Veterinary Information Network. http://goo.gl/M97qr

Haug, L. (2008). Canine aggression toward unfamiliar people and dogs. *Vet Clin NA: Sm Animal Pract* **38**: 1023–1041.

Howard, J.L., Ed. (1986). *Current Veterinary Therapy 2, Food Animal Practice*. Philadelphia, W.B. Saunders.

Ivey, E. & J. Morrisey (2000). Therapeutics for Rabbits. *Vet Clin NA: Exotic Anim Pract* 3:1(Jan): 183–216.

Kaiser–Klingler, S. (2009). Exotic animal anesthesia for the small animal practice. Proceedings: World Veterinary Congress. Accessed via: Veterinary Information Network. http://goo.gl/SdnQy

Knipe, M. (2006). Make it stop! Managing status epilepticus. Proceedings; Vet Neuro Symposium. Accessed via: Veterinary Information Network. http://goo.gl/sDYLA

Knipe, M. (2009). The short and long of seizure management. Proceedings: UCD Veterinary Neurology Symposium. Accessed via: Veterinary Information Network. http://goo.gl/N66kW

Lumb, W.V. & E.W. Jones (1984). *Veterinary Anesthesia, 2nd Ed*. Philadelphia, Lea & Febiger.

Mariani, C. (2010a). Maintenance therapy for the routine & difficult to control epileptic patient. Proceedings: ACVIM Forum. Accessed via: Veterinary Information Network. http://goo.gl/quX8P

Mariani, C. (2010b). Treatment of cluster seizures and stauts epilepticus. Proceedings: ACVIM Forum. Accessed via: Veterinary Information Network. http://goo.gl/QhJST

Mathews, N. (1999). Anesthesia in large animals—Injectable (field) anesthesia: How to make it better. Proceedings: Central Veterinary Conference, Kansas City.

Morrisey, J. & J. Carpenter (2004). Formulary. *Ferrets, Rabbits, and Rodents Clinical Medicine and Surgery 2nd ed*. K Quesenberry and J Carpenter Eds. St Louis, Saunders.

Munana, K. (2010). Current Approaches to Seizure Management. Proceedings: ACVIM Forum. Accessed via: Veterinary Information Network. http://goo.gl/vl8Lp

Neilson, J. (2009). Pharmacologic Interventions for Behavioral Problems. Proceedings: Western Veterinary Conference. Accessed via: Veterinary Information Network. http://goo.gl/HVVZL

Osborne, C., J. Kruger, et al. (2000). Feline Lower Urinary Tract Diseases. *Textbook of Veterinary Internal Medicine: Diseases of the Dog and Cat.* S Ettinger and E Feldman Eds. Philadelphia, WB Saunders. 2: 1710–1747.

Overall, K. (2000). Behavioral Pharmacology. Proceedings: American Animal Hospital Association 67th Annual Meeting, Toronto.

Platt, S. & J. McDonnell (2000). Status epilepticus: Managing refactroy cases and treating out–of–hospital patients. *Comp CE* 22:8(August).

Podell, M. (2006). Status epilepticus: Stopping seizures from the home to the hospital. Proceedings: ACVIM. Accessed via: Veterinary Information Network. http://goo.gl/hffM0

Podell, M. (2009). Status epilepticus: Stopping seizures from home to hospital. Proceedings: IVECCS. http://goo.gl/8bunc

Ralston, S.L. (1987). Feeding Problems. *Current Therapy in Equine Medicine.* NE Robinson Ed. Phialdelphia, WB Saunders: 123–126.

Reisner, I. & K. Houpt (2000). Behavioral Disorders. *Textbook of Veterinary Internal Medicine: Diseases of the Dog and Cat.* S Ettinger and E Feldman Eds. Philadelphia, WB Saunders. 1: 156–162.

Shell, L. (2000). Feline Seizure Disorders. *Kirk's Current Veterinary Therapy: XIII Small Animal Practice.* J Bonagura Ed. Philadelphia, WB Saunders: 963–966.

Sherman, B.L. & D.S. Mills (2008). Canine anxieties and phobias: An update on separation anxiety and noise aversions. *Veterinary Clinics of North America–Small Animal Practice* 38(5): 1081–+.

Sweeney, C.R. & T.O. Hansen (1987). Narcolepsy and epilepsy. *Current Therapy in Equine Medicine.* NE Robinson Ed. Phialdelphia, WB Saunders: 349–353.

Thurmon, J.C. & G.J. Benson (1987). Injectable anesthetics and anesthetic adjuncts. *Vet Clin North Am (Equine Practice)* 3(1): 15–36.

DIAZOXIDE, ORAL

(di-az-**ok**-side)   Proglycem®, Hyperstat IV®

DIRECT VASODILATOR/
HYPERGLYCEMIC

Prescriber Highlights

▶ Orally administered drug used to treat insulinomas in small animals

▶ Contraindications/Cautions: Functional hypoglycemia or hypoglycemia secondary to insulin overdosage (diabetics); hypersensitive to thiazide diuretics; CHF or renal disease

▶ Adverse Effects: Most likely are anorexia, vomiting &/or diarrhea (may be reduced by giving with food). Less likely: tachycardia, hematologic abnormalities, diabetes mellitus, cataracts, & sodium & water retention. Adverse effects are more likely in dogs with hepatic disease.

Uses/Indications

Oral diazoxide has been used in canine and ferret medicine for the treatment of hypoglycemia secondary to hyperinsulin secretion (*e.g.*, insulinoma). Insulinomas are apparently very rare in the cat; there is little experience with this drug in that species.

Pharmacology/Actions

Although related structurally to the thiazide diuretics, diazoxide does not possess any appreciable diuretic activity. By directly causing a vasodilatory effect on the smooth muscle in peripheral arterioles, diazoxide reduces peripheral resistance and blood pressure. To treat malignant hypertension, intravenous diazoxide is generally required for maximal response.

Diazoxide exhibits hyperglycemic activity by directly inhibiting pancreatic insulin secretion. This action may be a result of the drug's capability to decrease the intracellular release of ionized calcium, thereby preventing the release of insulin from the insulin granules. Diazoxide does not apparently affect the synthesis of insulin, nor does it possess any antineoplastic activity. Diazoxide also enhances hyperglycemia by stimulating the beta-adrenergic system thereby stimulating epinephrine release and inhibiting the uptake of glucose by cells.

Pharmacokinetics

The serum half-life of diazoxide has been reported to be about 5 hours in the dog; other pharmacokinetic parameters in the dog appear to be unavailable. In humans, serum diazoxide (at 10 mg/kg PO) levels peaked at about 12 hours after dosing with capsules. It is unknown what blood levels are required to obtain hyperglycemic effects. Highest concentrations of diazoxide are found in the kidneys with high levels also found in the liver and adrenal glands. Approximately 90% of the drug is bound to plasma proteins and it crosses the placenta and into the CNS. It is not known if diazoxide is distributed into milk. Diazoxide is partially metabolized in the liver and is excreted as both metabolites and unchanged drug by the kidneys. Serum half-life of the drug is prolonged in patients with renal impairment.

Contraindications/Precautions/Warnings

Diazoxide should not be used in patients with functional hypoglycemia or for treating hypoglycemia secondary to insulin overdosage in diabetic patients. Unless the potential advantages outweigh the risks, do not use in patients hypersensitive to thiazide diuretics.

Because diazoxide can cause sodium and water retention, use cautiously in patients with congestive heart failure or renal disease.

Adverse Effects

When used to treat insulinomas in dogs, the most commonly seen adverse reactions include hypersalivation, anorexia, vomiting and/or diarrhea; these effects may be lessened by administering the drug with food. Other effects that may be seen include: tachycardia, hematologic abnormalities (agranulocytosis, aplastic anemia, thrombocytopenia), diabetes mellitus, cataracts (secondary to hyperglycemia?), and sodium and water retention.

Administering the drug with meals or temporarily reducing the dose may alleviate the gastrointestinal side effects. Adverse effects may be more readily noted in dogs with concurrent hepatic disease.

Adverse effects reported with diazoxide use in ferrets include: inappetence, vomiting, diarrhea, malaise, and bone marrow suppression.

The drug is reportedly very bitter.

Reproductive/Nursing Safety

In humans, the FDA categorizes this drug as category **C** for use during pregnancy (*Animal studies have shown an adverse effect on the fetus, but there are no adequate studies in humans; or there are no animal reproduction studies and no adequate studies in humans.*)

It is unknown if diazoxide enters milk.

Overdosage/Acute Toxicity

Acute overdosage may result in severe hyperglycemia and ketoacidosis. Treatment should include insulin (see insulin monograph), fluids and electrolytes. Intensive and prolonged monitoring is recommended.

Drug Interactions

The following drug interactions have either been reported or are theoretical in humans or animals receiving diazoxide and may be of significance in veterinary patients:

- **ALPHA-ADRENERGIC AGENTS (e.g., phenoxy-benzamine):** May decrease the effectiveness of diazoxide in increasing glucose levels

- **HYPOTENSIVE AGENTS, OTHER (e.g., hydralazine, prazosin, etc.):** Diazoxide may enhance the hypotensive actions of other hypotensive agents

- **PHENOTHIAZINES (e.g., acepromazine, chlorpromazine):** May enhance the hyperglycemic effects of diazoxide

- **PHENYTOIN:** Diazoxide may increase the metabolism, or decrease the protein binding of phenytoin

- **THIAZIDE DIURETICS:** May potentiate the hyperglycemic effects of oral diazoxide. Some clinicians have recommended using hydrochlorothiazide (2–4 mg/kg/day PO) in combination with diazoxide, if diazoxide is ineffective alone to increase blood glucose levels; Caution: hypotension may occur

Laboratory Considerations

- Diazoxide will cause a false-negative insulin response to the **glucagon-stimulation** test.

- Diazoxide may displace **bilirubin** from plasma proteins

Doses

- **DOGS:**

For hypoglycemia secondary to insulin secreting islet cell tumors:

a Initially, 5 mg/kg PO twice daily; increase to a maximum of 30 mg/kg PO twice daily to control clinical signs (Meleo and Caplan 2000)

b) If after frequent feedings (4–6 small meals per day) and glucocorticoids (prednisone 1.1–4.4 mg/kg/day) alone fail to control hypoglycemia or dog develops "Cushingoid" appearance, add diazoxide (reduce prednisone dose if "Cushingoid") initially at 10 mg/kg divided twice a day. May gradually increase dosage to 60 mg/kg/day as tolerated and add hydrochlorothiazide (2–4 mg/kg/day). (Feldman & Nelson 1987)

For adjunctive therapy of hypoglycemia secondary to insulin secreting non-islet cell (extra-pancreatic) tumors:

a) Diazoxide 5–13 mg/kg PO three times daily (may add hydrochlorothiazide 2–4 mg/kg/day) (Weller 1988)

- **CATS:**

For hypoglycemia secondary to insulin secreting islet cell tumors:

a) Initially, 5 mg/kg PO twice daily; increase to a maximum of 30 mg/kg PO twice daily to control clinical signs (Meleo & Caplan 2000)

- **FERRETS:**

For hypoglycemia secondary to insulin secreting islet cell tumors:

a) After surgical resection of pancreatic nodules or partial pancreatectomy: Prednisone at 0.5–2 mg/kg PO q12h will usually control mild to moderate clinical signs. Begin at lowest dose and gradually increase as needed. Add diazoxide when clinical signs cannot be controlled with prednisone alone. Begin at 5–10 mg/kg PO q12h. At same time prednisone dosage may be lowered. (Johnson 2006)

Monitoring

■ Blood (serum) glucose

■ CBC (at least every 3–4 months)

■ Physical exam (monitor for clinical signs of other adverse effects—see above)

Client Information

■ Clients should be instructed to monitor for symptoms of hyper- or hypoglycemia, abnormal bleeding, GI disturbances, etc.

Chemistry/Synonyms

Related structurally to the thiazide diuretics, diazoxide occurs as an odorless, white to creamy-white, crystalline powder with a melting point of about 330°. It is practically insoluble to sparingly soluble in water and slightly soluble in alcohol.

Diazoxide may also be known as: diazoxidum, NSC-64198, Sch-6783, SRG-95213, *Eudemine®*, *Glicemin®*, *Hypertonalum®*, *Hyperstat IV®*, *Proglicem®*, *Sefulken®*, or *Tensuril®*.

Storage/Stability

Diazoxide capsules and oral suspensions should be stored at 2–30°C and protected from light. Protect solutions/suspensions from freezing. Do not use darkened solutions/suspensions, as they may be subpotent.

Compatibility/Compounding Considerations

Diazoxide has a very bitter taste and taste masking agents (preferably sugar free) may be useful in increasing patient acceptance of this medication.

Dosage Forms/Regulatory Status

VETERINARY-LABELED PRODUCTS: None

The ARCI (Racing Commissioners International) has designated this drug as a class 3 substance. See the appendix for more information.

HUMAN-LABELED PRODUCTS:

Diazoxide Oral Capsules: 50 mg; *Proglycem®* (Ivax); (Rx)

Diazoxide Oral Suspension: 50 mg; with sorbitol in 30 mL calibrated dropper; *Proglycem®* (Ivax); (Rx)

References

Feldman, E.C. & R.W. Nelson (1987). *Canine and Feline Endocrinology and Reproduction*. Philadelphia, WB Saunders.

Johnson, D. (2006). Ferrets: the other companion animal. Proceedings: ACVC. Accessed via: Veterinary Information Network. http://goo.gl/bSeol

Meleo, K. & E. Caplan (2000). Treatment of insulinoma in the dogs, cat, and ferret. *Kirk's Current Veterinary Therapy: XIII Small Animal Practice*. J Bonagura Ed. Philadelphia, WB Saunders: 357–361.

Weller, R.E. (1988). Paraneoplastic Syndromes. *Handbook of Small Animal Practice*. RV Morgan Ed. New York, Churchill Livingstone: 819–827.

DICHLORPHENAMIDE

(dye-klor-*fen*-a-mide)   Daranide®

CARBONIC ANHYDRASE INHIBITOR

Prescriber Highlights

▶ Used primarily for open angle glaucoma

▶ Contraindicated in patients with significant hepatic, renal, pulmonary or adrenocortical insufficiency, hyponatremia, hypokalemia, hyperchloremic acidosis or electrolyte imbalance

▶ Give oral doses with food if GI upset occurs

▶ Monitor with tonometry for glaucoma; check electrolytes

▶ Availability issues; may need to be obtained from a compounding pharmacy

Uses/Indications

Dichlorphenamide is used for the medical treatment of glaucoma. Because of availability issues and toxic effects associated with systemic therapy, human (and many veterinary) ophthalmologists are using topical carbonic anhydrase inhibitors (*e.g.,* dorzolamide or brinzolamide) in place of acetazolamide, dichlorphenamide or methazolamide.

Pharmacology/Actions

The carbonic anhydrase inhibitors act by a non-competitive, reversible inhibition of the enzyme carbonic anhydrase. This reduces the formation of hydrogen and bicarbonate ions from carbon dioxide and reduces the availability of these ions for active transport into body secretions.

Pharmacologic effects of the carbonic anhydrase inhibitors include decreased formation of aqueous humor, thereby reducing intraocular pressure; increased renal tubular secretion of sodium and potassium and, to a greater extent, bicarbonate, leading to increased urine alkalinity and volume; and anticonvulsant activity, which is independent of its diuretic effects (mechanism not fully understood, but may be due to carbonic anhydrase or a metabolic acidosis effect).

Pharmacokinetics

The pharmacokinetics of this agent have apparently not been studied in domestic animals. In small animals, onset of action is 30 minutes, maximal effect in 2–4 hours, and duration of action is 8–12 hours.

Contraindications/Precautions/Warnings

Carbonic anhydrase inhibitors are contraindicated in patients with significant hepatic disease (may precipitate hepatic coma), renal or adrenocortical insufficiency, hyponatremia, hypokalemia, hyperchloremic acidosis, or electrolyte imbalance. They should not be used in patients with severe pulmonary obstruction unable to increase alveolar ventilation or those who are hypersensitive to them. Long-term use of carbonic anhydrase inhibitors is contraindicated in patients with chronic, noncongestive, angle-closure glaucoma as angle closure may occur and the drug may mask the condition by lowering intra-ocular pressures.

Adverse Effects

Potential adverse effects that may be encountered include panting, GI disturbances (inappetence, vomiting, diarrhea), CNS effects (sedation, depression, excitement, etc.), hematologic effects (bone marrow depression), renal effects (crystalluria, dysuria, renal colic, polyuria), metabolic acidosis, hypokalemia, hyperglycemia, hyponatremia, hyperuricemia, hepatic insufficiency, dermatologic effects (rash, etc.), and hypersensitivity reactions.

Reproductive/Nursing Safety

In humans, the FDA categorizes this drug as category *C* for use during pregnancy (*Animal studies have shown an adverse effect on the fetus, but there are no adequate studies in humans; or there are no animal reproduction studies and no adequate studies in humans.*)

Overdosage/Acute Toxicity

Information regarding overdosage of this drug is not readily available. It is suggested to monitor serum electrolytes, blood gases, volume status, and CNS status during an acute overdose. Treat symptomatically and supportively.

Drug Interactions

The following drug interactions have either been reported or are theoretical in humans or animals receiving dichlorphenamide and may be of significance in veterinary patients:

- **ANTIDEPRESSANTS, TRICYCLIC:** Alkaline urine cause by dichlorphenamide may decrease excretion

- **ASPIRIN (or other salicylates):** Increased risk of dichlorphenamide accumulation and toxicity; increased risk for metabolic acidosis; dichlorphenamide increases salicylate excretion

- **DIGOXIN:** As dichlorphenamide may cause hypokalemia, increased risk for toxicity

- **INSULIN:** Rarely, carbonic anhydrase inhibitors interfere with the hypoglycemic effects of insulin

- **METHENAMINE COMPOUNDS:** Dichlorphenamide may negate effects in the urine

- **POTASSIUM, DRUGS AFFECTING (corticosteroids, amphotericin B, corticotropin, or other diuretics):** Concomitant use may exacerbate potassium depletion

- **PHENOBARBITAL:** Increased urinary excretion, may reduce phenobarbital levels

- **PRIMIDONE:** Decreased primidone concentrations

- **QUINIDINE:** Alkaline urine cause by dichlorphenamide may decrease excretion

Laboratory Considerations

- By alkalinizing the urine, carbonic anhydrase inhibitors may cause false positive results in determining **urine protein** using bromphenol blue reagent (*Albustix®*, *Albutest®*, *Labstix®*), sulfosalicylic acid (*Bumintest®*, Exton's Test Reagent), nitric acid ring test, or heat and acetic acid test methods.

- Carbonic anhydrase inhibitors may decrease **iodine uptake** by the thyroid gland in hyperthyroid or euthyroid patients.

Doses

- **DOGS:**

  For adjunctive treatment of glaucoma:

  a) 2.2–4.4 mg/kg PO two to three times daily (q8–12h) (Nasisse 2005), (Miller 2005)

  b) 10–15 mg/kg per day divided 2–3 times daily (Brooks 2002)

  c) 2–5 mg/kg PO q8–12h (Wilkie 2003)

- **CATS:**

  For adjunctive treatment of glaucoma:

  a) 0.5–1.5 mg/kg PO two to three times daily (Powell 2003)

  b) 1–2 mg/kg PO q8–12h (Miller 2005)

Monitoring

- Intraocular pressure/tonometry

- Serum electrolytes; may need to supplement potassium

- Baseline CBC with differential and periodic retests if using chronically

- Other adverse effects

Client Information

- If GI upset occurs, give with food.

- Notify veterinarian if abnormal bleeding or bruising occurs or if animal develops tremors or a rash.

Chemistry/Synonyms

A carbonic anhydrase inhibitor, dichlorphenamide occurs as a white or nearly white, crystalline powder with a melting range of 235–240°C, and pK_as of 7.4 and 8.6. It is very slightly soluble in water and soluble in alcohol.

Dichlorphenamide may also be known as: dichlorphenamide, diclofenamidum, *Antidrasi®*, *Fenamide®*, *Glaucol®*, *Glauconide®*, *Glaumid®*, *Oralcon®*, *Oratrol®*, or *Tensodilen®*.

Storage/Stability

Store tablets in well-closed containers and at room temperature. An expiration date of 5 years after the date of manufacture is assigned to the commercially available tablets.

Dosage Forms/Regulatory Status

VETERINARY-LABELED PRODUCTS: None

HUMAN-LABELED PRODUCTS: None

Dichlorphenamide availability has been an issue and it may not be available commercially; if not, contact a compounding pharmacy for information.

References

Brooks, D.E. (2002). Glaucoma–Medical and Surgical Treatment. Proceedings: Western Veterinary Conference. Accessed via: Veterinary Information Network. http://goo.gl/LwKdh

Miller, P. (2005). New drugs for glaucoma. Proceedings: Western Vet Conf. Accessed via: Veterinary Information Network. http://goo.gl/otZtU

Nasisse, M. (2005). Treatment of canine glaucoma, Proceedings: ACVIM. Accessed via: Veterinary Information Network. http://goo.gl/Uv8BB

Powell, C. (2003). Feline Glaucoma. Proceedings: Western Veterinary Conference. Accessed via: Veterinary Information Network. http://goo.gl/29jgx

Wilkie, D. (2003). Glaucoma. Proceedings: Atlantic Coast Veterinary Conference. Accessed via: Veterinary Information Network. http://goo.gl/mTse9

DICHLORVOS

(dye-**klor**-vose)   Atgard®

ORGANOPHOSPHATE ANTIPARASITIC

Prescriber Highlights

▶ Organophosphate used orally as a wormer (primarily roundworms) in pigs & as ectoparasiticide ("No Pest Strip") for small mammals, etc.

▶ Contraindications: Anticholinesterase drugs; do not allow fowl access to medicated feed or manure from treated animals

▶ Adverse Effects (dose related): Vomiting, tremors, bradycardia, respiratory distress, hyperexcitability, salivation, & diarrhea

▶ Drug Interactions

Uses/Indications

Dichlorvos is effective in swine against Ascaris, Trichuris, *Ascarops strongylina* and *Oesophagostomum* spp.

Dichlorvos as a "No Pest Strip" is used as an ectoparasiticide for small mammals. It is also used as a premise spray to keep fly populations controlled.

In horses, dichlorvos is labeled as being effective for the treatment and control of bots, pinworms, large and small bloodworms, and large roundworms, but no systemic equine products are currently being marketed in the USA.

Dichlorvos was available for use internally in dogs and cats for the treatment of roundworms and hookworms, but no products are currently being marketed since newer, safer and more effective anthelmintics have replaced dichlorvos.

Pharmacology/Actions

Like other organophosphate agents, dichlorvos inhibits acetylcholinesterase interfering with neuromuscular transmission in susceptible parasites.

Pharmacokinetics

Specific information was not located for this agent.

Contraindications/Precautions/Warnings

For the product (*Atgard*®) for use in swine, no adverse contraindications are labeled, but it should not be used within a few days of any other cholinesterase inhibiting drug, pesticide or chemical.

Do not allow fowl access to medicated feed or manure from treated animals.

Unused medication or medicated feed should be buried 18 inches below the ground and covered so that it is unavailable to any other animal.

Avoid contact with the skin and keep out of reach of children.

Adverse Effects

When used as labeled, there are no listed adverse effects in swine. Adverse effects are generally dose-related and may include those listed below in the Overdosage/Acute Toxicity section.

Reproductive/Nursing Safety

Studies performed in target species have demonstrated no teratogenic effects at usual doses. In pigs, no effects have been noted on reproductive capability, performance or litter survivability.

Overdosage/Acute Toxicity

If overdoses occur, vomiting, tremors, bradycardia, respiratory distress, hyperexcitability, salivation, and diarrhea may occur. Atropine (see atropine and pralidoxime monographs for more information) may be antidotal. Use of succinylcholine, theophylline, aminophylline, reserpine, or respiratory depressant drugs (*e.g.*, narcotics, phenothiazines) should be avoided in patients with organophosphate toxicity. If ingestion occurs by a human, contact a poison control center, physician, or hospital emergency room.

Drug Interactions

The following drug interactions have either been reported or are theoretical in humans or animals receiving dichlorvos and may be of significance in veterinary patients:

◼ **ACEPROMAZINE or other phenothiazines:** Should not be given within one month of worming with an organophosphate agent as their effects may be potentiated

◼ **ANTICHOLINESTERASE DRUGS (e.g., neostigmine, physostigmine, and pyridostigmine):** Avoid use when using organophosphates as they can inhibit cholinesterase

◼ **DMSO:** Because of its anticholinesterase activity, avoid the use of organophosphates with DMSO

◼ **MORPHINE:** Avoid use when using organophosphates as it can inhibit cholinesterase

◼ **PYRANTEL PAMOATE (or tartrate):** Adverse effects could be intensified if used concomitantly with an organophosphate

- **SUCCINYLCHOLINE:** Patients receiving organophosphate anthelmintics should not receive succinylcholine or other depolarizing muscle relaxants for at least 48 hours

Doses

- **RABBITS/RODENTS/SMALL MAMMALS:**
  a) **Mice, Rats, Gerbils, Hamsters, Guinea pigs, Chinchillas:** Hang 5 cm of a dichlorvos strip (*e.g., Vapona No Pest Strip*) 6 inches above cage for 24 hours, twice weekly for 3 weeks (Anderson 1994); (Adamcak & Otten 2000) or hang in room for 24 hours once a week for 6 weeks or a 1 inch square laid on cage for 24 hours once a week for 6 weeks (Adamcak & Otten 2000)

- **SWINE:**
  a) For *Atgard® Swine Wormer:* Dosing for pigs is accomplished by adding to feed (crumble-type or dry meal). Specific amounts of feed per packet are dependent on pig weight. See the label for specific recommendations.

Monitoring

- Efficacy
- Adverse effects

Client Information

- Keep out of reach of children. Handling of dichlorvos liquid preparations (*e.g.,* premise spray) must be done with extreme care; follow all label directions!
- Oral pellets are non-digestible and may be seen in the animals' feces.

Chemistry/Synonyms

An organophosphate insecticide, dichlorvos may also known as: 2,2,-dichlorovinyl dimethyl phosphate DDVP, NSC-6738, OMS-14, SD-1750, *Atgard®*, or *Ravap E.C.®*.

Storage/Stability

Store *Atgard®* swine wormer at less than 80°F. Dichlorvos feed additives should not be stored at temperatures below freezing. Dichlorvos is sensitive to hydrolysis if exposed to moisture or oxidizing agents.

Dosage Forms/Regulatory Status

VETERINARY-LABELED PRODUCTS:

Dichlorvos Feed Additives: *Atgard®* C (Boehringer Ingelheim); (OTC); *Atgard®* Swine Wormer (Boehringer Ingelheim); (OTC). When used as labeled there are no slaughter withdrawal times required in swine.

Dichlorvos with Tetrachlorvinphos (*Rabon®*) Premise and Topical Insecticide: *Ravap E.C.®* (Boehringer Ingelheim); (OTC)

Dichlorvos may also be found in premise insecticidal products.

HUMAN-LABELED PRODUCTS: None

References

Adamcak, A. & B. Otten (2000). Rodent Therapeutics. *Vet Clin NA: Exotic Anim Pract* 3:1(Jan): 221–240.
Anderson, N. (1994). Basic husbandry and medicine of pocket pets. *Saunders Manual of Small Animal Practice.* S Birchard and R Sherding Eds. Philadelphia, W.B. Saunders Company: 1363–1389.

DICLAZURIL

(dye-*klaz*-yoor-il)   Protazil®, Clinicox®

ANTIPROTOZOAL

Prescriber Highlights

➤ FDA-approved (in USA) for EPM in horses & as a coccidiostat in broiler chickens

➤ Adverse effect profile not well known

Uses/Indications

In the USA, diclazuril is FDA-approved for the treatment of equine protozoal myeloencephalitis (EPM) caused by *Sarcocystis neurona* and as a coccidiostat in broiler chickens.

In the U.K., oral diclazuril suspension is approved for the treatment and prevention of coccidial infections in lambs caused, in particular, by the more pathogenic *Eimeria* species *E. crandallis* and *E. ovinoidalis* and to aid in the control of coccidiosis in calves caused by *Eimeria bovis* and *Eimeria zuernii*. Recent studies, comparing diclazuril and toltrazuril have shown that toltrazuril is more effective in reducing oocyte shedding in lambs and calves than is diclazuril (Le Sueur *et al.* 2009), (Mundt *et al.* 2009), (Mundt *et al.* 2007).

Diclazuril could potentially be useful in treating coccidiosis, *Neospora caninum* and Toxoplasma infections in dogs or cats.

Pharmacology/Actions

The triazine class of antiprotozoals are believed to target the "plastid" body, an organelle found in the members of the Apicomplexa phylum, including *Sarcocystis neurona*. The actual mechanism of action is not well described. *In vitro* levels required to inhibit (95%) *Sarcocystis neurona* are about 1 ng/mL.

Pharmacokinetics

In horses, oral bioavailability is about 5%. CSF levels are approximately 1-5% of those found in plasma. Elimination half-life is prolonged (43–65 hours). Doses of 1 mg/kg/day should give mean steady-state plasma levels of about 2–2.5 mg/mL with corresponding CSF levels of 20–70 ng/mL which is in excess of the *in vitro* IC_{95} (1 ng/mL).

Contraindications/Precautions/Warnings

The drug is contraindicated in patients known to be hypersensitive to diclazuril.

The safe use of *Protazil®* in horses used for breeding purposes, during pregnancy, in lactation, or with other therapies has not been evaluated.

Adverse Effects

The adverse effect profile in horses is not well known. In field trials, no adverse effects could be ascribed to the drug.

On rare occasions, highly susceptible lambs may develop severe diarrhea (scour) after dosing; fluid therapy is required and antibiotics may be necessary.

Reproductive/Nursing Safety

The manufacturer states that the safe use of *Protazil®* in horses used for breeding purposes, during pregnancy, or in lactation has not been evaluated.

Overdosage/Acute Toxicity

Limited information is available, but the drug appears to have large safety margin in animals. Normal horses dosed up to 50 mg/kg/day (50X) for 42 days developed only marginal effects (decreased weight gain, increased creatinine, BUN). Doses of up to 60X in lambs and calves did not cause any demonstrable side effects.

Drug Interactions

■ None were noted. The manufacturer states that the safety of *Protazil®* with concomitant therapies in horses has not been evaluated.

Laboratory Considerations

■ None were noted.

Doses

■ **DOGS/CATS:**

a) For coccidiosis: 25 mg/kg PO once. (Greene *et al.* 2006)

b) For coccidiosis in kittens: 1 mL (2.5 mg) PO of the sheep solution per 4 kg body mass. (Miller 2007)

c) For *Isospora* spp. infections in cats: 25 mg/kg PO once. (Dubey *et al.* 2009)

■ **HORSES:**

a) For treatment of equine protozoal myeloencephalitis (*S. neurona*): Using the oral pellets and the provided cup: Top dress at the rate of 1 mg/kg bodyweight for 28 days. If horse's bodyweight is in between two graduations on the dosing cup, fill the cup to the higher of the two marks. (Label information; *Protazil®*—Schering-Plough)

■ **SHEEP (LAMBS):**

a) Therapeutic use: 1 mg/kg (1 mL of the 2.5mg/mL suspension per 2.5 kg bodyweight) PO once. For preventative use: 1 mg/kg PO at about 4-6 weeks of age at the time that coccidiosis can normally be expected on the farm. Under conditions of high infection pressure, a second treatment may be indicated about 3 weeks after the first dosing. Recommended to treat all lambs in flock. (Label Information; *Vecoxan®*—Janssen U.K.)

■ **CATTLE (CALVES):**

a) As an aid to control coccidiosis: 1 mg/kg (1 mL of the 2.5 mg/mL suspension per 2.5 kg bodyweight) PO as a single dose, 14 days after moving into a potentially high risk environment. If a satisfactory response is not observed, then further advice should be sought from your veterinary surgeon and the cause of the condition should be reviewed. It is good practice to ensure the cleanliness of calf housing. Recommended to treat all calves in pen (Label Information; *Vecoxan®*—Janssen U.K.)

Monitoring

■ Clinical efficacy (neuro exams)

Client Information

■ Must be dosed daily as prescribed to be effective

■ Will not necessarily return a horse to "normal"

■ If using oral suspension, shake well before use and store below 30°C.

Chemistry/Synonyms

Diclazuril occurs as a white to light yellow powder. It is practically insoluble in water and alcohol.

Diclazuril may also be known as diclazurilo, diclazurilum, R 64433 and by the trade names, *Clinicox®*, *Protazil®*, and *Vecoxan®*.

Storage/Stability

Diclazuril pellets should be stored at room temperature (15–30°C).

Dosage Forms/Regulatory Status

VETERINARY-LABELED PRODUCTS:

Diclazuril Oral Pellets 1.56% in 2 lb. and 10 lb. containers: *Protazil®* (Schering-Plough); (Rx). FDA-approved for use in horses not intended for food. One 2 lb. bucket will treat an 1100 lb. horse for 28 days.

Diclazuril 0.2% Type A Medicated Feed Article in 50 lb. containers; *Clinicox®* (Schering-Plough). FDA-approved for use in broiler chickens.

In the UK and other countries, diclazuril may be available as an oral suspension containing 2.5 mg/mL diclazuril. One trade name is *Vecoxan®* (Janssen). When used as labeled, no withdrawal time is required in the U.K.

HUMAN-LABELED PRODUCTS: None

References

Dubey, J., D. Lindsay, et al. (2009). Toxoplasmosis and other intestinal coccidial infections in cats and dogs. *Vet Clin Small Anim* 39: 1009–1034.

Greene, C., K. Hartmannn, et al. (2006). Appendix 8: Antimicrobial Drug Formulary. *Infectious Disease of the Dog and Cat.* C Greene Ed., Elsevier: 1186–1333.

Le Sueur, C., C. Mage, et al. (2009). Efficacy of toltrazuril (BaycoxA (R) 5% suspension) in natural infections with pathogenic Eimeria spp. in housed lambs. *Parasitology Research* 104(5): 1157–1162.

Miller, D. (2007). Kitten Diarrhoea. Proceedings: World Small Animal Association. Accessed via: Veterinary Information Network. http://goo.gl/P95JW

Mundt, H.C., K. Dittmar, et al. (2009). Study of the Comparative Efficacy of Toltrazuril and Diclazuril against Ovine Coccidiosis in Housed Lambs. *Parasitology Research* 105: S141–S150.

Mundt, H.C., F. Rodder, et al. (2007). Control of coccidiosis due to Eimeria bovis and Eimeria zuernii in calves with toltrazuril under field conditions in comparison with diclazuril and untreated controls. *Parasitology Research* 101: S93–S104.

DICLOFENAC SODIUM

(dye-*kloe*-fen-ak)   Surpass®

NON-STEROIDAL ANTIINFLAMMATORY (NSAID)

Prescriber Highlights

▶ NSAID FDA-approved for topical use in horses for local control of joint pain & inflammation

▶ Appears well-tolerated at recommended dosage

Uses/Indications

The equine topical cream (*Surpass®*) is labeled for the control of pain and inflammation associated with osteoarthritis in tarsal, carpal, metacarpophalangeal, metarsophalangeal, and proximal interphalangeal (hock, knee, fetlock, pastern) joints for use up to 10 days duration. While, theoretically, diclofenac could be used systemically (orally) in other veterinary species, there are FDA-approved and safer alternatives.

Pharmacology/Actions

Diclofenac is a non-specific inhibitor of cyclooxygenase (both COX-1 and COX-2). It may also have some inhibitory effects on lipooxygenase. By inhibiting COX-2 enzymes, diclofenac reduces the production of prostaglandins associated with pain, hyperpyrexia, and inflammation.

Pharmacokinetics

When diclofenac is administered topically to horses via the 1% liposomal cream, it is absorbed locally, but specific bioavailability data was not located. Peak levels in transudate obtained from tissue cages were about 80 ng/mL; levels stay increased from 6 hours to at least 18 hours after administration. At the dosages recommended for the topical cream, most of the drug remains in the tissues local to the administration point, but detectable levels in the systemic circulation may occur. In humans, diclofenac is more than 99% bound to plasma proteins. It is metabolized in the liver and the metabolites are excreted primarily into the urine.

Contraindications/Precautions/Warnings

Topical diclofenac should not be used in horses hypersensitive to it or any component of the cream. It has not been evaluated in horses less than one year old.

Exceeding the recommended dosage or treating multiple joints may cause adverse effects.

Do not use diclofenac in birds as it has been implicated in causing death in vultures.

Adverse Effects

The topical cream in horses appears to be well tolerated. One case of a horse developing colic during therapy has been reported. Other adverse effects that may be seen include weight loss, gastric ulcers, diarrhea, or uterine discharge. In the FDA's adverse reaction database local reactions (inflammation, swelling, alopecia) have been reported.

Reproductive/Nursing Safety

Reproductive safety for topical diclofenac has not been investigated in breeding, pregnant or lactating horses.

Overdosage/Acute Toxicity

When overdoses are administered topically to horses, adverse effects may occur including weight loss, gastric ulcers, colic, diarrhea, and uterine discharge. Treatment is supportive.

For small animals, There were 140 exposures to diclofenac sodium reported to the ASPCA Animal Poison Control Center (APCC) during 2008-2009. In these cases 131 were dogs with 37 showing clinical signs and the remaining 9 cases were cat exposures with 3 showing clinical signs. Common findings in dogs recorded in decreasing frequency included vomiting, diarrhea, bloody diarrhea, melena and polydipsia.

This medication is a NSAID. As with any NSAID, overdosage can lead to gastrointestinal and renal effects. Decontamination with emetics and/or activated charcoal is appropriate. For doses where GI effects are expected, the use of gastrointestinal protectants is warranted. If renal effects are also expected, fluid diuresis is warranted.

Diclofenac ingestion has caused death in vultures eating dead carcasses of animals that received diclofenac.

Drug Interactions

When used topically at recommended dosages, there are no reported drug interactions in horses.

Laboratory Considerations

■ No specific laboratory interactions or considerations were noted.

Doses

■ **HORSES:**

a) For the control of pain and inflammation associated with osteoarthritis in tarsal, carpal, metacarpophalangeal, metarsophalangeal, and proximal interphalangeal (hock, knee, fetlock, pastern) joints using *Surpass®* topical cream: Apply a five inch ribbon twice daily over the affected joint for up to 10 days. Wear rubber gloves and rub cream thoroughly into the hair covering the joint until cream disappears. (Label information; *Surpass®*—Idexx)

Monitoring

■ Efficacy

■ Adverse effects

Client Information

■ Clients should be instructed to use as directed, not to increase the dose (area applied) or duration (not too exceed 10 days), or adverse effects may occur.

■ Clients should wear protective gloves (non-permeable) when applying the cream.

■ A client information sheet is supplied with the medication and should be given to the client.

Chemistry/Synonyms

A phenyl-acetic acid derivative non-steroidal antiinflammatory agent, diclofenac sodium occurs as a white to off-white, hygroscopic, crystalline powder. It is sparingly soluble in water, soluble in alcohol and practically insoluble in chloroform and ether.

Diclofenac may also be known as: GP-45840, diclofenacum or diclophenac; many trade names are available for diclofenac products outside of the USA.

Storage/Stability

Unless otherwise labeled, diclofenac sodium products should be stored in airtight containers and protected from light. The commercially available 1% cream (*Surpass®*) should be stored at temperatures up to 25°C (77°F); protect from freezing.

Dosage Forms/Regulatory Status

VETERINARY-LABELED PRODUCTS:

Diclofenac sodium (liposomal) 1% topical cream in 124 g tubes, *Surpass®* (Idexx); (Rx). FDA-approved for use in horses.

Injectable forms of this medication are available in some countries.

HUMAN-LABELED PRODUCTS:

Diclofenac Tablets: 50 mg (as potassium); *Cataflam®* (Novartis); generic; (Rx)

Diclofenac Delayed-release Tablets: 25 mg, 50 mg, 75 mg & 100 mg (as sodium); *Voltaren-XR®* (Novartis); generic; (Rx)

Diclofenac Sodium Gel: 3% (1 g contains 30 mg diclofenac sodium) with benzyl alcohol in 25 g & 50 g; *Solaraze®* (SkyePharma); (Rx)

Diclofenac Sodium/Misoprostol Tablets: (each tablet consists of an enteric-coated core containing diclofenac sodium surrounded by an outer mantle containing misoprostol) 50 mg/misoprostol 200 mcg & 75 mg/misoprostol 200 mcg; *Arthrotec®* (Searle) (Rx)

Diclofenac sodium is also FDA-approved as a topical ophthalmic agent (see the ophthalmology drug appendix).

DICLOXACILLIN SODIUM

(di-klox-a-*sill*-in)   Dynapen®

ANTI-STAPHYLOCOCCAL PENICILLIN

Prescriber Highlights

▶ Oral isoxazolyl (anti-staphylococcal) penicillin

▶ Contraindications: hypersensitivity to penicillins; do not use oral medications in critically ill patients

▶ Most predominant adverse effects are GI in nature

▶ Must dose orally quite often (q6–8h); expense, efficacy & owner compliance may be issues

---

Uses/Indications

The veterinary use of dicloxacillin has been primarily in the PO treatment of bone, skin, and other soft tissue infections in small animals when penicillinase-producing Staphylococcus species have been isolated. Because of its low oral bioavailability and short half-life, other drugs with good staph coverage are usually employed.

Pharmacology/Actions

Cloxacillin, dicloxacillin and oxacillin have nearly identical spectrums of activity and can be considered therapeutically equivalent when comparing *in vitro* activity. These penicillinase-resistant penicillins have a narrower spectrum of activity than the natural penicillins. Their antimicrobial efficacy is aimed directly against penicillinase-producing strains of gram-positive cocci, particularly Staphylococcal species. They are sometimes called anti-staphylococcal penicillins. There are documented strains of Staphylococcus that are resistant to these drugs (so-called methicillin-resistant Staph, MRSA), but these strains have not yet been a major problem in veterinary species. While this class of penicillins does have activity against some other gram-positive and gram-negative aerobes and anaerobes, other antibiotics (penicillins and others) are usually better choices. The penicillinase-resistant penicillins are inactive against Rickettsia, mycobacteria, fungi, Mycoplasma and viruses.

Pharmacokinetics

Dicloxacillin is only available in oral dosage forms. Dicloxacillin sodium is resistant to acid inactivation in the gut but is only partially absorbed. The bioavailability after oral administration in dogs is only about 23% and in humans has been reported to range from 35–76%. If given with food, both the rate and extent of absorption is decreased.

The drug is distributed to the liver, kidneys,

bone, bile, pleural, synovial and ascitic fluids. However, one manufacturer states that levels of the drug that are achieved in ascitic fluid are not clinically therapeutic. As with the other penicillins, only minimal amounts are distributed into the CSF. In humans, approximately 95–99% of the drug is bound to plasma proteins.

Dicloxacillin is partially metabolized to both active and inactive metabolites. These metabolites and the parent compound are rapidly excreted in the urine via both glomerular filtration and tubular secretion mechanisms. A small amount of the drug is also excreted in the feces via biliary elimination. The serum half-life in humans with normal renal function ranges from about 24–48 minutes. In dogs, 20–40 minutes to 2.6 hours have been reported as the elimination half-life.

Contraindications/Precautions/Warnings

Penicillins are contraindicated in patients with a history of hypersensitivity to them. Because there may be cross-reactivity, use penicillins cautiously in patients who are documented hypersensitive to other beta-lactam antibiotics (e.g., cephalosporins, cefamycins, carbapenems).

Do not administer systemic antibiotics orally in patients with septicemia, shock, or other grave illnesses as absorption of the medication from the GI tract may be significantly delayed or diminished. Parenteral (preferably IV) routes should be used for these cases.

Adverse Effects

Adverse effects with the penicillins are usually not serious and have a relatively low frequency of occurrence.

Hypersensitivity reactions unrelated to dose can occur with these agents and can manifest as rashes, fever, eosinophilia, neutropenia, agranulocytosis, thrombocytopenia, leukopenia, anemias, lymphadenopathy, or full-blown anaphylaxis. In humans, it is estimated that 1–15% of patients hypersensitive to cephalosporins will also be hypersensitive to penicillins. The incidence of cross-reactivity in veterinary patients is unknown.

When given orally, penicillins may cause GI effects (anorexia, vomiting, diarrhea). Because the penicillins may also alter gut flora, antibiotic-associated diarrhea can occur and allow the proliferation of resistant bacteria in the colon (superinfections).

Neurotoxicity (e.g., ataxia in dogs) has been associated with very high doses or very prolonged use. Although the penicillins are not considered hepatotoxic, elevated liver enzymes have been reported. Other effects reported in dogs include tachypnea, dyspnea, edema, and tachycardia.

Reproductive/Nursing Safety

Penicillins have been shown to cross the placenta and safe use of them during pregnancy has not been firmly established, but neither have there been any documented teratogenic problems associated with these drugs. However, use only when the potential benefits outweigh the risks. In humans, the FDA categorizes this drug as category **B** for use during pregnancy (*Animal studies have not yet demonstrated risk to the fetus, but there are no adequate studies in pregnant women; or animal studies have shown an adverse effect, but adequate studies in pregnant women have not demonstrated a risk to the fetus in the first trimester of pregnancy, and there is no evidence of risk in later trimesters.*) In a separate system evaluating the safety of drugs in canine and feline pregnancy (Papich 1989), this drug is categorized as in class: **A** (*Probably safe. Although specific studies may not have proved the safety of all drugs in dogs and cats, there are no reports of adverse effects in laboratory animals or women.*)

Dicloxacillin is distributed into milk. While safety cannot be assured (may alter neonatal gut flora or cause hypersensitivity), it is unlikely to pose much risk to nursing offspring.

Overdosage/Acute Toxicity

Acute oral penicillin overdoses are unlikely to cause significant problems other than GI distress, but other effects are possible (see Adverse Effects). In humans, very high dosages of parenteral penicillins, especially in patients with renal disease, have induced CNS effects.

Drug Interactions

The following drug interactions have either been reported or are theoretical in humans or animals receiving dicloxacillin and may be of significance in veterinary patients:

- **AMINOGLYCOSIDES:** *In vitro* evidence of synergism with dicloxacillin against *S. aureus* strains
- **CYCLOSPORINE:** Dicloxacillin may reduce levels
- **PROBENECID:** Competitively blocks the tubular secretion of dicloxacillin, thereby increasing serum levels and serum half-lives
- **TETRACYCLINES:** Theoretical antagonism; use together usually not recommended
- **WARFARIN:** Dicloxacillin may cause decreased warfarin efficacy

Laboratory Considerations

- As penicillins and other beta-lactams can inactivate aminoglycosides *in vitro* (and *in vivo* in patients in renal failure), serum concentrations of aminoglycosides may be falsely decreased if the patient is also receiving beta-lactam antibiotics and the serum is stored prior to analysis. It is recommended that if the assay is delayed, samples be frozen and, if possible, drawn at times when the beta-lactam antibiotic is at a trough.

Doses

- **DOGS/CATS:**
  For susceptible infections:
  a) For localized soft tissue infections or skin

infections caused by susceptible (non-beta-lactamase producers) bacteria: 25 mg/kg PO q6h for 14−84 days. (Greene *et al.* 2006)

b) Dogs: For dermatologic infections: 22 mg/kg PO q8h (White 2003)

c) Dogs: For recurrent skin infections: 20−30 mg/kg PO three times daily; food may decrease absorption (Logas 2005)

Monitoring

■ Because penicillins usually have minimal toxicity associated with their use, monitoring for efficacy is usually all that is required unless toxic clinical signs develop. Serum levels and therapeutic drug monitoring are not routinely done with these agents.

Client Information

■ Owners should be instructed to give oral penicillins to animals with an empty stomach, unless using amoxicillin or if GI effects (anorexia, vomiting) occur.

■ Compliance with the therapeutic regimen should be stressed.

■ Reconstituted oral suspensions should be kept refrigerated and discarded after 14 days.

Chemistry/Synonyms

An isoxazolyl-penicillin, dicloxacillin sodium is a semisynthetic, penicillinase-resistant penicillin. It is available commercially as the monohydrate sodium salt that occurs as a white to off-white, crystalline powder that is freely soluble in water and has a pK_a of 2.7−2.8. One mg of dicloxacillin sodium contains not less than 850 micrograms of dicloxacillin.

Dicloxacillin Sodium may also be known as: sodium dicloxacillin, dichlorphenylmethyl isoxazolyl penicillin sodium, methyldichlorophenyl isoxazolyl penicillin sodium, dicloxacilina sodica, dicloxacillinum natricum, or P-1011; many trade names are available.

Storage/Stability

Dicloxacillin sodium capsules should be stored at temperatures less than 40°C and preferably at room temperature (15−30°C).

Dosage Forms/Regulatory Status

VETERINARY-LABELED PRODUCTS:

No products are apparently being currently marketed in the USA. The FDA's "Green Book" still lists 100 mg and 500 mg capsules; *Dicloxin*® (Fort Dodge) as approved for use in dogs.

HUMAN-LABELED PRODUCTS:

Dicloxacillin Sodium Capsules: 250 mg & 500 mg; generic; (Rx)

References

Greene, C., K. Hartmann, et al. (2006). Appendix 8: Antimicrobial Drug Formulary. *Infectious Disease of the Dog and Cat.* C Greene Ed., Elsevier: 1186−1333.

Logas, D. (2005). Superficial and Deep Pyoderma. Proceedings: Western Veterinary Conf. Accessed via: Veterinary Information Network. http://goo.gl/qMbzy

White, P. (2003). Medical management of canine pruritus. Proceedings: Western Veterinary Conf. Accessed via: Veterinary Information Network. http://goo.gl/2P8ET

DIETHYL-CARBAMAZINE CITRATE

(dye-ethel-kar-*bam*-a-zeen)
Hetrazan®, DEC

Prescriber Highlights

▶ Piperazine-derivative antiparasiticide used for daily heartworm prevention & at higher dosages for other parasites

▶ No veterinary-labeled commercial preparations in USA available

▶ Contraindications: Dogs with microfilaria

▶ Adverse Effects: Rarely, GI effects; combination product with oxibendazole (no longer marketed) was implicated in causing hepatopathy in dogs

Uses/Indications

Once the hallmark agent for heartworm disease prophylaxis in dogs, DEC is no longer commercially available in the USA (in oral veterinary dosage forms). DEC is FDA-approved for use for the prophylaxis of heartworm disease (*D. immitis*), and/or the treatment of ascariasis in dogs. The drug is also used in ferrets and zoo animals susceptible to heartworm. DEC is used in dogs at higher dosages as alternative therapy for several other parasites (see Dosage section below). Some products were labeled for use in cats to treat ascarid infections.

In cats, DEC may help alleviate the course (preventing lymphoma development) of FeLV infection.

In the U.K., DEC is used as an injectable product to control parasitic bronchitis (*Dictyocaulus viviparous*) in sheep and cattle.

In humans, DEC is indicated as a filaricidal for the treatment of *Wucheria bancrofti, Brugia malayi, Loa loa,* and *Onchocerca volvulus.*

Pharmacology/Actions

The exact mechanism of how DEC exerts its anti-filaricidal (early larval stages of *D. immitis*) and anti-nematodal effects in not clearly understood. It is believed that DEC acts on the parasite's nervous system in a nicotinic-like fashion, thereby paralyzing it. DEC also has immunomodulatory effects via an unknown mechanism.

Pharmacokinetics

DEC is rapidly absorbed after oral administration, with peak serum levels occurring in about 3 hours. The drug is distributed to all tissues and organs except fat. DEC is rapidly metabolized and is primarily excreted in the urine (70% of a dose within 24 hours) as metabolites or unchanged drug (10−25% of a dose).

Contraindications/Precautions/Warnings

Diethylcarbamazine is contraindicated in dogs with microfilaria, as a shock-like reaction can occur in dogs with microfilaria that are treated with DEC. This effect may only be seen in 0.3–5% of dogs, but the potential seriousness of the reaction precludes its use in all dogs with microfilaria. Dogs cleared of adult worms and microfilaria may be started on DEC therapy for prophylaxis. Microfilaria detected in dogs that have undergone adulticide and microfilaricide therapy, and are receiving DEC prophylaxis, should have the DEC stopped until existing microfilaria are eliminated.

DEC has been reported to cause infertility problems in male dogs, but these reports are rare. Controlled studies have not found any adverse effects on semen volume, pH, sperm counts, or motility.

Adverse Effects

When used at recommended doses for heartworm prophylaxis, adverse effects are very uncommon for DEC. Some dogs develop diarrhea or vomiting while on the drug, which may necessitate discontinuation. GI effects are more predominant when used at higher dosages for the treatment of ascarids or other susceptible parasites. Giving with food or soon after eating may alleviate GI disturbances. Case reports of fixed drug eruptions after DEC have also been reported in dogs.

In microfilaria positive dogs that receive DEC, an anaphylactoid reaction can be seen within 20 minutes of dosing. Systems affected or clinical signs seen may include GI (salivation, diarrhea, emesis), CNS (depression, ataxia, prostration, lethargy), shock (pale mucous membranes, weak pulses, tachycardia, dyspnea), hepatic (increased liver enzymes) or DIC. The reaction generally peaks within 1–2 hours after the dose and death can occur. Treatment is basically supportive, using fluid therapy and intravenous corticosteroids.

Cats have reportedly developed hepatic injury from DEC.

Reproductive/Nursing Safety

DEC alone is reportedly safe to use in pregnant dogs throughout the gestational period. In humans, the FDA categorizes this drug as category **C** for use during pregnancy (*Animal studies have shown an adverse effect on the fetus, but there are no adequate studies in humans; or there are no animal reproduction studies and no adequate studies in humans.*) In a separate system evaluating the safety of drugs in canine and feline pregnancy (Papich 1989), this drug is categorized as in class: **A** (*Probably safe. Although specific studies may not have proved the safety of all drugs in dogs and cats, there are no reports of adverse effects in laboratory animals or women.*)

Overdosage/Acute Toxicity

DEC is considered a relatively non-toxic compound, but quantitative data regarding its toxicity was not found. In dogs, large overdoses generally result in vomiting or depression. Inducement of vomiting or absorption reduction measures (activated charcoal, cathartics) could be considered for very large ingestions. Clinical signs, should they occur, should be handled in a supportive manner.

Drug Interactions

The following drug interactions have either been reported or are theoretical in humans or animals receiving DEC and may be of significance in veterinary patients:

■ **NICOTINE-LIKE COMPOUNDS, OTHER (e.g., pyrantel, morantel, levamisole):** If used with diethylcarbamazine, other nicotine-like compounds could theoretically enhance the toxic effects of each other; use with DEC only with intensified monitoring

Doses

■ **DOGS:**

For heartworm prophylaxis:

a) 6.6 mg/kg PO once a day preceding infection and for 60 days following last exposure to mosquitoes. In dogs that become microfilaremic while on DEC, may continue, but do not interrupt daily DEC therapy. (Knight 1989)

b) 6.6 mg/kg PO daily from beginning of mosquito season and for two months thereafter. Should be given year-round in areas where mosquitoes are active throughout the year. Re-examine 3 months after starting therapy and at 6-month intervals for microfilaria. (Todd *et al.* 1985)

c) 2.5–3 mg/kg PO daily; begin prior to mosquito season (Rawlings & Calvert 1989)

d) 5–7 mg/kg PO daily. Begin before infection is likely and continue 60 days after mosquito season. Some areas will require year-round treatment. (Calvert & Rawlings 1986)

For treatment of susceptible parasites (other than heartworm—must not be used in microfilaria positive patients):

a) For ascarids: 55–110 mg/kg PO; may be used as a preventative for ascaridiasis when dosed at 6.6 mg/kg PO per day (Todd *et al.* 1985)

b) For lungworms (*Crenosoma vulpis*): 80 mg/kg PO q12h for 3 days (Todd *et al.* 1985)

■ **CATS:**

a) For Ascarids: 55–110 mg/kg PO (Todd *et al.* 1985)

■ **FERRETS:**

a) For heartworm prophylaxis: 5.5 mg/kg PO once a day (Randolph 1986)

■ **CATTLE:**

a) For the treatment of early stages of *Dictyocaulus viviparous* infestations: 22 mg/kg IM for 3 successive days; or 44 mg/kg IM once. (**Note:** DEC is available in an injectable dosage form containing 400 mg/mL in the U.K., no FDA-approved injectable form is available in the U.S.A.) (Brander *et al.* 1982)

Monitoring

■ Microfilaria, when used for heartworm prophylaxis

■ Clinical efficacy, when used as an anthelmintic

Client Information

■ Give all doses as directed

■ Dogs must be checked for microfilaria before restarting DEC in the spring. Dogs receiving DEC year around should be checked every six months

Chemistry/Synonyms

A piperazine derivative, diethylcarbamazine citrate (DEC) occurs as a white, slightly hygroscopic, crystalline powder that is either odorless or has a slight odor and a melting point of approximately 138°C. It is very soluble in water and slightly soluble (1 g in 35 mL) in alcohol.

Diethylcarbamazine citrate may also be known as: diethylcarbamazine acid citrate, diethylcarbamazini citras; ditrazini citras, RP-3799, *Banocide®, Diethizine®, Filarcidan®, Hetrazan®,* or *Notezine®.*

Storage/Stability

Unless otherwise specified by the manufacturer, diethylcarbamazine products should be stored in tight containers at room temperature and protected from light.

Dosage Forms/Regulatory Status

VETERINARY-LABELED PRODUCTS: No products are apparently being currently marketed in the USA. However, the FDA's "Green Book" still lists 10 oral products that are approved for use in the USA.

HUMAN-LABELED PRODUCTS:

Diethylcarbamazine Citrate Tablets: 50 mg; *Hetrazan®* (Wyeth-Ayerst); (Rx) **Note:** This product is available from the manufacturer without charge for compassionate use (in humans) only.

References

Brander, C.G., D.M. Pugh, et al. (1982). *Veterinary Applied Pharmacology and Therapeutics.* London, Baillière Tindall.

Calvert, C.A. & C.A. Rawlings (1986). Therapy of canine heartworm disease. *Current Veterinary Therapy IX: Small Animal Practice.* RW Kirk Ed. Philadelphia, WB Saunders: 406–419.

Knight, D.H. (1989). Heartworm Disease. *Handbook of Small Animal Practice.* RV Morgan Ed. New York, Churchill Livingstone: 139–148.

Randolph, R.W. (1986). Preventive medical care for the pet ferret. *Current Veterinary Therapy IX: Small Animal*

Practice. RW Kirk Ed. Philadelphia, WB Saunders: 772–774.

Rawlings, C.A. & C.A. Calvert (1989). Heartworm Disease. *Textbook of Veterinary Internal Medicine.* SJ Ettinger Ed. Philadelphia, WB Saunders. 2: 1163–1184.

Todd, K.S., A.J. Paul, et al. (1985). Parasitic Diseases. *Handbook of Small Animal Therapeutics.* LE Davis Ed. New York, Churchill Livingstone: 89–126.

DIETHYLSTILBESTROL DES

(dye-ethel-stil-*bes*-tral)

HORMONAL AGENT

Prescriber Highlights

▶ Synthetic estrogen used in dogs primarily for estrogen responsive incontinence & other estrogen indications (prostatic hypertrophy, estrus induction, etc.)

▶ Prohibited for use in food animals (potential carcinogen)

▶ Teratogen

▶ Many potential adverse effects: blood dyscrasias, GI effects, cystic endometrial hyperplasia & pyometra (non-spayed females), feminization (males), neoplasia

▶ Availability issues; must be obtained via a compounding pharmacy

Uses/Indications

DES has been used in estrogen responsive incontinence in spayed female dogs and in the medical treatment of benign prostatic hypertrophy in male dogs. It has also been used for the prevention of pregnancy after mismating in female dogs and cats, but is typically no longer recommended because of serious side effects.

Pharmacology/Actions

Estrogens are necessary for the normal growth and development of the female sex organs and in some species contribute to the development and maintenance of secondary female sex characteristics. Estrogens cause increased cell height and secretions of the cervical mucosa, thickening of the vaginal mucosa, endometrial proliferation, and increased uterine tone.

Estrogens have effects on the skeletal system. They increase calcium deposition, accelerate epiphyseal closure and increase bone formation. Estrogens have a slight anabolic effect and can increase sodium and water retention.

Estrogens affect the release of gonadotropins from the pituitary gland, which can cause inhibition of lactation, inhibition of ovulation, and inhibition of androgen secretion.

Excessive estrogen will delay the transport of the ovum and prevent it from reaching the uterus at the appropriate time for implantation. DES also possesses antineoplastic activity against some types of neoplasias (perianal gland adenoma and prostatic hyperplasia). It affects mRNA and protein synthesis in the cell nucleus and is cell cycle nonspecific.

The mechanism of action for estrogen-responsive urinary incontinence is thought due to increasing sphincter sensitivity to norepinephrine.

Pharmacokinetics

DES is well absorbed from the GI tract of monogastric animals. It is slowly metabolized by the liver, primarily to a glucuronide form and then excreted in the urine and feces.

Contraindications/Precautions/Warnings

DES is prohibited by the FDA for use in food animals.

Because of potential effects on bone marrow, DES should be used with extreme caution in patients with preexisting anemias or leukopenias. DES is contraindicated in females with estrogen-sensitive neoplasms.

Adverse Effects

While adverse effects with estrogen therapy can be serious (see below) in small animals, when used for estrogen-responsive incontinence at the lowest effective dose, it is usually well-tolerated.

In cats and dogs, estrogens are considered toxic to the bone marrow and can cause blood dyscrasias. Blood dyscrasias are more prevalent in older animals and if higher dosages are used. Initially, a thrombocytosis and/or leukocytosis may be noted, but thrombocytopenia/leukopenias will gradually develop. Changes in a peripheral blood smear may be apparent within two weeks after estrogen administration. Chronic estrogen toxicity may be characterized by a normochromic, normocytic anemia, thrombocytopenia, and neutropenia. Bone marrow depression may be transient and begin to resolve within 30–40 days or may persist or progress to a fatal aplastic anemia. Doses of 2.2 mg/kg per day have caused death in cats secondary to bone marrow toxicity.

Estrogens may induce mammary neoplasias.

In cats, daily administration of DES has resulted in pancreatic, hepatic, and cardiac lesions.

Estrogens may cause cystic endometrial hyperplasia and pyometra. After therapy is initiated, an open-cervix pyometra may be noted 1–6 weeks after therapy.

When used chronically in male animals, feminization may occur. In females, signs of estrus may occur and persist for 7–10 days.

Experimental administration of DES to female dogs as young as 8 months of age have induced malignant ovarian adenocarcinomas. Doses ranging from 60 to 495 mg given over 1 month to 4 years were implicated in causing these tumors.

Reproductive/Nursing Safety

DES is contraindicated during pregnancy, as it can cause fetal malformations of the genitourinary system.

Estrogens have been documented to be carcinogenic at low levels in some laboratory animals. Because of the potential for danger to the public health, DES must not be used in animals to be used for human consumption.

Overdosage/Acute Toxicity

Acute overdosage in humans with estrogens has resulted in nausea, vomiting and withdrawal bleeding in females. No information was located regarding acute overdose in veterinary patients, however, the reader is referred to the warnings and adverse effects listed above.

Drug Interactions

The following drug interactions have either been reported or are theoretical in humans or animals receiving DES and may be of significance in veterinary patients:

- **ANTIFUNGALS, AZOLE (itraconazole, ketoconazole, etc.):** May increase estrogen levels
- **CIMETIDINE:** May decrease metabolism of estrogens
- **CORTICOSTEROIDS:** Enhanced glucocorticoid effects may result if estrogens are used concomitantly with corticosteroid agents. It has been postulated that estrogens may either alter the protein binding of corticosteroids and/or decrease their metabolism. Corticosteroid dosage adjustment may be necessary when estrogen therapy is either started or discontinued
- **ERYTHROMYCIN, CLARITHROMYCIN:** May decrease the metabolism of estrogens
- **PHENOBARBITAL:** May decrease estrogen concentrations
- **PHENYTOIN:** May decrease estrogen concentrations
- **RIFAMPIN:** May induce hepatic microsomal enzymes and decrease estrogen levels
- **WARFARIN:** Oral anticoagulant activity may be decreased if estrogens are administered concurrently; increases in anticoagulant dosage may be necessary if adding estrogens

Laboratory Considerations

- Estrogens in combination with progestins (*e.g.*, oral contraceptives) have been demonstrated in humans to increase thyroxine-binding globulin (TBG) with resultant increases in total circulating thyroid hormone. Decreased T3 resin uptake also occurs, but free T4 levels are unaltered.

Doses

- **DOGS:**

For treatment of primary sphincter mechanism incompetence (idiopathic incontinence, hormone-responsive incontinence):
a) As an alternative to phenylpropanolamine: 0.1–1 mg (total dose) per dog PO for 5 days followed by maintenance of 1 mg/week or a maximum of

0.1 mg/kg/week. Minimum effective dose should be used for maintenance. Do NOT give more than recommended. (Adams 2009)

b) In females: 0.1–1 mg (total dose) PO once daily for 5 days, then 1 mg once a week (Labato 2002)

c) 0.5–1 mg (0.02 mg/kg; maximum dose of 1 mg) for 3–5 days as an induction dose and then periodically decreased to every other day and then to the lowest dose that will maintain continence. In difficult cases, may be used with phenylpropanolamine. (Chew & DiBartola 2006)

Note: Because of the unavailability of commercial DES products, some clinicians have used conjugated estrogens (*e.g., Premarin®*) as a substitute: Example doses include: 20 micrograms/kg PO every 4 days (Grauer 2000); 20 micrograms/kg PO once daily for 5–7 days, then every 2–3 days as needed. (Lane 2006)

For estrus induction:

a) DES at 5 mg/day for a tentative 7 days. The first day of vulvar swelling is designated as Day 1. Continue DES on DAY 1 and Day 2. If no effect is seen in 7 days, give DES at 10 mg/day for another tentative 7 days. If vulvar swelling and bleeding detected, DES is continued on Day 1 and Day 2. If no effect seen in these 14 days, discontinue and restart in 30 days. Once proestrus initiated, on Day 5 give 5 mg of Luteinizing hormone (LH) if obtainable. If LH unavailable, give GnRH 3.3 micrograms/kg IM and FSH 10 mg IM in its place. Bitch is bred on Day 13. **Note:** Adjust dosages of LH and FSH for animal size—the above dosages are for a dog weighing 50–60 lbs. (Purswell 1999)

For treatment of prostatic hyperplasias:

a) For benign prostatic hypertrophy: 0.2–1 mg total dose PO for 5 days (Root Kustritz & Klausner 2000)

■ **CATS:**

For treatment of estrogen-responsive incontinence:

a) In females: 0.1–1 mg (total dose) PO once daily for 5 days, then 1 mg once a week (Labato 2002)

Monitoring

When therapy is either at high dosages or chronic; see Adverse Effects for more information.

Perform at least monthly:

■ Packed Cell Volumes (PCV)

■ White blood cell counts

■ Platelet counts

■ Perform liver function tests at baseline, and one month after therapy begins, repeat in 2 months after cessation of therapy if abnormal.

Client Information

■ Contact veterinarian if signs of lethargy, diarrhea, vomiting, abnormal discharge from vulva, excessive water consumption and urination or abnormal bleeding occur.

Chemistry/Synonym

A synthetic nonsteroidal estrogen agent, diethylstilbestrol occurs as an odorless, white, crystalline powder with a melting range of 169°–175°C. It is practically insoluble in water; soluble in alcohol or fatty oils.

Diethylstilbestrol may also be known as: DES, diethylstilbestrolum, diethylstilboestrol, NSC-3070, stilbestrol, stilboestrol, *Apstil®, Boestrol®, Destilbenol®*, or *Distilbene®*.

Storage/Stability

All commercially available DES tablets (plain tablets, enteric-coated tablets) should be stored at room temperature (15–30°C) in well-closed containers.

Dosage Forms/Regulatory Status

VETERINARY-LABELED PRODUCTS: None

HUMAN-LABELED PRODUCTS:

No commercially available regular oral DES products are available in the USA, however, compounded preparations may be available from compounding pharmacies.

References

Adams, L. (2009). Role of cystoscopy in diagnosis and treatment of urinary incontinence. Proceedings: ECVIM–CA Congress. Accessed via: Veterinary Information Network. http://goo.gl/8njWA

Chew, D. & S. DiBartola (2006). Tips for managing lower urinary tract disorders: Urinary incontinence. Proceedings: ACVIM. Accessed via: Veterinary Information Network. http://goo.gl/14GHP

Labato, M. (2002). Management of micturition disorders. Proceedings: Tufts Animal Expo. Accessed via: Veterinary Information Network. http://goo.gl/COfqD

Lane, I. (2006). Challenging incontinence cases. Proceedings: Western Vet Conf. Accessed via: Veterinary Information Network. http://goo.gl/0oDHc

Purswell, B. (1999). Pharmaceuticals used in canine theriogenology – Part 1 & 2. Proceedings: Central Veterinary Conference, Kansas City.

Root Kustritz, M. & J. Klausner (2000). Prostatic Diseases. *Textbook of Veterinary Internal Medicine: Diseases of the Dog and Cat.* S Ettinger and E Feldman Eds. Philadelphia, WB Saunders. 2: 1687–1698.

DIFLOXACIN HCL

(dye-*flox*-a-sin)   Dicural®

FLUOROQUINOLONE ANTIBIOTIC

Prescriber Highlights

▶ Veterinary-labeled fluoroquinolone antibiotic for dogs

▶ Labeled for once daily administration

▶ Contraindications: Hypersensitivity. Relatively contraindicated for young, growing animals due to cartilage abnormalities

▶ Caution: Seizure disorders, hepatic or renal insufficiency, dehydration

▶ Adverse Effects: GI distress, CNS stimulation, or hypersensitivity

▶ Administer PO preferably on an empty stomach, unless GI upset

Uses/Indications

Difloxacin is indicated for treatment in dogs for bacterial infections susceptible to it. In dogs with moderate to severe renal failure, difloxacin may have an advantage over the other FDA-approved fluoroquinolones as it has more extensive hepatobiliary excretion and may be less likely to accumulate to toxic levels.

Difloxacin tablets are not labeled for use in cats or other species.

Pharmacology/Actions

Like other drugs in its class, difloxacin is a concentration-dependent bactericidal agent. It acts by inhibiting bacterial DNA-gyrase (a type-II topoisomerase), thereby preventing DNA supercoiling and DNA synthesis. The net result is disruption of bacterial cell replication.

Difloxacin has good activity against many gram-negative and gram-positive bacilli and cocci, including most species and strains of *Klebsiella* spp., *Staphylococcus* spp., *E. coli*, Enterobacter, Campylobacter, Shigella, Proteus, and Pasturella species. Some strains of *Pseudomonas aeruginosa* and Pseudomonas species are resistant and most *Enterococcus* spp. are resistant. Like other fluoroquinolones, difloxacin has weak activity against most anaerobes and is not a good choice when treating known or suspected anaerobic infections.

Development of bacterial resistance to 4-fluoroquinolones can occur.

When comparing *in vitro* antibacterial activity against common porcine and bovine veterinary pathogens, difloxacin showed significantly less activity than enrofloxacin (Grobbel *et al.* 2007).

Pharmacokinetics

After oral administration in dogs, difloxacin serum levels peak about 3 hours post dosing. The drug is well absorbed (bioavailability >80%) and distributed (V_d=2.8–4.7 L/kg) in dogs and marginally bound to plasma proteins (16–52% in dogs). Difloxacin is eliminated by excretion in the bile and more than 80% of a dose is eliminated in the feces. Elimination half-life is about 9.3 hours. While excretion by the kidneys may only account for 5% of the total dose, urine levels remain well above MIC's for susceptible organisms for at least 24 hours after dosing.

In horses, oral bioavailability after intragastric administration of a 5 mg/kg oral suspension (100 mg/mL; in simple syrup:deionized water at 60:40) was approximately 70%. Peak levels were about 0.73 mg/L. After IV administration, volume of distribution (steady-state) was about 1 L/kg and terminal elimination half-life about 2.7 hours. Elimination half-life after IM injection was about 5.7 hours; after intragastric administration about 10.8 hours.

Contraindications/Precautions/Warnings

Difloxacin, like other fluoroquinolones can cause arthropathies in immature, growing animals. Because dogs appear to be more sensitive to this effect, the manufacturer states that the drug is contraindicated in immature dogs during the rapid growth phase (between 2–8 months in small and medium-sized breeds and up to 18 months in large and giant breeds). The drug should be considered contraindicated in dogs known to be hypersensitive to difloxacin or other drugs in its class (quinolones).

The manufacturer states that difloxacin should be used with caution in animals with known or suspected CNS disorders (*e.g.*, seizure disorders) as rarely drugs in this class have been associated with CNS stimulation and seizures.

While difloxacin may find use in other species, early anecdotal reports state that it can cause nausea and vomiting in cats. Its ophthalmic safety has not been determined in cats.

Adverse Effects

While the manufacturer reports that only self-limited gastrointestinal effects (anorexia, vomiting, diarrhea) were reported during clinical studies (at 5 mg/kg dosing) in adult animals, higher doses or additional experience with use of the drug may demonstrate additional adverse effects.

Reproductive/Nursing Safety

Safety in breeding or pregnant dogs has not been established. It is not known whether difloxacin is excreted into milk.

Overdosage/Acute Toxicity

Dogs receiving up to 2.5X (25 mg/kg) for 30 days did not demonstrate overly significant adverse effects. Facial erythema/edema, diarrhea, decreased appetite and weight loss were noted.

Drug Interactions

The manufacturer reports that difloxacin was used concurrently in field trials with a variety of drugs including heartworm preventative, thyroid hormones, ectoparasiticides, antiseizure drugs, anesthetics, antihistamines, and topical antibiotic/antiinflammatory preps without untoward effects.

However, the following drug interactions have either been reported or are theoretical in humans or animals receiving other oral fluoroquinolones and may be of significance in veterinary patients receiving difloxacin:

- **ANTACIDS/DAIRY PRODUCTS containing cations (Mg^{++}, Al^{+++}, Ca^{++}):** May bind to ciprofloxacin and prevent its absorption; separate doses of these products by at least 2 hours from difloxacin

- **ANTIBIOTICS, OTHER (aminoglycosides, 3rd-generation cephalosporins, penicillins—extended-spectrum):** Synergism may occur, but is not predictable, against some bacteria (particularly *Pseudomonas aeruginosa*) with these compounds. Although difloxacin has minimal activity against anaerobes, *in vitro* synergy has been reported when first generation fluoroquinolones have been used with **clindamycin** against strains of Peptostreptococcus, Lactobacillus and *Bacteroides fragilis*.

- **CYCLOSPORINE:** Fluoroquinolones may exacerbate the nephrotoxicity and reduce the metabolism of cyclosporine (used systemically)

- **GLYBURIDE:** Severe hypoglycemia possible

- **IRON, ZINC (oral):** Decreased difloxacin absorption; separate doses by at least two hours

- **METHOTREXATE:** Increased MTX levels possible with resultant toxicity

- **NITROFURANTOIN** may antagonize the antimicrobial activity of the fluoroquinolones and their concomitant use is not recommended

- **PHENYTOIN:** Difloxacin may alter phenytoin levels

- **PROBENECID:** Blocks tubular secretion of ciprofloxacin and may also increase the blood level and half-life of difloxacin

- **SUCRALFATE:** May inhibit absorption of difloxacin; separate doses of these drugs by at least 2 hours

- **THEOPHYLLINE:** Difloxacin may increase theophylline blood levels

- **WARFARIN:** Potential for increased warfarin effects

Laboratory Considerations
- In some human patients, the fluoroquinolones have caused increases in **liver enzymes, BUN,** and **creatinine** and decreases in **hematocrit**. The clinical relevance of these mild changes is not known at this time.

Doses

- **DOGS:**
  a) For susceptible infections: 5–10 mg/kg once daily PO for 2–3 days beyond the cessation of clinical signs to a maximum of 30 days therapy (Package Insert; *Dicural®*)

- **HORSES:**
  a) For susceptible infections (MIC ≤ 0.25 micrograms/mL): 7.5 mg/kg PO (non-fasted) once daily (q24h). Appears to be safe, adequately absorbed and well distributed. Further investigation is warranted to substantiate. Unknown whether administration of difloxacin to young, growing horses should be avoided. (Adams *et al.* 2005)

Monitoring/Client Information
- Efficacy is the most important monitoring parameter.
- Clients should be instructed on the importance of giving the medication as instructed and not to discontinue it on their own.

Chemistry/Synonyms
A 4-fluoroquinolone antibiotic, difloxacin HCl is poorly water soluble at neutral pH. At a pH of 5 solubility is increased and it is highly water soluble at a pH of 9.

Difloxacin HCl may also be known as: A-56619, Abbott-56619, or *Dicural®*.

Storage/Stability
Commercially available tablets should be stored between 15–30°C (59–86°F) and protected from excessive heat.

Dosage Forms/Regulatory Status
VETERINARY-LABELED PRODUCTS:
Difloxacin Oral Scored Tablets: 11.4 mg (single scored), 45.4 mg (single scored), & 136 mg (double scored); *Dicural®* (BIVI); (Rx). FDA-approved for use in dogs. Federal law prohibits the extra-label use of the drug in food-producing animals.

HUMAN-LABELED PRODUCTS: None

References
Adams, A., G. Haines, et al. (2005). Pharmacokinetics of difloxacin and its concentration in body fluids and endometrial tissues of mares after repeated intragastric administration. *Can J Vet Res* **69**: 229–235.

Grobbel, M., A. Lbbke–Becker, et al. (2007). Comparative quantification of the in vitro activity of veterinary fluoroquinolones. *Veterinary Microbiology* **124**(1–2): 73–81.

DIGOXIN

(di-**jox**-in)   Lanoxin®, Cardoxin®

CARDIAC GLYCOSIDE

Prescriber Highlights

▶ Oral & parenteral cardiac glycoside used for CHF & SVT's in many species; usually with other agents

▶ Contraindications: V-fib, digitalis intoxication; many veterinarians feel that digoxin is relatively contraindicated in cats with hypertrophic cardiomyopathy

▶ Extreme Caution: Patients with glomerulonephritis & heart failure or with idiopathic hypertrophic subaortic stenosis (IHSS)

▶ Caution: Severe pulmonary disease, hypoxia, acute myocarditis, myxedema, or acute MI, frequent VPC's V-tach, chronic constrictive pericarditis or incomplete AV block

▶ Adverse Effects usually associated with high or toxic blood levels: Cardiac effects may include almost every type of cardiac arrhythmia described with a resultant worsening of heart failure clinical signs. Extracardiac: mild GI upset, anorexia, weight loss & diarrhea

▶ Drug Interactions

▶ Monitoring of blood levels highly suggested

Uses/Indications

The veterinary indications for digoxin include treatment of congestive heart failure, atrial fibrillation or flutter, and supraventricular tachycardias.

In dogs with heart failure and a supraventricular arrhythmia such as atrial fibrillation, digoxin is often considered the drug of choice for treating the arrhythmias. Digoxin therapy is more controversial for treating heart failure without accompanying supraventricular arrhythmias. Today, many cardiologists no longer feel that digoxin is first line therapy for heart failure in dogs and cats, and with the availability of pimobendan this trend is expected to continue. Many state that digoxin can have beneficial effects in certain patients when used with diuretics and, possibly, ACE inhibitors, but digoxin alone is rarely, if ever, used for heart failure.

Pharmacology/Actions

The pharmacology of the digitalis glycosides have been extensively studied, but a thorough discussion is beyond the scope of this reference. Digitalis glycosides cause the following effects in patients with a failing heart: increased myocardial contractility (inotropism) with increased cardiac output; increased diuresis with reduction of edema secondary to a decrease in sympathetic tone; reduction in heart size, heart rate, blood volume, and pulmonary and venous pressures; and (usually) no net change in myocardial oxygen demand.

The digitalis glycosides have several electrocardiac effects, including: decreased conduction velocity through the AV node, and prolonged effective refractory period (ERP). They may increase the PR interval, decrease the QT interval and cause ST segment depression.

The exact mechanism of action of these agents has not been fully described, but their ability to increase the availability of Ca^{++} to myocardial fibers and to inhibit Na^+-K^+-ATPase with resultant increased intracellular Na^+ and reduced K^+ probably explains their actions.

For additional information, it is suggested to refer to a pharmacology text.

Pharmacokinetics

Absorption following oral administration occurs in the small intestine and is variable dependent upon the oral dosage form used (see Dosage Forms below). Food may delay, but not alter, the extent of absorption in most species studied. Food reportedly decreases the amount absorbed by 50% in cats after tablet administration. Peak serum levels generally occur within 45–60 minutes after oral elixir and about 90 minutes after oral tablet administration. In patients receiving an initial oral dose of digoxin, peak effects may occur in 6–8 hours after the dose.

The drug is distributed widely throughout the body with highest levels found in kidneys, heart, intestine, stomach, liver and skeletal muscle. Lowest concentrations are found in the brain and plasma. Digoxin does not significantly enter ascitic fluid, so dosage adjustments may be required in animals with ascites. At therapeutic levels, approximately 20–30% of the drug is bound to plasma proteins. Because only small amounts are found in fat, obese patients may receive dosages too high if dosing is based on total body weight versus lean body weight.

Digoxin is metabolized slightly, but the primary method of elimination is renal excretion both by glomerular filtration and tubular secretion. As a result, dosage adjustments must be made in patients with significant renal disease. Values reported for the elimination half-life of digoxin in dogs and cats have been highly variable, with values reported from 14.4–56 hours for dogs; 30–173 hours for cats. Elimination half-lives reported in other species include: Sheep≈7.15 hours; Horses≈16.9–28.8 hours; and Cattle≈7.8 hours.

Contraindications/Precautions/Warnings

Many cardiologists feel that digoxin is relatively contraindicated in cats with hypertrophic cardiomyopathy as it may increase myocardial oxygen demand and lead to dynamic outflow obstruction.

s actively transported by the p-
pump, but the Washington State
Clinical Pharmacology Lab reports
...s not documented any increased sensitivity to digoxin and does not recommend any
dose reductions in dogs with MDR1 mutations.
They do however, recommend therapeutic drug
monitoring (WSU-VetClinPharmLab 2009).

Digitalis cardioglycosides are contraindicated
in patients with ventricular fibrillation or in
digitalis intoxication. They should be used with
extreme caution in patients with glomerulonephritis and heart failure or with idiopathic
hypertrophic subaortic stenosis (IHSS). They
should be used with caution in patients with severe pulmonary disease, hypoxia, acute myocarditis, myxedema, or acute myocardial infarction,
frequent ventricular premature contractions,
ventricular tachycardias, chronic constrictive
pericarditis or incomplete AV block. They may
be used in patients with stable, complete AV
block or severe bradycardia with heart failure if
the block was not caused by the cardiac glycoside.

When used to treat atrial fibrillation or flutter prior to administration with an antiarrhythmic agent that has anticholinergic activity (e.g.,
quinidine, procainamide, disopyramide), digitalis glycosides will reduce, but not eliminate,
the increased ventricular rates that may be produced by those agents. Since digitalis glycosides
may cause increased vagal tone, they should be
used with caution in patients with increased carotid sinus sensitivity.

Elective cardioversion of patients with atrial
fibrillation should be postponed until digitalis
glycosides have been withheld for 1–2 days, and
should not be attempted in patients with signs
of digitalis toxicity.

Principally eliminated by the kidneys, digoxin should be used with caution and serum
levels monitored in patients with renal disease.
Animals that are hypernatremic, hypokalemic,
hypercalcemic, hyper- or hypothyroid may require smaller dosages; monitor carefully.

As digoxin does not distribute well into ascitic
fluid or fat, dosing is generally based upon lean
body weight.

Adverse Effects
Adverse effects of digoxin are usually associated
with high or toxic serum levels and are categorized into cardiac and extracardiac clinical signs.
There are species differences with regard to the
sensitivity to digoxin's toxic effects also. Cats are
relatively sensitive to digoxin while dogs tend to
be more tolerant of high serum levels.

Cardiac effects may be seen before other
extra-cardiac clinical signs and may include almost every type of cardiac arrhythmia described
with a resultant worsening of heart failure clinical signs. More common arrhythmias or ECG
changes observed include: complete or incomplete heart block, bigeminy, ST segment changes,
paroxysmal ventricular or atrial tachycardias
with block, and multifocal premature ventricular contractions. Because these effects can also
be caused by worsening heart disease, it may
be difficult to determine if they are a result of
the disease process or digitalis intoxication. If
in doubt, monitor serum levels or stop digoxin
therapy temporarily.

Extracardiac clinical signs most commonly
seen in veterinary medicine include mild GI
upset, anorexia, weight loss, and diarrhea.
Vomiting has been associated with IV injections
and should not cause anxiety or alarm. Ocular
and neurologic effects are routinely seen in humans, but are not prevalent in animals or are not
detected.

Reproductive/Nursing Safety
In humans, the FDA categorizes this drug as
category C for use during pregnancy (*Animal
studies have shown an adverse effect on the fetus,
but there are no adequate studies in humans; or
there are no animal reproduction studies and no
adequate studies in humans.*) In a separate system evaluating the safety of drugs in canine and
feline pregnancy (Papich 1989), this drug is categorized as in class: A (*Probably safe. Although
specific studies may not have proved the safety of
all drugs in dogs and cats, there are no reports of
adverse effects in laboratory animals or women.*)

Studies have shown that digoxin concentrations in mother's serum and milk are similar;
however, it is unlikely to have any pharmacological effect in nursing offspring.

Overdosage/Acute Toxicity
Clinical signs of chronic toxicity are discussed above. In dogs the acute toxic dose after IV administration has been reported to be
0.177 mg/kg.

Treatment of chronic digoxin toxicity is dictated by the severity of the clinical signs associated with it. Many patients will do well after
temporarily stopping the drug and reevaluating
the dosage regimen.

If an acute ingestion has recently occurred
and no present cardiotoxic or neurologic signs
(coma, seizures, etc.) have manifested, emptying the stomach may be indicated followed with
activated charcoal administration. Because digoxin can be slowly absorbed and there is some
enterohepatic recirculation of the drug, repeated
charcoal administration may be beneficial even
if the ingestion occurred well before treatment.
Anion-exchange resins such as colestipol or
cholestyramine have been suggested to reduce
the absorption and enterohepatic circulation of
digoxin, but are not readily available in most veterinary practices.

Dependent on the type of cardiotoxicity, supportive and symptomatic therapy should be
implemented. Serum electrolyte concentrations,
drug level if available on a "stat" basis, arterial
blood gases if available, and continuous ECG

monitoring should be instituted. Acid-base, hypoxia, and fluid and electrolyte imbalances should be corrected. The use of potassium in normokalemic patients is very controversial and should only be attempted with constant monitoring and clinical expertise.

The use of specific antiarrhythmic agents in treating life-threatening digitalis-induced arrhythmias may be necessary. Lidocaine and phenytoin are most commonly employed for these arrhythmias. Atropine may be used to treat sinus bradycardia, SA arrest, or 2nd or 3rd degree AV block.

Digoxin immune Fab is a promising treatment for digoxin or digitoxin life-threatening toxicity. It is produced from specific digoxin antibodies from sheep and will bind directly to the drug, inactivating it. It is very expensive however and veterinary experience with it is extremely limited.

Drug Interactions

There are many potential drug interactions associated with digoxin and the following list is not necessarily all inclusive. Because of the narrow therapeutic index associated with the drug, consider enhanced monitoring when these drugs (are those in the same class) are added to patients stabilized on digoxin.

The following drug interactions have either been reported or are theoretical in humans or animals receiving digoxin and may be of significance in veterinary patients:

The following drugs may **reduce digoxin serum levels**:

■ **AMINOSALICYLIC ACID**
■ **ANTACIDS**
■ **CHLORAMPHENICOL (DOGS)** (Pedersoli 1980)
■ **CHOLESTYRAMINE**
■ **CIMETIDINE**
■ **METOCLOPRAMIDE**
■ **NEOMYCIN (ORAL)**
■ **PHENOBARBITAL**
■ **ST JOHN'S WORT**
■ **SUCRALFATE**
■ **SULFASALAZINE**

The following drugs or herbs may **increase serum levels, decrease the elimination rate, or enhance the toxic effects** of digoxin:

■ **AMIODARONE**
■ **ANTICHOLINERGICS**
■ **CAPTOPRIL** (or other **ACEIs**)
■ **COLEUS**
■ **DIAZEPAM**
■ **DILTIAZEM** (data conflicts)
■ **ERYTHROMYCIN**
■ **FUROSEMIDE** (not significantly altered in cats receiving furosemide and aspirin)
■ **HAWTHORN**
■ **KETOCONAZOLE/ITRACONAZOLE**

■ **OMEPRAZOLE** (or other **PPIs**)
■ **QUINIDINE** (if used together the rule of thumb is to decrease digoxin dose by 50%)
■ **RESERPINE**
■ **SUCCINYLCHOLINE**
■ **TETRACYCLINE**
■ **VERAPAMIL**
■ **BETA-BLOCKERS:** Can have additive negative effects on AV conduction, complete heart block possible
■ **CALCIUM-CHANNEL BLOCKERS** (diltiazem, etc.): Can have additive negative effects on AV conduction
■ **PENICILLAMINE:** May decrease serum levels of digoxin independent of route of digoxin dosing.
■ **POTASSIUM/ELECTROLYTE BALANCE, DRUGS AFFECTING** (e.g., diuretics, amphotericin B, glucocorticoids, laxatives, sodium polystyrene sulfonate, glucagon, high dose IV dextrose, dextrose/insulin infusions, furosemide, thiazides): May predispose the patient to digitalis toxicity
■ **SPIRONOLACTONE:** May enhance or decrease the toxic effects of digoxin
■ **THYROID SUPPLEMENTS:** Patients on digoxin that receive thyroid replacement therapy may need their digoxin dosage adjusted

Laboratory Considerations

■ No specific laboratory test concerns
■ Digoxin can cause prolonged PR interval and ST segment depression, and false-positive changes on EKG ST-T in human patients during exercise testing

Doses

■ **DOGS:**

a) For CHF with atrial fibrillation in dogs with normal renal function: 0.005–0.0075 mg/kg PO q12h. Trough level of 0.8–1.2 nanograms/mL is the recommended target. (Keene & Bonagura 2009)

b) Because of the variability in pharmacokinetics in individual animals, administration to any animal should be viewed as a pharmacological "experiment":

Usually, in dogs weighing less than 20 kg (44 lbs.) give 0.005–0.011 mg/kg PO q12h. In dogs weighing more than 20 kg (44 lbs), initial dose is 0.22 mg/m² (NOT mg/kg) PO q12h. These doses result in a serum concentration in the therapeutic range by the second day of administration. If more rapid digitalization is required, the maintenance dose can be doubled for the first one or two doses. This method results in a therapeutic serum concentration within the first day. Monitor for signs of toxicity and efficacy and measure serum concentration 3–5 days later to determine if in therapeutic range. Readjust dosage accordingly. (Kittleson 2010)

c) For adjunctive treatment of dilated cardiomyopathy patients with atrial fibrillation; more caution in patients with ventricular arrhythmias. Given as much for its effects on baroreceptor sensitivity with resultant decrease in sympathetic outflow as for its positive inotropic action. Dose is 0.0025 mg/kg PO q12h; loading dose usually not given. Trough therapeutic level is 0.8–1.2 ng/mL. (Luis Fuentes 2009)

d) For adjunctive treatment of atrial fibrillation: 0.003–0.005 mg/kg PO q12h (Hogan 2004)

e) If pimobendan is not available or too expensive, especially if refractory heart failure exists or atrial fibrillation is observed: Start with a low dose (0.005 mg/kg PO twice a day) and round down if needed. (Meurs 2006)

f) For supraventricular arrhythmias: 0.22 mg/m^2 (NOT mg/kg) PO q12h (Smith 2009)

■ **CATS:**

For dilated cardiomyopathy or advanced atrioventricular valve insufficiency (**Note:** digoxin is generally contraindicated for feline hypertrophic cardiomyopathy):

a) Initial dose: 0.007 mg/kg PO every other day. Use lean body weight to determine dosage. Measure serum digoxin level 10+ days later. Draw level 8–10 hours after dosing. Therapeutic level: 1–2 ng/mL. If level is less than 0.8 ng/mL, increase dose up to 30% and repeat serum level monitoring as above. If toxicity is suspected, stop therapy for at least 1–2 days and then resume at a reduced dose (by 50%). (Ware & Keene 2000)

b) The starting dose for normal cats is ¼th of a 0.125 mg tablet administered every other day for cats weighing less than 3 kg, ¼th of a tablet every day for cats weighing 3 to 6 kg, and ¼th of a tablet every day to q12h for cats weighing more than 6 kg. Tablets are better tolerated than the alcohol-based elixir. (Kittleson 2010)

■ **FERRETS:**

For adjunctive therapy for heart failure:

a) For dilated cardiomyopathy: 0.01 mg/kg PO once daily initially (use oral liquid). May increase to twice daily if necessary. Monitor as per dogs and cats. (Hoeffer 2000)

b) 0.005–0.01 mg/kg PO once to twice daily using the elixir; for maintenance; monitor blood levels if possible (Williams 2000)

c) Treatment follows the same principles of other small animal medicine: Dilated cardiomyopathy long-term maintenance with furosemide (2 mg/kg q12h), enalapril (0.5 mg/kg q48h) and digoxin (0.01 mg/kg q24h). Monitor potassium if using diuretics longer than a few days. (Johnson-Delaney 2005b)

■ **RABBITS/RODENTS/SMALL MAMMALS:**

a) Hamsters: For dilated cardiomyopathy: 0.05–0.1 mg/kg PO q12h (Adamcak & Otten 2000)

■ **CATTLE:**

a) 0.25 mg/100 lbs body weight (not destroyed in rumen), titrate dose to normalize atrial rate; not excreted in milk (McConnell & Hughey 1987)

■ **HORSES:** (**Note:** ARCI UCGFS Class 4 Drug)

a) Loading dose: 11 micrograms/kg IV given slowly or in divided doses, *or* 44 micrograms/kg PO;

Maintenance Dose: 2.2 micrograms/kg IV every 12h or 11 micrograms/kg PO every 12 hours. Maintain plasma concentrations between 0.5–2 ng/mL. (Mogg 1999)

■ **BIRDS:**

a) Because of its very small therapeutic margin, it may be best to use digoxin to stabilize patients in an emergency rather than for long-term therapy; initial doses are 0.02–0.5 mg/kg q12h for 2–3 days, then decreased to 0.01 mg/kg q12–24h. Consider switching to an ACE inhibitor. (Johnson-Delaney 2005a)

Monitoring

■ Serum levels: Because of the significant interpatient pharmacokinetic variation seen with this drug, and its narrow therapeutic index, it is strongly recommended to monitor serum levels to help guide therapy. Unless the patient received an initial loading dose, at least 6 days should pass after beginning therapy to monitor serum levels to allow levels to approach steady-state. Historically, suggested therapeutic serum levels in the dog have ranged widely (0.8–3 ng/mL), but most now believe that levels above 2.5 ng/mL are "toxic." A recent reference (Luis Fuentes 2009) states that trough serum levels should be in the 0.9–1.2 ng/mL range that is lower than previously recommended. Therapeutic levels in cats are reported to be between 0.9–2 ng/mL (Lainesse 2009). For other species, values from 0.5–2 ng/mL can be used as guidelines. Levels at the higher end of the suggested range may be necessary to treat some atrial arrhythmias, but may also result in higher incidences of adverse effects. Usually a trough level (just before next dose or at least 8 hours after last dose) is recommended, but drawing a sample any-time is acceptable.

■ Appetite/weight
■ Cardiac rate, ECG changes
■ Serum electrolytes
■ Renal Function Tests
■ Clinical efficacy for CHF (improved perfusion, decreased edema, increased venous (or arterial) O2 levels).

Client Information
■ Contact veterinarian if animal demonstrates changes in behavior, vomits, has diarrhea, shows lack of appetite, clinical signs of colic (horses), or becomes lethargic or depressed.

Chemistry/Synonyms
A cardiac glycoside, digoxin occurs as bitter tasting, clear to white crystals or as white, crystalline powder. It is practically insoluble in water, slightly soluble in diluted alcohol, and very slightly soluble in 40% propylene glycol solution. Above 235°C, it melts with decomposition.

Digoxin may also be known as: digoxinum or digoxosidum; many trade names are available. Occasionally, digoxin is described as digitalis.

Storage/Stability
The commercial injection consists of a 40% propylene glycol, 10% alcohol solution having a pH of 6.6–7.4.

Digoxin tablets, capsules, elixir and injection should be stored at room temperature (15–30°C) and protected from light.

At pH's from 5–8, digoxin is stable, but in solutions with a pH of less than 3, it is hydrolyzed.

Compatibility/Compounding Considerations
The injectable product is **compatible** with most commercially available IV solutions, including lactated Ringer's, D_5W, and normal saline. To prevent the possibility of precipitation occurring, one manufacturer (GlaxoWellcome) recommends that the injection be diluted by a volume at least 4 times; with either sterile water, D_5W, or normal saline. Digoxin injection has been demonstrated to be **compatible** with bretylium tosylate, cimetidine HCl, lidocaine HCl, and verapamil HCl.

Digoxin is **incompatible** with dobutamine HCl, acids, and alkalies. The manufacturer does not recommend mixing digoxin injection with other medications. Compatibility is dependent upon factors such as pH, concentration, temperature and diluent used; consult specialized references or a hospital pharmacist for more specific information.

Dosage Forms/Regulatory Status
There are bioavailability differences between dosage forms and in tablets produced by different manufacturers. It is recommended that tablets be used from a manufacturer that the clinician has confidence in and that brands not be routinely interchanged. Should a change in

dosage forms be desired, the following bioavailability differences can be used as guidelines in altering the dose: Intravenous = 100%, IM ≈ 80%, Oral tablets ≈ 60%, Oral elixir ≈ 75%, Oral capsules ≈ 90–100%. The bioavailability of digoxin in veterinary species has only been studied in a limited manner. One study in dogs yielded similar values as those above for oral tablets and elixir, but in horses only about 20% of an intragastric dose was bioavailable.

VETERINARY-LABELED PRODUCTS:
The veterinary-labeled products are no longer available commercially in the USA.

The ARCI (Racing Commissioners International) has designated this drug as a class 4 substance. See the appendix for more information.

HUMAN-LABELED PRODUCTS:
Digoxin Solution for Injection: 250 micrograms/mL (0.25 mg/mL) in 2 mL amps, and 1 & 2 mL *Tubex* or *Carpuject*; Pediatric solution for Injection: 100 micrograms/mL (0.1 mg/mL) in 1 mL amps; *Lanoxin®* (GlaxoSmithKline); generic; (Rx)

Digoxin Oral Tablets: 125 micrograms (0.125 mg), and 250 micrograms (0.25 mg); *Lanoxin®* (GlaxoSmithKline); generic; (Rx)

Digoxin Oral Solution: 50 micrograms/mL (0.05 mg/mL) in 60 mL and UD 2.5 & 5 mL; generic; (Rx)

References
Adamcak, A. & B. Otten (2000). Rodent Therapeutics. *Vet Clin NA: Exotic Anim Pract* 3:1(Jan): 221–240.

Hoeffer, H. (2000). Heart Disease in Ferrets. *Kirk's Current Veterinary Therapy: XIII Small Animal Practice.* J Bonagura Ed. Philadelphia, WB Saunders: 1144–1148.

Hogan, D. (2004). Arrhythmias: diagnosis and treatment. Proceedings: ACVIM Forum. Accessed via: Veterinary Information Network. http://goo.gl/voENn

Johnson–Delaney, C. (2005a). Avian Cardiology for the Practitioner. Proceedings: Atlantic Coast Veterinary Conference. Accessed via: Veterinary Information Network. http://goo.gl/RgFh0

Johnson–Delaney, C. (2005b). Ferret Cardiology. Proceedings: Atlantic Coast Veterinary Conference. Accessed via: Veterinary Information Network. http://goo.gl/qiaGG

Keene, B.W. & J. Bonagura (2009). Management of heart failure in dogs. *Kirk's Current Veteinary Therapy XIV.* J Bonagura and D Twedt Eds., Saunders: 769–780.

Kittleson, M. (2010). Management of Heart Failure – Pharmacokinetics. *Small Animal Cardiovascular Medicine, 2nd Ed.* M Kittleson and R Kienle Eds., Accessed Online via the Veterinary Drug Information Network.

Lainesse, C. (2009). TDM: Basic Pharmacokinetics for Dosage Adjustements! Proceedings: WVC. Accessed via: Veterinary Information Network. http://goo.gl/Qmydz

Luis Fuentes, V. (2009). Treatment of Canine Heart Failure. Proceedings: WSAVA World Congress. Accessed via: Veterinary Information Network. http://goo.gl/mMzTS

McConnell, V.C. & T. Hughey (1987). *Formulary, The University of Georgia, Veterinary Medical Teaching Hospital.* Athens, GA.

Meurs, K. (2006). Therapeutic management of canine dilated cardiomyopathy. Proceedings: ACVIM. Accessed via: Veterinary Information Network. http://goo.gl/F2Rbt

Mogg, T. (1999). Equine Cardiac Disease: Clinical pharmacology and therapeutics. *The Veterinary Clinics of North America: Equine Practice* 15:3(December).

Pedersoli, W.M. (1980). Serum Digoxin Concentrations in Dogs Before and After Concomitant Treatment with Chloramphenicol. *Journal of the American Animal Hospital Association* 16(6): 839–844.

Smith, F. (2009). Update on Antiarrhythmic Therapy. Proceedings: Western Veterinary Conference. Accessed via: Veterinary Information Network. http://goo.gl/aiVDJ

Ware, W. & B. Keene (2000). Outpatient management of chronic heart failure. *Kirk's Current Veterinary Therapy: XIII Small Animal Practice*. J Bonagura Ed. Philadelphia, WB Saunders: 748–752.

Williams, B. (2000). Therapeutics in Ferrets. *Vet Clin NA: Exotic Anim Pract* 3:1(Jan): 131–153.

WSU–VetClinPharmLab (2009). "Problem Drugs." http://goo.gl/aIGlM.

DIHYDRO-TACHYSTEROL
DHT

(dye-*hye*-droe-*tak*-ee-ster-ole)
DHT®, Hytakerol®

VITAMIN D ANALOG

Prescriber Highlights

▶ Commercial dosage forms discontinued; may be available from compounding pharmacies

▶ Vitamin D analog for hypocalcemia secondary to hypoparathyroidism or renal disease; calcitriol more often recommended

▶ Raises calcium faster than ergocalciferol & effects dissipate more rapidly after the drug is stopped

▶ Contraindications: Hypercalcemia, vitamin D toxicity, malabsorption syndrome, or abnormal sensitivity to the effects of vitamin D. Extreme caution: Hyperphosphatemia, renal dysfunction (when receiving the drug for non-renal indications)

▶ Adverse Effects: Hypercalcemia (may present as polydipsia, polyuria & anorexia), nephrocalcinosis, & hyperphosphatemia

▶ Some animals are resistant to therapy

▶ Monitoring serum calcium mandatory

Uses/Indications

DHT is used in small animals to treat hypocalcemia secondary to hypoparathyroidism or severe renal disease. Because of availability issues and time to resolve hypercalcemia secondary to DHT toxicity, most are now recommending calcitriol.

Pharmacology/Actions

DHT is hydroxylated in the liver to 25-hydroxy-dihydrotachysterol that is the active form of the drug and is an analog of 1,25-dihydroxyvitamin D. Vitamin D is considered a hormone and, in conjunction with parathormone (PTH) and calcitonin, regulates calcium homeostasis in the body. Active analogues (or metabolites) of vitamin D enhance calcium absorption from the GI tract, promote reabsorption of calcium by the renal tubules, and increase the rate of accretion and resorption of minerals in bone.

Pharmacokinetics

If fat absorption is normal, vitamin D analogs are readily absorbed from the GI tract (small intestine). There are anecdotal reports of dogs and cats not responding to the oral tablets or capsule forms of the drug, but responding to the oral liquid dosage forms. Bile is required for adequate absorption and patients with steatorrhea, liver or biliary disease will have diminished absorption. DHT is hydroxylated in the liver to 25-hydroxy-dihydrotachysterol that is the active form of the drug. Unlike some other forms of vitamin D, DHT does not require parathormone activation in the kidneys. The time required for maximal therapeutic effect is usually seen within the first week of treatment. Unlike some other forms of vitamin D, DHT offloads relatively rapidly (1–3 weeks).

Contraindications/Precautions/Warnings

DHT is contraindicated in patients with hypercalcemia, vitamin D toxicity, malabsorption syndrome, or abnormal sensitivity to the effects of vitamin D. It should be used with extreme caution in patients with hyperphosphatemia (many clinicians believe hyperphosphatemia or a combined calcium/phosphorous product of >70 mg/dL is a contraindication to its use), or in patients with renal dysfunction (when receiving the drug for non-renal indications).

Adverse Effects

Hypercalcemia, nephrocalcinosis, and hyperphosphatemia are potential complications of DHT therapy. Clinical signs of hypercalcemia include polydipsia, polyuria, and anorexia. Monitoring of serum calcium levels is mandatory while using this drug.

Reproductive/Nursing Safety

Hypervitaminosis D has caused fetal abnormalities in a variety of species. In humans, the FDA categorizes this drug as category *C* for use during pregnancy (*Animal studies have shown an adverse effect on the fetus, but there are no adequate studies in humans; or there are no animal reproduction studies and no adequate studies in humans.*) Weigh the risks versus benefits of treating animal patients with this drug during pregnancy.

Vitamin D is excreted in breast milk in limited amounts; use with caution.

Overdosage/Acute Toxicity

Acute ingestions should be managed using established protocols for removal or prevention of the drug being absorbed from the GI. Orally administered mineral oil may reduce absorption and enhance fecal elimination.

Hypercalcemia secondary to chronic dosing of the drug should be treated by first temporarily discontinuing DHT and exogenous calcium therapy. If the hypercalcemia is severe, furosemide, calcium-free IV fluids (*e.g.*, normal saline), urine acidification, and corticosteroids may be employed. Because of the long duration of action of DHT (usually one week and potentially up to 3 weeks), hypercalcemia may persist. Restart DHT/calcium therapy at a reduced dosage with diligent monitoring when calcium serum levels return to the normal range.

Drug Interactions

The following drug interactions have either been reported or are theoretical in humans or animals receiving DHT and may be of significance in veterinary patients:

- **CALCIUM-CONTAINING PHOSPHORUS BINDING AGENTS (*e.g.*, calcium carbonate):** Use with vitamin D analogs may induce hypercalcemia

- **CORTICOSTEROIDS:** Can nullify the effects of vitamin D analogs

- **DIGOXIN or VERAPAMIL:** Patients on verapamil or digoxin are sensitive to the effects of hypercalcemia; intensified monitoring is required

- **MINERAL OIL, SUCRALFATE, CHOLESTYRAMINE:** May reduce the amount of drug absorbed

- **PHENYTOIN, BARBITURATES or PRIMIDONE:** May induce hepatic enzyme systems and increase the metabolism of Vitamin D analogs thus decreasing their activity

- **THIAZIDE DIURETICS:** May cause hypercalcemia when given in conjunction with Vitamin D analogs

Laboratory Considerations

- **Serum cholesterol** levels may be falsely elevated by vitamin D analogs when using the Zlatkis-Zak reaction for determination.

Doses

Vitamin D therapy for hypocalcemic conditions is often used with exogenously administered calcium products. Refer to the calcium monograph or the references cited below for further information.

- **DOGS:**

For hypocalcemia secondary to hypoparathyroidism:

a) Initially give 0.03 mg/kg PO for several days or until effect is demonstrated, then give 0.02 mg/kg for 2 days, then 0.01 mg/kg per day. Pet should remain hospitalized until serum calcium concentration remains stable between 8–9.5 mg/dL. Recheck serum calcium on a weekly basis during early stages of treatment; recheck every 2–3 months long-term. Some dogs and cats that appear to be resistant to treatment on tablets or capsules may respond to the liquid form. (Feldman 2005)

- **CATS:**

For hypocalcemia secondary to hypoparathyroidism:

a) Initially give 0.03 mg/kg PO for several days or until effect is demonstrated, then give 0.02 mg/kg for 2 days, then 0.01 mg/kg per day. Pet should remain hospitalized until serum calcium concentration remains stable between 8–9.5 mg/dL. Recheck serum calcium on a weekly basis during early stages of treatment; recheck every 2–3 months long-term. Some dogs and cats that appear to be resistant to treatment on tablets or capsules may respond to the liquid form. (Feldman 2005)

b) For chronic hypocalcemia with oral calcium tx: Initially: 0.02–0.03 mg/kg/day PO. Maintenance: 0.01–0.02 mg/kg PO q24-48h. (Kerl 2008)

Monitoring

- Serum calcium levels should be monitored closely (some clinicians recommend twice daily) during the initial treatment period. When the animal is stabilized, frequency may be reduced but never discontinued. All animals receiving DHT therapy should have calcium levels determined at least 2–4 times yearly

- Serum phosphorous (particularly in renal failure patients)

Client Information

- Clients should be briefed on the clinical signs of hypercalcemia (polydipsia, polyuria, anorexia) and hypocalcemia (muscle tremors, twitching, tetany, weakness, stiff gait, ataxia, behavioral changes, and seizures) and instructed to report these symptoms to the veterinarian.

Chemistry/Synonyms

A vitamin D analog, dihydrotachysterol (DHT) occurs as odorless, colorless or white crystals, or crystalline white powder. It is practically insoluble in water, sparingly soluble in vegetable oils, and soluble in alcohol.

Dihydrotachysterol may also be known as: DHT, dichysterol, or dihydrotachysterol$_2$, AT 10, Atiten, *DHT®*, *Dihydral®*, *Dygratyl®*, *Tachyrol®*, or *Tachystin®*.

Storage/Stability

All DHT products should be stored at room temperature (15–30°C). Capsules or tablets should be stored in well-closed, light-resistant containers and the oral concentrate should be stored in tight, light-resistant containers.

Dosage Forms/Regulatory Status

VETERINARY-LABELED PRODUCTS: None

HUMAN-LABELED PRODUCTS: None

Note: Dosage forms may be available from compounding pharmacies.

References

Feldman, E. (2005). Disorders of the parathyroid glands. *Textbook of Veterinary Internal Medicine, 6th Ed.* S Ettinger and E Feldman Eds., Elsevier: 1508–1535.

Kerl, M. (2008). Electrolyte Imbalances in the Cat. Proceedings: IVECCS. Accessed via: Veterinary Information Network. http://goo.gl/S3RxI

DILTIAZEM HCL

(dil-**tye**-a-zem)   Cardizem®, Dilacor XR®

CALCIUM CHANNEL BLOCKER

Prescriber Highlights

▶ Calcium channel blocker used in dogs, cats, & ferrets for SVT's, pulmonary hypertension, systemic hypertension, or hypertrophic cardiomyopathy; may prove useful in horses in combination with quinidine to treat atrial fibrillation

▶ Contraindications: Severe hypotension, sick sinus syndrome or 2nd or 3rd degree AV block, acute MI, radiographically documented pulmonary congestion, hypersensitivity

▶ Caution: Geriatric patients or those with heart failure (particularly if also receiving beta blockers), or hepatic or renal impairment

▶ Potential teratogen (high doses)

Uses/Indications

Diltiazem may be useful in the treatment of hypertension, atrial fibrillation, and supraventricular tachycardias.

Diltiazem is used for the treatment of feline hypertrophic cardiomyopathy, but enthusiasm for its use for this indication has cooled somewhat in recent years.

Pharmacology/Actions

Diltiazem is a calcium-channel blocker similar in action to drugs such as verapamil or nifedipine. While the exact mechanism remains unknown, diltiazem inhibits the transmembrane influx of extracellular calcium ions in myocardial cells and vascular smooth muscle, but does not alter serum calcium concentrations. The net effect of this action is to inhibit the cardiac and vascular smooth muscle contractility, thereby dilating main systemic and coronary arteries. Total peripheral resistance, blood pressure, and cardiac afterload are all reduced.

Diltiazem has effects on cardiac conduction. It slows AV node conduction and prolongs refractory times. Diltiazem rarely affects SA node conduction, but in patients with Sick Sinus Syndrome, resting heart rates may be reduced.

Although diltiazem can cause negative inotropic effects, it is rarely of clinical importance (unlike verapamil or nifedipine). Diltiazem apparently does not affect plasma renin, aldosterone, glucose, or insulin concentrations.

Pharmacokinetics

In humans after an oral dose, about 80% of the dose is absorbed rapidly from the gut, but because of a high first pass effect, only about half of the absorbed drug reaches the systemic circulation. Bioavailability in cats is reported to range from 50–80% with peak levels occurring about 45 minutes after oral dosing. In dogs, bioavailability may only be around 25%. Pharmacokinetics of a long acting product (*Cardizem® CD*) given at 10 mg/kg once daily to healthy cats were: bioavailability 22–59%; half-life 411 +/-59 minutes; peak levels achieved in 340 +/-140 minutes. A different sustained-release product (*Dilacor XR*) has a bioavailability of about 94% in cats and doses of 1 mg/kg PO q8h maintained the serum concentration within the suspected therapeutic range for 8 hours.

Approximately 70-75% of the drug is bound to serum proteins. Diltiazem enters milk in concentrations approximating those found in plasma. Diltiazem is rapidly and almost completely metabolized in the liver to several metabolites, including two that are active. Serum half-life in cats is about 2 hours, about 3 hours in dogs, and about 90 minutes in horses. In humans, elimination half-life ranges from 3.5 to 10 hours. Renal impairment may only slightly increase half-lives.

Contraindications/Precautions/Warnings

Diltiazem is contraindicated in patients with severe hypotension (<90 mm Hg systolic), sick sinus syndrome or 2nd or 3rd degree AV block (unless a functioning pacemaker is in place), acute MI, radiographically documented pulmonary congestion, or when the patient is hypersensitive to it.

Diltiazem should be used with caution in geriatric patients or those with heart failure (particularly if also receiving beta blockers), or hepatic or renal impairment.

If giving direct IV administration (push), give over at least two minutes.

Adverse Effects

At usual doses, bradycardia is the most prominent side effect reported in dogs. In cats, vomiting is reported as the most common side effect. Potentially, lethargy, GI distress (anorexia), hypotension, heart block or other rhythm disturbances, CNS effects, rashes, or elevations in liver function tests could occur in either species.

Cats receiving the 60 mg sustained-release pellet (found in 240 mg sustained-release capsules) are prone to developing significant adverse effects.

Reproductive/Nursing Safety

High doses in rodents have resulted in increased fetal deaths and skeletal abnormalities. Use during pregnancy only when the benefits outweigh the potential risks. In humans, the FDA categorizes this drug as category *C* for use during pregnancy (*Animal studies have shown an adverse effect on the fetus, but there are no adequate studies in humans; or there are no animal reproduction studies and no adequate studies in humans.*)

Diltiazem is excreted in milk and concentrations may approximate those found in the serum; use during nursing with caution.

Overdosage/Acute Toxicity

The oral LD_{50} in dogs has been reported as >50 mg/kg. Clinical signs noted after overdosage may include GI signs, heart block, bradycardia, hypotension, and heart failure. A dog who ingested approximately 100 mg/kg PO of a sustained release product developed bradycardia, hypotension, CNS depression, 2nd degree AV block with ventricular escape, and gastrointestinal effects. Ultimately the dog required a transvenous pacemaker for 19 hours, but recovered (Syring *et al.* 2008).

Treatment should consist of gut emptying protocols when warranted, and supportive and symptomatic treatment. Atropine may be used to treat bradycardias or 2nd or 3rd degree AV block. If these do not respond to vagal blockade, isoproterenol may be tried (with caution). Fixed block may require cardiac pacing. Inotropics (*e.g.*, dobutamine, dopamine, isoproterenol) and pressors (*e.g.*, dopamine, norepinephrine) may be required to treat heart failure and hypotension. A slow intravenous calcium infusion (1 mL/10 kg body weight of 10% calcium gluconate) may also be useful for severe acute toxicity.

Drug Interactions

The following drug interactions have either been reported or are theoretical in humans or animals receiving diltiazem and may be of significance in veterinary patients:

■ **ANESTHETICS, GENERAL:** May increase cardiac depressant effects of diltiazem

■ **BENZODIAZEPINES:** Diltiazem may increase benzodiazepine levels

■ **BETA-BLOCKERS:** Diltiazem may increase the likelihood of bradycardia, AV block or CHF developing in patients also receiving beta-blockers (including **ophthalmic beta-blockers**); additionally, diltiazem may substantially increase the bioavailability of propranolol

■ **BUSPIRONE:** Diltiazem may increase buspirone levels

■ **CISAPRIDE:** Diltiazem could potentially increase risk for increased QT intervals

■ **DIGOXIN:** While data conflicts regarding whether diltiazem affects digoxin pharmacokinetics, diligent monitoring of digoxin serum concentrations should be performed

■ **CIMETIDINE/RANITIDINE:** Cimetidine may increase plasma diltiazem concentrations; increased monitoring of diltiazem's effects is warranted. Ranitidine may also affect diltiazem concentrations, but to a lesser extent.

■ **CYCLOSPORINE:** Diltiazem may increase cyclosporine serum concentrations; increased monitoring and dosage adjustments may be required

■ **RIFAMPIN:** May decrease diltiazem levels

■ **QUINIDINE:** Diltiazem may increase quinidine serum concentrations; increased monitoring and dosage adjustments may be required

Doses

■ **DOGS:**

For treatment of supraventricular tachyarrhthymias:

a) For decreasing ventricular rate in dogs with atrial fibrillation: Digoxin most commonly used first and once a therapeutic serum concentration is achieved, if heart rate response is not adequate can add diltiazem: Initially, 0.5 mg/kg PO q8h, if response not adequate can increase to 1 mg/kg PO q8h and finally, to 1.5 mg/kg PO q8h. In general, do not use with beta blocker.

For acute treatment of supraventricular tachycardia: Generally, 0.05 mg/kg IV administered over 1-2 minutes. May repeat this dose up to two times, with 5 minutes between doses. Some cardiologists use a dose of 0.25 mg/kg administered over 5 minutes.

For chronic treatment of supraventricular tachycardia: Initially, 1 mg/kg PO q8h and titrated upward to a maximum of 4 mg/kg PO q8h. Doses from 2–4 mg/kg q8h should probably not be given to dogs that have moderate to severe myocardial failure or with significant cardiac compromise due to any reason. (Kittleson 2010)

b) For acute treatment of atrial tachycardia: 0.05–0.15 mg/kg slowly IV, repeat every 5 minutes to effect or until a total dose of 0.1–0.3 mg/kg; *OR* give 0.5 mg/kg PO followed by 0.25 mg/kg PO every hour until conversion or a total oral dose of 1.5–2 mg/kg has been given. Chronically: May give an initial dose of 0.5 mg/kg PO q8h up to 2 mg/kg. (Ware 2000)

c) For emergency treatment: Initially, 0.25 mg/kg IV bolus given over 2 minutes; subsequent 0.25 mg/kg boluses may be repeated at 15 minute intervals until conversion occurs or to a maximum (total) dose of 0.75 mg/kg. (Rush 2005)

For adjunctive treatment of pulmonary hypertension:

a) 1–2 mg/kg PO three times daily. (Oyama 2009)

For emergency management of hypertension when the capabilities for using nitroprusside are unavailable:

a) 0.5 mg/kg PO q6h (if blood pressure not

controlled, may add a beta-blocker (*e.g.*, atenolol) (Brown & Henik 2000)

■ **CATS:**

For treatment of hypertrophic cardiomyopathy:

a) 7.5 mg (total dose) PO q8–12h; Long-acting forms: *Cardizem® CD Capsules*: 10 mg/kg once daily. *Dilacor® XR Capsules*: 15–30 mg total dose q12–24h. Some cats tolerate 60 mg daily, but vomiting may be a problem. (Fox 2000)

b) 1.75–2.5 mg/kg PO q8h or sustained release (*Dilacor®*) dosed at 30 mg (total dose) PO q12h (Ware & Keene 2000)

c) 7.5–15 mg (total dose) per cat PO q8h. Alternatively, the sustained-release products *Cardizem® CD* at 45 mg (total dose) PO q24h or *Dilacor® XR* at 30 mg (total dose; 1/2 of one of the 60 mg tablets found within the capsule) PO q12h can be used. (Kittleson 2009), (Kittleson 2010)

d) If using standard release formulations: 1–2.5 mg/kg PO q8h; if using sustained release formations: 30–60 mg (total dose per cat) q24h. Also indicated for supraventricular arrhythmias. (Smith 2009)

e) If cat has minimal tachycardia and a loud S4 gallop, many prefer using diltiazem (over a beta blocker): *Dilacor® XR* 30 mg/cat PO q24h. (Lichtenberger 2009)

For treatment of supraventricular tachyarrhythmias:

a) For emergency treatment: Initially, 0.25 mg/kg IV bolus given over 2 minutes; subsequent 0.25 mg/kg boluses may be repeated at 15 minute intervals until conversion occurs or to a maximum (total) dose of 0.75 mg/kg. (Rush 2005)

b) For acute management: 0.125–0.35 mg/kg IV; for chronic management: 7.5 (per cat) PO q8h (used in combination with digoxin for patients. with CHF unless cat has hypertrophic cardiomyopathy and atrial fib, then digoxin not used) (Wright 2000)

For emergency management of hypertension when the capabilities for using nitroprusside are unavailable:

a) 0.5 mg/kg PO q6h (if blood pressure not controlled, may add a beta-blocker (*e.g.*, atenolol) (Brown & Henik 2000)

■ **FERRETS:**

For hypertrophic cardiomyopathy:

a) 2–7.5 mg/kg PO twice daily; adjust as necessary. May result in heart block. (Williams 2000)

Monitoring
■ ECG/Heart rate
■ Blood pressure
■ Adverse effects

Client Information
■ Inform clients of potential adverse effects. Stress adherence to dosing regimen.

Chemistry/Synonyms
A calcium channel blocker, diltiazem HCl occurs as a white to off-white crystalline powder having a bitter taste. It is soluble in water and alcohol. Potencies may be expressed in terms of base (active moiety) and the salt. Dosages are generally expressed in terms of the salt.

Diltiazem may also be known as: CRD-401, diltiazemi hydrochloridum, latiazem hydrochloride, and MK-793; many trade names are available.

Storage/Stability
Diltiazem oral products should be stored at room temperature in tight, light resistant containers.

The powder for injection should be stored between 15–30°C. After reconstituting, discard after 24 hours.

Compatibility/Compounding Considerations
Diltiazem is **compatible** with D5W and sodium chloride 0.9% digoxin, bumetanide, dobutamine, dopamine, epinephrine, lidocaine, morphine, nitroglycerin, potassium chloride, sodium nitroprusside, and vasopressin. It is **incompatible** with diazepam, furosemide, phenytoin and thiopental.

Dosage Forms/Regulatory Status
VETERINARY-LABELED PRODUCTS: None

The ARCI (Racing Commissioners International) has designated this drug as a class 4 substance. See the appendix for more information.

HUMAN-LABELED PRODUCTS:

Diltiazem Oral Tablets: 30 mg, 60 mg, 90 mg & 120 mg; *Cardizem®* (Biovail); generic; (Rx)

Diltiazem Tablet & Capsules Extended/Sustained Release: 60 mg, 90 mg, 120 mg, 180 mg, 240 mg, 300 mg, 360 mg and 420 mg; *Cardizem CD®* & *LA®* (Abbott); *Cartia XT®* (Andrx); *Dilacor XR®* (Watson); *Tiazac®* (Forest), *Diltia XT®* & *Taztia XT®* (Andrx); *Dilt-CD®* & *XR®* (Apotex USA); generic; (Rx)

Diltiazem Injection: 5 mg/mL in 5 mL, 10 mL and 25 mL vials; Powder for Injection: 25 mg in single-use containers (carton of 6 Lyo-Ject syringes with diluent); *Cardizem®* (Biovail); generic; (Rx)

References

Brown, S. & R. Henik (2000). Therapy for Systemic Hypertension in Dogs and Cats. *Kirk's Current Veterinary Therapy: XIII Small Animal Practice.* J Bonagura Ed. Philadelphia, WB Saunders: 838–841.

Fox, P. (2000). Feline Cardiomyopathies. *Textbook of Veterinary Internal Medicine: Diseases of the Dog and Cat.* S Ettinger and E Feldman Eds. Philadelphia, WB Saunders. 1: 896–923.

Kittleson, M. (2009). Treatment of feline hypertrophic cardiomyopathy (HCM)—Lost Dreams. Proceedings: ACVIM. Accessed via: Veterinary Information Network. http://goo.gl/XvCZt

Kittleson, M. (2010). "Chapt 29: Drugs used in treatment of cardiac arrhythmias– Drugs used to treat tachyarrythmias – part 6." *Small Animal Cardiovascular Medicine, 2nd Ed.* http://goo.gl/FXvDZ.

Lichtenberger, M. (2009). How I treat congestive heart failure II. Proceedings: WVC. Accessed via: Veterinary Information Network. http://goo.gl/neTT8

Oyama, M. (2009). Pulmonary Hypertension: What you can't see can kill you. Proceedings: ACVC. Accessed via: Veterinary Information Network. http://goo.gl/0jNQb

Rush, J. (2005). Treatment of life–threatening arrhythmias. Proceedings: IVECCS. Accessed via: Veterinary Information Network. http://goo.gl/UxBxv

Smith, F. (2009). Feline Cardiomyopathies: Diagnosis and treatment. Proceedings: WVC. Accessed via: Veterinary Information Network. http://goo.gl/w4AMz

Syring, R.S., M.F. Costello, et al. (2008). Temporary transvenous cardiac pacing in a dog with diltiazem intoxication. *Journal of Veterinary Emergency and Critical Care* **18**(1): 75–80.

Ware, W. (2000). Therapy for Critical Arrythmias: New Advances. Proceedings: The North American Veterinary Conference, Orlando.

Ware, W. & B. Keene (2000). Outpatient management of chronic heart failure. *Kirk's Current Veterinary Therapy: XIII Small Animal Practice.* J Bonagura Ed. Philadelphia, WB Saunders: 748–752.

Williams, B. (2000). Therapeutics in Ferrets. *Vet Clin NA: Exotic Anim Pract* 3:1(Jan): 131–153.

Wright, K. (2000). Assessment and treatment of supraventricular tachyarrhythmias. *Kirk's Current Veterinary Therapy: XIII Small Animal Practice.* J Bonagura Ed. Philadelphia, WB Saunders: 726–730.

DIMENHYDRINATE

(dye-men-*hye*-dri-nate)
Dramamine®, Gravol®

ANTIHISTAMINE

Prescriber Highlights

▶ Antihistamine used primarily for prevention of motion sickness in dogs & cats; may be useful as an adjunctive treatment for feline pancreatitis

▶ Contraindications: Hypersensitivity to it or others in class

▶ Caution: Angle closure glaucoma, GI or urinary obstruction, COPD, hyperthyroidism, seizure disorders, cardiovascular disease or hypertension; may mask clinical signs of ototoxicity

▶ Adverse Effects: CNS depression & anticholinergic effects. GI effects (diarrhea, vomiting, anorexia) are less common

Uses/Indications

In veterinary medicine, dimenhydrinate is used primarily for its antiemetic effects for vomiting and in the prophylactic treatment of motion sickness in dogs and cats. Because histamine is thought not to be an important mediator of vomiting in cats, other choices such as NK-1

antagonists (*e.g.,* maropitant) or M₁-cholinergic antagonists (*e.g.,* prochlorperazine, chlorpromazine) may be better choices for treating motion sickness or vomiting in cats. As dimenhydrinate is often thought of as "half-strength diphenhydramine" it can be employed whenever a histamine-1 blocker is desired.

Pharmacology/Actions

Dimenhydrinate has antihistaminic (H1), antiemetic, anticholinergic, CNS depressant and local anesthetic effects. These principle pharmacologic actions are thought to be a result of only the diphenhydramine moiety. Used most commonly for its antiemetic/motion sickness effects, dimenhydrinate's exact mechanism of action for this indication is unknown, but the drug does inhibit vestibular stimulation. The anticholinergic actions of dimenhydrinate may play a role in blocking acetylcholine stimulation of the vestibular and reticular systems. Tolerance to the CNS depressant effects can ensue after a few days of therapy and antiemetic effectiveness may also diminish with prolonged use.

Theoretically, histamine-1 (diphenhydramine, dimenhydrinate, etc.) and histamine-2 (ranitidine, famotidine, etc.) blockers may reduce histamine-mediated increases in microvasculature permeability that is associated with the development of hemorrhagic necrosis in feline pancreatitis.

Pharmacokinetics

The pharmacokinetics of this agent have apparently not been studied in veterinary species. In humans, the drug is well absorbed after oral administration with antiemetic effects occurring within 30 minutes of administration. Antiemetic effects occur almost immediately after IV injection. The duration of effect is usually 3–6 hours.

Diphenhydramine is metabolized in the liver, and the majority of the drug is excreted as metabolites into the urine. The terminal elimination half-life in adult humans ranges from 2.4–9.3 hours.

Contraindications/Precautions/Warnings

Dimenhydrinate is contraindicated in patients who are hypersensitive to it or to other antihistamines in its class. Because of their anticholinergic activity, antihistamines should be used with caution in patients with angle closure glaucoma, prostatic hypertrophy, pyloroduodenal or bladder neck obstruction, and COPD if mucosal secretions are a problem. Additionally, they should be used with caution in patients with hyperthyroidism, seizure disorders, cardiovascular disease or hypertension. It may mask the clinical signs of ototoxicity and should therefore be used with this knowledge when concomitantly administering with ototoxic drugs.

The sedative effects of antihistamines, may adversely affect the performance of working dogs.

Adverse Effects

Most common adverse reactions seen are CNS depression (lethargy, somnolence) and anticholinergic effects (dry mouth, urinary retention). GI effects (diarrhea, vomiting, anorexia) are less common, but have been noted. The sedative effects of antihistamines may diminish with time.

Reproductive/Nursing Safety

In humans, the FDA categorizes this drug as category **B** for use during pregnancy (*Animal studies have not yet demonstrated risk to the fetus, but there are no adequate studies in pregnant women; or animal studies have shown an adverse effect, but adequate studies in pregnant women have not demonstrated a risk to the fetus in the first trimester of pregnancy, and there is no evidence of risk in later trimesters.*) In a separate system evaluating the safety of drugs in canine and feline pregnancy (Papich 1989), this drug is categorized as in class: **B** (*Safe for use if used cautiously. Studies in laboratory animals may have uncovered some risk, but these drugs appear to be safe in dogs and cats or these drugs are safe if they are not administered when the animal is near term.*)

Small amounts of dimenhydrinate are excreted in milk; this is unlikely to pose much risk to nursing offspring.

Overdosage/Acute Toxicity

Overdosage may cause CNS stimulation (excitement to seizures) or depression (lethargy to coma), anticholinergic effects, respiratory depression and death. Treatment consists of emptying the gut if the ingestion was oral. Induce emesis if the patient is alert and CNS status is stable. Administration of a saline cathartic and/or activated charcoal may be given after emesis or gastric lavage. Treatment of other clinical signs should be performed using symptomatic and supportive therapies. Phenytoin (IV) is recommended in the treatment of seizures caused by antihistamine overdose in humans; use of barbiturates and diazepam are avoided.

Drug Interactions

Dimenhydrinate has been demonstrated to induce hepatic microsomal enzymes in animals (species not specified); the clinical implications of this effect are unclear.

The following drug interactions have either been reported or are theoretical in humans or animals receiving dimenhydrinate and may be of significance in veterinary patients:

- **ANTICHOLINERGIC DRUGS** (including **tricyclic antidepressants**): Dimenhydrinate may potentiate the anticholinergic effects of other anticholinergic drugs
- **CNS DEPRESSANT DRUGS:** Increased sedation can occur if dimenhydrinate (diphenhydramine) is combined with other CNS depressant drugs

Laboratory Considerations

- Antihistamines can decrease the wheal and flare response to **antigen skin testing**. In hu-

mans, it is suggested that antihistamines be discontinued at least 4 days before testing.

Doses

- **DOGS:**
  For prevention and treatment of motion sickness:
  a) As an antiemetic: 4–8 mg/kg PO three times daily. (Lichtenberger 2009)
  b) 4–8 mg/kg PO q8h (Washabau and Elie 1995), (Dowling 2003)
  As an antihistamine:
  a) 4–8 mg/kg q8–12h (Papich 2000)

- **CATS:**
  For prevention and treatment of motion sickness/vomiting:
  a) 8 mg/kg PO q8h (Scherk 2003)
  b) 4–8 mg/kg PO q8h (Dowling 2003)
  As an antihistamine:
  a) 4 mg per cat PO q8h (Scherk 2006)
  For adjunctive treatment of pancreatitis:
  a) 8 mg/kg PO q8h (Scherk 2005)

Monitoring

- Clinical efficacy
- Adverse effects (sedation, anticholinergic signs, etc.)

Chemistry/Synonyms

An ethanolamine derivative antihistamine, dimenhydrinate contains approximately 54% diphenhydramine and 46% 8-chlorotheophylline. It occurs as an odorless, bitter-tasting and numbing, white crystalline powder with a melting range of 102°–107°C. Dimenhydrinate is slightly soluble in water and is freely soluble in propylene glycol or alcohol. The pH of the commercially available injection ranges from 6.4 to 7.2.

Dimenhydrinate may also be known as: chloranautine, dimenhydrinatum, diphenhydramine teoclate, and diphenhydramine theoclate; many trade names are available.

Storage/Stability

Dimenhydrinate products should be stored at room temperature; avoid freezing the oral solution and injectable products. The oral solution should be stored in tight containers; tablets stored in well-closed containers.

Compatibility/Compounding Considerations

Dimenhydrinate injection is reportedly physically **compatible** with all commonly used intravenous replenishment solutions and the following drugs: amikacin sulfate, atropine sulfate, calcium gluconate, chloramphenicol sodium succinate, corticotropin, diatrizoate meglumine and sodium, diphenhydramine HCl, droperidol, fentanyl citrate, heparin sodium, iothalamate meglumine and sodium, meperidine HCl, methicillin sodium, metoclopramide, morphine sulfate, norepinephrine bitartrate, oxytetracycline HCl, penicillin G potassium, pentazocine

DIMERCAPROL 443

lactate, perphenazine, phenobarbital sodium, potassium chloride, scopolamine HBr, vancomycin HCl and vitamin B-complex with vitamin C.

The following drugs are either physically **incompatible** or **compatible only in certain concentrations** with dimenhydrinate: aminophylline, ammonium chloride, amobarbital sodium, butorphanol tartrate, glycopyrrolate, hydrocortisone sodium succinate, hydroxyzine, iodipamide meglumine, pentobarbital sodium, prochlorperazine edisylate, promazine HCl, promethazine HCl, tetracycline HCl, and thiopental sodium. Compatibility is dependent upon factors such as pH, concentration, temperature, and diluent used; consult a hospital pharmacist or specialized references for more specific information.

Dosage Forms/Regulatory Status

VETERINARY-LABELED PRODUCTS: None
HUMAN-LABELED PRODUCTS:
Dimenhydrinate Oral Tablets: 50 mg (regular & chewable); *Dramamine®* (Upjohn); *Dimetabs®* (Jones Medical); *Triptone®* (Del Pharmaceuticals); generic; [OTC & Rx (*Dimetabs®* only)]

Dimenhydrinate Oral Liquid: 12.5 mg/4 mL in 90 mL, pts and gals; 12.5 mg/5 mL in 120 mL; 15.62 mg/5 mL in 480 mL; *Dramamine®* and *Children's Dramamine®* (Upjohn); generic; (OTC)

Dimenhydrinate Injection: 50 mg/mL in 1 mL and 10 mL vials; *Dinate®* (Seatrace); *Dramanate®* (Pasadena); *Dymenate®* (Keene); generic (Abraxis); (Rx)

References

Dowling, P. (2003). GI Therapy: When what goes in won't stay down. Proceedings: Western Veterinary Conference. Accessed via: Veterinary Information Network. http://goo.gl/co8V8
Lichtenberger, M. (2009). How I treat congestive heart failure II. Proceedings: WVC. Accessed via: Veterinary Information Network. http://goo.gl/neTT8
Papich, M. (2000). Antihistamines: Current Therapeutic Use. *Kirk's Current Veterinary Therapy: XIII Small Animal Practice*. J Bonagura Ed. Philadelphia, WB Saunders: 49–53.
Scherk, M. (2003). Feline pancreatitis: underdiagnosed and overlooked. Proceedings: World Small Animal Veterinary Assoc World Congress. Accessed via: Veterinary Information Network. http://goo.gl/S8hdO
Scherk, M. (2005). Feline pancreatitis. Proceedings: Western Veterinary Conference. Accessed via: Veterinary Information Network. http://goo.gl/emF25
Scherk, M. (2006). Snots and Snuffles: Chronic Feline Upper Respiratory Syndrome. Proceedings: ACVIM. Accessed via: Veterinary Information Network. http://goo.gl/tWQ49

DIMERCAPROL
BAL

(dye-mer-*kap*-role)   BAL in Oil®
ANTIDOTE

Prescriber Highlights

▶ Chelating agent for arsenicals; sometimes used for lead, mercury, & gold compounds

▶ Contraindications: Patients with impaired hepatic function, unless secondary to acute arsenic toxicity, & in iron, cadmium, & selenium poisoning

▶ Caution: Patients with impaired renal function

▶ Alkalinize urine

▶ Administer deep IM (still painful)

▶ Adverse Effects: Usually transient & can include vomiting & seizures with higher dosages; increased blood pressure with tachycardia possible

Uses/Indications

The principal use of dimercaprol in veterinary medicine is in treating intoxications caused by arsenical compounds. It is occasionally used for lead, mercury and gold intoxication.

Pharmacology/Actions

The sulfhydryl groups found on dimercaprol form heterocyclic ring complexes with heavy metals, principally arsenic, lead, mercury and gold. This binding helps prevent or reduce heavy metal binding to sulfhydryl-dependent enzymes. Different metals have differing affinities for both dimercaprol and sulfhydryl-dependent enzymes and the drug is relatively ineffective in chelating some metals (*e.g.*, selenium). Chelation to dimercaprol is not irreversible and metals can dissociate from the complex as dimercaprol concentrations decrease, or in an acidic environment, or if oxidized. The dimercaprol-metal complex is excreted via renal and fecal routes.

Pharmacokinetics

After IM injection, peak blood levels occur in 30–60 minutes. The drug is slowly absorbed through the skin after topical administration. Dimercaprol is distributed throughout the body, including the brain. Highest tissue levels are found in the liver and kidneys.

Non-metal bound drug is rapidly metabolized to inactive compounds and excreted in the urine, bile and feces. In humans, the duration of action is thought to be about 4 hours with the drug completely eliminated within 6–24 hours.

Contraindications/Precautions/Warnings

Dimercaprol is contraindicated in patients with impaired hepatic function, unless secondary to acute arsenic toxicity. The drug is also contraindicated in iron, cadmium, and selenium poisoning, as the chelated complex can be more toxic than the metal alone.

Because dimercaprol is potentially nephrotoxic, it should be used cautiously in patients with impaired renal function. In order to protect the kidneys, the urine should be alkalinized to prevent the chelated drug from dissociating in the urine. Animals with diminished renal function or who develop renal dysfunction while on therapy should either have the dosage adjusted or discontinue therapy dependent on the clinical situation.

Adverse Effects

IM injections are necessary with this compound but can be very painful, particularly if the drug is not administered deeply. Vomiting and seizures can occur with higher dosages. Transient increases in blood pressure with concomitant tachycardia have been reported. Most adverse effects are transient in nature as the drug is eliminated rapidly.

Dimercaprol is potentially nephrotoxic.

Reproductive/Nursing Safety

In humans, the FDA categorizes this drug as category *C* for use during pregnancy (*Animal studies have shown an adverse effect on the fetus, but there are no adequate studies in humans; or there are no animal reproduction studies and no adequate studies in humans.*)

It is not known if dimercaprol is excreted in milk.

Overdosage/Acute Toxicity

Clinical signs of dimercaprol overdosage in animals include vomiting, seizures, tremors, coma, and death. No specific doses were located to correspond with these clinical signs, however.

Drug Interactions

The following drug interactions have either been reported or are theoretical in humans or animals receiving dimercaprol and may be of significance in veterinary patients:

■ **IRON or SELENIUM:** Because dimercaprol can form a toxic complex with certain metals (**cadmium, selenium, uranium, and iron**), do not administer with iron or selenium salts. At least 24 hours should pass after the last dimercaprol dose, before iron or selenium therapy can begin.

Laboratory Considerations

■ Iodine I[131] thyroidal uptake values may be decreased during or immediately following dimercaprol therapy as it interferes with normal iodine accumulation by the thyroid. (Osweiler, G. 2007)

Doses

■ **DOGS & CATS:**
For arsenic toxicity:

a) Intensive supportive care is required. Give dimercaprol as early as possible after exposure at 2.5–5 mg/kg IM. The 5 mg/kg dose should only be used for acute cases and only for the first day of therapy. Repeat doses at 4 hour intervals for the first 2 days; every 8 hours on the third day, and twice daily for the next 10 days until recovery. Give with sodium thiosulfate: 40–50 mg/kg IV as a 20% solution two to three times daily until recovery. (Neiger 1989)

b) Cats: If ingestion was recent, use emetics or gastric lavage to help prevent arsenic absorption. If clinical signs are present and ingestion was within 36 hours, begin dimercaprol therapy at 2.5–5 mg/kg IM q4h for the first 2 days, the q12h until recovery. Fluid therapy should be instituted to prevent dehydration and maintain renal function. (Reid & Oehme 1989)

c) 4 mg/kg IM q4–6h; do not give for more than 4 continuous days (Grauer & Hjelle 1988)(

d) Loading dose of 5 mg/kg IM (acute cases only) followed by 2.5 mg/kg IM q3–4h for two days, then progressively lengthen the dosing interval to q12h until recovery is evident (Mount 1989)

■ **FOOD ANIMALS:**

a) For arsenic toxicity: No clinical signs after exposure: 3 mg/kg IM q8h; Clinical signs after exposure: 6 mg/kg IM q8h for 3–5 days (Post & Keller 2000)

b) Ruminants: Traditional treatment for arsenic, lead or mercury poisonings: 2.5–5 mg/kg IM q4h for 2 days. Withdrawal information not available in food animals. Efficacy questionable unless given before signs appear or very early in clinical course. FDA has not exempted this drug for compounding from bulk supplies. (Osweiler, G. 2007)

c) For mercury toxicity for bovine or swine: 3 mg/kg IM four times daily for 3 days, then twice daily for 10 days. Treatment is often unsuccessful. (Osweiler, G.D. & Hook 1986)

■ **HORSES:**
For arsenic toxicity:

a) Dimercaprol therapy in horses is difficult because of the amounts of dimercaprol that are required, the necessity to inject the drug IM and that it must be used acutely and any substantial delays in treatment significantly decrease its effectiveness. If available, the dose is: 5 mg/kg IM initially, followed by 3 mg/kg IM q6h for the remainder of the first day, then 1 mg/kg IM q6h for two or more additional days, as needed. (Oehme 1987)

b) Wash off topically absorbable arsenic and empty the digestive tract with laxatives. Administer sodium thiosulfate at

50–75 grams PO every 6–8 hours to bind unabsorbed arsenic. IV thiosulfate (25–30 grams as a 20% solution in distilled water) may counter-absorb arsenic. Dimercaprol is effective if administered within hours of ingestion. Initial treatment is: 5 mg/kg IM, followed by 3 mg/kg IM q6h for the remainder of the first day, then 1 mg/kg IM q6h for the next 48 hours. IM injections are painful; identify source of arsenic and eliminate it. (Rees 2004)

Monitoring

- Liver function
- Renal function
- Hemogram
- Hydration and perfusion status
- Electrolytes and acid/base status
- Urinary pH

Client Information

- Because of the potential toxicity of this agent and the seriousness of most heavy metal intoxications, this drug should be used with close professional supervision only.
- Dimercaprol can impart a strong, unpleasant mercaptan-like odor to the animal's breath.

Chemistry/Synonyms

A dithiol chelating agent, dimercaprol occurs as a colorless or nearly colorless, viscous liquid that is soluble in alcohol, vegetable oils, and water, but is unstable in aqueous solutions. It has a very disagreeable mercaptan-like odor. The commercially available injection is a peanut oil and benzyl benzoate solution. Although the solution may be turbid or contain small amounts of flocculent material or sediment, this does not mean that the solution is deteriorating.

Dimercaprol may also be known as: BAL, British Anti-Lewisite, dimercaptopropanol, dithioglycerol dimercaprolum, *BAL® in Oil* or *Sulfactin Homburg®*.

Storage/Stability

Dimercaprol injection should be stored below 40°C; preferably at room temperature (15–30°C).

Compatibility/Compounding Considerations:

Dimercaprol is not on the FDA's CPG 608.400 list of drugs allowed to be compounded from bulk supplies.

Dosage Forms/Regulatory Status

VETERINARY-LABELED PRODUCTS: None

HUMAN-LABELED PRODUCTS:

Dimercaprol Injection: 100 mg/mL (10%) (for IM use only) in 3 mL amps; *BAL® in Oil* (Taylor); (Rx)

References

Grauer, G.F. & J.J. Hjelle (1988). Pesticides. *Handbook of Small Animal Practice*. RV Morgan Ed. New York, Churchill Livingstone: 1095–1100.

Mount, M.E. (1989). Toxicology. *Textbook of Veterinary Internal Medicine*. SJ Ettinger Ed. Philadelphia, WB Saunders. **1**: 456–483.

Neiger, R.D. (1989). Arsenic Poisoning. *Current Veterinary Therapy X: Small Animal Practice*. RW Kirk Ed. Philadelphia, WB Saunders: 159–161.

Oehme, F.W. (1987). Arsenic. *Current Therapy in Equine Medicine*. NE Robinson Ed. Philadelphia, WB Saunders: 668–670.

Osweiler, G. (2007). Detoxification and Antidotes for Ruminant Poisoning. Proceedings: ACVIM. Accessed via: Veterinary Information Network. http://goo.gl/h1YRI

Osweiler, G.D. & B.S. Hook (1986). Mercury. *Current Veterinary Therapy: Food Animal Practice 2*. JL Howard Ed. Philadelphia, W.B. Saunders: 440–442.

Post, L. & W. Keller (2000). Current status of food animal antidotes. *The Veterinary Clinics of North America: Food Animal Practice* **16**:3(November).

Rees, C. (2004). Disorders of the skin. *Equine Internal Medicine 2nd Ed*. S Reed, W Bayly and D Sellon Eds. Philadelphia, Saunders: 667–720.

Reid, F.M. & F.W. Oehme (1989). Toxicoses. *The Cat: Diseases and Clinical Management*. RG Sherding Ed. New York, Churchill Livingstone. **1**: 185–215.

DIMETHYL SULFOXIDE

DMSO

(dye-*meth*-el sul-*fox*-ide)   Domoso®

FREE RADICAL SCAVENGER

Prescriber Highlights

- Free radical scavenger that has anti-inflammatory, cryopreservative, anti-ischemic, & radioprotective effects
- Caution: Mastocytomas, dehydration/shock; may mask existing pathology
- Handle cautiously; will be absorbed through skin & can carry toxic compounds across skin
- May cause localized "burning" when administered topically
- Administer IV to horses slowly & at concentrations of 20% or preferably, less (10%); may occasionally cause diarrhea, tremors, & colic
- Odor may be an issue

Uses/Indications

Purported uses for DMSO are rampant, but the only FDA-approved veterinary indication for DMSO is: ". . . as a topical application to reduce acute swelling due to trauma" (Package Insert; *Domoso®*—Syntex). Other possible indications for DMSO include: adjunctive treatment in transient ischemic conditions, CNS trauma and cerebral edema, skin ulcers/wounds/burns, adjunctive therapy in intestinal surgeries, and analgesia for post-operative or intractable pain, amyloidosis in dogs, reduction of mammary engorgement in the nursing bitch, enhancement of antibiotic penetration in mastitis in cattle, and limitation of tissue damage following extravasation injuries secondary to chemotherapeutic agents.

DMSO's effect on alcohol dehydrogenase, may make it useful in the treatment of ethylene glycol poisoning, but this has not been sufficiently studied as of yet. DMSO's attributes as a potential carrier of therapeutic agents across the skin and into the systemic circulation and its synergistic effects with other agents are potentially exciting, but require much more study before they can be routinely recommended.

While the potential indications for DMSO are many, unfortunately, the lack of well-controlled studies leaves many more questions than answers regarding this drug.

Pharmacology/Actions

The pharmacologic effects of DMSO are diverse. DMSO traps free radical hydroxide and its metabolite, dimethyl sulfide (DMS), traps free radical oxygen. It appears that these actions help to explain some of the antiinflammatory, cryopreservative, antiischemic, and radioprotective qualities of DMSO.

DMSO will easily penetrate the skin. It serves as a carrier agent in promoting the percutaneous absorption of other compounds (including drugs and toxins) that normally would not penetrate. Drugs such as insulin, heparin, phenylbutazone, and sulfonamides may all be absorbed systemically when mixed with DMSO and applied to the skin.

DMSO has weak antibacterial activity when used clinically and possible clinical efficacy when used topically as an antifungal. The mechanism for these antimicrobial effects has not been elucidated.

The antiinflammatory/analgesic properties of DMSO have been thoroughly investigated. DMSO appears to be more effective as an antiinflammatory agent when used for acute inflammation versus chronic inflammatory conditions. The analgesic effects of DMSO have been compared to that produced by narcotic analgesics and is efficacious for both acute and chronic musculoskeletal pain.

DMSO decreases platelet aggregation but reports of its effects on coagulability have been conflicting, as has its effect on the myocardium. DMSO has diuretic activity independent of the method of administration. It provokes histamine release from mast cells, which probably contributes to the local vasodilatory effects seen after topical administration.

DMSO also apparently has some anticholinesterase activity and enhances prostaglandin E, but blocks the synthesis of prostaglandins E_2, F_2-alpha, H_2, and G_2. It inhibits the enzyme alcohol dehydrogenase, which not only is responsible for the metabolism of alcohol, but also the metabolism of ethylene glycol into toxic metabolites.

Pharmacokinetics

DMSO is well absorbed after topical administration, especially at concentrations between 80–100%. It is extensively and rapidly distributed to virtually every area of the body. After IV administration to horses, the serum half-life was approximately 9 hours. In dogs, the elimination half-life is approximately 1.5 days. DMSO is metabolized to dimethyl sulfide (DMS) and is primarily excreted by the kidneys, although biliary and respiratory excretion also takes place.

In cattle, the drug is eliminated quite rapidly and after 20 days no detectable drug or metabolites are found in milk, urine, blood, or tissues.

Contraindications/Precautions/Warnings

Wear rubber gloves when applying topically, and apply with clean or sterile cotton to minimize the chances for contaminating with potentially harmful substances. Apply only to clean, dry areas to avoid carrying other chemicals into the systemic circulation.

DMSO may mask existing pathology with its antiinflammatory and analgesic activity.

Because DMSO may degranulate mast cells, animals with mastocytomas should only receive DMSO with extreme caution. DMSO should be used cautiously in animals suffering from dehydration or shock as its diuretic and peripheral vasodilatory effects may exacerbate these conditions.

Adverse Effects

When used as labeled, DMSO appears to be an extremely safe drug. Local effects ("burning", erythema, vesiculation, dry skin, local allergic reactions) and garlic or oyster-like breath odor are the most likely adverse effects. They are transient and quickly resolve when therapy is discontinued. Lenticular changes, which may result in myopia, have been noted primarily in dogs and rabbits when DMSO is used chronically and at high doses. These effects are slowly reversible after the drug is discontinued.

When DMSO is administered intravenously to horses it may cause hemolysis and hemoglobinuria. While older dosage references often recommended 20% or less concentrations for IV use in horses, 10% solutions are more commonly recommended today as they are probably safer. Slow administration IV may also reduce adverse effects. Other adverse effects may include diarrhea, muscle tremors and colic.

Reports of hepatotoxicity and renal toxicity have also been reported for various species and dosages. These occur fairly rarely and some clinicians actually believe DMSO has a protective effect on ischemically insulted renal tissue.

Reproductive/Nursing Safety

At high doses, DMSO has been shown to be teratogenic in hamsters and chicks, but not mice, rats, or rabbits; weigh the risks versus benefits when using in pregnant animals. In humans, the FDA categorizes this drug as category *C* for use during pregnancy (*Animal studies have shown an adverse effect on the fetus, but there are no adequate studies in humans; or there are no animal reproduction studies and no adequate studies in humans.*). In a separate system evaluating the safety of drugs in canine and feline pregnancy (Papich 1989), this drug is categorized as in class: *C* (*These drugs may have potential risks. Studies in people or laboratory animals have uncovered risks, and these drugs should be used cautiously as a last resort when the benefit of therapy clearly outweighs the risks.*)

It is not known whether this drug is excreted in milk; use in nursing dams with caution.

Overdosage/Acute Toxicity

The reported LD_{50}'s following IV dosage in dogs and cats are: Cats ≈ 4 g/kg, and Dogs ≈ 2.5 g/kg. Signs of toxicity include: sedation and hematuria at non-lethal doses; coma, seizures, opisthotonus, dyspnea and pulmonary edema at higher dosages. Should an acute overdosage be encountered, treat supportively.

Drug Interactions

The following drug interactions have either been reported or are theoretical in humans or animals receiving DMSO and may be of significance in veterinary patients:

Because of its anticholinesterase activity, avoid the use of organophosphates or other cholinesterase inhibitors with DMSO. A fatality secondary to mercury intoxication was reported when DMSO was mixed with a mercury salt "red blister" and applied topically to the leg of a horse. Because it inhibits alcohol dehydrogenase, DMSO may prolong the effects of **alcohol. Insulin, corticosteroids,** (including endogenous steroids), and **atropine** may be potentiated by DMSO.

Doses

■ **DOGS:**

a) Liberal application should be administered topically to the skin over the affected area 3−4 times daily. Total daily dosage should not exceed 20 grams (or mL of liquid) and therapy should not exceed 14 days. (Package Insert; *Domoso®*—-Syntex Animal Health)

b) For calcinosis cutis: Dogs may "feel bad" if large areas are treated initially, but do not become hypercalcemic. Apply topically to a small area of the body initially (if extensive areas are involved) once daily; and as these areas improve, add new treatment areas. (Merchant 2000)

c) For bladder instillation to treat persistent cases of hemorrhagic cystitis (secondary to cyclophosphamide tx): 10 mL of DMSO medical grade 50% solution is diluted with 10 mL of water and instilled into bladder and removed after 20 minutes. (Blackwood 2008)

d) For doxorubicin extravasation—see the doxorubicin monograph for more information.

■ **HORSES: (Note:** ARCI UCGFS Class 5 Drug) While older dosage references often recommended 20% or less concentrations for IV use in horses, 10% solutions are more commonly recommended today as they are probably safer. Some recent references state unequivocally "do not exceed 10% concentrations".

a) Liberal application should be administered topically to the skin over the affected area 2−3 times daily. Total daily dosage should not exceed 100 grams (or mL of liquid) and therapy should not exceed 30 days. (Package Insert; *Domoso®*—Syntex Animal Health)

b) For adjunctive treatment with surgical colics: 25 mg/kg IV intra-operatively and continued twice daily for the first 24−48 hours post-op. (Hassel 2005)

c) For acute rhabdomyolysis: DMSO 1 g/kg in a 10% solution of lactated Ringer's or Multisol IV or orally. May be given in the acute stages of rhabdomyolysis once hydration status has been restored. (Hanson 1999)

d) As an adjunctive treatment for laminitis: 0.1−1 g/kg IV, 2−3 times daily (Brumbaugh *et al.* 1999)

Monitoring

■ Efficacy

■ Hemoglobinuria/hematocrit if indicated

■ Ophthalmic exams with high doses or chronic use in the dog

Client Information

■ Do not use non-medical grades of DMSO as they may contain harmful impurities. Wear rubber gloves when applying topically. DMSO should be applied with clean or sterile cotton to minimize the chances for contaminating with potentially harmful substances. Apply only to clean, dry skin. Use in well-ventilated area; avoid inhalation and contact with eyes. May damage some fabrics. Keep lid tightly on container when not in use. Keep out of reach of children. Do not mix with any other substance without veterinarian's approval.

■ Selected DMSO products are FDA-approved for use in dogs and in horses not intended for food purposes. It is a veterinary prescription (Rx) drug.

Chemistry/Synonyms

DMSO is a clear, colorless to straw-yellow liquid. It is dipolar, aprotic (acts as a Lewis base) and extremely hygroscopic. It has a melting/freezing point of 18.5°C, boiling point of 189°C, and a molecular weight of 78.1. It is miscible with water (heat is produced), alcohol, acetone, chloroform, ether and many organic solvents. A 2.15% solution in water is isotonic with serum.

Dimethylsulfoxide may also be known as: dimethyl sulphoxide, dimethylis sulfoxidum, DMSO, methyl sulphoxide, NSC-763, SQ-9453, sulphinylbismethane, *Domoso®, Kemsol®, Rheumabene®, Rimso®,* or *Synotic®.*

Storage/Stability

Must be stored in airtight containers away from light. As DMSO may react with some plastics, it should be stored in glass or in the container provided by the manufacturer. If DMSO is allowed to contact room air it will self-dilute to a concentration of 66–67%.

Compatibility/Compounding Considerations

DMSO is apparently compatible with many compounds, but because of the chances for accidental percutaneous absorption of potentially toxic compounds, the admixing of DMSO with other compounds is not to be done casually.

Dosage Forms/Regulatory Status

VETERINARY APPROVED PRODUCTS:

Dimethyl Sulfoxide Veterinary Gel 90%: *Domoso® Gel* (Pfizer) 90% (medical grade) in 60 g, and 120 g tubes, and 425 g containers. Labeled for use in dogs and horses. Do not administer to horses that are to be slaughtered for food.

Dimethyl Sulfoxide Veterinary Solution 90%: *Domoso® Solution* (Pfizer) 90% (medical grade) in 1 pint and 1 gallon bottles. Labeled for use in canines and equines. Do not administer to horses that are to be slaughtered for food.

The ARCI (Racing Commissioners International) has designated this drug as a class 5 substance. See the appendix for more information.

Note: A topical otic product, *Synotic®* (Pfizer) that contains: DMSO 60% and fluocinolone acetonide 0.01% is also available for veterinary use. Supplied in 8 mL and 60 mL dropper bottles.

HUMAN APPROVED PRODUCTS:

Dimethylsulfoxide Solution: 50% aqueous solution in 50 mL; *Rimso-50®* (Research Industries); generic (Bioniche); (Rx);

References

Blackwood, L. (2008). Problems with Chemotherapy of Lymphoma—How to Cope. Proceedings: World Small Afnimal Assoc World Congress. Accessed via: Veterinary Information Network. http://goo.gl/52Mc6

Brumbaugh, G., H. Lopez, et al. (1999). The pharmacologic basis for the treatment of laminitis. *The Veterinary Clinics of North America: Equine Practice* 15:2(August).

Hanson, R. (1999). Diagnosis and First Aid of Sporting Horse Injuries. Proceedings: Central Veterinary Conference, Kansas City.

Hassel, D. (2005). Post–operative complications in the colic. Proceedings: IVECCS. Accessed via: Veterinary Information Network. http://goo.gl/UDFPN

Merchant, S. (2000). New Therapies in Veterinary Dermatology. Proceedings: American Animal Hospital Association 67th Annual Meeting, Toronto.

DIMINAZENE ACETURATE

(dye-*min*-ah-zeen ass-ah-*toor*-ate)
Berenil®

ANTIPROTOZOAL

Prescriber Highlights

▶ Antiprotozoal agent used in several species for trypanosomiasis, babesiosis, or cytauxzoonosis

▶ Available in several countries, but not in USA

Uses/Indications

Diminazene is used to treat trypanosomiasis in dogs and livestock (sheep, goats, cattle), Babesia infections in dogs and horses, and cytauxzoonosis in cats. The drug is not commercially available in the USA, but is available and used in many countries.

Pharmacology/Actions

Diminazene's exact mechanism of action is not well understood. With Babesia, it is thought to interfere with aerobic glycolysis and DNA synthesis.

Diminazene may not completely eradicate the organism but because it is slowly metabolized, suppression of recurrence of clinical signs or prophylaxis can be attained for several weeks after a single dose.

Pharmacokinetics

Diminazene's pharmacokinetics have been investigated in several species. The drug is rapidly absorbed after IM administration in target species studied and distributed rapidly. High levels can be found in the liver and kidney. The drug appears to enter the CSF, but at levels significantly lower than that found in plasma in healthy animals. CSF levels are higher in infected dogs with African trypanosomiasis, probably due to meningeal inflammation. Diminazene apparently is metabolized somewhat in the liver, but identification and whether metabolites possess anti-protozoal activity is not known.

Elimination half-lives are reportedly widely variable. Reported values range from 10–30 hours in dogs, goats, and sheep, to over 200 hours in one study for cattle. Differences in assay methodology and study design may account for some of this variation, but even within an individual study in dogs using a modern assay (HPLC), wide inter-patient variability was noted.

Contraindications/Precautions/Warnings

Camels appear highly susceptible to the toxic effects of diminazene, and product labels may state the drug is contraindicated in camelids.

Adverse Effects

At usual dosages in domestic livestock, diminazene is reportedly relatively free of adverse effects. Adverse effects associated with therapeutic dosages of diminazene in dogs may include vomiting and diarrhea, pain and swelling at the injection site, and transient decreases in blood pressure. Very rarely (<0.1%) ataxia, seizures, or death have been reported.

Reproductive/Nursing Safety

Little information is available. Rats given up to 1 g/kg PO on days 8–15 demonstrated no teratogenic effects, but decreased body weights and increased resorptions were noted at the highest dose.

Diminazene is distributed into milk; safety for nursing offspring has not been established.

Overdosage/Acute Toxicity

Little information is available. Diminazene appears most toxic in dogs and camels. Dosages greater than 7 mg/kg can be very toxic to camels; dosages above 10 mg/kg IM in dogs can cause severe gastrointestinal, respiratory, nervous system, or musculoskeletal effects.

Drug Interactions

■ No significant drug interactions were identified

Laboratory Considerations

■ No issues were noted

Doses

Note: There is a multitude of protozoal diseases worldwide that may respond to diminazene. Depending on the species/strain (protozoan) and species of the patient treated, there may be local specific recommendations for chemotherapy treatment or prevention. The following should be used as general guidelines only.

■ **DOGS:**

For treatment of Babesia:

a) 3.5–5 mg/kg IM, once for *B. canis*, repeat in 24 hours for *B. gibsoni*. Risk for neurotoxicity higher when total dosages are 7 mg/kg or higher. (Toboada & Lobetti 2006)

b) For small Babesia (Okinawa): 3.5 mg/kg IM; repeat once in 24 hours. (Brosey 2003)

c) For treatment of Babesia (South Africa): 4.2 mg/kg IM. Do not repeat within a 21-day period. (Miller *et al.* 2005)

For treatment of African trypanosomiasis:

a) 3.6–7 mg/kg IM every 2 weeks as needed to control relapse or reinfection. (Barr 2006)

■ **CATS:**

For treatment of cytauxzoonosis:

a) 3–5 mg/kg IM one time, tick control remains the best means of preventing disease as treatment attempts meet with little success. (Blagburn 2005)

b) 2 mg/kg IM, repeat in one week. (Greene *et al.* 2006)

■ **HORSES, CATTLE, SHEEP, GOATS:**

For treatment of susceptible protozoal (Trypanosomes, Babesia) infections (West Africa):

a) In general, 3.5 mg/kg IM one time. Depending on susceptibility, dose can be increased to 8 mg/kg. Do not exceed 4 grams total dose per animal. (Label directions; *Berenil®*—Intervet West Africa)

Monitoring

■ For Babesia infections in dogs monitoring would include surveillance for potential adverse effects of diminazene and signs for clinical efficacy, including monitoring serial CBCs. Severe cases may have elevated BUN or liver enzymes and hypokalemia.

■ Current recommendation for determining "clearing" of the organism (*Babesia gibsoni*) is to perform a PCR test at 60 and 90 days post-therapy

Client Information

■ Clients should understand that depending on the species treated, parasites may not be completely eradicated and that retreatment may be required

Chemistry/Synonyms

Diminazene aceturate is an aromatic diamidine derivative chemically related to pentamidine. One gram of diminazene is soluble in approximately 14 mL of water and it is slightly soluble in alcohol.

Diminazene aceturate may also be known as: diminazene diaceturate, or diminazeno; many international trade names are available.

Storage/Stability

Read and follow label directions for storage and preparation of each product used; diminazene powder, granules, or packets for reconstitution for injection should generally be stored in a dry, cool place out of direct sunlight. Once reconstituted, the solution's stability is temperature dependent; up to 14 days when refrigerated, up to 5 days at 20°C and only for 24 hours at temperatures above 50°C.

Dosage Forms/Regulatory Status

VETERINARY-LABELED PRODUCTS: None in the USA.

Diminazene aceturate is available in many countries either alone, or in combination products (*e.g.*, with antipyrine), with the following trade names: *Azidine®, Azidin®, Babezeen®, Crede-Bab-Minazene®, Berenil®, Dimisol®, Dizine®, Ganaseng®, Ganasegur®, Pirocide®,* or *Veriben®.*

The FDA may allow legal importation of this medication for compassionate use in animals; for more information, see the *Instructions for Legally Importing Drugs for Compassionate Use in the USA* found in the appendix.

Withdrawal times may vary depending on the

product, dosage, and the country where it is used. In South Africa, *Berenil®* (Intervet), has an animal slaughter withdrawal period of 21 days.

The JECFA of FAO/WHO has established the following maximum residue limit recommendations for diminazene in cattle: muscle (500 micrograms/kg), liver (12000 micrograms/kg), kidney (6000 micrograms/kg), and milk (150 micrograms/L).

HUMAN-LABELED PRODUCTS: None

References

Barr, S. (2006). Trypanosomiasis. *Infectious Diseases of the Dog and Cat.* C Greene Ed., Elsevier: 676–685.

Blagburn, B. (2005). Treatment and control of tick borne diseases and other important parasites of companion animals. Proceedings: ACVC2005. Accessed via: Veterinary Information Network. http://goo.gl/Pexfa

Brosey, B. (2003). Babesia gibsoni: a clinical perspective from Southeast Asia. Proceedings: ACVIM2003. Accessed via: Veterinary Information Network. http://goo.gl/dbRSI

Greene, C., J. Meinkoth, et al. (2006). Cytauxzoonosis. *Infectious Diseases of the Dog and Cat.* C Greene Ed., Elsevier: 716–722.

Miller, D., G. Swan, et al. (2005). The pharmacokinetics of diminazene aceturate after intramuscular administration in healthy dogs. *J S Afr Vet Assoc* 76(3): 146–150.

Toboada, J. & R. Lobetti (2006). Babesiosis. *Infectious Diseases of the Dog and Cat.* C Greene Ed., Elsevier: 722–736.

DINOPROST TROMETHAMINE PROSTAGLANDIN F₂ALPHA TROMETHAMINE

(*dye*-noe-prost)   Lutalyse®

PROSTAGLANDIN

Prescriber Highlights

▶ (THAM) salt of the naturally occurring prostaglandin F_2alpha used as a luteolytic agent for estrous synchronization, pyometra treatment, & as an abortifacient

▶ Contraindications: Pregnancy (when abortion or induced parturition not wanted); manufacturer lists several contraindications for horses; has been associated with serious toxicity and death in camelids

▶ Do NOT administer IV; extreme caution in elderly or debilitated animals

▶ Pregnant women should not handle; humans with asthma & women of childbearing age should handle with caution

▶ Adverse effects (*Dogs/Cats*): Abdominal pain, emesis, defecation, urination, pupillary dilation followed by constriction, tachycardias, restlessness & anxiety, fever, hypersalivation, dyspnea & panting; fatalities possible (esp. dogs)

▶ Adverse Effects: (*Cattle*): Infection at injection site, salivation, & hyperthermia possible

▶ Adverse Effects (*Swine*): Erythema & pruritus, urination, defecation, slight ataxia, hyperpnea, dyspnea, nesting behavior, abdominal muscle spasms, tail movements, increased vocalization & salivation

▶ Adverse Effects (*Horses*): Body temperature changes/sweating; seen less frequently: increased respiratory & heart rates, ataxia, abdominal pain, & lying down; Usually has more side effects then cloprostenol

Uses/Indications

Lutalyse® (Upjohn) is labeled for use in cattle as a luteolytic agent for estrous synchronization, unobserved (silent) estrous in lactating dairy cattle, pyometra, and as an abortifacient in feedlot and non–lactating dairy cattle. It is labeled in swine to act as a parturient inducing agent. The product is labeled for use in mares as a luteolytic agent to control the time of estrus in cycling mares and to assist in inducing estrus in "difficult to breed mares."

Unlabeled uses of dinoprost include its use in small animals as an abortifacient agent and as adjunctive medical therapy in pyometra, but newer regimens for pyometra that combine aglepristone with cloprostenol or misoprostol appear to be effective without the side effects of dinoprost. Although not FDA-approved, dinoprost is used also in sheep and goat reproductive medicine.

Pharmacology/Actions

Prostaglandin F_2alpha has several pharmacologic effects on the female reproductive system, including stimulation of myometrial activity, relaxation of the cervix, and inhibition of steroidogenesis by corpora lutea; can potentially lyse corpora lutea.

Pharmacokinetics

In studies done in rodents, dinoprost was demonstrated to distribute very rapidly to tissues after injection. In cattle, the serum half-life of dinoprost has been stated to be only "minutes" long.

Contraindications/Precautions/Warnings

Unless being used as an abortifacient or parturition inducer, dinoprost should not be used during pregnancy in all species. Dinoprost is contraindicated in animals with bronchoconstrictive respiratory disease (*e.g.*, asthma, "heavey" horses). It should not be administered intravenously.

According to the manufacturer, dinoprost is contraindicated in mares with acute or subacute disorders of the vascular system, GI tract, respiratory system, or reproductive tract.

Dinoprost should be used with extreme caution, if at all, in dogs or cats greater than 8 years old, or with preexisting cardiopulmonary or other serious disease (liver, kidney, etc.). Some clinicians regard closed-cervix pyometra as a relative contraindication to the use of dinoprost.

Dinoprost has been associated with acute toxicity and death in camelids.

Adverse Effects

In cattle, increased temperature has been reported when administered in overdose (5–10X recommended doses) quantities. Limited salivation and bacterial infections at the injection site have been reported. If administered intravenously, increased heart rates have been noted.

In mares, transient decreased body (rectal) temperature and sweating have been reported most often. Less frequently, increased respiratory and heart rates, ataxia, abdominal pain, and lying down have also been noted. These effects are generally seen within 15 minutes of administration and resolve within an hour.

In swine, dinoprost has caused erythema and pruritus, urination, defecation, slight ataxia, hyperpnea, dyspnea, nesting behavior, abdominal muscle spasms, tail movements, increased vocalization and salivation. These effects may last up to 3 hours. At doses of 10 times recommended, vomiting may be seen.

In dogs and cats, dinoprost can cause abdominal pain, emesis, defecation, urination, pupillary dilation followed by constriction, tachycardias, restlessness and anxiety, fever, hypersalivation, dyspnea, and panting. Cats may also exhibit increased vocalization and intense grooming behavior. Severity of effects is generally dose dependent. Defecation can be seen even with very low dosages. Reactions generally appear in 5–120 minutes after administration and may persist for 20–30 minutes. Fatalities have occurred (especially in dogs) after use. Dogs and cats should be monitored for cardiorespiratory effects, especially after receiving higher dosages.

When used as an abortifacient in humans, dinoprost causes nausea, vomiting, or diarrhea in about 50% of patients.

Reproductive/Nursing Safety

Unless being used as an abortifacient or parturition inducer, dinoprost should not be used during pregnancy in all species. In swine, dinoprost should not be administered prior to 3 days of normal predicted farrowing as increased neonatal mortality may result.

Overdosage/Acute Toxicity

Dogs are apparently more sensitive to the toxic effects of dinoprost than other species. The LD_{50} in the bitch has been reported to be 5.13 mg/kg after SC injection, which may be only 5X greater than the recommended dose by some clinicians.

In cattle, swine, and horses, dinoprost's effects when administered in overdose quantities are outlined above in the Adverse Effects section. If clinical signs are severe in any species and require treatment; supportive therapy is recommended.

Drug Interactions

The following drug interactions have either been reported or are theoretical in humans or animals receiving dinoprost and may be of significance in veterinary patients:

■ **OTHER OXYTOCIC AGENTS:** Activity may be enhanced by dinoprost. Reduced effect of dinoprost would be expected with concomitant administration of a progestin.

Doses

■ **DOGS:**

For treatment of pyometra:

a) Use is restricted to bitches 6 years of age or younger who are not critically ill, do not have significant concurrent illness, do have an open cervix, and an owner who is adamant about saving the animal's reproductive potential. After making definitive diagnosis; use natural prostaglandin F_2alpha (*Lutalyse®*): Day 1: 0.1 mg/kg SC once; Day 2: 0.2 mg/kg SC once; Days 3–7: 0.25 mg/kg SC once daily. Use antibiotics (effective against *E.*

coli) concurrent with prostaglandin treatment and for 14 days after completion. Reevaluate at 7 and 14 days after treating with prostaglandin. Re-treat at 14 days if purulent discharge persists or fever, increased WBC and fluid filled uterus persist. (Feldman, E. 2000)

As an abortifacient:

a) After day 25 or 30: SC injections must be given at least twice a day, using a maximum dosage of 80–100 micrograms/kg, starting with half the dose for the first day (or first two administrations). Treatment must initially be done under the supervision of a clinician, after which the bitch can be sent home (with owner administration) once side effects have been carefully (monitored) after the first injection. Side effects include: emesis, salivation, defecation, urination and slight tachypnea. Treatment must continue (for 6 days or longer) until verification with ultrasound or palpation. (Romagnoli 2006)

b) As an adjunctive therapy for the termination of mid-term pregnancy in the bitch: Pregnancy is confirmed with ultrasound and begun no sooner than 30 days after breeding. 1–3 micrograms/kg misoprostol given intravaginally once daily concurrently with prostaglandin F$_2$alpha (*Lutalyse*®) at 0.1 mg/kg SC three times daily for 3 days and then 0.2 mg/kg SC three times daily to effect. Monitor efficacy with ultrasound. (Cain 1999)

■ **CATS:**

For treatment of pyometra:

a) Initially 0.1 mg/kg SC, then 0.25 mg/kg SC once a day for 5 days. Give bactericidal antibiotics concurrently. Not recommended in animals >8 yrs. old or if severely ill. Closed-cervix pyometra is a relative contraindication. Reevaluate in 2 weeks; retreat for 5 more days if necessary. (Nelson & Feldman 1988), (Feldman, E.C. & Nelson 1989)

As an abortifacient:

a) 2 mg (total dose) per cat IM once a day beginning at day 33. Side effects include prostration, vomiting and diarrhea. (Romagnoli 2006)

■ **CATTLE:**

For estrus synchronization in beef cattle and non-lactating dairy heifers:

a) 25 mg IM either once or twice at a 10–12 day interval. If using single injection method, breed at usual time relative to estrus. If using dual dose method, breed at either the usual time relative to estrus, or about 80 hours after the second injection. (Package Insert; *Lutalyse*®—Upjohn)

For unobserved (silent) estrus in lactating dairy cattle with a corpus luteum:

a) 25 mg IM. Breed cows as they are detected in estrus. If estrus not detected, breed at 80 hours post injection. If cow returns to estrus, breed at usual time relative to estrus. (Package Insert; *Lutalyse*®—Upjohn)

For pyometra/endometritis:

a) For pyometra: 25 mg IM twice, 8 hours apart; estrus usually ensues in 3–7 days, however evaluation of the uterus using palpation and/or ultrasonography is recommended before these cows are inseminated. For endometritis if a corpus luteum is present: Administration of PGF2a to cows 14 days apart places 90% of cows between days 5–10 of the estrus cycle, and a conception rate of 45% to the Ovsynch protocol started 12 days after the second injection. (Archbald *et al.* 2006)

b) For pyometra: 25 mg IM. Uterus begins evacuating within 24 hours of injection (McCormack 1986), (Package Insert; *Lutalyse*®—Upjohn)

As an abortifacient:

a) Between 5–150 days of gestation: 25–30 mg IM. After 150 days of gestation: 25 mg dexamethasone with 25 mg dinoprost (efficacy up to 95%) (Drost 1986)

b) 25 mg IM during the first 100 days of gestation (Package Insert; *Lutalyse*®—Upjohn)

To induce parturition:

a) 25–30 mg IM; delivery will occur in about 72 hours (Drost 1986)

■ **HORSES:**

For difficult to breed mares secondary to progesterone levels consistent with the presence of a functional corpus luteum: 1 mg per 45 kg body weight IM (Package Insert; *Lutalyse*®—Upjohn)

For controlling time of estrus of estrous cycling mares: 1 mg per 45 kg body weight IM. When treated during diestrus, most mares return to estrus in 2–4 days and ovulate 8–12 days after treatment (Package Insert; *Lutalyse*®—Upjohn)

For luteolysis and to stimulate uterine contractions: 10 mg (total dose) IM once. Cloprostenol has not been associated with as severe side effects. (Dascanio 2009)

As an abortifacient:

a) Prior to the 12th day of pregnancy: 5 mg IM. After the 4th month of pregnancy: 1 mg per 45 kg body weight (1 mg per 100 pounds) daily until abortion takes place (Lofstedt 1986)

b) From day 80–300: 2.5 mg q12h; approximately 4 injections required on average to induce abortion (Roberts 1986)

For estrus synchronization in normally cycling mares:

a) Three methods:

1) *Two injection method*: On day 1 give 5 mg dinoprost and again on day 16. Most (60%) mares will begin estrus 4 days after the second injection and about 90% will show estrous behavior by the 6th day after the second injection. Breed using AI every second day during estrus or inseminate at predetermined times without estrus detection. Alternatively, an IM injection of HCG (2500–3300 Units) can be added on the first or second day (usually day 21) of estrus to hasten ovulation. Breed using AI on days: 20, 22, 24, and 26. This may be of more benefit when used early in the breeding season.

2) *Progestagen/Prostaglandin method*: Give altrenogest (0.44 mg/kg) for 8–12 days PO. On last day of altrenogest therapy (usually day 10) give dinoprost (dose not noted, but suggest using same dose as "1" above). Majority of mares will show estrus 2–5 days after last treatment. Inseminate every 2 days after detection of estrus. Synchronization may be improved by giving 2500 Units of HCG IM on first or second day of estrus or 5–7 days after altrenogest is withdrawn.

3) On day 1, inject 150 mg progesterone and 10 mg estradiol-17beta daily for 10 days. On last day, also give dinoprost (dose not noted, but suggest using same dose as "1" above). Perform AI on alternate days after estrus detection or on days 19, 21, and 23. (Bristol 1987)

■ **SWINE:**

For estrus synchronization (grouping):

a) At 15–55 days of gestation 15 mg dinoprost IM, followed in 12 hours by 10 mg IM. Animals will abort and return to estrus in 4–5 days. Close observation of estrus over several days is needed. (Carson 1986)

As an abortifacient:

a) 5–10 mg IM; abortion occurs in 24–48 hours and estrus occurs 4–5 days later (Drost 1986)

To induce parturition:

a) 10–25 mg IM from 2–6 days before expected parturition; farrowing usually occurs 24–36 hours later (Drost 1986)

■ **SHEEP & GOATS:**

For estrus synchronization in cycling ewes and does:

a) Ewes: Give 8 mg IM on day 5 of estrous cycle and repeat in 11 days. Estrus will begin approximately 2 days after last injection. Does: Give 8 mg IM on day 4 of estrous cycle and repeat in 11 days. Estrus will begin approximately 2 days after last injection. (Carson 1986)

To treat pseudopregnancy (hydrometra/mucometra) in goats: 5 mg IM once. (Tibary 2009)

As an abortifacient:

a) Does: 5–10 mg IM throughout entire pregnancy; abortion takes place in 4–5 days.

Ewes (during first two months of pregnancy): 10–15 mg IM; abortion takes place within 72 hours (Drost 1986)

To induce parturition:

a) Does: 2.5–20 mg on days 144–149. Higher dosage (20 mg) yields more predictable interval from injection to delivery ($\approx$32 hours). (Ott 1986)

Monitoring

■ Depending on use, see above. Monitoring for adverse effects is especially important in small animals.

Client Information

■ Dinoprost should be used by individuals familiar with its use and precautions.

■ Pregnant women, asthmatics, or other persons with bronchial diseases should handle this product with extreme caution. Any accidental exposure to skin should be washed off immediately.

Chemistry/Synonyms

The tromethamine (THAM) salt of the naturally occurring prostaglandin F2alpha, dinoprost tromethamine occurs as a white to off-white, very hygroscopic, crystalline powder with a melting point of about 100°C. One gram is soluble in about 5 mL of water. 1.3 micrograms of dinoprost tromethamine is equivalent to 1 microgram of dinoprost.

Dinoprost and dinoprost tromethamine may also be known as: PGF(2alpha), prostaglandin F(2alpha), idinoprostum trometamoli, PGF(2alpha) THAM, prostaglandin F(2alpha) trometamol, U-14583E, U-14583, *Amtech Prostamate®, Lutalyse®, Enzaprost®, In-Synch®, Minprostin F(2)alpha®, Prostamate®, Prostin®, Prostin F2®, Prostin F2 Alpha®, Prostin F2 Alpha®, and Prostine F(2) Alpha®, Oriprost®, Glandin®, Noroprost®, Dinolytic®,* and *Prostarmon F®.*

Storage/Stability

Dinoprost for injection should be stored at room temperature (15–30°C) in airtight containers. The human FDA-approved product is recommended to be stored under refrigeration. Dinoprost is considered to be relatively insensitive to heat, light, and alkalis.

Dosage Forms/Regulatory Status

VETERINARY-LABELED PRODUCTS:

Dinoprost Tromethamine for injection, equivalent to 5 mg/mL of dinoprost in 10 mL and 30 mL vials; *Lutalyse® Sterile Solution* (Pharmacia and Upjohn); *Amtech Prostamate®* (IVX); *In-Synch®* (ProLabs); *Prostamate®* (various); (Rx). FDA-approved for use in beef and non-lactating dairy cattle, swine and mares. No preslaughter withdrawal or milk withdrawal is required when used as labeled; no specific tolerance for dinoprost residues has been published. It is not for use in horses intended for food.

HUMAN-LABELED PRODUCTS: None

References

Archbald, L., J. Bartolome, et al. (2006). Use of a prostaglandin (F2a) for the treatment of uterine infections. Proceedings: Western Vet Conf. Accessed via: Veterinary Information Network. http://goo.gl/anHWu

Bristol, F. (1987). Synchronization of estrus. *Current Therapy in Equine Medicine: 2.* NE Robinson Ed. Phialdelphia, WB Saunders: 495–498.

Cain, J. (1999). Canine reproduction: Commonly referred problems. Proceedings: American College of Veterinary Internal Medicine: 17th Annual Veterinary Medical Forum, Chicago.

Carson, R.L. (1986). Synchronization of estrus. *Current Veterinary Therapy: Food Animal Practice 2.* JL Howard Ed. Philadelphia, W.B. Saunders: 781–783.

Dascanio, J. (2009). Hormonal Control of Reproduction. Proceedings: ABVP. Accessed via: Veterinary Information Network. http://goo.gl/o2vHk

Drost, M. (1986). Elective termination of pregnancy. *Current Veterinary Therapy 2: Food Animal Practice.* JL Howard Ed. Philadelphia, WB Saunders: 797–798.

Feldman, E. (2000). The cystic endometrial hyperplasia/pyometra complex and infertility in female dogs. *Textbook of Veterinary Internal Medicine: Diseases of the Dog and Cat.* S Ettinger and E Feldman Eds. Philadelphia, WB Saunders. 2: 1549–1565.

Feldman, E.C. & R.W. Nelson (1989). Diagnosis and treatment alternatives for pyometra in dogs and cats. *Current Veterinary Therapy X: Small Animal Practice.* RW Kirk Ed. Philadelphia, WB Saunders: 1305–1310.

Lofstedt, R.M. (1986). Termination of unwanted pregnancy in the mare. *Current Therapy in Theriogenology 2: Diagnosis, Treatment and Prevention of Reproductive Diseases in Small and Large Animals.* DA Morrow Ed. Philadelphia, WB Saunders: 715–718.

Nelson, R.W. & E.C. Feldman (1988). Diseases of the Endocrine Pancreas. *Handbook of Small Animal Practice.* RV Morgan Ed. New York, Churchill Livingstone: 527–535.

Ott, R.S. (1986). Prostaglandins for induction of estrous, estrous synchronization, abortion and induction of parturition. *Current Therapy in Theriogenology 2: Diagnosis, Treatment and Prevention of Reproductive Diseases in Small and Large Animals.* DA Morrow Ed. Philadelphia, WB Saunders: 583–585.

Roberts, S.J. (1986). Abortion and other gestational diseases in mares. *Current Therapy in Theriogenology 2: Diagnosis, Treatment and Prevention of Reproductive Diseases in Small and Large Animals.* DA Morrow Ed. Philadelphia, WB Saunders: 705–710.

Romagnoli, S. (2006). Control of reproduction in dogs and cats: Use and misuse of hormones. Proceedings: WSAVA World Congress. Accessed via: Veterinary Information Network. http://goo.gl/aGuBF

Tibary, A. (2009). Infertility in goats: Individual & herd approach. Proceedings: WVC. Accessed via: Veterinary Information Network. http://goo.gl/yzHwv

DIPHENHYDRAMINE HCL

(dye-fen-*hye*-dra-meen)   Benadryl®

ANTIHISTAMINE

Prescriber Highlights

▶ Antihistamine used primarily for its antihistaminic effects, but with various indications (prevention of motion sickness, sedative, antiemetic, etc.)

▶ Caution: Angle closure glaucoma, GI or urinary obstruction, COPD, hyperthyroidism, seizure disorders, cardiovascular disease or hypertension. May mask clinical signs of ototoxicity.

▶ Adverse Effects: CNS depression & anticholinergic effects; GI effects (diarrhea, vomiting, anorexia) are less common

Uses/Indications

In veterinary medicine, diphenhydramine is used principally for its antihistaminic effects, but also for other pharmacologic actions. Its sedative effects can be of benefit in treating the agitation (pruritus, etc.) associated with allergic responses. It has also been used for treatment and prevention of motion sickness and as an antiemetic in small animals. Because histamine is thought not to be an important mediator of vomiting in cats, other choices such as NK-1 antagonists (*e.g.*, maropitant) or M_1-cholinergic antagonists (*e.g.*, prochlorperazine, chlorpromazine) may be better choices for treating motion sickness or vomiting in cats. It has been suggested for use as adjunctive treatment of aseptic laminitis in cattle and it may be useful as an adjunctive treatment for feline pancreatitis. For other suggested uses, refer to the Dosage section below.

Pharmacology/Actions

Like other antihistamines, diphenhydramine competitively inhibits histamine at H_1 receptors. In addition, it possesses substantial sedative, anticholinergic, antitussive, and antiemetic effects.

Pharmacokinetics

The pharmacokinetics of this agent have apparently not been studied in domestic animals. In humans, diphenhydramine is well absorbed after oral administration, but because of a relatively high first-pass effect, only about 40–60% reaches the systemic circulation.

Following IV administration in rats, diphenhydramine reaches its highest levels in the spleen, lungs and brain. The drug is distributed into milk, but has not been measured quantitatively. In humans, diphenhydramine crosses the placenta and is approximately 80% bound to plasma proteins.

Diphenhydramine is metabolized in the liver and the majority of the drug is excreted as metabolites into the urine. The terminal elimination half-life in adult humans ranges from 2.4–9.3 hours.

Contraindications/Precautions/Warnings

Diphenhydramine is contraindicated in patients who are hypersensitive to it or other antihistamines in its class. Because of their anticholinergic activity, antihistamines should be used with caution in patients with angle closure glaucoma, prostatic hypertrophy, pyloroduodenal or bladder neck obstruction, and COPD if mucosal secretions are a problem. Additionally, they should be used with caution in patients with hyperthyroidism, cardiovascular disease or hypertension.

Adverse Effects

The most commonly seen adverse effects are CNS depression (lethargy, somnolence), and anticholinergic effects (dry mouth, urinary retention). The sedative effects of antihistamines may diminish with time. GI effects (diarrhea, vomiting, anorexia) are a possibility.

The sedative effects of antihistamines may adversely affect the performance of working dogs.

Diphenhydramine may cause paradoxical excitement in cats. The liquid formulation is very distasteful.

Reproductive/Nursing Safety

In humans, the FDA categorizes this drug as category *B* for use during pregnancy (*Animal studies have not yet demonstrated risk to the fetus, but there are no adequate studies in pregnant women; or animal studies have shown an adverse effect, but adequate studies in pregnant women have not demonstrated a risk to the fetus in the first trimester of pregnancy, and there is no evidence of risk in later trimesters.*) In a separate system evaluating the safety of drugs in canine and feline pregnancy (Papich 1989), this drug is categorized as in class: *B* (*Safe for use if used cautiously. Studies in laboratory animals may have uncovered some risk, but these drugs appear to be safe in dogs and cats or these drugs are safe if they are not administered when the animal is near term.*)

Diphenhydramine is excreted milk. Use with caution, particularly in neonates.

Overdosage/Acute Toxicity

Overdosage can cause CNS stimulation (excitement to seizures) or depression (lethargy to coma), anticholinergic effects, respiratory depression and death. Treatment consists of emptying the gut after oral ingestion using standard protocols. Induce emesis if the patient is alert and CNS status is stable. Administration of a saline cathartic and/or activated charcoal may be given after emesis or gastric lavage. Treatment of other clinical signs should be performed using symptomatic and supportive therapies. Phenytoin (IV) is recommended in the treatment of seizures caused by antihistamine over-

dose in humans; barbiturates and diazepam should be avoided.

Drug Interactions

The following drug interactions have either been reported or are theoretical in humans or animals receiving diphenhydramine and may be of significance in veterinary patients:

■ **ANTICHOLINERGIC DRUGS** (including **tricyclic antidepressants**): Diphenhydramine may potentiate anticholinergic effects

■ **CNS DEPRESSANT DRUGS:** Increased sedation can occur

Laboratory Considerations

■ Antihistamines can decrease the wheal and flare response to antigen **skin testing**. In humans, it is suggested that antihistamines be discontinued at least 4 days before testing.

Doses

■ **DOGS:**

As an antihistamine:

a) 2–4 mg/kg q8–12h PO; 1 mg/kg q8–12h IM, SC, IV (do not exceed 40 mg total dose) (Papich 2000)

b) 2.2 mg/kg PO twice daily–three times daily (Peikes 2003)

c) For severe urticaria and angioedema: 2 mg/kg IM twice daily as needed (with steroids: prednisone 2 mg/kg IM twice daily and epinephrine 1:10,000: 0.5–2 mL SC) (Giger & Werner 1989)(

d) For canine atopic dermatitis: 25–50 mg (total dose) PO three times daily. (Hill 2007)

e) For treatment of anaphylaxis (associated with doxorubicin chemotherapy): 3–4 mg/kg IM with dexamethasone sodium phosphate (0.5–1 mg/kg IV) wait for reaction to subside before restarting infusion at slower rate. (Vail 2006)

f) For preoperative therapy for splenic mast cell tumors: 2 mg/kg PO three times daily with famotidine (0.5 mg/kg PO once daily) are used to prevent anaphylaxis. (Garrett 2006)

g) For adjunctive tx of pruritus: 2–4 mg/kg PO two to three times a day. (Marsella 2008)

Prevention of motion sickness/antiemetic:

a) 2–4 mg/kg PO, IM q8h (Washabau & Elie 1995), (Richter 2009)

For preoperative therapy for splenic mast cell tumors:

a) 2 mg/kg PO three times daily with famotidine (0.5 mg/kg PO once daily) are used to prevent anaphylaxis. (Garrett 2006)

For treatment of the reverse sneeze syndrome:

a) 25 mg PO three to four times a day, dosage is usually decreased to once or twice a week for maintenance (Prueter 1989)

■ **CATS:**

As an antihistamine:

a) 0.5 mg/kg PO q12h; liquid formulation is distasteful (Messinger 2000)

b) 2–4 mg (total dose) q12–24h (Hnilica 2003)

c) 2–4 mg/kg PO q8h (Scherk 2006)

d) For severe urticaria and angioedema: 2 mg/kg IM twice daily as needed (with steroids: prednisone 2 mg/kg IM twice daily and epinephrine 1:10,000 (0.5–2 mL SC) (Giger & Werner 1989)

For adjunctive treatment of pancreatitis:

a) 2–4 mg/kg PO q8h (Scherk 2005)

■ **FERRETS:**

a) Prevaccination: 2 mg/kg PO, IM or IV 10 minutes prior to vaccination (Williams 2000)

b) Pretreatment before doxorubicin: 5 mg (total dose) IM (Johnson 2006)

■ **RABBITS/RODENTS/SMALL MAMMALS:**

a) **Guinea pigs:** 7.5 mg/kg PO (Adamcak & Otten 2000)

b) **Rabbits:** 1–2 mg/kg PO twice daily as an antihistamine (Morrisey & Antinoff 2003), (Antinoff 2008)

■ **BIRDS:**

For adjunctive treatment of pruritus causing feather picking in Psittacines:

a) 2 mg/kg PO q12h (Siebert 2003)

■ **HORSES:** (**Note:** ARCI UCGFS Class 3 Drug)

As an antihistamine:

a) For adjunctive therapy of anaphylaxis: 0.25–1 mg/kg IV or IM (Evans 1996)

b) For allergic skin diseases (atopy): 1–2 mg/kg twice daily (route not specified) (Miller 2005)

c) For allergic skin diseases (atopy): 0.75–1 mg/kg PO q12h (Rees 2004)

d) For adjunctive tx of pruritus: 1–2 mg/kg PO two to three times a day. (Marsella 2008)

■ **CATTLE:**

a) For adjunctive therapy of anaphylaxis: 0.5–1 mg/kg IM or IV (used with epinephrine and steroids) (Clark 1986)

b) For adjunctive therapy of aseptic laminitis: During the acute phase (with corticosteroids): 55–110 mg/100 kg body weight (0.55–1.1 mg/kg) IV or IM (Berg 1986)

Monitoring

■ Clinical efficacy

■ Adverse effects

Client Information

■ Most commonly diphenhydramine causes sleepiness or lethargy, but it can cause dry mucous membranes and, particularly in cats, it can cause excitement.

Chemistry/Synonyms

An ethanolamine-derivative antihistamine, diphenhydramine HCl occurs as an odorless, white, crystalline powder which will slowly darken upon exposure to light. It has a melting range of 167–172°C. One gram is soluble in about 1 mL of water or 2 mL of alcohol. Diphenhydramine HCl has a pK_a of about 9; the commercially available injection has its pH adjusted to 5–6.

Diphenhydramine HCl may also be known as: chloranautine, dimenhydrinatum, diphenhydramine teoclate, and diphenhydramine theoclate; many trade names are available.

Storage/Stability

Preparations containing diphenhydramine should be stored at room temperature (15–30°C) and solutions should be protected from freezing. Tablets and oral solutions should be kept in well-closed containers. Capsules and the elixir should be stored in tight containers.

Compatibility/Compounding Considerations

Diphenhydramine for injection is reportedly physically **compatible** with all commonly used IV solutions and the following drugs: amikacin sulfate, aminophylline, ascorbic acid injection, atropine sulfate, bleomycin sulfate, butorphanol tartrate, cephapirin sodium, chlorpromazine HCl, colistimethate sodium, diatrizoate meglumine/sodium, dimenhydrinate, droperidol, erythromycin lactobionate, fentanyl citrate, glycopyrrolate, hydromorphone HCl, hydroxyzine HCl, iothalamate meglumine/sodium, lidocaine HCl, meperidine HCl, methicillin sodium, metoclopramide, methyldopate HCl, morphine sulfate, nafcillin sodium, netilmicin sulfate, penicillin G potassium/sodium, pentazocine lactate, perphenazine, polymyxin B sulfate, prochlorperazine edisylate, promazine HCl, promethazine HCl, scopolamine HBr, tetracycline HCl, and vitamin B complex with C. Compatibility is dependent upon factors such as pH, concentration, temperature, and diluent used; consult specialized references or a hospital pharmacist for more specific information.

Diphenhydramine is reportedly physically **incompatible** with the following drugs: amobarbital sodium, amphotericin B, cephalothin sodium, hydrocortisone sodium succinate, iodipamide meglumine, pentobarbital sodium, secobarbital sodium, and thiopental sodium.

Dosage Forms/Regulatory Status

VETERINARY-LABELED PRODUCTS:

No systemic products. A shampoo, topical spray and topical liquid are available. See the topical dermatology section in the appendix for more information.

The ARCI (Racing Commissioners International) has designated this drug as a class 3 substance. See the appendix for more information.

HUMAN-LABELED PRODUCTS:

Diphenhydramine HCl Capsules and Tablets: 12.5 mg (as hydrochloride, chewable), 25 mg (as either hydrochloride or tannate, chewable), 50 mg (as hydrochloride); *Banophen®* (Major); *Genahist®* (Goldline); *Benadryl® Allergy, Benadryl Allergy Kapseals, Benadryl Dye-Free Allergy Liqui Gels, Benadryl® Allergy Ultratabs & AllerMax® Caplets, Maximum Strength* (Pfizer); *Diphenhist®* & *Diphenhist® Captabs* (Rugby); *Dytan®* (Hawthorn); (OTC and Rx)

Diphenhydramine HCl Orally Disintegrating Tablets: 12.5 mg (equiv. to 19 mg citrate) with mannitol 4.5 mg *phenylalanine; Children's Benadryl Allergy Fastmelt®* (Pfizer); (OTC)

Diphenhydramine Orally Disintegrating Strips: 12.5 mg & 25 mg (as hydrochloride); *Benadryl® Allergy Quick Dissolve Strips* (Pfizer); (OTC)

Diphenhydramine HCl Oral Liquid, Solution, Suspension. Elixir or Syrup: 12.5 mg/5 mL (as hydrochloride) in 30 mL, 118 mL, 120 mL, 236 mL, 237 mL, 473 mL, and 3.8 L; 25 mg/5 mL (as tannate) in 118 mL; *Scot-Tussin Allergy Relief Formula Clear®* (Scot-Tussin); *AllerMax®* (Pfieffer); *Benadryl® Children's Allergy, Children's Pedia Care Nighttime Cough® & Benadryl® Children's Dye-Free Allergy* (Pfizer); *Diphen AF®* (Morton Grove); *Altaryl® Children's Allergy* (Altaire); *Diphenhist®* (Rugby); *Banophen® Allergy* (Major); *Siladryl®* (Silarx); *Tusstat®* (Century); *Genahist®* (Goldline); *Hydramine Cough* (various); (OTC and Rx)

Diphenhydramine Injection: 50 mg/mL (as hydrochloride) in 1 mL fill in 2 mL cartridges, 1 mL amps, 1 mL and 10 mL *Steri-vials* and 1 mL *Steri-dose* syringes; *Benadryl®* (Parke-Davis), generic; (Rx)

References

Adamcak, A. & B. Otten (2000). Rodent Therapeutics. *Vet Clin NA: Exotic Anim Pract* 3:1(Jan): 221–240.

Antinoff, N. (2008). Respiratory diseases of ferrets, rabbits, and rodents. Proceedings: IVECCS. Accessed via: Veterinary Information Network. http://goo.gl/JjmjJ

Berg, J.N. (1986). Aseptic laminitis in cattle. *Current Veterinary Therapy: Food Animal Practice 2*. JL Howard Ed. Philadelphia, W.B. Saunders: 896–898.

Clark, D.R. (1986). Diseases of the general circulation. *Current Veterinary Therapy: Food Animal Practice 2*. JL Howard Ed. Phialdelphia, W.B. Saunders: 694–696.

Evans, A. (1996). Hypersensitivity Reactions. *Large Animal Internal Medicine, 2nd Ed.* B Smith Ed. St Louis, Mosby: 1405–1411.

Garrett, L. (2006). Practical approach to treatment of canine mast cell tumors. Proceedings: ACVIM. Accessed via: Veterinary Information Network. http://goo.gl/q2HR8

Giger, U. & L.L. Werner (1989). Immune–Mediated Diseases. *Handbook of Small Animal Practice*. RV Morgan Ed. New York, Churchill Livingstone: 841–860.

Hill, P. (2007). Treatment of canine atopic dermatitis: balancing the three factors. *In Practice* 29(10): 566–+.

Hnilica, K. (2003). Eosinophilic dermatopathies in cats. Proceedings: Western Veterinary Conf. Accessed via: Veterinary Information Network. http://goo.gl/IiCOD

Johnson, D. (2006). Ferrets: the other companion animal. Proceedings: ACVC. Accessed via: Veterinary Information Network. http://goo.gl/bSeol

Marsella, R. (2008). Medical management of pruritus: Non–specific therapy for the pruritic dog or cat. Proceedings: ACVC. Accessed via: Veterinary Information Network. http://goo.gl/5qKrx

Messinger, L. (2000). Pruritis Therapy in the Cat. *Kirk's Current Veterinary Therapy: XIII Small Animal Practice*. J Bonagura Ed. Philadelphia, WB Saunders: 542–545.

Miller, W. (2005). Allergic Skin Diseases in 2005. Proceedings: ACVC. Accessed via: Veterinary Information Network. http://goo.gl/7Vxcs

Morrisey, J. & N. Antinoff (2003). Respiratory diseases of rabbits, ferrets, and rodents. Proceedings: IVECCS. Accessed via: Veterinary Information Network. http://goo.gl/OO1FA

Peikes, H. (2003). Approach to the pruritic dog. Proceedings: Atlantic Coast Veterinary Conference. Accessed via: Veterinary Information Network. http://goo.gl/WnfvD

Prueter, J.C. (1989). Diseases of the nasal cavity and sinus. *Handbook of Small Animal Practice*. RV Morgan Ed. New York, Churchill Livingstone: 167–172.

Rees, C. (2004). Disorders of the skin. *Equine Internal Medicine 2nd Ed.* S Reed, W Bayly and D Sellon Eds. Philadelphia, Saunders: 667–720.

Richter, K. (2009). Acute Vomiting: A Systemic Approach. Proceedings: ACVIM. Accessed via: Veterinary Information Network. http://goo.gl/VYeZ1

Scherk, M. (2005). Feline pancreatitis. Proceedings: Western Veterinary Conference. Accessed via: Veterinary Information Network. http://goo.gl/emF25

Scherk, M. (2006). Snots and Snuffles: Chronic Feline Upper Respiratory Syndrome. Proceedings: ACVIM. Accessed via: Veterinary Information Network. http://goo.gl/tWQ49

Siebert, L. (2003). Psittacine feather picking. Proceedings: Western Veterinary Conference. Accessed via: Veterinary Information Network. http://goo.gl/MCA9y

Vail, D. (2006). New supportive therapies for cancer patients. Proceedings: ACVIM. Accessed via: Veterinary Information Network. http://goo.gl/r4oMT

Washabau, R. & M. Elie (1995). Antiemetic therapy. *Kirk's Current Veterinary Therapy:XII.* J Bonagura Ed. Philadelphia, W.B. Saunders: 679–684.

Williams, B. (2000). Therapeutics in Ferrets. *Vet Clin NA: Exotic Anim Pract* 3:1(Jan): 131–153.

DIPHENOXYLATE HCL + ATROPINE SULFATE

(dye-fen-*ox*-i-late/at-roe-peen)　Lomotil®

OPIATE AGONIST/ANTICHOLINERGIC

Prescriber Highlights

▶ Opiate GI motility modifier used primarily in dogs; also has antitussive properties

▶ Contraindications: Known hypersensitivity to narcotic analgesics, patients receiving monoamine oxidase inhibitors (MAOIs), diarrhea caused by a toxic ingestion until the toxin is eliminated from the GI tract, intestinal obstruction

▶ Caution: Respiratory disease, hepatic encephalopathy, hypothyroidism, severe renal insufficiency, adrenocortical insufficiency (Addison's), head injuries, or increased intracranial pressure, acute abdominal conditions, & in geriatric or severely debilitated patients

▶ Adverse Effects: Constipation, bloat, & sedation. Potential for: paralytic ileus, toxic megacolon, pancreatitis, & CNS effects

▶ Dose carefully in small dogs; not advisable to use in very young kittens

▶ Diphenoxylate is a class-V controlled substance

Uses/Indications

Diphenoxylate is an opiate in combination with atropine in antidiarrheal products used primarily in dogs; it also has antitussive properties. Use in cats is controversial and many clinicians do not recommend its use in this species.

Pharmacology/Actions

Among their other actions, opiates inhibit GI motility and excessive GI propulsion. They decrease intestinal secretion induced by cholera toxin, prostaglandin E_2 and diarrheas caused by factors where calcium is the second messenger (non-cyclic AMP/GMP mediated). Opiates may also enhance mucosal absorption.

Pharmacokinetics

In humans, diphenoxylate is rapidly absorbed after administration of either the tablets or oral solution; bioavailability of the tablets is approximately 90% that of the solution. Generally, onset of action occurs within 45 minutes to one hour after dosing and is sustained for 3−4 hours. Diphenoxylate is metabolized into diphenoxylic acid, an active metabolite. The serum half-lives of diphenoxylate and diphenoxylic acid are approximately 2.5 hours and 3−14 hours, respectively.

Contraindications/Precautions/Warnings

All opiates should be used with caution in patients with hypothyroidism, severe renal insufficiency, adrenocortical insufficiency, (Addison's), and in geriatric or severely debilitated patients. Opiate antidiarrheals are contraindicated in cases where the patient is hypersensitive to narcotic analgesics, in patients receiving monoamine oxidase inhibitors (MAOIs), and patients with diarrhea caused by a toxic ingestion (until the toxin is eliminated from the GI tract).

Opiate antidiarrheals should be used with caution in patients with head injuries or increased intracranial pressure and acute abdominal conditions (*e.g.*, colic), as it may obscure the diagnosis or clinical course of these conditions. It should be used with extreme caution in patients suffering from respiratory disease or from acute respiratory dysfunction (*e.g.*, pulmonary edema secondary to smoke inhalation). Opiate antidiarrheals should be used with extreme caution in patients with hepatic disease with CNS clinical signs of hepatic encephalopathy; hepatic coma may result.

Many clinicians recommend not using diphenoxylate or loperamide in dogs weighing less than 10 kg, but this is probably a result of the potency of the tablet or capsule forms of the drugs. Dosage titration using the liquid forms of these agents should allow their safe use in dogs when indicated.

Adverse Effects

In dogs, constipation, bloat, and sedation are the most likely adverse reactions encountered when usual doses are used. Potentially, paralytic ileus, toxic megacolon, pancreatitis, and CNS effects could be seen.

Use of antidiarrheal opiates in cats is controversial; this species may react with excitatory behavior.

Opiates used in horses with acute diarrhea (or in any animal with a potentially bacterial-induced diarrhea) may have a detrimental effect. Opiates may enhance bacterial proliferation, delay the disappearance of the microbe from the feces, and prolong the febrile state.

Reproductive/Nursing Safety

Diphenoxylate/atropine is classified as category *C* for use during pregnancy (*Animal studies have shown an adverse effect on the fetus, but there are no adequate studies in humans; or there are no animal reproduction studies and no adequate studies in humans.*)

Exercise caution when administering diphenoxylate HCl with atropine to nursing patients. Diphenoxylic acid may be, and atropine is, excreted in maternal milk but effects on the infant may not be significant.

Overdosage/Acute Toxicity

Acute overdosage of the opiate antidiarrheals could result in CNS, cardiovascular, GI, or respiratory toxicity. Because the opiates may significantly reduce GI motility, absorption from the GI may be delayed and prolonged. For more information, refer to the meperidine and morphine monographs found in the CNS section. Naloxone may be necessary to reverse the opiate effects.

Massive overdoses of diphenoxylate/atropine sulfate may induce atropine toxicity. Refer to the atropine monograph for more information.

Drug Interactions
The following drug interactions have either been reported or are theoretical in humans or animals receiving opiate antidiarrheals and may be of significance in veterinary patients:

■ **CNS DEPRESSANT DRUGS:** Other CNS depressants (*e.g.*, **anesthetic agents, antihistamines, phenothiazines, barbiturates, tranquilizers, alcohol,** etc.) may cause increased CNS or respiratory depression when used with opiate antidiarrheal agents

■ **MONOAMINE OXIDASE INHIBITORS** (including **amitraz**, and possibly **selegiline**): Opiate antidiarrheal agents are contraindicated in human patients receiving systemic monoamine oxidase (MAO) inhibitors for at least 14 days after receiving MAO inhibitors

Laboratory Considerations
■ Plasma **amylase** and **lipase** values may be increased for up to 24 hours following administration of opiates.

Doses

■ **DOGS:**
As an antidiarrheal:
a) 0.1–0.2 mg/kg PO q12h (Marks 2008)
b) 0.05 mg/kg PO three times a day; probably should not be given longer than 5 days and are potentially contraindicated when diarrhea is suspected to be caused by enteric infections (Hall & Simpson 2000)
c) 0.05–0.2 mg/kg PO q8–12h (Willard 2003)
d) 0.05–0.1 mg/kg PO three to four times a day. (Washabau 2007)
As an antitussive:
a) Approximately 0.25 mg/kg PO q8–12h (Church 2006), (Schaer 2008)
b) Diphenoxylate at 0.2–0.5 mg/kg PO q12h until clinical signs subside. May be used for extended periods. Constipation is an occasional problem, but stool softeners can alleviate. (Hardie & Lascelles 2004)

■ **CATS:**
As an antidiarrheal:
a) 0.08–0.1 mg/kg PO q12h (Marks 2008)

Monitoring
■ Clinical efficacy
■ Fluid and electrolyte status in severe diarrhea

■ CNS effects, if using high dosages

Client Information
■ If diarrhea persists or if animal appears listless or develops a high fever, contact veterinarian
■ When used as antitussive (for cough) watch for constipation; contact veterinarian if this is a problem

Chemistry/Synonyms
Structurally related to meperidine, diphenoxylate HCl is a synthetic phenylpiperidine-derivative opiate agonist. It occurs as an odorless, white, crystalline powder that is slightly soluble in water and sparingly soluble in alcohol. Commercially available preparations also contain a small amount of atropine sulfate to discourage the abuse of the drug for its narcotic effects. At therapeutic doses, the atropine has no clinical effect.

This combination may be known as co-phenotrope in the U.K. and elsewhere. Other synonyms include: R 1132, NIH 7562 or difenoxilato. A commonly used trade name is *Lomotil®*.

Storage/Stability
Diphenoxylate/atropine tablets should be stored at room temperature in well-closed, light-resistant containers. Diphenoxylate/atropine oral solution should be stored at room temperature in tight, light-resistant containers; avoid freezing.

Dosage Forms/Regulatory Status

VETERINARY-LABELED PRODUCTS: None

HUMAN-LABELED PRODUCTS:

Diphenoxylate HCl Tablets: 2.5 mg with 0.025 mg Atropine Sulfate; *Logen®* (Goldline); *Lomotil®* (Searle); *Lonox®* (Sandoz); generic; (Rx, C-V)

Diphenoxylate HCl Liquid: 2.5 mg with 0.025 mg Atropine Sulfate per 5 mL in 60 mL with dropper and UD 4 mL & 10 mL; *Lomotil®* (Searle), *Lomanate®* (Qualitest); generic; (Rx, C-V)

References
Church, D. (2006). Drugs used in the management of respiratory diseases. Proceedings; WSAVA World Congress. Accessed via: Veterinary Information Network. http://goo.gl/QKV7b
Hall, E. & K. Simpson (2000). Diseases of the Small Intestine. *Textbook of Veterinary Internal Medicine: Diseases of the Dog and Cat*. S Ettinger and E Feldman Eds. Philadelphia, WB Saunders. 2: 1182–1238.
Hardie, E. & B. Lascelles (2004). The honking dog: Current controversies in collapsing tracheas. Proceedings: SeniorCare. Accessed via: Veterinary Information Network. http://goo.gl/OJ7ih
Marks, S. (2008). GI Therapeutics: Which Ones and When? Proceedings; IVECCS. Accessed via: Veterinary Information Network. http://goo.gl/rxwcs
Schaer, M. (2008). Differential Diagnosis and Clinical Management of Canine Respiratory Diseases. Proceedings: ACVC. Accessed via: Veterinary Information Network. http://goo.gl/QvuG4
Washabau, R. (2007). Evidence–Based Medicine: GI Drugs in the ICU. Proceedings: IVECCS. Accessed via: Veterinary Information Network. http://goo.gl/IHZon

Willard, M. (2003). Digestive system disorders. *Small Animal Internal Medicine, 3rd Ed.* R Nelson and C Couto Eds. St Louis, Mosby: 343–471.

Diphenylhydantoin–see Phenytoin Sodium

DIRLOTAPIDE

(dir-loe-ta-pyde)   Slentrol®

GUT MICROSOMAL TRIGLYCERIDE TRANSFER PROTEIN (GMTP) IN-HIBITOR

Prescriber Highlights

▶ Indicated for the management of obesity in dogs; not for cats

▶ Not recommended for dogs with liver disease, unmanaged Cushing's, or receiving corticosteroids

▶ Primary adverse effects are GI (vomiting, diarrhea); increased liver enzymes possible

▶ Safe use not established for treatment beyond one year

▶ Fairly complex dosing guidelines; regular monitoring & dosage adjustment required

Uses/Indications

Dirlotapide oral solution is indicated for the management of obesity in dogs.

Pharmacology/Actions

Dirlotapide is a selective microsomal triglyceride transfer protein inhibitor that blocks the formation and release of lipoproteins into the systemic circulation. The mechanism of action for weight reduction is not completely understood, but it seems to result from reduced fat absorption and a satiety signal (Peptide YY) from lipid-filled enterocytes.

Dirlotapide primarily acts locally in the gut to reduce appetite, increase fecal fat and produce weight loss in the management of obesity in dogs. Although systemic blood levels do not directly correlate with efficacy, they seem to correlate with the drug's systemic toxicity.

Pharmacokinetics

In dogs, dirlotapide is available systemically, but absorption is highly variable (22–41%). Presence of food in the gut apparently increases bioavailability. Dirlotapide in the circulation is highly protein bound and the volume of distribution is 1.3 L/kg. Systemically absorbed dirlotapide is metabolized in the liver. Dirlotapide and its metabolites are excreted in the bile and may undergo enterohepatic circulation. Nonlinear pharmacokinetics with less-than-proportional exposure, drug accumulation (at higher doses), and large inter-patient variability has been observed in multiple studies and at vari-

ous doses. The mean elimination half-life in dogs ranged between 5 and 18 hours, and may increase with dosage and after repeated dosing. The fecal and biliary routes are the predominant routes of elimination. Renal excretion accounts for less than 1% of the drug administered.

Contraindications/Precautions/Warnings

The manufacturer states that dirlotapide is not recommended for use in dogs currently receiving long-term corticosteroid therapy. Do not use in dogs with liver disease. Pre-existing endocrine disease, including hyperadrenocorticism (Cushing's disease), should be managed prior to use of dirlotapide.

Dirlotapide should not be used in cats; increases risk of hepatic lipidosis during weight loss in obese cats.

Safe use for longer than one year has not been evaluated.

Adverse Effects

Adverse effects most likely seen with dirlotapide in dogs include (in decreasing order of frequency): vomiting (especially during the first month of treatment and 3-4 hours after dosing), diarrhea, lethargy, anorexia, salivation, constipation and dehydration. As additional patients receive this medication, this profile could change.

During field trials, some dogs developed mild to moderate elevation in serum hepatic transaminase activity early in treatment that decreased over time while treatment continued.

Reproductive/Nursing Safety

Safety in breeding, pregnant, or lactating dogs has not been established.

Overdosage/Acute Toxicity

Oral doses of 0.5, 1 and 2 mL/kg (2.5X, 5X, 10X of maximum labeled dose) were administered to normal weight Beagles for two weeks. The drug was tolerated but vomiting, diarrhea, anorexia, lethargy, transient elevations in liver enzymes (transaminase) were noted. No histopathologic evidence of hepatic necrosis was seen.

Drug Interactions

Drug interactions with dirlotapide have not been reported at the time of writing, but the drug could potentially alter the oral absorption (rate and extent) of many drugs. Until safe concomitant use is determined with oral drugs with narrow therapeutic indexes, it is suggested to dose these drugs at least two hours prior to administering dirlotapide; additional monitoring may be required.

■ **FAT SOLUBLE VITAMINS (A, E, K):** During the first 6 months of treatment, plasma vitamin A and E concentrations of treated dogs were significantly below the vitamin A and E concentrations of the control dogs. Plasma vitamin A concentration was low after one month and the median values did not decline any further. Plasma vitamin E concentrations were lowest after 6 months of treatment but adipose tissue levels of vitamin E appeared to be increased compared to control dogs after 12 months of treatment. Plasma vitamin A and E concentrations appeared to increase during the weight stabilization phase (second 6 months of treatment) and returned to concentrations similar to the control dogs when treatment was discontinued. Prothrombin times were similar in the treated and the control dogs and there were no clinical signs of abnormal hemostasis observed during the 12-month study.

Laboratory Considerations

■ No specific alterations to laboratory tests have been noted; the drug can increase **serum transaminase** in some patients.

Doses

■ **DOGS:**

Weight Loss Phase:

Initial assessment and dosing in first month: Assess the dog prior to initiation of therapy to determine the desired weight and to assess the animal's general health (See Precautions). The initial dosage is 0.01 mL/kg (0.05 mg/kg) body weight, administered once daily, orally, for the first 14 days. After the first 14 days of treatment, the dose volume should be doubled to 0.02 mL/kg (0.1 mg/kg) of body weight, administered once daily for the next 14 days (days 15 to 28 of treatment).

Subsequent Monthly Dose Adjustments for Weight Loss: Dogs should be weighed monthly and the dose volume adjusted every month, as necessary, to maintain a target percent weight loss of ≥ 0.7% per week. To determine if a dose adjustment is necessary, compare the Actual % weight loss to the Target % weight loss and use the following guidelines. **Note:** All dose adjustments are based solely on volume (mL).

First (or Subsequent) Dose Adjustment Section: *If the dog has lost weight,* determine if an adjustment in dose is required using the following calculations: (Number of weeks between visits) X 0.7 % per week = Target % weight loss. Example–in 4 weeks (28 days) the Target weight loss would be 4 X 0.7% per week, or at least 2.8% of the total body weight. Compare the Target % weight loss (of ≥ 0.7% per week) with the Actual % weight loss for that dog.

Monthly weight loss rate achieved. If the Actual % weight loss is the same or greater than the Target % weight loss, the dose volume (number of mL administered each day) should remain the same for the next month of dosing until the next scheduled assessment.

Monthly weight loss not achieved. If the Actual % weekly weight loss is less than the Target % weight loss of 0.7% weekly, the following dose adjustment instructions apply:

First dose adjustment: The dose volume (number of mL administered each day) should be increased by 100%, resulting in an increase of the dose volume to 2 times the dose administered during the previous month of dosing. Only perform a 100% dose increase once during treatment after day 14.

Subsequent dose adjustments: If additional dose increases are necessary in the following months, the dose volume (number of mL administered each day) should be increased by 50%, resulting in an increase of the dose volume to 1.5 times the dose administered the previous month of dosing. Based on the dog's current body weight a daily dose of 0.2 mL/kg (0.09 mL/lb) should not be exceeded.

If a dog's food consumption is greatly reduced for several consecutive days, the dose may be withdrawn until the appetite returns (usually 1–2 days) and then resume dosing at the same volume.

The monthly adjustments should continue in this way until the desired weight determined at the start of therapy is reached. When the desired weight is reached, begin the weight management phase.

Weight Management Phase:

A 3-month weight management phase is recommended to successfully maintain the weight loss achieved with treatment. During the weight management phase, the veterinarian and the pet owner should establish the optimal level of food intake and physical activity needed. Dirlotapide administration should be continued during the weight management phase until the dog owner can establish the food intake and physical activity needed to stabilize body weight at the dog's desired weight. To dose for weight management, body weight should continue to be assessed at monthly intervals.

First dose adjustment:

If the dog lost ≥1% body weight per week in the last month of the weight loss phase, the dose volume (number of mL administered each day) should be decreased by 50% resulting in a decrease of the dose volume to 0.5 times the dose administered the previous month.

If the dog lost between 0 and 1% the dose should remain the same.

If the dog gained weight, the dose should

be increased by 50% resulting in an increase of the dose volume to 1.5 times the dose administered the previous month.

Subsequent dose adjustments:

In subsequent months the dose volume should be increased or decreased by 25% to maintain a constant weight.

If the dog is within -5% to +5% of the body weight at the end of the weight loss phase, the dose volume (number of mL administered each day) should remain unchanged.

If the dog lost >5% body weight, then the dose should be decreased by 25%.

If the dog gained > 5% body weight, then the dose should be increased by 25%. Based on the dog's current body weight a daily dose of 0.2 mL/kg (0.09 mL/lb) should not be exceeded.

When dirlotapide is discontinued, the daily amount of food offered and physical activity should be continued as established during the weight management phase. Reverting to previous food intake or physical activity levels at this point can contribute to a re-gain of some or all of the weight loss that has been achieved.

(Package Insert; *Slentrol®*—Pfizer)

Monitoring
■ Patient weight (see dosing)
■ Adverse effects
■ Liver enzymes (baseline, and occasional)

Client Information
■ Not a cure for obesity, dirlotapide decreases the food intake of the dog by decreasing appetite and associated begging behavior. Decreased appetite seen in treated dogs is only temporary and lasts no longer than 1–2 days beyond the cessation of therapy. Weight gain will occur if the amount of food offered is not limited at the time the drug is discontinued.

■ Successful, long-term weight management requires changes that extend beyond the period of drug therapy. To maintain weight loss; adjustments in dietary management and physical activity that were begun as part of the overall weight loss program must be continued.

■ If total lack of appetite (inappetence or anorexia) is observed for more than one day, contact veterinarian.

■ Almost 1 in 4 of dogs placed on therapy experienced occasional episodes of vomiting and diarrhea. In most cases these episodes lasted for one or two days. Vomiting occurred most often during the first month of treatment or within a week of a dose increase. If vomiting occurs it is recommended to continue dosing at the same dose volume, however, the time of day or method of administration (with or without food) may be changed. If vomiting is severe or lasts longer than 2 days, consult veterinarian

■ To prepare for oral administration, remove the bottle cap and insert the supplied oral dosing syringe through the membrane into the bottle. Invert the bottle and withdraw the appropriate volume required using the graduation marks on the side of the oral dosing syringe.

■ Can be administered directly into the dog's mouth or on a small amount of food; can be given with a meal or at a different time of day.

■ Wipe the oral dosing syringe clean after each use with a clean dry cloth or disposable towel; do not introduce water into the oral dosing syringe or the solution.

■ Not for use in humans. Keep this and all drugs out of reach of children.

■ If accidental eye exposure occurs, flush the eyes immediately with clean water.

Chemistry/Synonyms
Dirlotapide has the chemical name 5-[(4'-trifluoromethyl-biphenyl-2-carbonyl)-amino]-1H-indole-2-carboxylic acid benzylmethyl carbamoylamide. It has a molecular weight of 674.7. The commercial product is a liquid formulation containing 5 mg/mL of dirlotapide in medium chain triglyceride (MCT) oil.

Dirlotapide may also be known as CP-742,033 or by its trade name *Slentrol®*.

Storage/Stability
Dirlotapide liquid should be stored in the original container at room temperature 15–30°C (59–86°F).

Dosage Forms/Regulatory Status
VETERINARY-LABELED PRODUCTS:

Dirlotapide Oral Solution 5 mg/mL in 20 mL, 50 mL and 150 mL bottles; *Slentrol®* (Pfizer); (Rx). Labeled for use in dogs.

HUMAN-LABELED PRODUCTS: None

DISOPYRAMIDE PHOSPHATE

(dye-soe-*peer*-a-mide) Norpace®

ANTIARRHYTHMIC AGENT

Prescriber Highlights

▶ Rarely used 2nd or 3rd line antiarrhythmic for use in the dog; negative inotrope & can prolong QT interval

▶ Contraindications: Hypersensitivity to the drug, 2nd or 3rd degree AV block, cardiogenic shock, severe uncompensated or poorly compensated cardiac failure or hypotension, glaucoma (closed-angle), urinary retention, or myasthenia gravis

▶ Caution: Sick sinus syndrome, bundle branch block, or Wolff-Parkinson-White (WPW) syndrome, hepatic or renal disease

▶ Adverse effects most likely noted: Anticholinergic effects (dry mouth, eyes, nose; constipation; urinary hesitancy or retention) & cardiovascular effects (edema, hypotension, dyspnea, syncope, & conduction disturbances (AV block); can reduce serum glucose

▶ Drug interactions

Uses/Indications

Disopyramide may be indicated for the oral treatment or prevention of ventricular tachyarrhythmias in dogs. Because of its negative inotropic effects and short half-life, disopyramide is generally considered to be a 2nd or 3rd line agent for veterinary (canine) use. A controlled release product is available which may prove useful, but it has not been extensively evaluated in dogs.

Pharmacology/Actions

Considered to be a class Ia (membrane-stabilizing) antiarrhythmic with actions similar to either quinidine or procainamide, disopyramide reduces myocardial excitability and conduction velocity and also possesses anticholinergic activity (150 mg of disopyramide $\approx$0.09 mg of atropine) that may contribute to the effects of the drug.

The drug's exact mechanism of action has not been established. Disopyramide's cardiac electrophysiologic effects include: 1) shortened sinus node recovery time; 2) increased atrial and ventricular refractory times; 3) decreased conduction velocity through the atria and ventricles; 4) decreased automaticity of ectopic atrial or ventricular pacemakers.

Disopyramide has direct negative inotropic effects. It generally has minimal effects on resting heart rates or blood pressure. Systemic peripheral resistance may increase by 20%.

Pharmacokinetics

The half-life of the disopyramide is approximately 7 hours in humans with normal renal function, but only 2−3 hours in the dog. Oral bioavailability in dogs is about 70% and it is rapidly absorbed. In humans, disopyramide is rapidly absorbed following oral administration with peak levels occurring within 2−3 hours after the conventional capsules are administered. Peak levels occur at about 6 hours post dose with the controlled-release capsules.

Disopyramide is distributed throughout the body in the extracellular water and is not extensively bound to tissues. Binding to plasma proteins is variable and dependent on the drug's concentration. At therapeutic levels it is approximately 50−65% plasma protein bound (human data). Disopyramide crosses the placenta and milk concentrations may exceed those found in plasma.

Disopyramide is metabolized in the liver, but 40−65% of it is excreted unchanged in the urine. Patients with renal disease may need dosage adjustments made to prevent drug accumulation.

Contraindications/Precautions/Warnings

Disopyramide should usually not be used in patients with glaucoma (closed-angle), urinary retention, or myasthenia gravis because of its anticholinergic effects.

Disopyramide is contraindicated in 2nd or 3rd degree AV block (unless pacemaker inserted), cardiogenic shock, or if the patient is hypersensitive to the drug.

Disopyramide should not be used in patients with severe uncompensated or poorly compensated cardiac failure or hypotension because of its negative inotropic effects. Patients with atrial fibrillation or flutter must be digitalized before disopyramide therapy to negate increased ventricular response (beyond acceptable). Disopyramide should be used with caution in patients with sick sinus syndrome, bundle branch block, or Wolff-Parkinson-White (WPW) syndrome.

Use of disopyramide with other class 1A antiarrhythmics or propranolol may cause additive negative inotropic effects (see Drug Interactions).

Disopyramide should be used with caution (and possibly at a reduced dosage) in patients with hepatic or renal disease.

Adverse Effects

Most common adverse reactions are secondary to disopyramide's anticholinergic effects (*e.g.*, dry mouth, eyes, or nose; constipation; urinary hesitancy or retention) and cardiovascular effects (edema, hypotension, dyspnea, syncope, or conduction disturbances such as AV block. Other adverse effects that have been reported in humans include: GI effects (vomiting, diarrhea, etc.), intrahepatic cholestasis, hypoglycemia, fatigue, headache, muscle weakness and pain. In contrast to the urinary hesitancy effects, disopyramide can also cause urinary frequency and urgency.

Doses of 15 mg/kg q8h in dogs prolongs the QT interval and doses above 30 mg/kg widen the QRS complex.

Reproductive/Nursing Safety

In humans, the FDA categorizes this drug as category C for use during pregnancy (*Animal studies have shown an adverse effect on the fetus, but there are no adequate studies in humans; or there are no animal reproduction studies and no adequate studies in humans.*)

Disopyramide has been detected in milk at a concentration not exceeding that found in maternal plasma. Use with caution in nursing animals.

Overdosage/Acute Toxicity

Clinical signs of overdosage/toxicity include: anticholinergic effects, apnea, loss of consciousness, hypotension, cardiac conduction disturbances and arrhythmias, widening of the QRS complex and QT interval, bradycardia, congestive heart failure, seizures, asystole, and death.

Treatment consists initially of prompt gastric emptying, charcoal, and cathartics. Followed by vigorous symptomatic therapy using, if necessary, cardiac glycosides, vasopressors and sympathomimetics, diuretics, mechanically assisted respiration, and endocardial pacing. Disopyramide can be removed with hemodialysis.

Drug Interactions

The following drug interactions have either been reported or are theoretical in humans or animals receiving disopyramide and may be of significance in veterinary patients:

- ■ **ANTICHOLINERGIC DRUGS:** Additive anticholinergic effects may be encountered if disopyramide is used concomitantly with other anticholinergics (atropine, glycopyrrolate)

- ■ **CISAPRIDE:** Additional prolongation of QT interval

- ■ **MACROLIDE ANTIBIOTICS (erythromycin, clarithromycin):** Increased disopyramide levels; prolongation of QT interval may occur

- ■ **PHENOBARBITAL:** May increase disopyramide's metabolism, reduce levels

- ■ **PROCAINAMIDE, LIDOCAINE:** May be used with disopyramide, but widening of QRS and prolongation of QT interval may occur

- ■ **QUINIDINE:** May increase disopyramide levels; disopyramide may decrease quinidine levels

- ■ **RIFAMPIN:** May increase disopyramide's metabolism and reduce serum levels

- ■ **VERAPAMIL:** Because of additional negative inotropic effects, use of disopyramide within 48 hours of using verapamil is not recommended

Doses

- ■ **DOGS:**
  a) When used as an antiarrhythmic (almost never used): 7–30 mg/kg PO q4h (Kittleson 2006)

Monitoring

- ■ ECG

- ■ Blood pressure

- ■ Clinical signs of adverse effects (see above); liver function tests if chronic therapy

- ■ Serum levels if indicated (lack of efficacy, toxicity)

- ■ Therapeutic levels in humans have been reported to be between 2–7 micrograms/mL and toxic levels are considered to above 9 micrograms/mL. Levels of up to 7 micrograms/mL may be necessary to treat and prevent the recurrence of refractory ventricular tachycardias.

Client Information

- ■ Contact veterinarian if animal has persistent problems with difficult urination, dry mouth, vomiting, constipation, becomes lethargic or depressed, or has difficulty breathing.

Chemistry/Synonyms

Structurally dissimilar from other available antiarrhythmic agents, disopyramide phosphate occurs as a white or practically white crystalline powder with a pK_a of 10.4. It is freely soluble in water and slightly soluble in alcohol.

Disopyramide Phosphate may also be known as: disopyramidi phosphas, SC-13957, *Norpace®, Dicorantil®, Dirythmin®, Dirytmin®, Diso-Duriles®, Disomet®, Disonorm®, Durbis®, Durbis®, Isomide®, Isorythm®, Ritmodan®, Ritmoforine®, Rythmical®, Rythmodan®,* and *Rythmodul®.*

Storage/Stability

Disopyramide capsules should be stored at room temperature (15–30°C) in well-closed containers. An extemporaneously prepared suspension of 1–10 mg/mL of disopyramide (from capsules) in cherry syrup has been shown to be stable for one month if stored in amber bottles and refrigerated (2–8°C).

Dosage Forms/Regulatory Status

VETERINARY-LABELED PRODUCTS: None
The ARCI (Racing Commissioners International) has designated this drug as a class 4 substance. See the appendix for more information.

HUMAN-LABELED PRODUCTS:
Disopyramide Phosphate Capsules: 100 mg & 150 mg; *Norpace®* (Pharmacia); generic; (Rx)

Disopyramide Phosphate Capsules Extended-Release: 100 mg & 150 mg; *Norpace CR®* (Pharmacia); generic; (Rx)

References

Kittleson, M. (2006). "Chapt 29: Drugs used in the treatment of cardiac arrhythmias." *Small Animal Cardiology, 2nd Ed.*

dl-Methionine—see Methionine

DMSO—see Dimethyl Sulfoxide

DOBUTAMINE HCL

(*doe*-byoo-ta-meen)   Dobutrex®

PARENTERAL BETA ADRENERGIC INOTROPIC

Prescriber Highlights

▶ Parenteral, rapid acting inotropic agent

▶ Contraindications: Known hypersensitivity to the drug or the preservative (sodium bisulfite); or patients with IHSS

▶ Caution: Post MI

▶ Animals with atrial fibrillation should be digitalized prior to receiving dobutamine

▶ Most common adverse effects: facial twitching, tachycardia; higher doses can cause CNS effects (especially in cats)

▶ Use only in an "ICU" setting

Uses/Indications

Dobutamine is used as a rapid-acting injectable positive inotropic agent for short-term treatment of heart failure. It is also useful in shock patients when fluid therapy alone has not restored acceptable arterial blood pressure, cardiac output, or tissue perfusion.

Pharmacology/Actions

Dobutamine is considered a direct $beta_1$-adrenergic agonist. It also has mild $beta_2$- and $alpha_1$-adrenergic effects at therapeutic doses. These effects tend to balance one another and cause little direct effect on the systemic vasculature. In contrast to dopamine, dobutamine does not cause the release of norepinephrine. It has relatively mild chronotropic, arrhythmogenic, and vasodilative effects, but higher dosages can cause tachycardia.

Increased myocardial contractility and stroke volumes result in increased cardiac output. Decreases in left ventricular filling pressures (wedge pressures) and total peripheral resistance occur in patients with a failing heart. Blood pressure and cardiac rate generally are unaltered or slightly increased because of increased cardiac output. Increased myocardial contractility may increase myocardial oxygen demand and coronary blood flow.

Pharmacokinetics

Because it is rapidly metabolized in the GI tract and is not available after oral administration, dobutamine is only administered intravenously (as a constant infusion). After intravenous administration, the onset of action generally occurs within 2 minutes and peaks after 10 minutes.

Dobutamine is metabolized rapidly in the liver and other tissues and has a plasma half-life of approximately 2 minutes in humans. The drug's effects diminish rapidly after cessation of therapy.

Pharmacokinetic data for domestic animals is apparently unavailable. It is unknown if dobutamine crosses the placenta or into milk.

Contraindications/Precautions/Warnings

Dobutamine is contraindicated in patients with known hypersensitivity to the drug or with idiopathic hypertropic subaortic stenosis (IHSS). The injectable formulation contains sodium bisulfite as a preservative that has been documented to cause allergic-type reactions in some human patients. Hypovolemic states must be corrected before administering dobutamine. Because it may increase myocardial oxygen demand and increase infarct size, dobutamine should be used very cautiously after myocardial infarction.

Use with extreme caution in patients with ventricular tachyarrhythmias or atrial fibrillation. Dobutamine can enhance atrioventricular conduction; animals with atrial fibrillation should be digitalized prior to receiving dobutamine. In horses that will receive electrocardioversion for atrial fibrillation, it has been recommended to stop dobutamine for at least 5 minutes before shock delivery (McGurrin 2010).

Adverse Effects

Adverse effects reported in dogs include: tachycardia, facial twitching, seizures and tachyphylaxis (increasing dosages required over time). In cats, doses greater than 5 micrograms/kg/min may cause CNS effects such as tremors or seizures.

The most commonly reported adverse effects in humans are: ectopic beats, increased heart rate, increased blood pressure, chest pain, and palpitations. At usual doses these effects are generally mild and will not necessitate halting therapy, but dosage reductions should be performed. Other, more rare, adverse effects reported include: nausea, headache, vomiting, leg cramps, paresthesias, and dyspnea.

Reproductive/Nursing Safety

In humans, the FDA categorizes this drug as category *B* for use during pregnancy (*Animal studies have not yet demonstrated risk to the fetus, but there are no adequate studies in pregnant women; or animal studies have shown an adverse effect, but adequate studies in pregnant women have not demonstrated a risk to the fetus in the first trimes-*

ter of pregnancy, and there is no evidence of risk in later trimesters.)

No specific information on lactation safety for dobutamine was found.

Overdosage/Acute Toxicity

Clinical signs reported with excessive dosage include tachycardias, increased blood pressure, nervousness, and fatigue. Because of the drug's short duration of action, temporarily halting therapy is usually all that is required to reverse these effects.

Drug Interactions

The following drug interactions have either been reported or are theoretical in humans or animals receiving dobutamine and may be of significance in veterinary patients:

■ **ANESTHETICS, GENERAL HALOGENATED HYDROCARBON:** Use of halothane or cyclopropane with dobutamine may result in increased incidences of ventricular arrhythmias

■ **BETA-BLOCKERS (e.g., metoprolol, propranolol):** May antagonize the cardiac effects of dobutamine, and result in a preponderance of alpha-adrenergic effects and increased total peripheral resistance

■ **NITROPRUSSIDE:** Synergistic effects (increased cardiac output and reduced wedge pressure) can result if dobutamine is used with nitroprusside

■ **OXYTOCIC DRUGS:** May induce severe hypertension when used with dobutamine in obstetric patients

Doses

Dobutamine is administered as a constant rate intravenous infusion only.

■ **DOGS:**

a) For short-term treatment of acute heart failure: 5–40 micrograms/kg/minute IV; Doses of 5–20 micrograms/kg/minute are generally adequate for dogs. Infusions greater than 20 micrograms/kg/minute may cause tachycardia. (Kittleson 2006)

b) For shock where fluid therapy alone not adequate: 5–15 micrograms/kg/minute constant rate IV infusion (Haskins 2000)

c) For severe, decompensated, congestive heart failure: 2–20 micrograms/kg/min as a CRI. Start at low end and titrate to effect. Some patients may develop tachyphylaxis after 24-72 hours of therapy. (Erling & Mazzaferro 2008)

d) For short-term treatment of low cardiac output and acute heart failure: 2.5–10 micrograms/kg min IV. If tachycardia and arrhythmias occur, reduce dose or discontinue. (Reiser 2003)

e) 5–20 micrograms/kg/minute IV CRI. Increase dose rate over 48–72 hours. There is a prolonged, positive hemodynamic

effect that usually lasts for weeks after therapy is discontinued. (Kramer 2003)

f) 1–10 micrograms/kg/minute IV (DeFrancesco 2006)

g) For vasodilatory shock if fluid resuscitation is not successful: 2.5–10 micrograms/kg/min. (Scroggin & Quandt 2009)

■ **CATS:**

a) For short-term treatment of acute heart failure: 5–15 micrograms/kg/minute IV (Kittleson 2006)

b) 1–3 micrograms/kg/minute IV (DeFrancesco 2006)

c) 1–5 micrograms/kg/minute IV; start at 1 microgram/kg/minute and titrate until clinical effect. (Marks 2009)

■ **HORSES: (Note:** ARCI UCGFS Class 2 Drug)

a) 1–10 micrograms/kg/minute as an IV infusion (Mogg 1999)

b) **Foals** (after volume repletion): 2–20 micrograms/kg minute CRI (**Note:** another section of this reference states the dose is 3–40 micrograms/kg/minute). Follow the rule of "6": 6 times the weight of foal (in kg) = the number of mg to add to 100 mL of saline (1 mL/hr = 1 microgram/kg/minute). (Wilkins 2004)

Monitoring

■ Heart rate and rhythm, blood pressure

■ Mucous membrane color

■ Urine flow

■ Ideally, measurement of central venous or pulmonary wedge pressures and cardiac output

Client Information

■ This drug should only be used by professionals familiar with its use and in a setting where adequate patient monitoring can be performed.

Chemistry/Synonyms

Dobutamine HCl is a synthetic inotropic agent related structurally to dopamine. It occurs as a white, to off-white, crystalline powder with a pK_a of 9.4. Dobutamine is sparingly soluble in water and alcohol.

Dobutamine HCl may also be known as: 46236, compound 81929, dobutamini hydrochloridum, and LY-174008; many trade names are available.

Storage/Stability

Dobutamine injection should be stored at room temperature (15–30°C); diluted solutions should be used within 24 hours.

Compatibility/Compounding Considerations

Preparation for Injection: The solution for injection must be further diluted to a concentration no greater than 5 mg/mL (total of at least 50 mL of diluent) before administering.

Generally, dobutamine is added to D_5W, normal saline (if animal not severely sodium restricted) or other compatible IV solution. The following approximate concentrations will result if 1 vial (250 mg) is added either 250, 500, or 1000 mL IV solutions:

1 vial (250 mg) in:
    250 mL ≈ 1000 micrograms/mL
    500 mL ≈ 500 micrograms/mL
    1000 mL ≈ 250 micrograms/mL

A mechanical fluid administration control device should be used, if available, to administer dobutamine. When using a mini-drip IV administration set (60 drops ≈ 1 mL), 1 drop contains approximately 8.3 micrograms at the 500 micrograms/mL (one 250 mg vial in 500 mL IV fluids) concentration.

A formula for calculating dobutamine or dopamine CRI's has been published (Plunkett & McMichael 2008): 6 x body weight in kg = the number of milligrams of dobutamine or dopamine added to a total volume of 100 mL 0.9% NaCl. When delivered at a rate of 1 mL/hour IV, 1 microgram/kg/min is administered.

Dobutamine is physically **compatible** with the usually used IV solutions (D_5W, sodium chloride 0.45% and 0.9%, dextrose-saline combinations, lactated Ringer's) and is reported to be physically **compatible** with the following drugs: amiodarone HCl, atropine sulfate, dopamine HCl, epinephrine HCl, hydralazine HCl, isoproterenol HCl, lidocaine HCl, meperidine HCl, metaraminol bitartrate, morphine sulfate, nitroglycerin, norepinephrine (levarterenol) bitartrate, phentolamine mesylate, phenylephrine HCl, procainamide HCl, propranolol HCl, and verapamil HCl.

Dobutamine may be physically **incompatible** with the following agents: aminophylline, bretylium tosylate, bumetanide, calcium chloride or gluconate, diazepam, digoxin, furosemide, heparin (inconsistent results), regular insulin, magnesium sulfate, phenytoin sodium, potassium chloride (at high concentrations only— 160 mEq/L), potassium phosphate, and sodium bicarbonate.

Dosage Forms/Regulatory Status

VETERINARY-LABELED PRODUCTS: None
The ARCI (Racing Commissioners International) has designated this drug as a class 2 substance. See the appendix for more information.

HUMAN-LABELED PRODUCTS:

Dobutamine HCl Injection Concentrated Solution: 12.5 mg/mL in 20 mL & 40 mL single-use vials & 100 mL pharmacy bulk packages; generic; (Rx)

Dobutamine HCL Solution for Injection: 250 mg/250 mL (1 mg/mL) preservative free in 250 mL single use containers; 500 mg/500 mL (1 mg/mL) preservative free in 500 mg single-use containers; 500 mg/250 mL (2 mg/mL) preservative free in 250 mL single-use containers & 1,000 mg/250 mL (4 mg/mL) preservative free in 250 mL single-use containers; Dobutamine Hydrochloride in 5% Dextrose Injection (Baxter); (Rx)

References

DeFrancesco, T. (2006). Refractory heart failure. Proceedings: IVECCS 2006. Accessed via: Veterinary Information Network. goo.gl/WObuJ

Erling, P. & E.M. Mazzaferro (2008). Left–sided congestive heart failure in dogs: Treatment and monitoring of emergency patients. *Compendium—Continuing Education for Veterinarians* 30(2): 94–+.

Haskins, S. (2000). Therapy for Shock. *Kirk's Current Veterinary Therapy: XIII Small Animal Practice*. J Bonagura Ed. Philadelphia, WB Saunders: 140–147.

Kittleson, M. (2006). "Chapt 10: Management of Heart Failure." *Small Animal Cardiology, 2nd Ed*.

Kramer, G. (2003). Advances in the treatment of heart failure. part I and II. Proceedings: Atlantic Coast Veterinary Conference. Accessed via: Veterinary Information Network. http://goo.gl/MmkxH

Marks, S.L. (2009). A review of drugs for the ER. Proceedings: IVECCS. Accessed via: Veterinary Information Network. http://goo.gl/XI8qP

McGurrin, M. (2010). Therapeutic Options in Atrial Fibrillation. Proceedings: ACVIM. Accessed via: Veterinary Information Network. http://goo.gl/pFM13

Mogg, T. (1999). Equine Cardiac Disease: Clinical pharmacology and therapeutics. *The Veterinary Clinics of North America: Equine Practice* 15:3(December).

Plunkett, S.J. & M. McMichael (2008). Cardiopulmonary resuscitation in small animal medicine: An update. *Journal of Veterinary Internal Medicine* 22(1): 9–25.

Reiser, T. (2003). Emergency Management of Heart Failure. Proceedings: Western Veterinary Conference. Accessed via: Veterinary Information Network. http://goo.gl/Ecm6U

Scroggin, R.D. & J. Quandt (2009). The use of vasopressin for treating vasodilatory shock and cardiopulmonary arrest. *Journal of Veterinary Emergency and Critical Care* 19(2): 145–157.

Wilkins, P. (2004). Disorders of foals. *Equine Internal Medicine, 2nd Ed*. S Reed, W Bayly and D Sellon Eds. Philadelphia, Saunders: 1381–1431.

DOCUSATE SODIUM DOCUSATE CALCIUM

(**dok**-yoo-sate)   Colace®

SURFACTANT; STOOL SOFTENER

Prescriber Highlights

▶ Surfactant stool softener

▶ Caution: Fluid/electrolyte abnormalities

▶ Adverse Effects: Cramping, diarrhea, & GI mucosal damage

Uses/Indications

Docusate is used in small animals when feces are hard or dry, or in anorectal conditions when passing firm feces would be painful or detrimental. Docusate is used alone and in combination with mineral oil in treating fecal impactions in horses.

Pharmacology/Actions

Docusate salts reduce surface tension and allow water and fat to penetrate the ingesta and formed feces thereby softening the stool. Recent *in vivo* studies have demonstrated that docusate also increases cAMP concentrations in colonic mucosal cells that may increase both ion secretion and fluid permeability from these cells into the colon lumen.

Pharmacokinetics

It is unknown how much docusate is absorbed after oral administration, but it is believed that some is absorbed from the small intestine and then excreted into the bile.

Contraindications/Precautions/Warnings

Use with caution in patients with pre-existing fluid or electrolyte abnormalities; monitor.

Adverse Effects

At usual doses, clinically significant adverse effects should be very rare. Cramping, diarrhea, and intestinal mucosal damage are possible. The liquid preparations may cause throat irritation if administered by mouth. Docusate sodium is very bitter tasting.

Overdoses in horses may be serious.

Reproductive/Nursing Safety

In humans, the FDA categorizes this drug as category *C* for use during pregnancy (*Animal studies have shown an adverse effect on the fetus, but there are no adequate studies in humans; or there are no animal reproduction studies and no adequate studies in humans.*)

It is not known whether docusate calcium, docusate potassium, or docusate sodium are excreted in milk, but it is unlikely to be of concern.

Overdosage/Acute Toxicity

In horses, single doses of 0.65–1 g/kg have caused dehydration, intestinal mucosal damage, and death. Maximum therapeutic dosages of up to 0.2 g/kg have been reported. Signs of overdoses in horses can begin in 1–2 hours after dosing with initial signs including restlessness and increased intestinal sounds; increases in respiratory and cardiac rates can follow. Abdominal pain, watery diarrhea, and dehydration can occur with horses deteriorating over hours to several days to lateral recumbency and death. Because of the secretory effects that high dose docusate can produce, hydration and electrolyte status should be monitored and treated if necessary. Treatment is supportive; GI protectants, bicarbonate, corticosteroids, and antiendotoxemic agents (NSAIDs) have been suggested as being potentially helpful.

Drug Interactions

The following drug interactions have either been reported or are theoretical in humans or animals receiving docusate and may be of significance in veterinary patients:

■ **MINERAL OIL:** Theoretically, mineral oil should not be given with docusate (DSS) as enhanced absorption of the mineral oil could occur; however, this interaction does not appear to be of significant clinical concern with large animals. It is less clear whether there is a significant problem in using this combination in small animals and the concurrent use of these agents together in dogs or cats cannot be recommended. If it is deemed necessary to use both docusate and mineral oil in small animals, separate doses by at least two hours.

Doses

■ **DOGS:**
Docusate Sodium:
a) 50–100 mg (total dose) PO q12-24h (Jergens 2007)
b) **Small Dogs:** 25 mg PO once to twice daily
   Medium/large Dogs: 50 mg PO once to twice daily (Morgan 1988)
Docusate Calcium:
a) Two to three 50 mg capsules or one 240 mg capsule PO once daily (Burrows 1986)
b) One or two 50 mg capsules q12-24h PO (Kirk 1989)

■ **CATS:**
Docusate Sodium:
a) 50 mg PO per day; 5–10 mL of *Colace*® (strength not specified) as an enema (Sherding 1989)
b) 50 mg PO as needed; suppository: 1–2 pediatric suppositories as needed. (Washabau 2007)
c) 50 mg PO q12-24h (Jergens 2007)
Docusate Calcium:
a) 50 mg PO once daily (Washabau 2007)

■ **HORSES:**
a) For large colon impaction (to soften): 6–12 g/500 kg diluted in 2–4 liters of water by nasogastric tube q12-24h. (Blikslager & Jones 2004)

Monitoring

■ Clinical efficacy

■ Hydration and electrolyte status, if indicated

Client Information

■ Unless otherwise directed, give this medication to animal that has an empty stomach.

■ Do not give with other laxative agents without the approval of the veterinarian.

Chemistry/Synonyms

Docusate is available in sodium, and calcium salts. They are anionic, surface-active agents and possess wetting and emulsifying properties.

Docusate sodium (also known as dioctyl sodium succinate, DSS, or DOSS) occurs as a white, wax-like plastic solid with a characteristic odor. One g is soluble in approximately 70 mL of water and it is freely soluble in alcohol and glycerin. Solutions are clear and have a bitter taste.

Docusate calcium (also known as dioctyl calcium succinate) occurs as a white, amorphous solid with a characteristic odor (octyl alcohol). It is very slightly soluble in water, but freely soluble in alcohol.

Docusate sodium may also be known as: dioctyl sodium sulphosuccinate, dioctyl sodium sulfosuccinate, docusatum natricum, DSS, and sodium dioctyl sulphosuccinate; many trade names are available.

Storage/Stability

Capsules of salts of docusate should be stored in tight containers at room temperature. Temperatures above 86°F can soften or melt soft gelatin capsules. Docusate sodium solutions should be stored in tight containers and the syrup should be stored in tight, light-resistant containers.

Dosage Forms/Regulatory Status

VETERINARY APPROVED PRODUCTS:

There are several docusate products marketed for veterinary use; their approval status is unknown. Docusate products are available without prescription (OTC). Products include:

Docusate Sodium Bloat Preparation: 240 mg/1 fl. oz in 12 fl oz containers. FDA-approved for use in ruminants. Milk Withdrawal = 96 hours. Slaughter Withdrawal = 3 days. *Bloat Treatment®* (Durvet); (OTC).

Docusate Sodium Enema: 5% water miscible solution in 1 gal containers. FDA-approved for use in dogs, cats and horses. *Dioctynate®* (Butler); (OTC).

Docusate Sodium Enema: 250 mg in 12 mL syringes. FDA-approved for use in dogs and cats. *Disposable Enema®* (Vedco) (Rx), *Pet-Enema®* (Phoenix), (OTC); *Enema SA®* (Butler), (OTC); *Docu-Soft® Enema* (Life Science) (OTC)

Docusate sodium oral liquid 5% in gallons; various; generic. May also be called Veterinary Surfactant; (OTC)

HUMAN-LABELED PRODUCTS:

Docusate Sodium Oral Tablets: 100 mg; *ex-lax® Stool Softener* (Novartis Consumer Health); *Dioctyn®* (Dixon-Shane); (OTC)

Docusate Sodium Oral Capsules & Soft-gel Capsules: 50 mg, 100 mg, & 250 mg; *Colace®* (Purdue); *D-S-S®* (Magno-Humphries); *Non-Habit Forming Stool Softener®* and *Stool Softener®* (Rugby); *Phillips'® Liqui-Gels* (Bayer Consumer); *Sof-lax®* (Fleet); generic (OTC)

Docusate Sodium Oral Syrup: 20 mg/5 mL in 480 mL; 50 mg/15 mL in UD 15 & 30 mL; 60 mg/15 mL in 237 mL, 473 mL and 480 mL; 100 mg/30 mL in UD 15 & 30 mL; *Docu®* (Hi-Tech Pharmacal Co.); *Colace®* (Purdue); *Silace®* (Silarx) *Diocto* (various); generic (Roxane); (OTC)

Docusate Sodium Oral Liquid: 10 mg/mL in 473 mL; *Silace®* (Silarx); (OTC) & 150 mg/15 mL in 30 mL, & 480 mL; *Colace®* (Purdue); *Docu®* (Hi-Tech Pharmacal Co.), *Diocto* (various); (OTC).

Docusate Calcium Capsules: 240 mg (regular and soft gel), *Stool Softener®* (Apothecary), *Stool Softener DC®* (Rugby), *Surfak® Liquigels* (Pharmacia and Upjohn), *DC Softgels®* (Goldline); generic; (OTC).

References

Blikslager, A. & S. Jones (2004). Obstructive disorders of the gastrointestinal tract. *Equine Internal Medicine 2nd Ed.* S Reed, W Bayly and D Sellon Eds. Philadelphia, Saunders: 623–936.

Burrows, C.F. (1986). Constipation. *Current Veterinary Therapy IX: Small Animal Practice.* RW Kirk Ed. Philadelphia, WB Saunders: 904– 908.

Jergens, A. (2007). Constipation and Obstipation. *Blackwell's Five–Minute Veterinary Consult: Canine & Feline.* L Tilley and F Smith Eds., Blackwell Publishing: 294–295.

Kirk, R.W., Ed. (1989). *Current Veterinary Therapy X, Small Animal Practice.* Philadelphia, W.B. Saunders.

Morgan, R.V., Ed. (1988). *Handbook of Small Animal Practice.* New York, Churchill Livingstone.

Sherding, R.G. (1989). Diseases of the Intestines. *The Cat: Diseases and Clinical Management.* RG Sherding Ed. New York, Churchill Livingstone. 2: 955–1006.

Washabau, R. (2007). Evidence–Based Medicine: GI Drugs in the ICU. Proceedings: IVECCS. Accessed via: Veterinary Information Network. http://goo.gl/IHZon

DOLASETRON MESYLATE

(doe-*laz*-e-tron)   Anzemet®

ANTIEMETIC AGENT

Prescriber Highlights

▶ 5-HT$_3$ receptor antagonist antiemetic particularly useful for chemo-related nausea & vomiting in small animals

▶ Once daily administration for IV or PO doses

▶ Usually well tolerated; may cause dose-related ECG changes

▶ Oral human tablets not easily dosed in small animals (strength)

▶ Expense may be an issue; must be reformulated for PO use in cats

Uses/Indications

Dolasetron may be effective in treating severe nausea and vomiting in dogs and cats, particularly if caused by cancer chemotherapy drugs. Because it is given once a day, the injectable form of dolasetron is often preferred over ondansetron, a similarly effective antiemetic. However, for oral use in small animals, dolasetron tablets are too large (50 and 100 mg) to be practically administered.

Pharmacology/Actions

Dolasetron exerts its anti-nausea and antiemetic actions by selectively antagonizing 5-hydroxytryptamine$_3$ (5-HT$_3$) receptors. These receptors are found primarily in the CNS chemoreceptor trigger zone, on vagal nerve terminals and enteric neurons in the GI tract. Chemotherapy induced vomiting is believed to be caused principally by serotonin release from the mucosal enterochromaffin cells in the small intestine.

Pharmacokinetics

After dolasetron is administered IV to dogs, its half-life is only minutes long as it is rapidly reduced via carbonyl reductase to hydrodolasetron (also called reduced dolasetron or red-dolasetron). Hydrodolasetron is primarily responsible for the drug's pharmacologic effect. Oral dolasetron is also rapidly absorbed and converted to hydrodolasetron. Hydrodolasetron's volume of distribution in dogs is 8.5 L/kg; total body clearance is 25 mL/min/kg and half-life about 4 hours.

In humans, dolasetron is rapidly absorbed and converted to hydrodolasetron. Oral bioavailability is about 75%. Hydrodolasetron's half-life in humans is about 7−8 hours. The drug is partially metabolized in the liver, but 50−60% is excreted unchanged into the urine. Clearance may be reduced in patients with severe renal or hepatic impairment.

Contraindications/Precautions/Warnings

Dolasetron is contraindicated in patients hypersensitive to it, with atrioventricular block II to III, or with markedly prolonged QT_c. It should be given with caution to patients with, or susceptible to, developing prolongation of cardiac conduction intervals. This includes patients with hypokalemia, hypomagnesemia, receiving anti-arrhythmic drugs or diuretics that may induce electrolyte abnormalities, congenital QT syndrome, or a cumulative high dose of anthracycline chemotherapy.

These agents are generally ineffective when used for vomiting associated with feline hepatic lipidosis or GI obstruction.

Adverse Effects

Dolasetron appears to be well tolerated in the limited numbers of small animal patients that have received it. In humans, it has been associated with dose-related ECG interval prolongation (PR, QT_c, JT prolongation and QRS widening). Other adverse effects that have been reported in humans using the drug during chemotherapy include headache and dizziness.

Reproductive/Nursing Safety

In pregnant humans, dolasetron is designated by the FDA as a category *B* drug (*Animal studies have not demonstrated risk to the fetus, but there are no adequate studies in pregnant women; or animal studies have shown an adverse effect, but adequate studies in pregnant women have not demonstrated a risk to the fetus during the first trimester of pregnancy, and there is no evidence of risk in later trimesters.*) Teratogenicity studies in laboratory animals failed to demonstrate any teratogenic effects.

It is unknown if the drug enters milk; the manufacturer urges caution.

Overdosage/Acute Toxicity

There is very limited data available. One hu-

man patient who received 13 mg/kg of dolasetron developed severe hypotension and dizziness and was treated with pressors and fluids. The patient's blood pressure returned to baseline 3 hours after the dose was administered. It is suggested to manage overdoses with supportive therapy. The lethal intravenous doses in mice and rats were 160 mg/kg and 140 mg/kg respectively. This is equivalent to 6−12 times the human recommended dose when comparing equivalent body surface areas.

Drug Interactions

The following drug interactions have either been reported or are theoretical in humans or animals receiving dolasetron and may be of significance in veterinary patients:

- ■ **ATENOLOL:** May reduce the clearance and increase blood levels of hydrodolasetron
- ■ **CIMETIDINE:** May reduce the clearance and increase blood levels of hydrodolasetron
- ■ **KETOCONAZOLE:** May reduce the clearance and increase blood levels of hydrodolasetron
- ■ **PHENOBARBITAL:** Can reduce hydrodolasetron blood levels
- ■ **RIFAMPIN:** Can reduce hydrodolasetron blood levels

Laboratory Considerations

- ■ No dolasetron-related laboratory interactions were noted.

Doses

In humans, the injection can be given as rapidly as 100 mg over 30 seconds or diluted into 50 mL of a compatible IV solution and infused over a period of up to 15 minutes.

- ■ **DOGS:**
    a) As an anti-emetic, particularly for patients receiving chemotherapeutics: 0.6 mg/kg IV once daily. (Dowling 2003)
    b) 0.6 mg/kg IV q24h or 0.5 mg/kg PO, SC or IV q24h (Encarnacion *et al.* 2009)
    c) For vomiting disorders: 0.6−1 mg/kg PO q12h (Washabau 2006)
    d) To prevent vomiting: 0.6 mg/kg IV or PO once daily. To treat vomiting: 1 mg/kg PO or IV once daily (Marks 2008)

- ■ **CATS:**
    a) As an anti-emetic, particularly for patients receiving chemotherapeutics: 0.6 mg/kg IV once daily. (Dowling 2003)
    b) For vomiting disorders: 0.6−1 mg/kg PO q12h (Washabau 2006)
    c) To prevent vomiting: 0.6 mg/kg IV or PO once daily. To treat vomiting: 1 mg/kg PO or IV once daily (Marks 2008)
    d) 0.6 mg/kg IV q12h or 0.6−1 m g/kg PO q12h (Encarnacion *et al.* 2009)

Monitoring

- ■ Efficacy
- ■ Heart rhythm in at-risk patients

Client Information

■ The injectable form of this drug is most appropriately administered at the veterinary clinic/hospital. Oral forms of the drug will most likely need to be compounded to lesser strengths; maropitant or ondansetron tablets may be more practical for oral dosing in small animal patients.

Chemistry/Synonyms

A 5-HT$_3$ receptor antagonist antiemetic, dolasetron mesylate occurs as a white to off-white powder. It is freely soluble in water or propylene glycol, and slightly soluble in 0.9% sodium chloride solution or alcohol.

Dolasetron may also be known as *Anzemet®*, *Anemet®* or *Zamanon®*.

Storage/Stability

The commercially available tablets should be stored at room temperature 20–25°C (68–77°F) and protected from light. The commercially available injection should be stored at room temperature (20–25°C; 68–77°F) with excursions permitted to 15–30°C (59–86° F); protect from light.

Compatibility/Compounding Considerations

Dolasetron injection is reportedly **compatible** with the following injectable solutions: sodium chloride 0.9%, 5% dextrose, sodium chloride 0.45% with 5% dextrose, 5% dextrose and lactated Ringer's, lactated Ringer's, and mannitol 10% injection. After dilution, the injectable is stable under normal lighting at room temperatures for 24 hours; 48 hours if refrigerated. The manufacturer does not recommend mixing with other injectable drugs and states to flush the infusion line before and after administering dolasetron.

Dosage Forms/Regulatory Status

VETERINARY-LABELED PRODUCTS: None

HUMAN-LABELED PRODUCTS:

Dolasetron Tablets: 50 mg & 100 mg; *Anzemet®* (Aventis); (Rx)

Dolasetron Injection: 20 mg/mL with 38.2 mg/mL mannitol in single use 0.625 mL ampules, 0.625 mL fill in 2 mL *Carpuject*, single-use 5 mL vials & 25 mL multi-dose vials; *Anzemet®* (Aventis); (Rx)

References

Dowling, P. (2003). GI Therapy: When what goes in won't stay down. Proceedings: Western Veterinary Conference. Accessed via: Veterinary Information Network. http://goo.gl/co8V8

Encarnacion, H.J., J. Parra, et al. (2009). Vomiting. *Compendium–Continuing Education for Veterinarians* 31(3): 122–+.

Marks, S. (2008). GI Therapeutics: Which Ones and When? Proceedings; IVECCS. Accessed via: Veterinary Information Network. http://goo.gl/rxwcs

Washabau, R. (2006). Current anti–emetic therapy. Proceedings WVC 2006, Accessed via the Veterinary Information Network Jan 2007. Accessed via: Veterinary Information Network. http://goo.gl/LYKDB

DOMPERIDONE

(dohm-*pare*-i-dohne)   Motilium®

PROKINETIC (DOPAMINE-2 AGONIST) AGENT EQUIDONE®

Prescriber Highlights

▶ Dopamine-2 antagonist

▶ Used in: *Horses*: Tall fescue toxicity, as a diagnostic agent for PPID; *Small Animals*: Prokinetic agent

Uses/Indications

Domperidone is FDA-approved in the USA for prevention of fescue toxicosis in periparturient mares. It may also be useful as a prokinetic or antiemetic agent in small animals. It has more effect on conditions with delayed gastric emptying than other GI hypomotility conditions.

Via its effects on prolactin, domperidone may also be used to stimulate milk production in horses and small animals.

Domperidone has been shown to increase plasma ACTH in horses with equine pituitary pars intermedia dysfunction (PPID, Equine Cushing's) and may be useful in helping diagnose this condition.

Pharmacology/Actions

Domperidone is a dopamine antagonist (D2-receptors) with similar actions as metoclopramide. It has been stated that the drug does not cross the blood brain barrier and thus does not have CNS effects as does metoclopramide, but it may be more accurate to say that it does not readily cross into the CNS, as extrapyramidal adverse effects have been reported in some human patients.

Domperidone antagonizes dopamine in the GI tract and in the chemoreceptor trigger zone causing its prokinetic and antiemetic effects. It also is an antagonist for alpha$_2$ and beta$_2$ adrenergic receptors in the stomach.

Domperidone's apparent efficacy for the treatment of fescue toxicosis in pregnant mares is related to the fact that tall fescue toxicosis causes decreased prolactin levels. Dopamine is involved in the reduction of prolactin production and it is postulated that the alkaloids found in tall fescue act as dopamine-mimetic agents. Domperidone ostensibly blocks this effect.

Pharmacokinetics

Domperidone is absorbed from the GI tract, but its bioavailability in dogs is only about 20%, presumably due to a high first pass effect. Peak serum levels occur about 2 hours after oral dosing and the drug is highly bound (93%) to serum proteins. Domperidone is primarily metabolized and metabolites are excreted in the feces and urine.

Contraindications/Precautions/Warnings

Domperidone should not be used in animals with known hypersensitivity to it or when GI obstructions are present or suspected. Do not use in pregnant mares >15 days prior to the expected foaling date (see Reproductive Safety below). In horses, domperidone failure of passive transfer of immunoglobulins (IgG) may occur even in the absence of leakage of colostrum or milk. All foals born to mares treated with domperidone should be tested for serum IgG concentrations. Do not use in horses intended for human consumption.

Because domperidone is potentially a neurotoxic substrate of P-glycoprotein, it should be used with caution in those herding breeds (*e.g.*, Collies) that may have the gene mutation (MDR1) that causes a nonfunctional protein. Also see Drug Interactions.

Adverse Effects

Because plasma prolactin levels may be increased, galactorrhea or gynecomastia may result. In horses the most commonly reported adverse effects are premature lactation (dripping of milk prior to foaling) and failure of passive transfer. Injectable products (now withdrawn) have been associated with arrhythmias in human patients with heart disease or hypokalemia. Rarely, somnolence or dystonic reactions have occurred in people.

Reproductive/Nursing Safety

The equine product label states: *Equidone® Gel* may lead to premature birth, low birth weight foals or foal morbidity if administered >15 days prior to the expected foaling date. Accurate breeding date(s) and an expected foaling date are needed for the safe use of *Equidone® Gel*. The safety of *Equidone® Gel* has not been evaluated in breeding, pregnant and lactating mares other than in the last 45 days of pregnancy and the first 15 days of lactation (see Animal Safety). The safety in stallions has not been evaluated. The long-term effects on foals born to mares treated with *Equidone® Gel* have not been evaluated.

Domperidone has been shown to have teratogenic effects when used at high doses in mice, rats and rabbits. The drug's effect of causing prolactin release may impact fertility in both females and males.

Domperidone has been used to increase milk supply in women. In rats, it enters milk in small amounts with approximately 1/500th of the adult dose reaching the pups.

Overdosage/Acute Toxicity

There is no specific antidote for domperidone overdose. Use standard decontamination procedures and treat supportively.

Drug Interactions

The following drug interactions have either been reported or are theoretical in humans or animals receiving domperidone and may be of significance in veterinary patients:

- **AZOLE ANTIFUNGALS (ketoconazole, etc.):** May increase domperidone levels

- **ANTICHOLINERGIC DRUGS:** May reduce the efficacy of domperidone

- **BROMOCRIPTINE/CABERGOLINE:** Domperidone may antagonize effects on prolactin

- **MACROLIDE ANTIBIOTICS (erythromycin, clarithromycin):** May increase domperidone levels

- **OPIOIDS:** May reduce the efficacy of domperidone

- **SUSTAINED-RELEASE or ENTERIC-COATED ORAL MEDICATIONS:** Domperidone may alter the absorptive characteristics of these drugs by decreasing GI transit times

Laboratory Considerations

- Domperidone may increase **serum prolactin** levels

- Domperidone may increase **ALT and AST**

- Domperidone may cause a false positive result on the **milk calcium** test used to predict foaling.

Doses

- **DOGS:**

  As a prokinetic agent:

  a) 0.05–0.1 mg/kg PO once or twice a day. **Note:** Scant clinical experience; suggested dose based upon experimental data. (Hall & Washabau 1997)

  b) For vomiting due to gastritis: 2–5 mg (total dose) PO two to three times a day. (Bishop 2005)

- **CATS:**

  As a prokinetic agent:

  a) 0.05–0.1 mg/kg PO once or twice a day. **Note:** Scant clinical experience; suggested dose based upon experimental data. (Hall & Washabau 1997)

- **HORSES:**

  For fescue toxicity:

  a) 1.1 mg/kg PO once daily starting 10 to 15 days prior to Expected Foaling Date (EFD). Treatment may be continued for up to 5 days after foaling if mares are not producing adequate milk after foaling. (Label information—*Equidone Gel®*; Dechra)

Monitoring

- Clinical efficacy

Client Information

Pregnant and lactating women should use caution when handling the equine gel product. Systemic exposure to domperidone may affect reproductive hormones.

Chemistry/Synonyms

Domperidone maleate occurs as a white or almost white powder that exhibits polymorphism. It is very slightly soluble in water or alcohol.

Domperidone may also be known as domperidonum and R-33812. Common trade names include *Motilium®* or *Equidone®*, but many trade names are available internationally.

Storage/Stability

Domperidone gel should be stored at controlled room temperature 25°C (77°F) with excursions between 15°-30°C (59°-86°F) permitted. Recap after each use. Domperidone tablets should be stored at room temperature and protected from light and moisture.

Dosage Forms/Regulatory Status

VETERINARY-LABELED PRODUCTS: None
Domperidone Oral Gel 11% (110 mg/mL) in 25 mL multi-dose oral syringes; *Equidone® Gel* (Dechra); (Rx)

HUMAN-LABELED PRODUCTS: None in the USA. In Canada (10 mg tablet only) and in Europe, human oral tablets of 10 mg, suppositories and oral suspension may be available.

References

Bishop, Y. (2005). *The Veterinary Formulary, 6th Ed.* Cambridge, The Pharmaceutical Press.

Hall, J. & R. Washabau (1997). Gastrointestinal Prokinetic Therapy: Dopaminergic Antagonist Drugs. *Comp CE* 19(February): 214–221.

DOPAMINE HCL

(doe-pa-meen)   Intropin®

ADRENERGIC/DOPAMINERGIC INOTROPIC AGENT

Prescriber Highlights

▶ Catecholamine that in most species dilates the renal mesenteric, coronary, & intracerebral vascular beds at lower doses; at higher doses, systemic peripheral resistance is increased & hypotension treated

▶ Use in an "ICU" setting

▶ Contraindications: Pheochromocytoma, ventricular fibrillation, & uncorrected tachyarrhythmia

▶ Not a substitute for adequate reperfusion therapy

▶ Adverse Effects: Nausea/vomiting, ectopic beats, tachycardia, hypotension, hypertension, dyspnea, headache & vasoconstriction

▶ Avoid extravasation injuries

Uses/Indications

Dopamine should be used only in critical care settings where adequate monitoring can be provided. It is used to correct the hemodynamic imbalances present in shock after adequate fluid volume replacement, and as adjunctive therapy for the treatment of acute heart failure.

It has now been shown that low-dose dopamine for the treatment of oliguric renal failure is not efficacious in improving GFR in humans; its use for this purpose in dogs is unproven and somewhat controversial. In cats, low dose dopamine reportedly does not cause renal vasodilatation.

Pharmacology/Actions

Dopamine is a precursor to norepinephrine and acts directly and indirectly (by releasing norepinephrine) on both alpha- and beta$_1$-receptors. Dopamine also has dopaminergic effects.

While there are species differences, in general at very low IV doses, 0.5–2 micrograms/kg/min, dopamine acts predominantly on dopaminergic receptors and dilates the renal, mesenteric, coronary, and intracerebral vascular beds. At doses from 2–10 micrograms/kg/min, dopamine also stimulates alpha$_1$- and beta$_1$-adrenergic receptors. The net effect at this dosage range is to exert positive cardiac inotropic activity, increase organ perfusion, renal blood flow and urine production, but GFR does not appreciably improve. At these lower doses, systemic vascular resistance increases with the dose. At higher doses, >10–12 micrograms/kg/min, the dopaminergic effects are overridden by alpha effects. Systemic peripheral resistance is increased and hypotension may be corrected in cases where systemic vascular resistance is diminished; renal and peripheral blood flows are thus decreased. One study in cats showed that dopamine at 15 micrograms/kg/min did not increase systemic vascular resistance (Pascoe *et al.* 2006).

Pharmacokinetics

Dopamine is not administered orally as it is rapidly metabolized in the GI tract. After IV administration, the onset of action is usually within 5 minutes and persists for less than 10 minutes after the infusion has stopped.

Dopamine is widely distributed in the body, but does not cross the blood-brain barrier in appreciable quantities. It is unknown if dopamine crosses the placenta.

The plasma half-life of dopamine is approximately 2 minutes. It is metabolized in the kidney, liver, and plasma by monoamine oxidase (MAO) and catechol-O-methyltransferase (COMT) to inactive compounds. Up to 25% of a dose of dopamine is metabolized to norepinephrine in the adrenergic nerve terminals. In human patients receiving monoamine oxidase inhibitors, dopamine's duration of activity can be as long as one hour.

Contraindications/Precautions/Warnings

Dopamine is contraindicated in patients with pheochromocytoma, ventricular fibrillation, and uncorrected tachyarrhythmias. It is not a substitute for adequate fluid, electrolyte or blood product replacement therapy. Dopamine should be used with caution in patients with ischemic heart disease or an occlusive vascular disease. Decrease dose or discontinue the drug should clinical signs occur implicating dopamine as the cause of reduced circulation to the extremities or the heart. The drug should be discontinued or dosage reduced should arrhythmias (PVC's) occur.

Cats are unlikely to benefit (and it may be detrimental) from low dose dopamine therapy for oliguric renal failure.

Adverse Effects

Most frequent adverse effects seen include: nausea and vomiting, ectopic beats, tachycardia, palpitation, hypotension, hypertension, dyspnea, headache, and vasoconstriction.

Extravasation injuries with dopamine can be very serious with necrosis and sloughing of surrounding tissue. Patient's IV sites should be routinely monitored. Should extravasation occur, infiltrate the site (ischemic areas) with a solution of 5–10 mg phentolamine (*Regitine®*) in 10–15 mL of normal saline. A syringe with a fine needle should be used to infiltrate the site with many injections.

Reproductive/Nursing Safety

In humans, the FDA categorizes this drug as category *C* for use during pregnancy (*Animal studies have shown an adverse effect on the fetus, but there are no adequate studies in humans; or there are no animal reproduction studies and no adequate studies in humans.*) In a separate system evaluating the safety of drugs in canine and feline pregnancy (Papich 1989), this drug is categorized as in class: *B* (*Safe for use if used cautiously. Studies in laboratory animals may have uncovered some risk, but these drugs appear to be safe in dogs and cats or these drugs are safe if they are not administered when the animal is near term.*)

It is not known whether dopamine is excreted in breast milk.

Overdosage/Acute Toxicity

Accidental overdosage is manifested by excessive blood pressure elevation (see adverse effects above). Treatment consists only of temporarily discontinuing therapy since dopamine's duration of activity is so brief. Should the patient's condition fail to stabilize, phentolamine has been suggested for use.

Drug Interactions

The following drug interactions have either been reported or are theoretical in humans or animals receiving dopamine and may be of significance in veterinary patients:

- ■ **ALPHA-ADRENERGIC BLOCKERS (e.g., prazosin):** May antagonize the vasoconstrictive properties of dopamine (high-dose)
- ■ **ANESTHETICS, GENERAL HALOGENATED HYDROCARBON:** Use of halothane or cyclopropane with dopamine may result in increased incidences of ventricular arrhythmias
- ■ **ANTIDEPRESSANTS, TRICYCLIC:** May potentiate adverse cardiovascular effects

- ■ **BETA-BLOCKERS (e.g., metoprolol, propranolol):** May antagonize the cardiac effects of dopamine
- ■ **DIURETICS:** May potentiate urine production effects of low-dose dopamine
- ■ **MONOAMINE OXIDASE INHIBITORS:** Monoamine oxidase inhibitors can significantly prolong and enhance the effects on dopamine
- ■ **OXYTOCIC DRUGS:** May cause severe hypertension when used with dopamine
- ■ **PHENOTHIAZINES:** In animals (species not specified), the renal and mesenteric vasodilatation effects of dopamine have been antagonized by phenothiazines
- ■ **VASOPRESSORS/VASOCONSTRICTORS:** Use with dopamine may cause severe hypertension

Laboratory Considerations

Dopamine may:

- ■ Suppress **serum prolactin** secretion from the pituitary
- ■ Suppress **thyrotropin** secretion from the pituitary
- ■ Suppress **growth hormone** secretion from the pituitary

Doses

The dosage of dopamine is determined by its indication (for more information refer to the pharmacology section above). Use an IV pump or other flow-controlling device to increase precision in dosing.

a) For vasodilatory shock if fluid resuscitation and dobutamine is not successful: 2.5–10 micrograms/kg/min. If not successful may try adding norepinephrine. (Scroggin & Quandt 2009)

b) For adjunctive therapy for acute heart failure (dogs): IV infusion of 1–10 micrograms/kg/min (doses higher may increase peripheral vascular resistance and heart rate). Initially, a dose of 2 micrograms/kg/min is usually used and titrated upward to desired clinical effect (improved hemodynamics) (Kittleson 2006)

c) For treatment of severe hypotension/shock: (**Note:** Dopamine is not a substitute for adequate volume replacement therapy when indicated.) 1–3 micrograms/kg/minute CRI (constant rate IV infusion); higher dosages of 3–10 micrograms/kg/min CRI are indicated if greater cardiotonic and BP support are indicated (Haskins 2000)

d) For treatment of severe hypotension/shock after fluid correction and if dobutamine does not give desired effect: 1–10 micrograms/kg/min IV as a CRI titrated to effect. (Plunkett & McMichael 2008)

e) For adjunctive therapy for oliguric renal failure (usually for dogs only): Low doses (1–3 micrograms/kg/min) with diuretics (furosemide) are used to attempt to convert a patient from an oliguric state to a non-oliguric one (Elliott & Cowgill 2000) **Note:** Many now believe that dopamine is not indicated for treating acute renal failure.

Monitoring

■ Urine flow

■ Cardiac rate/rhythm

■ Blood pressure

■ IV site

Client Information

■ Dopamine should be used only in an intensive care setting or where adequate monitoring is possible

Chemistry/Synonyms

An endogenous catecholamine that is the immediate precursor to norepinephrine, dopamine (as the HCl salt) occurs as a white to off-white crystalline powder. It is freely soluble in water and soluble in alcohol. The injectable concentrated solution has a pH of 2.5–5.5 and may contain an antioxidant (sodium bisulfite). The pH's of the ready-to-use injectable products in dextrose range from 3–5.

Dopamine HCl may also be known as: ASL-279, dopamini hydrochloridum, and 3-hydroxytyramine hydrochloride; many trade names are available.

Storage/Stability/Preparation/ Compatibility

Dopamine injectable products should be protected from light. Solutions that are pink, yellow, brown, or purple indicate decomposition of the drug. Solutions that are darker than a light yellow should be discarded. Dopamine solutions should be stored at room temperature (15–30°C).

After dilution in a common IV solution (not 5% bicarbonate), dopamine is stable for at least 24 hours at room temperature, but it is recommended to dilute the drug just prior to use. Dopamine is stable in solutions with a pH of less than 6.4, and most stable at pH's less than 5. It is oxidized at alkaline pH.

Compatibility/Compounding Considerations

To prepare solution: Add contents of vial to either 250 mL, 500 mL, or 1000 mL of normal saline, D_5W, lactated Ringer's injection, or other compatible IV fluid. If adding a 200 mg vial (5 mL @ 40 mg/mL) to a one-liter bag, the resultant solution will contain an approximate concentration of 200 micrograms/mL. If using a mini-drip IV set (60 drops/mL), each drop will contain approximately 3.3 micrograms. In small dogs and cats, it may be necessary to use less dopamine so the final concentration will be less; in large animals, a higher concentration may be necessary.

A formula for calculating dobutamine or dopamine CRI's has been published (Plunkett & McMichael 2008): 6 x body weight in kg = the number of mgs of dobutamine or dopamine added to a total volume of 100 mL of 0.9% NaCl. When delivered at a rate of 1 mL/hour IV, 1 microgram/kg/min is administered.

Dopamine is reported to be physically **compatible** with the following IV fluids: D_5 in LRS, D_5 in half-normal saline, D_5 in normal saline, D_5W, mannitol 20% in water, lactated Ringer's, normal saline, and 1/6M sodium lactate. Dopamine is reported to be physically **compatible** with the following drugs: aminophylline, bretylium tosylate, calcium chloride, carbenicillin disodium, cephalothin sodium neutral, chloramphenicol sodium succinate, dobutamine HCl, gentamicin sulfate (gentamicin potency retained for only 6 hours), heparin sodium, hydrocortisone sodium succinate, kanamycin sulfate, lidocaine HCl, methylprednisolone sodium succinate, oxacillin sodium, potassium chloride, tetracycline HCl, and verapamil HCl.

Dopamine is reported to be physically **incompatible** with: amphotericin B, ampicillin sodium, iron salts, metronidazole with sodium bicarbonate, penicillin G potassium, and sodium bicarbonate. Compatibility is dependent upon factors such as pH, concentration, temperature, and diluent used; it is suggested to consult specialized references for more specific information.

Dosage Forms/Regulatory Status

VETERINARY-LABELED PRODUCTS: None
The ARCI (Racing Commissioners International) has designated this drug as a class 2 substance. See the appendix for more information.

HUMAN-LABELED PRODUCTS:
Dopamine HCl for Concentrated Solution for Injection: 40 mg/mL, 80 mg/mL and 160 mg/mL in 5 mL & 10 mL vials; generic; (Rx)

Dopamine HCl in Dextrose 5% Injection Solution: 200 mg/250 mL (0.8 mg/mL); 400 mg/500 mL (0.8 mg/mL); 400 mg/250 mL (1.6 mg/mL); 800 mg/500 mL (1.6 mg/mL); & 800 mg/250 mL (3.2 mg/mL) in 250 mL premixed single-use containers; generic; (Rx)

References

Elliott, D. & L. Cowgill (2000). Acute Renal Failure. *Kirk's Current Veterinary Therapy: XIII Small Animal Practice.* J Bonagura Ed.: 173–178.

Haskins, S. (2000). Therapy for Shock. *Kirk's Current Veterinary Therapy: XIII Small Animal Practice.* J Bonagura Ed. Philadelphia, WB Saunders: 140–147.

Kittleson, M. (2006). "Chapt 10: Management of Heart Failure." *Small Animal Cardiology, 2nd Ed.*

Pascoe, P.J., J.E. Ilkiw, et al. (2006). Effects of increasing infusion rates of dopamine, dobutamine, epinephrine, and phenylephrine in healthy anesthetized cats. *American Journal of Veterinary Research* 67(9): 1491–1499.

Plunkett, S.J. & M. McMichael (2008). Cardiopulmonary resuscitation in small animal medicine: An update. *Journal of Veterinary Internal Medicine* 22(1): 9–25.

Scroggin, R.D. & J. Quandt (2009). The use of vasopressin for treating vasodilatory shock and cardiopulmonary arrest. *Journal of Veterinary Emergency and Critical Care* 19(2): 145–157.

DORAMECTIN

(dor-a-**mek**-tin)   Dectomax®

AVERMECTIN ANTIPARASITIC AGENT

Prescriber Highlights

▶ Injectable (cattle, swine) & topical (cattle only) avermectin antiparasiticide

▶ Potentially useful for generalized demodicosis in small animals

▶ Manufacturer warns about using in other species

▶ IM injections may cause muscle blemishes

▶ Not labeled for female dairy cattle (20 months or older)

▶ Relatively long slaughter withdrawal times

Uses/Indications

Doramectin injection is indicated for the treatment and control of the following endo- and ectoparasites in cattle: roundworms (adults and some fourth stage larvae)—*Ostertagia ostertagi* (including inhibited larvae), *O. lyrata, Haemonchus placei, Trichostrongylus axei, T. colubriformis, T. longispicularis, Cooperia oncophora, C. pectinata, C. punctata, C. surnabada* (*syn. mcmasteri*), *Bunostomum phlebotomum, Strongyloides papillosus, Oesophagostomum radiatum, Trichuris* spp.; lungworms (adults and fourth stage larvae)—*Dictyocaulus viviparus*; eyeworms (adults)—*Thelazia* spp.; grubs (parasitic stages)—*Hypoderma bovis, H. lineatum*; lice—*Haematopinus eurysternus, Linognathus vituli, Solenopotes capillatus*; and mange mites—*Psoroptes bovis, Sarcoptes scabiei.*

In swine the injection is labeled for the treatment and control gastrointestinal roundworms (adults and 4th stage *Ascaris suum*, adults and 4th stage *Oesophagostomum dentatum, Oesophagostomum quadrispinolatum* adults, *Strongyloides ransomi* adults, and *Hydrostrongylus rubidus* adults), lungworms (*Stephanurus dentatus* adults), mange mites (adults and immature stages *Sarcoptes scabeii var. suis*), and sucking lice (adults and immature stages *Haematopinus suis*)

The manufacturer states the doramectin protects cattle against infection or reinfection with *Ostertagia ostertagi* for up to 21 days.

Doramectin topical (pour-on) is FDA-approved for use in cattle and has a similar spectrum of action against a variety of endo- and ectoparasites, including biting lice.

Injectable doramectin has been used for treating a variety of nematode and arthropod parasites in companion animals, including generalized demodicosis in dogs and cats and spirocercosis in dogs.

Pharmacology/Actions

The primary mode of action of avermectins like doramectin is to affect chloride ion channel activity in the nervous system of nematodes and arthropods. Doramectin binds to receptors that increase membrane permeability to chloride ions. This inhibits the electrical activity of nerve cells in nematodes and muscle cells in arthropods and causes paralysis and death of the parasites. Avermectins also enhance the release of gamma amino butyric acid (GABA) at presynaptic neurons. GABA acts as an inhibitory neurotransmitter and blocks the postsynaptic stimulation of the adjacent neuron in nematodes or the muscle fiber in arthropods. Avermectins are generally not toxic to mammals as they do not have glutamate-gated chloride channels and these compounds do not readily cross the blood-brain barrier where mammalian GABA receptors occur.

Pharmacokinetics

After subcutaneous injection, the time to peak plasma concentration in cattle is about 5 days. Bioavailability is, for practical purposes, equal with SC and IM injections in cattle.

Contraindications/Precautions/Warnings

The manufacturer warns to not use in other animal species as severe adverse reactions, including fatalities in dogs, may result.

It is recommended to use alternative treatments for demodicosis or spirocercosis in untested dogs of breeds susceptible to MDR1-allele mutation (Collies, Australian Shepherds, Shelties, Long-haired Whippet) as they are at higher risk for toxicity.

Adverse Effects

No listed adverse effects. Intramuscular injections may have a higher incidence of injection site blemishes at slaughter than do subcutaneous injections.

When used for demodicosis in dogs, adverse effects are uncommon but may include pupil dilation, lethargy, blindness, or coma.

Reproductive/Nursing Safety

In studies performed in breeding animals (bulls and cows in early and late pregnancy), at a dose of 3X recommended had no effect on breeding performance.

Overdosage/Acute Toxicity

In field trials, no toxic signs were seen in cattle given up to 25X the recommended dose. In breeding animals (bulls, and cows in early and late pregnancy), a dose 3 times the recommended dose had no effect on breeding performance.

Drug Interactions

■ None noted

Doses

■ **DOGS:**

For treatment of generalized demodicosis:

a) 600 micrograms/kg PO once daily has been utilized with success in some cases of canine generalized demodicosis. Once weekly subcutaneous injections at 600 micrograms/kg can also be used. If improvement is not seen after 60 days, an alternative therapy should be used. (Merchant 2009)

b) Get informed consent from owner for extra-label treatment. Give 600 micrograms/kg (0.6 mg/kg) SC once per week. (Hillier 2006)

For treatment of benign nodules secondary to *S. lupi*:

a) 400 micrograms/kg SC at two week intervals once; may use milbemycin in MDR-1 sensitive breeds. (Dvir & Clift 2009)

■ **CATS:**

For feline demodicosis (*D. cati, D. gatoi):*

a) Get informed consent from owner for extra-label treatment. Give 600 micrograms/kg (0.6 mg/kg) SC once per week. Alternative treatments include Lime sulfur dips or amitraz. (Hillier 2006)

■ **CATTLE:**

a) For labeled indications (Injectable): 200 micrograms/kg (1 mL per 110 lb. body weight) SC or IM. Injections should be made using 16 to 18 gauge needles. Subcutaneous injections should be administered under the loose skin in front of or behind the shoulder. Intramuscular injections should be administered into the muscular region of the neck. Beef Quality Assurance guidelines recommend subcutaneous administration as the preferred route. (Label Directions; *Dectomax®*—Pfizer)

b) For labeled indications (Pour-on): Topically at a dosage of 500 micrograms/kg (1 mL per 22 lb. body weight). Administer topically along the mid-line of the back in a narrow strip between the withers and tailhead. (Label Directions; *Dectomax® Pour-On*—Pfizer)

■ **SWINE:**

a) For labeled indications: 300 micrograms/kg (1 mL per 75 lb. body weight) IM. Injections should be made using 16 g x 1.5 inch needles for sows and boars and 18 g x 1 inch needle for young animals. Use a tuberculin syringe and a 20 g x 1 inch needle for piglets. Intramuscular injections should be administered into the muscular region of the neck. See the label for recommended treatment pro-

gram for sows, gilts, boars, feeder pigs, weaners, growers and finishers. (Label Directions; *Dectomax®*—Pfizer)

■ **RABBITS:**

a) For *P. cuniculi* infestations: 200 micrograms/kg IM once. (Kanbur *et al.* 2008)

Monitoring

■ Efficacy

Client Information

■ Read and follow all labeled instructions carefully.

■ Cattle must not be slaughtered for human consumption within 35 days of treatment.

■ Not for use in female dairy cattle 20 months of age or older.

■ A withdrawal period has not been established for this product in pre-ruminating calves.

■ Should not be used in calves to be processed for veal.

■ Swine should not be slaughtered for human consumption within 24 days of treatment.

Chemistry/Synonyms

An avermectin antiparasitic compound, doramectin is isolated from fermentations from the soil organism *Streptomyces avermitilis*.

Doramectin may also be known as UK-67994, or *Dectomax®*.

Storage/Stability

The commercially available injectable solution is a colorless to pale yellow, sterile solution. The injectable solution should be stored below 86°F (30°C). The topical pour on solution should be stored below 30°C (86°F) and protected from light.

Dosage Forms/Regulatory Status

VETERINARY-LABELED PRODUCTS:

Doramectin Injectable Solution: 10 mg/mL in 100 mL, 250 mL, and 500 mL multi-dose vials; *Dectomax®* (Pfizer); (OTC). FDA-approved for use in cattle and swine When used at labeled doses: Slaughter Withdrawal: cattle = 45 days, swine = 24 days. Do not use in female dairy cattle 20 months of age or older or in calves to be used for veal. A withdrawal period has not been established in preruminating calves.

Doramectin Pour-On Solution: 5 mg/mL in 250 mL, 1 L, 2.5 L and 5 L multi-dose containers; *Dectomax® Pour-On* (Pfizer); (OTC). FDA-approved for use in cattle. Slaughter withdrawal = 45 days. Not for use in female dairy cattle 20 months of age or older. A withdrawal period has not been established in preruminating calves. Do not use in calves to be used for veal.

HUMAN-LABELED PRODUCTS: None

References

Dvir, E. & S. Clift (2009). Update on spirocercosis–induced oesophageal sarcoma and Spirocerca lupi aberrant migration. Proceedings: ECVIM–CA Congress. Accessed

via: Veterinary Information Network. http://goo.gl/
EaEyz

Hillier, A. (2006). Update on canine demodicosis. Proceedings: ACVC. Accessed via: Veterinary
Information Network. http://goo.gl/O2tAz

Kanbur, M., O. Atalay, et al. (2008). The curative and an-
tioxidative efficiency of doramectin and doramectin
plus vitamin AD(3)E treatment on Psoroptes cuniculi
infestation in rabbits. *Research in Veterinary Science*
85(2): 291–293.

Merchant, S. (2009). Demodeciosis in the Dog: Diagnosis
and Management. Proceedings: ACVC. Accessed via:
Veterinary Information Network. http://goo.gl/Jk0zX

DOXAPRAM HCL

(***docks***-a-pram)   Dopram-V®

CNS/RESPIRATORY STIMULANT

Prescriber Highlights

▶ CNS stimulant usually used to stimulate respirations in newborns or after
anesthesia; also used for assessment
of laryngeal function in small animals;
use in small animal neonates is controversial

▶ Not a substitute for aggressive artificial (mechanical) respiratory support
when required

▶ Possible contraindications: Receiving
mechanical ventilation, hypersensitivity,
seizure disorders, head trauma/CVA,
uncompensated heart failure, severe
hypertension, respiratory failure secondary to neuromuscular disorders,
airway obstruction, pulmonary embolism, pneumothorax, acute asthma,
dyspnea, or whenever hypoxia is not
associated with hypercapnia.

▶ Caution: History of asthma, arrhythmias, or tachycardias. Use extreme
caution in patients with cerebral edema or increased CSF pressure, pheochromocytoma, or hyperthyroidism.

▶ Avoid IV extravasation or using a single
injection site for a prolonged period

▶ Adverse Effects: Hypertension, arrhythmias, seizures, & hyperventilation
leading to respiratory alkalosis

Uses/Indications

The manufacturer of *Dopram*®-*V* lists the following indications: For Dogs, Cats, and Horses:
To stimulate respiration during and after general anesthesia and/or to speed awakening and
reflexes after anesthesia. For Neonatal Dogs and
Cats: stimulate respirations following dystocia
or cesarean section. It is reported that in small
animals, doxapram is most likely to be beneficial in increasing respiratory efforts in neonates
with low-frequency, gasping, erratic pattern of
breathing after receiving oxygen therapy (Traas
2009).

Doxapram has been used for treatment of
CNS depression in food animals (not FDA-
approved) and has been suggested as a treatment of respiratory depression in small animals
caused by reactions to radiopaque contrast media or for barbiturate overdosage (see precautions below).

The use of doxapram to initiate and stimulate
respirations in newborns is somewhat controversial as the drug has been shown in experimental animals to increase myocardial oxygen
demand and reduce cerebral blood flow.

Doxapram has been shown to be useful to
offset suppression of general anesthetic agents
when laryngeal function is being assessed.

Pharmacology/Actions

Doxapram is a general CNS stimulant, with
all levels of the CNS affected. The effects of
respiratory stimulation are a result of direct
stimulation of the medullary respiratory centers and, possibly, through the reflex activation
of carotid and aortic chemoreceptors. Transient
increases in respiratory rate and volume occur,
but increases in arterial oxygenation usually do
not ensue. This is because doxapram usually
increases the work associated with respirations
with resultant increased oxygen consumption
and carbon dioxide production.

Pharmacokinetics

Little published pharmacokinetic data appears
for domestic animals. Onset of effect in humans
and animals after IV injection usually occurs
within 2 minutes. The drug is well distributed
into tissues. In dogs, doxapram is rapidly metabolized and most is excreted as metabolites in the
urine within 24–48 hours after administration.
Small quantities of metabolites may be excreted
up to 120 hours after dosing.

Contraindications/Precautions/Warnings

Doxapram should not be used as a substitute
for aggressive artificial (mechanical) respiratory support in instances of severe respiratory
depression.

In calves, doxapram has been reported as
contraindicated in premature calves or other
patients with clinical signs indicative of lung
immaturity as effects are only minimal and use
could lead to increased pulmonary blood pressure with fetal circulation persisting resulting
from a right-to-left shunt via the patent ductus
and foramen ovale. (Bleul *et al.* 2010)

Contraindications from the human literature
include: seizure disorders, head trauma, uncompensated heart failure, severe hypertension,
cardiovascular accidents, respiratory failure secondary to neuromuscular disorders, airway obstruction, pulmonary embolism, pneumothorax, acute asthma, dyspnea, or whenever hypoxia
is not associated with hypercapnia. Doxapram
should be used with caution in patients with
a history of asthma, arrhythmias, or tachycardias. It should be used with extreme caution in
patients with cerebral edema or increased CSF

pressure, pheochromocytoma or hyperthyroidism. Patients with a history of hypersensitivity to the drug or are receiving mechanical ventilation should not receive doxapram. The above contraindications/precautions are not listed in the veterinary product literature provided by the manufacturer.

Avoid the use of a single injection site for a prolonged period of time or extravasation when administering intravenously. Subcutaneous injection has been recommended however for use in neonatal feline and canine patients.

Repeated IV doses in neonates should be done with caution as the product contains benzyl alcohol.

Adverse Effects

Hypertension, arrhythmias, seizures, and hyperventilation leading to respiratory alkalosis has been reported. These effects appear most probable with repeated or high doses. The drug reportedly has a narrow margin of safety when used in humans.

Doxapram has been shown in experimental animals to increase myocardial oxygen demand and reduce cerebral blood flow.

Reproductive/Nursing Safety

Safety of doxapram has not been established in pregnant animals. The potential risks versus benefits should be weighed before using. In humans, the FDA categorizes this drug as category *B* for use during pregnancy (*Animal studies have not yet demonstrated risk to the fetus, but there are no adequate studies in pregnant women; or animal studies have shown an adverse effect, but adequate studies in pregnant women have not demonstrated a risk to the fetus in the first trimester of pregnancy, and there is no evidence of risk in later trimesters.*)

It is not known whether this drug is excreted in milk.

Overdosage/Acute Toxicity

Reported LD_{50} for IV administration in neonatal dogs and cats is approximately 75 mg/kg. Clinical signs of overdosage include: respiratory alkalosis, hypertension, skeletal muscle hyperactivity, tachycardia, and generalized CNS excitation including seizures. Treatment is supportive. Drugs such as short acting IV barbiturates may be used to help decrease CNS hyperactivity. Oxygen therapy may be necessary.

Drug Interactions

The following drug interactions have either been reported or are theoretical in humans or animals receiving doxapram and may be of significance in veterinary patients:

■ **ANESTHETICS, GENERAL:** Doxapram may increase epinephrine release; therefore, use should be delayed for approximately 10 minutes after discontinuation of anesthetic agents (*e.g.*, **halothane, enflurane**) that have been demonstrated to sensitize the myocardium to catecholamines

■ **MUSCLE RELAXANTS:** Doxapram may mask the effects of muscle relaxant drugs

■ **SYMPATHOMIMETIC AGENTS:** Additive pressor effects may occur with sympathomimetic agents

Doses

■ **DOGS:**
a) 1.1 mg/kg (for gas anesthesia) or 5.5–11 mg/kg (for barbiturate anesthesia) IV; adjust dosage for depth of anesthesia, respiratory volume and rate. Dosage may be repeated in 15–20 minutes if necessary.

To initiate or stimulate respirations in neonates after caesarian section or dystocia: May be administered either SC, sublingually, or via the umbilical vein in doses of 1–5 drops (1–5 mg) depending on size of neonate and degree of respiratory crisis. (Package Insert; *Dopram®-V*—Fort Dodge)

b) To stimulate respiratory function in neonates: 0.1 mL (2 mg) IV (IM or SL also possible); most likely to be beneficial to increase efforts in neonates with low-frequency, gasping, erratic pattern of breathing after receiving oxygen therapy (Traas 2009)

c) To assess laryngeal function: 2.2 mg/kg IV to stimulate respiration and increase intrinsic laryngeal motion. Onset of effect occurs within 15–30 seconds and persists for approximately 2 minutes. Anesthetic depth may lighten substantially. Prepare for immediate intubation should airway obstruction or laryngeal paralysis occur. (McKiernan 2007)

■ **CATS:**
a) 1.1 mg/kg (for gas anesthesia) or 5.5–11 mg/kg (for barbiturate anesthesia) IV; adjust dosage for depth of anesthesia, respiratory volume and rate. Dosage may be repeated in 15–20 minutes if necessary.

To initiate or stimulate respirations in neonates after caesarian section or dystocia: May be administered either SC, or sublingually in doses of 1–2 drops (1–2 mg) depending on severity of respiratory crisis. (Package Insert; *Dopram®-V*—Fort Dodge)

b) To stimulate respiratory function in neonates: 0.1 mL (2 mg) IV (IM or SL also possible); most likely to be beneficial to increase efforts in neonates with low-frequency, gasping, erratic pattern of breathing after receiving oxygen therapy. (Traas 2009)

■ **RABBITS/RODENTS/SMALL MAMMALS:**
For respiratory depression:
a) **Rabbits:** 2–5 mg/kg SC or IV q15 minute

b) **Rodents:** 2–5 mg/kg S C q15 minutes (Huerkamp 1995)

c) **Mice, Rats, Gerbils, Hamsters:** 5–10 mg/kg IV; **Guinea pigs:** 5 mg/kg IV; **Chinchillas:** 2–5 mg/kg IV (Adamcak & Otten 2000)

■ **BIRDS:**

a) For respiratory depression: 5–10 mg/kg IM or IV (Harris 2003)

■ **REPTILES:**

a) To stimulate respiration after general anesthesia: 5 mg/kg IV (Wilson 2002)

■ **CATTLE & SWINE:**

a) For primary apnea in asphyxic calves when intubation and mechanical ventilation are not feasible: 2 mg/kg IV. Contraindicated in premature calves or other patients with clinical signs indicative of lung immaturity. (Bleul *et al.* 2010)

b) For primary apnea in newborn calves: 2 mg/kg IV (Constable 2006)

■ **HORSES:** (**Note:** ARCI UCGFS Class 2 Drug)

a) 0.44 mg/kg (for halothane, methoxyflurane anesthesia) or 0.55 mg/kg (for chloral hydrate ± magnesium sulfate anesthesia) IV; adjust dosage for depth of anesthesia, respiratory volume and rate. Dosage may be repeated in 15–20 minutes if necessary. (Package Insert; *Dopram®-V*—Fort Dodge)

b) For adjunctive treatment to stimulate respirations in foals with sepsis or hypoxic-ischemic encephalopathy: 0.02–0.05 mg/kg/hr IV CRI; foals with significant hypercapnia and hypoxia despite O_2 tx require positive pressure ventilation (Giguere *et al.* 2008), (McKenzie 2009).

Monitoring

■ Respiratory rate

■ Cardiac rate and rhythm

■ Blood gases if available and indicated

■ CNS level of excitation; reflexes

■ Blood pressure if indicated

Client Information

■ This agent should be used in an inpatient setting or with direct professional supervision.

Chemistry/Synonyms

Doxapram HCl is a white to off-white, odorless, crystalline powder that is stable in light and air. It is soluble in water, sparingly soluble in alcohol and practically insoluble in ether. Injectable products have a pH from 3.5–5. Benzyl alcohol or chlorobutanol is added as a preservative agent in the commercially available injections.

Doxapram HCl may also be known as: AHR-619, doxaprami hydrochloridum, *Docatone®*, *Dopram ®*, *Doxapril®*, or *Respiram®*.

Storage/Stability

Store at room temperature and avoid freezing solution. Do not mix with alkaline solutions (*e.g.*, thiopental, aminophylline, sodium bicarbonate). Doxapram is physically **compatible** with D_5W or normal saline.

Dosage Forms/Regulatory Status

VETERINARY-LABELED PRODUCTS:

Doxapram HCl for Injection: 20 mg/mL; 20 mL multi-dose vial; *Dopram-V®* (BIVI); *Respiram®* (MVT); (Rx). FDA-approved for use in dogs, cats and horses.

The ARCI (Racing Commissioners International) has designated this drug as a class 2 substance. See the appendix for more information.

HUMAN-LABELED PRODUCTS:

Doxapram HCl for Injection: 20 mg/mL in 20 mL multi-dose vials; *Dopram®* (Baxter Healthcare Corp); generic; (Bedford); (Rx)

References

Adamcak, A. & B. Otten (2000). Rodent Therapeutics. *Vet Clin NA: Exotic Anim Pract* **3**:1(Jan): 221–240.

Bleul, U., B. Bircher, et al. (2010). Respiratory and cardiovascular effects of doxapram and theophylline for the treatment of asphyxia in neonatal calves. *Theriogenology* 73(5): 612–619.

Constable, P. (2006). Resuscitation of calves after dystocia. Proceedings: ACVIM. Accessed via: Veterinary Information Network. http://goo.gl/oDa1I

Giguere, S., J.K. Slade, et al. (2008). Retrospective comparison of caffeine and doxapram for the treatment of hypercapnia in foals with hypoxic–ischemic encephalopathy. *Journal of Veterinary Internal Medicine* 22(2): 401–405.

Harris, D. (2003). Emergency management of acute illness and trauma in avian patients. Proceedings: Atlantic Coast Veterinary Conference. Accessed via: Veterinary Information Network. http://goo.gl/EdaFf

Huerkamp, M. (1995). Anesthesia and postoperative management of rabbits and pocket pets. *Kirk's Current Veterinary Therapy:XII.* J Bonagura Ed. Philadelphia, W.B. Saunders: 1322–1327.

McKenzie, E. (2009). Management of the Septic Foal. Proceedings: WVC. Accessed via: Veterinary Information Network. http://goo.gl/CXM0Q

McKiernan, B. (2007). Laryngeal function and doxapram HCl (Dopram). Proceedings: Veterinary Information Network MEDFAQ. Accessed via: Veterinary Information Network. http://goo.gl/vwBTL

Traas, A. (2009). Pediatric Emergencies. Proceedings: IVECCS. Accessed via: Veterinary Information Network. http://goo.gl/DZjjO

Wilson, H. (2002). Reptile anesthesia and surgery. Proceedings: Atlantic Coast Veterinary Conference. Accessed via: Veterinary Information Network. http://goo.gl/OyUg6

DOXEPIN HCL

(**dox**-e-pin)   Sinequan®

TRICYCLIC ANTIDEPRESSANT/
ANTIHISTAMINE

Prescriber Highlights

▶ Tricyclic antidepressant used primarily in small animals for adjunctive therapy of psychogenic dermatoses, particularly those that have an anxiety component; also has antihistaminic (H-1) properties

▶ Contraindications: Prior sensitivity to tricyclics; concomitant use with MAOIs (selegiline?); probably contraindicated in dogs with urinary retention or glaucoma

▶ Most likely adverse effects: Hyperexcitability, GI distress, or lethargy; ventricular arrhythmias after overdoses possible

Uses/Indications

The primary use for doxepin in veterinary medicine is the adjunctive therapy of psychogenic dermatoses, particularly those that have an anxiety component. Its efficacy as an antihistamine for atopic dermatoses is in question.

Pharmacology/Actions

Doxepin is a tricyclic agent that has antihistaminic, anticholinergic, and alpha$_1$-adrenergic blocking activity. In the CNS, doxepin inhibits the reuptake of norepinephrine and serotonin (5-HT) by the presynaptic neuronal membrane, thereby increasing their synaptic concentrations. Doxepin is considered a moderate inhibitor of norepinephrine and weak inhibitor of serotonin.

Pharmacokinetics

Doxepin appears to be well absorbed after oral administration. The drug is extensively metabolized in the liver.

Contraindications/Precautions/Warnings

These agents are contraindicated if prior sensitivity has been noted with any other tricyclic. Concomitant use with monoamine oxidase inhibitors is generally contraindicated. Doxepin is probably contraindicated in dogs with urinary retention or glaucoma.

Adverse Effects

While doxepin has less potential for cardiac adverse effects than many other tricyclics, it can cause ventricular arrhythmias, particularly after overdoses. In dogs, it may also cause hyperexcitability, GI distress, or lethargy. However, potential adverse effects can run the entire gamut of systems. Refer to other human drug references for additional information.

Reproductive/Nursing Safety

Rodent studies have demonstrated no teratogenic effects, but safety during pregnancy has not been established. In humans, the FDA categorizes this drug as category *C* for use during pregnancy (*Animal studies have shown an adverse effect on the fetus, but there are no adequate studies in humans; or there are no animal reproduction studies and no adequate studies in humans.*)

Doxepin and its N-demethylated active metabolite are distributed into milk. One case report of sedation and respiratory depression in a human infant has been reported. Exercise caution when using in a nursing patient.

Overdosage/Acute Toxicity

Overdosage with tricyclics can be life-threatening (arrhythmias, cardiorespiratory collapse). Because the toxicities and therapies for treatment are complicated and controversial, it is recommended to contact an animal poison control center for further information in any potential overdose situation.

Drug Interactions

The following drug interactions have either been reported or are theoretical in humans or animals receiving doxepin and may be of significance in veterinary patients:

■ **ANTICHOLINERGIC AGENTS:** Because of additive effects, use with doxepin cautiously

■ **CIMETIDINE:** May inhibit tricyclic antidepressant metabolism and increase the risk of toxicity

■ **CNS DEPRESSANTS:** Because of additive effects, use with doxepin cautiously

■ **MEPERIDINE, PENTAZOCINE, DEXTROMETHORPHAN:** Increased risk for serotonin syndrome

■ **MONOAMINE OXIDASE INHIBITORS (including amitraz, and possibly selegiline):** Concomitant use (within 14 days) of tricyclics with monoamine oxidase inhibitors is generally contraindicated (serotonin syndrome)

■ **QUINIDINE:** Increased risk for QTc interval prolongation and tricyclic adverse effects

■ **SSRIs (e.g., fluoxetine, paroxetine, sertraline, etc.):** Increased risk for serotonin syndrome

■ **SYMPATHOMIMETIC AGENTS:** Use in combination with tricyclic agents may increase the risk of cardiac effects (arrhythmias, hypertension, hyperpyrexia)

Laboratory Considerations

■ Tricyclics can widen QRS complexes, prolong PR intervals and invert or flatten T-waves on **ECG**.

■ Tricyclics may alter (increase or decrease) **blood glucose** levels.

Doses

■ **DOGS:**

For treatment of psychogenic dermatoses:

a) 3–5 mg/kg PO q12h; maximum dose is 150 mg (per dog) q12h (Shanley & Overall 1992)(Shanley and Overall 1992)

b) 3–5 mg/kg, PO q8–12h. Begin at 3 mg/kg PO q12h for 2 weeks, then increase by 1 mg/kg PO q12h for 2 weeks up to the maximum dosage as needed; if no clinical response after at least 3–4 weeks of therapy, decrease dosage by 1 mg/kg PO q12h for 2 weeks until at the initial dosage (Virga 2003), (Virga 2005)

For antihistaminic effects in treatment of atopy:

a) 2.2 mg/kg PO three times daily (White 2007)

b) 3–5 mg/kg twice daily; used especially if dog has anxiety or other behavioral condition (Peikes 2003)

c) 0.5–2 mg/kg PO q12h; may be best in nervous or highly strung dogs (Hillier 2006)

d) 1–2 mg/kg PO q12h (Thomas 2005)

For treatment of behavior problems where tricyclics may be of benefit (e.g., obsessive/compulsive disorders, acral lick granulomas):

a) For OCD: 0.5–1 mg/kg PO twice daily; for acral lick granulomas: doses as above for psychogenic dermatoses. (Seksel 2008)

■ **CATS:**

For treatment of psychogenic dermatoses:

a) 0.5–1 mg/kg PO q12–24h. Up to 25–50 mg (total dose) per cat. Allow 3–4 weeks for initial trial. (Virga 2003), (Virga 2005)

b) For excessive grooming: 0.5–1 mg/kg PO q12h. (Siebert 2003a)

c) For treatment of behavior problems where tricyclics may be of benefit (e.g., overgrooming, intercat aggression, etc.): 0.5–1 mg/kg PO once to twice daily. (Seksel 2008)

■ **BIRDS:**

For treatment of anxiety, pruritus caused feather plucking in psittacines:

a) 1–2 mg/kg PO q12h (Siebert 2003b)

b) 0.5–1 mg/kg PO twice daily (Rich 2005)

Monitoring

■ Efficacy

■ Adverse effects

Client Information

■ Inform clients that several weeks may be required before efficacy is noted and to continue dosing as prescribed.

■ All tricyclics should be dispensed in child-resistant packaging and kept well away from children or pets.

Chemistry/Synonyms

A dibenzoxazepine derivative tricyclic antidepressant, doxepin HCl occurs as a white powder that is freely soluble in alcohol.

Doxepin may also be known as: doxepini hydrochloridum, NSC-108160, P-3693A, *Adapin®*, *Anten®*, *Aponal®*, *Deptran®*, *Desidoxepin®*, *Doneurin®*, *Doxal®*, *Doxepia®*, *Gilex®*, *Mareen®*, *Quitaxon®*, *Sinequan®*, *Triadapin®*, *Xepin®*, and *Zonalon®*.

Storage/Stability

Store hydroxyzine products protected from direct sunlight in tight, light-resistant containers at room temperature.

Dosage Forms/Regulatory Status

VETERINARY-LABELED PRODUCTS: None

The ARCI (Racing Commissioners International) has designated this drug as a class 2 substance. See the appendix for more information.

HUMAN-LABELED PRODUCTS:

Doxepin Capsules: 10 mg, 25 mg, 50 mg, 75 mg, 100 mg & 150 mg; *Sinequan®* (Roerig); generic; (Rx)

Doxepin Oral Concentrate: 10 mg/mL in 120 mL; generic; (Rx)

References

Hillier, A. (2006). Therapeutic options for atopic dermatitis. Proceedings: ACVC. Accessed via: Veterinary Information Network. http://goo.gl/dtZEv

Peikes, H. (2003). Approach to the pruritic dog. Proceedings: Atlantic Coast Veterinary Conference. Accessed via: Veterinary Information Network. http://goo.gl/WnfvD

Rich, G. (2005). Top ten causes of feather picking. Proceedings: Western Vet Conf. Accessed via: Veterinary Information Network. http://goo.gl/sKaGX

Seksel, K. (2008). To medicate or not to medicate—That is the question! What to use, when and why. Proceedings: World Veterinary Congress. Accessed via: Veterinary Information Network. http://goo.gl/KjRxj

Shanley, K. & K. Overall (1992). Psychogenic dermatoses. *Current Veterinary Therapy XI: Small Animal Practice*. R Kirk and J Bonagura Eds. Philadelphia, W.B. Saunders Company: 552–558.

Siebert, L. (2003a). Antidepressants in behavioral medicine. Proceedings: Western Veterinary Conference. Accessed via: Veterinary Information Network. http://goo.gl/HHo8w

Siebert, L. (2003b). Psittacine feather picking. Proceedings: Western Veterinary Conference. Accessed via: Veterinary Information Network. http://goo.gl/MCA9y

Thomas, R. (2005). Canine atopic dermatitis II: Treatment. Proceedings: WVC2005. Accessed via: Veterinary Information Network. http://goo.gl/Zi2W7

Virga, V. (2003). Use of Analgesic Anxiolytics. Proceedings: Western Veterinary Conference. Accessed via: Veterinary Information Network. http://goo.gl/SJ1Rj

Virga, V. (2005). Psychopharmacology for anxiety disorders. Proceedings: Western Vet Cong 2005. Accessed via: Veterinary Information Network. http://goo.gl/4uZW3

White, S. (2007). Atopic dermatitis and its secondary infections. Proceedings: Canine Medicine Symposium. Accessed via: Veterinary Information Network. http://goo.gl/upBF7

DOXORUBICIN HCL

(dox-oh-*roo*-bi-sin)   Adriamycin®, Doxil®

ANTINEOPLASTIC

Prescriber Highlights

▶ Injectable antibiotic antineoplastic widely used alone or in combination protocols for small animals

▶ Relatively contraindicated in patients with myelosuppression, impaired cardiac function, or who have reached the total cumulative dose level of doxorubicin &/or daunorubicin

▶ Caution: Patients with hyperuricemia/ hyperuricuria, or impaired hepatic function (dosage adjustments necessary)

▶ Breeds predisposed to developing cardiomyopathy (Doberman pinchers, Great Danes, Rottweilers, Boxers); monitor carefully

▶ Handle very carefully

▶ Teratogenic & embryotoxic

▶ Adverse Effects include bone marrow suppression, cardiac toxicity, nephrotoxicity (esp. cats), alopecia, gastroenteritis (vomiting, diarrhea), & stomatitis

▶ Immediate-hypersensitivity reported (primarily in dogs); potentially brand specific

▶ Extravasation injuries can be serious

Uses/Indications

Doxorubicin is perhaps the most widely used antineoplastic agent at present in small animal medicine. It may be useful in the treatment of a variety of lymphomas, carcinomas, leukemias, and sarcomas in both the dog and cat, either alone or in combination protocols.

Pharmacology/Actions

Although possessing antimicrobial properties, doxorubicin's cytotoxic effects precludes its use as an anti-infective agent. The drug causes inhibition of DNA synthesis, DNA-dependent RNA synthesis and protein synthesis, but the precise mechanisms for these effects are not well understood. The drug acts throughout the cell cycle and also possesses some immunosuppressant activity.

Doxorubicin is most cytotoxic to cardiac cells, followed by melanoma, sarcoma cells, and normal muscle and skin fibroblasts. Other rapidly proliferating "normal" cells, (such as bone marrow, hair follicles, GI mucosa), may also be affected by the drug.

Pharmacokinetics

Doxorubicin must be administered IV as it is not absorbed from the GI tract and is extremely ir-

ritating to tissues if administered SC or IM. After IV injection, the drug is rapidly and widely distributed, but does not appreciably enter the CSF. It is highly bound to tissue and plasma proteins, probably crosses the placenta and is distributed into milk.

Doxorubicin is metabolized extensively by the liver and other tissues via aldo-keto reductase primarily to doxorubicinol, which is active; other inactive metabolites are also formed. Doxorubicin and its metabolites are primarily excreted in the bile and feces. Only about 5% of the drug is excreted in the urine within 5 days of dosing. Doxorubicin is eliminated in a triphasic manner. During the first phase ($t_{1/2} \approx 0.6$ hours) doxorubicin is rapidly metabolized, via the "first pass" effect followed by a second phase ($t_{1/2} \approx$ 3.3 hours). The third phase has a much slower elimination half-life (17 hours for doxorubicin; 32 hours for metabolites), presumably due to the slow release of the drug from tissue proteins.

Contraindications/Precautions/Warnings

Doxorubicin is contraindicated or relatively contraindicated (measure risk vs. benefit) in patients with myelosuppression, impaired cardiac function, have reached the total cumulative dose level of doxorubicin and/or daunorubicin. It is also contraindicated in cats with preexisting renal insufficiency. It should be used with caution in patients with hyperuricemia/ hyperuricuria, or impaired hepatic function. Dosage adjustments are necessary in patients with hepatic impairment. Breeds predisposed to developing cardiomyopathy (Doberman pinchers, Great Danes, Rottweilers, Boxers) should be monitored carefully while receiving doxorubicin therapy.

Doxorubicin is actively transported by the p-glycoprotein pump and certain breeds susceptible to MDR1-allele mutation (Collies, Australian Shepherds, Shelties, Long-haired Whippet) may be at higher risk for toxicity. Bone marrow suppression (decreased blood cell counts, particularly neutrophils) and GI toxicity (anorexia, vomiting, diarrhea) are more likely to occur at normal doses in dogs with the *ABCB1* mutation. To reduce the likelihood of severe toxicity in these dogs (mutant/normal or mutant/ mutant), the Veterinary Clinical Pharmacology Laboratory at Washington State University recommends reducing the dose by 25–30% and carefully monitoring these patients (WSU-VetClinPharmLab 2009).

Because doxorubicin can be very irritating to skin, gloves should be worn when administering or preparing the drug. Ideally, doxorubicin injection should be prepared in a biological safety cabinet. Should accidental skin or mucous membrane contact occur, wash the area immediately using soap and copious amounts of water.

Adverse Effects

Doxorubicin may cause several adverse effects including bone marrow suppression, cardiac toxicity, alopecia, gastroenteritis (vomiting, diarrhea), and stomatitis.

Myelosuppression nadirs are generally 5–10 days after treatment.

An immediate hypersensitivity reaction may be seen (particularly in dogs) characterized by urticaria, facial swelling, vomiting, arrhythmias (see below), and/or hypotension. The rate of infusion can have a direct impact on this effect. Pretreatment with a histamine$_1$ blocker such as diphenhydramine (IV prior to treatment at 10 mg for dogs up to 9 kg; 20 mg for dogs 9–27 kg; and 30 mg for dogs over 27 kg) or alternatively, dexamethasone (0.55 mg/kg IV), is often recommended to reduce or eliminate these effects. There is some evidence to suggest that a given brand of doxorubicin may be more allergenic than another. Patients that have developed hypersensitive reactions to one brand, may not react, if switched to another.

Cardiac toxicity of doxorubicin falls into two categories, acute and cumulative. Acute cardiac toxicity may occur during IV administration or several hours subsequent, and is manifested by cardiac arrest preceded by ECG changes (T-wave flattening, S-T depression, voltage reduction, arrhythmias). Rarely, an acute hypertensive crisis has been noted after infusion. Acute cardiac toxicity does not preclude further use of the drug, but additional treatment should be delayed. The administration of diphenhydramine and/or glucocorticoids before doxorubicin administration may prevent these effects.

Cumulative cardiac toxicity requires halting any further therapy and can be extremely serious. Diffuse cardiomyopathy with severe congestive heart failure refractory to traditional therapies is generally noted. It is believed that the risk of cardiac toxicity is greatly increased in dogs when the cumulative dose exceeds 240 mg/m^2, but may be seen at doses as low as 90 mg/m^2. Therefore, it is not recommended to exceed 240 mg/m^2, total dose, in dogs. It is unknown what the incidence of cardiotoxicity or the dosage ceiling for doxorubicin is in cats, but most clinicians believe that 240 mg/m^2 should also be used as the upper limit cumulative dose in cats.

In cats, doxorubicin is a potential nephrotoxin and they should have renal function monitored both before and during therapy.

Doxorubicin should be administered IV slowly, over at least 10 minutes, in a free flowing line.

Extravasation injuries secondary to perivascular administration of doxorubicin can be quite serious, with severe tissue ulceration and necrosis possible. Prevention of extravasation should be a priority and animals should be frequently checked during the infusion. Should extravasation occur, it is suggested to treat as per the human recommendations. There are currently two treatments recommended for doxorubicin extravasation injuries. Both have been shown to be effective, but no comparative trials have been published. **1)** Apply dimethyl sulfoxide (DMSO) 99% by saturating a gauze pad and painting on an area twice the size of the extravasation. Allow the site to air dry and repeat the application every 6 hours for 14 days. Do not cover the area with dressing. **2)** Dexrazoxane is FDA-approved for the treatment of extravasation resulting from anthracycline IV therapy, refer to the dexrazoxane monograph for more information. Additionally, ice compresses applied to the affected area for 15 minutes every 6 hours for 48 hours may be useful.

Reproductive/Nursing Safety

Doxorubicin is teratogenic and embryotoxic in laboratory animals. It is unknown if it affects male fertility. In humans, the FDA categorizes this drug as category *D* for use during pregnancy (*There is evidence of human fetal risk, but the potential benefits from the use of the drug in pregnant women may be acceptable despite its potential risks.*). In a separate system evaluating the safety of drugs in canine and feline pregnancy (Papich 1989), this drug is categorized as in class: *C* (*These drugs may have potential risks. Studies in people or laboratory animals have uncovered risks, and these drugs should be used cautiously as a last resort when the benefit of therapy clearly outweighs the risks.*)

Doxorubicin is excreted in milk in concentrations that may exceed those found in plasma. Because of risks to nursing offspring, consider using milk replacer if the dam is receiving doxorubicin.

Overdosage/Acute Toxicity

Inadvertent acute overdosage may be manifested by exacerbations of the adverse effects outlined above. A lethal dose for dogs has been reported as 72 mg/m^2 (O'Keefe and Harris 1990). Supportive and symptomatic therapy is suggested should an overdose occur. Dexrazoxane may be useful to help prevent cardiac toxicity.

Drug Interactions

The following drug interactions have either been reported or are theoretical in humans or animals receiving doxorubicin and may be of significance in veterinary patients:

■ **ANTINEOPLASTIC AGENTS, OTHER:** May potentiate the toxic effects of doxorubicin

■ **CALCIUM-CHANNEL BLOCKERS:** Potentially could increase risk for cardiotoxicity associated with doxorubicin

■ **CARBAMAZEPINE:** Decreased carbamazepine levels

■ **CISPLATIN:** Increased risk of toxicity for both agents; carefully weigh risks versus benefits

■ **CYCLOPHOSPHAMIDE:** May increase doxorubicin blood levels (AUC); doxorubicin may potentiate and prolong hematologic toxicity; coma and seizures have been reported in human patients

■ **CYCLOSPORINE:** Cyclosporine can increase doxorubicin and doxorubicinol (active metabolite) levels

■ **GLUCOSAMINE:** May reduce doxorubicin effectiveness; use together not recommended in humans

■ **PHENYTOIN:** Doxorubicin may decrease phenytoin levels

■ **PHENOBARBITAL:** May increase elimination and reduce blood levels of doxorubicin

■ **STREPTOZOCIN:** May inhibit doxorubicin metabolism

■ **VERAPAMIL:** May increase doxorubicin levels

■ **WARFARIN:** Increased risk for bleeding

■ **ZIDOVUDINE:** Increased risk for neutropenia

Laboratory Considerations
■ Doxorubicin may significantly increase both blood and urine concentrations of **uric acid**

Doses
Note: Because of the potential toxicity of this drug to patients, veterinary personnel and clients, and since chemotherapy indications, treatment protocols, monitoring and safety guidelines often change, the following dosages should be used only as a general guide. Consultation with a veterinary oncologist and referral to current veterinary oncology references [*e.g.*, (Henry & Higginbotham 2009); (Argyle *et al.* 2008); (Withrow & Vail 2007); (Villalobos 2007); (Ogilvie & Moore 2006); (Ogilvie & Moore 2001)] is *strongly recommended.*

■ **DOGS:**
Depending on the protocol used, doxorubicin is usually dosed at 30 mg/m^2 (**NOT** mg/kg) IV every 2-3 weeks. Maximum cumulative dose = 240 mg/m^2.

■ **CATS:**
Depending on the protocol used, doxorubicin is usually dosed at 20-30 mg/m^2 (**NOT** mg/kg) IV every 2-4 weeks. Maximum cumulative dose is usually 240 mg/m^2.

■ **FERRETS:**
Depending on the protocol used, doxorubicin is usually dosed at 30 mg/m^2 (**NOT** mg/kg) IV every 3 weeks.

Monitoring
■ Efficacy
■ Toxicity:
  a) CBC with platelets
  b) Dogs with pre-existing heart disease should be monitored with regular ECG's (insensitive to early toxic changes caused doxorubicin) and/or echocardiogram
  c) Evaluate hepatic function prior to therapy

  d) Urinalyses and serum creatinine/BUN in cats

Client Information
■ Clients must be briefed on the possibilities of severe toxicity developing from this drug, including drug-related mortality. Clients should contact the veterinarian should the animal exhibit any clinical signs of profound depression, abnormal bleeding (including bloody diarrhea) and/or bruising.

■ Doxorubicin may cause urine to be colored orange to red for 1-2 days after dosing; although uncommon in veterinary patients, it is not harmful should it occur.

■ Mild anorexia and occasional vomiting are commonly seen 2-5 days post-therapy.

■ Avoid skin contact with urine or feces of treated animals. After treatment, doxorubicin drug residues may be found in treated dog's urine up to 21 days and in feces for several days. (Knobloch et al. 2010)

■ Although it is unknown how much drug is found in the saliva of treated animals, do not allow treated animals to lick human skin while receiving chemotherapy treatment.

Chemistry/Synonyms
An anthracycline glycoside antibiotic antineoplastic, doxorubicin HCl occurs as a lyophilized, red-orange powder that is freely soluble in water, slightly soluble in normal saline, and very slightly soluble in alcohol. The commercially available powder for injection also contains lactose and methylparaben to aid dissolution. After reconstituting, the solution has a pH from 3.8-6.5. The commercially available solution for injection has a pH of approximately 3.

Doxorubicin HCl may also be known as: cloridrato de doxorrubicina, doxorubicin hydrochloride liposome, doxorubicini hydrochloridum, liposomal doxorubicin hydrochloride, NSC-123127, *Adriamycin RDF®, Adriblastin®, Adriblastina®, Adriblastine®, Adrim®, Adrimedac®, Biorrub®, Caelyx®, DOXO-cell®, Doxolem®, Doxorbin®, Doxorubin®, Doxotec®, Doxtie®, Farmiblastina®, Fauldoxo®, Flavicina®, Ifadox®, Myocet®, Neoxan®, Ranxas®, Ribodoxo-L®,* and *Rubex®.*

Storage/Stability
Lyophilized powder for injection should be stored away from direct sunlight in a dry place. After reconstituting with sodium chloride 0.9%, the single-use lyophilized powder product is reportedly stable for 24 hours at room temperature and 48 hours when refrigerated. The manufacturer recommends protecting from sunlight, not freezing the product and discarding any unused portion. However, one study found that powder reconstituted with sterile water to a concentration of 2 mg/mL lost only about 1.5% of its potency per month over 6 months when

stored in the refrigerator. When frozen at -20°C, no potency loss after 30 days was detected and sterility was maintained by filtering the drug through a 0.22-micron filter before injection.

The commercially available solution for injection is stable for 18 months when stored in the refrigerator (2–8°C) and protected from light.

The manufacturer states that after reconstitution, the multi-dose vials may be stored for up to 7 days at room temperature in normal room light, and for up to 15 days in the refrigerator.

Compatibility/Compounding Considerations
Doxorubicin HCl is reportedly physically **compatible** with the following intravenous solutions and drugs: dextrose 3.3% in sodium chloride 3%, D_5W, Normosol R (pH 7.4), lactated Ringer's injection, and sodium chloride 0.9%. In syringes with: bleomycin sulfate, cisplatin, cyclophosphamide, droperidol, fluorouracil, leucovorin calcium, methotrexate sodium, metoclopramide HCl, mitomycin, and vincristine sulfate. The drug is physically **compatible during Y-site injection** with bleomycin sulfate, cisplatin, cyclophosphamide, droperidol, fluorouracil, leucovorin calcium, methotrexate sodium, metoclopramide HCl, mitomycin, vinblastine sulfate and vincristine sulfate.

Doxorubicin HCl **compatibility information conflicts** or is dependent on diluent or concentration factors with the following drugs or solutions: vinblastine sulfate (in syringes and as an IV additive). Compatibility is dependent upon factors such as pH, concentration, temperature and diluent used; consult specialized references or a hospital pharmacist for more specific information

Doxorubicin HCl is reportedly physically **incompatible** with the following solutions or drugs: aminophylline, cephalothin sodium, dexamethasone sodium phosphate, diazepam, fluorouracil (as an IV additive only), furosemide, heparin sodium, and hydrocortisone sodium succinate.

Dosage Forms/Regulatory Status

VETERINARY-LABELED PRODUCTS: None

HUMAN-LABELED PRODUCTS:

Doxorubicin HCl (Conventional) Lyophilized Powder for Injection, (conventional): 10 mg, 20 mg, 50 mg, and 150 mg vials; *Adriamycin RDF®* (Pharmacia & Upjohn); generic (Bedford); (Rx). Reconstitute with appropriate amount of 0.9% sodium chloride for final concentration of 2 mg/mL.

Doxorubicin HCl (Conventional) Injection (aqueous): 2 mg/mL in 5 mL, 10 mL, 25 mL, and 100 mL; *Adriamycin PFS®* (Bedford), generic; (Rx)

Doxorubicin, Liposomal Injection: 20 mg in 10 mL & 50 mg in 30 mL single-use vials; *Doxil®* (Ortho Biotech); (Rx)

References

Argyle, D., M. Brearly, et al. (2008). *Decision Making in Small Animal Oncology,* Wiley–Blackwell.

Henry, C. & M. Higginbotham (2009). *Cancer Management in Small Animal Practice,* Saunders.

Knobloch, A., S. Mohring, et al. (2010). Cytotoxic Drug Residues in Urine of Dogs Receiving Anticancer Chemotherapy. *J Vet Intern Med* **24**: 384–390.

Ogilvie, G. & A. Moore (2001). *Feline Oncology: A Comprehensive Guide to Compassionate Care,* Veterinary Learning Systems.

Ogilvie, G. & A. Moore (2006). *Managing the Canine Cancer Patient: A Practical Guide to Compassionate Care,* Veterinary Learning Systems.

Villalobos, A. (2007). *Canine and Feline Geriatric Oncology.* Ames, Blackwell.

Withrow, S. & D. Vail (2007). *Withrow and MacEwen's Small Animal Clinical Oncology 4th Ed.* Philadelphia, Elsevier.

WSU—VetClinPharmLab (2009). "Problem Drugs." http://goo.gl/aIGIM.

DOXYCYCLINE CALCIUM
DOXYCYCLINE HYCLATE
DOXYCYCLINE MONOHYDRATE

(dox-i-sye-kleen)   Vibramycin®

TETRACYCLINE ANTIBIOTIC

Prescriber Highlights

▶ Oral & parenteral tetracycline antibiotic

▶ Bone & teeth abnormalities are less likely to be caused then with other tetracyclines, but use with caution in pregnant & young animals

▶ May be used in patients with renal insufficiency

▶ Not for IV injection in horses; do not give IM or SC to any species

▶ Most common adverse effects are GI, but increased liver enzymes can occur

▶ Esophagitis and strictures possible; must follow oral doses with sufficient fluid to get medication into stomach

▶ Drug Interactions

Uses/Indications

Although there are no veterinary FDA-approved doxycycline products available, its favorable pharmacokinetic parameters (longer half-life, higher CNS penetration) when compared to either tetracycline HCl or oxytetracycline HCl make it a reasonable choice to use in small animals when a tetracycline is indicated, particularly when a tetracycline is indicated in an azotemic patient. It is commonly used in small animals to treat a variety of infections caused by several different microorganisms that include

Borrelia, Leptospira, Rickettsiae, Chlamydia, Mycoplasma, Bartonella, and Bordetella.

At the time of writing (2010) there is considerable interest in using ivermectin or another macrocyclic lactone with doxycycline for several months prior to melarsomine adulticide therapy in dogs. Ivermectin can kill *D. immitis* larval stages 3 & 4, kill microfilaria, and reduce lifespan of adult heartworms. Doxycycline treatment can potentially reduce adult worm populations by eliminating *Wolbachia*, a bacterium associated with *D. immitis*. The American Heartworm Society has stated; ". . . it is beneficial to administer a macrocyclic lactone for up to three months prior to administration of melarsomine, when the clinical presentation does not demand immediate intervention" and "Doxycycline administered at 10 mg/kg twice daily for four weeks has been shown to eliminate over 90% of the *Wolbachia* organisms and the levels remain low for three to four months." (American-Heartworm-Society 2010)

In avian species, some clinicians feel that doxycycline is the drug of choice in the oral treatment of chlamydiosis, particularly when treating only a few birds.

Pharmacology/Actions

Tetracyclines generally act as bacteriostatic antibiotics and inhibit protein synthesis by reversibly binding to 30S ribosomal subunits of susceptible organisms, thereby preventing binding to those ribosomes of aminoacyl transfer-RNA. Tetracyclines also are believed to reversibly bind to 50S ribosomes and, additionally, alter cytoplasmic membrane permeability in susceptible organisms. In high concentrations, tetracyclines can also inhibit protein synthesis by mammalian cells.

As a class, the tetracyclines have activity against most mycoplasma, spirochetes (including the Lyme disease organism), Chlamydia and Rickettsia. Against gram-positive bacteria, the tetracyclines have activity against some strains of staphylococcus and streptococci, but resistance by these organisms is increasing. Gram-positive bacteria that are usually covered by tetracyclines include: *Actinomyces* spp., *Bacillus anthracis, Clostridium perfringens* and *tetani, Listeria monocytogenes* and Nocardia. Among gram-negative bacteria that tetracyclines usually have *in vitro* and *in vivo* activity against, include *Bordetella* spp., Brucella, Bartonella, *Haemophilus* spp., *Pasturella multocida*, Shigella, and *Yersinia pestis*. Many or most strains of *E. coli*, Klebsiella, Bacteroides, Enterobacter, Proteus and *Pseudomonas aeruginosa* are resistant to the tetracyclines.

Doxycycline generally has very similar activity as other tetracyclines against susceptible organisms, but some strains of bacteria may be more susceptible to doxycycline or minocycline and additional *in vitro* testing may be required.

Pharmacokinetics

Doxycycline is well absorbed after oral administration. Bioavailability is 90–100% in humans and it is thought that the drug is also readily absorbed in most monogastric animals. Unlike tetracycline HCl or oxytetracycline, doxycycline absorption in humans may only be reduced by 20% by either food or dairy products in the gut. But in horses, giving orally in fed state may reduce bioavailability to less than 5%. This may be due to the high fiber content in most equine diets.

Tetracyclines, as a class, are widely distributed to the heart, kidney, lungs, muscle, pleural fluid, bronchial secretions, sputum, bile, saliva, synovial fluid, ascitic fluid, and aqueous and vitreous humor. When doxycycline was dosed to horses at 10 mg/kg PO q12h, it did not yield appreciable levels in the aqueous or vitreous humor (Gilmour *et al.* 2005). In horses, doxycycline has been shown to penetrate into the synovial fluid with an AUC synovial fluid:plasma factor of 4.6 and is eliminated from synovial fluid more slowly than plasma (Schnabel *et al.* 2010).

Doxycycline is more lipid-soluble and penetrates body tissues and fluids better than tetracycline HCl or oxytetracycline, including into the CSF, prostate, and eye. While CSF levels are generally insufficient to treat most bacterial infections, doxycycline has been shown to be efficacious in the treatment of the CNS effects associated with Lyme disease in humans. The volume of distribution at steady-state in dogs is approximately 1.5 L/kg. Doxycycline is bound to plasma proteins in varying amounts dependent upon species. The drug is approximately 25–93% bound to plasma proteins in humans, 75–86% in dogs, 82% in horses, and about 93% in cattle and pigs. Cats have higher binding to plasma proteins than dogs. Doxycycline accumulates intracellularly and concentrates in equine PMNs (Davis *et al.* 2006).

Doxycycline's elimination from the body is relatively unique. The drug is primarily excreted into the feces via non-biliary routes in an inactive form. It is thought that the drug is partially inactivated in the intestine by chelate formation and then excreted into the intestinal lumen. In dogs, about 75% of a given dose is handled in this manner. Renal excretion of doxycycline can only account for about 25% of a dose in dogs, and biliary excretion less than 5%. The serum half-life of doxycycline in dogs is approximately 10–12 hours and a clearance of about 1.7 mL/kg/min. In calves, the drug has similar pharmacokinetic values. In horses, elimination half-life is about 12 hours and clearance is approximately 0.7 mL/kg/min. Doxycycline does not accumulate in patients with renal dysfunction.

Contraindications/Precautions/Warnings

Doxycycline is contraindicated in patients hypersensitive to the drug. Because tetracyclines can retard fetal skeletal development and discolor deciduous teeth, they should only be used in the last half of pregnancy when the benefits outweigh the fetal risks. Doxycycline is considered to be less likely to cause these abnormalities than other more water-soluble tetracyclines (*e.g.*, tetracycline, oxytetracycline). Unlike either oxytetracycline or tetracycline, doxycycline can be used in patients with renal insufficiency. As increases in hepatic enzymes have been documented in some dogs after doxycycline treatment, use with caution in dogs with significant liver dysfunction.

Until further studies documenting the safety of intravenous doxycycline in horses are done, the parenteral route of administering this drug in horses should be considered contraindicated.

Doxycycline is pumped by P-glycoprotein, but the Washington State University Clinical Pharmacology Lab reports that it has not seen any increased sensitivity to doxycycline and does not recommend any dose alterations in dogs with MDR1 mutations. (WSU-VetClinPharmLab 2009)

Adverse Effects

The most commonly reported side effects of oral doxycycline therapy in dogs and cats are vomiting, diarrhea and anorexia. Giving the drug with food may help alleviate these GI effects without significantly reducing drug absorption. Increased liver enzymes (ALT, ALP) have been reported in up to 40% of dogs treated. The clinical significance of increased liver enzymes has not been determined.

Oral doxycycline has been implicated in causing esophageal strictures in cats. If using oral tablets, be sure that "pilling" is followed by at least 6 mL of water. Do not dry pill.

Tetracycline therapy (especially long-term) may result in overgrowth (superinfections) of non-susceptible bacteria or fungi.

In humans, doxycycline (or other tetracyclines) has also been associated with photosensitivity reactions and, rarely, hepatotoxicity or blood dyscrasias.

Intravenous injection of even relatively low doses of doxycycline has been associated with cardiac arrhythmias, collapse, and death in horses.

Reproductive/Nursing Safety

In humans, the FDA categorizes this drug as category *D* for use during pregnancy (*There is evidence of human fetal risk, but the potential benefits from the use of the drug in pregnant women may be acceptable despite its potential risks.*) In a separate system evaluating the safety of drugs in canine and feline pregnancy (Papich 1989), this drug is categorized as in class: *D* (*Contraindicated. These drugs have been shown to cause congenital malformations or embryotoxicity.*)

Tetracyclines are excreted in milk. Milk:plasma ratios vary between 0.25 and 1.5. Avoid nursing if the dam requires doxycycline.

Overdosage/Acute Toxicity

With the exception of intravenous dosing in horses (see above), doxycycline is apparently quite safe in most mild overdose situations. Oral overdoses would most likely be associated with GI disturbances (vomiting, anorexia, and/or diarrhea). Although doxycycline is less vulnerable to chelation with cations than other tetracyclines, oral administration of divalent or trivalent cation antacids may bind some of the drug and reduce GI distress. Should the patient develop severe emesis or diarrhea, fluids and electrolytes should be monitored and replaced if necessary.

Rapid intravenous injection of doxycycline has induced transient collapse and cardiac arrhythmias in several species, presumably due to chelation with intravascular calcium ions. If overdose quantities are inadvertently administered, these effects may be more pronounced.

Drug Interactions

The following drug interactions have either been reported or are theoretical in humans or animals receiving doxycycline and may be of significance in veterinary patients:

- **ANTACIDS, ORAL:** When orally administered, tetracyclines can chelate divalent or trivalent cations that can decrease the absorption of the tetracycline or the other drug if it contains these cations. Oral antacids, saline cathartics, or other GI products containing aluminum, calcium, magnesium, zinc, or bismuth cations are most commonly associated with this interaction. Doxycycline has a relatively low affinity for calcium ions, but it is recommended that all oral tetracyclines be given at least 1–2 hours before or after the cation-containing product.
- **BISMUTH SUBSALICYLATE, KAOLIN, PECTIN:** May reduce absorption
- **IRON, ORAL:** Oral iron products are associated with decreased tetracycline absorption, and administration of iron salts should preferably be given 3 hours before or 2 hours after the tetracycline dose.
- **PENICILLINS:** Bacteriostatic drugs, like the tetracyclines, may interfere with bactericidal activity of the penicillins, cephalosporins, and aminoglycosides. There is a fair amount of controversy regarding the actual clinical significance of this interaction, however.
- **PHENOBARBITAL:** May decrease doxycycline half-life and reduce levels
- **WARFARIN:** Tetracyclines may depress plasma prothrombin activity and patients on anticoagulant (*e.g.*, warfarin) therapy may need dosage adjustment.

Laboratory Considerations

- Tetracyclines (not minocycline) may cause falsely elevated values of **urine catecholamines** when using fluorometric methods of determination.

■ Tetracyclines reportedly can cause false-positive **urine glucose** results if using the cupric sulfate method of determination (Benedict's reagent, *Clinitest®*), but this may be the result of ascorbic acid that is found in some parenteral formulations of tetracyclines. Tetracyclines have also reportedly caused false-negative results in determining urine glucose when using the glucose oxidase method (*Clinistix®*, *Test-Tape®*).

Doses

■ **DOGS:**

For susceptible infections:

a) General use for infection: 3–5 mg/kg PO q12h for 7–14 days;

For soft tissue, urinary tract: 4.4–11 mg/kg PO or IV q12h for 7–14 days;

For acute *E. canis* infection: 5 mg/kg PO q12h or 10 mg/kg PO q24h for 14–16 days;

For chronic *E. canis* infection: 10 mg/kg PO q24h for 30–42 days. (Greene *et al.* 2006)

b) For canine granulocytic anaplasmosis (*Anaplasma phagocytotophilum*): 5 mg/kg PO q12h for 14 days; most dogs show clinical improvement in 24–48 hours. (Carrade *et al.* 2009)

c) For Lyme disease: 10 mg/kg PO q24h for 21–28 days (Appel & Jacobson 1995)

d) For Ehrlichiosis (*E. canis*) in dogs with a positive test result and clinical signs consistent with the infection: 10 mg/kg PO (rarely IV) q12-24h for 28 days. (Ford 2009b)

e) For leptospirosis: 5–10 mg/kg PO twice daily for 2 weeks. Management of underlying renal disease is a must. Regardless 10-30% of patients die. (Ford 2009a)

f) For *Toxoplasma gondii*: 5–10 mg/kg PO q12h for 4 weeks (Lappin 2000a)

g) For Rocky Mountain Spotted-Fever (*Rickettsia rickettsii*): 5 mg/kg PO q12h (Breitschwerdt 2000)

h) For idiopathic lymphoplasmacytic (chronic) rhinitis: Long term administration of antibiotics having immunomodulatory effects combined with nonsteroidal antiinflammatory agents can be helpful in some dogs. Doxycycline 3–5 mg/kg PO q12h, or azithromycin 5 mg/kg PO q24h in combination with piroxicam 0.3 mg/kg PO q24h. (Kuehn 2010)

i) For uncomplicated infectious tracheobronchitis (*B. bronchiseptica*): 5–10 mg/kg PO once daily for a minimum of 2 weeks; treatment for up to 3 months should be considered, particularly when managing simultaneous infections in multiple dogs in the same environment. (Ford 2009a)

j) In combination with ivermectin as an adulticide for *D. immitis*: In this study doxycycline was administered at 10 mg/kg PO once daily for 30 days along with ivermectin/pyrantel pamoate with the ivermectin dose at 6–14 micrograms/kg PO once every 15 days for 6 months. 100% (total of 11 dogs) were negative for circulating microfilaria by day 90. 74% of dogs were negative for circulating antigens at day 300 (4-months post ivermectin). (Grandi *et al.* 2010)

k) For salmon poisoning (*Neorickettsia helmintheca*): 10 mg/kg IV twice a day for at least 7 days (Rikihisa & Zimmerman 1995)

For its antiarthritic effect:

a) 3–4 mg/kg PO once daily for 7–10 days. (Greene *et al.* 2006)

■ **CATS:**

Do not dry pill cats with oral doxycycline; follow with at least 6 mL of water or use a compounded slurry ("triple fish" or similar) to administer.

For susceptible infections:

a) For Hemotropic mycoplasmosis: 5–10 mg/kg PO once daily for 14 days; round dose to nearest whole tablet or capsule;

For Bartonellosis: 50 mg (total dose) PO q12h for 14–28 days;

For systemic infections, bacteremia: 5–11 mg/kg PO or IV q12h as long as necessary;

For Ehrlichiosis or Anaplasmosis: 5–10 mg/kg PO q12h for 21 days. (Greene *et al.* 2006)

b) For clinical hemoplasmosis or bartonellosis: 10 mg/kg PO q12–24h (Lappin 2006)

c) For *Toxoplasma gondii*: 5–10 mg/kg PO q12h for 4 weeks (Lappin 2000b)

d) For susceptible mycobacterial, L-Forms, or mycoplasma infections: 5–10 mg/kg PO q12h. (Bonenberger 2009)

e) For treatment of *Nocardia* (*N. nova*) infections: Combination therapy with: amoxicillin 20 mg/kg PO twice daily with clarithromycin 62.5–125 mg (total dose per cat) PO twice daily and/or doxycycline 5 mg/kg or higher PO twice daily. (Malik 2006)

f) For feline chlamydial infections (*C. felis*): 10 mg/kg PO once daily for a minimum of 3–4 weeks; additional topical ocular treatment may reduce ocular discomfort. (Gruffyd-Jones 2009)

■ **HORSES:**

Warning: Doxycycline intravenously in horses has been associated with fatalities. Until further work is done demonstrating the safety of this drug, it cannot be recommended for parenteral use in this species.

a) For Lyme disease: 10 mg/kg PO once to twice daily for up to 30 days (Divers 1999)

b) For equine granulocytic ehrlichiosis (anaplasmosis; EGE) as an alternative to oxytetracycline: 10 mg/kg PO q12h for 10-14 days. (Lewis *et al.* 2009)

c) For organisms with an MIC ≤ 0.25 micrograms/mL (including many susceptible *Streptococcus* spp, *Staphylococcus* spp, *Pasteurella* spp, *Rhodococcus equi*, *Actinobacillus equuli*, and most ehrlichial organisms), a dose of 20 mg/kg PO q24h; preferably food should be withheld for at least 8 hours before and 2 hours after dosing. For bacteria with an MIC of 0.5-1 micrograms/mL, 20 mg/kg PO q12h is necessary to maintain adequate trough levels. Feeding should ideally be withheld as above, but may not be practically possible. One horse in the study developed a severe, acute colitis and the authors recommended that further clinical and safety studies be performed before using this regimen. (Davis *et al.* 2006)

■ **RABBITS/RODENTS/SMALL MAMMALS:**

a) **Mice, Rats:** For mycoplasmal pneumonia: 5 mg/kg PO twice daily with enrofloxacin (10 mg/kg PO twice daily) (Burke 1999)

b) **Chinchillas, Gerbils, Guinea Pigs, Hamsters, Mice, Rats:** 2.5-5 mg/kg PO q12h. Do not use in young or pregnant animals. (Adamcak & Otten 2000)

■ **BIRDS:**

For Psittacosis (Chlamydiosis):

a) Study done in experimentally infected cockatiels: Doxycycline 35 mg/kg PO once daily for 21 days. Birds were dosed via metallic feeding tube into crop using the commercially available (*Vibramycin*®) human oral suspension. (Guzman *et al.* 2010)

b) Routes of treatment include intramuscular injections, oral dosage with a suspension, medicated mash (approximately 1000 mg per kg of feed), and water-soluble approaches.

IM: 75-100 mg/kg IM every 5-7 days for the first 4 weeks and subsequently every 5 days for the duration of a 45 day treatment.

PO: 40-50 mg/kg PO once daily for cockatiels, Senegal parrots, Blue fronted and Orange winged amazons, 25 mg/kg PO once daily for African Grey parrots, Goffin's cockatoos, Blue and gold macaws and Green winged macaws. Empirically: 25-50 mg/kg PO once a day is the recommended starting dosage for unstudied avian species. (Speer 1999)

c) Using the oral liquid/suspension: 50 mg/kg PO every 24 hours, or divided every 12 hours (use less for macaws). Using the hyclate salt on corn, beans, rice and oatmeal: 1 gram per kg of feed. Using the injectable product (*Vibaravenos*®— may not be available commercially in the USA): 100 mg/kg IM once weekly (75 mg/kg IM once weekly in macaws and lovebirds) (Bauck & Hoefer 1993)

d) Ratites: 2-3.5 mg/kg PO twice daily (Jenson 1998)

■ **REPTILES:**

For susceptible infections:

a) For chelonians: 10 mg/kg PO once daily for 4 weeks. Useful for bacterial respiratory infections in tortoises having suspected Mycoplasma infections.

b) In most species: 10 mg/kg PO once daily for 10-45 days (Gauvin 1993)

Monitoring

■ Clinical efficacy

■ Adverse effects

Client Information

■ Do not "dry pill" as esophageal damage can occur; if using oral tablets or capsules, especially in cats, give medication followed by at least one 6 mL (a little more than a teaspoonful) of liquid. In cats, buttering the lips after administration to induce salivation and reduce esophageal transit time has been suggested.

■ Oral doxycycline products may be administered without regard to feeding, but giving with some food may reduce gastrointestinal effects. Milk or other dairy products do not significantly alter the amount of doxycycline absorbed.

Chemistry/Synonyms

A semi-synthetic tetracycline that is derived from oxytetracycline, doxycycline is available as hyclate, calcium and monohydrate salts. The hyclate salt is used in the injectable dosage form and in oral tablets and capsules. It occurs as a yellow, crystalline powder that is soluble in water and slightly soluble in alcohol. After reconstitution with sterile water, the hyclate injection has a pH of 1.8-3.3. Doxycycline hyclate may also be known as doxycycline hydrochloride.

The monohydrate salt is found in the oral powder for reconstitution. It occurs as a yellow, crystalline powder that is very slightly soluble in water and sparingly soluble in alcohol. The calcium salt is formed *in situ* during manufacturing. It is found in the commercially available oral syrup.

Doxycycline may also be known as: doxycycline monohydrate, doxycyclinum, and GS-3065; many trade names are available.

Storage/Stability

Doxycycline hyclate tablets and capsules should be stored in tight, light resistant containers at temperatures less than 30°C, and preferably at room temperature (15–30°C). After reconstituting with water, the monohydrate oral suspension is stable for 14 days when stored at room temperature.

The hyclate injection when reconstituted with a suitable diluent (*e.g.*, D₅W, Ringer's injection, Sodium Chloride 0.9%, or Plasma-Lyte 56 in D₅W) to a concentration of 0.1 to 1 mg/mL may be stored for 72 hours if refrigerated. Frozen reconstituted solutions (10 mg/mL in sterile water) are stable for at least 8 weeks if kept at -20°C, but should not be refrozen once thawed. If solutions are stored at room temperature, different manufacturers give different recommendations regarding stability, ranging from 12–48 hours. Infusions should generally be completed within 12 hours of administration.

Compatibility/Compounding Considerations

Doxycycline hyclate for injection is reportedly physically **compatible** with the following IV infusion solutions and drugs: D₅W, Ringer's injection, sodium chloride 0.9%, or Plasma-Lyte 56 in D₅W, Plasma-Lyte 148 in D₅W, Normosol M in D₅W, Normosol R in D₅W, invert sugar 10%, acyclovir sodium, hydromorphone HCl, magnesium sulfate, meperidine HCl, morphine sulfate, perphenazine and ranitidine HCl. Compatibility is dependent upon factors such as pH, concentration, temperature, and diluent used; consult specialized references or a hospital pharmacist for more specific information.

One study examining doxycycline blood levels in birds following injection of commercially available (not in USA) intramuscular formulation (*Vibravenös®*; Pfizer Switz.) and two concentrations of a pharmacist compounded product, showed variable blood levels and a high incidence of localized tissue reactions, including necrosis, with the compounded products (Flammer & Papich 2005).

Doxycycline administered to budgerigars at 250–300 ppm in a hulled seed diet has been shown to maintain doxycycline levels sufficient to treat chlamydiosis.

Doxycycline oral suspensions should be stored in the refrigerator, protected from light and used within 7 days. Although some compounding pharmacies claim stability of 6 months for compounded doxycycline suspensions, others have demonstrated that compounded doxycycline suspensions degrade rapidly between 7 and 14 days even if refrigerated. One study (Sadrieh *et al.* 2005) demonstrated that doxycycline tablets

mixed with water or foods (*e.g.*, milk, pudding, yogurt, apple sauce, jellies) lose more than 10% potency after 24 hours.

Dosage Forms/Regulatory Status

VETERINARY-LABELED PRODUCTS: None for systemic use.

Doxycycline gel: 8.5% activity once mixed. (2 syringe system); *Doxirobe®* (Pfizer); (Rx). FDA-approved for dogs; oral application for the prevention and treatment of periodontal disease.

HUMAN-LABELED PRODUCTS:

Doxycycline (as the hyclate) Tablets & Capsules: 20 mg, 50 mg, & 100 mg; *Periostat®* (CollaGenex), *Alodox Convenience Kit®* (OCuSOFT, Inc); *Vibramycin®* & *Vibra-Tabs®* (Pfizer); *Oraxyl®* (E5 Pharma); generic; (Rx)

Doxycycline (as the hyclate) Delayed-Release Tablets & Capsules: 75 mg, 100 mg & 150 mg, & 40 mg (30 mg immediate release & 10 mg delayed release); *Doryx®* (Warner Chilcott); *Oracea®* (CollaGenex); (Rx)

Doxycycline (as monohydrate) Tablets and Capsules: 50 mg, 75 mg, 100 mg & 150 mg; *Monodox®* (Oclassen); *Adoxa®* (Doak); generic; (Rx)

Doxycycline Capsules (coated-pellets) (as hyclate): 75 mg & 100 mg; *Doryx®* (Warner Chilcott); generic (Eon); (Rx)

Doxycycline (as the monohydrate) Powder for Oral Suspension: 5 mg/mL after reconstitution in 60 mL; *Vibramycin®* (Pfizer); Doxycycline (Teva); (Rx)

Doxycycline (as the calcium salt) Oral Syrup: 10 mg/mL in 473 mL; *Vibramycin®* (Pfizer); (Rx)

Doxycycline Injection: 42.5 mg (as hyclate, 10%) in vials; *Atridox®* (CollaGenex); (Rx)

Doxycycline (as the hyclate) Lyophilized Powder for Injection: 100 mg & 200 mg with 300 mg & 600 mg mannitol respectively in vials; *Doxy®-100* & *-200* (AAP); generic; (Rx)

References

Adamcak, A. & B. Otten (2000). Rodent Therapeutics. *Vet Clin NA: Exotic Anim Pract* 3:1(Jan): 221–240.

American–Heartworm–Society (2010). "Canine Guidlines." 2010, http://www.heartwormsociety.org/veterinary–resources/canine–guidelines.html#9.

Appel, M. & R. Jacobson (1995). CVT Update: Canine Lyme Disease. *Kirk's Current Veterinary Therapy:XII*. J Bonagura Ed. Philadelphia, W.B. Saunders: 303–309.

Bauck, L. & H. Hoefer (1993). Avian antimicrobial therapy. *Seminars in Avian & Exotic Med* 2(1): 17–22.

Bonenberger, T. (2009). Typical Cat Bite Abscess, or Not: Chronic Draining Tracts & Nodules. Proceedings: WVC. Accessed via: Veterinary Information Network. http://goo.gl/sNkTB

Breitschwerdt, E. (2000). Rocky Mountain Spotted Fever. Proceedings: American Animal Hospital Association 67th Annual Meeting, Toronto.

Burke, T. (1999). Husbandry and Medicine of Rodents and Lagomorphs. Proceedings: Central Veterinary Conference, Kansas City.

Carrade, D.D., J.E. Foley, et al. (2009). Canine Granulocytic Anaplasmosis: A Review. *Journal of Veterinary Internal Medicine* 23(6): 1129–1141.

Davis, J.L., J.H. Salmon, et al. (2006). Pharmacokinetics and tissue distribution of doxycycline after oral administration of single and multiple doses in horses. *American Journal of Veterinary Research* 67(2): 310–316.

Divers, T. (1999). Lyme disease in horses – Diagnosis and treatment. Proceedings: The North American Veterinary Conference, Orlando.

Flammer, K. & M. Papich (2005). Assessment of plasma concentrations and effects of injectable doxycycline in three psittacine species. *Journal of Avian Medicine and Surgery* 19(3): 216–224.

Ford, R. (2009a). Canine infectious disease update. Proceedings: ACVC. Accessed via: Veterinary Information Network. http://goo.gl/XVqzQ

Ford, R. (2009b). Tick–Borne Disease Diagnosis: Moving from 3Dx to 4Dx. Proceedings: ACVC. Accessed via: Veterinary Information Network. http://goo.gl/0Pb6s

Gauvin, J. (1993). Drug therapy in reptiles. *Seminars in Avian & Exotic Med* 2(1): 48–59.

Gilmour, M.A., C.R. Clarke, et al. (2005). Ocular penetration of oral doxycycline in the horse. *Veterinary Ophthalmology* 8(5): 331–335.

Grandi, G., C. Quintavalla, et al. (2010). A combination of doxycycline and ivermectin is adulticidal in dogs with naturally acquired heartworm disease (Dirofilaria immitis). *Veterinary Parasitology* 169(3–4): 347–351.

Greene, C., K. Hartmannn, et al. (2006). Appendix 8: Antimicrobial Drug Formulary. *Infectious Disease of the Dog and Cat*. C Greene Ed., Elsevier: 1186–1333.

Gruffyd–Jones, T. (2009). Chlamydial infections of cats. Proceedings: WSAVA. Accessed via: Veterinary Information Network. http://goo.gl/mMifv

Guzman, D.S.M., O. Diaz–Figueroa, et al. (2010). Evaluating 21–day Doxycycline and Azithromycin Treatments for Experimental Chlamydophila psittaci Infection in Cockatiels (Nymphicus hollandicus). *Journal of Avian Medicine and Surgery* 24(1): 35–45.

Jenson, J. (1998). Current ratite therapy. *The Veterinary Clinics of North America: Food Animal Practice* 16:3(November).

Kuehn, N. (2010). Chronic Nasal Disease in Dogs: Diagnosis & Treatment. Proceedings: ACVIM. Accessed via: Veterinary Information Network. http://goo.gl/2OQgm

Lappin, M. (2000a). Infectious causes of feline diarrhea. The North American Veterinary Conference, Orlando.

Lappin, M. (2000b). Protozoal and Miscellaneous Infections. *Textbook of Veterinary Internal Medicine: Diseases of the Dog and Cat*. S Ettinger and E Feldman Eds. Philadelphia, WB Saunders. 1: 408–417.

Lappin, M. (2006). Chronic feline infectious disease. Proceedings: Western Vet Conf. Accessed via: Veterinary Information Network. http://goo.gl/wZ7Kh

Lewis, S.R., L. Zimmerman, et al. (2009). Equine Granulocytic Anaplasmosis: A Case Report and Review. *Journal of Equine Veterinary Science* 29(3): 160–166.

Malik, R. (2006). Nocardia infections in cats. Proceedings Western Vet Conf. Accessed via: Veterinary Information Network. http://goo.gl/bY0lh

Rikihisa, Y. & G. Zimmerman (1995). Salmon Poisoning Disease. *Kirk's Current Veterinary Therapy:XII*. J Bonagura Ed. Philadelphia, W.B. Saunders: 297–300.

Sadrieh, N., J. Brower, et al. (2005). Stability, dose uniformity, and palatability of three counterterrorism drugs – Human subject and electronic tongue studies. *Pharmaceutical Research* 22(10): 1747–1756.

Schnabel, L.V., M.G. Papich, et al. (2010). Orally administered doxycycline accumulates in synovial fluid compared to plasma. *Equine Veterinary Journal* 42(3): 208–212.

Speer, B. (1999). An update on avian chlamydiosis. Proceedings: Central Veterinary Conference, Kansas City.

WSU–VetClinPharmLab (2009). "Problem Drugs." http://goo.gl/aIGlM.

EDETATE CALCIUM DISODIUM CALCIUM EDTA

(**ed**-a-tayt)   Calcium Disodium Versenate®

ANTIDOTE

Prescriber Highlights

▶ Heavy metal chelator used primarily for lead or zinc toxicity

▶ Contraindications: Patients with anuria; Extreme Caution: Patients with decreased renal function

▶ Recommend using SC route when treating small animals; do not give PO

▶ Adverse Effects: Renal toxicity (renal tubular necrosis); may cause depression & GI clinical signs in dogs

Uses/Indications

CaEDTA is used as a chelating agent in the treatment of lead poisoning. Succimer is more commonly recommended today for treating lead poisoning in dogs and cats.

CaEDTA may used in combination with dimercaprol treatment.

Pharmacology/Actions

The calcium in CaEDTA can be displaced by divalent or trivalent metals to form a stable water soluble complex that can be excreted in the urine. One gram of CaEDTA can theoretically bind 620 mg of lead, but in reality only about 5 mg per gram is actually excreted into the urine in lead poisoned patients. In addition to chelating lead, CaEDTA chelates and eliminates zinc from the body. CaEDTA also binds cadmium, copper, iron, and manganese, but to a much lesser extent than either lead or zinc. CaEDTA is relatively ineffective for use in treating mercury, gold, or arsenic poisoning.

There is some evidence that thiamine supplementation may increase the clinical efficacy of CaEDTA in treating acute lead poisoning in cattle.

Pharmacokinetics

CaEDTA is well absorbed after either IM or SC administration. It is distributed primarily in the extracellular fluid. Unlike dimercaprol, CaEDTA does not penetrate erythrocytes or enter the CNS in appreciable amounts. The drug is rapidly excreted renally, either as unchanged drug or chelated with metals. Changes in urine pH or urine flow do not significantly alter the rate of excretion. Decreased renal function can cause accumulation of the drug and can increase its nephrotoxic potential. In humans with normal renal function, the average elimination half-life of CaEDTA is 20–60 minutes after IV administration, and 1.5 hours after IM administration.

Contraindications/Precautions/Warnings

CaEDTA is contraindicated in patients with anuria. It should be used with extreme caution and with dosage adjustment in patients with diminished renal function.

Most small animal clinicians recommend using the SC route when treating small animals, as IV administration of CaEDTA has been associated with abrupt increases in CSF pressure and death in children with lead-induced cerebral edema.

Lead should be removed from the GI tract before using CaEDTA. Do not administer CaEDTA orally as it may increase the amount of lead absorbed from the GI tract.

Animals with clinical signs of cerebral edema should not be over hydrated.

Adverse Effects

The most serious adverse effect associated with this compound is renal toxicity (renal tubular necrosis), but in dogs, CaEDTA can cause depression, vomiting, and diarrhea. GI clinical signs may be alleviated by zinc supplementation.

Chronic therapy may lead to zinc deficiency; zinc supplementation should be considered in these animals.

Reproductive/Nursing Safety

In humans, the FDA categorizes this drug as category *B* for use during pregnancy (*Animal studies have not yet demonstrated risk to the fetus, but there are no adequate studies in pregnant women; or animal studies have shown an adverse effect, but adequate studies in pregnant women have not demonstrated a risk to the fetus in the first trimester of pregnancy, and there is no evidence of risk in later trimesters*).

It is not known whether this drug is excreted in milk.

Overdosage/Acute Toxicity

Doses greater than 12 g/kg are lethal in dogs; refer to Adverse Effects for more information.

Drug Interactions

The following drug interactions have either been reported or are theoretical in humans or animals receiving CaEDTA and may be of significance in veterinary patients:

■ **GLUCOCORTICOIDS:** The renal toxicity of CaEDTA may be enhanced by the concomitant administration of glucocorticoids

■ **INSULIN (NPH, PZI):** Concurrent administration of CaEDTA with zinc insulin preparations (NPH, PZI) will decrease the sustained action of the insulin preparation

■ **NEPHROTOXIC DRUGS, OTHER:** Use with caution with other nephrotoxic compounds (*e.g.*, **aminoglycosides, amphotericin B**)

Laboratory Considerations

■ CaEDTA may cause increased urine glucose values and/or cause inverted T-waves on ECG

Doses

The manufacturer of the injectable (human) product recommends diluting the injection to a concentration of 2–4 mg/mL with either normal saline or 5% dextrose when used for intravenous use. Because the injection is painful when given IM, it is recommended to add 1 mL of procaine HCl 1% to each mL of injection before administering IM.

■ **DOGS & CATS:**

For lead poisoning:

a) Be sure there is no lead in GI tract before using. Give 100 mg/kg SC divided into 4 daily doses in 5% dextrose for 5 days. May require second course of treatment, particularly if blood lead levels >0.10 ppm. Do not exceed 2 g/day and do not treat for more than 5 consecutive days. (Grauer & Hjelle 1988)

b) 25 mg/kg SC four times daily for 5 days. Give as 1% solution in D$_5$W. Provide a 5–7 day rest period between courses of treatment to minimize potential for nephrotoxicity. Succimer is now the treatment of choice for lead in small animals. (Poppenga 2002)

c) Cats: 27.5 mg/kg in 15 mL D$_5$W SC four times daily for 5 days. Recheck blood lead 2–3 weeks later and repeat therapy (with either CaEDTA or penicillamine) if greater than 0.2 ppm. (Reid & Oehme 1989)

For zinc toxicity:

a) 100 mg/kg divided into four SC doses per day. Dilute in D5W to reduce local irritation at site of injection. Exact dosage is not known nor how long therapy should continue. If possible, monitor serum zinc concentrations and maintain animal's hydration status. (Meurs & Breitschwerdt 1995)

■ **RABBITS/RODENTS/SMALL MAMMALS:**

a) **Chinchillas:** 30 mg/kg SC q12h (Adamcak & Otten 2000)

■ **HORSES:**

For lead poisoning:

a) Remove animal from source of lead. If severely affected give CaEDTA at 75 mg/kg IV slowly in D$_5$W or saline daily for 4–5 days (may divide daily dose into 2–3 administrations per day). Stop therapy for 2 days and repeat for another 4–5 days. Give adequate supportive and nutritional therapy. (Oehme 1987)

■ **FOOD ANIMALS:**

Note: FARAD recommends a 2 day meat and milk withdrawal time after use in food animals. (Haskell *et al.* 2005)

For lead poisoning:

a) 110 mg/kg per day in 3–4 divided doses; dilute to 1 gram/mL in D5W; first dose IV, then subcutaneously (Post & Keller 2000)

b) **Cattle:** 67 mg/kg slow IV twice daily for 2 days; withhold dose for 2 days and then give again for 2 days. Cattle may require 10–14 days to recover and may require several series of treatments. (Bailey 1986)

c) **Cattle:** 73.3 mg/kg/day slow IV divided 2–3 times a day for 3–5 days. If additional therapy is required, a 2-day rest period followed by another 5-day treatment regimen is recommended. (Sexton & Buck 1986)

■ **BIRDS:**
For lead poisoning:

a) In psittacines: 35 mg/kg IM twice daily for 5–7 days. After initial therapy, may give orally until all lead fragments are dissolved and/or passed from GI tract. (McDonald 1989)

b) In raptors (falcons): In this study, 25% CaEDTA was given undiluted IM at a dose of 100 mg/kg q12h for 5–25 consecutive days. Falcons were treated if blood lead was >65 micrograms/dL for 5 day courses, until blood lead was <20 micrograms/dL. No evidence of muscle damage, nephrotoxicity or hepatotoxicity seen. (Samour & Naldo 2004)

c) For lead or zinc poisoning: 30–35 mg/kg IM q12h x 3-5 days, off 3-5 days, may repeat and/or use another chelator. Maintain hydration. Do not give orally or may increase lead absorption from GI tract. Can be used IV short term (48 hrs) at 20–35 mg/kg diluted in saline. Many published regimens. (Johnson-Delaney & Reavill 2009)

Monitoring

■ Blood lead or zinc (serial), and/or urine d-ALA

■ Renal function tests, urinalyses, hydration status

■ Serum phosphorus and calcium values

■ Periodic cardiac rate/rhythm monitoring may be warranted during administration

Client Information

■ Because of the potential toxicity of this agent and the seriousness of most heavy metal intoxications, this drug should be used with close professional supervision only.

Chemistry/Synonyms

A heavy metal chelating agent, edetate calcium disodium (CaEDTA) occurs as an odorless, white, crystalline powder or granules and is a mixture of dihydrate and trihydrate forms. It has a slight saline taste and is slightly hygroscopic. CaEDTA is freely soluble in water and very slightly soluble in alcohol. The commercially available injection (human) has a pH of 6.5–8 and has approximately 5.3 mEq of sodium per gram of CaEDTA.

Edetate calcium disodium may also be known as: sodium calcium edetate, calcium disodium edathamil, calcium disodium edetate, calcium disodium ethylenediaminetetra-acetate, calcium disodium versenate, calcium EDTA, disodium calcium tetracemate, E385, natrii calcii edetas, sodium calciumedetate, *Calcium Disodium Versenate®*, *Calcium Vitis®*, *Calciumedetat-Heyl®*, *Chelante®*, *Chelintox®*, or *Ledclair®*.

Storage/Stability

CaEDTA should be stored at temperatures less than 40°, and preferably at room temperature (15–30°C). The injection can be diluted with either normal saline or 5% dextrose.

Dosage Forms/Regulatory Status

Note: Do not confuse with Edetate Disodium which should *not* be used for lead poisoning as it may cause severe hypocalcemia.

VETERINARY-LABELED PRODUCTS:

None in the USA; may be available from compounding pharmacies.

HUMAN-LABELED PRODUCTS:

Edetate Calcium Disodium Injection Solution: 200 mg/mL in 5 mL amps (1 gram/amp); *Calcium Disodium Versenate®* (Graceway); (Rx)

References

Adamcak, A. & B. Otten (2000). Rodent Therapeutics. *Vet Clin NA: Exotic Anim Pract* 3:1(Jan): 221–240.

Bailey, E.M. (1986). Management and treatment of toxicosis in cattle. *Current Veterinary Therapy 2: Food Animal Practice.* JL Howard Ed. Philadelphia, WB Saunders: 341–354.

Grauer, G.F. & J.J. Hjelle (1988). Household Toxins. *Handbook of Small Animal Practice.* RV Morgan Ed. New York, Churchill Livingstone: 1109–1114.

Haskell, S., M. Payne, et al. (2005). Farad Digest: Antidotes in Food Animal Practice. *JAVMA* 226(6): 884–887.

Johnson-Delaney, C. & D. Reavill (2009). Toxicoses in Birds: Ante- and Postmortem Findings for Practitioners. Proceedings: AAV. Accessed via: Veterinary Information Network. http://goo.gl/LVYYE

McDonald, S.E. (1989). Summary of medications for use in psittacine birds. *JAAV* 3(3): 120–127.

Meurs, K. & E. Breitschwerdt (1995). CVT Update: Zinc Toxicity. *Kirk's Current Veterinary Therapy:XII.* J Bonagura Ed. Philadelphia, W.B. Saunders: 238–239.

Oehme, F.W. (1987). LEad. *Current Therapy in Equine Medicine.* NE Robinson Ed. Philadelphia, WB Saunders: 667–668.

Poppenga, R. (2002). Decontaminating and detoxifying the poisoned patient. Proceedings: Western Veterinary Conf. Accessed via: Veterinary Information Network. http://goo.gl/Hq3dC

Post, L. & W. Keller (2000). Current status of food animal antidotes. *The Veterinary Clinics of North America: Food Animal Practice* 16:3(November).

Reid, F.M. & F.W. Oehme (1989). Toxicoses. *The Cat: Diseases and Clinical Management.* RG Sherding Ed. New York, Churchill Livingstone. 1: 185–215.

Samour, J. & J. Naldo (2004). The use of Ca Na2 EDTA in the treatment of lead toxicosis in falcons. Proceedings: AAV. Accessed via: Veterinary Information Network. http://goo.gl/jq2ur

Sexton, J.W. & W.B. Buck (1986). Lead. *Current Veterinary Therapy: Food Animal Practice 2.* JL Howard Ed. Philadelphia, W.B. Saunders: 439–440.

EDROPHONIUM CHLORIDE

(ed-roe-*foe*-nee-um)   Tensilon®, Enlon®

CHOLINERGIC (ANTICHOLINESTERASE)
AGENT

Prescriber Highlights

▶ Short-acting parenteral quanternary
ammonium cholinergic used primarily
to test for myasthenia gravis

▶ Secondary indications are to reverse
nondepolarizing agents or to treat
some SVT's

▶ Relatively contraindicated: Asthma or
mechanical urinary or intestinal tract
obstruction

▶ Caution: Bradycardias or atrioventricular block

▶ Overdoses can cause cholinergic crisis

Uses/Indications

The primary use for edrophonium is in the presumptive diagnosis of myasthenia gravis (MG).
The so-called "Tensilon Test" for MG has a fair
percentage of false-positives and false-negatives
associated with it and is probably best to use
while awaiting results from a more specific and
sensitive test such as the acetylcholine receptor
antibody test.

Edrophonium can also be used for the reversal of nondepolarizing agents (*e.g.*, vecuronium,
pancuronium, metocurine, atracurium, gallamine or tubocurarine). Because of its short
duration of action, its clinical usefulness for this
indication is questionable as longer acting drugs
such as neostigmine or pyridostigmine may be
more useful. Edrophonium, in a controlled intensive care-type setting, may also be useful in
the diagnosis and treatment of some supraventricular arrhythmias, particularly when other
more traditional treatments are ineffective.

Pharmacology/Actions

Edrophonium is an anticholinesterase agent that
is very short acting. It briefly attaches to acetylcholinesterase thereby inhibiting its hydrolytic
activity on acetylcholine. As acetylcholine accumulates, the following clinical signs may be
noted: miosis, increased skeletal and intestinal
muscle tone, bronchoconstriction, ureter constriction, salivation, sweating (in animals with
sweat glands), and bradycardia.

Pharmacokinetics

Edrophonium is only effective when given parenterally. After IV administration, it begins to
have effects on skeletal muscle within one minute and effects may persist for up to 10 minutes.
Myasthenic patients may have effects persisting
longer after the first dose. Edrophonium's exact
metabolic fate and excretion characteristics have
not been well described.

Contraindications/Precautions/Warnings

Edrophonium is considered relatively contraindicated in patients with bronchial asthma, or
mechanical urinary or intestinal tract obstruction. It should be used with caution (with adequate monitoring and treatment available) in
patients with bradycardias or atrioventricular
block. Some human patients are documented to
be hypersensitive to the drug and exhibit severe
cholinergic reactions.

It is recommended to have IV atropine and an
endotracheal tube readily available before using
edrophonium.

Adverse Effects

Adverse effects associated with edrophonium are
generally dose related and cholinergic in nature
(urination, lacrimation, vomiting, defecation,
bradycardia, bronchospasm). Although usually
mild and easily treated with a "tincture of time",
pre-treatment or treatment with an anticholinergic drug (*e.g.*, atropine) can help prevent or
alleviate these effects. Severe adverse effects are
possible with large overdoses (see below).

Reproductive/Nursing Safety

Edrophonium's safety profile during pregnancy
is not established; use only when necessary.
While no problems have been documented in
nursing humans or animals, its safety has not
been established. In humans, the FDA categorizes this drug as category *C* for use during pregnancy (*Animal studies have shown an adverse effect on the fetus, but there are no adequate studies
in humans; or there are no animal reproduction
studies and no adequate studies in humans.*)

It is unknown whether edrophonium enters
maternal milk.

Overdosage/Acute Toxicity

Overdosage of edrophonium may induce a
cholinergic crisis. Clinical signs of cholinergic
toxicity can include: GI effects (nausea, vomiting, diarrhea), salivation, sweating (in animals
able to do so), respiratory effects (increased
bronchial secretions, bronchospasm, pulmonary
edema, respiratory paralysis), ophthalmic effects
(miosis, blurred vision, lacrimation), cardiovascular effects (bradycardia or tachycardia, cardiospasm, hypotension, cardiac arrest), muscle
cramps and weakness.

Treatment of edrophonium overdose consists of both respiratory and cardiac supportive
therapy and, atropine, if necessary. Refer to the
atropine monograph for more information on
its use for cholinergic toxicity.

Drug Interactions

The following drug interactions have either been
reported or are theoretical in humans or animals
receiving edrophonium and may be of significance in veterinary patients:

◼ **ATROPINE:** Atropine will antagonize the
muscarinic effects of edrophonium and

some clinicians routinely use the two together, but concurrent use should be used cautiously as atropine can mask the early clinical signs of cholinergic crisis

■ **DEXPANTHENOL:** Theoretically, dexpanthenol may have additive effects when used with edrophonium

■ **DIGOXIN:** Edrophonium's cardiac effects may be increased in patients receiving digoxin; excessive slowing of heart rate may occur

■ **MUSCLE RELAXANTS:** Edrophonium may prolong the Phase I block of depolarizing muscle relaxants (*e.g.*, **succinylcholine, decamethonium**) and edrophonium antagonizes the actions of non-depolarizing neuromuscular blocking agents (*e.g.*, **pancuronium, tubocurarine, gallamine, vecuronium, atracurium**, etc.)

Doses

■ **DOGS:**

For presumptive diagnosis of myasthenia gravis (MG):

a) This test is easiest to assess in patients with the generalized form of MG, those who tire with exercise. The patient is gently exercised until fatigued. Place indwelling catheter. Edrophonium dose is 0.1–0.2 mg/kg IV. (Have atropine drawn up so that if cholinergic signs (SLUD) develop, it can be given at 0.02–0.04 mg/kg IV). The catheter is flushed with sterile saline, and then the patient is immediately lightly exercised, or if non-ambulatory, encouraged to rise. In patients with focal MG such as facial muscle weakness, the palpebral reflex may be assessed after IV edrophonium. Patients are assessed as having a positive or negative "Tensilon Test". (Vernau 2009)

b) 1–10 mg (total dose) IV; presumptive positive test results in transient improvement in clinical weakness; sometimes objective criteria for this test are difficult to establish. (LeCouteur 2005)

c) 0.1–0.2 mg/kg IV; have atropine and endotracheal tube readily available in case of overdose. (Abramson 2005)

d) Pre-treat with atropine (0.02–0.04 mg/kg IM or SC); then give edrophonium at 0.1 mg/kg IV. In affected animals, paresis should resolve within one minute and effects should last for up to 15 minutes. (Kornegay 2006)

■ **CATS:**

For presumptive diagnosis of myasthenia gravis (MG):

a) This test is easiest to assess in patients with the generalized form of MG, who tire with exercise. The patient is gently exercised until fatigued. Place indwell-

ing catheter. Edrophonium dose is 0.25 to 0.5 mg (total dose) IV. (Have atropine drawn up so that if cholinergic signs (SLUD) develop, it can be given at 0.02–0.04 mg/kg IV). The catheter is flushed with sterile saline and then the patient is immediately lightly exercised, or if non-ambulatory, encouraged to rise. In patients with focal MG such as facial muscle weakness, the palpebral reflex may be assessed after IV edrophonium. Patients are assessed as having a positive or negative "Tensilon Test". (Vernau 2009)

b) Pre-treat with atropine (0.02–0.04 mg/kg IM or SC); then give edrophonium at 0.1 mg/kg IV. In affected animals, paresis should resolve within one minute and effects should last for up to 15 minutes. (Kornegay 2006)

Monitoring

■ Cholinergic adverse effects

■ Improvement (for 1–15 minutes) of paresis for presumptive diagnosis of MG

Client Information

■ Edrophonium is a drug that should be used in a controlled clinical setting

■ Clients should be briefed on the side effects that can occur with its use

Chemistry/Synonyms

A synthetic quarternary ammonium cholinergic (parasympathomimetic) agent, edrophonium chloride occurs as a white crystalline powder having a bitter taste. Approximately 2 grams are soluble in 1 mL of water. The injection has a pH of approximately 5.4.

Edrophonium chloride may also be known as: edrophonii chloridum, *Anticude*®, *Camsilon*®, *Enlon*®, *Reversol*®, or *Tensilon*®.

Storage/Stability

Edrophonium chloride injection should be stored at room temperature.

It is reportedly physically **compatible** at Y-site injections with heparin sodium, hydrocortisone sodium succinate, potassium chloride and vitamin B complex with C. Compatibility is dependent upon factors such as pH, concentration, temperature and diluent used; consult specialized references or a hospital pharmacist for more specific information.

Dosage Forms/Regulatory Status

VETERINARY-LABELED PRODUCTS: None

HUMAN-LABELED PRODUCTS:

Edrophonium Chloride Solution for Injection: 10 mg/mL in 10 mL & 15 mL vials; *Enlon*® (Bioniche); *Reversol*® (Organon); (Rx)

Edrophonium Chloride/Atropine Sulfate for Injection: 10 mg/mL with 0.14 mg/mL atropine sulfate in 5 mL single-dose amps & 15 mL multi-dose vials; *Enlon-Plus*® (Bioniche); (Rx)

References

Abramson, C. (2005). Neuromuscular disease. Proceedings: Western Vet Conf. Accessed via: Veterinary Information Network. http://goo.gl/72wwm

Kornegay, J. (2006). Neuromuscular disease I & II. Proceedings: Western Vet Conf. Accessed via: Veterinary Information Network. http://goo.gl/plFca

LeCouteur, R. (2005). Neuropathies, junctionopathies & myopathies of dogs and cats: 1–5. Proceedings: Veterinary Neurology Seminar. Accessed via: Veterinary Information Network. http://goo.gl/jUyAu

Vernau, K. (2009). Beyond Tensilon and Titers: Myasthenia Gravis. Veterinary Neurology Symposium; Univ. of Calif.-Davis. Accessed via: Veterinary Information Network. http://goo.gl/UHXuc

EFA-Caps®–see Fatty Acids

EMODEPSIDE + PRAZIQUANTEL

(ee-moe-*dep*-side + pra-zi-*kwon*-tel)
Profender®

TOPICAL ANTIPARASITIC (NEMATOCIDE; CESTOCIDE)

Prescriber Highlights

▶ Topical cestocide & nematocide labeled for cats

▶ Appears safe in cats >1 kg & at least 8 weeks old

▶ Applied to back of cat's neck; do not allow patient or other cats to lick area of application for at least one hour

Uses/Indications

Emodepside/Praziquantel topical solution (*Profender®*) is indicated for the treatment and control of hookworm infections caused by *Ancylostoma tubaeforme* (adults, immature adults, and fourth stage larvae), roundworm infections caused by *Toxocara cati* (adults and fourth stage larvae), and tapeworm infections caused by *Dipylidium caninum* (adults) and *Taenia taeniaeformis* (adults) in cats.

Topical *Profender®* may also be of use in treating other species (*e.g.*, reptiles) where oral dosing may be overly stressful.

There are also oral products available (not in USA) for use in dogs.

Pharmacology/Actions

Emodepside has a unique mode of action in comparison to other antiparasitic compounds. The drug attaches pre-synaptically at the neuromuscular junction to a latrophilin-like receptor, resulting in an increase in intracellular calcium and diacylglycerol levels. At the end of the signal transduction cascade, vesicles containing inhibitory neuropeptide fuse with pre-synaptic membranes. Inhibitory neuropeptides such as PF1- and/or PF2-like receptor are then released into the synaptic cleft, stimulating postsynaptic receptors and resulting in an inhibition of pha-

ryngeal pumping and locomotion of the nematode. The end result is flaccid paralysis and death of the parasite.

Praziquantel's exact mechanism of action against cestodes has not been determined, but it may be the result of interacting with phospholipids in the integument causing ion fluxes of sodium, potassium and calcium. At low concentrations *in vitro*, the drug appears to impair the function of their suckers and stimulates the worm's motility. At higher concentrations *in vitro*, praziquantel increases the contraction (irreversibly at very high concentrations) of the worm's strobilla (chain of proglottids). In addition, praziquantel causes irreversible focal vacuolization with subsequent cestodal disintegration at specific sites of the cestodal integument.

Pharmacokinetics

Following dermal application of the product (*Profender®*) to cats, emodepside and praziquantel are absorbed through the skin and into the systemic circulation. Absorption of both active ingredients through the skin is relatively rapid, with serum concentrations detectable within 2 hours for emodepside and within 1 hour for praziquantel. Peak concentrations occur within 6 hours for praziquantel and 2 days for emodepside. After a single application, both emodepside and praziquantel were detectable for up to 28 days following treatment were noted.

A study looking at topical absorption in a variety of reptiles found variability in blood levels that was associated with skin thickness (Schilliger *et al.* 2009).

Contraindications/Precautions/Warnings

There are no absolute contraindications for use of this product on cats noted on the label. However, safe use has not been evaluated in cats: less than 8 weeks of age or weighing less than 2.2 lb (1 kg), used for breeding, during pregnancy, or in lactating queens. Use with caution in sick or debilitated, or heartworm positive cats.

Adverse Effects

In pre-approval efficacy studies, the most common side effects observed were dermal- and gastrointestinal-related. In a field study, adverse reactions reported by cat owners included licking/excessive grooming (3%), scratching treatment site (2.5%), salivation (1.7%), lethargy (1.7%), alopecia (1.3%), agitation/nervousness (1.2%), vomiting (1%), diarrhea (0.5%), eye irritation in 3 cats (0.5%), respiratory irritation (0.2%) and shaking/tremors (0.2%). All adverse reactions were self-limiting. The following adverse events were reported voluntarily during post-approval use of the product in foreign markets: application site reaction (hair loss, dermatitis, pyoderma, edema, and erythema), salivation, pruritus, lethargy, vomiting, diarrhea, dehydration, ataxia, loss of appetite, facial swelling, rear leg paralysis, seizures, hyperesthesia, twitching, and death. A case report of one cat developing

498 EMODEPSIDE + PRAZIQUANTEL

a morphea-like (scleroderma) lesion after application has been reported (Seixas & Taboada 2009).

Reproductive/Nursing Safety
Safe use has not been evaluated in cats used for breeding, during pregnancy, or in lactating queens. Studies performed in laboratory animals (rats, rabbits) suggest that emodepside may interfere with fetal development in those species.

Overdosage/Acute Toxicity
Oral doses of emodepside of 200 mg/kg were tolerated by rats without mortalities. The oral LD50 in rats is >500 mg/kg; in mice >2,500 mg/kg. The acute dermal toxicity dose of emodepside in rats is high; a dose of 2,000 mg/kg was tolerated without mortality.

Praziquantel has a wide margin of safety. In rats and mice, the oral LD$_{50}$ is at least 2 g/kg. An oral LD$_{50}$ could not be determined in dogs, as at doses greater than 200 mg/kg, the drug induced vomiting. Parenteral doses of 50–100 mg/kg in cats caused transient ataxia and depression. Injected doses at 200 mg/kg were lethal in cats.

Kittens approximately 8 weeks of age were treated topically with the combination product up to 5X at 2 week intervals for treatments. Clinical signs of transient salivation and/or tremors were seen in a few animals in the 5X group, all of which were self-limiting.

Seven- to eight-month-old cats treated topically with the topical solution at 10X developed transient salivation, tremor, and lethargy.

Studies where the product was administered orally in cats have caused salivation, vomiting, anorexia, tremors, abnormal respirations, and ataxia. Adverse effects in all animals treated in these studies resolved without treatment.

Drug Interactions
No drug interactions have been documented for this product, but emodepside is reportedly a substrate for P-glycoprotein. Use with other drugs that are P-glycoprotein substrates or inhibitors (e.g., **ivermectin, erythromycin, prednisolone, cyclosporine**) could cause pharmacokinetic drug interactions.

Doses
- **CATS:**
  For labeled indications:
  a) Minimum dose is 3 mg/kg emodepside & 12 mg/kg praziquantel applied to the skin on the back of the neck as a single topical dose. A second treatment should not be necessary. If re-infection occurs, the product can be re-applied after 30 days. (Label information; *Profender®*—Bayer)

- **REPTILES:**
  a) Serum levels vary between species, but a dose of 4 drops/100 g body weight appears to be effective. Aquatic species must be kept in a dry place for 48 hours after treatment. Caution is advised until further studies verify safety and efficacy, particularly in sick animals. (Schilliger *et al.* 2009)

Monitoring
- Clinical efficacy

Client Information
- Do not apply to broken skin or if hair coat is wet.
- Do not get in the cat's mouth or eyes or allow the cat to lick the application site for one hour. Oral exposure can cause salivation and vomiting; treatment at the base of the head will minimize the opportunity for ingestion while grooming.
- In households with multiple pets, keep animals separated to prevent licking of the application site.
- Not for human use. Keep out of reach of children. To prevent accidental ingestion of the product, children should not come in contact with the application site for 24 hours while the product is being absorbed. Pregnant women, or women who may become pregnant, should avoid direct contact with, or wear disposable gloves when applying, this product.

Chemistry/Synonyms
Emodepside is an N-methylated 24-membered cyclooctadepsipeptide, consisting of four alternating residues of N-methyl-L-leucine, two residues of D-lactate, and two residues of D-phenylacetate.

Praziquantel occurs as a white to practically white, hygroscopic, bitter tasting, crystalline powder, either odorless or having a faint odor. It is very slightly soluble in water and freely soluble in alcohol.

Praziquantel may also be known as: EMBAY-8440, or praziquantelum.

Storage/Stability
Store product at or below 25°C (77°F); do not allow to freeze.

Dosage Forms/Regulatory Status
VETERINARY-LABELED PRODUCTS:
Emodepside (1.98% w/w; 21.4 mg/mL) and Praziquantel (7.94% w/w; 85.8 mg/mL) Topical Solution in 0.35 mL (cats 2.2–5.5 lb.), 0.7 mL (cats >5.5–11 lb.) & 1.12 mL (cats >11–17.6 lb.) tubes: *Profender®* (Bayer); (Rx). FDA-approved for use on cats.

An oral product for dogs, *Profender® for Dogs* is available in many countries, but is not currently FDA-approved in the USA.

HUMAN-LABELED PRODUCTS: None

References
Schilliger, L., O. Betremieux, et al. (2009). Absorption and efficacy of a spot-on combination containing emodepside plus praziquantel in reptiles. *Revue de Medecine Veterinaire* **160**(12): 557–561.

Seixas, G. & P. Taboada (2009). Morphea-Like Lesion Following Topical Application of an Endectocide in a Cat. Proceedings: WSAVA. Accessed via: Veterinary Information Network. http://goo.gl/EtGuR

ENALAPRIL MALEATE
ENALAPRILAT

(e-*nal*-a-pril)   Enacard®, Vasotec®

ANGIOTENSIN-CONVERTING ENZYME (ACE) INHIBITOR

Prescriber Highlights

▶ Veterinary & human ACE inhibitor used primarily as a vasodilator in the treatment of heart failure or hypertension; may also be of benefit in the treatment of chronic renal failure or protein losing nephropathies

▶ Caution: pregnancy, renal insufficiency (doses may need to be reduced), patients with hyponatremia, coronary or cerebrovascular insufficiency, preexisting hematologic abnormalities or a collagen vascular disease (e.g., SLE)

▶ Adverse Effects: GI distress (anorexia, vomiting, diarrhea); Potentially: weakness, hypotension, renal dysfunction & hyperkalemia

Uses/Indications

The principle use of enalapril/enalaprilat in veterinary medicine at present is as a vasodilator in the treatment of heart failure. Recent studies have demonstrated that enalapril, particularly when used in conjunction with furosemide, does improve the quality of life in dogs with heart failure. There is now reasonable evidence that ACE inhibitors can modestly increase survival times in dogs with Class II-IV heart failure, but further studies are required to clarify any benefits. Enalapril may also be of benefit in treating the effects associated with valvular heart disease (mitral regurgitation) and left to right shunts.

Enalapril and ACE inhibitors decrease efferent glomerular resistance and may reduce proteinuria and have renoprotective effects; they are being explored for adjunctive treatment in idiopathic glomerulonephritis, chronic renal failure and protein losing nephropathies in small animals.

ACE inhibitors are used in treating feline hypertrophic cardiomyopathy and may be of benefit, but at present there is not good evidence that they prolong survival times.

While ACE inhibitors are a mainstay for treating hypertension in humans, they have not been particularly useful when used alone in treating hypertension in dogs or cats.

Pharmacology/Actions

Enalapril is converted in the liver to the active compound enalaprilat. Enalaprilat prevents the formation of angiotensin-II (a potent vasoconstrictor) by competing with angiotensin-I for the enzyme angiotensin-converting enzyme

(ACE). ACE has a much higher affinity for enalaprilat than for angiotensin-I. Because angiotensin-II concentrations are decreased, aldosterone secretion is reduced and plasma renin activity is increased.

The cardiovascular effects of enalaprilat in patients with CHF include: decreased total peripheral resistance, pulmonary vascular resistance, mean arterial and right atrial pressures, and pulmonary capillary wedge pressure, no change or decrease in heart rate, and increased cardiac index and output, stroke volume, and exercise tolerance.

ACE inhibitors increase renal blood flow and decrease glomerular efferent arteriole resistance. In animals with glomerular disease, ACE inhibitors decrease proteinuria and may help to preserve renal function. Enalapril, at least partially blocks amlodipine's activation of the renin-angiotensin-aldosterone system (RAAS) in dogs (Atkins *et al.* 2007).

Pharmacokinetics

Enalapril/enalaprilat has different pharmacokinetic properties than captopril in dogs. It has a slower onset of action (4−6 hours) but a longer duration of action (12−14 hours). In dogs, approximately 95% of enalapril is cleared via renal routes and reduced renal function can impact elimination rates.

In humans, enalapril is well absorbed after oral administration, but enalaprilat is not. Approximately 60% of an oral dose is bioavailable. Both enalapril and enalaprilat are distributed poorly into the CNS and are distributed into milk in trace amounts. Enalaprilat crosses the placenta. In humans, the half-life of enalapril is about 2 hours; enalaprilat about 11 hours. Half-lives are increased in patients with renal failure or severe CHF.

Contraindications/Precautions/Warnings

Enalaprilat is contraindicated in patients who have demonstrated hypersensitivity to the ACE inhibitors. It should be used with caution and close supervision in patients with renal insufficiency and doses may need to be reduced.

Enalaprilat should also be used with caution in patients with hyponatremia or sodium depletion, coronary or cerebrovascular insufficiency, preexisting hematologic abnormalities, or a collagen vascular disease (*e.g.*, SLE). Patients with severe CHF should be monitored very closely upon initiation of therapy.

Adverse Effects

Enalapril/enalaprilat's adverse effect profile in dogs is principally GI distress (anorexia, vomiting, diarrhea). Potentially, weakness, hypotension, renal dysfunction and hyperkalemia could occur. Because it lacks a sulfhydryl group (unlike captopril), there is less likelihood that immune-mediated reactions will occur, but rashes, neutropenia, and agranulocytosis have been reported in humans. In humans, ACE inhibitors commonly cause coughs, but this occurs rarely in dogs or cats.

Adverse effects associated with enalapril in cats include lethargy and inappetence.

Reproductive/Nursing Safety

Enalapril crosses the placenta. High doses in rodents have caused decreased fetal weights and increases in fetal and maternal death rates; teratogenic effects have not been reported. In humans, the FDA categorizes this drug as *category C for use during pregnancy in the first trimester* (*Animal studies have shown an adverse effect on the fetus, but there are no adequate studies in humans; or there are no animal reproduction studies and no adequate studies in humans.*) In humans, the FDA categorizes this drug as *category D for use during pregnancy in second and third trimesters* (*There is evidence of human fetal risk, but the potential benefits from the use of the drug in pregnant women may be acceptable despite its potential risks.*) as ACE inhibitors may cause abnormal fetal and postnatal kidney development.

Enalapril/enalaprilat is excreted into milk. Safe use during nursing cannot be assumed.

Overdosage/Acute Toxicity

In dogs, a dose of 200 mg/kg was lethal, but 100 mg/kg was not. In overdose situations, the primary concern is hypotension; supportive treatment with volume expansion with normal saline is recommended to correct blood pressure. Because of the drug's long duration of action, prolonged monitoring and treatment may be required. Recent overdoses should be managed by using gut emptying protocols when warranted.

Drug Interactions

The following drug interactions have either been reported or are theoretical in humans or animals receiving enalaprilat and may be of significance in veterinary patients:

■ **ANTIDIABETIC AGENTS (insulin, oral agents):** Possible increased risk for hypoglycemia; enhanced monitoring recommended

■ **DIURETICS (e.g., furosemide, hydrochlorothiazide):** Potential for increased hypotensive effects; some veterinary clinicians recommend reducing furosemide doses (by 25–50%) when adding enalapril or benazepril to therapy in CHF.

■ **DIURETICS, POTASSIUM-SPARING (e.g., spironolactone, triamterene):** Increased hyperkalemic effects, enhanced monitoring of serum potassium recommended

■ **HYPOTENSIVE AGENTS, OTHER:** Potential for increased hypotensive effect

■ **LITHIUM:** Increased serum lithium levels possible; increased monitoring required

■ **NSAIDS:** May reduce the anti-hypertensive or positive hemodynamic effects of enalapril; may increase risk for reduced renal function, but clinical significance has not been demonstrated in dogs receiving enalapril and an NSAID.

■ **POTASSIUM SUPPLEMENTS:** Increased risk for hyperkalemia

Laboratory Considerations

■ When using iodohippurate sodium I^{123}/I^{134} or Technetium Tc^{99} pententate **renal imaging** in patients with renal artery stenosis, ACE inhibitors may cause a reversible decrease in localization and excretion of these agents in the affected kidney which may lead to confusion in test interpretation.

Doses

■ **DOGS:**

a) As a vasodilator in heart failure: 0.5 mg/kg PO twice daily (Kittleson 2000)

b) For adjunctive treatment of heart failure: 0.5 mg/kg once daily initially with or without food. If response is inadequate increase to 0.5 mg/kg twice daily (Package Insert; *Enacard®*—Merial)

For adjunctive treatment of glomerular disease:

a) 0.5 mg/kg PO q12–24h (Grauer & DiBartola 2000)

b) 0.5 mg/kg PO once daily. If no reduction in proteinuria after 2–4 weeks, increase to twice daily. (Vaden 2003)

c) 0.25–1 mg/kg PO q12-24h. (Bartges 2009)

As an adjunctive treatment for ureteroliths:

a) 0.25–0.5 mg/kg PO q12–24h; may potentially reduce interstitial expansion and fibrosis. (Lulich 2006)

For systemic hypertension:

a) As a first step drug for systolic hypertension >160 mmHg, diastolic >120 mmHg; after **1)** enalapril/benazepril (0.5 mg/kg q12h); **2)** amlodipine (0.1 mg/kg q24h); **3)** amlodipine (0.2 mg/kg q24h); **4)** spironolactone (1–2 mg/kg twice daily); **5)** hydralazine 0.5 mg/kg PO twice daily. Each step added (except when increasing amlodipine dose) if after 1-2 weeks systolic BP > 160 mmHg. (Henik 2007)

■ **CATS:**

For adjunctive treatment of heart failure due to hypertrophic cardiomyopathy:

a) 1.25–2.5 mg (total dose) PO once daily (q24h). (Kittleson 2009)

b) 0.25–0.5 mg/kg (roughly 1.25–2.5 mg per cat) PO once a day (q24h) (Meurs 2006)

c) 0.5 mg/kg PO once daily, twice daily if necessary (Ware & Keene 2000)

For proteinuria, hypertension in chronic kidney disease:

a) 0.25 mg/kg PO once daily to 0.5 mg/kg PO twice daily; rarely higher (Polzin 2006)

For systemic hypertension:

a) As a 2nd step drug when systolic BP >160 mmHg, diastolic >120 mmHg: **1)** amlodipine (0.625 mg per cat q24h, if cat greater then 6 kg, 1.25 mg/cat q24h), add ACE inhibitor if proteinuric; **2)** ACE inhibitor (benazepril/enalapril 0.5 mg/kg q12h); **3)** spironolactone (1–2 mg/kg twice daily); **4)** hydralazine 0.5 mg/kg PO twice daily. Each step added (except when increasing amlodipine dose) if after 1–2 weeks systolic BP > 160 mmHg. (Henik 2007)

■ **FERRETS:**

For adjunctive therapy for heart failure:

a) 0.5 mg/kg PO once every other day (q48h) initially and may be increased to once a day if tolerated. Dissolve tablet(s) in distilled water and add a methylcellulose suspending agent (e.g., Ora-Plus®) and cherry syrup for flavor. (Hoeffer 2000)

b) For dilative cardiomyopathy: 0.25–0.5 mg/kg PO once a day to every other day (Williams 2000)

■ **BIRDS:**

For adjunctive therapy for heart failure:

a) 1.25 mg/kg PO two to three times daily (Pees *et al.* 2006)

b) 0.25–0.5 mg/kg PO q24-48h with furosemide. (Oglesbee 2009)

Monitoring

■ Clinical signs of CHF

■ Serum electrolytes, creatinine, BUN, urine protein

■ CBC with differential, periodic

■ Blood pressure (if treating hypertension or clinical signs associated with hypotension arise)

Client Information

■ May be given with or without food

■ Do not abruptly stop or reduce therapy without veterinarian's approval

■ Contact veterinarian if vomiting or diarrhea persist or are severe or if animal's condition deteriorates

Chemistry/Synonyms

Angiotensin-converting enzyme (ACE) inhibitors, enalapril maleate and enalaprilat are structurally related to captopril. Enalapril is a prodrug and is converted *in vivo* by the liver to enalaprilat. Enalapril maleate occurs as a white to off white crystalline powder. 25 mg are soluble in one mL of water. Enalaprilat occurs as a white to off white crystalline powder and is slightly soluble in water.

Enalapril maleate may also be known as: enalaprili maleas, and MK-421; many trade names are available. Enalaprilat may also be known as: enalaprilic acid, MK-422, *Enacard®, Glioten®,*

Lotrial®, Pres®, Renitec®, Reniten®, Vasotec®, and *Xanef®.*

Storage/Stability

The commercially available tablets should be stored at temperatures less than 30°C in tight containers. When stored properly, the tablets have an expiration date of 30 months after manufacture.

Enalaprilat injection should be stored at temperatures less than 30°C. After dilution with D_5W, normal saline, or D_5 in lactated Ringer's it is stable for up to 24 hours at room temperature.

Compatibility/Compounding Considerations

Enalaprilat has been documented to be physically **incompatible** with amphotericin B or phenytoin sodium. Many other medications have been noted to be compatible with enalaprilat at various concentrations. Compatibility is dependent upon factors such as pH, concentration, temperature and diluent used; consult specialized references or a hospital pharmacist for more specific information.

Compounded preparation stability: Enalapril oral suspension compounded from commercially available tablets has been published (Allen & Erickson 1998). Triturating six (6) enalapril 20 mg tablets with 60 mL of Ora-Plus® and qs ad to 120 mL with Ora-Sweet® (or Ora-Sweet® SF) yields a 1 mg/mL oral suspension that retains >90% potency for 60 days stored at both 5°C and 25°C. Degradation of enalapril is pH dependent with maximum stability at pH 3 and increased decomposition above pH 5. Compounded preparations of enalapril should be protected from light.

Dosage Forms/Regulatory Status

VETERINARY-LABELED PRODUCTS:

Enalapril Maleate Tablets: 1 mg, 2.5 mg, 5 mg, 10 mg, & 20 mg; *Enacard®* (Merial); (Rx). FDA-approved for use in dogs.

The ARCI (Racing Commissioners International) has designated this drug as a class 3 substance. See the appendix for more information.

HUMAN-LABELED PRODUCTS:

Enalapril Maleate Tablets: 2.5 mg, 5 mg, 10 mg & 20 mg; *Vasotec®* (Biovail); generic (Rx).

Enalaprilat Injection: (for IV use) equivalent to 1.25 mg/mL in 1 mL & 2 mL vials; generic; (Rx)

References

Allen, L.V. & M.A. Erickson (1998). Stability of alprazolam, chloroquine phosphate, cisapride, enalapril maleate, and hydralazine hydrochloride in extemporaneously compounded oral liquids. *Am J Health Syst Pharm* 55(18): 1915–1920.

Atkins, C.E., W.P. Rausch, et al. (2007). The effect of amlodipine and the combination of amlodipine and enalapril on the renin-angiotensin-aldosterone system in the dog. *Journal of Veterinary Pharmacology and Therapeutics* 30(5): 394–400.

Bartges, J. (2009). Update on management of proteinuria. Proceedings: WVC. Accessed via: Veterinary Information Network. http://goo.gl/D50Km

Grauer, G. & S. DiBartola (2000). Glomerular Disease. *Textbook of Veterinary Internal Medicine: Diseases of the Dog and Cat.* S Ettinger and E Feldman Eds. Philadelphia, WB Saunders. 2: 1662–1678.

Henik, R. (2007). Stepwise therapy of systemic hypertension. Proceedings: IVECCS. Accessed via: Veterinary Information Network. http://goo.gl/nofKU

Hoeffer, H. (2000). Heart Disease in Ferrets. *Kirk's Current Veterinary Therapy: XIII Small Animal Practice.* J Bonagura Ed. Philadelphia, WB Saunders: 1144–1148.

Kittleson, M. (2009). Treatment of feline hypertrophic cardiomyopathy (HCM)--Lost Dreams. Proceedings: ACVIM. Accessed via: Veterinary Information Network. http://goo.gl/XvCZt

Lulich, J. (2006). Managment of Nephroliths in Dogs and Cats. Proceedings: ECVIM-CA Congress. Accessed via: Veterinary Information Network. http://goo.gl/VFfjp

Meurs, K. (2006). Therapeutic management of feline cardiomyopathy. Proceedings: ACVIM. Accessed via: Veterinary Information Network. http://goo.gl/TNXxJ

Oglesbee, B. (2009). Working up the pet bird with lower respiratory tract disorders. Proceedings: WVC. Accessed via: Veterinary Information Network. http://goo.gl/4nQwK

Pees, M., K. Kuhring, et al. (2006). Bioavailability and compatibility of enalapril in birds. Accessed via: Veterinary Information Network. http://goo.gl/EKDS2

Polzin, D. (2006). Treating feline renal failure: an evidenced-based approach. Proceedings: WVC. Accessed via: Veterinary Information Network. http://goo.gl/C2JgZ

Vaden, S. (2003). Glomerulopathy in dogs. Proceedings: ACVIM Forum. Accessed via: Veterinary Information Network. http://goo.gl/AYZ8l

Ware, W. & B. Keene (2000). Outpatient management of chronic heart failure. *Kirk's Current Veterinary Therapy: XIII Small Animal Practice.* J Bonagura Ed. Philadelphia, WB Saunders: 748–752.

Williams, B. (2000). Therapeutics in Ferrets. *Vet Clin NA: Exotic Anim Pract* **3**:1(Jan): 131–153.

ENOXAPARIN SODIUM

(en-*ocks*-a-par-in)   Lovenox®

ANTICOAGULANT

Prescriber Highlights

▶ Low molecular weight (fractionated) heparin that may be useful for treatment or prophylaxis of thromboembolic disease

▶ Preferentially inhibits factor Xa & only minimally impacts thrombin & clotting time (TT or aPTT)

▶ Hemorrhage unlikely, but possible

▶ Must be given subcutaneously, potentially every 6 hours; fair amount of uncertainty about effective dosing requirements for dogs or cats

▶ Expense may be an issue, particularly in large dogs or horses

Uses/Indications

Enoxaparin may be useful for prophylaxis or treatment of deep vein thrombosis or pulmonary embolus. Recent pharmacokinetic work in dogs and cats, raises questions whether the drug can be effectively and practically administered long-term. In humans, it is also indicated for prevention of ischemic complications associated with unstable angina/non Q-wave MI.

Pharmacology/Actions

By binding to and accelerating antithrombin III, low molecular weight heparins (LMWHs) enhance the inhibition of factor Xa and thrombin. The potential advantage to using these products over standard (unfractionated) heparin is that they preferentially inhibit factor Xa; only minimally impacting thrombin and clotting times (TT or aPTT). Recent work in cats (Van De Wiele *et al.* 2010), has suggested that anti-Xa activity may not be an accurate determiner for predicting antithrombotic activity.

Pharmacokinetics

In dogs after SC administration, enoxaparin has a shorter duration of anti-Xa activity than in humans and probably must be dosed more frequently. A study examining enoxaparin dose response (anti-Xa activity) in dogs, showed that an enoxaparin dose of 0.8 mg/kg SC q6h would be required to effectively and consistently inhibit factor Xa activity in dogs (Lunsford, K.V. *et al.* 2009).

Cats appear to have a much shorter duration of activity (anti-Xa) associated with LMWHs than do humans and to maintain a therapeutic target of anti-XA activity of 0.5–1 IU/mL requires 1.5 mg/kg SC q6h dosing of enoxaparin (Alwood, A. *et al.* 2007). However, a recently published study (Van De Wiele *et al.* 2010) has suggested that anti-Xa activity may not be an accurate determiner for antithrombotic activity of enoxaparin in cats. In their venous stasis model, antithrombotic activity persisted well beyond the time after anti-Xa levels were below what are thought to be therapeutic.

After subcutaneous injection in humans, enoxaparin is absorbed rapidly, with a bioavailability of about 92%; peak plasma levels (activity) occur in 3–5 hours. Anti-factor Xa activity persists for up to 24 hours; doses are usually given once to twice a day. Enoxaparin is metabolized in the liver and excreted in the urine as both unchanged drug and metabolites; elimination half-life is about 4–5 hours.

Contraindications/Precautions/Warnings

Enoxaparin is contraindicated in patients who are hypersensitive to it, other LMWHs, heparin, or porcine products. Use enoxaparin cautiously in patients with significant renal dysfunction as drug accumulation could result.

Do not administer via IM or IV routes; enoxaparin must be given via deep subcutaneous injection only. Enoxaparin cannot be used interchangeably with other LMWHs or heparin sodium because the dosages differ for each.

Adverse Effects

In humans, adverse effects do not routinely occur; hemorrhage is a possibility and has been reported in up to 13% of patients in one study.

Injection site hematoma, anemia, thrombocytopenia, nausea, and fever have also been reported.

Reproductive/Nursing Safety

In humans, enoxaparin is designated by the FDA as a category **B** drug (*Animal studies have not demonstrated risk to the fetus, but there are no adequate studies in pregnant women; or animal studies have shown an adverse effect, but adequate studies in pregnant women have not demonstrated a risk to the fetus during the first trimester of pregnancy, and there is no evidence of risk in later trimesters.*)

Overdosage/Acute Toxicity

Overdosage may lead to hemorrhagic complications. If treatment is necessary, protamine sulfate may be administered via slow IV. One mg of protamine sulfate can inhibit the effects of one mg of enoxaparin.

Drug Interactions

The following drug interactions have either been reported or are theoretical in humans or animals receiving enoxaparin and may be of significance in veterinary patients:

■ **ANTICOAGULANTS, ORAL (warfarin):** Increased risk for hemorrhage

■ **PLATELET-AGGREGATION INHIBITORS (aspirin, clopidogrel):** Increased risk for hemorrhage

■ **THROMBOLYTIC AGENTS:** Increased risk for hemorrhage

Laboratory Considerations

■ Low molecular weight heparins may cause asymptomatic, fully reversible increases in AST or ALT; bilirubin is only rarely increased in these patients. Therefore, interpret these tests with caution; increases do not necessarily indicate hepatic damage or dysfunction.

Doses

■ **DOGS:**

a) 0.8 mg/kg SC q6h appears to effectively and consistently maintain therapeutic levels of anti-Xa in normal dogs. (Lunsford, K. et al. 2005), (Lunsford, K.V. et al. 2009)

b) 0.8–1 mg/kg SC q6-8h. (Alwood, A.J. 2008)

■ **CATS:**

a) From a study done in healthy cats: Doses of 1 mg/kg SC q12h results in a measurable antithrombotic effect. (Van De Wiele et al. 2010)

b) Cats appear to have a much shorter duration of activity (anti-Xa) associated with LMWHs than do humans; to maintain a therapeutic target of anti-XA activity of 0.5–1 IU/mL requires 1.5 mg/kg SC q6h dosing of enoxaparin. Based on this research in healthy cats, current recommendations are to dose at 1.25 mg/kg SC

q6h (Alwood, A. et al. 2007), (Alwood, A.J. 2008)

■ **HORSES:**

a) No published dosage recommendation at the time of writing. A study (Schwarzwald et al. 2002) investigating the pharmacokinetic variables of enoxaparin in horses demonstrated that the drug has similar activity (effect, duration) as in humans and the once daily SC injections may be useful for anticoagulant therapy.

Monitoring

■ CBC (with platelet count); baseline and ongoing during therapy

■ Urinalysis

■ Stool occult blood test

■ Routine coagulation tests (aPTT, PT) are usually insensitive measures of activity and usually not warranted

■ Factor Xa activity (available at Cornell Coagulation Laboratory) may be useful, particularly if bleeding occurs or patient has renal dysfunction

Client Information

■ If this drug is to be used on an outpatient basis, clients must be instructed in proper injection technique for subcutaneous injection. If not using the pre-filled syringes, use a very small gauge insulin or tuberculin syringe and needle (e.g., 27 g).

■ Clients should immediately report any signs associated with bleeding or pulmonary thrombosis.

■ Clients should understand that if they do not use the drug regularly (as prescribed), clots may form.

Chemistry/Synonyms

A low molecular weight heparin (LMWH), enoxaparin sodium is obtained by alkaline depolymerization of heparin derived from pork intestinal mucosa. The average molecular weight is about 4500 and ranges from 3500–5500 (heparin sodium has a molecular weight around 12000). 1 mg of enoxaparin is equivalent to 100 Units of anti-factor Xa.

Enoxaparin sodium may also be known as: Enoxaparinum natricum, PK-10169, RP-54563, *Clexane®, Decipar®, Klexane®, Lovenox®, Plaucina®*, and *Trombenox®*.

Storage/Stability

The commercially available injection should be stored at room temperature (25°C, 77°F); excursions permitted to 15–30°C (59–86°F).

One study showed that diluting 100 mg/mL commercially available solution with sterile water to 20 mg/mL was stable for 4 weeks when stored in a glass vial or in plastic syringes at room temperature or refrigerated. (Dager et al. 2004)

Dosage Forms/Regulatory Status

VETERINARY-LABELED PRODUCTS: None

HUMAN-LABELED PRODUCTS:

Enoxaparin Sodium for Injection: 30 mg/0.3 mL, 40 mg/0.4 mL, 60 mg/0.6 mL, 80 mg/0.8 mL, 100 mg/1 mL, 120 mg/0.8 mL, & 150 mg/1 mL preservative free in single-dose prefilled syringes; 300 mg/3 mL containing 15 mg/mL benzyl alcohol in 3 mL multidose vials; *Lovenox®* (Sanofi-Aventis); (Rx)

References

Alwood, A., A. Downend, et al. (2007). Anticoagulant effects of low -molecular weight heparins in healthy cats. *J Vet Intern Med* 21(3): 378–387.

Alwood, A.J. (2008). Heparin Therapy in Critical Care-- Should We Be Using Low Molecular Weight Heparins? Proceedings: IVECCS. Accessed via: Veterinary Information Network. http://goo.gl/LrRcQ

Dager, W., R. Gosselin, et al. (2004). AntiXa stability of enoxaparin for use in pediatrics. *Ann Pharmacother* 38(4): 569–573.

Lunsford, K., A. Mackin, et al. (2005). Pharmacokinetics of the biological effects of subcutaneous enoxaparin in dogs. Proceedings: ACVIM. Accessed via: Veterinary Information Network. http://goo.gl/KhynL

Lunsford, K.V., A.J. Mackin, et al. (2009). Pharmacokinetics of Subcutaneous Low Molecular Weight Heparin (Enoxaparin) in Dogs. *Journal of the American Animal Hospital Association* 45(6): 261–267.

Schwarzwald, C., K. Feige, et al. (2002). Comparison of pharmacokinetic variables for two low-molecular-weight heparins after subcutaneous administration of a single dose to horses. *Am J Vet Res* 63(Jun): 868–873.

Van De Wiele, C.M., D.F. Hogan, et al. (2010). Antithrombotic Effect of Enoxaparin in Clinically Healthy Cats: A Venous Stasis Model. *Journal of Veterinary Internal Medicine* 24(1): 185–191.

ENROFLOXACIN

(en-roe-*flox*-a-sin)   Baytril®

FLUOROQUINOLONE ANTIBIOTIC

Prescriber Highlights

▶ Veterinary oral & injectable fluoro-quinolone antibiotic effective against a variety of pathogens; not effective against anaerobes

▶ In dogs, oral bioavailability is better than ciprofloxacin

▶ Relatively contraindicated for young, growing animals due to cartilage abnormalities

▶ FDA prohibits extra-label use in food animals

▶ Caution: Hepatic or renal insufficiency, dehydration

▶ Higher doses (>5 mg/kg/day) not recommended in cats; may cause blindness

▶ Adverse Effects: GI distress, CNS stimulation, crystalluria, or hypersensitivity; IV administration can potentially be very risky in small animals

▶ Administer PO (to dogs/cats) preferably on an empty stomach (unless vomiting occurs)

▶ Drug interactions

▶ Should not be used in humans (CNS effects)

Uses/Indications

Enrofloxacin is FDA-approved for use in dogs and cats (oral only) for the management of diseases associated with bacteria susceptible to enrofloxacin. Because of the dosage restriction (5 mg/kg) for cats, enrofloxacin is generally used in this species only for the most susceptible bacterial infections. It is also FDA-approved for use in cattle (not dairy cattle or veal calves), but extra-label use is prohibited.

Pharmacology/Actions

Enrofloxacin is a bactericidal agent. The bactericidal activity of enrofloxacin is concentration dependent, with susceptible bacteria cell death occurring within 20–30 minutes of exposure. Enrofloxacin has demonstrated a significant post-antibiotic effect for both gram-negative and -positive bacteria and is active in both stationary and growth phases of bacterial replication.

Its mechanism of action is believed to act by inhibiting bacterial DNA-gyrase (a type-II topoisomerase), thereby preventing DNA supercoiling and DNA synthesis.

Both enrofloxacin and ciprofloxacin have similar spectrums of activity. These agents have good activity against many gram-negative bacilli and cocci, including most species and strains of *Pseudomonas aeruginosa*, *Klebsiella* spp., *E. coli*, Enterobacter, Campylobacter, Shigella, Salmonella, Aeromonas, Haemophilus, Proteus, Yersinia, Serratia, and Vibrio species. Of the currently commercially available quinolones, ciprofloxacin and enrofloxacin have the lowest MIC values for the majority of these pathogens treated. Other organisms that are generally susceptible include *Brucella* spp., *Chlamydia trachomatis*, Staphylococci (including penicillinase-producing and methicillin-resistant strains), Mycoplasma, and *Mycobacterium* spp. (not the etiologic agent for Johne's Disease).

The fluoroquinolones have variable activity against most streptococci and are not usually recommended for use in these infections. These drugs have weak activity against most anaerobes and are ineffective in treating anaerobic infections.

Bacterial resistance development is an ongoing concern, as many isolates of *Pseudomonas aeruginosa* are now resistant to enrofloxacin. Resistance occurs by mutation, particularly with *Pseudomonas aeruginosa*, *Klebsiella pneumonia*, Acinetobacter and enterococci, but plasmid-mediated resistance is not thought to commonly occur.

Pharmacokinetics

Enrofloxacin is well absorbed after oral administration in most species. In dogs, enrofloxacin's bioavailability (approximately 80%) is about twice that of ciprofloxacin after oral dosing. Oral bioavailability in horses is between 60-80%. 50% of Cmax is reportedly attained within 15 minutes of dosing and peak levels (Cmax) occur within one hour of dosing. The presence of food in the stomach may delay the rate, but not the extent of absorption. In sheep, enrofloxacin administered orally is about 65-75% bioavailable.

Enrofloxacin is distributed throughout the body. Volume of distribution in dogs is approximately 3-4 L/kg. Only about 27% is bound to canine plasma proteins. Highest concentrations are found in the bile, kidney, liver, lungs, and reproductive system (including prostatic fluid and tissue). Enrofloxacin reportedly concentrates in macrophages. Therapeutic levels are also attained in bone, synovial fluid, skin, muscle, aqueous humor and pleural fluid. In hospitalized horses, volume of distribution was about 1.25 L/kg. After mechanical disruption of the blood-aqueous humor barrier (BAB) in horses, 7.5 mg/kg IV produced levels in the aqueous humor sufficient to treat *Leptospira pomona* (Divers *et al.* 2008). Low concentrations are found in the CSF; levels may only reach 6–10% of those found in the serum. In cattle, the volume of distribution is about 1.5 L/kg and in sheep, 0.4 L/kg.

Enrofloxacin is eliminated via both renal and non-renal mechanisms. Approximately 15–50% of the drug is eliminated unchanged into the urine, by both tubular secretion and glomerular filtration. Enrofloxacin is metabolized to various metabolites, most of which are less active than the parent compounds. Approximately 10–40% of circulating enrofloxacin is metabolized to ciprofloxacin in most species including humans, dogs, cats, adult horses, cattle, turtles, and snakes. Foals, pigs, and some lizards apparently do not convert much enrofloxacin, if any, to ciprofloxacin. These metabolites are eliminated both in the urine and feces. Because of the dual (renal and hepatic) means of elimination, patients with severely impaired renal function may have slightly prolonged half-lives and higher serum levels that may not require dosage adjustment. The approximate elimination half-lives in various species are: dogs 4–5 hours; cats 6 hours; sheep 1.5–4.5 hours; horses 5-10 hours, turtles 18 hours; and alligators 55 hours.

Contraindications/Precautions/Warnings

Enrofloxacin is labeled as contraindicated in small and medium breed dogs from 2 to 8 months of age. Bubble-like changes in articular cartilage have been noted when the drug was given at 2–5 times recommend doses for 30 days, although clinical signs have only been seen at the 5X dose. To avoid cartilage damage, large and giant breed dogs may need to wait longer than the recommended 8 months before treatment since they may be in the rapid-growth phase past 8 months of age. Quinolones are contraindicated in patients hypersensitive to them.

Because ciprofloxacin has occasionally been reported to cause crystalluria in humans, animals should not be allowed to become dehydrated during therapy with either ciprofloxacin or enrofloxacin. Enrofloxacin may cause CNS stimulation and should be used with caution in patients with seizure disorders. Patients with severe renal or hepatic impairment may require dosage adjustments to prevent drug accumulation.

Use of the canine or bovine injectable products in cats or administered to dogs via other non-FDA-approved parenteral routes (IV, SC) is controversial and may result in significant adverse effects. Parenteral administration in cats at doses less than 5 mg/kg have reportedly caused ophthalmic toxicity (blindness). Because of the high pH (approx. 11) of the solution, subcutaneous administration in any species may cause pain and tissue damage. If administered rapidly or undiluted IV to dogs, there is an increased risk for cardiac arrhythmias, hypotension, vomiting, and mast cell degranulation (histamine and other mediator release).

The extra-label use in dogs of the IM 22.7 mg/mL (2.27%) product diluted 1:1 to 1:10 with sodium chloride 0.9% for slow IV administration (over at least 10 minutes; some give over 30–45 minutes) has anecdotally been described. However, the rapid absorption of enrofloxacin after IM administration in dogs (peak levels in about 30 minutes) questions the necessity of using this non-approved route (IV) of administration. Injectable enrofloxacin must not be mixed with, or come into contact with any IV solution containing magnesium (*e.g.*, *Normosol-R*, *Plasmalyte-R, -A*, or *−56*); morbidity and mortality secondary to micro-precipitants lodging in patient lungs have been reported. Dilution and extra-label use in small animals of the large animal product (100 mg/mL; 10%) via any route is discouraged.

Do not use in foals as they appear to be highly susceptible to the fluoroquinolone's arthropathic effects. Do not give rapidly IV to horses as ataxia and other neurologic effects may occur. IM injections are not recommended in horses as localized tissue reactions can occur.

Extra-label use of fluoroquinolones is prohibited in animals to be used for food.

Enrofloxacin should not be used by humans; it may cause hallucinations, vivid dreams, and headache.

Adverse Effects

With the exception of potential cartilage abnormalities in young animals (see Contraindications above), the adverse effect profile of enrofloxacin is usually limited to GI distress (vomiting, anorexia). In dogs, rare incidences of elevated hepatic enzymes, ataxia, seizures, depression, lethargy, and nervousness have also been reported. Hypersensitivity reactions or crystalluria could potentially occur.

In cats, rare incidences of ocular toxicity have been reported characterized by mydriasis, retinal degeneration, and blindness. These effects were generally seen at higher dosage ranges (>15 mg/kg) and have necessitated a reduction in dosage recommendations in cats to a maximum of 5 mg/kg/day. Other rare adverse effects seen in cats may include: vomiting, anorexia, elevated hepatic enzymes, diarrhea, ataxia, seizures, depression/lethargy, vocalization, and aggression.

While enrofloxacin has been implicated in causing antibiotic-associated diarrhea/enterocolitis in horses, due its poor activity against anaerobes, oral or parenterally administered enrofloxacin appears to carry a low risk of causing antibiotic-associated diarrhea.

Reproductive/Nursing Safety

The safety of enrofloxacin in pregnant dogs has been investigated. Breeding, pregnant, and lactating dogs receiving up to 15 mg/kg day demonstrated no treatment related effects. However, because of the risks of cartilage abnormalities in young animals, the fluoroquinolones are not generally recommended for use during pregnancy unless the benefits of therapy clearly outweigh the risks. Limited studies in male dogs at various dosages have indicated no effects on male breeding performance.

Safety in breeding, pregnant, or lactating cats has not been established.

Overdosage/Acute Toxicity

It is unlikely an acute overdose in dogs with enrofloxacin would result in clinical signs more serious than either anorexia or vomiting, but the adverse effects noted above could occur. Dogs receiving 10X the labeled dosage rate of enrofloxacin for at least 14 days developed only vomiting and anorexia. Death occurred in some dogs when fed 25 times the labeled rate for 11 days, however.

In cats overdoses can be serious (blindness, seizures); 20 mg/kg or more can cause retinopathy and blindness which can be irreversible.

There were 322 exposures to enrofloxacin reported to the ASPCA Animal Poison Control Center (APCC) during 2008-2009. In these cases 301 were dogs with 85 showing clinical signs and the remaining 21 cases were cats with 6 showing clinical signs. Common findings in dogs recorded in decreasing frequency included vomiting, lethargy, seizures, anorexia, depression, and diarrhea. Findings in cats recorded in decreasing frequency included seizures and recumbency.

Drug Interactions

The following drug interactions have either been reported or are theoretical in humans or animals receiving ciprofloxacin or enrofloxacin and may be of significance in veterinary patients:

- ■ **ANTACIDS/DAIRY PRODUCTS:** Containing cations (Mg^{++}, Al^{+++}, Ca^{++}) may bind to enrofloxacin and prevent its absorption; separate doses of these products by at least 2 hours

- ■ **ANTIBIOTICS, OTHER (aminoglycosides, 3rd-generation cephalosporins, penicillins—extended-spectrum:** Synergism may occur, but is not predictable against some bacteria (particularly *Pseudomonas aeruginosa*) with these compounds. Although enrofloxacin/ciprofloxacin has minimal activity against anaerobes, *in vitro* synergy has been reported when used with **clindamycin** against strains of Peptostreptococcus, Lactobacillus and *Bacteroides fragilis*.

- ■ **CYCLOSPORINE:** Fluoroquinolones may exacerbate the nephrotoxicity and reduce the metabolism of cyclosporine (used systemically)

- ■ **FLUNIXIN:** Has been shown in dogs to increase the AUC and elimination half-life of enrofloxacin and enrofloxacin increases the AUC and elimination half-life of flunixin; it is unknown if other NSAIDs interact with enrofloxacin in dogs

- ■ **GLYBURIDE:** Severe hypoglycemia possible

- ■ **IRON, ZINC (oral):** Decreased enrofloxacin/ciprofloxacin absorption; separate doses by at least two hours

- ■ **METHOTREXATE:** Increased MTX levels possible with resultant toxicity

- ■ **NITROFURANTOIN:** May antagonize the antimicrobial activity of the fluoroquinolones and their concomitant use is not recommended

■ **PHENYTOIN:**   Enrofloxacin/ciprofloxacin may alter phenytoin levels

■ **PROBENECID:** Blocks tubular secretion of ciprofloxacin and may increase its blood level and half-life

■ **QUINIDINE:** Increased risk for cardiotoxicity

■ **SUCRALFATE:** May inhibit absorption of enrofloxacin; separate doses of these drugs by at least 2 hours

■ **THEOPHYLLINE:**   Enrofloxacin/ciprofloxacin may increase theophylline blood levels; in dogs theophylline levels may be increased by about 30-50% (Trepanier 2008).

■ **WARFARIN:** Potential for increased warfarin effects

Laboratory Considerations

■ Enrofloxacin may cause false-positive **urine glucose** determinations when using cupric sulfate solution (Benedict's Solution, *Clinitest*®). Tests utilizing glucose oxidase (*Tes-Tape*®, *Clinistix*®) are not affected by enrofloxacin

■ In some human patients, the fluoroquinolones have caused increases in **liver enzymes, BUN,** and **creatinine** and decreases in **hematocrit**. The clinical relevance of these mild changes is not known at this time.

Doses

■ **DOGS:**
For susceptible infections:

a) 5–20 mg/kg per day PO, may be given once daily or divided and given twice daily (q12h). Treatment should continue for at least 2–3 days beyond cessation of clinical signs, to a maximum duration of therapy is 30 days. (Package insert; *Baytril*®—Bayer)

b) For sepsis: 5–20 mg/kg IV q12h (Hardie 2000)

c) For skin, urinary infections: 2.5–5 mg/kg PO q12h for 7–14 days;

For deep pyodermas, complicated urinary infections: 5 mg/kg PO once daily (q24h) for 7–14 days (treatment may be required for 10–12 weeks for deep pyoderma, especially in German shepherds);

For lower respiratory tract infections: 5–10 mg/kg PO once daily (q24h) for 7–84 days;

For prostate infections: 5 mg/kg PO twice daily (q12h) for 7–14 days;

For histiocytic ulcerative colitis: 5 mg/kg PO twice daily (q12h) for 21–90 days;

For hemotropic mycoplasmosis: 5 mg/kg PO, IM q12h for 7–14 days;

For   systemic   orthopedic   infections:

5–11 mg/kg PO, IV, IM, SC q12h for 10 days;

For Pseudomonas infections in soft tissues: 11–20 mg/kg PO, IM, SC q12h for 7 days minimum, treat as long as necessary;

For bacteremia, sepsis: 11 mg/kg PO, IV, IM, SC q12h for as long as necessary. (Greene *et al.* 2006)

d) For   histiocytic   ulcerative   colitis: 5–10 mg/kg PO once daily for at least 4-6 weeks. (Burgener 2010)

■ **CATS:**
For susceptible infections:

a) 5 mg/kg per day PO, may be given once daily or divided and given twice daily (q12h). Treatment should continue for at least 2–3 days beyond cessation of clinical signs, to a maximum duration of therapy is 30 days. (Package insert; *Baytril*®—Bayer)

b) For hemoplasmosis: 5–10 mg/kg PO q24h for 14 days. (Dowers 2009)

■ **HORSES:**
Note: Usage of enrofloxacin in horses remains somewhat controversial. While there has been much discussion regarding the potential for cartilage abnormalities or other arthropathies in horses, objective data are lacking. At present, however, enrofloxacin probably should only be used in adult horses when other antibiotics are inappropriate. If using *Baytril*® injection orally in horses, it can be very irritating to the mouth. This may be alleviated by coating the liquid with molasses or preparing a gel (see Compounding Considerations below) and rinsing the horse's mouth with water after administration.

a) 5 mg/kg IV q24h; 5–7.5 mg/kg PO q24h. (Haggett & Wilson 2008)

b) 7.5 mg/kg PO or IV once daily for susceptible respiratory infections (Ainsworth & Hackett 2004)

c) Using the compounded gel as described below   (Compatibility/Compounding Considerations): 7.5 mg/kg PO once daily. Horses should be fasted for 11–14 hours prior to dosing and for 1–2 hours after dosing, but should have access to water. Rinse horse's mouth with water after dosing to reduce risks for oral ulceration. (Epstein *et al.* 2004)

■ **CATTLE:**
a) Enrofloxacin (*Baytril*® 100) is FDA-approved for the treatment of bovine respiratory disease associated with *Pasteurella haemolytica, Pasteurella multocida,* and *Haemophilus sommus.* It is administered by injection and is intended for the treatment of individual animals. The labeled dosage is: 2.5–5 mg/kg SC once daily for

3–5 days or 7.5–12.5 mg/kg SC once. The product is prescription only and is not for use in cattle intended for dairy production or in veal calves. Animals intended for human consumption must not be slaughtered within 28 days from the last treatment. Extralabel use of fluoroquinolones in food animals is prohibited by the FDA.

■ **FERRETS:**

For susceptible infections:

a) 10–20 mg/kg PO, IM, SC twice daily (Williams 2000)

■ **RABBITS/RODENTS/SMALL MAMMALS:**

a) For Pasteurella upper respiratory infections in rabbits: 15–20 mg/kg PO twice daily for a minimum of 14 days in mild cases and up to several months for chronic infections; first dose may be made by SC injection (do NOT give subsequent doses SC or severe tissue reactions can occur). (Antinoff 2008)

b) **Rabbits:** 5 mg/kg PO, SC, IM or IV q12h for 14 days. Drug of choice for Pasteurella. If giving SC, dilute or skin may slough. Do not give injectable product PO because it is very unpalatable (Ivey & Morrisey 2000)

c) **Hedgehogs:** 5–10 mg/kg PO or SC q12h (Smith 2000)

d) **Chinchillas:** 5–10 mg/kg PO, IM q12h (Hayes 2000)

e) For mycoplasmal pneumonia in mice and rats: 10 mg/kg PO twice daily with doxycycline (5 mg/kg PO twice daily) (Burke 1999)

f) **Chinchillas, Gerbils, Guinea Pigs, Hamsters, Mice, Rats:** 5–10 mg/kg PO or IM q12h or 5–20 mg/kg PO or SC q24h. In drinking water: 50–200 mg/liter for 14 days. Do not use in young animals. (Adamcak & Otten 2000)

g) Chronic respiratory disease in rats: 10–25 mg/kg PO twice daily. If using theophylline concurrently, reduce the ophylline dose by 30%. (Monks & Cowan 2009)

■ **CAMELIDS:**

For susceptible infections in alpacas:

a) 5 mg/kg SC or 10 mg/kg PO once daily (Gandolf *et al.* 2005)

■ **BIRDS:**

For susceptible gram-negative infections:

a) For empirical treatment in Psittacines. For stable, immunocompetent birds: 20 mg/kg PO once daily with amoxicillin/clavulanate (125 mg/kg PO three times daily). For debilitated immunocompetent birds: 15–20 mg/kg SC in fluid pocket once daily. For debilitated, immunocompromised birds:

15–20 mg/kg SC in fluid pocket twice daily. When used orally, compounding the liver-flavored tablets grape syrup (*Syrpalta®*; Humco Labs) may improve acceptance. (Flammer 2006)

b) **Ratites:** 1.5–2.5 mg/kg PO or SC twice daily. Drinking water: 10% solution, 10 mg/kg for 3 days; 5 mg/kg IM (IM injections cause severe muscle necrosis) twice daily for 2 days (Jenson 1998)

■ **REPTILES:**

For susceptible respiratory infections for most species:

a) 5 mg/kg IM every 5 days for 25 days; For chronic respiratory infections in tortoises: 15 mg/kg IM every 72 hours for 5–7 treatments (Gauvin 1993)

Monitoring

■ Clinical efficacy

■ Adverse effects

■ In cats, monitor for mydriasis and/or retinal changes.

Client Information

■ Do not crush film-coated tablets, as drug is very bitter tasting

■ Animals should have access to water at all times

■ Do not exceed dosage recommendations in cats; blindness can occur

Chemistry/Synonyms

A fluoroquinolone antibiotic, enrofloxacin occurs as a pale yellow, crystalline powder. It is slightly soluble in water. Enrofloxacin is related structurally to the human-FDA-approved drug ciprofloxacin (enrofloxacin has an additional ethyl group on the piperazinyl ring)

Enrofloxacin may also be known as: Bay-Vp-2674 or *Baytril®*.

Storage/Stability

Unless otherwise directed by the manufacturer, enrofloxacin tablets should be stored in tight containers at temperatures less than 30°C. Protect from strong UV light. Enrofloxacin has been reported to be soluble and stable in water, but solubility is pH dependent and altering the pH of the commercially available injections can cause precipitation.

The canine FDA-approved product (2.27%) for IM injection should be stored protected from light; do not freeze.

The cattle FDA-approved product (10%) injectable solution should be stored protected from sunlight. It should not be refrigerated, frozen or stored above 40°C (104°F). If exposed to cold temperatures, precipitation may occur; to redissolve, warm and then shake the vial.

Injectable enrofloxacin must not be mixed with, or come into contact with any IV solution containing magnesium (*e.g., Normosol-R, Plasmalyte-R, -A,* or *-56*); morbidity and mortality secondary to micro-precipitants lodging in patient lungs have been reported.

Compatibility/Compounding Considerations

For horses an oral gel formulated from the bovine injectable product has been described (Epstein *et al.* 2004). 100 mL of the 100 mg/mL bovine injection (*Baytril®* 100) is used. Stevia (0.35 g) is mixed with approximately 15 mL of liquid enrofloxacin until dissolved. Apple flavoring 0.6 mL is added until dissolved. Sodium carboxymethylcellulose (2 g) is sprinkled over the mixture and stirred until incorporated. Immediately begin gradually adding the remaining enrofloxacin (85 mL) before the mixture solidifies. Approximate concentration is 100 mg/mL. Stable for up to 84 days if kept in the refrigerator and protected from light.

Because the oral tablets taste "terrible", birds may better accept enrofloxacin orally by compounding the liver-flavored tablets with grape syrup (*Syrpalta®*; Humco Labs) (Flammer 2006).

A method to make a 10.2 mg/mL oral suspension of enrofloxacin has been described: Make a stock solution of "HMC 0.15%" by mixing 7.5 mL of *Lubrivet®* with 92.5 mL of water. Crush three (3) whole 68 mg tablets with a "pinch" of citric acid. Add crushed mixture to a dispensing vial and add 15 mL of "HMC 0.15%." Shake well to dissolve tablet coating; add a sufficient quantity of "HMC 0.15%" to a total of 20 mL and allow to stand at room temperature for 30 minutes to allow tablet coating to completely dissolve. Shake well before use and keep refrigerated. A 14-day expiration date has been assigned. By crushing six (6) tablets, a 20.4 mg/mL suspension may be compounded using the same technique.

Dosage Forms/Regulatory Status

VETERINARY-LABELED PRODUCTS:

Enrofloxacin Tablets (Film-Coated) & Oral Taste Tablets: 22.7 mg, 68 mg, 136 mg; *Baytril®* (Bayer Corp); (Rx). FDA-approved for use in dogs and cats.

Enrofloxacin Injection: 22.7 mg/mL (2.27%) in 20 mL vials; *Baytril®* (Bayer Corp); (Rx). FDA-approved for use in dogs.

Enrofloxacin Injection: 100 mg/mL in 100 mL and 250 mL bottles. FDA-approved for use in cattle only. Not for use in cattle intended for dairy production or in calves to be processed for veal. Any extra-label use in food animals is banned by the FDA. Slaughter Withdrawal = 28 days when used as labeled. A withdrawal period has not been established in pre-ruminating calves. *Baytril 100®* (Bayer); (Rx)

HUMAN-LABELED PRODUCTS: None.

Note: Use of enrofloxacin by humans cannot be recommended due to a high degree of CNS effects.

References

Adamcak, A. & B. Otten (2000). Rodent Therapeutics. *Vet Clin NA: Exotic Anim Pract* 3:1(Jan): 221–240.

Ainsworth, D. & R. Hackett (2004). Disorders of the Respiratory System. *Equine Internal Medicine 2nd Ed.* M Reed, W Bayly and D Sellon Eds. Phila., Saunders: 289–354.

Antinoff, N. (2008). Respiratory diseases of ferrets, rabbits, and rodents. Proceedings: IVECCS. Accessed via: Veterinary Information Network. http://goo.gl/JjmjJ

Burgener, I. (2010). Approach to Canine and Feline Colitis. Proceedings: World Small Animal Assoc. Accessed via: Veterinary Information Network. http://goo.gl/Re0LK

Burke, T. (1999). Husbandry and Medicine of Rodents and Lagomorphs. Proceedings: Central Veterinary Conference, Kansas City.

Divers, T.J., N.L. Irby, et al. (2008). Ocular penetration of intravenously administered enrofloxacin in the horse. *Equine Veterinary Journal* 40(2): 167–170.

Dowers, K. (2009). Causes of feline anemia: old and new? Proceedings: ACVIM. Accessed via: Veterinary Information Network. http://goo.gl/N1GTZ

Epstein, K., N. Cohen, et al. (2004). Pharmacokinetics, stability, and retrospective analysis of use of an oral gel formulation of the bovine injectable enrofloxacin in horses. *Vet Therapeutics* 5(2): 155–167.

Flammer, K. (2006). Antibiotic drug selection in companion birds. *Journal of Exotic Pet Medicine* 15(3): 166–176.

Gandolf, A., M. Papich, et al. (2005). Pharmacokinetics after intravenous, subcutaneous and oral administration of enrofloxacin to alpacas. *AJVR* 66(5): 767–771.

Gauvin, J. (1993). Drug therapy in reptiles. *Seminars in Avian & Exotic Med* 2(1): 48–59.

Greene, C., K. Hartmannn, et al. (2006). Appendix 8: Antimicrobial Drug Formulary. *Infectious Disease of the Dog and Cat.* C Greene Ed., Elsevier: 1186–1333.

Haggett, E.F. & W.D. Wilson (2008). Overview of the use of antimicrobials for the treatment of bacterial infections in horses. *Equine Veterinary Education* 20(8): 433–448.

Hardie, E. (2000). Therapeutic Mangement of Sepsis. *Kirk's Current Veterinary Therapy: XIII Small Animal Practice.* J Bonagura Ed. Philadelphia, WB Saunders: 272–275.

Hayes, P. (2000). Diseases of Chinchillas. *Kirk's Current Veterinary Therapy: XIII Small Animal Practice.* J Bonagura Ed. Philadelphia, WB Saunders: 1152–1157.

Ivey, E. & J. Morrisey (2000). Therapeutics for Rabbits. *Vet Clin NA: Exotic Anim Pract* 3:1(Jan): 183–216.

Jenson, J. (1998). Current ratite therapy. *The Veterinary Clinics of North America: Food Animal Practice* 16:3(November).

Monks, D. & M. Cowan (2009). Chronic respiratory disease in rats. Proceedings: AAVC-UEP. Accessed via: Veterinary Information Network. http://goo.gl/BPUjq

Smith, A. (2000). General husbandry and medical care of hedgehogs. *Kirk's Current Veterinary Therapy: XIII Small Animal Practice.* J Bonagura Ed. Philadelphia, WB Saunders: 1128–1133.

Trepanier, L. (2008). Top Ten Potential Drug Interactions in Dogs and Cats. Proceedings: WSAVA. Accessed via: Veterinary Information Network. http://goo.gl/CRszS

Williams, B. (2000). Therapeutics in Ferrets. *Vet Clin NA: Exotic Anim Pract* 3:1(Jan): 131–153.

EPHEDRINE SULFATE

(e-*fed*-rin)

SYMPATHOMIMETIC
   BRONCHODILATOR/VASOPRESSOR

Prescriber Highlights

▶ Sympathomimetic used primarily for oral treatment of urinary incontinence & topically for nasal uses; parenterally as an indirect acting catecholamine pressor agent

▶ Contraindications: Severe CV disease, especially with arrhythmias

▶ Caution: Patients with glaucoma, prostatic hypertrophy, hyperthyroidism, diabetes mellitus, cardiovascular disorders or hypertension

▶ Adverse Effects: CNS stimulation, tachycardia, hypertension, or anorexia

▶ Excreted into milk, may affect neonates

Uses/Indications

Ephedrine is used chiefly for the treatment of urethral sphincter hypotonus and resulting incontinence in dogs and cats. It has also been used in an attempt to treat nasal congestion and/or bronchoconstriction in small animals. It can also be used parenterally as a pressor agent in the treatment of shock or anesthesia-associated hypotension.

Pharmacology/Actions

While the exact mechanism of ephedrine's actions are undetermined, it is believed that it indirectly stimulates both alpha-, beta$_1$-, beta$_2$-adrenergic receptors by causing the release of norepinephrine. Prolonged use or excessive dosing frequency can deplete norepinephrine from its storage sites and tachyphylaxis (decreased response) may ensue. Tachyphylaxis has not been documented in dogs or cats, however, when used for urethral sphincter hypotonus.

Pharmacologic effects of ephedrine include: increased vasoconstriction, heart rate, coronary blood flow, blood pressure, mild CNS stimulation, and decreased bronchoconstriction, nasal congestion and appetite. Ephedrine can also increase urethral sphincter tone and produce closure of the bladder neck; its principle veterinary indications are as a result of these effects.

Pharmacokinetics

Ephedrine is rapidly absorbed after oral or parenteral administration. Although not confirmed, ephedrine is thought to cross both the blood-brain barrier and the placenta. Ephedrine is metabolized in the liver and excreted unchanged in the urine. Urine pH may significantly alter excretion characteristics. In humans: at urine pH of 5, half-life is about 3 hours; at urine pH of 6.3, half-life is about 6 hours.

Contraindications/Precautions/Warnings

Ephedrine is contraindicated in patients with severe cardiovascular disease, particularly with arrhythmias. Ephedrine should be used with caution in patients with glaucoma, prostatic hypertrophy, hyperthyroidism, diabetes mellitus, cardiovascular disorders or hypertension.

When administered IV, administration rate should not exceed 10 mg/minute (in humans); it is suggested to scale the rate for veterinary patients.

Adverse Effects

Most likely side effects include restlessness, irritability, tachycardia, or hypertension. Anorexia may be a problem in some animals.

Tachyphylaxis (decreased response to subsequent doses) secondary to depleted stores of endogenous norepinephrine can occur with repeated doses.

Reproductive/Nursing Safety

Ephedrine's effects on fertility, pregnancy or fetal safety are not known. Use with caution during pregnancy. The drug is excreted in milk and may have deleterious effects on nursing animals. In humans, the FDA categorizes this drug as category *C* for use during pregnancy (*Animal studies have shown an adverse effect on the fetus, but there are no adequate studies in humans; or there are no animal reproduction studies and no adequate studies in humans.*)

Ephedrine is excreted in milk. If ephedrine is absolutely necessary for the dam, consider using milk replacer.

Overdosage/Acute Toxicity

Clinical signs of overdosage may consist of an exacerbation of the adverse effects listed above or, if a very large overdose, severe cardiovascular (hypertension to rebound hypotension, bradycardias to tachycardias, and cardiovascular collapse) or CNS effects (stimulation to coma) can be seen.

If the overdose was recent, empty the stomach using the usual precautions and administer charcoal and a cathartic. Treat clinical signs supportively as they occur.

Drug Interactions

The following drug interactions have either been reported or are theoretical in humans or animals receiving ephedrine and may be of significance in veterinary patients:

■ **ACEPROMAZINE (and other PHENOTHIAZINES):** Phenothiazines block alpha-adrenergic receptors; concomitant epinephrine or ephedrine can lead to unopposed beta-activity causing vasodilation and increased cardiac rate.

■ **ALPHA-BLOCKERS (***e.g.***, phentolamine, prazosin):** May negate the therapeutic effects of ephedrine

■ **ANESTHETICS, GENERAL:** An increased risk of arrhythmias developing can occur if ephedrine is administered to patients who have received cyclopropane or a halogenated hydrocarbon anesthetic agent. Propranolol may be administered should these occur.

■ **BETA-BLOCKERS:** Concomitant use of ephedrine with beta-blockers may diminish the effects of both drugs

■ **DIGOXIN:** An increased risk of arrhythmias may occur if ephedrine is used concurrently with digitalis glycosides.

■ **MONAMINE OXIDASE INHIBITORS** (including **amitraz**): Ephedrine should not be given within two weeks of a patient receiving monoamine oxidase inhibitors; severe hypertension, hyperpyrexia possible

■ **SYMPATHOMIMETIC AGENTS, OTHER:** Ephedrine should not be administered with other sympathomimetic agents (**e.g., phenylpropanolamine**) as increased toxicity may result

■ **RESERPINE:** May reverse the pressor effects of ephedrine

■ **THEOPHYLLINE:** Ephedrine may increase the risk for theophylline toxicity

■ **TRICYCLIC ANTIDEPRESSANTS:** May decrease the pressor effects of ephedrine

■ **URINARY ALKALINIZERS (e.g., sodium bicarbonate, citrates, carbonic anhydrase inhibitors):** May reduce the urinary excretion of ephedrine and prolong its duration of activity. Dosage adjustments may be required to avoid toxic clinical signs.

■ **Laboratory Considerations**

■ Beta-adrenergic agonists may decrease **serum potassium** concentrations. Clinical relevance is unknown.

Doses

■ **DOGS:**

For treatment of bronchospasm:

a) For maintenance therapy: 1–2 mg/kg PO q8–12h (McKiernan 1992)

b) 2 mg/kg PO q8–12h (Bonagura 1994)

For treatment of urinary incontinence responsive to adrenergic drugs:

a) 5–15 mg (total dose) PO q8h (Labato 1994)

b) 1.2 mg/kg PO q8h or 5–15 mg (total dose) PO q8h (Bartges 2003)

For treatment of hypotension associated with anesthesia:

a) 0.03–0.1 mg/kg IV bolus. Dilute 5 mg in 10 mL of saline and give the lower dosage first as sinus tachycardia may accompany the higher dose. May repeat in 5 minutes after first dose if hypotension does not improve. (Pablo 2003)

b) 0.1–0.25 mg/kg IV bolus (Mazzaferro 2005)

c) For relatively short procedures in ASA I or II patients when hypotension is not

responsive to 1 or 2 crystalloid boluses: 0.1–0.2 mg/kg IV bolus; duration of action is approximately 15-60 minutes after a single bolus. (Teixereia Neto 2009)

d) Can give 0.15–0.25 mg/kg diluted into 5 mL of a balanced electrolyte solution or saline and give small increment IV boluses until desirable blood pressure achieved. Can also give as a CRI at 5–10 micrograms/kg/minute. (Ko 2009)

■ **CATS:**

For treatment of bronchospasm:

a) For emergency treatment 2–5 mg PO (McKiernan 1992)

For treatment of urinary incontinence responsive to adrenergic drugs:

a) 2–4 mg (total dose) PO q8h (Labato 1994)

b) 2–4 mg/kg PO q6–12h or 2–4 mg (total dose) PO q8h (Bartges 2003)

c) 2–4 mg per cat PO q8–12h (Polzin 2005)

For treatment of hypotension associated with anesthesia:

a) Can give 0.15–0.25 mg/kg diluted into 5 mL of a balanced electrolyte solution or saline and give small increment IV boluses until desirable blood pressure achieved. Can also give as a CRI at 5–10 micrograms/kg/minute. (Ko 2009)

Monitoring

■ Clinical effectiveness

■ Adverse effects (see above)

Client Information

■ In order for this drug to be effective, it must be administered as directed by the veterinarian; missed doses will negate its effect. It may take several days for the full benefit of the drug to take place.

■ Contact veterinarian if the animal demonstrates ongoing changes in behavior (restlessness, irritability) or if incontinence persists or increases.

Chemistry/Synonyms

A sympathomimetic alkaloid, ephedrine sulfate occurs as fine, odorless, white crystals or powder. Approximately 770 mg are soluble in one mL of water. The commercially available injection has a pH of 4.5–7.

Ephedrine sulfate may also be known as ephedrine sulphate.

Storage/Stability

Store ephedrine sulfate products in tight, light resistant containers at room temperature unless otherwise directed.

When used parenterally, ephedrine sulfate is usually administered directly and not diluted.

Dosage Forms/Regulatory Status

VETERINARY-LABELED PRODUCTS: None
The ARCI (Racing Commissioners Interna-

tional) has designated this drug as a class 2 substance. See the appendix for more information.

HUMAN-LABELED PRODUCTS:

Ephedrine Sulfate Capsules: 25 mg; generic (West-Ward); (OTC)

Ephedrine Sulfate Injection: 50 mg/mL in 1 mL single-dose vials & preservative free in 1 mL single-dose amps; generic; (Rx)

In the USA, ephedrine sulfate is classified as a list 1 chemical (drugs that can be used as precursors to manufacture methamphetamine) and in some states it may be a controlled substance or have other restrictions placed upon its sale. Be alert to persons desiring to purchase this medication.

References

Bartges, J. (2003). Canine lower urinary tract cases. Proceedings: ACVIM Forum. Accessed via: Veterinary Information Network. http://goo.gl/HH41u

Bonagura, J. (1994). Bronchopulmonary disorders. *Saunders Manual of Small Animal Practice.* S Birchard and R Sherding Eds. Philadelphia, W.B. Saunders Company: 561–573.

Ko, J. (2009). Anesthesia monitoring techniques and management. Proceedings: ACVC. Accessed via: Veterinary Information Network. http://goo.gl/ff1Ab

Labato, M. (1994). Micturition Disorders. *Saunders Manual of Small Animal Practice.* S Birchard and R Sherding Eds. Philadelphia, W.B. Saunders Company: 857–864.

Mazzaferro, E. (2005). Anesthesia in critically ill patients. Proceedings: Western Vet Conf. Accessed via: Veterinary Information Network. http://goo.gl/rIa30

McKiernan, B. (1992). Current uses and hazards of bronchodilator therapy. *Current Veterinary Therapy XI: Small Animal Practice.* R Kirk and J Bonagura Eds. Philadelphia, W.B. Saunders Company: 515–518.

Pablo, L. (2003). Management of anesthesia complications. Proceedings: World Small Animal Veterinary Assoc World Congress. Accessed via: Veterinary Information Network. http://goo.gl/2H0bU

Polzin, D. (2005). Urinary Tract Therapeutics--What, When & How. Proceedings: ACVC. Accessed via: Veterinary Information Network. http://goo.gl/jRZ0n

Teixereia Neto, F. (2009). Intraoperative hypotension: a stepwise approach to treatment. Proceedings: WSAVA. Accessed via: Veterinary Information Network. http://goo.gl/B9VL9

EPINEPHRINE

(ep-i-*nef*-rin)   Adrenalin®

ALPHA- & BETA-ADRENERGIC AGONIST

Prescriber Highlights

▶ Alpha- & beta-adrenergic agonist agent used systemically for treating anaphylaxis & cardiac resuscitation

▶ Contraindications: Narrow-angle glaucoma, hypersensitivity to epinephrine, shock due to non-anaphylactoid causes, during general anesthesia with halogenated hydrocarbons, during labor (may delay the second stage), cardiac dilatation or coronary insufficiency; cases where vasopressor drugs are contraindicated (e.g., thyrotoxicosis, diabetes, hypertension, toxemia of pregnancy)

▶ Use extreme caution patients with a prefibrillatory cardiac rhythm

▶ Caution: Hypovolemia (not a substitute for adequate volume replacement)

▶ Do not inject with local anesthetics into small appendages of the body (e.g., toes, ears, etc.); may cause necrosis/sloughing

▶ Adverse Effects: Anxiety, tremor, excitability, vomiting, hypertension (overdosage), arrhythmias, hyperuricemia, & lactic acidosis (prolonged use or overdosage)

▶ Concentrations must not be confused

▶ Drug interactions

Uses/Indications

Epinephrine is employed primarily in veterinary medicine as a treatment for anaphylaxis or cardiac resuscitation. Because of its vasoconstrictive properties, epinephrine is added to local anesthetics to retard systemic absorption and prolong effect.

Pharmacology/Actions

Epinephrine is an endogenous adrenergic agent that has both alpha and beta activity. It relaxes smooth muscle in the bronchi and the iris, antagonizes the effects of histamine, increases glycogenolysis, and raises blood sugar. If given by rapid IV injection it causes direct stimulation of the heart (increased heart rate and contractility), and increases systolic blood pressure. If given slowly IV, it usually produces a modest rise in systolic pressure and a decrease in diastolic blood pressure. Total peripheral resistance is decreased because of beta effects.

Pharmacokinetics

Epinephrine is well-absorbed following IM or SC administration. IM injections are slightly faster absorbed than SC administration; absorption can be expedited by massaging the injection site. Epinephrine is rapidly metabolized in the GI tract and liver after oral administration and is not effective via this route. Following SC injection, the onset of action is generally within 5–10 minutes. The onset of action following IV administration is immediate and intensified.

Epinephrine does not cross the blood-brain barrier, but does cross the placenta and is distributed into milk.

Epinephrine's actions are ended primarily by the uptake and metabolism of the drug into sympathetic nerve endings. Metabolism takes place in both the liver and other tissues by monoamine oxidase (MAO) and catechol-O-methyltransferase (COMT) to inactive metabolites.

Contraindications/Precautions/Warnings

Epinephrine is contraindicated in patients with narrow-angle glaucoma, hypersensitivity to epinephrine, shock due to non-anaphylactoid causes, during general anesthesia with halogenated hydrocarbons or cyclopropane, during labor (may delay the second stage), and cardiac dilatation or coronary insufficiency. Epinephrine should also not be used in cases where vasopressor drugs are contraindicated (*e.g.*, thyrotoxicosis, diabetes, hypertension, toxemia of pregnancy). It should not be injected with local anesthetics into small appendages of the body (*e.g.*, toes, ears, etc.) because of the chance of necrosis and sloughing.

Use epinephrine with caution in cases of hypovolemia; it is not a substitute for adequate fluid replacement therapy. It should be used with extreme caution in patients with a prefibrillatory cardiac rhythm, because of its excitatory effects on the heart. While epinephrine's usefulness in asystole is well documented, it can cause ventricular fibrillation; use cautiously in cases of ventricular fibrillation.

Adverse Effects

Epinephrine can induce feelings of fear or anxiety, tremor, excitability, vomiting, hypertension (overdosage), arrhythmias (especially if patient has organic heart disease or has received another drug that sensitizes the heart to arrhythmias), hyperuricemia, and lactic acidosis (prolonged use or overdosage). Repeated injections can cause necrosis at the injection site.

Reproductive/Nursing Safety

In humans, the FDA categorizes this drug as category *C* for use during pregnancy (*Animal studies have shown an adverse effect on the fetus, but there are no adequate studies in humans; or there are no animal reproduction studies and no adequate studies in humans.*)

It is not known if this drug is excreted in milk.

Overdosage/Acute Toxicity

Clinical signs seen with overdosage or inadvertent IV administration of SC or IM dosages can include: sharp rises in systolic, diastolic, and venous blood pressures, cardiac arrhythmias, pulmonary edema and dyspnea, vomiting, headache, and chest pain. Cerebral hemorrhages may result because of the increased blood pressures. Renal failure, metabolic acidosis and cold skin may also result.

Because epinephrine has a relatively short duration of effect, treatment is mainly supportive. If necessary, the use an alpha-adrenergic blocker (*e.g.*, phentolamine) or a beta-adrenergic blocker (*e.g.*, propranolol) can be considered to treat severe hypertension and cardiac arrhythmias. Prolonged periods of hypotension may follow, which may require treatment with norepinephrine.

Drug Interactions

The following drug interactions have either been reported or are theoretical in humans or animals receiving epinephrine and may be of significance in veterinary patients:

- **ALPHA-BLOCKERS (*e.g.*, phentolamine, phenoxybenzamine, prazosin):** May negate the therapeutic effects of epinephrine

- **ALPHA-2 AGONISTS (*e.g.*, detomidine, dexmedetomidine, medetomidine, xylazine):** As epinephrine possesses alpha agonist effects, do NOT use to treat cardiac effects caused by alpha2 agonists

- **ANESTHETICS, GENERAL:** An increased risk of arrhythmias developing can occur if epinephrine is administered to patients who have received cyclopropane or a halogenated hydrocarbon anesthetic agent. Propranolol may be administered should these occur.

- **ANTIHISTAMINES:** Certain antihistamines (**diphenhydramine, chlorpheniramine, etc.**) may potentiate the effects of epinephrine

- **BETA-BLOCKERS:** Propranolol (or other beta-blockers) may potentiate hypertension, and antagonize epinephrine's cardiac and bronchodilating effects by blocking the beta effects of epinephrine

- **DIGOXIN:** An increased risk of arrhythmias may occur if epinephrine is used concurrently with digitalis glycosides

- **NITRATES:** May reverse the pressor effects of epinephrine

- **LEVOTHYROXINE:** May potentiate the effects of epinephrine

- **OXYTOCIC AGENTS:** Hypertension may result if epinephrine is used with oxytocic agents

- **SYMPATHOMIMETIC AGENTS, OTHER:** Epinephrine should not be administered with other sympathomimetic agents (*e.g.*, **isoproterenol**) as increased toxicity may result

- **PHENOTHIAZINES:** May reverse the pressor effects of epinephrine

- **RESERPINE:** May potentiate the pressor effects of epinephrine

■ **TRICYCLIC ANTIDEPRESSANTS:** May potentiate the effects of epinephrine

Doses

Note: Be certain when preparing injection that you do not confuse 1:1000 (1 mg/mL) with 1:10,000 (0.1 mg/mL) concentrations. To convert a 1:1000 solution to a 1:10,000 solution for IV or intratracheal use, dilute each mL with 9 mL of normal saline for injection. Epinephrine is only one aspect of treating cardiac arrest; refer to specialized references or protocols for more information.

■ **DOGS:**

Cardiac resuscitation (asystole):

a) Using the epinephrine first protocol: After the "ABC's" (airway, breathing, compressions) give epinephrine 0.01 mg/kg IV, continue ABCs for 3–5 minutes. If no response (return to spontaneous circulation; ROSC), vasopressin at 0.2–0.8 Units/kg IV, continue ABC's for 3–5 minutes. If no ROSC, epinephrine 0.01 mg/kg IV, continue ABC's for 3–5 minutes.

Using the vasopressin first protocol: After the "ABC's" (airway, breathing, compressions) give vasopressin 0.2–0.8 Units/kg IV, continue ABCs for 3-5 minutes. If no response (return to spontaneous circulation; ROSC), epinephrine 0.01 mg/kg IV, continue ABC's for 3 -5 minutes. If no ROSC, repeat epinephrine 0.01 mg/kg IV, continue ABC's for 3 -5 minutes.

For either protocol, the authors suggest trying atropine 0.04 mg/kg IV and/or naloxone 0.02–0.04 mg/kg IV. (Scroggin & Quandt 2009)

b) Both high dose (0.1–0.2 mg/kg) and low dose (0.01–0.02 mg/kg) IV or IO epinephrine have been advocated. In human medicine, generally the low dose is attempted first and if no response go to the high dose. In veterinary medicine (at present), either dose seems acceptable. Doses may be repeated at 3–5 minute intervals if there is no response. (Drobatz 2004)

c) 0.01–0.02 mg/kg IV every 3-5 minutes or 0.03–0.1 mg/kg IT (dilute in 5-10 mL of sterile water or normal saline). (Lopez Quintana 2009)

d) Neonates, when respiratory support and chest compression fails to elicit a heartbeat: Epinephrine at 0.1–0.3 mg/kg IV or IO. (Traas 2009)

For anaphylaxis:

a) 0.01–0.02 mg/kg IV; or the dosage may be doubled and given via the endotracheal tube if IV line is not yet established. In less severe cases, may be given IM or SC (Cohen 1995)

b) 0.2–0.5 mg (total dose) SC or IM (Wohl 2005)

c) For bronchoconstriction: 20 micrograms/kg (0.02 mg/kg) IV, IM, SC, or IT (Johnson 2000)

For treatment of hypotension associated with anesthesia:

a) As a last line of defense: 1–10 micrograms/kg/minute CRI. (Ko 2009)

b) 0.05–0.4 micrograms/kg/min IV (Dodam 2005), (Mazzaferro 2005)

■ **CATS:**

For cardiopulmonary-cerebral resuscitation:

a) See the Dog dose (Scroggin & Quandt 2009) above.

b) Neonates, when respiratory support and chest compression fails to elicit a heartbeat: Epinephrine at 0.1–0.3 mg/kg IV or IO. (Traas 2009)

For bronchoconstriction/anaphylaxis:

a) 0.01–0.02 mg/kg IV; or the dosage may be doubled and given via the endotracheal tube if IV line is not yet established. In less severe cases, may be given IM or SC. (Cohen 1995)

b) 20 micrograms/kg (0.02 mg/kg) IV, IM, SC, or IT (Johnson 2000)

■ **BIRDS:**

a) 0.1 mg/kg IV or intracardiac (Harris 2003)

■ **HORSES:** (**Note:** ARCI UCGFS Class 2 Drug)

For anaphylaxis:

a) 3–5 mL of 1:1,000 per 450 kg of body weight either IM or SC; For foal resuscitation: 0.1 mL/kg of 1:1,000 IV (preferably diluted with saline) (Robinson 1987)

For cardiopulmonary resuscitation of newborn foals:

a) 0.01–0.02 mg/kg (0.5–1 mL of a 1:1000 solution for a 50 kg foal) IV every 3 minutes until return of spontaneous circulation. If given intratracheally (IT), dose is 0.1–0.2 mL/kg. (Corley 2003)

■ **RUMINANTS, SWINE:**

For treatment of anaphylaxis:

a) 0.5–1 mL/100 lbs. body weight of 1:1,000 SC or IM; dilute to 1:10,000 if using IV; may be repeated at 15 minute intervals Often used in conjunction with corticosteroids and diphenhydramine (Clark 1986)

Monitoring

■ Cardiac rate/rhythm
■ Respiratory rate/auscultation during anaphylaxis
■ Urine flow, if possible
■ Blood pressure and blood gases, if indicated and possible

Client Information

■ Pre-loaded syringes containing an appropriate amount of epinephrine may be dispensed to clients for treatment of anaphylaxis in animals with known hypersensitivity.

■ Anaphylactic clinical signs (depending on species) should be discussed.

■ Clients should be instructed in proper injection technique (IM or SC) and storage conditions for epinephrine.

■ Do not use epinephrine if it is outdated, discolored, or contains a precipitate.

Chemistry/Synonyms

An endogenous catecholamine, epinephrine occurs as white to nearly white, microcrystalline powder or granules. It is only very slightly soluble in water, but it readily forms water-soluble salts (e.g., HCl) when combined with acids. Both the commercial products and endogenous epinephrine are in the Levo form, which is about 15 times more active than the dextro-isomer. The pH's of commercial injections are from 2.5–5.

Epinephrine is commonly called adrenalin.

Storage/Stability

Epinephrine HCl for injection should be stored in tight containers protected from light. Epinephrine will darken (oxidation) upon exposure to light and air. Do not use the injection if it is pink, brown, or contains a precipitate. The stability of the injection is dependent on the form and the preservatives present and may vary from one manufacturer to another. Epinephrine is rapidly destroyed by alkalies, or oxidizing agents.

Compatibility/Compounding Considerations

Epinephrine HCl is reported to be physically **compatible** with the following intravenous solutions and drugs: Dextran 6% in dextrose 5%, Dextran 6% in normal saline, dextrose-Ringer's combinations, dextrose-lactated Ringer's combinations, dextrose-saline combinations, dextrose 2.5%, dextrose 5% (becomes unstable at a pH >5.5), dextrose 10%, Ringer's injection, lactated Ringer's injection, normal saline, and sodium lactate 1/6 M, amikacin sulfate, cimetidine HCl, dobutamine HCl, metaraminol bitartrate, and verapamil HCl.

Epinephrine HCl is reported to be physically **incompatible** with the following intravenous solutions and drugs: Ionosol-D-CM, Ionosol-PSL (Darrow's), Ionosol-T with dextrose 5% (**Note:** other Ionosol products are compatible), sodium chloride 5%, and sodium bicarbonate 5%, aminophylline, cephapirin sodium, hyaluronidase, mephentermine sulfate, sodium bicarbonate, and warfarin sodium. Compatibility is dependent upon factors such as pH, concentration, temperature, and diluent used; consult specialized references or a hospital pharmacist for more specific information.

Dosage Forms/Regulatory Status

VETERINARY-LABELED PRODUCTS:

Epinephrine HCl for Injection 1 mg/mL (1:1,000) in 1 mL amps and syringes and 10 mL, 30 mL and 100 mL vials; *Amtech® Epinephrine Injection USP* (Phoenix Scientific); *Am-Vet® Epinephrine 1:000* (Neogen); Epinephrine (Vedco, Vet Tek); *Epinject®* (Vetus); *Epinephrine 1:000* (AgriPharm, Durvet, Bimeda, Butler, Phoenix Pharmaceutical); Epinephrine Injection (AgriLabs); (Rx). Labeled for dogs, cats, cattle, horses, sheep and swine.

The ARCI (Racing Commissioners International) has designated this drug as a class 2 substance. See the appendix for more information.

HUMAN-LABELED PRODUCTS:

Epinephrine HCl Solution for Injection: 1 mg/mL (1:1,000) in 1 mL amps & 30 mL vials (may contain sulfites);& 1 mL (with sodium bisulfite) & 30 mL (with chlorobutanol & sodium bisulfate) vials; *Adrenalin Chloride®* (JHP); generic; (Abbott); (Rx)

Epinephrine HCl Solution for Injection: 1:1,000 (0.3 mg/0.3 mL); in prefilled single-dose syringes (may contain sodium metabisulfite); 0.3 mL single-dose auto-injectors with sodium bisulfite; in dual-dose auto-injectors with chlorobutanol & sodium bisulfite; *EpiPen®* (Dey); *Twinject®* (Sciele); generic; (Rx)

Epinephrine HCl Solution for Injection: 1:1,000 (0.15 mg/0.15 mL) in dual-dose auto-injectors with chlorobutanol & sodium bisulfite; *Twinject®* (Sciele); (Rx)

Epinephrine HCl Solution for Injection: 1:2,000 (0.15 mg/0.3 mL) with sodium metabisulfite in 0.3 mL single dose auto-injectors; *EpiPen Jr®* (Dey); (Rx)

Epinephrine HCl Solution for Injection: 1:10,000 (0.1 mg/mL as hydrochloride & may contain sulfites in 10 mL syringes & vials; generic; (Rx)

Epinephrine bitartrate is available as a powder form (aerosol) for inhalation, topical solution and a solution for nebulization; ophthalmic preparations are available.

References

Clark, D.R. (1986). Diseases of the general circulation. *Current Veterinary Therapy: Food Animal Practice 2.* JL Howard Ed. Phialdelphia, W.B. Saunders: 694–696.

Cohen, R. (1995). Systemic Anaphylaxis. *Kirk's Current Veterinary Therapy:XII.* J Bonagura Ed. Philadelphia, W.B. Saunders: 150–152.

Corley, K. (2003). Cardiopulmonary resuscitation of the newborn foal. Proceedings: ACVIM Forum. Accessed via: Veterinary Information Network. http://goo.gl/ UGiTA

Dodam, J. (2005). Recognizing and treating hypotension. Proceedings: Western Vet Conf. Accessed via: Veterinary Information Network. http://goo.gl/x7pFx

Drobatz, K. (2004). Cardiopulmonary/cerebral resuscitation. Proceedings: ACVC. Accessed via: Veterinary Information Network. http://goo.gl/jOhPz

Harris, D. (2003). Emergency management of acute illness

and trauma in avian patients. Proceedings: Atlantic Coast Veterinary Conference. Accessed via: Veterinary Information Network. http://goo.gl/EdaFf

Johnson, L. (2000). Diseases of the Bronchus. *Textbook of Veterinary Internal Medicine: Diseases of the Dog and Cat.* S Ettinger and E Feldman Eds. Philadelphia, WB Saunders. 2: 1055–1061.

Ko, J. (2009). Anesthesia monitoring techniques and management. Proceedings: ACVC. Accessed via: Veterinary Information Network. http://goo.gl/ff1Ab

Lopez Quintana, A. (2009). What's new in CPCR? Proceedings: WSAVA. Accessed via: Veterinary Information Network. http://goo.gl/qQZxB

Mazzaferro, E. (2005). Anesthesia in critically ill patients. Proceedings: Western Vet Conf. Accessed via: Veterinary Information Network. http://goo.gl/rIa30

Robinson, N.E. (1987). Table of Common Drugs: Approximate Doses. *Current Therapy in Equine Medicine, 2.* NE Robinson Ed. Philadelphia, W.B. Saunders: 761.

Scroggin, R.D. & J. Quandt (2009). The use of vasopressin for treating vasodilatory shock and cardiopulmonary arrest. *Journal of Veterinary Emergency and Critical Care* 19(2): 145–157.

Traas, A. (2009). Pediatric Emergencies. Peroceedings: IVECCS. Accessed via: Veterinary Information Network. http://goo.gl/DZjjO

Wohl, J. (2005). Vasopressors in vasodilatory shock. Proceedings: IVECCS. Accessed via: Veterinary Information Network. http://goo.gl/dWIKx

EPOETIN ALFA
ERYTHROPOIETIN

(eh-*poe*-ee-tin *al*-fah)
EPO, rHuEPO, Epogen®, Procrit®
ERYTHROPOETIC AGENT

Prescriber Highlights

▶ Hormone that regulates erythropoiesis; used for anemia associated with chronic renal failure

▶ Contraindications: Patients with uncontrolled hypertension or in those who are hypersensitive to it; formation of significant autoantibodies with prior treatment

▶ Adverse Effects: Autoantibodies with resultant resistance to treatment, vomiting, hypertension, seizures, uveitis, iron depletion (iron supplementation often used), local reactions at injection sites, fever, arthralgia, & mucocutaneous ulcers

▶ Adequate monitoring vital

Uses/Indications

rHuEPO (human recombinant erythropoietin has been used to treat dogs and cats for anemia associated with chronic renal failure. Some clinicians state that because of the expense and potential risks (especially formation of antibodies to erythropoietin) associated with its use, it is more often now considered a "last ditch effort" and PCV's should be in the "teens" before considering EPO therapy. It is hoped that canine

and feline recombinant products will become available commercially in the future to reduce autoantibody formation concerns. Additionally, EPO may be demonstrated in the future to have benefits in reducing the number or volume of transfusions, or as a neuroprotective agent.

Pharmacology/Actions

Erythropoietin is a naturally occurring substance produced in the kidney and considered a hormone as it regulates erythropoiesis. It stimulates erythrocyte production by stimulating the differentiation and proliferation of committed red cell precursors. EPO also stimulates the release of reticulocytes.

Recombinant Human EPO alfa (r-HuEPO-alpha) serves as a substitute for endogenous EPO, primarily in patients with renal disease. Various uremic toxins may be responsible for the decreased production of EPO by the kidney.

Pharmacokinetics

EPO is only absorbed after parenteral administration. It is unclear whether the drug crosses the placenta or enters milk. The drug's metabolic fate is unknown. In patients with chronic renal failure, half-lives are prolonged approximately 20% over those with normal renal function. Depending on initial hematocrit and dose, correction of hematocrit may require 2–8 weeks.

Contraindications/Precautions/Warnings

EPO is contraindicated in patients with uncontrolled hypertension or in those who are hypersensitive to it (see Adverse Effects below). EPO cannot be recommended for use in equines. In animals with moderate to severe hypertension or iron deficiency, therapy should be started with caution or withheld until corrected.

Patients receiving EPO, generally require exogenous administration of iron supplements.

Adverse Effects

In dogs and cats, the most troublesome aspect of EPO therapy is the development of autoantibodies (20–70% incidence) with resultant resistance to further treatment. Perhaps up to 30% of all patients will develop antibodies significant enough to cause profound anemia, arrestment of erythropoiesis, and transfusion dependency. Should a patient develop refractory anemia while receiving adequate EPO doses and have normal iron metabolism, a bone marrow aspirate should be considered. A myeloid:erythroid ratio of greater than 6 predicts significant autoantibody formation and contraindicates further EPO therapy. Some clinicians believe that the drug (EPO) should be withdrawn if PCV starts to drop while on therapy.

Other effects reported include: systemic hypertension, high blood viscosity, seizures, and iron depletion. Local reactions at injection sites (which may be a predictor of antibody formation), fever, arthralgia, and mucocutaneous ulcers are also possible. Other effects that have been noted that may be a result of the animal's disease (or compounded by such), include cardiac disease (may be related to hypertension associated with chronic renal failure). In humans, hyperkalemia, seizures, and iron deficiency have been reported.

Therapy should be discontinued if any of the following are recognized: polycythemia, fever, anorexia, joint pain, cellulitis, cutaneous or mucosal ulceration (Cowgill 2002).

Reproductive/Nursing Safety

Some teratogenic effects (decrease in body weight gain, delayed ossification, etc.) have been noted in pregnant rats given high dosages. Rabbits receiving 500 mg/kg during days 6–18 of gestation showed no untoward effects on offspring; however, use during pregnancy only when benefits outweigh the potential risks. In humans, the FDA categorizes this drug as category *C* for use during pregnancy (*Animal studies have shown an adverse effect on the fetus, but there are no adequate studies in humans; or there are no animal reproduction studies and no adequate studies in humans.*)

It is not known whether epoetin alfa is excreted in milk, but it is unlikely to pose much risk to nursing offspring.

Overdosage/Acute Toxicity

Acute overdoses appear to be relatively free of adverse effects. Single doses of up to 1600 Units per kg in humans demonstrated no signs of toxicity. Chronic overdoses may lead to polycythemia or other adverse effects. Cautious phlebotomy may be employed should polycythemia occur.

Drug Interactions

The following drug interactions have either been reported or are theoretical in humans or animals receiving EPO and may be of significance in veterinary patients:

■ **ANDROGENS:** May increase the sensitivity of erythroid progenitors; this interaction has been used for therapeutic effect; (**Note:** This effect has not been confirmed in well-controlled studies nor has the safety of this combination been determined.)

■ **DESMOPRESSIN:** With EPO can decrease bleeding times

■ **PROBENECID:** Probenecid has been demonstrated to reduce the renal tubular excretion of EPO; clinical significance remains unclear at this time

Laboratory Considerations

■ No laboratory interactions of major clinical importance have been described.

Doses

■ **DOGS:**

As adjunctive therapy for the treatment of anemia associated with end-stage renal disease:

a) Initially, 100 Units/kg SC 3 times weekly, until the bottom of the target hematocrit

range of 37–45% is attained. Once the lower range of the target hematocrit is attained, the dosing interval is changed to twice weekly. As the hematocrit approaches the upper target value, reduce to once weekly. The dosage schedule is then further modified as required and EPO administered between one and three times weekly to maintain hematocrit within the target range.

A lower initial dosage of 50–100 Units/kg 3 times weekly may be used if slower response is acceptable and appropriate for the patient. If adequate control is not achieved within 8–12 weeks, then dose can be increased by an additional 25–50 Units/kg every 3–4 weeks while maintaining dosing interval at 3 times a week. Withhold treatment temporarily if hematocrit exceeds target range. Once hematocrit is reestablished at the upper limit of the target range, re-institute treatment at a lower dosing schedule. Do not adjust dosage or dosing interval more often than once every three weeks (due to the long lag time for a response). Generally, a maintenance dose of 75–100 Units/kg SC 1–2 times weekly is sufficient (not less than once per week, and not more than 3 times a week). Iron supplementation required. (Cowgill 2002)

b) Initially, 48.4–145 Units/kg SC three times a week. Most dogs and cats should be started at 97 Units/kg SC 3 times a week. Use high end dose initially when anemia is severe (HCT less than 14%) and low end dose if hypertension is present or when anemia is not severe. Monitor hematocrit weekly until a target hematocrit of 37–45% is reached. When hematocrit reaches low end of target decrease dosing to two times weekly. Continue monitoring and adjusting dose and frequency as necessary, but take lag phase into account and do not adjust too rapidly. If animal requires >145 Units/kg three times a week, evaluate for epoetin resistance. Oral iron supplements recommended for all patients on epoetin. (Polzin *et al.* 2000)

■ **CATS:**

As adjunctive therapy for the treatment of anemia associated with end-stage renal disease:

a) As above (for each specific author), but the target hematocrit is: 30–40%. (Cowgill 2002), (Polzin *et al.* 2000)

b) Consider using epoetin when PCV is <20%; dose at 75–100 Units/kg SC three times a week until PCV is in the low normal range (35%), then reduce dose and frequency to 50–75 Units/kg two times per week. Monitor PCV and blood pressure. It is important to administer iron at start of regime and until appetite is good. (Scherk 2003)

c) Cats with problematic clinical signs and PCV <20%: Initially, 100 Units/kg SC 3 times per week. Iron deficiency is avoided by monitoring serum iron and total iron binding capacity and providing oral supplementation with ferrous sulfate (5–50 mg per cat per day). When lower end of the target PCV range (30-40%) is reached, reduce to twice per week. Depending upon the severity of anemia, it may require 3-4 weeks for the PCV to enter the target range. Up to 50% of treated dogs and cats develop antibodies after 1 to 3 months of treatment. (Chew 2009)

■ **FERRETS:**
a) 50–150 Units/kg IM 3 times weekly; may decrease to once weekly if RBC indices are significantly improved (Williams 2000)

■ **RABBITS/RODENTS/SMALL MAMMALS:**
a) **Rabbits:** 50–150 Units/kg SC every 2–3 days until PVC is normal; then once weekly (q7 days) for at least 4 weeks (Ivey & Morrisey 2000)

Monitoring

■ Hematocrit; PCV; (Initially weekly to every other week for 2–4 months, then when dose and Hct are stable, at 1–2 month intervals)

■ Blood Pressure (initially, at least monthly then every 1–2 months thereafter)

■ Renal Function Status

■ Iron status (serum iron, TIBC), RBC indices (initially and regularly during therapy to insure adequate iron availability)

Client Information

■ For outpatient administration, training in proper injection techniques, drug handling and storage should be performed

Chemistry/Synonyms

A biosynthetic form of the glycoprotein human hormone erythropoietin, epoetin alfa (EPO) has a molecular weight of approximately 30,000. It is commercially available as a sterile, preservative-free, colorless solution. Sodium chloride solution is added to adjust tonicity and is buffered with sodium citrate or citric acid. Human albumin (2.5 mg per vial) is also added to the solution.

Epoetins may also be known by the following synonyms and internationally registered trade names: erythropoietin, r-HuEPO, BI-71.052 (epoetin gamma), BM-06.019 (epoetin beta), EPO (epoetin alfa), EPOCH (epoetin beta), *Bioyetin®*, *Culat®*, *Epogin®*, *Epomax®*, *Epopen®*, *Epotin®*, *Epoxitin®*, *Eprex®*, *Erantin®*, *Eritina®*, *Eritrogen®*, *Eritromax®*, *Erypo®*, *Espo®*, *Exetin-A®*, *Globuren®*, *Hemax®*, *Hemax-Eritron®*, *Hypercri®*, *Mepotin®*, *NeoRecormon®*,

Neorecormon®, *Procrit®*, *Pronivel®*, *Recormon®*, *Repotin®*, *Tinax®*, and *Wepox®*.

Storage/Stability

The injectable solution should be stored in the refrigerator (2-8°C); do not freeze. Do not shake the solution as denaturation of the protein with resultant loss of activity may occur. If light exposure is limited to 24 hours or less, no effects on potency should occur. When stored as directed, the solution has an expiration date of 2 years after manufacture. Do not mix with other drugs or use the same IV tubing with other drugs running. Because the solution contains no preservatives, the manufacturer recommends using each vial only as a single use.

Compatibility/Compounding Considerations

A method of diluting the Amgen product to facilitate giving very small dosages has been described (Grodsky 1994). Using a 1:20 dilution (1 part *Epogen®* to 19 parts bacteriostatic normal saline does not require any additional albumin to prevent binding of the drug to container). No data is available commenting on this dilution's stability.

Dosage Forms/Regulatory Status

VETERINARY-LABELED PRODUCTS: None
The ARCI (Racing Commissioners International) has designated this drug as a class 2 substance. It is also prohibited on the premises of a racing facility.

HUMAN-LABELED PRODUCTS:
Epoetin Alfa, Solution for Injection: 2000 Units/mL, 3000 Units/mL, 4000 Units/mL, 10,000 Units/mL, 20,000 Units/mL and 40,000 Units/mL in 1 mL and 2 mL (10,000 U only) both single-dose and multidose vials; *Epogen®* (Amgen), *Procrit®* (Ortho Biotech); (Rx)

References

Chew, D. (2009). Updates in treatment of chronic renal disease: What is most important? Proceedings: WVC. Accessed via: Veterinary Information Network. http://goo.gl/uJWQr

Cowgill, L. (2002). Anemia and hypertension: The ignored consequences of chronic renal failure, Proceedings: Tufts Animal Expo. Accessed via: Veterinary Information Network. http://goo.gl/AofHC

Grodsky, B. (1994, Last Update). "Personal Communication."

Ivey, E. & J. Morrisey (2000). Therapeutics for Rabbits. *Vet Clin NA: Exotic Anim Pract* 3:1(Jan): 183–216.

Polzin, D., C. Osborne, et al. (2000). Chronic renal failure. *Textbook of Veterinary Internal Medicine: Diseases of the Dog and Cat*. S Ettinger and E Feldman Eds. Philadelphia, WB Saunders. 2: 1634–1662.

Scherk, M.A. (2003). Therapeutic implications of recent findings in feline renal insufficiency. Proceedings: ACVIM Forum. Accessed via: Veterinary Information Network. http://goo.gl/bNxMX

Williams, B. (2000). Therapeutics in Ferrets. *Vet Clin NA: Exotic Anim Pract* 3:1(Jan): 131–153.

EPRINOMECTIN

(e-pri-no-*mek*-tin)   Ivomec® Eprinex®

TOPICAL AVERMECTIN ANTIPARASITIC AGENT

Prescriber Highlights

➤ Topically applied avermectin antiparasiticide for cattle

➤ Used as labeled; there are no milk or meat withdrawal times required

Uses/Indications

In cattle, eprinomectin is indicated for a variety gastrointestinal roundworms including adult and L4 stages of *Haemonchus placei, Ostertagia ostertagi, Trichostrongylus axei* and *colubriformis, Cooperia oncophora/punctata/surnabada, Nematodirus helvetianus, Oesophagostomum radiatum, Bunostomum phlebotomum,* and *Trichuris* spp. (adults only); cattle grubs; lice; mange mites; horn flies (for 7 days after treatment), and lungworms (*Dictyocaulus vivaparus*—for 21 days after treatment).Topical eprinomectin may be useful for the topical treatment of Psoroptic mange (*P. equi*) in horses or ear mites (*Psoroptes cuniculi*) in rabbits. One small study (6 subjects) showed partial response when rabbits were dosed at 5 mg/kg topically, twice at 14 day intervals. (Ulutas *et al.* 2005)

Pharmacology/Actions

Eprinomectin binds selectively to glutamate-gated chloride ion channels that occur in invertebrate nerve and muscle cells. This leads to an increase in cell membrane permeability to chloride ions, leading to paralysis and death of the parasite. Like ivermectin, eprinomectin enhances the release of gamma amino butyric acid (GABA) at presynaptic neurons. GABA acts as an inhibitory neurotransmitter and blocks the post-synaptic stimulation of the adjacent neuron in nematodes or the muscle fiber in arthropods. These compounds are generally not toxic to mammals as they do not have glutamate-gated chloride channels and do not readily cross the blood-brain barrier.

Pharmacokinetics

No information noted.

Contraindications/Precautions/Warnings

Do not give orally or intravenously.

Adverse Effects

No adverse reactions are listed on the product label. On the FDA's Cumulative Adverse Drug Experience database for topical administration on cattle, the three most common adverse experiences reported are: Ineffectiveness for parasite control, anorexia, and udder hypogalactia (Anon 2009). It must be noted that incidence rates are not listed and causal effect is not established for listings on this database.

Overdosage/Acute Toxicity

Calves given up to 5X dosage showed no signs of adverse effects. One subject (of 6) showed signs of mydriasis when given a 10X dose.

Drug Interactions

■ No interactions noted

Doses

■ **CATTLE:**
For labeled indications:
a) 1 mL per 10 kg (22 lb) body weight applied topically along backline in a narrow strip from the withers to the tailhead (Package Insert; *Ivomec® Eprinex®*—Merial)

■ **HORSES:**
For treatment of psoroptic (*P. equi*) mange:
a) 500 micrograms/kg (0.5 mg/kg) topically once weekly for 4 treatments. Author's suggest getting informed consent before use. (Ural *et al.* 2008)

Client Information

■ When used as labeled, there are no milk or meat withdrawal times required.

■ Weather conditions (including rainfall) during administration do not affect efficacy.

■ Do not apply to backline if covered with mud or manure.

■ Dispose of containers in an approved landfill or by incineration; do not contaminate water as eprinomectin may adversely affect fish and aquatic organisms.

Chemistry/Synonyms

A member of the avermectin-class of antiparasitic agents, eprinomectin is also known as MK-397 or 4-epi-acetylamino-4-deoxy-avermectin B1.

Storage/Stability

The commercially available product should be stored protected from light and kept at 86°F (30°C) or less. Storage up to 104°F (40°C) is permitted for a short period.

Dosage Forms/Regulatory Status

VETERINARY-LABELED PRODUCTS:

Eprinomectin Topical (Pour-On) Solution: 5 mg/mL in 250 mL/8.5 fl oz and 1 L/33.8 fl oz bottle with a squeeze-measure-pour-system, or a 2.5 L/84.5 fl oz and 5 L/169 fl oz collapsible pack for use with appropriate automatic dosing equipment; *Ivomec® Eprinex®* (Merial); (OTC). FDA-approved for use in beef or dairy cattle.

HUMAN-LABELED PRODUCTS: None

References

Anon (2009). "Cumulative Veterinary Adverse Drug Experience (ADE) Reports." 2010, http://www.fda.gov/AnimalVeterinary/SafetyHealth/ProductSafetyInformation/ucm055394.htm.

Ulutas, B., H. Voyvoda, et al. (2005). Efficacy of topical administration of eprinomectin for treatment of ear mite infestation in six rabbits. *Vet Derm* 16: 334–337.

Ural, K., B. Ulutas, et al. (2008). Eprinomectin treatment of psoroptic mange in hunter jumper and dressage horses: A prospective, randomized, double-blinded, placebo-controlled clinical trial. *Veterinary Parasitology* 156(3–4): 353–357.

Epsom Salts–see Magnesium Sulfate

EPSIPRANTEL

(ep-si-*pran*-tel)   Cestex®

CESTOCIDAL ANTIPARASITIC AGENT

Prescriber Highlights

▶ Oral cestocide for dogs & cats

▶ Not appreciably absorbed when given orally

▶ Not FDA-approved in puppies or kittens less than 7 weeks old

▶ Adverse Effects: GI (vomiting, diarrhea) possible

Uses/Indications

Epsiprantel is indicated for the treatment (removal) of *Dipylidium caninum* and *Taenia pisiformis* in dogs, and *Dipylidium caninum* and *Taenia taeniaeformis* in cats.

Pharmacology/Actions

Epsiprantel's exact mechanism of action against cestodes has not been determined. The tapeworm's ability to regulate calcium is apparently affected, causing tetany and disruption of attachment to the host. Alteration to the integument makes the worm vulnerable to digestion by the host animal.

Pharmacokinetics

Unlike praziquantel, epsiprantel is absorbed very poorly after oral administration and the bulk of the drug is eliminated in the feces. Less than 0.1% of the drug is recovered in the urine after dosing. No metabolites have thus far been detected.

Contraindications/Precautions/Warnings

There are no labeled contraindications to this drug, but the manufacturer states not to use it in puppies or kittens less than 7 weeks of age.

Adverse Effects

Adverse effects would be unexpected with this agent, although vomiting and/or diarrhea could potentially occur.

Reproductive/Nursing Safety

Safety for use in pregnant or breeding animals has not been determined, but teratogenic effects would be highly unlikely since the drug is so poorly absorbed.

Overdosage/Acute Toxicity

Acute toxicity resulting from an inadvertent overdose is highly unlikely. Doses as high as 36X the recommended dose resulted in vomiting in some of the kittens tested. Single doses of 36X

those recommended in dogs caused no adverse effects.

Drug Interactions/Laboratory Considerations

■ None reported; theoretically, prokinetic agents or fast acting laxatives may reduce the drug's efficacy

Doses

■ **DOGS:**

  a) 5.5 mg/kg (2.5 mg/lb) PO once; round up to the next larger tablet size (Package insert; *Cestex*®—Pfizer)

■ **CATS:**

  a) 2.75 mg/kg PO once. Cats up to 10 lb. should receive one 12.5 mg tablet; cats 11–20 lb. should receive one 25 mg tablet (Package insert; *Cestex*®—Pfizer)

Monitoring

■ Clinical efficacy

Client Information

■ Fasting is not required nor is it recommended before dosing

■ Because the worm may be partially or completely digested, worm fragments may not be seen in the feces after treatment.

■ A single dose is usually effective, but measures should be taken to prevent reinfection, particularly against *D. caninum*.

Chemistry/Synonyms

A pyrazino-benzazepine oral cesticide, epsiprantel occurs as a white powder that is sparingly soluble in water.

Epsiprantel may also be known as BRL-38705 or *Cestex*®.

Storage/Stability

Tablets should be stored at room temperature.

Dosage Forms/Regulatory Status

VETERINARY-LABELED PRODUCTS:

Epsiprantel Oral Tablets (Film-coated): 12.5 mg, 25 mg, 50 mg & 100 mg; *Cestex*® (Pfizer); (Rx). FDA-approved for use in dogs and cats.

HUMAN-APPROVED PRODUCTS: None

ERGOCALCIFEROL

(er-goh-kal-*sif*-er-ole)

Vitamin D2, Calciferol, Drisdol®

VITAMIN D ANALOG

Prescriber Highlights

▶ May be used to treat hypocalcemia associated with hypoparathyroidism, but DHT or calcitriol usually recommended first

▶ Less expensive than DHT or calcitriol, but takes large initial doses for effect, effects take longer to be seen, & if hypercalcemia develops, takes longer (up to 18 weeks) for toxicity relief

Uses/Indications

Ergocalciferol is sometimes used in dogs or cats to treat hypocalcemia secondary to parathyroid gland failure, particularly when dihydrotachysterol or calcitriol are too expensive for the owner. When compared to those agents, ergocalciferol takes longer to have a maximal effect on serum calcium. Additionally, if hypercalcemia should develop, ergocalciferol's effects persist longer than either calcitriol or dihydrotachysterol.

Pharmacology/Actions

Ergocalciferol is first hydroxylated in the liver to 25-hydroxyvitamin D (has some activity) and then activated in the kidneys to 1,25-dihydroxyvitamin D, the primary active form of the drug. Vitamin D is considered a hormone and, in conjunction with parathormone (PTH) and calcitonin, regulates calcium homeostasis in the body. Active analogues (or metabolites) of vitamin D enhance calcium and phosphate absorption from the GI tract, promote reabsorption of calcium by the renal tubules, and increase the rate of accretion and resorption of minerals in bone.

Pharmacokinetics

Specific pharmacokinetic values for dogs and cats were not located. But the following information (human-based) generally applies: In the presence of bile salts, ergocalciferol is absorbed from the small intestine; after conversion to its 25-hydroxylated form in the liver and kidneys, it is stored in the liver and fat. Cats do not appear to convert ergocalciferol to its 25-hydroxylate form as well as cholecalciferol. Several days of therapy may be required until distribution steady state is achieved. In dogs and cats, maximal effect on calcium homeostasis is usually noted from 5–21 days after treatment was begun; effects may persist for up to 18 weeks once treatment is discontinued (Feldman 2005).

Contraindications/Precautions/Warnings

Ergocalciferol, at therapeutic dosages, is contraindicated in patients with hypercalcemia, vitamin D toxicity, malabsorption syndrome, or abnormal sensitivity to the effects of vitamin D. It should be used with extreme caution in patients with hyperphosphatemia. As patients with kidney dysfunction may not convert ergocalciferol into the primary active metabolite, calcitriol or DHT would be preferred since they do not require activation by the kidney. Chronic therapy should not be initiated unless owners are willing to commit to ongoing patient monitoring.

Adverse Effects

The primary concern with using ergocalciferol is "overshooting" the dosage with resultant hypercalcemia and, potentially, hyperphosphatemia or nephrocalcinosis. Hypercalcemia can persist for weeks to months.

Reproductive/Nursing Safety

Hypervitaminosis D in pregnant females has been implicated in causing teratogenic effects in animals and infants. Potential benefits of therapy must be weighed against the risks if considering use in pregnant dogs or cats.

As large doses of vitamin D can be excreted into milk, consider using milk replacer in offspring of dams receiving therapeutic dosages of ergocalciferol.

Overdosage/Acute Toxicity

Because of the potential serious ramifications of overdoses, contacting an animal poison control center is strongly recommended. The toxic acute oral dose of ergocalciferol in dogs is reported as 4 mg/kg (160,000 Units/kg).

Acute ingestions should be managed using established protocols for removal or prevention of the drug being absorbed from the GI. Orally administered mineral oil may reduce absorption and enhance fecal elimination.

Hypercalcemia secondary to chronic dosing of the drug should be treated by first temporarily discontinuing it and exogenous calcium therapy. If the hypercalcemia is severe, furosemide, calcium-free IV fluids (*e.g.,* normal saline), urine acidification, and corticosteroids may be employed. Because of the long duration of action of ergocalciferol (potentially up to 18 weeks), hypercalcemia may persist. Restart therapy (if desired) at a reduced dosage only when calcium serum levels return to the normal range. Diligent monitoring is required.

Drug Interactions

The following drug interactions have either been reported or are theoretical in humans or animals receiving ergocalciferol and may be of significance in veterinary patients:

- **CORTICOSTEROIDS:** Can reduce the effects of vitamin D analogs
- **DIGOXIN or VERAPAMIL:** Patients on these drugs are sensitive to the effects of hypercalcemia; intensified monitoring is required
- **MINERAL OIL:** May reduce the amount of ergocalciferol absorbed
- **THIAZIDE DIURETICS:** May cause hypercalcemia when given in conjunction with Vitamin D analogs

Laboratory Considerations

- **Serum cholesterol** levels may be falsely elevated by vitamin D analogs when using the Zlatkis-Zak reaction for determination.

Doses

- **DOGS/CATS:**

  For maintenance therapy of parathyroid failure after using parenteral calcium to control hypocalcemic tetany:

  a) Dihydrotachysterol or calcitriol are preferred, but ergocalciferol is less expensive. If using ergocalciferol, patient should be hospitalized. Initially give ergocalcifer~~ ~~ 4000–6000 Units/kg PO once da~~ ~~ 1–5 days, parenteral calcium c~~ ~~ be discontinued. Patient sho~~ ~~

hospitalized until serum calcium concentration remains between 8–10 mg/dL without parenteral calcium support, then patient can be discharged. Continue ergocalciferol, but administer every other day. Weekly serum calcium concentrations should be performed and ergocalciferol dosage adjusted to maintain serum calcium concentrations between 8–9.5 mg/dL. Maintenance doses usually range from 1000–2000 Units/kg PO once daily to once weekly. Goal is to prevent hypocalcemic tetany, but not induce hypercalcemia. Once animal is stable, monthly rechecks for 6 months are strongly advised; then every 2–3 months thereafter. (Feldman 2005)

Monitoring

■ See dosage information above

Client Information

■ While ergocalciferol is less expensive than DHT or calcitriol, it is usually not recommended as it takes longer to have an effect and can persist in the body longer than DHT or calcitriol

■ Using vitamin D products may require lifelong treatment and regular laboratory monitoring

■ While this agent can treat low calcium, it can cause calcium levels in the blood to become too high; this effect can last for many weeks, even after the medication is discontinued

Chemistry/Synonyms

Ergocalciferol is obtained by irradiating (with ultraviolet light) ergosterol, a sterol present in fungi and yeasts. It occurs as white or almost white crystals or yellowish crystalline powder and is practically insoluble in water, but is soluble in fatty oils. One mg of ergocalciferol provides 40,000 Units of vitamin D activity.

Ergocalciferol may be known as calciferol, vitamin D2, viosterol, activated ergosterol, or irradiated ergosterol; there are many international trade names.

Storage/Stability

Ergosterol is sensitive to light, heat and air. Store capsules or liquid at room temperature (15–30°C) and protect from light.

Dosage Forms/Regulatory Status

VETERINARY-LABELED PRODUCTS: None

HUMAN-LABELED PRODUCTS:

Ergocalciferol Oral Liquid (Drops): 8,000 Units/mL (200 micrograms/mL) in 60 mL; *Drisdol® Drops* (Sanofi), *Calciferol® Drops* (Schwarz); generic; (OTC)

Ergocalciferol Oral Capsules: 50,000 Units (1.25 mg); *Drisdol®* (Sanofi), generic; (Rx)

References

Feldman, E. (2005). Disorders of the parathyroid glands. *Textbook of Veterinary Internal Medicine, 6th Ed.* S Ettinger and E Feldman Eds., Elsevier: 1508–1535.

ERTAPENEM SODIUM

(er-ta-*pen*-um)   Invanz®

CARBAPENEM ANTIBIOTIC

Prescriber Highlights

▶ Carbapenem antibiotic similar to imipenem & meropenem, but has narrower spectrum of activity

▶ Not effective against Pseudomonas or Acinetobacter

▶ May only need to be dosed once daily

▶ Very limited information available for use in dogs or cats; must be considered investigational

Uses/Indications

Ertapenem may be useful in treating resistant gram-negative bacterial infections, particularly when aminoglycoside use would be risky (*i.e.*, renal failure) or not effective (*i.e.*, resistance or CNS infections), and when meropenem is not available. While ertapenem has a broad spectrum, it is not active against *Pseudomonas aeruginosa*. It potentially could be useful against mixed anaerobic/gram-negative aerobic infections when *Pseudomonas* is not considered a likely pathogen.

Pharmacology/Actions

Ertapenem is a carbapenem antibiotic similar to imipenem and meropenem. Like other beta-lactams, it inhibits bacterial cell wall synthesis and is usually bactericidal.

Ertapenem has a broad antibacterial spectrum similar to that of imipenem, but it is more active against *Enterobacteriaceae* and anaerobes, has equivalent activity against gram-positive bacteria, and minimal activity against *Pseudomonas aeruginosa* and *Acinetobacter*. Methicillin-resistant *Staphylococci* and *Enterococcus* are usually resistant to ertapenem. Because ertapenem, like meropenem, is more stable than imipenem to renal dehydropeptidase I, it does not require the addition of cilastatin to inhibit that enzyme.

Pharmacokinetics

At the time of writing, no pharmacokinetic data was available for dogs or cats.

In humans, the drug must be administered parenterally as it is not appreciably absorbed after oral administration. Intramuscular bioavailability is about 90% and peak plasma levels occur in approximately 2.3 hours. Ertapenem exhibits concentration-dependent binding to human plasma proteins. At plasma concentrations of <100 micrograms/mL it is 95% bound; at 300 micrograms/mL, 85% bound. Ertapenem biotransformation is not dependent on hepatic mechanisms as the major metabolite (inactive) is formed by hydrolysis of the beta-lactam ring. Approximately 80% of an IV dose is excreted in the urine, evenly split between inactive metabolites and unchanged drug. Approximately 10% is excreted in the feces. In young, healthy adults, elimination half-life is about 4 hours; about 2.5 hours in pediatric patients.

Contraindications/Precautions/Warnings

Ertapenem is contraindicated in patients hypersensitive to it or other carbapenems and those that have developed anaphylaxis after receiving any beta-lactam antibiotic. It is contraindicated in patients hypersensitive to lidocaine or other amide-type local anesthetics (if used IM with 1% lidocaine as the diluent).

As ertapenem has not been widely used clinically in veterinary medicine and little information for use in dogs or cats is published, consider its use investigational.

Adverse Effects

The adverse effect profile for ertapenem in dogs or cats is unknown. In humans, intravenous injection site reactions are the most common adverse reaction. Gastrointestinal effects (nausea, vomiting, diarrhea), headache, or tachycardia have occasionally been reported. Rarely, hypersensitivity or CNS effects (hallucinations, agitation, seizures, etc.) have been seen.

Reproductive/Nursing Safety

Ertapenem has been shown to cross the placenta in rats, but no teratogenic effects have been reported. In humans, ertapenem is designated by the FDA as a category *B* drug (*Animal studies have not demonstrated risk to the fetus, but there are no adequate studies in pregnant women; or animal studies have shown an adverse effect, but adequate studies in pregnant women have not demonstrated a risk to the fetus during the first trimester of pregnancy, and there is no evidence of risk in later trimesters.*)

Although risk cannot be ruled out, it is likely that ertapenem is safe to use while nursing.

Overdosage/Acute Toxicity

Inadvertent overdoses are unlikely. Humans receiving 3 grams intravenously had an increased incidence of nausea and diarrhea. Should an overdose occur and adverse effects noted, treat supportively.

Drug Interactions

The following drug interactions have either been reported or are theoretical in humans or animals receiving ertapenem and may be of significance in veterinary patients:

■ **PROBENECID:** In humans, coadministration of ertapenem with probenecid can increase ertapenem AUC by 25% and elimination half-life by about 20%. Because of these relatively small effects, the manufacturer does not recommend using probenecid to extend the half-life of ertapenem.

Laboratory Considerations

■ No specific laboratory interactions or concerns were noted.

Doses

■ **DOGS/CATS:**
Note: There is very little information available regarding ertapenem use in dogs or cats and, therefore use must be considered investigational. If the drug is to be administered, it is suggested to use the human pediatric dose of 15 mg/kg IV or IM every 12 hours (not to exceed a daily dosage of 1 gram). Monitor the literature for additional data and recommendations.

Monitoring

■ Clinical efficacy (WBC, fever, etc.)

■ Adverse effects (potentially: GI, neurotoxicity, hypersensitivity); in humans receiving ertapenem for a prolonged period, hepatic, hematopoietic, and renal function are suggested for periodic assessment

Client Information

■ Clients should understand the investigational nature of using this drug in animals and that it should be administered only by veterinary professionals

Chemistry/Synonyms

Ertapenem sodium is a synthetic 1-(beta) methyl carbapenem antibiotic that occurs as a white to off-white, hygroscopic, crystalline powder. It is soluble in water and normal saline.

Ertapenem may also be known as L-749345, ML-0826, ZD-4433, ertapenemum or *Invanz®*.

Storage/Stability

The 1 gram injectable product contains approximately 6 mEq of sodium and 175 mg of sodium bicarbonate (as an excipient). It should be stored at temperatures at, or below, 25°C.

Compatibility/Compounding Considerations

For intravenous use, vial contents can be reconstituted with 10 mL of water for injection, bacteriostatic water for injection, or 0.9% sodium chloride injection. After shaking to dissolve the powder, immediately transfer to a 50 mL bag of 0.9% sodium chloride. Do not use diluents containing dextrose. Once reconstituted and diluted in normal saline for IV use, ertapenem is stable at room temperature for 6 hours. If refrigerated, it can be stored for 24 hours and used within 4 hours after removal from the refrigerator. Do not freeze reconstituted solutions.

If ertapenem is to be given IM, dilute the vial with 3.2 mL of 1% lidocaine HCl injection (*without epinephrine*). Use within one hour. Do not give IV.

Do not mix ertapenem with other medications or use IV solutions containing dextrose.

Dosage Forms/Regulatory Status

VETERINARY-LABELED PRODUCTS: None

HUMAN-LABELED PRODUCTS:

Ertapenem Sodium Lyophilized Powder for Injection: 1 g (as 1.045 g ertapenem) in single-dose vials; *Invanz®* (Merck); (Rx)

ERYTHROMYCIN
ERYTHROMYCIN ESTOLATE
ERYTHROMYCIN ETHYLSUCCINATE
ERYTHROMYCIN LACTOBIONATE

(er-ith-roe-*mye*-sin)   Gallimycin®

MACROLIDE ANTIBIOTIC

Prescriber Highlights

▶ Macrolide antibiotic; also used as a prokinetic agent

▶ Contraindicated in rabbits, gerbils, guinea pigs, & hamsters; oral use in ruminants, adult horses (?), hypersensitivity

▶ Adverse Effects: GI distress (oral), pain on IM injection; thrombophlebitis (IV), hyperthermia (foals). May cause neurological signs in dogs with MDR1 mutation.

▶ Many drug interactions possible

Uses/Indications

Erythromycin is FDA-approved for use to treat infections caused by susceptible organisms in swine, sheep, and cattle. It is often employed when an animal is hypersensitive to penicillins or if other antibiotics are ineffective against a certain organism.

Erythromycin, is still one of the treatments (with rifampin) for the treatment of *C. (Rhodococcus) equi* infections in foals, but many now use other macrolides (clarithromycin, azithromycin ± rifampin/rifampicin). Erythromycin estolate and microencapsulated base appear to be the most efficacious forms of the drug in foals due to better absorption and less frequent adverse effects.

Erythromycin may be used as a prokinetic agent to increase gastric emptying in dogs and cats. It may also be beneficial in treating reflux esophagitis.

Pharmacology/Actions

Erythromycin is usually a bacteriostatic agent, but in high concentrations or against highly susceptible organisms it may be bactericidal. The macrolides (erythromycin and tylosin) are believed to act by binding to the 50S ribosomal subunit of susceptible bacteria, thereby inhibiting peptide bond formation.

Erythromycin has *in vitro* activity against gram-positive cocci (staphylococci, streptococci), gram-positive bacilli (*Bacillus anthracis*, Corynebacterium, *Clostridium* spp.—not *C. difficile*, Listeria, Erysipelothrix), and some strains of gram-negative bacilli, including Haemophilus, Pasturella, and Brucella. Some strains of Actinomyces, Mycoplasma, Chlamydia, Ureaplasma, and Rickettsia are also inhibited by erythromycin. Most strains of the family Enterobacteriaceae (Pseudomonas, *E. coli*, Klebsiella, etc.) are resistant to erythromycin.

Erythromycin is less active at low pHs and many clinicians suggest alkalinizing the urine if using the drug to treat UTI's.

At sub-antimicrobial doses, erythromycin mimics the effects of motilin (cats, humans, rabbits) or 5-hydroxytryptophan$_3$ (5-HT$_3$) and stimulates migrating motility complexes and antegrade peristalsis. By inducing antral contractions, gastric emptying is enhanced. Erythromycin also increases lower esophageal pressure. Erythromycin is reported to stimulate colonic activity in dogs, but not in cats. Erythromycin's prokinetic mechanism of action in dogs is not completely understood, but probably is via activation of 5-HT$_3$ receptors. Prokinetic activity may diminish with chronic use (tachyphylaxis). It has been suggested that combining erythromycin with metoclopramide may be associated with less tachyphylaxis.

Pharmacokinetics

Erythromycin is absorbed after oral administration in the upper small intestine. Several factors can influence the bioavailability of erythromycin, including salt form, dosage form, GI acidity, food in the stomach, and stomach emptying time. Both erythromycin base and stearate are susceptible to acid degradation; enteric coatings are often used to alleviate this. Both the ethylsuccinate and estolate forms are dissociated in the upper small intestine and then absorbed. After IM or SC injection of the polyethylene-based veterinary product (*Erythro®-200; Gallimycin®-200*) in cattle, absorption is very slow. Bioavailabilities are only about 40% after SC injection and 65% after IM injection.

Erythromycin is distributed throughout the body into most fluids and tissues including the prostate, macrophages, and leukocytes. CSF levels are poor. In foals, erythromycin levels in bronchiolar lavage cells are equivalent to those found in the serum, but concentrations in pulmonary epithelial lining fluid are lower. Erythromycin may be 73–81% bound to serum proteins and the estolate salt, 96% bound. Erythromycin will cross the placenta; fetal serum levels are 5–20% of maternal levels. Erythromycin levels of about 50% of those found in the serum can be detected in milk. The volume of distribution for erythromycin in dogs is reportedly 2 L/kg; 3.7–7.2 L/kg in foals; 2.3 L/kg in mares; and 0.8–1.6 L/kg in cattle. In lactating dairy cattle, the milk to plasma ratio about 6–7.

Erythromycin is primarily excreted unchanged in the bile, but is also partly metabolized by the liver via N-demethylation to inactive metabolites. Some of the drug is reabsorbed after biliary excretion. Only about 2–5% of a dose is excreted unchanged in the urine.

The reported elimination half-life of erythromycin in various species is: 60–90 minutes in dogs and cats, 60–70 minutes in foals and mares, and 190 minutes in cattle.

Contraindications/Precautions/Warnings

Erythromycin is contraindicated in patients hypersensitive to it. In humans, the estolate form has been associated rarely with the development of cholestatic hepatitis. This effect has not apparently been reported in veterinary species, but the estolate should probably be avoided in patients with preexisting liver dysfunction.

As it may induce a toxic enterocolitis, erythromycin (and other macrolides) is contraindicated in rabbits, gerbils, guinea pigs, and hamsters.

Many clinicians believe that erythromycin is contraindicated in adult horses (see Adverse Effects below), and oral erythromycin should not be used in ruminants as severe diarrhea may result. Unless *R. equi* is confirmed, erythromycin should be used with caution in horses greater than 4 months old (Divers 2009).

Because erythromycin is implicated in causing hyperthermia/fatal respiratory distress in foals treated during hot weather, provision of shade and close observation is advised.

Adverse Effects

Adverse effects are relatively infrequent with erythromycin when used in small animals, swine, sheep, or cattle. When injected IM, local reactions and pain at the injection site may occur. Oral erythromycin may occasionally cause GI disturbances such as diarrhea, anorexia, and vomiting. Rectal edema and partial anal prolapse have been associated with erythromycin in swine. Intravenous injections must be given very slowly, as they can readily cause thrombophlebitis. Allergic reactions can occur but are thought to be rare.

A case of a dog with the mdr1 mutation developing neurological signs after receiving erythromycin has been reported.

Oral erythromycin should not be used in ruminants as severe diarrheas may result.

In foals treated with erythromycin, a mild, self-limiting diarrhea can occur; however, severe enterocolitis is possible. Erythromycin may alter temperature homeostasis in foals. Foals between the ages of 2–4 months old have been reported to develop hyperthermia with associated respiratory distress and tachypnea. Physically cooling off these animals has been successful in controlling this effect.

Adult horses may develop severe, sometimes fatal, diarrheas from erythromycin making the use of the drug in adults very controversial. Mares of foals treated with erythromycin have, on occasion, developed severe diarrhea/fatal colitis, possibly through contamination of feeders, water buckets, or via coprophagia.

When used as prokinetic agent, erythromycin may actually increase clinical signs of intestinal distress as it can stimulate emptying of larger food particles into the intestine than is normal.

Reproductive/Nursing Safety

While erythromycin has not demonstrated teratogenic effects in rats, and the drug is not thought to possess serious teratogenic potential, it should only be used during pregnancy when the benefits outweigh the risks. In humans, the FDA categorizes erythromycin and its salts, except ethylsuccinate, as category *B* for use during pregnancy (*Animal studies have not yet demonstrated risk to the fetus, but there are no adequate studies in pregnant women; or animal studies have shown an adverse effect, but adequate studies in pregnant women have not demonstrated a risk to the fetus in the first trimester of pregnancy, and there is no evidence of risk in later trimesters.*) In a separate system evaluating the safety of drugs in canine and feline pregnancy (Papich 1989), this drug is categorized as in class: *A* (*Probably safe. Although specific studies may not have proved the safety of all drugs in dogs and cats, there are no reports of adverse effects in laboratory animals or women.*)

In humans, the FDA categorizes erythromycin ethylsuccinate as category *C* for use during pregnancy (*Animal studies have shown an adverse effect on the fetus, but there are no adequate studies in humans; or there are no animal reproduction studies and no adequate studies in humans.*)

Erythromycin is excreted in milk and may concentrate (observed milk:plasma ratio of 0.5). Erythromycin is considered compatible with breastfeeding by the American Academy of Pediatrics.

Overdosage/Acute Toxicity

With the exception of the adverse effects outlined above, erythromycin is relatively non-toxic; however, shock reactions have been reported in baby pigs receiving erythromycin overdosages.

Drug Interactions

The following drug interactions have either been reported or are theoretical in humans or animals receiving erythromycin and may be of significance in veterinary patients:

- **AZOLE ANTIFUNGALS (ketoconazole, fluconazole, itraconazole):** Possible increased erythromycin levels

- **CISAPRIDE:** Erythromycin can inhibit the metabolism of cisapride and the manufacturer states that use of these drugs together (in humans) is contraindicated; however it has been reported that in one study in dogs, erythromycin did not alter the pharmacodynamics of cisapride (Trepanier 2008).

- **CHLORAMPHENICOL:** *in vitro* evidence of antagonism

- **CLINDAMYCIN, LINCOMYCIN:** *in vitro* evidence of antagonism

- **DIGOXIN:** Erythromycin may increase the serum level of digoxin
- **DILTIAZEM, VERAPAMIL:** May increase erythromycin levels
- **ERGOT ALKALOIDS:** Acute ergot toxicity possible
- **OMEPRAZOLE:** Erythromycin and omeprazole can increase the plasma levels of one another
- **SUCRALFATE:** May reduce the absorption of erythromycin; separate doses by two hours if possible
- **WARFARIN:** Erythromycin may potentiate the effects of oral anticoagulant drugs

Erythromycin can inhibit the metabolism of other drugs that use the CYP3A subfamily of the cytochrome P450 enzyme system. Depending on the therapeutic index of the drug(s) involved, therapeutic drug monitoring and/or dosage reduction may be required if the drugs must be used together. These drugs include:

- **ALFENTANIL**
- **BROMOCRIPTINE**
- **BUSPIRONE**
- **CARBAMAZEPINE**
- **CYCLOSPORINE**
- **DISOPYRAMIDE** (also risk of increased QT interval)
- **METHYLPREDNISOLONE**
- **MIDAZOLAM, ALPRAZOLAM, TRIAZOLAM**
- **QUINIDINE** (also risk of increased QT interval)
- **SILDENAFIL**
- **TACROLIMUS (systemic)**
- **THEOPHYLLINE**

Laboratory Considerations

- Erythromycin may cause falsely elevated values of **AST** (SGOT), and **ALT** (SGPT) when using colorimetric assays.
- Fluorometric determinations of **urinary catecholamines** can be altered by concomitant erythromycin administration.

Doses

- **DOGS:**
  For susceptible infections:
  a) 10−20 mg/kg PO three times daily (Aucoin 2000)
  b) For localized, soft tissue infections: 10−15 mg/kg PO q8h or 15−25 mg/kg PO q12h for 7−10 days;
  For systemic, bacteremia infections: 22 mg/kg PO or IV q8h for as long as necessary (Greene & Watson 1998)

  As a prokinetic agent:
  a) 0.5−1 mg/kg PO q8h (Hall & Washabau 2000), (Twedt 2008)

- **CATS:**
  For susceptible infections:
  a) 10−20 mg/kg PO three times daily (Aucoin 2000)
  b) For localized, soft tissue infections: 10−15 mg/kg PO q8h or 15−25 mg/kg PO q12h for 7−10 days;
  For systemic, bacteremia infections: 22 mg/kg PO or IV q8h for as long as necessary (Greene & Watson 1998)

  As a prokinetic agent:
  a) 0.5−1 mg/kg PO q8h (Hall & Washabau 2000)

- **FERRETS:**
  For susceptible infections:
  a) 10 mg/kg PO 4 times daily (Williams 2000)

- **BIRDS:**
  For susceptible infections:
  a) Oral suspension: 60 mg/kg PO q12h (Hoeffer 1995)
  b) **Ratites:** 5−10 mg/kg PO 3 times daily (Jenson 1998)

- **CATTLE:**
  For susceptible infections:
  a) 4−8 mg/kg IM q12−24h (Jenkins 1987)
  b) For bronchopneumonia and fibrinous pneumonia in cattle associated with bacteria sensitive to erythromycin and resistant to sulfas, penicillin G and tetracyclines: Using *Erythro-200*®: 44 mg/kg IM q24h usually for a maximum of 4 days. Inject no more than 10 mL at any one site. Do not inject at any site previously used. Severe local tissue reactions may occur. Recommend a 30-day slaughter withdrawal at this dosage. (Hjerpe 1986)

  For mastitis:
  a) Dry cow (using dry cow formula): Milk out affected quarter, clean and disinfect. Infuse contents of one syringe into each affected quarter at time of drying off. Close teat orifice with gentle pressure and massage udder.
  b) Lactating cow (using lactating cow formula): As above, but repeat after each milking for 3 milkings (Label directions; *Erythro*®-*Dry* and *Erythro*®-*36*—Ceva)

- **HORSES:**
  For treatment of *C. (Rhodococcus) equi* infections in foals:
  a) Erythromycin:15−25 mg/kg PO q12−24h daily, with Rifampin (5 mg/kg, PO q12h). Treatment may be necessary for 1−3 months. (Chaffin 2006)
  b) Erythromycin: 25 mg/kg PO q12h with rifampin: 3−5 mg/kg PO q12h. If rifampin use becomes cost prohibitive, use erythromycin alone. Treat for 4−6 weeks

or until lungs are clear of abscesses on radiographs. (Foreman 1999)

c) 20–25 mg/kg PO q6-8h (estolate or microencapsulated base are preferred) (Haggett & Wilson 2008)

For treatment of proliferative enteropathy caused by *L. intracellularis* infections in foals:

a) Erythromycin estolate: 25 mg/kg PO q6-8h, with rifampin: 10 mg/kg PO q12h for a minimum of 21 days (Lavoie & Drolet 2003)

■ **SWINE:**

For susceptible infections:

a) For respiratory infections: 2.2–6.6 mg/kg IM once daily

b) For scours in young pigs: 22 mg/kg IM in one or more daily doses (Label directions; *Erythro®-100* and *Erythro®-200*—Ceva)

■ **SHEEP:**

For susceptible infections:

a) For respiratory infections in older animals: 2.2 mg/kg IM once daily as indicated.

b) For prevention of "dysentery" in newborn lambs when the likely causative agent is susceptible to erythromycin: 123 mg/kg IM once soon after birth (Label directions; *Erythro®-100* and *Erythro®-200*—Ceva)

Monitoring

■ Clinical efficacy

■ Adverse effects (periodic liver function tests if patient receiving erythromycin estolate long-term; may not be necessary for foals receiving erythromycin and rifampin for Rhodococcus infections)

Client Information

■ The intramuscular 100 mg/mL (*Erythro-100®*) product (*Erythro-200®*) has quite specific instructions on where and how to inject the drug. Refer to the label directions or package insert for more information before using.

■ When administering orally to small animals, give on an empty stomach unless gastrointestinal signs (vomiting, lack of appetite, diarrhea) occur, then give with food. The estolate, ethylsuccinate or enteric-coated forms of erythromycin may be given with or without food.

■ If gastrointestinal adverse effects are severe or persist, contact veterinarian.

Chemistry/Synonyms

A macrolide antibiotic, produced from *Streptomyces erythreus*, erythromycin is a weak base that is available commercially in several salts and esters. It has a pK_a of 8.9.

Erythromycin base occurs as a bitter tasting, odorless or practically odorless, white to slight yellow, crystalline powder. Approximately

1 mg is soluble in 1 mL of water; it is soluble in alcohol.

Erythromycin estolate occurs as a practically tasteless and odorless, white, crystalline powder. It is practically insoluble in water and approximately 50 mg are soluble in 1 mL of alcohol. Erythromycin estolate may also be known as erythromycin propionate lauryl sulfate.

Erythromycin ethylsuccinate occurs as a practically tasteless and odorless, white to slight yellow, crystalline powder. It is very slightly soluble in water and freely soluble in alcohol.

Erythromycin lactobionate occurs as white to slightly yellow crystals or powder. It may have a faint odor and is freely soluble in water and alcohol.

Erythromycin may also be known as: eritromicina, and erythromycinum; many trade names are available.

Storage/Stability

Erythromycin (base) capsules and tablets should be stored in tight containers at room temperature (15–30°C). Erythromycin estolate preparations should be protected from light. To retain palatability, the oral suspensions should be refrigerated.

Erythromycin ethylsuccinate tablets and powder for oral suspension should be stored in tight containers at room temperature. The commercially available oral suspension should be stored in the refrigerator to preserve palatability. After dispensing, the oral suspensions are stable for at least 14 days at room temperature, but individual products may have longer labeled stabilities.

Erythromycin lactobionate powder for injection should be stored at room temperature. For initial reconstitution (vials), only sterile water for injection should be used. After reconstitution, the drug is stable for 24 hours at room temperature and 2 weeks if refrigerated. To prepare for administration via continuous or intermittent infusion, the drug is further diluted in 0.9% sodium chloride, Lactated Ringer's, or Normosol-R. Other infusion solutions may be used, but first must be buffered with 4% sodium bicarbonate injection (1 mL per 100 mL of solution). At pH's of <5.5, the drug is unstable and loses potency rapidly.

Compatibility/Compounding Considerations

Many drugs are physically **incompatible** with erythromycin lactobionate; it is suggested to consult specialized references or a hospital pharmacist for more specific information.

Dosage Forms/Regulatory Status

VETERINARY-LABELED PRODUCTS:

Erythromycin 100 mg/mL for IM Injection (with 2% butyl aminobenzoate as a local anesthetic) in 100 mL vials; *Gallimycin®-100* (Cross); (OTC). FDA-approved for use in cattle, sheep, and swine. Milk withdrawal (when used as labeled) = 72 hours. Slaughter withdrawal (when used as labeled) for cattle = 14 days, sheep = 3 days, swine = 7 days.

There may also be erythromycin premixes alone and in combination with other drugs for use in swine and/or poultry.

HUMAN-LABELED PRODUCTS:

Erythromycin Base Delayed-release Oral Tablets enteric-coated: 250 mg, 333 mg & 500 mg; *Ery-Tab®* (Abbott); (Rx)

Erythromycin Base Tablets Film-coated: 250 mg, & 500 mg; *Erythromycin Filmtabs®* (Abbott); (Rx)

Erythromycin Base Delayed-release Oral Capsules enteric-coated pellets: 250 mg; generic (Abbott); (Rx)

Erythromycin Stearate Film-coated tablets: 250 mg; generic (Abbott); (Rx)

Erythromycin Ethylsuccinate Tablets: 400 mg; *E.E.S. 400®* (Abbott); generic (Abbott); (Rx)

Erythromycin Ethylsuccinate Powder for Oral Suspension: 200 mg/5 mL when reconstituted 100 mL & 200; *EryPed® 200* (Abbott); (Rx)

Erythromycin Ethylsuccinate Granules for Oral Suspension: 200 mg/5 mL in 100 & 200 mL; *E.E.S. Granules®* (Abbott)(Rx)

Erythromycin Ethylsuccinate Powder for Oral Suspension: 400 mg/5 mL in 100, 200, & UD 5 mL; *EryPed 400®* (Abbott); (Rx)

Erythromycin Ethylsuccinate Powder for Oral Suspension: 100 mg/2.5 mL in 50 mL *EryPed Drops®* (Abbott); (Rx)Erythromycin Lactobionate Lyophilized Powder for Injection Solution: 500 mg & 1 g (as lactobionate) in vials; *Eythrocin®* (Hospira); (Rx)

Erythromycin & Sulfisoxazole Granules for Oral Suspension: erythromycin ethylsuccinate (equivalent to 200 mg erythromycin activity) and sulfisoxazole acetyl (equivalent to 600 mg sulfisoxazole) per 5 mL when reconstituted in 100 mL, 150 mL & 200 mL; *Eryzole®* (Alra); *Pediazole®* (Ross); generic; (Rx)

Topical and ophthalmic preparations are also available.

References

Aucoin, D. (2000). Antimicrobial Drug Formulary. *Target: The antimicrobial guide to effective treatment* Port Huron, MI, North American Compendiums Inc: 93–142.

Chaffin, M. (2006). Treatment and chemoprophylaxis of Rhodococcus equi pneumonia in foals. Proceedings: ACVIM. Accessed via: Veterinary Information Network. http://goo.gl/wuP4O

Divers, T.J. (2009). Diagnosing, treating and preventing Rhodococcus equi. Proceedings: WVC. Accessed via: Veterinary Information Network. http://goo.gl/rG-GeM

Foreman, J. (1999). Equine respiratory pharmacology. *The Veterinary Clinics of North America: Equine Practice* 15:3(December): 665–686.

Greene, C. & A. Watson (1998). Antimicrobial Drug Formulary. *Infectious Diseases of the Dog and Cat.* C Greene Ed. Philadelphia, WB Saunders: 790–919.

Haggett, E.F. & W.D. Wilson (2008). Overview of the use of antimicrobials for the treatment of bacterial infections in horses. *Equine Veterinary Education* 20(8): 433–448.

Hall, J. & R. Washabau (2000). Gastric Prokinetic Agents. *Kirk's Current Veterinary Therapy: XIII Small Animal Practice.* J Bonagura Ed. Philadelphia, WB Saunders: 609–617.

Hjerpe, C.A. (1986). The bovine respiratory disease complex. *Current Veterinary Therapy: Food Animal Practice 2.* JL Howard Ed. Philadelphia, W.B. Saunders: 670–681.

Hoeffer, H. (1995). Antimicrobials in pet birds. *Kirk's Current Veterinary Therapy:XII.* J Bonagura Ed. Philadelphia, W.B. Saunders: 1278–1283.

Jenkins, W.L. (1987). Chloramphenicol, Macrolides, Lincosamides,Vancomycin, Polymyxins, Rifamycins. *The Bristol Handbook of Antimicrobial Therapy.* DE Johnston Ed. Evansville, Veterinary Learning Systems: 261–265.

Jenson, J. (1998). Current ratite therapy. *The Veterinary Clinics of North America: Food Animal Practice* 16:3(November).

Lavoie, J.-P. & R. Drolet (2003). Proliferative enteropathy in foals. Proceedings: ACVIM Forum. Accessed via: Veterinary Information Network. http://goo.gl/Q17MH

Trepanier, L. (2008). Top Ten Potential Drug Interactions in Dogs and Cats. Proceedings: WSAVA. Accessed via: Veterinary Information Network. http://goo.gl/CRszS

Twedt, D. (2008). Antiemetics, prokinetics & antacids. Proceedings: ACVIM. Accessed via: Veterinary Information Network. http://goo.gl/bRKsO

Williams, B. (2000). Therapeutics in Ferrets. *Vet Clin NA: Exotic Anim Pract* 3:1(Jan): 131–153.

ESMOLOL HCL

(ess-moe-lol)   Brevibloc®

BETA-$_1$ BLOCKER

Prescriber Highlights

▶ Ultra-short acting beta$_1$-blocker used IV for short-term treatment of SVT's or to determine if beta-blockers are effective for controlling arrhythmias

▶ Contraindications: Patients with overt cardiac failure, 2nd or 3rd degree AV block, sinus bradycardia, or in cardiogenic shock

▶ Caution: Patients with CHF, bronchoconstrictive lung disease, or diabetes mellitus

▶ Adverse Effects: Hypotension & bradycardia are the effects most likely seen

Uses/Indications

Esmolol may be used as test drug to indicate whether beta-blocker therapy is warranted as an antiarrhythmic agent, particularly in cats with hypertrophic cardiomyopathy, or as an infusion in the short-term treatment of supraventricular tachyarrhythmias (*e.g.*, atrial fibrillation/flutter, sinus tachycardia).

Pharmacology/Actions

Esmolol primarily blocks both beta$_1$-adrenergic receptors in the myocardium. At clinically used doses, esmolol does not have any intrinsic sympathomimetic activity (ISA) and unlike propranolol, does not possess membrane-stabilizing effects (quinidine-like) or bronchoconstrictive effects. Cardiovascular effects secondary to esmolol include negative inotropic and chronotropic activity that can lead to reduced myocardial oxygen demand. Systolic and diastolic blood pressures are reduced at rest and during exercise. Esmolol's antiarrhythmic effect is thought to be due to its blockade of adrenergic stimulation of cardiac pacemaker potentials. Esmolol increases sinus cycle length, slows AV node conduction, and prolongs sinus node recovery time.

Pharmacokinetics

After IV injection esmolol is rapidly and widely distributed but not appreciably to the CNS, spleen or testes. The distribution half-life is about 2 minutes. Steady-state blood levels occur in about 5 minutes if a loading dose was given or about 30 minutes if no load was given. It is unknown whether the drug crosses the placenta or enters milk. Esmolol is rapidly metabolized in the blood by esterases to a practically inactive metabolite. Renal or hepatic dysfunction do not appreciably alter elimination characteristics. Terminal half-life is about 10 minutes and duration of action after discontinuing IV infusion is usually about 20 minutes post-infusion in dogs.

Contraindications/Precautions/Warnings

Esmolol is contraindicated in patients with overt cardiac failure, 2nd or 3rd degree AV block, sinus bradycardia, or in cardiogenic shock. It should be used with caution (weigh benefit vs. risk) in patients with CHF, bronchoconstrictive lung disease, or diabetes mellitus.

Adverse Effects

At usual doses adverse effects are uncommon and generally are an extension of the drug's pharmacologic effects. Hypotension (with resultant clinical signs) and bradycardia are the most likely adverse effects seen. These usually prove mild and transient in nature. Esmolol may mask certain clinical signs of developing hypoglycemia (such as increased heart rate or blood pressure).

Reproductive/Nursing Safety

Studies done in rats and rabbits demonstrated no teratogenic effects at doses up to 3 times the maximum human maintenance dose (MHMD). Higher doses (8 times or more MHMD) demonstrated some maternal death and fetal resorption.

It is unknown if esmolol is excreted in milk.

Overdosage/Acute Toxicity

The IV LD_{50} in dogs is approximately 32 mg/kg. Dogs receiving 2 mg/kg per minute for one hour showed no adverse effects; doses of 3 mg/kg/minute for one hour produced ataxia and salivation and 4 mg/kg/minute for one hour caused muscular rigidity, tremors, seizures, ptosis, vomiting, hyperpnea, vocalizations, and prostration. These effects all resolved within 90 minutes of the end of infusion. Because of the short duration of action of the drug, discontinuation or dosage reduction may be all that is required; otherwise, symptomatic and supportive treatment may be initiated.

Drug Interactions

The following drug interactions have either been reported or are theoretical in humans or animals receiving esmolol and may be of significance in veterinary patients:

- **DIGOXIN:** Esmolol may increase serum digoxin levels up to 20%, but these drugs have been used together safely and effectively

- **MONOAMINE OXIDASE INHIBITORS:** Concurrent use of monoamine oxidase inhibitors with esmolol is not recommended due to potential risk of hypertension

- **MORPHINE:** Titrate esmolol dosage carefully in patients also receiving morphine as it may increase steady-state esmolol serum concentrations up to 50%.

- **RESERPINE:** May see additive effects (hypotension, bradycardia) if used with esmolol

- **VASOCONSTRICTORS/INOTROPES (e.g., dopamine, epinephrine, norepinephrine):** If systemic vascular resistance is high, there is an increase risk for blocked cardiac contractility; esmolol is not recommended to control SVT's in patients receiving these drugs

- **VERAPAMIL:** In humans, particularly with severe cardiomyopathy, cardiac arrest has occurred (rarely)

Doses

- **DOGS:**

  For ultra-short acting beta blockade (for treating or assisting in treatment of ventricular arrhythmias):
  a) Can be administered two ways: **1)** An initial loading dose of 0.25–0.5 mg/kg (250–500 micrograms/kg) administered IV as slow bolus over 1–2 minutes, then followed by a constant rate infusion of 10–200 micrograms/kg/minute; or **2)** Start CRI at 10–200 micrograms/kg/minute without the bolus loading dose. If no loading dose, maximal effect should occur in 10–20 minutes.

  Use of a loading dose and the high end of the infusion rate dose should only be used in dogs with normal cardiac function. In dogs with severe dilated cardiomyopathy or severe mitral regurgitation do not give loading dose and start CRI at 10–20 micrograms/kg/min and titrate upward every 10 minutes to an effective endpoint. (Kittleson 2006)

  b) For SVTs: 0.05–0.1 mg/kg (50–100 micrograms/kg) IV bolus over 2 minutes; repeat every 5 minutes to a maximum of 0.5 mg/kg (500 micrograms/kg). (Fine 2006), (Rush 2005)

c) Give in incremental IV bolus doses of 0.05–0.1 mg/kg every 5 minutes up to a maximum dose of 0.5 mg/kg. Because esmolol's effects are short-lived, if arrhythmia conversion does not occur, other negative inotropes (*e.g.*, diltiazem, or verapamil) can be safely used 30 minutes after esmolol. (Smith 2009)

■ **CATS:**

For ultra-short acting beta blockade for treating or assisting in treatment of ventricular arrhythmias, or in cats with HCM to determine if beta-blockers will reduce the dynamic left-ventricular outflow tract obstruction resulting from systolic anterior motion of the mitral valve:

a) In cats with HCM: An initial loading dose of 0.25–0.5 mg/kg (250–500 micrograms/kg) administered IV as slow bolus over 1–2 minutes, then followed by a constant rate infusion of 10–200 micrograms/kg/minute. (Kittleson 2006)

b) Loading dose of 200–500 micrograms/kg IV over 1 minute; followed by a constant rate IV infusion of 25–200 micrograms/kg/minute (Ware 2000)

Monitoring

■ Blood Pressure

■ ECG

■ Heart Rate

Client Information

■ Esmolol should only be used in an in-patient setting where appropriate monitoring is available.

Chemistry/Synonyms

A short acting beta$_1$-adrenergic blocker, esmolol occurs as white or off white crystalline powder. It is not as lipophilic as either labetolol or propranolol, but is comparable to acebutolol. 650 mg are soluble in one mL of water and 350 mg are soluble in one mL of alcohol.

Esmolol HCl may also be known as ASL-8052, *Brevibloc®* or *Miniblock®*.

Storage/Stability

The concentrate for injection should be stored at room temperature; do not freeze and protect from excessive heat. It is a clear, colorless to light yellow solution. Expiration dates of 3 years are assigned after manufacture.

After diluted to a concentration of 10 mg/mL esmolol HCl is stable (at refrigeration temperatures or room temperature) for at least 24 hours in commonly used IV solutions.

Compatibility/Compounding Considerations

Esmolol may be diluted in standard D5, LRS or saline (or combinations thereof) IV fluids. At this concentration it is reportedly physically **compatible** with digoxin, dopamine, fentanyl, lidocaine, morphine sulfate, nitroglycerin, and nitroprusside. Compatibility is dependent upon factors such as pH, concentration, temperature, and diluent used; consult specialized references or a hospital pharmacist for more specific information.

Dosage Forms/Regulatory Status

VETERINARY-LABELED PRODUCTS: None

The ARCI (Racing Commissioners International) has designated this drug as a class 3 substance. See the appendix for more information.

HUMAN-LABELED PRODUCTS:

Esmolol HCl Injection: 10 mg/mL regular & preservative free in 10 mL vials; 20 mg/mL preservative free in 5 mL vials & 100 mL bags; and 250 mg/mL in 10 mL amps; *Brevibloc®* (Baxter); generic; (Rx)

References

Fine, D. (2006). Emergency management of cardiac arrhythmias. Proceedings: ACVIM. Accessed via: Veterinary Information Network. http://goo.gl/ieCZL

Kittleson, M. (2006). "Chapt 29: Drugs used in the treatment of cardiac arrhythmias." *Small Animal Cardiology, 2nd Ed.*

Rush, J. (2005). Treatment of life-threatening arrhythmias. Proceedings: IVECCS. Accessed via: Veterinary Information Network. http://goo.gl/UxBxv

Smith, F. (2009). Update on Antiarrhythmic Therapy. Proceedings: Western Veterinary Conference. Accessed via: Veterinary Information Network. http://goo.gl/aiVDJ

Ware, W. (2000). Therapy for Critical Arrythmias: New Advances. Proceedings: The North American Veterinary Conference, Orlando.

ESTRADIOL CYPIONATE

(ess-tra-**dye**-ole)   ECP®

HORMONAL AGENT (ESTROGEN)

Prescriber Highlights

▶ Natural estrogen salt used primarily to induce estrus; has been used as an abortifacient (but rarely recommended today)

▶ Contraindications: Pregnancy (abortifacient, teratogen); the FDA has stated that the use of ECP in food animals is illegal

▶ Adverse Effects: In *cats & dogs*: Bone marrow toxicity, cystic endometrial hyperplasia, pyometra;

▶ In male animals, feminization may occur; in females, signs of estrus may occur;

▶ In *cattle*: Prolonged estrus, genital irritation, decreased milk flow, precocious development, & follicular cysts may develop

▶ Drug Interactions

Uses/Indications

For mares, indications for the use of estradiol include enhancing estrus behavior and receptivity in ovariectomized mares and to treat estrogen-responsive incontinence. Historically, estradiol cypionate has been used as an abortifacient agent in cattle, cats and dogs, but estrogens are no longer recommended by most theriogenologists for use as an abortifacient in small animals and the FDA stated (April 5, 2006): "The use of ECP in food-producing animals is illegal, and manufacturing and compounding of ECP for such use is illegal."

Pharmacology/Actions

The most active endogenous estrogen, estradiol possesses the pharmacologic profile expected of the estrogen class. Estrogens are necessary for the normal growth and development of the female sex organs and in some species contribute to the development and maintenance of secondary female sex characteristics. Estrogens cause increased cell height and secretions of the cervical mucosa, thickening of the vaginal mucosa, endometrial proliferation, and increased uterine tone.

Estrogens have effects on the skeletal system. They increase calcium deposition, accelerate epiphyseal closure, and increase bone formation. Estrogens have a slight anabolic effect and can increase sodium and water retention.

Estrogens affect the release of gonadotropins from the pituitary gland. This can cause inhibition of lactation, ovulation, and androgen secretion.

Pharmacokinetics

No specific information was located regarding the pharmacokinetics of estradiol in veterinary species. In humans, estrogen in oil solutions after IM administration are absorbed promptly and absorption continues over several days. Esterified estrogens (*e.g.*, estradiol cypionate) have delayed absorption after IM administration. Estrogens are distributed throughout the body and accumulate in adipose tissue. Elimination of the steroidal estrogens occurs principally by hepatic metabolism. Estrogens and their metabolites are primarily excreted in the urine, but are also excreted into the bile where most is reabsorbed from the GI.

Contraindications/Precautions/Warnings

Estradiol is contraindicated during pregnancy as it can cause fetal malformations of the genitourinary system and induce bone marrow depression in the fetus.

Estradiol cypionate should not be used to treat estrogen–responsive incontinence in small animals; other estrogens (DES, conjugated estrogens) are less toxic.

In cases of prolonged corpus luteum in cows, a thorough uterine exam should be completed to determine if endometritis or a fetus is present.

Estradiol is reportedly very toxic (bone marrow) to ferrets.

Adverse Effects

Estrogens have been associated with severe adverse reactions in small animals. In cats and dogs, estrogens are considered toxic to the bone marrow and can cause blood dyscrasias. Blood dyscrasias are more prevalent in older animals and if higher dosages are used. Initially, a thrombocytosis and/or leukocytosis may be noted, but thrombocytopenia/leukopenias will gradually develop. Changes in a peripheral blood smear may be apparent within two weeks after estrogen administration. Chronic estrogen toxicity may be characterized by a normochromic, normocytic anemia, thrombocytopenia, and neutropenia. Bone marrow depression may be transient and begin to resolve within 30–40 days or may persist or progress to a fatal aplastic anemia.

Estrogens may cause cystic endometrial hyperplasia and pyometra. After therapy is initiated, an open-cervix pyometra may be noted 1–6 weeks after therapy.

Estrogens may induce mammary neoplasia.

When used chronically in male animals, feminization may occur. In females, signs of estrus may occur and persist for 7–10 days.

In cattle, prolonged estrus, genital irritation, decreased milk-flow, precocious development, and follicular cysts may develop after estrogen therapy. These effects may be secondary to overdosage and dosage adjustment may reduce or eliminate them.

Reproductive/Nursing Safety

Estradiol is contraindicated during pregnancy. In humans, the FDA categorizes this drug as category **X** for use during pregnancy (*Studies in animals or humans demonstrate fetal abnormalities or adverse reaction; reports indicate evidence of fetal risk. The risk of use in pregnant women clearly outweighs any possible benefit.*) In a separate system evaluating the safety of drugs in canine and feline pregnancy (Papich 1989), this drug is categorized as in class: **D** (*Contraindicated. These drugs have been shown to cause congenital malformations or embryotoxicity.*)

Estrogens have been shown to decrease the quantity and quality of maternal milk.

Overdosage/Acute Toxicity

No reports of inadvertent acute overdosage in veterinary patients were located; see Adverse Effects above.

Drug Interactions

The following drug interactions have either been reported or are theoretical in humans or animals receiving estradiol and may be of significance in veterinary patients:

■ **AZOLE ANTIFUNGALS (fluconazole, itraconazole, ketoconazole):** May increase estrogen levels

■ **CORTICOSTEROIDS:** Enhanced glucocorticoid effects may result if estrogens are used concomitantly with corticosteroid agents. It has been postulated that estrogens may either alter the protein binding of corticosteroids and/or decrease their metabolism; corticosteroid dosage adjustment may be necessary when estrogen therapy is either started or discontinued

■ **MACROLIDE ANTIBIOTICS (erythromycin, clarithromycin):** May increase estrogen levels

■ **PHENOBARBITAL:** May decrease estrogen activity if administered concomitantly

■ **RIFAMPIN:** May decrease estrogen activity if administered concomitantly

■ **ST. JOHN'S WORT:** May decrease estrogen activity if administered concomitantly

■ **WARFARIN:** Oral anticoagulant activity may be decreased if estrogens are administered concurrently; increases in anticoagulant dosage may be necessary if adding estrogens

Laboratory Considerations

■ Estrogens in combination with progestins (*e.g.*, oral contraceptives) have been demonstrated in humans to increase **thyroxine-binding globulin (TBG)** with resultant increases in total circulating thyroid hormone. Decreased T_3 resin uptake also occurs, but free T_4 levels are unaltered. It is unclear if estradiol affects these laboratory tests in veterinary patients.

Doses

■ **DOGS:**

For pregnancy avoidance after mismating:
Note: This drug is rarely used for this indication today as there are safer, more effective treatments.
a) 44 micrograms/kg (0.044 mg/kg) IM once; during day 4 estrus to day 2 of diestrus, toxic at ≥100 micrograms/kg. (Wiebe & Howard 2009)

■ **CATS:**

For pregnancy avoidance after mismating:
Note: This drug is rarely used for this indication today as there are safer, more effective treatments.
a) 250 micrograms/kg (0.25 mg/kg) IM once 6 days after coitus; or 0.25 mg/cat IM at 40 hours after coitus. (Wiebe & Howard 2009)

■ **CATTLE:**

The FDA has stated that the use of ECP in food-producing animals is illegal.

■ **HORSES:**

To enhance estrus behavior and receptivity in ovariectomized mares:
a) 5–10 mg (total dose) IM once. (Dascanio 2009)

For treatment of mares with estrogen-responsive incontinence:
a) 4–10 micrograms/kg estradiol cypionate IM daily for three days and then every other day. Some mares will improve, but does not "cure." (Schott II & Carr 2003)

Monitoring

When therapy is either at high dosages or chronic, see adverse effects for more information. Done at least monthly:

■ Packed Cell Volumes (PCV)

■ White blood cell counts (CBC)

■ Platelet counts; Baseline, one month after therapy, and repeated two months after cessation of therapy if abnormal

■ Liver function tests

Chemistry/Synonyms

Estradiol is a naturally occurring steroidal estrogen. Estradiol cypionate is produced by esterifying estradiol with cyclopentanepropionic acid, and occurs as a white to practically white, crystalline powder. It is either odorless or may have a slight odor and has a melting range of 149–153°C. Less than 0.1 mg/mL is soluble in water and 25 mg/mL is soluble in alcohol. Estradiol cypionate is sparingly soluble in vegetable oils.

Estradiol may also be known as: beta-oestradiol, dihydrofolliculin, dihydrotheelin, dihydroxyoestrin, estradiolum, NSC-9895, NSC-20293 (alpha-estradiol), and oestradiol; many trade names are available.

Estradiol Cypionate may also be known as: oestradiol cyclopentylpropionate, oestradiol cypionate, *Delestrogen®*, *Depo-Estradiol®*, *Depogen®*, *Dura-Estrin®*, *ECP®*, *E-Cypionate®*, *Estra-D®*, *Estrace®*, *Estro-Cyp®*, *Estroject®*, *dep-Gynogen®*, *Femtrace®*, or *Gynodiol®*.

Storage/Stability

Estradiol cypionate should be stored in light-resistant containers at temperatures of less than 40°C, preferably at room temperature (15–30°C); avoid freezing.

Commercially available injectable solutions of estradiol cypionate are sterile solutions in a vegetable oil (usually cottonseed oil); they may contain chlorobutanol as a preservative.

Compatibility/Compounding Considerations

It is not recommended to mix estradiol cypionate with other medications.

In the USA it is illegal to compound estradiol for use in food producing animals.

Dosage Forms/Regulatory Status

VETERINARY-LABELED PRODUCTS:

There are several estradiol-containing implants for use in beef cattle.

HUMAN-LABELED PRODUCTS:

Estradiol Cypionate in Oil for Injection: 5 mg/mL in 5 mL vials; *Depo-Estradiol®* (Pfizer); (Rx)

Estradiol Valerate in Oil for Injection: 10 mg/mL, 20 mg/mL & 40 mg/mL in 5 mL multi-dose vials; *Delestrogen®* (JHP); generic; (Rx)

Estradiol Tablets: 0.45 mg, 0.5 mg, 0.9 mg, 1 mg, 1.5 mg, 1.8 mg & 2 mg micronized estradiol; *Estrace®* (Warner Chilcott), *Gynodiol®* (Novavax), *Femtrace®* (Warner Chilcott); generic; (Rx)

References

Dascanio, J. (2009). Hormonal Control of Reproduction. Proceedings: ABVP. Accessed via: Veterinary Information Network. http://goo.gl/o2vHk

Schott II, H. & E. Carr (2003). Urinary incontinence in horses. Proceedings: ACVIM Forum. Accessed via: Veterinary Information Network. http://goo.gl/q7Uo2

Wiebe, V.J. & J.P. Howard (2009). Pharmacologic Advances in Canine and Feline Reproduction. *Topics in Companion Animal Medicine* 24(2): 71–99.

ETHAMBUTOL HCL

(e-*tham*-byoo-tole)   Myambutol®, Etibi®

ORAL ANTIMYCOBACTERIAL ANTIBIOTIC

Prescriber Highlights

► Can be used as an ingredient in an antimycobacterial "cocktail" for dogs, cats, birds

► Treating these infections is controversial because of potential public health risks associated with the infections

► Optic or neuro toxicity greatest concern

Uses/Indications

In combination with other antimycobacterial drugs, ethambutol may be useful in treating mycobacterial infections caused by *M. bovis, M. tuberculosis, M. genavense, M. avium-intracellulare* complex (MAC) in dogs or cats, particularly when the organism is resistant to treatment with other drug combinations (rifampin, enrofloxacin, azithromycin). In birds, ethambutol has been used in combination with other agents for treating mycobacterial (*e.g., M. avium*) infections.

Because of public health risks, particularly in the face of increased populations of immunocompromised people, treatment of mycobacterial (*M. bovis, M. tuberculosis,* etc.) infections in domestic or captive animals is controversial.

Pharmacology/Actions

A synthetic, bacteriostatic, antimycobacterial agent, ethambutol is only active against actively dividing mycobacteria. It enters mycobacterial cells and interferes with RNA synthesis and appears to interfere with the incorporation of mycolic acid into cell walls, allowing other antimycobacterial agents to penetrate the cell wall. Ethambutol does not have appreciable activity against other bacteria or fungi. Resistance can occur and is thought to develop in a step-wise manner. Cross-resistance with other antimycobacterial agents has not been reported.

Pharmacokinetics

Pharmacokinetic values for cats or birds were not located. In dogs, ethambutol is reported to have a volume of distribution of 3.8 L/kg, a total body clearance of 13.2 mL/min/kg, and an elimination half-life of 4.1 hours. Nephrectomized dogs had an elimination half-life of 5 hours.

In humans, ethambutol is rapidly absorbed after PO administration and bioavailability is around 75%. The drug is distributed widely in the body, but CSF levels only range from 10–50% of those found in serum. Erythrocyte concentrations are about twice that of the serum and can serve as a depot for the drug. About 15% of absorbed drug is hepatically metabolized to inactive metabolites. The majority of the drug is eliminated both by tubular secretion and glomerular filtration as unchanged drug in the urine. Elimination half-life in humans with normal renal function is about 3–4 hours; up to 8 hours if renal function is impaired.

Contraindications/Precautions/Warnings

Ethambutol should not be used in patients with a history of prior hypersensitivity reactions to it.

Patients with markedly reduced renal function may need dosage adjustment.

Adverse Effects

Well-described adverse effect profiles for ethambutol in dogs, cats or birds are not available. Because ethambutol is used in combination with other medications, adverse effects associated with treatment may not be a result of ethambutol. In pre-clinical studies, some dogs receiving ethambutol over prolonged periods developed non-dose related degenerative changes in the central nervous system. In toxicology studies, dogs receiving large, prolonged doses developed signs of myocardial toxicity and depigmentation of the tapetum lucidum of the eyes. However, doses as large as 400 mg/kg/day for 4 weeks in dogs demonstrated no significant abnormalities in electroretinogram or visual evoked potential. In humans, optic neuritis (usually reversible after drug discontinuation) causing decreased visual acuity has been reported; routine ophthalmologic exams are recommended for humans taking this medication long-term.

Because antimycobacterial therapy involves multiple drugs for extended periods of time, bacterial or fungal overgrowth infections can occur. Antifungal medications may be required.

Reproductive/Nursing Safety

Ethambutol crosses the placenta; fetal levels are reported to range from 30–75% of that found in maternal serum. Teratogenic effects associated with ethambutol have not been reported in humans, but studies in mice, rats, and rabbits given high doses yielded a variety of abnormalities in offspring. Although risks exist, most believe that ethambutol is relatively safe to use during human pregnancy and untreated tuberculosis poses a much greater risk to the fetus.

Ethambutol is excreted into milk in levels approximating those found in maternal serum. While no problems have been documented and it is most likely safe, risk to offspring cannot be ruled out.

Overdosage/Acute Toxicity

Very limited information exists. Acute overdoses of greater than 10 grams in humans have caused optic neuritis. Other adverse effects noted with human overdoses can include: CNS effects (confusion, visual hallucinations), abdominal pain, nausea, fever and headache; treatment is supportive.

Drug Interactions
The following drug interactions have either been reported or are theoretical in humans or animals receiving ethambutol and may be of significance in veterinary patients:

■ **ALUMINUM-CONTAINING ANTACIDS:** In humans, it has been documented that co-administration can reduce oral absorption of ethambutol; it is suggested to separate dosing by at least 4 hours if both drugs are necessary

Laboratory Considerations
■ No specific concerns; in humans, increased **serum uric acid** levels have been noted

Doses

■ **DOGS:**
a) For treatment of disseminated *M. tuberculosis*: Ethambutol: 10–25 mg/kg PO once daily, in combination with rifampin (5–10 mg/kg PO q12–24h; maximum of 600 mg/day) and isoniazid (10–20 mg/kg PO once daily; maximum of 300 mg/day). May also add pyrizinamide at 15–40 mg/kg PO once daily. **Note:** pyrizinamide is ineffective for *M. bovis*. Treatment must continue for more than 9 months. (Greene & Gunn-Moore 2006)

■ **CATS:**
a) For treatment of feline tuberculosis: Initial treatment phase with rifampin (10–20 mg/kg PO q12–24h); enrofloxacin (5 mg/kg PO q12–24h); azithromycin (5–10 mg/kg PO q12–24h) for the first two months, then continuation phase (for approximately another 4 months) with rifampin and either enrofloxacin or azithromycin. If resistance develops, rifampin, isoniazid (10–20 mg/kg PO once daily) and ethambutol (15 mg/kg PO once daily) may be considered. If only two drugs are required, suggest using only rifampin and isoniazid. (Hartmannn & Greene 2005)

■ **BIRDS:**
a) For treatment of *M. avium* infections in caged birds: Several protocols have been used, but controlled trials have not been performed. Combination therapy and treatment for 6–12 months is required.
Protocol 1: Ciprofloxacin 20 mg/kg PO q12h or Enrofloxacin 15 mg/kg PO or IM (**Note:** repeated IM injections can cause muscle necrosis) for 10 days; Clofazimine 1.5 mg/kg PO once daily; Cycloserine 5 mg/kg PO q12h; and Ethambutol 20 mg/kg PO q12h.

Protocol 2: Clofazimine 6 mg/kg PO once daily; Ethambutol 30 mg/kg PO once daily; Rifampin 45 mg/kg PO once daily.
Protocol 3: Ciprofloxacin 80 mg/kg PO once daily or Enrofloxacin 30 mg/kg PO once daily; Ethambutol 30 mg/kg PO once daily; Rifampin 45 mg/kg PO once daily or Rifabutin 15 mg/kg PO once daily. (Phalen 2006)
b) For Avian mycobacteriosis: All are dosed PO once daily for 9–12 months: Rifabutin 45–55 mg/kg; Clarithromycin 60–85 mg/kg; Ethambutol 30–85 mg/kg; Enrofloxacin 20 mg/kg. (Flammer 2006)

Monitoring
■ Clinical efficacy
■ With long-term therapy, consider periodic monitoring of visual, liver, and renal function; CBC
■ Monitor for fungal or bacterial overgrowth infections

Client Information
■ Clients must be informed of the potential public health issues associated with mycobacterium infections and should be encouraged to contact a physician, preferably an infectious disease specialist for guidance
■ Treatment can be very prolonged (many months) and expensive
■ May be administered with or without food
■ Report any changes noted with patient's eyes or vision to the veterinarian

Chemistry/Synonyms
Ethambutol HCl occurs as a white, crystalline powder that is freely soluble in water and soluble in alcohol.

Ethambutol may also be known as: CL-40882, etambutol, or ethambutoli; there are many trade names for international products.

Storage/Stability
Ethambutol tablets should be stored below 40°C and preferably, between 15–30°C in well-closed containers.

Dosage Forms/Regulatory Status
VETERINARY-LABELED PRODUCTS: None
HUMAN-LABELED PRODUCTS:
Ethambutol HCl Tablets: 100 mg, & 400 mg (scored); *Myambutol®* (X-Gen); generic; (Rx)

References
Flammer, K. (2006). Managing Avian Bacterial Diseases II. Proceedings: WVC2006. Accessed via: Veterinary Information Network. http://goo.gl/wPvdh
Greene, C. & D. Gunn-Moore (2006). Mycobacterial Infections: Infections caused by slow-growing mycobacteria. *Infectious Diseases of the Dog and Cat, 3rd Ed.* C Greene Ed., Elsevier: 462–477.
Hartmannn, K. & C. Greene (2005). Diseases caused by systemic bacterial infections. *Textbook of Veterinary Internal Medicine, 6th Ed.* S Ettinger and E Feldman Eds., Elsevier: 616–631.

Phalen, D. (2006). Selected Infectious Diseases: A Review
for the ABVP V. Proceedings: ABVP 2006. Accessed via:
Veterinary Information Network. http://goo.gl/SZvGQ

ETHANOL
ALCOHOL, ETHYL

(*eth*-a-nol)   Alcohol

ANTIDOTE

Prescriber Highlights

▶ Used for treatment of ethylene glycol
  or methanol toxicity

▶ Contraindications: None (above are life
  threatening)

▶ Adverse Effects: CNS depression,
  diuresis, pain, & infection at the injection site.

▶ Avoid extravasation

▶ Monitor fluid & electrolyte status,
  alcohol & toxin levels (if possible)

Uses/Indications

The principal use of ethanol in veterinary medicine is for the treatment of ethylene glycol or
methanol toxicity. While fomepizole (4-methyl
pyrazole) is now the treatment of choice for ethylene glycol poisoning, alcohol is a readily available and an economical alternative when patients present within a few hours after ingestion.

Percutaneous injection of ethanol 95% has
been used successfully to treat feline hyperthyroidism.

Ethyl alcohol has also been used in aerosol
form as a mucokinetic agent in horses.

Pharmacology/Actions

By competitively inhibiting alcohol dehydrogenase, alcohol can prevent the formation of
ethylene glycol to its toxic metabolites (glycoaldehyde, glycolate, glyoxalate, and oxalic acid).
This allows the ethylene glycol to be principally
excreted in the urine unchanged. A similar sce-
nario exists for the treatment of methanol poisoning. For alcohol to be effective, however, it
must be given very early after ingestion; it is sel-
dom useful if started 8 hours after a significant
ingestion.

Pharmacokinetics

Alcohol is well absorbed orally, but is administered intravenously for toxicity treatment. It
rapidly distributes throughout the body and
crosses the blood-brain barrier. Alcohol crosses
the placenta.

Contraindications/Precautions/Warnings

Because ethylene glycol and methanol intoxications are life threatening, there are no absolute
contraindications to ethanol's use for these
indications.

Use of ethanol with fomepizole is usually
contraindicated; see drug interactions for more
information.

Adverse Effects

The systemic adverse effects of alcohol are quite
well known. The CNS depression and respiratory depression associated with the high levels used to treat ethylene glycol and methanol
toxicity can confuse the clinical monitoring of
these toxicities. Ethanol's affects on antidiuretic
hormone (vasopressin) may enhance diuresis.
As both ethylene glycol and methanol may also
cause diuresis, fluid and electrolyte therapy requirements need to be monitored and managed.
Hypocalcemia and metabolic acidosis may be
noted and pulmonary edema can occur. Other
adverse affects include pain and infection at the
injection site and phlebitis. Extravasation should
be watched for and avoided. When aerosolized
in horses, irritation and bronchoconstriction
may result.

Reproductive/Nursing Safety

Alcohol's safety during pregnancy has not been
established for short-term use. Use only when
necessary. In humans, the FDA categorizes this
drug as category *C* for use during pregnancy
(*Animal studies have shown an adverse effect on
the fetus, but there are no adequate studies in humans; or there are no animal reproduction studies
and no adequate studies in humans.*)

Alcohol passes freely into milk in levels that
approximate maternal serum levels, but it is
unlikely to have negative effects on nursing offspring.

Overdosage/Acute Toxicity

If clinical signs of overdosage occur (lateral
nystagmus, respiratory depression, profound
obtundation), either slow the infusion or discontinue temporarily. Alcohol blood levels may
be used to monitor both efficacy and toxicity of
alcohol.

Drug Interactions

The following drug interactions have either been
reported or are theoretical in humans or animals
receiving ethanol and may be of significance in
veterinary patients:

■ **BROMOCRIPTINE:** Alcohol may increase the
  severity of side effects seen with bromocriptine

■ **CHARCOAL, ACTIVATED:** Will inhibit absorption of orally administered ethanol; do not
  use activated charcoal if administering ethanol orally for methanol or ethylene glycol
  intoxication

■ **CNS DEPRESSANT DRUGS (*e.g.*, barbiturates,
  benzodiazepines, phenothiazines, etc.):** Alcohol may cause additive CNS depression
  when used with other CNS depressant drugs

■ **FOMEPIZOLE (4-MP):** Inhibits alcohol dehydrogenase; ethanol metabolism is reduced
  significantly and alcohol poisoning (CNS
  depression, coma, death) can occur. Use together is generally not recommended, but if
  both drugs are used, monitoring of ethanol
  blood levels is mandatory.

■ **INSULIN and other antidiabetic drugs:** Alcohol may affect glucose metabolism and the actions of insulin or oral antidiabetic agents

■ A disulfiram reaction (increased acetaldehyde with tachycardia, vomiting, weakness) may occur if alcohol is used concomitantly with the following drugs: **chlorpropamide, furazolidone, metronidazole.**

Laboratory Considerations

Ethylene Glycol Testing Kits: Ethanol may cause false positive reports on ethylene glycol screening tests. Refer to the product used, for more information.

Doses

■ **DOGS:**

For ethylene glycol poisoning:

a) As a 20% solution, give 5.5 mL/kg IV q4h for 5 treatments, then q6h for four additional treatments; dosed as a CRI over 1 hour (Forrester & Lees 1994), (Hall 2009)

b) Make a 7% ethanol solution (see Compatibility/Compounding below) and give 8.6 mL/kg slowly IV followed by a CRI of 1.43 mL/kg/hr for at least 36 hours although 48 hours is probably better. If the EG test was positive initially, then check it before stopping treatment; discontinue treatment if it reverts to negative. (Shell 2006)

■ **CATS:**

For ethylene glycol poisoning:

a) As a 20% solution, give 5 mL/kg IV q6h for 5 treatments, then q8h for four additional treatments; dosed as a CRI over 1 hour (Forrester & Lees 1994), (Hall 2009)

b) Make a 7% ethanol solution (see Compatibility/Compounding below) and give 8.6 mL/kg slowly IV followed by a CRI of 1.43 mL/kg/hr for at least 36 hours although 48 hours is probably better. If the EG test was positive initially, then check it before stopping treatment; discontinue treatment if it reverts to negative. (Shell 2006)

Monitoring

■ Alcohol blood levels (and ethylene glycol or methanol levels). **Note:** In humans, blood alcohol levels should be maintained at 100 to 130 mg/deciliter (21.7 to 28.2 milliMoles/liter). It is safer to maintain a blood ethanol concentration greater than 130 mg/deciliter than to have it fall below 100 mg/deciliter. (*POISINDEX® Managements*, Thompson; MICROMEDEX® Healthcare Series, 2007)

■ Degree of CNS effect

■ Fluid/electrolyte status

Client Information

■ Systemically administered alcohol should be given in a controlled clinical environment.

Chemistry/Synonyms

A transparent, colorless, volatile liquid having a characteristic odor and a burning taste, ethyl alcohol is miscible with water and many other solvents.

"Proof" is considered 2X the percentage of ethanol. For example, a 100 proof vodka is 50% ethanol; an 80 proof vodka is 40% ethanol. In some states, pure grain alcohol (often called "Everclear") can be purchased which is a 95% ethanol (190 proof) product.

Ethanol may also be known as aethanolum, alcool, grain alcohol, ethanolum, and ethyl alcohol.

Storage/Stability/Preparation

Alcohol should be protected from extreme heat or freezing. Do not use unless the solution is clear. Alcohol may precipitate many drugs; do not administer other medications in the alcohol infusion solution unless compatibility is documented (consult specialized references or a hospital pharmacist for more specific information).

Compatibility/Compounding Considerations

Note: Since alcohol infusions are generally only used in veterinary medicine for the treatment of ethylene glycol/methanol toxicity and obtaining medical or laboratory grade alcohol or pharmaceutical grade products can be very difficult in an emergency, veterinarians have often had to improvise. One method that has been successful, albeit not pharmaceutically elegant, is to use commercially available vodka (40%–80 proof; 50%-100 proof) or grain alcohol ("Everclear"; 95%-190 proof) diluted in an appropriate IV solution (*e.g.*, LRS, D5W, etc.).

■ To make an ethanol solution of a lesser concentration than the stock solution:

■ Choose the percentage you want (5%–20%) to administer

■ Divide this number by the % (NOT proof) of ethanol of the stock solution

■ Multiply this amount by the total volume of the IV bag that will be used (250 mL–1000 mL) to determine the mLs of stock solution to use.

■ Remove this amount from the fluid bag and add the appropriate amount of alcohol solution to make a solution of the desired alcohol percentage

Examples:

■ To make a 20% ethanol solution using 80 proof (40%) vodka in a one liter bag of fluids: 20% ÷ 40% = 0.5; multiply by 1000 = 500 mL. Remove 500 mL of fluids from the bag and add 500 mL of 80 proof vodka = 1000 mL of a 20% ethanol solution

■ To make a 5% solution using 100 proof (50%) vodka in a 500 mL bag of fluids: 5% ÷ 50% = 0.1; multiply by 500 = 50 mL. Remove 50 mL of fluids from the bag and add 50 mL of 100 proof vodka = 500 mL of a 5% ethanol solution

■ To make a 7% ethanol solution from 190 proof (95%) "Everclear" in a 250 mL bag of fluids: 7% ÷ 95% = 0.074; multiply by 250 = 18.5 mL. Remove 18.5 mL of fluids from the bag and add 18.5 mL of 190 proof (95%) grain alcohol = 250 mL of a 7% ethanol solution

Regardless of the product used, it is recommended that an in-line filter be used for the IV and the client give informed consent for the use of this non-pharmaceutical product.

Dosage Forms/Regulatory Status

VETERINARY-LABELED PRODUCTS: None
HUMAN-LABELED PRODUCTS:
Alcohol (Ethanol) in Dextrose Infusions:

5% Alcohol and 5% Dextrose in Water (450 Cal/L, 1114 mOsm/L) in 1000 mL; generic; (Rx)
5% Alcohol and 5% Dextrose in Water (450 Cal/L, 1125 mOsm/L) in 1000 mL; (McGaw); (Rx)
10% Alcohol and 5% Dextrose in Water (720 Cal/L, 1995 mOsm/L) in 1000 mL; (McGaw) (Rx)

For information on obtaining tax-free alcohol for medicinal purposes, contact a regional office of the Bureau of Alcohol, Tobacco, and Firearms.

References

Forrester, S. & G. Lees (1994). Disease of the Kidney and Ureter. *Saunders Manual of Small Animal Practice*. S Birchard and R Sherding Eds. Philadelphia, W.B. Saunders Company: 799–820.

Hall, K. (2009). Toxicosis Treatments. *Kirk's Current Veterinary Therapy XIV*. J Bonagura and D Twedt Eds. 112–116, Saunders Elsevier: 112–116.

Shell, L. (2006). "Ethylene Glycol Toxicity." *Associate Database*. 2010, http://goo.gl/qHd1h.

ETIDRONATE DISODIUM

(e-*ti*-droe-nate)   Didronel®

ORAL BISPHOSPHONATE BONE
RESORPTION INHIBITOR

Prescriber Highlights

▶ Biphosphonate that reduces calcium resorption from bone; used primarily to treat hypercalcemia associated with malignancy

▶ Contraindications: Treatment of hypercalcemia in patients with severe renal function impairment

▶ Caution in patients with bone fractures, enterocolitis, cardiac failure, or moderate renal function impairment

▶ Adverse Effects: Potentially, diarrhea, nausea, or bone pain/tenderness

▶ Do not confuse etidronate with etretinate or etomidate

▶ Expense may be an issue

Uses/Indications

Etidronate is a first generation bisphosphonate that may be useful for the treatment of severe hypercalcemia associated with neoplastic disease. Its use in human medicine has been largely replaced with newer, more potent bisphosphonates that can be dosed less often or have fewer adverse effects. Etidronate is also indicated in humans for the treatment of Paget's disease and heterotopic ossification (*e.g.*, after total hip replacement).

Pharmacology/Actions

Etidronate's primary site of action is bone. It reduces normal and abnormal bone resorption. This effect can reduce hypercalcemia associated with malignant neoplasms. Etidronate can also increase serum phosphate concentrations, presumably by increasing the renal tubular reabsorption of phosphate. Some early studies in lab animals suggest that etidronate may inhibit the formation of bone metastases with some tumor types.

Pharmacokinetics

Oral absorption is poor and dose dependent. As little as 1% of a dose (smaller doses) may be absorbed; with higher doses, up to 20% may be absorbed. Food substantially reduces the amount absorbed. After oral dosing, the drug is rapidly cleared from blood and 50% of the absorbed goes into bone. At usual doses, it appears that etidronate does not cross the placenta. Duration of effect may be very prolonged. In humans, effects have persisted for up to one year after discontinuation in patients with Paget's disease. Effects for hypercalcemia may last for 11 days. Absorbed etidronate is excreted unchanged by the kidneys. Approximately 50% of the absorbed dose is excreted within 24 hours; the remainder is chemisorbed to bone and then slowly eliminated.

Contraindications/Precautions/Warnings

Etidronate is considered contraindicated for the treatment of hypercalcemia in patients with renal function impairment (serum creatinines >5 mg/dL). Risk vs. benefit should be carefully considered in patients with bone fractures (delays healing), enterocolitis (higher risk of diarrhea), cardiac failure (especially with parenteral etidronate as patients may not tolerate the extra fluid load), or those with renal function impairment (serum creatinines 2.5–5 mg/dL).

Do not confuse etidronate with etretinate or etomidate.

Adverse Effects

Adverse effects are not well described in small animals. In humans, diarrhea, nausea (with higher oral doses), and bone pain/tenderness are most the likely adverse effects reported. Increases in serum creatinine are possible.

A syndrome called "frozen bone" has been reported in dogs on moderately high doses of etidronate or other non-amino bisphosphonates (clodronate). Bone remodeling and repair are inhibited enough that bones can weaken and fracture. Newer bisphosphonates appear to be much safer with respect to this syndrome.

Reproductive/Nursing Safety

Etidronate's safety during pregnancy has not been established. Rabbits given oral doses 5X those recommended in humans, demonstrated no overt problems with offspring. Rats, given very large doses IV, showed skeletal malformations. In humans, the FDA categorizes this drug as category *C* for use during pregnancy (*Animal studies have shown an adverse effect on the fetus, but there are no adequate studies in humans; or there are no animal reproduction studies and no adequate studies in humans.*)

It is unknown if the drug enters milk.

Overdosage/Acute Toxicity

Very little information is available at this time. Overdoses may result in hypocalcemia (ECG changes may occur), bleeding problems (secondary to rapid chelation of calcium) and proximal renal tubule damage.

Use standard gut emptying protocols after oral ingestion when warranted. IV calcium administration (*e.g.,* calcium gluconate) may be used to reverse hypocalcemia. Intensive monitoring is suggested.

Drug Interactions

The following drug interactions have either been reported or are theoretical in humans or animals receiving etidronate and may be of significance in veterinary patients:

■ **ANTACIDS, DIARY PRODUCTS, MINERAL SUPPLEMENTS**, and medications containing **iron, magnesium, calcium** or **aluminum:** Absorption of oral etidronate may be inhibited; separate etidronate doses from these substances by at least two hours.

Laboratory Considerations

■ Etidronate may interfere with bone uptake of technetium **Tc 99m** medronate or technetium Tc 99m oxidronate

Doses

■ **DOGS:**

For severe hypercalcemia associated with neoplastic disease:

a) 5–15 mg/kg daily to twice daily PO; for moderate to severe hypercalcemia (Chew *et al.* 2003)

■ **CATS:**

For severe hypercalcemia associated with neoplastic disease:

a) 5–20 mg/kg/day PO (Ward 1999)

Monitoring

■ Serum calcium

■ Serum protein

Client Information

■ Recommended to give dose to animal that has an empty stomach.

■ If anorexia or vomiting occur, notify veterinarian.

Chemistry/Synonyms

An analog of pyrophosphate, etidronate disodium (also known as EHDP, Na_2EHDP, or sodium etidronate) is a biphosphonate agent that occurs as a white powder and is freely soluble in water. Unlike pyrophosphate, etidronate is resistant to enzymatic degradation in the gut.

Etidronate disodium may also be known as: EHDP, disodium etidronate, etidronate disodium, *Anfozan®, Bonemass®, Didronate®, Didronel®, Difosfen®, Diphos®, Dralen®, Dronate-OS®, Etidrate®, Etidron®, Etiplus®, Feminoflex®, Ostedron®, Osteodidronel, Osteum®, Ostogene®, Ostopor®, Somaflex®,* and *Sviroxit®.*

Storage/Stability

Store tablets in tight containers at room temperature.

Dosage Forms/Regulatory Status

VETERINARY-LABELED PRODUCTS: None

HUMAN-LABELED PRODUCTS:

Etidronate Disodium Tablets: 200 mg, & 400 mg; *Didronel®* (Procter & Gamble Pharm.); generic (Genpharm); (Rx)

References

Chew, D., P. Schenck, et al. (2003). Assessment and treatment of clinical cases with elusive disorders of hypercalcemia. Proceedings: ACVIM Forum. Accessed via: Veterinary Information Network. http://goo.gl/goje1

Ward, H. (1999). Management of cancer-associated hypercalcemia. Proceedings: The North American Veterinary Conference, Orlando.

ETODOLAC

(ee-toe-*doe*-lak)   EtoGesic®, Lodine®

NON-STEROIDAL ANTIINFLAMMATORY AGENT

Prescriber Highlights

▶ NSAID (SC, oral) used in dogs, relatively few adverse effects & labeled for once daily

▶ Contraindications: Hypersensitivity

▶ Caution: Patients with preexisting or occult GI, hepatic, renal, cardiovascular, or hematologic abnormalities

▶ Safe use not established for dogs less than 12 months of age or in breeding, pregnant, or lactating dogs

▶ Adverse Effects: Vomiting, diarrhea, lethargy, hypoproteinemia; keratoconjunctivitis sicca possible; localized pain or tissue reactions at injection site

▶ Drug interactions

Uses/Indications

Etodolac is labeled for the management of pain and inflammation associated with osteoarthritis in dogs. It may find uses, however, for a variety of conditions where pain and/or inflammation should be treated.

Pharmacology/Actions

Like other NSAIDs, etodolac has analgesic, anti-inflammatory, and antipyretic activity. Etodolac appears to be more selective for inhibition of cyclooxygenase-2 than cyclooxygenase-1, but studies conflict and a definitive answer is not presently agreed upon. It may be better to describe etodolac as a COX-1 sparing drug, rather than a COX-2 selective drug. In dogs, etodolac dose also affects whether the drug causes gastrointestinal adverse effects. Doses as little as 2.7X can produce gastrointestinal lesions. Etodolac is also thought to inhibit macrophage chemotaxis, which may explain some of its antiinflammatory activity.

In horses, etodolac does not exhibit much COX-2 selectivity.

Pharmacokinetics

The S(+) enantiomer is thought to provide the bulk of the pharmacologic activity, but the drug is supplied as a racemic mixture. Pharmacokinetic studies that measure both forms as one are not very relevant clinically. After oral administration to healthy dogs, etodolac is rapidly and nearly completely absorbed. The presence of food may alter the rate, but not the extent, of absorption. Peak serum levels occur about 2 hours post dosing. Etodolac is highly bound to serum proteins. The drug is primarily excreted via the bile into the feces. Glucuronide conjugates have been detected in the bile but not the urine. Elimination half-life in dogs varies depending whether food is present in the gut, which may affect the rate of enterohepatic circulation of the drug. These values range from about 8 hours (fasted) to 12 hours (non-fasted). Serum half-life is not necessarily a good predictor for duration of efficacy, possibly due to the drug's high protein binding.

In horses, etodolac has an oral bioavailability of about 77%. After IV dosing, volume of distribution was 0.29 L/kg and the clearance was 235 mL/hr/kg. Elimination half-life (after IV dosing) was approximately 2.5–3 hours.

Contraindications/Precautions/Warnings

Etodolac is contraindicated in dogs previously found to be hypersensitive to it. It should be used with caution in dogs with preexisting or occult GI, hepatic, cardiovascular, or hematologic abnormalities as NSAIDs may exacerbate these conditions. Patients may be more susceptible to renal injury from etodolac if they are dehydrated, on diuretics, or have preexisting renal, hepatic, or cardiovascular dysfunction.

Safety of etodolac has not been established in dogs less than 12 months of age.

Adverse Effects

In clinical field studies, etodolac's primary adverse effect was vomiting/regurgitation, reported in about 5% of dogs tested. Diarrhea, lethargy, and hypoproteinemia have also been reported in dogs. Urticaria, behavioral changes, and inappetence were reported in less than 1% of dogs treated. Potentially, hepatotoxicity and/or nephrotoxicity are possible, but are not well-documented problems in dogs.

Etodolac injection may cause localized pain or tissue reactions at injection site.

Etodolac may decrease total serum T4 in some dogs. Clinical significance is unclear.

Etodolac appears to have less impact on clotting times than other canine-FDA-approved NSAIDs.

Cases have been reported of dogs developing keratoconjunctivitis sicca (KCS) after receiving etodolac treatment. Incidence rate is unknown at this time.

The manufacturer warns to terminate therapy if inappetence, vomiting, fecal abnormalities, or anemia are observed.

Reproductive/Nursing Safety

Safe use has not been established in breeding, pregnant, or lactating dogs; use only when the benefits clearly outweigh the potential risks in these animals. In humans, the FDA categorizes this drug as category *C* for use during pregnancy (*Animal studies have shown an adverse effect on the fetus, but there are no adequate studies in humans; or there are no animal reproduction studies and no adequate studies in humans.*)

Most NSAIDs are excreted in milk; use with caution.

Overdosage/Acute Toxicity

Limited information is available, but in a safety study where dogs were given 40 mg/kg/day (2.7X) GI ulcers, weight loss, emesis and local occult blood were noted. Doses of 80 mg/kg/day (5.3X), caused 6 of 8 dogs to either die or become moribund secondary to GI ulceration. It should be noted that these were not single dose overdoses. However, they demonstrate that there is a relatively narrow therapeutic window for the drug in dogs and that doses should be carefully determined (*i.e.*, do not confuse mg/kg dosages with mg/lb).

There were 39 exposures to etodolac reported to the ASPCA Animal Poison Control Center (APCC) during 2006-2009. In these cases 4 were cats with 2 showing clinical signs and the remaining 35 cases were dogs with 5 showing clinical signs. Common findings in theses cats are recorded in decreasing frequency including acute renal failure, anorexia, collapse, hyperkalemia and hypersalivation. As with any NSAID, overdosage can lead to gastrointestinal and renal effects. Decontamination with emetics and/or activated charcoal may be appropriate. For doses where GI effects are expected, the use of gastrointestinal protectants is warranted. If renal effects are also expected, fluid diuresis is warranted.

Drug Interactions

Note: Although the manufacturer does not list any specific drug interactions in the package insert, it does caution to avoid or closely monitor etodolac's use with other drugs, especially those that are also highly protein bound. It also recommends close monitoring, or to **avoid using etodolac with any other ulcerogenic drugs** (*e.g.*, **corticosteroids, other NSAIDs**). While some advocate a multi-day washout period when switching from one NSAID to another (not aspirin—see below), there does not appear to be any credible evidence that this is required. Until so, consider starting the new NSAID when the next dose would be due for the old one.

The following drug interactions have either been reported or are theoretical in humans or animals receiving etodolac and may be of significance in veterinary patients:

- **ACE INHIBITORS (enalapril, benazepril,** etc.): Etodolac may reduce the antihypertensive effects of ACE inhibitors. Because ACE inhibitors potentially can reduce renal blood flow, use with NSAIDs could increase the risk for renal injury. However, one study in dogs receiving tepoxalin did not show any adverse effect. It is unknown what effects, if any, occur if other NSAIDs and ACE inhibitors are used together in dogs.

- **ASPIRIN:** When aspirin is used concurrently with etodolac, plasma levels of etodolac could decrease and an increased likelihood of GI adverse effects (blood loss) could occur; concomitant administration of aspirin with etodolac cannot be recommended. Washout periods of several days is probably warranted when switching from an NSAID to aspirin therapy in dogs.

- **CYCLOSPORINE:** Etodolac may increase cyclosporine blood levels and increase the risk for nephrotoxicity

- **DIGOXIN:** Etodolac may increase serum levels of digoxin. Use with caution in patients with severe cardiac failure

- **FUROSEMIDE & OTHER DIURETICS:** Etodolac may reduce the saluretic and diuretic effects of furosemide

- **METHOTREXATE:** Serious toxicity has occurred when NSAIDs have been used concomitantly with methotrexate; use together with caution

- **NEPHROTOXIC AGENTS** (*e.g.*, **amphotericin B, aminoglycosides, cisplatin,** etc.): Potential for increased risk of nephrotoxicity if used with NSAIDs

- **PHENOBARBITAL:** May increase the metabolism of etodolac in dogs

- **PROBENECID:** May cause a significant increase in serum levels and half-life of etodolac

- **WARFARIN:** Etodolac may increase the risk for bleeding

Laboratory Considerations

- Etodolac may cause false-positive determinations of **urine bilirubin.**

- Etodolac therapy may alter **thyroid function tests** and their interpretation; falsely low values may occur in dogs receiving etodolac.

Doses

- **DOGS:**
  a) For treatment of pain and inflammation associated with osteoarthritis: Oral Tablets: 10–15 mg/kg PO once daily. Dogs less than 5 kg cannot be accurately dosed with EtoGesic® tablets. Adjust dose to obtain satisfactory response, but do not exceed 15 mg/kg. For long-term therapy, reduce dose level to minimum effective dosage.

  Injection: 10–15 mg/kg as a dorsoscapular subcutaneous (SC) injection. If needed, daily doses of tablets may begin 24 hours after the last injectable treatment. Use alternate injection sites. The likelihood of injection site reactions increases when administered near previous injection sites. (Package Insert; *EtoGesic® Tablets; Injection*—BIVI)

Monitoring

- Baseline (especially in geriatric dogs or dogs with chronic diseases or those where prolonged treatment is likely): physical exam, CBC, Serum chemistry panel (including liver and renal function tests), UA. It is recommended to reassess liver enzymes at one week of therapy. Should elevation occur, recommend discontinuing the drug

- Tear production prior to, and during therapy

- Clinical efficacy

- Signs of potential adverse reactions: inappetence, diarrhea, mucoid feces, vomiting, melena, polyuria/polydipsia, anemia, jaundice, lethargy, behavior changes, ataxia, or seizures

- Chronic therapy: Consider repeating CBC, UA, and serum chemistries on an ongoing basis.

Client information

- Give the client written information on the proper use and monitoring for etodolac

Chemistry/Synonyms

An indole acetic acid derivative non-steroidal antiinflammatory agent (NSAID), etodolac occurs as a white, crystalline compound that is insoluble in water, but soluble in alcohol or DMSO. Etodolac has a chirally active center with a corresponding S (+) enantiomer and an R (-) enantiomer. The commercially available product is supplied as a racemic mixture of the forms.

Etodolac may also be known as: AY-24236, etodolacum, etodolic acid, *Acudor®, Articulan®, Dualgan®, Eccoxolac®, Edolan®, Elderin®,*

EtoGesic®, Etonox®, Etopan®, Flancox®, Hypen®, Lodot®, Lonine®, Metazin®, Sodolac®, Todolac®, Ultradol®, and *Zedolac®.*

Storage/Stability

The commercially available veterinary tablets should be stored at controlled room temperature (15–30°C).

The commercially available injection should be stored at or below 77°F (25°C).

Dosage Forms/Regulatory Status

VETERINARY-LABELED PRODUCTS:

Etodolac Scored Tablets: 150 mg & 300 mg in bottles of 30 & 90; *EtoGesic®* (BIVI); (Rx). FDA-approved for use in dogs. Do not use in cats.

Etodolac Injection 10% (100 mg/mL) in 50 mL vials; *EtoGesic® Injectable* (BIVI); (Rx). FDA-approved for use in dogs. The ARCI (Racing Commissioners International) has designated this drug as a class 4 substance. See the appendix for more information.

HUMAN-LABELED PRODUCTS:

Etodolac Tablets: 400 mg & 500 mg; Capsules: 200 mg & 300 mg; and 400 mg, 500 mg & 600 mg extended-release tablets; generic; (Rx)

ETOMIDATE

(ee-toe-*mi*-date)   Amidate®

INJECTABLE ANESTHETIC

Prescriber Highlights

▶ Injectable non-barbiturate anesthetic agent that may be useful as an alternative to thiopental or propofol for induction, particularly in patients with preexisting cardiac dysfunction, head trauma, or that are critically ill

▶ Can inhibit cortisol production; may need to supplement corticosteroids in critically ill patients

▶ Not a controlled substance

▶ Relatively expensive, especially in large dogs

Uses/Indications

Etomidate may be useful as an alternative to thiopental or propofol for anesthetic induction in small animals, particularly in patients with preexisting cardiac dysfunction, head trauma, or that are critically ill.

Pharmacology/Actions

The exact mechanism of action of etomidate is not well defined. Etomidate causes minimal hemodynamic changes and little effect on the cardiovascular system when compared to other injectable anesthetic agents. At usual doses, etomidate has little effect on respiratory rate or rhythm. Etomidate decreases cerebral blood flow and oxygen consumption. It usually lowers intraocular pressure and causes slight decreases

in intracranial pressure. Etomidate reportedly does not induce malignant hyperthermia, but can speed its onset in susceptible patients secondary to a triggering agent.

The reported therapeutic index (toxic dose/therapeutic dose) for etomidate is 16. Therapeutic indexes for propofol and thiopental are 3 and 5 respectively.

In comparing etomidate with propofol when used for inductions in dogs, patients receiving etomidate had higher systolic arterial pressures and mean arterial pressures, but it caused longer and poorer recoveries than propofol (Sams *et al.* 2008).

Pharmacokinetics

No specific information on the pharmacokinetics of etomidate in domesticated animals was located. In humans, after intravenous injection etomidate is rapidly distributed into the CNS and then rapidly cleared from the brain back into systemic tissues. Duration of hypnosis is short (3–5 minutes) and dependent upon dose. Recovery from anesthesia appears to be as fast as with thiopental, but slower than propofol. Etomidate is 75% bound to plasma proteins. The drug is rapidly metabolized in the liver primarily via hydrolysis or glucuronidation to inactive metabolites. The majority of the drug and metabolites are excreted into the urine with the remainder into the bile and feces. Elimination half-life ranges from 1.25–5 hours.

Contraindications/Precautions/Warnings

Etomidate is contraindicated in patients known to be hypersensitive to it.

Etomidate can inhibit adrenocortical function; it should not be used for purposes other than induction, and with caution in patients whose adrenocortical function is impaired. Exogenous glucocorticoid administration should be considered in severely compromised animals.

Etomidate does not provide significant analgesia.

Limited studies in patients with impaired hepatic or renal function have shown that elimination half-lives may be significantly increased in these patients and the propylene glycol carrier in the injection may be problematic in patients with liver dysfunction.

Adverse Effects

Common adverse effects include pain at intravenous injection site, vomiting, skeletal muscle movements (myoclonus), eye movements, and post-operative retching. Preanesthetic medications and a benzodiazepine (diazepam, midazolam) just prior to etomidate can minimize these effects.

Some hemolysis may occur due to the propylene glycol content of the injection. Some anesthesiologists recommend injecting etomidate into a running IV line to decrease the pain associated with injection and, potentially, reduce hemolysis.

While etomidate causes minimal cardiopulmonary depression, a brief period of hypoventilation and decreased arterial blood pressure can occur after administration.

Apnea, laryngospasm, hiccups, hyperventilation, hypoventilation, hypertension, hypotension, lactic acidosis, arrhythmias, and postoperative vomiting have all been reported in human patients that have received the drug. Seizures have been reported in a few human patients receiving etomidate; this adverse effect may be reduced if an opiate premed is first administered.

Reproductive/Nursing Safety

In humans, the FDA categorizes etomidate as a category *C* drug for use during pregnancy (*Animal studies have shown an adverse effect on the fetus, but there are no adequate studies in humans; or there are no animal reproduction studies and no adequate studies in humans*). Etomidate has caused embryocidal effects in rats and maternal toxicity in rabbits and rats.

Some etomidate is excreted into maternal milk; use with caution in nursing patients.

Overdosage/Acute Toxicity

Acute overdoses would be expected to cause enhanced pharmacologic effects of the drug. Treatment would be supportive (*i.e.*, mechanical ventilation), until the effects of the medication are diminished.

Drug Interactions

The following drug interactions have either been reported or are theoretical in humans or animals receiving etomidate and may be of significance in veterinary patients:

■ **CNS/RESPIRATORY DEPRESSANTS (e.g., barbiturates, opiates, anesthetics, etc.):** Additive pharmacological effects can occur if etomidate is used concurrently with other drugs that can depress CNS or respiratory function

■ **VERAPAMIL:** Has been associated with potentiating the anesthetic and respiratory depressant effects of etomidate

Laboratory Considerations

■ Etomidate's effects on inhibiting cortisol may invalidate **ACTH stimulation** and **glucose tolerance** tests. In dogs, cortisol function may be affected up to 3 hours after an etomidate dose.

Doses

■ **DOGS & CATS:**
  a) As an induction agent: etomidate 1 mg/kg IV plus diazepam 0.5 mg/kg IV (Cornell 2004)

  b) As an induction agent: 1–2 mg/kg rapidly IV (Heath 2003)

  c) As an induction agent: 0.5–2 mg/kg IV. Pre-medication is highly recommended to reduce incidence of side effects (my-

oclonus, vomiting). Alternatively or additionally, etomidate may be given with a benzodiazepine. Because of its effects on cortisol, administration of a physiologic dose of dexamethasone or another short-acting glucocorticoid prior to etomidate is suggested. (Mama 2002)

■ **FERRETS:**
  a) As an induction agent in the cardiovascular unstable patient: etomidate 1–2 mg/kg IV after diazepam (0.5 mg/kg IV) (Lichtenberger 2006)

■ **SMALL MAMMALS:**
  a) **Rabbits:** As an induction agent in the cardiovascular unstable patient: etomidate 1–2 mg/kg IV after diazepam (0.5 mg/kg IV) (Lichtenberger 2006)

Monitoring

As per any anesthetic agent:
■ Level of consciousness
■ Respiration rate and depth
■ Cardiovascular function

Client Information

■ Etomidate is a potent sedative-hypnotic that should only be used by professionals in a setting where adequate patient monitoring is available.

Chemistry/Synonyms

An injectable, carboxylic imidazole anesthetic, etomidate occurs as a white or almost white powder. It is very slightly soluble in water and freely soluble in alcohol. The commercially available injection has a pH of 8.1, contains 35% propylene glycol, and is hyperosmolar (4640 mosm/l).

Etomidate may also be known as: R-16659, *Amidate®*, *Hypnomidate®*, *Radenarcon®*, or *Sibul®*.

Storage/Stability

Unless otherwise labeled, store etomidate injection at room temperature and protect from light.

Dosage Forms/Regulatory Status

VETERINARY-LABELED PRODUCTS: None
HUMAN-LABELED PRODUCTS:
Etomidate Injection: 2 mg/mL in 10 mL & 20 mL single-dose vials, 10 mL & 20 mL amps and 20 mL *Abboject* syringes; *Amidate®* (Hospira); generic; (Rx)

References

Cornell, C. (2004). Anesthetic Drugs. Proceedings: ACVIM Forum. Accessed via: Veterinary Information Network. http://goo.gl/edDP1

Heath, D. (2003). Anesthesia in the critical patient. Proceedings: ACVIM Forum. Accessed via: Veterinary Information Network. http://goo.gl/RfcDQ

Lichtenberger, M. (2006). Anesthesia Protocols and Pain Management for Exotic Animal Patients. Proceedings: Western Vet Conf. Accessed via: Veterinary Information Network. http://goo.gl/hB5Kt

Mama, K. (2002). Injectable anesthesia: Pharmacology and clinical use of contemporary agents. Proceedings:

World Small Animal Veterinary Association. Accessed via: Veterinary Information Network. http://goo.gl/1Z7Iy

Sams, L., C. Braun, et al. (2008). A comparison of the effects of propofol and etomidate on the induction of anesthesia and on cardiopulmonary parameters in dogs. *Veterinary Anaesthesia and Analgesia* 35(6): 488–494.

Etretinate–see Acitretin

EUTHANASIA AGENTS WITH PENTOBARBITAL

(yoo-thon-*ayzh*-ya; pen-toe-*barb*-i-tal)

For therapeutic uses (other than euthanasia) of pentobarbital, see the main pentobarbital monograph for this agent. The sections on chemistry, storage, pharmacokinetics, overdosage, drug interactions, and monitoring parameters can be found in the main pentobarbital monograph.

Prescriber Highlights

▶ Used for humane euthanasia for animals not to be used for food

▶ Store so that it will not be confused with therapeutic agents; keep out of reach of children

▶ Use care in handling filled syringes & dispose of used injection equipment properly

▶ Avoid any contact with open wounds or accidental injection

▶ Tranquilizing agent may be necessary when the animal is in pain or agitated

▶ Renderers may not accept carcasses euthanized with pentobarbital

Uses/Indications

For rapid, humane euthanasia in animals not intended for food purposes. Individual products may be approved for use in specific species.

"The advantages of using barbiturates for euthanasia in small animals far outweigh the disadvantages. Intravenous injection of a barbituric acid derivative is the preferred method for euthanasia of dogs, cats, other small animals, and horses. Intraperitoneal injection may be used in situations when an intravenous injection would be distressful or even dangerous. Intracardiac injection must only be used if the animal is heavily sedated, unconscious, or anesthetized." (AVMA Guidelines on Euthanasia, 2007)

Pharmacology/Actions

Pentobarbital causes death by severely depressing the medullary respiratory and vasomotor centers when administered at high doses. Cardiac activity may persist for several minutes following administration.

Phenytoin is added to *Beuthanasia®-D Special* (Schering) for its added cardiac depressant effects and to denature the compounds from a Class-II controlled substance to Class-III drugs.

Contraindications/Precautions/Warnings

Must not be used in animals to be used for food purposes (human or animal consumption). Should be stored in such a manner that these products will not be confused with therapeutic agents. Extreme care in handling filled syringes and proper disposal of used injection equipment must be undertaken. Avoid any contact with open wounds or accidental injection. Keep out of reach of children.

Prior use of a tranquilizing agent may be necessary when the animal is in pain or agitated.

Adverse Effects

Minor muscle twitching may occur after injection. Death may be delayed or not accomplished if injection given perivascularly.

Doses

Because different products have different concentrations, please refer to the information provided with the product in use.

■ **DOGS:**

a) Pentobarbital sodium (as a single agent): Approximately 120 mg/kg for the first 4.5 kg of body weight, and 60 mg/kg for every 4.5 kg of body weight thereafter. Preferably administer IV.

b) Pentobarbital sodium with phenytoin (*Beuthanasia®-D Special*): 1 mL for each 4.5 kg of body weight.

■ **CATS:**

a) Pentobarbital sodium (as a single agent): Approximately 120 mg/kg for the first 4.5 kg of body weight, and 60 mg/kg for every 4.5 kg of body weight thereafter. Administer IV.

b) Pentobarbital sodium with phenytoin: (*Beuthanasia®-D Special*): 1 mL for each 4.5 kg of body weight (not FDA-approved for use in this species)

■ **LARGE ANIMALS:**
Note: Must not be used in animals to be consumed by either humans or other animals.

a) Depending on product concentration, most animals require 10–15 mL per 100 pounds of body weight.

Monitoring
■ Respiratory rate
■ Cardiac rate
■ Corneal reflex

Client Information
■ Must be administered by an individual familiar with its use.
■ Animals must be restrained during administration.
■ Inform clients observing euthanasia that

animal may give a terminal gasp after becoming unconscious.

Dosage Forms/Regulatory Status

See other pentobarbital dosage forms under the main pentobarbital monograph for lower concentration products that are used therapeutically.

VETERINARY-LABELED PRODUCTS:

Pentobarbital Sodium 390 mg/mL & Phenytoin Sodium 50 mg/mL for Injection (Euthanasia) in 100 mL vials; *Beuthanasia®-D Special* (Schering-Plough); *Euthasol®* (Virbac); *Euthanasia-III® Solution* (Med-Pharmex); *Somnasol®* (Butler); (Rx, C-III). Approved for use in dogs.

Pentobarbital Sodium Powder:

392 mg/mL when constituted with 250 mL of water. *Fatal-Plus® Powder* (Vortech), *Pentasol® Powder* (Virbac); (Rx, C-II) Approved for use in animals regardless of species.

Pentobarbital Sodium for Injection (Euthanasia):

260 mg/mL: *Sleepaway®* (Pfizer) 26%: in 100 mL bottles; (Rx, C-II). Labeled for use in dogs and cats.

324 mg/mL: *SP5®* (Vedco) in 100 mL vials; (Rx, C-II). Labeled for use in dogs and cats.

389 mg/mL: *Socumb-6gr®* (ButlerSchein), *Somlethol®* (Webster), *SP6®* (Vedco); 100 mL & 250 mL vials; (Rx, C-II). Labeled for use in dogs and cats.

390 mg/mL: *Fatal-Plus® Solution* (Vortech); in 250 mL vials (Rx, C-II). Labeled for use in animals regardless of species.

HUMAN-LABELED PRODUCTS: None

FAMCICLOVIR

(fam-sye-*klow*-veer)   Famvir®

ANTIVIRAL (HERPES)

Prescriber Highlights

▶ May be effective in treating feline herpes (FHV-1) infections

▶ Limited experience and information available in using this medication in cats

▶ Appears to be well tolerated when used short-term (2–3 weeks)

▶ Relatively expensive, but prices may decrease now that generics are available

Uses/Indications

Famciclovir may be of benefit in treating feline herpes infections.

Pharmacology/Actions

In most species, famciclovir is rapidly converted *in vivo* to penciclovir. In cells infected with susceptible Herpes virus or varicella zoster virus, viral thymidine kinase phosphorylates penciclovir to penciclovir monophosphate. Cellular kinases further convert this compound to penciclovir triphosphate which inhibits herpes virus DNA polymerase via competition with deoxyguanosine triphosphate, thereby selectively inhibiting herpes viral DNA synthesis.

Viral resistance can occur by mutation.

Pharmacokinetics

The pharmacokinetics of famciclovir in cats is complex and not well understood. After oral administration of famciclovir (62.5 mg), penciclovir peak levels were less than the *in vitro* inhibitory concentration 50 (IC-50) for FHV-1. In humans, conversion of famciclovir to penciclovir requires oxidation by hepatic aldehyde oxidase. As cats possess little hepatic aldehyde oxidase they may require higher dosages than are used in humans or other species. (Thomasy *et al.* 2006), (Maggs 2009)

In humans, famciclovir is well absorbed after oral administration, but undergoes extensive first pass metabolism (not by CYP enzymes). Food can decrease peak levels, but does not significantly impact clinical efficacy. Penciclovir (active metabolite) is only marginally bound to plasma proteins. In humans, penciclovir elimination half-life is about 2–3 hours; excretion is primarily via renal mechanisms. Intracellular half-lives of penciclovir in infected cells are significantly longer.

Contraindications/Precautions/Warnings

Famciclovir is contraindicated in patients known to be hypersensitive to it or penciclovir.

It should be used with caution (and dosage adjustment) in patients with renal dysfunction. In humans patients with CrCl <40 mL/min, dosage adjustments are recommended.

Adverse Effects

Adverse effects in cats are not well documented, but the drug appears to be tolerated quite well when used for up to 3 weeks. At doses of 90 mg/kg PO q8h, anorexia and polydipsia have been noted in some cats.

In humans, famciclovir can cause nausea, vomiting, diarrhea, and headache. Neutropenia has been reported and renal failure can occur, particularly when doses are not adjusted in patients with renal dysfunction.

Reproductive/Nursing Safety

In laboratory animals, doses of up to 1,000 mg/kg/day did not cause any observed effects on developing embryos or fetuses. In humans, the FDA categorizes this drug as category *B* for use during pregnancy (*Animal studies have not yet demonstrated risk to the fetus, but there are no adequate studies in pregnant women; or animal studies have shown an adverse effect, but adequate studies in pregnant women have not demonstrated a risk to the fetus in the first trimester of pregnancy, and there is no evidence of risk in later trimesters.*)

Famciclovir (as penciclovir) is excreted in the milk of rats. It is unclear if there is any clinical significance for nursing offspring.

Overdosage/Acute Toxicity

Little information is available. Supportive treatment has been recommended. Penciclovir can be removed by hemodialysis.

Drug Interactions

The following drug interactions have either been reported or are theoretical in humans or animals receiving famciclovir and may be of significance in veterinary patients:

■ **PROBENECID:** Can reduce the amount of penciclovir excreted by the kidneys, increase penciclovir plasma levels can occur

Laboratory Considerations

■ No concerns noted

Doses

■ **CATS:**

For feline herpes virus (FHV-1):

Note: There is a considerable amount of uncertainty at present how to dose cats with famciclovir, but because the drug looks promising, there will be more data forthcoming.

a) There is a wide range of doses used; author's choice: 125 mg (total dose) PO 2-3 times a day. (Ketring 2009)

b) For adjunctive treatment of FHV-1 rhinotracheitis: 31.25 mg (1/4 of one 125 mg tablet) PO q12h for 14 days. Has not been evaluated for long-term therapy. (Lappin 2007)

c) For chronic, recurrent and/or severe herpes viral infection: Dose range is variable! Kittens: ⅛th of one 125 mg tablet PO once daily (q24h) for 2 weeks; adult cats: 1/4 of one 250 mg tablet once daily (q24h) for 3 weeks. (Diehl 2007)

d) 1/4 of one 125 mg tablet PO twice daily (q12h) for 10−14 days; may continue once daily for up to 30 days. (Ramsey 2006)

e) For adjunctive treatment (with interferon and lysine) of herpes virus-associated ulcerative facial dermatitis & stomatitis: 125 mg PO q12h. (Hillier 2006)

Monitoring

■ Clinical efficacy

■ Adverse effects (most likely GI)

■ Consider occasional CBC's and creatinine to monitor for neutropenia or renal dysfunction if using the drug chronically

Client Information

■ May be administered with food

■ There is limited experience with this drug in cats, report any unusual effects to the veterinarian

■ FHV-1 infections are controlled, not cured, and recurrence may occur even if the cat is treated life-long

Chemistry/Synonyms

A prodrug, famciclovir is a purine-derived, synthetic, acyclic purine nucleoside analog.

Famciclovir may also be known as AV 42810, BRL 42810, famciclovirum, or by the trade name *Famvir®*.

Storage/Stability

Famciclovir tablets should be stored at room temperature (15−30°C).

Dosage Forms/Regulatory Status

VETERINARY-LABELED PRODUCTS: None

HUMAN-LABELED PRODUCTS:

Famciclovir Oral Tablets (film-coated) 125 mg, 250 mg, & 500 mg: *Famvir®* (Novartis); generic; (Rx)

References

Diehl, K. (2007). Pink and puffy: What the cat conjunctiva is trying to tell you. Proceedings: Western Vet Conf. Accessed via: Veterinary Information Network. http://goo.gl/p6cEV

Hillier, A. (2006). Emerging feline skin diseases. Proceedings: ACVC. Accessed via: Veterinary Information Network. http://goo.gl/IBxXq

Ketring, K. (2009). Feline Herpes--New Drugs and New Thoughts. Proceedings: WVC. Accessed via: Veterinary Information Network. http://goo.gl/yn5WW

Lappin, M. (2007). Treating feline sinusitis. Proceedings: Western Vet Conf. Accessed via: Veterinary Information Network. http://goo.gl/uy82F

Maggs, D. (2009). Update on the diagnosis and treatment of feline herpesvirus. Proceedings: World Small Animal Veterinary Assoc. World Congress. Accessed via: Veterinary Information Network. http://goo.gl/1Zyak

Ramsey, D. (2006). Ocular manifestations of feline herpesvirus. Proceedings: ACVO. Accessed via: Veterinary Information Network. http://goo.gl/YhLHv

Thomasy, S., D. Maggs, et al. (2006). Pharmacokinetics of penciclovir following oral administration of famciclovir to cats. Proceedings: ACVIM. Accessed via: Veterinary Information Network. http://goo.gl/TyzvN

FAMOTIDINE

(fa-*moe*-ti-deen)   Pepcid®

H2-RECEPTOR ANTAGONIST

Prescriber Highlights

▶ H2-receptor antagonist used to reduce GI acid production

▶ Longer duration of action & fewer drug interactions than cimetidine

▶ Contraindications: Hypersensitivity to H2 blockers

▶ Caution: Patients with cardiac disease, significantly impaired hepatic or renal function; (consider dosage reduction)

▶ Adverse Effects: Too rapid IV infusion may cause bradycardia. Potentially: GI effects, headache, or dry mouth or skin; rarely, intravascular hemolysis anecdotally reported when given IV to cats

Uses/Indications

In veterinary medicine, famotidine may be useful for the treatment and/or prophylaxis of gastric, abomasal and duodenal ulcers, uremic gastritis, stress-related or drug-induced erosive gastritis, esophagitis, duodenal gastric reflux, and esophageal reflux. It has been recommended in dogs as an "... excellent drug for routine prophylaxis where cost is a concern and where an injectable drug is preferred or ... in dogs requiring extended therapy (a minimum of one week), since its effects will improve with time and become comparable to the more expensive PPIs" (Bersenas 2007).

Famotidine has significantly fewer drug interactions than cimetidine and activity may persist longer.

In dogs, famotidine did not improve outcomes (eradication) of Helicobacter infections when added to triple antibiotic therapy (Leib *et al.* 2007). Omeprazole was superior to famotidine when used to prevent exercise-induced gastritis in racing Alaskan sled dogs (Williamson *et al.* 2010).

Pharmacology/Actions

At the H_2 receptors of the parietal cells, famotidine competitively inhibits histamine, thereby reducing gastric acid output both during basal conditions and when stimulated by food, pentagastrin, histamine or insulin. Gastric emptying time, pancreatic or biliary secretion, and lower esophageal pressures are not altered by famotidine. By decreasing the amount of gastric juice produced, H_2-blockers also decreases the amount of pepsin secreted.

Pharmacokinetics

Famotidine is not completely absorbed after oral administration, but undergoes only minimal first-pass metabolism. In humans, systemic bioavailability is about 40–50%. Distribution characteristics are not well described. In rats, the drug concentrates in the liver, pancreas, kidney and submandibular gland. Only about 15–20% is bound to plasma proteins. In rats, the drug does not cross the blood brain barrier or the placenta. It is distributed into milk. When the drug is administered orally, about 1/3 is excreted unchanged in the urine and the remainder primarily metabolized in the liver and then excreted in the urine. After intravenous dosing, about 2/3's of a dose is excreted unchanged.

The pharmacokinetics of famotidine, ranitidine, and cimetidine have been investigated in horses. (Duran and Ravis 1993) After a single IV dosage, elimination half-lives of cimetidine, ranitidine, and famotidine all were in the 2–3 hour range and were not significantly different. Of the three drugs tested, famotidine had a larger volume of distribution (4.28 L/kg) than either cimetidine (1.14 L/kg) or ranitidine (2.04 L/kg). Bioavailability of each of the drugs was low; famotidine (13%), ranitidine (13.5%) and cimetidine (30%).

Contraindications/Precautions/Warnings

Famotidine is contraindicated in patients with known hypersensitivity to the drug.

Famotidine should be used cautiously in geriatric patients and patients with significantly impaired hepatic or renal function. Consider dosage reduction in patients with significant renal dysfunction. Famotidine may have negative inotropic effects and have some cardioarrhythmogenic properties. Use with caution in patients with cardiac disease.

Adverse Effects

Too rapid IV infusion may cause bradycardia. Other H_2-blockers have been demonstrated to be relatively safe and exhibit minimal adverse effects. Potential adverse effects (documented in humans) that could be seen include GI effects (anorexia, vomiting, diarrhea), headache, or dry mouth or skin. Rarely, agranulocytosis may develop particularly when used concomitantly with other drugs that can cause bone marrow depression.

There are rare anecdotal reports of famotidine causing intravascular hemolysis when given intravenously to cats. It is believed this is probably an idiosyncratic reaction that occurs in a small percentage of cats treated. A retrospective study evaluating IV famotidine in 56 hospitalized cats did not show any evidence of hemolysis. The authors concluded that the IV route appeared safe in cats when famotidine was administered over 5 minutes (Galvao & Trepanier 2008).

Reproductive/Nursing Safety

In lab animal studies, famotidine demonstrated no detectable harm to offspring. Large doses could affect the mother's food intake and weight gain during pregnancy that could indirectly be harmful. Use in pregnancy when potential benefits outweigh the risks. In rats, nursing from mothers receiving very high doses of famotidine, transient decreases in weight gain occurred. In humans, the FDA categorizes this drug as category *B* for use during pregnancy (*Animal studies have not yet demonstrated risk to the fetus, but there are no adequate studies in pregnant women; or animal studies have shown an adverse effect, but adequate studies in pregnant women have not demonstrated a risk to the fetus in the first trimester of pregnancy, and there is no evidence of risk in later trimesters.*)

Famotidine is excreted in the milk of rats. It is unclear if there is any clinical significance for nursing offspring with H_2-blockers in milk.

Overdosage/Acute Toxicity

The minimum acute lethal dose in dogs is reported to be >2 grams/kg for oral doses and approximately 300 mg/kg for intravenous doses. IV doses in dogs ranging from 5–200 mg/kg IV caused: vomiting, restlessness, mucous membrane pallor and redness of the mouth and ears. Higher doses caused hypotension, tachycardia and collapse.

Because of this wide margin of safety associated with the drug, most overdoses should require only monitoring. In massive oral overdoses, gut-emptying protocols should be considered and supportive therapy initiated when warranted.

Drug Interactions
The following drug interactions have either been reported or are theoretical in humans or animals receiving famotidine and may be of significance in veterinary patients:

■ **AZOLE ANTIFUNGALS (ketoconazole, itraconazole, fluconazole):** By raising gastric pH, famotidine may decrease the absorption of these agents; if both drugs are required, administer the azole one hour prior to famotidine

■ **CEFPODOXIME, CEFUROXIME:** Famotidine may decrease the absorption of these cephalosporins; taking with food may alleviate this effect

■ **IRON SALTS (ORAL):** Famotidine may decrease the absorption of oral iron; administer iron at least one hour prior to famotidine

Unlike cimetidine or ranitidine, famotidine does not appear to inhibit hepatic cytochrome P-450 enzyme systems and dosage adjustments of other drugs (*e.g.*, warfarin, theophylline, diazepam, procainamide, phenytoin) that are metabolized by this metabolic pathway should usually not be required.

Laboratory Considerations
■ Histamine$_2$-blockers may antagonize the effects of **histamine** and **pentagastrin** in the evaluation gastric acid secretion.

■ After using allergen extract **skin tests**, histamine$_2$ antagonists may inhibit histamine responses. It is recommended that histamine$_2$ blockers be discontinued at least 24 hours before performing either of these tests.

Doses
■ **DOGS:**
To reduce gastric acid production:
a) 0.1–0.2 mg/kg PO, SC, IM, IV q12h (Marks 2008)
b) 0.5 mg/kg PO, SC, IM, IV q12–24 hours (Matz 1995)
c) For esophagitis: 0.5–1 mg/kg PO q12h (Glazer & Walters 2008)
d) 0.55–1.1 mg/kg PO q24h (or every 12 hours if there is severe esophagitis) for 2–3 weeks in dogs with acute reflex esophagitis (Tams 2003)
e) For adjunctive treatment (to prevent/treat gastric ulcers) of mast cell tumors: 0.5 mg/kg once daily (route not specified). (Garrett 2006)
f) For adjunctive treatment of GI effects (anorexia, nausea, vomiting) associated with chronic kidney disease: 0.5 mg/kg PO once daily (q24h) Effective evidence grade: 3. (Polzin 2005)

■ **CATS:**
Note: See the warning (in the adverse effects section) about IV use in cats.
To reduce gastric acid production:
a) 0.2 mg/kg PO, SC, IM, IV q24h (Marks, 2008)
b) 0.5 mg/kg PO, SC, IM, IV q12–24 hours (Matz, 1995)
c) For esophagitis: 0.5 mg/kg PO q12h (Glazer & Walters 2008)
d) 0.55–1.1 mg/kg PO q24h (or every 12 hours if there is severe esophagitis) for 2–3 weeks in cats with acute reflex esophagitis (Tams 2003)

For adjunctive treatment of GI effects (anorexia, nausea, vomiting) associated with chronic progressive renal disease:
a) 1 mg/kg PO once daily (q24h) (Wolf 2006)
b) 0.5–1 mg/kg PO once or twice daily (q12–24h) (Zoran 2006)

■ **FERRETS:**
a) For stress induced ulcers: 0.25–0.5 mg/kg PO, IV once daily (Williams 2000)
b) In combination with antibiotics for Helicobacter treatment: 0.25–0.5 mg/kg PO, IV q24h (Fisher 2005)

■ **SMALL MAMMALS:**
Rabbits: For stress induced ulcer prevention once critically ill animal has stabilized:
a) 1 mg/kg IV once daily (q24h) (Johnston 2006)

■ **HORSES:** (**Note:** ARCI UCGFS Class 5 Drug)
As an adjunct in ulcer treatment:
a) IV doses: 0.23 mg/kg, IV q8h or 0.35 mg/kg IV q12h.
Oral doses: 1.88 mg/kg, PO q8h or 2.8 mg/kg PO q12h (Duran & Ravis 1993)

Monitoring
■ Clinical efficacy (dependent on reason for use); monitored by decrease in symptomatology, endoscopic examination, blood in feces, etc.

■ Adverse effects, if noted

Client Information
■ To maximize the benefit of this medication, it must be administered as prescribed by the veterinarian

■ Clinical signs may reoccur if dosages are missed

Chemistry/Synonyms
An H$_2$-receptor antagonist, famotidine occurs as a white to pale yellow, crystalline powder. It is odorless, but has a bitter taste. 740 micrograms are soluble in one mL of water.

Famotidine may also be known as: famotidinum, L-643341, MK-208, and YM-11170; many trade names are available.

Storage/Stability

Tablets should be stored in well-closed, light-resistant containers at room temperature. Tablets are assigned an expiration date of 30 months after date of manufacture.

The powder for oral suspension should be stored in tight containers at temperatures less than 40°C. After reconstitution, the resultant suspension is stable for 30 days when stored at temperatures less than 30°C.; do not freeze.

Famotidine injection should be stored in the refrigerator (2–8°C).

Compatibility/Compounding Considerations

Famotidine is physically **compatible** with most commonly used IV infusion solutions and is stable for 48 hours at room temperature when diluted in these solutions.

Compounded preparation stability: Famotidine oral suspension compounded from commercially available tablets has been published (Dentinger *et al.* 2000). Triturating twenty-four (24) famotidine 40 mg tablets with 60 mL of *Ora-Plus®* and qs ad to 120 mL with *Ora-Sweet®* (or *Ora-Sweet®* SF) brought to a favorable pH of 5.8 yields an 8 mg/mL oral suspension that retains >90% potency for 95 days stored at 25°C. Famotidine is stable in buffered solutions at pH 4-6, but rapid and extensive drug degradation occurs at pH less than 2.

Another "recipe" to make a 4 mg/mL flavored, oral aqueous-based suspension from 10 mg tablets: To make a 30 mL suspension: Pulverize twelve 10 mg tabs (0.12 g) to a fine powder in a mortar and pestle. Wet with glycerin (1–2 mL) to make a thick paste. Add up to 1 mL of a water-soluble flavoring agent. Add enough oral suspending vehicle—OSV (*e.g.*, *Ora-Plus®*, *Ora-Sweet®*, etc.) and mix to allow transfer to an amber prescription bottle. May need to repeat this process several times to "wash" the mortar. "q.s ad" to 30 mL with additional OSV. Shake well before use, store in the refrigerator and dispose any unused amount after 30 days.

Dosage Forms/Regulatory Status

VETERINARY-LABELED PRODUCTS: None
The ARCI (Racing Commissioners International) has designated this drug as a class 5 substance. See the appendix for more information.

HUMAN-LABELED PRODUCTS:

Famotidine Oral Tablets (plain, film-coated, chewable & orally disintegrating) & Gelcaps: 10 mg & 20 mg, & 40 mg; *Pepcid®*, *Pepcid AC® Maximum Strength* & *Pepcid RPD®* (Merck); (Rx); *Pepcid AC®* (J & J Merck); generic; (Rx & OTC)

Famotidine Powder for Oral Suspension: 8 mg/mL when reconstituted in 400 mg bottles; *Pepcid®* (Merck); (Rx)

Famotidine Injection: 10 mg/mL in 1 & 2 mL single dose vials and 4 mL, 20 mL & 50 mL multidose vials (may contain mannitol or benzyl alcohol); 20 mg/50 mL premixed in 50 mL single-dose *Galaxy* containers; generic; (Rx)

References

Bersenas, A. (2007). Antacids: What is the evidence? Proceedings: IVECCS. Accessed via: Veterinary Information Network. http://goo.gl/YZKJB

Dentinger, P.J., C.F. Swenson, et al. (2000). Stability of famotidine in an extemporaneously compounded oral liquid. *Am J Health Syst Pharm* 57(14): 1340–1342.

Duran, S. & W. Ravis (1993). Comparative pharmacokinetics of H2 antagonists in horses. Proceedings of the Eleventh Annual Veterinary Medical Forum, Washington D.C., American College of Veterinary Internal Medicine.

Fisher, P. (2005). Ferret Medicine I. Proceedings: Western Vet Conf. Accessed via: Veterinary Information Network. http://goo.gl/bSPRO

Galvao, J. & L.A. Trepanier (2008). Risk of hemolytic anemia with intravenous administration of famotidine to hospitalized cats. *Journal of Veterinary Internal Medicine* 22(2): 325–329.

Garrett, L. (2006). Practical approach to treatment of canine mast cell tumors. Proceedings: ACVIM. Accessed via: Veterinary Information Network. http://goo.gl/q2HR8

Glazer, A. & P. Walters (2008). Esophagitis and esophageal strictures. *Comp CE*(May): 281–292.

Johnston, M. (2006). Clinical monitoring of the critically ill rabbit. Proceedings: IVECCS. Accessed via: Veterinary Information Network. http://goo.gl/3NEfN

Leib, M.S., R.B. Duncan, et al. (2007). Triple antimicrobial therapy and acid suppression in dogs with chronic vomiting and gastric Helicobacter spp. *Journal of Veterinary Internal Medicine* 21(6): 1185–1192.

Marks, S. (2008). GI Therapeutics: Which Ones and When? Proceedings: IVECCS. Accessed via: Veterinary Information Network. http://goo.gl/rxwcs

Matz, M. (1995). Gastrointestinal ulcer therapy. *Kirk's Current Veterinary Therapy:XII*. J Bonagura Ed. Philadelphia, W.B. Saunders: 706–710.

Polzin, D. (2005). Treating kidney disease in dogs—standards of care. Proceedings: ACVC. Accessed via: Veterinary Information Network. http://goo.gl/Lg0mN

Tams, T. (2003). Disorders of the esophagus. Proceedings: Atlantic Coast Veterinary Conf. Accessed via: Veterinary Information Network. http://goo.gl/LqV3V

Williams, B. (2000). Therapeutics in Ferrets. *Vet Clin NA: Exotic Anim Pract* 3:1(Jan): 131–153.

Williamson, K.K., M.D. Willard, et al. (2010). Efficacy of Omeprazole versus High-Dose Famotidine for Prevention of Exercise-Induced Gastritis in Racing Alaskan Sled Dogs. *Journal of Veterinary Internal Medicine* 24(2): 285–288.

Wolf, A. (2006). Chronic progressive renal disease in the cat: Recognition and management. Proceedings: ABVP2006. Accessed via: Veterinary Information Network. http://goo.gl/1q5Bq

Zoran, D. (2006). Feline CPRD: Therapeutic keys. Proceedings: Western Vet Conf. Accessed via: Veterinary Information Network. http://goo.gl/a3Itm

FAT EMULSION, INTRAVENOUS

Intralipid®, Liposyn®, Intravenous Lipid
Emulsion

**PARENTERAL NUTRITIONAL AGENT;
ANTIDOTE (FAT-SOLUBLE TOXINS)**

Prescriber Highlights

▶ Parenteral calorie and fatty acid
source;

▶ Potentially useful in overdose situations to reduce free-drug levels
of fat-soluble drugs; may be particularly useful in veterinary medicine for
toxicities associated with high morbidity or mortality, particularly when
traditional therapies have failed or are
cost-prohibitive

▶ When used for parenteral nutrition, use
is controversial in critically ill patients

*Monograph reviewed by Justine Lee, DVM,
DACVECC*

Uses/Indications

Intravenous fat emulsions (IFE; intravenous
lipid emulsion; ILE) can be used as a source of
calories or essential fatty acids when parenteral
feeding is required.

IFE can be considered as a rescue treatment
for intoxications caused by fat-soluble drugs/
toxins when traditional treatments are not effective (Fernandez *et al.* 2011). At present, this
use is extra-label and good evidence is scant in
veterinary medicine supporting this use clinically, but research is ongoing and some evidence
exists that IFE is, or theoretically could be useful
for reducing free-drug levels for drugs or drug
classes such as local anesthetics (bupivacaine,
mepivacaine, ropivacaine, lidocaine) (O'Brien
et al. 2010), macrocyclic lactones (ivermectin,
moxidectin) (Crandell & Weinberg 2009), calcium channel blockers (verapamil, amlodipine), beta-blockers (propranolol, carvedilol),
antidepressants (bupropion, doxepin, sertraline,
clomipramine), antipsychotics (chlorpromazine, quetiapine), antiepileptics (carbamazepine, lamotrigine), muscle relaxants (baclofen,
cyclobenzaprine), and flecainide. As certain
treatments available for humans (*e.g.*, hemoperfusion, hemodialysis, long-term ventilator
or intensive care) are either unavailable or cost
prohibitive in veterinary medicine, early intervention with IFE in the poisoned patient with
severe clinical signs may be a relatively low cost
and safe method to effectively treat veterinary
patients for fat-soluble intoxications.

Pharmacology/Actions

Intravenously administered lipid emulsions can
provide an efficient method (1 mL of a 20%

emulsion provides approximately 2 kCal) of
providing calories, and serve as a source of essential fatty acids. In addition, intravenous lipids
can have immunosuppressive effects, increase
pro-inflammatory cytokines, and affect pulmonary function.

When used for toxicologic indications, IFE's
exact mechanism of action is unknown, but it
may serve as a "lipid sink" for fat soluble compounds, reducing the amount of free drug in
the circulation and thereby reducing the drug's
toxic effects. Other hypotheses include: improving cardiac performance/function by increasing
intracellular calcium and/or providing myocytes
an energy substrate, or increasing the pool of
fatty acids thus overcoming the inhibition of mitochondrial fatty acid metabolism by drugs such
as bupivacaine.

Pharmacokinetics

IFE appears to be removed from the blood
stream about as rapidly as chylomicrons, but the
rate of removal requires prior lipolysis of IFE
into free fatty acids and seems to be increased
with heparin activated lipoprotein. In humans,
elimination half-life is about 30 minutes.

Contraindications/Precautions/Warnings

Intravenous lipids are contraindicated in patients with severe egg yolk allergies or abnormal
fat metabolism.

Strict aseptic technique and good IV catheter care are imperative when using IFE with or
without amino acids and dextrose. When used
alone, IFE may be administered via a peripheral line, but when combined with amino acids/
dextrose as total parenteral nutrition (TPN), a
dedicated central line is required due to the solution's hypertonicity.

Use of IFE in critically ill animals is somewhat controversial. While there are no studies
specifically addressing the role or safety of lipids in critically ill animals, human data suggests
that lipid administration may be associated with
significant immunosuppression, exacerbation
of pre-existing pulmonary pathology, and increasing infection rates. Data also supports that
withholding lipids for moderate periods of time
is not associated with an increase in morbidity
or mortality administration (Crandell 2005). In
humans, intravenous lipids are used with caution in premature and low-birth weight infants
(Black Box Warning; lipemia), patients with
blood coagulation disorders, pulmonary disease, renal impairment, severe liver damage, and
those at risk for fat emboli.

Adverse Effects

While IFE's adverse effect profile/incidence rates
have not been reported in veterinary patients,
they are likely similar to those seen in human
patients.

In humans, adverse effects associated with IFE
are infrequent and are primarily reported when
intravenous lipids are used for nutritional sup-

port. Most common are sepsis or thrombophlebitis secondary to IV administration, but these can occur whether intravenous lipids are used or not in parenteral nutrition therapy. Fat overload syndrome (hyperlipidemia, hepatomegaly, icterus, splenomegaly, fat embolism, thrombocytopenia, hemolysis, and prolonged clotting times) can occur, particularly if doses are too high or administration is too fast. More rarely (<1%), IFE can cause pulmonary toxicity, GI effects, somnolence, headache, flushing, fat emboli, hyperlipemia, pancreatitis, hypercoagulability, and hypersensitivity. IFE effects on pulmonary function and oxygenation are temporary and resolve after discontinuation.

Reproductive/Nursing Safety

When used when clearly needed, the benefits of using intravenous lipids during pregnancy would likely outweigh the risks. However, the FDA has placed them in category *C* (*Animal studies have shown an adverse effect on the fetus, but there are no adequate studies in humans; or there are no animal reproduction studies and no adequate studies in humans.*). No data regarding the safe use of IFE during lactation is available, but while likely safe, the risks of nursing in patients that require IFE may outweigh the benefits to offspring.

Overdosage/Acute Toxicity

In the case of an inadvertent overdose, stop the infusion until the lipid has cleared. This can be evaluated in a gross manner by visually inspecting the plasma (hematocrit tubes), or by laboratory methods (triglyceride concentrations, plasma light-scattering activity by nephelometry).

When using IFE for drug toxicity, heparin therapy (75–250 Units/kg SQ q6h) can be considered in cases where severe hyperlipidemia is present as it may increase lipid clearance. However, heparin's direct effect on IFE clearance is not proven. Weigh the risks of treating with heparin versus the effects of the target toxin, as the use of heparin may potentially affect the mechanism of action of IFE with fat-soluble toxicosis. Although there is no direct proof that hyperlipidemia secondary to IFE increases the risk for pancreatitis, some advocate using heparin when hyperlipemia occurs in dog breeds susceptible to pancreatitis (*e.g.*, Shetland sheepdog, miniature schnauzer, Yorkshire terrier, obesity, etc.). Otherwise, heparin therapy is not recommended unless clinical signs or advanced diagnostics indicate otherwise. Monitor partial thromboplastin time (PTT) prior to use of heparin to ensure the patient is not already coagulopathic. If PTT exceeds 2-2.5X normal, the use of heparin should be either lowered (75 Units/kg SQ q. 6-8) or discontinued. (Lee 2010).

Drug Interactions

The following drug interactions have either been reported or are theoretical in humans or animals receiving IFE and may be of significance in veterinary patients:

- ■ **LIPID SOLUBLE DRUGS:** Intravenous lipids (IFE) may affect the pharmacokinetics of lipid soluble drugs by serving as a "lipid sink" for free drug in the circulation. At present, clinical significance is not clear. However, when IFE is used (as a nutritional agent) concurrently with a fat soluble drug, monitor for decreased efficacy of the drug.

Laboratory Considerations

- ■ Blood samples for diagnostics should be collected prior to administration of IFE to minimize affects from hyperlipidemia.

- ■ Falsely high hemoglobin, MCH and MCHC values can occur if samples are drawn during or shortly after fat emulsion infusion.

- ■ Serum bilirubin values may be affected by IFE.

Doses

As a nutritional agent for parenteral nutrition (PN):

Note: If using IFE for parenteral nutrition, the reader is advised to consult with a veterinary nutritionist and refer to more detailed references on the subject including: (Thomovsky, Backus *et al.* 2007), (Thomovsky, Reniker *et al.* 2007), (Chandler *et al.* 2008), (Campbell *et al.* 2006), (Freeman & Chan 2006)

a) Most recommendations are to consider intravenous lipids as energy substrates, and to administer them at 30-40% of total calories. In veterinary medicine, lipid administration ranges from 25-60% of calories administered. (Crandell 2005). Traditionally, IFE administration is not recommended at > 2 g/kg/day for TPN therapy. (Lee 2011).

b) There are two strategies employed by nutritionists to supply calories. One approach is to provide daily resting energy requirements (RER) with a mixture of all three nutrients (protein, dextrose, lipids) starting with provision of adequate protein (4-6 grams/100 kcal). Other nutritionists advocate supplying the daily RER in dextrose and lipids and adding protein "on top." This approach asserts that proteins not catabolized for energy can be used to maintain protein synthesis. Hyperalimentation may be more frequent with the second approach. Generally, either approach can be used for total parenteral nutrition (TPN), but with partial parenteral nutrition (PPN) care should be taken with the second approach to keep the solution below 600 mOsm/L. Some nutritionists will supplement lipids alone for up to 3 days at RER. For example, a 10 kg dog with RER of 370 kcal/day. *Intralipid®* 20% solution (2 kcal/mL) could supply RER peripherally at 8 mL/hr. The lipid component of PN is controversial and some nutritionists do not include lipids in PN for critically ill patients because of concerns of increases in infection complications, immunosuppression, free radical generation and inflammation. Author recommends using caution when using imbalanced strategies. (Waldrop 2009)

As a rescue agent for fat-soluble drug/toxin intoxication:

a) In a study evaluating the evidence for using IFE for treating intoxications *in humans*, the authors concluded: Pending new evidence, IFE should be used in local anesthetic toxicosis at the onset of neurological or cardiovascular signs. Also reasonable to administer IFE in any other hemodynamically significant intoxication from fat-soluble drugs after general supportive measures and recognized antidotes have been attempted unsuccessfully. All efforts to maximize oxygenation and perfusion should be provided before administration of ILE. No optimal regimen has been established to this date, but until then: IFE 20% via a sterile, peripheral IV catheter as a 1.5 mL/kg bolus over 1–3 minutes, then 0.25–0.5 mL/kg/min for 30–60 min. The bolus could be repeated in case of cardiac arrest. Titrating the infusion rate to the clinical response and repeating IFE administration at the onset of any recurrent deterioration appear reasonable. (Jamaty *et al.* 2010)

b) Currently, dose recommendations for IFE 20% are extrapolated from human medicine as noted in dose "a" above with a goal not to exceed 8 mL/kg/day. However, this dose has been exceeded in clinical recommendations by Pet Poison Helpline without ill effect and the use of IFE in an acute setting for toxicosis likely can exceed the current human recommendations. In a patient that continues to be symptomatic after traditional dosing (listed in dose "a" above), consider additional doses of 1.5 mL/kg IV over 30 min q4-6h for 24-36 hours until clinical signs resolve (based on clinical judgment), or maintaining a CRI of 0.5 mL/kg/hour until clinical signs resolve. (Lee 2010)

Monitoring

■ When used for toxicology indications: drug levels (serum or plasma) to evaluate the response to IFE therapy. This will aid in data collection for future retrospective study analysis. General recommended time frames for drug levels include: time 0 (at the time of presentation to the health care facility), 30 minutes after administration of IFE, 1 hour post, 6, hours post, 12 hours post, and 24 hours post. (Lee 2010) However, this should be based on the pharmacokinetics of said drug. (Lee 2010)

■ When used for nutrition support; monitoring can be very involved and can include: blood glucose, serum triglycerides/lipemia, PCV, total protein, catheter and catheter site status, hydration status, vital signs (temperature, respiration rate, cardiac rate), serum electrolytes (including phosphorous), renal and liver function tests, CBC, etc. It is recommended to consult with a veterinary nutritionist and refer to a more detailed reference (see references in Doses above) for more information.

Chemistry/Synonyms

Fat Emulsion, intravenous are emulsified soybean (*Intralipid®*, *Liposyn® III*), or soybean and safflower (*Liposyn® II*) oils that provide the fatty acids: linoleic, stearic, linolenic, oleic and palmitic acids. Egg yolk phospholipids serve as the primary emulsifying agent and glycerol is used to adjust tonicity. Osmolarity varies with product, but range from 200–293 mOsm/L. The pH of IFE is between 6 and 9. Initially the pH is around 9, but secondary to hydrolysis of triglycerides into free fatty acids (FFA), the pH decreases to 6 at the end of the product's shelf-life.

Storage/Stability

Unopened IFE products should be stored at room temperature (not above 25°C, 77°F) and not allowed to freeze. If accidentally frozen, it should be discarded. If a partial amount of a bag or bottle is used, the remaining product should be stored protected in the refrigerator (2-8°C), and discarded 24 hours after opening. A new bag or vial must be used every 24 hours.

Compatibility/Compounding Considerations

IFE is compatible when mixed with the usual components used in parenteral nutrition (dextrose, amino acids, parenteral multivitamins and trace elements), but it is advisable to contact a hospital pharmacist or refer to a drug compatibility reference for more information, as concentrations and mixing order can affect compatibility. This is particularly important as the opaque nature of IFE makes detection of precipitates very difficult.

Admixtures must be prepared with strict aseptic technique. Do not add additives directly to IFE, and in no case add fat emulsion to the total parenteral nutrition container first. The proper order of mixing: **1)** transfer dextrose to the admixture container; **2)** transfer amino acid solution; then **3)** transfer fat emulsion. Alternatively, amino acids, dextrose, and fat emulsion may be simultaneously transferred to the admixture container; gently agitate the mixture. Use these admixtures promptly; store under refrigeration (2° to 8°C; 36° to 46°F) for 24 hours or less and use within 24 hours after removal from refrigeration.

Dosage Forms/Regulatory Status

VETERINARY-LABELED PRODUCTS: None

HUMAN-LABELED PRODUCTS:

Fat Emulsion, Intravenous 10%, 20%, 30%; depending on product, in 50 mL, 100 mL, 200 mL, 250 mL, & 500 mL bottles or bags; *Intralipid®* (Baxter); *Liposyn® II* & *Liposyn® III* (Hospira); (Rx)

References

Campbell, S., M. Karriker, et al. (2006). Central and peripheral parenteral nutrition. *Waltham Focus* 16(3): 22–30.

Chandler, M., W. Guilford, et al. (2008). Parenteral Nutrition. *Small Animal Critical Care Medicine*. D Silverstein and K Hopper Eds. St Louis, Elsevier: 58–62.

Crandell, D.E. & G.L. Weinberg (2009). Moxidectin toxicosis in a puppy successfully treated with intravenous lipids. *Journal of Veterinary Emergency and Critical Care* 19(2): 181–186.

Fernandez, A., J.A. Lee, et al. (2011). The Use of Intravenous Lipid Emulsion as an Antidote in Toxicology: A Review. *J Vet Emerg Crit Care* Pending Publication.

Freeman, L. & D. Chan (2006). Total parenteral nutrition. *Fluid, Electrolyte, and Acid-base Disorders in Small Animal Practice*. SP DiBartola Ed. St Louis, Elsevier: 584–600.

Jamaty, C., B. Bailey, et al. (2010). Lipid emulsions in the treatment of acute poisoning: a systematic review of human and animal studies. *Clinical Toxicology* 48(1): 1–27.

Lee, J.A. (2010). Advances in Toxicology: The Use of Intra-Lipid Therapy & High-Dextrose Insulin Therapy. Proceedings: ACVIM. Accessed via: Veterinary Information Network. http://goo.gl/fuZdi

Lee, J.A. (2011, Last Update). "Personal Communication."

O'Brien, T.Q., S.C. Clark-Price, et al. (2010). Infusion of a lipid emulsion to treat lidocaine intoxication in a cat. *Javma-Journal of the American Veterinary Medical Association* 237(12): 1455–1458.

Thomovsky, E., R. Backus, et al. (2007). Parenteral nutrition: Formulation, monitoring, and complications. *Compendium on Continuing Education for the Practicing Veterinarian* 29(2): 88–103.

Thomovsky, E., A. Reniker, et al. (2007). Parenteral nutrition: Uses, indications, and compounding. *Compendium on Continuing Education for the Practicing Veterinarian* 29(2): 76–+.

Waldrop, J. (2009). Parenteral Nutrition in Real Practice. Proceedings: IVECCS. Accessed via: Veterinary Information Network. http://goo.gl/ruxoo

FATTY ACIDS, ESSENTIAL/OMEGA FISH OIL/VEGETABLE OIL

NUTRITIONAL

Prescriber Highlights

▶ Used for treatment of dogs with pruritus associated with atopy, idiopathic seborrhea; in cats for pruritus associated with miliary dermatitis & eosinophilic granuloma complex; may be useful in cats with heart failure.

▶ May also be useful in other species & for other disease states

▶ Safety in pregnancy not established; use caution in patients with coagulopathies

▶ Adverse Effects: High doses may cause GI distress; rarely some dogs may become lethargic or more pruritic

Uses/Indications

These products are usually used for the treatment of pruritus associated with atopy, idiopathic seborrhea, miliary dermatitis and eosinophilic granuloma complex. In cats, omega-3 fatty acids may be helpful to reduce cytokines, and improve appetite in cats with heart failure. Fatty acids may improve coat quality and be helpful for adjunctive therapy for arthropathies such as hip dysplasia.

When used for pruritus, significant therapeutic effects may be noted in only 25–50% of patients treated and require 2–3 months of treatment before evaluating efficacy. Antihistamine and fatty acid therapy may be synergistic for treatment of pruritus.

Polyunsaturated fatty acids, particularly the omega-3's may prove to be useful for a variety of conditions, including renal failure, arthritis (both degenerative and autoimmune), cardiovascular disease (hypercoagulable states, heart failure, dysrhythmias), and some neoplastic diseases.

One study suggested that dogs with chronic osteoarthritis fed a diet supplemented with fish oil omega-3 fatty acids could allow reductions in carprofen dosage (Fritsch *et al.* 2010). In another, dogs with osteoarthritis fed a diet with a very high omega-3 to omega-6 ratio (compared with the control diet, omega-3 levels were 31X greater, and omega-6 levels were 34X lower) had significantly lower serum levels of arachadonic acid and owners reported subjective improvement in arthritic condition (Roush *et al.* 2010).

The ACVIM consensus statement on proteinuria in dogs and cats (Lees *et al.* 2005), states:

"The treatment strategies to be considered are to feed an appropriate diet (one with reduced quantity but high-quality protein with omega-3 fatty acid supplementation), to administer an angiotensin-converting-enzyme inhibitor drug or both."

Fish oil (but not Flax oil) significantly reduced VPCs in Boxer dogs with arrhythmogenic right ventricular cardiomyopathy (Smith, C.E. *et al.* 2007).

Pharmacology/Actions
The exact pharmacologic actions of these products are not well described; particularly in light of the combination nature of the commercial products being marketed, it is difficult to ascertain which compounds may be responsible for their proposed efficacy. The particular therapeutic benefits and ratios of omega-3 versus omega-6 fatty acids are still being debated.

Fish oils affect arachidonic acid levels in plasma lipids and platelet membranes. They may affect production of inflammatory prostaglandins in the body, thereby reducing inflammation and pruritus. Linolenic or linoleic acids may be used as essential fatty acid sources which are necessary for normal skin and haircoats.

Contraindications/Precautions/Warnings
Because of potential affects on bleeding times, use with caution in patients with coagulation disorders or those receiving anticoagulant medications. Use with caution in patients with non-insulin dependent diabetes as omega-3 fatty acids have impaired insulin secretion with resultant increased glucose levels in humans with type-2 diabetes. Fatty acids should be used with caution in dogs that have had previous bouts with pancreatitis or protracted diarrhea.

Adverse Effects
At high dosages, GI disturbances (*e.g.*, vomiting, diarrhea) may be seen. Rarely, some dogs become lethargic or more pruritic. In human patients, increased bleeding times and decreased platelet aggregation have been noted with use of fish oils; use with caution in patients with coagulopathies.

Reproductive/Nursing Safety
Safe use in pregnancy has not been established; these products are not recommended for use in pregnant human patients. Use cautiously in veterinary patients.

Overdosage/Acute Toxicity
With products containing vitamin A, acute toxicosis may result after accidental overdoses. Contact a poison control center for additional information.

Drug Interactions
The following drug interactions have either been reported or are theoretical in humans or animals receiving fatty acids/fish oils and may be of significance in veterinary patients:

■ **ANTICOAGULANTS:** Because of potential af-

fects on bleeding times, use with caution in patients receiving anticoagulant medications such as aspirin, warfarin, or heparin

Doses
Because of the unique nature of each commercially available product, see the actual label directions of that product for specific dosage recommendations.

■ **DOGS:**
   a) A few published clinical articles suggest that (for pruritus in dogs) a beneficial dose for eicosapentanoic acid (EPA) is around 22 mg/kg /day. (White 2003)

   b) For adjunctive treatment of heart failure (particularly in dogs with cachexia or anorexia): The recommended daily dosage for fish oil is 40 mg/kg of eicosapentaenoic acid (EPA) or 25 mg/kg of docosahexaenoic acid (DHA). (*Note: the "or" in the previous sentence may be a typo and perhaps should be an "and" as fish oil supplements generally contain both EPA and DHA—Plumb*) The amount of these specific fatty acids vary with different fish oil supplements, so check the label for recommending how many capsules to take. (Smith, F. 2009)

   c) In Boxers with arrhythmogenic right ventricular cardiomyopathy (ARVC): Fish oil capsules containing a total of 390 mg EPA and 248.5 mg DHA were used in the study and dosed at PO once daily over 6 weeks. (Smith, C.E. *et al.* 2007)

■ **CATS:**
   a) For adjunctive treatment in cats with CHF: Optimal dose of omega-3 fatty acids for cats is not yet known, author currently recommends 40 mg/kg EPA and 25 mg/kg DHA in cats. Fish oil supplements vary widely in the amount of EPA and DHA they contain so know the exact amount in supplements recommended. Capsules that contain approximately 180 mg EPA and 120 mg DHA can be purchased OTC at human pharmacies and administered at a dose of 1 capsule per 10 pounds body weight. Fish oil should contain vitamin E as an antioxidant, but supplements that contain other nutrients are not recommended to avoid toxicities. Cod liver oil and flax oil should not be used. (Freeman 2010)

Monitoring
■ Efficacy
■ Adverse effects

Chemistry/Synonyms/Storage/Stability
The commercially available veterinary products generally contain a combination of fish oil (eicosapentanoic and docosahexanoic acids) and vegetable oil (gamma linolenic acid) that serve as essential fatty acids. They may also

contain vitamin E (d-alpha tocopherol) and vitamin A.

The oral capsules should be stored in tight containers and protected from heat (cool, dry place).

Dosage Forms/Regulatory Status

VETERINARY-LABELED PRODUCTS:

There are many combination products available without prescription having various trade names, including (partial listing): *Dermapet Eicosderm®, Dermapet OFA plus EZ-C Caps®, F.A. Caps®, F.A. Caps ES®, Omega EFA® Capsules, Omega EFA® Capsules XS, Performer® OFA Gel Capsules Extra Strength, etc.*

HUMAN-LABELED PRODUCTS:

There are many fish oil or flaxseed oil capsules available without prescription having various trade names.

References

Freeman, L. (2010). Optimal Nutrition for Feline Cardiac Patients. Proceedings: ACVIM. Accessed via: Veterinary Information Network. http://goo.gl/MsZct

Fritsch, D.A., T.A. Allen, et al. (2010). A multicenter study of the effect of dietary supplementation with fish oil omega-3 fatty acids on carprofen dosage in dogs with osteoarthritis. *Javma-Journal of the American Veterinary Medical Association* 236(5): 535–539.

Lees, G., S. Brown, et al. (2005). Assessment and Management of Proteinuria in Dogs and Cats: 2004 ACVIM Forum Consensus Statement (Small Animal). *J Vet Intern Med* 19: 377–385.

Roush, J.K., C.E. Dodd, et al. (2010). Multicenter veterinary practice assessment of the effects of omega-3 fatty acids on osteoarthritis in dogs. *Javma-Journal of the American Veterinary Medical Association* 236(1): 59–66.

Smith, C.E., L.M. Freeman, et al. (2007). Omega-3 fatty acids in boxer dogs with arrhythmogenic right ventricular cardiomyopathy. *Journal of Veterinary Internal Medicine* 21(2): 265–273.

Smith, F. (2009). Alternative therapies for the cardiac diseases. Proceedings: WVC. Accessed via: Veterinary Information Network. http://goo.gl/HwxlW

White, P. (2003). Medical management of canine pruritus. Proceedings: Western Veterinary Conf. Accessed via: Veterinary Information Network. http://goo.gl/2P8ET

Febantel–See the product Drontal® Plus listed in the Praziquantel and Pyrantel monographs

FELBAMATE

(*fell*-ba-mate)   Felbatol®

ANTICONVULSANT

Prescriber Highlights

▶ 2nd or 3rd line antiseizure medication for dogs

▶ Appears relatively safe to use in dogs, but because of limited use, adverse effect profile may be incomplete

▶ Cost & accessibility may be issues

Uses/Indications

Felbamate is an anticonvulsant agent that may useful for treating seizure disorders (generalized seizures, but especially complex partial seizures) in dogs. A potential advantage of felbamate therapy is that when used alone or in combination with phenobarbital and/or bromides, it does not appear to cause additive sedation.

Pharmacology/Actions

Felbamate's anticonvulsant activity is thought to be due its ability to reduce excitatory neurotransmission; its exact mechanism is unknown, but it is believed to increase activation of sodium channels thereby decreasing sustained high-frequency firing of action potentials.

Pharmacokinetics

Felbamate is well absorbed after oral administration in dogs. Felbamate is both excreted unchanged and as metabolites in the urine (about 50:50). The half-life in dogs may range from 5–14 hours, but averages around 6 hours. Because the drug can induce liver enzyme induction, half-lives may decrease with time and dosages may need adjustment.

Contraindications/Precautions/Warnings

Felbamate is contraindicated in patients hypersensitive to it or other carbamates (meprobamate). In humans, felbamate should not be used in patients with a history of blood dyscrasias or hepatic dysfunction. In dogs, however, these are probably only cautions since dogs who require felbamate are often close to euthanasia due to the refractoriness of their conditions and a lack of evidence that felbamate causes liver toxicity in dogs.

Adverse Effects

Adverse reactions in the dog include KCS, liver enzyme induction, tremor, limb rigidity, salivation, restlessness and agitation (at high doses). In humans, aplastic anemia and hepatic necrosis have been noted and could be a factor in canine medicine. There apparently have not been any case reports yet of aplastic anemia in dogs, but blood dyscrasias (thrombocytopenia, lymphopenia, and leukopenia) have been reported. Additionally, sedation, and vomiting/nausea have been reported in dogs, but usually in those receiving other anticonvulsants as well.

Reproductive/Nursing Safety

Although no overt teratogenicity has been documented, felbamate should only be used during pregnancy when its potential benefits outweigh its potential risks. In humans, the FDA categorizes this drug as category *C* for use during pregnancy (*Animal studies have shown an adverse effect on the fetus, but there are no adequate studies in humans; or there are no animal reproduction studies and no adequate studies in humans.*)

The drug is excreted into maternal milk, but adverse consequences to nursing puppies appear remote.

Overdosage/Acute Toxicity

Limited information is available. One human subject taking 12 grams over 12 hours only developed mild gastric distress and a slightly increased heart rate.

Drug Interactions

The following drug interactions have either been reported or are theoretical in humans or animals receiving felbamate and may be of significance in veterinary patients:

■ **PHENOBARBITAL:** When felbamate is added to patients taking phenobarbital it may cause increases in phenobarbital levels. When phenobarbital is added to patients taking felbamate, felbamate levels may decrease. The same effect can occur with **phenytoin**.

■ **VALPROATE:** Felbamate can cause increases in valproic acid levels

Doses

■ **DOGS:**

For seizures:

a) As either add-on therapy or monotherapy: Starting dose is 15 mg/kg PO q8h. Dose can be increased in 15 mg/kg increments every 2 weeks until seizures are controlled. Doses as high as 70 mg/kg q8h are required and tolerated in some dogs. (Thomas 2010)

b) As a third choice antiepileptic agent: 15–65 mg/kg PO q8h. Steady state reached after 4th oral dose. Monitor CBC and liver function tests as you would for phenobarbital. Therapeutic serum concentration reported to be 15–100 micrograms/mL. (Quesnel 2000)

c) For patients on phenobarb and bromides (both in therapeutic range) and seizure activity unchanged or having intolerable side effects with this combination: If intolerable side effects, do levels and decrease the dose of the one that is in the high end of the range. Then add felbamate at 5–20 mg/kg PO three times daily. (Neer 2000)

Monitoring

■ There is some controversy about monitoring felbamate use in dogs, probably since there is such limited experience with its use. Some clinicians state that liver function tests and CBC's should be regularly assessed (q2–3 months). Others state that the drug is very safe in dogs and that monitoring does not appear to be necessary. Clearly, if the dog is receiving other drugs (especially phenobarbital), monitoring is essential.

■ Therapeutic drug levels for felbamate in dogs are not truly known, but appear to be in the 25–100 micrograms/mL range. The usefulness of monitoring serum levels is questionable at this point.

Client Information

■ Clients must understand the importance of giving doses as prescribed. Because of its short half-life, three times daily administration is routinely administered to adequately judge the efficacy of this drug.

■ Because felbamate use in dogs has been limited, the adverse effect profile and possible incidence of serious effects (liver, blood) is not truly known.

Chemistry/Synonyms

Felbamate is a unique dicarbamate anticonvulsant agent, that is slightly soluble in water.

Felbamate may also be known by as: AD-03055, W-554, *Felbamyl®*, *Felbatol®*, *Taloxa®*, and *Taloxa®*.

Storage/Stability

Felbamate preparations should be stored at room temperature. The suspension should be shaken well before use.

Dosage Forms/Regulatory Status

VETERINARY-LABELED PRODUCTS: None

The ARCI (Racing Commissioners International) has designated this drug as a class 3 substance. See the appendix for more information.

HUMAN-LABELED PRODUCTS:

Felbamate Tablets: 400 mg, & 600 mg; *Felbatol®* (Wallace Labs); (Rx)

Felbamate Suspension: 120 mg/mL in 240 & 960 mL; *Felbatol®* (Wallace Labs); (Rx)

References

Neer, T. (2000). The refractory seizure patient: What should be my diagnostic and therapeutic approach? American Animal Hospital Assoc, Toronto.

Quesnel, A. (2000). Seizures. *Textbook of Veterinary Internal Medicine: Diseases of the Dog and Cat.* S Ettinger and E Feldman Eds. Philadelphia, WB Saunders. **1**: 148–152.

Thomas, W. (2010). Idiopathic epilepsy in dogs and cats. *Vet Clin NA: Sm Anim Pract* **40**(1): 161–179.

FENBENDAZOLE

(fen-*ben*-da-zole)   Panacur®, Safe-Guard®

ANTIPARASITIC AGENT

Prescriber Highlights

▶ Anthelmintic useful for a variety of parasites in dogs, cats, cattle, horses, swine, etc

▶ Adverse Effects: Antigen release by dying parasites may occur; particularly at high dosages; vomiting may occur infrequently in dogs or cats

▶ In dogs, give with food

Uses/Indications

Fenbendazole is indicated (labeled) for the removal of the following parasites in dogs: ascarids (*Toxocara canis, T. leonina*), Hookworms (*Ancylostoma caninum, Uncinaria stenocephala*), whipworms (*Trichuris vulpis*), and tapeworms (*Taenia pisiformis*). It is not effective against *Dipylidium caninum*. Fenbendazole has also been used clinically to treat *Capillaria aerophilia*, *Filaroides hirthi*, and *Paragonimus kellicotti* infections in dogs.

Fenbendazole is indicated (labeled) for the removal of the following parasites in cattle: Adult forms of: *Haemonchus contortus, Ostertagia ostertagi, Trichostrongylus axei, Bunostomum phlebotomum, Nematodirus helvetianus, Cooperia* spp., *Trichostrongylus colubriformis, Oesophagostomum radiatum*, and *Dictyocaulus vivaparus*. It is also effective against most immature stages of the above listed parasites. Although not FDA-approved, it has good activity against *Moniezia* spp., and arrested 4th stage forms of *Ostertagia ostertagi*.

Fenbendazole is indicated (labeled) for the removal of the following parasites in horses: large strongyles (*S. edentatus, S. equinus, S. vulgaris*), small strongyles (*Cyathostomum* spp., *Cylicocylus* spp., *Cylicostephanus* spp., *Triodontophorus spp.)*, and pinworms (*Oxyuris equi*).

Fenbendazole is indicated (labeled) for the removal of the following parasites in swine: large roundworms (*Ascaris suum*), lungworms (*Metastrongylus pair*), nodular worms (*Oesophagostomum dentatum, O. quadrispinolatum*), small stomach worms (*Hyostrongylus rubidus*), whipworms (*Trichuris suis*), and kidney worms (*Stephanurus dentatus*; both mature and immature).

Although not FDA-approved, fenbendazole has been used in cats, sheep, goats, pet birds, and llamas. See Dosage section for more information.

Pharmacology/Actions

Fenbendazole is a methylcarbamate benzimidazole antiparasitic agent and has a broad spectrum of activity against a variety of pathogenic internal parasites. In susceptible parasites, benzimidazole mechanism of action is believed due to disrupting intracellular microtubular transport systems by binding selectively and damaging tubulin, preventing tubulin polymerization, and inhibiting microtubule formation. Benzimidazoles also act at higher concentrations to disrupt metabolic pathways within the helminth, and inhibit metabolic enzymes, including malate dehydrogenase and fumarate reductase. Benzimidazoles may be considered time-dependent antiparasitic agents.

Pharmacokinetics

Fenbendazole is only marginally absorbed after oral administration. The amount absorbed from the gut is apparently more associated with the solubility of the drug and not the dose given. In dogs, when doses ranging from 25–100 mg/kg were administered, the area-under-the-curves were similar. Bioavailability is increased in dogs when fenbendazole is administered with food. Fat content of food does not significantly alter bioavailability (McKellar *et al.* 1993).

After oral dosing in calves and horses, peak blood levels of 0.11 micrograms/mL and 0.07 micrograms/mL, respectively, were measured. Absorbed fenbendazole is metabolized (and vice-versa) to the active compound, oxfendazole (sulfoxide) and the sulfone. In sheep, cattle, and pigs, 44–50% of a dose of fenbendazole is excreted unchanged in the feces, and <1% in the urine.

Contraindications/Precautions/Warnings

Fenbendazole is not FDA-approved for use in horses intended for food purposes.

Adverse Effects

At usual doses, fenbendazole generally does not cause any adverse effects. Hypersensitivity reactions secondary to antigen release by dying parasites may occur, particularly at high dosages. Salivation, vomiting, and diarrhea may infrequently occur in dogs or cats receiving fenbendazole. Pancytopenia has been reported in one dog (Gary *et al.* 2004).

Single doses (even at exaggerated doses) are not effective in dogs and cats; must treat for at least 3 days.

Reproductive/Nursing Safety

Fenbendazole is considered safe to use in pregnant bitches and is generally considered safe to use in pregnancy for all species. It is the drug of choice for treating giardia in pregnant animals (Tams 2007). In a system evaluating the safety of drugs in canine and feline pregnancy (Papich 1989), this drug is categorized as in class: *A (Probably safe. Although specific studies may not have proved the safety of all drugs in dogs and cats, there are no reports of adverse effects in laboratory animals or women.)*

Overdosage/Toxicity

Fenbendazole is apparently well tolerated at doses up to 100X recommended. The LD_{50} in laboratory animals exceeds 10 grams/kg when administered PO. It is unlikely an acute overdosage would lead to clinical signs.

Drug Interactions

■ **BROMSALAN FLUKICIDES (dibromsalan, tribromsalan**; not available in the USA): Oxfendazole or fenbendazole should not be given concurrently with the bromsalan flukicides; abortions in cattle and death in sheep have been reported after using these compounds together

Doses

■ **DOGS:**

For susceptible ascarids, hookworms, whipworms, and tapeworms (*Taenia* spp. only):

a) 50 mg/kg, PO for 3 consecutive days (Package insert; *Panacur®*—Hoechst), (Cornelius & Roberson 1986)

b) 55 mg/kg, PO for 3 days (5 days for Taenia) (Chiapella 1989), (Reinemeyer, C.R. 1985)

For Giardia:

a) 50 mg/kg PO once daily for 3 consecutive days; if this does not clear the infection a longer course of therapy (5-7 days) is used (Tams 2007)

To prevent transplacental and transmammary transmission of somatic *T. canis* and *A. caninum*:

a) 50 mg/kg PO once daily from the 40th day of gestation to the 14th day of lactation. (Kazacos 2002)

For *Capillaria plica*:

a) 50 mg/kg once daily for 3 days; repeat a single 50 mg/kg dose 3 weeks later (Todd *et al.* 1985)

b) 50 mg/kg, PO daily for 3-10 days (Brown & Prestwood 1986)

For *Capillaria aerophilia*:

a) 25-50 mg/kg q12h for 10-14 days (Hawkins, E.C. *et al.* 1989), (Hawkins, E. 2000)

b) 50 mg/kg PO once daily for 10-14 days (Reinemeyer, C. 1995)

For *Filaroides hirthi*:

a) 50 mg/kg, PO once daily for 14 days. Symptoms may worsen during therapy, presumably due to a reaction when the worm dies. (Hawkins, E.C. *et al.* 1989)

b) 50 mg/kg PO once daily for 10-14 days (Reinemeyer, C. 1995)

For *Paragonimus kellicotti*:

a) 25-50 mg/kg PO twice daily for 10-14 days (Todd *et al.* 1985), (Hawkins, E. 2000)

b) 50 mg/kg PO once daily for 10-14 days (Reinemeyer, C. 1995)

c) 50 mg/kg, PO once daily for 3 consecutive days; repeat in 2-3 weeks and again in 2 months (DeNovo 1988)

For *Crenosoma vulpis*:

a) 50 mg/kg PO once daily for 3 days (Reinemeyer, C. 1995); (Hawkins, E. 2000)

For *Eucoleus boehmi*:

a) 50 mg/kg PO once daily for 10-14 days; improvement may only be temporary (Reinemeyer, C. 1995)

■ **CATS, DOMESTIC:**

For susceptible ascarids, hookworms, strongyloides, and tapeworms (*Taenia* spp. only):

a) 50 mg/kg, PO for 5 days (Dimski 1989)

For Giardia:

a) 50 mg/kg PO once daily for 3 consecutive days; if this does not clear the infection, a longer course of therapy (5-7 days) is used (Tams 2007)

b) 50 mg/kg PO q24h for 3-5 days (Vasilopulos 2006)

For lungworms (*Aelurostrongylus abstrusus*):

a) 25-50 mg/kg q12h for 10-14 days (Hawkins, E.C. *et al.* 1989); (Hawkins, E. 2000)

b) 50 mg/kg, PO for 10 days (Pechman 1989)

c) 20 mg/kg PO once daily for 5 days; repeat in 5 days (Reinemeyer, C. 1995))

For lungworms (*Capillaria aerophilia*):

a) 50 mg/kg, PO for 10 days (Pechman 1989)

b) 50 mg/kg PO once daily for 10-14 days (Reinemeyer, C. 1995)

For *Capillaria feliscati*:

a) 25 mg/kg, twice daily PO for 3-10 days (Brown & Prestwood 1986)

b) 25 mg/kg, PO q12h for 10 days (Brown & Barsanti 1989)

For *Paragonimus kellicotti*:

a) 25-50 mg/kg PO twice daily for 10-14 days (Hawkins, E. 2000)

b) 50 mg/kg PO once daily for 10-14 days (Reinemeyer, C. 1995)

For *Eurytrema procyonis* (pancreatic fluke):

a) 30 mg/kg, PO daily for 6 days (Steiner & Williams 2000)

■ **CATS, LARGE (EXOTIC):**

For labeled parasites:

a) 10 mg/kg PO once daily for 3 consecutive days. (Label information; *Panacur® 22.25 Granules*—Intervet)

■ **BEARS (URSIDAE):**

For labeled parasites:

a) 10 mg/kg PO once daily for 3 consecutive days. (Label information; *Panacur® 22.25 Granules*—Intervet)

■ **SMALL MAMMALS/RODENTS:**

a) For pinworms in mice, rats, hamsters, gerbils and rabbits: 50 mg/kg PO once (Burke 1999)

b) For Giardia in Chinchillas: 25 mg/kg PO once a day for 3 days (Hayes 2000)

c) **Mice, Rats, Gerbils, Hamsters, Guinea pigs, Chinchillas:** 20-50 mg/kg PO once daily for 5 days (Higher dose is for Giardia) (Adamcak & Otten 2000)

■ **CATTLE:**

For removal/control of *Haemonchus contortus, Ostertagia ostertagi, Trichostrongylus axei, Bunostomum phlebotomum, Nematodirus helvetianus, Cooperia* spp., *Trichostrongylus colubriformis, Oesophagostomum radiatum*, and *Dictyocaulus vivaparus*:

a) 5 mg/kg, PO (Paul 1986)

b) 7.5 mg/kg, PO (Roberson 1988)

c) 4 mg/kg PO; under conditions of continuous exposure to parasites, animals may need to be retreated after 4–6 weeks, (Label information *Panacur® Paste*—Intervet)

For *Moniezia* spp., and arrested 4th stage forms of *Ostertagia ostertagi*:

a) 10 mg/kg, PO (Paul 1986), (Roberson 1988)

For giardiasis in calves:

a) 15 mg/kg PO for 3 successive days and then moved to a pen that was thoroughly cleaned and disinfected with 10% ammonia. (Claerebout 2006)

■ **HORSES:**

For susceptible parasites:

a) For control of large and small strongyles, and pinworms in adult horses: 5 mg/kg PO;

For foals and weanlings (less than 18 months of age) where ascarids are a common problem: 10 mg/kg PO;

For control of encysted early 3rd stage, late 3rd stage and 4th stage cyathostome larvae and 4th stage *Strongylus vulgaris* larvae) 10 mg/kg PO for 5 consecutive days. (Label information *Panacur® Paste*—Intervet)

For treatment of migrating large strongyles:

a) 50 mg/kg PO for 3 consecutive days, or 10 mg/kg for 5 consecutive days (Herd 1987)

For mucosal stage of small strongyles:

a) 7.5–10 mg/kg PO once daily for 5 days; a single dose of 30 mg/kg is effective against older encysted stages (Lyons & Drudge 2000)

■ **SWINE:**

For susceptible parasites:

a) 5 mg/kg PO; 3 mg/kg in feed for 3 days; 10 mg/kg for ascarids (Roberson 1988)

b) For whipworms in potbellied pigs: 9 mg/kg PO for days (Braun 1995)

■ **SHEEP & GOATS:**

For susceptible parasites:

a) 5 mg/kg in feed for 3 days (Roberson 1988)

■ **CAMELIDS:**

For susceptible parasites in new world camelids:

a) 10–20 mg/kg PO for 3–5 days (Wolff 2009)

b) For adjunctive treatment of meningeal worm infestation (*Parelaphostrongylus tenius*): Fenbendazole 50 mg/kg PO for 5 days with ivermectin 0.3 mg/kg SC for 5 days. Also use prophylactic treatment for stress ulcers (*e.g.,* ranitidine, omeprazole), antiinflammatories (*e.g.,* flunixin, dexamethasone, DMSO), fluids, nutritional support, etc. (Edmondson 2009)

■ **BIRDS:**

a) For Ascarids: 10–50 mg/kg PO once; repeat in 10 days. Do not use during molt (may cause stunted feathers) or while nesting.

For flukes or microfilaria: 10–50 mg/kg PO once daily for 3 days

For *Capillaria*: 10–50 mg/kg PO once daily for 5 days. Is not effective against gizzard worms in finches. (Clubb 1986)

b) For nematodes, some trematodes: 10–50 mg/kg PO once daily for 3–5 days; 20–100 mg/kg oral single dose range; 125 mg/L of drinking water for 5 days (50 mg/L for 5 days in finches); or 100 mg/kg of feed for 5 days. Not recommended to be used in breeding season during molting. (Marshall 1993)

c) **Ratites:** 15 mg/kg PO once daily for 3 days. Has efficacy against ostrich tapeworm. (*Houttuynia struthionus*) (Jenson 1998)

■ **REPTILES:**

For susceptible infections:

a) For most species: 50–100 mg/kg PO once; repeat in 2–3 weeks; very effective against Strongyloides. (Gauvin 1993)

Chemistry/Synonyms

A benzimidazole anthelmintic, fenbendazole occurs as a white, crystalline powder. It is only slightly soluble in water.

Fenbendazole may also be known as: Hoe-881V, *Panacur®*, and *Safe-Guard®*.

Storage/Stability

Fenbendazole products should be stored at room temperature.

Dosage Forms/Regulatory Status

VETERINARY-LABELED PRODUCTS:

Fenbendazole Granules: 222 mg/gram (22.2%) in 0.18 oz and 1 g, 2 g, 4 g packets and 1 lb jars; *Panacur® Granules 22.2%* (Intervet); (Rx); *Safeguard® Canine Dewormer* (Intervet), (OTC). FDA-approved for use in dogs, large exotic cats (lions, etc.), and bears (black bears, polar bears, etc.)

Fenbendazole Granules: 222 mg/gram (22.2%); *Panacur® Granules 22.2%* (Intervet). (OTC). FDA-approved for use in horses not intended for food.

Fenbendazole Suspension: 100 mg/mL (10%); available in both equine and bovine labeled products; *Panacur® Suspension* (Intervet); (Rx). FDA-approved for use in horses (not intended for food) and cattle. Slaughter withdrawal = 8 days (cattle*). Safe-Guard® Suspension* (Intervet); (OTC). FDA-approved for use in beef and dairy cattle. Slaughter withdrawal at labeled doses = 8 days

Fenbendazole Paste: 100 mg/gram (10%);

available in both equine and bovine labeled products and sizes. *Panacur® Paste* (Intervet); (OTC). FDA-approved for use in horses (not intended for food) and cattle. Slaughter withdrawal at labeled doses = 8 days (cattle). *Safe Guard® Paste* (Intervet); (OTC). FDA-approved for use in horses not intended for food and cattle. Slaughter withdrawal at labeled doses = 8 days; no milk withdrawal time at labeled doses.

Fenbendazole Type B Medicated Feed
Safe-Guard® EZ Scoop Swine Dewormer (Intervet) (OTC). 1.8% Fenbendazole No slaughter withdrawal time required at labeled doses
Safe-Guard® 0.96% Scoop Dewormer (Intervet); (OTC). FDA-approved for use in cattle. No milk withdrawal time; slaughter withdrawal time at labeled doses = 13 days
Fenbendazole Type C Medicated Feed
Safe-Guard® Free-choice Cattle Dewormer (Intervet); (OTC); 0.50% Fenbendazole (2.27 g/lb). FDA-approved for use in beef and dairy cattle. No milk withdrawal time.
Safe-Guard® 35% Salt Free-choice Cattle Dewormer (Intervet); (OTC); 1.9 g/lb Fenbendazole. FDA-approved for use in dairy and beef cattle. Slaughter withdrawal time at labeled doses = 13 days; no milk withdrawal time.
Fenbendazole Pellets
Safe-Guard® 0.5% Cattle Top Dress (Intervet); (OTC). At labeled dose, slaughter withdrawal time = 13 days; no milk withdrawal period at labeled doses
Safe-Guard® 1.96% Scoop Dewormer Mini Pellets (Intervet); (OTC). FDA-approved for use in beef and dairy cattle. No milk withdrawal time at labeled doses; slaughter withdrawal time at labeled doses = 13 days
Fenbendazole Premix 20% Type A (200 mg/gram)
Safe-Guard® Premix (Intervet); (OTC). FDA-approved for use in swine, growing turkeys, dairy and beef cattle, zoo and wildlife animals. Slaughter withdrawal for cattle = 13 days; no milk withdrawal time. Slaughter withdrawal for swine at labeled doses = none. Wildlife animal slaughter (hunting) withdrawal = 14 days at labeled doses.

Combination Products:

Fenbendazole 454 mg, Ivermectin 27 mcg, & Praziquantel 23 mg (2.16 g small chews) Chewable Tablets; *Panacur Plus® Soft Chews* (Intervet); (Rx). FDA-approved for use in adult dogs.

Fenbendazole 1.134 g, Ivermectin 68 mcg, & Praziquantel 57 mg (5.4 g large chews) Chewable Tablet; *Panacur Plus® Soft Chews* (Intervet); (Rx). FDA-approved for use in adult dogs.

HUMAN-LABELED PRODUCTS: None

References

Adamcak, A. & B. Otten (2000). Rodent Therapeutics. *Vet Clin NA: Exotic Anim Pract* 3:1(Jan): 221–240.

Braun, W. (1995). Potbellied pigs: General medical care. *Kirk's Current Veterinary Therapy:XII.* J Bonagura Ed. Philadelphia, W.B. Saunders: 1388–1389.

Brown, S.A. & J.A. Barsanti (1989). Diseases of the bladder and urethra. *Textbook of Veterinary Internal Medicine.* SJ Ettinger Ed. Philadelphia, WB Saunders. 2: 2108–2141.

Brown, S.A. & A.K. Prestwood (1986). Parasites of the urinary tract. *Current Veterinary Therapy IX, Small Animal Practice.* RW Kirk Ed. Philadelphia, W.B. Saunders: 1153–1155.

Burke, T. (1999). Husbandry and Medicine of Rodents and Lagomorphs. Proceedings: Central Veterinary Conference, Kansas City.

Chiapella, A.M. (1989). Diseases of the Small Intestine. *Handbook of Small Animal Practice.* RV Morgan Ed. New York, Churchill Livingstone: 395–420.

Claerebout, E. (2006). New therapeutic approaches to Cryptosporidiosis and Giardiasis. Proceedings: ACVIM. Accessed via: Veterinary Information Network. http://goo.gl/JHGD3

Clubb, S.L. (1986). Therapeutics: Individual and Flock Treatment Regimens. *Clinical Avian Medicine and Surgery.* GJ Harrison and LR Harrison Eds. Philadelphia, W.B. Saunders: 327–355.

Cornelius, L.M. & E.L. Roberson (1986). Treatment of gastrointestinal parasitism. *Current Veterinary Therapy IX: Small Animal Practice.* K R.W. Ed. Philadelphia, W.B. Saunders: 921–924.

DeNovo, R.C. (1988). Diseases of the Large Bowel. *Handbook of Small Animal Practice.* RV Morgan Ed. New York, Churchill Livingstone: 421–439.

Dimski, D.S. (1989). Helminth and noncoccidial protozoan parasites of the gastrointestinal tract. *The Cat: Diseases and Clinical Management.* RG Sherding Ed. New York, Churchill Livingstone. 1: 459–477.

Edmondson, M. (2009). Internal parasites of goats, sheep, and camelids. ABVP. http://goo.gl/41DcU

Gary, A.T., M.E. Kerl, et al. (2004). Bone marrow hypoplasia associated with fenbendazole administration in a dog. *Journal of the American Animal Hospital Association* 40(3): 224–229.

Gauvin, J. (1993). Drug therapy in reptiles. *Seminars in Avian & Exotic Med* 2(1): 48–59.

Hawkins, E. (2000). Pulmonary Parenchymal Diseases. *Textbook of Veterinary Internal Medicine: Diseases of the Dog and Cat.* S Ettinger and E Feldman Eds. Philadelphia, WB Saunders. 2: 1061–1091.

Hawkins, E.C., S.J. Ettinger, et al. (1989). Diseases of the lower respiratory tract (lung) and pulmonary edema. *Textbook of Veterinary Internal Medicine.* SJ Ettinger Ed. Philadelphia, WB Saunders. 1: 816–866.

Hayes, P. (2000). Diseases of Chinchillas. *Kirk's Current Veterinary Therapy: XIII Small Animal Practice.* J Bonagura Ed. Philadelphia, WB Saunders: 1152–1157.

Herd, R.P. (1987). Chemotherapy of Migrating Strongyles. *Current Therapy in Equine Medicine, 2.* NE Robinson Ed. Philadelphia, W.B. Saunders: 331–332.

Jenson, J. (1998). Current ratite therapy. *The Veterinary Clinics of North America: Food Animal Practice* 16:3(November).

Kazacos, K. (2002). Treatment and control of gastrointestinal helminths. Proceedings: Western Veterinary Conference. Accessed via: Veterinary Information Network. http://goo.gl/USGQR

Lyons, E. & J. Drudge (2000). Larval Cyathostomiasis. *The Veterinary Clinics of North America: Equine Practice* 16:3(December).

Marshall, R. (1993). Avian anthelmintics and antiprotozoals. *Seminars in Avian & Exotic Med* 2(1): 33–41.

McKellar, Q.A., E.A. Galbraith, et al. (1993). Oral Absorption and Bioavailability of Fenbendazole in the Dog and the Effect of Concurrent Ingestion of Food. *Journal of Veterinary Pharmacology and Therapeutics* 16(2): 189–198.

Paul, J.W. (1986). Anthelmintic Therapy. *Current Veterinary Therapy: Food Animal Practice 2.* JL Howard Ed. Philadelphia, W.B. Saunders: 39–44.

Pechman, R.D. (1989). Respiratory Parasites. *The Cat: Diseases and Clinical Management.* RG Sherding Ed.

New York, Churchill Livingstone. 1: 485–494.

Reinemeyer, C. (1995). Parasites of the respiratory system. *Kirk's Current Veterinary Therapy:XII.* J Bonagura Ed. Philadelphia, W.B. Saunders: 895–898.

Reinemeyer, C.R. (1985). Strategies for management of gastrointestinal parasitism of small animals. *Eith Annual Kal Kan Symposium for the Treatment of Small Animal Diseases* Vernon, Kal Kan Foods, Inc.: 25–32.

Roberson, E.L. (1988). Antinematodal Agents. *Veterinary Pharmacology and Therapeutics.* NH Booth and LE McDonald Eds. Ames, Iowa State University Press: 882–927.

Steiner, J. & D. Williams (2000). Feline Exocrine Pancreatic Disease. *Kirk's Current Veterinary Therapy: XIII Small Animal Practice.* J Bonagura Ed. Philadelphia, WB Saunders: 701–705.

Tams, T. (2007). Acute diarrhea in dogs and cats. Proceedings: ACVC. Accessed via: Veterinary Information Network. http://goo.gl/nPF2I

Todd, K.S., A.J. Paul, et al. (1985). Parasitic Diseases. *Handbook of Small Animal Therapeutics.* LE Davis Ed. New York, Churchill Livingstone: 89–126.

Vasilopulos, R. (2006). Advances in diagnosis and treatment of feline protozoal diarrhea. Proceedings: ACVIM 2006. Accessed via: Veterinary Information Network. http://goo.gl/FYwOW

Wolff, P. (2009). Camelid Medicine. Proceedings: AAZV. Accessed via: Veterinary Information Network. http://goo.gl/4TEAy

FENTANYL, TRANSDERMAL FENTANYL CITRATE

(fen-ta-nil)   Sublimaze®, Duragesic®

OPIATE

Prescriber Highlights

▶ Class-II opiate analgesic used parenterally & transdermally in small animals

▶ Contraindications: Use extreme caution when additional respiratory, or CNS depression would be deleterious

▶ Use caution in geriatric, very ill or debilitated patients & those with a preexisting respiratory problem

▶ Adverse Effects: Dose related respiratory, CNS & circulatory depression (bradycardia); also, rashes at the patch site, urine retention, constipation, dysphoria, or agitation

▶ Lag time before effective analgesia with patches; dispose of properly

▶ Lab values (amylase, lipase) may be altered

Uses/Indications

In veterinary medicine, fentanyl injection and transdermal patches are used primarily in dogs and cats and have been shown to be useful for the adjunctive control of postoperative pain and in the control of severe pain associated with chronic pain, dull pain, and non-specific, widespread pain (*e.g.*, associated with cancer, pancreatitis, aortic thromboemboli, peritonitis, etc.). Perioperative injectable fentanyl may also reduce the requirements for inhalational anesthetics during surgery, which could be particularly advantageous in patients with compromised cardiac function. Because of its short duration of action, fentanyl CRI's are particularly useful in critically ill or post-surgical patients as it can be adjusted to meet the analgesia needs of the patient, minimize adverse effects and temporarily halted to assess neurologic status. Injectable fentanyl may be particularly useful in cats, especially when higher analgesic doses are required, as it appears to have fewer adverse effects than either hydromorphone or morphine.

Transdermal fentanyl has been clinically effective overall and has not demonstrated substantial adverse effects. However, one study in dogs comparing transdermal fentanyl versus IM morphine for pain control during the first 24 hours post-orthopedic surgery did not show any significant pain control benefit and was considerably more expensive, then IM morphine (Egger *et al.* 2007).

In humans, significant respiratory depression with use of the patches after surgery has precluded post-operative use, but this has not been a significant problem in veterinary medicine.

Pharmacology/Actions

Fentanyl is a *mu* opiate agonist that is very short acting and approximately 100 times more potent than morphine. *Mu* receptors are found primarily in the pain regulating areas of the brain. They are thought to contribute to the analgesia, euphoria, respiratory depression, physical dependence, miosis, and hypothermic actions of opiates. Receptors for opiate analgesics are found in high concentrations in the limbic system, spinal cord, thalamus, hypothalamus, striatum, and midbrain. They are also found in tissues such as the gastrointestinal tract, urinary tract, and in other smooth muscle.

The pharmacology of the opiate agonists is discussed in more detail in the monograph, Narcotic (opiate) Agonist Analgesics.

Pharmacokinetics

When used via a single dose IV injection, fentanyl has a relatively short duration of effect (15–30 minutes.)

When administered to dogs as 10 micrograms/kg IV bolus, fentanyl rapidly distributes and exhibits a large volume of distribution (5 L/kg). The terminal elimination half life is about 45 minutes; total clearance is 78 mL/min/kg. After a 10 micrograms/kg bolus, dogs administered a constant rate intravenous infusion of 10 mcg/kg/hr were able to maintain blood levels around 1 ng/mL (the assumed—but not verified therapeutic analgesic level). (Sano *et al.* 2006)

Half-life after IV administration in cats is approximately 2.5 hours.

There have been limited pharmacokinetic

studies performed with transdermal fentanyl patches in dogs, cats, and horses. While therapeutic levels of fentanyl are usually attained, there is a significant interpatient variability with both the time to achieve therapeutic levels and the levels themselves. Some animals may not achieve serum levels that are thought to be therapeutic (1 ng/mL). Cats tend to achieve therapeutic levels faster than do dogs; in dogs, the patch should be applied 24 hours in advance of need if possible; minimum of 12 hours preneed. Most cats attain therapeutic benefit in about 6 hours after application. While applied, duration of action persists for at least 72 hours (usually for at least 104 hours). Duration of action is generally longer in cats than in dogs. For continued use, patches may need to be changed every 48 hours in dogs or horses.

In horses, fentanyl from patches is rapidly absorbed with therapeutic levels (thought to be 1 ng/mL) achieved in about 6 hours after application and persists for 48+ hours. However, in about one-third of the horses in the study, plasma levels never reached ≥ 1 ng/mL (Orsini *et al.* 2006).

Contraindications/Precautions/Warnings

Fentanyl is contraindicated in patients with known hypersensitivity to it or any component of the product (including the adhesive for the patch).

When transdermal patches are used, absorption and efficacy can be highly patient variable; injectable rescue analgesia should be available.

Because of its potency, fentanyl injection should be used only by professionals familiar with its use in circumstances where patients can be adequately monitored and supported.

Use cautiously with other CNS depressants. Dosages of other opiates may need to be reduced when given with fentanyl transdermal, particularly several hours after application of the patch. Transdermal fentanyl should be used cautiously in geriatric, very ill or debilitated patients and those with a preexisting respiratory problem. Febrile patients may have increased absorption of fentanyl and will require increased monitoring.

Because opioids may cause mydriasis in cats, approach slowly so as not to startle, and keep animal out of very bright light or sunlight while pupils are dilated.

In the past, fentanyl patches were only available in a gel form that could not be cut. Now, other brands are available that potentially can be cut, but with the availability of 12 mg patches there is little therapeutic reason to do so. It is advised to obtain a pharmacist's advice before cutting patches. Do not allow applied fentanyl patch to be exposed to exogenous heat sources (heating pads, etc.). Increased drug release and absorption have occurred with fatal results.

Adverse Effects

Dose related respiratory, CNS and circulatory depression (bradycardia) are the primary adverse effects with fentanyl injection. Anticholinergic agents may be required to treat bradycardia, when fentanyl is used intraoperatively. Dogs and cats appear less prone, but not immune to opiate-induced respiratory depression, than are humans.

Respiratory depression and bradycardia associated with fentanyl patches are the most concerning adverse effects, but incidence of these effects have not been widespread thus far when used alone (without other opiates or other respiratory and cardiodepressant medications). Rashes at the patch site have been reported and should they occur, the patch should be removed; if an additional patch is warranted, a different site should be chosen. Urine retention and constipation may occur. Consider removing patch in patients developing a fever after application, as fentanyl absorption may increase. Some patients exhibit dysphoria or agitation after application; acepromazine or other mild tranquilizer may alleviate dysphoria.

Reproductive/Nursing Safety

Safe use in pregnancy has not been established. In humans, the FDA categorizes fentanyl as category *C* for use during pregnancy (*Animal studies have shown an adverse effect on the fetus, but there are no adequate studies in humans; or there are no animal reproduction studies and no adequate studies in humans.*) In a separate system evaluating the safety of drugs in canine and feline pregnancy (Papich 1989), this drug is categorized as in class: *B* (*Safe for use if used cautiously. Studies in laboratory animals may have uncovered some risk, but these drugs appear to be safe in dogs and cats or these drugs are safe if they are not administered when the animal is near term.*)

Most narcotic agonist analgesics are excreted into milk, but effects on nursing offspring may not be significant.

Overdosage/Acute Toxicity

Overdosage may produce profound respiratory and/or CNS depression in most species. Newborns may be more susceptible to these effects than adult animals. Other toxic effects may include cardiovascular collapse, tremors, neck rigidity, and seizures. There were 374 exposures to fentanyl reported to the ASPCA Animal Poison Control Center (APCC) during 2008-2009. In these cases, 362 were dogs with 295 showing clinical signs, and 12 were cats with 5 showing clinical signs. Common findings in dogs recorded in decreasing frequency included lethargy, hypersalivation, ataxia, bradycardia, hypothermia, depression, and diarrhea.

Naloxone is the agent of choice in treating respiratory depression. In massive overdoses, naloxone doses may need to be repeated; animals should be closely observed as naloxone's effects sometimes diminish before sub-toxic levels of fentanyl are attained. Mechanical respiratory support should also be considered in cases of severe respiratory depression.

Drug Interactions

The following drug interactions have either been reported or are theoretical in humans or animals receiving fentanyl and may be of significance in veterinary patients:

▪ **AZOLE ANTIFUNGALS (ketoconazole, itraconazole, fluconazole):** May inhibit fentanyl metabolism

▪ **CNS DEPRESSANTS, OTHER:** Additive CNS effects possible

▪ **DIURETICS:** Opiates may decrease efficacy in CHF patients

▪ **MACROLIDE ANTIBIOTICS (erythromycin, clarithromycin):** May inhibit fentanyl metabolism

▪ **MONOAMINE OXIDASE INHIBITORS (e.g., amitraz, and possibly selegiline):** Severe and unpredictable opiate potentiation may be seen; not recommended (in humans) if MAO inhibitor has been used within 14 days)

▪ **MUSCLE RELAXANTS, SKELETAL:** Fentanyl may enhance neuromuscular blockade

▪ **NITROUS OXIDE:** High fentanyl doses may cause cardiovascular depression

▪ **PHENOBARBITAL, PHENYTOIN:** May increase the metabolism of fentanyl

▪ **RIFAMPIN:** May increase the metabolism of fentanyl

▪ **TRICYCLIC ANTIDEPRESSANTS (clomipramine, amitriptyline, etc.):** Fentanyl may exacerbate the effects of tricyclic antidepressants

▪ **WARFARIN:** Opiates may potentiate anticoagulant activity

Laboratory Considerations

▪ As they may increase biliary tract pressure, opiates can increase plasma amylase and lipase values up to 24 hours following their administration.

Doses

WARNING: Do not confuse doses listed as micrograms/kg with those that are listed as mg/kg. Always double-check dosages and resulting volumes when using fentanyl.

▪ **DOGS:**

Fentanyl Injectable:

a) For perioperative pain: The combination of a 10 micro-grams/kg loading dose IV followed by a CRI of 10 micrograms/kg/hour investigated in this study might be a guideline for a CRI dose of fentanyl during general anesthesia to provide analgesia in dogs. (Sano *et al.* 2006)

b) Loading dose: 2–5 micrograms/kg IV, followed by a CRI at 2–5 micrograms/kg/hr for pain management; CRI

at 10–45 micrograms/kg/hr for surgical analgesia. (Wagner 2002)

c) For analgesia: 2–6 micrograms/kg/hour (Hansen 2008)

d) For induction: 0.001–0.005 mg/kg IV. For MAC reduction during general anesthesia: 10–45 micrograms/kg/hr CRI. (Mama 2002)

e) For severe to excruciating pain in the emergent patient: Fentanyl at 10–50 micrograms/kg, administered IV titrated to effect; use the effective dose as an hourly CRI. NSAIDs when not contraindicated. Ketamine at 4 mg/kg as a bolus, use with fentanyl. Lidocaine at 2–4 mg/kg bolus, followed by 2–4-mg/kg/hr CRI; caution with respect to overdose if local anesthetics have been administered by means of a different route. Tachycardia may persist and it may be impossible to control the pain. Consider combining these analgesics with epidurally placed analgesics or local blocks, or anesthetize the patient while attempting to find or treat the inciting cause. Remove the inciting cause immediately. This degree of pain can cause death. (Dyson 2008)

f) As an epidural for pain control: 0.004 mg/kg (4 micrograms/kg), diluted with 0.2 mL with preservative-free saline or local anesthetic. Has predominantly supraspinal effects. Onset in less than 10 minutes and duration of ½ hour. (Valverde 2008)

g) For maintenance analgesia/heavy sedation in critically ill animals who become hypotensive animals when exposed to inhalant anesthetics: See cat dose "g" below. (Brainard 2009)

Fentanyl Transdermal:

Note: There is significant interpatient variability on the response of the transdermal product. When used as the primary analgesic for post-operative pain, application prior to surgery is advised as many hours may be required for "therapeutic" levels to be achieved. Generally in dogs = 12–24 hours may be necessary; cats = 6–24 hours; and horses = 6+ hours.

The following dosage regimen has been used at the University of Minnesota Veterinary Medical Center and is adapted from information provided by Dr. Lynelle Graham:

Choose your patient carefully, realizing that the fentanyl patch alone may not provide sufficient analgesia. Fentanyl patches are effective for relief of chronic pain, dull pain and non-specific, widespread pain (peritonitis, pancreatitis, cancer, aortic thromboemboli, declaws, etc.) In the face of acute surgical pain or severe traumatic pain (fractures, thoracotomies, HBC/traumatic injuries/head trauma), analgesia provided by a fentanyl patch tends to be inadequate. Therefore, the patch should be used as an adjunctive measure for pain relief in these patients. If the patient is febrile, do not use fentanyl patch.

Choose your Patch Size:

Patient	Dose (Patch Size)	Fentanyl Content
Small Dogs (<5kg) ** and Cats**	**25 mcg/hr or 12.5 mcg/hr**	**2.5 mg; 1.25 mg**
Dogs: 5–10 kg	25 mcg/hr	2.5 mg
Dogs: 10–20 kg	50 mcg/hr	5 mg
Dogs: 20–30 kg	75 mcg/hr	7.5 mg
Dogs: >30 kg	100 mcg/hr	10 mg
Horses: 350–500 kg	2 x 100 mcg/hr	20 mg
Pigs: 17–25 kg	50–100 mcg/hr	5–10 mg
Sheep	1–3 x 50 mcg/hr	5–15 mg
Goats	50 mcg/hr	5 mg
Rabbits	25 mcg/hr	2.5 mg

**These patients can be dosed with 1/2 of a 25 mcg/hr patch, i.e., only half of the membrane is exposed to the patient's skin (cover the other half with tape); depending on the brand used. DO NOT CUT the patch in half, as this will alter the drug releasing membrane and allow evaporation of the fentanyl-containing alcohol-cellulose gel. Obtain a pharmacist's advice before cutting the patch. Current research suggests dosing with a whole 25 mcg/hr patch in otherwise healthy patients of this size (i.e., fractures, declaws). However, in order to avoid sedation, "half-patch" dosing may be desired for pediatric, geriatric, and systemically ill cats and very small dogs, but this is controversial.

Choose your location:

■ **Dog:** Thorax, inguinal area, metatarsal/carpal areas, base of tail (dorsal or lateral cervical area has been used, but leashes must not be placed around the neck if fentanyl patches are in place)

■ **Cat:** Lateral thorax, inguinal area, metatarsal/carpal areas; base of tail (the cervical area is NOT recommended, as the patch tends not to remain on)

■ **Horse:** Neck, antebrachium

■ **Pig; Rabbit:** Lateral thorax

■ **Sheep, Goat:** Abdomen, cervical area

Note: Direct patch contact with heating pads can significantly increase fentanyl absorption and risk toxicity. The patch should be kept dry; be aware of potential surgical clip sites.

1) Clip close, but don't shave, the site. DO NOT use depilatory agents in preparation of the site. Clip at least a 1 cm margin around the patch.

2) Wipe the site with a damp cloth and allow the skin to dry. This step is absolutely necessary, or patch will not stick to the skin. DO NOT wipe the area with alcohol or surgical scrub solution. Alcohol and surgical scrubs may "de-fat" the skin and alter drug absorption.

3) Place the patch on the skin and hold it in place with the palm of your hand for 2–3 minutes. The heat of your hand will help the adhesive bond to the skin. Failure to perform this step will allow the patch to fall off. If patch is not fully adhered to the skin, fentanyl will not be absorbed properly.

4) Cover the patch with a light bandage or clear adhesive bandage (i.e., Bioclusive®, Johnson and Johnson, Arlington, TX). If you choose to use Bioclusive®, apply the fentanyl patch as described above. Spray around the perimeter and over the patch with medical adhesive spray (Medical Adhesive®, Hollister, Libertyville, IL). Place the Bioclusive® over the site and press it down firmly. Be sure to clip an area large enough so that the Bioclusive® can adhere to the patch and the skin. If the Bioclusive® can only adhere to the patch and fur, without good adherence to skin, the patch will tend to peel up and dislodge.

5) Label the site with the size of patch (25, 50, 75 or 100 mcg/hr) and the date and time the patch was placed. Patches have shown to release effective fentanyl levels for up to five days in cats, three days in dogs and two days in horses. Potentially, the patches could be left longer, especially in dogs; this decision can be made by the attending clinician.

6) Potential side effects include bradycardia, respiratory depression, urinary retention, and constipation. All patients with fentanyl patches should be monitored accordingly. If a patient with a patch develops a fever, consider patch removal. If the patch is left in place, the patient must be closely monitored since the rate of fentanyl absorption may increase.

7) Person applying or removing the patch must gently, but thoroughly rinse their hands with water to remove any drug residue. Soap, cleansers or solvents should not be used. Surgical gloves may be worn to place or remove patches, as skin contact does occur when handling the adhesive edges.

8) Dispose of used patches in a safe and effective manner.

■ **CATS:**

Fentanyl Injectable:

a) For perioperative pain: 2–3 micrograms/kg IV plus 2–3 micrograms/kg/hour IV infusion (Pascoe 2000)

b) Loading dose: 1–3 micrograms/kg IV, followed by a CRI at 1–4 micrograms/kg/hr for pain management; CRI at 10–30 micrograms/kg/hr for surgical analgesia. (Wagner 2002)

c) For analgesia: 2–4 micrograms/kg/hour

d) For induction: 0.001–0.002 mg/kg IV. For MAC reduction during general anesthesia: 10–20 micrograms/kg/hr CRI. (Mama 2002)

e) For severe to excruciating pain in the emergent patient: Fentanyl at 10–50 micrograms/kg, administered IV titrated to effect; use the effective dose as an hourly CRI. NSAIDs when not contraindicated. Ketamine at 4 mg/kg, as a bolus (used with fentanyl). Lidocaine at 0.25–1 mg/kg bolus and then 0.5–2 mg/kg/hr CRI; caution with respect to overdose if local anesthetics have been administered by means of a different route. Tachycardia may persist and it may be impossible to control the pain. Consider combining these analgesics with epidurally placed analgesics or local blocks, or anesthetize the patient while attempting to find or treat the inciting cause. Remove the inciting cause immediately. This degree of pain can cause death. (Dyson 2008)

f) As an epidural for pain control: 0.004 mg/kg (4 micrograms/kg), diluted 0.2 mL with preservative-free saline or local anesthetic. Has predominantly supraspinal effects. Onset in less than 10 minutes and duration of ½ hour. (Valverde 2008)

g) For maintenance analgesia/heavy sedation in critically ill animals who become hypotensive animals when exposed to inhalant anesthetics: In addition to a local line block, fentanyl at 0.5–0.8 micrograms/kg/minute (equivalent to 30–50 micrograms/kg/hr). Intermittent IV bolus or a CRI of midazolam (0.1 mg/kg single bolus or given over an hour) will boost sedation to a neuroleptic state. 100% O_2 provided via the anesthetic circuit. Monitor ventilation using end-tidal CO_2 monitoring, or blood gases if ventilation not being assisted. Nitrous oxide can also be used to cause a neuroleptic effect and offset hypotension. (Brainard 2009)

Fentanyl Transdermal:

a) See above in dog dose section (Graham)

b) To transition to a fentanyl patch: Adjust CRI infusion rate to reach optimal effect before patch is applied; after patch applied, the infusion is then tapered and discontinued over the next 8-24 hours while observing patient response. If the patient does well on the infusion, but poorly on the patch, then failure of the patch is suspected. In cats, fentanyl delivery from the patch is highly variable. A 25 microgram patch provides approximately 10 micrograms/hr. 12 mg patches are available for very small cats. (Hansen 2008)

■ **FERRETS:**

Fentanyl Injectable:

a) Pre-op dose: 5–10 micrograms/kg IV; Intra-operatively: CRI at 10–20 micrograms/kg/hr with a ketamine CRI (0.3–0.4 mg/kg/hr); Post-operatively: 2–5 micrograms/kg/hr with a ketamine CRI. (Lichtenberger 2006)

■ **RABBITS/RODENTS/SMALL MAMMALS:**

Fentanyl Injectable:

a) For perioperative pain: 5–20 micrograms/kg IV bolus (30–60 minute duration; causes sedation and respiratory depression) (Ivey & Morrisey 2000)

Fentanyl Transdermal:

a) **Rabbits** for postoperative analgesia: 1/2 small patch (25 micrograms/hr) per medium sized rabbit (3 kg) every 3 days. Do not cut patch (Ivey & Morrisey 2000)

b) **Rabbits:** See above in dog dose section

■ **HORSES: (Note:** ARCI UCGFS Class 1 Drug)

Fentanyl Transdermal: See above in dog dose section

■ **SHEEP, GOATS & SWINE:**

Fentanyl Transdermal: See above in dog dose section

Monitoring

■ Analgesic efficacy

■ Heart rate and respiratory rate

Client Information

■ Fentanyl injection should be used only by professionals familiar with its use in a setting where adequate monitoring can occur.

■ Fentanyl Patches: Explain carefully to clients how to apply (if applicable), remove and dispose of patches. Consider making application, removal, and disposal an outpatient procedure, thereby bypassing concerns with clients.

■ Should accidental human skin contact occur with the patch, wash with water only (no soap, etc.). Use cautiously in households where young children or animals could remove and ingest or be exposed to patches.

Chemistry/Synonyms

Fentanyl citrate, a very potent opiate agonist, occurs as a white, crystalline powder. It is sparingly soluble in water and soluble in alcohol. It is odorless and tasteless (not recommended for taste test because of extreme potency) with a pK_a of 8.3 and a melting point between 147°–152°C.

Fentanyl and fentanyl citrate may also be known as: fentanylum, fentanyli citras, McN-JR-4263-49, phentanyl citrate, R-4263, *Actiq®*, *Fenodid®*, *Fenta-Hameln®*, *Fentabbott®*, *Fentanest®*, *Fentax®*, *Fentora®*, *Haldid®*, *Ionsys®*, *Leptanal®*, *Nafluvent®*, *Sintenyl®*, *Sublimaze®*, *Tanyl®*, and *Trofentyl®*.

Storage/Stability

Fentanyl transdermal patches should be stored at temperatures less than 25°C and applied immediately after removing from the individually sealed package. Do not cut patches.

The transmucosal (buccal) tablets should be stored at room temperature; do not refrigerate or freeze.

Fentanyl injection should be stored protected from light. It is hydrolyzed in an acidic solution.

Compatibility/Compounding Considerations

The injection is **compatible** with normal saline and D5W.

Dosage Forms/Regulatory Status

VETERINARY-LABELED PRODUCTS: None

The ARCI (Racing Commissioners International) has designated this drug as a class 1 substance. See the appendix for more information.

HUMAN-LABELED PRODUCTS:

Fentanyl Buccal Tablets: 100 mcg, 200 mcg, 400 mcg, 600 mcg, & 800 mcg with mannitol in color-coded blister packs; *Fentora®* (Cephalon); (Rx, C-II)

Fentanyl Injectable: 0.05 mg/mL (50 micrograms/mL) in 2 mL, 5 mL, 10 mL, & 20 mL amps; 30 mL and 50 mL vials; preservative free in 2 mL, 5 mL, 10 mL, & 20 mL amps; *Sublimaze®* (Akorn); generic; (Rx, C-II)

Fentanyl Transdermal System:

1.25 (5 cm^2; **12 mcg/hr**);

2.5 to 2.75 (6.25–10 cm^2; **25 mcg/hr**);

2.5 to 5.5 (12.5–20 cm^2; **50 mcg/hr**);

7.5 to 8.25 (18.75–30 cm^2; **75 mcg/hr**);

10 to 11 (25–40 cm^2; **100 mcg/hr**);

Duragesic®-12, -25, -50, -75 and -100 (Janssen); generic; (Rx, C-II)

Fentanyl Iontophoretic Transdermal System: 40 mcg/dose fentanyl hydrochloride (equivalent to 44.4 mcg of fentanyl) delivered over a 10-minute period upon each activation of the dose button; Each system contains fentanyl hydrochloride 10.8 mg; *Ionsys®* (Ortho-McNeil); (Rx; C-II)

Fentanyl Transmucosal System: Lozenges on a stick: 200 mcg, 400 mcg, 600 mcg, 800 mcg, 1200 mcg and 1600 mcg (as base); *Actiq®* (Cephalon); generic; (Rx, C-II)

All fentanyl products are Class-II controlled substances.

References

Brainard, B. (2009). Anesthetic approaches for critically ill animals. Proceedings: ACVC. Accessed via: Veterinary Information Network. http://goo.gl/JPELT

Dyson, D. (2008). Analgesia and Chemical Restraint for the Emergent Veterinary Patient. *Vet Clin Small Anim* 38: 1329–1352.

Egger, C.M., L. Glerum, et al. (2007). Efficacy and cost-effectiveness of transdermal fentanyl patches for the relief of post-operative pain in dogs after anterior cruciate ligament and pelvic limb repair. *Veterinary Anaesthesia and Analgesia* 34(3): 200–208.

Hansen, B. (2008). Analgesia for the critically ill dog or cat: An update. *Vet Clin NA: Sm Anim Pract* 38: 1353–1363.

Ivey, E. & J. Morrisey (2000). Therapeutics for Rabbits. *Vet Clin NA: Exotic Anim Pract* 3:1(Jan): 183–216.

Lichtenberger, M. (2006). Clinical monitoring of the critically ill ferret. Proceedings: IVECCS. Accessed via: Veterinary Information Network. http://goo.gl/MMCIj

Mama, K. (2002). Use of opioids in anesthesia practice. Proceeedings: World Small Animal Veterinary Association.

Orsini, J.A., P.J. Moate, et al. (2006). Pharmacokinetics of fentanyl delivered transdermally in healthy adult horses - variability among horses and its clinical implications. *Journal of Veterinary Pharmacology and Therapeutics* 29(6): 539–546.

Pascoe, P. (2000). Perioperative pain management. *Vet Clin NA: Small Anim Pract* 30:4(July): 917–932.

Sano, T., R. Nishimura, et al. (2006). Pharmacokinetics of fentanyl after single intravenous injection and constant rate infusions in dogs. *Vet Anaesth Analg* 33: 266–273.

Valverde, A. (2008). Epidural analgesia and anesthesia in dogs and cats. *Vet Clin NA: Sm Anim Pract* 38: 1205–1230.

Wagner, A. (2002). Opioids. *Handbook of Veterinary Pain Management*. J Gaynor and W Muir Eds., Mosby: 164–183.

FERROUS SULFATE

(*fer*-us sul-*fayte*)   Fer-In-Sol®, Feosol®

NUTRITIONAL/HEMATINIC

Prescriber Highlights

▶ Oral iron supplement for the treatment of iron-deficiency anemias

▶ Contraindications: Patients with hemosiderosis, hemochromatosis, hemolytic anemias, or known hypersensitivity; some consider it contraindicated with GI ulcers

▶ Adverse Effects: With non-toxic doses, mild gastrointestinal upset

▶ May be very toxic (life threatening) if OD'd

Uses/Indications

While iron is a necessary trace element in all hemoglobin-utilizing animals, the use of therapeutic dosages of ferrous sulfate (or other oral iron) preparations in veterinary medicine is limited primarily to the treatment of iron-deficiency anemias in dogs (usually due to chronic blood loss), and as adjunctive therapy in cats when receiving epoetin (erythropoietin) therapy. Injectable iron products are usually used in the treatment of iron deficiency anemias associated with newborn animals.

Pharmacology/Actions

Iron is necessary for myoglobin and hemoglobin in the transport and utilization of oxygen. While neither stimulating erythropoiesis nor correcting hemoglobin abnormalities not caused by iron deficiency, iron administration does correct both physical signs and decreased hemoglobin levels secondary to iron deficiency.

Ionized iron is a component in the enzymes cytochrome oxidase, succinic dehydrogenase, and xanthine oxidase.

Pharmacokinetics

Oral absorption of iron salts is complex and determined by a variety of factors including diet, iron stores present, degree of erythropoiesis, and dose. Iron is thought to be absorbed throughout the GI tract, but is most absorbed in the duodenum and proximal jejunum. Food in the GI tract may reduce the amount absorbed.

After absorption, the ferrous iron is immediately bound to transferrin, transported to the bone marrow and eventually incorporated into hemoglobin. Iron metabolism occurs in a nearly closed system. Because iron liberated by the destruction of hemoglobin is reused by the body and only small amounts are lost by the body via hair and nail growth, normal skin desquamation and GI tract sloughing, normal dietary intake usually is sufficient to maintain iron homeostasis.

Contraindications/Precautions/Warnings

Ferrous sulfate (or other oral iron products) are considered contraindicated in patients with hemosiderosis, hemochromatosis, hemolytic anemias, or known hypersensitivity to any component of the product. Because of the GI irritating properties of the drugs, oral iron products are considered contraindicated by some clinicians in patients with GI ulcerative diseases.

Adverse Effects

Adverse effects associated with non-toxic doses are usually limited to mild gastrointestinal upset. Division of the daily dosage may reduce this effect, but dosage reduction may also be necessary in some animals.

Reproductive/Nursing Safety

In humans, the FDA categorizes this drug as category *A* for use during pregnancy (*Adequate studies in pregnant women have not demonstrated a risk to the fetus in the first trimester of pregnancy, and there is no evidence of risk in later trimesters.*)

Overdosage/Acute Toxicity

Ingestion of iron containing products may result in serious toxicity. While lethal doses are not readily available in domestic species, as little as 400 mg (of elemental iron) is potentially fatal in a child. Initial clinical signs of acute iron poisoning usually present with an acute onset of gastrointestinal irritation and distress (vomiting—possibly hemorrhagic, abdominal pain, diarrhea). The onset of these effects can be seen within 30 minutes of ingestion, but can be delayed for several hours. Peripheral vascular collapse may rapidly follow with clinical signs of depression, weak and/or rapid pulse, hypotension, cyanosis, ataxia, and coma possible. Some patients do not exhibit this phase of toxicity and may be asymptomatic for 12–48 hours after ingestion, when another critical phase may occur. This phase may be exhibited by pulmonary edema, vasomotor collapse, cyanosis, pulmonary edema, fulminant hepatic failure, coma and death. Animals that survive this phase may exhibit long-term sequelae, including gastric scarring and contraction and have persistent digestive disturbances.

Because an acute onset of gastroenteritis may be associated with a multitude of causes, diagnosis of iron intoxication may be difficult unless the animal has been observed ingesting the product or physical evidence suggests ingestion. Ferrous sulfate (and gluconate) tablets are radiopaque and often can be observed on abdominal radiographs. Serum iron levels and total iron binding capacity (TIBC) may also be helpful in determining the diagnosis, but must be done on an emergency basis to have any clinical benefit.

Treatment of iron intoxication must be handled as an emergency. In humans who have ingested 10 mg/kg or more of elemental iron within 4 hours of presentation, the stomach is emptied, preferably using gastric lavage with a large bore tube to remove tablet fragments. It is generally recommended to avoid using emetics in patients who already have had episodes of hemorrhagic vomiting. These patients are lavaged using tepid water or 1–5% sodium bicarbonate solution.

In dogs, one author (Mount 1989), has recommended using oral milk of magnesia to help bind the drug, administering apomorphine if appropriate to help dislodge tablets, and to instill a gastric lavage slurry of 50% sodium bicarbonate with a portion left in the stomach. Deferoxamine is useful in chelating iron that has been absorbed. See that monograph for further information.

In addition to chelation therapy, other supportive measures may be necessary including treatment of acidosis, prophylactic antibiotics, oxygen, treatment for shock, coagulation abnormalities, seizures, and/or hyperthermia. After the acute phases have resolved, dietary evaluation and management may be required.

Drug Interactions

The following drug interactions have either been reported or are theoretical in humans or animals receiving ferrous sulfate and may be of significance in veterinary patients:

- ■ **ANTACIDS:** May bind to iron and decrease oral absorption; administer at least two hours apart

■ **CALCIUM (ORAL):** May bind to iron and decrease oral absorption; administer at least two hours apart

■ **CHLORAMPHENICOL:** Because chloramphenicol may delay the response to iron administration, avoid using chloramphenicol in patients with iron deficiency anemia

■ **FLUOROQUINOLONES (enrofloxacin, etc.):** Iron may reduce the absorption of oral fluoroquinolones; administer at least two hours apart

■ **H2-RECEPTOR ANTAGONISTS (e.g., ranitidine, famotidine, etc.):** Increased gastric pH may decrease iron absorption

■ **PENICILLAMINE:** Iron can decrease the efficacy of penicillamine, probably by decreasing its absorption; if both drugs are required, space doses of the two drugs as far apart as possible

■ **PROTON-PUMP INHIBITORS (e.g., omeprazole):** Increased gastric pH may decrease iron absorption

■ **TETRACYCLINES:** Oral iron preparations can bind to orally administered tetracyclines, thereby decreasing the absorption of both compounds

■ **THYROXINE:** Iron may reduce the absorption of oral thyroxine; administer at least two hours apart

■ **VITAMIN C:** May enhance the absorption of iron

Laboratory Considerations
■ Large doses of oral iron can color the feces black and cause false-positives with the guaiac test for occult blood in the feces.
■ Iron does not usually affect the benzidine test for occult blood.

Doses

Caution: Unless otherwise noted, doses are for ferrous sulfate (regular—not dried). Dosing of oral iron products can be confusing; some authors state doses in terms of the iron salt and some state doses in terms of elemental iron. For the doses below, assume that the doses are for ferrous sulfate and not elemental iron, unless specified.

■ **DOGS:**
For iron deficiency anemia:
a) 100–300 mg (total dose) PO once a day. (Jutkowitz 2009)
b) First correct underlying cause of blood loss, then give ferrous sulfate at 100–300 mg per day (total dose) PO. Absorption is enhanced if administered 1 hour before or several hours after feeding. Reduce dosage if GI side effects occur. (Harvey *et al.* 1982)

For patients to be treated with epoetin (erythropoietin):

a) 100–300 mg (total dose) PO per day (Cowgill 2002); (Vaden 2006)

■ **CATS:**
For iron deficiency anemia:
a) 50–100 mg (total dose) PO once daily (Macintire 2009), (Jutkowitz 2009)
b) 30–200 mg (total dose) PO per day for 2 weeks or more (Adams 1988)

For patients to be treated with epoetin (erythropoietin):
a) 50–100 mg (total dose) PO per day. Many cats do not tolerate oral iron therapy and are better treated with iron dextran at 50 mg IM q3–4 weeks. (Cowgill 2002)
b) 5–50 mg per cat PO once daily (DiBartola & Chew 2006)
c) 50–100 mg per cat PO once daily (Vaden 2006)
d) 10 mg/kg PO once daily (Macintire 2009)

■ **CATTLE:**
As a hematinic:
a) 8–15 g PO per day for 2 weeks or more (Adams 1988)

■ **HORSES:**
As a hematinic:
a) 2–8 g PO per day for 2 weeks or more (Adams 1988)

■ **SWINE:**
As a hematinic:
a) 0.5–2 g PO per day for 2 weeks or more (Adams 1988)

■ **SHEEP:**
As a hematinic:
a) 0.5–2 g PO per day for 2 weeks or more (Adams 1988)

Monitoring
■ Efficacy; adverse effects:
a) Hemograms
b) Serum iron and total iron binding capacity, if necessary. Normal serum iron values for dogs and cats are reported as 80–180 micrograms/dL and 70–140 micrograms/dL, respectively. Total iron binding for dogs and cats are reported as 280–340 micrograms/dL and 270–400 micrograms/dL, respectively. (Morgan 1988). Serum transferrin saturation can estimated by dividing serum iron by total iron binding capacity.

Client Information
■ Because of the potential for serious toxicity when overdoses of oral iron-containing products are ingested by either children or animals, these products should be kept well out of reach of children and pets.

Chemistry/Synonyms
An orally available iron supplement, ferrous sulfate occurs as odorless, pale-bluish-green, crystals or granules having a saline, styptic taste.

In dry air the drug is efflorescent. If exposed to moisture or moist air, the drug is rapidly oxidized to a brownish-yellow ferric compound that should not be used medicinally. Exposure to light or an alkaline medium will enhance the conversion from the ferrous to ferric state.

Ferrous sulfate is available commercially in two forms, a "regular" and a "dried" form. Regular ferrous sulfate contains 7 molecules of water of hydration and is freely soluble in water and insoluble in alcohol. Ferrous sulfate contains approximately 200 mg of elemental iron per gram. Dried ferrous sulfate consists primarily of the monohydrate with some tetrahydrate. It is slowly soluble in water and insoluble in water. Dried ferrous sulfate contains 300 mg of elemental iron per gram. Ferrous sulfate, dried may also be known as ferrous sulfate, exsiccated.

Ferrous sulfate may also be known as: eisen(II)-sulfat, ferreux (sulfate), ferrosi sulfas heptahydricus, ferrous sulphate, ferrum sulfuricum oxydulatum, iron (II) sulphate heptahydrate, iron sulphate; many trade names are available.

Storage/Stability

Unless otherwise instructed, store ferrous sulfate preparations in tight, light-resistant containers.

Dosage Forms/Regulatory Status

VETERINARY-LABELED PRODUCTS:

No veterinary-FDA-approved products containing only ferrous sulfate could be located, but there are many multivitamin with iron containing products available.

HUMAN-LABELED PRODUCTS:

Ferrous Sulfate Oral Tablets: 325 mg (65 mg iron); *Feosol®* (GlaxoSmithKline); *FeroSul®* (Major); generic; (OTC)

Ferrous Sulfate Oral Elixir/Liquid: 220 mg/5mL (44 mg iron/5 mL), 300 mg/5 mL (60 mg iron/5 mL) in 5 mL; generic; (OTC)

Ferrous Sulfate Oral Drops: 15 mg iron/mL & 75 mg/0.6 mL (15 mg iron/0.6 mL) in 50 mL; *Enfamil Fer-In-Sol®* (Mead Johnson Nutritionals); *Fer-Gen-Sol®* (Goldline); generic; (OTC)

References

Adams, H.R. (1988). Antianemic Drugs. *Veterinary Pharmacology and Therapeutics*. NH Booth and LE McDonald Eds. Ames, Iowa State University Press: 469–481.

Cowgill, L. (2002). Anemia and hypertension: The ignored consequences of chronic renal failure. Proceedings: Tufts Animal Expo. Accessed via: Veterinary Information Network. http://goo.gl/AofHC

DiBartola, S. & D. Chew (2006). Tips for managing chronic renal failure. Proceedings: ACVIM. Accessed via: Veterinary Information Network. http://goo.gl/hf5C4

Harvey, J.W., T.W. French, et al. (1982). Chronic Iron Deficiency in Dogs. *JAAHA* 18: 946–960.

Jutkowitz, L. (2009). Clinical approach to the anemic patient. Proceedings: WVC. Accessed via: Veterinary Information Network. http://goo.gl/9y9Hw

Macintire, D. (2009). ANEMIA IN FELINE CRITICAL ILLNESS. Proceedings: IVECCS. Accessed via: Veterinary Information Network. http://goo.gl/7GSxX

Morgan, R.V., Ed. (1988). *Handbook of Small Animal Practice*. New York, Churchill Livingstone.

Vaden, S. (2006). Management of Chronic Renal Failure. Proceedings: Western Vet Conf. Accessed via: Veterinary Information Network. http://goo.gl/86oQf

FILGRASTIM (GRANULOCYTE COLONY STIMULATING FACTOR; GCSF)

(fill-*grass*-stim)   Neupogen®

CYTOKINE HEMATOPOIETIC AGENT

Prescriber Highlights

▶ Cytokine that in the bone marrow primarily increases the proliferation, differentiation, & activation of progenitor cells in the neutrophil-granulocyte line

▶ Human origin product; antibodies may form that can cause prolonged neutropenia

▶ Treatment is very expensive

Uses/Indications

Filgrastim may be of benefit in treating neutropenias in dogs or cats when the intrinsic response to endogenously produced cytokines is thought to be inadequate and there is evidence that there are precursors in the bone marrow available. Because of the drug's cost, potential for antibody development and the lack of good evidence for its efficacy in reducing mortality versus using antibiotic therapy alone, its use in small animal medicine is controversial.

Pharmacology/Actions

Filgrastim is a hematopoietic agent that primarily affects the bone marrow to increase the proliferation, differentiation, and activation of progenitor cells in the neutrophil-granulocyte line. While derived from human DNA, the product is not species specific and also affects canine and feline bone marrow.

Pharmacokinetics

After subcutaneous injection, filgrastim is rapidly absorbed and distributed with highest concentrations found in the bone marrow, liver, kidneys and adrenal glands. It is unknown if it crosses the blood-brain barrier, placenta, or enters maternal milk. The elimination pathways of filgrastim are still under investigation.

Contraindications/Precautions/Warnings

Filgrastim is contraindicated in patients hypersensitive to it. Dogs or cats that have developed antibodies to filgrastim with resultant neutropenia should probably not receive it in the future.

Adverse Effects

Because the human DNA origin product can be immunogenic to dogs and cats, some patients may develop severe neutropenia by mounting an immune response against both endogenously produced and exogenously administered G-CSF. Studies in cats have demonstrated that short pulse doses of 3–5 days at the time of neutropenia may be safe and minimize the development of neutrophil neutralizing antibodies. Preliminary studies using canine origin G-CSF have not demonstrated autoantibody formation in either dogs or cats.

Additionally, there are concerns that exogenously administered filgrastim can elicit undesirable responses in other tissues, including causing myelofibrosis and medullary histiocytosis.

Occasionally irritation at the injection site may occur. Bone pain, splenomegaly, and hypotension have been reported in humans.

Reproductive/Nursing Safety
Adverse effects in females and offspring have been demonstrated after filgrastim was administered to pregnant laboratory animals at high dosages. To interpret this data for use in a clinical setting is difficult, but filgrastim should be used in pregnant females only when the benefits of treating outweigh the potential risks. In humans, the FDA categorizes this drug as category *C* for use during pregnancy (*Animal studies have shown an adverse effect on the fetus, but there are no adequate studies in humans; or there are no animal reproduction studies and no adequate studies in humans.*)

It is not known whether filgrastim is excreted in milk, but it is unlikely to pose significant risk to nursing offspring.

Overdosage/Acute Toxicity
Limited information is available. Because of the expense of the drug and its apparent limited acute toxic potential, clinically significant overdoses are unlikely.

Drug Interactions
The following drug interactions have either been reported or are theoretical in humans or animals receiving filgrastim and may be of significance in veterinary patients:

■ **ANTINEOPLASTICS:** While filgrastim was developed primarily to prevent the neutropenias associated with some chemotherapeutic agents, some controversy exists about using filgrastim within 24 hours of a dose of antineoplastic agents that target rapidly proliferating cells; generally, in human medicine, use is avoided within 24 hours of such antineoplastics

Doses
Note: To avoid the development of autoantibody formation, most clinicians using this agent recommend using filgrastim in dogs or cats using a "pulse" therapy of no more than 5 days in duration.

■ **DOGS:**
a) For adjunctive therapy of neutropenia

(secondary to drug induced aplastic pancytopenia): 5 micrograms/kg SC daily (Ruiz de Gopegui & Feldman 2000)

b) For neutropenia: 1–5 micrograms/kg SC daily (Ritt & Modiano 1999)

■ **CATS:**
a) For neutropenia secondary to drug toxicity, infectious diseases, FeLV-associated cyclic neutropenia or idiopathic causes: 5 micrograms/kg SC twice daily. Cost and/or development of antibodies usually limit usefulness to a few weeks, but often it is effective for acute or life-threatening neutropenia. (Levy, JK 2000)

b) For neutropenia: 1–5 micrograms/kg SC daily (Ritt & Modiano 1999)

c) For adjunctive therapy of neutropenia: 5 micrograms/kg SC daily until neutrophil count exceeds 3,000/mcl for 2 days (Levy, J 2002)

Monitoring
■ CBC with platelets, routinely

Client Information
■ Clients should be briefed on the cost of this agent as well as the possibility that it may cause antibodies to form against endogenously produced G-CSF, thereby causing a potentially life threatening neutropenia.

Chemistry/Synonyms
Prepared via recombinant DNA technology from human DNA, filgrastim is a single chain polypeptide containing 175 amino acids with a molecular weight of about 18,800 daltons. The commercially available injection occurs as a clear solution; buffered to a pH of 4.

Filgrastim may also be known as: granulocyte colony-stimulating factor, G-CSF, recombinant methionyl human GCS-F, r-metHuG-CSF, *Filgen®*, *Gran®*, *Granulen®*, *Granulokine®*, *Neulasta®*, *Neupogen®*, and *Neutromax®*.

Storage/Stability
Injection should be stored in the refrigerator (2–8°C). Do not freeze or shake contents of vial. The drug should never be diluted with saline as a precipitate may form. If necessary it may be diluted into 5% dextrose for injection, but if diluted to concentrations between 5 and 15 micrograms/mL, it is recommended that albumin be added to the solution to a concentration of 2 mg/mL to reduce adsorption to plastic IV tubing. It is not recommended to dilute to a concentration of less than 5 micrograms/mL.

Dosage Forms/Regulatory Status
VETERINARY-LABELED PRODUCTS: None

HUMAN-LABELED PRODUCTS:

Filgrastim Injection: 300 micrograms/mL preservative free in 1 mL and 1.6 mL single dose vials; 300 micrograms/0.5 mL preservative free in 0.5 mL and 0.8 mL prefilled syringes; *Neupogen®* (Amgen); (Rx)

References

Levy, J. (2000). FeLV and Non-Neoplastic FeLV-related Disease. *Textbook of Veterinary Internal Medicine: Diseases of the Dog and Cat.* S Ettinger and E Feldman Eds. Philadelphia, WB Saunders. **1**: 424–432.

Levy, J. (2002). Management of the immunosuppressed cat. Proceedings: Waltham Feline Medicine Symposium. Accessed via: Veterinary Information Network. http://goo.gl/Nz3a5

Ritt, M. & J. Modiano (1999). Hematopoietic growth factors in health and disease. American College of Veterinary Internal Medicine: 17th Annual Veterinary Medical Forum, Chicago.

Ruiz de Gopegui, R. & B. Feldman (2000). Platelets and von Willebrand's Disease. *Textbook of Veterinary Internal Medicine: Diseases of the Dog and Cat.* S Ettinger and E Feldman Eds. Philadelphia, WB Saunders. **2**: 1817–1828.

FINASTERIDE

(fin-**as**-te-ride)   Proscar®, Propecia®

5-ALPHA-REDUCTASE INHIBITOR

Prescriber Highlights

▶ 5-alpha-reductase inhibitor potentially useful for dogs with benign prostatic hypertrophy & ferrets with adrenal disease

▶ Contraindications: Hypersensitivity to finasteride; sexually developing animals

▶ Caution: Patients with significant hepatic impairment

▶ Adverse Effects: Potentially may cause some minor sexual side effects

▶ Expense may be an issue, but generics now available

Uses/Indications

Finasteride may be useful in treating the benign prostatic hypertrophy in canine patients, particularly those that are used for breeding. Because of the drug's relative expense and the long duration of therapy required to see a response, its usefulness may be limited in veterinary medicine.

It may also be useful in the adjunctive treatment of adrenal disease in ferrets.

Pharmacology/Actions

Finasteride specifically and totally inhibits 5-alpha-reductase. This enzyme is responsible for metabolizing testosterone to dihydrotestosterone (DHT) in the prostate, liver and skin. DHT is a potent androgen and is the primary hormone responsible for the development of the prostate.

Pharmacokinetics

Finasteride is absorbed after oral administration and in humans about 65% is bioavailable. The presence of food does not affect absorption. It is distributed across the blood-brain barrier and is found in seminal fluid. In humans, about 90% is bound to plasma proteins. Finasteride is metabolized in the liver and the half-life is about 6 hours. Metabolites are excreted in the urine and feces. In humans, a single daily dose suppresses DHT concentrations for 24 hours.

Contraindications/Precautions/Warnings

Finasteride is contraindicated in patients hypersensitive to it. It should be used with caution in patients with significant hepatic impairment as metabolism of the drug may be reduced. Finasteride should be used in males only; do not use in sexually developing animals.

Adverse Effects

One study done in dogs reported no adverse effects or irreversibility of effects after treating for 21 weeks at 1 mg/kg. The adverse effects reported in humans have been very limited, mild and transient. Decreased libido, decreased ejaculate volume, and impotence have been reported.

Reproductive/Nursing Safety

In humans, the FDA categorizes this drug as category **X** for use during pregnancy (*Studies in animals or humans demonstrate fetal abnormalities or adverse reaction; reports indicate evidence of fetal risk. The risk of use in pregnant women clearly outweighs any possible benefit.*)

Finasteride is not indicated for use in females. It is not known whether finasteride is excreted in milk.

Overdosage/Acute Toxicity

Limited information is available; gastrointestinal effects may be noted.

Drug Interactions

The following drug interactions have either been reported or are theoretical in humans or animals receiving finasteride and may be of significance in veterinary patients:

■ **ANTICHOLINERGIC DRUGS:** May precipitate or aggravate urinary retention thereby negating the effects of the drug when used for BPH

Doses

■ **DOGS:**
   a) For benign prostatic hyperplasia: 0.1–0.5 mg/kg once daily PO; for a 10–50 kg dog, one 5 mg tablet daily (Sirinarumitr *et al.* 2001), (Bartges 2006)

   b) For dogs <15 kg: 1.5 mg (approx. 1/3 of a 5 mg tablet); for dogs 15–30 kg = 2.5 mg (1/2 tablet); for dogs >30 kg = 5 mg (one tablet). Given PO daily. (Romagnoli 2006)

■ **FERRETS:**
   a) For adjunctive treatment of adrenal disease: 5 mg (total dose) tablet once daily (Johnson 2006a), (Johnson 2006b)

Monitoring

■ Efficacy: Prostate exam

Client Information

■ Clients should understand that therapy might be prolonged before efficacy can be determined and regular dosing compliance is mandatory. Once the drug is stopped, the prostate will start growing again.

■ Pregnant women should be advised to guard against exposure to this drug as it may cause birth defects.

Chemistry/Synonyms

Finasteride is a 4-azasteroid synthetic drug that inhibits 5 alpha-dihydroreductase (DH), and has a molecular weight of 372.55.

Finasteride may also be known as: finasteridum, MK-0906, and MK-906; many trade names are available.

Storage/Stability

Store tablets below 30°C in tight containers and protected from light.

Dosage Forms/Regulatory Status

VETERINARY-LABELED PRODUCTS: None
HUMAN-LABELED PRODUCTS:
Finasteride Oral Tablets: 1 mg & 5 mg; *Proscar®*, *Propecia®* (Merck); generic; (Rx)

References

Bartges, J. (2006). The State of the Prostate: Canine Prostate Disease. Proceedings: ACVC 2006. Accessed via: Veterinary Information Network. http://goo.gl/nE9jU

Johnson, D. (2006a). Current Therapies for Ferret Adrenal Disease. Proceedings: ACVC. Accessed via: Veterinary Information Network. http://goo.gl/pOMYy

Johnson, D. (2006b). Ferrets: the other companion animal. Proceedings: ACVC. Accessed via: Veterinary Information Network. http://goo.gl/bSeol

Romagnoli, S. (2006). Two common causes of infertility in the male dog. Proceedings: WSAVA World Congress. Accessed via: Veterinary Information Network. http://goo.gl/dh8Sa

Sirinarumitr, K., S.D. Johnston, et al. (2001). Effects of finasteride on size of the prostate gland and semen quality in dogs with benign prostatic hypertrophy. *Journal of the American Veterinary Medical Association* 218(8): 1275–1280.

Fipronil–See the listing in the Dermatological Agents, Topical Appendix

FIROCOXIB

(feer-oh-**koks**-ib)   Previcox®, Equioxx®
ORAL COX-2 INHIBITOR NSAID

Prescriber Highlights

▶ Oral COX-2 NSAID labeled for the control of pain & inflammation associated with osteoarthritis in dogs & horses

▶ Adverse effect profile not fully determined; in *dogs:* GI effects (vomiting, anorexia) most likely, but serious effects are possible

▶ Adverse effects in horses include mouth ulcers, facial skin lesions, excitation (rare)

Uses/Indications

Firocoxib is indicated in dogs and horses for the control of pain and inflammation associated with osteoarthritis and in dogs for the control of post-operative pain and inflammation associated with orthopedic surgery. A chewable tablet form for dogs and an oral paste for horses are available.

Like other NSAIDs, firocoxib can be useful for treating fever, pain, and/or inflammation associated with other conditions, post-surgery, trauma, etc.

Firocoxib may also be useful in other species, but information is scant regarding its safety and efficacy. One study in cats (McCann *et al.* 2005) evaluating firocoxib in experimentally induced pyrexia, demonstrated that the drug was effective after a single oral dose in preventing or attenuating pyrexia at all doses studied (0.75–3 mg/kg).

Pharmacology/Actions

Firocoxib is a coxib-class, nonsteroidal anti-inflammatory drug (NSAID). It is believed to predominantly inhibit cyclooxygenase-2 (COX-2) and spare COX-1 at therapeutic dosages. This theoretically would inhibit production of the prostaglandins that contribute to pain and inflammation (COX-2) and spare those that maintain normal gastrointestinal, platelet and renal function (COX-1). However, COX-1 and COX-2 inhibition studies are done *in vitro* and do not necessarily correlate perfectly with clinical effects seen in actual patients.

Firocoxib also has some anti-tumor activity and it may find a role in treating cancer in animals.

Pharmacokinetics

In dogs, firocoxib absorption after oral dosing varies among individuals. Oral bioavailability with the chewable tablets, on average, is about 38%. Food will delay, but not affect the amount absorbed. Peak levels occur about 1 hour after dosing if fasted, and 5 hours if the patient is fed. Volume of distribution at steady state is about 3 L/kg; it is 96% bound to plasma proteins. Biotransformation occurs predominantly via dealkylation and glucuronidation in the liver; elimination is principally in the bile and feces. Elimination half-life in dogs is approximately 6–8 hours.

In horses, oral availability after administering the paste is approximately 79%. Peak levels occur 4–12 hours after dosing. Volume of distribution at steady state is about 1.7-2.3 L/kg and it is 98% bound to plasma proteins. Biotransformation in horses occurs primarily via decyclopropylmethylation and then glucuronidation. Metabolites are primarily excreted in the urine. Elimination half-life is approximately 30–40 hours.

Pharmacokinetics of firocoxib have only been reported in two cats studied (McCann *et al.* 2005). Oral bioavailability after administering an oral suspension was about 60% and the volume of distribution, between 2–3 L/kg. Elimination half-life in the two cats studied averaged about 10 hours.

Contraindications/Precautions/Warnings

Firocoxib should not be used in animals hypersensitive to it or other NSAIDs. The drug should be used with caution and enhanced monitoring in patients with preexisting renal, hepatic or cardiovascular dysfunction, and those that are dehydrated, hypovolemic, hypotensive, or on concomitant diuretic therapy. Because geriatric patients have reduced renal function and firocoxib is often used for osteoarthritis in this patient population, ongoing monitoring for adverse effects is mandatory.

Because all NSAIDs can potentially cause GI toxicity, firocoxib is relatively contraindicated in dogs with active GI ulcerative conditions. As it may affect platelet function, it is relatively contraindicated in patients with bleeding disorders or thrombocytopenia, but one study done in dogs did not show any changes on platelet aggregation (Roiz Martin *et al.* 2009).

The safety of firocoxib in horses less than one year old has not been established.

A chronic dosing (5 mg/kg for 6 months) study performed in puppies 10–13 weeks old, showed subclinical periportal hepatic fatty changes in half the dogs studied. Higher doses (15–25 mg/kg; 3–5X) in this age range caused increased rates of hepatic fatty changes; some dogs died or were euthanized due to moribund conditions. The manufacturer states in the package insert: "Use of this product at doses above the recommended 5 mg/kg in puppies less than 7 months old has been associated with serious adverse reactions, including death" and ". . . this product cannot be accurately dosed in dogs weighing less than seven pounds in body weight." The labeling in the UK states that it should not be used in dogs "less than 10 weeks of age."

If changing from one NSAID to another in dogs for reasons of efficacy, consider a washout period between agents. While the actual length of time between agents is controversial and opinions vary widely, often a 24-hour washout period between COX-2 selective agents is recommended. Recommendations for washout periods before starting a COX-2 selective agent after using a non-selective agent or aspirin are usually much longer (72 hours–1 week).

Adverse Effects

Because firocoxib is a relatively new product, its adverse effect profile in dogs is yet to be fully determined. In pre-approval studies (128 dogs treated), vomiting and decreased appetite/anorexia were the most common adverse effects noted with an approximate incidence rate of 4% and 2%, respectively. The drug sponsor has a toll-free overdose hotline in the USA: 877-217-3543.

In the FDA's CVM Cumulative Adverse Drug Experiences (ADE) Summaries Report (through 12/06/2006) for firocoxib in dogs, the most prevalent ADE reported was vomiting. On the list of 10 most reported ADE's for firocoxib, the second most reported event was anorexia. Other effects on this list included: diarrhea, increases in BUN, creatinine, alkaline phosphatase and ALT, depression/lethargy, and ataxia. Melena, GI ulcers, bloody vomiting and GI perforation were included within the 25 most reported events listed. It should be noted that this data reflects voluntary reporting to the FDA and does not reflect actual incidence rates, nor is causation necessarily proven.

In pre-approval studies done in horses treated for 14 days, diarrhea/loose stools were seen in about 2%. Excitation was rarely (<1%) detected. In safety studies, oral lesions/ulcers were seen in some horses after dosages of 1–5X were given.

Reproductive/Nursing Safety

Information on the safety of firocoxib in breeding, pregnant or lactating dogs or horses is not available. Studies performed in pregnant rabbits at dosages approximating those given to dogs, demonstrated maternotoxic and fetotoxic effects.

Overdosage/Acute Toxicity

Limited information is available for acute overdoses in animals. The reported oral LD50 for rats is > 2 grams per kg. Should an overdose occur, contacting an animal poison control center or the manufacturer (1-877-217-3543) is highly recommended. Use of gut emptying protocols and supportive treatment (IV fluids, oral sucralfate, etc.) may be useful in managing the case.

Drug Interactions

In the package insert for *Previcox*, the manufacturer states the following (**Note: bold** mine—Plumb): "As a class, cyclooxygenase inhibitory NSAIDs may be associated with renal and gastrointestinal toxicity. Sensitivity to drug-associated adverse events varies with the individual patient. Patients at greatest risk for renal toxicity are those that are dehydrated, on concomitant **diuretic therapy**, or those with existing renal, cardiovascular, and/or hepatic dysfunction. Concurrent administration of **potentially nephrotoxic drugs** should be carefully approached. NSAIDs may inhibit the prostaglandins that maintain normal homeostatic function. Such antiprostaglandin effects may result in clinically significant disease in patients with underlying or pre-existing disease that has not been previously diagnosed. Since many NSAIDs possess the potential to produce gastrointestinal ulcerations, concomitant use with other antiinflammatory drugs, such as **NSAIDs** or **corticosteroids**, should be avoided or closely monitored. The concomitant use of **protein bound drugs** with *Previcox*® Chewable Tablets has not been studied in dogs. Commonly used **protein-bound drugs** include cardiac, anticonvulsant, and behavioral medications. The influence of concomitant drugs that may inhibit the metabolism of *Previcox®* Chewable Tablets has not been evaluated."

Drug interactions reported in humans taking NSAIDS, that may be of significance in veterinary patients receiving firocoxib include:

■ **ACE INHIBITORS (e.g., enalapril, benazepril):** Some NSAIDs can reduce effects on blood pressure

■ **ASPIRIN:** May increase the risk of gastrointestinal toxicity (*e.g.*, ulceration, bleeding, vomiting, diarrhea)

■ **CORTICOSTEROIDS (e.g., prednisone):** May increase the risk of gastrointestinal toxicity (*e.g.*, ulceration, bleeding, vomiting, diarrhea)

■ **DIGOXIN:** NSAIDS may increase serum levels

■ **FLUCONAZOLE:** Administration has increased plasma levels of celecoxib in humans and potentially could also affect firocoxib levels in dogs

■ **FUROSEMIDE:** NSAIDs may reduce the saluretic and diuretic effects

■ **HIGHLY PROTEIN BOUND DRUGS (phenytoin, valproic acid, oral anticoagulants, other antiinflammatory agents, salicylates, sulfonamides, sulfonylurea antidiabetic agents):** As firocoxib is highly bound to plasma proteins (95–98%), it may displace other highly bound drugs or these agents could displace firocoxib. Increased serum levels, duration of actions and toxicity could occur.

■ **METHOTREXATE:** Serious toxicity has occurred when NSAIDs have been used concomitantly with **methotrexate**; use together with extreme caution

■ **NEPHROTOXIC DRUGS (e.g., furosemide, aminoglycosides, amphotericin B, etc.):** May enhance the risk of nephrotoxicity development

Laboratory Considerations
■ No specific laboratory concerns; see Monitoring

Doses

■ **DOGS:**
For the control of pain and inflammation associated with osteoarthritis (labeled indication):

a) 5 mg/kg (2.27 mg/lb) PO once daily. Dosage should be calculated in half tablet increments and can be administered with or without food. (Package insert; *Previcox®*—Merial)

■ **CATS:**
Caution: While firocoxib may ultimately be shown to be safe for use in cats, supporting information (or FDA approval) is not currently available for it to be recommended.

■ **HORSES:**
For the control of pain and inflammation associated with osteoarthritis (labeled indication):

a) 0.1 mg/kg (0.045 mg/lb) body weight PO daily for up to 14 days (Package insert; *Equioxx®*—Merial)

Monitoring
■ Baseline and periodic physical exam including clinical efficacy and adverse effect queries

■ Baseline and periodic: CBC, liver function, renal function, and electrolytes; urinalysis

Client Information
■ The manufacturer provides a client handout that is recommended to be distributed each time the drug is dispensed

■ May be administered with or without food

■ Contact veterinarian if any of the following occur in dogs: vomiting, decreased appetite/weight loss, diarrhea or loose stools, changes in behavior or activity, changes in water consumption or urination, or yellowing of whites of eyes or mucous membranes

■ For horses, contact veterinarian if patient develops ulcers or sores on tongue or in mouth, sores or lesions on facial skin or lips, diarrhea/loose stools, changes in behavior/activity, changes in feed or water consumption, or yellowing of whites of eyes or mucous membranes

Chemistry/Synonyms
Firocoxib occurs a white crystalline powder.

Firocoxib may also be known as: 3-(cyclopropylmethoxy)-5,5-dimethyl-4-(4-methylsulfonyl) phenylfuran-2(5H)-on or ML-1,785,713, *Equioxx®*, and *Previcox®*.

Storage/Stability
Commercially available tablets and oral paste should be stored at room temperature (15–30°C); brief excursions are permitted up to 40°C (104°F).

Dosage Forms/Regulatory Status
VETERINARY-LABELED PRODUCTS:

Firocoxib Chewable Tablets (scored): 57 mg, & 227 mg; *Previcox®* (Merial); (Rx). FDA-approved for use in dogs.

Firocoxib Oral Paste: 0.82% w/w (8.2 mg firocoxib per gram of paste) in a 6.93 gram oral syringe (total of 56.8 mg of firocoxib per syringe); *Equioxx®* (Merial); (Rx).

HUMAN-LABELED PRODUCTS: None

References
McCann, M., E. Rickes, et al. (2005). In vitro effects and in vivo efficacy of a novel cyclooxygenase-2 inhibitor in cats with lipopolysaccharide-induced pyrexia. *AJVR* 66(7): 1278–1284.

Roiz Martin, S., L. Palacio Garcia, et al. (2009). Evaluation of the Effects of Firocoxib on Platelet Function of Healthy Dogs Studied By PFA-100. Proceedings: ECVIM. Accessed via: Veterinary Information Network. http://goo.gl/UBcpL

Fish Oil—See Fatty Acids

FLAVOXATE HCL

(fla-**vox**-ate) Urispas®

PARASYMPATHETIC BLOCKER; URINARY ANTISPASMODIC

Prescriber Highlights

▶ Alternative medication to treat with detrusor hyperspasticity (hyperactive bladder; urge incontinence) in dogs

▶ Not commonly used; little information available on veterinary use

▶ Most likely adverse effect is weakness

Uses/Indications

Flavoxate may be considered for treating dogs with detrusor hyperspasticity (hyperactive bladder, urge incontinence). Flavoxate, propantheline or oxybutynin can be particularly useful in dogs where phenylpropanolamine alone has not resulted in continence.

Pharmacology/Actions

Flavoxate has direct smooth muscle relaxing properties and antimuscarinic effects.

Pharmacokinetics

No information was located for dogs or cats. In humans, the drug's onset of action is within an hour with peak effects at around 2 hours post dose. 57% of a dose is excreted in the urine within 24 hours.

Contraindications/Precautions/Warnings

Flavoxate is contraindicated in human patients with pyloric or duodenal obstruction, obstructive intestinal lesions or ileus, achalasia, GI hemorrhage or obstructive uropathies of the lower urinary tract. It is to be given with caution in patients with suspected glaucoma.

Adverse Effects

Weakness is the most likely adverse effect seen in dogs treated with flavoxate.

Reproductive/Nursing Safety

In laboratory animals, doses of up to 34X (human dose) demonstrated no harm to fetuses or impaired fertility. In humans, flavoxate is designated by the FDA as a category *B* drug (*Animal studies have not demonstrated risk to the fetus, but there are no adequate studies in pregnant women; or animal studies have shown an adverse effect, but adequate studies in pregnant women have not demonstrated a risk to the fetus during the first trimester of pregnancy, and there is no evidence of risk in later trimesters.*)

It is not known whether this drug is excreted into milk. Use with caution in nursing mothers.

Overdosage/Acute Toxicity

The approximate oral LD-50 for rats and mice are 4300 mg/kg and 1800 mg/kg respectively.

Drug Interactions

■ No significant drug interactions with flavoxate were located; however, concomitant use with other **anticholinergic drugs** may cause additive effects.

Laboratory Considerations

■ No concerns noted

Doses

■ **DOGS:**
To decrease urinary bladder contractility:
a) 100–200 mg (per dog) PO q6–8h (Bartges 2006)

Monitoring

■ Clinical efficacy

■ Adverse effects (most likely GI)

■ Consider occasional CBC's and creatinine to monitor for neutropenia or renal dysfunction if using the drug chronically

Client Information

■ May cause weakness or changes in activity level in treated dogs; if these become a problem, contact veterinarian

Chemistry/Synonyms

Flavoxate HCl occurs as a white or almost white crystalline powder. It is slightly soluble in water or alcohol.

Flavoxate may also be known as flavoxato, AK 123, or Rec 7-0040. A common trade name is *Urispas®*.

Storage/Stability

Flavoxate tablets should be stored at room temperature (15–30°C).

Dosage Forms/Regulatory Status

VETERINARY-LABELED PRODUCTS: None

HUMAN-LABELED PRODUCTS:

Flavoxate HCl Oral Tablets (film-coated) 100 mg: *Urispas®* (Ortho-McNeil), generic (Global); (Rx)

References

Bartges, J. (2006). Broken plumbing: urinary incontinence. Proceedings: ACVC 2006. Accessed via: Veterinary Information Network. http://goo.gl/XgEUd

FLORFENICOL

(flor-**fen**-i-col)   NuFlor®
ANTIBIOTIC

Prescriber Highlights

▶ Broad spectrum antibiotic FDA-approved for use in cattle, swine, & fish, but may be useful in other species (e.g., dogs, cats)

▶ Contraindications: Do not give IV, to veal calves or cattle of breeding age (per manufacturer)

▶ Adverse Effects: Cattle: Anorexia, decreased water consumption, diarrhea, injection site reactions (may result in trim loss); IM injection may be painful in small animals

▶ Slaughter withdrawals depend upon route of administration (IM shorter than SC)

Uses/Indications

The drug is FDA-approved for use in cattle only (in the USA) for the treatment of bovine respiratory disease (BRD) associated with *Mannheimia haemolytica*, *Pasteurella multocida*, *Histophilus somni*, and *Mycoplasma bovis*.

Because florfenicol has activity against a wide range of microorganisms, it may be useful for treating other infections in cattle (or other species) as well, but specific data is limited.

The combination product containing florfenicol and flunixin (*Resflor Gold®*) is FDA-approved for SC use in beef and non-lactating dairy cattle (not veal calves) for treatment of BRD associated with *Mannheimia haemolytica, Pasteurella multocida, Histophilus somni, Mycoplasma bovis* and control BRD-associated pyrexia.

Pharmacology/Actions

Like chloramphenicol, florfenicol is a broad-spectrum antibiotic that has activity against many bacteria. It acts by binding to the 50S ribosome, thereby inhibiting bacterial protein synthesis.

Pharmacokinetics

After IM injection in cattle, approximately 79% of the dose is bioavailable. The drug appears to be well distributed throughout the body, including achievement of therapeutic levels in the CSF. In cattle, the volume of distribution is about 0.7 L/kg and only about 13% is bound to serum proteins. Mean serum half-life is 18 hours, but wide interpatient variation exists. When dosed at 40 mg/kg IM, serum levels are above the MIC_{90} (1 microgram/mL) for *M. haemolytica* for 72 hours and above MIC_{90} (0.5 micrograms/mL) for *P. multocida* and *H. somnus* for 96 hours.

In dogs, florfenicol is absorbed poorly after subcutaneous injection and has an elimination half-life of less than 5 hours. After IV administration, total body clearance is approximately 1 L/kg/hr. PO administration results in good bioavailability (95%), but the drug is eliminated rapidly (elimination half-life 1.25 hours) (Park *et al.* 2008).

Cats, however, have high absorption of a 100 mg/mL solution when either given IM or orally and have an elimination half-life of less than 5 hours. Times above an MIC of 2 mg/mL were 12 hours (IM) and 18 hours (PO); and an MIC of 8 mg/mL were 10 hours (IM) and 6 hours (PO), respectively, in cats.

Contraindications/Precautions/Warnings

Not for use in animals intended for breeding purposes. The effects of florfenicol on bovine reproductive performance, pregnancy, and lactation have not been determined. Also see the residue warnings (in Dosage Forms).

Caution: Do not give this drug IV.

Adverse Effects

Noted transient adverse reactions in cattle include anorexia, decreased water consumption, or diarrhea. Injection site reactions can occur that may result in trim loss. Reactions may be more severe if injected at sites other than the neck. Anaphylaxis and collapse have been reported in cattle.

When used in other species (mammals), gastrointestinal effects, including severe diarrheas are potentially possible.

Reproductive/Nursing Safety

Safety or effects when used in breeding cattle or swine, during pregnancy, or during lactation are unknown and the manufacturer states that the drug is not for use in cattle of breeding age or in swine intended for breeding.

Overdosage/Acute Toxicity

In toxicology studies where feeder calves were injected with up to 10X the recommended dosage, the adverse effects noted above were seen, plus increased serum enzymes. These effects were generally transient in nature. Long-term (43 day) standard dosage studies showed a transient decrease in feed consumption, but no long-term negative effects were noted.

Drug Interactions

No specific drug interactions for florfenicol were located, but the drug may behave similarly to chloramphenicol. If so, florfenicol could antagonize the bactericidal activity of the **penicillins** or **aminoglycosides**. This antagonism has not been demonstrated *in vivo*, and these drug combinations have been used successfully many times clinically. Other antibiotics that bind to the 50S ribosomal subunit of susceptible bacteria (**erythromycin, clindamycin, lincomycin, tylosin,** etc.) may potentially antagonize the activity of chloramphenicol or vice versa, but the clinical significance of this potential interaction has not been determined. For other drug interactions that florfenicol may share with chloramphenicol, see the monograph for chloramphenicol or refer to other drug information resources.

Doses

■ **CATTLE:**

a) For treatment of BRD: 20 mg/kg IM (in neck muscle only); repeat in 48 hours. Alternatively, a single 40 mg/kg SC dose (in neck) may be used. **Note:** 20 mg/kg equates to 3 mL of the injection per 100 lb. of body weight. Do not exceed 10 mL per injection site. (Package Insert; *Nuflor®* —Schering Plough)

b) For treatment of BRD: 40 mg/kg (6 mL/100 lb B.W.) administered once by subcutaneous injection. Do not administer more than 15 mL at each site. The injection should be given only in the neck. Injection sites other than the neck have not been evaluated. (Label Information; *Nuflor Gold®*—Intervet Schering)

c) Using the combination product containing florfenicol/flunixin (*Resflor Gold®*): 40 mg/kg florfenicol/2.2 mg/kg flunixin (6 mL/100 lb. B.W.) SC once. Do not administer more than 10 mL at each site. The injection should be given only in the neck. Injection sites other than the neck have not been evaluated. (Label Information—*Resflor Gold®*; Intervet Schering)

■ **DOGS:**

a) For susceptible systemic (bacterial or rickettsial) infections when myelotoxic potential (in humans or animals) of chloramphenicol is to be avoided: 20 mg/kg IM q8h for 3–5 days. (Greene *et al.* 2006)

■ **CATS:**

a) For susceptible systemic infections (bacterial or rickettsial) infections when myelotoxic potential (in humans or animals) of chloramphenicol is to be avoided: 22 mg/kg IM, PO q12h for 3–5 days (**Note:** Oral dosage form not available, but solution given orally to experimental cats was well absorbed) (Greene *et al.* 2006)

■ **SHEEP & GOATS:**

a) For respiratory disease complex in kids: 20 mg/kg a day (route not specified; assume IM) for 2 days (de la Concha 2002)

■ **SWINE:**

a) For swine respiratory disease: In water at a concentration of 400 mg/gallon (100 ppm). Use as only source of drinking water for 5 days. For bulk tank add one gallon concentrate to 128 gallons of water; for proportioner set to 1:128 (0.8%). (Label information; *NuFlor® Concentrate Solution*—Schering-Plough)

Monitoring

■ Clinical efficacy

■ Injection site reactions

Client Information

■ Residue Warnings: When administered as labeled, cattle slaughter withdrawal is 28 days post injection if using the IM route; 38 days after the SC route. Swine (in drinking water) = 16 days.

■ Not to be used in female dairy cattle 20 months of age or older.

■ A withdrawal period has not been established in preruminating calves. Do not use in calves to be processed for veal.

■ Do not give IV.

Chemistry/Synonyms

A fluorinated analog of thiamphenicol, florfenicol is commercially available as light yellow to straw-colored injectable solution also containing n-ethyl-2-pyrrolidone, propylene glycol, and polyethylene glycol. The commercially available products range from a bright yellow to straw color. Color does not affect potency.

Florfenicol may also be known as Sch-25298 and *NuFlor®*.

Storage/Stability

Florfenicol injection (*Nuflor®*, *Nuflor Gold®*) should be stored between 2°–30°C (36°–86°F). Use within 28 days of first use.

The oral solution (swine) should be stored between 2°–26°C (36°–77°F).

The combination product with flunixin (*Resflor Gold®*) should not be stored above 30°C (86°F) and used within 28 days. The 500 mL vial should not be punctured more than 10 times.

Dosage Forms/Regulatory Status/ Withdrawal Times

VETERINARY-LABELED PRODUCTS:

Florfenicol Injection: 300 mg/mL in 100 mL, 250 mL and 500 mL multi-dose vials; *NuFlor®* (Intervet Schering); (Rx). FDA-approved for use in cattle; see residue warnings above. Slaughter withdrawal (at labeled dosages) = 28 days (IM treatment), 38 days (subcutaneous treatment). Do not use in female dairy cattle 20 months of age or older. A withdrawal period has not been established in preruminating calves. Do not use in calves to be processed for veal.

Florfenicol Injection: 300 mg/mL (also contains 300 mg of 2-pyrrolidone, and triacetin) in 100 mL, 250 mL, & 500 mL vials; *Nuflor Gold®* (Intervet Schering); (Rx). FDA-approved for use in beef and non-lactating dairy cattle. Do not slaughter within 44 days of last treatment. Do not use in female dairy cattle 20 months of age or older. Use may cause milk residues. A withdrawal period has not been established in preruminating calves.

Florfenicol 2.3% (23 mg/mL) Concentrate Solution in 2.2 btls; *NuFlor® Concentrate Solution* (Schering-Plough); (Rx). FDA-approved for use in swine; Slaughter withdrawal (at labeled dosages) = 16 days.

There are florfenicol products for addition to catfish or salmonid feeds (*Aquaflor®*) and to feed for swine.

Florfenicol 300 mg/mL with Flunixin 16.5 mg/mL Injection in 100 mL, 250 mL and 500 mL vials; *Resflor Gold®* (Intervet Schering); (Rx). FDA-approved for use in beef and non-lactating dairy cattle. Do not slaughter within 38 days of last treatment. Not for use in female dairy cattle 20 months of age or older or in calves to be processed for veal. Use may cause milk residues. A withdrawal period has not been established in preruminating calves.

HUMAN-LABELED PRODUCTS: None

References

de la Concha, A. (2002). Diseases of kids. Proceedings: Western Veterinary Conference. Accessed via: Veterinary Information Network. http://goo.gl/t2w7e

Greene, C., K. Hartmannn, et al. (2006). Appendix 8: Antimicrobial Drug Formulary. *Infectious Disease of the Dog and Cat.* C Greene Ed., Elsevier: 1186–1333.

Park, B.K., J.H. Lim, et al. (2008). Pharmacokinetics of florfenicol and its metabolite, florfenicol amine, in dogs. *Research in Veterinary Science* **84**(1): 85–89.

FLUCONAZOLE

(floo-**kon**-a-zole)   Diflucan®

ANTIFUNGAL

Prescriber Highlights

▶ Oral or parenteral antifungal particularly useful for CNS infections

▶ Caution: Renal failure (dosage adjustment needed), pregnancy (safety not established), hepatic failure

▶ Adverse Effects: Occasional GI effects (inappetence) in cats or dogs; in humans: headache &, rarely, increased liver enzymes & hepatic toxicity

▶ Expensive, but price is decreasing now that it is available as a generic

▶ Drug Interactions

Uses/Indications

Fluconazole may have use in veterinary medicine in the treatment of systemic mycoses, including cryptococcal meningitis, blastomycosis, and histoplasmosis. It may also be useful for superficial candidiasis or dermatophytosis. Because of the drug's unique pharmacokinetic qualities, it is probably more useful in treating CNS infections or fungal urinary tract infections than other azole derivatives. Fluconazole does not have appreciable effects (unlike ketoconazole) on hormone synthesis and may have fewer side effects than ketoconazole in small animals.

Pharmacology/Actions

Fluconazole is a fungistatic triazole compound. Triazole-derivative agents, like the imidazoles (clotrimazole, ketoconazole, etc.), presumably act by altering the cellular membranes of susceptible fungi, thereby increasing membrane permeability and allowing leakage of cellular contents and impaired uptake of purine and pyrimidine precursors. Fluconazole has efficacy against a variety of pathogenic fungi including yeasts and dermatophytes. *In vivo* studies using laboratory models have shown that fluconazole has fungistatic activity against some strains of Candida, Cryptococcus, Histoplasma, and Blastomyces. *In vivo* studies of efficacy against Aspergillus strains have been conflicting.

Pharmacokinetics

Fluconazole is rapidly and nearly completely absorbed (90%) after oral administration. Gastric pH or the presence of food, do not appreciably alter fluconazole's oral bioavailability. It has low protein binding and is widely distributed throughout the body and penetrates well into the CSF, eye, and peritoneal fluid. Fluconazole is eliminated primarily via the kidneys and achieves high concentrations in the urine. In humans, fluconazole's serum half-life is about 30 hours in patients with normal renal function. Because of it's long half-life, fluconazole does not reach steady state plasma levels for 6–14 days after beginning therapy, unless loading doses are given. Patients with impaired renal function may have half-lives extended significantly and dosage adjustment may be required.

Contraindications/Precautions/Warnings

Fluconazole should not be used in patients hypersensitive to it or other azole antifungal agents. In patients with hepatic impairment it should be used only when the potential benefits outweigh the risks. Because fluconazole is eliminated primarily by the kidneys, fluconazole doses or dosing intervals may need to be adjusted in patients with renal impairment.

Fluconazole is reportedly toxic to budgerigars.

Adverse Effects

There is limited experience with this drug in domestic animals. Thus far, it appears to be safe to use in dogs and cats. Occasionally, inappetence, vomiting, or diarrhea may be reported. Hepatotoxicity is possible.

In humans, the side effects have been generally limited to occasional GI effects (vomiting, diarrhea, anorexia/nausea) and headache. Rarely, increased liver enzymes and hepatic toxicity, exfoliative skin disorders, and thrombocytopenia have been reported in humans. Thrombocytopenia has not been reported thus far in animals.

Reproductive/Nursing Safety

Safety during pregnancy has not been established and it is not recommended for use in pregnant animals unless the benefits outweigh the risks. In humans, the FDA categorizes this drug as category *C* for use during pregnancy (*Animal studies have shown an adverse effect on the fetus, but there are no adequate studies in humans; or there are no animal reproduction studies and no adequate studies in humans.*)

Fluconazole is excreted in milk at concentrations similar to plasma. Use with caution in nursing dams.

Overdosage/Acute Toxicity

There is very limited information on the acute toxicity of fluconazole. Rats and mice survived doses of 1 g/kg, but died within several days after receiving 1–2 g/kg. Rats and mice receiving very high dosages demonstrated respiratory depression, salivation, lacrimation, urinary incontinence, and cyanosis. If a massive overdose occurs, consider gut emptying and give supportive therapy as required. Fluconazole may be removed by hemodialysis or peritoneal dialysis.

Drug Interactions

The following drug interactions have either been reported or are theoretical in humans or animals receiving fluconazole and may be of significance in veterinary patients:

■ **AMPHOTERICIN B:** Lab animal studies have shown that fluconazole used concomitantly with amphotericin B may be antagonistic against Aspergillus or Candida; the clinical importance of these findings is not yet clear

■ **BUSPIRONE:** Plasma concentrations may be elevated

■ **CISAPRIDE:** Fluconazole may increase cisapride levels and the possibility for toxicity

■ **CORTICOSTEROIDS:** Fluconazole may inhibit the metabolism of corticosteroid; potential for increased adverse effects

■ **CYCLOPHOSPHAMIDE:** Fluconazole may inhibit the metabolism of cyclophosphamide and its metabolites; potential for increased toxicity

■ **CYCLOSPORINE:** Fluconazole increases cyclosporine levels. In normal dogs, fluconazole at 5 mg/kg once daily decreased cyclosporine dosages by 29%-51% to achieve similar therapeutic trough levels. In renal transplant dogs (also on mycophenolate), fluconazole decreased cyclosporine dose requirements 33% on average (Katayama *et al.* 2010).

■ **DIURETICS, THIAZIDES:** Increased fluconazole concentrations

■ **FENTANYL/ALFENTANIL:** Fluconazole may increase fentanyl levels

■ **MIDAZOLAM:** Increased midazolam levels and effects

■ **NSAIDS:** Fluconazole may increase plasma levels; increased risk for adverse effects

■ **QUINIDINE:** Increased risk for cardiotoxicity

■ **RIFAMPIN:** May decrease fluconazole efficacy; fluconazole may increase rifampin levels

■ **THEOPHYLLINE/AMINOPHYLLINE:** Increased theophylline concentrations

■ **TRICYCLIC ANTIDEPRESSANTS (clomipramine, amitriptyline, etc.):** Fluconazole may exacerbate the effects of tricyclic antidepressants

■ **SULFONYLUREA ANTIDIABETIC AGENTS (e.g., glipizide, glyburide):** Fluconazole may increase levels; hypoglycemia possible

■ **VINCRISTINE/VINBLASTINE:** Fluconazole may inhibit vinca alkaloid metabolism

■ **WARFARIN:** Fluconazole may cause increased prothrombin times in patients receiving warfarin or other coumarin anticoagulants

Doses

■ **DOGS:**

a) General dosing guidelines: Give twice calculated daily dose for the first day of treatment; give for 2–3 days if rapidly advancing or severe disseminated mycosis. Give IV solution over 1–2 hours.

For cryptococcosis, candidiasis, systemic mycoses, nasal aspergillosis: 2.5–5 mg/kg PO or IV q12–24h for 56–84 days. Often treat neurologic ocular cryptococcosis for at least 12 weeks or 2 weeks after CSF exam shows resolution of inflammation and antigen test results on serum and CSF are negative.

For fungal meningitis: 5–8 mg/kg PO or IV q12h OR 8–12 mg/kg PO or IV once daily (q24h) for 56–84 days;

For urinary candidiasis: 5–10 mg/kg PO q24h for 21–42 days;

For urinary *Candida glabrata* infection: 12 mg/kg PO once daily for 21–42 days. (Greene *et al.* 2006)

b) For cryptococcosis: 5 mg/kg PO once or twice daily. Treatment should continue for at least 2 months beyond resolution of clinical signs. (Taboada 2000)

c) For blastomycosis: 5 mg/kg PO q12h for 60 days

For cryptococcosis: 5–15 mg/kg PO q12–24h for 6–10 months (Lemarie 2003)

d) For treatment of *Malassezia* (may be safer than itraconazole or ketoconazole in dogs with hepatic disease): 5 mg/kg PO once daily. (Thomas 2005)

e) For systemic treatment of *Malassezia* dermatitis: 5 mg/kg PO once daily; for recurrent *Malassezia* dermatitis: 5 mg/kg PO 3 times per week. (Ihrke 2008)

f) For systemic treatment of *Malassezia* dermatitis: 2–5 mg/kg PO once daily (q24h). (Beale & Murphy 2006)

g) As an alternative to itraconazole or terbinafine for nasal aspergillosis (with topical agents when the cribriform plate is penetrated): 2.5–5 mg/kg PO q12h for 3-6 months. Cure rates up to 60%. (Kuehn 2010)

■ **CATS:**

a) General dosing guidelines: Give twice calculated daily dose for the first day of treatment; give for 2–3 days if rapidly advancing or severe disseminated mycosis. For cryptococcosis or other systemic infections, treatment should continue until antigen testing results of blood or CSF are negative, this is usually at least 2 months beyond clinical resolution (mean time of 8 months treatment).

For nasal or dermal cryptococcosis: 5–10 mg/kg PO q12–24h, or 10 mg/kg PO q24h; for most infections, 50 mg/cat PO once daily achieves adequate therapeutic levels.

For CNS, intraocular, or multisystemic cryptococcosis: 50–100 mg/cat PO or IV q12h. Often treat neurologic ocular cryptococcosis for at least 12 weeks or 2 weeks after CSF exam shows resolution of inflammation and antigen test results on serum and CSF are negative.

For CNS, intraocular, or multisystemic mycoses: 50 mg/cat PO once daily (q24h); (Greene *et al.* 2006)

b) For cryptococcosis: 50 mg (total dose) PO twice daily. Treatment should continue for 1 month beyond resolution of clinical signs. (Legendre 1995)

c) For cryptococcosis: 50 mg (total dose) PO twice daily. Treatment should continue for at least 2 months beyond resolution of clinical signs. (Taboada 2000)

■ **HORSES:**

a) For *C. immitis* infection or *Candida* bacteremia: Loading dose of 14 mg/kg followed by 5 mg/kg PO once daily. Anecdotal reports of successful treatment of fungal keratitis using 1 mg/kg PO q24h. (Stewart *et al.* 2008)

■ **RABBITS/RODENTS/SMALL MAMMALS:**

a) **Rabbits:** 25–43 mg/kg slow IV q12h (Ivey & Morrisey 2000)

■ **BIRDS:**

a) For treating candidiasis: A report where fluconazole pharmacokinetics were determined in Goffin's cockatoos, Timneh African grey parrots, and orange-winged Amazon parrots showed that fluconazole dosed at 20 mg/kg PO q24-48h or 10 mg/kg PO q24h would likely be effective for treating *C. albicans*. *C. galabrata*

and *C. papasilosis* may have MIC's greater than this dose could effectively treat. (Flammer 2008)

b) For treating candidiasis in cockatiels: In this report, both a 10 mg/kg fluconazole PO suspension and 100 mg/mL fluconazole treated drinking water maintained plasma levels above the MIC for most strains of *Candida albicans*. (Ratzlaff & Flammer 2009)

c) As an alternate treatment of aspergillosis: 5–10 mg/kg PO once daily for up to 6 weeks, with or after amphotericin B. (Oglesbee & Bishop 1994)

Monitoring
■ Clinical Efficacy
■ With long-term therapy, occasional liver function tests are recommended

Client Information
■ Cost of this drug may be an issue. Fluconazole therapy may be prolonged (several weeks to months) and an average dosage in a cat (50 mg twice a day) may be very expensive
■ Compliance with treatment recommendations must be stressed.
■ Have clients report any potential adverse effects.

Chemistry/Synonyms
A synthetic triazole antifungal agent, fluconazole occurs as a white crystalline powder. It is slightly soluble (8 mg/mL) in water.

Fluconazole may also be known as UK-49858; many trade names are available.

Storage/Stability
Fluconazole tablets should be stored at temperatures less than 30°C in tight containers. Fluconazole injection should be stored at temperatures from 5–30°C (5–25°C for the *Viaflex®* bags); avoid freezing. Do not add additives to the injection.

Dosage Forms/Regulatory Status
VETERINARY-LABELED PRODUCTS: None
HUMAN-LABELED PRODUCTS:
Fluconazole Oral Tablets: 50 mg, 100 mg, 150 mg, & 200 mg; *Diflucan®* (Pfizer); generic; (Rx)

Fluconazole Powder for Oral Suspension: 10 mg/mL & 40 mg/mL (when reconstituted) in 35 mL; *Diflucan®* (Pfizer); generic; (Rx)

Fluconazole Injection: 2 mg/mL in 100 mL or 200 mL bottles or *Viaflex Plus* (available with sodium chloride or dextrose diluents); *Diflucan®* (Pfizer); generic; (Rx)

References
Beale, K. & M. Murphy (2006). Selecting appropriate antimicrobial therapy for infections of the skin of the dog. Proceedings: Western Vet Conf. Accessed via: Veterinary Information Network. http://goo.gl/jHBLR
Flammer, K. (2008). Avian Mycoses: Managing those difficult cases. Proceedings: AAV. Accessed via: Veterinary Information Network. http://goo.gl/iDsnR

Greene, C., K. Hartmannn, et al. (2006). Appendix 8: Antimicrobial Drug Formulary. *Infectious Disease of the Dog and Cat.* C Greene Ed., Elsevier: 1186–1333.

Ihrke, P. (2008). Malassezia dermatitis: Diagnosis and management. Proceedings: WSAVA. Accessed via: Veterinary Information Network. http://goo.gl/F13JR

Ivey, E. & J. Morrisey (2000). Therapeutics for Rabbits. *Vet Clin NA: Exotic Anim Pract* 3:1(Jan): 183–216.

Katayama, M., H. Igarashi, et al. (2010). Fluconazole decreases cyclosporine dosage in renal transplanted dogs. *Research in Veterinary Science* 89(1): 124–125.

Kuehn, N. (2010). Chronic Nasal Disease in Dogs: Diagnosis & Treatment. Proceedings: ACVIM. Accessed via: Veterinary Information Network. http://goo.gl/2OQgm

Legendre, A. (1995). Antimycotic Drug Therapy. *Kirk's Current Veterinary Therapy:XII.* J Bonagura Ed. Philadelphia, W.B. Saunders: 327–331.

Lemarie, S. (2003). Fungal dermatopathies. Proceedings: Western Veterinary Conference. Accessed via: Veterinary Information Network. http://goo.gl/e5Zb6

Oglesbee, B. & C. Bishop (1994). Avian Infectious Diseases. *Saunders Manual of Small Animal Practice.* S Birchard and R Sherding Eds. Philadelphia, W.B. Saunders Company: 1257–1270.

Ratzlaff, K. & K. Flammer (2009). Fluconazole in cockatiels. Proceedings: AAV. Accessed via: Veterinary Information Network. http://goo.gl/witAd

Stewart, A., E. Welles, et al. (2008). Pulmonary and systemic fungal infections. *Compendium Equine*(June): 260–272.

Taboada, J. (2000). Systemic Mycoses. *Textbook of Veterinary Internal Medicine: Diseases of the Dog and Cat.* S Ettinger and E Feldman Eds. Philadelphia, WB Saunders. 1: 453–476.

Thomas, R. (2005). Malassezia dermatitis in the dog. Proceedings: WVC2005. Accessed via: Veterinary Information Network. http://goo.gl/okHO0

FLUCYTOSINE

(floo-sye-toe-seen)   Ancobon®

ANTIFUNGAL

Prescriber Highlights

▶ Infrequently used antifungal used in combination with other drugs (to reduce resistance development)

▶ Extreme Caution: Renal impairment, preexisting bone marrow depression, hematologic diseases, or receiving other bone marrow suppressant drugs

▶ Caution: Hepatic disease

▶ Adverse Effects: Most common: GI disturbances; Potentially: dose dependent bone marrow depression, cutaneous eruption & rash primarily seen on the scrotum & nasal planum (in dogs), oral ulceration, increased hepatic enzymes, CNS effects in cats

▶ Dogs may not tolerate therapy for more than 10–14 days

▶ Teratogenic in rats

Uses/Indications

Flucytosine is principally active against strains of Cryptococcus and Candida. When used alone, resistance can develop quite rapidly to flucytosine, particularly with Cryptococcus.

Because it penetrates relatively well into the CNS, it has been used in combination for the treatment of CNS cryptococcosis. Some cases of subcutaneous and systemic chromoblastosis may also respond to flucytosine. The drug can have synergistic efficacy when used with amphotericin B. Clinically, it is used primarily with amphotericin B in the treatment of cryptococcosis.

Pharmacology/Actions

Flucytosine penetrates fungal cells where it is deaminated by cytosine deaminase to fluorouracil. Fluorouracil acts as an antimetabolite by competing with uracil, thereby interfering with pyrimidine metabolism and eventually RNA and protein synthesis. It is thought that flucytosine is converted to fluorodeoxyuredylic acid that inhibits thymidylate synthesis and ultimately DNA synthesis.

In human cells, cytosine deaminase is apparently not present or only has minimal activity. Rats apparently metabolize some of the drug to fluorouracil, which may explain the teratogenic effects seen in this species. It is unclear how much cytosine deaminase activity dog and cat cells possess.

Pharmacokinetics

Flucytosine is well absorbed after oral administration. The rate, but not extent, of absorption will be decreased if given with food.

Flucytosine is distributed widely throughout the body. CSF concentrations may be 60−100% of those found in the serum. In healthy humans, the volume of distribution is about 0.7 L/kg. Only about 2−4% of the drug is bound to plasma proteins. It is unknown if flucytosine is distributed into milk.

Absorbed flucytosine is excreted basically unchanged in the urine via glomerular filtration. In humans, the half-life is about 3−6 hours in patients with normal renal function, but may be significantly prolonged in patients with renal dysfunction.

Contraindications/Precautions/Warnings

Flucytosine is contraindicated in patients hypersensitive to it.

Flucytosine should be used with extreme caution in patients with renal impairment. Some clinicians recommend monitoring serum flucytosine levels in these patients and adjusting dosage (or dosing interval) to maintain serum levels at less than 100 micrograms/mL. One clinician (Macy, 1987) recommends dividing the flucytosine dose by the serum creatinine level if azotemia develops.

Use flucytosine with extreme caution in patients with preexisting bone marrow depression, hematologic diseases, or receiving other bone marrow suppressant drugs. Flucytosine should also be used cautiously (with enhanced monitoring) in patients with hepatic disease.

Adverse Effects

Most common adverse effects seen with flucytosine are GI disturbances (nausea, vomiting, diarrhea). Other potential adverse effects include a dose dependent bone marrow depression (anemia, leukopenia, thrombocytopenia), cutaneous eruption and rash primarily seen on the scrotum and nasal planum (occurring in dogs), oral ulceration and increased levels of hepatic enzymes. Dogs receiving flucytosine often develop a severe drug reaction within 10–14 days of treatment.

Reports of aberrant behavior and seizures in a cat without concurrent CNS infection have been noted after flucytosine use. There are anecdotal reports of toxic epidermal necrolysis occurring in cats treated with flucytosine.

Reproduction/Nursing Safety

Flucytosine has caused teratogenic effects in rats. It should be used in pregnant animals only when the benefits of therapy outweigh the risks. In humans, the FDA categorizes this drug as category *C* for use during pregnancy (*Animal studies have shown an adverse effect on the fetus, but there are no adequate studies in humans; or there are no animal reproduction studies and no adequate studies in humans.*)

It is not known whether this drug is excreted in milk. Because there are potential serious adverse reactions in nursing offspring, consider using milk replacer.

Overdosage/Acute Toxicity

No specifics regarding flucytosine overdosage were located. It is suggested that a substantial overdose be handled with gut emptying, charcoal and cathartic administration unless contraindicated.

Drug Interactions

The following drug interactions have either been reported or are theoretical in humans or animals receiving flucytosine and may be of significance in veterinary patients:

■ **AMPHOTERICIN B:** When used with amphotericin B, synergism against Cryptococcus and Candida has been demonstrated *in vitro*. However, if amphotericin B induces renal dysfunction, toxicity of flucytosine may be enhanced if it accumulates. Should clinically significant renal toxicity develop, flucytosine dosage may need to be adjusted.

Laboratory Considerations

■ When determining **serum creatinine** using the **Ektachem®** analyzer, false elevations in levels may be noted if patients are also taking flucytosine.

Doses

■ **DOGS:**

For cryptococcosis:

a) 50–75 mg/kg PO q8h; treatment requires 1–12 months. Must be given with a poly-

ene or azole antifungal agent. (Malik *et al.* 2006)

For candidiasis:

a) 25–50 mg/kg PO q6h or 50–65 mg/kg PO q8h for 42 days. Must be given with a polyene or azole antifungal agent. (Greene & Watson 1998)

■ **CATS:**

For cryptococcosis:

a) Flucytosine at 30 mg/kg PO q6h or 50 mg/kg PO q8h or 75 mg/kg PO q12h). Cats 3.5 kg or greater should receive 250 mg (total) q6–8h. Must be given with a polyene (amphotericin B) or azole antifungal agent. Treatment requires 1–9 months. (Malik *et al.* 2006)

For candidiasis:

a) 25–50 mg/kg PO q6h or 50–65 mg/kg PO q8h for 42 days. Must be given with a polyene or azole antifungal agent (Greene & Watson 1998)

■ **BIRDS:**

For susceptible fungal infections:

a) In Psittacines: 250 mg/kg twice daily as a gavage. May be used for extended periods of time for aspergillosis. May cause bone marrow toxicity; periodic hematologic assessment is recommended.

In raptors: 18–30 mg/kg q6h as a gavage

In Psittacines and Mynahs: 100–250 mg/lb in feed for flock treatment of severe aspergillosis or Candida (especially respiratory Candida). Apply to favorite food mix or mixed with mash. (Clubb 1986)

b) Ratites: 80–100 mg/kg PO twice daily (Jenson 1998)

Monitoring

■ Renal function (at least twice weekly if also receiving amphotericin B)

■ CBC with platelets

■ Hepatic enzymes at least monthly

Client Information

■ Clients should report any clinical signs associated with hematologic toxicity (abnormal bleeding, bruising, etc.).

■ Prolonged treatment times, as well as costs of medication and associated monitoring, require substantial client commitment.

Chemistry/Synonyms

A fluorinated pyrimidine antifungal agent, flucytosine occurs as a white to off-white, crystalline powder that is odorless or has a slight odor with pK_as of 2.9 and 10.71. It is sparingly soluble in water and slightly soluble in alcohol.

Flucytosine may also be known as: 5-FC, 5-fluorocytosine, flucytosinum, Ro-2-9915, *Alcobon®*, and *Ancotil®*.

Storage/Stability

Store flucytosine capsules in tight, light-resistant containers at temperatures less than 40°C, and preferably at room temperature (15–30°C). The commercially available capsules are assigned an expiration date of 5 years from the date of manufacture.

Compatibility/Compounding Considerations

Compounded preparation stability: Flucytosine oral suspension compounded from commercially available capsules has been published (Allen & Erickson 1996). Triturating four (4) flucytosine 250 mg capsules with 50 mL of *Ora-Plus®* and *qs ad* to 100 mL with *Ora-Sweet®* (or *Ora-Sweet® SF*) yields a 10 mg/mL oral suspension that retains >95% potency for 60 days stored at both 5°C and 25°C.

Dosage Forms/Regulatory Status

VETERINARY-LABELED PRODUCTS: None

HUMAN-LABELED PRODUCTS:

Flucytosine Oral Capsules: 250 mg & 500 mg; *Ancobon®* (ICN); (Rx)

References

Allen, L.V. & M.A. Erickson (1996). Stability of acetazolamide, allopurinol, azathioprine, clonazepam, and flucytosine in extemporaneously compounded oral liquids. *Am J Health Syst Pharm* 53(16): 1944–1949.

Clubb, S.L. (1986). Therapeutics: Individual and Flock Treatment Regimens. *Clinical Avian Medicine and Surgery*. GJ Harrison and LR Harrison Eds. Philadelphia, W.B. Saunders: 327–355.

Greene, C. & A. Watson (1998). Antimicrobial Drug Formulary. *Infectious Diseases of the Dog and Cat*. C Greene Ed. Philadelphia, WB Saunders: 790–919.

Jenson, J. (1998). Current ratite therapy. *The Veterinary Clinics of North America: Food Animal Practice* 16:3(November).

Malik, R., M. Krockenberger, et al. (2006). Cryptococcosis. *Infectious Diseases of the Dog and Cat, 3rd Ed.* C Greene Ed., Elsevier: 584–598.

FLUDROCORTISONE ACETATE

(flue-droe-*kor*-ti-sone) **Florinef®**
MINERALOCORTICOID

Prescriber Highlights

▶ Oral mineralocorticoid alternative to DOCP used to treat adrenal insufficiency in small animals; may be useful to treat hyperkalemia as well

▶ Also has some glucocorticoid effect which may cause adverse effects

▶ Adverse Effects: Dosage related; PU/PD, hypertension, edema, & hypokalemia possible

▶ May be excreted in significant quantities in milk

▶ Patients may require supplemental glucocorticoids

▶ Expense may be an issue, especially in larger dogs

Uses/Indications

Fludrocortisone is used in small animal medicine for the treatment of adrenocortical insufficiency (Addison's disease). It can also be used as adjunctive therapy in hyperkalemia.

Additionally, in humans, fludrocortisone has been used in salt-losing, congenital adrenogenital syndrome and in patients with severe postural hypotension.

Pharmacology/Actions

Fludrocortisone acetate is a potent corticosteroid that possesses both glucocorticoid and mineralocorticoid activity. It is approximately 10–15 times as potent a glucocorticoid agent as hydrocortisone, but is a much more potent mineralocorticoid (125 times that of hydrocortisone). It is only used clinically for its mineralocorticoid effects.

The site of action of mineralocorticoids is at the renal distal tubule where they increase the absorption of sodium. Mineralocorticoids also enhance potassium and hydrogen ion excretion.

Pharmacokinetics

In humans, fludrocortisone is well absorbed from the GI with peak levels occurring in approximately 1.7 hours; plasma half-life is about 3.5 hours, but biologic activity persists for 18–36 hours.

Contraindications/Precautions/Warnings

Fludrocortisone is contraindicated in patients known to be hypersensitive to it.

Some dogs or cats may require additional supplementation with a glucocorticoid agent on an ongoing basis. All animals with hypoadrenocorticism should receive additional glucocorticoids (2–10 times basal) during periods of stress or acute illness.

Adverse Effects

Adverse effects of fludrocortisone are generally a result of chronic, excessive dosage (see Overdosage below) or if withdrawal is too rapid. Since fludrocortisone also possesses glucocorticoid activity, it theoretically could cause the adverse effects associated with those compounds and polyuria/polydipsia may be a problem for some dogs. (See the section on the glucocorticoids for more information.)

Reproductive/Nursing Safety

In humans, the FDA categorizes this drug as category **C** for use during pregnancy (*Animal studies have shown an adverse effect on the fetus, but there are no adequate studies in humans; or there are no animal reproduction studies and no adequate studies in humans.*)

Fludrocortisone may be excreted in clinically significant quantities in milk. Puppies or kittens of mothers receiving fludrocortisone should receive milk replacer after colostrum is consumed.

Overdosage/Acute Toxicity

Overdosage may cause hypertension, edema, and hypokalemia. Electrolytes should be aggressively monitored and potassium may need to be supplemented. Patients should have the drug discontinued until clinical signs associated with overdosage have resolved; then restart the drug at a lower dosage.

Drug Interactions

The following drug interactions have either been reported or are theoretical in humans or animals receiving fludrocortisone and may be of significance in veterinary patients:

- ■ **AMPHOTERICIN B:** Patients may develop hypokalemia if fludrocortisone is administered concomitantly with amphotericin B

- ■ **ASPIRIN:** Fludrocortisone may reduce salicylate levels

- ■ **DIURETICS, POTASSIUM-DEPLETING (e.g., thiazides, furosemide):** Patients may develop hypokalemia if fludrocortisone is administered concomitantly with diuretics; diuretics can cause a loss of sodium, and may counteract the effects of fludrocortisone

- ■ **INSULIN:** Potentially, fludrocortisone could increase the insulin requirements of diabetic patients

Doses

- ■ **DOGS:**

    For hypoadrenocorticism:

    a) Initial dose of 0.01 mg/kg PO twice daily. Adjust dose based on monitoring serum electrolyte concentrations every 1-2 weeks until stable. Once stable, recheck serum chemistry profile including electrolytes every 3-4 months. Many dogs need an increase in the dose with time. Many dogs do well on fludrocortisone alone, but some dogs require additional glucocorticoid treatment. Polyuria, polydipsia, and other signs of Cushing's syndrome can be a problem in some dogs on fludrocortisone and can occur even when hyponatremia and, less frequently, hyperkalemia persist. Addition of NaCl (0.1 g/kg/day) can be useful in reducing the dose of fludrocortisone, maintaining a normal serum sodium, and possibly reduce the PU/PD. (Panciera 2009)

    b) For maintenance: Initially, 0.01–0.02 mg/kg/day PO and adjusted by 0.05–0.1 mg (total dose) increments based on serial electrolyte determinations. Electrolytes are initially checked weekly until stabilized in normal range. In many dogs, dose requirements increase incrementally over the first 6–24 months. Most dogs will ultimately require 0.02–0.03 mg/kg/day. (Kintzer 2004)

    c) 0.01 mg/kg PO twice daily. Titrate dose to effect; typically dose needs to be increased over time. For glucocorticoid replacement, starting dose of prednisone

is 0.1–0.22 mg/kg initially, but then taper to lowest dose that will control clinical signs. Only 50% of dogs on fludrocortisone require supplemental prednisone. (Scott-Moncrieff 2010)

- ■ **CATS:**

    For maintenance therapy of hypoadrenocorticism:

    a) 0.02 mg/kg PO once daily. Prednisone or prednisolone (1.25 mg per cat PO once daily) can be used for glucocorticoid replacement. (Scott-Moncrieff 2010)

    b) Maintenance therapy: 0.1 mg total dose/cat PO once daily with prednisolone (0.2 mg/kg PO once daily). (Caney 2009)

- ■ **FERRETS:**

    For hypoadrenocorticism:

    a) For those animals that still exhibit Addisonian signs even with prednisone therapy: 0.05–0.1 mg/kg PO q24h or divided q12h. (Johnson 2006)

Monitoring

- ■ Serum electrolytes, BUN, creatinine; initially every 1–2 weeks, then every 3–4 months once stabilized

- ■ Weight, PE for edema

Client Information

- ■ Clients should be familiar with the signs associated with both hypoadrenocorticism (e.g., weakness, depression, anorexia, vomiting, diarrhea, etc.) and fludrocortisone overdosage (e.g., edema) and report these to the veterinarian immediately.

Chemistry/Synonyms

A synthetic glucocorticoid with significant mineralocorticoid activity, fludrocortisone acetate occurs as hygroscopic, fine, white to pale yellow powder or crystals. It is odorless or practically odorless and has a melting point of approximately 225°C. Fludrocortisone is insoluble in water and slightly soluble in alcohol.

Fludrocortisone acetate may also be known as: fluohydrisone acetate, fluohydrocortisone acetate, 9alpha-fluorohydrocortisone acetate, fludrocortisoni acetas, 9alpha-fluorohydrocortisone 21-acetate, *Astonin®, Astonin H®, Florinef®, Florinefe®,* and *Lonikan®.*

Storage/Stability

Fludrocortisone acetate tablets should be stored at room temperature (15–30°C) in well-closed containers; avoid excessive heat. The drug is relatively stable in light and air.

Dosage Forms/Regulatory Status

VETERINARY-LABELED PRODUCTS: None

HUMAN-LABELED PRODUCTS:

Fludrocortisone Acetate Tablets: 0.1 mg; *Florinef® Acetate* (Monarch); generic; (Rx)

References

Caney, S. (2009). Feline adrenal disease: Diagnosis and management. Proceedings: BSAVA. Accessed via: Veterinary Information Network. http://goo.gl/iY5jX

Johnson, D. (2006). Current Therapies for Ferret Adrenal Disease. Proceedings: ACVC. Accessed via: Veterinary Information Network. http://goo.gl/pOMYy

Kintzer, P. (2004). Unmasking the imposter: diagnosis and treatment of canine hypoadrenocorticism. Proceedings: ACVIM Forum. Accessed via: Veterinary Information Network. http://goo.gl/Ad7h0

Panciera, D. (2009). Diagnosis and management of hypoadrenocorticism. Proceedings: ACVC. Accessed via: Veterinary Information Network. http://goo.gl/bqWai

Scott-Moncrieff, J.C. (2010). Hypoadrenocorticism in dogs and cats: Update on diagnosis & treatment. Proceedings: ACVIM Forum. Accessed via: Veterinary Information Network. http://goo.gl/DV3Xh

FLUMAZENIL

(floo-*maz*-eh-nill)   Romazicon®

BENZODIAZEPINE ANTAGONIST

Prescriber Highlights

▶ Benzodiazepine antagonist to reverse either OD's or therapeutic effects

▶ Contraindications: Known hypersensitivity, when benzodiazepines are treating life-threatening conditions (e.g., status epilepticus, increased CSF pressure), during tricyclic antidepressant OD treatment

▶ Use extreme caution in mixed overdoses

▶ Adverse Effects: Potentially injection site reactions, vomiting, cutaneous vasodilatation, vertigo, ataxia, & blurred vision; seizures have been reported in humans

▶ Potentially teratogenic at high dosages

Uses/Indications

Flumazenil may be useful for the reversal of benzodiazepine effects after either therapeutic use or overdoses. Flumazenil may be of benefit in the treatment of encephalopathy in patients with severe hepatic failure or in treating overdoses with zolpidem (*Ambien*®) or other imidazopyridine hypnotic agents.

A report of using flumazenil to reverse the anesthetic effects of tiletamine-zolazepam in dogs, demonstrated that analgesia, posture, and auditory effects were reversed, but it had no effect on sedation or muscle relaxation. Recovery times (head up, sternal recumbency, standing, walking) from anesthesia were reduced in the flumazenil treated dogs. Heart rates, glucose levels, body temperature were significantly higher in the flumazenil treated group. (Kim *et al.* 2009).

Pharmacology/Actions

Flumazenil is a competitive blocker of benzodiazepines at benzodiazepine receptors in the CNS. It antagonizes the sedative and amnestic qualities of benzodiazepines.

Pharmacokinetics

Flumazenil is administered by rapid IV injection. Therapeutic effect may occur within 1–2 minutes of administration. It is rapidly distributed and metabolized in the liver. In humans, the average half-life is about one hour.

Contraindications/Precautions/Warnings

Flumazenil is contraindicated in patients hypersensitive to it or other benzodiazepines or in patients with where benzodiazepines are being used to treat a potentially life-threatening condition (*e.g.*, status epilepticus, increased CSF pressure). It should not be used in patients with a serious tricyclic antidepressant overdose. Flumazenil should not be used, or used with extreme caution, in patients with mixed overdoses where benzodiazepine reversal may lead to seizures or other complications.

While flumazenil has been tried as treatment for overdoses of baclofen or carisoprodol, it may actually be contraindicated as it may cause worsening of clinical signs (Mazzaferro 2008). Flumazenil does not alter benzodiazepine pharmacokinetics. Effects of long-acting benzodiazepines may recur after flumazenil's effects subside.

Adverse Effects

In some human patients, flumazenil use has been associated with seizures. These patients usually have a long history of benzodiazepine use or are showing signs of serious tricyclic antidepressant toxicity. Adverse effects reported in humans include injection site reactions, vomiting, cutaneous vasodilatation, vertigo, ataxia and blurred vision. Deaths have been associated with its use in humans having serious underlying diseases.

Overdosage/Acute Toxicity

Large IV overdoses have rarely caused symptoms in otherwise healthy humans. Seizures, if precipitated, have been treated with barbiturates, benzodiazepines and phenytoin, usually with prompt responses.

Drug Interactions

The following drug interactions have either been reported or are theoretical in humans or animals receiving flumazenil and may be of significance in veterinary patients:

■ **CYCLIC (tri-, tetra-) ANTIDEPRESSANTS (e.g., clomipramine, amitriptyline, etc.):** Increased risk for seizures; use contraindicated

■ **NEUROMUSCULAR BLOCKING AGENTS:** Not recommended to use flumazenil until neuromuscular blockade has been fully reversed

Doses

■ **DOGS & CATS:**

As an antagonist for benzodiazepines:
a) Dogs: 0.01 mg/kg IV (Bunch 2003)
b) Dogs/Cats: 0.01 mg/kg IV; may need to be repeated as half-life is only about an hour.

May also be administered intratracheally in an emergency. (Wismer 2004)

For adjunctive therapy to improve neurologic function in dogs with severe hepatic encephalopathy:

a) 0.02 mg/kg IV (one time) (Bunch 2003)

b) 0.02 mg/kg IV; if animal responds, safe to use repeatedly (Michel 2003)

■ **ZOO, EXOTIC, WILDLIFE SPECIES:**

For use of flumazenil in zoo, exotic and wildlife medicine refer to specific references, including:

a) *Zoo Animal and Wildlife Immobilization and Anesthesia.* West, G, Heard, D, Caulkett, N. (eds.). Blackwell Publishing, 2007.

b) *Handbook of Wildlife Chemical Immobilization, 3rd Ed.* Kreeger, T.J. and J.M. Arnemo. 2007.

c) *Restraint and Handling of Wild and Domestic Animals.* Fowler, M (ed.), Iowa State University Press, 1995

d) *Exotic Animal Formulary, 3rd Ed.* Carpenter, J.W., Saunders. 2005

e) The 2009 American Association of Zoo Veterinarian Proceedings by D. K. Fontenot also has several dosages listed for restraint, anesthesia, and analgesia for a variety of drugs for carnivores and primates. VIN members can access them at: http://goo.gl/BHRih or http://goo.gl/9UJse

Monitoring
■ Efficacy
■ Monitor for seizures in susceptible patients

Client Information
■ Flumazenil should only be used in a controlled environment by clinically experienced professionals.

Chemistry/Synonyms
A benzodiazepine antagonist, flumazenil is a 1,4-imidazobenzodiazepine derivative.

Flumazenil may also be known as: flumazenilum, flumazepil, Ro-15-1788, Ro-15-1788/000, *Anexate®, Fadaflumaz®, Flumage®, Flumanovag®, Flumazen®, Fluxifarm®, Lanexat®* and *Romazicon®*.

Storage/Stability
Store flumazenil at 25°C (77°F); excursions are permitted from 15° to 30°C (59° to 86°F). Once drawn into a syringe or mixed with the above solutions, discard after 24 hours.

Compatibility/Compounding Considerations
Flumazenil is physically **compatible** with lactated Ringer's, D5W, or normal saline solutions.

Dosage Forms/Regulatory Status
VETERINARY-LABELED PRODUCTS: None
HUMAN-LABELED PRODUCTS:
Flumazenil Injection: 0.1 mg/mL in 5 mL &

10 mL vials; *Romazicon®* (Hoffman-LaRoche); generic; (Rx)

References
Bunch, S. (2003). Hepatobiliary and exocrine pancreatic disorders. *Small Animal Internal Medicine, 3rd Ed.* R Nelson and C Couto Eds. St Louis, Mosby: 472–567.
Kim, M., H. Won, et al. (2009). Antagonistic Effects of Flumazenil on Tiletamine-Zolazepam Induced Anesthesia in Dogs. Proceedings: WSAVA. Accessed via: Veterinary Information Network. http://goo.gl/wUJL2
Mazzaferro, E. (2008). Emergency Intoxications. Proceedings: WVC. Accessed via: Veterinary Information Network. http://goo.gl/L9tAS
Michel, K. (2003). Nutritional intervention: hepatic failure. Proceedings: IVECCS Symposium. Accessed via: Veterinary Information Network. http://goo.gl/Stixz
Wismer, T. (2004). Newer antidotal therapies. Proceedings: IVECC Symposium. Accessed via: Veterinary Information Network. http://goo.gl/jNp8A

FLUMETHASONE

(floo-*meth*-a-sone)   Flucort®

GLUCOCORTICOID

Prescriber Highlights

▶ Injectable & oral glucocorticoid (oral may not be available commercially in USA)

▶ Long-acting; 15–30X more potent than hydrocortisone; no appreciable mineralocorticoid activity

▶ Therapy goal is to use as much as is required & as little as possible for as short an amount of time as possible

▶ Primary adverse effects are "Cushingoid" in nature with sustained use

▶ Many potential drug & lab interactions

Uses/Indications
Flumethasone injection is available commercially as a free steroid alcohol solution. While it does not work quite as rapidly as the corticosteroid phosphate and succinate esters (methylprednisolone sodium succinate, prednisolone sodium succinate, or dexamethasone sodium phosphate), it can be given either IM or IV and is useful for acute reactions such as insect bite hypersensitivity or vaccine reactions (Dowling 2007).

Flumethasone injection (*Flucort®*) is labeled in horses as indicated for: 1) Musculoskeletal conditions due to inflammation, where permanent structural changes do not exist, such as bursitis, carpitis, osselets and myositis. Following therapy an appropriate period of rest should be instituted to allow a more normal return to function of the affected part. 2) In allergic states such as hives, urticaria and insect bites.

Flumethasone injection (*Flucort®*) is labeled in dogs as indicated for: 1) Musculoskeletal conditions due to inflammation of muscles or joints and accessory structures, where permanent structural changes do not exist, such as arthritis, osteoarthritis, the disc syndrome and myositis. In septic arthritis appropriate antibacterial therapy should be concurrently administered. 2) In certain acute and chronic dermatoses of varying etiology to help control the pruritus, irritation and inflammation associated with these conditions. The drug has proven useful in otitis externa in conjunction with topical medication for similar reasons. 3) In allergic states such as hives, urticaria and insect bites. 4) Shock and shock-like states, by intravenous administration.

Flumethasone injection (*Flucort®*) is labeled in cats as indicated for certain acute and chronic dermatoses of varying etiology to help control the pruritus, irritation and inflammation associated with these conditions.

Pharmacology/Actions

For more information refer to the Glucocorticoids, General Information monograph.

Pharmacokinetics

No information was located for this agent.

Contraindications/Precautions/Warnings

Flumethasone is contraindicated during the last trimester of pregnancy. Systemic use of glucocorticoids is generally considered contraindicated in systemic fungal infections (unless used for replacement therapy in Addison's), when administered IM in patients with idiopathic thrombocytopenia, and in patients hypersensitive to a particular compound. Use of sustained-release, injectable glucocorticoids is contraindicated for chronic corticosteroid therapy of systemic diseases.

Animals that have received glucocorticoids systemically, other than with "burst" therapy, should be tapered off the drugs. Patients who have received the drugs chronically should be tapered off slowly as endogenous ACTH and corticosteroid function may return slowly. Should the animal undergo a "stressor" (*e.g.*, surgery, trauma, illness, etc.) during the tapering process or until normal adrenal and pituitary function resume, additional glucocorticoids should be administered.

Adverse Effects

Adverse effects are generally associated with long-term administration of these drugs, especially if given at high dosages or not on an alternate day regimen. Effects generally manifest as clinical signs of hyperadrenocorticism. When administered to young, growing animals, glucocorticoids can retard growth. Many of the potential effects, adverse and otherwise, are outlined above in the Pharmacology section.

In dogs, polydipsia (PD), polyphagia (PP), and polyuria (PU) may all be seen with short-term "burst" therapy as well as with alternate-day maintenance therapy on days when giving the drug. Adverse effects in dogs can include: dull, dry haircoat, weight gain, panting, vomiting, diarrhea, elevated liver enzymes, pancre-atitis, GI ulceration, lipidemias, activation or worsening of diabetes mellitus, muscle wasting and behavioral changes (depression, lethargy, viciousness). Discontinuation of the drug may be necessary; changing to an alternate steroid may also alleviate the problem. With the exception of PU/PD/PP, adverse effects associated with anti-inflammatory therapy are relatively uncommon. Adverse effects associated with immunosuppressive doses are more common and potentially more severe.

Cats generally require higher dosages than dogs for clinical effect, but tend to develop fewer adverse effects. Occasionally, polydipsia, polyuria, polyphagia with weight gain, diarrhea, or depression can be seen. Long-term, high dose therapy can lead to "Cushingoid" effects, however.

Reproductive/Nursing Safety

Corticosteroid therapy may induce parturition in large animal species during the latter stages of pregnancy. In a system evaluating the safety of drugs in canine and feline pregnancy (Papich 1989), this drug is categorized as in class: *C* (*These drugs may have potential risks. Studies in people or laboratory animals have uncovered risks, and these drugs should be used cautiously as a last resort when the benefit of therapy clearly outweighs the risks.*)

Overdosage/Acute Toxicity

Glucocorticoids when given short-term are unlikely to cause harmful effects, even in massive dosages. One incidence of a dog developing acute CNS effects after accidental ingestion of glucocorticoids has been reported. Should clinical signs occur, use supportive treatment if required.

Chronic usage of glucocorticoids can lead to serious adverse effects. Refer to Adverse Effects above for more information.

Drug Interactions

The following drug interactions have either been reported or are theoretical in humans or animals receiving flumethasone and may be of significance in veterinary patients:

- ■ **AMPHOTERICIN B:** Administered concomitantly with glucocorticoids may cause hypokalemia
- ■ **ANTICHOLINESTERASE AGENTS (e.g., pyridostigmine, neostigmine, etc.):** In patients with myasthenia gravis, concomitant glucocorticoid and anticholinesterase agent administration may lead to profound muscle weakness. If possible, discontinue anticholinesterase medication at least 24 hours prior to corticosteroid administration.
- ■ **ASPIRIN:** Glucocorticoids may reduce salicylate blood levels
- ■ **BARBITURATES:** May increase the metabolism of glucocorticoids and decrease flumethasone blood levels

■ **CYCLOPHOSPHAMIDE:** Glucocorticoids may inhibit the hepatic metabolism of cyclophosphamide; dosage adjustments may be required

■ **CYCLOSPORINE:** Concomitant administration of glucocorticoids and cyclosporine may increase the blood levels of each by mutually inhibiting the hepatic metabolism of each other; the clinical significance of this interaction is not clear

■ **DIAZEPAM:** Flumethasone may decrease diazepam levels

■ **DIURETICS, POTASSIUM-DEPLETING (e.g., spironolactone, triamterene):** Administered concomitantly with glucocorticoids may cause hypokalemia

■ **EPHEDRINE:** May reduce flumethasone blood levels

■ **INSULIN:** Insulin requirements may increase in patients receiving glucocorticoids

■ **KETOCONAZOLE AND OTHER AZOLE ANTIFUNGALS:** May decrease the metabolism of glucocorticoids and increase flumethasone blood levels; ketoconazole may induce adrenal insufficiency when glucocorticoids are withdrawn by inhibiting adrenal corticosteroid synthesis

■ **MACROLIDE ANTIBIOTICS (erythromycin, clarithromycin):** May decrease the metabolism of glucocorticoids and increase flumethasone blood levels

■ **MITOTANE:** May alter the metabolism of steroids; higher than usual doses of steroids may be necessary to treat mitotane-induced adrenal insufficiency

■ **NSAIDS:** Administration of ulcerogenic drugs with glucocorticoids may increase the risk of gastrointestinal ulceration

■ **PHENYTOIN:** May increase the metabolism of glucocorticoids and decrease flumethasone blood levels

■ **RIFAMPIN:** May increase the metabolism of glucocorticoids and decrease flumethasone blood levels

■ **VACCINES:** Patients receiving corticosteroids at immunosuppressive dosages should generally not receive live attenuated-virus vaccines as virus replication may be augmented; a diminished immune response may occur after vaccine, toxoid, or bacterin administration in patients receiving glucocorticoids

Laboratory Considerations

■ Glucocorticoids may increase **serum cholesterol**

■ Glucocorticoids may increase **urine glucose** levels

■ Glucocorticoids may decrease **serum potassium**

■ Glucocorticoids can suppress the release of thyroid stimulating hormone (TSH) and reduce T_3 & T_4 values. Thyroid gland atrophy has been reported after chronic glucocorticoid administration. Uptake of I^{131} by the thyroid may be decreased by glucocorticoids.

■ Reactions to **skin tests** may be suppressed by glucocorticoids

■ False-negative results of the **nitroblue tetrazolium** test for systemic bacterial infections may be induced by glucocorticoids

■ Glucocorticoids may cause **neutrophilia** within 4–8 hours after dosing and return to baseline within 24–48 hours after drug discontinuation

■ Glucocorticoids can cause **lymphopenia** which can persist for weeks after drug discontinuation in dogs

Doses

■ **DOGS:**
For labeled indications (musculoskeletal conditions due to inflammation . . . , certain acute and chronic dermatoses . . . when given orally, and also for allergic states or shock when given intravenously). Treat and adjust dosage on an individual basis:
a) Orally: 0.0625–0.25 mg daily in divided doses. Dosage is dependent on size of animal, stage and severity of disease. **Note:** Tablets no longer marketed in the USA
Parenterally: 0.0625–0.25 mg IV, IM, SC daily; may repeat;
Intra-articularly: 0.166–1 mg;
Intra-lesionally: 0.125–1 mg (Package insert; *Flucort®*—Fort Dodge)
b) 0.06–0.25 mg IV, IM, SC, or PO once daily (Kirk 1989)

■ **CATS:**
For labeled indications (certain acute and chronic dermatoses . . .): Treat and adjust dosage on an individual basis:
a) Orally: 0.03125–0.125 mg daily in divided doses; **Note:** Tablets no longer marketed in the USA
Parenterally: 0.03125–0.125 mg IV, IM, or SC. If necessary, may repeat. (Package insert; *Flucort®*—Fort Dodge)
b) 0.03–0.125 mg IV, IM, SC, or PO once daily (Kirk 1989)

■ **HORSES:** (**Note:** ARCI UCGFS Class 4 Drug)
For labeled indications (musculoskeletal conditions due to inflammation, where permanent changes do not exist; and also for allergic states such as hives, urticaria and insect bites):
a) 1.25–2.5 mg daily by IV, IM or intra-articular injection. If necessary, the dose may be repeated. (Package insert; *Flucort®*—Fort Dodge)
b) 1–2.5 mg/450 kg IV or IM (Robinson 1987)

Monitoring

Monitoring of glucocorticoid therapy is dependent on its reason for use, dosage, agent used (amount of mineralocorticoid activity), dosage schedule (daily versus alternate day therapy), duration of therapy, and the animal's age and condition. The following list may not be appropriate or complete for all animals; use clinical assessment and judgment should adverse effects be noted:

- Weight, appetite, signs of edema
- Serum and/or urine electrolytes
- Total plasma proteins, albumin
- Blood glucose
- Growth and development in young animals
- ACTH stimulation test if necessary

Client Information

- Clients should carefully follow the dosage instructions and should not discontinue the drug abruptly without consulting with veterinarian beforehand.
- Clients should be briefed on the potential adverse effects that can be seen with these drugs and instructed to contact the veterinarian should these effects become severe or progress.

Chemistry/Synonyms

Flumethasone occurs as an odorless, white to creamy white, crystalline powder. Its chemical name is 6alpha, 9alpha-difluoro-16alpha methylprednisolone.

Flumethasone may also be known as: flumetasone, glumetasoni pivalas, NSC-107680, *Cerson®*, *Flucort®*, *Locacorten®*, *Locacortene®*, *Locorten®*, *Locortene®*, and *Lorinden®*.

Storage/Stability

Flumethasone injection should be stored at room temperature; avoid freezing.

Dosage Forms/Regulatory Status

VETERINARY-LABELED PRODUCTS:

Flumethasone Injection: 0.5 mg/mL in 100 mL vials; *Flucort® Solution* (Pfizer); (Rx). FDA-approved for use in dogs, cats, and horses.

The ARCI (Racing Commissioners International) has designated this drug as a class 4 substance. See the appendix for more information.

HUMAN-LABELED PRODUCTS: None

References

Dowling, P. (2007). Corticosteroids: The wonderful, terrible drugs. Proceedings: AAFP. Accessed via: Veterinary Information Network. http://goo.gl/qMSfj

Kirk, R.W., Ed. (1989). *Current Veterinary Therapy X, Small Animal Practice*. Philadelphia, W.B. Saunders.

Robinson, N.E. (1987). Table of Common Drugs: Approximate Doses. *Current Therapy in Equine Medicine, 2*. NE Robinson Ed. Philadelphia, W.B. Saunders: 761.

FLUNIXIN MEGLUMINE

(floo-*nix*-in)   Banamine®

NON-STEROIDAL ANTIINFLAMMATORY AGENT

Prescriber Highlights

▶ Veterinary-only non-steroidal antiinflammatory agent used in a variety of species

▶ Caution in patients with preexisting GI ulcers, renal, hepatic, or hematologic diseases; in horses with colic, flunixin may mask the behavioral & cardiopulmonary signs associated with endotoxemia or intestinal devitalization

▶ Use in small animals largely supplanted by FDA-approved agents or those with better adverse effect profile in target species

▶ If first dose is ineffective for pain control, subsequent doses unlikely to be of benefit

▶ Adverse Effects in Horses & Cattle: Rare anaphylaxis (especially after rapid IV administration); IM injections (extra-label in food animals) may cause pain/swelling

Uses/Indications

In the United States, flunixin meglumine is FDA-approved for use in horses, cattle and swine; however, it is approved for use in dogs in other countries. The FDA-approved indications for its use in the horse are for the alleviation of inflammation and pain associated with musculoskeletal disorders and alleviation of visceral pain associated with colic. In cattle it is FDA-approved for the control of pyrexia associated with bovine respiratory disease and endotoxemia, and control of inflammation in endotoxemia. In swine, flunixin is FDA-approved for use to control pyrexia associated with swine respiratory disease. In ruminants, there is some evidence that flunixin is a better analgesic for visceral pain rather than musculoskeletal pain.

Flunixin has been suggested for many other indications in various species, including: Horses: foal diarrheas, shock, colitis, respiratory disease, post-race treatment, and pre- and post ophthalmic and general surgery; Dogs: disk problems, arthritis, heat stroke, diarrhea, shock, ophthalmic inflammatory conditions, pre- and post ophthalmic and general surgery, and treatment of parvovirus infection; Cattle: acute respiratory disease, acute coliform mastitis with endotoxic shock, pain (downer cow), and calf diarrheas; Swine: agalactia/hypogalactia, lameness, and piglet diarrhea. It should be noted that the evidence supporting some of these indications is equivocal and flunixin may not be appropriate for every case.

The combination product containing florfenicol and flunixin (*Resflor Gold®*) is FDA-approved for SC use in beef and non-lactating dairy cattle (not veal calves) for treatment of BRD associated with *Mannheimia haemolytica, Pasteurella multocida, Histophilus somni, Mycoplasma bovis* and control BRD-associated pyrexia.

Pharmacology/Actions

Flunixin is a very potent inhibitor of cyclooxygenase and, like other NSAIDs, it exhibits analgesic, antiinflammatory, and antipyretic activity. Flunixin does not appreciably alter GI motility in horses and may improve hemodynamics in animals with septic shock.

Pharmacokinetics

In the horse, flunixin is rapidly absorbed following oral administration with an average bioavailability of 80% and peak serum levels in 30 minutes. Oral bioavailability is good when the injection is mixed with molasses and given orally. The onset of action is generally within 2 hours; peak response occurs between 12–16 hours and the duration of action lasts up to 30 hours. Flunixin is highly bound to plasma proteins (>99% cattle, 92% dogs, 87% horses). Volume of distributions ranges from approximately 0.15 L/kg in horses to 0.78 L/kg in cattle. Elimination is primarily via hepatic routes by biliary excretion. Serum half-lives have been determined in horses $\approx$ 1.6–4.2 hours, dogs $\approx$ 3.7 hours; cattle $\approx$ 3.1–8.1 hours. Flunixin is detectable in equine urine for at least 48 hours after a dose.

Contraindications/Precautions/Warnings

The only contraindication the manufacturer lists for flunixin's use in horses is for patients with a history of hypersensitivity reactions to it. It is suggested, however, that flunixin be used cautiously in animals with renal, hepatic, or hematologic diseases. When using to treat colic, flunixin may mask the behavioral and cardiopulmonary signs associated with endotoxemia or intestinal devitalization and must be used with caution.

In horses with known or suspected EGUS, use should be avoided; single doses of flunixin will probably not result in catastrophic consequences, but repeated doses can exacerbate gastric ulcers (Videla & Andrews 2009).

In cattle, the drug is contraindicated in animals that have shown prior hypersensitivity reactions. The IM route is extra-label in cattle and should only be used when the IV route is not feasible for use. Longer withdrawal times would be required after IM use. Flunixin should not be used in an attempt to ambulate cattle to be shipped for slaughter.

Flunixin is usually considered contraindicated in cats, but some clinicians have used it short-term. However, FDA-approved (and safer?) NSAIDs are available for cats.

Adverse Effects

When used for pain, if the animal does not respond to an initial dose, it is unlikely additional doses will be effective and may result in increased chance for toxicity. In horses following IM injection, reports of localized swelling, induration, stiffness, and sweating have been reported. Do not inject intra-arterially as it may cause CNS stimulation (hysteria), ataxia, hyperventilation, and muscle weakness. Clinical signs are transient and generally do not require any treatment. Flunixin appears to be a relatively safe agent for use in the horse, but the potential exists for GI intolerance, hypoproteinemia, and hematologic abnormalities to occur. Flunixin is not to be used in horses intended for food.

Horses have developed oral and gastric ulcers, anorexia, and depression when given high doses for prolonged periods (>2 weeks). Although gastric ulceration is frequently observed in adult horses and foals, evidence of an association between this disease and administration of NSAIDs such as flunixin at recommended dosages is lacking. On the basis of current evidence, prophylactic anti-ulcer medications to horses receiving therapeutic doses of NSAIDs is probably unnecessary in horses that are otherwise at low risk for gastric ulceration (Fennell & Franklin 2009).

In horses and cattle, rare anaphylactic-like reactions have been reported, primarily after rapid IV administration. IM injections may rarely be associated with clostridial myonecrosis.

Hematochezia and hematuria have been reported in cattle treated for longer than the 3-day recommendation.

In dogs, GI distress is the most likely adverse reaction. Clinical signs may include, vomiting, diarrhea, and ulceration with very high doses or chronic use. There have been anecdotal reports of flunixin causing renal shutdown in dogs when used at higher dosages pre-operatively.

In birds, flunixin has been shown to cause dose-related, significant renal ischemia and nephrotoxicity.

Reproductive/Nursing Safety

Although reports of teratogenicity, effects on breeding performance, or gestation length have not been noted, flunixin should be used cautiously in pregnant animals. Flunixin is not recommended for use in breeding bulls (lack of reproductive safety data).

In a system evaluating the safety of drugs in canine and feline pregnancy (Papich 1989), this drug is categorized as in class: **C** (*These drugs may have potential risks. Studies in people or laboratory animals have uncovered risks, and these drugs should be used cautiously as a last resort when the benefit of therapy clearly outweighs the risks.*)

Overdosage/Acute Toxicity

No clinical case reports of flunixin overdoses were discovered. It is suggested that acute overdosage be handled by using established protocols of emptying the gut (if oral ingestion and practical or possible) and treating the patient supportively.

Gastric ulceration is a distinct possibility in horses that have received overdoses of flunixin. Consider using anti-ulcer medications in overdosed horses.

Drug Interactions

Drug/drug interactions have not been appreciably studied for flunixin and the label does not mention any drug interactions. However, the following drug interactions have either been reported or are theoretical in humans or animals receiving other NSAIDs and may be of significance in veterinary patients receiving flunixin:

■ **ASPIRIN:** When aspirin is used concurrently with NSAIDs, plasma levels of the NSAID could decrease and an increased likelihood of GI adverse effects (blood loss) could occur

■ **CYCLOSPORINE:** NSAIDs may increase cyclosporine blood levels and increase the risk for nephrotoxicity

■ **DIGOXIN:** NSAIDs may increase serum levels of digoxin; use with caution in patients with severe cardiac failure

■ **ENROFLOXACIN:** Has been shown in dogs to increase the AUC and elimination half-life of flunixin and flunixin increases the AUC and elimination half-life of enrofloxacin; it is unknown if other NSAIDs interact with enrofloxacin in dogs. Enrofloxacin and flunixin did not interact in rabbits.

■ **FUROSEMIDE & OTHER DIURETICS:** NSAIDs may reduce the saluretic and diuretic effects of furosemide

■ **METHOTREXATE:** Serious toxicity has occurred when NSAIDs have been used concomitantly with methotrexate; use together with caution

■ **NEPHROTOXIC AGENTS (e.g., amphotericin B, aminoglycosides, cisplatin, etc.):** Potential for increased risk of nephrotoxicity if used with NSAIDs

■ **PROBENECID:** May cause a significant increase in serum levels and half-life of some NSAIDs

■ **WARFARIN:** Use with NSAIDs may increase the risk for bleeding

Doses

■ **DOGS:**
Note: There are many canine doses published from a time when there were no FDA-approved NSAIDs for dogs; using FDA-approved drugs first is recommended.

a) As an antidiarrheal/antipyretic: 1 mg/kg IV (do not administer more than once in an animal that has received corticosteroids (Tams 1999)

b) For surgical pain: 1 mg/kg IV, SC or IM initially once; 1 mg/kg subsequent daily doses
For pyrexia: 0.25 mg/kg IV, SC or IM once, may be repeated in 12–24 hours if needed
For ophtho procedures: 0.25–1 mg/kg IV, IM or SC once; may be repeated in 12–24 hours if needed (Johnson 1996)

■ **FERRETS:**
a) 0.5–2 mg/kg PO or IM one time daily (Williams 2000)

■ **RABBITS/RODENTS/SMALL MAMMALS:**
a) **Rabbits:** 1.1 mg/kg SC, IM, IV q12–24h (Ivey & Morrisey 2000)
b) **Rabbits:** 1.1 mg/kg SC or IM q12h
Rodents: 2.5 mg/kg SC or IM q12h (Huerkamp 1995)
c) **Chinchillas:** 1–3 mg/kg SC q12h **Guinea pigs:** 2.5–5 mg/kg SC q12h **Gerbils, Mice, Rats, Hamsters:** 2.5 mg/kg SC q12–24h (Adamcak & Otten 2000)

■ **CATTLE:**
a) For labeled indications: 1.1–2.2 mg/kg (1–2 mL per 100 lbs. BW) given slow IV either once a day as a single dose or divided into two doses q12h for up to 3 days. Avoid rapid IV administration. (Package Insert; *Banamine®*—Schering).

b) As an analgesic: 1.1–2.2 mg/kg IV q6–12 hours; recommend 72 hour milk withdrawal at this dose rate. (Walz 2006)

c) As an analgesic for visceral pain: 0.25–1 mg/kg IV q12–24h. (Anderson 2006)

d) Using the combination product containing florfenicol/flunixin (*Resflor Gold®*): 40 mg/kg florfenicol/2.2 mg/kg flunixin (6 mL/100 lb. B.W.) SC once. **Do not administer more than 10 mL at each site. The injection should be given only in the neck. Injection sites other than the neck have not been evaluated.** (Label Information—*Resflor Gold®* ; Intervet Schering)

■ **HORSES:** (**Note:** ARCI UCGFS Class 4 Drug)
a) Injectable: 1.1 mg/kg IV or IM once daily for up to 5 days. For colic cases, use IV route and may redose when necessary.
Oral Paste: 1.1 mg/kg PO (see markings on syringe—calibrated in 250 lb. weight increments) once daily. One syringe will treat a 1000 lb. horse for 3 days. Do not exceed 5 days of consecutive therapy.
Oral Granules: 1.1 mg/kg PO once daily. One packet will treat 500 lbs of body weight. May apply on feed. Do not exceed 5 consecutive days of therapy. (Package Inserts; *Banamine®*—Schering Animal Health)

b) For adjunctive treatment of medical colic: 0.25–1.1 mg/kg IV q8–12h; usually 1.1 mg/kg IV q12h. (Blikslager 2006)

c) To decrease pain, inflammation, and edema in laminitis: 0.5–1.1 mg/kg IV or PO q8–12 hours. A dose of 0.25 mg/kg can be administered IV q8h to interrupt eicosanoid production associated with endotoxemia. (Moore 2003)

d) For adjunctive treatment of patients with, or at risk for laminitis: 1.1 mg/kg IV three times daily with proper monitoring for hydration and renal status and monitoring for gastrointestinal ulceration. (Belknap 2008)

e) For adjunctive treatment of uveitis in foals: 0.5–1 mg/kg (route not noted) twice daily (Cutler 2003)

■ **SHEEP, GOATS:**
a) As an analgesic: 1–2 mg/kg IV q24h; oral paste has also been at 1–4 mg/kg PO once daily. (Snyder 2009)

■ **SWINE:**
a) To control pyrexia associated with swine respiratory disease: 2.2 mg/kg IM once, only in the neck musculature with a maximum of 10 mL per site. (Label information; *Banamine®*-S—Schering-Plough)

■ **BIRDS:**
a) As an antiinflammatory analgesic: 1–10 mg/kg IM once daily. **Note:** Renal disease and death occur occasionally in psittacines after repeated doses of flunixin. Use the lowest possible dose for the shortest duration of time. Recommend supplemental hydration. (Clyde & Paul-Murphy 2000)

■ **ZOO, EXOTIC, WILDLIFE SPECIES:**
For use of flunixin in zoo, exotic and wildlife medicine refer to specific references, including:

a) *Zoo Animal and Wildlife Immobilization and Anesthesia.* West, G, Heard, D, Caulkett, N. (eds.). Blackwell Publishing, 2007.

b) *Handbook of Wildlife Chemical Immobilization, 3rd Ed.* Kreeger, T.J. and J.M. Arnemo. 2007.

c) *Restraint and Handling of Wild and Domestic Animals.* Fowler, M (ed.), Iowa State University Press, 1995

d) *Exotic Animal Formulary, 3rd Ed.* Carpenter, J.W., Saunders. 2005

e) The 2009 American Association of Zoo Veterinarian Proceedings by D. K. Fontenot also has several dosages listed for restraint, anesthesia, and analgesia for a variety of drugs for carnivores and primates. VIN members can access them at: http://goo.gl/BHRih or http://goo.gl/9UJse

Monitoring
■ Analgesic/antiinflammatory/antipyretic effects

■ GI effects in dogs
■ CBC's, occult blood in feces with chronic use in horses

Client Information
■ If injecting IM, do not inject into neck muscles.
■ The IM route is extra-label in cattle and should only be used when the IV route is not feasible for use. Longer withdrawal times would be required after IM use.
■ Flunixin should not be used in an attempt to ambulate cattle to be shipped for slaughter.

Chemistry/Synonyms
Flunixin meglumine, a nonsteroidal antiinflammatory agent is a highly substituted derivative of nicotinic acid, and is unique structurally when compared to other NSAIDs. It occurs as a white to off-white powder that is soluble in water and alcohol. The chemical name for flunixin is 3-pyridine-carboxylic acid.

Flunixin may also be known as 3-pyridine-carboxylic acid, flunixin meglumine, Sch-14714, *Banamine®*, *Flumeglumine®*, and *Finadyne®*, *Flu-Nix®D*, *Flunixamine®*, *Flunixiject®*, *Flunizine®*, *Prevail®*, *Suppressor®*, and *Vedagesic®*.

Storage/Stability
All flunixin products should be stored between 2–30°C (36–86°F). It has been recommended that flunixin meglumine injection not be mixed with other drugs because of unknown compatibilities.

The combination product with florfenicol (*Resflor Gold®*) should not be stored above 30°C (86°F). Once the vial is entered it should be used within 28 days. The 500 mL vial should not be punctured more than 10 times.

Dosage Forms/Regulatory Status

VETERINARY-LABELED PRODUCTS:
Note: Individual products may be FDA-approved and be labeled for different species, lactation status, different routes of administration (IV, IM). Flunixin is also FDA-approved only for use in horses not intended for food. Refer to the specific product label for more information

Flunixin Meglumine for Injection: 50 mg/mL in 50 mL, 100 mL and 250 mL vials; At the time of writing, the following products are FDA-approved for use in horses and use in beef and dairy cattle (not for use in dry dairy cows or veal calves): *Banamine®* (Schering-Plough), *Flunixin Meglumine Injection* (IVX, Vet Tek, Aspen), *Flumeglumine®* (Phoenix Pharmaceuticals), *Flunixamine®* (Fort Dodge), *Flunixiject®* (Butler), *Prevail®* (VetOne), *Suppressor® Dairy* (RXV), *Flunizine®* (Bimeda), *Vedagesic®* (Vedco); *Flu-Nix®D* (AgriLabs); (Rx). Depending on product, when used as labeled: withdrawal (Cattle): Milk 36 hours; Slaughter 4 days.

Flunixin Meglumine for Injection: 50 mg/mL

in 100 mL vials; At the time of writing, the following product is FDA-approved for IM use in swine: *Banamine®-S* (Schering-Plough); (Rx) Withdrawal: Slaughter = 12 days.

Flunixin Meglumine for Injection: 50 mg/mL in 100 mL vials; At the time of writing, the following product is FDA-approved for use in horses: *Suppressor®* (RXV); (Rx)

Flunixin Meglumine Oral Paste: 1500 mg/syringe in 30 gram syringes in boxes of 6; *Banamine® Paste* (Schering-Plough); (Rx). FDA-approved for use in horses.

Flunixin Meglumine Oral Granules: 250 mg in 10 gram sachets in boxes of 50; 20 g sachets containing 500 mg flunixin in boxes of 25; *Banamine® Granules* (Schering-Plough); (Rx). FDA-approved for use in horses.

Flunixin 16.5 mg/mL with Florfenicol 300 mg/mL Injection in 100 mL, 250 mL and 500 mL vials; *Resflor Gold®* (Intervet Schering); (Rx). FDA-approved for use in beef and non-lactating dairy cattle. Do not slaughter within 38 days of last treatment. Not for use in female dairy cattle 20 months of age or older or in calves to be processed for veal. Use may cause milk residues. A withdrawal period has not been established in preruminating calves. The ARCI (Racing Commissioners International) has designated this drug as a class 4 substance. See the appendix for more information.

HUMAN-LABELED PRODUCTS: None

References

Adamcak, A. & B. Otten (2000). Rodent Therapeutics. *Vet Clin NA: Exotic Anim Pract* 3:1(Jan): 221–240.

Anderson, D. (2006). Bovine Pain Management I & II. Proceedings: Western Vet Conf. Accessed via: Veterinary Information Network. http://goo.gl/r5BZ7

Belknap, J. (2008). Treatment of the horse at risk of laminitis. Proceedings: IVECCS. Accessed via: Veterinary Information Network. http://goo.gl/svItq

Blikslager, A. (2006). What's new in medicating for equine colic. Proceedings: Western Vet Conf. Accessed via: Veterinary Information Network. http://goo.gl/pw0Gq

Clyde, V. & J. Paul-Murphy (2000). Avian Analgesia. *Kirk's Current Veterinary Therapy: XIII Small Animal Practice*. J Bonagura Ed. Philadelphia, WB Saunders: 1126–1128.

Cutler, T. (2003). Neonatal foals: beyond corneal ulcers. Proceedings: ACVIM Forum. Accessed via: Veterinary Information Network. http://goo.gl/HiUNP

Fennell, L.C. & R.P. Franklin (2009). Do nonsteroidal anti-inflammatory drugs administered at therapeutic dosages induce gastric ulcers in horses? *Equine Veterinary Education* 21(12): 660–662.

Huerkamp, M. (1995). Anesthesia and postoperative management of rabbits and pocket pets. *Kirk's Current Veterinary Therapy:XII*. J Bonagura Ed. Philadelphia, W.B. Saunders: 1322–1327.

Ivey, E. & J. Morrisey (2000). Therapeutics for Rabbits. *Vet Clin NA: Exotic Anim Pract* 3:1(Jan): 183–216.

Johnson, S. (1996). Nonsteroidal antiinflammatory analgesics to manage acute pain in dogs and cats. *Comp CE*(October 1996): 1117–1123.

Moore, R. (2003). New developments in the treatment of reperfusion injury and acute laminitis in horses. Proceedings: ACVIM Forum. Accessed via: Veterinary Information Network. http://goo.gl/eqELM

Snyder, J. (2009). Anestheisa and pain management: Minor surgeries. Proceedings: WVC. Accessed via: Veterinary Information Network. http://goo.gl/ljAl5

Tams, T. (1999). Acute Diarrheal Diseases of the Dog and Cat. Proceedings: The North American Veterinary Conference, Orlando.

Videla, R. & F.M. Andrews (2009). New Perspectives in Equine Gastric Ulcer Syndrome. *Veterinary Clinics of North America-Equine Practice* 25(2): 283–+.

Walz, P. (2006). Practical management of pain in cattle. Proceedings: ABVP. Accessed via: Veterinary Information Network. http://goo.gl/hScVv

Williams, B. (2000). Therapeutics in Ferrets. *Vet Clin NA: Exotic Anim Pract* 3:1(Jan): 131–153.

5-Fluorocytosine–see Flucytosine

FLUOROURACIL (5-FU)

(flure-oh-**yoor**-a-sill)   Adrucil®

ANTINEOPLASTIC AGENT

Prescriber Highlights

▶ Antineoplastic agent used in dogs for susceptible tumors (see doses) & intra-lesionally in horses for skin tumors

▶ Contraindications: Do NOT use in any form on cats; Patients hypersensitive to it, in poor nutritional states, depressed bone marrow, serious infections

▶ Known teratogen

▶ Adverse Effects: Dose-dependent myelosuppression, GI toxicity, & neurotoxicity

Uses/Indications

Chemotherapeutic agent that has been used for canine mammary carcinoma (in combination with doxorubicin and cyclophosphamide—FAC protocol), dermal squamous cell carcinoma and GI tract tumors. It is also used topically and for intralesional injection with epinephrine into certain skin neoplasms (squamous cell carcinoma, melanoma, sarcoid) in horses.

Pharmacology/Actions

Fluorouracil is converted via intracellular mechanisms to active metabolites (fluoruridine monophosphate—FUMP and fluoruridine triphosphate—FUTP). FUMP inhibits the synthesis of deoxythymidine triphosphate thereby interfering with DNA synthesis. FUTP incorporates into RNA and inhibits cell function.

Pharmacokinetics

Fluorouracil is administered systemically via the IV route. It rapidly disappears from the systemic circulation (plasma half live is about 15 minutes in humans) and is primarily distributed into tumor cells, intestinal mucosa, liver, and bone marrow. While some of the drug is converted to active metabolites, (see Pharmacology above), the majority of it is metabolized by the liver. A small amount (about 15% of dose) is excreted unchanged into the urine.

Contraindications/Precautions/Warnings

Cats develop a severe, potentially fatal neurotoxicity when given fluorouracil. It is *contraindicated in cats* in any form (including topical).

5-FU is contraindicated in patients hypersensitive to it, in poor nutritional states, with depressed or reduced bone marrow function or concurrent serious infections.

Adverse Effects

In dogs, 5-FU causes a dose-dependent myelosuppression, GI toxicity (diarrhea, GI ulceration/sloughing, stomatitis), and neurotoxicity (seizures). Fluorouracil has a very narrow therapeutic index and should be used only by clinicians with experience using cancer chemotherapeutic agents.

Reproductive/Nursing Safety

The drug is a known teratogen and its use should be weighed against any risks to offspring. In humans, the FDA categorizes this drug as category *D* for use during pregnancy (*There is evidence of human fetal risk, but the potential benefits from the use of the drug in pregnant women may be acceptable despite its potential risks.*)

It is not known whether fluorouracil is excreted in milk. Because fluorouracil inhibits DNA, RNA and protein synthesis, milk replacer should be considered if the dam requires 5-FU.

Overdosage/Acute Toxicity

While overdoses are possible with IV use, careful checking of dosages and preparation should minimize the risks. Oral ingestions of topical products have occurred with dogs and cats and can be very serious The lowest reported toxic dose at which dogs show adverse signs is 8.6 mg/kg. Signs at lower doses include mild GI irritation and vomiting. Seizures and death have been reported at doses as low as 10.3 mg/kg (APCC database) and survival in dogs may be as low as 25% Very small ingestions can reportedly cause death in cats. Clinical signs may be seen within 30 minutes to 6 hours after ingestion; death has been reported in 7 hours. Clinical signs include acute nausea, vomiting, hemorrhagic diarrhea, abdominal pain, GI sloughing, ataxia, severe and non-responsive seizures, and severe dose-dependent myelosuppression affecting all cell lines. Severe metabolic acidosis and signs of multi-organ failure can be seen. (Lee 2010)

There were 90 exposures to fluorouracil reported to the ASPCA Animal Poison Control Center (APCC) during 2008–2009. In these cases 89 were dogs with 72 showing clinical signs and the remaining 1 case was a cat showing no clinical signs. Common findings in dogs recorded in decreasing frequency included vomiting, seizures, ataxia, disorientation, euthanasia, lethargy, and death.

Should an oral ingestion occur, aggressive GI decontamination with GI protection should be done, especially if the ingestion was very recent.

However, decontamination may not be effective due to the rapid onset of toxicity. Treatment is primarily supportive and can include antiemetics, anticonvulsants, fluid support, etc. Intensive monitoring is required. Seizure control with diazepam is often unrewarding and a barbiturate or general anesthesia is often required. Control of pain and body temperature are important. Use broad-spectrum antibiotics to prevent secondary bacterial infections. If bone marrow suppression develops, filgrastim (*Neupogen®*) can be considered to stimulate bone marrow stem cell proliferation in dogs. Complete blood counts should be routinely performed (every 3-4 days) for at least 18 days, as it may take up to 3 weeks before all cell lines return to normal (Lee 2010).

Patients given an accidental parenteral overdose should undergo intensive hematologic monitoring for at least 4 weeks and be supported as required.

Drug Interactions

The following drug interactions have either been reported or are theoretical in humans or animals receiving fluorouracil and may be of significance in veterinary patients:

■ **LEUCOVORIN:** May increase the GI toxic effects of 5-FU

Laboratory Considerations

■ Fluorouracil may cause increases in alkaline phosphatase, serum transaminase, serum bilirubin, and lactic dehydrogenase

Doses

Note: Because of the potential toxicity of this drug to patients, veterinary personnel and clients, and since chemotherapy indications, treatment protocols, monitoring and safety guidelines often change, the following dosages should be used only as a general guide. Consultation with a veterinary oncologist and referral to current veterinary oncology references [*e.g.*, (Henry & Higginbotham 2009); (Argyle *et al.* 2008); (Withrow & Vail 2007); (Villalobos 2007); (Ogilvie & Moore 2006); (Ogilvie & Moore 2001)] is *strongly recommended.*

■ **DOGS:**

a) For canine mammary carcinoma (in combination with doxorubicin and cyclophosphamide—FAC protocol), dermal squamous cell carcinoma and GI tract tumors: 150 mg/m^2 IV weekly, or 5–10 mg/kg IV weekly (Kitchell & Dhaliwal 2000)

■ **CATS:**

5-FU is CONTRAINDICATED in cats in any form (including topical)

■ **HORSES:**

a) For intratumoral injection with epinephrine into certain skin neoplasms (squamous cell carcinoma, melanoma, sarcoid): 0.3 mL of 1:1000 epinephrine is added to each mL of 5-FU solution up to a maximum of 3 mL of epinephrine per total volume of 5-FU injected. Epinephrine may result in white hair growth and can cause transient excitation, tachycardia, and shaking if absorbed systemically in sufficient quantities. (Moll 2002)

Monitoring

■ CBC's (nadirs usually occur between days 9–14 with recovery by day 30; no dog info located)

■ GI and CNS adverse effects

■ Efficacy

Client Information

■ Clients should understand the serious potential effects of the drug (including death) and be committed for follow-up monitoring

Chemistry/Synonyms

A pyrimidine antagonist antineoplastic agent, fluorouracil (5-FU) occurs as a white, practically odorless, crystalline powder. It is sparingly soluble in water and slightly soluble in alcohol. The commercially available injection has its pH adjusted to 8.6–9.4 and may be colorless or slightly yellow in color.

Fluorouracil may also be known as 5-fluorouracil, fluorouracilo, fluorouracilum, 5-FU, NSC-19893, Ro-2-9757, and WR-69596; many trade names are available.

Storage/Stability

The injection should be stored between 15–30°C; avoid freezing and exposure to light. Slight color changes in the solution can be ignored. If a precipitate forms, the solution can be heated to 60°C and shaken vigorously to redissolve the drug. Cool to body temperature before administering. If unsuccessful in redissolving the drug, it should not be used.

Dosage Forms/Regulatory Status

VETERINARY-LABELED PRODUCTS: None

HUMAN-LABELED PRODUCTS:

Fluorouracil Injection: 50 mg/mL in 10 mL, 20 mL, 50 mL, & 100 mL vials and 10 mL amps; *Adrucil*® (Gensia Sicor); generic; (Rx)

Also available in topical creams and solutions in concentrations ranging from 0.5% to 5%. These are indicated in humans for treating multiple actinic or solar keratoses, and superficial basal cell carcinomas (5%) when other treatments are impractical.

References

Argyle, D., M. Brearly, et al. (2008). *Decision Making in Small Animal Oncology*, Wiley-Blackwell.
Henry, C. & M. Higginbotham (2009). *Cancer Management in Small Animal Practice*, Saunders.
Kitchell, B. & R. Dhaliwal (2000). CVT Update: Anticancer Drugs and Protocols Using Traditional Drugs. *Kirk's Current Veterinary Therapy: XIII Small Animal Practice*. J Bonagura Ed. Philadelphia, WB Saunders: 465–473.
Lee, J.A. (2010). Top Ten Small Animal Toxins: Recognition, Diagnosis, Treatment. Proceedings: ACVIM. Accessed

via: Veterinary Information Network. http://goo.gl/KM7ta
Moll, H. (2002). Skin tumor management. Proceedings: Western Veterinary Conference. Accessed via: Veterinary Information Network. http://goo.gl/xtUEh
Ogilvie, G. & A. Moore (2001). *Feline Oncology: A Comprehensive Guide to Compassionate Care*, Veterinary Learning Systems.
Ogilvie, G. & A. Moore (2001). *Managing the Canine Cancer Patient: A Practical Guide to Compassionate Care*, Veterinary Learning Systems.
Villalobos, A. (2007). *Canine and Feline Geriatric Oncology*. Ames, Blackwell.
Withrow, S. & D. Vail (2007). *Withrow and MacEwen's Small Animal Clinical Oncology 4th Ed.* Philadelphia, Elsevier.

FLUOXETINE HCL

(**floo-ox**-e-teen)   Prozac®, Reconcile®

SELECTIVE SEROTONIN-REUPTAKE INHIBITOR (SSRI)

Prescriber Highlights

▶ A selective-serotonin reuptake inhibitor antidepressant used in dogs & cats for a variety of behavior disorders

▶ Contraindications: Patients with known hypersensitivity or receiving monoamine oxidase inhibitors

▶ Caution: Patients with diabetes mellitus or seizure disorders; dosages may need to be reduced in patients with severe hepatic impairment

▶ Adverse Effects: *Dogs:* Anorexia, lethargy, GI effects, anxiety, irritability, insomnia/hyperactivity, or panting, & aggressive behavior in previously unaggressive dogs is possible; *Cats:* May exhibit behavior changes (anxiety, irritability, sleep disturbances), anorexia, & changes in elimination patterns

▶ Drug Interactions

Uses/Indications

Fluoxetine may be beneficial for the treatment of canine aggression, stereotypic behaviors (and other obsessive-compulsive behaviors), and anxiety. It may be useful in cats for the aforementioned behaviors and, additionally, for inappropriate elimination.

The veterinary FDA-approved product (*Reconcile®*) has a labeled indication for the treatment of canine separation anxiety in conjunction with a behavior modification plan.

Pharmacology/Actions

Fluoxetine is a highly selective inhibitor of the reuptake of serotonin in the CNS thereby potentiating the pharmacologic activity of serotonin. Fluoxetine apparently has little effect on other neurotransmitters (*e.g.*, dopamine or norepinephrine). In dogs and cats, fluoxetine has anxiolytic and anticompulsive effects, and may also reduce aggressive behaviors.

Pharmacokinetics

Fluoxetine is apparently well absorbed after oral administration. In a study done in beagles, approximately 70% of an oral dose reached the systemic circulation. The presence of food altered the rate, but not the extent, of absorption. The oral capsules and oral liquid apparently are bioequivalent. When applied transdermally (15% in a PLO gel) to cats, bioavailability was approximately 10% of the oral route (Ciribassi *et al.* 2003).

Fluoxetine and its principal metabolite, norfluoxetine (active), are apparently distributed throughout the body with highest levels found in the lungs and the liver. CNS concentrations are detected within one hour of dosing. In humans, fluoxetine is approximately 95% bound to plasma proteins. Fluoxetine crosses the placenta in rats, but it is unknown if it does so in other species. Fluoxetine enters maternal milk in concentrations about 20–30% of those found in plasma.

Fluoxetine is primarily metabolized in the liver to a variety of metabolites, including norfluoxetine (active). Both fluoxetine and norfluoxetine are eliminated slowly. In humans, the elimination half-life of fluoxetine is about 2–3 days and norfluoxetine, about 7–9 days. In dogs, elimination half-life average for fluoxetine is about 6+ hours and for norfluoxetine, about 2 days; wide interpatient variation does occur, however. Renal impairment does not apparently affect elimination rates substantially, but liver impairment will decrease clearance rates.

Contraindications/Precautions/Warnings

The labeling for the veterinary (canine) FDA-approved drug states that fluoxetine should not be used in dogs with epilepsy or a history of seizures, and should not be given with drugs that lower the seizure threshold (*e.g.*, acepromazine, chlorpromazine). Fluoxetine is contraindicated in patients with known hypersensitivity to it, as well as those receiving monoamine oxidase inhibitors (see Drug Interactions below).

Fluoxetine should be used with caution in patients with diabetes mellitus as it may alter blood glucose. Dosages may need to be reduced in patients with severe hepatic impairment.

Because of the long half-life of norfluoxetine, tapering off the drug is probably only necessary when a patient has been on the drug long-term (>8 weeks) (Landsberg 2008).

Adverse Effects

In multi-site field trials in dogs, seizures were reported in some of the dogs treated with fluoxetine. Absolute causality and incidence rate has not been determined. Fluoxetine may cause lethargy, GI effects, anxiety, irritability, insomnia/hyperactivity, or panting. Anorexia is a common side-affect in dogs (usually transient and may be negated by temporarily increasing the palatability of food and/or hand feeding). Some dogs have persistent anorexia that precludes further treatment. Aggressive behavior in previously unaggressive dogs has been reported. Cats may exhibit behavior changes (anxiety, irritability, sleep disturbances), anorexia, and changes in elimination patterns.

In humans, potential adverse effects are extensive and diverse, but most those most commonly noted include anxiety, nervousness, insomnia, drowsiness, fatigue, dizziness, anorexia, nausea, rash, diarrhea, and sweating; seizures or hepatotoxicity are possible. About 15% of human patients discontinue treatment due to adverse effects.

Reproductive/Nursing Safety

Fluoxetine's safety during pregnancy has not been established. The canine FDA-approved product states that studies to determine the effects of fluoxetine in breeding, pregnant, or lactating dogs or in patients less than 6 months of age have not been conducted. Preliminary studies done in rats demonstrated no overt teratogenic effects. In humans, the FDA categorizes this drug as category **C** for use during pregnancy (*Animal studies have shown an adverse effect on the fetus, but there are no adequate studies in humans; or there are no animal reproduction studies and no adequate studies in humans.*)

The drug is excreted into milk (20–30% of plasma levels), so caution is advised in nursing patients. Clinical implications for nursing offspring are not clear.

Overdosage/Acute Toxicity

The LD_{50} for rats is 452 mg/kg. Five of six dogs given an oral "toxic" dose developed seizures that immediately stopped after giving IV diazepam. The dog having the lowest plasma level of fluoxetine that developed seizures had a level twice that expected of a human taking 80 mg day (highest recommended dose.)

There were 363 exposures to fluoxetine reported to the ASPCA Animal Poison Control Center (APCC) during 2008-2009. In these cases 293 were dogs with 59 showing clinical signs, 68 were cats with 17 showing clinical signs. The remaining reported cases were 2 birds showing no clinical signs. Common findings in dogs recorded in decreasing frequency included vomiting, mydriasis, lethargy, and hyperactivity. Common findings in cats recorded in decreasing frequency included hypersalivation, vomiting, mydriasis, and vocalization.

Treatment of fluoxetine overdoses consists of symptomatic and supportive therapy. Gut emptying techniques should be employed when warranted and otherwise not contraindicated. Diazepam should be considered to treat seizures. Cyproheptadine can be used as a serotonin antagonist.

Drug Interactions

The following drug interactions have either been reported or are theoretical in humans or animals

596 FLUOXETINE HCL

receiving fluoxetine and may be of significance in veterinary patients:

- **BUSPIRONE:** Increased risk for serotonin syndrome
- **CYPROHEPTADINE:** May decrease or reverse the effects of SSRIs
- **DIAZEPAM, ALPRAZOLAM:** Fluoxetine may increase diazepam levels
- **DIURETICS:** Increased risk for hyponatremia
- **INSULIN:** May alter insulin requirements
- **ISONIAZID:** Increased risk for serotonin syndrome
- **MAO INHIBITORS** (including **amitraz** and potentially, **selegiline**): High risk for serotonin syndrome; use contraindicated; in humans, a 5 week washout period is required after discontinuing fluoxetine and a 2 week washout period if first discontinuing the MAO inhibitor
- **PENTAZOCINE:** Serotonin syndrome-like adverse effects possible
- **PHENYTOIN:** Increased plasma levels of phenytoin possible
- **PROPRANOLOL, METOPROLOL:** Fluoxetine may increase these beta-blocker's plasma levels; atenolol may be safer to use if fluoxetine required
- **TRAMADOL:** SSRI's can inhibit the metabolism of tramadol to the active metabolites decreasing its efficacy and increasing the risk of toxicity (serotonin syndrome, seizures).
- **TRICYCLIC ANTIDEPRESSANTS (e.g., clomipramine, amitriptyline):** Fluoxetine may increase TCA blood levels and may increase the risk for serotonin syndrome
- **TRAZODONE:** Increased plasma levels of trazodone possible
- **WARFARIN:** Fluoxetine may increase the risk for bleeding

Doses

- **DOGS:**
  For the adjunctive treatment of behavior disorders (see Indications above):
  a) For the treatment of canine separation anxiety in conjunction with a behavior modification plan: 1–2 mg/kg PO once daily (Label Information; *Reconcile®*—Lilly)
  b) For separation anxiety and noise aversions: 1–2 mg/kg PO once daily with behavioral therapy. May use long-term. Continue medication until 2 months after a satisfactory response and then discontinue gradually if possible; behavioral management program should continue. Animals that relapse may resume therapy. Some dogs may require life-long treatment at the lowest effective dose. During seasonal noise fears, may add a benzodiazepine. (Sherman & Mills 2008)

c) For adjunctive pharmacological intervention for conflict-related aggression: 1–2 mg/kg PO once a day. May take up to 4 weeks for efficacy. (Luescher & Reisner 2008)
d) For compulsive disorders: 1–2 mg/kg PO once daily (Irimajiri *et al.* 2009)
e) 1–1.5 mg/kg PO once daily (Seibert 2003)
f) 1 mg/kg PO once daily (up to 3 mg/kg PO once daily) (Landsberg 2004)

- **CATS:**
  a) For adjunctive treatment of aggression: 0.5–1.5 mg/kg PO once daily. (Curtis 2008)
  b) To help control urine marking or separation anxiety: 0.5–1 mg/kg (2.5–5 mg per cat) PO once daily. (Levine 2008), (Neilson 2006b); (Neilson 2006a)
  c) To control pruritus when other therapies have failed: 1–5 mg/cat PO once daily; advise obtaining baseline lab work. Assess therapy after 1–4 weeks. Taper off dose over 6–8 weeks. (Messinger 2000)
  d) For generalized anxiety disorder: 0.5–1.5 mg/kg PO once daily (Crowell-Davis 2009), (Landsberg 2004)

Monitoring
- Efficacy
- Adverse effects; including appetite (weight)

Client Information
- This medication is most effective when used with a behavior modification program
- Keep this medication away from children and other pets
- Most commonly reported adverse effects with use of this medication include: lethargy/depression, decreased appetite, vomiting, shaking, tremor, restlessness, diarrhea, and excessive vocalization (whining); if these are severe or persist, contact your veterinarian
- Do not stop this medication abruptly without veterinarian's guidance
- Rarely, dogs may develop seizures (convulsion) while receiving this medication; contact veterinarian immediately should this occur

Chemistry/Synonyms
A member of the phenylpropylamine-derivative antidepressant group, fluoxetine differs both structurally and pharmacologically from either the tricyclic or monoamine oxidase inhibitor antidepressants. Fluoxetine HCl occurs as a white to off-white crystalline solid. Approximately 50 mg are soluble in 1 mL of water.

Fluoxetine may also be known as: fluoxetini hydrochloridum, and LY-110140; many trade names are available.

Storage/Stability

Capsules and tablets should be stored in well-closed containers at room temperature. The oral liquid should be stored in tight, light-resistant containers at room temperature.

Dosage Forms/Regulatory Status

VETERINARY-LABELED PRODUCTS:

Fluoxetine Chewable Tablets: 8 mg, 16 mg, 32 mg, & 64 mg; *Reconcile®* (Lilly); (Rx). FDA-approved for use in dogs.

The ARCI (Racing Commissioners International) has designated this drug as a class 2 substance. See the appendix for more information.

HUMAN-LABELED PRODUCTS:

Fluoxetine HCl Oral Tablets: 10 mg, 15 mg & 20 mg; generic; (Rx)

Fluoxetine HCl Oral Capsules: 10 mg, 20 mg, 40 mg & 90 mg (delayed-release only); *Prozac® Pulvules* & *Prozac® Weekly* (Eli Lilly/Dista); *Sarafem® Pulvules* (Warner Chilcott); generic; (Rx)

Fluoxetine HCl Oral Solution 20 mg/5 mL (may contain alcohol, sucrose) in 120 mL & 473 mL; *Prozac®* (Eli Lilly/Dista); generic; (Rx)

References

Ciribassi, J., A. Luescher, et al. (2003). Comparative bioavailability of fluoxetine after transdermal and oral administration to healthy cats. *American Journal of Veterinary Research* 64(8): 994–998.

Crowell-Davis, S.L. (2009). Generalized Anxiety Disorder. *Compendium-Continuing Education for Veterinarians* 31(9): 427–430.

Curtis, T. (2008). Human-directed aggression in the cat. *Vet Clin NA: Sm Anim Pract* 38: 1131–1143.

Irimajiri, M., A.U. Luescher, et al. (2009). Randomized, controlled clinical trial of the efficacy of fluoxetine for treatment of compulsive disorders in dogs. *Javma-Journal of the American Veterinary Medical Association* 235(6): 705–709.

Landsberg, G. (2004). A behaviorists approach to compulsive disorders. Proceedings: ACVIM Forum, Minneapolis. Accessed via: Veterinary Information Network. http://goo.gl/eRUh2

Landsberg, G. (2008). Treating canine and feline anxiety: Drug therapy and pheromones. Proceedings: BSAVA. Accessed via: Veterinary Information Network. http://goo.gl/3ci5J

Levine, E. (2008). Feline Fear and Anxiety. *Vet Clin NA: Sm Anim Pract* 38: 1065–1079.

Luescher, A.U. & I.R. Reisner (2008). Canine aggression toward familiar people: A new look at an old problem. *Vet Clin NA: Sm Anim Pract* 38: 1107–1130.

Messinger, L. (2000). Pruritis Therapy in the Cat. *Kirk's Current Veterinary Therapy: XIII Small Animal Practice.* J Bonagura Ed. Philadelphia, WB Saunders: 542–545.

Neilson, J. (2006a). The fearful feline. BSAV Congress Proceedings. Accessed via: Veterinary Information Network. http://goo.gl/SHfh5

Neilson, J. (2006b). Pee-Mail: The ultimate form of feline communication. BSAV Congress Proceedings. Accessed via: Veterinary Information Network. http://goo.gl/RtUry

Seibert, L. (2003). Antidepressants in behavioral medicine. Proceedings: Western Veterinary Conference. Accessed via: Veterinary Information Network. http://goo.gl/LyQ8m

Sherman, B.L. & D.S. Mills (2008). Canine anxieties and phobias: An update on separation anxiety and noise aversions. *Veterinary Clinics of North America-Small Animal Practice* 38(5): 1081–+.

FLUTICASONE PROPIONATE

(floo-*ti*-ca-sone) Flovent®

GLUCOCORTICOID, INHALED/TOPICAL

Prescriber Highlights

▶ Glucocorticoid used most commonly in veterinary medicine as an inhaled aerosol

▶ Has shown efficacy in treating feline asthma, dogs with chronic cough, & in horses for recurrent airway obstruction or inflammatory airway disease

▶ May be useful as a nasally inhaled treatment for allergy-related rhinosinusitis

▶ Appears to be well tolerated; suppression of HPA axis possible

■ Must be used with a species-appropriate delivery device

▶ Expense may be an issue

Uses/Indications

While there are topical forms of fluticasone, most veterinary interests are in the inhaled versions of the drug. The aerosol for pulmonary inhalation appears to be effective in treating feline asthma, recurrent airway obstruction (RAO, heaves) or inflammatory airway disease (IAD) in horses, and dogs with chronic tracheobronchial disease. While the majority of small animal use has been with fluticasone, there are several other aerosol corticosteroids for inhalation (beclomethasone dipropionate, flunisolide, and triamcinolone acetonide) that theoretically could be used for the same purpose. The nasal inhalation corticosteroid products may be useful for allergy-related chronic rhinosinusitis in cats and dogs.

Pharmacology/Actions

Like other glucocorticoids, fluticasone has potent antiinflammatory activity. Fluticasone has an affinity 18X that of dexamethasone for human glucocorticoid receptors. For a more thorough discussion of glucocorticoid effects, refer to the Glucocorticoids, General Information monograph.

Pharmacokinetics

In humans, when fluticasone aerosol is administered via the lung, about 30% is absorbed into the systemic circulation. In humans, a dose of 880 micrograms (4 puffs of the 220 microgram aerosol) showed peak plasma concentrations of 0.1 to 1 ng/mL. Volume of distribution averages 4.2 L/kg and it is 91% bound to human plasma proteins. Fluticasone is metabolized via cytochrome P450 3A4 isoenzymes to a metabolite with negligible pharmacologic activity. Terminal elimination half-life is about 8 hours. Most of the drug is excreted in the feces as parent drug and metabolites.

Contraindications/Precautions/Warnings

Fluticasone is contraindicated when patients are hypersensitive to it or during acute bronchospasm (status asthmaticus).

Adverse Effects

In humans, the most likely adverse effects are pharyngitis and upper respiratory infections. While inhaled steroids generally cause significantly fewer adverse effects than injectable or oral therapy, suppression of the HPA axis can potentially occur. However, one study in cats using different concentrations of inhaled fluticasone, did not show any significant HPAA suppression at any of the doses used (Cohn *et al.* 2010). When transferring patients from systemic steroid therapy to inhaled steroids, wean slowly off systemic therapy to avoid acute adrenal insufficiency. Prepare to cover patients with additional steroid therapy during periods of acute stress, severe asthma attacks occurring during the withdrawal stage, or after transfer to inhaled steroids. Fluticasone is not useful for acute bronchospasm; cases of fluticasone-induced bronchospasm have been reported in humans.

Reproductive/Nursing Safety

In humans, the FDA categorizes inhaled fluticasone as a category *C* drug for use during pregnancy (*Animal studies have shown an adverse effect on the fetus, but there are no adequate studies in humans; or there are no animal reproduction studies and no adequate studies in humans*). When given subcutaneously to laboratory animals, fluticasone caused a variety of teratogenic effects, including growth retardation, cleft palate, omphalocele and retarded cranial ossification. It should be used during pregnancy only when the benefits clearly outweigh the risks of therapy.

It is not known if the drug enters maternal milk; use with caution in nursing dams.

Overdosage/Acute Toxicity

Acute overdoses of this medication are unlikely, but there have been reported cases of dogs puncturing canisters of albuterol and developing adverse effects. A similar occurrence with fluticasone would unlikely require treatment. Chronic overdoses could result in significant HPA axis suppression and cushinoid effects.

Drug Interactions

While the manufacturer states that due to the low systemic plasma levels associated with inhalational therapy clinically significant drug interactions are unlikely, use caution when used in conjunction with other drugs (such as **ketoconazole**) that can inhibit CYP 3A4 isoenzymes; theoretically, fluticasone levels could be increased.

Laboratory Considerations

- No specific laboratory interactions or considerations were noted.

Doses

■ CATS:

For treatment of feline "asthma":

a) Initially, try the 44 micrograms/puff MDI: one puff q12h. In the study, all three dosages (44 micrograms, 110 micrograms and 220 micrograms) significantly reduced the proportion of eosinophils in airway lavage fluid. (Cohn *et al.* 2010)

b) For cats with signs of bronchial disease that occur more than once per week:

Give prednisolone at 1–2 mg/kg PO twice daily for 5-7 days. Most newly diagnosed cats will have greatly diminished signs; then the dose is slowly tapered over at least 2-3 months. Some cats are effectively managed by low dose, alternate day corticosteroids, but most will continue to wheeze/cough. For those, encourage inhaled corticosteroids such as fluticasone.

Use a delivery device (*e.g.*, AeroKat®) in combination with a spacer and 110 micrograms fluticasone metered dose inhaler (MDI) and administer one puff twice daily. Cats with more serious disease may require the 220 micrograms MDI. Author has not found the 44 microgram inhaler to provide consistent clinical results.

Attach MDI and the facemask to the spacer. Place facemask gently over cats mouth and nose and actuates the MDI to fill the spacer with medication. The cat breathes in and out for 7–10 times with the mask in place. (Padrid 2006), (Padrid 2008)

■ DOGS:

For adjunctive treatment of chronic tracheobronchial disease:

a) In dogs with excessive side effects associated with oral steroids therapy: Use a delivery device (*e.g.*, AeroDawg®) in combination with either fluticasone 220 microgram or 110 microgram (1 puff) twice daily. Ensure a tightly fitting face mask and counting 7–10 respirations after actuating the MDI into the spacer is important for optimizing therapy. (Johnson 2007)

b) Using the 220 micrograms/puff MDI: 2 puffs q12h. (Hawkins 2009)

■ HORSES:

Use a delivery device (*e.g.*, Aeromask® or Equine-haler®) in combination with a metered dose inhaler:

a) For the prototypical young racehorse with IAD: Weeks 1 and 2: Fluticasone 2200 micrograms (10 puffs) twice daily or beclomethasone HFA 1000 mg (5 puffs) twice daily with albuterol 450 micrograms (5 puffs) prior to steroid inhaler and at approximately 30 minutes before exercise. Weeks 3 and 4: Fluticasone 2200 micrograms (10 puffs) once daily or beclomethasone HFA 1000 mg (5 puffs) twice daily. Recheck in 4 weeks to determine further treatment.

For the typical horse with moderate RAO (heaves): Begin stringent control of environment and a course of systemic prednisone therapy. (**Note:** Reference does not state when oral prednisone should be discontinued.) At week 3 add fluticasone 2200 micrograms (10 puffs) twice daily with salmeterol 210 micrograms (10 puffs) twice daily. Week 4: fluticasone 2200 micrograms (10 puffs) once daily with salmeterol 210 micrograms (10 puffs) once daily. If lung function shows a good response at end of 4 weeks: fluticasone 2200 micrograms (10 puffs) once every other day with salmeterol 210 micrograms (10 puffs) once daily. (Mazan 2002); (Mazan 2003)

b) Using the EquineHaler: 6 mg q12h. In the study this dose was as effective as dexamethasone (0.1 mg/kg IV) for prevention of exacerbations, but not as effective as dexamethasone for short-term treatment. It is highly likely that a lower dose of fluticasone can be used. (Robinson *et al.* 2009)

Monitoring

■ Efficacy

Client Information

■ Before using, shake well and, if possible, bring canister to room temperature. Do not puncture or incinerate can. Must be used with a spacer device appropriate for the species being treated.

■ Allow animal to breath with the mask on for 7–10 times before removing

■ One puff twice a day will last approximately 2 months

Chemistry/Synonyms

A trifluorinated glucocorticoid, fluticasone propionate occurs as a white to off-white powder that is practically insoluble in water and slightly soluble in ethanol.

Fluticasone may also be known as: CCI-18781, fluticasoni propionas, *Advair Diskus®*, *Cutovate®*, *Flixotide®*, *Flixonase®*, *Flovent®*, and *Flutivate®*.

Storage/Stability

Fluticasone propionate aerosol for inhalation (*Flovent®*) should be stored between 2–30°C (36–86°F); protect from freezing and direct sunlight. Store canister with the mouthpiece down.

Dosage Forms/Regulatory Status

VETERINARY-LABELED PRODUCTS: None
HUMAN-LABELED PRODUCTS:

Fluticasone Propionate aerosol for inhalation: 44 micrograms per actuation, 110 micrograms per actuation, 220 micrograms per actuation in 10.6 g & 12 g canisters with actuator. Each canister contains approximately 120-metered inhalations; *Flovent® HFA & Diskus* (GlaxoSmithKline); (Rx)

Fluticasone is also available commercially in combination as:

Fluticasone Propionate/Salmeterol Powder for Inhalation: 100 mcg fluticasone propionate, 50 mcg salmeterol; 250 mcg fluticasone propionate, 50 mcg salmeterol; & 500 mcg fluticasone propionate, 50 mcg salmeterol) in color-coded blisters; *Advair Diskus®* (GlaxoSmithKline); (Rx)

Fluticasone Propionate/Salmeterol Aerosol for Inhalation: 45 mcg fluticasone propionate/salmeterol 21 mcg per actuation; 115 mcg fluticasone propionate /salmeterol 21 mcg per actuation & 230 mcg fluticasone propionate/salmeterol 21 mcg per actuation equiv. to salmeterol xinafoate 30.45 mcg in 12 g pressurized canisters containing 120 metered inhalations.

Nasal solutions, topical creams and ointments containing fluticasone are also available.

References

Cohn, L.A., A.E. DeClue, et al. (2010). Effects of fluticasone propionate dosage in anexperimental model of feline asthma. *Jnl Fel Med Surg* 12: 91–96.

Hawkins, E. (2009). Treating Canine Chronic Bronchitis: Revisiting the Basics. Proceedings: WVC. Accessed via: Veterinary Information Network. http://goo.gl/R2I3v

Johnson, L. (2007). The coughing dog. Proceedings: Univ Cal-Davis Canine Medicine Symposium. Accessed via: Veterinary Information Network. http://goo.gl/GmC6o

Mazan, M. (2002). Inhaled Drugs: The hows, whys, and whens in prescribing. Proceedings: TUFTS 2002. Accessed via: Veterinary Information Network. http://goo.gl/2W58M

Mazan, M. (2003). Use of aerosolized bronchodilators and corticosteroids. *Current Therapy in Equine Medicine 5.* N Robinson Ed., Saunders: 440–445.

Padrid, P. (2006). Diagnosis and therapy of feline asthma. Proceedings: ACVIM 2006. http://goo.gl/ovF3z

Padrid, P. (2008). Inhaled Steroids to Treat Feline Lower Airway Disease: 300 Cases 1995–2007. Proceedings: ACVIM. Accessed via: Veterinary Information Network. http://goo.gl/zHJyO

Robinson, N.E., C. Berney, et al. (2009). Fluticasone Propionate Aerosol is More Effective for Prevention than Treatment of Recurrent Airway Obstruction. *Journal of Veterinary Internal Medicine* 23(6): 1247–1253.

FLUVOXAMINE MALEATE

(floo-vox-a-meen) Luvox®

SELECTIVE SEROTONIN-REUPTAKE INHIBITOR (SSRI)

Prescriber Highlights

▶ A selective-serotonin reuptake inhibitor (SSRI) antidepressant similar to fluoxetine; used in dogs & cats for a variety of behavior disorders

▶ Not commonly used

▶ Contraindications: Patients with known hypersensitivity or receiving MAOIs

▶ Must treat for 6–8 weeks before evaluating efficacy

▶ Caution: Patients with severe cardiac, renal or hepatic disease; dosages may need to be reduced in patients with severe renal or hepatic impairment

▶ Adverse effect profile not well established: Potentially, Dogs: Anorexia, lethargy, GI effects, anxiety, irritability, insomnia/hyperactivity, or panting; aggressive behavior in previously non-aggressive dogs possible. Cats: May exhibit sedation, decreased appetite/anorexia, vomiting, diarrhea, behavior changes (anxiety, irritability, sleep disturbances), & changes in elimination patterns

▶ Drug-drug interactions

Uses/Indications

Fluvoxamine may be considered for use in treating a variety of behavior-related diagnoses in dogs and cats, including aggression and stereotypic behaviors (and other obsessive-compulsive behaviors).

Pharmacology/Actions

Fluvoxamine is a highly selective inhibitor of the reuptake of serotonin in the CNS thereby potentiating the pharmacologic activity of serotonin. Fluvoxamine apparently has little effect on dopamine or norepinephrine, and apparently no effect on other neurotransmitters.

Pharmacokinetics

There is limited data on the pharmacokinetics of fluvoxamine in domestic animals. In dogs, fluvoxamine appears to be completely absorbed; only about 10% of a dose is excreted unchanged in the urine. Half-life appears to be similar to humans (15 hours).

In humans, fluvoxamine is absorbed after oral administration, but bioavailability is only around 50%. Peak plasma concentrations occur between 3–8 hours post-dose. Food does not appear to affect the absorptive characteristics of the drug. Fluvoxamine is widely distributed in the body and about 80% bound to plasma proteins. The drug is extensively metabolized in the liver to non-active metabolites and eliminated in the urine. Plasma half-life is about 15 hours.

Contraindications/Precautions/Warnings

Fluvoxamine is contraindicated in patients hypersensitive to it or any SSRI or if the patient is receiving a monoamine oxidase inhibitor (MAOI) or cisapride. Consider using a lower dosage in patients with hepatic impairment or in geriatric patients.

Adverse Effects

The adverse effect profile of fluvoxamine in dogs or cats has not been well established. In dogs, SSRIs can cause lethargy, GI effects, anxiety, irritability, insomnia/hyperactivity, or panting. Anorexia is a common side effect in dogs (usually transient and may be negated by temporarily increasing the palatability of food and/or hand feeding). Some dogs have persistent anorexia that precludes further treatment. Aggressive behavior in previously non-aggressive dogs has been reported. SSRIs in cats can cause sedation, decreased appetite/anorexia, vomiting, diarrhea, behavior changes (anxiety, irritability, sleep disturbances), and changes in elimination patterns.

In humans, common adverse reactions (>10%) include sexual side effects (abnormal ejaculation, anorgasmia), agitation/nervousness, insomnia, nausea, dry mouth, constipation/diarrhea, dyspepsia, dizziness, headache, and somnolence

Reproductive/Nursing Safety

In humans, the FDA categorizes fluvoxamine as a category *C* drug for use during pregnancy (*Animal studies have shown an adverse effect on the fetus, but there are no adequate studies in humans; or there are no animal reproduction studies and no adequate studies in humans*). In rats, fluvoxamine reportedly increased pup mortality at birth and was associated with decreased birth weights.

Fluvoxamine enters maternal milk, although it appears unlikely to be of significant clinical concern.

Overdosage/Acute Toxicity

Limited data exists for animals. Reportedly, any dosage over 10 mg/kg can cause tremors and lethargy. Other signs associated with overdoses may include vomiting, somnolence/coma, tremors, diarrhea, hypotension, heart rate/rhythm disturbances (bradycardia/tachycardia, ECG changes), seizures, etc.

Cyproheptadine may be useful in the adjunctive treatment of serotonin syndrome.

Fatalities have been reported in human overdoses; the highest reported dose where the patient survived was 10,000 mg. Treatment recommendations include standard protocols for drug adsorption/removal from the GI for potentially dangerous overdoses and symptomatic and supportive therapy. Serotonin effects may be negated somewhat by administration (oral or rectal) with cyproheptadine at a dose of 1.1 mg/kg. Seizures or other neurologic signs may be treated with diazepam. The drug has an elimination half-life of approximately 15 hours in dogs.

Drug Interactions

The following drug interactions have either been reported or are theoretical in humans or animals receiving fluvoxamine and may be of significance in veterinary patients:

- **BUSPIRONE:** Fluvoxamine may paradoxically decrease the clinical efficacy of buspirone
- **CISAPRIDE:** Fluvoxamine may increase plasma levels of cisapride leading to toxicity
- **CYPROHEPTADINE:** May decrease or reverse the effects of SSRIs
- **DIAZEPAM, ALPRAZOLAM, MIDAZOLAM:** Fluvoxamine may increase diazepam levels
- **DILTIAZEM:** Fluvoxamine may increase the effects of diltiazem; bradycardia has been reported in humans taking this drug combination
- **MAO INHIBITORS (including amitraz and potentially, selegiline):** High risk for serotonin syndrome; use contraindicated; in humans, a 5 week washout period is required after discontinuing fluvoxamine and a 2 week washout period if first discontinuing the MAO inhibitor
- **METHADONE:** Fluvoxamine may increase plasma levels of methadone, leading to toxicity
- **PHENYTOIN:** Increased plasma levels of phenytoin possible
- **PROPRANOLOL, METOPROLOL:** Fluvoxamine may increase these beta-blocker's plasma levels; atenolol may be safer to use if fluoxetine required
- **THEOPHYLLINE:** Fluvoxamine may increase plasma levels of theophylline
- **TRAMADOL:** SSRI's can inhibit the metabolism of tramadol to the active metabolites decreasing its efficacy and increasing the risk of toxicity (serotonin syndrome, seizures)
- **TRICYCLIC ANTIDEPRESSANTS (e.g., clomipramine, amitriptyline):** Fluvoxamine may increase TCA blood levels and may increase the risk for serotonin syndrome
- **WARFARIN:** Fluvoxamine may increase the risk for bleeding

Laboratory Considerations

No fluvoxamine-related laboratory interactions noted.

Doses

- **DOGS:**
  a) For treatment of compulsive disorders: 0.5–2 mg/kg PO twice daily (Landsberg 2004)
  b) 1–3 mg/kg PO once daily (q24h); (allow 8 weeks for initial trial). (Virga 2007)

  c) For treatment of behavioral diagnoses: 1 mg/kg PO q12–24h (once to twice a day); must treat for 3–5 weeks minimum to assess effects; then treat until "well" and either have no signs associated with diagnosis or some low, consistent level (a minimum of another 1–2 months). Continue to treat for another 1–2 months (minimum) so that reliability of assessment is reasonably assured. If weaning off the drug, do so over 3–5 weeks (or longer). Treatment should last for a minimum 4–6 months once initiating therapy. (Overall 2001)

- **CATS:**
  a) For treatment of compulsive disorders: 0.25–0.5 mg/kg PO once daily (Landsberg 2004)
  b) For treatment of behavioral diagnoses: 0.25–0.5 mg/kg PO q24h (once a day); must treat for 3–5 weeks minimum to assess effects; then treat until "well" and either have no signs associated with diagnosis or some low, consistent level (a minimum of another 1–2 months). Continue to treat for another 1–2 months (minimum) so that reliability of assessment is reasonably assured. If weaning off the drug, do so over 3–5 weeks (or longer). Treatment should last for a minimum 4–6 months once initiating therapy. (Overall 2001)
  c) For spraying: 0.25 mg/kg PO q12h; avoid use with benzodiazepines (Seksel 2006)
  d) 0.5–1 mg/kg PO once daily (q24h); (allow 8 weeks for initial trial) (Virga 2007)

Monitoring

- Efficacy
- Adverse Effects; including appetite (weight)
- Consider doing baseline liver function tests and ECG and re-test as needed

Client Information

- This medication is most effective when used with a behavior modification program
- Keep this medication away from children and other pets
- Because there has not been widespread use of fluvoxamine in dogs or cats, its adverse effect and efficacy profiles have not been yet fully determined; clients should be briefed to report any significant abnormal findings to the veterinarian.
- Clients must understand that this drug is unlikely to have effect immediately or even in the short term, and must commit to using the drug for months so that an adequate trial can occur.

Chemistry/Synonyms

A selective serotonin-reuptake inhibitor (SSRI), fluvoxamine maleate occurs as a white to almost white crystalline powder. It is freely soluble in alcohol and sparingly soluble in water.

Fluvoxamine may also be known as DU-23000, desifluvoxamin, *Dumirox®*, *Dumyrox®*, *Faverin®*, *Favoxil®*, *Felixsan®*, *Fevarin®*, *Flox-ex®*, *Floxyfral®*, *Fluvohexal®*, *Fluvosol®*, *Fluvoxadura®*, *Fluvoxin®*, *Luvox®*, and *Maveral®*.

Storage/Stability
The commercially available tablets should be stored in tight containers at room temperatures of 15–30° C (59–86° F) and protected from high humidity.

Dosage Forms/Regulatory Status

VETERINARY-LABELED PRODUCTS: None
The ARCI (Racing Commissioners International) has designated this drug as a class 2 substance. See the appendix for more information.

HUMAN-LABELED PRODUCTS:
Fluvoxamine Oral Tablets: 25 mg, 50 mg, & 100 mg; *Luvox®* (Jazz); generic; (Rx)
Fluvoxamine Oral Extended-release Capsules: 100 mg & 150 mg; *Luvox CR®* (Jazz); (Rx)

References

Landsberg, G. (2004). A behaviorists approach to compulsive disorders. Proceedings: ACVIM Forum, Minneapolis. Accessed via: Veterinary Information Network. http://goo.gl/eRUh2
Overall, K. (2001). Pharmacology and Behavior: Practical Applications. Proceedings: Atlantic Coast Veterinary Conference. Accessed via: Veterinary Information Network. http://goo.gl/7RRam
Seksel, K. (2006). Anxiety disorders in cats. Proceedings: Western Vet Conf. Accessed via: Veterinary Information Network. http://goo.gl/IyuKJ
Virga, V. (2007). Veterinary Psychopharmacology: Applications in Clinical Practice. Proceedings: ACVC. Accessed via: Veterinary Information Network. http://goo.gl/84nue

FOLIC ACID

(*foe*-lik *ass*-id)   Folate, Folacin

WATER-SOLUBLE "B" VITAMIN

Prescriber Highlights

- ▶ "B" Vitamin necessary for nucleoprotein synthesis & normal erythropoiesis
- ▶ Injectable or oral dosage forms
- ▶ Folic acid deficiency may be seen in animals (especially cats) with proximal or diffuse small intestinal inflammatory disease
- ▶ May be used when dihydrofolate reductase inhibitor drugs (e.g., trimethoprim, ormetoprim, pyrimethamine) are used for a prolonged period
- ▶ Very safe

Uses/Indications

Folic acid is used to treat folic acid deficiency in dogs, cats, and horses (theoretically in other animal species as well) often due to small intestinal disease. Cats with exocrine pancreatic insufficiency appear to be most at risk for folate and cobalamin deficiencies secondary to malabsorption of folic acid in the diet. Dogs with exocrine pancreatic insufficiency often are noted to have increased folate levels secondary to overgrowths of folate-synthesizing bacteria in the proximal small intestine. Chronic administration of dihydrofolate reductase inhibiting drugs such as pyrimethamine, ormetoprim or trimethoprim can potentially lead to reduced activated folic acid (tetrahydrofolic acid); folic acid supplementation is sometimes prescribed in an attempt to alleviate this situation.

Pharmacology/Actions

Folic acid is required for several metabolic processes. It is reduced via dihydrofolate reductase in the body to tetrahydrofolate (5-methyltetrahydrofolate) which acts as a coenzyme in the synthesis of purine and pyrimidine nucleotides that are necessary for DNA synthesis. Folic acid is also required for maintenance of normal erythropoiesis.

Pharmacokinetics

Therapeutically administered folic acid is primarily absorbed in the proximal small intestine via carrier-mediated diffusion. In humans, synthetic folic acid is nearly completely absorbed after oral administration while folate in foodstuffs is about 50% bioavailable. Folic acid is converted to its active form, tetrahydrofolic acid, principally in the liver and plasma. Folate is distributed widely throughout the body and is stored in the liver. Erythrocyte and CSF levels can be significantly higher than those found in serum. It can undergo enterohepatic recirculation and is excreted primarily in the urine either as metabolites or unchanged drug (when administered in excess of body requirements).

Contraindications/Precautions/Warnings

Folic acid treatment is contraindicated only when known intolerance to the drug is documented. In humans, cobalamin (B-12) levels may be reduced with megaloblastic anemias; folic acid therapy may mask the signs associated with it. Folic acid doses in people above 0.4 mg/day (except during pregnancy and lactation) are not to be used until pernicious anemia has been ruled out.

As dogs may have increased, normal, or decreased folate levels associated with enteropathies, do not administer therapeutic doses until folate and cobalamin levels have been determined.

Adverse Effects

Folic acid is quite non-toxic and should not cause significant adverse effects. Rarely in humans, folic acid tablets or injection have reportedly caused hypersensitivity reactions or gastrointestinal effects. Very high oral doses in humans (15 mg/day) have occasionally caused

CNS effects (*e.g.*, difficulty sleeping, excitement, confusion, etc.).

Reproductive/Nursing Safety

Folic acid is safe to use during pregnancy and in humans it is routinely prescribed as part of prenatal vitamin supplementation as folate deficiency can increase the risk for fetal neural tube defects. In humans, the FDA categorizes this drug as category *A* for use during pregnancy (*Adequate studies in pregnant women have not demonstrated a risk to the fetus in the first trimester of pregnancy, and there is no evidence of risk in later trimesters.*)

Folic acid is distributed into milk, but is safe. Folic acid requirements may be increased in lactating animals.

Overdosage/Acute Toxicity

Folic acid is relatively non-toxic and no treatment should be required if an inadvertent overdose occurs. Excess drug is metabolized or rapidly excreted unchanged in the urine.

Drug Interactions

The following drug interactions or have been reported in humans and may be of significance in veterinary patients receiving folic acid or may alter patient folic acid requirements:

■ **CHLORAMPHENICOL:** May delay response to folic acid

■ **METHOTREXATE, TRIMETHOPRIM, PYRI-METHAMINE (drugs that inhibit dihydrofolate reductase):** May interfere with folic acid utilization

■ **PHENYTOIN:** May decrease serum folate levels, and phenytoin dosage may need to be increased; increased frequency in seizures can occur

■ **SULFASALAZINE, BARBITURATES, NITROFU-RANTOIN, PRIMIDONE:** May increase risk for folate deficiency

Laboratory Considerations

■ Serum samples to be analyzed for cobalamin and/or folate should be protected from bright light and excessive heat

■ Hemolysis can cause falsely elevated serum concentrations of folate

■ Potentially, decreased cobalamin serum levels (B-12) can occur in patients receiving prolonged folic acid supplementation

Doses

■ **DOGS/CATS:**

a) For severe folate deficiency: 0.5–2 mg (total dose) once daily for 1 month. (Williams 2000)

b) For cats with folate deficiency secondary to exocrine pancreatic insufficiency: 400 micrograms (0.4 mg) PO once daily. (Steiner & Williams 2005)

c) For cats on long-term use of high dose trimethoprim/sulfa (for treating *Nocardia*): 2 mg (total dose) PO once daily. (Wolf 2006)

d) For dogs with folate and cobalamin deficiency secondary to inflammatory bowel disease: folic acid at 5 mg (total dose) PO once daily for 1–6 months and cyanocobalamin 750 micrograms (total dose) parenterally once per month. (Hoskins 2005)

e) For adjunctive therapy in cats with inflammatory bowel disease: 0.5–1 mg PO q24h (once daily) with cobalamin at 125–250 micrograms (total dose) SC or IM once a week for 4-6 weeks. (Boothe 2009)

■ **HORSES:**

a) Prolonged therapy with antifolate medications (*e.g.*, trimethoprim, pyrimethamine): Sometimes recommend folic acid at 20–40 mg (total dose) PO per day. Pregnant mares should routinely receive folic acid supplementation during treatment with antifolates. (Granstrom & Saville 1998)

Monitoring

■ Small Animals: folate & cobalamin levels (serum); before and after treatment

■ Clinical signs associated with deficiency

■ CBC, baseline and ongoing if abnormal

Client Information

■ When used to treat folate deficiency associated with small intestinal disease or pancreatic insufficiency, lifelong monitoring and periodic replacement therapy may be required

Chemistry/Synonyms

Folic acid occurs as a yellow, yellow-brownish, or yellowish-orange, odorless crystalline powder. It is very slightly soluble in water and insoluble in alcohol. Commercially available folic acid is obtained synthetically.

Folic acid may also be known as: folate, folacin, vitamin B9, acidum folicum, pteroylglutamic acid, pteroylmonoglutamic acid, *Folvite*® and vitamin B11.

Storage/Stability

Folic acid tablets should be stored in well-closed containers below 40°C (104°F), preferably between 15–30°C; protect from light and moisture. The injection should be stored protected from light below 40°C (104°F), preferably between 15–30°C. Do not allow to freeze.

Dosage Forms/Regulatory Status

VETERINARY-LABELED PRODUCTS:

None as sole ingredient products. There are many products available that contain folic acid as one of the ingredients. If using one of these products, be certain it has enough folic acid to treat folate deficiency without overdosing fat soluble vitamins A or D.

HUMAN-LABELED PRODUCTS:

Folic Acid Tablets: 0.4 mg, & 0.8 mg; generic

(OTC); 1 mg, 7.5 mg, & 15 mg; *Deplin®* (Pamlab); generic; (Rx)

Folic Acid Injection: 5 mg/mL in 10 mL vials; *Folvite®* (Lederle), generic (American Pharmaceutical Partners); (Rx)

References

Boothe, D.M. (2009). Control of Inflammatory Allergic Disease in Cats II. Proceedings; WVC. http://goo.gl/q6uOz

Granstrom, D. & W. Saville (1998). Equine Protozoal Myeloencephalitis. *Equine Internal Medicine.* S Reed and W Bayly Eds., Saunders: 486–491.

Hoskins, J. (2005). Geriatric medicine: Gastrointestinal tract diseases. Proceedings: ACVC 2006, Accessed from the Veterinary Information Network, Jan 2007. Accessed via: Veterinary Information Network. http://goo.gl/x1SyS

Steiner, J. & D. Williams (2005). Feline Exocrine Pancreatic Disease. *Textbook of Veterinary Internal Medicine; Diseases of the Dog and Cat, 6th Ed.* S Ettinger and E Feldman Eds., Elsevier: 1489–1495.

Williams, D. (2000). Cobalamin and Folate, Serum. *The 5-Minute Veterinary Consult: Canine and Feline 2nd Edition.* L Tilley and F Smith Eds., Lippincott: 254–255.

Wolf, A. (2006). Chronic draining tracts and nodules in cats. Proceedings: ABVP2006, Accessed from the Veterinary information Network, Jan 2007. Accessed via: Veterinary Information Network. http://goo.gl/Xronr

FOMEPIZOLE
4-METHYLPYRAZOLE
(4-MP)

(foe-*me*-pi-zole)   Antizol-Vet®

ANTIDOTE

Prescriber Highlights

▶ Synthetic alcohol dehydrogenase inhibitor used to treat dogs and cats for ethylene glycol poisoning

▶ May be efficacious in cats at high dosages, if given within 3 hours of ingestion

▶ Adverse Effects: Rapid IV infusion may cause vein irritation & phlebosclerosis; anaphylaxis is potentially possible

▶ Dilute as directed in the commercially available kit

▶ Monitor & treat acid/base, fluid, electrolyte imbalances

▶ May inhibit elimination of ethanol (& vice versa)

▶ Expense & rapid availability may be issues

Uses/Indications

Fomepizole is used for the treatment of known or suspected ethylene glycol toxicity in dogs (and humans). Fomepizole, at high doses, may be efficacious in treating recent (within 3 hours) ingestion of ethylene glycol in cats. Ethanol treatment has been recommended as the drug of choice for ethylene glycol toxicity in cats, but a recent study demonstrated that high dose fomepizole was more effective. (Connally, H.E. *et al.* 2010)

Pharmacology/Actions

Ethylene glycol itself is only mildly toxic in dogs, but when it is metabolized to glycoaldehyde, glycolate, glyoxalic acid, and oxalic acid, the resultant metabolic acidosis and renal tubular necrosis can be fatal. Fomepizole is a competitive inhibitor of alcohol dehydrogenase, the primary enzyme that converts ethylene glycol into glycoaldehyde and other toxic metabolites. This allows ethylene glycol to be excreted primarily unchanged in the urine decreasing the morbidity and mortality associated with ethylene glycol ingestion.

Pharmacokinetics

Fomepizole is excreted primarily by the kidneys and apparently exhibits a dose-dependent accumulation of the drug over time; therefore, a reduction in subsequent doses can safely occur.

Contraindications/Precautions/Warnings

There are no labeled contraindications to fomepizole's use. In dogs, fomepizole treatment may be successful as late as 8 hours post-ingestion, but if azotemia is noted, treatment is less successful and the prognosis is poor. If so, treatment should still be considered up to 36 hours post-ingestion, as fomepizole can potentially prevent further renal damage and some dogs may survive with dialysis and supportive therapy.

Fomepizole has been shown to be effective in treating ethylene glycol in cats, but a high dosage is required and treatment should be started within 3 hours of ingestion.

Adverse Effects

Giving concentrated drug rapidly intravenously may cause vein irritation and phlebosclerosis. Dilute as directed in the commercially available kit.

One dog during clinical trials was reported to develop anaphylaxis.

Cats may develop mild sedation when receiving fomepizole.

Use of fomepizole alone without adequate monitoring and adjunctive supportive care (*e.g.*, correction of acid/base, fluid, electrolyte imbalances) may lead to therapeutic failure. If animal presents within 1–2 hours post ingestion, consider inducing vomiting and/or gastric lavage with activated charcoal to prevent further absorption.

Reproductive/Nursing Safety

Fomepizole's safe use during pregnancy, lactation or in breeding animals has not been established. However, because of the morbidity and mortality associated with ethylene glycol toxicity, the benefits of fomepizole should generally outweigh its risks. In humans, the FDA categorizes this drug as category *C* for use during pregnancy (*Animal studies have shown an adverse ef-*

fect on the fetus, but there are no adequate studies in humans; or there are no animal reproduction studies and no adequate studies in humans.)

It is not known whether this drug is excreted in milk.

Overdosage/Acute Toxicity

Overdosage may cause significant CNS depression. No specific treatment is recommended.

Drug Interactions

The following drug interactions have either been reported or are theoretical in humans or animals receiving fomepizole and may be of significance in veterinary patients:

■ **ETHANOL:** Fomepizole inhibits alcohol dehydrogenase; ethanol metabolism is reduced significantly and alcohol poisoning (CNS depression, coma, death) can occur. Use together is generally not recommended, but if both drugs are used, monitoring of ethanol blood levels is mandatory.

Laboratory Considerations

Ethylene Glycol Testing Kits: Fomepizole may cause false readings on ethylene glycol screening tests. Refer to the product used, for more information.

Doses

■ **DOGS:**

a) For treatment of ethylene glycol toxicity: Initially load at 20 mg/kg IV; at 12 hours post initial dose give 15 mg/kg IV; at 24 hours post initial dose give another 15 mg/kg IV and at 36 hours after initial dose give 5 mg/kg; may give additional 5 mg/kg doses as necessary (animal has not recovered or has additional ethylene glycol in blood). (Package Insert; *Antizol-Vet®*)

■ **CATS:**

a) For treatment of ethylene glycol toxicity: Initially, 125 mg/kg slow IV; at 12, 24, 36 hours give 31.25 mg/kg IV. In addition, treat supportively with supplemental fluids. Cats must be treated within 3 hours of ingestion. Cats whose treatment began 4 hours post ethylene glycol had 100% mortality with either fomepizole or ETOH therapy. (Connally, H. & Thrall 2002), (Connally, H.E. *et al.* 2010)

Monitoring

■ Ethylene glycol blood levels (mostly important to document diagnosis if necessary and to determine if therapy can be discontinued after 36 hours of treatment.)

■ Blood gases and serum electrolytes

■ Hydration status

■ Renal function tests (*e.g.*, Urine output and urinalysis; BUN or serum creatinine)

■ Cats: body temperature

Client Information

■ Clients should be informed that treatment of serious ethylene glycol toxicity is an "intensive care" admission and that appropriate monitoring and therapy can be quite expensive, particularly when fomepizole is used in large dogs.

■ Because time is of the essence in this therapy, clients will need to make an informed decision rapidly. Dogs treated within 8 hours post ingestion have a significantly better prognosis than those treated after 10–12 hours post ingestion. Cats must be treated within 3 hours of ingestion with high dosages.

Chemistry/Synonyms

A synthetic alcohol dehydrogenase inhibitor, fomepizole is commonly called 4-methylpyrazole (4-MP). Its chemical name is 4-methyl-1H-pyrazole. It has a molecular weight of 81; it is soluble in water and very soluble in ethanol.

Fomepizole may also be known as: 4-methylpyrazole, 4-MP, fomepisol, fomepizolum, and *Antizol®*.

Storage/Stability

Commercially available solutions should be stored at room temperature. The concentrate for injection may solidify at temperatures less than 25°C. Should this occur, resolubolize by running warm water over the vial. Solidification or resolubolization does not affect drug potency or stability. Store reconstituted vial at room temperature and discard after 72 hours.

Compatibility/Compounding Considerations

Preparation: If drug has solidified, run warm water over vial; Add entire contents to 30 mL vial of 0.9% NaCl (in kit), mix well. Resultant solution is: 50 mg/mL. Reconstituted solutions may be further diluted in D_5W or normal saline for IV infusion.

Dosage Forms/Regulatory Status

VETERINARY-LABELED PRODUCTS:

Fomepizole 1.5 g Kit for Injection; *Antizol-Vet®* (Paladin); (Rx). FDA-approved for use in dogs. **Note:** At recommended doses 1 kit will treat a 26 kg dog (up to 58 lb.); larger dogs will require additional kits

HUMAN-LABELED PRODUCTS:

Fomepizole Injection Concentrate: 1 g/mL preservative free (must be diluted) in 1.5 mL vials; *Antizol®* (Paladin); generic (X-Gen Pharm.); (Rx)

References

Connally, H. & M. Thrall (2002). Safety and efficacy of high dose fomepizole therapy for EG intoxication in cats. Proceedings: 8th IVECCS.

Connally, H.E., M.A. Thrall, et al. (2010). Safety and efficacy of high-dose fomepizole compared with ethanol as therapy for ethylene glycol intoxication in cats. *Journal of Veterinary Emergency and Critical Care* 20(2): 191–206.

FOSFOMYCIN TROMETHAMINE

(fos-foe-*my*-sin)   Monurol®

PHOSPHONIC ACID ANTIMICROBIAL

Prescriber Highlights

▶ Human phosphonic acid derivative urinary antibiotic; only oral dose form (granules) available in USA

▶ Potentially could be useful in dogs for UTI, especially multi-drug resistant E.coli; may be useful for systemic infections, but data supporting clinical use is lacking

▶ Appears to be nephrotoxic in cats; use with extreme caution in this species

▶ Currently, very expensive

Uses/Indications

Fosfomycin, is an antibacterial agent that may be useful for treating multi-drug resistant urinary tract infections in dogs. Very little information has been published for this agent in veterinary medicine and its use must be considered as investigational for treating UTI's when other antibiotics are not effective.

Pharmacology/Actions

Fosfomycin is a phosphonic acid derivative, synthetic, antibacterial agent. It irreversibly inhibits phosphoenol pyruvate transferase, an enzyme that catalyzes the formation of uridine diphosphate-N-acetylmuramic acid, which is the first step of microbial cell wall peptidoglycan synthesis. Additionally, it reduces adherence of bacteria to uroepithelial cells. Fosfomycin is primarily a time-dependent antibacterial, but it also exhibits some characteristics of a concentration–dependent agent. It is bactericidal in urine (at therapeutic doses) against susceptible bacteria. It has activity (*in vitro*) against a variety of gram-positive and gram-negative bacteria, including multi-drug resistant isolates of *E.coli* and enterococcus. Cross resistance apparently does not occur with beta-lactams or aminoglycosides. Resistance to fosfomycin, when it occurs, is via hydrolysis secondary to FosX or FosA enzymes that are chromosomally mediated.

Pharmacokinetics

Fosfomycin tromethamine is rapidly converted to the free acid fosfomycin after absorption. Fosfomycin is distributed into the kidneys, bladder wall, and prostate, and crosses the placenta. Primary route of elimination is as unchanged drug in urine (38% of an oral dose in humans). Renal dysfunction can substantially increase half-life and reduce urine levels.

In dogs, fosfomycin (disodium salt) is rapidly absorbed after oral administration; peak levels occur about 2 hours in dogs after oral dosing. Bioavailability in dogs is about 29% which is similar to the values reported for humans (tromethamine salt). Volume of distribution (steady-state) is about 0.7 L/kg and protein binding is very low; clearance is approximately 15 mL/kg/hour, and terminal half-life is approximately 2 hours (Gutierrez *et al.* 2008).

In horses (using fosfomycin disodium), SC bioavailability is about 85%. Peak levels occur about 3.25 hours after SC dosing. Mean volume of distribution (steady-state) is 0.21 L/kg; clearance 16-24 mL/kg/hour; and terminal half-life about 1.3 hours (Zozaya *et al.* 2008).

Contraindications/Precautions/Warnings

Because of concerns that fosfomycin may be nephrotoxic in cats, it presently should be considered contraindicated in young cats and used with caution in adult cats. In a study where cats where given 20 mg/kg of fosfomycin (as the calcium or sodium salt) once daily for 3 days, all young cats (actual age not noted) given the drug orally had significant increases in serum creatinine. Tubular necrosis, disappearance of tubular cells and rearrangement of eosinophilic non-structural material were observed in the kidneys of all the young and adult cats (Fukata *et al.* 2008).

In humans, this drug is used as a one-time dose; multiple doses do not enhance efficacy and increase incidence of adverse events.

Adverse Effects

There is very little information available on this drug's adverse effect profile in animals. In humans, the most common adverse effect is diarrhea. In cats, renal tubular damage is possible (see contraindications above).

Reproductive/Nursing Safety

In humans, fosfomycin is listed as a category *B* drug (*Animal studies have not demonstrated risk to the fetus, but there are no adequate studies in pregnant women; or animal studies have shown an adverse effect, but adequate studies in pregnant women have not demonstrated a risk to the fetus during the first trimester of pregnancy, and there is no evidence of risk in later trimesters.*)

It is unknown if fosfomycin is distributed into milk; use with caution in nursing dams.

Overdosage/Acute Toxicity

No information was located. Single overdoses would most likely cause GI effects. Overdoses in cats may cause nephrotoxicity.

Drug Interactions

The following drug interactions have either been reported or are theoretical in humans or animals receiving fosfomycin and may be of significance in veterinary patients:

■ **METOCLOPRAMIDE:** Can decrease serum concentrations and reduce urine levels. Although no interactions have been reported, other drugs that can increase GI motility (*e.g.,* **bethanechol, cisapride, domperidone, ranitidine, laxatives**) may have a similar effect.

Laboratory Considerations

■ No specific concerns noted

Doses

■ **DOGS:**

For UTI:

a) Until scientific evidence defines the most appropriate dose, interval and duration, the use of fosfomycin might be prudently reserved for treatment of MDR-*E. coli* for which no other alternative exists and the risk of not treating the infection presents harm to the patient. Use of fosfomycin should be based on susceptibility testing only. If the decision is made to use fosfomycin, re-culture and supportive care are indicated. A single dose of 40 mg/kg (disodium salt) PO was well tolerated in dogs in a pharmacokinetic study. Future studies should determine pharmacokinetic data for the commercially available preparation (tromethamine salt), time or concentration dependency, and evidence of safety. These should be followed by multi-center randomized clinical trials involving dogs with spontaneous UTI associated with *E. coli*. (Boothe & Hubka 2010), (Hubka & Boothe 2010)

■ **HORSES:**

a) Based on their pharmacokinetic study, the authors concluded that clinically effective plasma concentrations might be obtained for up to 10 hours administering 20 mg/kg SC. (Zozaya *et al.* 2008) (*Note:* In this study, fosfomycin disodium was used. This salt is not currently commercially available in the USA)

Monitoring

■ Adverse Effects: GI

■ Standard monitoring for UTI treatment (*i.e.*, before and after culture and susceptibility, clinical signs, urinalysis)

■ Cats: Renal function tests

Client Information

■ There is little clinical experience with this drug in animals; report any possible side effects to the veterinarian immediately

■ It is likely that this drug will be provided to you as a compounded product; follow the directions for using it exactly as prescribed. For human use, the granules are to be diluted in water (not hot water) just prior to dosing. The drug can be given regardless of feeding status (full or empty stomach).

Chemistry/Synonyms

Fosfomycin tromethamine (also known as fosfomycin trometamol) is an antibacterial isolated from *Streptomyces fradiae*. It occurs as a white or almost white, hygroscopic powder that is very soluble in water, slightly soluble in alcohol or methyl alcohol, and practically insoluble in ac-etone. A 5% solution in water has a pH of 3.5 to 5.5.

Fosfomycin may also be known as MK-955, phosphomycin, phosphonomycin, fosfomicina, fosfomycine, fosfomycinum, or fosfomysiini. Its chemical name is cis-1, 2-epoxyphosphonic acid.

Storage/Stability

Fosfomycin tromethamine granules should be stored at room temperature (25°C).

Compatibility/Compounding Considerations

The product's label (for human use) states: Pour the entire contents of a single-dose sachet of fosfomycin into 90 to 120 mL of water (1/2 cup) and stir to dissolve. Do not use hot water. Fosfomycin should be taken immediately after dissolving in water.

Dosage Forms/Regulatory Status

VETERINARY-LABELED PRODUCTS: None

HUMAN-LABELED PRODUCTS:

Fosfomycin Tromethamine 3 grams per packet (for dilution and oral use); *Monurol*® (Forest); (Rx)

References

Boothe, D. & P. Hubka (2010). Fosfomycin: An Alternative Drug for Treatment of E. coli Urinary Tract Infections? Proceedings: ACVIM. Accessed via: Veterinary Information Network. http://goo.gl/wV5LL

Fukata, T., N. Imai, et al. (2008). Acute renal insufficiency in cats after fosfomycin administration. *Veterinary Record* 163(11): 337–338.

Gutierrez, O.L., C.L. Ocampo, et al. (2008). Pharmacokinetics of disodium-fosfomycin in mongrel dogs. *Research in Veterinary Science* 85(1): 156–161.

Hubka, P. & D.M. Boothe (2010). In vitro susceptibility of canine and feline Escherichia coli to fosfomycin. *Veterinary Microbiology* In Press, Corrected Proof.

Zozaya, D.H., O.L. Gutierrez, et al. (2008). Pharmacokinetics of a single bolus intravenous, intramuscular and subcutaneous dose of disodium fosfomycin in horses. *Journal of Veterinary Pharmacology and Therapeutics* 31(4): 321–327.

FURAZOLIDONE

(fyoor-a-**zoe**-li-done)   Furoxone®

ANTIBACTERIAL/ANTIPROTOZOAL

Prescriber Highlights

▶ Antibacterial/antiprotozoal nitrofuran that has been used in dogs & cats; availability is an issue

▶ Contraindications: Known hypersensitivity; food animals

▶ Adverse Effects: GI effects (anorexia, vomiting, cramping & diarrhea) possible

▶ May innocuously discolor urine to a dark yellow to brown color

▶ Drug Interactions

Uses/Indications

Furazolidone is usually a drug of second choice in small animals to treat enteric infections caused by the organisms listed below. Because it is no longer commercially available (in the USA), it may be difficult to locate.

Pharmacology/Actions

Furazolidone interferes with susceptible bacterial enzyme systems. Its mechanism against susceptible protozoa is not well determined. Furazolidone has activity against Giardia, Vibrio cholerae, Trichomonas, Coccidia, and many strains of E. coli, Enterobacter, Campylobacter, Salmonella, and Shigella. Not all strains are sensitive, but resistance is usually limited and develops slowly. Furazolidone also inhibits monoamine oxidase.

Pharmacokinetics

Conflicting information on furazolidone's absorption characteristics are published. As colored metabolites are found in the urine, it is clearly absorbed to some extent. Because furazolidone is used to treat enteric infections, absorption becomes important only when discussing adverse reactions and drug interaction issues. Furazolidone reportedly distributes into the CSF. Absorbed furazolidone is rapidly metabolized in the liver and the majority of absorbed drug is eliminated in the urine.

Contraindications/Precautions/Warnings

Furazolidone is contraindicated in patients hypersensitive to it.

The FDA has prohibited the extralabel use of furazolidone in food animals.

Adverse Effects

Adverse effects noted with furazolidone are usually minimal. Anorexia, vomiting, cramping, and diarrhea may occasionally occur. Some human patients are reported to be hypersensitive to the drug. Because furazolidone also inhibits monoamine oxidase it may, potentially, interact with several other drugs and foods (see Drug Interactions below). The clinical significance of these interactions remains unclear, particularly in light of the drug's poor absorptive characteristics.

Reproductive/Nursing Safety

While the safe use of furazolidone during pregnancy has not been established, neither were there any teratogenic issues located for it. However, one reference (Tams 2003) states that furazolidone should not be used in pregnant queens. In humans, the FDA categorizes this drug as category **C** for use during pregnancy (*Animal studies have shown an adverse effect on the fetus, but there are no adequate studies in humans; or there are no animal reproduction studies and no adequate studies in humans.*)

It is unknown if furazolidone enters maternal milk.

Overdosage/Acute Toxicity

No information was located; but moderate overdoses are unlikely to cause significant toxicity. Gut emptying may be considered for large overdoses.

Drug Interactions

The following drug interactions have either been reported or are theoretical in humans or animals receiving furazolidone and may be of significance in veterinary patients:

- ■ **ALCOHOL:** With furazolidone may cause a disulfiram-like reaction.

Because furazolidone inhibits monoamine oxidase, its use concurrently with the following drugs is not recommended because dangerous hypertension could occur:

- ■ **AMITRAZ**
- ■ **BUSPIRONE**
- ■ **SELEGILINE**
- ■ **SYMPATHOMIMETIC AMINES (phenylpropanolamine, ephedrine, etc.)**
- ■ **TRICYCLIC ANTIDEPRESSANTS**
- ■ **FISH OR POULTRY (high tyramine content)**

Laboratory Considerations

- ■ Furazolidone may cause a false-positive urine glucose determination when using the cupric sulfate solution test (*e.g., Clinitest®*).

Doses

- ■ **DOGS:**
  a) For *amebic colitis*: 2.2 mg/kg PO q8h for 7 days;

     For coccidiosis: 8–20 mg/kg PO for one week (Sherding & Johnson 1994)
  b) For treatment of Giardia: 4 mg/kg PO twice daily (q12h) for 7 days

     For *Cystoisospora* spp.: 8–20 mg/kg PO q12–24h for 5 days (Lappin 2000)
  c) For coccidiosis: 8–20 mg/kg PO once daily for 7 days

     For entamebiasis: 2.2 mg/kg PO q8h for 7 days (Greene & Watson 1998)

- ■ **CATS:**
  a) For treatment of Giardia: 4 mg/kg PO twice daily (q12h) for 7–10 days; if retreatment is required, elevated dosages or lengthened treatment regimens may provide better results. (Reinemeyer 1992)
  b) For treatment of Giardia: 4 mg/kg, PO twice daily (q12h) for 7 days

     For *Cystoisospora* spp.: 8–20 mg/kg PO q12–24h for 5 days (Lappin 2000)
  c) For coccidiosis: 8–20 mg/kg PO once daily for 7 days

     For giardiasis: 4 mg/kg PO q12h for 5–10 days

     For amebiasis: 2.2 mg/kg PO q8h for 7 days (Greene & Watson 1998)
  d) For *amebic colitis*: 2.2 mg/kg PO q8h for 7 days; For coccidiosis: 8–20 mg/kg PO for one week; for Giardia: 4 mg/kg PO q12h for 5 days (Sherding & Johnson 1994)

- ■ **HORSES:**
  a) 4 mg/kg PO three times daily (Robinson 1992)

Monitoring

■ Efficacy (stool exams for parasitic infections)

Client Information

■ Furazolidone may discolor urine to a dark yellow to brown color; this is not significant.

■ Have clients report prolonged or serious GI effects.

Chemistry/Synonyms

A synthetic nitrofuran-derivative antibacterial/antiprotozoal, furazolidone occurs as a bitter-tasting, yellow, crystalline powder. It is practically insoluble in water.

Furazolidone may also be known as: nifurazolidonum, *Enterolidon®*, *Exofur®*, *Furasian®*, *Furion®*, *Furoxona®*, *Fuxol®*, *Giarcid®*, *Giardil®*, *Giarlam®*, *Neo Furasil®*, *Nifuran®*, *Novafur®*, *Salmocide®*, and *Seforman®*.

Storage/Stability

Store protected from light in tight containers.

Dosage Forms/Regulatory Status

VETERINARY-LABELED PRODUCTS:

No systemic products are available; a 4% topical powder/spray is available. The FDA prohibits its use on food producing animals.

HUMAN-LABELED PRODUCTS:

None; the human product *Furoxone®* has apparently been withdrawn from the USA market. Preparations may be available from compounding pharmacies.

References

Greene, C. & A. Watson (1998). Antimicrobial Drug Formulary. *Infectious Diseases of the Dog and Cat.* C Greene Ed. Philadelphia, WB Saunders: 790–919.

Lappin, M. (2000). Protozoal and Miscellaneous Infections. *Textbook of Veterinary Internal Medicine: Diseases of the Dog and Cat.* S Ettinger and E Feldman Eds. Philadelphia, WB Saunders. 1: 408–417.

Reinemeyer, C. (1992). Feline Gastrointestinal Parasites. *Current Veterinary Therapy XI: Small Animal Practice.* R Kirk and J Bonagura Eds. Philadelphia, W.B. Saunders Company: 626–630.

Robinson, N. (1992). Table of Drugs: Approximate Doses. *Current Therapy in Equine Medicine 3.* N Robinson Ed. Philadelphia, W.B. Saunders Co.: 815–821.

Sherding, R. & S. Johnson (1994). Diseases of the intestines. *Saunders Manual of Small Animal Practice.* S Birchard and R Sherding Eds. Philadelphia, W.B. Saunders Company: 687–714.

Tams, T. (2003). Giardiasis, Clostridium perfringens enterotoxicosis, and cryptosporidiosis. Proceedings: Atlantic Coast Veterinary Conference. Accessed via: Veterinary Information Network. http://goo.gl/DjFbK

FUROSEMIDE

(fur-*oh*-se-mide)   Lasix®

LOOP DIURETIC

Prescriber Highlights

▶ A loop diuretic commonly used in many species for treatment of congestive cardiomyopathy, pulmonary edema, udder edema, hypercalcuric nephropathy, uremia, as adjunctive therapy in hyperkalemia &, occasionally, as an antihypertensive agent

▶ Used in racehorses to prevent/reduce EIPH

▶ Contraindications: Patients with anuria, hypersensitivity, or seriously depleted electrolytes

▶ Caution: Patients with pre-existing electrolyte or water balance abnormalities, impaired hepatic function, & diabetes mellitus

▶ Adverse Effects: Fluid & electrolyte (esp. hyponatremia) abnormalities, others included: ototoxicity, GI distress, hematologic effects, ototoxicity, weakness, & restlessness

▶ Pre-renal azotemia if dehydration occurs

▶ Encourage normal food & water intake

Uses/Indications

Furosemide is used for its diuretic activity in all species. It is used in small animals for the treatment of congestive cardiomyopathy, pulmonary edema, hypercalcuric nephropathy, uremia, as adjunctive therapy in hyperkalemia and, occasionally, as an antihypertensive agent. In cattle, it is FDA-approved for use for the treatment of post-parturient udder edema. It has been used to help prevent or reduce epistaxis (exercise-induced pulmonary hemorrhage; EIPH) in racehorses.

Pharmacology/Actions

Furosemide reduces the absorption of electrolytes in the ascending section of the loop of Henle, decreases the reabsorption of both sodium and chloride and increases the excretion of potassium in the distal renal tubule, and directly effects electrolyte transport in the proximal tubule. The exact mechanisms of furosemide's effects have not been fully established. It has no effect on carbonic anhydrase nor does it antagonize aldosterone.

Furosemide increases renal excretion of water, sodium, potassium, chloride, calcium, magnesium, hydrogen, ammonium, and bicarbonate. In dogs, excretion of potassium is affected much less so than is sodium; hyponatremia may be more of a concern than hypokalemia. It causes some renal venodilation and transiently increases glomerular filtration rates (GFR). Renal blood flow is increased and decreased peripheral resistance may occur. While furosemide increases renin secretion, due to its effects on the nephron, increases in sodium and water retention do not occur. Furosemide can cause hyperglycemia, but to a lesser extent than the thiazides.

At high doses (10–12 mg/kg), thoracic duct lymph flow is increased in dogs. In horses, guinea pigs and humans, furosemide has some bronchodilative effects. Cats are reportedly more sensitive than other species to the diuretic effects of furosemide.

Pharmacokinetics

The pharmacokinetics of furosemide have been studied in a limited fashion in domestic animals. In dogs, the oral bioavailability is approximately 77% and the elimination half-life approximately 1–1.5 hours.

In humans, furosemide is 60–75% absorbed following oral administration. The diuretic effect takes place within 5 minutes after IV administration and within one hour after oral dosing. Peak effects occur approximately 30 minutes after IV dosing, and 1–2 hours after oral dosing. The drug is approximately 95% bound to plasma proteins in both azotemic and normal patients. The serum half-life is about 2 hours, but prolonged in patients with renal failure, uremia, CHF, and in neonates.

Contraindications/Precautions/Warnings

Furosemide is contraindicated in patients with anuria or who are hypersensitive to the drug. The manufacturer states that the drug should be discontinued in patients with progressive renal disease if increasing azotemia and oliguria occur during therapy.

Furosemide should be used with caution in patients with preexisting electrolyte or water balance abnormalities, impaired hepatic function (may precipitate hepatic coma), and diabetes mellitus. Patients with conditions that may lead to electrolyte or water balance abnormalities (*e.g.*, vomiting, diarrhea, etc.) should be monitored carefully. Patients hypersensitive to sulfonamides may also be hypersensitive to furosemide (not documented in veterinary species).

Adverse Effects

Furosemide may induce fluid and electrolyte abnormalities. Patients should be monitored for hydration status and electrolyte imbalances (especially potassium, calcium, magnesium and sodium). Prerenal azotemia may result if moderate to severe dehydration occurs. Hyponatremia is probably the greatest concern, but hypocalcemia, hypokalemia, and hypomagnesemia may all occur. Animals that have normal food and water intake are much less likely to develop water and electrolyte imbalances than those who do not.

Other potential adverse effects include ototoxicity, especially in cats with high dose IV

therapy. Dogs reportedly require dosages greater than 22 mg/kg IV to cause hearing loss. Other effects include gastrointestinal disturbances, hematologic effects (anemia, leukopenia), weakness, and restlessness.

Reproductive/Nursing Safety

In humans, the FDA categorizes this drug as category **C** for use during pregnancy (*Animal studies have shown an adverse effect on the fetus, but there are no adequate studies in humans; or there are no animal reproduction studies and no adequate studies in humans.*) In a separate system evaluating the safety of drugs in canine and feline pregnancy (Papich 1989), this drug is categorized as in class: **B** (*Safe for use if used cautiously. Studies in laboratory animals may have uncovered some risk, but these drugs appear to be safe in dogs and cats or these drugs are safe if they are not administered when the animal is near term.*)

Furosemide appears in milk; clinical significance to nursing offspring is unknown.

Overdosage/Acute Toxicity

The LD_{50} in dogs after oral administration is >1000 mg/kg; after IV injection >300 mg/kg. Chronic overdosing at 10 mg/kg for six months in dogs led to development of calcification and scarring of the renal parenchyma.

Acute overdosage may cause electrolyte and water balance problems, CNS effects (lethargy to coma and seizures) and cardiovascular collapse.

Treatment consists of emptying the gut after recent oral ingestion, using standard protocols. Avoid giving concomitant cathartics as they may exacerbate the fluid and electrolyte imbalances that can occur. Aggressively monitor and treat electrolyte and water balance abnormalities supportively. Additionally, monitor respiratory, CNS, and cardiovascular status. Treat supportively and symptomatically if necessary.

Drug Interactions

The following drug interactions have either been reported or are theoretical in humans or animals receiving furosemide and may be of significance in veterinary patients:

- **ACE INHIBITORS (*e.g.*, enalapril, benazepril):** Increased risks for hypotension, particularly in patients who are volume or sodium depleted secondary to diuretics

- **AMINOGLYCOSIDES (gentamicin, amikacin, etc.):** Increased risk for ototoxicity

- **AMPHOTERICIN B:** Loop diuretics may increase the risk for nephrotoxicity development; hypokalemia

- **CORTICOSTEROIDS:** Increased risk for GI ulceration; hypokalemia

- **DIGOXIN:** Furosemide-induced hypokalemia may increase the potential for digoxin toxicity

- **INSULIN:** Furosemide may alter insulin requirements

■ **MUSCLE RELAXANTS, NON-DEPOLARIZING** (*e.g.*, **atracurium, tubocurarine**)**:** Furosemide may prolong neuromuscular blockade

■ **PROBENECID:** Furosemide can reduce uricosuric effects

■ **SALICYLATES:** Loop diuretics can reduce the excretion of salicylates

■ **SUCCINYLCHOLINE:** Furosemide may potentiate

■ **THEOPHYLLINE:** Pharmacologic effects of theophylline may be enhanced when used with furosemide

Laboratory Considerations

■ **Free T4:** Furosemide can result in an increased free T4 fraction; furosemide inhibits T4 binding to canine serum *in vitro*

Doses

■ **DOGS & CATS:**

As a general diuretic:

a) 2.5–5 mg/kg (lower dose suggested for cats) once or twice daily at 6–8 hour intervals PO, IV or IM (Package Insert; *Salix®*—Intervet)

For cardiogenic or pulmonary edema:

a) *For severe acute pulmonary edema* (parenteral dosing)

Dogs: Up to 8 mg/kg IV or IM every 1–2 hours until respiratory rate and/or respiratory character improves; alternately a CRI of 0.66 mg/kg/hr may be used and potentially can produce greater diuresis, natriuresis and less kaliuresis.

Cats: Initially 2- 4 mg/kg IV or IM; cats that can tolerate an IV injection may benefit from a faster onset of action (5 minutes IV vs 30 minutes IM). The dose may be repeated within 1-2 hours. To avoid severe dehydration, dosing must be reduced sharply once respiratory rate starts to decrease.

For heart failure (oral dosing; often in combination with an ACE inhibitor and digoxin):

Dogs: Dosage ranges from 1 mg/kg PO every other day for very mild heart failure to 4 mg/kg PO q8h for severe heart failure;

Cats: Currently, author still recommends using an ACE inhibitor with furosemide in cats with HCM. Maintenance dose of furosemide usually ranges from 6.25 mg once a day to 12.5 mg PO q8h (higher doses, up to 37.5 mg PO q12h have been used in some cats not responding to conventional treatment without severe consequences as long as they were eating and drinking.) Doses must be titrated carefully in each patient and the owner should be instructed how to count sleeping respiration rates at home and to do a daily log of respiratory rate (normal sleeping respiration rates are 15-30 per minute, but some cats will go up to 40 per minute.)

Animals must drink adequate amounts of water or severe dehydration may result. (Kittleson 2000), (Kittleson 2006), (Kittleson 2009)

b) For chronic therapy: Most cardiologists now recommend using ACE inhibitors and diuretics in animals with CHF, but it is difficult to define the exact dose of furosemide required by the patient as the dose required to clear significant edema and allow the animal to be minimally symptomatic is often close to a dose that may result in electrolyte disturbances. Some degree of experimentation must be performed to best evaluate an individual animal's needs. In most instances, dogs are given less than 2 mg/kg PO q12h and cats, initially, try 6.25 mg/cat/day for chronic therapy. Some cats require higher doses and some can be maintained on 6.25 mg every other day. Goal is to give the "lowest possible dose of furosemide". It can be helpful to give owners a dosage range with upper and lower limits of furosemide doses and have them "give more for difficulty breathing or rapid respirations, and give less if the animal appears weak, lethargic, anorexic or depressed." Measure renal function prior to therapy and 5-10 days after starting drugs. (Rush 2008)

c) In combination with rest, vasodilators and rate-control: 1–4 mg/kg IV, IM or PO q1-12 hours. (Rozanski 2009)

For hypercalcemia/hypercalciuric nephropathy:

a) For adjunctive treatment of moderate to severe hypercalcemia: Volume expansion is necessary prior to use of furosemide; 2–4 mg/kg two to three times daily, IV, SC or PO. (Chew *et al.* 2003)

For acute oliguric renal failure:

a) Initially 2 mg/kg IV; if no substantial diuresis develops in one hour, the dose may be doubled to 4 mg/kg. If this dose fails to induce diuresis, may increase to 6 mg/kg. If diuresis still does not ensue, very large doses of furosemide, an alternative diuretic (*e.g.*, mannitol), or the combination of furosemide and dopamine may be considered. If furosemide successfully induces diuresis, it may be repeated at 8 hour intervals as needed to sustain diuresis and promote potassium secretion. The need for continued furosemide therapy must be considered in light of its potential side effects. (Polzin 2005), (Polzin 2009)

b) In fluid replete patients, furosemide as a bolus at 1–6 mg/kg IV. If adequate diuresis is not evident in 30 minutes, re-administer initial or higher dose. If diuresis ensues, can repeat dose every 6-8 hours or a CRI at 0.1–1 mg/kg/hr. Fluid balances must be carefully monitored to prevent dehydration and further renal compromise. (Silverstein 2009)

■ **FERRETS:**

For adjunctive therapy for heart failure:

a) 2–3 mg/kg IM or IV initially for fulminant CHF; 1–2 mg/kg PO q12h for long-term maintenance therapy (Hoeffer 2000)

b) 1–4 mg/kg PO, SC, IM or IV 2–3 times a day (Williams 2000)

■ **RABBITS/RODENTS/SMALL MAMMALS:**

a) **Rabbits:** For CHF: 2–5 mg/kg PO, SC, IM or IV q12h; For pulmonary edema: 1–4 mg/kg IV or IM q4–6h (Ivey & Morrisey 2000)

b) **Mice, Rats, Gerbils, Hamsters, Guinea pigs, Chinchillas:** 5–10 mg/kg q12h (Adamcak & Otten 2000)

■ **CATTLE:**

a) 500 mg once daily or 250 mg twice daily; 2 grams PO once daily. Treatment not to exceed 48 hours post-partum (for udder edema). Package Insert; *Lasix*®–Hoechst)

b) 2.2–4.4 mg/kg IV q12h (Howard 1986)

■ **HORSES:** (**Note:** Refer to state guidelines for use of furosemide in racing animals)

As a diuretic:

a) For adjunctive therapy for congestive heart failure: Initially, 1–2 mg/kg IM or IV q6–12h to control edema. Long-term therapy: 0.5–2 mg/kg PO or IM q8–12h (Mogg 1999)

b) For adjunctive therapy of acute renal failure: 2–4 mg/kg q6h (Jose-Cunilleras & Hinchcliff 1999)

For epistaxis/EIPH prevention:

a) 500 mg (total dose) 4 hours prior to race. (Hinchcliff *et al.* 2009)

b) 250 mg IV 4 hours prior to racing (Foreman 1999)

■ **BIRDS:**

As a diuretic:

a) 0.05 mg/300 grams body weight IM twice daily (**Note:** Lories are very sensitive to this agent and can be easily overdosed) (Clubb 1986)

■ **REPTILES:**

For most species:

a) 5 mg/kg IV or IM as needed (Gauvin 1993)

Monitoring

■ Serum electrolytes, BUN, creatinine, glucose

■ Hydration status

■ Blood pressure, if indicated

■ Clinical signs of edema, patient weight, if indicated

■ Evaluation of ototoxicity, particularly with prolonged therapy or in cats

Client Information

■ Clients should contact veterinarian if clinical signs of water or electrolyte imbalance occur, such as excessive thirst, lethargy, lassitude, restlessness, reduced urination, GI distress or fast heart rate.

Chemistry/Synonyms

A loop diuretic related structurally to the sulfonamides, furosemide occurs as an odorless, practically tasteless, white to slightly yellow, fine, crystalline powder. Furosemide has a melting point between 203°–205°C with decomposition, and a pK_a of 3.9. It is practically insoluble in water, sparingly soluble in alcohol, and freely soluble in alkaline hydroxides. The injectable product has its pH adjusted to 8–9.3 with sodium hydroxide.

Furosemide may also be known as: frusemide, furosemidum, and LB-502; many trade names are available.

Storage/Stability

Furosemide tablets should be stored in light-resistant, well-closed containers. The oral solution should be stored at room temperature and protected from light and freezing. Furosemide injection should be stored at room temperature. A precipitate may form if the injection is refrigerated, but will resolubolize when warmed without alteration in potency. The human injection (10 mg/mL) should not be used if it has a yellow color. The veterinary injection (50 mg/mL) normally has a slight yellow color. Furosemide is unstable at an acid pH, but is very stable under alkaline conditions.

Compatibility/Compounding Considerations

Furosemide injection (10 mg/mL) is reportedly physically **compatible** with all commonly used intravenous solutions and the following drugs: amikacin sulfate, cimetidine HCl, kanamycin sulfate, tobramycin sulfate, and verapamil.

It is reportedly physically **incompatible** with the following agents: ascorbic acid solutions, dobutamine HCl, epinephrine, gentamicin sulfate, netilmicin sulfate and tetracyclines. It should generally not be mixed with antihistamines, local anesthetics, alkaloids, hypnotics, or opiates.

Dosage Forms/Regulatory Status

VETERINARY-LABELED PRODUCTS:

Furosemide Tablets: 12.5 mg, & 50 mg; *Salix*®, *Disal*®, generic; (Rx). Products may be FDA-approved for use in dogs and cats.

Furosemide Oral Solution (Syrup): 10 mg/mL in 60 mL; generic; (Rx). FDA-approved for use in dogs.

Furosemide for Injection: 50 mg/mL (5%) in 50 mL & 100 mL vials; *Disal® Injection, Salix® Injection*, generic; (Rx). Products may be FDA-approved for use in dogs, cats and horses.

HUMAN-LABELED PRODUCTS:

Furosemide Oral Tablets: 20 mg, 40 mg, & 80 mg; *Lasix®* (Aventis); generic; (Rx)

Furosemide Oral Solution: 10 mg/mL in 60 mL & 120 mL; 40 mg/5 mL in 500 mL & UD 5 mL & 10 mL; generic; (Rx)

Furosemide Injection: 10 mg/mL in 2 mL (20 mg), 4 mL (40 mg) & 10 mL (100 mg) single-dose vials; generic; (Rx)

References

Adamcak, A. & B. Otten (2000). Rodent Therapeutics. *Vet Clin NA: Exotic Anim Pract* 3:1(Jan): 221–240.
Chew, D., P. Schenck, et al. (2003). Assessment and treatment of clinical cases with elusive disorders of hypercalcemia. Proceedings: ACVIM Forum. Accessed via: Veterinary Information Network. http://goo.gl/goje1
Clubb, S.L. (1986). Therapeutics: Individual and Flock Treatment Regimens. *Clinical Avian Medicine and Surgery*. GJ Harrison and LR Harrison Eds. Philadelphia, W.B. Saunders: 327–355.
Foreman, J. (1999). Equine respiratory pharmacology. *The Veterinary Clinics of North America: Equine Practice* 15:3(December): 665–686.
Gauvin, J. (1993). Drug therapy in reptiles. *Seminars in Avian & Exotic Med* 2(1): 48–59.
Hinchcliff, K.W., P.S. Morley, et al. (2009). Efficacy of furosemide for prevention of exercise-induced pulmonary hemorrhage in Thoroughbred racehorses. *Javma-Journal of the American Veterinary Medical Association* 235(1): 76–82.
Hoeffer, H. (2000). Heart Disease in Ferrets. *Kirk's Current Veterinary Therapy: XIII Small Animal Practice*. J Bonagura Ed. Philadelphia, WB Saunders: 1144–1148.
Howard, J.L., Ed. (1986). *Current Veterinary Therapy 2, Food Animal Practice*. Philadelphia, W.B. Saunders.
Ivey, E. & J. Morrisey (2000). Therapeutics for Rabbits. *Vet Clin NA: Exotic Anim Pract* 3:1(Jan): 183–216.
Jose-Cunilleras, E. & K. Hinchcliff (1999). Renal pharmacology. *The Veterinary Clinics of North America: Equine Practice* 15:3(December): 647–664.
Kittleson, M. (2000). Therapy of Heart Failure. *Textbook of Veterinary Internal Medicine: Diseases of the Dog and Cat*. S Ettinger and E Feldman Eds. Philadelphia, WB Saunders. 1: 713–737.
Kittleson, M. (2006). "Chapt 10: Management of Heart Failure." *Small Animal Cardiology, 2nd Ed*.
Kittleson, M. (2009). Treatment of feline hypertrophic cardiomyopathy (HCM)--Lost Dreams. Proceedings: ACVIM. Accessed via: Veterinary Information Network. http://goo.gl/XvCZt
Mogg, T. (1999). Equine Cardiac Disease: Clinical pharmacology and therapeutics. *The Veterinary Clinics of North America: Equine Practice* 15:3(December).
Polzin, D. (2005). Managing the acute uremic crisis. Proceedings: ACVC. Accessed via: Veterinary Information Network. http://goo.gl/iav1L
Polzin, D. (2009). How I treat uremic crisis in dogs and cats with chronic kidney disease. Proceedings: WSAVA. Accessed via: Veterinary Information Network. http://goo.gl/xtcpx
Rozanski, E. (2009). Diagnosis and management of pulmonary edema. Proceedings: WVC. Accessed via: Veterinary Information Network. http://goo.gl/66Jz1
Rush, J. (2008). Heart failure in dogs and cats. Proceedings: IVECCS. Accessed via: Veterinary Information Network. http://goo.gl/cFKka
Silverstein, D. (2009). Diagnosis and management of acute renal failure. Proceedings: Western Veterinary Conf. Accessed via: Veterinary Information Network. http://goo.gl/Wgq77
Williams, B. (2000). Therapeutics in Ferrets. *Vet Clin NA: Exotic Anim Pract* 3:1(Jan): 131–153.

GABAPENTIN

(gab-ah-*pen*-tin)   Neurontin®

ANTICONVULSANT; NEUROPATHIC PAIN ANALGESIC

Prescriber Highlights

▶ May be useful in dogs & cats as adjunctive therapy for refractory or complex partial seizures or the treatment of pain

▶ Caution in patients with diminished renal function, but dogs partially (30–40%) metabolize the drug (humans do not)

▶ Avoid use of xylitol-containing oral liquid in dogs

▶ Sedation or ataxia most likely adverse effects

▶ Three times a day dosing in dogs may be problematic

Uses/Indications

Gabapentin may be useful as adjunctive therapy for refractory or complex partial seizures. As an analgesic, gabapentin has been demonstrated to be most useful in treating chronic pain, particularly neuropathic pain in small animals. Gabapentin does not appear to be of significant use for treating acute pain, but it may be of benefit when given preemptively for acute pain (*e.g.*, before surgery); studies are ongoing to evaluate this indication for small animals.

Pharmacology/Actions

Gabapentin has analgesic effects and can prevent allodynia (sensation of pain resulting from a normally non-noxious stimulus) or hyperalgesia (exaggerated response to painful stimuli). It also has anticonvulsant activity. The mechanism of action of gabapentin, for either its anticonvulsant or analgesic actions is not fully understood, but it appears to bind to CaVa2-d (alpha2-delta subunit of the voltage-gated calcium channels). By decreasing calcium influx, release of excitatory neurotransmitters (*e.g.*, substance P, glutamate, norepinephrine) are inhibited. While gabapentin is structurally related to GABA, it does not appear to alter GABA binding, reuptake, or degradation, or serve as a GABA agonist *in vivo*.

Pharmacokinetics

In dogs, oral bioavailability is about 80% at a dose of 50 mg/kg. Peak plasma levels occur about 2 hours post dose. Elimination is primarily via renal routes, but gabapentin is partially metabolized to N-methyl-gabapentin. Elimination half-life is approximately 2–4 hours in dogs.

In cats, gabapentin is well absorbed after oral dosing with a bioavailability average of 90%, but there was significant interpatient variation (50%-120%). Peak levels occurred about 100 minutes after dosing. Volume of distribution is relatively low (apparent Vd_{ss} of 0.65 L/kg.) Clearance was about 3 mL/min/kg and mean elimination half-life of 2.8 hours is similar to that of dogs. (Siao *et al.* 2010)

In four horses given single oral doses of 5 mg/kg, gabapentin was rapidly absorbed with peak levels noted within 2 hours (mean 1.4 hours). Plasma elimination half-life was about 3.4 hours. (Dirikolu *et al.* 2008)

In humans, gabapentin bioavailability decreases as dosage increases. At doses of 900 mg/day, 60% of the dose is absorbed. Percentage absorbed is reduced as doses are increased to a minimum of 27% of the dose being absorbed when 4800 mg/day is administered. Presence of food only marginally alters absorption rate and extent of absorption. Gabapentin is only minimally bound to plasma proteins; CSF levels are approximately 20% of those in plasma. The drug is not significantly metabolized and is almost exclusively excreted unchanged into the urine. Elimination half-lives in humans are approximately 5-7 hours.

Contraindications/Precautions/Warnings

Gabapentin is considered contraindicated in patients hypersensitive to it. Because gabapentin is eliminated via renal routes (practically 100% in humans), it should be used with caution in patients with renal insufficiency; if required, dosage adjustment should be considered. In dogs, the drug is also metabolized (30-40%) of a dose, so dosage adjustment may not be required in dogs with mild to moderate renal dysfunction.

In general, avoid the use of the commercially available human oral solution (*Neurontin*®) in dogs as it reportedly contains 300 mg/mL xylitol. As the threshold dose that can cause hypoglycemia in dogs is approximately 100 mg/kg, doses of up to 15 mg/kg in dogs using the solution should be safe, but further data is needed to confirm this. Additionally, xylitol may be hepatotoxic in dogs. Doses of 500 mg/kg of xylitol are currently thought to be the threshold for this toxicity, but there have been anecdotal reports of it occurring at much lower doses. In cats, at the dosages used presently, xylitol toxicity does not appear to be a problem with gabapentin oral solution, but use with caution.

Adverse Effects

Sedation or ataxia are probably the most likely adverse effects seen in small animals. Starting the dose at the lower end of the range and increasing with time, may alleviate this effect. In humans, the most common adverse effects associated with gabapentin therapy are dizziness, somnolence, and peripheral edema.

Gabapentin was associated with an increased rate of pancreatic adenocarcinoma in male rats. It is unknown if this effect crosses into other species.

Abrupt discontinuation of the drug has lead to withdrawal-precipitated seizures. In humans, it is recommended to wean off the drug when it is used for epilepsy treatment.

Reproductive/Nursing Safety

In humans, the FDA categorizes gabapentin as a category *C* drug for use during pregnancy (*Animal studies have shown an adverse effect on the fetus, but there are no adequate studies in humans; or there are no animal reproduction studies and no adequate studies in humans*). At high dosages (at or above human maximum dosages), gabapentin was associated with a variety of fetotoxic and teratogenic effects (*e.g.*, delayed ossification, hydronephrosis, fetal loss) in rats, mice and rabbits.

Gabapentin enters maternal milk. It has been calculated that a nursing human infant could be exposed to a maximum dosage of 1 mg/kg/day. This is 5-10% of the usual pediatric (>3 yrs old) therapeutic dose. In veterinary patients, this appears unlikely to be of significant clinical concern.

Overdosage/Acute Toxicity

In humans, doses of up to 49 grams have been reported without fatality. Most likely effects include ataxia, lethargy/somnolence, diarrhea, etc.

The commercially available oral solution contains 300 mg/mL of xylitol; doses of 0.33 mL/kg may cause hypoglycemia or liver toxicity in dogs.

There were 232 exposures to gabapentin reported to the ASPCA Animal Poison Control Center (APCC) during 2008-2009. In these cases 188 were dogs with 31 showing clinical signs and 43 cases were cats with 13 showing clinical signs. The remaining 1 case involved a bird that did not show any clinical signs. Common findings in dogs recorded in decreasing frequency included lethargy, ataxia, vomiting and somnolence. Common findings in cats recorded in decreasing frequency included ataxia, lethargy, and sedation.

Treatment is basically supportive with general decontamination procedures including emesis, activated charcoal, and cathartics. The drug can be removed with hemodialysis. Should xylitol toxicity be suspected secondary to the human liquid formulation, contact an animal poison control center for further guidance.

Drug Interactions

The following drug interactions have either been reported or are theoretical in humans or animals receiving gabapentin and may be of significance in veterinary patients:

- ■ **ANTACIDS:** Oral antacids given concurrently with gabapentin may decrease oral bioavailability by 20%; if antacids are required, separate doses at least 2 hours from gabapentin
- ■ **HYDROCODONE:** Co-administration of ga-

bapentin and hydrocodone may increase the AUC (area under the curve) of gabapentin and increase the efficacy and/or adverse effects of the drug. Gabapentin can reduce the AUC of hydrocodone, potentially reducing the drug's effectiveness.

■ **MORPHINE:** May increase gabapentin levels

Laboratory Considerations

■ There are reports of gabapentin causing false-positive **urinary protein** readings on *Ames N-Multistix SG* dipstick tests. The use of a sulfosalicylic acid precipitation test to determine presence of urine protein is recommended for patients receiving gabapentin.

Doses

■ **DOGS:**

For ancillary therapy of refractory seizures:

a) 10–20 mg/kg q6-8h. In author's experience, gabapentin is the least effective of the newer antiepileptic drugs, particularly in dogs. (Munana 2010)

b) 10–30 mg/kg PO q8–12h (Podell 2006)

c) 25–60 mg/kg/day PO *divided* q6–8h, the author initially uses 10 mg/kg PO q8h. (Dewey 2005)

d) Study was done in dogs with uncontrolled seizures (at least 2 per month and at least 6 over the prior 3 months) when phenobarbital and potassium bromide levels were therapeutic, or subtherapeutic but had unacceptable side effects: Dogs were dosed at approximately 10 mg/kg PO q8h for 3 months. Six of eleven dogs had a minimum of 50 % reduction in seizures per week. (Platt *et al.* 2006)

e) 10–30 mg/kg PO q8h (Mariani 2010)

As an analgesic:

a) For adjunctive treatment of chronic or cancer pain: 3 mg/kg PO once a day (Lascelles 2003)

b) 1.25–10 mg/kg PO q24h (once daily) (Hardie 2006)

c) Most VIN consultants recommend doses of 5–10 mg/kg PO 2-3 times a day for analgesia. (Rishniw 2007)

d) 2.5–10 mg/kg (up to 15 mg/kg) PO 1-3 times a day. (Posner & papich 2009)

■ **CATS:**

For ancillary therapy of refractory seizures:

a) 5–10 mg/kg PO q8–12h (Podell 2006), (Munana 2010)

b) 5 mg/kg PO three times daily (Pearce 2006)

c) 10–30 mg/kg PO q8-12h (Mariani 2010)

As an analgesic:

a) 1.25–10 mg/kg PO q24h (once daily) (Hardie 2006)

b) For adjunctive treatment of chronic or cancer pain: 3 mg/kg PO once a day (Lascelles 2003), (Hardie *et al.* 2003)

c) For adjunctive analgesia associated with neuropathic pain: While suggested range in cats is 2.5–5 mg/kg PO q12h, this author starts at 5 mg/kg and increases (up to 10 mg/kg) if no effect seen in two hours. May be a higher requirement in cats for post-seizure or CPR vocalization and thrashing. Wean off slowly or patient may experience worse pain. Reduce in renal insufficiency. Usually the limit of dosing is reached when patient is sedated. (Mathews 2006)

d) Most VIN consultants recommend doses of 5–10 mg/kg PO 2-3 times a day for analgesia. (Rishniw 2007)

e) 50 mg (total dose) per cat 1-3 times a day. (Posner & papich 2009)

Monitoring

■ **Note:** Gabapentin serum levels are usually not monitored; therapeutic levels are thought to be 4-16 micrograms/mL.

■ Clinical efficacy and adverse effects should be monitored.

Client Information

■ Clients should report any significant adverse effects such as ataxia or hypersomnolence

Chemistry/Synonyms

Gabapentin occurs as white to off-white crystalline solid that is freely soluble in water. It has a pK_{a1} of 3.7 and a pK_{a2} of 10.7. It is structurally related to GABA (gamma-aminobutyric acid).

Gabapentin may also be known as: CI-945, GOE-3450, *Aclonium®, Equipax®, Gantin®, Gabarone®, Neurontin®, Neurostil®* and *Progresse®*.

Storage/Stability

The commercially available capsules and tablets should be stored at room temperature (25°C, 77°F); excursions permitted to 15–30°C (59–86°F). The oral liquid should be stored in the refrigerator at 2–8°C (36–46°F).

Compatibility/Compounding Considerations

Compounded preparation stability: Commercially available gabapentin solutions contain amounts of xylitol which may be toxic to canine patients. Gabapentin oral suspension compounded from commercially available tablets has been published (Nahata 1999). Triturating twenty (20) gabapentin 600 mg tablets with 60 mL of *Ora-Plus®* and *qs ad* to 120 mL with *Ora-Sweet®* (or *Ora-Sweet® SF*) yields a 100 mg/mL oral suspension that retains >90% potency for 56 days stored at both 4°C and 25°C. Liquid formulations of gabapentin are most stable in the pH range of 5.5 to 6.5

Dosage Forms/Regulatory Status

VETERINARY-LABELED PRODUCTS: None
The ARCI (Racing Commissioners International) has designated this drug as a class 4 substance. See the appendix for more information.

HUMAN-LABELED PRODUCTS:
Gabapentin Oral Capsules & Tablets: 100 mg, 300 mg, 400 mg; 600 mg, & 800 mg (film-coated); *Neurontin®* (Pfizer); generic; (Rx)

Gabapentin Oral Solution: 250 mg/5mL (50 mg/mL) in 470 mL; *Neurontin®* (Pfizer); (Rx) **Note:** Contains xylitol. Use with caution in dogs.

References

Dewey, C. (2005). Managing the Seizure Patient. Proceedings: IVECCS. Accessed via: Veterinary Information Network. http://goo.gl/rmkrc

Dirikolu, L., A. Dafalla, et al. (2008). Pharmacokinetics of gabapentin in horses. *Journal of Veterinary Pharmacology and Therapeutics* 31(2): 175–177.

Hardie, E. (2006). Managing intractable pain. Proceedings: Western Vet Conf 2006. Accessed via: Veterinary Information Network. http://goo.gl/sED8X

Hardie, E., D. Lascelles, et al. (2003). Managing Chronic Pain in Dogs: The Next Level. Proceedings: Pain Management 2003. Accessed via: Veterinary Information Network. http://goo.gl/mAki4

Lascelles, B. (2003). Case examples in the management of cancer pain in dogs and cats, and the future of cancer pain alleviation. Proceedings: American College of Veterinary Internal Medicine. Accessed via: Veterinary Information Network. http://goo.gl/Yxog0

Mariani, C. (2010). Maintenance therapy for the routine & difficult to control epileptic patient. Proceedings: ACVIM Forum. Accessed via: Veterinary Information Network. http://goo.gl/quX8P

Mathews, K. (2006). How do you know your patient hurts? Assessment, recognition & treatment of pain in cats. Proceedings: AAFP. Accessed via: Veterinary Information Network. http://goo.gl/5knAj

Munana, K. (2010). Current Approaches to Seizure Management. Proceedings: ACVIM Forum. Accessed via: Veterinary Information Network. http://goo.gl/vl8Lp

Nahata, M.C. (1999). Development of two stable oral suspensions for gabapentin. *Pediatr Neurol* 20(3): 195–197.

Pearce, L. (2006). Seizures in cats; Why they are not little dogs. Proceedings: Western Vet Conf. Accessed via: Veterinary Information Network. http://goo.gl/dnvl3

Platt, S.R., V. Adams, et al. (2006). Treatment with gabapentin of 11 dogs with refractory idiopathic epilepsy. *Veterinary Record* 159(26): 881–884.

Podell, M. (2006). New Horizons in the treatment of epilepsy. Proceedings: ACVIM. Accessed via: Veterinary Information Network. http://goo.gl/PlHdG

Posner, L.P. & M.G. papich (2009). Your patient is still in pain--Now what? "Rescue analgesia". Proceedings: WVC. Accessed via: Veterinary Information Network. http://goo.gl/WMON9

Rishniw, M. (2007). "Gabapentin Analgesia." *Medical FAQs.* http://goo.gl/aZ7Al.

Siao, K.T., B.H. Pypendop, et al. (2010). Pharmacokinetics of gabapentin in cats. *American Journal of Veterinary Research* 71(7): 817–821.

GEMCITABINE HCL

(jem-*site*-ah-ben)   Gemzar®

ANTINEOPLASTIC

Prescriber Highlights

▶ Antineoplastic agent that may potentially be useful for treating several cancers in dogs or cats

▶ Very limited clinical use & research performed thus far

▶ Myelosuppression most likely adverse effect

▶ Very expensive

Uses/Indications

Very limited clinical use and research performed with this drug to date have demonstrated limited clinical efficacy. However, it potentially may be useful as a radiosensitizer for non-resectable tumors, as part of combination protocols, or as a single agent for tumors not amenable to more accepted therapies. Follow research reports for the most up-to-date information.

In humans, gemcitabine has shown some efficacy in treating pancreatic carcinoma, small-cell lung carcinoma, lymphoma, bladder and other soft tissue carcinomas.

Pharmacology/Actions

Gemcitabine exhibits cell phase specificity and acts primarily on the S phase. It also inhibits cell progression through the G1/S-phase boundary.

Gemcitabine is metabolized intracellularly to diflurodeoxycytidine monophosphate (dFdCMP) that is then converted into diphosphate (dFdCDP) and triphosphate (dFdCTP) forms, the metabolites that give the drug its activity. The diphosphate inhibits ribonucleotide reductase. The triphosphate competes with deoxycytidine triphosphate (dTCP; the "normal" nucleotide) for incorporation into DNA strands.

Pharmacokinetics

In dogs, gemcitabine exhibits first order elimination and has a terminal half-life of about 1.5–3.2 hours. Volume of distribution (steady-state) is around 1 L/kg. Approximately 80% of the drug is excreted in the urine within 24 hours of dosing, primarily as the uracil metabolite.

In humans, gemcitabine levels achieve steady state in about 15 minutes during a 30 minute infusion. Protein binding is negligible. Volume of distribution is about 50 L/m^2. Less than 10% of the drug is excreted unchanged in the urine.

Contraindications/Precautions/Warnings

Gemcitabine is contraindicated in patients hypersensitive to it. It should be used with caution in patients with diminished renal or hepatic function.

Adverse Effects

Gemcitabine may cause myelosuppression and can affect red cell, white cell, and platelet cell lines, but neutrophils and platelets appear to be most affected. Neutrophil nadirs usually occur 3–7 days post treatment. GI effects have been reported in animals receiving the drug, but are usually mild. Retinal hemorrhage could occur in animals receiving gemcitabine.

In a pilot study (Kosarek et al. 2005) in 19 dogs receiving up to 675 mg/m^2 biweekly demonstrated "minimal and acceptable toxicity." Another study (Turner et al. 2006) where dogs with lymphoma were given gemcitabine as single agent therapy at 400 mg/m^2 weekly for 3 weeks and then off one week, showed significant decreases in neutrophils and platelets 7 days post treatment. 15 of the 21 dogs in the study required dosage reduction or delay in retreatment. Only 7 of the 21 dogs finished the initial 4 week cycle and a second cycle did not result in any objective therapeutic response. In a study where gemcitabine was combined with carboplatin treatment for carcinomas in dogs adverse effects included mild to moderate GI and hematologic toxicity; 32% of dogs developed grade 3 or 4 neutropenia, 24% developed thrombocytopenia and 73% developed mild to moderate, self-limiting GI toxicity. (Dominguez et al. 2009)

In cats treated with double therapy (carboplatin/gemcitabine), 21% or 50% of treated cats, depending on the dosing protocol used, developed grade 3 or 4 neutropenia or thrombocytopenia and 7% developed grade 3 or 4 GI toxicity. (Martinez-Ruzafa et al. 2009)

Reproductive/Nursing Safety

In pregnant humans, gemcitabine is designated by the FDA as a category *D* drug (*There is evidence of human fetal risk, but the potential benefits from the use of the drug in pregnant women may be acceptable despite its potential risks.*)

It is unknown whether gemcitabine is excreted in maternal milk.

Overdosage/Acute Toxicity

There is no known antidote to gemcitabine in an overdose situation. Myelosuppression should be expected. Treatment is supportive.

Drug Interactions

No specific drug interactions were noted, but toxic effects (myelosuppression, GI) could be additive when used with other drugs that also cause those effects.

Laboratory Considerations

■ No specific laboratory interactions or considerations noted.

Doses

Note: Because of the potential toxicity of this drug to patients, veterinary personnel and clients, and since chemotherapy indications, treatment protocols, monitoring and safety guidelines often change, the following dosages should be used only as a general guide. Consultation with a veterinary oncologist and referral to current veterinary oncology references [*e.g.*, (Henry & Higginbotham 2009); (Argyle et al. 2008); (Withrow & Vail 2007); (Villalobos 2007); (Ogilvie & Moore 2006); (Ogilvie & Moore 2001)] is *strongly recommended.*

■ **DOGS/CATS:**
Depending on the study, gemcitabine doses for dogs and cats have ranged widely from 45 mg/m^2–800 mg/m^2. Recent studies combining it with carboplatin in dogs and cats have used 2 mg/kg IV over 20-30 minutes no more than once every 7 days.

Monitoring

■ CBC before each treatment

■ Fundic exam weekly while on therapy

■ Prior to therapy, baseline renal and hepatic function and periodically thereafter

Client Information

■ Owners should understand that veterinary experience with this drug is limited and it must be considered an "investigational" treatment.

■ Gemcitabine residues can be detected in urine up to 7 days after a dose. If owners must clean up urine from treated dogs, they should take proper precautions, such as wearing gloves.

Chemistry/Synonyms

A synthetic pyrimidine nucleoside cytarabine analog antineoplastic agent, gemcitabine HCl occurs as white to off-white solid. It is soluble in water and practically insoluble in ethanol or polar organic solvents. Its chemical name is 2,2'-diflurodeoxycytidine.

Gemcitabine may also be known as: dFdC, LY-288022, *Abine®*, *Antoril®*, *Gemcite®*, or *Gemtrol®* and *Gemzar®*.

Storage/Stability

Store unreconstituted gemcitabine at controlled room temperature (20–25°C; 68–77°F). After reconstitution with 0.9% sodium chloride injection without preservatives, the resulting solution may be stored at room temperature for up to 24 hours. Reportedly, when frozen at -20°C, the reconstituted solution is stable for 7 days. Do not refrigerate or re-crystallization may occur. Reconstituted solution should not be greater than 40 mg/mL (at least 5 mL of diluent for 200 mg vial; 25 mL diluent for 1 gram vial). Additional diluent may be added to yield concentrations as low as 0.1 mg/mL.

Compatibility/Compounding Considerations

Gemcitabine injection is reportedly physically **incompatible** with the following medications when used via Y-site injection: acyclovir, amphotericin B, cefoperazone, cefotaxime sodium, furosemide, imipenem, methotrexate, methylprednisolone sodium succinate, mitomycin, piperacillin, and prochlorperazine.

Dosage Forms/Regulatory Status

VETERINARY-LABELED PRODUCTS: None

HUMAN-LABELED PRODUCTS:

Gemcitabine HCl lyophilized Powder for Injection: 200 mg (in 10 mL single-use vials) and 1 g (in 50 mL single-use vials); *Gemzar®* (Lilly); (Rx)

References

Argyle, D., M. Brearly, et al. (2008). *Decision Making in Small Animal Oncology*, Wiley-Blackwell.

Dominguez, P.A., N.G. Dervisis, et al. (2009). Combined Gemcitabine and Carboplatin Therapy for Carcinomas in Dogs. *Journal of Veterinary Internal Medicine* 23(1): 130–137.

Henry, C. & M. Higginbotham (2009). *Cancer Management in Small Animal Practice*, Saunders.

Kosarek, C., W. Kissabeth, et al. (2005). Clinical evaluation of gemcitabine in dogs with spontaneously occurring malignancies. *J Vet Intern Med* 19(1): 81–86.

Martinez-Ruzafa, I., P.A. Dominguez, et al. (2009). Tolerability of Gemcitabine and Carboplatin Doublet Therapy in Cats with Carcinomas. *Journal of Veterinary Internal Medicine* 23(3): 570–577.

Ogilvie, G. & A. Moore (2001). *Feline Oncology: A Comprehensive Guide to Compassionate Care*, Veterinary Learning Systems.

Ogilvie, G. & A. Moore (2006). *Managing the Canine Cancer Patient: A Practical Guide to Compassionate Care*, Veterinary Learning Systems.

Turner, A., K. Hahn, et al. (2006). Single agent gemcitabine chemotherapy in dogs with spontaneously occurring lymphoma. *J Vet Intern Med* 20(6): 1384–1388.

Villalobos, A. (2007). *Canine and Feline Geriatric Oncology.* Ames, Blackwell.

Withrow, S. & D. Vail (2007). *Withrow and MacEwen's Small Animal Clinical Oncology 4th Ed.* Philadelphia, Elsevier.

GEMFIBROZIL

(jem-*fih*-broh-zil)   Lopid®

ORAL ANTIHYPERLIPIDEMIC

Prescriber Highlights

▶ May be useful as adjunctive therapy (with low fat diet) to treat hypertriglyceridemia in dogs or cats

▶ Very limited experience & no published clinical studies in dogs or cats; efficacy or safety is not established

Uses/Indications

Gemfibrozil may be useful to reduce serum triglycerides in those dogs or cats with hypertriglyceridemia and when diet modifications alone have been unsuccessful. One reference (Elliott 2005) suggests not adding drug therapy to treat hypertriglyceridemia unless the serum triglyceride concentration exceeds 500 mg/dL with associated clinical signs. Another states that because side effects are believed to occur rarely, gemfibrozil is commonly recommended in dogs in combination with dietary therapy when the latter fails to lower triglyceride levels below 5.65 mmol/L (500 mg/dL) (Xenoulis & Steiner 2010).

Gemfibrozil has been shown to reduce influenza-related mortality in mice and may become an adjunctive treatment for severe influenza.

Pharmacology/Actions

Gemfibrozil inhibits lipolysis in adipose issue and reduces hepatic uptake of plasma free fatty acids causing reduced production of triglycerides. Secondarily, gemfibrozil inhibits the synthesis of very low-density lipoprotein (VLDL) carrier apolipoprotein B, which reduces VLDL production and incorporation of long-chain fatty acids into triglycerides.

Pharmacokinetics

No pharmacokinetic data for dogs or cats was found. In humans, gemfibrozil is rapidly and completely absorbed from the GI tract. The rate and extent of absorption are greatest when administered 30 minutes before a meal. It is highly bound to plasma protein and highest concentrations of the drug are found in the liver and kidneys. In the liver, 4 major metabolites are formed in humans, which are primarily excreted in the urine. Elimination half-life is about 1.5 hours. Reductions in plasma VDL levels are noted within 5 days; peak reductions occur about 4 weeks after starting therapy.

Contraindications/Precautions/Warnings

Contraindications for using gemfibrozil in dogs or cats are not known. In humans, gemfibrozil is contraindicated in patients with severe hepatic or renal dysfunction or with known hypersensitivity to gemfibrozil.

Use with caution in dogs or cats as very limited safety data is available for this medication.

Adverse Effects

Because no clinical studies have been published regarding gemfibrozil use in dogs and cats and clinical use has been quite limited, an accurate adverse effect profile is not known. Anecdotal reports are that the drug has been well tolerated in the few patients that have received the medication, but abdominal pain, vomiting, diarrhea, and abnormal liver function tests have been reported.

In humans, the most common adverse effects reported are GI related (dyspepsia, nausea, vomiting, diarrhea, etc.) and CNS related (headache, paresthesias, somnolence, dizziness, fatigue). Other adverse effects reported include myositis, taste alterations, blurred vision, eczema and decreased libido/impotence. Rarely, hypersensitivity reactions, bone marrow depression, and increases in liver function test values (AST, ALT, Alk Phos, bilirubin) have been reported. Long-term studies in rats have demonstrated an increased rate of benign and malignant liver tumors when doses were approximately 1.3X of the human dose.

Reproductive/Nursing Safety

Gemfibrozil administered to female rats prior to and during gestation at 0.6–2X the human dose, showed decreased fertility rates and their offspring had an increased incidence of skeletal abnormalities. When given to pregnant rabbits at 1–3X the human dose, litter sizes were decreased and at the highest dose (3X), parietal bone variations were noted. In humans, the FDA categorizes gemfibrozil as category *C* for use during pregnancy (*Animal studies have shown an adverse effect on the fetus, but there are no adequate studies in humans; or there are no animal reproduction studies and no adequate studies in humans.*)

It is not known if gemfibrozil enters milk and safe use during nursing cannot be assured.

Overdosage/Acute Toxicity

Limited information is available. One 7-year-old child ingested up to 9 grams and recovered with supportive treatment. The reported LD50 (oral) in rats is 1414 mg/kg. Consider gut-emptying protocols for recent large oral ingestions and support as required. Monitor for dehydration and electrolyte imbalance if vomiting and/or diarrhea is severe or persists. Monitor liver function tests.

Drug Interactions

The following drug interactions have either been reported or are theoretical in humans or animals receiving gemfibrozil and may be of significance in veterinary patients:

■ **THIAZIDE DIURETICS, BETA-BLOCKERS, ESTROGENS:** May possibly increase triglyceride concentrations

■ **URSODIOL:** May reduce effectiveness of gemfibrozil

■ **WARFARIN:** Gemfibrozil may potentiate anticoagulant effects

Laboratory Considerations

■ No specific concerns associated with gemfibrozil; see Monitoring

Doses

■ **DOGS/CATS:**
For hypertriglyceridemia that has not been controlled with diet alone:
a) **Dogs:** 150 mg–300 mg (total dose) PO q12h;
Cats: 7.5–10 mg/kg PO q12h
b) **Dogs:** 200 mg (total dose) PO once daily;
Cats: 10 mg/kg PO q12h (Elliott 2005)

Monitoring

■ Plasma triglycerides; realistic goal for therapy is 400 mg/dL or less
■ Baseline and periodic: CBC, liver function tests
■ Adverse effects
■ If treatment is less effective than hoped, assure that clients have adhered to prescribed diet and dosing schedule before altering dosage

Client Information

■ Clients must understand the use of this drug in animals is "investigational"; although FDA-approved for use in people, little information is known about it for use in dogs or cats
■ Gemfibrozil is used in conjunction with diet modification; lack of adherence to dietary recommendations will likely negate the benefits of using this medication
■ Report any significant adverse effects to the veterinarian, including changes in behavior, activity level, gastrointestinal effects (vomiting, diarrhea, lack of appetite), yellowish eyes or mucous membranes, etc.

Chemistry/Synonyms

Gemfibrozil is a fibric acid derivative that occurs as a waxy, crystalline solid that is practically insoluble in water, but soluble in alcohol.

Gemfibrozil may also be known as: CI-719, gemfibrozilo, or gemfibrozilium; many international trade names are available.

Storage/Stability

Gemfibrozil tablets or capsules should be stored below 30°C in tight containers.

Dosage Forms/Regulatory Status

VETERINARY-LABELED PRODUCTS: None
HUMAN-LABELED PRODUCTS:
Gemfibrozil Oral Tablets: 600 mg; *Lopid*® (Parke-Davis); generic (Rx). **Note:** 300 mg capsules are available in Canada

References

Elliott, D. (2005). Dietary and medical considerations in hyperlipidemia. *Textbook of Veterinary Internal Medicine.* S Ettinger and E Feldman Eds., Elsevier: 592–595.
Xenoulis, P.G. & J.M. Steiner (2010). Lipid metabolism and hyperlipidemia in dogs. *Veterinary Journal* 183(1): 12–21.

GENTAMICIN SULFATE

(jen-ta-*mye*-sin)   Gentocin®, Garamycin®
AMINOGLYCOSIDE ANTIBIOTIC

Prescriber Highlights

▶ Parenteral-aminoglycoside antibiotic that has "good" activity against a variety of bacteria, predominantly gram-negative aerobic bacilli, but also many staphylococci strains
▶ Because of potential adverse effects, usually reserved for serious infections when given systemically
▶ Adverse effect profile: Nephrotoxicity, ototoxicity, neuromuscular blockade
▶ Cats may be more sensitive to toxic effects
▶ Risk factors for nephrotoxicity: Pre-existing renal disease, age (both neonatal & geriatric), fever, sepsis, & dehydration
▶ Usually dosed once daily

Uses/Indications

The inherent toxicity of the aminoglycosides limit their systemic (parenteral) use to the treatment of serious gram-negative infections when there is either a documented lack of susceptibility to other less toxic antibiotics or when the clinical situation dictates immediate treatment of a presumed gram-negative infection before culture and susceptibility results are reported.

Various gentamicin products are FDA-approved for parenteral use in dogs, cats, chickens, turkeys, and swine, although the injectable small animal products appear to be no longer marketed. Although routinely used parenterally in horses, gentamicin is only FDA-approved for intrauterine infusion in this species. Oral products are FDA-approved for gastrointestinal infections in swine and turkeys. For more information, refer to the Dosage section below.

Pharmacology/Actions

Gentamicin has a mechanism of action and spectrum of activity (primarily gram-negative aerobes) similar to the other aminoglycosides. Like the other aminoglycoside antibiotics, it acts on susceptible bacteria presumably by irreversibly binding to the 30S ribosomal subunit thereby inhibiting protein synthesis. It is considered a bactericidal concentration-dependent antibiotic.

Gentamicin's spectrum of activity includes coverage against many aerobic gram-negative and some aerobic gram-positive bacteria, including most species of *E. coli, Klebsiella, Proteus, Pseudomonas, Salmonella, Enterobacter, Serratia,* and *Shigella, Mycoplasma,* and *Staphylococcus* (strains of MRSA are often resistant). Several strains of *Pseudomonas aeruginosa, Proteus,* and *Serratia* that are resistant to gentamicin may still be treated with amikacin.

Antimicrobial activity of the aminoglycosides is enhanced in an alkaline environment.

The aminoglycoside antibiotics are inactive against fungi, viruses and most anaerobic bacteria.

Pharmacokinetics

Gentamicin, like other aminoglycosides, is not appreciably absorbed after oral or intrauterine administration, but is absorbed from topical administration (not skin or urinary bladder) when used in irrigations during surgical procedures. Patients receiving oral aminoglycosides with hemorrhagic or necrotic enteritises may absorb appreciable quantities of the drug. After IM administration to dogs and cats, peak levels occur from 1/2 to 1 hour later. Subcutaneous injection results in slightly delayed peak levels and with more variability than after IM injection. Bioavailability from extravascular injection (IM or SC) is greater than 90%.

After absorption, aminoglycosides are distributed primarily in the extracellular fluid. They are found in ascitic, pleural, pericardial, peritoneal, synovial and abscess fluids and high levels are found in sputum, bronchial secretions and bile. Aminoglycosides are minimally protein bound (<20%, streptomycin 35%) to plasma proteins. Aminoglycosides do not readily cross the blood-brain barrier or penetrate ocular tissue. CSF levels are unpredictable and range from 0−50% of those found in the serum. Therapeutic levels are found in bone, heart, gallbladder and lung tissues after parenteral dosing. Aminoglycosides tend to accumulate in certain tissues, such as the inner ear and kidneys, which may help explain their toxicity. Volumes of distribution have been reported to be 0.15−0.3 L/kg in adult cats and dogs, and 0.26−0.58 L/kg in horses. Volumes of distribution may be significantly larger in neonates and juvenile animals due to their higher extracellular fluid fractions. Aminoglycosides cross the placenta, but one study showed no detectable levels in foals when gentamicin was administered to mares at term. In other species, fetal concentrations range from 15−50% of those found in maternal serum.

Elimination of aminoglycosides after parenteral administration occurs almost entirely by glomerular filtration. The elimination half-lives for gentamicin have been reported to be 1.82−3.25 hours in horses, 2.2−2.7 hours in calves, 2.4 hours in sheep, 1.8 hours in cows, 1.9 hours in swine, 1 hour in rabbits, and 0.5−1.5 hours in dogs and cats. Patients with decreased renal function can have significantly prolonged half-lives. In humans with normal renal function, elimination rates can be highly variable with the aminoglycoside antibiotics.

Contraindications/Precautions/Warnings

Aminoglycosides are contraindicated in patients who are hypersensitive to them. Because these drugs are often the only effective agents in severe gram-negative infections there are no other absolute contraindications to their use. However, they should be used with extreme caution in patients with preexisting renal disease with concomitant monitoring and dosage interval adjustments made. Other risk factors for the development of toxicity include age (both neonatal and geriatric patients), fever, sepsis and dehydration.

Because aminoglycosides can cause irreversible ototoxicity, they should be used with caution in "working" dogs (e.g., "seeing-eye", herding, dogs for the hearing impaired, etc.).

Aminoglycosides should be used with caution in patients with neuromuscular disorders (e.g., myasthenia gravis) due to their neuromuscular blocking activity. They should not be used in animals with botulism.

Sighthound dogs may require reduced dosages of aminoglycosides as they have significantly smaller volumes of distribution.

Because aminoglycosides are eliminated primarily through renal mechanisms, they should be used cautiously, preferably with serum monitoring and dosage adjustment in neonatal or geriatric animals.

IM injections in horses have caused muscle irritation and IV injections are preferred. The risk for antibiotic associated diarrhea/colitis in horses due to gentamicin is thought to be low. But gentamicin may promote Beta-2 toxin production by *C. perfringens* and may increase the severity of colitis (McGorum & Pirie 2010).

Aminoglycosides are often considered contraindicated in rabbits as they adversely affect the GI flora balance in these animals, but dosages are listed below. Use with caution.

Adverse Effects

The aminoglycosides are infamous for their nephrotoxic and ototoxic effects. The nephrotoxic (tubular necrosis) mechanisms of these drugs are not completely understood, but are probably related to interference with phospholipid metabolism in the lysosomes of proximal renal tubular cells, resulting in leakage of proteolytic enzymes into the cytoplasm. Nephrotoxicity is usually manifested by increases in: BUN, creatinine, non-protein nitrogen in the serum, and decreases in urine specific gravity and creatinine clearance. Proteinuria and cells or casts may also be seen in the urine. Nephrotoxicity is usually reversible once the drug is discontinued. While gentamicin may be more nephrotoxic than the other aminoglycosides, the incidences of nephrotoxicity with all of these agents require equal caution and monitoring.

Ototoxicity (8th cranial nerve toxicity) of the aminoglycosides can manifest by either auditory and/or vestibular clinical signs and may be irreversible. Vestibular clinical signs are more frequent with streptomycin, gentamicin, or tobramycin. Auditory clinical signs are more frequent with amikacin, neomycin, or kanamycin, but other forms can occur with any of the drugs. Cats are apparently very sensitive to the vestibular effects of the aminoglycosides.

The aminoglycosides can also cause neuromuscular blockade, facial edema, pain/inflammation at injection site, peripheral neuropathy, and hypersensitivity reactions. Rarely, GI clinical signs, hematologic and hepatic effects have been reported.

Reproductive/Nursing Safety

Aminoglycosides can cross the placenta and, while rare, may cause 8th cranial nerve toxicity or nephrotoxicity in fetuses. Because the drug should only be used in serious infections, the benefits of therapy may exceed the potential risks. In humans, the FDA categorizes this drug as category *D* for use during pregnancy (*There is evidence of human fetal risk, but the potential benefits from the use of the drug in pregnant women may be acceptable despite its potential risks.*). In a separate system evaluating the safety of drugs in canine and feline pregnancy (Papich 1989), this drug is categorized as in class: *C* (*These drugs may have potential risks. Studies in people or laboratory animals have uncovered risks, and these drugs should be used cautiously*

as a last resort when the benefit of therapy clearly outweighs the risks.)

While small amounts of gentamicin may be excreted into milk, the risk to nursing offspring appears minimal.

Overdosage/Acute Toxicity

Should an inadvertent overdosage be administered, three treatments have been recommended. **1)** Hemodialysis is very effective in reducing serum levels of the drug, but is not a viable option for most veterinary patients. **2)** Peritoneal dialysis also will reduce serum levels, but is much less effective. **3)** Complexation of drug with ticarcillin (12–20 g/day in humans) is reportedly nearly as effective as hemodialysis.

Drug Interactions

The following drug interactions have either been reported or are theoretical in humans or animals receiving gentamicin and may be of significance in veterinary patients:

- **BETA-LACTAM ANTIBIOTICS (penicillins, cephalosporins):** May have synergistic effects against some bacteria; some potential for inactivation of aminoglycosides *in vitro* (do not mix together) and *in vivo* (patients in renal failure)

- **CEPHALOSPORINS:** The concurrent use of aminoglycosides with cephalosporins is somewhat controversial. Potentially, cephalosporins could cause additive nephrotoxicity when used with aminoglycosides, but this interaction has only been well documented with cephaloridine and cephalothin (both no longer marketed).

- **DIURETICS, LOOP (e.g., furosemide, torsemide) or OSMOTIC (e.g., mannitol):** Concurrent use with loop or osmotic diuretics may increase the nephrotoxic or ototoxic potential of the aminoglycosides

- **NEPHROTOXIC DRUGS, OTHER (e.g., cisplatin, amphotericin b, polymyxin B, or vancomycin):** Potential for increased risk for nephrotoxicity

- **NEUROMUSCULAR BLOCKING AGENTS & ANESTHETICS, GENERAL:** Concomitant use with general anesthetics or neuromuscular blocking agents could potentiate neuromuscular blockade

Laboratory Considerations

- **Gentamicin serum concentrations** may be falsely decreased if the patient is also receiving beta-lactam antibiotics and the serum is stored prior analysis. It is recommended that if assay is delayed, samples be frozen and, if possible, drawn at times when the beta-lactam antibiotic is at a trough.

Doses

Note: Most infectious disease clinicians now agree that aminoglycosides should be dosed once a day in most patients (mammals). This dosing regimen yields higher peak levels with resultant greater bacterial kill, and as aminoglyco-sides exhibit a "post-antibiotic effect", surviving susceptible bacteria generally do not replicate as rapidly even when antibiotic concentrations are below MIC. Periods where levels are low may decrease the "adaptive resistance" (bacteria take up less drug in the presence of continuous exposure) that can occur. Once daily dosing may also decrease the toxicity of aminoglycosides as lower urinary concentrations may mean less-uptake into renal tubular cells. However, patients who are neutropenic (or otherwise immunosuppressed) may benefit from more frequent dosing (q8h).

■ **DOGS:**

For susceptible infections:

a) For empiric therapy: 10–14 mg/kg once a day *(route not specified; assume IV, SC, IM—Plumb)* (Autran de Morais 2009)

b) For localized, urinary infections: First dose of 4.4 mg/kg IM, SC and then 2.2 mg/kg IM, SC once daily (q24h) for 7–10 days;

For orthopedic and soft tissue infections: 4.4–6.6 mg/kg IV, IM, SC once daily (q24h) for <7 days.

For bacteremia, sepsis: 6.6 mg/kg IV, IM, SC once daily (q24h) for <7 days.

Monitor renal function by urine sediment examination and serum urea nitrogen levels. (Greene *et al.* 2006)

c) For Brucellosis: Gentamicin 5 mg/kg SC once daily (q24h) for 7 days; 2-courses of treatment, treating on weeks one and four; plus Minocycline at 25 mg/kg PO once daily (q24h) for 4 weeks. Eventually, doxycycline can be substituted for minocycline at the same dosage to lower cost. Infected animals may need to be treated for two or more 4-week courses. Sequential antibody tests at 3 to 6 monthly intervals are recommended to monitor treatment. Monitor renal function secondary to gentamicin therapy. (Hartmannn & Greene 2005)

d) For Greyhounds and probably other Sighthound breeds: 6 mg/kg IV q24h or 9 mg/kg SC/IM q24h. (KuKanich 2008)

■ **CATS:**

For susceptible infections:

a) For empiric therapy: 5–8 mg/kg once a day *(route not specified; assume IV, SC, IM—Plumb)* (Autran de Morais 2009)

b) 6–8 mg/kg (route not specified) once daily (q24h). Neutropenic or immunocompromised patients may still need to be dosed q8h (dose divided). (Trepanier 1999)

c) 8 mg/kg once daily or 2–4 mg/kg q8h IV, IM or SC (Aucoin 2002)

d) For localized, urinary infections: 2.2 mg/kg IV, IM, SC once daily (q24h) for <7 days;

For bacteremia, sepsis: 4.4 mg/kg IV, IM, SC once daily (q24h) for <7 days.

Monitor renal function by urine sediment examination and serum urea nitrogen levels. (Greene *et al.* 2006)

■ **FERRETS:**

For susceptible infections:

a) 5 mg/kg SC, IM q24h; use with caution or avoid use. (Morrisey & Carpenter 2004)

b) 4–8 mg/kg IM, SC, IV divided and given 2–3 times daily. Use only when culture and sensitivity dictates. (Williams 2000)

■ **RABBITS/RODENTS/SMALL MAMMALS:**

a) **Rabbits:** 5–8 mg/kg daily dose (may divide into q8h–q24h) SC, IM or IV. Increased efficacy and decreased toxicity if given once daily. If given IV, dilute into 4 mL/kg of saline and give over 20 minutes (Ivey & Morrisey 2000)

b) **Chinchillas, Gerbils, Guinea pigs, Hamsters, Mice, Rats:** 2–4 mg/kg SC or IM q8–24h (Adamcak & Otten 2000)

c) **Chinchillas:** 2–4 mg/kg SC, IM q8–24h (Hayes 2000)

■ **HORSES:**

For susceptible infections:

a) Foals: 11–15 mg/kg q24h *(route not listed; assume IV—Plumb)*. Ideally, TDM should be used to reduce risk for nephrotoxicity and optimizing efficacy. (Corley & Hollis 2009)

b) Adults: 6.6 mg/kg IV or IM—(because IM administration may cause muscle irritation in some horses most prefer using IV) once daily (q24h) (Foreman 1999), (Chaffin 2006), (Haggett & Wilson 2008)

c) For systemic treatment of susceptible bacterial infections of the reproductive tract: gentamicin 6.6 mg/kg IV (slow infusion) once daily (q24h). For intrauterine infusion: Irrigate uterus (Morresey & Waldridge 2010) for 2-3 days prior to antibiotic infusion to remove inflammatory debris. Gentamicin dosed at 1–2 grams IU. Buffer with bicarbonate (equal volume of 7.5% bicarbonate and diluted in saline) or large volume (200 mL) of saline. Mares with bacterial endometritis should be treated with IU antibiotics for 3-7 days. Treatment length dependent on history, chronicity of infection, bacteria isolated, and mare's ability to clear uterine fluid. (LeBlanc 2009)

d) For pleuropneumonia in adults: Initial dose 8 mg/kg IV, adjust as needed based upon therapeutic drug monitoring; or 6.6 mg/kg IV or IM q24h. (Sprayberry 2009)

e) From a case report of successful treatment of an adult horse with *R. equi*: ceftiofur (2 mg/kg IV q12h) and gentamicin 6.6. mg/kg IV q24h for 14 days. Thereafter, treatment was changed to doxycycline (10 mg/kg PO q12h for 28 days.) (Morresey & Waldridge 2010)

■ **SWINE:**

For susceptible infections:

a) For colibacillosis in neonates: 5 mg PO or IM once (Label directions; *Garacin*® *Pig Pump* and *Piglet Injection*—Schering)

b) For weanlings and other swine:

Colibacillosis: 1.1 mg/kg/day in drinking water (concentration of 25 mg/gallon) for 3 days.

Swine dysentery (*Treponema hyodysenteriae*): 2.2 mg/kg/day in drinking water (concentration of 50 mg/gallon) for 3 days (Label directions; *Garacin*® *Soluble Powder* and *Oral Solution*—Schering)

■ **BIRDS:**

For susceptible infections:

a) In companion birds: Amikacin is the preferred aminoglycoside, but gentamicin can be used to reduce expense: 2.5–5 mg/kg once per day (*Note: route not listed, IM assumed as author lists IM doses for amikacin—Plumb*). In severely immunocompromised birds, twice daily administration with a beta-lactam antibiotic may improve treatment success. Birds often show polyuria during treatment, but it usually resolves after short duration (<7 days) of therapy. Concurrent SC fluids may reduce nephrotoxicity. (Flammer 2006)

b) Ratites: 5 mg/kg IM once daily; **Note:** use only as a last resort as it causes visceral gout (Jenson 1998)

■ **REPTILES:**

For susceptible infections:

a) For bacterial gastritis in snakes: gentamicin 2.5 mg/kg IM every 72 hours with oral neomycin 15 mg/kg plus oral live lactobacillus. (Burke 1986)

b) For bacterial shell diseases in turtles: 5–10 mg/kg daily in water turtles, every other day in land turtles and tortoises for 7–10 days. Used commonly with a beta-lactam antibiotic. Recommend beginning therapy with 20 mL/kg fluid injection. Maintain hydration and monitor uric acid levels when possible. (Rosskopf 1986)

Monitoring (Parenteral use)

■ Efficacy (cultures, clinical signs associated with infection)

■ Renal toxicity; baseline urinalysis, serum creatinine/BUN. Casts in the urine are often the initial sign of impending nephrotoxicity. Casts or increased serum creatinine may not be good markers in neonates. Frequency of monitoring during therapy is controversial. Frequency of monitoring during therapy is controversial, but daily urinalysis and serum creatinine may not be too frequent.

■ Gross monitoring of vestibular or auditory toxicity is recommended

■ Serum levels, if possible. Draw levels at 1, 2, and 4 hours post dose. Peak should be at least 20 micrograms/mL and 4 hour sample should be less than 10 micrograms/mL (Papich 2003).

Client Information

■ With appropriate training, owners may give subcutaneous injections at home, but routine monitoring of therapy for efficacy and toxicity must still be done.

■ Clients should understand that the potential exists for severe toxicity (nephrotoxicity, ototoxicity) developing from this medication.

Chemistry/Synonyms

An aminoglycoside obtained from cultures of *Micromonaspora purpurea*, gentamicin sulfate occurs as a white to buff powder that is soluble in water and insoluble in alcohol. The commercial product is actually a combination of gentamicin sulfate C_1, C_2, and C_3, but all these compounds apparently have similar antimicrobial activities. Commercially available injections have a pH from 3–5.5.

Gentamicin may also be known as: gentamicin sulphate, gentamicini sulfas, NSC-82261, and Sch-9724; many trade names are available.

Storage/Stability

Gentamicin sulfate for injection and the oral solution should be stored at room temperature (15–30°C); freezing or temperatures above 40°C should be avoided. The soluble powder should be stored from 2–30°C. Do not store or offer medicated-drinking water in rusty containers or the drug may be destroyed.

Compatibility/Compounding Considerations

While the manufacturer does not recommend that gentamicin be mixed with other drugs, it is reportedly physically **compatible** and stable in all commonly used intravenous solutions and with the following drugs: bleomycin sulfate, cefoxitin sodium, cimetidine HCl, clindamycin phosphate, methicillin sodium, metronidazole (with and without sodium bicarbonate), penicillin G sodium, and verapamil HCl.

The following drugs or solutions are reportedly physically **incompatible** or only compatible in specific situations with gentamicin: amphotericin B, ampicillin sodium, carbenicillin disodium, cefamandole naftate, cephalothin sodium, cephapirin sodium, dopamine HCl, furosemide, and heparin sodium. Compatibility is depen-

624 GENTAMICIN SULFATE

dent upon factors such as pH, concentration, temperature and diluent used; consult specialized references or a hospital pharmacist for more specific information.

In vitro inactivation of aminoglycoside antibiotics by beta-lactam antibiotics is well documented. Gentamicin is very susceptible to this effect and it is recommended to avoid mixing these compounds together.

Dosage Forms/Regulatory Status

VETERINARY-LABELED PRODUCTS:

Gentamicin Sulfate Injection: 100 mg/mL in 100 mL and 250 mL vials; *Amtech® Gentamax 100* (IVX), *Gentafuse®* (Butler), *Gentamax® 100* (Phoenix Pharmaceutical), *Gentaved® 100* (Vedco), *Gentozen®* (Schering-Plough), *Legacy®* (AgriLabs); generic; (Rx). FDA-approved for horses.

Gentamicin Sulfate Injection: 100 mg/mL (poultry only) in 100 mL vials; *Garasol® Injection* (Schering-Plough); *Amtech® Gentapoult* (IVX); (OTC) For use in day-old chickens (slaughter withdrawal = 5 weeks) and 1–3 day-old turkeys (slaughter withdrawal=9 weeks) only.

Gentamicin Sulfate Injection: 5 mg/mL in 250 mL vials; *Garacin® Piglet Injection* (Schering-Plough); (OTC). FDA-approved for use in piglets up to 3 days of age. Slaughter (when used as labeled) = 40 days.

Gentamicin Sulfate Oral Solution: 5 mg/mL in 118 mL bottles with pump applicator; generic; (Rx); FDA-approved for use in neonatal swine only. Slaughter withdrawal = 14 days.

Gentamicin Soluble Powder: 333.33 mg/g in 360 gram jars. FDA-approved for use in weanling swine. Slaughter withdrawal = 10 days. *Gen-Gard® Soluble Powder* (AgriLabs); (OTC)

Gentamicin Sulfate Soluble Powder: 2 g gentamicin/30 grams of powder in 360-gram jar; *Garacin® Soluble Powder* (Schering-Plough); (OTC). FDA-approved for use in swine. Slaughter (when used as labeled) = 10 days.

Veterinary FDA-approved injections for chickens and turkeys plus a water additive for egg dipping may also be available. Ophthalmic, otic, and topical preparations are available with veterinary labeling.

HUMAN-APPROVED PRODUCTS (partial listing):

Gentamicin Sulfate Injection: 40 mg/mL (as sulfate) in 2 mL & 20 mL vials and 1.5 mL & 2 mL cartridge-needle Units; 10 mg/mL (as sulfate) in 2 mL vials & ADD-Vantage 60 mg, 80 mg & 100 mg vials; 0.8 mg/mL, 0.9 mg/mL, & 1 mg/mL (as gentamicin base) in 100 mL single-dose containers; 1.2 mg/mL, 1.4 mg/mL & 1.6 mg/mL (as gentamicin base) in 50 mL single-dose containers; Pediatric Gentamicin Sulfate (Abraxis); Gentamicin Sulfate in 0.9% Sodium Chloride (Hospira); generic; (Rx)

Topical, otic and ophthalmic labeled products are also available.

References

Adamcak, A. & B. Otten (2000). Rodent Therapeutics. *Vet Clin NA: Exotic Anim Pract* 3:1(Jan): 221–240.

Aucoin, D. (2002). Rational approach to antimiocrobial therapy in companion animals. Proceedings: Atlantic Coast Veterinary Conference. Accessed via: Veterinary Information Network. http://goo.gl/5atZq

Autran de Morais, H. (2009). Empiric Antibiotic Therapy. Proceedings: WSAVA. Accessed via: Veterinary Information Network. http://goo.gl/Cl3HM

Burke, T.J. (1986). Regurgitation in snakes. *Current Veterinary Therapy in Small Animal Practice.* RW Kirk Ed. Philadelphia, WB Saunders: 749–750.

Chaffin, M. (2006). Bacterial pneumonia and lung abscesses of adult horses. Proceedings: Western Vet Conf. Accessed via: Veterinary Information Network. http://goo.gl/4r0d0

Corley, K.T.T. & A.R. Hollis (2009). Antimicrobial therapy in neonatal foals. *Equine Veterinary Education* 21(8): 436–448.

Flammer, K. (2006). Antibiotic drug selection in companion birds. *Journal of Exotic Pet Medicine* 15(3): 166–176.

Foreman, J. (1999). Equine respiratory pharmacology. *The Veterinary Clinics of North America: Equine Practice* 15:3(December): 665–686.

Greene, C., K. Hartmannn, et al. (2006). Appendix 8: Antimicrobial Drug Formulary. *Infectious Disease of the Dog and Cat.* C Greene Ed., Elsevier: 1186–1333.

Haggett, E.F. & W.D. Wilson (2008). Overview of the use of antimicrobials for the treatment of bacterial infections in horses. *Equine Veterinary Education* 20(8): 433–448.

Hartmannn, K. & C. Greene (2005). Diseases caused by systemic bacterial infections. *Textbook of Veterinary Internal Medicine, 6th Ed.* S Ettinger and E Feldman Eds., Elsevier: 616–631.

Hayes, P. (2000). Diseases of Chinchillas. *Kirk's Current Veterinary Therapy (CVT) IX Small Animal Practice.* J Bonagura Ed. Philadelphia, WB Saunders: 1152–1157.

Ivey, E. & J. Morrisey (2000). Therapeutics for Rabbits. *Vet Clin NA: Exotic Anim Pract* 3:1(Jan): 183–216.

Jenson, J. (1998). Current ratite therapy. *The Veterinary Clinics of North America: Food Animal Practice* 16:3(November).

KuKanich, B. (2008). Canine breed specific differences in clinical pharmacology. Proceedings: WVC. Accessed via: Veterinary Information Network. http://goo.gl/GCUEn

LeBlanc, M.M. (2009). The current status of antibiotic use in equine reproduction. *Equine Veterinary Education* 21(3): 156–167.

McGorum, B.C. & R.S. Pirie (2010). Antimicrobial associated diarrhoea in the horse. Part 2: Which antimicrobials are associated with AAD in the horse? *Equine Veterinary Education* 22(1): 43–50.

Morresey, P.R. & B.M. Waldridge (2010). Successful Treatment of Rhodococcus equi Pneumonia in an Adult Horse. *Journal of Veterinary Internal Medicine* 24(2): 436–438.

Morrisey, J. & J. Carpenter (2004). Formulary. *Ferrets, Rabbits, and Rodents Clinical Medicine and Surgery 2nd ed.* K Quesenberry and J Carpenter Eds. St Louis, Saunders.

Papich, M. (2003). Problems in drug therapy for rabbits: How diseases, physiologic condition, and body composition can alter drug therapy. Proceedings: ACVIM Forum. Accessed via: Veterinary Information Network. http://goo.gl/R8Zmz

Rosskopf, W.J. (1986). Shell diseases in turtles and tortoises. *Current Veterinary Therapy (CVT) IX Small Animal Practice.* RW Kirk Ed. Philadelphia, WB Saunders: 751–759.

Sprayberry, K. (2009). Pleuropneumonia. *Compendium Equine*(May): 166–175.

Trepanier, L. (1999). Management of resistant infections in small animal patients. Proceedings: American Veterinary Medical Association: 16th Annual Convention, New Orleans.

Williams, B. (2000). Therapeutics in Ferrets. *Vet Clin NA: Exotic Anim Pract* 3:1(Jan): 131–153.

GLIMEPIRIDE

(glye-*meh*-per-ide)   Amaryl®

SULFONYLUREA ANTIDIABETIC AGENT

Prescriber Highlights

▶ Oral, once-daily, anti-hyperglycemic agent; could be useful in the adjunctive treatment of non-insulin dependent diabetes mellitus (NIDDM) in cats

▶ Very limited experience in cats

▶ Contraindicated: Patients hypersensitive to it or with diabetic ketoacidosis

▶ Hypoglycemia may occur

▶ Potentially, significant drug interactions

▶ Do not confuse glipizide, glimepiride & glyburide

Uses/Indications

Glimepiride may potentially be a useful adjunct in the treatment of non-insulin dependent diabetes mellitus (NIDDM) in cats. Its duration of action in humans allows it to be dosed once daily, which could be of benefit in cats. It may also have fewer side effects than glipizide in cats.

Pharmacology/Actions

Glimepiride is a medium- to long-acting secretagogue sulfonylurea. It increases pancreatic release of insulin from functioning beta cells and, with continued use, may also increase peripheral tissue sensitivity to insulin. The exact mechanism for these effects is not well understood.

Pharmacokinetics

No pharmacokinetic data for cats was located. But when 0.5 mg glimepiride was administered orally to healthy cats followed by an intravenous glucose tolerance test 3-6 hours later (Mori *et al.* 2009), glucose levels were lowest at 3 hours post dose and insulin levels peaked twice, first at 60 minutes and a smaller peak at 4 hours.

In humans, glimepiride is completely absorbed from the GI tract. Peak levels occur in 2–3 hours; food delays the peak somewhat and lowers AUC by about 9%. Volume of distribution is 0.11 L/kg; the drug is greater than 99% bound to plasma proteins. Glimepiride is hepatically metabolized to at least two major metabolites. One of these, M1, has activity at about 1/3 that of the parent compound; clearance is 48 mL/min and elimination half-life about 9 hours. Approximately 60% of the drug (as metabolites) are excreted into the urine and the remainder in the feces. The drug has a 24-hour duration of activity in humans.

Contraindications/Precautions/Warnings

Glimepiride is contraindicated in patients hypersensitive to it or with diabetic ketoacidosis.

Adverse Effects

Hypoglycemia has been reported in about 1% of human patients taking the drug. Dizziness and asthenia have been reported; rarely, liver function impairment, allergic respiratory reactions, dermatologic reactions, or hematologic reactions have been reported in humans.

Reproductive/Nursing Safety

In humans, the FDA categorizes glimepiride as a category *C* drug for use during pregnancy (*Animal studies have shown an adverse effect on the fetus, but there are no adequate studies in humans; or there are no animal reproduction studies and no adequate studies in humans*). In rabbits and rats, glimepiride did not cause teratogenic effects when given at high dosages. There were some intrauterine deaths when maternal hypoglycemia was induced by the drug.

Some glimepiride is excreted into maternal milk of rats. The manufacturer states to discontinue the drug in nursing, human mothers.

Overdosage/Acute Toxicity

Overdoses may result in hypoglycemia, ranging from mild to severe. Treatment consists of glucose administration and intensive monitoring. Because of the drug's long duration of activity, patients may need to be supported with glucose for a least 48 hours post-ingestion, even after apparent recovery.

Drug Interactions

The following drug interactions have either been reported or are theoretical in humans or animals receiving glimepiride and may be of significance in veterinary patients:

■ **ANTIFUNGALS, AZOLE (ketoconazole, itraconazole, fluconazole):** May increase plasma levels of glimepiride

■ **BETA-BLOCKERS:** May potentiate hypoglycemic effect

■ **CHLORAMPHENICOL:** May displace glimepiride from plasma proteins

■ **CORTICOSTEROIDS:** May reduce efficacy

■ **DIURETICS, THIAZIDE:** May reduce hypoglycemic efficacy

■ **ISONIAZID:** May reduce hypoglycemic efficacy

■ **NIACIN:** May reduce hypoglycemic efficacy

■ **PHENOTHIAZINES:** May reduce hypoglycemic efficacy

■ **PHENYTOIN:** May reduce hypoglycemic efficacy

■ **SULFONAMIDES:** May displace glimepiride from plasma proteins

■ **SYMPATHOMIMETIC AGENTS:** May reduce hypoglycemic efficacy

■ **WARFARIN:** May displace glimepiride from plasma proteins

Laboratory Considerations

■ No specific laboratory interactions or considerations were noted.

Doses

◼ **CATS:**

For treatment of NIDDM:

a) 2 mg (total dose) per cat once daily (Bruyette 2004)

b) 1–2 mg (total dose per cat) PO once daily (Scherk 2005)

Monitoring

◼ Efficacy: Standard methods of monitoring efficacy treatment should be followed (*e.g.*, fasting blood glucose, appetite, attitude, body condition, PU/PD resolution and, perhaps, serum fructosamine and/or glycosylated hemoglobin levels)

◼ Adverse effects

Client Information

◼ Clients should understand the "investigational" nature of using this drug in cats and report any untoward effects to the veterinarian.

Chemistry/Synonyms

A sulfonylurea antidiabetic agent, glimepiride occurs as a white to yellowish-white, crystalline, odorless to practically odorless powder. It is practically insoluble in water.

Glimepiride may also be known as: HOE-490, *Amarel®, Amaryl®, Amarylle®, Euglim®, Glimepil®, Solosa®*, and *Roname®*.

Storage/Stability

Glimepiride tablets should be stored between 15–30°C (59–86°F) in well closed containers.

Dosage Forms/Regulatory Status

VETERINARY-LABELED PRODUCTS: None

HUMAN-LABELED PRODUCTS:

Glimepiride Oral Tablets: 1 mg, 2 mg, & 4 mg; *Amaryl®* (Sanofi-Aventis); generic; (Rx)

References

Bruyette, D. (2004). Diabetes Mellitus in dogs and cats. Proceedings: Northeast Vet Conf. Accessed via: Veterinary Information Network. http://goo.gl/QzvHS

Mori, A., P. Lee, et al. (2009). Effect of glimepiride and nateglinide on serum insulin and glucose concentration in healthy cats. *Veterinary Research Communications* 33(8): 957–970.

Scherk, M. (2005). Management of the Diabetic Cat. Proceedings: Western Veterinary Conference. Accessed via: Veterinary Information Network. http://goo.gl/dGiYr

GLIPIZIDE

(**glip**-i-zide)   Glucotrol®

SULFONYLUREA ANTIDIABETIC AGENT

Prescriber Highlights

▶ Human oral antidiabetic agent (Type II) that may be useful in cats

▶ May take 4 to 8 weeks before full effects are seen

▶ Contraindications: Severe burns/trauma/infection, diabetic coma or other hypoglycemic conditions, major surgery, ketosis, ketoacidosis or other significant acidotic conditions

▶ Caution: Untreated adrenal or pituitary insufficiency; thyroid, renal or hepatic function impairment; prolonged vomiting; high fever; malnourishment or debilitated condition

▶ Adverse Effects: *Cats:* GI (*i.e.*, anorexia, vomiting), hypoglycemia, liver toxicity

▶ Drug interactions

▶ Do not confuse glipizide, glimepiride & glyburide

Uses/Indications

Glipizide may be of benefit in treating cats with type II diabetes if they have a population of functioning beta cells. Perhaps 20%-30% of newly diagnosed cats may benefit (improvement in hyperglycemia) from glipizide, but there is not a way to predict which cats will benefit in advance of a trial. It has been suggested that there are two situations when a glipizide trial can be recommended, 1) If an owner refuses to consider using insulin usually due to a fear of needles, and 2) the cat appears to be relatively well controlled on quite small doses of insulin and the owner would strongly prefer to no longer give insulin (Feldman 2005).

While glipizide potentially could be useful in treating canine patients with type II or III diabetes, however, by the time dogs present with hyperglycemia, they are absolutely or relatively insulinopenic and glipizide would unlikely be effective.

Pharmacology/Actions

Glipizide is a second generation sulfonylurea. Sulfonylureas lower blood glucose concentrations in both diabetics and non-diabetics. The exact mechanism of action is not known, but these agents are thought to exert the effect primarily by stimulating the beta cells in the pancreas to secrete additional endogenous insulin. Extrapancreatic effects include enhanced tissue sensitivity of circulating insulin. Ongoing use of the sulfonylureas appears to enhance peripheral sensitivity to insulin and reduce the production of hepatic basal glucose. The mechanisms causing these effects are yet to be fully explained, however.

Prolonged hyperglycemia may cause beta cell "exhaustion" and permanent damage to beta cells contributing to their death. It has been suggested that by treating all cats initially with insulin to rapidly reduce hyperglycemia may allow increases in beta cell sensitivity and insulin release to occur with time and potentially increase success with glipizide (Sparkes 2009).

Pharmacokinetics

Glipizide is rapidly and practically completely absorbed after oral administration. Transdermal administration on cats does not appear to be adequately absorbed to be useful. The absolute bioavailability reported in humans ranges from 80–100%. Food will alter the rate, but not the extent, of absorption. Glipizide is very highly bound to plasma proteins. It is primarily biotransformed in the liver to inactive metabolites that are then excreted by the kidneys. In humans, half-life is about 2–4 hours. Effects on insulin levels in cats tend to be short-lived. Effects peak in about 15 minutes and return to baseline after about 60 minutes.

Contraindications/Precautions/Warnings

Oral antidiabetic agents are considered contraindicated with the following conditions: severe burns, severe trauma, severe infection, diabetic coma or other hypoglycemic conditions, major surgery, ketosis, ketoacidosis or other significant acidotic conditions. Glipizide should only be used when its potential benefits outweigh its risks during untreated adrenal or pituitary insufficiency; thyroid, renal or hepatic function impairment; prolonged vomiting; high fever; malnourishment or debilitated condition is present.

While glipizide may initially be effective, it may become ineffective in weeks to months after starting therapy; insulin will then be required.

Some patients with type II or type III diabetes may have their disease complicated by the production of excessive amounts of cortisol or growth hormone which may antagonize insulin's effects. These causes should be ruled out before initiating oral antidiabetic therapy.

Adverse Effects

Approximately 15% of cats receiving glipizide develop gastrointestinal adverse effects (i.e., anorexia, vomiting). Vomiting usually occurs shortly after dosing and will subside in 2–5 days. If it persists or is severe, decrease dose or frequency and, if necessary, discontinue.

Some cats receiving this drug have developed hypoglycemia, but severe hypoglycemia appears to be rare. Should hypoglycemia occur, discontinue glipizide and recheck glucose in one week; may restart at a lower dose or dosing frequency if hyperglycemia is noted.

Increased amyloid deposit formation can occur with glipizide which can potentially cause further destruction of functional beta cells.

Effects on the liver have been reported. Approximately 8% of cats treated with glipizide may develop cholestatic jaundice and have increases in liver enzymes. Serum hepatic enzymes should be checked every 1–2 weeks initially. Discontinue glipizide in cats with elevated enzymes if they develop lethargy, anorexia, vomiting, or if ALT exceeds 500 IU/L; should icterus occur, discontinue glipizide and restart at a lower dose once icterus resolves; discontinue use should icterus reoccur.

Other adverse effects that are possible (noted in humans) include: allergic skin reactions, and bone marrow suppression.

Glipizide does not appear to be effective in cats demonstrating insulin resistance.

Reproductive/Nursing Safety

Safe use during pregnancy has not been established. Glipizide was found to be mildly fetotoxic in rats when given at doses at 5–50 mg/kg; however, no other teratogenic effects were noted. Use in pregnancy only when benefits outweigh potential risks. In humans, the FDA categorizes this drug as category *C* for use during pregnancy (*Animal studies have shown an adverse effect on the fetus, but there are no adequate studies in humans; or there are no animal reproduction studies and no adequate studies in humans.*)

It is unknown if glipizide enters milk.

Overdosage/Acute Toxicity

Oral LD_{50}'s are greater than 4 g/kg in all animal species tested. Profound hypoglycemia is the greatest concern after an overdose. Gut emptying protocols should be employed when warranted. Because of its shorter half-life than chlorpropamide, prolonged hypoglycemia is less likely with glipizide, but blood glucose monitoring and treatment with parenteral glucose may be required for several days. Massive overdoses may also require additional monitoring (blood gases, serum electrolytes) and supportive therapy.

Drug Interactions

The following drug interactions have either been reported or are theoretical in humans or animals receiving glipizide and may be of significance in veterinary patients:

- ◼ **ALCOHOL:** A disulfiram-like reaction (anorexia, nausea, vomiting) has been reported in humans who have ingested alcohol within 48–72 hours of receiving glipizide

- ◼ **ANTIFUNGALS, AZOLE (ketoconazole, itraconazole, fluconazole):** May increase plasma levels of glipizide

- ◼ **BETA-BLOCKERS:** May potentiate hypoglycemic effect

- ◼ **CHLORAMPHENICOL:** May displace glipizide from plasma proteins

- ◼ **CIMETIDINE:** May potentiate hypoglycemic effect

■ **CORTICOSTEROIDS:** May reduce efficacy

■ **DIURETICS, THIAZIDE:** May reduce hypoglycemic efficacy

■ **ISONIAZID:** May reduce hypoglycemic efficacy

■ **MOA INHIBITORS:** May potentiate hypoglycemic effect

■ **NIACIN:** May reduce hypoglycemic efficacy

■ **PHENOTHIAZINES:** May reduce hypoglycemic efficacy

■ **PHENYTOIN:** May reduce hypoglycemic efficacy

■ **PROBENECID:** May potentiate hypoglycemic effect

■ **SULFONAMIDES:** May displace glipizide from plasma proteins

■ **SYMPATHOMIMETIC AGENTS:** May reduce hypoglycemic efficacy

■ **THYROID AGENTS:** May reduce hypoglycemic effect

■ **WARFARIN:** May displace glipizide from plasma proteins

Doses

■ **CATS:**

For diabetes mellitus:

a) In non-ketotic cats that are relatively healthy: Initially monitor weight, urine/glucose/ketones, and several blood glucose measurements. Then give 2.5 mg PO per cat twice daily in conjunction with a meal. During first 24 hours of therapy perform spot blood glucose measurements (every 3-4 hours for the initial 12-18 hours) to check for hypoglycemia. After 2 weeks, monitor again and if hyperglycemia is still present and adverse reactions (vomiting, icterus) have not occurred, increase dose to 5 mg twice daily. Therapy is continued as long as cat is stable. If euglycemic or hypoglycemia develop, the dosage may be tapered down or discontinued, and blood glucose concentrations re-evaluated 1 week later to assess the need for the drug. If hyperglycemia recurs, the dosage is increased or glipizide is reinitiated, with a reduction in dosage in those cats previously developing hypoglycemia. Discontinue and initiate insulin therapy if clinical signs continue to worsen, the cat becomes ill, develops ketoacidosis, blood glucose concentrations remain greater than 15 mmol/L (270 mg/dL) after one or two months of therapy, or the owners become dissatisfied with the treatment. (Herrtage 2009)

b) 2.5–5 mg per cat PO twice a day when combined with dietary fiber therapy. Evaluate every one to two weeks for a period of 2–3 months. If fasting blood glucose decreases to less than 200 mg/dL, continue at same dosage and reevaluate in 3–6 months. If fasting blood glucose remains greater than 200 mg/dL after 2–3 months, discontinue and institute insulin therapy (Greco 2000)

c) If cat is generally well, weight loss is mild, not ketoacidotic, and does not have peripheral neuropathy, may try glipizide at: 2.5 mg (total dose) PO twice a day. (Daminet 2003)

d) 5 mg per cat twice daily, may decrease dose if hypoglycemia occurs or increase to 7.5 mg (maximum) twice daily if not controlled. Slightly less than 50% of cats may tolerate the drug, have improved clinical signs and blood glucose levels. Response may be delayed, so it should be given for 4–8 weeks before deciding if it was efficacious (owner opinion, body weight, blood glucose determinations over a one-day period every 4 weeks.) (Feldman 2005)

Monitoring

■ Weekly exams during first month of therapy, including PE, body weight, urine glucose/ketones, and several blood glucose exams.

■ Adverse effects (anorexia, vomiting, icterus), and occasional liver enzymes and CBC.

Client Information

■ Clients should be informed of clinical signs to watch for that would indicate either hypoglycemia or hyperglycemia and be instructed to report these to the veterinarian.

■ Compliance with dosing regimen should also be stressed.

Chemistry/Synonyms

A sulfonylurea antidiabetic agent, glipizide (also known as glydiazinamide) occurs as a whitish powder. It is practically insoluble in water and has pK_a of 5.9.

Glipizide may also be known as: CP-28720, glipizidum, glydiazinamide, or K-4024; many international trade names are available.

Storage/Stability

Tablets should be stored in tight, light-resistant containers at room temperature.

Dosage Forms/Regulatory Status

VETERINARY-LABELED PRODUCTS: None

HUMAN-LABELED PRODUCTS:

Glipizide Oral Tablets: 5 mg, & 10 mg; *Glucotrol®* (Pfizer); generic (Rx)

Glipizide Oral Extended Release Tablets: 2.5 mg, 5 mg, & 10 mg; *Glucotrol XL®* (Pfizer); generic; (Rx)

Glipizide/Metformin Hydrochloride Tablets (film-coated): 2.5 mg glipizide/250 mg or 500 mg metformin; 5 mg glipizide/500 mg metformin; *Metaglip®* (Bristol-Myers Squibb); generic (Sandoz); (Rx)

References

Daminet, S. (2003). Canine and Feline Diabetes Mellitus. Proceedings: World Small Animal Veterinary Assoc. World Congress. Accessed via: Veterinary Information Network. http://goo.gl/YRCPp

Feldman, E. (2005). Management of Diabetes Mellitus in Dogs and Cats: I, II, & III. Proceedings: Western Vet Conf. Accessed via: Veterinary Information Network. http://goo.gl/XhKAK

Greco, D. (2000). Treatment of non-insulin-dependent diabetes mellitus in cats using oral hypoglycemic agents. *Kirk's Current Veterinary Therapy: XIII Small Animal Practice.* J Bonagura Ed. Philadelphia, WB Saunders: 350–357.

Herrtage, M. (2009). New Strategies in the Management of Feline Diabetes Mellitus. Proceedings: WSAVA. Accessed via: Veterinary Information Network. http://goo.gl/b2CzL

Sparkes, A. (2009). Long-Term Care of Diabetic Cats: Home Monitoring and Hospital. Proceedings: BSAVA. Accessed via: Veterinary Information Network. http://goo.gl/mivpR

GLUCAGON

(*gloo*-ka-gon)   GlucoGen®

HORMONAL AGENT

Prescriber Highlights

▶ Hormone to increase blood glucose that may be useful for treating hypoglycemia in small animals & potentially fatty liver syndrome in dairy cows

▶ May be effective in treating beta-blocker or calcium channel overdoses

▶ Must be parenterally administered

▶ When used as CRI, must be in a setting where blood glucose can be monitored

▶ Unlikely to cause adverse effects

Uses/Indications

In small animals, the primary use for glucagon is to increase blood glucose in patients with excessive insulin levels, either endogenously produced (insulinoma) or exogenously administered (insulin overdose). Glucagon has potential in the treatment of fatty liver syndrome in dairy cattle.

In human medicine, glucagon has been used in treating the cardiac manifestations of beta-blocker and calcium-channel blocker overdoses. One study (Kerns *et al.* 1997) in dogs, however, demonstrated insulin to be superior to glucagon in treating experimental propranolol overdoses in dogs.

Pharmacology/Actions

Glucagon's main pharmacologic activities are to increase blood glucose and relax smooth muscle of the GI tract. It primarily increases blood glucose by stimulating hepatic glycogenolysis. The mechanisms of action for its GI effects are poorly understood.

Pharmacokinetics

Glucagon must be administered parenterally; it is destroyed in the gut after oral dosing. After intravenous injection, maximum glucose levels are attained within 30 minutes; hyperglycemic effects persist up to 90 minutes after dosing. Glucagon is degraded in the plasma, liver and kidneys; in humans, plasma half-life is around 10 minutes.

Contraindications/Precautions/Warnings

Glucagon should usually not be used in patients with pheochromocytoma as catecholamines may be released leading to hypertension. When used for insulinoma, it must be in a setting where blood glucose can be closely monitored. While glucagon may be useful for blood glucose elevation in insulinoma patients, in humans its use for this is cautioned as it can increase insulin production, leading to greater hypoglycemia once the drug is discontinued.

Adverse Effects

Glucagon is usually well tolerated, but potentially nausea and vomiting could occur after administration. Hypokalemia and hypersensitivity reactions (very rare) are also possible.

Reproductive/Nursing Safety

In humans, glucagon is designated by the FDA as a category *B* drug (*Animal studies have not demonstrated risk to the fetus, but there are no adequate studies in pregnant women; or animal studies have shown an adverse effect, but adequate studies in pregnant women have not demonstrated a risk to the fetus during the first trimester of pregnancy, and there is no evidence of risk in later trimesters.*) As an endogenously produced hormone, it is unlikely to cause significant risk to offspring.

It is unknown if glucagon enters maternal milk, but it is unlikely to cause harm to nursing offspring.

Overdosage/Acute Toxicity

Adverse effects seen with overdose include nausea, vomiting, diarrhea, gastric hypotonicity and, possibly, hypokalemia. Because glucagon's elimination half-life is so short, treatment may not be necessary and would be symptomatic in nature. If the patient is also receiving beta-blockers, greater increases in blood pressure and heart rate may be seen.

Drug Interactions

The following drug interactions have either been reported or are theoretical in humans or animals receiving glucagon and may be of significance in veterinary patients:

■ **ANTICOAGULANTS:** May have their effects increased when glucagon is concurrently administered; this effect may be delayed. It is suggested to monitor for bleeding and pro-thrombin activity if glucagon is necessary.

Laboratory Considerations

■ No glucagon-related laboratory interactions noted.

Doses

■ **DOGS:**

a) For hypoglycemic (neuroglycopenic) crises in patients with "insulinomas": 1 mg of glucagon is reconstituted per manufacturer directions and then added to 1000 mL of 0.9% Sodium Chloride; this results in a 1000 ng/mL (nanograms/mL) solution. [**Note:** Some references state to not mix or dilute with saline solutions, but to use D5W only.] Initially give a 50 ng/kg bolus IV and then administer at a constant rate infusion (CRI) using a suitable pump at a rate of 10–15 ng/kg/minute. May need to increase up to 40 ng/kg/min to maintain euglycemia. (Smith 2002)

b) For refractory hypoglycemic patients with insulinoma: Prepare solution as in "a" above. Give at an initial infusion rate of 5 ng/kg/min and increase as needed. (Garrett 2003)

■ **CATS:**

a) For hypoglycemic (neuroglycopenic) crises in patients with "insulinomas": 1 mg of glucagon is reconstituted per manufacturer directions and then added to 1000 mL of 0.9% Sodium Chloride; this results in a 1000 ng/mL solution. [**Note:** Some references state to not mix or dilute with saline solutions, but to use D5W only.] Initially give a 50 ng/kg bolus IV and then administer at a constant rate infusion (CRI) using a suitable pump at a rate of 10–15 ng/kg/minute. May need to increase up to 40 ng/kg/min to maintain euglycemia. (Smith 2002)

■ **CATTLE:**

a) For treatment of fatty liver in early lactation dairy cows older than 3.5 years: 5 mg glucagon in 60 mL of normal saline SC q8h (15 mg/day) for 14 days (Bobe *et al.* 2003)

Monitoring

■ Blood glucose

■ Serum potassium if used other than for acute treatment

Client Information

■ Glucagon could potentially be used for outpatient emergency initial treatment of hypoglycemia, but oral glucose is probably more appropriate for use by clients.

■ Glucagon should be used as a CRI only in a setting where blood glucose can be adequately monitored.

Chemistry/Synonyms

A hormone secreted by the alpha$_2$ cells of the pancreas, glucagon is a straight chain polypeptide that contains 29 amino acids whose sequence is consistent throughout mammalian species. It has a molecular weight of 3483. When in crystalline form it is a white- to off-white powder that is relatively insoluble in water at physiologic pH, but is soluble at pH of less than 3 and greater than 9.5. Glucagon may be expressed in terms of International Units (IU; expressed as Units in this reference) or by weight. One International Unit is equivalent to one milligram of glucagon. Commercially available glucagon is now obtained via recombinant DNA sources.

Glucagon may also be known as glucagonum or HGF, and *GlucaGen®*.

Storage/Stability

The commercially available powder for reconstitution should be stored at room temperature between 20–25°C (68–77°F); avoid freezing and protect from light. Once reconstituted with the supplied diluent the solution should be clear with a water-like consistency and used immediately; any unused portion should be discarded. If the solution contains any gel formation or particles, it should be discarded.

Compatibility/Compounding Considerations

To prepare glucagon for a continuous rate infusion, dilute 1 mg with the supplied diluent or sterile water; roll gently until dissolved, this may then be further diluted in D5W. May be given through a Y-tube or 3-way stopcock if a dextrose solution is running.

Dosage Forms/Regulatory Status

VETERINARY-LABELED PRODUCTS: None

HUMAN-LABELED PRODUCTS:

Glucagon Powder for Injection: 1 mg (1 unit) with 1 mL diluent in vials & syringes; *GlucaGen® Diagnostic Kit* & *GlucaGen HypoKit®* (Novo Nordisk); *Glucagon Emergency Kit®* (Eli Lilly); (Rx)

References

Bobe, G., B. Ametaj, et al. (2003). Potential treatment of fatty liver with 14–day subcutaneous injections of glucagon. *J Dairy Sci* **86**: 3138–3147.

Garrett, L. (2003). Insulinomas: A review and what's new. Proceedings: ACVIM. Accessed via: Veterinary Information Network. http://goo.gl/KgsDV

Kerns, W., S. D, et al. (1997). Insulin improves survival in a canine model of acute beta-blocker toxicity. *Ann Emerg Med.* **29**(6): 748–757.

Smith, S. (2002). The hypoglycemic crisis: When dextrose fails. ACVIM.

GLUCOCORTICOID AGENTS, GENERAL INFORMATION

Glucocorticoid Comparison Table

DRUG	EQUIV. ANTI-INFLAMMATORY DOSE (MG)	RELATIVE ANTI-INFLAMMATORY POTENCY	RELATIVE MINERAL-CORTICOID ACTIVITY	PLASMA HALF-LIFE DOGS (MIN) [HUMANS]	DURATION OF ACTION AFTER ORAL/IV	ESTER FORM: SOLUBILITY/RELEASE DURATIONS (IM)
Hydrocortisone (Cortisol)	20	1	1–2	52–57 [90]	<12 hrs (8-12)	Sodium Succinate: Very/Minutes
Betamethasone	0.6	25	0	[300+]	>36 (36-54) hrs	Sodium Succinate or phosphate: Very/Minutes
Dexamethasone	0.75	30	0	119–136 [200–300+]	>36 hours (36-54) hrs	Sodium Succ or Sod. Phos: Very/Minutes Phenylpropionate or Isonicotinate: Mod./Days to weeks
Flumethasone	1.5	15–30	?	?		Very/Minutes
Isoflupredone		17				Acetate: Duration of action up to 48 hours
Methylprednisolone	4	5	0	91 [200]	12–36 hrs	Sod. Succinate: Very/Minutes Acetate: Mod./Days to weeks
Prednisolone	5	4	1	69–197 [115–212]	12–36 hrs	Sodium Succinate: Very/Minutes Acetate: Mod./Days to weeks
Prednisone	5	4	1	[60]	12–36 hrs	
Triamcinolone	4	5	0	[200+]	24-48 hrs	Acetonide: Poorly/Weeks

Uses/Indications

Glucocorticoids have been used in an attempt to treat practically every malady that afflicts man or animal, but there are four broad uses and dosage ranges for use of these agents. **1)** Replacement of glucocorticoid activity in patients with adrenal insufficiency, **2)** as an antiinflammatory agent, **3)** as a cytotoxic/antineoplastic agent, and **4)** as an immunosuppressive. Among some of the uses for glucocorticoids include treatment of: endocrine conditions (*e.g.*, adrenal insufficiency), rheumatic diseases (*e.g.*, rheumatoid arthritis), collagen diseases (*e.g.*, systemic lupus), allergic states, respiratory diseases (*e.g.*, asthma), dermatologic diseases (*e.g.*, pemphigus, allergic dermatoses), hematologic disorders (*e.g.*, thrombocytopenias, autoimmune hemolytic anemias), neoplasias, nervous system disorders, GI diseases (*e.g.*, ulcerative colitis exacerbations), and renal diseases (*e.g.*, nephrotic syndrome). Some glucocorticoids are used topically in the eye and skin for various conditions or are injected intra-articularly or intra-lesionally. The above listing is certainly not complete. For specific dosages and indications refer to the Doses section for each glucocorticoid drug monograph.

Glucocorticoids have been used for CNS trauma (especially spinal chord injury) or shock, but their use for these indications are controversial as there is little evidence supporting their use. Relative adrenal insufficiency may occur in critically ill animals, and low or physiologic doses of corticosteroids (having both glucocorticoid and mineralocorticoid activity, *e.g.*, hydrocortisone) may be indicated in patients that have not responded to pressor agents.

Pharmacology/Actions

Glucocorticoids have effects on virtually every cell type and system in mammals. An overview of the effects of these agents follows:

Cardiovascular System: Glucocorticoids can reduce capillary permeability and enhance vasoconstriction. A relatively clinically insignificant positive inotropic effect can occur after glucocorticoid administration. Increased blood pressure can result from both the drugs' vasoconstrictive properties and increased blood volume that may be produced.

Cells: Glucocorticoids inhibit fibroblast proliferation, macrophage response to migration inhibiting factor, sensitization of lymphocytes and the cellular response to mediators of inflammation. Glucocorticoids stabilize lysosomal membranes.

CNS/Autonomic Nervous System: Glucocorticoids can lower seizure threshold, alter mood and behavior, diminish the response to pyrogens, stimulate appetite and maintain alpha rhythm. Glucocorticoids are necessary for normal adrenergic receptor sensitivity.

Endocrine System: When animals are not stressed, glucocorticoids will suppress the release of ACTH from the anterior pituitary, thereby reducing or preventing the release of endogenous corticosteroids. Stress factors (*e.g.,* renal disease, liver disease, diabetes) may sometimes nullify the suppressing aspects of exogenously administered steroids. Release of thyroid-stimulating hormone (TSH), follicle-stimulating hormone (FSH), prolactin, and luteinizing hormone (LH) may all be reduced when glucocorticoids are administered at pharmacological doses. Conversion of thyroxine (T_4) to triiodothyronine (T_3) may be reduced by glucocorticoids; and plasma levels of parathyroid hormone increased. Glucocorticoids may inhibit osteoblast function. Vasopressin (ADH) activity is reduced at the renal tubules and diuresis may occur. Glucocorticoids inhibit insulin binding to insulin-receptors and the post-receptor effects of insulin.

Hematopoietic System: Glucocorticoids can increase the numbers of circulating platelets, neutrophils and red blood cells, but platelet aggregation is inhibited. Decreased amounts of lymphocytes (peripheral), monocytes and eosinophils are seen as glucocorticoids can sequester these cells into the lungs and spleen and prompt decreased release from the bone marrow. Removal of old red blood cells becomes diminished. Glucocorticoids can cause involution of lymphoid tissue.

GI Tract and Hepatic System: Glucocorticoids increase the secretion of gastric acid, pepsin, and trypsin. They alter the structure of mucin and decrease mucosal cell proliferation. Iron salts and calcium absorption are decreased while fat absorption is increased. Hepatic changes can include increased fat and glycogen deposits within hepatocytes, increased serum levels of alanine aminotransferase (ALT), and gamma-glutamyl transpeptidase (GGT). Significant increases can be seen in serum alkaline phosphatase levels. Glucocorticoids can cause minor increases in BSP (bromosulfophthalein) retention time.

Immune System (also see Cells and Hematopoietic System): Glucocorticoids can decrease circulating levels of T-lymphocytes; inhibit lymphokines; inhibit neutrophil, macrophage, and monocyte migration; reduce production of interferon; inhibit phagocytosis and chemotaxis; antigen processing; and diminish intracellular killing. Specific acquired immunity is affected less than nonspecific immune responses. Glucocorticoids can also antagonize the complement cascade and mask the clinical signs of infection. Mast cells are decreased in number and histamine synthesis is suppressed. Many of these effects only occur at high or very high doses and there are species differences in response.

Metabolic effects: Glucocorticoids stimulate gluconeogenesis. Lipogenesis is enhanced in certain areas of the body (*e.g.,* abdomen) and adipose tissue can be redistributed away from the extremities to the trunk. Fatty acids are mobilized from tissues and their oxidation is increased. Plasma levels of triglycerides, cholesterol, and glycerol are increased. Protein is mobilized from most areas of the body (not the liver).

Musculoskeletal: Glucocorticoids may cause muscular weakness (also caused if there is a lack of glucocorticoids), atrophy, and osteoporosis. Bone growth can be inhibited via growth hormone and somatomedin inhibition, increased calcium excretion and inhibition of vitamin D activation. Resorption of bone can be enhanced. Fibrocartilage growth is also inhibited.

Ophthalmic: Prolonged corticosteroid use (both systemic or topically to the eye) can cause increased intraocular pressure and glaucoma, cataracts, and exophthalmos.

Renal, Fluid, & Electrolytes: Glucocorticoids can increase potassium and calcium excretion, sodium and chloride reabsorption, and extracellular fluid volume. Hypokalemia and/or hypocalcemia rarely occur. Diuresis may develop following glucocorticoid administration.

Skin: Thinning of dermal tissue and skin atrophy can be seen with glucocorticoid therapy. Hair follicles can become distended and alopecia may occur.

Contraindications/Precautions/Warnings

Systemic use of glucocorticoids is generally considered contraindicated in systemic fungal infections (unless used for replacement therapy in Addison's), when administered IM in patients with idiopathic thrombocytopenia, and in patients hypersensitive to a particular compound. Use of sustained-release injectable glucocorticoids is considered contraindicated for chronic corticosteroid therapy of systemic diseases.

Animals that have received glucocorticoids systemically, other than with "burst" therapy, should be tapered off the drugs. Patients who have received the drugs chronically should be tapered off slowly as endogenous ACTH and corticosteroid function may return slowly. Should the animal undergo a "stressor" (*e.g.,* surgery, trauma, illness, etc.) during the tapering process or until normal adrenal and pituitary function resume, additional glucocorticoids should be administered.

Adverse Effects

Adverse effects are generally associated with long-term administration of these drugs, especially if given at high dosages or not on an alternate day regimen. Effects generally manifest as clinical signs of hyperadrenocorticism. When administered to young, growing animals, glucocorticoids can retard growth. Many of the potential effects, adverse and otherwise, are outlined above in the Pharmacology section.

In dogs, polydipsia (PD), polyphagia (PP), and polyuria (PU) may all be seen with short-term "burst" therapy as well as with alternate-day maintenance therapy on days when the drug is given. Adverse effects in dogs can include: dull, dry haircoat, weight gain, panting, vomiting, diarrhea, elevated liver enzymes, pancreatitis, GI ulceration, lipidemias, activation or worsening of diabetes mellitus, muscle wasting and behavioral changes (depression, lethargy, viciousness). Discontinuation of the drug may be necessary; changing to an alternate steroid may also alleviate the problem. With the exception of PU/PD/PP, adverse effects associated with short-term antiinflammatory therapy occur relatively uncommonly. Adverse effects associated with immunosuppressive doses are more common and potentially more severe.

In dogs, glucocorticoids can increase liver enzymes (SAP>ALT) and cause vacuolar hepatopathy. Cats may show mild vacuolar changes, but enzymes are generally not affected.

Cats generally require higher dosages than dogs for clinical effect, but tend to develop fewer adverse effects. Occasionally, polydipsia, polyuria, polyphagia with weight gain, diarrhea, or depression can be seen. Long-term, high dose therapy can lead to "Cushingoid" effects, however.

Administration of dexamethasone or triamcinolone may play a role in the development of laminitis in horses.

Reproductive/Nursing Safety

Glucocorticoids are probably necessary for normal fetal development. They may be required for adequate surfactant production, myelin, retinal, pancreatic, and mammary development. Excessive dosages early in pregnancy may lead to teratogenic effects. In horses and ruminants, exogenous steroid administration may induce parturition when administered in the latter stages of pregnancy.

Glucocorticoids unbound to plasma proteins will enter milk. High dosages or prolonged administration to mothers may potentially inhibit the growth of nursing newborns. In humans, several studies suggest that amounts excreted in human breast milk are negligible with prednisone or prednisolone doses of 20 mg/day or less, or methylprednisolone doses less than or equal to 8 mg/day. Large doses for short periods may not harm the infant. Waiting 3–4 hours after the dose before nursing and using prednisolone rather than prednisone may result in a lower corticosteroid dose to offspring.

Overdosage/Acute Toxicity

Glucocorticoids when given short-term are unlikely to cause harmful effects, even in massive dosages. One incidence of a dog developing acute CNS effects after accidental ingestion of glucocorticoids has been reported. Should clinical signs occur, use supportive treatment if required.

Chronic usage of glucocorticoids can lead to serious adverse effects. Refer to Adverse Effects above for more information.

Drug Interactions

The following drug interactions have either been reported or are theoretical in humans or animals receiving glucocorticoids and may be of significance in veterinary patients:

- **AMPHOTERICIN B:** When administered concomitantly with glucocorticoids may cause hypokalemia

- **ANTICHOLINESTERASE AGENTS (e.g., pyridostigmine, neostigmine, etc.):** In patients with myasthenia gravis, concomitant glucocorticoid with these agents may lead to profound muscle weakness. If possible, discontinue anticholinesterase medication at least 24 hours prior to corticosteroid administration.

- **ASPIRIN (salicylates):** Glucocorticoids may reduce salicylate blood levels

- **CYCLOPHOSPHAMIDE:** Glucocorticoids may also inhibit the hepatic metabolism of cyclophosphamide; dosage adjustments may be required.

- **CYCLOSPORINE:** Concomitant administration of may increase the blood levels of each, by mutually inhibiting the hepatic metabolism of each other; clinical significance of this interaction is not clear

- **DIGOXIN:** Secondary to hypokalemia, increased risk for arrhythmias

- **DIURETICS, POTASSIUM-DEPLETING (furosemide, thiazides):** When administered concomitantly with glucocorticoids may cause hypokalemia

- **EPHEDRINE:** May increase metabolism

- **ESTROGENS:** The effects of hydrocortisone, and possibly other glucocorticoids, may be potentiated by concomitant administration with estrogens

- **INSULIN:** Requirements may increase in patients receiving glucocorticoids

- **KETOCONAZOLE:** May decrease metabolism

- **MITOTANE:** May alter the metabolism of steroids; higher than usual doses of steroids may be necessary to treat mitotane-induced adrenal insufficiency

- **NSAIDS:** Administration of other ulcerogenic drugs with glucocorticoids may increase risk

- **PHENOBARBITAL:** May increase the metabolism of glucocorticoids

■ **PHENYTOIN:** May increase the metabolism of glucocorticoids

■ **RIFAMPIN:** May increase the metabolism of glucocorticoids

■ **VACCINES:** Patients receiving corticosteroids at immunosuppressive dosages should generally not receive live attenuated-virus vaccines as virus replication may be augmented; a diminished immune response may occur after vaccine, toxoid, or bacterin administration in patients receiving glucocorticoids

Laboratory Considerations

■ Glucocorticoids may increase serum **cholesterol** and **urine glucose** levels.

■ Glucocorticoids may decrease serum **potassium**.

■ Glucocorticoids can suppress the release of thyroid stimulating hormone (TSH) and reduce T_3 & T_4 values. Thyroid gland atrophy has been reported after chronic glucocorticoid administration. Uptake of I^{131} by the thyroid may be decreased by glucocorticoids.

■ Reactions to **skin tests** may be suppressed by glucocorticoids.

■ False-negative results of the **nitroblue tetrazolium test for systemic bacterial infections** may be induced by glucocorticoids.

Monitoring

Monitoring of glucocorticoid therapy is dependent on its reason for use, dosage, agent used (amount of mineralocorticoid activity), dosage schedule (daily versus alternate day therapy), duration of therapy, and the animal's age and condition. The following list may not be appropriate or complete for all animals; use clinical assessment and judgment should adverse effects be noted:

■ Weight, appetite, signs of edema

■ Serum and/or urine electrolytes

■ Total plasma proteins, albumin

■ Blood glucose

■ Growth and development in young animals

■ ACTH stimulation test if necessary

Client Information

■ Clients should carefully follow the dosage instructions and should not discontinue the drug abruptly without consulting with veterinarian beforehand.

■ Clients should be briefed on the potential adverse effects that can be seen with these drugs and instructed to contact the veterinarian should these effects progress or become severe.

GLUCOSAMINE/ CHONDROITIN SULFATE

(gloo-*kose*-a-meen/kon-*droy*-tin *sul*-fayt)
Cosequin®

NUTRITIONAL SUPPLEMENT

Prescriber Highlights

▶ So-called nutraceutical that can be used as an adjunctive treatment for osteoarthritis or other painful conditions in horses, cats, dogs, etc; FLUTD in cats

▶ Well tolerated, but efficacy is uncertain

▶ Not a regulated drug; choose products carefully; large variation in commercially available products

Uses/Indications

These compounds may be useful in treating osteoarthritis or other painful conditions in domestic animals, but large, well-designed controlled clinical studies proving efficacy were not located. Additionally, since there is no FDA-approval process or oversight for these products, product quality and bioavailability may be highly variable. One study in dogs (McCarthy *et al.* 2007) showed some positive effect, but this study was not placebo controlled and compared responses versus carprofen. Another placebo-controlled, blinded study in dogs (Moreau *et al.* 2003), did not demonstrate statistically significant improvement after 60 days of treatment. An article reviewing the quality of evidence supporting the use of glucosamine-based nutraceuticals in equine joint disease, concluded that ". . . the quality of these studies is generally low. A poorly defined experimental paradigm makes balanced interpretation of individual studies difficult, and analysis of the body of literature as a whole virtually impossible." (Pearson & Lindinger 2009)

These compounds potentially could be of benefit in cats with FLUTD (feline lower urinary tract disease) because of the presence of glycosaminoglycans as part of the protective layer of the urinary tract. Controlled studies have shown some positive effects in some cats, but overall did not appear to make a significant difference.

Pharmacology/Actions

Cartilage cells use glucosamine to produce glycosaminoglycans and hyaluronan. Glucosamine also regulates synthesis of collagen and proteoglycans in cartilage and has mild antiinflammatory effects due to its ability to scavenge free radicals. Chondrocytes normally produce ample quantities of glucosamine from glucose and amino acids, but this ability may diminish with age, disease, or trauma. Exogenously administered glucosamine appears to be able to be utilized by chondrocytes.

Chondroitin sulfate possesses several pharmacologic effects. It appears to inhibit destructive enzymes in joint fluid and cartilage. Thrombi formation in microvasculature may be reduced. In joint cartilage, it stimulates the production of glycosaminoglycans and proteoglycans.

While *in vitro* evidence exists, there is not solid evidence that using these compounds together improves clinical effect over either alone, but *in vivo* studies are ongoing.

Pharmacokinetics

The pharmacokinetics of these compounds are hard to evaluate due to the different salts, lack of standards, etc. Both glucosamine HCl and glucosamine sulfate are absorbed in the gut after the salt is cleaved in the stomach. There exists controversy as to whether either salt of glucosamine is superior to the other. Theoretically, if the amount of glucosamine base contained in the product is equivalent, the amount absorbed should be as well. Most clinical studies in veterinary species have been done with the HCl salt. Purified, low molecular weight chondroitin appears to be absorbed from the gut. Reported bioavailability in horses for chondroitin sulfate is about 25%; glucosamine, about 2%; bioavailability in dogs is reportedly about 5% for chondroitin sulfate and 12% for glucosamine.

Onset of any clinical efficacy may require 2–6 weeks of treatment.

Contraindications/Precautions/Warnings

No absolute contraindications were located for these compounds. As hypersensitivity reactions are a theoretical possibility, animals demonstrating prior hypersensitivity reactions to these compounds should not receive them.

In humans, glucosamine may exacerbate symptoms associated with asthma. Although this has not yet been reported in veterinary patients, caution is advised in patients with bronchoconstrictive conditions.

Adverse Effects

These products appear to be very well tolerated in dogs, cats, and horses. Adverse effects could potentially include some minor gastrointestinal effects (flatulence, stool softening). Since these products are often derived from natural sources, hypersensitivity reactions could occur.

Reproductive/Nursing Safety

No studies on the safety of these compounds in pregnant or lactating animals have been performed.

Overdosage/Acute Toxicity

Oral overdosage is unlikely to cause significant problems. The LD_{50} for the combined compound in rats is greater than 5 g/kg. Gastrointestinal effects may result. Changes in coagulation parameters could occur, but have not been documented to date.

Products that contain manganese could lead to manganese toxicity if given in very high dosages (above label recommendations) chronically.

Drug Interactions

No clinically significant drug interactions have been reported to date in animals. By reducing **doxorubicin** or **etoposide** inhibition of topoisomerase II, glucosamine may induce resistance to these agents. High dose chondroitin sulfate and/or glucosamine potentially could enhance the effects of **warfarin, heparin**, or other drugs that affect coagulation.

Laboratory Considerations

■ High dose chondroitin and glucosamine theoretically could increase International Normalized Ratio (**INR**) in patients taking warfarin.

Doses

Note: Because of the variability in products available, it is recommended to choose a product that has been tested in the species for which it is marketed; consult the product label.

■ **DOGS:**

a) For adjunctive treatment of chronic pain: Glucosamine/chondroitin: 13–15 mg/kg (of the chondroitin component) PO once daily (q24h). (Hardie *et al.* 2003)

b) For adjunctive treatment of cancer pain: Glucosamine/chondroitin: 15–30 mg/kg (of the chondroitin component) PO once daily (q24h) for 4–6 weeks then half the dose. (Lascelles 2003)

c) For adjunctive treatment of chronic pain: Glucosamine/chondroitin: 13–15 mg/kg (of the chondroitin component) PO once daily or every other day (q24–48h). (Hansen 2003)

d) Label Recommendation as a Dietary Supplement for *Cosequin®*:

For Small Dogs (under 25 lbs): Initially, using Regular Strength capsules for cats and small dogs: under 10 lb.: ½ to 1 capsule daily; 10–24 lb.: 2 capsules daily (1 in AM; 1 in PM). Maintenance Administration (after initial 4–6 week period): under 10 lb. can often have their dosage reduced to ½ capsule daily or 1 capsule every other day. 10 to 24 lb. can often have their dosage reduced to 1 capsule daily.

For Medium and Large Dogs (>25 lbs.): Initially, using *Cosequin®DS* (double strength) tablets or capsules: 25–49 lb.: 2 capsules daily (1 in AM; 1 in PM); 50–100 lb.: 3 capsules daily (2 in AM; 1 in PM); over 100 lb.: 4 capsules daily (2 in AM; 2 in PM). Maintenance Admin-

636   GLUCOSAMINE/CHRONDROITIN SULFATE

istration (after initial 4–6 week period): dogs can have their total daily dosage gradually lowered until maintenance level is reached.

Amount can be increased at any time depending on the pet's needs. Tablets can be given as a treat or crumbled and mixed with the pet's food. The capsules can be pulled apart and the contents sprinkled on the pet's food. Wet or moist food works best. As an alternative, pets can be pilled or the capsules administered by wrapping in a small piece of food. (Label recommendations; *Cosequin*®—Nutramax)

■ **CATS:**

a) For adjunctive treatment of cancer pain: Glucosamine/chondroitin: 15–30 mg/kg (of the chondroitin component) PO once daily (q24h) for 4–6 weeks then half the dose. (Lascelles 2003)

b) For adjunctive treatment of chronic pain: Glucosamine/chondroitin: 15–20 mg/kg (of the chondroitin component) PO once daily or every other day (q24–48h). (Hansen 2003)

c) Label Recommendation as a Dietary Supplement for *Cosequin*® *For Cats*: Initially: under 10 lb.: 1 capsule sprinkled on food daily; over 10 lb.: 2 capsules sprinkled on food daily (1 in AM/1 in PM). Maintenance Administration (after initial 4–6 week period): once desired response is obtained, capsules may be administered every other day.

Number of capsules can be increased at any time depending on the pet's needs. The capsules contain a flavored powder. The capsules should be opened and the contents mixed with or sprinkled over the food. Dry food may be moistened with a small amount of water so that the powder sticks. Alternatively, the contents of the capsules may be mixed with a small amount (*i.e.*, tablespoon) of wet or moist food. As an alternative, cats can be pilled. (Label recommendations; *Cosequin*® *For Cats*—Nutramax)

■ **HORSES:**

a) For navicular syndrome: Using *Cosequin*® *Concentrated Powder* labeled for horses: 16.5 grams (5 scoops) in feed twice daily. (Hanson *et al.* 2001)

b) Label Recommendation as a Dietary Supplement for *Cosequin*® *Concentrated Powder*: Initially: for horses under 600 lb., 2 scoops in AM and 2 scoops in PM; horses 600–1,200 lb., 3 scoops in AM and 3 scoops in PM; horses over 1,200 lb., 4 scoops in AM and 4 scoops in PM. The initial administration period is 2 to 4 weeks; if horse shows little or no re-

sponse, extend initial amount for two more weeks.

Transition Period: Do not lower amount until horse has begun to respond. After achieving a good response, reduce total daily amount by one level scoop each week. Gradually reducing the amount will help find an individual maintenance level. Suggested Maintenance Administration: horses under 600 lb., 1 scoop daily; horses 600–1,200 lb., 1–2 scoops daily; horses over 1,200 lb., 2 scoops daily. Amount can be increased at any time.

May be top dressed on sweet feed. Add a small amount of water or molasses to get the powder to stick to dry feed. (Label and insert recommendations; *Cosequin*® *Concentrated Powder*—Nutramax Labs)

Monitoring
■ Clinical efficacy

Client Information
■ Onset of any clinical improvement may require 2–6 weeks of treatment.
■ Do not switch brands from that prescribed without first contacting your veterinarian.
■ Side effects are unlikely, but mild gastrointestinal upset has been reported in small animals. Should this be troublesome, contact your veterinarian.

Chemistry/Synonyms
Glucosamine is most often available as either glucosamine HCl or glucosamine sulfate. It is an amino sugar that is synthesized *in vivo* by animal cells from glucose and glutamine.

Glucosamine (HCl or Sulfate) may also be known as: chitosamine, NSC-758, 2-amino-2-deoxy-beta-D-glucopyranose, G6SD-glucosamine, glucose-6-phosphate, or amino monosaccharide.

Chondroitin sulfate is an acid mucopolysaccharide/glycosaminoglycan that is found in most cartilaginous tissues. It is a long chain compound that contains Units of galactosamine and glucuronic acid.

Chondroitin sulfate may also be known as chondroitin 4-sulfate, chondroitin sulfate A, chondroitin sulfate B, chondroitin sulfate C, chondroitin sulfate sodium, CSA, sodium chondroitin sulfate, chondroitin polysulfate, CDA, CSCSC, GAG, or galactosaminogluconoglycan sulfate.

Storage/Stability
Because of the multiple products and product formulations available, check label for storage and stability (expiration date) information. Chondroitin sulfate is an extremely hygroscopic compound and, generally, these products should be stored in tight containers at room temperature. Avoid storing in direct sunlight.

Dosage Forms/Regulatory Status

VETERINARY-LABELED PRODUCTS:

None as pharmaceuticals. Supplements are available from a wide variety of sources and dosage forms include tablets, capsules and powder in a variety of concentrations. There are specific products marketed for use in animals, including *Cosequin®, Restor-A-Flex®, OsteO-3®, Arthri-Nu®, ProMotion®, Seraquin®, Oste-O-Guard®, Caniflex®, Equi-Phar Flex®*, etc.

Glucosamine and chondroitin sulfate are considered nutritional supplements by the FDA. No standards have been accepted for potency, purity, safety or efficacy by regulatory bodies.

Bioequivalence between products cannot be assumed and independent analysis has shown a wide variation in products.

HUMAN-LABELED PRODUCTS: None as pharmaceuticals

References

Hansen, B. (2003). Updated opinions on analgesic techniques. Proceedings: ACVIM Forum. Accessed via: Veterinary Information Network. http://goo.gl/EPWL2

Hanson, R., W. Brawner, et al. (2001). Oral treatment with nutraceutical (Cosequin) for ameliorating signs of navicular syndrome in horses. *Vet Therapeutics* 2: 148–159.

Hardie, E., D. Lascelles, et al. (2003). Managing Chronic Pain in Dogs: The Next Level. Proceedings: Pain Management 2003. Accessed via: Veterinary Information Network. http://goo.gl/mAki4

Lascelles, B. (2003). Case examples in the management of cancer pain in dogs and cats, and the future of cancer pain alleviation. Proceedings: American College of Veterinary Internal Medicine. Accessed via: Veterinary Information Network. http://goo.gl/Yxog0

McCarthy, G., J. O'Donovan, et al. (2007). Randomised double-blind, positive-controlled trial to assess the efficacy of glucosamine/chondroitin sulfate for the treatment of dogs with osteoarthritis. *Vet J* 174(1): 54–61.

Moreau, M., J. Dupuis, et al. (2003). Clinical evaluation of a nutraceutical, carprofen and meloxicam for the treatment of dogs with osteoarthritis. *Vet Rec* 152(11): 323–329.

Pearson, W. & M. Lindinger (2009). Low quality of evidence for glucosamine-based nutraceuticals in equine joint disease: Review of in vivo studies. *Equine Veterinary Journal* 41(7): 706–712.

GLUTAMINE

*(gloo-*ta-meen)

NUTRITIONAL

Prescriber Highlights

▶ Amino acid that may be useful in preventing/treating GI epithelium damage or pancreatitis (exocrine function)

▶ Little documentation for efficacy, but adverse effects unlikely

Uses/Indications

Glutamine has been used as a GI protectant and in an attempt to enhance GI healing in conditions where GI epithelium is damaged (Parvo enteritis, chemotherapy, etc.), pancreatitis, or when patients are under severe stress (critically ill). Animals that have an adequate dietary protein intake, are unlikely to benefit from exogenously administered glutamine.

A study that evaluated the efficacy of glutamine supplementation in cats with methotrexate-induced enteritis found no difference between cats supplemented with glutamine and those that were not. (Marks *et al.* 1999)

Pharmacology/Actions

Glutamine is a conditionally essential amino acid that is produced primarily in skeletal muscle and then released into the circulation. Glutamine is required for proper function of the immune system, GI tract, kidneys, and liver. Glutamine also serves as a precursor for glutathione, glutamate, purines, pyrimidines, and other amino acids.

Glutamine's effects on the gastrointestinal tract are one of the primary areas of interest for its therapeutic use as an exogenously administered drug. When the body is under severe stress, it consumes more glutamine than it can produce and progressive muscle wasting occurs as it tries to meet glutamine requirements. There is some evidence that glutamine may have a role in intestinal cell proliferation and determination. When glutamine is depleted, intestinal epithelium can atrophy, ulcerate, or become necrotic. In patients undergoing cancer chemotherapy or radiotherapy, diminished glutamine levels in the gastrointestinal tract can cause increased GI toxicity. Supplementation of exogenous glutamine may help protect the GI from these effects.

Pharmacokinetics

Little information was located outside of what is described in the pharmacology section.

Contraindications/Precautions/Warnings

Because it is partially metabolized into ammonia and glutamate, use with caution in patients with severe hepatic insufficiency, severe behavior disorders or epilepsy.

Adverse Effects

Glutamine is well tolerated when used orally or intravenously. Potentially, it may have some CNS effects at high dosages.

Reproductive/Nursing Safety

There is insufficient data available documenting the safe use of glutamine during pregnancy or nursing.

Overdosage/Acute Toxicity

Overdosages are unlikely to be harmful. Doses of up to 40 grams per day IV have been tolerated in humans without ill effects. Because glutamine is partially metabolized to ammonia, patients with hepatic insufficiency may be adversely affected.

Drug Interactions

The following drug interactions have either been reported or are theoretical in humans or animals receiving glutamine and may be of significance in veterinary patients:

■ **ANTICONVULSANT MEDICATIONS:** Glutamine could potentially affect the efficacy of antiseizure medications (**phenobarbital, potassium bromide,** etc.). It is partially converted into glutamate, which can act as an excitatory neurotransmitter.

■ **LACTULOSE:** Theoretically, glutamine may antagonize the effects of lactulose in patients with hepatic encephalopathy.

Laboratory Considerations

■ Glutamine may increase **serum ammonia** or **glutamate** levels.

Doses

■ **DOGS & CATS:**

For adjunctive treatment of GI inflammatory conditions:

a) 0.5 grams/kg PO daily (Wynn 2002)

b) 0.5 gram/kg/day PO divided twice a day in the water or food. (Silverstein 2003)

c) Animals not eating may benefit from 0.5 grams/kg per day divided into 2-3 doses and dissolved in drinking water. (Laflamme 2009)

Monitoring

■ Efficacy

Client Information

■ May be administered with food.

Chemistry/Synonyms

Glutamine is an aliphatic amino acid. It occurs as white crystals or crystalline powder and is soluble in water and practically insoluble in alcohol.

Glutamine may also be known as: glutamic acid, GLN, glutamate, glutaminate, levoglutamide, levoglutamine, L-glutamic acid, L-glutamic acid 5-amide, l-glutamine, L-glutamine, and Q.

Storage/Stability

Glutamine tablets and powder should be stored in tight containers at room temperature.

Dosage Forms/Regulatory Status

VETERINARY-LABELED PRODUCTS: None

HUMAN-LABELED PRODUCTS:

Glutamine is considered a nutrient. Glutamine may be purchased as L-glutamine 500 mg tablets, glutamine powder, or glutamic acid in 500 mg tablets, powder. Glutamic acid is rapidly degraded in the body to glutamine. Parenteral forms of glutamate may be available in other countries.

References

Laflamme, D. (2009). Dietary management of gastrointestinal disease. Proceedings: Western Vet Conference. Accessed via: Veterinary Information Network. http://goo.gl/gKXEa

Marks, S., A. Cook, et al. (1999). Effects of glutamine supplementation of an an amino acid-based purified diet on intestinal mucosal integrity in cats with methotrexate-induced enteritis. Am J Vet Res 60(6): 755–773.

Silverstein, D. (2003). Intensive care treatment of severe Parvovirus enteritis. Proceedings: IVECCS. Accessed via: Veterinary Information Network. http://goo.gl/S5gKe

Wynn, S. (2002). Nutraceutical options in veterinary medicine. Proceedings Western Veterinary Conference. Accessed via: Veterinary Information Network. http://goo.gl/JdSbp

GLYBURIDE

(*glye*-byoor-ide)   DiaBeta®, Micronase®

SULFONYLUREA ANTIDIABETIC AGENT

Prescriber Highlights

▶ Human oral antidiabetic agent (Type II) that may be useful in cats

▶ Glipizide used more often when oral hypoglycemics are tried; glyburide may be useful if glipizide unavailable or if once a day dosing is important

▶ Contraindications: Severe burns, severe trauma, severe infection, diabetic coma or other hypoglycemic conditions, major surgery, ketosis, ketoacidosis or other significant acidotic conditions

▶ Caution: Untreated adrenal or pituitary insufficiency; thyroid, renal, or hepatic function impairment; prolonged vomiting; high fever; malnourishment or debilitated condition

▶ Adverse Effects: *Cats:* GI (*i.e.*, vomiting), hypoglycemia, liver toxicity

▶ Drug interactions

▶ Do not confuse glipizide, glimepiride & glyburide

Uses/Indications

Glyburide is an alternative oral treatment for non-insulin dependent diabetes mellitus (NIDDM) in cats, particularly if glipizide is unavailable or if twice daily administration of glipizide is not tolerated (by cat or owner). Insulin therapy for cats with diabetes is generally preferred over oral treatments.

Pharmacology/Actions

Like glipizide and other oral sulfonylureas, glyburide lowers blood glucose concentrations in both diabetic and normal patients. While it is unknown how glyburide precisely lowers glucose, it initially stimulates secretion of endogenous functional beta cells in the pancreas. It also may enhance insulin activity at post receptor sites and reduce basal hepatic glucose production that may explain its effectiveness with long-term administration.

Pharmacokinetics

Glyburide appears to be well absorbed but bioavailability data is lacking. Food apparently does not have an effect on the absorptive characteristics of the drug. Glyburide is distributed throughout the body, including into the brain and across the placenta. Glyburide is apparently completely metabolized, presumably in the liver. Metabolites are excreted in both the feces and the urine. While its elimination half-life in cats is not known, once a day dosing appears to be effective in cats with NIDDM.

Contraindications/Precautions/Warnings
Oral antidiabetic agents are considered contraindicated with the following conditions: severe burns, severe trauma, severe infection, diabetic coma or other hypoglycemic conditions, major surgery, ketosis, ketoacidosis or other significant acidotic conditions. Glyburide should only be used when its potential benefits outweigh its risks in patients with untreated adrenal or pituitary insufficiency; thyroid, renal, or hepatic function impairment; prolonged vomiting; high fever; malnourishment or in debilitated condition.

Some patients with type II diabetes may have their disease complicated by the production of excessive amounts of cortisol or growth hormone that may antagonize insulin's effects. These causes should be ruled out before initiating oral antidiabetic therapy.

Adverse Effects
Experience with glyburide is limited in veterinary medicine. Hypoglycemia, vomiting, icterus, and increased ALT (SGPT) levels are all potentially possible. Should toxicity develop, reinstitution of drug therapy may be attempted at a lower dosage after clinical signs resolve.

Other adverse effects that are possible (noted in humans) include: allergic skin reactions, arthralgia, bone marrow suppression, or cholestatic jaundice.

Glyburide may not be effective in cats demonstrating insulin resistance.

Reproductive/Nursing Safety
In humans, the FDA categorizes this drug as category *C* for use during pregnancy (*Animal studies have shown an adverse effect on the fetus, but there are no adequate studies in humans; or there are no animal reproduction studies and no adequate studies in humans.*)

It is unknown if glyburide is excreted in milk.

Overdosage/Acute Toxicity
Profound hypoglycemia is the greatest concern after an overdose. In humans, severe hypoglycemia has occurred at relatively low dosages. Gut emptying protocols should be employed when warranted. Because its half-life is longer than glipizide, prolonged hypoglycemia may occur and blood glucose monitoring and treatment with parenteral glucose may be required for several days. Massive overdoses may also require additional monitoring (blood gases, serum electrolytes) and supportive therapy.

Drug Interactions
The following drug interactions have either been reported or are theoretical in humans or animals receiving glyburide and may be of significance in veterinary patients:

- **ALCOHOL:** A disulfiram-like reaction (anorexia, nausea, vomiting) is possible
- **ANTIFUNGALS, AZOLE (ketoconazole, itraconazole, fluconazole):** May increase plasma levels of glyburide
- **BETA-BLOCKERS:** May potentiate hypoglycemic effect
- **CHLORAMPHENICOL:** May displace glyburide from plasma proteins
- **CIMETIDINE:** May potentiate hypoglycemic effect
- **CORTICOSTEROIDS:** May reduce efficacy
- **DIURETICS, THIAZIDE:** May reduce hypoglycemic efficacy
- **ISONIAZID:** May reduce hypoglycemic efficacy
- **MOA INHIBITORS:** May potentiate hypoglycemic effect
- **NIACIN:** May reduce hypoglycemic efficacy
- **PHENOTHIAZINES:** May reduce hypoglycemic efficacy
- **PHENYTOIN:** May reduce hypoglycemic efficacy
- **PROBENECID:** May potentiate hypoglycemic effect
- **SULFONAMIDES:** May displace glyburide from plasma proteins
- **SYMPATHOMIMETIC AGENTS:** May reduce hypoglycemic efficacy
- **THYROID AGENTS:** May reduce hypoglycemic effect
- **WARFARIN:** May displace glyburide from plasma proteins

Doses

- **CATS:**
  For NIDDM:
  a) Initial dose at 0.625 mg (1/2 of a 1.25 mg tablet) PO once daily. (Nelson 2000)
  b) If cat is generally well, weight loss is mild, is not ketoacidotic, and does not have peripheral neuropathy, may try glyburide at: 2.5 mg (total dose) PO twice a day. (Daminet 2003)

Monitoring
- Weekly exams during first month of therapy including PE, body weight, urine glucose/ketones and several blood glucose exams.
- Adverse effects (vomiting, icterus), and occasional liver enzymes and CBC.

Client Information
- Clients should be informed of clinical signs to watch for that would indicate either hypoglycemia or hyperglycemia and be instructed to report these to the veterinarian.
- Compliance with dosing regimen should also be stressed.

Chemistry/Synonyms

An oral sulfonylurea antidiabetic agent, glyburide occurs as a white or nearly white, odorless or almost odorless, crystalline powder. As pH increases, solubility increases. At a pH of 4, solubility in water is about 4 micrograms/mL and at a pH of 9,600 micrograms/mL. Glyburide has a pKa of 6.8.

Glyburide may also be known as: glibenclamide, glibenclamidum, glybenclamide, glybenzcyclamide, HB-419, and U-26452; many trade names are available.

Storage/Stability

Glyburide oral tablets should be stored in well-closed containers at room temperature.

Dosage Forms/Regulatory Status

VETERINARY-LABELED PRODUCTS: None

HUMAN-LABELED PRODUCTS:

Glyburide Oral Tablets: 1.25 mg, 2.5 mg, & 5 mg; micronized tablets: 1.5 mg, 3 mg, 4.5 mg & 6 mg; *Glynase® PresTab* (Pharmacia & Upjohn); *DiaBeta®* (Hoechst Marion Roussel); generic; (Rx)

Fixed dose combinations of glyburide and metformin are also available.

References

Daminet, S. (2003). Canine and Feline Diabetes Mellitus. Proceedings: World Small Animal Veterinary Assoc. World Congress. Accessed via: Veterinary Information Network. http://goo.gl/YRCPp

Nelson, R. (2000). Diabetes Mellitus. *Textbook of Veterinary Internal Medicine: Diseases of the Dog and Cat.* S Ettinger and E Feldman Eds. Philadelphia, WB Saunders. 2: 1438–1460.

GLYCERIN, ORAL

(*gli*-ser-in)   Osmoglyn®

OSMOTIC AGENT

Prescriber Highlights

▶ Oral osmotic that reduces intraocular & CSF pressure

▶ Contraindications: Patients with known hypersensitivity, anuria (well established), severe dehydration, severe cardiac decompensation, acute pulmonary edema

▶ Caution: Hypovolemia, cardiac disease, or diabetes

▶ Adverse Effects: Vomiting (most common)

Uses/Indications

Oral glycerin is used primarily for the short-term reduction of IOP in small animals with acute glaucoma. It may also be considered for use to reduce increased CSF pressure.

The IOP-lowering effect of glycerin may be more variable than with mannitol, but since it may be given orally, it may be more advantageous to use in certain cases.

Pharmacology/Actions

Glycerin in therapeutic oral doses increases the osmotic pressure of plasma so that water from extracellular spaces is drawn into the blood. This can decrease intraocular pressure (IOP). The amount of decrease in IOP is dependent upon the dose of glycerin, and the cause and extent of increased IOP. Glycerin also decreases extracellular water content from other tissues and can cause dehydration and decreased CSF pressure.

Pharmacokinetics

Glycerin is rapidly absorbed from the GI tract and decreases in IOP can be seen within 30 minutes; peak serum levels generally occur within 90 minutes and maximum decreases in IOP usually occur within an hour of dosing and persist for up to 10 hours. Glycerin is distributed throughout the blood and is primarily metabolized by the liver. About 10% of the drug is excreted unchanged in the urine. Serum half-life in humans is about 30–45 minutes.

Contraindications/Precautions/Warnings

Glycerin is contraindicated in patients hypersensitive to it. It is also contraindicated in patients with well-established anuria, that are severely dehydrated, severely cardiac decompensated, or with frank or impending acute pulmonary edema.

Glycerin should be used with caution in animals when the blood:ocular barrier is not intact (hyphema, uveitis), and those with hypovolemia, cardiac disease, or diabetes. One reference states that glycerine is contraindicated in dogs with diabetes mellitus, dehydration, and cardiac or renal disease (Reinstein *et al.* 2009). Another states that heart failure is a contraindication and use should be avoided in patients with chronic renal failure or compromised renal function (Pickett 2009). Acute urinary retention should be avoided during the preoperative period.

Adverse Effects

Vomiting after dosing is the most common adverse effect seen with glycerin use. In humans, headache, nausea, thirst, and diarrhea have also been reported.

Reproductive/Nursing Safety

The safety of this drug in pregnant animals is unknown; use only when potential benefits outweigh the risks of therapy. In humans, the FDA categorizes this drug as category *C* for use during pregnancy (*Animal studies have shown an adverse effect on the fetus, but there are no adequate studies in humans; or there are no animal reproduction studies and no adequate studies in humans.*)

No specific information on glycerin was located for lactation safety.

Overdosage/Acute Toxicity

No specific information was located, but cardiac arrhythmias, non-ketotic hyperosmolar coma, and severe dehydration have been reported with the drug.

Drug Interactions

The following drug interactions have either been reported or are theoretical in humans or animals receiving glycerin and may be of significance in veterinary patients:

■ **CARBONIC ANHYDRASE INHIBITORS (e.g., acetazolamide, dichlorphenamide):** Concomitant administration of carbonic anhydrase inhibitors or topical miotic agents may prolong the IOP-reducing effects of glycerin.

■ **MIOTIC AGENTS, TOPICAL:** Concomitant administration topical miotic agents may prolong the IOP-reducing effects of glycerin

Doses

■ **DOGS/CATS:**

For acute glaucoma:

a) 1–2 g/kg PO as a 50% oral solution (Herring 2003), (Reinstein *et al.* 2009)

b) 1–2 mL/kg (of a 90% solution) PO usually as a single dose; withhold water for 3–4 hours after administration. Author uses glycerin often because it is quicker and easier to administer than mannitol and is usually effective. (Collins 2006)

c) As an "emergency drug" in place of aqueous centesis to rapidly reduce IOP: Using glycerin syrup (90%) at 1.1–2.2 mL/kg (0.5–1 mL/lb); mixing with an equal volume of ice cream or milk will help reduce vomiting. (Pickett 2009)

Monitoring

■ IOP

■ Urine output

■ Hydration status

Chemistry/Synonyms

A trihydric alcohol, glycerin occurs as clear, sweet-tasting, syrupy, hygroscopic liquid that has a characteristic odor. It is miscible with water and alcohol, but not miscible in oils. Glycerin solutions are neutral to litmus.

Glycerin may also be known as: E422, glycerol, glicerol, glycerin, glycerine, and glycerolum; many trade names are available.

Storage/Stability

Glycerin oral solution should be stored in tight containers at room temperature; protect from freezing.

Dosage Forms/Regulatory Status

VETERINARY-LABELED PRODUCTS: None for systemic use.

HUMAN-LABELED PRODUCTS:

Glycerin Oral Liquid: 50% (0.6 g glycerin/mL) in 220 mL; *Osmoglyn®* (Alcon); (Rx)

Glycerin is also available in a topical ophthalmic solution and as suppositories or liquid for rectal laxative use. USP glycerin 90% could be used for oral use in small animals (see doses above).

References

Collins, B. (2006). Update for glaucoma. Proceedings; Western Vet Conf. Accessed via: Veterinary Information Network. http://goo.gl/2uZWc

Herring, I. (2003). Glaucoma. *Handbook of Small Animal Practice, 4th Ed.* R Morgan, R Bright and M Swartout Eds. Phila., Saunders: 988–994.

Pickett, J. (2009). The canine glaucomas. Proceedings; ABVP. Accessed via: Veterinary Information Network. http://goo.gl/GmzfP

Reinstein, S.L., A.J. Rankin, et al. (2009). Canine Glaucoma: Medical and Surgical Treatment Options. *Compendium-Continuing Education for Veterinarians* 31(10): 454–458.

Glyceryl Guaiacolate; GG–see Guaifenesin

GLYCOPYRROLATE

(glye-koe-*pye*-roe-late)   Robinul®

ANTICHOLINERGIC (ANTIMUSCARINIC)

Prescriber Highlights

▶ Synthetic antimuscarinic agent similar to atropine available both orally & parenterally; used for a variety of indications (bradycardia, premed, antidote, etc.)

▶ Contraindicated in conditions where anticholinergic effects would be detrimental (e.g., narrow angle glaucoma, tachycardias, ileus, urinary obstruction, etc.)

▶ Adverse effects are dose related & anticholinergic in nature, including: dry secretions; initial bradycardia, then tachycardia; slowing of gut & urinary tract motility; mydriasis/cycloplegia

▶ Drug interactions

Uses/Indications

Glycopyrrolate injection is FDA-approved for use in dogs and cats. The FDA-approved indication for these species is as a preanesthetic anticholinergic agent. The drug is also used to treat sinus bradycardia, sinoatrial arrest, and incomplete AV block, where anticholinergic therapy may be beneficial. When cholinergic agents such as neostigmine or pyridostigmine are used to reverse neuromuscular blockade due to nondepolarizing muscle relaxants, glycopyrrolate may be administered simultaneously to prevent the peripheral muscarinic effects of the cholinergic agent.

Pharmacology/Actions

An antimuscarinic with similar actions as atropine, glycopyrrolate is a quaternary ammonium compound and, unlike atropine, does not cross appreciably into the CNS. It, therefore, should not exhibit the same extent of CNS adverse effects that atropine possesses. For further information, refer to the atropine monograph.

Pharmacokinetics

Quaternary anticholinergic agents are not completely absorbed after oral administration, but quantitative data reporting the rate and extent of absorption of glycopyrrolate is not available. In dogs, following IV administration, the onset of action is generally within one minute. After IM or SC administration, peak effects occur approximately 30–45 minutes post injection. The vagolytic effects persist for 2–3 hours and the antisialagogue (reduced salivation) effects persist for up to 7 hours. After oral administration, the anticholinergic effects of glycopyrrolate may persist for 8–12 hours.

Little information is available regarding the distributory aspects of glycopyrrolate. Being a quaternary ammonium compound, glycopyrrolate is completely ionized; therefore, it has poor lipid solubility and does not readily penetrate into the CNS or eye. Glycopyrrolate crosses the placenta only marginally; it is unknown if it is excreted into milk.

Glycopyrrolate is eliminated rapidly from the serum after IV administration and virtually no drug remains in the serum 30 minutes to 3 hours after dosing. Only a small amount is metabolized and the majority is eliminated unchanged in the feces and urine.

Contraindications/Precautions/Warnings

One manufacturer (Fort Dodge) of the veterinary product lists contraindications to glycopyrrolate's use in dogs and cats hypersensitive to it and that it should not be used in pregnant animals.

Antimuscarinic agents should be used with extreme caution in patients with known or suspected GI infections. Atropine or other antimuscarinic agents can decrease GI motility and prolong retention of the causative agent(s) or toxin(s) resulting in prolonged clinical signs. Antimuscarinic agents must also be used with extreme caution in patients with autonomic neuropathy.

Antimuscarinic agents should be used with caution in patients with hepatic or renal disease, geriatric or pediatric patients, hyperthyroidism, hypertension, CHF, tachyarrhythmias, prostatic hypertrophy, or esophageal reflux. These drugs can produce sinus tachycardia and predispose hypotensive patients to cardiac arrhythmias (including ventricular fibrillation).

Adverse Effects

With the exceptions of rare CNS adverse effects and being slightly less arrhythmogenic, glycopyrrolate can be expected to have a similar adverse effect profile as atropine. The manufacturer of the veterinary product (Fort Dodge) lists only mydriasis, tachycardia, and xerostomia as adverse effects in dogs and cats at the doses they recommend. For more information, refer to the atropine monograph.

Reproductive/Nursing Safety

In humans, the FDA categorizes this drug as category *B* for use during pregnancy *(Animal studies have not yet demonstrated risk to the fetus, but there are no adequate studies in pregnant women; or animal studies have shown an adverse effect, but adequate studies in pregnant women have not demonstrated a risk to the fetus in the first trimester of pregnancy, and there is no evidence of risk in later trimesters.)* In a separate system evaluating the safety of drugs in canine and feline pregnancy (Papich 1989), this drug is categorized as in class: *B (Safe for use if used cautiously. Studies in laboratory animals may have uncovered some risk, but these drugs appear to be safe in dogs and cats or these drugs are safe if they are not administered when the animal is near term.)*

No specific lactation safety information was found; however, it is unlikely to be excreted into milk in substantial quantities because of its quaternary structure.

Overdosage/Acute Toxicity

In dogs, the LD_{50} for glycopyrrolate is reported to be 25 mg/kg IV. Doses of 2 mg/kg IV daily for 5 days per week for 4 weeks demonstrated no signs of toxicity. In the cat, the LD_{50} after IM injection is 283 mg/kg. Because of its quaternary structure, it would be expected that minimal CNS effects would occur after an overdose of glycopyrrolate when compared to atropine. See the information listed in the atropine monograph for more information.

Drug Interactions

Glycopyrrolate would be expected to have a similar drug interaction profile as atropine. The following drug interactions have either been reported or are theoretical in humans or animals receiving atropine or glycopyrrolate and may be of significance in veterinary patients:

The following drugs may enhance the activity or toxicity of atropine and its derivatives:

- **AMANTADINE**
- **ANTICHOLINERGIC AGENTS (other)**
- **ANTICHOLINERGIC MUSCLE RELAXANTS**
- **ANTIHISTAMINES (e.g., diphenhydramine)**
- **DISOPYRAMIDE**
- **MEPERIDINE**
- **PHENOTHIAZINES**
- **PROCAINAMIDE**
- **PRIMIDONE**
- **TRICYCLIC ANTIDEPRESSANTS (e.g., amitriptyline, clomipramine)**
- **AMITRAZ:** Atropine may aggravate some signs seen with amitraz toxicity; leading to hypertension and further inhibition of peristalsis
- **ANTACIDS:** May decrease PO atropine absorption; give oral atropine at least 1 hour prior to oral antacids
- **CORTICOSTEROIDS (long-term use):** may increase intraocular pressure

■ **DIGOXIN (slow-dissolving):** Atropine may increase serum digoxin levels; use regular digoxin tablets or oral liquid

■ **KETOCONAZOLE:** Increased gastric pH may decrease GI absorption; administer atropine 2 hours after ketoconazole

■ **METOCLOPRAMIDE:** Atropine and its derivatives may antagonize the actions of metoclopramide

Doses

■ **DOGS:**

As an adjunct to anesthesia:

a) 0.011 mg/kg IV, IM, or SC (Package Insert; *Robinul®-V* —Fort Dodge)

b) 0.01−0.02 mg/kg SC or IM (Bellah 1989)

For adjunctive therapy of bradyarrhythmias:

a) 0.011 mg/kg IV or IM (Russell & Rush 1995)

b) Associated with anesthesia: 0.005−0.01 mg/kg IV (Pablo 2003)

c) For bradyarrhythmias (sinus bradycardia, high-grade 2nd-degree and 3rd-degree AV block) produced by increased vagal tone: 0.05−0.1 mg/kg IV. (Muir 2008)

To reduce hypersialism:

a) 0.01 mg/kg SC as needed (Krahwinkel 1989)

■ **CATS:**

As an adjunct to anesthesia:

a) 0.011 mg/kg IM, for maximum effect give 15 minutes prior to anesthetic administration (Package Insert; *Robinul®-V*— Fort Dodge)

For bradyarrhythmias:

a) 0.005−0.01 mg/kg IV or IM, 0.01−0.02 mg/kg SC (Tilley & Miller 1986)

b) Associated with anesthesia: 0.005−0.01 mg/kg IV (Pablo 2003)

■ **FERRETS:**

As a premed:

a) 0.01 mg/kg SC or IM (Williams 2000)

b) 0.01−0.02 mg/kg IM or IV (Vella 2009)

■ **RABBITS/RODENTS/SMALL MAMMALS:**

a) **Rabbits:** For prevention of bradycardia and to decrease airway and salivary secretions: 0.01−0.1 mg/kg IM, SC; 0.01 mg/kg IV (Ivey & Morrisey 2000)

b) **Rabbits:** As adjunct to anesthesia: 0.01− 0.02 mg/kg SC as needed (Huerkamp 1995)

c) As a preanesthetic: Rodents: 0.01−0.02 mg/kg SC or IM. Rabbits: 0.01−0.1 mg/kg IM or SC. As part of an injectable anesthesia protocol in rabbits: acepromazine (0.2 mg/kg), plus oxymorphone (0.1 mg/kg), plus glycopyrrolate (0.01 mg/kg) IM. (Bennett 2009)

■ **HORSES: (Note:** ARCI UCGFS Class 3 Drug)

For treatment of bradyarrhythmias:

a) 0.005−0.01 mg/kg (5−10 micrograms/kg) IV (Mogg 1999)

As a bronchodilator:

a) Initially, 2−3 mg IM two to three times daily for a 450 kg animal (Beech 1987)

To control muscarinic adverse effects associated with imidocarb therapy:

a) 0.0025 mg/kg IV (Donnellan *et al.* 2003)

■ **REPTILES:**

a) For bradycardia (prolonged or profound) associated with anesthesia: 0.01 mg/kg IM, IV or IC (intracoelemic). (Mehler 2009)

Monitoring

■ Dependent on route of administration, dose, and reason for use. See the atropine monograph for more information.

Client Information

■ Parenteral glycopyrrolate administration is best performed by professional staff and where adequate cardiac monitoring is available.

■ If animal is receiving glycopyrrolate tablets, allow animal free access to water and encourage drinking if dry mouth is a problem.

Chemistry/Synonyms

A synthetic quaternary ammonium antimuscarinic agent, glycopyrrolate occurs as a bitter-tasting, practically odorless, white, crystalline powder with a melting range of 193−198°C. One gram is soluble in 20 mL of water; 30 mL of alcohol. The commercially available injection is adjusted to a pH of 2−3 and contains 0.9% benzyl alcohol as a preservative.

Glycopyrrolate may also be known as: glycopyrronium bromide, AHR-504, *Acpan®*, *AmTech®*, *Gastrodyn®*, *Glycostigmin®*, and *Robinul®*.

Storage/Stability

Glycopyrrolate tablets should be stored in tight containers and both the injection and tablets should be stored at room temperature (15−30°C).

Glycopyrrolate is stable under ordinary conditions of light and temperature. It is most stable in solution at an acidic pH and undergoes ester hydrolysis at pH's above 6.

Compatibility/Compounding Considerations

Although stability information was not located: glycopyrrolate injection has been mixed in syringes with acepromazine, buprenorphine, morphine and ketamine.

Glycopyrrolate injection is physically **stable** in the following IV solutions: D_5W, D_5/half normal saline, Ringer's injection, and normal saline. Glycopyrrolate may be administered via the tubing of an IV running lactated Ringer's, but rapid hydrolysis will occur if it is added to an IV bag of LRS. The following drugs are reportedly physically **compatible** with glycopyrrolate: atropine sulfate, benzquinamide, chlorpromazine HCl, codeine phosphate, diphenhydramine HCl, droperidol, droperidol/fentanyl, hydromorphone, hydroxyzine HCl, lidocaine HCl, meperidine HCl, meperidine HCl/promethazine HCl, morphine sulfate, neostigmine methylsulfate, oxymorphone HCl, procaine HCl, prochlorperazine HCl, promazine HCl, promethazine HCl, pyridostigmine Br, scopolamine HBr, and trimethobenzamide HCl.

The following drugs are reportedly physically **incompatible** with glycopyrrolate: chloramphenicol sodium succinate, dexamethasone sodium phosphate, diazepam, dimenhydrinate, methohexital sodium, methylprednisolone sodium succinate, pentazocine lactate, pentobarbital sodium, secobarbital sodium, sodium bicarbonate, and thiopental sodium. Other alkaline drugs (*e.g.*, thiamylal) would also be **expected to be incompatible** with glycopyrrolate. Compatibility is dependent upon factors such as pH, concentration, temperature, and diluent used; consult specialized references for more specific information.

Dosage Forms/Regulatory Status

VETERINARY-LABELED PRODUCTS:

Glycopyrrolate for Injection: 0.2 mg/mL in 20 mL vials; *Robinul®-V* (Pfizer), generic; (Rx). FDA-approved for use in dogs and cats.

The ARCI (Racing Commissioners International) has designated this drug as a class 3 substance. See the appendix for more information.

HUMAN-LABELED PRODUCTS:

Glycopyrrolate Tablets: 1 mg & 2 mg; *Robinul®* & *Robinul Forte®* (Horizon); generic; (Rx)

Glycopyrrolate Injection: 0.2 mg/mL in 1 mL, 2 mL, 5 mL, & 20 mL vials; *Robinul®* (Robins); generic; (Rx)

References

Beech, J. (1987). Drug therapy of respiratory disorders. *Vet Clin North Am (Equine Practice)* 3(1): 59–80.

Bellah, J.R. (1989). Acute gastric dilatation-volvulus. *Handbook of Small Animal Practice.* RV Morgan Ed. New York, Churchill Livingstone: 385–394.

Bennett, R. (2009). Small Mammal Anesthesia--Rabbits and Rodents. Proceedings: ACVC. Accessed via: Veterinary Information Network. http://goo.gl/hRqTS

Donnellan, C., P. Page, et al. (2003). Effect of atropine and glycopyrrolate in ameliorating the side effects caused by imidocarb dipropionate administration in horses. Proceedings: ACVIM Forum. Accessed via: Veterinary Information Network. http://goo.gl/ylpBJ

Huerkamp, M. (1995). Anesthesia and postoperative management of rabbits and pocket pets. *Kirk's Current Veterinary Therapy:XII.* J Bonagura Ed. Philadelphia, W.B. Saunders: 1322–1327.

Ivey, E. & J. Morrisey (2000). Therapeutics for Rabbits. *Vet Clin NA: Exotic Anim Pract* 3:1(Jan): 183–216.

Krahwinkel, D.J. (1989). Disease of the salivary glands. *Handbook of Small Animal Practice.* RV Morgan Ed. New York, Churchill Livingstone: 347–356.

Mehler, S. (2009). Anaesthesia and care of the reptile. Proceedings: BSAVA. Accessed via: Veterinary Information Network. http://goo.gl/2QYZU

Mogg, T. (1999). Equine Cardiac Disease: Clinical pharmacology and therapeutics. *The Veterinary Clinics of North America: Equine Practice* 15:3(December).

Muir, W. (2008). New Approaches to Cardiopulmonary Cerebral Resuscitation. Proceedings: IVECCS. Accessed via: Veterinary Information Network. http://goo.gl/NE4oz

Pablo, L. (2003). Management of anesthesia complications. Proceedings: World Small Animal Veterinary Assoc World Congress. Accessed via: Veterinary Information Network. http://goo.gl/2H0bU

Russell, L. & J. Rush (1995). Cardiac Arrhythmias in Systemic Disease. *Kirk's Current Veterinary Therapy:XII.* J Bonagura Ed. Philadelphia, W.B. Saunders: 161–166.

Tilley, L.P. & M.S. Miller (1986). Antiarrhythmic drugs and management of cardiac arrhythmias. *Current Veterinary Therapy IX: Small Animal Practice.* RV Kirk Ed. Philadelphia, WB Saunders: 346–360.

Vella, D. (2009). Rabbit General Anesthesia. Proceedings: AAVAC-UEP. Accessed via: Veterinary Information Network. http://goo.gl/XKsCh

Williams, B. (2000). Therapeutics in Ferrets. *Vet Clin NA: Exotic Anim Pract* 3:1(Jan): 131–153.

GOLD SALTS, INJECTABLE GOLD SODIUM THIOMALATE

(*gold* soe-*dee*-um thye-*oh*-mal-ate) Aurothiomalate, Aurolate®, Myochrisine®

AUROTHIOGLUCOSE

(aur-oh-*thye*-oh-*gloo*-kose)   Solganal®

INJECTABLE GOLD IMMUNOSUPPRESSIVES

Prescriber Highlights

▶ Aurothioglucose may no longer be available commercially; potentially may substitute with gold sodium thiomalate (aurothiomalate)

▶ Injectable administered gold; for pemphigus complex in small animals or plasmacytic stomatitis/pyodermatitis in cats; may also be useful for pemphigus in goats or horses

▶ Can be quite toxic & expensive, intensive ongoing monitoring required

▶ Considered contraindicated in SLE (exacerbates), renal or hepatic disease, preexisting hematologic abnormalities, severe debilitation, or uncontrolled diabetes

▶ Possible teratogen

▶ Litany of serious adverse effects possible; pain on injection

Note: Aurothioglucose has traditionally been the injectable gold compound used in veterinary medicine, but it is no longer commercially available. Some now use gold sodium thiomalate (aurothiomalate) in its place. The following monograph primarily applies to aurothioglucose, but the two drugs are thought to have similar actions, adverse effects, etc. Doses specific for gold sodium thiomalate are noted in the dosage section.

Uses/Indications

In human medicine, gold compounds are used primarily as a treatment for rheumatoid arthritis that has not adequately responded to less toxic treatment modalities. In veterinary medicine (primarily small animal medicine), its use has been generally for treating immune-mediated serious skin disorders such as pemphigus complex in dogs or cats and plasmacytic stomatitis/pyodermatitis in cats. Gold salts have also been used to treat goats and horses with pemphigus.

Pharmacology/Actions

Injectable gold compounds have antiinflammatory, antirheumatic, immunomodulating, and antimicrobial (*in vitro*) effects. The exact mechanisms for these actions are not well understood. Gold is taken up by macrophages where it inhibits phagocytosis and may inhibit lysosomal enzyme activity. Gold also inhibits the release of histamine, and production of prostaglandins. While gold does have antimicrobial effects *in vitro*, it is not clinically useful for this purpose.

Pharmacokinetics

After IM injection, aurothioglucose is quite rapidly absorbed and peak serum concentrations are reached in 4-6 hours. It is distributed to several tissues (liver, kidney, spleen, bone marrow, adrenals, and lymph nodes), but highest levels are found in the synovium. In plasma, 95% is bound to plasma proteins. Gold salts may be found in the epithelial cells in the renal tubules years after dosing has ended. Plasma half-lives increase in length after multiple doses have been given. These values have ranged from 21-168 hours in humans. Approximately 70% of a dose is excreted by the kidneys, while the remaining 30% is excreted in the feces.

There appears to be no correlation with serum levels and efficacy. It usually takes from 6-12 weeks for a beneficial effect to be noted after beginning therapy.

Contraindications/Precautions/Warnings

Contraindications for chrysotherapy (gold therapy) include patients with renal or hepatic disease, SLE (lupus erythematosus, diabetes mellitus (uncontrolled), severe debilitation, and preexisting hematologic disorders.

Do not administer these compounds intravenously.

Adverse Effects

Veterinary experience with these agents is limited. Pain at the injection site is common and some animals may develop thrombocytopenia with petechia and ecchymoses. One author (Kummel 1995), reports that four pemphigus canine cases treated with aurothioglucose given immediately after cessation of azathioprine, developed a fatal toxic epidermal necrolysis. Other adverse effects noted in cats or dogs include stomatitis, hepatic necrosis or renal dysfunction.

Adverse reactions seen in people include: mucocutaneous reactions, which are fairly common (15-20%) and are characterized by rashes, (with or preceded by pruritus), and mucosal lesions (usually seen as a stomatitis). Hematologic reactions (thrombocytopenia, leukopenia, aplastic anemias), although rare in humans, can be life threatening. Renal effects are generally mild and if noted early, reversible with cessation of therapy. Proteinuria is an early sign associated with the proximal tubule damage that gold can cause. Reversible pulmonary infiltrates have been noted, but are reversible when therapy is discontinued. Enterocolitis, which may be fatal, has been reported in rare instances.

Because of the serious nature of these adverse reactions, adequate patient monitoring is essential.

Reproductive/Nursing Safety

The safety of aurothioglucose or gold sodium thiomalate has not been established during pregnancy, and these drugs should only be used when the potential benefits outweigh the risks involved. In humans, the FDA categorizes them as category *C* for use during pregnancy (*Animal studies have shown an adverse effect on the fetus, but there are no adequate studies in humans; or there are no animal reproduction studies and no adequate studies in humans.*)

Injectable gold is excreted in milk. Trace amounts appear in the serum and red blood cells of nursing offspring. As this may cause adverse effects in nursing offspring, switching to milk replacer is recommended if gold therapy is to be continued in the dam. Because gold is slowly excreted, persistence in milk will occur even after the drug is discontinued.

Overdosage/Acute Toxicity

Overdosages resulting from a too rapid increase in dosage are exhibited by rapid development of toxic signs, primarily renal (hematuria, proteinuria) and hematologic (thrombocytopenia, granulocytopenia) effects. Other clinical signs include: nausea, vomiting, diarrhea, skin lesions, and fever.

Treat with dimercaprol (BAL) to chelate the gold and treat the hematologic and renal effects supportively.

Drug Interactions

The following drug interactions have either been reported or are theoretical in humans or animals receiving injectable gold compounds and may be of significance in veterinary patients:

- **CYTOTOXIC AGENTS** (including high dose corticosteroids): Auranofin's safety when used with these agents has not been established; use with caution

- **PENICILLAMINE or ANTIMALARIAL DRUGS:** Use with gold salts is not recommended due to the increased potential for hematologic or renal toxicity

Doses

Note: Dosages below are for the product aurothioglucose, unless otherwise noted; however, dosing for both drugs appear to be equivalent.

■ **DOGS:**

For canine pemphigus foliaceus/vulgaris:

a) Gold sodium thiomalate: 1–5 mg IM as a test dose then 1 mg/kg IM once weekly. Need to use initially with corticosteroids as gold therapy may take 6–8 weeks to take effect. Side effects include skin lesions, thrombocytopenia and toxic epidermal necrolysis. (Logas 2005)

b) Gold sodium thiomalate: 1–5 mg (1 mg for small patients; 5 mg for large patients) IM as a test dose then 1 mg/kg IM once weekly until remission, then taper to monthly. (Morris 2004)

c) For those cases where corticosteroids and/or azathioprine are ineffective or causing unacceptable adverse effects: Discontinue azathioprine for one month and then give 1 mg/5 kg of body weight IM weekly for 10 weeks and then monthly thereafter. **Note:** Before treating, the reader is advised to refer to the full reference for additional information. (Kummel 1995)

d) 1 mg/kg IM (the paraspinal muscles work best) weekly for 6–12 weeks; then decrease to every other week and if possible, once monthly. Rarely, may be able to discontinue injections if free from clinical signs for 6 months after switching to once monthly injections. Corticosteroids must usually be used with gold therapy. (White 2000)

■ **CATS:**

a) For pemphigus complex or plasmacytic/pododermatitis: Gold sodium thiomalate: 1–5 mg IM as a test dose then 1 mg/kg IM once weekly. Need to use initially with glucocorticoids as gold therapy may take 6–8 weeks to take effect. Side effects include skin lesions, thrombocytopenia and toxic epidermal necrolysis. (Logas 2005)

b) For pemphigus complex (rescue drug) or plasmacytic/pododermatitis: Gold sodium thiomalate: 1–5 mg (1 mg for small patients; 5 mg for large patients) IM as a test dose then 1 mg/kg IM once weekly until remission, then taper to monthly. (Morris 2004)

c) 1 mg/kg IM per week. Clinical response may take 6–8 weeks and combination with glucocorticoids is recommended. May be associated with renal dysfunction, drug eruptions, hepatic necrosis and thrombocytopenia. (Shaw 2003)

d) For idiopathic pruritus when nothing else works: 1 mg/kg IM every 7 days until remission (8–20 weeks), then 1 mg/kg IM every 4 weeks (Hnilica 2003)

■ **HORSES:**

a) Give 20 mg IM and then 40 mg IM one week apart. If no adverse effects (stomatitis, urticaria, sloughing, blood dyscrasias), give 1 mg/kg IM weekly until observing a response (6–12 weeks). Tailor maintenance therapy to the individual, which may involve biweekly or monthly therapy. Treatment can be very expensive. Perform weekly CBC/urinalysis for the first month, then monthly if no abnormalities. (Rees 2004)

Monitoring

■ Urinalysis—baseline, then weekly

■ CBC–baseline, then every 2 weeks; **Note:** eosinophilia may denote impending reactions

■ Renal and hepatic function tests; baseline and periodic. After the patient is on maintenance therapy, hemograms and urinalyses may be done every month or two.

Client Information

■ Clients should be instructed to notify the veterinarian if pruritus, rash, or diarrhea develops, or if the animal becomes ill or depressed

Chemistry/Synonyms

Gold sodium thiomalate occurs as an odorless, or practically odorless, yellow powder containing approximately 50% gold. It is very soluble in water. The injection is a light yellow to yellow solution with a pH of 5.8–6.5 and contains benzyl alcohol as a preservative.

Gold sodium thiomalate may also be known as aurothiomalate, *Aurolate®*, and *Myochrisine®*.

Storage/Stability

Protect these products from light and store between 15–30° C; avoid freezing. A five-year expiration date is assigned after manufacture. Do not mix with any other compound when injecting.

Dosage Forms/Regulatory Status

VETERINARY-LABELED PRODUCTS: None

HUMAN-LABELED PRODUCTS:

Gold Sodium Thiomalate Injection: 50 mg/mL in 2 mL &10 mL vials, and 2 mL & 1 mL fill in 2 mL single-dose vials & 10 mL multiple-dose vials; *Aurolate®* (Pasadena); *Myochrisine®* (Taylor); generic; (Rx)

References

Hnilica, K. (2003). Managing Feline Pruritus. Proceedings: Western Veterinary Conference. Accessed via: Veterinary Information Network. http://goo.gl/U19xu

Kummel, B. (1995). Medical treatment of canine pemphigus-pemphigoid. *Kirk's Current Veterinary Therapy:XII.* J Bonagura Ed. Philadelphia, W.B. Saunders: 636–638.

Logas, D. (2005). Overview of immunosuppressive drugs. Proceedings: Western Veterinary Conf. Accessed via: Veterinary Information Network. http://goo.gl/HUfaF

Morris, D. (2004). Immunomodulatory drugs in veterinary dermatology. Proceedings: Western Veterinary Conf 2004. Accessed via: Veterinary Information Network. http://goo.gl/PiK89

Rees, C. (2004). Disorders of the skin. *Equine Internal Medicine 2nd Ed.* S Reed, W Bayly and D Sellon Eds. Philadelphia, Saunders: 667–720.

Shaw, S. (2003). Immune-mediated skin diseases in cats. Proceedings: World Small Animal Veterinary Association World Congress. Accessed via: Veterinary Information Network. http://goo.gl/l7O6r

White, S. (2000). Nonsteroidal Immunosuppressive Therapy. *Kirk's Current Veterinary Therapy: XIII Small Animal Practice.* J Bonagura Ed. Philadelphia, WB Saunders: 536–538.

GONADORELIN

(goe-*nad*-oe-rell-in)

Cystorelin®, Fertagyl®, Factrel®

HORMONAL AGENT

Prescriber Highlights

▶ Hypothalamic hormone used to treat ovarian cysts & other reproductive disorders in a variety of species

▶ Duration of action is very short (minutes)

▶ Contraindications & adverse effects: None reported

▶ No slaughter or milk withdrawal when used as labeled

Uses/Indications

Gonadorelin is indicated (FDA-approved) for the treatment of ovarian follicular cysts in dairy cattle. Additionally, gonadorelin has been used in cattle to reduce the time interval from calving to first ovulation and to increase the number of ovulations within the first 3 months after calving. This may be particularly important in increasing fertility in cows with retained placenta.

In dogs, gonadorelin has been used experimentally to help diagnose reproductive disorders or to identify intact animals versus castrated ones by maximally stimulating FSH and LH production. It has also been used experimentally in dogs to induce estrus through pulsatile dosing. While apparently effective, specialized administration equipment is required for this method.

Gonadorelin has been used in cats as an alternate therapy to FSH or hCG to induce estrus in cats with prolonged anestrus.

In Europe, a synthetic analogue buserelin has been used in horses to stimulate cyclic estrus. Its efficacy rates poorly when compared to an artificial light program, however.

In human medicine, gonadorelin has been used for the diagnosis of hypothalamic-pituitary dysfunction, cryptorchidism, and depression secondary to prolonged severe stress.

Pharmacology/Actions

Gonadorelin is a synthetic form of GnRH and stimulates the production and the release of FSH and LH from the anterior pituitary. Secretion of endogenous GnRH from the hypothalamus is thought to be controlled by several factors, including circulating sex hormones.

Gonadorelin causes a surge-like release of FSH and LH after a single injection. In cows and ewes, this can induce ovulation, but not in estrus mares. A constant infusion of gonadorelin will initially stimulate LH and FSH release, but after a period of time, levels will return to baseline.

Pharmacokinetics

After intravenous injection in pigs, gonadorelin is rapidly distributed to extracellular fluid, with a distribution half-life of about 2 minutes. The elimination half-life of gonadorelin is approximately 13 minutes in the pig.

After intravenous injection in humans, gonadorelin reportedly has a plasma half-life of only a few minutes. Within one hour, approximately half the dose is excreted in the urine as metabolites.

Contraindications/Precautions/Warnings

None are noted on the label.

Adverse Effects

No reported adverse reactions were located for this agent. Synthetically prepared gonadorelin should not cause any hypersensitivity reactions. This may not be the case with pituitary-obtained LH preparations or hCG.

Reproductive/Nursing Safety

In humans, the FDA categorizes this drug as category *B* for use during pregnancy (*Animal studies have not yet demonstrated risk to the fetus, but there are no adequate studies in pregnant women; or animal studies have shown an adverse effect, but adequate studies in pregnant women have not demonstrated a risk to the fetus in the first trimester of pregnancy, and there is no evidence of risk in later trimesters.*)

No specific lactation safety information was listed for this drug.

Overdosage/Acute Toxicity

In doses of up to 120 micrograms/kg, no untoward effects were noted in several species of test animals. Gonadorelin is unlikely to cause significant adverse effects after inadvertent overdosage.

Drug Interactions

■ None noted

Doses

■ DOGS:

a) GnRH stimulation test to differentiate castration from cryptorchidism: Take pre-sample, give 50 micrograms gonadorelin (GnRH) IM, 2–3 hours later take post-injection sample. Castrated dogs have testosterone concentrations <0.1 ng/mL and GnRH does not stimulate. (Pinto 2007)

b) GnRH stimulation test to determine if dog has retained testicle: Take pre-sample, give gonadorelin 2.5 micrograms IM (if very small dog use 25 micrograms total dose instead) and take second sample in 60-90 minutes. (Freshman 2009)

c) To aid in the descent of cryptorchid testes: 50–100 micrograms SC or IV; if no response give additional dose in 4–6 days (Cox 1986)

d) To increase libido in male dogs: Anecdotally, 50–100 micrograms IM weekly for 4 to 6 weeks may improve libido. (Freshman 2002)

e) For cystic ovarian disease in bitches: 3.3 micrograms/kg IM once daily for 3 days. An elevated progesterone level (>2 ng/mL) measured 1–2 weeks post treatment verifies success. (Purswell 1999)

■ **CATS:**

a) To stimulate ovulation after mating: 25 micrograms IM after mating (Morgan 1988)

b) For infertility, reduced libido, testis descent in male cats: 1 microgram/kg every 2–3 days (Verstegen 2000)

c) To detect ovarian remnants in queens after ovariohysterectomy: 25 micrograms per cat. A progesterone level (>1 ng/mL) measured 1–2 weeks post treatment verifies presence of ovarian tissue in the abdomen. (Purswell 1999)

■ **FERRETS:**

a) 20 micrograms IM; repeat in one week as necessary. Most effective 14 days after onset of estrus (Williams 2000)

■ **CATTLE:**

To treat of ovarian cysts in cattle:

a) 100 micrograms IM or IV (Package Insert; *Cystorelin®*—Ceva)

b) 100 micrograms IM per cow (Package insert; *Factrel®*—Fort Dodge)

■ **SHEEP & GOATS:**

a) To induce ovulation outside of the breeding season in the doe: 100 micrograms injected daily for 4–5 days (Smith 1986)

Chemistry/Synonyms

A hormone produced by the hypothalamus, gonadorelin is obtained from natural sources or is synthetically produced. It is a decapeptide that occurs as white or faintly yellowish-white powder. One gram is soluble in 25 mL of water or in 50 mL of methyl alcohol. 50 micrograms of gonadorelin acetate is approximately equivalent to 31 Units. The commercially available products in the United States are the diacetate decahydrate (*Cystorelin®*, others) and HCl (*Factrel®*) salts.

Gonadorelin may also be known as: follicle stimulating hormone-releasing factor, GnRH, gonadoliberin, gonadorelinum, gonadotropin-releasing hormone, Hoe-471, LH/FSH-RF, LH/FSH-RH, LH-RF, LH-RH, luliberin, luteinising hormone-releasing factor, *Cryptocur®, Cystorelin®, Factrel®, Fertagyl®, Fertiral®, HRF®, Kryptocur®, LRH®, Luforan®, Luteoliberina®, Lutrefact®, Ovacyst®, Parlib®, Pulsil®, Relefact LH-RH®*, and *Stimu-LH®*.

Storage/Stability

The manufacturers recommend storing gonadorelin in the refrigerator (2-8°C). There is very little information available on the stability and compatibility of gonadorelin. Because bacterial contamination can inactivate the product, it has been recommended that multi-dose vials be used completely and as rapidly as possible.

Dosage Forms/Regulatory Status

VETERINARY-LABELED PRODUCTS:

Gonadorelin (diacetate tetrahydrate) for Injection: 50 micrograms/mL, 2 mL single-use or 10 mL multi-dose vials; *Cystorelin®* (Merial); *Fertagyl®* (Intervet); *Fertalin®, Ovacyst®*, (Teva); (Rx). FDA-approved for use in dairy cattle. There are no withdrawal times required for either milk or slaughter.

Gonadorelin HCl Solution for Injection: 50 micrograms/mL in 2 mL single-use, and 20 mL multi-dose vials; *Factrel®* (Pfizer); (Rx). FDA-approved for use in cattle. No withdrawal period required.

HUMAN-LABELED PRODUCTS:

Gonadorelin HCl Powder for Injection (lyophilized): 100 micrograms/vial & 500 micrograms/vial (as hydrochloride) with 2 mL sterile diluent; *Factrel®* (Wyeth-Ayerst); (Rx)

References

Cox, V.S. (1986). Cryptorcidism in the dog. *Current Therapy in Theriogenology 2: Diagnosis, Treatment and Prevention of Reproductive Diseases in Small and Large Animals.* DA Morrow Ed. Philadelphia, WB Saunders: 541–544.

Freshman, J. (2002). When Boys Won't Be Boys: Clinical Diagnosis Of Infertility In The Stud Dog. Proceedings: ACVIM. Accessed via: Veterinary Information Network. http://goo.gl/6nSMO

Freshman, J. (2009). "Dosage for gonadotropin releasing hormone stimulation test to determine if dog is cryptorchid." VIN Boards. http://goo.gl/IScA0.

Morgan, R.V., Ed. (1988). *Handbook of Small Animal Practice.* New York, Churchill Livingstone.

Pinto, C. (2007). Cryptorchidism. *Blackwell's Five-Minute Veterinary Consult: Canine & Feline.* L Tilley and F Smith Eds., Blackwell: 318.

Purswell, B. (1999). Pharmaceuticals used in canine theriogenology - Part 1 & 2. Proceedings: Central Veterinary Conference, Kansas City.

Smith, M.C. (1986). Synchronization of estrus and the use of implants and vaginal sponges. *Current Therapy in Theriogenology 2: Diagnosis, Treatment and Prevention of Reproductive Diseases in Small and Large Animals.* DA Morrow Ed. Philadelphia, WB Saunders: 582–583.

Verstegen, J. (2000). Feline Reproduction. *Textbook of Veterinary Internal Medicine: Diseases of the Dog and Cat.* S Ettinger and E Feldman Eds. Philadelphia, WB Saunders. 2: 1585–1598.

Williams, B. (2000). Therapeutics in Ferrets. *Vet Clin NA: Exotic Anim Pract* 3:1(Jan): 131–153.

Gonadotropin, Chorionic—See
Chorionic Gonadotropin

GRANISETRON HCL

(gran-*iss*-eh-tron)   Kytril®

5-HT3 ANTAGONIST ANTIEMETIC

Prescriber Highlights

▶ 5-HT3 receptor antagonist for the treatment of severe vomiting or emesis prophylaxis before chemotherapy

▶ Appears to be safe

▶ Relatively expensive

Uses/Indications

Granisetron is an alternative to other 5-HT3 receptor antagonists (*e.g.*, ondansetron or dolasetron) for the treatment of severe vomiting or prophylaxis before administering antineoplastic drugs such as cisplatin that can cause severe vomiting.

Pharmacology/Actions

Granisetron, like ondansetron or dolasetron, exerts its anti-nausea and antiemetic actions by selectively antagonizing 5-hydroxytryptamine3 (5-HT3; serotonin3) receptors. These receptors are found primarily in the CNS chemoreceptor trigger zone, on vagal nerve terminals and enteric neurons in the GI tract. Chemotherapy associated vomiting in cats is believed primarily due to activation of 5-HT3 receptors in the chemoreceptor trigger zone (CTZ), but in dogs, enteric and vagal receptors may be more important.

Pharmacokinetics

No pharmacokinetic data for dogs or cats was located. In humans, granisetron is rapidly absorbed after oral dosing and peak levels occur in about 2 hours. Oral bioavailability is only 60% due to first-pass metabolism in the liver. The presence of food can decrease AUC by 5%, but increase peak levels by 30%. Granisetron has a volume of distribution of about 3 L/kg and plasma protein binding is approximately 65%. The drug is metabolized in the liver, primarily via demethylation and oxidation and then conjugation. Less than 20% is excreted unchanged in the urine; the remainder is eliminated in the urine and feces as metabolites. Elimination half-life varies considerably, with reported values from about 1–30 hours. Cancer patients appear to have longer elimination half-lives than do healthy adults.

Contraindications/Precautions/Warnings

There are no known contraindications to using this medication in dogs or cats. In humans, granisetron is contraindicated in patients hypersensitive to it and it should not be used to treat vomiting associated with apomorphine (see Drug Interactions).

No dosage adjustments are required in elderly patients or those with impaired renal or hepatic function. Granisetron may mask the signs associated with progressive ileus and/or gastric distention; it should not replace required nasogastric suction.

Adverse Effects

Because of limited use in dogs and cats, a comprehensive adverse effect profile for granisetron is not known, however, it appears to be tolerated well.

In humans, the most common adverse effect reported is headache. Other adverse effects that may occur include abdominal pain, constipation or diarrhea, asthenia, or somnolence. Rarely, hypersensitivity reactions or cardiovascular effects (arrhythmias, chest pain, hypotension) have been reported.

Reproductive/Nursing Safety

Safety in pregnancy is not clearly established, but high dose studies in rodents and rabbits did not demonstrate overt fetal toxicity or teratogenicity. In humans, the FDA categorizes this drug as category *B* for use during pregnancy (*Animal studies have not yet demonstrated risk to the fetus, but there are no adequate studies in pregnant women; or animal studies have shown an adverse effect, but adequate studies in pregnant women have not demonstrated a risk to the fetus in the first trimester of pregnancy, and there is no evidence of risk in later trimesters.*)

It is not known if granisetron enters milk, but it is probably safe to use during nursing.

Overdosage/Acute Toxicity

Limited information is available. An overdose of 38.5 mg in a person caused only a slight headache. Observation and, if required, supportive treatment are suggested.

Drug Interactions

The following drug interactions have either been reported or are theoretical in humans or animals receiving granisetron and may be of significance in veterinary patients:

▪ **APOMORPHINE:** Profound hypotension can occur

▪ **KETOCONAZOLE:** May inhibit the metabolism of granisetron

▪ **PHENOBARBITAL:** Can induce the metabolism of granisetron

Laboratory Considerations

▪ No specific laboratory concerns associated with granisetron

Doses

▪ **DOGS/CATS:**

a) Cats (with pancreatitis): 0.1–0.5 mg/kg PO or IV q12–24h. (Zoran 2006), (Washabau 2006b)

b) Dogs or Cats: 0.1–0.5 mg/kg PO or IV twice daily. (Washabau 2006a)

Monitoring

■ Clinical efficacy

Client Information

■ This drug is usually used on an inpatient basis or during outpatient visits for chemotherapy

■ If used orally on an outpatient basis, have client contact veterinarian for further instructions if vomiting is not controlled or if the dose is vomited up after administrating

Chemistry/Synonyms

Granisetron HCl occurs as a white or almost white powder that is freely soluble in water. Dosages are expressed in terms of the base; 1.12 mg of granisetron HCl is equivalent to 1 mg of granisetron base.

Granisetron may also be known as: granistroni, granisetrono, or BRL-43694A, *Aludal®*, *Eumetic®*, *Granicip®*, *Granitron®*, *Kytril®*, *Kevatril®*, *Rigmoz®* or *Setron®*.

Storage/Stability

The commercially available tablets and oral solution should be stored at room temperature (15–30°C) in tight containers and protected from light. The oral solution should be stored in an upright position. The injectable solution should be stored between 15–30°C; preferably at 25°C. Protect from light and do not freeze solution. Once the multi-dose vial is penetrated, it must be used within 30 days.

Compatibility/Compounding Considerations

The injectable solution is **compatible** with sodium chloride 0.9%, dextrose 5% in sodium chloride 0.45% or 0.9%, and dextrose 5% in water. It is compatible with many drugs at intravenous Y-sites, but is **incompatible** with amphotericin B.

Dosage Forms/Regulatory Status

VETERINARY-LABELED PRODUCTS: None

HUMAN-LABELED PRODUCTS:

Granisetron Oral Tablets: 1 mg (1.12 mg as HCl); *Kytril®* (Roche); (Rx)

Granisetron Oral Solution: 1 mg/5 mL (1.12 mg/5 mL as HCl; orange flavor; contains sorbitol) in 30 mL bottles; *Kytril®* (Roche); *Granisol®* (Hawthorn); (Rx)

Granisetron Injection Solution: 0.1 mg/mL (0.112 mg/mL as HCl) preservative-free, may contain sodium chloride 9 mg in 1 mL single-use vials; 1 mg/mL (1.12 mg/mL as HCl), regular & preservative-free, in 1 mL single-dose & 4 mL multi-dose vials; *Kytril®* (Roche); generic; (Rx)

Granisetron Transdermal Patch: 3.1 mg/24 hours (34.3 mg/52 cm^2); *Sancuso®* (ProStrakan); (Rx)

References

Washabau, R. (2006a). Current anti-emetic therapy. Proceedings WVC 2006, Accessed via the Veterinary Information Network Jan 2007. Accessed via: Veterinary Information Network. http://goo.gl/LYKDB

Washabau, R. (2006b). Feline Exocrine Pancreatic Disease. Proceedings WVC 2006, Accessed via the Veterinary Information Network Jan 2007. Accessed via: Veterinary Information Network. http://goo.gl/LqLIU

Zoran, D. (2006). Pancreatitis in cats: diagnosis and treatment for a complicated disease. Proceedings: ABVP 2006, Accessed via the Veterinary Information Network Jan 2007. Accessed via: Veterinary Information Network. http://goo.gl/wvApB

GRISEOFULVIN (MICROSIZE) GRISEOFULVIN (ULTRAMICROSIZE)

(gri-see-oh-*ful*-vin)   Fulvicin®

ANTIFUNGAL AGENT

Prescriber Highlights

▶ Fungistatic antibiotic used primarily for ringworm & other dermatophytic infections; no effect on other fungi

▶ Contraindications: Pregnancy, known hypersensitivity, or hepatocellular failure

▶ Caution: Kittens may be overly sensitive to the drug; cats with FIV

▶ Adverse Effects: Anorexia, vomiting, diarrhea, anemia, neutropenia, leukopenia, thrombocytopenia, depression, ataxia, hepatotoxicity, or dermatitis/photosensitivity

▶ Known teratogen in cats

▶ Only new hair & nail growth resistant to fungi after treating

▶ Dosing is different for microsize & ultramicrosize forms

▶ Availability becoming an issue

Uses/Indications

In veterinary species, griseofulvin is FDA-approved for use in dogs and cats to treat dermatophytic fungal (see below) infections of the skin, hair and claws, and to treat ringworm (caused by *T. equinum* and *M. gypseum*) in horses. It has also been used in laboratory animals and ruminants for the same indications. The oral tablets FDA-approved for dogs and cats are no longer marketed in the USA, but human dosage forms are available.

Pharmacology/Actions

Griseofulvin acts on susceptible fungi by disrupting the structure of the cell's mitotic spindle, arresting the metaphase of cell division. Griseofulvin has activity against species of *Trichophyton*, *Microsporum* and *Epidermophyton*. Only new hair and nail growth is resistant to infection. It has no antibacterial activity and is not clinically useful against other pathogenic fungi, including Malassezia yeasts.

Pharmacokinetics

The microsized form of the drug is absorbed variably (25–70%); dietary fat will enhance absorption. The ultramicrosize form of the drug may be nearly 100% absorbed. Generally, the ultramicrosize form is absorbed 1.5 times as well as the microsized form for a given patient.

Griseofulvin is concentrated in skin, hair, nails, fat, skeletal muscle, and the liver, and can be found in the stratum corneum within 4 hours of dosing.

Griseofulvin is metabolized by the liver via oxidative demethylation and glucuronidation to 6-desmethylgriseofulvin, which is not active. In humans, the half-life is 9–24 hours. A serum half-life of 47 minutes has been reported for dogs. Less than 1% of the drug is excreted unchanged in the urine.

Contraindications/Precautions/Warnings

Griseofulvin is contraindicated in patients hypersensitive to it or with hepatocellular failure. It should not be used in pregnant animals. It must not be used in horses intended for food.

Because kittens may be overly sensitive to the adverse effects associated with griseofulvin, they should be monitored carefully if treatment is instituted. Cats should be tested for FIV before using griseofulvin because of the possible neutropenic or panleukopenic effects of the drug.

Adverse Effects

Griseofulvin can cause anorexia, vomiting, diarrhea, anemia, neutropenia, leukopenia, thrombocytopenia, depression, ataxia, hepatotoxicity, dermatitis/photosensitivity and toxic epidermal necrolysis. With the exception of GI clinical signs, adverse effects are uncommon at usual doses. Cats, particularly kittens, may be more susceptible to adverse effects (*e.g.*, bone marrow depression) than other species. This could be due to this species' propensity to more slowly form glucuronide conjugates and thus metabolize the drug at a slower rate than either dogs or humans.

Reproductive/Nursing Safety

Griseofulvin is a known teratogen in cats and, probably, in dogs and horses as well. Dosages of 35 mg/kg given to cats during the first trimester caused cleft palate and other skeletal and brain malformations in kittens. Griseofulvin may also inhibit spermatogenesis. Because dermatophytic infections are not generally life-threatening and alternative therapies are available, use of the drug should be considered contraindicated during pregnancy. However, griseofulvin has been used in mares during the later stages of pregnancy without noted ill effect. (Davis 2008).

In humans, the FDA categorizes this drug as category *C* for use during pregnancy (*Animal studies have shown an adverse effect on the fetus, but there are no adequate studies in humans; or there are no animal reproduction studies and no adequate studies in humans.*) In a separate system evaluating the safety of drugs in canine and feline pregnancy (Papich 1989), this drug is categorized as in class: *D* (*Contraindicated. These drugs have been shown to cause congenital malformations or embryotoxicity.*)

No lactation safety information was found.

Overdosage/Acute Toxicity

No specifics regarding griseofulvin overdosage or acute toxicity were located. It is suggested that significant overdoses be handled with gut emptying, charcoal and cathartic administration unless contraindicated. Contact a poison control center for more information.

Horses have received 100 mg/kg PO for 20 days without apparent ill effect.

Drug Interactions

The following drug interactions have either been reported or are theoretical in humans or animals receiving griseofulvin and may be of significance in veterinary patients:

- ◼ **ALCOHOL:** Griseofulvin may potentiate the effects of alcohol

- ◼ **ASPIRIN:** Griseofulvin may decrease salicylate levels

- ◼ **CYCLOSPORINE:** Griseofulvin may decrease cyclosporine levels

- ◼ **PHENOBARBITAL:** Phenobarbital and other barbiturates have been implicated in causing decreased griseofulvin blood concentrations, presumably by inducing hepatic microsomal enzymes and/or reducing absorption. If phenobarbital and griseofulvin are given concurrently, griseofulvin dosage adjustment may be necessary.

- ◼ **THEOPHYLLINE:** In some patients, griseofulvin may decrease theophylline half-life and levels

- ◼ **WARFARIN:** Coumarin anticoagulants may have their anticoagulant activity reduced by griseofulvin; anticoagulant adjustment may be required

Doses

Note: all doses are for microsize preparations unless otherwise indicated.

- ◼ **DOGS:**

   For susceptible dermatophytic infections:

   a) Microsize: 25 mg/kg q12h PO for 42–56 days; Ultramicrosize: 5–10 mg/kg PO once daily for 42 days. May need to treat longer for Trichophyton than for Microsporum. Give following a fatty meal or administration of corn oil. Continue for at least 2 weeks after resolution of signs and at least 5 months for onychomycosis. (Greene *et al.* 2006)

   b) Microsize: 50 mg/kg PO once daily with fatty meal. Used with topical therapy (see references). May double dose in resistant cases. If GI distress occurs may divide dose and give twice daily with food. Prolonged course of therapy required. Begin taking cultures after 4 weeks of treatment. Continue therapy for 2 weeks beyond clinical cure *and* when 2–3 negative cultures are obtained at weekly intervals. (Frank 2000)

■ **CATS:**
For susceptible dermatophytic infections:

a) Microsize: 50–120 mg/kg PO; divided daily. Give with a fatty meal. Ultramicrosize: 10–15 mg/kg PO twice daily. Give for 4–6 weeks or longer, until culture is negative. (Foil 2003)

b) Microsize: 50 mg/kg PO once daily or 25 mg/kg PO q12h for 42–70 days; Ultramicrosize: 5–10 mg/kg PO once daily for 42 days. Give following a fatty meal or administration of corn oil. Continue for at least 2 weeks after resolution of signs and at least 5 months for onychomycosis. (Greene *et al.* 2006)

c) Microsize: 50 mg/kg PO once daily with fatty meal. Used with topical therapy (see references). May double dose in resistant cases. If GI distress occurs may divide dose and give twice daily with food. Prolonged course of therapy required. Begin taking cultures after 4 weeks of treatment. Continue therapy for 2 weeks beyond clinical cure *and* when 2–3 negative cultures are obtained at weekly intervals. (Frank 2000)

d) For feline eosinophilic granuloma complex: Microsize: 25 mg/kg PO twice daily with food. Give at least for one month to judge efficacy. (White 2003)

■ **RABBITS/RODENTS/SMALL MAMMALS:**

a) **Rabbits** for advanced dermatophytosis: Ultramicrosize 6.25 mg/kg PO q12h for 4–6 weeks. Microsize: 25 mg/kg PO q12–24h for one month (Ivey & Morrisey 2000)

b) **Chinchillas:** 25 mg/kg PO once daily for 30–60 days (Hayes 2000)

c) **Gerbils, Guinea pigs, Hamsters, Rats:** 25 mg/kg PO q24h for 14–28 days; **Mice:** 25 mg/kg PO q24h for 14 days; **Chinchillas:** 25 mg/kg PO q24h for 28–40 days (Adamcak & Otten 2000)

d) **Guinea pigs** for dermatophytosis: 25 mg/kg PO (as a suspension) once daily for 28 days. (Johnson 2006b)

e) **Chinchillas:** 25 mg/kg PO once daily (q24h) for 30 days (Johnson 2006a)

■ **CATTLE** (and other ruminants):
For susceptible dermatophytic infections:

a) Ultramicrosize: 10–20 mg/kg PO once daily for 1–2 weeks. 100 mg/kg PO given twice (or more) 1 week apart may also be effective. Not FDA-approved for use in

food animals and can be very expensive. (Pier 1986)

b) 20 mg/kg PO once daily for 6 weeks (Howard 1986)

■ **HORSES:**
For susceptible dermatophytic infections:

a) Using the microsize (not ultra-microsize) products: 5 mg/kg PO once daily. Smaller doses (1.25 grams) should be used for foals or ponies. If using ultra-microsize (human) formulations the dose should be reduced by 50%. (Davis 2008)

■ **SWINE:**
For susceptible dermatophytic infections:

a) 20 mg/kg PO once daily for 6 weeks (Howard 1986)

■ **BIRDS:**
a) **Ratites:** 35–50 mg/kg PO once daily (Jenson 1998)

Monitoring
■ Clinical efficacy; culture
■ Adverse effects
■ CBC; before therapy and q1–3 weeks during therapy
■ Liver enzymes (if indicated)

Client Information
■ Clients should be instructed in procedures used to prevent reinfection (destruction of old bedding, disinfection, periodic re-examinations, hair clipping, etc.), and the importance of compliance with the dosage regimen.
■ Should animal develop adverse effects other than mild GI disturbances, they should contact their veterinarian.

Chemistry/Synonyms
A fungistatic antibiotic produced by species of Penicillium (primarily *P. griseofulvum*), griseofulvin occurs as an odorless or nearly odorless, bitter tasting, white to creamy white powder. It is very slightly soluble in water and sparingly soluble in alcohol.

Two forms of the drug are available commercially. Microsize griseofulvin contains particles with a predominant size of 4 micrometers in diameter, while the ultramicrosize form particle size averages less than 1 micron in diameter.

Griseofulvin may also be known as: curling factor, griseofulvina, and griseofulvinum; many trade names are available.

Storage/Stability
Although griseofulvin is relatively thermostable, products should be stored at less than 40°C, preferably at 15–30°C. Griseofulvin suspension should be stored in tight, light-resistant containers. Microsize tablets and capsules should be stored in tight containers; the ultramicrosize tablets should be stored in well-closed containers.

Dosage Forms/Regulatory Status

VETERINARY-LABELED PRODUCTS:

Griseofulvin (Microsize) Powder: 2.5 g griseofulvin in 15 g sachets; *AmTech® Griseofulvin Powder* (Teva); (Rx). FDA-approved for use in horses not intended for food.

The FDA's "Green Book" still lists several other veterinary FDA-approved griseofulvin products, but it does not appear they are presently being marketed.

HUMAN-LABELED PRODUCTS:

Griseofulvin Microsize Oral Tablets: 500 mg; *Grifulvin V®* (Ortho); (Rx)

Griseofulvin Microsize Oral Suspension: 125 mL/5 mL in 120 mL; generic; (Rx)

Griseofulvin Ultramicrosize Tablets: 125 mg & 250 mg; *Gris-PEG®* (Pedinol); (Rx)

References

Adamcak, A. & B. Otten (2000). Rodent Therapeutics. *Vet Clin NA: Exotic Anim Pract* 3:1(Jan): 221-240.

Davis, J. (2008). The use of antifungals. *Comp Equine*(April): 128-133.

Foil, C. (2003). Ringworm update. Proceedings: Western Veterinary Conf. Accessed via: Veterinary Information Network. http://goo.gl/O9j3A

Frank, L. (2000). Dermatophytosis. *Kirk's Current Veterinary Therapy: XIII Small Animal Practice.* J Bonagura Ed. Philadelphia, WB Saunders: 577-580.

Greene, C., K. Hartmannn, et al. (2006). Appendix 8: Antimicrobial Drug Formulary. *Infectious Disease of the Dog and Cat.* C Greene Ed., Elsevier: 1186-1333.

Hayes, P. (2000). Diseases of Chinchillas. *Kirk's Current Veterinary Therapy: XIII Small Animal Practice.* J Bonagura Ed. Philadelphia, WB Saunders: 1152-1157.

Howard, J.L., Ed. (1986). *Current Veterinary Therapy 2, Food Animal Practice.* Philadelphia, W.B. Saunders.

Ivey, E. & J. Morrisey (2000). Therapeutics for Rabbits. *Vet Clin NA: Exotic Anim Pract* 3:1(Jan): 183-216.

Jenson, J. (1998). Current ratite therapy. *The Veterinary Clinics of North America: Food Animal Practice* 16:3(November).

Johnson, D. (2006a). Chinchilla Care. Proceedings: ACVC. Accessed via: Veterinary Information Network. http://goo.gl/ikSGV

Johnson, D. (2006b). Guinea Pig Medicine Primer. Proceedings: ACVC. Accessed via: Veterinary Information Network. http://goo.gl/WmWhU

Pier, A.C. (1986). Dermatophytosis. *Current Veterinary Therapy: Food Animal Practice 2.* JL Howard Ed. Philadelphia, W.B. Saunders: 924-927.

White, S. (2003). Eosinophilic granuloma complex in cats and dogs. Proceedings: World Animal Veterinary Assoc. World Congress. Accessed via: Veterinary Information Network. http://goo.gl/VVE6L

GUAIFENESIN

(gwye-*fen*-e-sin) GG, Guailaxin®

PARENTERAL MUSCLE RELAXANT/ORAL EXPECTORANT

Prescriber Highlights

▶ An expectant (oral) & muscle relaxant (parenteral) adjunctive to anesthesia

▶ Contraindications: None noted except concurrent use with physostigmine

▶ Adverse Effects: Mild hypotensive effect & increase in cardiac rate, thrombophlebitis possible

▶ Availability an issue for the injection

Uses/Indications

In veterinary medicine, guaifenesin is used to induce muscle relaxation and restraint as an adjunct to anesthesia for short procedures (30–60 minutes) in large and small animal species. There are combination oral products containing guaifenesin for treating respiratory conditions in horses.

In human medicine, guaifenesin has long been touted as an oral expectorant, but definitive proof of its efficacy is lacking.

Pharmacology/Actions

While the exact mechanism of action for the muscle relaxant effect is not known, it is believed that guaifenesin acts centrally by depressing or blocking nerve impulse transmission at the internuncial neuron level of the subcortical areas of the brain, brainstem and spinal cord. It relaxes both the laryngeal and pharyngeal muscles, thus allowing easier intubation. Guaifenesin also has mild intrinsic analgesic and sedative qualities.

Guaifenesin causes an excitement-free induction and recovery from anesthesia in horses. It produces relaxation of skeletal muscles but does not affect diaphragmatic function and has little, if any, effect on respiratory function at usual doses. Possible effects on the cardiovascular system include transient mild decreases in blood pressure and increases in cardiac rate. Gastrointestinal motility may be increased, but generally no adversity is seen with this.

Guaifenesin potentiates the activity of preanesthetic and anesthetic agents.

Pharmacokinetics

The pharmacokinetics of guaifenesin have not been thoroughly studied in most species. When administered alone to horses IV, recumbency usually occurs within 2 minutes and light (not surgical level) restraint persists for about 6 minutes. Muscle relaxation reportedly persists for 10–20 minutes after a single dose.

Guaifenesin is conjugated in the liver and excreted into the urine. A gender difference in the elimination half-life of guaifenesin in ponies has been demonstrated, with males having a $t_{1/2}$ of approximately 85 minutes, and females a $t_{1/2}$ of about 60 minutes. Guaifenesin reportedly crosses the placenta, but adverse effects in newborns of mothers who received guaifenesin have not been described.

Contraindications/Precautions/Warnings

The manufacturer states that the use of physostigmine is contraindicated with guaifenesin (see Drug Interactions).

Avoid giving ruminants concentrations of guaifenesin greater than 5% as hemolysis can occur.

Adverse Effects

At usual doses, side effects are transient and generally minor. A mild decrease in blood pressure and increase in cardiac rate can be seen. Thrombophlebitis has been reported after IV injection, and perivascular administration may cause some tissue reaction. Hemolysis may occur in solutions containing greater than a 5% concentration of guaifenesin, but some sources state this is insignificant at even a 15% concentration. Hemolysis may be more of an issue in ruminants then in horses.

Reproductive/Nursing Safety

In humans, the FDA categorizes this drug as category *C* for use during pregnancy *(Animal studies have shown an adverse effect on the fetus, but there are no adequate studies in humans; or there are no animal reproduction studies and no adequate studies in humans.)*

It is not known whether guaifenesin is excreted in milk.

Overdosage/Acute Toxicity

The margin of safety is reportedly 3 times the usual dose. Clinical signs of apneustic breathing, nystagmus, hypotension, and contradictory muscle rigidity are associated with toxic levels of the drug.

There were 64 exposures to guaifenesin reported to the ASPCA Animal Poison Control Center (APCC) during 2005-2009. In these cases 64 were dogs with only 5 showing clinical signs and 6 cases were cats with only 3 showing clinical signs. The dog received a dosage estimated between 415 and 830 mg/kg and exhibited hypothermia, mild tremors, ataxia and vomiting. The cat received a dosage of 132 mg/kg and exhibited lethargy and anorexia.

No specific antidote is available. It is suggested that treatment be supportive until the drug is cleared to sub-toxic levels.

Drug Interactions

Drug interactions with guaifenesin are not well studied. The following drug interactions have either been reported or are theoretical in animals receiving guaifenesin and may be of significance in veterinary patients:

▪ **PHYSOSTIGMINE:** The manufacturer (Robins) states that physostigmine is contraindicated in horses receiving guaifenesin, but does not elucidate on the actual interaction. It may be logical to assume that other anticholinesterase agents (**neostigmine, pyridostigmine, edrophonium**) may also be contraindicated.

Doses

▪ **DOGS:**
a) 110 mg/kg IV for muscle relaxation during certain toxicoses (e.g., strychnine) or tetanus (Morgan 1988)

b) For chemical restraint for ventilatory support: Combination of guaifenesin 50 mg/mL, ketamine 1 mg/mL, and xylazine 0.25 mg/mL; give 0.55 mL bolus initially followed by 2.2 mL/kg/hr thereafter (Pascoe 1986)

▪ **CATTLE:**
a) 55–110 mg/kg IV (Mandsager 1988)

▪ **HORSES:** (**Note:** ARCI UCGFS Class 4 Drug)
a) 110 mg/kg IV, give first ⅓–½ of dose until horse falls gently, then give remainder unless respiratory or cardiovascular effects are observed (Package Insert; *Guailaxin®*—Robins)

b) To provide muscle relaxation in balanced anesthesia:

A CRI of ketamine at 0.8–2.3 mg/kg/hr with guaifenesin at 18–60 mg/kg/hr may reduce MAC requirements by 50%.

A CRI of ketamine 1 mg/kg/hr with medetomidine at 0.00125 mg/kg/hr and guaifenesin at 25 mg/kg/hr may reduce MAC requirements by 50%. (Driessen 2008)

c) In field anesthesia:
To augment muscle relaxation in horses that are too light or too tense after alpha-2 agonist + ketamine ± diazepam induction, and do not respond sufficiently to additional increments of alpha-2 agonist or ketamine: Approximately 25–50 mg/kg (250–500 mL of a 5% solution) IV.

For long-term IV (>30 minutes) anesthesia using "GKX" or "triple-drip": Guaifenesin (50 mg/mL), ketamine (1–2 mg/mL; 2 mg/mL concentration used for more painful or noxious procedures), and xylazine (0.5 mg/mL). Most practitioners prefer to induce with xylazine/ketamine or xylazine/diazepam/ketamine and then use GKX for maintenance. Typically the CRI runs at 1.5–2.2 mL /kg/hr depending on the procedure, patient response and ketamine concentration.

An alternative to "GKX" is "GKD" where detomidine is substituted for the xylazine and the concentrations of guaifenesin and ketamine are increased. Guaifenesin (100 mg/mL), ketamine (4 mg/mL), and detomidine (0.04 mg/mL). The CRI runs at 0.8 mL/kg/hr for the first hour and 0.6 mL/kg/hour for the final 30 minutes.

(Wagner 2009b)

d) For equine intravenous anesthesia:

For normal healthy patients: Administer xylazine (0.44–0.66 mg/kg IV, or 200–300 mg/450 kg horse). *Wait* for sedation and muscle relaxation to occur (approximately 5 minutes). Guaifenesin (5% solution, or 50 mg/mL) is then rapidly infused using pressurization until marked sedation and muscle relaxation is achieved (generally a total dose of 30–50 mg/kg). Ketamine (2.2 mg/kg IV, 1000 mg/450 kg) should be administered at a point that allows for its slow onset to occur without the patient becoming excessively weak and collapsing from effects of guaifenesin. Recumbency generally occurs approximately 60 seconds following ketamine administration. The slow administration of guaifenesin described below can also be used in normal healthy patients in place of a supplemental dose of xylazine when the level of initial sedation is inadequate.

For compromised patients: Try to use a very modest dose of xylazine (0.22–0.44 mg/kg IV, or 100–200 mg/450 kg horse) depending on status and demeanor to minimize its cardiovascular effects in compromised patients. Slow administration of guaifenesin (5% solution) can be used to gradually create the desired level of sedation. It is still important to allow adequate time for centralization of cardiac output to progress sufficiently prior to initiating the rapid phase of guaifenesin administration that precedes the induction bolus. Guaifenesin has a slow onset of action, when used to augment the level of pre-induction sedation. SLOW administration is important to avoid creating an overly weak and ataxic patient while waiting for centralization to progress sufficiently. Guaifenesin is then rapidly infused using pressurization until marked sedation and muscle relaxation is achieved (generally a total dose of 30–50 mg/kg IV). Ketamine (dose decreases as degree of compromise increases, 1.34–1.55 mg/kg IV, or 600–700 mg/450 kg) for extremely compromised patients should be administered at a point that allows for its slow onset to occur without the patient becoming excessively weak and collapsing

from the growing effects of guaifenesin. Experience may be required to get the timing right. Recumbency takes even longer (up to a couple minutes) when ketamine dose is reduced in compromised patients. (Abrahamsen 2007)

e) For adjunctive symptomatic treatment of strychnine poisoning: 110 mg/kg IV; repeated as necessary (Schmitz 2004)

■ **SHEEP, GOATS:**

a) Using "GKX" for induction/maintenance: Mix 1000 mL of 5% (50 mg/mL) guaifenesin with 1000 mg of ketamine ± 0–100 mg of xylazine. Induce with 2.2 mL/kg IV (calculate dose; do NOT overdose!). Maintain with approximately 2.2 mL/kg/hr IV (calculate drip rate, adjust as needed). (Wagner 2009a)

b) Using "GKX": To a 500 mL bag of 5% guaifenesin, add 50 mg of xylazine and 500 mg ketamine. Administer at a rate of 2–4 mL/kg IV. Given rapidly until animal is recumbent and then slowed to maintain desired anesthesia plane. Monitor drip to prevent overdosing. (Rings 2005)

■ **CAMELIDS:**

a) Using "GKX" for induction/maintenance: Mix 1000 mL of 5% (50 mg/mL) guaifenesin with 1000 mg of ketamine ± 200 mg of xylazine. Induce with 2.2 mL/kg IV (calculate dose; do NOT overdose!). Maintain with approximately 2.2 mL/kg/hr IV (calculate drip rate, adjust as needed). (Wagner 2009a)

Monitoring

■ Level of muscle relaxation
■ Cardiac and respiratory rate

Chemistry/Synonyms

Formerly known as glyceryl guaiacolate, guaifenesin occurs as a white to slightly gray, crystalline powder that may have a characteristic odor. It is nonhygroscopic and melts between 78°–82°C. One g is soluble in 15 mL of water and soluble in alcohol, propylene glycol and glycerin.

Guaifenesin may also be known as: GG, glyceryl guaiacolate, glycerylguayacolum, guaiacol glycerol ether, guaiacyl glyceryl ether, guaifenesina, guaifenesinum, guaiphenesin, and guajacolum glycerolatum; many trade names are available.

Storage/Stability

Guaifenesin is stable in light and heat (less than melting point). It should be stored in well-closed containers.

When dissolved into aqueous solutions, guaifenesin may slightly precipitate out of solution when the temperature is less than 22°C (72°F). Slight warming and agitation generally resolubilizes the drug. A microwave oven has been suggested for heating and dissolving the drug. It is recommended that the solution be prepared freshly before use, but a 10% solution (in sterile water) may apparently be stored safely at room temperature for up to one week with only slight precipitation occurring.

Compatibility/Compounding Considerations
Guaifenesin is physically **compatible** with sterile water or D₅W. It is also reportedly **compatible** with ketamine, pentobarbital, thiamylal, thiopental, and xylazine.

As there are apparently no commercially available injections being marketed in the USA, compounding an injection product from a USP grade powder is the only way to obtain a parenteral dosage form. Compounding pharmacies may be able to prepare a sterile product. The commercially available products contained per mL: Guaifenesin 50 mg, Dextrose (anhydrous) 50 mg, Propylene Glycol 20 mg, Dimethyl acetamide 50 mg, Edetate Disodium 0.75 mg, Water for Injection q.s. For stability, it is highly recommended that the compounding pharmacy use this formula.

Dosage Forms/Regulatory Status

VETERINARY-LABELED PRODUCTS:
Guaifenesin Injection 50 mg/mL in 500 mL & 1000 mL. There are several GG 5% injection products still listed as FDA-approved in the FDA's Green Book, but it is believed that there are no products presently being marketed commercially

There are several oral products containing guaifenesin in combination with an antihistamine (pyrilamine) labeled for use in horses, including *Anhist®* (AHC), & *Hist-EQ® Powder* (Butler); (OTC)

There are oral products containing guaifenesin and other expectorants (potassium iodide, ammonium chloride) labeled for use in horses, cattle, and sheep, including *Spect-Aid®* (AHC), and *Spec-Tuss®* (Neogen); (OTC)

There may be veterinary oral cough syrups or tablets containing guaifenesin available labeled for use in small animals.

The ARCI (Racing Commissioners International) has designated this drug as a class 4 substance. See the appendix for more information.

HUMAN-LABELED PRODUCTS:
Guaifenesin Oral Tablets: 200 mg & 400 mg; 600 mg & 1200 mg (extended-release); *Organidin NR®* (Medpointe); *Liquibid®* (Capellon); generic; (Rx); *Mucinex®* (Reckitt Benkhiser); *Humibid® Maximum Strength* (Adams); generic; (OTC)

Guaifenesin Oral Granules: 50 mg/packet & 100 mg/packet; *Mucinex® Mini-Melts for Kids* (Reckitt Benkhiser); (OTC)

Guaifenesin Syrup/Liquid: 100 mg/5mL in 118 mL, 237 mL & 473 mL; 200 mg/5 mL in 120 mL; *Buckley's Chest Congestion Mixture®* (Novartis); *Mucinex for Kids®* (Reckitt Benk-

hiser); *Diabetic Tussin®* (Health Care Products); *Robitussin®* (Wyeth); *Siltussin DAS®* & *SA®* (Silarx); *Scot-Tussin Expectorant®* (Scot-Tussin); *Naldecon Senior EX®* (Sandoz); generic; (OTC); *Ganidin NR®* (Cypress); *Guaifenesin NR®* (Silarx); (Rx)

No parenteral preparations are FDA-approved. There are many OTC oral expectorant/cough preparations on the market.

References

Abrahamsen, E. (2007). Analgesia in equine practice. Proceedings: Western Vet Conference. Accessed via: Veterinary Information Network. http://goo.gl/PpibC

Driessen, B. (2008). Balanced Anesthesia in the Equine: Techniques That Work in Practice. Proceedings: IVECCS. Accessed via: Veterinary Information Network. http://goo.gl/9ykAr

Mandsager, R.E. (1988, Last Update). "Personal Communication."

Morgan, R.V., Ed. (1988). *Handbook of Small Animal Practice.* New York, Churchill Livingstone.

Pascoe, P.J. (1986). Short-term ventilatory support. *Current Veterinary Therapy IX: Small Animal Practice.* RV Kirk Ed. Philadelphia, WB Saunders: 269–277.

Rings, D. (2005). Anesthesia and Surgical Procedures for Small Ruminants I & II. *Proceedings: WVC.*

Schmitz, D. (2004). Toxicologic problems. *Equine Internal Medicine 2nd Ed.* S Reed, W Bayly and D Sellon Eds. Philadelphia, Saunders: 1441–1512.

Wagner, A.E. (2009a). Anaesthesia for Small Ruminants and Camelids. Proceedings: AVA. Accessed via: Veterinary Information Network. http://goo.gl/XH3dN

Wagner, A.E. (2009b). Injectable Field Anaesthesia in the Horse. Proceedings: AVA. Accessed via: Veterinary Information Network. http://goo.gl/iAYqq

HALOTHANE

(ha-loe-thane)   Fluothane®

GENERAL ANESTHETIC

Prescriber Highlights

▶ Classic inhalant general anesthetic; no longer available in many countries

▶ Contraindications: History or predilection towards malignant hyperthermia; significant hepatotoxicity after previous exposure

▶ Caution in patients with hepatic function impairment, cardiac arrhythmias, increased CSF or head injury, myasthenia gravis, or pheochromocytoma

▶ Adverse Effects: Dose related hypotension, malignant hyperthermia-stress syndrome, cardiac depression & dysrhythmias, hepatotoxicity

▶ May be teratogenic; use with caution in pregnancy

▶ Drug interactions

Uses/Indications

Halothane in the past was a mainstay general anesthetic in veterinary medicine due to its relative safety, potency, controllability, non-flammability, and comparatively low cost. However, it is no longer available commercially in many countries as it has been replaced by agents that have less cardiodepressant effects such as isoflurane, desflurane and sevoflurane.

Pharmacology/Actions
While the precise mechanism that inhalant anesthetics exert their general anesthetic effect is not precisely known, they may interfere with functioning of nerve cells in the brain by acting at the lipid matrix of the membrane. Some key pharmacologic effects noted with halothane include: CNS depression, depression of body temperature regulating centers, increased cerebral blood flow, respiratory depression (pronounced in ruminants), hypotension, vasodilatation, and myocardial depression.

Minimal Alveolar Concentration (MAC; %) in oxygen reported for halothane in various species: Dog = 0.76; Cat = 0.82; Horse = 0.88; Human = 0.76. Several factors may alter MAC (acid/base status, temperature, other CNS depressants on board, age, ongoing acute disease, etc.).

Pharmacokinetics
Halothane is rapidly absorbed through the lungs. About 12% of absorbed drug is metabolized by the liver to trifluoroacetic acid (only small amounts), chlorine, and bromine radicals that are excreted in the urine. The bulk of the absorbed drug is re-excreted by the lungs and eliminated with expired air. Halothane is distributed into milk.

Contraindications/Precautions/Warnings
Halothane is contraindicated in patients with a history or predilection towards malignant hyperthermia or significant hepatotoxicity after previous halothane exposure (see Adverse Effects below). It should be used with caution (benefits vs. risks) in patients with hepatic function impairment, cardiac arrhythmias, increased CSF or head injury, myasthenia gravis, or pheochromocytoma (cardiac arrhythmias due to catecholamines).

Adverse Effects
Hypotension may occur and is considered dose-related. A malignant hyperthermia-stress syndrome has been reported in pigs, horses, dogs, and cats. Halothane may cause cardiac depression and dysrhythmias. Halothane-induced hypotension may be treated by volume expansion and dobutamine. Lidocaine has been used to treat or prevent halothane-induced cardiac dysrhythmias. In humans, jaundice and a postanesthetic fatal liver necrosis have been reported rarely. The incidence of this effect in veterinary species is not known, however, halothane should be considered contraindicated for future use if unexplained fever, jaundice, or other clinical signs associated with hepatotoxicity occur.

Reproductive/Nursing Safety
Some animal studies have shown that halothane may be teratogenic; use only when benefits outweigh potential risks. In a system evaluating the safety of drugs in canine and feline pregnancy (Papich 1989), this drug is categorized as in class: *C* (*These drugs may have potential risks. Studies in people or laboratory animals have uncovered risks, and these drugs should be used cautiously as a last resort when the benefit of therapy clearly outweighs the risks.*)

Drug Interactions
The following drug interactions have either been reported or are theoretical in humans or animals receiving halothane and may be of significance in veterinary patients:

■ **ACETAMINOPHEN:** Is not recommended for use for post-operative analgesia in patients that have received halothane anesthesia

■ **ACEPROMAZINE:** Can decrease requirements of halothane by up to 40%

■ **AMINOGLYCOSIDES:** Use with caution with halogenated anesthetic agents as additive neuromuscular blockade may occur

■ **LINCOSAMIDES:** Use with caution with halogenated anesthetic agents as additive neuromuscular blockade may occur

■ **NON-DEPOLARIZING   NEUROMUSCULAR BLOCKING AGENTS:** Additive neuromuscular blockade may occur

■ **SUCCINYLCHOLINE:** With inhalation anesthetics, may induce increased incidences of cardiac effects (bradycardia, arrhythmias, sinus arrest and apnea) and, in susceptible patients, malignant hyperthermia

■ **SYMPATHOMIMETICS (dopamine, epinephrine, norepinephrine, ephedrine, metaraminol, etc.):** Because halothane sensitizes the myocardium to the effects of sympathomimetics, especially catecholamines, severe ventricular arrhythmias may result. If these drugs are needed, they should be used with caution and in significantly reduced dosages with intensive monitoring

■ **D-TUBOCURARINE:** May cause significant hypotension if used with halothane

Laboratory Considerations
■ Halothane may transiently increase values of **liver function tests.**

Doses
■ **DOGS/CATS:**
Note: Concentrations are dependent upon fresh gas flow rate; the lower the flow rate, the higher the concentration required.
a) 3% (induction); 0.5–1.5% (maintenance) (Papich 1992)
b) 0.5–3.5%, inhaled (Hubbell 1994)

■ **RABBITS/RODENTS/SMALL MAMMALS:**
a) **Mice, Rats, Gerbils, Hamsters, Guinea pigs, Chinchillas:** Using a non-rebreathing system: Induction: 2%–4%, maintenance: 0.25%–2% (Anderson 1994); (Adamcak & Otten 2000)

■ **BIRDS:**

a) Using an anesthetic vaporizer, induction usually occurs in 2–4 minutes at a concentration of 2% for small birds and 2.5%–3% for large birds. Maintenance can generally be maintained at concentrations of 0.5%–1.5%. Recovery usually takes 3–5 minutes. Bradycardia, hypotension and hypothermia may occur, but rapidly resolve once halothane is discontinued. (Bennett 2002)

■ **HORSES:**

a) For draft horses: Following induction, the largest ET tube that will comfortably fit (20–40 mm) should be placed and cuff inflated. In an oxygen-enriched semi-closed large animal circle system 4%–5% of halothane is administered initially and is reduced as indicated by physical monitoring of neural reflexes and cardio-pulmonary parameters. The goal should be the lowest concentration inhalant anesthetic that provides adequate surgical anesthesia and restraint. Most draft horses can be maintained on 2.5%–3% halothane. (See reference for more information on monitoring and use.) (Geiser 1992)

Monitoring

■ Respiratory and ventilatory status

■ Cardiac rate/rhythm; blood pressure (particularly with "at risk" patients)

■ Level of anesthesia

Chemistry/Synonyms

An inhalant general anesthetic agent, halothane occurs as a colorless, nonflammable, heavy liquid. It has a characteristic odor resembling chloroform and a sweet, burning taste. Halothane is slightly soluble in water and miscible with alcohol. At 20°C, halothane's specific gravity is 1.872–1.877 and vapor pressure is 243 mmHg.

Halothane may also be known as: phthorothanum, *Fluothane®*, and *Ineltano®*.

Storage/Stability

Store halothane below 40°C in a tight, light-resistant container. Halothane stability is maintained by the addition of thymol and ammonia. The thymol does not vaporize so it may accumulate in the vaporizer causing a yellow discoloration. Do not use discolored solutions. Discolored vaporizer and wick may be cleaned with diethyl ether (all ether must be removed before reuse).

In the presence of moisture, halothane vapor can react with aluminum, brass, and lead (not copper). Rubber and some plastics are soluble in halothane leading to their rapid deterioration.

Dosage Forms/Regulatory Status

VETERINARY-LABELED PRODUCTS: None

HUMAN-LABELED PRODUCTS: None in USA

References

Adamcak, A. & B. Otten (2000). Rodent Therapeutics. *Vet Clin NA: Exotic Anim Pract* 3:1(Jan): 221–240.

Bennett, R. (2002). Avian Anesthesia. Proceedings: Western Veterinary Conference. Accessed via: Veterinary Information Network. http://goo.gl/pXOp9

http://goo.gl/BWb4f

Geiser, D. (1992). Chemical restraint and anesthesia of the draft horse. *Current Therapy in Equine Medicine 3.* N Robinson Ed. Philadelphia, W.B. Saunders Co.: 95–101.

Hubbell, J. (1994). PRactical methods of anesthesia. *Saunders Manual of Small Animal Practice.* S Birchard and R Sherding Eds. Philadelphia, W.B. Saunders Company: 31–21.

Papich, M. (1992). Table of Common Drugs: Approximate Dosages. *Current Veterinary Therapy XI: Small Animal Practice.* R Kirk and J Bonagura Eds. Philadelphia, W.B. Saunders Company: 1233–1249.

HCG–see Chorionic Gonadotropin

HEMOGLOBIN GLUTAMER-200 (BOVINE)

(hee-moe-*gloe*-bin *gloo*-ta-mer)

HG-200, HBOC-301, Oxyglobin®

SEMI-SYNTHETIC HEMOGLOBIN REPLACER; COLLOID

Prescriber Highlights

▶ Bovine-source polymerized hemoglobin product for the treatment of anemias

▶ Contraindications: Advanced cardiac disease, renal impairment with oliguria or anuria

▶ Many potential adverse effects; most are not serious (see below)

▶ Potential drug-lab interactions

▶ Availability has been an issue

Uses/Indications

Hemoglobin glutamer-200 [bovine] (HG-200, HBOC-301, *Oxyglobin®*) is indicated for the treatment of dogs with anemia, regardless of the cause of anemia (hemolysis, blood loss, or ineffective erythropoiesis). From a prognostic standpoint, the drug should be more valuable in dogs with regenerative anemias (versus nonregenerative anemias). It has also been used extra-label in other species as well, such as cats or foals for neonatal isoerythrolysis.

Its primary benefit is for the patient that is anemic and difficult to transfuse due to unavailability of blood, or when no suitable donors are identified on crossmatch. (Jandrey 2007)

Pharmacology/Actions

The bovine hemoglobin in the product is polymerized into larger molecules to increase safety, efficacy, and intravascular persistence, is shipped in a deoxygenated state and becomes oxygenated once circulated through the lungs. HG-200 does not contain red blood cells and is stroma free. HG-200 releases oxygen to tissue in a mechanism similar to endogenous hemoglobin; thereby increasing plasma and total hemoglobin concentrations, and systemic oxygen content. Because of its small size (in comparison to normal RBC's), it may better deliver oxygen to cells supplied by severely constricted arteries. HG-200 shifts the oxygen dissociation curve to the right, so oxygen is transferred to tissues more easily. In experimentally-induced hypovolemic shock in dogs, HG-200 caused severe vasoconstriction and decreased cardiac output (Driessen *et al.* 2001).

HG-200 also has colloidal properties similar to dextran 70 and hetastarch.

Pharmacokinetics

In dogs receiving 15 mL/kg: peak plasma hemoglobin concentrations increased approximately 2.5 g/dL; at 30 mL/kg, approximately 4 mg/dL. Duration of effect continues for at least 24 hours. The plasma half-life in dogs at present labeled dosages is approximately 18–43 hours and HG-200 can be detected in plasma for 5–7 days after a single dose.

As with endogenous hemoglobin, HG-200 is metabolized and eliminated by the reticuloendothelial system. Small amounts of unstabilized hemoglobin (<5%) may be excreted through the kidneys, causing discoloration (red) of the urine.

Contraindications/Precautions/Warnings

As safe use of *Oxyglobin®* has not been tested for the following conditions and plasma expanders are generally contraindicated in them, the product is labeled as contraindicated in dogs with advanced cardiac disease (*i.e.*, congestive heart failure) or otherwise severely impaired cardiac function or renal impairment with oliguria or anuria. The safety and efficacy of *Oxyglobin®* has not been evaluated in dogs with DIC, thrombocytopenia with active bleeding, hemoglobinemia and hemoglobinuria, or autoagglutination.

HG-200 is a potent colloid and can cause vasoconstriction. Care must be taken not to volume overload patients when receiving this drug as hydrostatic pressures may be increased and cause pulmonary overload (pleural effusion, pulmonary edema). This is particularly important in cats.

Because of its vasoconstrictive properties, the amount of HG-200 required for fluid resuscitation in trauma patients is approximately 1/3 that of hetastarch (Rudloff & Devey 2009).

Administration of any foreign protein has the potential to cause immunologic reactions. While low levels of IgG antibodies have been detected after multiple dosages, no anaphylactic reactions have been reported thus far. If an immediate hypersensitivity reaction occurs, infusion should be immediately discontinued and appropriate treatment administered. If a delayed type of hypersensitivity reaction occurs, immunosuppressant therapy is recommended.

Adverse Effects

The package insert lists the following frequency of adverse reactions that occurred in greater than 4% of dogs treated with *Oxyglobin®* (**Note:** first figure is % of dogs treated; in parentheses: % treated having hemolytic anemia): Discolored mucous membranes 69% (47%); discolored sclera (yellow, red, brown) 56% (48%); discolored urine (orange, red, brown) 52% (41%); discolored skin (yellow) 12% (83%); increased central venous pressure (CVP) 33% (47%); ventricular arrhythmias (AV block, tachycardia, ventricular premature contractions) 15% (78%); ecchymosis/petechiae 8% (50%); bradycardia 6% (67%); vomiting 35% (72%); diarrhea 15% (50%); anorexia 8% (25%); tachypnea 15% (50%); dyspnea 14% (71%); pulmonary edema 12% (67%); harsh lung sounds/crackles 8% (50%); pleural effusion 6% (67%); fever 17% (40%); death/euthanasia 15% (63%); peripheral edema 8% (25%); hemoglobinuria 6% (67%); dehydration 6% (33%).

Adverse reactions occurring in 4% of the dogs treated with *Oxyglobin®* include: coughing, disseminated intravascular coagulopathy, melena, nasal discharge/crusts (red), peritoneal effusion, respiratory arrest, and weight loss (5–7% body weight). Adverse reactions occurring in less than 2% of the dogs treated with *Oxyglobin®* included: abdominal discomfort on palpation, acidosis, cardiac arrest, cardiovascular volume overload (by echocardiography), collapse, cystitis, dark stool, discolored soft stool (red-brown) and tongue (purple), focal hyperemic areas on gums, forelimb cellulitis/lameness, hematemesis or hemoptysis (unable to differentiate), hypernatremia, hypotension, hypoxemia, lack of neurologic responses, left forebrain signs, nystagmus, pancreatitis, pendulous abdomen, polyuria, pulmonary thromboembolism, ptosis, reddened pinnae with papules/head shaking, reduction in heart rate, thrombocytopenia (worsening), and venous thrombosis.

Increases in IgG antibodies have been detected in dogs receiving multiple courses of HG-200, but no documented cases of anaphylaxis have been reported.

Small amounts of unstabilized hemoglobin (<5%) may be excreted through the kidneys, resulting in transient discoloration (red) of the urine following the infusion. This discoloration of the urine should not be interpreted as due to intravascular hemolysis and has no effect on renal function.

In clinical use, *Oxyglobin®* has not been demonstrated to affect platelet function or impair coagulation.

Increases in aspartate aminotransferase (AST) and alanine aminotransferase (ALT) not associated with histopathologic changes in the liver, increase in serum total protein, and hemoglobinuria may also be seen.

Reproductive/Nursing Safety

Safe use in breeding dogs and pregnant or lactating bitches has not been determined.

Overdosage/Acute Toxicity

The clinical signs associated with *Oxyglobin®* administered at 1, 2, and 3 times the recommended dose twice, 3 days apart include yellow-orange discoloration of skin, ear canals, pinnae, mucous membranes (gums), and sclera, red-dark-green-black discoloration of feces, brown-black discoloration of urine, red spotting of skin and/or lips (less common), decreased appetite and thirst, vomiting, diarrhea, and decreased skin elasticity. The frequency and/or intensity of these signs increased with repeated and increasing doses. Healthy dogs administered 3X overdoses twice, all survived.

Overdosage or an excessively rapid administration rate (*i.e.*, >10 mL/kg/hr) may result in circulatory overload.

Drug Interactions

Other than concerns with compatibility, (no specific drug interactions have been noted.

Laboratory Considerations

■ Hemoglobin-based oxygen carriers (HBOCs) can impact several laboratory tests. The manufacturer maintains a website: www.HBOCLab.com to help guide laboratories and clinicians.

■ The presence of HG-200 in serum may cause artifactual increases or decreases in the results of **serum chemistry tests**, depending on the type of analyzer and reagents used. May cause false increases in **AST**, or **creatinine**. May cause false decreases in **LDH**. May cause unacceptable interference with **GGT, albumin**, or **bilirubin**.

■ There is reportedly no interference with directly measured hemoglobin tests, but due to the dilutional effects of HG-200, PCV and RBC count are not accurate measures of the degree of anemia for 24 hours following administration. **Prothrombin time** (PT) and **activated partial thromboplastin time** (aPTT) determined using methods that are mechanical, magnetic and light scattering are accurate, but optical methods are not reliable while HG-200 is present.

■ **Urine dipstick** measurements (*i.e.*, pH, glucose, ketones, protein) are inaccurate while gross discoloration of the urine is present.

Doses

■ **DOGS:**

a) For labeled indications: One-time dose of 10–30 mL/kg IV at a rate of up to 10 mL/kg/hr.

May be warmed to 37°C prior to administration. Blood transfusions are not contraindicated in dogs which receive *Oxyglobin®* nor is *Oxyglobin®* contrain-

dicated in dogs which have previously received a blood transfusion. There is no need for typing or crossmatching before use. Should be administered using aseptic technique via a standard intravenous infusion set and catheter through a central or peripheral vein at a rate of 10 mL/kg/hr. Do not administer with other fluids or drugs via the same infusion set. Do not add medications or other solutions to the bag. Do not combine the contents of more than one bag. (Package Insert; *Oxyglobin®*—Biopure)

b) For resuscitation of trauma patients in shock with or without hemorrhage: Empirically, 3–5 mL/kg with concurrent crystalloid at 1/2 to 2 times maintenance. (Gfeller 2002)

c) To provide a "bridge" until immunosuppressive drugs take effect in dogs with IMHA with a transfusion reaction: 7–10 mL/kg q12h can maintain hemoglobin levels above 3.5 g/dL; higher doses 30 mL/kg may provide oxygen carrying support for 48–72 hours. (Macintire 2006)

d) As an option to provide oxygen carrying capacity in the trauma patient: 10–15 mLs/kg IV given over several hours. Care must be taken not to cause fluid overload. (Waddell 2009)

e) As a vasopressor once there is adequate intravascular volume in trauma patients: 3–5 mL/kg IV. (Rudloff & Devey 2009)

■ **CATS:**

a) As an option to provide oxygen carrying capacity in the trauma patient: 5–10 mLs/kg IV given over several hours. Care must be taken not to cause fluid overload especially in cats. (Waddell 2009)

Monitoring

■ Hgb; clinical signs of adequate tissue oxygenation

■ Signs of circulatory overload (CVP)

■ Other adverse effects (see above)

Client Information

■ Clients should be informed of the cost/risk/benefit profile for this agent before use.

Chemistry/Synonyms

Oxyglobin® is a sterile, clear, dark purple solution containing 13 g/dL purified, polymerized hemoglobin of bovine origin in a modified lactated Ringer's solution. It has an osmolality of 300 mOsm/kg and a pH of 7.8. Less than 5% of the hemoglobin are as unstabilized tetramers, and approximately 50% have a molecular weight between 65 & 130 kD, with no more than 10% having a molecular weight >500 kD. The product contains less than the detectable level of 3.5 micrograms/mL free-glutaraldehyde and 0.05 EU/mL, endotoxin.

Hemoglobin glutamer-200 (bovine) may also be known as HBOC-301, Hb-200, or HG-200.

Storage/Stability

The product remains stable at room temperature or refrigerated (2°–30°C) for up to 3 years; expiration date is printed on the bag. Outdated product is not returnable. Do not freeze. It must remain in its over wrap during storage; once removed, it should be used within 24 hours. The foil over wrap serves as an oxygen barrier, protecting the hemoglobin from conversion to methemoglobin.

The manufacturer states that *Oxyglobin®* is physically **compatible** with any other IV fluid, but should not be mixed with other solutions or medications in the bag; other intravenous solutions and medications may be administered via a separate site and line, however.

Dosage Forms/Regulatory Status

VETERINARY-LABELED PRODUCTS:

Hemoglobin Glutamer-200 (bovine) in 60 mL and 125 mL ready to use infusion bags; *Oxyglobin®* (OPK Biotech); (Rx). FDA-approved for use in dogs.

The ARCI (Racing Commissioners International) has designated this drug as a class 2 substance. It is prohibited to be at racing premises. See the appendix for more information.

HUMAN-LABELED PRODUCTS: None in USA at present

References

Driessen, B., J.S. Jahr, et al. (2001). Inadequacy of low-volume resuscitation with hemoglobin-based oxygen carrier hemoglobin glutamer-200 (bovine) in canine hypovolemia. *Journal of Veterinary Pharmacology and Therapeutics* 24(1): 61–71.

Gfeller, R. (2002). Traumatic shock resuscitation-What now? Proceedings: ACVIM Forum. Accessed via: Veterinary Information Network. http://goo.gl/dMFhE

Jandrey, K. (2007). Principles and practice of transfusion medicine. Proceedings: UCD Canine Medicine Symposium. Accessed via: Veterinary Information Network. http://goo.gl/g6J5x

Macintire, D. (2006). Immune-mediated hemolytic anemia--a metabolic disaster. Proceedings: ACVC. Accessed via: Veterinary Information Network. http://goo.gl/08aII

Rudloff, E. & J. Devey (2009). Assessment and Management of the Multi-trauma Patient. Proceedings: IVECCS. Accessed via: Veterinary Information Network. http://goo.gl/nWAjU

Waddell, L.S. (2009). Fluid therapy in the trauma patient. *Proceedings: WVC.*

HEPARIN SODIUM

(**hep**-ah-rin)   Unfractionated Heparin, UHF

ANTICOAGULANT

Prescriber Highlights

▶ Parenteral anticoagulant used primarily for treatment of DIC (use controversial) & thromboembolic disease

▶ Contraindications: Known hypersensitivity, severe thrombocytopenia, or uncontrollable bleeding (caused by something other than DIC)

▶ Adverse Effects: Most common are bleeding & thrombocytopenia

▶ Protamine may reverse effects

▶ Intensive monitoring required

Uses/Indications

Heparin's primary uses in small animal medicine have been treatment of disseminated intravascular coagulation (DIC) and prophylaxis of thromboembolic disease. The most recent evidence is strong that prophylactic heparin can reduce incidence in patients at high risk for developing macrovascular thromboembolism. Use for treating DIC has become increasingly controversial and current evidence suggests that heparin should not be used during DIC in patients with concurrent inflammatory processes.

In horses, it has been used in the treatment of DIC and as prophylactic therapy for laminitis. To date, there are no controlled prospective studies that demonstrate efficacy for these indications. Heparin has also been administered systemically (IV, SC) or as a intraperitoneally administered lavage solution to prevent intestinal adhesion formation after surgery. Its efficacy for this indication is questionable.

Pharmacology/Actions

Heparin acts on coagulation factors in both the intrinsic and extrinsic coagulation pathways. Low concentrations of heparin when combined with antithrombin III inactivate factor X_a and prevent the conversion of prothrombin to thrombin. In higher doses, heparin inactivates thrombin, blocks the conversion of fibrinogen to fibrin and when combined with antithrombin III inactivates factors IX, X, XI, XII. By inhibiting the activation of factor XIII (fibrin stabilizing factor), heparin prevents the formation of stable fibrin clots. While heparin will inhibit the reactions that lead to clotting, it does not significantly change the concentrations of clotting factors. Heparin does not lyse clots, but it can prevent the growth of existing clots.

Heparin causes increased release of lipoprotein lipase, thereby increasing the clearance of circulating lipids and boosting plasma levels of free fatty acids.

Pharmacokinetics

Heparin is not absorbed by the gut when administered orally; it must be given parenterally to be effective. Anticoagulant activity begins immediately after direct IV bolus injection, but may take up to one hour after deep SC injection. When heparin is given by continuous IV infusion, an initial bolus must be administered for full anticoagulant activity to begin.

Heparin is extensively protein bound, primarily to fibrinogen, low-density lipoproteins and globulins. It does not appreciably cross the placenta or enter milk.

Heparin's metabolic fate is not completely understood. The drug is apparently partially metabolized by the liver and also inactivated by the reticuloendothelial system. Serum half-lives in humans averages 1–2 hours.

In healthy dogs, bioavailability after subcutaneous injection is about 50%. When 200 Units/kg were administered to healthy dogs SC, plasma heparin concentrations were in the therapeutic range between 1 and 6 hours after administration. (Diquelou *et al.* 2005)

Contraindications/Precautions/Warnings

Heparin is contraindicated in patients hypersensitive to it, having severe thrombocytopenia or uncontrollable bleeding (caused by something other than DIC). One author (Green 1989) states that with DIC "heparin should not be given to actively bleeding patients that have severe factor depletion and thrombocytopenia, as fatal hemorrhage may result."

Use for treating DIC has become increasingly controversial. The most recent evidence suggests that heparin should not be used during DIC in patients with concurrent inflammatory processes. Until further evidence suggests practices to the contrary, heparin should be used with extreme caution in both human and veterinary patients with dysfunctional interactions between inflammatory and hemostatic systems and the endothelium. (Bateman 2005)

Do not administer IM as heparin may cause hematoma formation. Hematomas, pain, and irritation may occur after deep SC dosing.

Dogs with renal insufficiency may have lower plasma levels and faster elimination rates of heparin; dosage adjustment may be required.

Adverse Effects

Bleeding and thrombocytopenia are the most common adverse effects associated with heparin therapy. Because heparin is derived from bovine or porcine tissues, hypersensitivity reactions may be possible. Less commonly encountered adverse effects that have been reported in animals and/or humans include vasospastic reactions (after several days of therapy), osteoporosis and diminished renal function (after long-term, high-dose therapy), rebound hyperlipidemia, hyperkalemia, alopecia, suppressed aldosterone synthesis and priapism.

The most common adverse effect associated with heparin therapy in horses is anemia which is probably due to erythrocyte agglutination. Erythrocyte counts return to normal within 96 hours after heparin is stopped. Other adverse effects reported in horses include hemorrhage, thrombocytopenia, and pain at injection sites.

Reproductive/Nursing Safety

While heparin does not cross the placenta and is generally felt to be the anticoagulant of choice during pregnancy, its safe use in pregnancy has not been firmly established and pregnancy outcomes may be unfavorable. It should be used cautiously and only when clearly necessary. In humans, the FDA categorizes this drug as category *C* for use during pregnancy (*Animal studies have shown an adverse effect on the fetus, but there are no adequate studies in humans; or there are no animal reproduction studies and no adequate studies in humans.*)

Heparin is not excreted into milk.

Overdosage/Acute Toxicity

Overdosage of heparin is associated with bleeding. Clinical signs that could be seen before frank bleeding occurs include hematuria, tarry stools, petechiae, bruising, etc. Protamine can reverse heparin's effects; see the Protamine monograph for more information.

Drug Interactions

The following drug interactions have either been reported or are theoretical in humans or animals receiving heparin and may be of significance in veterinary patients:

- ■ **ASPIRIN:** May increase the risk for hemorrhage

- ■ **DEXTRAN:** May increase the risk for hemorrhage

- ■ **NSAIDS:** May increase the risk for hemorrhage

- ■ **WARFARIN:** May increase the risk for hemorrhage

- ■ The following drugs may partially counteract heparin's anticoagulant effects: **ANTIHISTAMINES, NITROGLYCERIN** (IV), **PROPYLENE GLYCOL, DIGOXIN,** and **TETRACYCLINES.**

Laboratory Considerations

- ■ Unless heparin is administered by continuous infusion, it can alter prothrombin time, (**PT**), which can be misleading in patients also receiving a coumarin or an indanedione anticoagulant.

- ■ Heparin can interfere with the results of the **BSP** (sulfobromophthalein, bromosulfophthalein) test by changing the color intensity of the dye and shifting the absorption peak from 580 nm to 595 nm.

- ■ Heparin can cause falsely elevated values of serum **thyroxine** if using competitive protein binding methods of determination. Radioimmunoassay (RIA) and protein bound iodine methods are apparently unaffected by heparin.

■ When heparin is used as an anticoagulant *in vitro* (*e.g.*, in **blood collection containers**), white cell counts should be performed within 2 hours of collection. Do not use heparinized blood for platelet counts, erythrocyte sedimentation rates, erythrocyte fragmentation tests, or for any tests involving complement or isoagglutinins. Errors in blood gas determinations for CO_2 pressure, bicarbonate concentration, or base excess may occur if heparin encompasses 10% or more of the blood sample.

Doses

■ **DOGS/ CATS:**

For adjunctive treatment of DIC (See Contraindications/Warnings above): **Note:** Heparin therapy may be only one aspect of successful treatment of DIC. Alleviation of the precipitating causes, administration of fluids, blood, aspirin, and diligent monitoring of coagulation tests (aPTT, PT), fibrin degradation products, and fibrinogen may all be important factors in the treatment of DIC. Doses of heparin are controversial; dosage ranges and methods may vary widely depending on the clinician/author.

a) 75 Units/kg SC three times daily (Wingfield & Van Pelt 1989)

b) After pH has been corrected and perfusion maximized, transfuse heparinized whole fresh blood or plasma (75 Units/kg heparin) one time. Then begin mini-dose heparin therapy at 5–10 Units/kg/hour by continuous IV infusion or 75 Units/kg SC q8h. Continue without interruption until DIC has completely disappeared. With these doses, bleeding risk is negligible and aPTT monitoring not necessary, although thrombocytopenia may develop. (Slappendel 1989)

c) Before administering heparin, provide sufficient fresh whole blood to maintain platelet counts above 30,000/microliter and fibrinogen levels over 50 mg/dL. Then give heparin at 50–100 Units/kg SC q6h. Alternatively, dose heparin sufficiently to increase aPTT to 1.5–2 times normal (may be more effective in patients susceptible to thromboembolization). (Green 1989)

For adjunctive treatment of thromboembolic disease:

a) For feline arterial thromboembolism: 250–300 Units/kg SC q8h. First dose is administered IV to cats showing signs of shock. Monitoring aPTT (1.5–2.5 fold) and ACT (15–20 sec) should be regarded as rough guidelines only, as these may still result in heparin levels below the recommended therapeutic range. (Smith 2004)

b) Dogs: For "bridging therapy" while dog is started on warfarin for maintenance therapy for pulmonary thromboembolism: Heparin in 200–500 Units/kg SC q8h initially and then adjusted to reach a target aPTT of 1.5-2 times the treatment values or anti-factor Xa activity between 0.35-0.7 Units/mL. Treat for the first 5-7 days of warfarin therapy or until monitoring has documented adequate prolongation of PT. (Lunsford, K.V. & Mackin, A.J. 2007)

c) For maintenance therapy for arterial thromboembolic disease in cats: 250–300 Units/kg SC every 8 hours for the initial in-hospital therapy. (Lunsford, K. & Mackin, A. 2007)

d) Dogs: To cause anticoagulation without an excessive risk of bleeding: 150–300 Units/kg SC q6-8h. Each animal is individual and may respond differently to this dose, and must be monitored by serial physical examination and by PTT or other coagulation assay (e.g., thromboelastography). In critically ill animals, constant rate IV infusion of UFH is more likely to result in consistent anti-coagulation and prolongation of PTT. A loading dose of 100 Units/kg is followed by a CRI from 20-50 Units/kg/hr. Small changes in the dose can result in large changes in PTT, and it is recommended to start at a low dose and slowly titrate higher in increments of 5 Units/kg/hr. To help prevent rebound hypercoagulability, it is recommended to taper the dose gradually, decreasing by 50 Units/kg per dose day over 3-4 days. (Brainard 2008)

To prevent clots forming when performing closed chest lavage with pyothorax:

a) Add 1000 U of heparin per liter of lavage fluid (warm normal saline). This fluid is instilled at 20 mL/kg twice daily for 5–7 days. Antibiotics (often penicillin) or enzymes (*e.g.*, streptokinase) may also be added to fluid. (Berkwitt & Berzon 1989)

For hyperadrenocorticoid dogs undergoing adrenalectomy:

a) At anesthetic induction, give heparinized plasma at a rate of 35 Units/kg, followed on the day of surgery by two doses 8 hours apart of 35 Units/kg. Next day give 25 Units/kg SC and taper over the next 4 days. (Lunsford, K.V. & Mackin, A.J. 2007)

For detection of lipoprotein lipase activity (heparin stimulation test):

a) Measure serum lipids just before and 15 minutes after heparin at 100 Units/kg IV. Lack of increase in lipolytic activity is suggestive of lipoprotein lipase deficiency. (Kay & Richter 1988)

■ **HORSES:**

For prevention of complications (*e.g.*, venous thrombosis, laminitis, DIC) associated with hypercoagulable states:

a) Initially 150 Units/kg SC. Then 125 Units/kg q12h for 6 doses and then decreased to 100 Units/kg SC every 12 hours. (Rush Moore & Hinchcliff 1994)

For adjunctive treatment of DIC: **Note:** Heparin therapy may be only one aspect of successful treatment of DIC. Alleviation of the precipitating causes, administration of fluids, blood, aspirin, and diligent monitoring of coagulation tests (APTT, PT), fibrin degradation products, and fibrinogen may all be important factors in the treatment of DIC.

a) Heparin at 80–100 Units/kg IV q4–6h (may be added to fluids and given as a slow drip). Low grade DIC may be treated with 25–40 Units/kg SC 2–3 times a day. (Byars 1987)

As adjunctive therapy in endotoxic shock:

a) 40 Units/kg IV or SC 2–3 times a day may prevent the development of microthrombi; additional studies are required to confirm positive benefits (Semrad & Moore 1987)

As adjunctive therapy in the prevention of laminitis:

a) 25–100 Units/kg subcutaneously 3 times daily. Higher doses used when a thrombotic event is underway, lower dosages should have fewer adverse effects and still have antithrombotic activity. Ideally, APTT and ACT should be monitored. Targets are 1.5–2.5 times baseline for APTT and 1.2–1.4 times baseline for ACT. (Brumbaugh *et al.* 1999)

In an attempt to prevent abdominal adhesions:

a) 30,000–50,000 Units heparin in 10 L of lavage fluid (warm LRS) and administered intraperitoneally via a 32 french fenestrated trocar catheter placed in the right ventral abdomen at the time of surgery. Lavage performed at 12, 18, 36, and 48 hours post-surgery and allowed to drain through a Heimlich valve. Drain removed after final lavage or it becomes occluded. (Eggleston & Mueller 2003)

Monitoring

Note: The frequency of monitoring is controversial and is dependent on several factors, including heparin dose, patient's condition, concomitant problems, etc. Because of the high incidence of hemorrhage associated with heparin use, frequent monitoring of aPTT is essential early in therapy (particularly using higher dosages) and in critically ill animals.

■ While whole blood clotting time (WBCT), partial thromboplastin time (PTT), and activated partial thromboplastin times (aPTT) may all be used to monitor therapy, aPTT is most often recommended, but newer tests (*e.g.*, thromboelastography) are being utilized.

■ Platelet counts and hematocrit (PCV) should be done periodically;

■ Occult blood in stool and urine; other observations for bleeding;

■ Clinical efficacy

Client Information

■ Because of the intense monitoring necessary with heparin's use and the serious nature of the disease states in which it is used, this drug should be utilized only by professionals familiar with it, preferably in an inpatient setting.

Chemistry/Synonyms

Heparin is an anionic, heterogeneous sulfated glycosaminoglycan molecule with an average molecular weight of 12,000 that is found naturally in mast cells. It is available commercially as the sodium salt and is obtained from either porcine intestinal mucosa or from bovine lung tissue (sodium salt only). Heparin sodium occurs as white or pale-colored, amorphous, hygroscopic powder having a faint odor. It is soluble in water and practically insoluble in alcohol; the commercial injections have a pH of 5–7.5. Heparin potency is expressed in terms of USP Heparin Units and values are obtained by comparing against a standard reference from the USP. The USP requires that potencies be not less than 120 Units/mg on a dried basis for heparin derived from lung tissue, and 140 Units/mg when derived from all other tissue sources.

Heparin sodium may also be as: heparinum natricum, sodium heparin, and soluble heparin; many trade names are available.

Storage/Stability

Heparin solutions should be stored at room temperature (15–30°C) and not frozen. Avoid excessive exposure to heat.

Compatibility/Compounding Considerations

Heparin sodium is reportedly physically **compatible** with the following intravenous solutions and drugs: amino acids 4.25%-dextrose 25%, dextrose-Ringer's combinations, dextrose-lactated Ringer's solutions, fat emulsion 10%, Ringer's injection, *Normosol®*, aminophylline, amphotericin B with or without hydrocortisone sodium phosphate, ascorbic acid injection, bleomycin sulfate, calcium gluconate, cephapirin sodium, chloramphenicol sodium succinate, clindamycin phosphate, dimenhydrinate, dopamine HCl, erythromycin gluceptate, isoproterenol HCl, lidocaine HCl, methylprednisolone sodium succinate, metronidazole with sodium succinate, nafcillin sodium, norepinephrine bitartrate, potassium chloride, prednisolone sodium succinate, promazine HCl, sodium bicarbonate, verapamil HCl, and vitamin B-complex with or without vitamin C.

Heparin **compatibility information conflicts** or is dependent on diluent or concentration factors with the following drugs or solutions: dextrose-saline combinations, dextrose in water, lactated Ringer's injection, saline solutions, ampicillin sodium, cephalothin sodium, dobutamine HCl, hydrocortisone sodium succinate, methicillin sodium, oxytetracycline HCl, penicillin G sodium/potassium, and tetracycline HCl. Compatibility is dependent upon factors such as pH, concentration, temperature and diluent used; consult specialized references or a hospital pharmacist for more specific information.

Heparin sodium is reported physically **incompatible** when mixed with the following solutions or drugs: sodium lactate 1/6 M, amikacin sulfate, chlorpromazine HCl, codeine phosphate, cytarabine, daunorubicin HCl, diazepam, doxorubicin HCl, droperidol HCl with and without fentanyl citrate, erythromycin lactobionate, gentamicin sulfate, hyaluronidase, kanamycin sulfate, levorphanol bitartrate, meperidine HCl, methadone HCl, morphine sulfate, pentazocine lactate, phenytoin sodium, polymyxin B sulfate, streptomycin sulfate, and vancomycin HCl.

Dosage Forms/Regulatory Status

VETERINARY-LABELED PRODUCTS: None
HUMAN-LABELED PRODUCTS:

Heparin Sodium Injection: 1000 Units/mL, 2000 Units/mL, 2500 Units/mL, 5000 Units/mL, 10,000 Units/mL, 20,000 Units/mL, & 40,000 Units/mL in 0.5 mL, 1 mL, 2 mL, 4 mL, 5 mL, 10 mL, and 30 mL vials; generic; (Rx).

Heparin Unit-Dose Sodium Injection: 1000 Units/dose, 2500 Units/dose, 5000 Units/dose, 7500 Units/dose, 10,000 Units/dose and 20,000 Units/dose in 1 mL, 10 mL, & 30 mL *Dosette* vials, 0.5 mL & 1 mL *Tubex*, 0.5 mL, 1 mL, 4 mL & 10 mL vials, and 1 mL fill in 2 mL *Carpuject* (depending on concentration and manufacturer); generic; (Rx)

Heparin Sodium and 0.9% Sodium Chloride Injection: 1000 & 2000 Units in 500 mL and 1000 mL, respectively; generic; (Rx)

Heparin Sodium and 0.45% Sodium Chloride Injection: 12,500 in 250 mL & 25,000 Units in 250 mL & 500 mL; generic (Abbott); (Rx)

Heparin Sodium Lock Flush (IV use) Injection: 1 unit/mL in 1, 2, 2.5, 5 & 10 mL syringes; 10 Units/mL and 100 Units/mL in 1, 2, 5, 10 mL (regular and preservative free), 30 mL & 50 mL vials; 1 mL (regular and preservative free) & 2 mL *Dosette* vials; 1 mL & 2.5 mL *Dosette* cartridge needle Units; 1 mL amps; 1 mL, 2 mL, 2.5 mL, 3 mL, and 5 mL disposable syringes; *Hep-Lock®* and *Hep-Loc® U/P* (various); *Hep-flush-10®* (American Pharmaceutical Partners); Heparin I.V. Flush (Medefil); generic; (Rx)

References

Bateman, S. (2005). DIC and Heparin. Proceedings: IVECCS. Accessed via: Veterinary Information Network. http://goo.gl/rSri0

Berkwitt, L. & J.L. Berzon (1989). Pleural cavity diseases. *Handbook of Small Animal Practice*. RV Morgan Ed. New York, Churchill Livingstone: 215–225.

Brainard, B. (2008). Practical anticoagulation. Proceedings: IVECCS. Accessed via: Veterinary Information Network. http://goo.gl/1odyW

Brumbaugh, G., H. Lopez, et al. (1999). The pharmacologic basis for the treatment of laminitis. *The Veterinary Clinics of North America: Equine Practice* 15:2(August).

Byars, T.D. (1987). Disseminated Intravascular Coagulation. *Current Therapy in Equine Medicine 2*. NE Robinson Ed. Phialdelphia, WB Saunders: 306–309.

Diquelou, A., C. Barbaste, et al. (2005). Pharmacokinetics and pharmacodynamics of a therapeutic dose of unfractionated heparin (200 I/kg) administered subcutaneously or intravenous to healthy dogs. *Vet Clin Path* 34(3): 237–242.

Eggleston, R.B. & P.O.E. Mueller (2003). Prevention and treatment of gastrointestinal adhesions. *Veterinary Clinics of North America-Equine Practice* 19(3): 741–+.

Green, R.A. (1989). Hemostatic disorders: Coagulation and thrombotic disorders. *Textbook of Veterinary Internal Medicine*. SJ Ettinger Ed. Philadelphia, WB Saunders: 2: 2246–2264.

Kay, A.D. & K.P. Richter (1988). Diseases of the parathyroid glands. *Handbook of Small Animal Practice*. RV Morgan Ed. New York, Churchill Livingstone: 521–526.

Lunsford, K. & A. Mackin (2007). Evidence-based veterinary medicine: Thromboembolic therapies in dogs and cats and evidence-based approach. *Vet Clin NA: Sm Anim Pract* 37(3): 579–609.

Lunsford, K.V. & A.J. Mackin (2007). Thromboembolic therapies in dogs and cats: An evidence-based approach. *Veterinary Clinics of North America-Small Animal Practice* 37(3): 579–+.

Rush Moore, B. & K.W. Hinchcliff (1994). Heparin: A Review of its Pharmacology and Therapeutic Use in Horses. *J Vet Intern Med* 8: 26–35.

Semrad, S.D. & J.N. Moore (1987). Endotoxemia. *Current Therapy in Equine Medicine 2*. NE Robinson Ed. Philadelphia, WB Saunders: 81–87.

Slappendel, R.J. (1989). Disseminated intravascular coagulation. *Current Veterinary Therapy X: Small Animal Practice*. RW Kirk Ed. Philadelphia, WB Saunders: 451–457.

Smith, S. (2004). Feline arterial thromboembolism: An update. Proceedings: ACVIM Forum. Accessed via: Veterinary Information Network. http://goo.gl/fJeSR

Wingfield, W.E. & D. Van Pelt (1989). Abnormal Bleeding. *Vet Clin of North Amer: Sm Anim Pract: Critical Care* 19(6).

HYALURONATE SODIUM
SODIUM HYALURONATE
HYALURONAN

(hy-al-yoo-*ron*-nate)
Hyalovet®, Hyvisc®, Legend®

MUCOPOLYSACCHARIDE

Prescriber Highlights

▶ Parenteral, high viscosity mucopolysaccharide used for synovitis

▶ Contraindications: None on label

▶ Adverse Effects: Local reactions possible

▶ Different products have different dosages, etc; check label before using

Uses/Indications

Hyaluronate sodium (HS) is useful in the treatment of synovitis not associated with severe degenerative joint disease. It may be helpful to treat secondary synovitis in conditions where full thickness cartilage loss exists.

The choice of a high molecular weight product (MW >1x10^6) versus a low molecular weight one is quite controversial. One author (Nixon 1992) states that ". . . low molecular weight products (which tend to be less expensive) can be equally efficacious in ameliorating signs of joint disease. When synovial adhesions and pannus are to be avoided (as in most surgeries for carpal and fetlock fracture fragment removal), higher molecular weight preparations are recommended because they inhibit proliferation of synovial fibroblasts." However, at the time of writing, there are no controlled studies directly comparing the various products for treating joint disease and product choice is primarily a result of a clinician's personal preference.

There is considerable interest in oral hyaluronate administration for treating equine joint disease. One blinded, controlled study found the use of an oral gel "nutraceutical" significantly reduced synovial effusion in tarsocrural joints post-arthroscopic surgery for osteochondritis dissecans (OCD) (Bergin *et al.* 2006).

Pharmacology/Actions

Hyaluronate sodium (HS) is found naturally in the connective tissue of both man and animals and is identical chemically regardless of species. Highest concentrations found naturally are in the synovial fluid, vitreous of the eye and umbilical cord. Surfaces of articular cartilage are covered with a thin layer of a protein-hyaluronate complex; hyaluronate is also found in synovial fluid and the cartilage matrix. The net effects in joints include a cushioning effect, reduction of protein and cellular influx into the joint, and a lubricating effect. Hyaluronate has a direct anti-inflammatory effect in joints by scavenging free radicals and suppressing prostaglandins.

Pharmacokinetics

In the equine joint the half life of hyaluronate has been reported to be 96 hours.

Contraindications/Precautions/Warnings

No contraindications to HS's use are noted on the label. HS should not be used as a substitute for adequate diagnosis; radiographic examinations should be performed to rule out serious fractures. Do not perform intra-articular injections through skin that has been recently fired or blistered, or that has excessive scurf and counterirritants on it.

Adverse Effects

Some patients may develop local reactions manifested by heat, swelling, and/or effusion. Effects generally subside within 24–48 hours; some animals may require up to 96 hours for resolution. No treatment for this effect is recommended.

When used in combination with other drugs, incidence of flares may actually be higher. No systemic adverse effects have been noted.

Reproductive/Nursing Safety

While HS is unlikely to cause problems, safe use in breeding animals has not been established and most manufacturers caution against its use in these animals.

Overdosage/Acute Toxicity

Acute toxicology studies performed in horses have demonstrated no systemic toxicity associated with overdoses.

Drug Interactions/Laboratory Considerations

None were noted.

Doses

■ **HORSES:**

a) Because of the differences in the commercially available products, see each individual product's label for specific dosing information. The following are recommended doses from a review article (Goodrich & Nixon 2006) on the medical treatment of osteoarthritis in the horse:

Hylartin-V®: 20 mg IA

Hyvisc®: 20 mg IA

Equron®: 10 mg IA

Synacid®: 50 mg IA

Hyalovet®: 20 mg IA

Legend®: 40 mg IV (also labeled for IA injection: 20 mg)

b) To reduce joint effusion post-arthroscopic surgery for osteochondritis dissecans (OCD): 100 mg PO (as an oral gel; *Conquer®*) once daily for 30 days. (Bergin *et al.* 2006)

■ **DOGS:**

a) For the adjunctive treatment of synovitis (rather than the presence of a damaged articular cartilage): Using a high molecular weight compound: 3–5 mg intra-articularly using sterile technique at weekly intervals. Long-term effects are not achieved. (Bloomberg 1992)

Client Information

■ HS should be administered by a veterinarian only, using aseptic technique.

Chemistry/Synonyms

Hyaluronate sodium (HS) is the sodium salt of hyaluronic acid which is a naturally occurring high-viscosity mucopolysaccharide. Much of the commercially available hyaluronic acid products are derived from the combs of roosters.

Hyaluronate sodium may also be known as: HA, hyaluronan, "rooster juice", hyaluronic acid, and natrii hyaluronas; many trade names are available.

Storage/Stability

Store at room temperature or refrigerate depending on the product used—check label; do not freeze. Protect from light.

Dosage Forms/Regulatory Status

VETERINARY-LABELED PRODUCTS:

Hyaluronate Sodium: (average MW of 500,000–730,000) 20 mg/mL in 2 mL disposable syringes; *Hyalovet®* (BIVI); (Rx). FDA-approved for use in horses not intended for food.

Hyaluronate Sodium Injection: 2 mL vial for IA administration; 4 mL, & 20 mL vials for IV administration; *Legend®* (Bayer); (Rx). FDA-approved for use in horses not intended for food.

Hyaluronate Sodium Injection: 11 mg/mL in 2 mL syringes; *Hyvisc®* (BIVI); (Rx). FDA-approved for use in horses not intended for food.

Hyaluronate Sodium: 10 mg/mL (MW 3.5×10^6) in 2 mL disposable syringes; *Hylartin®V* (Pfizer); (Rx). FDA-approved for use in horses not intended for food.

Hyaluronate Sodium Oral Gel: 10 mg/mL (100 mg/10 mL) (apple-flavored) in 60 mL tubes; *Conquer® Equine Gel* (Kinetic). This product is labeled as a nutritional supplement and is not FDA-approved.

There may also be other hyaluronate products marketed as topical solutions, semen extenders, and oral supplements. These products are not necessarily approved by the FDA.

HUMAN-LABELED PRODUCTS: None

References

Bergin, B.J., S.W. Pierce, et al. (2006). Oral hyaluronan gel reduces post operative tarsocrural effusion in the yearling Thoroughbred. *Equine Veterinary Journal* **38**(4): 375–378.

Bloomberg, M. (1992). Pharmacokinetics of musculoskeletal drugs (Polysulfated Glycosaminoglycans, DMSO, Orgotein, and Hyaluronic Acid). Minnesota Veterinary Medicine Association: Annual Conference, Bloomington.

Goodrich, L.R. & A.J. Nixon (2006). Medical treatment of osteoarthritis in the horse - A review. *Veterinary Journal* **171**(1): 51–69.

HYDRALAZINE HCL

(hye-*dral*-a-zeen)   Apresoline®

VASODILATOR

Prescriber Highlights

▶ Vasodilator drug used primarily for hypertension or adjunctive treatment of heart failure

▶ Contraindications: Known hypersensitivity, coronary artery disease, hypovolemia or preexisting hypotension

▶ Caution: Severe renal disease, intracerebral bleeding, preexisting autoimmune diseases

▶ Adverse Effects: Hypotension, reflex tachycardia, sodium/water retention (if not given concurrently with a diuretic), or GI distress (vomiting, diarrhea)

▶ Drug interactions

Uses/Indications

Primary use of hydralazine in veterinary medicine is as an afterload reducer for the adjunctive treatment in CHF in small animals, particularly if mitral valve insufficiency is the primary cause. It is also useful in dogs and cats with large septal defects or severe aortic regurgitation. Hydralazine is usually used in cases where enalapril or another ACE inhibitor is not effective in clinical improving dogs with mitral insufficiency. It is used to treat systemic hypertension, particularly in combination with other drugs (*e.g.*, beta-blockers) to offset hydralazine's tendency to cause reflex tachycardia and fluid retention. Hydralazine is not particularly useful in treating heart failure when myocardial disease is present.

Pharmacology/Actions

Hydralazine acts upon vascular smooth muscle and reduces peripheral resistance and blood pressure. Hydralazine is a semicarbazide-sensitive amine oxidase (SSAO) inhibitor. It is believed that hydralazine alters cellular calcium metabolism in smooth muscle, thereby interfering with calcium movements and preventing the initiation and maintenance of the contractile state. Hydralazine has more effect on arterioles than on veins.

In patients with CHF, hydralazine significantly increases cardiac output, and decreases systemic vascular resistance. Cardiac rate may be slightly increased or unchanged, while blood pressure, pulmonary venous pressure, and right atrial pressure may be decreased or unchanged.

When used to treat hypertensive patients (without CHF), increased heart rate, cardiac output and stroke volume can be noted. The renin-angiotensin system can be activated with a resultant increase in sodium and water retention if not given with diuretics or sympathetic blocking drugs.

Parenteral hydralazine administration can cause respiratory stimulation.

Pharmacokinetics

In dogs, hydralazine is rapidly absorbed after oral administration with an onset of action within one hour and peak effects at 3–5 hours. There is a high first-pass effect after oral administration. The presence of food may enhance the bioavailability of hydralazine tablets.

Hydralazine is widely distributed in body tissues. In humans, approximately 85% of the drug in the blood is bound to plasma proteins. Hydralazine crosses the placenta and very small amounts are excreted into the milk.

Hydralazine is extensively metabolized in the liver and approximately 15% is excreted unchanged in the urine. The half-life in humans is usually 2–4 hours, but may be as long as 8 hours.

Specific pharmacokinetic parameters for this drug in veterinary species are limited, but the duration of action of hydralazine in dogs after oral administration is reportedly 11–13 hours. Vasodilating effects occur within one hour and peak within 3 hours of dosing. Food decreases oral bioavailability in dogs by about 63%. At lower doses there is relatively high first pass effect, but this is apparently a saturable process as bioavailability increases with dose. N-acetylation is a primary enzymatic pathway for hydralazine metabolism and this pathway is mostly absent in dogs leading to concerns for increased risks for toxicity.

Contraindications/Precautions/Warnings

Hydralazine is contraindicated in patients hypersensitive to it and those with coronary artery disease. The drug is listed as contraindicated in human patients with mitral valvular rheumatic disease, but it has been recommended for use in small animal patients with mitral valve insufficiency. It is not recommended to use the drug in patients with hypovolemia or preexisting hypotension.

Doses need to be titrated upwards carefully as severe hypotension can result.

Hydralazine should be used with caution in patients with renal disease. Secondary to reduced renal blood flow, hydralazine can activate the renin angiotensin aldosterone system (RAAS) and exacerbate renal injury; pretreatment with an ACE inhibitor and spironolactone is often advised to reduce this risk.

Hydralazine should be used with caution in patients with intracerebral bleeding. In humans, a syndrome resembling systemic lupus erythematosus (SLE) has been documented after hydralazine use. While this syndrome has not been documented in veterinary patients, the drug should be used with caution in patients with preexisting autoimmune diseases.

Adverse Effects

The most prevalent adverse effects seen in small animals are hypotension, weakness/lethargy and syncope particularly when doses are increased too fast. Reflex tachycardia, sodium/water retention (if not given concurrently with a diuretic), and GI distress (vomiting, diarrhea) can also occur. Hydralazine can increase creatinine levels. Other adverse effects documented in humans that could occur include: an SLE-like syndrome, lacrimation, conjunctivitis, peripheral neuritis, blood dyscrasias, urinary retention, constipation, and hypersensitivity reactions.

Tachycardias may be treated with concomitant digitalis treatment or a beta-blocker (Caution: beta-blockers may reduce cardiac performance).

Reproductive/Nursing Safety

In humans, the FDA categorizes this drug as category *C* for use during pregnancy (*Animal studies have shown an adverse effect on the fetus, but there are no adequate studies in humans; or there are no animal reproduction studies and no adequate studies in humans*). In a separate system evaluating the safety of drugs in canine and feline pregnancy (Papich 1989), this drug is categorized as in class: *B* (*Safe for use if used cautiously. Studies in laboratory animals may have uncovered some risk, but these drugs appear to be safe in dogs and cats or these drugs are safe if they are not administered when the animal is near term.*)

Hydralazine is excreted in milk. According to the American Academy of Pediatrics, hydralazine is compatible with breastfeeding, but exercise caution.

Overdosage /Acute Toxicity

Overdoses may be characterized by severe hypotension, tachycardia or other arrhythmias, skin flushing, and myocardial ischemia. Cardiovascular system support is the primary treatment modality. Evacuate gastric contents and administer activated charcoal using standard precautionary measures if the ingestion was recent and cardiovascular status has been stabilized. Treat shock using volume expanders without using pressor agents if possible. If a pressor agent is required to maintain blood pressure, the use of a minimally arrhythmogenic agent (*e.g.*, phenylephrine or methoxamine) is recommended. Digitalis agents may be required. Monitor blood pressure and renal function diligently.

Drug Interactions

The following drug interactions have either been reported or are theoretical in humans or animals receiving hydralazine and may be of significance in veterinary patients:

- **ACE-INHIBITORS:** May cause additive hypotensive effect; usually used for therapeutic advantage

- **BETA-BLOCKERS:** May cause additive hypotensive effect; usually used for therapeutic advantage

- **DIAZOXIDE:** Potentially could cause profound hypotension

■ **DIURETICS:** May cause additive hypotensive effect; usually used for therapeutic advantage

■ **FUROSEMIDE:** Hydralazine may increase furosemide's renal effects

■ **MAO INHIBITORS:** May cause additive hypotensive effect

■ **SYMPATHOMIMETICS (e.g., epinephrine):** Hydralazine may cause decreased pressor effect and may cause additive tachycardia

Doses

Because of the sodium/water retention associated with this drug it is often used concurrently with a diuretic when used for adjunctive treatment of heart failure. When used for hypertension, a diuretic may not be required. Many clinicians recommend adding a venous dilating agent (*e.g.*, nitroglycerin ointment) to reduce preload.

■ **DOGS:**

For adjunctive therapy in treatment of heart failure:

a) Effective dose is 0.5–3 mg/kg PO q12h. Dose must be titrated, starting with a low dose and titrating upwards.

In dogs *not receiving ACE inhibitors:* Get initial baseline assessment (mucous membrane color, capillary refill time, murmur intensity, cardiac size on radiographs, and severity of pulmonary edema). Starting dose is 1 mg/kg PO q12h and repeat assessments made in 12–48 hours. If no response identified, increase dosage to 2 mg/kg q12h. Repeat assessments as above and increase to 3 mg/kg PO q12h if no response. Can be titrated with or without blood pressure monitoring. If BP cannot be monitored titration is performed more slowly and clinical and radiographic signs are monitored.

If blood pressure measurement available, dosage titration can be made more rapidly than above: Measure baseline blood pressure. Administer 1 mg/kg PO. Repeat BP in 1–2 hours and if it has decreased by at least 15 mmHg, administer q12h from then on. If response inadequate, give another 1 mg/kg and repeat BP measurement in 1–2 hours. This may be repeated until a cumulative dose of 3 mg/kg has been given within a 12 hour period. The resulting cumulative dose becomes the dosage to be given q12h.

For dogs with acute, fulminant heart failure due to severe mitral regurgitation and not receiving ACE inhibitors: 2 mg/kg along with IV furosemide. May cause hypotension, but the risks of not effectively treating fulminant pulmonary edema outweigh the risks of treatment.

For dogs *receiving ACE inhibitors:* Give

hydralazine with caution as severe hypotension may occur if dosage not titrated carefully. Begin dosing at 0.5 mg/kg with blood pressure monitoring and increase in 0.5 mg/kg increments until a response is identified to a maximum of 3 mg/kg. Consider referral. (Kittleson, M., 2007)

b) For short-term treatment of CHF secondary to valve disease: Initial dose of 1 mg/kg PO. Blood pressure should be monitored; if the desired goal (MAP of 60-80 mmHg) is not achieved with the first 1 mg/kg dose (clinical effects noted within 1 hour and peak levels at 3 hours), an additional 0.5–1 mg/kg can be administered, to a maximum cumulative dose of 3 mg/kg. Once the desired blood pressure has been achieved, the dose can be administered PO q12h. (Erling & Mazzaferro 2008)

For treatment of systemic hypertension:

a) As a fifth step drug for systolic hypertension >160 mmHg, diastolic >120 mmHg; after **1)** enalapril/benazepril (0.5 mg/kg q12h); **2)** amlodipine (0.1 mg/kg q24h); **3)** amlodipine (0.2 mg/kg q24h); **4)** spironolactone (1–2 mg/kg twice daily); **5)** hydralazine 0.5 mg/kg PO twice daily. Each step added (except when increasing amlodipine dose) if after 1-2 weeks systolic BP > 160 mmHg. (Henik 2007)

■ **CATS:**

For adjunctive therapy in treatment of heart failure:

a) See (a) above "For adjunctive therapy in treatment of heart failure in dogs:", but start titration at 2.5 mg (total dose) and if necessary, increase up to 10 mg. (Kittleson, M.D. 1985)

For treatment of systemic hypertension:

a) As a fourth step drug when systolic BP >160 mmHg, diastolic >120 mmHg: **1)** amlodipine (0.625 mg per cat q24h, if cat greater then 6 kg, 1.25 mg/cat q24h), add ACE inhibitor if proteinuric; **2)** ACE inhibitor (benazepril/enalapril 0.5 mg/kg q12h); **3)** spironolactone (1–2 mg/kg twice daily); **4)** hydralazine 0.5 mg/kg PO twice daily. Each step added (except when increasing amlodipine dose) if after 1-2 weeks systolic BP > 160 mmHg. (Henik 2007)

■ **HORSES: (Note:** ARCI UCGFS Class 3 Drug) For adjunctive therapy in treatment of heart failure (afterload reducer:)

a) 0.5 mg/kg IV; for long-term therapy use 0.5–1.5 mg/kg PO q12h (Mogg 1999)

Monitoring

■ Baseline thoracic radiographs

■ Mucous membrane color

■ Serum electrolytes

■ If possible, arterial blood pressure and venous PO$_2$. A mean arterial pressure (MAP) of between 60-80 mmHg has been recommended when used in dogs for the short-term treatment of CHF secondary to valve disease (Erling & Mazzaferro 2008).

■ Because blood dyscrasias are a possibility, an occasional CBC should be considered.

Client Information

■ Compliance with directions is necessary to maximize the benefits from this drug.

■ Notify veterinarian if the animal's condition deteriorates or if it becomes lethargic, weak or depressed, (signs of hypotension).

Chemistry/Synonyms

A phthalazine-derivative antihypertensive and vasodilating agent, hydralazine HCl occurs as an odorless, white to off-white crystalline powder with a melting point between 270−280°C and a pK$_a$ of 7.3. One gram is soluble in approximately 25 mL of water or 500 mL of alcohol. The commercially available injection has a pH of 3.4−4.

Hydralazine may also be known as: apressinum, hydralazini, hydrallazine, idralazina, *Alphapress®*, *Apresolin®*, *Apresolina®*, *Bionobal®*, *Cesoline®*, *Hidral®*, *Hydrapres®*, *Hyperex®*, *Hyperphen®*, *Ipolina®*, *Nepresol®*, *Novo-Hylazin®*, *Nu-Hydral®*, *Rolazine®*, *Slow-Apresoline®*, and *Supres®*.

Storage/Stability

Hydralazine tablets should be stored in tight, light resistant containers at room temperature. The injectable product should be stored at room temperature; avoid refrigeration or freezing.

When mixed with most infusion solutions a color change can occur which does not necessarily indicate a loss in potency (if occurred over 8−12 hours).

Compatibility/Compounding Considerations

Hydralazine is reported to be physically **compatible** with the following infusion solutions/drugs: dextrose-Ringer's combinations, dextrose-saline combinations, Ringer's injection, lactated Ringer's injection, sodium chloride solutions, and dobutamine HCl.

Hydralazine is reported to be physically **incompatible** when mixed with 10% dextrose or fructose and is reported to be physically incompatible when mixed with the following drugs: aminophylline, ampicillin sodium, chlorothiazide sodium, edetate calcium disodium, hydrocortisone sodium succinate, mephentermine sulfate, methohexital sodium, phenobarbital sodium, and verapamil HCl. Compatibility is dependent upon factors such as pH, concentration, temperature, and diluent used; consult specialized references for more specific information.

Dosage Forms/Regulatory Status

VETERINARY-LABELED PRODUCTS: None

The ARCI (Racing Commissioners International) has designated this drug as a class 3 substance. See the appendix for more information.

HUMAN-LABELED PRODUCTS:

Hydralazine HCl Oral Tablets: 10 mg, 25 mg, 50 mg & 100 mg; *Apresoline®* (Novartis); generic; (Rx)

Hydralazine Injection: 20 mg/mL in 1 mL vials; generic; (Solopak); (Rx)

References

Erling, P. & E.M. Mazzaferro (2008). Left-sided congestive heart failure in dogs: Treatment and monitoring of emergency patients. *Compendium-Continuing Education for Veterinarians* 30(2): 94−+.

Henik, R. (2007). Stepwise therapy of systemic hypertension. Proceedings: IVECCS. Accessed via: Veterinary Information Network. http://goo.gl/nofKU

Kittleson, M. (2007). Management of Heart Failure. *Small Animal Medicine Cardiology Textbook, 2nd Ed.*, Accessed Online via the Veterinary Drug Information Network.

Kittleson, M.D. (1985). Pathophysiology and treatment of heart failure. *Manual of Small Animal Cardiology*. LP Tilley and JM Owens Eds. New York, Churchill Livingstone: 308−33pp.

Mogg, T. (1999). Equine Cardiac Disease: Clinical pharmacology and therapeutics. *The Veterinary Clinics of North America: Equine Practice* 15:3(December).

HYDROCHLORO-THIAZIDE

(hye-*droe*-klor-oh-*thye*-a-zide)
HydroDIURIL®

THIAZIDE DIURETIC

Prescriber Highlights

▶ Thiazide diuretic used for nephrogenic diabetes insipidus, hypertension, calcium oxalate uroliths, hypoglycemia, & diuretic for heart failure

▶ Contraindications: Hypersensitivity; pregnancy (relative contraindication)

▶ Extreme Caution/Avoid: Severe renal disease, preexisting electrolyte/water balance abnormalities, impaired hepatic function, hyperuricemia, SLE, diabetes mellitus

▶ Adverse Effects: Hypokalemia, hypochloremic alkalosis, other electrolyte imbalances, hyperuricemia, GI effects

▶ Many possible drug interactions; lab test interactions

Uses/Indications

In veterinary medicine, furosemide has largely supplanted the use of thiazides as a general diuretic (edema treatment). But there are times when they can be very useful drugs. Thiazides are still used for the treatment of systemic hypertension, ascites, hypermagnesemia, neph-rogenic diabetes insipidus, and to help prevent the recurrence of calcium oxalate uroliths in dogs, and potentially cats. In horses, hydro-chlorothiazide may be used as an alternative to acetazolamide for HyPP in horses where dietary therapy alone does not control episodes.

Pharmacology/Actions

Thiazide diuretics act by interfering with the transport of sodium ions across renal tubular epithelium possibly by altering the metabolism of tubular cells. The principle site of action is at the cortical diluting segment of the nephron. Enhanced excretion of sodium, chloride, and water results. Thiazides increase the excretion of potassium, magnesium, phosphate, iodide, and bromide and decrease the glomerular fil-tration rate (GFR). Plasma renin and resulting aldosterone levels are increased which contrib-ute to the hypokalemic effects of the thiazides. Bicarbonate excretion is increased, but effects on urine pH are usually minimal. Thiazides initially have a hypercalciuric effect, although with continued therapy calcium excretion this is significantly decreased. Uric acid excretion is decreased by the thiazides. Thiazides can cause or exacerbate hyperglycemia in diabetic patients or induce diabetes mellitus in predia-betic patients.

The antihypertensive effects of thiazides are well known and these agents are used extensively in human medicine for treating essential hyper-tension. The exact mechanism for this effect has not been established.

Thiazides paradoxically reduce urine output in patients with diabetes insipidus (DI). They have been used as adjunctive therapy in patients with neurogenic DI and are the only drug thera-py for nephrogenic DI.

Pharmacokinetics

The pharmacokinetics of the thiazides have ap-parently not been studied in domestic animals. In humans, hydrochlorothiazide is about 65–75% absorbed after oral administration. The on-set of diuretic activity occurs in 2 hours; peaks at 4–6 hours. The serum half-life is approximately 5.6–14.8 hours and the duration of activity is 6–12 hours. The drug is apparently not metabo-lized and is excreted unchanged into the urine. Like all thiazides, the antihypertensive effects of hydrochlorothiazide may take several days to occur.

Contraindications/Precautions/Warnings

Thiazides are contraindicated in patients hyper-sensitive to any one of these agents or to sulfon-amides, and in patients with anuria. In humans, their use is inappropriate during pregnancy in women who are otherwise healthy and have only mild edema.

Do not use in dogs with absorptive (intesti-nal) hypercalcuria as hypercalcemia may result.

Thiazides should be used with extreme cau-tion, if at all, in patients with severe renal dis-ease or with preexisting electrolyte (including hypercalcemia) or water balance abnormalities, impaired hepatic function (may precipitate hepatic coma), hyperuricemia, lupus (SLE), or diabetes mellitus. Patients with conditions that may lead to electrolyte or water balance abnor-malities (e.g., vomiting, diarrhea, etc.) should be monitored carefully.

Adverse Effects

Hypokalemia is one of the most common ad-verse effects associated with the thiazides but rarely causes clinical signs or progresses, how-ever, monitoring of potassium is recommended with chronic therapy.

Hypochloremic alkalosis (with hypokalemia) may develop, especially if there are other causes of potassium and chloride loss (e.g., vomit-ing, diarrhea, potassium-losing nephropathies, etc.) or the patient has cirrhotic liver disease. Dilutional hyponatremia and hypomagnesemia may occur. Hyperparathyroid-like effects of hy-percalcemia and hypophosphatemia have been reported in humans, but have not led to effects such as nephrolithiasis, bone resorption, or pep-tic ulceration.

Hyperuricemia can occur, but is usually as-ymptomatic.

Other possible adverse effects include: GI re-actions (vomiting, diarrhea, etc.), hypersensitiv-ity/dermatologic reactions, GU reactions (poly-uria), hematologic toxicity, hyperglycemia, hyperlipidemias, and orthostatic hypotension.

Reproductive/Nursing Safety

In humans, the FDA categorizes this drug as cat-egory *B* for use during pregnancy (*Animal stud-ies have not yet demonstrated risk to the fetus, but there are no adequate studies in pregnant women; or animal studies have shown an adverse effect, but adequate studies in pregnant women have not demonstrated a risk to the fetus in the first trimes-ter of pregnancy, and there is no evidence of risk in later trimesters.*) In a separate system evaluating the safety of drugs in canine and feline preg-nancy (Papich 1989), thiazides are categorized as in class: *C* (*These drugs may have potential risks. Studies in people or laboratory animals have un-covered risks, and these drugs should be used cau-tiously as a last resort when the benefit of therapy clearly outweighs the risks.*)

Thiazides may appear in milk and there have been case reports of newborn human infants de-veloping thrombocytopenia when their mothers received thiazides.

Overdosage/Acute Toxicity

Acute overdosage may cause electrolyte and wa-ter balance problems, CNS effects (lethargy to coma and seizures), and GI effects (hypermotil-ity, GI distress). Transient increases in BUN have been reported.

Treatment consists of emptying the gut after recent oral ingestion using standard protocols.

Avoid giving concomitant cathartics as they may exacerbate the fluid and electrolyte imbalances that may ensue. Monitor and treat electrolyte and water balance abnormalities supportively. Additionally, monitor respiratory, CNS, and cardiovascular status; treat supportively and symptomatically if required.

Drug Interactions

The following drug interactions have either been reported or are theoretical in humans or animals receiving hydrochlorothiazide and may be of significance in veterinary patients:

- **AMPHOTERICIN B:** Use with thiazides can lead to an increased risk for severe hypokalemia
- **CORTICOSTEROIDS, CORTICOTROPIN:** Use with thiazides can lead to an increased risk for severe hypokalemia
- **DIAZOXIDE:** Increased risk for hyperglycemia, hyperuricemia, and hypotension
- **DIGOXIN:** Thiazide-induced hypokalemia, hypo-magnesemia, and/or hypercalcemia may increase the likelihood of digitalis toxicity
- **INSULIN:** Thiazides may increase insulin requirements
- **LITHIUM:** Thiazides can increase serum lithium concentrations
- **METHENAMINE:** Thiazides can alkalinize urine and reduce methenamine effectiveness
- **NSAIDS:** Thiazides may increase risk for renal toxicity and NSAIDs may reduce diuretic actions of thiazides
- **NEUROMUSCULAR BLOCKING AGENTS:** Tubocurarine or other nondepolarizing neuromuscular blocking agents response or duration of effect may be increased
- **PROBENECID:** Blocks thiazide-induced uric acid retention (used to therapeutic advantage)
- **QUINIDINE:** Half-life may be prolonged by thiazides (thiazides can alkalinize the urine)
- **VITAMIN D OR CALCIUM SALTS:** Hypercalcemia may be exacerbated if thiazides are concurrently administered

Laboratory Considerations

- **AMYLASE:** Thiazides can increase serum amylase values in asymptomatic patients and those in the developmental stages of acute pancreatitis (humans)
- **CORTISOL:** Thiazides can decrease the renal excretion of cortisol
- **ESTROGEN, URINARY:** Hydrochlorothiazide may falsely decrease total urinary estrogen when using a spectrophotometric assay
- **HISTAMINE:** Thiazides may cause false-negative results when testing for pheochromocytoma
- **PARATHYROID-FUNCTION TESTS:** Thiazides may elevate serum calcium; recommend to discontinue thiazides prior to testing

- **PHENOLSULFONPHTHALEIN (PSP):** Thiazides can compete for secretion at proximal renal tubules
- **PHENTOLAMINE TEST:** Thiazides may give false-negative results
- **PROTEIN-BOUND IODINE:** Thiazides may decrease values
- **TRIIODOTHYRONINE RESIN UPTAKE TEST:** Thiazides may slightly reduce uptake
- **TYRAMINE:** Thiazides can cause false-negative results

Doses

- **DOGS:**

For treatment of nephrogenic diabetes insipidus:

a) Based on a case report: 2 mg/kg PO twice daily with a low sodium diet. (Takemura 1998)

b) 2.5–5 mg/kg PO twice daily (Nichols 1989)

For treatment of systemic hypertension:

a) As a second choice agent, 1 mg/kg PO q12–24h; may combine with spironolactone (1–2 mg/kg PO q12 hours) to reduce potassium loss (Brown & Henik 2000), (Brown 2008)

For prevention of recurrent calcium oxalate uroliths with renal hypercalcuria (usually added when dietary therapy does not adequately control calcium oxalate crystalluria):

a) 2 mg/kg q12h PO (Polzin & Osborne 1985), (Adams 2009)

b) 2.2 mg/kg PO q12h; repeat urinalysis q2–4 weeks and monitor serum electrolytes within several weeks of initial dose and within 2 weeks of dosage adjustment (Lulich et al. 2000)

c) 2–4 mg/kg PO q12h (Bartges 2006)

As a diuretic:

a) For heart failure In combination with furosemide in patients who have become refractory to furosemide alone: 2–4 mg/kg PO q12h (Kittleson 2000), (Kittleson 2006)

b) For adjunctive treatment of heart failure when a dog requires 4–5 mg/kg PO q8h of furosemide and continues to exhibit clinical signs of congestion, reduce the furosemide dose by 50% and add hydrochlorothiazide at 2 mg/kg PO q12h. (Saunders 2008)

c) For ascites secondary to right-sided heart failure; In addition to furosemide (4–6 mg/kg PO q8h), spironolactone (1–2 mg/kg PO q12h), ACE inhibitors, dietary sodium restriction, etc consider: hydrochlorothiazide at 2 mg/kg initially on an every other day bases; monitor electrolytes and renal function. (Connolly 2006)

d) For ascites in patients with liver disease: Using the fixed-dose combination with spironolactone (*aka Aldactazide®*): Dosed empirically based on the spironolactone content at 0.5–1 mg/kg PO twice daily. (Trepanier 2008)

e) 1–4 mg/kg PO q12h (Haskins 2007)

■ **CATS:**

For treatment of systemic hypertension:

a) As a second choice agent, 1 mg/kg PO q12–24h; may combine with spironolactone (1–2 mg/kg PO q12 hours) to reduce potassium loss (Brown & Henik 2000), (Brown, 2008)

b) 2–4 mg/kg PO q12h. Not effective as a single agent in cats, and may be contraindicated (*e.g.*, chronic renal failure). Possibly helpful acutely with retinal detachment. (Sparkes, 2003)

As a diuretic:

a) For heart failure: In combination with furosemide in patients who have become refractory to furosemide alone: 1–2 mg/kg PO q12h (Kittleson 2000). (Kittleson 2006)

b) For ascites in patients with liver disease: Using the fixed-dose combination with spironolactone (*aka Aldactazide®*): Dosed empirically based on the spironolactone content at 0.5–1 mg/kg PO twice daily. (Trepanier 2008)

To reduce calcium oxalate saturation in urine:

a) Study done in normal cats, unknown what effect HCTZ will have in cats with spontaneously occurring calcium oxalate urolithiasis: 1 mg/kg PO q12h. (Hezel *et al.* 2007)

■ **HORSES: (Note:** ARCI UCGFS Class 4 Drug)

For adjunctive therapy of hyperkalemic periodic paralysis (HyPP):

a) 0.5–1 mg/kg PO q12h when diet adjustment does not control episodes. (Valberg 2008)

Client Information

■ Clients should contact veterinarian if clinical signs of water or electrolyte imbalance occur. Clinical signs such as excessive thirst, lethargy, lassitude, restlessness, oliguria, GI distress, or tachycardia may indicate electrolyte or water balance problem.

Chemistry/Synonyms

Hydrochlorothiazide occurs as a practically odorless, slightly bitter-tasting, white, or practically white, crystalline powder with pK_as of 7.9 and 9.2. It is slightly soluble in water and soluble in alcohol.

Hydrochlorothiazide may also be known as: HCTZ, hidroclorotiazida, or hydrochlorothiazidum; many trade names are available.

Storage/Stability

Hydrochlorothiazide capsules and tablets should be stored at room temperature in well-closed containers.

Compatibility/Compounding Considerations

Compounded preparation stability: Spironolactone and hydrochlorothiazide oral suspension compounded from commercially available tablets has been published (Allen & Erickson 1996). Triturating twenty-four (24) spironolactone and hydrochlorothiazide 25/25 mg tablets with 60 mL of *Ora-Plus®* and qs ad to 120 mL with *Ora-Sweet®* (or *Ora-Sweet® SF*) yields a 5 mg/mL suspension of both spironolactone and hydrochlorothiazide that retains >90% potency for 60 days stored at both 5°C and 25°C. Compounded preparations of hydrochlorothiazide should be protected from light.

Dosage Forms/Regulatory Status

VETERINARY-LABELED PRODUCTS:
None. The ARCI (Racing Commissioners International) has designated this drug as a class 4 substance. See the appendix for more information.

HUMAN-LABELED PRODUCTS:
Hydrochlorothiazide Oral Tablets: 25 mg, 50 mg, & 100 mg; *HydroDIURIL®* (Merck); *Hydro-Par®* (Parmed); *Ezide®* (Econo Med); generic; (Rx)

Hydrochlorothiazide Oral Capsules: 12.5 mg; *Microzide® Capsules* (Watson); generic; (Rx)

Spironolactone/Hydrochlorothiazide Oral Tablets: 25 mg/25 mg & 50 mg/50 mg; *Aldactazide®* (Searle), generic; (Rx)

There are other fixed dose combinations available with hydrochlorothiazide, including: hydralazine, amiloride, propranolol, triamterene, captopril, reserpine, enalapril, guanethidine, metoprolol, timolol, methyldopa or labetolol.

References

Adams, L. (2009). Minimally Invasive Management of Uroliths: To Cut or Not to Cut. Proceedings: WVC. Accessed via: Veterinary Information Network. http://goo.gl/ERRua

Allen, L.V. & M.A. Erickson (1996). Stability of labetalol hydrochloride, metoprolol tartrate, verapamil hydrochloride, and spironolactone with hydrochlorothiazide in extemporaneously compounded oral liquids. . *Am J Health Syst Pharm* 53(19): 2304–2309.

Bartges, J. (2006). Rock 'N' Roll Cats: Urolithiasis. Proceedings: ACVC 2006. Accessed via: Veterinary Information Network. http://goo.gl/EADQy

Brown, S. (2008). Current Knowledge in the Field of Renoprotection: Blood Pressure Control. Proceedings: ECVIM. Accessed via: Veterinary Information Network. http://goo.gl/qv8nM

Brown, S. & R. Henik (2000). Therapy for Systemic Hypertension in Dogs and Cats. *Kirk's Current Veterinary Therapy: XIII Small Animal Practice.* J Bonagura Ed. Philadelphia, WB Saunders: 838–841.

Connolly, D. (2006). The ascitic dog. Proceedings: BSAVA Congress. Accessed via: Veterinary Information Network. http://goo.gl/BB9AX

Haskins, S. (2007). Diuretics and the critical patient. Proceedings: IVECCS. Accessed via: Veterinary Information Network. http://goo.gl/TDpTX

Hezel, A., J. Bartges, et al. (2007). Influence of Hydrochlorothiazide on Urinary Calcium Oxalate Relative Supersaturation in Healthy Young Adult Female Domestic Shorthaired Cats.

Kittleson, M. (2000). Therapy of Heart Failure. *Textbook of Veterinary Internal Medicine: Diseases of the Dog and Cat.* S Ettinger and E Feldman Eds. Philadelphia, WB Saunders. 1: 713–737.

Kittleson, M. (2006). "Chapt 10: Management of Heart Failure." *Small Animal Cardiology, 2nd Ed.*

Lulich, J., C. Osborne, et al. (2000). Canine Lower Urinary Tract Disorders. *Textbook of Veterinary Internal Medicine: Diseases of the Dog and Cat.* S Ettinger and E Feldman Eds. WB Saunders. 2: 1747–1781.

Nichols, R. (1989). Diabetes Insipidus. *Current Veterinary Therapy X: Small Animal Practice.* RW Krik Ed. Philadeliphia, WB Saunders: 974–978.

Polzin, D.J. & C.A. Osborne (1985). Diseases of the Urinary Tract. *Handbook of Small Animal Therapeutics.* LE Davis Ed. New York, Churchill Livingstone: 333–395.

Saunders, A.B. (2008). Diagnosis & Therapy for Canine Heart Failure. *Peroceedings: WVC.*

Sparkes, A. (2003). Feline systemic hypertension–A hidden killer. Proceedings: World Small Animal Veterinary Assoc. Accessed via: Veterinary Information Network. http://goo.gl/QgVkr

Takemura, N. (1998). Successful long-term treatment of congenital nephrogenic diabetes insipidus in a dog. *Journal of Small Animal Practice* 39(12): 592–594.

Trepanier, L. (2008). Choosing therapy for chronic liver disease. Proceedings: WSAVA. Accessed via: Veterinary Information Network. http://goo.gl/NLh4X

Valberg, S. (2008). Muscle Tremors in Horses. Proceedings: Western Veterinary Conference. Accessed via: Veterinary Information Network. http://goo.gl/xNHsO

HYDROCODONE BITARTRATE

(hye-droe-*koe*-done)   Tussigon®, Hycodan®

OPIATE

Prescriber Highlights

▶ Opiate agonist used primarily as an antitussive in dogs. Also potentially useful as an oral analgesic for moderate pain in dogs.

▶ Contraindications: Hypersensitivity to narcotic analgesic, patients receiving monoamine oxidase inhibitors (MAOIs; Selegiline?), diarrhea caused by a toxic ingestion. Any combination product containing acetaminophen must NOT be used in cats.

▶ Caution: Patients with hypothyroidism, severe renal insufficiency, adrenocortical insufficiency (Addison's), head injuries or increased intracranial pressure, acute abdominal conditions, & geriatric or severely debilitated patients

▶ Use extreme caution in patients suffering from respiratory diseases when respiratory secretions are increased or when liquids are nebulized into the respiratory tract

▶ Adverse Effects: Sedation, constipation (with chronic therapy), vomiting, or other GI disturbances

▶ May mask the clinical signs (cough) of respiratory disease

▶ Combination products are C-III controlled substances

Uses/Indications

Used principally in canine medicine as an antitussive for cough secondary to conditions such as collapsing trachea, bronchitis, or canine upper respiratory infection complex (C-URI, "kennel cough", canine infectious tracheobronchitis). Its use is generally reserved for harsh, dry, nonproductive coughs. Hydrocodone may be useful in treating opioid-related behavior problems in dogs and cats (lick granuloma, stereotypies) by providing an exogenous source of opioid, thereby reducing the need for the self-stimulating behavior.

The human combination products containing hydrocodone and acetaminophen potentially could be useful oral analgesics in dogs (NOT cats).

Pharmacology/Actions

While hydrocodone exhibits the characteristics of other opiate agonists, it tends to have a slightly greater antitussive effect than codeine (on a weight basis). The mechanism of this effect is thought to be as a result of direct suppression of the cough reflex on the cough center in the medulla. Hydrocodone tends to have a drying effect on respiratory mucosa and the viscosity of respiratory secretions may be increased; the addition of homatropine MBr (in *Hycodan®* and others) may enhance this effect. Hydrocodone may also be more sedating than codeine, but it is not more constipating.

Pharmacokinetics

In humans, hydrocodone is well absorbed after oral administration and has a serum half-life of about 3.8 hours; antitussive effect usually lasts 4–6 hours in adults.

Hydrocodone has an oral bioavailability of 40%-80% in dogs. Hydrocodone is partially metabolized to hydromorphone. The antitussive and analgesic actions of hydrocodone generally persist for 6–12 hours.

Contraindications/Precautions/Warnings

Hydrocodone is contraindicated in cases where the patient is hypersensitive to narcotic analgesics, and those with diarrhea caused by a toxic ingestion (until the toxin is eliminated from the GI tract). All opiates should be used with caution in patients with hypothyroidism, severe renal insufficiency, adrenocortical insufficiency (Addison's), and geriatric or severely debilitated patients.

Hydrocodone products containing acetaminophen (*e.g., Vicodin®, Lortab®*, etc.) must not be used in cats.

Hydrocodone should be used with caution in patients with head injuries or increased intracranial pressure and acute abdominal conditions as it may obscure the diagnosis or clinical course of these conditions. It should be used with extreme caution in patients suffering from respiratory diseases when respiratory secretions are increased or when liquids are nebulized into the respiratory tract.

Hydrocodone products have a relatively high abuse potential in humans and veterinarians are advised to be on the lookout for drug seeking clients.

Adverse Effects

Side effects that may be encountered with hydrocodone therapy in dogs include sedation, constipation (with chronic therapy), vomiting or other GI disturbances.

Hydrocodone may mask the clinical signs (cough) of respiratory disease and should not take the place of appropriate specific treatments for the underlying cause of coughs.

Reproductive/Nursing Safety

In humans, the FDA categorizes this drug as category *C* for use during pregnancy (*Animal studies have shown an adverse effect on the fetus, but there are no adequate studies in humans; or there are no animal reproduction studies and no adequate studies in humans*).

It is unknown if hydrocodone enters milk; use with caution.

Overdosage/Acute Toxicity

The initial concern with a very large overdose of *Hycodan®* (or equivalent) would be the CNS, cardiovascular and respiratory depression secondary to the opiate effects.

There were 21 exposures to hydrocodone bitartrate reported to the ASPCA Animal Poison Control Center (APCC; www.apcc.aspca.org) during 2001–2006. In these cases 18 were dogs and 3 were cats. No clinical signs were reported in these cases.

If the ingestion was recent, emptying the gut using standard protocols should be performed and treatment with naloxone instituted as necessary. The homatropine ingredient may give rise to anticholinergic effects that may complicate the clinical picture, but its relatively low toxicity may not require any treatment. For further information on handling opiate or anticholinergic overdoses, refer to the meperidine and atropine monographs, respectively.

Drug Interactions

The following drug interactions have either been reported or are theoretical in humans or animals receiving hydrocodone and may be of significance in veterinary patients:

- ■ **ACEPROMAZINE:** Acepromazine and hydrocodone may cause additive hypotension in dogs with collapsing trachea
- ■ **ANTICHOLINERGIC DRUGS:** May cause additive anticholinergic effects
- ■ **ANTIDEPRESSANTS, TRICYCLIC & MOA INHIBITORS:** Use with hydrocodone may potentiate the adverse effects associated with the antidepressant
- ■ **CNS DEPRESSANTS, OTHER:** Other CNS depressants (*e.g.*, anesthetic agents, antihistamines, phenothiazines, barbiturates, tranquilizers, alcohol, etc.) may cause increased CNS or respiratory depression when used with hydrocodone.

Doses

- ■ **DOGS:**
  a) For cough: 0.22 mg/kg PO q6–12h; goal is to suppress coughing without causing excessive sedation (Johnson 2000)
  b) As an analgesic using the fixed dose combination products with acetaminophen: 0.22–0.5 mg/kg of the hydrocodone component PO q8-12h. Do not exceed 15 mg/kg of the acetaminophen component q8h. (KuKanich 2008)
  c) For cough using *Hycodan®* (or equivalent): ¼ to 1 tablet (5 mg) once to 4 times daily in small and medium sized dogs. For lick granulomas: 5–10 mg (1–2 tablets) per 20 kg of body weight PO three times daily. (Trepanier 1999)
  d) For adjunctive treatment of opioid-related stereotypies, lick granuloma: 0.22–0.25 mg/kg PO q8–12h. Supplies

exogenous opioids to decrease the need for self-stimulation. (Siebert 2003)

■ **CATS:**

a) For adjunctive treatment of opioid-related stereotypies: 1.25–5 mg per cat PO q12h. Supplies exogenous opioids to decrease the need for self-stimulation. *(NOTE: Do NOT use any product that contains acetaminophen—Plumb)* (Siebert 2003)

Monitoring

■ Clinical efficacy

■ Adverse effects

Chemistry/Synonyms

A phenanthrene-derivative opiate agonist, hydrocodone bitartrate occurs as fine, white crystals or crystalline powder. One gram is soluble in about 16 mL of water; it is slightly soluble in alcohol.

Hydrocodone bitartrate may also be as: hydrocodone tartrate, dihydrocodeinone acid tartrate, hydrocodone acid tartrate, hydrocodoni bitartras, hydrocone bitartrate, *Biocodone®*, *Dicodid®*, *Hydrokon®*, and *Robidone®*.

Storage/Stability

Products should be protected from light.

Dosage Forms/Regulatory Status

VETERINARY-LABELED PRODUCTS: None

The ARCI (Racing Commissioners International) has designated this drug as a class 1 substance. See the appendix for more information.

HUMAN-LABELED PRODUCTS:

Hydrocodone Bitartrate Oral Tablets: 5 mg, Homatropine MBr 1.5 mg; *Tussigon®* (Daniels); *Hycodan®* (Endo); (Rx, C-III)

Hydrocodone Bitartrate Oral Syrup: 5 mg, Homatropine MBr 1.5 mg (per 5 mL) in 473 mL and 3.8 L; *Hycodan® Syrup* (Endo); *Hydromet® Syrup* (Alpharma); *Hydromide® Syrup* (Major); *Hydropane® Syrup* (Watson); (Rx, C-III)

The following are representative oral dosage forms containing hydrocodone and acetaminophen and include those most likely to be of benefit in treating dogs (higher ratios of hydrocodone:acetaminophen) and are usually stocked at human pharmacies. **WARNING:** These products must NOT be used in cats:

Hydrocodone/Acetaminophen Oral Tablets: 5 mg/325mg, 5 mg/500 mg (also available in capsules), 7.5 mg/325mg, & 10 mg/325mg. An oral elixir containing hydrocodone 2.5mg/5 mL and acetaminophen 167 mg/5 mL (0.5 mg/mL hydrocodone and 33.3 mg/mL of acetaminophen) is also readily available. Commonly used trade names for these products include: *Vicodin®*, *Norco®*, and *Lortabs®*.

There are also oral tablets and liquids with hydrocodone available in combination with

decongestants (pseudoephedrine, phenylephrine, or phenylpropanolamine), antihistamines (chlorpheniramine), analgesics (ibuprofen or aspirin) or expectorants (guaifenesin). In the USA, there are no hydrocodone products available as a sole ingredient. All commercially available products containing hydrocodone are Class-III controlled substances.

References

Johnson, L. (2000). Diseases of the Bronchus. *Textbook of Veterinary Internal Medicine: Diseases of the Dog and Cat.* S Ettinger and E Feldman Eds. Philadelphia, WB Saunders. 2: 1055–1061.

KuKanich, B. (2008). Beyond NSAIDs and Opioids. Proceedings: WVC. Accessed via: Veterinary Information Network. http://goo.gl/tY3VR

Siebert, L. (2003). Antidepressants in behavioral medicine. Proceedings: Western Veterinary Conference. Accessed via: Veterinary Information Network. http://goo.gl/HHo8w

Trepanier, L. (1999). Fifteen Drugs Useful in Dogs. American Animal Hospital Association: Proceedings from the 1999 Annual Meeting, Denver.

HYDROCORTISONE
HYDROCORTISONE SODIUM SUCCINATE

(hye-droe-*kor*-ti-zone)

Cortef®, Solu-Cortef®

GLUCOCORTICOID

Prescriber Highlights

▶ "Benchmark" injectable, oral, & topical glucocorticoid (depending on salt)

▶ Has both mineralocorticoid & glucocorticoid activity

▶ If using for therapy, goal is to use as much as is required & as little as possible, for as short an amount of time as possible

▶ Primary adverse effects are "Cushingoid" in nature with sustained use

▶ Many potential drug & lab interactions

Uses/Indications

Because of its rapid effect and relatively high mineralocorticoid effect, hydrocortisone sodium succinate (*Solu-Cortef®*) is the most commonly used form of this medication when an acute glucocorticoid/mineralocorticoid effect is desired (*e.g.*, acute adrenal insufficiency). Corticosteroids have not been shown beneficial in treating hypovolemic shock, but low dose glucocorticoids probably reduce mortality associated with septic shock.

Glucocorticoids have been used in an attempt to treat practically every malady that afflicts man or animal, but there are three broad uses and dosage ranges for use of these agents. 1) Replacement of glucocorticoid activity in patients with adrenal insufficiency, 2) as an antiinflammatory agent, and 3) as an immunosuppressive. Among some of the uses for gluco-corticoids include treatment of: endocrine conditions (*e.g.*, adrenal insufficiency), rheumatic diseases (*e.g.*, rheumatoid arthritis), collagen diseases (*e.g.*, systemic lupus), allergic states, respiratory diseases (*e.g.*, asthma), dermatologic diseases (*e.g.*, pemphigus, allergic dermatoses), hematologic disorders (*e.g.*, thrombocytopenias, autoimmune hemolytic anemias), neoplasias, nervous system disorders (increased CSF pressure), GI diseases (*e.g.*, ulcerative colitis exacerbations), and renal diseases (*e.g.*, nephrotic syndrome). Some glucocorticoids are used topically in the eye and skin for various conditions or are injected intra-articularly or intra-lesionally. The above listing is certainly not complete.

Pharmacology/Actions
Glucocorticoids have effects on virtually every cell type and system in mammals. See the Glucocorticoid General Information monograph for more information.

Pharmacokinetics
In humans, hydrocortisone is readily absorbed after oral administration. Hydrocortisone sodium succinate is administered parenterally, and absorption is rapid after IM administration. Duration of activity is 8-12 hours.

Contraindications/Precautions/Warnings
Systemic use of glucocorticoids are generally considered contraindicated in systemic fungal infections (unless used for replacement therapy in Addison's), when administered IM in patients with idiopathic thrombocytopenia, and in patients hypersensitive to a particular compound. Use of sustained-release injectable glucocorticoids is considered contraindicated for chronic corticosteroid therapy of systemic diseases.

Animals that have received glucocorticoids systemically other than with "burst" therapy, should be tapered off the drugs. Patients who have received the drugs chronically should be tapered off slowly as endogenous ACTH and corticosteroid function may return slowly. Should the animal undergo a "stressor" (*e.g.*, surgery, trauma, illness, etc.) during the tapering process or until normal adrenal and pituitary function resume, additional glucocorticoids should be administered.

Adverse Effects
Adverse effects are generally associated with long-term administration of these drugs, especially if given at high dosages or not on an alternate day regimen. Effects generally manifest as clinical signs of hyperadrenocorticism. When administered to young, growing animals, glucocorticoids can retard growth. Many of the potential effects, adverse and otherwise, are outlined above in the Pharmacology section.

In dogs, polydipsia (PD), polyphagia (PP), and polyuria (PU), may all be seen with short-term "burst" therapy as well as with alternate-day maintenance therapy on days when drug is given. Adverse effects in dogs can include: dull, dry haircoat, weight gain, panting, vomiting, diarrhea, elevated liver enzymes, pancreatitis, GI ulceration, lipidemias, activation or worsening of diabetes mellitus, muscle wasting and behavioral changes (depression, lethargy, viciousness). Discontinuation of the drug may be necessary; changing to an alternate steroid may also alleviate the problem. With the exception of PU/PD/PP, adverse effects associated with antiinflammatory therapy are relatively uncommon. Adverse effects associated with immunosuppressive doses are more common and potentially more severe.

Cats generally require higher dosages than dogs for clinical effect, but tend to develop fewer adverse effects. Occasionally, polydipsia, polyuria, polyphagia with weight gain, diarrhea, or depression can be seen. Long-term, high dose therapy can lead to "Cushingoid" effects.

Reproductive/Nursing Safety
Glucocorticoids are probably necessary for normal fetal development. They may be required for adequate surfactant production, myelin, retinal, pancreatic, and mammary development. Excessive dosages early in pregnancy may lead to teratogenic effects. In horses and ruminants, exogenous steroid administration may induce parturition when administered in the latter stages of pregnancy. In humans, the FDA categorizes this drug as category *C* for use during pregnancy (*Animal studies have shown an adverse effect on the fetus, but there are no adequate studies in humans; or there are no animal reproduction studies and no adequate studies in humans.*)

Glucocorticoids unbound to plasma proteins will enter milk. High dosages or prolonged administration to mothers may potentially inhibit the growth of nursing newborns.

Overdosage/Acute Toxicity
Glucocorticoids when given short-term are unlikely to cause harmful effects, even in massive dosages. One incidence of a dog developing acute CNS effects after accidental ingestion of glucocorticoids has been reported. Should clinical signs occur, use supportive treatment if required.

Chronic usage of glucocorticoids can lead to serious adverse effects. Refer to Adverse Effects above for more information.

Drug Interactions
The following drug interactions have either been reported or are theoretical in humans or animals receiving hydrocortisone and may be of significance in veterinary patients:

- ■ **AMPHOTERICIN B:** Administered concomitantly with glucocorticoids may cause hypokalemia; in humans, there have been cases of CHF and cardiac enlargement reported after using hydrocortisone to treat Amphotericin B adverse effects

- ■ **ANTICHOLINESTERASE AGENTS (*e.g.*, pyr-**

idostigmine, neostigmine, etc.): In patients with myasthenia gravis, concomitant glucocorticoid and anticholinesterase agent administration may lead to profound muscle weakness. If possible, discontinue anticholinesterase medication at least 24 hours prior to corticosteroid administration

■ **ASPIRIN:** Glucocorticoids may reduce salicylate blood levels and increase risk for GI ulceration/bleeding

■ **BARBITURATES:** May increase the metabolism of glucocorticoids and decrease flumethasone blood levels

■ **CYCLOPHOSPHAMIDE:** Glucocorticoids may inhibit the hepatic metabolism of cyclophosphamide; dosage adjustments may be required

■ **CYCLOSPORINE:** Concomitant administration of glucocorticoids and cyclosporine may increase the blood levels of each by mutually inhibiting the hepatic metabolism of each other; the clinical significance of this interaction is not clear

■ **DIURETICS, POTASSIUM-DEPLETING (e.g., spironolactone, triamterene):** Administered concomitantly with glucocorticoids may cause hypokalemia

■ **EPHEDRINE:** May reduce hydrocortisone blood levels

■ **ESTROGENS:** The effects of hydrocortisone and, possibly, other glucocorticoids, may be potentiated by concomitant administration with estrogens

■ **INSULIN:** Insulin requirements may increase in patients receiving glucocorticoids

■ **KETOCONAZOLE AND OTHER AZOLE ANTI-FUNGALS:** May decrease the metabolism of glucocorticoids and increase hydrocortisone blood levels; ketoconazole may induce adrenal insufficiency when glucocorticoids are withdrawn by inhibiting adrenal corticosteroid synthesis

■ **MACROLIDE ANTIBIOTICS (erythromycin, clarithromycin):** May decrease the metabolism of glucocorticoids and increase hydrocortisone blood levels

■ **MITOTANE:** May alter the metabolism of steroids; higher than usual doses of steroids may be necessary to treat mitotane-induced adrenal insufficiency

■ **NSAIDS:** Administration of ulcerogenic drugs with glucocorticoids may increase the risk of gastrointestinal ulceration

■ **PHENOBARBITAL:** May increase the metabolism of glucocorticoids and decrease hydrocortisone blood levels

■ **RIFAMPIN:** May increase the metabolism of glucocorticoids and decrease hydrocortisone blood levels

■ **VACCINES:** Patients receiving corticosteroids at immunosuppressive dosages should generally not receive live attenuated-virus vaccines as virus replication may be augmented; a diminished immune response may occur after vaccine, toxoid, or bacterin administration in patients receiving glucocorticoids

■ **WARFARIN:** Hydrocortisone may affect INR's; monitor

Laboratory Considerations

■ Hydrocortisone can cross react with cortisol in ACTH response test. This test must be performed before hydrocortisone is administered. (**Note:** Dexamethasone does not cross react)

■ Glucocorticoids may increase **serum cholesterol**

■ Glucocorticoids may increase **urine glucose** levels

■ Glucocorticoids may decrease **serum potassium**

■ Glucocorticoids can suppress the release of thyroid stimulating hormone (TSH) and reduce T_3 & T_4 values. Thyroid gland atrophy has been reported after chronic glucocorticoid administration. Uptake of I^{131} by the thyroid may be decreased by glucocorticoids.

■ Reactions to **skin tests** may be suppressed by glucocorticoids

■ False-negative results of the **nitroblue tetrazolium** test for systemic bacterial infections may be induced by glucocorticoids

■ Glucocorticoids may cause **neutrophilia** within 4–8 hours after dosing and return to baseline within 24–48 hours after drug discontinuation

■ Glucocorticoids can cause **lymphopenia** which can persist for weeks after drug discontinuation in dogs

Doses

■ **DOGS:**

For adjunctive therapy for adrenocortical insufficiency:

a) For adjunctive treatment for acute hypoadrenocortical crisis: Hydrocortisone sodium succinate 0.5 mg/kg/hr as an IV infusion until GI function has returned, the dog is eating and drinking normally and can be changed to oral steroid supplementation. (Church 2009)

b) For adjunctive treatment of acute crisis: Hydrocortisone sodium succinate as a constant CRI of 0.3 mg/kg IV. May also be given IV at 2 mg/kg IV q6h or 2-4 mg/kg IV q8h. (Panciera 2009)

For adjunctive therapy of septic shock:

a) 0.08 mg/kg/hr IV. Low-dose hydrocortisone infusions can reduce the time that vasopressors are required and lead to earlier resolution of sepsis-induced organ dysfunction. (Crowe 2002)

■ **CATS:**

For adjunctive therapy of septic shock:

a) 0.08 mg/kg/hr IV. Low-dose hydrocortisone infusions can reduce the time that vasopressors are required and lead to earlier resolution of sepsis-induced organ dysfunction. (Crowe 2002)

■ **CATTLE:**

For adjunctive treatment of photosensitization reactions:

a) 100–600 mg (salt not specified) in 1000 mL of 10% dextrose saline IV or SC. (Black 1986)

■ **HORSES: (Note:** ARCI UCGFS Class 4 Drug) As a glucocorticoid:

a) Hydrocortisone sodium succinate: 1–4 mg/kg as an IV infusion (Robinson 1987)

Monitoring

Monitoring of glucocorticoid therapy is dependent on its reason for use, dosage, agent used (amount of mineralocorticoid activity), dosage schedule (daily versus alternate day therapy), duration of therapy, and the animal's age and condition. The following list may not be appropriate or complete for all animals; use clinical assessment and judgment should adverse effects be noted:

■ Weight, appetite, signs of edema

■ Serum and/or urine electrolytes

■ Total plasma proteins, albumin

■ Blood glucose

■ Growth and development in young animals

■ ACTH stimulation test if necessary

Client Information

■ Clients should carefully follow the dosage instructions and should not discontinue the drug abruptly without consulting with the veterinarian beforehand.

■ Clients should be briefed on the potential adverse effects that can be seen with these drugs and instructed to contact the veterinarian should these effects become severe or progress.

Chemistry/Synonyms

Also known as compound F or cortisol, hydrocortisone is secreted by the adrenal gland. Hydrocortisone occurs as an odorless, white to practically white, crystalline powder. It is very slightly soluble in water and sparingly soluble in alcohol. Hydrocortisone is administered orally.

Hydrocortisone sodium succinate occurs as an odorless, white to nearly white, hygroscopic, amorphous solid. It is very soluble in both water and alcohol. Hydrocortisone sodium succinate injection is administered via IM or IV routes.

Hydrocortisone may also be known as: antiin-

flammatory hormone, compound F, cortisol, hydrocortisonum, 17-hydroxycorticosterone, and NSC-10483; many trade names are available.

Storage/Stability

Hydrocortisone sodium succinate (HSS) in intact containers should be stored at controlled room temperatures of 68-77°F (20–25°C). After reconstitution, solutions are stable if protected from light and kept at, or below controlled room temperature. The solution should only be used if clear; discard unused solutions after three days. Hydrocortisone sodium succinate is heat labile and cannot be autoclaved. Reconstituted HSS 500 mg/4 mL solution kept frozen for 4 weeks showed no loss of potency.

Hydrocortisone tablets should be stored in well-closed containers. The cypionate oral suspension should be stored in tight, light resistant containers. All products should be stored at room temperature (15–30°C); avoid freezing the suspensions or solutions. After reconstituting solutions, only use products that are clear. Discard unused solutions after 3 days.

Compatibility/Compounding Considerations

Hydrocortisone sodium succinate is reportedly physically **compatible** with the following solutions and drugs: dextrose-Ringer's injection combinations, dextrose-Ringer's lactate injection combinations, dextrose-saline combinations, dextrose injections, Ringer's injection, lactated Ringer's injection, sodium chloride injections, amikacin sulfate, aminophylline, amphotericin B (limited quantities), calcium chloride/gluconate, cephalothin sodium (not in combination with aminophylline), cephapirin sodium, chloramphenicol sodium succinate, clindamycin phosphate, corticotropin, daunorubicin HCl, dopamine HCl, erythromycin gluceptate, erythromycin lactobionate, lidocaine HCl, mephentermine sulfate, metronidazole with sodium bicarbonate, netilmicin sodium, penicillin G potassium/sodium, piperacillin sodium, polymyxin B sulfate, potassium chloride, prochlorperazine edisylate, sodium bicarbonate, thiopental sodium, vancomycin HCl, verapamil HCl, and vitamin B-complex with C.

Hydrocortisone sodium succinate is reportedly physically **incompatible** when mixed with the following solutions and drugs: ampicillin sodium, bleomycin sulfate, colistimethate sodium, dimenhydrinate, diphenhydramine HCl, doxorubicin HCl, ephedrine sulfate, heparin sodium, hydralazine HCl, metaraminol bitartrate, methicillin sodium, nafcillin sodium, oxytetracycline HCl, pentobarbital sodium, phenobarbital sodium, promethazine HCl, secobarbital sodium, and tetracycline HCl.

Compatibility is dependent upon factors such as pH, concentration, temperature and diluent used; consult specialized references or a hospital pharmacist for more specific information.

Dosage Forms/Regulatory Status

VETERINARY-LABELED PRODUCTS:

There are no products containing hydrocortisone (or its salts) known for systemic use. There are a variety of hydrocortisone veterinary products for topical use. A 10 ppb tolerance has been established for hydrocortisone (as the succinate or acetate) in milk.

The ARCI (Racing Commissioners International) has designated this drug as a class 4 substance. See the appendix for more information.

HUMAN-LABELED PRODUCTS:

Hydrocortisone Oral Tablets: 5 mg, 10 mg, & 20 mg; *Cortef®* (Upjohn); generic; (Rx)

Hydrocortisone Sodium Succinate Injection: 100 mg/vial, 250 mg/vial, 500 mg/vial, 1000 mg/vial (as sodium succinate) in 2 mL, 4 mL and 8 mL *Univials*, fliptop vials, *Act-O-Vials* and vials; *Solu-Cortef®* (Pfizer); *A-Hydrocort®* (Hospira); (Rx)

There are many OTC and Rx topical and anorectal products available in a variety of dosage forms.

References

Black, L. (1986). Environmental skin conditions: Photosensitization with gangrene. *Current Veterinary Therapy: Food Animal Practice 2*. JL Howard Ed. Philadelphia, W.B. Saunders: 932–933.

Church, D.B. (2009). Management of Hypoadrenocorticism. Proceedings: WSAVA. Accessed via: Veterinary Information Network. http://goo.gl/1YHrT

Crowe, D. (2002). On the cutting edge of emergency and critical care. Proceedings: Western Veterinary Conference. Accessed via: Veterinary Information Network. http://goo.gl/j2w3I

Panciera, D. (2009). Diagnosis and management of hypoadrenocorticism. Proceedings: ACVC. Accessed via: Veterinary Information Network. http://goo.gl/bqWai

Robinson, N.E. (1987). Table of Common Drugs: Approximate Doses. *Current Therapy in Equine Medicine, 2*. NE Robinson Ed. Philadelphia, W.B. Saunders: 761.

HYDROGEN PEROXIDE 3% (ORAL)

(*hye*-droe-jen per-*oks*-ide)

ORAL EMETIC, TOPICAL ANTISEPTIC

Also see the Decontamination information in the appendix

Prescriber Highlights

▶ Topical antiseptic that is used orally as an emetic in dogs & sometimes cats particularly when clients cannot transport the patient to a veterinary hospital in a timely manner

▶ Many contraindications to use (for emesis)

Uses/Indications

Hydrogen peroxide 3% solution can be used as an orally administered emetic in dogs, cats, pigs and ferrets. It is best reserved for those cases when animals cannot be transported to a veterinary hospital in a timely way and immediate emesis is required. Apomorphine for dogs and cats (apomorphine is somewhat controversial for cats), or xylazine for cats are generally preferred emetic agents to be administered in a veterinary practice.

Pharmacology/Actions

Orally administered hydrogen peroxide solution (3%) induces a vomiting reflex via direct irritant effects of the oropharynx and gastric lining. After administering PO to dogs or cats, emesis usually ensues within 10 minutes.

Pharmacokinetics

No pharmacokinetic information located.

Contraindications/Precautions/Warnings

Do not induce emesis in those dogs or cats that are already vomiting, severely lethargic, comatose, debilitated (*e.g.*, respiratory distress, decreased swallowing reflex, bradycardia, etc.), seizuring or hyperactive, have had recent abdominal surgery or with megaesophagus. Emesis is generally contraindicated after ingestions of corrosives/caustics (*e.g.*, acids, alkalis), sharp objects, or bagged illicit drugs. Emesis is usually contraindicated after ingestion of a hydrocarbon or petroleum distillate.

Use caution when attempting to induce emesis in a dog that has ingested a compound that can cause seizures or CNS depression as CNS status may rapidly deteriorate.

Before inducing emesis, obtain a complete history of the ingestion and ensure that vital signs are stable.

Administration and emesis generally must occur within 4 hours (some say 2 hours or 6 hours maximum) of the toxic ingestion.

Do not use emetics in rodents or rabbits.

If home administration of hydrogen peroxide is necessary, be sure that clients use only the 3% medical grade solution and not another more concentrated hydrogen peroxide product.

Because aspiration and/or bradycardia are possible, animals should be closely observed after administration. Suctioning, respiratory and cardiovascular support (*e.g.*, atropine) should be available. Do not allow animal to re-ingest vomitus.

Successful induction of emesis does not ensure that stomach contents have been emptied and significant quantities of the ingested drug/toxin may remain or already been absorbed.

Adverse Effects

Aspiration of hydrogen peroxide solution during administration or stomach contents after inducing emesis is possible. Inducing emesis in animals with cardiovascular compromise may cause a vasovagal (bradycardic) response.

Gastric ulceration in cats and gastric-dilatation-volvulus in dogs have been reported.

Reproductive/Nursing Safety

No specific information was located. While orally administered 3% hydrogen peroxide is unlikely to cause reproductive harm, weigh the risks to the dam and offspring of the ingested toxin versus the risks associated with inducing emesis.

Overdosage/Acute Toxicity

Hydrogen peroxide 3% solution is relatively non-toxic (see Adverse Effects) after oral ingestion. Hydrogen peroxide in concentrations of 10% or greater can be very corrosive (severe burns to oral/gastric mucosa) and induce oxygen emboli after oral ingestion.

Drug Interactions

- **ACETYLCYSTEINE (oral):** Hydrogen peroxide can oxidize acetylcysteine in the gut and although clinical significance is unclear, alternative emetics (*e.g.,* apomorphine, xylazine) are preferred for acetaminophen overdoses

- **ANTIEMETICS (e.g., ondansetron, maropitant, etc.):** Preadministration or ingestion of these products may negate the emetic effects of hydrogen peroxide

Laboratory Considerations

- No specific concerns were noted.

Doses

- **DOGS/CATS:** (**Note:** May also be effective in pot-bellied pigs and ferrets):
  As an emetic:

  a) 1 teaspoon (5 mL) per 5 lbs. (2.3 kg) of body weight (approximately 2 mL/kg) not to exceed 3 tablespoons (45 mL). Vomiting usually occurs within minutes and can be repeated once if not initially successful. (Richardson 2009)

  b) 1–2 mL/kg PO up to 2–3 times (Rudloff 2006)

  c) 1–5 mL/kg PO; generally not to exceed 50 mL for dogs and 10 mL for cats; may repeat one time if after 10 minutes emesis does not occur. Inducing emesis is most effective if administered after a small meal. (Peterson 2006)

Monitoring

- Efficacy (emesis, signs associated with toxicity of the substance ingested, blood levels of toxicants if applicable)

- Heart rate/respiration rate & auscultation after emesis

Client Information

- Use only under the direct instructions of a veterinarian or a poison control center

- Only use hydrogen peroxide 3%; stronger concentrations can be very toxic

- Carefully administer; do not allow patient to "inhale" the liquid

- Observe animal after administration, do not allow them to re-ingest the vomited material (vomitus)

- Save all vomitus for the veterinarian to examine

Chemistry/Synonyms

Hydrogen peroxide 3% solution is a clear, colorless liquid containing 2.5–3.5% w/v hydrogen peroxide. Up to 0.05% of the liquid may contain preservatives.

Hydrogen peroxide 3% solution may also be known as dilute hydrogen peroxide solution, hydrogen peroxide solution 10-volume (**Note:** NOT 10%), or hydrogen peroxide topical solution.

Storage/Stability

Store 3% solutions in airtight containers at room temperature and protected from light.

Hydrogen peroxide 3% can deteriorate with time; outdated or improperly stored products may not be effective as an emetic.

Dosage Forms/Regulatory Status

VETERINARY-LABELED PRODUCTS:
None as an oral emetic

HUMAN-LABELED PRODUCTS:
None as an oral emetic. Hydrogen Peroxide 3% Solution is readily available over-the-counter from a variety of manufacturers. It is usually sold in pint bottles.

References

Peterson, M. (2006). Toxicological decontamination. *Small Animal Toxicology, 2nd Ed.* M Peterson and P Talcott Eds., Elsevier: 127–141.

Richardson, J.A. (2009). Managing toxicoses in dogs and cats. Proceedings: ACVC. Accessed via: Veterinary Information Network. http://goo.gl/qqcjl

Rudloff, E. (2006). Poisonings and intoxications. Proceedings: Western Veterinary Conference. Accessed via: Veterinary Information Network. http://goo.gl/bFWOg

HYDROMORPHONE

(hye-droe-*mor*-fone)   Dilaudid®

OPIATE AGONIST

Prescriber Highlights

▶ Injectable opiate sedative/restraining agent, analgesic, & preanesthetic similar to oxymorphone

▶ Significantly less expensive than oxymorphone

▶ Contraindications: Hypersensitivity to it, diarrhea caused by a toxic ingestion, prior to GI obstructive surgery (may cause vomiting)

▶ Extreme caution: Respiratory disease or acute respiratory dysfunction

▶ Caution: Hypothyroidism, severe renal insufficiency (acute uremia), adrenocortical insufficiency, geriatric or severely debilitated patients, head injuries or increased intracranial pressure & acute abdominal conditions (e.g., colic)

▶ Adverse Effects *Dogs:* Nausea/vomiting, defecation, panting, vocalization, & sedation are common. CNS depression, respiratory depression, & bradycardia; decreased GI motility with resultant constipation (with chronic use) possible

▶ Adverse Effects *Cats:* Nausea common. Ataxia, hyperesthesia, hyperthermia, & behavioral changes (without concomitant tranquilization) possible.

▶ Drug-drug; drug-lab interactions

▶ C-II controlled substance

Uses/Indications

Like oxymorphone, hydromorphone is used in dogs and cats as a sedative/restraining agent, analgesic and preanesthetic. It may also be useful in other species, but little data or experience is available. Because of expense and availability issues with oxymorphone, hydromorphone is rapidly replacing it in veterinary medicine. In dogs and cats, hydromorphone is generally less sedating that morphine, usually causes minimal histamine release after IV administration, and rarely causes vasodilation and hypotension. One randomized, blinded, clinical trial in dogs and cats found hydromorphone's analgesic efficacy and duration of action similar to oxymorphone, but the incidence of nausea and vomiting was higher with hydromorphone (Bateman *et al.* 2008).

Pharmacology/Actions

Receptors for opiate analgesics are found in high concentrations in the limbic system, spinal cord,

thalamus, hypothalamus, striatum, and midbrain. They are also found in tissues such as the gastrointestinal tract, urinary tract, and in other smooth muscle.

The morphine-like agonists (morphine, meperidine, oxymorphone, hydromorphone) have primary activity at the *mu* receptors, with some activity possible at the delta receptor. The primary pharmacologic effects of these agents include: analgesia, antitussive activity, respiratory depression, sedation, emesis, physical dependence, and intestinal effects (constipation/defecation). Secondary pharmacologic effects include: CNS: euphoria, sedation, and confusion. Cardiovascular: bradycardia due to central vagal stimulation, alpha-adrenergic receptors may be depressed resulting in peripheral vasodilation, decreased peripheral resistance, and baroreceptor inhibition. Orthostatic hypotension and syncope may occur. Urinary: Increased bladder sphincter tone can induce urinary retention.

Various species may exhibit contradictory effects from these agents. For example, horses, cattle, swine, and cats may develop excitement and dogs may defecate after morphine injections. These effects are in contrast to the expected effects of sedation and constipation. Dogs and humans may develop miosis, while other species (especially cats) may develop mydriasis.

Hydromorphone is approximately 5 times more potent an analgesic on a per weight basis when compared to morphine and approximately equal in potency to oxymorphone. At the usual doses employed, hydromorphone alone has good sedative qualities in the dog. Respiratory depression can occur especially in debilitated, neonatal, or geriatric patients. Bradycardia, as well as a slight decrease in cardiac contractility and blood pressure, may be seen. Like oxymorphone, hydromorphone does initially increase the respiratory rate (panting in dogs) while actual oxygenation may be decreased and blood CO_2 levels may increase by 10 mmHg or more. Gut motility is decreased with resultant increases in stomach emptying times. Unlike either morphine or meperidine, hydromorphone may only infrequently cause mild histamine release in dogs or cats after IV injection.

Pharmacokinetics

Hydromorphone is absorbed when given by IV, IM, SC, and rectal routes. After hydromorphone is administered subcutaneously to dogs, peak levels occur between 10-30 minutes after dosing. The volume of distribution in dogs is high; > 4 L/kg both with IV and SC dosing. Terminal half-lives are rapid and appear to be route and dose dependent; half-lives are about 35 minutes to an hour long (KuKanich *et al.* 2008).

The drug is metabolized in the liver, primarily by glucuronidation. Because cats are deficient in this metabolic pathway, half-lives in cats are probably prolonged. The glucuronidated metabolite is excreted by the kidney.

Contraindications/Precautions/Warnings

All opiates should be used with caution in patients with hypothyroidism, severe renal insufficiency, adrenocortical insufficiency (Addison's), and geriatric or severely debilitated patients. Hydromorphone is contraindicated in patients hypersensitive to narcotic analgesics, and those with diarrhea caused by a toxic ingestion (until the toxin is eliminated from the GI tract). All opiates should be used with caution in patients with hypothyroidism, severe renal insufficiency, adrenocortical insufficiency (Addison's), and geriatric or severely debilitated patients.

Because it may cause vomiting, hydromorphone use should be considered contraindicated as a preanesthetic med in animals with suspected gastric dilation, volvulus, or intestinal obstruction.

Hydromorphone should be used with extreme caution in patients with head injuries, increased intracranial pressure, and acute abdominal conditions (*e.g.*, colic) as it may obscure the diagnosis or clinical course of these conditions. It should be used with extreme caution in patients suffering from respiratory disease or acute respiratory dysfunction (*e.g.*, pulmonary edema secondary to smoke inhalation).

Hydromorphone can cause bradycardia and therefore should be used cautiously in patients with preexisting bradyarrhythmias.

Neonatal, debilitated, or geriatric patients may be more susceptible to the effects of hydromorphone and may require lower dosages. Patients with severe hepatic disease may have prolonged duration of action of the drug.

Hyperthermia has been reported in cats with hydromorphone use and some recommend to avoid the use of this drug in cats (Hansen, B. 2008). If used in cats at high dosages, the drug has been recommended to be given along with a tranquilizing agent, as hydromorphone can produce bizarre behavioral changes in this species. This also is true in cats for the other opiate agents, such as morphine.

Opiate analgesics are contraindicated in patients who have been stung by the scorpion species *Centruroides sculpturatus Ewing* and *C. gertschi Stahnke* as it may potentiate these venoms.

Adverse Effects

Hydromorphone has a similar adverse effect profile to oxymorphone or morphine in dogs and cats. In dogs, sedation, panting, whining/vocalization, vomiting and defecation are often noted. Vomiting, nausea and defecation may occur more frequently with SC dosing versus intravenous dosing. CNS depression may be greater than desired, particularly when treating moderate to severe pain. In dogs, constant rate IV infusions of >0.05 mg/kg/hr administered for more than 12 hours may cause sedation and adverse effects severe enough to require reducing the rate (Hansen, B. 2008). Dose related respiratory depression is possible, and more likely during general anesthesia. Panting (may occur more often than with oxymorphone) and cough suppression (may be of benefit) may occur.

Opioids can increase body temperature in cats. One study done in eight cats showed that hydromorphone, morphine, butorphanol, and buprenorphine all cause an increase in body temperature in cats and that hydromorphone increased body temperature equivalently to those other drugs. The increased body temperature in all of the experimental treatments was self limiting, and the majority returned to normal within 5 hours. No apparent morbidity or mortality was noted. Administration of ketamine or isoflurane in addition to hydromorphone did not produce a clinically relevant increase in body temperature compared with that of administration of hydromorphone alone (Posner *et al.* 2010). Should hyperthermia occur, naloxone has been used to rapidly reduce body temperature in cats.

Secondary to enhanced vagal tone, hydromorphone can cause bradycardia. This apparently occurs on par with morphine or oxymorphone. Hydromorphone may cause histamine release that, while significantly less then with morphine and usually clinically insignificant, may be significant in critically ill animals. Constipation is possible with chronic dosing.

Reproductive/Nursing Safety

In humans, the FDA categorizes this drug as category **C** for use during pregnancy (*Animal studies have shown an adverse effect on the fetus, but there are no adequate studies in humans; or there are no animal reproduction studies and no adequate studies in humans.*)

Most opiates are excreted into milk, but effects on nursing offspring may not be significant.

Overdosage/Acute Toxicity

Massive overdoses may produce profound respiratory and/or CNS depression in most species. Other effects may include cardiovascular collapse, hypothermia, and skeletal muscle hypotonia. Mania may be seen in cats. Naloxone is the agent of choice in treating respiratory depression. In massive overdoses, naloxone doses may need to be repeated, and animals should be closely observed as naloxone's effects can diminish before sub-toxic levels of oxymorphone are attained. Mechanical respiratory support should be considered in cases of severe respiratory depression.

In susceptible patients, moderate overdoses may require naloxone and supportive treatment as well.

Drug Interactions

The following drug interactions have either been reported or are theoretical in humans or animals receiving hydromorphone and may be of significance in veterinary patients:

■ **BUTORPHANOL, NALBUPHINE:** Potentially could antagonize opiate effects

■ **CNS DEPRESSANTS, OTHER:** Additive CNS effects possible

■ **DIURETICS:** Opiates may decrease efficacy in CHF patients

■ **MONOAMINE OXIDASE INHIBITORS (e.g., amitraz and potentially, selegiline):** Severe and unpredictable opiate potentiation may be seen; not recommended (in humans) if MAO inhibitor has been used within 14 days

■ **MUSCLE RELAXANTS, SKELETAL:** Hydromorphone may enhance effects

■ **PHENOTHIAZINES:** Some phenothiazines may antagonize analgesic effects and increase risk for hypotension

■ **TRICYCLIC ANTIDEPRESSANTS (clomipramine, amitriptyline, etc.):** Hydromorphone may exacerbate the effects of tricyclic antidepressants

■ **WARFARIN:** Opiates may potentiate anticoagulant activity

Laboratory Considerations

■ As they may increase biliary tract pressure, opiates can increase plasma amylase and lipase values up to 24 hours following their administration.

Doses

■ **DOGS:**

a) As an analgesic: 0.1 mg/kg IV or SC q2h or as a CRI at 0.03 mg/kg/hr are suggested doses based on the results of pharmacokinetic study. (KuKanich *et al.* 2008)

b) For cancer pain: 0.08–0.2 mg/kg IV, IM, or SC (Lester & Gaynor 2000)

c) As an analgesic: 0.05–0.2 mg/kg IV, IM, SC q2–4h (Hansen, B 2003), (Hardie 2006)

d) As an analgesic: 0.2–0.6 mg/kg PO q6–8h; For perioperative pain: 0.1–0.2 mg/kg IV, IM, SC q2–4h (Pascoe 2006)

e) As a premed prior to moderately painful procedures: 0.1 mg/kg; may be combined with acepromazine (0.02–0.05 mg/kg) in young, healthy patients. As a sedative/restraint agent for fractious or aggressive dogs: 0.1–0.2 mg/kg mixed with acepromazine (0.05 mg/kg) IM. Maximal effect usually reached in about 15 minutes, but an additional wait of another 15 minutes may be necessary in some dogs.

As an alternate induction method (especially in critical patients): hydromorphone 0.05–0.2 mg/kg IV, slowly to effect followed by diazepam 0.02 mg/kg IV (do not mix two drugs together). Endotracheal intubation may be possible after administration, if not, delivery of an

inhalant by facemask will give a greater depth of anesthesia. Positive pressure ventilation likely will be necessary. If bradycardia requires treatment, use either glycopyrrolate (0.01–0.02 mg/kg IV) or atropine (0.02–0.04 mg/kg IV). (Pettifer & Dyson 2000)

■ **CATS:**

a) As an analgesic: 0.05–0.1 mg/kg IM, IV or SC q2–6 hours (Wagner 2002)

b) For cancer pain: 0.08–0.2 mg/kg IV, IM, or SC (Lester & Gaynor 2000)

c) For moderate to severe pain: 0.08–0.3+ mg/kg IV, IM or SC q2–6 hours (Mathews 2000)

d) As a premed prior to moderately painful procedures: 0.1 mg/kg; may be combined with acepromazine (0.05–0.2 mg/kg) in young, healthy patients.

As an alternate induction method (especially in critical patients): hydromorphone 0.05–0.2 mg/kg IV, slowly to effect followed by diazepam 0.02 mg/kg IV (do not mix two drugs together). Endotracheal intubation may be possible after administration, if not, delivery of an inhalant by facemask will give a greater depth of anesthesia. Positive pressure ventilation likely will be necessary. If bradycardia requires treatment, use either glycopyrrolate (0.01–0.02 mg/kg IV) or atropine (0.02–0.04 mg/kg IV). (Pettifer & Dyson 2000)

■ **FERRETS:**

a) As a pre-op: 0.05–0.1 mg/kg IV; as a CRI post-op: 0.05 mg/kg IV loading dose, then 0.05–0.1 mg/kg/hr (Lichtenberger 2006)

■ **SMALL MAMMALS:**

a) **Rabbits:** 0.05–0.1 mg/kg IV; as a CRI post-op: 0.05 mg/kg IV loading dose, then 0.05–0.1 mg/kg/hr (Lichtenberger 2006)

Monitoring

■ Respiratory rate/depth (pulse oximetry highly recommended)

■ CNS level of depression/excitation

■ Blood pressure (especially with IV use)

■ Cardiac rate

■ Analgesic efficacy

Client Information

■ When given parenterally, this agent should be used in an inpatient setting or with direct professional supervision

Chemistry/Synonyms

A semi-synthetic phenanthrene-derivative opiate related to morphine, hydromorphone HCl occurs as white, fine, crystalline powder. It is freely soluble in water. The commercial injection has a pH of 4–5.5.

Hydromorphone may also be known as: dihydromorphinone hydrochloride, *Dolonovag®*, *Hydal®*, *HydroStat IR®*, *Hydromorph®*, *Opidol®*, *Palladon®*, *Palladone®*, and *Sophidone®*.

Storage/Stability

The injection should be stored at room temperature and protected from light. A slight yellowish tint to the solution may occur, but does not indicate loss of potency. The injection remains stable for at least 24 hours when mixed with commonly used IV fluids if protected from light.

Hydromorphone tablets should be stored at room temperature in tight, light resistant containers. The suppositories should be kept in the refrigerator.

Compatibility/Compounding Considerations

Hydromorphone injection is **compatible** in commonly used IV fluids (for 24 hours when protected from light at 25°C) and with midazolam, ondansetron, potassium chloride, and heparin sodium. Hydromorphone injection mixed in the same syringe with atropine and medetomidine (*Domitor®*) for use as a pre-op in dogs prior to sevoflurane or propofol anesthesia has been described (Ko 2005). Hydromorphone is **incompatible** with sodium bicarbonate, or thiopental.

Dosage Forms/Regulatory Status

VETERINARY-LABELED PRODUCTS: None

HUMAN-LABELED PRODUCTS:

Hydromorphone HCl Injection: 1 mg/mL in 1 mL amps & syringes, 2 mg/mL in 1 mL vials, amps & syringes, 20 mL vials & multidose vials; 4 mg/mL in1 mL amps & syringes; and 10 mg/mL (concentrate) in 1 mL, & 5 mL, single-dose vials & amps and 50 mL single-dose vials; *Dilaudid®* and *Dilandid-HP®* (Abbott); generic; (Rx, C-II)

Hydromorphone HCl Powder for Injection, lyophilized: 250 mg (10 mg/mL after reconstitution) preservative-free in single-dose vials; *Dilaudid-HP®* (Abbott); (Rx, C-II)

Hydromorphone HCl Oral Tablets: 2 mg, 4 mg, & 8 mg; *Dilaudid®* (Abbott); generic; (Rx, C-II)

Hydromorphone HCl Oral Capsules (extended-release): 8 mg, 12 mg, & 16 mg; *Exalgo®* (Alza); (Rx, C-II)

Hydromorphone HCL Oral Liquid: 1 mg/1 mL in 4 mL & 8 mL UD patient cups; 250 mL & 473 mL (may contain sodium metabisulfite); *Dilaudid®* (Abbott); generic; (Rx, C-II)

Hydromorphone Suppositories: 3 mg; Hydromorphone HCl (Paddock); *Dilaudid®* (Abbott); (Rx, C-II)

References

Bateman, S.W., S. Haldane, et al. (2008). Comparison of the analgesic efficacy of hydromorphone and oxymorphone in dogs and cats: a randomized blinded study. *Veterinary Anaesthesia and Analgesia* 35(4): 341–347.

Hansen, B. (2003). Updated opinions on analgesic techniques. Proceedings: ACVIM Forum. Accessed via: Veterinary Information Network. http://goo.gl/EPWL2

Hansen, B. (2008). Analgesia for the Critically III Dog or Cat: An Update. *Veterinary Clinics of North America-Small Animal Practice* 38(6): 1353–+.

Hardie, E. (2006). Managing intractable pain. Proceedings: Western Vet Conf 2006. Accessed via: Veterinary Information Network. http://goo.gl/sED8X

Ko, J. (2005). New anesthesia-analgesia injectable combinations in dogs and cats. Proceedings: ACVC. Accessed via: Veterinary Information Network. http://goo.gl/Yklxx

KuKanich, B., B.K. Hogan, et al. (2008). Pharmacokinetics of hydromorphone hydrochloride in healthy dogs. *Veterinary Anaesthesia and Analgesia* 35(3): 256–264.

Lester, P. & J. Gaynor (2000). Management of cancer pain. *Vet Clin NA: Small Anim Pract* 30(July): 951–966.

Lichtenberger, M. (2006). Anesthesia Protocols and Pain Management for Exotic Animal Patients. Proceedings: Western Vet Conf. Accessed via: Veterinary Information Network. http://goo.gl/hB5Kt

Mathews, K. (2000). Pain assessment and general approach to management. *Vet Clin NA: Small Anim Pract* 30:4(July): 729–756.

Pascoe, P. (2006). Pain management in the canine patient. Proceedings: UCD Canine Medicine Conference. Accessed via: Veterinary Information Network. http://goo.gl/hjQru

Pettifer, G. & D. Dyson (2000). Hydromorphone: A cost-effective alternative to the use of oxymorphone. *Can Vet Jnl* 41(2): 135–137.

Posner, L.P., A.A. Pavuk, et al. (2010). Effects of opioids and anesthetic drugs on body temperature in cats. *Veterinary Anaesthesia and Analgesia* 37(1): 35–43.

Wagner, A. (2002). Opioids. *Handbook of Veterinary Pain Management*. J Gaynor and W Muir Eds., Mosby: 164–183.

HYDROXYETHYL STARCH (HES) HETASTARCH (HES 450/0.7) IN SALINE

Hespan®

HETASTARCH (HES 670/0.75) IN LACTATED ELECTROLYTE

Hextend®

TETRASTARCH (HES 130/0.4) IN SALINE

Voluven®
(**het**-uh-starch), (**te**-truh-starch)

COLLOID VOLUME EXPANDER

Prescriber Highlights

▶ Volume expanders used to treat hypovolemia where colloidal therapy required

▶ Different HES molecular weight/degree of substitution products available

▶ Contraindications: Severe heart failure, severe bleeding disorders, & patients in oliguric or anuric renal failure

▶ Caution: Thrombocytopenia, patients undergoing CNS surgery; liver disease

▶ May cause volume overload: Use with caution in patients with renal dysfunction, congestive heart failure, or pulmonary edema

▶ Adverse Effects: Coagulopathies possible; too rapid administration to small animals (especially cats) may cause nausea/vomiting; hypersensitivity reactions possible but very rare

Note: Nomenclature for these products can be confusing. Hydroxyethyl starch and hetastarch are often used interchangeably, but this is not necessarily true. It is best when examining references to determine not only the % HES used and the fluid in which it is diluted, but the molecular weight/degree of substitution. Be certain when using HES products that you are familiar with the specific product and its respective cautions and uses. The bulk of this monograph pertains to the HES 450/0.7 product which has been used most frequently in veterinary medicine.

Uses/Indications

There are two principle reasons to choose HES colloid therapy over crystalloid therapy. The first is their better intravascular persistence and more prolonged volume expanding effects, and secondly, in patients with "capillary leak syndromes" where they can reduce vascular permeability and down-regulate expression of pro-inflammatory mediators (Boag 2007). Often, in hypovolemic patients where total protein is less than 3.5 g/dL and crystalloid therapy is likely to reduce this level further, colloid therapy (plasma, dextran or hetastarch) is considered as part of intravascular volume restoration oftentimes when colloid therapy is required and blood products are unavailable, or time is of the essence and the wait for crossmatching is unacceptable.

In experimental isoflurane-induced hypotension in dogs, hetastarch administration was found superior to LRS (Aarnes *et al.* 2009).

In horses, hetastarch may be useful in increasing plasma oncotic pressure and volume expansion in hypoproteinemic conditions (*e.g.,* acute colitis) and may reduce endotoxin-induced vascular permeability better then plasma.

The most commonly used hydroxyethyl starch (HES) solution in North America has been the high molecular weight (MW) product, hetastarch (6% HES 450/0.7) in normal saline with the trade name, *Hespan®*. The low-MW product, tetrastarch (*Voluven®*, 6% HES 130/0.4) in normal saline was recently FDA-approved in the USA for use in humans. It potentially may cause less coagulation altering effects then the high-MW product. There is also a very high-MW product, (HES 670/0.75) in LRS, *Hextend®*. The clinical use in veterinary medicine of these latter two products has been limited to date. In many European countries, an HES 200/0.5 product, often called pentastarch, is commonly used.

Pharmacology/Actions

HES acts as a plasma volume expander by increasing the oncotic pressure within the intravascular space similarly to either dextran or albumin. Maximum volume expansion occurs within a few minutes of the completion of infusion. Duration of effect is variable, but may persist for 24 hours or more. When added to whole blood in humans, hetastarch causes an increase in erythrocyte sedimentation rate.

Pharmacokinetics

Lower molecular weight molecules, (less than 50,000) are rapidly excreted by the kidneys; larger molecules are slowly degraded enzymatically to a size where they then can be excreted. About 40% of a dose is excreted in the first 24 hours after infusion. After about 2 weeks, practically all the drug is excreted. In hypoproteinemic horses, colloidal pressure may be increased up to 24 hours after dosing.

Contraindications/Precautions/Warnings

It is believed that significant bleeding can occur if hetastarch is used in animals with compromised coagulation systems. For example, use in patients with von Willebrand's disease could significantly increase the risk for bleeding. Because of its effect on platelets, hetastarch should be used with caution in patients with thrombocytopenia and with extreme caution in patients undergoing CNS surgery.

As it has no oxygen carrying capacity, hetastarch is not a replacement for whole blood or red blood cells.

In humans, there is a potential of risk for acute kidney injury with HES, particularly in acute sepsis patients. It is unknown if this risk also occurs in veterinary patients. Use hetastarch with caution in patients with liver disease due to its effects on indirect serum bilirubin levels.

Because of the danger of volume overload, use of HES for the treatment of shock not accompanied by hypovolemia may be hazardous; it should be used in caution in patients with renal dysfunction, congestive heart failure or pulmonary edema. Additionally, animals with sepsis, systemic inflammatory response syndrome (SIRS) or severe trauma may extravasate colloids such as hetastarch into the lungs which could potentially, cause or worsen pulmonary edema. Monitoring for clinical signs of pulmonary edema and if possible, blood gases is mandatory in these circumstances.

In humans, HES is contraindicated in patients with severe heart failure, severe bleeding disorders and patients in oliguric or anuric renal failure.

Adverse Effects

HES can affect platelet function and coagulation times. It can alter Factor VIII (FVIII) and von Willebrand Factor. At recommended dosages, hetastarch may cause changes in clotting times and platelet counts due to direct (precipitation of factor VIII) and dilutional causes. A retrospective study in dogs, showed that hetastarch can significantly increase PTT's, but did not affect survival rates (Helmbold *et al.* 2009). Clinically, these effects may be insignificant, but patients with preexisting coagulopathies may be predisposed to further bleeding. Potentially, tetrastarch may have less effect on coagulation then hetastarch.

HES is less antigenic than dextran, but can cause sensitivity reactions and interfere with antigen-antibody testing. Anaphylactic reactions and severe coagulopathies are thought to occur rarely, however.

When given via rapid infusion to cats, hetastarch may cause signs of nausea and vomiting; if administered over 15–30 minutes, these signs are eliminated.

Circulatory overload leading to pulmonary edema is possible, particularly when large dosages are administered to patients with diminished renal function. Do not give intramuscularly as bleeding, bruising, or hematomas may occur.

When hetastarch infusions are stopped a "rebound effect" can occur; colloid that has leaked into interstitial spaces can pull additional fluid from the intravascular space.

In humans, increases in serum indirect bilirubin have occurred occasionally. No effect on other liver function tests were noted and the increases subsided over several days. Serum amylase levels may be falsely elevated for several days after hetastarch is administered. While clinically insignificant, the changes may preclude using serum amylase to diagnosis or monitor patients with acute pancreatitis.

Reproductive/Nursing Safety

Hetastarch's safety during pregnancy has not been established, but no untoward effects have apparently been reported. In humans, the FDA categorizes this drug as category *C* for use during pregnancy (*Animal studies have shown an adverse effect on the fetus, but there are no adequate studies in humans; or there are no animal reproduction studies and no adequate studies in humans.*)

It is not known whether hetastarch is excreted in milk, but it is unlikely to pose much risk to offspring.

Overdosage/Acute Toxicity

Overdosage could result in volume overload in susceptible patients. Dose and monitor fluid status carefully.

Drug Interactions

None reported.

Laboratory Considerations

■ Hetastarch (670/0.75) can falsely elevate **urine** concentration **(specific gravity)** in dogs (Smart *et al.* 2009).

Doses

■ **DOGS/CATS: Note:** All doses are for hetastarch (6% HES 450/0.7; *Hespan®*) unless otherwise noted.

For use as a plasma volume expander in shock: **Note:** Rate of administration is determined by individual patient requirements (*i.e.*, blood volume, indication, and patient response); adequate monitoring for successful treatment of shock is mandatory. The following dosages are NOT "Give and forget"; they should be used as general guidelines for treatment.

a) Shock bolus (resuscitation): 10–20 mL/kg in dogs and 5–10 mL/kg in cats. (Petrollini 2003)

b) Shock bolus (resuscitation): 10–20 mL/kg in dogs and 5–10 mL/kg in cats.

As an infusion: Dogs: 1–2 mL/kg/hr; not to exceed 20 mL/kg in a 24 hour period; Cats: 1–2 mL/kg/hr; not to exceed 10 mL/kg in a 24 hour period (Hopper 2006)

c) Dogs: 20 mL/kg /day; cats: 10/mL/kg/day. Rate of administration depends on the condition treated. For emergent situations, it can be given as a slow bolus over 15–30 minutes. For supporting colloid oncotic pressure in hypoalbuminemic patients, it can be given as a 24-hour infusion with low-rate crystalloid infusion. (Martin 2004)

d) For shock resuscitation, standard dose is 20 mL/kg. The dose is given as an IV bolus (slower in the cat). When used for colloid oncotic support the dose is given over 24 hours. Rapid administration to cats can cause nausea and vomiting. Patients may have elevations in prothrombin time and activated partial thromboplastin time without evidence of bleeding. (Barton 2002)

■ **HORSES:**

a) Adult horses: 8–10 mL/kg/day. Foals who require rapid volume support: 3–5 mL/kg in addition to crystalloids. May also be used in horses that are hypo-oncotic, but well hydrated at: 0.5–1 mL/kg per hour, up to 10 mL/kg/day. (Magdesian, K. 2004)

b) When colloids are selected for volume replacement, hetastarch at 3–10 mL/kg can be used. Total daily doses of 10 mL/kg should not be exceeded due to risk for coagulopathies. (Magdesian, K.G. 2010)

c) For colloidal support for fluid resuscitation and management of hypoproteinemia: 8–10 mL/kg IV bolus or as a CRI at 0.5–1 mL/kg/hr (max. of 10 mL/kg/day). (Naylor & Dunkel 2009)

■ **BIRDS:**

a) 10–15 mL/kg over 20-40 minutes, up to four times daily, OR 10–15 mL/kg bolus over 20-40 minutes followed by 1–2 mL/kg/hr continuous rate infusion. Recommended maximum dose is 20 mL/kg/24 hours, but author notes that she has exceeded this dose with no side effects noted.

For small volume replacement/CPCR resuscitation: For the shocky debilitated patient, hypertonic saline is administered (3–5 mL/kg) over 5 minutes, followed by hetastarch (3–5 mL/kg over 5 min). This combination prior to crystalloid administration enables fluids to stay within the vascular space. Blood pressure should be monitored closely. Follow with small boluses of crystalloid fluids (LRS, Plasma-Lyte at 15–20 mL/kg) along with hetastarch at 3–5 mL/kg) over 15 minutes, and reassess the bird every 15 minutes. The crystalloids and hetastarch can be combined in the same syringe or bag. This process is repeated every 15-20 minutes until temperature normalizes and blood pressure is over 120 mmHg (Antinoff 2009)

b) 3–5 mL/kg IV or IO over 10 minutes, one to two boluses. (Lennox 2009)

■ **CAMELIDS:**

a) A study done in healthy llamas showed that 15 mL/kg significantly increased COP for up to 96 hours. Transient, mild hemodilution and mild increases in PT and PTT were noted. (McKenzie et al. 2009)

Monitoring

■ Other than the regular monitoring performed in patients that would require volume expansion therapy, there is no inordinate monitoring required specific to hetastarch therapy, but consider monitoring coagulation parameters particularly in high risk patients or when using high dosages of hetastarch

Client Information

■ As hetastarch is used in an in-patient setting only, the two factors to consider when communicating with clients are the drug's cost and the reasons for using colloid therapy.

Chemistry/Synonyms

A synthetic polymer derived from a waxy starch, HES is composed primarily of amylopectin. Hetastarch occurs as a white powder. It is very soluble in water and insoluble in alcohol.

To avoid degradation by serum amylase, hydroxyethyl ether groups are added to the glucose Units. Commercially available HES solutions are classified by their mean molecular weight (MW) and degree of substitution (DS). The DS refers to the average number of hydroxyethyl groups per glucose unit within the branched-chain polymer. The most commonly used HES solution is HES 450/0.7 (*Hespan®*) and therefore has an average MW of 670 kD and a DS of 0.75. While the average molecular weight is 450,000, commercial HES solutions contain a vide variation in molecule sizes, ranging from a few thousand to a few million Daltons distributed in a concentration/size ratio more or less as a bell-shaped curve.

The commercially available colloidal solution appears as a clear, pale yellow to amber solution. In 500 mL of the commercial preparation containing HES (450/0.7) 6% and 0.9% sodium chloride, there are 77 mEq of sodium and chloride. It has an osmolality of 310 mOsm/L and a pH of about 5.5.

The HES (670/0.75) product in lactated electrolyte solution (*Hextend®*) contains 143 mEq/L of sodium, 124 mEq/L of chloride, 28 mEq/L of lactate, 5 mEq/L of calcium, 3 mEq/L of potassium, 0.9 mEq/L of magnesium, and 0.99 grams/L of dextrose. These values approximate what is found in human plasma.

Hetastarch may also be known by the following synonyms: etherified starches, HES, and hydroxyethyl starch; many trade names are available.

Storage/Stability

Hetastarch 6% in 0.9% NaCl or lactated electrolyte should be stored at temperatures less than 40°C; freezing should be avoided. Exposure to temperature extremes may result in formation of a crystalline precipitate or a color change to a turbid deep brown. Do not use should this occur.

Compatibility/Compounding Considerations

The following drugs are reported **compatible** at Y-sites with hetastarch (450/0.7) 6% in normal saline: cimetidine, diltiazem, enalaprilat, and ertapenem. For *Hextend®*: Do not administer simultaneously with blood through the same administration set as there is a risk of coagulation.

Dosage Forms/Regulatory Status

VETERINARY-LABELED PRODUCTS: None

HUMAN-LABELED PRODUCTS:

Hetastarch Injection: 6% (6 g/100 mL) HES (450/0.7) in 0.9% sodium chloride in 500 mL IV infusion bottles, polyolefin bags & single-dose containers; *Hespan®* (B. Braun Medical); 6% Hetastarch (Hospira); (Rx)

Hetastarch Injection: 6% (6 g/100 mL) HES (670/0.75) in lactated electrolyte in 500 mL IV infusion single-dose containers; *Hextend®* (Hospira), generic; (Rx)

Tetrastarch Injection: 6% (6 g/100 mL) HES (130/0.4) in 0.9% sodium chloride in 500 mL polyolefin bags; *Voluven®* (Hospira); (Rx)

References

Aarnes, T.K., R.M. Bednarski, et al. (2009). Effect of intravenous administration of lactated Ringer's solution or hetastarch for the treatment of isoflurane-induced hypotension in dogs. *American Journal of Veterinary Research* 70(11): 1345–1353.

Antinoff, N. (2009). Avian Critical Care: What's Old, What's New. Proceedings: IVECCS. Accessed via: Veterinary Information Network. http://goo.gl/WVvLn

Barton, L. (2002). Fluid therapy for the acute patient. Proceedings: Atlantic Coast Veterinary Conference. Accessed via: Veterinary Information Network. http://goo.gl/F95t6

Boag, A. (2007). Hetastarch: Not All Starches Are the Same. Proceedings: IVECCS. Accessed via: Veterinary Information Network. http://goo.gl/k12Mg

Helmbold, K., K. Hall, et al. (2009). Effects of hetastarch on coagulation parameters and clinical outcome in dogs. Proceedings: IVECC. Accessed via: Veterinary Information Network. http://goo.gl/vjn0j

Hopper, K. (2006). Hetastarch: The pros and cons. Proceedings: Western Vet Conf. Accessed via: Veterinary Information Network. http://goo.gl/L9czg

Lennox, A. (2009). Avian advanced anaesthesia, monitoring and critical care. Proceedings: BSAVA. Accessed via: Veterinary Information Network. http://goo.gl/er09t

Magdesian, K. (2004). Volume replacement in the critical equine: Colloids. Proceedings: ACVIM Forum. Accessed via: Veterinary Information Network. http://goo.gl/wbtIi

Magdesian, K.G. (2010). Replacement Fluid Therapy for the Critical Equine Patient. Proceedings: ACVIM. Accessed via: Veterinary Information Network. http://goo.gl/z8QYy

Martin, L. (2004). Plasma vs Synthetic Colloids: Do you know which to use? Proceedings: ACVIM Forum. Accessed via: Veterinary Information Network. http://goo.gl/rba5H

McKenzie, E., K. Carney, et al. (2009). Hetastarch on the colloid osmotic pressure of healthy llamas. Proceedings: IVECC. Accessed via: Veterinary Information Network. http://goo.gl/NlA0Q

Naylor, R.J. & B. Dunkel (2009). The treatment of diarrhoea in the adult horse. *Equine Veterinary Education* 21(9): 494–504.

Petrollini, E. (2003). Synthetic colloids. Proceedings: IVECCS. Accessed via: Veterinary Information Network. http://goo.gl/Rl594

Smart, L., K. Hopper, et al. (2009). The Effect of Hetastarch (670/0.75) on Urine Specific Gravity and Osmolality in the Dog. *Journal of Veterinary Internal Medicine* 23(2): 388–391.

HYDROXYUREA

(hye-drox-ee-yor-ee-a)
Hydrea®, Droxia®, Mylocel®
ANTINEOPLASTIC

Prescriber Highlights

▶ Antineoplastic used for treatment of polycythemia vera, mastocytomas, & leukemias in dogs & cats

▶ Caution: Anemia, bone marrow depression, history of urate stones, infection, impaired renal function, or in patients who have received previous chemotherapy or radiotherapy

▶ Adverse Effects: GI effects, stomatitis, sloughing of nails, alopecia, & dysuria; most serious are bone marrow depression & pulmonary fibrosis

▶ Proven teratogen

Uses/Indications

Hydroxyurea may be useful in the treatment of polycythemia vera, mastocytomas, and leukemias in dogs and cats. It is often used to treat dogs with chronic myelogenous leukemia no longer responsive to busulfan. Hydroxyurea, potentially, may be of benefit in the treatment of feline hypereosinophilic syndrome and in the adjunctive treatment of canine meningiomas. It can also be used in dogs for the adjunctive medical treatment (to reduce hematocrit) of right to left shunting patent ductus arteriosus or tetralogy of Fallot.

Pharmacology/Actions

While the exact mechanism of action for hydroxyurea has not been determined, it appears to interfere with DNA synthesis without interfering with RNA or protein synthesis. Hydroxyurea apparently inhibits thymidine incorporation into DNS and may directly damage DNA. It is an S-phase inhibitor, but may also arrest cells at the G_1-S border.

Hydroxyurea inhibits urease, but is less potent than acetohydroxamic acid. Hydroxyurea can stimulate production of fetal hemoglobin.

Pharmacokinetics

Hydroxyurea is well absorbed after oral administration and crosses the blood-brain barrier.

Approximately 50% of an absorbed dose is excreted unchanged in the urine and about 50% is metabolized in the liver and then excreted in the urine.

Contraindications/Precautions/Warnings

Risk versus benefit should be considered before using hydroxyurea in patients with the following conditions: anemia, bone marrow depression, history of urate stones, current infection, impaired renal function, or in patients who have received previous chemotherapy or radiotherapy.

Adverse Effects

Potential adverse effects include GI effects (anorexia, vomiting, diarrhea), stomatitis, sloughing of nails, alopecia, and dysuria. The most serious adverse effects associated with hydroxyurea are bone marrow depression (anemia, thrombocytopenia, leukopenia) and pulmonary fibrosis. If myelotoxicity occurs, it is recommended to halt therapy until values return to normal. Methemoglobinemia has been reported in cats given high dosages (>500 mg).

Reproductive/Nursing Safety

Hydroxyurea is a teratogen. Use only during pregnancy when the benefits to the mother outweigh the risks to the offspring. Hydroxyurea can suppress gonadal function; arrest of spermatogenesis has been noted in dogs. In humans, the FDA categorizes this drug as category *D* for use during pregnancy (*There is evidence of human fetal risk, but the potential benefits from the use of the drug in pregnant women may be acceptable despite its potential risks.*)

Although hydroxyurea distribution into milk has not been documented, nursing puppies or kittens should receive milk replacer when the dam is receiving hydroxyurea.

Overdosage/Acute Toxicity

Cats given hydroxyurea in doses greater than 500 mg (total) may develop methemoglobinemia. Because of the potential toxicity of the drug, overdoses should be treated aggressively with gut emptying protocols employed when possible. For further information, refer to an animal poison control center.

Drug Interactions

The following drug interactions have either been reported or are theoretical in humans or animals receiving hydroxyurea and may be of significance in veterinary patients:

■ **BONE MARROW DEPRESSANT DRUGS, OTHER (e.g., other antineoplastics, chloramphenicol, flucytosine, amphotericin B, or colchicine):** Other bone marrow depressant drugs may cause additive myelosuppression when used with hydroxyurea

Laboratory Considerations

■ Hydroxyurea may raise serum **uric acid** levels; drugs such as allopurinol may be required to control hyperuricemia

Doses

Note: Because of the potential toxicity of this drug to patients, veterinary personnel and clients, and since chemotherapy indications, treatment protocols, monitoring and safety guidelines often change, the following dosages should be used only as a general guide. Consultation with a veterinary oncologist and referral to current veterinary oncology references [*e.g.,* (Henry & Higginbotham 2009); (Argyle *et al.* 2008); (Withrow & Vail 2007); (Villalobos 2007); (Ogilvie & Moore 2006); (Ogilvie & Moore 2001)] is *strongly recommended*.

■ **DOGS:**
For polycythemia vera; chronic myelogenous leukemia:

a) 50 mg/kg 3 times per week (Jacobs *et al.* 1992)

For polycythemia vera:

a) Initially at 20–25 mg/kg PO twice daily; once the hematocrit is below 60% give every other day. (Vail & Thamm 2005)

b) 30 mg/kg once daily for one week, then 15 mg/kg once daily until remission; then taper to lowest effective frequency by monitoring hematocrit (Raskin 1994)

c) 50–80 mg/kg PO every 3 days (Kitchell & Dhaliwal 2000)

For chronic myelogenous leukemia:

a) 50 mg/kg PO q24h for 1–2 weeks, then every other day (Couto 2003)

■ **CATS:**
For polycythemia vera; chronic myelogenous leukemia:

a) 25 mg/kg 3 times per week (Jacobs *et al.* 1992)

For polycythemia vera:

a) Initially at 10–15 mg/kg PO twice daily; once the hematocrit is below 60% give every other day. (Vail & Thamm 2005)

b) 30 mg/kg once daily for one week, then 15 mg/kg once daily until remission; then taper to lowest effective frequency by monitoring hematocrit. Cats must be monitored more frequently than dogs as they have a greater risk of developing bone marrow toxicity. (Raskin 1994)

Monitoring

■ CBC with platelets at least every 1–2 weeks until stable; then every 3 months

■ BUN/Serum Creatinine; initially before starting treatment and then every 3–4 months

Chemistry/Synonyms

Structurally similar to urea and acetohydroxamic acid, hydroxyurea occurs as white, crystalline powder that is freely soluble in water. It is moisture labile.

Hydroxyurea may also be known as: hydroxy-carbamide, hydroxycarbamidum, NSC-32065, SQ-1089, WR-83799, *Dacrodil®*, *Droxiurea®*, *Hydrea®*, *Droxia®*, *Hydrine®*, *Litalir®*, *Medroxyurea®*, *Neodrea®*, *Onco-Carbide®*, *Oxeron®*, and *Syrea®*.

Storage/Stability

Capsules should be stored in tight containers at room temperature. Avoid excessive heat.

Compatibility/Compounding Considerations

Compounded preparation stability: Hydroxyurea oral suspension compounded from commercially available capsules has been published (Heeney *et al.* 2004). Triturating ten (10) hydroxyurea 500 mg capsules with room temperature water, stirring, filtering and bringing to a final volume of 50 mL with *Syrpalta®* yields a 100 mg/mL suspension that retains >95% potency for 180 days stored at 25°C. Suspensions of hydroxyurea heated to 41°C result in an immediate 40% loss of drug potency. Compounded preparations of hydroxyurea should be protected from light.

Dosage Forms/Regulatory Status

VETERINARY-LABELED PRODUCTS: None

HUMAN-LABELED PRODUCTS:

Hydroxyurea Oral Capsules: 200 mg, 300 mg, 400 mg & 500 mg; *Hydrea®* (Bristol-Myers Squibb); *Droxia®* (Bristol-Myers Squibb Oncology); generic; (Rx)

References

Argyle, D., M. Brearly, et al. (2008). *Decision Making in Small Animal Oncology*, Wiley-Blackwell.

Couto, C. (2003). Oncology. *Small Animal Internal Medicine, 3rd Ed.* R Nelson and C Couto Eds. St Louis, Mosby: 1093–1155.

Heeney, M.M., M.R. Whorton, et al. (2004). Chemical and functional analysis of hydroxyurea oral solutions. *J Pediatr Hematol Oncol* 26(3): 179–184.

Henry, C. & M. Higginbotham (2009). *Cancer Management in Small Animal Practice*, Saunders.

Jacobs, R., J. Lumsden, et al. (1992). Canine and Feline Reference Values. *Current Veterinary Therapy XI: Small Animal Practice*. R Kirk and J Bonagura Eds. Philadelphia, W.B. Saunders Company: 1250–1277.

Kitchell, B. & R. Dhaliwal (2000). CVT Update: Anticancer Drugs and Protocols Using Traditional Drugs. *Kirk's Current Veterinary Therapy: XIII Small Animal Practice*. J Bonagura Ed. Philadelphia, WB Saunders: 465–473.

Ogilvie, G. & A. Moore (2001). *Feline Oncology: A Comprehensive Guide to Compassionate Care*, Veterinary Learning Systems.

Ogilvie, G. & A. Moore (2006). *Managing the Canine Cancer Patient: A Practical Guide to Compassionate Care*, Veterinary Learning Systems.

Raskin, R. (1994). Erythrocytes, leukocytes and platelets. *Saunders Manual of Small Animal Practice*. S Birchard and R Sherding Eds. Philadelphia, W.B. Saunders Company: 147–163.

Vail, D. & D. Thamm (2005). Hematopoietic tumors. *Textbook of Veterinary Internal Medicine, 6th Ed.* S Ettinger and E Feldman Eds., Elsevier: 732–747.

Villalobos, A. (2007). *Canine and Feline Geriatric Oncology*. Ames, Blackwell.

Withrow, S. & D. Vail (2007). *Withrow and MacEwen's Small Animal Clinical Oncology 4th Ed*. Philadelphia, Elsevier.

HYDROXYZINE HCL
HYDROXYZINE PAMOATE

(hye-*drox*-i-zeen)   Atarax®, Vistaril®

ANTIHISTAMINE

Prescriber Highlights

▶ Used principally for antihistaminic, antipruritic, & sedative/tranquilization qualities, often in atopic patients

▶ Contraindications: Hypersensitivity to the drug

▶ Caution in patients with prostatic hypertrophy, bladder neck obstruction, severe cardiac failure, angle-closure glaucoma, or pyeloduodenal obstruction

▶ Adverse Effects: Sedation most likely; Dogs (rarely): Tremors, seizures; Cats: Polydipsia, depression, or behavioral changes.

Uses/Indications

Hydroxyzine is used principally for its antihistaminic, antipruritic, and sedative/tranquilization qualities, often in atopic patients.

Pharmacology/Actions

Like other H_1-receptor antihistamines, hydroxyzine acts by competing with histamine for sites on H_1-receptor sites on effector cells. Antihistamines do not block histamine release, but can antagonize its effects. In addition to its antihistaminic effects, hydroxyzine possesses anticholinergic, sedative, tranquilizing, antispasmodic, local anesthetic, mild bronchodilative, and antiemetic activities.

Pharmacokinetics

Hydroxyzine is rapidly and well absorbed after oral administration. Effects generally persist for 6–8 hours in dogs and up to 12 hours in cats. Hydroxyzine is apparently metabolized in liver.

Contraindications/Precautions/Warnings

Hydroxyzine is contraindicated in patients hypersensitive to it. It should be used with caution in patients with prostatic hypertrophy, bladder neck obstruction, severe cardiac failure, angle-closure glaucoma, or pyeloduodenal obstruction.

Adverse Effects

The most likely adverse effect associated with hydroxyzine is sedation. In dogs, this is usually mild and transient. Occasionally antihistamines can cause a hyperexcitability reaction. Dogs have reportedly developed fine rapid tremors, whole body tremors and, rarely, seizures while receiving this drug. Cats may develop polydipsia, depression, or behavioral changes while on this medication.

Reproductive/Nursing Safety

At doses substantially greater than those used therapeutically, hydroxyzine has been shown to be teratogenic in lab animals. Use during pregnancy (particularly during the first trimester) only when the benefits outweigh the risks. In humans, the FDA categorizes this drug as category *C* for use during pregnancy (*Animal studies have shown an adverse effect on the fetus, but there are no adequate studies in humans; or there are no animal reproduction studies and no adequate studies in humans.*)

It is unknown if hydroxyzine enters maternal milk; cetirizine a metabolite of hydroxyzine, has been detected in milk.

Overdosage/Acute Toxicity

Overdoses would be expected to cause increased sedation and perhaps, hypotension. At high doses, fine rapid tremors and rarely seizures have been reported. There were 109 exposures to hydroxyzine reported to the ASPCA Animal Poison Control Center (APCC) during 2008-2009. In these cases, 105 were dogs with 39 showing clinical signs, and 4 were cats that showed no clinical signs. Common findings in dogs recorded in decreasing frequency included hyperthermia, lethargy, tachycardia, trembling, tremors, ataxia, and somnolence.

There are no specific antidotes available. Gut emptying protocols should be considered with large or unknown quantity overdoses. Supportive and symptomatic treatment is recommended if necessary.

Drug Interactions

The following drug interactions have either been reported in humans or animals or are theoretical in humans or animals receiving hydroxyzine and may be of significance in veterinary patients:

■ **ANTICHOLINERGIC AGENTS:** Additive anticholinergic effects may occur when hydroxyzine is used concomitantly with other anticholinergic agents

■ **CNS DEPRESSANT DRUGS, OTHER:** Additive CNS depression may be seen if combining hydroxyzine with other CNS depressant medications, such as barbiturates, tranquilizers, etc.

■ **EPINEPHRINE:** Hydroxyzine may inhibit or reverse the vasopressor effects of epinephrine; use norepinephrine or metaraminol instead

Laboratory Considerations

■ False increases have been reported in **17-hydroxycorticosteroid** urine values after hydroxyzine use

■ Because antihistamines can decrease the wheal and flair response to skin **allergen testing**, antihistamines should be discontinued from 3–7 days (depending on the antihistamine used and the reference) before intradermal skin tests

Doses

■ **DOGS:**
As an antipruritic/antihistamine:
a) 2.2 mg/kg PO three times daily (q8h) (Gershwin 1992), (Paradis & Scott 1992), (White 2007)
b) For flea allergy dermatitis: 2 mg/kg q8h PO (Griffen 1994)

■ **CATS:**
As an antipruritic/antihistamine:
a) For pruritus: 1–2 mg/kg or 5–10 mg/cat PO q8–12h (Messinger 2000)
b) For pruritus: 5–10 mg (total dose) or 2.2 mg/kg PO q8–12h (Hnilica 2003)
For frequently recurrent idiopathic lower urinary tract disease:
a) 5–10 mg (total dose) per cat PO q12h (Lane 2002)

■ **FERRETS:**
a) 2 mg/kg PO 3 times daily (Williams 2000)

■ **HORSES:** (**Note:** ARCI UCGFS Class 2 Drug)
a) 0.5–1 mg/kg IM or PO twice daily (Robinson 1992)
b) Using the pamoate salt: 0.67 mg/kg PO twice daily (Duran 1992)

■ **BIRDS:**
For pruritus associated with allergies, feather picking, or self-mutilation:
a) 2 mg/kg q8h PO or 1.5–2 mg per 4 oz of drinking water daily; adjust dose to minimize drowsiness and maximize effect (Hillyer 1994)
b) 2 mg/kg PO q12h (Siebert 2003)

Monitoring
■ Efficacy
■ Adverse effects

Client Information
■ May cause drowsiness and impede working dogs' abilities

Chemistry/Synonyms

A piperazine-derivative antihistamine, hydroxyzine HCl occurs as a white, odorless powder. It is very soluble in water and freely soluble in alcohol. Hydroxyzine pamoate occurs as a light yellow, practically odorless powder. It is practically insoluble in water and alcohol.

Hydroxyzine may also be known as: hydroxyzine embonate, hydroxyzine pamoate, hydroxyzine HCl, hydroxyzini HCl, *Vistaril®*, *Atarax®* or *Masmoran®*.

Storage/Stability

Hydroxyzine oral products should be stored at room temperature in tight, light-resistant containers. Avoid freezing all liquid products.

Compatibility/Compounding Considerations

The HCl injection has been reported to be physically **compatible** with the following drugs

when mixed in syringes: atropine sulfate, benzquinamide HCl, butorphanol tartrate, chlorpromazine HCl, cimetidine HCl, codeine phosphate, diphenhydramine HCl, doxapram HCl,
droperidol, fentanyl citrate, glycopyrrolate,
hydromorphone HCl, lidocaine HCl, meperidine HCl, methotrimeprazine, metoclopramide
HCl, midazolam HCl, morphine sulfate, oxymorphone HCl, pentazocine lactate, procaine
HCl, prochlorperazine edisylate, promazine
HCl, promethazine HCl, and scopolamine HBr.
Compatibility is dependent upon factors such
as pH, concentration, temperature and diluent
used; consult specialized references or a hospital
pharmacist for more specific information.

Dosage Forms/Regulatory Status

VETERINARY-LABELED PRODUCTS: None

The ARCI (Racing Commissioners International) has designated this drug as a class 2
substance. See the appendix for more information.

HUMAN-LABELED PRODUCTS:

Hydroxyzine HCl Oral Tablets: 10 mg, 25 mg, &
50 mg; generic; (Rx)

Hydroxyzine HCl Oral Syrup: 10 mg/5 mL in
118 mL & 473 mL (may contain alcohol); generic; (Rx)

Hydroxyzine HCl Injection: 25 mg/mL (may
contain benzyl alcohol) in 1 mL & 2 mL vials
and 50 mg/mL (may contain benzyl alcohol) in
1 mL, 2 mL & 10 mL vials; generic; (Rx)

Hydroxyzine Pamoate Oral Capsules (equivalent to hydroxyzine HCl): 25 mg, 50 mg, & 100
mg (as pamoate); generic; (Rx)

Hydroxyzine Pamoate Suspension (equivalent
to hydroxyzine HCl): 25 mg/5 mL (as pamoate)
in 120 mL & 473 mL; *Vistaril®* (Pfizer); (Rx)

References

Duran, S. (1992, Last Update). "Personal Communication."
Gershwin, L. (1992). Treatment of hypersensitiv-
    ity: General guidelines. *Current Veterinary Therapy
    XI: Small Animal Practice.* R Kirk and J Bonagura Eds.
    Philadelphia, W.B. Saunders Company: 54–59.
Griffen, C. (1994). Flea allergy dermatitis. *Saunders
    Manual of Small Animal Practice.* S Birchard and R
    Sherding Eds. Philadelphia, W.B. Saunders Company:
    299–301.
Hillyer, E. (1994). Avian dermatology. *Saunders Manual of
    Small Animal Practice.* S Birchard and R Sherding Eds.
    Philadelphia, W.B. Saunders Company: 1271–1281.
Hnilica, K. (2003). Managing Feline Pruritus. Proceedings:
    Western Veterinary Conference. Accessed via:
    Veterinary Information Network. http://goo.gl/U19xu
Lane, J. (2002). Feline urology update. Proceedings:
    Western Veterinary Conference. Accessed via:
    Veterinary Information Network. http://goo.gl/
    GNVpX
Messinger, L. (2000). Pruritis Therapy in the Cat. *Kirk's
    Current Veterinary Therapy: XIII Small Animal Practice.*
    J Bonagura Ed. Philadelphia, WB Saunders: 542–545.
Paradis, M. & D. Scott (1992). Nonsteroidal therapy for
    canine and feline pruritis. *Current Veterinary Therapy
    XI: Small Animal Practice.* R Kirk and J Bonagura Eds.
    Philadelphia, W.B. Saunders Company: 563–566.
Robinson, N. (1992). Table of Drugs: Approximate Doses.
    Current Therapy in Equine Medicine 3. N Robinson Ed.
    Philadelphia, W.B. Saunders Co.: 815–821.
Siebert, L. (2003). Psittacine feather picking. Proceedings:
    Western Veterinary Conference. Accessed via:
    Veterinary Information Network. http://goo.gl/
    MCA9y
White, S. (2007). Atopic dermatitis and its secondary in-
    fections. Proceedings: Canine Medicine Symposium.
    Accessed via: Veterinary Information Network. http://
    goo.gl/upBF7
Williams, B. (2000). Therapeutics in Ferrets. *Vet Clin NA:
    Exotic Anim Pract* 3:1(Jan): 131–153.

HYOSCYAMINE SULFATE

(hye-oh-*sye*-ah-meen or hye-*ah*-ska-meen)
Levsin®

**ORAL AND INJECTABLE
ANTICHOLINERGIC**

Prescriber Highlights

▶ Anticholinergic that may be useful for
treating hypermotile GI conditions such
as irritable bowel syndrome or bradycardia in dogs

▶ Limited use in veterinary medicine

▶ Adverse effects can include mydriasis,
xerostomia, constipation, urinary retention, & xerophthalmia

Uses/Indications

Although not commonly used in veterinary
medicine, hyoscyamine may be useful as an alternative to other anticholinergic drugs such as
glycopyrrolate for treating bradycardia or hypermotile GI conditions such as irritable bowel
syndrome in dogs. It, potentially, could be useful for treating hypersalivation, urinary spasms,
vomiting, or reducing secretions peri-operative-
ly, but little is known regarding safety and efficacy in animals when used for these conditions.

In humans, hyoscyamine is used primarily
for its effects in reducing GI tract motility or
to decrease pharyngeal, bronchial and tracheal
secretions.

Pharmacology/Actions

Hyoscyamine is an anticholinergic agent similar to atropine, but more potent both in central
and peripheral effects. It inhibits acetylcholine
at tissues innervated by postganglionic nerves
and smooth muscles that respond to acetylcholine but do not have cholinergic innervation.
It does not have action on autonomic ganglia.
Pharmacologic effects include dose-related
reductions in secretions, gastrointestinal and
urinary tract motility, mydriasis, and increased
heart rate.

Pharmacokinetics

No pharmacokinetic data was located for veterinary species. In humans, hyoscyamine is rap-

idly and nearly completely absorbed after oral or sublingual administration. Extended release oral dosage forms may have somewhat reduced oral bioavailability. It is distributed throughout the body, enters the CNS and crosses the placenta. Hyoscyamine is partially hydrolyzed in the liver to tropic acid and tropine. The majority of the drug is excreted unchanged in the urine. Elimination half-life is about 3.5 hours; about 7 hours for the sustained-release product, *Levsinex®*. Average duration of action in humans is approximately 4–6 hours.

Contraindications/Precautions/Warnings

Hyoscyamine is contraindicated in patients hypersensitive to it. Patients sensitive to one belladonna alkaloid or derivative may be sensitive to another.

Use with caution in patients with renal dysfunction as hyoscyamine elimination may be reduced. Use of anticholinergics should be carefully considered in patients with tachyarrhythmias, cardiac valve disease or congestive heart failure. Patients with myasthenia gravis may have their condition aggravated with concurrent use of hyoscyamine. Other contraindications for using hyoscyamine in humans include: glaucoma (narrow or wide angle), intestinal obstruction, toxic megacolon, intestinal atony, severe ulcerative colitis, obstructive uropathy, or acute hemorrhage.

Adverse Effects

Adverse effects can include mydriasis, xerostomia, constipation, urinary retention, and xerophthalmia. Higher dosages may cause CNS effects (somnolence or excitement) or tachycardia.

Reproductive/Nursing Safety

There is limited information available on the drug's use during pregnancy. While hyoscyamine crosses the placenta, reproductive studies in animals have not been performed. Two limited studies (322 & 281 pregnancies) in humans have been published evaluating hyoscyamine safety during pregnancy. One study showed no increase in congenital malformations, but the other showed a slight increase above normally expected malformations in infants. In humans, the FDA categorizes hyoscyamine as category *C* for use during pregnancy (*Animal studies have shown an adverse effect on the fetus, but there are no adequate studies in humans; or there are no animal reproduction studies and no adequate studies in humans.*)

Only traces of hyoscyamine are detected in milk. While no problems have been reported and risk to offspring cannot be ruled out, it is probably safe to use in nursing patients.

Overdosage/Acute Toxicity

The LD50 for hyoscyamine in rats is 375 mg/kg. Significant overdosage in animals may be serious and contacting an animal poison control center is advised. Toxicity is exhibited by intensified and prolonged anticholinergic effects; signs include: increased heart rate, CNS effects (behavior changes, depression, seizures), urinary retention, decreased gut sounds/motility, and mydriasis. Protocols to decrease oral absorption should be considered if overdose was recent. Severe anticholinergic effects can be treated with physostigmine or neostigmine, but it is suggested to do so only under the guidance of an animal poison control center. In humans, delirium or excitement has been treated with small doses of short-acting barbiturates or benzodiazepines. Hyoscyamine can be removed by hemodialysis.

Drug Interactions

The following drug interactions have either been reported or are theoretical in humans or animals receiving hyoscyamine and may be of significance in veterinary patients:

- ◼ **ANTACIDS containing magnesium, aluminum or calcium salts:** May interfere with hyoscyamine absorption

- ◼ **ANTICHOLINERGICS, OTHER (atropine, glycopyrrolate, etc.):** Additive actions and adverse effects can occur

- ◼ **ANTIHISTAMINES, FIRST GENERATION (e.g., diphenhydramine):** Additive actions and adverse effects can occur

- ◼ **PROKINETIC AGENTS (e.g., cisapride, metoclopramide):** Hyoscyamine may counteract their effects

Laboratory Considerations

- ◼ No specific concerns noted with hyoscyamine

Doses

- ◼ **DOGS:**

  Note: The following dosages are assumed to be for the immediate release oral dosage forms. Potentially, the extended release tablets or capsules could be effective and reduce dosing frequency, particularly in larger dogs, but no data is available for using them.

  a) For irritable bowel syndrome: 0.003–0.006 mg/kg PO two to three times a day (Leib 2005)

  b) For long-term management of symptomatic patients with sinus node disease: 0.003–0.006 mg/kg PO q8h (Smith 2004)

Monitoring

- ◼ Clinical efficacy

- ◼ Adverse effects (*e.g.*, heart rate, bowel or urinary elimination difficulties)

Client Information

- ◼ Contact the veterinarian if patient has difficulty urinating or defecating, dry eyes, difficulty swallowing, or demonstrates changes in behavior or activity

Chemistry/Synonyms

Hyoscyamine sulfate is a tertiary amine that occurs as white, odorless, crystals or crystalline powder. One gram is soluble in 0.5 mL of water or in 1 mL of alcohol. It is practically insoluble in ether.

Hyoscyamine may also be known as: daturin, duboisine, tropine-L-tropate. International trade names include: *Egazil Duretter®* and *Neo-Allospasmin®*.

Storage/Stability

Unless otherwise advised by the manufacturer, hyoscyamine sulfate oral products should be stored at room temperature, in tight containers, and protected from light. The injectable product should be stored at room temperature and protected from freezing.

Dosage Forms/Regulatory Status

VETERINARY-LABELED PRODUCTS:

None as single ingredient products.

HUMAN-LABELED PRODUCTS:

Hyoscyamine Oral Tablets: 0.125 mg (regular & chewable), & 0.15 mg; *Anaspaz®* (Ascher), *ED-SPAZ®* (Edwards), *HyoMax®* and *HyoMax-FT®* (Aristos); *Levsin®* (Alaven), *Cystospaz®* (Poly-Medica), generic; (Rx)

Hyoscyamine Orally Disintegrating Tablets: 0.125 mg, & 0.25 mg; *Neosol®* (Breckenridge), *NuLev®* (Schwarz), *Symax FasTab®* (Capellon), *Mar-Spas®* (Marnel); (Rx)

Hyoscyamine Sublingual Oral Tablets: 0.125 mg; *Levsin/SL®* (Alaven); *Symax-SL®* (Capellon); generic; (Rx)

Hyoscyamine Extended/Sustained-Release Oral Tablets: 0.25 mg (0.125 mg immediate-release) & 0.375 mg; *Levbid®* (Alaven), *Symax-SR®* and *Symax Duotab®* (Capellon); generic; (Rx)

Hyoscyamine Extended/Timed-Release Oral Capsules: 0.375 mg; *Levsinex®* (Alaven); generic; (Rx)

Hyoscyamine Oral Solution: 0.125 mg/mL in 15 mL; generic; (Rx)

Hyoscyamine Oral Elixir: 0.025 mg/mL (0.125mg/5mL) in pint bottles generic; (Rx)

Hyoscyamine Oral Spray: 0.125 mg/spray in 30 mL; *IB-Stat®* (InKline); (Rx)

Hyoscyamine Injection: 0.05 mg/mL in 1 mL amps & 10 mL vials; *Levsin®* (Alaven); (Rx)

References

Leib, M. (2005). Idiopathic large intestinal diarrhea in dogs. Proceedings: Western Veterinary Conference 2005, Accessed via the Veterinary Information Network Jan 2007. Accessed via: Veterinary Information Network. http://goo.gl/rYA0d

Smith, F. (2004). Update on antiarrhythmic therapy. Proceedings: Western Veterinary Conference 2005, Accessed via the Veterinary Information Network Jan 2007. Accessed via: Veterinary Information Network. http://goo.gl/HPzaA

IBAFLOXACIN

(ih-bah-*floks*-ah-sin)   Ibaflin®

ORAL FLUOROQUINOLONE ANTIBIOTIC

Prescriber Highlights

▶ Oral fluoroquinolone used in dogs & cats primarily in Europe (not available in USA); oral dosage form is a gel in a "dial" syringe

▶ Similar to other veterinary fluoroquinolones, but may not be as effective against Pseudomonas

▶ Adverse effects can include diarrhea/soft feces, vomiting, dullness, anorexia & salivation

▶ No indication of causing ocular toxicity in cats

Uses/Indications

Ibafloxacin is used in dogs and cats to treat infections susceptible to it. It is labeled (in the UK) for treating dogs with dermal infections (superficial and deep pyoderma, wounds, abscesses) and in cats for treating dermal infections (soft tissue infections—wounds, abscesses) and upper respiratory tract infections caused by susceptible bacteria. Ibafloxacin may also be useful in treating urinary tract infections in dogs.

Pharmacology/Actions

Ibafloxacin is a bactericidal fluoroquinolone antibiotic and acts by inhibiting bacterial DNA-gyrase (a type-II topoisomerase), preventing DNA supercoiling and synthesis. It has a similar spectrum of activity as other veterinary commercially available agents (*Enterobacteriaceae*, *Staphylococcus* spp), but is not very effective against *Pseudomonas* spp, *Streptococcus* spp, or *Proteus mirabilis*.

Ibafloxacin's primary metabolites, 8-hydroxy-ibafloxacin and 7-hydroxy-ibafloxacin, are also active (but less so than ibafloxacin) and contribute to the drug's overall efficacy.

Pharmacokinetics

In dogs, oral bioavailability is about 70–80% with peak levels occurring around 1.5 hours after dosing. At 15 mg/kg, Cmax was 6 micrograms/mL; volume of distribution at steady state was 1.1 L/kg. Ibafloxacin is presumably metabolized in the liver to at least two metabolites, 8-hydroxy-ibafloxacin and 7-hydroxy-ibafloxacin. Both metabolites have been shown to be active, but less so than the parent compound. Elimination occurs in both the urine and feces as unchanged drug and glucuronidated metabolites. Total clearance is 8.7 mL/min/kg and elimination half-life, 5.2 hours (Coulet *et al.* 2002).

In cats, ibafloxacin is rapidly absorbed after oral dosing. After dosing with food, peak levels occur in about 2–3 hours. Food slightly delays absorption, but peak levels are doubled and AUC increased when compared to fasted administration. Cats appear to metabolize and eliminate ibafloxacin in a similar manner as dogs; with repeated dosing, cats, unlike dogs, apparently show significant increases over time in both AUC and Cmax of the parent drug and active metabolites (Coulet *et al.* 2005).

In goats, ibafloxacin has a steady state volume of distribution of 1.65 L/kg and an elimination half-life of 3.76 hours. Clearance was 1.05 L/hr/kg. The milk:plasma ratio of drug concentration under the curve was 0.2 (Marin *et al.* 2007).

Contraindications/Precautions/Warnings
The label (UK) states that for the majority of breeds, use is contraindicated in dogs less than 8 months of age and in giant breeds less than 18 months old. It is contraindicated in cats less than 8 months of age. It is also contraindicated in dogs or cats with known quinolone hypersensitivity. It is stated that the product should only be used based upon susceptibility testing.

Adverse Effects
Adverse effects reported in dogs and cats include diarrhea, soft feces, vomiting, dullness, anorexia and salivation. These reportedly are mild and transient and occur with low frequency. No reports of ibafloxacin-associated ocular toxicity in cats were found.

In dogs, other fluoroquinolones have, in rare incidences, caused elevated hepatic enzymes, ataxia, seizures, depression, lethargy, or nervousness; these could potentially also occur with ibafloxacin.

Reproductive/Nursing Safety
The label (UK) states that ibafloxacin can be used during pregnancy in dogs, but that safety has not been established in pregnant cats or in lactating dogs and cats.

After dosing to goats, ibafloxacin was detected in milk only in scant quantities.

Overdosage/Acute Toxicity
Specific information not located for ibafloxacin. It is unlikely an acute overdose of ibafloxacin would result in signs more serious than anorexia or vomiting, but the adverse effects noted above could occur. If the overdose occurs in cats, ophthalmic monitoring is recommended. In dogs doses of 75 mg/kg/day (5X) were apparently well tolerated; cats receiving up to 75 mg/kg/day demonstrated salivation and vomiting.

Drug Interactions
Drug interactions associated with other fluoroquinolones would also be expected with ibafloxacin. The label states that ibafloxacin should not be used with **NSAIDs** in dogs with a history of seizures.

Other drug interactions with oral fluoroquinolones include:

■ **ANTACIDS or Supplements containing cations (iron, zinc, magnesium, aluminum, calcium):** May bind to ibafloxacin and prevent its absorption

■ **CYCLOSPORINE:** Fluoroquinolones may exacerbate the nephrotoxicity of cyclosporine (used systemically)

■ **NITROFURANTOIN:** May antagonize the antimicrobial activity of the fluoroquinolones; concomitant use is not recommended

■ **QUINIDINE:** Increased risk for cardiotoxicity

■ **SUCRALFATE:** May inhibit absorption of ibafloxacin, separate doses of these drugs by at least 2 hours

■ **THEOPHYLLINE:** Ibafloxacin may increase theophylline blood levels

Laboratory Considerations
■ No specific laboratory concerns noted

Doses

■ **DOGS/CATS:**

For susceptible infections:

a) Using the 3% oral gel for labeled indications (dogs: dermal infections; cats: dermal or respiratory tract infections): 15 mg/kg PO once daily. The syringe should be adjusted to the calculated dosage by setting the syringe ring (steps of 0.5 mL for the 15 mL syringe). Give at time of feeding. Duration treatment depends upon infection nature and severity; usually a 10-day course is sufficient, but can be extended until response is considered adequate. Reconsider treatment if no improvement in clinical response is seen after 5 days of therapy. In cases of deep pyoderma, reconsider treatment if sufficient improvement not seen in 21 days of treatment. (Label Information; *Ibaflin®*—Intervet UK)

Monitoring
■ Clinical efficacy

■ Adverse effects—GI (vomiting, hypersalivation, diarrhea, anorexia)

Client Information
■ Give at the time of feeding

■ Contact veterinarian if vomiting, diarrhea or lack of appetite persist or are severe

■ Give as directed for the period the veterinarian specifies, even if the patient seems well

Chemistry/Synonyms
Ibafloxacin is a fluoroquinolone with a molecular weight of 275.28 and is available commercially as the racemate.

Ibafloxacin may also be known as S-25030 or *Ibaflin®*.

Storage/Stability
The oral gel should not be stored at temperatures more than 25°C. Once opened, it is recommended that the syringe be used within 8 weeks. Once a course of treatment is completed, dispose of unused product.

Dosage Forms/Regulatory Status

VETERINARY-LABELED PRODUCTS: None in the USA

A 3% Oral Gel (30 mg ibafloxacin per gram of gel; 30.9 mg per mL of gel) in 15 mL syringes with 0.5 mL steps is available and labeled for use in dogs and cats in the UK, and in several other EU countries; *Ibaflin®* (Intervet); (Rx).

Depending on the market, 7.5% oral gel, 30 mg, 150 mg, 300 mg, and 900 mg tablets may be available for use in dogs.

HUMAN-LABELED PRODUCTS: None

References

Coulet, M., C. Morello, et al. (2005). Pharmacokinetics of ibafloxacin in healthy cats. Journal of Veterinary Pharmacology and Therapeutics 28(1): 37–44.

Coulet, M., M.V. Waalkes, et al. (2002). Pharmacokinetics of ibafloxacin following intravenous and oral administration to healthy Beagle dogs. Journal of Veterinary Pharmacology and Therapeutics 25(2): 89–97.

Marin, P., C.M. Carceles, et al. (2007). Pharmacokinetics and milk penetration of ibafloxacin after intravenous administration to lactating goats. Canadian Journal of Veterinary Research-Revue Canadienne De Recherche Veterinaire 71(1): 74–76.

IFOSFAMIDE

(eye-*foss*-fa-mide)   Ifex®

ANTINEOPLASTIC

Prescriber Highlights

▶ Alkylating agent that may be useful in treating lymphomas & sarcomas in dogs & cats

▶ Limited veterinary clinical experience to date

▶ May be very toxic (myelosuppression, nephrotoxic, bladder toxicity, neurotoxicity, GI, etc.)

▶ Must be given with saline diuresis & bladder-protective agent (mesna)

Uses/Indications

In small animals, ifosfamide may be of benefit as part of treatment protocols for a variety of neoplasms. Treatment of lymphomas and soft tissue sarcomas with ifosfamide in dogs and cats has been investigated to some extent; some efficacy has been demonstrated. A phase II study in cats with vaccine associated sarcoma, demonstrated a measurable response in 41% of treated cats (Rassnick, Rodriguez et al. 2006).

In humans, ifosfamide is used in various treatment protocols for testicular neoplasms, bone and soft tissue sarcomas, bladder cancer, lung cancer, cervical cancer, ovarian cancer, and some types of lymphomas.

Pharmacology/Actions

Ifosfamide appears to act similarly to other alkylating agents. Its active metabolites interfere with DNA replication and transcription of RNA,

thereby disrupting nucleic acid function. It is cycle-phase nonspecific.

Pharmacokinetics

As ifosfamide is a prodrug and does not have pharmacologic activity, it must be biotransformed into active metabolites. Ifosfamide's pharmacokinetics are very complex and are not well understood. While normally given IV, it is well absorbed after SC injection or oral administration; bioavailabilities via these routes are 90% or greater. Ifosfamide and its metabolites are widely distributed and enter into both bone and CNS. Ifosfamide is converted into its metabolites primarily via oxidative pathways found in the liver and, to a smaller extent, in the lungs. It then is catalyzed (primarily in cells) into the primary active alkylating agent, ifosfamide mustard. Ifosfamide and its metabolites are primarily excreted via the kidney into urine.

Contraindications/Precautions/Warnings

Because of its toxicity, ifosfamide should only be used by clinicians experienced with the use of cytotoxic agents and able to adequately monitor the effects of therapy. Ifosfamide is contraindicated in patients hypersensitive to it or with severely depressed bone marrow function or active hemorrhagic cystitis. Ifosfamide should be used with extreme caution in patients with impaired renal function.

Ifosfamide must be used in conjunction with mesna to reduce the risk for hemorrhagic cystitis.

Adverse Effects

Dose related myelosuppression occurs with ifosfamide use; neutropenia generally occurs at 5−7 days post treatment, but may be delayed (14−21 days) particularly with repeated dosing. Nadirs in cats are seen typically at day 7 or 8. Platelets can also be significantly impacted. Ifosfamide can damage bladder epithelium, and cause nephrotoxicity with resultant electrolyte abnormalities. Renal toxicity is primarily focused on proximal and distal tubular damage, but glomerular effects may occur. To reduce the incidence of nephrotoxicity and bladder toxicity, saline diuresis is performed (see dosages) and mesna given concomitantly to reduce bladder epithelial toxicity (see below). Volume overload with pulmonary edema may result however, particularly in patients with preexisting cardiac disease. Other adverse effects that may occur include: hypersensitivity reactions, nausea, particularly during infusion, vomiting, neurotoxicity (somnolence to confusion, coma, encephalopathy), alopecia, and abnormal liver function tests.

In studies in cats, when doses were at 900 mg/m^2 or less, neutrophil counts of <1,000 cells/microL were seen in about 33% of treated cats, but no secondary infections were noted. Some cats did show some mild, self-limiting GI effects (lack of appetite, vomiting, diarrhea).

Signs of nausea during IV infusion were seen in about ⅓rd of those treated; pulmonary edema, and hypersensitivity were seen in single cats. Nephrotoxicity was seen in two cats. (Rassnick, Moore et al. 2006), (Rassnick, Rodriguez et al. 2006).

Administering mesna with ifosfamide significantly reduces the incidence and severity of ifosfamide-induced hemorrhagic cystitis and hematuria. Mesna interacts with metabolites of ifosfamide that cause the toxicity. Because mesna is hydrophilic, it does not enter most cells and, therefore, does not appear to significantly reduce the anti-tumor efficacy of ifosfamide. Mesna does not prevent or reduce the incidence of other adverse effects associated with ifosfamide (e.g., myelosuppression, GI effects, neurotoxicity, renal toxicity).

Like other cytotoxic drugs, ifosfamide should be handled and disposed of appropriately.

Reproductive/Nursing Safety

In pregnant humans, ifosfamide is designated by the FDA as a category **D** drug (*There is evidence of human fetal risk, but the potential benefits from the use of the drug in pregnant women may be acceptable despite its potential risks.*) Teratogenic and fetotoxic effects have been demonstrated at usual doses in humans and laboratory animals.

Ifosfamide is excreted in maternal milk. If this drug is being used in lactating mothers, consider using milk replacer.

Overdosage/Acute Toxicity

There is limited information available on acute overdoses. It would be expected that toxicity would be exacerbations of the adverse effects seen at usual doses. No specific antidote (including mesna) is known; treatment is supportive. Methylene blue (50 mg in a 1–2% aqueous solution IV over 5 minutes) has been suggested to treat ifosfamide-induced encephalopathy in humans.

Drug Interactions

The following drug interactions have either been reported or are theoretical in humans or animals receiving ifosfamide and may be of significance in veterinary patients:

■ **BENZODIAZEPINES:** A study where mice received benzodiazepines (**diazepam, chlordiazepoxide, oxazepam**) prior to receiving ifosfamide had increased concentrations of active ifosfamide and showed increased toxicity to the drug; clinical significance has not been determined for human (or dog or cat) patients

■ **CISPLATIN:** Ifosfamide may enhance cisplatin-induced ototoxicity and nephrotoxicity

■ **MYELOSUPPRESSIVE DRUGS, Other (e.g., other antineoplastics, chloramphenicol, flucytosine, amphotericin B, or colchicine):** Other bone marrow depressant drugs may cause additive myelosuppression when used with ifosfamide

Laboratory Considerations

■ No specific laboratory interactions or considerations were noted.

Doses

Note: Because of the potential toxicity of this drug to patients, veterinary personnel and clients, and since chemotherapy indications, treatment protocols, monitoring and safety guidelines often change, the following dosages should be used only as a general guide and not as a dosage protocol. Consultation with a veterinary oncologist and referral to current veterinary oncology references [*e.g.,* (Henry & Higginbotham 2009); (Argyle *et al.* 2008); (Withrow & Vail 2007); (Villalobos 2007); (Ogilvie & Moore 2006); (Ogilvie & Moore 2001)] is *strongly recommended.*

■ **DOGS:**

a) For treating lymphomas and soft tissue sarcomas: Give IV saline at 18.3 mL/kg/hr for 6 hours. Give ifosfamide at 350 mg/m² (if patient weighs less than 10 kg), 375 mg/m² (if greater than 10 kg) IV during the second 30 minutes of the 6-hour infusion. Mesna at a dose of 20% of the ifosfamide dose is given as an IV bolus at the start of the IV infusion and again 2 and 5 hours after the ifosfamide infusion. Repeat every 3 weeks. (Brewer 2003)

b) As cat dose "b" below, but dog dose: 375 mg/m². (Kitchell 2008)

■ **CATS:**

a) Based upon a phase I safety study and a phase II trial for vaccine-related sarcomas, the authors recommend a dose of 900 mg/m² every 3 weeks. Mesna bolus and saline diuresis (30 minutes at 18.3 mL/kg/hr) were first given, then ifosfamide and saline diuresis continued for 5 hours after ifosfamide administration completed. (Rassnick, Moore et al. 2006; Rassnick, Rodriguez et al. 2006)

b) Normal (0.9%) saline IV diuresis at a fluid rate of 6 times maintenance over 30 minutes.

Ifosfamide 900 mg/m² diluted to 20 mg/mL or less, IV over 20 minutes.

Normal saline IV diuresis at 6 times maintenance over 5 hours

Mesna urothelial protectant at ⅕ the patient's calculated mg dose at time zero (immediately before ifosfamide administration), and repeated 2 and 5 hours after ifosfamide This therapy may be repeated on a 21 day basis. (Kitchell 2008)

Monitoring

■ CBC with platelets (baseline and before re-dosing)

■ Renal function with electrolytes (baseline and before re-dosing)

- Urinalysis baseline and periodic)
- Liver function (baseline and periodic)
- Other adverse effects (volume overload/pulmonary edema, neurotoxicity, GI toxicity)
- Efficacy

Client Information

- Clients should understand the relative investigational nature of using ifosfamide in dogs or cats and accept the possibility of severe adverse effects due to its use.
- Owners should be instructed to avoid contact with animal's saliva or urine for at least 24 hours after dosing.

Chemistry/Synonyms

An alkylating agent structurally related to cyclophosphamide, ifosfamide occurs as a white, crystalline powder with a melting point of 40°C. It is freely soluble in water and very soluble in alcohol. A 10% solution in water has a pH between 4 and 7.

Ifosfamide may also be known as: MJF-9325, NSC-109724, Z-4942, *Ifex®, Asoifos®, Cuantil®, Duvaxan®, Fentul®, Holoxan®, Holaxane®, Ifex®, IFO-cell®, IFX®, Ifocris®, Ifolem®, Ifomida®, Ifos®, Ifosmixan®, Ifoxan®, Mitoxana®, Seromida®,* or *Troxanol®.*

Storage/stability

Ifosfamide powder for injection should be stored at 20–25°C (68–77°F). It should be protected from temperatures greater than 30°C (86°F) as the drug may liquefy at temperatures greater than 35°C (95°F). Once reconstituted with sterile water for injection or bacteriostatic water for injection the solution is stable for 24 hours when refrigerated. (**Note:** One reference states that bacteriostatic water for injection containing benzyl alcohol caused the solution to become turbid at concentrations of ifosfamide greater than 60 mg/mL. No such incompatibility occurred when using bacteriostatic water for injection containing parabens.)

Compatibility/Compounding Considerations

The reconstituted drug is **compatible** with D_5W, normal saline, or lactated Ringer's and is stable for up to 24 hours when refrigerated. Ifosfamide is **compatible** and stable when mixed with mesna in D_5W or lactated Ringer's.

Dosage Forms/Regulatory Status

VETERINARY-LABELED PRODUCTS: None

HUMAN-LABELED PRODUCTS:

Ifosfamide Powder: for IV infusion 1 gram with 200 mg amps of Mesnex (mesna) in single dose vials; 3 grams with 400 mg amps of Mesnex (mesna) in single dose vials; *Ifex®* (Baxter Medication Delivery); Ifosfamide (American Pharmaceutical Partners); (Rx)

References

Argyle, D. M. Brearly, et al. (2008). *Decision Making in Small Animal Oncology,* Wiley-Blackwell.

Brewer, W. (2003). New, Promising Chemotherapy Agents. Proceedings: Western Veterinary Conference. Accessed via: Veterinary Information Network. http://goo.gl/Ffkz3

Henry, C. & M. Higginbotham (2009). *Cancer Management in Small Animal Practice,* Saunders.

Kitchell, B. (2008). Advances in feline oncology. Proceedings: WSAVA. Accessed via: Veterinary Information Network. http://goo.gl/SeFV3

Ogilvie, G. & A. Moore (2001). *Feline Oncology: A Comprehensive Guide to Compassionate Care,* Veterinary Learning Systems.

Ogilvie, G. & A. Moore (2006). *Managing the Canine Cancer Patient: A Practical Guide to Compassionate Care,* Veterinary Learning Systems.

Rassnick, K.M., A.S. Moore, et al. (2006). Phase I trial and pharmacokinetic analysis of ifosfamide in cats with sarcomas. *American Journal of Veterinary Research* **67**(3): 510–516.

Rassnick, K.M., C.O. Rodriguez, et al. (2006). Results of a phase II clinical trial on the use of ifosfamide for treatment of cats with vaccine-associated sarcomas. *American Journal of Veterinary Research* **67**(3): 517–523.

Villalobos, A. (2007). *Canine and Feline Geriatric Oncology.* Ames, Blackwell.

Withrow, S. & D. Vail (2007). *Withrow and MacEwen's Small Animal Clinical Oncology 4th Ed.* Philadelphia, Elsevier.

Imidacloprid—See the listing in the Topical Dermatologic section in the appendix

IMIDOCARB DIPROPINATE

(i-*mid*-oh-karb)   Imizol®

ANTIPROTOZOAL

Prescriber Highlights

- Antiprotozoal useful against Babesia & related parasites
- Contraindications: Patients exposed to cholinesterase-inhibiting drugs (e.g., pyridostigmine), pesticides, or chemicals
- Caution: Impaired lung, hepatic or renal function; safety in puppies, pregnant, lactating, or breeding animals has not been established
- Adverse Effects: Most common are pain during injection & mild cholinergic signs (salivation, nasal drip, & brief episodes of vomiting); less common: panting, diarrhea, injection site inflammation (rarely ulceration), & restlessness
- Not for intravenous administration

Uses/Indications

Imidocarb is FDA-approved for use to treat *Babesia canis* infections (babesiosis) in dogs, but the drug may also be efficacious against other babesia species (*B. Conradae* and North Carolina Babesia species). Imidocarb appears to be more effective against *B. canis* than *B. gibsoni.*

Imidocarb has been used to treat ehrlichiosis (*E. canis*) but one study found that when used alone, it did not clear the organism (Eddlestone, S.M. *et al.* 2006). Imidocarb appears to be effective for hepatozoonosis (*H. canis*) in dogs and it has also been suggested as a treatment for American canine hepatozoonosis (*H. americanum*), but it does not clear the encysted stage.

In cats, imidocarb therapy has been recommended for treating cytauxzoonosis (*C. felis*) and a prospective study is ongoing, but the results are presently unavailable.

Imidocarb may be of benefit in treating Babesia and related parasitic diseases in a variety of domestic and exotic animals.

Pharmacology/Actions

Imidocarb is thought to act by combining with nucleic acids of DNA in susceptible organisms, causing the DNA to unwind and denature. This damage to DNA is believed to inhibit cellular repair and replication.

Pharmacokinetics

No specific information was located for this drug.

Contraindications/Precautions/Warnings

Do not use imidocarb in patients exposed to cholinesterase-inhibiting drugs, pesticides, or chemicals. The manufacturer states to consider risks versus benefits before treating dogs with impaired lung, hepatic, or renal function. Donkeys appear to be sensitive to the toxic effects of the drug.

Do *not* administer intravenously. In cats, puppies and debilitated dogs, pretreatment with atropine or glycopyrrolate has been advised.

Adverse Effects

Most commonly reported adverse effects in dogs include pain during injection and mild cholinergic signs (salivation, nasal drip and brief episodes of vomiting). Less commonly reported effects include panting, diarrhea, injection site inflammation (rarely ulceration), and restlessness. Rarely, severe renal tubular or hepatic necrosis has occurred. Imidocarb has reportedly caused an increase incidence of tumor formation in rats. Cholinergic adverse effects can be treated with an antimuscarinic (*e.g.*, atropine, glycopyrrolate) if necessary.

Horses given high therapeutic dosages (4 mg/kg) develop lacrimation, sweating, and serous nasal discharge for 30 minutes after treatment.

Reproductive/Nursing Safety

Safety in puppies, pregnant, lactating, or breeding animals has not been established.

Overdosage/Acute Toxicity

Dogs receiving a dosage of 9.9 mg/kg (1.5X labeled dose) showed signs of liver injury (slightly increased liver enzymes), pain and swelling at the injection site, and vomiting. Overdoses or chronic toxicity may present with cholinergic signs (vomiting, weakness, lethargy, salivation)

or adverse changes in liver, kidney, lung, or intestinal function. Treatment with atropine may be useful to treat cholinergic signs associated with imidocarb.

The LD-50 in horses is reportedly 16 mg/kg.

Drug Interactions

The manufacturer warns not use imidocarb in patients exposed to **cholinesterase-inhibiting drugs, pesticides, or chemicals**.

Laboratory Considerations

▪ Imidocarb IM injections may cause significant increases in **creatine kinase (CK)**.

Doses

▪ **DOGS:**

For treatment of babesiosis:

a) 6.6 mg/kg IM or SC; repeat dose in 2 weeks (Package Insert; *Imizol®*—Schering)

b) 5–6.6 mg/kg IM or SC; repeat in 14 days *or* 7.5 mg/kg IM or SC once. A single dose of 6 mg/kg the day following a dose of diminazene at 3.5 mg/kg has also been shown to clear the infection. (Taboada & Lobetti 2006)

For treatment of Ehrlichiosis:

Note: A study (Eddlestone, S. *et al.* 2005; Eddlestone, S.M. *et al.* 2006) demonstrated that imidocarb alone was *not* effective in clearing *Ehrlichia canis* from the blood of experimentally infected dogs.

a) In particularly severe cases, imidocarb at 5 mg/kg SC (in a single injection or two injections 15 days apart) with doxycycline at 10 mg/kg/day for 28 days (Sainz 2002)

For treatment of hepatozoonosis (*H. canis*):

a) 5 mg/kg IM or SC; every 14 days until parasitemia clears. Usually 1–2 injections are sufficient. (Macintire 1999)

▪ **CATS:**

For treatment of *Cytauxzoon felis*:

a) 3–4 mg/kg IM; repeated 7 days after initial dose. Efficacy not proven. Cholinergic effects can be mitigated by pre-treating with atropine. Must also give supportive therapy (IV fluids, prophylactic heparin, nutritional/nursing care, analgesia, and potentially transfusion). This dose is from a prospective clinical trial to determine efficacy and adverse effects. (Cohn, L. 2006; Cohn, L.A. 2009)

b) 5 mg/kg IM once and then 14 days later. (Greene *et al.* 2006)

For treatment of feline hemoplasmosis (Haemobartonellosis; *Mycoplasma haemofelis, Mycoplasma Haemominutum*):

a) Doxycycline is preferred, but in cats intolerant of doxycycline the following alternatives may be effective: imidocarb can be used at 5 mg/kg IM, SC every 14 days until able to maintain a normal PCV. Other optional treatment includes enrofloxacin at 5 mg/kg PO daily or marbofloxacin at 2.75 mg/kg PO daily. (Lappin, M. 2002), (Lappin, M. 2006)

For treatment of feline clinical ehrlichiosis or anaplasmosis:

a) As an alternative to doxycycline, imidocarb can be used at 5 mg/kg IM every 14 days for at least 2-4 treatments. (Lappin, M.R. 2008)

■ HORSES:

For treatment of equine piroplasmosis (*Babesia caballi; Babesia equi*):

a) 2.2 mg/kg IM will generally allow clinical signs to subside. To eliminate *B. caballi* inject 2 mg/kg IM once a day for 2 days. *B. equi* more difficult to eliminate; there has been some success reported when imidocarb is given at 4 mg/kg IM at 72 hour intervals for 4 doses. (Sellon 2004)

■ SHEEP:

For treatment of babesiosis:

a) 1.2 mg/kg IM; repeat in 10–14 days (McHardy *et al.* 1986)

Monitoring

■ Efficacy

■ Adverse effect profile

Chemistry/Synonyms

Imidocarb dipropinate is a diamidine of the carbanalide series of antiprotozoal compounds.

Imidocarb may also be known as 4A65 (imidocarb hydrochloride) and *Imizol®*.

Storage/Stability

The injection should be stored between 2°–25°C (36°–77°F) and protected from light.

Dosage Forms/Regulatory Status

VETERINARY-LABELED PRODUCTS:

Imidocarb Dipropinate for IM or SC Injection: 120 mg/mL in 10 mL multi-dose vials; *Imizol®* (Schering-Plough); (Rx). FDA-approved for use in dogs.

HUMAN-LABELED PRODUCTS: None

References

Cohn, L. (2006). Update on Feline Cytauxzoonosis. Proceedings: ACVIM Forum. Accessed via: Veterinary Information Network. http://goo.gl/Q27Kv

Cohn, L.A. (2009). Update on the Epidemiology & Treatment of Feline Cytauxzoonosis. Peroceedings: ACVIM. Accessed via: Veterinary Information Network. http://goo.gl/Di1Nk

Eddlestone, S., M. Neer, et al. (2005). Failure of imidocarb dipropionate to clear experimentally induced Ehrlichia canis in dogs. Proceedings: ACVIM. Accessed via: Veterinary Information Network. http://goo.gl/huSS2

Eddlestone, S.M., T.M. Neer, et al. (2006). Failure of imidocarb dipropionate to clear experimentally induced Ehrlichia canis infection in dogs. Journal of Veterinary Internal Medicine 20(4): 840–844.

Greene, C., J. Meinkoth, et al. (2006). Cytauxzoonosis. Infectious Diseases of the Dog and Cat. C Greene Ed., Elsevier: 716–722.

Lappin, M. (2002). Imidocarb dipropionate for the treatment of recurrent Haemobartonellosis in cats. Proceedings: ACVIM Forum. Accessed via: Veterinary Information Network. http://goo.gl/OSWUf

Lappin, M. (2006). Update on Flea-associated agents of cats: Bartonella Spp., Hemoplasma Spp., and Rickettsia felis. Proceedings: WSAVA World Congress. Accessed via: Veterinary Information Network. http://goo.gl/0yYU8

Lappin, M.R. (2008). Schering-Plough's Update on Blood Borne Diseases in the Cat. Proceedings; WVC. Accessed via: Veterinary Information Network. http://goo.gl/16fHX

Macintire, D. (1999). Canine Hepatazoonosis. American College of Veterinary Internal Medicine: 17th Annual Veterinary Medical Forum, Chicago.

McHardy, N., R. Woolon, et al. (1986). Efficacy, toxicity and metabolism of imidocarb dipropionate in the treatment of Babesia ovis infection in sheep. Res Vet Sci 41((1)): 14–20.

Sainz, A. (2002). Clinical and therapeutic aspects of canine ehrlichiosis. Proceedings: World Small Animal Veterinary Association World Congress. Accessed via: Veterinary Information Network. http://goo.gl/TMwwb

Sellon, D. (2004). Disorders of the hematopoietic system. Equine Internal Medicine, 2nd Ed. M Reed, W Bayly and D Sellon Eds. Phila., Saunders: 721–768.

Taboada, J. & R. Lobetti (2006). Babesia. Infectious Diseases of the Dog and Cat, 3rd Ed. C Greene Ed., Elsevier: 722–736.

IMIPENEM-CILASTATIN SODIUM

(ih-me-*peh*-nem sye-la-*sta*-tin)   Primaxin®

CARBAPENEM ANTIBIOTIC

Prescriber Highlights

▶ Broad spectrum antibiotic/deactivating enzyme inhibitor combination used for serious infections where a single agent is desired

▶ Contraindications/Cautions: Patients hypersensitive to it or other beta-lactams, patients with renal impairment (dosages adjustment may be required), CNS disorders (*e.g.*, seizures, head trauma)

▶ Adverse Effects: GI effects, CNS toxicity (seizures, tremors), hypersensitivity, & infusion reactions (thrombophlebitis)

▶ Too rapid IV infusions may cause GI or CNS toxicity, or other untoward effects; Rarely: increases in renal or hepatic function tests; hypotension or tachycardia

▶ Separate dosage forms for IM or IV use

▶ Can be expensive

Uses/Indications

Imipenem may be useful in equine or small animal medicine to treat serious infections when other less expensive antibiotics are ineffective or have unacceptable adverse effect profiles. The carbapenems, including imipenem, ertapenem, and meropenem are particularly valuable when treating serious multi-drug resistant gram-negative infections.

Pharmacology/Actions

This fixed combination of a carbapenem antibiotic (imipenem) and an inhibitor (cilastatin) of dehydropeptidase I (DHP I) has a very broad spectrum of activity. Imipenem is generally considered to be a bactericidal agent, but may be static against some bacteria. It has an affinity for and binds to most penicillin-binding protein sites, thereby inhibiting bacterial cell wall synthesis.

Imipenem has activity against a wide variety of bacteria, including gram-positive aerobic cocci (including some bacteriostatic activity against some enterococci), gram-positive aerobic bacilli (including static activity against Listeria), gram-negative aerobic bacteria (Haemophilus, Enterobacteriaceae, many strains of *Pseudomonas aeruginosa*), and anaerobes (including some strains of Bacteroides).

Imipenem is not efficacious for treating infections caused by methicillin-resistant staphylococci or resistant strains of *Enterococcus faecium*.

Cilastatin inhibits the metabolism of imipenem by DHP 1 on the brush borders of renal tubular cells. This serves two functions: it allows higher urine levels and may protect against proximal renal tubular necrosis that can occur when imipenem is used alone.

Pharmacokinetics

Neither drug is absorbed appreciably from the GI tract and, therefore, they are given parenterally. Bioavailability after IM injection is approximately 95% for imipenem and 75% for cilastatin. In dogs, bioavailability of imipenem after SC injection is complete. Imipenem is distributed widely throughout the body, with the exception of the CSF. Imipenem crosses the placenta and is distributed into milk. When given with cilastatin, imipenem is eliminated by both renal and non-renal mechanisms. Approximately 75% of a dose is excreted in the urine and about 25% is excreted by unknown non-renal mechanisms. Half-lives in patients with normal renal function range from 1–3 hours on average. In horses average elimination time is 70 minutes; 60 minutes in dogs.

Contraindications/Precautions/Warnings

The potential risks versus benefits should be carefully weighed before using imipenem/cilastatin in patients hypersensitive to it or other beta-lactam antibiotics (*e.g.*, penicillins, cephalosporins as partial cross-reactivity may occur), with renal function impairment (dosages may need to be reduced or time between doses lengthened), or with CNS disorders (*e.g.*, seizures, head trauma) as CNS adverse effects may be more likely to occur.

Do not give this drug via rapid IV infusion as seizures are possible. In humans, it is recommended to give doses of 500 mg or less over 20–30 minutes, and doses over 500 mg over 40–60 minutes. If given IM (or SC), the specific IM product should be used.

Adverse Effects

Potential adverse effects include: GI effects (vomiting, anorexia, diarrhea), CNS toxicity (seizures, tremors), hypersensitivity (pruritus, fever to anaphylaxis) and infusion reactions (thrombophlebitis; too rapid IV infusions may cause GI or CNS toxicity. Rapid IV infusion or multiple high doses to animals with reduced renal function (including neonates and geriatric animals) may increase the risk for seizures.

Imipenem may be administered IM (and some have used it SC), but it can cause severe pain at the injection site and neurovascular damage. It is suggested to dilute the IM form in 1% lidocaine to relieve the associated pain. Rarely, transient increases in renal (BUN or serum creatinine values) or hepatic (AST/ALT/ Alk Phosphatase) function tests may be noted, as well as, hypotension or tachycardias.

Reproductive/Nursing Safety

While no teratogenic effects have been noted in animal studies, safe use during pregnancy has not been firmly established. In humans, the FDA categorizes this drug as category *C* for use during pregnancy (*Animal studies have shown an adverse effect on the fetus, but there are no adequate studies in humans; or there are no animal reproduction studies and no adequate studies in humans.*)

While imipenem enters milk, no adverse effects attributable to it have been noted in nursing offspring.

Overdosage/Acute Toxicity

Little information is available. The LD_{50} of imipenem:cilastatin in a 1:1 ratio in mice and rats is approximately 1 gram/kg/day. Acute overdoses should be handled by halting therapy then treating supportively and symptomatically.

Drug Interactions

The following drug interactions have either been reported or are theoretical in humans or animals receiving imipenem-cilastatin and may be of significance in veterinary patients:

- **■ AMINOGLYCOSIDES:** Additive effects or synergy may result when aminoglycosides are added to imipenem/cilastatin therapy, particularly against Enterococcus, *Staph. aureus*, and *Listeria monocytogenes*. There is apparently neither synergy nor antagonism when used in combination against Enterobacteriaceae, including *Pseudomonas aeruginosa*.

- **■ BETA-LACTAM ANTIBIOTICS:** Antagonism may occur when used in combination with other beta lactam antibiotics against several Enterobacteriaceae (including many strains of *Pseudomonas aeruginosa* and some strains of Klebsiella, Enterobacter, Serratia, Enterobacter, Citrobacter, and Morganella); clinical importance of this interaction is unclear, but at present it is not recommended to use imipenem in conjunction with other beta-lactam antibiotics.

■ **CHLORAMPHENICOL:** May antagonize the antibacterial effects of imipenem (*in vitro* evidence)

■ **PROBENECID:** May increase concentrations and elimination half-life of cilastatin, but not imipenem; concurrent use not recommended

■ **TRIMETHOPRIM/SULFA:** Synergy may occur against *Nocardia asteroides* when imipenem is used in combination with trimethoprim/sulfa

Laboratory Considerations

■ Imipenem may cause a false-positive **urine glucose** determination when using the cupric sulfate solution test (*e.g.*, *Clinitest®*), Benedict' solution or Fehling's solution. Enzymatic glucose oxidase based tests are not affected (*e.g.*, *Tes-Tape®, Clinistix®*).

Doses

Note: When giving IM, the manufacturer recommends a 21g needle (deep IM) with aspiration, to avoid IV administration.

■ **DOGS/CATS:**

For susceptible infections:

a) 5−10 mg/kg IV, SC or IM (IM form is different) q8h (Aucoin 2002)

b) 5−10 mg/kg IV (given over 30 minutes) q6h or IM q6h (mixed with 1% lidocaine to reduce pain). **Note:** Cannot interchange IV and IM dosage forms. (Trepanier 1999)

c) For tissue infections: 3−7.5 mg/kg IV, SC or IM q4−6h for 3−5 days; for sepsis, more resistant organisms give 5 mg/kg IV q4h (multi-drug resistant bacteria may require q2h dosing) for 3−5 days (Greene *et al.* 2006)

d) For treatment of Nocardiosis: 2−5 mg/kg IV q8h (Lemarie 2003)

■ **HORSES:**

For susceptible infections:

a) Adult horses: 10−20 mg/kg via slow IV (over a 10 minute period) q6h; alternatively a CRI of 16 micrograms/kg/minute should maintain synovial concentrations greater than 1 microgram/mL. (Orsini *et al.* 2005)

b) **Foals:** 10−20 mg/kg IV q6h (Haggett & Wilson 2008; Wilkins 2004)

c) **Foals:** 10−15 mg/kg IV q6-12h; IM if diluted into 1% lidocaine. May give as a CRI at 0.4−0.8 mg/kg/hr. (Corley & Hollis 2009)

Monitoring

■ Efficacy

■ Adverse effects (including renal and hepatic function tests if treatment is prolonged or patient's renal or hepatic functions are in question)

Client Information

■ Imipenem/cilastatin should be administered in an inpatient setting.

■ Clients should be informed of the cost of using this medication.

Chemistry/Synonyms

Imipenem monohydrate is a carbapenem antibiotic that occurs as white or off-white, non-hygroscopic, crystalline compound. At room temperature, 11 mg are soluble in 1 mL of water. Cilastatin sodium, an inhibitor of dehydropeptidase I (DHP I), occurs as an off-white to yellowish, hygroscopic, amorphous compound. More than 2 grams are soluble in 1 mL of water.

The commercially available injections are available in a 1:1 fixed dose ratio. The solutions are clear to yellowish in color. pH after reconstitution ranges from 6.5 to 7.5. These products have sodium bicarbonate added as a buffer. The suspensions for IM use are white to light tan in color.

Imipenem may also be known as: N-formimidoyl thienamycin, imipemide, MK-787, and MK-0787; multi-ingredient preparations: *Imipem®, Klonam®, Primaxin®, Tenacid®, Tienam®, Tracix®,* and *Zienam®*.

Storage/stability

Commercially available sterile powders for injection should be stored at room temperature (<25°C). After reconstitution, the solution is stable for 4 hours at room temperature; 10 hours when refrigerated. If other diluents are used, stability times may be reduced (see package insert). Do not freeze solutions. The manufacturer does not recommend admixing with other drugs.

After reconstitution the sterile powder for suspension with 1% lidocaine HCl injection, the suspension should be used within one hour.

Compatibility/Compounding Considerations

The following drugs are reportedly **compatible** with imipenem/cilastatin for IV infusion at a Y-site: aztreonam, cefepime, diltiazem, famotidine, insulin, ondansetron, and propofol.

To dilute the IM form of the drug with lidocaine: Use 1% lidocaine solution (without epinephrine). Prepare the 500 mg vial with 2 mL lidocaine and the 750 mg vial with 3 mL lidocaine.

Dosage Forms/Regulatory Status

VETERINARY-LABELED PRODUCTS: None

HUMAN-LABELED PRODUCTS:

Imipenem Cilastatin Powder for Injection: 250 mg imipenem equivalent and 250 mg cilastatin equivalent (0.8 mEq sodium); 500 mg imipenem equivalent and 500 mg cilastatin equivalent (1.6 mEq sodium) in vials, infusion bottles and *ADD-Vantage* vials; *Primaxin® I.V.* (Merck); (Rx)

Imipenem Cilastatin Powder for Injection: 500 mg imipenem equivalent and 500 mg cilastatin equivalent (1.4 mEq sodium) in vials; *Primaxin® I.M.* (Merck); (Rx)

References

Aucoin, D. (2002). Rational approach to antimicrobial therapy in companion animals. Proceedings: Atlantic Coast Veterinary Conference. Accessed via: Veterinary Information Network. http://goo.gl/5atZq

Corley, K.T.T. & A.R. Hollis (2009). Antimicrobial therapy in neonatal foals. *Equine Veterinary Education* 21(8): 436–448.

Greene, C., K. Hartmannn, et al. (2006). Appendix 8: Antimicrobial Drug Formulary. *Infectious Disease of the Dog and Cat*. C Greene Ed., Elsevier: 1186–1333.

Haggett, E.F. & W.D. Wilson (2008). Overview of the use of antimicrobials for the treatment of bacterial infections in horses. *Equine Veterinary Education* 20(8): 433–448.

Lemarie, S. (2003). Cutaneous mycobacterium, nocardia and actinomyces. Proceedings Western Veterinary Conf. http://goo.gl/xhbNj

Orsini, J., P. Moate, et al. (2005). Pharmacokinetics of imipenem-cilastatin following intravenous administration in healthy horses. *J Vet Phamacol Ther* 28: 355–361.

Trepanier, L. (1999). Treating resistant infections in small animals. Proceedings: 17th Annual American College of Veterinary Internal Medicine Meeting, Chicago.

Wilkins, P. (2004). Disorders of foals. *Equine Internal Medicine, 2nd Ed.* S Reed, W Bayly and D Sellon Eds. Philadelphia, Saunders: 1381–1431.

IMIPRAMINE HCL
IMIPRAMINE PAMOATE

(im-*ip*-ra-meen)   Tofranil®

TRICYCLIC ANTIDEPRESSANT

Prescriber Highlights

▶ Tricyclic "antidepressant" used primarily for cataplexy & urinary incontinence (dogs/cats) narcolepsy & ejaculatory dysfunction (horses)

▶ May reduce seizure thresholds in epileptic animals

▶ Very toxic in overdoses to both animals & humans

▶ May be teratogenic

▶ Adverse Effects: Sedation & anticholinergic effects (tachycardia, hyperexcitability, tremors) most likely

Uses/Indications

In dogs and cats, imipramine has been used to treat cataplexy and urinary incontinence. In horses, imipramine has been used to treat narcolepsy and ejaculatory dysfunction (no parenteral dosage forms available).

Pharmacology/Actions

Imipramine and its active metabolite, desipramine, have a complicated pharmacologic pro-file. From a slightly oversimplified viewpoint, they have 3 main characteristics: blockage of the amine pump, thereby increasing neurotransmitter levels (principally serotonin, but also norepinephrine), sedation, and central and peripheral anticholinergic activity. While not completely understood, it is thought that the antienuretic activity of imipramine is related to its anticholinergic effects, but imipramine may also have some alpha adrenergic agonist activity. In animals, tricyclic antidepressants are similar to the actions of phenothiazines in altering avoidance behaviors.

Pharmacokinetics

Imipramine is rapidly absorbed from both the GI tract and from parenteral injection sites. Peak levels occur within 1−2 hours after oral dosing. Imipramine and desipramine enter the CNS and maternal milk in levels equal to that found in maternal serum. The drug is metabolized in the liver to several metabolites, including desipramine, which is active. In humans the terminal half-life is approximately 8−16 hours.

Contraindications/Precautions/Warnings

These agents are contraindicated if prior sensitivity has been noted with any other tricyclic. Concomitant use with monoamine oxidase inhibitors is generally contraindicated.

Use with caution in patients with seizure disorders. Imipramine may lower seizure threshold.

Adverse Effects

While there is little experience with this drug in domestic animals, the most predominant adverse effects seen with the tricyclics are related to their sedating and anticholinergic (dry mouth, constipation, tachycardia, hyperexcitability, tremors) properties. They can cause CNS stimulation (seizures) however, and adverse effects can run the entire gamut of systems including hematologic (bone marrow suppression), GI (diarrhea, vomiting), endocrine, etc.

Reproductive/Nursing Safety

Isolated reports of limb reduction abnormalities have been noted; restrict use to pregnant animals when the benefits clearly outweigh the risks. In humans, the FDA categorizes this drug as category *D* for use during pregnancy (*There is evidence of human fetal risk, but the potential benefits from the use of the drug in pregnant women may be acceptable despite its potential risks.*)

Imipramine is excreted into milk in low concentrations (approximate milk:plasma ratio of 0.4 to 1.5).

Overdosage/Acute Toxicity

Overdosage with tricyclics can be life-threatening (arrhythmias, cardiorespiratory collapse). Because the toxicities and therapies for treatment are complicated and controversial, it is recommended to contact a poison control center for further information in any potential overdose situation.

Drug Interactions

The following drug interactions have either been reported or are theoretical in humans or animals receiving imipramine and may be of significance in veterinary patients:

■ **ANTICHOLINERGIC AGENTS:** Because of additive effects, use with imipramine cautiously

■ **CIMETIDINE:** May inhibit tricyclic antidepressant metabolism and increase the risk of toxicity

■ **CISAPRIDE:** Increased risk for prolonged QT interval

■ **CLONIDINE:** Tricyclics may increase blood pressure

■ **CNS DEPRESSANTS:** Because of additive effects, use with imipramine cautiously

■ **LEVODOPA:** Imipramine may decrease levodopa oral absorption

■ **PHENOBARBITAL:** May decrease tricyclic levels

■ **QUINIDINE:** Increased risk for QTc interval prolongation and tricyclic adverse effects

■ **RIFAMPIN:** May decrease tricyclic blood levels

■ **SSRIS (e.g., fluoxetine, paroxetine, sertraline, etc.):** Increased risk for serotonin syndrome

■ **SYMPATHOMIMETIC AGENTS:** Use in combination with sympathomimetic agents may increase the risk of cardiac effects (arrhythmias, hypertension, hyperpyrexia)

■ **MONOAMINE OXIDASE INHIBITORS (including amitraz, and possibly selegiline):** Concomitant use (within 14 days) with monoamine oxidase inhibitors is generally contraindicated (serotonin syndrome)

■ **THYROID AGENTS:** May increase risk for cardiac arrhythmias

Laboratory Considerations

■ **ECG:** Tricyclics can widen QRS complexes, prolong PR intervals and invert or flatten T-waves on ECG

■ **GLUCOSE, BLOOD:** Tricyclics may alter (increase or decrease) blood glucose levels

Doses

■ **DOGS:**

For urethral incompetence:

a) 5–15 mg (total dose) PO q12h (Labato 1994), (Bartges 2006)

b) For urinary incontinence when other agents fail: 5–20 mg (total dose) PO q12h (Lane 2000)

For cataplexy:

a) 0.5–1 mg/kg PO q8h; titrate dose based on clinical effect (Fenner 1994); (Coleman 1999)

For behavior-related conditions:

a) For adjunctive treatment of separation anxiety or other tricyclic antidepressant-responsive behavior disorders: 2.2–4.4 mg/kg PO once to twice daily (Marder 1991)

For adjunctive treatment of pain:

a) For adjunctive cancer pain treatment: 0.5–1 mg/kg PO q8h (Lester & Gaynor 2000)

■ **CATS:**

For urethral incompetence:

a) 2.5–5 mg (total dose) PO q12h (Labato 1994)(Bartges 2006)

For adjunctive cancer pain treatment:

a) 2.5–5 mg (total dose) PO q12h (Lester & Gaynor 2000)

■ **HORSES: (Note:** ARCI UCGFS Class 2 Drug) **Note:** The injectable product is no longer marketed in the USA.

a) For pharmacologic induced ejaculation: 2 mg/kg IV. If imipramine alone does not induce erection and ejaculation in 10–15 minutes, give xylazine 0.2–0.3 mg/kg IV. (Samper 2004)

b) For narcolepsy/cataplexy: 0.55 mg/kg IV or 250–750 mg (total dose) orally. PO administration produces inconsistent results. (Andrews & Matthews 2004)

Monitoring

■ Efficacy

■ Adverse effects

Client Information

■ All tricyclics should be dispensed in child-resistant packaging and kept well away from children or pets.

■ Inform clients that several weeks may be required before efficacy is noted and to continue dosing as prescribed.

Chemistry/Synonyms

A tricyclic antidepressant agent, imipramine is available commercially in either the hydrochloride or pamoate salts. Imipramine HCl occurs as an odorless or practically odorless, white to off-white crystalline powder that is freely soluble in water or alcohol. Imipramine pamoate occurs as a fine yellow powder that is practically insoluble in water, but soluble in alcohol. The HCl injection has a pH of 4–5.

Imipramine HCl may also be known as: imipramini chloridum, imipramini hydrochloridum, imizine, *Antidep®*, *Celamine®*, *Depramina®*, *Depsonil®*, *Elepsin®*, *Ethipramine®*, *Impra®*, *Imiprex®*, *Imiprin®*, *Imp-Tab®*, *Impril®*, *Janimine®*, *Melipramine®*, *Mipralin®*, *Novo-Pramine®*, *Praminan®*, *Primonil®*, *Pryleugan®*, *Sermonil®*, *Surplix®*, *Talpramin®*, and *Tofranil®*.

Storage/Stability

Imipramine HCl tablets and the pamoate capsules should be stored in tight, light resistant containers, preferably at room temperature. The

HCl injection should be stored at temperatures less than 40°C and freezing should be avoided. Expiration dates for oral HCL products are from 3–5 years after manufacture; for the pamoate, 3 years.

Imipramine HCl will turn yellow to reddish on exposure. Slight discoloration will not affect potency, but marked changes in color are associated with a loss of potency.

Dosage Forms/Regulatory Status

VETERINARY-LABELED PRODUCTS: None

The ARCI (Racing Commissioners International) has designated this drug as a class 2 substance. See the appendix for more information.

HUMAN-LABELED PRODUCTS:

Imipramine HCl Tablets: 10 mg, 25 mg & 50 mg; *Tofranil*® (Norvartis), generic; (Rx)

Imipramine Pamoate Capsules: 75 mg, 100 mg, 125 mg & 150 mg; *Tofranil*®-*PM* (Norvartis), generic; (Rx)

References

Andrews, F. & H. Matthews (2004). Seizures, narcoplexy, and cataplexy. *Equine Internal Medicine, 2nd Ed.* S Reed, W Bayly and D Sellon Eds. Philadelphia, Saunders: 560–579.

Bartges, J. (2006). Broken plumbing: urinary incontinence. Proceedings: ACVC 2006. Accessed via: Veterinary Information Network. http://goo.gl/XgEUd

Coleman, E. (1999). Canine narcolepsy and the role of the nervous system. Comp CE 21(7): 641-650.

Labato, M. (1994). Micturition Disorders. *Saunders Manual of Small Animal Practice.* S Birchard and R Sherding Eds. Philadelphia, W.B. Saunders Company: 857–864.

Lane, I. (2000). Use of anticholinergic agents in lower urinary tract disease. Kirk's Current Veterinary Therapy: XIII Small Animal Practice. J Bonagura Ed. Philadelphia, WB Saunders: 899- 902.

Lester, P. & J. Gaynor (2000). Management of cancer pain. *Vet Clin NA: Small Anim Pract* **30**:4(July): 951–966.

Marder, A. (1991). Psychotropic drugs and behavioral therapy. *Veterinary Clinics of North America: Small Animal Practice* **21**(2): 329–342.

Samper, J. (2004). The stallion. *Equine Internal Medicine, 2nd Ed.* S Reed, W Bayly and D Sellon Eds. Philadelphia, Saunders: 1135–1168.

Imiquimod—see the Topical Dermatologic section in the appendix

IMMUNE GLOBULIN (HUMAN), INTRAVENOUS

(im-*myoon glob*-yoo-lin)   IGIV, IVIG, hIVIG

IMMUNE SERUM

Prescriber Highlights

▶ Potentially useful for canine immune-mediated diseases (e.g., IMHA, pIMT, immune-mediated dermatopathies)

▶ Limited experience in dogs

▶ Hypersensitivity reactions possible

▶ Very expensive

Uses/Indications

In veterinary medicine, intravenous immune globulin (human) or IVIG has been used, and may be useful for treating immune-mediated hemolytic (IMHA), immune-mediated dermatopathies, and immune-mediated thrombocytopenia (pIMT) particularly in patients that have failed other treatments. Limited retrospective and prospective studies have demonstrated mixed results, but the data, while very limited, suggests that IVIG may be most useful in treating primary immune-mediated thrombocytopenia in dogs. Definitive studies evaluating the safety and efficacy of IVIG in veterinary patients are not available and because of the drug's significant expense are unlikely in the foreseeable future. Some question whether the drug should be used at all in veterinary patients as supply is limited and some countries ration its use in humans.

A prospective, randomized, double-blinded, controlled trial of IVIG (with glucocorticoids) in 28 dogs with recently diagnosed IMHA was recently published (Whelan *et al.* 2009). There were no statistically significant differences between the treated and placebo groups in survival, length of hospitalization, time to hematocrit stabilization, and transfusion requirements. While the study population was relatively small, the authors concluded that the cost of the treatment does not lend support to its use as an early intervention treatment in dogs.

In humans, IVIG has been used for a variety of immune system-related conditions including primary and secondary immunodeficiencies, graft versus host disease, Guillain-Barre syndrome, chronic inflammatory demyelinating polyneuropathy, autoimmune hemolytic anemia, juvenile idiopathic arthritis, myasthenia gravis, toxic epidermal necrolysis, systemic vasculitis, and sepsis.

Pharmacology/Actions

Immunoglobulins are produced by B lymphocytes as part of the humoral response to foreign antigens. IVIG antibodies act through a variety of mechanisms, including antimicrobial or antitoxin neutralization. Its efficacy for treating autoimmune disorders may be due to: providing anti-idiotypic antibodies that neutralize autoantibodies; negative feedback and down-regulation of antibody production; binding to CD5 receptors, interleukin (IL)-1a, IL-6, tumor necrosis factor-alpha, and T-cell receptors; and suppressing pathogenic cytokines and phagocytes.

Pharmacokinetics

Elimination half-life in dogs is reported to be 7–9 days. In humans, the onset of actions is rapid. Immunoglobulins are primarily eliminated by catabolism and the mean half-life is about 3 weeks. Fever or infection may decrease antibody half-life because of increased catabolism or consumption.

Contraindications/Precautions/Warnings

Dogs that have had prior hypersensitivity reactions after receiving human albumin, should not receive IVIG. Trace amounts of human albumin may be found in IVIG.

In humans, many adverse reactions are associated with administering IVIG at rates higher than recommended. Follow infusion rate guidelines carefully. At doses used in dogs (0.5–1.5 grams/kg), IVIG is generally infused over a 6–12 hour period.

The FDA has placed a "Black Box Warning" on the labeling of IVIG for use in humans as IVIG has been associated with renal dysfunction, acute renal failure, osmotic nephrosis, and death.

Adverse Effects

In dogs, IVIG can cause increased blood pressure. Local reactions at or near the injection site are possible. Anecdotal reports of anaphylaxis have been reported in dogs receiving IVIG. IVIG can contain trace amounts of human albumin that has been associated with hypersensitivity reactions in dogs. As IVIG can have colloid-like properties, volume overload is possible. Thrombotic events have been reported in humans and are possible in dogs.

In humans, adverse effects of IVIG in people are relatively uncommon and most are transient, self-limiting and include fever, chills, facial flushing, headache, and nausea. Thrombotic events have been reported. Rarely, acute renal failure, acute tubular necrosis, osmotic nephrosis, and proximal tubular nephropathy have been reported in humans. Increases in creatinine and BUN have been seen as soon as 1-2 days following infusion. Hypersensitivity reactions, including anaphylaxis have been reported, but are very rare in human patients.

Reproductive/Nursing Safety

In humans, the FDA has placed IVIG in category C for use during pregnancy (*Animal studies have shown an adverse effect on the fetus, but there are no adequate studies in humans; or there are no animal reproduction studies and no adequate studies in humans*. However, there does not appear to be a significant risk to offspring.

The drug appears to be safe for use during lactation and nursing.

Overdosage/Acute Toxicity

Fluid volume overload is possible. Other reactions could include pain and tenderness at the injection site.

Drug Interactions

The following drug interactions have either been reported or are theoretical in humans or animals receiving IVIG and may be of significance in veterinary patients:

■ **VACCINES, LIVE:** IVIG may interfere with immune response and efficacy

Laboratory Considerations

■ **BLOOD GLUCOSE:** Falsely elevated blood glucose measurements can occur when using the glucose dehydrogenase pyrroloquinoline quinone (GDH-PQQ) based test. Consider using tests that are not affected, including the glucose oxidase, glucose dehydrogenase nicotine adenine dinucleotide (GDH-NAD), or glucose dehydrogenase flavin adenine dinucleotide (GDH-FAD) methods

■ **COOMBS TEST:** In humans, the transitory rise of the various passively transferred antibodies may cause positive serological testing results, potentially altering the test's results and interpretation

Doses

■ **DOGS:**

a) Various dosages have been used in dogs ranging from 0.3–1.5 grams/kg which translates into an estimated $400 to $1500 associated with the cost of the drug alone. Recommendations that IVIG should be considered when dogs with IMHA or ITP fail to respond to conventional therapy must be weighed against the additional cost after clients have already spent a considerable amount of money during initial treatment. From a healthcare system point of view this would appear to be unjustifiable and probably would not be recommended, however, on an individual patient basis, clients and clinicians may find such therapy offers some degree of hope and cost-analyses may not dissuade its usage. (Chan 2009)

b) IVIG has shown some benefit in IMHA patients that are refractory to conventional treatment. It is given at a dose of 0.5–1.5 grams/kg IV over 12 hours.(Macintire 2006)

c) For primary immune-mediated thrombocytopenia (pIMT): In the study, dogs in the treatment group received a single

IV infusion of IVIG at 0.5 grams/kg. (Bianco *et al.* 2007)

d) For refractory cases of erythema multiforme, Stevens-Johnson syndrome/toxic epidermal necrolysis, and other cutaneous adverse drug reactions, treatment with human IVIG may be effective. A 5–6% solution is given at 0.5–1 gram/kg IV over a 4-6 hour period, 1-2 times, 24 hours apart. This treatment may need to be repeated for 3-4 days in a row. Further study is needed. (Jazic 2010)

Monitoring
■ Vital signs: including blood pressure, temperature
■ Lung auscultation to assess for volume overload
■ Renal function tests and urine output
■ Efficacy (depending on purpose for use)

Client Information
■ It is imperative that before use, clients understand that this drug is not commonly used in veterinary medicine, and the costs and risks associated with its use.

Chemistry/Synonyms
IVIG consists of fractionated immunoglobulins, and is primarily intact IgG. It is obtained from pooled human plasma (1,000–60,000 human donors). It may also contain trace amounts of IgM, IgA, soluble CD4, CD8 and HLA molecules, and some cytokines. Further processing is performed to inactivate viruses and remove IgG aggregates and other contaminants. Stabilizing agents can include polyethylene glycol, glycine, sorbitol, polysorbate 80, and sugars (maltose, glucose, sucrose).

Immune globulin (human) may also be known as hIVIG, IVIG, IGIV, immunoglobulin, immunglobuline, or immunoglobulinas.

Storage/Stability
IVIG products are usually stored at room temperature, but specific storage requirements may vary with each product; refer to the label. These products should not be frozen.

Compatibility/Compounding Considerations
IVIG should not be mixed with other medications. One product's label (*Privigen®*) states that it can be diluted with 5% dextrose in water (D5W) if necessary.

Dosage Forms/Regulatory Status
VETERINARY-LABELED PRODUCTS: None

HUMAN-LABELED PRODUCTS:

Immune Globulin (Human) Injection 5% (50 mg/mL) preservative-free in 10 mL, 20 mL, 50 mL, 100 mL, & 200 mL (0.5 gram, 1 gram, 2.5 grams, 5 grams, & 10 grams—depending on product) single use bottles; *Felbogamma®* (Grifols), *Octagam®* (Octapharm), *Gammaplex®* (FFF); (Rx)

Immune Globulin (Human) Injection 10% (100 mg/mL) preservative-free in 10 mL, 20 mL, 50 mL, 100 mL, & 200 mL (1 gram, 2 grams, 10 grams, & 20 grams—depending on product) single use bottles; *Gamunex®* (Talecris), *Gammagard®* (Baxter), *Privigen®* (AventisB); (Rx)

Immune Globulin (Human) Lyophilized Powder for Solution 0.5 gram, 3 grams, 6 grams & 12 grams—depending on product); *Carimune NF®* (ZLB), *Gammagard S/D®* (Baxter); (Rx)

References
Bianco, D., P.J. Armstrong, et al. (2007). Treatment of severe immune-mediated thrombocytopenia with human IV immunoglobulin in 5 dogs. Journal of Veterinary Internal Medicine 21(4): 694–699.

Chan, D. (2009). Immunoglobulin Therapy: Worth the Cost? Proceedings: IVECCS. Accessed via: Veterinary Information Network. http://goo.gl/Gul8O

Jazic, E. (2010). The Great Chameleon: Diagnosis and Management of Cutaneous Adverse Drug Reactions in Dogs and Cats. Proceedings: WVC. Accessed via: Veterinary Information Network. http://goo.gl/Ab7pq

Macintire, D. (2006). New therapies for immune-mediated hemolytic anemia. Proceedings: ACVIM 2006. Accessed via: Veterinary Information Network. http://goo.gl/ILCPS

Whelan, M.F., T.E. O'Toole, et al. (2009). Use of human immunoglobulin in addition to glucocorticoids for the initial treatment of dogs with immune-mediated hemolytic anemia. Journal of Veterinary Emergency and Critical Care 19(2): 158–164.

INAMRINONE LACTATE

(in-*am*-ri-none)   Amrinone, Inocor®

INOTROPIC AGENT

Prescriber Highlights

▶ Second-line agent for short-term management of CHF
▶ Contraindicated with severe aortic or pulmonic valve disease; use extreme caution with hypertrophic cardiomyopathy
▶ Monitoring of cardiac effects & adverse effects mandatory
▶ Very Expensive

Uses/Indications
Inamrinone is considered a second line agent for the short-term management of CHF. It was originally called amrinone, but was changed to inamrinone presumably to avoid confusion with amiodarone.

Pharmacology/Actions
The exact mechanisms of amrinone's cardiac effects are not well understood. It is thought the primary effects are due to its vasodilatory effects, thereby reducing both preload and afterload. Because it inhibits phosphodiesterase, it may directly stimulate cardiac contractility.

Pharmacokinetics
Although no oral commercial dosage forms are available, inamrinone is rapidly absorbed after

oral administration. After initial intravenous injection, effects begin within 2–3 minutes and peak effects occur within 10 minutes. Cardiac effects generally correlate with the drug's serum level. Amrinone's distribution characteristics are not well described. In humans, it has an apparent volume of distribution of 1.2 L/kg. It exhibits low to moderate protein binding (10–49%). It is unknown if it crosses the placenta, blood-brain barrier, or enters into maternal milk. Inamrinone is eliminated primarily via the kidneys. About 63% of a dose is excreted (10–40% unchanged) into the urine. The duration of effect (in humans) is dose related with a single dose lasting from 30 minutes after a 0.75 mg/kg IV dose to 2 hours after a 3 mg/kg dose. Plasma half-lives may be prolonged in patients with CHF.

Contraindications/Precautions/Warnings

Inamrinone is considered contraindicated when severe aortic or pulmonic valve disease is present or in patients hypersensitive to it or bisulfites. The potential risks versus benefits of therapy with inamrinone should be carefully considered in patients with hypertrophic cardiomyopathy.

Adverse Effects

Use in domestic animals is very limited. Adverse effects that potentially could be seen include arrhythmias (drug is not inherently arrhythmogenic, but CHF patients are more susceptible to arrhythmias secondary to any drug), hypotension, GI effects (vomiting, diarrhea), thrombocytopenia (particularly with prolonged therapy), hepatotoxicity, and hypersensitivity reactions (variable symptomatology: pericarditis to myositis, etc.). Inamrinone should only be used in settings where appropriate monitoring may be employed.

Reproductive/Nursing Safety

Reproductive safety data are conflicting; use only when benefits outweigh risks. In humans, the FDA categorizes this drug as category **C** for use during pregnancy (*Animal studies have shown an adverse effect on the fetus, but there are no adequate studies in humans; or there are no animal reproduction studies and no adequate studies in humans.*)

It is not known whether inamrinone is secreted in milk; exercise caution.

Overdosage/Acute Toxicity

Only one case (human) of accidental massive overdose resulting in death has been reported (causal relationship not unequivocally established). Because hypotension is the primary problem that would generally be seen, circulatory support should be instituted.

Drug Interactions

The following drug interactions have either been reported or are theoretical in humans or animals receiving inamrinone lactate and may be of significance in veterinary patients:

- ■ **DIGOXIN:** Digoxin and other inotropic cardiac glycosides have an additive effect with inamrinone; this is generally considered a positive drug interaction.
- ■ **DISOPYRAMIDE:** May cause excessive hypotension when used with inamrinone

Doses

■ **DOGS:**

As a positive inotropic agent:

a) 1–3 mg/kg IV as a slow IV bolus followed by a 10–100 micrograms/kg/min IV CRI; ½ the initial bolus may be administered 20–30 minutes after the first bolus. (Kittleson 2006)

b) 1–3 mg/kg IV followed by a 30–100 micrograms/kg/min IV CRI (Muir & Bonagura 1994)

c) 2 mg/kg bolus IV, followed by 30–300 micrograms/kg/min IV infusion (Fox 2003)

d) For patients coming off cardiopulmonary bypass with poor cardiac contractility: 0.25–0.6 mg/kg loading, then 5–45 micrograms/kg/min CRI (Nelson 2003)

e) As an alternative to dopamine or dobutamine for the adjunctive treatment (with fluids, IV calcium, and potentially glucagon) for calcium channel blocker overdose: 30–100 micrograms/kg/min CRI. (Holder 2000)

■ **CATS:**

a) 1–3 mg/kg IV followed by 30–100 micrograms/kg/min IV infusion (Muir & Bonagura 1994)

b) 1–3 mg/kg IV as a slow IV bolus followed by a 10–100 micrograms/kg/min IV CRI; ½ the initial bolus may be administered 20–30 minutes after the first bolus. (Kittleson 2006)

Monitoring

- ■ Blood pressure
- ■ Heart rate/rhythm; continuous ECG recommended
- ■ Body weight
- ■ Platelet counts

Client Information

- ■ Clients should be made aware of the "investigational nature" of the use of this drug in dogs or cats

Chemistry/Synonyms

Formerly known as amrinone lactate, inamrinone is unrelated structurally to cardiac glycosides or catecholamines, and is a bipyrdine cardiac inotropic agent. It occurs as a pale yellow, crystalline powder and is insoluble in water and slightly soluble in alcohol. The commercially available injection has a pH adjusted to 3.2–4 and an osmolality of 101 mOsm/L.

Inamrinone may also be known as: amrinone,

Win-40680, *Amcoral®, Inocor®, Vesistol®,* and
Wincoram®.

Storage/Stability

The commercially available injection should be
stored at room temperature and protected from
light. It is stable for 2 years after manufacture.

Compatibility/Compounding Considerations

Inamrinone lactate for injection is reportedly
compatible with 0.45% or 0.9% sodium chloride injection, propranolol HCl, and verapamil
HCl. It is reportedly **incompatible** with solutions
containing dextrose or sodium bicarbonate.
Compatibility is dependent upon factors such
as pH, concentration, temperature and diluent
used; consult specialized references or a hospital
pharmacist for more specific information.

Dosage Forms/Regulatory Status

VETERINARY-LABELED PRODUCTS: None

HUMAN-LABELED PRODUCTS:

Inamrinone Lactate for Injection: 5 mg/mL (as
lactate) in 20 mL amps; generic (Abbott Hospital); (Rx)

References

Fox, P. (2003). Congestive heart failure: Clinical ap-
proach and management. Proceedings: World Small
Animal Veterinary Assoc World Congress. Accessed
via: Veterinary Information Network. http://goo.gl/
xMFKn
Holder, T. (2000). Toxicology Brief: Calcium Channel
Blocker Toxicosis. Veterinary Medicine(December).
Kittleson, M. (2006). "Chapt 10: Management of Heart
Failure." Small Animal Cardiology, 2nd Ed.
Muir, W. & J. Bonagura (1994). Drugs for the treatment
of cardiovascular disease. Saunders Manual of Small
Animal Practice. S Birchard and R Sherding Eds.
Philadelphia, W.B. Saunders Company: 436–443.
Nelson, D. (2003). Post operative management of the car-
diopulmonary bypass patient. Proceedings: IVECCS
Symposium. Accessed via: Veterinary Information
Network. http://goo.gl/RqXIT

INSULIN
REGULAR
(CRYSTALLINE ZINC)
LISPRO
ISOPHANE (NPH)
PROTAMINE ZINC (PZI)
PORCINE ZINC (LENTE)
GLARGINE
DETEMIR

(*in*-su-lin)

HORMONE

Note: *Insulin preparations available to the
practitioner are in a constant state of change.
It is highly recommended to review current
references or sources of information pertaining to insulin therapy for dogs and cats to
maximize efficacy of therapy and reduce the
chance for errors.*

Prescriber Highlights

▶ Pancreatic hormone used to treat
  diabetic ketoacidosis, uncomplicated
  diabetes mellitus, & as adjunctive
  therapy in treating hyperkalemia

▶ Contraindications: No absolute contraindications except during episodes of
  hypoglycemia

▶ Adverse Effects: Hypoglycemia, insulin-
  induced hyperglycemia ("Somogyi
  effect"), insulin antagonism/resistance,
  rapid insulin metabolism, & local reactions to the "foreign" proteins

▶ Do not confuse insulin types, strengths,
  syringes

▶ Drug Interactions

*Monograph by Dinah Jordan, PharmD,
DICVP*

Uses/Indications

Insulin preparations are used for the adjunctive treatment of diabetic ketoacidosis (DKA),
uncomplicated diabetes mellitus, and as adjunctive therapy in treating hyperkalemia. Veterinary
use of insulin has been primarily in dogs and
cats, although there are documented reports in
a number of other species, including, but not
limited to, birds, guinea pigs, ferrets, horses, and
cattle.

Regular insulin is commonly used for stabilization of the diabetic patient and is the only
formulation labeled for intravenous administration (IV); it is also administered by intramuscular (IM) and subcutaneous (SC) injection.

Intravenous administration of regular insulin is recommended in patients with poor tissue perfusion, shock, or cardiovascular collapse, or in patients requiring insulin for the treatment of severe, life-threatening hyperkalemia causing cardiotoxicity (*i.e*, >8 mEq/L). While historically, regular insulin was the only insulin preparation recommended for treatment of DKA in veterinary patients, new information suggests that other preparations may be equally effective. A study demonstrated that lispro insulin administered as an intravenous continuous rate infusion was a safe and effective alternative to regular insulin treatment in dogs with DKA (Sears *et al.* 2009). Another study demonstrated that intramuscular administration of glargine is effective for treatment of feline DKA (Marshall *et al.* 2010) and another study showed that a combination of glargine administered subcutaneously every 12 hours and regular insulin administered IM up to every 8 hours resolved DKA faster in cats than a protocol using regular insulin in a CRI (Buob *et al.* 2010). Once the patient is stabilized, longer acting insulin products are given subcutaneously for maintenance insulin therapy.

Pharmacology

Insulin is a hormone secreted by the beta cells of the pancreatic islets of Langerhans. Eliciting multiple biological responses, insulin initiates its actions by binding to cell-surface receptors, present in varying numbers in virtually all mammalian cells. This binding results in a cascade of intracellular events which can be studied in detail by consulting a physiology text.

Insulin is the primary hormone responsible for controlling the uptake, utilization, and storage of cellular nutrients. Insulin affects primarily liver, muscle, and adipose tissues, but also exerts potent regulatory effects on other cell types as well. Insulin stimulates carbohydrate metabolism in cardiac, skeletal, and adipose tissue by facilitating the uptake of glucose by these cells. Other tissues, such as brain, nerve, intestinal, liver, and kidney tubules, do not require insulin for glucose transport. Liver cells do need insulin to convert glucose to glycogen (for storage), and the hypothalamus requires insulin for glucose entry into the satiety center. Insulin has a direct effect on fat and protein metabolism. The hormone stimulates lipogenesis, increases protein synthesis, and inhibits lipolysis and free fatty acid release from adipose tissues. Insulin promotes an intracellular shift of potassium and magnesium. Exogenous insulin elicits all the pharmacologic responses usually produced by endogenous insulin.

Pharmacokinetics

Insulin is metabolized mainly by the liver and kidneys (also muscle and fat to a lesser degree) by enzymatic reduction to form peptides and amino acids. About 50% of the insulin that reaches the liver via the portal vein is destroyed and never reaches the general circulation. Insulin is filtered by the renal glomeruli and is reabsorbed by the tubules, which also degrade it. Severe impairment of renal function appears to affect the rate of clearance of circulating insulin to a greater extent than hepatic disease. Hepatic degradation of insulin operates near its maximal capacity and cannot compensate for diminished renal breakdown of the hormone. The half-life of endogenous insulin is less than ten minutes in normal subjects and in patients with uncomplicated diabetes.

Note: The pharmacokinetics of various insulin formulations can vary widely from published values between species, among individuals within a species, and within the same individual patient from day to day. Therefore, the values should only be used as a general reference guide.

Regular insulin injection: When the recombinant human insulin product is given IV to dogs and cats, it has an immediate onset of action, with maximum effects occurring at 0.5–2 hours; duration of action is 1–4 hours. Following IM administration, onset is 10–30 minutes; peak 1–4 hours; and duration 3–8 hours. After subcutaneous administration, onset is generally 10–30 minutes; peak from 1–5 hours; duration 4–10 hours.

Although the kinetics of all insulin products vary markedly for the individual product between species, regular insulin appears to exhibit the most similar properties.

Insulin lispro injection: While published studies are lacking, the pharmacokinetics of lispro and regular insulin in dogs and cats when administered intravenously appear to be comparable to humans.

Isophane insulin suspension (NPH): NPH is administered by the subcutaneous route only. Following SC administration of the recombinant human insulin product, onset is 0.5–2 hours in dogs and cats; peak is 2–10 hours in dogs and 2–8 hours in cats; and duration is 6–18 hours in dogs and 4–12 hours in cats.

Porcine insulin zinc suspension (Lente): Lente is classified as intermediate-acting; it has two peaks of activity following subcutaneous administration (the first at around 4 hours and the second at around 11 hours). The duration of activity varies between 14 and 24 hours. The peak(s), duration of activity, and dose required to adequately control diabetic signs will vary between dogs. Following SC administration of the recombinant human insulin lente product, onset is 0.5–2 hours in dogs and cats. Pharmacokinetics of the purified pork product are similar to the human product.

Protamine zinc suspension (PZI): Following SC administration, onset is 1–4 hours in dogs and cats; peak is 4–8 hours; duration is 6–28 hours in dogs; 6–24 hours in cats.

Insulin glargine injection: Following subcutaneous injection, the acidic solution is neutralized and microprecipitates are formed that slowly release small amounts of insulin glargine. This action results in a relatively constant concentration/time profile over 24 hours with no pronounced peak in humans. A small study compared equal doses of insulin glargine, PZI (mixed beef/pork), and purified pork lente insulin in 9 healthy cats. Results showed no significant difference in onset of action or nadir glucose concentrations among the insulins; time to reach nadir glucose concentration was longer for glargine (~16 hours) vs. PZI (~6 hours) and lente (~4.5 hours). Duration was significantly shorter for lente than for glargine or PZI, with glargine and PZI not significantly different. The study in healthy cats also showed there were definite peaks in insulin concentration and glucose lowering effects of glargine. (Marshall & Rand 2004) If glargine is diluted or administered either IM or IV, microprecipitates are not formed producing a rapid release of insulin similar to regular insulin.

Insulin detemir injection: A comparison study of glargine and detemir in 10 young healthy cats showed that following administration of 0.5 Units/kg SC, the onset of action was 1.8 ± 0.8 and 1.3 ± 0.5 hours for insulin detemir and insulin glargine respectively. End of action of insulin detemir was reached at 13.5 ± 3.5 hours and for insulin glargine at 11.3 ± 4.5 hours. Time-to-peak action of insulin detemir was reached at 6.9 ± 3.1 hours and for insulin glargine at 5.3 ± 3.8 hours. The time-action curves of both insulin analogs varied between relatively flat curves in some cats and peaked curves in others (Gilor *et al.* 2010).

Contraindications/Precautions/Warnings

Because there are no alternatives for insulin when it is used for diabetic indications, there are no absolute contraindications to its use except during episodes of hypoglycemia. If animals develop hypersensitivity (local or otherwise) or should insulin resistance develop, a change in type or species of insulin should be tried. Pork insulin is identical to canine insulin and is considered the insulin source of choice for diabetic dogs. Human insulin has a low potential for producing insulin antibodies in dogs (~5%), while beef/pork insulin produces antibody formation in a higher percentage of dogs (~45%) and is associated with insulin resistance and poor or erratic glycemic control. Dogs known to have a systemic allergy to pork or pork products should not be treated with *Vetsulin®*. The incidence of insulin antibody production related to insulin source is low in cats, and overt insulin resistance occurs in less than 5% of cats treated with recombinant human insulin; approximately the same rate as in cats treated with beef/pork insulin.

Do not inject insulin at the same site day after day or lipodystrophic reactions can occur.

Do not abbreviate Units as "U" as it has been shown to increase the rate of transcription and dosage errors.

Adverse Effects

Adverse effects of insulin therapy may include hypoglycemia (see overdosage below), insulin-induced hyperglycemia ("Somogyi effect"), insulin antagonism/resistance, rapid insulin metabolism, and local reactions to the "foreign" proteins.

Reproductive/Nursing Safety

In humans, the FDA categorizes purified pork, all human insulin, and human insulin analog lispro as category *B* for use during pregnancy (*Animal studies have not yet demonstrated risk to the fetus, but there are no adequate studies in pregnant women; or animal studies have shown an adverse effect, but adequate studies in pregnant women have not demonstrated a risk to the fetus in the first trimester of pregnancy, and there is no evidence of risk in later trimesters.*) In humans, the FDA categorizes insulin glargine and detemir as category *C* for use during pregnancy (*Animal studies have shown an adverse effect on the fetus, but there are no adequate studies in humans; or there are no animal reproduction studies and no adequate studies in humans.*)

Insulin is compatible with nursing.

Overdosage/Acute Toxicity

Overdosage of insulin can lead to various degrees of hypoglycemia. Signs may include weakness, shaking, head tilting, lethargy, ataxia, seizures, blindness, bizarre behavior, and coma. Other signs may include restlessness, hunger, and muscle fasciculations. Prolonged hypoglycemia can result in permanent brain damage or death.

Mild hypoglycemia may be treated by offering the animal its usual food. More serious symptoms (such as seizure) should be treated with oral dextrose solutions (*e.g., Karo®* syrup) rubbed on the oral mucosa (not poured down the throat) or by intravenous injections of 50% dextrose solutions (small amounts, slowly administered—usually $2-15$ mL). If the animal is seizuring, fingers should not be placed in the animal's mouth. Once the animal's hypoglycemia is alleviated (response usually occurs within $1-2$ minutes), it should be closely monitored (both by physical observation and serial blood glucose levels) to prevent a recurrence of hypoglycemia (especially with the slower absorbed products) and to prevent hyperglycemia from developing. Future insulin dosages or feeding habits should be adjusted to prevent further occurrences of hypoglycemia.

Drug Interactions

The following drug interactions have either been reported or are theoretical in humans or animals receiving insulin and may be of significance in veterinary patients:

■ **BETA-ADRENERGIC BLOCKERS (*e.g.*, propranolol):** Can have variable effects on glycemic control and can mask the signs associated with hypoglycemia

- **CLONIDINE; RESERPINE:** Can mask the signs associated with hypoglycemia

- **DIGOXIN:** Because insulin can alter serum potassium levels, patients receiving concomitant cardiac glycoside (*e.g.,* digoxin) therapy should be closely monitored; especially true in patients receiving concurrent diuretic therapy

The following drugs or drug classes may *potentiate* the hypoglycemic activity of insulin:

- **ALCOHOL**
- **ANABOLIC STEROIDS (e.g., stanozolol, boldenone)**
- **ANGIOTENSIN CONVERTING ENZYME INHIBITORS (e.g., captopril, enalapril)**
- **ASPIRIN or other salicylates**
- **DISOPYRAMIDE**
- **FLUOXETINE**
- **MONOAMINE OXIDASE INHIBITORS**
- **SOMATOSTATIN DERIVATIVES (e.g., octreotide)**
- **SULFONAMIDES**

The following drugs or drug classes may *decrease* the hypoglycemic activity of insulin:

- **CALCIUM CHANNEL BLOCKERS (e.g., diltiazem)**
- **CORTICOSTEROIDS**
- **DANAZOL**
- **DIURETICS**
- **ISONIAZID**
- **NIACIN**
- **PHENOTHIAZINES**
- **THYROID HORMONES** (can elevate blood glucose levels in diabetic patients when thyroid hormone therapy is first initiated)

Doses

Note: Treatment of diabetes mellitus and in particular, diabetic ketoacidosis is complex. Insulin is only one component of therapy; fluid and electrolytes, acid/base, and if necessary, antimicrobial therapy must also be employed. Adequate patient monitoring is mandatory. The reader is strongly encouraged to refer to more thorough discussions of treatment in veterinary endocrinology or internal medicine references for additional information.

- **DOGS:**

    For adjunctive therapy of diabetic ketoacidosis:

    a) Using regular insulin, choose either the intermittent IM technique or low-dose IV infusion technique.

    Intermittent IM technique: Initial Dose: 0.2 Units/kg IM into muscles of the rear legs; repeat IM doses of 0.1 Units/kg hourly. Initial doses (first 2 to 3 injections) may be reduced by 25–50% in

animals with severe hypokalemia. Goal is to slowly lower blood glucose to 200–250 mg/dL over a 6–10 hour period. As blood glucose approaches 250 mg/dL, switch to IM regular insulin at 0.1–0.3 Units/kg q4–6h or subcutaneous (if hydration status is good) q6–8h. Goal is to keep blood glucose in the 150–300 mg/dL range. Giving 5% dextrose IV is necessary during this stage.

Constant Low-Dose Infusion Technique: Administer insulin infusion in an IV line separate from that for fluid therapy. Initial doses may be reduced by 25–50% in animals with severe hypokalemia. Adjust infusion rate based upon hourly blood glucose determinations. An hourly reduction in blood glucose by 50–100 mg/dL is ideal. Once blood glucose approaches 250 mg/dL switch to IM regular insulin every 4–6 hours or to subcutaneous regular insulin at 0.1–0.4 Units/kg q6–8h if hydration status is good. Goal is to keep blood glucose in the 150–300 mg/dL range. Giving 5% dextrose IV is necessary during this stage. Alternatively, may continue IV infusion at a decreased rate until exchanged for a longer-acting product. (Nelson 2008; Nelson & Elliott 2003a)

b) For IV infusion: Preparation of insulin infusion by adding 2.2 Units/kg *regular insulin* to 250 ml of 0.9% sterile saline for injection. Run approximately 50 mL of the insulin-containing fluid through the drip set prior to administration (See adsorption). (Hess, R.S. 2008)

Blood Glucose Concentration (mg/dL)	IV Fluid	Rate of Administration (mL/hr)
>250	0.9% NaCl	10
200-250	0.45% NaCl + 2.5% dextrose	7
150-200	0.45% NaCl + 2.5% dextrose	5
100-150	0.45% NaCl + 5% dextrose	5
<100	0.45% NaCl + 5% dextrose	Stop fluid administration

For adjunctive treatment of severe hyperkalemia (>8 mEq/L):

a) Give *regular insulin* 0.25–0.5 Units/kg slow IV bolus followed by 50% dextrose (4 mL/U of administered insulin); or give regular 0.5–1 Units/kg in parenteral fluids plus 2 grams dextrose per unit insulin administered (Nelson & Elliott 2003b)

For initial insulin treatment of uncomplicated diabetes mellitus:

a) *Using Vetsulin®:* 0.5 Units/kg SC once daily concurrently with or right after a meal. Revaluate at appropriate intervals and adjust dose based on clinical signs, urinalysis results, and glucose curve values until adequate glycemic control has been attained. Twice daily therapy should be initiated if the duration of insulin action is determined to be inadequate. If twice daily treatment is initiated, the two doses should be 25% less than the once daily dose required to attain an acceptable nadir. For example, if a dog receiving 20 units of *Vetsulin®* once daily has an acceptable nadir but inadequate duration of activity, the *Vetsulin®* dose should be changed to 15 units twice daily. (*Vetsulin®* product package insert)

b) *Vetsulin®*: 0.5 Units/kg SC twice daily. (Bruyette 2010)

c) Intermediate-acting insulin (*i.e, NPH, Lente*) is the initial insulin of choice for establishing control of glycemia in diabetic dogs. Recombinant human or porcine source insulin should be used to minimize development of insulin antibodies. Insulin therapy is begun with recombinant human NPH or porcine Lente (*Vetsulin®*) at an approximate dosage of 0.25 Units/kg twice a day. Insulin *glargine* (*Lantus®*) is used in poorly-controlled diabetic dogs where NPH and Lente insulin are ineffective because of problems with too short a duration of insulin effect. (Nelson 2006)

d) *Glargine*: 0.25–0.5 Units/kg SC q12h. (Fracassi *et al.* 2010)

e) *Insulin detemir:* 0.1–0.2 Units/kg SC q 12 hours. Note the lower starting dose for detemir. Canine insulin receptors appear to be 4x more sensitive than human receptors to detemir. (Ford *et al.* 2010)

■ **CATS:**

For adjunctive therapy of diabetic ketoacidosis:

a) Use the same protocol using *regular insulin* as described above in "a" for dogs (Hess, R. 2010; Nelson & Elliott 2003a)

b) Using *insulin glargine*: 2 Units per cat SC and 1 Unit per cat IM (regardless of body weight) initially; repeat the IM dose 4 or more hours later if the blood glucose concentration is greater than 14 to 16 mMol/L (250-290 mg/dL); repeat the SC dose every 12 hours. (Rand 2010a)

For adjunctive treatment of severe hyperkalemia:

a) 0.5 to 1 Unit/kg IM *regular insulin* plus 2 grams dextrose per unit of insulin IV (Feldman & Church 2010)

For initial insulin treatment of uncomplicated diabetes mellitus:

Note: Cats are very unpredictable in their response to insulin therapy, and no single type of insulin is routinely effective in maintaining glycemic control, even with twice daily dosing. Cats should be closely monitored during the first month of insulin therapy.

a) Using *glargine, detemir, or PZI insulin*:

Blood glucose <360 mg/dL (<20mmol/L): 0.25 Units/kg of ideal body weight SC every 12 hours;

Blood glucose ≥360 mg/dL (>20mmol/L): 0.5 Units/kg of ideal body weight SC every 12 hours;

Monitor response to therapy for first 3 days then increase or decrease the insulin dose weekly as needed. If no monitoring is occurring in the first week, begin with 1 Unit per cat every 12 hours (Rand 2010b)

b) Using *ProZinc®*: starting dose is 0.2–0.7 Units/kg SC every 12 hours given concurrently with or right after a meal. Monitor clinical signs & blood glucose nadirs. Goal: glucose nadir (9 hr glucose curve) between 80 & 150 mg/dL & improvement in clinical signs (*ProZinc®* product package insert)

c) Using *Vetsulin®*: Starting dose: 0.5 Units/kg SC once daily (*Vetsulin®* product package insert)

d) Other recommended starting doses for *porcine insulin zinc (lente):*

1 Unit per cat SC twice daily for cats <4kg & 1.5–2 Units/cat twice daily for cats >4kg. (Behrend 2007; Reusch 2005)

0.25 Units/kg SC twice daily if BG between 216-342 mg/dL; 0.5 Units/kg SC twice daily if BS>360mg/dL. (Behrend 2007)

■ **BIRDS:**

Diabetes mellitus is most common in budgies, cockatiels, and toucans. Blood glucose levels in diabetic birds range from 600–2000 mg/dL (Definitive diagnosis requires persistently elevated blood glucose levels >800 mg/dL). Insulin therapy is sometimes hindered by the highly variable dose needed for individual birds, the development of insulin resistance, and the development of pancreatic atrophy and pancreatic insufficiency.

a) Insulin dose: Initially, 0.1–0.2 Units/kg regular insulin. When stabilized, NPH insulin can be started. Dose range is 0.067–3.3 Units/kg IM every 12–24 hours. (Oglesbee 2003)

b) A blood glucose curve should be obtained. Determine blood glucose levels initially, then every 2–3 hours for 12–24 hours. The dose is adjusted based on blood glucose levels. Frequency varies from twice daily to once every several days. Bird should be placed on a low-car-bohydrate diet. Clinical sign of successful treatment is weight gain. Monitor for hypoglycemia. Treat hypoglycemia with oral or injectable dextrose or oral corn syrup. (Rupley 1997)

■ **FERRETS:**

Treatment of diabetes mellitus:

a) NPH: 0.5–1 Unit per ferret SC twice daily. Goal of therapy is negative ketones and a small amount of glucose in the urine. (Quesenberry & Carpenter 2003)

b) NPH: 0.1–0.5 Units/kg IM or SC twice daily to start; adjust to optimal dose. May require insulin to be diluted; monitor urine for glucose/ketones. (Williams 2000)

■ **CATTLE:**

For adjunctive treatment of ketosis:

a) PZI insulin 200 Units (total dose) SC once every 48 hours (Smith 2002)

■ **HORSES:**

For diabetes mellitus:

a) True diabetes mellitus rarely occurs in horses. Most cases are a result of pituitary tumors that cause hyperglycemia secondary to excessive ACTH or growth hormone. A case is cited where an animal received 0.5–1 Unit/kg of PZI insulin and the hyperglycemia was controlled. Patients with hyperglycemia secondary to a pituitary tumor are apparently insulin-resistant (Merritt 1987)

b) PZI insulin 0.15 Units/kg IM or SC twice daily (Robinson 1987)

For treatment of hyperlipemia in ponies:

a) For a 200 kg pony: PZI 30 Units (total dose) IM every 12 hours on odd days (given with 100 grams glucose orally once daily); PZI 15 Units (total dose) IM every 12 hours on even days (given with 100 grams galactose orally once daily) until hyperlipemia resolves. (Smith 2002)

Monitoring Parameters

■ Blood glucose

■ Patient weight, appetite, fluid intake/output

■ Blood, urine ketones (if warranted)

■ Glycosylated hemoglobin and fructosamine [goal = fructosamine <450 micromol/L] (if available and warranted)

Client Information

■ Keep insulin products away from temperature extremes. If stored in the refrigerator, allow to come to room temperature in syringe before injecting.

■ Clients must be instructed in proper techniques for withdrawing insulin into the syringe, including rolling the vial, not shaking before withdrawing into syringe, and using the proper syringe size with insulin concentration (*e.g.*, not confusing U-40 insulin/syringes with U-100 insulin/syringes).

■ Proper injection techniques should be taught and practiced with the client before the animal's discharge.

■ The symptoms of hypoglycemia should be thoroughly reviewed with the owner.

■ A written protocol outlining monitoring procedures and treatment steps for hypoglycemia should be sent home with the owner.

■ When traveling, insulin should not be left in carry-on luggage that will pass through airport surveillance equipment. Generally, insulin stability is not affected by a single pass through surveillance equipment; however, longer than normal exposure or repeated passes through surveillance equipment may alter insulin potency.

Chemistry and Biosynthesis

The endocrine component of the pancreas is organized as discrete islets (islets of Langerhans) that contain four cell types, each of which produces a different hormone. Insulin is produced in the beta cells, which comprise 60–80% of the islet. Insulin is a protein consisting of two chains, designated A and B, with 21 and 30 amino acids respectively that are connected by two disulfide bonds. The amino acid composition of insulin has been determined in various species of animals. The insulin of dogs, pigs, and certain whales (sperm and fin) is identical in structure; sheep insulin is identical to goat. Cattle, sheep, horses, and dogs differ only in positions 8, 9, and 10 of the A chain. Porcine insulin differs from human insulin by one amino acid [alanine instead of threonine at the carboxy terminal of the B chain (*i.e.*, in position B 30)], and bovine insulin differs by two additional alterations in the A chain (threonine and isoleucine in positions A8 and A10 are replaced by alanine and valine, respectively). Of the domestic species, feline insulin is most similar to bovine insulin, differing by only 1 amino acid (at position 18 of the A chain). Human insulin differs from rabbit insulin by a single amino acid. There is a single insulin gene and a single protein product in most mammalian species (multiple insulins appear to occur frequently among fishes).

For therapeutic purposes, doses and concentrations of insulin are expressed in Units. This is sometimes abbreviated as "U", but this practice is discouraged to reduce the chance for transcription and dosage errors. One unit of insulin is equal to the amount required to reduce the concentration of blood glucose in a fasting rabbit to 45 mg/dL (2.5 mM). All commercial preparations of human insulin currently manufactured in the U.S. are supplied in solution or suspension at a concentration of 100 Units/mL, which is approximately 3.6 mg of insulin per milliliter; likewise, one unit of insulin equals about 36 micrograms of insulin.

Insulin is a small protein; human insulin has a molecular weight of 5808. Insulin secretion is a tightly regulated process designed to provide stable concentrations of glucose in blood during fasting and feeding. This regulation is achieved by the coordinated interplay of various nutrients, gastrointestinal and pancreatic hormones, and autonomic neurotransmitters. The primary stimulus for secretion of endogenous insulin is glucose.

Regular insulin is a rapid-acting sterile solution prepared by precipitating insulin in the presence of zinc chloride to form zinc insulin crystals. Regular insulin 100 Units/mL is a clear and colorless or almost colorless solution. Discoloration, turbidity, or unusual viscosity indicates deterioration or contamination.

Insulin lispro injection, USP (rDNA origin) is a human insulin analog that is rapid-acting and is synthesized in a special non-pathogenic laboratory strain of *Escherichia coli* that has been genetically altered. The sterile solution consists of zinc-insulin lispro crystals dissolved in a clear aqueous fluid.

Isophane insulin, more commonly known as *NPH*, is an intermediate-acting, sterile suspension of zinc insulin crystals and protamine sulfate in buffered water for injection.

Porcine Lente insulin is a sterile aqueous suspension of purified pork Lente insulin consisting of 30% amorphous zinc insulin and 70% crystalline zinc insulin. It is available only as a U-40 insulin concentration and is a cloudy or milky suspension of a mixture of characteristic crystals and particles with no uniform shape.

Protamine zinc suspension (PZI) is composed of 90% beef/10% pork insulin combined with zinc and protamine (a protein extracted from salmon testes), which slow the release of the insulin into tissues. PZI is clear (not cloudy) with white sediment (no clumps), that when mixed gently, looks like watery milk. It is available only as a U-40 insulin concentration.

Insulin glargine is a long-acting human insulin analog produced by recombinant DNA technology utilizing a non-pathogenic laboratory strain of *E. coli*. It differs from human insulin in that the amino acid asparagine at position A21 is replaced by glycine, and two arginines are added to the C-terminus of the B chain. The injection consists of insulin glargine dissolved in a clear aqueous fluid. It is available only as a U-100 insulin concentration.

Insulin detemir is a long-acting human insulin analog produced by recombinant DNA technology using a genetically modified strain of *Saccharomyces cerevisiae*. Insulin detemir differs from human insulin in that the amino acid threonine in position B30 has been omitted, and a C14 fatty acid chain has been attached to the amino acid B29. It is a clear, colorless, aqueous solution.

All human, purified pork, and beef/pork insulin products have a neutral pH of approximately 7–7.8, while insulin glargine has an acidic pH of approximately 4.

Stability/Storage

Manufacturers of insulin recommend that all insulin products be stored in the refrigerator but protected from freezing temperatures (do not store at temperatures <36°F or <2°C). Freezing may alter the protein structure, decreasing potency. Particle aggregation and crystal damage may be visible to the naked eye or may require microscopic examination. Higher temperature (>86°F or >30°C) extremes and direct exposure to sunlight should be avoided (such as might occur when insulin is stored in a car glove compartment or on a window sill), since insulin transformation products and fibril formation may occur. Although the manufacturers recommend a maximum of 30 days storage at room temperature (except for detemir, which is 42 days), studies have actually shown that regular insulin maintains stability of 24–30 months at 25°C. One study showed a 5% loss of biological potency after about 36 months at 25°C.

According to the manufacturer's label, insulin glargine has a discard date of 28 days after the initial puncture of the vial (consistent with all human-labeled insulin products except for detemir, which has a discard date of 42 days) and stored at room temperature, although clinical reports indicate that opened vials stored in the refrigerator can be used for up to 6 months; discard vial immediately if there is any discoloration. Bacterial contamination and precipitation associated with pH change can cause cloudiness (Rand 2010b).:

For animals requiring small doses of glargine, the 3 mL cartridge may be preferable to the 10 mL vial to prevent the need for extended use beyond the recommended discard date.

Flocculation of NPH human insulin may appear 3–6 weeks after opening the vial. Deterioration in glycemic control may appear before frosting of the vial. If unexplained hyperglycemia is observed, a new vial of insulin should be used.

Regular and NPH insulin may be stored in plastic or glass syringes under refrigeration for 5–7 days without loss of potency. One study found no degradation after 14 days storage under refrigeration. Other sources state that prefilled insulin syringes are stable for 30 days when stored in the refrigerator. It is generally accepted that syringes of insulin can be stored for 28 days under refrigeration without fear of potency loss.

Compatibility/Compounding Considerations

Regular insulin is reportedly physically **compatible** with following drugs/solutions: normal saline, TPN solutions (4% amino acids, 25% dextrose with electrolytes and vitamins; must occasionally shake bag to prevent separation), bretylium tosylate, cimetidine HCl, lidocaine HCl, oxytetracycline HCl, and verapamil HCl.

Regular insulin may be mixed with other insulin products (except for glargine) used in veterinary medicine (*e.g.*, NPH, PZI, etc.).

Regular insulin is reportedly physically **incompatible** when mixed with the following drugs/solutions: aminophylline, amobarbital sodium, chlorothiazide sodium, cytarabine, dobutamine HCl, nitrofurantoin sodium, pentobarbital sodium, phenobarbital sodium, phenytoin sodium, secobarbital sodium, sodium bicarbonate, sulfisoxazole sodium, and thiopental sodium. Compatibility is dependent upon factors such as pH, concentration, temperature, and diluent used; consult specialized references for more specific information.

Diluting insulin: Other than for immediate use, insulin should only be diluted using product-specific sterile diluents supplied by the manufacturer. Diluents for Regular insulin (*Humulin R*) and NPH insulin (*Humulin N*) and sterile vials can be obtained by telephoning the manufacturer. Diluted insulin is stable for 4 (preferred) to 6 weeks and should be stored in the refrigerator. For immediate use, insulin products (except glargine) can be diluted with normal saline for injection, but the potency cannot be predicted after 24 hours. **Insulin glargine must not be diluted or mixed** with any other insulin or solution because the prolonged action is dependent on its pH.

Adsorption: The adsorption of regular insulin to the surfaces of IV infusion solution containers, glass and plastic (including PVC, ethylene vinyl acetate, polyethylene, and other polyolefins), tubing, and filters has been demonstrated. Estimates of loss of potency range from 20–80%, although reports of 20–30% are more common. The percent adsorbed is inversely proportional to the concentration of the insulin, and may include other factors such as the amount of container surface area, the fill volume of the solution, the type of solution, type and length of administration set, temperature, previous exposure of tubing to insulin, and the presence of other drugs, blood, etc. The adsorption process is instantaneous, with the bulk of insulin adsorption occurring within the first 30–60 minutes. To saturate binding sites and deliver a more predictable dose to the patient through an IV infusion, it is recommended that the first 50 mL be run through the IV tubing and discarded.

Insulin Syringes: Syringes are designed for use with a specific strength of insulin, with the needle covers color-coded according to strength. U-40 syringes have a red top, while U-100 syringes have an orange top. U-40 syringes contain ½ cc (equivalent to 0.5 mL) and have 20 unit marks. Measuring U-40 insulin to the one unit mark in a U-40 syringe will contain 1 Unit of insulin. U-100 syringes are available in $^3/_{10}$ cc, ½cc, and 1cc size. Measuring U-100 insulin to one mark in a U-100 syringe will contain 1 Unit of insulin.

Tuberculin syringes can also be used, but are not generally recommended because the potential for confusion is substantial. If using 100 Units/mL or TB syringes to measure 40 Units/mL insulin doses:

- ■ Determine the required dose in units.
- ■ If using U-100 insulin syringes (orange top), multiply the required Units of U-40 insulin by 2.5 (*e.g.* If required dose is 10 units, 10 x 2.5=25 units).
- ■ If using TB syringes, multiply the required Units of U-40 insulin x 0.025 (*e.g.*, If the required dose is 10 Units, 10 x 0.025= 0.25 mL).

Reuse of Insulin Syringes: Reuse of disposable insulin syringes has been suggested to reduce client costs. However, disposable insulin syringes are usually siliconized, and reuse can result in contamination of vials of insulin with silicone oil, causing a white precipitate and impairment of biological effects. Also, needles become dull with more than one use and can cause pain at the injection site.

Dosage Forms/Regulatory Status

VETERINARY-LABELED PRODUCTS:

Porcine insulin zinc suspension 40 Units/mL in 10 mL vials, intermediate-acting; *Vetsulin*® (Intervet/Schering Plough); (Rx). FDA-approved for use in dogs and cats. Note: *Vetsulin*® not currently (February 2011) available in the USA due to manufacturing issues. *Caninsulin*® (Intervet/Schering Plough) is available in Canada & Europe.

Protamine zinc (recombinant human) insulin (PZI) aqueous suspension 40 Units/mL in 10 mL vials; *ProZinc*® (BIVI); Rx. FDA-approved for use in cats.

HUMAN-LABELED PRODUCTS:

Note: Partial listing; includes only those products generally used in veterinary medicine.

Short-Acting:

Insulin, Regular Injection Human (rDNA): 100 Units/mL in 10 mL vials; *Humulin*®R (Lilly); *Novolin*®R (Novo Nordisk); (OTC)

Insulin Lispro Injection Human (rDNA): 100 Units/mL in 3 mL & 10 mL vials, *Humalog*® (Lilly); (Rx)

Intermediate-Acting:

Isophane (Neutral Protamine Hagedorn; NPH) Human (rDNA): 100 Units/mL in 10 mL vials, 5 x 1.5 mL prefilled syringes & 5 x 3 mL pen insulin delivery devices; *Humulin*®N (Lilly); *Novolin*®N & Prefilled (Novo Nordisk); (OTC)

NPH/Regular Insulin Mixtures: Human (rDNA) 100 Units/mL 70% isophane insulin (NPH) & 30 % insulin injection (regular) in 5 x 3 mL disposable pen insulin delivery devices, 10 mL vials & 5 x 1.5 mL prefilled syringes; *Humulin*® 70/30 (Lilly); *Novolin*® 70/30 & Prefilled (Novo Nordisk); (OTC)

Human (rDNA) Injection (suspension): 100 Units/mL; 50% isophane insulin (NPH) & 50% insulin injection (regular) in 10 mL vials; *Humulin®* 50/50 (Lilly); (OTC)

Long-Acting:

Insulin Glargine Injection Human (rDNA) 100 Units/mL in 10 mL vials & 3 mL cartridge system; *Lantus®* (Aventis); (Rx)

Insulin Detemir Injection Human (rDNA) 100 Units/mL in 10 mL vials; *Levemir®* (Novo Nordisk); (Rx)

References

Behrend, E.N. (2007). Current therapies for diabetes mellitus. Proceedings: WVC. http://goo.gl/uKI2N

Bruyette, D. (2010). Treatment Canine Diabetes Mellitus: What Are My Options Proceedings; WVC. Accessed via: Veterinary Information Network. http://goo.gl/0vIAO

Buob, S., O. Mahony, et al. (2010). An Intermittent Insulin Protocol Improves Metabolic Acidosis Faster Than a Continuous Rate Infusion of Regular Insulin in Feline Diabetic Ketoacidosis. Proceedings: ACVIM. Accessed via: Veterinary Information Network. http://goo.gl/OxRYE

Feldman, E. & D. Church (2010). Electrolyte Disorders: Potassium (Hyper/Hypokalemia). *Textbook of Veterinary Internal Medicine, 7th Ed.* S Ettinger and E Feldman Eds. St Louis, Saunders: 303–308.

Ford, S., J. Rand, et al. (2010). Evaluation of Detemir Insulin in Diabetic Dogs Managed with Home Blood Glucose Monitoring Proceedings: ACVIM. Accessed via: Veterinary Information Network. http://goo.gl/juIFq

Fracassi, F., F.S. Boretti, et al. (2010). Use of Insulin Glargine in Dogs with Diabetes Mellitus. Proceedings: ECVIM. Accessed via: Veterinary Information Network. http://goo.gl/tQgcd

Gilor, C., T.K. Ridge, et al. (2010). Pharmacodynamics of Insulin Detemir and Insulin Glargine Assessed by an Isoglycemic Clamp Method in Healthy Cats. *Journal of Veterinary Internal Medicine* **24**(4): 870–874.

Hess, R. (2010). Diabetic Emergencies. *Consultations in Feline Internal Medicine.* J August Ed. St Louis, Saunders: 297–303.

Hess, R.S. (2008). Canine Diabetic Ketoacidosis. Proceedings: ACVIM. Accessed via: Veterinary Information Network. http://goo.gl/WZGYc

Marshall, R. & J. Rand (2004). Comparison of the pharmacokinetics and pharmacodynamics of glargine, protamine zinc and porcine lente insulins in normal cats. Proceedings: ACVIM Forum. Accessed via: Veterinary Information Network. http://goo.gl/SjRN4

Marshall, R., J. Rand, et al. (2010). Glargine Administered Intramuscularly is Effective for Treatment of Feline Diabetic Ketoacidosis. Proceedings: ACVIM. Accessed via: Veterinary Information Network. http://goo.gl/KFXiO

Merritt, A.M. (1987). Diabetes Mellitus. *Current Therapy in Equine Medicine, 2.* NE Robinson Ed. Philadelphia, W.B. Saunders: 181–182.

Nelson, R. (2006). Canine Diabetes Mellitus. Proceedings: UCDCMC2006. http://goo.gl/Z1iKt

Nelson, R. (2008). Managing Diabetic Ketoacidosis. Proceedings: WVC. Accessed via: Veterinary Information Network. http://goo.gl/7bBTN

Nelson, R. & D. Elliott (2003a). Endocrine disorders. *Small Animal Internal Medicine, 3rd Ed.* R Nelson and C Couto Eds. St Louis, Mosby: 660–815.

Nelson, R. & D. Elliott (2003b). Metabolic and electrolyte disorders. *Small Animal Internal Medicine, 3rd Ed.* R Nelson and C Couto Eds. St Louis, Mosby: 816–846.

Quesenberry, K. & J. Carpenter (2003). *Ferrets, Rabbits, and Rodents Clinical Medicine and Surgery 2nd ed.* St Louis, Saunders.

Rand, J. (2010a). Diabetes Mellitus: Ketoacidosis. *The Feline Patient, 4th Ed.* G Norsworthy, S Grace, M Crystal and L Tilley Eds., Wiley-Blackwell.

Rand, J. (2010b). Use of Longa-Acting Insulin in the Treatment of Diabetes Mellitus. *Consultations in Feline Internal Medicine.* J August Ed. St Louis, Saunders: 286–296.

Reusch, C.E. (2005). Monitoring and Treatment of the Diabetic Cat. Proceedings: ECVIM. Accessed via: Veterinary Information Network. http://goo.gl/oDYll

Robinson, N.E. (1987). Table of Common Drugs: Approximate Doses. *Current Therapy in Equine Medicine, 2.* NE Robinson Ed. Philadelphia, W.B. Saunders: 761.

Rupley, A. (1997). *Manual of Avian Practice.* Philadelphia, Saunders.

Sears, K., K.J. Drobatz, et al. (2009). Use of Lispro Insulin for Treatment of Dogs with Diabetic Ketoacidosis. Proceedings: ACVIM. Accessed via: Veterinary Information Network. http://goo.gl/9BQCE

Smith, B. (2002). *Large Animal Internal Medicine, 3rd edition.* St Louis, Mosby.

Williams, B. (2000). Therapeutics in Ferrets. *Vet Clin NA: Exotic Anim Pract* **3**:1(Jan): 131–153.

INTERFERON ALFA, HUMAN RECOMBINANT

(in-ter-*feer*-on)   Roferon-A®, Intron-A®

IMMUNOMODULATOR

Prescriber Highlights

▶ Cytokine used to alleviate clinical effects of certain viral diseases; little scientific info available to document safety/efficacy in small animals

▶ Cautions: Preexisting autoimmune disease, severe cardiac disease, pulmonary disease, "brittle" diabetes, Herpes infections, hypersensitivity to the drug, or CNS disorders

▶ Adverse Effects: In cats, adverse effects are apparently uncommon with PO; higher dosages given parenterally may cause malaise; fever, allergic reactions, myelotoxicity & myalgia are possible

Uses/Indications

Interferon alfa use in veterinary medicine has primarily been centered on its SC, or oral/buccal administration in cats to treat a variety of virus-induced diseases. Despite rapid antibody development when injected parenterally and little, if any, absorption after oral administration, the drug does appear to have some efficacy for certain diseases, either via direct antiviral action or more likely, an immunomodulatory effect. Interferon-alfa has been used in dogs for the adjunctive treatment of viral- or immunosuppression-related conditions, such as papillomas, pododermatitis, or digital keratomas. Some work has been done in dogs evaluating it as an adjunctive treatment for certain neoplastic diseases (*e.g.*, hemangiosarcoma).

In summarizing the *in vitro*, controlled study and clinical efficacy status *in vivo* for human interferon-alfa use in virus infected cats, one author (Hartmann 2008) reports: High dose SC administration to cats does not appear to be clinically effective for FIV or FeLV infections. Low dose oral treatment does appear to have some efficacy for FIV in cats. Low dose oral therapy does not appear to be effective for FeLV, FHV-1, or FCV (feline calicivirus), and is contraindicated in FIP. Topical administration to FHV-1 infected cats may have some efficacy (see topical ophthalmology section). Feline interferon-omega has recently become available in several countries and it may be useful in treating viral diseases in both cats and dogs. A separate monograph for that agent follows this one.

Pharmacology/Actions

The pharmacologic effects of the interferons are widespread and complex. Suffice it to say, that interferon alfa has antiviral, antiproliferative, and immunomodulating effects. Its antiproliferative and antiviral activities are thought to be due to its effects on the synthesis of RNA, DNA, and cellular proteins (oncogenes included). The mechanisms for its antineoplastic activities are not well understood, but are probably related these effects as well.

Pharmacokinetics

Interferon alfa is poorly absorbed after oral administration due to its degradation by proteolytic enzymes and studies have not detected measurable levels in the systemic circulation, however, there may be some absorption via upper GI mucosa. It may have some immunomodulating effect via stimulation of local lymphoid tissues.

Interferon alfa is widely distributed throughout the body, although it does not penetrate into the CNS well. It is unknown if it crosses the placenta. Interferon alfa is freely filtered by the glomeruli, but is absorbed by the renal tubules where it is metabolized by brush border or lysosomes. Hepatic metabolism is of minor importance. The plasma half-life in cats has been reported as 2.9 hours.

Contraindications/Precautions/Warnings

When used parenterally, consider the risks versus benefits in patients with preexisting autoimmune disease, severe cardiac disease, pulmonary disease, "brittle" diabetes, Herpes infections, hypersensitivity to the drug, or CNS disorders.

One author states that low dose oral therapy is contraindicated in cats with FIP (Hartmann 2008).

Adverse Effects

When used orally in cats, adverse effects are apparently uncommon. Higher dosages given parenterally to cats may cause malaise; fever, allergic reactions, myelotoxicity, and myalgia are possible. Cats given human interferon-alfa parenterally may develop significant antibodies to

it after 3-7 weeks of treatment with resultant loss of efficacy.

When used systemically in humans, adverse effects have included anemia, leukopenias, thrombocytopenia, hepatotoxicity, neurotoxicity, taste sensation changes, anorexia, nausea, vomiting, diarrhea, dizziness, "flu-like" syndrome, transient hypotension, skin rashes, and dry mouth. Except for the "flu-like "syndrome, most adverse effects are dose-related and may vary depending on the condition treated.

Reproductive/Nursing Safety

Safety during pregnancy has not been established; high parenteral doses in monkeys did not cause teratogenic effects, but did increase abortifacient activity. In humans, the FDA categorizes this drug as category **C** for use during pregnancy (*Animal studies have shown an adverse effect on the fetus, but there are no adequate studies in humans; or there are no animal reproduction studies and no adequate studies in humans.*)

It is not known whether this drug is excreted in milk.

Overdosage/Acute Toxicity

No information was located. Determine dosages carefully.

Drug Interactions

The following drug interactions have either been reported or are theoretical in humans or animals receiving interferon and may be of significance in veterinary patients:

■ **ACYCLOVIR, ZIDOVUDINE, VIDARABINE:** Additive or synergistic antiviral effects may occur when interferon alfa is used in conjunction with zidovudine (AZT) or acyclovir. This effect does not appear to occur with vidarabine, although increased toxicities may occur. The veterinary significance of these potential interactions is unclear.

Doses

■ **DOGS:**

a) For cutaneous T-cell lymphoma and severe cases of oral/cutaneus papillomas: 1.5–2 million Units/m^2 SC 3 times weekly (White 2000)

b) As an immunostimulant for the adjunctive treatment of certain dermatologic conditions (*e.g.*, pododermatitis, papillomas, digital keratomas): 1000 Units PO once daily (given as 1000 Unit/mL solution). (Yu 2008)

■ **CATS:**

For treatment of virus infections:

a) FeLV-infected cats: Low dose: 30 Units/cat PO daily; 7 days on, 7 days off); Hi dose: 10,000–1,000,000 Units/kg SC once daily. Little in the way of large, controlled trials to determine which, if any, immunomodulating therapies (interferon or other agents) are likely to benefit FeLV-infected cats. (Levy 2004)

b) For FIV: 30 Units per cat PO daily; 7 days on, 7 days off (Barr & Phillips 2000)

c) For chronic FHV-1 infections: 30 Units per cat PO daily; 7 days on, 7 days off; repeat cycle. May also use topical ophthalmic therapy: one drop of 25–50 Units/mL of saline in affected eye(s) q4–6 hours. (Powell 2002)

d) For acute life-threatening FHV-1 infections in kittens: 10,000 Units/kg SC daily for up to 3 weeks (Lappin 2003)

Client Information

■ Owners should be made aware of the "investigational" nature of this compound and understand that efficacy and safety have not necessarily been established.

Chemistry/Synonyms

Prepared from genetically engineered cultures of E. coli with genes from human leukocytes, interferon alfa-2a is commercially available as a sterile solution or sterile powder. Human interferon alfa is a complex protein that contains 165 or 166 amino acids.

Interferon may also be known as: IFN-alpha, interferon-alpha, Ro-22-8181 (interferon alfa-2a), Sch-30500 (interferon alfa-2b); there are many internationally registered trade names available.

Storage/stability

Commercially available products should be stored in the refrigerator; do not freeze the accompanying diluent. Do not expose solutions to room temperature for longer than 24 hours. Do not vigorously shake solutions.

An article proposing using this product in cats for the treatment of FeLV states that after dilution of 3 million Units in one liter of sterile saline the resultant solution remains active for years if frozen or for months if refrigerated. However, data corroborating this is apparently not available.

Compatibility/Compounding Considerations

To prepare a *3 Unit/mL solution for oral administration*: Using the 3 million Unit vial (see below), dilute the entire contents into 100 mL of sterile water; mix well. Resulting solution contains approximately 30,000 Units/mL. Take 0.1 mL of this solution and add to one liter of sterile saline that has 4 mL of 25% albumin added to it. Albumin is optional but adds stability. Solution is now 3 Units/mL. Divide into aliquots of 15 mL and freeze, preferably at −70°C. Thaw as needed and keep refrigerated. Discard unused portion after 60 days. Discard unused 30,000 Units/mL solution within 2–3 hours of making initial dilutions.

Preparation of solution for *30 Units/mL oral administration*: Using the 3 million Unit vial (see below), dilute the entire contents into a 1 L bag of sterile normal saline; mix well. Resulting solution contains approximately 3,000 Units/mL. Divide into aliquots of either 1 or 10 mL and freeze. By diluting further 100 fold (1 mL of 3000 Units/mL solution with 100 mL of sterile saline, or 10 mL with 1000 mL of sterile saline) a 30 Units/mL solution will result. Some have advised aliquoting the diluted solution into 1 mL volumes for freezing up to a year; defrost as necessary. Once defrosted, the drug can be refrigerated up to one week. Freezing the most dilute solutions is associated with loss in activity unless protein such as albumin (see above) is added during dilution. (Greene *et al.* 2006)

Dosage Forms/Regulatory Status

VETERINARY-LABELED PRODUCTS: None

HUMAN-LABELED PRODUCTS:

Interferon Alfa-2a (recombinant rIFN-A; IF-LrA) Injection: Prefilled syringes: 3 million I.U./syringe (0.5 mL single-use syringes); 6 million I.U./syringe (0.5 mL single-use syringes); 9 million I.U./syringe (0.5 mL single-use syringes); *Roferon-A®* (Hoffman La-Roche); (Rx)

Interferon Alfa-2b (recombinant (IFN-alpha2; rIFN-a2; a-2-interferon) Powder for Injection: 5 million Units/vial; 10 million Units/vial; 18 million Units/vial; 25 million Units/vial & 50 million Units/vial in vials with a mL, 2 mL or 5 mL diluent/vial; *Intron A®* (Schering); (Rx)

Interferon Alfa-2b (recombinant (IFN-alpha2; rIFN-a2; a-2-interferon) Injection: 3 million Units/dose; 5 million Units/dose, & 10 million Units/dose in multidose pens; *Intron A®* (Schering); (Rx)

Interferon Alfa-2b (recombinant (IFN-alpha2; rIFN-a2; a-2-interferon) Solution for Injection: 3 million Units/vial, 5 million Units/vial; 10 million Units/vial; 18 million Units/vial & 25 million Units/vial in vials, Pak-3, -5, -10 (vials & syringes); & in multidose vials (22.8 million Units/3.8 mL/vial or 32 million Units/3.2 mL/vial); *Intron A®* (Schering); (Rx)

Interferon Alfa-N3 (human leukocyte derived) Injection: 5 million Units/mL (8 mg NaCl, 1.74 mg Na phosphate dibasic, 0.2 mg K phosphate monobasic, 0.2 mg KCl) in 1 mL vials; *Alferon N®* (Interferon Sciences Inc.); (Rx)

References

Barr, M. & T. Phillips (2000). FIV and FIV-related Disease. *Textbook of Veterinary Internal Medicine: Diseases of the Dog and Cat.* S Ettinger and E Feldman Eds. Philadelphia, WB Saunders. **1:** 433–438.

Greene, C., K. Hartmannn, et al. (2006). Appendix 8: Antimicrobial Drug Formulary. *Infectious Disease of the Dog and Cat.* C Greene Ed., Elsevier: 1186–1333.

Hartmann, K. (2008). Antiviral chemotherapy in veterinary medicine. Proceedings: ACVIM. Accessed via: Veterinary Information Network. http://goo.gl/0SrWH

Lappin, M. (2003). Infectious upper respiratory diseases I and II. Proceedings: Western Veterinary Conference. Accessed via: Veterinary Information Network. http://goo.gl/qsOaI

Levy, J. (2004). FELV: Afraid of a positive? Proceedings: ACVIM Forum. Accessed via: Veterinary Information Network. http://goo.gl/gGs7t

Powell, C. (2002). Feline Herpesvirus Ocular Disease. Proceedings: Western Veterinary Conference. Accessed via: Veterinary Information Network. http://goo.gl/4PIL9

White, S. (2000). Veterinary Dermatology: New Treatments, 'New' Diseases. Proceedings: The North American Veterinary Conference, Orlando.

Yu, A. (2008). Pododermatitis I: Infectious. Proceedings: WVC. Accessed via: Veterinary Information Network. http://goo.gl/V08U0

INTERFERON-Ω (OMEGA)

(in-ter-*feer*-on oh-*may*-ga)
Virbagen Omega®

Recombinant Omega Interferon of Feline Origin, rFeIFN-w

IMMUNOMODULATOR

Prescriber Highlights

▶ Immunomodulating cytokine labeled for treating FeLV & FIV in cats & Parvo in dogs; not commercially available in USA. May potentially be effective in treating canine atopic dermatitis.

▶ Appears to be well tolerated; adverse effects include: hyperthermia, vomiting, diarrhea (cats), fatigue (cats)

▶ Increases in ALT & decreases in RBC, WBC, & platelet counts have been seen

▶ Treatment may be very expensive

Uses/Indications

Omega interferon (feline) is labeled (in the EU) for dogs 1 month of age or older for the reduction in mortality and clinical signs of parvovirus (enteric form). In cats 9 weeks of age or older, it is labeled for treating FeLV and/or FIV, in non-terminal clinical stages. It may be of benefit in treating canine distemper, canine atopic dermatitis, acute feline calicivirus infections, FIP, or topically for feline herpetic keratitis, but data is still being gathered to document efficacy.

In summarizing the *in vitro*, controlled study and clinical efficacy status *in vivo* for feline interferon-omega use in virus infected cats and dogs, one author (Hartmann 2008) reports: that controlled studies have been done for FIV (ineffective), FeLV (some effect), and canine parvovirus (effective). Controlled studies have not been performed for FHV-1 (possibly effective), FCV (possibly effective), FIP (possibly effective) or feline panleukovirus (likely effective).

Pharmacology/Actions

Omega interferon is a type 1 interferon related to alpha interferon. Its principle action is not as a direct anti-viral, but by acting on virus-infected cells inhibiting mRNA and translation proteins thereby inhibiting viral replication. It may also nonspecifically enhance immune defense mechanisms.

Pharmacokinetics

It has been stated that omega interferon pharmacokinetics in dogs and cats is similar to that of human interferons. After intravenous injection, omega interferon is rapidly bound to specific receptor sites on a variety of cells. Highest tissue levels are found in the liver and kidneys. Interferon is filtered in the renal glomeruli and catabolized in the kidneys. In dogs, volume of distribution at steady state is about 0.1L/kg. Biphasic elimination occurs with an alpha half-life of 3.14 hours and a beta half-life of 0.24 hours. Total body clearance is 6.9 mL/min/kg.

Contraindications/Precautions/Warnings

The manufacturer cautions against vaccinating dogs currently being treated with omega interferon and not to vaccinate until the patient appears to have recovered. As both FeLV and FIV infections are known to be immunosuppressive, the manufacturer states that cat vaccinations are contraindicated during and after omega interferon treatment.

There are several different interferons available for use in humans (several sub-types of alpha, beta, or gamma interferon); one cannot be substituted for another.

Adverse Effects

In cats and dogs, hyperthermia (3–6 hours postdose) and vomiting have been reported. Slight decreases in RBCs, platelets and WBCs, and increased ALT have been observed but, reportedly, these indices return to normal within a week of the last injection.

Additionally, soft feces/mild diarrhea and transient fatigue may be noted in cats. Intravenous administration to cats may cause increased incidence and severity of adverse effects, but in cats, adverse effects occur uncommonly.

Dogs may develop antibodies to interferon omega if treatment is prolonged (beyond labeled dosage period) or repeated.

Reproductive/Nursing Safety

Safety during pregnancy or lactation has not been established.

Overdosage/Acute Toxicity

10X overdoses in dogs and cats caused mild lethargy/somnolence, slight hyperthermia, slight increases in respiratory and heart rates. In animals tested, signs resolved within 7 days and no treatment was required.

Drug Interactions

No reported drug interactions at the time of writing, but use caution when using other drugs that can be hepatotoxic or myelosuppressive.

Laboratory Considerations

■ No specific concerns were noted

Doses

■ DOGS:

a) For treatment of parvovirus as labeled: 2.5 million Units/kg IV once daily for 3 days. The earlier the dog is treated, the more likely of success. (Label information; *Virbagen Omega®*—Virbac UK)

b) For treatment of atopic dermatitis: Per injection: Dogs 8-15 kg = 1 million Units; 15-29 kg = 2 million Units; 29–40 kg = 3 million Units; 29–40 kg = 4 million Units. In the study, doses were administered. In the study, dogs were dosed SC on days: 0, 3, 7, 14, 21, 35, 56, 90, 120, & 150. Further larger-scale studies needed to confirm that low dose rFeIFN-omega is cost-effective and safe option for long-term treatment. (Carlotti *et al.* 2009)

■ **CATS:**

a) For treatment of FeLV or FV as labeled: 1 million Units/kg SC once daily for 5 days. Three separate 5-day treatments performed at day 0, day 14, and day 60. (Label information; *Virbagen Omega®*—Virbac UK)

b) From a case report treating a cat with FHV-1 facial dermatitis: Day 0: Cat sedated with propofol and rFeIFN-ω 1.5 million Units/kg injected, half of which was injected peri-lesionally and intradermally and the other half subcutaneously on the lateral thorax. Day 2 and day 9: 1.5 million Units/kg injected SC on the lateral thorax. On days 19, 21, and 23: 0.75 million Units/kg injected peri-lesionally and intradermally as well as 0.75 million Units/kg SC on the lateral thorax. The cat was sedated as described above when peri-lesional and intradermal injections made. (Gutzwiller *et al.* 2007)

Monitoring

■ Monitor for efficacy for infection treated

■ CBC and hepatic function tests suggested

Client Information

■ This drug is best administered on an in-patient basis where the patient may be observed and supported

Chemistry/Synonyms

Interferon omega of feline origin is a type 1 recombinant interferon obtained from silkworms after inoculation with a recombinant baculovirus. It is provided commercially as a lyophilisate powder with a separate solvent.

Recombinant omega interferon of feline origin may also be known as: Interferon omega, omega interferon, interferon-ω, IFN-ω, IFN-ω (feline recombinant), rFeIFN-ω, and *Virbagen Omega®*.

Storage/stability

The commercial veterinary product should be stored in its original carton refrigerated (4°C ± 2°C) and protected from freezing. It has a designated shelf life of 2 years when properly stored. Once reconstituted with the supplied isotonic sodium chloride solution, it should be used immediately as it contains no preservative, however, the solution is reported to be stable for at least 3 weeks when refrigerated. No data was located on the stability of the reconstituted solution when frozen.

Compatibility/Compounding Considerations

The manufacturer states: Do not mix with any other vaccine/immunological product, except the solvent supplied for use with the product.

Dosage Forms/Regulatory Status

VETERINARY-LABELED PRODUCTS: None in the USA

In the EU:

Recombinant Omega Interferon of Feline Origin 10 million Units/vial; *Virbagen Omega®* (Virbac); (Rx). Licensed for dogs and cats. A 5 million Unit vial may be available in some countries.

The FDA may allow legal importation into the USA of this medication for compassionate use in animals; for more information, see the *Instructions for Legally Importing Drugs for Compassionate Use in the USA* found in the appendix.

HUMAN-LABELED PRODUCTS: None

References

Carlotti, D.N., M. Boulet, et al. (2009). The use of recombinant omega interferon therapy in canine atopic dermatitis: a double-blind controlled study. *Veterinary Dermatology* **20**(5–6): 405–411.

Gutzwiller, M.E.R., C. Brachelente, et al. (2007). Feline herpes dermatitis treated with interferon omega. *Veterinary Dermatology* **18**(1): 50–54.

Hartmann, K. (2008). Antiviral chemotherapy in veterinary medicine. Proceedings: ACVIM. Accessed via: Veterinary Information Network. http://goo.gl/0SrWH

IODIDE, SODIUM
IODIDE, POTASSIUM

(eye-oh-dide)   SSKI, Iodoject®

ANTIFUNGAL, NUTRITIONAL

Prescriber Highlights

▶ Iodides used for actinobacillosis in ruminants, sporotrichosis in horses, dogs, & cats

▶ Contraindications: Iodide hypersensitivity, lactating animals, hyperthyroidism, renal failure, or dehydration

▶ Do not inject IM; give IV slowly & with caution to horses as severe generalized reactions have been reported

▶ May cause abortion in cattle

▶ Adverse Effects: Iodism: Excessive tearing, vomiting, anorexia nasal discharge, muscle twitching, cardiomyopathy, scaly haircoats/dandruff, hyperthermia, decreased milk production & weight gain, coughing, inappetence, & diarrhea

▶ Cats more prone to developing toxicity

Uses/Indications

The primary use for sodium iodide is in the treatment of actinobacillosis and actinomycosis in cattle. It has been used as an expectorant with little success in a variety of species and occasionally as a supplement for iodine deficiency disorders. In horses, dogs and cats, oral sodium or potassium iodide has been used in the treatment of sporotrichosis. Use in cats is controversial as they may be prone to developing adverse effects; cats may require other antifungal (*e.g.*, itraconazole) therapy. Potassium iodide has also been used as an expectorant, but documentation of efficacy is lacking.

Pharmacology/Actions

While the exact mode of action for its efficacy in treating actinobacillosis is unknown, iodides probably have some effect on the granulomatous inflammatory process. Iodides have little, if any, *in vitro* antibiotic activity.

Pharmacokinetics

Little published information appears to be available. Therapeutic efficacy of intravenous sodium iodide for actinobacillosis is rapid, with beneficial effects usually seen within 48 hours of therapy.

Contraindications/Precautions/Warnings

Sodium iodide injection labels state that it should not be given to lactating animals or to animals with hyperthyroidism. Do not inject intramuscularly (IM).

Iodides given parenterally should be administered slowly and with caution to horses; severe generalized reactions have been reported.

Should not be used in animals in renal failure or that are severely dehydrated.

Adverse Effects

In ruminants, the adverse effect profile is related to excessive iodine (see Overdosage below). Young animals may be more susceptible to iodism than adults.

Foals have developed goiter when mares have been excessively supplemented.

Chronic use or overdoses may cause iodism. Cats are apparently more prone to developing this than other species. Signs can include vomiting, inappetence, depression, twitching, hypothermia, and cardiovascular failure.

The taste of the liquid is very unpleasant and animals may avoid dosing. Giving with food or a fatty liquid (whole milk, ice cream) may improve palatability and reduce nausea and vomiting. Cats reportedly tolerate the taste of sodium iodide better then potassium iodide. There are potassium iodide oral tablets 130 mg available (OTC, for reducing risk for thyroid cancer after radioactive isotope exposure) that may be useful in small dogs or cats that cannot tolerate oral solutions.

Reproductive/Nursing Safety

Anecdotal reports that iodides can cause abortion in cattle persist and label information of some veterinary products state not to use in pregnant animals. Clearly, potential risks versus benefits of therapy must be weighed. In humans, the FDA categorizes this drug as category **D** for use during pregnancy (*There is evidence of human fetal risk, but the potential benefits from the use of the drug in pregnant women may be acceptable despite its potential risks.*)

Iodides are excreted in milk. If iodides are required in the nursing dam, switch to milk replacer.

Overdosage/Acute Toxicity

Excessive iodine in animals can cause excessive tearing, vomiting, anorexia, nasal discharge, muscle twitching, cardiomyopathy, scaly haircoats/dandruff, hyperthermia, decreased milk production and weight gain, coughing, inappetence, and diarrhea.

Drug Interactions

The following drug interactions have either been reported or are theoretical in humans or animals receiving iodide and may be of significance in veterinary patients:

■ **ANTITHYROID MEDICATIONS:** Iodides may decrease the efficacy of antithyroid medications

■ **THYROID SUPPLEMENTS:** Iodides may enhance the efficacy of thyroid medications

Doses

■ **DOGS:**
For Sporotrichosis:
a) Using SSKI: 40 mg/kg PO q8h for at least 60 days (Greene & Watson 1998)
b) Using SSKI: 40 mg/kg PO q12h with food; itraconazole less likely to have adverse effects (Grooters 2005)

■ **CATS:**
For Sporotrichosis:
a) 20 mg/kg PO q12–24h for at least 60 days (Greene & Watson 1998)
b) Using SSKI: 20 mg/kg PO q12–24h with food; itraconazole less likely to cause adverse effects (Grooters 2005)

■ **CATTLE, SHEEP & GOATS:**
a) For treatment of actinobacillosis (woody tongue): 70 mg/kg IV given as a 10% or 20% solution; repeat at least one more time at a 7–10 day interval. Refractory cases may require more frequent (2–3 day intervals) treatment. Severe, generalized, or refractory cases may require adjunctive treatment with antibiotics (sulfas, aminoglycoside or tetracyclines). (Smith 1996)

■ **HORSES:**

a) For treatment of sporotrichosis: Sodium iodide 20–40 mg/kg orally daily for several weeks (Fadok 1992)

b) Loading dose of sodium iodide at 20–40 mg/kg IV for 2–5 days, then 20–40 mg/kg PO once daily for at least 3 weeks after all clinical lesions disappear. May administer via oral syringe or mixed in sweet feed. Topical hot packs of 20% sodium iodide may be used on open wounds. (Rees 2004)

c) For Conidiobolomycosis: A mare with *C. coronatus* granulomatous tracheitis was successfully treated with 20% sodium iodide at 44 mg/kg IV for 7 days, then ethylenediamine dihydroiodide (iodide powder, granules) at 1.3 mg/kg PO q12h for 4 months, then q24h for 1 year, then once per week. Excessive lacrimation was occasionally noted, but resolved if the drug was held for one day. (Stewart & Salazar 2005)

Monitoring

■ Clinical efficacy

■ Signs of iodism (excessive tearing, nasal discharge, scaly haircoats/dandruff, hyperthermia, decreased milk production and weight gain, coughing, inappetence, and diarrhea

Client Information

■ Although formal withholding times were not located, there is concern about using this product in food animals about to be slaughtered. In the interest of public health, contact FARAD (see appendix) for guidance.

■ When giving orally in small animals, give with food or a fatty liquid (whole milk, cream) as the taste is extremely unpleasant and nausea or vomiting may otherwise occur.

Chemistry/Synonyms

Sodium iodide occurs as colorless, odorless crystals or white crystalline powder. It develops a brown tint upon degradation. Approximately 1 gram is soluble in 0.6 mL of water and 2 mL of alcohol.

Potassium iodide occurs as a clear to white granular powder. Approximately 1 gram is soluble in 0.7 mL of water. One gram (one mL) of SSKI contains 6 mEq of potassium.

Potassium iodide oral solution may also be known as SSKI (super saturated potassium iodide), or *Pima*®.

Storage/stability

Commercially available veterinary injectable products should generally be stored at room temperature (15–30° C).

Supersaturated potassium iodide (SSKI) solution should be stored below 40°C (104°F) and preferably between 15–30°C (59–86°F) in a tight, light-resistant container; protect from freezing. Crystallization can occur, particularly

if stored at low temperatures; re-warming the contents and shaking will usually redissolve the crystals. If oxidation occurs, the solution will turn brownish yellow in color; discard should this occur.

Compatibility/Compounding Considerations

Sodium iodide injection is reportedly physically **incompatible** with vitamins B and C injection.

Dosage Forms/Regulatory Status

VETERINARY-LABELED PRODUCTS:

Sodium Iodide Injection: 20 grams/100 mL (20%; 200 mg/mL) in 250 mL vials—available as multi- or single use vials; generic; (Rx). Labeled for use in non-lactating cattle.

Oral iodide powders/granules for addition to feeds are available. Active ingredient is ethylenediamine dihydroiodide.

HUMAN-LABELED PRODUCTS:

Potassium Iodide Solution: 1 gram potassium iodide/mL; 325 mg potassium iodide/5 mL in 30 mL, pt & gal; *SSKI*® (Upsher-Smith); generic; (Rx)

Potassium Iodide Oral Syrup: 62.5 mg potassium iodide/mL in pints and gallons; *Pima*® (Fleming); (Rx)

Potassium Iodide Oral Tablets 65 mg, & 130 mg; *Thyrosafe*® (Recip), *Iosat*® (Anbex); (OTC)

There are also radioactive iodine compounds available for thyroid diagnostic and treatment.

References

Fadok, V. (1992). Appendicular Inflammatory Disorders. Current Therapy in Equine Medicine 3. N Robinson Ed. Philadelphia, W.B. Saunders Co.: 161–165.

Greene, C. & A. Watson (1998). Antimicrobial Drug Formulary. Infectious Diseases of the Dog and Cat. C Greene Ed. Philadelphia, WB Saunders: 790–919.

Grooters, A. (2005). Deep fungal infections. Proceedings; ACVIM. Accessed via: Veterinary Information Network. http://goo.gl/wV8J7

Rees, C. (2004). Disorders of the skin. Equine Internal Medicine 2nd Ed. S Reed, W Bayly and D Sellon Eds. Philadelphia, Saunders: 667–720.

Smith, B. (1996). Actinomycosis. Large Animal Internal Medicine 2nd Ed. B Smith Ed. St Louis, Mosby: 796–797.

Stewart, A. & T. Salazar (2005). Fungal infections of the respiratory tract. Proceedings: ACVIM. Accessed via: Veterinary Information Network. http://goo.gl/w5oUA

IOHEXOL

(eye-oh-*hex*-ol)   Omnipaque®

CONTRAST AGENT

Prescriber Highlights

▶ Contrast agent used in medical imaging and to determine GFR

▶ Fewer adverse effects than with older ionic iodine contrast agents

Uses/Indications

Iohexol can be used as a contrast agent for variety of radiographic imaging procedures in veterinary patients, and can be used as a marker agent for estimating glomerular filtration rates (GFR) in dogs or cats. The current usual laboratory measures of renal function (plasma/serum creatinine, plasma/blood urea nitrogen) are not very sensitive indicators for detecting early kidney disease or monitoring real-time renal function status, so other tests are needed. This is an area of intense research interest; it is hoped that, ultimately, results from a simple one or two sample test incorporated with patient characteristics that estimate extra-cellular fluid volume (e.g., age, weight, breed, etc.) can be inserted into an equation that then can be used to reasonably estimate renal function status. Iohexol clearance closely mimics inulin clearance, but iohexol has the advantages of being readily available in dosage forms amenable for clinical use, less expensive than inulin, and being stable in plasma or urine.

Iohexol, when used as a contrast agent can be administered (depending on product and procedure) via intravascular (venous and arterial), intrathecal, intracavitary, or oral routes.

Pharmacology/Actions

Iohexol is a near ideal marker for measuring glomerular filtration rate and thereby, renal function. Its protein binding is negligible, it is nearly 100% excreted unchanged in the urine within 24 hours and can be measured in plasma using a variety of assays.

When used as a radio contrast agent, organic iodine is relatively radiopaque and can help define adjacent structures.

Iohexol has a lower osmolality when compared with conventional (ionic) radio contrast agents, and has been associated with (in humans) a lower incidence of side effects such as pain, heat sensations, adverse hemodynamic changes, EKG changes, endothelial and erythrocyte damage.

Pharmacokinetics

After intravascular administration, iohexol is rapidly distributed throughout the circulation. Protein binding is very low (<1%). Within 24 hours, nearly 100% of a dose is excreted in the urine in patients with normal renal function. In dogs, mean pharmacokinetic parameters reported include: volume of distribution (Vd_{ss}): 221 mL/kg; clearance in dogs is about 2.5−2.9 mL/kg/minute; mean residence time: 82 minutes; elimination half-life: 75 minutes (Heiene *et al.* 2010), (Goy-Thollot *et al.* 2006). Mean clearance of iohexol in cats reported include: 2.3 mL/kg/minute (Heiene *et al.* 2009), and 2.75 mL/kg/minute (Goy-Thollot *et al.* 2006).

Iohexol has an elimination half-life of about 2 hours in human patients.

Contraindications/Precautions/Warnings

Iohexol is contraindicated in patients with a prior hypersensitivity reaction.

Adverse Effects

When used intravascularly, iohexol appears to be well tolerated, but usage in dogs or cats has been limited. Hypersensitivity reactions with iohexol can occur, but in humans, only very rarely. Nephrotoxicity from iohexol is potentially possible, but the risk appears slight. Iohexol is considered to be one of the agents used for contrast studies with the lowest toxicity for humans.

Reproductive/Nursing Safety

While iohexol use in the latter stages of pregnancy potentially carries some fetal risk (thyroid function in newborns), the FDA has designated it as a category *B* drug (*Animal studies have not demonstrated risk to the fetus, but there are no adequate studies in pregnant women; or animal studies have shown an adverse effect, but adequate studies in pregnant women have not demonstrated a risk to the fetus during the first trimester of pregnancy, and there is no evidence of risk in later trimesters.*)

Iohexol is distributed into milk in very low quantities, but no adverse effects have been seen in breastfeeding infants whose mothers received iohexol; the American Academy of Pediatrics considers that iohexol is usually compatible with breastfeeding.

Overdosage/Acute Toxicity

The adverse effects of intravenous overdosage can be serious and life-threatening and primarily affect the pulmonary and cardiovascular systems. Clinical signs can include: cyanosis, bradycardia, acidosis, pulmonary hemorrhage, convulsions, coma, and cardiac arrest. Treatment is supportive.

Drug Interactions

The following drug interactions have either been reported or are theoretical in humans or animals receiving iohexol and may be of significance in veterinary patients:

- ■ **DRUGS THAT MAY PROLONG QTc INTERVALS (e.g., amiodarone, cisapride, procainamide, quinidine, sotalol, cisapride, dolasetron, moxifloxacin):** Iohexol may cause additive prolongation of QTc interval. Iohexol does not cause as much QTc prolongation (in humans) as diatrizoate.

- ■ **IODINE ISOTOPES:** Iohexal may alter binding to thyroid tissue for up to two weeks

- ■ **PHENOTHIAZINES:** Iohexal (especially when used intrathecally) may increase risk for lowering seizure threshold

Laboratory Considerations

- ■ **Thyroid Function Tests:** If iodine-containing isotopes are to be used for diagnosing thyroid disease, prior use of iohexol can reduce the iodine-binding capacity of thyroid tissue for up to 2 weeks. Thyroid function tests that do not depend on iodine estimation are not affected.

Doses

■ **DOGS/CATS:**

To estimate GFR: At the time of writing, the widespread clinical use or usefulness for limited-sample iohexol clearance determination in dogs and cats has yet to be realized, but the following illustrate that significant work is being performed and results are promising for use in clinical settings. Follow the current literature and scientific proceedings for more information as it becomes available.

a) Dogs: Comparing iohexol clearance using a limited sampling (2-4 sample) method versus a 9-sample method; study done in healthy dogs: Using iohexol 300 mg/mL given IV over a minute. Doses administered varied from 129–658 mg/kg of iohexol. The lower doses were initially given to dogs early in the study due to concerns for toxicity, but resulted in many samples with plasma concentrations too low for accurate analysis. No toxicity was seen at the higher dose. Using the 2-sample method, samples were obtained at 2 and 3 hours post dose; 3-sample method at 2, 3, and 4 hours post-dose. Clearance was predicted via a trapezoidal method using an empirical polynomial regression equation. Authors concluded that limited sample methods for iohexol clearance may be acceptable in most situations in which available resources do not allow determination of the complete plasma disappearance curve. (Heiene *et al.* 2010)

b) Dogs and Cats: Using a single sampling method to estimate iohexol clearance: In the study, dogs were administered iohexol 300 mg/mL at a dose of 90 mg iodine content/kg in non-azotemic animals and 45 mg iodine content/kg in azotemic animals IV. Three samples were drawn (at 120, 180, & 240 minutes in non-azotemic animals; 120, 240, & 360 minutes in azotemic animals). The 120 minute sample was used to assess the validity of a single-sample method. After receiver operating characteristics (ROC) analysis was performed to assess the sensitivity and specificity of the single sampling methods for detection of decreasing GFR in dogs and cats, results for sensitivity and specificity for dogs were 98% and 93%, respectively, and in cats, the sensitivity and specificity were 98% and 93%, respectively. No adverse effects were seen in the dogs or cats studied (N = 779 dogs; 339 cats). (Miyagawa *et al.* 2010)

As a contrast agent:

a) For patients with suspected GI perforation: Newer non-ionic iodinated contrast media (*e.g.,* iohexol) with lower osmolality (520 mOsm/mL, undiluted iohexol, 240 mg Iodine/mL) are now recommended for patients with suspected GI perforation. In cats, the recommended dose is a 1:3 dilution of iohexol 240 at 10 mL/kg of body weight. In dogs, a similar dosage is recommended (700–875 mg Iodine/kg, 10 mL/kg). Best administered via orogastric tube (dogs) or nasogastric/nasoesophogeal tube (cats). Radiographs should be obtained immediately following the administration of contrast material; additional sets of radiographs can be obtained at 15, 30, and 60 minutes. (Saunders 2008)

■ **BIRDS:**

As a contrast agent:

a) Indications for contrast imaging may include differentiation of abdominal masses, organ placement or displacement, assessment of GI abnormalities (perforation, foreign body), or GI transit time (proventricular dilatation disease). Contrast agents safe for use in the avian patient include barium sulfate or iohexol administered directly into the crop by gavage. (Retrograde administration of contrast medium directly into the cloaca may help to evaluate cloacal abnormalities.) Survey radiographs (without contrast) should precede the use of contrast agents. The number of images and intervals are based on the agent used and the purpose of the study. If perforation is suspected, iohexol is preferred over barium sulfate. Dosing is based on the estimated crop volume of 25-30 mL/kg. Iohexol may be diluted 1:1 with water. (Murray 2008)

Monitoring

■ No specific monitoring outside of adverse effects

Chemistry/Synonyms

Iohexol is a nonionic iodinated contrast agent that occurs as a white to off-white, hygroscopic, odorless powder; it is very soluble in water and in methyl alcohol; practically insoluble or insoluble in chloroform and ether. Commercial products list the concentration of the product as organic iodine concentration per mL. For example, *Omnipaque® 180* contains iohexol 288 mg/mL, equivalent to 180 mg/mL of organic iodine content. Physical properties of iohexol injection include:

Concentration (mg/mL) organic iodine	Osmolality (mOsm/ kg H_2O)	Viscosity		Specific Gravity (grams/mL) @37°C
		@ 20°C	@ 37°C	
180	408	3.1	2	1.209
210	460	4.2	2.5	1.244
240	520	5.8	3.4	1.280
300	672	11.8	6.3	1.349
350	844	20.4	10.4	1.406

Iohexol may also be known as WIN-39424, iohexolum, ioheksoli, or ioheksolis. A common trade name is *Omnipaque®*.

Storage/Stability

Iohexol should be stored at room temperature 25°C (68°F); excursions permitted between 15°-30°C. Protect from light.

Compatibility/Compounding Considerations

Depending on concentration, the following drugs are reported **compatible** with iohexol: ampicillin, chloramphenicol sodium succinate, cimetidine, diazepam, diphenhydramine, epinephrine, gentamicin, heparin, hydrocortisone sodium succinate, lidocaine, methylprednisolone sodium succinate, nitroglycerin, protamine, and vasopressin. Because compatibility depends on several factors and is time dependent, it is advisable to contact a hospital pharmacist before admixing drugs.

Dosage Forms/Regulatory Status

VETERINARY-LABELED PRODUCTS: None

HUMAN-LABELED PRODUCTS:

Iohexol Injection (preservative-free; concentrations are listed as organic iodine content per mL) 180 mg/mL, 240 mg/mL, 300 mg/mL & 350 mg/mL in 10 mL, 20 mL, 30 mL, 50 mL, 100 mL, 150 mL, 200 mL, & 500 mL vials, bottles, syringes or cartridges (depending on concentration); *Omnipaque®* (GE Healthcare); (Rx)

References

Goy-Thollot, I., C. Chafotte, et al. (2006). Iohexol plasma clearance in healthy dogs and cats. *Veterinary Radiology & Ultrasound* 47(2): 168–173.

Heiene, R., K.A. Eliassen, et al. (2010). Glomerular filtration rate in dogs as estimated via plasma clearance of inulin and iohexol and use of limited-sample methods. *American Journal of Veterinary Research* 71(9): 1100–1107.

Heiene, R., B.S. Reynolds, et al. (2009). Estimation of glomerular filtration rate via 2-and 4–sample plasma clearance of iohexol and creatinine in clinically normal cats. *American Journal of Veterinary Research* 70(2): 176–185.

Miyagawa, Y., N. Takemura, et al. (2010). Assessments of Factors that Affect Glomerular Filtration Rate and Indirect Markers of Renal Function in Dogs and Cats. *Journal of Veterinary Medical Science* 72(9): 1129–1136.

Murray, J. (2008). Avian Radiographic Imaging. Proceedings: AAV. Accessed via: Veterinary Information Network. http://goo.gl/HInKN

Saunders, A.B. (2008). Team Approach to Treating the Emergency Patient with GI Emergencies: Imaging. Proceedings: IVECCS. Accessed via: Veterinary Information Network. http://goo.gl/bu8ER

IPODATE SODIUM

(eye-*poe*-date)

ANTITHYROID AGENT

Prescriber Highlights

▶ Organic iodine compound that may be useful in some cats for medical treatment of hyperthyroidism

▶ Very limited experience

▶ Less effective for cats with severe hyperthyroidism

▶ Efficacy may be transient

▶ Dosage forms must be compounded

Uses/Indications

Ipodate may be useful in some cats for the medical treatment of hyperthyroidism when methimazole (or carbimazole) cannot be tolerated. Because it uses a different mechanism of action than methimazole, ipodate may, potentially, be useful in reducing methimazole dosages (and hence toxicity).

Pharmacology/Actions

Ipodate's efficacy in treating hyperthyroidism is thought to be primarily due to inhibition of the conversion of T_4 to T_3. Ipodate may also block T_3 receptors and thereby protecting the heart from the hypertrophic effects of hyperthyroidism. It may block the actions of TSH.

Pharmacokinetics

The drug is well absorbed after oral administration. Other pertinent pharmacokinetic data for cats is unavailable.

Contraindications/Precautions/Warnings

Ipodate is contraindicated in patients with known hypersensitivity to it. It should be used with caution in patients who have had previous reactions to iodine compounds. Humans with hepatic dysfunction should not receive multiple doses of the drug as renal toxicity has resulted in a few patients. It is recommended for use with caution in human patients with hyperuricemia (possible uric acid nephropathy).

Adverse Effects

Cats reportedly tolerate ipodate well, but may become refractory to treatment after a relatively short time. Oral iodine containing products can cause GI distress (nausea, vomiting, diarrhea, cramping, inappetence). Drug-induced pemphigus is a possibility. Skin rashes, itching, dizziness and headache have been reported by human patients.

Reproductive/Nursing Safety

If administered to pregnant cats, congenital hypothyroidism is a possibility.

Overdosage/Acute Toxicity

No specific information located. Cats have reportedly tolerated daily doses up to 400 mg.

Drug Interactions

The following drug interactions have either been reported or are theoretical in humans or animals receiving ipodate and may be of significance in veterinary patients:

■ **IODINE, RADIOACTIVE:** Ipodate may interfere with radioactive iodine therapy. It is suggested to treat no sooner than 2 weeks after discontinuing ipodate (3–4 weeks or more if possible).

Laboratory Considerations

■ Ipodate may increase **BSP** retention times and **serum bilirubin** levels

■ False positive **urine protein** determinations may occur

■ Ipodate can interfere with thyroid scanning

Doses

■ **CATS:**

For medical treatment of hyperthyroidism in patients who cannot tolerate methimazole and whose owners will not permit surgery or radioiodine therapy:

a) 100–200 mg (total dose; empiric) PO once daily (Lorenz & Melendez 2002; Trepanier 2006)

b) 50 mg per cat PO twice daily, if "good" clinical response not obtained, at 2 week intervals may increase dose to 150 mg/day (100 mg AM, 50 mg PM) and then to 200 mg/day (100 mg twice daily). Cats with severe hyperthyroidism are less likely to respond. (Murray & Peterson 1997)

c) For use before surgery: 15 mg/kg PO q12h. (Jones 2006)

Monitoring

■ Clinical efficacy (heart rate, body weight, etc.)

■ Serum T_3 (**Note:** T4 did not change—remained high in study group)

Client Information

■ It must be stressed to owners that this drug will decrease excessive thyroid hormones, but does not cure the condition and that compliance with the treatment regimen is necessary for success.

■ Long-term efficacy is questionable.

Chemistry/Synonyms

An orally administered radiopaque organic iodine compound, ipodate sodium occurs as a white to off-white, fine crystalline powder. It is freely soluble in alcohol and water. Each 500 mg capsule contains 61.4% (or 333.4 mg) of iodine.

Ipodate calcium may also be known as: calcium iopodate, calcium ipodate, ipodate calcium, *Solu-Biloptin®*, and *Solubiloptine®*.

Ipodate sodium may also be known as: sodium iopodate, sodium ipodate, NSC-106962, *Bilivist®*, *Biloptin®*, and *Oragrafin®*.

Storage/Stability

Store capsules in tight containers and protect from light.

Dosage Forms/Regulatory Status

VETERINARY-LABELED PRODUCTS: None

HUMAN-LABELED PRODUCTS:

None; must obtained via a compounding pharmacy.

Note: Most of the studies using ipodate in cats have been done with calcium ipodate. It is likely that sodium ipodate would be fairly equivalent. If the compounding pharmacy has access to calcium ipodate, it is suggested to use that form. Other options that have been used anecdotally in cats at similar dosages include iopanoic acid or diatrizoate meglumine (Trepanier 2006).

References

Jones, B. (2006). Feline Hyperthyroidism. Proceedings: WSAVA World Congress. Accessed via: Veterinary Information Network. http://goo.gl/QvHL1

Lorenz, M. & L. Melendez (2002). Diagnosis and treatment options for feline hyperthyroidism. Proceedings: Western Veterinary Conference. Accessed via: Veterinary Information Network. http://goo.gl/0byKN

Murray, L. & M. Peterson (1997). Ipodate treatment of hyperthyroidism in cats. *JAVMA* **211**(1): 63–67.

Trepanier, L.A. (2006). Medical management of hyperthyroidism. *Clinical Techniques in Small Animal Practice* **21**(1): 22–28.

IPRATROPIUM BROMIDE

(eye-prah-*troh*-pee-um)   Atrovent®

INHALED ANTIMUSCARINIC

Prescriber Highlights

▶ Inhaled antimuscarinic agent for adjunctive treatment of bronchoconstrictive conditions

▶ Very little information available for use in small animals

▶ Likely safe

▶ May need to be administered quite often, duration of activity is relatively short

Uses/Indications

Locally administered (inhaled) ipratropium bromide can be used for the adjunctive treatment of bronchospastic conditions.

Pharmacology/Actions

Ipratropium inhibits vagally mediated reflexes by antagonizing acetylcholine. Increases in intracellular concentrations of cyclic guanosine monophosphate (cyclic GMP) secondary to acetylcholine are prevented, thereby reducing bronchial smooth muscle constriction. Unlike atropine, ipratropium does not reduce mucociliary clearance.

Pharmacokinetics

Because the medication is inhaled, minimal drug is absorbed in the systemic circulation. In humans, elimination half-life is about 2 hours. In healthy cats with experimentally induced bronchospasm, inhaled (neb) ipratropium gave maximal efficacy for about 4 hours. When combined with albuterol (salbutamol), increased efficacy resulted. (Leemans *et al.* 2006) In horses, onset of action is approximately 30 minutes and duration of effect is approximately 4–6 hours.

Contraindications/Precautions/Warnings

Ipratropium is contraindicated in patients hypersensitive to it or other atropine derivatives.

It should be used with caution in other conditions where antimuscarinics may be harmful, including narrow-angle glaucoma, bladder-neck obstruction, or prostatic hypertrophy.

Adverse Effects

Adverse effects are unlikely to be significant. Tracheal or bronchial irritation (coughing) have been reported on occasion. Allergic responses are possible and some patients develop anticholinergic effects.

Reproductive/Nursing Safety

Large oral dosages in laboratory animals did not cause teratogenic effects. In humans, the FDA categorizes ipratropium as category *B* for use during the first two trimesters of pregnancy (*Animal studies have not yet demonstrated risk to the fetus, but there are no adequate studies in pregnant women; or animal studies have shown an adverse effect, but adequate studies in pregnant women have not demonstrated a risk to the fetus in the first trimester of pregnancy, and there is no evidence of risk in later trimesters.*)

Ipratropium is likely to be safe to use during nursing.

Overdosage/Acute Toxicity

Overdosage is unlikely to be a cause for concern. The drug is not well absorbed orally or after inhalation and oral LD50 values for laboratory animals were greater than 1 gram/kg.

Drug Interactions

The following drug interactions have either been reported or are theoretical in humans or animals receiving ipratropium and may be of significance in veterinary patients:

- **ANTICHOLINERGIC DRUGS:** May cause additive antimuscarinic effects
- **BETA-ADRENERGIC AGONISTS (e.g., albuterol):** May have additive therapeutic effects

Laboratory Considerations

- No specific concerns were noted

Doses

- **HORSES:**
  - a) For adjunctive treatment of RAO, heaves (mild to moderate disease): 180 micrograms inhaled aerosol q4-6h for 14 days. (Rush, B & Grady 2008)

  - b) For adjunctive treatment of RAO/heaves (moderate to severe disease): 90–180 micrograms inhaled via Equine Aeromask or Equine Haler every 6 hours. (Beard 2008)
  - c) For adjunctive treatment of foals with severe bronchospasm: 2–3 micrograms/kg via aerosol q6-8h. (Rush, BR 2007)

- **SMALL MAMMALS:**
  - a) As a bronchodilator in rats: one puff into nebulization chamber twice daily. (Monks & Cowan 2009)

Monitoring

- Clinical efficacy

Client Information

- If using the aerosol metered dose inhalers, do not use after 200 inhalations (puffs) even if there appears to be medication remaining; active ingredient cannot be assured; do not shake the HFA canister before using
- This medication is not for treating an acute asthma attack, it is for maintenance treatment

Chemistry/Synonyms

Ipratropium bromide occurs as a white or almost white crystalline powder. It is soluble in water and slightly soluble in alcohol The pH of a 1% solution is between 5 and 7.5.

Ipratropium bromide may also be known as Sch-1000; many trade names are available including *Atrovent.*®

Storage/stability

The solution for inhalation should be stored at room temperature and protected from light. Keep in foil pouch until time of use. The metered dose inhalers should be stored at room temperature.

Compatibility/Compounding Considerations

The solution for nebulization may be mixed with albuterol or metaproterenol if used within one hour.

Dosage Forms/Regulatory Status

VETERINARY-LABELED PRODUCTS: None

HUMAN-LABELED PRODUCTS:

Ipratropium Bromide Solution for Inhalation: 0.02% (500 micrograms/vial) preservative free in 25 & 60 unit-dose vials (2.5 mL UD "nebs"); generic (Dey); (Rx)

Ipratropium Bromide Aerosol for Inhalation: each actuation delivers 17 micrograms in 12.9 grams metered dose inhaler w/mouthpiece (approx 200 inhalations); *Atrovent*® HFA (BI); (Rx)

Nasal sprays are available, and in combination with albuterol as nebs: *DuoNeb*® (Dey) and as a metered dose inhaler, *Combivent*® (BI).

References

Beard, L. (2008). Consequences of the geriatric mouth. Proceedings: WVC. Accessed via: Veterinary Information Network. http://goo.gl/wTOGw

Leemans, J., N. Kischvink, et al. (2006). Bronchoprotective effect of inhaled salmeterol, salbutamol and ipratropium bromide using different devices on muscarinic bronchoconstriction in healthy cats. Proceedings: ECVIM. Accessed via: Veterinary Information Network. http://goo.gl/kWgMx

Monks, D. & M. Cowan (2009). Chronic respiratory disease in rats. Proceedings: AAVC-UEP. Accessed via: Veterinary Information Network. http://goo.gl/BPUjq

Rush, B. (2007). Foal Pneumonia. Proceedings: ABVP. Accessed via: Veterinary Information Network. http://goo.gl/XHcba

Rush, B. & J.A. Grady (2008). Recurrent airway obstruction (Heaves). *Compendium Equine*(May): 198–205.

IRBESARTAN

(ihr-beh-*sar*-tan)   Avapro®

ANGIOTENSIN-II RECEPTOR BLOCKER (ARB)

Prescriber Highlights

▶ ARB that may be useful in treating dogs with hypertension secondary to renal insufficiency

▶ Very limited experience in veterinary medicine

▶ Not safe during pregnancy

Uses/Indications

Although experience in veterinary medicine is minimal irbesartan may be useful in treating canine hypertension associated with renal insufficiency. It possibly is effective in treating heart failure when dogs are unable to tolerate ACE inhibitors, but documentation for this use is lacking. One study, using very high irbesartan dosages (60 mg/kg PO twice daily) in dogs with subacute mitral regurgitation, demonstrated no improvement in left ventricular function or prevention of left ventricular remodeling (Perry *et al.* 2002).

Pharmacology/Actions

Irbesartan is an angiotensin-II receptor blocker (ARB). By selectively blocking the AT1 receptor, aldosterone synthesis and secretion is reduced causing vasodilation and decreased potassium and increased sodium excretion. While plasma concentrations of renin and angiotensin-II are increased, this does not counteract the blood pressure lowering effects of irbesartan. Irbesartan does not interfere with substance P or bradykinin responses.

Irbesartan does not need to be converted to an active metabolite as does the ARB, losartan (*Cozaar*®). Dogs, unlike humans, reportedly do not covert losartan to the active metabolite.

Pharmacokinetics

After single 30 mg/kg oral doses in dogs with experimentally induced renal hypertension, irbesartan peak levels occurred between 3–4 hours later and elimination half-life was approximately 9 hours. After 30 mg/kg doses PO once daily for 8 days, the elimination half-life was approximately 21 hours (Huang *et al.* 2005).

In humans, absorption is rapid and bioavailability ranges from 60–80%. Peak levels occur in about 1.5–2 hours. Bioavailability is not altered by the presence of food. The drug is 90% bound to plasma proteins and crosses the blood-brain barrier and placenta in small quantities. Irbesartan is metabolized in the liver via glucuronidation and oxidation; metabolites are not active. Both metabolites and unchanged drug are eliminated primarily in the feces and to a lesser extent, in urine. Terminal elimination half-life ranges from 11–15 hours. Dosages do not need to be adjusted in patients with renal dysfunction.

Contraindications/Precautions/Warnings

Patients who are volume or sodium depleted should have these corrected before starting therapy. Do not use in hypotensive patients. In humans, the drug is contraindicated in patients hypersensitive to it. It should not be used during pregnancy (see Reproductive Safety).

Adverse Effects

An adverse effect profile for dogs is not known due to limited use of this medication. In humans, the most commonly reported adverse effects include diarrhea, dyspepsia, fatigue, and orthostatic dizziness/hypotension.

Reproductive/Nursing Safety

Irbesartan is not safe to use during pregnancy. Studies in pregnant rats given high doses demonstrated a variety of fetal abnormalities (renal pelvic cavitation, hydroureter, absence of renal papilla). Smaller doses in rabbits caused increased maternal death and spontaneous abortion. In humans, the drug is considered teratogenic, particularly during the 2nd and 3rd trimesters. During this time, the FDA categorizes irbesartan as category *D* for use during pregnancy (*There is evidence of human fetal risk, but the potential benefits from the use of the drug in pregnant women may be acceptable despite its potential risks.*) If pregnancy is detected in patients receiving irbesartan, the drug should be discontinued as soon as possible.

Because small amounts of irbesartan have been detected in rat milk, and there is significant concern about the safety of the drug in neonates, the manufacturer recommends that it not be used in nursing women.

Overdosage/Acute Toxicity

Rats and mice survived acute oral overdoses in excess of 2000 mg/kg. Likely effects seen in an overdose situation include hypotension and either bradycardia or tachycardia; treatment is supportive. Contact an animal poison control center for further information.

Drug Interactions

In humans or veterinary patients, no clinically significant drug interactions have been reported. Because of the drug's pharmacologic actions, use caution with other drugs that can reduce blood pressure.

Laboratory Considerations

■ No specific concerns were noted

Doses

■ **DOGS:**

a) As an alternative to ACE inhibitors for treatment of hypertension associated with renal insufficiency: 5 mg/kg PO q12–24 hours. (Brown 2004)

Monitoring

■ Blood pressure, heart rate

■ Serum electrolytes, BUN, creatinine

■ Adverse Effects: possibly GI (diarrhea), somnolence/activity changes

Client Information

■ Clients should understand that veterinary experience with this medication is limited and that the adverse effect profile is not well known; anything unusual should be reported to the veterinarian

■ May be given with food or on an empty stomach

Chemistry/Synonyms

Irbesartan is a nonpeptide angiotensin-II antagonist and occurs as white to off-white, crystalline powder. It is practically insoluble in water and slightly soluble in alcohol.

Irbesartan may also be known as: BMS 186295, SR 47436, *Irbesartanum*, *Aprovel®*, *Arbit®*, *Avalide®*, *Avapro®*, *Cavapro®*, *Coaproval®*, *Ecard®*, *Ibsan®*, *Irban®*, *Irbes®*, *Iretensa®*, *Irovel®*, *Irvell®*, *Isart®*, and *Karvea®*.

Storage/Stability

Irbesartan tablets should be stored at room temperature (15–30°C).

Dosage Forms/Regulatory Status

VETERINARY-LABELED PRODUCTS: None

The ARCI (Racing Commissioners International) has designated this drug as a class 3 substance.

HUMAN-LABELED PRODUCTS:

Irbesartan Tablets: 75 mg, 150 mg, & 300 mg; *Avapro®* (Bristol-Meyers Squibb); (Rx)

Irbesartan 150 mg with Hydrochlorothiazide 12.5 mg Tablets, Irbesartan 300 mg with Hydrochlorothiazide 12.5 mg or 25 mg Tablets; *Avalide®*; (Bristol-Myers Squibb); (Rx)

References

Brown, S. (2004). Renoprotective mechanisms of angiotensin inhibition. Proceedings: ACVIM 2004, Accessed via the Veterinary Information Network Jan 2007. Accessed via: Veterinary Information Network. http://goo.gl/iVlmZ

Huang, X., F. Qiu, et al. (2005). Pharmacokinetic and pharmacodynamic interaction between irbesartan and hydrochlorothiazide in renal hypertensive dogs. *J Cardiovasc Pharmacol* 46(6): 863–869.

Perry, G., C. Wei, et al. (2002). Angiotensin II receptor blockade does not improve left ventricular function and remodeling in subacute mitral regurgitation in the dog. *J AM Coll Cardiol* 39(8): 1374–1379.

IRON DEXTRAN

(*eye*-urn *dex*-tran)

INJECTABLE HEMATINIC

Prescriber Highlights

▶ Injectable hematinic

▶ Contraindications: Known hypersensitivity to iron dextran, or with any anemia other than iron deficiency anemia; acute renal infections, in conjunction with oral iron supplements

▶ Adverse Effects: Prostration & muscular weakness, anaphylactoid reactions

▶ High dosages may cause increased incidences of teratogenicity & embryotoxicity

▶ Pigs born of vitamin E/selenium-deficient sows may demonstrate nausea, vomiting, & sudden death within 1 hour of injection

▶ IM use in pigs after 4 weeks of age may cause muscle tissue staining

Uses/Indications

Iron dextran is used in the treatment and prophylaxis of iron deficiency anemias, primarily in neonatal food-producing animals.

Pharmacology/Actions

Iron is necessary for myoglobin and hemoglobin in the transport and utilization of oxygen. While neither stimulating erythropoiesis nor correcting hemoglobin abnormalities not caused by iron deficiency, iron administration does correct both physical signs and decreased hemoglobin levels secondary to iron deficiency.

Ionized iron is a component in the enzymes cytochrome oxidase, succinic dehydrogenase, and xanthine oxidase.

Pharmacokinetics

After IM injection, iron dextran is slowly absorbed primarily via the lymphatic system. About 60% of the drug is absorbed within 3 days of injection and up to 90% of the dose is absorbed after 1–3 weeks. The remaining drug may be absorbed slowly over several months.

After absorption, the reticuloendothelial cells of the liver, spleen, and bone marrow gradually clear the drug from plasma. The iron is cleaved from the dextran component and the dextran is then metabolized or excreted. The iron is immediately bound to protein elements to form hemosiderin, ferritin or transferrin. Iron crosses the placenta, but in what form is unknown. Only traces of iron are excreted in milk.

Iron is not readily eliminated from the body. Iron liberated by the destruction of hemoglobin is reused by the body and only small amounts are lost by the body via hair and nail growth, normal skin desquamation, and GI tract sloughing. Accumulation can result with repeated dosing as only trace amounts of iron are eliminated in the feces, bile, or urine.

Contraindications/Precautions/Warnings

Iron dextran is contraindicated in patients with known hypersensitivity to it or with any anemia other than iron deficiency anemia. It is not to be used in patients with acute renal infections, and should not be used in conjunction with oral iron supplements.

Adverse Effects

The manufacturers of iron dextran injection for use in pigs state that occasionally pigs may react after injection with iron dextran, characterized by prostration and muscular weakness. Rarely, death may result from an anaphylactoid reaction. Iron dextran used in pigs born of vitamin E/selenium-deficient sows may demonstrate nausea, vomiting, and sudden death within 1 hour of injection. Iron dextran injected IM in pigs after 4 weeks of age may cause muscle tissue staining.

Large SC doses have been associated with the development of sarcomas in laboratory animals (rabbits, mice, rats, and hamsters).

Reproductive/Nursing Safety

High dosages may cause increased incidences of teratogenicity and embryotoxicity. Use only when clearly necessary at recommended doses in pregnant animals. In humans, the FDA categorizes this drug as category *C* for use during pregnancy (*Animal studies have shown an adverse effect on the fetus, but there are no adequate studies in humans; or there are no animal reproduction studies and no adequate studies in humans.*)

Traces of unmetabolized iron dextran are excreted in milk.

Overdosage/Acute Toxicity

Depending on the size of the dose, inadvertent overdose injections may require chelation therapy. For more information, refer to the Ferrous Sulfate monograph for information on using deferoxamine and other treatments for iron toxicity.

Drug Interactions

The following drug interactions have either been reported or are theoretical in humans or animals receiving iron and may be of significance in veterinary patients:

- **CHLORAMPHENICOL:** Because chloramphenicol may delay the response to iron administration, avoid using chloramphenicol in patients with iron deficiency anemia

Laboratory Considerations

- Large doses of injectable iron may discolor the serum brown which can cause falsely elevated **serum bilirubin** values and falsely decreased **serum calcium** values.

- After large doses of iron dextran, **serum iron** values may not be meaningful for up to 3 weeks.

Doses

- **DOGS:**
  a) For iron deficiency anemia: Iron dextran 10–20 mg/kg once, followed by oral therapy with ferrous sulfate (see ferrous sulfate monograph) (Weiser 1989)

- **CATS:**
  a) For prevention of transient neonatal iron deficiency anemia: 50 mg iron dextran injection at 18 days of age (Weiser 1989)
  b) For adjunctive therapy with erythropoietin treatment: 10 mg/kg IM every 3-4 weeks. (Grauer 2008)
  c) For adjunctive therapy with erythropoietin treatment in cats who cannot tolerate oral iron therapy: 50 mg IM q3–4 weeks (Hoskins 2005)

- **FERRETS:**
  a) 10 mg/kg IM once weekly (Williams 2000)

- **SWINE:**
  a) For prevention of iron deficiency anemia in baby pigs (2–4 days of age): Administer an initial intramuscular injection of 100 mg of elemental iron to each animal at 2 to 4 days of age. Dosage may be repeated in 14 to 21 days. (Label directions; *Ferrextran-100®*—Fort Dodge)

- **BIRDS:**
  For iron deficiency anemia or following hemorrhage:
  a) 10 mg/kg IM; repeat in 7–10 days if PCV fails to return to normal (Clubb 1986)
  b) 10 mg/kg IM; repeat weekly (McDonald 1989)

Monitoring

- If indicated: CBC, RBC indices
- Adverse reactions

Client Information

- In pigs, inject IM in the back of the ham

Chemistry/Synonyms

Iron dextran is a complex of ferric oxyhydroxide and low molecular weight partially hydrolyzed dextran derivative. The commercially available injection occurs as a dark brown, slightly viscous liquid that is completely miscible with water or normal saline and has a pH of 5.2–6.5.

Iron dextran may also be known as: iron-dextran complex, *Cosmofer®, DexFerrum®, Dexiron®, Driken®, Fercayl®, Ferrocel®, Ferroin®, Ferrum Hausmann®, Fexiron®, Imferdex®, Imferon®, InFeD®,* and *Infufer®.*

Storage/stability

Iron dextran injection should be stored at room temperature (15–30°C); avoid freezing.

Compatibility/Compounding Considerations

Iron dextran injection is reportedly physically **incompatible** when mixed with oxytetracycline HCl and sulfadiazine sodium.

Dosage Forms/Regulatory Status/Withdrawal Times

VETERINARY-LABELED PRODUCTS:

Iron Dextran Injection: 100 mg of elemental iron/mL and 200 mg of elemental iron/mL in 100 mL vials; various manufacturers and trade names; (OTC). FDA-approved for use in swine. No slaughter withdrawal time required.

HUMAN-LABELED PRODUCTS:

Iron Dextran Injection: 50 mg of elemental iron/mL (as dextran) in 1 mL & 2 mL single-dose vials; *InFeD®* (Watson); *DexFerrum®* (American Regent); (Rx)

References

Clubb, S.L. (1986). Therapeutics: Individual and Flock Treatment Regimens. *Clinical Avian Medicine and Surgery.* GJ Harrison and LR Harrison Eds. Philadelphia, W.B. Saunders: 327–355.

Grauer, G.F. (2008). Staging and Management of Feline Chronic Kidney Disease. Proceedings: AAFP. Accessed via: Veterinary Information Network. http://goo.gl/WO1yI

Hoskins, J. (2005). Geriatric medicine: Kidney diseases. Proceedings: ACVC 2006, Accessed from the Veterinary Information Network, Jan 2007. http://goo.gl/eLSHI

McDonald, S.E. (1989). Summary of medications for use in psittacine birds. *JAAV* **3**(3): 120–127.

Weiser, M.G. (1989). Erythrocytes and Associated Disorders. *The Cat: Diseases and Clinical Management.* RG Sherding Ed. New York, Churchill Livingstone. **1:** 529–556.

Williams, B. (2000). Therapeutics in Ferrets. *Vet Clin NA: Exotic Anim Pract* **3:1**(Jan): 131–153.

ISOFLUPREDONE ACETATE

(eye-so-*floo*-preh-dohn)   Predef 2X®

INJECTABLE GLUCOCORTICOID

For topical or otic use of isoflupredone, see the Topical Dermatological Agents, and Otic Appendixes

Prescriber Highlights

▶ Injectable glucocorticoid labeled for use in cattle, horses & swine for antiinflammatory & immunosuppressive effects

▶ Less likely to cause early parturition than dexamethasone or betamethasone, but avoid use in pregnancy

▶ May have mineralocorticoid effects in horses & cattle; hypokalemia has been noted

Uses/Indications

Isoflupredone acetate is a potent glucocorticoid and like other glucocorticoids can be used for its antiinflammatory or immunosuppressive effects. Labeled indications for isoflupredone include: adjunctive treatment of bovine ketosis, alleviating pain and lameness associated with musculoskeletal conditions, acute hypersensitivity reactions, adjunctive treatment of over-whelming infections with severe toxicity, shock, supportive therapy in the treatment of stress conditions (*e.g.*, surgery), dystocia, retained placenta, inflammatory ocular conditions, snakebite and parturient paresis.

A study evaluating the effects of isoflupredone (20 mg IM) with or without insulin (ultralente 100 Units) on energy metabolism, milk production and overall health in dairy cows during the early lactation phase showed that isoflupredone with or without insulin "offered no metabolic, production, or reproductive benefits in lactating dairy cattle." (Seifi *et al.* 2007)

In horses, isoflupredone has been used parenterally to reduce inflammation associated with recurrent airway obstruction (RAO, "heaves," COPD).

While the drug could be used in small animals, it is recommended to use other glucocorticoid agents instead, where there has been more experience and other FDA-approved products for dogs and cats are available.

Pharmacology/Actions

Isoflupredone's antiinflammatory potency is approximately 17 times that of hydrocortisone (cortisol). The label states that the glucocorticoid activity of isoflupredone is 50 times that of hydrocortisone and 10 times that of prednisolone as measured by liver glycogen deposition in rats. Isoflupredone reportedly has some mineralocorticoid effects, and can cause hypokalemia.

For more information on the pharmacologic actions associated with glucocorticoids, see the *Glucocorticoid Agents, General Information* monograph.

Pharmacokinetics

No specific pharmacokinetic values were located. The manufacturer states that gluconeogenic activity persists for 48 hours after dosing in cattle.

Contraindications/Precautions/Warnings

Systemic use of glucocorticoids is generally considered contraindicated in systemic fungal infections (unless used for replacement therapy in Addison's), when administered IM in patients with idiopathic thrombocytopenia, and in patients hypersensitive to a particular compound. Because of their ulcerogenic potential, glucocorticoids should be used with extreme caution in patients with active GI ulcers or those susceptible to them. Use cautiously in patients with diabetes mellitus.

Because it can cause hypokalemia, it should not be used in downer cows or animals susceptible to the effects of hypokalemia.

Chronic use in young, growing animals must be undertaken cautiously, as decreased growth may occur.

Not to be used in calves to be processed into veal.

See Reproductive Safety for information on use during pregnancy.

Adverse Effects

Adverse effects are generally associated with long-term administration of glucocorticoids, particularly if given at higher dosages; these effects generally are manifested as signs of hyperadrenocorticism. Recent research has indicated, however, that even single doses administered to dairy cattle can cause hypokalemia. Potential adverse effects include: reduced milk production, hypokalemia, delayed wound healing, GI ulceration, increased infection rates, diabetes mellitus exacerbation/hyperglycemia, pancreatitis, hepatopathy, renal dysfunction, osteoporosis, laminitis (horses), hypothyroidism, and hyperlipidemia. When administered to young, growing animals, glucocorticoids can retard growth.

Reproductive/Nursing Safety

Avoid using isoflupredone during pregnancy. Glucocorticoids can induce abortion or early parturition in the later stages of pregnancy; most commonly seen in ruminants. While isoflupredone appears to have a much lower abortifacient potential (like hydrocortisone, prednisolone, & triamcinolone) than steroids such as dexamethasone, betamethasone or flumethasone; it may induce premature parturition with retained placenta and its use should generally be avoided during the later stages of pregnancy.

Glucocorticoids used during the first trimester have been linked to a variety of teratogenic effects in dogs and laboratory animals.

Glucocorticoid administration may reduce milk production. Glucocorticoids unbound to plasma proteins will enter milk. High dosages or prolonged administration to mothers may potentially inhibit the growth of nursing newborns.

Overdosage/Acute Toxicity

A single overdose of isoflupredone is unlikely to cause harmful effects. Should clinical signs require intervention, use supportive treatment.

Chronic usage of glucocorticoids can lead to serious adverse effects. Refer to the Adverse Effects section for more information.

Drug Interactions

The following drug interactions have either been reported or are theoretical in humans or animals receiving isoflupredone or other glucocorticoids and may be of significance in veterinary patients:

■ **DIGITALIS GLYCOSIDES (digoxin):** Increased chance of digitalis toxicity may occur should hypokalemia develop; diligent monitoring of potassium and digitalis glycoside levels is recommended

■ **POTASSIUM-DEPLETING DIURETICS (furosemide, thiazides):** Administered concomitantly with glucocorticoids may cause hypokalemia

■ **SALICYLATES:** Glucocorticoids may reduce salicylate blood levels

■ **ULCEROGENIC DRUGS (e.g., NSAIDs):** With glucocorticoids may increase the risk of gastrointestinal ulceration

■ **VACCINES, TOXOIDS, BACTERINS:** A diminished immune response may occur after vaccine, toxoid, or bacterin administration; patients receiving corticosteroids at immunosuppressive dosages should generally not receive live attenuated-virus vaccines as virus replication may be augmented

Laboratory Considerations

■ Glucocorticoids may increase **serum cholesterol** and **serum** and **urine glucose** levels

■ Isoflupredone may decrease **serum potassium**

■ Glucocorticoids can suppress the release of thyroid stimulating hormone (TSH) and reduce T_3 & T_4 values; thyroid gland atrophy has been reported after chronic glucocorticoid administration

■ Reactions to **skin tests** may be suppressed by glucocorticoids.

■ Glucocorticoids may cause false-negative results of the **nitroblue tetrazolium test** for systemic bacterial infections.

Doses

■ **CATTLE:**

a) For labeled systemic indications: 10–20 mg (total dose) IM, according to the size of the animal and severity of the condition. The dose may be repeated in 12 to 24 hours if indicated. (Label information; *Predef 2X®*—Pharmacia & Upjohn)

■ **HORSES: (Note:** RCI Class 4)

a) For labeled systemic indications: 5–20 mg (total dose) IM repeated as necessary. For intrasynovial administration: 5–20 mg or more depending on the size of the joint cavity. (Label information; *Predef 2X®*—Pharmacia & Upjohn)

b) For intraarticular administration: 4–20 mg; has a short to medium duration of action. (Goodrich 2006)

c) For treatment of "heaves" (RAO): 10–14 mg (total dose) IM once daily for a horse weighing between 450–500 kg. (Lavoie 2003)

d) For treatment of recurrent airway obstruction (RAO): 0.03 mg/kg IM once daily. Patients were treated for 14 days and developed significant decreases in serum potassium. (Picandet *et al.* 2003)

■ **SWINE:**

a) For labeled systemic indications: 5 mg (total dose) IM for a 300 lb. animal. Adjust dose proportionally for a smaller or larger animal. (Label information; *Predef 2X®*—Pharmacia & Upjohn)

Monitoring

■ Single injections may not require monitoring beyond observation of the patient for efficacy and adverse effects, but consider evaluating serum potassium

■ Ongoing usage requires enhanced monitoring including: renal and liver function, CBC, blood glucose and serum electrolytes

■ ACTH stimulation tests may be indicated to determine extent of HPA axis suppression

■ Consider thyroid hormone monitoring if use is prolonged or patient exhibits signs associated with thyroid hormone deficiency

Client Information

■ If used in dairy cattle, warn producer that milk production may be affected

■ If owners are to administer the medication, caution them to only administer as the veterinarian directs

Chemistry/Synonyms

Isoflupredone acetate is a fluorinated synthetic corticosteroid with a molecular weight of 420.5. The commercial injection is in an aqueous suspension that also contains sodium citrate, polyethylene glycol 3350, and povidone.

Isoflupredone acetate may also be known as: U-6013, 9alpha-fluoroprednisolone acetate, and *Predef 2x®*.

Storage/Stability

The injection should be stored at controlled room temperature 20°–25°C.

Dosage Forms/Regulatory Status

VETERINARY-LABELED PRODUCTS:

Isoflupredone acetate 2 mg/mL aqueous suspension for injection in 10 mL and 100 mL vials; *Predef 2x®* (Pfizer); (Rx). In the USA, *Predef 2x®* is FDA-approved for use in cattle, horses and swine.

Meat withdrawal time is 7 days; it is not to be used in calves to be processed for veal. There is no milk withdrawal time for isoflupredone in the USA, but in Canada a 72-hour withdrawal time is specified.

Isoflupredone is also found in some topical and otic products. For more information see the *Dermatological Agents, Topical* and *Otic* Appendixes.

The ARCI (Racing Commissioners International) has designated this drug as a class 4 substance.

HUMAN-LABELED PRODUCTS: None

References

Goodrich, L. (2006). Current therapies for osteoarthritis. Proceedings: Western Veterinary Conf 2006, Accessed via the Veterinary Information Network Jan 2007. Accessed via: Veterinary Information Network. http://goo.gl/APgPD

Lavoie, J.-P. (2003). Heaves (recurrent airway obstruction): practical management of acute episodes and prevention of exacerbations. *Current Therapy in Equine Medicine 5*. N Robinson Ed., Saunders: 417–421.

Picandet, V., R. Leguillette, et al. (2003). Comparison of efficacy and tolerability of isoflupredone and dexamethasone in the treatment of horses affected with recurrent airway obstruction (RAO). *Equine Vet J* 35(4): 419–424.

Seifi, H.A., S.J. LeBlanc, et al. (2007). Effect of isoflupredone acetate with or without insulin on energy metabolism, reproduction, milk production, and health in dairy cows in early lactation. *Journal of Dairy Science* 90(9): 4181–4191.

ISOFLURANE

(eye-soe-*flure*-ane)   Isoflo®, Iso-Thesia®

GENERAL ANESTHETIC, INHALANT

Prescriber Highlights

▶ Inhalant general anesthetic

▶ Contraindications: History or predilection towards malignant hyperthermia

▶ Caution with increased CSF or head injury, or myasthenia gravis

▶ Adverse Effects: Dose related hypotension, respiratory depression, & GI effects (nausea, vomiting, ileus); cardiodepression generally is minimal at doses causing surgical planes of anesthesia. Arrhythmias are rare.

▶ May be fetotoxic

▶ Drug interactions

Uses/Indications

As halothane is no longer available, isoflurane is now the primary inhalant anesthetic used in veterinary medicine. When compared with older anesthetics such as halothane or methoxyflurane, isoflurane has less myocardial depressant and catecholamine sensitizing effects, and it can be used safely in patients with hepatic or renal disease. The newer inhalant anesthetics, sevoflurane (ability to change depth of anesthesia faster; not as respiratory irritating; mask inductions possible) and desflurane (very fast onset, faster recoveries) have some advantages over isoflurane, but are more expensive

Pharmacology/Actions

While the precise mechanism that inhalant anesthetics exert their general anesthetic effects is not precisely known, they may interfere with functioning of nerve cells in the brain by acting at the lipid matrix of the membrane. Some key pharmacologic effects noted with isoflurane include: CNS depression, depression of body temperature regulating centers, increased cerebral blood flow, respiratory depression, hypotension, vasodilatation, myocardial depression (less so than with halothane), and muscular relaxation.

Minimal Alveolar Concentration (MAC; %) in oxygen reported for isoflurane in various species: Dog = 1.5; Cat = 1.2; Horse = 1.31; Human = 1.2. Several factors may alter MAC (acid/base status, temperature, other CNS depressants on board, age, ongoing acute disease, etc.).

Pharmacokinetics

Isoflurane is rapidly absorbed from the alveoli. It is rapidly distributed into the CNS and crosses the placenta. The vast majority of the drug is eliminated via the lungs; only about 0.17% is metabolized in liver and only very small amounts of inorganic fluoride is formed.

Contraindications/Precautions/Warnings

Isoflurane is contraindicated in patients with a history or predilection towards malignant hyperthermia. It should be used with caution (benefits vs. risks) in patients with increased CSF or head injury, or myasthenia gravis.

Because of its respiratory depressant effects, intermittent positive pressure ventilation may be required to achieve anesthesia, particularly in horses; overdose risks are increased, however.

Both isoflurane and desflurane can be irritating to the respiratory system and are not recommended for mask induction (Clarke 2008).

Adverse Effects

Hypotension (secondary to vasodilation, not cardiodepression) may occur and is considered to be dose related. Hypotension usually responds to fluids, but profound hypotension may require the use of vasopressors.

Dose-dependent respiratory depression, and GI effects (nausea, vomiting, ileus) have been reported. While cardiodepression generally is minimal at doses causing surgical planes of anesthesia, it may occur. Arrhythmias have rarely been reported.

Reproductive/Nursing Safety

Some animal studies have indicated that isoflurane may be fetotoxic. Use during pregnancy with caution. In a system evaluating the safety of drugs in canine and feline pregnancy (Papich 1989), this drug is categorized as in class: *B (Safe for use if used cautiously. Studies in laboratory animals may have uncovered some risk, but these drugs appear to be safe in dogs and cats or these drugs are safe if they are not administered when the animal is near term.)*

Drug Interactions

The following drug interactions have either been reported or are theoretical in humans or animals receiving isoflurane and may be of significance in veterinary patients:

- ■ **AMINOGLYCOSIDES:** Use with caution with halogenated anesthetic agents as additive neuromuscular blockade may occur

- ■ **ACE INHIBITORS OR OTHER HYPOTENSIVE AGENTS:** Concomitant use may increase risks for hypotension. Enalapril caused significant decreases in systolic blood pressure in cats and dogs undergoing isoflurane anesthesia (Ishikawa, Uechi & Ishikawa 2007), (Ishikawa, Uechi & Hori 2007)

- ■ **LINCOSAMIDES:** Use with caution with halogenated anesthetic agents as additive neuromuscular blockade may occur

- ■ **NON-DEPOLARIZING NEUROMUSCULAR BLOCKING AGENTS:** Additive neuromuscular blockade may occur

- ■ **SUCCINYLCHOLINE:** With inhalation anesthetics, may induce increased incidences of cardiac effects (bradycardia, arrhythmias, sinus arrest and apnea) and, in susceptible patients, malignant hyperthermia

- ■ **SYMPATHOMIMETICS (dopamine, epinephrine, norepinephrine, ephedrine, metaraminol, etc.):** While isoflurane sensitizes the myocardium to the effects of sympathomimetics less so than halothane, arrhythmias may still result. If these drugs are needed, they should be used with caution and in significantly reduced dosages with intensive monitoring

Doses

- ■ **DOGS/CATS:**
   (**Note:** Concentrations are dependent upon fresh gas flow rate; the lower the flow rate, the higher the concentration required.)
   a) 5% induction; 1.5–2.5% maintenance (Papich 1992)
   b) 0.5–3%, inhaled (Hubbell 1994)

- ■ **FERRETS/SMALL MAMMALS:**
   a) **Mice, Rats, Gerbils, Hamsters, Guinea pigs, Chinchillas:** Using a non-rebreathing system: Induction: 2–3%, maintenance: 0.25–2% (Anderson 1994); (Adamcak & Otten 2000)
   b) **Ferrets:** After premed with medetomidine at 50–100 micrograms/kg. Atropine at 0.05 mg/kg SC is used to counteract hypersalivation and bradycardia. Starting isoflurane at 1–2% will be less irritating to the ferret and cause less of a struggle. Use a non-rebreathing system. Consider intubation in procedures lasting longer than 30 minutes. For post-op pain either butorphanol at 0.1 mg/kg SC or buprenorphine at 0.02 mg/kg SC. (Johnson 2006)

- ■ **REPTILES:**
   a) Give 5% isoflurane and oxygen in a clear plastic bag or induction chamber. Fill chamber with gas and seal. Induction time may take 30–60 minutes, but can be shortened to 15–30 minutes with increased depth of anesthesia if animal is injected with 10–20 mg/kg of ketamine (SC or IM). Patient should be kept warm by placing on a water blanket. Surgical anesthesia can be determined by the loss of righting reflex. After induction, use either a mask, ET tube, or leave head in chamber. Maintenance levels are 3–5% (if isoflurane used alone). If apnea occurs during or after anesthesia, discontinue gas anesthetic and apply gentle manual ventilation 2–4 times per minute with small doses of doxapram IV. Normal respiration generally resumes in 3–5 minutes. Righting reflex generally recovers in

an hour, but animal may be tranquilized for up to 24 hours. (Gillespie 1994)

b) Anesthetic gas of choice for reptiles. Induction can be with a face mask, or with a "cat box." Animal may be intubated, especially if has been preanesthetized with ketamine or *Telazol*®, and "bag" it down with positive pressure ventilation. Maintenance is usually 1.5–3%. (Funk 2002)

■ **BIRDS:**

a) Small birds can be anesthetized safely in 15–30 seconds at 4% (Ludders 1992)

b) Induction occurs within 1–2 minutes at a concentration of 3–5%. Maintenance at 1.5–2% is adequate for most birds. Anesthetic of choice for birds; heart rate may decrease, but not to the same degree as halothane. Recovery very rapid; most patients are standing and cage safe within 5 min. after anesthesia discontinued, but there seems to be a direct relationship between anesthesia time and recovery time. (Bennett 2002)

Monitoring
■ Respiratory and ventilatory status
■ Cardiac rate/rhythm; blood pressure (particularly with "at risk" patients
■ Level of anesthesia

Chemistry/Synonyms
An inhalant general anesthetic agent, isoflurane occurs as a colorless, nonflammable, stable liquid. It has a characteristic mildly pungent musty, ethereal odor. At 20°C, isoflurane's specific gravity is 1.496 and vapor pressure is 238 mm Hg. Its boiling point is 48.5°C and solubility coefficients are blood-gas: 1.4; and oil-gas: 91.

Isoflurane may also be known as: compound 469, isofluranum, *AErrane*®, *Forene*®, *Forenium*®, *Forthane*®, *Isoflo*®, *Isofor*®, *Isoforine*®, *Isosol*®, *Isothane*®, *Iso-Thesia*®, *Lisorane*®, *Sofloran*®, *Tensocold*®, *Terrell*® and *Zuflax*®.

Storage/stability
Isoflurane should be stored at room temperature; it is relatively unaffected by exposure to light, but should be stored in a tight, light-resistant container. Isoflurane does not attack aluminum, brass, tin, iron, or copper.

Dosage Forms/Regulatory Status
VETERINARY-LABELED PRODUCTS:
Isoflurane Inhalation Anesthetic: 99.9%/mL in 100 mL and 250 mL bottles; *Isoflo*® (Abbott), *Isosol*® (Vedco), *Iso-Thesia*® (Butler), generic, (Halocarbon, VetOne, Phoenix Pharmaceutical); (Rx). FDA-approved for use in horses (those not intended for food) and dogs.

HUMAN-LABELED PRODUCTS:
Isoflurane Liquid for inhalation in 100 mL and 250 mL; *Forane*® (Baxter Healthcare); *Terrell*® (Minrad); generic (Abbott); (Rx)

References
Adamcak, A. & B. Otten (2000). Rodent Therapeutics. *Vet Clin NA: Exotic Anim Pract* **3:1**(Jan): 221–240.
Anderson, N. (1994). Basic husbandry and medicine of pocket pets. *Saunders Manual of Small Animal Practice*. S Birchard and R Sherding Eds. Philadelphia, W.B. Saunders Company: 1363–1389.
Bennett, R. (2002). Avian Anesthesia. Proceedings: Western Veterinary Conference. Accessed via: Veterinary Information Network. http://goo.gl/pXOp9
Clarke, K.W. (2008). Options for inhalation anaesthesia. *In Practice* **30**(9): 513–518.
Funk, R. (2002). Anesthesia in reptiles. Proceedings: Western Veterinary Conf. Accessed via: Veterinary Information Network. http://goo.gl/9l98U
Gillespie, D. (1994). Reptiles. *Saunders Manual of Small Animal Practice*. S Birchard and R Sherding Eds. Philadelphia, W.B. Saunders Company: 1390–1411.
Hubbell, J. (1994). PRactical methods of anesthesia. *Saunders Manual of Small Animal Practice*. S Birchard and R Sherding Eds. Philadelphia, W.B. Saunders Company: 31–21.
Ishikawa, Y., M. Uechi, et al. (2007). Effect of Isoflurane Anesthesia on Hemodynamics Following Administration of an Angiotensin-Converting Enzyme Inhibitor in Dogs. Proceedings: ACVIM. Accessed via: Veterinary Information Network. http://goo.gl/2p2Ev
Ishikawa, Y., M. Uechi, et al. (2007). Effect of Isoflurane Anesthesia on Hemodynamics Following Administration of an Angiotensin-Converting Enzyme Inhibitor in Cats. Proceedings: ACVIM. Accessed via: Veterinary Information Network. http://goo.gl/0ZZ3x
Johnson, D. (2006). Ferrets: the other companion animal. Proceedings: ACVC. Accessed via: Veterinary Information Network. http://goo.gl/bSeol
Ludders, J. (1992). Advantages and guidelines for using isoflurane. *The Veterinary Clinics of North America; Small Animal Practice* **22**(2: March): 328–331.
Papich, M. (1989). Effects of drugs on pregnancy. *Current Veterinary Therapy X: Small Animal Practice*. R Kirk Ed. Philadelphia, Saunders: 1291–1299.
Papich, M. (1992). Table of Common Drugs: Approximate Dosages. *Current Veterinary Therapy XI: Small Animal Practice*. R Kirk and J Bonagura Eds. Philadelphia, W.B. Saunders Company: 1233–1249.

ISONIAZID (INH)
(eye-so-*nye*-ah-zid)
Isonicotinic acid hydrazide
ANTIMYCOBACTERIAL

Prescriber Highlights
▶ Antimycobacterial that may be used for chemoprophylaxis of M. bovis or M. tuberculosis in small animals
▶ Treating active infections is controversial because of potential public health risks associated with the infections
▶ Hepatotoxicity & neurotoxicity possible; narrow therapeutic index

Uses/Indications
Isoniazid (INH) is sometimes used for chemoprophylaxis in small animals in households having a human with tuberculosis. It potentially can be used in combination with other antimycobacterial drugs to treat infections of *M. bovis* or *M. tuberculosis* in dogs or cats. But because of the public health risks, particularly in the face of

increased populations of immunocompromised people, treatment of mycobacterial (*M. bovis, M. tuberculosis*) infections in domestic or captive animals is controversial. In addition, INH has a narrow therapeutic index and toxicity is a concern (see Adverse Effects).

In humans, isoniazid (INH) is routinely used alone to treat latent tuberculosis infections (positive tuberculin skin test) and in combination with other antimycobacterial agents to treat active disease.

Pharmacology/Actions

Isoniazid inhibits the synthesis of mycoloic acids, a component of mycobacterial cell walls; its exact mechanism is not well understood. It is most active against mycobacteria that are actively dividing and affects both extracellular and intracellular mycobacteria.

Isoniazid is only active against *M. tuberculosis, M. bovis* and some strains of *M. kansasii*. In humans, resistance develops rapidly if used alone against active clinical disease, but not when used for prophylactic treatment.

Pharmacokinetics

No information was located on the pharmacokinetics of INH in dogs or cats.

In humans, isoniazid is rapidly absorbed after oral administration; food can decrease absorption somewhat and INH may undergo significant first pass metabolism. The drug is highly distributed in the body and crosses into the CSF and caseous material. It is distributed into milk and crosses the placenta. It is only slightly (10%) bound to plasma proteins. In humans, the drug is initially primarily acetylated in the liver. The N-acetylated form is then further biotransformed to isonicotinic acid and monoacetylhydrazine. Monoacetylhydrazine is thought to play a role in the drug's hepatic toxicity. As dogs, like some humans, lack N-acetyltransferase, increased potential for INH toxicity may occur in this species. Elimination half-life in fast acetylators (humans) is 0.5–1.6 hours and 2–5 hours in slow acetylators. Patients with acute or chronic liver disease may have substantially longer half-lives (2X). The drug is mostly eliminated in the urine as inactive metabolites.

Contraindications/Precautions/Warnings

Isoniazid is contraindicated in patients with acute liver disease or those that developed hepatopathy while taking the medication in the past.

It should be used with caution in patients with decreased hepatic function or severe renal disease.

Adverse Effects

The primary adverse effects associated with INH is hepatotoxicity with increased serum liver enzymes. Additional adverse effects reported in dogs include CNS stimulation, peripheral neuropathy and thrombocytopenia. Ataxia, seizures, salivation, diarrhea, vomiting and arrhythmias have been reported after overdoses in dogs.

Adverse effects reported in cats include hepatotoxicity and peripheral neuritis In humans, urticaria, hepatotoxicity and peripheral neuropathy are commonly reported; rarely, blood dyscrasias, SLE, and seizures have been reported.

Reproductive/Nursing Safety

Isoniazid crosses the placenta and has been found to be embryocidal in some laboratory species, but teratogenic effects have not been detected in mice, rabbits, or rats. In humans, the FDA categorizes isoniazid as category **C** for use during pregnancy (*Animal studies have shown an adverse effect on the fetus, but there are no adequate studies in humans; or there are no animal reproduction studies and no adequate studies in humans.*)

Isoniazid is excreted in milk in low concentrations (approx. 1–2% of maternal serum concentrations in humans) and it is thought to be safe to use during nursing. Ingested levels via milk are not high enough to serve as prophylaxis for tuberculosis in nursing infants.

Overdosage/Acute Toxicity

Overdosage of INH can be very serious. In dogs, the reported LD50 is 50 mg/kg; serious toxicity can occur with as little as one 300 mg tablet ingested. Ataxia, seizures, myocardial necrosis, metabolic acidosis, rhabdomyolysis, salivation, diarrhea, vomiting, and arrhythmias have been reported after overdoses in dogs; it is strongly recommended to contact an animal poison control center in the event of any inadvertent ingestion. Treatment may include enterogastric lavage, activated charcoal and drugs such as diazepam or phenobarbital to control seizures. Fluids and acidemia may need correction.

Pyridoxine (Vitamin B-6) has been suggested to be administered intravenously (preferably over 30–60 minutes) on a mg per mg of INH-ingested basis. It is commercially available as a 100 mg/mL 1 mL vial, but it may be difficult to obtain in an emergency situation. A local human hospital may stock it.

Drug Interactions

Drug interactions have not been reported with isoniazid in animals. The following drug interactions have either been reported or are theoretical in humans receiving INH and may be of significance in veterinary patients:

- ■ **ALFENTANIL:** Prolonged alfentanil duration of action
- ■ **ANTACIDS (especially those containing aluminum):** Decreased INH absorption
- ■ **BENZODIAZEPINES:** INH may reduce benzodiazepine metabolism
- ■ **CORTICOSTEROIDS:** May reduce INH efficacy
- ■ **KETOCONAZOLE:** INH may reduce ketoconazole serum concentrations
- ■ **OTHER HEPATOTOXIC DRUGS (e.g., acetaminophen, itraconazole, fluconazole, methimazole, ketoconazole, phenothiazines,**

sulfonamides, estrogens, etc.): increased risk of hepatotoxicity

■ **OTHER NEUROTOXIC DRUGS:** Increased risk of neurotoxicity

■ **PYRIDOXINE:** INH may antagonize or increase the excretion of pyridoxine, increased pyridoxine may be required; increased peripheral neuritis may occur secondary to pyridoxine/INH interaction

■ **PHENYTOIN:** INH may inhibit metabolism and increase risks for phenytoin toxicity

■ **RIFAMPIN:** Increased risk for hepatotoxicity

■ **THEOPHYLLINE:** Increased risk of theophylline toxicity

■ **FOOD INTERACTIONS** in humans: **cheese** (Swiss, Cheshire, etc.) or **fish** (Tuna, Skipjack, Sardinella): INH may interfere with metabolism of tyramine and histamine found in fish and cheese

Laboratory Considerations

■ INH may cause false-positive **urine glucose determinations** when using cupric sulfate solution (Benedict's Solution, *Clinitest®*); tests utilizing glucose oxidase (*Tes-Tape®*, *Clinistix®*) are not affected

Doses

■ **DOGS:**

a) For *M. tuberculosis* chemoprophylaxis: 10 mg/kg PO once daily. Drug can be hepatotoxic and dose is extrapolated from human data. Treatment *of M. tuberculosis* or *M. bovis* infections in dogs and cats is not recommended. (Greene & Gunn-Moore 2006)

■ **CATS:**

a) As a second-line treatment (reserved for resistant infections) for feline TB: 10–20 mg/kg PO once daily. (Gunn-Moore 2008)

Monitoring

■ Baseline and periodic physical exam, including clinical efficacy and adverse effect queries

■ Baseline and periodic: CBC, liver function, renal function

Client Information

■ Best to administer on an empty stomach

■ If this medication is to be effective, it must be given regularly as directed

■ If a dose is missed, do not double the next dose

■ Store well out of reach of children or pets; overdoses can be very serious

■ Contact veterinarian if any of the following occur: vomiting, decreased appetite/weight loss, diarrhea or loose stools, changes in behavior or activity, yellowing of whites of eyes or mucous membranes, or difficulty running or going up/down stairs

Chemistry/Synonyms

Isoniazid occurs as colorless, or white, odorless crystals. It is freely soluble in water and sparingly soluble in alcohol. It is recommended not to use sugars such as glucose, fructose or sucrose in compounded oral solutions, as a condensation product can be formed that can impair absorption.

Isoniazid may also be known as: INH, INAH, isonicotinic acid hydrazide, isonicotinylhydrazide, isonicotinylhydrazine, or tubazid. INH is available throughout the world in many trade names, some of the more commonly used names include *Isotamine®, Laniazid®,* or *Nydrazid®.* **Caution:** *Isopyrin®* is one isoniazid trade name that in some countries contains ramifenazone and not isoniazid.

Storage/Stability

Isoniazid tablets should be stored at temperatures below 40°C, preferably between 15–30°C, in well-closed, light-resistant containers. The oral syrup should be stored at temperatures below 40°C, preferably between 15–30°C, in well-closed, light-resistant containers protected from freezing. The injection should be stored at temperatures below 40°C, preferably between 15–30°C; protected from light and freezing. At low temperatures, crystals may form in the injectable solution; crystals should redissolve upon warming to room temperature.

Dosage Forms/Regulatory Status

VETERINARY-LABELED PRODUCTS: None

HUMAN-LABELED PRODUCTS:

Isoniazid Oral Tablets: 100 mg & 300 mg; generic; (Rx)

Isoniazid Oral Syrup: 10 mg/mL in pints; generic; (Rx)

Isoniazid Injection Solution: 100 mg/mL in 10 mL multidose vials; *Nydrazid®* (Apothecon); generic; (Rx)

Combination Products:

Tablets: Rifampin 120 mg, Isoniazid 50 mg, & Pyrazinamide 300 mg; *Rifater®* (Aventis); (Rx)

Capsules: Rifampin 300 mg & Isoniazid 150 mg; *IsonaRif®* (VersaPharm), *Rifamate®* (Aventis); (Rx)

References

Greene, C. & D. Gunn-Moore (2006). Mycobacterial Infections: Infections caused by slow-growing mycobacteria. Infectious Diseases of the Dog and Cat, 3rd Ed. C Greene Ed., Elsevier: 462–477.

Gunn-Moore, D. (2008). Feline Mycobacterial Infections. Proceedings: WSAVA. Accessed via: Veterinary Information Network. http://goo.gl/DPklQ

ISOPROTERENOL HCL

(eye-soe-proe-*ter*-e-nole)   Isuprel®

BETA-ADRENERGIC AGONIST

Prescriber Highlights

▶ Non-specific beta agonist used rarely for acute bronchial constriction, cardiac arrhythmias (complete AV block), & as adjunctive therapy in shock or heart failure

▶ Contraindications: Tachycardias or AV block caused by cardiac glycoside intoxication, ventricular arrhythmias that do not require increased inotropic activity

▶ Caution: Coronary insufficiency, hyperthyroidism, renal disease, hypertension, or diabetes; not a substitute for adequate fluid replacement in shock

▶ Adverse Effects: Tachycardia, anxiety, tremors, excitability, headache, weakness, & vomiting; more arrhythmogenic than dopamine or dobutamine

▶ Short duration of activity (including adverse effects)

Uses/Indications

Isoproterenol is infrequently used in veterinary medicine in the treatment of acute bronchial constriction, cardiac arrhythmias (complete AV block) and, occasionally, as adjunctive therapy in shock or heart failure (limited use because of increases in heart rate and ventricular arrhythmogenicity).

Pharmacology/Actions

Isoproterenol is a synthetic beta$_1$- and beta$_2$-adrenergic agonist that has no appreciable alpha activity at therapeutic doses. It is thought that isoproterenol's adrenergic activity is a result of stimulating cyclic-AMP production. Its primary actions are increased inotropism and chronotropism, relaxation of bronchial smooth muscle, and peripheral vasodilatation. Isoproterenol may increase perfusion to skeletal muscle (at the expense of vital organs in shock). Isoproterenol will inhibit the antigen-mediated release of histamine and slow releasing substance of anaphylaxis (SRS-A).

Hemodynamic effects noted include decreased total peripheral resistance, increased cardiac output, increased venous return to the heart, and increased rate of discharge by cardiac pacemakers.

Pharmacokinetics

Isoproterenol is rapidly inactivated by the GI tract and metabolized by the liver after oral administration. Sublingual administration is not reliably absorbed and effects may take up to 30 minutes to be seen. Intravenous administration results in immediate effects, but only persists for a few minutes after discontinuation.

It is unknown if isoproterenol is distributed into milk. The pharmacologic actions of isoproterenol are ended primarily through tissue uptake. Isoproterenol is metabolized in the liver and other tissues by catechol-O-methyltransferase (COMT) to a weakly active metabolite.

Contraindications/Precautions/Warnings

Isoproterenol is contraindicated in patients that have tachycardias or AV block caused by cardiac glycoside intoxication. It is also contraindicated in ventricular arrhythmias that do not require increased inotropic activity.

Use isoproterenol with caution in patients with coronary insufficiency, hyperthyroidism, renal disease, hypertension or diabetes. Isoproterenol is not a substitute for adequate fluid replacement in shock.

Adverse Effects

Isoproterenol can cause tachycardia, anxiety, tremors, excitability, headache, weakness, and vomiting. Because of isoproterenol's short duration of action, adverse effects are usually transient and do not require cessation of therapy, but may require lowering the dose or infusion rate. Isoproterenol is considered more arrhythmogenic than either dopamine or dobutamine, so it is rarely used in the treatment of heart failure.

Reproductive/Nursing Safety

In humans, the FDA categorizes this drug as category **C** for use during pregnancy. (*Animal studies have shown an adverse effect on the fetus, but there are no adequate studies in humans; or there are no animal reproduction studies and no adequate studies in humans.*) In a separate system evaluating the safety of drugs in canine and feline pregnancy (Papich 1989), this drug is categorized as in class: **C** (*These drugs may have potential risks. Studies in people or laboratory animals have uncovered risks, and these drugs should be used cautiously as a last resort when the benefit of therapy clearly outweighs the risks.*)

No specific lactation safety information was found, however, as isoproterenol is rapidly deactivated in the gut, it is unlikely to pose much risk to nursing offspring.

Overdosage/Acute Toxicity

In addition to the signs listed in the Adverse Effects section, high doses may cause an initial hypertension, followed by hypotension as well as tachycardias and other arrhythmias. Besides halting or reducing the drug, treatment is considered to be supportive. Should tachycardias persist, a beta-blocker could be considered for treatment (if patient does not have a bronchospastic disease).

Drug Interactions

The following drug interactions have either been reported or are theoretical in humans or animals receiving isoproterenol and may be of significance in veterinary patients:

■ **ANESTHETICS, GENERAL:** An increased risk of arrhythmias developing can occur if isoproterenol is administered to patients who have received cyclopropane or a halogenated hydrocarbon anesthetic agent. Propranolol may be administered should these occur.

■ **BETA-BLOCKERS:** May antagonize isoproterenol's cardiac, bronchodilating, and vasodilating effects by blocking the beta effects of isoproterenol. Beta-blockers may be administered to treat the tachycardia associated with isoproterenol use, but use with caution in patient's with bronchospastic disease.

■ **DIGOXIN:** An increased risk of arrhythmias may occur if isoproterenol is used concurrently with digitalis glycosides.

■ **OXYTOCIC AGENTS:** Hypertension may result if isoproterenol is used with oxytocic agents.

■ **SYMPATHOMIMETIC AGENTS, OTHER:** Isoproterenol should not be administered with other sympathomimetic agents (*e.g.*, **phenylpropanolamine**) as increased toxicity may result.

■ **THEOPHYLLINE:** Isoproterenol may increase the risk for theophylline toxicity.

Doses

Note: Because of the cardiostimulatory properties of isoproterenol, its parenteral use in human medicine for the treatment of bronchospasm has been largely supplanted by other more beta$_2$ specific drugs (*e.g.*, terbutaline) and administration methods (nebulization). Use with care.

■ **DOGS:**
For sinoatrial arrest, sinus bradycardia, complete AV block:

a) 0.4 mg in 250 mL D$_5$W drip slowly to effect; or *Isuprel*® Glossets 5–10 mg sublingually or rectally q 4–6h (Tilley & Miller 1986)

b) 0.04–0.08 micrograms/kg/min IV infusion; or 0.1–0.2 mg IM, SC q4h; or 0.4 mg in 250 mL D$_5$W IV slowly (Morgan 1988)

c) As an alternative to atropine for the adjunctive treatment for bradycardia associated with calcium channel blocker overdose: Mix 0.4 mg in 250 mL of D5W and give via slow IV drip to effect. (Holder 2000)

■ **CATS:**
For sinoatrial arrest, sinus bradycardia, complete AV block:

a) 0.4 mg in 250 mL D$_5$W drip slowly to effect (Tilley & Miller 1986)

■ **HORSES:** (**Note:** ARCI UCGFS Class 2 Drug)
For short-term bronchodilatation:

a) Dilute 0.2 mg in 50 mL of saline and administer 0.4 micrograms/kg as an IV infusion, monitor heart rate continuously and discontinue when heart rate doubles. Effects may only last for an hour. (Derksen 1987)

Monitoring
■ Cardiac rate/rhythm
■ Respiratory rate/auscultation during anaphylaxis
■ Urine flow if possible
■ Blood pressure, and blood gases if indicated and possible

Client Information
■ Isoproterenol for injection should be used only by trained personnel in a setting where adequate monitoring can be performed.

Chemistry/Synonyms
Isoproterenol HCl is a synthetic beta-adrenergic agent that occurs as a white to practically white, crystalline powder that is freely soluble in water and sparingly soluble in alcohol. The pH of the commercially available injection is 3.5–4.5.

Isoproterenol HCl may also be known as: isoprenaline hydrochloride, isopropylarterenol hydrochloride, isopropylnoradrenaline hydrochloride, *Imuprel*®, *Isolin*®, *Isuprel*®, *Lenoprel*®, *Norisodrine Aerotrol*®, *Proterenal*, *Saventrine*®, and *Vapo-iso*®.

Storage/stability
Store isoproterenol preparations in tight, light-resistant containers. It is stable indefinitely at room temperature. Isoproterenol salts will darken with time upon exposure to air, light, or heat. Sulfites or sulfur dioxide may be added to preparations as an antioxidant. Solutions may become pink or brownish-pink if exposed to air, alkalies, or metals. Do not use solutions that are discolored or contain a precipitate. If isoproterenol is mixed with other drugs or fluids that result in a solution with a pH greater than 6, it is recommended that it be used immediately.

Compatibility/Compounding Considerations
Isoproterenol for injection is reported to be physically **compatible** with all commonly used IV solutions (except 5% sodium bicarbonate), and the following drugs: calcium chloride/gluceptate, cephalothin sodium, cimetidine HCl, dobutamine HCl, heparin sodium, magnesium sulfate, multivitamin infusion, netilmicin sulfate, oxytetracycline HCl, potassium chloride, succinylcholine chloride, tetracycline HCl, verapamil HCl, and vitamin B complex with C.

It is reported to be physically **incompatible** when mixed with: aminophylline or sodium bicarbonate. Compatibility is dependent upon factors such as pH, concentration, temperature, and diluent used; consult specialized references for more specific information.

Dosage Forms/Regulatory Status
VETERINARY-LABELED PRODUCTS: None

Isoproterenol HCl for Injection: 1:5000 solution (0.2 mg/mL) 5 mL & 10 mL vials; generic; (Rx)

References

Derksen, F.J. (1987). Chronic obstructive pulmonary disease. *Current Therapy in Equine Medicine*. NE Robinson Ed. Philadelphia, WB Saunders: 596–602.

Holder, T. (2000). Toxicology Brief: Calcium Channel Blocker Toxicosis. *Veterinary Medicine*(December).

Morgan, R.V., Ed. (1988). *Handbook of Small Animal Practice*. New York, Churchill Livingstone.

Papich, M. (1989). Effects of drugs on pregnancy. *Current Veterinary Therapy X: Small Animal Practice*. R Kirk Ed. Philadelphia, Saunders: 1291–1299.

Tilley, L.P. & M.S. Miller (1986). Antiarrhythmic drugs and management of cardiac arrhythmias. *Current Veterinary Therapy IX: Small Animal Practice*. RV Kirk Ed. Philadelphia, WB Saunders: 346–360.

ISOSORBIDE DINITRATE
ISOSORBIDE MONONITRATE

(eye-soe-*sor*-bide)   Isordil®, Ismo®, Imdur®

VASODILATOR

Prescriber Highlights

▶ Limited clinical experience; but may have some utility in small animal medicine for adjunctive treatment of heart failure

Uses/Indications

Isosorbide mononitrate (ISMN) and dinitrate (ISDN) are organic nitrates potentially useful as preload reducing agents in treating heart failure in small animals, however, research and clinical experience demonstrating clinical efficacy are lacking in dogs or cats. Limited research indicates that dogs may require much higher dosages of isosorbide to achieve therapeutic effects than do humans.

In humans, isosorbide nitrates are used for treating or preventing angina, treating esophageal spasm, and as an adjunctive treatment in CHF.

Pharmacology/Actions

Organic nitrates (*e.g.*, isosorbide nitrates, nitroglycerin) share a similar pharmacologic profile. They relax vascular smooth muscle causing vasodilation, predominantly on the venous side, but somewhat on arteries/arterioles as well. The mechanism of action is related to their conversion to free radical nitric oxide. Nitric acid is thought to activate guanylate cyclase, thus increasing cyclic GMP and eventually leading to dephosphorylating light chain myosin, causing vasodilation. In humans, nitrates reduce myocardial oxygen demand, but the exact mechanism for this effect is not well understood. Nitrates functionally antagonize the effects of

acetylcholine, norepinephrine and histamine. Additionally, nitrates relax all smooth muscle including biliary (including biliary ducts, sphincter of Oddi), bronchial, GI (including the esophagus), ureteral and uterine.

Serum concentrations of isosorbide mononitrate above 100 ng/mL minimum concentration of the drug are believed required for hemodynamic effects in dogs and humans. However, a study (Adin *et al.* 2001) in both normal dogs and those with CHF, demonstrated no hemodynamic effects (blood pressure, heart rate, PCV, thoracic blood volume percentage, abdominal blood volume percentage) at doses that yielded peak levels as high as $2,352 \pm 701$ ng/mL.

In a study (Nagasawa *et al.* 2003) performed in dogs with experimentally induced mitral regurgitation, oral dosages of a sustained-release isosorbide dinitrate product at 8 mg/kg and above resulted in significant decreases in preload and afterload with increased cardiac output. Effects were sustained for at least 10 hours after dosing.

Pharmacokinetics

In dogs, isosorbide mononitrate oral bioavailability is approximately 70% after oral administration. Oral doses with standard tablets above 2 mg/kg yield peak plasma levels above 100 ng/mL, which is believed to be the minimum concentration of the drug required for hemodynamic effects in dogs and humans. Elimination half-life in dogs with standard tablets is about 1.5 hours. Dogs (24–31kg BW) given 60 mg sustained-release tablets (*Imdur®*) had peak plasma levels of approximately 550 ng/mL 3 hours after dosing. No pharmacokinetic information was located for cats.

Limited information on isosorbide dinitrate pharmacokinetics in small animals is available; it is reported that pharmacokinetics are similar in dogs and humans. In humans, both isosorbide dinitrate and mononitrate are well absorbed after oral administration. Food may delay the rate, but not the extent, of absorption. Isosorbide dinitrate undergoes extensive first-pass metabolism primarily to isosorbide mononitrate. Isosorbide mononitrate is metabolized primarily in the liver, but does not undergo first pass metabolism. Metabolites do not appear to have pharmacologic activity and are principally excreted in the urine.

Contraindications/Precautions/Warnings

Isosorbide nitrates should not be used in patients in shock or used alone in treating heart failure. Use with extreme caution in patients with low blood pressure or hypovolemia.

Adverse Effects

As there is limited experience in using these drugs in animals an adverse effect profile is not well known.

In humans, the most common adverse effects are headache and postural hypotension.

Tachycardia, restlessness or gastrointestinal effects are not uncommon. There have been rare cases of patients who are hypersensitive to organic nitrates.

Reproductive/Nursing Safety

Isosorbide nitrates are probably safe to use at therapeutic dosages during pregnancy. Dose-related increases in embryotoxicity occurred in rabbits given isosorbide dinitrate at 35–150X human dosages and there were some effects noted in rats (litter size, pup survival, prolonged gestation/parturition) given 125X doses of isosorbide mononitrate. Isosorbide mononitrate administered to rats and rabbits at 250 mg/kg/day (75X human dose) demonstrated no untoward effects. In humans, the FDA categorizes isosorbide nitrates as category **C** for use during pregnancy (*Animal studies have shown an adverse effect on the fetus, but there are no adequate studies in humans; or there are no animal reproduction studies and no adequate studies in humans.*)

It is unknown if isosorbide nitrates enter milk. Safe use during lactation cannot be guaranteed, but it is unlikely these drugs would pose significant risk to nursing offspring.

Overdosage/Acute Toxicity

Isosorbide mononitrate caused significant lethality in rats and mice at dosages of 2000 mg/kg and 3000 mg/kg, respectively. The primary concerns with an overdosage of isosorbide nitrates would be venous pooling, decreased cardiac output, and hypotension. Treatment is basically supportive; drug therapies with agents such as epinephrine are not recommended. Increasing central fluid volume may be useful but in patients with CHF, must be used with extreme caution.

Drug Interactions

The following drug interactions have either been reported or are theoretical in humans or animals receiving isosorbide and may be of significance in veterinary patients:

- ■ **ANTIHYPERTENSIVE DRUGS:** Possible additive hypotensive effects
- ■ **PHENOTHIAZINES:** Possible additive hypotensive effects
- ■ **SELECTIVE PHOSPHODIESTERASE INHIBITORS (e.g., sildenafil):** Profound hypotension (use is contraindicated)

Laboratory Considerations

- ■ **Serum cholesterol** levels may be falsely decreased by nitrates when using the Zlatkis-Zak color reaction method

Doses

- ■ **DOGS/CATS:**
  a) Cats: For adjunctive treatment of heart failure associated with thyroid storm: Isosorbide dinitrate at 0.5–2 mg/kg PO q8–12h. Start at lowest level and titrate upward. (Ward 2006)

  b) Dogs/Cats: Efficacy is unknown, but isosorbide dinitrate at 0.5–2 mg/kg PO twice daily or isosorbide mononitrate at 0.25–2 mg/kg PO twice daily are occasionally used for refractory heart failure or in combination with hydralazine or amlodipine in patients unable to tolerate ACE inhibitors. It is unknown if nitrate-free periods are required to prevent nitrate tolerance. (Bulmer & Sisson 2005)

Monitoring

- ■ Clinical efficacy

Client Information

- ■ Inform clients of the limited experience in veterinary medicine with this medication
- ■ May be given with or without meals

Chemistry/Synonyms

To minimize the risk for explosion, dry isosorbide dinitrate is mixed with lactose, mannitol or other inert excipients. To further stabilize the mixture, up to 1% ammonium phosphate or other suitable stabilizer can be used. The resultant dry mixture contains approximately 25% isosorbide dinitrate and is called diluted isosorbide dinitrate. It is an ivory-white, odorless powder that is very slightly soluble in water and sparingly soluble in alcohol.

Undiluted isosorbide mononitrate occurs as a white, crystalline powder that is freely soluble in water or alcohol. It is diluted with lactose or another suitable excipient to stabilize the powder and permit safe handling.

Isosorbide dinitrate may also be known as: ISD, ISDN, EV-151, or sorbide nitrate, *Dilatrate-SR®*, *Isochron®*, *Isordil®* and *Titradose®*; many international trade name products are available.

Isosorbide mononitrate may also be known as: AHR-4698, BM-22145, IS-5-MN, or isosorbide-5-mononitrate, *Imdur®*, *Ismo®*, and *Monoket®*; many international trade name products are available.

Storage/Stability

Isosorbide dinitrate oral tablets, chewable tablets, extended-release tablets, and sublingual tablets should be stored in well-closed containers, below 40°C and preferably between 15°–30°C. Heat and moisture accelerates loss of potency.

Isosorbide mononitrate tablets should be stored in tight containers, below 40°C and preferably between 15°–30°C. Isosorbide mononitrate extended-release tablets should be stored in tight containers, between 2°–30°C. Heat and moisture accelerates loss of potency.

Dosage Forms/Regulatory Status

VETERINARY-LABELED PRODUCTS: None

The ARCI (Racing Commissioners International) has designated this drug as a class 4 substance.

HUMAN-LABELED PRODUCTS:

Isosorbide Dinitrate Oral Tablets: 5 mg, 10 mg, 20 mg, 30 mg, & 40 mg; generic, *Isordil Titradose®* (Wyeth); (Rx)

Isosorbide Dinitrate Sublingual Oral Tablets: 2.5 mg, & 5 mg; generic; (Rx)

Isosorbide Dinitrate Extended-Release Oral Tablets: 40 mg; *Isochron®* (Forest), generic; (Corepharma); (Rx)

Isosorbide Dinitrate Sustained-Release Oral Capsules: 40 mg; *Dilatrate-SR®* (Schwarz Pharma); (Rx)

Isosorbide Mononitrate Tablets: 10 mg, & 20 mg; generic, *Monoket®* (Schwarz Pharma); *Ismo®* (Reddy); (Rx)

Isosorbide Mononitrate Extended-Release Tablets: 30 mg, 60 mg, & 120 mg; generic, *Imdur®* (Key); (Rx)

References

Adin, D., M. Kittleson, et al. (2001). Efficacy of a single oral dose of isosorbide 5–mononitrate in normal dogs and in dogs with congestive heart failure. *J Vet Intern Med* **15**: 105–111.

Bulmer, B. & D. Sisson (2005). Therapy of heart failure. *Textbook of Veterinary Internal Medicine 6th Ed.* S Ettinger and E Feldman Eds., Elsevier: 948–972.

Nagasawa, Y., K. Takashima, et al. (2003). Effect of sustained release isosorbide dinitrate (EV151) in dogs with experimentally-induced mitral insufficiency. *J Vet Med Sci* **65**(5): 615–618.

Ward, C. (2006). Thyroid storm in cats: fact or fiction. Proceedings: ACVIM 2006, Accessed via the Veterinary Information Network. Accessed via: Veterinary Information Network. http://goo.gl/7P0oA

ISOTRETINOIN

(eye-so-***tret***-i-noyn)   Accutane®

RETINOID

Prescriber Highlights

▶ Synthetic retinoid that may be useful in treatment a variety of dermatology diseases associated with epithelial cell proliferation & differentiation

▶ Cautions (risk vs. benefit): Serum hypertriglyceridemia, hypersensitivity to drug; known teratogen

▶ Adverse Effects: Most common adverse effect seen in dogs is keratoconjunctivitis sicca (KCS); apparently not a problem in cats. Other potential adverse effects in small animals include: GI effects (anorexia, vomiting, abdominal distention), CNS effects (lassitude, hyperactivity, collapse), pruritus, erythema of feet & mucocutaneous junctions, polydipsia, swollen tongue

▶ Obtaining the medication for veterinary patients may be difficult

▶ Pregnant women should avoid contact with medication

Uses/Indications

Isotretinoin may be useful in treating a variety of dermatologic-related conditions, including canine lamellar ichthyosis, cutaneous T-cell lymphoma, intracutaneous cornifying epitheliomas, multiple epidermal inclusion cysts, comedo syndrome in Schnauzers, and sebaceous adenitis seen in standard poodles.

Because of the concerns of teratogenic effects in humans, availability to veterinarians may be restricted by the manufacturers and drug distributors; obtaining the medication for veterinary patients may be difficult.

Pharmacology/Actions

A retinoid, isotretinoin's major pharmacologic effects appear to be regulation of epithelial cell proliferation and differentiation. It affects monocyte and lymphocyte function, which can cause changes in cellular immune responses. The effects on skin include reduction of sebaceous gland size and activity, thereby reducing sebum production. It also has anti-keratinization and antiinflammatory activity and may indirectly reduce bacterial populations in sebaceous pores.

Pharmacokinetics

Isotretinoin is rapidly absorbed from the gut once the capsule disintegrates and the drug is dispersed in the GI contents. This may require up to 2 hours after dosing. Animal studies have shown that only about 25% of a dose reaches the systemic circulation, but food or milk in the gut may increase this amount. Isotretinoin is distributed into many tissues, but is not stored in the liver (unlike vitamin A). It crosses the placenta and is highly bound to plasma proteins. It is unknown if it enters milk. Isotretinoin is metabolized in the liver and is excreted in the urine and feces. In humans, terminal half-life is about 10–20 hours.

Contraindications/Precautions/Warnings

Isotretinoin should only be used when the potential benefits outweigh the risks when the following conditions exist: hypertriglyceridemia, severe renal or hepatic disease, or sensitivity to isotretinoin.

Isotretinoin is a known teratogen. Major anomalies have been reported in children of women taking the medication and it is not advised to use the medication in households were pregnant women are present.

Adverse Effects

There appears to be a low incidence of adverse effects, particularly in dogs. The most common adverse effect seen in dogs is keratoconjunctivitis sicca (KCS). This apparently is not a problem in cats. Other potential adverse effects include: GI effects (anorexia, vomiting, diarrhea, abdominal distention), CNS effects (lassitude, hyperactivity, behavioral changes, collapse), stiffness of limbs, pruritus, exfoliative dermatitis, erythema of feet and mucocutaneous junctions/cheilitis, polydipsia, and swollen tongue.

Incidence of adverse effects may be higher in cats. Effects reported include: blepharospasm, periocular crusting, erythema, diarrhea and, especially, weight loss secondary to anorexia. If cats develop adverse effects, the time between doses may be prolonged (*e.g.*, every other week give every other day) to reduce the total dose given.

Reproductive/Nursing Safety

Isotretinoin is a known teratogen. Major anomalies have been reported in children of women taking the medication. It is absolutely contraindicated in pregnant veterinary patients as well. Isotretinoin also appears to inhibit spermatogenesis. In humans, the FDA categorizes this drug as category *X* for use during pregnancy (*Studies in animals or humans demonstrate fetal abnormalities or adverse reaction; reports indicate evidence of fetal risk. The risk of use in pregnant women clearly outweighs any possible benefit.*)

It is not known whether this drug is excreted in breast milk. At this time, it is not recommended for use in nursing mothers.

Overdosage/Acute Toxicity

There were 147 exposures to isotretinoin reported to the ASPCA Animal Poison Control Center (APCC) during 2008–2009. In these cases 140 were dogs with 5 showing clinical signs and the remaining 7 reported cases were cats showing no clinical signs. Common findings in dogs included hypersalivation. Because of the drug's potential adverse effects, gut emptying should be considered with acute overdoses when warranted.

Drug Interactions

The following drug interactions have either been reported or are theoretical in humans or animals receiving isotretinoin and may be of significance in veterinary patients:

■ **VITAMIN A or OTHER RETINOIDS:** Isotretinoin used with other retinoids (**etretinate, tretinoin,** or **vitamin A**) may cause additive toxic effects.

■ **CYCLOSPORINE:** Isotretinoin may increase cyclosporine levels

■ **TETRACYCLINES:** Use with tetracyclines may increase the potential for the occurrence of pseudotumor cerebri (cerebral edema and increased CSF pressure).

Laboratory Considerations

■ Increases in serum **triglyceride** and **cholesterol** levels may be noted which can be associated with corneal lipid deposits

■ **Platelets** may be increased

■ **ALT** (SGOT), **AST** (SGPT), and **LDH** levels may be increased

Doses

■ **DOGS:**

a) For sebaceous adenitis when more conservative treatments have failed: 1 mg/kg PO q12h for one month; if improvement is noted reduce dose to 1 mg/kg PO once daily; long-term goal is to treat with either 1 mg/kg PO every other day or 0.5 mg/kg once daily (Rosser 1992)

b) For sebaceous adenitis: 1–3 mg/kg PO once a day to twice daily (Bloom 2006)

c) For treatment of Schnauzer comedo syndrome: 1 mg/kg once daily or divided q12h PO;

For sebaceous adenitis in poodles; granulomatous sebaceous adenitis in viszlas: 1–2 mg/kg once daily or divided q12h PO;

For epitheliotrophic lymphoma, cutaneus lymphoma: 2 mg/kg once daily or divided q12h PO (Power & Ihrke 1995)

d) For schnauzer comedo syndrome, sebaceous adenitis in poodles, ichthyosis, keratocanthoma, epitheliotropic lymphoma, and sebaceous gland hyperplasia and adenoma: 1–3 mg/kg q12–24h PO (Kwochka 2003)

e) For cutaneous lymphosarcoma: Isotretinoin at 3–4 mg/kg PO daily. Prednisone (1 mg/kg/day) may be useful to alleviate pruritus. Lomustine at 50 mg/m^2 q21–30 days may be effective (see lomustine monograph for more information) (White 2005)

■ **CATS:**

For feline acne:

a) 5 mg/kg PO once daily (Hall & Campbell 1994)

b) 10 mg per cat once daily PO (Power & Ihrke 1995)

c) 1–3 mg/kg q12–24h PO (Kwochka 2003)

For epitheliotrophic lymphoma, cutaneus lymphoma:

a) 10 mg/cat once daily PO (Power & Ihrke 1995)

Monitoring

See Lab Considerations and Adverse Effects.

■ Efficacy

■ Liver function tests (baseline and if signs appear)

■ Dogs: Schirmer Tear tests (monthly—especially in older dogs)

■ Cats: Weight

Client Information

■ Isotretinoin should not be handled by pregnant females and use in households with pregnant women present is ill advised. Veterinarians must take the personal responsibility to educate clients of the potential risk of ingestion by pregnant females.

■ Milk or high fat foods will increase the absorption of isotretinoin. To reduce variability of absorption, either have clients consistently give with meals or not.

◼ Avoid prolonged or excessive exposure to sunlight as UV light effects can be enhanced.

◼ Long-term therapy can be quite expensive.

Chemistry/Synonyms

A synthetic retinoid, isotretinoin occurs as a yellow-orange to orange, crystalline powder. It is insoluble in both water and alcohol. Commercially, it is available in soft gelatin capsules as a suspension in soybean oil.

Isotretinoin may also be known as: isotretinoinum, 13-cis-retinoic acid, Ro-4-3780, *Accure®*, *Accutane®*, *Accutin®*, *Amnesteem®*, *Claravis®*, *Curatane®*, *Isoacne®*, *Isohexal®*, *Isotrex®*, *Liderma®*, *Nimegen®*, *Oratane®*, *Procuta®*, *Roaccutan®*, *Roaccutane®*, *Roacutan®*, *Sotret®*, *Stiefotrex®*, and *Tretin®*.

Storage/Stability

Capsules should be stored at room temperature in tight, light resistant containers. The drug is photosensitive and will degrade with light exposure. Expiration dates of 2 years are assigned after manufacture.

Dosage Forms/Regulatory Status

VETERINARY-LABELED PRODUCTS: None

HUMAN-LABELED PRODUCTS:

Isotretinoin Oral Capsules: 10 mg, 20 mg, 30 mg & 40 mg (regular & soft gel); *Claravis®* (Teva); *Amnesteem®* (Mylan); *Sotret®* (Ranbaxy); (Rx)

Note: Because of the concerns of teratogenic effects in humans, availability to veterinarians may be restricted by the manufacturers and drug distributors; obtaining the medication for veterinary patients may be difficult.

References

Bloom, P. (2006). Nonpruritic alopecia in the dog. Proceedings: Western Vet Conf 2006. Accessed via: Veterinary Information Network. http://goo.gl/Qh57f

Hall, I. & K. Campbell (1994). Antibiotic-responsive dermatoses. *Consultations in Feline Internal Medicine: 2.* J August Ed. Philadelphia, W.B. Saunders Company: 233–239.

Kwochka, K. (2003). Treatment of scaling disorders in dogs. Proceedings: Atlantic Coast Veterinary Conference. Accessed via: Veterinary Information Network. http://goo.gl/CnVgl

Power, H. & P. Ihrke (1995). The use of synthetic retinoids in veterinary medicine. *Kirk's Current Veterinary Therapy:XII.* J Bonagura Ed. Philadelphia, W.B. Saunders: 585–590.

Rosser, E. (1992). Sebaceous adenitis. *Current Veterinary Therapy XI: Small Animal Practice.* R Kirk and J Bonagura Eds. Philadelphia, W.B. Saunders Company: 534–539.

White, S. (2005). Cutaneous paraneoplastic syndromes. Proceedings: ACVIM. Accessed via: Veterinary Information Network. http://goo.gl/2tNkb

ISOXSUPRINE HCL

(eye-*sox*-suh-preen)   Vasodilan®

Prescriber Highlights

▶ Peripheral vasodilator that may have some efficacy in treatment of navicular disease in horses; efficacy in doubt when used orally

▶ May be beneficial for Raynaud's-like syndrome in dogs

▶ Contraindications: Immediately postpartum or in the presence of arterial bleeding

▶ Adverse Effects: After injection, CNS stimulation (uneasiness, hyperexcitability, nose-rubbing) or sweating. Adverse effects are unlikely after oral administration.

Uses/Indications

Isoxsuprine is used in veterinary medicine principally for the treatment of navicular disease in horses; however, recent studies have shown disappointing efficacy when used orally. It has been used in humans for the treatment of cerebral vascular insufficiency, dysmenorrhea, and premature labor, but efficacies are unproven for these indications.

There have been anecdotal reports of isoxsuprine being helpful for treating dogs with a Raynaud's-like syndrome (periodic digital cyanosis, onychogryphosis) (Carlotti 2002) and to improve microcirculation in birds.

Pharmacology/Actions

Isoxsuprine causes direct vascular smooth muscle relaxation primarily in skeletal muscle. While it stimulates beta-adrenergic receptors it is believed that this action is not required for vasodilatation to occur. In horses with navicular disease, isoxsuprine will raise distal limb temperatures significantly. Isoxsuprine will relax uterine smooth muscle and may have positive inotropic and chronotropic effects on the heart. At high doses, isoxsuprine can decrease blood viscosity and reduce platelet aggregation. Isoxsuprine does not appear to possess significant analgesia properties in horses (Lizarraga *et al.* 2004).

Pharmacokinetics

In humans, isoxsuprine is almost completely absorbed from the GI tract, but in one study that looked at the cardiovascular and pharmacokinetic effects of isoxsuprine in horses (Matthews 1986), bioavailability was low after oral administration, probably due to a high first-pass effect. After oral dosing of 0.6 mg/kg, the drug was non-detectable in plasma and no cardiac changes were detected. This study did not evaluate cardiovascular effects in horses with navicular disease, nor did it attempt to measure changes in distal limb blood flow. After IV administration in horses, the elimination half-life is between 2.5–3 hours.

Contraindications/Precautions/Warnings

Isoxsuprine should not be administered to animals immediately post-partum or in the presence of arterial bleeding.

Adverse Effects

After parenteral administration, horses may show signs of CNS stimulation (uneasiness, hyperexcitability, nose-rubbing) or sweating. Adverse effects are unlikely after oral administration, but hypotension, tachycardia, and GI effects are possible.

Reproductive/Nursing Safety

In humans, the FDA categorizes this drug as category *C* for use during pregnancy (*Animal studies have shown an adverse effect on the fetus, but there are no adequate studies in humans; or there are no animal reproduction studies and no adequate studies in humans.*)

No specific lactation safety information was found.

Overdosage/Acute Toxicity

Serious toxicity is unlikely in horses after an inadvertent oral overdose, but signs listed in the Adverse Effects section could be seen. Treat signs if necessary. CNS hyperexcitability could be treated with diazepam, and hypotension with fluids.

Drug Interactions

No clinically significant drug interactions have been reported for this agent.

Laboratory Considerations

■ None were noted

Doses

■ **HORSES: (Note:** ARCI UCGFS Class 4 Drug) For treatment of orthopedic conditions, such as navicular disease:

a) For long break-over if therapeutic shoeing does not correct: Initially, 1.2 mg/kg PO q8h for 3 weeks. The dose is decreased as soundness improves, to 1.2 mg/kg PO once daily for 6 weeks, then every other day until heel first landing occurs. Phenylbutazone is added if lameness is greater than grade II on a scale of I–V, or until recheck occurs.

To increase the circulation to the podotrochlea: 0.6–1.2 mg/kg twice daily until sound, then decreased to once daily for 2 weeks then further decreased to every other day. The drug is classified as a "blocking" agent by the AHSA. (Turner 1999)

b) 0.6–2 mg/kg PO q12h (Brumbaugh *et al.* 1999)

As a tocolytic agent:

a) 0.4–0.6 mg/kg IM or PO twice daily. Efficacy is unproven and oral bioavailability appears highly variable. (Wilkins 2004)

■ **DOGS:**

For treatment of "Raynaud-like" disease:

a) 1 mg/kg/day PO (Carlotti 2002),

Monitoring

■ Clinical efficacy
■ Adverse effects (tachycardia, GI disturbances, CNS stimulation)

Client Information

■ To be maximally effective, doses must be given routinely as directed.
■ Tablets may be crushed and made into a slurry, suspension, or paste by adding corn syrup, cherry syrup, etc., just before administration.

Chemistry/Synonyms

A peripheral vasodilating agent, isoxsuprine occurs as an odorless, bitter-tasting, white, crystalline powder with a melting point of about 200°C. It is slightly soluble in water and sparingly soluble in alcohol.

Isoxsuprine HCl may also be known as: Caa-40, isoxsuprini hydrochloridum, phenoxyisopropylnorsuprifen, *Dilum®, Duvadilan®, Fadaespasmol®, Fenam®, Inibina®, Isodilan®, Isotenk®, Uterine®, Vadosilan®, Vasodilan®, Vasolan®, Vasosuprina Ilfi®, Voxsuprine®,* and *Xuprin®.*

Storage/Stability

Tablets should be stored in tight containers at room temperature (15–30°C).

Dosage Forms/Regulatory Status

VETERINARY-LABELED PRODUCTS: None

The ARCI (Racing Commissioners International) has designated this drug as a class 4 substance. See the appendix for more information.

HUMAN-LABELED PRODUCTS:

Isoxsuprine HCl Tablets: 10 mg & 20 mg; *Vasodilan®* (Mead Johnson); *Voxsuprine®* (Major); generic; (Rx)

References

Brumbaugh, G., H. Lopez, et al. (1999). The pharmacologic basis for the treatment of laminitis. The Veterinary Clinics of North America: Equine Practice 15:2(August).

Carlotti, D.-N. (2002). Claw diseases in dogs and cats. Proceedings: World Small Animal Veterinary Association World Congress. Accessed via: Veterinary Information Network. http://goo.gl/PoVcE

Lizarraga, I., F. Castillo, et al. (2004). An analgesic evaluation of isoxsuprine in horses. Journal of Veterinary Medicine Series a-Physiology Pathology Clinical Medicine 51(7–8): 370–374.

Matthews, H. (1986). Cardiovascular and pharmacokinetic effects of isoxsuprine in the horse. Am J Vet Res 47(10): 2110–2113.

Turner, T. (1999). Diagnosing lower limb lameness in the horse. Proceedings: Central Veterinary Conference, Kansas City.

Wilkins, P. (2004). Disorders of foals. Equine Internal Medicine, 2nd Ed. S Reed, W Bayly and D Sellon Eds. Philadelphia, Saunders: 1381–1431.

ITRACONAZOLE

(ey-tra-*kon*-a-zole)   Sporanox®

ANTIFUNGAL

Prescriber Highlights

▶ Synthetic oral triazole antifungal used for systemic mycoses, including aspergillosis, cryptococcal meningitis, blastomycosis, & histoplasmosis

▶ Not amenable to compounding; be wary of compounded itraconazole dosage forms as bulk powder itraconazole may not be absorbed

▶ Contraindications (relative: risk vs. benefit): Hypersensitivity to it or other azole antifungal agents, hepatic impairment, or achlorhydria (or hypochlorhydria)

▶ Adverse Effects: *Dogs:* Anorexia is the most common, but hepatic toxicity most significant adverse effect. At the higher dosage rate, some develop ulcerative skin lesions/vasculitis & limb edema. Rare, serious erythema multiforme or toxic epidermal necrolysis

▶ Adverse Effects: *Cats:* Dose related; GI effects (anorexia, weight loss, vomiting), hepatotoxicity (increased ALT, jaundice), & depression

▶ May be more efficacious than ketoconazole, but is also more expensive; long-term treatment may be required

▶ Maternotoxicity, fetotoxicity, & teratogenicity in lab animals at high dosages (5–20 times labeled)

▶ Drug interactions

Uses/Indications

Itraconazole may have use in veterinary medicine in the treatment of systemic mycoses, including aspergillosis, cryptococcal meningitis, blastomycosis, and histoplasmosis. Itraconazole is probably more effective than ketoconazole, but is significantly more expensive. It may also be useful for superficial candidiasis or dermatophytosis. Itraconazole does not have appreciable effects (unlike ketoconazole) on hormone synthesis and may have fewer side effects than ketoconazole in small animals.

It is considered by many to be the drug of choice for treating blastomycosis, unless moderate or severe hypoxemia is present (than amphotericin B).

In horses, itraconazole may be useful in the treatment of sporotrichosis and *Coccidioides immitis* osteomyelitis.

Pharmacology/Actions

Itraconazole is a fungistatic triazole compound. Triazole-derivative agents, like the imidazoles (clotrimazole, ketoconazole, etc.), presumably act by altering the cellular membranes of susceptible fungi, thereby increasing membrane permeability and allowing leakage of cellular contents and impaired uptake of purine and pyrimidine precursors. Itraconazole has efficacy against a variety of pathogenic fungi, including yeasts and dermatophytes. *In vivo* studies using laboratory models have shown that itraconazole has fungistatic activity against many strains of Candida, Aspergillus, Cryptococcus, Histoplasma, Blastomyces, and *Trypanosoma cruzi.*

Itraconazole has immune-suppressing activity, probably via suppressing T-lymphocyte proliferation.

Pharmacokinetics

Itraconazole absorption is highly dependent on gastric pH and presence of food. When given on an empty stomach, bioavailability may only be 50% or less; with food, it may approach 100%. In cats, the oral solution is more bioavailable and probably has fewer GI effects. The commercially available capsules are specially formulated to increase oral bioavailability. Compounding capsules from bulk powders may not yield a dosage form that is absorbed. The commercially available liquid preparation possesses adequate oral bioavailability in dogs and other species. The oral solution appears to be much better absorbed than capsules in horses.

Itraconazole has very high protein binding and is widely distributed throughout the body, particularly to tissues high in lipids (drug is highly lipophilic). Skin, sebum, female reproductive tract, and pus all have concentrations greater than those found in the serum. Only minimal concentrations are found in CSF, urine, aqueous humor, and saliva. However, many fungal infections in the CNS, eye, or prostate can be effectively treated with itraconazole.

Itraconazole is metabolized by the liver to many different metabolites, including to hydroxyitraconazole, which is active. In humans, itraconazole's serum half-life ranges from 21–64 hours. Elimination may be a saturable process. Because of its long half-life, itraconazole does not reach steady state plasma levels for at least 6 days after starting therapy. If loading doses are given, levels will approach those of steady-state sooner.

Contraindications/Precautions/Warnings

Itraconazole should not be used in patients hypersensitive to it or other azole antifungal agents.

Use itraconazole in patients with hepatic impairment or achlorhydria (or hypochlorhydria) only when the potential benefits outweigh the risks.

Itraconazole may have a negative inotropic effect; use with caution in animals with reduced cardiac function.

African grey Parrots appear to be extremely sensitive to itraconazole and can develop anorexia and depression. Other antifungals or reduced dosage of itraconazole are recommended for use in this species.

Compounding capsules from bulk powders may not yield a dosage form that is absorbed.

Adverse Effects
In dogs, anorexia is the most common adverse effect seen, especially at higher dosages, but hepatic toxicity appears to be the most significant adverse effect. Approximately 10% of dogs receiving 10 mg/kg/day and 5% of dogs receiving 5 mg/kg/day developed hepatic toxicosis serious enough to discontinue treatment (at least temporarily). Hepatic injury is determined by an increased ALT activity. Anorexia is often the symptomatic marker for toxicity and usually occurs in the second month of treatment. Some dogs (7%) given itraconazole at the higher dosage rate (10 mg/kg/day) may develop ulcerative skin lesions/vasculitis and limb edema that may require dosage reduction. These generally resolve following drug discontinuation. Rarely, serious erythema multiforme or toxic epidermal necrolysis reactions have been noted.

In cats, adverse effects appear to be dose related. GI effects (anorexia, weight loss, vomiting), hepatotoxicity (increased ALT, jaundice) and depression have been noted. Should adverse effects occur and ALT is elevated, the drug should be discontinued. Increased liver enzymes in the absence of other signs do not necessarily mandate dosage reduction or drug discontinuation. Once ALT levels return to normal and other adverse effects have diminished, if necessary, the drug may be restarted at a lower dosage or use longer dosing intervals with intense monitoring.

Reproductive/Nursing Safety
In laboratory animals, itraconazole has caused dose-related maternotoxicity, fetotoxicity and teratogenicity at high dosages (5–20 times labeled). As safety has not been established, use only when the benefits outweigh the potential risks. In humans, the FDA categorizes this drug as category *C* for use during pregnancy (*Animal studies have shown an adverse effect on the fetus, but there are no adequate studies in humans; or there are no animal reproduction studies and no adequate studies in humans.*)

Itraconazole enters maternal milk; significance is unknown.

Overdosage/Acute Toxicity
There is very limited information on the acute toxicity of itraconazole. Giving oral antacids may help reduce absorption. If a large overdose occurs, consider gut emptying and give supportive therapy as required. Itraconazole is not removed by dialysis.

In chronic toxicity studies, dogs receiving 40 mg/kg PO daily for 3 months demonstrated no overt toxicity.

Drug Interactions
The following drug interactions have either been reported or are theoretical in humans or animals receiving itraconazole and may be of significance in veterinary patients:

- **AMPHOTERICIN B:** Lab animal studies have shown that itraconazole used concomitantly with amphotericin B may be antagonistic against Aspergillus or Candida; the clinical importance of these findings is not yet clear

- **ANTACIDS:** May reduce oral absorption of itraconazole; administer itraconazole at least 1 hour before or 2 hours after antacids

- **BENZODIAZEPINES (alprazolam, diazepam, midazolam, triazolam):** Itraconazole may increase levels

- **BUSPIRONE:** Plasma concentrations may be elevated

- **BUSULFAN:** Itraconazole may increase levels

- **CALCIUM-CHANNEL BLOCKING AGENTS (amlodipine, verapamil):** Itraconazole may increase levels

- **CISAPRIDE:** Itraconazole may increased cisapride levels and possibility for toxicity; use together contraindicated in humans

- **CLOMIPRAMINE:** Itraconazole may decrease metabolism and increase clomipramine levels

- **CORTICOSTEROIDS:** Itraconazole may inhibit the metabolism of corticosteroids; potential for increased adverse effects

- **CYCLOPHOSPHAMIDE:** Itraconazole may inhibit the metabolism of cyclophosphamide and its metabolites; potential for increased toxicity

- **CYCLOSPORINE:** Increased cyclosporine levels

- **DIGOXIN:** Itraconazole may increase digoxin levels; use together considered contraindicated in humans

- **FENTANYL/ALFENTANIL:** Itraconazole may increase fentanyl or alfentanil levels

- **H2-BLOCKERS (ranitidine, famotidine, etc.):** Increased gastric pH may reduce itraconazole absorption

- **IVERMECTIN:** Itraconazole may increase risk for neurotoxicity

- **MACROLIDE ANTIBIOTICS (erythromycin, clarithromycin):** May increase itraconazole concentrations

- **PHENOBARBITAL/PHENYTOIN:** May decrease itraconazole levels

- **PROTON-PUMP INHIBITORS (omeprazole, etc.):** Increased gastric pH may reduce itraconazole absorption

- **QUINIDINE:** Increased risk for quinidine toxicity

- **RIFAMPIN:** May decrease itraconazole levels; itraconazole may increase rifampin levels

■ **SULFONYLUREA ANTIDIABETIC AGENTS (e.g., glipizide, glyburide):** Itraconazole may increase levels; hypoglycemia possible

■ **VINCRISTINE/VINBLASTINE:** Itraconazole may inhibit vinca alkaloid metabolism and increase levels

■ **WARFARIN:** Itraconazole may cause increased prothrombin times in patients receiving warfarin or other coumarin anticoagulants

Laboratory Considerations

■ Itraconazole may cause **hypokalemia** or increases in **liver function tests** in a small percentage of patients.

Doses

■ **DOGS:**

For systemic mycoses:

a) For Malassezia dermatitis: 5 mg/kg PO once daily for 3 weeks. (Fair evidence supports recommendation) (Negre *et al.* 2009)

b) Pulse therapy for Malassezia dermatitis: 5 mg/kg for 2 consecutive days per week for 3 weeks (Foil 2003a)

c) For dermatophytosis: 5 mg/kg PO once daily. Prolonged course of therapy required. Begin taking cultures after 4 weeks of treatment. Continue therapy for 2 weeks beyond clinical cure *and* when 2–3 negative cultures are obtained at weekly intervals. (Frank 2000)

d) For dermatophytosis: 5 mg/kg PO once daily on an every other week schedule. Treatment is generally continued for three "pulses" of one week on, one week off. Toxicity problems are rare with this protocol. (DeBoer 2006)

e) For Blastomycosis: 5 mg/kg PO once daily for at least 30 days after all signs of disease have resolved (treatment must persist for at least 60–90 days). Give with food. (Davidson & Mathews 2000)

f) For Histoplasmosis: 10 mg/kg daily PO; given with food; if dog has intestinal histoplasmosis, treat with amphotericin B (0.5 mg/kg IV over 3–4 hours in D5W every other day) initially. Usually after six doses of amphotericin B, may switch to itraconazole. Total treatment times (amphotericin B and itraconazole) should be for at least 30 days after all signs of disease have resolved (treatment must persist for at least 90 days). (Legendre & Toal 2000)

g) For Blastomycosis: 5 mg/kg PO once a day or divided twice a day. Continue for 2–3 months or until active disease is not apparent. A loading dose of 10 mg/kg once a day (or divided twice a day) for the first three days may reduce the "lag" phase of effectiveness.

For coccidiomycosis: 5–10 mg/kg PO once daily; may need to treat for 6–12 months (Taboada 2000)

h) For sporotrichosis: 5–10 mg/kg once daily for 30 days beyond complete resolution of detectable lesions.

For pythiosis or lagendiosis (after lesion resection): 10 mg/kg PO once daily (with terbinafine at 5–10 mg/kg PO q24h) for at least 2 months after surgery.

For zygomycosis (after aggressive surgical resection: 5–10 mg/kg PO q24h. For non-resectable lesions, either itraconazole for 3–6 months or amphotericin B lipid complex. Recurrence is possible with either surgical or medical therapy. (Grooters 2005)

i) For idiopathic lymphoplasmacytic (chronic) rhinitis (LPR): 5 mg/kg PO q12h for a minimum of 3-6 months has shown dramatic beneficial improvement in some dogs.

For nasal aspergillosis: 5 mg/kg PO q12h for 3-6 months may cure up to 60–70% of dogs with aspergillosis, although some studies have shown only marginal efficacy. (Kuehn 2010)

j) For coccidioidomycosis: 5–10 mg/kg PO q24h or 5 mg/kg PO q12h. (Graupmann-Kuzma *et al.* 2008)

■ **CATS:**

For susceptible systemic mycoses:

a) For Histoplasmosis: 10 mg/kg daily PO; given with food

For Cryptococcosis: 50–100 mg per cat per day PO for many months. Mean treatment time is 8.5 months. If response inadequate, may add flucytosine (at 100–125 mg/kg divided into three doses per day). (Legendre & Toal 2000)

b) For Blastomycosis: 10 mg/kg PO once a day or divided twice a day. Continue for 2–3 months or until active disease is not apparent (**Note:** cats usually require longer treatment than dogs)

For Histoplasmosis: 10 mg/kg once daily or divided twice daily PO; at least 2–4 months of treatment required

For coccidiomycosis: 5–10 mg/kg PO once daily; may need to treat for 6–12 months (Taboada 2000)

c) For sporotrichosis: 5–10 mg/kg once daily for 30 days beyond complete resolution of detectable lesions. (Grooters 2005)

d) For Cryptococcosis: For mild to moderate disease where cats are eating and do not have CNS involvement: Cats weighing 3.5 kg or less receive 50 mg PO once daily or 100 mg PO every other day; medium to large cats get 100 mg PO once daily. Give with food; may be mixed with tasty food treat. Monitor ALT; itraconazole hepatotoxicity is reversible upon discontinuation of the drug and it can usually be restarted safely at 50% of the original dose. Continue treatment until cat appears completely normal; generally takes 3–12 months. Then obtain serum sample to determine decline in antigen titer. A 4–5 fold reduction suggests successful therapy. Then restart therapy (possibly at a reduced dose) or change to ketoconazole (50 mg/day) until antigen level declines to zero. (Malik 2006)

e) For coccidioidomycosis: 25–50 mg (total dose) per cat q12-24h (**Note:** *reference lists dosing frequency as q12-14h, but it is believed that this is a typo—Plumb*). (Graupmann-Kuzma *et al.* 2008)

For generalized dermatophytosis:

a) Caused by *Microsporum canis*: 5 mg/kg PO once daily preferably between meals for 7 days on, 7 days off; repeat 3 times. Cats must be treated during weeks 1, 3 and 5 and left untreated during weeks 2 and 4. In cases where a positive culture is obtained 4 weeks after the end of administration, the treatment should be repeated once at the same dosage regimen. In such cases where the cat is also immunosuppressed, treatment should be repeated and the underlying disease addressed. (Label Information—*Intrafungol®*; Janssen. U.K.)

b) 5 mg/kg PO twice daily or 10 mg/kg with food. Give until culture is negative 2 times at two week intervals; generally 3–5 weeks. Open capsule and measure out calculated portion; give in butter or *a/d®*. Can be stored in the freezer.

Pulse therapy: 5 mg/kg PO for 2 consecutive days per week, increasing interval gradually is useful in the management of dermatophytosis in longhaired cats and in cats in a heavily contaminated environment.

For dermatophyte granuloma (TOC): 10 mg/kg PO once daily for weeks to months, at least one month beyond clinical resolution and until brush culture is negative x 2. (Foil 2003b)

c) For dermatophytosis: 5 mg/kg PO once daily on an every other week schedule. Treatment is generally continued for three "pulses" of one week on, one week off. Toxicity problems are rare with this protocol. (DeBoer 2006)

■ **RABBITS, RODENTS, SMALL MAMMALS:**

a) **Mice:** For blastomycosis: 50–150 mg/kg q24h; **Rats:** For vaginal candidiasis: 2.5–10 mg/kg q24h; **Guinea pigs:** 5 mg/kg

q24h for systemic candidiasis (Adamcak & Otten 2000)

■ **HORSES:**

a) For guttural pouch mycosis, mycotic rhinitis or osteomyelitis: Using the oral solution at 5 mg/kg PO q24h should be sufficient for treatment. (Davis 2007)

■ **BIRDS:**

a) Ratites: 6–10 mg/kg PO once daily; if neuro signs develop reduce dose or discontinue (Jenson 1998)

b) 5–10 mg/kg PO q12-24h. Use with caution in African grey parrots. (Tully 2008)

c) For aspergillosis: 5–10 mg/kg PO once daily in Amazon parrots; 2.5–5 mg/kg PO once daily in African grey Parrots. (Oglesbee 2009)

Monitoring

■ Clinical Efficacy

■ With long-term therapy, routine liver function tests are recommended (monthly ALT)

■ Appetite

■ Physical assessment for ulcerative skin lesions in dogs

Client Information

■ Compliance with treatment recommendations must be stressed

■ Have clients report any potential adverse effects

■ Give capsules with food. Preferably, give oral solution on an empty stomach in mammals.

■ For cats and small dogs, capsules can be opened and the appropriate dose measured proportionally. Pellets from within the capsule can be added to a food the animal will readily eat (cheese, butter, etc).

■ Do not give with any other medications without veterinarian's approval

Chemistry/Synonyms

A synthetic triazole antifungal, itraconazole is structurally related to fluconazole. It has a molecular weight of 706 and a pKa of 3.7. It is practically insoluble in water and highly lipophilic.

Itraconazole may also be known as: itraconazolum, oriconazole, R-51211, or *Sporanox®*; many other trade names are available.

Storage/stability

Itraconazole capsules should be stored between 15–25°C and protected from light and moisture.

Itraconazole oral solution should be stored at temperatures less than 26°C, and protected from freezing.

Compatibility/Compounding Considerations

Compounding capsules or solutions from bulk chemicals or powders likely will not yield dosage forms that are absorbed. The oral bioavailability and solubility of itraconazole is dependent upon complexation with cyclodextran molecules, a technology used in the brand (*Sporanox®*) and generic commercially produced human drug products for itraconazole, but not in compounded dosage forms. A recent study (Smith *et al.* 2010) demonstrated that itraconazole compounded from the bulk chemical produces inferior blood levels in Black-footed penguins compared to FDA-approved itraconazole products. Inferior blood levels of itraconazole may contribute to treatment failure and fatality if compounded itraconazole is utilized in life-threatening infections such as blastomycosis or pythiosis. Unless itraconazole dosage forms are formulated from FDA-approved dosage forms, it is recommended *not to use compounded* itraconazole products unless prepared from commercial capsules or documented bioavailability and stability data are provided.

Compounded preparation stability: Two methods of preparing a stable (not necessarily bioavailable) itraconazole oral suspension prepared from commercially available capsules have been published. **1)** Triturating twenty-four (24) itraconazole 100 mg capsules with 5 mL ethanol 95%, allowing to stand 3–4 minutes, grinding to paste and then bringing to a final volume of 60 mL with simple syrup yields a 40 mg/mL oral suspension that retains >95% potency for 35 days stored at 4°C and protected from light (Jacobson *et al.* 1995). **2)** Triturating forty (40) itraconazole 100 mg capsules with 15 mL of ethanol 95%, allowing to stand 3-4 minutes, grinding to paste, adding 100 mL of *Ora-Plus*® and bringing to volume of 200 mL *Ora-Sweet*® yields a 20 mg/mL itraconazole suspension (Abdel-Rahmen & Nahata 1998). Solutions of itraconazole have a pH of 2.

Dosage Forms/Regulatory Status

VETERINARY-LABELED PRODUCTS: None in the USA.

In several countries, itraconazole oral liquid 10 mg/mL in 52 mL bottles with dosing syringe; *Intrafungol*® (Janssen); (Rx). Labeled for use in cats (in the UK).

HUMAN-LABELED PRODUCTS:

Itraconazole Capsules: 100 mg; *Sporanox*® (Janssen); generic; (Rx)

Itraconazole Oral Solution: 10 mg/mL in 150 mL; *Sporanox*® (Ortho Biotech); (Rx)

References

Abdel-Rahmen, S. & M.C. Nahata (1998). Stability of itraconazole in an extemporaneous suspension. *J Pediatr Pharm Pract* **3**: 115–118.

Adamcak, A. & B. Otten (2000). Rodent Therapeutics. *Vet Clin NA: Exotic Anim Pract* **3:1**(Jan): 221–240.

Davidson, A. & K. Mathews (2000). CVT Update: Therapy for Nasal Aspergillosis. *Kirk's Current Veterinary Therapy: XIII Small Animal Practice*. J Bonagura Ed. Philadelphia, WB Saunders: 315–317.

Davis, J.L. (2007). Update on Antifungal Therapies in Horses. Proceedings: ACVIM. Accessed via: Veterinary Information Network. http://goo.gl/F1BCZ

DeBoer, D. (2006). Dermatophytosis: Recent advances in treatment and control. Proceedings: NA Vet Derm Forum.

Foil, C. (2003a). New drugs in dermatology. Proceedings: Western Veterinary Conf. Accessed via: Veterinary Information Network. http://goo.gl/iEYic

Foil, C. (2003b). Ringworm update. Proceedings: Western Veterinary Conf. Accessed via: Veterinary Information Network. http://goo.gl/O9j3A

Frank, L. (2000). Dermatophytosis. *Kirk's Current Veterinary Therapy: XIII Small Animal Practice*. J Bonagura Ed. Philadelphia, WB Saunders: 577–580.

Graupmann-Kuzma, A., B.A. Valentine, et al. (2008). Coccidioidomycosis in dogs and cats: A review. *Journal of the American Animal Hospital Association* **44**(5): 226–235.

Grooters, A. (2005). Deep fungal infections. Proceedings; ACVIM. Accessed via: Veterinary Information Network. http://goo.gl/wV8J7

Jacobson, P.A., C.E. Johnson, et al. (1995). Stability of Itraconazole in an Extemporaneously Compounded Oral Liquid. *American Journal of Health-System Pharmacy* **52**(2): 189–191.

Jenson, J. (1998). Current ratite therapy. *The Veterinary Clinics of North America: Food Animal Practice* **16:3**(November).

Kuehn, N. (2010). Chronic Nasal Disease in Dogs: Diagnosis & Treatment. Proceedings: ACVIM. Accessed via: Veterinary Information Network. http://goo.gl/2OQgm

Legendre, A. & R. Toal (2000). Diagnosis and Treatment of Fungal Diseases of the Respiratory System. *Kirk's Current Veterinary Therapy: XIII Small Animal Practice*. J Bonagura Ed. Philadelphia, WB Saunders: 815–819.

Malik, R. (2006). Treatment of Cryptococcosis in Cats. Proceedings: Western Vet Conf. Accessed via: Veterinary Information Network. http://goo.gl/qxQAx

Negre, A., E. Bensignor, et al. (2009). Evidence-based veterinary dermatology: a systematic review of interventions for Malassezia dermatitis in dogs. *Veterinary Dermatology* **20**(1): 1–12.

Oglesbee, B. (2009). Working up the pet bird with upper respiratory tract disorders. Proceedings: WVC. Accessed via: Veterinary Information Network. http://goo.gl/fh5gC

Smith, J.A., M.G. Papich, et al. (2010). Effects Of Compounding On Pharmacokinetics Of Itraconazole In Black-Footed Penguins (Spheniscus Demersus). *Journal of Zoo and Wildlife Medicine* **41**(3): 487–495.

Taboada, J. (2000). Systemic Mycoses. *Textbook of Veterinary Internal Medicine: Diseases of the Dog and Cat*. S Ettinger and E Feldman Eds. Philadelphia, WB Saunders. **1**: 453–476.

Tully, T. (2008). Treating avian fungal diseases. Proceedings: Atlantic Coast Veterinary Conf. Accessed via: Veterinary Information Network. http://goo.gl/PrjeG

IVERMECTIN

(eye-ver-*mek*-tin)   Heartgard®, Ivomec®

ANTIPARASITIC

Prescriber Highlights

▶ Prototype avermectin drug used in variety of species as an antiparasiticide

▶ Contraindications: Label specific due to lack of safety data (foals, puppies, etc.) or public health safety (lactating dairy animals)

▶ Caution in breeds susceptible to *ABCB1*-1Δ (formerly MDR1-allele) mutation (Collies, Australian Shepherds, Shelties, Long-haired Whippet, "white feet"); at higher risk for CNS toxicity

▶ Adverse Effects: *Horses:* Swelling & pruritus at the ventral mid-line can be seen approximately 24 hours after ivermectin administration due to a hypersensitivity reaction to dead *Onchocerca* spp. microfilaria. *Dogs:* May exhibit a shock-like reaction when ivermectin is used as a microfilaricide, presumably due to a reaction associated with the dying microfilaria. *Cattle:* Ivermectin can induce serious adverse effects by killing the larva when they are in vital areas; may also cause discomfort or transient swelling at the injection site. *Mice & rats:* May cause neurologic toxicity at doses slightly more than usually prescribed. *Birds:* Death, lethargy, or anorexia may be seen. Orange-cheeked Waxbill Finches & budgerigars may be more sensitive to ivermectin than other species

Uses/Indications

Ivermectin is FDA-approved in horses for the control of: large strongyles (adult) (*Strongylus vulgaris, S. edentatus, S. equinus, Triodontophorus* spp.), small strongyles, pinworms (adults and 4th stage larva), ascarids (adults), hairworms (adults), large-mouth stomach worms (adults), neck threadworms (microfilaria), bots (oral and gastric stages), lungworms (adults and 4th stage larva), intestinal threadworms (adults), and summer sores (cutaneous 3rd stage larva) secondary to *Hebronema* or *Draschia* Spp.

In cattle, ivermectin is FDA-approved for use in the control of gastrointestinal roundworms (adults and 4th stage larva), lungworms (adults and 4th stage larva), cattle grubs (parasitic stages), sucking lice, and mites (scabies). For a listing of individual species covered, refer to the product information.

In swine, ivermectin is FDA-approved for use to treat GI roundworms, lungworms, lice, and mange mites. For a listing of individual species covered, refer to the product information.

In reindeer, ivermectin is FDA-approved for use in the control of warbles.

In American Bison, ivermectin is FDA-approved for use in the control of grubs.

In dogs and cats, ivermectin is FDA-approved only for use as a preventative for heartworm. It has also been used as a microfilaricide, slow-kill adulticide, ectoparasiticide, and endoparasiticide. At the time of writing (2010) there is considerable interest in using ivermectin or another macrocyclic lactone with doxycycline for several months prior to melarsomine adulticide therapy in dogs. Ivermectin can kill *D. immitis* larval stages 3 & 4, kill microfilaria, and reduce the lifespan of adult heartworms. Doxycycline treatment can potentially reduce adult worm populations by eliminating *Wolbachia*, a bacterium associated with *D. immitis*. The American Heartworm Society has stated; ". . . it is beneficial to administer a macrocyclic lactone for up to three months prior to administration of melarsomine, when the clinical presentation does not demand immediate intervention" and "Doxycycline administered at 10 mg/kg twice daily for four weeks has been shown to eliminate over 90% of the *Wolbachia* organisms and the levels remain low for three to four months." (American-Heartworm-Society 2010)

Pharmacology/Actions

Ivermectin enhances the release of gamma amino butyric acid (GABA) at presynaptic neurons. GABA acts as an inhibitory neurotransmitter and blocks the post-synaptic stimulation of the adjacent neuron in nematodes or the muscle fiber in arthropods. By stimulating the release of GABA, ivermectin causes paralysis of the parasite and eventual death. As liver flukes and tapeworms do not use GABA as a peripheral nerve transmitter, ivermectin is ineffective against these parasites.

Pharmacokinetics

In simple-stomached animals, ivermectin is up to 95% absorbed after oral administration. Ruminants only absorb ¼–⅓ of a dose due to inactivation of the drug in the rumen. While there is greater bioavailability after SC administration, absorption after oral dosing is more rapid than SC. It has been reported that ivermectin's bioavailability is lower in cats than in dogs, necessitating a higher dosage for prophylaxis of heartworm in this species.

Ivermectin is well distributed to most tissues, but does not readily penetrate into the CSF, thereby minimizing its toxicity. Collie-breed dogs with a specific gene defect allow more ivermectin into the CNS than other breeds/species.

Ivermectin has a long terminal half-life in most species (see below). It is metabolized in the liver via oxidative pathways and is primarily excreted in the feces. Less than 5% of the drug (as parent compound or metabolites) is excreted in the urine.

Pharmacokinetic parameters of ivermectin have been reported for various species:

Cattle: Volume of distribution = 0.45–2.4 L/kg; elimination half-life = 2–3 days; total body clearance = 0.79 L/kg/day.

Dogs: Bioavailability = 0.95; volume of distribution = 2.4 L/kg; elimination half-life = 2 days.

Swine: Volume of distribution = 4 L/kg; elimination half-life = 0.5 days.

Sheep: Bioavailability = 1 (intra-abomasal), 0.25 (intra-ruminal); volume of distribution = 4.6 L/kg; elimination half-life = 2–7 days.

Contraindications/Precautions/Warnings

The manufacturer recommends that ivermectin not be used in foals less than 4 months old, as safety of the drug in animals this young has not been firmly established. However, foals less than 30 days of age have tolerated doses as high as 1 mg/kg without signs of toxicity.

Ivermectin is not recommended for use in puppies less than 6 weeks old. After receiving heartworm prophylaxis doses, the manufacturer recommends observing Collie-type breeds for at least 8 hours after administration. Most clinicians feel that ivermectin should not be used in breeds susceptible (Collies, Shelties, Australian shepherds, etc.) to the *ABCB1*-1Δ (formerly MDR1-allele) mutation at the doses specified for treating microfilaria or other parasites unless the patient has been tested and found not to have the gene defect. A specific test for identifying dogs that have the gene defect (deletion mutation of the *ABCB1*-1Δ (formerly MDR1 gene) is now available. Contact the veterinary clinical pharmacology lab at www.vetmed.wsu.edu.

Ivermectin is reportedly contraindicated in chelonians, Indigo snakes and skinks. Milbemycin has reportedly been given safely to chelonians.

Because milk withdrawal times have not been established, the drug is not FDA-approved for use in lactating dairy animals or females of breeding age.

The injectable products for use in cattle and swine should be given subcutaneously only; do not give IM or IV.

If using a product in a species not labeled for that product (extra-label), be certain of the dosage and/or dilutions. There are many reports of overdoses in small animals when large animal products have been used.

Adverse Effects

In horses, swelling and pruritus at the ventral mid-line can be seen approximately 24 hours after ivermectin administration due to a hypersensitivity reaction to dead *Onchocerca* spp. microfilaria. The reaction is preventable by administering a glucocorticoid just prior to, and for 1–2 days after ivermectin. If untreated, swelling usually subsides within 7–10 days and pruritus will resolve within 3 weeks.

Dogs may exhibit a shock-like reaction when ivermectin is used as a microfilaricide, presumably due to a reaction associated with the dying microfilaria. Other adverse effects when used as a microfilaricide include depression, hypothermia, and vomiting. Pretreatment with diphenhydramine (2 mg/kg IM) and dexamethasone (0.25 mg/kg IV) can help prevent adverse reactions (Atkins 2005).

When used to treat *Hypoderma bovis* larva (Cattle grubs) in cattle, ivermectin can induce serious adverse effects by killing the larva when they are in vital areas. Larva killed in the vertebral canal can cause paralysis and staggering. Larva killed around the gullet can induce salivation and bloat. These effects can be avoided by treating for grubs immediately after the Heal fly (Warble fly) season or after the stages of grub development where these areas would be affected. Cattle may experience discomfort or transient swelling at the injection site. Using a maximum of 10 mL at any one-injection site can help minimize these effects.

Neurotoxicity is possible in dogs, particularly in those with the gene defect (deletion mutation of the *ABCB1*Δ (formerly MDR1) gene) that has been seen in certain genetic lines of Collie-type breeds. There are case reports of dogs without the *ABCB1*Δ mutation developing neurotoxicity after receiving ivermectin at demodicosis doses.

There are case reports of horses developing neurotoxicity after receiving recommended oral dosages (Swor *et al.* 2009).

In mice and rats, ivermectin may cause neurologic toxicity at doses slightly more than usually prescribed (less than 0.5 mg/kg).

In birds, death, lethargy or anorexia may be seen. Orange-cheeked Waxbill Finches and budgerigars may be more sensitive to ivermectin than other species.

For additional information refer to the Overdosage/Acute Toxicity section below.

Reproductive/Nursing Safety

Ivermectin is considered safe to use during pregnancy. Reproductive studies performed in dogs, horses, cattle and swine have not demonstrated adverse effects to fetuses. Reproductive performance in male animals is apparently unaltered. In humans, the FDA categorizes this drug as category **C** for use during pregnancy (*Animal studies have shown an adverse effect on the fetus, but there are no adequate studies in humans; or there are no animal reproduction studies and no adequate studies in humans.*) In a separate system evaluating the safety of drugs in canine and feline pregnancy (Papich 1989), this drug is categorized as in class: **A** (*Probably safe. Although specific studies may not have proved the safety of all drugs in dogs and cats, there are no reports of adverse effects in laboratory animals or women.*)

Ivermectin is excreted in milk in low concentrations; it is unlikely to pose significant risk to nursing offspring.

Overdosage/Acute Toxicity

There were 318 exposures to ivermectin reported to the ASPCA Animal Poison Control Center (APCC) during 2008-2009. In these cases 282 were dogs with 203 showing clinical signs, 24 cats with 15 showing clinical signs, 3 were cows with 3 showing clinical signs, and there was one reported turtle that showed clinical signs. The remaining 8 cases consisted of two rodents, two ovines, and 4 equines, none of which showed clinical signs. Common findings in dogs recorded in decreasing frequency included vomiting, ataxia, lethargy, tachycardia, hypersalivation, mydriasis, and seizures. Common findings in cats recorded in decreasing frequency included ataxia, diarrhea, hypersensitivity, and vomiting. Common findings in bovines recorded included diarrhea.

In dogs (non-sensitive breeds), signs of acute toxicity rarely occur at single dosages of 1 mg/kg (1000 micrograms/kg) or less. At 2.5 mg/kg, mydriasis occurs, and at 5 mg/kg, tremors occur. At doses of 10 mg/kg, severe tremors and ataxia are seen. Deaths occurred when dosages exceeded 40 mg/kg, but the LD50 is 80 mg/kg. Dogs (Beagles) receiving 0.5 mg/kg PO for 14 weeks developed no signs of toxicity, but at 1–2 mg/kg for the same time period, developed mydriasis and had some weight decreases. Half of the dogs receiving 2 mg/kg/day for 14 weeks developed signs of depression, tremors, ataxia, anorexia, and dehydration.

Ivermectin is actively transported by the p-glycoprotein pump and certain breeds susceptible to MDR1-allele mutation (Collies, Australian Shepherds, Shelties, Long-haired Whippets, etc.) are at higher risk for CNS toxicity. At the dosage recommended for heartworm prophylaxis, it is generally believed that the drug is safe to use in these animals. In cases of overdoses signs can develop within 4 hours in sensitive breeds. In cases of overdoses in these dogs, clinical signs can appear within 4 hours of exposure.

Dogs who receive an overdosage of ivermectin or develop signs of acute toxicity (CNS effects, GI, cardiovascular) should receive supportive and symptomatic therapy. Emptying the gut should be considered for recent massive oral ingestions in dogs or cats. For both oral and injected ivermectin overdoses, the use of repeated activated charcoal doses is advised to interrupt enterohepatic recirculation. Although the therapy is still in the experimental stages, some veterinarians have administered intravenous fat emulsion to patients after large overdoses. This therapy may facilitate the clearance of the ivermectin due to its highly lipophilic nature.

Ivermectin has a large safety margin in cats. Kittens receiving doses of at least 110 mcg/kg and adult cats receiving at least 750 mcg/kg showed no untoward effects. The margin of safety is narrower in kittens as significant clinical signs have been seen at 300 micrograms/kg. Acute toxic signs associated with massive overdoses in cats will appear within 10 hours of ingestion. Signs may include agitation, vocalization, anorexia, mydriasis, rear limb paresis, tremors, and disorientation. Blindness, head pressing, wall climbing, absence of oculomotor menace reflex, and a slow and incomplete response to pupillary light may also be seen. Neurologic signs usually diminish over several days and most animals completely recover within 2–4 weeks. Symptomatic and supportive care is recommended.

In horses, doses of 1.8 mg/kg (9x recommended dose) PO did not produce signs of toxicity, but doses of 2 mg/kg caused signs of visual impairment, depression and ataxia. In cattle, toxic effects generally do not appear until dosages of 30x those recommended are injected. At 8 mg/kg, cattle showed signs of ataxia, listlessness, and occasionally, death.

Sheep have shown signs of ataxia and depression at ivermectin doses of 4 mg/kg.

Swine have shown signs of toxicosis (lethargy, ataxia, tremors, lateral recumbency, and mydriasis) at doses of 30 mg/kg. Neonatal pigs may be more susceptible to ivermectin overdosages, presumably due to a more permeable blood-brain barrier. Accurate dosing practices are recommended.

Drug Interactions

The following drug interactions have either been reported or are theoretical in humans or animals receiving ivermectin and may be of significance in veterinary patients:

- ■ **BENZODIAZEPINES:** Effects may be potentiated by ivermectin; use together not advised in humans

- ■ **KETAMINE:** It has been recommended not to use ivermectin in reptiles within 10 days of ketamine (Bays 2009)

- ■ **SPINOSAD** (*Comfortis®*): It has been recommended not to use with the high extra-label doses of ivermectin (Kuhl 2009)

Caution is advised if using other drugs that can inhibit **p-glycoprotein.** Those dogs at risk for *ABCB1-1Δ* (formerly MDR1 allele) mutation (Collies, Australian Shepherds, Shelties, Long-haired Whippet, etc., "white feet") should probably not receive ivermectin with the following drugs, unless tested "normal"; at least one reference states that ivermectin should never be used with ketoconazole in dogs (Waisglass 2009). Drugs and drug classes involved include:

- ■ **AMIODARONE**
- ■ **CARVEDILOL**
- ■ **CLARITHROMYCIN**
- ■ **CYCLOSPORINE**
- ■ **DILTIAZEM**
- ■ **ERYTHROMYCIN**
- ■ **ITRACONAZOLE**

- **■ KETOCONAZOLE**
- **■ QUINIDINE**
- **■ SPIRONOLACTONE**
- **■ TAMOXIFEN**
- **■ VERAPAMIL**

Laboratory Considerations

- ■ When used at microfilaricide dosages, ivermectin may yield false-negative results in animals with occult heartworm infection.

Doses

■ DOGS:

Note: When used for prophylaxis or treatment of dirofilariasis it is suggested to review the guidelines published by the American Heartworm Society at www.heartwormsociety.org for more information.

As a preventative for heartworm:

a) 6–12 micrograms/kg PO once monthly (Knight 2000)

b) Minimum dosage of 6 micrograms/kg (0.006 mg/kg) PO per month. (Package insert; *Heartgard30®*—Merial)

As a microfilaricide:

a) When used to kill third, fourth, and young fifth stage larvae for prophylaxis or to kill these larval stages prior to adulticide therapy along with microfilariae, ivermectin is dosed at 6–12 micrograms/kg PO once a month. When only used to kill circulating microfilariae, ivermectin can be administered at 6 micrograms/kg (the FDA-approved prophylactic dose) or at a dose of 50 micrograms/kg (approximately 10 times the prophylactic dose). Microfilariae numbers decrease gradually to, or close to, zero within several months at the lower dose. The chance of adverse reactions with this approach is minimal. The higher dose results in a rapid kill that is associated with more adverse effects. (Kittleson 2006)

As an adulticide or pre-adulticide for heartworm:

a) In combination with doxycycline as an adulticide for *D. immitis*: In this study, doxycycline was administered at 10 mg/kg PO once daily for 30 days along with ivermectin/pyrantel pamoate with the ivermectin dose at 6–14 micrograms/kg PO once every 15 days for 6 months. 100% (total of 11 dogs) were negative for circulating microfilaria by day 90. 74% of dogs were negative for circulating antigens at day 300 (4-months post ivermectin). (Grandi *et al.* 2010)

As an ectoparasiticide (miticide):

a) For generalized demodicosis: **Note:** Do not consider use in *ABCB1-1Δ* (formerly MDR1-allele) mutation susceptible breeds unless tested "normal/normal"

for mutation (www.vetmed.wsu.edu). If normal/normal, drug reaction is very unlikely. Start at low dosage and increase:

Day 1: 100 micrograms/kg PO q24h,

Day 4: 200 micrograms/kg PO q24h,

Day 7: 300 micrograms/kg; continue to increase by 100 micrograms/kg every 3rd day until reach target dose of 600 micrograms/kg PO daily and continue treatment 1–2 months after 2 negative skin scrapes. Treatment usually requires 10–33 weeks. (Hillier 2006)

b) For demodicosis: Start at a trial dose of 0.05 mg/kg (50 micrograms/kg) day 1. Then increase the dose to 0.12 mg/kg for the next week (this was the "test dose" that we used to use, as sensitive Collies generally react at this dose). If all is well, go up to 0.2 mg/kg for the next 3 days, and then increase the dose weekly by 0.1 mg/kg until you reach 0.6 mg/kg. Advise the owner to discontinue immediately if there is evidence of ivermectin toxicosis (especially lethargy, ataxia, mydriasis and gastrointestinal signs). If there is no reaction at a lower, but therapeutic, dose (above 0.3 mg/kg), author usually will try again at that lower dose but on an alternate day treatment schedule. Continue treatment for 2 months past negative scrapings (3-7 months of treatment). (Waisglass 2009)

c) As scabicide: 300–400 micrograms/kg PO or SC once weekly for weeks. If using the 1% injection, 1 mL = 10,000 micrograms. Beware in sensitive breeds (*e.g.*, Collies, etc.; "white feet, don't treat"). Check heartworm status prior to treatment. Adverse effects are rare outside of sensitive breeds. (Foil 2003)

As an endoparasiticide:

a) For treatment of parasitic lung disease (*Capillaria* spp.): 0.2 mg/kg PO once (Bauer 1988)

b) For *Oslerus osleri*: 0.4 mg/kg SC once (Reinemeyer 1995)

c) For *Eucoleus boehmi*: 0.2 mg/kg PO once (Reinemeyer 1995)

d) For *Pneumonyssoides caninum*: 0.2 mg/kg SC once (Reinemeyer 1995)

■ CATS:

Note: When used for prophylaxis or treatment of dirofilariasis it is suggested to review the guidelines published by the American Heartworm Society at www.heartwormsociety.org for more information

As a preventative for heartworm:

a) Minimum effective dosage: 0.024 mg/kg (24 micrograms/kg) PO every 30–45 days (**Note:** also controls hookworms at this dosage) (Knight 1995)

For *Aelurostrongylus abstrusus*:

a) 0.4 mg/kg SC once (Reinemeyer 1995); (Hawkins 2000)

■ **FERRETS:**

a) For prevention of heartworm disease: 0.02 mg/kg PO monthly (Hoeffer 2000)

b) To treat heartworm disease using the very slow protocol: 50 micrograms PO once a month. (Hernandez-Divers 2007)

■ **RABBITS/RODENTS/SMALL MAMMALS:**

a) **Rabbits:** For *Sarcoptes scabiei, Notoedres cati*: 0.3–0.4 mg/kg SC, repeat in 14 days. For ear mites (Psoroptes) 0.2–0.44 mg/kg PO, SC repeat in 8–18 days (Ivey & Morrisey 2000)

b) **Rabbits:** For treatment of ear mites: 200 micrograms/kg SC and repeated in two weeks. All rabbits in colony should be treated and cages cleaned and disinfected. (Burke 1999)

c) **Rodents and lagomorphs:** For treatment of sarcoptoid and some fur mites: 200–250 micrograms/kg SC. Cages should be thoroughly cleaned and disinfected. (Burke 1999)

d) **Mice, Rats, Gerbils, Guinea pigs, Chinchillas:** 200 micrograms/kg SC or PO every 7 days for 3 weeks Hamsters: 200–500 micrograms/kg SC or PO every 14 days for 3 weeks (Adamcak & Otten 2000)

e) **Guinea pigs** for *Trixacarus caviae* mites: 500 micrograms/kg SC, repeated at 14 and 28 days. (Johnson 2006)

■ **CATTLE:**

For susceptible parasites:

a) 200 micrograms/kg SC. Doses greater than 10 mL should be given at two separate sites. (Paul 1986)

b) For psoroptic mange: 200 mg/kg IM (**Note:** Reference was written before approval of the SC labeled bovine product); isolate from other cattle for at least 5 days after treatment. (Mullowney 1986)

c) 200 micrograms/kg (0.2 mg/kg) SC under the loose skin in front of or behind the shoulder (Product Information; *Ivomec® Inj. for Cattle 1%*—MSD)

■ **HORSES:**

For susceptible parasites:

a) 200 micrograms/kg (0.2 mg/kg) PO using oral paste or oral liquid (Product Information; *Eqvalan®*—MSD)

b) 0.2 mg/kg PO; 0.2 mg/kg PO at 4 day intervals for lice and mange (Robinson 1987)

c) As a larvicidal for arterial stages of *S. vulgaris*: 0.2 mg/kg once (Herd 1987)

■ **SWINE:**

For susceptible parasites:

a) 300 micrograms/kg (0.3 mg/kg) SC in the neck immediately behind the ear (Product Information; *Ivomec® Inj. for Swine 1%*—MSD)

b) For general control of endo- and ectoparasites in potbellied pigs: 300 micrograms/kg SC or IM once for internal parasites and repeated in 10–14 days for external parasites (only partially effective against whipworms—see fenbendazole) (Braun 1995)

■ **SHEEP/GOATS:**

For susceptible parasites:

a) 200 micrograms/kg for nasal bot infection (Bennett 1986)

b) 200 micrograms/kg SC for one dose (goats also) (Upson 1988)

c) For adjunctive treatment of meningeal worm (*Parelaphostrongylus tenuis*): To prevent further migration: Ivermectin at 0.3 mg/kg SC once daily for 5 days with fenbendazole (50 mg/kg PO once daily for 5 days). (Edmondson 2009)

■ **CAMELIDS:**

For susceptible parasites:

a) New world camelids: 0.2 mg/kg PO or SC for one dose (Cheney & Allen 1989)

b) For GI helminths in new world camelids: 0.2 mg/kg PO once. (Wolff 2009)

c) For adjunctive treatment of meningeal worm (*Parelaphostrongylus tenuis*): To prevent further migration: Fenbendazole at 50 mg/kg PO once daily for 5 days and ivermectin at 0.3 mg/kg SC once daily for 5 days. Camelids very susceptible to GI ulcers; give prophylaxis or treat with omeprazole or ranitidine. (Edmondson 2009)

■ **BIRDS:**

For susceptible parasites:

a) For ascarids, Capillaria and other intestinal worms, *Knemidocoptes pilae* (scaly face and leg mites): Dilute to a 2 mg/mL concentration. After diluting product, use immediately.

Most birds: Inject 220 micrograms/kg IM;

Amazons: 0.1 mg IM;

Macaws: 0.2 mg IM;

Finches: 0.02 mg (Stunkard 1984)

b) For ascarids, coccidia and other intestinal nematodes, Oxysipura, gapeworms, *Knemidocoptes pilae* (scaly face and leg mites): Dilute bovine preparation (10 mg/mL) 1:4 with propylene glycol.

For most species: 200 micrograms/kg IM or orally; repeat in 10–14 days.

Budgerigars: 0.01 mL of diluted product (see above) IM or PO (Clubb 1986)

c) 200 micrograms/kg (0.2 mg/kg) SC; dilute using propylene glycol. (Sikarskie 1986)

d) **Ratites:** 200 micrograms/kg PO, IM or SC. Has efficacy against *Chandlerella quiscali* in emus. (Jenson 1998)

■ **REPTILES:**

For most nematodes, ectoparasites:

a) **Lizards, snakes, and alligators:** 0.2 mg/kg (200 micrograms/kg) IM, SC, or PO once; repeat in 2 weeks. A third treatment can be given if still positive after the second treatment. **Note:** Ivermectin is toxic to chelonians, indigo snakes, skinks (de la Navarre 2003; Gauvin 1993)

Monitoring

■ Clinical efficacy

■ Adverse effects/toxicity (see Adverse Effects and Overdosage Sections)

Client Information

■ When using large animal products the manufacturer recommends not eating or smoking and to wash hands after use. Avoid contact with eyes.

■ Dispose of unused products and containers by incineration or in approved-landfills. Ivermectin may adversely affect fish or other water-borne organisms if disposed in water.

■ Contact veterinarian if any treated animal exhibits signs of toxicity (see Adverse effects and Overdosage sections above).

Chemistry/Synonyms

An avermectin anthelmintic, ivermectin occurs as an off-white to yellowish powder. It is very poorly soluble in water (4 micrograms/mL), but is soluble in propylene glycol, polyethylene glycol, and vegetable oils.

Ivermectin may also be known as MK 933, Ivermectine, Ivermectinum or Ivermectina; many trade names are available.

Storage/Stability

Ivermectin is photolabile in solution; protect from light. Unless otherwise specified by the manufacturer, store ivermectin products at room temperature (15–30°C).

Ivermectin 1% oral solution (equine tube wormer product) is stable at 1:20 and 1:40 dilutions with water for 72 hours when stored in a tight container, at room temperature, and protected from light.

Dosage Forms/Regulatory Status

VETERINARY FDA-APPROVED PRODUCTS:

Note: As ivermectin is no longer patent protected in the USA, there are a variety of "generic" products available with many trade names. The following may not be a complete listing.

Ivermectin for Injection: 10 mg/mL (1%) in 50 mL, 200 mL and 500 mL packs; *Ivomec®* (Merial); (OTC); FDA-approved for use in swine. Slaughter withdrawal (at labeled doses) = 18 days.

Ivermectin for Injection: 10 mg/mL (1%) in 50 mL, 200 mL, 500 mL bottles; *Ivomec® 1% Injection for Cattle* and *Swine* (Merial), *Double Impact®* (AgriLabs); *Ultramectrin® Injection* (RXV); (OTC). FDA-approved for use in cattle (not female dairy cattle of breeding age) and swine. Slaughter (when used as labeled): cattle = 35 days, swine = 18 days, reindeer = 56 days, bison = 56 days. No milk withdrawal time has been established.

Ivermectin for Injection: 2.7 mg/mL (0.27%) in 200 mL bottles; *Ivomec® 0.27% Injection for Feeder* and *Grower Pigs* (Merial); (OTC). FDA-approved for use in swine. Slaughter (when used as labeled) = 18 days

Ivermectin Oral Paste: 1.87% (18.7 mg/gram) in 6.08 gram syringes; *Equimectrin® Paste 1.87%* (Farnam), *Eqvalan® Paste 1.87%* (Merial), *Rotectin® 1 Paste 1.87%* (Farnam), *Zimectrin® Paste* (Farnam); (OTC). FDA-approved for use in horses (not intended for food purposes).

Oral Paste: containing 1.87% ivermectin and 14.03% of praziquantel in oral syringes (sufficient to treat one 1320 lb horse); *Equimax®*(Pfizer); (OTC). FDA-approved for use in horse or ponies not intended for food purposes.

Oral Paste: containing 1.55% ivermectin and 7.75% of praziquantel in oral syringes; *Zimecterin Gold®*(Merial); (OTC). FDA-approved for use in horse or ponies not intended for food purposes.

Ivermectin Liquid: 1% (10 mg/mL) in 50 mL and 100 mL btls (for tube administration; **not** for injection); *Amtech Phoenectin® Liquid for Horses* (Phoenix Scientific), *Eqvalan® Liquid* (Merial), *Ivercide® Liquid for Horses* (Phoenix Pharmaceutical); (Rx). FDA-approved for use in horses (not intended for food purposes).

Ivermectin Oral Tablets: 68 mcg, 136 mcg, 272 micrograms (Plain or Chewable) in 6 chewables in carton in 10 carton trays, *Heartgard® Tablets* (Merial), *Heartgard® Chewables* (Merial); (Rx). FDA-approved for use in dogs.

Ivermectin Oral Chewable Tablets: 55 micrograms or 165 micrograms in cartons of 6 in 10 cartons per tray. *Heartgard® for Cats* (Merial); (Rx) FDA-approved for use in cats.

Ivermectin Oral Solution: 0.08% in 960 mL and 4,800 mL containers; *Ivomec® Sheep Drench* (Merial); (OTC); FDA-approved for use in sheep. Slaughter withdrawal time = 11 days.

Ivermectin Bolus: 1.72 gram; *Ivomec® SR Bolus* (Merial); (OTC). FDA-approved for use in cattle (not female dairy cattle of breeding age). Slaughter withdrawal time = 180 days. No milk withdrawal time has been established.

Ivermectin Medicated feeds: *Ivomec® Premix for Swine Type A Medicated Article* (Merial) 0.6% in 50 lb. *Ivomec® Premix for Swine Type C Medicated Feed 0.02%* (Merial) in 20 lb one-ton bag and 40 lb two-ton bag, *Ivomec® Premix for Swine Type C medicated feed 0.1%* (Merial) in 20 lb one-ton bag. FDA-approved for use in swine. Slaughter withdrawal = 5 days

Ivermectin Topical Parasiticide Pour-on for Cattle: 5 mg/mL 250 mL, 500 mL, 1 liter and 1 gallon bottles. FDA-approved for use in cattle (not female dairy cattle of breeding age). Slaughter withdrawal time = 48 days, milk withdrawal has not been established. *Amtech Phoenectin® Pour-on for Cattle* (Phoenix Scientific), *Bimectin® Pour-On* (Bimeda), *Ivercide® Pour-On for Cattle* (Phoenix Pharmaceutical), *Ivermectin® Pour-On* (Aspen, Durvet), *Ivomec® Eprinex® Pour-on for Beef and Dairy Cattle* and *Ivomec® Pour-on for Cattle* (Merial), *Prozap® Ivermectin Pour-on* (Loveland), *Top Line®* (AgriLabs), *Ultramectrin® Pour-On* (RXV); (OTC)

Combination Products:

Ivermectin for Injection: 10 mg/mL (1%) and Clorsulon 100 mg/mL; *Ivomec® Plus Injection for Cattle* (Merial); (OTC). FDA-approved for use in cattle (not female dairy cattle of breeding age). Slaughter withdrawal (at labeled doses) = 40 days. No milk withdrawal has been established.

Ivermectin/Pyrantel Oral Tablets: 68 micrograms/57 mg, 136 micrograms/114 mg, 272 micrograms/228 mg); *Heartgard® Plus Chewables* (Merial); *Tri-Heart® Plus Chewable Tablets* (Schering); (Rx). FDA-approved for use in dogs.

Fenbendazole 454 mg, Ivermectin 27 mcg, & Praziquantel 23 mg (2.16g small chews) Chewable Tablets; *Panacur Plus® Soft Chews* (Intervet); (Rx). FDA-approved for use in adult dogs.

Fenbendazole 1.134 g, Ivermectin 68 mcg, & Praziquantel 57 mg (5.4g large chews) Chewable Tablet; *Panacur Plus® Soft Chews* (Intervet); (Rx). FDA-approved for use in adult dogs.

An otic product *Acarexx®* is also available.

HUMAN-LABELED PRODUCTS:

Ivermectin Tablets: 3 mg and 6 mg; *Stromectol®* (Merck); (Rx)

References

Adamcak, A. & B. Otten (2000). Rodent Therapeutics. *Vet Clin NA: Exotic Anim Pract* 3:1(Jan): 221–240.
American-Heartworm-Society (2010). "Canine Guidlines." 2010, http://www.heartwormsociety.org/veterinary-resources/canine-guidelines.html#9.
Atkins, C. (2005). Recent Advances, Controversies and Complications with Canine Heartworm Disease. Proceedings: ACVIM. Accessed via: Veterinary Information Network. http://goo.gl/3Stls
Bauer, T.G. (1988). Pulmonary parenchymal disorders. *Handbook of Small Animal Practice.* RV Morgan Ed. New York, Churchill Livingstone: 195–213.
Bays, T. (2009). Practice tips for exotic animals. Proceedings: WVC. Accessed via: Veterinary Information Network. http://goo.gl/faYZP
Bennett, D.G. (1986). Parasites of the respiratory system. *Current Veterinary Therapy: Food Animal Practice 2.* JL Howard Ed. Phialdelphia, W.B. Saunders: 684–687.
Braun, W. (1995). Potbellied pigs: General medical care. *Kirk's Current Veterinary Therapy:XII.* J Bonagura Ed. Philadelphia, W.B. Saunders: 1388–1389.
Burke, T. (1999). Husbandry and Medicine of Rodents and Lagomorphs. Proceedings: Central Veterinary Conference, Kansas City.
Cheney, J.M. & G.T. Allen (1989). Parasitism in Llamas. *Vet Clin North America: Food Animal Practice 5*(1): 217–232.
Clubb, S.L. (1986). Therapeutics: Individual and Flock Treatment Regimens. *Clinical Avian Medicine and Surgery.* GJ Harrison and LR Harrison Eds. Philadelphia, W.B. Saunders: 327–355.
de la Navarre, B. (2003). Common parasitic diseases of reptiles and amphibians. Proceedings: Western Veterinary Conf. Accessed via: Veterinary Information Network. http://goo.gl/ZafJD
Edmondson, M. (2009). Internal parasites of goats, sheep, and camelids. ABVP. http://goo.gl/41DcU
Foil, C. (2003). Update on treating scabies and cheyletiella. Proceedings: Western Veterinary Conference. Accessed via: Veterinary Information Network. http://goo.gl/lXjUF
Gauvin, J. (1993). Drug therapy in reptiles. *Seminars in Avian & Exotic Med 2*(1): 48–59.
Grandi, G., C. Quintavalla, et al. (2010). A combination of doxycycline and ivermectin is adulticidal in dogs with naturally acquired heartworm disease (Dirofilaria immitis). *Veterinary Parasitology* 169(3–4): 347–351.
Hawkins, E. (2000). Pulmonary Parenchymal Diseases. *Textbook of Veterinary Internal Medicine: Diseases of the Dog and Cat.* S Ettinger and E Feldman Eds. Philadelphia, WB Saunders. 2: 1061–1091.
Herd, R.P. (1987). Chemotherapy of Migrating Strongyles. *Current Therapy in Equine Medicine, 2.* NE Robinson Ed. Philadelphia, W.B. Saunders: 331–332.
Hernandez-Divers, S.J. (2007). Conundrums in Ferret Medicine. Proceedings: ACVC. http://goo.gl/LVIgo
Hillier, A. (2006). Update on canine demodicosis. Proceedings: ACVC. Accessed via: Veterinary Information Network. http://goo.gl/O2tAz
Hoeffer, H. (2000). Heart Disease in Ferrets. *Kirk's Current Veterinary Therapy: XIII Small Animal Practice.* J Bonagura Ed. Philadelphia, WB Saunders: 1144–1148.
Ivey, E. & J. Morrisey (2000). Therapeutics for Rabbits. *Vet Clin NA: Exotic Anim Pract* 3:1(Jan): 183–216.
Jenson, J. (1998). Current ratite therapy. *The Veterinary Clinics of North America: Food Animal Practice* 16:3(November).
Johnson, D. (2006). Guinea Pig Medicine Primer. Proceedings: ACVC. Accessed via: Veterinary Information Network. http://goo.gl/WmWhU
Kittleson, M. (2006). "Chapt 23: Heartworm Infection and Disease (Dirofilariasis)." *Small Animal Cardiology, 2nd Ed.*
Knight, D. (1995). Guidelines for diagnosis and management of heartworm (Dirofilaria Immitis) infection. *Kirk's Current Veterinary Therapy:XII.* J Bonagura Ed. Philadelphia, W.B. Saunders: 879–887.
Kuhl, K. (2009). Integrated Parasite Control in Dogs. Proceedings: WVC. Accessed via: Veterinary Information Network. http://goo.gl/7yKXe
Mullowney, P.C. (1986). Bovine Mange. *Current Veterinary Therapy: Food Animal Practice 2.* JL Howard Ed. Philadelphia, W.B. Saunders: 920–924.
Papich, M. (1989). Effects of drugs on pregnancy. *Current Veterinary Therapy X: Small Animal Practice.* R Kirk Ed. Philadelphia, Saunders: 1291–1299.
Paul, J.W. (1986). Anthelmintic Therapy. *Current Veterinary Therapy: Food Animal Practice 2.* JL Howard Ed. Philadelphia, W.B. Saunders: 39–44.
Reinemeyer, C. (1995). Parasites of the respiratory system. *Kirk's Current Veterinary Therapy:XII.* J Bonagura Ed. Philadelphia, W.B. Saunders: 895–898.
Robinson, N.E. (1987). Table of Common Drugs:

Approximate Doses. *Current Therapy in Equine Medicine, 2*. NE Robinson Ed. Philadelphia, W.B. Saunders: 761.

Sikarskie, J.G. (1986). The use of ivermectin in birds, reptiles, and small mammals. *Current Veterinary Therapy (CVT) IX Small Animal Practice*. RW Kirk Ed. Philadelphia, W.B. Saunders: 743–745.

Stunkard, J.M. (1984). *Diagnosis, Treatment and Husbandry of Pet Birds*. Edgewater, MD, Stunkard Publishing.

Swor, T.M., J.L. Whittenburg, et al. (2009). Ivermectin toxicosis in three adult horses. *Javma-Journal of the American Veterinary Medical Association* **235**(5): 558–562.

Upson, D.W. (1988). *Handbook of Clinical Veterinary Pharmacology*. Manhattan, Dan Upson Enterprises.

Waisglass, S. (2009). Demodicosis Update—Some Considerations to Increase Your Success Rate. Proceedings: WVC. Accessed via: Veterinary Information Network. http://goo.gl/4R2el

Wolff, P. (2009). Camelid Medicine. Proceedings: AAZV. Accessed via: Veterinary Information Network. http://goo.gl/4TEAy

KAOLIN/PECTIN

(*kay*-oh-lin/*pek*-tin)   Kaopectolin

GI ADSORBENT/PROTECTANT

Prescriber Highlights

▶ Adsorbent for treatment of diarrhea & GI toxins; questionable efficacy

▶ Contraindications: Should not be relied on to control severe diarrheas or to replace adequate fluid/electrolyte monitoring or as replacement therapy in severe or chronic diarrheas

▶ Adverse Effects: Transient constipation

▶ Drug Interactions

Uses/Indications

Although its efficacy is in question, kaolin/pectin is used primarily in veterinary medicine as an oral anti-diarrheal agent. It has also been used as an adsorbent agent following the ingestion of certain toxins. Administration may be difficult due to the large volumes that may be necessary to give orally.

Pharmacology/Actions

Kaolin/pectin is thought to possess adsorbent and protective qualities. Presumably, bacteria and toxins are adsorbed in the gut and the coating action of the suspension may protect inflamed GI mucosa. The pectin component, by forming galacturonic acid, has been demonstrated to decrease pH in the intestinal lumen.

In one study in children with acute nonspecific diarrhea, stool fluidity was decreased, but stool frequency, water content, and weight remained unchanged. No studies documenting the clinical efficacy of this combination in either human or veterinary species were located.

Pharmacokinetics

Neither kaolin nor pectin are absorbed after oral administration. Up to 90% of the pectin administered may be decomposed in the gut.

Contraindications/Precautions/Warnings

There are no absolute contraindications to kaolin/pectin therapy, but it should not be relied on to control severe diarrheas. Kaolin/pectin should not replace adequate fluid/electrolyte monitoring or replacement therapy in severe or chronic diarrheas.

Adverse Effects

At usual doses, kaolin/pectin generally has no adverse effects. Constipation may occur, but is usually transient and associated with high dosages. High doses in debilitated, or in very old or young patients may rarely cause fecal impaction. In rats, kaolin/pectin has been demonstrated to increase fecal sodium loss in diarrhea.

In humans, kaolin/pectin is recommended for use only under the direct supervision of a physician, in patients less than 3 years of age or for longer than 48 hours.

Reproductive/Nursing Safety

Adsorbent (only) anti-diarrheal products should be safe to use during pregnancy and lactation. The addition of other active ingredients (*e.g.*, as opiates) may alter this recommendation.

Overdosage/Acute Toxicity

Overdosage is unlikely to cause any serious effects, but constipation requiring treatment may occur.

Drug Interactions

The following drug interactions have either been reported or are theoretical in humans or animals receiving kaolin/pectin and may be of significance in veterinary patients:

▮ **DIGOXIN:** Some evidence exists that kaolin/pectin may impair the oral absorption of digoxin. Separate doses by at least two hours.

▮ **LINCOMYCIN:** Kaolin/pectin may inhibit the oral absorption of lincomycin. If both drugs are to be used, administer kaolin/pectin at least 2 hours before or 3–4 hours after the lincomycin dose.

Doses

▪ **DOGS:**

For diarrhea:

a) 1–2 mL/kg PO q2–6h (Kirk 1986)

For enterotoxins secondary to garbage ingestion:

a) 2–5 mL/kg PO q1–6 hours (Coppock & Mostrom 1986)

b) 10–15 grams of kaolin/kg PO four times daily (Grauer & Hjelle 1988)

▪ **CATS:**

For diarrhea:

a) 1–2 mL/kg PO q2–6h (Kirk 1986)

▪ **FERRETS:**

a) 1–2 mL/kg PO 3–4 times daily (Williams 2000)

▪ **RABBITS/RODENTS/SMALL MAMMALS:**

a) **Guinea pigs:** 0.2 mL PO 3–4 times a day (Adamcak & Otten 2000)

■ **CATTLE:**
   a) Adult: 4–10 fl. oz. PO; Calves: 2–3 fl. oz PO; repeat every 2–4 hours or as indicated until condition improves. If no improvement in 48 hours additional treatment is indicated. (Label Directions; *Kao-Forte®*—Vet-A-Mix)

■ **HORSES:**
   For diarrhea:
   a) 2–4 quarts PO per 450 kg body weight twice daily (Robinson 1987)
   b) 1 oz. per 8 kg body weight PO 3–4 times a day (Clark & Becht 1987)
   c) Foals: 3–4 oz PO q6–8h (authors believe that bismuth subsalicylate is superior) (Martens & Scrutchfield 1982)

■ **SWINE:**
   a) ½–2 fl. oz PO; repeat every 2–4 hours or as indicated until condition improves. If no improvement in 48 hours additional treatment is indicated. (Label Directions; *Kao-Forte®*—Vet-A-Mix)

■ **SHEEP:**
   a) 3–4 oz PO q2–3h (McConnell & Hughey 1987)

■ **BIRDS:**
   a) **Canary or parakeet:** 1 drop PO twice daily; or 1 and ½ dropperful placed in ⅔ oz. drinking water.

   Medium-sized birds: 0.5 mL PO

   Large birds: 1 mL PO 1 to 4 times a day (Stunkard 1984)
   b) 2 mL/kg PO two to four times a day (Clubb 1986)

Monitoring
■ Clinical efficacy
■ Fluid and electrolyte status in severe diarrhea

Client Information
■ Shake well before using
■ If diarrhea persists, or if animal appears listless or develops a high fever, contact veterinarian

Chemistry/Synonyms
Kaolin is a naturally occurring hydrated aluminum silicate that is powdered and refined for pharmaceutical use. Kaolin is a white/light, odorless, almost tasteless powder that is practically insoluble in water.

Pectin is a carbohydrate polymer consisting primarily of partially methoxylated polygalacturonic acids. Pectin is a course or fine, yellowish-white, almost odorless with a mucilaginous flavor. It is obtained from the inner rind of citrus fruits or from apple pomace. One gram of pectin is soluble in 20 mL of water and forms a viscous, colloidal solution.

In the United States, the two compounds generally are used together in an oral suspension formulation in most proprietary products.

Kaolin may also be known as: bolus alba, E559, weisser ton, *Childrens Diarrhoea Mixture®*, *Entrocalm®*, *Kao-Pec®*, *Kao-Pect®*, *Kao-Pront®*, *Kaogel®*; many multi-ingredient trade names are available.

Storage/Stability
Kaolin/pectin should be stored in airtight containers; protect from freezing.

Compatibility/Compounding Considerations
It is physically **incompatible** when mixed with alkalis, heavy metals, salicylic acid, tannic acid, or strong alcohol.

Dosage Forms/Regulatory Status
There are a variety of kaolin/pectin products available without prescription. Several products are labeled for veterinary use; their approval status is not known. Many products that formerly contained kaolin (*e.g.*, *Kaopectate®*) no longer contain any kaolin. In the USA, *Kaopectate®* now contains bismuth subsalicylate as its active ingredient. In Canada, *Kaopectate®* reportedly contains attapulgite..

VETERINARY-LABELED PRODUCTS:

Kaolin Pectin 90 gr kaolin/2 grams pectin per fluid oz. in 1 quart and 1 gallon containers. generic, (Bimeda, Durvet), *Kaolin Pectin Plus®* (AgriPharm), *Kao-Pec®* (AgriLabs), *Kao-Pect®* (Phoenix Pharmaceutical), Kaopectolin (Aspen, Butler); (OTC). Products may be labeled for use in horses, dogs and cats.

Kaolin Pectin 90 grams kaolin/4 grams pectin per fl oz. in 1 gallon containers. Kaolin Pectin Suspension (Vedco); (OTC)

HUMAN-LABELED PRODUCTS:

Kaolin, Pectin Antidiarrheal Suspension: 90 grams kaolin, 2 grams pectin/30 mL in 180 mL and 360 mL, pt and UD 30 mL; Kapectolin (various); generic; (OTC)

References

Adamcak, A. & B. Otten (2000). Rodent Therapeutics. *Vet Clin NA: Exotic Anim Pract* 3:1(Jan): 221–240.

Clark, E.S. & J.L. Becht (1987). Clinical Pharmacology of the Gastrointestinal Tract. *Vet Clin North Am (Equine Practice)* 3(1): 101–122.

Clubb, S.L. (1986). Therapeutics: Individual and Flock Treatment Regimens. *Clinical Avian Medicine and Surgery*. GJ Harrison and LR Harrison Eds. Philadelphia, W.B. Saunders: 327–355.

Coppock, R.W. & M.S. Mostrom (1986). Intoxication Due to Contaminated Garbage, Food, and Water. *Current Veterinary Therapy IX: Small Animal Practice*. K R.W. Ed. Philadelphia, W.B. Saunders: 221–225.

Grauer, G.F. & J.J. Hjelle (1988). Household Drugs. *Handbook of Small Animal Practice*. RV Morgan Ed. New York, Churchill Livingstone: 1115–1118.

Kirk, R.W., Ed. (1986). *Current Veterinary Therapy IX, Small Animal Practice*. Philadelphia, W.B. Saunders.

Martens, R.J. & W.L. Scrutchfield (1982). Foal Diarrhea: Pathogenesis, Etiology, and Therapy. *Comp Cont Ed* 4(4): S175–S186.

McConnell, V.C. & T. Hughey (1987). *Formulary, The University of Georgia, Veterinary Medical Teaching Hospital*. Athens, GA.

Robinson, N.E. (1987). Table of Common Drugs: Approximate Doses. *Current Therapy in Equine Medicine, 2*. NE Robinson Ed. Philadelphia, W.B. Saunders: 761.

Stunkard, J.M. (1984). *Diagnosis, Treatment and Husbandry of Pet Birds*. Edgewater, MD, Stunkard Publishing.

Williams, B. (2000). Therapeutics in Ferrets. *Vet Clin NA: Exotic Anim Pract* 3:1(Jan): 131–153.

KETAMINE HCL

(**kee**-ta-meen)   Ketaset®, Ketaflo®, Vetalar®

DISSOCIATIVE GENERAL ANESTHETIC;
NMDA-RECEPTOR ANTAGONIST

Prescriber Highlights

▶ Dissociative general anesthetic; also inhibits NMDA-receptors so may be adjunctively useful to control pain

▶ Contraindications: Prior hypersensitivity reactions; animals to be used for human consumption, alone for general anesthesia, increased CSF pressure/head trauma

▶ Relative contraindications: Significant blood loss, malignant hyperthermia, increased intra-ocular pressure or open globe injuries; procedures involving the pharynx, larynx, or trachea

▶ Caution: Significant hypertension, heart failure, & arterial aneurysms, hepatic or renal insufficiency, seizure disorders

▶ Adverse Effects: Hypertension, hypersalivation, respiratory depression, hyperthermia, emesis, vocalization, erratic & prolonged recovery, dyspnea, spastic jerking movements, seizures, muscular tremors, hypertonicity, opisthotonos, & cardiac arrest; pain after IM injection may occur

▶ Cats' eyes remain open after ketamine; protect

▶ Minimize exposure to handling or loud noises during the recovery period, but monitor adequately

▶ Drug interactions

Uses/Indications

Ketamine has been FDA-approved for use in humans, sub-human primates, and cats, although it has been used in many other species (see Dosage section). The FDA-approved indications for cats include, "for restraint, or as the sole anesthetic agent for diagnostic, or minor, brief, surgical procedures that do not require skeletal muscle relaxation . . . and in subhuman primates for restraint." (Package Insert; *Ketaset®*—Bristol).

Ketamine can inhibit NMDA receptors in the CNS and can decrease "wind-up" effect. There is increasing interest in using it to prevent exaggerated pain associated with surgery or chronic pain states in animals.

Pharmacology/Actions

Ketamine is a rapid acting general anesthetic that has significant analgesic activity and a relative lack of cardiopulmonary depressant effects in healthy animals. It is thought to induce both anesthesia and amnesia by functionally disrupting the CNS through over stimulating the CNS or inducing a cataleptic state. Ketamine inhibits GABA, and may block serotonin, norepinephrine, and dopamine in the CNS. The thalamoneocortical system is depressed while the limbic system is activated. It induces anesthetic stages I and II, but not stage III. In cats, it causes a slight hypothermic effect as body temperatures decrease on average by 1.6°C after therapeutic doses.

Effects on muscle tone are described as being variable, but ketamine generally either causes no changes in muscle tone or increased tone. Ketamine does not abrogate the pinnal and pedal reflexes, nor the photic, corneal, laryngeal or pharyngeal reflexes.

Ketamine's effects on the cardiovascular system include increased cardiac output, heart rate, mean aortic pressure, pulmonary artery pressure, and central venous pressure. Its effects on total peripheral resistance are described as being variable. Cardiovascular effects are secondary to increased sympathetic tone; ketamine has negative inotropic effects if the sympathetic system is blocked.

Ketamine can cause apneustic breathing (rapid breaths followed by breath-holding). It does not cause significant respiratory depression at usual doses, but at higher doses it can cause respiratory rates to decrease. Ketamine can cause bronchodilation and in humans with asthma, ketamine causes decreased airway resistance.

Pharmacokinetics

After IM injection in the cat, peak levels occur in approximately 10 minutes. Administration of a ketamine spray sublingually to cats appears to be absorbed enough to have pharmacologic action (Issabeagloo 2008). Ketamine is distributed into all body tissues rapidly, with highest levels found in the brain, liver, lung, and fat. Plasma protein binding is approximately 50% in the horse, 53% in the dogs, and 37–53% in the cat.

In most species, ketamine is metabolized in the liver principally by demethylation and hydroxylation and these metabolites, along with unchanged ketamine, are eliminated in the urine. One active metabolite, nor-ketamine, has 10-30% of the activity of the parent compound. In cats, ketamine is almost exclusively excreted unchanged in the urine. Ketamine will induce hepatic microsomal enzymes, but there appears to be little clinical significance associated with this effect. The elimination half-life in the cat, calf, and horse is approximately 1 hour, in humans it is 2–3 hours. Like the thiobarbiturates, the redistribution of ketamine out of the CNS is more of a factor in determining duration of anesthesia than is the elimination half-life.

By increasing the dose, the duration of anesthesia will increase, but not the intensity.

Contraindications/Precautions/Warnings

Ketamine is contraindicated in patients who have exhibited prior hypersensitivity reactions to it and animals to be used for human consumption. Use in patients with significant hypertension, heart failure, and arterial aneurysms could be hazardous. The manufacturer warns against its use in patients with hepatic or renal insufficiency but in humans with renal insufficiency, the duration of action is not prolonged. Because ketamine does not provide good muscle relaxation, it is contraindicated when used alone for major surgery.

Ketamine can cause increases in CSF pressure and it should not be used in cases with elevated pressures or when head trauma has occurred. Because of its supposed epileptogenic potential, it should generally not be used (unless very cautiously) in animals with preexisting seizure disorders. As myelography can induce seizures, ketamine should be used cautiously in animals undergoing this procedure.

Ketamine is considered to be relatively contraindicated when increased intra-ocular pressure or open globe injuries exist, and for procedures involving the pharynx, larynx, or trachea. Animals that have lost significant amounts of blood, may require significantly reduced ketamine dosages.

While ketamine has been used safely in humans with malignant hyperthermia, its use in animals susceptible to this condition is controversial.

Ketamine can increase heart rate, increase blood pressure and myocardial oxygen consumption; its use should be avoided in cats with hypertrophic cardiomyopathy (HCM) or in other patients where an increase in heart rate, blood pressure and myocardial oxygen consumption can be detrimental (*e.g.*, unstable shock or congestive heart failure). Its effects on respiratory function may be enhanced in patients with unstable cardiopulmonary function. Because of ketamine's tendencies to increase sympathetic tone (increased norepinephrine release), it should be used with caution in animals where increased sympathetic tone concurrently exists (*e.g.*, pheochromocytoma, hyperthyroidism). Hyperthyroid human patients (and those receiving exogenous thyroid replacement) may be susceptible to developing severe hypertension and tachycardia when given ketamine. The veterinary significance of this potential problem is unknown.

Cats' eyes remain open after receiving ketamine, and should be protected from injury plus an ophthalmic lubricant (*e.g.*, *Lacri-Lube*®) should be applied to prevent excessive drying of the cornea.

Because ketamine is excreted almost exclusively via renal mechanisms, it should be used with caution in cats with reduced renal function.

To minimize the incidences of emergence reactions, it is recommended to minimize exposure to handling or loud noises during the recovery period. The monitoring of vital signs should still be performed during the recovery phase, however.

Because ketamine can increase blood pressure, careful control of post-surgical hemorrhage (*e.g.*, declawing) should be managed. It is not essential to withhold food or water prior to surgery, but in elective procedures, it is recommended to withhold food for 6 hours prior to surgery.

Adverse Effects

In species where the drug is FDA-approved, the following adverse reactions are listed by the manufacturer: "respiratory depression . . . following high doses, emesis, vocalization, erratic and prolonged recovery, dyspnea, spastic jerking movements, convulsions, muscular tremors, hypertonicity, opisthotonos and cardiac arrest. In the cat, myoclonic jerking and/or tonic/clonic convulsions can be controlled by ultrashort-acting barbiturates or acepromazine. These latter drugs must be given intravenously, cautiously, and slowly, to effect (approximately $1/6$ to $1/4$ the normal dose may be required)." (Package Insert; *Ketaset*®—Fort Dodge)

Seizures have been reported to occur in up to 20% of cats that receive ketamine at therapeutic dosages. Diazepam is suggested if treatment is necessary. It has been reported to rarely cause a variety of other CNS effects (mild CNS effects to blindness and death). Ketamine has been documented to cause hyperthermia in cats; low doses of acepromazine (0.01–0.02 mg/kg IV) may alleviate. Anecdotal reports of ketamine causing acute, CHF in cats with mild to moderate heart disease have been reported.

Pain after IM injection may occur.

To reduce the incidence of hypersalivation and other autonomic signs, atropine or glycopyrrolate is often administered.

Reproductive/Nursing Safety

In humans, the FDA categorizes this drug as category **C** for use during pregnancy (*Animal studies have shown an adverse effect on the fetus, but there are no adequate studies in humans; or there are no animal reproduction studies and no adequate studies in humans.*) In a separate system evaluating the safety of drugs in canine and feline pregnancy (Papich 1989), this drug is categorized as class: **B** (*Safe for use if used cautiously. Studies in laboratory animals may have uncovered some risk, but these drugs appear to be safe in dogs and cats or these drugs are safe if they are not administered when the animal is near term.*)

No specific lactation information was found.

Overdosage/Acute Toxicity

Ketamine is considered to have a wide therapeutic index (approximately 5 times greater when compared to pentobarbital). When given too rapidly or in excessive doses, significant respiratory depression may occur. Treatment using mechanically assisted respiratory support is recommended versus the use of analeptic agents. In cats, yohimbine with 4-aminopyridine has been suggested for use as a partial antagonist.

Drug Interactions

The following drug interactions have either been reported or are theoretical in humans or animals receiving ketamine and may be of significance in veterinary patients:

- **CHLORAMPHENICOL (parenteral):** May prolong the anesthetic actions of ketamine
- **CNS DEPRESSANTS:** Narcotics, barbiturates, or diazepam may prolong the recovery time after ketamine anesthesia
- **HALOTHANE:** When used with halothane, ketamine recovery rates may be prolonged and the cardiac stimulatory effects of ketamine may be inhibited; close monitoring of cardiac status is recommended when using ketamine with halothane
- **IVERMECTIN:** It has been recommended not to use ivermectin in reptiles within 10 days of ketamine (Bays 2009)
- **NEUROMUSCULAR BLOCKERS (e.g., succinylcholine and tubocurarine):** May cause enhanced or prolonged respiratory depression
- **THYROID HORMONES:** When given concomitantly with ketamine, thyroid hormones have induced hypertension and tachycardia in humans; beta-blockers (e.g., propranolol) may be of benefit in treating these effects

Doses

Note: Ketamine is used in many different combinations with other agents. The following are representative, but not necessarily inclusive; it is suggested to refer to a recent veterinary anesthesia reference for more information.

- **DOGS:**

  As an adjunct to anesthesia:

  a) For use in combination with an opioid and ketamine (so-called "doggie magic") to provide anesthesia and pain management (**Note:** reference has dosing tables for conversion of patient weight to various micrograms/m^2 doses of dexmedetomidine; opioid concentrations used in the reference are: Butorphanol 10 mg/mL, Hydromorphone 2 mg/mL, Morphine 15 mg/mL, & Buprenorphine 0.3 mg/mL. Ketamine concentration is 100 mg/mL. As these drugs may be available in other concentrations, only use those products with the above concentrations if using this protocol.):

  For geriatric dogs, dogs with renal or liver dysfunction as a premed prior to propofol or face mask induction, followed by maintenance on isoflurane or sevoflu-

rane: dexmedetomidine at 62.5 micrograms/m^2. Combine with equal volumes of one of the opioids noted above and ketamine. May administer IM or IV.

For slightly heavier sedation in ASA class II or II dogs requiring sedation for radiographic procedures: Dexmedetomidine at 125 micrograms/m^2. Combine with equal volumes of one of the opioids noted above and ketamine. May administer IM or IV.

For dogs undergoing minor surgery, Penn hip or OFA-types of radiographic procedures that require significant muscle relaxation: Dexmedetomidine at 250 micrograms/m^2. Combine with equal volumes of one of the opioids noted above and ketamine. May administer IM or IV.

To induce a surgical plane of anesthesia for OHE, castration, or other abdominal surgery: Dexmedetomidine at 375 micrograms/m^2. Combine with equal volumes of one of the opioids noted above and ketamine. May administer IM or IV. Provides rapid immobilization; lateral recumbency in 5-8 minutes. Dogs can be intubated and maintained on oxygen. Supplemental low doses of isoflurane (0.5%) or sevoflurane (1%) can be used.

For immobilizing extremely fractious dogs and wolf-hybrid dogs: Dexmedetomidine at 500 micrograms/m^2. Combine with equal volumes of one of the opioids noted above and ketamine. Administer IM. This dose is rarely required.

To reverse above, atipamezole IM at the same volume as the dexmedetomidine. (Ko 2009)

As an NMDA antagonist for adjunctive pain control:

a) 0.1−1 mg/kg PO, IM or SC q4−6h for mild to moderate pain in conjunction with opioids. (Nieves 2002)

b) For intraoperative use: If anesthesia was induced with a drug other than ketamine, give a loading dose of 0.5 mg/kg IV, then an infusion of 10−20 micrograms/kg/minute. A CRI of 2−10 micrograms/kg/minute can be used post-op. (Hellyer 2006)

c) In combination with opioids or lidocaine: 0.5 mg/kg IV loading bolus followed by 10 micrograms/kg/min CRI during surgery and 2 micrograms/kg/min for 24 hrs following surgery. (Shaffran 2009)

- **CATS:**

  Most clinicians recommend giving atropine or glycopyrrolate before use to decrease hypersalivation.

a) 11 mg/kg IM for restraint; 22–33 mg/kg for diagnostic or minor surgical procedures not requiring skeletal muscle relaxation (Package Insert; *Ketaset®*—Bristol)

b) For use in combination with an opioid and ketamine (so-called "kitty magic", "DKT" or "Triple Combination") to provide sedation and analgesia (**Note:** Opioid concentrations used in the reference are: Butorphanol 10 mg/mL, Hydromorphone 2 mg/mL, Morphine 15 mg/mL, & Buprenorphine 0.3 mg/mL. Ketamine concentration is 100 mg/mL. Dexmedetomidine concentration is 0.5 mg/mL. As these drugs may be available in other concentrations, only use those products with the above concentrations if using this protocol.):

For the chart below: MILD = For sedation or as a premed prior to propofol or face mask induction; MODERATE = For castration or minor surgical procedures; PROFOUND = Invasive surgical procedures including OHE and declaws. Cats can be reversed immediately with an equal volume (of the dexmedetomidine dose) of atipamezole.

Cat Weight		Volume (of each) of: Dexmedetomidine-Opioid-Ketamine			IM Route
Lbs	Kg	MILD	MODERATE	PROFOUND	
4-7	2-3	0.025 mL	0.05 mL	0.1–0.15 mL	
7-9	3-4	0.05 mL	0.1 mL	0.2–0.25 mL	
9-13	4-6	0.1 mL	0.2 mL	0.3–0.35 mL	
14-15	6-7	0.2 mL	0.3 mL	0.4–0.45 mL	
15-18	7-8	0.3 mL	0.4 mL	0.5–0.55 mL	

(Ko 2009)

c) In combination as an immobilizing agent: For cats requiring more sedation when insufficient sedation from opioid, higher doses of medetomidine, and midazolam: butorphanol 0.2 mg/kg; medetomidine 0.015–0.02 mg/kg; midazolam 0.05–0.2 mg/kg; ketamine 1–5 mg/kg; all are given IM. For painful procedures consider adding buprenorphine at 0.02–0.04 mg/kg or substituting butorphanol or buprenorphine with either morphine 0.5 mg/kg or hydromorphone 0.1 mg/kg. More information available from: www.vsag.org.

For highly aggressive cats, 1 mL of ketamine can be sprayed into the open mouth or directed into the cat's mouth using a feline urethral catheter through the cage bars. The drug should be sprayed quickly so the cat does not chew and swallow the catheter. (Moffat 2008)

As an NMDA antagonist for adjunctive pain control:

a) 0.1–1 mg/kg IM or SC q4–6h for mild to moderate pain in conjunction with opioids. (Nieves 2002)

b) For intraoperative use: If anesthesia was induced with a drug other than ketamine, give a loading dose of 0.5 mg/kg IV, then an infusion of 10–20 micrograms/kg/minute. A CRI of 2–10 micrograms/kg/minute can be used post-op. (Hellyer 2006)

c) In combination with opioids or lidocaine: 0.5 mg/kg IV loading bolus followed by 10 micrograms/kg/min CRI during surgery and 2 micrograms/kg/min for 24 hrs following surgery.

Using the MLK (morphine/lidocaine/ketamine) mixture: To a 500 mL bag of LRS add 10 mg morphine sulfate, 120 mg lidocaine, and 100 mg ketamine. Infuse at a rate of 10 mL/kg/hr (will provide morphine at 0.2 mg/kg/hr, lidocaine 40 micrograms/kg/minute, and ketamine 2 mg/kg/hr). Can add dexmedetomidine if needed. (Shaffran 2009)

■ **RABBITS/RODENTS/SMALL MAMMALS:**

For chemical restraint:

a) **Mice:** Alone: 50 –100 mg/kg IM or IP, 50 mg/kg IV;
In combination with diazepam: Ketamine 200 mg/kg with Diazepam 5 mg/kg IM or IP;
In combination with xylazine: Ketamine 100 mg/kg with Xylazine 5–15 mg/kg IM or IP (Burke 1999)

b) **Rats:** Alone: 50 –100 mg/kg IM or IP, 40–50 mg/kg IV;
In combination with diazepam: Ketamine 40–60 mg/kg with Diazepam 5–10 mg/kg IP;
In combination with xylazine: Ketamine 40–75 mg/kg with Xylazine 5–12 mg/kg IM or IP (Burke 1999)

c) **Hamsters/Gerbils:** 100 mg/kg IM;
In combination with diazepam: Ketamine 50 mg/kg with Diazepam 5 mg/kg IM;
In combination with xylazine: Not recommended (Burke 1999)

d) **Guinea pig:** Alone: 10–30 mg/kg IM;
In combination with diazepam: Ketamine 60–100 mg/kg with Diazepam 5–8 mg/kg IM;
In combination with xylazine: Ketamine 85 mg/kg with Xylazine 12–13 mg/kg IM (Burke 1999)

e) **Rabbits:** Alone: 20–60 mg/kg IM or IV;
In combination with diazepam: Ketamine 60–80 mg/kg with Diazepam 5–10 mg/kg IM;
In combination with xylazine: Ketamine 10 mg/kg with Xylazine 3 mg/kg IV (Burke 1999)

f) **Rabbits:** Alone: 20–50 mg/kg IM or 15–20 mg/kg IV

In combination with diazepam for induction: Diazepam 5–10 mg/kg IM give ketamine 30 minutes after diazepam at 20–40 mg/kg IM or Diazepam 0.2–0.5 mg/kg and Ketamine 10–15 mg/kg (to effect) IV;

In combination with diazepam for anesthesia without inhalants: Diazepam 5–10 mg/kg IM plus ketamine 60–80 mg/kg IM 30 minutes later;

In combination with xylazine: Not recommended for pet rabbits (Ivey & Morrisey 2000)

g) Injectable anesthesia: **Rodents:** midazolam (5 mg/kg) + ketamine (100 mg/kg) + buprenorphine (0.05 mg/kg) IP.

Rabbits: Midazolam (0.05 mg/kg) + buprenorphine (0.03 mg/kg) + ketamine (10 mg/kg) IM. (Bennett 2009)

■ **FERRETS:**

a) For injectable anesthesia: Butorphanol 0.1 mg/kg, Ketamine 5 mg/kg, medetomidine 80 micrograms/kg. Combine in one syringe and give IM. May need to supplement with isoflurane (0.5–1.5%) for abdominal surgery. (Finkler 1999)

■ **CATTLE:**

a) Premedicate with atropine and xylazine, then ketamine 2 mg/kg IV bolus (Thurmon & Benson 1986)

b) After sedation, 2.2 mg/kg IV (Mandsager 1988)

c) As a CRI for adjunctive analgesia: 0.4–1.2 mg/kg/hr. (Miesner 2009)

■ **HORSES: (Note:** ARCI UCGFS Class 2 Drug)

a) For field anesthesia: Sedate with xylazine (1 mg/kg IV; 2 mg/kg IM) given 5–10 minutes (longer for IM route) before induction of anesthesia with ketamine (2 mg/kg IV). Horse must be adequately sedated (head to the knees) before giving the ketamine (ketamine can cause muscle rigidity and seizures). If adequate sedation does not occur, either: **1)** Redose xylazine: up to half the original dose, or **2)** Add butorphanol (0.02–0.04 mg/kg IV). Butorphanol can be given with the original xylazine if you suspect that the horse will be difficult to tranquilize (e.g., high-strung Thoroughbreds) or added before the ketamine. This combination will improve induction, increase analgesia and increase recumbency time by about 5–10 minutes, or **3)** Diazepam (0.03 mg/kg IV). Mix the diazepam with the ketamine. This combination will improve induction when sedation is marginal, improve muscle relaxation during anesthesia and prolong anesthesia by

about 5–10 minutes, or **4)** Guaifenesin (5% solution administered IV to effect) can also be used to increase sedation and muscle relaxation. (Mathews 1999)

b) Initially give xylazine 1.1 mg/kg IV and wait for full sedative effect (4–8 minutes); then give ketamine 2.2–2.75 mg/kg IV only (the higher dose may be necessary for ponies, young "high-strung" Arabians, Hackneys, and Thoroughbreds) as a bolus. Do not administer to an "excited" horse. If surgery time requires additional anesthesia, ⅓–½ of the original xylazine/ketamine doses may be given IV. For procedures where better muscle relaxation is required, use guaifenesin-thiobarbiturate. Do not disturb horse until fully recovered. (Thurmon & Benson 1987)

c) For foals and ponies: Add 500 mg ketamine and 250 mg xylazine to 500 mL of 5% guaifenesin solution. For induction, give 1.1 mL/kg IV rapidly. Anesthesia may be maintained by constant IV infusion of 2–3 mL/kg/hr. Lower doses for foals, higher doses for ponies. (Thurmon & Benson 1987)

d) For induction of surgical colic patients: Use guaifenesin to effect, than 1.6–2.2 mg/kg ketamine (Mandsager 1988)

e) 200 mg bolus (in a 454 kg horse) intraoperatively to reduce movement with light general anesthesia (Mandsager 1988)

■ **SWINE:**

a) Give atropine, then ketamine at 11 mg/kg IM. To prolong anesthesia and increase analgesia give additional ketamine 2–4 mg/kg IV. Local anesthetics injected at the surgical site (e.g., 2% lidocaine) may enhance analgesia. (Thurmon & Benson 1986)

b) Ketamine (22 mg/kg) combined with acepromazine (1.1 mg/kg) IM (Swindle 1985)

c) 4.4 mg/kg IM or IV after sedation (Mandsager 1988)

■ **SHEEP:**

a) Premedicate with atropine (0.22 mg/kg) and acepromazine (0.55 mg/kg; then ketamine 22 mg/kg IM. To extend anesthetic time, may give ketamine intermittently IV at 2–4 mg/kg. (Thurmon & Benson 1986)

b) 2 mg/kg IV for induction, then 4 mL/minute constant infusion of ketamine in a concentration of 2 mg/mL in D_5W (Thurmon & Benson 1986)

■ **GOATS:**

a) Give atropine 0.4 mg/kg, followed by xylazine 0.22 mg/kg IM 20–25 minutes later. Approximately 10 minutes after xylazine give ketamine 11 mg/kg IM. To extend anesthesia give ketamine 2–4 mg/kg IV (shorter extension) or 6 mg/kg (longer extension). (Thurmon & Benson 1986)

■ **CAMELIDS (llamas and alpacas):**

a) As an anesthetic: butorphanol 0.07–0.1 mg/kg; ketamine 0.2–0.3 mg/kg; xylazine 0.2–0.3 mg/kg IV or butorphanol 0.05–0.1 mg/kg; ketamine 0.2–0.5 mg/kg; xylazine 0.2–0.5 mg/kg IM (Wolff 2009)

b) For procedural pain (*e.g.*, castrations) when recumbency (up to 30 minutes) is desired: Alpacas: butorphanol 0.046 mg/kg; xylazine 0.46 mg/kg; ketamine 4.6 mg/kg. Llamas: butorphanol 0.037 mg/kg; xylazine 0.37 mg/kg; ketamine 3.7 mg/kg. All drugs are combined in one syringe and given IM. May administer 50% of original dose of ketamine and xylazine during anesthesia to prolong effect up to 15 minutes.

If doing mass castrations on 3 or more animals, can make up bottle of the "cocktail". Add 10 mg (1 mL) of butorphanol and 100 mg (1 mL) xylazine to a 1 gram (10 ml) vial of ketamine. This mixture is dosed at 1 mL/40 lbs. (18 kg) for alpacas, and 1 mL per 50 lbs. (22 kg) for llamas. Handle quietly and allow plenty of time before starting procedure. Expect 20 minutes of surgical time; patient should stand 45 minutes to 1 hour after injection. (Miesner 2009)

■ **REPTILES:**

a) **Medium to small land Tortoises:** Medetomidine 100–150 micrograms/kg with ketamine 5–10 mg/kg IV or IM;

Freshwater Turtles: Medetomidine 150–300 micrograms/kg with ketamine 10–20 mg/kg IV or IM;

Giant Land Tortoises: 200 kg Aldabra tortoise: Medetomidine 40 micrograms/kg with ketamine 4 mg/kg IV or IM

Smaller Aldabra tortoises: Medetomidine 40–80 micrograms/kg with ketamine 4–8 mg/kg IV or IM. Wait 30–40 minutes for peak effect;

Iguanas: Medetomidine 100–150 micrograms/kg with ketamine 5–10 mg/kg IV or IM;

Reversal of all dosages with atipamezole is 4–5 times the medetomidine dose (Heard 1999)

■ **BIRDS:**

a) Birds weighing:

<100 grams (canaries, finches, budgies): 0.1–0.2 mg/gm IM;

250–500 grams (parrots, pigeons): 0.05–0.1 mg/gm IM;

500 grams–3 kg (chickens, owls, hawks): 0.02–0.1 mg/gm IM;

>3 kg (ducks, geese, swans): 0.02–0.05 mg/gm IM (Booth 1988)

b) In combination with xylazine: Ketamine 10–30 mg/kg IM; Xylazine 2–6 mg/kg IM; birds less than 250 grams require a higher dosage (per kg) than birds weighing greater than 250 g. Xylazine is not recommended to be used in debilitated birds because of its cardiodepressant effects.

In combination with diazepam: Ketamine 10–50 mg/kg IM; Diazepam 0.5–2 mg/kg IM or IV; doses can be halved for IV use.

In combination with acepromazine: Ketamine 25–50 mg/kg IM; Acepromazine 0.5–1 mg/kg IM (Wheler 1993)

■ **ZOO, EXOTIC, WILDLIFE SPECIES:**

For use of ketamine in zoo, exotic and wildlife medicine refer to specific references, including:

a) *Zoo Animal and Wildlife Immobilization and Anesthesia.* West, G, Heard, D, Caulkett, N. (eds.). Blackwell Publishing, 2007.

b) *Handbook of Wildlife Chemical Immobilization, 3rd Ed.* Kreeger, T.J. and J.M. Arnemo. 2007.

c) *Restraint and Handling of Wild and Domestic Animals.* Fowler, M (ed.), Iowa State University Press, 1995

d) *Exotic Animal Formulary, 3rd Ed.* Carpenter, J.W., Saunders. 2005

e) The 2009 American Association of Zoo Veterinarian Proceedings by D. K. Fontenot also has several dosages listed for restraint, anesthesia, and analgesia for a variety of drugs for carnivores and primates. VIN members can access them at: http://goo.gl/BHRih or http://goo.gl/9UJse

Monitoring

■ Level of anesthesia/analgesia

■ Respiratory function; cardiovascular status (rate, rhythm, BP if possible)

■ Monitor eyes to prevent drying or injury;

■ Body temperature

Client Information

■ Should only be administered by individuals familiar with its use.

Chemistry/Synonyms

A congener of phencyclidine, ketamine HCl occurs as white, crystalline powder. It has a melting point of 258–261°C, a characteristic odor, and will precipitate as the free base at high pH. One gram is soluble in 5 mL of water, and 14 mL of alcohol. The pH of the commercially-available injections are between 3.5–5.5.

Ketamine HCl may also be known as: CI-581, CL-369, CN-52372-2, ketamini hydrochloridum, *Amtech®, Brevinaze®, Calypsol®, Cost®, Inducmina®, Keta®, Keta-Hameln®, Ketaject®, Ketalin®, Ketanest®, Ketaset®, Ketasthesia®, Ketasthetic®, Ketava®, Ketina®, Ketmin®, Ketolar®, Velonarcon®, VetaKet®,* and *Vetalar®.*

Storage/Stability

Ketamine injection should be stored between 15–30°C (59–86°C) and protected from light.

Solution may darken upon prolonged exposure to light which does not affect the drug's potency. Do not use if precipitates appear.

Ketamine may be mixed with sterile water for injection, D_5W, and normal saline for diluent purposes. Do not mix ketamine with barbiturates or diazepam in the same syringe or IV bag as precipitation may occur.

Compatibility/Compounding Considerations

Ketamine may be mixed with sterile water for injection, D_5W, and normal saline for diluent purposes. Ketamine is physically **compatible in the same syringe** with xylazine, morphine, fentanyl, dexamethasone sodium phosphate, lidocaine, bupivacaine and doxapram (if used within 9 hours).

Mixing ketamine with barbiturates or diazepam in the same syringe or IV bag is not recommended as precipitation may occur. Although there are many anecdotal reports of mixing ketamine with diazepam, or ketamine with midazolam in the same syringe just prior to injection there does not appear to be any published information documenting the stability of the drugs after mixing. Do not use if a visible precipitate forms.

A study (Taylor *et al.* 2009) evaluating the stability, sterility, pH, particulate formation and efficacy in laboratory rodents of compounded ketamine, acepromazine and xylazine ("KAX") supported the finding that the drugs are stable and efficacious for at least 180 days after mixing if stored in the dark at room temperature.

Information "on file" with the manufacturer states that dexmedetomidine 0.5 mg/mL solution for injection can be mixed with butorphanol 2 mg/mL or with ketamine 50 mg/mL solution, or with butorphanol 2 mg/mL solution and ketamine 50 mg/mL solution, in the same syringe and possesses no pharmacological risk.

Dosage Forms/Regulatory Status

VETERINARY-LABELED PRODUCTS:

Ketamine HCl for Injection: 100 mg/mL in 10 mL vials; *Ketaject®* (Phoenix Pharmaceutical), *Ketaset®* (Pfizer), *Keta-sthetic®* (RXV), *Vetalar®* (BIVI), *VetaKet®* (Lloyd), generic; (Rx, C-III). FDA-approved for use in cats and sub-human primates.

The ARCI (Racing Commissioners International) has designated this drug as a class 2 substance. See the appendix for more information.

HUMAN-LABELED PRODUCTS:

Ketamine HCl Injection: 10 mg/mL in 20 mL vials; 50 mg/mL in 10 mL vials & 100 mg/mL in 5 mL vials; *Ketalar®* (JHP); generic; (Rx, C-III)

References

Bays, T. (2009). Practice tips for exotic animals. Proceedings: WVC. Accessed via: Veterinary Information Network. http://goo.gl/faYZP

Bennett, R. (2009). Small Mammal Anesthesia—Rabbits and Rodents. Proceedings: ACVC. Accessed via: Veterinary Information Network. http://goo.gl/hRqTS

Booth, N.H. (1988). Drugs Acting on the Central Nervous System. Veterinary Pharmacology and Therapeutics–6th Ed. NH Booth and LE McDonald Eds. Ames, Iowa State University Press: 153–408.

Burke, T. (1999). Husbandry and Medicine of Rodents and Lagomorphs. Proceedings: Central Veterinary Conference, Kansas City.

Finkler, M. (1999). Anesthesia in Ferrets. Proceedings: Central Veterinary Conference, Kansas City.

Heard, D. (1999). Advances in Reptile Anesthesia. The North American Veterinary Conference, Orlando.

Hellyer, P. (2006). Pain assessment and multimodal analgesic therapy in dogs and cats. Proceedings: ABVP. Accessed via: Veterinary Information Network. http://goo.gl/LMXcX

Issabeagloo, E. (2008). Comparison of sedative effects of oral ketamine and alprazolam in cat (Poster Session). Intl Jnl Psychophysiology 69: 276–316.

Ivey, E. & J. Morrisey (2000). Therapeutics for Rabbits. Vet Clin NA: Exotic Anim Pract 3:1(Jan): 183–216.

Ko, J. (2009). Dexmedetomidine and its injectable anesthetic-pain management combinations. Proceedings: ACVC. Accessed via: Veterinary Information Network. http://goo.gl/8UTsp

Mandsager, R.E. (1988, Last Update). "Personal Communication."

Mathews, N. (1999). Anesthesia in large animals—Injectable (field) anesthesia: How to make it better. Proceedings: Central Veterinary Conference, Kansas City.

Miesner, M. (2009). Field anesthesia techniques in camelids. Proceedings: WVC. Accessed via: Veterinary Information Network. http://goo.gl/aYHQB

Moffat, K. (2008). Addressing canine and feline aggression in the veterinary clinic. Vet Clin NA: Sm Anim Pract 38: 983–1003.

Nieves, M. (2002). Pain management in the orthopedic patient. Proceedings: Western Veterinary Conference. Accessed via: Veterinary Information Network. http://goo.gl/udPdg

Papich, M. (1989). Effects of drugs on pregnancy. Current Veterinary Therapy X: Small Animal Practice. R Kirk Ed. Philadelphia, Saunders: 1291–1299.

Shaffran, N. (2009). Leaps and Bounds in Pain Management with CRIS. Proceedings: IVECCS. Accessed via: Veterinary Information Network. http://goo.gl/8N6sW

Swindle, M.M. (1985). Anesthesia in Swine. Charles River Tech Bul 3(3).

Taylor, B.J., S.A. Orr, et al. (2009). Beyond-Use Dating of Extemporaneously Compounded Ketamine, Acepromazine, and Xylazine: Safety, Stability, and Efficacy over Time. Journal of the American Association for Laboratory Animal Science 48(6): 718–726.

Thurmon, J.C. & G.J. Benson (1986). Anesthesia in ruminants and swine. Current Veterinary Therapy 2: Food Animal Practice. JL Howard Ed. Philadelphia, WB Saunders: 51–71.

Thurmon, J.C. & G.J. Benson (1987). Injectable anesthetics and anesthetic adjuncts. Vet Clin North Am (Equine Practice) 3(1): 15–36.

Wheler, C. (1993). Avian anesthetics, analgesics, and tranquilizers. Seminars in Avian & Exotic Med 2(1): 7–12.

Wolff, P. (2009). Camelid Medicine. Proceedings: AAZV. Accessed via: Veterinary Information Network. http://goo.gl/4TEAy

KETOCONAZOLE

(kee-toe-*kah*-na-zole)   Nizoral®

AZOLE ANTIFUNGAL

Prescriber Highlights

▶ Original imidazole oral antifungal used for systemic mycoses, including aspergillosis, cryptococcal meningitis, blastomycosis, & histoplasmosis; also used to reduce dose/costs of cyclosporine therapy and as an alternative treatment of hyperadrenocorticism in dogs.

▶ Contraindications: Known hypersensitivity; some believe ketoconazole is contraindicated in cats

▶ Caution: Hepatic disease or thrombocytopenia

▶ Potentially teratogenic & embryotoxic; weigh risks vs. benefits

▶ May cause infertility in male dogs by decreasing testosterone synthesis.

▶ Adverse Effects: GI (anorexia, vomiting, &/or diarrhea) most common & more prevalent in cats; hepatic toxicity, thrombocytopenia, reversible lightening of haircoat, transient dose-related suppressant effect on gonadal & adrenal steroid synthesis

▶ Long-term treatment may be required

▶ Many drug interactions

Uses/Indications

Because of its comparative lack of toxicity when compared to amphotericin B, oral administration, and relatively good efficacy, ketoconazole has been used to treat several fungal infections in dogs, cats, and other small species. Ketoconazole is often employed with amphotericin B to enhance the efficacy of ketoconazole, and by reducing the dose of amphotericin B, decreasing its risk of toxicity. See the Dosage section or Pharmacology section for specifics. Newer antifungal agents (fluconazole, itraconazole) have advantages over ketoconazole, primarily less toxicity and/or enhanced efficacy; however, ketoconazole can be significantly less expensive than the newer agents. Ketoconazole is considered by some to still be the drug of choice for treating histoplasmosis in dogs.

Use of ketoconazole in cats is controversial and some say it should never be used that species.

Ketoconazole is also used clinically for the medical treatment of hyperadrenocorticism in dogs. Ketoconazole appears to be a viable option, although it's relatively expensive and less effective when compared with mitotane. However, it may be particularly useful for palliative therapy in dogs with large, malignant, or invasive tumors where surgery is not an option. Ketoconazole is also used frequently in dogs for stabilization prior to surgery. As it is a reversible inhibitor of steroidogenesis, it is usually not a viable option for long-term treatment.

Because it interferes with the metabolism of cyclosporine, ketoconazole has been used to reduce cyclosporine dosage and costs in dogs.

Pharmacology/Actions

At usual doses and serum concentrations, ketoconazole is fungistatic against susceptible fungi. At higher concentrations for prolonged periods of time or against very susceptible organisms, ketoconazole may be fungicidal. It is believed that ketoconazole increases cellular membrane permeability and causes secondary metabolic effects and growth inhibition. The exact mechanism for these effects has not been determined, but may be due to ketoconazole interfering with ergosterol synthesis. The fungicidal action of ketoconazole may be due to a direct effect on cell membranes.

Ketoconazole has activity against most pathogenic fungi, including Blastomyces, Coccidioides, Cryptococcus, Histoplasma, Microsporum, and Trichophyton. Higher levels are necessary to treat most strains of Aspergillus and Sporothrix. Resistance to ketoconazole has been documented for some strains of *Candida albicans*.

Ketoconazole has *in vitro* activity against *Staphylococcus aureus* and *epidermidis*, Nocardia, enterococci, and herpes simplex virus types 1 and 2. The clinical implications of this activity are unknown.

Via inhibition of 5-lipooxygenase, ketoconazole possesses some antiinflammatory activity. The drug can suppress the immune system, probably by suppressing T-lymphocytes proliferation.

Ketoconazole also has endocrine effects as steroid synthesis is directly inhibited by blocking several P-450 enzyme systems. Measurable reductions in testosterone or cortisol synthesis can occur at dosages used for antifungal therapy, but higher dosages are generally required to reduce levels of testosterone or cortisol to be clinically useful in the treatment of prostatic carcinoma or hyperadrenocorticism. Effects on mineralocorticoids are negligible.

Pharmacokinetics

Although it is reported that ketoconazole is well absorbed after oral administration, oral bioavailability of ketoconazole tablets in dogs is highly variable. One study (Baxter et al. 1986) in six normal dogs, found bioavailabilities ranging from 0.04−0.89 (4−89%) after 400 mg (19.5−25.2 mg/kg) was administered to fasted dogs. Peak serum concentrations occur between 1 and 4.25 hours after dosing and peak serum levels ranged from 1.1–45.6 micrograms/mL. This wide interpatient variation may have significant clinical implications from both a toxicity and efficacy standpoint, particularly since ketoconazole is often used in life-threatening infections, and assays for measuring serum levels are not readily available. Administration with food may increase absorption.

Oral absorption of tablets in horses is poor. Single doses of 30 mg/kg yielded nondetectable blood levels. But if given via NG tube in a 0.2 Normal hydrochloric acid solution, bioavailability increased to 23%. The commercially available oral solution is reportedly 60% bioavailable.

Ketoconazole absorption is enhanced in an acidic environment and should not be administered (at the same time) with H_2 blockers or antacids (see Drug Interactions below). Whether to administer ketoconazole with meals or during a fasted state to maximize absorption is controversial. The manufacturer recommends giving with food in human patients. Dogs or cats that develop anorexia/vomiting during therapy may benefit from administration with meals.

After absorption, ketoconazole is distributed into the bile, cerumen, saliva, urine, synovial fluid, and CSF. CSF levels are generally less than 10% of those found in the serum, but may be increased if the meninges are inflamed. High levels of the drug are found in the liver, adrenals, and pituitary gland, while more moderate levels are found in the kidneys, lungs, bladder, bone marrow, and myocardium. At usual doses (10 mg/kg), attained levels are probably inadequate in the brain, testis, and eyes to treat most infections; higher dosages are required. Ketoconazole is 84–99% bound to plasma proteins and crosses the placenta (at least in rats). The drug is found in bitch's milk.

Ketoconazole is metabolized extensively by the liver into several inactive metabolites. These metabolites are excreted primarily into the feces via the bile. About 13% of a given dose is excreted into the urine and only 2–4% of the drug is excreted unchanged in the urine. Half-life in dogs is about 1–6 hours (avg. 2.7 hours).

Contraindications/Precautions/Warnings

Ketoconazole is contraindicated in patients with known hypersensitivity to it. It should be used with caution in patients with hepatic disease or thrombocytopenia.

Adverse Effects

Gastrointestinal signs of anorexia, vomiting, and/or diarrhea are the most common adverse effects seen with ketoconazole therapy and are more prevalent in cats. Anorexia may be minimized by dividing the dose and/or giving it with meals. Appetite stimulants such as oxazepam or cyproheptadine may also be of benefit in cats.

Hepatic toxicity consisting of cholangio-hepatitis and increased liver enzymes has been reported with ketoconazole, and may be either idiosyncratic in nature or a dose-related phenomenon. Cats may be more prone to developing hepatotoxicity than dogs. While liver enzymes should be monitored during therapy, an increase does not necessarily mandate dosage reduction or discontinuation unless concomitant anorexia, vomiting, diarrhea, or abdominal pain is present. Thrombocytopenia has also been reported with ketoconazole therapy, but is rarely encountered. A reversible lightening of haircoat may also occur in patients treated with ketoconazole.

Ketoconazole has a transient dose-related suppressant effect on gonadal and adrenal steroid synthesis. Doses as low as 10 mg/kg depressed serum testosterone levels in dogs within 3–4 hours after dosing, but levels returned to normal within 10 hours. Doses of 30 mg/kg/day have been demonstrated to suppress serum cortisol levels in dogs with hyperadrenocorticism (see Dosages section). Dogs undergoing high dose antifungal therapy may need additional glucocorticoid support during periods of acute stress.

Reproductive/Nursing Safety

Ketoconazole is a known teratogen and embryotoxin in rats. There have been reports of mummified fetuses and stillbirths in dogs who have been treated. Ketoconazole should not be considered absolutely contraindicated in pregnant animals, however, as it is often used in potentially life-threatening infections. The benefits of therapy should be weighed against the potential risks. Ketoconazole may cause infertility in male dogs by decreasing testosterone synthesis. Testosterone production rebounds once the drug is discontinued.

In humans, the FDA categorizes this drug as category **C** for use during pregnancy (*Animal studies have shown an adverse effect on the fetus, but there are no adequate studies in humans; or there are no animal reproduction studies and no adequate studies in humans.*) In a separate system evaluating the safety of drugs in canine and feline pregnancy (Papich 1989), this drug is categorized as in class: **B** (*Safe for use if used cautiously. Studies in laboratory animals may have uncovered some risk, but these drugs appear to be safe in dogs and cats or these drugs are safe if they are not administered when the animal is near term.*)

Ketoconazole is excreted in milk; use with caution in nursing dams.

Overdosage/Acute Toxicity

No reports of acute toxicity associated with overdosage were located. The oral LD_{50} in dogs after oral administration is >500 mg/kg. Should an acute overdose occur, the manufacturer recommends employing supportive measures, including gastric lavage with sodium bicarbonate.

Drug Interactions

The following drug interactions have either been reported or are theoretical in humans or animals receiving ketoconazole and may be of significance in veterinary patients:

- **ALCOHOL:** Ethanol may interact with ketoconazole and produce a disulfiram-like reaction (vomiting)
- **ANTACIDS:** May reduce oral absorption of ketoconazole; administer ketoconazole at least 1 hour before or 2 hours after
- **ANTIDEPRESSANTS, TRICYCLIC (amitriptyline, clomipramine):** Ketoconazole may reduce metabolism and increase adverse effects
- **BENZODIAZEPINES (MIDAZOLAM, TRIAZOLAM):** Ketoconazole may increase levels
- **BUSPIRONE:** Plasma concentrations may be elevated
- **BUSULFAN:** Ketoconazole may increase levels
- **CALCIUM-CHANNEL BLOCKING AGENTS (amlodipine, verapamil):** Ketoconazole may increase levels
- **CISAPRIDE:** Ketoconazole may increase cisapride levels and possibility for toxicity; use together contraindicated in humans
- **CORTICOSTEROIDS:** Ketoconazole may inhibit the metabolism of corticosteroids; potential for increased adverse effects
- **CYCLOPHOSPHAMIDE:** Ketoconazole may inhibit the metabolism of cyclophosphamide and its metabolites; potential for increased toxicity
- **CYCLOSPORINE:** Increased cyclosporine levels
- **DIGOXIN:** Ketoconazole may increase digoxin levels
- **FENTANYL/ALFENTANIL:** Ketoconazole may increase fentanyl or alfentanil levels
- **H2-BLOCKERS (ranitidine, famotidine, etc.):** Increased gastric pH may reduce ketoconazole absorption
- **HEPATOTOXIC DRUGS, OTHER:** Because ketoconazole can cause hepatotoxicity, it should be used cautiously with other hepatotoxic agents
- **ISONIAZID:** May affect ketoconazole levels and concomitant use not recommended in humans
- **IVERMECTIN:** Ketoconazole may increase risk for neurotoxicity. At least one reference states that ivermectin should never be used with ketoconazole in dogs (Waisglass 2009).
- **MACROLIDE ANTIBIOTICS (erythromycin, clarithromycin):** May increase ketoconazole concentrations
- **MITOTANE:** Mitotane and ketoconazole are not recommended for use together to treat hyperadrenocorticism as the adrenolytic effects of mitotane may be inhibited by ketoconazole's inhibition of cytochrome P450 enzymes
- **PHENYTOIN:** May decrease ketoconazole levels
- **PROTON-PUMP INHIBITORS (omeprazole, etc.):** Increased gastric pH may reduce ketoconazole absorption
- **QUINIDINE:** Ketoconazole may increase quinidine levels
- **RIFAMPIN:** May decrease ketoconazole levels; ketoconazole may increase rifampin levels
- **SUCRALFATE:** May reduce absorption of ketoconazole
- **SULFONYLUREA ANTIDIABETIC AGENTS (e.g., glipizide, glyburide):** Ketoconazole may increase levels; hypoglycemia possible
- **THEOPHYLLINE:** Ketoconazole may decrease serum theophylline concentrations in some patients; theophylline levels should be monitored
- **VINCRISTINE/VINBLASTINE:** Ketoconazole may inhibit vinca alkaloid metabolism and increase levels
- **WARFARIN:** Ketoconazole may cause increased prothrombin times in patients receiving warfarin or other coumarin anticoagulants

Laboratory Considerations

- Ketoconazole can reduce serum cortisol levels and affect adrenal function tests. After stopping ketoconazole, cortisol levels usually return to baseline within 24 hours.

Doses

Note: Clinical antifungal effects may require 10−14 days of therapy

- **DOGS:**

  For coccidioidomycosis:

  a) For the systemic form of the disease: 5−10 mg/kg PO twice daily; For the CNS form: 15−20 mg/kg PO twice daily. Treatment should persist for a minimum of 3−6 months. Animals with bony lesions or relapses after discontinuing therapy, give lifelong therapy at 5 mg/kg PO every other day. (Macy 1989)

  b) 10−30 mg/kg PO divided twice a day, most animals need to be treated for 6−12 months (Taboada 2000)

  For blastomycosis:

  a) 10 mg/kg PO twice daily (15−20 mg/kg PO twice daily if CNS involvement) for at least 3 months with amphotericin B: initially at 0.25−0.5 mg/kg every other day IV. If tolerated, increase dose to 1 mg/kg until 4−5 mg/kg total dose is administered. See amphotericin B monograph for more information. (Macy 1989)

b) Ketoconazole 20 mg/kg/day PO once daily or divided twice daily; 40 mg/kg divided twice daily for ocular or CNS involvement (for at least 2–3 months or until remission then start maintenance) with amphotericin B 0.15–0.5 mg/kg IV 3 times a week. When a total dose of amphotericin B reaches 4–6 mg/kg, start maintenance dosage of amphotericin B at 0.15–0.25 mg/kg IV once a month or use ketoconazole at 10 mg/kg PO either once daily, divided twice daily or ketoconazole at 2.5–5 mg/kg PO once daily. If CNS/ocular involvement, use ketoconazole at 20–40 mg/kg PO divided twice daily (Greene, C.E. *et al.* 1984)

For histoplasmosis:

a) 10 mg/kg PO once a day or twice a day for at least 3 months. Treat at least 30 days after complete resolution of clinical disease. If patient relapses, retreat as above then put on maintenance 5 mg/kg PO every other day indefinitely. For acute cases: use with amphotericin B (see blastomycosis recommendation by same author above) (Macy 1988)

b) Ketoconazole 10–20 mg/day PO once daily or divided twice daily (for at least 2–3 months or until remission then start maintenance) with amphotericin B at 0.15–0.5 mg/kg IV 3 times a week. When a total dose of amphotericin B reaches 2–4 mg/kg start maintenance dosage of amphotericin B at 0.15–0.25 mg/kg IV once a month or use ketoconazole at 10 mg/kg PO either once daily, divided twice daily or at 2.5–5 mg/kg PO once daily (Greene, C.E. *et al.* 1984)

For aspergillosis:

a) 20 mg/kg PO for at least 6 weeks; may require long-term/maintenance therapy (Macy 1989)

b) For nasal aspergillosis: 10 mg/kg PO once daily (q24h) or 5 mg/kg PO q12h. Treatment requires many weeks and should continue for 1 month beyond last detection of infection. Itraconazole somewhat more effective. (Greene, C. *et al.* 2006)

For cryptococcosis:

a) Amphotericin B 0.15–0.4 mg/kg IV 3 times a week with flucytosine 150–175 mg/kg PO divided three to four times a day. When a total dose of amphotericin B reaches 4–6 mg/kg start maintenance dosage of amphotericin B at 0.15–0.25 mg/kg IV once a month with flucytosine at dosage above or with ketoconazole at 10 mg/kg PO once daily or divided twice daily (Greene, C.E. *et al.* 1984)

For fungal myocarditis:

a) 10 mg/kg PO three times daily (Ogburn 1988)

For Candidiasis:

a) 10 mg/kg PO once daily (q24h) or 5 mg/kg PO q12h. Treatment requires many weeks and should continue for 1 month beyond last detection of infection. Itraconazole somewhat more effective. (Greene, C. *et al.* 2006)

For Sporotrichosis:

a) 15 mg/kg PO q12h. Treatment requires many weeks and should continue for 1 month beyond last detection of infection. (Greene, C. *et al.* 2006)

For Malassezia dermatitis:

a) For severe cases: Dosing of oral ketoconazole ranges from 5 mg/kg PO once daily to 10 mg/kg twice daily. Improvement (but usually not cure) should be noted in 2 weeks. If a low dose of ketoconazole is given and improvement is not noted in 2 weeks, a higher dose should be given before the diagnosis is reconsidered; administer until the clinical signs have abated and no organisms are seen on cytologic evaluations. (Merchant 2009b)

b) 5–10 mg/kg PO twice a day for 30 days. Often used with therapeutic shampoos containing selenium disulfide, miconazole, ketoconazole or chlorhexidine. Underlying conditions must be identified and remedied or condition will recur. (Noxon 1997)

c) 5–10 mg/kg PO daily for 10 days, then every other day for an additional 10 days. This regimen resolves the majority of cases, but some may need higher dosages. (Muse 2000)

d) Initial dose is 5 mg/kg twice daily for 21–30 days, may increase to 10 mg/kg PO twice daily if poor response. Absorption is enhanced when administered with food and is ideal in an acid environment. (McDonald 1999)

e) 2.5–10 mg/kg PO once daily (q24h) for 7–14 days; once a good response is seen taper to every other day (q48h) and continue until a complete remission occurs. In the rare case when ketoconazole is ineffective or intolerance or toxicity is seen, itraconazole or fluconazole can be used. (Rosenkrantz 2006)

For treatment of hyperadrenocorticism:

a) Author usually uses mitotane therapy, but if animal fails to respond can try ketoconazole: Initiate therapy at 5–10 mg/kg PO twice daily. The patient is monitored as for mitotane—water consumption or first sign of side effects (vomiting, diarrhea or anorexia) which can be seen as a result of the drug or secondary to hypocortisolemia. An idiosyncratic hepatopathy can also be seen (rare?). If no side effects are seen or the patient was not PU/PD initially, then the medication is given for 7 to 14 days and the patient is reevaluated with an ACTH stimulation test. The goal of therapy is to have an ACTH stimulation test in the low normal range to slightly below normal. If there is a continued exaggerated response, then ketoconazole dose is increased to 15 mg/kg PO twice daily and the patient reevaluated as above. The patient is maintained on the same dose that brought the ACTH stimulation test into the normal or subnormal range (*e.g.*, 5−15 mg/kg PO twice daily). The ACTH stimulation test is then performed every 3-4 months. (Merchant 2009a)

b) Begin with a dose of 5 mg/kg q12h for 5−7 days and if there are no side effects (usually GI-related), increase dose to 10 mg/kg q12h for 10−14 days and perform ACTH stimulation test. Plasma cortisol levels should be between 0.7−1.8 micrograms/dL if ketoconazole is to be effective. Over 25% of cases do not respond to ketoconazole and many cases that do respond, require doses of between 15−20 mg/kg q12h. Because of unpredictable efficacy, high occurrence of adverse effects, twice daily dosing, and expense, ketoconazole usage for PDH has been limited. (Church 2004)

c) For palliative treatment of canine Cushing's syndrome: 15 mg/kg PO q12h (Lorenz & Melendez 2002)

To reduce the dosage requirements of cyclosporine:

a) Ketoconazole at 5−10 mg/kg PO per day can be administered concurrently with cyclosporine; in these patients the cyclosporine dose can be reduced (approximately half) or possibly tapered sooner than in patients not receiving the combination. Addition of ketoconazole is particularly useful in allergic patients with concurrent Malassezia dermatitis or otitis. (Hnilica 2006)

b) To treat perianal fistula: ketoconazole 7.5 mg/kg PO twice daily; cyclosporine 0.5−0.75 mg PO twice daily. (O'Neill *et al.* 2001)

c) For atopic dermatitis: Cyclosporine at 5−7 mg/kg/day or less. Ideally should be given on an empty stomach, but if causes GI upset administration with food may help. In large dogs, administration of cyclosporine at 2.5 mg/kg/day with ketoconazole (5 mg/kg/day) may give good results and reduce expenses. (White 2007)

d) As an alternative immunosuppressive agent for refractory IMHA, especially those that are non-regenerative: Cyclosporine at 5−10 mg/kg PO divided twice daily to achieve plasma trough levels of >200 ng/mL (**Note:** reference states >200 mg/mL, but it is believed this is a typo). Large breed dogs can be dosed concurrently with ketoconazole (10 mg/kg/day) to allow reduction of cyclosporine dose. (Macintire 2006)

■ **CATS:**

Note: Use of ketoconazole in cats is somewhat controversial and some clinicians recommend that it not be used in this species because of its toxic potential. Consider using itraconazole in its place.

a) For coccidioidomycosis: 10−30 mg/kg PO divided twice a day, most animals need to be treated for 6−12 months (Taboada 2000)

b) For coccidioidomycosis: 50 mg per cat PO once daily; or 25−75 mg per cat q12−48h. Treatment requires many months (9−12 on average) and should continue for 1 month beyond last detection of infection. (Greene, C. *et al.* 2006)

c) For blastomycosis: 10 mg/kg q12h PO (for at least 60 days) with amphotericin B: 0.25 mg/kg in 30 mL D_5W IV over 15 minutes q48h. Continue amphotericin B therapy until a cumulative dose of 4 mg/kg is given or until BUN >50 mg/dL. If renal toxicity does not develop, may increase dose to 0.5 mg/kg of amphotericin B. (Legendre, A.M. 1989)

d) For cryptococcosis: 10 mg/kg twice daily. Very useful for this condition in cats, but at this dosage can produce anorexia and debility. (Legendre, A. 1995)

e) For aspergillosis: 10 mg/kg PO q12h (Legendre, A.M. 1989)

f) For dermatophytosis: Usually reserved for when griseofulvin ineffective or not tolerated. 10 mg/kg PO once daily with an acidic meal. Prolonged course of therapy required. Begin taking cultures after 4 weeks of treatment. Continue therapy for 2 weeks beyond clinical cure *and* when 2−3 negative cultures are obtained at weekly intervals. (Frank 2000)

g) For Sporotrichosis: 5−10 mg/kg PO q12−24h. Treatment requires many weeks (2−4 months on average) and should continue for 1 month beyond last detection of infection. (Greene, C. *et al.* 2006)

■ **HORSES:**

a) For susceptible yeasts and *Aspergillus* spp: Using the commercial oral solution

(*Note: Not marketed in the USA*): 5 mg/kg PO once daily.

For *Scopulariopsis* pneumonia: Oral tablets may be administered via NG tube by mixing them with 0.2 Normal hydrochloric acid and dosed at 30 mg/kg q12h. (Stewart *et al.* 2008a; Stewart *et al.* 2008b)

■ **RABBITS/RODENTS/SMALL MAMMALS:**

a) **Rabbits:** 10–40 mg/kg per day PO for 14 days (Ivey & Morrisey 2000)

b) **Hamsters, Gerbils, Mice, Rats, Guinea pigs, Chinchillas:** For systemic mycoses/candidiasis: 10–40 mg/kg per day PO for 14 days (Adamcak & Otten 2000)

■ **BIRDS:**

For susceptible fungal infections:

a) For severe refractory candidiasis in Psittacines: 5–10 mg/kg as a gavage twice daily for 14 days. For local effect in crop dissolve ¼ tablet (50 mg) in 0.2 mL of 1 N hydrochloric acid and add 0.8 mL of water. Solution turns pale pink when dissolved. Add mixture to food for gavage.

To add to water for most species: 200 mg/L for 7–14 days. As drug is not water soluble at neutral pH, dissolve in acid prior to adding to water (see above).

To add to feed for most species: 10–20 mg/kg for 7–14 days. Add to favorite food or add to mash. (Clubb 1986)

b) 20–30 mg/kg PO twice daily (based on the kinetics determined in a single trial of Moluccan Cockatoos) (Flammer 2003)

c) **Ratites:** 5–10 mg/kg PO once daily (Jenson 1998)

■ **REPTILES:**

a) For susceptible infections: For most species: 15–30 mg/kg PO once daily for 2–4 weeks (Gauvin 1993)

b) For fungal shell diseases in turtles/tortoises: 25 mg/kg PO once a day for 2–4 weeks (Rosskopf 1986)

Monitoring

■ Liver enzymes with chronic therapy (at least every 2 months; some clinicians say monthly)

■ CBC with platelets

■ Efficacy and other adverse effects

Client Information

■ If animal develops gastrointestinal signs divide dose and administer with meals.

■ Long-term therapy with adequate dosing compliance is usually necessary for successful results

■ Clients must be committed for both the financial and dosing burdens associated with therapy.

Chemistry/Synonyms

An imidazole antifungal agent, ketoconazole occurs as a white to slightly beige powder with pK_as of 2.9 and 6.5. It is practically insoluble in water.

Ketoconazole may also be known as ketoconazolum, and R-41400; many trade names are available.

Storage/Stability

Ketoconazole tablets should be stored at room temperature in well-closed containers.

Compatibility/Compounding Considerations

Compounded preparation stability: Ketoconazole oral suspension compounded from the commercially available tablets has been published (Allen & Erickson 1996). Triturating twelve (12) ketoconazole 200 mg tablets with 60 mL of *Ora Plus®* and *qs ad* to 120 mL with *Ora Sweet®* or *Ora-Sweet-SF®* yields a 20 mg/mL ketoconazole oral suspension that retains >95% potency for 60 days when stored at both 5°C and 25°C and protected from light.

Dosage Forms/Regulatory Status

VETERINARY-LABELED PRODUCTS: None for systemic use.

HUMAN-LABELED PRODUCTS:

Ketoconazole Tablets: 200 mg (scored); generic; (Rx)

Topical forms are also available.

References

Adamcak, A. & B. Otten (2000). Rodent Therapeutics. Vet Clin NA: Exotic Anim Pract 3:1(Jan): 221–240.

Allen, L.V. & M.A. Erickson (1996). Stability of ketoconazole, metolazone, metronidazole, procainamide hydrochloride, and spironolactone in extemporaneously compounded oral liquids. Am J Health Syst Pharm 53(17): 2073–2078.

Church, D. (2004). Managing canine hyperadrenocorticism without mitotane-Practical, achievable alternatives. Proceedings: ACVIM Forum. Accessed via: Veterinary Information Network. http://goo.gl/YHqmA

Clubb, S.L. (1986). Therapeutics: Individual and Flock Treatment Regimens. Clinical Avian Medicine and Surgery. GJ Harrison and LR Harrison Eds. Philadelphia, W.B. Saunders: 327–355.

Flammer, K. (2003). Antifungal therapy in avian medicine. Proceedings: Western Veterinary Conference. Accessed via: Veterinary Information Network. http://goo.gl/rgOfo

Frank, L. (2000). Dermatophytosis. Kirk's Current Veterinary Therapy: XIII Small Animal Practice. J Bonagura Ed. Philadelphia, WB Saunders: 577–580.

Gauvin, J. (1993). Drug therapy in reptiles. Seminars in Avian & Exotic Med 2(1): 48–59.

Greene, C., K. Hartmannn, et al. (2006). Appendix 8: Antimicrobial Drug Formulary. Infectious Disease of the Dog and Cat. C Greene Ed., Elsevier: 1186–1333.

Greene, C.E., K.G. O'Neal, et al. (1984). Antimicrobial chemotherapy. Clinical Microbiology and INfectious Diseases of the Dog and Cat. CE Greene Ed. Philadelphia, WB Saunders: 144–188.

Hnilica, K. (2006). Cyclosporine Therapy. Proceedings: Western Vet Conf. Accessed via: Veterinary Information Network. http://goo.gl/gJGzD

Ivey, E. & J. Morrisey (2000). Therapeutics for Rabbits. Vet Clin NA: Exotic Anim Pract 3:1(Jan): 183–216.

Jenson, J. (1998). Current ratite therapy. The Veterinary Clinics of North America: Food Animal Practice 16:3(November).

Legendre, A. (1995). Antimycotic Drug Therapy. Kirk's Current Veterinary Therapy:XII. J Bonagura Ed. Philadelphia, W.B. Saunders: 327–331.

Legendre, A.M. (1989). Systemic mycotic infections. The Cat: Diseases and Clinical Management. RG Sherding Ed. New York, Churchill Livingstone. 1: 427–457.

Lorenz, M. & L. Melendez (2002). Hyperadrenocorticism (Canine Cushing;s Syndrome, CCS). Proceedings: Western Veterinary Conference. Accessed via: Veterinary Information Network. http://goo.gl/

Macintire, D. (2006). New therapies for immune-mediated hemolytic anemia. Proceedings: ACVIM 2006. Accessed via: Veterinary Information Network. http://goo.gl/ILCPS

Macy, D.W. (1989). Systemic Mycoses. Handbook of Small Animal Practice. RV Morgan Ed. New York, Churchill Livingstone: 963–973.

McDonald, J. (1999). Cutaneous Mallassezia. Proceedings: Central Veterinary Conference, Kansas City.

Merchant, S. (2009a). Diagnosis and Long Term Management of Canine Cushing's Disease. Proceedings: ACVC. Accessed via: Veterinary information Network. http://goo.gl/peR8M

Merchant, S. (2009b). Diagnosis and management of the pruritic dog. Proceedings: ACVC. Accessed via: Veterinary information Network. http://goo.gl/LWWtF

Muse, R. (2000). Malassezia Dermatitis. Kirk's Current Veterinary Therapy: XIII Small Animal Practice. J Bonagura Ed. Philadelphia, WB Saunders: 574–577.

Noxon, J. (1997). Bacterial and Fungal Diseases of the Skin. Practical Small Animal Internal Medicine. M Leib and M WE Eds. Philadelphia, Saunders: 33–48.

O'Neill, T., G. Edwards, et al. (2001). Clinical use of cyclosporin A and ketoconazole in the treatment of perianal fistula. Proceedings: World Small Animal Association World Congress. Accessed via: Veterinary Information Network. http://goo.gl/hs2Rj

Ogburn, P.N. (1988). Myocardial Diseases. Handbook of Small Animal Practice. RV Morgan Ed. New York, Churchill Livingstone: 109–128.

Papich, M. (1989). Effects of drugs on pregnancy. Current Veterinary Therapy X: Small Animal Practice. R Kirk Ed. Philadelphia, Saunders: 1291–1299.

Rosenkrantz, W. (2006). Appropriate therapy for Malassezia dermatitis. Proceedings: Western Vet Conf. Accessed via: Veterinary Information Network. http://goo.gl/ri2z1

Rosskopf, W.J. (1986). Shell diseases in turtles and tortoises. Current Veterinary Therapy (CVT) IX Small Animal Practice. RW Kirk Ed. Philadelphia, WB Saunders: 751–759.

Stewart, A., E. Welles, et al. (2008a). Fungal infections of the upper respiratory tract. Compendium Equine(May): 208–.

Stewart, A., E. Welles, et al. (2008b). Pulmonary and systemic fungal infections. Compendium Equine(June): 260–272.

Taboada, J. (2000). Systemic Mycoses. Textbook of Veterinary Internal Medicine: Diseases of the Dog and Cat. S Ettinger and E Feldman Eds. Philadelphia, WB Saunders. 1: 453–476.

Waisglass, S. (2009). Demodicosis Update—Some Considerations to Increase Your Success Rate. Proceedings: WVC. Accessed via: Veterinary Information Network. http://goo.gl/4R2el

White, S. (2007). Atopic dermatitis and its secondary infections. Proceedings: Canine Medicine Symposium. Accessed via: Veterinary Information Network. http://goo.gl/upBF7

KETOPROFEN

(kee-toe-*proe*-fen)   Ketofen®, Anafen®

NON-STEROIDAL ANTIINFLAMMATORY AGENT

Prescriber Highlights

▶ Nonsteroidal antiinflammatory agent used in horses, cats (short-term) & dogs

▶ Cautions: GI ulceration or bleeding, hypoproteinemia, breeding animals (especially late in pregnancy), significant renal or hepatic impairment; may mask the signs of infection (inflammation, hyperpyrexia)

▶ Adverse Effects: *Horses:* Potentially, gastric mucosal damage & GI ulceration, renal crest necrosis, & mild hepatitis may occur. *Dogs:* Vomiting, anorexia, & GI ulcers

▶ Do not administer intra-arterially & avoid SC injections

▶ Drug-drug; drug-lab interactions

Uses/Indications

Ketoprofen is labeled for use in horses for the alleviation of inflammation and pain associated with musculoskeletal disorders. Like flunixin (and other NSAIDs), ketoprofen potentially has many other uses in a variety of species and conditions.

Some consider ketoprofen to be the NSAID of choice for use short-term for analgesia in cats. There are approved dosage forms for dogs and cats in Europe and Canada. In Canada, ketoprofen has labeled indications for use in dogs and cats for the alleviation of inflammation, lameness and pain due to osteoarthritis, hip dysplasia, disc disease, spondylosis, panosteitis, trauma, and related musculoskeletal diseases; for the management of post-surgical pain; and for the symptomatic treatment of fever. It is labeled to be used with appropriate antiinfective therapy when inflammation and/or fever are associated with a primary infectious process.

Pharmacology/Actions

Ketoprofen exhibits actions similar to that of other nonsteroidal antiinflammatory agents in that it possesses antipyretic, analgesic and antiinflammatory activity. Its purported mechanism of action is the inhibition of cyclooxygenase catalysis of arachidonic acid to prostaglandin precursors (endoperoxides), thereby inhibiting the synthesis of prostaglandins in tissues. Ketoprofen purportedly has inhibitory activity on lipoxygenase, whereas flunixin reportedly does not at therapeutic doses, but the evidence for this action is weak as *in vitro* studies have not confirmed lipoxygenase activity in studied species.

The S (+) enantiomer is associated with anti-prostaglandin activity and toxicity and the R (-) form analgesia without the GI effects.

Pharmacokinetics

In species studied (rats, dog, man), ketoprofen is rapidly and nearly completely absorbed after oral administration. The presence of food or milk decreases oral absorption. Oral absorption is poor in horses. It has been reported that when comparing IV vs. IM injections in horses, the areas under the curve are relatively equivalent. Volume of distribution is low in adult horses. Volume of distribution is reportedly higher in foals and doses may need to be higher (1.5X) with longer durations between doses in neonates (Wilcke et al. 1998). The drug enters synovial fluid and is highly bound to plasma proteins (99% in humans, and approximately 93% in horses). In horses, the manufacturer reports that the onset of activity is within 2 hours and peak effects 12 hours post dose.

Ketoprofen is eliminated via the kidneys both as a conjugated metabolite (primarily glucuronidation in dogs and horses) and unchanged drug. In cats, thioesterification is proposed as a major elimination mechanism. The elimination half-life in horses is about 1.5 hours and in adult cats it is approximately 1-1.5 hours. The S- form half-life in dogs is about 1.6 hours.

Contraindications/Precautions/Warnings

While the manufacturer states that there are no contraindications to the drug's use (other than previous hypersensitivity to ketoprofen), it should be used only when the potential benefits outweigh the risks in cases where GI ulceration or bleeding is evident or in patients with significant renal or hepatic impairment. Ketoprofen may mask the clinical signs of infection (inflammation, hyperpyrexia). Because ketoprofen is highly protein bound, patients with hypoproteinemia may have increased levels of free drug, thereby increasing the risks for toxicity.

Adverse Effects

Ketoprofen appears to have low toxicity in horses and reports indicate that ketoprofen appears relatively safe to use in horses and may have a lower incidence of adverse effects than either phenylbutazone or flunixin. Potentially, gastric mucosal damage and GI ulceration, renal crest necrosis, and mild hepatitis may occur.

Do not administer intra-arterially and avoid SC injections. While not labeled for IM use in horses, it reportedly is effective and may only cause occasional inflammation at the injection site.

In dogs or cats, ketoprofen may cause vomiting, anorexia, and GI ulcers.

Reproductive/Nursing Safety

The manufacturer cautions against ketoprofen's use in breeding horses because effects on fertility, pregnancy, or fetal health have not been established. However, rat and mice studies have not demonstrated increased teratogenicity or embryotoxicity. Rabbits receiving twice the human dose exhibited increased embryotoxicity, but not teratogenicity. Because non-steroidal antiinflammatory agents inhibit prostaglandin synthesis, adversely affecting neonatal cardiovascular systems (premature closure of patent ductus), ketoprofen should not be used late in pregnancy. Studies in male rats demonstrated no changes in fertility. In humans, the FDA categorizes this drug as category *B* for use during the first two trimesters of pregnancy (*Animal studies have not yet demonstrated risk to the fetus, but there are no adequate studies in pregnant women; or animal studies have shown an adverse effect, but adequate studies in pregnant women have not demonstrated a risk to the fetus in the first trimester of pregnancy, and there is no evidence of risk in later trimesters.*)

It is presently unknown whether ketoprofen enters equine milk. Ketoprofen does enter canine milk; use with caution.

Overdosage/Acute Toxicity

Humans have survived oral ingestions of up to 5 grams. The LD_{50} in dogs after oral ingestion has been reported to be 2000 mg/kg, but exposures as low as 0.44 mg/kg in dogs have caused GI ulcers. Cats have developed renal toxicity at doses as low as 0.7 mg/kg. Horses given ketoprofen at doses up to 11 mg/kg administered IV once daily for 15 days exhibited no signs of toxicity. Severe laminitis was observed in a horse given 33 mg/kg/day (15X over labeled dosage) for 5 days. Anorexia, depression, icterus, and abdominal swelling were noted in horses given 55 mg/kg/day (25X labeled dose) for 5 days. Upon necropsy, gastritis, nephritis, and hepatitis were diagnosed in this group.

There were 16 exposures to ketoprofen reported to the ASPCA Animal Poison Control Center (APCC) during 2008-2009. In these cases 9 were dogs with 2 showing clinical signs and the remaining 7 cases with 2 showing clinical signs. Common findings in dogs recorded included vomiting.

This medication is a NSAID. As with any NSAID, overdosage can lead to gastrointestinal and renal effects. Decontamination with emetics and/or activated charcoal is appropriate. For doses where GI effects are expected, the use of gastrointestinal protectants is warranted. If renal effects are also expected, fluid diuresis is warranted.

Drug Interactions

The following drug interactions have either been reported or are theoretical in humans or animals receiving ketoprofen and may be of significance in veterinary patients:

- ■ **AMINOGLYCOSIDES (gentamicin, amikacin, etc.):** Increased risk for nephrotoxicity
- ■ **ANTICOAGULANTS (heparin, LMWH, warfarin):** Increased risk for bleeding possible

■ **ASPIRIN:** When aspirin is used concurrently with ketoprofen, plasma levels of ketoprofen could decrease and an increased likelihood of GI adverse effects (blood loss) could occur. Concomitant administration of aspirin with ketoprofen cannot be recommended.

■ **BISPHOSPHONATES (alendronate, etc.):** May increase risk for GI ulceration

■ **CORTICOSTEROIDS:** Concomitant administration with NSAIDs may significantly increase the risks for GI adverse effects

■ **CYCLOSPORINE:** May increase risk for nephrotoxicity

■ **FLUCONAZOLE:** May increase NSAID levels

■ **FUROSEMIDE:** Ketoprofen may reduce the saluretic and diuretic effects of furosemide

■ **HIGHLY PROTEIN BOUND DRUGS (e.g., phenytoin, valproic acid, oral anticoagulants, other antiinflammatory agents, salicylates, sulfonamides, and the sulfonylurea antidiabetic agents):** Because ketoprofen is highly bound to plasma proteins (99%), it potentially could displace other highly bound drugs; increased serum levels and duration of actions may occur. Although these interactions are usually of little concern clinically, use together with caution.

■ **METHOTREXATE:** Serious toxicity has occurred when NSAIDs have been used concomitantly with methotrexate; use together with extreme caution.

■ **PROBENECID:** May cause a significant increase in serum levels and half-life of ketoprofen

Laboratory Considerations
Ketoprofen may cause:

■ Falsely elevated **blood glucose** values when using the glucose oxidase and peroxidase method using ABTS as a chromogen;

■ Falsely elevated **serum bilirubin** values when using DMSO as a reagent;

■ Falsely elevated **serum iron** concentrations using the Ramsey method, or falsely decreased serum iron concentrations when using bathophenanthroline disulfonate as a reagent

Doses
■ **DOGS:**
As an antiinflammatory/analgesic:

a) Injection at a dose of 2 mg/kg (0.2 mL/kg) IM, IV or SC injection for one day, and continue with ketoprofen tablets PO at a lower maintenance dose of 1 mg/kg once a day for four more days. (Adapted from label information—*Anafen®*; Merial-Canada)

b) For post-operative pain control: 1–2 mg/kg IV, IM once daily for 2–3 days duration (Tranquilli 2003)

c) For post-operative pain control: 1–2 mg/kg IV, SC once daily for 3 days duration after surgery; or 1 mg/kg PO once daily for 5 days, after surgery (Hansen 2003)

d) For acute indications: 2 mg/kg SC, IM, IV once daily for up to 3 consecutive day. If preferred after one injection treatment may be followed on the next day with tablets at 1 mg/kg PO per day and continued on successive days for up to 4 days (*i.e.,* up to 5 days in total). For chronic pain: 0.25 mg/kg PO once daily for up to 30 days. (Label Information *Ketofen 1%*; *Ketofen® Tablets*—Merial U.K.)

■ **CATS:**
As an antiinflammatory/analgesic:

a) Injection at a dose of 2 mg/kg (0.2 mL/kg) SC for one day, and continue with ketoprofen tablets PO at a lower maintenance dose of 1 mg/kg once a day for four more days. In severe cases, the parenteral loading dose of 2 mg/kg can be given for up to three consecutive days. (Label information; *Anafen®*—Merial-Canada)

b) 1 mg/kg PO or SC once daily for up to 5 days, or 2 mg/kg SC as a single injection. (Duncan *et al.* 2007)

c) For post-operative pain control: 1–2 mg/kg IV, SC once daily for 3 days duration after surgery; or 1 mg/kg PO once daily for 3 days, after surgery (Hansen 2003)

d) 2 mg/kg SC once daily for up to 3 consecutive days. If preferred after one injection treatment may be followed on the next day with tablets at 1 mg/kg and continued on successive days for up to 4 days (*i.e.,* up to 5 days in total). (Label Information *Ketofen® 1%*; *Ketofen® Tablets*—Merial U.K.)

■ **FERRETS:**
a) As a post-operative analgesic: 1–2 mg/kg *(route not indicted; suggest SC or IM as per cats—Plumb)* q24h. (Lichtenberger 2008)

■ **RABBITS/RODENTS/SMALL MAMMALS:**
a) **Rabbits:** For chronic pain/antiinflammatory: 1 mg/kg IM q12–24h (Ivey & Morrisey 2000)

b) **Rats:** 5 mg/kg SC (Adamcak & Otten 2000)

c) **Rabbits:** 3 mg/kg IM, estimated duration of action 12-24 hours. (Flecknell 2008)

■ **HORSES:** (**Note:** ARCI UCGFS Class 4 Drug)
a) For labeled indications: 2.2 mg/kg (1 mL/100 lbs) IV once daily for up to 5 days (Package insert; *Ketofen®*)

b) As an adjunctive treatment for laminitis: 2.2 mg/kg IV once daily (Brumbaugh *et al.* 1999)

■ **CATTLE:**

a) 3 mg/kg IV or deep IM once daily for up to 3 days; withdrawal times (U.K.) are meat: 4 days; milk: 0 days (Label information *Comforion Vet®*—Merial U.K.)

b) 3.3 mg/kg; duration of effect 24 hours; appropriate withdrawal times: 24 hours for milk; 7 days for meat. (Walz 2006)

■ **SWINE:**

a) 3 mg/kg IM once daily for up to 3 days; withdrawal times (U.K.) for meat: 4 days (Label information *Comforion Vet®*—Merial U.K.)

■ **BIRDS:**

As an antiinflammatory analgesic:

a) 2 mg/kg IM q8–24 hours (Clyde & Paul-Murphy 2000)

b) 2 mg/kg IM or SC q8-24h (Echols 2008)

■ **ZOO, EXOTIC, WILDLIFE SPECIES:**

For use of ketoprofen in zoo, exotic and wildlife medicine refer to specific references, including:

a) *Exotic Animal Formulary, 3rd Ed.* Carpenter JW. Saunders. 2005

b) The 2009 American Association of Zoo Veterinarian Proceedings by D. K. Fontenot also has several dosages listed for restraint, anesthesia, and analgesia for a variety of drugs for carnivores and primates. VIN members can access them at: http://goo.gl/BHRih or http://goo.gl/9UJse

Monitoring

■ Efficacy

■ Adverse Effects (occasional liver or renal function tests are recommended with long-term therapy)

Chemistry/Synonyms

A propionic acid derivative nonsteroidal antiinflammatory agent (NSAID), ketoprofen occurs as an off-white to white, fine to granular powder. It is practically insoluble in water, but freely soluble in alcohol at 20°C. Ketoprofen has a pK_a of 5.9 in a 3:1 methanol:water solution. Ketoprofen has both an S enantiomer and R enantiomer. The commercial product contains a racemic mixture of both. The S (+) enantiomer has greater antiinflammatory potency than the R (-) form.

Ketoprofen may also be known as ketoprofenum and RP-19583; many trade names are available.

Storage/Stability

Ketoprofen oral capsules should be stored at room temperature in tight, light resistant containers. The veterinary injection should be stored at room temperature. Compatibility studies with injectable ketoprofen and other compounds have apparently not been published.

Dosage Forms/Regulatory Status

VETERINARY-LABELED PRODUCTS:

Ketoprofen Injection: 100 mg/mL in 50 mL and 100 mL multi-dose vials; *Ketofen®* (Pfizer), generic (Phoenix), (Rx). FDA-approved for use in horses not intended for food.

In Canada and the U.K., there are FDA-approved oral dosage forms (5, 10, 20 mg tablets) and an injectable form (10 mg/mL) for use in dogs and cats. Trade names include *Anafen®* and *Ketofen®*.

The ARCI (Racing Commissioners International) has designated this drug as a class 4 substance. See the appendix for more information.

HUMAN-LABELED PRODUCTS:

Ketoprofen Capsules: 50 mg & 75 mg; generic; (Rx)

Ketoprofen Extended-Release Capsules: 100 mg, 150 mg and 200 mg; generic; (Rx)

References

Adamcak, A. & B. Otten (2000). Rodent Therapeutics. Vet Clin NA: Exotic Anim Pract 3:1(Jan): 221–240.

Brumbaugh, G., H. Lopez, et al. (1999). The pharmacologic basis for the treatment of laminitis. The Veterinary Clinics of North America: Equine Practice 15:2(August).

Clyde, V. & J. Paul-Murphy (2000). Avian Analgesia. Kirk's Current Veterinary Therapy: XIII Small Animal Practice. J Bonagura Ed. Philadelphia, WB Saunders: 1126–1128.

Duncan, A., X. Lascelles, et al. (2007). Nonsteroidal antiinflammatory drugs in cats: a review. Veterinary Anaesthesia and Analgesia 34(4): 228–250.

Echols, M. (2008). Avian Anesthesia and Analgesia. Proceedings: IVECCS. Accessed via: Veterinary Information Network. http://goo.gl/kSQMJ

Flecknell, P. (2008). Analgesia and perioperative care. Proceedings: World Veterinary Congress. Accessed via: Veterinary Information Network. http://goo.gl/dLHJR

Hansen, B. (2003). Updated opinions on analgesic techniques. Proceedings: ACVIM Forum. Accessed via: Veterinary Information Network. http://goo.gl/EPWL2

Ivey, E. & J. Morrisey (2000). Therapeutics for Rabbits. Vet Clin NA: Exotic Anim Pract 3:1(Jan): 183–216.

Lichtenberger, M. (2008). Anesthesia and Analgesia for the Exotic Pets. Proceedings: WVC. Accessed via: Veterinary Information Network. http://goo.gl/dIduT

Tranquilli, W. (2003). Pain management alternatives for common surgeries. Proceedings: PAIN 2003. Accessed via: Veterinary Information Network. http://goo.gl/UCsTh

Walz, P. (2006). Practical management of pain in cattle. Proceedings: ABVP. Accessed via: Veterinary Information Network. http://goo.gl/hScVv

Wilcke, J.R., M.V. Crisman, et al. (1998). Pharmacokinetics of ketoprofen in healthy foals less than twenty-four hours old. American Journal of Veterinary Research 59(3): 290–292.

KETOROLAC TROMETHAMINE

(**kee**-toe-role-ak)   Toradol®

NON-STEROIDAL ANTIINFLAMMATORY
AGENT

Prescriber Highlights

▶ NSAID used primarily for short-term analgesia

▶ Contraindications: Active GI ulcers or history of hypersensitivity to the drug

▶ Relatively contraindicated: Hematologic, renal, or hepatic disease

▶ Caution: History of gastric ulcers, heart failure

▶ Adverse Effects: GI ulcers & perforation, renal effects possible with chronic use; consider co-dosing with misoprostol/sucralfate in dogs to reduce chances of ulcers

Uses/Indications

Ketorolac is used primarily for its analgesic effects for short-term treatment of mild to moderate pain in dogs and rodents. The duration of analgesic effect in dogs is about 8–12 hours, but because of the availability of approved, safer NSAIDs for dogs, its use is questionable.

Pharmacology/Actions

Like other NSAIDs, ketorolac exhibits analgesic, antiinflammatory, and antipyretic activity probably through its inhibition of cyclooxygenase with resultant impediment of prostaglandin synthesis. Ketorolac may exhibit a more potent analgesic effect than some other NSAIDs. It inhibits both COX-1 and COX-2 receptors.

Pharmacokinetics

After oral administration, ketorolac is rapidly absorbed; in dogs peak levels occur in about 50 minutes and oral bioavailability is about 50–75%.

Ketorolac is distributed marginally through the body. It does not appear to cross the blood-brain barrier and is highly bound to plasma proteins (99%). The volume of distribution in dogs is reported to be about 0.33–0.42 L/kg (similar in humans). The drug does cross the placenta.

Ketorolac is primarily metabolized via glucuronidation and hydroxylation. Both unchanged drug and metabolites are excreted mainly in the urine. Patients with diminished renal function will have longer elimination times than normal. In normal dogs, the elimination half-life is between 4–8 hours.

Contraindications/Precautions/Warnings

Ketorolac is relatively contraindicated in patients with a history of, or preexisting, hematologic, renal or hepatic disease. It is contraindicated in patients with active GI ulcers or with a history of hypersensitivity to the drug. It should be used cautiously in patients with a history of GI ulcers, or heart failure (may cause fluid retention), and in geriatric patients. Animals suffering from inflammation secondary to concomitant infection, should receive appropriate antimicrobial therapy.

Because ketorolac has a tendency to cause gastric erosion and ulcers in dogs, long-term use (>3 days) is not recommended in this species.

Adverse Effects

Ketorolac use is limited in domestic animals because of its adverse effect profile and a lack of veterinary-labeled products. The primary issue in dogs is its GI toxicity. GI ulceration can be common if the drug is used chronically. Most clinicians who have used this medication in dogs limit treatment to less than 3 days and give misoprostol with or without sucralfate concurrently. Like other NSAIDS, platelet inhibition, renal, and hepatic toxicity are also possible with this drug.

Reproductive/Nursing Safety

Ketorolac does cross the placenta. In humans, the FDA categorizes this drug as category *C* for use during the *first two trimesters of pregnancy* (*Animal studies have shown an adverse effect on the fetus, but there are no adequate studies in humans; or there are no animal reproduction studies and no adequate studies in humans.*) In humans, all NSAIDs are assigned to category *D* for use during pregnancy during the *third trimester* or near delivery (*There is evidence of human fetal risk, but the potential benefits from the use of the drug in pregnant women may be acceptable despite its potential risks.*)

Most NSAIDs are excreted in milk. Ketorolac was detected in human breast milk at a maximum milk:plasma ratio of 0.037. It is unlikely to pose great risk to nursing offspring.

Overdosage/Acute Toxicity

Limited information is available. Cats have developed renal toxicity at doses as low as 0.7 mg/kg. The oral LD_{50} is 200 mg/kg in mice. GI effects, including GI ulceration are likely in overdoses in small animals. Metabolic acidosis was reported in one human patient. Consider GI emptying in large overdoses; patients should be monitored for GI bleeding. Treat ulcers with sucralfate; consider giving misoprostol early.

Drug Interactions

The following drug interactions have either been reported or are theoretical in humans or animals receiving ketorolac and may be of significance in veterinary patients:

■ **ACE INHIBITORS:** Increased risk for nephrotoxicity

■ **ALPRAZOLAM:** Hallucinations reported in some human patients taking with ketorolac

■ **AMINOGLYCOSIDES (gentamicin, amikacin, etc.):** Increased risk for nephrotoxicity

■ **ANTICOAGULANTS (heparin, LMWH, warfarin):** Increased risk for bleeding possible

■ **ASPIRIN:** Increased likelihood of GI adverse effects (blood loss)

■ **BISPHOSPHONATES (alendronate, etc.):** May increase risk for GI ulceration

■ **CORTICOSTEROIDS:** Concomitant administration with NSAIDs may significantly increase the risks for GI adverse effects

■ **CYCLOSPORINE:** May increase risk for nephrotoxicity

■ **FLUCONAZOLE:** May increase NSAID levels

■ **FLUOXETINE:** Hallucinations reported in some human patients taking with ketorolac

■ **FUROSEMIDE:** Ketorolac may reduce the saluretic and diuretic effects of furosemide

■ **METHOTREXATE:** Serious toxicity has occurred when NSAIDs have been used concomitantly with methotrexate; use together with extreme caution

■ **MUSCLE RELAXANTS, NONDEPOLARIZING:** Ketorolac may potentiate effects

■ **PROBENECID:** May cause a significant increase in serum levels and half-life of ketorolac

Doses

■ **DOGS:**

a) As an analgesic: 0.5 mg/kg IV three times daily or 0.3 mg/kg PO twice daily. Repeated doses have considerable potential for causing GI or renal toxicity. Treated dogs should receive misoprostol. (Dowling 2000)

b) As an analgesic: 0.3–0.5 mg/kg IV, IM q8–12h for one or two doses (Scherk 2003)

■ **CATS:**

a) As an analgesic: 0.25 mg/kg IM q8–12h for one or two doses (Scherk 2003)

■ **GOATS:**

a) As an analgesic: 0.3–0.7 mg/kg IV, IM, SC, PO three times daily (Resources 2000)

■ **RABBITS/RODENTS/SMALL MAMMALS:**

a) As an analgesic: Mice: 0.7–10 mg/kg PO once daily. Rats: 3–5 mg/kg PO once to twice a day; 1 mg/kg IM once to twice a day (Huerkamp 2000)

Monitoring

■ Analgesic/antiinflammatory efficacy

■ GI: appetite, feces (occult blood, diarrhea)

Client Information

■ Notify veterinarian if signs of GI distress (anorexia, vomiting, diarrhea, black feces, or blood in stool) occur, or if the animal becomes depressed.

Chemistry/Synonyms

A carboxylic acid derivative nonsteroidal antiinflammatory agent, ketorolac tromethamine occurs as an off-white crystalline powder with a pKa of 3.54 (in water). More than 500 mg are soluble in one mL of water at room temperature. The commercially available injection is a clear, slightly yellow solution with a pH of 6.9–7.9. Sodium chloride is added to make the solution isotonic.

Ketorolac tromethamine may also be known as RS-37619-00-31-3; many trade names are available.

Storage/Stability

Both the tablets and injection should be stored at room temperature and protected from light. Protect the tablets from excessive humidity. The injection is stable for at least 48 hours in commonly used IV solutions.

Compatibility/Compounding Considerations

It is recommended to not mix the injection with other drugs in the same syringe.

Dosage Forms/Regulatory Status

VETERINARY-LABELED PRODUCTS: None

The ARCI (Racing Commissioners International) has designated this drug as a class 3 substance. See the appendix for more information.

HUMAN-LABELED PRODUCTS:

Ketorolac Tromethamine Tablets: 10 mg; generic; (Rx)

Ketorolac Tromethamine Injection: 15 mg/mL & 30 mg/mL in 1 mL, 2 mL single-dose vials, & 10 mL multiple-dose vials; generic; (Rx)

A topical ophthalmic preparation is also available; see the ophthalmology section in the appendix for further information.

References

Dowling, P. (2000). Non-steroidal anti-inflammatory drugs for small animal practitioners. District of Columbia Academy of Veterinary Medicine, Fairfax VA.

Huerkamp, M. (2000). The use of analgesics in rodents and rabbits. Emory University, Division of Animal Resources.

Resources, R.A. (2000). Veterinary Formulary. Minneapolis, University of Minnesota.

Scherk, M. (2003). Feline analgesia in 2003. Proceedings: World Small Animal Veterinary Assoc World Congress. Accessed via: Veterinary Information Network. http://goo.gl/nXadm

L-Asparaginase—see Asparaginase

L-Thyroxine—see Levothyroxine Sodium

Lactated Ringer's—see the appendix section on intravenous fluids

LACTULOSE

(*lak*-tyoo-lose)   Cephulac®

DISACCHARIDE LAXATIVE/AMMONIA
  REDUCER

Prescriber Highlights

▶ Disaccharide laxative & reducer of
  blood ammonia levels

▶ Adverse Effects: Flatulence, gastric
  distention, cramping, etc.; diarrhea &
  dehydration are signs of overdosage

▶ Cats dislike the taste of lactulose liquid & administration may be difficult;
  lactulose crystals (*Kristalose*®) mixed
  into cats' food may be more accepted

▶ May alter insulin requirements in
  diabetics

Uses/Indications

The primary use of lactulose in veterinary medicine is to reduce ammonia blood levels in the
prevention and treatment of hepatic encephalopathy (portal-systemic encephalopathy; PSE)
in small animals and pet birds. It is also used as a
laxative in small animals.

Pharmacology/Actions

Lactulose is a disaccharide (galactose/fructose)
that is not hydrolyzable by mammalian and,
probably, avian gut enzymes. Upon reaching
the colon, lactulose is metabolized by the resident bacteria resulting in the formation of low
molecular weight acids (lactic, formic, acetic)
and CO_2. These acids have a dual effect; they increase osmotic pressure drawing water into the
bowel causing a laxative effect and also acidify
colonic contents. The acidification causes ammonia NH_3 (ammonia) to migrate from the
blood into the colon where it is trapped as
$[NH_4]^+$ (ammonium ion) and expelled with the
feces.

Pharmacokinetics

In humans, less than 3% of an oral dose of lactulose in absorbed (in the small intestine). The
absorbed drug is not metabolized and excreted
unchanged in the urine within 24 hours.

Contraindications/Precautions/Warnings

Lactulose syrup contains some free lactose and
galactose, and may alter the insulin requirements in diabetic patients. In patients with preexisting fluid and electrolyte imbalances, lactulose may exacerbate these conditions if it causes
diarrhea; use cautiously.

Adverse Effects

Signs of flatulence, gastric distention, cramping, etc. are not uncommon early in therapy, but
generally abate with time. Diarrhea and dehydration are signs of overdosage; dosage should
be reduced.

Cats dislike the taste of lactulose syrup and

administration may be difficult. Lactulose granules (crystals) have been more successfully administered after mixing into food.

Reproductive/Nursing Safety

In humans, the FDA categorizes this drug as category **B** for use during pregnancy (*Animal studies have not yet demonstrated risk to the fetus, but
there are no adequate studies in pregnant women;
or animal studies have shown an adverse effect,
but adequate studies in pregnant women have not
demonstrated a risk to the fetus in the first trimester of pregnancy, and there is no evidence of risk in
later trimesters.*)

It is not known whether lactulose is excreted
in milk, but it would be unexpected.

Overdosage/Acute Toxicity

Excessive doses may cause flatulence, diarrhea,
cramping, and dehydration. Replace fluids and
electrolytes if necessary.

Drug Interactions

The following drug interactions have either been
reported or are theoretical in humans or animals
receiving lactulose and may be of significance in
veterinary patients:

◼ **ANTACIDS, ORAL:** Antacids (non-adsorb-
  able) may reduce the colonic acidification
  effects (efficacy) of lactulose

◼ **LAXATIVES, OTHER:** Do not use lactulose
  with other laxatives as the loose stools that
  are formed can be falsely attributed to the
  lactulose with resultant inadequate therapy
  for hepatic encephalopathy

◼ **NEOMYCIN:** Theoretically, orally administered antibiotics (*e.g.*, neomycin) could
  eliminate the bacteria responsible for metabolizing lactulose, thereby reducing its
  efficacy. However, some data suggests that
  synergy may occur when lactulose is used
  with an oral antibiotic (*e.g.*, neomycin) for
  the treatment of hepatic encephalopathy;
  enhanced monitoring of lactulose efficacy is
  probably warranted in cases where an oral
  antibiotic is added to the therapy

Doses

◾ **DOGS:**

  If using the crystals for oral solution: one
  gram of the crystals is equivalent to 1.5 mL
  of the liquid.

  For hepatic encephalopathy:

  a) 15–30 mL PO four times a day; adjust the
    dosage to produce 2–3 soft stools per day
    (Cornelius & Bjorling 1989)

  b) Give 5 mL per 2.5 lbs. of body weight di-
    vided three times a day, may increase as
    necessary to achieve 2–3 soft stools per
    day. If patient is in hepatic encephalopa-
    thy crisis, may give 20–60 mL via stomach
    tube every 4–6 hours or may give as an
    intermittent enema (diluted with water)
    to total 200–300 mL (300–450 grams).
    (Tams 2000)

c) 1–10 mL PO three times daily; adjust dose to give 3–4 soft stools per day; reduce dose if diarrhea develops. May also give via enema in treating severe hepatic encephalopathy. (Twedt 2005)

d) 0.5 mL/kg PO two to three times a day with dietary adjustments. (Favier 2009)

For constipation:

a) 1 mL per 4.5 kg of body weight PO q8h initially, then adjust as needed (Kirk 1986)

■ **CATS:**

If using the crystals for oral solution: one gram of the crystals is equivalent to 1.5 mL of the liquid. An anecdotal suggested dose for constipation in cats is ½ to ¾ of a teaspoonful twice daily.

For hepatic encephalopathy:

a) 0.25–1 mL PO; individualize dosage until semi-formed stools are produced (Center *et al.* 1986)

For constipation:

a) As an enema: 5–10 mL per cat; administered slowly with a well-lubricated 10-12 (french) rubber catheter or feeding tube. Orally: 0.5 mL/kg PO two to three times a day. (Washabau 2007)

b) For maintaining soft stools in cats with chronic constipation: 0.5 mL/kg PO two to three times daily. Dosage is adjusted to obtain the stool quality desired. (Carr 2009)

■ **BIRDS:**

For hepatic encephalopathy; to stimulate appetite, improve intestinal flora:

a) **Cockatiel:** 0.03 mL PO two to three times a day; **Amazon:** 0.1 mL PO two to three times a day. Reduce dosage if diarrhea develops. May be used for weeks. (Clubb 1986)

■ **REPTILES:**

As a laxative:

a) **Green Iguana:** 0.3 mL/kg PO q12h (Wilson 2002)

Monitoring

■ Clinical efficacy (2–3 soft stools per day) when used for PSE

■ In long-term use (months) or in patients with preexisting fluid/electrolyte problems, serum electrolytes should be monitored.

Client Information

■ Contact veterinarian if diarrhea develops.

■ When lactulose is used for hepatic encephalopathy, contact veterinarian if signs worsen or less than 2–3 soft stools are produced per day.

Chemistry/Synonyms

A synthetic derivative of lactose, lactulose is a disaccharide containing one molecule of galactose and one molecule of fructose. It occurs as a white powder that is very slightly soluble in alcohol and very soluble in water. The commercially available solutions are viscous, sweet liquids with an adjusted pH of 3–7.

One gram of the lactulose crystals for oral solution (*Kristalose®*) is equivalent to 1.5 mL of the liquid.

Lactulose may also be known as lactulosum; many trade names are available.

Storage/Stability

Lactulose syrup should be stored in tight containers, preferably at room temperature; avoid freezing. If exposed to heat or light, darkening or cloudiness of the solution may occur, but apparently this does not affect drug potency.

Dosage Forms/Regulatory Status

VETERINARY-LABELED PRODUCTS: None

HUMAN-LABELED PRODUCTS:

Lactulose Solution: 10 grams lactulose per 15 mL (<1.6 grams galactose, <1.2 grams lactose and ≤1.2 grams of other sugars) in 237 mL, 473 mL, 946 mL, 960 mL, 1893 mL, 1.89 L, 1.9 L, & UD 30 mL; *Cephulac®* (Hoechst-Marion Roussel); *Constulose®* and *Enulose®* (Alpharma); generic; (Rx)

Lactulose Crystals for Oral Solution: Lactulose (<0.3 grams galactose and lactose/10 g) in 10 grams and 20 grams; *Kristalose®* (Bertek); (Rx)

Lactulose Solution for oral or rectal use: 10 grams/15 mL in 473 mL & 1,892 mL; *Generiac®* (Morton Grove Pharmaceuticals); (Rx)

References

Carr, A. (2009). Managing Constipation in Cats. Proceedings: ACVIM. Accessed via: Veterinary Information Network. http://goo.gl/BIOaz

Center, S.A., W.E. Hornbuckle, et al. (1986). Congenital Portosystemic Shunts in Cats. *Current Veterinary Therapy (CVT) IX Small Animal Practice.* RW Kirk Ed. Philadelphia, WB Saunders: 825–830.

Clubb, S.L. (1986). Therapeutics: Individual and Flock Treatment Regimens. *Clinical Avian Medicine and Surgery.* GJ Harrison and LR Harrison Eds. Philadelphia, W.B. Saunders: 327–355.

Cornelius, L.M. & D.E. Bjorling (1989). Diseases of the Liver and Biliary System. *Handbook of Small Animal Practice.* RV Morgan Ed. New York, Churchill Livingston: 441–464.

Favier, R.P. (2009). Idiopathic Hepatitis and Cirrhosis in Dogs. *Veterinary Clinics of North America-Small Animal Practice* **39**(3): 481–+.

Kirk, R.W., Ed. (1986). *Current Veterinary Therapy IX, Small Animal Practice.* Philadelphia, W.B. Saunders.

Tams, T. (2000). Diagnosis and Management of Liver Disease in Dogs. Proceedings: American Animal Hospital Association 67th Annual Meeting, Toronto.

Twedt, D. (2005). Treating liver disease. Proceedings: Western Vet Conf. Accessed via: Veterinary Information Network. http://goo.gl/eaI27

Washabau, R. (2007). Evidence-Based Medicine: GI Drugs in the ICU. Proceedings: IVECCS. Accessed via: Veterinary Information Network. http://goo.gl/IHZon

Wilson, H. (2002). Disease management of the Green Iguana. Proceedings: Atlantic Coast Veterinary Conference. Accessed via: Veterinary Information Network. http://goo.gl/N4Ey2

LANTHANUM CARBONATE

(*lan*-tha-num)   Fosrenol®, Lantharenol®

PHOSPHATE BINDING AGENT

Prescriber Highlights

▶ Orally administered phosphate binder; products labeled for use in cats in some countries

▶ Limited experience and relatively little published in veterinary literature

▶ Appears safe; vomiting nausea/inappetence possible

Uses/Indications

Lanthanum carbonate is potentially useful as an orally administered phosphate binding agent for patients with end stage renal disease. While phosphorous dietary restrictions are the mainstay of controlling hyperphosphatemia in small animals, binding agents such as aluminum, sevelamer, or lanthanum can be considered for use in patients whose phosphate levels are not controlled with diet alone or they will not consume very-low phosphorous diets.

Pharmacology/Actions

Lanthanum carbonate's mechanism of action to reduce hyperphosphatemia is by dissociating in the acid environment of the upper GI tract to release lanthanum ions. These ions bind to dietary phosphate and form highly insoluble lanthanum phosphate complexes that are then eliminated in the feces.

Pharmacokinetics

Following oral doses, lanthanum bioavailability is very low (less than 0.002%). In humans, systemically available lanthanum is very highly bound to plasma proteins (>99%). Studies in dogs, mice, and rats have shown that lanthanum levels in tissues increase over time and can be several orders of magnitude higher than that found in the plasma. Highest tissue levels are found in the GI tract, bone, and liver. In rats, absorbed lanthanum is cleared primarily via biliary excretion into the feces. In dogs, mean recovery of an oral dose of lanthanum averages 94%.

Contraindications/Precautions/Warnings

There are no listed contraindications for lanthanum carbonate, but it should be used with caution in patients where the GI tract is not intact (*e.g.*, GI ulcers, colitis, etc.) as there is an increased chance for oral absorption.

Adverse Effects

Limited information is available for dogs and cats but it appears that lanthanum is well tolerated. Vomiting has been reported in cats.

In humans, adverse effects most commonly reported include nausea and vomiting. These are generally self-limiting and usually abate with continued use.

Reproductive/Nursing Safety

It is likely that lanthanum is safe to use during pregnancy. For humans, the FDA has placed it in category *C* for use during pregnancy (*Animal studies have shown an adverse effect on the fetus, but there are no adequate studies in humans; or there are no animal reproduction studies and no adequate studies in humans. However, there does not appear to be a significant risk to offspring.*)

Lanthanum should be safe to use in nursing dams.

Overdosage/Acute Toxicity

No specific information was located. It is likely that an acute overdose would be tolerated, with the chance that it might cause GI effects. Only supportive treatment should be required. In a poster presentation of a dose escalation study in cats, cats tolerated oral dosages up to 1 gram/kg, but vomited repeatedly after receiving 2 grams/kg (Schmidt & Spiecker-Hauser 2009).

Drug Interactions

Drug interactions with lanthanum carbonate have not been reported, but as it is a binding agent similar to aluminum, it seems prudent to separate by two hours dosing lanthanum and the following:

▧ **ALLOPURINOL**

▧ **CHLOROQUINE**

▧ **CORTICOSTEROIDS**

▧ **DIGOXIN**

▧ **ETHAMBUTOL**

▧ **FLUOROQUINOLONES**

▧ **H-2 ANTAGONISTS (ranitidine, famotidine, etc.)**

▧ **IRON SALTS**

▧ **ISONIAZID**

▧ **PENICILLAMINE**

▧ **PHENOTHIAZINES**

▧ **TETRACYCLINES**

▧ **THYROID HORMONES**

Laboratory Considerations

▧ No specific concerns

Doses

▧ **CATS:**

As a phosphate binder:

a) Relatively little is known about use of sevalamer and lanthanum in dogs and cats; anecdotally they appear to be both safe and effective. Both have been used in cats at a dose of 200 mg (total dose) PO (on/in food) 2–3 times daily. (Sparkes 2006)

b) Using the proprietary product *Renalzin®*: The standard recommended dosage is 2 mLs (400 mg) applied in the cat's food, once or twice daily depending on the cat's feeding regimen. (*Renalzin®*—Bayer-UK)

Monitoring
- Serum phosphorous (and other electrolytes such as potassium, calcium, bicarbonate, chloride)

Client Information
- As the human dosing recommendations are to chew tablets and not to swallow whole tablets intact, crush and place on the animal's food. If using a veterinary commercial product containing lanthanum carbonate, follow the administration directions.

Chemistry/Synonyms
Lanthanum is a chemical element with the symbol La and atomic number 57. When used pharmacologically, it is administered as lanthanum carbonate. Lanthanum carbonate may also be known as: Bay-78-1887, and by the trade names *Lantharenol®*, *Renalzin®*, and *Fosrenol®*.

Storage/Stability
Store tablets at room temperature (25°C, 77°F); excursions are permitted to 15°–30°C (59°–86°F). Protect from moisture.

Dosage Forms/Regulatory Status
VETERINARY-LABELED PRODUCTS: None in USA

A lanthanum carbonate (octa-hydrate), kaolin, and vitamin E labeled product (*Renalzin®*) for use in cats is available in several countries (not USA or Canada at time of writing). It does not appear to be a licensed product, but is a food additive/supplement in those countries. Confirmed concentrations of the ingredients were not found, but it has been reported that 1 mL contains 200 mg of lanthanum carbonate. Available as a pump gel/paste in 50 mL and 150 mL pump containers; *Renalzin®* (Bayer)

HUMAN-LABELED PRODUCTS:

Lanthanum Carbonate Oral Chewable Tablet 500 mg, 750 mg, & 1,000 mg; *Fosrenol®* (Rexar); (Rx)

References
Schmidt, B.H. & U. Spiecker-Hauser (2009). Overdose acceptance and tolerance of Lantharenol (R) in adult healthy cats. Journal of Veterinary Pharmacology and Therapeutics 32: 129–129.
Sparkes, A. (2006). Chronic renal failure in the cat. Proceedings: WSAVA Congress. Accessed via: Veterinary Information Network. http://goo.gl/xrddI

LAXATIVES, HYPEROSMOTIC MAGNESIUM SALTS PEG 3350 PRODUCTS SORBITOL

GoLYTELY®, Epsom Salts, Glauber's Salt

LAXATIVES

Prescriber Highlights

▶ Saline/hyperosmotic agents for constipation, bowel "cleansing", & to increase elimination of GI toxins

▶ Contraindications: PEG 3350 solutions are contraindicated in patients with GI obstruction, gastric retention, bowel perforation, toxic colitis, or megacolon (humans). Saline cathartics should be used with extreme caution in patients with renal insufficiency, pre-existing water-balance or electrolyte abnormalities, or cardiac disease.

▶ Adverse Effects: Cramping, nausea possible. Electrolyte disturbances possible, particularly with repeated use

▶ If magnesium salts used chronically: Hypermagnesemia (muscle weakness, ECG changes & CNS effects)

▶ Drug Interactions

Also see the preceding monograph for Lactulose

Uses/Indications
The hyperosmotic laxatives are used for their cathartic action to relieve constipation. They are also used to reduce intestinal transit time thereby reducing the absorption of orally ingested toxicants. Commonly, or historically used hyperosmotic laxatives include: magnesium sulfate, magnesium oxide (milk of magnesia), sodium sulfate, sorbitol, and polyethylene glycol 3350 products.

Pharmacology/Actions
Although unproven, it is commonly believed that the hyperosmotic effect of the poorly absorbed magnesium cation causes water retention, stimulates stretch receptors and enhances peristalsis in the small intestine and colon. Recent data, however, suggests that magnesium ions may directly decrease transit times and increase cholecystokinin release.

Sorbitol is a non-absorbable sugar alcohol that acts as an osmotic laxative.

Polyethylene glycol (PEG) 3350 is a non-absorbable compound that when used alone (*MiraLax®*, etc.) acts as an osmotic laxative agent. When used as a bowel cleansing solution

(*CoLyte®*, *GoLytely®*, etc.), additional electrolytes are added to help prevent electrolyte imbalances from occurring. Sodium sulfate is the primary sodium source so sodium absorption is minimized. Other electrolytes (bicarbonate potassium and chloride) are also added so that no net change occurs with either absorption or secretion of electrolytes or water in the gut.

Pharmacokinetics

When magnesium salts are administered, up to 30% of the magnesium dose of magnesium can be absorbed.

Generally, the onset of action of saline cathartics (characterized by a loose, watery stool) occurs in 3–12 hours after dosing in monogastric animals and within 18 hours in ruminants. Depending on dose and additional fluid consumed, polyethylene glycol (PEG) and sorbitol laxatives can have an effect within one hour of dosing.

Contraindications/Precautions/Warnings

Saline cathartics are contraindicated in dehydrated patients or for long-term use. Sodium containing laxatives are contraindicated in patients with congestive heart failure or congenital megacolon. In humans, PEG 3350 and sorbitol solutions are contraindicated in patients with GI obstruction, gastric retention, bowel perforation, toxic colitis, or megacolon. Saline cathartics should be used with extreme caution in patients with renal insufficiency, pre-existing water-balance or electrolyte abnormalities, or cardiac disease.

Adverse Effects

Except for possible cramping and nausea, adverse effects in otherwise healthy patients generally occur only with the saline cathartics with chronic use or overdoses.

When magnesium salts are used, hypermagnesemia manifested by muscle weakness, ECG changes and CNS effects can occur.

Sorbitol may cause vomiting, dehydration, secondary hypernatremia, abdominal cramping or pain, and possible hypotension.

In one small study (N=6) in cats where PEG 3350 with electrolytes (*e.g.*, *CoLyte®*) was given long-term (powder in food and dose titrated to produce soft, but formed stools), one cat sporadically vomited after dosing, mild erythrocytosis was noted in one cat, and 3 cats developed mild hyperkalemia. The authors concluded that PEG 3350 was a safe and palatable oral laxative in cats for long-term use; potential side effects include hyperkalemia and subclinical dehydration (Tam *et al.* 2010). In humans, polyethylene glycol 3350 has rarely caused hyponatremia secondary to syndrome of inappropriate vasopressin release (SIADH).

Reproductive/Nursing Safety

In humans, the FDA categorizes magnesium sulfate as category *B* for use during pregnancy (*Animal studies have not yet demonstrated risk to the fetus, but there are no adequate studies in pregnant women; or animal studies have shown an adverse effect, but adequate studies in pregnant women have not demonstrated a risk to the fetus in the first trimester of pregnancy, and there is no evidence of risk in later trimesters.*) Other saline or hyperosmolar cathartics should be safe to use in pregnancy when used infrequently.

Magnesium emulsions administered orally did not affect the stools of nursing infants, although magnesium content in breast milk was slightly elevated compared with untreated patients. In veterinary patients, it should be safe to use during nursing when used infrequently.

Overdosage/Acute Toxicity

Clinical signs of overdosage of magnesium containing laxatives are described above. Treatment should consist of monitoring and correcting any fluid imbalances that occur with parenteral fluids.

If hypermagnesemia occurs, furosemide may be used to enhance the renal excretion of the excess magnesium. Calcium has been suggested to help antagonize the CNS effects of magnesium.

Drug Interactions

All orally administered saline laxatives may alter the rate and extent of absorption of **other orally administered drugs** by decreasing intestinal transit times. The extent of these effects has not been well characterized for individual drugs, however.

■ **TETRACYCLINES:** Magnesium laxatives should **not** be administered with tetracycline products

Doses

■ **DOGS:**

Magnesium hydroxide (Milk of Magnesia) as a cathartic:

a) 5–10 mL (Davis, L.E. 1985)

b) 1–20 mL PO (Rossoff 1974)

Magnesium sulfate:

a) 5–25 grams PO (Davis, L.E. 1985)

b) 2–60 grams PO (Rossoff 1974)

Sorbitol (70%):

a) As a cathartic with activated charcoal in intoxications: If activated charcoal does not contain a pre-existing cathartic (for the first dose administered), one can potentially add in sorbitol (70% solution) for a one dose dosing at: 1–2 mL/kg, PO, given within 60 minutes of toxin ingestion. (Lee 2010)

Polyethylene Glycol-Electrolyte Solution:

a) For colonic cleansing prior to colonoscopy using *Go-Lytely®*: Keep animal from food for 24–36 hours. On the evening prior to a morning colonoscopy (or the morning for an afternoon colonoscopy), give 60 mL/kg via orogastric tube. Repeat in 2 hours. A warm water enema should follow each dose and a third enema given prior to anesthesia. (Leib 2003), (Leib 2006)

b) For colonic cleansing prior to colonoscopy using *Go-Lytely*®: 12–18 hours prior to colonoscopy give 25 mL/kg via orogastric tube three to five times, one hour apart. Give enema shortly after last *Go-Lytely*® dose and one to two hours prior to endoscopy procedure. (Richter 2003)

c) For colonic cleansing prior to colonoscopy using *Go-Lytely*®: Withhold food for 18–24 hours. Give two doses of 20 mL/kg *Go-Lytely*® 4–6 hours apart the afternoon before an AM endoscopy. The morning of procedure, a warm-water enema is administered. (Jergens 2003)

d) For mechanical bowel cleansing prior to (antibiotics and) colonic surgery: *Go-Lytely*® (or similar osmotic cathartic): 50–75 mL/kg by stomach tube or NE tube the evening prior to surgery. (Trepanier 2003)

■ **CATS:**

Magnesium hydroxide (Milk of Magnesia) as a cathartic:

a) 2–6 mL (Davis, L.E. 1985)

b) 1–5 mL PO (Rossoff 1974)

Magnesium sulfate:

a) 2–5 grams PO (Davis, L.E. 1985), (Rossoff 1974)

Sorbitol (70%):

a) As a cathartic with activated charcoal in intoxications: If activated charcoal does not contain a pre-existing cathartic (for the first dose administered), one can potentially add in sorbitol (70% solution) for a one dose dosing at: 1–2 mL/kg, PO, given within 60 minutes of toxin ingestion. (Lee 2010)

Polyethylene Glycol 3350 (*e.g.*, *MiraLax*®):

a) As a laxative: ⅛th to ¼ teaspoonful twice daily in food. (Scherk 2010)

Polyethylene Glycol-Electrolyte Solution:

a) For colonic cleansing prior to colonoscopy using *Go-Lytely*®: Keep animal from food for 24–36 hours. On the evening prior to a morning colonoscopy (or the morning for an afternoon colonoscopy), give 60 mL/kg via nasogastric tube. Repeat in 2 hours. A warm water enema should follow each dose and a third enema given prior to anesthesia. Metoclopramide (0.2 mg/kg SC 15–20 minutes before the first *Go-Lytely*® dose is given to reduce vomiting. (Leib 2003), (Leib 2006)

■ **HORSES:**

a) As a cathartic for plant intoxications: Activated charcoal (AC) slurry dosage range of 1–5 grams/kg (~1 gram of activated charcoal per 5 ml of water). Multi-dose activated charcoal is beneficial for a number of plant intoxications, including oleander. Administration of a cathartic mixed in the AC slurry helps to hasten elimination of contents from the gastrointestinal tract. Commonly used cathartics include sodium sulfate (Glauber's salts), magnesium sulfate (Epsom salts), and sorbitol. Sodium or magnesium sulfate can be administered at 250–500 mg/kg mixed in the AC slurry. Sorbitol (70%), also mixed in the AC slurry, can be administered at 3 mL/kg. There is little need to administer a cathartic if significant diarrhea is already present. (Puschner 2010)

Magnesium sulfate (Epsom salt):

a) 0.2 grams/kg diluted in 4 L of warm water administered via nasogastric tube. Administer only to well-hydrated animals (ideally in conjunction with IV fluid therapy). Do not treat longer than 3 days or there is an increased risk of enteritis or magnesium toxicity occurring. (Clark & Becht 1987)

b) As a laxative: 1 gram/kg PO every 1–2 days; in colic delay treatment until rehydrated (Moore 1999)

c) To reduce absorption of toxicants and GI transit time: 500 grams (as a 20% solution) PO. If mineral oil has been used initially, give saline cathartic 30–45 minutes after mineral oil. (Oehme 1987)

d) For cecal impactions: 1 gram/kg dissolved in water dissolved in water and given via NG tube. Give with a balanced electrolyte solution IV to stimulate secretion into the dehydrated ingesta. (White 2005)

■ **CATTLE:**

a) Sodium sulfate (as a cathartic) 500–750 grams PO as a 6% solution via stomach tube (Davis, L. 1993) **Note:** When used in food animals, FARAD states that this salt is rapidly excreted and not considered a residue concern in animal tissues; therefore, a 24 hour preslaughter withdrawal interval (WDI) would be sufficient. (Haskell *et al.* 2005)

b) See the reference by Puschner in the horse section above.

Magnesium sulfate (as a cathartic):

a) 0.5–1 kg/500 kg orally (Whitlock 1986)

b) 1–2 grams/kg PO (Howard 1993)

Magnesium oxide:

a) 0.5–1 kg/500 kg orally (Whitlock 1986)

■ **SHEEP & GOATS:**

a) Sodium sulfate (as a cathartic) 60 grams PO as a 6% solution via stomach tube (Davis, L. 1993)

■ **SWINE:**

a) Magnesium sulfate (as a cathartic): 1–2 grams/kg PO (Howard 1993)

b) Sodium sulfate (as a cathartic): 30–60 grams PO as a 6% solution via stomach tube (Davis, L. 1993)

■ **BIRDS:**

Magnesium sulfate:

a) To act as a cathartic and reduce lead absorption: 0.5–1 gram/kg PO as a 5% solution in drinking water (McDonald 1986)

Monitoring

■ Fluid and electrolyte status in susceptible patients, high doses, or chronic use

■ Clinical efficacy

Client Information

■ Do not give dosages greater than, or for periods longer than those recommended by veterinarian

■ Contact veterinarian if patient begins vomiting

Chemistry/Synonyms

Magnesium cation containing solutions of magnesium citrate, magnesium hydroxide, or magnesium sulfate act as saline laxatives. Magnesium citrate solutions contain 4.71 mEq of magnesium per 5 mL. Magnesium hydroxide contains 34.3 mEq of magnesium per gram and milk of magnesia contains 13.66 mEq per 5 mL. One gram of magnesium sulfate (Epsom salt) contains approximately 8.1 mEq of magnesium.

Sodium sulfate (hexahydrate form) occurs as large, colorless, odorless, crystals or white crystalline powder. It will effloresce in dry air and partially dissolve in its own water of crystallization at about 33°C. 1 gram is soluble in about 2.5 mL of water. Sodium sulfate may also be known as E514, Glauber's Salt, natrii sulphas, natrio sulfata, or natrium sulfuricum.

Polyethylene glycol 3350 is a non-absorbable compound that acts as an osmotic agent.

Storage/Stability

Magnesium citrate solutions should be stored at 2–30°C. Store milk of magnesia at temperatures less than 35°C, but do not freeze. PEG 3350 reconstituted (from powder by the pharmacy, client, clinic, etc.) solutions should be kept refrigerated and used within 24 hours.

Dosage Forms/Regulatory Status

Saline cathartic products have apparently not been formally FDA-approved for use in domestic animals. They are available without prescription (OTC).

VETERINARY-LABELED PRODUCTS: None located

HUMAN-LABELED PRODUCTS:

Saline/Hyperosmotic Laxatives (not an inclusive list):

Magnesium Hydroxide Suspension (Milk of Magnesia): equiv. to 30 mL milk of magnesia in 100 mL, 400 mL & UD 10 mL; magnesium hydroxide 160 mg/mL & 80 mg/mL in 180 mL, 240 mL, 360 mL, 400 mL, 480 mL, 780 mL, UD 30 mL; *Milk of Magnesia Concentrated*® (Roxane); *Phillips'*® *Milk of Magnesia* and *Phillips'*® *Milk of Magnesia Concentrated* (Bayer); generic; (OTC)

Magnesium Sulfate (Epsom Salt) Granules: in 120 g, 1lb and 4lbs; generic; (OTC)

Sodium sulfate (hexahydrate) is available from chemical supply houses.

Sorbitol 70% in pints; generic; (OTC). Sorbitol is also included in several activated charcoal products.

Polyethylene Glycol 3350 Powder for solution: *MiraLax*® (Plough); *GlycoLax*® (K-U); *ClearLax*® (Perrigo); *Dulcolax Balance*® (BI); generic. Available in either pre-measured 17 gram packets or bulk powder and are OTC.

Polyethylene Glycol 3350 and Electrolyte Solutions (Rx):

OCL® Solution (Abbott); (Rx) Oral Solution in 1500 mL: 146 mg sodium chloride, 168 mg sodium bicarbonate, 1.29 grams sodium sulfate decahydrate, 75 mg potassium chloride, 6 grams PEG-3350.

CoLyte® (Schwartz Pharma); (Rx); 1 gallon of Powder for Oral Solution in bottles: 227.1 grams PEG 3350, 5.53 grams sodium chloride, 6.36 grams sodium bicarbonate, 21.5 grams sodium sulfate, 2.82 grams potassium chloride; 4L of solution: 240 grams PEG 3350, 22.72 grams sodium sulfate, 6.72 grams sodium bicarbonate, 5.84 grams NaCl, 2.98 grams KCL

GoLYTELY® (Braintree Labs); (Rx); Powder for Oral Solution in jugs: 5.86 grams sodium chloride, 6.74 grams sodium bicarbonate, 22.74 grams sodium sulfate, 2.97 grams potassium chloride, 236 grams PEG 3350; Packets: 227.1 grams PEG 3350, 21.5 grams sodium sulfate, 6.36 grams sodium bicarbonate, 5.53 grams NaCl, 2.82 grams KCl

NuLytely® (Braintree Labs); *TriLyte*® (Schwarz Pharma); (Rx); Powder for Reconstitution in 4 L jugs: 420 grams PEG 3350, 5.72 grams sodium bicarbonate, 11.2 grams NaCl, 1.48 grams KCL

MoviPrep® (Salix); (Rx); Powder for Reconstitution in pouches: 100 grams PEG 3350, 7.5 grams sodium sulfate, 2.691 grams NaCl, 1.015 grams KCl.

References

Clark, E.S. & J.L. Becht (1987). Clinical Pharmacology of the Gastrointestinal Tract. Vet Clin North Am (Equine Practice) 3(1): 101–122.

Davis, L. (1993). Drugs Affecting the Digestive System. Current Veterinary Therapy 3: Food Animal Practice. J Howard Ed. Philadelphia, W.B. Saunders Co.

Davis, L.E. (1985). General Care of the Patient. Handbook of Small Animal Therapeutics. LE Davis Ed. New York, Churchill Livingstone: 1–20.

Haskell, S., M. Payne, et al. (2005). Farad Digest: Antidotes in Food Animal Practice. JAVMA 226(6): 884–887.

Howard, J. (1993). Table of Common Drugs: Approximate Doses. Current Veterinary Therapy 3: Food Animal Practice. J Howard Ed. Philadelphia, W.B. Saunders Co.: 930–933.

Jergens, A. (2003). Practical tips for maximizing endoscopic biopsy of the GI tract. Proceedings: Western Veterinary Conference. Accessed via: Veterinary Information Network. http://goo.gl/7M4IG

Lee, J.A. (2010). Complications & Controversies of Decontamination: Activated Charcoal—To Use or Not To Use? Proceedings: ACVIM. Accessed via: Veterinary Information Network. http://goo.gl/TA6xo

Leib, M. (2003). Chronic diarrhea in dogs and cats: Parts 1 & 2. Proceedings: Atlantic Coast Veterinary Conference. Accessed via: Veterinary Information Network. http://goo.gl/amUiP

Leib, M. (2006). Colonoscopy. Proceedings: WVC. Accessed via: Veterinary Information Network. http://goo.gl/cW3op

McDonald, S.E. (1986). Lead Poisoning in Psittacine Birds. Current Veterinary Therapy IX: Small Animal Practice. RW Kirk Ed. Philadelphia, WB Saunders: 713–718.

Moore, R. (1999). Medical treatment of abdominal pain in the horse: Enteric treatment and motility modifiers. Proceedings: The North American Veterinary Conference, Orlando.

Oehme, F.W. (1987). General Principles in Treatment of Poisoning. Current Therapy in Equine Medicine 2. NE Robinson Ed. Philadelphia, W.B. Saunders: 653–656.

Puschner, B. (2010). Diagnostic and therapeutic approach to plant poisonings in large animals. Accessed via: Veterinary Information Network. http://goo.gl/WFJfn

Richter, K. (2003). Colonoscopy. Proceedings: Western Veterinary Conf. Accessed via: Veterinary Information Network. http://goo.gl/Lr28K

Rossoff, I.S. (1974). Handbook of Veterinary Drugs. New York, Springer Publishing.

Scherk, M. (2010). Megacolon: Which Cats are Predisposed? The Hard Facts. Proceedings: WVC. Accessed via: Veterinary Information Network. http://goo.gl/rvFew

Tam, F., A. Carr, et al. (2010). Safety and palatability of polyethylene glycol 3350 as an oral laxative in cats. Proceedings: ACVIM. Accessed via: Veterinary Information Network. http://goo.gl/KAkKH

Trepanier, L. (2003). Perioperative antimicrobial prophylaxis. Proceedings: International Veterinary Emergency and Critical Care Symposium. Accessed via: Veterinary Information Network. http://goo.gl/Ixsc6

White, N. (2005). Intestinal diseases. Western Veterinary Conference: Proceedings. Accessed via: Veterinary Information Network. http://goo.gl/RHnOz

Whitlock, R.H. (1986). Constipation. Current Veterinary Therapy 2: Food Animal Practice. JL Howard Ed. Philadelphia, WB Saunders: 711.

LEFLUNOMIDE

(le-*floo*-noh-myde)   Arava®

IMMUNOMODULATING AGENT

Prescriber Highlights

▶ Immunomodulating drug that may be useful in dogs for treating a variety of immune-mediated conditions such as IMHA, systemic & cutaneous reactive histiocytosis, granulomatous meningoencephalitis, etc.; can be used as part of transplant rejection protocols in dogs. Has been used with methotrexate to treat rheumatoid arthritis in cats.

▶ Appears well-tolerated in dogs and cats, but numbers treated are low

▶ Teratogenic (Category X)

▶ Active metabolite can persist in body for years

▶ Treatment can be very expensive, but prices dropping secondary to generic availability

Uses/Indications

Leflunomide is an immunomodulating drug that may be useful in dogs for treating a variety of immune-related conditions such as IMHA, systemic and cutaneous reactive histiocytosis, granulomatous meningoencephalitis, etc; it can be used as part of transplant rejection protocols in dogs.

Leflunomide has been used with methotrexate to treat rheumatoid arthritis in cats.

Pharmacology/Actions

Leflunomide inhibits autoimmune T-cell proliferation and autoantibody production by B cells. Leflunomide acts almost exclusively via its active metabolite A77 1726 (M1). This metabolite reversibly inhibits the mitochondrial enzyme dihydroorotate dehydrogenase thereby preventing the formation of ribonucleotide uridine monophosphate (rUMP). This causes decreased DNA and RNA synthesis, inhibition of cell proliferation, and G1 cell cycle arrest.

Pharmacokinetics

Specific information on the pharmacokinetics of leflunomide in dogs and cats was not located, but it has been reported that the conversion to a toxic metabolite is slower in cats then in dogs. In humans, leflunomide is rapidly converted to A77 1726 (active metabolite; M1) in the GI mucosa and liver. Peak levels of A77 1726 occur between 6–12 hours after an oral dose. The presence of food in the gut does not appear to affect oral bioavailability. A77 1726 Is highly bound to albumin >99%). A77 1726 is further degraded in the liver as glucuronides and an oxalinic acid compound which are excreted in the urine and bile. Half-life is about 15 days, but the metabolite (A77 1726) can be detectable in patients up to 2 years after it is discontinued.

Contraindications/Precautions/Warnings

Leflunomide is contraindicated during pregnancy and in patients hypersensitive to it. It should be used with extreme caution in patients with immunodeficiency and in patients with significant renal impairment.

Adverse Effects

Leflunomide appears to be well tolerated by dogs. Adverse effects reported include decreased appetite, lethargy, vomiting, lymphopenia, and anemia.

In humans, gastrointestinal effects (diarrhea, nausea), alopecia and rash are most commonly reported. Serious adverse effects that have been reported include hematologic toxicity, dermatologic effects (TEN, Stevens-Johnson, etc.), and hepatotoxicity.

Reproductive/Nursing Safety

Leflunomide should not be used during pregnancy. A variety of teratogenic effects in laboratory animals have been detailed at doses used clinically. In humans, the FDA categorizes this drug as category *X* for use during pregnancy (*Studies in animals or humans demonstrate fetal abnormalities or adverse reaction; reports indicate evidence of fetal risk. The risk of use in pregnant women clearly outweighs any possible benefit.*)

It is not known whether leflunomide is excreted in milk; it is suggested to use milk replacer if the dam is receiving the drug.

Overdosage/Acute Toxicity

Acute toxicologic studies in mice and rats have demonstrated that the minimally toxic dose is 200 mg/kg and 100 mg/kg, respectively. Cholestyramine or activated charcoal are recommended to accelerate elimination. Contact an animal poison control center for more information.

Drug Interactions

The following drug interactions have either been reported or are theoretical in humans or animals receiving leflunomide and may be of significance in veterinary patients:

- **CHARCOAL, ACTIVATED:** Can increase elimination and decrease A77 1726 drug concentrations; may be used when more rapid elimination is desirable

- **CHOLESTYRAMINE:** Can increase elimination and decrease A77 1726 drug concentrations; may be used when more rapid elimination is desirable

- **HEPATOTOXIC AGENTS, OTHER:** Increased risk for toxicity

- **METHOTREXATE:** Increased adverse effects and ALT possible

- **PHENYTOIN:** Leflunomide can increase phenytoin levels

- **RIFAMPIN:** Can increase A77 1726 peak levels

- **VACCINES, LIVE VIRUS:** Live virus vaccines should be used with caution, if at all, during leflunomide therapy

- **WARFARIN:** Leflunomide may increase INR

Doses

- **DOGS:**

  a) As an immunosuppressive as part of a protocol (with cyclosporine) following organ transplant: Leflunomide 4–6 mg/kg PO q24h and then to maintain trough plasma levels of 20 micrograms/mL. (Sykes 2007)

  b) As an adjunctive immunosuppressive for immune-mediated hemolytic anemia: 4 mg/kg PO q24h. (Chabanne 2006)

  c) For treatment of systemic and cutaneous reactive histiocytosis: 2–4 mg/kg PO once daily to attain trough levels of 20 micrograms/mL. (Foil 2003)

  d) For treatment of Evans' Syndrome in a diabetic dog (from a case report): In combination with human intravenous immunoglobulin (hIVIg), leflunomide was initiated at a dosage of 2 mg/kg PO q12h (based on the nontoxic dosage of 4 mg/kg per day used in studies of the canine renal transplantation model). Leflunomide dosage was decreased by 25% every 4 weeks for the first 4 months in order to achieve a trough level of approximately 20 micrograms/mL (leflunomide trough levels were based on studies of the canine renal transplantation model); then the dosage was decreased every 8 weeks until discontinuation after 10 months of therapy. (Bianco & Hardy 2009)

- **CATS:**

  a) For rheumatoid arthritis: Initially, leflunomide at 10 mg (total dose) PO once daily and methotrexate at 2.5 mg (total dose) PO three times on *one day per week*. When significant improvement occurs, reduce doses of leflunomide to 10 mg PO twice weekly and methotrexate to 2.5 mg PO once weekly. (Bennett 2005)

Monitoring

- Adverse effects (CBC, liver enzymes)
- Trough levels of A771 1726 (20 micrograms/mL is target)

Client Information

- Relatively experimental when used in veterinary patients; contact veterinarian if any unusual effects are noted
- Treatment can be very expensive

Chemistry/Synonyms

Leflunomide has a melting point of 165–166°C. It is poorly soluble in water (21 mg/L).

Leflunomide may also be known as HWA 486, RS 34821, or SU 101; a common trade name is *Arava®*.

Storage/Stability
Leflunomide tablets should be stored at room temperature (15–30°C) and protected from light.

Dosage Forms/Regulatory Status
VETERINARY-LABELED PRODUCTS: None

HUMAN-LABELED PRODUCTS:

Leflunomide Tablets: 10 mg & 20 mg; *Arava®* (Hoechst Marion Roussel); generic; (Rx)

References

Bennett, D. (2005). Immune-mediated and infective arthritis. Textbook of Veterinary Internal Medicine, 6th Ed. S Ettinger and E Feldman Eds., Elsevier: 1958–1965.

Bianco, D. & R.M. Hardy (2009). Treatment of Evans' Syndrome With Human Intravenous Immunoglobulin and Leflunomide in a Diabetic Dog. Journal of the American Animal Hospital Association 45(3): 147–150.

Chabanne, L. (2006). Immune-Mediated Hemolytic Anemia In the Dog. Proceedings: WSAVA Congress. Accessed via: Veterinary Information Network. http://goo.gl/LICvo

Foil, C. (2003). New drugs in dermatology. Proceedings: Western Veterinary Conf. Accessed via: Veterinary Information Network. http://goo.gl/iEYic

Sykes, J. (2007). Infections in renal transplant patients. Proceedings: ACVIM. Accessed via: Veterinary Information Network. http://goo.gl/5EFbQ

LEUCOVORIN CALCIUM

(loo-koe-*vor*-in)
Folinic Acid, Citrovorum Factor

ORAL OR INJECTABLE FOLIC ACID DERIVATIVE

Prescriber Highlights

▶ Primarily used in veterinary medicine to help reverse neurotoxicity or hematologic toxicity associated with dihydrofolate reductase inhibitors (e.g., pyrimethamine, trimethoprim, or ormetoprim)

▶ Leucovorin does not require conversion by dihydrofolate reductase for it to be active

Uses/Indications
Leucovorin calcium is the calcium salt of folinic acid and is used as an antidote for toxicity from folic acid antagonists (*e.g.*, methotrexate, pyrimethamine, trimethoprim, ormetoprim). It is used routinely in human medicine as a rescue agent for high-dose methotrexate chemotherapy, but the drug is rarely used for this in veterinary medicine. More commonly, it is used in dogs, cats or horses to help reverse or prevent hematologic toxicity associated with pyrimethamine, trimethoprim, or ormetoprim.

Pharmacology/Actions
Reduced folates act as coenzymes in the synthesis of purine and pyrimidine nucleotides that are necessary for DNA synthesis. Folates are also required for maintenance of normal erythropoiesis.

Leucovorin is a reduced form of folic acid that does not require dihydrofolate reductase conversion, as does folic acid, for it to become biologically active. It is further converted to active reduced forms, of which 5-methyltetrahdyrofolate (5-methyl THF) is predominantly responsible for its activity. Although, leucovorin is a mixture of diastereoisomers, only the (-)-L-isomer (citrovorum factor) becomes biologically active.

Leucovorin inhibits thymidylate synthase by stabilizing the binding of fluorodeoxyuredylic acid to the enzyme. This can potentiate the activity, but also the toxicity of fluorouracil (5-FU).

Pharmacokinetics
There is limited information available on the pharmacokinetics of leucovorin in animals. In dogs, the elimination half-life of the L-isomer (active) of leucovorin is about 50 minutes. It is extensively metabolized and then excreted into the urine. The D-form (not biologically active) elimination half-life is about 2.5 hours. Apparent volume of distribution for both forms is about 0.6 L/kg.

In humans, oral bioavailability of leucovorin is reduced as dosage is increased above 25 mg. A 25 mg dose in an adult has a bioavailability of 97%, while 50 mg and 100 mg doses have bioavailabilities of 75% and 37%, respectively. IM bioavailability is similar to IV. Oral doses of 25 mg yield peak levels of leucovorin in about an hour and peaks of the active reduced folates occur between 1.7 and 2.4 hours after dosing. After intravenous administration, peak total reduced folate levels occur in about 10 minutes. About 50% of oral body stores of reduced folates are found in the liver. Elimination occurs in the urine, primarily as 10-formyl-THF or 5,10-methyl-THF. Elimination half-life is approximately 5–6 hours for total reduced folates.

Contraindications/Precautions/Warnings
Leucovorin is contraindicated only when known intolerance to the drug is documented. In humans, cobalamin (B-12) levels may be reduced with megaloblastic anemias and folinic acid therapy may mask the signs associated with it.

Use with extreme caution in patients receiving systemic fluorouracil (see Drug Interactions).

Because of its calcium content, large intravenous doses should be given slowly and not bolused.

Reproductive/Nursing Safety
Leucovorin reproductive studies have not been performed nor is it known if it enters milk, however, it is likely safe to administer during pregnancy or nursing.

Adverse Effects
Adverse effects have not been noted when leucovorin has been used in animals. In humans, gastrointestinal effects can be seen when the drug is given orally and, very rarely, seizures or hypersensitivity reactions may occur.

Overdosage/Acute Toxicity

Except in situations where drug interactions are possible, an inadvertent overdose is unlikely to be of concern.

Drug Interactions

The following drug interactions have either been reported or are theoretical in humans or animals receiving leucovorin and may be of significance in veterinary patients:

■ **BARBITURATES, PRIMIDONE, PHENYTOIN:** Large doses of leucovorin may reduce the antiseizure efficacy of these agents

■ **FLUOROURACIL:** Leucovorin may increase both the antineoplastic efficacy and toxicity of 5-FU

■ **TRIMETHOPRIM, ORMETOPRIM, PYRIMETHAMINE** (drugs that inhibit dihydrofolate reductase): Leucovorin may reduce efficacy somewhat, however, protozoa cannot utilize leucovorin

Laboratory Considerations

■ No specific concerns were noted

Doses

■ **DOGS/CATS:**

a) For folate deficiency associated with pyrimethamine use: 5–15 mg (total dose) PO or parenterally once daily. (Greene *et al.* 2006)

b) Cats: For bone marrow suppression associated with pyrimethamine or trimethoprim/sulfa: 5 mg (route not specified) once daily. (Lindsay 2004)

c) Cats: To prevent bone marrow toxicity associated with pyrimethamine: 1 mg/kg (route not specified) once daily. (Inzana 2002)

d) For methotrexate overdose: Most effective if given within 48 hours of overdose. The dose of leucovorin is dependent on the serum methotrexate concentration. Dogs with serum methotrexate levels greater than 10^{-7} M at 48 hours have toxic reactions. Leucovorin dosage ranges from 25–200 mg/m^2 parenterally every 6 hours until methotrexate levels are less than 1 X 10^{-8} M. In one study, dogs tolerated methotrexate dosages up to 3 grams/m^2 when leucovorin was given at 15 mg/m^2 IV q 3 hours for 8 doses, then IM q6h hours for 8 doses. Higher doses of methotrexate may be tolerated if higher doses of leucovorin are given. (O'Keefe & Harris 1990)

■ **HORSES:**
For macrocytic anemia and neutropenia associated with pyrimethamine and/or trimethoprim (especially in pregnant mares): 0.1–0.3 mg/kg PO once daily. A more practical approach would be to ensure that the horse receives green hay or pasture (high tetrahydrofolate levels in green roughage) (Divers 2002)

Monitoring

■ CBC

■ Methotrexate serum levels (contact a local human hospital) if used for methotrexate overdoses

Client Information

■ If being used for methotrexate toxicity, this medication should only be administered in an inpatient setting

■ Oral leucovorin may be administered with or without meals.

■ Stress adherence to dosage schedule in order to adequately treat or prevent hematologic toxicity

Chemistry/Synonyms

Leucovorin calcium occurs as a yellowish-white or yellow, odorless powder. It is very soluble in water and practically insoluble in alcohol. It is a mixture of diasterioisomers of 5-formyl tetrahydrofolic acid.

Leucovorin calcium may also be known as: folinic acid, citrovorum factor, 5-formyl tetrahydrofolate, citrovorin, folidan, folinic, FTHF, NSC-3590, calcium folinate, calcifolin, calfonat, or folinic acid calcium salt; many international trade names are available.

Storage/Stability

Leucovorin calcium tablets should be stored below 40°C, preferably between 15–30°C in a well-closed container; protect from light.

Leucovorin solution for injection should be stored refrigerated between 2°–8°C; protect from light.

Leucovorin Powder for reconstitution and injection should be stored below 40°C, preferably between 15–30°C; protect from light.

Compatibility/Compounding Considerations

The powder for injection is reconstituted by adding 5 or 10 mL of bacteriostatic water for injection or sterile water for injection. As bacteriostatic water for injection contains benzyl alcohol, it is not recommended in neonates or very small animals. If reconstituting with sterile water for injection, the resulting solution should be administered immediately; solutions made with bacteriostatic water for injection are stable up to 7 days.

Intravenous solutions containing leucovorin calcium in Ringer's lactate, Ringer's, or 0.9% sodium chloride are stable up to 24 hours at room temperature. Leucovorin calcium is **not compatible** with solutions containing fluorouracil.

Dosage Forms/Regulatory Status

VETERINARY-LABELED PRODUCTS: None

HUMAN-LABELED PRODUCTS:

Note: Strengths listed are in terms of leucovorin base.

Leucovorin Calcium Oral Tablets: 5 mg, 15 mg, & 25 mg; generic; (Rx)

Leucovorin Calcium Injection Solution: 10 mg/mL in 5 mg single dose vials; generic; (Rx)

Leucovorin Calcium Powder for Injection: 50 mg, 100 mg, 200 mg & 350 mg in vials; generic; (Rx)

References

Divers, T. (2002). Management and treatment of equine protozoal myeloencephalitis (EPM). Proceedings: ACVIM 2002. Accessed via: Veterinary Information Network. http://goo.gl/HQWw0

Greene, C., K. Hartmannn, et al. (2006). Appendix 8: Antimicrobial Drug Formulary. Infectious Disease of the Dog and Cat. C Greene Ed., Elsevier: 1186–1333.

Inzana, K. (2002). Infectious and inflammatory encephalopathies I and II. Proceedings: Western Veterinary Conference. Accessed via: Veterinary Information Network. http://goo.gl/enVkm

Lindsay, D. (2004). Toxoplasma gondii and feline toxoplasmosis. Proceedings: Western Veterinary Conference 2004. Accessed via: Veterinary Information Network. http://goo.gl/Sb23p

O'Keefe, D.A. & C.L. Harris (1990). Toxicology of Oncologic Drugs. Vet Clinics of North America: Small Animal Pract 20(2): 483–504.

LEUPROLIDE

(loo-*proe*-lide)   Lupron®

HORMONAL AGONIST

Prescriber Highlights

▶ For medical treatment of adrenal associated endocrinopathy in ferrets, & to treat inappropriate egg laying in captive birds

▶ Depot form must not be confused with once a day injectable, doses below are for depot (IM suspension)

▶ Teratogenic, contraindicated in pregnancy

▶ Extremely costly (especially for ferrets); may be obtained in smaller aliquots from compounding pharmacies

▶ Lab considerations

Uses/Indications

The primary uses for leuprolide at present are for the medical treatment of adrenal associated endocrinopathy in ferrets, and to treat inappropriate egg laying in captive cockatiels. In ferrets, it may be more effective in treating clinical signs associated with adrenal hyperplasia or adenomas than with adenocarcinomas.

Pharmacology/Actions

Leuprolide is a luteinizing hormone-releasing hormone agonist. Via negative feedback, leuprolide inhibits the release of luteinizing hormone and follicle stimulating hormone from the pituitary. Both estrogen and androgen levels are decreased in the serum.

Pharmacokinetics

No veterinary data was located. The depot forms appear to have sustained effects in birds and ferrets.

Contraindications/Precautions/Warnings

Contraindicated in pregnancy.

Adverse Effects

In ferrets, adverse effects reported include pain/irritation at injection site, dyspnea, and lethargy. Tachyphylaxis (higher dosages required over time to obtain same effect) has been reported when using leuprolide in ferrets.

Little information is available on the adverse effect profile of leuprolide birds. At this point, it appears safe at the recommended doses.

Reproductive/Nursing Safety

Leuprolide is considered contraindicated in pregnancy. Major fetal abnormalities may result. In humans, the FDA categorizes this drug as category *X* for use during pregnancy (*Studies in animals or humans demonstrate fetal abnormalities or adverse reaction; reports indicate evidence of fetal risk. The risk of use in pregnant women clearly outweighs any possible benefit.*)

It is not known whether leuprolide is excreted in milk; use with caution.

Overdosage/Acute Toxicity

Because of its expense and method of dosing, it is unlikely an acute overdose would occur. Studies in lab animals at dosages of up to 5 grams/kg IM produced no untoward effects.

Drug Interactions

No documented adverse drug interactions with leuprolide were located.

Laboratory Considerations

■ Diagnostic tests measuring **pituitary gonadotrophic** and **gonadal functions** may be misleading during, and for several months after discontinuing therapy

Doses

■ **FERRETS:**

For treatment of adrenal associated endocrinopathy:

a) Leuprolide acetate (Lupron Depot 30 day formulation): 100 micrograms/kg IM for females, 200 micrograms/kg IM for males q30 days has been proven effective in ferrets for management of the disease.

Leuprolide acetate (Lupron Depot 3 month formulation): 1 mg (total dose) IM every 60-75 days (length of control in intact ferrets in Spring; may be useful for annual Dec/Feb suppression).

Leuprolide acetate (Lupron Depot 4 month formulation): 2 mg (total dose) IM every 70-80 days (anecdotal time before signs reappear; may be useful for annual Dec/Feb suppression. (Johnson-Delaney 2009)

b) Using the 30 day depot form: If ferret

weighs less than 1 kg: 100 micrograms IM q30 days. If weighs >1 kg: 200 micrograms IM q30 days. Generally, the drug is diluted from its original concentration to negate the muscle necrosis problem that has been reported. The diluted form appears to remain active after being stored in the freezer for a year. (Murray 2002) **(Note:** *The manufacturer states that the depot form is not to be frozen and no studies are known that support the stability of the depot activity when frozen and thawed—Plumb)*

c) Using the one month depot form: 100–250 micrograms/kg IM every 4 weeks until signs resolve, then every 4–8 weeks as needed, lifelong. Larger ferrets may require the higher dosage range. (Johnson 2006)

■ **BIRDS:**

a) For inappropriate egg laying in Cockatiels if management changes, such as conversion to a pelleted diet, decreasing photoperiod, and reducing 'mate' interactions can be helpful. However, if unsuccessful, leuprolide acetate (*Lupron Depot®*) 800 micrograms/kg IM every 2 weeks for 3 injections, is often effective at reducing reproduction at least in the short-term. (Hernandez-Divers 2009)

b) To inhibit egg laying in pet birds: 100 micrograms/kg per day. Multiply dose by number of days for effect and give once monthly. Example: 100 micrograms/kg for 28 days = 2800 micrograms/kg dose (Olsen & Orosz 2000)

c) For macroorchidism: Treatment protocol of 3 injections of leuprolide acetate (using the 7.5 mg 1-month form) at 2,300 micrograms/kg for psittacine birds weighing <50 grams and 1,500 micrograms/kg for species weighing >50 grams at 3-week intervals gave the best overall response. If there was a favorable clinical response, radiographic evaluation at 12 weeks demonstrated the best radiographic quantitative improvement. (Nernetz 2009)

Monitoring

■ Clinical effects Birds: decreased egg-laying; Ferrets: decreases in vulvar swelling, pruritus, undesirable sexual behaviors, aggression, and increased hair regrowth

Client Information

■ Relatively experimental in birds or ferrets. Long-term safety is not known.

■ Can be extremely expensive to treat.

Chemistry/Synonyms

A synthetic nonapeptide analog of GnRH (gonadotropin releasing hormone, gonadorelin, luteinizing hormone-releasing hormone),

leuprolide acetate occurs as a white to off-white powder. In water more than 250 mg are soluble in one mL.

Leuprolide may also be known as: leuproprelin, leuprorelinum, abbott-43818, leuprolide acetate, TAP-144, *Carcinil®, Daronda®, Eligard®, Elityran®, Enanton®, Enantone®, Enantone-Gyn®, Ginecrin®, Lectrum®, Leuplin®, Lucrin®, Lupride®, Lupron®, Procren®, Procrin®, Prostap®, Reliser®, Trenantone®, Uno-Enantone®,* and *Viadur®.*

Storage/Stability

The injection should be stored below room temperature (<78°F); do not freeze and protect from light (store in carton until use). The depot form may be stored at room temperature. After reconstituting the suspension is stable for 24 hours, but as it contains no preservative it is recommended for immediate use.

Compatibility/Compounding Considerations

The issue whether the solution containing microspheres (depot forms) can be frozen for later use is somewhat controversial as some have frozen the solution and state that it is still effective. However, the manufacturer states that the depot form is not to be frozen as the microspheres are destroyed and no studies are known that support the stability of the depot activity when frozen and thawed. Some compounding pharmacies may divide the lyophilized powder into individual dosages in vials. If it is decided to freeze the solution, most recommend putting individual aliquots into tuberculin syringes before freezing; do not re-freeze once thawed.

Dosage Forms/Regulatory Status

VETERINARY-LABELED PRODUCTS: None

HUMAN-LABELED PRODUCTS:

Leuprolide Acetate Injection: 5 mg/mL in 2.8 mL multi-dose vials; *Lupron® Lupron® for Pediatric Use* (TAP Pharm); generic; (Rx)

Leuprolide Acetate Injection: 22.5 mg in single-use kits with a 2-syringe mixing system and needle; 30 mg & 45 mg in single-use kit with 2-syringe mixing system and syringe containing *Atrigel®; Eligard®* (Sanofi-Synthelabo); (Rx)

Leuprolide Powder for Injection: lyophilized 7.5 mg in single-use kits with a 2-syringe mixing system and needle; *Eligard®* (Sanofi-Synthelabo); (Rx)

Leuprolide Acetate Microspheres for Injection, lyophilized and preservative free with mannitol: 3.75 mg, 7.5 mg, 11.25 mg (regular—30 day & 3 month), 15 mg, 22.5 mg (3 month), & 30 mg (4 month) in single dose kits and pre-filled dual-chamber syringes; *Lupron® Depot* and *Lupron® Depot-Ped* and *Lupron® Depot-3* or *-4 Month* (TAP Pharm); (Rx)

References

Hernandez-Divers, S. (2009). Avian reproductive medicine and surgery. Proceedings: AAZV. Accessed via: Veterinary Information Network. http://goo.gl/6ZiLH

Johnson, D. (2006). Current Therapies for Ferret Adrenal Disease. Proceedings: ACVC. Accessed via: Veterinary Information Network. http://goo.gl/pOMYy

Johnson-Delaney, C. (2009). Endocrine System and Diseases of Exotic Companion Mammals. Proceedings: ABVP. Accessed via: Veterinary Information Network. http://goo.gl/Tozhd

Murray, M. (2002). Ferret Geriatrics. Proceedings: Western Veterinary Conference. Accessed via: Veterinary Information Network. http://goo.gl/nZpzX

Nernetz, L. (2009). Management of Macroorchidism Using Leuprolide Acetate. Proceedings: AAV. Accessed via: Veterinary Information Network. http://goo.gl/zIT43

Olsen, G. & S. Orosz (2000). Manual of Avian Medicine. St Louis, Mosby.

LEVAMISOLE

(leh-*vam*-i-sole)   Levasole®, Tramisol®

ANTIPARASITIC, IMMUNE STIMULANT

Prescriber Highlights

▶ Antinematodal parasiticide that also may be useful as an immune stimulant

▶ Contraindications: Milk-producing animals (not approved)

▶ Very cautiously, if at all: Severely debilitated, or significant renal or hepatic impairment; in cattle that are stressed due to vaccination, dehorning, or castration

▶ Not usually used in horses; infrequently used in small animals today as an antiparasitic agent

▶ Numerous adverse effects

Uses/Indications

Depending on the product licensed, levamisole is indicated for the treatment of many nematodes in cattle, sheep and goats, swine, poultry. In sheep and cattle, levamisole has relatively good activity against abomasal nematodes, small intestinal nematodes (not particularly good against *Strongyloides* spp.), large intestinal nematodes (not *Trichuris* spp.), and lungworms. Adult forms of species that are usually covered by levamisole, include: *Haemonchus* spp., *Trichostrongylus* spp., *Osteragia* spp., *Cooperia* spp., *Nematodirus* spp., *Bunostomum* spp., *Oesophagostomum* spp., *Chabertia* spp., and *Dictyocaulus vivaparus*. Levamisole is less effective against the immature forms of these parasites, and is generally ineffective in cattle (but not sheep) against arrested larval forms. Resistance of parasites to levamisole is a growing concern.

In swine, levamisole is indicated for the treatment of *Ascaris suum*, *Oesophagostomum* spp., *Strongyloides*, *Stephanurus*, and *Metastrongylus*.

Levamisole has been used in dogs as a microfilaricide to treat *Dirofilaria immitis* infection in the past, but is rarely used today. It has also garnered some interest as an immunostimulant in the adjunctive therapy of various neoplasms.

Because of its narrow margin for safety and limited efficacy against many equine parasites, levamisole is not generally used in horses as an antiparasitic agent. It has been tried as an immune stimulant, however.

Pharmacology/Actions

Levamisole stimulates the parasympathetic and sympathetic ganglia in susceptible worms. At higher levels, levamisole interferes with nematode carbohydrate metabolism by blocking fumarate reduction and succinate oxidation. The net effect is a paralyzing effect on the worm that is then expelled alive. Levamisole's effects are considered to be nicotine-like in action.

Levamisole's mechanism of action for its immunostimulating effects are not well understood. It is believed it restores cell-mediated immune function in peripheral T-lymphocytes and stimulates phagocytosis by monocytes. Its immune stimulating effects appear to be more pronounced in animals that are immune-compromised.

Pharmacokinetics

Levamisole is absorbed from the gut after oral dosing and through the skin after dermal application, although bioavailabilities are variable. It is reportedly distributed throughout the body. Levamisole is primarily metabolized with less than 6% excreted unchanged in the urine. Plasma elimination half-lives have been determined for several veterinary species: Cattle, 4–6 hours; Dogs, 1.8–4 hours; and Swine, 3.5–6.8 hours. Metabolites are excreted in both the urine (primarily) and feces.

Contraindications/Precautions/Warnings

Levamisole is contraindicated in lactating animals (not approved). It should be used cautiously, if at all, in animals that are severely debilitated, or significant renal or hepatic impairment.

Use cautiously or, preferably, delay use in cattle that are stressed due to vaccination, dehorning, or castration.

Levamisole is not indicated for use as a dirofilarial adulticide.

Avoid, if possible, administering levamisole intramuscularly to birds.

One reference states that levamisole is contraindicated in cats with FIV or FIP and likely ineffective in cats with FeLV (Hartmann 2009).

Adverse Effects

Adverse effects that may be seen in cattle can include muzzle foaming or hypersalivation, excitement or trembling, lip-licking and head shaking. These effects are generally noted with higher than recommended doses or if levamisole is used concomitantly with organophosphates. Signs generally subside within 2 hours. When injecting into cattle, swelling may occur at the injection site. This will usually abate in 7–14 days, but may be objectionable in animals that are close to slaughter.

In sheep, levamisole may cause a transient excitability in some animals after dosing. In goats, levamisole may cause depression, hyperesthesia, and salivation. Injecting levamisole SC in goats apparently causes a stinging sensation.

In swine, levamisole may cause salivation or muzzle foaming. Swine infected with lungworms may develop coughing or vomiting.

Adverse effects that may be seen in dogs include GI disturbances (usually vomiting, diarrhea), neurotoxicity (panting, shaking, agitation or other behavioral changes), immune-mediated anemia, agranulocytosis, dyspnea, pulmonary edema, immune-mediated skin eruptions (erythroedema, erythema multiforme, toxic epidermal necrolysis), and lethargy.

Adverse effects seen in cats include hypersalivation, excitement, mydriasis, and vomiting.

Reproductive/Nursing Safety

There is little information available regarding the safety of this drug in pregnant animals. Levamisole has been implicated in causing abortion in goats. Although levamisole is considered relatively safe to use in large animals that are pregnant, use only if the potential benefits outweigh the risks. In humans, the FDA categorizes this drug as category **C** for use during pregnancy (*Animal studies have shown an adverse effect on the fetus, but there are no adequate studies in humans; or there are no animal reproduction studies and no adequate studies in humans.*) In a separate system evaluating the safety of drugs in canine and feline pregnancy (Papich 1989), this drug is categorized as in class: **C** (*These drugs may have potential risks. Studies in people or laboratory animals have uncovered risks, and these drugs should be used cautiously as a last resort when the benefit of therapy clearly outweighs the risks.*)

Levamisole is excreted in cows' milk; use with caution in nursing dams.

Overdosage/Toxicity

Signs of levamisole toxicity often mimic those of organophosphate toxicity. Signs may include hypersalivation, hyperesthesias and irritability, clonic seizures, CNS depression, dyspnea, defecation, urination, and collapse. These effects are best treated by supportive means as animals generally recover within hours of dosing. Acute levamisole overdosage can result in death due to respiratory failure. Should respiratory failure occur, artificial ventilation with oxygen should be instituted until recovery occurs. Cardiac arrhythmias may also be seen. If the ingestion was oral, emptying the gut and/or administering charcoal with cathartics may be indicated.

Levamisole is considered to be more dangerous when administered parenterally than when given orally or topically. Intravenous administration is particularly hazardous, and is never recommended.

In pet birds (cockatoos, budgerigars, Mynah birds, parrots, etc.), 40 mg/kg has been reported as a toxic dose when administered SC. IM injections may cause more severe toxicity. Depression, ataxia, leg and wing paralysis, mydriasis, regurgitation, and death may be seen after a toxic dose in birds.

Drug Interactions

The following drug interactions have either been reported or are theoretical in humans or animals receiving levamisole and may be of significance in veterinary patients:

■ **ASPIRIN:** Levamisole may increase salicylate levels

■ **CHLORAMPHENICOL:** Fatalities have been reported after concomitant levamisole and chloramphenicol administration; avoid using these agents together

■ **CHOLINESTERASE-INHIBITING DRUGS (e.g., organophosphates, neostigmine):** Could theoretically enhance the toxic effects of levamisole; use together with caution

■ **NICOTINE-LIKE COMPOUNDS (e.g., pyrantel, morantel, diethylcarbamazine):** Could theoretically enhance the toxic effects of levamisole; use together with caution.

■ **WARFARIN:** Increased risk for bleeding

Doses

■ **DOGS:**

As an immune stimulant:

a) For recurrent cutaneous infections: 2.2 mg/kg PO every other day, with appropriate antimicrobial therapy (Rosenkrantz 1989)

b) 0.5–2 mg/kg PO 3 times a week (Kirk 1989)

c) For adjunctive therapy in dogs with chronic pyoderma: 0.5–1.5 mg/kg PO 2–3 times a week (efficacy not established) (Lorenz 1984)

d) For adjunctive therapy in dogs with chronic pyoderma: 2.2 mg/kg PO every other day (may only be efficacious in 10% of cases) (Ihrke 1986)

As an alternative treatment for SLE:

a) 3–7 mg/kg PO every other day for 4 months; alone or in combination with corticosteroids (Marks & Henry 2000)

As a microfilaricide (**Note:** Rarely recommended today):

a) 11 mg/kg PO for 6–12 days. Examine for microfilaria within 7–10 days and at weekly intervals until eliminated or treatment is halted. Retching and vomiting are common. Avoid giving on an empty stomach or immediately after drinking water. A "conditioning" dose of 5 mg/kg PO once a day may be necessary. Stop therapy if abnormal behavior or ataxia develops. (Knight 1989)

For treatment of *Angiostrongylus vasorum*:

a) 7.5 mg/kg (route not specified) for two consecutive days, followed by 10 mg/kg for 2 days; if the infection is not cleared, the regimen is repeated. (Bowman 2006)

For the treatment of lungworms:

a) For *Crenosoma vulpis*: 8 mg/kg once (Todd *et al.* 1985)

b) For Capillaria: 7–12 mg/kg once daily PO for 3–7 days

For *Filaroides osleri*: 7–12 mg/kg once daily PO for 20–45 days (Roudebush 1985)

c) 7.5 mg/kg PO twice daily or 25 mg/kg PO every other day for 10 days (Bauer 1988)

d) For *Capillaria aerophilia*: 10 mg/kg PO once daily for 5 days; repeat in 9 days (Reinemeyer 1995)

■ **CATS:**

For the treatment of lungworms:

a) 20–40 mg/kg PO every other day for 5–6 treatments (Kirk 1989)

b) For *Aelurostrongylus abstrusus*: 100 mg PO daily every other day for 5 treatments; give atropine (0.5 mg SC, 15 minutes before administering); or 15 mg/kg PO every other day for 3 treatments, then 3 days later: 30 mg/kg PO, then 2 days later: 60 mg/kg.

For *Capillaria aerophilia*: 4.4 mg/kg SC for 2 days, then 8.8 mg/kg once 2 weeks later; or 5 mg/kg PO once daily for 5 days, followed by 9 days of no therapy, repeat two times (Todd *et al.* 1985)

c) 25 mg/kg every other day for 10–14 days (Roudebush 1985)

d) For *Capillaria aerophilia*: 10 mg/kg PO once daily for 5 days; repeat in 9 days (Reinemeyer 1995)

For treatment of *Ollulanus tricuspis*:

a) 5 mg/kg SC (Todd *et al.* 1985)

As a microfilaricide:

a) 10 mg/kg PO for 7 days (Dillon 1986)

As an immune-stimulant:

a) For adjunctive therapy of feline plasma-cell gingivitis/pharyngitis: 25 mg PO every other day for 3 doses (DeNovo *et al.* 1989)

■ **RABBITS/RODENTS/SMALL MAMMALS:**

a) **Rabbits:** For nematodes: 12.5–20 mg/kg PO (for gastric nematodes) or SC (for extragastric nematodes) (Ivey & Morrisey 2000)

■ **HORSES:**

As an immunostimulant:

a) Dosages have ranged from 2.5 mg/kg injected at 7 day intervals, and 2.2 mg/kg PO every 24 hours for 3 days, then off for 4 days for a period of 4–6 weeks.

Anecdotal reports of beneficial effects in the treatment of nasal viral papillomas, COPD, and EPM have been suggested. (Bentz 2006)

b) As adjunctive therapy for EPM: 1–2 mg/kg per day PO (MacKay 2008)

■ **CATTLE:**

For treatment of susceptible nematodes (also refer to specific label directions for FDA-approved products):

a) For removal of mature and immature *Dictyocaulus vivaparus*: 5.5–11 mg/kg PO, either given in feed or as a drench or oral bolus. May also be administered SC at 3.3–8 mg/kg. (Bennett 1986)

b) 7.5 mg/kg PO (Brander *et al.* 1982)

■ **CAMELIDS:**

For treatment of susceptible nematodes:

a) **Llamas:** 5–8 mg/kg IM, or PO (Fowler 1989)

b) **Llamas:** 5–8 mg/kg PO or SC for 1 day (Cheney & Allen 1989)

■ **SWINE:**

For treatment of susceptible nematodes (refer to specific label directions for FDA-approved products):

a) For removal of mature and immature Metastrongylus: 8 mg/kg PO in feed or water (Bennett 1986)

■ **SHEEP & GOATS:**

For treatment of susceptible nematodes (also refer to specific label directions for FDA-approved products):

a) For removal of mature and immature *Dictyocaulus vivapurus*: 8 mg/kg PO (Bennett 1986)

b) 7.5 mg/kg PO (Brander *et al.* 1982)

■ **BIRDS:**

a) Using 13.65% injectable:

For intestinal nematodes: 5–15 mL/gallon of drinking water for 1–3 days; repeat in 10 days. If birds refuse to drink, withhold water prior to treating.

For gavage in Australian Parakeets (or desert species that refuse to drink water): 15 mg/kg; repeat in 10 days

For parenteral use: 4–8 mg/kg IM or SC; repeat in 10–14 days. May cause vomiting, ataxia, or death. Do not use in debilitated birds.

For immunostimulation: 0.3 mL/gallon of water for several weeks

As a parenteral immunostimulant: 2 mg/kg IM or SC. 3 doses at 14 day intervals (Clubb 1986)

b) As a nebulized immunostimulant: 1 mL (of 13.65% levamisole phosphate) in 15 mL saline (Spink 1986)

c) For Capillaria infections: 15–30 mg/kg orally as a single bolus or through a crop tube; or 2.25 mg/gallon of drinking water for 4–5 days. Repeat treatment in 10–14 days. (Flammer 1986)

d) Poultry: 18–36 mg/kg, PO (Brander et al. 1982)

e) **Ratites:** For *Libyastrongylus douglassi*: Give 30 mg/kg PO or IM at one month of age, then once a month for 7 treatments, then 4 times yearly (Jenson 1998)

■ **REPTILES:**

a) As an anthelmintic: Nematodes: 5–10 mg/kg PO; repeat in two weeks followed by a fecal exam 14 days after the second dose. If positive, a third dose is given. Acanthocephalans, or Pentastomes: as above, but may also be given SC or ICe. (de la Navarre 2003)

Monitoring
■ Clinical efficacy
■ Adverse effects/toxicity observation

Client Information
■ Levamisole is not FDA-approved for use in dairy animals of breeding age.
■ Follow directions on the product label unless otherwise directed by veterinarian. Animals that are severely parasitized or in conditions with constant helminth exposure should be retreated 2–4 weeks after initial treatment.
■ Do not administer injectable products IV.
■ Report serious adverse effects to veterinarian.

Chemistry/Synonyms
The levo-isomer of dl-tetramisole, levamisole has a greater safety margin than does the racemic mixture. It is available commercially in two salts, a phosphate and a hydrochloride. Levamisole hydrochloride occurs as a white to pale cream colored, odorless or nearly odorless, crystalline powder. One gram is soluble in 2 mL of water.

Levamisole HCl may also be known as: cloridrato de levamizol, ICI-59623, levamisoli hydrochloridum, NSC-177023, R-12564, RP-20605, l-tetramisole hydrochloride, *Amtech®*, *Ascaridil®*, *Decaris®*, *Ergamisol®*, *Immunol®*, *Ketrax®*, *Levasole®*, *Meglum®*, *Prohibit®*, *Solaskil®*, *Vermisol®*, and *Vizole®*.

Storage/Stability
Levamisole hydrochloride products should be stored at room temperature (15–30°C), unless otherwise instructed by the manufacturer; avoid temperatures greater than 40°C. Levamisole phosphate injection should be stored at temperatures at or below 21°C (70°F); refrigeration is recommended and freezing should be avoided.

Compatibility/Compounding Considerations
Compounded preparation stability: Levamisole oral solution compounded from the commercially available tablets and active pharmaceutical ingredient powder has been published (Chiadmi *et al.* 2005). Triturating 2500 mg (2.5 grams) of levamisole hydrochloride powder with 100 mL sterile water yields a 25 mg/mL levamisole hydrochloride oral solution that retains >97% potency for 90 days when stored at both 4°C and 25°C and protected from light

Dosage Forms/Regulatory Status/Withdrawal Times
In cattle, sheep, and swine a level of 0.1 ppm has been established for negligible residues in edible tissues.

VETERINARY-LABELED PRODUCTS:

Note: marketing status of these products is not known; it has been reported that levamisole is "getting harder to find."

Levamisole Phosphate Injection: 136.5 mg/mL (13.65%) in 500 mL vials. Levamisole Injectable (AgriLabs), *Levasole® Injectable Solution 13.65%* (Schering Plough); FDA-approved for use in cattle. Slaughter withdrawal (at labeled dosages) = 7 days. To prevent residues in milk, do not administer to dairy animals of breeding age.

Levamisole Hydrochloride Water Medication: 18.15 grams in 0.71 oz bottle. *Levamisole Soluble Pig Wormer®* (AgriLabs, Durvet, Aspen); (OTC); *Levasole® Soluble Pig Wormer* (Schering-Plough), generic; (OTC). FDA-approved for use in swine. Slaughter withdrawal (at labeled dosages) = 72 hours

Levamisole Hydrochloride Antihelmintic Oral: *Levasole® Soluble Drench Powder* 46.8g/packet (Schering-Plough); (OTC). FDA-approved for use in cattle (Not in dairy animals of breeding age), and sheep. Slaughter withdrawal (at labeled dosages) = 48 hours (cattle); 72 hours (sheep)

Levamisole Hydrochloride Soluble Drench Powder 46.8 grams/packet; 544.5 grams/21.34 oz bottle. *Prohibit®* (AgriLabs) (OTC). FDA-approved for use in cattle and sheep. Slaughter withdrawal (at labeled dosages) cattle = 48 hours, sheep = 72 hours. To prevent residues in milk, do not administer to dairy animals of breeding age.

Levamisole HCl Oral Tablets/Boluses: 184 mg bolus: *Levasole® Sheep Wormer Bolus* (Schering Plough); (OTC). FDA-approved for use in sheep. Slaughter withdrawal (at labeled dosages) = 72 hours.

Levamisole 2.19 gram bolus: *Levasole® Cattle Wormer Boluses* (Schering-Plough); (OTC). FDA-approved for use in beef (not for use in dairy animals of breeding age). Slaughter withdrawal (at labeled dosages) = 48 hours.

HUMAN-LABELED PRODUCTS: None

References

Bauer, T.G. (1988). Pulmonary parnechymal disorders. Handbook of Small Animal Practice. RV Morgan Ed. New York, Churchill Livingstone: 195–213.

Bennett, D.G. (1986). Parasites of the respiratory system. Current Veterinary Therapy: Food Animal Practice 2. JL Howard Ed. Philadelphia, W.B. Saunders: 684–687.

Bentz, B. (2006). Antiviral therapies in the horse. Proceedings: ABVP. Accessed via: Veterinary Information Network. http://goo.gl/50Z0J

Bowman, D. (2006). Canine respiratory parasites—a review. Proceedings: ACVC. Accessed via: Veterinary Information Network. http://goo.gl/g5qQR

Brander, C.G., D.M. Pugh, et al. (1982). Veterinary Applied Pharmacology and Therapeutics. London, Baillière Tindall.

Cheney, J.M. & G.T. Allen (1989). Parasitism in Llamas. Vet Clin North America: Food Animal Practice 5(1): 217–232.

Chiadmi, F., A. Lyer, et al. (2005). Stability of levamisole oral solutions prepared from tablets and powder. J Pharm Pharm Sci 8(2): 322–325.

Clubb, S.L. (1986). Therapeutics: Individual and Flock Treatment Regimens. Clinical Avian Medicine and Surgery. GJ Harrison and LR Harrison Eds. Philadelphia, W.B. Saunders: 327–355.

de la Navarre, B. (2003). Common parasitic diseases of reptiles and amphibians. Proceedings: Western Veterinary Conf. Accessed via: Veterinary Information Network. http://goo.gl/ZafJD

DeNovo, R.C., K.A. Potter, et al. (1989). Diseases of the oral cavity and pharynx. Handbook of Small Animal Practice. RV Morgan Ed. New York, Churchill Livingstone: 327–345.

Dillon, R. (1986). Feline heartworm disease. Current Veterinary Therapy IX: Small Animal Practice. RW Kirk Ed. Philadelphia, WB Saunders: 420–425.

Flammer, K. (1986). Oropharyngeal diseases in caged birds. Current Veterinary Therapy IX: Small Animal Practice. RW Kirk Ed. Philadelphia, W.B. Saunders: 699–702.

Fowler, M.E. (1989). Medicine and Surgery of South American Camelids. Ames, Iowa State University Press.

Hartmann, K. (2009). Immunomodulators in Veterinary Medicine—Is There Evidence of Efficacy? Proceedings: ACVIM. Accessed via: Veterinary Information Network. http://goo.gl/WplyC

Ihrke, P.J. (1986). Antibacterial therapy in dermatology. Current Veterinary Therapy IX: Small Animal Practice. RW Kirk Ed. Philadelphia, W.B. Saunders: 566–571.

Ivey, E. & J. Morrisey (2000). Therapeutics for Rabbits. Vet Clin NA: Exotic Anim Pract 3:1(Jan): 183–216.

Jenson, J. (1998). Current ratite therapy. The Veterinary Clinics of North America: Food Animal Practice 16:3(November).

Kirk, R.W., Ed. (1989). Current Veterinary Therapy X, Small Animal Practice. Philadelphia, W.B. Saunders.

Knight, D.H. (1989). Heartworm Disease. Handbook of Small Animal Practice. RV Morgan Ed. New York, Churchill Livingstone: 139–148.

Lorenz, M.D. (1984). Integumentary Infections. Clinical Microbiology and INfectious Diseases of the Dog and Cat. CE Greene Ed. Philadelphia, WB Saunders: 189–207.

MacKay, R. (2008). Equine Protozoal Myeloencephalitis: Managing Relapses. Comp Equine(Jan/Feb): 24–27.

Marks, S. & C. Henry (2000). CVT Update: Diagnosis and Treatment of Systemic Lupus Erythematosus. Kirk's Current Veterinary Therapy: XIII Small Animal Practice. J Bonagura Ed. Philadelphia, WB Saunders: 514–516.

Papich, M. (1989). Effects of drugs on pregnancy. Current Veterinary Therapy X: Small Animal Practice. R Kirk Ed. Philadelphia, Saunders: 1291–1299.

Reinemeyer, C. (1995). Parasites of the respiratory system. Kirk's Current Veterinary Therapy:XII. J Bonagura Ed. Philadelphia, W.B. Saunders: 895–898.

Rosenkrantz, W. (1989). Immunomodulating drugs in dermatology. Current Veterinary Therapy X: Small Animal Practice. RW Kirk Ed. Philadelphia, WB Saunders: 570–577.

Roudebush, P. (1985). Respiratory Diseases. Handbook of Small Animal Therapeutics. LE Davis Ed. New York, Churchill Livingstone: 287–332.

Spink, R.R. (1986). Aerosol Therapy. Clinical Avian Medicine and Surgery. GJ Harrison and LR Harrison Eds. Philadelphia, W.B. Saunders: 376–379.

Todd, K.S., A.J. Paul, et al. (1985). Parasitic Diseases. Handbook of Small Animal Therapeutics. LE Davis Ed. New York, Chirchill Livingstone: 89–126.

LEVETIRACETAM

(lee-ve-tye-*ra*-se-tam)   Keppra®

ANTICONVULSANT

Prescriber Highlights

▶ In dogs, may be useful as a third drug adjunct for refractory canine epilepsy or when either phenobarbital or bromides are not tolerated. Dogs may become refractory to therapy with time.

▶ In cats, probably a second-line drug when phenobarbital alone does not control seizures, but can be tried as sole therapy when phenobarbital is not tolerated

▶ Appears to be well tolerated; adverse effects (may be transient) include sedation in dogs, and lethargy and decreased appetite in cats

▶ Phenobarbital may cause significant drug interaction with levetiracetam in dogs

▶ Dosage frequency (three times daily) problematic

▶ Cost has been an issue, but costs decreasing with availability of generics

Uses/Indications

Levetiracetam may be useful as a third antiseizure medication in dogs that are not well controlled with phenobarbital and bromides or when either bromides or phenobarbital are not tolerated. Some evidence suggests that in dogs suffering from phenobarbital liver toxicity, the addition of levetiracetam will allow reduction of their phenobarbital dosage without increasing seizure frequency. Recent reports in dogs of reduced efficacy with time ("honeymoon effect") and that phenobarbital can significantly affect levetiracetam pharmacokinetics in dogs is concerning.

Levetiracetam may also be useful as add-on therapy in cats when phenobarbital does not control seizures. It can be tried as sole therapy when phenobarbital is not tolerated.

Pharmacology/Actions

The exact mechanism for levetiracetam's antiseizure activity is not well understood. It may selectively prevent hypersynchronization of epileptiform burst-firing and propagation of seizure activity. It does not affect normal neuronal excitability.

Pharmacokinetics

In dogs and cats levetiracetam is well absorbed after oral dosing and peak levels occur in about 2 hours. In dogs, levetiracetam elimination half-life is about 2-5 hours and volume of distribution is about 0.9 L/kg. In cats, levetiracetem half-life is around 3 hours, but there can be wide inter-patient variation.

In humans, levetiracetam is rapidly, and nearly completely, absorbed after oral administration. Peak levels occur about one hour after dosing. Presence of food in the gut delays the rate, but not the extent of drug absorbed and it can be administered without regard to feeding status. Less than 10% of the drug is bound to plasma proteins. While not extensively metabolized, the drug's acetamide group is enzymatically hydrolyzed to the carboxylic acid metabolite that is apparently not active. Hepatic CYP P450 isoenzymes are not involved. Half-life in humans is about 7 hours; about 66% of a given dose is excreted unchanged via renal mechanisms, primarily glomerular filtration and active tubular secretion. Clearance can be significantly reduced in patients with impaired renal function.

Contraindications/Precautions/Warnings

Levetiracetam is contraindicated in patients who have previously exhibited hypersensitivity to it or any of its components. It should be used with caution in patients with renal impairment; dosage amounts or dosing frequency changes should be considered. In humans, renal elimination of levetiracetam correlates with creatinine clearance.

Adverse Effects

Levetiracetam appears to be very well tolerated in dogs and cats. Most common adverse effects reported include sedation in dogs and reduced appetite and lethargy in cats. These effects may be transient. Changes in behavior, and gastrointestinal effects could occur.

In humans, it is recommended to withdraw the drug slowly to prevent "withdrawal" seizures.

Reproductive/Nursing Safety

In pregnant dogs or cats, levetiracetam should be used with caution. In humans, the FDA categorizes levetiracetam as a category *C* drug for use during pregnancy (*Animal studies have shown an adverse effect on the fetus, but there are no adequate studies in humans; or there are no animal reproduction studies and no adequate studies in humans*). At high dosages, levetiracetam has caused increased embryofetal mortality in rabbits and rats. At dosages equivalent to the maximum human therapeutic dose, levetiracetam caused minor skeletal abnormalities and retarded offspring growth in rats.

Levetiracetam is excreted into maternal milk and its safety in nursing offspring is unknown. Use with caution in nursing patients.

Overdosage/Acute Toxicity

Levetiracetam is a relatively safe agent. Dogs given 1200 mg/kg/day (approximately 20 times therapeutic dosage) developed only salivation and vomiting. Human patients given 6000 mg/kg during drug testing developed only drowsiness. Other effects noted in human overdoses (doses not specified) after the drug was released include depressed levels of consciousness, agitation, aggression and respiratory depression. Treatment is basically supportive; the drug can be removed with hemodialysis. In the circumstance of a significant overdose in animals, contact an animal poison control center for further recommendations.

Drug Interactions

■ **NSAIDS:** In humans, naproxen and ketorolac have been implicated with increasing the risk for seizures in patients with epilepsy. Veterinary significance is not clear.

■ **PHENOBARBITAL:** In dogs, ongoing (21 days in the study) phenobarbital use significantly increased levetiracetam clearance and reduced half-life (from 3.43 hrs without phenobarbital to 1.73 hrs after 21 days of phenobarbital); dosage adjustments may be required. (Moore *et al.* 2009)

Laboratory Considerations

■ No specific laboratory interactions or considerations noted.

Doses

■ **DOGS:**

a) As an add-on treatment for epilepsy in dogs refractory to phenobarbital and bromides: 20 mg/kg PO every 8 hours (Munana, K 2004), (Munana, KR 2010)

b) As an add-on treatment for epilepsy in dogs refractory to phenobarbital and/or bromides: 7.1–23.8 mg/kg PO every 8 hours (Steinberg & Faissler 2004)

c) 10–20 mg/kg PO q8h (Dickinson 2007)

d) Initially, 20 mg/kg PO q8h. May increase dose in 20 mg/kg increments until efficacy achieved, side effects become apparent, or the drug becomes cost prohibitive. (Dewey, C. 2005)

e) 20 mg/kg PO q8h; may also be given as an IV bolus (20 mg/kg). (Fletcher 2009)

f) From a single-dose pharmacokinetic study: In normal dogs, a 60 mg/kg IV bolus dose of levetiracetam is well tolerated and achieves plasma drug concentrations within or above the therapeutic range reported for humans for at least 8 hours after administration. (Dewey, C.W. *et al.* 2008)

g) For status epilepticus: Initially, lorazepam at 0.2 mg/kg IV once, followed by a bolus IV loading dose of levetiracetam at 60 mg/kg. (Podell 2009)

■ **CATS:**

a) As an add-on to phenobarbital treatment for epilepsy: Initially, 20 mg/kg PO three times daily; slowly increase to effect (Pearce 2006)

b) As an adjunct to phenobarbital in suspected idiopathic epilepsy: Initially, 20 mg/kg PO three times daily. Monitor as below. If ineffective, increase dose in 20 mg/kg increments. (Bailey & Dewey 2009)

Monitoring

■ The therapeutic range for animals has not been specifically determined, but it is thought that it is similar to humans, 5–45 micrograms/mL. Monitoring is recommended approximately one week after starting levetiracetam and then every 6-12 months. Because the drug appears to be very safe, therapeutic drug monitoring is used primarily to adjust dosage (Bailey & Dewey 2009).

■ Veterinarians should have the owner keep a record of seizure activity to document efficacy and report any potential levetiracetam-associated adverse effects.

■ Routine CBC, basic metabolic panel every 6 months

Client Information

■ Clients should understand that limited experience has occurred with levetiracetam in dogs and cats. Although it appears to be well tolerated, information on its safety and efficacy profile is still being generated.

■ The current dosage frequency recommendation (q8h) may be difficult to adhere to, but the drug may not be effective if not followed.

Chemistry/Synonyms

A pyrrolidone-derivative antiepileptic agent, levetiracetam occurs as an odorless, bitter-tasting, white to off-white crystalline powder. It is very soluble in water and soluble in ethanol. It is a chiral molecule with one asymmetric carbon atom. Levetiracetam is not related chemically to other antiseizure medications.

Levetiracetam may also be known as: S-Etriacetam, UCB-22059, UCB-L059, and *Keppra®*.

Storage/Stability

Levetiracetam tablets or oral solution should be stored at 25°C (77°F); excursions permitted to 15–30°C (59–86°F).

Dosage Forms/Regulatory Status

VETERINARY-LABELED PRODUCTS: None

HUMAN-LABELED PRODUCTS:

Levetiracetam Oral Tablets (film-coated, scored): 250 mg, 500 mg, 750 mg & 1000 mg; *Keppra®* (UCB); generic; (Rx)

Levetiracetam Extended-Release Oral Tablets: 500 mg & 750 mg; *Keppra XR®* (UCB); (Rx)

Levetiracetam Oral Solution: 100 mg/mL in 473 mL, 480 mL & 500 mL; *Keppra®* (UCB); generic; (Rx)

Levetiracetam Concentrate for Injection: 100 mg/mL in 5 mL single-use vials; *Keppra®* (UCB); (Rx)

References

Bailey, K.S. & C.W. Dewey (2009). The Seizuring Cat. Diagnostic work-up and therapy. Journal of Feline Medicine and Surgery 11(5): 385–394.

Dewey, C. (2005). Advances in the treatment of canine seizure disorders. Proceedings: ACVIM. Accessed via: Veterinary Information Network. http://goo.gl/Wh7WY

Dewey, C.W., K.S. Bailey, et al. (2008). Pharmacokinetics of single-dose intravenous levetiracetam administration in normal dogs. Journal of Veterinary Emergency and Critical Care 18(2): 153–157.

Dickinson, P. (2007). Seizures—The Good, The Bad and the Ugly. Proceedings: Western Vet Conf. Accessed via: Veterinary Information Network. http://goo.gl/3fTPH

Fletcher, D. (2009). Seizure Management and Anticonvulsant Therapy. Proceedings: ACVC. Accessed via: Veterinary Information Network. http://goo.gl/U6s6B

Moore, S., K. Munana, et al. (2009). The Pharmacokinetics of Levetiracetam in Dogs Concurrently Receiving Phenobarbital. Proceedings: ACVIM. Accessed via: Veterinary Information Network. http://goo.gl/McGT7

Munana, K. (2004). Managing the Refractory Epileptic. Proceedings: ACVIM Forum, Minneapolis. Accessed via: Veterinary Information Network. http://goo.gl/nQ9ba

Munana, K. (2010). Current Approaches to Seizure Management. Proceedings: ACVIM Forum. Accessed via: Veterinary Information Network. http://goo.gl/vI8Lp

Pearce, L. (2006). Seizures in cats; Why they are not little dogs. Proceedings: Western Vet Conf. Accessed via: Veterinary Information Network. http://goo.gl/dnvI3

Podell, M. (2009). Status epilepticus: Stopping seizures from home to hospital. Proceedings: IVECCS. http://goo.gl/8bunc

Steinberg, M. & D. Faissler (2004). Levetiracetam therapy for long-term idiopathic epileptic dogs. Proceedings: ACVIM Forum, Minneapolis. Accessed via: Veterinary Information Network. http://goo.gl/SYQvG

LEVOTHYROXINE SODIUM

(lee-voe-thye-*rox*-een)
Soloxine®, Synthroid®

THYROID HORMONE

Prescriber Highlights

▶ Thyroid hormone for hypothyroidism in all species

▶ Contraindications: Acute myocardial infarction, thyrotoxicosis, or untreated adrenal insufficiency

▶ Caution: Concurrent hypoadrenocorticism (treated), cardiac disease, diabetes, or elderly patients

▶ Adverse Effects: Only associated with OD's (tachycardia, polyphagia, PU/PD, excitability, nervousness, & excessive panting); some cats may appear apathetic

▶ Drug-drug; drug-lab interactions

Uses/Indications

Levothyroxine sodium is indicated for the treatment of hypothyroidism in all species.

Pharmacology/Actions

Thyroid hormones affect the rate of many physiologic processes including: fat, protein, and carbohydrate metabolism, increasing protein synthesis, increasing gluconeogenesis, and promoting mobilization and utilization of glycogen stores. Thyroid hormones also increase oxygen consumption, body temperature, heart rate and cardiac output, blood volume, enzyme system activity, and growth and maturity. Thyroid hormone is particularly important for adequate development of the central nervous system. While the exact mechanisms how thyroid hormones exert their effects are not fully understood, it is known that thyroid hormones (primarily triiodothyronine) act at the cellular level.

In humans, triiodothyronine (T_3) is the primary hormone responsible for activity. Approximately 80% of T_3 found in the peripheral tissues is derived from thyroxine (T_4) which is the principle hormone released by the thyroid.

Pharmacokinetics

In dogs, peak plasma concentrations after oral dosing reportedly occur 4–12 hours after administration and the serum half-life is approximately 12–16 hours. There is wide variability from animal to animal, however.

Contraindications/Precautions/Warnings

Levothyroxine (and other replacement thyroid hormones) are contraindicated in patients with acute myocardial infarction, thyrotoxicosis, or untreated adrenal insufficiency. It should be used with caution, and at a lower initial dosage, in patients with concurrent hypoadrenocorticism (treated), cardiac disease, diabetes, or in those who are aged.

Adverse Effects

When administered at an appropriate dose to patients requiring thyroid hormone replacement, there should not be any adverse effects associated with therapy. For adverse effects associated with overdosage, see below.

Reproductive/Nursing Safety

In humans, the FDA categorizes this drug as category *A* for use during pregnancy (*Adequate studies in pregnant women have not demonstrated a risk to the fetus in the first trimester of pregnancy, and there is no evidence of risk in later trimesters.*)

Minimal amounts of thyroid hormones are excreted in milk and should not affect nursing offspring.

Overdosage/Acute Toxicity

Chronic overdosage will produce signs of hyperthyroidism, including tachycardia, polyphagia, PU/PD, excitability, nervousness and excessive panting. Dosage should be reduced and/or temporarily withheld until signs subside. Some (10%?) cats may exhibit signs of "apathetic" (listlessness, anorexia, etc.) hyperthyroidism.

A single acute overdose in small animals is less likely to cause severe thyrotoxicosis than with chronic overdosage. Vomiting, diarrhea, hyperactivity to lethargy, hypertension, tachycardia, tachypnea, dyspnea, and abnormal pupillary light reflexes may be noted in dogs and cats. In dogs, clinical signs may appear within 1–9 hours after ingestion. If ingestion occurred within 2 hours, treatment to reduce absorption of drug should be accomplished using standard protocols (emetics, cathartics, charcoal) unless contraindicated by the patient's condition. Treatment is supportive and symptomatic. Oxygen, artificial ventilation, cardiac glycosides, beta-blockers (*e.g.*, propranolol), fluids, dextrose, and antipyretic agents have all been suggested for use if necessary; contact an animal poison control center for further guidance.

Drug Interactions

The following drug interactions have either been reported or are theoretical in humans or animals receiving levothyroxine and may be of significance in veterinary patients:

■ **AMIODARONE:** May decrease the metabolism of T4 to T3

■ **ANTACIDS, ORAL:** May reduce levothyroxine absorption; separate doses by 4 hours

■ **ANTIDEPRESSANTS, TRICYCLIC/TETRACYCLIC:** Increased risk for CNS stimulation and cardiac arrhythmias

■ **ANTIDIABETIC AGENTS (insulin, oral agents):** Levothyroxine may increase requirements for insulin or oral agents

■ **CHOLESTYRAMINE:** May reduce levothyroxine absorption; separate doses by 4 hours

- **CORTICOSTEROIDS (high dose):** Decreased conversion of T4 to T3
- **DIGOXIN:** Potential for reduced digoxin levels
- **FERROUS SULFATE:** May reduce levothyroxine absorption; separate doses by 4 hours
- **HIGH FIBER DIET:** May reduce levothyroxine absorption
- **KETAMINE:** May cause tachycardia and hypertension
- **PHENOBARBITAL:** Possible increased metabolism of thyroxine; dosage adjustments may be needed
- **PROPYLTHIOURACIL:** Decreased conversion of T4 to T3
- **RIFAMPIN:** Possible increased metabolism of thyroxine; dosage adjustments may be needed
- **SERTRALINE:** May increase levothyroxine requirements
- **SUCRALFATE:** May reduce levothyroxine absorption; separate doses by 4 hours
- **SYMPATHOMIMETIC AGENTS (epinephrine, norepinephrine, etc.):** Levothyroxine can potentiate effects
- **WARFARIN:** Thyroid hormones increase the catabolism of vitamin K-dependent clotting factors that may increase the anticoagulation effects in patients on warfarin

Laboratory Considerations

- **Renal Function Tests:** Hypothyroid dogs can have decreased GFR (creatinine clearance); restoration to a euthyroid state can increase GFR and reduce serum creatinine levels

The following drugs may have effects on thyroid function tests; evaluate results accordingly:

- *Effects on serum T_4:* aminoglutethimide↓, anabolic steroids/androgens↓, antithyroid drugs (PTU, methimazole)↓, asparaginase↓, barbiturates↓, corticosteroids↓, danazol↓, diazepam↓, estrogens↑ (**Note:** estrogens may have no effect on canine T_3 or T_4 concentrations), fluorouracil↑, heparin↓, insulin↑, lithium carbonate↓, mitotane (o,p-DDD)↓, nitroprusside↓, phenylbutazone↓, phenytoin↓, propranolol↑, salicylates (large doses)↓, sulfonamides↓, and sulfonylureas↓.

- *Effects on serum T_3:* antithyroid drugs (PTU, methimazole)↓, barbiturates↓, corticosteroids↓, estrogens↑, fluorouracil↑, heparin↓, lithium carbonate↓, phenytoin↓, propranolol↓, salicylates (large doses)↓, sulfonamides↓, and thiazides↑.

- *Effects on T_3 uptake resin:* anabolic steroids/androgens↑, antithyroid drugs (PTU, methimazole)↓, asparaginase↑, corticosteroids↓, danazol↑, estrogens↓, fluorouracil↓, heparin↑, lithium carbonate↓, phenylbutazone↑, and salicylates (large doses)↑.

- *Effects on serum TSH:* aminoglutethimide↑, antithyroid drugs (PTU, methimazole)↑, corticosteroids↓, danazol↓, lithium carbonate↑, and sulfonamides↑.

- *Effects on Free Thyroxine Index (FTI):* antithyroid drugs (PTU, methimazole)↓, barbiturates↓, corticosteroids↓, heparin↑, lithium carbonate↓, and phenylbutazone↓.

Doses

- **DOGS:**

For hypothyroidism:

a) Use a trade name product. Initially give 20 micrograms/kg (0.02 mg/kg) body weight PO twice daily with a maximum dose of 0.8 mg twice daily. Four to eight weeks later evaluate clinical response and draw a T4 level 4–6 hours post dosing.

If positive clinical response and **1)** low normal T4: increase dose and recheck in 4 weeks; **2)** high normal to slightly higher than normal T4: no change in dosing and recheck in 6 months; **3)** 40% or more greater than high normal: decrease dose or consider once a day therapy and recheck in 4 weeks (if once a day dosing get a level prior to dosing as well).

If a negative clinical response and **1)** low normal T4: increase dose and recheck in 8 weeks (may need to increase dose again, change to 3 times a day dosing, or reevaluate diagnosis); **2)** high normal to 40% or more greater than high normal: re-evaluate diagnosis.

For myxedema coma: 5 micrograms/kg IV q12h initially as oral administration may be poorly absorbed (Scott-Moncrieff & Guptill-Yoran 2000)

b) Initial treatment dosages vary from 10–22 micrograms/kg q12h or q24h according to the author and the formulation used, with a maximum of 0.8 mg of levothyroxine q12h. Patient is revaluated 1 to 2 months after initiating therapy and dosage is adjusted based on clinical response and results of the TT4. When interpreting the result of TT4, time of sampling compared to the administration of the medication should be taken into consideration. Most commonly, blood is taken 3 to 6 hours after the last medication is administered (post-tablet test) and peak concentrations are measured. In this case, TT4 is expected to be within the reference range (upper half limit), and a TT4 value just above the reference range is acceptable. In most patients, follow-up of TSH does not offer a significant advantage over a measurement of T4 solely. (Daminet 2010)

c) 0.02 mg/kg PO twice daily to start; (0.02–0.04 mg/kg PO once daily or, if necessary divided twice daily to maintain). Alternatively, give 0.5 mg/m^2 which may prevent hyperthyroid effects, particularly in large breed dogs. (Ferguson 2002)

d) To confirm diagnosis of hypothyroidism using a trial of levothyroxine: It is not recommended to initiate treatment without performing thyroid function testing, but if this is to be done, the following protocol should provide the most accurate assessment of response to treatment. Obtain history and physical examination after treatment for 6-8 weeks of levothyroxine treatment (0.02 mg/kg q12h). If a positive response has occurred, treatment should be withdrawn and the dog re-examined in 4-6 weeks. A diagnosis of hypothyroidism is made when the clinical signs improve or resolve during treatment and reoccur after cessation of treatment. Other treatment should be avoided during this trial period. (Panciera 2009)

■ **CATS:**

For hypothyroidism:

a) 0.05–0.1 mg per cat PO once daily. Monitoring and dosage adjustments as above for dogs. (Scott-Moncrieff & Guptill-Yoran 2000)

b) Initially, 0.05–0.1 mg once daily. Wait a minimum of 4–6 weeks to assess cat's clinical response to treatment. Then obtain a serum T$_4$ level prior to, and 6–8 hours after, dosing. Increase or decrease dose and/or dosing frequency after reviewing these values and clinical response. If levothyroxine is ineffective, may try liothyronine. (Feldman & Nelson 1987)

c) Post thyroidectomy: Initially, 0.1–0.2 mg (total dose) PO once daily beginning 24-48 hours post-op for several weeks or months. Monitor T4 levels, to determine when this supplementation can be ceased. (Scherk 2009)

■ **HORSES:**

For hypothyroidism:

a) 10 mg in 70 mL of corn syrup once daily. Monitor T$_4$ levels one week after initiation of therapy. Obtain one blood sample just before administration and on sample 2–3 hours after dosing. (Chen & O.W.I. 1987)

For adjunctive treatment of equine metabolic syndrome:

a) Using the *Thyro-L®* product (Lloyd, Inc): Approximate dosage of 0.1 mg/kg PO once daily, initiate treatment at 48 mg/day (with restricted caloric intake) and then increase to 72 mg/day after 3 months if the horse remains obese. Weight loss is enhanced by restricting caloric intake and increasing exercise at the same time that levothyroxine is administered. Horses should not be allowed free access to pasture during treatment because levothyroxine is likely to induce hyperphagia, which offsets the effects of treatment. Most horses are treated for 6 months and then taken off the drug by administering 24 mg/day for 2 weeks and then 12 mg/day for 2 weeks. A level scoop of *Thyro-L®* powder contains 12 mg levothyroxine. Some horse owners and veterinarians leave horses on a "maintenance" dose of levothyroxine (12 to 24 mg/day), but there is no scientific evidence to support this approach. (Frank 2010)

■ **BIRDS:**

For hypothyroidism:

a) One 0.1 mg tablet in 30 mL–120 mL of water daily; stir water and offer for 15 minutes and remove. Use high dose for budgerigars and low dose for water drinkers. Used for respiratory clicking, vomiting in budgerigars and thyroid responsive problems. (Clubb 1986)

■ **REPTILES:**

For hypothyroidism in tortoises:

a) 0.02 mg/kg PO every other day (Gauvin 1993)

Monitoring

■ Therapeutic efficacy should be judged first via clinical effects, and, if necessary serum T4

■ Serum T$_4$; after therapy is started wait at a week before measuring T$_4$. Draw level preferably just prior to the next dose. Dosage should generally be reduced if serum thyroxine levels exceed 100 ng/mL or signs of thyrotoxicosis develop.

Client Information

■ Clients should be instructed in the importance of compliance with therapy as prescribed.

■ Also, review the signs that can be seen with too much thyroid supplementation (see Overdosage section above).

Chemistry/Synonyms

Prepared synthetically for commercial use, levothyroxine sodium is the levo isomer of thyroxine that is the primary secretion of the thyroid gland. It occurs as an odorless, light yellow to buff-colored, tasteless, hygroscopic powder that is very slightly soluble in water and slightly soluble in alcohol. The commercially available powders for injection also contain mannitol.

100 micrograms of levothyroxine is approximately equivalent to 65 mg (1 grain) of desiccated thyroid.

Levothyroxine sodium may also be known as: T$_4$, T$_4$ thyroxine sodium, levothyroxin natrium, levothyroxinum natricum, 3,5,3',5'-tetra-iodo-L-thyronine sodium, thyroxine sodium, L-thyroxine sodium, thyroxinum natricum, tirossina, and tiroxina sodica; many trade names are available.

Storage/Stability

Levothyroxine sodium preparations should be stored at room temperature in tight, light-resistant containers. The injectable product should be reconstituted immediately before use; unused injection should be discarded after reconstituting. Do not mix levothyroxine sodium injection with other drugs or IV fluids.

Levothyroxine sodium is reportedly unstable in aqueous solutions. If using a commercial liquid preparation, it is suggested to obtain validated stability data for the product.

Dosage Forms/Regulatory Status

All levothyroxine products require a prescription, but are not necessarily FDA-approved. There have been bioavailability differences between products reported. It is recommended to use a reputable product and not to change brands indiscriminately.

VETERINARY-LABELED PRODUCTS:

Levothyroxine Sodium Tablets: 0.1 mg, 0.2 mg, 0.3 mg, 0.4 mg, 0.5 mg, 0.6 mg, 0.7 mg, 0.8 mg, (1 mg *Soloxine®*); *Levosyn®* (V.E.T.); *Soloxine®* (Virbac); *Thyro-Tabs®* (Vet-A-Mix); *Thyrosyn®* (Vedco); *Thyroxine-L Tablets®* (Butler); *Thyrozine®* (Phoenix Pharmaceutical); *Thyrokare® Tablets* (Neogen); generic; (Rx). Labeled for use in dogs.

Levothyroxine Sodium Tablets Chewable (Veterinary) 0.1 mg, 0.2 mg, 0.3 mg, 0.4 mg, 0.5 mg, 0.6 mg, 0.7 mg, 0.8 mg; *Canine Thyroid Chewable Tablets®* (Pala-Tech); *Nutrived® T-4 Chewable Tablets* (Vedco); *Heska Thyromed® Chewable Tablets* (Heska); (Rx). Labeled for use in dogs.

Levothyroxine Oral Solution: 1 mg/mL in 30 mL bottles: *Leventa® Oral Solution* (Virbac); (Rx) Labeled for use in dogs.

Levothyroxine Sodium Powder (Veterinary): 0.22% (1 gram of T$_4$ in 454 grams of powder): One level teaspoonful contains 12 mg of T$_4$. Available in 1 lb. and 10 lb. containers: *Equine Thyroid Supplement®* (Pala-Tech); *Thyrozine Powder®* (Phoenix Pharmaceutical); *Levoxine® Powder* (First Priority); *Thyro-L®* (Lloyd); *Throxine-L® Powder* (Butler); *Equi-Phar Thyrosyn Powder®* (Vedco); *Thyrokare® Powder* (Neogen); (Rx). Labeled for use in horses.

HUMAN-LABELED PRODUCTS:

Levothyroxine Sodium Tablets: 0.025 mg (25 micrograms), 0.05 mg (50 micrograms), 0.075 mg (75 micrograms), 0.088 mg (88 micrograms), 0.1 mg (100 micrograms), 0.112 mg (112 micrograms), 0.125 mg (125 micrograms), 0.137 mg (137 micrograms), 0.15 mg (150 micrograms), 0.175 mg

(175 micrograms), 0.2 mg (200 micrograms) & 0.3 mg (300 mcg); *Synthroid®* (Abbott); *Levothroid®* (Forest); *Levoxyl®* (Jones Pharma); *Thyro-Tabs®* (Lloyd); *Unithroid®*; generic; (Rx)

Levothyroxine Sodium Liquid-filled Oral Capsules: 13 micrograms (0.013 mg), 25 micrograms (0.025 mg), 50 micrograms (0.05 mg), 75 micrograms (0.075 mg), 88 micrograms (0.088 mg), 100 micrograms (0.1 mg), 112 micrograms (0.112 mg), 125 micrograms (0.125 mg), 137 micrograms (0.137 mg) & 150 micrograms (0.15 mg) in blister 56s; *Tirosint®* (Akrimax); (Rx)

Levothyroxine Powder for Injection lyophilized: 200 micrograms (0.2 mg) & 500 micrograms (0.5 mg) in 10 mL vials; generic; (Rx)

References

Chen, D.C.L. & L. O.W.I. (1987). Hypothyroidism. Current Therapy in Equine Medicine 2. NE Robinson Ed. Philadelphia, W.B. Saunders: 185–187.

Clubb, S.L. (1986). Therapeutics: Individual and Flock Treatment Regimens. Clinical Avian Medicine and Surgery. GJ Harrison and LR Harrison Eds. Philadelphia, W.B. Saunders: 327–355.

Daminet, S. (2010). Canine Hypothyroidism: Update on Diagnosis and Treatment. Proceedings: WSAVA. Accessed via: Veterinary Information Network. http://goo.gl/mMcuX

Feldman, E.C. & R.W. Nelson (1987). Hypothyroidism. Canine and Feline Endocrinology and Reproduction Philadelphia, WB Saunders: 55–90.

Ferguson, D. (2002). Thyroid hormone replacement therapy-The numbers game. A physiological perspective. Proceedings: ACVIM Forum. Accessed via: Veterinary Information Network.

Frank, N. (2010). Which Endocrine Disorder Are We Dealing With? Pituitary Pars Intermedia Dysfunction versus Equine Metabolic Syndrome: Treatment Options. Proceedings: ACVIM. Accessed via: Veterinary Information Network. http://goo.gl/i9mON

Gauvin, J. (1993). Drug therapy in reptiles. Seminars in Avian & Exotic Med 2(1): 48–59.

Panciera, D. (2009). Diagnostic Testing and Treatment Options for Canine Hypothyroidism: Proceedings: ACVC. Accessed via: Veterinary Information Network. http://goo.gl/wCImP

Scherk, M. (2009). Endocrine Update: There's More to Cats Than Thyroids and Diabetes. Proceedings: UC-Davis Feline Medicine Symposium. Accessed via: Veterinary Information Network. http://goo.gl/C3ACD

Scott-Moncrieff, J. & L. Guptill-Yoran (2000). Hypothyroidism. Textbook of Veterinary Internal Medicine: Diseases of the Dog and Cat. S Ettinger and E Feldman Eds. Philadelphia, WB Saunders. 2: 1419–1429.

LIDOCAINE HCL (SYSTEMIC)

(*lye*-doe-kane)   Xylocaine®

ANTIARRHYTHMIC/LOCAL ANESTHETIC

Prescriber Highlights

▶ Local anesthetic & antiarrhythmic agent; may be useful to prevent post-operative ileus, reperfusion injury in horses

▶ Low dose IV constant-rate and intermittent or constant regional infusions been found useful to treat hyperalgesia and neuropathic pain induced by trauma or surgical procedures

▶ Contraindications: Known hypersensitivity to the amide-class local anesthetics, severe degree of SA, AV, or intraventricular heart block (if not being artificially paced), or Adams-Stokes syndrome

▶ Caution: Cats appear more sensitive to cardiodepressant and CNS effects of lidocaine; use with caution in patients with liver disease, congestive heart failure, shock, hypovolemia, severe respiratory depression, marked hypoxia, bradycardia, or incomplete heart block having VPC's, unless the heart rate is first accelerated

▶ Patients susceptible to malignant hyperthermia should receive intensified monitoring

▶ Adverse Effects: Most common adverse effects reported are dose related (serum level) & mild. CNS signs include drowsiness, depression, ataxia, muscle tremors, etc.; nausea & vomiting (usually transient). Adverse cardiac effects usually only at high plasma concentrations in most species, but cats are susceptible.

▶ When an IV bolus is given too rapidly, hypotension may occur

▶ Do NOT use the product containing epinephrine intravenously

▶ Drug interactions

Uses/Indications

Besides its use as a local and topical anesthetic agent, lidocaine is used to treat ventricular arrhythmias, principally ventricular tachycardia and ventricular premature complexes in all species. Cats may be more sensitive to the drug and some clinicians feel that it should not be used in this species as an antiarrhythmic, but this remains controversial. In horses, lidocaine may be useful to prevent post-operative ileus and reperfusion injury.

Low dose intravenous lidocaine infusions for hyperalgesia and neuropathic pain states induced by trauma or surgical procedures have been documented to be useful.

Pharmacology/Actions

Lidocaine is considered to be a class IB (membrane-stabilizing) antidysrhythmic agent. It is thought that lidocaine acts by combining with fast sodium channels when inactive which inhibits recovery after repolarization. Class IB agents demonstrate rapid rates of attachment and dissociation to sodium channels. At therapeutic levels, lidocaine causes phase 4 diastolic depolarization attenuation, decreased automaticity, and either a decrease or no change in membrane responsiveness and excitability. These effects will occur at serum levels that will not inhibit the automaticity of the SA node, and will have little effect on AV node conduction or His-Purkinje conduction.

Lidocaine's analgesic effects are not well understood but are likely via several mechanisms, including reducing ectopic activity of damaged afferent neurons.

Lidocaine apparently has some enhancing effects on intestinal motility in patients with postoperative ileus. The mechanism for this effect is not well understood, but probably involves more than just blocking increased sympathetic tone.

Lidocaine has been shown to be a scavenger of reactive oxygen species (ROS) and lipid peroxidation.

Pharmacokinetics

Lidocaine is not effective orally as it has a high first-pass effect. If very high oral doses are given, toxic signs occur (due to active metabolites?) before therapeutic levels can be reached. Following a therapeutic IV bolus dose, the onset of action is generally within 2 minutes and has duration of action of 10–20 minutes. If a constant infusion is begun without an initial IV bolus, it may take up to an hour for therapeutic levels to be reached. IM injections may be given every 1.5 hours in the dog, but because monitoring and adjusting dosages are difficult, it should be reserved for cases where IV infusions are not possible.

After injection, the drug is rapidly redistributed from the plasma into highly perfused organs (kidney, liver, lungs, heart) and distributed widely throughout body tissues. It has a high affinity for fat and adipose tissue and is bound to plasma proteins, primarily alpha$_1$-acid glycoprotein. It has been reported that lidocaine binding to this protein is highly variable and concentration dependent in the dog and may be higher in dogs with inflammatory disease. Lidocaine is distributed into milk. The apparent volume of distribution (V_d) has been reported to be 4.5 L/kg in the dog.

Lidocaine is rapidly metabolized in the liver to active metabolites (MEGX and GX). The terminal half-life of lidocaine in humans is 1.5–2 hours and has been reported to be 0.9 hours in the dog. The half-lives of lidocaine and MEGX may be prolonged in patients with cardiac failure or hepatic disease. Less than 10% of a parenteral dose is excreted unchanged in the urine.

Contraindications/Precautions/Warnings

Cats tend to be more sensitive to the CNS and cardiodepressant effects of lidocaine; use with caution. Cats with concurrent illnesses or under general anesthesia may be particularly sensitive to lidocaine's effects.

Lidocaine is contraindicated in patients with known hypersensitivity to the amide-class local anesthetics, a severe degree of SA, AV or intraventricular heart block (if not being artificially paced), or Adams-Stokes syndrome. The use of lidocaine in patients with Wolff-Parkinson-White (WPW) syndrome is controversial. Some manufacturers state its use is contraindicated, but several physicians have used the drug in people.

Lidocaine should be used with caution in patients with liver disease, congestive heart failure, shock, hypovolemia, severe respiratory depression, or marked hypoxia. It should also be used with caution in patients with bradycardia or incomplete heart block having VPC's, unless the heart rate is first accelerated. Patients susceptible to developing malignant hyperthermia should receive lidocaine with intensified monitoring.

When preparing lidocaine for intravenous injection, be certain of the concentration and do not use products containing epinephrine.

Adverse Effects

At usual doses and if the serum level remains within the proposed therapeutic range (1–5 micrograms/mL), serious adverse reactions are quite rare. The most common adverse effects reported are dose related (serum level) and mild. CNS signs include drowsiness, depression, ataxia, muscle tremors, etc. Nausea and vomiting may occur, but are usually transient. Adverse cardiac effects generally only occur at high plasma concentrations and are usually associated with PR and QRS interval prolongation and QT interval shortening. Lidocaine may increase ventricular rates if used in patients with atrial fibrillation. If an IV bolus is given too rapidly, hypotension may occur.

Be certain not to use the product that contains epinephrine intravenously.

Reproductive/Nursing Safety

In humans, the FDA categorizes systemic lidocaine as category *B* for use during pregnancy (*Animal studies have not yet demonstrated risk to the fetus, but there are no adequate studies in pregnant women; or animal studies have shown an adverse effect, but adequate studies in pregnant women have not demonstrated a risk to the fetus in the first trimester of pregnancy, and there is no evidence of risk in later trimesters.*) In a separate system evaluating the safety of drugs in canine

and feline pregnancy (Papich 1989), systemic lidocaine is categorized as in class: *B* (*Safe for use if used cautiously. Studies in laboratory animals may have uncovered some risk, but these drugs appear to be safe in dogs and cats or these drugs are safe if they are not administered when the animal is near term.*)

Lidocaine is excreted in concentrations of approximately 40% of that found in the serum and would unlikely to pose significant risk to nursing offspring.

Overdosage/Acute Toxicity

In dogs, if serum levels of >8 micrograms/mL are attained, toxicity may result. Signs may include ataxia, nystagmus, depression, seizures, bradycardia, hypotension and, at very high levels, circulatory collapse. Because lidocaine is rapidly metabolized, cessation of therapy or reduction in infusion rates with monitoring may be all that is required for minor signs. Seizures or excitement may be treated with diazepam, or a short or ultrashort acting barbiturate. Longer acting barbiturates (*e.g.*, pentobarbital) should be avoided. Should circulatory depression occur, treat with fluids, pressor agents and, if necessary, begin CPR.

Drug Interactions

The following drug interactions have either been reported or are theoretical in humans or animals receiving lidocaine and may be of significance in veterinary patients:

- **ANESTHETICS, GAS:** Lidocaine infusions perioperatively have been shown to reduce MAC requirements in dogs, horses and cats. In dogs and horses, this may be of benefit, but in cats, additive cardiodepression has been shown.

- **ANTIARRHYTHMICS, OTHER (e.g., procainamide, quinidine, propranolol, phenytoin):** When administered with lidocaine may cause additive or antagonistic cardiac effects and toxicity may be enhanced

- **CIMETIDINE:** Lidocaine levels or effects may be increased

- **FUROSEMIDE (or other drugs that can cause hypokalemia):** Hypokalemia may reduce the antiarrhythmic effects of lidocaine

- **PHENOBARBITAL, PHENYTOIN:** May increase lidocaine metabolism; decrease levels

- **PROPRANOLOL:** Lidocaine levels or effects may be increased

- **SUCCINYLCHOLINE:** Large doses of lidocaine may prolong succinylcholine-induced apnea

Laboratory Considerations

- Lidocaine may cause increased **creatine kinase** levels (CK).

Doses

- **DOGS:**

  As an antiarrhythmic agent:

  a) For immediate treatment of ventricular

tachycardia in dogs, lidocaine is the drug of choice. For sustained VT, use lidocaine at 2–4 mg/kg bolus given over a minute and repeat up to 8 mg/kg (total dose over 10 minutes). If successful, perform constant rate infusion (CRI) of lidocaine at 40–80 micrograms/kg/min. (Schwartz 2009)

b) For rapid conversion of life-threatening, incessant, unstable ventricular tachycardia: Initial IV bolus of 1–2 mg/kg preferably over 30 seconds to judge response, higher doses may be required but rarely need to give 4 mg/kg. Once effectiveness determined, begin constant rate infusion at 25–80 micrograms/kg/minute. Adjust dose to attain efficacy but without side effects. To prevent adverse effects total dose should not exceed 8 mg/kg over approximately one hour. Alternatively may give lidocaine at 4 mg/kg IM, but not if shock is present. Effects generally are seen in 10–15 minutes, and persist for about 90 minutes. (Moise 2000)

c) For ventricular arrhythmias: Initial dosage of 2–8 mg/kg IV slowly is given to effect while monitoring ECG; then following by a CRI of 25–75 micrograms/kg/minute starting at a high dose and tapering down when possible. (Macintire 2006)

As an analgesic agent:

a) CRI: 2–4 mg/kg/hour. **Note:** *also see the "recipe" for combination with morphine, ketamine and medetomidine in the Compatibility/Compounding Considerations section below.* (Hansen 2008)

b) Using the MLK (morphine/lidocaine/ketamine) mixture: To a 500 mL bag of LRS add 10 mg morphine sulfate, 120 mg lidocaine, and 100 mg ketamine. Infuse at a rate of 10 mL/kg/hr (will provide morphine at 0.2 mg/kg/hr, lidocaine 40 micrograms/kg/minute, and ketamine 2 mg/kg/hr). Can add dexmedetomidine if needed. (Shaffran 2009)

c) 1–4 mg/kg IV bolus, followed by a CRI of 1–5 mg/kg/hr depending on severity of pain. (Dyson 2008)

d) Initial bolus of 2 mg/kg IV given over 2–3 minutes, then a CRI of 50–100 micrograms/kg/min (3–6 mg/kg hr) (Grint 2008)

As an epidural:

a) 4–5 mg/kg epidurally. Onset of action <10 minutes; duration 1.5 hours. Can be combined with alpha2 agonists or opioids. Adding epinephrine prolongs duration of action. (Valverde 2008)

■ **CATS:**
Caution: Cats are reportedly very sensitive to

the CNS effects of lidocaine and can develop cardiodepression. There are several sources that state that lidocaine should not be used in cats as an injectable analgesic. If lidocaine is to be used, monitor carefully.

As an antiarrhythmic:

a) Initially, IV bolus of 0.25–0.5 mg/kg given slowly; can repeat at 0.15–0.25 mg/kg in 5–20 minutes; if effective, 10–20 micrograms/kg/minute (0.01–0.02 mg/kg/min) as a constant rate IV infusion (Ware 2000)

b) 0.25–0.5 mg/kg slow IV, with the possibility of repeating up to twice more if needed. If diluting for accurate dosing, use an insulin/tuberculin syringe. May be used as first-line therapy, or after propranolol, if it was ineffective. (Cote 2004)

As an epidural:

a) 4–5 mg/kg epidurally. Onset of action <10 minutes; duration 1.5 hours. Can be combined with alpha2 agonists or opioids. Adding epinephrine prolongs duration of action. (Valverde 2008)

■ **HORSES:** (**Note:** ARCI UCGFS Class 2 Drug)
For ventricular tachyarrhythmias:

a) Initially IV bolus of 1–1.5 mg/kg. Will generally distinguish between ventricular tachyarrhythmias (effective) and supraventricular tachyarrhythmias (no effect). To maintain effect, a constant IV infusion will be required. (Hilwig 1987)

b) 0.25–0.5 mg/kg IV (slowly) every 5–10 minutes up to a total dose of 1.5 mg/kg (Mogg 1999)

For postoperative ileus:

a) Initially, IV bolus of 1.3 mg/kg followed by a IV infusion of 0.05 mg/kg/minute for 24 hours (Malone *et al.* 1999)(Valverde 2008)

For colic patients:

a) Lidocaine has anti-endotoxic, analgesic and anti-ileus properties. Can be dosed as an initial IV bolus at 1.4 mg/kg, then as a CRI at 0.03–0.05 mg/kg/min (1.8–3 mg/kg/hr). (Hallowell 2008)

Monitoring

■ ECG

■ Signs of toxicity (see Adverse Effects and Overdosage)

■ If available and indicated, serum levels may be monitored. Therapeutic levels are considered to range from 1–6 micrograms/mL.

Client Information

■ This drug should only be used systemically by professionals familiar with its use and in a setting where adequate patient monitoring can be performed.

Chemistry/Synonyms

A potent local anesthetic and antiarrhythmic agent, lidocaine HCl occurs as a white, odorless, slightly bitter tasting, crystalline powder with a melting point between 74°–79°C and a pK_a of 7.86. It is very soluble in water and alcohol. The pH of the commercial injection is adjusted to 5–7, and the pH of the commercially available infusion in dextrose 5% is adjusted to 3.5–6.

Lidocaine may also be known as: lidocaini hydrochloridum, and lignocaine hydrochloride; many trade names are available; a common trade name is *Xylocaine*® (Astra).

Storage/Stability/Preparation

Lidocaine for injection should be stored at temperatures less than 40°C and preferably between 15–30°C; avoid freezing.

Compatibility/Compounding Considerations

Lidocaine is physically **compatible** with most commonly used IV infusion solutions, including D5W, lactated Ringer's, saline, and combinations of these. It is also reportedly physically **compatible** with: aminophylline, bretylium tosylate, calcium chloride/gluceptate/gluconate, carbenicillin disodium, chloramphenicol sodium succinate, chlorothiazide sodium, cimetidine HCl, dexamethasone sodium phosphate, dexmedetomidine, digoxin, diphenhydramine HCl, dobutamine HCl, ephedrine sulfate, erythromycin lactobionate, fentanyl, glycopyrrolate, heparin sodium, hydrocortisone sodium succinate, hydroxyzine HCl, ketamine, insulin (regular), mephentermine sulfate, metaraminol bitartrate, methicillin sodium, metoclopramide HCl, morphine sulfate, nitrofurantoin sodium, oxytetracycline HCl, penicillin G potassium, pentobarbital sodium, phenylephrine HCl, potassium chloride, procainamide HCl, prochlorperazine edisylate, promazine HCl, sodium bicarbonate, sodium lactate, tetracycline HCl, verapamil HCl, and Vitamin B-Complex with C.

Lidocaine **may not be compatible** with dopamine, epinephrine, isoproterenol, or norepinephrine as these require low pH's for stability. Lidocaine is reportedly physically **incompatible** when mixed with ampicillin sodium, cefazolin sodium, methohexital sodium, or phenytoin sodium. Compatibility is dependent upon factors such as pH, concentration, temperature, and diluent used; consult specialized references or a hospital pharmacist for more specific information.

To prepare IV infusion solution using the veterinary 2% solution add 1 gram (50 mL of 2% solution to 1 liter of D_5W or other compatible solution, this will give an approximate concentration of 1 mg/mL (1000 micrograms/mL). When using a mini-drip (60 drops/mL) IV set, each drop will contain approximately 17 micrograms. In small dogs and cats, a less concentrated solution may be used for greater dosage accuracy. When preparing solutions be certain that you are not using the lidocaine product that contains epinephrine.

A combination intravenous infusion for analgesia and sedation in vigorous postoperative patients (dogs, NOT cats) that require sedation to sleep the night after surgery is described (Hansen 2008): For this technique, plan on adding the drugs to a bag of fluids for which the administration rate will not change, which usually means picking a fluid and administration rate calculated to provide maintenance needs for water. For example, to calculate a drug plan for a 20-kg dog that is to receive morphine, lidocaine, ketamine, and medetomidine for the first 8 to 24 hours postoperatively, drug doses to consider might include:

Morphine: 0.1 mg/kg/hr x 20 kg = 2 mg/hr
Lidocaine: 2.5 mg/kg/hr x 20 kg = 50 mg/hr
Ketamine: 0.1 mg/kg/hr x 20 kg = 2 mg/hr
Medetomidine: 2 micrograms/kg/hr x 20 kg = 40 micrograms/hr (**Note:** This is *not* the dose for *dexmedetomidine*)

The maintenance fluid administration rate for a dog this size lying quietly in a cage is roughly 800 mL/day or 33 mL/hr. Therefore, a 1-L bag contains approximately 30 hour's worth of treatment, and to a 1-L bag one must add:

Morphine: 2 mg/hr x 30 hours = 60 mg = 4 mL (if using 15 mg/mL morphine)
Lidocaine: 50 mg/hr x 30 hours = 1500 mg = 75 mL (if using 20 mg/mL lidocaine)
Ketamine: 2 mg/hr x 30 hours = 60 mg = 0.6 mL (if using 100 mg/mL ketamine)
Medetomidine: 40 micrograms/hr x 30 hours = 1200 micrograms = 1.2 mL (if using 1000 micrograms/mL medetomidine)

If the drugs are added to a 1-L bag of fluid, the final volume is greater than a liter—in this case 1081 mL. Therefore, 81 mL should be removed from the bag before addition of the medications.

Dosage Forms/Regulatory Status

VETERINARY-LABELED PRODUCTS:

There are injectable lidocaine products labeled for use in veterinary medicine (dogs, cats, horses, and cattle) as an injectable anesthetic, but it is not FDA-approved for use as an antiarrhythmic agent. Information regarding its use in food-producing species is conflicting; when using a food animal it is suggested to contact FARAD (see appendix).

Lidocaine HCl for Injection: 2% (20 mg/mL) in 100 mL & 250 mL multi-use vials; (contains preservatives); generic; (Rx)

The ARCI (Racing Commissioners International) has designated this drug as a class 2 substance. See the appendix for more information.

HUMAN-LABELED PRODUCTS:

Lidocaine Hydrochloride Injection: 0.5%, 1%, 1.5%, 2% & 4% in 5 mL, 10 mL, 20 mL, 30 mL & 50 mL single- & multi-dose vials, 2 mL &

5 mL amps, 5 mL syringes & cartridges (with or without laryngotracheal cannula); 10 mL & 20 mL *PolyAmp DuoFit* & 1.8 mL cartridges; *Xylocaine®* & *Xylocaine MPF®* (AstraZeneca); generic; (Rx)

Lidocaine Hydrochloride with Dextrose Injection: 1.5% with 7.5% dextrose & 5% with 7.5 % dextrose in 2 mL amps & single-dose amps; *Xylocaine MPF®* (APP Pharmaceutical); generic; (Abbott); (Rx)

Premixed with D5W for IV infusion in concentrations of 2 mg/mL, 4 mg/mL, and 5 mg/mg, injections with epinephrine, topical liquids, patches, ointment, cream, lotion, gel, spray, & jelly available.

References

Cote, E. (2004). Feline arrhythmias. Proceedings: ACVIM Forum. Accessed via: Veterinary Information Network. http://goo.gl/jiqyx

Dyson, D.H. (2008). Analgesia and Chemical Restraint for the Emergent Veterinary Patient. Veterinary Clinics of North America-Small Animal Practice 38(6): 1329-+.

Grint, N. (2008). Constant Rate Infusions (CRIS) in Pain Management. Proceedings: BSAVA. Accessed via: Veterinary Information Network. http://goo.gl/CIXUX

Hallowell, G. (2008). Update on Current and New Treatments for Colic Patients. Proceedings: ACVIM. Accessed via: Veterinary Information Network. http://goo.gl/D04NS

Hansen, B. (2008). Analgesia for the Critically III Dog or Cat: An Update. Veterinary Clinics of North America-Small Animal Practice 38(6): 1353-+.

Hilwig, R.W. (1987). Cardiac arrhythmias. Current Therapy in Equine Medicine. NE Robinson Ed. Philadelphia, WB Saunders: 154–164.

Macintire, D. (2006). Cardiac Emergencies. Proceedings: ACVC 2006. Accessed via: Veterinary Information Network. http://goo.gl/KxqeK

Malone, E., T. Turner, et al. (1999). Intravenous lidocaine for the treatment of equine ileus (abstract). Proceedings: American College of Veterinary Internal Medicine: 17th Annual Veterinary Medical Forum, Chicago.

Mogg, T. (1999). Equine Cardiac Disease: Clinical pharmacology and therapeutics. The Veterinary Clinics of North America: Equine Practice 15:3(December).

Moise, N. (2000). CVT Update: Ventricular Arrhythmias. Kirk's Current Veterinary Therapy: XIII Small Animal Practice. J Bonagura Ed. Philadelphia, WB Saunders: 733–737.

Papich, M. (1989). Effects of drugs on pregnancy. Current Veterinary Therapy X: Small Animal Practice. R Kirk Ed. Philadelphia, Saunders: 1291–1299.

Schwartz, D. (2009). This Dog Has Ventricular Arrhythmias—What Do I Do? Proceedings: WSAVA. Accessed via: Veterinary Information Network. http://goo.gl/ij2xD

Shaffran, N. (2009). Leaps and Bounds in Pain Management with CRIS. Proceedings: IVECCS. Accessed via: Veterinary Information Network. http://goo.gl/8N6sW

Valverde, A. (2008). Epidural Analgesia and Anesthesia in Dogs and Cats. Vet Clin NA: Sm Anim Pract 38: 1205–1230.

Ware, W. (2000). Therapy for Critical Arrythmies: New Advances. Proceedings: The North American Veterinary Conference, Orlando.

LINCOMYCIN HCL

(lin-koe-*mye*-sin)   Lincocin®, Lincomix®

LINCOSAMIDE ANTIBIOTIC

Prescriber Highlights

▶ Lincosamide antibiotic similar to clindamycin; broad spectrum against many anaerobes, gram-positive aerobic cocci, Toxoplasma, etc.

▶ Contraindications: Horses, Rodents, Ruminants, Lagomorphs; Hypersensitivity to lincosamides

▶ Caution: Liver or renal dysfunction; consider reducing dosage if severe

▶ Adverse Effects: Gastroenteritis, pain at injection site if given IM; rapid IV administration can cause hypotension & cardiopulmonary arrest

▶ Distributed into milk; may cause diarrhea in nursing animals

▶ Drug interactions

Uses/Indications

Lincomycin has dosage forms FDA-approved for use in dogs, cats, swine, and in combination with other agents for chickens. Because clindamycin is generally better absorbed, more active, and probably less toxic, it has largely supplanted the use of lincomycin for oral and injectable therapy in small animals, but some clinicians believe that clindamycin does not offer enough clinically significant improvements over lincomycin to justify its higher cost. For further information, refer to the Pharmacology or Doses sections.

Pharmacology/Actions

The lincosamide antibiotics lincomycin and clindamycin, share mechanisms of action and have similar spectrums of activity although lincomycin is usually less active against susceptible organisms. Complete cross-resistance occurs between the two drugs; at least partial cross-resistance occurs between the lincosamides and erythromycin. They may act as bacteriostatic or bactericidal agents, depending on the concentration of the drug at the infection site and the susceptibility of the organism. The lincosamides are believed to act by binding to the 50S ribosomal subunit of susceptible bacteria, thereby inhibiting peptide bond formation.

Most aerobic gram-positive cocci are susceptible to the lincosamides (*Strep. faecalis* is not), including staphylococcus and streptococci. Other organisms that are generally susceptible include: *Corynebacterium diphtheriae, Nocardia asteroides,* Erysepelothrix, *and Mycoplasma* spp. Anaerobic bacteria that may be susceptible to the lincomycin include: *Clostridium perfringens. C. tetani* (not *C. difficile*), Bacteroides (including many strains of *B. fragilis*), Fusobacterium,

Peptostreptococcus, Actinomyces, and Peptococcus.

Pharmacokinetics

The pharmacokinetics of lincomycin have not apparently been extensively studied in veterinary species. Unless otherwise noted, the following information applies to humans. The drug is rapidly absorbed from the gut, but only about 30–40% of the total dose is absorbed. Food both decreases the extent and the rate of absorption. Peak serum levels are attained about 2–4 hour after oral dosing. IM administration gives peak levels about double those reached after oral dosing, and peak at about 30 minutes post injection.

Lincomycin is distributed into most tissues. Therapeutic levels are achieved in bone, synovial fluid, bile, pleural fluid, peritoneal fluid, skin, and heart muscle. CNS levels may reach 40% of those in the serum if meninges are inflamed. Lincomycin is bound from 57–72% to plasma proteins, depending on the drug's concentration. The drug crosses the placenta and can be distributed into milk at concentrations equal to those found in plasma.

Lincomycin is partially metabolized in the liver. Unchanged drug and metabolites are excreted in the urine, feces and bile. Half-lives can be prolonged in patients with renal or hepatic dysfunction. The elimination half-life of lincomycin is reportedly 3–4 hours in small animals.

Contraindications/Precautions/Warnings

Although there have been case reports of parenteral administration of lincosamides to horses, cattle and sheep, the lincosamides are considered *contraindicated* for use in **rabbits, hamsters, guinea pigs, horses,** and **ruminants** because of serious gastrointestinal effects that may occur, including death.

Lincomycin is contraindicated in patients with known hypersensitivity to it or having a preexisting monilial infection.

Lincomycin is generally not recommended for use in neonatal animals because of its effects on gut flora.

Adverse Effects

Adverse effects reported in dogs and cats include gastroenteritis (emesis, loose stools, and infrequently bloody diarrhea in dogs). IM injections reportedly cause pain at the injection site. Rapid intravenous administration can cause hypotension and cardiopulmonary arrest.

Swine may develop gastrointestinal disturbances while receiving the medication.

Reproductive/Nursing Safety

Lincomycin crosses the placenta and cord blood concentrations are approximately 25% of those found in maternal serum. Safe use during pregnancy has not been established, but neither has the drug been implicated in causing teratogenic effects.

In humans, the FDA categorizes this drug as category **B** for use during pregnancy (*Animal studies have not yet demonstrated risk to the fetus, but there are no adequate studies in pregnant women; or animal studies have shown an adverse effect, but adequate studies in pregnant women have not demonstrated a risk to the fetus in the first trimester of pregnancy, and there is no evidence of risk in later trimesters.*) In a separate system evaluating the safety of drugs in canine and feline pregnancy (Papich 1989), this drug is categorized as in class: **A** (*Probably safe. Although specific studies may not have proved the safety of all drugs in dogs and cats, there are no reports of adverse effects in laboratory animals or women.*)

Because lincomycin is distributed into milk, nursing animals of mothers given lincomycin may develop diarrhea.

Overdosage/Acute Toxicity

There is little information available regarding overdoses of this drug. In dogs, oral doses of up to 300 mg/kg/day for up to one year or parenterally at 60 mg/kg/day apparently did not result in toxicity.

Drug Interactions

The following drug interactions have either been reported or are theoretical in humans or animals receiving lincomycin and may be of significance in veterinary patients:

- **CYCLOSPORINE:** Lincomycin may reduce levels

- **ERYTHROMYCIN:** *In vitro* antagonism when used with lincomycin; concomitant use should probably be avoided

- **KAOLIN:** Kaolin (found in several over-the-counter antidiarrheal preparations) has been shown to reduce the absorption of lincomycin by up to 90% if both are given concurrently; if both drugs are necessary, separate doses by at least 2 hours

- **NEUROMUSCULAR BLOCKING AGENTS (e.g., pancuronium):** Lincomycin possesses intrinsic neuromuscular blocking activity and should be used cautiously with other neuromuscular blocking agents

Laboratory Considerations

- Slight increases in **liver function tests** (AST, ALT, Alk. Phosph.) may occur. There is apparently not any clinical significance associated with these increases.

Doses

- **DOGS:**

  For susceptible infections:

  a) For skin and soft tissue infections: 15.4 mg/kg PO q8h or 22 mg/kg PO q12h. Treatment for superficial pyoderma 21–42 days; for deep, resistant pyoderma 56 days;

    For systemic infections: 22 mg/kg IM, SC, or IV (must be diluted and given as a slow drip infusion) q24h or 11 mg/kg IM or SC q12h for 12 days or less.

For bacteremia, sepsis: 11–22 mg/kg IV q8h for 12 days or less. (Greene *et al.* 2006)

b) For pyoderma: 40–50 mg/kg/day PO divided into two or three doses per day. (Carlotti 2008)

c) For superficial pyodermas: 20 mg/kg PO q12h (White 2007)

d) For pyoderma: 22 mg/kg PO twice daily; good for first time pyodermas. (Logas 2005)

■ **CATS:**

For susceptible infections:

a) For skin and soft tissue infections: 11 mg/kg IM q12h or 22 mg/kg IM q24h. Treatment for 12 days or less;

For systemic infections: 15 mg/kg PO q8h or 22 mg/kg PO q12h. Treatment for 12 days or less. (Greene *et al.* 2006)

■ **FERRETS:**

For susceptible infections:

a) 10–15 mg/kg PO three times daily; 10 mg/kg IM twice daily (Williams 2000)

■ **SWINE:**

For susceptible infections:

a) For mycoplasmal (*M. hyopneumoniae*) pneumonia: Fed at 200 grams per ton of feed for 21 days or 11 mg/kg IM once daily (Amass 1999)

b) 11 mg/kg IM once daily for 3–7 days; or added to drinking water at a rate of 250 mg/gallon (average of 8.36 mg/kg/day) (Label directions; *Lincocin®*—Upjohn)

Monitoring

■ Clinical efficacy

■ Adverse effects; particularly severe diarrheas

Client Information

■ Clients should be instructed to report the incidence of severe, protracted, or bloody diarrhea to the veterinarian.

Chemistry/Synonyms

An antibiotic obtained from cultures of *Streptomyces lincolnensis*, lincomycin is available commercially as the monohydrate hydrochloride. It occurs as a white to off-white, crystalline powder that is freely soluble in water. The powder may have a faint odor and has a pK_a of 7.6. The commercially available injection has a pH of 3–5.5 and occurs as a clear to slightly yellow solution.

Lincomycin may also be as: U-10149, NSC-70731, *Anbycin®*, *Frademicina®*, *Fredcina®*, *Linco®*, *Lincocin®*, *LincoMed®*, *Lincomix®*, *Linco-Ped®*, *Lincono®*, and *Macrolin®*.

Storage/Stability

Lincomycin capsules, tablets and soluble powder should be stored at room temperature (15–30°C) in tight containers. Lincomycin injectable products should be stored at room temperature; avoid freezing.

Lincomycin HCl for injection is reportedly physically **compatible** for at least 24 hours in the following IV infusion solutions and drugs: D_5W, D_5W in sodium chloride 0.9%, $D_{10}W$, sodium chloride 0.9%, Ringer's injection, amikacin sulfate, cephalothin sodium, chloramphenicol sodium succinate, cimetidine HCl, cytarabine, heparin sodium, penicillin G potassium/sodium (4 hours only), polymyxin B sulfate, tetracycline HCl, and vitamin B-complex with C.

Drugs that are reportedly physically **incompatible** when mixed with lincomycin, data conflicts, or compatibility is concentration and/or time dependent include: ampicillin sodium, carbenicillin disodium, methicillin sodium, and phenytoin sodium. Compatibility is dependent upon factors such as pH, concentration, temperature and diluent used; consult specialized references or a hospital pharmacist for more specific information.

Dosage Forms/Regulatory Status

VETERINARY-LABELED PRODUCTS:

Lincomycin Oral Tablets: 100 mg, 200 mg, 500 mg; *Lincocin®* (Pfizer); (Rx). FDA-approved for use in dogs and cats.

Lincomycin Oral Solution: 50 mg/mL in 20 mL dropper bottles; *Lincocin® Aquadrops* (Pfizer); (Rx). FDA-approved for use in dogs and cats.

Lincomycin Sterile Injection: 100 mg/mL in 20 mL vials; *Lincocin®* (Pfizer); (Rx). FDA-approved for use in dogs and cats.

Lincomycin Sterile Injection: 25 mg/mL, 100 mg/mL & 300 mg/mL in 100 mL vials; FDA-approved for use in swine. Slaughter withdrawal (when used as labeled) = 48 hours. *Lincocin® Sterile Solution* (Pfizer); *Lincomix® Injectable* (Pfizer); generic; (OTC)

There are also several lincomycin combination feed/water additive products for use in swine and/or poultry.

HUMAN-LABELED PRODUCTS:

Lincomycin Injection: 300 mg (as hydrochloride)/mL in 2 mL & 10 mL vials; *Lincocin®* (Upjohn), (Rx)

References

Amass, S. (1999). A review of mycoplasmal pneumonia. Proceedings: The North American Veterinary Conference, Orlando.

Carlotti, D.-N. (2008). Canine recurrent and resistant pyoderma. Proceedings: World Veterinary Congress. Accessed via: Veterinary Information Network. http://goo.gl/ol64c

Greene, C., K. Hartmannn, et al. (2006). Appendix 8: Antimicrobial Drug Formulary. Infectious Disease of the Dog and Cat. C Greene Ed., Elsevier: 1186–1333.

Logas, D. (2005). Superficial and Deep Pyoderma. Proceedings: Western Veterinary Conf. Accessed via: Veterinary Information Network. http://goo.gl/qMbzy

Papich, M. (1989). Effects of drugs on pregnancy. Current Veterinary Therapy X: Small Animal Practice. R Kirk Ed. Philadelphia, Saunders: 1291–1299.

White, S. (2007). Atopic dermatitis and its secondary infections. Proceedings: Canine Medicine Symposium. Accessed via: Veterinary Information Network. http://goo.gl/upBF7

Williams, B. (2000). Therapeutics in Ferrets. Vet Clin NA: Exotic Anim Pract 3:1(Jan): 131–153.

LIOTHYRONINE SODIUM

(lye-oh-*thye*-roe-neen)   Cytomel®, Triostat®

THYROID HORMONE

Prescriber Highlights

▶ Form of T3 (active thyroid hormone) used for hypothyroidism particularly in animals unresponsive to T4

▶ Shorter duration of effect than levothyroxine

▶ Contraindications: Acute myocardial infarction, thyrotoxicosis, or untreated adrenal insufficiency

▶ Caution: Concurrent hypoadrenocorticism (treated), cardiac disease, diabetes, or elderly

▶ Adverse Effects: Only associated with OD's (tachycardia, polyphagia, PU/PD, excitability, nervousness, & excessive panting); some cats may appear apathetic

▶ Drug-drug; drug-lab interactions

Uses/Indications

Because of its shorter duration of action, liothyronine is generally not considered the drug of first choice in treating hypothyroidism. Infrequently, animals not responding to levothyroxine may respond to liothyronine. Liothyronine is not recommended for initial therapy because only serum T3 concentrations are normalized while T4 levels remain low.

Pharmacology/Actions

Thyroid hormones affect the rate of many physiologic processes including: fat, protein, and carbohydrate metabolism, increasing protein synthesis, increasing gluconeogenesis, and promoting mobilization and utilization of glycogen stores. Thyroid hormones also increase oxygen consumption, body temperature, heart rate and cardiac output, blood volume, enzyme system activity, and growth and maturity. Thyroid hormone is particularly important for adequate development of the central nervous system. While the exact mechanisms how thyroid hormones exert their effects are not well understood, it is known that thyroid hormones (primarily triiodothyronine) act at the cellular level.

In humans, triiodothyronine (T_3) is the primary hormone responsible for activity. Approximately 80% of T_3 found in the peripheral tissues is derived from thyroxine (T_4) which is the principle hormone released by the thyroid.

Pharmacokinetics

In dogs, peak plasma levels of liothyronine occur 2–5 hours after oral dosing. The plasma half-life is approximately 5–6 hours. In contrast to levothyroxine, it is believed that liothyronine is nearly completely absorbed by dogs and absorption is not as affected by stomach contents, intestinal flora changes, etc.

Contraindications/Precautions/Warnings

Liothyronine (and other replacement thyroid hormones) are contraindicated in patients with acute myocardial infarction, thyrotoxicosis, or untreated adrenal insufficiency. It should be used with caution, and at a lower initial dosage, in patients with concurrent hypoadrenocorticism (treated), cardiac disease, diabetes, or in elderly patients.

Adverse Effects

When administered at an appropriate dose to patients requiring thyroid hormone replacement, there should not be any adverse effects associated with therapy. For adverse effects associated with overdosage, see below.

Reproductive/Nursing Safety

In humans, the FDA categorizes this drug as category *A* for use during pregnancy (*Adequate studies in pregnant women have not demonstrated a risk to the fetus in the first trimester of pregnancy, and there is no evidence of risk in later trimesters.*)

Minimal amounts of thyroid hormones are excreted in milk and should not adversely affect nursing offspring.

Overdosage/Acute Toxicity

Chronic overdosage will produce signs of hyperthyroidism, including tachycardia, polyphagia, PU/PD, excitability, nervousness, and excessive panting. Dosage should be reduced and/or temporarily withheld until signs subside. Some (10%?) cats may exhibit signs of "apathetic" (listlessness, anorexia, etc.) hyperthyroidism.

Acute massive overdosage can produce signs resembling thyroid storm. After oral ingestion, treatment to reduce absorption of drug should be accomplished using standard protocols (emetics or gastric lavage, cathartics, charcoal) unless contraindicated by the patient's condition. Treatment is supportive and symptomatic. Oxygen, artificial ventilation, cardiac glycosides, beta-blockers (*e.g.*, propranolol), fluids, dextrose, and antipyretic agents have all been suggested for use if necessary.

Drug Interactions

The following drug interactions have either been reported or are theoretical in humans or animals receiving liothyronine and may be of significance in veterinary patients:

■ **ANTIDEPRESSANTS, TRICYCLIC/TETRACYCLIC:** Increased risk for CNS stimulation and cardiac arrhythmias

- ■ **ANTIDIABETIC AGENTS (insulin, oral agents):** Levothyroxine may increase requirements for insulin or oral agents
- ■ **CHOLESTYRAMINE:** May reduce liothyronine absorption; separate doses by 4 hours
- ■ **DIGOXIN:** Potential for reduced digoxin levels
- ■ **KETAMINE:** May cause tachycardia and hypertension
- ■ **SYMPATHOMIMETIC AGENTS (epinephrine, norepinephrine, etc.):** Levothyroxine can potentiate effects
- ■ **WARFARIN:** Thyroid hormones increase the catabolism of vitamin K-dependent clotting factors that may increase the anticoagulation effects in patients on warfarin

Laboratory Considerations The following drugs may have effects on thyroid function tests; evaluate results accordingly:

- ■ *Effects on serum T_4:* aminoglutethimide↓, anabolic steroids/androgens↓, antithyroid drugs (PTU, methimazole)↓, asparaginase↓, barbiturates↓, corticosteroids↓, danazol↓, diazepam↓, estrogens↑ (**Note:** estrogens may have no effect on canine T_3 or T_4 concentrations), fluorouracil↑, heparin↓, insulin↑, lithium carbonate↓, mitotane (o,p-DDD)↓, nitroprusside↓, phenylbutazone↓, phenytoin↓, propranolol↑, salicylates (large doses)↓, sulfonamides↓, and sulfonylureas↓.
- ■ *Effects on serum T_3:* antithyroid drugs (PTU, methimazole)↓, barbiturates↓, corticosteroids↓, estrogens↑, fluorouracil↑, heparin↓, lithium carbonate↓, phenytoin↓, propranolol↓, salicylates (large doses)↓, sulfonamides↓, and thiazides↑.
- ■ *Effects on T_3 uptake resin:* anabolic steroids/androgens↑, antithyroid drugs (PTU, methimazole)↓, asparaginase↑, corticosteroids↑, danazol↑, estrogens↓, fluorouracil↓, heparin↑, lithium carbonate↑, phenylbutazone↑, and salicylates (large doses)↑.
- ■ *Effects on serum TSH:* aminoglutethimide↑, antithyroid drugs (PTU, methimazole)↑, corticosteroids↓, danazol↓, lithium carbonate↑, and sulfonamides↑.
- ■ *Effects on Free Thyroxine Index (FTI):* antithyroid drugs (PTU, methimazole)↓, barbiturates↓, corticosteroids↓, heparin↑, lithium carbonate↓, and phenylbutazone↓.

Doses

- ■ **DOGS:**
  For hypothyroidism:
  a) Initially, 4–6 micrograms/kg PO q8h. Some dogs may require less frequent dosing (Nelson 1989)

  b) Initial starting dose is 4–6 micrograms/kg PO q8h. Liothyronine is only indicated in those few situations when T4 supplementation has failed to achieve a response in a dog with confirmed hypothyroidism, perhaps due to impaired GI T4 absorption. Dogs receiving T3 supplementation may be more susceptible to iatrogenic thyrotoxicosis since serum T4 concentrations are important in the feedback regulation of the hypothalamic-pituitary-thyroid axis. Combination products that contain both T3 and T4 should be avoided for similar reasons. (Scott-Moncrieff, J. & Guptill-Yoran 2000)(Scott-Moncrieff, J.C. 2009)

- ■ **CATS:**
  For hypothyroidism:
  a) Initially, 4.4 micrograms/kg PO 2–3 times a day (Feldman & Nelson 1987)

Monitoring

- ■ Similar to levothyroxine, but T_4 levels will remain low. When monitoring T_3 levels, draw serum just prior to dosing and again 2–4 hours after administering the drug.

Client Information

- ■ Clients should be instructed in the importance of compliance with therapy as prescribed
- ■ Also, review the signs that can be seen with too much thyroid supplementation

Chemistry/Synonyms
A synthetically prepared sodium salt of the naturally occurring hormone T_3, liothyronine sodium occurs as an odorless, light tan crystalline powder. It is very slightly soluble in water and slightly soluble in alcohol. Each 25 micrograms of liothyronine is approximately equivalent to 60–65 mg (1 grain) of thyroglobulin or desiccated thyroid and 100 micrograms or less of levothyroxine.

Liothyronine sodium may also be known as: T_3, T_3 thyronine sodium, L-triiodothyronine, sodium L-triiodothyronine, liothyroninum natricum, sodium liothyronine, l-tri-iodothyronine sodium, *Cynomel®*, *Cytomel®*, *Dispon®*, *Neo-Tiroimade®*, *T3®*, *Tertroxin®*, *Thybon®*, *Thyrotardin N®*, *Ti-Tre®*, *Triiodothyronine Injection®*, *Triostat®*, *Triyodisan®*, and *Triyotex®*.

Storage/Stability
Liothyronine tablets should be stored at room temperature (15–30°C) in tight containers.

The injection should be stored refrigerated (2–8°C).

Dosage Forms/Regulatory Status
VETERINARY-LABELED PRODUCTS: None
HUMAN-LABELED PRODUCTS:

Liothyronine Sodium Tablets: 5 mcg, 25 mcg & 50 mcg; *Cytomel®* (Monarch); generic; (Rx)

Liothyronine Sodium Injection Solution: 10 micrograms/mL in 1 mL vials; *Triostat®* (JHP Pharmaceuticals); generic; (Rx)

References

Feldman, E.C. & R.W. Nelson (1987). Hypothyroidism. Canine and Feline Endocrinology and Reproduction Philadelphia, WB Saunders: 55–90.

Nelson, R.W. (1989). Treatment of canine hypothyroidism. Current Veterinary Therapy X: Small Animal Practice. RW Kirk Ed. Philadelphia, WB Saunders: 993–997.

Scott-Moncrieff, J. & L. Guptill-Yoran (2000). Hypothyroidism. Textbook of Veterinary Internal Medicine: Diseases of the Dog and Cat. S Ettinger and E Feldman Eds. Philadelphia, WB Saunders. 2: 1419–1429.

Scott-Moncrieff, J.C. (2009). Canine Hypothyroidism. Proceedings: WVC. Accessed via: Veterinary Information Network. http://goo.gl/cyqRl

LISINOPRIL

(lye-*sin*-oh-pril)   Prinivil®, Zestril®

ANGIOTENSIN-CONVERTING ENZYME (ACE) INHIBITOR

Prescriber Highlights

▶ ACE inhibitor used primarily as a vaso-dilator in the treatment of heart failure or hypertension; may also be of benefit in the treatment of chronic renal failure or protein losing nephropathies

▶ May be less expensive than other ACE inhibitors & probably can be dosed once daily

▶ Not as much information available or experience as enalapril or benazepril in dogs or cats

▶ Caution: Renal insufficiency (doses may need to be reduced), patients with hyponatremia, coronary or cerebrovas-cular insufficiency, preexisting hema-tologic abnormalities, or a collagen vascular disease (e.g., SLE)

▶ Adverse Effects: GI distress (anorexia, vomiting, diarrhea); Potentially: weak-ness, hypotension, renal dysfunction, & hyperkalemia

Uses/Indications

The principle uses of lisinopril in veterinary medicine at present are as a vasodilator in the treatment of heart failure or hypertension. Recent studies have demonstrated that ACE inhibitors, particularly when used in conjunc-tion with furosemide, do improve the quality of life in dogs with heart failure. It is not clear, however, whether it has any significant effect on survival times. Lisinopril may also be of bene-fit in treating the effects associated with valvular heart disease (mitral regurgitation) and left to right shunts. It is being explored as adjunctive treatment in chronic renal failure and in protein losing nephropathies.

Lisinopril may have advantages over other ACE inhibitors in that it may be dosed dai-ly and less expensive. Disadvantages are that it is only available in human labeled dosage forms and there is much less published information on its use (efficacy, safety, dosing) in veterinary species.

Pharmacology/Actions

Unlike enalapril, lisinopril does not need to be converted in the liver to an active metabolite. Lisinopril prevents the formation of angioten-sin-II (a potent vasoconstrictor) by competing with angiotensin-I for the enzyme angiotensin-converting enzyme (ACE). ACE has a much higher affinity for lisinopril than for angioten-sin-I. Because angiotensin-II concentrations are decreased, aldosterone secretion is reduced and plasma renin activity is increased. Lisinopril has a higher affinity for ACE than either enalaprilat or captopril.

The cardiovascular effects of lisinopril in pa-tients with CHF include decreased total periph-eral resistance, pulmonary vascular resistance, mean arterial and right atrial pressures, and pul-monary capillary wedge pressure, no change or decrease in heart rate, and increased cardiac in-dex and output, stroke volume, and exercise tol-erance. Renal blood flow can be increased with little change in hepatic blood flow. In animals with glomerular disease, ACE inhibitors proba-bly decrease proteinuria and help to preserve renal function.

Pharmacokinetics

In dogs, lisinopril's bioavailability ranges from 25–50% with peak levels occurring about 4 hours after dosing. Lisinopril is distributed poorly into the CNS. It is unknown if it is dis-tributed into maternal milk, but it does cross the placenta. Half-lives are increased in patients with renal failure or severe CHF. Duration of action in dogs has been described as being 24 hours, but effects tend to drop off with time.

Contraindications/Precautions/Warnings

Lisinopril is contraindicated in patients who have demonstrated hypersensitivity to the ACE inhibitors. It should be used with caution and close supervision in patients with renal insuffi-ciency and doses may need to be reduced.

Lisinopril should be used with caution in patients with hyponatremia or sodium deple-tion, coronary or cerebrovascular insufficiency, preexisting hematologic abnormalities, or a col-lagen vascular disease (*e.g.*, SLE). Patients with severe CHF should be monitored very closely upon initiation of therapy.

Adverse Effects

Lisinopril's adverse effect profile in dogs is re-portedly similar to other ACE inhibitors, princi-pally GI distress (anorexia, vomiting, diarrhea). Potentially, cough, weakness, hypotension, renal dysfunction, and hyperkalemia could oc-cur. Because it lacks a sulfhydryl group (unlike captopril), there is less likelihood that immune-mediated reactions will occur, but rashes, neutropenia, and agranulocytosis have been reported in humans.

Reproductive/Nursing Safety

Lisinopril crosses the placenta. High doses in rodents have caused decreased fetal weights and increases in fetal and maternal death rates; teratogenic effects have not been reported.

Current recommendations for humans are to discontinue ACE inhibitors as soon as pregnancy is detected. In humans, the FDA categorizes this drug as category *C* for use during the *first trimester* of pregnancy (*Animal studies have shown an adverse effect on the fetus, but there are no adequate studies in humans; or there are no animal reproduction studies and no adequate studies in humans.*) In humans, the FDA categorizes this drug as category *D* for use during the *second and third trimesters* of pregnancy (*There is evidence of human fetal risk, but the potential benefits from the use of the drug in pregnant women may be acceptable despite its potential risks.*)

It is not known whether lisinopril is excreted in milk; use with caution.

Overdosage/Acute Toxicity

There were 688 exposures to lisinopril reported to the ASPCA Animal Poison Control Center (APCC) during 2008-2009. In these cases 654 were dogs with 58 showing clinical signs, 31 were cats with 2 showing clinical signs, and the remaining cases were 3 birds with 1 showing clinical signs. Common findings in dogs recorded in decreasing frequency included hypotension, lethargy, vomiting, and tachycardia.

The ASPCA Animal Poison Control Center (APCC) has over 3500 lisinopril exposure cases in its files, mostly involving dogs, but some birds and cats. The lowest dosage documented to cause hypotension in dogs is 27 mg/kg. Generally dosages below 20 mg/kg cause mild signs only, most commonly vomiting and lethargy. Higher dosages warrant decontamination. Only a single cat out of 218 cats developed hypotension at a dosage of 4.9 mg/kg. In birds, only mild somnolence occurred at 41 mg/kg.

In overdose situations, the primary concern is hypotension; supportive treatment with volume expansion with normal saline is recommended to correct blood pressure. Because of the drug's long duration of action, prolonged monitoring and treatment may be required. Recent overdoses should be managed using gut-emptying protocols when warranted.

Drug Interactions

The following drug interactions have either been reported or are theoretical in humans or animals receiving lisinopril and may be of significance in veterinary patients:

■ **ANTIDIABETIC AGENTS (insulin, oral agents):** Possible increased risk for hypoglycemia; enhanced monitoring recommended

■ **DIURETICS (e.g., furosemide, hydrochlorothiazide):** Potential for increased hypotensive effects; some veterinary clinicians recommend reducing furosemide doses (by 25-50%) when adding ACE-inhibitors to therapy in CHF

■ **DIURETICS, POTASSIUM-SPARING (e.g., spironolactone, triamterene):** Increased hyperkalemic effects, enhanced monitoring of serum potassium recommended

■ **HYPOTENSIVE AGENTS, OTHER:** Potential for increased hypotensive effect

■ **LITHIUM:** Increased serum lithium levels possible; increased monitoring required

■ **NSAIDS:** May reduce the anti-hypertensive or positive hemodynamic effects of enalapril; may increase risk for reduced renal function

■ **POTASSIUM SUPPLEMENTS:** Increased risk for hyperkalemia

Laboratory Considerations

■ ACE inhibitors may cause a reversible decrease in localization and excretion of **iodohippurate sodium** I^{123}/I^{134}, or **Technetium** Tc^{99} pententate renal imaging in the affected kidney in patients with renal artery stenosis, which may lead to confusion in test interpretation.

Doses

■ **DOGS:**
For adjunctive treatment of heart failure:
a) 0.5 mg/kg PO q12-24 hours (Ware & Keene 2000)
b) 0.5 mg/kg PO q24h (Fuentes 2003)
c) 0.25-0.5 mg/kg PO once daily (q24h); highest recommended doses should be used unless not tolerated by patient. (Rishniw 2008)

■ **CATS:**
For adjunctive treatment of heart failure:
a) 0.25-0.5 mg/kg PO once daily (Fox 2000)

Monitoring

■ Clinical signs of CHF
■ Serum electrolytes, creatinine, BUN, urine protein
■ CBC with differential, periodic
■ Blood pressure (if treating hypertension or signs associated with hypotension arise)

Client Information

■ Do not abruptly stop or reduce therapy without veterinarian's guidance
■ Contact veterinarian if vomiting or diarrhea persist or are severe or if animal's condition deteriorates

Chemistry/Synonyms

An oral angiotensin-converting enzyme inhibitor (ACE inhibitor) lisinopril is directly active and not a prodrug like enalapril. It occurs as a white crystalline powder. One mg is soluble in 10 mL of water; 70 mL of methanol. It is practically insoluble in alcohol, chloroform, or ether.

Lisinopril may also be known as: L-154826, lisinoprilum, and MK-521; many trade names are available.

Storage/Stability

Store lisinopril tablets at room temperature in tight containers, unless otherwise directed by manufacturer.

Compatibility/Compounding Considerations

Compounded preparation stability: Lisinopril oral suspension compounded from the commercially available tablets has been published (Nahata & Morosco 2004). Triturating ten (10) lisinopril 10 mg tablets with 50 mL of *Ora Plus*® and qs ad to 100 mL with *Ora Sweet*® yields a 1 mg/mL lisinopril oral suspension that retains >95% potency for 91 days when stored at 4°C and protected from light.

Dosage Forms/Regulatory Status

VETERINARY-LABELED PRODUCTS: None

The ARCI (Racing Commissioners International) has designated this drug as a class 3 substance. See the appendix for more information.

HUMAN-LABELED PRODUCTS:

Lisinopril Oral Tablets: 2.5 mg, 5 mg, 10 mg, 20 mg, 30 mg & 40 mg; *Prinivil*® (Merck); *Zestril*® (AstraZeneca); generic; (Rx)

Also available are fixed dose combinations of lisinopril with hydrochlorothiazide.

References

Fox, P. (2000). CVT Update: Therapy for Feline Myocardial Diseases. Kirk's Current Veterinary Therapy: XIII Small Animal Practice. J Bonagura Ed. Philadelphia, WB Saunders: 762–767.

Fuentes, V. (2003). Juggling furosemide and ACE inhibitors. Proceedings: Western Veterinary Conference. Accessed via: Veterinary Information Network. http://goo.gl/l2riv

Nahata, M.C. & R.S. Morosco (2004). Stability of lisinopril in two liquid dosage forms. Ann Pharmacother 38(3): 396–399.

Rishniw, M. (2008). "Treatment of Heart Failure." Canine Associate Databse. http://goo.gl/MDgCr.

Ware, W. & B. Keene (2000). Outpatient management of chronic heart failure. Kirk's Current Veterinary Therapy: XIII Small Animal Practice. J Bonagura Ed. Philadelphia, WB Saunders: 748–752.

LOMUSTINE (CCNU)

(loe-*mus*-teen)   CeeNu®

Prescriber Highlights

▶ Antineoplastic usually used for CNS neoplasms, mast cell tumors, histiocytic sarcomas or as a rescue agent for lymphoma

▶ Cautions (risk vs. benefit): Anemia, bone marrow depression, pulmonary function impairment, current infection, impaired renal function, sensitivity to lomustine, or patients that have received previous chemotherapy or radiotherapy

▶ Adverse Effects: GI effects (anorexia, vomiting, diarrhea), stomatitis, alopecia, corneal de-epithelization, &, rarely, renal toxicity, hepatotoxicity, & pulmonary infiltrates or fibrosis. Most serious: bone marrow depression (anemia, thrombocytopenia, leukopenia); nadirs in dogs generally occur about 1–3 weeks after treatment

▶ Teratogenic

Uses/Indications

Lomustine may be useful in the adjunctive treatment of CNS neoplasms, lymphomas, and mast cell tumors in dogs and cats.

Pharmacology/Actions

While lomustine's mechanism of action is not totally understood, it is believed it acts as an alkylating agent; however, other mechanisms such as carbamoylation and cellular protein modification may be involved; net effects are DNA and RNA synthesis inhibition. Lomustine is cell cycle-phase nonspecific.

Pharmacokinetics

Lomustine is absorbed rapidly and extensively from the GI tract and some absorption occurs after topical administration. Lomustine or its active metabolites are widely distributed in the body. While lomustine is not detected in the CSF, its active metabolites are detected in substantial concentrations. Lomustine is metabolized extensively in the liver to both active and inactive metabolites that are then eliminated primarily in the urine. Lomustine half-life in humans is very short (about 15 minutes), but its biologic activity is significantly longer due to the longer elimination times of active metabolites.

Contraindications/Precautions/Warnings

Lomustine should be used only when its potential benefits outweigh its risks with the following conditions: anemia, bone marrow depression, pulmonary function impairment, current infection, impaired renal function, sensitivity to lomustine, or patients who have received previous chemotherapy or radiotherapy.

Adverse Effects

The most serious adverse effects are bone marrow depression (anemia, thrombocytopenia, leukopenia) and hepatotoxicity. CBC nadirs in dogs generally occur about 1–6 weeks after treatment has begun. In dogs, lomustine may cause delayed, cumulative dose-related, chronic, irreversible hepatotoxicity (Kristal *et al.* 2004). There are some anecdotal reports of SAMe and silymarin being successfully used to treat or prevent lomustine hepatotoxicity. Other potential adverse effects include GI effects (anorexia, vomiting, diarrhea), stomatitis, alopecia, corneal de-epithelization and rarely, renal toxicity, and pulmonary infiltrates or fibrosis.

Cross-resistance may occur between lomustine and carmustine.

Reproductive/Nursing Safety

Lomustine is a teratogen in lab animals. Use only during pregnancy when the benefits to the mother outweigh the risks to the offspring. Lomustine can suppress gonadal function. In humans, the FDA categorizes this drug as category *D* for use during pregnancy (*There is evidence of human fetal risk, but the potential benefits from the use of the drug in pregnant women may be acceptable despite its potential risks.*)

Lomustine and its metabolites have been detected in maternal milk. Nursing puppies should receive milk replacer when the bitch is receiving lomustine.

Overdosage/Acute Toxicity

No specific information was located. Because of the potential toxicity of the drug, overdoses should be treated aggressively with gut emptying protocols employed when possible. For further information, refer to an animal poison control center.

Drug Interactions

The following drug interactions have either been reported or are theoretical in humans or animals receiving lomustine and may be of significance in veterinary patients:

- **IMMUNOSUPPRESSIVE DRUGS, OTHER (e.g., azathioprine, cyclophosphamide, corticosteroids):** Use with other immunosuppressant drugs may increase the risk of infection.

- **MYELOSUPPRESSIVE DRUGS, OTHER (e.g., chloramphenicol, flucytosine, amphotericin B, or colchicine):** The principal concern with lomustine is with its concurrent use with other drugs that are also myelosuppressive, including many of the other antineoplastics and other bone marrow depressant drugs. Bone marrow depression may be additive.

- **VACCINES, LIVE VIRUS:** Live virus vaccines should be used with caution, if at all, during lomustine therapy.

Doses

NOTE: Because of the potential toxicity of this drug to patients, veterinary personnel and clients, and since chemotherapy indications, treatment protocols, monitoring and safety guidelines often change, the following dosages should be used only as a general guide. Consultation with a veterinary oncologist and referral to current veterinary oncology references [*e.g.*, (Henry & Higginbotham 2009); (Argyle *et al.* 2008); (Withrow & Vail 2007); (Villalobos 2007); (Ogilvie & Moore 2006); (Ogilvie & Moore 2001)] is *strongly recommended*.

- **DOGS/CATS:**
  The following is a usual dose or dose range for this drug and should be used only as a general guide: Depending on the indication and protocol, lomustine is usually dosed in dogs from 50–90 mg/m^2 (**NOT** mg/kg) every 2–6 weeks and in cats at 60 mg/m^2 every 6 weeks or as a single 10 mg dose every 3 weeks.

Monitoring

- CBC with platelets one week after dosing and prior to next dose; If platelets less than 200,000/mcl; stop therapy until thrombocytopenia is resolved

- Liver function tests; initially before starting treatment and then every 3–4 months

Client Information

- Lomustine or its metabolites can be detected in the urine up to 24 hours after a dose. If urine must be cleaned up, use appropriate protection to avoid skin contact.

- Liver and bone marrow toxicity are possible; contact veterinarian immediately if patient develops an infection, runs a fever, bleeds, has yellowing of the whites of the eyes, has persistent vomiting or becomes ill.

Chemistry/Synonyms

A nitrosourea derivative alkylating agent, lomustine occurs as a yellow powder that is practically insoluble in water and soluble in alcohol.

Lomustine may also be known as: CCNU, lomustinum, NSC-79037, RB-1509, WR-139017, *Belustine®*, *CCNU®*, *Cecenu®*, *CeeNu®*, *CiNU®*, *Citosta®*, *Lomeblastin®*, *Lucostin®*, *Lucostine®*, and *Prava®*.

Storage/Stability

Store capsules in well-closed containers at room temperature. Expiration dates of two years are assigned after manufacture.

Dosage Forms/Regulatory Status

VETERINARY-LABELED PRODUCTS: None

HUMAN-LABELED PRODUCTS:

Lomustine Capsules: 10 mg, 40 mg & 100 mg with mannitol; *CeeNu®* (Bristol Labs Oncology); (Rx)

References

Argyle, D., M. Brearly, et al. (2008). Decision Making in Small Animal Oncology, Wiley-Blackwell.

Henry, C. & M. Higginbotham (2009). Cancer Management in Small Animal Practice, Saunders.

Kristal, O., K. Rassnick, et al. (2004). Hepatotoxicity associated with CCNU (lomustine) Chemotherapy in Dogs. J Vet Intern Med 18: 75–80.

Ogilvie, G. & A. Moore (2001). Feline Oncology: A Comprehensive Guide to Compassionate Care, Veterinary Learning Systems.

Ogilvie, G. & A. Moore (2006). Managing the Canine Cancer Patient: A Practical Guide to Compassionate Care, Veterinary Learning Systems.

Villalobos, A. (2007). Canine and Feline Geriatric Oncology. Ames, Blackwell.

Withrow, S. & D. Vail (2007). Withrow and MacEwen's Small Animal Clinical Oncology 4th Ed. Philadelphia, Elsevier.

LOPERAMIDE HCL

(loe-*per*-a-mide)   Imodium®

OPIATE ANTIDIARRHEAL

Prescriber Highlights

▶ Synthetic opiate GI motility modifier used for symptomatic treatment of diarrhea, primarily in dogs

▶ Contraindications: Dogs with ABCB1-1Δ (MDR1) mutation. Known hypersensitivity to narcotic analgesics, diarrhea caused by a toxic ingestion until the toxin is eliminated from the GI tract

▶ Caution: Respiratory disease, hepatic encephalopathy, hypothyroidism, severe renal insufficiency, adrenocortical insufficiency (Addison's), head injuries, or increased intracranial pressure, & acute abdominal conditions (*e.g.*, colic), & in geriatric or severely debilitated patients; avoid use in untested dogs of breeds ("white-feet") susceptible to MDR1 mutation

▶ Adverse Effects: *Dogs:* Constipation, bloat, & sedation. Potential for: paralytic ileus, toxic megacolon, pancreatitis, & CNS effects. *Cats:* Use is controversial, may exhibit excitatory behavior.

▶ Dose very carefully in small dogs and cats

Uses/Indications

Loperamide is used as a GI motility modifier in small animals. Some have found that loperamide is useful for treating or helping to reduce chemotherapy-induced (*e.g.*, toceranib) diarrhea in dogs (London 2010), (Vail 2009). Use in cats is controversial and many clinicians do not recommend using in cats.

Pharmacology/Actions

Among their other actions, opiates inhibit GI motility and excessive GI propulsion. They also decrease intestinal secretion induced by cholera toxin, prostaglandin E_2 and diarrheas caused by factors in which calcium is the second messenger (non-cyclic AMP/GMP mediated). Opiates may also enhance mucosal absorption.

Pharmacokinetics

In dogs, loperamide reportedly has a faster onset of action and longer duration of action than diphenoxylate, but clinical studies confirming this appear to be lacking. In humans, loperamide's half-life is about 11 hours. It is unknown if the drug enters milk or crosses the placenta.

Contraindications/Precautions/Warnings

All opiates should be used with caution in patients with hypothyroidism, severe renal insufficiency, adrenocortical insufficiency, (Addison's), and in geriatric or severely debilitated patients.

Opiate antidiarrheals should be used with caution in patients with head injuries or increased intracranial pressure and acute abdominal conditions (*e.g.*, colic), as it may obscure the diagnosis or clinical course of these conditions. It should be used with extreme caution in patients suffering from respiratory disease or from acute respiratory dysfunction (*e.g.*, pulmonary edema secondary to smoke inhalation). Opiate antidiarrheals should be used with extreme caution in patients with hepatic disease with CNS clinical signs of hepatic encephalopathy. Hepatic coma may result.

Many clinicians recommend not using diphenoxylate or loperamide in dogs weighing less than 10 kg, but this is probably a result of the potency of the tablet or capsule forms of the drugs. Dosage titration using the liquid forms of these agents should allow their safe use in dogs when indicated.

Because loperamide is potentially a neurotoxic substrate of P-glycoprotein, it is contraindicated in dogs tested positive for the *ABCB1*-1Δ (MDR1) mutation. Alternative antidiarrheals should be considered in untested dogs of herding breeds (*e.g.*, Collies, Shelties, Australian shepherds, etc.) that may have the gene mutation.

Adverse Effects

In dogs, constipation, bloat, and sedation are the most likely adverse reactions encountered when usual doses are used. Potentially, paralytic ileus, toxic megacolon, pancreatitis, and CNS effects could be seen.

Use of antidiarrheal opiates in cats is controversial; this species may react with excitatory behavior.

Reproductive/Nursing Safety

In humans, the FDA categorizes loperamide as category ***B*** for use during pregnancy (*Animal studies have not yet demonstrated risk to the fetus, but there are no adequate studies in pregnant women; or animal studies have shown an adverse effect, but adequate studies in pregnant women have not demonstrated a risk to the fetus in the first trimester of pregnancy, and there is no evidence of risk in later trimesters.*)

It is not known whether loperamide is excreted in maternal milk. Safety during nursing has not been established.

Overdosage/Acute Toxicity

In dog toxicity studies, doses of 1.25–5 mg/kg/day produced vomiting, depression, severe salivation, and weight loss. Breeds with a defective MDR-1 gene are more sensitive to CNS depression with loperamide than other breeds and have shown signs at 0.06 mg/kg per the APCC database.

There were 376 exposures to loperamide reported to the ASPCA Animal Poison Control Center (APCC) during 2008-2009. In these cases 358 were dogs with 231 showing clinical signs and 14 cats with 1 showing clinical signs. The remaining cases were 4 birds with 1 showing clinical signs. Common findings in dogs recorded in decreasing frequency included diarrhea, vomiting, lethargy, anorexia, weakness, and hypersalivation.

Treatment should follow standard decontamination protocols, although the use of apomorphine for emesis should be avoided since it can have additive CNSA or respiratory depressant effects. Naloxone may be used to treat severe depression; higher than usual doses may be required.

Drug Interactions

The following drug interactions have either been reported or are theoretical in humans or animals receiving loperamide and may be of significance in veterinary patients:

- **AMIODARONE:** By inhibiting P-gp may increase loperamide plasma concentrations
- **CARVEDILOL:** By inhibiting P-gp may increase loperamide plasma concentrations
- **ERYTHROMYCIN:** By inhibiting P-gp may increase loperamide plasma concentrations
- **KETOCONAZOLE, ITRACONAZOLE:** By inhibiting P-gp may increase loperamide plasma concentrations
- **QUINIDINE:** By inhibiting P-gp may increase loperamide plasma concentrations
- **TAMOXIFEN:** By inhibiting P-gp may increase loperamide plasma concentrations
- **VERAPAMIL:** By inhibiting P-gp may increase loperamide plasma concentrations

Laboratory Considerations

- Plasma **amylase** and **lipase** values may be increased for up to 24 hours following administration of opiates.

Doses

- **DOGS:**
  As an antidiarrheal:
  Note: Collies and related breeds (MDR1 mutation) may be overly sensitive to loperamide
  a) 0.08 mg/kg, PO three times daily (DeNovo 1988; Washabau 2004)
  b) 0.1–0.2 mg/kg PO q8–12h (Willard 2003)
  c) 0.1 mg/kg PO three times a day; probably

should not be given longer than 5 days and is potentially contraindicated when diarrhea is suspected to be caused by enteric infections (Hall & Simpson 2000)
  d) As adjunctive treatment for diarrhea associated with chemotherapy: 0.08 mg/kg PO three times daily. (Vail 2009)
  e) 0.08 mg/kg PO 3–4 times a day (Cote 2000)
  f) 0.1–0.2 mg/kg PO q6–12h (Leib 2004)

- **CATS:**
  Note: Use of antidiarrheal opiates in cats is controversial; this species may react with excitatory behavior.
  a) For Diarrhea: Using the suspension 0.04–0.06 mg/kg PO twice daily (Tams 1999)
  b) 0.08–0.16 mg/kg PO q12h (Willard 2003)

- **RABBITS, RODENTS, SMALL MAMMALS:**
  a) **Rabbits:** 0.1 mg/kg in 1 mL of water PO q8h for 3 days, then once daily for 2 days (Ivey & Morrisey 2000)
  b) **Mice, Rats, Gerbils, Hamsters, Guinea pigs, Chinchillas:** 0.1 mg/kg PO q8h for 3 days, then once daily for 2 days; give in 1 mL of water (Adamcak & Otten 2000)

Monitoring

- Clinical efficacy
- Fluid and electrolyte status in severe diarrhea
- CNS effects if using high dosages

Client Information

- If diarrhea persists or if animal appears listless or develops a high fever, contact veterinarian.

Chemistry/Synonyms

A synthetic piperidine-derivative antidiarrheal, loperamide occurs as a white to faintly yellow powder with a pK_a of 8.6 that is soluble in alcohol and slightly soluble in water.

Loperamide may also be known as PJ 185, or R 18553; a common trade name is *Imodium*®.

Storage/Stability

Loperamide capsules or oral solution should be stored at room temperature in well-closed containers. It is recommended that the oral solution not be diluted with other solvents.

Dosage Forms/Regulatory Status

VETERINARY-LABELED PRODUCTS: None

HUMAN-LABELED PRODUCTS:

Loperamide HCl Oral Liquid: 1 mg/5 mL (0.2 mg/mL), & 1 mg/7.5 mL in 60 mL, 90 mL, 118 mL and 120 mL; *Imodium*® *A-D* (McNeil-CPC); generic; (OTC)

Loperamide HCl Capsules and Tablets: 2 mg; *Imodium*® *A-D Caplets* (McNeil-CPC); *Neo-Diaral*® (Roberts); *K-Pek II*® (Rugby); generic; (OTC & Rx)

References

Adamcak, A. & B. Otten (2000). Rodent Therapeutics. Vet Clin NA: Exotic Anim Pract 3:1(Jan): 221–240.

Cote, E. (2000). Over-the-Counter Pharmaceuticals. Textbook of Veterinary Internal Medicine: Diseases of the Dog and Cat. S Ettinger and E Feldman Eds. Philadelphia, WB Saunders. 1: 318–320.

DeNovo, R.C. (1988). Diseases of the Large Bowel. Handbook of Small Animal Practice. RV Morgan Ed. New York, Churchill Livingstone: 421–439.

Hall, E. & K. Simpson (2000). Diseases of the Small Intestine. Textbook of Veterinary Internal Medicine: Diseases of the Dog and Cat. S Ettinger and E Feldman Eds. Philadelphia, WB Saunders. 2: 1182–1238.

Ivey, E. & J. Morrisey (2000). Therapeutics for Rabbits. Vet Clin NA: Exotic Anim Pract 3:1(Jan): 183–216.

Leib, M. (2004). Diagnostic approach to acute diarrhea in dogs. Proceedings: Western Vet Conf. Accessed via: Veterinary Information Network. http://goo.gl/w0Z4q

London, C.A. (2010). Tyrosine Kinase Inhibitor (TKI) Therapy in Companion Animals: Year One. Proceedings: ACVIM. Accessed via: Veterinary Information Network. http://goo.gl/v01GA

Tams, T. (1999). Acute Diarrheal Diseases of the Dog and Cat. Proceedings: The North American Veterinary Conference, Orlando.

Vail, D.M. (2009). Supporting the Veterinary Cancer Patient on Chemotherapy: Neutropenia and Gastrointestinal Toxicity. Topics in Companion Animal Medicine 24(3): 122–129.

Washabau, R. (2004). Canine Diarrheal Disorders: Therapy. Proceedings: ACVC. Accessed via: Veterinary Information Network. http://goo.gl/753DU

Willard, M. (2003). Digestive system disorders. Small Animal Internal Medicine, 3rd Ed. R Nelson and C Couto Eds. St Louis, Mosby: 343–471.

LORAZEPAM

(lor-*ayz*-eh-pam)   Ativan®

BENZODIAZEPINE

Prescriber Highlights

▶ Benzodiazepine that can be useful as an anxiolytic in dogs & cats or as an alternative to diazepam for treating status epilepticus

▶ Can be administered intranasally or IV for status epilepticus

▶ Adverse Effects (most likely): Increased appetite, activity or behavior changes (lethargy/somnolence to hyperexcitability/aggression)

Uses/Indications

Lorazepam may be useful in treating status epilepticus in dogs and the adjunctive treatment of behavior disorders (fears, phobias, anxiety) in dogs and cats. Although, in veterinary medicine, when compared with diazepam, there is much less experience using lorazepam, it has some advantages. Lorazepam is not metabolized by the liver into active metabolites so it can be used more safely in patients with liver dysfunction, obese, or geriatric patients. It appears as effective as diazepam, may have longer anticonvulsant duration of action (not proven in dogs), and can be easier to administer (intranasal, IM, sublingual/buccal).

In human medicine, lorazepam is now frequently used in place of diazepam for treating status epilepticus and anxiolytic indications. It is also used for treating cancer chemotherapy-induced nausea and emesis, alcohol withdrawal, and akathisia secondary to antipsychotic medications.

Pharmacology/Actions

Lorazepam and other benzodiazepines depress the subcortical levels (primarily limbic, thalamic, and hypothalamic) of the CNS thus producing anxiolytic, sedative, skeletal muscle relaxant, and anticonvulsant effects. The exact mechanism of action is unknown, but postulated mechanisms include: antagonism of serotonin, increased release of and/or facilitation of gamma-aminobutyric acid (GABA) activity, and diminished release or turnover of acetylcholine in the CNS. Benzodiazepine specific receptors have been located in the mammalian brain, kidney, liver, lung, and heart. Receptors are lacking in the white matter In all species studied.

Pharmacokinetics

In dogs, intravenous administration of 0.2 mg/kg gave peak levels of about 165 ng/mL and remained above 30 ng/mL (considered necessary for anticonvulsant activity in humans) for 60 minutes. After intranasal administration of 0.2 mg/kg to dogs (Mariani *et al.* 2003), peak levels of about 106 ng/mL were achieved; in 3/6 dogs studied, levels stayed above 30 ng/mL for 60 minutes. Levels reached 30 ng/mL between 3–9 minutes after intranasal administration. While elimination half-life has been reported as approximately 1 hour in dogs, concentrations in the brain may persist longer than in the serum as lorazepam has a high affinity for benzodiazepine receptors in the CNS. Rectal administration of lorazepam in dogs does not appear to yield serum concentrations high enough for efficacious treatment of status epilepticus due to a high first-pass effect. Lorazepam is converted into glucuronide forms in the liver in most species. These metabolites are not active. Primary elimination route is via the urine in dogs. In cats, elimination is approximately 50% in the urine (primarily as the glucuronide) and 50% in the feces.

In humans, absolute bioavailability is about 90% after oral administration and, unlike diazepam, it is relatively rapidly and completely absorbed after IM dosing. Sublingual administration has similar bioavailability as oral dosing, but serum levels peak sooner. Elimination half-life appears to be much longer in humans (12 hours) than in dogs (≈1 hour).

Contraindications/Precautions/Warnings

Lorazepam is contraindicated in patients known to be hypersensitive to benzodiazepines, or with severe respiratory insufficiency unless being mechanically ventilated.

When using for negative behaviors, withdraw

the drug gradually or a rebound effect may occur. Physical dependency has been induced in dogs. If long-term regular usage has occurred, withdraw the drug gradually.

Injectable lorazepam must not be given intraarterially; arteriospasm may occur resulting in necrosis.

Adverse Effects

In small animals, benzodiazepines can cause increased appetite, aggression, increased activity/excitement, and vocalization. With initiation of therapy, dosage increases, or at higher dosages, ataxia, somnolence and lethargy can occur.

Reproductive/Nursing Safety

For humans, lorazepam is designated by the FDA as category *D* for use during pregnancy (*There is evidence of human fetal risk, but the potential benefits from the use of the drug in pregnant women may be acceptable despite its potential risks.*) However, studies in animals generally suggest that the drug is relatively safe for use during pregnancy at usual dosages. Except in one study in mice that were given approximately 400X the human dose producing offspring with an increased rate of cleft palate formation, animal studies have not shown significant increased rates of teratogenicity. If high doses are used just prior to delivery, "floppy infant" syndrome has been seen in humans.

Small amounts of lorazepam are distributed into milk, but it should be safe to use during nursing.

Overdosage/Acute Toxicity

Overdoses of lorazepam are generally limited to CNS depression (confusion, lethargy, somnolence, decreased reflexes, etc.). Very large overdoses can cause ataxia, hypotension, coma, and death (very rare).

Treatment of acute orally-ingested toxicity consists of standard protocols for removing and/or binding the drug in the gut and supportive systemic measures. In patients with normal renal function, forced diuresis with intravenous fluids/electrolytes and mannitol may enhance excretion of lorazepam. The use of analeptic agents (CNS stimulants such as caffeine) is generally not recommended. Flumazenil may be considered for adjunctive treatment of serious overdoses of benzodiazepines, but its use does not replace proper supportive therapy. Flumazenil is not recommended in patients with seizure-disorders as it may induce seizures.

Drug Interactions

The following drug interactions have either been reported or are theoretical in humans or animals receiving lorazepam and may be of significance in veterinary patients:

- ◾ **CNS DEPRESSANTS (e.g., opiates, barbiturates, sedatives, anticonvulsants):** Additive CNS effects
- ◾ **PROBENECID:** Decreased renal clearance of lorazepam

- ◾ **SCOPOLAMINE:** Increased CNS depression, irrational behavior
- ◾ **THEOPHYLLINE:** Decreased sedation from lorazepam
- ◾ **VALPROATE:** Increased lorazepam serum concentration

Laboratory Considerations
- ◾ No specific concerns noted

Doses
- ◾ **DOGS:**

For status epilepticus:
- a) As an alternative to diazepam for status epilepticus: 0.2 mg/kg IV, IM or intranasal once. (Hopper 2006)
- b) Lorazepam 0.2 mg/kg IV once, followed by a bolus IV loading dose of levetiracetam at 60 mg/kg. (Podell 2009)

For behavior indications:
- a) For fears, anxieties, phobias: 0.02–0.1 mg/kg PO once daily to three times a day; may be used on an as needed basis. (Landsberg 2005)
- b) As an anxiolytic: 0.05–0.25 mg/kg PO q12–24h. (Virga 2005)
- c) For fears/anxiety: 0.02–0.5 mg/kg PO q8h. The lowest dose and frequency that alleviate the fear should be used. (Crowell-Davis 2008)
- d) For fears, anxieties, phobias, aversions: 0.02–0.1 mg/kg PO q8-24h; minimally sedating, may require 4 weeks to peak effect. (Sherman & Mills 2008)

- ◾ **CATS:**
- a) For fears/anxiety: 0.03–0.08 mg/kg PO q12h. The lowest dose and frequency that alleviate the fear should be used. (Crowell-Davis 2008)
- b) For fears, anxieties, phobias: 0.125 mg–0.25 mg total dose (¼–½ of a 0.5 mg tablet) once to twice a day; may be used on an as needed basis. (Landsberg 2005)
- c) As an anxiolytic: 0.05–0.25 mg/kg PO q12–24h. (Virga 2005)

Monitoring
- ◾ No specific monitoring is required beyond clinical efficacy and adverse effects

Client Information
- ◾ This medication may increase appetite, diligent food restriction may be required
- ◾ May cause changes in activity levels and can cause either lethargy or increased activity/excitement
- ◾ Do not stop treatment abruptly without veterinarian's guidance; animals receiving this medication on a regular basis for a prolonged period of time may develop withdrawal signs if not "weaned off" the drug
- ◾ Although liver toxicity has not yet been reported in animals receiving this medication,

a drug (diazepam) similar to lorazepam has rarely caused liver toxicity in cats. If vomiting, lack of appetite, or yellowing of the whites of eyes or mucous membranes occur contact veterinarian immediately.

■ Tablets are relatively tasteless and readily disintegrate in saliva. If pilling is difficult, place inside the patient's cheek and follow in a minute or so with a small treat to facilitate swallowing of saliva/medication.

Chemistry/Synonyms

Lorazepam occurs as a white or practically white, practically odorless powder. It is insoluble in water and sparingly soluble in alcohol.

Lorazepam may also be known as BRN-07599084, CB-8133, Ro-7-8408, Wy-4036, lorazapamum, anxiedin, azurogen, bonatranquan, delormetazepam, lorazin, lorazon, lorenin, norlormetazepam, novhepar, novolorazem, o-Chloroxazepam, sinestron, *Ativan®*, and *Lorazepam Intensol®*; many international trade names are available.

Storage/Stability

Lorazepam tablets should be stored in well-closed containers at room temperature (20–25°C). The oral solution and injection should be stored refrigerated (2–8°C) and protected from light.

The injection must be further diluted just prior before to intravenous injection with an equal volume of D5W, normal saline, or sterile water for injection. Do not shake the syringe vigorously, but gently invert repeatedly until the injection is diluted and completely mixed in solution. Do not use if solution is discolored or a precipitate forms. IV injections should be administered slowly, 2 mg over 2–5 minutes.

Although not part of the label information, lorazepam can be further diluted in D5W or NS for IV infusion. When used in this manner, lorazepam injection is most soluble in final concentrations from 0.1–0.2 mg/mL. For example, if using the 2 mg/mL injection, further dilution with 9 mL or 19 mL of D5W or NS would yield a final concentration of 0.2 or 0.1 mg/mL. The injection is very viscous; mix well before use. As precipitation/crystallization can occur, observe the solution before and during the infusion. D5W may be less prone to crystallization formation than is NS. Solutions for infusion mixed in this manner should be used within 12 hours of preparation.

Compatibility/Compounding Considerations

Medications reported to be **compatible** (partial listing):

■ **Syringe:** hydromorphone

■ **Y-Site:** albumin, amikacin, amphotericin B cholesteryl, atracurium, cefotaxime, ciprofloxacin, cisplatin, dexamethasone, diltiazem, dobutamine, doxorubicin, famotidine, fentanyl, gentamicin, heparin, morphine, propofol, ranitidine, and vancomycin

Dosage Forms/Regulatory Status

VETERINARY-LABELED PRODUCTS: None

The ARCI (Racing Commissioners International) has designated this drug as a class 2 substance. See appendix for more information.

HUMAN-LABELED PRODUCTS:

Lorazepam Tablets: 0.5 mg, 1 mg, & 2 mg; generic; (Rx; C-IV)

Lorazepam Concentrated Oral Solution: 2 mg/mL in 10 mL and 30 mL with dropper; *Lorazepam Intensol®* (Roxane); (Rx; C-IV)

Lorazepam Injection: 2 mg/mL & 4 mg/mL in 1 mL prefilled syringes, 1 mL single use vials & 10 mL multidose vials; *Ativan®* (Baxter), generic; (Rx; C-IV)

References

Crowell-Davis, S.L. (2008). Benzodiazepines: Pros and Cons for Fear and Anxiety. Compendium-Continuing Education for Veterinarians 30(10): 526–+.

Hopper, K. (2006). Emergency management of the seizuring patient. Proceedings: Western Veterinary Conf. Accessed via: Veterinary Information Network. http://goo.gl/2tfAN

Landsberg, G. (2005). Fear, anxiety and phobias—Diagnosis and treatment. Proceedings: ACVC 2005. Accessed via: Veterinary Information Network. http://goo.gl/HXM4j

Mariani, C., R. Clemmons, et al. (2003). A comparison of intranasal and intravenous lorazepam in normal dogs. Proceedings: ACVIM 2003. Accessed via: Veterinary Information Network. http://goo.gl/sbt5j

Podell, M. (2009). Status epilepticus: Stopping seizures from home to hospital. Proceedings: IVECCS. http://goo.gl/8bunc

Sherman, B.L. & D.S. Mills (2008). Canine anxieties and phobias: An update on separation anxiety and noise aversions. Veterinary Clinics of North America-Small Animal Practice 38(5): 1081–+.

Virga, V. (2005). Psychopharmacology for anxiety disorders. Proceedings: Western Vet Cong 2005. Accessed via: Veterinary Information Network. http://goo.gl/4uZW3

LUFENURON

(loo-*fen*-yur-on)   Program®, Sentinel®
CHITIN SYNTHESIS INHIBITOR

Prescriber Highlights

▶ Used for flea control in dogs & cats; potentially an antifungal agent

▶ Adverse Effects: None at recommended doses

Uses/Indications

Lufenuron is FDA-approved for use in dogs and cats 6 weeks of age and older for the control of flea populations. The combination product of lufenuron and milbemycin (*Sentinel®*) is indicated for use in puppies and dogs 4 weeks and older for prevention and control flea populations, prevention of heartworm disease, control of adult hookworms, and the removal and control of adult roundworms and whipworms.

In evaluating lufenuron as an ectoparasiticide, advantages include: convenient, can be administered orally, safe environmentally and to patient. Disadvantages: Treated animals must not come into contact with any untreated animal, must be given with food, no repellant activity, does not kill adult fleas of pupae, adult flea must feed on animal to ingest, no activity on ticks, lag period of several weeks to months (often 60-90 days), can be expensive in multi-pet households. One author (Ihrke 2009) recommends lufeneron to be used with spot-ons or with newer oral products for long-term control, not for use as sole therapy unless very closed environment.

Lufeneron has been proposed as a potential treatment or preventative for *E. cuniculi* infections in rabbits, but no studies are available evaluating its use for this indication.

Lufeneron showed initial promise as a treatment for fungal infections, but the early enthusiasm has dampened considerably as efficacy appears doubtful.

Pharmacology/Actions

Lufenuron acts by inhibiting chitin synthesis, polymerization, and deposition in fleas, thereby preventing eggs from developing into adults. It is believed that lufeneron's nonspecific effect on chitin synthesis is related to serine protease inhibition. Lufeneron's mechanism of action, theoretically, would also have effect on fungi.

Lufenuron does not kill adult fleas.

Pharmacokinetics

Approximately 40% of an oral dose is absorbed with the remainder eliminated in the feces. To maximize oral absorption, the manufacturer recommends administering in conjunction with or immediately after (within 30 minutes) a full meal. The drug is absorbed in the small intestine and stored in lipose tissue that acts as depot reservoir to slowly redistribute the drug back into the circulation. While the drug concentrates in the milk of lactating animals, it apparently does not cause ill effects in nursing animals.

After cats receive the injectable product, 2–3 weeks are required before blood levels attain effective concentrations. Cats require a substantially higher oral dosage per kg than do dogs for equivalent efficacy. The drug is apparently not metabolized, but excreted unchanged into the bile and eliminated in the feces.

Contraindications/Precautions/Warnings

The cat labeled injectable product should not be used in dogs; severe local reactions are possible.

Adverse Effects

Adverse effects reported in dogs and cats after oral lufenuron include: vomiting, lethargy/depression, pruritus/urticaria, diarrhea, dyspnea, anorexia, and reddened skin. The manufacturer reports that the adverse reaction rate is less than 5 animals in one million doses.

After receiving the injectable product, a small lump at the injection site has been noted in some cats. A few weeks may be required for this to dissipate.

Reproductive/Nursing Safety

The oral lufenuron products are considered safe to use in pregnant, breeding, or lactating animals; safety of the injectable product in reproducing cats has not been formally established at this time.

Overdosage/Acute Toxicity

Growing puppies were dosed at levels up to 30X for 10 months without overt effect on growth or viability noted. Cats receiving oral dosages of up to 17X apparently were unaffected.

Drug Interactions

Limited data available; the manufacturer states that when used with a variety of adulticides, vaccines, antibiotics, anthelmintics, and steroids no adverse effects or interactions were noted in either dogs or cats.

Doses

* **DOGS:**
  a) For control of flea populations: See the label directions for *Program with Capstar* for using lufenuron with nitenpyram.

     For control of fleas, heartworm prevention, hookworm, ascarid or whipworms: see the label directions for Lufenuron/Milbemycin with Nitenpyram (*Sentinel®* and *Capstar®*—Novartis)

  b) For adjunctive therapy for dermatophytosis: 50–100 mg/kg PO once every 14 days for two treatments, then once a month until at least two negative fungal cultures are obtained (Mantousek 2003)

* **CATS:**
  a) For control of flea populations: See the label directions *Program* and *Program with Capstar* for using lufenuron with or without nitenpyram.

  b) For adjunctive therapy for dermatophytosis: 50–100 mg/kg PO once every 14 days for two treatments, then once a month until at least two negative fungal cultures are obtained. (Mantousek 2003)

* **RABBITS/RODENTS/SMALL MAMMALS:**
  a) **Rabbits:** 30 mg/kg PO every month (Ivey & Morrisey 2000)

Monitoring

* Efficacy

Client Information

* Must be used every 30 days to maximize efficacy.

* All animals in a household should be treated.

* Absorption of the drug is enhanced if given with a fatty meal. If animal vomits within 2 hours after dosing, the drug should be re-dosed. If a dose is missed, re-dose and then resume a monthly dosage regimen (dogs receiving the lufenuron/milbemycin product should be tested in 6 months or more for heartworm exposure with an antigen test).

* Do not split tablets.

Chemistry/Synonyms

A benzoylphenylurea derivative, lufenuron is classified as an insect development inhibitor. The drug is lipophilic.

Lufenuron may also be known as CGA-184699, *Capstar®*, *Program®* and *Sentinel®*.

Storage/Stability

The commercially available tablets and suspension should be stored at room temperature (15–30°C). The manufacturer states that intermittent exposure or exposure less than 48 hours to temperatures outside of storage recommendations for the tablets or suspension should not affect potency. Lufenuron tablets are assigned a 4 year expiration date after manufacture; the suspension 3 years after manufacture; and *Sentinel®* tablets 3 years after manufacture. Opened pouches of the suspension are not recommended for storage or use for the following dosing cycle.

Dosage Forms/Regulatory Status

VETERINARY-LABELED PRODUCTS:

Lufenuron Oral Suspension: in six tube packs; 135 mg (for cats up to 10 lb,—orange), 270 mg (for cats 11–20 lb,—green), cats over 20 lbs are provided the appropriate combination of packs.; *Program® Suspension* (Novartis); (Rx). FDA-approved for use in cats and kittens (6 weeks of age or older).

Lufenuron 6 Month Injectable for Cats: 100 mg/mL in 10 syringe packages: 0.4 mL (40 mg) prefilled syringe (for cats up to 8.8 lb), 0.8 mL (80 mg) prefilled syringe (for cats 8.9–17.6 lb); *Program® 6 Month Injectable* (Novartis); (Rx). FDA-approved for use in cats and kittens 6 weeks of age or older.

Lufenuron Oral Flavor Tabs for Dogs and Cats: For dogs up to 10 lb: 45 mg; For dogs 11 to 20 lb: 90 mg; For dogs 21 to 45 lb: 204.9 mg; For dogs 46 to 90 lb: 409.8 mg; Dogs over 90 lbs receive the appropriate combination of lufeneron tablets; For cats up to 6 lbs. 90 mg; 7–15 lb: 204.9 mg; cats over 15 lb. receive the appropriate combination of lufeneron tablets *Program® Flavor Tabs* (Novartis); (OTC). FDA-approved for use in dogs, puppies, cats, & kittens (4 weeks of age or older).

Lufenuron and Nitenpyram Oral Tablets for Dogs: For dogs up to 10 lb: 45 mg Lufeneron, 11.4 mg nitenpyram; For dogs 11 to 20 lb: 90 mg lufenuron, 11.4 mg nitenpyram; For dogs 21 to 25 lb: 204.9 mg lufenuron, 11.4 mg nitenpyram; For dogs 26 to 45 lb: 204.9 mg lufenuron, 57 mg nitenpyram; For dogs 46 to 90 lb: 409.8 mg lufenuron, 57 mg nitenpyram; Dogs over 90 lbs receive the appropriate combination of Lufeneron tablets and 57 mg nitenpyram tablets; *Program® Flavor Tabs* and *Capstar® Flea Management System for Dogs* (Novartis); (OTC). FDA-approved for use in dogs and puppies (6 weeks of age or older).

Lufenuron and Nitenpyram Oral Tablets for Cats: For cats 2 to 6 lb: 90 mg lufenuron, 11.4 mg nitenpyram; For cats 7 to 15 lb: 204.9 mg lufenuron, 11.4 mg nitenpyram; For cats 16 to 25 lb: appropriate combination of tabs provided lufenuron, 11.4 mg nitenpyram; *Program® Flavor Tabs* (OTC); and *Capstar® Flea Management System for Cats* (Novartis); (OTC)

Milbemycin/Lufenuron Oral Tablets with Nitenpyram Oral Tablets for Dogs: For dogs 2 to 10 lb: 46 mg milbemycin/Lufeneron, 11.4 mg nitenpyram; For dogs 11 to 25 lb: 115 mg milbemycin/lufenuron, 11.4 mg nitenpyram; For dogs 26–50 lb: 230 mg milbemycin/lufenuron, 57 mg nitenpyram; For dogs 51 to 100 lb: 460 mg milbemycin/lufenuron, 57 mg nitenpyram; For dogs100 to125 lb: (appropriate number supplied) milbemycin/lufenuron, 57 mg nitenpyram; *Sentinel® Flavor Tabs with Capstar®* (Novartis); (Rx). FDA-approved for use in dogs and puppies 4 weeks of age or older.

HUMAN-APPROVED PRODUCTS: None

References

Ihrke, P. (2009). Managing flea allergy- Where are we in 2009? Proceedings: WVC. Accessed via: Veterinary Information Network. http://goo.gl/7zZ05

Ivey, E. & J. Morrisey (2000). Therapeutics for Rabbits. Vet Clin NA: Exotic Anim Pract 3:1(Jan): 183–216.

Mantousek, J. (2003). Infectious skin diseases. Handbook of Small Animal Practice 4th ed. R Morgan, R Bright and M Swartout Eds. Philadelphia, Saunders: 842–857.

LYSINE
L-LYSINE

(*lye*-seen)

NUTRITIONAL AMINO ACID

Prescriber Highlights

▶ Amino acid that may be effective in suppressing FHV-1 infections in cats; efficacy in doubt

▶ Adverse effects unlikely if mixed with food

▶ Long-term treatment required

Uses/Indications

Lysine may be effective in suppressing FHV-1 infections in cats. Three recently published studies (Drazenovich *et al.* 2009), (Maggs *et al.* 2007), (Rees & Lubinski 2008) however, have not shown lysine to be effective to prevent or reduce the recurrence of upper respiratory tract infections in shelter cats and in two of these studies, cats receiving lysine supplementation had increases in disease severity and detection of FHV-1 DNA.

Pharmacology/Actions

Lysine is an amino acid that is thought to compete with arginine for incorporation into many herpes viruses. As it is believed that arginine is required for producing infective viral particles, when lysine is incorporated, the virus becomes less infective.

Pharmacokinetics
No specific information was located.

Contraindications/Precautions/Warnings
No specific contraindications.

Adverse Effects
Adverse effects are unlikely when mixed with food. Patients (human) taking lysine have occasionally complained of abdominal pain and diarrhea; one patient developing tubulointerstitial nephritis has been reported.

Reproductive/Nursing Safety
Lysine showed no teratogenic effects when given to pregnant rats, although safety has not been established in other species.

Overdosage/Acute Toxicity
Significant toxicity is unlikely. Gastrointestinal effects (nausea, vomiting, diarrhea) may occur.

Drug Interactions
The following drug interactions have either been reported or are theoretical in humans or animals receiving lysine and may be of significance in veterinary patients:

■ **ARGININE:** Arginine may negate the anti-herpesvirus effects of lysine

■ **CALCIUM, ORAL:** Concomitant use with calcium supplements may increase calcium absorption from the gut and decrease calcium loss in the urine

Laboratory Considerations
■ No specific concerns noted

Doses
■ **CATS:**

To prevent or reduce recurrent feline herpesvirus ocular infections:

a) 500 mg PO twice daily for life (Glaze 2002)

b) 500 mg mixed with food daily (Nasisse 2002)

c) 250 mg PO twice daily (Powell 2002), (August 2007)

As adjunctive therapy for feline herpesvirus dermatologic infections:

a) 250 mg PO twice daily (Griffies 2002)

b) 250 mg PO once to twice daily (Boord 2002)

Monitoring
■ No specific monitoring is required for lysine except those that would be required to monitor the herpes infection in the patient.

Client Information
■ Lysine is easiest to administer by crushing tablets or emptying capsules and then mixing with food.

■ Clients should understand that lysine does not cure the infection, but helps to control

it (reduces the severity and frequency) and that lifetime therapy may be required.

■ When purchasing, avoid products that contain propylene glycol.

Chemistry/Synonyms
An aliphatic amino acid, lysine has the chemical name L-2,6-diaminohexanoic acid and has a molecular weight of 146.2. It may be commercially available as the acetate or hydrochloride salts, or as the base.

Lysine may also be known as: L-lysine, *L-Lysine Powder-Pure®*, *Lys*, *K*, *Enisyl®*, *Incremin®*, and *Viralys®*.

Storage/Stability
Unless otherwise specified on the label, lysine should be stored at room temperature in tight containers.

Dosage Forms/Regulatory Status
VETERINARY-LABELED PRODUCTS:

Note: There are many products containing lysine as one of many ingredients. The following products were located with veterinary labeling where lysine is the sole active ingredient:

L-lysine Gel: 250 mg per 1.25 mL: *Viralys® Gel* (Vet Solutions); (OTC). Labeled for use in cats and kittens.

L-lysine Powder: (in a palatable base) approximately 250 mg per rounded scoop: *Viralys® Powder* (Vet Solutions); (OTC). Labeled for use in cats and kittens.

L-Lysine Powder Feed Additive: in 16 oz. jars and 5 lb. pails; *L-Lysine Powder-Pure®* (AHC); (OTC) Labeled for use in horses.

HUMAN-LABELED PRODUCTS:

L-Lysine Tablets & Capsules: 312 mg, 334 mg, 500 mg & 1000 mg; *Enisyl®* (Person & Covey); generic; (OTC)

Lysine is considered a nutrient in the USA, therefore, it is exempt from FDA approval requirements. There are many products available including tablets and capsules that usually range in strengths from 250 mg to 1000 mg. Combination products are also available.

References
August, J. (2007). Antimicrobial therapy in cats: Meeting the needs of a unique species. Proceedings: Western Vet Conf. Accessed via: Veterinary Information Network. http://goo.gl/sCaFg

Boord, M. (2002). What's new in feline facial dermatitis. Proceedings: Western Veterinary Conference. Accessed via: Veterinary Information Network. http://goo.gl/XUYgL

Drazenovich, T.L., A.J. Fascetti, et al. (2009). Effects of dietary lysine supplementation on upper respiratory and ocular disease and detection of infectious organisms in cats within an animal shelter. American Journal of Veterinary Research 70(11): 1391–1400.

Glaze, M. (2002). Feline Corneal Disease. Proceedings: Atlantic Coast Veterinary Conference. Accessed via: Veterinary Information Network. http://goo.gl/6Piou

Griffies, J. (2002). Viral Dermatitis, Not as rare as you think. Proceedings: Western Veterinary Conference. Accessed via: Veterinary Information Network. http://goo.gl/t40yV

Maggs, D.J., J.E. Sykes, et al. (2007). Effects of dietary lysine supplementation in cats with enzootic upper respiratory disease. Journal of Feline Medicine and Surgery 9(2): 97–108.

Nasisse, M. (2002). Conjunctival and Corneal Diseases of Cats. Proceedings: Tufts 2002. Accessed via: Veterinary Information Network. http://goo.gl/GY3yZ

Powell, C. (2002). Feline Herpesvirus Ocular Disease. Proceedings: Western Veterinary Conference. Accessed via: Veterinary Information Network. http://goo.gl/4PIL9

Rees, T.M. & J.L. Lubinski (2008). Oral supplementation with L-lysine did not prevent upper respiratory infection in a shelter population of cats. Journal of Feline Medicine and Surgery 10(5): 510–513.

Magnesium-containing Laxatives (Magnesium Sulfate; Magnesium Oxide)—see Laxatives, Hyperosmotic

MAGNESIUM HYDROXIDE MAGNESIUM/ ALUMINUM ANTACIDS

(mag-*nee*-zee-um hye-*droks*-ide)

ORAL ANTACID/LAXATIVE

Prescriber Highlights

▶ Used as a gastric antacid for ulcers, etc., but use largely supplanted by newer agents

▶ In ruminants, can be useful to increase rumen pH; powder much more effective than boluses

▶ Magnesium salts contraindicated in patients with renal disease; in cattle, rumen pH should be measured before use

▶ Magnesium salts may cause diarrhea

▶ Chronic use may lead to electrolyte abnormalities

▶ Many potential drug interactions

Uses/Indications

Magnesium hydroxide in combination with aluminum salts have been used in veterinary medicine for the adjunctive treatment of esophagitis, gastric hyperacidity, peptic ulcer and gastritis. In foals and small animals, because of difficulty in administration, the frequent dosing that is often required, and availability of the histamine-2 blocking agents (cimetidine, ranitidine, etc.), proton-pump inhibitors (*e.g.*, omeprazole) and sucralfate, antacids have largely been relegated to adjunctive roles in therapy for these indications.

Magnesium hydroxide alone (milk of magnesia) is sometimes used as an oral laxative in small animals.

In ruminants, magnesium hydroxide is used to increase rumen pH and as a laxative in the treatment of rumen overload syndrome (*aka* acute rumen engorgement, rumen acidosis, grain overload, engorgement toxemia, rumen impaction).

Pharmacology/Actions

Oral antacids used in veterinary medicine are generally relatively non-absorbable salts of aluminum, calcium or magnesium. Up to 20% of an oral dose of magnesium can be absorbed, however. Antacids decrease HCl concentrations in the GI. One gram of these compounds generally neutralizes 20–35 mEq of acid (*in vitro*). Although the pH of the gastric fluid can rarely be brought to near-neutral conditions, at a pH of 3.3, 99% of all gastric acid is neutralized, thereby reducing gastric acid back-diffusion through the gastric mucosa and reducing the amount of acid presented to the duodenum. Pepsin proteolytic activity is reduced by raising the pH and can be minimized if the pH of the gastric contents is increased to >4.

In cattle, orally administered magnesium hydroxide can act as a rumen alkalinizing agent and decrease rumen antimicrobial activity.

Contraindications/Precautions/Warnings

Magnesium-containing antacids are contraindicated in patients with renal disease. Some products have significant quantities of sodium or potassium and should be used cautiously in patients who should have these electrolytes restricted in their diet. Aluminum-containing antacids may inhibit gastric emptying; use cautiously in patients with gastric outlet obstruction.

Oral magnesium hydroxide should only be used clinically in ruminants with documented rumen acidosis and should not be used for treatment of other suspected rumen disorders or hypomagnesemia. (Smith & Correa 2004).

Adverse Effects

In monogastric animals, the most common side effects of antacid therapy are constipation with aluminum- and calcium-containing antacids, and diarrhea or frequent loose stools with magnesium containing antacids. Many products contain both aluminum and magnesium salts in the attempt to balance the constipating and laxative actions of the other.

If the patient is receiving a low phosphate diet, hypophosphatemia can develop if the patient chronically receives aluminum antacids. Magnesium-containing antacids can cause hypermagnesemia in patients with severe renal insufficiency.

In ruminants, alkalinization of the rumen may enhance the absorption of ammonia, histamine or other basic compounds.

Reproductive/Nursing Safety

In a system evaluating the safety of drugs in canine and feline pregnancy (Papich 1989), these drugs are categorized as class: *A* (*Probably safe. Although specific studies may not have proved the safety of all drugs in dogs and cats, there are no reports of adverse effects in laboratory animals or women.*)

Overdosage/Acute Toxicity

See the Adverse Effects section above. If necessary, GI and electrolyte imbalances that can occur with chronic or acute overdose should be treated symptomatically.

Drug Interactions

The following drug interactions have either been reported or are theoretical in humans or animals receiving oral magnesium hydroxide and may be of significance in veterinary patients:

- ■ **QUINIDINE:** Increased absorption or pharmacologic effect may occur

- ■ **SODIUM POLYSTYRENE SULFONATE** (*Kayexalate®*): Antacids may decrease the potassium lowering effectiveness of the drug and in patients in renal failure may cause metabolic alkalosis

- ■ **SUSTAINED- or EXTENDED-RELEASE MEDICATIONS:** When magnesium hydroxide is used at laxative dosages, it may alter the absorption of these drugs by altering GI transit times

- ■ **SYMPATHOMIMETIC AGENTS:** Increased absorption or pharmacologic effect may occur

Oral magnesium salts can **decrease** the amount absorbed or the pharmacologic effect the drugs listed below; separate oral doses of oral magnesium salts and these drugs by two hours to help reduce this interaction.

- ■ **ALLOPURINOL**
- ■ **AZOLE ANTIFUNGALS (Ketoconazole, Itraconazole)**
- ■ **CHLOROQUINE**
- ■ **CORTICOSTEROIDS**
- ■ **DIGOXIN**
- ■ **ETHAMBUTOL**
- ■ **FLUOROQUINOLONES**
- ■ **H-2 ANTAGONISTS (Ranitidine, Famotidine, etc.)**
- ■ **IRON SALTS**
- ■ **ISONIAZID**
- ■ **PENICILLAMINE**
- ■ **PHENOTHIAZINES**
- ■ **TETRACYCLINES**
- ■ **THYROID HORMONES**

Doses

- ■ **DOGS:**

  For adjunctive treatment of hypomagnesemia in dogs with GI disease and severe hypocalcemia:

a) Oral magnesium hydroxide (milk of magnesia) at 5–15 mL/per dog per 24 hours. If giving parenterally: magnesium (magnesium sulfate) at 1 mEq/kg/day. (Marks 2009)

For adjunctive therapy for gastric ulcers:

a) Aluminum hydroxide suspension or aluminum hydroxide/magnesium hydroxide suspension: 2–10 mL PO q2–4h (Hall & Twedt 1989)

As an antacid:

a) Magnesium hydroxide (Milk of Magnesia): 5–30 mL PO once to twice daily (Morgan 1988)

- ■ **CATS:**

  As an antacid:

a) Magnesium hydroxide (Milk of Magnesia): 5–15 mL PO once to twice daily (Morgan 1988)

- ■ **CATTLE:**

  For rumen overload syndrome:

a) For adult animals: Up to 1 gram/kg (MgOH) mixed in 2–3 gallons of warm water and given PO per tube. May repeat (use smaller doses) at 6–12 hour intervals. If the rumen has been evacuated, do not exceed 225 grams initially. Dehydration and systemic acidosis must be concomitantly corrected.

   Calves: As above but use ⅛th–¼th the amount (Wass *et al.* 1986)

- ■ **HORSES:**

  For adjunctive gastroduodenal ulcer therapy in foals:

a) Aluminum/magnesium hydroxide suspension: 15 mL 4 times a day (Clark & Becht 1987)

- ■ **SHEEP & GOATS:**

  For rumen overload syndrome:

a) As above for cattle, but use ⅛th–¼th the amount (Wass *et al.* 1986)

Monitoring

- ■ Monitoring parameters are dependent upon the indication for the product. Patients receiving high dose or chronic therapy should be monitored for electrolyte imbalances outlined above.

Client Information

- ■ Oral magnesium hydroxide products are available without prescription (OTC); do not give on a regular basis without veterinary supervision

Dosage Forms/Regulatory Status

VETERINARY-LABELED PRODUCTS:

Oral Boluses 17.9–27 grams of magnesium hydroxide (**Note:** products may also contain ginger, capsicum and methyl salicylate); *Magnalax®* (Aspen), *Carmilax®* (Pfizer), *Polymag®* (Butler), *Rumen Bolus®* (Durvet), *Instamag®*

(Vedco), *Magnalax®* (Phoenix), *Polyox®II* (Bimeda), *Laxade®* (AgriPharm); (OTC)

Oral Powder, each pound of powder contains: 350–361 grams of magnesium hydroxide (**Note:** products may also contain ginger, capsicum and methyl salicylate); *Carmilax Powder®* (Pfizer), *Magnalax®* (Phoenix), *Polyox®* (Bimeda), *Laxade®* (AgriPharm); (OTC)

Milk of Magnesia (Magnesium Hydroxide) 80 mg/mL in gallons; generic, (Neogen); (OTC)

HUMAN-LABELED PRODUCTS:

The following is a list of some magnesium hydroxide products available, it is not meant to be all-inclusive.

Magnesium Hydroxide

Tablets chewable: 311 mg & 400 mg; *Phillips' Chewable®* (Bayer Consumer); *Pedia-Lax®* (Fleet); (OTC)

Liquid, Oral (also called Milk of Magnesia): 400 mg/5 mL in 129 mL, 355 mL, 360 mL, 780 mL, pt, gal and UD 15 mL & 30 mL; liquid concentrate: 800 mg/5 mL in 240 mL & 1,200 mg/5 mL in 400 mL; generic; (OTC)

Aluminum Hydroxide and Magnesium Hydroxide

Suspension (**NOTE:** There are too many products and concentrations to list in this reference; a representative product is *Maalox® Suspension* (Rorer) which contains 225 mg aluminum hydroxide and 200 mg magnesium hydroxide per 5 mL.

All aluminum and magnesium hydroxide preparations are OTC. Other dosage forms that are available commercially include: tablets, chewable tablets, and aerosol foam suspension.

References

Clark, E.S. & J.L. Becht (1987). Clinical Pharmacology of the Gastrointestinal Tract. Vet Clin North Am (Equine Practice) 3(1): 101–122.

Hall, J.A. & D.C. Twedt (1989). Diseases of the Stomach. Handbook of Small Animal Practice. RV Morgan Ed. New York, Churchill LIvingstone: 371–384.

Marks, S.L. (2009). Diagnosis and management of protein-losing enteropathies. Proceedings: WVC. Accessed via: Veterinary Information Network. http://goo.gl/1gowF

Morgan, R.V., Ed. (1988). Handbook of Small Animal Practice. New York, Churchill Livingstone.

Papich, M. (1989). Effects of drugs on pregnancy. Current Veterinary Therapy X: Small Animal Practice. R Kirk Ed. Philadelphia, Saunders: 1291–1299.

Smith, G.W. & M.T. Correa (2004). The effects of oral magnesium hydroxide administration on rumen fluid in cattle. Journal of Veterinary Internal Medicine 18(1): 109–112.

Wass, W.M., J.R. Thompson, et al. (1986). Diseases of the ruminant forestomach. Current Veterinary Therapy 2: Food Animal Practice. JL Howard Ed. Philadelphia, WB Saunders: 715–723.

MAGNESIUM MAGNESIUM SULFATE, PARENTERAL MAGNESIUM CHLORIDE, PARENTERAL

(mag-*nee*-zee-um)

PARENTERAL ELECTROLYTE

For information on the use of oral magnesium hydroxide, refer to the previous monograph. Magnesium oxide and oral magnesium sulfate are also detailed in the monograph for Saline/Hyperosmotic laxatives.

Prescriber Highlights

▶ Parenteral electrolyte for hypomagnesemia, for adjunctive therapy of malignant hyperthermia in swine, as an anticonvulsant, & for refractory ventricular arrhythmias

▶ Contraindications: Significant myocardial damage or heart block

▶ Caution: Impaired renal function

▶ Adverse Effects: Usually as a result of OD (drowsiness or other CNS depressant effects, muscular weakness, bradycardia, hypotension, respiratory depression, & increased Q-T intervals on ECG). Very high levels: Neuromuscular blocking activity &, eventually, cardiac arrest

▶ Must monitor to avoid hypermagnesemia

▶ Do not confuse mEq/mL & mg/mL concentrations & dosages

Uses/Indications

Parenteral magnesium sulfate is used as a source of magnesium in magnesium deficient states (hypomagnesemia), for adjunctive therapy of malignant hyperthermia in swine, and also as an anticonvulsant. It may be of benefit in the treatment of refractory ventricular fibrillation.

Pharmacology/Actions

Magnesium is used as a cofactor in a variety of enzyme systems and plays a role in muscular excitement and neurochemical transmission.

Pharmacokinetics

IV magnesium results in immediate effects; IM administration may require about 1 hour for effect. Magnesium is about 30–35% bound to proteins and the remainder exists as free ions. It is excreted by the kidneys at a rate proportional to the serum concentration and glomerular filtration.

Contraindications/Precautions/Warnings

Parenteral magnesium is contraindicated in patients with myocardial damage or heart block. Magnesium should be given with caution to patients with impaired renal function. Patients receiving parenteral magnesium should be observed and monitored carefully to avoid hypermagnesemia.

Adverse Effects

Magnesium sulfate (parenteral) adverse effects are generally the result of magnesium overdosage and may include drowsiness or other CNS depressant effects, muscular weakness, bradycardia, hypotension, hypocalcemia, respiratory depression and increased Q-T intervals on ECG. Very high magnesium levels may cause neuromuscular blocking activity and, eventually, cardiac arrest.

When using IV for hypomagnesemia, reduce potassium supplementation or hyperkalemia may result.

Reproductive/Nursing Safety

In humans, the FDA categorizes this drug as category *C* for use during pregnancy (*Animal studies have shown an adverse effect on the fetus, but there are no adequate studies in humans; or there are no animal reproduction studies and no adequate studies in humans.*) The possibility of fetal harm appears remote; however, use only if clearly needed.

Magnesium is excreted in milk, but is unlikely to pose significant risk to nursing offspring.

Overdosage/Acute Toxicity

See Adverse Effects above. Treatment of hypermagnesemia is dependent on the serum magnesium level and any associated clinical effects. Ventilatory support and administration of intravenous calcium [10–50 mg/kg IV; (Macintire 2003)] may be required for severe hypermagnesemia.

Drug Interactions

The following drug interactions have either been reported or are theoretical in humans or animals receiving parenteral magnesium sulfate or HCl and may be of significance in veterinary patients:

- ■ **CALCIUM:** Concurrent use of calcium salts may negate the effects of parenteral magnesium

- ■ **CNS DEPRESSANT DRUGS (e.g., barbiturates, general anesthetics):** Additive CNS depression may occur.

- ■ **DIGOXIN:** Because serious conduction disturbances can occur, parenteral magnesium should be used with extreme caution with digitalis cardioglycosides

- ■ **NEUROMUSCULAR BLOCKING AGENTS:** Excessive neuromuscular blockade possible

Doses

Note: Do not confuse mEq/mL and mg/mL concentrations and dosages; One gram of mag-

nesium sulfate hexahydrate contains 8.1 mEq of magnesium. Magnesium chloride contains 9.25 mEq of magnesium per gram.

■ **DOGS/CATS:**

For hypomagnesemia:

a) Use magnesium sulfate as an IV CRI at 1 mEq/kg/24 hours; often seen in refractory hypokalemic patients (Reiser 2006)

b) For chronic hypomagnesemia (once parenteral repletion has occurred): Using oxide or hydroxide salts, 1–2 mEq/kg/day PO. Diarrhea may occur. (Fascetti 2003)

c) For hypomagnesemia associated with diabetic ketoacidosis in cats: Total magnesium concentrations of less than 1.5 mg/dL should be treated with magnesium sulfate as an IV CRI of 0.5–1 mEq/kg administered over 24 hours. (Waddell 2007)

d) For adjunctive treatment of hypomagnesemia in dogs with GI disease and severe hypocalcemia: Parenterally: magnesium (magnesium sulfate) at 1 mEq/kg/day. Oral treatment: magnesium hydroxide (milk of magnesia) at 5–15 mL/per dog per 24 hours. (Marks 2009)

e) For hypomagnesemia in cats: Mild hypomagnesemia may be treated by administering isotonic replacement crystalloid solutions that contain magnesium (*Plasma-Lyte 148®*). For severe hypomagnesemia (serum magnesium <1.2 mg/dL), an infusion of magnesium sulfate can be made by adding to 5% dextrose in water at an initial dose of 0.75–1 mEq/kg/day CRI for the first 24 hours, then reducing the dose by 50% for the next 3–5 days. (Kerl 2008)

For refractory ventricular arrhythmias:

a) Magnesium sulfate: 30 mg/kg slowly IV (**Note:** This converts to a dose of 0.243 mEq/kg—Plumb) (Macintire 2006)

b) If needed for life-threatening ventricular arrhythmias: 0.15–0.3 mEq/kg may be administered over 5–15 minutes. (Holland & Chastain 1995)

■ **HORSES:**

For hypomagnesemia:

a) Magnesium sulfate and magnesium chloride are the solutions of choice for intravenous administration. For oral treatment, magnesium oxide, magnesium carbonate and magnesium sulfate can be used. For magnesium sulfate, a dose of 100 mg/kg will provide 9.7 mg/kg of Mg^{++} while for magnesium chloride a dose of 100 mg/kg will provide 25.5 mg/kg of Mg^{++}. This is critical as overdosing can be fatal. Excessive oral (nasogastric) supplementation with magnesium sulfate can act as a laxative and induce CNS depression. Recommended IV dose rates for magnesium sulfate in adult horses are 25–150 mg/kg/IV/day diluted in 0.9% NaCl, dextrose or polyionic isotonic solutions. Constant rate infusions (CRI) of magnesium sulfate at 100–150 mg/kg/day should meet the daily requirements of foals and adult horses. Magnesium sulfate is also used to treat ventricular arrhythmias, in particular quinidine intoxication (torsades de pointes), and should be considered in horses with refractory ileus and synchronous diaphragmatic flutter. Doses of 50–100 mg/kg over 30 minutes are considered safe. This is equivalent to 25–50 grams of magnesium sulfate for an adult horse. In foals with ischemic encephalopathy, an initial magnesium sulfate dose of 50 mg/kg in the first hour, followed by a CRI of 25 mg/kg/hr has been proposed. This regime can be continued for several days, adjusting the dose based on serum magnesium concentrations. Oral supplementation with magnesium oxide, magnesium carbonate or magnesium sulfate should be considered in animals with chronic hypomagnesemia, malabsorption, renal disease, and exercise-associated hypomagnesemia. Recommended doses are 30–50 mg/kg/day for magnesium oxide, 60–80 mg/kg/day for magnesium carbonate, or 80–100 mg/kg/day for magnesium sulfate. These doses are safe for horses, particularly when compared to the cathartic doses of magnesium sulfate (0.5–1 gram/kg). (Toribio 2009)

For VTach:

a) 4 mg/kg IV boluses every 2 minutes or a 2 mg/kg/min IV infusion to a total dose of 50 mg/kg (**Note:** Do not use magnesium plus calcium containing solutions) (Mogg 1999)

For adjunctive treatment of perinatal asphyxia syndrome in foals:

a) Magnesium sulfate 50 mg/kg diluted to 1% and given IV over one hour, then decrease to 25 mg/kg/hr as a constant rate infusion for 24 hours (Vaala 2003)

b) As above in "a", but after the first hour: 25 mg/kg/hr CRI for 1–3 days. (Bentz 2006)

■ **RUMINANTS:**

For hypomagnesemia (grass and other magnesium-related tetanies):

a) **Cattle** (presentation was specifically on beef cattle): A typical treatment to an adult cow has been slow intravenous administration (over at least 5 minutes) of 100 mL of the 25% Epsom salt solution, this provides 2.5 grams of magnesium

(0.025 grams of magnesium/mL of solution). This solution is highly hypertonic (2028 mOsm/L). Hypomagnesemia is most commonly treated using commercially available combined calcium, magnesium, and phosphorous solutions, 500 mL of these solutions typically contain 1.6 to 2.7 grams of magnesium in the form of a borogluconate, chloride, or hypophosphite salt (the phosphorous in hypophosphite salt form is unavailable to ruminants and therefore worthless). Combined calcium and magnesium solutions are preferred for intravenous administration to 25% Epsom salt solution because ruminants with hypomagnesemia frequently have hypocalcemia, and hypercalcemia provides some protection against the toxic effects of hypermagnesemia. The maximum safe rate of administration of magnesium in cattle is 0.04 mL of 25% Epsom salt solution/kg body weight/minute. For a 500 kg cow with hypomagnesemia, this corresponds to a maximum safe rate of administration of 20 mL/minute.

Subcutaneous administration can cause necrosis of the skin. Only combined solutions containing calcium and magnesium solutions should be given subcutaneously.

In a seizuring, hypomagnesemic beef cow, rectal administration may be the only safe and practical way to administer magnesium. After evacuating the rectal contents, an enema containing 60 grams of Epsom Salts (magnesium sulfate heptahydrate) or magnesium chloride in 200 mL of water can be placed in the descending colon (NOT the rectum) and the tail held down for 5 minutes; this increases plasma magnesium concentrations within 10 minutes. Enema solutions can be prematurely evacuated, eliminating the chance for therapeutic success, and some degree of colonic mucosal injury is expected because of the high osmolarity of 30% solutions (approximately 2400 mOsm/L). (Constable 2008)

b) **Cattle:** 350 mL (250 mL of 25% calcium borogluconate and 100 mL of 10% of magnesium sulfate) by slow IV. If not a proprietary mixture, give calcium first. Relapses occur frequently after IV therapy, and 350 mL SC of magnesium sulfate 20% may give more sustained magnesium levels. Alternating calcium and magnesium may prevent adverse effects. Continue control measures for 4–7 days to prevent relapse. (Merrall & West 1986)

c) **Sheep and Goats:** 50–100 mL of above solution (calcium/magnesium). (Merrall & West 1986)

For whole milk tetany in calves 2–4 months of age:

a) Magnesium sulfate 10% 100 mL; followed by oral magnesium oxide at daily doses of 1 gram PO (0–5 weeks old), 2 grams PO (5–10 weeks old), and 3 grams PO (10–15 weeks old) (Merrall & West 1986)

■ **SWINE:**

For adjunctive therapy of malignant hyperthermia syndrome:

a) Magnesium sulfate 50%: Incremental doses of 1 gram injected slowly IV until heart rate and muscle tone are reduced. Use calcium if magnesium-related cardiac arrest occurs. (Booth & McDonald 1988)

Monitoring

■ Toxicity, including serum magnesium

■ Physical signs associated with hypomagnesemia

■ Serum calcium, potassium if indicated

Chemistry/Synonyms

Magnesium sulfate occurs as small, usually needle-like, colorless crystals with a cool, saline, bitter taste. It is freely soluble in water and sparingly soluble in alcohol. Magnesium sulfate injection has a pH of 5.5–7. One gram of magnesium sulfate hexahydrate contains 8.1 mEq of magnesium. Magnesium chloride contains 9.25 mEq of magnesium per gram.

Magnesium Sulfate may also be known as: 518, epsom salts, magnesii sulfas, magnesium sulfuricum heptahydricum, magnesium sulphate, sal amarum, sel anglais, and sel de sedlitz; many trade names are available.

Storage/Stability

Magnesium sulfate and magnesium chloride for injection should be stored at room temperature (15–30°C); avoid freezing. Refrigeration may result in precipitation or crystallization.

Compatibility/Compounding Considerations

Magnesium sulfate is reportedly physically **compatible** with the following intravenous solutions: dextrose 5%, LRS, and Normal saline. It is also **compatible** with calcium gluconate, cephalothin sodium, chloramphenicol sodium succinate, cisplatin, hydrocortisone sodium succinate, isoproterenol HCl, methyldopate HCl, metoclopramide HCl (in syringes), norepinephrine bitartrate, penicillin G potassium, potassium phosphate, and verapamil HCl. Additionally, at Y-sites: acyclovir sodium, amikacin sulfate, ampicillin sodium, carbenicillin disodium, cefamandole naftate, cefazolin sodium, cefoperazone sodium, ceforanide, cefotaxime sodium, cefoxitin sodium, cephalothin sodium, cephapirin sodium, clindamycin phosphate, doxycycline phosphate, erythromycin lactobionate, esmolol HCl, gentamicin sulfate, heparin sodium, ka-

namycin sulfate, labetolol HCl, metronidazole (RTU), moxalactam disodium, nafcillin sodium, oxacillin sodium, piperacillin sodium, potassium chloride, tetracycline HCl, ticarcillin disodium, tobramycin sulfate, trimethoprim/sulfamethoxazole, vancomycin HCl, and vitamin B-complex with C.

Magnesium sulfate is reportedly physically **incompatible** when mixed with alkali hydroxides, alkali carbonates, salicylates and many metals, including the following solutions or drugs: fat emulsion 10 %, calcium glucceptate, dobutamine HCl, polymyxin B sulfate, procaine HCl, and sodium bicarbonate. Compatibility is dependent upon factors such as pH, concentration, temperature and diluent used; consult specialized references or a hospital pharmacist for more specific information.

Dosage Forms/Regulatory Status

VETERINARY-LABELED PRODUCTS:

There are no parenteral magnesium-only products FDA-approved for veterinary medicine. There are, however, several proprietary magnesium-containing products available that may also include calcium, phosphorus, potassium, and/or dextrose; refer to the individual product's labeling for specific dosage information. Trade names for these products include: *Norcalciphos®* (Pfizer); *Cal-Dextro® Special*, and *#2* (Fort Dodge); and *CMPK®*; and *Cal-Phos® #2* (TechAmerica). They are legend (Rx) drugs.

HUMAN-LABELED PRODUCTS:

Magnesium Sulfate Injection, Solution in 5% Dextrose: 1% (10 mg/mL; 0.081 mEq/mL) in single-dose containers; 2% (20 mg/mL; 0.162 mEq/mL) in 500 mL & 1,000 mL single-dose containers; generic; (Rx)

Magnesium Sulfate Injection, solution: 4% (40 mg/mL; 0.325 mEq/mL) in 50 mL, 100 mL, 500 mL & 1,000 mL; 8% (80 mg/mL; 0.65 mEq/mL) in 50 mL; 50% (500 mg/mL; 4 mEq/mL) in 2 mL, 10 mL, 20 mL & 50 mL vials; generic; (Rx)

Magnesium Chloride Injection: 20% (200 mg/mL; 1.97 mEq/mL) in 50 mL multidose vials; generic; (Rx)

There are many oral magnesium products in various dosage forms available.

References

Bentz, B. (2006). Current management practices for critically ill foals. Proceedings: ABVP. Accessed via: Veterinary Information Network. http://goo.gl/wFEGR

Booth, N.H. & L.E. McDonald, Eds. (1988). *Veterinary Pharmacology and Therapeutics*. Ames, Iowa State University Press.

Constable, P.D. (2008). Metabolic Disease of Beef Cattle: Diagnosis, Treatment, & Prevention. Western Veterinary Conference. Accessed via: Veterinary Information Network. http://goo.gl/vmVKl

Fascetti, A. (2003). Magnesium: pathophysiological, clinical and therapeutic aspects. Proceedings: ACVIM

Forum. Accessed via: Veterinary Information Network. http://goo.gl/9YLJ7

Holland, M. & C. Chastain (1995). Uses & misuses of aspirin. *Kirk's Current Veterinary Therapy:XII*. J Bonagura Ed. Philadelphia, W.B. Saunders: 70–73.

Kerl, M. (2008). Electrolyte Imbalances in the Cat. Proceedings: IVECCS. Accessed via: Veterinary Information Network. http://goo.gl/S3RxI

Macintire, D. (2003). Metabolic derangements in critical patients. Proceedings: ACVIM Forum. Accessed via: Veterinary Information Network. http://goo.gl/LPqrD

Macintire, D. (2006). Cardiac Emergencies. Proceedings: ACVC 2006. Accessed via: Veterinary Information Network. http://goo.gl/KxqeK

Marks, S.L. (2009). Diagnosis and management of protein-losing enteropathies. Proceedings: WVC. Accessed via: Veterinary Information Network. http://goo.gl/1gowF

Merrall, M. & D.M. West (1986). Rumiant hypomagnesemic tetanies. *Current Veterinary Therapy: Food Animal Practice 2*. JL Howard Ed. Philadelphia, W.B. Saunders: 328–332.

Mogg, T. (1999). Equine Cardiac Disease: Clinical pharmacology and therapeutics. *The Veterinary Clinics of North America: Equine Practice* **15**:3(December).

Reiser, T. (2006). Challenging electrolyte disturbances. Proceedings: ACVIM. Accessed via: Veterinary Information Network. http://goo.gl/qm0tH

Toribio, R. (2009). Disorders of the Equine Calcium & Magnesium Metabolism. Proceedings: ACVIM. Accessed via: Veterinary Information Network. http://goo.gl/eaEne

Vaala, W. (2003). Perinatal asphyxia syndrome in foals. *Current Therapy in Equine Medicine 5*. N Robinson and E Carr Eds. Phila., Saunders: 644–649.

Waddell, L. (2007). Diabetic ketoacidosis in cats. Proceedings: Western Vet Conference. Accessed via: Veterinary Information Network. http://goo.gl/YKWAL

MANNITOL

(man-i-tole)

OSMOTIC DIURETIC

Prescriber Highlights

▶ Osmotic diuretic used for acute oliguric renal failure, to reduce intraocular & intracerebral pressures, to enhance urinary excretion of some toxins &, with other diuretics, to rapidly reduce edema or ascites (caution)

▶ Contraindications: Anuria secondary to renal disease, severe dehydration, severe pulmonary congestion, or pulmonary edema

▶ Halt treatment if progressive heart failure, pulmonary congestion, or progressive renal failure/damage develop

▶ Adverse Effects: Fluid & electrolyte imbalances, GI (nausea, vomiting), cardiovascular (pulmonary edema, CHF, tachycardia), & CNS effects (dizziness, headache, etc.)

▶ Adequate urine output, fluid, & electrolyte monitoring & treatment mandatory

▶ Be certain crystals are dissolved in solution before administering; in-line IV filter (5 micron) is recommended

Uses/Indications

Mannitol is used to promote diuresis in acute oliguric renal failure, reduce intraocular and intracerebral pressures, enhance urinary excretion of some toxins, (*e.g.*, aspirin, some barbiturates, bromides, ethylene glycol) and, in conjunction with other diuretics, to rapidly reduce edema or ascites when appropriate (see Contraindications-Precautions below). In humans, it is also used as an irrigating solution during transurethral prostatic resections.

Pharmacology/Actions

After intravenous administration, mannitol is freely filtered at the glomerulus and poorly reabsorbed in the tubule. The increased osmotic pressure prevents water from being reabsorbed at the tubule. To be effective, there must be sufficient renal blood flow and filtration for mannitol to reach the tubules. Although water is proportionately excreted at a higher rate, sodium, other electrolytes, uric acid, and urea excretions are also enhanced.

Mannitol may have a nephro-protective effect by preventing the concentration of nephrotoxins from accumulating in the tubular fluid. Additionally, it may minimize renal tubular swelling via its osmotic properties, increase renal blood flow and glomerular filtration by causing renal arteriole dilatation, decreased vascular resistance, and decreased blood viscosity.

Mannitol does not appreciably enter the eye or the CNS, but can decrease intraocular and CSF pressure through its osmotic effects. Rebound increases in CSF pressures may occur after the drug is discontinued. Mannitol can reduce intracranial pressure for 2-5 hours and intraocular pressure is reduced usually for 4-12 hours.

Pharmacokinetics

Although long believed to be unabsorbed from the GI, up to 17% of an oral dose is excreted unchanged in the urine after oral dosing in humans. After intravenous dosing, mannitol is distributed to the extracellular compartment and does not penetrate the eye. Unless the patient has received very high doses, is acidotic, or there is loss of integrity of the blood-brain barrier, it does not cross into the CNS.

Only 7–10% of mannitol is metabolized, the remainder is excreted unchanged in the urine. The elimination half-life of mannitol is approximately 100 minutes in adult humans. Half-lives in cattle and sheep are reported to be between 40–60 minutes.

Contraindications/Precautions/Warnings

Mannitol is contraindicated in patients with anuria secondary to renal disease, severe dehydration, severe pulmonary congestion or pulmonary edema. In humans, mannitol is labeled as contraindicated in patients with intracranial bleeding (unless during craniotomy), but there does not appear to be any clinical evidence to support this contraindication.

Use mannitol with caution when treating ethylene glycol toxicity or other hyperosmolar states as it can add to intravascular hyperosmolarity.

When using for increased CSF pressure, an intact capillary membrane is required for efficacy. If this membrane is disrupted, mannitol can leak into the brain interstitium and increase cerebral edema.

It has been reported that manitol caused harmful effects when used in a feline model of acute spinal cord trauma.

Mannitol therapy should be stopped if progressive heart failure, pulmonary congestion, progressive renal failure or damage (including increasing oliguria and azotemia) develops after mannitol therapy is instituted.

Use with caution in hypovolemic patients as mannitol can enhance hypotension. Hypertonic saline may be a better choice to treat increased CSF pressure and increase intravascular volume in these patients.

Mannitol is relatively contraindicated for treating secondary glaucomas, as it may cross the damaged "blood-aqueous barrier" and increase intraocular pressure (IOP).

Do not administer more than a test dose of mannitol until determining whether the patient has some renal function and urine output. Adequate fluid replacement must be administered to dehydrated animals before mannitol therapy is begun. Do not give mannitol with whole blood products, unless at least 20 mEq/L of sodium chloride is added to the solution or pseudo-agglutination may result.

Be certain any crystals in solution are redissolved before administering; an in-line IV filter (5 micron) is also recommended.

Adverse Effects

Fluid and electrolyte imbalances are the most severe adverse effects generally encountered during mannitol therapy. Mannitol can promote hypernatremia. Adequate monitoring and support are imperative.

When used for oliguric renal failure, the potential exists for volume overload should oliguria persist.

Other adverse effects that may be encountered include GI (nausea, vomiting), cardiovascular (pulmonary edema, CHF, tachycardia), and CNS effects (dizziness, headache, etc.).

Reproductive/Nursing Safety

In humans, the FDA categorizes this drug as category *C* for use during pregnancy (*Animal studies have shown an adverse effect on the fetus, but there are no adequate studies in humans; or there are no animal reproduction studies and no adequate studies in humans.*)

It is not known whether this drug is excreted in milk, but it is unlikely that it would pose significant risk to nursing offspring.

Overdosage/Acute Toxicity

Inadvertent overdosage can cause excessive excretion of sodium, potassium, and chloride. If urine output is inadequate, water intoxication or pulmonary edema may occur. Treat by halting mannitol administration and monitoring and correcting electrolyte and fluid imbalances. Hemodialysis is effective in clearing mannitol.

Drug Interactions

The following drug interactions have either been reported or are theoretical in humans or animals receiving mannitol and may be of significance in veterinary patients:

- **LITHIUM:** Mannitol can increase the renal elimination of lithium
- **SOTALOL:** Mannitol's effects on potassium and magnesium may increase the risk for QT prolongation

Laboratory Considerations

- Mannitol can interfere with **blood inorganic phosphorus** concentrations and **blood ethylene glycol** determinations.

Doses

- **DOGS/CATS:**

  For treatment of oliguric renal failure:

  a) After correcting fluid, electrolyte, acid/base balance and determining that the patient is not anuric: Mannitol (20–25% solution) 0.25–0.5 gram/kg IV over 5–10 minutes. If substantial diuresis occurs, may repeat q4–6 hours or administered as a constant infusion (8–10% solution) for first 12–24 hours of therapy. Mannitol has at least three theoretical advantages over furosemide: **1)** it may enhance renal function by minimizing renal tubular cell swelling via its osmotic properties, **2)** mannitol exerts its diuretic effects along the entire nephron and therefore may directly affect the proximal tubule, and **3)** mannitol may expand the extracellular fluid volume. The major disadvantage of mannitol is the potential for vascular overload if oliguria persists. Therefore, mannitol should be avoided in over hydrated oliguric patients. (Polzin 2005; Polzin 2009)

  b) After rehydration, but not fluid overloaded give mannitol at 0.25–0.5 gram/kg IV slowly over 5–10 minutes; repeat dose at 30–40 minute intervals up to 1.5 gram/kg total. Author prefers using furosemide for ARF. (Bersenas 2007)

  c) In fluid replete animals: 0.5 gram/kg IV over 20–30 minutes; if significant diuresis is accomplished within 30 minutes, may administer as a CRI of 60–120 mg/kg/hr IV or as intermittent boluses repeated every 4–6 hours. Mannitol is contraindicated in patients who are still dehydrated, hypervolemic, or anuric. (Waddell 2007)

d) Mannitol (10-25%) is given to fluid replete animals as an initial slow bolus of
0.5 gram/kg IV over 20-30 minutes to
promote diuresis. If significant diuresis is
accomplished within 30 minutes, mannitol can then be started as a constant rate
infusion (CRI) at 60-120 mg/kg/hour IV
or as intermittent repeated boluses every
4-6 hours (as above). Mannitol is contraindicated in patients who are hypervolemic or have evidence of cardiac failure
or pulmonary edema. Fluid balances
must be carefully monitored to prevent
dehydration and further renal compromise. (Silverstein 2009)

For adjunctive treatment of acute glaucoma:

a) Drug of first choice in the acute patient;
0.5-1 gram/kg IV given over 15-20 minutes; withhold water for 3-4 hours. IOP
reduction begins in 20-30 minutes and
has a 4-6 hour duration of effect. Efficacy
reduced in patients with anterior uveitis.
(Wilkie 2002)

b) If latanoprost (*Xalatan*®) has not affected
pupil size and started to reduce IOP after one hour, give mannitol (20%) at
1-2 grams/kg IV over a period of 20 minutes and withhold water for 1-2 hours.
Peak effect is about 90 minutes after administration. (Millichamp 2006)

c) Greatest value is in acute primary angle-
closure glaucoma and pre-op in lens
luxations. Give 1 gram/kg of mannitol
20% for injection IV over 20 min. May
repeat in 4 hours if needed but chronic
use is not advised. Should heat/filter
(5 micron filters) to avoid giving crystals IV. Withhold water for several hours
post-dose. Mannitol can lower IOP from
60-80 mm Hg to normal in 1-2 hours and
keep IOP low for 12-24 hrs. Toxicity limits its use to eyes that have vision or the
potential for vision. Side effects include
headache, osmotic diuresis and worsening of dehydration, renal failure, or cardiovascular disease. Fatalities may occur
with IV crystals and from pulmonary
edema if given with methoxyflurane.
Use with caution in uveitis or hyphema.
(Miller 2009)

For adjunctive treatment of increased CSF
pressure/cerebral edema:

a) 0.5-1.5 grams/kg IV over 10-20 minutes.
Maximum effect occurs 10-20 minutes
after administration and the effects last
for 2-5 hours. May repeat every 6-8
hours based on clinical response and
intracranial pressure monitoring. Do
not use if patient hypovolemic. Monitor serum osmolality and electrolytes.
(McDonnell 2004)

b) Mannitol should be administered as a
bolus over a 15-minute period, rather
than as an infusion in order to obtain
the plasma expanding effect; its effect on
decreasing brain edema takes approximately 15-30 minutes to establish and
lasts between 2-5 hours. Administering
doses of 0.25 gram/kg appear equally effective in lowering ICP as doses as large as
1 gram/kg, but may last a shorter time.
Repeated administration of mannitol can
cause an accompanying diuresis, which
may result in volume contraction, intracellular dehydration and the concomitant
risk of hypotension and ischemia. It is
therefore recommended that mannitol
use be reserved for the critical patient
(Glasgow coma score of < 8) or for the
deteriorating patient. (Platt 2008)

c) 0.5-1.5 grams/kg intravenously over
10-20 minutes. Serum osmolality and
electrolytes should be monitored with
repeated mannitol use; osmolality should
be maintained at or below 320 mOsm/L
(to reduce the risk of renal failure due
to renal vasoconstriction) and electrolytes should be kept within normal
limits. Although monitoring measured
(not calculated) osmolality and osmolal
gap (the difference between measured
and calculated osmolality) and avoiding
large changes in either is recommended,
a recent retrospective study of 95 human
patients with head trauma showed that
neither was correlated with the development of acute renal insufficiency. A useful
guideline to prevent possible unwanted
side effects of mannitol use is to limit
administration of mannitol to three boluses in a 24-hr period. However, due to
the conflicting evidence in the literature
regarding the potential for patients to develop renal failure secondary to mannitol
infusion, the authors recommend that
mannitol be aggressively administered to
patients with progressive neurologic signs
that are responding to it. Since mannitol
tends to crystallize at room temperature,
it should be warmed to approximately
37°C (99°F) and administered through
an in-line filter. (Dewey 2008)

d) Secondary to trauma: 0.5-1 gram/kg IV
followed 20 minutes later by furosemide
(1 mg/kg IV). Potential risk for worsening intracranial hemorrhage, but patients
that are dying before your eyes can benefit from this aggressive therapy. (Mazzaferro 2007)

■ **CATTLE, SWINE, SHEEP, GOATS:**
For adjunctive treatment of cerebral edema:

a) 1-3 gram/kg IV (usually with steroids
and/or DMSO) (Dill 1986)

As a diuretic for oliguric renal failure:

a) 1–2 gram/kg (5–10mL of 20% solution) IV after rehydration; monitor urine flow and fluid balance (Osweiler 1986)

■ **HORSES:**

a) 0.25–2 gram/kg as a 20% solution by slow IV infusion (Schultz 1986)

b) For increased intracranial pressure from traumatic brain injury (TBI): Intermittent IV bolus doses of 0.25–1 gram/kg. Mannitol produces immediate reduction of ICP by decreasing hematocrit and viscosity, improving CBF, and decreasing blood vessel diameter. Cerebral oxygenation improves because of improved red cell oxygen transport. These effects are best accomplished with rapid bolus administration rather than continuous administration. The patient must be monitored to avoid hypovolemia and hypotension. Risks of mannitol therapy are the development of acute renal failure, rebound cerebral edema, and blood brain barrier disruption with repeated or high dosages. The efficacy of mannitol wanes with repeated administration. In humans, mannitol is avoided if serum osmolality is >320 mOsm/L to prevent the risk of acute renal failure. (Aleman 2007)

Monitoring

■ Serum electrolytes (especially sodium), osmolality

■ BUN, serum creatinine

■ Urine output

■ Central venous pressure, if possible

■ Lung auscultation

Client Information

■ Mannitol should be administered by professional staff in a setting where adequate monitoring can occur.

Chemistry/Synonyms

An osmotic diuretic, mannitol occurs as an odorless, sweet-tasting, white, crystalline powder with a melting range of 165°–168° and a pK_a of 3.4. One gram is soluble in about 5.5 mL of water (at 25°C); it is very slightly soluble in alcohol. The commercially available injectable products have approximate pH's of 4.5–7.

Mannitol may also be known as: cordycepic acid, E421, manita, manitol, manna sugar, mannite, mannitolum, Eufusol M 20, *Am-Vet® Mannitol Injection 20%, Isotol®, Manicol®, Manniject®, Maniton®, Mannistol®, Mannit-Losung®, Mannite®, Mede-Prep®, Osmofundin 15% N®, Osmofundin 20%, Osmofundina®, Osmofundina® Concentrada, Osmorol®, Osmosteril® 20%, Resectisol®* and *Thomaemannit®*.

Storage/Stability

Mannitol solutions are recommended to be stored at room temperature; avoid freezing.

Crystallization may occur at low temperatures in concentrations greater than 15%. Resolubolization of the crystals can be accomplished by heating the bottle in hot (up to 80°C) water. Cool to body temperature before administering. An in-line IV filter is recommended when administering concentrated mannitol solutions. Alternatively, heated storage chambers (35°–50°C) have been suggested to assure that soluble product is available at all times. Microwaving glass ampules/vials has been suggested, but explosions have been documented and this procedure cannot be recommended. Supersaturated solutions of mannitol in PVC bags may show a white flocculent precipitate that will tend to reoccur even after heating.

Compatibility/Compounding Considerations

Drugs reported to be physically **compatible** with mannitol include: amikacin sulfate, bretylium tosylate, cefamandole naftate, cefoxitin sodium, cimetidine HCl, dopamine HCl, gentamicin sulfate, metoclopramide HCl, netilmicin sulfate, tobramycin sulfate, and verapamil HCl.

Mannitol should NOT be added to whole blood products to be used for transfusion. Sodium or potassium chloride can cause mannitol to precipitate out of solution when mannitol concentrations are 20% or greater. Mannitol may be physically **incompatible** when mixed with strongly acidic or alkaline solutions.

Mannitol is reportedly stable when mixed with cisplatin for a short period of time, but advanced premixing of the drugs should be avoided because a complex may form between them.

Dosage Forms/Regulatory Status

VETERINARY-LABELED PRODUCTS:

There are no FDA-approved products listed in the "Green Book" (on date of review: 09/2010). Unapproved, veterinary-labeled products may be available.

HUMAN-LABELED PRODUCTS:

Mannitol for Injection

Mannitol Injection: 5% (50 mg/mL; 275 mOsm/L) in 1000 mL;

10% (100 mg/mL; 550 mOsm/L) in 500 mL and 1000 mL;

15% (150 mg/mL; 825 mOsm/L) in 500 mL;

20% (200 mg/mL; 1100 mOsm/L) in 250 mL and 500 mL;

25% (250 mg/mL; 1375 mOsm/L) in 50 mL vials and syringes (12.5 grams/vial); generic; (Rx)

Mannitol Solution: 5 grams/100 mL in distilled water (275 mOsm/L) in 2000 mL; generic; (Rx)

References

Aleman, M. (2007). Pharmacotherapy for neurologic disorders. Proceedings: IVECCS. Accessed via: Veterinary Information Network. http://goo.gl/I8kGM

Bersenas, A. (2007). Renal failure and peritoneal dialysis. Proceedings: Western Vet Conf. Accessed via: Veterinary Information Network. http://goo.gl/j4nE3

Dewey, C.W. (2008). CNS Trauma: The First 48 Hours.

Proceedings: IVECCS. Accessed via: Veterinary Information Network. http://goo.gl/LKyC2

Dill, S.G. (1986). Polioencephalomalacia in Ruminants. Current Veterinary Therapy: Food Animal Practice 2. JL Howard Ed. Philadelphia, W.B. Saunders: 868–869.

Mazzaferro, E. (2007). Triage and approach to trauma. Proceedings: Western Vet Conf. Accessed via: Veterinary Information Network. http://goo.gl/f72CT

McDonnell, J. (2004). Head trauma pathophysiology and treatment. Proceedings: ACVIM Forum. Accessed via: Veterinary Information Network. http://goo.gl/SBWYl

Miller, P. (2009). Ophthalmic Drugs: Keepers and Losers. Proceedings: WVC. Accessed via: Veterinary Information Network. http://goo.gl/JI79J

Millichamp, N. (2006). Glaucoma: The worst ocular disease? Proceedings: IVECCS. Accessed via: Veterinary Information Network. http://goo.gl/cMnwT

Osweiler, G.D. (1986). Nephrotoxic Plants. Current Veterinary Therapy: Food Animal Practice 2. JL Howard Ed. Philadelphia, W.B. Saunders: 401–404.

Platt, S.R. (2008). Assessment & Management of Head Trauma. Proceedings: ACVIM. Accessed via: Veterinary Information Network. http://goo.gl/xZsQv

Polzin, D. (2005). Managing the acute uremic crisis. Proceedings: ACVC. Accessed via: Veterinary Information Network. http://goo.gl/iav1L

Polzin, D. (2009). How I treat uremic crisis in dogs and cats with chronic kidney disease. Proceedings: WSAVA. Accessed via: Veterinary Information Network. http://goo.gl/xtcpx

Schultz, C.S. (1986). Formulary, Veterinary Hospital Pharmacy, Washington State University. Pullman, Washington, Washington State University Press.

Silverstein, D. (2009). Diagnosis and management of acute renal failure. Proceedings: Western Veterinary Conf. Accessed via: Veterinary Information Network. http://goo.gl/Wgq77

Waddell, L. (2007). Acute renal failure. Proceedings: Western Vet Conference. Accessed via: Veterinary Information Network. http://goo.gl/RlcNc

Wilkie, D. (2002). Glaucoma. Proc: Western Veterinary Conference.

MARBOFLOXACIN

(mar-boe-*flox*-a-sin)   Zeniquin®

FLUOROQUINOLONE ANTIBIOTIC

Prescriber Highlights

▶ Veterinary oral fluoroquinolone antibiotic effective against a variety of pathogens

▶ Not effective against anaerobes

▶ Contraindications: Hypersensitivity to fluoroquinolones; Relatively contraindicated for young, growing animals due to cartilage abnormalities

▶ Caution: Hepatic or renal insufficiency, seizure patients, or dehydration

▶ Adverse Effects: GI distress; does not appear to cause ocular toxicity in cats

▶ Drug interactions

Uses/Indications

Marbofloxacin is labeled for the treatment of susceptible bacterial infections in dogs and cats.

Pharmacology/Actions

Marbofloxacin is a bactericidal agent. The bactericidal activity of marbofloxacin is concentration dependent, with susceptible bacteria cell death occurring within 20–30 minutes of exposure. Like other fluoroquinolones, marbofloxacin has demonstrated a significant post-antibiotic effect for both gram − and + bacteria and is active in both stationary and growth phases of bacterial replication.

Its mechanism of action is not thoroughly understood, but it is believed to act by inhibiting bacterial DNA-gyrase (a type-II topoisomerase), preventing DNA supercoiling and DNA synthesis.

Marbofloxacin has a similar spectrum of activity as the other veterinary commercially available agents. These agents have good activity against many gram-negative bacilli and cocci, including most species and strains of *Pseudomonas aeruginosa, Klebsiella* spp., *E. coli,* Enterobacter, Campylobacter, Shigella, Salmonella, Aeromonas, Haemophilus, Proteus, Yersinia, Serratia, and Vibrio species. Other organisms that are generally susceptible include *Brucella* spp., *Chlamydia trachomatis,* Staphylococci (including penicillinase-producing and methicillin-resistant strains), Mycoplasma, and *Mycobacterium* spp. (not the etiologic agent for Johne's Disease).

The fluoroquinolones have variable activity against most streptococci and are not usually recommended to use for these infections. These drugs have weak activity against most anaerobes and are ineffective in treating anaerobic infections.

Resistance does occur by mutation, particularly with *Pseudomonas aeruginosa, Klebsiella pneumonia,* Acinetobacter, and Enterococci, but plasmid-mediated resistance is thought to occur only rarely.

Pharmacokinetics

In dogs, marbofloxacin is characterized as being rapidly absorbed after oral administration with a bioavailability of 94%. Peak plasma levels occur in about 1.5 hours. Protein binding is low and the apparent volume of distribution is 1.2–1.9 L/kg. Elimination half-life averages 9–12 hours. The drug is eliminated unchanged in the urine (40%) and bile/feces. Only about 15% of a dose is metabolized in the liver.

In cats, absorption after oral dosing is nearly complete and peak serum levels occur about 1–2 hours post-dose. Terminal elimination half-life is about 13 hours.

Renal impairment does not significantly alter dosing requirements.

Contraindications/Precautions/Warnings

Like other quinolones, marbofloxacin is labeled as contraindicated in small and medium breed dogs up to 8 months of age, large breeds to 12 months old, and giant breeds to 18 months old. It is also labeled as contraindicated in cats under 12 months of age. Quinolones are also contraindicated in patients hypersensitive to them.

Marbofloxacin can (rarely) cause CNS stimulation and should be used with caution in patients with seizure disorders.

The FDA has prohibited the use of this drug in food-producing animals.

Adverse Effects

With the exception of potential cartilage abnormalities in young animals (see Contraindications above), the adverse effect profile of marbofloxacin is usually limited to GI distress (vomiting, anorexia, soft stools, diarrhea) and decreased activity.

Other fluoroquinolones have, in rare incidences, caused elevated hepatic enzymes, ataxia, seizures, depression, lethargy, and nervousness in dogs. Hypersensitivity reactions or crystalluria could potentially occur.

It is not known if marbofloxacin can also cause the ocular toxicity that has been reported with high dose enrofloxacin in cats. While unlikely, FDA's Adverse Drug Reaction database has received 14 reports (as of July 3, 2007) of blindness associated with marbofloxacin. Causal effect cannot be proven, but use higher dosages carefully.

Reproductive/Nursing Safety

Safety of marbofloxacin during pregnancy has not been established.

Overdosage/Acute Toxicity

It is unlikely an acute overdose of marbofloxacin would result in signs more serious than either anorexia or vomiting, but the adverse effects noted above could occur. Dogs receiving 55 mg/kg per day for 12 days developed anorexia, vomiting, dehydration, tremors, red skin, facial swelling, lethargy, and weight loss.

Drug Interactions

The following drug interactions have either been reported or are theoretical in humans or animals receiving marbofloxacin or related fluoroquinolones and may be of significance in veterinary patients:

- **ANTACIDS/DAIRY PRODUCTS:** Containing cations (Mg^{++}, Al^{+++}, Ca^{++}) may bind to marbofloxacin and prevent its absorption; separate doses of these products by at least 2 hours

- **ANTIBIOTICS, OTHER (aminoglycosides, 3rd-generation cephalosporins, penicillins—extended-spectrum):** Synergism may occur, but is not predictable, against some bacteria (particularly *Pseudomonas aeruginosa*) with these compounds. Although marbofloxacin has minimal activity against anaerobes, *in vitro* synergy has been reported when used with **clindamycin** against strains of Peptostreptococcus, Lactobacillus and *Bacteroides fragilis*.

- **CYCLOSPORINE:** Fluoroquinolones may exacerbate the nephrotoxicity and reduce the metabolism of cyclosporine (used systemically)

- **FLUNIXIN:** Has been shown in dogs to increase the AUC and elimination half-life of enrofloxacin and enrofloxacin increases the AUC and elimination half-life of flunixin; it is unknown if marbofloxacin also causes this effect or if other NSAIDs interact with marbofloxacin in dogs

- **GLYBURIDE:** Severe hypoglycemia possible

- **IRON, ZINC (oral):** Decreased marbofloxacin absorption; separate doses by at least two hours

- **METHOTREXATE:** Increased MTX levels possible with resultant toxicity

- **NITROFURANTOIN:** May antagonize the antimicrobial activity of the fluoroquinolones and their concomitant use is not recommended

- **PHENYTOIN:** Marbofloxacin may alter phenytoin levels

- **PROBENECID:** Blocks tubular secretion of ciprofloxacin and may also increase the blood level and half-life of marbofloxacin

- **QUINIDINE:** Increased risk for cardiotoxicity

- **SUCRALFATE:** May inhibit absorption of marbofloxacin; separate doses of these drugs by at least 2 hours

- **THEOPHYLLINE:** Marbofloxacin may increase theophylline blood levels; this interaction is more likely with enrofloxacin than with marbofloxacin (Martin-Jimenez 2009)

- **WARFARIN:** Potential for increased warfarin effects

Laboratory Considerations

- In some human patients, the fluoroquinolones have caused increases in liver enzymes, BUN, and creatinine and decreases in hematocrit. The clinical relevance of these mild changes is not known at this time.

Doses

- **DOGS:**

  a) For susceptible infections (urinary tract, skin and soft tissue): 2.75–5.5 mg/kg PO once daily. Give for 2–3 days beyond cessation of clinical signs (skin/soft tissue infections); and for at least 10 days (urinary tract). If no improvement noted after 5 days, reevaluate diagnosis. Maximum duration of treatment is 30 days. (Package insert; *Zeniquin®*—Pfizer)

  b) For susceptible *Pseudomonas* otitis in patients with otitis media, patients with severe proliferative chronic otitis externa, patients with ulcerative otitis externa, patients where inflammatory cells are seen cytologically (indicating deeper skin involvement) and in patients where owners cannot administer topical therapy or where a patient has had an adverse reaction to topically administered antimicrobial agents: Dose at the high end of the flexible dosing label (**Note:** high end = 5.5 mg/kg PO once daily). (Cole 2008)

■ **CATS:**

a) For susceptible infections (urinary tract, skin and soft tissue): 2.75–5.5 mg/kg PO once daily. Give for 2–3 days beyond cessation of clinical signs (skin/soft tissue infections); and for at least 10 days (urinary tract). If no improvement noted after 5 days, reevaluate diagnosis. Maximum duration of treatment is 30 days. (Package insert; *Zeniquin®*—Pfizer)

b) First-line treatment (pending definitive diagnosis) for feline tuberculosis (if decision is made to treat in cases of localized cutaneous infections) or non-tuberculous mycobacteria (NTM; not effective against MAC infection): 2 mg/kg PO once daily. (Gunn-Moore 2008)

c) For hemoplasmosis: 2.75 mg/kg PO once daily (q24h). (Dowers 2009)

■ **REPTILES:**

a) Study done in Ball pythons (*Python regius*): 10 mg/kg PO at least every 48 hours. Further studies required to determine effective doses and toxicity. (Coke *et al.* 2006)

Monitoring

■ Clinical efficacy

■ Adverse effects

Client Information

■ Give as the veterinarian prescribes; do not stop treating just because the animal appears well.

Chemistry/Synonyms

A synthetic fluoroquinolone antibiotic, marbofloxacin is soluble in water, but solubility decreases as pH increases.

Marbofloxacin may also be known as Ro 9-1168, *Marbocyl®*, or *Zeniquin®*.

Storage/Stability

Marbofloxacin tablets should be stored below 30°C.

Dosage Forms/Regulatory Status

VETERINARY-LABELED PRODUCTS:

Marbofloxacin Oral Tablets: 25 mg, 50 mg, 100 mg, 200 mg; *Zeniquin®* (Pfizer); (Rx). FDA-approved for use in dogs and cats. Must not be used in food animals.

HUMAN-LABELED PRODUCTS: None

References

Coke, R.L., R. Isaza, et al. (2006). Preliminary single-dose pharmacokinetics of marbofloxacin in ball pythons (Python regius). Journal of Zoo and Wildlife Medicine 37(1): 6–10.

Cole, L. (2008). Pseudomonas Otitis: Diagnosis, Treatment, and Prognosis. Peroceedings: AVA. Accessed via: Veterinary Information Network. http://goo.gl/j5eAX

Dowers, K. (2009). Causes of feline anemia: old and new? Proceedings: ACVIM. Accessed via: Veterinary Information Network. http://goo.gl/N1GTZ

Gunn-Moore, D. (2008). Feline Mycobacterial Infections. Proceedings: WSAVA. Accessed via: Veterinary Information Network. http://goo.gl/DPklQ

Martin-Jimenez, T. (2009). Antimicrobial Drug-Drug Interactions—Synergy & Antagonism. Proceedings: ACVIM. Accessed via: Veterinary Information Network. http://goo.gl/rNCxB

MAROPITANT CITRATE

(mar-*oh*-pit-ent)   Cerenia®

NEUROKININ (NK₁) RECEPTOR ANTAGONIST ANTIEMETIC

Prescriber Highlights

▶ Veterinary FDA-approved antiemetic for use in dogs 16 weeks of age & older; also used extra-label in cats (little published information available for cats, but appears well tolerated)

▶ Acts at the emetic center; therefore effective for emesis mediated via either peripheral or central mechanisms

▶ Subcutaneous injection is FDA-approved for the prevention & treatment of acute vomiting; SC injections may cause pain and swelling at injection site

▶ Oral form is FDA-approved for the prevention of acute vomiting & the prevention of vomiting due to motion sickness; different oral dosages for each indication

▶ Oral dose is higher than subcutaneous dose due to decreased bioavailability of the oral tablet

Uses/Indications

Maropitant citrate injectable solution is indicated for the prevention and treatment of acute vomiting in dogs; maropitant citrate tablets are indicated for the prevention of acute vomiting and the prevention of vomiting due to motion sickness in dogs. Both are also used extra-label in cats.

Maropitant has been effective to control vomiting secondary to a variety of stimuli, including cisplatin (chemotherapy)—induced vomiting, copper sulfate and apomorphine-induced vomiting, and ipecac induced vomiting.

Pharmacology/Actions

Maropitant is a neurokinin-1 (NK₁) receptor antagonist, which acts in the central nervous system by inhibiting Substance P, the key neurotransmitter involved in vomiting. Maropitant suppresses both peripheral & centrally mediated emesis. Maropitant has been shown to reduce the MAC requirements of sevoflurane and reduce visceral pain in dogs as NK-1 receptors are stimulated by substance P (Boscan *et al.* 2009). Maropitant does not affect gastric emptying times or intestinal transit times, but it can decrease small intestine contraction pressure patterns (McCord *et al.* 2009).

Pharmacokinetics

In dogs, maropitant is rapidly absorbed after oral (PO) & subcutaneous (SC) administration. Peak plasma concentrations (Tmax) occur in less than 1 hour following 1 mg/kg subcutaneous administration and less than 2 hours after oral administration of 2 or 8 mg/kg. After oral administration bioavailability is 24% (2 mg/kg) and 37% (8 mg/kg), suggesting first pass metabolism that becomes saturated at the higher dose. Feeding status does not affect bioavailability.

Maropitant follows non-linear pharmacokinetics (PK) at oral therapeutic doses but approximately linear PK at higher doses (20–50 mg/kg). Bioavailability is 91% following subcutaneous administration of 1 mg/kg. An accumulation ratio of 1.5 occurs after once daily use of maropitant for 5 consecutive days at 1 mg/kg SC or 2 mg/kg PO. Accumulation ratio is 2.18 after 2 consecutive days at 8 mg/kg PO daily.

Hepatic metabolism of maropitant involves two cytochrome P450 enzymes: CYP2D15 (low capacity, high affinity) and CYP 3A12 (high capacity, low affinity). The non-linear kinetics at oral doses of 2–16 mg/kg may be due to saturation of the low capacity enzyme and increased involvement of CYP3A12 at higher doses. Twenty-one metabolites have been identified with the major (pharmacologically active) metabolite being CJ-18,518, a product of hydroxylation. Plasma protein binding of maropitant is high (99.5%). Half-life is 8.84 hours (range: 6.07–17.7 hrs) for 1 mg/kg SC; 4.03 hours (range: 2.58–7.09 hrs) for 2 mg/kg. Maropitant is eliminated primarily by the liver. Urinary recovery of maropitant and its major metabolite is minimal (<1%). Large inter-patient pharmacokinetic variations have been observed.

In cats, bioavailability is about 50% (PO) and 100+% (SC). Terminal elimination half-life is approximately 15 hours (Hickman *et al.* 2008).

Contraindications/Precautions/Warnings

Use with caution in dogs with hepatic dysfunction as maropitant is hepatically metabolized.

Use with caution with other medications that are highly protein bound, although clinical significance has not been determined.

Use with caution in puppies less than 11 weeks old, a higher frequency and greater severity of histological evidence of bone marrow hypoplasia was seen in puppies treated with maropitant than in control puppies.

Adverse Effects

Maropitant is well tolerated in dogs. Pre-travel vomiting and hypersalivation are the two most common side effects seen after administration of the tablets at the higher dosage required for prevention of motion sickness. Swelling or pain at the injection site has been reported following SC administration of the drug. While the label states that the drug should be stored at room temperature, one study found that when the injection was stored in the refrigerator and immediately injected, dogs had less pain at the injection site (Narishetty *et al.* 2007). Diarrhea (4–8%) & anorexia (1.5–5.2%) were the most common side effects noted during U.S. field studies.

Very limited information is available for cats, but in a study in 30 cats at various dosages (0.5–5 mg/kg SC over 15 days) was well tolerated. Localized reactions at injection sites were noted in some cats (Hickman *et al.* 2008).

Reproductive/Nursing Safety

The safe use of maropitant has not been evaluated in dogs used for breeding, pregnant or lactating bitches. Maropitant should only be used in pregnant or lactating bitches following a benefit/risk assessment by the veterinarian.

Overdosage/Acute Toxicity

Single dose toxicity was studied in mice and rats after oral and intravenous administration. No adverse events were reported after oral administration of up to 30 mg/kg (mice) and 100 mg/kg (rats) and after IV administration of 6.5 mg/kg (mice) and 2.5 mg/kg (rats). The clinical signs of overdosage in mice and rats were similar and independent from the route of administration and included decreased activity, irregular or labored respiration, ataxia and tremors. Salivation, nasal discharge and "raspy" breathing were also noted in rats after oral dosing, while the excretion of reddish urine was observed in some mice and rats following intravenous administration.

In dogs, tolerance has been confirmed in doses of up to 3 times the recommended oral dose of 8 mg/kg, for 3 times longer than the proposed maximum duration of treatment. A GLP compliant study revealed no adverse events in dogs after repeated oral doses delivered by oral gavage (5 mg/kg PO q 24h x 93 days). In the same study at 20 mg/kg/day, effects included emesis in two females on day 1, body weights losses of 8–15% when compared to those at start of study, ECG changes (slight increases in P-R interval, P wave duration and QRS amplitude were noted over the course of treatment), slightly lower serum albumin and slightly higher adrenal weights (females) at 20 mg/kg/day in both sexes.

Oral toxicokinetic studies with the primary metabolite were conducted in mice, rats, rabbits and dogs, indicating that the metabolite was well tolerated.

Drug Interactions

During field safety and efficacy studies, a number of medications were used concomitantly with maropitant. Many dogs received multiple medications. The most common concomitant medication was metronidazole. Other commonly used concomitant medications included: dextrose/Ringers solution IV, sodium chloride

IV, amoxicillin, ampicillin, cefazolin, cephalexin, enrofloxacin, sulfamethoxazole/trimethoprim, famotidine, sucralfate, cimetidine, dexamethasone, ivermectin, ivermectin/pyrantel, pyrantel, lufenuron/milbemycin, milbemycin, moxidectin, vitamin B, and vaccines. There were no problems observed with any of these drugs in conjunction with maropitant.

Laboratory Considerations
■ No specific concerns noted.

Doses
■ **DOGS:**
Prevention of acute vomiting:

1 mg/kg SC given at least one hour prior to anticipated emetogenic event and q24h thereafter for up to 5 consecutive days.

2 mg/kg PO given at least two hours prior to anticipated emetogenic event and q24h thereafter for up to 5 consecutive days.

Treatment of acute vomiting:

1 mg/kg SC q24h for up to 5 consecutive days.

Note: If a longer duration of therapy is needed, a 48 hour washout period is recommended due to accumulation of the drug.

Prevention of vomiting due to motion sickness:

8 mg/kg (minimum dose) PO given at least two hours prior to travel and q24h for up to 2 consecutive days;

Note: If a longer duration of therapy is needed, a 72 hour washout period is recommended.

(Label Information; *Cerenia*®—Pfizer)

■ **CATS:**
a) As an antiemetic: One pharmacokinetic study suggests a dose of 1 mg/kg SC or PO. (Richter 2009)

b) As an antiemetic: 0.5−1 mg/kg SC once daily for up to 5 days. (Marks 2008)

Monitoring
■ Clinical efficacy measured by decreased episodes of vomiting
■ Adverse effects

Client Information
■ Tablets should not be tightly wrapped or embedded in food/snacks as this may delay dissolution of tablets

■ Avoid prolonged fasting before administration of tablets

■ Feeding a small meal or snack one hour before administration of tablets for motion sickness will minimize the occurrence of pre-trip vomiting following administration of tablets

Chemistry/Synonyms
Classified as a substituted quinuclidine, maropitant's molecular weight is 678.81. The chemical name is (2S,3S)-2-benzhydryl-N-(5-tert-butyl-2-methoxybenzyl) quinuclidin-3-amine citrate.

Maropitant may also be known as CJ-11,972.

Storage/Stability
Maropitant injectable solution contains a preservative and is designed for multi-dose use. The product label states that the vial should be stored at controlled room temperature 20−25°C (68−77°F) with excursions permitted between 15−30°C (59−86°F) and be used within 28 days of first vial puncture in accordance with FDA requirements. Although the product may be chemically stable beyond this time, multiple punctures may lead to contamination of the product; therefore, extended use beyond the labeled discard date is discouraged.

Maropitant tablets are packaged in foil to protect them from moisture uptake, which was observed in less-protective packaging. A European stability study indicated that tablets removed from the blister pack and halved showed no loss of potency during the 48 hour testing period.

Compatibility/Compounding Considerations
No drug-drug compatibility information was located for maropitant.

Dosage Forms/Regulatory Status
VETERINARY-LABELED PRODUCTS:

Maropitant Citrate Injectable Solution: 10 mg/mL in 20 mL multidose vials; *Cerenia*® (Pfizer); (Rx). Labeled for use in dogs.

Maropitant Citrate Oral Tablets: 16, 24, 60, and 160 mg in blister packs (4 tablets per pack; carton of 10); Tablets are peach-colored and scored with the tablet strength and MPT imprinted on one side and the Pfizer logo imprinted on the other side; *Cerenia*® (Pfizer); (Rx). Labeled for use in dogs.

HUMAN-LABELED PRODUCTS: None

References
Boscan, P., E. Monnet, et al. (2009). Maropitant, a NK-1 Antagonist Decreases the Sevoflurane MAC During Visceral Stimulation in Dogs. Proceedings: IVECCS. Accessed via: Veterinary Information Network. http://goo.gl/kK7Cg

Hickman, M.A., S.R. Cox, et al. (2008). Safety, pharmacokinetics and use of the novel NK-1 receptor antagonist maropitant (Cerenia(TM)) for the prevention of emesis and motion sickness in cats. Journal of Veterinary Pharmacology and Therapeutics 31(3): 220–229.

Marks, S. (2008). GI Therapeutics: Which Ones and When? Proceedings: IVECCS. Accessed via: Veterinary Information Network. http://goo.gl/rxwcs

McCord, K., P. Boscan, et al. (2009). Comparison of Gastrointestinal Motility in Dogs Treated with Metoclopramide, Cisapride, Erythromycin or Maropitant Using theSmartpillTM. Proceedings: ACVIM. Accessed via: Veterinary Information Network. http://goo.gl/uIOkZ

Narishetty, S., B. Galvan, et al. (2007). "Effect of Refrigeration of the Antiemetic Cerenia (Maropitant) on Pain on Injection."

Richter, K. (2009). Acute Vomiting: A Systemic Approach. Proceedings: ACVIM. Accessed via: Veterinary Information Network. http://goo.gl/VYeZ1

MAVACOXIB

(mav-ah-*cox*-ib)   Trocoxil®

LONG-ACTING NSAID

Prescriber Highlights

▶ Very long acting NSAID for dogs; half life averages 16–17 days

▶ At time of writing not available in the USA.

▶ Limited clinical experience, but appears to be relatively safe and effective

▶ Adverse effect profile expected to be similar to other canine-approved NSAIDs

▶ Primary benefit appears to be for patients whose owners have difficulty adhering to a daily oral dosing regimen; but adverse effects may persist as well

Uses/Indications

Mavacoxib is a very long acting oral NSAID that is licensed for use in dogs in the UK, Europe and elsewhere. In the UK it is labeled "for the treatment of pain and inflammation associated with degenerative joint disease in dogs aged 12 months or more in cases where continuous treatment exceeding one month is indicated." At present, its place in the NSAID armamentarium for canine use is to be determined. It could be of benefit in those cases where owners have difficulty adhering to a daily oral dosing regimen, but because of its long half-life and duration of action, adverse effects could persist for many weeks after the drug was last given.

In a study comparing the safety and efficacy of mavacoxib with carprofen in 124 dogs, efficacy comparing the two were statistically equivalent and each had a similar rate and profile of adverse effects (Johnson *et al.* 2009).

Pharmacology/Actions

In dogs, mavacoxib appears to be a relative selective inhibiting cyclooxygenase (COX)-1 versus COX-2. It is believed to predominantly inhibit cyclooxygenase-2 (COX-2) and spare COX-1 at therapeutic dosages. This, theoretically, would inhibit production of the prostaglandins that contribute to pain and inflammation (COX-2) and spare those that maintain normal gastrointestinal and renal function (COX-1). However, COX-1 and COX-2 inhibition studies are done *in vitro* and do not necessarily correlate perfectly with clinical effects seen in actual patients.

Pharmacokinetics

Pharmacokinetic values for mavacoxib in dogs are widely patient variable. Average bioavailability after oral dosing is about 46% when fasted, but nearly doubles (87%) when given with food. Peak levels occur in about 11 hours, but range widely. In most dogs, blood levels of those thought to be therapeutic occur in approximately one hour after dosing when given with food. Apparent volume of distribution (steady-state) averaged 1.6 L/kg and the drug is highly bound to canine plasma proteins (98%). Total body clearance was a very low 2.7 mL/hour/kg and it is primarily cleared by biliary excretion. The average terminal half-life was 16.6 days (range: 8-39 days) (Cox *et al.* 2010).

Contraindications/Precautions/Warnings

The UK labels lists the following contraindications: Dogs less than 12 months of age and/or less than 5 kg body weight; dogs with GI disorders including ulceration and bleeding, evidence of a hemorrhagic disorder, impaired renal or hepatic function, cardiac insufficiency, (history of) hypersensitivity to the active substance, sulfonamides or to any of the excipients. Do not use in pregnant, breeding or lactating animal or use concomitantly with glucocorticoids or other NSAIDs. Do not administer other NSAIDs within 1 month of the last administration of mavacoxib. It also states to avoid use in any dehydrated, hypovolemic or hypotensive animal, as there is a potential risk of increased renal toxicity. Concurrent administration of potentially nephrotoxic medicinal products should be avoided.

Animals should not become dehydrated when receiving this or other NSAIDs.

Adverse Effects

As mavacoxib is a new agent, its adverse effect profile has not been fully determined in dogs; field studies have indicated that it causes similar adverse effects seen with other NSAIDs, but it is not known if this drug will have fewer or greater incidences of adverse effects when compared with other FDA-approved NSAIDs. NSAID adverse effects in dogs can include: inappetence, diarrhea, vomiting, depression and renal toxicity.

Reproductive/Nursing Safety

The safety of mavacoxib has not been established during pregnancy and lactation. The UK label states: Do not use in pregnant, breeding or lactating animals. Studies in pregnant rabbits with another coxib-class NSAID (firocoxib) at dosages approximating those given to dogs, demonstrated maternotoxic and fetotoxic effects.

Overdosage/Acute Toxicity

In overdose safety studies performed in dogs, repeated doses (at labeled dosage frequency) of 5 and 10 mg/kg did not demonstrate adverse events, abnormal clinical chemistry or significant histological abnormalities. At 15 mg/kg, vomiting, and softened/mucoid feces and increases in clinical chemistry parameters reflecting decreased renal function were noted. Doses of 25 mg/kg cause GI ulceration. One study dog died from GI perforation and peritonitis at the 25 mg/kg dose (Krautmann *et al.* 2009).

Oral acute overdoses of mavacoxib, should be managed as with other NSAID toxicity, but because of the drug's very long duration of effect, prolonged monitoring and treatment may be required; consulting a veterinary poison center or the drug sponsor's hotline seems prudent until more experience has been gained with this agent.

As with any NSAID, overdosage can lead to gastrointestinal and renal effects. The ASPCA Animal Poison Control Center (APCC) has not yet set a dosage level of concern for renal damage for dogs or cats. Decontamination with emetics and/or activated charcoal is appropriate. For doses where GI effects are expected, the use of gastrointestinal protectants is warranted. If renal effects are also expected, fluid diuresis is warranted.

Drug Interactions

At the time of writing, no drug interactions have been reported with mavacoxib, but the manufacturer warns that use in conjunction with other **NSAIDs** or **corticosteroids** be avoided. It is also possible mavacoxib could cause increased renal dysfunction if used with other drugs that can cause or contribute to **renal dysfunction** (*e.g.*, **diuretics, aminoglycosides**), but the clinical significance of this potential interaction is unclear. The following drug interactions are either expected or are for dogs receiving mavacoxib and may be of clinical significance:

- **ACE INHIBITORS (*e.g.*, enalapril, benazepril):** Some NSAIDs can reduce effects on blood pressure. Because ACE inhibitors potentially can reduce renal blood flow, use with NSAIDs could increase the risk for renal injury. However, one study in dogs receiving tepoxalin did not show any adverse effect. It is unknown what effects, if any, occur if other NSAIDs and ACE inhibitors are used together in dogs.

- **ASPIRIN:** May increase the risk of gastrointestinal toxicity (*e.g.*, ulceration, bleeding, vomiting, diarrhea). Washout periods several weeks long are probably warranted when switching from mavacoxib to aspirin therapy in dogs.

- **CORTICOSTEROIDS (*e.g.*, prednisone):** May increase the risk of gastrointestinal toxicity (*e.g.*, ulceration, bleeding, vomiting, diarrhea)

- **DIGOXIN:** NSAIDs may increase serum levels

- **FLUCONAZOLE:** Administration has increased plasma levels of celecoxib in humans and potentially could also affect mavacoxib levels in dogs

- **FUROSEMIDE:** NSAIDs may reduce saluretic and diuretic effects

- **METHOTREXATE:** Serious toxicity has occurred when NSAIDs have been used concomitantly with methotrexate; use together with extreme caution

- **NEPHROTOXIC DRUGS (*e.g.*, furosemide, aminoglycosides, amphotericin B, etc.):** May enhance the risk of nephrotoxicity development

- **NSAIDs, OTHER:** May increase the risk of gastrointestinal toxicity (*e.g.*, ulceration, bleeding, vomiting, diarrhea)

Laboratory Considerations

- None identified

Doses

- **DOGS:**

   a) For the treatment of pain and inflammation associated with degenerative joint disease in dogs aged 12 months or more in cases where continuous treatment exceeding one month is indicated: 2 mg/kg PO given immediately before or with the dog's main meal. Care should be taken to ensure that the tablet is ingested. The treatment should be repeated 14 days later; thereafter the dosing interval is **one month.** A treatment cycle should not exceed 7 consecutive doses (6.5 months). THIS IS **not a daily NSAID.** (Label Information—*Trocoxil®*; Pfizer U.K.)

Monitoring

- Baseline and periodic CBC and serum chemistry (including BUN/serum creatinine, and liver function assessment)

- Baseline history and physical

- Efficacy of therapy

- Adverse effect monitoring via client

Client Information

- Give doses exactly as directed by veterinarian, do not give extra doses or increase the dose without veterinarian's guidance

- Give the medication with the dog's largest meal of the day. The drug is much better absorbed from the stomach if given with food.

- Contact the veterinarian if any of the following adverse effects persist or are severe: loss of appetite, vomiting, change in bowel movements (*e.g.*, stool color), change in behavior, decrease in water consumption, or urination; these could potentially occur after many weeks after the last dose was given. Immediately report to the veterinarian if any of the following adverse effects occur: bloody stool/diarrhea, bloody vomiting, or allergic reaction (facial swelling face, hives, red, itchy skin)

- Since dogs may find the chewable tablets' taste desirable, the drug should be stored out of reach of animals and children

Chemistry/Synonyms

Mavacoxib is structurally related to the human NSAID celecoxib and categorized as a diaryl substituted pyrazole. Its chemical name is 4-[5-(4-fluorophenyl)-3-(trifluoromethyl)-

1H-pyrazol-1-yl]- benzenesulfonamide. Mavacoxib's solubility in water is relatively low (0.006 mg/mL).

Mavacoxib may also be known as mavacoxibum; PHA 739,521; or UNII-YFT7X7SR77. A common trade name is *Trocoxil®*.

Storage/Stability

Store in the original packaging at room temperature out of reach of pets and children.

Dosage Forms/Regulatory Status

VETERINARY-LABELED PRODUCTS: None in USA at time of writing.

In the UK and elsewhere: Mavacoxib Oral Chewable Tablets® 6 mg, 20 mg, 30 mg, 75 mg, & 95 mg; *Trocoxil®* (Pfizer); (Rx)

HUMAN-LABELED PRODUCTS: None

References

Cox, S., S. Lesman, et al. (2010). The pharmacokinetics of mavacoxib, a long-acting COX-2 inhibitor, in young adult laboratory dogs. J Vet Pharmacol Ther 33: 461–470.

Johnson, M., J. Boucher, et al. (2009). Determination of the Efficacy and Safety of Mavacoxib Tablets Administered Monthly at 2 mg/Kg BW in the Treatment of Pain and Inflammation Associated with Osteoarthritis in Dogs. Proceedings: BSAVA. Accessed via: Veterinary Information Network. http://goo.gl/GWMUb

Krautmann, M., J.F. Boucher, et al. (2009). Target animal safety studies of mavacoxib in dogs. J Vet Pharmacol Ther 32(Suppl.1): 46–47.

MECHLORETHAMINE HCL

(me-klor-*eth*-a-meen)   Mustargen®

ANTINEOPLASTIC

Prescriber Highlights

▶ Antineoplastic for lymphoreticular neoplasms or pleural & peritoneal effusions (intracavitary)

▶ Contraindications (relative; risk vs. benefit): Anemia, bone marrow depression, tumor cell infiltration into bone marrow, current infection, sensitivity to mechlorethamine, or patients who have received previous chemotherapy or radiotherapy

▶ Adverse Effects: Bone marrow depression, GI effects (vomiting, nausea), ototoxicity (high dosages or regional perfusions); Potentially: alopecia, hyperuricemia, hepatotoxicity, peripheral neuropathy, & GI ulcers

▶ Teratogen

▶ Avoid extravasation

Uses/Indications

In small animals, mechlorethamine may be useful for the adjunctive treatment of lymphoreticular neoplasms or, with intracavitary administration, for treating pleural and peritoneal effusions. A change in owners of the pharmaceutical product has reportedly resulted in very large price increases for this medication and some veterinary oncologists are substituting dactinomycin for the mechlorethamine in MOPP rescue protocols.

Pharmacology/Actions

Mechlorethamine is an alkylating agent, thereby interfering with DNA replication, RNA transcription, and protein synthesis. It is cell cycle-phase nonspecific.

With intracavitary administration, mechlorethamine causes sclerosing and an inflammatory response on serous membranes, thereby causing adherence of serosal surfaces.

Pharmacokinetics

Because mechlorethamine is so irritating to tissues it must be given IV for systemic use. It is incompletely absorbed after intracavitary administration. After injection, mechlorethamine is rapidly (within minutes) inactivated.

Contraindications/Precautions/Warnings

Mechlorethamine is contraindicated in patients with a known infection or have had a prior anaphylactic reaction to the drug.

Mechlorethamine should be used only when its potential benefits outweigh its risks with the following conditions: anemia, bone marrow depression, tumor cell infiltration into bone marrow, sensitivity to mechlorethamine, or patients who have received previous chemotherapy or radiotherapy.

Adverse Effects

Bone marrow depression (leukopenia, thrombocytopenia) and GI effects (vomiting, nausea) are quite common and can be serious enough to halt therapy. Ototoxicity may occur with either high dosages or regional perfusions. Other potential effects include alopecia, hyperuricemia, hepatotoxicity, peripheral neuropathy, and GI ulcers.

Because severe tissue sloughing may occur, avoid extravasation.

Reproductive/Nursing Safety

Mechlorethamine is a teratogen in lab animals. Use only during pregnancy when the benefits to the mother outweigh the risks to the offspring. Mechlorethamine can suppress gonadal function. In humans, the FDA categorizes this drug as category *D* for use during pregnancy (*There is evidence of human fetal risk, but the potential benefits from the use of the drug in pregnant women may be acceptable despite its potential risks.*)

While it is not known whether mechlorethamine enters maternal milk, nursing puppies or kittens should receive milk replacer when the dam is receiving mechlorethamine.

Overdosage/Acute Toxicity

Because of the toxic potential of this agent, overdoses must be avoided. Determine dosages carefully.

Drug Interactions

The following drug interactions have either been reported or are theoretical in humans or animals receiving mechlorethamine and may be of significance in veterinary patients:

■ **IMMUNOSUPPRESSANT DRUGS (e.g., azathioprine, cyclophosphamide, corticosteroids):** Use with other immunosuppressant drugs may increase the risk of infection.

■ **MYELOSUPPRESSIVE DRUGS (e.g., chloramphenicol, flucytosine, amphotericin B, or colchicine):** Use extreme caution when used concurrently with other drugs that are also myelosuppressive, including many of the other antineoplastics and other bone marrow depressant drugs. Bone marrow depression may be additive.

■ **VACCINES, LIVE:** Live virus vaccines should be used with caution, if at all, during therapy.

Laboratory Considerations

■ Mechlorethamine may raise **serum uric acid** levels. Drugs such as allopurinol may be required to control hyperuricemia.

Doses

NOTE: Because of the potential toxicity of this drug to patients, veterinary personnel and clients, and since chemotherapy protocols, treatment protocols, monitoring and safety guidelines often change, the following dosages should be used only as a general guide and not as a dosage protocol. Consultation with a veterinary oncologist and referral to current veterinary oncology references [e.g., (Henry & Higginbotham 2009); (Argyle *et al.* 2008); (Withrow & Vail 2007); (Villalobos 2007); (Ogilvie & Moore 2006); (Ogilvie & Moore 2001)] is *strongly recommended*.

■ **DOGS/CATS:**

Mechlorethamine is usually dosed as part of a lymphoma rescue protocol that includes vincristine (or vinblastine), procarbazine and prednisone (or prednisolone), the so-called MOPP protocol. Doses of mechlorethamine are usually 3 mg/m^2 IV given on days 0 and 7 of a 28 day protocol, but some are giving it on days 0 and 14 to better allow bone marrow to recover.

Monitoring

■ CBC with platelets at least every 1–2 weeks until stable; then every 3 months

■ Liver function tests; initially before starting treatment and then every 3–4 months

■ Injection site for signs of extravasation

Chemistry/Synonyms

A bifunctional alkylating agent, mechlorethamine occurs as a hygroscopic, white, crystalline powder that is very soluble in water. After reconstitution with sterile water or sterile saline, the resultant solution is clear and has a pH of 3–5.

Mechlorethamine may also be known as: nitrogen mustard, mustine, HN$_2$, chlormethine hydrochloride, chlorethazine hydrochloride, HN2 (mustine [chlormethine]), mechlorethamine hydrochloride, mustine hydrochloride, nitrogen mustard (mustine [chlormethine]), NSC-762, WR-147650, *Caryolisine*®, *Mustargen*® and *Onco-Cloramin*®.

Storage/Stability

Store the powder for injection at room temperature. Mechlorethamine is highly unstable in neutral or alkaline aqueous solutions and rapidly degrades. While more stable in an acidic environment, the drug should be administered immediately after preparation.

Compatibility/Compounding Considerations

It is NOT recommended to mix mechlorethamine with any other medication or to dilute further beyond what is described in the package insert.

Drugs that have been reported to be **compatible** with mechlorethamine when given via an IV Y-site include aztreonam, filgrastim, granisetron, melphalan, and ondansetron.

Unused portions of reconstituted drug can be neutralized by adding equal volumes of 5% sodium thiosulfate and 5% sodium bicarbonate. This solution is allowed to stand for 45 minutes and then can be discarded appropriately.

Dosage Forms/Regulatory Status

VETERINARY-LABELED PRODUCTS: None

HUMAN-LABELED PRODUCTS:

Mechlorethamine Powder for Injection: 10 mg; *Mustargen*® (Lundbeck); (Rx)

References

Argyle, D., M. Brearly, et al. (2008). Decision Making in Small Animal Oncology, Wiley-Blackwell.

Henry, C. & M. Higginbotham (2009). Cancer Management in Small Animal Practice, Saunders.

Ogilvie, G. & A. Moore (2001). Feline Oncology: A Comprehensive Guide to Compassionate Care, Veterinary Learning Systems.

Ogilvie, G. & A. Moore (2006). Managing the Canine Cancer Patient: A Practical Guide to Compassionate Care, Veterinary Learning Systems.

Villalobos, A. (2007). Canine and Feline Geriatric Oncology. Ames, Blackwell.

Withrow, S. & D. Vail (2007). Withrow and MacEwen's Small Animal Clinical Oncology 4th Ed. Philadelphia, Elsevier.

MECLIZINE HCL

(**mek**-li-zeen)   Antivert®

ANTIHISTAMINE, ANTIEMETIC

Prescriber Highlights

▶ Antihistamine with sedative & antiemetic effects, used primarily for motion sickness

▶ Caution: Prostatic hypertrophy, bladder neck obstruction, severe cardiac failure, angle-closure glaucoma, or pyeloduodenal obstruction

▶ Adverse Effects: Sedation; less frequently anticholinergic effects may be noted (dry mucous membranes, eyes, tachycardia, etc.); contradictory CNS stimulation possible

Uses/Indications

Meclizine is principally used in small animals as an antiemetic and for the treatment and prevention of motion sickness.

Pharmacology/Actions

Meclizine is a piperazine antihistamine and, beside its antihistamine activity, it also possesses antiemetic, CNS depressant, antispasmodic, and local anesthetic effects. The exact mechanisms of action for its antiemetic and anti-motion-sickness effects are not completely understood, but it is thought they are as a result of the drug's central anticholinergic and CNS depressant activity. The antiemetic effect is probably mediated through the chemoreceptor trigger zone (CTZ).

Pharmacokinetics

Very little information is available. Meclizine is metabolized in the liver and has a serum half-life of about 6 hours.

Contraindications/Precautions/Warnings

Meclizine is contraindicated in patients hypersensitive to it. It should be used with caution in patients with prostatic hypertrophy, bladder neck obstruction, severe cardiac failure, angle-closure glaucoma, or pyeloduodenal obstruction.

Adverse Effects

The usual adverse effect noted with meclizine is sedation; less frequently anticholinergic effects may be noted (dry mucous membranes, eyes, tachycardia, etc.). Contradictory CNS stimulation has also been reported. Cats may develop inappetence while receiving this medication.

Reproductive/Nursing Safety

Meclizine is considered teratogenic at high dosages in laboratory animals and cleft palates have been noted in rats at 25–50 times higher than labeled dosages. However, in humans, it has been suggested that meclizine possesses the lowest risk for teratogenicity for antiemetic drugs and that it is the drug of first choice to treat nausea/vomiting associated with pregnancy. In humans, the FDA categorizes this drug as category *B* for use during pregnancy (*Animal studies have not yet demonstrated risk to the fetus, but there are no adequate studies in pregnant women; or animal studies have shown an adverse effect, but adequate studies in pregnant women have not demonstrated a risk to the fetus in the first trimester of pregnancy, and there is no evidence of risk in later trimesters.*)

It is unknown if meclizine enters milk; its anticholinergic activity may, potentially, inhibit lactation.

Overdosage/Acute Toxicity

Moderate overdosage may result in drowsiness alternating with hyperexcitability. Massive overdosages may result in profound CNS depression, hallucinations, seizures and other anticholinergic effects (tachycardia, urinary retention, etc.). Treatment is considered symptomatic and supportive. Consider gut emptying when patients present soon after ingestion. Avoid respiratory depressant medications.

Drug Interactions

The following drug interactions have either been reported or are theoretical in humans or animals receiving meclizine and may be of significance in veterinary patients:

■ **CNS DEPRESSANTS:** Use with other CNS depressants may cause additive sedation

■ **ANTICHOLINERGIC DRUGS:** Other anticholinergic drugs may cause additive anticholinergic effects

Laboratory Considerations

■ Because these drugs are antihistamines, they may affect the results of **skin tests** using allergen extracts. Do not use within 3–7 days before testing.

Doses

■ **DOGS:**

a) For supportive treatment of peripheral vestibular disease: 25 mg per dog PO once daily. Treatment is usually unnecessary after 72–96 hours. (Hoskins 2005)

b) As a vestibular suppressant: 12.5–50 mg (total dose per dog) PO twice daily. (Podell 2009)

c) As anti-emetic: 4 mg/kg PO once a day (Dowling 2003)

d) For palliative treatment of vertigo: 25 mg per dog PO once daily. (Schubert 2007)

■ **CATS:**

a) 12.5 mg per cat PO once daily (Pearce 2006)

b) 6.25 mg/5 kg of body weight PO (Day 1993)

c) As anti-emetic: 4 mg/kg PO once a day (Dowling 2003)

d) For palliative treatment of vertigo:

12.5 mg per cat PO once daily. (Schubert 2007)

■ **RABBITS, RODENTS, SMALL MAMMALS:**

a) **Rabbits:** For Rolling, torticollis, motion sickness: 2−12 mg/kg PO once daily (Ivey & Morrisey 2000)

b) **Rabbits:** For adjunctive treatment of torticollis, head tilt ("wry neck"): 12.5 mg (total dose) PO q12−24h. (Johnson 2006)

Monitoring
■ Efficacy

■ Adverse effects

Client Information
■ When using for motion sickness prevention, instruct client to give medication 30−60 minutes before travel.

Chemistry/Synonyms
Meclizine HCl is a piperazine derivative antiemetic antihistamine.

Meclizine may also be known as: meclozine hydrochloride, meclizine hydrochloride; meclizinium chloride; meclozini hydrochloridum; parachloramine hydrochloride, *Agyrax®, Ancolan®, Antivert®, Antrizine®, Bonamine®, Bonine®, Calmonal®, Chiclida®, D-Vert 30®, Dizmiss®, Dramamine II®, Dramine®, Duremesan®, Emetostop®, Marevit®, Meni-D®, Navicalm®, Neo-Istafene®, Nico-Vert®, Peremesin®, Peremesin N®, Peremesine®, Postadoxin N®, Postafen®, Postafene®, Ru-Vert-M®, Sea-Legs®, Suprimal®, Vergon®,* and *Vertin®.*

Storage/Stability
Meclizine products should be stored at room temperature in well-closed containers.

Dosage Forms/Regulatory Status
VETERINARY-LABELED PRODUCTS: None

The ARCI (Racing Commissioners International) has designated this drug as a class 4 substance. See the appendix for more information.

HUMAN-LABELED PRODUCTS:

Meclizine HCl Oral Tablets: 12.5 mg, 25 mg (plain and chewable) & 50 mg; *Antivert®* & *Antivert/25®* (Pfizer US); *Antrizine®* (Major); *Dramamine® Less Drowsy Formula* (Pharmacia & Upjohn); *Bonine®* (Pfizer); generic; (Rx and OTC).

Meclizine Oral Capsules: 25 mg; *Meni-D®* (Seatrace); (Rx)

References

Day, K. (1993, Last Update). "Personal Communication."
Dowling, P. (2003). GI Therapy: When what goes in won't stay down. Proceedings: Western Veterinary Conference. Accessed via: Veterinary Information Network. http://goo.gl/co8V8
Hoskins, J. (2005). Geriatric medicine: Nervous System. Proceedings: ACVC 2006. Accessed via: Veterinary Information Network. http://goo.gl/LHU4m
Ivey, E. & J. Morrisey (2000). Therapeutics for Rabbits. Vet Clin NA: Exotic Anim Pract 3:1(Jan): 183−216.
Johnson, D. (2006). Rabbit Medicine and Surgery. Proceedings: ACVC. Accessed via: Veterinary Information Network. http://goo.gl/Ualte
Pearce, L. (2006). Feline balance disorders: diagnostic tricks and common disorders. Proceedings: Western Vet Conf. Accessed via: Veterinary Information Network. http://goo.gl/Vdtih
Podell, M. (2009). From Ear to Brain: A Short Pathway to Disaster. Proceedings: IVECCS. Accessed via: Veterinary Information Network. http://goo.gl/qX57E
Schubert, T. (2007). Diagnosis and management of vestibular disease in dogs and cats. Proceedings: ACVIM. Accessed via: Veterinary Information Network. http://goo.gl/UGHV6

MEDETOMIDINE HCL

(mee-de-*toe*-mi-deen)   Domitor®

ALPHA-2 ADRENERGIC AGONIST

Prescriber Highlights

▶ Alpha2-adrenergic sedative analgesic used primarily in dogs & cats, but also may be useful in small mammals, exotics, etc.

▶ Contraindications: Cardiac disease, respiratory disorders, liver or kidney diseases, shock, severe debilitation, or animals stressed due to heat, cold or fatigue. Caution in very old or young animals

▶ NOT recommended for use during pregnancy

▶ Adverse Effects: Bradycardia, occasional AV blocks, decreased respiration, hypothermia, urination, vomiting, hyperglycemia, & pain on injection (IM). Rarely: prolonged sedation, paradoxical excitation, hypersensitivity, apnea & death from circulatory failure

▶ Drug interactions

▶ Do NOT confuse with detomidine or dexmedetomidine

Uses/Indications
Medetomidine is labeled for use as a sedative and analgesic in dogs over 12 weeks of age to facilitate clinical examinations and procedures, minor surgical procedures not requiring muscle relaxation, and minor dental procedures not requiring intubation. The manufacturer recommends the IV route of administration for dental procedures.

Medetomidine has also been used in cats, primarily in Europe. But there is apparently much less data available to evaluate its use; caution is advised.

Pharmacology/Actions
An alpha adrenergic receptor, medetomidine has an $alpha_2$:$alpha_1$ selectivity factor of 1620, and when compared to xylazine is reportedly 10X more specific for $alpha_2$ receptors versus $alpha_1$ receptors. The pharmacologic effects of medetomidine include: depression of CNS

(sedation, anxiolysis), GI (decreased secretions, varying affects on intestinal muscle tone) and endocrine functions, peripheral and cardiac vasoconstriction, bradycardia, respiratory depression, diuresis, hypothermia, analgesia (somatic and visceral), muscle relaxation (but not enough for intubation), and blanched or cyanotic mucous membranes. Effects on blood pressure are variable, but medetomidine can cause hypertension longer than does xylazine. Medetomidine also induces sedation for a longer period than does xylazine. Sedative effects persist longer than analgesic effects.

Pharmacokinetics

After IV or IM injection, onset of effect is rapid (5 min. for IV; 10–15 min. for IM). After SC injection, responses are unreliable and this method of administration cannot be recommended. The drug is absorbed via the oral mucosa when administered sublingually in dogs, but efficacy at a given dose may be less than IM dosing.

Contraindications/Precautions/Warnings

The label states that medetomidine is contraindicated in dogs having the following conditions: cardiac disease, respiratory disorders, liver or kidney diseases, shock, severe debilitation, or dogs stressed due to heat, cold, or fatigue.

Dogs that are extremely agitated or excited may have a decreased response to medetomidine; the manufacturer suggests allowing these dogs to rest quietly before administration of the drug. Dogs not responding to medetomidine should not be re-dosed. Use in very young or older dogs should be done with caution.

Adverse Effects

The adverse effects reported with medetomidine are essentially extensions of its pharmacologic effects including bradycardia, occasional AV blocks, decreased respiration, hypothermia, urination, vomiting, hyperglycemia, and pain on injection (IM). Rare effects have also been reported, including prolonged sedation, paradoxical excitation, hypersensitivity, apnea, and death from circulatory failure.

Reproductive/Nursing Safety

The drug is not recommended for use in pregnant dogs or those used for breeding purposes because safety data for use during pregnancy is insufficient; therefore, use only when the benefits clearly outweigh the drug's risks.

Overdosage/Acute Toxicity

Single doses of up to 5X (IV) and 10X (IM) were tolerated in dogs, but adverse effects can occur (see above). Death has occurred rarely in dogs (1 in 40,000) receiving 2X doses.

Because of the potential of additional adverse effects occurring (heart block, PVC's, or tachycardia), treatment of medetomidine-induced bradycardia with anticholinergic agents (atropine or glycopyrrolate) is usually not recommended. Atipamezole is probably a safer choice to treat any medetomidine-induced effect.

Drug Interactions

The following drug interactions have either been reported or are theoretical in humans or animals receiving medetomidine and may be of significance in veterinary patients:

Note: Before attempting combination therapy with medetomidine, it is strongly advised to access references from veterinary anesthesiologists familiar with the use of this product.

- ■ **ATROPINE, GLYCOPYRROLATE:** The use of atropine or glycopyrrolate to prevent or treat medetomidine-caused bradycardia is controversial as tachycardia and hypertension may result. This is more important when using higher doses of medetomidine (>20 micrograms/kg) and concomitant use is discouraged.

- ■ **OPIATES:** Enhancement of sedation and analgesia may occur when medetomidine is used concurrently with fentanyl, butorphanol, or meperidine, but adverse effects may be pronounced as well. Reduced dosages and monitoring is advised if contemplating combination therapy.

- ■ **PROPOFOL:** When propofol is used after medetomidine, hypoxemia may occur. Dosage adjustments may be required along with adequate monitoring.

- ■ **YOHIMBINE:** May reverse the effects of medetomidine; but atipamezole is preferred for clinical use to reverse the drug's effects

Laboratory Considerations

- ■ Medetomidine can inhibit ADP-induced **platelet aggregation** in cats.

Doses

- ■ **DOGS:**

  For sedation/analgesia:

  a) 10–40 micrograms/kg IM; higher doses do not cause greater sedation, but increase the duration of effect (McGrath & Ko 1997)

  b) For use with an IM opioid: 5–10 micrograms/kg. (Hardie 2000)

  c) In the cardiovascular-stable patient, as a constant rate infusion for analgesia with an initial loading dose of 1 microgram/kg IV, then CRI of 1 to 3 micrograms/kg/hour. (Quandt 2009)

- ■ **CATS:**

  For sedation/analgesia:

  a) 40–80 micrograms/kg IM; higher doses do not cause greater sedation, but increase the duration of effect (McGrath & Ko 1997)

  b) For use with an IM opioid: 5–10 micrograms/kg (Hardie 2000)

  c) 0.001–0.01 mg/kg (1–10 micrograms/kg) IV, IM or SC (Carroll 1999)

  d) For large, exotic cat (tigers, etc.) immobilization: Midazolam (0.1 mg/kg) plus medetomidine (0.05–0.07 mg/kg) IM followed by ketamine (4–10 mg/kg) IM, if needed. May antagonize with atipamezole (0.25–0.35 mg/kg) IV, SC. (Curro 2002)

■ **SMALL MAMMALS/RODENTS:**

For chemical restraint:

a) **Rats:** 0.25–0.5 mg/kg IM;

Guinea pig: 0.5 mg/kg IM;

Rabbits: 0.25–0.5 mg/kg IM (Burke 1999)

■ **FERRETS:**

As a sedative/analgesic:

a) 15 minutes prior to medetomidine, give atropine (0.05 mg/kg) or glycopyrrolate (0.01 mg/kg) then give medetomidine at 60–80 micrograms/kg IM or SC. Sedation lasts for up to 3 hours. May be reversed with atipamezole (400 micrograms/kg IM);

For injectable anesthesia: Butorphanol 0.1 mg/kg, Ketamine 5 mg/kg, Medetomidine 80 micrograms/kg. Combine in one syringe and give IM. May need to supplement with isoflurane (0.5–1.5%) for abdominal surgery. (Finkler 1999)

■ **BIRDS:**

For sedation/analgesia:

a) 0.1 mg/kg IM; limited data available on duration of effect, adverse effects, etc. (Clyde & Paul-Murphy 2000)

■ **REPTILES:**

a) Medium to small land Tortoises: Medetomidine 100–150 micrograms/kg with ketamine 5–10 mg/kg IV or IM;

Freshwater Turtles: Medetomidine 150–300 micrograms/kg with ketamine 10–20 mg/kg IV or IM;

Giant Land Tortoises: 200 kg Aldabra tortoise: Medetomidine 40 micrograms/kg with ketamine 4 mg/kg IV or IM;

Smaller Aldabra tortoises: Medetomidine 40–80 micrograms/kg with ketamine 4–8 mg/kg IV or IM. Wait 30–40 minutes for peak effect.

Iguanas: Medetomidine 100–150 micrograms/kg with ketamine 5–10 mg/kg IV or IM;

Reversal of all dosages with atipamezole is 4–5 times the medetomidine dose. (Heard 1999)

■ **ZOO, EXOTIC, WILDLIFE SPECIES:**

For use of medetomidine in zoo, exotic and wildlife medicine refer to specific references, including:

a) *Zoo Animal and Wildlife Immobilization and Anesthesia.* West, G, Heard, D, Caulkett, N. (eds.). Blackwell Publishing, 2007.

b) *Handbook of Wildlife Chemical Immobilization, 3rd Ed.* Kreeger, T.J. and J.M. Arnemo. 2007.

c) *Restraint and Handling of Wild and Domestic Animals.* Fowler, M (ed.), Iowa State University Press, 1995

d) *Exotic Animal Formulary, 3rd Ed.* Carpenter, J.W., Saunders. 2005

e) The 2009 American Association of Zoo Veterinarian Proceedings by D. K. Fontenot also has several dosages listed for restraint, anesthesia, and analgesia for a variety of drugs for carnivores and primates. VIN members can access them at: http://goo.gl/BHRih or http://goo.gl/9UJse

Monitoring

■ Level of sedation and analgesia; heart rate; body temperature

■ Heart rhythm, blood pressure, respiration rate, and pulse oximetry should be considered, particularly in higher risk patients if the drug is to be used

Client Information

■ This drug should be administered and monitored by veterinary professionals only

■ Clients should be made aware of the potential adverse effects associated with its use, particularly in dogs at risk (older, preexisting conditions)

Chemistry/Synonyms

An alpha$_2$-adrenergic agonist, medetomidine occurs as a white or almost white crystalline substance. It is soluble in water. While the compound exists as two stereoisomers, only the D-isomer is active.

Medetomidine HCl may also be known as MPV-785 and *Domitor®*.

Storage/Stability

The commercially available injection should be stored at room temperature (15–30°C) and protected from freezing.

Dosage Forms/Regulatory Status

VETERINARY-LABELED PRODUCTS:

Medetomidine HCl for Injection: 1 mg/mL in 10 mL multidose vials; *Domitor®* (Pfizer); (Rx). FDA-approved for use in dogs over 12 weeks of age. Although still listed in the FDA's Green Book, it may not be currently marketed in the USA.

The ARCI (Racing Commissioners International) has designated this drug as a class 3 substance. See the appendix for more information.

HUMAN-LABELED PRODUCTS: None

References

Burke, T. (1999). Husbandry and Medicine of Rodents and Lagomorphs. Proceedings: Central Veterinary Conference, Kansas City.

Carroll, G. (1999). Common Premedications for pain management: Pain management made simple. Proceedings: The North American Veterinary Conference, Orlando.

Clyde, V. & J. Paul-Murphy (2000). Avian Analgesia. Kirk's Current Veterinary Therapy: XIII Small Animal Practice. J Bonagura Ed. Philadelphia, WB Saunders: 1126–1128.

Curro, T. (2002). Large cat anesthesia. Proceedings: Western Veterinary Conference. Accessed via: Veterinary Information Network. http://goo.gl/jcIOK

Finkler, M. (1999). Anesthesia in Ferrets. Proceedings: Central Veterinary Conference, Kansas City.

Hardie, E. (2000). Pain: Management. Textbook of Veterinary Internal Medicine: Diseases of the Dog and Cat. S Ettinger and E Feldman Eds. Philadelphia, WB Saunders. 1: 23–25.

Heard, D. (1999). Advances in Reptile Anesthesia. The North American Veterinary Conference, Orlando.

McGrath, C. & J. Ko (1997). How to use medetomidine (Domitor®) in dogs. Virgina Veterinary Notes, Veterinary Teaching Hospital.

Quandt, J. (2009). Sedation and analgesia for the critically ill patient: Comprehensive review. Proceedings; ACVIM. Accessed via: Veterinary Information Network. http://goo.gl/wfkfQ

MEDIUM CHAIN TRIGLYCERIDES (MCT OIL)

NUTRITIONAL

Prescriber Highlights

▶ Lipid sometimes used to provide calories & fatty acids to dogs with restricted fat intake due to chronic infiltrative disease of small intestine or fat malabsorption syndromes present.

▶ Most clinicians use dietary therapy instead of MCT oil today

▶ Cautions: Significant hepatic disease (e.g., portacaval shunts, cirrhosis, etc.)

▶ Adverse Effects: Unpalatability (dogs), bloating, flatulence, & diarrhea

Uses/Indications

MCT oil as a separate compound (not as an ingredient in commercial foods) is sometimes used to offset the caloric reduction when long-chain triglycerides found in dietary fat are restricted, usually in chronic infiltrative diseases of the small intestine or when there is fat malabsorption of any cause. Because of expense and unpalatability to dogs, many clinicians are bypassing MCT oil and having their clients prepare homemade, highly digestible, ultra-low fat diets (e.g., white turkey meat plus rice/potato) or using very low fat prescription diets.

MCT oil may be useful as a base-vehicle to administer drugs to cats. A study evaluating the acceptance of low-dose (0.1 mL/kg) MCT oil, gelatin capsules, or thin-film dissolving strips, found that owner-perceived acceptability by cats of MCT oil and thin-film strips cats was significantly higher than gelatin capsules (Traas et al. 2010).

Pharmacology/Actions

Medium chain triglycerides (MCT) are more readily hydrolyzed than conventional food fat. They also require less bile acids for digestion, are not dependent for chylomicron formation or lymphatic transport, and are transported by the portal vein. Medium chain triglycerides are not a source for essential fatty acids.

MCT oil supplementation (as coconut oil) to the diet of cats did not cause food aversion or significant effects on lipid metabolism (Trevizan et al. 2010).

Pharmacokinetics

No specific information located; see Pharmacology above.

Contraindications/Precautions/Warnings

MCT oil should be used with caution in patients with significant hepatic disease (e.g., portacaval shunts, cirrhosis, etc.). Medium chain triglycerides are rapidly absorbed via the portal vein and if their hepatic clearance is impaired, significantly high systemic blood and CSF levels of medium chain fatty acids can occur. This may precipitate or exacerbate hepatic coma.

Adverse Effects

Adverse effects seen with MCT oil in small animals include unpalatability, bloating, flatulence, and diarrhea. These may be transient and minimized by starting doses at the low end of the spectrum and then gradually increasing the dose. Fat-soluble vitamin supplementation (Vitamins A, D, E, and K) by using a commercial feline or canine vitamin-mineral supplement has been recommended.

Reproductive/Nursing Safety

Although, no reproductive safety data was located, MCT oil would likely not cause problems.

Overdosage/Acute Toxicity

Overdosage would likely exacerbate the GI adverse effects noted above. Treat severe diarrhea supportively if necessary.

Drug Interactions

■ None listed, but MCT oil could, theoretically, affect absorption of drugs that are dependent on fat for oral absorption (e.g., griseofulvin, fat soluble vitamins, etc.).

Doses

■ **DOGS:**

To offset the caloric reduction when long-chain triglycerides found in dietary fat are restricted:

a) Orally ½–4 teaspoons divided per day with food (Williams 2000)

b) 0.5–2 mL/kg per day added to food. (Simpson 2009)

c) 1–2 mL/kg per day (Steiner 2003)

Monitoring

■ Adverse Effects

■ Efficacy (weight, stool consistency)

Client Information

■ Because of the unpalatability of the oil, it should be mixed with small quantities of food before offering to the patient.

Chemistry/Synonyms

MCT Oil is a lipid fraction of coconut oil consisting principally of the triglycerides C_8 (approx. 67%) and C_{10} (approx. 23%) saturated fatty acids. Each 15 mL contains 115 kCal (7.67 kCal/mL).

Medium chain triglycerides may also be known as: triglycerida saturata media, *Alembicol D®*, *Liprocil®*, *Liquigen®*, *MCT®*, *Mytic 810®*, *Structolipid®*, and *Teceeme®*.

Storage/Stability

Unless otherwise noted by the manufacturer, store at room temperature in glass bottles.

Dosage Forms/Regulatory Status

VETERINARY-LABELED PRODUCTS: None

HUMAN-LABELED PRODUCTS:

Medium Chain Triglycerides Oil: in quart bottles; *MCT®* (Mead Johnson Nutritionals); (OTC)

References

Simpson, K. (2009). Nutritional Management of Gastrointestinal Disease. Proceedings: WVC. Accessed via: Veterinary Information Network. http://goo.gl/UA5ew

Steiner, J. (2003). Protein-losing enteropathies in dogs. Proceedings: World Small Animal Veterinary Association World Congress. Accessed via: Veterinary Information Network. http://goo.gl/OyTGT

Traas, A.M., T. Fleck, et al. (2010). Ease of oral administration and owner-perceived acceptability of triglyceride oil, dissolving thin film strip, and gelatin capsule formulations to healthy cats. American Journal of Veterinary Research 71(6): 610–614.

Trevizan, L., A.D. Kessler, et al. (2010). Effects of dietary medium-chain triglycerides on plasma lipids and lipoprotein distribution and food aversion in cats. American Journal of Veterinary Research 71(4): 435–440.

Williams, D. (2000). Exocrine Pancreatic Disease. Textbook of Veterinary Internal Medicine: Diseases of the Dog and Cat. S Ettinger and E Feldman Eds. Philadelphia, WB Saunders. 2: 1345–1367.

MEDROXY-PROGESTERONE ACETATE

(me-*drox*-ee-proe-*jess*-te-rone)　　Provera®

PROGESTIN

Prescriber Highlights

▶ Synthetic progestin used primarily to treat sexually dimorphic behavior problems such as roaming, inter-male aggressive behaviors, spraying, mounting, etc.; sometimes used to treat feline psychogenic dermatitis & alopecia

▶ Because of its serious adverse effect profile, particularly in small animals, consider safer alternatives first

▶ Contraindications: Do not use in pre-pubescent cats or dogs, diabetics, pseudopregnant bitches, females in diestrus or with prolonged heat, uterine hemorrhage or discharge

▶ Adverse Effects: Increased thirst, appetite, weight gain, depression, lethargy, personality changes, adrenocortical depression, mammary changes (including enlargement, milk production, & neoplasms), diabetes mellitus, pyometra, & temporary inhibition of spermatogenesis

▶ SC injection may cause permanent local alopecia, atrophy & depigmentation may occur

▶ Drug-lab (including pathology) interactions

Uses/Indications

In cats, medroxyprogesterone acetate (MPA) has been used when either castration is ineffective or undesirable to treat sexually dimorphic behavior problems such as roaming, inter-male aggressive behaviors, spraying, mounting, etc. MPA has also been used as a tranquilizing agent to treat syndromes such as feline psychogenic dermatitis and alopecia, but treatment with "true" tranquilizing agents may be preferable.

In dogs, MPA may be useful for treating progestin-responsive dermatitis, aggressive behaviors, long-term reproductive control, treatment of young German shepherd dwarfs, short-term treatment of benign prostatic hypertrophy, and luteal insufficiency.

Progesterones have been used in horses for many purposes, including management of the spring transition period, prevention of estrus behavior, induction of estrous cycle synchrony, pregnancy maintenance, and modification of stallion behavior (Dascanio 2009). MPA does not appear to effectively suppress estrous behavior or follicular activity in normal cycling mares (Gee *et al.* 2008).

In humans, parenteral MPA has been used as a long-acting contraceptive in females, to decrease sexually deviant behavior in males, and as an antineoplastic agent for some carcinomas (see Pharmacology section above). Oral MPA is used in human females to treat secondary amenorrhea and to treat abnormal uterine bleeding secondary to hormone imbalances.

Pharmacology/Actions

Progestins are primarily produced endogenously by the corpus luteum. They transform proliferative endometrium to secretory endometrium, enhance myometrium hypertrophy and inhibit spontaneous uterine contraction. Progestins have a dose-dependent inhibitory effect on the secretion of pituitary gonadotropins and can have an anti-insulin effect. Medroxyprogesterone has exhibited a pronounced adrenocorticoid effect in animals (species not listed) and can suppress ACTH and cortisol release. MPA is anti-estrogenic and will also decrease plasma testosterone levels in male humans and dogs.

MPA has antineoplastic activity against endometrial carcinoma and renal carcinoma (efficacy in doubt) in human patients. The mechanism for this activity is not known.

Pharmacokinetics

No specific pharmacokinetic parameters in veterinary species were located for this drug. It has been reported (Beaver 1989) that injectable MPA has an approximate duration of action of 30 days when used to treat behavior disorders in cats. When administered IM to women, MPA has contraceptive activity for at least 3 months.

Contraindications/Precautions/Warnings

Progestagen therapy can cause serious adverse effects (see below). Safer alternative treatments should be considered when possible, otherwise, weigh the potential risks versus benefits before instituting therapy. Many clinicians believe that progestogens are grossly overused.

Do not use MPA prior to puberty in cats, as chronic, severe, mammary hypertrophy may result. Use in dogs before puberty may precipitate subclinical uterine or endocrine conditions (*e.g.*, cystic endometrial hyperplasia-pyometra; diabetes).

This agent should not be used during pregnancy or to treat bitches with pseudo-pregnancy. Females should not be treated during diestrus, or with uterine hemorrhage. Do not use in females with prolonged heat unless cystic ovarian disease is confirmed and surgery or GNRH or hCG are not viable options. Animals with diabetes should not receive medroxyprogesterone.

Because this drug can suppress adrenal function, exogenous steroids may need to be administered if the patient is stressed (*e.g.*, surgery, trauma).

When used for reproductive control, patients should **1)** undergo a thorough reproductive history to rule out occurrence of estrus within the last 1–2 months (female in diestrus); **2)** complete physical exam; **3)** palpation of mammary glands to rule out mammary nodules; **4)** vaginal smear to rule out presence of estrus (Romagnoli 2002)

Adverse Effects

If MPA is administered subcutaneously, permanent local alopecia, atrophy, and depigmentation may occur. If injecting SC, it is recommended to use the inguinal area to avoid these manifestations. Adverse reactions that are possible in dogs and cats include: increased appetite with increases in body weight and/or thirst, depression, lethargy, personality changes, adrenocortical depression, mammary changes (including enlargement, milk production, and neoplasms), diabetes mellitus, hypothyroidism, pyometra, and temporary inhibition of spermatogenesis. In dogs, acromegaly and increased growth hormone levels have been seen when used in patients with diabetes mellitus.

Reproductive/Nursing Safety

See the dog dose "a", and the horse dose below, for more information on use of MPA during canine or equine pregnancy.

In humans, the FDA categorizes this drug as category **X** for use during pregnancy—especially the first 4 months: (*Studies in animals or humans demonstrate fetal abnormalities or adverse reaction; reports indicate evidence of fetal risk. The risk of use in pregnant women clearly outweighs any possible benefit.*)

Medroxyprogesterone can be detected in maternal milk, but in humans, no adverse effects in nursing infants have been noted.

Overdosage/Acute Toxicity

No reports or information was located on inadvertent overdosage with this agent. Refer to the Adverse Effects section above.

Drug Interactions

The following drug interactions have either been reported or are theoretical in humans or animals receiving medroxyprogesterone and may be of significance in veterinary patients:

■ **AMINOGLUTETHIMIDE:** May decrease medroxyprogesterone effects

■ **FELBAMATE:** May increase medroxyprogesterone metabolism

■ **RIFAMPIN:** A potential interaction exists with rifampin, which may decrease progestin activity if administered concomitantly. This is presumably due to microsomal enzyme induction with resultant increase in progestin metabolism. The clinical significance of this potential interaction is unknown.

Laboratory Considerations

■ In humans, progestins in combination with estrogens (*e.g.*, oral contraceptives) have been demonstrated to increase thyroxine-binding globulin (TBG) with resultant increases in total circulating thyroid hormone. Decreased T_3 resin uptake also occurs, but free T_4 levels are unaltered. Liver function tests may also be altered.

■ The manufacturer recommends notifying the pathologist of patient medroxyprogesterone exposure when submitting relevant specimens.

Doses

■ DOGS:

a) For apparent luteal insufficiency in bitches: 0.1 mg/kg PO once daily. Treatment is discontinued several days prior to the expected due date to avoid prolonged gestation. In humans, progestins have caused congenital heart defects, limb-reduction deformities, hypospadias in male fetuses, and mild virilization of the external genitalia of female fetuses, especially when administered to women during the first 4 months of pregnancy. Facial deformities were reported in one of the four pups in a litter from a bitch treated with MPA for hypoluteoidism. In most instances, the potential benefits of progesterone treatment for hypoluteoidism during the second half of pregnancy outweigh the maternal and fetal risks. (Gorlinger *et al.* 2005), (Johnson 2008)

b) For long-term reproductive control: 2.5–3 mg/kg IM q5 months (Romagnoli 2002; Romagnoli 2006; Romagnoli 2009)

c) For adjunctive treatment of aggressive behaviors: 10 mg/kg IM or SC (see Adverse Effects above) as necessary; works best when combined with behavior modification. To treat inter-male aggression: as above, but do not exceed 3 treatments per year. (Voith & Marder 1988)

d) For treatment of young German shepherd dwarfs: medroxyprogesterone acetate at 2.5–5 mg/kg initially at 3 week intervals and subsequently at 6 week intervals has resulted in some increase in body size and development of an adult hair coat. (Kooistra 2006)

e) For treatment of benign prostatic hypertrophy; best used to maintain breeding potential for short time prior to castration; use with caution: MPA at 0.3 mg/kg SC once; effects last approximately 10 months. (Lane 2006)

f) For progestin-responsive dermatitis: 20 mg/kg IM; May repeat in 3–6 months if needed (Kunkle 1986)

■ CATS:

a) To treat behavioral disorders: To reduce marking in neutered male cats when all other drugs have been unsuccessful: Me-

droxyprogesterone acetate at 5–20 mg/kg SC or IM three to four times yearly. (Landsberg 2007)

b) For feline psychogenic alopecia and dermatitis: 75–150 mg IM or SC (see Adverse Effects above); repeat as necessary, but never more often than every 2–3 months (Walton 1986)

c) For progestagen-responsive dermatitis: 50–100 mg IM; may repeat in 3–6 months if needed (Kunkle 1986)

d) To treat recurrent abortion secondary to progesterone-deficiency: 1–2 mg/kg IM once weekly, stop treatment 7–10 days prior to parturition (Barton & Wolf 1988)

For long-term reproductive control:

a) 2.5–5 mg PO once weekly; 25 mg injected every 6 months to postpone estrus (Henik *et al.* 1985)

b) 2 mg/kg IM q5 months (Romagnoli 2002; Romagnoli 2006; Romagnoli 2009)

■ HORSES:

a) Progesterones have been used in horses for many purposes, including management of the spring transition period, prevention of estrus behavior, induction of estrous cycle synchrony, pregnancy maintenance, and modification of stallion behavior. MPA (*Depo-Provera®*) is dosed at about 500 to 800 mg IM. The interval between shots varies between horses. Most injections last 2 to 3 months. This drug will not prevent pregnancy loss and does not stop cyclicity. (Dascanio 2009)

■ BIRDS:

a) As an antipruritic and to suppress ovulation: 0.025–1 mL (3 mg/100 grams body weight) IM once every 4–6 weeks. May cause obesity, fatty liver, polydipsia/polyuria and lethargy if used repeatedly. (Clubb 1986)

Monitoring

■ Weight

■ Blood glucose (draw baseline before therapy)

■ Mammary gland development

■ Adrenocortical function

■ Efficacy

Chemistry/Synonyms

A synthetic progestin, medroxyprogesterone acetate (MPA) occurs as an odorless, white to off-white, crystalline powder. It is insoluble in water and sparingly soluble in alcohol. It has a melting range of 200°–210°C.

Medroxyprogesterone acetate may also be known as: MPA, MAP, acetoxymethylprogesterone, medroxyprogesteroni acetas, methylacetoxyprogesterone, metipregnone, and NSC-26386; many trade names are available.

Storage/Stability

Medroxyprogesterone acetate suspensions for injection should be stored at room temperature (15 – 30°C); avoid freezing and temperatures above 40°C. MPA tablets should be stored in well-closed containers at room temperature.

Dosage Forms/Regulatory Status

VETERINARY-LABELED PRODUCTS: None

HUMAN-LABELED PRODUCTS:

Medroxyprogesterone Acetate Tablets (scored): 2.5 mg, 5 mg & 10 mg; *Provera®* (Pharmacia & Upjohn); generic; (Rx)

Medroxyprogesterone Acetate Injection: 104 mg (160 mg/mL) in 0.65 mL prefilled syringes; 150 mg/mL in 1 mL vials; 400 mg/mL in 2.5 mL & 10 mL vials and 1 mL *U-ject; depo-subQ provera 104®* (Pfizer); *Depo-Provera®* (Pharmacia); generic; (Rx)

References

Barton, C.L. & A.M. Wolf (1988). Disorders of Reproduction. *Handbook of Small Animal Practice.* RV Morgan Ed. New York, Churchill Livingstone: 679–700.

Clubb, S.L. (1986). Therapeutics: Individual and Flock Treatment Regimens. *Clinical Avian Medicine and Surgery.* GJ Harrison and LR Harrison Eds. Philadelphia, W.B. Saunders: 327–355.

Dascanio, J. (2009). Hormonal Control of Reproduction. Proceedings: ABVP. Accessed via: Veterinary Information Network. http://goo.gl/o2vHk

Gee, E.K., P.M. McCue, et al. (2008). Efficacy of medroxyprogesterone acetate in suppression of estrous behavior and follicular activity. *Theriogenology* 70(3): 588–588.

Gorlinger, S., S. Galac, et al. (2005). Hypoluteoidism in a bitch. *Theriogenology* 64(1): 213–219.

Henik, R.A., P.N. Olson, et al. (1985). Progestagen Therapy in Cats. *Comp CE* 7(2): 132–141.

Johnson, C.A. (2008). High-risk pregnancy and hypoluteoidism in the bitch. *Theriogenology* 70(9): 1424–1430.

Kooistra, H. (2006). Growth hormomne disorders in dogs. Proceedings: WSAVA World Congress. Accessed via: Veterinary Information Network. http://goo.gl/qzgGi

Kunkle, G.A. (1986). Progestagens in Dermatology. *Current Veterinary Therapy IX: Small Animal Practice.* RW Kirk Ed. Philadelphia, WB Saunders: 601–605.

Landsberg, G. (2007). Drug and natural alternatives for marking cats. Proceedings: Western Vet Conference. Accessed via: Veterinary Information Network. http://goo.gl/ro1SR

Lane, I. (2006). Update on prostatic disorders. Proceedings: Western Vet Conf. Accessed via: Veterinary Information Network. http://goo.gl/aeEgg

Romagnoli, S. (2002). Clinical use of hormones in the control of reproduction in the bitches and queens. Proceedings: World Small Animal Veterinary Association World Congress. Accessed via: Veterinary Information Network. http://goo.gl/jLusn

Romagnoli, S. (2006). Control of reproduction in dogs and cats: Use and misuse of hormones. Proceedings: WSAVA World Congress. Accessed via: Veterinary Information Network. http://goo.gl/aGuBF

Romagnoli, S. (2009). Non-Surgical Contraception in Dogs and Cats. Proceedings: WSAVA World Congress. Accessed via: Veterinary Information Network. http://goo.gl/ajvCN

Voith, V.L. & A.R. Marder (1988). Canine Behavioral Disorders. *Handbook of Small Animal Practice.* RV Morgan Ed. New York, Churchill Livingstone: 1033–1043.

Walton, D.K. (1986). Psychodermatoses. *Current Veterinary Therapy IX: Small Animal Practice.* RW Kirk Ed. Philadelphia, WB Saunders: 557–559.

MEGESTROL ACETATE

(me-*Jess*-trole)   Ovaban®, Megace®

PROGESTIN

Prescriber Highlights

▶ Synthetic progestin used in *dogs (female):* for postponement of estrus & the alleviation of false pregnancy; *Dogs (male):* benign prostatic hypertrophy. *Cats:* Many dermatologic & behavior-related conditions

▶ Contraindications: Pregnant animals or with uterine disease, diabetes mellitus, or mammary neoplasias; should not be used treat bitches with pseudopregnancy; females should not be treated during diestrus, or with uterine hemorrhage

▶ Caution: Thrombophlebitis

▶ Adverse Effects: *Cats:* Profound adrenocortical suppression, adrenal atrophy, transient diabetes mellitus, polydipsia/polyuria, personality changes, increased weight, endometritis, cystic endometrial hyperplasia, mammary hypertrophy, neoplasias, & hepatotoxicity possible. *Dogs:* Increased appetite & weight gain, lethargy, change in behavior or hair color, mucometra, endometritis, cystic endometrial hyperplasia, mammary enlargement & neoplasia, acromegaly, adrenocortical suppression, or lactation (rare)

Uses/Indications

Megestrol acetate (*Ovaban®*—Schering) is FDA-approved for use in dogs only for the postponement of estrus and the alleviation of false pregnancy. In male dogs, it has been used for benign prostatic hypertrophy. It is used clinically for many dermatologic and behavior-related conditions, primarily in the cat. See the Dosage section for specific indications and dosages for both dogs and cats.

Megestrol acetate is indicated in humans for the palliative treatment of advanced carcinoma of the breast or endometrium.

Pharmacology/Actions

Megestrol acetate possesses the pharmacologic actions expected of the other progestationals discussed (*e.g.*, medroxyprogesterone acetate). It has significant anti-estrogen and glucocorticoid activity (with resultant adrenal suppression). It does not have anabolic or masculinizing effects on the developing fetus.

Pharmacokinetics

Megestrol acetate is well absorbed from the GI tract and appears to be metabolized completely in the liver to conjugates and free steroids.

The half-life of megestrol acetate is reported to be 8 days in the dog.

Contraindications/Precautions/Warnings

Megestrol acetate is contraindicated in pregnant animals or in animals with uterine disease, diabetes mellitus, or mammary neoplasias. It has been recommended that MA not be used in dogs prior to their first estrous cycle or for anestrus therapy in dogs with abnormal cycles. The manufacturer (Schering) recommends that mating be prevented should estrus occur within 30 days of cessation of MA therapy.

This agent should not be used during pregnancy or to treat bitches with pseudo-pregnancy. Females should not be treated during diestrus, or with uterine hemorrhage. Do not use in females with prolonged heat unless cystic ovarian disease is confirmed and surgery or GNRH or hCG are not viable options. Animals with diabetes should not receive megestrol.

Because this drug can suppress adrenal function, exogenous steroids may need to be administered if the patient is stressed (*e.g.,* surgery, trauma).

For estrus control, the manufacturer recommends that drug must be given for the full treatment regimen to be effective. The package insert states that "*Ovaban®* should not be given for more than two consecutive treatments," but the reasons for this are unclear; some theriogenologists question the need for this precaution.

When used for reproductive control, it has been recommended that patients: **1)** undergo a thorough reproductive history to rule out occurrence of estrus within the last 1-2 months (female in diestrus); **2)** complete physical exam; **3)** palpation of mammary glands to rule out mammary nodules; **4)** vaginal smear to rule out presence of estrus (Romagnoli 2002; Romagnoli 2009)

In humans, megestrol acetate is to be used with caution in patients with thrombophlebitis and is contraindicated as a test for pregnancy.

Adverse Effects

In cats, megestrol acetate can induce a profound adrenocortical suppression, adrenal atrophy, and an iatrogenic "Addison's" syndrome can develop at "standard" dosages (2.5–5 mg every other day) within 1-2 weeks. Once the drug has been discontinued, serum cortisol levels (both resting and ACTH-stimulated) will return to normal levels within a few weeks. Clinical signs of adrenocortical insufficiency (*e.g.,* vomiting, lethargy) are uncommon, but exogenous steroid support should be considered if the animal is stressed (surgery, trauma, etc.). Cats may develop a transient diabetes mellitus while receiving MA. Polydipsia/polyuria, personality changes, increased weight, endometritis, cystic endometrial hyperplasia, mammary hypertrophy and neoplasias may also occur. Increased appetite and weight gain is not consistently seen, but MA is occasionally used as an appetite stimulant. Rarely, megestrol acetate can cause hepatotoxicity (increased alkaline phosphatase) in cats. Megestrol potentially can exacerbate latent viral infections (*e.g.,* FHV-1).

Limited clinical studies have suggested that megestrol acetate may cause less cystic endometrial hyperplasia than other progestational agents, but cautious use and vigilant monitoring is still warranted.

In dogs, increased appetite and weight gain, lethargy, change in behavior or hair color, mucometra, endometritis, cystic endometrial hyperplasia, mammary enlargement and neoplasia, acromegaly, adrenocortical suppression or lactation (rare) may occur. One dog reportedly developed diabetes mellitus after use.

Reproductive/Nursing Safety

No effects were noted in either the bitch or litter when pregnant dogs received 0.25 mg/kg/day for 32 days during the first half of pregnancy; reduced litter sizes and puppy survival were detected when the dose was given during the last half of pregnancy. Fetal hypospadias are possible if progestational agents are administered during pregnancy.

During the *first 4 months of pregnancy* in humans, the FDA categorizes this drug as category *X* for use during pregnancy (*Studies in animals or humans demonstrate fetal abnormalities or adverse reaction; reports indicate evidence of fetal risk. The risk of use in pregnant women clearly outweighs any possible benefit.*) During the *last 5 months* of pregnancy in humans, the FDA categorizes this drug as category *D* for use during pregnancy (*There is evidence of human fetal risk, but the potential benefits from the use of the drug in pregnant women may be acceptable despite its potential risks.*)

Detectable amounts of progestins enter the milk of mothers receiving these agents. Effects on nursing infants have not been established.

Overdosage/Acute Toxicity

No information was located regarding acute overdosage of megestrol acetate. In humans, dosages of up to 800 mg/day caused no observable adverse reactions.

Toxicity studies performed in dogs at dosages of 0.1–0.25 mg/kg/day PO for 36 months yielded no gross abnormalities in the study population. Histologically, cystic endometrial hyperplasia was noted at 36 months, but resolved when therapy was discontinued. At dosages of 0.5 mg/kg/day PO for 5 months, a reversible uterine hyperplasia was seen in treated dogs. Dosages of 2 mg/kg/day demonstrated early cystic endometritis in biopsies done on dogs at 64 days.

Drug Interactions

■ **CORTICOSTEROIDS:** Megestrol used with corticosteroids (long-term) may exacerbate adrenocortical suppression and diabetes mellitus.

■ **RIFAMPIN:** May decrease progestin activity if administered concomitantly. This is presumably due to microsomal enzyme induction with resultant increase in progestin metabolism. The clinical significance of this potential interaction is unknown.

Doses

■ **DOGS:**

For estrus control:

a) To halt cycle in proestrus: 2.2 mg/kg once daily for 8 days starting during the first 3 days of proestrus. While the timing of the next cycle is variable, it may be prolonged with 2.2 mg/kg/day for 4 days, then 0.55 mg/kg/day for 16–20 days.

To postpone an anticipated cycle: 0.55 mg/kg/day for 32 days, beginning at least 7 days prior to proestrus (Burke 1985)

b) For suppression during proestrus (first 3 days): 2.2 mg/kg once daily for 8 days (92% efficacy). Bitch must be controlled until behavioral signs of estrus disappear. If mating occurs during first 3 days of therapy, stop treatment and consider mismating therapy. There is an increased likelihood of pyometra developing if progestins are used concomitantly with estrogens. If mating occurs after 3 or more days of therapy continue at a dosage rate of 3–4 mg/kg PO.

To delay an anticipated heat during anestrus: 0.55 mg/kg PO for 32 days initiated 7 days prior to proestrus. Recommend doing vaginal cytology prior to therapy. If no erythrocytes are seen, initiate therapy if cycle time frame is appropriate. If erythrocytes are seen, delay therapy until proestrus therapy can be instituted. Do not repeat therapy more often than once every 6 months. (Woody 1989)

c) 2 mg/kg (or less) administered for <2 weeks in proestrus, or <2 mg/kg administered for a longer duration in anestrus. A typical dose for estrus suppression is 2 mg/kg PO once daily for 8 consecutive days, while a typical dose for temporary postponement is 0.5 mg/kg PO once daily in late anestrus. (Romagnoli 2002; Romagnoli 2006; Romagnoli 2009)

For benign prostatic hypertrophy:

a) 0.5 mg/kg PO daily for 4–8 weeks (Root Kustritz & Klausner 2000)

b) 0.55 mg/kg PO daily (Purswell 1999)

c) 0.1–0.5 mg/kg per day for 3–8 weeks; best used to maintain breeding potential for short time prior to castration; use with caution. (Lane 2006)

For pseudocyesis (false pregnancy):

a) 0.5 mg/kg PO once daily for 8 days (Barton & Wolf 1988)

To prevent vaginal hyperplasia development:

a) 2.2 mg/kg PO for 7 days early in proestrus (Wykes 1986)

For treatment of severe galactorrhea:

a) 0.55 mg/kg PO once daily for 7 days (Olson & Olson 1986)

For behavior disorders:

a) For adjunctive treatment of aggressive or unacceptable masculine behavior: 1.1–2.2 mg/kg PO once daily for 2 weeks, then 0.5–1.1 mg/kg once daily for 2 weeks. Should be used with behavior modification. (Voith & Marder 1988)

■ **CATS:**

For suppression of estrus:

a) In anestrus: 5 mg/cat PO every 2 weeks or 2.5 mg/cat per week (better if divided into 2 doses given every 3.5 days); In proestrus: 5 mg/cat per day for 4 days, then 5 mg PO every 2 weeks. (Romagnoli 2006; Romagnoli 2009)

b) If in behavioral estrus, signs may be inhibited by giving 5 mg/day PO until estrus stops (generally within 3–5 days), then 2.5–5 mg PO once weekly for 10 weeks

Postponement of estrus (if started during diestrus): 2.5 mg PO daily for 8 weeks

Postponement of estrus (if started during anestrus): 2.5 mg PO once weekly for up to 18 months. Recommend allowing cat to have a cycle (unmedicated) before beginning another treatment cycle. (Woody 1989)

c) If started in diestrus: 2.5 mg per day PO for up to 2 months

If started in anestrus: 2.5 mg per week for up to 18 months

For prevention of estrus: 5 mg daily PO for 3 days as soon as behavioral signs of estrus are seen; next estrus period will occur in approximately 4 weeks (Romatowski 1989) (information from package insert; *Ovarid®*—Glaxovet)

For treatment of idiopathic feline miliary dermatitis:

a) 2.5–5 mg once every other day, followed by weekly maintenance dosages. May be necessary to treat for animal's lifetime. Reserve use for severe cases; explain risks to owner and do not exceed 2.5 mg per week during maintenance phase. (Kwochka 1986)

As appetite stimulant:

a) 0.25–0.5 mg/kg q24h for 3–5 days, then q48–72h (Smith 2003)

As an alternative treatment for immune-mediated skin diseases:

a) 2.5–5 mg PO once daily for 10 days, then every other day (Giger & Werner 1989)

For adjunctive therapy of eosinophilic granulomas:

a) 0.5 mg/kg PO once daily for 2 weeks, then twice weekly as needed (Coppoc 1988)

For eosinophilic ulcers:

a) Alone or in combination with methyl-prednisolone acetate (*Depo-Medrol®*): 5–10 mg PO every other day for 10–14 doses, then every 2 weeks as needed (De-Novo *et al.* 1989)

As a "last ditch" (because of potential side effects) alternative for treating feline atopy:

a) Remission of clinical signs can often be achieved with an oral dose of 2.5–5 mg per cat PO every 48 hours for 1-3 weeks. This dose is then used once weekly. (Rosychuk 2007)

For feline plasma cell gingivitis:

a) 2.5 mg PO once daily for 10 days, then once every other day for 5 treatments, then as needed (Morgan 1988)

As a secondary therapy (thyroid hormone replacement first choice) for treatment of feline endocrine alopecia (FEA):

a) 5 mg PO every second to third day initially, then 2.5 mg PO once to twice weekly (Thoday 1986)

For feline psychogenic alopecia and dermatitis:

a) 2.5–5 mg every other day initially, then taper to the lowest maintenance dosage possible, given weekly as needed (Walton 1986)

For adjunctive therapy (with urine acidification, increased urine crystalloid solubility, and antispasmodics if required) for persistent hematuria and urethritis in a non-obstructed cat:

a) 2.5–5 mg PO once daily to every other day (with prednisone: 2.5–5 mg PO daily) (Lage *et al.* 1988)

For urine marking, intraspecies aggression, anxiety:

a) 2 mg/kg/day for 5 days, then 1 mg/kg/day for 5 days, then 0.5 mg/kg/day for 5 days (Romatowski 1989) (information from package inserts; *Ovarid®*—Glaxovet)

b) To reduce marking in neutered male cats when all other drugs have been unsuccessful: megestrol acetate at 2.5–10 mg (total dose) per cat PO daily for one week, then reduce to once or twice weekly. (Landsberg 2007)

c) 5 mg per cat once daily for 2 weeks, then wean to lowest effective maintenance

dose. Has poor efficacy in neutered males (50%) and spayed females (10%); many potential adverse effects. (Levine 2008)

Monitoring

- ■ Weight
- ■ Blood glucose (draw baseline before therapy)
- ■ Mammary gland development and appearance
- ■ Adrenocortical function
- ■ Liver enzymes if long-term treatment
- ■ Efficacy

Client Information

- ■ The client should fully understand the potential risks of therapy (see Adverse Effects above) before starting therapy and should report changes in mammary glands or other signs associated with adverse reactions (*e.g.*, PU/PD, extreme lethargy, behavior changes, etc.) to the veterinarian.

Chemistry/Synonyms

A synthetic progestin, megestrol acetate (MA) occurs as an essentially odorless, tasteless, white to creamy white, crystalline powder that is insoluble in water, sparingly soluble in alcohol, and slightly soluble in fixed oils. It has a melting range of 213°–219°C over a 3° range and a specific rotation of +8° to +12°.

Megestrol acetate may also be known as: BDH-1298, compound 5071, megestroli acetas, NSC-71423, SC-10363, *Acestrol®*, *Borea®*, *Endace®*, *Gynodal®*, *Maygace®*, *Megace®*, *Megastrol®*, *Megefren®*, *Megestat®*, *Megestil®*, *Megestin®*, *Megostat®*, *Meltonar®*, *Meprogest®*, *Mestrel®*, *Nia®*, *Niagestin®*, *Niagestine®*, *Ovaban®*, *Prazoken®*, and *Varigestrol®*.

Storage/Stability

Megestrol acetate tablets should be stored in well-closed containers at a temperature of less than 40°C. The tablets may be crushed and administered with food. The veterinary manufacturer recommends storing the tablets from 2°–30°C (36°–86°F).

Dosage Forms/Regulatory Status

VETERINARY-LABELED PRODUCTS:

Megestrol Acetate Oral Tablets: 5 mg, 20 mg; available in bottles of 250 and 500 tablets, and in 30 foil strips of 8 and packaged in cartons of 240 tablets; *Ovaban®* (Schering-Plough); (Rx). FDA-approved for use in dogs only.

HUMAN-LABELED PRODUCTS:

Megestrol Acetate Tablets: 20 mg & 40 mg; *Megace®* (Bristol-Meyers Oncology); generic; (Rx)

Megestrol Acetate Suspension: 40 mg/mL in 240 mL & 125 mg/mL in 150 mL; *Megace®* (Bristol-Meyers Oncology); *Megace ES®* (Par Pharmaceutical Inc); (Rx)

References

Barton, C.L. & A.M. Wolf (1988). Disorders of Reproduction. *Handbook of Small Animal Practice.* RV Morgan Ed. New York, Churchill Livingstone: 679–700.

Burke, T.J. (1985). Reproductive Disorders. *Handbook of Small Animal Therapeutics.* LE Davis Ed. New York, Churchill Livingstone: 605–616.

Coppoc, G.L. (1988). Chemotherapy of neoplastic diseases. *Veterinary Pharmacology and Therapeutics.* NH Booth and LE McDonald Eds. Ames, Iowa State University Press: 861–876.

DeNovo, R.C., K.A. Potter, et al. (1989). Diseases of the oral cavity and pharynx. *Handbook of Small Animal Practice.* RV Morgan Ed. New York, Churchill Livingstone: 327–345.

Giger, U. & L.L. Werner (1989). Immune-Mediated Diseases. *Handbook of Small Animal Practice.* RV Morgan Ed. New York, Churchill Livingstone: 841–860.

Kwochka, K.W. (1986). Differential diagnosis of feline miliary dermatitis. *Current Veterinary Therapy (CVT) IX Small Animal Practice.* RW Kirk Ed. Philadelphia, W.B. Saunders: 538–544.

Lage, A.L., D. Polzin, et al. (1988). Diseases of the Bladder. *Handbook of Small Animal Practice.* RV Morgan Ed. New York, Churchill Livingstone: 605–620.

Landsberg, G. (2007). Drug and natural alternatives for marking cats. Proceedings: Western Vet Conference. Accessed via: Veterinary Information Network. http://goo.gl/ro1SR

Lane, I. (2006). Update on prostatic disorders. Proceedings: Western Vet Conf. Accessed via: Veterinary Information Network. http://goo.gl/aeEgg

Levine, E. (2008). Feline fear and anxiety. *Veterinary Clinics Small Animal* 38: 1065–1079.

Morgan, R.V., Ed. (1988). *Handbook of Small Animal Practice.* New York, Churchill Livingstone.

Olson, J.D. & P.N. Olson (1986). Disorders of the canine mammary gland. *Current Therapy in Theriogenology 2: Diagnosis, Treatment and Prevention of Reproductive Diseases in Small and Large Animals.* DA Morrow Ed. Philadelphia, WB Saunders: 506–509.

Purswell, B. (1999). Pharmaceuticals used in canine theriogenology–Part 1 & 2. Proceedings: Central Veterinary Conference, Kansas City.

Romagnoli, S. (2002). Clinical use of hormones in the control of reproduction in the bitches and queens. Proceedings: World Small Animal Veterinary Association World Congress. Accessed via: Veterinary Information Network. http://goo.gl/jLusn

Romagnoli, S. (2006). Control of reproduction in dogs and cats: Use and misuse of hormones. Proceedings: WSAVA World Congress. Accessed via: Veterinary Information Network. http://goo.gl/aGuBF

Romagnoli, S. (2009). Non-Surgical Contraception in Dogs and Cats. Proceedings: WSAVA World Congress. Accessed via: Veterinary Information Network. http://goo.gl/ajvCN

Root Kustritz, M. & J. Klausner (2000). Prostatic Diseases. *Textbook of Veterinary Internal Medicine: Diseases of the Dog and Cat.* S Ettinger and E Feldman Eds. Philadelphia, WB Saunders. 2: 1687–1698.

Rosychuk, R. (2007). Dermatologic Diseases of the Head–Part I. Proceedings: AAFP. Accessed via: Veterinary Information Network. http://goo.gl/5fg7d

Smith, A. (2003). Special concerns in cat chemotherapy. Proceedings: ACVIM Forum. Accessed via: Veterinary Information Network. http://goo.gl/dnmJ3

Thoday, K.L. (1986). Differential diagnosis of symetric alopecia in the cat. *Current Veterinary Therapy IX: Small Animal Practice.* RV Kirk Ed. Philadelphia, WB Saunders: 545–553.

Voith, V.L. & A.R. Marder (1988). Canine Behavioral Disorders. *Handbook of Small Animal Practice.* RV Morgan Ed. New York, Churchill Livingstone: 1033–1043.

Walton, D.K. (1986). Psychodermatoses. *Current Veterinary Therapy IX: Small Animal Practice.* RW Kirk Ed. Phialdelphia, WB Saunders: 557–559.

Woody, B.J. (1989). Prevention of estrus and pregnancy. *Handbook of Small Animal Practice.* RV Morgan Ed. New York, Churchill Livingstone: 701–705.

Wykes, P.M. (1986). Diseases of the vagina and vulva in the bitch. *Current Therapy in Theriogenology 2: Diagnosis, Treatment and Prevention of Reproductive Diseases in Small and Large Animals.* DA Morrow Ed. Philadelphia, WB Saunders: 476–481.

MEGLUMINE ANTIMONIATE

(*meg*-loo-meen an-tih-*mohne*-ee-ate)

Glucantime®, Gulcantim®

PENTAVALENT ANTIMONY ANTILEISHMANIAL

Prescriber Highlights

▶ Pentavalent antimony compound used for treating leishmaniasis (with or without allopurinol) in dogs

▶ Not available in USA

▶ Extreme caution (relatively contraindicated) in patients with cardiac, hepatic or renal insufficiency

▶ Primary adverse effects noted in dogs with meglumine antimoniate are injection site reactions, lethargy & gastrointestinal effects (inappetence, vomiting)

▶ Resistance to treatment has been reported

▶ Treatment is prolonged & cost may be substantial

Uses/Indications

Meglumine antimoniate is used alone or in combination with allopurinol to treat leishmaniasis in dogs. It is available commercially in some Mediterranean and South American countries but not in the USA.

Pharmacology/Actions

Pentavalent antimony compounds such as meglumine antimoniate and sodium stibogluconate selectively inhibit the leishmanial enzymes required for glycolytic and fatty acid oxidation. Pentavalent antimony compounds rarely are successful in eradicating *Leishmania* organisms completely in infected dogs. When used with allopurinol, synergy for treating leishmaniasis and reduced risk for antimonial drug-resistance development may occur.

Pharmacokinetics

After subcutaneous or intramuscular injections in dogs systemic bioavailability is about 92%; highest tissue concentrations are found in the liver, spleen, and skin. Within 9 hours of dosing, 80% of the antimony is excreted in the urine. Reduced renal function can cause increased antimoniate half-lives.

Contraindications/Precautions/Warnings

Patients with renal, hepatic or cardiac failure are more likely to develop serious adverse effects with this agent; weigh the potential risks versus benefits carefully before treating. Decreased renal function in particular, may lead to drug accumulation and an increased risk for toxicity. In dogs with severe renal failure (IRIS stages III-IV) the correction of fluid and acid-base imbalances prior to treatment with allopurinol alone has been recommended (Koutinas & Koutinas 2007).

Hypersensitivity reactions have been reported in people, and any patient with previous hypersensitivity to meglumine antimoniate should not receive the drug.

Adverse Effects

Primary adverse effects noted in dogs are injection site reactions (cutaneous abscesses/cellulitis), lethargy, and gastrointestinal effects (inappetence, vomiting). Transient increases in liver enzymes have been reported.

Potentially, the drug may be nephrotoxic in dogs, but this is difficult to evaluate in clinically-infected dogs as renal dysfunction is one of the likely consequences of the infection. A study done in healthy dogs showed diffuse proximal tubule cell vacuolization and multifocal areas with coagulative necrosis under light microscopy. Electron microscopy showed reduced organellar content, loss or attenuation of brush border, cellular detachment from the basement membrane, apical blebbing and individual cell necrosis. The authors concluded that meglumine antimoniate caused severe tubular damage (Brovida *et al.* 2009).

Drug resistance may occur. After several courses of treatment, decreased sensitivity of *L. infantum* to meglumine antimoniate or antimonials has been reported.

In humans, increased serum lipase, amylase, creatinine, urea nitrogen, and increased QT interval on ECG, have been reported. Occasionally, decreases in white blood cell counts and hemoglobin have been reported in humans.

Reproductive/Nursing Safety

There is limited information available. Pregnant rats given up to 300 mg/kg on days 6–15 caused increased fetal resorptions and increased rates of abnormalities of the atlas bone. Weigh the risks versus benefits when deciding to treat during pregnancy. It is unknown if the drug enters maternal milk.

Overdosage/Acute Toxicity

No specific overdose information was located. Depending on the dosage, a single overdose could potentially cause renal, hepatic, pancreatic, and hematologic effects, but gastrointestinal effects (vomiting) and lethargy would be the most likely outcomes. It is recommended to observe the patient and contact an animal poison control center for further guidance with an overdose situation.

Drug Interactions

The following drug interactions have either been reported or are theoretical in humans or animals receiving meglumine antimoniate and may be of significance in veterinary patients (dogs):

■ **AGENTS THAT CAN PROLONG QT INTERVAL (e.g., tricyclic antidepressants, disopyramide, quinidine, procainamide, etc.):** meglumine antimoniate may prolong QT interval further with increased risk for arrhythmias

Laboratory Considerations

■ No specific laboratory interactions or considerations noted

Doses

■ **DOGS:**

For leishmaniasis:

a) As first line treatment: meglumine antimoniate at 75–100 mg/kg SC once daily for 4–8 weeks, with allopurinol (10 mg/kg PO twice daily for at least 6–12 months. (Solano-Gallego *et al.* 2009)

b) Meglumine antimoniate at a minimum dosage of 100 mg/kg SC daily for 3–4 weeks; better results are obtained with longer durations (4–6 weeks) of treatment. Protocol with allopurinol may reduce relapse rates: meglumine antimoniate as above with allopurinol at 20–40 mg/kg PO daily for a minimum of 3 weeks. Followed with long-term treatment with allopurinol (alone) at 20–40 mg/kg PO daily or intermittently (one week treatment per month). (Noli & Auxilia 2005)

c) Meglumine antimoniate (100 mg/kg/day SC) until resolution; with allopurinol at 20 mg/kg PO q12h for 9 months. (Brosey 2005)

Monitoring

■ Efficacy (PCR preferred)

■ CBC (baseline and periodic)

■ Liver enzymes; renal function tests (serum creatinine, BUN); serum lipase and amylase (baseline and periodic)

■ Urinalysis (baseline and periodic)

Client Information

■ Clients should understand that treatment with this drug can be prolonged and expensive, and that a "cure" (complete eradication) is unlikely

Chemistry/Synonyms

Meglumine antimoniate is 1-Deoxy-1-methylamino-D-glucitol antimoniate. It has a molecular weight of 366. One gram contains approximately 272 mg of antimony.

Meglumine antimoniate may also be known as: meglumine antimonate, N-methylglucamine antimoniate, RP-2168, antimony meglumine, Protostib, 1-Deoxy-1-methylamino-D-glucitol antimoniate, *Glucantime*® and *Glucantim*®.

Storage/Stability

Unless otherwise specified by the manufacturer, commercially available ampules should be stored below 40°C, preferably between 15°–30°C; protect from freezing.

Dosage Forms/Regulatory Status

VETERINARY-LABELED PRODUCTS: None in the USA.

May be available via the CDC, see: http://www.cdc.gov/ncidod/srp/drugs/drug-service.html

HUMAN-LABELED PRODUCTS: None in the USA

Meglumine antimoniate may be available in several countries, including Brazil, Venezuela, and in Europe; trade names include: *Glucantime®* and *Glucantim®*. Commercially it is available as a solution containing 1.5 grams of meglumine antimoniate (425 mg pentavalent antimony) per 5 mL.

The FDA may allow legal importation of this medication for compassionate use in animals; for more information, see the *Instructions for Legally Importing Drugs for Compassionate Use in the USA* found in the appendix.

References

Brosey, B. (2005). Leishmaniasis. Proceedings: ACVIM 2005. Accessed via: Veterinary Information Network. http://goo.gl/qQ0Yr

Brovida, C., P. Bianciardi, et al. (2009). Evaluation of Nephrotoxic Effects of Miltefosine and Meglumine Antimonate in 8 Healthy Beagles. Proceedings: ECVIM. Accessed via: Veterinary Information Network. http://goo.gl/n9S6x

Koutinas, A. & C. Koutinas (2007). Renal function in canine leishmaniasis. Proceedings: ECVIM. Accessed via: Veterinary Information Network. http://goo.gl/MrZ0T

Noli, C. & S. Auxilia (2005). Review: Treatment of canine Old World visceral leishmaniasis: a systematic review. *Vet Dermatology* **16**: 213–232.

Solano-Gallego, L., A. Koutinas, et al. (2009). Directions for the diagnosis, clinical staging, treatment and prevention of canine leishmaniosis. *Veterinary Parasitology* **165**(1–2): 1–18.

MELARSOMINE

(mee-*lar*-soe-meen)   Immiticide®

ARSENICAL ANTIPARASITIC

Prescriber Highlights

▶ Organic arsenical for heartworm disease

▶ Contraindications: Class IV (very severe) heartworm disease; weigh risk vs. potential benefits in pregnant, lactating, or breeding dogs

▶ Reportedly very toxic to cats; not currently recommended

▶ Adverse Effects: Many possible, most common are: Injection site reactions coughing/gagging, depression/lethargy, anorexia/inappetence, excessive salivation, fever, lung congestion, vomiting, pulmonary thromboembolism

▶ Special IM injection technique; do not give IV or SC

▶ Avoid human exposure

▶ Calculate dosages very carefully

▶ Strict cage rest after treatment recommended

Uses/Indications

Melarsomine is indicated for the treatment of stabilized class I, II, and III heartworm disease caused by immature (4 month old, stage L$_5$) to mature adult infections of *D. immitis* in dogs. When compared with thiacetarsamide, melarsomine appears to be more efficacious, less irritating to tissues, and does not cause hepatic necrosis.

At the time of writing (2010) there is considerable interest in using ivermectin or another macrocyclic lactone with doxycycline for several months prior to melarsomine adulticide therapy. Ivermectin can kill *D. immitis* larval stages 3 & 4, kill microfilaria, and reduce lifespan of adult heartworms. Doxycycline treatment can potentially reduce adult worm populations by eliminating *Wolbachia*, a bacterium associated with *D. immitis*. The American Heartworm Society has stated; "…it is beneficial to administer a macrocyclic lactone for up to three months prior to administration of melarsomine, when the clinical presentation does not demand immediate intervention" and "Doxycycline administered at 10 mg/kg twice daily for four weeks has been shown to eliminate over 90% of the *Wolbachia* organisms and the levels remain low for three to four months." (American-Heartworm-Society 2010)

Melarsomine may also be useful for treating ferrets; it has been suggested to contact the manufacturer before using the drug in this species.

Pharmacology/Actions

While melarsomine is an arsenical compound, its exact mechanism of action is not known. Both laboratory and field studies have demonstrated that melarsomine is 90−99% effective in killing adult and L5 larvae of *D. immitis* in dogs at recommended dosages.

Pharmacokinetics

Melarsomine is reportedly rapidly absorbed after IM injection in dogs; time to peak plasma concentration is about 11 minutes. The apparent volume of distribution is about 0.7 L/kg; terminal half-life is approximately 3 hours.

Contraindications/Precautions/Warnings

Melarsomine is contraindicated in dogs with class IV (very severe) heartworm disease. Class IV is having caval syndrome (heartworms present in venae cavae and right atrium). Melarsomine is reportedly very toxic to cats and its use cannot be recommended for this species at this time.

Older dogs (>8 years) may be more susceptible to adverse effects than younger dogs.

Do NOT give IV or SC; significant toxicity or tissue damage may occur. Administer only deep IM as directed (lumbar epaxial muscles (L3-L5). Do not administer at any other site.

While all dogs with heartworm disease are at risk for post-treatment pulmonary thromboembolism, those with severe pulmonary artery disease are at increased risk for post treatment morbidity and mortality. Strict exercise restriction after administration can decrease the severity associated with thromboembolic events. Cage rest (2-4 weeks) in the veterinary clinic is recommended if feasible. If clinic cage rest and observation are not possible, owners should be advised that unless the patient's exercise is restricted, thrombolic events are more likely and can be fatal. Wash hands after use or wear gloves. Avoid drug contact with animal's eyes; if exposed wash with copious amounts of water. Avoid human exposure. If human exposure occurs, contact a physician.

Adverse Effects

Approximately ⅓ of dogs show signs of injection site reactions (pain, swelling, tenderness, reluctance to move) after receiving melarsomine. Most of these signs resolve within weeks, but, rarely, severe injection reactions can occur. Firm nodules at the injection site can persist indefinitely. SC or IV injections must be avoided. The most severe local reactions are usually seen if the drug leaks back from the injection site into subcutaneous tissues. Applying firm pressure to the injection site after administration may reduce the risk for this problem.

Other reactions reported in 5% or more dogs treated include: coughing/gagging (22% incidence; average day of onset after treatment = 10); depression/lethargy (15% incidence; average day of onset after treatment = 5); anorexia/inappetence (13% incidence; average day of onset after treatment = 5); fever (7%); lung congestion (6%); vomiting (5%). There is significant interpatient variance in both the date of onset and duration for the above effects. Dogs may also exhibit excessive salivation after dosing.

There are a plethora of other adverse effects in dogs with reported incidences less than 3%, including paresis and paralysis. Refer to the package insert for specifics.

Animals not exhibiting adverse effects after the first dose or course of therapy may demonstrate them after the second dose or course of therapy.

Reproductive/Nursing Safety

Safety has not been established for use in pregnant, lactating, or breeding dogs. Risks versus potential benefits of therapy should be weighed before use.

Overdosage/Acute Toxicity

There is low margin of safety with melarsomine dosages. A 3X dose (7.5 mg/kg) in healthy dogs have demonstrated respiratory inflammation and distress, excessive salivation, restlessness, panting, vomiting, edema, tremors, lethargy, ataxia, cyanosis, stupor, and death. Signs of diarrhea, excessive salivation, restlessness, panting, vomiting, and fever have been noted in infected dogs that have received inadvertent overdoses (2X).

Treatment with dimercaprol (BAL in Oil) may be considered to treat melarsomine overdoses. Clinical efficacy of melarsomine may be reduced, however.

Drug Interactions

The manufacturer reports that during clinical field trials, melarsomine was given to dogs receiving antiinflammatory agents, antibiotics, insecticides, heartworm prophylactic medications, and various other drugs commonly used to stabilize and support dogs with heartworm disease and that no adverse drug interactions were noted.

■ **ASPIRIN:** Has been shown not to reduce adverse effects and may complicate therapy; use is not recommended

■ **CNS DEPRESSANT DRUGS:** Drugs that have similar adverse effects (*e.g.*, depression caused by CNS depressants, etc.) may cause additive adverse effects or increase their incidence when used with melarsomine

Doses

CAUTION: Because of the low margin of safety; calculate dosages very carefully. Do not confuse mg/lb with mg/kg!

■ **DOGS:**

For treatment of dirofilariasis it is suggested to review the guidelines published by the American Heartworm Society at www.heartwormsociety.org for more information.

Immiticide® (Merial) product support phone number: 888-637-4251

For treatment of heartworm disease:

a) After diagnosis, determine the class (stage) of the disease. **Note:** The manufacturer provides worksheets that assist in the classification and treatment regime determination. It is highly recommended to use these treatment records to avoid confusion and document therapy.

Class I, & II: 2.5 mg/kg deep IM as directed (lumbar epaxial muscles (L3-L5) twice 24 hours apart and rest. Use alternating sides with each administration. In 4 months, the regimen may be repeated.

Class III: 2.5 mg/kg deep IM as directed (lumbar epaxial muscles (L3-L5). Strict rest and give all necessary systemic treatment. One month later, give 2.5 mg/kg deep IM as directed (lumbar epaxial muscles (L3-L5) twice 24 hours apart.

Note: Recommended needle size for dogs 10 kg or less = 23 gauge 1 inch; 10 kg or more body weight = 22 gauge 1.5 inch. (Package Insert; *Immiticide*®—Merial)

b) The three-injection alternative protocol 2.5 mg/kg deep IM as directed (lumbar epaxial muscles; L3-L5). Strict rest and give all necessary systemic treatment. One month later, give 2.5 mg/kg deep IM as directed (lumbar epaxial muscles; L3-L5) twice 24 hours apart] is the treatment of choice of the American Heartworm Society and several university teaching hospitals, regardless of stage of disease, due to the increased safety and efficacy benefits and subsequently fewer dogs that require further treatment with melarsomine. (American Heartworm Society; www. heartwormsociety.org; accessed 2010)

Monitoring/Client Information
- Clinical efficacy
- Adverse effects; dogs should be observed for 24 hours after the last injection
- Strict exercise restriction after dosing is extremely important
- Because of the seriousness of the disease and the potential for morbidity and mortality associated with the treatment, clients should give informed consent before electing to treat.

Chemistry/Synonyms
An organic arsenical compound, melarsomine dihydrochloride has a molecular weight of 501 and is freely soluble in water.

Melarsomine may also be known as *Immiticide*®. Its CAS registry is 128470-15-5.

Storage/Stability/Preparation
The unreconstituted powder should be stored upright at room temperature. Once reconstituted, the solution should be kept in the origi-

nal container and kept refrigerated for up to 24 hours. Do not freeze. Do not mix with any other drug.

Reconstitute with 2 mL of the diluent provided (sterile water for injection) with a resultant concentration of 25 mg/mL. Once reconstituted, the solution should be kept in the original container and kept refrigerated for up to 24 hours. Do not freeze.

Dosage Forms/Regulatory Status
VETERINARY-LABELED PRODUCTS:

Melarsomine Dihydrochloride Powder for Injection: 50 mg/vial; *Immiticide*® (Merial); (Rx). FDA-approved for use in dogs.

HUMAN-LABELED PRODUCTS: None

References
American-Heartworm-Society (2010). "Canine Guidlines." 2010, http://www.heartwormsociety.org/veterinary-resources/canine-guidelines.html#9.

MELATONIN

(mel-a-*tone*-in)   Regulin®

HORMONE

Prescriber Highlights

▶ Oral & implantable pineal gland hormone

▶ Potential uses include: As a reversible estrus suppression agent in cats, treatment of alopecia in dogs, sleep & behavior disorders in cats & dogs, adjust seasonally controlled fertility in sheep, goats, & horses, & adjunctive treatment for adrenal disease in ferrets

▶ Adverse effects appear to be minimal, but little experience

▶ Potential contraindications include: Pregnancy, sexually immature animals, & liver dysfunction

Uses/Indications
Melatonin may be useful to treat Alopecia-X in Nordic breeds, canine pattern baldness, or canine recurrent flank alopecia in dogs. It has been used anecdotally for the treatment of sleep cycle disorders in cats and geriatric dogs and to treat phobias and separation anxiety in dogs. Melatonin implants are used in the mink and fox pelt industries to promote the development of luxurious hair coats. Implants are also used to improve early breeding and ovulation rates in sheep and goats. Preliminary research is being done for this purpose in horses also. Preliminary evidence suggests that melatonin implants (18 mg) can provide short-term estrus control in cats. Melatonin may also have beneficial effects in treating hyperadrenocorticism, some types of hepatopathies, and colitis.

In pigs, one study (Bubenik, Ayles et al. 1998) demonstrated that 5 mg/kg in feed reduced the incidence of gastric ulcers in young pigs.

Pharmacology/Actions

Melatonin is involved with the neuroendocrine control of photoperiod dependent molting, hair growth and pelage color. Melatonin stimulates winter coat growth and spring shedding occurs when melatonin decreases. The mechanism of how melatonin induces these effects is not well understood. It may have direct effects on the hair follicle or alter the secretion of prolactin and/or melanocyte stimulating hormone.

Melatonin also increases serum prolactin levels, growth hormone, and increases response to growth hormone releasing hormone. Long-term use may decrease luteinizing hormone. Melatonin is also ostensibly a free radical scavenger.

Pharmacokinetics

No specific information was located.

Contraindications/Precautions/Warnings

Melatonin implants are considered contraindicated in pregnant or sexually immature animals. There are very specific times for administration depending on latitude, hemisphere, and breed. Animals that are nursing young may not benefit from implant therapy.

In humans, melatonin is considered contraindicated in patients with hepatic insufficiency as it is cleared hepatically. Use with caution in patients with renal impairment. Because of its CNS depressant qualities, melatonin is sometimes stated that it should be used with caution in patients with a history of cerebrovascular disease, depression or neurological disorders.

Adverse Effects

Melatonin appears to be quite safe in dogs. Side effects in dogs when given orally are rare but the hormone may cause sedation, and affect sex hormone secretion and fertility. Subcutaneous implants in dogs have been associated with sterile abscesses.

Adverse effects in ferrets have not been reported.

Adverse effects reported in humans include altered sleep patterns, hypothermia, sedation, tachycardia, confusion, headache, and pruritus.

Reproductive/Nursing Safety

No information was located; use with caution.

Overdosage/Acute Toxicity

Little information is available; unlikely to cause significant morbidity after a single overdose.

Drug Interactions

The following drug interactions have either been reported or are theoretical in humans or animals receiving melatonin and may be of significance in veterinary patients:

- ◼ **BENZODIAZEPINES:** Melatonin may potentiate effects

- ◼ **SUCCINYLCHOLINE:** Melatonin may potentiate effects

Laboratory Considerations

- ◼ Melatonin can reduce cortisol and estradiol levels

Doses

- ◼ **DOGS:**

  For dermatologic conditions:

  a) For experimental treatment of Alopecia-X in Nordic breeds, canine pattern baldness, or canine recurrent flank alopecia: Empirical dose of one to four 12 mg implants SC. Retreatment may be necessary once or twice a year. If implants are unavailable, oral melatonin at 3–6 mg every 8–12 hours may be tried. Although appears to be safe, recommend having owners sign a release form noting the "experimental" nature of treatment. (Paradis 2000)

  b) For treatment of canine recurrent flank alopecia or seasonal flank alopecia: 2–3 mg per dog PO once daily for 3–5 days weekly or monthly or this as a daily dose. Doses of up to 10 mg per dog have used. Improvement is usually seen in one month with maximal improvement in 3 months. (Merchant 2000)

  c) For treatment of Alopecia X: Neutering is recommended initially. If this fails to be of benefit (or the patient must be left intact), try melatonin for a 3-month period at 3–6 mg (total dose) PO 2-3 times a day. Treat until maximal response is noted and discontinue. Re-institute therapy if and when signs recur.

  Canine recurrent flank alopecia: 3–6 mg (total dose) PO 2-3 times a day for 2–3 months (until hair loss is not noted as expected as the season changes or until good hair regrowth is noted). Therapy is stopped once hair growth has been attained; re-institute for recurrences.

  Color dilution alopecia: 1.5–6 mg PO 2–3 times a day, stop when good regrowth occurs and restart if needed. (Rosychuk 2008)

  d) For treatment of Alopecia-X: Empirical dose is 3 mg–12 mg (depending on the dog's size) PO 2 to 3 times a day. Perform a trial for at least 4 months before evaluating response; only reported side effect is drowsiness. (Torres 2007)

  For sleep disorders (nocturnal activity):

  a) 3–6 mg (total dose) PO q12–24h (Virga 2002)

  b) 0.1 mg/kg PO q8h. May be useful as a sleep aid and for canine fears and phobias. (Landsberg 2008)

For idiopathic vacuolar hepatopathy:

a) Some have suggested administering melatonin 4–6 mg/day PO in dogs weighing 15 kg or less may improve liver enzymes and hepatic changes. More studies are required to confirm this finding. (Twedt 2009)

■ **CATS:**

For sleep disorders (nocturnal activity):

a) 3–12 mg (total dose) PO q12–24h (Virga 2002)

For suppression of estrus:

a) 18 mg implant SC suppressed estrus for 2-4 months. (Gimenez et al. 2009)

■ **FERRETS:**

For adjunctive treatment of adrenal disease:

a) 0.5–1 mg per ferret PO once daily 7–9 hours after sunrise has been anecdotally effective in alleviating alopecia, aggressive behavior, vulvar swelling and prostatomegaly. Improvement more likely in patients with adrenal hyperplasia or adenoma; less likely if adenocarcinoma. Has no effect on tumor growth or metastasis. The implant form (5.4 mg) releases melatonin over a 3–4 month period. Response to melatonin, in general, is better in fall and winter. Can be used with other treatments (e.g., leuprolide, anastrozole, bicalutamide, finasteride). (Johnson 2006)

b) 1–2 mg per ferret PO once daily; or use 5.4 mg implant. May allow hair growth, refractory in a few months; implant may work better, does not control tumor growth. If ferret weighs under 600 grams may cause excessive drowsiness. (Johnson-Delaney 2009)

Monitoring

■ Clinical efficacy

Client Information

■ For use in small animals, must be administered as directed to be effective.

■ Relatively "experimental"; safety and efficacy are not clearly established.

Chemistry/Synonyms

A naturally occurring hormone produced in the pineal gland, melatonin occurs as a pale yellow, crystalline solid and has a molecular weight of 232. It can be derived from natural sources or by synthetic means.

Melatonin may also be known as: n-acetyl-5-methoxytryptamine, MEL, MLT, pineal hormone, *Benedorm®, Buenas Noches®, Cronocaps®, Dermatonin®, Ferretonin®, HT90®, Melapure®, Melatol®, Regulin®, Repentil®, Revenox®,* and *Transzone®.*

Storage/Stability

Unless otherwise labeled, store at room temperature in tight containers.

Dosage Forms/Regulatory Status

VETERINARY-LABELED PRODUCTS:

Melatonin 5.4 mg implant product marketed for ferrets; *Ferretonin®* (Melatek); 1-877-635-2835; www.melatek.net; Approval status is not known

Melatonin 8 mg, 12 mg, 18 mg implant product marketed for dogs; *Dermatonin®* (Melatek); Approval status not known

An 18 mg implant for sustained subcutaneous release is available in a variety of countries. One trade name is *Regulin®.* It is labeled for use in sheep (UK and NZ) and goats (NZ) to improve early breeding and ovulation rates.

There reportedly are mink implants available in the United States from Neo-Dynamics (800-206-7227).

HUMAN-LABELED PRODUCTS:

Melatonin tablets are available in a variety of strengths from a variety of sources. Common strengths available range from 0.5 mg to 3 mg tablets. Sustained release capsules (3 mg) and oral liquid (500 micrograms/mL) may also be available. Because melatonin is considered a "nutrient" there is no official labeling or central quality control systems for it in the USA. Purchase from reputable sources.

References

Gimenez, F., M.C. Stornelli, et al. (2009). Suppression of estrus in cats with melatonin implants. *Theriogenology* 72(4): 493–499.
Johnson, D. (2006). Current Therapies for Ferret Adrenal Disease. Proceedings: ACVC. Accessed via: Veterinary Information Network. http://goo.gl/pOMYy
Johnson-Delaney, C. (2009). Endocrine System and Diseases of Exotic Companion Mammals. Proceedings: ABVP. Accessed via: Veterinary Information Network. http://goo.gl/Tozhd
Landsberg, G. (2008). Treating canine and feline anxiety: Drug therapy and pheromones. Proceedings: BSAVA. Accessed via: Veterinary Information Network. http://goo.gl/3ci5J
Merchant, S. (2000). New Therapies in Veterinary Dermatology. Proceedings: American Animal Hospital Association 67th Annual Meeting, Toronto.
Paradis, M. (2000). Melatonin therapy for canine alopecia. *Kirk's Current Veterinary Therapy: XIII Small Animal Practice.* J Bonagura Ed. Philadelphia, WB Saunders: 546–549.
Rosychuk, R. (2008). Canine Alopecias: What's New? Proceeedings: WVC. Accessed via: Veterinary Information Network. http://goo.gl/cleWh
Torres, S. (2007). Alopecia X. Proceedings: Western Vet Conf. Accessed via: Veterinary Information Network. http://goo.gl/8QI6E
Twedt, D. (2009). Common liver diseases in the dog. Proceedings: ACVC. Accessed via: Veterinary Information Network. http://goo.gl/fl9Qp
Virga, V. (2002). Which drug and why: An update on psychopharmacology. Proceedings: Atlantic Coast Veterinary Conference. Accessed via: Veterinary Information Network. http://goo.gl/m8qr4

MELOXICAM

(mel-ox-i-kam)   Metacam®

NONSTEROIDAL ANTIINFLAMMATORY AGENT

Prescriber Highlights

▶ NSAID used in dogs & cats; COX-2 preferential

▶ May be useful as low-cost oral analgesic antiinflammatory for treating pain in calves after dehorning or castration

▶ Available as both an injectable & oral product

▶ GI adverse effects can occur

Uses/Indications

Meloxicam is principally used for the symptomatic treatment of osteoarthritis in dogs. Short-term (single dose injectable) use is also FDA-approved (in the USA) for cats for the control of postoperative pain and inflammation associated with orthopedic surgery, ovariohysterectomy and castration when administered prior to surgery.

Recent work in calves suggests that oral meloxicam may be a cost-effective agent to treat painful procedures such as castration or dehorning (Coetzee *et al.* 2009).

Pharmacology/Actions

Meloxicam has antiinflammatory, analgesic, and antipyretic activity similar to other NSAIDs. Like other NSAIDs, meloxicam exhibits analgesic, antiinflammatory, and antipyretic activity probably through its inhibition of cyclooxygenase, phospholipase A_2, and inhibition of prostaglandin synthesis. It is considered COX-2 preferential (not COX-2 specific) as at higher dosages its COX-2 specificity is diminished.

Acute dosing studies in dogs have not demonstrated any untoward renal or hepatic toxicity.

Pharmacokinetics

In dogs, meloxicam is well absorbed after oral administration. Food does not alter absorption. Peak blood levels occur in about 7–8 hours after administration. The volume of distribution in dogs is 0.3 L/kg and about 97% is bound to plasma proteins. Meloxicam is extensively biotransformed to several different metabolites in the liver; none of these appear to have pharmacologic activity. The majority of these (and unchanged drug) are eliminated in the feces. A significant amount of enterohepatic recirculation occurs. Elimination half-life is species specific. The elimination half-life in dogs averages 24 hours (range: 12–36 hours); other species: pigs: 4 hours; horses: 3 hours; cattle: 13 hours.

In cats, subcutaneous injection is nearly completely absorbed. Peak levels occur about 1.5 hours after injection. Meloxicam is relatively highly bound to feline plasma proteins (97%) and volume of distribution is about 0.27 L/kg. After a single dose, total systemic clearance is approximately 130 mL/hr/kg and elimination half life is approximately 15 hours. Major pathway for biotransformation is oxidation and the major elimination route is fecal.

In ruminant calves (approx. 3 months old) oral meloxicam at 1 mg/kg was well absorbed and had an elimination half-life of about one day (Coetzee *et al.* 2009).

Contraindications/Precautions/Warnings

Meloxicam is contraindicated in dogs hypersensitive to it. Safe use has not been evaluated in dogs less than 6 months old. The European label states that safe use has not been evaluated in dogs less than 6 weeks old. Although not part of the label, it should probably not be used in dogs with active GI ulceration or bleeding. It should be used with caution in patients with impaired hepatic, cardiac or renal function and hemorrhagic disorders.

Due to its long half-life in dogs, a 5–7 day washout period after stopping meloxicam has been recommended before starting a new NSAID (KuKanich 2008).

Meloxicam is contraindicated in cats with known hypersensitivity to meloxicam or other NSAIDs. The manufacturer warns that additional doses of meloxicam or other NSAIDs are contraindicated as no safe dosage for repeated NSAID administration has been established. Use in cats less than 4 months of age has not been established. Use preoperatively for cats undergoing major surgery where hypotensive episodes are possible; may be at higher risk for renal damage.

The human label states that no dosage adjustment is necessary in patients with mild to moderate hepatic or renal impairment. Use extreme caution in dehydrated, hypovolemic, or hypotensive animals as there is a potential increased risk of renal toxicity developing.

Adverse Effects

Experience in Europe and Canada has demonstrated a relatively safe adverse effect profile for meloxicam in dogs. GI distress is the most commonly reported adverse effect, and in US field trials vomiting, soft stools, diarrhea, and inappetence were the most common adverse effects reported. Renal toxicity appears to be quite low. Post-approval adverse effects reported have included GI effects (vomiting, anorexia, diarrhea, melena, ulceration), elevated liver enzymes, pruritus, azotemia, elevated creatinine, and renal failure.

In cats, single doses of meloxicam appear relatively safe. In field trials some cats developed elevated BUN, post-treatment anemia and, rarely, residual pain at the injection site. In other studies, meloxicam has caused GI effects (vomiting, diarrhea, inappetence), behavior changes, and lethargy. Repeated use of meloxicam in cats is controversial, as repeated doses have been associated with renal failure and death. Recently, the FDA has changed the label in the USA to warn against repeated doses in cats. However, low dose chronic use is licensed in some countries and the ISFM & AAFP guidelines for long-term NSAID use in cats suggests that benefits of treatment often outweigh the risks (Sparkes *et al.* 2010).

Reproductive/Nursing Safety

Safe use has not been established in dogs or cats used for breeding, or in pregnant or lactating animals. In humans, the FDA categorizes this drug as category *C* for use during pregnancy (*Animal studies have shown an adverse effect on the fetus, but there are no adequate studies in humans; or there are no animal reproduction studies and no adequate studies in humans.*)

Most NSAIDs are excreted in milk; use cautiously.

Overdosage/Acute Toxicity

The manufacturer warns to prevent accidental overdosing in small dogs, and to administer drops on food and not directly into the mouth. Treat symptomatically and supportively.

Drug Interactions

The following drug interactions have either been reported or are theoretical in humans or animals receiving meloxicam and may be of significance in veterinary patients:

- **ACE INHIBITORS (*e.g.*, enalapril, benazepril):** Some NSAIDs can reduce effects on blood pressure
- **ANTICOAGULANTS (*e.g.*, heparin, warfarin, etc.):** Increased chance for bleeding
- **ASPIRIN:** May increase the risk of gastrointestinal toxicity (*e.g.*, ulceration, bleeding, vomiting, diarrhea)
- **CORTICOSTEROIDS (*e.g.*, prednisone):** May increase the risk of gastrointestinal toxicity (*e.g.*, ulceration, bleeding, vomiting, diarrhea)
- **DIGOXIN:** NSAIDS may increase serum levels
- **FLUCONAZOLE:** Administration has increased plasma levels of celecoxib in humans and potentially could also affect meloxicam levels in dogs
- **FUROSEMIDE:** NSAIDs may reduce saluretic and diuretic effects
- **METHOTREXATE:** Serious toxicity has occurred when NSAIDs have been used concomitantly with methotrexate; use together with extreme caution
- **NEPHROTOXIC DRUGS (*e.g.*, furosemide, aminoglycosides, amphotericin B, etc.):** May enhance the risk of nephrotoxicity
- **NSAIDS, OTHER:** May increase the risk of gastrointestinal toxicity (*e.g.*, ulceration, bleeding, vomiting, diarrhea)

Doses

When doses are listed in "drops" use with caution, as drug concentration per drop may be different in products marketed in various countries.

- **DOGS:**

For FDA-approved indications (osteoarthritis, analgesia, inflammatory conditions):

a) Initially 0.2 mg/kg PO, IV or SC on the first day of treatment, subsequent doses of 0.1 mg/kg PO once daily in food or placed directly into mouth (not when dosing by the drop). (Package Insert; *Metacam® Injection/Oral Suspension*)

- **CATS:**

For pain:

a) For labeled indications: 0.3 mg/kg as a single one-time administration subcutaneous dose that should not be followed by additional doses of meloxicam or other NSAIDs. (Label information; *Metacam® Injection for Cats*—BI)

Note: The following dosages are extra-label in the USA and in 2010 the drug sponsor (BIVI-USA) and the FDA issued the following: *WARNING: Repeated use of meloxicam in cats has been associated with acute renal failure and death. Do not administer additional doses of injectable or oral meloxicam to cats. See Contraindications, Warnings and Precautions for detailed information.*

However, in another document published in 2010, the *ISFM and AAFP Consensus Guidelines: Long-Term Use of NSAIDs in Cats*, in their summary points they state: "It is only recently that NSAIDs have become licensed for long-term use in cats in some countries. The panel believe that these drugs have a major role to play in the management of chronic pain in cats, but at present only limited feline-specific data are available. To date, published studies of the medium- to long-term use of the COX-1 sparing drug meloxicam in older cats and cats with chronic kidney disease provide encouraging data that these drugs can be used safely and should be used to relieve pain when needed. While further data are needed, and would undoubtedly lead to refinement of the guidelines presented here, the panel hope that these recommendations will encourage rational and safe long-term use of NSAIDs in cats, thereby improving patients' quality of life in the face of painful disease conditions." (Sparkes *et al.* 2010)

b) 0.2 mg/kg PO initially, followed by 0.1 mg/kg PO (in food) once daily for 2 days and then 0.025 mg/kg 2–3 times a week (McLaughlin 2000)

c) Chronic musculoskeletal disorders: Initial treatment is a single oral dose of 0.1 mg meloxicam/kg body weight on the first day. Treatment is to be continued once daily by oral administration (at 24-hour intervals) at a maintenance dose of 0.05 mg meloxicam/kg body weight. A clinical response is normally seen within 7 days. Treatment should be discontinued after 14 days at the latest if no clinical improvement is apparent. (*Metacam®* Oral Suspension for Cats—BIVI-U.K.

d) For surgical pain: 0.2 mg/kg (or less) PO or SC once; 0.1 mg/kg (or less) SC, PO daily for 3–4 days

For chronic pain: 0.2 mg/kg (or less) PO, SC once; 0.1 mg/kg (or less) PO for 3–4 days; 0.025 mg/kg PO (0.1 mg maximum dose per cat) 2–3 times weekly (Mathews 2000)

■ **HORSES:**

For inflammation and pain associated with musculoskeletal disorders or colic pain (IV):

a) IV: Single intravenous injection at a dosage of 0.6/kg bodyweight (*i.e* 3 mL/100kg bodyweight); may follow with oral dosing after 24 hours. Oral: Either mixed with food or directly into the mouth at a dosage of 0.6 mg/kg bodyweight, once daily, up to 14 days. Where the product is mixed with food, it should be added to a small quantity of food, prior to feeding. Withdrawal periods: Meat/Offal: 5 days (Label Directions; *Metacam®* Injection & Oral Suspension for Horses—BIVI-UK)

■ **CATTLE:**

For use in acute respiratory infection with appropriate antibiotic therapy to reduce clinical signs in cattle. For use in diarrhea, in combination with oral rehydration therapy, to reduce clinical signs in calves of over one week of age and young non-lactating cattle. For adjunctive therapy in the treatment of acute mastitis, in combination with antibiotic therapy:

a) Single SC or IV injection at a dose rate of 0.5 mg/kg bodyweight (*i.e* 2.5 mL/100 kg bodyweight) in combination with antibiotic therapy or with oral rehydration therapy as appropriate. U.K. Withdrawal periods: Meat/Offal: 15 days; Milk: 120 hours. (*Metacam®* Injection—BIVI-UK)

■ **SWINE:**

For use in non-infectious locomotor disorders to reduce the symptoms of lameness and inflammation. For adjunctive therapy in the treatment of puerperal septicemia and toxemia (mastitis-metritis-agalactia syndrome) with appropriate antibiotic therapy:

a) Single IM injection at a dosage of 0.4 mg/kg bodyweight (*ie:* 2 mL/100 kg bodyweight) in combination with antibiotic therapy, as appropriate. If required, a second administration of meloxicam can be given after 24 hours. Withdrawal periods: Meat/Offal: 5 days (*Metacam®* Injection—BIVI-UK)

■ **FERRETS:**

a) For post-surgical pain: 0.2 mg/kg PO or SC once. (Schoemaker 2008)

For musculoskeletal and mild visceral pain:

a) 0.2 mg/kg PO or SC once daily. Has a duration of action for 24–48 hours in most species; may be used for prolonged periods of time; also very effective when used in combination with opioids. (Mayer 2007)

b) 0.2–0.3 mg/kg PO once daily (q24h). Doses of 0.2 mg/kg once daily for 10 days was well tolerated by rabbits studied. (Carpenter *et al.* 2009)

■ **BIRDS:**

a) As an analgesic: 0.5 mg/kg IM is also commonly used in birds and may be the safest of the NSAID analgesics for avian species. As the side effects of all analgesics have not been studied in birds, these drugs should be used carefully in avian patients. (Echols 2008)

b) As adjunctive treatment for proventricular dilatation disease (PDD): 0.1–0.5 mg/kg PO q12h. (Oglesbee 2009)

■ **ZOO, EXOTIC, WILDLIFE SPECIES:**

For use of meloxicam in zoo, exotic and wildlife medicine refer to specific references, including:

a) *Exotic Animal Formulary, 3rd Ed.* Carpenter JW. Saunders. 2005

b) The 2009 American Association of Zoo Veterinarian Proceedings by D. K. Fontenot also has several dosages listed for restraint, anesthesia, and analgesia for a variety of drugs for carnivores and primates. VIN members can access them at: http://goo.gl/BHRih or http://goo.gl/9UJse

Monitoring

■ Clinical efficacy

■ Adverse effects

■ Renal function and hepatic function if used chronically

Client Information

■ Shake oral liquid well before using.

■ Carefully measure dose (oral liquid); do not confuse the markings on the syringe (provided by the manufacturer) with mL or kgs. If using drops to measure dose in small dogs, do not place drops directly into dog's mouth; mix with food. Otherwise, may place oral syringe into dogs mouth or mix with food.

■ If animal develops adverse effects, contact the veterinarian

■ If dispensed for outpatient use, obtain client information sheet for this medication

Chemistry/Synonyms

A COX-2 receptor preferential NSAID, meloxicam occurs as a pale yellow powder. It is in the oxicam class, related to piroxicam.

Meloxicam may also be known as: UH-AC-62, and UH-AC-62XX; many trade names are available.

Storage/Stability

Unless otherwise labeled, store the injection and oral liquid at room temperature.

Dosage Forms/Regulatory Status

VETERINARY-LABELED PRODUCTS:

Meloxicam Oral Suspension: 1.5 mg/mL (0.05 mg per drop in the USA product) in a honey-flavored base: 10 mL, 32 mL, 100 mL dropper bottles with measuring syringe (marked in 5 lb body weight increments); *Metacam®* (BIVI); (Rx). FDA-approved for use in dogs.

Meloxicam 5 mg/mL for Injection: 10 mL vial; *Metacam® Injection for Dogs* (BIVI); (Rx). FDA-approved for use in dogs.

Meloxicam 5 mg/mL for Injection: 10 mL vial; *Metacam® Injection for Cats* (BIVI); (Rx). FDA-approved for use in cats.

The ARCI (Racing Commissioners International) has designated this drug as a class 3 substance. See the appendix for more information.

HUMAN-LABELED PRODUCTS:

Meloxicam Tablets: 7.5 mg & 15 mg; *Mobic®* (Boehringer Ingelheim/Abbott); generic; (Rx)

Meloxicam Oral Suspension: 7.5 mg/5 mL in 100 mL; *Mobic®* (Boehringer Ingelheim/Abbott); Meloxicam (Roxane); (Rx)

In Canada, *Mobicox®* (Boehringer Ingelheim); (Rx)

References

Carpenter, J.W., C.G. Pollock, et al. (2009). Single And Multiple-Dose Pharmacokinetics Of Meloxicam After Oral Administration To The Rabbit (Oryctolagus Cuniculus). Journal of Zoo and Wildlife Medicine 40(4): 601–606.

Coetzee, J., B. KuKanich, et al. (2009). Pharmacokinetics of intravenous and oral meloxicam in ruminant calves. Vet Therapeutics 10(4).

Echols, M. (2008). Avian Anesthesia and Analgesia. Proceedings: IVECCS. Accessed via: Veterinary Information Network. http://goo.gl/kSQMJ

KuKanich, B. (2008). NSAIDs in Dogs. Proceedings: WVC. Accessed via: Veterinary Information Network. http://goo.gl/EZ6lK

Mathews, K. (2000). Non-steroidal antiinflammatory analgesics: Indications and contraindications for pain management in dogs and cats. Vet Clin NA: Small Anim Pract 30:4(July): 783–804.

Mayer, J. (2007). Analgesia and Anesthesia in Rabbits & Rodents. Proceedings: Western Vet Conf. Accessed via: Veterinary Information Network. http://goo.gl/2uzPu

McLaughlin, R. (2000). Management of Osteoarthritic Pain. Vet ClinNA: Small Anim Pract 30:4(July): 933–947.

Oglesbee, B. (2009). Vomiting & Diarrhea in Pet Birds: Where do I Start? Proceedings: WVC. Accessed via: Veterinary Information Network. http://goo.gl/waFP2

Schoemaker, N. (2008). What every veterinarian should know about ferret medicine. Proceedings: BSAVA. Accessed via: Veterinary Information Network. http://goo.gl/xqCHt

Sparkes, A.H., R. Heiene, et al. (2010). ISFM AND AAFP CONSENSUS GUIDELINES Long-term use of NSAIDs in cats. Journal of Feline Medicine and Surgery 12(7): 521–538.

MELPHALAN

(*mel*-fa-lan)   Alkeran®

ANTINEOPLASTIC

Prescriber Highlights

▶ Alkylating agent antineoplastic used for ovarian carcinoma, lymphoreticular neoplasms, osteosarcoma, mammary or pulmonary neoplasms, & multiple myeloma

▶ Contraindications (relative; risk vs. benefit): Anemia, bone marrow depression, current infection, impaired renal function, tumor cell infiltration of bone marrow, sensitivity to drug, or patients who have received previous chemotherapy or radiotherapy

▶ Adverse Effects: GI effects (anorexia, vomiting, diarrhea), pulmonary infiltrates or fibrosis, bone marrow depression (anemia, thrombocytopenia, leukopenia)

▶ Potential teratogen

▶ Determine dosages carefully

Uses/Indications

Melphalan may be useful in the treatment of a variety of neoplastic diseases, including ovarian carcinoma, lymphoreticular neoplasms, osteosarcoma, and mammary or pulmonary neoplasms. When combined with prednisone, it is considered the drug of choice for treating multiple myeloma. It has been used successfully in a rescue protocol combining dexamethasone, melphalan, dactinomycin and cytarabine to treat relapsed multicentric lymphoma in dogs.

Pharmacology/Actions

Melphalan is a bifunctional alkylating agent and interferes with RNA transcription and DNA replication, thereby disrupting nucleic acid function. Because it is bifunctional, it has affect on both dividing and resting cells. Melphalan does not require activation by the liver (unlike cyclophosphamide).

Pharmacokinetics

Melphalan absorption is variable and often incomplete. It is distributed throughout the body water, but it is unknown whether it crosses the placenta, blood brain barrier or enters maternal milk. Melphalan is eliminated principally by hydrolysis in plasma. In humans, terminal half-lives average about 90 minutes.

Contraindications/Precautions/Warnings

Melphalan should be used with the following conditions only when its potential benefits outweigh its risks: anemia, bone marrow depression, current infection, impaired renal function, tumor cell infiltration of bone marrow, sensitivity to melphalan or patients who have received previous chemotherapy or radiotherapy.

Adverse Effects

The most serious adverse effect likely with melphalan is bone marrow depression (anemia, thrombocytopenia, leukopenia). Potential adverse effects include GI effects (anorexia, vomiting, diarrhea), pulmonary infiltrates or fibrosis, or neurotoxic effects.

Reproductive/Nursing Safety

Safe use of melphalan during pregnancy has not been established; other alkylating agents are known teratogens. Use only during pregnancy when the benefits to the mother outweigh the risks to the offspring. Melphalan can suppress gonadal function.

While it is unknown whether melphalan enters maternal milk, nursing puppies or kittens should receive milk replacer when the bitch or queen is receiving melphalan.

Overdosage/Acute Toxicity

Because of the toxic potential of this agent, overdoses must be avoided. Determine dosages carefully.

Drug Interactions

The following drug interactions have either been reported or are theoretical in humans or animals receiving melphalan and may be of significance in veterinary patients:

■ **CYCLOSPORINE:** There are anecdotal reports of melphalan causing increased nephrotoxicity associated with systemic cyclosporine use in humans.

■ **IMMUNOSUPPRESSANT DRUGS (e.g., azathioprine, cyclophosphamide, corticosteroids):** Use with other immunosuppressant drugs may increase the risk of infection.

■ **MYELOSUPPRESSIVE DRUGS (e.g., chloramphenicol, flucytosine, amphotericin B, or colchicine):** Use extreme caution when used concurrently with other drugs that are also myelosuppressive, including many of the other antineoplastics and other bone marrow depressant drugs. Bone marrow depression may be additive.

■ **VACCINES, LIVE:** Live virus vaccines should be used with caution, if at all, during therapy.

Laboratory Considerations

■ Melphalan may raise serum **uric acid** levels. Drugs such as allopurinol may be required to control hyperuricemia.

Doses

Note: Because of the potential toxicity of this drug to patients, veterinary personnel and clients, and since chemotherapy indications, treatment protocols, monitoring and safety guidelines often change, *the following dosages should be used only as a general guide. Consultation with a veterinary oncologist and referral to current veterinary oncology references* [e.g., (Henry & Higginbotham 2009); (Argyle et al. 2008); (Withrow & Vail 2007); (Villalobos 2007); (Ogilvie & Moore 2006); (Ogilvie & Moore 2001)] *is strongly recommended.*

a) For multiple myeloma: Several dosing schedules have been developed to treat canine multiple myeloma with melphalan. One recommended dosing regimen is 0.1 mg/kg PO q24h for 10 days, followed by 0.05 mg/kg PO q48h thereafter. Another source recommends 0.25 mg/kg/day PO for 4 days and 2 to 4 mg/day PO maintenance. Pulse therapy is another reported option (7 mg/m^2 PO q24h for 5 days every 21 days). The recommended intravenous dose is 16 mg/m^2 every 2 weeks for 4 doses and then every 4 weeks. A 50% dose reduction is recommended for animals with preexisting renal insufficiency. Clinical response can be assessed by improved clinical signs and reduced serum immunoglobulin. Melphalan should be administered indefinitely until clinical relapse, which may involve worsened bone pain, recurrence of bleeding diathesis, funduscopic changes, or elevated serum immunoglobulins. (Kitchell & Wiedemann 2004)

b) As part of a rescue protocol (DMAC) to treat relapsed multicentric lymphoma: Dactinomycin (0.75 mg/m^2 IV), Cytarabine (300 mg/m^2 IV over 4 hours or SC) and dexamethasone (1 mg/kg PO) on day 0 and melphalan (20 mg/m^2 PO) and dexamethasone (1 mg/kg PO) on day 7. The cycle is repeated continuously every 2 weeks as long as a complete or partial remission is achieved. After four cycles, chlorambucil was substituted for melphalan at the same dose. If complete remission achieved, protocol was discontinued after 5–8 cycles and maintenance therapy with the LMP (chlorambucil, methotrexate, prednisone) or lomustine/prednisone protocols were instituted. If dogs developed grades 3 or 4 toxicosis, DMAC was discontinued and maintenance protocol was started. (Alvarez et al. 2006; Rassnick 2006)

■ **CATS:**

For chronic lymphocytic leukemia:

a) 2 mg/m^2 PO every other day with or without prednisone at 20 mg/m^2 PO every other day (Peterson and Couto 1994)

Monitoring

■ CBC with platelets at least every week for 2 weeks and then monthly thereafter. Significant myelosuppression requires an alteration in dose or frequency of administration.

Client Information

■ Clients must understand the importance of both administering melphalan as directed and immediately reporting any signs associated with toxicity (*e.g.*, abnormal bleeding, bruising, urination, depression, infection, shortness of breath, etc.).

Chemistry/Synonyms

A nitrogen mustard derivative, melphalan occurs as an off-white to buff-colored powder that is practically insoluble in water.

Melphalan may also be known as: CB-3025, NSC-8806, PAM, L-PAM, L-phenylalanine mustard, phenylalanine mustard, phenylalanine nitrogen mustard, L-sarcolysine, WR-19813, *Alkeran®* or *Alkerana®*.

Storage/Stability

Store melphalan tablets in well-closed, light-resistant, glass containers in the refrigerator (2–8°C). It is recommended to dispense the tablets in glass containers.

Once reconstituted, the injectable product should not be refrigerated or a precipitate may form. It is stable at room temperature for 90 minutes after reconstitution. For administration, the reconstituted solution should be further diluted with sterile 0.9% sodium chloride to a concentration of not more than 0.45 mg/mL. This diluted solution is stable for 60 minutes at room temperature.

Dosage Forms/Regulatory Status

VETERINARY-LABELED PRODUCTS: None

HUMAN-LABELED PRODUCTS:

Melphalan Oral Tablets: 2 mg; *Alkeran®* (GlaxoSmithKline); (Rx)

Melphalan Powder for Injection (lyophilized): 50 mg in single use vials with 10 mL vial of sterile diluent; *Alkeran®* (GlaxoSmithKline); (Rx)

References

Alvarez, F., W. Kisseberth, et al. (2006). Dexamethasone, melphalan, actinomycin D, cytosine arabinoside (DMAC) protocol for dogs with relapsed lymphoma. *J Vet Intern Med* **20**: 1178–1183.

Argyle, D., M. Brearly, et al. (2008). *Decision Making in Small Animal Oncology*, Wiley-Blackwell.

Henry, C. & M. Higginbotham (2009). *Cancer Management in Small Animal Practice*, Saunders.

Kitchell, B. & A. Wiedemann (2004). "Pharm Profile: Melphalan."

Ogilvie, G. & A. Moore (2001). *Feline Oncology: A Comprehensive Guide to Compassionate Care*, Veterinary Learning Systems.

Ogilvie, G. & A. Moore (2006). *Managing the Canine Cancer Patient: A Practical Guide to Compassionate Care*, Veterinary Learning Systems.

Rassnick, K. (2006). Rescue chemotherapy protocols for dogs with lymphoma. Proceedings: ACVIM. Accessed via: Veterinary Information Network. http://goo.gl/soSsv

Villalobos, A. (2007). *Canine and Feline Geriatric Oncology*. Ames, Blackwell.

Withrow, S. & D. Vail (2007). *Withrow and MacEwen's Small Animal Clinical Oncology 4th Ed.* Philadelphia, Elsevier.

MEPERIDINE HCL

(me-*per*-i-deen)   Demerol®, Pethidine

OPIATE AGONIST

Prescriber Highlights

▶ Opiate analgesic; infrequently used as it has a short duration of analgesia & may cause more adverse effects than other commonly used injectable opiates

▶ Contraindications: Hypersensitivity to it, diarrhea caused by a toxic ingestion

▶ Extreme Caution: Respiratory disease or acute respiratory dysfunction

▶ Caution: Hypothyroidism, severe renal insufficiency, adrenocortical insufficiency, geriatric or severely debilitated patients, head injuries or increased intracranial pressure, & acute abdominal conditions (*e.g.*, colic)

▶ Adverse Effects: Respiratory depression, histamine release, bronchoconstriction, CNS depression, GI (nausea, vomiting, & decreased intestinal peristalsis), mydriasis (dogs), salivation (esp. cats); physical dependence (chronic use). Horses (in addition): Tachycardia with PVC's, profuse sweating, hyperpnea; may potentiate intestinal obstruction secondary to reduced intestinal motility

▶ Give very slowly if using IV (many state not to use IV), may be irritating if given SC

▶ C-II controlled substance

Uses/Indications

Although no product is licensed in the United States for veterinary use, this agent has been used as an analgesic in several different species. It has been used as sedative/analgesic in small animals for both post-operative pain and for medical conditions such as acute pancreatitis and thermal burns, but usually other opiates are preferred as the drug has a short analgesic duration of activity and can cause significant histamine release. It is occasionally used in equine medicine in the treatment of colic and in other large animal species for pain control.

Pharmacology/Actions

Receptors for opiate analgesics are found in high concentrations in the limbic system, spinal cord, thalamus, hypothalamus, striatum, and midbrain. They are also found in tissues such as the gastrointestinal tract, urinary tract, and in other smooth muscle.

The morphine-like agonists (morphine, meperidine, oxymorphone) have primary activity at the *mu* receptors, with some activity possible at the delta receptor. The primary pharmacologic effects of these agents include: analgesia, antitussive activity, respiratory depression, sedation, emesis, physical dependence, and intestinal effects (constipation/defecation). Secondary pharmacologic effects include: *CNS*: euphoria, sedation, and confusion. *Cardiovascular*: bradycardia due to central vagal stimulation, alpha-adrenergic receptors may be depressed resulting in peripheral vasodilation, decreased peripheral resistance, and baroreceptor inhibition. Orthostatic hypotension and syncope may occur. *Urinary*: Increased bladder sphincter tone can induce urinary retention.

Meperidine is primarily a *Mu* agonist. It is approximately ⅓–⅛th as potent as morphine, but produces equivalent respiratory depression at equi-analgesic doses as morphine. Like morphine, it can cause histamine release. It does not have antitussive activity at doses lower than those causing analgesia. Meperidine is the only used opioid that has vagolytic and negative inotropic properties at clinically used doses. One study in ponies demonstrated changes in jejunal activity after meperidine administration, but no effects on transit time or colonic electrical activity were noted.

Refer to the monograph: *Narcotic (opiate) Analgesic Agonists, Pharmacology of*, for more information.

Pharmacokinetics

Although generally well absorbed orally, a marked first-pass effect limits the oral effectiveness of meperidine. After injection by IM or subcutaneous routes the peak analgesic effects occur between 30–60 minutes, with the IM route having a slightly faster onset. Duration of action is variable with effects generally lasting from 1–6 hours in most species. In dogs and cats, analgesic duration of only <2 hours and often less than 1 hour at clinically used doses. The drug is metabolized primarily in the liver (mostly hydrolysis with some conjugation) and approximately 5% is excreted unchanged in the urine.

Contraindications/Precautions/Warnings

Meperidine is contraindicated in cases where the patient is hypersensitive to narcotic analgesics, or in patients receiving monamine oxidase inhibitors (MAOIs). It is also contraindicated in patients with diarrhea caused by a toxic ingestion until the toxin is eliminated from the GI tract. All opiates should be used with caution in patients with hypothyroidism, severe renal insufficiency, adrenocortical insufficiency (Addison's disease), and in geriatric or severely debilitated patients.

Many clinicians state that meperidine should not be administered intravenously. If given IV, it must be given very slowly or severe hypotension can result.

Meperidine should be used with caution in patients with head injuries or increased intracranial pressure and acute abdominal conditions (*e.g.*, colic) as it may obscure the diagnosis or clinical course of these conditions. It should be used with extreme caution in patients suffering from respiratory disease or from acute respiratory dysfunction (*e.g.*, pulmonary edema secondary to smoke inhalation).

Opiate analgesics are also contraindicated in patients who have been stung by the scorpion species *Centruroides sculpturatus Ewing* and *C. gertschi Stahnke* as they may potentiate these venoms. Meperidine should not be used for pain secondary to envenomations from Gila monsters or Mexican beaded lizards (Hackett 2007).

Adverse Effects

Meperidine may be irritating when administered subcutaneously and must be given very slowly IV or it may cause severe hypotension. It can cause pronounced histamine release, particularly with IV administration. At usual doses, the primary concern is the effect the opioids have on respiratory function. Decreased tidal volume, depressed cough reflex, and the drying of respiratory secretions may all have a detrimental effect on a susceptible patient. Bronchoconstriction following IV doses has been noted in dogs. Gastrointestinal effects may include: nausea, vomiting, and decreased intestinal peristalsis. In dogs, meperidine causes mydriasis (unlike morphine). If given orally, the drug may be irritating to the buccal mucosa and cause salivation; this is of particular concern in cats. Chronic administration can lead to physical dependence.

In horses undergoing general anesthesia, meperidine has been associated with a reaction that manifests as tachycardia with PVC's, profuse sweating, and hyperpnea.

Reproductive/Nursing Safety

In humans, the FDA categorizes this drug as category *C* for use during pregnancy (*Animal studies have shown an adverse effect on the fetus, but there are no adequate studies in humans; or there are no animal reproduction studies and no adequate studies in humans.*) In a separate system evaluating the safety of drugs in canine and feline pregnancy (Papich 1989), this drug is categorized as class: *B* (*Safe for use if used cautiously. Studies in laboratory animals may have uncovered some risk, but these drugs appear to be safe in dogs and cats or these drugs are safe if they are not administered when the animal is near term.*)

Most opiates are excreted into milk. Meperidine enters human breast milk at concentrations slightly higher than those found in serum, but effects on nursing offspring may not be significant.

Overdosage/Acute Toxicity

In most species, overdosage may produce profound respiratory and/or CNS depression. Other effects can include cardiovascular collapse, hypothermia, and skeletal muscle hypotonia. Some species (especially cats) may demonstrate CNS excitability (hyperreflexia, tremors) and seizures at doses greater than 20 mg/kg. Naloxone is the agent of choice in treating respiratory depression. In massive overdoses, naloxone doses may need to be repeated, and animals should be closely observed as naloxone's effects can diminish before subtoxic levels of meperidine are attained. Mechanical respiratory support should also be considered in cases of severe respiratory depression.

Pentobarbital has been suggested as a treatment for CNS excitement and seizures in cats. Caution must be used as barbiturates and narcotics can have additive effects on respiratory depression.

Drug Interactions

The following drug interactions have either been reported or are theoretical in humans or animals receiving meperidine and may be of significance in veterinary patients:

- **CNS DEPRESSANTS, OTHER (e.g., anesthetic agents, antihistamines, phenothiazines, barbiturates, tranquilizers, alcohol, etc.):** May cause increased CNS or respiratory depression when used with meperidine

- **DIURETICS:** Opiates may decrease efficacy in CHF patients

- **ISONIAZID:** Meperidine may enhance INH adverse effects

- **MONAMINE OXIDASE (MAO) INHIBITORS (e.g., amitraz, possibly selegiline):** Meperidine is contraindicated in patients receiving monamine oxidase (MAO) inhibitors for at least 14 days after receiving MAO inhibitors in humans. Some human patients have exhibited signs of opiate overdose after receiving therapeutic doses of meperidine while taking MAOIs.

- **MUSCLE RELAXANTS, SKELETAL:** Meperidine may enhance neuromuscular blockade

- **TRICYCLIC ANTIDEPRESSANTS (clomipramine, amitriptyline, etc.):** Meperidine may exacerbate the effects of tricyclic antidepressants

- **WARFARIN:** Opiates may potentiate anticoagulant activity

Laboratory Considerations

- As they may increase biliary tract pressure, opiates can increase plasma amylase and lipase values up to 24 hours following their administration.

Doses

- **DOGS:**
  Analgesic duration in dogs usually lasts 45 minutes to 1 hour.
  a) 5–10 mg/kg IM, SC. Duration of effect is short (30–60 minutes) (Mama 2002)
  b) For perioperative pain: 3–5 mg/kg IM or

SC. Duration of action 1–2 hours (Pascoe 2000)
  c) In healthy dogs: 3–4 mg/kg IM as a premed; 1–2 mg/kg IM post-op. (Trim 2008)

- **CATS:**
  For perioperative pain:
  a) 3–5 mg/kg IM or SC. Duration of action 1–2 hours (Pascoe 2000)
  b) 2–5 mg/kg IM, SC. Duration of effect is short (30 minutes to an hour) (Mama 2002)
  c) In healthy cats: 3–4 mg/kg IM as a premed; 1–2 mg/kg IM post-op. (Trim 2008)
  Not recommended for cats. (Scherk 2003)

- **FERRETS:**
  a) 5–10 mg/kg SC or IM every 2–3 hours (Williams 2000)

- **RABBITS, RODENTS, SMALL MAMMALS:**
  a) Rabbits: For moderate pain: 5–10 mg/kg SC, IM q2–3h. Using Banana flavored oral syrup: 0.2 mg/mL in drinking water (Ivey & Morrisey 2000)
  b) Analgesic (patient administered moderate pain relief): 0.2 mg/mL in drinking water (Huerkamp 1995)

- **CATTLE:**
  As an analgesic:
  a) 3.3–4.4 mg/kg SC or IM (Jenkins 1987)
  b) 500 mg IM (Booth 1988)
  c) 150–200 mg/100 lbs IM or SC (or slow IV) (McConnell & Hughey 1987)

- **HORSES:**
  Note: Narcotics (meperidine included) may cause CNS excitement in the horse. Some recommend pretreatment with acepromazine (0.02–0.04 mg/kg IV), or xylazine (0.3–0.5 mg/kg IV) to reduce the behavioral changes caused by these drugs. **Warning:** Narcotic analgesics can mask the behavioral and cardiovascular signs associated with mild colic.
  As an analgesic:
  a) 2–4 mg/kg IM or IV (may cause excitement and hypotension with IV use) (Jenkins 1987)
  b) 500 mg (total dose) IV (slowly, CNS excitement may occur) or 1000 mg (total dose) IM (Booth 1988)

- **SWINE:**
  As a restraining agent:
  a) Given alone the drug does not give much restraint in large animals. Has been used in combination with promazine (2 mg/kg IM) and atropine (0.07–0.09 mg/kg IM) at a dose of 1–2 mg/kg IM as a preanesthetic 45–60 minutes before barbiturate/inhalant anesthesia. All the above should be given in separate sites (Booth 1988)

As an analgesic:

a) 2 mg/kg IM q4h IM as needed (Jenkins 1987)

■ **SHEEP & GOATS:**

As an analgesic:

a) Up to 200 mg total dose IM (Jenkins 1987)

Monitoring

■ Respiratory rate/depth
■ CNS level of depression/excitation
■ Blood pressure (especially with IV use)
■ Analgesic activity

Client Information

■ Oral dosage forms may cause mouth irritation.
■ When given parenterally, this agent should be used in an inpatient setting or with direct professional supervision.

Chemistry/Synonyms

A synthetic opiate analgesic, meperidine HCl is a fine, white, crystalline, odorless powder that is very soluble in water, sparingly soluble in ether and soluble in alcohol. It has a pK_a of 7.7–8.15 and a melting range of 186–189°C. The pH of the commercially available injectable preparation is between 3.5 and 6.

Meperidine HCl may also be known as: pethidine HCl, isonipecaine, meperidine hydrochloride, pethidini hydrochloridum; *Alodan®*, *Centralgine®*, *Demerol®*, *Dolantin®*, *Dolantina®*, *Dolantine®*, *Dolestine®*, or *Dolosal®*.

Storage/Stability

Meperidine is stable at room temperature. Avoid freezing the injectable solution and protect from light during storage. Meperidine has not exhibited significant adsorption to PVC IV bags or tubing in studies to date.

Compatibility/Compounding Considerations

Meperidine is reported to be physically **compatible** with the following fluids and drugs: sodium chloride 0.45 and 0.9%, Ringer's injection, lactated Ringer's injection, dextrose 2.5, 5 and 10% for injection, dextrose/saline combinations, dextrose/Ringers lactated solutions, atropine, benzquinamide, butorphanol, chlorpromazine, dimenhydrinate, diphenhydramine HCl, dobutamine, droperidol, fentanyl citrate, glycopyrrolate, metoclopramide, pentazocine lactate, promazine HCl, succinylcholine, and verapamil HCl.

Meperidine is reported to be physically **incompatible** when mixed with the following agents: aminophylline, amobarbital sodium, heparin sodium, hydrocortisone sodium succinate, methicillin, methylprednisolone sodium succinate, morphine sulfate, nitrofurantoin sodium, oxytetracycline HCl, pentobarbital sodium, phenobarbital sodium, phenytoin sodium, sodium iodide, tetracycline HCl, thiopental sodium, and thiamylal sodium.

Dosage Forms/Regulatory Status

VETERINARY-LABELED PRODUCTS: None

HUMAN-LABELED PRODUCTS:

Meperidine HCl Injection: 25 mg/mL in 1 mL vials, amps & 1mL *Carpuject* syringes; 50 mg/mL in 1 mL vials, 0.5 mL, 1 mL, 1.5 mL and 2 mL amps, 30 mL multi-dose vials and 1 mL *Carpuject* syringes; 75 mg/mL in 1 mL vials, amps & 1 mL *Carpuject* syringes; 100 mg/mL in 1 mL vials & amps, 20 mL multidose vials and 1 mL *Carpuject* syringes; *Demerol®* (Abbott); generic, (Rx, C-II)

Meperidine HCl Tablets: 50 mg & 100 mg; *Demerol®* (Sanofi-Synthelabo); generic; (Rx, C-II)

Meperidine HCl Syrup/Oral Solution: 50 mg/5 mL in 473 mL & 500 mL, *Demerol®* (Sanofi-Synthelabo); generic (Roxane); (Rx, C-II)

Note: Meperidine is listed as a Class-II controlled substance and all products require a prescription. Very accurate record keeping is required as to use and disposition of stock.

References

Booth, N.H. (1988). Drugs Acting on the Central Nervous System. *Veterinary Pharmacology and Therapeutics–6th Ed.* NH Booth and LE McDonald Eds. Ames, Iowa State University Press: 153–408.

Hackett, T. (2007). Spiders and Snakes: Recognizing and Treating Envenomations.

Huerkamp, M. (1995). Anesthesia and postoperative management of rabbits and pocket pets. *Kirk's Current Veterinary Therapy:XII.* J Bonagura Ed. Philadelphia, W.B. Saunders: 1322–1327.

Ivey, E. & J. Morrisey (2000). Therapeutics for Rabbits. *Vet Clin NA: Exotic Anim Pract* **3:**1(Jan): 183–216.

Jenkins, W.L. (1987). Pharmacologic aspects of analgesic drugs in animals: An overview. *JAVMA* **191**(10): 1231–1240.

Mama, K. (2002). Use of opioids in anesthesia practice. Proceeedings: World Small Animal Veterinary Association.

McConnell, V.C. & T. Hughey (1987). *Formulary, The University of Georgia, Veterinary Medical Teaching Hospital.* Athens, GA.

Papich, M. (1989). Effects of drugs on pregnancy. *Current Veterinary Therapy X: Small Animal Practice.* R Kirk Ed. Philadelphia, Saunders: 1291–1299.

Pascoe, P. (2000). Perioperative pain management. *Vet Clin NA: Small Anim Pract* **30:**4(July): 917–932.

Scherk, M. (2003). Feline analgesia in 2003. Proceedings: World Small Animal Veterinary Assoc World Congress. Accessed via: Veterinary Information Network. http://goo.gl/nXadm

Trim, C. (2008). Opioid Analgesia. Proceedings: WVC. Accessed via: Veterinary Information Network. http://goo.gl/VACG6

Williams, B. (2000). Therapeutics in Ferrets. *Vet Clin NA: Exotic Anim Pract* **3:**1(Jan): 131–153.

MERCAPTOPURINE

(mer-kap-toe-*pyoor*-een)   Purinethol®

ANTINEOPLASTIC;
IMMUNOSUPPRESSANT

Prescriber Highlights

▶ Oral antineoplastic/immunosuppressant used for adjunctive treatment of lymphosarcoma, acute leukemias, & severe rheumatoid arthritis or other autoimmune conditions (*e.g.*, unresponsive ulcerative colitis)

▶ Caution (risk versus benefit): In patients with hepatic dysfunction, bone marrow depression, infection, renal function impairment (adjust dosage), or with a history of urate urinary stones

▶ Adverse Effects: GI effects (nausea, anorexia, vomiting, diarrhea) most likely; bone marrow suppression, hepatotoxicity, pancreatitis, GI (including oral) ulceration &, potentially, dermatologic reactions.

▶ Teratogenic; use milk replacer in nursing animals

▶ Drug interactions

Uses/Indications

Rarely used in veterinary medicine. Veterinary uses of mercaptopurine have included adjunctive therapy of lymphosarcoma, acute leukemias, and severe rheumatoid arthritis. It may have potential benefit in treating other autoimmune conditions (*e.g.*, unresponsive ulcerative colitis) as well.

Pharmacology/Actions

Intracellularly, mercaptopurine is converted into a ribonucleotide that acts as a purine antagonist, thereby inhibiting RNA and DNA synthesis. Mercaptopurine acts as an immunosuppressant, primarily inhibiting humoral immunity.

Pharmacokinetics

Absorption after oral dosing is variable and incomplete. Absorbed drug and its metabolites are distributed throughout the total body water. The drug crosses the blood-brain barrier, but not in levels significant enough to treat CNS neoplasms. It is unknown whether mercaptopurine enters milk.

Via the enzyme, xanthine oxidase, mercaptopurine is rapidly metabolized in the liver to 6-thiouric acid, which along with the parent compound and other metabolites are principally excreted in the urine.

Contraindications/Precautions/Warnings

Mercaptopurine is contraindicated in patients hypersensitive to it. The drug should be used cautiously (risk versus benefit) in patients with hepatic dysfunction, bone marrow depression, infection, renal function impairment (adjust dosage), or a history of urate urinary stones.

Adverse Effects

At usual doses, GI effects (nausea, anorexia, vomiting, diarrhea) are most likely seen in small animals. However, bone marrow suppression, hepatotoxicity, pancreatitis, GI (including oral) ulceration, and dermatologic reactions are, potentially, possible.

Reproductive/Nursing Safety

Mercaptopurine is mutagenic and teratogenic and is not recommended for use during pregnancy. In humans, the FDA categorizes this drug as category *D* for use during pregnancy (*There is evidence of human fetal risk, but the potential benefits from the use of the drug in pregnant women may be acceptable despite its potential risks.*)

It is not known whether mercaptopurine is excreted in milk, but use of milk replacer is recommended for nursing bitches or queens.

Overdosage/Acute Toxicity

Toxicity may present acutely (GI effects) or be delayed (bone marrow depression, hepatotoxicity, gastroenteritis). It is suggested to use standard protocols to empty the GI tract if ingestion was recent and to treat supportively.

Drug Interactions

The following drug interactions have either been reported or are theoretical in humans or animals receiving mercaptopurine and may be of significance in veterinary patients:

■ **ALLOPURINOL:** The hepatic metabolism of mercaptopurine may be decreased by concomitant administration of allopurinol. In humans, it is recommended to reduce the mercaptopurine dose to ¼–⅓ usual if both drugs are to be used together.

■ **AMINOSALICYLATES (mesalamine, sulfasalazine):** May increase risk for mercaptopurine toxicity

■ **HEPATOTOXIC DRUGS (*e.g.*, halothane, ketoconazole, valproic acid, phenobarbital, primidone, etc.):** Mercaptopurine should be used cautiously with other drugs that can cause hepatotoxicity. In humans, one study demonstrated increased hepatotoxicity when mercaptopurine was used in conjunction with doxorubicin.

■ **IMMUNOSUPPRESSIVE DRUGS (*e.g.*, azathioprine, cyclophosphamide, corticosteroids):** Use with other immunosuppressant drugs may increase the risk of infection.

■ **MYELOSUPPRESSIVE DRUGS (*e.g.*, antineoplastics, chloramphenicol, flucytosine, amphotericin B, colchicine, etc.):** Use extreme caution when used concurrently with other drugs that are also myelosuppressive, including many of the other antineoplastics and other bone marrow depressant drugs; bone marrow depression may be additive. In humans, enhanced bone marrow depression has occurred when used concomitantly with **trimethoprim/sulfa.**

■ **VACCINES, LIVE:** Live virus vaccines should be used with caution, if at all, during therapy

■ **WARFARIN:** Mercaptopurine may reduce anticoagulant effect

Laboratory Considerations

■ Mercaptopurine may give falsely elevated **serum glucose** and **uric acid** values when using a SMA (sequential multiple analyzer) 12/60.

Doses

■ **DOGS:**

a) As an immunosuppressant in combination with corticosteroids for treating bullous pemphigoid: 2.2 mg/kg once daily (q24h), then q48h. (Swartout 2004)

b) For erosive, immune-mediated polyarthritis in combination with corticosteroids: 2 mg/kg PO once daily (q24h) for 14–21 days, then q48h (every other day). (Beale & Worley 2004)

c) For treatment of immune-mediated diseases or acute lymphocytic and granulocytic leukemias: 50 mg/m^2 PO once daily (q24h) to effect, then every other day (q48h) or as needed. (Jacobs *et al.* 1992)

Monitoring

■ Hemograms (including platelets) should be monitored closely; initially every 1–2 weeks and every 1–2 months once on maintenance therapy. It is recommended by some clinicians that if the WBC count drops to between 5,000–7,000 cells/mm^3 the dose be reduced by 25%. If WBC count drops below 5,000 cells/mm^3 treatment should be discontinued until leukopenia resolves.

■ Liver function tests; serum amylase, if indicated

■ Efficacy

Client Information

■ Clients must be briefed on the possibilities of severe toxicity developing from this drug, including drug-related neoplasms or mortality.

■ Clients should contact veterinarian should the animal exhibit signs of abnormal bleeding, bruising, anorexia, vomiting, or infection.

■ Although, no special precautions are necessary with handling intact tablets, it is recommended to wash hands after administering the drug.

Chemistry/Synonyms

A purine analog, mercaptopurine occurs as a slightly yellow, crystalline powder. It is insoluble in water and has a pKa of 7.6.

Mercaptopurine may also be known as: 6-mercaptopurine, 6-MP, 6MP, mercaptopurinum, NSC-755, purinethiol, WR-2785, *Flocofil®, Ismipur®, Mercap®, Mercaptina®, Puri-Nethol®, Purinethol®,* and *Varimer®.*

Storage/Stability

Mercaptopurine tablets should be stored at room temperature in well-closed containers.

Dosage Forms/Regulatory Status

VETERINARY-LABELED PRODUCTS: None

HUMAN-LABELED PRODUCTS:

Mercaptopurine Tablets: 50 mg; *Purinethol®* (Gate Pharmaceuticals); generic (Par); (Rx)

References

Beale, B. & D. Worley (2004). Polyarthritis, erosive, immune-mediated. *The 5–MInute Veterinary Consult: Canine & Feline, 3rd Ed.* P Shires Eds., Lippincott: 1040–1041.

Jacobs, R., J. Lumsden, et al. (1992). Canine and Feline Reference Values. *Current Veterinary Therapy XI: Small Animal Practice.* R Kirk and J Bonagura Eds. Philadelphia, W.B. Saunders Company: 1250–1277.

Swartout, M. (2004). Bullous pemphigoid. *The 5–MInute Veterinary Consult: Canine & Feline, 3rd Ed.* K Rhodes Ed., Lippincott: 128–129.

MEROPENEM

(mare-oh-*pen*-ehm)   Merrem I.V.®

CARBAPENEM ANTIBIOTIC

Prescriber Highlights

▶ Carbapenem antibiotic similar to imipenem, but does not cause seizures & may be more effective against some resistant gram-negative infections

▶ Can be administered more rapidly and with less volume than imipenem

▶ Use should be reserved for documented resistant infections &/or when aminoglycosides not indicated (renal dysfunction, CNS infections)

▶ Seems well-tolerated in animal patients

▶ Must be given IV or SC

▶ Price is decreasing as now available as a generic

Uses/Indications

Meropenem may be useful in treating resistant gram-negative bacterial infections, particularly when aminoglycoside use would be risky (*i.e.,* renal failure) or not effective (*i.e.,* resistance or CNS infections).

Pharmacology/Actions

Meropenem has a broad antibacterial spectrum similar to that of imipenem, but meropenem is more active against Enterobacteriaceae and less so against gram-positive bacteria. Oxacillin-resistant Staphylococcus are usually resistant to meropenem. Because meropenem is more stable to renal dehydropeptidase-I than is imipenem, it does not require the addition of cilastatin to inhibit that enzyme. Meropenem may also have less potential to induce seizures than imipenem or ertapenem.

Pharmacokinetics

Meropenem must be administered via parenteral means. After SC injection in dogs, bioavailability is 84%. After IV injection in dogs, meropenem's volume of distribution is approximately 0.37 L/kg and protein binding about 12%; half-life $\approx$ 40 minutes, and clearance $\approx$ 6.5 mL/min/kg. Concentrations of unbound drug in tissue fluid and plasma are similar.

In ewes, after IM injection meropenem was rapidly absorbed and had a bioavailability equal to that of intravenous dosing. Volume of distribution at steady state was 0.06 L/kg and protein binding about 43%; elimination half-life was about 43 minutes. 91% of the drug was recovered in the urine over 24 hours after IM injection.

Pharmacokinetic data for humans include: wide distribution in body tissues and fluids, including into the CSF and bile; very low protein binding $\approx$ 2%; in patients with normal renal function, elimination half-life is about an hour. One inactive metabolite has been identified, but the majority of the drug is eliminated via renal mechanisms (tubular secretions and glomerular filtration) and 70% of a dose is recovered unchanged in the urine over 12 hours.

Contraindications/Precautions/Warnings

Meropenem is contraindicated in patients hypersensitive to it or other carbapenems, and those that have developed anaphylaxis after receiving any beta-lactam antibiotic.

Adverse Effects

Meropenem is usually very well tolerated. Animals given the drug SC may show slight hair loss over injection sites. In human patients receiving meropenem, only GI effects (nausea, vomiting, diarrhea) have been reported to occur in greater than 1% of patients treated.

Reproductive/Nursing Safety

In humans, meropenem is designated by the FDA as a category *B* drug (*Animal studies have not demonstrated risk to the fetus, but there are no adequate studies in pregnant women; or animal studies have shown an adverse effect, but adequate studies in pregnant women have not demonstrated a risk to the fetus during the first trimester of pregnancy, and there is no evidence of risk in later trimesters.*)

Meropenem is likely safe to use during lactation.

Overdosage/Acute Toxicity

Overdoses of meropenem are unlikely to occur in patients with normal renal function. In human trials, doses of 2 grams every 8 hours failed to demonstrate any significant adversity. Should an overdose occur, the drug can be discontinued if necessary or the next dose could be delayed by a few hours. Meropenem can be removed via hemodialysis when necessary.

Drug Interactions

The following drug interactions have either been reported or are theoretical in humans or animals receiving meropenem and may be of significance in veterinary patients:

- ■ **AMINOGLYCOSIDES:** *In vitro* evidence of synergy against *Pseudomonas aeruginosa*
- ■ **PROBENECID:** May increase serum concentrations and elimination half-life of meropenem

Laboratory Considerations

- ■ No specific laboratory interactions were noted for meropenem.

Doses

- ■ **DOGS/CATS:**

  For treatment of susceptible infections:
  a) For bacteremia/sepsis: 24 mg/kg IV q24h (once daily) or 12 mg/kg SC q8h;

  For UTI: 12 mg/kg SC q12h;

  For CNS infections: 40 mg/kg IV or SC q8h. This dose is extrapolated from children and maximum dose per administration is 2 grams. To help prevent development of resistant strains that might infect humans, use should be limited or avoided unless ultimately necessary. (Greene *et al.* 2006)

  b) For systemic infections: 12 mg/kg q8h SC or 24 mg/kg IV q24h (once daily); for urinary tract infections 12 mg/kg q12h SC (Papich 2002)

  c) 125 mg (total dose) for small dogs and cats q8h IV or SC; 250 mg q8h IV or SC for medium dogs; 500 mg q8h IV or SC for large (>100 lbs.) dogs. **Note:** If serum creatinine greater than 4, may be given q12h. (Aucoin 2002)

  d) Cats: 8 mg/kg IV or SC q8h. (Hawkins 2009)

Monitoring

- ■ There are no specific monitoring requirements for meropenem except to monitor for clinical efficacy.

Client Information

- ■ This drug is generally used on an inpatient basis usually because of the seriousness of the infections treated, but clients could give SC injections at home, particularly when treating urinary tract infections.

Chemistry/Synonyms

A synthetic carbapenem antibiotic, meropenem occurs as a clear to white to pale yellow powder or crystals. It is very slightly soluble in water or hydrated alcohol and practically insoluble in acetone or ether. When the commercially available injection is reconstituted the resulting pH is between 7.3 and 8.3.

Meropenem may also be known as: ICI-194660, SM-7338, *Meronem®*, *Meropen®*, *Merrem®*, *Optinem®*, or *Zeropenem®*.

Storage/Stability

The powder for injection should be stored at controlled room temperature (20–25°C; 69–77°F). When the commercially available powder for injection is reconstituted with sterile water for injection (up to a concentration of 50 mg/mL), it is stable (per the manufacturer) for up to 2 hours at room temperature; up to 12 hours when refrigerated. The package insert lists several options for dilution with several different solutions in plastic IV bags, syringes, minibags, etc. The longest time the drug the manufacturer states the drug is stable, is 48 hours when diluted in normal saline or sterile water for injection at concentrations from 1–20 mg/mL in plastic syringes and kept refrigerated.

The manufacturer recommends that solutions of meropenem not be frozen, but meropenem concentrations of 1 and 22 mg/mL in dextrose 5% and sodium chloride 0.9% have been stored frozen at -20°C for up to 14 days with a calculated loss of potency of 10%.

For subcutaneous administration in veterinary patients, meropenem has been diluted to a concentration of 20 mg/mL in sterile sodium chloride 0.9%. The solution should be protected from light and is reportedly stable if kept refrigerated for up to 96 hours. Once the refrigerated solution is brought back to room temperature it should be used within 6 hours. (Jordan 2004)

Compatibility/Compounding Considerations

Meropenem has been reported **compatible** with vancomycin, ranitidine, morphine sulfate, metoclopramide, heparin, gentamicin, furosemide, dopamine, dobutamine, dexamethasone sodium phosphate, atropine, and aminophylline. Compatibility is dependent upon factors such as pH, concentration, temperature and diluent used; consult specialized references or a hospital pharmacist for more specific information.

Dosage Forms/Regulatory Status

VETERINARY-LABELED PRODUCTS: None

HUMAN-LABELED PRODUCTS:

Meropenem Powder for solution for Injection: 500 mg & 1 gram in 20 mL, & 30 mL vials; *Merrem® I.V*; (AstraZeneca); generic (Rx)

References

Aucoin, D. (2002). Rational approach to antimicrobial therapy in companion animals. Proceedings: Atlantic Coast Veterinary Conference. Accessed via: Veterinary Information Network. http://goo.gl/5atZq

Greene, C., K. Hartmannn, et al. (2006). Appendix 8: Antimicrobial Drug Formulary. *Infectious Disease of the Dog and Cat.* C Greene Ed., Elsevier: 1186–1333.

Hawkins, E. (2009). Dyspneic Cats: Infections You Are Missing. Proceedings: WVC. Accessed via: Veterinary Information Network. http://goo.gl/Lvhqi

Jordan, D. (2004, Last Update). "Personal Communication."

Papich, M. (2002). New advances in antibiotic treatment for animals. Proceedings: WSAVA 2002 Congress. Accessed via: Veterinary Information Network. http://goo.gl/2mqTW

METERGOLINE

(meh-*tir*-goe-leen)   Contralac®, Liserdol®

SEROTONIN ANTAGONIST; PROLACTIN INHIBITOR

Prescriber Highlights

▶ Serotonin antagonist prolactin inhibitor used primarily for pseudopregnancy in dogs

▶ Not available commercially in USA

▶ Primary adverse effects are GI (esp. vomiting) and behavior-related

Uses/Indications

Metergoline is an ergot-derivative drug that is used for pseudopregnancy in dogs. It is available as a veterinary product in several European and South American countries. It has been investigated as an abortifacient in dogs at high doses (0.4–0.6 mg/kg), similar to other ergot prolactin inhibitors it can only used reliably for this effect during the last 3 weeks of gestation (Nothling *et al.* 2003).

In humans, metergoline has been used for hyperprolactemia, prolactinomas, and for the prophylactic treatment of migraine headaches.

Pharmacology/Actions

Metergoline reduces prolactin primarily via its serotonin antagonism effects. It differs from cabergoline and bromocriptine in that it has both strong central and peripheral anti-serotonin effects, and only weak direct dopamine-2 agonist effects. Like those drugs, it also is an antagonist at dopamine-1 receptors. Potentially, metergoline could be used to induce estrus or treat pyometra in bitches.

Pharmacokinetics

Little information was located for dogs. Metergoline half-life is reportedly quite short (approx. 4 hours) and twice daily dosing is required.

In humans, metergoline oral bioavailability is about 25% and volume of distribution is 0.8 L/kg. It is metabolized in the liver to at least one active metabolite (1-desmethylmetergoline) which attains plasma levels higher than that of the parent drug. Elimination half-life of the parent drug is about 50 minutes; 1-desmethylmetergoline, 80-100 minutes.

Contraindications/Precautions/Warnings

Metergoline is contraindicated in dogs and cats that are pregnant unless abortion is desired (see indications). It should not be used in patients who are hypersensitive to ergot derivatives. Patients that do not tolerate cabergoline or bromocriptine may or may not tolerate metergoline. Patients with significantly impaired liver function should receive the drug with caution and, if required, possibly at a lower dosage.

Adverse Effects

Reported adverse effects for metergoline in dogs include behavior-related effects (anxiety, aggressiveness, depression, hyperexcitation, whining and escaping) and GI effects (anorexia, vomiting, nausea).

Reproductive/Nursing Safety

Metergoline is contraindicated in dogs and cats that are pregnant unless abortion is desired (see indications). Because it suppresses prolactin, it should not be used in nursing mothers.

Overdosage/Acute Toxicity

Little information is available. Vomiting is the most likely effect that would be seen in overdose situations.

Drug Interactions

The following drug interactions have either been reported or are theoretical in humans or animals receiving metergoline and may be of significance in veterinary patients:

■ **BROMOCRIPTINE, CABERGOLINE:** May cause additive effects if used with metergoline

■ **CYPROHEPTADINE:** May cause additive effects if used with metergoline

■ **METOCLOPRAMIDE:** Use with metergoline may reduce the efficacy of both drugs and should be avoided

■ **SSRIS (e.g., fluoxetine, paroxetine, sertraline, etc.):** Potentially could reduce the efficacy of each drug

Laboratory Considerations

■ No particular laboratory interactions or considerations were located for this drug.

Doses

■ **DOGS:**

For treatment of pseudopregnancy:

a) 0.5 mg/kg (500 micrograms/kg) PO twice a day. Administration for 4-5 days is effective in treating pseudopregnancy signs and reducing milk production in most bitches. Occasional failures can be dealt with by repeating the treatment protocol and extending it to 8 to 10 days, or by using joint protocols of cabergoline plus metergoline or cabergoline plus bromocriptine. (Romagnoli 2009)

b) The recommended dose is 0.1 mg/kg, PO twice a day for 8 to 10 days. (Gobello *et al.* 2001)

c) In the study, dogs were given 0.1 mg/kg q12h PO with food for 10 days. At day 14 in the treatment group, 10 of 14 dogs had a full remission, and 3 of 14 dogs had partial (intermediate) remission of signs. In the treatment group, side effects were limited to hyperexcitation and nausea, did not lead to termination of therapy, and gradually dissipated during the second week of the protocol. (Castex *et al.* 2002)

To induce estrus:

a) Cabergoline and bromocriptine have consistently given positive results, while metergoline's results have been more variable depending on dosage. Using low dose (0.1 mg/kg PO twice a day) the commercial oral preparation of metergoline administered from 100 days after ovulation until the following proestrus, the interoestrous interval can be significantly shortened (Romagnoli 2006).

■ **CATS:**

For treatment of pseudopregnancy or to halt post-partum lactation:

a) 0.125 mg/kg PO twice a day for 4–8 days. (Label Information—*Contralac®*; Virbac-Switzerland)

Monitoring

■ Efficacy and adverse effects

■ If used long term, liver function tests

Client Information

■ Give this medication with food; contact veterinarian if vomiting persists

■ Keep this an all medications away from pets and animals

Chemistry/Synonyms

Metergoline is an ergot derivative and has the chemical name: Benzyl (8S,10S)-(1,6-dimethylergolin-8-ylmethyl)carbamate.

Metergoline may also be known as: FI-6337, MCE, Metergoliini, Metergolin, Metergolina, Métergoline, Metergolinum, or Methergoline. A common trade name is *Contralac®* (veterinary) and *Liserdol®* (human).

Storage/Stability

Metergoline tablets should be stored at room temperature; protected from light.

Dosage Forms/Regulatory Status

VETERINARY-LABELED PRODUCTS:

None in the USA, in several countries in Europe and South America: Metergoline 0.5 mg & 2 mg oral tablets are available; *Contralac®* (Virbac)

HUMAN-LABELED PRODUCTS:

None in USA. In some countries: Metergoline 4 mg tablets are available.

References

Castex, G., Y. Corrada, et al. (2002). A clinical trial of the prolactin inhibitor metergoline in the treatment of canine pseudopregnancy. *Revista Científica-Facultad De Ciencias Veterinarias* 12(6): 712–714.

Gobello, C., C. Concannon, et al. (2001). Canine Pseudopregnancy: A Review. *Recent Advances in Small Animal Reproduction.* C Concannon, G England, J Verstegen and C Linde-Forsberg Eds. Ithaca, IVIS.

Nothling, J.O., D. Gerber, et al. (2003). Abortifacient and endocrine effects of metergoline in beagle bitches during the second half of gestation. *Theriogenology* 59(9): 1929–1940.

Romagnoli, S. (2006). Control of reproduction in dogs and cats: Use and misuse of hormones. Proceedings: WSAVA World Congress. Accessed via: Veterinary Information Network. http://goo.gl/aGuBF

Romagnoli, S. (2009). An update on pseudopregnancy. Proceedings: WSAVA. Accessed via: Veterinary Information Network. http://goo.gl/1CpI2

METFORMIN HCL

(met-*fore*-min)   Glucophage®

ANTIHYPERGLYCEMIC

Prescriber Highlights

▶ Oral anti-hyperglycemic agent that potentially could be useful in the adjunctive treatment of non-insulin dependent diabetes mellitus (NIDDM) in cats; use is controversial and unlikely to be of benefit

▶ Potentially useful for treating insulin resistance in horses, but has a negative pharmacokinetic profile (low PO bioavailability; fast half-life)

▶ Contraindicated in patients hypersensitive to it; with renal dysfunction, metabolic acidosis, or temporarily when iodinated contrast agents are to be used (see Drug Interactions)

▶ Adverse effects may include lethargy, inappetence, vomiting, & weight loss

▶ Potentially significant drug interactions

▶ Human dosage forms may be difficult to accurately dose in cats

Uses/Indications

Metformin may be useful in the adjunctive treatment of non-insulin dependent diabetes mellitus in cats. Only limited trials of the drug have been performed in cats, with only very limited success when the drug is used alone. Studies comparing its safety and efficacy with other oral antihyperglycemics (*e.g.*, glipizide or insulin) were not located.

There has been some research evaluating metformin for treating insulin resistance in horses.

Pharmacology/Actions

Metformin's actions are multifaceted. At usual dosages, it increases insulin's ability to transport glucose across cell membranes in skeletal muscle without increasing lactate production and inhibits formation of advanced glycosylation end-products. Metformin decreases hepatic glucose production, and may decrease intestinal absorption of glucose. It does not stimulate insulin production or release from the pancreas and, therefore, does not cause hypoglycemia.

Pharmacokinetics

A pharmacokinetic study done in cats (Chastain *et al.* 1999) showed that metformin is variably absorbed after oral administration 35–67%. In cats, steady-state volume of distribution was 0.55 L/kg; elimination half-life about 12 hours and total clearance was 0.15 L/hr/kg. Metformin is primarily eliminated via the kidneys. The authors concluded that the drug's pharmacokinetics are similar to that seen in humans, and that a dosage of 2 mg/kg twice daily would give plasma concentrations known to be effective in humans.

In a small (4 subjects) pharmacokinetic study in horses, metformin demonstrated very low oral bioavailability (4% fed, 7% fasted). Maximum blood levels were around 0.4 micrograms/mL. Elimination half-life after IV dosing was about 25 minutes. (Hustace *et al.* 2009)

Contraindications/Precautions/Warnings

In humans (and presumably cats), metformin is contraindicated in patients hypersensitive to it, with renal dysfunction or metabolic acidosis. It is also temporarily contraindicated when iodinated contrast agents are to be used (see Drug Interactions).

Adverse Effects

In cats, metformin may cause lethargy, inappetence, vomiting, and weight loss. In a study evaluating metformin in diabetic cats (Nelson *et al.* 2004), 1 of 5 diabetic cats studied died 11 days after receiving metformin. As the cause of death was undetermined, metformin could not be ruled out as a causative factor. Hypoglycemia would not be an expected adverse effect when metformin is used as a single agent.

Reproductive/Nursing Safety

In pregnant humans, metformin is designated by the FDA as a category *B* drug (*Animal studies have not demonstrated risk to the fetus, but there are no adequate studies in pregnant women; or animal studies have shown an adverse effect, but adequate studies in pregnant women have not demonstrated a risk to the fetus during the first trimester of pregnancy, and there is no evidence of risk in later trimesters.*)

Metformin is excreted in maternal milk in levels equivalent to those found in plasma. While adverse effects in nursing kittens would be unlikely, use with caution in lactating queens.

Overdosage/Acute Toxicity

Massive overdoses in humans (100 grams) caused hypoglycemia only 10% of the time, but lactic acidosis occurred. Lactic acidosis has been seen in human overdoses of 7 and 20 grams (total dose). It is unknown at what dose acidosis may occur in domestic animals. Ingestion of up to 1700 mg by children is not usually associated with significant toxicity.

There were 243 exposures to metformin reported to the ASPCA Animal Poison Control Center (APCC) during 2008-2009. In these cases 231 were dogs with 27 showing clinical signs and the remaining 12 cases were cats with 2 showing clinical signs. Common findings in dogs recorded in decreasing frequency included vomiting and diarrhea.

In small animals hypoglycemia is not commonly seen in overdoses of metformin alone. It has a narrow margin of safety regarding GI upset. GI upset commonly occurs with ingestions of metformin in small animals.

Drug Interactions

The following drug interactions have either been reported or are theoretical in humans or animals receiving metformin and may be of significance in veterinary patients:

- **ACE INHIBITORS:** May increase risk for hypoglycemia
- **CIMETIDINE:** In humans, cimetidine can cause a 60% increase in peak metformin plasma levels and a 40% increase in AUC
- **CORTICOSTEROIDS:** May reduce efficacy
- **DIURETICS, THIAZIDE:** May reduce hypoglycemic efficacy
- **FUROSEMIDE:** Can increase the AUC and plasma levels of metformin by 22% in humans; metformin can decrease the peak plasma concentrations and AUC of furosemide
- **IODINATED CONTRAST AGENTS, PARENTERAL:** May cause acute renal failure and lactic acidosis if used within 48 hours of a metformin dose
- **ISONIAZID:** May reduce hypoglycemic efficacy
- **SYMPATHOMIMETIC AGENTS:** May reduce hypoglycemic efficacy

Laboratory Considerations

- No specific laboratory interactions or considerations noted.

Doses

- **CATS:**
  a) The author states that "*metformin has been shown toxic to cats and should not be used. It is also ineffective.*" (Greco 2007)
  b) For cats with non-insulin dependent diabetes mellitus (patients with detectable concentrations of insulin): 50 mg (total dose) per cat PO twice daily; may be efficacious only in cats with detectable concentrations of insulin at time of treatment (Nelson *et al.* 2004)
  c) For early NIDDM: 2 mg/kg PO q12h (Melendez & Lorenz 2002)

- **BIRDS:**
  a) Recommended dosages include 100–500 mg/L of drinking water. (Lightfoot 2008)

Monitoring

- Efficacy: Standard methods of monitoring efficacy for diabetes treatment should be followed (*e.g.*, fasting blood glucose, appetite, attitude, body condition, PU/PD resolution, and perhaps serum fructosamine and/or glycosylated hemoglobin levels)
- Renal function (baseline and annually)
- Adverse effects

Client Information

- Clients should understand the relative "investigational" nature of using this compound in cats and report any untoward effects to the veterinarian.

Chemistry/Synonyms

A biguanide oral anti-hyperglycemic agent, metformin HCl occurs as white to off-white crystals that are slightly soluble in alcohol and freely soluble in water. It is a weak base; a 1% aqueous solution of metformin HCl has a pKa of 6.68 and metformin base has a pKa of 12.4.

Metformin HCl may also be known as dimethylbiguanide HCl or metforimini hydrochloridium. There are many proprietary names outside of the USA for this drug.

Storage/Stability

Metformin HCl oral products (oral tablets, sustained-release tablets, and fixed dose combination products with glipizide or rosiglitazone) should be stored protected from light at a controlled room temperature of 20–25°C (68–77°F), excursions permitted to 15–30°C (59–86°F). The combination product containing metformin HCL and glyburide should be stored at temperatures up to 25°C (77°F) and protected from light.

Dosage Forms/Regulatory Status

VETERINARY-LABELED PRODUCTS: None

HUMAN-LABELED PRODUCTS:

Metformin HCl Oral Tablets: 500 mg, 850 mg & 1000 mg; *Glucophage®* (Bristol-Myers Squibb); generic; (Rx)

Metformin HCl Extended-Release Oral Tablets: 500 mg, 750 mg & 1000 mg; *Glucophage XR®* (Bristol-Myers Squibb); *Glumetza®* (Depomed); *Fortamet®* (First Horizon); generic; (Rx)

Metformin HCl Oral Solution: 500 mg/5 mL in 118 mL & 473 mL; *Riomet®* (Ranbaxy); (Rx)

The are also fixed-dose oral tablet combination products available containing metformin and glyburide or glipizide.

References

Chastain, C., D. Panciera, et al. (1999). Pharmacokinetics of the antihyperglycemic agent metformin in cats. *Am Jnl Vet Res* **60**: 738–742.

Greco, D. (2007). Roles of Diet and Drugs in Feline Diabetes Mellitus. Proceedings Western Vet Conf. Accessed via: Veterinary Information Network. http://goo.gl/qfJiP

Hustace, J.L., A.M. Firshman, et al. (2009). Pharmacokinetics and bioavailability of metformin in horses. *American Journal of Veterinary Research* **70**(5): 665–668.

Lightfoot, T. (2008). Avian Pancreas: Anatomy, Physiology and Disease. Proceedings: ABVP. Accessed via: Veterinary Information Network. http://goo.gl/yYJGi

Melendez, L. & M. Lorenz (2002). Feline Insulin Resistance and Diabetes Mellitus. Proceedings: Western Veterinary Conference. Accessed via: Veterinary Information Network. http://goo.gl/PrwTk

Nelson, R., D. Spann, et al. (2004). Evaluation of the oral antihyperglycemic drug metformin in normal and diabetic cats. *J Vet Intern Med* **18**(1): 18–24.

METHADONE HCL

(*meth*-a-done)   Dolophine®

OPIATE AGONIST

Prescriber Highlights

▶ Narcotic agonist that may be used as an alternative to morphine in dogs, cats

▶ Causes less histamine-release (with IV), sedation & vomiting than morphine

▶ Depending on country, may be significantly more expensive than morphine

▶ C-II controlled substance in USA

Uses/Indications

Methadone may be used as an alternative opioid preanesthetic or analgesic in dogs or cats. It is also being investigated for epidural use for horses. Poor oral bioavailability precludes oral dosing in dogs.

Pharmacology/Actions

In small animals methadone acts similarly to morphine with regard to its degree of analgesia and duration of action. Methadone is a *mu*-receptor agonist that also is a non-competitive inhibitor of NMDA (n-methyl-d-aspartate) receptors. Methadone can also reduce re-uptake of norepinephrine and serotonin which may contribute to its analgesic effects. Due to these other actions, methadone potentially may be more efficacious than other *mu* agonists (*e.g.*, morphine) particularly for neuropathic or chronic pain. Methadone is more lipid-soluble than is morphine and approximately 1–1.5 times as potent. It does not cause significant histamine release when administered intravenously.

Refer to the monograph: *Narcotic (opiate) Analgesic Agonists, Pharmacology of*, for more information.

Pharmacokinetics

Limited information is available on the pharmacokinetics of methadone in domestic animals. In dogs, methadone has poor oral bioavailability and ketoconazole or omeprazole do not significantly affect oral bioavailability. Unlike in humans, CYP3A does not appear to be a major metabolic pathway for methadone biotransformation in dogs (KuKanich *et al.* 2005). Subcutaneous administration has a bioavailability of about 80% and peak levels occur around an hour after dosing. Terminal elimination half-life after intravenous dosing is about 1.75–4 hours in dogs; clearance is about 25-30 mL/kg/min. After SC administration, half-life is closer to 11 hours, but there was wide interpatient variation. (Ingvast-Larsson *et al.* 2010).

In horses, orally administered methadone appears to be well absorbed, but is rapidly eliminated (half-life around 1 hour) (Linardi *et al.* 2008).

In humans, methadone is well absorbed from the GI tract (PO), and after subcutaneous or intramuscular injection. It is widely distributed and extensively bound to plasma proteins (60–90%). Methadone is metabolized in the liver primarily by the cytochrome P450 CYP3A isoenzyme, but other isoenzymes also play a role. Metabolites do not have activity. Methadone half-life is widely variable in humans (15–60 hours); elimination half-lives may be extended if giving multiple doses.

Contraindications/Precautions/Warnings

All opiates should be used with caution in patients with heart failure, hypertension, head injuries, elevated CSF pressures, and in geriatric or severely debilitated patients.

Adverse Effects

Adverse effects from methadone can include panting, whining, sedation, defecation, constipation, bradycardia, and respiratory depression. Methadone tends to cause less sedation or vomiting than morphine.

Methadone in cats appears to cause less excitation or vomiting than some other *mu* agonists.

In horses, methadone at IV doses of 0.1 mg/kg or greater has caused pronounced CNS excitement.

Reproductive/Nursing Safety

Methadone is relatively safe to use at low dosages for short periods during the first two trimesters of pregnancy, but it should be avoided late in term as significant respiratory depression and increased rates of stillbirths have been noted in humans. Infants of humans who have been taking methadone for opiate addiction, have shown high rates of moderate to severe opiate withdrawal signs during the neonatal period, and long-term developmental problems.

Although methadone enters maternal milk, the American Academy of Pediatrics considers methadone compatible with breast-feeding in women.

Overdosage/Acute Toxicity

Overdosage may produce profound respiratory and/or CNS depression in most species. Newborns may be more susceptible to these effects than adult animals. Other toxic effects can include cardiovascular collapse, hypothermia, and skeletal muscle hypotonia. Naloxone is the agent of choice in treating respiratory depression. In massive overdoses, naloxone doses may need to be repeated. Animals should be closely observed since naloxone's effects might diminish before sub-toxic levels of methadone are attained. Mechanical respiratory support should be considered in cases of severe respiratory depression. Dialysis, charcoal hemoperfusion, or forced diuresis do not appear to be beneficial in treating methadone overdoses.

Drug Interactions

The following drug interactions have either been reported or are theoretical in humans or animals

receiving methadone and may be of significance in veterinary patients:

- ◼ **ANTIARRHYTHMICS, CLASS I & III (e.g., lidocaine, procainamide, quinidine, amiodarone):** Use with methadone may increase risks for arrhythmias

- ◼ **ALPHA2-AGONISTS (e.g., medetomidine, xylazine):** In a small study done in dogs, methadone potentiated the sedative and analgesic effects of medetomidine in dogs, but severe hypoxemia was seen in dogs breathing room air (Raekallio *et al.* 2009). Results from another study combining xylazine and methadone, suggested that methadone is a good alternative for sedation in dogs when combined with acepromazine or xylazine. A satisfactory degree of sedation was achieved with both combinations. The combination of methadone and xylazine appeared to result in better analgesia compared to xylazine alone (Monteiro *et al.* 2008).

- ◼ **AZOLE ANTIFUNGALS (fluconazole, itraconazole, ketoconazole):** May increase methadone levels (Does not appear to be true for dogs)

- ◼ **CALCIUM CHANNEL BLOCKERS:** Use with methadone may increase risks for arrhythmias

- ◼ **CNS DEPRESSANTS, OTHER (e.g., anesthetic agents, antihistamines, phenothiazines, barbiturates, tranquilizers, alcohol, etc.):** May cause increased CNS or respiratory depression when used with methadone

- ◼ **CORTICOSTEROIDS (MINERALOCORTICOIDS):** Use with methadone may increase potential for electrolyte abnormalities

- ◼ **DIURETICS:** Opiates may decrease efficacy in CHF patients

- ◼ **MACROLIDE ANTIBIOTICS (erythromycin, clarithromycin):** May inhibit metabolism of methadone and increase levels (Does not appear to be true for dogs)

- ◼ **MONAMINE OXIDASE (MAO) INHIBITORS (e.g., amitraz, possibly selegiline):** Meperidine with MAOIs in humans has caused severe CNS/behavior reactions and potentially could do the same with methadone; avoid concomitant use

- ◼ **MUSCLE RELAXANTS, SKELETAL:** Methadone may enhance neuromuscular blockade

- ◼ **PHENOBARBITAL, PHENYTOIN:** May decrease methadone levels (Probably does not affect dogs)

- ◼ **RIFAMPIN:** May decrease methadone levels (Probably does not affect dogs)

- ◼ **SSRI ANTIDEPRESSANTS (fluoxetine, sertraline, etc.):** May increase methadone levels

- ◼ **ST JOHN'S WORT:** May decrease methadone levels (Probably does not affect dogs)

- ◼ **TRICYCLIC ANTIDEPRESSANTS (clomipramine, amitriptyline, etc.):** Methadone may exacerbate the effects of tricyclic antidepressants

- ◼ **WARFARIN:** Opiates may potentiate anticoagulant activity

- ◼ **ZIDOVUDINE:** Methadone may increase zidovudine levels

Laboratory Considerations

- ◼ As they may increase biliary tract pressure, opiates can increase plasma **amylase** and **lipase** values up to 24 hours following their administration.

Doses

- ◼ **DOGS:**
  a) As a pre-anesthetic: 0.2–0.5 mg/kg SC, IM; or a combination of methadone 0.1–0.3 mg/kg with acepromazine 0.02–0.05 mg/kg SC, IM (Cornell 2004)
  b) For pain: 0.1–0.25 mg/kg IM, SC, IV. Duration of effect 4–6 hours. (Otero 2006)
  c) For perioperative pain control: 0.1–0.5 mg/kg IM or SQ; duration of effect is 2–4 hours. (Pascoe 2006)
  d) For analgesia: 0.5 mg/kg IV q6h or 0.5–1 mg/kg q6-8h IV, IM or SC. (Posner & Papich 2009)

- ◼ **CATS:**
  a) For perioperative pain control: 0.05–0.5 mg/kg IV, IM or SC q4–6h (Tranquilli 2003)
  b) As a pre-anesthetic: 0.1–0.2 mg/kg SC, IM; or a combination of methadone 0.1–0.3 mg/kg with acepromazine 0.02–0.05 mg/kg SC, IM (Cornell 2004)
  c) For moderate to severe pain: 0.1–0.2+ mg/kg IM or SQ; duration of effect is 2–6 hours. For IV dosing use ½ the low end dose, titrate over 3–5 minutes; duration of effect is 1–4 hours. (Mathews 2006)
  d) For pain: 0.1–0.2 mg/kg SC, IV. Duration of effect 2–3 hours. (Otero 2006)

- ◼ **HORSES:**
  a) As an analgesic: 0.1–0.2 mg/kg PO. Anecdotal; author has not prescribed this drug. (Sellon 2007)

Monitoring

- ◼ Analgesic or preanesthetic efficacy
- ◼ At higher dosages, monitor for respiratory depression

Client Information

- ◼ When given parenterally, this agent should be used in an inpatient setting or with direct professional supervision.
- ◼ If being used orally for pain control, be sure to keep out of reach of children and pets.

Chemistry/Synonyms

A synthetic diphenylheptane-derivative narcotic agonist, methadone HCl occurs as an odorless, colorless or white crystalline powder. It is freely soluble in water, chloroform, or alcohol and practically insoluble in ether or glycerol. The pH of a 1% solution in water is between 4.5 and 6.5. The commercially available injection has a pH from 3–6.5. The dispersible tablet formulation (*Diskets®*) contains insoluble ingredients that deter their use for injection.

Methadone may also be known as: Amidine HCl, amidone HCl, methadoni hydrochloridum, Phenadone, *Adolan®, Biodone®, Cloro Nona®, Dolmed®, Eptadone®, Gobbidona®, Heptadon®, Ketalgine®, Metadol®, Metasedin®, Methaddict®, Methadose®, Methatabs®, Methex®, Pallidone®, Phymet®, Physeptone®, Pinadone®, Sedo®, Symoron®,* or *Synastone®.*

Storage/Stability

Unless otherwise labeled, methadone products should be stored at room temperature and protected from light.

Compatibility/Compounding Considerations

Methadone injection is reportedly **stable** when mixed in a syringe with acepromazine. The injection is reportedly **not compatible** with pentobarbital, phenobarbital, amobarbital, or thiopental.

Dosage Forms/Regulatory Status

VETERINARY-LABELED PRODUCTS: None

The ARCI (Racing Commissioners International) has designated this drug as a class 1 substance. See the appendix for more information.

HUMAN-LABELED PRODUCTS:

Methadone HCl Injection: 10 mg/mL in 20 mL multidose vials; generic; (Rx, C-II)

Methadone HCl Oral Tablets: 5 mg & 10 mg; Dispersible Tablets 40 mg; *Dolophine®* Hydrochloride (Roxane); *Methadose®* (Mallinckrodt); generic; (Rx, C-II)

Methadone HCl Oral Solution/Liquid Concentrate: 1 mg/mL, 2 mg/mL & 10 mg/mL in 30 mL (w/calibrated dropper), 500 mL, 946 mL, 1 L & 15 L; generic; *Methadose®* (Mallinckrodt); (Rx, C-II)

All methadone-containing products are C-II controlled substances in the USA. When used as an analgesic, methadone may be dispensed by any pharmacy or practitioner registered with the DEA for Class-II narcotics. When methadone is used to treat narcotic addiction, specialized approval must be obtained from the FDA and, usually, state regulators.

References

Cornell, C. (2004). Anesthetic Drugs. Proceedings: ACVIM Forum. Accessed via: Veterinary Information Network. http://goo.gl/edDP1

Ingvast-Larsson, C., A. Holgersson, et al. (2010). Clinical pharmacology of methadone in dogs. *Veterinary Anaesthesia and Analgesia* 37(1): 48–56.

KuKanich, B., B.D.X. Lascelles, et al. (2005). The effects of inhibiting cytochrome P450 3A, p-glycoprotein, and gastric acid secretion on the oral bioavailability of methadone in dogs. *Journal of Veterinary Pharmacology and Therapeutics* 28(5): 461–466.

Linardi, R., S. Barker, et al. (2008). Oral Absorption and Pharmacokinetics of Methadone HCl in Horses. Proceedings: IVECCS. Accessed via: Veterinary Information Network. http://goo.gl/INMzV

Mathews, K. (2006). How do you know your patient hurts? Assessment, recognition & treatment of pain in cats. Proceedings: AAFP. Accessed via: Veterinary Information Network. http://goo.gl/5knAj

Monteiro, E.R., D.N. Figueroa, et al. (2008). Effects of methadone, alone or in combination with acepromazine or xylazine, on sedation and physiologic values in dogs. *Veterinary Anaesthesia and Analgesia* 35(6): 519–527.

Otero, P. (2006). Acute pain management in emergency. Proceedings: WSAVA World Congress. Accessed via: Veterinary Information Network. http://goo.gl/vB0IV

Pascoe, P. (2006). Pain management in the canine patient. Proceedings: UCD Canine Medicine Conference. Accessed via: Veterinary Information Network. http://goo.gl/hjQru

Posner, L.P. & M.G. Papich (2009). Your patient is still in pain—Now what? "Rescue analgesia". Proceedings: WVC. Accessed via: Veterinary Information Network. http://goo.gl/WMON9

Raekallio, M.R., M.P. Raiha, et al. (2009). Effects of medetomidine, l-methadone, and their combination on arterial blood gases in dogs. *Veterinary Anaesthesia and Analgesia* 36(2): 158–161.

Sellon, D. (2007). New Alternatives for Pain Management in Horses. Proceedings: New Alternatives for Pain Management in Horses. Accessed via: Veterinary Information Network. http://goo.gl/gXMfb

Tranquilli, W. (2003). Pain management alternatives for common surgeries. Proceedings: PAIN 2003. Accessed via: Veterinary Information Network. http://goo.gl/UCsTh

---

METHAZOLAMIDE

(meth-a-**zoe**-la-mide)   Neptazane®

CARBONIC ANHYDRASE INHIBITOR

Prescriber Highlights

▶ Oral carbonic anhydrase inhibitor used primarily for open angle glaucoma

▶ Contraindicated in patients with significant hepatic, renal, pulmonary or adrenocortical insufficiency, hyponatremia, hypokalemia, hyperchloremic acidosis or electrolyte imbalance

▶ Primary adverse effects are GI-related, hypokalemia, metabolic acidosis

▶ Give oral doses with food if GI upset occurs

▶ Monitor with tonometry for glaucoma; check electrolytes

Uses/Indications

Orally administered methazolamide is used for the medical treatment of glaucoma. Topical carbonic anhydrase inhibitors (*e.g.,* dorzolamide) are more commonly used today as they can lower IOP as well as systemic drugs and have fewer adverse effects.

Pharmacology/Actions

The carbonic anhydrase inhibitors act by a non-competitive, reversible inhibition of the enzyme carbonic anhydrase. This reduces the formation of hydrogen and bicarbonate ions from carbon dioxide and reduces the availability of these ions for active transport into body secretions.

Pharmacologic effects of the carbonic anhydrase inhibitors include decreased formation of aqueous humor, thereby reducing intraocular pressure; increased renal tubular secretion of sodium and potassium and, to a greater extent, bicarbonate, leading to increased urine alkalinity and volume; anticonvulsant activity, which is independent of its diuretic effects (mechanism not fully understood, but may be due to carbonic anhydrase or a metabolic acidosis effect).

Pharmacokinetics

Little information is available. Methazolamide is absorbed from the GI tract albeit more slowly than acetazolamide. It is distributed throughout the body, including the CSF and aqueous humor. Methazolamide is at least partially metabolized in the liver.

Contraindications/Precautions/Warnings

Carbonic anhydrase inhibitors are contraindicated in patients with significant hepatic disease (may precipitate hepatic coma), renal or adrenocortical insufficiency, hyponatremia, hypokalemia, hyperchloremic acidosis or electrolyte imbalance. They should not be used in patients with severe pulmonary obstruction unable to increase alveolar ventilation or those who are hypersensitive to them. Long-term use of carbonic anhydrase inhibitors is contraindicated in patients with chronic, noncongestive, angle-closure glaucoma as angle closure may occur and the drug may mask the condition by lowering intra-ocular pressures.

Adverse Effects

Potential adverse effects that may be encountered include GI disturbances (vomiting, diarrhea, inappetence), metabolic acidosis (with heavy panting), CNS effects (sedation, depression, disorientation, excitement, etc.), hematologic effects (bone marrow depression, thrombocytopenia), renal effects (crystalluria, dysuria, renal colic, polyuria, polydipsia), hypokalemia, hyperglycemia, hyponatremia, hyperuricemia, hepatic insufficiency, dermatologic effects (rash, etc.), and hypersensitivity reactions. Electrolyte imbalances may manifest as weakness or cardiac arrhythmias.

Combining methazolamide (oral dosing) with topical (ophthalmic) dorzolamide does not apparently yield additive reductions in intraocular pressure and may cause increased adverse effects.

Reproductive/Nursing Safety

In humans, the FDA categorizes this drug as category **C** for use during pregnancy (*Animal studies have shown an adverse effect on the fetus,* *but there are no adequate studies in humans; or there are no animal reproduction studies and no adequate studies in humans.*)

Safety for use during nursing has not been established. But a related compound, acetazolamide, is excreted in the milk in concentrations unlikely to have pharmacologic effect.

Overdosage/Acute Toxicity

Information regarding overdosage of this drug is not readily available. It is suggested to monitor serum electrolytes, blood gases, volume status, and CNS status during an acute overdose. Treat symptomatically and supportively.

Drug Interactions

The following drug interactions have either been reported or are theoretical in humans or animals receiving methazolamide and may be of significance in veterinary patients:

- ■ **ANTIDEPRESSANTS, TRICYCLIC:** Alkaline urine caused by methazolamide may decrease excretion

- ■ **ASPIRIN (or other salicylates):** Increased risk of methazolamide accumulation and toxicity; increased risk for metabolic acidosis; methazolamide increases salicylate excretion

- ■ **DIGOXIN:** As methazolamide may cause hypokalemia, increased risk for toxicity

- ■ **INSULIN:** Rarely, carbonic anhydrase inhibitors interfere with the hypoglycemic effects of insulin

- ■ **METHENAMINE COMPOUNDS:** Methazolamide may negate effects in the urine

- ■ **POTASSIUM, DRUGS AFFECTING (corticosteroids, amphotericin B, corticotropin, or other diuretics):** Concomitant use may exacerbate potassium depletion

- ■ **PHENOBARBITAL:** Increased urinary excretion, may reduce phenobarbital levels

- ■ **PRIMIDONE:** Decreased primidone concentrations

- ■ **QUINIDINE:** Alkaline urine caused by methazolamide may decrease excretion

Laboratory Considerations

- ■ By alkalinizing the urine, carbonic anhydrase inhibitors may cause false positive results in determining **urine protein** using bromphenol blue reagent (*Albustix®, Albutest®, Labstix®*), sulfosalicylic acid (*Bumintest®, Exton's® Test Reagent*), nitric acid ring test, or heat and acetic acid test methods.

- ■ Carbonic anhydrase inhibitors may **decrease iodine uptake** by the thyroid gland in hyperthyroid or euthyroid patients.

Doses

- ■ **DOGS:**
  For medical treatment of glaucoma:
  a) 2.5–5 mg/kg PO q8–12h (Reinstein *et al.* 2009)

b) 2–4 mg/kg PO two to three times a day (Diehl 2007)

c) 3–5 mg/kg *divided q12h* PO (Millichamp 2006)

d) 2–5 mg/kg PO two to three times a day (Collins 2006; WIlkie 2007)

e) 2.2–4.4 mg/kg PO two to three times a day. (Pickett 2009)

f) 2–10 mg/kg PO two to three times a day. (Giuliano 2009)

■ **CATS:**

For medical treatment of glaucoma:

a) 3–4 mg/kg PO twice a day. Cats may not tolerate oral carbonic anhydrase inhibitors (CAIs) as well as dogs. Reported side effects include lethargy, inappetence, vomiting. Topical CAIs may be better tolerated. (Powell 2003)

b) 1–2 mg/kg PO q8-12h (Miller 2009)

Monitoring

■ Intraocular pressure/tonometry

■ Serum electrolytes, pH

■ Baseline CBC with differential and periodic retests if using chronically

■ Other adverse effects

Client Information

■ If GI upset occurs, give with food.

■ Notify veterinarian if abnormal bleeding or bruising occurs or if animal develops tremors or a rash.

Chemistry/Synonyms

A carbonic anhydrase inhibitor similar to dichlorphenamide, methazolamide occurs as a white to slightly yellow crystalline powder. It is very slightly soluble in water.

Methazolamide may also be known as: *GlaucTabs®, Glaumetax®, MZM®,* and *Neptazane®.*

Storage/Stability

Methazolamide tablets should be stored at room temperature in well-closed containers. Methazolamide tablets have an expiration date of 5 years after manufacture.

Dosage Forms/Regulatory Status

VETERINARY-LABELED PRODUCTS: None

The ARCI (Racing Commissioners International) has designated this drug as a class 4 substance. See the appendix for more information.

HUMAN-LABELED PRODUCTS:

Methazolamide Tablets: 25 mg & 50 mg; generic; (Rx)

References

Collins, B. (2006). Update for glaucoma. Proceedings; Western Vet Conf. Accessed via: Veterinary Information Network. http://goo.gl/2uZWc

Diehl, K. (2007). How to stay calm when the pressure is ris-
ing: Glaucoma I & II. Proceedings: Western Vet Conf. Accessed via: Veterinary Information Network. http://goo.gl/5g9Hr

Giuliano, E. (2009). Uveitis and Glaucoma: Part II. Procedings: IVECCS. Accessed via: Veterinary Information Network. http://goo.gl/qkTMf

Miller, P. (2009). Ophthalmic Drugs: Keepers and Losers. Proceedings: WVC. Accessed via: Veterinary Information Network. http://goo.gl/Jl79J

Millichamp, N. (2006). Glaucoma: The worst ocular disease? Proceedings: IVECCS. Accessed via: Veterinary Information Network. http://goo.gl/cMnwT

Pickett, J. (2009). The canine glaucomas. Proceedings: ABVP. Accessed via: Veterinary Information Network. http://goo.gl/GmzfP

Powell, C. (2003). Feline Glaucoma. Proceedings: Western Veterinary Conference. Accessed via: Veterinary Information Network. http://goo.gl/29jgx

Reinstein, S.L., A.J. Rankin, et al. (2009). Canine Glaucoma: Medical and Surgical Treatment Options. *Compendium-Continuing Education for Veterinarians* 31(10): 454–458.

WIlkie, D. (2007). Glaucoma. Proceedings: ACVC. Accessed via: Veterinary Information Network. http://goo.gl/afFvr

METHENAMINE HIPPURATE

(meth-*en*-a-meen)   Hiprex®, Urex®

URINARY ANTISEPTIC

Prescriber Highlights

▶ Theoretically, converted into an urinary antiseptic; efficacy somewhat questionable in small animals

▶ Contraindications: Metabolic acidosis, hypersensitivity to it, renal insufficiency, severe hepatic impairment (due to ammonia production), or severe dehydration

▶ Adverse Effects: GI irritation; dysuria possible if used long-term

▶ Urine pH must be below 6.5 and ideally less than 6, to be effective

Uses/Indications

Methenamine is used as an antimicrobial agent for prophylaxis of recurrent urinary tract infection. It is not commonly used in veterinary medicine and little good evidence is available to confirm its efficacy in dogs or cats.

Pharmacology/Actions

In an acidic urinary environment (pH <6.5), methenamine is converted to formaldehyde. Formaldehyde is a non-specific antibacterial agent that exerts a bactericidal effect. It has activity on a variety of bacteria, including both gram-positive (*Staphylococcus aureus, S. epidermidis,* Enterococcus) and gram-negative organisms (*E. Coli,* Enterobacter, Klebsiella, Proteus, and *Pseudomonas aeruginosa*). Reportedly, methenamine has activity against fungal urinary tract infections.

Hippuric acid is added primarily to help acidify the urine, but it also has some non-specific antibacterial activity. Bacterial resistance to formaldehyde or hippuric acid does not usually occur.

Pharmacokinetics

Human data: While methenamine and its salts are well absorbed from the GI tract, up to 30% of a dose may be hydrolyzed by gastric acid to ammonia and formaldehyde. With enteric-coated tablets, the amount hydrolyzed in the gut is reduced. While absorbed, plasma concentrations of both formaldehyde and methenamine are very low and have negligible systemic antibacterial activity. Methenamine does cross the placenta and is distributed into milk.

Within 24 hours, 70–90% of a dose is excreted unchanged into the urine. In acidic urine, conversion to ammonia and formaldehyde takes place, maximal hydrolysis occurs at urine pH's of 5.5 or less, but at pH's below 6.5 some conversion occurs. Peak formaldehyde concentrations occur in the urine at about 2 hours post-dose (3–8 hours with enteric-coated tablets).

Contraindications/Precautions/Warnings

Methenamine and its salts are contraindicated in patients known to be hypersensitive to it, with renal insufficiency, metabolic acidosis, severe hepatic impairment (due to ammonia production), or severe dehydration.

Adverse Effects

The most likely adverse effect noted is gastrointestinal upset, with nausea, vomiting, and anorexia predominant. Some patients may develop dysuria, probably secondary to irritation due to high formaldehyde concentrations. Cats reportedly do not tolerate methenamine as well as dogs. Lipoid pneumonitis has been reported in some humans receiving prolonged therapy with the suspension. Potentially, systemic acidosis could occur.

Because methenamine requires acid urine to be beneficial, urine pH should ideally be kept at or below 5.5. Some urea-splitting bacteria (e.g., Proteus and some strains of staphylococci, Enterobacter and Pseudomonas) may increase urine pH. Addition of a urinary acidification program may be required using dietary modification and acidifying drugs (e.g., ascorbic acid, methionine, sodium biphosphate, ammonium chloride).

Reproductive/Nursing Safety

While methenamine crosses the placenta and lab animal studies have not demonstrated any teratogenic effects, it should be used with caution during pregnancy. In humans, the FDA categorizes this drug as category C for use during pregnancy (*Animal studies have shown an adverse effect on the fetus, but there are no adequate studies in humans; or there are no animal reproduction studies and no adequate studies in humans.*)

Methenamine enters milk but no adverse effects have not been reported in nursing children of mothers taking methenamine.

Overdosage/Acute Toxicity

Dogs have received single IV dosages of up to 600 mg/kg of methenamine hippurate without overt toxic effects. Large oral overdoses should be handled using established gut emptying protocols, maintaining hydration status and supporting as required.

Drug Interactions

The following drug interactions have either been reported or are theoretical in humans or animals receiving methenamine and may be of significance in veterinary patients:

■ **SULFAMETHIAZOLE:** Use of methenamine with sulfamethiazole is not recommended. An insoluble precipitate may form.

■ **URINE ALKALINIZING DRUGS (e.g., calcium or magnesium containing antacids, carbonic anhydrase inhibitors, citrates, sodium bicarbonate, thiazide diuretics):** Use of urinary alkalinizing drugs may reduce the efficacy of the methenamine

Laboratory Considerations

■ Urinary values of the following compounds may be falsely elevated: **catecholamines, vanillylmandelic acid (VMA), 17-hydrocorticosteroid**

■ Falsely decreased urinary values of **estriol** or **5-HIAA** may occur

■ Methenamine may cause may cause false-positive **urine glucose determinations** when using cupric sulfate solution (Benedict's Solution, *Clinitest*®) and false-negative tests utilizing the glucose oxidase (*Tes-Tape*®, *Clinistix*®) method

Doses

■ **DOGS:**

Note: Methenamine mandelate has been discontinued in the USA, there does not appear to be a compelling reason that methenamine hippurate could not be substituted.

a) Methenamine mandelate: 10 mg/kg PO q6h; use with ammonium chloride to acidify urine and increase effectiveness (Grauer 2003)

b) Methenamine mandelate: 10 mg/kg PO q6h (Bartges 2007)

c) Methenamine mandelate: The dose is not well established but recommended doses are 10–20 mg/kg PO q 8-12h. If necessary, urine pH may need to be lowered by use of an acidifying diet and/or urinary acidifiers. (Adams 2009)

■ **CATS:**

a) Methenamine hippurate: 250 mg PO q12h (Papich 1992)(Bartges 2007)

Monitoring

■ Urine pH
■ Efficacy

Client Information

■ Give after meals if GI distress occurs

■ Encourage compliance

Chemistry/Synonyms

Methenamine is chemically unrelated to other anti-infective agents. It is commercially available as methenamine hippurate. Methenamine hippurate occurs as a white, crystalline powder with a sour taste and contains approximately 44% methenamine and 56% hippuric acid. It is freely soluble in water.

Methenamine may also be known as: hexamine amygdalate, hexamine mandelate, mandelato de metenamina, *Aci-steril®*, *Hiprex®*, *Reflux®*, *Urocedulamin®*, and *Urex®*.

Storage/Stability

Commercially available methenamine products should be stored at room temperature. Because acids hydrolyze methenamine to formaldehyde and ammonia, do not mix with acidic vehicles before administering.

Compatibility/Compounding Considerations

Methenamine is physically **incompatible** when mixed with most alkaloids and metallic salts (*e.g.*, ferric, mercuric or silver salts). Ammonium salts or alkalis will darken methenamine.

Dosage Forms/Regulatory Status

VETERINARY-LABELED PRODUCTS: None

HUMAN-LABELED PRODUCTS:

Methenamine Hippurate Oral Tablets: 1 gram; *Hiprex®* (Hoechst Marion Roussel); *Urex®* (3M Pharm); (Rx)

Note: For many years methenamine mandelate dosage forms were available commercially in the USA, but these products have reportedly been discontinued.

References

Adams, L. (2009). Recurrent Urinary Tract Infections: Bad Bugs That Won't Go Away. Proceedings: WVC. Accessed via: Veterinary Information Network. http://goo.gl/eX3w6

Bartges, J. (2007). Urinary tract infections: Which antimicrobials work best? Proceedings: Western Vet Conf. Accessed via: Veterinary Information Network. http://goo.gl/vZZDm

Grauer, G. (2003). Urinary Tract Disorders. *Small Animal Internal Medicine 3rd Edition*. R Nelson and C Couto Eds. Phila, Saunders: 568–659.

METHIMAZOLE

(meth-*im*-a-zole)   Tapazole®

Prescriber Highlights

▶ Used for medical treatment of feline hyperthyroidism

▶ Potentially, transdermal gels with methimazole may have efficacy in cats (or owners) that cannot tolerate oral dosing

▶ Contraindications: Hypersensitivity to it

▶ Caution: History of or concurrent hematologic abnormalities, liver disease, or autoimmune disease

▶ Adverse Effects: Most occur within first 3 mos. of treatment: vomiting, anorexia, & depression most frequent. Eosinophilia, leukopenia, & lymphocytosis are usually transient. Rare, but serious: self-induced excoriations, bleeding, hepatopathy, thrombocytopenia, agranulocytosis, positive direct antiglobulin test, & acquired myasthenia gravis

▶ Place kittens on milk replacer if mother receiving drug

▶ Very bitter taste

Uses/Indications

Methimazole is considered by most clinicians in North America the agent of choice when using drugs to treat feline hyperthyroidism. Sustained-release carbimazole is not presently available commercially and propylthiouracil has significantly higher incidences of adverse reactions when compared to methimazole and is rarely used today. Transdermal methimazole (in PLO gel; 2.5 mg twice daily) has been used with some therapeutic success in cats that do not tolerate oral dosing. Efficacy may require four or more weeks to detect. Studies are ongoing.

Methimazole appears to be useful for the prophylactic prevention of cisplatin-induced nephrotoxicity in dogs.

Pharmacology/Actions

Methimazole interferes with iodine incorporation into tyrosyl residues of thyroglobulin, thereby inhibiting the synthesis of thyroid hormones. It also inhibits iodinated tyrosyl residues from coupling to form iodothyronine. Methimazole has no effect on the release or activity of thyroid hormones already formed or in the general circulation.

Pharmacokinetics

Information on the pharmacokinetics of methimazole in cats is available (Trepanier, Peterson, and Aucoin 1989). These researchers reported that in normal cats, the bioavailability of the drug is highly variable (45−98%), as is the volume of distribution (0.12−0.84 L/kg).

After oral dosing, plasma elimination half-life ranges from 2.3–10.2 hours. There is usually a 1–3 week lag time between starting the drug and significant reductions in serum T_4. In dogs, methimazole has a serum half-life of 8–9 hours. Methimazole apparently concentrates in thyroid tissue.

Contraindications/Precautions/Warnings

Methimazole is contraindicated in patients who are hypersensitive to it, carbimazole or the excipient, polyethylene glycol. The veterinary label also states that it is contraindicated in cats with autoimmune disease, primary liver disease, renal failure, hematologic disorders or coagulopathies, or pregnant or lactating queens.

Adverse Effects

Most adverse effects associated with methimazole use in cats occur within the first three months of therapy, with vomiting, anorexia, and depression/lethargy occurring most frequently. GI effects occur in about 10% of treated cats may be related to the drug's bitter taste or direct gastric irritation and are usually transient. Eosinophilia, leukopenia, thrombocytopenia, and lymphocytosis may be noted in approximately 15% of cats treated within the first 8 weeks of therapy. These hematologic effects usually are also transient and generally do not require drug withdrawal. Other more serious but rare adverse effects include: self-induced facial excoriations secondary to facial pruritus (2.3%), bleeding (2.3%), hepatopathy (1.5%), thrombocytopenia (2.7%), agranulocytosis (1.5%), and positive direct antiglobulin test (1.9%). These effects generally require withdrawal of the drug and adjunctive therapy. Up to 50% of cats receiving methimazole chronically (>6 months) will develop a positive ANA, requiring dosage reduction. Rarely cats will develop an acquired myasthenia gravis that requires either withdrawal or concomitant glucocorticoid therapy.

Reproductive/Nursing Safety

High levels of methimazole cross the placenta and may induce hypothyroidism in kittens born of queens receiving the drug. The veterinary label states that the drug should not be used in pregnant or lactating queens as laboratory studies in mice and rats have shown evidence of teratogenic and embryotoxic effects.

In humans, the FDA categorizes this drug as category **D** for use during pregnancy (*There is evidence of human fetal risk, but the potential benefits from the use of the drug in pregnant women may be acceptable despite its potential risks.*)

Levels higher than those found in plasma are detected in human breast milk. It is suggested that kittens be placed on a milk replacer after receiving colostrum from mothers on methimazole.

Overdosage/Acute Toxicity

Acute toxicity that may be seen with overdosage include those that are listed above under Adverse Effects. Agranulocytosis, hepatopathy, and thrombocytopenias are perhaps the most serious effects that may be seen. Treatment consists of following standard protocols in handling an oral ingestion (empty stomach, if not contraindicated, administer charcoal, etc.) and to treat symptomatically and supportively.

Drug Interactions

The following drug interactions have either been reported or are theoretical in humans or animals receiving methimazole and may be of significance in veterinary patients:

- ■ **BENZIMIDAZOLE ANTIPARASITICS:** Methimazole can reduce hepatic oxidation of benzimidazoles and increase blood levels

- ■ **BETA-BLOCKERS:** Veterinary label states: A reduction in dose may be needed when the patient becomes euthyroid

- ■ **BUPROPION:** Potential for increased risk for hepatotoxicity; increased monitoring (LFT's) necessary

- ■ **DIGOXIN:** Methimazole may decrease digoxin efficacy, but the veterinary label states: A reduction in dose may be needed when the patient becomes euthyroid.

- ■ **PHENOBARBITAL:** Veterinary label states: Concurrent use of phenobarbital may reduce the clinical effectiveness

- ■ **THEOPHYLLINE:** Veterinary label states: A reduction in dose may be needed when the patient becomes euthyroid

- ■ **WARFARIN:** In human hyperthyroid patients, the metabolism of vitamin K clotting factors is increased, resulting in increased sensitivity to oral anticoagulants. By reducing the effects of hyperthyroidism, methimazole may decrease clotting factor metabolism reduce the effects of warfarin. However, patients euthyroid on methimazole and receiving warfarin may develop hypoprothrombinemia if methimazole is stopped and they become thyrotoxic again. The veterinary label states: Anticoagulants may be potentiated by methimazole. Recommendation: If methimazole and warfarin are used together, increased monitoring anticoagulant effect is warranted.

Doses

- ■ **DOGS:**

  As an investigative method to reduce nephrotoxicity associated with cisplatin therapy:
  a) 40 mg/kg IV over one minute prior to cisplatin. (Kitchell & Dhaliwal 2000) **Note:** No commercially available parenteral product in USA at time of writing.

- ■ **CATS:**

  For hyperthyroidism:
  a) The starting dose is 2.5 mg administered every 12 hours. Following 3 weeks of treatment, the dose should be titrated to

effect based on individual serum total T4 (TT4) levels and clinical response. Dose adjustments should be made in 2.5 mg increments. The maximum total dosage is 20 mg per day divided, not to exceed 10 mg as a single administration. (Label Information; *Felimazole®*—Dechra)

b) For cats with azotemia or for clients declining radioiodine: 1.25–5 mg per cat twice daily (start at lower end. (Trepanier 2007). Methimazole (50 mg/mL; 5 mg/0.1 mL) in PLO for *transdermal administration*: 2.5 mg to inner pinna q12h. Person applying should wear gloves or finger cots. Somewhat lower efficacy than PO (67% vs 82% euthyroid at 4 weeks). Lower incidence of GI effects with transdermal (4% vs. 24%). No difference in facial excoriation, neutropenia, hepatotoxicity, or thrombocytopenia. Drawbacks for transdermal administration include: erythema at application site, increased cost, and stability of compounded medication (2 weeks guaranteed stable). (Trepanier 2006)

c) Initially, 2.5 mg (total dose) PO once a day for 2 weeks. If adverse reactions not noted by owner, physical exam reveals no new problems, CBC and platelets are within normal limits, and serum T4 concentration is greater than 26 nmol/L after 2 weeks of therapy, the dose is increased to 2.5 mg PO twice daily and the same parameters are checked in another 2 weeks. The dosage should then be increased every 2 weeks by 2.5 mg per day until serum T4 is between 13 and 26 nmol/L or adverse effects develop. Serum T4 concentrations decline into the reference range within 1–2 weeks, once the cat is receiving an effective dose. (Nelson 2003)

d) If no signs of renal insufficiency/failure, begin at 5 mg (total dose) PO twice daily in cases with severely increased T4 levels. If renal insufficiency present (or not sure), start at 2.5 mg twice daily. If azotemia and overt renal insufficiency, start at 1.25 mg twice a day. Monitor in 1–2 weeks (T4, CBC with platelet count, renal blood parameters, urinalysis). Monitor for other signs of adverse effects. Based on clinical signs and bloodwork, dose can be increased slowly. Monitor every 2–3 weeks for the first 3 months, then every 3–6 months thereafter. (Ward 2003)

Monitoring

During first 3 months of therapy (baseline values and every 2–3 weeks):

■ CBC, platelet count

■ Serum T_4

■ If indicated by symptomatology: liver function tests, ANA

After stabilized (at least 3 months of therapy):

■ T_4 at 3–6 month intervals

■ Other diagnostic tests as dictated by adverse effects

■ The label for the feline-approved product states: Hematology, biochemistry, and TT4 should be evaluated prior to initiating treatment and monitored after 3 weeks and 6 weeks of treatment. Thereafter, bloodwork should be monitored every 3 months and the dose adjusted as necessary. Cats receiving doses greater than 10 mg per day should be monitored more frequently.

Client Information

■ It must be stressed to owners that this drug will decrease excessive thyroid hormones, but does not cure the condition and that compliance with the treatment regimen is necessary for success.

■ The manufacturer warns that: Pregnant women or women who may become pregnant, and nursing mothers should wear gloves when handling tablets, litter or bodily fluids of treated cats.

Chemistry/Synonyms

A thioimidazole-derivative antithyroid drug, methimazole occurs as a white to pale buff crystalline powder, having a faint characteristic odor and a melting point of 144–147°C. It is freely soluble (1 gram in 5 mL) in water or alcohol.

Methimazole may also be known as: thiamazole, mercazolylum, methylmercaptoimidazole, thiamazolum; tiamazol, *Antitiroide®*, *Danantizol®*, *Favistan®*, *Felimazole®*, *Mercaptizol®*, *Metibasol®*, *Strumazol®*, *Tapazol®*, *Thacapzol®*, *Thycapzol®*, *Thyrozol®*, *Tirodril®*, and *Unimazole®*.

Storage/Stability

Methimazole tablets should be stored in well-closed, light-resistant containers at room temperature; protect from moisture.

Dosage Forms/Regulatory Status

VETERINARY-LABELED PRODUCTS:

Methimazole Tablets (sugar-coated): 2.5, & 5 mg; *Felimazole®* (Dechra); (Rx). FDA-approved (USA) for use in cats.

HUMAN-LABELED PRODUCTS:

Methimazole Tablets (plain & scored): 5 mg, 10 mg, 15 mg & 20 mg; *Tapazole®* (Monarch); *Northyx®* (Centrix); generic; (Rx)

References

Kitchell, B. & R. Dhaliwal (2000). CVT Update: Anticancer Drugs and Protocols Using Traditional Drugs. *Kirk's Current Veterinary Therapy: XIII Small Animal Practice.* J Bonagura Ed. Philadelphia, WB Saunders: 465–473.

Nelson, R. (2003). Diagnostic and Treatment Options for Feline Hyperthyroidism. Proceedings: World Small Animal Veterinary Association. Accessed via: Veterinary Information Network. http://goo.gl/ZmFDc

Trepanier, L. (2006). Transdermal medication in cats: Can it be done? Proceedings: ECVIM-CA Congress.

Accessed via: Veterinary Information Network. http://
goo.gl/SKfqL

Trepanier, L. (2007). Pharmacologic management of feline hyperthyrodism. *Vet Clin NA: Sm Anim Pract* **37**:
775–788.

Ward, C. (2003). Manifestations and management of the
hyperthyroid cat. Proceedings: IVECCS Symposium.
Accessed via: Veterinary Information Network. http://
goo.gl/wvc0o

METHIONINE
DL-METHIONINE
RACEMETHIONINE

(me-*thye*-oh-neen)   Ammonil®

URINARY ACIDIFIER; NUTRITIONAL

Prescriber Highlights

▶ Used primarily as a urinary acidifier;
questionable efficacy in reducing stone
formation

▶ Contraindications: Renal failure, pancreatic disease, hepatic insufficiency,
preexisting acidosis, oxalate or urate
calculi; not recommended for kittens

▶ Adverse Effects: Gastrointestinal distress (food may alleviate), Heinz-body
hemolytic anemia (cats)

▶ Drug interactions

Uses/Indications

In small animals, methionine has been used
primarily for its urine acidification effects in
the treatment and prevention of certain types
(*e.g.*, struvite) of stone formation and to reduce ammoniacal urine odor. Use is generally
not recommended unless urine pH is >6.5. In
food animals, it has been used as a nutritional
supplement in swine and poultry feed and in the
treatment of ketosis in cattle. It has been touted
as a treatment for laminitis in horses and cattle
(purportedly provides a disulfide bond substrate
to maintain the hoof-pedal bone bond), but definitive studies demonstrating its effectiveness
for this indication are lacking.

The drug is used in humans to reduce urine
ammonia (pH) and odor.

Pharmacology/Actions

Methionine has several pharmacologic effects.
It is an essential amino acid (l-form) and nutrient, a lipotrope (prevents or corrects fatty liver
in choline deficiency), and a urine acidifier. Two
molecules of methionine can be converted to 1
molecule of cysteine. Methionine supplies both
sulfhydryl and methyl groups to the liver for
metabolic processes. Choline is formed when
methionine supplies a methyl group to ethanolamine. After methionine is metabolized, sulfate
is excreted in the urine as sulfuric acid, thereby
acidifying it.

Pharmacokinetics

No information is available on the pharmacokinetics of this agent in veterinary species or
humans.

Contraindications/Precautions/Warnings

Methionine (in therapeutic doses) is contraindicated in patients with renal failure or pancreatic
disease. If used in patients with frank hepatic
insufficiency, methionine can cause increased
production of mercaptan-like compounds and
intensify the signs of hepatic dementia or coma.
Methionine should not be given to animals with
preexisting acidosis, oxalate or urate calculi. It is
not recommended for use in kittens.

Adverse Effects

At usual doses, gastrointestinal distress can occur; give with food to alleviate this effect and to
enhance efficacy. Methionine may cause Heinz-
body hemolytic anemia in cats. See Overdosage
(below) for other potential adverse effects.

Unmonitored use with an acidifying diet (*e.g.*,
s/d, c/d), may lead to signs associated with overdose.

Reproductive/Nursing Safety

No specific information was located; methionine could, potentially, cause fetal acidosis.

Overdosage/Acute Toxicity

Methionine may be toxic to kittens who consume other cats' food in which methionine has
been added. When methionine was administered at a dose of 2 grams orally per day to mature cats, anorexia, methemoglobinemia, Heinz
body formation (with resultant hemolytic anemia), ataxia and cyanosis were noted. Metabolic
acidosis, particularly in combination with an
acidifying diet may occur with overdoses in any
species. No specific information was located on
the treatment of methionine overdose.

Drug Interactions

The following drug interactions have either been
reported or are theoretical in humans or animals
receiving methionine and may be of significance
in veterinary patients:

■ **AMINOGLYCOSIDES (gentamicin, amikacin,
etc):** The aminoglycosides are more effective in an alkaline medium; urine acidification may diminish these drugs effectiveness
in treating bacterial urinary tract infections

■ **ERYTHROMYCIN:** Is more effective in an alkaline medium; urine acidification may diminish erythromycin effectiveness in treating bacterial urinary tract infections

■ **QUINIDINE:** Urine acidification may increase
the renal excretion of quinidine

Doses

■ **DOGS:**

For urine acidification:

a) At approximately 100 mg/kg PO q12h
methionine is safe and effective in dissolving presumed infection-induced
struvite uroliths in dogs in combination

with an appropriate anti-microbial agent without using a struvite dissolution diet. Successful dissolution occurs when uroliths decrease in size by at least 50% at the 1 month re-evaluation. If uroliths do not decrease in size by at least 50% at the 1 month re-evaluation, then consideration should be given to (1) lack of compliance, (2) inappropriate dosage, (3) difficulty in controlling the bacterial urinary tract infection, or (4) uroliths being composed of other minerals, most likely calcium oxalate, in addition to or instead of struvite. (Bartges & Moyers 2010)

b) In struvite dissolution therapy if diet and antimicrobials do not result in acid urine: 0.2–1 gram PO q8h (Kirk 1986; Lage *et al.* 1988)

■ **CATS:**

For urine acidification:

a) 1000–1500 mg per day given in the food once daily (if diet and antimicrobials do not reduce pH) (Lewis *et al.* 1987)

b) 0.2–1 gram PO once daily (Lage *et al.* 1988)

■ **CATTLE:**

a) 20–30 grams PO (Jenkins 1988)

■ **HORSES:**

a) 22 mg/kg PO once daily for one week; then 11 mg/kg PO once daily for 1 week; then 5.5 mg/kg PO once daily for one week (Robinson 1987)(

b) 12.5 grams IV in one liter saline/dextrose solution (may be effective in Senecio-induced liver damage (Rossoff 1974)

Monitoring

■ Urine pH (Urine pH's of ≤6.5 have been recommended as goal of therapy)

■ Blood pH if signs of toxicity are present

■ CBC in cats exhibiting signs of toxicity

Client Information

■ Give with meals or mixed in food, unless otherwise instructed by veterinarian.

Chemistry/Synonyms

A sulfur-containing amino acid, methionine occurs as a white, crystalline powder with a characteristic odor. One gram is soluble in about 30 mL of water and it is very slightly soluble in alcohol. 74.6 mg is equivalent to 1 mEq of methionine.

Methionine may also be known as: dl-methionine, racemethionine, M, s-methionine, l-methioninum, *Acimethin®, Acimol®, Ammonil®, DL-Methionine Tablets®, M-Caps®, Methigel®, Methio-Form®, Methiotrans®, Methnine®, Neutrodor®, Pedameth®, Uracid®,* and *Uromethin®*.

Storage/Stability

Methionine should be stored at room temperature.

Dosage Forms/Regulatory Status

VETERINARY-LABELED PRODUCTS:

Methionine is labeled for use in dogs, cats, and horses in pharmaceutical dosage forms, but at the time of review 02/11, there were no methionine products listed in the FDA's "Green Book" of approved products. Products labeled as nutritionals may be approved for use in other species. Depending on the product, methionine may be available without prescription. Methionine is an ingredient in many other nutritional products.

Methionine Tablets: 200 mg and 500 mg; *Ammonil® Tablets* (Virbac), *DL-Methionine Tablets®* (V.E.T.); (Rx). Labeled for use in cats and dogs.

Methionine Tablets Chewable: 500 mg; *Methio-Form®* (Vet-A-Mix); (Rx). Labeled for use in cats and dogs.

Methionine Powder (concentration varies with product); Trade Names/Products include: d-l-methionine Powder (Butler, First Priority). Labeled for use in dogs and cats.

Methionine Gel: 400 mg (8%) in 120.5 gram tubes. *Methigel®* (Vetoquinol); (OTC). Labeled for use in cats and dogs.

HUMAN-LABELED PRODUCTS:

Methionine Capsules: 500 mg; generic; (Rx)

Topical Ointments, cream, lotion, pads and powder available.

References

Bartges, J. & T. Moyers (2010). Evaluation of D, L-Methionine and Antimicrobial Agents for Medical Dissolution of Spontaneously Occurring Infection-Induced Struvite Urocystoliths in Dogs. Proceedings: ACVIM. Accessed via: Veterinary Information Network. http://goo.gl/aHu0O

Jenkins, W.L. (1988). Drugs affecting gastrointestinal functions. *Veterinary Pharmacology and Therapeutics 6th Ed.* NH Booth and LE McDonald Eds. Ames, Iowa Stae Univ. Press: 657–671.

Kirk, R.W., Ed. (1986). *Current Veterinary Therapy IX, Small Animal Practice.* Philadelphia, W.B. Saunders.

Lage, A.L., D. Polzin, et al. (1988). Diseases of the Bladder. *Handbook of Small Animal Practice.* RV Morgan Ed. New York, Churchill Livingstone: 605–620.

Lewis, L.D., M.L. Morris, Jr., et al. (1987). Feline Urological Syndrome. *Small Animal Clinician Nutrition III* Topeka, Mark Morris Assoc.

Robinson, N.E. (1987). Table of Common Drugs: Approximate Doses. *Current Therapy in Equine Medicine, 2.* NE Robinson Ed. Philadelphia, W.B. Saunders: 761.

Rossoff, I.S. (1974). *Handbook of Veterinary Drugs.* New York, Springer Publishing.

METHOCARBAMOL

(meth-oh-*kar*-ba-mole)   Robaxin®

MUSCLE RELAXANT

Prescriber Highlights

▶ Oral & injectable centrally acting muscle relaxant; appears useful in treating muscle tremors associated with toxic agents

▶ Contraindications: Food animals, renal disease (injectable only), hypersensitivity to it

▶ Adverse Effects: Sedation, salivation, emesis, lethargy, weakness, & ataxia

▶ Give IV slowly (don't exceed 2 mL/min); avoid extravasation; do not give SC

Uses/Indications

In dogs and cats, methocarbamol is indicated (FDA approved) "as adjunctive therapy of acute inflammatory and traumatic conditions of the skeletal muscle and to reduce muscular spasms." In horses, intravenous use is indicated (FDA approved) "as adjunctive therapy of acute inflammatory and traumatic conditions of the skeletal muscle to reduce muscular spasms, and effect striated muscle relaxation." (Package insert; *Robaxin®V*—Robins). Intravenous methocarbamol has been found useful in treating tremors associated with various toxicities in dogs and cats.

Pharmacology/Actions

Methocarbamol's exact mechanism of causing skeletal muscle relaxation is unknown. It is thought to work centrally, perhaps by general depressant effects. It has no direct relaxant effects on striated muscle, nerve fibers, or the motor endplate. It will not directly relax contracted skeletal muscles. The drug has a secondary sedative effect.

Pharmacokinetics

Limited pharmacokinetic data is available in veterinary species. In humans, methocarbamol has an onset of action of about 30 minutes after oral administration. Peak levels occur approximately 2 hours after dosing. Serum half-life is about 1–2 hours. The drug is metabolized and the inactive metabolites are excreted into the urine and the feces (small amounts).

In horses, plasma clearances appear to be dose dependent after IV administration (Muir, Sams, and Ashcraft 1984), lower clearances were measured after higher doses were given. The serum half-life of methocarbamol in the horse is approximately 60–70 minutes. Guaifenesin is a minor metabolite of methocarbamol, but because of very low concentrations, it probably has no clinical effect in the horse.

Contraindications/Precautions/Warnings

Because the injectable product contains polyethylene glycol 300, the manufacturer lists known or suspected renal pathology as a contraindication to injectable methocarbamol therapy. Polyethylene glycol 300 has been noted to increase preexisting acidosis and urea retention in humans with renal impairment.

Methocarbamol should not be used in patients hypersensitive to it or in animals to be used for food purpose.

Do not administer subcutaneously and avoid extravasation. Do not exceed 2 mL per minute when injecting IV in dogs and cats.

Adverse Effects

Side effects can include sedation, salivation, emesis, lethargy, weakness, and ataxia in dogs and cats. Sedation and ataxia are possible in horses. Because of its CNS depressant effects, methocarbamol may impair the abilities of working animals.

Reproductive/Nursing Safety

Methocarbamol should be used with caution during pregnancy as studies demonstrating its safety during pregnancy are lacking. In humans, the FDA categorizes this drug as category *C* for use during pregnancy (*Animal studies have shown an adverse effect on the fetus, but there are no adequate studies in humans; or there are no animal reproduction studies and no adequate studies in humans.*). In a separate system evaluating the safety of drugs in canine and feline pregnancy (Papich 1989), this drug is categorized as class: *C* (*These drugs may have potential risks. Studies in people or laboratory animals have uncovered risks, and these drugs should be used cautiously as a last resort when the benefit of therapy clearly outweighs the risks.*)

It is not known whether methocarbamol is excreted in milk. Exercise caution, but the American Academy of Pediatrics classifies methocarbamol as compatible with women breastfeeding.

Overdosage/Acute Toxicity

Overdosage is generally characterized by CNS depressant effects (loss of righting reflex, prostration). Excessive doses in dogs and cats may be represented by emesis, salivation, weakness, and ataxia. If the overdose is after oral administration, emptying the gut may be indicated if the overdose was recent. Do not induce emesis if the patient's continued consciousness is not assured. Other clinical signs should be treated if severe and in a supportive manner.

Drug Interactions

The following drug interactions have either been reported or are theoretical in humans or animals receiving methocarbamol and may be of significance in veterinary patients:

■ **CNS DEPRESSANTS, OTHER:** Additive depression may occur when given with other CNS depressant agents

■ **PYRIDOSTIGMINE:** One human patient, with myasthenia gravis and taking pyridostigmine, developed severe weakness after receiving methocarbamol

Laboratory Considerations

■ Urinary values of the following compounds may be falsely elevated: **vanillylmandelic acid (VMA), or 5-HIAA**

Doses

■ **DOGS:**

a) Injectable: For relief of moderate conditions: 44 mg/kg IV; For controlling severe effects of strychnine and tetanus: 55–220 mg/kg IV, do not exceed 330 mg/kg/day. Administer half the estimated dose rapidly, then wait until animal starts to relax and continue administration to effect.

Tablets: Initially, 132 mg/kg/day PO divided q8h–q12h, then 61–132 mg/kg divided q8–12h. If no response in 5 days, discontinue. (Package insert; *Robaxin®-V*—Fort Dodge)

b) For muscle relaxation for intervertebral disk disease: 15–20 mg/kg PO three times daily.

For muscle relaxation for certain toxicosis (*e.g.*, strychnine, metaldehyde, tetanus): 150 mg/kg IV (Morgan 1988)

c) To help control severe tremors associated with tremorgenic Mycotoxin intoxication: 55–220 mg/kg IV to effect at a rate no more than 2 mL/minute (Schell 2000)

d) To help control tremors associated with Guarna (*Paillinia* spp.; caffeine) toxicity: 50–220 mg/kg IV, administered slowly and to effect; do not exceed 330 mg/kg/day. (Atkins 2006)

■ **CATS:**

a) Injectable: For relief of moderate conditions: 44 mg/kg IV; For controlling severe effects of strychnine and tetanus: 55–220 mg/kg IV, do not exceed 330 mg/kg/day. Administer half the estimated dose rapidly, then wait until animal starts to relax and continue administration to effect.

Tablets: Initially, 132 mg/kg/day PO divided q8h–q12h, then 61–132 mg/kg divided q8–12h. If no response in 5 days, discontinue. (Package insert, *Robaxin®-V*—Fort Dodge)

b) For adjunctive treatment (control of seizures/muscle tremors) of permethrin toxicity: initially administered at 50–150 mg/kg IV. First half is given IV slowly over approximately 5-10 minutes and the second half is given as needed to effect. The dose can be repeated up to a maximum of 330 mg/kg/day; in severely affected cases, the total daily dose can be calculated and given over 24 hours as a constant rate infusion. (Boag 2009)

■ **CATTLE:**

a) For treatment of CNS hyperactivity: 110 mg/kg IV (Bailey 1986)

■ **HORSES:** (**Note:** ARCI UCGFS Class 4 Drug)

a) For moderate conditions: 4.4–22 mg/kg IV to effect; for severe conditions: 22–55 mg/kg IV (Package insert, *Robaxin®-V*— Fort Dodge)

b) 15–25 mg/kg IV by slow infusion (Robinson 1987)

c) To give orally: Use 2–3 times the recommended IV dose (Cunningham *et al.* 1992)

d) For acute rhabdomyolysis: 15–25 mg/kg slow IV infusion. May repeat up to four times daily if needed to decrease muscle cramping. (Hanson 1999)

Monitoring

■ Level of muscle relaxation/sedation

Client Information

■ Animal's urine color may darken, but need not be a concern.

Chemistry/Synonyms

A centrally acting muscle relaxant related structurally to guaifenesin, methocarbamol occurs as a fine, white powder with a characteristic odor. In water, it has a solubility of 25 mg/mL. The pH of commercial injection is approximately 4–5.

Methocarbamol may also be known as: guaiphenesin carbamate, *Labycarbol®*, *Laxan®*, *Lumirelax®*, *Miowas®*, *Musxan®*, *Myocin®*, *Myomethol®*, *Ortoton®*, *Remisol®*, *Rexivin®*, *Robinax®*, and *Traumacut®*.

Storage/Stability

Methocarbamol tablets should be stored at room temperature in tight containers; the injection should be stored at room temperature and not frozen. Solutions prepared for IV infusion should not be refrigerated as a precipitate may form. Because a haze or precipitate may form, all diluted intravenous solutions should be physically inspected before administration.

Dosage Forms/Regulatory Status

VETERINARY-LABELED PRODUCTS:

Note: As of autumn 2010, the two veterinary products below are still listed in the FDA's Green Book, but their marketing status is uncertain. The injectable is listed in the "Fort Dodge to Pfizer" acquired product listing, but is not listed on the Pfizer Animal Health website.

Methocarbamol Tablets: 500 mg; *Robaxin®V* (Pfizer); (Rx). FDA-approved for use in dogs and cats.

Methocarbamol Injection: 100 mg/mL in vials of 20 mL and 100 mL; *Robaxin®-V* (Pfizer);

(Rx). FDA-approved for use in dogs, cats, and horses not intended for food.

The ARCI (Racing Commissioners International) has designated this drug as a class 4 substance. See the appendix for more information.

HUMAN-LABELED PRODUCTS:

Methocarbamol Tablets: 500 mg & 750 mg; *Robaxin® Robaxin-750®* (Schwarz Pharma); generic; (Rx)

Methocarbamol Injection: 100 mg/mL in 10 mL vials; *Robaxin®* (Baxter); (Rx)

References

Atkins, L. (2006). Toxicology: Looking for Zebras. Proceedings: Western Vet Conf. Accessed via: Veterinary Information Network. http://goo.gl/zGfZ8

Bailey, E.M. (1986). Management and treatment of toxicosis in cattle. *Current Veterinary Therapy 2: Food Animal Practice.* JL Howard Ed. Philadelphia, WB Saunders: 341–354.

Boag, A. (2009). Dealing with Poison Cases in ER. Accessed via: Veterinary Information Network. http://goo.gl/qMAXf

Cunningham, F., J. Fisher, et al. (1992). The pharmacokinetics of methocarbamol in the thoroughbred race horse. *J Vet Pharmacol Therap* **15**: 96–100.

Hanson, R. (1999). Diagnosis and First Aid of Sporting Horse Injuries. Proceedings: Central Veterinary Conference, Kansas City.

Morgan, R.V., Ed. (1988). *Handbook of Small Animal Practice.* New York, Churchill Livingstone.

Papich, M. (1989). Effects of drugs on pregnancy. *Current Veterinary Therapy X: Small Animal Practice.* R Kirk Ed. Philadelphia, Saunders: 1291–1299.

Robinson, N.E. (1987). Table of Common Drugs: Approximate Doses. *Current Therapy in Equine Medicine, 2.* NE Robinson Ed. Philadelphia, W.B. Saunders: 761.

Schell, M. (2000). Tremorgenic Mycotoxin Intoxication. *Vet Med* **95**: 285–286.

METHOHEXITAL SODIUM

(meth-oh-*hex*-i-tal)   Brevital®

ULTRA-SHORT ACTING BARBITURATE

Prescriber Highlights

▶ Infrequently used ultra-short acting barbiturate for anesthesia induction, or for anesthesia for very short procedures, especially in sight hounds.

▶ Can cause very rough recoveries in dogs if used alone; premed or continuation of gas anesthesia during methohexital recovery may help reduce/prevent rough recoveries.

▶ Contraindications: Absolute contraindications: absence of suitable veins for IV administration, history of hypersensitivity reactions to barbiturates, status asthmaticus. Relative contraindications: severe cardiovascular disease or preexisting ventricular arrhythmias, shock, increased intracranial pressure, myasthenia gravis, asthma, & conditions where hypnotic effects may be prolonged (e.g., severe hepatic disease, myxedema, severe anemia, excessive premedication, etc.)

▶ NOT recommended for use in cattle

▶ Avoid extravasation

▶ No analgesic or muscle relaxant properties

▶ Adverse Effects: Apnea, hypotension, tremors, or seizures during recovery

▶ C-IV Controlled Substance; relatively expensive

Uses/Indications

Methohexital is sometimes used in small animals as an ultrashort acting anesthetic agent, but, propofol has largely supplanted methohexital's use in small animals. However, because it is not dependent on redistribution to fat to reverse its effect, it may be useful in canine sight hound breeds. Because methohexital can induce anesthesia very rapidly, it may also be useful when general anesthesia must be administered to a patient with a full stomach, as an ET tube may be placed rapidly before aspiration of vomitus can occur.

Pharmacology/Actions

Methohexital is an ultra-short acting methylated oxybarbiturate anesthetic agent. It is about twice as potent as thiopental and has a duration of action about ½ as long. Like all the barbiturates, methohexital acts by depressing the reticular activating center of the brain.

Pharmacokinetics

After IV injection, methohexital rapidly causes anesthesia (15–60 seconds). Its distribution half-life is 5–6 minutes. When used alone, a single dose will cause surgical anesthesia for 5–15 minutes. Unlike the thiobarbiturates, methohexital is rapidly metabolized by the liver and is not dependent on redistribution to fat to reverse its effects. No drug is detectable in the body 24 hours after administration. Its elimination half-life is reported to be 3–5 hours. Recovery times in small animals average 30 minutes.

Contraindications/Precautions/Warnings

Contraindicated in patients hypersensitive to barbiturates or who do not have adequate veins for safe IV administration. Relative contraindications include: seizure-prone animals, severe cardiovascular disease or preexisting ventricular arrhythmias, shock, increased intracranial pressure, myasthenia gravis, asthma, and conditions where hypnotic effects may be prolonged (e.g., severe hepatic disease, myxedema, severe anemia, excessive premedication, etc.). These relative contraindications do not preclude the use of methohexital, but dosage adjustments must be considered and the drug must be given slowly and cautiously.

Repeated dosing or using an IV infusion are not recommended as recovery times can be significantly prolonged and increase the risk for complications.

Because of its unpredictability in cattle, it is not recommended for use in this species.

Adverse Effects

Methohexital can cause profound respiratory depression. The lethal dose may only be 2–3 times that of the anesthetic dose. Because excitation (including muscle tremors and seizures) can occur upon recovery, methohexital is generally recommended for use with a premed. Postoperative seizures have been reported and can be treated with IV diazepam.

In small animals (especially dogs), methohexital may induce rougher recoveries when compared to thiopental or other anesthetics. Premedication or using gas anesthetics during methohexital recovery phase may be helpful to reduce or prevent this occurrence.

Because of its rapid elimination and very short action, there is a possibility that methohexital's effects may diminish before inhalant anesthesia takes full effect.

Too rapid an injection may lead to apnea and hypotension. Barbiturates do not provide analgesia or any muscle relaxation.

Because it can be very irritating to tissues and localized necrosis can occur in soft tissue, methohexital solutions must be only given IV, and perivascular injection must be avoided. Extravasation injuries can be treated with multiple infiltrates of sterile normal saline. Lidocaine can be injected to reduce pain.

Reproductive/Nursing Safety

While safety of methohexital has not been established in pregnancy, doses of up to 7 times those of humans given to pregnant rabbits and rats resulted in no overt teratogenicity or fetal harm. In humans, the FDA categorizes this drug as category *B* for use during pregnancy (*Animal studies have not yet demonstrated risk to the fetus, but there are no adequate studies in pregnant women; or animal studies have shown an adverse effect, but adequate studies in pregnant women have not demonstrated a risk to the fetus in the first trimester of pregnancy, and there is no evidence of risk in later trimesters.*)

Small amounts of thiopental have been detected in milk following administration of large doses to humans. It is unlikely that methohexital poses much risk to nursing offspring.

Overdosage/Acute Toxicity

See Adverse Effects above; figure dosages carefully.

Drug Interactions

The following drug interactions have either been reported or are theoretical in humans or animals receiving methohexital and may be of significance in veterinary patients:

■ **CNS DEPRESSANT DRUGS (e.g., ALPHA2-AGONISTS, OPIOIDS, etc):** When used with other CNS depressant drugs, methohexital may have additive effects. Use with a premed is usually preferred to reduce methohexital dosage required for inductions and to decrease rough recoveries.

Doses

■ **DOGS:**

a) For induction with premedication: 5 mg/kg; give ½ to ¾ of dose over 10 seconds. In 30 seconds if adequate plane is not reached to allow intubation, give additional drug. Delay will result in poor induction due to rapid redistribution. (McKelvey & Hollingshead 2000)

b) For induction or sole anesthetic in non-premedicated dogs or cats: 11 mg/kg IV, give approximately ½ the dose rapidly and then titrate to effect. If premedicated, give 5.5–6.6 mg/kg IV, 10–30% is given rapidly IV and then the remainder titrated to effect. (Paddleford 1999)

■ **CATS:**

a) For induction or sole anesthetic in non-premedicated dogs or cats: 11 mg/kg IV, give approximately ½ the dose rapidly and then titrate to effect. If premedicated, give 5.5–6.6 mg/kg IV, 10–30% is given rapidly IV and then the remainder titrated to effect. (Paddleford 1999)

Monitoring

■ Plane of anesthesia

■ Respiratory rate/depth

■ Cardiac rate, rhythm and blood pressure

■ Upon recovery, monitor for CNS stimulation (seizures)

Client Information

■ Methohexital should be used in a setting only where adequate monitoring and support are available.

Chemistry/Synonyms

An ultra-short acing barbiturate agent, methohexital occurs as a white, crystalline powder. It is freely soluble in water.

Methohexital sodium may also be known as: compound 25398, enallynymalnatrium, methohexitone sodium, *Brevimytal®*, *Brevital®*, and *Brietal®*.

Storage/Stability

Methohexital sodium powder for injection should be stored at room temperature (less than 25°C). Preferably, reconstitute the powder for injection with sterile water for injection. D₅W or 0.9% sodium chloride may also be used, particularly when making concentrations of 0.2% (to avoid extreme hypotonicity). While the manufacturer states not to make concentrations greater than 1%, some veterinary anesthesiologists will make concentrations of up 6% (especially when using in large animals). Do not use solutions with bacteriostatic agents to prepare the solution.

The labeling for this product was changed to reduce the permitted time after reconstitution to 24 hours primarily since the product did not contain preservatives. Formerly, the labeling stated that after reconstituting with sterile water for injection, solutions are stable for at least 6 weeks at room temperature and as long as the solution remains clear and colorless, it is permissible to use. Solutions of D₅W or normal saline are not stable for much more than 24 hours after reconstituting. A study demonstrated that solutions reconstituted with sterile water to a concentration of 10 mg/mL were stable up to 6 weeks when refrigerated and did not show any antimicrobial growth (Beeman *et al.* 1994).

Compatibility/Compounding Considerations

Methohexital solutions are alkaline. Do NOT mix with acidic drugs (*e.g.,* atropine or succinylcholine). Refer to specialized references before attempting to mix methohexital with another drug. Methohexital is **incompatible** with silicone. Do not allow contact with silicone-treated rubber stoppers or silicone treated parts of disposable syringes.

Dosage Forms/Regulatory Status

VETERINARY-LABELED PRODUCTS: None

The ARCI (Racing Commissioners International) has designated this drug as a class 2 substance. See the appendix for more information.

HUMAN-LABELED PRODUCTS:

Methohexital Sodium Powder for Injection: 500 mg & 2.5 grams in 50 mL multiple dose vials; *Brevital® Sodium* (JHP Pharm); (Rx, C-IV)

References

Beeman, C.S., J. Dembo, et al. (1994). Stability Of Reconstituted Methohexital Sodium. *Journal of Oral and Maxillofacial Surgery* 52(4): 393–396.

McKelvey, D. & K. Hollingshead (2000). *Small Animal Anesthesia and Analgesia*. St Louis, Mosby.

Paddleford, R. (1999). *Manual of Small Animal Anesthesia*. Philadelphia, WB Saunders.

METHOTREXATE
METHOTREXATE SODIUM

(meth-oh-*trex*-ate)   MTX, Amethopterin

ANTINEOPLASTIC, IMMUNOSUPPRESSIVE

Prescriber Highlights

▶ Antineoplastic/immunosuppressant used primarily for lymphomas & some solid tumors in dogs & cats

▶ Contraindications: Preexisting bone marrow depression, severe hepatic or renal insufficiency, or hypersensitivity to the drug

▶ Caution: If patient susceptible or has preexisting clinical signs associated with the adverse reactions associated with this drug (see below)

▶ Adverse Effects: GI (diarrhea, nausea, & vomiting); Higher dosage: listlessness, GI toxicity (ulcers, mucosal sloughing, stomatitis), hematopoietic toxicity (nadir at 4–6 days), hepatopathy, renal tubular necrosis, alopecia, depigmentation, pulmonary infiltrates & fibrosis; anaphylaxis (rare)

▶ Avoid human exposure

▶ Teratogenic; may affect spermatogenesis

▶ Determine dosages accurately

▶ Drug interactions

Uses/Indications

Indicated for lymphomas and some solid tumors in dogs and cats.

Low-dose methotrexate has been used in some cats with lymphatic cholangitis that have not responded to prednisolone or chlorambucil. In human medicine, methotrexate is also being used to treat refractory rheumatoid arthritis and severe psoriasis.

Pharmacology/Actions

An S-phase specific antimetabolite antineoplastic agent, methotrexate competitively inhibits folic acid reductase, preventing the reduction of dihydrofolate to tetrahydrofolate and affecting production of purines and pyrimidines. Rapidly proliferating cells (*e.g.*, neoplasms, bone marrow, GI tract epithelium, fetal cells, etc.) are most sensitive to the drug's effects.

Dihydrofolate reductase has a much greater affinity for methotrexate than either folic acid or dihydrofolic acid and coadministration of folic acid will not reduce methotrexate's effects. Leucovorin calcium, a derivative of tetrahydrofolic acid, can block the effects of methotrexate.

Methotrexate also has immunosuppressive activity, possibly due to its effects on lymphocyte replication. Tumor cells have been noted to develop resistance to methotrexate that may be due to decreased cellular uptake of the drug.

Pharmacokinetics

Methotrexate is well absorbed from the GI tract after oral administration of dosages <30 mg/m^2 with a bioavailability of about 60%. In humans, peak levels occur within 4 hours after oral dosing, and between 30 minutes and 2 hours after IM injection.

Methotrexate is widely distributed in the body and is actively transported across cell membranes. Highest concentrations are found in the kidneys, spleen, gallbladder, liver, and skin. When given orally or parenterally, methotrexate does not reach therapeutic levels in the CSF. When given intrathecally, methotrexate attains therapeutic levels in the CSF and also passes into the systemic circulation. Methotrexate is about 50% bound to plasma proteins and crosses the placenta.

Methotrexate is excreted almost entirely by the kidneys via both glomerular filtration and active transport. Serum half-life is less than 10 hours and generally between 2–4 hours.

Contraindications/Precautions/Warnings

Methotrexate is contraindicated in patients with preexisting bone marrow depression, severe hepatic or renal insufficiency, or hypersensitivity to the drug. It should be used with caution in patients who are susceptible to, or have preexisting clinical signs associated with, the adverse reactions associated with this drug.

When administering MTX, either wear gloves or immediately wash hands after handling. Gloves are particularly important if handling split, broken, or crushed tablets. Preparation of intravenous solutions should ideally be performed in a vertical laminar flow hood.

Adverse Effects

In dogs and cats, gastrointestinal side effects are most prevalent with diarrhea, nausea, inappetence (especially cats) and vomiting (especially dogs) seen. Higher dosages may lead to listlessness, GI toxicity (ulcers, mucosal sloughing, stomatitis), hematopoietic toxicity (nadir at 4–6 days), hepatopathy, renal tubular necrosis, alopecia, depigmentation, pulmonary infiltrates, and fibrosis. CNS toxicity (encephalopathy) may be noted if methotrexate is given intrathecally. Rarely, anaphylaxis may be seen.

Reproductive/Nursing Safety

Methotrexate is teratogenic, embryotoxic, and may affect spermatogenesis in male animals. In humans, the FDA categorizes this drug as category **X** for use during pregnancy (*Studies in animals or humans demonstrate fetal abnormalities or adverse reaction; reports indicate evidence of fetal risk. The risk of use in pregnant women clearly outweighs any possible benefit.*) In a separate system evaluating the safety of drugs in canine and feline pregnancy (Papich 1989), this drug is categorized as class: *C* (*These drugs may have potential risks. Studies in people or laboratory animals have uncovered risks, and these drugs should be used cautiously as a last resort when the benefit of therapy clearly outweighs the risks.*)

Methotrexate is contraindicated in nursing mothers. It is excreted in breast milk in low concentrations with a milk:plasma ratio of 0.08:1. Nursing offspring should be switched to milk replacer if the dam requires methotrexate.

Overdosage/Acute Toxicity

Acute overdosage in dogs is associated with exacerbations of the adverse effects outlined above, particularly myelosuppression and acute renal failure. Acute tubular necrosis is secondary to drug precipitation in the tubules. In dogs, the maximally tolerated dose is reported to be 0.12 mg/kg q24h for 5 days. 10 mg/kg is considered a lethal dose if leucovorin rescue is not performed.

Treatment of acute oral overdoses include emptying the gut and preventing absorption using standard protocols if the ingestion is recent. Additionally, oral neomycin has been suggested to help prevent absorption of MTX from the intestine. In order to minimize renal damage, forced alkaline diuresis should be considered. Urine pH should be maintained between 7.5–8 by the addition of 0.5–1 mEq/kg of sodium bicarbonate per 500 mL of IV fluid.

Leucovorin calcium is specific therapy for methotrexate overdoses. It should be given as soon as possible, preferably within the first hour and, definitely, within 48 hours. Doses of leucovorin required are dependent on the MTX serum concentration. Humans having serum concentrations greater than 5 x 10^{-7} M at 48 hours are likely to develop severe toxicity. Leucovorin in doses ranging from 25–200 mg/m^2 every 6 hours doses is given until serum levels fall below 1 x 10^{-8} M. Dogs treated with leucovorin at 15 mg/m^2 every 3 hours IV for 8 doses, then IM q6h for 8 doses were able to tolerate very high MTX doses.

Drug Interactions

The following drug interactions have either been reported or are theoretical in humans or animals receiving methotrexate (MTX) and may be of significance in veterinary patients:

- **AMIODARONE:** Prolonged PO administration of amiodarone (>2 weeks) may inhibit MTX metabolism

- **ASPARAGINASE:** Asparaginase given concomitantly with MTX may decrease MTX efficacy

- **AZATHIOPRINE:** Potential for increased risk for hepatic toxicity

- **CHLORAMPHENICOL:** May displace MTX from plasma proteins increasing risk for toxicity, but also may reduce MTX absorption and enterohepatic recirculation

- **CISPLATIN:** May have synergistic action with MTX, but alter the renal elimination of MTX

- **CYCLOSPORINE:** May increase MTX levels

- **FOLIC ACID:** May reduce MTX efficacy, but folate deficiency increases MTX toxicity

- **NEOMYCIN (oral):** Oral neomycin may decrease the absorption of oral methotrexate if given concomitantly

- **NSAIDS, SALICYLATES:** In humans, severe hematologic and GI toxicity has resulted in patients receiving both MTX and non-steroidal antiinflammatory agents; use caution in dogs also on MTX

- **PENICILLINS:** May decrease MTX renal elimination

- **PROBENECID:** May inhibit the tubular secretion of MTX and increase its half-life

- **PYRIMETHAMINE:** Pyrimethamine, a similar folic acid antagonist, may increase MTX toxicity and should not be given to patients receiving MTX

- **RETINOIDS:** Potential for increased risk for hepatic toxicity

- **SULFASALAZINE:** Potential for increased risk for hepatic toxicity

- **SULFONAMIDES:** May displace MTX from plasma proteins increasing risk for toxicity

- **TETRACYCLINES:** May displace MTX from plasma proteins increasing risk for toxicity, but also may reduce MTX absorption and enterohepatic recirculation

- **THEOPHYLLINES:** MTX may reduce theophylline elimination

- **TRIMETHOPRIM/SULFA:** Rarely, may increase myelosuppression of MTX

- **VACCINES, LIVE:** Live virus vaccines should be used with caution, if at all during therapy

Laboratory Considerations
- Methotrexate may interfere with the microbiologic assay for **folic acid.**

Doses

Dosages of methotrexate sodium are expressed in terms of methotrexate as are the dosage forms. **Note:** Because of the potential toxicity of this drug to patients, and potentially, veterinary personnel and clients, and since chemotherapy indications, treatment protocols, monitoring and safety guidelines often change, the following dosages should be used only as a general guide and not as a dosage protocol. When using MTX as part of chemotherapy protocols, consultation with a veterinary oncologist and referral to current veterinary oncology references [*e.g.*, (Henry & Higginbotham 2009); (Argyle *et al.* 2008); (Withrow & Vail 2007); (Villalobos 2007); (Ogilvie & Moore 2006); (Ogilvie & Moore 2001)] is *strongly recommended*.

- **DOGS:**

  For susceptible neoplastic diseases (usually as part of a multi-drug protocol):

  a) As part of the LMP protocol for maintenance of canine lymphoma: Chlorambucil 20 mg/m^2 PO every 15 days; Methotrexate 2.5–5 mg/m^2 PO twice a week; Prednisone 20 mg/m^2 PO every other day. When Vincristine is added it is at a dose of 0.5–0.7 mg/m^2 and is given every 15 days alternating weeks with the chlorambucil. (Berger 2005)

  b) In combination with other antineoplastics (per protocol) 5 mg/m^2 PO twice weekly or 0.8 mg/kg IV every 21 days; alternatively 2.5 mg/m^2 PO daily (USPC 1990)

- **CATS:**

  a) For susceptible neoplastic diseases (usually as part of a multi-drug protocol): 2.5 mg/m^2 PO 2–3 times weekly; 0.3–0.8 mg/m^2 IV every 7 days (O'Keefe & Harris 1990)

  b) For non-suppurative cholangitis/cholangiohepatitis (CCHC) syndrome with fibrosis: A total dose of 0.4 mg per cat total dose given on one day in three divided doses: 0.26 mg at hour zero, 0.13 mg at the 12 and 24 hour dosing. Repeat every 7-10 days. Use in conjunction with ursodeoxycholic acid (15 mg/kg PO q24h) and folate (0.25 mg/kg PO q24h). (Scherk 2007)

Monitoring
- Efficacy
- Toxicity:

  a) Monitor for clinical signs of GI irritation and ulceration

  b) Complete blood counts (with platelets) should be performed weekly early in therapy and eventually every 4–6 weeks when stabilized. If WBC is <4000/mm^3 or platelet count is <100,000/mm^3 therapy should be discontinued

  c) Baseline renal function tests. Continue to monitor if abnormal

  d) Baseline hepatic function tests. Monitor liver enzymes on a regular basis during therapy.

Client Information

■ Clients must be briefed on the possibilities of severe toxicity developing from this drug, including drug-related mortality.

■ Clients should contact the veterinarian if the patient exhibits clinical signs of profound depression, abnormal bleeding (including bloody diarrhea) and/or bruising.

■ Wear gloves when administering tablets (particularly if crushed or split); if gloves are not used, wash hands thoroughly after handling tablets.

Chemistry/Synonyms

A folic acid antagonist, methotrexate is available commercially as the sodium salt. It occurs as a yellow powder that is soluble in water. Methotrexate sodium injection has a pH of 7.5–9.

Methotrexate and methotrexate sodium may also be known as: MTX, amethopterin, 4-Amino-4-deoxy-10-methylpteroyl-L-glutamic acid, 4-Amino-10-methylfolic acid, CL-14377, alpha-methopterin, methotrexatum, metotrexato, NSC-740, WR-19039; there are many trade names available.

Storage/Stability

Methotrexate sodium tablets should be stored at room temperature (15–30°C) in well-closed containers and protected from light. The injection and powder for injection should be stored at room temperature (15–30°C) and protected from light.

Compatibility/Compounding Considerations

Methotrexate sodium is reportedly physically **compatible** with the following intravenous solutions and drugs: Amino acids 4.25%/dextrose 25%, D$_5$W, sodium bicarbonate 0.05 M, cephalothin sodium, cytarabine, 6-mercaptopurine sodium, sodium bicarbonate, and vincristine sulfate. In syringes, methotrexate is physically **compatible** with: bleomycin sulfate, cyclophosphamide, doxorubicin HCl, fluorouracil, furosemide, leucovorin calcium, mitomycin, vinblastine sulfate, and vincristine sulfate.

Methotrexate sodium **compatibility information conflicts** or is dependent on diluent or concentration factors with the following drugs or solutions: heparin sodium and metoclopramide HCl. Compatibility is dependent upon factors such as pH, concentration, temperature and diluent used; consult specialized references or a hospital pharmacist for more specific information.

Methotrexate sodium is reportedly physically **incompatible** when mixed with the following solutions or drugs: bleomycin sulfate (as an IV additive only; **compatible** in syringes and Y-lines), fluorouracil (as an IV additive only; **compatible** in syringes and Y-lines), prednisolone sodium phosphate, droperidol, and ranitidine HCl.

Dosage Forms/Regulatory Status

VETERINARY-LABELED PRODUCTS: None

The ARCI (Racing Commissioners International) has designated this drug as a class 2 substance. See the appendix for more information.

HUMAN-LABELED PRODUCTS:

Methotrexate Sodium Tablets (plain & scored): 2.5 mg, 5 mg, 7.5 mg, 10 mg & 15 mg; *Rheumatrex® Dose Pack* (STADA); *Trexal®* (Barr); generic; (Rx)

Methotrexate Sodium Injection: 25 mg/mL (as base) in 2 mL & 10 mL vials; preservative-free in 2 mL, 4 mL, 8 mL, 10 mL, 20 mL, & 40 mL single-use vials; *Methotrexate LPF® Sodium* (Xanodyne); generic; (Rx)

Methotrexate Powder for Injection, lyophilized: 1 gram preservative free in single-use vials; generic; (Rx)

References

Argyle, D., M. Brearly, et al. (2008). *Decision Making in Small Animal Oncology*, Wiley-Blackwell.

Berger, F. (2005). Rescue treatment of canine lymphoma. Proceedings: WSAVA World Congress. Accessed via: Veterinary Information Network. http://goo.gl/obkhZ

Henry, C. & M. Higginbotham (2009). *Cancer Management in Small Animal Practice*, Saunders.

O'Keefe, D.A. & C.L. Harris (1990). Toxicology of Oncologic Drugs. *Vet Clinics of North America: Small Animal Pract* **20**(2): 483–504.

Ogilvie, G. & A. Moore (2001). *Feline Oncology: A Comprehensive Guide to Compassionate Care*, Veterinary Learning Systems.

Ogilvie, G. & A. Moore (2006). *Managing the Canine Cancer Patient: A Practical Guide to Compassionate Care*, Veterinary Learning Systems.

Papich, M. (1989). Effects of drugs on pregnancy. *Current Veterinary Therapy X: Small Animal Practice.* R Kirk Ed. Philadelphia, Saunders: 1291–1299.

Scherk, M. (2007). Cholangitis/Cholangiohepatitis Complex (CCHC). Proceedings: ACVC. Accessed via: Veterinary Information Network. http://goo.gl/LX3c3

USPC (1990). Veterinary Information- Appendix III. *Drug Information for the Health Professional* Rockville, United States Pharmacopeial Convention. **2**: 2811–2860.

Villalobos, A. (2007). *Canine and Feline Geriatric Oncology.* Ames, Blackwell.

Withrow, S. & D. Vail (2007). *Withrow and MacEwen's Small Animal Clinical Oncology 4th Ed.* Philadelphia, Elsevier.

METHYLENE BLUE

(*meth*-i-leen)

ANTIDOTE

Prescriber Highlights

▶ Thiazine dye used to primarily treat methemoglobinemia in ruminants

▶ Contraindications: Cats (most agree), lactating dairy animals, renal insufficiency; hypersensitive to methylene blue; or given as an intraspinal (intrathecal) injection

▶ Not very effective in horses

▶ Adverse Effects: Heinz body anemia or other red cell morphological changes, methemoglobinemia, & decreased red cell life spans. Cats most sensitive, but to a lesser degree, dogs & horses also.

▶ A 180-day slaughter withdrawal time has been suggested, but 14 days may be sufficient (see doses)

Uses/Indications

Methylene blue is used primarily for treating methemoglobinemia secondary to oxidative agents (nitrates, chlorates) in ruminants. It is also employed occasionally as adjunctive or alternative therapy for cyanide toxicity.

Intra-operative methylene blue is also being used to preferentially stain islet-cell tumors of the pancreas in dogs in order to aid in their surgical removal or in determining the animal's prognosis.

Pharmacology/Actions

Methylene blue is rapidly converted to leucomethylene blue in tissues. This compound serves as a reducing agent that helps to convert methemoglobin (Fe^{+++}) to hemoglobin (Fe^{++}). Methylene blue is an oxidating agent, and, if high doses (species dependent) are administered, may actually cause methemoglobinemia.

Pharmacokinetics

Methylene blue is absorbed from the GI tract, but is usually administered parenterally in veterinary medicine. It is excreted in the urine and bile, primarily in the colorless form, but some unchanged drug may be also excreted.

Contraindications/Precautions/Warnings

Methylene blue is contraindicated in patients with renal insufficiency, or are hypersensitive to methylene blue. It cannot be given as an intraspinal (intrathecal) injection. Because cats may develop Heinz body anemia and methemoglobinemia secondary to methylene blue, it is considered contraindicated in this species by most clinicians. Methylene blue is considered relatively ineffective in reducing methemoglobin in horses.

Adverse Effects

The greatest concern with methylene blue therapy is the development of Heinz body anemia or other red cell morphological changes, methemoglobinemia, and decreased red cell life spans. Cats tend to be very sensitive to these effects; the drug is usually considered contraindicated in them, but dogs and horses can also develop these effects at relatively low dosages.

When injected SC or if extravasation occurs during IV administration, necrotic abscesses may develop.

Reproductive/Nursing Safety

Safe use of this agent during pregnancy has not been demonstrated. In humans, the FDA categorizes this drug as category *C* for use during pregnancy (*Animal studies have shown an adverse effect on the fetus, but there are no adequate studies in humans; or there are no animal reproduction studies and no adequate studies in humans.*)

No information on lactation safety was found.

Overdosage/Acute Toxicity

The LD_{50} for IV administered 3% methylene blue is approximately 43 mg/kg in sheep.

Drug Interactions

■ None reported

Laboratory Considerations

■ Methylene blue can cause a green-blue color in urine and may affect the accuracy of **urinalysis**.

Doses

■ **DOGS:**

To preferentially stain islet-cell tumors of the pancreas:

a) 3 mg/kg in 250 mL sterile normal saline and administered IV over 30–40 minutes intraoperatively. Initial tumor staining requires approximately 20 minutes after infusion has begun and is maximal at about 25–35 minutes after infusion is started. Tumors generally appear to be a reddish-violet in color versus a dusky blue (background staining). (Fingeroth & Smeak 1988)

To treat methemoglobinemia:

a) Secondary to phenol exposure: A single, slow IV infusion of 4 mg/kg of methylene blue; may use with 20 mg/kg ascorbic acid PO (Dorman & Clark 2000)

b) For severe methemoglobinemia: 1 mg/kg as a 1% solution given slowly IV over several minutes. A dramatic response should occur during the first 30 minutes after treatment. It may be repeated if necessary, but it should be used cautiously as can cause Heinz body anemia. Measure hematocrit for 3 days after treatment. (Harvey 2006)

■ **CATS:**

To treat methemoglobinemia:

a) Secondary to phenol exposure: A single,

slow IV infusion of 1.5 mg/kg of methylene blue, may use with 20 mg/kg ascorbic acid PO (Dorman & Clark 2000)

b) 1–1.5 mg/kg IV one time only (Christopher 2000)

c) For severe methemoglobinemia: 1 mg/kg as a 1% solution given slowly IV over several minutes. A dramatic response should occur during the first 30 minutes after treatment. It may be repeated if necessary, but it should be used cautiously as can cause Heinz body anemia. Measure hematocrit for 3 days after treatment. (Harvey 2006)

■ **RUMINANTS:**

Note: When used in food animals, FARAD recommends a minimum milk withdrawal time of 4 days after the last treatment. Because of concerns of carcinogenicity, an extremely conservative withdrawal time for meat of 180 days has been recommended; however, available data suggest that a much shorter withdrawal time of 14 days would be sufficient. (Haskell *et al.* 2005)

For methemoglobin-producing toxins (nitrites, nitrates, chlorates):

a) Using a 1% solution, methylene blue is given at 4–15 mg/kg IV q6h. (Osweiler 2007)

b) For nitrate poisoning in cattle: 5–15 mg/kg as a 1% solution in physiologic saline. With severe cases, repeat treatment at a lower dose may be required. In animals that do not succumb, recovery occurs by 24 hours. (Hall 2006)

For cyanide toxicity:

a) 4–6 grams IV per 454 kg (1000 lb.) of body weight (Oehme 1986)

■ **HORSES:**

For methemoglobinemia secondary to chlorate toxicity:

a) 4.4 mg/kg as 1% solution by intravenous drip; may repeat in 15–30 minutes if clinical response is not obtained. (Schmitz 2004)

Monitoring
■ Methemoglobinemia
■ Red cell morphology, red cell indices, hematocrit, hemoglobin

Client Information
■ Because of the potential toxicity of this agent and the seriousness of methemoglobin-related intoxications, this drug should be used with close professional supervision only.
■ Methylene blue may be very staining to clothing or skin. Removal may be accomplished using hypochlorite solutions (bleach).

Chemistry/Synonyms
A thiazine dye, methylene blue occurs as dark green crystals or crystalline powder that has a bronze-like luster. It may have a slight odor and is soluble in water and sparingly soluble in alcohol. When dissolved, a dark blue solution results. Commercially available methylene blue injection (human-labeled) has a pH from 3–4.5.

Methylene blue may also be known as: methylthioninium chloride, azul de metileno, blu di metilene, CI basic blue 9, colour index no. 52015, methylene blue, methylenii caeruleum, methylthioninii chloridum, schultz no. 1038, tetramethylthionine chloride trihydrate, *Azul Metile®, Collubleu®, Desmoidpillen®, Vitableu®, Urolene Blue®* and *Zumetil®.*

Storage/Stability
Unless otherwise instructed by the manufacturer, store methylene blue at room temperature.

Compatibility/Compounding Considerations
Methylene blue is reportedly physically **incompatible** when mixed with caustic alkalies, dichromates, iodides, and oxidizing or reducing agents.

Dosage Forms/Regulatory Status
VETERINARY-LABELED PRODUCTS:

None FDA-approved as pharmaceuticals for internal use. A 1% (10 mg/mL) methylene blue solution (Centaur) is labeled for animal use as a dye, laboratory indicator and reagent. It is available in pint and gallon bottles. Methylene Blue, USP powder may be available from chemical supply houses

HUMAN-LABELED PRODUCTS:

Methylene Blue Injection: 10 mg/mL in 1 mL & 10 mL amps; generic; (Rx)

References
Christopher, M. (2000). Disorders of Feline Red Blood Cells. *Kirk's Current Veterinary Therapy: XIII Small Animal Practice.* J Bonagura Ed. Philadelphia, WB Saunders: 421–424.

Dorman, D. & J. Clark (2000). Common Household Chemical Hazards. *Kirk's Current Veterinary Therapy: XIII Small Animal Practice.* J Bonagura Ed. Philadelphia, WB Saunders: 223–227.

Fingeroth, J.M. & D.D. Smeak (1988). Intravenous methylene blue infusion for intraoperative identification of pancreatic islet-cell tumors in dogs. Part II: Clinical trials and results in four dogs. *J Am Anim Hosp Assoc* **24**(2): 175–182.

Hall, J. (2006). Urea and Nitrate Poisoning of Ruminants. Proceedings: Western Veterinary Conference. Accessed via: Veterinary Information Network. http://goo.gl/7CdEa

Harvey, J. (2006). Toxic hemolytic anemias. Proceedings: ACVIM. Accessed via: Veterinary Information Network. http://goo.gl/lATcp

Haskell, S., M. Payne, et al. (2005). Farad Digest: Antidotes in Food Animal Practice. *JAVMA* **226**(6): 884–887.

Oehme, F.W. (1986). Cyanogenic Plants. *Current Veterinary Therapy: Food Animal Practice 2.* JL Howard Ed. Philadelphia, W.B. Saunders: 390–392.

Osweiler, G. (2007). Detoxification and Antidotes for Ruminant Poisoning. Proceedings: ACVIM. Accessed via: Veterinary Information Network. http://goo.gl/h1YRI

Schmitz, D. (2004). Toxicologic problems. *Equine Internal Medicine 2nd Ed.* S Reed, W Bayly and D Sellon Eds. Philadelphia, Saunders: 1441–1512.

METHYLPHENIDATE

(meth-ill-*fen*-i-date)   Ritalin®
CNS STIMULANT

Prescriber Highlights

▶ Amphetamine-like drug that may be useful for treating cataplexy/narcolepsy or hyperkinesis/hyperactivity in dogs

▶ Use with caution in dogs with seizure disorders, cardiac disease/hypertension, or in aggressive animals

▶ Adverse effects are primarily CNS stimulation-related

▶ Class-II controlled drug in USA

Uses/Indications

Methylphenidate may be useful for diagnosing and treating cataplexy/narcolepsy or hyperactivity in dogs.

Pharmacology/Actions

Methylphenidate has stimulating effects on the central nervous and respiratory systems similar to that of amphetamines. It also has weak sympathomimetic activity, and at normal dosages has little effect on peripheral circulation.

Pharmacokinetics

In dogs, there is limited information available. Single PO doses of immediate-release 20 mg tablets to 7–19 kg beagles gave peak levels of about 60 micrograms/mL in about 15 minutes after dosing. Clearance was about 0.27 L/hr and elimination half-life around an hour. With 20 mg sustained-release tablets there was much more inter-patient variation, serum concentrations peaked around 30 minutes after dosing, peak levels of 19 micrograms/mL were much lower then the immediate-release tablets. Clearance was about 0.97 L/hr and elimination half-life was approximately 40 minutes. For reference, the therapeutic plasma concentration of methylphenidate is thought to be between 1–10 micrograms/mL. (Giorgi *et al.* 2010)

In humans, methylphenidate (regular tablets) is rapidly and well absorbed from the GI tract. Food in the GI tract may increase the rate, but not the extent, of drug absorbed. Peak levels occur about 2 hours post-dose. The drug is extensively metabolized during the first-pass; protein binding is low. Terminal elimination half-life is approximately 3 hours; less than 1% is excreted unchanged in the urine.

Contraindications/Precautions/Warnings

The risks associated with methylphenidate should be carefully considered before using this drug in dogs with seizure disorders, cardiac disease/hypertension, or in aggressive animals.

Adverse Effects

Most likely adverse effects to be encountered include increased heart and respiratory rates, anorexia, tremors and hyperthermia (particularly exercised-induced).

Reproductive/Nursing Safety

In humans, the FDA categorizes methylphenidate as a category *C* drug for use during pregnancy (*Animal studies have shown an adverse effect on the fetus, but there are no adequate studies in humans; or there are no animal reproduction studies and no adequate studies in humans*). Methylphenidate was associated with teratogenic effects in rabbits, but at massive dosages (200 mg/kg/day).

It is unknown if methylphenidate enters maternal milk.

Overdosage/Acute Toxicity

In dogs, dosages of 1 mg/kg (or below) can cause toxic reactions; there is one report of a fatality after a dog ingested 3.1 mg/kg, but research dogs have survived doses of 20 mg/kg/day for 90 days. A cat given a 5 mg tablet of methylphenidate, showed signs of tremors, agitation, mydriasis, tachycardia, tachypnea and hypertension; signs resolved 25 hours post-ingestion with supportive care (dark cage, diazepam, fluids).

Expected signs associated with an overdose in dogs are generally CNS over-stimulation and excessive sympathomimetic effects and can include: hyperactivity, salivation, diarrhea, head bobbing, agitation, tachycardia, hypertension, tremors, seizures, and hyperthermia. Consider the dosage form (extended-release vs. regular tablets) when considering treatment options and expected onset and duration of effects. Employ treatment using standard gut detoxification techniques (emetic, activated charcoal, cathartic, etc.); however, emesis should be avoided in animals displaying signs associated with toxicity or that are otherwise at risk for emesis-related adverse effects. Treatment is basically supportive by controlling signs associated with toxicity. Phenothiazines (*e.g.,* acepromazine, chlorpromazine) may be useful in controlling agitation; beta-blockers can help control tachycardia; external cooling may be used for hyperthermia; and cyproheptadine may help prevent serotonin syndrome.

Drug Interactions

The following drug interactions have either been reported or are theoretical in humans or animals receiving methylphenidate and may be of significance in veterinary patients:

◼ **ANTICONVULSANTS (phenobarbital, primidone, phenytoin):** Methylphenidate may increase serum levels

◼ **CLONIDINE:** Rare cases (in humans) of cardiovascular effects (including death); mechanism not understood and causality not established

◼ **HYPOTENSIVE DRUGS:** Methylphenidate may reduce effects

■ **MAO INHIBITORS (including amitraz and potentially, selegiline):** Could lead to hypertensive crisis

■ **SSRI ANTIDEPRESSANTS (e.g., fluoxetine, sertraline, etc.):** Methylphenidate may inhibit metabolism and increase levels

■ **TRICYCLIC ANTIDEPRESSANTS (e.g., amitriptyline, clomipramine, etc.):** Methylphenidate may inhibit metabolism and increase levels

■ **WARFARIN:** Methylphenidate may inhibit warfarin metabolism and increase INR

Laboratory Considerations

■ No specific laboratory interactions were noted for this drug.

Doses

■ **DOGS:**

a) For treatment of narcolepsy/cataplexy: 5–10 mg (total dose) PO once daily. (Joseph 2000)

b) For treatment of narcolepsy/cataplexy (to supplement imipramine at 0.5–1 mg/kg PO q8–12h): Methylphenidate: 0.25–0.5 mg/kg PO or 5–10 mg (total dose) PO q12–24h (Shell 2003)

c) For diagnosis and treatment of hyperkinesis: 5–20 mg (total dose) q8–12h; give for 3 days and assess for improvement of target behaviors (anxiety, overactivity, learning ability) (Siebert 2003)

d) For hyperkinesis-hyperactivity: Small dogs: 5+ mg total dose PO q12h; Large Dogs: 20–40 mg total dose PO q12h (Virga 2002)

Monitoring

■ Clinical efficacy

■ Occasional physical exam to monitor vital signs, body weight

■ In humans, it is recommended to do periodic CBC with differential and platelet counts during prolonged therapy.

Client Information

■ Clients should understand that this drug has significant potential for abuse by humans and to keep it safely secure.

■ Clients should report untoward stimulatory effects to the veterinarian.

■ If using an extended-release product, do not crush tablet or capsule.

Chemistry/Synonyms

A CNS stimulant related to amphetamines, methylphenidate HCl occurs as fine, white odorless, crystalline powder. It is feely soluble in water and soluble in alcohol.

Methylphenidate may also be known as: *Attenta®, Daytrana®, Equasym®, Focalin®, Metadate ER®, Methylin®, Rilatine®, Riphenidate®, Ritalina®, Ritalin®, Ritaline®, Ritaphen®, Rubifen®,* or *Tranquilyn®.*

Storage/Stability

Unless otherwise noted on the label, methylphenidate tablets and extended-release tablets and capsules should be stored in tight, light-resistant containers at room temperature.

Dosage Forms/Regulatory Status

VETERINARY-LABELED PRODUCTS: None

The ARCI (Racing Commissioners International) has designated this drug as a class 1 substance. See the appendix for more information.

HUMAN-LABELED PRODUCTS:

Methylphenidate Oral Tablets: 5 mg, 10 mg & 20 mg; Chewable Tablets: 2.5 mg, 5 mg & 10 mg; Extended-Release Tablets: 10 mg, 18 mg, 20 mg, 27 mg, 36 mg & 54 mg; Extended-Release Capsules: 20 mg, 30 mg, 40 mg, 50 mg & 60 mg; *Methylin®* (Mallinckrodt); *Ritalin®, Ritalin® LA, & Ritalin-SR®* (Novartis); *Metadate ER®* & *Metadate CD®* (UCB); *Concerta®* (Janssen); (Rx; C-II)

Methylphenidate Oral Solution: 5 mg/5 mL & 10 mg/5 mL in 500 mL; *Methylin®* (Sciele); (Rx; C-II)

Methylphenidate Transdermal Patch: 10 mg/9 h (1.1 mg/h; 27.5 mg total), 15 mg/9 h (1.6 mg/h; 41.3 mg total), 20 mg/9 h (2.2 mg/h; 55 mg total) & 30 mg/9 h (3.3 mg/h; 82.5 mg total); *Daytrana®* (Shire); (Rx; C-II)

References

Giorgi, M., U. Prise, et al. (2010). Pharmacokinetics of methylphenidate following two oral formulations (immediate and sustained release) in the dog. *Veterinary Research Communications* **34**: S73–S77.

Joseph, R. (2000). Seizures and other episodic disorders, Veterinary Information Network, Rounds Presentation.

Shell, L. (2003). "Narcolepsy/Cataplexy."

Siebert, L. (2003). Psychoactive drugs in behavioral medicine. Western Veterinary Conference.

Virga, V. (2002). Which drug and why: An update on psychopharmacology. Proceedings: Atlantic Coast Veterinary Conference. Accessed via: Veterinary Information Network. http://goo.gl/m8qr4

METHYLPRED-NISOLONE
METHYLPRED-NISOLONE ACETATE
METHYLPRED-NISOLONE SODIUM SUCCINATE

(meth-ill-pred-*niss*-oh-lone)
Medrol®, Depo-Medrol®

GLUCOCORTICOID

Prescriber Highlights

▶ Oral & parenteral glucocorticoid that is 4–5X more potent than hydrocortisone; no appreciable mineralocorticoid activity

▶ Contraindicated (relatively): Systemic fungal infections, manufacturer lists: "in viral infections . . . animals with arrested tuberculosis, peptic ulcer, acute psychoses, corneal ulcer, & Cushingoid syndrome. The presence of diabetes, osteoporosis, chronic psychotic reactions, predisposition to thrombophlebitis, hypertension, CHF, renal insufficiency, & active tuberculosis necessitates carefully controlled use."

▶ Acetate can cause significant HPA axis suppression. In cats, extracellular hyperglycemia can cause volume expansion and may predispose cats to congestive heart failure. IM administration generally reserved when owners cannot adhere to oral treatment regimens

▶ Usual therapy goal is to use as much as is required & as little as possible for as short an amount of time as possible

▶ Primary adverse effects are "Cushingoid" in nature with sustained use

▶ Many potential drug & lab interactions

Uses/Indications

Glucocorticoids have been used in an attempt to treat practically every malady that afflicts man or animal, but there are three broad uses and dosage ranges for use of these agents. **1)** Replacement of glucocorticoid activity in patients with adrenal insufficiency, **2)** as an antiinflammatory agent, and **3)** as an immunosuppressive. Among some of the uses for glucocorticoids include treatment of: endocrine conditions (*e.g.*, adrenal insufficiency), rheumatic diseases (*e.g.*, rheumatoid arthritis), collagen diseases (*e.g.*, systemic lupus), allergic states, respiratory diseases (*e.g.*, asthma), dermatologic diseases (*e.g.*, pemphigus, allergic dermatoses), hematologic disorders (*e.g.*, thrombocytopenias, autoimmune hemolytic anemias), neoplasias, nervous system disorders (increased CSF pressure), GI diseases (*e.g.*, ulcerative colitis exacerbations), and renal diseases (*e.g.*, nephrotic syndrome). Some glucocorticoids are used topically in the eye and skin for various conditions or are injected intra-articularly or intra-lesionally.

High dose fast-acting corticosteroid use for shock or CNS trauma is controversial; recent studies have not demonstrated significant clinical benefit and it actually may cause increased deleterious effects.

Pharmacology/Actions

Methylprednisolone may be administered either orally or parenterally. Its relative antiinflammatory potency is approximately 5 times that of cortisol. It has negligible to very slight mineralocorticoid activity. Once in the systemic circulation it has an approximate duration of activity of 12–36 hours. Duration of activity is not dependent on elimination half-life.

Glucocorticoids have effects on virtually every cell type and system in mammals. For more information, refer to the Glucocorticoid Agents, General Information monograph.

Pharmacokinetics

Methylprednisolone administered orally is relatively well absorbed and extensively distributed. The liver is the primary site for metabolism (oxidation); most of the drug is excreted renally as metabolites. Elimination half-life is multiphasic and does not appreciably effect duration of action.

The sodium succinate IV injection is water soluble and considered very fast acting.

The acetate IM injection is slowly absorbed and can have a duration of effect of weeks to months.

Contraindications/Precautions/Warnings

The original manufacturer (Upjohn Veterinary) states that the drug (tablets) should not be used in dogs or cats "in viral infections, . . . animals with arrested tuberculosis, peptic ulcer, acute psychoses, corneal ulcer, and Cushingoid syndrome. The presence of diabetes, osteoporosis, chronic psychotic reactions, predisposition to thrombophlebitis, hypertension, CHF, renal insufficiency, and active tuberculosis necessitates carefully controlled use."

The injectable acetate product is contraindicated as outlined above when used systemically. When injected intrasynovially, intratendinously, or by other local means, it is contraindicated in the "presence of acute local infections."

Systemic use of glucocorticoids is generally considered contraindicated in systemic fungal infections (unless used for replacement therapy in Addison's), when administered IM in patients with idiopathic thrombocytopenia, and in patients hypersensitive to a particular compound. Use of sustained-release injectable glucocorticoids is considered contraindicated for chronic corticosteroid therapy of systemic diseases.

Animals that have received glucocorticoids systemically other than with "burst" therapy, should be tapered off the drugs. Patients who have received the drugs chronically should be tapered off slowly as endogenous ACTH and corticosteroid function may return slowly. Should the animal undergo a "stressor" (*e.g.*, surgery, trauma, illness, etc.) during the tapering process or until normal adrenal and pituitary function resume, additional glucocorticoids should be administered.

Adverse Effects

Adverse effects are generally associated with long-term administration of these drugs, especially if given at high dosages or not on an alternate day regimen, but high-dose short-term adverse effects can occur. With long-term use adverse effects generally are manifested as clinical signs of hyperadrenocorticism. When administered to young, growing animals, glucocorticoids can retard growth. In dogs, high-dose methylprednisolone sodium succinate has been associated with diarrhea, blood in stools (melena, hematochezia) vomiting, GI bleeding, and anorexia. Many other potential effects, adverse and otherwise, are outlined above in the Pharmacology section.

In dogs, polydipsia (PD), polyphagia (PP), and polyuria (PU) may all be seen with short-term "burst" therapy as well as with alternate-day maintenance therapy on days when administering the drug. Adverse effects in dogs can include dull, dry haircoat, weight gain, panting, vomiting, diarrhea, elevated liver enzymes, pancreatitis, GI ulceration, lipidemias, activation or worsening of diabetes mellitus, muscle wasting, and behavioral changes (depression, lethargy, viciousness). Discontinuation of the drug may be necessary; changing to an alternate steroid may also alleviate the problem. With the exception of PU/PD/PP, adverse effects associated with anti-inflammatory therapy are relatively uncommon. Adverse effects associated with immunosuppressive doses are more common and, potentially, more severe.

Cats generally require higher dosages than dogs for clinical effect, but tend to develop fewer adverse effects. Occasionally, polydipsia, polyuria, polyphagia with weight gain, diarrhea, or depression can be seen. Long-term high dose therapy can lead to "Cushingoid" effects, however. In cats, the long-acting acetate salt has been implicated in causing extracellular hyperglycemia leading to volume expansion and may predispose patients to congestive heart failure; however, current evidence for this effect is not strong.

Corticosteroid-related diabetes mellitus may be related to increased urinary excretion of chromium and potentially could respond to chromium supplementation.

Reproductive/Nursing Safety

Glucocorticoids are probably necessary for normal fetal development. They may be required for adequate surfactant production, myelin, retinal, pancreas and mammary development. Excessive dosages early in pregnancy may lead to teratogenic effects. In horses and ruminants, exogenous steroid administration may induce parturition when administered in the latter stages of pregnancy. The FDA categorizes this drug as category *C* for use during pregnancy (*Animal studies have shown an adverse effect on the fetus, but there are no adequate studies in humans; or there are no animal reproduction studies and no adequate studies in humans.*)

Use with caution in nursing dams. Glucocorticoids unbound to plasma proteins will enter milk. High dosages or prolonged administration to mothers may, potentially, inhibit growth, interfere with endogenous corticosteroid production or cause other unwanted effects in nursing offspring. However, in humans, several studies suggest that amounts excreted in breast milk are negligible when methylprednisolone doses are less than or equal to 8 mg/day. Larger doses for short periods may not harm the infant.

Overdosage/Acute Toxicity

Glucocorticoids when given short-term are unlikely to cause harmful effects, even in massive dosages. One incidence of a dog developing acute CNS effects after accidental ingestion of glucocorticoids has been reported. Should clinical signs occur, use supportive treatment if required.

Chronic usage of glucocorticoids can lead to serious adverse effects. Refer to Adverse Effects above for more information.

Drug Interactions

The following drug interactions have either been reported or are theoretical in humans or animals receiving methylprednisolone and may be of significance in veterinary patients:

■ **AMPHOTERICIN B:** Administered concomitantly with glucocorticoids may cause hypokalemia; in humans, there have been cases of CHF and cardiac enlargement reported after using methylprednisolone to treat Amphotericin B adverse effects

■ **ANALGESICS, OPIATE and/or ANESTHETICS, LOCAL (epidural injections):** Combination with glucocorticoids in epidurals has caused serious CNS injuries and death; do not use more volume than very small intrathecal test doses of these agents with glucocorticoids

■ **ANTICHOLINESTERASE AGENTS (e.g., pyridostigmine, neostigmine, etc.):** In patients with myasthenia gravis, concomitant glucocorticoid and anticholinesterase agent administration may lead to profound muscle weakness. If possible, discontinue anticholinesterase medication at least 24 hours prior to corticosteroid administration

■ **ASPIRIN:** Glucocorticoids may reduce salicylate blood levels

■ **BARBITURATES:** May increase the metabolism of glucocorticoids and decrease blood levels

■ **CYCLOPHOSPHAMIDE:** Glucocorticoids may inhibit the hepatic metabolism of cyclophosphamide; dosage adjustments may be required

■ **CYCLOSPORINE:** Concomitant administration of glucocorticoids and cyclosporine may increase the blood levels of each, by mutually inhibiting the hepatic metabolism of each other; the clinical significance of this interaction is not clear

■ **DIURETICS, POTASSIUM-DEPLETING (e.g., spironolactone, triamterene):** Administered concomitantly with glucocorticoids may cause hypokalemia

■ **EPHEDRINE:** May reduce methylprednisolone blood levels

■ **ESTROGENS:** The effects of methylprednisolone, and possibly other glucocorticoids, may be potentiated by concomitant administration with estrogens

■ **INSULIN:** Insulin requirements may increase in patients receiving glucocorticoids

■ **KETOCONAZOLE and other AZOLE ANTIFUNGALS:** May decrease the metabolism of glucocorticoids and increase methylprednisolone blood levels; ketoconazole may induce adrenal insufficiency when glucocorticoids are withdrawn by inhibiting adrenal corticosteroid synthesis

■ **MACROLIDE ANTIBIOTICS (erythromycin, clarithromycin):** May decrease the metabolism of glucocorticoids and increase methylprednisolone blood levels

■ **MITOTANE:** May alter the metabolism of steroids; higher than usual doses of steroids may be necessary to treat mitotane-induced adrenal insufficiency

■ **NSAIDS:** Administration of ulcerogenic drugs with glucocorticoids may increase the risk of gastrointestinal ulceration

■ **PHENOBARBITAL:** May increase the metabolism of glucocorticoids and decrease methylprednisolone blood levels

■ **RIFAMPIN:** May increase the metabolism of glucocorticoids and decrease methylprednisolone blood levels

■ **VACCINES:** Patients receiving corticosteroids at immunosuppressive dosages should generally not receive live attenuated-virus vaccines as virus replication may be augmented; a diminished immune response may occur after vaccine, toxoid, or bacterin administration in patients receiving glucocorticoid

■ **WARFARIN:** Methylprednisolone may affect INR's; monitor

Laboratory Considerations

■ Methylprednisolone acetate may reduce **post-ACTH cortisol** concentrations by 20–50%.

■ Glucocorticoids may increase **serum cholesterol**

■ Glucocorticoids may increase **serum and urine glucose** levels

■ Glucocorticoids may decrease **serum potassium**

■ Glucocorticoids can suppress the release of thyroid stimulating hormone (TSH) and reduce T_3 & T_4 values. Thyroid gland atrophy has been reported after chronic glucocorticoid administration. Uptake of I^{131} by the thyroid may be decreased by glucocorticoids.

■ Reactions to **skin tests** may be suppressed by glucocorticoids

■ False-negative results of the **nitroblue tetrazolium** test for systemic bacterial infections may be induced by glucocorticoids

■ Glucocorticoids may cause **neutrophilia** within 4–8 hours after dosing and return to baseline within 24–48 hours after drug discontinuation

■ Glucocorticoids can cause **lymphopenia** which can persist for weeks after drug discontinuation in dogs

Doses

There are a plethora of doses and protocols associated with many specific indications for systemic administration of glucocorticoids, but there are four primary uses and dose ranges: **1)** replacement or supplementation (*e.g.*, relative adrenal insufficiency associated with septic shock) of glucocorticoid effects secondary to hypoadrenocorticism, **2)** as an antiinflammatory, **3)** as an immunosuppressive, and **4)** as an antineoplastic agent. Current evidence does not support high dose use for hemorrhagic or hypovolemic shock, head trauma, spinal cord trauma, or sepsis.

■ **DOGS:**
Note: *If using methylprednisolone tablets or methylprednisolone sodium succinate for IV injection, refer to the prednis(ol)one dose section to determine an appropriate dose for the condition treated using prednisone or prednisolone. That dose can be converted to a near equivalent dose for methylprednisolone by dividing it by 1.25 (e.g., if the dose is 5 mg of prednisone or prednisolone, the methylprednisolone dose would be 4 mg).*

For labeled uses:

a) Oral: Dogs weighing 5–15 lbs: 2 mg; Dogs weighing 15–40 lbs: 2–4 mg; Dogs weighing 40–80 lbs: 4–8 mg; these total daily doses should be divided and given

6–10 hours apart. (Label information; *Medrol®*—Pfizer)

Intramuscularly: 2–120 mg IM (average 20 mg); depending on breed (size), severity of condition, and response. May repeat at weekly intervals or in accordance with the severity of the condition and the response. (Package insert; *Depo-Medrol®*—Upjohn) The manufacturer has specific directions for use of the drug intrasynovially. It is recommended to refer directly to the package insert for more information.

For intralesional (sub-lesional) use:

a) A sufficient volume of 20 mg/mL methylprednisolone acetate is used to undermine the lesion (10–40 mg total dose) (Scott 1982)

■ **CATS:**
Note: If using methylprednisolone tablets or methylprednisolone sodium succinate for IV injection, refer to the prednisolone dose section to determine an appropriate dose for the condition treated using prednisone or prednisolone. That dose can be converted to a near equivalent dose for methylprednisolone by dividing it by 1.25 (e.g., if the dose is 5 mg of prednisolone, the methylprednisolone dose would be 4 mg).

For labeled uses:

a) Oral: Cats weighing 5–15 lbs: 2 mg; Cats weighing >15 lbs: 2–4 mg. These total daily doses should be divided and given 6–10 hours apart. (Label information; *Medrol®*—Pfizer)

Intramuscularly using methylprednisolone acetate (*Depo-Medrol®*): up to 20 mg (average 10 mg) IM; depending on breed (size), severity of condition, and response. May repeat at weekly intervals or in accordance with the severity of the condition and the response. (Package insert; *Depo-Medrol®*—Upjohn)

For intralesional (sub-lesional) use:

a) A sufficient volume of 20 mg/mL methylprednisolone acetate is used to undermine the lesion (10–40 mg total dose) (Scott 1982)

■ **HORSES:**
As an antiinflammatory (glucocorticoid effects):

a) For labeled uses: Methylprednisolone acetate 200 mg IM repeated as necessary (Package insert; *Depo-Medrol®*—Upjohn). The manufacturer has specific directions for use of the drug intrasynovially. It is recommended to refer directly to the package insert for more information.

b) For intra-articular use: Methylprednisolone acetate 100 mg IA (McClure 2002)

Monitoring
Monitoring of glucocorticoid therapy is dependent on its reason for use, dosage, agent used (amount of mineralocorticoid activity), dosage schedule (daily versus alternate day therapy), duration of therapy, and the animal's age and condition. The following list may not be appropriate or complete for all animals; use clinical assessment and judgment should adverse effects be noted:

■ Weight, appetite, signs of edema
■ Serum and/or urine electrolytes
■ Total plasma proteins, albumin
■ Blood glucose
■ Growth and development in young animals
■ ACTH stimulation test if necessary

Client Information
■ Clients should carefully follow the dosage instructions and should not discontinue the drug abruptly without consulting with veterinarian beforehand.
■ Clients should be briefed on the potential adverse effects that can be seen with these drugs and instructed to contact the veterinarian should these effects become severe or progress.

Chemistry/Synonyms
Methylprednisolone is a synthetically produced glucocorticoid. Both the free alcohol and the acetate ester occur as odorless, white or practically white, crystalline powder. They are practically insoluble in water and sparingly soluble in alcohol.

Methylprednisolone sodium succinate occurs as an odorless, white or nearly white, hygroscopic, amorphous solid. It is very soluble in both water and alcohol.

Methylprednisolone may also be known as: 6alpha-methylprednisolone, methylprednisolonum, NSC-19987, *A-Methapred®*, *Alergolon®*, *Caberdelta M®*, *Cipridanol®*, *Cortisolona®*, *Depo-Medrol®*, *Esametone®*, *Firmacort®*, *Medrate®*, *Medrol®*, *Medrone®*, *Mega-Star®*, *Metilpren®*, *Metisona®*, *Methapred®*, *Metypred®*, *Metysolon®*, *Predni M®*, *Prednilen®*, *Reactenol®*, *Sieropresol®*, *Solomet®*, *Solu-Medrol®*, *Summicort®* and *Urbason®*.

Storage/Stability
Commercially available products of methylprednisolone should be stored at room temperature (15–30°C); avoid freezing the acetate injection. After reconstituting the sodium succinate injection, store at room temperature and use within 48 hours; only use solutions that are clear.

Compatibility/Compounding Considerations
Methylprednisolone sodium succinate injection is reportedly physically **compatible** with the following fluids and drugs: amino acids 4.25%/dextrose 25%, amphotericin B (limited amounts), chloramphenicol sodium succinate,

cimetidine HCl, clindamycin phosphate, dopamine HCl, heparin sodium, metoclopramide, norepinephrine bitartrate, penicillin G potassium, sodium iodide/aminophylline, and verapamil.

The following drugs and fluids have either been reported to be physically **incompatible** when mixed with methylprednisolone sodium succinate, compatible dependent upon concentration, or **data conflicts**: D_5/half normal saline, D_5 normal saline (80 mg/L reported compatible), D_5W (up to 5 grams/L reported compatible), Lactated Ringer's (up to 80 mg/L reported compatible), normal saline (data conflicts; some reports of up to 60 grams/Liter compatible), calcium gluconate, cephalothin sodium (up to 500 mg/L in D5W or NS compatible), glycopyrrolate, insulin, metaraminol bitartrate, nafcillin sodium, penicillin G sodium, and tetracycline HCl. Compatibility is dependent upon factors such as pH, concentration, temperature, and diluent used; consult specialized references or a hospital pharmacist for more specific information.

Dosage Forms/Regulatory Status

VETERINARY-LABELED PRODUCTS:

Methylprednisolone Tablets: 4 mg tablets, *Medrol®*; (Pfizer); (Rx). FDA-approved for use in dogs and cats.

Methylprednisolone Acetate Injection: 20 mg/mL in 10 mL and 20 mL vials, and 40 mg/mL in 5 mL vials; *Depo-Medrol®* (Pfizer); generic; (Rx). FDA-approved for IM and intrasynovial injection in dogs and horses; for IM injection in cats.

The ARCI (Racing Commissioners International) has designated this drug as a class 4 substance. See the appendix for more information.

A 10 ppb tolerance has been established for methylprednisolone in milk.

HUMAN-LABELED PRODUCTS:

Methylprednisolone Oral Tablets: 2 mg, 4 mg, 8 mg, 16 mg, 24 mg & 32 mg; *Medrol®* (Upjohn); generic; (Rx)

Methylprednisolone Acetate Injection: 20 mg/mL, 40 mg/mL, 80 mg/mL suspension in 1 mL (40 & 80 mg only), 5 mL & 10 mL vials; *Depo-Medrol®* (Pfizer); generic; (Rx)

Methylprednisolone Sodium Succinate Powder for Injection: 40 mg/vial in 1 mL & 3 mL vials and 1 mL *Univials* and *Act-O-Vials*; 125 mg/vial in 2 mL & 5 mL vials and 2 mL *Univials* and *Act-O-Vials*; 500 mg/vial in 1 mL, 4 mL, 8mL (with or without diluent) and 20 mL vials; 1 gram/vial in 1 mL, 8 mL, 50 mL, & 1 gram vials (with or without diluent), 8 mL *Act-O-Vials*; 2 grams/vial in 2 grams vials with diluent; *Solu-Medrol®* (Pfizer); *A-Methapred®* (Hospira); generic; (Rx)

References

McClure, S. (2002). An opinion on joint therapy. Proceedings: Western Veterinary Conf. Accessed via: Veterinary Information Network. http://goo.gl/wVJwW

Scott, D.W. (1982). Dermatologic Use of Glucocorticoids: Systemic and Topical. *Vet Clin of North America: Small Anim Prac* **12**(1): 19–32.

4-Methylpyrazole—see Fomepizole

METHYLTESTOSTERONE

(meth-ill-tess-**toss**-ter-ohn)
Android®, Methitest®

ANDROGENIC/ANABOLIC

Prescriber Highlights

▶ Androgenic & anabolic agent that may be useful to suppress estrus, treat testosterone-responsive alopecia, & pseudopregnancy in dogs

▶ Use in cats is controversial as hepatotoxicity may be more prevalent

▶ Contraindicated in pregnancy or hepatic dysfunction

▶ Most serious adverse effect is hepatotoxicity

Uses/Indications

In female dogs, methyltestosterone may be useful for suppression of estrus, treating estrogen-dependent mammary tumors, pseudopregnancy, or certain hormonal-dependent alopecias. In male dogs, it may be useful for treating deficient libido and certain hormonal alopecias. In cats, methyltestosterone may be useful for certain hormonal-dependent alopecias and to increase libido in toms. Because of the potential for abuse by humans, and potential toxicity (especially hepatotoxicity) in animals, use of methyltestosterone is somewhat controversial in veterinary medicine, particularly in racing Greyhounds and cats.

Pharmacology/Actions

Methyltestosterone is an androgen with anabolic effects. It has a methyl-group at the 17 position of the steroid nucleus of testosterone, resulting in better oral absorption and slower hepatic metabolism than testosterone. Androgens are required for both the development and maintenance of male sexual characteristics and function. The anabolic effects of methyltestosterone include stimulating erythropoiesis, enhancing nitrogen balance and protein anabolism (in the presence of sufficient protein and calories) and retention of potassium, sodium, and phosphorus.

Pharmacokinetics

Methyltestosterone is absorbed from the GI tract and oral mucosa. It undergoes less first pass metabolism than orally administered testosterone. In dogs, methyltestosterone is metabolized in the liver. Principle metabolites found in urine are glucuronidated forms (both conjugated and free) of methyltestosterone. Unlike in humans, sulfated forms are not a major metabolic component.

In humans, peak levels occur about 2 hours after oral dosing; elimination half-life is approximately 3 hours.

Contraindications/Precautions/Warnings

Methyltestosterone is contraindicated in patients with hepatic dysfunction and during pregnancy (see Reproductive Safety). It should be used with extreme caution in animals with heart failure. Prolonged use in young animals can cause premature epiphyseal closure.

Adverse Effects

Adverse effects in animals include: hepatotoxicity, virilization of females (clitoral hypertrophy), vaginal discharge, prostatic hyperplasia and increased aggression in males. Chronic dosing in dogs of 2–6 mg/kg/day for 27 weeks caused hepatotoxicity characterized by enlarged periportal hepatocytes, and hemosiderin in macrophages. Cats may be more susceptible to hepatic injury than are dogs.

Reproductive/Nursing Safety

Spermatogenesis suppression in males may occur with high dosage methyltestosterone secondary to a negative feedback mechanism. Methyltestosterone may suppress estrus in females (see Uses). After the drug is discontinued, normal reproductive function usually returns in both males and females.

Methyltestosterone is contraindicated during pregnancy. Dose-related genital masculinization of female fetuses is well described. In humans, the FDA categorizes this drug as category **X** for use during pregnancy (*Studies in animals or humans demonstrate fetal abnormalities or adverse reaction; reports indicate evidence of fetal risk. The risk of use in pregnant women clearly outweighs any possible benefit.*)

Overdosage/Acute Toxicity

Information on the acute toxicity of methyltestosterone is limited. Nausea and edema are the most likely effects of a single overdose. Consider liver function monitoring with large overdoses.

Drug Interactions

The following drug interactions have either been reported or are theoretical in humans or animals receiving methyltestosterone and may be of significance in veterinary patients:

■ **CYCLOSPORINE:** Methyltestosterone may increase serum cyclosporine levels

■ **INSULIN; ORAL ANTIDIABETIC AGENTS:** Methyltestosterone may decrease serum glucose levels

■ **WARFARIN:** Methyltestosterone may increase anticoagulant effects

Laboratory Considerations

■ Methyltestosterone or other androgens can decrease **thyroxine-binding globulin** concentrations. This can cause decreased serum levels of **total T4** and increased resin uptake of T4 and T3. Clinically, this is unimportant, as free thyroid hormone concentrations are not affected.

Doses

■ **DOGS/CATS:**

a) Dogs: For Alopecia X when melatonin fails: 1 mg/kg to a maximum dose of 30 mg (total dose) PO once daily. Generally tolerated well, but can cause hepatotoxicity, aggressive behavior and/or seborrhea. Get baseline liver profile and then again one and two months after starting treatment. Stop after maximal hair regrowth is noted. (Rosychuk 2008)

b) Dogs: For treatment of testosterone-responsive dermatosis: 1 mg/kg PO every other day, to a maximum dose of 30 mg. Once dog responds, then every 4–7 days. (Nelson & Elliott 2003)

c) Dogs: To suppress estrus in Greyhounds: 5 mg (total dose) once weekly or divided, two times a week. (Eilts 2005)

d) Dogs: For estrus suppression: 25–50 mg (total dose) twice weekly PO. (Romagnoli 2003)

e) Dogs/Cats: For anti-estrogenic activity, development of male sexual characteristics (anatomical and behavioral), negative feedback on gonadotropin release from pituitary, and anabolic effects: 0.5 mg/kg PO once daily; dose may need to be adjusted, but should not exceed 1 mg/kg. (Label information; *Orandrone®*—Intervet UK. **Note:** This product has reportedly been withdrawn from the U.K. market.)

Monitoring

■ Hepatic function (liver enzymes, icterus, anorexia/weight loss/vomiting)

Client Information

■ Potential adverse effects include: liver toxicity, masculinization or vaginal discharge in females, prostate problems and aggression in males

■ Contact veterinarian if any of the following occur: changes in behavior, anorexia/weight loss/vomiting, or signs of icterus

Chemistry/Synonyms

Methyltestosterone occurs as white or creamy-white, odorless, crystals or crystalline powder. It is slightly hygroscopic, practically insoluble in water, freely soluble in alcohol, and sparingly soluble in vegetable oils.

Methyltestosterone may also be known as NSC-9701 or by its chemical name, 17beta-Hydroxy-17alpha-methyladrost-4-ene-3one, *Android®*, *Methitest®*, *Testred®* and *Virilon®*. A tradename for a veterinary product formerly available in the U.K. is *Orandrone®* (Intervet).

Storage/Stability

Unless otherwise specified by the manufacturer, methyltestosterone tablets or capsules should be stored below 40°C, preferably between 15°–30°C in well-closed containers.

Dosage Forms/Regulatory Status

VETERINARY-LABELED PRODUCTS: None

The ARCI (Racing Commissioners International) has designated this drug as a class 4 substance. See appendix for more information.

HUMAN-LABELED PRODUCTS:

Methyltestosterone Tablets: 10 mg & 25 mg; *Methitest®* (Global), generic; (Rx, C-III)

Methyltestosterone Buccal Tablets: 10 mg; generic; (Rx, C-III)

Methyltestosterone Capsules: 10 mg; *Testred®* & *Android®* (Valeant), *Virilon®* (Star); (Rx, C-III)

References

Eilts, B. (2005). Contraception and pregnancy termination in the dog and cat. *Textbook of Veterinary Internal Medicine 6th Ed.* S Ettinger and E Feldman Eds., Elsevier: 1669–1676.

Nelson, R. & D. Elliott (2003). Endocrine disorders. *Small Animal Internal Medicine, 3rd Ed.* R Nelson and C Couto Eds. St Louis, Mosby: 660–815.

Romagnoli, S. (2003). Control of the estrous cycle in the bitch and queen (including the use of progestins and GnRH agonists). Proceedings: WSAVA2003. Accessed via: Veterinary Information Network. http://goo.gl/rlMEm

Rosychuk, R. (2008). Canine Alopecias: What's New? Proceeedings: WVC. Accessed via: Veterinary Information Network. http://goo.gl/cIeWh

METOCLOPRAMIDE HCL

(met-oh-kloe-*pra*-mide)   Reglan®

GI PROKINETIC AGENT

Prescriber Highlights

▶ Stimulates upper GI motility & has antiemetic properties; more potent as an antiemetic (in dogs) than a prokinetic agent. May be a poor antiemetic in cats.

▶ Contraindications: GI hemorrhage, obstruction or perforation, hypersensitivity

▶ Relatively contraindicated: Seizure disorders, pheochromocytoma

▶ Adverse Effects: Dogs: Changes in mentation & behavior, constipation; Cats: Signs of frenzied behavior or disorientation, constipation; Horses: IV use, severe CNS effects, behavioral changes & abdominal pain; Foals: Adverse effects less common

Uses/Indications

Metoclopramide has been used in veterinary species for both its GI stimulatory and antiemetic properties. It has been used clinically for gastric stasis disorders, gastroesophageal reflux, to allow intubation of the small intestine, as a general antiemetic (for parvovirus, uremic gastritis, etc.), and an antiemetic to prevent or treat chemotherapy-induced vomiting.

Pharmacology/Actions

The primary pharmacologic effects of metoclopramide are associated with the GI tract and the CNS. In the GI tract, metoclopramide stimulates motility of the upper GI without stimulating gastric, pancreatic or biliary secretions. While the exact mechanisms for these actions are unknown, it appears that metoclopramide sensitizes upper GI smooth muscle to the effects of acetylcholine. Intact vagal innervation is not necessary for enhanced motility, but anticholinergic drugs will negate metoclopramide's effects. Gastrointestinal effects seen include increased tone and amplitude of gastric contractions, relaxed pyloric sphincter, and increased duodenal and jejunal peristalsis. Gastric emptying and intestinal transit times can be significantly reduced. There is little or no effect on colon motility. Additionally, metoclopramide will increase lower esophageal sphincter pressure and prevent or reduce gastroesophageal reflux. The above actions evidently give metoclopramide its local antiemetic effects.

Cats reportedly have few CNS dopamine receptors and therefore metoclopramide may be a poor antiemetic choice in that species (Twedt 2008).

In a study in horses comparing the effects of certain drugs (metoclopramide, cisapride, mosapride) on gastric emptying, and small intestinal and cecal motility, metoclopramide promoted jejunal motility, but did not significantly affect gastric emptying or cecal motility (Okamura *et al.* 2009).

In the CNS, metoclopramide apparently antagonizes dopamine at the receptor sites. This action can explain its sedative, central antiemetic (blocks dopamine in the chemo-receptor trigger zone), extrapyramidal, and prolactin secretion stimulation effects.

Pharmacokinetics

Metoclopramide is absorbed well after oral administration, but a significant first-pass effect in some human patients may reduce systemic bioavailability to 30%. There apparently is a great deal of interpatient variation with this effect. Bioavailability after intramuscular administration has been measured to be 74–96%. After oral dosing, peak plasma levels generally occur within 2 hours.

The drug is well distributed in the body and enters the CNS. Metoclopramide is only weakly bound to 13–22% of plasma proteins. The drug also crosses the placenta and enters the milk in concentrations approximately twice those of plasma.

Metoclopramide is primarily excreted in the urine in humans. Approximately 20–25% of the drug is excreted unchanged in the urine. The majority of the rest of the drug is metabolized to glucuronidated or sulfated conjugate forms and then excreted in the urine. Approximately 5% is excreted in the feces. The half-life of metoclopramide in the dog has been reported to be approximately 90 minutes.

Contraindications/Precautions/Warnings

Metoclopramide is contraindicated in patients with GI hemorrhage, obstruction or perforation, and in those hypersensitive to it. It is relatively (some say absolutely) contraindicated in patients with seizure disorders or head trauma. In patients with pheochromocytoma, metoclopramide may induce a hypertensive crisis. Several veterinary references state that metoclopramide is contraindicated with concurrent phenothiazine therapy (see Drug Interactions).

Metoclopramide should be avoided in dogs with pseudopregnancy as it can cause prolactin release (Romagnoli 2009).

Dosage adjustment may be required when used as a CRI in patients with renal failure. One reference suggests based upon anecdotal experience, reducing the CRI 25-50% of standard dosage (Trepanier, L. 2008).

Adverse Effects

In dogs, the most common (although infrequent) adverse reactions seen are changes in mentation and behavior (motor restlessness, involuntary spasms, aggression, and hyperactivity to drowsiness/depression). Cats may exhibit signs of frenzied behavior or disorientation. Both species can develop constipation while receiving this medication.

In adult horses, IV metoclopramide administration has been associated with the development of severe CNS effects. Alternating periods of sedation and excitement, behavioral changes and abdominal pain have been noted. These effects appear to be less common in foals.

Other adverse effects that have been reported in humans and are potentially plausible in animals include extrapyramidal effects, nausea, diarrhea, transient hypertension, and elevated prolactin levels.

Reproductive/Nursing Safety

In humans, the FDA categorizes this drug as category *B* for use during pregnancy (*Animal studies have not yet demonstrated risk to the fetus, but there are no adequate studies in pregnant women; or animal studies have shown an adverse effect, but adequate studies in pregnant women have not demonstrated a risk to the fetus in the first trimester of pregnancy, and there is no evidence of risk in later trimesters.*) In a separate system evaluating the safety of drugs in canine and feline pregnancy(Papich 1989), this drug is categorized as class: *B* (*Safe for use if used cautiously. Studies in laboratory animals may have uncovered some risk, but these drugs appear to be safe in dogs and cats or these drugs are safe if they are not administered when the animal is near term.*)

Metoclopramide is excreted into milk and may concentrate at about twice the plasma level, but there does not appear to be significant risk to nursing offspring.

Overdosage/Acute Toxicity

The oral LD_{50} doses of metoclopramide in mice, rats, and rabbits are 465 mg/kg, 760 mg/kg and 870 mg/kg, respectively. Because of the high dosages required for lethality, it is unlikely an oral overdose will cause death in a veterinary patient. Likely clinical signs of overdosage include sedation, ataxia, agitation, extrapyramidal effects, nausea, vomiting, and constipation.

There is no specific antidotal therapy for metoclopramide intoxication. If an oral ingestion was recent, the stomach should be emptied using standard protocols. Anticholinergic agents (diphenhydramine 2.2 mg/kg IV, benztropine, etc.) that enter the CNS may be helpful in controlling extrapyramidal effects. Peritoneal dialysis or hemodialysis is not thought to be effective in enhancing the removal of the drug.

Drug Interactions

The following drug interactions have either been reported or are theoretical in humans or animals receiving oral metoclopramide and may be of significance in veterinary patients:

■ **ASPIRIN, ACETAMINOPHEN, ALCOHOL:** In overdose situations in humans, metoclopramide has enhanced absorption of these agents

■ **ANESTHETICS:** If metoclopramide is used concurrently IV, acute hypotension has been reported

■ **ATROPINE (and related anticholinergic compounds):** May antagonize the GI motility effects of metoclopramide

■ **CEPHALEXIN:** In dogs, oral metoclopramide was shown to increase cephalexin peak plasma concentrations and area under the curve. No dosage adjustments are required. (Prados *et al.* 2007)

■ **CHOLINERGIC DRUGS (e.g., bethanechol):** May enhance metoclopramide's GI effects

■ **CNS DEPRESSANTS (e.g., anesthetic agents, antihistamines, phenothiazines, barbiturates, tranquilizers, alcohol, etc.):** Metoclopramide may enhance CNS depressant effects

■ **CYCLOSPORINE:** Metoclopramide increase the rate and extent of GI absorption

■ **OPIATE ANALGESICS:** May antagonize the GI motility effects of metoclopramide and enhance metoclopramide's CNS effects.

■ **MAO INHIBITORS (including amitraz and potentially, selegiline):** Could cause hypertension

■ **PHENOTHIAZINES (e.g., acepromazine, chlorpromazine, etc.) and BUTYROPHENONES (e.g., droperidol, azaperone):** May potentiate the extrapyramidal effects of metoclopramide.

■ **PROPOFOL:** In humans, metoclopramide reduces induction requirements of propofol by 20-25%.

■ **SSRI ANTIDEPRESSANTS (e.g., fluoxetine, sertraline, paroxetine):** Potential for enhanced extrapyramidal effects

■ **TETRACYCLINES:** Metoclopramide increase the rate and extent of GI absorption

Doses

■ **DOGS:**
  a) As an antiemetic: 0.1–0.4 mg/kg q6h PO, SC or IM; or 1–2 mg/kg/day as a continuous IV infusion (Washabau & Elie 1995)
  b) As an antiemetic: Best results are observed when given as a CRI at 0.01–0.02 mg/kg every hour or 1 to 2 mg/kg every 24 hours. (Twedt 2008)
  c) To treat vomiting associated with pancreatitis: 0.01–0.02 mg/kg/hr IV as a CRI or 0.1–0.5 mg/kg IM q8h (Waddell 2007)
  d) For vomiting disorders, gastroesophageal reflux, delayed gastric emptying, ileus, intestinal pseudo-obstruction: 0.2–0.5 mg/kg PO q8h PO or parenterally (may be given as a constant rate IV infusion at 0.01–0.02 mg/kg/hr) (Hall 2008)

  e) For adjunctive treatment of esophagitis: 0.2–0.4 mg/kg PO q8h. Metoclopramide has a limited effect on esophageal motility. (Glazer & Walters 2008)
  f) For post-operative ileus: 0.2–0.5 mg/kg PO or SC at least 30 minutes prior to a meal and at bedtime, or as an IV CRI of 0.01–0.02 mg/kg/hour. (Dowling 2007)
  g) As an antiemetic/prokinetic: 0.2–1 mg/kg PO, SC, IM 4 times a day, or as a CRI at 0.08–0.16 mg/kg/hour (2–4 mg/kg/day). For chemotherapy-induced vomiting, maropitant or drugs like ondansetron are more effective, but metoclopramide is much less expensive. If using metoclopramide, use high dosages (1mg/kg). (Richter 2009)
  h) To induce milk let-down for secondary agalactia: oxytocin 0.25–1 Unit (total dose) SC q2h. Neonates are removed for 30 minutes post-injection, and then encouraged to suckle, or gentle stripping of the glands performed. Metoclopramide at 0.1–0.2 mg/kg SC q12h (dopamine antagonist) can be used to promote milk production. Therapy is usually rewarding within 24 hours. (Davidson 2009)

To increase bladder contractility:
  a) 0.2–0.5 mg/kg PO q8h (Lane 2000)

■ **CATS:**
  a) As a prokinetic for adjunctive treatment of esophagitis: 0.2–0.4 mg/kg PO q8h. Cisapride considered superior. (Glazer & Walters 2008)
  b) 0.2–0.4 mg/kg PO, SC 3–4 times daily; or as a continuous IV infusion (1–2 mg/kg per day) (Trepanier, LA 1999)
  c) 0.2–0.5 mg/kg q8h PO or parenterally (may be given as a constant rate IV infusion at 0.01–0.02 mg/kg/hr) (Hall & Washabau 2000)
  d) To increase bladder contractility: 0.2–0.5 mg/kg PO q8h (Lane 2000)
  e) To induce milk let-down for secondary agalactia: oxytocin 0.25–1 Unit (total dose) SC q2h. Neonates are removed for 30 minutes post injection, and then encouraged to suckle, or gentle stripping of the glands performed. Metoclopramide at 0.1–0.2 mg/kg SC q12h (dopamine antagonist) can be used to promote milk production. Therapy is usually rewarding within 24 hours. (Davidson 2009)

■ **RABBITS, RODENTS, SMALL MAMMALS:**
  a) **Rabbits:** 0.2–1 mg/kg PO or SC q6–8h (Ivey & Morrisey 2000)
  b) **Rabbits:** To assist in removing gastric hairballs: 0.5 mg/kg PO once a day (up to three times a day) (Burke 1999)
  c) **Rabbits:** 0.5 mg/kg SC or PO q8-24h.

Useful pro-motile drug in rabbits with ileus. Do not administer in the presence of an obstruction. (Bryan 2009)

d) **Mice, Rats, Gerbils, Hamsters, Guinea pigs, Chinchillas:** 0.2–1 mg/kg PO, SC, IM q12h (Adamcak & Otten 2000)

■ **HORSES: (Note:** ARCI UCGFS Class 4 Drug) To stimulate the gastrointestinal tract:

a) 0.04 mg/kg/hr as a CRI (Lester 2004)

b) For reflux esophagitis: 0.02–0.1 mg/kg SC q4–12 hours; horses may be prone to the extrapyramidal neurologic side effects of metoclopramide. (Jones & Blikslager 2004)

Monitoring

■ Clinical efficacy
■ Adverse effects

Client Information

■ Contact veterinarian if animal develops clinical signs of involuntary movement of eyes, face, or limbs; or develops a rigid posture.

Chemistry/Synonyms

A derivative of para-aminobenzoic acid, metoclopramide HCl occurs as an odorless, white, crystalline powder with pK_as of 0.6 and 9.3. One gram is approximately soluble in 0.7 mL of water or 3 mL of alcohol. The injectable product has a pH of 3–6.5.

Metoclopramide HCl may also be known as: AHR-3070-C, DEL-1267, metoclopramidi hydrochloridum, and MK-745; many trade names are available.

Storage/Stability

Metoclopramide is photosensitive and must be stored in light resistant containers. All metoclopramide products should be stored at room temperature. Metoclopramide tablets should be kept in tight containers.

The injection is reportedly stable in solutions of a pH range of 2–9 and with the following IV solutions: D_5W, 0.9% sodium chloride, D_5-½ normal saline, Ringer's, and lactated Ringer's injection.

Compatibility/Compounding Considerations

The following drugs have been stated to be physically **compatible** with metoclopramide for at least 24 hours: aminophylline, ascorbic acid, atropine sulfate, benztropine mesylate, chlorpromazine HCl, cimetidine HCl, clindamycin phosphate, cyclophosphamide, cytarabine, dexamethasone sodium phosphate, dimenhydrinate, diphenhydramine HCl, doxorubicin HCl, droperidol, fentanyl citrate, heparin sodium, hydrocortisone sodium phosphate, hydroxyzine HCl, insulin (regular), lidocaine HCl, magnesium sulfate, mannitol, meperidine HCl, methylprednisolone sodium succinate, morphine sulfate, multivitamin infusion (MVI), pentazocine lactate, potassium acetate/chloride/

phosphate, prochlorperazine edisylate, TPN solution (25% dextrose with 4.25% *Travasol*® with or without electrolytes), verapamil, and vitamin B-complex with vitamin C.

Metoclopramide is reported to be physically **incompatible** when mixed with the following drugs: ampicillin sodium, calcium gluconate, cephalothin sodium, chloramphenicol sodium succinate, cisplatin, erythromycin lactobionate, methotrexate sodium, penicillin G potassium, sodium bicarbonate, and tetracycline. Compatibility is dependent upon factors such as pH, concentration, temperature, and diluent used; consult specialized references or a hospital pharmacist for more specific information.

Dosage Forms/Regulatory Status

VETERINARY-LABELED PRODUCTS: None

The ARCI (Racing Commissioners International) has designated this drug as a class 4 substance. See the appendix for more information.

HUMAN-LABELED PRODUCTS:

All doses expressed in terms of metoclopramide monohydrate.

Metoclopramide HCl Oral Tablets: 5 mg & 10 mg; Disintegrating Tablets: 5 mg & 10 mg; *Reglan*® (Alaven); *Metozolv*® (Salix); generic; (Rx)

Metoclopramide HCl Oral Syrup: 1 mg/mL in 480 mL and UD 10 mL; generic; (Rx)

Metoclopramide HCl Injection Solution: 5 mg/mL in 2 mL, 10 mL, 20 mL, & 30 mL vials; and 2 mL amps; preservative free in 2 mL, 10 mL & 30 mL vials; and 2 mL & 10 mL amps; *Reglan*® (Wyeth-Ayerst); generic; (Rx)

References

Adamcak, A. & B. Otten (2000). Rodent Therapeutics. *Vet Clin NA: Exotic Anim Pract* **3:1**(Jan): 221–240.

Bryan, J. (2009). Rabbit GI Physiology: What do I do now? Proceedings: WVC. Accessed via: Veterinary Information Network. http://goo.gl/cAD9L

Burke, T. (1999). Husbandry and Medicine of Rodents and Lagomorphs. Proceedings: Central Veterinary Conference, Kansas City.

Davidson, A. (2009). Postpartum disorders in the bitch and queen. Proceedings: WVC. Accessed via: Veterinary Information Network. http://goo.gl/Z6o5F

Dowling, P. (2007). Therapy of Gastrointestinal (GI) Motility Disorders. Proceedings: AAFP. Accessed via: Veterinary Information Network. http://goo.gl/PHTRM

Glazer, A. & P. Walters (2008). Esophagitis and esophageal strictures. *Comp CE*(May): 281–292.

Hall, J. (2008). Gastric Motility Disorders & Prokinetic Therapies in Small Animals. Proceedings: ACVIM. Accessed via: Veterinary Information Network. http://goo.gl/4D9L

Hall, J. & R. Washabau (2000). Gastric Prokinetic Agents. *Kirk's Current Veterinary Therapy: XIII Small Animal Practice*. J Bonagura Ed. Philadelphia, WB Saunders: 609–617.

Ivey, E. & J. Morrisey (2000). Therapeutics for Rabbits. *Vet Clin NA: Exotic Anim Pract* **3:1**(Jan): 183–216.

Jones, S. & A. Blikslager (2004). Esophageal diseases. *Equine Internal Medicine, 2nd Ed.* S Reed, W Bayly and D Sellon Eds. Philadelphia, Saunders: 855–863.

Lane, I. (2000). Urinary Obstruction and Functional Urine Retention. *Textbook of Veterinary Internal Medicine: Diseases of the Dog and Cat.* S Ettinger and E Feldman Eds. Philadelphia, WB Saunders. 1: 93–96.

Lester, G. (2004). Gastrointestinal ileus. *Equine Internal Medicine, 2nd Ed.* S Reed, W Bayly and D Sellon Eds. Philadelphia, Saunders: 815–821.

Okamura, K., N. Sasaki, et al. (2009). Effects of mosapride citrate, metoclopramide hydrochloride, lidocaine hydrochloride, and cisapride citrate on equine gastric emptying, small intestinal and caecal motility. *Research in Veterinary Science* 86(2): 302–308.

Papich, M. (1989). Effects of drugs on pregnancy. *Current Veterinary Therapy X: Small Animal Practice.* R Kirk Ed. Philadelphia, Saunders: 1291–1299.

Prados, A.P., V. Kreil, et al. (2007). Metoclopramide modifies oral cephalexin pharmacokinetics in dogs. *Journal of Veterinary Pharmacology and Therapeutics* 30(2): 127–131.

Richter, K. (2009). Acute Vomiting: A Systemic Approach. Proceedings: ACVIM. Accessed via: Veterinary Information Network. http://goo.gl/VYeZ1

Romagnoli, S. (2009). An update on pseudopregnancy. Proceedings: WSAVA. Accessed via: Veterinary Information Network. http://goo.gl/1CpI2

Trepanier, L. (1999). Fifteen Drugs Useful in Cats. American Animal Hospital Association: Proceedings from the 1999 Annual Meeting, Denver.

Trepanier, L. (2008). Case presentations: Drug dose adjustments. Proceedings: ACVIM. Accessed via: Veterinary Information Network. http://goo.gl/nRhTT

Twedt, D. (2008). Antiemetics, prokinetics & antacids. Proceedings: ACVIM. Accessed via: Veterinary Information Network. http://goo.gl/bRKsO

Waddell, L. (2007). Diagnosis and management of acute pancreatitis. Proceedings: Western Vet Conference. Accessed via: Veterinary Information Network. http://goo.gl/24TqH

Washabau, R. & M. Elie (1995). Antiemetic therapy. *Kirk's Current Veterinary Therapy:XII.* J Bonagura Ed. Philadelphia, W.B. Saunders: 679–684.

METOPROLOL TARTRATE
METOPROLOL SUCCINATE

(me-*toe*-pro-lole)   Lopressor®, Toprol XL®

BETA-ADRENERGIC BLOCKER

Prescriber Highlights

▶ Beta$_1$-blocker used for supraventricular tachyarrhythmias, premature ventricular contractions (PVC's, VPC's), systemic hypertension, & treatment in cats with hypertrophic cardiomyopathy

▶ Probably safer to use than propranolol in animals with bronchoconstrictive disease

▶ Contraindications: Overt or unstable heart failure, hypersensitivity beta-blockers, greater than first-degree heart block, or sinus bradycardia

▶ Caution: Significant hepatic insufficiency, bronchospastic lung disease, CHF, hyperthyroidism (masks clinical signs, but may be useful for treatment), labile diabetics, & sinus node dysfunction

▶ Adverse Effects: Most common in geriatric animals or those that have acute decompensating heart disease, include: bradycardia, lethargy & depression, impaired AV conduction, CHF or worsening of heart failure, hypotension, hypoglycemia, bronchoconstriction, syncope, & diarrhea

▶ Try to wean off drug gradually

Uses/Indications

Because metoprolol is relatively safe to use in animals with bronchospastic disease, it is often chosen over propranolol. It may be effective in supraventricular tachyarrhythmias, premature ventricular contractions (PVC's, VPC's), systemic hypertension, and treating cats with hypertrophic cardiomyopathy. There is increasing interest in using beta blockers in heart failure in dogs; one retrospective study showed increased survival times when dogs were given metoprolol, but definitive prospective, double-blinded studies have not been reported documenting the benefit (increased survival) of beta-blockers in dogs with heart failure.

Pharmacology/Actions

Metoprolol is a relatively specific beta$_1$-blocker and is sometimes characterized as a second generation beta blocker. At higher dosages, this specificity may be lost and beta$_2$ blockade can occur. Metoprolol does not possess any intrinsic sympathomimetic activity like pindolol nor does it possess membrane-stabilizing activity like pindolol or propranolol. Cardiovascular effects secondary to metoprolol's negative inotropic and chronotropic actions include: decreased sinus heart rate, slowed AV conduction, diminished cardiac output at rest and during exercise, decreased myocardial oxygen demand, reduced blood pressure, and inhibition of isoproterenol-induced tachycardia.

Pharmacokinetics

Metoprolol tartrate is rapidly and nearly completely absorbed from the GI tract, but it has a relatively high first pass effect (50%) so systemic bioavailability is reduced. The drug has very low protein binding characteristics (5–15%) and is distributed well into most tissues. Metoprolol crosses the blood-brain barrier and CSF levels are about 78% of those found in the serum. It crosses the placenta and levels in milk are higher (3-4X) than those found in plasma. Metoprolol is primarily biotransformed in the liver; unchanged drug and metabolites are then principally excreted in the urine. Reported half-lives in various species: Dogs: 1.6 hours; Cats: 1.3 hours; Humans 3–4 hours.

Contraindications/Precautions/Warnings

Metoprolol is contraindicated in patients with overt or unstable heart failure, hypersensitivity to this class of agents, greater than first-degree heart block, or sinus bradycardia. Non-specific beta-blockers are generally contraindicated in patients with CHF unless secondary to a tachyarrhythmia responsive to beta-blocker therapy. They are also relatively contraindicated in patients with bronchospastic lung disease.

Metoprolol should be used cautiously in patients with significant hepatic insufficiency or sinus node dysfunction.

Metoprolol (at high dosages) can mask the clinical signs associated with hypoglycemia. It can also cause hypoglycemia or hyperglycemia and, therefore, should be used cautiously in labile diabetic patients.

Metoprolol can mask the clinical signs associated with thyrotoxicosis, but it may be used clinically to treat the clinical signs associated with this condition.

Adverse Effects

It is reported that adverse effects most commonly occur in geriatric animals or those that have acute decompensating heart disease. Adverse effects considered clinically relevant include: bradycardia, lethargy, weakness and depression, impaired AV conduction, CHF or worsening of heart failure, hypotension, hypoglycemia, and bronchoconstriction (less so with $beta_1$ specific drugs like metoprolol). Syncope and diarrhea have also been reported in canine patients with beta-blockers.

Exacerbation of clinical signs has been reported following abrupt cessation of beta-blockers in humans. It is recommended to withdraw therapy gradually in patients who have been receiving the drug chronically.

Reproductive/Nursing Safety

Safe use during pregnancy has not been established, but adverse effects to fetuses have apparently not been documented. In humans, the FDA categorizes this drug as category *C* for use during pregnancy (*Animal studies have shown an adverse effect on the fetus, but there are no adequate studies in humans; or there are no animal reproduction studies and no adequate studies in humans.*)

Metoprolol is excreted in milk in very small quantities and is unlikely to pose significant risk to nursing offspring.

Overdosage/Acute Toxicity

There is limited information available on metoprolol overdosage. Humans have apparently survived dosages of up to 5 grams. The most predominant clinical signs expected would be extensions of the drug's pharmacologic effects: hypotension, bradycardia, bronchospasm, cardiac failure, and, potentially, hypoglycemia.

There were 8 exposures to metoprolol reported to the ASPCA Animal Poison Control Center (APCC) during 2005–2006. In these cases 7 were dogs with 1 showing clinical signs and the remaining case was a cat that showed no clinical signs. Common findings in dogs recorded in decreasing frequency included lethargy and tachycardia.

If overdose is secondary to a recent oral ingestion, emptying the gut and charcoal administration may be considered. Use caution inducing emesis as coma and seizures may develop rapidly. Monitor: ECG; blood glucose, potassium, and, blood pressure. Treatment of the cardiovascular effects is symptomatic. Use fluids and pressor agents to treat hypotension. Bradycardia may be treated with atropine. If atropine fails, isoproterenol, given cautiously, has been recommended. Use of a transvenous pacemaker may be necessary. Cardiac failure can be treated with a digitalis glycosides, diuretics, and oxygen. Glucagon (5–10 mg IV—Human dose) may increase heart rate and blood pressure and reduce the cardiodepressant effects of metoprolol.

Drug Interactions

The following drug interactions have either been reported or are theoretical in humans or animals receiving metoprolol and may be of significance in veterinary patients:

■ **ANESTHETICS, GENERAL (with myocardial depressant effects):** Increased risk for heart failure and hypotension

■ **CALCIUM-CHANNEL BLOCKERS (e.g., diltiazem, verapamil, amlodipine):** Concurrent use of beta-blockers with calcium channel blockers (or other negative inotropics) should be done with caution, particularly in patients with preexisting cardiomyopathy or CHF

■ **DIGOXIN:** Use with metoprolol may increase negative effects on SA or AV node conduction

■ **DIURETICS (thiazides, furosemide):** May increase hypotensive effect of metoprolol

■ **HYDRALAZINE:** May increase the risks for pulmonary hypertension in uremic patients

■ **QUINIDINE:** May increase metoprolol plasma concentrations

■ **RESERPINE:** Potential for additive effects (hypotension, bradycardia)

■ **SSRI ANTIDEPRESSANTS (e.g., fluoxetine, sertraline, paroxetine):** May increase metoprolol plasma concentrations

■ **SYMPATHOMIMETICS (metaproterenol, terbutaline, beta-effects of epinephrine, phenylpropanolamine, etc.):** May have their actions blocked by metoprolol and they may, in turn, reduce the efficacy of atenolol

Doses

■ **DOGS:**

As an oral beta blocker:

a) For rate control in chronic atrial fibrillation: 0.25–1 mg/kg PO q12-24h. (Saunders *et al.* 2009)

b) For CHF: The role of beta-blocker therapy in dogs with congestive heart failure is unclear. Beta-blockers are best employed in animals that are minimally symptomatic with early/mild heart failure, or in animals in later stages of CHF that are already well controlled on a stable cardiac drug regimen. Metoprolol has been used at 0.2 mg/kg PO twice daily, with slow titration upwards every 2–3 weeks up to 0.4–6.6 mg/kg PO three times a day. Many dogs will not tolerate this upward titration. (Rush 2008)

c) To decrease the incidence atrial fibrillation and flutter in dogs undergoing valve surgery: Using sustained release metoprolol (*Toprol-XR®*) at 0.4–1 mg/kg PO q24h administered before and as soon as feasible after surgery. (Orton 2006)

■ **CATS:**

As an oral beta blocker:

a) 2–15 mg (total dose) PO q8h (Brovida 2002)

Monitoring

■ Cardiac function, pulse rate, ECG if necessary, BP if indicated

■ Toxicity (see Adverse Effects/Overdosage)

Client Information

■ To be effective, the animal must receive all doses as prescribed

■ Notify veterinarian if animal becomes lethargic or exercise intolerant, has shortness of breath or cough, or develops a change in behavior or attitude

Chemistry/Synonyms

A beta$_1$ specific adrenergic blocker, metoprolol tartrate occurs as a white, crystalline powder having a bitter taste. It is very soluble in water. Metoprolol succinate occurs as a white, crystalline powder and is freely soluble in water.

Metoprolol may also be known as: CGP-2175E; H-93/26, and metoprolol; many trade names are available.

Storage/Stability

Store all products protected from light. Store tablets in tight, light-resistant containers at room temperature. Avoid freezing the injection.

Compatibility/Compounding Considerations

The injection is **compatible** with D5W and normal saline, and at Y-sites with morphine sulfate.

Compounded preparation stability: Metoprolol oral suspension compounded from the commercially available tablets has been published (Allen & Erickson 1996). Triturating twelve (12) metoprolol tartrate 100 mg tablets with 60 mL of *Ora-Plus®* and *qs ad* to 120 mL with *Ora-Sweet®* or *Ora-Sweet SF®* yields a 10 mg/mL metoprolol tartrate oral suspension that retains >95% potency for 60 days when stored at both 4°C and 25°C and protected from light.

Dosage Forms/Regulatory Status

VETERINARY-LABELED PRODUCTS: None

The ARCI (Racing Commissioners International) has designated this drug as a class 3 substance. See the appendix for more information.

HUMAN-LABELED PRODUCTS:

Metoprolol Tartrate Oral Tablets: 25 mg, 50 mg & 100 mg; *Lopressor®* (Novartis); generic; (Rx)

Metoprolol Succinate Extended-Release Tablets: 25 mg, 50 mg, 100 mg & 200 mg; *Toprol XL®* (AstraZeneca); generic; (Rx)

Metoprolol Tartrate Injection: 1 mg/mL in 5 mL amps and *Carpuject* sterile cartridge units; *Lopressor®* (Novartis); generic; (Rx)

References

Allen, L.V. & M.A. Erickson (1996). Stability of labetalol hydrochloride, metoprolol tartrate, verapamil hydrochloride, and spironolactone with hydrochlorothiazide in extemporaneously compounded oral liquids. *Am J Health Syst Pharm* 53(19): 2304–2309.

Brovida, C. (2002). Hypertension in renal diseases and failure. The practical aspect. Proceedings: World Small Animal Association. Accessed via: Veterinary Information Network. http://goo.gl/5iMw3

Orton, E. (2006). Supportive care after cardiac surgery. Proceedings: IVECCS. Accessed via: Veterinary Information Network. http://goo.gl/lwYUE

Rush, J. (2008). Heart failure in dogs and cats. Proceedings: IVECCS. Accessed via: Veterinary Information Network. http://goo.gl/cFKka

Saunders, A., S. Gordon, et al. (2009). Canine Atrial Fibrillation. *Comp CE*(November): E1–E!).

METRONIDAZOLE
METRONIDAZOLE
BENZOATE

(me-troe-*ni*-da-zole)   Flagyl®

ANTIBIOTIC, ANTIPARASITIC

Prescriber Highlights

▶ Injectable & oral antibacterial (anaerobes) & antiprotozoal agent

▶ Prohibited by the FDA for use in food animals

▶ Contraindications: Hypersensitivity to it or nitroimidazole derivatives. Extreme caution: in severely debilitated, pregnant or nursing animals; hepatic dysfunction.

▶ Adverse Effects: Neurologic disorders, lethargy, weakness, neutropenias, hepatotoxicity, hematuria, anorexia, nausea, vomiting, & diarrhea

▶ May be a teratogen, especially in early pregnancy

Uses/Indications

Although there are no veterinary-approved metronidazole products, the drug has been used extensively in the treatment of Giardia in both dogs and cats. It is also used clinically in small animals for the treatment of other parasites (Trichomonas and *Balantidium coli*) as well as treating both enteric and systemic anaerobic infections.

In horses, metronidazole has been used clinically for the treatment of anaerobic infections.

Pharmacology/Actions

Metronidazole is a concentration-dependent bactericidal agent against susceptible bacteria. Its exact mechanism of action is not completely understood, but it is taken-up by anaerobic organisms where it is reduced to an unidentified polar compound. It is believed that this compound is responsible for the drug's antimicrobial activity by disrupting DNA and nucleic acid synthesis in the bacteria.

Metronidazole has activity against most obligate anaerobes including *Bacteroides* spp. (including *B. fragilis*), Fusobacterium, Veillonella, *Clostridium* spp., Peptococcus, and Peptostreptococcus. Actinomyces is frequently resistant to metronidazole.

Metronidazole is also trichomonacidal and amebicidal in action and acts as a direct amebicide. Its mechanism of action for its antiprotozoal activity is not understood. It has therapeutic activity against *Entamoeba histolytica*, Trichomonas, Giardia, and *Balantidium coli*. It acts primarily against the trophozoite forms of Entamoeba rather than encysted forms.

Finally, metronidazole has some inhibitive actions on cell-mediated immunity.

Pharmacokinetics

Metronidazole is relatively well absorbed after oral administration. Metronidazole is rather lipophilic and is rapidly and widely distributed after absorption. It is distributed to most body tissues and fluids, including bone, abscesses, the CNS, and seminal fluid. It is less than 20% bound to plasma proteins in humans. Metronidazole is primarily metabolized in the liver via several pathways. Both the metabolites and unchanged drug are eliminated in the urine and feces.

The oral bioavailability in dogs is high, but interpatient variable, with ranges from 50–100% reported. If given with food, absorption is enhanced in dogs, but delayed in humans. Peak levels occur about one hour after oral dosing.

In a single-dose study in cats (Sekis *et al.* 2009), the oral bioavailability of metronidazole benzoate is variable, but averages around 65%. Peak levels after oral dosing appear to be highly variable in cats (ranging from 1–8 hours) and peak serum concentrations are somewhat lower in cats than in dogs or humans. Mean systemic clearance is slower in cats than dogs (2.49 mL/kg/min vs. 1.53 mL/kg/min). Despite the concern that glucuronidation is a metabolic pathway for metronidazole, terminal elimination half-life is only slightly (not significantly) longer (5-6 hours) in cats.

The oral bioavailability of the drug in horses averages about 80% (range 57–100%). If administered rectally to horses, bioavailability is decreased by about 50%. Elimination half-life in the horse is about 2.9-4.3 hours.

Contraindications/Precautions/Warnings

Metronidazole is prohibited for use in food animals by the FDA.

Metronidazole is contraindicated in animals hypersensitive to the drug or nitroimidazole derivatives. It has been recommended not to use the drug in severely debilitated, pregnant or nursing animals. Metronidazole should be used with caution in animals with hepatic dysfunction. If the drug must be used in animals with significant liver impairment, consider using only 25–50% of the usual dose.

Because of the risk for neurotoxicity in dogs, total daily doses of metronidazole should not exceed 65 mg/kg per day (Tams 2007).

Adverse Effects

Adverse effects reported in dogs include neurologic disorders, lethargy, weakness, neutropenias, hepatotoxicity, hematuria, anorexia, nausea, vomiting, and diarrhea. Neurologic toxicity in dogs may be manifested after acute high dosages or, more likely, with chronic moderate to high-dose therapy. Clinical signs reported are described below in the Overdosage section.

In cats, vomiting, inappetence, hepatotoxicity and rarely, central nervous toxicity can occur with metronidazole therapy (Scorza & Lappin 2004). Genotoxicity was detected in peripheral blood mononuclear cells collected from cats after 7 days of oral metronidazole, but resolved within 6 days of discontinuing the drug. Clinical significance, particularly with chronic therapy, is yet to be determined. (Sekis *et al.* 2009)

In horses, metronidazole may occasionally cause anorexia, ataxia and depression, particularly when used at higher dosages. There have been reported cases of *C. difficile* and *C. perfringens* diarrhea and death after use of metronidazole.

Metronidazole tablets have a sharp, metallic taste that animals find unpleasant. Placing in capsules or using compounded oral suspensions may alleviate the problem of dosing avoidance.

Reproductive/Nursing Safety

Metronidazole's potential for teratogenicity is somewhat controversial; some references state that it has been teratogenic in some laboratory animal studies, but others state that it has not. However, unless the benefits to the mother outweigh the risks to the fetus(es), it should not be used during pregnancy, particularly during the first 3 weeks of gestation. In humans, the FDA categorizes this drug as category *B* for use during pregnancy (*Animal studies have not yet demonstrated risk to the fetus, but there are no adequate studies in pregnant women; or animal studies have shown an adverse effect, but adequate studies in pregnant women have not demonstrated a risk to the fetus in the first trimester of pregnancy, and there is no evidence of risk in later trimesters.*) In a separate system evaluating the safety of drugs in canine and feline pregnancy (Papich 1989), this drug is categorized as class: *C* (*These drugs may have potential risks. Studies in people or laboratory animals have uncovered risks, and these drugs should be used cautiously as a last resort when the benefit of therapy clearly outweighs the risks.*)

Because of the potential for tumorigenicity, consider using alternative therapy or switching to milk replacer for nursing patients.

Overdosage/Acute Toxicity

Signs of intoxication associated with metronidazole in dogs and cats, include anorexia and/or vomiting, depression, mydriasis, nystagmus, ataxia, head-tilt, deficits of proprioception, joint knuckling, disorientation, tremors, seizures, bradycardia, rigidity and stiffness. These effects may be seen with acute overdoses, doses in dogs above 60 mg/kg per day, or in some animals on chronic therapy when using "recommended" doses (*e.g.*, 30 mg/kg/day).

In dogs, common signs of metronidazole toxicity include generalized ataxia with a very rapid positional nystagmus. Most often, dogs have neurological deficits localized to the central vestibular system and/or cerebellum. Dogs with mild to moderate clinical signs usually improve rapidly within 1-2 days, once metronidazole has been discontinued. (Vernau 2009).

Diazepam has been used successfully to decrease the CNS effects associated with metronidazole toxicity, but has not been evaluated in a controlled manner. See the Diazepam monograph or the reference by Evans, Levesque, et al for more information (Evans *et al.* 2002).

Acute overdoses should be handled by attempting to limit the absorption of the drug using standard protocols. Extreme caution should be used before attempting to induce vomiting in patients demonstrating CNS effects or aspiration may result. If acute toxicity is seen after chronic therapy, the drug should be discontinued and the patient treated supportively and symptomatically. Neurologic clinical signs may require several days before showing signs of resolving.

Drug Interactions

The following drug interactions have either been reported or are theoretical in humans or animals receiving metronidazole and may be of significance in veterinary patients:

- ■ **ALCOHOL:** May induce a disulfiram-like (nausea, vomiting, cramps, etc.) reaction when given with metronidazole.

- ■ **CIMETIDINE:** May decrease the metabolism of metronidazole and increase the likelihood of dose-related side effects.

- ■ **PHENOBARBITAL or PHENYTOIN:** May increase the metabolism of metronidazole, thereby decreasing blood levels.

- ■ **WARFARIN:** Metronidazole may prolong the PT in patients receiving warfarin or other coumarin anticoagulants. Avoid concurrent use if possible; otherwise, intensify monitoring.

Laboratory Considerations

- ■ Metronidazole can cause falsely decreased readings of **AST** (SGOT) and **ALT** (SGPT) when determined using methods measuring decreases in ultraviolet absorbance when NADH is reduced to NAD.

Doses

- ■ **DOGS:**

    Note: Doses are for metronidazole base unless otherwise noted. If using metronidazole benzoate adjust dosages unless provided by pharmacy as "mg/mL of the base". 1 mg of metronidazole base = 1.6 mg of metronidazole benzoate.

    For treatment of Giardia:

    a) 15–25 mg/kg PO q12–24h daily for 5–7 days (Lappin 2006)

    b) 22 mg/kg PO twice daily for 5 days. May be combined with fenbendazole (50 mg/kg PO once daily for 3 or 5 days) to relieve clinical signs and eliminate parasites. (Payne & Artzer 2009)

For other protozoal infections:

a) *Entamoeba histolytica* or *Pentatrichomas hominis*: 25 mg/kg PO q12h for 8 days (Lappin 2000)

For anaerobic infections:

a) For sepsis: 15 mg/kg IV q12h (Hardie 2000)

For eliminating Helicobacter gastritis infections:

a) Using triple therapy: Metronidazole 15.4 mg/kg q8h, amoxicillin 11 mg/kg q8h and bismuth subsalicylate (original *Pepto-Bismol®*) 0.22 mL/kg PO q4–6h. Give each for 3 weeks. (Hall 2000)

For adjunctive therapy of plasmacytic/lymphocytic enteritis:

a) 10–30 mg/kg PO q8–24h for 2–4 weeks in refractory cases (Leib, M.S. *et al.* 1989)

For *Clostridium perfringens* enterotoxicosis:

a) 10–20 mg/kg PO twice daily for 7–28 days. (Tams 2007)

For inflammatory bowel disease:

a) 10–20 mg/kg PO two to three times a day has been used in the treatment of mild to moderate cases of large bowel IBD. (Washabau 2009)

b) For ulcerative colitis in dogs refractory to other therapies (*e.g.*, sulfasalazine, immunosuppressants, diet, etc.): 10–20 mg/kg PO twice daily–three times a day; may be beneficial in treating for 2–4 weeks those dogs with chronic colitis having unexplained diarrhea (Leib, M. 2000).

c) 10–15 mg/kg PO q8–12h; combine with prednisone to manage moderate to severe cases. (Marks 2007)

d) In cases of predominantly large bowel diarrhea (colitis with typical clinical presentation) if parasiticide treatment and elimination diet fail, a therapeutic trial can be made: metronidazole 20–25 mg/kg PO twice daily for 5-10 days with the addition of fiber to the diet (*e.g.*, psyllium at 0.5 tablespoon for toy breeds, 1 tablespoon for small dogs, 2 tablespoons for medium dogs, and 3 tablespoons for large dogs. However, sampling of mucosal biopsies prior to further treatment may be the best course of action. (Gaschen 2008)

For treatment of medial canthus syndrome (tear staining):

a) 100–200 mg (total dose) PO once per day for 10 days each month. (Krohne 2008)

■ **CATS:**
Note: Doses are for metronidazole base unless otherwise noted. If using metronidazole benzoate adjust dosages unless provided by pharmacy as "mg/mL of the base". 1 mg of

metronidazole base = 1.6 mg of metronidazole benzoate.

For treatment of Giardia:

a) 15–25 mg/kg PO q12–24h daily for 5–7 days (Lappin 2006)

b) 25 mg/kg PO q12h for 7 days (Zoran 2007)

c) 22 mg/kg PO twice daily for 5 days. May be combined with fenbendazole (50 mg/kg PO once daily for 3 or 5 days) to relieve clinical signs and eliminate parasites. (Payne, 2009)

For other protozoal infections:

a) *Entamoeba histolytica* or *Pentatrichomas hominis*: 25 mg/kg PO q12h for 8 days (Lappin, 2000)

For treating *H. pylori*:

a) Metronidazole 10–15 mg/kg PO two times a day; clarithromycin 7.5 mg/kg PO two times a day; amoxicillin 20 mg/kg PO twice daily for 14 days (Simpson 2003)

For anaerobic infections:

a) For sepsis: 15 mg/kg IV q12h (Hall 2000)

For adjunctive therapy of GI conditions:

a) 10–20 mg/kg PO two to three times a day has been used in the treatment of mild to moderate cases of large bowel IBD. (Washabau 2009)

b) For inflammatory bowel disease: With a change of diet to "hypoallergenic", may give metronidazole at 62.5 mg (total dose) PO per cat once daily for 10–20 days. Resistant cats or those with severe disease are given immunosuppressive doses of prednisolone (1–2 mg/kg initially twice daily). (Gaschen 2006)

c) 10–15 mg/kg PO q8–12h; combine with prednisone to manage moderate to severe cases. (Marks 2007)

d) For hepatic encephalopathy: 7.5 mg/kg PO q8–12h (Cornelius *et al.* 2000)

■ **FERRETS:**
Note: Doses are for metronidazole base unless otherwise noted. If using metronidazole benzoate adjust dosages unless provided by pharmacy as "mg/mL of the base". 1 mg of metronidazole base = 1.6 mg of metronidazole benzoate.

For eliminating *Helicobacter mustelae* gastritis infections:

a) Using triple therapy: Metronidazole 22 mg/kg, amoxicillin 22 mg/kg and bismuth subsalicylate (original *Pepto-Bismol®*) 17.6 mg/kg PO. Give each 3 times daily for 3–4 weeks. (Hall 2000)

b) Amoxicillin 30 mg/kg PO q8h, metronidazole 20 mg/kg PO q8h, & bismuth subsalicylate 7.5 mg/kg PO q8h. All are given for 21-28 days. (Johnson-Delaney 2008)

For susceptible infections:

a) 10–30 mg/kg PO once to twice daily. Very bitter; mask flavor. (Williams 2000)

For inflammatory bowel disease:

a) 50 mg/kg PO once daily. (Johnson-Delaney 2008)

■ **RABBITS, RODENTS, SMALL MAMMALS:**

Note: Doses are for metronidazole base unless otherwise noted. If using metronidazole benzoate adjust dosages unless provided by pharmacy as "mg/mL of the base". 1 mg of metronidazole base = 1.6 mg of metronidazole benzoate.

a) **Rabbits:** For anaerobic infections: 20 mg/kg PO q12h for 3–5 days or 40 mg/kg PO once daily; 5 mg/kg slow IV q12h (Ivey & Morrisey 2000)

b) **Chinchillas:** 10–40 mg/kg PO once daily as an antimicrobial; 50–60 mg/kg PO twice daily for 5 days as an antiparasiticide (Giardia) (Hayes 2000)

c) **Chinchillas, Gerbils, Guinea Pigs, Hamsters, Mice, Rats:** 20–60 mg/kg PO q8–12h. Mice: 3.5 mg/mL in water for 5 days. Rats: 10–40 mg per rat PO once daily. Chinchillas, Guinea pigs: 10–40 mg/kg PO once daily. Gerbils, Hamsters: 7.5 mg/70–90 grams of body weight PO q8h. Add sucrose to improve palatability. (Adamcak & Otten 2000)

■ **HORSES:**

For susceptible anaerobic infections:

a) 20–25 mg/kg PO q8–12h; for treatment of colitis due to *Clostridium* spp., may dose at 15 mg/kg PO q8h. Can also dose at same dosages rectally if unable to dose PO. Metronidazole is uncommonly associated with diarrhea and neurologic side effects. (Bentz 2007)

b) For metritis secondary to *B. fragilis*: 15–25 mg/kg PO q12h. (LeBlanc 2009)

c) Foals: Oral metronidazole therapy should be strongly considered for all foals with severe diarrhea as about 35% of foals tested are positive for toxins associated with clostridia. Oral metronidazole is typically administered at 15–25 mg/kg PO q8h, but doses of 25 mg/kg q12h have recently also been recommended. May also give IV; authors use a loading dose of 15 mg/kg, and then give 7.5 mg/kg q6h based on the human dose recommendation. (Corley & Hollis 2009)

d) Foals with *C. perfringens*: 10–15 mg/kg PO 3–4 times a day (dose depends on severity); if animal has an ileus and is intolerant of oral feeding give IV at 10 mg/kg IV 4 times a day (Slovis 2003)

e) For *L. intracellularis* infections: metronidazole 10–15 mg/kg PO q8–12h with either oxytetracycline (10–18 mg/kg

via slow IV q24h) or chloramphenicol (44 mg/kg PO q6–8h). (Frazer 2007)

■ **BIRDS:**

For susceptible infections (anaerobes; giardia):

a) 10–50 mg/kg PO q12h. (Oglesbee 2009)

b) Ratites (not to be used for food): 20–25 mg/kg PO twice daily (Jenson 1998)

■ **REPTILES/AMPHIBIANS:**

a) For anaerobic infections in most reptile species: 150 mg/kg PO once; repeat in one week

For amoebae and flagellates in most species: 100–275 mg/kg PO once; repeat in 1–2 weeks.

In *Drymarchon* spp., *Lampropeltis pyromelana*, and *L. zonata*: 40 mg/kg PO once; repeat in 2 weeks (Gauvin 1993)

b) In reptiles and amphibians treatment for amoebae, flagellates and ciliates is typically with metronidazole 100 mg/kg PO repeated in 2 weeks; or 50 mg/kg PO once daily for 3-5 days; repeat prn. As is the case with all medications used in reptiles and amphibians, each animal has to be treated on a case-by-case basis for all medications; in the literature there are several different doses as well as treatment schedules listed. (de la Navarre 2003)

Monitoring

■ Clinical efficacy

■ Adverse effects (clients should report any neurologic signs)

Client Information

■ Report any neurologic clinical signs to veterinarian (see Overdose section).

Chemistry/Synonyms

A synthetic, nitroimidazole antibacterial and antiprotozoal agent, metronidazole occurs as white to pale yellow crystalline powder or crystals with a pK_a of 2.6. It is sparingly soluble in water or alcohol. Metronidazole base is commercially available as tablets or solution for IV injection and metronidazole HCl is available as injectable powder for reconstitution. The hydrochloride is very soluble in water.

Metronidazole benzoate is the benzoic ester of metronidazole. It occurs as a white to slightly yellow, crystalline powder that is practically insoluble in water, slightly soluble in alcohol, and soluble in acetone. As it is less soluble in aqueous solutions than is the base, it does not taste as bad.

Metronidazole may also be known as: Bayer-5360, metronidazolum, SC-32642, NSC-50364, RP-8823, and SC-10295; many trade names are available.

Storage/Stability

Metronidazole tablets and HCl powder for injection should be stored at temperatures less than 30°C and protected from light. The injection should be protected from light and freezing and stored at room temperature.

Specific recommendations on the reconstitution, dilution, and neutralization of metronidazole HCl powder for injection are detailed in the package insert of the drug and should be referred to if this product is used. Do not use aluminum hub needles to reconstitute or transfer this drug as a reddish-brown discoloration may result in the solution.

Compatibility/Compounding Considerations

The following drugs and solutions are reportedly physically **compatible** with metronidazole ready-to-use solutions for injection: amikacin sulfate, aminophylline, carbenicillin disodium, cefazolin sodium, cefotaxime sodium, cefoxitin sodium, cefuroxime sodium, cephalothin sodium, chloramphenicol sodium succinate, clindamycin phosphate, disopyramide phosphate, gentamicin sulfate, heparin sodium, hydrocortisone sodium succinate, hydromorphone HCl, magnesium sulfate, meperidine HCl, morphine sulfate, moxalactam disodium, multielectrolyte concentrate, multivitamins, netilmicin sulfate, penicillin G sodium, and tobramycin sulfate. Compatibility is dependent upon factors such as pH, concentration, temperature, and diluent used; consult specialized references or a hospital pharmacist for more specific information.

The following drugs and solutions are reportedly physically **incompatible** (or compatibility data conflicts) with metronidazole ready-to-use solutions for injection: aztreonam, cefamandole naftate, and dopamine HCl.

Metronidazole hydrochloride is very bitter tasting and even with taste masking or flavoring agents is universally unpalatable to veterinary patients. Although not commercially available in the United States, the metronidazole ester of benzoic acid, metronidazole benzoate, is relatively palatable to animal patients and is often used in extemporaneously compounded suspensions, particularly for cats to reduce the drug's bitterness. If using metronidazole benzoate adjust dosages from those for the base unless provided by pharmacy as "mg/mL of the base". 1 mg of metronidazole base ≈ 1.6 mg of metronidazole benzoate. Crystallization and sedimentation can occur in aqueous metronidazole benzoate suspensions when conversion from the anhydrous to the monohydrate form occurs.

Compounded preparation stability: One method for compounding a metronidazole benzoate suspension (80 mg/mL) that is stable (when protected from light, ambient temperature) for at least a year, has been published (Vu et al. 2008). To make 750 mL of an 80 mg/mL suspension: Place metronidazole benzoate powder 60 grams in a suitable mortar. The powder is then triturated with 1.25 grams of Propylene Glycol, NF to a smooth paste, then add increasing amounts of *SyrSpend SF* (Gallipot) until the suspension is pour-able. The liquid suspension should then be transferred to a suitable graduated container and the mortar rinsed with three small aliquots of *SyrSpend SF*, which are then added to the suspension. Add additional *SyrSpend SF* to bring the suspension to the final volume of 750 mL. Store in light-resistant containers refrigerated or at room temperature.

Another published method is to triturate 9.6 grams (9,600 mg) of metronidazole benzoate powder with 60 mL of *Ora-Plus*® and *qs ad* to 120 mL with *Ora-Sweet*® or *Ora-Sweet SF*® to yield a 80 mg/mL metronidazole benzoate oral suspension (equivalent to 50 mg/mL metronidazole hydrochloride) that retains >90% potency for 90 days when stored at both 4°C and 25°C and protected from light (Mathew *et al.* 1994).

Dosage Forms/Regulatory Status

VETERINARY-LABELED PRODUCTS: None

Metronidazole is prohibited for use in food animals by the FDA.

HUMAN-LABELED PRODUCTS:

Metronidazole Oral Tablets: 250 mg & 500 mg; *Flagyl*® (Pfizer); generic; (Rx)

Metronidazole Oral Capsules: 375 mg; *Flagyl 375*® (Pfizer); generic; (Rx)

Metronidazole Extended-Release Oral Tablets: 750 mg; *Flagyl ER*® (Pfizer); (Rx)

Metronidazole Injection: 5 mg/mL in 100 mL vials and single-dose containers; generic; (B. Braun); Metronidazole in Sodium Chloride (Claris Lifesciences); (Rx)

Bismuth Subsalicylate, Metronidazole & Tetracycline HCl Combination Tablets & Capsules: 262.4 mg bismuth subsalicylate, 250 mg metronidazole; 500 mg tetracycline; *Helidac*® (Procter & Gamble); (Rx)

Lotions, gels, vaginal products and creams also available.

References

Adamcak, A. & B. Otten (2000). Rodent Therapeutics. *Vet Clin NA: Exotic Anim Pract* 3:1(Jan): 221–240.

Bentz, B. (2007). Antimicrobial selections for foals. Proceedings: Western Vet Conf. Accessed via: Veterinary Information Network. http://goo.gl/bA5Ny

Corley, K.T.T. & A.R. Hollis (2009). Antimicrobial therapy in neonatal foals. *Equine Veterinary Education* 21(8): 436–448.

Cornelius, L., J. Bartges, et al. (2000). CVT Update: Therapy for Hepatic Lipidosis. *Kirk's Current Veterinary Therapy: XIII Small Animal Practice*. J Bonagura Ed. Philadelphia, WB Saunders: 686–690.

de la Navarre, B. (2003). Common parasitic diseases of reptiles and amphibians. Proceedings: Western Veterinary Conf. Accessed via: Veterinary Information Network. http://goo.gl/ZafJD

Evans, J., D. Levesque, et al. (2002). The use of diazepam in the treatment of metronidazole toxicosis in the dog.

Proceedings: ACVIM Forum. Accessed via: Veterinary Information Network. http://goo.gl/M97qr

Frazer, M. (2007). A review of Lawsonia intracellularis: A significant equine pathogen. Proceedings: ACVIM. Accessed via: Veterinary Information Network. http://goo.gl/xyEwh

Gaschen, F. (2006). Small Intestinal Diarrhea—Causes and Treatment. Proceedings: WSAVA. Accessed via: Veterinary Information Network. http://goo.gl/eKjft

Gaschen, F. (2008). How I Treat Chronic Canine Enteropathies. Peroceedings: WSAVA. Accessed via: Veterinary Information Network. http://goo.gl/cGz2Y

Gauvin, J. (1993). Drug therapy in reptiles. *Seminars in Avian & Exotic Pet Med* 2(1): 48–59.

Hall, J. (2000). Diseases of the Stomach. *Textbook of Veterinary Internal Medicine: Diseases of the Dog and Cat.* S Ettinger and E Feldman Eds. Philadelphia, WB Saunders. **2**: 1154–1182.

Hardie, E. (2000). Therapeutic Mangement of Sepsis. *Kirk's Current Veterinary Therapy: XIII Small Animal Practice.* J Bonagura Ed. Philadelphia, WB Saunders: 272–275.

Hayes, P. (2000). Diseases of Chinchillas. *Kirk's Current Veterinary Therapy: XIII Small Animal Practice.* J Bonagura Ed. Philadelphia, WB Saunders: 1152–1157.

Ivey, E. & J. Morrisey (2000). Therapeutics for Rabbits. *Vet Clin NA: Exotic Anim Pract* 3:1(Jan): 183–216.

Jenson, J. (1998). Current ratite therapy. *The Veterinary Clinics of North America: Food Animal Practice* 16:3(November).

Johnson-Delaney, C. (2008). Gastrointestinal Diseases in Ferrets. Proceedings: WVC. Accessed via: Veterinary Information Network. http://goo.gl/UC3zs

Krohne, S. (2008). Tear Staining & Pigment & Hairs—Oh My: Treating Medial Canthus Syndrome in Dogs. Proceedings: World Veterinary Conference. Accessed via: Veterinary Information Network. http://goo.gl/gjJG3

Lappin, M. (2000). Protozoal and Miscellaneous Infections. *Textbook of Veterinary Internal Medicine: Diseases of the Dog and Cat.* S Ettinger and E Feldman Eds. Philadelphia, WB Saunders. **1**: 408–417.

Lappin, M. (2006). Giardia infections. Proceedings: WSAVA World Congress. Accessed via: Veterinary Information Network. http://goo.gl/aywXP

LeBlanc, M.M. (2009). The current status of antibiotic use in equine reproduction. *Equine Veterinary Education* 21(3): 156–167.

Leib, M. (2000). Chronic Colitis in Dogs. *Kirk's Current Veterinary Therapy: XIII Small Animal Practice.* J Bonagura Ed. Philadelphia, WB Saunders: 643–648.

Leib, M.S., W.H. Hay, et al. (1989). Plasmacytic-Lymphocytic colitis in dogs. *Current Veterinary Therapy X: Small Animal Practice.* RW Kirk Ed. Philadelphia, Saunders: 939–944.

Marks, S. (2007). Inflammatory Bowel Disease—More than a garbage can diagnosis. Proceedings: UCD Canine Medicine Symposium. Accessed via: Veterinary Information Network. http://goo.gl/ZGPg1

Mathew, M., V. Das Gupta, et al. (1994). Stability of metronidazole benzoate in suspensions. *J Clin Pharm Ther* 19(1): 31–34.

Oglesbee, B. (2009). Vomiting & Diarrhea in Pet Birds: Where do I Start? Proceedings: WVC. Accessed via: Veterinary Information Network. http://goo.gl/waFP2

Papich, M. (1989). Effects of drugs on pregnancy. *Current Veterinary Therapy X: Small Animal Practice.* R Kirk Ed. Philadelphia, Saunders: 1291–1299.

Payne, P.A. & M. Artzer (2009). The Biology and Control of Giardia spp and Tritrichomonas foetus. *Veterinary Clinics of North America-Small Animal Practice* 39(6): 993–+.

Scorza, A.V. & M.R. Lappin (2004). Metronidazote for the treatment of fetine giardiasis. *Journal of Feline Medicine and Surgery* 6(3): 157–160.

Sekis, I., K. Ramstead, et al. (2009). Single-dose pharmacokinetics and genotoxicity of metronidazole in cats. *Journal of Feline Medicine and Surgery* 11(2): 60–68.

Simpson, K. (2003). Intragastric warfare in Helicobacter infected cats. Proceedings: ACVIM Forum. Accessed via: Veterinary Information Network. http://goo.gl/gSR3T

Slovis, N. (2003). Infectious diarrhea in foals. Proceedings: ACVIM Forum. Accessed via: Veterinary Information Network. http://goo.gl/JllC0

Tams, T. (2007). Giardiasis, Clostridium perfringens Enterotoxicosis, Tritrichomonas foetus, and Cryptosporidiosis. Prpoceedings: ABVP. Accessed via: Veterinary Information Network. http://goo.gl/YEJXk

Vernau, K. (2009). Cerebellar Disease. Veterinary Neurology Symposium; Univ. of Calif.-Davis. Accessed via: Veterinary Information Network.

Vu, N., V. Aloumanis, et al. (2008). Stability of Metronidazole Benzoate in SyrSpend SF One-Step Suspension System. *Intl Jnl Pharmaceutical Cmpd* 12(6): 558–564.

Washabau, R. (2009). Principles in the therapy of canine inflammatory bowel disease. Proceedings: WSAVA. Accessed via: Veterinary Information Network. http://goo.gl/L5Asz

Williams, B. (2000). Therapeutics in Ferrets. *Vet Clin NA: Exotic Anim Pract* 3:1(Jan): 131–153.

Zoran, D. (2007). Diarrhea in kittens and cats: What can you do? Proceedings; Western Vet Conf. Accessed via: Veterinary Information Network. http://goo.gl/oC0Qg

METYRAPONE

(me-*teer*-a-pone)   Metopirone®

ADRENAL STEROID INHIBITOR

Prescriber Highlights

▶ Adrenal steroid synthesis inhibitor primarily used in cats with hyperadrenocorticism; may be most useful for short-term treatment to stabilize patient before adrenalectomy

▶ Seems well tolerated in cats at recommended doses

▶ May alter insulin requirements; monitor blood glucose closely

▶ Has had availability issues

Uses/Indications

Metyrapone may be useful to treat cats with hyperadrenocorticism, especially short-term in an attempt to stabilize the patient prior to adrenalectomy. Clinical experience is quite limited, but it appears to give consistent results and not be overly toxic to cats. Resolving hypercortisolism should reduce insulin antagonism and reduce or eliminate the need for exogenous insulin in some cats (Feldman 2009). Metyrapone may potentially be useful in treating hyperadrenocorticism in ferrets and small mammals (*e.g.*, hamsters), but there is little, if any, information available on its use in these species.

In humans, metyrapone is used with other biochemical and laboratory evaluations in the diagnostic evaluation of hypothalamic-pituitary adrenal corticotropin hormone-function. It is also used for treatment of Cushing's Syndrome (not an FDA-approved indication).

Pharmacology/Actions

Metyrapone reduces cortisol and corticosterone production by inhibiting hydroxylation of 11-deoxycortisol to cortisol in the adrenal cortex. ACTH production can increase as the negative feedback mechanism is inhibited. With time, this may override the effects of metyrapone on the adrenal gland. Metyrapone can also suppress synthesis of aldosterone, and cause a mild natriuresis. Continued inhibition stimulates increased ACTH production that can ultimately override the inhibitory effects. Mineralocorticoid deficiency does not usually occur with long-term metyrapone therapy because inhibition of the 11-beta-hydroxylation reaction increases production of 11-desoxycorticosterone, a mineralocorticoid that can cause hypertension in patients receiving long-term metyrapone therapy.

Pharmacokinetics

No information on the pharmacokinetics of metyrapone was located for cats. In humans, metyrapone is well absorbed after oral administration. Peak levels occur in about an hour; however, pharmacological response to metyrapone does not occur immediately. It is rapidly cleared from the plasma and has an average elimination half-life of around 2 hours. Metyrapone's major metabolite, metyrapol, is active and formed via reduction; it has a half-life about twice as long as metyrapone. Both metyrapol and metyrapone are conjugated with glucuronide in humans. As cats are unable to effectively glucuronidate, it is unclear what metabolic path(s) metyrapone takes in this species.

Contraindications/Precautions/Warnings

Metyrapone should not be used in animals that are hypersensitive to it or have adrenal cortical insufficiency.

Use cautiously (enhanced monitoring) in cats with concurrent diabetes; monitor blood glucose closely as hypoglycemia can develop rapidly.

Adverse Effects

Metyrapone appears be relatively well tolerated in cats. Dosages ranging from 195–250 mg/cat/day (divided) have been used in cats with hyperadrenocorticism without observed toxicity (Bruyette 2010). The following adverse effects have been reported in human patients taking metyrapone: headache, dizziness, sedation, allergic rash, nausea, vomiting, and abdominal pain. Rarely, metyrapone can cause bone marrow depression.

Reproductive/Nursing Safety

Metyrapone should be given to pregnant queens only if clearly needed. Animal reproduction studies have not been conducted with metyrapone. In women given the drug in the 2nd and 3rd trimester, evidence of fetal pituitary response to the enzymatic block was detected. The FDA has assigned metyrapone to category **C** for use during pregnancy (*Animal studies have shown an adverse effect on the fetus, but there are no adequate studies in humans; or there are no animal reproduction studies and no adequate studies in humans.*)

Metyrapone's safety in lactating animals and their offspring is not known.

Overdosage/Acute Toxicity

The oral LD_{50} in rats (mg/kg) was 521 mg/kg. Metyrapone overdoses likely would cause GI effects and, possibly, acute adrenocortical insufficiency. Other effects that may be seen include: hypoglycemia, hyponatremia, hypochloremia, hyperkalemia, cardiac arrhythmias, hypotension, dehydration, and impairment of consciousness. There is no specific antidote. Standard decontamination protocols should be considered with intravenous hydrocortisone, saline and glucose. Monitoring and support for several days may be required. Contact an animal poison control center for more information and guidance.

Drug Interactions

The following drug interactions have either been reported or are theoretical in humans or animals receiving metyrapone and may be of significance in veterinary patients:

■ **ACETAMINOPHEN (Do NOT use in cats):** In humans, there is an increased risk for acetaminophen toxicity

■ **CORTICOSTEROIDS:** Decreases the efficacy of metyrapone.

Laboratory Considerations

■ In humans, the following drugs have been reported to interfere with the results of the metyrapone test: antidepressants such as amitriptyline, antithyroid drugs, phenothiazines, barbiturates, corticosteroids, cyproheptadine, and hormones such as estrogens and progesterone.

■ The metyrapone test may not be reliable in humans with hyper- or hypothyroidism.

Doses

■ **CATS:**

For treatment of hyperadrenocorticism:

a) Metyrapone has been used to successfully treat hyperadrenocorticism in the cat; recommended dose is 65 mg/kg PO every 8 to 12 hours. (Scott-Moncrieff 2010)

Monitoring

■ Blood glucose should be closely monitored in cats, particularly those that are diabetic

■ Clinical signs associated with hyperadrenocorticism or hypoadrenocorticism

Client Information

■ Metyrapone will likely need to compounded from the commercially available capsule, follow specific storage requirements.

■ To reduce the chances for vomiting, give this medication with food.

■ Contact veterinarian immediately if cat develops any of the following signs: will not eat, weakness or lack of normal energy, vomiting, excessive drinking or urinating, or diarrhea.

Chemistry/Synonyms

Metyrapone occurs as a white to light amber, fine, crystalline powder, with a characteristic odor. It is sparingly soluble in water; soluble in chloroform and methyl alcohol.

Metyrapone may also be known as SU-4885, metirapon, metirapona, or metyraponum. A common trade name is *Metopirone®*.

Storage/Stability

Store metyrapone at room temperature in a well-closed, light-resistant container.

Dosage Forms/Regulatory Status

VETERINARY-LABELED PRODUCTS: None

HUMAN-LABELED PRODUCTS:

Metyrapone Oral Capsules: 250 mg; *Metopirone®* (Ciba-Geigy); (Rx)

References

Bruyette, D. (2010). Feline Adrenal Disease: Exploring the Unexplored. Proceedings: WVC. Accessed via: Veterinary Information Network. http://goo.gl/BcIAo

Feldman, E.C. (2009). Diagnosis & Treatment of Hyperadrenocorticism in Cats. Proceedings: Western Veterinary Conference. Accessed via: Veterinary Information Network. http://goo.gl/6JxRm

Scott-Moncrieff, J.C. (2010). Update on treatment of hyperadrenocorticism: What is the current recommendation? Proceedings: ACVIM Forum. Accessed via: Veterinary Information Network. http://goo.gl/OsV6A

MEXILETINE HCL

(mex-*ill*-i-teen)   Mexitil®

ORAL ANTIARRHYTHMIC

Prescriber Highlights

▶ Oral antiarrhythmic with similar effects as lidocaine; used for V tach, PVC's; often used with atenolol

▶ Extreme caution: Pre-existing 2nd or 3rd degree AV block (without pacemaker), or in patients with cardiogenic shock

▶ Caution: Severe congestive heart failure or acute myocardial infarction, hepatic function impairment, hypotension, intraventricular conduction abnormalities, sinus node function impairment, seizure disorder, or sensitivity to the drug

▶ Adverse Effects: GI distress, including vomiting (give with meals to alleviate); Potentially: CNS effects (trembling, unsteadiness, dizziness, depression), shortness of breath, PVC's & chest pain could occur; rarely (reported in humans): seizures, agranulocytosis, & thrombocytopenia

▶ Relatively expensive (compared to quinidine)

▶ Drug-drug; drug-lab interactions

Uses/Indications

Mexiletine may be useful to treat some ventricular arrhythmias, including PVC's and ventricular tachycardia in small animals. Ventricular tachycardias that have responded to lidocaine usually (but not always) respond to mexiletine as well. Mexiletine may have less cardiodepressant effects and appears to have fewer adverse effects than either procainamide or quinidine, but it is much more costly.

Mexiletine may be useful treating certain myopathies in dogs such as myotonia congenita (most studied in miniature schnauzers and Chow Chows) and myokymia in Jack Russell Terriers.

Pharmacology/Actions

Mexiletine is considered a class IB antiarrhythmic agent and is similar to lidocaine in its mechanism of antiarrhythmic activity. It inhibits the inward sodium current (fast sodium channel), thereby reducing the rate of rise of the action potential, Phase O. In the Purkinje fibers, automaticity is decreased, action potential is shortened and, to a lesser extent, effective refractory period is decreased. Usually conduction is unaffected, but may be slowed in patients with preexisting conduction abnormalities.

Pharmacokinetics

Mexiletine is relatively well absorbed from the gut and has a low first-pass effect. In humans, it is moderately bound to plasma proteins (60–75%), and is metabolized in the liver to inactive metabolites with an elimination half-life of about 10–12 hours. Half-lives may be significantly increased in patients with moderate to severe hepatic disease, or in those having severely reduced cardiac outputs. Half-lives may be slightly prolonged in patients with severe renal disease or after acute myocardial infarction.

Contraindications/Precautions/Warnings

Mexiletine should be used with extreme caution, if at all, in patients with pre-existing 2nd or 3rd degree AV block (without pacemaker), or with cardiogenic shock. It should be used only when the benefits of therapy outweigh the risks when the following medical conditions exist: severe congestive heart failure or acute myocardial infarction, hepatic function impairment, hypotension, intraventricular conduction abnormalities, sinus node function impairment, seizure disorder, or sensitivity to the drug.

Adverse Effects

The most likely adverse effect noted in animals is GI distress, including vomiting. Giving with meals may alleviate this. Potentially (reported in humans): CNS effects (trembling, unsteadiness, dizziness, depression), shortness of breath, PVC's and chest pain could occur. Rarely, seizures, agranulocytosis, and thrombocytopenia have been reported in humans.

Reproductive/Nursing Safety

Lab animal studies have not demonstrated teratogenicity. In humans, the FDA categorizes this drug as category *C* for use during pregnancy (*Animal studies have shown an adverse effect on the fetus, but there are no adequate studies in humans; or there are no animal reproduction studies and no adequate studies in humans.*)

Because mexiletine is secreted into maternal milk, it has been recommended to use milk replacer if the mother is receiving the drug.

Overdosage/Acute Toxicity
Toxicity associated with overdosage may be significant. Case reports in humans have noted that CNS signs always preceded cardiovascular signs. Treatment should consist of GI tract emptying protocols when indicated, acidification of the urine to enhance urinary excretion, and supportive therapy. Atropine may be useful if hypotension or bradycardia occur.

Drug Interactions
The following drug interactions have either been reported or are theoretical in humans or animals receiving mexiletine and may be of significance in veterinary patients:

■ **ANTACIDS, ALUMINUM-MAGNESIUM:** May slow the absorption of mexiletine

■ **ATROPINE:** May reduce the rate of oral absorption

■ **CIMETIDINE:** May increase or decrease mexiletine blood levels

■ **GRISEOFULVIN:** May accelerate the metabolism of mexiletine

■ **LIDOCAINE:** May cause additive adverse effects

■ **METOCLOPRAMIDE:** May accelerate the absorption of mexiletine.

■ **OPIATES:** May slow the absorption of mexiletine

■ **PHENOBARBITAL, PRIMIDONE, PHENYTOIN:** May accelerate the metabolism of mexiletine

■ **RIFAMPIN:** May accelerate the metabolism of mexiletine

■ **THEOPHYLLINE (aminophylline):** Metabolism may be reduced by mexiletine, thereby leading to theophylline toxicity

■ **URINARY ACIDIFYING DRUGS (e.g., methionine, ammonium chloride, potassium phosphate, sodium phosphate):** May accelerate the renal excretion of mexiletine

■ **URINARY ALKALINIZING DRUGS (e.g., citrates, bicarb, carbonic anhydrase inhibitors):** May reduce the urinary excretion of mexiletine

Laboratory Considerations
■ Some human patients (1–3%) have had **AST** values increase by as much as three times or more above the upper limit of normal. This is reportedly a transient effect and asymptomatic.

Doses
■ **DOGS:**
For treating or assisting in treatment of ventricular arrhythmias:
a) 5–8 mg/kg PO q8h (Fox 2003)
b) 4–10 mg/kg PO q8h (Hogan 2004)
c) For Boxers with ventricular arrhythmias: mexiletine at 5–7.5 mg/kg three times daily with sotalol at 1.5–3 mg/kg twice daily; was successful in 7/8 dogs treated in study, warrants further investigation. (Prosek *et al.* 2006)
d) 4–8 mg/kg PO q8h, combined with atenolol (0.5 mg/kg PO q12–24h) (Moise 2000)
e) For familial arrhythmic cardiomyopathy of Boxers: 5–8 mg/kg PO q8h with atenolol at 12.5 mg (total dose) q12h (Meurs 2003)
f) 5–6 mg/kg PO q8h; always give with food to avoid nausea. (Meurs 2006)

For treating myotonia congenital (most studied in Chow Chows and miniature schnauzers) or myokymia in Jack Russell terriers:
a) 8.3 mg/kg PO q8h (Lorenz 2007)

Monitoring
■ In humans, therapeutic plasma concentrations are: 0.5–2 micrograms/mL; toxicity may be noted at therapeutic levels
■ ECG
■ Adverse effects

Client Information
■ Give with food to reduce risk for vomiting or nausea
■ Reinforce adherence to prescribed therapy.

Chemistry/Synonyms
A class IB antiarrhythmic, mexiletine HCl occurs as a white or almost white, odorless, crystalline powder. It is freely soluble in water.

Mexiletine may also be known as: Ko-1173, mexiletini hydrochloridum, *Mexilen®*, *Mexitil®*, *Mexitilen®*, *Myovek®*, and *Ritalmex®*.

Storage/Stability
Mexiletine capsules should be stored in tight containers at room temperature.

Dosage Forms/Regulatory Status
VETERINARY-LABELED PRODUCTS: None

The ARCI (Racing Commissioners International) has designated this drug as a class 4 substance. See the appendix for more information.

HUMAN-LABELED PRODUCTS:

Mexiletine Oral Capsules: 150 mg, 200 mg & 250 mg; generic; (Rx)

References
Fox, P. (2003). Congestive heart failure: Clinical approach and management. Proceedings: World Small

Animal Veterinary Assoc World Congress. Accessed via: Veterinary Information Network. http://goo.gl/xMFKn

Hogan, D. (2004). Arrhythmias: diagnosis and treatment. Proceedings: ACVIM Forum. Accessed via: Veterinary Information Network. http://goo.gl/voENn

Lorenz, M. (2007). Section 1: Motor unit disorders/Peripheral neuropathies/Myopathies. Proceedings: Western Vet Conference. Accessed via: Veterinary Information Network. http://goo.gl/yY82X

Meurs, K. (2003). Familial arrhythmic cardiomyopathy of Boxers (ARVC). Proceedings: ACVIM Forum. Accessed via: Veterinary Information Network. http://goo.gl/BHNF9

Meurs, K. (2006). Canine cardiomyopathies: Dilated and arrythmogenic. Proceedings: Western Vet Conf. Accessed via: Veterinary Information Network. http://goo.gl/oiMqC

Moise, N. (2000). CVT Update: Ventricular Arrhythmias. *Kirk's Current Veterinary Therapy: XIII Small Animal Practice.* J Bonagura Ed. Philadelphia, WB Saunders: 733–737.

Prosek, R., A. Estrada, et al. (2006). Comparison of sotalol and mexiletine versus stand alone sotalol in treatment of Boxer dogs with ventricular arrhythmias. Proceedings: ACVIM. Accessed via: Veterinary Information Network. http://goo.gl/wnpJV

MIBOLERONE

(mye-*boe*-le-rone)   Cheque® Drops

ANDROGEN; ANABOLIC

Prescriber Highlights

▶ Availability an issue; now a controlled substance in the USA

▶ Androgenic, anabolic, antigonadotropic used to suppress estrus, treat pseudocyesis (false pregnancy) or severe galactorrhea in dogs

▶ Contraindications: Perianal adenoma, perianal adenocarcinoma or other androgen-dependent neoplasias, pregnant or lactating bitches, ongoing or history of liver or kidney disease. The manufacturer also recommends not using the drug in Bedlington terriers.

▶ NOT for use in cats

▶ Adverse Effects: Prepubescent females: premature epiphyseal closure, clitoral enlargement, & vaginitis. Adult bitch: mild clitoral hypertrophy, vulvovaginitis, increased body odor, abnormal behavior, urinary incontinence, voice deepening, riding behavior, enhanced clinical signs of seborrhea oleosa, epiphora (tearing), hepatic changes (intranuclear hyaline bodies), & increased kidney weight (without pathology), hepatic dysfunction (rare)

Uses/Indications

Cheque® Drops was labeled as indicated "for estrous (heat) prevention in adult female dogs not intended primarily for breeding purposes." In clinical trials it was 90% effective in suppressing estrus.

Although not approved, mibolerone at dosages of 50 micrograms per day will prevent estrus in the cat, but its use is generally not recommended because of the very narrow therapeutic index of the drug in this species (see the Adverse Effects and Overdosage sections for more information).

Pharmacology/Actions

Mibolerone acts by blocking the release of luteinizing hormone (LH) from the anterior pituitary via a negative feedback mechanism. Because of the lack of LH, follicles will develop to a certain point, but will not mature and hence no ovulation or corpus luteum development occurs. The net result is a suppression of the estrous cycle if the drug is given prior to (as much as 30 days) the onset of proestrus. After discontinuation of the drug, the next estrus may occur within 7-200 days (avg. 70 days).

Pharmacokinetics

Mibolerone is reported to be well absorbed from the intestine after oral administration and is rapidly metabolized in the liver to over 10 separate metabolites. Excretion is apparently equally divided between the urine and feces.

Contraindications/Precautions/Warnings

Mibolerone is contraindicated in female dogs with perianal adenoma, perianal adenocarcinoma or other androgen-dependent neoplasias. It is also contraindicated in patients with ongoing, or a history of, liver or kidney disease. The manufacturer recommends not using the drug in Bedlington Terriers.

Adverse Effects

Immature females (dogs) may be more prone to develop adverse reactions than more mature females. In prepubescent females, mibolerone can induce premature epiphyseal closure, clitoral enlargement, and vaginitis. Adverse effects that may be seen in the adult bitch include mild clitoral hypertrophy (may be partially reversible), vulvovaginitis, increased body odor, abnormal behavior, urinary incontinence, voice deepening, riding behavior, enhanced clinical signs of seborrhea oleosa, epiphora (tearing), hepatic changes (intranuclear hyaline bodies), and increased kidney weight (without pathology). Although reported, overt hepatic dysfunction would be considered to occur rarely in dogs. With the exception of residual mild clitoral hypertrophy, adverse effects will generally resolve after discontinuation of therapy.

In the cat, dosages of 60 micrograms/day have caused hepatic dysfunction and 120 micrograms/day have caused death. Other adverse effects that have been noted in cats include clitoral hypertrophy, thyroid dysfunction, os clitorides formation, cervical dermis thickening, and pancreatic dysfunction.

Reproductive/Nursing Safety

Mibolerone should not be used in pregnant bitches; masculinization of the female fetuses will occur. Alterations seen may include: changes in vagina patency, multiple urethral openings in the vagina, a phallus-like structure instead of a clitoris, formation of testes-like structures, and fluid accumulation in the vagina and uterus. Because it may inhibit lactation, it should not be used in nursing bitches.

The manufacturer recommends discontinuing the product after 24 months of use. It should not be used to try to attempt to abbreviate an estrous period or in bitches prior to their first estrous period.

Overdosage/Acute Toxicity

Many toxicology studies have been performed in dogs. The drug did not cause death in doses up to 30,000 micrograms/kg/day when administered to beagles for 28 days. For a more detailed discussion of the toxicology of the drug, the reader is referred to the package insert for *Cheque® Drops*.

In the cat, dosages as low as 120 micrograms/day have resulted in fatalities.

Drug Interactions

Increased seizure activity has been reported in a dog after receiving mibolerone who was previously controlled on **phenytoin**. Mibolerone should generally not be used concurrently with **progestins** or **estrogens**.

Laboratory Considerations

■ Mibolerone has been reported to cause **thyroid** dysfunction in cats.

Doses

■ **DOGS:**

For suppression of estrus (treatment must begin at least 30 days prior to proestrus):
a) Bitches weighing:

   0.5–11 kg: 30 micrograms (0.3 mL) PO per day

   12–22 kg: 60 micrograms (0.6 mL) PO per day

   23–45 kg: 120 micrograms (1.2 mL) PO per day

   >45 kg: 180 micrograms (1.8 mL) PO per day

   German shepherds or German shepherd crosses: 180 micrograms (1.8 mL) PO per day; regardless of weight (Package Insert; *Cheque® Drops*—Upjohn)

b) As above, but should dog come into estrus after receiving the drug for 30 or more days, stop drug and determine that the dog is not pregnant before resuming therapy. If owner compliance has been determined, increase dosage by 20–50%. (Burke 1985; Woody 1989)

For pseudocyesis (false pregnancy):
a) Use 10 times the dosage listed above for suppression of estrus PO once daily for 5 days (Barton & Wolf 1988)

b) 16 micrograms/kg PO once daily for 5 days (Concannon 1986)

For cystic endometrial hyperplasia (CEH):
a) 30 micrograms/25lb. body weight PO daily during 6 months. (Fontbonne 2006)

For treatment of severe galactorrhea:
a) 8–18 micrograms/kg PO once a day for 5 days. Once discontinued, prolactin may surge and galactorrhea resume. (Olson *et al.* 1986)

■ **CATS:**

WARNING: Because of the very low margin of safety with this drug in cats, it cannot be recommended for use in this species.

Monitoring

■ Clinical signs of estrus

■ Liver function tests (baseline, annual, or as needed)

■ Physical examination of genitalia

Client Information

■ It must be stressed to owners that compliance with dosage and administration direction is crucial for this agent to be effective.

Chemistry/Synonyms

A non-progestational, androgenic, anabolic, antigonadotropic, 19-nor-steroid, mibolerone occurs as a white, crystalline solid.

Mibolerone may also be known as: dimethyl-nortestosterone, NSC-72260, and U-10997.

Storage/Stability

The original manufacturer (Upjohn) states that the compound in *Cheque® Drops* is stable under ordinary conditions and temperatures. If using a compounded preparation, follow specific instructions from the pharmacy.

Dosage Forms/Regulatory Status

VETERINARY-LABELED PRODUCTS:

Commercially prepared mibolerone preparations are apparently no longer being marketed. Mibolerone may be available from compounding pharmacies. Mibolerone is now categorized as a Class-III controlled substance in the USA.

HUMAN-LABELED PRODUCTS: None

References

Barton, C.L. & A.M. Wolf (1988). Disorders of Reproduction. *Handbook of Small Animal Practice.* RV Morgan Ed. New York, Churchill Livingstone: 679–700.

Burke, T.J. (1985). Reproductive Disorders. *Handbook of Small Animal Therapeutics.* LE Davis Ed. New York, Churchill Livingstone: 605–616.

Concannon, P.W. (1986). Clinical and endocrine correlates of canine and ovarian cycles and pregnancy. *Current Veterinary Therapy IX, Small Animal Practice.* RW Kirk Ed. Philadelphia, W.B. Saunders: 1214–1224.

Fontbonne, A. (2006). Infertility in the bitch. Proceedings: WSAVA. Accessed via: Veterinary Information Network. http://goo.gl/au0Du

Olson, P.N., R.A. Bowen, et al. (1986). Terminating canine and feline pregnancies. *Current Veterinary Therapy IX: Small Animal Practice.* RW Kirk Ed. Phialdelphia, WB Saunders: 1236–1240.

Woody, B.J. (1989). Prevention of estrus and pregnancy. *Handbook of Small Animal Practice.* RV Morgan Ed. New York, Churchill Livingstone: 701–705.

MIDAZOLAM HCL

(mid-*ay*-zoe-lam)   Versed®

PARENTERAL BENZODIAZEPINE

Prescriber Highlights

▶ Injectable benzodiazepine used primarily as a pre-op med; unlike diazepam may be given IM

▶ Contraindications: Hypersensitivity to benzodiazepines; acute narrow-angle glaucoma. Caution: Hepatic or renal disease, debilitated or geriatric patients, & those in coma, shock, or with significant respiratory depression.

▶ Adverse Effects: Potential for respiratory depression is of most concern

▶ Avoid intra-carotid injection

▶ Drug interactions

Uses/Indications

In veterinary patients, midazolam is used principally as a premedicant for general anesthesia. Alone, it does not appear to provide predictable sedation in animals. Animals may become sedated or dysphoric and excited. Cats may be more prone to develop the "excited" effect more than dogs. When used in combination with other drugs (*i.e.*, opioids or ketamine), midazolam does provide more predictable sedation.

Midazolam may also be of benefit to treat status epilepticus when given either IV or IM (not rectally).

In humans, midazolam has been suggested for use as a premedicant before surgery, and as a conscious sedative when combined with potent analgesic/anesthetic drugs (*e.g.*, ketamine or fentanyl). In humans, midazolam reduces the incidences of "dreamlike" emergence reactions and increases in blood pressure and cardiac rate caused by ketamine.

When compared to the thiobarbiturate induction agents (*e.g.*, thiamylal, thiopental), midazolam has less cardiopulmonary depressant effects, is water-soluble, can be mixed with several other agents, and does not tend to accumulate in the body after repeated doses.

Pharmacology/Actions

Midazolam exhibits similar pharmacologic actions as other benzodiazepines. The subcortical levels (primarily limbic, thalamic, and hypothalamic), of the CNS are depressed by the benzodiazepines thus producing the anxiolytic, sedative, skeletal muscle relaxant, and anticonvulsant effects seen. The exact mechanism of action is unknown, but postulated mechanisms include: antagonism of serotonin, increased release and/or facilitation of gamma-aminobutyric acid (GABA) activity, and diminished release or turnover of acetylcholine in the CNS.

Benzodiazepine specific receptors have been located in the mammalian brain, kidney, liver, lung, and heart. In all species studied, receptors are lacking in the white matter.

Midazolam's unique solubility characteristics (water soluble injection but lipid soluble at body pH) give it a very rapid onset of action after injection. When compared to diazepam, midazolam has approximately twice the affinity for benzodiazepine receptors, is nearly 3 times as potent, and has a faster onset of action and a shorter duration of effect.

Pharmacokinetics

Following IM injection, midazolam is rapidly and nearly completely (91%) absorbed. Midazolam is well absorbed after oral administration (no oral products are marketed), but because of a rapid first-pass effect, bioavailabilities suffer (31–72%). The onset of action following IV administration is very rapid due to the high lipophilicity of the agent. In humans, the loss of the lash reflex or counting occurs within 30–97 seconds of administration.

In dogs, midazolam is absorbed when the commercially available injection is administered intranasally and peak levels are higher than when it is administered rectally. A 50 mg/mL compounded gel (0.2% hydroxypropylmethylcellulose) demonstrated significantly higher peak levels after intranasal administration than when the injection was administered rectally or intranasally to dogs (Eagleson *et al.* 2010).

The drug is highly protein bound (94–97%) and rapidly crosses the blood-brain barrier. Because only unbound drug will cross into the CNS, changes in plasma protein concentrations and resultant protein binding may significantly alter the response to a given dose.

Midazolam is metabolized in the liver, principally by microsomal oxidation. An active metabolite (alpha-hydroxymidazolam) is formed, but because of its very short half-life and lower pharmacologic activity, it probably has negligible clinical effects. The serum half-life and duration of activity of midazolam in humans is considerably shorter than that of diazepam. Elimination half-lives in dogs average 77 minutes; in humans, approximately 2 hours (vs. approx. 30 hrs for diazepam).

In dogs, rectal bioavailability of midazolam is very low and this route is not useful clinically.

Contraindications/Precautions/Warnings

The manufacturer lists the following contraindications for use in humans: hypersensitivity to benzodiazepines, or acute narrow-angle glaucoma. Additionally, intra-carotid artery injections must be avoided.

Use cautiously in patients with hepatic or renal disease, and in debilitated or geriatric patients. Patients with congestive heart failure may eliminate the drug more slowly. The drug should be administered to patients in coma, shock, or with significant respiratory depression very cautiously.

When used alone, midazolam does not possess significant effects on cardiorespiratory function, but in combination with other agents, cardiorespiratory effects may be noted. Increased heart rate and blood pressure may be noted when used with ketamine. If this combination is used after an opioid has been administered, these effects may be diminished. If isoflurane will be used as the general anesthetic, use ketamine/midazolam with caution as bradycardia, hypotension and reduced cardiac output are possible.

Midazolam/opioid combinations can cause less cardiovascular depression, but greater respiratory depression, than acepromazine/opioid.

Midazolam and butorphanol used during isoflurane anesthesia can cause decreased blood pressure, heart rate and enhanced respiratory depression.

Adverse Effects

The primary concern using midazolam in veterinary patients is the possibility of respiratory depression.

In dogs, after morphine/acepromazine pre-op, midazolam given at 0.2 mg/kg IV prior to propofol anesthesia caused excitement in some patients (Covey-Crump & Murison 2008).

Few adverse effects have been reported in human patients receiving midazolam. Most frequently, effects on respiratory rate, cardiac rate and blood pressure have been reported. Respiratory depression has been reported in patients who have received narcotics or have COPD. The following adverse effects have been reported in more than 1%, but less than 5% of patients receiving midazolam: pain on injection, local irritation, headache, nausea, vomiting, and hiccups.

Reproductive/Nursing Safety

Although midazolam has not been demonstrated to cause fetal abnormalities, in humans, other benzodiazepines have been implicated in causing congenital abnormalities if administered during the first trimester of pregnancy. Infants born of mothers receiving large doses of benzodiazepines shortly before delivery have been reported to suffer from apnea, impaired metabolic response to cold stress, difficulty in feeding, hyperbilirubinemia, hypotonia, etc. Withdrawal symptoms have occurred in infants whose mothers chronically took benzodiazepines during pregnancy. The veterinary significance of these effects is unclear, but the use of these agents during the first trimester of pregnancy should only occur when the benefits clearly outweigh the risks associated with their use. In humans, the FDA categorizes this drug as category *D* for use during pregnancy (*There is evidence of human fetal risk, but the potential benefits from the use of the drug in pregnant women may be acceptable despite its potential risks.*)

Midazolam is excreted in milk and may cause CNS effects in nursing neonates. Exercise caution when administering to a nursing mother.

Overdosage/Acute Toxicity

Very limited information is currently available. The IV LD_{50} in mice has been reported to be 86 mg/kg. It is suggested that accidental overdoses be managed in a supportive manner, similar to diazepam. Flumazenil could be used to antagonize midazolam effects, but because of midazolam's short duration of effect and flumazenil's high cost, supportive therapy may be more suitable in all but the largest overdoses.

Drug Interactions

See the precautions noted above (Contraindications/Precautions) when using midazolam with other agents for preoperative use in small animals. The following drug interactions have either been reported or are theoretical in humans or animals receiving midazolam and may be of significance in veterinary patients:

- ■ **ANESTHETICS, INHALATIONAL:** Midazolam may decrease the dosages required
- ■ **AZOLE ANTIFUNGALS (ketoconazole, itraconazole, fluconazole):** May increase midazolam levels
- ■ **CALCIUM CHANNEL BLOCKERS (diltiazem, verapamil):** May increase midazolam levels
- ■ **CIMETIDINE:** May increase midazolam levels
- ■ **CNS DEPRESSANTS, OTHER:** May increase the risk of respiratory depression
- ■ **MACROLIDES (erythromycin, clarithromycin):** May increase midazolam levels
- ■ **OPIATES:** May increase the hypnotic effects of midazolam and hypotension has been reported when used with meperidine
- ■ **PHENOBARBITAL:** May decrease peak levels and AUC of midazolam
- ■ **RIFAMPIN:** May decrease peak levels and AUC of midazolam
- ■ **THIOPENTAL:** Midazolam may decrease the dosages required

Doses

- ■ **DOGS:**

  As a preoperative agent:
  a) 0.2–0.4 mg/kg IV or IM with an opioid such as hydromorphone (0.1 mg/kg IV or 0.2 mg/kg IM) (Day 2002)
  b) 0.1–0.3 mg/kg; may be used in combination with ketamine in a 50:50 mixture (volume/volume) at a dose of 1 mL/9.1 kg (1 mL/20 lb), this equates to a dose of 0.28 mg/kg of midazolam and 5.5 mg/kg of ketamine (Reed 2002)
  c) 0.1–0.5 mg/kg IV (Hellyer 2005)

  For status epilepticus:
  a) 0.25 mg/kg IV (Knipe 2006)
  b) 0.2–0.4 mg/kg IV or IM (not per rectum); may repeat once. (Hopper 2006)

c) 0.07–0.2 mg/kg IV or IM; effects are short-lived, so if seizures recur a CRI can be helpful given at 0.05–0.5 mg/kg/hour. (Thomas 2010)

■ **CATS:**

As a preoperative agent:

a) 0.2–0.4 mg/kg IV or IM with an opioid such as hydromorphone (0.1 mg/kg IV or 0.2 mg/kg IM) (Day 2002)

b) 0.05–0.5 mg/kg; a dose of 0.3 mg/kg being the most effective when mixed with ketamine to allow for intubation. May be used in combination with ketamine in a 50:50 mixture (volume/volume) at a dose of 1 mL/9.1 kg (1 mL/20 lb), this equates to a dose of 0.28 mg/kg of midazolam and 5.5 mg/kg of ketamine. (Reed 2002)

c) 0.1–0.5 mg/kg IV (Hellyer 2005)

For status epilepticus:

a) 0.07–0.2 mg/kg IV or IM; effects are short-lived, so if seizures recur a CRI can be helpful given at 0.05–0.5 mg/kg/hour. (Thomas 2010)

■ **RABBITS, RODENTS, SMALL MAMMALS:**

a) **Rabbits:** As a tranquilizer (to increase relaxation of lightly anesthetized animals and permit ET intubation): 1 mg/kg IV as needed (Huerkamp 1995)

b) **Rabbits:** 1–2 mg/kg IM, IV. (Ivey & Morrisey 2000)

c) **Hamsters, Gerbils, Mice, Rats, Guinea pigs, Chinchillas:** 1–2 mg/kg IM (Adamcak & Otten 2000)

d) As a preanesthetic: **Rabbits:** 0.5–5 mg/kg IM or IV; **Rodents:** 3–5 mg/kg IM or IV; often beneficial to minimize stress, anxiety and patient struggling. May be reversed with flumazenil if necessary (0.1 mg/kg IV, but may precipitate seizures)

Injectable anesthesia: **Rodents:** midazolam (5 mg/kg) + ketamine (100 mg/kg) + buprenorphine (0.05 mg/kg) IP.

Rabbits: Midazolam (0.05 mg/kg) + buprenorphine (0.03 mg/kg) + ketamine (10 mg/kg) IM (Bennett 2009)

e) As an induction agent in rabbits: 0.05–0.5 mg/kg IV (typically via a marginal ear vein). The low end of the dosage range is usually given and topped up as necessary. In non-sedated animals, prior preparation of the area with topical local anesthetics may be useful. Intravenous midazolam leads to further sedation of the patient, sufficient to allow intubation, but may also induce apneic side effects. This, together with fentanyl's respiratory depression, can potentially compound the possibility of hypoxia. It is important therefore, that midazolam is

given to effect and that pre-oxygenation is performed. Intubation is considered essential when using this protocol. **Note:** Not all patients require midazolam induction for purposes of intubation. An assessment of the patient can be made in the first 10 minutes post premedicant delivery. Some rabbits may be sufficiently sedated to allow intubation at this point. (Vella 2009)

■ **HORSES:**

As a preoperative agent:

a) 0.011–0.0.44 mg/kg IV (Mandsager 1988)

For seizure control in foals:

a) 2–5 mg (total dose) for a 50 kg foal given IV; rapid IV administration may result in apnea and hypotension. A CRI may be used at a dose of 1–3 mg/hour for a 50 kg foal. (Bentz 2006)

b) 2–5 mg (total dose) for a 50 kg foal given IV or IM; may be repeated to effect. (Toppin 2007)

■ **BIRDS:**

a) For adjunctive use (with an analgesic) for pain control: 1–2 mg/kg IM or IV (Clyde & Paul-Murphy 2000)

b) As a pre-med for anxious or easily stressed birds (*e.g.*, macaws, African greys, raptors and many wild birds) midazolam at 1 mg/kg IM is used. This will cause mild sedation and relaxation. Doses as high as 6 mg/kg have been reported resulting in considerable sedation.

As part of an injectable anesthetic regimen: Injectable anesthetics are only occasionally used in birds for short procedures or in situations where inhalant anesthetics are not available. Ketamine at 10–30 mg/kg and midazolam at 2–6 mg/kg can be used. The midazolam can be reversed with flumazenil (0.1 mg/kg) if necessary. Butorphanol can be added for analgesia at a dose of 1–2 mg/kg. (Morrisey 2010)

■ **ZOO, EXOTIC, WILDLIFE SPECIES:**

For use of midazolam in zoo, exotic and wildlife medicine refer to specific references, including:

a) *Zoo Animal and Wildlife Immobilization and Anesthesia.* West, G, Heard, D, Caulkett, N. (eds.). Blackwell Publishing, 2007.

b) *Handbook of Wildlife Chemical Immobilization, 3rd Ed.* Kreeger, T.J. and J.M. Arnemo. 2007.

c) *Restraint and Handling of Wild and Domestic Animals.* Fowler, M (ed.), Iowa State University Press, 1995

d) *Exotic Animal Formulary, 3rd Ed.* Carpenter, J.W., Saunders. 2005

e) The 2009 American Association of Zoo Veterinarian Proceedings by D. K. Fontenot also has several dosages listed for restraint, anesthesia, and analgesia for a variety of drugs for carnivores and primates. VIN members can access them at: http://goo.gl/BHRih or http://goo.gl/9UJse

Monitoring

■ Level of sedation

■ Respiratory and cardiac signs

Client Information

■ This agent should be used in an inpatient setting only or with direct professional supervision where cardiorespiratory support services are available.

Chemistry/Synonyms

Midazolam HCL is a benzodiazepine that occurs as a white or yellowish crystalline powder. Solubility in water is dependent upon pH. At a pH of 3.4 (approximately the pH of commercial injection), 10.3 mg are soluble in one mL of water.

Midazolam HCl may also be known as Ro-21-3981/003, *Versed®*, *Dormicum®*, *Dormonid®*, *Fulsed®*, *Hypnovel®*, *Midaselect®*, and *Zolamid®*.

Storage/Stability

It is recommended to store midazolam injection at room temperature (15°–30°C) and protected from light. After being frozen for 3 days and allowed to thaw at room temperature, the injectable product was physically stable. Midazolam is stable at a pH from 3–3.6.

Compatibility/Compounding Considerations

Midazolam is reportedly physically **compatible** when mixed with the following products: D_5W, normal saline, lactated Ringer's, atropine sulfate, fentanyl citrate, glycopyrrolate, hydroxyzine HCl, ketamine HCl, meperidine HCl, morphine sulfate, nalbuphine HCl, and promethazine HCl, sufentanil citrate, and scopolamine HBr. Compatibility is dependent upon factors such as pH, concentration, temperature, and diluent used; consult specialized references or a hospital pharmacist for more specific information.

Compounded preparation stability: Midazolam hydrochloride oral suspension compounded from the commercially available injectable solution has been published (Steedman *et al.* 1992). Diluting midazolam 5 mg/mL injection in a 1:1 ratio with *Syrpalta®* yields a 2.5 mg/mL midazolam hydrochloride oral solution that retains >90% potency for 56 days when stored at both 7°C, 20°C, and 40°C and protected from light.

Dosage Forms/Regulatory Status

VETERINARY-LABELED PRODUCTS: None

The ARCI (Racing Commissioners International) has designated this drug as a class 2 substance. See the appendix for more information.

HUMAN-LABELED PRODUCTS:

Midazolam HCl Injection: 1 mg (as HCl)/mL in 2 mL, 5 mL vials and *Carpuject* vials, 10 mL vials; 5 mg (as HCl)/mL in 1 mL, 2 mL, 5 mL vials and *Carpuject* vials, 10 mL vials, & 2 mL syringes; generic; (Rx, C-IV)

Midazolam HCl Syrup: 2 mg/mL in 118 mL; generic (Roxane); (Rx, C-IV)

References

Adamcak, A. & B. Otten (2000). Rodent Therapeutics. *Vet Clin NA: Exotic Anim Pract* **3:**1(Jan): 221–240.

Bennett, R. (2009). Small Mammal Anesthesia—Rabbits and Rodents. Proceedings: ACVC. Accessed via: Veterinary Information Network. http://goo.gl/hRqTS

Bentz, B. (2006). Current management practices for critically ill foals. Proceedings: ABVP. Accessed via: Veterinary Information Network. http://goo.gl/wFEGR

Clyde, V. & J. Paul-Murphy (2000). Avian Analgesia. *Kirk's Current Veterinary Therapy: XIII Small Animal Practice.* J Bonagura Ed. Philadelphia, WB Saunders: 1126–1128.

Covey-Crump, G.L. & P.J. Murison (2008). Fentanyl or midazolam for co-induction of anaesthesia with propofol in dogs. *Veterinary Anaesthesia and Analgesia* **35**(6): 463–472.

Day, T. (2002). Injectable anesthesia for emergency and critical care patients. Proceedings: Western Veterinary Conference. Accessed via: Veterinary Information Network. http://goo.gl/Umu85

Eagleson, J., S. Platt, et al. (2010). Pharmacokinetics of a Novel Intranasal Midazolam Gel in Dogs. Proceedings: ACVIM. Accessed via: Veterinary Information Network. http://goo.gl/SzD6r

Hellyer, P. (2005). Anesthetic Premedications. Proceedings: Western Vet Conf. Accessed via: Veterinary Information Network. http://goo.gl/iatkR

Hopper, K. (2006). Emergency management of the seizuring patient. Proceedings: Western Veterinary Conf. Accessed via: Veterinary Information Network. http://goo.gl/2tfAN

Huerkamp, M. (1995). Anesthesia and postoperative management of rabbits and pocket pets. *Kirk's Current Veterinary Therapy:XII.* J Bonagura Ed. Philadelphia, W.B. Saunders: 1322–1327.

Ivey, E. & J. Morrisey (2000). Therapeutics for Rabbits. *Vet Clin NA: Exotic Anim Pract* **3:**1(Jan): 183–216.

Knipe, M. (2006). Make it stop! Managing status epilepticus. Proceedings; Vet Neuro Symposium. Accessed via: Veterinary Information Network. http://goo.gl/sDYLA

Mandsager, R.E. (1988, Last Update). "Personal Communication."

Morrisey, J.K. (2010). Avian Analgesia and Anesthesia. Procededings: WVC. Accessed via: Veterinary Information Network. http://goo.gl/o4VUa

Reed, M. (2002). Midazolam. *Comp CE* **24**(10): 774–777.

Steedman, S.L., J.R. Koonce, et al. (1992). Stability of midazolam hydrochloride in a flavored, dye-free oral solution. *Am J Hosp Pharm* **49**(3): 615–618.

Thomas, W.B. (2010). Idiopathic Epilepsy in Dogs and Cats. *Veterinary Clinics of North America-Small Animal Practice* **40**(1): 161–+.

Toppin, S. (2007). ICU activities and procedures for the newborn foal: I-III. Proceedings: Western Vet Conf. Accessed via: Veterinary Information Network. http://goo.gl/IgLvy

Vella, D. (2009). Rabbit General Anesthesia. Proceedings: AAVAC-UEP. Accessed via: Veterinary Information Network. http://goo.gl/XKsCh

MILBEMYCIN OXIME

(mil-beh-*my*-sin)   Interceptor®, Sentinel®

MACROLIDE ANTIPARASITIC

For information on the combination product with lufenuron (Sentinel®), see the lufenuron monograph

Prescriber Highlights

▶ GABA inhibitor in invertebrates used for heartworm prophylaxis, microfilaricide, & treat demodicosis, etc.

▶ Contraindications: No absolute contraindications

▶ Adverse Effects: Animals with circulating microfilaria may develop a transient shock-like syndrome; at higher doses, neuro signs become more likely

▶ When used for demodicosis in dogs, very expensive

Uses/Indications

Milbemycin tablets are labeled as a once-a-month heartworm preventative (*Dirofilaria immitis*) and for hookworm control (*Ancylostoma caninum*). It has activity against a variety of other parasites, including adult hookworms (*A. caninum*), adult roundworms (*T. canis, T. leonina*) and whipworms (*Trichuris vulpis*). Monthly administered milbemycin does not appear to be as effective as ivermectin as an adulticide, especially against older heartworms. In cats, milbemycin has been used successfully to prevent larval infection of *Dirofilaria immitis*.

Milbemycin, like ivermectin can be used for treatment of generalized demodicosis in dogs, but treatment can be significantly more expensive. It is likely safer to use in breeds susceptible to *ABCB1*-1Δ (formerly MDR1-allele) genetic mutation (Collies, Shelties, Australian shepherds, etc.) at the doses used for this indication, but neuro toxicity is possible. Older dogs, those that have had a long duration of disease prior to treatment, and dogs with pododemodicosis appear have a lower success rate with milbemycin treatment.

Pharmacology/Actions

Milbemycin is thought to act by disrupting the transmission of the neurotransmitter gamma amino butyric acid (GABA) in invertebrates.

Pharmacokinetics

No specific information was located. At labeled doses, milbemycin is considered effective for at least 45 days after infection by *D. immitis* larva.

Contraindications/Precautions/Warnings

Because some dogs with a high number of circulating microfilaria will develop a transient, shock-like syndrome after receiving milbemycin, the manufacturer recommends testing for preexisting heartworm infections.

If using milbemycin at doses greater than labeled in breeds susceptible to the *ABCB1* genetic mutation, genetic testing is recommended before initiating therapy.

The manufacturer states to not use the product (*Interceptor®*) in puppies less than 4 weeks of age or less than 2 lbs. of body weight or in kittens less than 6 weeks of age or less than 1.5 lbs. of body weight.

Adverse Effects

At labeled doses, adverse effects appear to be infrequent in microfilaria-free dogs, including breeds susceptible to neurologic toxicity (see Overdosage below). In a recent study where dogs of breeds susceptible to the *ABCB1* mutation were given milbemycin at doses from 1–2.2 mg/kg PO daily, all *ABCB1* mutant/mutant dogs experienced CNS toxicity, while no *ABCB1* wild-type/wild-type or *ABCB1* mutant/wild-type dogs experienced toxicity (Barbet *et al*. 2009).

Eight week old puppies receiving 2.5 mg/kg (5X label) for 3 consecutive days showed no clinical signs after the first day, but after the second or third consecutive dose, showed some ataxia and trembling.

Reproductive/Nursing Safety

The manufacturer states that safety in breeding, pregnant, and lactating queens and breeding toms has not been established.

Studies in pregnant dogs at daily doses 3X those labeled showed no adverse effects to offspring or bitch.

Milbemycin does enter maternal milk; at standard doses, no adverse effects have been noted in nursing puppies.

Overdosage/Acute Toxicity

Beagles have tolerated a single oral dose of 200 mg/kg (200 times monthly rate). Rough-coated collies have tolerated doses of 10 mg/kg (20 times labeled) without adversity. Toxic doses can cause mydriasis, hypersalivation, lethargy, ataxia, pyrexia, seizures, coma and death. There is no specific antidotal treatment and supportive therapy is recommended.

Drug Interactions

The manufacturer states that the drug was used safely during testing in dogs receiving other frequently used veterinary products, including vaccines, anthelmintics, antibiotics, steroids, flea collars, shampoos and dips.

The following drug interactions have either been reported or are theoretical in humans or animals receiving GABA agonists and may be of significance in veterinary patients:

■ **BENZODIAZEPINES:** Effects may be potentiated by milbemycin; use together not advised in humans

Caution is advised if using other drugs that can inhibit **p-glycoprotein** particularly in those dogs at risk for *ABCB1*-1Δ (formerly MDR1-allele) mutation (Collies, Australian Shepherds,

Shelties, Long-haired Whippet, etc. "white feet"), unless tested "normal": Drugs and drug classes involved include:

- ☒ **AMIODARONE**
- ☒ **AZOLE ANTIFUNGALS (e.g., ketoconazole)**
- ☒ **CARVEDILOL**
- ☒ **CYCLOSPORINE**
- ☒ **DILTIAZEM**
- ☒ **ERYTHROMYCIN; CLARITHROMYCIN**
- ☒ **QUINIDINE**
- ☒ **SPIRONOLACTONE**
- ☒ **TAMOXIFEN**
- ☒ **VERAPAMIL**

Doses

- ☒ **DOGS:**

For prophylaxis and treatment of dirofilariasis it is suggested to review the guidelines published by the American Heartworm Society at www.heartwormsociety.org for more information

As a parasiticide:

a) For heartworm prophylaxis, control of adult hookworms (*A. caninum*), adult roundworms (*T. canis, T. leonina*) and whipworms (*Trichuris vulpis*) in dogs 4 weeks of age or older and at least 2 lbs. body weight: Minimum dosage is 0.5 mg/kg PO once a month. (Label information; *Interceptor®*—Novartis)

b) 0.5–0.99 mg/kg PO once monthly (also controls hookworm, roundworm and whipworm infestations) (Calvert 1994)

c) For control of fleas (prevents egg development), heartworm prophylaxis, control of adult hookworms (*A. caninum*), adult roundworms (*T. canis, T. leonina*) and whipworms (*Trichuris vulpis*) in dogs 4 weeks of age or older and at least 2 lbs. body weight: Minimum dosage is 0.5 mg/kg PO once a month. (Label directions; *Sentinel®*—Novartis) [**Note:** when used with nitenpyram (*Capstar®*) adult fleas are controlled as well]

For microfilaricide chemotherapy:

a) In adulticide-pretreated dogs: Use preventative/prophylaxis dosage; repeat in 2 weeks if necessary. If heartworm transmission season has started, continue monthly prophylaxis. (Knight 1995)

b) In adulticide-pretreated dogs: Approximately one month after melarsomine give milbemycin at 0.5 mg/kg PO. (Legendre & Toal 2000)

For treatment of generalized demodicosis:

a) Recommend a microfilaria check prior to therapy. Begin at a dose of 1 mg/kg/day PO with a skin scraping after 30 days. If minimal improvement is seen, the dosage should be increased to 2 mg/kg. If no

improvement is seen after a second thirty days, either an increase to 3 mg/kg/day of milbemycin can be tried or an alternative therapy should be used. Most clients will not be able to afford this drug if it is priced at the monthly heartworm preventative price. Ivermectin sensitive breeds may be able to tolerate this therapy better than ivermectin, but side effects still can be seen that include ataxia, tremors and stupor. Dogs homozygous for the MDR1-1 delta gene mutation can show neurologic side effects at doses between 1 and 2.2 mg/kg/day. (Merchant 2009)

For treatment of cheyletiellosis:

a) 2 mg/kg PO every 7 days for 3 doses (White 2000)

For treatment of scabies:

a) 2 mg/kg PO every 7 days for 3 doses or 0.75 mg/kg once daily for 30 days (White 2000)

For chronic rhinitis caused by (*Pneumonyssus caninum*):

a) 1 mg/kg PO once every 10 days for 3 treatments. (Kuehn 2010)

- ☒ **CATS:**

For prevention of heartworm; treat adult hookworm and adult roundworms:

a) 2 mg/kg PO once monthly (Label directions; *Interceptor® Flavor Tabs for Cats*—Novartis)

- ☒ **REPTILES:**

For nematodes:

a) 0.5–1 mg/kg PO; repeat in 2 weeks. If 14 days after second dose, fecal is positive a third dose is given and the cycle continued until parasites are cleared. Milbemycin appears to be safe in chelonians (unlike ivermectin). (de la Navarre 2003)

Client Information

- ☒ Review importance of compliance with therapy and to be certain that the dose was consumed.

Chemistry/Synonyms

Milbemycin oxime consists of approximately 80% of the A_4 derivatives and 20% of the A_3 derivatives of 5-didehydromilbemycin. Milbemycin is considered to be a macrolide antibiotic structurally.

Milbemycin may also be known as CGA-179246, *Interceptor®* and *Sentinel®*.

Storage/Stability

Store milbemycin oxime tablets at room temperature.

Dosage Forms/Regulatory Status

VETERINARY-LABELED PRODUCTS:

Milbemycin Oxime Oral Tablets: 2.3 mg (brown, 2–10 lbs), 5.75 mg (green, 11–25 lbs), 11.5 mg (yellow, 26–50 lbs), 23 mg (white,

51–100 lbs), dogs >100 lbs are provided the appropriate combination of tablets; *Interceptor® Flavor Tabs*; (Novartis); (Rx). FDA-approved for use in dogs and puppies >4 weeks of age and 2 lbs or greater.

Milbemycin Oxime Oral Tablets: 5.75 mg (1.5–6 lbs), 11.5 mg (6.1–12 lbs), 23 mg (white, 12.1–25 lbs); *Interceptor® Flavor Tabs*; (Novartis); (Rx). FDA-approved for cats and kittens >6 wks old and >1.5 lbs.

Milbemycin/Lufenuron Oral Tablets (with Nitenpyram Oral Tablets in the combination flea management system) for Dogs:

For dogs 2–10 lb: 46 mg milbemycin/lufeneron, (11.4 mg nitenpyram)

For dogs 11–25 lb: 115 mg milbemycin/lufenuron, (11.4 mg nitenpyram)

For dogs 26–50 lb: 230 mg milbemycin/lufenuron, (57 mg nitenpyram)

For dogs 51–100 lb: 460 mg milbemycin/lufenuron, (57 mg nitenpyram)

For dogs 100–125 lb: (appropriate number supplied) milbemycin/lufenuron, (57 mg nitenpyram)

Sentinel® Flavor Tabs & Sentinel® Flavor Tabs with Capstar® Flea Management System (Novartis); (Rx). FDA-approved for use in dogs and puppies 4 weeks of age or older.

There is also a milbemycin 0.1% otic solution (*Milbemite®*) available.

HUMAN-LABELED PRODUCTS: None

References

Barbet, J.L., T. Snook, et al. (2009). ABCB1–1 Delta (MDR1–1 Delta) genotype is associated with adverse reactions in dogs treated with milbemycin oxime for generalized demodicosis. Veterinary Dermatology 20(2): 111–114.

Calvert, C. (1994). Heartworm Disease. Saunders Manual of Small Animal Practice. S Birchard and R Sherding Eds. Philadelphia, W.B. Saunders Company: 487–493.

de la Navarre, B. (2003). Common parasitic diseases of reptiles and amphibians. Proceedings: Western Veterinary Conf. Accessed via: Veterinary Information Network. http://goo.gl/ZafJD

Knight, D. (1995). Guidelines for diagnosis and management of heartworm (Dirofilaria Immitis) infection. Kirk's Current Veterinary Therapy:XII. J Bonagura Ed. Philadelphia, W.B. Saunders: 879–887.

Kuehn, N. (2010). Chronic Nasal Disease in Dogs: Diagnosis & Treatment. Proceedings: ACVIM. Accessed via: Veterinary Information Network. http://goo.gl/2OQgm

Legendre, A. & R. Toal (2000). Diagnosis and Treatment of Fungal Diseases of the Respiratory System. Kirk's Current Veterinary Therapy: XIII Small Animal Practice. J Bonagura Ed. Philadelphia, WB Saunders: 815–819.

Merchant, S. (2009). Demodicosis in the Dog: Diagnosis and Management. Proceedings: ACVC. Accessed via: Veterinary Information Network. http://goo.gl/Jk0zX

White, S. (2000). Veterinary Dermatology: New Treatments, 'New' Diseases. Proceedings: The North American Veterinary Conference, Orlando.

Milk Thistle—see Silymarin

MILTEFOSINE

(mil-*tef*-oh-seen)   Milteforan®

ANTILEISHMANIAL

Prescriber Highlights

▶ Oral treatment for canine leishmaniasis

▶ Not available commercially in USA (human orphan drug)

▶ Vomiting very common

▶ Like other drugs, unlikely to fully clear the organism, but can reduce clinical implications

▶ Appears to be more effective when used with allopurinol

Uses/Indications

Originally developed as an antineoplastic agent, miltefosine can be used alone or with allopurinol to treat canine leishmaniasis (CanL). Like other drugs, it does not completely clear the organism in dogs, but can substantially reduce the parasitic load. Clinical efficacy is improved when used with allopurinol.

Pharmacology/Actions

While the exact mechanism of action for miltefosine against *Leishmania infantum* is not understood, it is thought that it inhibits the penetration of the organism into macrophages by interacting with glycosomes and glycosylphosphatidyl-inositol anchors that are essential for the survival of Leishmania intracellularly. Also by inhibiting phospholipase, miltefosine disrupts Leishmania membrane signal transduction. Miltefosine also has antineoplastic, immunomodulatory, and antiviral activity.

Pharmacokinetics

After oral administration in dogs, miltefosine has a bioavailability of 94% with peak plasma levels occurring around 5 hours post-dose. The drug is distributed throughout the major organs, including the brain. Intravascularly, it is approximately equally distributed in the plasma and erythrocytes. Miltefosine is mainly eliminated via the feces, with approximately 10% of a dose eliminated unchanged. Renal elimination appears negligible. Miltefosine has a very long half-life of around 6.5 days.

Contraindications/Precautions/Warnings

Miltefosine is labeled as contraindicated in patients hypersensitive to it and in pregnant, lactating or breeding animals.

Use with caution in patients with severe hepatic dysfunction. Do not under dose as it may increase the risk for drug resistance to occur.

Adverse Effects

Vomiting is the most common adverse effect seen in dogs. Other GI signs (inappetence, diarrhea) may also be seen. Miltefosine potentially may cause nephrotoxicity and/or hepatotoxicity, but as leishmaniasis can cause kidney and liver damage, it is difficult to ascribe any specific risk for these potential adverse effects in dogs. One study in healthy Beagles, found that 2 mg/kg/day PO of miltefosine in 8 dogs did not cause renal tubular damage, but 100 mg/kg/day SC of meglumine antimoniate caused severe tubular damage (cell necrosis and apoptosis) (Bianciardi *et al.* 2009).

In humans, the most common (>10%) adverse effects are vomiting, diarrhea and an increase in liver enzymes. Nephrotoxicity has also been reported in humans treated with miltefosine for leishmaniasis.

Reproductive/Nursing Safety

Miltefosine is labeled as contraindicated in pregnant, lactating and breeding animals and during pregnancy and breastfeeding in humans. When pregnant rats were dosed at 1.2 mg/kg/day and higher during the early embryonic development (up to day 7 of pregnancy), an increased risk for embryotoxic, fetotoxic and teratogenic effects was determined. In pregnant rabbits given 2.4 mg/kg/day and higher during the organogenesis phase, embryotoxic and fetotoxic effects were also seen.

Male rats given miltefosine daily at 8.25 mg/kg showed testicular atrophy and impaired fertility; this was reversible within 10 weeks.

It is not known if miltefosine is excreted into milk. The canine and human labels state that it should not be used in nursing mothers.

Overdosage/Acute Toxicity

Overdoses likely would cause GI signs (vomiting, etc.). Potentially, hepatic, renal, and retinal toxicity are possible in large overdoses. A specific antidote for miltefosine overdose is not known.

Drug Interactions

No drug interactions have been reported for miltefosine at present.

Laboratory Considerations

■ No specific concerns noted.

Doses

■ **DOGS:**

For canine leishmaniasis:

a) The product should be administered at 2 mg/kg PO, poured onto food, with a full or partial meal once a day for 28 days. (From the translated label Information—*Milteforan®*; Virbac-France)

b) As an alternative treatment to meglumine antimoniate and allopurinol: Miltefosine 2 mg/kg PO once daily for 28 days with allopurinol (10 mg/kg PO q12h, orally for at least 6 months). (Zini 2010)

Monitoring

■ Baseline and periodic renal function and hepatic enzymes

■ Adverse effects (especially vomiting); patient weight

Client Information

■ Give with food, to help reduce the chance for vomiting

■ If vomiting or severe diarrhea occur, contact veterinarian

■ Wear disposable gloves when administering this product as it has caused skin reactions

■ Because this drug has caused birth defects, it should not be handled by pregnant women

■ Do not allow treated dogs to lick persons immediately after intake of the medication

■ To avoid foaming, do not shake the vial

Chemistry/Synonyms

Miltefosine is a phospholipid derivative (alkylphosphocholine) that is structurally related to the phospholipid components of cell membranes. The commercially available canine product (*Milteforan®*) is a clear, colorless, viscous solution containing 20 mg/mL of miltefosine. Excipients in the solution include hydroxypropylcellulose, propylene glycol, and water.

Miltefosine may also be known as D-18506, HDPC, hexadecilfosfocolina, hexadecylphosphocholine, miltefosiini, miltefosina, miltéfosine, or miltefosinum. Trade names include: *Milteforan®*, *Miltex®* and *Impavido®*.

Storage/Stability

This veterinary medicinal product does not require any special storage conditions. Avoid freezing the solution.

Dosage Forms/Regulatory Status

VETERINARY-LABELED PRODUCTS:

None in the USA. Elsewhere, a canine licensed product may be available. Miltefosine Oral Solution: 20 mg/mL in 30 mL, 50 mL & 90 mL vials; *Milteforan®* (Virbac); (Rx)

HUMAN-LABELED PRODUCTS:

Impavido® is approved as an orphan drug by FDA. In countries where leishmaniasis in humans is endemic, 10 mg and 50 mg capsules (*Impavido®*) may be marketed.

References

Bianciardi, P., C. Brovida, et al. (2009). Administration of Miltefosine and Meglumine Antimoniate in Healthy Dogs: Clinicopathological Evaluation of the Impact on the Kidneys. *Toxicologic Pathology* 37(6): 770–775.

Zini, E. (2010). Canine Leishmaniasis–Challenging Treatment of a Multifaceted Disease. Proceedings: ECVIM. http://goo.gl/X6q3S

MINERAL OIL

White Petrolatum

LUBRICANT LAXATIVE

Prescriber Highlights

▶ Lubricant laxative

▶ Cautions: Debilitated or pregnant patients, & patients with hiatal hernia, dysphagia, esophageal or gastric retention

▶ Use caution when administering by tube to avoid aspiration

▶ Adverse Effects: Lipid pneumonitis if aspirated; granulomatous reactions in liver etc. if significant amounts are absorbed from gut; oil leakage from the anus; long-term use may lead to decreased absorption of fat-soluble vitamins (A, D, E, & K)

▶ Drug interactions

Uses/Indications

Mineral oil is commonly used in horses to treat constipation and fecal impactions. It is also employed as a laxative in other species as well, but used less frequently. Mineral oil has been administered after ingesting lipid-soluble toxins (e.g., kerosene, metaldehyde) to retard the absorption of these toxins through its laxative and solubility properties.

Petrolatum containing products (e.g., Felaxin®, Laxatone®, Kat-A-Lax®, etc.) may be used in dogs and cats as a laxative or to prevent/reduce "hair-balls" in cats.

Pharmacology/Actions

Mineral oil and petrolatum act as laxatives by lubricating fecal material and the intestinal mucosa. They also reduce reabsorption of water from the GI tract, thereby increasing fecal bulk and decreasing intestinal transit time.

Pharmacokinetics

It has been reported that after oral administration, emulsions of mineral oil may be up to 60% absorbed, but most reports state that mineral oil preparations are only minimally absorbed from the gut.

Contraindications/Precautions/Warnings

No specific contraindications were noted with regard to veterinary patients. In humans, mineral oil (orally administered) is considered contraindicated in patients less than 6 yrs. old, debilitated or pregnant patients, and patients with hiatal hernia, dysphagia, esophageal or gastric retention. Use caution when administering by tube to avoid aspiration, especially in debilitated or recalcitrant animals. To avoid aspiration in small animals, orally administered mineral oil should not be attempted when there is an increased risk of vomiting, regurgitation, or other preexisting swallowing difficulty. Many clinicians believe that mineral oil should not be administered orally to small animals due to the risk for aspiration and, if used as a laxative, should be administered rectally.

Adverse Effects

When used on a short-term basis and at recommended doses, mineral oil or petrolatum should cause minimal adverse effects. The most serious effect that could be encountered is aspiration of the oil with resultant lipid pneumonitis; prevent this by using the drug only in appropriate cases, when "tubing", ascertain that the tube is in the stomach, and administrate the oil at a reasonable rate.

Granulomatous reactions have occurred in the liver, spleen and mesenteric lymph nodes when significant quantities of mineral oil are absorbed from the gut. Oil leakage from the anus may occur and be of concern in animals with rectal lesions or in house pets. Long-term administration of mineral oil/petrolatum may lead to decreased absorption of fat-soluble vitamins (A, D, E, and K). No reports were found documenting clinically significant hypovitaminosis in cats receiving long-term petrolatum therapy, however.

Reproductive/Nursing Safety

In humans, the FDA categorizes this drug as category C for use during pregnancy (Animal studies have shown an adverse effect on the fetus, but there are no adequate studies in humans; or there are no animal reproduction studies and no adequate studies in humans.)

Oral mineral oil should be safe to use during nursing.

Overdosage/Acute Toxicity

No specific information was located regarding overdoses of mineral oil; but it would be expected that with the exception of aspiration, the effects would be self-limiting. See adverse effects section for more information.

Drug Interactions

The following drug interactions have either been reported or are theoretical in humans or animals receiving mineral oil and may be of significance in veterinary patients:

■ DOCUSATE: Theoretically, mineral oil should not be given with docusate (DSS) as enhanced absorption of the mineral oil could occur. However, this does not appear to be of significant clinical concern with large animals.

■ VITAMINS A, D, E, K: Chronic administration of mineral oil may affect Vitamin K and other fat-soluble vitamin absorption. It has been recommended to administer mineral oil products between meals to minimize this problem.

Doses

■ **DOGS:**

Note: Because of the risk for aspiration, liquid mineral oil is rarely recommended for PO administration today.

As a laxative:

a) 2–60 mL PO (Jenkins 1988; Kirk 1989)

b) 5–30 mL PO (Davis 1985)

c) 5–25 mL PO (Burrows 1986)

■ **CATS:**

Note: Because of the risk for aspiration, liquid mineral oil is rarely recommended for PO administration today.

As a laxative (See specific label directions for "Cat Laxative" Products):

a) 2–10 mL PO (Jenkins 1988), (Kirk 1989)

b) 2–6 mL PO (Davis 1985)

c) 5 mL per day with food (Sherding 1989)

■ **RABBITS, RODENTS, SMALL MAMMALS:**

a) **Rabbits:** As a laxative/remove hairballs: Using feline laxative product: 1–2 mL/day for 3–5 days (Ivey & Morrisey 2000)

■ **CATTLE:**

Note: Administer via stomach tube.

As a laxative:

a) 1–4 liters (Howard 1986)

b) Adults: 0.5–2 liters; Calves: 60–120 mL (Jenkins 1988)

For adjunctive treatment of metaldehyde poisoning:

a) 8 mL/kg; may be used with a saline cathartic (Smith 1986)

For adjunctive treatment of nitrate poisoning:

a) 1 liter per 400 kg body weight (Osweiler & Ruhr 1986)

■ **HORSES:**

As a laxative (Administer via stomach tube):

a) For large colon impactions: 2–4 quarts q12–24 hours, may take up to 5 gallons. Mix 1–2 quarts of warm water with the oil to ease administration and give more fluid to the horse. Pumping in at a moderate speed is desirable over gravity flow. (Sellers & Lowe 1987)

b) For sand colic: In this experimental study, 0.5 kg psyllium was mixed with 1 liter of mash and given twice daily and 2 liters of mineral oil via NG tube were administered once daily. This combination was more effective (measured ash content of feces) than giving mineral oil alone. (Hotwagner, 2008)

c) Adults: 2–4 liters, may be repeated daily; Foals: 240 mL (Clark, 1987)

d) Adults: 0.5–2 liters; Foals: 60–120 mL (Jenkins 1988)

■ **SWINE:**

a) As a laxative: 50–100 mL; administer via stomach tube (Howard 1986)

■ **SHEEP & GOATS:**

a) As a laxative: 100–500 mL; administer via stomach tube (Howard 1986)

■ **BIRDS:**

Use as a laxative and to aid in the removal of lead from the gizzard:

a) 1–3 drops per 30 grams of body weight or 5 mL/kg PO once. Repeat as necessary. Give via tube or slowly to avoid aspiration. (Clubb 1986)

Monitoring

■ Clinical efficacy

■ If possibility of aspiration: auscultate, radiograph if necessary

Client Information

■ Follow veterinarian's instructions or label directions for "cat laxative" products.

■ Do not increase dosage or prolong treatment beyond veterinarian's recommendations.

Chemistry/Synonyms

Mineral oil, also known as liquid petrolatum, liquid paraffin or white mineral oil occurs as a tasteless, odorless (when cold), transparent, colorless, oily liquid that is insoluble in both water and alcohol. It is a mixture of complex hydrocarbons and is derived from crude petroleum. For pharmaceutical purposes, heavy mineral oil is recommended over light mineral oil, as it is believed to have a lesser tendency to be absorbed in the gut or aspirated after oral administration.

White petrolatum, also known as white petroleum jelly or white soft paraffin, occurs as a white or faintly yellow unctuous mass. It is insoluble in water and almost insoluble in alcohol. White petrolatum differs from petrolatum only in that it is further refined to remove more of the yellow color.

Mineral Oil may also be known as: liquid paraffin, 905 (mineral hydrocarbons), dickflussiges paraffin, heavy liquid petrolatum, huile de vaseline epaisse, liquid petrolatum, oleum petrolei, oleum vaselini, paraffinum liquidum, paraffinum subliquidum, vaselinol, vaselinum liquidum, and white mineral oil; many trade names are available.

Storage/Stability

Petrolatum products should be stored at temperatures less than 30°C.

Dosage Forms/Regulatory Status

VETERINARY-LABELED PRODUCTS:

Mineral oil products have not been formally FDA-approved for use in food animals. These products and preparations are available without a prescription (OTC).

Petrolatum Oral Preparations

Liquid Mineral Oil: available in gallons or 55 gallon drums.

Cat "Laxative" Products: Products may vary

in actual composition; some contain liquid petrolatum in place of white petrolatum and may have various flavors (tuna, caviar, malt, etc.). Trade names include (not necessarily complete): *Laxatone®*, *Laxa-Stat®* (Evsco and Tomlyn Health); *Vedalax®* (Vedco); *Cat Lax®* (Pharmaderm); *Vetscription® Hairball Remedy* (Sergeant's); *Hairball Preparation®* (Vet Solutions); *Hartz® Health Measures Hairball Remedy* (Hartz Mountain); *Petromalt®* (Virbac); *Petrotone®* (Butler); *Felilax®* (Vetus)

HUMAN-LABELED PRODUCTS:

Mineral Oil Liquid: in 180 mL and 473 mL; generic; (OTC)

Mineral Oil Emulsions:

There are several products available that are emulsions of mineral oil and may be more palatable for oral administration. Because of expense and with no increase in efficacy, they are used only in small animals. They may be dosed as described above, factoring in the actual percentage of mineral oil in the preparation used. Trade names include: *Kondremul® Plain* (Heritage Consumer Prod); (OTC) Various generic products are available.

References

Burrows, C.F. (1986). Constipation. *Current Veterinary Therapy IX: Small Animal Practice.* RW Kirk Ed. Philadelphia, WB Saunders: 904–908.

Clark, E.S. & J.L. Becht (1987). Clinical Pharmacology of the Gastrointestinal Tract. *Vet Clin North Am* (Equine Practice) 3(1): 101-122.

Clubb, S.L. (1986). Therapeutics: Individual and Flock Treatment Regimens. *Clinical Avian Medicine and Surgery.* GJ Harrison and LR Harrison Eds. Saunders: 327-355.

Davis, L.E. (1985). General Care of the Patient. *Handbook of Small Animal Therapeutics.* LE Davis Ed. New York, Churchill Livingstone: 1-20.

Hotwagner, K. & C. Iben (2008). Evacuation of sand from the equine intestine with mineral oil, with and without psyllium. *Journal of Animal Physiology and Animal Nutrition* 92(1): 86-91.

Howard, J.L., Ed. (1986). *Current Veterinary Therapy 2, Food Animal Practice.* Saunders.

Ivey, E. & J. Morrisey (2000). Therapeutics for Rabbits. *Vet Clin NA: Exotic Anim Pract* 3:1(Jan): 183-216.

Jenkins, W.L. (1988). Drugs affecting gastrointestinal functions. *Veterinary Pharmacology and Therapeutics 6th Ed.* NH Booth and LE McDonald Eds. Ames, ISU Press: 657- 671.

Kirk, R.W., Ed. (1989). *Current Veterinary Therapy X, Small Animal Practice.*

Osweiler, G.D. & L.P. Ruhr (1986). Plants affecting blood coagulation. *Current Veterinary Therapy: Food Animal Practice 2.* JL Howard Ed. Philadelphia, W.B. Saunders: 404-406.

Sellers, A.F. & J.E. Lowe (1987). Large Colon Impaction. *Current Therapy in Equine Medicine 2.* NE Robinson Ed. Phialdelphia, WB Saunders: 53-55.

Sherding, R.G. (1989). Diseases of the Intestines. *The Cat: Diseases and Clinical Management.* RG Sherding Ed. New York, Churchill Livingstone. 2: 955-1006.

Smith, J.A. (1986). Toxic encephalopathies in cattle. *Current Veterinary Therapy 2: Food Animal Practice.* JL Howard Ed. Philadelphia, WB Saunders: 855-86

MINOCYCLINE HCL

(mi-noe-sye-kleen)   Minocin®, Dynacin®

TETRACYCLINE ANTIBIOTIC

Prescriber Highlights

▶ Oral & parenteral tetracycline antibiotic

▶ Less likely to cause bone & teeth abnormalities than other tetracyclines, but avoid use in pregnancy & young animals

▶ May be used in patients with renal insufficiency

▶ Adverse Effects are most commonly GI-related

▶ Drug-drug; drug-lab interactions

Uses/Indications

Minocycline may be useful for treating Brucellosis (in combination with aminoglycosides), Lyme disease, and certain nosocomial infections where other more commonly used drugs are ineffective. It has been investigated as adjunctive therapy for treating hemangiosarcomas, but early results have been disappointing.

Pharmacology/Actions

Tetracyclines generally act as bacteriostatic antibiotics and inhibit protein synthesis by reversibly binding to 30S ribosomal subunits of susceptible organisms, thereby preventing binding to those ribosomes of aminoacyl transfer-RNA. Tetracyclines are believed to reversibly bind to 50S ribosomes and additionally alter cytoplasmic membrane permeability in susceptible organisms. In high concentrations, tetracyclines can also inhibit protein synthesis by mammalian cells.

As a class, the tetracyclines have activity against most mycoplasma, spirochetes (including the Lyme disease organism), Chlamydia, and Rickettsia. Against gram-positive bacteria, the tetracyclines have activity against some strains of staphylococci and streptococci, but resistance of these organisms is increasing. Gram-positive bacteria that are usually covered by tetracyclines, include *Actinomyces* spp., *Bacillus anthracis*, *Clostridium perfringens* and tetani, *Listeria monocytogenes*, and Nocardia. Among gram-negative bacteria that tetracyclines usually have *in vitro* and *in vivo* activity include *Bordetella* spp., Brucella, Bartonella, *Haemophilus* spp., *Pasturella multocida*, Shigella, and *Yersinia pestis*. Many or most strains of *E. coli*, Klebsiella, Bacteroides, Enterobacter, Proteus, and *Pseudomonas aeruginosa* are resistant to the tetracyclines.

Pharmacokinetics

Minocycline is well absorbed after oral absorption regardless of the presence of food.

Minocycline is highly lipid soluble and is distributed widely throughout the body. Therapeutic levels can be found in the CSF (whether meninges are inflamed or not), prostate, saliva, and eye. Minocycline is extensively metabolized in the liver and primarily excreted as inactive metabolites in the feces and urine. Less than 20% is excreted unchanged in the urine. The half-life in dogs is about 7 hours.

Contraindications/Precautions/Warnings

Minocycline should be considered contraindicated in patients hypersensitive to tetracyclines, those that are pregnant or nursing, or in animals less than 6 months old. Minocycline is considered to be less likely to cause these abnormalities than other more water-soluble tetracyclines (*e.g.*, tetracycline, oxytetracycline). Unlike either oxytetracycline or tetracycline, minocycline can be used in patients with moderate renal insufficiency without dosage adjustment. Oliguric renal failure may require dosage adjustment.

Adverse Effects

The most commonly reported side effects of oral minocycline therapy in dogs and cats are nausea and vomiting. To alleviate these effects, the drug could be given with food without clinically significant reductions in drug absorption. Dental or bone staining can occur when minocycline exposure occurs in utero or in early life. More rarely, increases in hepatic enzymes and ototoxicity are possible.

IV injections of minocycline in dogs have caused urticaria, shivering, hypotension, dyspnea, cardiac arrhythmias, and shock when given rapidly. Give IV slowly.

Tetracycline therapy (especially long-term) may result in overgrowth (superinfections) of non-susceptible bacteria or fungi.

In humans, minocycline (or other tetracyclines) has also been associated with photosensitivity reactions and, rarely, hepatotoxicity or blood dyscrasias. CNS effects (dizziness, lightheadedness) have been reported in people taking minocycline. A blue-gray pigmentation of skin and mucous membranes may occur.

Reproductive/Nursing Safety

Because tetracyclines can retard fetal skeletal development and discolor deciduous teeth, they should only be used in the last half of pregnancy when the benefits outweigh the fetal risks. Minocycline has been shown to impair fertility in male rats. In humans, the FDA categorizes this drug as category *D* for use during pregnancy (*There is evidence of human fetal risk, but the potential benefits from the use of the drug in pregnant women may be acceptable despite its potential risks.*)

Tetracyclines are excreted in milk. Milk:plasma ratios vary between 0.25 and 1.5. While minocycline probably has less effect on teeth and bones than other tetracyclines, its use should be avoided during nursing.

Overdosage/Acute Toxicity

Minocycline oral overdoses would most likely be associated with GI disturbances (vomiting, anorexia, and/or diarrhea). Although it is less vulnerable to chelation with cations than other tetracyclines, oral administration of divalent or trivalent cation antacids may bind some of the drug and reduce GI distress. Should the patient develop severe emesis or diarrhea, fluids and electrolytes should be monitored and replaced if necessary.

Drug Interactions

The following drug interactions have either been reported or are theoretical in humans or animals receiving minocycline and may be of significance in veterinary patients:

■ **ANTACIDS, ORAL:** When orally administered, tetracyclines can chelate divalent or trivalent cations that can decrease the absorption of the tetracycline or the other drug if it contains these cations. Oral antacids, saline cathartics, or other GI products containing aluminum, calcium, magnesium, zinc, or bismuth cations are most commonly associated with this interaction. Minocycline has a relatively low affinity for divalent or trivalent cations, but it is recommended that all oral tetracyclines be given at least 1–2 hours before or after the cation-containing product.

■ **BISMUTH SUBSALICYLATE, KAOLIN, PECTIN:** May reduce absorption

■ **IRON, ORAL:** Oral iron products are associated with decreased tetracycline absorption, and administration of iron salts should preferably be given 3 hours before or 2 hours after the tetracycline dose.

■ **ISOTRETINOIN:** When used with minocycline may increase the risk for nervous system effects

■ **PENICILLINS:** Bacteriostatic drugs, like the tetracyclines, may interfere with bactericidal activity of the penicillins, cephalosporins, and aminoglycosides. There is a fair amount of controversy regarding the actual clinical significance of this interaction, however.

■ **WARFARIN:** Tetracyclines may depress plasma prothrombin activity and patients on anticoagulant therapy may need dosage adjustment.

Laboratory Considerations

■ Tetracyclines reportedly can cause false-positive **urine glucose** results if using the cupric sulfate method of determination (Benedict's reagent, *Clinitest®*), but this may be the result of ascorbic acid that is found in some parenteral formulations of tetracyclines.

■ Tetracyclines reportedly have caused false-negative results in determining **urine glucose** when using the glucose oxidase method (*Clinistix®, Tes-Tape®*).

Doses

■ **DOGS:**

a) For susceptible soft tissue and urinary tract infections: 5–12 mg/kg PO or IV q12h for 7–14 days. (Greene *et al.* 2006)

b) For Brucellosis: Gentamicin 5 mg/kg SC once daily (q24h) for 7 days; 2-courses of treatment, treating on weeks one and four; plus Minocycline at 25 mg/kg PO once daily (q24h) for 4 weeks. Eventually, doxycycline can be substituted for minocycline at the same dosage to lower cost. Infected animals may need to be treated for two or more 4-week courses. Sequential antibody tests at 3 to 6 monthly intervals are recommended to monitor treatment. Monitor renal function secondary to gentamicin therapy. (Hartmannn & Greene 2005)

c) For adjunctive treatment of Nocardiosis, Actinomycosis: 5–25 mg/kg PO, IV q12h (Lemarie 2003)

d) For Brucellosis in animals that are housed singly and neutered: Minocycline at 25 mg/kg PO once daily for 14 days with dihydrostreptomycin (**Note:** not currently available in the USA) at 5 mg/kg IM twice daily for 7 days. (Root Kustritz 2007)

e) For Ehrlichiosis (*E. canis*) in dogs with a positive test result and clinical signs consistent with the infection: 10 mg/kg PO (rarely IV) q12h for 28 days. (Ford 2009)

■ **CATS:**

a) For hemotropic mycoplasmosis: 6–11 mg/kg PO q12h for 21 days. (Greene *et al.* 2006)

b) For adjunctive treatment atypical mycobacterial dermal infections: 5–12.5 mg/kg PO, IV q12h (Hnilica 2003)

c) For adjunctive treatment of Nocardiosis, Actinomycosis: 5–25 mg/kg PO, IV q12h (Lemarie 2003)

d) For susceptible mycobacterial, L-Forms, or mycoplasma infections: 5–12.5 mg/kg PO q12h. (Bonenberger 2009)

Monitoring

■ Clinical efficacy

■ Adverse effects

Client Information

■ Oral minocycline products may be administered without regard to feeding. Milk or other dairy products do not significantly alter the amount of minocycline absorbed.

■ Give as prescribed for as long as veterinarian recommends even if animal appears well.

Chemistry/Synonyms

A semisynthetic tetracycline, minocycline HCl occurs as a yellow, crystalline powder. It is soluble in water and slightly soluble in alcohol.

Minocycline may also be known as: minocyclini hydrochloridum, *Asolmicina®*, *Cyclimycin®*, *Cyclomin®*, *Dermirex®*, *Meibi®*, *Minogal®*, and *Minox®*; many other trade names are available.

Storage/Stability

Store the oral preparations at room temperature in tight containers. Do not freeze the oral suspension. The injectable should be stored at room temperature and protected from light. After reconstituting with sterile water for injection, solutions with a concentration of 20 mg/mL are stable for 24 hours at room temperature.

Compatibility/Compounding Considerations

While minocycline is **compatible** with the usual intravenous fluids (including Ringer's and lactated Ringer's) do not add any other calcium containing fluid as precipitation could result.

Dosage Forms/Regulatory Status

VETERINARY-LABELED PRODUCTS: None

HUMAN-LABELED PRODUCTS:

Minocycline HCl Oral Tablets: 50 mg, 75 mg & 100 mg; Extended-Release: 45 mg, 65 mg, 90 mg, 115 mg & 135 mg; *Dynacin®* (Medicis); *Myrac®* (Glades); *Solodyn®* (Medicis); generic; (Rx)

Minocycline HCl Oral Capsules: 50 mg, 75 mg & 100 mg; *Dynacin®* (Medicis); generic; (Rx)

Minocycline HCl Pellet-filled Oral Capsules: 50 mg & 100 mg; *Minocin®* (Lederle); (Rx)

Minocycline HCl Oral Suspension: 50 mg/5 mL in 60 mL; *Minocin®* (Lederle); (Rx)

Minocycline HCl Powder for Injection lyophilized for solution: 100 mg in vials; *Minocin®* (Triax); (Rx)

Minocycline HCl Powdered Microspheres, Extended-Release, dental: 1 mg; *Arestin®* (Cord Logistics); (Rx)

References

Bonenberger, T. (2009). Typical Cat Bite Abscess, or Not: Chronic Draining Tracts & Nodules. Proceedings: WVC. Accessed via: Veterinary Information Network. http://goo.gl/sNkTB

Ford, R. (2009). Tick-Borne Disease Diagnosis: Moving from 3Dx to 4Dx. Proceedings: ACVC. Accessed via: Veterinary Information Network. http://goo.gl/0Pb6s

Greene, C., K. Hartmannn, et al. (2006). Appendix 8: Antimicrobial Drug Formulary. *Infectious Disease of the Dog and Cat.* C Greene Ed., Elsevier: 1186–1333.

Hartmannn, K. & C. Greene (2005). Diseases caused by systemic bacterial infections. *Textbook of Veterinary Internal Medicine, 6th Ed.* S Ettinger and E Feldman Eds., Elsevier: 616–631.

Hnilica, K. (2003). Atypical presentations in feline dermatology. Proceedings: Western Veterinary Conf. Accessed via: Veterinary Information Network. http://goo.gl/Brs6Q

Lemarie, S. (2003). Cutaneous mycobacterium, nocardia and actinomyces. Proceedings Western Veterinary Conf. http://goo.gl/xhbNj

Root Kustritz, M. (2007). Canine Brucellosis. Proceedings: Western Vet Conf. Accessed via: Veterinary Information Network. http://goo.gl/GQJgb

MIRTAZAPINE

(mir-*taz*-ah-peen)   Remeron®

TETRACYCLIC ANTIDEPRESSANT;
5-HT3 ANTAGONIST

Prescriber Highlights

▶ Used in veterinary medicine primarily
   as an appetite stimulant & antiemetic
   in dogs & cats

▶ Can be used in conjunction with other
   antiemetics

▶ Primary side effect is sedation. In cats
   vocalization and increased affection
   can be noted.

▶ Use lowest effective dose to reduce
   sedative properties

▶ Do not exceed 30 mg per day when
   used for appetite stimulation

Uses/Indications

Veterinary uses of mirtazapine include treatment of chemotherapy-induced nausea and vomiting (CINV); anorexia associated with renal failure (azotemia), congestive heart failure, gastro-intestinal disorders, liver disease, or neoplasia. Other suggested uses include stress induced diseases; insomnia; post-pyometra symptoms; and post-operative inappetence.

Pharmacology/Actions

The antidepressant activity of mirtazapine appears to be mediated by antagonism at central pre-synaptic alpha$_2$-receptors, which normally acts as a negative feedback mechanism that inhibits further norepinephrine (NE) release. By blocking these receptors, mirtazapine overcomes the negative feedback loop and results in a net increase in NE. This mechanism may also contribute to the appetite stimulating effects of the medication since NE acts at other a-receptors to increase appetite. Additionally, mirtazapine antagonizes several serotonin (5HT) receptor subtypes. The drug is a potent inhibitor of the 5HT$_2$ and 5HT$_3$ receptors and of histamine (H$_1$) receptors. Antagonism at the 5HT$_3$ receptors accounts for the anti-nausea and antiemetic effects of the drug, and its action at H$_1$-receptors produces prominent sedative effects. It is a moderate peripheral alpha$_1$ adrenergic antagonist, a property that may explain the occasional orthostatic hypotension associated with its use; it is a moderate antagonist of muscarinic receptors, which may explain the relatively low incidence of anticholinergic effects.

Pharmacokinetics

In cats after oral dosing of either 1.88 mg (low dose; LD) or 3.75 mg (high dose, HD), mean elimination half-lives were between 10.2–15.4 hours. Mean clearance was 10.5 mL/kg/min (LD) and 18 mL/kg/min (HD). A single low

dose of mirtazapine was well tolerated and resulted in a half-life that is compatible with 24 hour dosing intervals in healthy cats (Quimby *et al.* 2009).

Following oral administration in humans, mirtazapine is rapidly and completely absorbed. Studies in rats showed a linear relationship between the effects of mirtazapine and measured plasma and brain concentrations. Peak plasma concentrations are reached within about 2 hours after an oral dose in humans. Food has minimal effects on both the rate and extent of absorption and does not require adjustments in the dose. Oral bioavailability of mirtazapine is about 20% for rats and dogs, and about 50% for humans.

Mirtazapine is metabolized via multiple pathways and varies by species. In all species tested (humans and laboratory animals), the drug was metabolized via the following mechanisms: 8-hydroxlaton followed by conjugation, N-oxidation, and demethylation followed by conjugation. Humans and guinea pigs also produce metabolites via N+-glucuronidation, whereas mice were the only species found to utilize demethylation followed by CO_2 addition and conjugation, and 13-hydroxylation followed by conjugation as methods of mirtazapine breakdown. These processes are conducted primarily by CYP2D6, CYP1A2, and CYP3A4, yet mirtazapine exerts minimal inhibition on any of these cytochromes. Several metabolic pathways of mirtazapine involve conjugation with glucuronide (glucuronidation). Since cats have a limited capacity for glucuronidation, mirtazapine is cleared less rapidly from the system and, therefore, an extended dosing may be required.

It is estimated that the active metabolite of mirtazapine contributes only 3–6% of the total pharmacodynamic profile of the drug since it is approximately 10-fold less active than mirtazapine and affects the AUC minimally. Therefore, only the levels of the parent compound are considered clinically relevant.

The extent of binding of drugs to plasma proteins sometimes differs considerably among animal species. Plasma protein binding (PPB) for mirtazapine appears to be approximately 70–72% for mice, rats, and dogs, whereas for humans and rabbits it is approximately 85%. Despite the interspecies differences in PPB, no displacement interactions or dosage adjustments for mirtazapine are expected due to its large therapeutic window and nonspecific and relative low affinity for plasma proteins.

Human literature documents that elimination occurs via the urine (75%) and the feces (15%), renal impairment may reduce elimination by 30–50% compared to normal subjects, and hepatic impairment may reduce clearance by up to 30%. Human studies show the elimination half-life of mirtazapine to be long and range from 20–40 hours across age and gender subgroups, so dosage increases should take place no sooner than every 7–14 days. Females (both human and animal) of all ages exhibit significantly longer elimination half-lives than males (mean half-life of 37 hours for females vs. 26 hours for males in humans).

Contraindications/Precautions/Warnings

Mirtazapine is contraindicated in patients with hypersensitivity to mirtazapine or who have taken monoamine oxidase inhibitors (*e.g.,* selegiline) in the past 14 days.

Mirtazapine has been associated with orthostatic hypotension in humans and should, therefore, be used with caution in patients with known cardiac disease or cerebrovascular disease that could be exacerbated by hypotension. Patients with renal impairment, renal failure, or hepatic disease should be monitored while on mirtazapine therapy.

Abrupt discontinuation of mirtazapine after long-term administration has resulted in withdrawal symptoms such as nausea, headache and malaise in humans. In general, antidepressants may affect blood glucose concentrations because of their indirect effects on the endocrine system; use with caution in patients with diabetes mellitus.

Mirtazapine exhibits very weak anticholinergic activity, consequently, vigilance should be used in patients who might be more susceptible to these effects, such as those with urinary retention, prostatic hypertrophy, acute, untreated closed-angle glaucoma or increased intraocular pressure, or GI obstruction or ileus. Also, effects of mirtazapine may be additive to anticholinergic medications.

Extra care should be taken with active animals as mirtazapine may impair concentration and alertness. Although extremely rare, mirtazapine has been associated with blood dyscrasias in humans and should be used cautiously in patients with pre-existing hematological disease, especially leukopenia, neutropenia, or thrombocytopenia.

Adverse Effects

Mirtazapine appears to be well tolerated in both dogs and cats, but use has been limited and controlled trials are lacking. Besides the desirable side effect of appetite stimulation, other currently reported side effects in animals include drowsiness/sedation, vocalization, increased affection in cats, hypotension, and tachycardia (all dose-dependent).

Reproductive/Nursing Safety

In humans, mirtazapine is FDA pregnancy category C (*animal studies have shown an adverse effect on the fetus, but there are no adequate studies in humans; or there are no animal reproduction studies and no adequate studies in humans*). However, reproductive studies in rats, rabbits, and dogs have shown no evidence of teratogenicity. Additional studies in hamsters, rabbits, and rats showed no evidence of fetal genetic mutation or reduction in parental fertility, although there were increases in post-implantation losses and pup deaths, as well as decreased pup birth weight. No fetal harm was reported in any of several case reports of mirtazapine use during pregnancy nor in animal studies.

In animals, mirtazapine is excreted in very small amounts in milk, the implications of which are currently unknown; consequently, it may be prudent to use caution in nursing mothers. Mirtazapine is distributed into human breast milk and safe use in humans during nursing cannot be assured. In one case report mirtazapine concentrations were detected in breast milk, but the examining neuropediatrician detected no adverse effects (including weight gain or sedation) in the infant.

Overdosage/Acute Toxicity

Mirtazapine ingestion of upwards of 10-fold therapeutic dose in humans exhibits minimal toxicity requiring no acute intervention and only 6 hours of observation. Similar effects were seen in patients receiving up to 30 times the recommended dose. Despite these reports, the package insert for mirtazapine recommends that activated charcoal be administered in addition to other standard monitoring activities in an overdose situation.

Drug Interactions

The following drug interactions have either been reported or are theoretical in humans or animals receiving mirtazapine and may be of significance in veterinary patients:

■ **CLONIDINE:** Mirtazapine may cause increases in blood pressure

■ **DIAZEPAM (and other benzodiazepines):** Minimal effects on mirtazapine blood levels, but may cause additive impairment of motor skills

■ **FLUVOXAMINE:** May cause increased serum concentrations of mirtazapine

■ **LINEZOLID:** Increased risk for serotonin syndrome

■ **SELEGILINE, AMITRAZ:** Increased risk for serotonin syndrome; MAO inhibitors considered contraindicated with mirtazapine

■ **TRAMADOL:** Increased risk for serotonin syndrome

In vitro studies identify mirtazapine as a substrate for several hepatic cytochrome CYP450 isoenzymes including 2D6, 1A2, and 3A4. Mirtazapine is not a potent inhibitor of any of these enzymes; clinically significant pharmacokinetic interactions are not likely with drugs metabolized by CYP enzymes.

Laboratory Considerations

■ No specific concerns noted.

Doses

Since no safety or efficacy trials have been performed in animals to date, currently recommended doses are based on extrapolations from human medicine and clinical experience in veterinary practice. According to the product package insert and several anecdotal reports, no adjustment is needed in liver disease or kidney dysfunction, although starting at the lower end of the dosage range and titrating up if needed is recommended in such situations.

Note: At doses exceeding 30 mg per day, mirtazapine loses its appetite stimulating properties in humans. Since the ceiling dose for cats and dogs is not currently known, total daily doses ≤30 mg are recommended for appetite stimulation depending upon the weight of the pet.

■ **DOGS:**

As an appetite stimulant and/or antiemetic:

a) 0.6 mg/kg PO q 24 h not to exceed 30 mg per day for appetite stimulation (Jordan 2007)

Dogs <20 lb. = 3.75 mg PO q24h;

21–50 lb. = 7.5 mg PO q 24h;

50–75 lb. = 15 mg PO q24h;

>75 lb. = 15 mg PO q12h or 30 mg PO q24h (once daily) (Jordan 2007)

■ **CATS:**

As an appetite stimulant and/or antiemetic:

a) 3.75 mg (¼ of a 15 mg tablet) PO q72h (every 3 days) (Jordan 2007)

b) 3 mg per cat PO q72h (every 3 days) (Churchill 2006)

c) 3–4 mg per cat PO q72h (every 3 days) (Scherk 2006)

Monitoring

■ Clinical efficacy measured by the following parameters: increased appetite, decreased episodes of vomiting, and weight gain

■ Adverse Effects

Client Information

■ Give only the prescribed dose.

■ Report excessive drowsiness or vocalization to your veterinarian.

■ If your animal is receiving the orally disintegrating tablets, make sure hands are dry before handling the tablet. Place the tablet under the animal's tongue and hold mouth closed for several seconds to allow it to dissolve (should occur quickly). After the tablet has melted, offer the patient water.

■ May be given without regard to food.

Chemistry/Synonyms

A member of the piperazino-azepine group of compounds, mirtazapine is classified as an atypical tetracyclic antidepressant and is not chemically related to other antidepressants. Mirtazapine, with a molecular weight of 265.36, occurs as a white to creamy white crystalline powder that is slightly soluble in water.

Mirtazapine may also be known as 6-azamianserin, Org-3770, mepirzapine and *Remeron®*;

many trade names for international products are available.

Storage/Stability

The coated tablets and the orally disintegrating tablets should be stored at 25°C (77°F) with excursions permitted to 15–30°C (59–86°F). Protect from light and moisture. The stability of the orally disintegrating tablets once removed from the tablet blister is unknown and immediate use is recommended.

Dosage Forms/Regulatory Status

VETERINARY-LABELED PRODUCTS: None

HUMAN-LABELED PRODUCTS:

Mirtazapine Oral Tablets: 7.5 mg 15 mg, 30 mg & 45 mg; *Remeron®* (Organon), generic; (Rx)

Mirtazapine Orally Disintegrating Tablets: 15 mg, 30 mg & 45 mg; *Remeron SolTab®* (Organon), generic; (Rx)

References

Churchill, J. (2006). Pleasing geriatric palates–Nutritional management of the finicky senior cat. Proceedings: AAFP Fall Meeting. Accessed via: Veterinary Information Network. http://goo.gl/p7Thu

Jordan, D. (2007, Last Update). "Personal Communication."

Quimby, J., D. Gustafson, et al. (2009). The Pharmacokinetics of Mirtazapine in Healthy Cats. Proceedings: ACVIM. Accessed via: Veterinary Information Network. http://goo.gl/9t5ll

Scherk, M. (2006). Snots and Snuffles: Chronic Feline Upper Respiratory Syndrome. Proceedings: ACVIM. Accessed via: Veterinary Information Network. http://goo.gl/tWQ49

MISOPROSTOL

(mye-soe-***prost***-ole)   Cytotec®

PROSTAGLANDIN E$_1$ ANALOG

Prescriber Highlights

▶ Prostaglandin E$_1$ analog for treating or preventing gastric ulcers, especially associated with NSAIDs; may also be useful as an abortifacient, & to treat atopy or cyclosporine-induced nephrotoxicity

▶ Contraindications: Pregnancy, nursing mothers (diarrhea in the nursing offspring)

▶ Caution: Sensitivity to prostaglandins or prostaglandin analogs; patients with cerebral or coronary vascular disease

▶ Adverse Effects: GI distress (diarrhea, abdominal pain, vomiting, & flatulence); Potentially, uterine contractions & vaginal bleeding in female dogs

▶ Pregnant women should handle with caution

Uses/Indications

Misoprostol may be useful as primary or adjunctive therapy in treating or preventing gastric ulceration, especially when caused or aggravated by non-steroidal antiinflammatory drugs (NSAIDs). Misoprostol is most useful to prevent GI ulceration or GI adverse effects (anorexia, vomiting) associated with NSAID therapy. While it can be used for treating gastric ulcers, other drugs are probably just as effective and less expensive. It does not appear to be very effective in reducing gastric ulceration secondary to high dose corticosteroid therapy.

Misoprostol may be efficacious in reducing or reversing cyclosporine-induced nephrotoxicity. More data is needed to confirm this effect.

There is some evidence for efficacy for pentoxifylline and misoprostol as antiallergic medications in dogs, but due to the modest benefits, relatively high costs and adverse effects associated with these medications, they probably should not be used as first line medications to treat dogs with atopic dermatitis (Olivry, T. *et al.* 2010).

Misoprostol's effects on uterine contractibility and cervical softening/opening make it effective as an adjunctive treatment in pregnancy termination.

Pharmacology/Actions

Misoprostol has two main pharmacologic effects that make it a potentially useful agent. By a direct action on parietal cells, it inhibits basal and nocturnal gastric acid secretion as well as gastric acid secretions that are stimulated by food, pentagastrin or histamine. Pepsin secretion is decreased under basal conditions, but not when stimulated by histamine.

Misoprostol also has a cytoprotective effect on gastric mucosa. Probably by increasing production of gastric mucosa and bicarbonate, increasing turnover and blood supply of gastric mucosal cells, misoprostol enhances mucosal defense mechanisms and healing in response to acid-related injuries.

Other pharmacologic effects of misoprostol include increased amplitude and frequency of uterine contractions, stimulating uterine bleeding, and causing total or partial expulsion of uterine contents in pregnant animals.

Pharmacokinetics

Approximately 88% of an oral dose of misoprostol is rapidly absorbed from the GI tract, but a significant amount is metabolized via the first-pass effect. The presence of food and antacids will delay the absorption of the drug. Misoprostol is rapidly de-esterified to misoprostol acid which is the primary active metabolite. Misoprostol and misoprostol acid are thought equal in their effects on gastric mucosa. Both misoprostol and the acid metabolite are fairly well bound to plasma proteins (approximately 90% bound). It is not believed that misoprostol enters maternal milk, but it is unknown whether the acid enters milk.

Misoprostol acid is further biotransformed via oxidative mechanisms to pharmacologically inactive metabolites. These metabolites, the free acid and small amounts of unchanged drug are principally excreted into the urine. In humans, the serum half-life of misoprostol is about 30 minutes and its duration of pharmacological effect is about 3–6 hours.

Contraindications/Precautions/Warnings

It should be used in patients with the following conditions only when its potential benefits outweigh the risks: Sensitivity to prostaglandins or prostaglandin analogs; patients with cerebral or coronary vascular disease (although not reported with misoprostol, some prostaglandins and prostaglandin analogs have precipitated seizures in epileptic human patients, and have caused hypotension which may adversely affect these patients).

Adverse Effects

The most prevalent adverse effect seen with misoprostol is GI distress, usually manifested by diarrhea, abdominal pain, vomiting, and flatulence. Adverse effects are often transient and resolve over several days or may be minimized by dosage adjustment or giving doses with food. Potentially, uterine contractions and vaginal bleeding could occur in female dogs.

Reproductive/Nursing Safety

Misoprostol is contraindicated during pregnancy due to its abortifacient activity. In humans, the FDA categorizes this drug as category *X* for use during pregnancy (*Studies in animals or humans demonstrate fetal abnormalities or adverse reaction; reports indicate evidence of fetal risk. The risk of use in pregnant women clearly outweighs any possible benefit.*) In a separate system evaluating the safety of drugs in canine and feline pregnancy (Papich 1989), this drug is categorized as class: *D* (*Contraindicated. These drugs have been shown to cause congenital malformations or embryotoxicity.*)

It is unlikely that misoprostol is excreted in milk because it is rapidly metabolized, however, it is not known if the active metabolite (misoprostol acid) is excreted in milk. Misoprostol is not recommended for nursing mothers as it potentially could cause significant diarrhea in the nursing offspring.

Overdosage/Acute Toxicity

There is limited information available. Overdoses in laboratory animals have produced diarrhea, GI lesions, emesis, tremors, focal cardiac, hepatic or renal tubular necrosis, seizures, and hypotension.

There were 11 exposures to misoprostol reported to the ASPCA Animal Poison Control Center (APCC) during 2008–2009. In these cases, all 11 were dogs with 4 showing clinical signs.

Overdoses should be treated seriously and standard gut emptying techniques employed when applicable. Resultant toxicity should be treated symptomatically and supportively.

Drug Interactions

The following drug interactions have either been

reported or are theoretical in humans or animals receiving misoprostol and may be of significance in veterinary patients:

■ **ANTACIDS, MAGNESIUM-CONTAINING:** Magnesium-containing antacids may aggravate misoprostol-induced diarrhea. If an antacid is required, an aluminum-only antacid may be a better choice. Antacids and food do reduce the rate of misoprostol absorption and may reduce the systemic availability, but probably do not affect therapeutic efficacy.

Doses

■ **DOGS:**
For the prevention and treatment of GI ulcers:

a) For prevention of aspirin-induced gastric injury: Study suggests that misoprostol 3 micrograms/kg PO q12h is as effective as misoprostol 3 micrograms/kg PO q8h. (Ward *et al.* 2003)

b) 2–5 micrograms/kg P0 four times daily. The main indication for misoprostol use is the prevention or treatment of gastric ulceration from NSAIDs. It is uncertain if misoprostol will improve healing of established gastric ulcers and apparently does not have distinct advantages over other antacids in treating ulcers not associated with NSAIDs. (Twedt 2008)

c) 2–5 micrograms/kg PO q8–12h (Dowling 2003; Marks 2008; Valdes 2009)

d) Major indication is preventing GI mucosal injury in dogs with arthritis that require long-term NSAID therapy; can also be used to treat cases of gastro-duodenal ulcer disease caused by NSAIDS: 3 micrograms/kg PO three times a day. (Leib 2008)

For reproductive system indications:

a) As an adjunctive therapy for the termination of mid-term pregnancy in the bitch: Pregnancy is confirmed with ultrasound and begun no sooner than 30 days after breeding. 1–3 micrograms/kg misoprostol given intravaginally once daily concurrently with prostaglandin F2alpha (*Lutalyse®*) at 0.1 mg/kg SC three times daily for 3 days and then 0.2 mg/kg SC three times daily to effect. Monitor efficacy with ultrasound. (Cain 1999)

b) For treating pyometra/metritis: Give aglepristone 10 mg/kg SC on days 1, 2, 8, 15, 29. Give misoprostol 10 micrograms/kg PO twice daily on days 3 through 12. Approximately 75% of cases show significant clinical improvement without developing the adverse effects associated with the prostaglandins (PG-F2alpha, cloprostenol). (Fontbonne 2007)

c) As part of an abortifacient protocol after mismating: Misoprostol 1–3 micro-

grams/kg once daily administered as a vaginal suppository to promote cervical dilation. This allows for a reduced dinoprost (PGF2 alpha) dose (0.1 mg/kg SC q8h for 2 days, then 0.2 mg/kg q8hh SC to effect). Abortion usually occurs after 5 days. (Shaw 2007)

As an adjunctive therapy for atopic dermatitis:

a) Target dosage of 5 micrograms/kg PO three times daily. Modest improvement in clinical signs. (Olivry, T *et al.* 2003)

b) 6 micrograms/kg q8h PO for 30 days (Campbell 1999)

■ **HORSES:**

a) For adjunctive treatment of acute colitis: 5 micrograms/kg q8h (*route not listed; assume PO—Plumb*). (Atherton *et al.* 2009)

b) For equine gastric ulcer syndrome: 5 micrograms/kg PO q8h. (Buchanan & Andrews 2003)

c) To induce cervical relaxation: From a case report of post-breeding endometritis in a maiden mare in which the cervix remained closed during estrus and acted as a barrier to uterine clearance: After uterus was lavaged and catheter removed, 1000 micrograms (total dose) of misoprostol as a compounded cream was applied to the caudal os and lumen of the cervix. Oxytocin (20 Units IM) was administered immediately following lavage and again every 6 hours until the following morning. (Nie & Barnes 2003)

Monitoring
■ Efficacy
■ Adverse effects

Client Information
■ Pregnant women should handle the drug with caution.
■ If diarrhea or other GI adverse effects become severe or persist, reduce dose or give with food or aluminum antacids to alleviate. Severe diarrheas may require supportive therapy.

Chemistry/Synonyms
A synthetic prostaglandin E_1 analog, misoprostol occurs as a yellow, viscous liquid having a musty odor.

Misoprostol may also be known as: SC-29333, *Arthotec®, Arthrotec®, Artotec®, Artrenac Pro®, Artrotec®, Condrotec®, Corrigast®, Cyprostol®, Cytotec®, Cytolog®, Diclotec®, Glefos®, Menpros®, Misodex®, Misofenac®, Napratec®, Normulen®, Oxaprost®,* and *Symbol®.*

Storage/Stability
Misoprostol tablets should be stored in well-closed containers at room temperature. After manufacture, misoprostol has an expiration date of 18 months.

Dosage Forms/Regulatory Status

VETERINARY-LABELED PRODUCTS: None

The ARCI (Racing Commissioners International) has designated this drug as a class 5 substance. See the appendix for more information.

HUMAN-LABELED PRODUCTS:

Misoprostol Tablets: 100 micrograms & 200 micrograms; *Cytotec®* (Pfizer); generic; (Rx)

References

Atherton, R., H. McKenzie, et al. (2009). Treating acute colitis. *Comp Equine*(Nov/Dec 2009): 416–427.

Buchanan, B. & F. Andrews (2003). Treatment and prevention of equine gastric ulcer syndrome. *Vet Clin Equine* **19**: 575–597.

Cain, J. (1999). Canine reproduction: Commonly referred problems. Proceedings: American College of Veterinary Internal Medicine: 17th Annual Veterinary Medical Forum, Chicago.

Campbell, K. (1999). New Drugs in Veterinary Dermatology. Proceedings: Central Veterinary Conference, Kansas City.

Dowling, P. (2003). GI Therapy: When what goes in won't stay down. Proceedings: Western Veterinary Conference. Accessed via: Veterinary Information Network. http://goo.gl/co8V8

Fontbonne, A. (2007). Anti-Progestins Compounds in Reproduction. Proceedings: World Small Animal Veterinary Association Congress. Accessed via: Veterinary Information Network. http://goo.gl/vbjmP

Leib, M.S. (2008). Drugs used to treat vomiting and upper GI diseases in dogs and cats. Proceedings: ACVC. Accessed via: Veterinary Information Network. http://goo.gl/R5KCS

Marks, S. (2008). GI Therapeutics: Which Ones and When? Proceedings: IVECCS. Accessed via: Veterinary Information Network. http://goo.gl/rxwcs

Nie, G.J. & A.J. Barnes (2003). Use of prostaglandin E-1 to induce cervical relaxation in a maiden mare with post breeding endometritis. *Equine Veterinary Education* **15**(4): 172–174.

Olivry, T., D.J. DeBoer, et al. (2010). Treatment of canine atopic dermatitis: 2010 clinical practice guidelines from the International Task Force on Canine Atopic Dermatitis. *Veterinary Dermatology* **21**(3): 233–248.

Olivry, T., S. Dunston, et al. (2003). A randomized controlled trial of misoprostol monotherapy for canine atopic dermatitis: effects on dermal cellularity and cutaneous tumor necrosis factor-alpha. *Vet Derm* **14**: 37–46.

Papich, M. (1989). Effects of drugs on pregnancy. *Current Veterinary Therapy X: Small Animal Practice*. R Kirk Ed. Philadelphia, Saunders: 1291–1299.

Shaw, S. (2007). Dealing with Reproductive Emergencies. Proceedings: IVECCS. Accessed via: Veterinary Information Network. http://goo.gl/EG5rA

Twedt, D. (2008). Antiemetics, prokinetics & antacids. Proceedings: ACVIM. Accessed via: Veterinary Information Network. http://goo.gl/bRKsO

Valdes, A. (2009). Anti-Emetics and Anti-Ulcers Drugs: When Are They Useful? Accessed via: Veterinary Information Network. http://goo.gl/W6fu6

Ward, D.M., M.S. Leib, et al. (2003). The effect of dosing interval on the efficacy of misoprostol in the prevention of aspirin-induced gastric injury. *Journal of Veterinary Internal Medicine* **17**(3): 282–290.

MITOTANE

(*mye*-toe-tane)   Lysodren®, o,p'–DDD

ADRENAL CYTOTOXIC;
ANTINEOPLASTIC

Prescriber Highlights

▶ Adrenal cytotoxic agent used for medical treatment of pituitary-dependent hyperadrenocorticism

▶ Caution: Pregnancy, diabetes, & preexisting renal or hepatic disease

▶ Adverse Effects: Lethargy, ataxia, weakness, anorexia, vomiting, &/or diarrhea; liver changes possible

▶ Relapses are not uncommon

▶ All dogs receiving mitotane therapy should receive additional glucocorticoid supplementation if undergoing a stress (e.g., surgery, trauma, acute illness)

▶ Monitoring is mandatory

▶ Avoid human exposure

Uses/Indications

In veterinary medicine, mitotane is used primarily for the medical treatment of pituitary-dependent hyperadrenocorticism (PDH), principally in dogs. When the specific cause of hyperadrenocorticism cannot be identified, mitotane is the preferred treatment as its cytotoxic effects may cause adrenal tumor shrinkage. It has also been used for the palliative treatment of adrenal carcinoma in humans and dogs.

Pharmacology/Actions

While mitotane is considered an adrenal cytotoxic agent, it apparently can also inhibit adrenocortical function without causing cell destruction. The exact mechanisms of action for these effects are not clearly understood.

In dogs with pituitary-dependent hyperadrenocorticism (PDH), mitotane has been demonstrated to cause severe, progressive necrosis of the zona fasciculata and zona reticularis. These effects occur quite rapidly (usually within 5–10 days of starting therapy). It has been stated that mitotane spares the zona glomerulosa and therefore aldosterone synthesis is unaffected. This is only partially true, as the zona glomerulosa may also be affected by mitotane therapy, but it is uncommon for clinically significant effects on aldosterone production to be noted with therapy.

Pharmacokinetics

In dogs, the systemic bioavailability of mitotane is poor. Oral absorption can be enhanced by giving the drug with food (especially food high in oil/fat content). In humans, approximately 40% of an oral dose of mitotane is absorbed after dosing, with peak serum levels occurring about 3–5 hours after a single dose. Distribution of the drug occurs to virtually all tissues in the body. The drug is stored in the fat and does not accumulate in the adrenal glands. A small amount may enter the CSF. It is unknown if the drug crosses the placenta or is distributed into milk.

Mitotane has a very long plasma half-life in humans, with values ranging from 18–159 days being reported. Serum half-lives may increase in a given patient with continued dosing, perhaps due to a depot effect from adipose tissue releasing the drug. The drug is metabolized in the liver and is excreted as metabolites in the urine and bile. Approximately 15% of an oral dose is excreted in the bile, and 10% in the urine within 24 hours of dosing.

Contraindications/Precautions/Warnings

Mitotane is contraindicated in patients known to be hypersensitive to it. Patients with concurrent diabetes mellitus may have rapidly changing insulin requirements during the initial treatment period. These animals should be closely monitored until they are clinically stable.

Dogs with preexisting renal or hepatic disease should receive the drug with caution and with more intense monitoring. It has been stated (Scott-Moncrieff 2010) that "Mitotane should never be administered in animals that are not eating well."

It has been stated that ". . . hyperadrenocorticism is a clinical condition. No dog should be treated for this condition unless there are obvious clinical signs, consistent with the diagnosis, that are worrisome to the owner." (Feldman, E. 2007)

Some clinicians recommend giving prednisolone at 0.2 mg/kg/day during the initial treatment period (0.4 mg/kg/day to diabetic dogs) to reduce the potential for side effects from acute endogenous steroid withdrawal. Other clinicians have argued that routinely administering steroids masks the clinical markers that signify when the endpoint of therapy has been reached and must be withdrawn 2–3 days before ACTH stimulation tests can be done. Since in adequately observed patients adverse effects requiring glucocorticoid therapy may only be necessary in 5% of patients, the benefits of routine glucocorticoid administration may not be warranted.

Adverse Effects

Most common adverse effects seen with initial therapy in dogs include lethargy, ataxia, weakness, anorexia, vomiting, and/or diarrhea. Neurologic signs can be seen, but are not common. Adverse effects are commonly associated with plasma cortisol levels of less than 1 microgram/dL or a too rapid decrease of plasma cortisol levels into the normal range. Adverse effects may also be more commonly seen in dogs weighing less than 5 kg, which may be due to the inability to accurately dose. The incidence

of one or more of these effects is approximately 25% and they are usually mild. If adverse effects are noted, it is recommended to temporarily halt mitotane therapy and supplement with glucocorticoids. Owners should be provided with a small supply of predniso(lo)ne tablets to initiate treatment. Should the clinical signs persist 3 hours after steroids are supplemented, consider other medical problems.

Liver changes (congestion, centrolobular atrophy, and moderate to severe fatty degeneration) have been noted in dogs given mitotane. Although not commonly associated with clinical symptomatology, these effects may be more pronounced with long-term therapy or in dogs with preexisting liver disease.

In perhaps 5% of dogs treated, long-term glucocorticoid and sometimes mineralocorticoid replacement therapy may be required. All dogs receiving mitotane therapy should receive additional glucocorticoid supplementation if undergoing a stress (*e.g.*, surgery, trauma, acute illness).

Relapses are not uncommon in canine patients treated for Cushing's with mitotane.

Reasons for treatment failure include misdiagnosis (*e.g.*, iatrogenic hyperadrenocorticism), adrenal tumors unresponsive to mitotane, loss of drug potency, or inadequate dose for that particular patient.

Reproductive/Nursing Safety

In humans, the FDA categorizes this drug as category *C* for use during pregnancy (*Animal studies have shown an adverse effect on the fetus, but there are no adequate studies in humans; or there are no animal reproduction studies and no adequate studies in humans.*) In a separate system evaluating the safety of drugs in canine and feline pregnancy (Papich 1989), this drug is categorized as class: *D* (*Contraindicated. These drugs have been shown to cause congenital malformations or embryotoxicity.*)

It is not known whether this drug is excreted in maternal milk. Because of the potential for adverse reactions in nursing offspring, decide whether to discontinue nursing or discontinue the drug.

Overdosage/Acute Toxicity

No specific recommendations were located regarding overdoses of this medication. Because of the drug's toxicity and long half-life, emptying the stomach and administering charcoal and a cathartic should be considered after a recent ingestion. It is recommended that the patient be closely monitored and given glucocorticoids if necessary.

Drug Interactions

The following drug interactions have either been reported or are theoretical in humans or animals receiving mitotane and may be of significance in veterinary patients:

■ **CNS DEPRESSANT DRUGS:** If mitotane is

used concomitantly with drugs that cause CNS depression, additive depressant effects may be seen

◼ **INSULIN:** Diabetic dogs receiving insulin may have their insulin requirements decreased when mitotane therapy is instituted

◼ **PHENOBARBITAL:** Can induce enzymes and reduce the efficacy of mitotane, conversely mitotane can induce hepatic microsomal enzymes and increase the metabolism of phenobarbital

◼ **SPIRONOLACTONE:** In dogs, spironolactone has been demonstrated to block the action of mitotane; it is recommended to use an alternate diuretic if possible

Laboratory Considerations

◼ Mitotane will bind competitively to thyroxine-binding globulin and decreases the amount of serum protein-bound iodine. Serum **thyroxine** concentrations may be unchanged or slightly decreased, but free thyroxine values remain in the normal range. Mitotane does not affect the results of the resin triiodothyronine uptake test.

◼ Mitotane can reduce the amounts measurable **17-OHCS** in the urine, which may or may not reflect a decrease in serum cortisol levels or adrenal secretion.

Doses

◼ **DOGS:**

For medical treatment of pituitary-dependent hyperadrenocorticism (bilateral adrenal hyperplasia): **Note:** The information provided below (in "a and b") is a synopsis of the referenced authors' treatment protocols. It is strongly recommended to refer to the original references or other detailed discussions on the treatment of hyperadrenocorticism before instituting therapy for the first time.

a) Beginning by reducing dog's food allotment by one-third the day before (Saturday) therapy. Owners should give ⅓ the daily allotment that morning and ⅓ the daily allotment that evening. This should make the dog quite hungry. No dog with a poor appetite should ever be treated medically for pituitary-dependent hyperadrenocorticism (PDH). Initiate therapy at home (on Sunday): 25 mg/kg twice a day, PO with food. Glucocorticoids are not routinely administered nor dispensed. Give until one of the following occurs: Polydipsic dogs' water consumption approaches 60 mL/kg/day of water, dog takes longer to consume a meal or it develops partial or complete anorexia, dog vomits, is unusually listless, or has diarrhea. Any of these observations demand the owner stop therapy and have the dog examined by a veterinarian. Any reduction in appetite indicates that the

induction phase of therapy is completed. Water intake is a less-consistent parameter in determining therapeutic end-point. Beginning on 2nd day of therapy, contact owner daily during the induction phase to monitor the situation and encourage.

When dog's appetite is reduced or 8 days of induction therapy have occurred (whichever comes first), history and physical repeated, ACTH response test, BUN, serum sodium, and potassium redone. If the dog has responded clinically, stop mitotane until ACTH response test can be evaluated. Successful therapy is indicated by pre- and post-ACTH serum cortisol concentrations >1.5mcg/dL and <5 micrograms/dL. Goals of therapy are to achieve resolution of clinical signs. Most dogs respond between 4 and 9 days of therapy.

Maintenance therapy: Is begun once dog seems much improved or normal to owner or if post-ACTH serum cortisol is <5 micrograms/dL (**Note:** reference states 54g/dL, but this is an obvious "typo"). Each dog must be treated individually. Dogs generally receive 25–50 mg/kg per week. If <1 microgram/dL, withhold medication for 2 weeks and restart at 25 micrograms/kg/week. Whenever possible, the weekly dose of medication should be divided in as many doses as possible (*e.g.*, if dog receiving 500 mg/week; divide tablet into quarters and give 4 times a week). Four weeks after therapy started, ACTH stimulation test rechecked. If post-ACTH results are 1–3.5 micrograms/dL, dog receives 25 mg/kg/week and recheck in 4 weeks. If 3.5–7.5 micrograms/dL, dog receives 50 mg/kg/week and recheck in 4 weeks. If >7.5 micrograms/dL be sure the drug is being administered properly. If given properly, may mix with corn oil and mixed with food. These animals should also be evaluated for other conditions (*e.g.*, renal disease, diabetes mellitus). ACTH stimulation results should be used as a guide for dosage adjustment, but owner opinion is the most important factor. (Feldman, B.F. 1989; Feldman, E. 2000)(Feldman, E. 2007)

b) Induction phase 30–50 mg/kg/day PO with a meal once daily or divided q12h for 7–10 days. If adverse effects (lethargy, vomiting, weakness, diarrhea) occur, discontinue mitotane and give glucocorticoids (prednis(ol)one at 0.15–0.25 mg/kg/day) until dog can be evaluated. If decreased appetite occurs discontinue mitotane and evaluate with an ACTH stimulation test.

Perform ACTH stimulation test at end of 10 day period or sooner if adverse effects occur. Goal is to have basal and post-ACTH cortisol between 1-5 micrograms/dL (normal for most labs). If basal and post ACTH cortisol falls below 1 microgram/dL, temporarily suspend mitotane and supplement with glucocorticoids until circulating cortisol normalizes (usually 2–4 weeks, but may take several weeks to months). If basal or post ACTH cortisol is above normal, continue daily mitotane and recheck ACTH stimulation tests at 5–10 day intervals until serum cortisol falls within normal resting range.

Begin maintenance when desired cortisol concentrations are documented by ACTH stimulation testing. Mitotane given initially at 35–50 mg/kg per week in 2–3 divided doses. Should adverse effects, discontinue mitotane and supplement with glucocorticoids until dog can be evaluated by serum electrolytes and ACTH stimulation test. (Kintzer, P. 2007)

c) Initial dose of 50 mg/kg divided q12h. Glucocorticoids are not usually administered concurrently, but a small supply of prednisone should be made available to the owner for emergencies. Continue until water consumption decreases to <100 mL/kg/day, or until a decreased appetite, depression, diarrhea, or vomiting are observed. The time for clinical response is quite variable but most dogs respond within 3-7 days. At this point the dog should be reevaluated and an ACTH stimulation test performed. Prednisone treatment (0.2 mg/kg) should be initiated in patients that are showing clinical signs of hypocortisolemia, until the results of the ACTH stimulation test are known. In patients that are not polydipsic prior to therapy, patients where water consumption cannot be monitored, and in patients whose polydipsia is due to another cause (*e.g.*, diabetes mellitus), mitotane should be administered for a maximum of 5-7 days prior to ACTH stimulation testing. The goal of treatment is to have both the pre- and post-cortisol measurement in the normal resting range (2–6 micrograms/dL). Maintenance therapy (50 mg/kg every 7–10 days) is started once the ACTH stimulation test shows adequate suppression and prednisone therapy (if necessary) has been discontinued. Failure to use maintenance therapy will result in re-growth of the adrenal cortex and recurrence of clinical signs. Efficacy of maintenance therapy is monitored by an ACTH stimulation test after one month of maintenance

treatment and then every 3 months. The dose of mitotane required for long term maintenance is very variable (26–330 mg/kg/week). (Scott-Moncrieff 2010)

d) Intentionally causing complete destruction of the adrenal cortex as an alternative to the traditional mitotane treatment: Mitotane at 75–100 mg/kg per day for 25 consecutive days, given in 3–4 doses per day with food. Lifelong prednisone at 0.1–0.5 mg/kg PO twice daily initially and mineralocorticoid therapy is begun at the start of mitotane therapy. Prednisone dose is tapered after completion of the 25-day protocol. Relapse is common and periodic ACTH stimulation testing is necessary. May be considerably more expensive than traditional therapy because of the expense associated with treating Addisonian dogs. (Nelson 2003)

e) For total adrenal ablation for management of Cushing's: Mitotane 100 mg/kg/day divided twice daily for 30 days. Supplemental cortisone acetate 2 mg/kg/day divided twice daily and fludrocortisone acetate 0.1 mg/ 10 lb of body weight PO once daily are begun on day 1 of mitotane therapy. Diet is supplemented with 1–5 grams of sodium chloride per day. One week after induction phase with mitotane, cortisone acetate is reduced to 1 mg/kg/day. Electrolytes and ACTH stimulation test are performed at end of induction, every 6 months, and at any time animal demonstrates signs compatible with either hypo- or hyperadrenocorticism. This form of management requires close patient monitoring and life-long daily therapy. Close attention during stress and non-adrenal illnesses required. (Bruyette 2002)

For palliative medical treatment of adrenal carcinomas or medical treatment of adrenal adenomas:

Initially, 50–75 mg/kg PO in daily divided doses for 10–14 days. May supplement with predniso(lo)ne at 0.2 mg/kg/day. Stop therapy and evaluate dog if adverse effects occur. After initial therapy run ACTH-stimulation test (do not give predniso(lo)ne the morning of the test). If basal or post-ACTH serum cortisol values are decreased, but still above the therapeutic end-point (<1 micrograms/dL), repeat therapy for an additional 7–14 days and repeat testing. If post-ACTH serum cortisol values remain greatly elevated or unchanged, increase mitotane to 100 mg/kg/day and repeat ACTH-stimulation test at 7–14 day intervals. If ACTH continues to remain greatly elevated, increase dosage by 50 mg/kg/day every 7–14 days until response occurs or drug intolerance ensues. Adjust dosage as necessary as patient tolerates or ACTH-responsive dictates. Once undetectable or low-normal post-ACTH cortisol levels are attained, continue mitotane at 100–200 mg/kg/week in divided doses with glucocorticoid supplementation (predniso(lo)ne 0.2 mg/kg/day). Repeat ACTH-stimulation test in 1–2 months. Continue at present dose if cortisol remains below 1 micrograms/dL. Should cortisol increase to 1–4 micrograms/dL, increase maintenance dose by 50%. If basal or post-ACTH cortisol goes above 4 micrograms/dL, restart daily treatment (50–100 mg/kg/day) as outlined above. Once patient is stabilized, repeat ACTH-stimulation tests at 3–6 month intervals. (Kintzer, P.P. & Peterson 1989)

■ **FERRETS:**

For medical treatment of hyperadrenocorticism where surgery has not been performed or tumor has not been fully resected:

a) 50 mg per ferret PO once daily for one week, then 50 mg PO 2–3 times per week. Have a compounding pharmacy make 50 mg capsules. Capsules can be easily administered if coated with a substance such as *Nutrical*. (Rosenthal & Peterson 2000)

Monitoring

Initially and as needed (see doses above):

■ Physical exam and history (including water and food consumption, weight)

■ BUN, CBC, Liver enzymes, Blood glucose, ACTH response test, serum electrolytes (Na$^+$/K$^+$)

Client Information

■ Clients must be clearly instructed in the adverse effects of the drug and the clinical signs of acute hypoadrenocorticism

■ This medication is best administered immediately after a meal

■ Because of the potential severe toxicity associated with this agent, clients should be instructed to wear gloves or wash their hands after administering and to keep the tablets out of reach of children or pets.

Chemistry/Synonyms

Mitotane, also commonly known in veterinary medicine as o,p'-DDD, is structurally related to the infamous insecticide, chlorophenothane (DDT). It occurs as a white, crystalline powder with a slightly aromatic odor. It is practically insoluble in water and soluble in alcohol.

Mitotane may also be known as: CB-313, o,p'DDD, NSC-38721, WR-13045, and *Lisodren*®.

Storage/Stability

Mitotane tablets should be stored at room temperature (15–30°C), in tight, light resistant containers.

Dosage Forms/Regulatory Status

VETERINARY-LABELED PRODUCTS: None

HUMAN-LABELED PRODUCTS:

Mitotane Tablets (scored): 500 mg; *Lysodren*® (Bristol-Myers Squibb Oncology); (Rx)

References

Bruyette, D. (2002). Diagnosis and Treatment of Canine Cushing's Syndrome. Western Veterinary Conference.

Feldman, B.F. (1989). Disorders of Platelets. *Current Veterinary Therapy X: Small Animal Practice*. RW Kirk Ed. Philadelphia, WB Saunders: 457–464.

Feldman, E. (2000). Hyperadrenocorticism. *Textbook of Veterinary Internal Medicine: Diseases of the Dog and Cat*. S Ettinger and E Feldman Eds. Philadelphia, WB Saunders. 2: 1460–1488.

Feldman, E. (2007). Medical management of canine hyperadrenocorticism: A comparison of trilostane to mitotane. Proceedings: UCD Canine Medicine Symposium. Accessed via: Veterinary Information Network. http://goo.gl/WbO8k

Kintzer, P. (2007). Treatment challenges in canine hyperadrenocorticism. Proceedings: Western Vet Conference. Accessed via: Veterinary Information Network. http://goo.gl/C723n

Kintzer, P.P. & M.E. Peterson (1989). Mitotane (o,p'-DDD) treatment of cortisol-secreting adrenocortical neoplasia. *Current Veterinary Therapy X: Small Animal Practice*. RW Kirk Ed. Philadelphia, WB Saunders: 1034–1037.

Nelson, R. (2003). Treatment Options for Canine Cushing's Disease. Proceedings: World Small Animal Veterinary Association. Accessed via: Veterinary Information Network. http://goo.gl/1uLx9

Papich, M. (1989). Effects of drugs on pregnancy. *Current Veterinary Therapy X: Small Animal Practice*. R Kirk Ed. Philadelphia, Saunders: 1291–1299.

Rosenthal, K. & M. Peterson (2000). Hyperadrenocorticism in the ferret. *Kirk's Current Veterinary Therapy: XIII Small Animal Practice*. J Bonagura Ed. Philadelphia, WB Saunders: 372–374.

Scott-Moncrieff, J.C. (2010). Update on treatment of hyperadrenocorticism: What is the current recommendation? Proceedings: ACVIM Forum. Accessed via: Veterinary Information Network. http://goo.gl/OsV6A

MITOXANTRONE HCL

(mye-toe-*zan*-trone)   Novantrone®
ANTINEOPLASTIC

Prescriber Highlights

▶ Antineoplastic that may be useful for a variety of neoplastic diseases

▶ Contraindications (relative): Myelosuppression, concurrent infection, impaired cardiac function; those who have received prior cytotoxic drug or radiation exposure

▶ Caution: Sensitivity to drug, hyperuricemia or hyperuricuria, impaired hepatic function

▶ Adverse Effects: Dose-dependent GI distress, bone marrow depression, lethargy, & seizures (cats)

▶ Relatively expensive

▶ Renal clearance of drug is minimal

Uses/Indications

Mitoxantrone may be useful in the treatment of several neoplastic diseases in dogs and cats, including lymphosarcoma mammary adenocarcinoma, squamous cell carcinoma, renal adenocarcinoma, fibroid sarcoma, thyroid or transitional cell carcinomas, and hemangiopericytoma.

Because renal clearance of the drug is minimal (10%), it may be administered to cats with renal insufficiency much more safely than doxorubicin.

Pharmacology/Actions

By intercalation between base pairs and a non-intercalative electrostatic interaction, mitoxantrone binds to DNA and inhibits both DNA and RNA synthesis. Mitoxantrone is not cell-cycle phase specific, but appears to be most active during the S phase.

Pharmacokinetics

Mitoxantrone is rapidly and extensively distributed after intravenous infusion. Highest concentrations of the drug are found in the liver, heart, thyroid, and red blood cells. In humans, it is approximately 78% bound to plasma proteins. Mitoxantrone is metabolized in the liver, but the majority of the drug is excreted unchanged in the urine. Half-life of the drug in humans averages about 5 days as a result of the drug being taken up, bound by, and then slowly released by tissues.

Contraindications/Precautions/Warnings

Mitoxantrone is relatively contraindicated (weigh risk vs. benefit) in patients with myelosuppression, concurrent infection, impaired cardiac function, or those who have received prior cytotoxic drug or radiation exposure. It should be used with caution in patients with sensitivity to mitoxantrone, hyperuricemia or hyperuricuria, or impaired hepatic function.

Adverse Effects

In dogs and cats, effects include dose-dependent GI distress (vomiting, anorexia, diarrhea) and bone marrow depression (sepsis). Non-regenerative anemias may be detected and white cell nadirs generally occur on day 10. Some evidence exists that by giving recombinant granulocyte-colony stimulating factor bone marrow depression severity and duration may be reduced. Lethargy may also be noticed. Some cats receiving this drug have developed seizures.

Unlike doxorubicin, cardiotoxicity has not yet been reported in dogs and only rarely occurs in humans. Other adverse effects less frequently or rarely noted in humans and, potentially possible in dogs, include conjunctivitis, jaundice, renal failure, seizures, allergic reactions, thrombocytopenia, irritation or phlebitis at injection site. Tissue necrosis associated with extravasation has only been reported in a few human cases.

Reproductive/Nursing Safety

In humans, the FDA categorizes this drug as category **D** for use during pregnancy (*There is evidence of human fetal risk, but the potential benefits from the use of the drug in pregnant women may be acceptable despite its potential risks.*)

Mitoxantrone is excreted in maternal milk and significant concentrations (18 ng/mL) have been reported for 28 days after the last administration to humans. Because of the potential for serious adverse reactions in offspring, it is recommended to use milk replacer if mitoxantrone is administered.

Overdosage/Acute Toxicity

Because of the potential serious toxicity associated with this agent, dosage determinations must be made carefully.

Drug Interactions

The following drug interactions have either been reported or are theoretical in humans or animals receiving mitoxantrone and may be of significance in veterinary patients:

■ **DOXORUBICIN, DAUNORUBICIN, or RADIATION THERAPY:** Cardiotoxicity risks may be enhanced in patients that have previously received doxorubicin, daunorubicin, or radiation therapy to the mediastinum

■ **IMMUNOSUPPRESSANT DRUGS (e.g., azathioprine, cyclophosphamide, corticosteroids):** Use with other immunosuppressant drugs may increase the risk of infection

■ **MYELOSUPPRESSIVE DRUGS (e.g., chloramphenicol, flucytosine, amphotericin B, or colchicine):** Use extreme caution when used concurrently with other drugs that are also myelosuppressive, including many of the other antineoplastics and other bone marrow depressant drugs; bone marrow depression may be additive

■ **VACCINES, LIVE:** Live virus vaccines should be used with caution, if at all, during therapy

Laboratory Considerations

■ Mitoxantrone may raise serum **uric acid** levels. Drugs such as allopurinol may be required to control hyperuricemia.

■ **Liver function tests** may become abnormal, indicating hepatotoxicity.

■ Mitoxantrone may discolor **urine** a green-blue.

Doses

Note: Because of the potential toxicity of this drug to patients, and potentially, veterinary personnel and clients, and since chemotherapy indications, treatment protocols, monitoring and safety guidelines often change, the following dosages should be used only as a general guide and not as a dosage protocol. When using mitoxantrone as part of chemotherapy protocols, consultation with a veterinary oncologist and referral to current veterinary oncology references [*e.g.*, (Henry & Higginbotham 2009); (Argyle *et al.* 2008); (Withrow & Vail 2007); (Villalobos 2007); (Ogilvie & Moore 2006); (Ogilvie & Moore 2001)] is *strongly recommended*.

■ **DOGS:**
As an alternative agent for the treatment of a variety of neoplastic diseases (see Indications above):

a) For transitional cell carcinoma: 5 mg/m^2 IV every 21 days with piroxicam (0.3 mg/kg PO once daily). (Chun 2007)

b) For lymphoma, squamous cell carcinoma, transitional cell carcinoma, mammary gland tumors, etc.: Effective dose is 6 mg/m^2 IV every 2–3 weeks (Ogilvie 2003)

c) As a single rescue agent for lymphoma: 5.5–6 mg/m^2 IV every 3 weeks (Meleo 2003)

d) As a rescue agent for canine lymphoma: 6 mg/m^2 IV every 2–3 weeks. Check CBC on day 7 after treatment and the protocol can be repeated on day 14 or 21 if the dog attains complete or partial response. Combining with DTIC (dacarbazine) may improve the response rate for dogs with refractory lymphoma, but there are no available studies. (Rassnick 2006)

e) For transitional cell carcinoma after laser ablation of the primary tumor: Mitoxantrone at 5 mg/m^2 IV every 3 weeks for 4 treatments. Piroxicam was given at a dosage of 0.3 mg/kg PO once daily for the remaining life of the dog. (Upton *et al.* 2006)

■ **CATS:**
a) For soft-tissue sarcomas: 6–6.5 mg/m^2 IV given every 3–4 weeks for 4–6 treatments. (Keller & Helfand 1994)

b) Effective dose: 6.5 mg/m^2 IV every 2–3 weeks (Ogilvie 2003)

c) As a single rescue agent for lymphoma: 6–6.5 mg/m^2 IV every 3 weeks (Meleo 2003)

Monitoring

■ CBC with differential and platelets (see Adverse Effects section)

■ Efficacy

■ Chest radiographs, ECG or other cardiac function tests if cardiac symptomatology present

■ Liver function tests if jaundice or other clinical signs of hepatotoxicity present

■ Serum uric acid levels for susceptible patients

Client Information

■ Clients should understand the potential costs and toxicities associated with therapy

■ A blue-green color to urine or a bluish color to sclera may be noted but is of no concern

■ Have clients report any clinical signs associated with toxicity immediately to veterinarian

■ Mitoxantrone or its metabolites may be detected in urine up to 6 days, and in feces up to 7 days after administration. Use appropriate precautions when cleaning up animal waste.

Chemistry/Synonyms

Mitoxantrone HCl is a synthetic anthracenedione antineoplastic. It occurs as a dark-blue powder and is sparingly soluble in water, practically insoluble in acetone, acetonitrile, and chloroform, and slightly soluble in methyl alcohol.

Mitoxantrone may also be known as: L-232315, DHAD, dihydroxyanthracenedione dihydrochloride, mitoxantroni hydrochloridum, NSC-301739, *Formyxan®*, *Genefadrone®*, *Micraleve®*, *Misostol®*, *Mitoxal®*, *Mitoxgen®*, *Mitroxone®*, *Neotalem®*, *Novantron®*, *Novantrone®*, *Oncotron®*, *Onkotrone®*, or *Pralifan®*.

Storage/Stability

Mitoxantrone HCl should be stored at room temperature. While the manufacturer recommends not to freeze, one study (Mauldin 2002) demonstrated that the drug maintained its cytotoxic effects when frozen and thawed at various intervals over a 12 month period. Do not mix or use the same IV line with heparin infusions (precipitate may form). At present, it is not recommended to mix with other IV drugs.

Compatibility/Compounding Considerations

Do not mix or use the same IV line with heparin infusions (precipitate may form). At present, it is recommended to not mix with other IV drugs.

Dosage Forms/Regulatory Status

VETERINARY-LABELED PRODUCTS: None

HUMAN-LABELED PRODUCTS:

Mitoxantrone HCl for Injection Solution Concentrate: 2 mg/mL, preservative free in 10 mL, 12.5 mL, & 15 mL multi-dose vials; *Novantrone®* (Serono); generic; (Rx)

References

Argyle, D., M. Brearly, et al. (2008). *Decision Making in Small Animal Oncology*, Wiley-Blackwell.

Chun, R. (2007). Canine transitional cell carcinoma. Proceedings; Western Vet Conference. Accessed via: Veterinary Information Network. http://goo.gl/VQ162

Henry, C. & M. Higginbotham (2009). *Cancer Management in Small Animal Practice*, Saunders.

Keller, E. & S. Helfand (1994). Clinical management of soft-tissue sarcomas. *Consultations in Feline Internal Medicine: 2.* J August Ed. Philadelphia, W.B. Saunders Company: 557–566.

Mauldin, G. (2002). Evaluation of the in vitro cytotoxicity of mitoxantrone following repeated freeze-thaw cycles. *Vet Therapeutics* 3(3): 290–296.

Meleo, K. (2003). Rescue protocols for lymphoma. Proceedings: Western Veterinary Conference. Accessed via: Veterinary Information Network. http://goo.gl/gQJgU

Ogilvie, G. (2003). Care beyond cure: Advances in compassionate chemotherapy. Proceedings: Atlantic Coast Veterinary Conference. Accessed via: Veterinary Information Network. http://goo.gl/rVZxd

Ogilvie, G. & A. Moore (2001). *Feline Oncology: A Comprehensive Guide to Compassionate Care*, Veterinary Learning Systems.

Ogilvie, G. & A. Moore (2006). *Managing the Canine Cancer Patient: A Practical Guide to Compassionate Care*, Veterinary Learning Systems.

Rassnick, K. (2006). Rescue chemotherapy protocols for dogs with lymphoma. Proceedings: ACVIM. Accessed via: Veterinary Information Network. http://goo.gl/soSsv

Upton, M., C. Tanger, et al. (2006). Evaluation of carbon dioxide laser ablation combined with mitoxantrone and piroxicam treatment in dogs with transitional cell carcinoma. *JAVMA* 228(4): 549–552.

Villalobos, A. (2007). *Canine and Feline Geriatric Oncology.* Ames, Blackwell.

Withrow, S. & D. Vail (2007). *Withrow and MacEwen's Small Animal Clinical Oncology 4th Ed.* Philadelphia, Elsevier.

MONTELUKAST SODIUM

(mon-teh-*loo*-kast)   Singulair®

LEUKOTRIENE ANTAGONIST

Prescriber Highlights

▶ Leukotriene inhibitor; potentially may be useful in cats for feline asthma, IBD, upper respiratory disease, and heartworm-associated respiratory disease syndrome

▶ Good evidence not yet available to support use in cats

▶ No significant adverse effects reported in cats to date

Uses/Indications

In veterinary medicine, montelukast has been used primarily in cats. Potential indications include: feline asthma, upper respiratory disease, inflammatory bowel disease and heartworm disease. Its use in treating feline asthma has been disappointing, and few recommend it for this purpose. At the time of writing, only anecdotal evidence exists for efficacy for this class of drugs in cats. A small trial in horses with RAO did not show efficacy (Robinson 2010).

In humans, montelukast is FDA-approved for allergic rhinitis and asthma. It is used off-label for atopic dermatitis, urticaria (chronic and NSAID-induced), and eosinophilic esophagitis.

Pharmacology/Actions

Montelukast is a leukotriene antagonist that inhibits at the cysteinyl leukotriene (CysLT1) receptor. The cysteinyl leukotrienes (LTC4, LTD4, LTE4) are pro-inflammatory products of arachidonic acid metabolism released from certain cells, including mast cells and eosinophils.

Pharmacokinetics

No pharmacokinetic information for cats was located.

In humans, oral bioavailability is 64% and peak levels occur 3-4 hours after dosing. The presence of food does not affect bioavailability. Montelukast is highly bound (99+%) to human plasma proteins. It is extensively metabolized in the liver via cytochrome P450 isoenzymes CYP3A4, CYP2A6, and CYP2C9. Based on *in vitro* studies in human liver microsomes, therapeutic plasma concentrations of montelukast do not inhibit CYP-450 isoenzymes 3A4, 2C9, 1A2, 2A6, 2C19, or 2D6. Metabolites are excreted primarily in the bile and eliminated in the feces. In healthy young adults, plasma half-life averages around 4 hours.

Contraindications/Precautions/Warnings

Montelukast is contraindicated in patients hypersensitive to it or to any component of the product. Humans are warned not use it to attempt to reverse acute bronchospasm.

Adverse Effects

No adverse effects were noted for cats but the drug has not been extensively studied or used in cats.

In humans, the drug is usually well tolerated with minimal adverse effects reported. Rarely, behavioral effects (aggression, suicidal thoughts), palpitations, cholestatic hepatitis and allergic granulomatous angiitis have been reported.

Reproductive/Nursing Safety

Montelukast appears safe to use during pregnancy. No teratogenicity was observed in rats at oral dosages of up to 100X; or rabbits at 110X the human dose. The FDA has designated it as a category *B* drug (*Animal studies have not demonstrated risk to the fetus, but there are no adequate studies in pregnant women; or animal studies have shown an adverse effect, but adequate studies in pregnant women have not demonstrated a risk to the fetus during the first trimester of pregnancy, and there is no evidence of risk in later trimesters.*)

While studies in rats have shown that montelukast is excreted in milk, it is likely safe to use during nursing.

Overdosage/Acute Toxicity

Montelukast is relatively safe in overdose situations. Rats and mice survived oral doses of approximately 230X and 335X and 230X of the usual human adult dose. Reports of human adults and children receiving doses as high as 1,000 mg have been reported and the majority of overdoses had no adverse effects. The most frequent adverse experiences observed in humans are: headache, vomiting, psychomotor hyperactivity, thirst, somnolence, mydriasis, hyperkinesia, and abdominal pain. Treatment is basically supportive.

Drug Interactions

The following drug interactions have either been reported or are theoretical in humans receiving montelukast and may be of significance in veterinary patients:

■ **CYP-450 ENZYME INDUCERS (e.g., phenobarbital, rifampin):** May reduce the montelukast plasma concentrations and efficacy

■ **PREDNISONE, PREDNISOLONE:** Severe peripheral edema has been reported in a human receiving both drugs, presumably due to increased renal tubular sodium and fluid retention. After prednisone was discontinued, edema resolved; clinical significance is not clear.

Laboratory Considerations

■ None

Doses

■ **CATS:**

a) For feline asthma: There are some anecdotal reports of efficacy of montelukast at 0.5–1 mg/kg PO once daily (q24h) and zafirlukast (1–2 mg/kg PO q12h) in the treatment of feline asthma, but more conclusive evidence is needed before these agents can be used regularly. (Martín-Jiménez 2010)

b) For adjunctive treatment of the chronic "snuffler": 0.25–0.5 mg/kg PO q24h (i.e, ⅛th of a 10 mg *Singulair*® tablet). (Scherk 2010)

c) For IBD: For mild cases of IBD involving eosinophils and lymphocytes, leukotriene antagonists should be considered; either montelukast at 0.5–1 mg/kg PO once daily or zafirlukast (0.15 to 0.2 mg/kg orally PO once daily). Alternatively, these drugs might be used in combination with other drugs in any stage. (Boothe 2009)

d) For adjunctive treatment of feline heartworm: There is anecdotal evidence that anti-leukotrienes (e.g., montelukast) at 2 mg total dose (PO) once daily may help to thwart an acute, fatal lung injury when an adult worm dies. (Nelson 2008)

Monitoring

■ Clinical efficacy

Client Information

■ May be given with or without food

■ This drug is not for the immediate treatment of asthma or other signs or symptoms

■ This drug has not been used often in animals; report any adverse effects to the veterinarian immediately

Chemistry/Synonyms

Montelukast is a cyclopropaneacetic acid derivative leukotriene inhibitor. It is freely soluble in ethanol, methanol, and water.

Montelukast may also be known as MK-476, L-706631, or montelukastum.

Storage/Stability

Store tablets or granules at room temperature; excursions are permitted to 15°-30°C (59°–86°F). Protect from moisture and light.

Dosage Forms/Regulatory Status

VETERINARY-LABELED PRODUCTS: None

HUMAN-LABELED PRODUCTS:

Montelukast Sodium Oral Tablets: 4 mg (chewable), 5 mg (chewable), 10 mg; oral granules 4 mg/packet; *Singulair*® (Merck); (Rx)

References

Boothe, D.M. (2009). Control of Inflammatory Allergic Disease in Cats II. Proceedings; WVC. http://goo.gl/q6uOz

Martín-Jiménez, T. (2010). Update of Therapies for Feline Asthma. Proceedings: WVC. Accessed via: Veterinary Information Network. http://goo.gl/bZ92B

Nelson, C. (2008). Dirofilaria immitis in Cats: Diagnosis and Management. *Comp CE*(July): 393–399.

Robinson, N.E. (2010). Airway Obstructive Disorders: Are Humans Good Models for Horses? Proceedings: ACVIM. Accessed via: Veterinary Information Network. http://goo.gl/vWrGH

Scherk, M. (2010). Snots and Snuffles: Rational approach to chronic feline upper respiratory syndromes. *Journal of Feline Medicine and Surgery* 12(7): 548–557.

MORANTEL TARTRATE

(mor-*an*-tel)   Rumatel®

ANTIPARASITIC AGENT

Prescriber Highlights

▶ Infrequently used anthelmintic for ruminants

▶ Contraindications: None

▶ Adverse Effects: Large safety margin; clinical signs of OD include increased respiratory rates, profuse sweating, ataxia or other cholinergic effects

Uses/Indications

Morantel is labeled for the removal of the following parasites in cattle: Mature forms of: *Haemonchus* spp., *Ostertagia* spp., *Trichostrongylus* spp., *Nematodirus* spp.,

Cooperia spp. and *Oesophagostomum radiatum*. It is also used in other ruminant species.

Pharmacology/Actions

Like pyrantel, morantel acts as a depolarizing neuromuscular blocking agent in susceptible parasites, thereby paralyzing the organism. The drug possesses nicotine-like properties and acts similarly to acetylcholine. Morantel also inhibits fumarate reductase in *Haemonchus* spp.

Morantel is slower than pyrantel in its onset of action, but is approximately 100 times as potent.

Pharmacokinetics

After oral administration, morantel is absorbed rapidly from the upper abomasum and small intestine. Peak levels occur about 4–6 hours after dosing. The drug is promptly metabolized in the liver. Within 96 hours of administration, 17% of the drug is excreted in the urine with the remainder in the feces.

Contraindications/Precautions/Warnings

There are no absolute contraindications to using this drug.

Adverse Effects

At recommended doses, adverse effects are not commonly seen. For more information, see Overdosage section below.

Reproductive/Nursing Safety

Morantel is considered generally safe to use during pregnancy.

Overdosage/Acute Toxicity

Morantel tartrate has a large safety margin. In cattle, dosages of up to 200 mg/kg (20 times recommended dose) resulted in no toxic reactions. The LD_{50} in mice is 5 grams/kg. Clinical signs of toxicity that might possibly be seen include increased respiratory rates, profuse sweating (in species with sweat glands), ataxia or other cholinergic effects.

Chronic toxicity studies have been conducted in cattle and sheep. Doses of 4 times recommended were given to sheep with no detectable deleterious effects. Cattle receiving 2.5 times recommended dose for 2 weeks showed no toxic signs.

Drug Interactions

■ **BENTONITE:** Do not add to feeds containing bentonite.

■ **LEVAMISOLE, PYRANTEL:** Because of similar mechanisms of action (and toxicity), morantel is not recommended for use concurrently with pyrantel or levamisole.

■ **ORGANOPHOSPHATES, DIETHYLCARBAM-AZINE:** Observation for adverse effects should be intensified if used concomitantly with an organophosphate or diethylcarbamazine.

■ **PIPERAZINE:** Has antagonistic mechanism of action; do not use with morantel.

Doses

■ **CATTLE:**

For susceptible parasites:
a) 9.68 mg/kg PO (Paul 1986)
b) Feed at the rate of 0.44 grams of morantel tartrate per 100 lbs of body weight. 10 lbs of premix per ton of food per 100 lbs of body weight. (Label Directions; *Rumatel®*—Philbro)
c) 8.8 mg/kg PO (Roberson 1988)

■ **SHEEP & GOATS:**

For susceptible parasites:
a) **Goats:** As a single therapeutic treatment at 0.44 grams morantel tartrate per 100 lb. body weight. Fresh water should be available at all times. Conditions of constant worm exposure may require retreatment in 2–4 weeks. (Label directions; *Goat Care-2X®*—Durvet)
b) **Sheep:** 10 mg/kg PO (Roberson 1988)
c) **Goats:** 10 mg/kg PO (de la Concha 2002)

Chemistry/Synonyms

A tetrahydropyrimidine anthelmintic, morantel tartrate occurs as a practically odorless, off-white to pale yellow, crystalline solid that is soluble in water. It has a melting range of 167–171°C. The tartrate salt is equivalent to 59.5% of base activity.

Morantel tartrate may also be known as: CP-12009-18, moranteli hydrogenotartras, or UK-2964-18, *Goat Care-2X®* and *Rumatel®*.

Storage/Stability

Morantel tartrate products should be stored at room temperature (15–30°C, 59–86°F) and protected from light unless otherwise instructed by the manufacturer.

Dosage Forms/Regulatory Status

VETERINARY-LABELED PRODUCTS:

Morantel Tartrate Medicated Pellets: 0.194% (880 mg/lb) in 3 lb (treats 12–50 lb goats) and 10 lb. (treats 40–50 lb. goats). *Goat Care-2X®* (Durvet); (OTC); No withdrawal time noted on label. Do not mix in feeds containing bentonite.

Morantel Tartrate Medicated Premix: 88 grams morantel tartrate per lb. in 25 lb bags: *Rumatel® Medicated Premix-88* (Philbro); (OTC). FDA-approved for use in beef or dairy cattle. Milk withdrawal (at labeled doses) = none; Slaughter withdrawal (at labeled doses) = 14 days

HUMAN-LABELED PRODUCTS: None

References

de la Concha, A. (2002). Diseases of kids. Proceedings: Western Veterinary Conference. Accessed via: Veterinary Information Network. http://goo.gl/t2w7e
Paul, J.W. (1986). Anthelmintic Therapy. *Current Veterinary Therapy: Food Animal Practice 2*. JL Howard Ed. Philadelphia, W.B. Saunders: 39–44.
Roberson, E.L. (1988). Antinematodal Agents. *Veterinary Pharmacology and Therapeutics*. NH Booth and LE McDonald Eds. Ames, Iowa State University Press: 882–927.

MORPHINE SULFATE

(*mor*-feen)

OPIATE AGONIST

Prescriber Highlights

▶ Classic opiate analgesic

▶ Contraindications: Hypersensitivity to morphine, diarrhea caused by a toxic ingestion

▶ Extreme Caution: Respiratory disease or from acute respiratory dysfunction

▶ Caution: Hypothyroidism, severe renal insufficiency (acute uremia), adrenocortical insufficiency, geriatric or severely debilitated patients, head injuries or increased intracranial pressure, & acute abdominal conditions (e.g., colic)

▶ Adverse Effects: Histamine release, respiratory depression, bronchoconstriction, CNS depression, physical dependence (chronic use), hyperthermia (cattle, goats, horses & cats), hypothermia (dogs, rabbits); GI Gastrointestinal effects may include: (nausea, vomiting, & decreased intestinal peristalsis), defecation (dogs)

▶ C-II controlled substance

Uses/Indications

Morphine is used for the treatment of acute pain in dogs, cats, horses, swine, sheep, and goats. It may be used as a preanesthetic agent in dogs and swine. Additionally, it has been used as an antitussive, antidiarrheal, and as adjunctive therapy for some cardiac abnormalities (see doses) in dogs. Due to its poor oral bioavailability in dogs, oral morphine is not recommended in canines.

Intra-articular administration of morphine as part of a balanced analgesic protocol, may be beneficial in horses (and other species) for synovitis or after joint surgery.

Pharmacology/Actions

The morphine-like agonists (morphine, meperidine, oxymorphone) have primary activity at the *mu* receptors, with some activity possible at the delta receptor. The primary pharmacologic effects of these agents include: analgesia, antitussive activity, respiratory depression, sedation, emesis, physical dependence, and intestinal effects (constipation/defecation). Secondary pharmacologic effects include: *CNS*: euphoria, sedation, and confusion. *Cardiovascular*: bradycardia due to central vagal stimulation, alpha-adrenergic receptors may be depressed resulting in peripheral vasodilation, decreased peripheral resistance, and baroreceptor inhibition. Orthostatic hypotension and syncope may occur. *Urinary*: Increased bladder sphincter tone can induce urinary retention.

When administered intra-articularly in horses with experimentally-induced synovitis, morphine demonstrated antiinflammatory effects (reduced swelling, reduced synovial total protein, serum amyloid and white blood cell counts) (Lindegaard *et al.* 2010).

Morphine's CNS effects are irregular and are species specific. Cats, horses, sheep, goats, cattle, and swine may exhibit stimulatory effects after morphine injection, while dogs, humans, and other primates exhibit CNS depression. Both dogs and cats are sensitive to the emetic effects of morphine, but significantly higher doses are required in cats before vomiting occurs. This effect is a result of a direct stimulation of the chemoreceptor trigger zone (CTZ). Other species (horses, ruminants, and swine) do not respond to the emetic effects of morphine. Like meperidine, morphine can affect the release of histamine from mast cells.

Morphine is an effective centrally acting antitussive in dogs. Following morphine administration, hypothermia may be seen in dogs and rabbits, while hyperthermia may be seen in cattle, goats, horses, and cats. Morphine can cause miosis (pinpoint pupils) in humans and rabbits. While miosis is listed as a pharmacologic effect of morphine in dogs, in a recent study in normal dogs, intravenous doses of morphine (dose not specified), did not significantly affect pupil size or intraocular pressure (Pirie *et al.* 2008).

While morphine is considered a respiratory depressant, respirations are stimulated initially in dogs. Panting may ensue which may be a result of increased body temperature. Often however, body temperature may be reduced due to a resetting of the "body's thermostat." As CNS depression increases and the hyperthermia resolves, respirations can become depressed. Morphine at moderate to high doses can also cause bronchoconstriction in dogs.

The cardiovascular effects of morphine in dogs are in direct contrast to its effects on humans. In dogs, morphine causes coronary vasoconstriction with resultant increase in coronary vascular resistance, and a transient decrease in arterial pressure. Both bradycardias and tachycardias have been reported in dogs. While morphine has been used for years as a sedative/analgesic in the treatment of myocardial infarction and congestive heart failure in humans, its effects on dogs make it a less than optimal choice in canine patients with clinical signs of cardiopulmonary failure.

The effects of morphine on the gastrointestinal (GI) tract consist primarily of a decrease in motility and secretions. The dog, however, will immediately defecate following an injection of morphine, then exhibit the signs of decreased intestinal motility and, ultimately, constipation can result. Both biliary and gastric secretions are reduced following administration of morphine, but gastric secretion of HCl will later be compensated by increased (above normal) acid secretion.

Initially, morphine can induce micturition, but with higher doses (>2.4 mg/kg IV) urine secretion can be substantially reduced by an increase in anti-diuretic hormone (ADH) release. Morphine may cause bladder hypertonia which can lead to increased difficulty in urination.

Pharmacokinetics

Morphine is absorbed when given by IV, IM, SC, and rectal routes. Although absorbed when given orally, bioavailability is reduced, probably because of a high first-pass effect. Very low oral bioavailability (<20%) in dogs, limits the clinical usefulness of orally administered morphine in canines. Morphine concentrates in the kidney, liver, and lungs; lower levels are found in the CNS. Although at lower levels then in the parenchymatous tissues, the majority of free morphine is found in skeletal muscle. Morphine crosses the placenta and narcotized newborns can result if mothers are given the drug before giving birth. These effects can be rapidly reversed with naloxone. Small amounts of morphine will also be distributed into the milk of nursing mothers.

The major route of elimination of morphine is by metabolism in the liver, primarily by glucuronidation. Because cats are deficient in this metabolic pathway, half-lives in cats are probably prolonged (reported to be approximately 3 hours). The glucuronidated metabolite M6G (active), is excreted by the kidney.

After IV administration in dogs, morphine has a volume of distribution of about 7.5 L/kg and a clearance of approximately 83 mL/min/kg. Its elimination half-life is slightly longer than 1 hour. The oral bioavailability of the extended release tablets is widely variable and this dosage form of the drug is erratically absorbed in dogs.

In horses, the serum half-life of morphine has been reported to be 88 minutes after a dose of 0.1 mg/kg IV. At this dose the drug was detectable in the serum for 48 hours and in the urine for up to 6 days. When morphine was administered epidurally to horses, rapid, short-lasting serum concentrations and delayed, long-lasting CSF concentrations (elimination half-life of approx. 8 hours) resulted. Isoflurane anesthesia did not significantly alter values (Bellei *et al.* 2008).

Contraindications/Precautions/Warnings

All opiates should be used with caution in patients with hypothyroidism, severe renal insufficiency, adrenocortical insufficiency (Addison's), and in geriatric or severely debilitated patients. Morphine is contraindicated in cases where the patient is hypersensitive to narcotic analgesics, receiving monamine oxidase inhibitors (MAOIs), or with diarrhea caused by a toxic ingestion until the toxin is eliminated from the GI tract.

Morphine should be used with extreme caution in patients with head injuries, increased intracranial pressure, and acute abdominal conditions (*e.g.*, colic) as it may obscure the diagnosis or clinical course of these conditions. Morphine may also increase intracranial pressure secondary to cerebral vasodilatation as a result of increased p_aCO_2 stemming from respiratory depression. It should be used with extreme caution in patients suffering from respiratory disease or from acute respiratory dysfunction (*e.g.*, pulmonary edema secondary to smoke inhalation).

Because of its effects on vasopressin (ADH), morphine must be used cautiously in patients suffering from acute uremia. Urine flow has been reported to decrease by as much as 90% in dogs given large doses of morphine. If administering IV, morphine must be given slowly or significant hypotension can result.

Neonatal, debilitated, or geriatric patients may be more susceptible to the effects of morphine and may require lower dosages. Patients with severe hepatic disease may have prolonged duration of action of the drug.

Morphine should be avoided in envenomation situations, as clinical signs associated with histamine-release can be confused with anaphylaxis. Opiate analgesics are contraindicated in patients who have been stung by the scorpion species *Centruroides sculpturatus Ewing* and *C. gertschi Stahnke* as they can potentiate these venoms.

Adverse Effects

At usual doses, the primary concern is the effect the opioids have on respiratory function. Decreased tidal volume, depressed cough reflex, and the drying of respiratory secretions may all have a detrimental effect on a susceptible patient. Bronchoconstriction (secondary to histamine release?) following IV doses has been noted in dogs. Significant hypotension can occur if administered rapidly IV. Panting is often seen in dogs after morphine administration.

Gastrointestinal effects may include: nausea, vomiting, and decreased intestinal peristalsis. Dogs will usually defecate after an initial dose of morphine, but this is not usually seen when used post-operatively. Horses exhibiting signs of mild colic may have their clinical signs masked by the administration of narcotic analgesics.

The CNS effects of morphine are dose and species specific. Animals that are stimulated by morphine may elucidate changes in behavior, appear restless and, at very high doses, have convulsions. The CNS depressant effects seen in dogs may encumber the abilities of working animals.

Body temperature changes may be seen. Cattle, goats, horses, and cats may exhibit signs of hyperthermia, while rabbits and dogs may develop hypothermia.

Chronic administration may lead to physical dependence.

Reproductive/Nursing Safety

Placental transfer of opiates is rapid. In humans, the FDA categorizes this drug as category *C* for use during pregnancy (*Animal studies have shown an adverse effect on the fetus, but there are no adequate studies in humans; or there are no animal reproduction studies and no adequate studies in humans.*) In a separate system evaluating the safety of drugs in canine and feline pregnancy (Papich 1989), this drug is categorized as class: *B* (*Safe for use if used cautiously. Studies in laboratory animals may have uncovered some risk, but these drugs appear to be safe in dogs and cats or these drugs are safe if they are not administered when the animal is near term.*)

Morphine appears in maternal milk, but effects on offspring may not be significant when used for short periods. Withdrawal symptoms have occurred however in breastfeeding infants when maternal administration of an opioid-analgesic stopped. Decide whether to accept the risks, discontinue nursing or to discontinue the drug, taking into account the importance of the drug to the mother.

Overdosage/Acute Toxicity

Overdosage may produce profound respiratory and/or CNS depression in most species. Newborns may be more susceptible to these effects than adult animals. Parenteral doses greater than 100 mg/kg are thought to be fatal in dogs. Other toxic effects can include cardiovascular collapse, hypothermia, and skeletal muscle hypotonia. Some species such as horses, cats, swine, and cattle may demonstrate CNS excitability (hyperreflexia, tremors) and seizures at high doses or if given rapidly intravenously. Naloxone is the agent of choice in treating respiratory depression. In massive overdoses, naloxone doses may need to be repeated. Animals should be closely observed as naloxone's effects might diminish before sub-toxic levels of morphine are attained. Mechanical respiratory support should be considered in cases of severe respiratory depression.

Pentobarbital has been suggested as a treatment for CNS excitement and seizures in cats. Extreme caution should be used as barbiturates and narcotics can have additive effects on respiratory depression.

Drug Interactions

The following drug interactions have either been reported or are theoretical in humans or animals receiving morphine and may be of significance in veterinary patients:

- ■ **CNS DEPRESSANTS, OTHER (e.g., anesthetic agents, antihistamines, phenothiazines, barbiturates, tranquilizers, alcohol, etc.):** May cause increased CNS or respiratory depression when used with morphine

- ■ **DIURETICS:** Opiates may decrease efficacy in CHF patients

- ■ **MONAMINE OXIDASE (MAO) INHIBITORS (e.g., amitraz, possibly selegiline):** Use MAOI's with morphine with extreme caution as meperidine (a related opiate) is contraindicated in human patients receiving monamine oxidase (MAO) inhibitors for at least 14 days after receiving MAO inhibitors. Some human patients have exhibited signs of opiate overdose after receiving therapeutic doses of meperidine while taking MAOIs.

- ■ **MUSCLE RELAXANTS, SKELETAL:** Morphine may enhance neuromuscular blockade

- ■ **TRICYCLIC ANTIDEPRESSANTS (clomipramine, amitriptyline, etc.):** Morphine may exacerbate the effects of tricyclic antidepressants

- ■ **WARFARIN:** Opiates may potentiate anticoagulant activity

Laboratory Considerations

- ■ As they may increase biliary tract pressure, opiates can increase plasma amylase and lipase values up to 24 hours following their administration.

Doses

For additional doses/protocols for using morphine in combination with other drugs (*e.g.*, ketamine, lidocaine, dexmedetomidine) for pain/sedation in dogs or cats, see the doses and their accompanying references in the dexmedetomidine, ketamine, and lidocaine monographs.

- ■ **DOGS:**

  For analgesia (acute pain):

  a) For post-op pain: 0.25–2 mg/kg IM, SQ; or as a CRI at 0.05–0.2 mg/kg/hr. (Grubb 2007)

  b) As a CRI for acute pain: 0.05–0.2 mg/kg hr. Morphine tends to produce increased sedation and side effects when used at a dosage of >0.1 mg/kg/h for more than 12 hours; therefore, the infusion rate must often be reduced by that time. (Hansen, B. 2008)

  c) 0.5–2.2 mg/kg SC, IM q 4–6h; 0.1–0.2 mg/kg IV q1–2h (Gaynor 2007)

  d) 0.2–0.5 mg/kg IM, SC or IV (slowly because of histamine release). Easily titrated to effect. Morphine is given every 4 hours to dogs or as required at author's hospital. (Self 2008)

  e) As a CRI for pain: Give a loading dose of 0.3 mg/kg slowly over 2-3 minutes IV, then a CRI of 0.1–0.2 mg/kg/hour. (Grint 2008)

  Epidural administration for pain control:

  a) 0.1 mg/kg preservative free morphine; duration of action 12–24 hours (Thomas 2000)

  b) Using regular morphine injection: 0.1 mg/kg once; using preservative-free morphine: epidural at 0.1–0.2 mg/kg q8h; spinal at 0.05 mg/kg q8h. (Hansen, B 2007)

c) Epidural: Morphine (use preservative-free if possible): 0.1 mg/kg in 0.3 mL/kg (max of 6 mL). Opioids provide analgesia without loss of hind limb function or muscle tone. Analgesia has a fairly long duration and can be maintained with an epidural catheter (although placement and maintenance of the catheter may be difficult). One advantage of epidural morphine is that the analgesia will migrate cranially and be effective up to about 18 hrs. (Matthews 2008)

As a preanesthetic:

a) As a premedicant with acepromazine: acepromazine 0.05 mg/kg IM; morphine 0.5 mg/kg IM (Pablo 2003)

b) In a healthy large breed dog acepromazine at 0.03 mg/kg IM, with morphine at 0.5 mg/kg IM (onset of action 40 minutes after dose); can induce heavy sedation. Giving the acepromazine 20 minutes before morphine (or hydromorphone) can significantly reduce vomiting.

Severe sedation and sedation/analgesia sufficient for minor surgical procedures can be achieved by IM administration of an opioid. If using morphine: 0.02–0.5 mg/kg with medetomidine (20–40 micrograms/kg), and either ketamine (4.4 mg/kg) or Telazol® (4 mg/kg). (Trim 2008)

c) In critical patients: 0.5–2 mg/kg IM. Use with diazepam, midazolam, or acepromazine. Caution with IV use due to histamine release. (Raffe 2008)

For adjunctive treatment of cardiogenic pulmonary edema:

a) 0.05–1 mg/kg IV q1–4 hours, or 0.1–0.5 mg/kg hr IV infusion, or 0.2–2 mg/kg IM or SC q2–4hr (Hansen, B 2003)

For treatment of hypermotile diarrhea:

a) 0.25 mg/kg (Jones 1985)

As an antitussive:

a) 0.1 mg/kg q6–12h SC (Roudebush 1985)

■ **CATS:**

For analgesia:

a) For post-op pain: 0.1–0.3 mg/kg IM, SC (Grubb 2007)

b) 0.1–0.2 mg/kg IM, SC or IV (slowly because of histamine release). Easily titrated to effect. Morphine is given every 6 hours to cats or as required at author's hospital. (Self 2008)

c) 0.1–0.4 mg/kg IM, SC q3–6h; concomitant tranquilization recommended (Hendrix & Hansen 2000)

d) 0.02–0.1 mg/kg IV q1–4hrs; 0.2–0.5 mg/kg IM, SC q3–4h; 0.2–0.5 mg/kg PO q6–8h. (Hansen, B 2007)

Epidural administration for pain control:

a) Using preservative-free morphine: epidural at 0.1–0.2 mg/kg q8h; spinal at 0.05 mg/kg q8h. (Hansen, B 2007)

As a preanesthetic:

a) In critical patients: 0.5–2 mg/kg IM. Use with diazepam or midazolam in cats. Caution with IV use due to histamine release. (Raffe 2008)

For adjunctive treatment of cardiogenic pulmonary edema:

a) 0.02–0.1 mg/kg IV q1–4 hours, or 0.2–0.5 mg/kg IM or SC q3–4hr (Hansen, B 2003)

■ **RABBITS, RODENTS, SMALL MAMMALS:**

a) Rabbits: 2–5 mg/kg IM or SC q2–4h for sedation and analgesia (Ivey & Morrisey 2000)

■ **HORSES: (Note:** ARCI UCGFS Class 1 Drug) **Note:** Narcotics may cause CNS excitement in the horse. Some clinicians recommend pretreatment with acepromazine, detomidine, or xylazine to reduce the behavioral changes these drugs can cause. **Warning:** Narcotic analgesics can mask the behavioral and cardiovascular clinical signs associated with mild colic.

For analgesia:

a) 0.1 mg/kg IM q4h; this dose reduces morphine's impact on GI motility, but patients must be observed for problems following morphine use. To cover the excitatory effects of morphine, small doses of acepromazine (0.011–0.022 mg/kg IM, or 5–10 mg/450 kg) are generally included with the morphine injection. (Abrahamsen 2007)

b) For epidural: Adult horses: 0.1–0.2 mg/kg using conventional morphine injection (15 mg/mL). Use a freshly opened vial. Suggest diluting with saline to a total volume of 0.04 mL/kg or 20 mL/450kg.

Foals: Using preservative free morphine at 0.1 mg/kg. If no preservative free morphine available, dilute to a volume of 0.2 mL/kg. (Abrahamsen 2007)

c) Morphine may be used IV (0.012–0.66 mg/kg) as an analgesic agent in combination with alpha2 agonists. When used IV as a sole analgesic agent, it may result in profound excitation. Anecdotally, IM morphine use is not associated with CNS excitation and this may represent an under-appreciated analgesic option.

Epidural: Morphine may be administered epidurally on its own or in combination with detomidine (0.03–0.06 mg/kg) to provide effective analgesia of the caudal half of the body. Morphine is typically used at doses of 0.1 to 0.2 mg/kg diluted to 10–20 mL with 0.9% saline (total volume of 0.04 mL/kg body weight). Analgesic effects are seen within 20-30 minutes and may last 8-24 hours without adverse effects on motor function. (Sellon 2007)

■ **SWINE:**

As a preanesthetic/analgesic (prior to chloralose, barbiturate):

a) 0.2–0.9 mg/kg IM. **Note:** may cause undesirable stimulation. (Booth 1988)

As an analgesic:

a) 0.2 mg/kg up to 20 mg total dose IM (Jenkins 1987)

■ **SHEEP & GOATS:**

As an analgesic:

a) Up to 10 mg total dose, IM (Jenkins 1987)

■ **CAMELIDS:**

a) Epidural: 0.1–0.3 mg/kg of preservative-free morphine diluted to 12 mL. (Cebra 2009)

■ **ZOO, EXOTIC, WILDLIFE SPECIES:**

For use of morphine in zoo, exotic and wildlife medicine refer to specific references, including:

a) *Zoo Animal and Wildlife Immobilization and Anesthesia.* West, G, Heard, D, Caulkett, N. (eds.). Blackwell Publishing, 2007.

b) *Handbook of Wildlife Chemical Immobilization, 3rd Ed.* Kreeger, T.J. and J.M. Arnemo. 2007.

c) *Restraint and Handling of Wild and Domestic Animals.* Fowler, M (ed.), Iowa State University Press, 1995

d) *Exotic Animal Formulary, 3rd Ed.* Carpenter, J.W., Saunders. 2005

e) The 2009 American Association of Zoo Veterinary Proceedings by D. K. Fontenot also has several dosages listed for restraint, anesthesia, and analgesia for a variety of drugs for carnivores and primates. VIN members can access them at: http://goo.gl/BHRih or http://goo.gl/9UJse

Monitoring

■ Respiratory rate/depth

■ CNS level of depression/excitation

■ Blood pressure (especially with IV use)

■ Analgesic activity

Client Information

■ When given parenterally, this agent should be used in an inpatient setting or with direct professional supervision.

Chemistry/Synonyms

The sulfate salt of a natural (derived from opium) occurring opiate analgesic, morphine sulfate occurs as white, odorless, crystals. Solubility: 1 gram in 16 mL of water (62.5 mg/mL), 570 mL

(1.75 mg/mL) of alcohol. It is insoluble in chloroform or ether. The pH of morphine sulfate injection ranges from 2.5–6.

Morphine sulfate may also be known as morphini sulfas, *Astramorph PF®, Avinza®, DepoDur®, Infumorph®, Kadian®, MSIR®, MS Contin®, Oramorph SR, RMS®,* and *Roxanol®.*

Storage/Stability

Oral morphine products should be stored at in tight, light-resistant containers at room temperature unless otherwise labeled. Morphine injection should be stored at room temperature, protected from light; do not freeze. Morphine gradually darkens in color when exposed to light; protect from prolonged exposure to bright light. Morphine does not appear to adsorb to plastic or PVC syringes, tubing or bags.

Compatibility/Compounding Considerations

Morphine sulfate has been shown to be physically **compatible** at a concentration of 16.2 mg/L with the following intravenous fluids: Dextrose 2.5%, 5%, 10% in water; Ringer's injection and Lactated Ringer's injection; Sodium Chloride 0.45% and 0.9% for injection. Compatibility is dependent upon factors such as pH, concentration, temperature, and diluent used; consult specialized references or a hospital pharmacist for more specific information.

The following drugs have been shown to be physically **incompatible** when mixed with morphine sulfate: aminophylline, chlorothiazide sodium, heparin sodium, meperidine, pentobarbital sodium, phenobarbital sodium, phenytoin sodium, sodium bicarbonate, and thiopental sodium. Morphine sulfate has been demonstrated to be generally physically **compatible** when mixed with the following agents: Atropine sulfate, benzquinamide HCl, butorphanol tartrate, chlorpromazine HCl, diphenhydramine HCl, dobutamine HCl, droperidol, fentanyl citrate, glycopyrrolate, hydroxyzine HCl, metoclopramide, pentazocine lactate, promazine HCl, scopolamine HBr, and succinylcholine chloride.

Dosage Forms/Regulatory Status

VETERINARY-LABELED PRODUCTS: None

The ARCI (Racing Commissioners International) has designated this drug as a class 1 substance. See the appendix for more information.

HUMAN-LABELED PRODUCTS:

Morphine Sulfate for Injection: 1 mg/mL, 2 mg/mL, 4 mg/mL, 5 mg/mL, 8 mg/mL, 10 mg/mL, 15 mg/mL, 25 mg/mL, 50 mg/mL in amps, vials, syringes, and pre-filled IV bags in sizes that range from 1 mL to 250 mL depending on manufacturer and concentration. (Rx; C-II)

Morphine Sulfate Liposomal Extended-release Injection: 10 mg/mL in 1 mL, 1.5 mL, & 2 mL single-use vials; *DepoDur®* (Endo); (Rx, C-II)

Morphine Sulfate for Injection (preservative-free): 0.5 mg/mL: 2 mL amps, & 10 mL amps and vials; 1 mg/mL: 10 mL amps and vials; 10 mg/mL (200 mg) in 20 mL amps; 25 mg/mL (500 mg) in 20 mL amps; *Infumorph®* (Baxter); *Astramorph PF®* (AstraZeneca); (Rx, C-II)

Morphine Sulfate Soluble Tablets for Injection: 10 mg, 15 mg & 30 mg; generic; (Ranbaxy); (Rx, C-II)

Morphine Sulfate Oral Tablets: 15 mg & 30 mg; generic; (Rx, C-II)

Morphine Sulfate Extended/Controlled Release Tablets: 15 mg, 30 mg, 60 mg, 100 mg & 200 mg; *MS Contin®* (Purdue Frederick); *Oramorph SR®* (aaiPharma); generic; (Rx, C-II)

Morphine Sulfate Extended/Sustained Release Capsules: 20 mg, 30 mg, 45 mg, 50 mg, 60 mg, 75 mg, 80 mg, 90 mg, 100 mg, 120 mg & 200 mg; *Avinza®* (King Pharmaceuticals); *Kadian®* (Actavis); (Rx, C-II)

Morphine Sulfate Oral Solution: 2 mg/mL in 100 mL, 500 mL and UD 5mL & 10 mL; 4 mg/mL in 100mL, 120 mL & 500 mL; 20 mg/mL (concentrate) in 15 mL, 30 mL, 120 mL & 240 mL/calibrated dropper or spoon; *MSIR®* (Purdue Frederick); Morphine Sulfate (Roxane); *Roxanol®, -T, & -100* (aaiPharma); generic; (Rx; C-II)

Morphine Sulfate Rectal Suppositories: 5 mg, 10 mg, 20 mg, & 30 mg; *RMS®* (Upsher-Smith); generic; (various); (Rx, C-II)

Note: All morphine products are Rx and a Class-II controlled substance. Very accurate record keeping is required as to use and disposition of stock.

References

Abrahamsen, E. (2007). Analgesia in equine practice. Proceedings: Western Vet Conference. Accessed via: Veterinary Information Network. http://goo.gl/PpibC

Bellei, M., C. Kerr, et al. (2008). Pharmacokinetics of Epidural Morphine in Awake and Isoflurane-Anesthetized Horses. Proceedings: IVECCS. Accessed via: Veterinary Information Network. http://goo.gl/oZswE

Booth, N.H. (1988). Drugs Acting on the Central Nervous System. *Veterinary Pharmacology and Therapeutics—6th Ed.* NH Booth and LE McDonald Eds. Ames, Iowa State University Press: 153–408.

Cebra, C.K. (2009). Abdominal Discomfort in Llamas & Alpacas: Diagnosis & Treatment. Proceedings: ACVIM. Accessed via: Veterinary Information Network. http://goo.gl/flIBS

Gaynor, J. (2007). Small Animal Acute Pain Control—NSAIDs and more. Proceedings: Western Vet Conference. Accessed via: Veterinary Information Network. http://goo.gl/9K2oy

Grint, N. (2008). Constant Rate Infusions (CRIS) in Pain Management. Proceedings: BSAVA. Accessed via: Veterinary Information Network. http://goo.gl/CIXUX

Grubb, T. (2007). The postanesthetic period and pain management. Proceedings: Western Vet Conf. Accessed via: Veterinary Information Network. http://goo.gl/h3Tjt

Hansen, B. (2003). Opiate use in cardiovascular medicine. Proceedings: ACVIM Forum.

Hansen, B. (2007). Pain management in emergency and critical care. Proceedings: Western Vet Conf. Accessed via: Veterinary Information Network. http://goo.gl/xgQQG

Hansen, B. (2008). Analgesia for the Critically Ill Dog or Cat: An Update. *Veterinary Clinics of North America-Small Animal Practice* **38**(6): 1353–+.

Hendrix, P. & B. Hansen (2000). Acute Pain Management. *Kirk's Current Veterinary Therapy: XIII Small Animal Practice.* J Bonagura Ed. Philadelphia, WB Saunders: 57–61.

Ivey, E. & J. Morrisey (2000). Therapeutics for Rabbits. *Vet Clin NA: Exotic Anim Pract* **3:1**(Jan): 183–216.

Jenkins, W.L. (1987). Pharmacologic aspects of analgesic drugs in animals: An overview. *JAVMA* **191**(10): 1231–1240.

Jones, B.D. (1985). Gastrointestinal disorders. *Handbook of Small Animal Therapeutics.* LE Davis Ed. New York, Churchill Livingston: 397–462.

Lindegaard, C., K.B. Gleerup, et al. (2010). Anti-inflammatory effects of intra-articular administration of morphine in horses with experimentally induced synovitis. *American Journal of Veterinary Research* **71**(1): 69–75.

Matthews, N. (2008). Perioperative Analgesia: Part 1. Concepts and Drugs. Proceedings: ACVC. Accessed via: Veterinary Information Network. http://goo.gl/HgU4D

Pablo, L. (2003). Total IV anesthesia in small animals. Proceedings: World Small Animal Veterinary Assoc World Congress. Accessed via: Veterinary Information Network. http://goo.gl/e1v31

Papich, M. (1989). Effects of drugs on pregnancy. *Current Veterinary Therapy X: Small Animal Practice.* R Kirk Ed. Philadelphia, Saunders: 1291–1299.

Pirie, C., C. Blaze, et al. (2008). The Effect of Intravenous Hydromorphone, Butorphanol, Morphine, and Buprenorphine on Pupil Size and Intraocular Pressure in Normal Dogs. Proceedings: ACVO. Accessed via: Veterinary Information Network. http://goo.gl/mqbPE

Raffe, M. (2008). Anesthesia and Analgesia of the Critical Patient. Proceedings: IVECCS. Accessed via: Veterinary Information Network. http://goo.gl/zEzFc

Roudebush, P. (1985). Respiratory Diseases. *Handbook of Small Animal Therapeutics.* LE Davis Ed. New York, Churchill Livingston: 287–332.

Self, I. (2008). 'Ouch That Hurts'—Post Operative Pain Assessment and Treatment Options. Proceedings: WSAVA. Accessed via: Veterinary Information Network. http://goo.gl/tDtje

Sellon, D. (2007). New Alternatives for Pain Management in Horses. Proceedings: New Alternatives for Pain Management in Horses. Accessed via: Veterinary Information Network. http://goo.gl/gXMfb

Thomas, W. (2000). Idiopathic epilepsy in dogs. *Vet Clin NA: Small Anim Pract* **30:1**(Jan): 183–206.

Trim, C. (2008). Opioid Analgesia. Proceedings: WVC. Accessed via: Veterinary Information Network. http://goo.gl/VACG6

MOXIDECTIN

(mox-i-**dek**-tin)   Cydectin®, ProHeart®,
Advantage® Multi

AVERMECTIN ANTIPARASITIC

Prescriber Highlights

▶ Avermectin antiparasitic with products
   FDA-approved for cattle, dogs, cats,
   sheep, & horses

▶ Labeling and use of *ProHeart®6* is
   presently dynamic; get most current
   info from label/manufacturer

▶ Contraindications (oral; topical): *Dogs:*
   Hypersensitive to drug; *Cattle:* Female
   dairy cattle of breeding age; *Horses:*
   Intended for food purposes or in foals
   younger than 4 months of age

▶ Adverse Effects (topical; oral): *Dogs*
   (potentially): Lethargy, vomiting, ataxia,
   anorexia, diarrhea, nervousness, weakness, increased thirst, & itching. *Cattle:*
   Adverse effects minimal. *Horses:* At
   labeled doses, appear minimal.

▶ Apparently safe to use in *ABCB1-1Δ*
   (formerly MDR1-allele) gene mutation
   dog breeds at labeled doses; higher
   doses may cause neurotoxicity in
   these dogs

Uses/Indications

In dogs and cats, moxidectin with lufenuron is
indicated as a once a month topical preventative
for the prevention of heartworm, flea adulticide,
ear mites (cats) and treatment for hookworms,
roundworms, and whipworms (dogs). It has also
been successfully used as a treatment for generalized demodicosis.

In dogs, a 6 month injectable product
(*ProHeart®6*) is FDA-approved for use (in the
USA) for use in dogs six months of age and
older for the prevention of heartworm disease
caused by *Dirofilaria immitis* and for the treatment of existing larval and adult hookworm
(*Ancylostoma caninum* and *Uncinaria stenocephala*) infections. At the time of writing (2010),
this product is currently available only through a
restricted distribution program, but this is likely
to change in forthcoming months.

In cattle, moxidectin is indicated for the
treatment and control of the following internal [adult and fourth stage larvae (L4)] and
external parasites: Gastrointestinal roundworms: *Ostertagia ostertagi* (adult and L4,
including inhibited larvae), *Haemonchus placei* (adult), *Trichostrongylus axei* (adult and
L4), *Trichostrongylus colubriformis* (adult),
Cooperia oncophora (adult), *Cooperia punctata* (adult), *Bunostomum phlebotomum*
(adult), *Oesophagostomum radiatum* (adult),
Nematodirus helvetianus (adult); Lungworm:
Dictyocaulus viviparus (adult and L4); Cattle
Grubs: *Hypoderma bovis, Hypoderma lineatum*
Mites: *Chorioptes bovis, Psoroptes ovis* (*Psoroptes
communis var. bovis*); Lice: *Linognathus vituli,
Haematopinus eurysternus, Solenopotes capillatus, Damalinia bovis*; Horn flies: *Haematobia ir-
ritans*. To control infections and to protect from
reinfection from *Ostertagia ostertagi* for 28 days
after treatment and from *Dictyocaulus viviparus*
for 42 days after treatment.

In sheep, oral moxidectin is indicated for
the control of *Haemonchus contortus* (adult
and L4), *Teladosrsagia circumcincta* & *trifurcata*
(adult and L4), *Trichostrongylus colubriformis,
axei,* & *vitrinius* (adult & L4), *Cooperia curticei*
& *oncophora* (adult and L4), *Oesophagostomum
columbianum* & *venolosum* (adult & L4), and
Nematodirus battus, filicollis, & *spathiger* (adult
& L4).

In horses and ponies, moxidectin is indicated
for the treatment and control of the following
stages of gastrointestinal parasites: Large strongyles: *Strongylus vulgaris* (adults and L4L5 arterial stages); *Strongylus edentatus* (adults and tissue stages); *Triodontophorus brevicauda* (adults);
Triodontophorus serratus (adults); Small
strongyles (adults and larvae): *Cyathostomum
spp. (adults); Cylicocyclus* spp. (adults);
Cylicostephanus spp. (adults); *Gyalocephalus
capitatus* (adults); undifferentiated lumenal larvae; Encysted cyathostomes: late L3 and L4 mucosal cyathostome larvae; Ascarids: *Parascaris
equorum* (adults and L4 larval stages); Pin
worms: *Oxyuris equi* (adults and L4 larval stages); Hair worms: Trichostrongylus axei (adults);
Large-mouth stomach worms: *Habronema mus-
cae* (adults); Horse stomach bots: *Gasterophilus
intestinalis* (2nd and 3rd instars). When combined with praziquantel, additional coverage
against *Anoplocephala* spp. occurs. Resistance to
antiparasitic agents is an ongoing problem. It is
recommended to perform fecal egg count reduction testing (FECRT) for strongyle nematodes.
A value of less than 95% in 5-10 horses is the
suggested cut-off for determining resistance on
a given farm (Nielsen & Kaplan 2009).

Pharmacology/Actions

The primary mode of action of avermectins like
moxidectin is to affect chloride ion channel activity in the nervous system of nematodes and
arthropods. The drug binds to receptors that increase membrane permeability to chloride ions.
This inhibits the electrical activity of nerve cells
in nematodes and muscle cells in arthropods
and causes paralysis and death of the parasites.
Avermectins also enhance the release of gamma
amino butyric acid (GABA) at presynaptic neurons. GABA acts as an inhibitory neurotransmitter and blocks the post-synaptic stimulation of the adjacent neuron in nematodes or
the muscle fiber in arthropods. Avermectins
are generally not toxic to mammals, since they

do not have glutamate-gated chloride channels and these compounds do not readily cross the blood-brain barrier where mammalian GABA receptors occur.

Pharmacokinetics

Minimal information was located. In cattle, the drug apparently has a long duration of plasma residence (14–15 days). After SC injection, approximately 5% of the dose given to the cow can be passed to the suckling calf.

In horses, moxidectin may have a period of action of up to 12 weeks.

Moxidectin is very lipophilic (100 times that of ivermectin), so volumes of distribution would likely be very high. Animals with very low body fat (neonates, cachexia) could potentially have serum levels much higher than normal patients.

Contraindications/Precautions/Warnings

Dogs: Contraindicated in dogs hypersensitive to it. The manufacturer warns to only use the oral product in dogs tested negative for heartworm infection. Adult heartworms and microfilaria should be removed prior to therapy. If more than two months pass between dosages of this or other once a month heartworm preventative medications, the dog should be tested for heartworm infection before receiving the next dose. Oral formulation doses (3 mg/kg/month) and topical formulation heartworm prevention doses (2500 micrograms/kg/month) are safe for all *ABCB1* genotypes (Mealey 2008).

For the 6-month injectable product (*ProHeart*®6; June 2010): Contraindicated in patients previously found hypersensitive to the drug, or are sick, debilitated, underweight or who have a history of weight loss. Use with caution in dogs with pre-existing allergic disease, including food allergy, atopy, and flea allergy dermatitis. Caution should be used when administering concurrently with vaccinations. Adverse reactions, including anaphylaxis, have been reported following the concomitant use of *ProHeart*®6 and vaccinations. Caution should be used when administering to heartworm positive dogs; prior to administration, dogs should be tested for existing heartworm infections. Safety and effectiveness has not been evaluated in dogs less than 6 months of age.

Cattle: Not for use in female dairy cattle of breeding age.

Horses: Not for horses intended for food purposes and is not labeled for use in foals younger than 4 months of age.

Animals with very low body fat (neonates, cachexia) could be more prone to develop adverse reactions.

Adverse Effects

Dogs: The topically applied product (w/imidacloprid) appears to be very well tolerated in dogs, regardless of their *ABCB1* genotype.

The injectable product (*ProHeart*®6) has been

implicated in serious adverse effects in the past. In 2004, at the request FDA, the manufacturer instituted a voluntary recall of *ProHeart*®6, after reports of serious adverse events in dogs that included anaphylaxis, liver disease, autoimmune hemolytic disease, convulsions and death. After evaluation of additional data and changes in the manufacturing process, a risk minimization plan (RISKmap) was instituted by the manufacturer. In a 2010 review of the adverse effect data associated with the RISKmap, adverse effect rates were very low. Anaphylaxis/anaphylactoid reactions were the prevalent ADRs reported, but at a rate of 1.24 cases per 10,000 doses administered. The RISKmap plan is at present (summer 2010) still in effect, but may be altered in the future. Contact the manufacturer (Pfizer Animal Health) for more information.

When used orally at demodicosis doses (0.2–0.4 mg/kg PO once daily), vomiting, ataxia, lethargy, and inappetence can be seen.

Cattle: Thus far at labeled doses, adverse effects appear to nonexistent or minimal.

Horses: Thus far at labeled doses, adverse effects appear to be nonexistent or minimal. A case report where three foals developed CNS depression and coma after receiving high dosages has been reported. Two of these three animals were less than 2 weeks of age and all received much higher than labeled dosages.

Reproductive/Nursing Safety

Dogs, Cats: Reproductive studies have demonstrated no evidence of adverse effects on fertility, reproductive performance, or offspring.

Cattle & Horses: Reproductive studies performed thus far have demonstrated no evidence of adverse effects on fertility, reproductive performance, or offspring in cattle or horses treated.

Overdosage/Acute Toxicity

Dogs: The drug apparently has a very wide margin of safety in dogs when administered orally at the appropriate dosage. Dosages of up to 300X (1120 micrograms/kg) demonstrated little or no effects. In *ABCB1* wild-type dogs, a single oral dose of 200 mg/kg did not cause neurologic toxicity. At 90 micrograms/kg, dogs with the *ABCB1* (mutant/mutant) genotype have shown signs of neurologic toxicity. Dogs administered inadvertent overdoses during a clinical study treating demodicosis showed signs of dysorexia, hypersalivation, mydriasis, and fasiculations and ataxia of the pelvic limbs.

There were 172 exposures to moxidectin reported to the ASPCA Animal Poison Control Center (APCC) during 2005–2006. In these cases, 171 were dogs with 42 showing clinical signs and the remaining case was 1 cat that showed clinical signs. Common findings in dogs recorded in decreasing frequency included tremors, ataxia, seizures, vomiting and hyperesthesia. Common findings in cats recorded included recumbency.

Cattle: In studies done on cattle, application of the pour-on solution at 5X the recommended dose for five consecutive days, 10X for two consecutive days and 25X for one day did not produce any significant adverse clinical or pathological effects.

Horses: In one study, three of eight foals given the 3X dose became depressed or ataxic after one treatment. The author has received an anecdotal report of a miniature horse developing seizures after receiving a full tube of *Quest®*.

Intravenous fat emulsion has been used to treat toxicity associated with macrocyclic lactones and other highly lipid soluble drugs.

Drug Interactions
While no specific drug interactions for moxidectin have been reported, the following drug interactions have either been reported or are theoretical in humans or animals receiving ivermectin (a related compound) and may be of significance in veterinary patients:

■ **BENZODIAZEPINES:** Effects may be potentiated by moxidectin; use together not advised in humans

Caution is advised if using other drugs that can inhibit **p-glycoprotein**. Those dogs at risk for *ABCB*1-1Δ (formerly MDR1-allele) mutation (Collies, Australian Shepherds, Shelties, Long-haired Whippet, etc. "white feet") should probably not receive moxidectin with the following drugs, unless tested "normal". Drugs and drug classes involved include:

■ **AMIODARONE**

■ **CARVEDILOL**

■ **CLARITHROMYCIN**

■ **CYCLOSPORINE**

■ **DILTIAZEM**

■ **ERYTHROMYCIN**

■ **ITRACONAZOLE**

■ **KETOCONAZOLE**

■ **QUINIDINE**

■ **SPIRONOLACTONE**

■ **TAMOXIFEN**

■ **VERAPAMIL**

Doses
■ **DOGS:**
a) For labeled indications (prevention of heartworm disease, adult fleas, adult and immature hookworms, adult roundworms, and adult whipworms) for *Advantage Multi®*: Recommended minimum dose is 10 mg/kg imidacloprid with 2.5 mg/kg moxidectin once a month by topical administration (**Note:** See package insert for specific instructions on application and safety). For dogs 3−9 lb = 0.4 mL; 9.1−20 lb = 1 mL; 20.1−55 lb = 2.5 mL, 55.1−88 lb = 4 mL; dogs over 88 lb should be treated with appropriate combination for their weight. (Label directions; *Advantage Multi® for Dogs*—Bayer)

b) For labeled indications (heartworm prevention, hookworms) **Note:** Current as of June 2010; see actual package insert for most up-to-date information): Owners should be given the Client Information Sheet for *ProHeart®6* to read before the drug is administered and should be advised to observe their dogs for potential drug toxicity described in the sheet.

The recommended subcutaneous dose is 0.05 mL of the constituted suspension/kg body weight. This provides 0.17 mg moxidectin/kg bodyweight. To ensure accurate dosing, calculate each dose based on the dog's weight at the time of treatment. Do not overdose growing puppies in anticipation of their expected adult weight. A dosage chart is found in the package insert that may be used as a guide. Injection Technique: The two-part sustained release product must be mixed at least 30 minutes prior to the intended time of use. Once constituted, swirl the bottle gently before every use to uniformly re-suspend the microspheres. Withdraw 0.05 mL of suspension/kg body weight into an appropriately sized syringe fitted with an 18G or 20G hypodermic needle. Dose promptly after drawing into dosing syringe. If administration is delayed, gently roll the dosing syringe prior to injection to maintain a uniform suspension and accurate dosing. Using aseptic technique, inject the product subcutaneously in the left or right side of the dorsum of the neck cranial to the scapula. No more than 3 mL should be administered in a single site. The location(s) of each injection (left or right side) should be noted so that prior injection sites can be identified and the next injection can be administered on the opposite side. Frequency of Treatment: *ProHeart®* 6 prevents infection by *D. immitis* for six months. It should be administered within one month of the dog's first exposure to mosquitoes. Follow-up treatments may be given every six months if the dog has continued exposure to mosquitoes and continues to be healthy without weight loss. When replacing another heartworm preventive product, *ProHeart®* 6 should be given within one month of the last dose of the former medication. (Label Information; *ProHeart®6*—Pfizer)

c) For scabiocidal therapy: Where *Cydectin®* is available for injection: 0.25 mg/kg SC every 7 days for three treatments. If using oral therapy 0.4 mg/kg PO every 3−4 days for 3−6 weeks. (Foil 2003) **Note:** These doses may cause toxicity in *ABCB*1 mutant genotype dogs.

d) For generalized demodicosis: 0.2–0.4 mg/kg PO once a day. Clinical cure averages 75 days; parasitic cure averages 112 days. (Carlotti 2008; Merchant 2000) **Note:** These doses may cause toxicity in *ABCB*1 mutant genotype dogs.

■ **CATS:**

a) For labeled indications (prevention of heartworm disease, adult fleas, ear mites, adult and immature hookworms, and adult roundworms: Recommended minimum dose is 10 mg/kg imidacloprid/1 mg/kg moxidectin once a month by topical administration (**Note:** See package insert for specific instructions on application and safety). For cats 2–5 lb = 0.23 mL; 5.1–9 lb = 0.4 mL; 9.1–18 lb = 0.8 mL; cats over 18 lb should be treated with appropriate combination for their weight. (Label directions; *Advantage Multi® for Cats*—Bayer)

b) For feline Aelurostrongylosis (*Aelurostrongylus abstrusus*): One to three topical applications of 1 mg/kg moxidectin (in combination with imidacloprid) appeared to be effective in the treatment of eight cats infected with *A. abstrusus*. (Conboy 2009)

■ **CATTLE:**

a) For labeled indications: 1 mL (5 mg)/10 kg (22 lb) bodyweight applied directly to the hair and skin along the top of the back from the withers to the base of the tail. Application should be made to healthy skin avoiding mange scabs, skin lesions or extraneous foreign matter. (Label Directions; *Cydectin® Pour-On*—Fort Dodge)

b) 0.2 mg/kg [1 mL for each 110 lb (50 kg) of bodyweight] subcutaneously under the loose skin in front of or behind the shoulder. Needles ½–¾ inch in length and 16–18 gauge are recommended. (Label Directions; *Cydectin® Injection*—Fort Dodge)

■ **SHEEP/GOATS:**

a) Sheep: For labeled indications: 0.2 mg/kg [1 mL per 11 lb (1 mL per 5 kg) bodyweight] PO (drench); *Cydectin® Oral Drench for Sheep*—Fort Dodge)

b) Goats: Moxidectin should be used at twice the sheep dose if it is deemed necessary for use. (Snyder 2009)

■ **HORSES:**

a) For labeled indications using the combination oral gel with praziquantel: Dial in the weight of the animal on the syringe. Administer gel by inserting the syringe applicator into the animal's mouth through the interdental space and depositing the gel in the back of the mouth near the base of the tongue. Once the syringe is removed, the animal's head should be raised to insure proper swallowing of the gel. Horses weighing more than 1250 lb require additional gel from a second syringe. (Label Directions; *Quest® Plus*—Fort Dodge)

b) For mucosal stages of small strongyles: 400 micrograms/kg PO (Lyons & Drudge 2000)

■ **CAMELIDS (NWC):**

a) Oral treatment with ivermectin or moxidectin at 0.2 mg/kg is generally felt to be the regimen of choice for gastrointestinal helminthes. (Wolff 2009)

Chemistry/Synonyms

An avermectin-class antiparasitic agent, moxidectin is a semi-synthetic methoxime derivative of nemadectin.

Moxidectin may also be known as CL-301423, *Advantage Multi®, ComboCare®, Cydectin®,* and *Quest®.*

Storage/Stability

For the sustained-release injection (*ProHeart®*6), store the unconstituted product at or below 25°C (77°F). Do not expose to light for extended periods of time. After constitution, the product is stable for 4 weeks stored under refrigeration at 2°-8°C (36°-46°F).

The commercially available injection and the oral drench for sheep should be stored at, or below 77°F (25°C) and protected from light.

The topical solution for cattle should be stored at or below room temperature. Do not allow prolonged exposure to temperatures above 77°F. If product becomes frozen, thaw completely and shake well before using.

The oral gel for horses should be stored at or near room temperature (59°F–86°F); avoid freezing. If product becomes frozen, thaw completely before using. Partially used syringes should have the cap tightly secured.

Compatibility/Compounding Considerations

When constituting the sustained-release injectable product (*ProHeart®*6) the provided diluent must be used and there are very specific direction for proper preparation. Refer to the package insert for more information.

Dosage Forms/Regulatory Status

VETERINARY-LABELED PRODUCTS:

Moxidectin 10% Sustained-Release (microspheres) Injectable 598 mg/vial with 17 mL diluent vial: *ProHeart®*6 (Pfizer); (Rx). FDA-Approved for use in dogs 6 weeks or older. See the package insert for the most up-to-date information for this product.

Moxidectin 0.5% (5 mg/mL) Pour-On for Cattle in 500 mL, 1 L, 2.5 L, 5 L, and 10 L containers; *Cydectin®* (BIVI); (OTC). FDA-approved for use in cattle; not to be used in veal calves. No meat or milk withdrawal times required, but FDA has established tolerances of 50 ppb and

200 ppb for parent moxidectin in muscle and liver, respectively, for cattle.

Moxidectin 10 mg/mL Injectable Solution in 200 mL and 500 mL; *Cydectin® Injectable Solution* (BIVI); (OTC). FDA-approved for cattle. Not to be used in female dairy cattle of breeding age, veal calves, and calves less than 8 weeks of age. Meat withdrawal = 21 days.

Moxidectin 1 mg/mL Oral Drench Solution in 1 L and 4 L; *Cydectin® Oral Drench for Sheep* (BIVI); (OTC). FDA-approved for sheep. Not to be used in female sheep providing milk for human consumption. Meat withdrawal = 7 days.

Moxidectin Oral Gel containing 20 mg/mL in 11.3 gram syringes (sufficient to treat one 1150 lb horse); *Quest®* (Pfizer); (OTC). FDA-approved for use in horse or ponies not intended for food purposes.

Oral Gel containing 20 mg/mL moxidectin and 125 mg/mL of praziquantel in 11.6 gram syringes (sufficient to treat one 1150 lb horse); *Quest Plus®*(Pfizer). FDA-approved for use in horse or ponies not intended for food purposes.

Moxidectin 1% (10 mg/mL) and Imidacloprid 10% (100 mg/mL) Topical Solution in 3—0.23mL tubes, 6—0.4mL tubes & 6—0.8mL tubes; *Advantage Multi® for Cats* (Bayer); (Rx). FDA-approved for use on cats 9 weeks of age or greater, and more than 2 lb body weight.

Moxidectin 2.5% (25 mg/mL) and Imidacloprid 10% (100 mg/mL) Topical Solution in 6—0.4mL tubes, 6—1mL tubes, 6—2.5 mL tubes, & 6—4mL tubes; *Advantage Multi® for Dogs* (Bayer); (Rx). FDA-approved for use on dogs 7 weeks of age or greater, and more than 3 lb body weight.

HUMAN-LABELED PRODUCTS: None

References

Carlotti, D.-N. (2008). Canine and Feline Demodicosis. Proceedings: WSAVA. Accessed via: Veterinary Information Network. http://goo.gl/yiNDm

Conboy, G. (2009). Helminth Parasites of the Canine and Feline Respiratory Tract. *Veterinary Clinics of North America-Small Animal Practice* 39(6): 1109–+.

Foil, C. (2003). Update on treating scabies and cheyletiella. Proceedings: Western Veterinary Conference. Accessed via: Veterinary Information Network. http://goo.gl/lXjUF

Lyons, E. & J. Drudge (2000). Larval Cyathostomiasis. *The Veterinary Clinics of North America: Equine Practice* 16:3(December).

Mealey, K.L. (2008). Canine ABCB1 and macrocyclic lactones: Heartworm prevention and pharmacogenetics. *Veterinary Parasitology* 158(3): 215–222.

Merchant, S. (2000). New Therapies in Veterinary Dermatology. Proceedings: American Animal Hospital Association 67th Annual Meeting, Toronto.

Nielsen, M. & R.M. Kaplan (2009). Diagnosis & Management of Anthelmintic Resistance in Equid Parasites. Proceedings: ACVIM. Accessed via: Veterinary Information Network. http://goo.gl/oIqSj

Snyder, J. (2009). Management of Internal Parasites in Sheep I & II. Proceedings: WVC. Accessed via: Veterinary Information Network. http://goo.gl/9cpiM

Wolff, P. (2009). Camelid Medicine. Proceedings: AAZV. Accessed via: Veterinary Information Network. http://goo.gl/4TEAy

---

MYCOBACTERIAL CELL WALL FRACTION IMMUNO-MODULATOR

(my-koe-bak-*tear*-ee-al)
Regressin®-V, Equimune® I.V.

IMMUNOSTIMULANT

Prescriber Highlights

▶ Biologic used in dogs as a locally infiltrated injection for immunotherapy treatment of mixed mammary tumor & mammary adenocarcinomas

▶ In horses, used for immunotherapy treatment of sarcoids (local infiltration), ERCD (IV) or as an aid in the treatment of equine metritis caused by *Streptococcus zooepidemicus* (IV, IU)

▶ Adverse effects include: Transient fever, depression, decreased appetite, localized pain. Hypersensitivity & systemic inflammatory reactions possible.

▶ Efficacy for systemic use is not well established

Uses/Indications

Mycobacterial cell wall fraction immunomodulator is commercially available as three products with veterinary labeling, *Regressin®-V*, *Equimune®-IV* and *Settle®*. *Regressin®-V* is labeled as a locally infiltrated injection for immunotherapy treatment of mixed mammary tumor and mammary adenocarcinomas in dogs, and for immunotherapy treatment of sarcoids in horses. *Equimune®-IV* is labeled for use in horses only as an immunotherapeutic agent for the treatment of Equine Respiratory Disease Complex (ERDC). *Settle®* is labeled as an aid in the treatment of equine metritis caused by *Streptococcus zooepidemicus* (IV, IU) in horses.

Although not labeled indications, *Equimune®-IV* has reportedly been used in horses as an adjuvant for EPM treatment and as an adjuvant for herpesvirus vaccines when injected IM at a separate site from the vaccine. Documentation of efficacy for these uses was not located.

Pharmacology/Actions

Mycobacterial fractionated compounds require a functional immune system for efficacy. They have a non-specific immune stimulatory primarily on cell-mediated immune mechanisms and macrophage activation. Interleukin-1 release from macrophages is thought to be the primary mediator for their actions.

Pharmacokinetics

No information was located.

Contraindications/Precautions/Warnings

These drugs should not be used in patients with prior hypersensitivity to mycobacterial cell wall compounds or those with mycobacterial infections.

The manufacturer warns that patients receiving cortisone or ACTH may not respond to treatment; in case of an anaphylactic reaction, administer epinephrine.

Adverse Effects

Horses: Adverse effects include fever, drowsiness and diminished appetite for 1–2 days after injection. Local infiltrations can cause pain and tenderness at injection site. Anaphylaxis and severe respiratory inflammatory reactions have also been reported.

Dogs: Adverse effects include fever, drowsiness and diminished appetite for 1–2 days after injection. Local infiltrations can cause pain and tenderness at injection site. Later necrosis and draining may occur. Anaphylaxis or hypersensitivity reactions are possible.

Reproductive/Nursing Safety

The manufacturer states that *Regressin®-V* and *Equimune®-I.V.* are safe to use in pregnant mares. No other information was located.

Overdosage/Acute Toxicity

No information was located.

Drug Interactions

■ **CORTICOSTEROIDS, ACTH, IMMUNOSUPPRESSIVE DRUGS (e.g., cyclosporine):** May reduce the effectiveness of mycobacterial cell wall immunostimulants.

Laboratory Considerations

■ None identified

Doses

■ **DOGS:**

a) Using *Regressin®-V* for immunotherapy of mixed mammary tumor and mammary adenocarcinoma: Using no larger than a 20-gauge needle, infiltrate entire tumor and a small region of adjacent and underlying tissue. Dosage varies with tumor size, but 1 mL should be considered a minimum dose. Be certain the emulsion is mixed thoroughly and inject quickly as emulsion can separate rapidly (see Stability information for more information on mixing.) As pain may occur, additional anesthetics or analgesics may be used. Tumors may be treated once, 2–4 weeks before surgery. If surgery is not to be used, repeat treatment every 1–3 weeks. If no response after 4 treatments, discontinue. (Label information; *Regressin®-V*—Bioniche)

■ **HORSES:**

a) Using *Regressin®-V* for immunotherapy of sarcoids: Large pedunculated sarcoids should be de-bulked by partial excision prior to treatment. Using no larger than a 20-gauge needle, infiltrate entire tumor and a small region of adjacent and underlying tissue. Dosage varies with tumor size, but 1 mL should be considered a minimum dose. Be certain the emulsion is mixed thoroughly and inject quickly as emulsion can separate rapidly (see Stability information for more information on mixing.) As pain may occur, additional anesthetics or analgesics may be used. Repeat treatment every 1–3 weeks. If no response after 4 treatments, discontinue. (Label information; *Regressin®-V*—Bioniche)

b) Using *Equimune®I.V.* as an immunotherapeutic agent for the treatment of Equine Respiratory Disease Complex (ERDC): 1.5 mL (one syringe) IV into the jugular vein. May be repeated in 1–3 weeks. (Label information; *Equimune®I.V.*—Bioniche)

c) Using *Settle®* as an aid in the treatment of equine metritis caused by *Streptococcus zooepidemicus*: Intravenous use: 1.5 mL (one syringe) IV into the jugular vein during the early estrus period. Or administer via intrauterine instillation: Dilute 1.5 mL of *Settle®* in sterile LRS, normal saline, water for injection or semen extender to provide a final volume of 25–50 mL. Aseptically administer the diluted solution into the uterus using a sterile catheter. (Label information; *Settle®*—Bioniche)

Monitoring

■ Clinical Efficacy (tumor size, metritis improvement, or respiratory infection improvement)

■ Adverse Effects (fever, local reactions, appetite)

Client Information

■ Intratumoral injection may cause pain or tenderness at the injection site. Tumors may drain or become necrotic indicating effectiveness; if this occurs and is bothersome, contact veterinarian for further instructions on management.

■ Treated animals may be depressed, develop fever, or have reduced appetite for a few days after treatment; if these persist or are severe, contact veterinarian

Chemistry/Synonyms

Regressin®-V, *Equimune®-I.V.* and *Settle®* are oil-in-water emulsions containing purified cell wall fractions obtained from Mycobacteria (species not described) that are non-pathogenic. Concentration is not listed for either product. *Regressin®-V* also contains procaine

HCl 0.2% w/v as a local anesthetic and a green tracking dye solution (not identified) 0.1% w/v used to indicate area infiltrated.

Mycobacterial cell wall fraction may also be known as mycobacterial cell wall extract, bacillus Calmette-Guerin, or BCG, *Equimune®*, *Regressin®*, and *Settle®*.

Storage/Stability

These products should be stored refrigerated (2–7°C), but not frozen. Unused product from vials not labeled for multi-dose use should be discarded after use.

The emulsion "breaks" upon standing and the product must be re-emulsified before administration. To re-emulsify to a milky appearance, shake vial, roll syringe between hands, or heat in hot water (150°F, 65°C).

Dosage Forms/Regulatory Status

VETERINARY-LABELED PRODUCTS:

Mycobacterial Cell Wall Fraction Immunomodulator for IV Injection in 1.5 mL single use vials and 4.5 mL multi-dose vials; *Equimune®I.V.* (Bioniche). Labeled for use in horses.

Mycobacterial Cell Wall Fraction Immunomodulator for IV injection of Intrauterine installation in 1.5 mL single use vials; *Settle®* (Bioniche). Contains gentamicin as a preservative. Labeled for use in horses.

Mycobacterial Cell Wall Fraction Immunomodulator for Tumor Infiltration in 10 mL vials; *Regressin®-V* (Bioniche). Also contains procaine and a green dye. Labeled for use in horses and dogs.

Note: These products are USDA-licensed biologics and are not FDA-approved products. *Equimune®I.V.* and *Regressin®-V* are not to be used in food producing animals. The label for *Settle®* states that it should not be administered to horses within 21 days of slaughter.

HUMAN-LABELED PRODUCTS: None

MYCOPHENOLATE MOFETIL

(my-koh-*fen*-oh-layt)   Cellcept®, MMF

IMMUNOSUPPRESSANT

Prescriber Highlights

▶ Immunosuppressive drug that may be useful for treating dogs with IMHA, glomerulonephritis, myasthenia gravis, pemphigus folacious or inflammatory bowel disease in dogs; potentially useful in cats, but little information available on safety or efficacy

▶ Very limited experience in veterinary medicine

▶ Gastrointestinal effects (diarrhea, vomiting, anorexia) most likely adverse effects & can be severe

▶ Treatment may be very expensive

Uses/Indications

While there has been very limited experience using mycophenolate in veterinary medicine, it potentially could be useful in the treatment of a variety of autoimmune diseases, including immune-mediated hemolytic anemia (IMHA), myasthenia gravis, glomerulonephritis, and pemphigus foliaceous. While mycophenolate has been suggested for use in treating inflammatory bowel disease in dogs, the drug's primary adverse effects in dogs are gastritis, diarrhea, and intestinal inflammation. Mycophenolate is also used in anti-rejection protocols for organ transplants in animals.

In humans, although it is used "off label" for a variety of autoimmune disease indications, the drug is only labeled for use to prevent transplant rejection.

Pharmacology/Actions

Mycophenolate mofetil (MMF) is a prodrug that must be converted (hydrolyzed) *in vivo* to mycophenolic acid (MPA) for it to be pharmacologically active. MPA non-competitively, but reversibly, inhibits inosine monophosphate dehydrogenase (IMPDHA). This is the rate-limiting enzyme in *de novo* synthesis of guanosine nucleotides. As T- and B-cells are dependent on *de novo* synthesis of purines (*e.g.*, guanosine) and unlike other cells cannot use salvage pathways, proliferative responses of T- and B-cells are inhibited and suppression of B-cell formation of antibodies occur. Via its effects, MPA can inhibit leukocyte recruitment to inflammatory sites and allotransplant tissues.

Pharmacokinetics

After oral administration mycophenolate mofetil is absorbed, but limited bioavailability studies in dogs have shown both a wide inter-patient and inter-dose variation. One study done in a single dog showed bioavailabilities of

54%, 65%, and 87% after doses of 10, 15, and 20 mg/kg of MMF were administered (Lupu *et al.* 2006). In humans, oral bioavailability averages 94%; food reduces peak levels of MPA by up to 40%. After absorption, MMF is rapidly hydrolyzed to mycophenolic acid.

In a study in dogs comparing mycophenolic acid's (MPA) pharmacokinetic parameters with its pharmacodynamic effects on inosine monophosphate dehydrogenase activity in lymphocytes (Langman *et al.* 1996), volume of distribution at steady-state was approximately 5 L/kg, but there was wide inter-patient variability (±4.5). Elimination half-life for MPA was about 8 hours (±4 hours). Mycophenolic acid is primarily excreted in the urine, both unchanged (approximately 5%) and as the glucuronide metabolite (approximately 90%). In this study, the authors concluded that the pharmacokinetic/pharmacodynamic profile of MMF in dogs suggests that an every 8-hour dosing schedule would be required for optimization of immunosuppressive efficacy.

Contraindications/Precautions/Warnings

Do not use in patients with documented hypersensitivity reactions to mycophenolate. Patients with severe renal dysfunction may require dosage adjustment.

Intravenous mycophenolate must be administered over at least two hours; it is not to be given as an IV bolus or via rapid IV infusion.

In humans, the active metabolite, MPA is primarily excreted as the MPA-glucuronide metabolite. As cats are deficient in this metabolic process, it should be used with caution in this species.

For humans, mycophenolate has a "black box" warning regarding potential increased risk for lymphoma associated with its use.

Adverse Effects

Because of the limited numbers of veterinary patients who have received this drug, the adverse effect profile is not well established. The primary adverse effects reported in dogs thus far include diarrhea, vomiting, anorexia, lethargy/reduced activity, lymphopenia, and increased rates of dermal infections. Because of the drug's immunosuppressive actions, increased systemic infection and malignancy rates are possible.

A study (Chanda *et al.* 2002) comparing adverse effects in dogs with mycophenolate mofetil capsules and mycophenolate sodium enteric-coated tablets demonstrated significantly greater occurrences and severity of diarrhea, weight loss and hypo-activity in the dogs that received the sodium salt enteric-coated tablets.

In humans, the most common adverse effects include GI effects (constipation, diarrhea, nausea, vomiting) and headache. Hypertension and peripheral edema occur in about 30% of patients. Leukopenia has been reported in 25–45% of patients taking the medication. Other effects

that occur more rarely include: GI bleeding, severe neutropenia, cough, confusion, tremor, infection and malignant lymphoma (0.4–1%).

Reproductive/Nursing Safety

At doses significantly lower than those used in humans, increased resorptions and malformations were noted in rabbits and rats; it is recommended that the drug be avoided, if at all possible, during pregnancy.

Mycophenolic acid is distributed in rat milk. It is unknown if it is safe to use during nursing.

Overdosage/Acute Toxicity

In oral acute studies performed in mice and monkeys, no deaths occurred in dosages up to 4,000 mg/kg and 1,000 mg/kg, respectively. In small animals, acute GI disturbances could be expected. Treat supportively, if required.

Drug Interactions

The following drug interactions have either been reported or are theoretical in humans or animals receiving mycophenolate mofetil and may be of significance in veterinary patients:

■ **ACYCLOVIR:** Increased serum concentrations of acyclovir and the phenolic glucuronide of mycophenolic acid

■ **ANTACIDS (aluminum or magnesium containing):** Decreased absorption of mycophenolate; separate dosing by at least 2 hours

■ **ASPIRIN (or other salicylates):** Potentially increased concentrations of free mycophenolic acid

■ **AZATHIOPRINE:** Increased risk for bone marrow suppression; use together not recommended in humans

■ **IRON (oral):** Decreased absorption of mycophenolate; separate dosing by at least 2 hours

■ **PROBENECID:** Potentially increased serum levels of mycophenolic acid and the phenolic glucuronide of mycophenolic acid

■ **VACCINES (live virus):** May be less effective; avoid use

Laboratory Considerations

■ No issues noted

Doses

■ **DOGS:**

For immune-mediated hemolytic anemia:

a) 12–17 mg/kg PO once daily or divided twice daily. Given with prednisolone (at 2 mg/kg q12–24h). Dogs also received ranitidine and sucralfate in the study. (Nielsen *et al.* 2005)

b) Limited use has shown a beneficial response in dogs with IMHA, myasthenia gravis or glomerulonephritis: 12–17 mg/kg PO once daily or divided twice daily. Given with prednisone (at 2.2 mg/kg q12–24h). (Macintire 2006)

c) Dose is unknown, and extrapolated from

human medicine, with reports of starting dosages of 400–600 mg/m^2 orally twice daily. Gastrointestinal side effects are common and dose limiting. (Noonan 2009)

d) For adjunctive treatment of glomerulonephritis: 10–20 mg/kg PO q12h. Immunosuppressive treatment is controversial. Other immunosuppressive drugs suggested include: glucocorticoids, cyclophosphamide, azathioprine, and cyclosporine. Trial of single drug therapy for 3–4 weeks recommended. (Labato 2006)

For pemphigus foliaceous:

a) For pemphigus foliaceous: 22–39 mg/kg/day divided into 3 daily doses. Success rates (limited use) of approximately 50%; most dogs require glucocorticoids to control signs. (Rosenkrantz 2004)

b) For pemphigus foliaceous: 20–40 mg/kg/day PO divided q8h; steroid-sparing only. (Scott 2008)

Miscellaneous indications:

a) For adjunctive treatment of glomerulonephritis: 10–20 mg/kg PO q12h. Immunosuppressive treatment is controversial. Other immunosuppressive drugs suggested include: glucocorticoids, cyclophosphamide, azathioprine, and cyclosporine. Trial of single drug therapy for 3–4 weeks recommended. (Labato 2006)

b) From a case report for treating aplastic anemia: 10 mg/kg PO q12h. The first effects (improvements in hematocrit) were observed 2 weeks later, and complete remission of all blood cell counts were obtained in approximately 3 weeks. (Yuki *et al.* 2007)

c) From a case report in 3 dogs as a rescue agent for generalized myasthenia gravis: Initially, dogs received 500 mg (15-20 mg/kg) diluted and given IV over 2–4 hours. Dogs were given daily IV treatments for 1–3 days until they could adequately swallow oral meds. They were then switched to oral mycophenolate at doses between 10–11 mg/kg PO q12h. Subsequently, doses were adjusted based upon clinical response and AChR titers. (Abelson *et al.* 2009)

■ **CATS:**
a) For IMHA: 10 mg/kg PO q12h. (Macintire 2009)

Monitoring

■ Efficacy

■ CBC, renal and hepatic function, serum electrolytes; baseline and periodically (frequency depending on reason for treatment)

■ Gastrointestinal effects (weight, client's report)

Client Information

■ Preferably give on an empty stomach; if vomiting or lack of appetite occurs, give with food to see if it improves

■ Because of concerns that this drug can cause birth defects, the manufacturer recommends that tablets or capsules not be crushed, split, or opened.

■ If diarrhea persists or is severe, contact veterinarian

Chemistry/Synonyms

Mycophenolate mofetil occurs as a white or almost white, crystalline powder. It is practically insoluble in water and sparingly soluble in alcohol.

Mycophenolate mofetil may also be known as: RS-61443 or MMF. International trade names include: *CellCept®, Cellmune®, Imuxgen®, Munotras®, Mycept®, Myfortic®,* and *Refrat®.*

Storage/Compatibility

Mycophenolate mofetil tablets and capsules should be stored between 15–30°C and protected from light.

Mycophenolate mofetil powder for oral suspension should be stored between 15–30°C; preferably at 25°C. Once reconstituted with 94 mL of water it may be stored at room temperature or in the refrigerator; do not freeze. Unused drug should be discarded after 60 days.

The injectable product should be stored between 15–30°C; preferably at 25°C. Each vial should be reconstituted with 14 mL of 5% dextrose injection; final volume is approximately 15 mL. Gently agitate to dissolve the powder. For human use, the manufacturer recommends further diluting with dextrose 5% to a concentration of 6 mg/mL for IV administration. This would be an additional 70 mL of dextrose 5% per vial. Mycophenolate injection should not be mixed or given with any other medication or diluent. It is recommended to administer within 6 hours of dilution. The drug must be administered over at least two hours and is not to be given as an IV bolus or via rapid IV infusion.

Compatibility/Compounding Considerations

Mycophenolate injection should not be mixed or given with any other medication or diluent.

Dosage Forms/Regulatory Status

VETERINARY-LABELED PRODUCTS: None

HUMAN-LABELED PRODUCTS:

Mycophenolate Mofetil Oral Capsules: 250 mg; *CellCept®* (Roche); generic (Rx)

Mycophenolate Mofetil Oral Tablets: 500 mg; *CellCept®* (Roche); (Rx)

Mycophenolate Mofetil Powder for Oral Suspension: 200 mg/mL (reconstituted) in 225 mL bottles; *CellCept®* (Roche); (Rx)

Mycophenolate Mofetil Lyophilized Powder for Injection: 500 mg in 20 mL vials; *CellCept®* (Roche); (Rx)

Mycophenolate is also available as the sodium salt in oral, delayed-release tablets in 180 mg and 360 mg strengths. Trade name is *Myfortic®* (Novartis); (Rx). It does not appear that this dosage form will be useful for veterinary patients.

References

Abelson, A.L., G.D. Shelton, et al. (2009). Use of mycophenolate mofetil as a rescue agent in the treatment of severe generalized myasthenia gravis in three dogs. *Journal of Veterinary Emergency and Critical Care* 19(4): 369–374.

Chanda, S., J. Sellin, et al. (2002). Comparative gastrointestinal effects of mycophenolate mofetil capsules and enteric-coated tablets of sodium mycophenolic acid in beagle dogs. *Transplantation Proceedings* 34(8): 3387–3392.

Labato, M. (2006). Improving survival for dogs with protein-losing nephropathies. Proceedings: ACVIM 2006. Accessed via: Veterinary Information Network. http://goo.gl/0jeng

Langman, L., A. Shapiro, et al. (1996). Pharmacodynamic assessment of mycophenolic acid-induced immunosuppression by measurement of inosine monophosphate dehydrogenase activity in a canine model. *Transplantation* 61(1): 87–92.

Lupu, M., J. McCune, et al. (2006). Pharmacokinetics of oral mycophenolate mofetil in dog: Bioavailability studies and the impact of antibiotic therapy. *Biology of Blood and Marrow Transplantation* 12(12): 1352–1354.

Macintire, D. (2006). New therapies for immune-mediated hemolytic anemia. Proceedings: ACVIM 2006. Accessed via: Veterinary Information Network. http://goo.gl/ILCPS

Macintire, D. (2009). Anemia In Feline Critical Illness. Proceedings: IVECCS. Accessed via: Veterinary Information Network. http://goo.gl/7GSxX

Nielsen, L., S. Niessen, et al. (2005). The Use of Mycophenolate Mofetil in Eight Dogs with Idiopathic Immune Mediated Haemolytic Anaemia. Proceedings ECVIM 2005. Accessed via: Veterinary Information Network. http://goo.gl/PgbJs

Noonan, M. (2009). Immune Mediated Hemolytic Anemia. Proceedings: IVECC. Accessed via: Veterinary Information Network. http://goo.gl/EaAXT

Rosenkrantz, W. (2004). Pemphigus: current therapy. *Vet Derm* 15: 90–98.

Scott, D.W. (2008). Pemphigus 2008: Pathogenesis, Presentation, & Management. Proceedings: ACVIM. Accessed via: Veterinary Information Network. http://goo.gl/Ygmbn

Yuki, M., N. Sugimoto, et al. (2007). Recovery of a dog from aplastic anaemia after treatment with mycophenolate mofetil. *Australian Veterinary Journal* 85(12): 495–497.

NALOXONE HCL

(nal-**ox**-one)   Narcan®

ANTIDOTE; OPIATE ANTAGONIST

Prescriber Highlights

▶ Injectable opiate antagonist

▶ Caution: Preexisting cardiac abnormalities or opioid dependent

▶ Reversal effect may last for a shorter time than opioid effect; monitor & re-dose as needed

Uses/Indications

Naloxone is used in veterinary medicine almost exclusively for its opiate reversal effects, but the drug is being investigated for treating other conditions (*e.g.*, septic, hypovolemic or cardiogenic shock). Naloxone may also be employed as a test drug to see if endogenous opiate blockade will result in diminished tail chasing or other self-mutilating behaviors. It, potentially, could be useful for treating overdoses of clonidine or the CNS effects of benzodiazepines (ivermectin?), but more research is necessary before recommending its use.

Pharmacology/Actions

Naloxone is considered a pure opiate antagonist and it has no analgesic activity. The exact mechanism for its activity is not understood, but it is believed that the drug acts as a competitive antagonist by binding to the *mu*, *kappa*, and *sigma* opioid receptor sites. The drug apparently has its highest affinity for the *mu* receptor.

Naloxone reverses the majority of effects associated with high-dose opiate administration (respiratory and CNS depression). In dogs, naloxone apparently does not reverse the emetic actions of apomorphine.

Naloxone may be useful in treating adverse effects associated with overdoses of propoxyphene, pentazocine, buprenorphine and loperamide, but larger naloxone doses may be required.

Naloxone has other pharmacologic activity at high doses, including effects on dopaminergic mechanisms (increases dopamine levels) and GABA antagonism.

Pharmacokinetics

Naloxone is only minimally absorbed when given orally as it is rapidly destroyed in the GI tract. Much higher doses are required if using this route of administration for any pharmacologic effect. When given IV, naloxone has a very rapid onset of action (usually 1–2 minutes). If given IM, the drug generally has an onset of action within 5 minutes of administration. The duration of action usually persists from 45–90 minutes, but may act for up to 3 hours.

Naloxone is distributed rapidly throughout the body with high levels found in the brain, kidneys, spleen, skeletal muscle, lung, and heart. The drug also readily crosses the placenta.

Naloxone is metabolized in the liver, principally via glucuronidative conjugation, with metabolites excreted into the urine. In humans, the serum half-life is approximately 60–100 minutes.

Contraindications/Precautions/Warnings

Naloxone is contraindicated in patients hypersensitive to it. It should be used cautiously in animals that have preexisting cardiac abnormalities or that may be opioid dependent. The veterinary manufacturer of the product once marketed for veterinary use states to use the drug ". . . cautiously in animals who have received exceedingly large doses of narcotics . . . it may produce an acute withdrawal syndrome and smaller doses should be employed." (Package Insert; *P/M® Naloxone HCl Injection*—Mallinckrodt)

In humans, naloxone is reportedly not effective for reversing meperidine-induced seizures. Benzodiazepines and/or barbiturates may be necessary.

In a case of a dog that received an overdose (10X) of meperidine, naloxone administration elicited CNS excitement. The authors recommend that naloxone (and butorphanol) should be avoided when normeperidine (active metabolite of meperidine) excitotoxicity is suspected, unless severe respiratory depression is present without a method of ventilatory support (Golder *et al.* 2010).

Naloxone has not been shown to be an effective therapy to reverse apnea of newborns and its routine use is not recommended. However, if the dam received opiates during parturition, it may reverse opiate-induced respiratory depression. Naloxone is not a good reversal agent for buprenorphine. Doses of 100X-usual have been required to reverse effects in a normal dog.

Adverse Effects

At usual doses, naloxone is relatively free of adverse effects in non-opioid dependent patients; however, when using to reverse opiates' effects, it can also reverse any analgesic activity of the opiate.

Because the duration of action of naloxone may be shorter than that of the narcotic being reversed, animals that are being treated for opioid intoxication or with clinical signs of respiratory depression should be closely monitored as additional doses of naloxone and/or ventilatory support may be required.

Reproductive/Nursing Safety

In humans, the FDA categorizes this drug as category *B* for use during pregnancy (*Animal studies have not yet demonstrated risk to the fetus, but there are no adequate studies in pregnant women; or animal studies have shown an adverse effect, but adequate studies in pregnant women have not demonstrated a risk to the fetus in the first trimester of pregnancy, and there is no evidence of risk in later trimesters.*) In a separate system evaluating the safety of drugs in canine and feline pregnancy (Papich 1989), this drug is categorized as class: *A* (*Probably safe. Although specific studies may not have proved he safety of all drugs in dogs and cats, there are no reports of adverse effects in laboratory animals or women.*)

It is not known whether the drug is excreted in maternal milk. Use caution when administering to nursing patients.

Overdosage/Acute Toxicity

Naloxone is considered a very safe agent with a very wide margin of safety, but very high doses have initiated seizures (secondary to GABA antagonism?) in a few patients.

Drug Interactions

The following drug interactions have either been reported or are theoretical in humans or animals receiving naloxone and may be of significance in veterinary patients:

- **OPIOID PARTIAL-AGONISTS (e.g., butorphanol, pentazocine, or nalbuphine):** Naloxone may also antagonize the effects these agents (respiratory depression, analgesia). It should not be relied upon to treat respiratory depression caused by **buprenorphine**.

- **CLONIDINE:** Naloxone may reduce the hypotensive and bradycardic effects of clonidine; potentially useful for clonidine overdoses

- **YOHIMBINE:** Naloxone may increase the CNS effects of yohimbine (anxiety, tremors, nausea, palpitations) and increase plasma cortisol levels

Doses

- **DOGS/CATS:**

For opioid reversal:

a) 0.01−0.02 mg/kg IM, IV, or SC. (Trim 2008)

b) Dogs: 0.04 mg/kg IV, IM or SC (Package Insert; *P/M® Naloxone HCl Injection*—Mallinckrodt), (Kirk 1989)

c) For dysphoria associated with postsurgical opioids: If the patient is clearly dysphoric or returns to a whining state shortly after additional opioid administration, or if suspicion exists related to the use of high doses of opioid during surgery, a slow titration of naloxone can be given to effect (4 micrograms/kg diluted to 10 mL and given in 1-mL increments every minute). (Dyson 2008)

d) Following caesarian sections when puppies or kittens are sedated or have respiratory depression from the expected placental transfer of the opioid: 1 drop of naloxone (0.4 mg/mL from a 1-mL syringe) can be administered under the tongue, and repeat doses can be sent home with the owner if longer acting opioids are involved. (Dyson 2008)

For adjunctive treatment of pulseless electrical activity (PEA) in CPCR:

a) 0.02−0.04 mg/kg IV may be effective in augmenting cardiac output by blocking endogenous endorphins or exogenous narcotics. (Scroggin & Quandt 2009)

For adjunctive treatment of hyperthermia in cats:

a) Authors have treated cats with body temperatures exceeding 41.1°C (106° F) following anesthesia with naloxone at 0.01 mg/kg IM or SC and have seen body temperature return to normal range in <30 minutes. (Posner *et al.* 2010)

- **RABBITS, RODENTS, SMALL MAMMALS:**

a) For opioid reversal in **rodents:**

0.01–0.1 mg/kg SC or IP as needed (Huerkamp 1995)

b) **Rabbits:** 0.005–0.1 mg/kg IM or IV (Ivey & Morrisey 2000)

c) **Hamsters, Gerbils, Mice, Rats, Guinea pigs, Chinchillas:** 0.01–0.1 mg/kg SC, IP (Adamcak & Otten 2000)

■ **HORSES: (Note:** ARCI UCGFS Class 3 Drug) For opioid reversal:

a) 0.01–0.022 mg/kg to reverse sedative and excitatory effects of narcotic agonists (Clark & Becht 1987)

b) 0.01 mg/kg IV to limit increases in locomotor activity secondary to narcotic agonists (Muir 1987)

c) For treatment of opioid gastrointestinal tract dysfunction: 10–50 micrograms/kg (*route not specified, assume IV—Plumb*) will induce movement and passage of contents. (Boscan 2009)

Monitoring

■ Respiratory rate/depth

■ CNS function

■ Pain associated with opiate reversal

Client Information

■ Should be used with direct professional supervision only

Chemistry/Synonyms

An opiate antagonist, naloxone HCl is structurally related to oxymorphone. It occurs as a white to slightly off-white powder with a pK_a of 7.94. Naloxone is soluble in water and slightly soluble in alcohol. The pH ranges of commercially available injectable solutions are from 3–4.5.

Naloxone HCl may also be known as: N-allylnoroxymorphone, naloxona, EN-15304, naloxoni and by the trade name, *Narcan®*.

Storage/Stability

Naloxone HCl for injection should be stored at room temperature (15–30°C) and protected from light.

Sterile water for injection is the recommended diluent for naloxone injection. When given as an IV infusion, either D_5W or normal saline should be used.

Compatibility/Compounding Considerations

Naloxone HCl injection **should not** be mixed with solutions containing sulfites, bisulfites, long-chain or high molecular weight anions or any solutions at alkaline pH.

Dosage Forms/Regulatory Status

VETERINARY-LABELED PRODUCTS: None

The ARCI (Racing Commissioners International) has designated this drug as a class 3 substance. See the appendix for more information.

HUMAN-LABELED PRODUCTS:

Naloxone HCl Injection: 0.4 mg/mL (400 micrograms/mL) in 1 mL amps, syringes and 1 mL, 2 mL, & 10 mL vials; *Narcan®* (DuPont Pharm.); generic; (Rx)

Naloxone HCl Neonatal Injection: 0.02 mg/mL in 2 mL vials; generic; (Rx)

References

Adamcak, A. & B. Otten (2000). Rodent Therapeutics. *Vet Clin NA: Exotic Anim Pract* **3:**1(Jan): 221–240.

Boscan, P. (2009). Opioid Agonists and Antagonists in the Gastrointestinal Tract. Proceedings: IVECCS. Accessed via: Veterinary Information Network. http://goo.gl/3dzv6

Clark, E.S. & J.L. Becht (1987). Clinical Pharmacology of the Gastrointestinal Tract. *Vet Clin North Am (Equine Practice)* **3**(1): 101–122.

Dyson, D.H. (2008). Perioperative Pain Management in Veterinary Patients. *Veterinary Clinics of North America-Small Animal Practice* **38**(6): 1309–+.

Golder, F.J., J. Wilson, et al. (2010). Suspected acute meperidine toxicity in a dog. *Veterinary Anaesthesia and Analgesia* **37**(5): 471–477.

Huerkamp, M. (1995). Anesthesia and postoperative management of rabbits and pocket pets. *Kirk's Current Veterinary Therapy:XII.* J Bonagura Ed. Philadelphia, W.B. Saunders: 1322–1327.

Ivey, E. & J. Morrisey (2000). Therapeutics for Rabbits. *Vet Clin NA: Exotic Anim Pract* **3:**1(Jan): 183–216.

Kirk, R.W., Ed. (1989). *Current Veterinary Therapy X, Small Animal Practice.* Philadelphia, WB Saunders.

Muir, W.W., III (1987). Analgesics in the treatment of colic. *Current Therapy in Equine Medicine.* NE Robinson Ed. Philadelphia, WB Saunders: 27–29.

Papich, M. (1989). Effects of drugs on pregnancy. *Current Veterinary Therapy X: Small Animal Practice.* R Kirk Ed. Philadelphia, Saunders: 1291–1299.

Posner, L.P., A.A. Pavuk, et al. (2010). Effects of opioids and anesthetic drugs on body temperature in cats. *Veterinary Anaesthesia and Analgesia* **37**(1): 35–43.

Scroggin, R.D. & J. Quandt (2009). The use of vasopressin for treating vasodilatory shock and cardiopulmonary arrest. *Journal of Veterinary Emergency and Critical Care* **19**(2): 145–157.

Trim, C. (2008). Opioid Analgesia. Proceedings: WVC. Accessed via: Veterinary Information Network. http://goo.gl/VACG6

NALTREXONE HCL

(nal-***trex***-ohne)   Trexan®, ReVia®

OPIATE ANTAGONIST

Prescriber Highlights

▶ Oral opiate antagonist that might be useful in determining if adverse behaviors have a significant endorphin component & for the short-term treatment of same

▶ Contraindications: Patients physically dependent on opiate drugs, in hepatic failure, or with acute hepatitis. Caution: hepatic dysfunction or who have had a history of allergic reaction to naltrexone or naloxone.

▶ Adverse Effects: Relatively free of adverse effects. Potentially: Abdominal cramping, nausea & vomiting, nervousness, insomnia, joint or muscle pain, skin rashes, & pruritus. Dose-dependent hepatotoxicity is possible.

▶ May cause withdrawal clinical signs in physically dependent patients

▶ Expensive

Uses/Indications

Naltrexone might be useful in determining if adverse behaviors (*e.g.*, self-mutilating or tail-chasing) in dogs or cats have a significant endorphin component. Its relative expense and other more accepted treatments have largely supplanted the use of this drug in animals for treatment of behavioral disorders.

Pharmacology/Actions

Naltrexone is an orally available narcotic antagonist. It competitively binds to opiate receptors in the CNS, thereby preventing both endogenous opiates (*e.g.*, endorphins) and exogenously administered opiate agonists or agonist/antagonists from occupying the site. Naltrexone may be more effective in blocking the euphoric aspects of the opiates and less effective at blocking the respiratory depressive or miotic effects.

Naltrexone may also increase plasma concentrations of luteinizing hormone (LH), cortisol, and ACTH. In dogs with experimentally-induced hypovolemic shock, naltrexone (like naloxone) given IV in high dosages increased mean arterial pressure, cardiac output, stroke volume, and left ventricular contractility.

Pharmacokinetics

In humans, naltrexone is rapidly and nearly completely absorbed, but undergoes a significant first-pass effect as only 5–12% of a dose reaches the systemic circulation. Naltrexone circulates throughout the body and CSF levels are approximately 30% of those found in plasma. Only about 20–30% is bound to plasma proteins. It is unknown whether naltrexone crosses the placenta or enters milk. Naltrexone is metabolized in the liver primarily to 6-beta-naltrexol, which has some opiate blocking activity. Naltrexone's metabolites are eliminated primarily via the kidney. In humans, serum half-life of naltrexone is about 4 hours and about 13 hours for 6-beta-naltrexol.

Contraindications/Precautions/Warnings

Naltrexone is contraindicated in patients physically dependent on opiate drugs, in hepatic failure, or with acute hepatitis. The benefits of the drug versus its risks should be weighed in patients with hepatic dysfunction or with a history of allergic reaction to naltrexone or naloxone.

Adverse Effects

At usual doses, naltrexone is relatively free of adverse effects in non-opioid dependent patients. Some human patients have developed abdominal cramping, nausea and vomiting, nervousness, insomnia, joint or muscle pain, skin rashes, and pruritus. Dose-dependent hepatotoxicity has been described in humans on occasion.

Naltrexone will block the analgesic, antidiarrheal, and antitussive effects of opiate agonist or agonist/antagonist agents. Withdrawal clinical signs may be precipitated in physically dependent patients.

Reproductive/Nursing Safety

In humans, the FDA categorizes this drug as category **D** for use during pregnancy (*There is evidence of human fetal risk, but the potential benefits from the use of the drug in pregnant women may be acceptable despite its potential risks.*) Very high doses have caused increased embryotoxicity in some laboratory animals. It should be used during pregnancy only when the benefits outweigh any potential risks.

Naltrexone enters into milk of humans and sheep. Use caution when administering to nursing patients.

Overdosage/Acute Toxicity

Naltrexone appears to be relatively safe even after very large doses. The LD_{50} in dogs after subcutaneous injection has been reported to be 200 mg/kg. Oral LD_{50}'s in species tested range from 1.1 grams/kg in mice to 3 grams/kg in monkeys (dogs or cats not tested). Deaths at these doses were a result of respiratory depression and/or tonic-clonic seizures. Massive overdoses should be treated using gut-emptying protocols when warranted and giving supportive treatment.

Drug Interactions

The following drug interactions have either been reported or are theoretical in humans or animals receiving naltrexone and may be of significance in veterinary patients:

■ **OPIOID PARTIAL-AGONISTS (e.g., butorphanol, pentazocine, or nalbuphine):** Naloxone may also antagonize the effects these agents (respiratory depression, analgesia).

■ **CLONIDINE:** Naltrexone may reduce the hypotensive and bradycardic effects of clonidine

■ **YOHIMBINE:** Naltrexone may increase the CNS effects of yohimbine (anxiety, tremors, nausea, palpitations) and increase plasma cortisol levels

Laboratory Considerations

■ Naltrexone reportedly does not interfere with TLC, GLC, or HPLC methods of determining **urinary opiates**, or quinine, but can interfere with some enzymatic assays

■ Naltrexone may cause increases in **hepatic function tests** (*e.g.*, AST, ALT) (see Adverse Effects above).

Doses

■ **DOGS:**

As adjunctive therapy in behavior disorders:

a) For tail chasing or excessive licking: First give 0.01 mg/kg SC of naloxone to determine if narcotic antagonists may be effective, if so give naltrexone PO at 1–2 mg/kg daily. Long-term therapy may be required. (Crowill-Davis 1992)

b) 2–5 mg/kg, PO once daily (Line 2000)

c) 1–2.2 mg/kg, PO q8–12h (Crowell-Davis 1999)

For the adjunctive treatment of acral pruritic dermatitis:

a) 2.2 mg/kg, PO once daily for one-month trial. Some dogs exhibit drowsiness and minor changes in behavior. 50–60% of patients have benefited. Expense is of concern. (Rosychuck 1991)

■ **CATS:**

As adjunctive therapy in behavior disorders:

a) 25–50 mg/cat PO q24h. **Note:** has a bitter taste (Crowell-Davis 1999)

■ **ZOO, EXOTIC, WILDLIFE SPECIES:**

For use of naltrexone in zoo, exotic and wildlife medicine refer to specific references, including:

a) *Zoo Animal and Wildlife Immobilization and Anesthesia*. West, G, Heard, D, Caulkett, N. (eds.). Blackwell Publishing, 2007.

b) *Handbook of Wildlife Chemical Immobilization, 3rd Ed*. Kreeger, T.J. and J.M. Arnemo. 2007.

c) *Restraint and Handling of Wild and Domestic Animals*. Fowler, M (ed.), Iowa State University Press, 1995

d) *Exotic Animal Formulary, 3rd Ed*. Carpenter, J.W., Saunders. 2005

e) The 2009 American Association of Zoo Veterinarian Proceedings by D. K. Fontenot also has several dosages listed for restraint, anesthesia, and analgesia for a variety of drugs for carnivores and primates. VIN members can access them at: http://goo.gl/BHRih or http://goo.gl/9UJse

Monitoring

■ Efficacy

■ Liver enzymes if using very high dose with prolonged therapy

Client Information

■ Stress the importance of compliance with prescribed dosing regimen

■ Additional behavior modification techniques may be required to alleviate clinical signs

Chemistry/Synonyms

A synthetic opiate antagonist, naltrexone HCl occurs as white crystals having a bitter taste. 100 mg are soluble in one mL of water.

Naltrexone may also be known as EN-1639A, *ReVia®* and *Vivitrol®*.

Storage/Stability

Naltrexone tablets should be stored at room temperature in well-closed containers.

Dosage Forms/Regulatory Status

VETERINARY-LABELED PRODUCTS: None

The ARCI (Racing Commissioners International) has designated this drug as a class 3 substance. See the appendix for more information.

HUMAN-LABELED PRODUCTS:

Naltrexone HCl Oral Tablets: 50 mg; *ReVia®* (Duramed); generic; (Rx)

Naltrexone HCl Powder for Suspension Extended-Release Injection: 380 mg/vial in single-use vials w/4 mL diluent; *Vivitrol®* (Alkermes); (Rx)

References

Crowell-Davis, S. (1999). Behavior Psychopharmacology Part 2: Anxiolytics, hormones, narcotic antagonists and Miscellaneous. Proceedings: Central Veterinary Conference, Kansas City.

Crowill-Davis, S. (1992). Tail chasing in dogs. *Current Veterinary Therapy XI: Small Animal Practice*. R Kirk and J Bonagura Eds. Philadelphia, W.B. Saunders Company: 995–997.

Line, S. (2000). Sensory Mutilation and Related Behavior Syndromes. *Kirk's Current Veterinary Therapy: XIII Small Animal Practice*. J Bonagura Ed. Philadelphia, WB Saunders: 90–93.

Rosychuck, R. (1991). Newer therapies in veterinary dermatology. Proceedings of the Ninth Annual Veterinary Medical Forum, New Orleans, American College of Veterinary Internal Medicine.

NANDROLONE DECANOATE

(*nan*-droe-lone)   Deca-Durabolin®

PARENTERAL ANABOLIC STEROID

Prescriber Highlights

▶ Injectable anabolic steroid; may be useful to stimulate erythropoiesis or to stimulate appetite. Rarely recommended or used today.

▶ Contraindications: Hepatic dysfunction, hypercalcemia, history of myocardial infarction, pituitary insufficiency, prostate carcinoma, mammary carcinoma, benign prostatic hypertrophy, & during the nephrotic stage of nephritis

▶ Adverse Effects: Sodium, calcium, potassium, water, chloride, & phosphate retention; hepatotoxicity, behavioral (androgenic) changes, & reproductive abnormalities (oligospermia, estrus suppression)

▶ Known teratogen

▶ Drug Interactions

▶ C-III Controlled Substance. No FDA-approved products marketed in USA; may be available from compounding pharmacies.

Uses/Indications

The principle use of nandrolone in veterinary medicine has been to stimulate erythropoiesis in patients with certain anemias (*e.g.*, secondary to renal failure, aplastic anemias). It has also been suggested for use as an appetite stimulant. Anabolic steroids are rarely recommended or used today in veterinary medicine.

Pharmacology/Actions

Nandrolone exhibits similar actions as other anabolic agents. In the presence of adequate protein and calories, anabolic steroids promote body tissue building processes and can reverse catabolism. As these agents are either derived from or closely related to testosterone, the anabolics have varying degrees of androgenic effects. Endogenous testosterone release may be suppressed by inhibiting luteinizing hormone (LH). Large doses can impede spermatogenesis by negative feedback inhibition of FSH.

Anabolic steroids can stimulate erythropoiesis. The mechanism for this effect may occur by stimulating erythropoietic stimulating factor. Anabolics can cause nitrogen, sodium, potassium, and phosphorus retention and decrease the urinary excretion of calcium. Many veterinary and human clinicians feel that nandrolone is clinically superior to other anabolics in its ability to stimulate erythropoiesis. It is believed that nandrolone may enhance red cell counts by directly stimulating red cell precursors in the bone marrow, increasing red cell 2,3-diphosphoglycerate and erythropoietin production in the kidney.

Pharmacokinetics

No specific information was located for this agent. It is generally recommended for both small animals and humans to be dosed on a weekly basis.

Contraindications/Precautions/Warnings

No specific recommendations were located for this agent in veterinary species.

In humans, anabolic agents are contraindicated in patients with hepatic dysfunction, hypercalcemia, patients with a history of myocardial infarction (can cause hypercholesterolemia), pituitary insufficiency, prostate carcinoma, in selected patients with breast carcinoma, benign prostatic hypertrophy, and during the nephrotic stage of nephritis.

Adverse Effects

Potential (from human data) adverse reactions of the anabolic agents in dogs and cats include: sodium, calcium, potassium, water, chloride, and phosphate retention; hepatotoxicity, behavioral (androgenic) changes, and reproductive abnormalities (oligospermia, estrus suppression).

Reproductive/Nursing Safety

In humans, the FDA categorizes this drug as category *X* for use during pregnancy (*Studies in animals or humans demonstrate fetal abnormalities or adverse reaction; reports indicate evidence of fetal risk. The risk of use in pregnant women clearly outweighs any possible benefit.*) Anabolic steroids can cause masculinization of the fetus.

It is not known whether anabolic steroids are excreted in maternal milk. Because of the potential for serious adverse reactions in nursing offspring, decide whether to discontinue nursing or the drug.

Overdosage/Acute Toxicity

No information was located for this specific agent. In humans, sodium and water retention can occur after overdosage of anabolic steroids. It is suggested to treat supportively and monitor liver function should an inadvertent overdose be administered.

Drug Interactions

The following drug interactions have either been reported or are theoretical in humans or animals receiving nandrolone and may be of significance in veterinary patients:

- **ANTICOAGULANTS (warfarin):** Anabolic agents as a class may potentiate the effects of anticoagulants; monitoring of INR and dosage adjustment of the anticoagulant (if necessary) are recommended

- **CORTICOSTEROIDS, ACTH:** Anabolics may enhance the edema that can be associated with ACTH or adrenal steroid therapy

- **INSULIN:** Diabetic patients receiving insulin may need dosage adjustments if anabolic therapy is added or discontinued; anabolics may decrease blood glucose and decrease insulin requirements

Laboratory Considerations

- Concentrations of **protein bound iodine (PBI)** can be decreased in patients receiving androgen/anabolic therapy, but the clinical significance of this is probably not important

- Androgen/anabolic agents can decrease amounts of **thyroxine-binding globulin** and decrease **total T_4** concentrations and increase **resin uptake of T_3 and T_4**; free thyroid hormones are unaltered and, clinically, there is no evidence of dysfunction

- Both **creatinine** and **creatine excretion** can be decreased by anabolic steroids

- Anabolic steroids can increase the urinary excretion of **17-ketosteroids**

- Androgenic/anabolic steroids may alter **blood glucose** levels.

- Androgenic/anabolic steroids may suppress **clotting factors II, V, VII, and X.**

- Anabolic agents can affect **liver function tests** (BSP retention, SGOT, SGPT, bilirubin, and alkaline phosphatase)

Doses

- **DOGS:**

For adjunctive treatment of chronic idiopathic myelofibrosis:

a) Prednisolone at 2–3 mg/kg PO once daily for 3–4 weeks, then every other day with a tapering of the dose as the anemia resolves. Nandrolone decanoate may be used at 2 mg/kg IM weekly for 3 weeks. If anemia does not respond to initial treatments, azathioprine at 2 mg/kg PO every other day can be given. (Raskin 2006)

For disuse muscle atrophy secondary to immobilization:

a) 1.5 mg/kg IM once weekly from the day of surgery/immobilization for up to 8 weeks. (Yun *et al.* 2005)

For treatment of anemia in patients with chronic renal failure:

a) 1–1.5 mg/kg IM once weekly; may require 2–3 months to achieve beneficial effects. Evidence to support use is poor. (Polzin, D. *et al.* 1992; Polzin, D.J. & Osborne 1985)

b) 5 mg/kg IM (maximum of 200 mg/week) every 2–3 weeks (Ross *et al.* 1989)

For treatment of metabolic and endocrine anemias:

a) 5 mg/kg IM once weekly (maximum of 200 mg); most resolve with correction of underlying disease process (Maggio-Price 1988)

For aplastic anemia:

a) 1–3 mg/kg IM weekly (Weiss 1986)

As an appetite stimulant:

a) 5 mg/kg IM (max. 200 mg/week) weekly (Macy & Ralston 1989)

■ **CATS:**

For FeLV-induced anemia or as a general bone marrow stimulant:

a) 10–20 mg IM once weekly (is of questionable benefit) (Maggio-Price 1988)

For chronic anemia secondary to feline cardiomyopathy:

a) 50 mg IM weekly (Harpster 1986)

■ **REPTILES:**

To reduce protein catabolism in renal disease of lizard species:

a) 1 mg/kg IM every 7–28 days (de la Navarre 2003)

Monitoring

■ Androgenic side effects

■ Fluid and electrolyte status, if indicated

■ Liver function tests if indicated

■ Red blood cell count, indices, if indicated

■ Weight, appetite

Client Information

■ Because of the potential for abuse of anabolic steroids by humans, this agent is a controlled (C-III) drug. It should be kept in a secure area and out of the reach of children.

Chemistry/Synonyms

An injectable anabolic steroid, nandrolone decanoate occurs as a white, to creamy white, crystalline powder. It is odorless or may have a slight odor and melts between 33–37°C. Nandrolone decanoate is soluble in alcohol and vegetable oils and is practically insoluble in water. The commercial injectable products were generally solutions of nandrolone decanoate dissolved in sesame oil.

Nandrolone decanoate may also be known as: nortestosterone decanoate, or nortestosterone decylate.

Storage/Stability

Nandrolone decanoate for injection should be stored at temperatures less than 40°C and preferably between 15–30°C (59–86°F); protect from freezing and light.

Dosage Forms/Regulatory Status

VETERINARY-LABELED PRODUCTS:

There are no commercial products available in the USA. Potentially, it may be available from compounding pharmacies. The ARCI (Racing Commissioners International) has designated this drug as a class 4 substance. See the appendix for more information.

HUMAN-LABELED PRODUCTS: None

References

de la Navarre, B. (2003). Acute and chronic renal disease (specifically in lizard species). Proceedings: Western Veterinary Conference. Accessed via: Current Veterinary Information Network. http://goo.gl/coWpS

Harpster, N.K. (1986). Feline myocardial diseases. *Current Veterinary Therapy IX: Small Animal Practice.* RW Kirk Ed. Philadelphia, WB Saunders: 380– 398.

Macy, D.W. & S.L. Ralston (1989). Cause and control of decreased appetite. *Current Veterinary Therapy X: Small Animal Practice.* RW Kirk Ed. Philadelphia, WB Saunders: 18–24.

Maggio-Price, L. (1988). Disorders of Red Blood Cells. *Handbook of Small Animal Practice.* RV Morgan Ed. New York, Churchill Livingstone: 725–748.

Polzin, D., C.A. Osborne, et al. (1992). Medical management of feline chronic renal failure. *Current Veterinary Therapy XI: Small Animal Practice.* C Kirk and J Bonagura Eds., Saunders: 848.

Polzin, D.J. & C.A. Osborne (1985). Diseases of the Urinary Tract. *Handbook of Small Animal Therapeutics.* LE Davis Ed. New York, Churchill Livingstone: 333–395.

Raskin, R. (2006). Chronic idiopathic myelofibrosis—diagnosis and treatment. Proceedings: WSAVA World Congress. Accessed via: Veterinary Information Network. http://goo.gl/QXjmL

Ross, L.A., E.B. Breitschwerdt, et al. (1989). Diseases of the Kidney. *Handbook of Small Animal Practice.* RV Morgan Ed. New York, Churchill Livingstone: 567–593.

Weiss, D.J. (1986). Therapy for disorders of erythropoiesis. *Current Veterinary Therapy IX: Small Animal Practice.* RW Kirk Ed. Philadelphia, WB Saunders: 490–495.

Yun, S., J. Lim, et al. (2005). Effect of nandrolone decanoate on disuse muscle atrophy and bone healing in dogs. Proceedings: WSAVA World Congress. Accessed via: Veterinary Information Network. http://goo.gl/2qrlW

NAPROXEN

(na-*prox*-en)   Naprosyn®, Aleve®

NONSTEROIDAL ANTIINFLAMMATORY AGENT

Prescriber Highlights

▶ NSAID; use largely superceded by newer, less GI-toxic NSAIDs in dogs & by other NSAIDs in horses as the equine product is no longer marketed (in USA)

▶ Contraindications: Active GI ulcers or history of hypersensitivity to the drug. Relatively Contraindicated: Hematologic, renal or hepatic disease. Caution: History of gastric ulcers, heart failure

▶ Because of difficulty in accurately dosing, adverse effects, & safer alternatives, usually not used in dogs

▶ Adverse Effects: Relatively uncommon in *Horses:* Possible GI (distress, diarrhea, ulcers), hematologic (hypoproteinemia, decreased hematocrit), renal (fluid retention), & CNS (neuropathies) *Dogs:* GI ulcers & perforation, renal effects (nephritis/nephrotic syndrome), & hepatic (increased liver enzymes) effects

▶ Drug Interactions

Uses/Indications

The former manufacturer listed the following indications: ". . . for the relief of inflammation and associated pain and lameness exhibited with myositis and other soft tissue diseases of the musculoskeletal system of the horse." (Package Insert; *Equiproxen®*—Syntex). It has also been used as an antiinflammatory/analgesic in dogs for the treatment of osteoarthritis and other musculoskeletal inflammatory diseases (see adverse reactions below).

Pharmacology/Actions

Like other NSAIDs, naproxen exhibits analgesic, antiinflammatory, and antipyretic activity probably through its inhibition of cyclooxygenase with resultant impediment of prostaglandin synthesis.

Pharmacokinetics

In horses, the drug is reported to have a 50% bioavailability after oral dosing and a half-life of approximately 4 hours. Absorption does not appear to be altered by the presence of food. It may take 5–7 days to see a beneficial response after starting treatment. Following a dose, the drug is metabolized in the liver. It is detectable in the urine for at least 48 hours in the horse after an oral dose.

In dogs, absorption after oral dosing is rapid and bioavailability is between 68–100%. The drug is highly bound to plasma proteins. The average half-life in dogs is very long at 74 hours.

In humans, naproxen is highly bound to plasma proteins (99%). It crosses the placenta and enters milk in levels of about 1% of those found in serum.

Contraindications/Precautions/Warnings

Naproxen is relatively contraindicated in patients with a history of or preexisting hematologic, renal, or hepatic disease. It is contraindicated in patients with active GI ulcers, or with a history of hypersensitivity to the drug. It should be used cautiously in patients with a history of GI ulcers, or heart failure (may cause fluid retention). Animals suffering from inflammation secondary to concomitant infection, should receive appropriate antimicrobial therapy.

Adverse Effects

Adverse effects are apparently uncommon in horses. The possibility exists for GI (distress, diarrhea, ulcers), hematologic (hypoproteinemia, decreased hematocrit), renal (fluid retention), and CNS (neuropathies) effects.

Reports of GI ulcers and perforation associated with naproxen have occurred in dogs. Dogs may also be overly sensitive to the adverse renal (nephritis/nephrotic syndrome) and hepatic effects (increased liver enzymes) of naproxen. Because of the apparently very narrow therapeutic index and the seriousness of the potential adverse reactions that can be seen in dogs, many clinicians feel that the drug should not be used in this species.

Reproductive/Nursing Safety

In humans, the FDA categorizes this drug as category *B* for use during pregnancy (*Animal studies have not yet demonstrated risk to the fetus, but there are no adequate studies in pregnant women; or animal studies have shown an adverse effect, but adequate studies in pregnant women have not demonstrated a risk to the fetus in the first trimester of pregnancy, and there is no evidence of risk in later trimesters.*) In studies in rodents and in limited studies in horses, no evidence of teratogenicity or adverse effects in breeding performance have been detected following the use of naproxen. Weigh the potential benefits of therapy against the potential risks of its use in pregnant animals.

Most NSAIDs are excreted in maternal milk. Naproxen appears at approximately 1% of maternal serum concentration.

Overdosage/Acute Toxicity

There is very limited information regarding acute overdoses of this drug in humans and domestic animals. The reported oral LD_{50} in dogs is >1000 mg/kg. In dogs, PO ingestions of >5 mg/kg can cause gastrointestinal signs and GI ulceration; >25 mg/kg (some dogs as low as 10 mg/kg) can cause significant renal damage, and >50 mg/kg can result in neuro signs.

One report of a dog that received 5.6 mg/kg

for 7 days has been published (Gilmour and Walshaw 1987). The dog presented with clinical signs of melena, vomiting, depression, regenerative anemia, and pale mucous membranes. Laboratory indices of note included neutrophilia with a left shift, BUN of 66 mg/dL, serum creatinine of 2.1 mg/dL, serum protein to albumin ratio of 4.0:2.1 grams/dL. The dog recovered following treatment with fluids/blood, antibiotics, vitamin/iron supplementation, oral antacids, and cimetidine.

There were 817 exposures to naproxen reported to the ASPCA Animal Poison Control Center (APCC) during 2008-2009. In these cases 764 were dogs with 335 dogs showing clinical signs, 49 cats with 13 showing clinical signs, 2 rodents with 1 showing clinical signs and the remaining 2 cases were 1 bird and 1 bovine showing no clinical signs. Common findings in dogs recorded in decreasing frequency included vomiting, lethargy, anorexia, bloody vomitus, diarrhea, melena, and anemia. Common findings in cats recorded in decreasing frequency included vomiting, lethargy, and anorexia.

As with any NSAID, overdosage can lead to gastrointestinal and renal effects. Decontamination with emetics and/or activated charcoal is appropriate. For doses where GI effects are expected, the use of gastrointestinal protectants, including misoprostol and sucralfate should be considered GI protectant treatment is generally recommended for 10-14 days post-exposure. If renal effects are also expected, fluid diuresis should be considered. Supportive treatment should be instituted as necessary. Monitor electrolyte and fluid balance carefully and manage renal failure using established guidelines.

Drug Interactions
The following drug interactions have either been reported or are theoretical in humans or animals receiving naproxen and may be of significance in veterinary patients:

- **AMINOGLYCOSIDES (gentamicin, amikacin, etc.):** Increased risk for nephrotoxicity
- **ANTICOAGULANTS (heparin, LMWH, warfarin):** Increased risk for bleeding possible
- **ASPIRIN:** When aspirin is used concurrently with naproxen, plasma levels of naproxen could decrease and an increased likelihood of GI adverse effects (blood loss) could occur. Concomitant administration of aspirin with naproxen cannot be recommended.
- **BISPHOSPHONATES (alendronate, etc.):** May increase risk for GI ulceration
- **CORTICOSTEROIDS:** Concomitant administration with NSAIDs may significantly increase the risks for GI adverse effects
- **FUROSEMIDE:** Naproxen may reduce the saluretic and diuretic effects of furosemide
- **HIGHLY PROTEIN BOUND DRUGS (e.g., phenytoin, valproic acid, oral anticoagulants,**

other antiinflammatory agents, salicylates, sulfonamides, and the **sulfonylurea antidiabetic agents**): Because naproxen is highly bound to plasma proteins (99%), it potentially could displace other highly bound drugs; increased serum levels and duration of actions may occur. Although these interactions are usually of little concern clinically, use together with caution.

- **METHOTREXATE:** Serious toxicity has occurred when NSAIDs have been used concomitantly with methotrexate; use together with extreme caution.
- **PROBENECID:** May cause a significant increase in serum levels and half-life of naproxen.

Doses

- **DOGS:**
  Note: Because of the difficulty in accurately dosing naproxen and its potential for adverse effects, the use of this drug in dogs should only be considered when FDA-approved and safer NSAIDs have been ineffective.
  a) 2 mg/kg PO every other day (q48h). (Hansen 2003; Hardie & Grauer 2007; Hardie et al. 2003)
- **RABBITS, RODENTS, SMALL MAMMALS:**
  a) Rabbits: For septic arthritis pain; inflammation: 2.4 mg/mL in drinking water for 21 days (Ivey & Morrisey 2000)
- **HORSES: (Note:** ARCI UCGFS Class 4 Drug)
  a) 5 mg/kg by slow IV, then 10 mg/kg, PO (top dressed in feed) twice daily for up to 14 days or 10 mg/kg, PO (top dressed in feed) twice daily for up to 14 consecutive days. (Package Insert; *Equiproxen®*—Syntex Animal Health; **Note:** No longer commercially available)
  b) 10 mg/kg PO daily (Trumble & Kawcak 2003)

Monitoring
- Analgesic/antiinflammatory efficacy
- GI: appetite, feces (occult blood, diarrhea)
- PCV (packed cell volume), hematocrit if indicated or on chronic therapy
- WBC's if indicated or on chronic therapy

Client Information
- Notify veterinarian if clinical signs of GI distress (anorexia, vomiting, diarrhea, black feces, or blood in stool) occur, or if animal becomes depressed.

Chemistry/Synonyms
Naproxen is a propionic acid derivative, having similar structure and pharmacologic profiles as ibuprofen and ketoprofen. It is a white to off-white crystalline powder with an apparent pK_a of 4.15. It is practically insoluble in water and freely soluble in alcohol. The sodium salt is also available commercially for human use.

Naproxen may also be known as: naproxen-um, RS-3540, RS-3650, *Aleve®*, *Anaprox®*, *EC-Naprosyn®*, *Midol®*, *Naprelan®* and *Naprosyn®*.

Storage/Stability

Naproxen should be stored in well-closed, light resistant containers at room temperature. Temperatures above 40° C (104°F) should be avoided.

Dosage Forms/Regulatory Status

VETERINARY-LABELED PRODUCTS:

None; the equine product is no longer marketed in the USA. The ARCI (Racing Commissioners International) has designated this drug as a class 4 substance. See the appendix for more information.

HUMAN-LABELED PRODUCTS:

Naproxen Oral Tablets/Gelcaps/Capsules: 200 mg (220 mg naproxen sodium), 250 mg (275 mg naproxen sodium), 375 mg, 500 mg (550 mg naproxen sodium); *Naprosyn®* (Roche); *Anaprox®* and *Anaprox DS®* (Roche); *Aleve®* & *Midol®* *Extended Relief* (Bayer Consumer); generic; (Rx and OTC)

Naproxen Delayed/Controlled-release Tablets: 375 mg, 500 mg & 750 mg; *EC-Naprosyn®* (Roche); *Naprelan®* (Victory Pharma); generic; (Rx)

Naproxen Oral Suspension: 125 mg/5 mL in 15 mL, 20 mL, 473 mL & 500 mL; *Naprosyn®* (Roche); generic; (Rx)

References

Hansen, B. (2003). Updated opinions on analgesic techniques. Proceedings: ACVIM Forum.

Hardie, E. & G. Grauer (2007). Treating the dog with osteoarthritis and chronic kidney disease. Proceedings: Western Vet Conf. Accessed via: Veterinary Information Network. http://goo.gl/572Rl

Hardie, E., D. Lascelles, et al. (2003). Managing Chronic Pain in Dogs: The Next Level. Proceedings: Pain Management 2003. Accessed via: Veterinary Information Network. http://goo.gl/mAki4

Ivey, E. & J. Morrisey (2000). Therapeutics for Rabbits. *Vet Clin NA: Exotic Anim Pract* **3:**1(Jan): 183–216.

Trumble, T. & C. Kawcak (2003). Systemic therapies for joint disease. *Current Therapy in Equine Medicine 5.* C Kollias-Baker Ed. Philadelphia, Saunders: 558–561.

NARCOTIC (OPIATE) AGONIST ANALGESICS, PHARMACOLOGY OF

Receptors for opiate analgesics are found in high concentrations in the limbic system, spinal cord, thalamus, hypothalamus, striatum, and midbrain. They are also found in tissues such as the gastrointestinal tract, urinary tract, and in other smooth muscle.

Opiate receptors are further broken down into five main sub-groups. *Mu* receptors are found primarily in the pain regulating areas of the brain. They are thought to contribute to the analgesia, euphoria, respiratory depression, physical dependence, miosis, and hypothermic actions of opiates. *Kappa* receptors are located primarily in the deep layers of the cerebral cortex and spinal cord. They are responsible for analgesia, sedation, and miosis. *Sigma* receptors are thought to be responsible for the dysphoric effects (struggling, whining), hallucinations, respiratory and cardiac stimulation, and mydriatic effects of opiates. *Delta* receptors, located in the limbic areas of the CNS, and epsilon receptors have also been described, but their actions have not been well explained at this time.

The morphine-like agonists (morphine, meperidine, oxymorphone) have primary activity at the *mu* receptors, with some activity possible at the *delta* receptor. The primary pharmacologic effects of these agents include: analgesia, antitussive activity, respiratory depression, sedation, emesis, physical dependence, and intestinal effects (constipation/defecation). Secondary pharmacologic effects include, *CNS*: euphoria, sedation, and confusion. *Cardiovascular*: bradycardia due to central vagal stimulation, alpha-adrenergic receptors may be depressed resulting in peripheral vasodilation, decreased peripheral resistance, and baroreceptor inhibition. Orthostatic hypotension and syncope may occur. *Urinary*: Increased bladder sphincter tone can induce urinary retention.

Various species may exhibit contradictory effects from these agents. For example, horses, cattle, swine, and cats may develop excitement after morphine injections and dogs may defecate after morphine. These effects are in contrast to the expected effects of sedation and constipation. Dogs and humans may develop miosis, while other species (especially cats) may develop mydriasis. For more information see the individual monographs for each agent.

N-BUTYLSCOPOL-AMMONIUM BROMIDE (HYOSCINE BUTYLBROMIDE)

(en-*byoo*-tel-skoe-*pahl*-ah-*moe*-nee-um **broe**-mide)   Buscopan®

QUATERNARY AMMONIUM ANTISPASMODIC & ANTICHOLINERGIC

Prescriber Highlights

▶ Injectable anticholinergic used in horses for treating colic associated with spasmodic colic, flatulent colic, & simple impactions

▶ Shorter acting than atropine; only labeled for a single (one-time) dose IV

▶ Not for use in patients with ileus or when decreased GI motility may be harmful

▶ Adverse effects include transient tachycardia, pupil dilation, decreased secretions & dry mucous membranes

Uses/Indications

N-butylscopolammonium bromide (NBB) injection is indicated (per the label) for control of abdominal pain (colic) associated with spasmodic colic, flatulent colic, and simple impactions in horses. It may also be of benefit in horses in combination with oxytocin to treat esophageal obstruction (choke), and as an aid to performing rectal exams, including colonoscopy.

Pharmacology/Actions

N-butylscopolammonium reduces gastrointestinal peristalsis and rectal pressure via its anticholinergic actions by competitively inhibiting muscarinic receptors on smooth muscle. N-butylscopolammonium has shorter duration of action than atropine. It appears to have brief (15-20 minutes) visceral colorectal distention antinociceptive effects in horses (Sanchez *et al.* 2008).

Pharmacokinetics

Limited information is available for horses. After an intravenous dose, the drug is eliminated within 48 hours in urine and feces equally. Estimated elimination half-life is approximately 6 hours.

Contraindications/Precautions

N-butylscopolammonium is labeled as contraindicated in horses with impaction colics associated with ileus or those with glaucoma.

This medication is not to be used in horses intended for food purposes.

The manufacturer has not studied the safety of IM administration.

Adverse Effects

Adverse effects include transient tachycardia and decreased borborygmal sounds that last for approximately 20-30 minutes after IV dosing. Transient pupil dilation can be noted. Other effects include decreased secretions and dry mucous membranes.

Because this drug can cause increases in heart rate, heart rate cannot be used as a valid pain indicator for 30 minutes after injection.

When used for labeled indications, a lack of response may indicate a more serious problem that may require surgery or more aggressive care (White 2005).

Reproductive/Nursing Safety

As no data is available to document safety, the manufacturer does not recommend use in nursing foals or pregnant or lactating mares.

Overdosage/Acute Toxicity

Dosages up to 10X (3 mg/kg) were administered to horses as part of pre-approval studies. Clinical effects noted included dilated pupils (returned to normal in 4-24 hours), tachycardia (returned to normal within 4 hours) and dry mucous membranes (returned to normal in 1-2 hours). Gut motility was inhibited, but returned to baseline within 4 hours and normal feces were seen within 6 hours. Two of the four horses treated at 10X dosage developed mild signs of colic which resolved without further treatment.

Drug Interactions

The following drug interactions have either been reported or are theoretical in animals receiving N-butylscopolammonium bromide and may be of significance in veterinary patients:

■ **ATROPINE or other anticholinergic agents:** May cause additive effects if used with N-butylscopolammonium

■ **METOCLOPRAMIDE and other drugs that have cholinergic-like actions on the GI tract:** These drugs and N-butylscopolammonium may counteract one another's actions on GI smooth muscle

Laboratory Considerations

■ No specific concerns noted.

Doses

■ **HORSES:**

For labeled indications:

a) 0.3 mg/kg (30 mg or 1.5 mL per 100 kg of body weight) via slow IV, one time (Label Dosage; *Buscopan*®—BI)

b) To treat esophageal obstruction: 0.3 mg/kg IV once with oxytocin (0.11-0.22 Units/kg IV once). Oxytocin use should be avoided in mares, or dose significantly reduced. Do not use in pregnant mares. (Beard 2008)

Monitoring

■ Heart rate (**Note:** heart rate cannot be used as indicator for pain for the first 30 minutes after administration)

■ GI motility via gut sounds and feces output

Client Information

■ Because an accurate patient assessment must be performed prior to the use of this medication and intravenous administration and subsequent monitoring are required, this drug should only be administered by veterinarians

Chemistry/Synonyms

N-butylscopolammonium bromide, a derivative of scopolamine, is a synthetic, quaternary ammonium antispasmodic-anticholinergic agent. It occurs as a white crystalline substance that is soluble in water.

N-butylscopolammonium bromide may also be known as: butylscopolamine bromide, hyoscine butylbromide, hysocine N-butylbromide, scopolamini butylbromidum, hyoscini butylbromidum, *Buscopan*® or *Buscapina*®.

Storage/Stability

The commercially available injection should be stored at room temperature (15−30°C).

Dosage Forms/Regulatory Status

VETERINARY-LABELED PRODUCTS:

N-butylscopolammonium bromide Injection: 20 mg/mL in 50 mL multi-dose vials, *Buscopan*® (BIVI); (Rx). FDA-approved for use in horses.

In the UK, *Buscopan Compositum*® (BI) is commercially available. This product contains metamizole (a form of dipyrone) 500 mg/mL and hyoscine butylbromide (synonym for N-butylscopolammonium Br) 4 mg/mL. It is labeled for use in horses, cattle and dogs.

HUMAN-LABELED PRODUCTS:

None in the USA. There are several products with the trade name *Buscopan*® or *Buscapina*® available in many countries. Refer to actual product labels as ingredients and concentrations may vary.

References

Beard, L. (2008). Respiratory disease in the geriatric patient. Proceedings: WVC. Accessed via: Veterinary Information Network. http://goo.gl/mNYAX

Sanchez, L.C., J.R. Elfenbein, et al. (2008). Effect of acepromazine, butorphanol, or N-butylscopolammonium bromide on visceral and somatic nociception and duodenal motility in conscious horses. *American Journal of Veterinary Research* 69(5): 579–585.

White, N. (2005). Medical Treatment of Colic. Western Veterinary Conference: Proceedings. Accessed via: Veterinary Information Network. http://goo.gl/MFP8L

NEOMYCIN SULFATE

(nee-o-*mye*-sin)   Biosol®, Neomix®

AMINOGLYCOSIDE ANTIBIOTIC

Prescriber Highlights

▶ Aminoglycoside antibiotic usually used orally (gut "sterilization") or in topical formulations

▶ Contraindications: Oral: Hypersensitive to aminoglycosides, intestinal blockage; rabbits

▶ Adverse Effects: Parenteral use can be very toxic (nephrotoxic) & is not recommended. Chronic use can lead to GI superinfections. Rarely, oral neomycin may cause ototoxicity, nephrotoxicity, severe diarrhea, & intestinal malabsorption

▶ Minimal amounts absorbed via GI (if intact)

Uses/Indications

Because neomycin is more nephrotoxic and less effective against several bacterial species than either gentamicin or amikacin, its use is generally limited to topical formulations for skin, eyes, and ears, oral treatment of enteric infections, to reduce microbe numbers in the colon prior to colon surgery, and oral or enema administration to reduce ammonia-producing bacteria in the treatment of hepatic encephalopathy. Doses for parenteral administration are listed below, but should be used only with extreme caution due to the drug's toxic potential.

Pharmacology/Actions

Neomycin has a mechanism of action and spectrum of activity (primarily gram-negative aerobes) similar to the other aminoglycosides, but in comparison to either gentamicin or amikacin, it is significantly less effective against several species of gram-negative organisms, including strains of Klebsiella, *E. coli*, and Pseudomonas. However, most strains of neomycin-resistant bacteria of these species remain susceptible to amikacin. More detailed information on the aminoglycosides mechanism of action and spectrum of activity is outlined in the amikacin monograph.

Pharmacokinetics

Approximately 3% of a dose of neomycin is absorbed after oral or rectal (retention enema) administration, but this can be increased if gut motility is slowed or if the bowel wall is damaged. Therapeutic levels are not attained in the systemic circulation after oral administration.

After IM administration, therapeutic levels can be attained with peak levels occurring within 1 hour of dosing. The drug apparently distributes to tissues and is eliminated like the other aminoglycosides (refer to Amikacin monograph for more details). Orally administered neomycin is nearly all excreted unchanged in the feces.

Contraindications/Precautions/Warnings

Oral neomycin is contraindicated in the presence of intestinal obstruction or if the patient is hypersensitive to aminoglycosides.

In neonates, orally administered neomycin can yield high systemic levels; avoid use in neonatal patients.

Chronic usage of oral aminoglycosides may result in bacterial or fungal superinfections.

Because aminoglycosides can cause irreversible ototoxicity when administered parenterally, they should be used with caution in "working" dogs.

Aminoglycosides should be used with caution in patients with neuromuscular disorders (e.g., myasthenia gravis) due to their neuromuscular blocking activity.

Because aminoglycosides are eliminated primarily through renal mechanisms, when administered parenterally they should be used cautiously, preferably with serum monitoring and dosage adjustment in neonatal or geriatric animals. When neomycin is given orally, only perhaps 3% of a dose is absorbed, but use with caution in patients with renal dysfunction.

Aminoglycosides are generally considered contraindicated in rabbits/hares, as they adversely affect the GI flora balance in these animals. Oral neomycin has been associated with antibiotic-associated diarrhea (enterocolitis) in horses and it is not commonly used in this species.

Adverse Effects

Refer to the amikacin monograph for more information regarding these topics with parenteral neomycin; however, parenterally administered neomycin is much more nephrotoxic than is amikacin.

Rarely, oral neomycin may cause ototoxicity, nephrotoxicity, severe diarrhea, and intestinal malabsorption.

Reproductive/Nursing Safety

In humans, the FDA categorizes this drug as category *C* for use during pregnancy (*Animal studies have shown an adverse effect on the fetus, but there are no adequate studies in humans; or there are no animal reproduction studies and no adequate studies in humans.*) In a separate system evaluating the safety of drugs in canine and feline pregnancy (Papich 1989), this drug is categorized as class: *A* (*Probably safe. Although specific studies may not have proved he safety of all drugs in dogs and cats, there are no reports of adverse effects in laboratory animals or women.*)

Neomycin is excreted in cow's milk following a single IM injection. If used orally, it is unlikely neomycin poses significant systemic risk to nursing offspring, but may negatively alter gut flora and cause diarrhea.

Drug Interactions

The following drug interactions have either been reported or are theoretical in humans or animals receiving oral neomycin and may be of significance in veterinary patients:

■ **DIGOXIN:** Oral neomycin with orally administered digoxin may result in decreased absorption. Separating the doses of the two medications may not alleviate this effect. Some human patients (<10%) metabolize digoxin in the GI tract and neomycin may increase serum digoxin levels in these patients. It is recommended that enhanced monitoring be performed if oral neomycin is added or withdrawn from the drug regimen of a patient stabilized on a digitalis glycoside.

■ **METHOTREXATE:** Absorption may be reduced by oral neomycin but is increased by oral kanamycin (found in *Amforal®*)

■ **OTOTOXIC, NEPHROTOXIC DRUGS:** Although only minimal amounts of neomycin are absorbed after oral or rectal administration, the concurrent use of other ototoxic or nephrotoxic drugs with neomycin should be done with caution

■ **PENICILLIN VK (oral):** Oral neomycin should not be given concurrently with oral penicillin VK as malabsorption of the penicillin may occur

■ **WARFARIN:** Oral neomycin may decrease the amount of vitamin K absorbed from the gut; this may have ramifications for patients receiving oral anticoagulants

Refer to the amikacin monograph for more information regarding drug interactions with parenteral neomycin.

Laboratory Considerations

No specific concerns noted

Doses

■ **DOGS:**

For treatment of hepatic encephalopathy:

a) A check list for acute management of hepatic encephalopathy includes: **1)** Lactulose (orally, or by enema if stupor or seizures); **2)** NPO for 12 to 24 hours; **3)** If no response, add metronidazole orally at 15 mg/kg/day; **4)** If no response, add neomycin orally at 20 mg/kg PO three times daily. **5)** Provide IV fluids with potassium (and dextrose for patients with portosystemic shunts or severe cirrhosis). **6)** Add anti-ulcer therapy (GI bleeding is a protein load in hepatic encephalopathy), and add vitamin K_1 if jaundiced. **7)** Withhold any glucocorticoids until encephalopathy is resolved! **8)** Give as much dietary protein as tolerated; increase the lactulose dosage if needed. (Trepanier 2008)

b) For adjunctive management of portosystemic shunts: 10−20 mg/kg PO two to three times a day. (Twedt 2009)

c) Animals that are neurologically and systemically stable should be treated with orally-administered nonabsorbable antibiotics in order to decrease the numbers of urease-producing bacteria within the gastrointestinal tract. If using neomycin: 20 mg/kg PO q12h. Avoid neomycin if any evidence of intestinal bleeding, ulcerations, or renal failure. The use of oral lactulose therapy, in conjunction with or as an alternative to antibiotics, is also beneficial in neurologically stable animals. The combination of neomycin and lactulose may be synergistic. (Silverstein 2009)

d) 15 mg/kg as an enema every 6 hours after a cleansing enema or 10–20 mg/kg, PO every 6 hours. May be used with lactulose. (Johnson 1986)

For GI tract infections:

a) For campylobacteriosis: 20 mg/kg PO q12h (Willard 2003)

For systemic therapy (**Caution:** Very nephrotoxic):

a) 3.5 mg/kg IV, IM or SC q8h (Kirk 1989)

■ **CATS:**

For treatment of hepatic encephalopathy:

a) See "A check list for acute management of hepatic encephalopathy" in Dog dose section above.

b) 22 mg/kg q8h PO (Cornelius, Bartges et al. 2000)

c) Lactulose at 0.5–1 mg/kg PO q8h with or without neomycin at 20 mg/kg PO q8–12h. (Marks 2004)

d) Animals that are neurologically and systemically stable should be treated with orally-administered nonabsorbable antibiotics in order to decrease the numbers of urease-producing bacteria within the gastrointestinal tract. If using neomycin: 20 mg/kg PO q12h. Avoid neomycin if any evidence of intestinal bleeding, ulcerations, or renal failure. The use of oral lactulose therapy, in conjunction with or as an alternative to antibiotics, is also beneficial in neurologically stable animals. The combination of neomycin and lactulose may be synergistic. (Silverstein 2009)

For GI tract infections: For campylobacteriosis:

a) 20 mg/kg PO q12h (Willard 2003)

For systemic therapy (**Caution:** Very nephrotoxic):

a) 3.5 mg/kg IV, IM or SC q8h (Kirk 1989)

■ **FERRETS:**

For susceptible enteric infections:

a) 10–20 mg/kg, PO twice to four times daily (Williams 2000)

■ **RODENTS, SMALL MAMMALS:**

Note: Contraindicated in rabbits/hares

a) **Chinchillas:** 15 mg/kg, PO once daily. **Gerbils:** 100 mg/kg, PO once daily, **Guinea Pigs:** 8 mg/kg, PO once daily. **Hamsters:** 100 mg/kg, PO once daily, or 0.5 mg/mL in drinking water. **Mice, Rats:** 50 mg/kg, PO once daily (Adamcak & Otten 2000)

■ **CATTLE:**

For oral administration to treat susceptible enteral infections:

a) 4–7.5 grams/day PO divided 2–4 times daily at regular intervals. Calves: 2–3 grams/day, PO divided 2–4 times daily at regular intervals. Doses are not standardized; use for general guidance only. (Brander et al. 1982)

b) 10–20 mg/kg q12h (general guideline only). (Jenkins 1986)

c) 7–12 mg/kg, PO q12h (Howard 1986)

d) Feed at levels of 70–140 grams/ton of feed or mix the appropriate dose in the drinking water which will be consumed by animals in 12 hours to provide 11 mg/kg or mix with reconstituted milk replacers to provide 200–400 mg/gallon. (Label directions; *Neomix Ag® 325*—Upjohn)

■ **HORSES:**

For oral administration to treat susceptible enteral infections:

a) Adults: 4–7.5 grams/day PO divided 2–4 times daily at regular intervals. Foals: 2–3 grams/day PO divided 2–4 times daily at regular intervals. Doses are not standardized; use for general guidance only. (Brander et al. 1982)

b) 5–15 mg/kg PO once daily (Robinson 1987)

For intrauterine infusion:

a) Neomycin alone: 3–4 grams. Combination of neomycin (2 grams) and procaine penicillin G (3,000,000 IU), Combination of Neomycin (1grams) and Polymyxin B (40,000 IU), Furaltadone (600 mg) and penicillin G (Sodium or potassium, 3,000,000–5,000,000 IU). Little science is available for recommending doses, volume infused, frequency, diluents, etc. Most intrauterine treatments are commonly performed every day or every other day for 3–7 days. (Perkins 1999)

■ **SWINE:**

For oral administration to treat susceptible enteral infections:

a) **Young pigs:** 0.75–1 grams/day, PO divided 2–4 times daily at regular intervals. Doses are not standardized; use for general guidance only. (Brander, Pugh, and Bywater 1982)

b) 7–12 mg/kg, PO q12h (Howard 1986)

■ **SHEEP & GOATS:**

For oral administration to treat susceptible enteral infections:

a) **Lambs:** 0.75–1 grams/day PO divided 2–4 times daily at regular intervals. Doses are not standardized; use for general guidance only. (Brander *et al.* 1982)

b) Feed at levels of 70–140 grams/ton of feed or mix the appropriate dose in the drinking water which will be consumed by animals in 12 hours to provide 11 mg/kg or mix with reconstituted milk replacers to provide 200–400 mg/gallon. (Label directions; *Neomix Ag® 325*—Upjohn)

■ **BIRDS:**

For bacterial enteritis:

a) **Chickens, turkeys, ducks:** Feed at levels of 70–140 grams/ton of feed or mix the appropriate dose in the drinking water which will be consumed by animals in 12 hours to provide 11 mg/kg (Label directions; *Neomix Ag® 325*—Upjohn)

■ **SNAKES:**

For susceptible infections:

a) For bacterial gastritis: gentamicin 2.5 mg/kg IM every 72 hours with oral neomycin 15 mg/kg plus oral live lactobacillus (Burke 1986)

Monitoring

For oral use:

■ Clinical efficacy

■ Systemic and GI adverse effects with prolonged use.

For parenteral use: Refer to Amikacin monograph

Client Information

■ Clients should understand that the potential exists for severe toxicity (nephrotoxicity, ototoxicity) developing from this medication when used parenterally.

Chemistry/Synonyms

An aminoglycoside antibiotic obtained from *Streptomyces fradiae*, neomycin is actually a complex of three separate compounds, neomycin A (neamine; inactive), neomycin C, and neomycin B (framycetin). The commercially available product almost entirely consists of the sulfate salt of neomycin B. It occurs as an odorless or almost odorless, white to slightly yellow, hygroscopic powder or cryodessicated solid. It is freely soluble in water and very slightly soluble in alcohol. One mg of pure neomycin sulfate is equivalent to not less than 650 Units. Oral or injectable (after reconstitution with normal saline) solutions of neomycin sulfate have a pH from 5–7.5.

Neomycin sulfate may also be known as: fradiomycin sulfate, neomycin sulphate, or neomycini sulfas, *Neo-325®*, *Neo-fradin®*, *Neo-Sol 50®*, and *Neovet®*.

Storage/Stability

Neomycin sulfate oral solution should be stored at room temperature (15–30°C) in tight, light-resistant containers. Unless otherwise instructed by the manufacturer, oral tablets/boluses should be stored in tight containers at room temperature. The sterile powder should be stored at room temperature and protected from light.

In the dry state, neomycin is stable for at least 2 years at room temperature.

Dosage Forms/Regulatory Status

VETERINARY-LABELED PRODUCTS:

Neomycin Sulfate Oral Liquid: 200 mg/mL (140 mg neomycin base/mL); generic; (OTC). Depending on labeling FDA-approved for use in cattle, swine, sheep, goats, turkeys, laying hens, and broilers. Check labels for slaughter withdrawals; may vary with product. General withdrawal times (when used as labeled): Cattle = 1 day; Sheep = 2 days and swine and goats = 3 days. Withdrawal period has not been established in pre-ruminating calves. Do not use in calves to be processed for veal. A milk discard period has not been established in lactating dairy cattle. Do not use in female dairy cattle 20 months of age or older.

Neomycin Sulfate Soluble Powder: 325 grams/lb: *Neo-325® Soluble Powder* (Bimeda); *Neovet® 325/100* & *NeoVet® 325 AG Grade* (includes turkey label); (AgriPharm) *Neo-Sol 50®* (Alpharma); (OTC). FDA-approved for use in cattle and goats (not veal calves), swine, sheep, goats and turkeys (some products). Check labels for slaughter withdrawals; may vary with product. General slaughter withdrawal times (when used as labeled): Cattle = 1 day; Turkeys = 0 days; Sheep = 2 days; Swine and Goats = 3 days.

HUMAN-LABELED PRODUCTS:

Neomycin Sulfate Tablets: 500 mg; generic; (Rx)

Neomycin Sulfate Oral Solution: 25 mg/mL in 480 mL; *Neo-fradin®* (Pharma-Tek); (Rx)

References

Adamcak, A. & B. Otten (2000). Rodent Therapeutics. *Vet Clin NA: Exotic Anim Pract* **3:**1(Jan): 221–240.

Brander, C.G., D.M. Pugh, et al. (1982). *Veterinary Applied Pharmacology and Therapeutics*. London, Baillière Tindall.

Burke, T.J. (1986). Regurgitation in snakes. *Current Veterinary Therapy (CVT) IX Small Animal Practice*. RW Kirk Ed. Philadelphia, WB Saunders: 749–750.

Howard, J.L., Ed. (1986). *Current Veterinary Therapy 2, Food Animal Practice*. Philadelphia, W.B. Saunders.

Jenkins, W.L. (1986). Antimicrobial Therapy. *Current Veterinary Therapy: Food Animal Practice 2*. JL Howard Ed. Philadelphia, W.B. Saunders: 8–23.

Johnson, S.E. (1986). Acute hepatic failure. *Current Veterinary Therapy (CVT) IX Small Animal Practice*. RW Kirk Ed. Philadelphia, WB Saunders: 945–952.

Kirk, R.W., Ed. (1989). *Current Veterinary Therapy X, Small Animal Practice*. Philadelphia, W.B. Saunders.

Marks, S. (2004). Dietary and therapeutic approach to commmon canine and feline liver diseases. Proceedings: IVECCS. Accessed via: Veterinary Information Network. http://goo.gl/JKrfA

Papich, M. (1989). Effects of drugs on pregnancy. *Current*

Veterinary Therapy X: Small Animal Practice. R Kirk Ed. Philadelphia, Saunders: 1291–1299.

Perkins, N. (1999). Equine reproductive pharmacology. *The Veterinary Clinics of North America: Equine Practice* 15:3(December): 687–704.

Robinson, N.E. (1987). Table of Common Drugs: Approximate Doses. *Current Therapy in Equine Medicine, 2*. NE Robinson Ed. Philadelphia, W.B. Saunders: 761.

Silverstein, D. (2009). Management of hepatic encephalopathy. Proceedings: Western Veterinary Conf. Accessed via: Veterinary Information Network. http://goo.gl/o0ODJ

Trepanier, L. (2008). Choosing therapy for chronic liver disease. Proceedings: WSAVA. Accessed via: Veterinary Information Network. http://goo.gl/NLh4X

Twedt, D. (2009). Treatment of liver disease. Proceedings: ACVC. Accessed via: Veterinary Information Network. http://goo.gl/7SUeb

Willard, M. (2003). Disorders of the intestinal tract. *Small Animal Internal Medicine, 3rd Ed*. R Nelson and C Couto Eds. St Louis, Mosby: 431–465.

Williams, B. (2000). Therapeutics in Ferrets. *Vet Clin NA: Exotic Anim Pract* 3:1(Jan): 131–153.

NEOSTIGMINE BROMIDE NEOSTIGMINE METHYLSULFATE

(nee-oh-**stig**-meen)   Prostigmin®

PARASYMPATHOMIMETIC (CHOLINERGIC)

Prescriber Highlights

▶ Parasympathomimetic used to initiate peristalsis, empty the bladder, & stimulate skeletal muscle contractions. Also for diagnosis & treatment of myasthenia gravis & treatment of non-depolarizing neuromuscular blocking agents (curare-type) overdose; has been used for treating massive ivermectin overdoses in cats

▶ Contraindications: Peritonitis, mechanical intestinal or urinary tract obstructions, late stages of pregnancy, hypersensitivity to this class of compounds, or if treated with other cholinesterase inhibitors

▶ Adverse Effects: Cholinergic in nature & dose related (nausea, vomiting, diarrhea, excessive salivation & drooling, sweating, miosis, lacrimation, increased bronchial secretions, bradycardia or tachycardia, cardiospasm, bronchospasm, hypotension, muscle cramps & weakness, agitation, restlessness, or paralysis)

▶ Cholinergic crisis & myasthenic crisis must not be confused

Uses/Indications

Neostigmine is indicated for rumen atony, initiating peristalsis, emptying the bladder, and stimulating skeletal muscle contractions in cattle, horses, sheep, and swine (Package insert; *Stiglyn® 1:500-P/M*—Mallinckrodt). It has been used in the diagnosis and treatment of myasthenia gravis and in treating non-depolarizing neuromuscular blocking agents (curare-type) overdoses in dogs. Neostigmine has also been used to treat massive ivermectin overdoses in cats.

Pharmacology/Actions

Neostigmine competes with acetylcholine for acetylcholinesterase. As the neostigmine-acetylcholinesterase complex is hydrolyzed at a slower rate than that of the acetylcholine-enzyme complex, acetylcholine will accumulate with a resultant exaggeration and prolongation of its effects. These effects can include increased tone of intestinal and skeletal musculature, stimulation of salivary and sweat glands, bronchoconstriction, ureter constriction, miosis and bradycardia. Neostigmine also has a direct cholinomimetic effect on skeletal muscle.

In horses, neostigmine may decrease jejunal activity and delay gastric emptying. Its use in treating colon impactions and ileus is controversial.

Pharmacokinetics

Information on the pharmacokinetics of neostigmine in veterinary species was not located. In humans, neostigmine bromide is poorly absorbed after oral administration with only 1–2% of the dose absorbed. Neostigmine effects on peristaltic activity in humans begin within 10–30 minutes after parenteral administration and can persist for up to 4 hours.

Neostigmine is 15–25% bound to plasma proteins. It has not been detected in human milk nor would it be expected to cross the placenta when given at usual doses.

In humans, the half-life of the drug is approximately one hour. It is metabolized in the liver and hydrolyzed by cholinesterases to 3-OH PTM, which is weakly active. When administered parenterally, approximately 80% of the drug is excreted in the urine within 24 hours, with 50% excreted unchanged.

Contraindications/Precautions/Warnings

Neostigmine is contraindicated in patients with peritonitis, mechanical intestinal or urinary tract obstructions, in animals hypersensitive to this class of compounds, or treated with other cholinesterase inhibitors.

Use neostigmine with caution in patients with epilepsy, peptic ulcer disease, bronchial asthma, cardiac arrhythmias, hyperthyroidism, vagotonia, or megacolon.

Adverse Effects

Adverse effects of neostigmine are dose-related and cholinergic in nature. See overdosage section below.

Reproductive/Nursing Safety

In humans, the FDA categorizes this drug as category *C* for use during pregnancy (*Animal studies have shown an adverse effect on the fetus, but there are no adequate studies in humans; or there are no animal reproduction studies and no adequate studies in humans.*)

Because it is ionized at physiologic pH, neostigmine would not be expected to be excreted in maternal milk.

Overdosage/Acute Toxicity

Overdosage of neostigmine can induce a cholinergic crisis. Clinical signs can include: nausea, vomiting, diarrhea, excessive salivation and drooling, sweating (in animals with sweat glands), miosis, lacrimation, increased bronchial secretions, bradycardia or tachycardia, cardiospasm, bronchospasm, hypotension, muscle cramps and weakness, agitation, restlessness, or paralysis. In patients with myasthenia gravis, it may be difficult to distinguish between a cholinergic crisis and myasthenic crisis. A test dose of edrophonium should differentiate between the two.

Treat cholinergic crisis by temporarily ceasing neostigmine therapy and instituting treatment with atropine (doses are listed in the Atropine monograph). Maintain adequate respirations using mechanical assistance if necessary.

Drug Interactions

The following drug interactions have either been reported or are theoretical in humans or animals receiving neostigmine and may be of significance in veterinary patients:

- ■ **ATROPINE:** Atropine will antagonize the muscarinic effects of neostigmine and some clinicians routinely use the two together, but concurrent use should be used cautiously as atropine can mask the early clinical signs of cholinergic crisis

- ■ **CORTICOSTEROIDS:** May decrease the anticholinesterase activity of neostigmine; after stopping corticosteroid therapy, neostigmine may cause increased anticholinesterase activity

- ■ **DEXPANTHENOL:** Theoretically, dexpanthenol may have additive effects when used with neostigmine

- ■ **MAGNESIUM:** Anticholinesterase therapy may be antagonized by administration of parenteral magnesium therapy, as it can have a direct depressant effect on skeletal muscle

- ■ **MUSCLE RELAXANTS:** Neostigmine may prolong the Phase I block of depolarizing muscle relaxants (*e.g.,* **succinylcholine, decamethonium**) and edrophonium antagonizes the actions of non-depolarizing neuromuscular blocking agents (*e.g.,* **pancuronium, tubocurarine, gallamine, vecuronium, atracurium,** etc.)

Doses

- ■ **DOGS:**
  a) For treatment of myasthenia gravis:

0.04 mg/kg IM q6h to bypass the problem of oral medication in actively regurgitating animals (Inzana 2000)

b) For diagnosis of myasthenia gravis: 0.05 mg/kg IM (diagnostic for MA if clinical improvement occurs in 15–30 minutes; pre-treat with atropine) (LeCouteur 1989)

c) For treatment of curare overdoses: 0.001 mg/kg SC, follow with IV injection of atropine (0.04 mg/kg) (Bailey 1986)

- ■ **CATS:**

For treatment of myasthenia gravis:

a) 0.04 mg/kg IM q6h to bypass the problem of oral medication in actively regurgitating animals (Inzana 2000)

- ■ **CATTLE:**
  a) 1 mg/100 lbs of body weight SC; repeat as indicated (Package Insert; *Stiglyn® 1:500-P/M*—Mallinckrodt)

- ■ **HORSES: (Note:** ARCI UCGFS Class 3 Drug)
  a) 1 mg/100 lbs of body weight SC; repeat as indicated (Package Insert; *Stiglyn® 1:500-P/M*—Mallinckrodt)

For treatment of ileus:

a) 0.022 mg/kg IV or 0.044 mg/kg SC, IM. This drug has no therapeutic value for small intestinal ileus. (White 2007)

b) For ileus with marked colonic distension in foals secondary to *C. perfringens* type C: 1–2 mg (2 mg for foals greater than 250 lb) SC, 2–3 doses at 1–hour intervals then as needed. (Slovis 2003)

c) 0.025 mg/kg SC q2–6h (Hassel 2005)

d) May be beneficial for treatment of small intestinal ileus at 2 mg per 500 kg adult horse administered SC or IV every 30 to 60 minutes to a maximum dose of 10 mg. Side effects include colic signs. (Hallowell 2008)

- ■ **SWINE:**
  a) 2–3 mg/100 lbs of body weight IM; repeat as indicated (Package Insert; *Stiglyn® 1:500-P/M*—Mallinckrodt)

  b) 0.03 mg/kg (Davis 1986)

- ■ **SHEEP:**
  a) 1–1.5 mg/100 lbs of body weight SC; repeat as indicated (Package Insert; *Stiglyn® 1:500-P/M*—Mallinckrodt)

  b) 0.01–0.02 mg/kg (goats also) (Davis 1986)

Monitoring

Dependent on reason for use.

- ■ Adverse reactions (see Adverse Effects and Overdosage above)

- ■ Clinical efficacy

Client Information

■ This product should only be used by professionals in locations where the drug's effects can be monitored.

Chemistry/Synonyms

Synthetic quaternary ammonium parasympathomimetic agents, neostigmine bromide and neostigmine methylsulfate both occur as odorless, bitter-tasting, white, crystalline powders that are very soluble in water and soluble in alcohol. The melting point of neostigmine methylsulfate is from 144–149°. The pH of the commercially available neostigmine methylsulfate injection is from 5–6.5.

Neostigmine methylsulfate may also be known as: neostigmine metilsulfate, neostigmine methylsulphate, neostigmini metilsulfas, proserinum, *Glycostigmin®*, *Intrastigmina®*, *Neostig-Reu®*, *Normastigmin®*, *Prostigmin®*, *Prostigmina®*, *Prostigmine®*, *Stiglyn®*, or *Tilstigmin®*.

Storage/Stability

Neostigmine bromide tablets should be stored at room temperature in tight containers. Neostigmine methylsulfate injection should be stored at room temperature and protected from light; avoid freezing.

Neostigmine methylsulfate injection is reportedly physically **compatible** with the commonly used IV replacement solutions and the following drugs: glycopyrrolate, pentobarbital sodium, and thiopental sodium.

Dosage Forms/Regulatory Status

VETERINARY-LABELED PRODUCTS: None

The ARCI (Racing Commissioners International) has designated this drug as a class 3 substance. See the appendix for more information.

HUMAN-LABELED PRODUCTS:

Neostigmine Methylsulfate Injection: 1:1000 (1 mg/mL) in 10 mL vials, 1:2000 (0.5 mg/mL) in 1 mL amps & 10 mL vials, 1:4000 (0.25 mg/mL) in 1 mL amps; *Prostigmin®* (ICN); generic; (Rx)

Neostigmine Bromide Oral Tablets: 15 mg; *Prostigmin®* (Valeant Pharmaceuticals); (Rx)

References

Bailey, E.M. (1986). Emergency and general treatment of poisonings. *Current Veterinary Therapy (CVT) IX Small Animal Practice*. RW Kirk Ed. Philadelphia, W.B. Saunders: 135–144.

Davis, L.E. (1986). Drugs affecting the digestive system. *Curret Veterinary Therapy 2: Food Animal Practice*. JL Howard Ed. Philadelphia, WB Saunders: 760–763.

Hallowell, G. (2008). Update on Current and New Treatments for Colic Patients. Proceedings: ACVIM. Accessed via: Veterinary Information Network. http://goo.gl/D004NS

Hassel, D. (2005). Post-operative complications in the colic. Proceedings: IVECCS. Accessed via: Veterinary Information Network. http://goo.gl/UDFPN

Inzana, K. (2000). Peripheral Nerve Disorders. *Textbook of Veterinary Internal Medicine: Diseases of the Dog and Cat*. S Ettinger and E Feldman Eds. Philadelphia, WB Saunders. 1: 662–684.

LeCouteur, R.A. (1989). Disorders of peripheral nerves. *Handbook of Small Animal Practice*. RV Morgan Ed. New York, Churchill Livingstone: 299–318.

Slovis, N. (2003). Infectious diarrhea in foals. Proceedings: ACVIM Forum. Accessed via: Veterinary Information Network. http://goo.gl/JllC0

White, N. (2007). Treatment of GI Motility Disorder: Are We Moving Along? Proceedings: IVECCS. Accessed via: Veterinary Information Network. http://goo.gl/GIdno

NIACINAMIDE (NICOTINAMIDE)

(nye-a-*sin*-a-mide)

IMMUNOMODULATOR; NUTRITIONAL

Prescriber Highlights

▶ Used in canine medicine in combination with tetracycline for treatment of discoid lupus erythematosus; may be useful in other immune-mediated dermatologic conditions such as sterile pyogranulomas, idiopathic onychodystrophy, pemphigus foliaceous, & pemphigus erythematosus. Not believed to be effective (w/tetracycline) for atopic dermatitis.

▶ Possible Contraindications: Liver disease, active peptic ulcers, or hypersensitivity to it

▶ Adverse Effects: Anorexia, vomiting, & lethargy; occasionally increases in liver enzymes seen

▶ Improvement may be gradual & take 6–8 weeks

▶ Inexpensive

Uses/Indications

When used in conjunction with tetracycline in dogs, niacinamide may be useful in controlling discoid lupus erythematosus (subacute cutaneous lupus) and pemphigus erythematosus in 25% to 65% of affected dogs. Can also be used for adjunctive therapy for pemphigus foliaceus (with prednisone and azathioprine). May also be effective in other dermatoses such as: vesicular cutaneous lupus erythematosus, lupoid onychodystrophy, dermatomyositis, German Shepherd Dog metatarsal fistulae, sterile granulomatous and/or pyogranulomatous dermatitis and/or panniculitis, vasculitis, cutaneous histiocytosis, sebaceous adenitis, and arteritis of the nasal philtrum (Bruner 2006).. It may make take 1–2 months before efficacy is noted.

Pharmacology/Actions

While niacinamide is an essential nutrient in humans (necessary for lipid metabolism. tissue respiration, and glycogenolysis) its primary pharmacologic use (in combination with tetracycline for discoid lupus erythematosus) in dogs is secondary to its action of blocking IgE-induced histamine release and degranulation of mast cells. When used with tetracycline, niacinamide may suppress leukocyte chemotaxis secondary to complement activation by antibody-antigen complexes. It also inhibits phosphodiesterases and decreases the release of proteases. In combination with tetracycline's immunomodulating and antiinflammatory effects, efficacy has been noted in up to two-thirds of dogs treated for DLE. While niacinamide and niacin act identically as vitamins, niacinamide does not affect blood lipid levels or the cardiovascular system.

Pharmacokinetics

Niacinamide is absorbed well after oral administration and widely distributed to body tissues. Niacinamide is metabolized in the liver to several metabolites that are excreted into the urine. At physiologic doses, only a small amount of niacinamide is excreted into the urine unchanged, but as dosages increase, larger quantities are excreted unchanged.

Contraindications/Precautions/Warnings

In humans, niacinamide therapy is contraindicated in patients with liver disease, active peptic ulcers, or hypersensitivity to the drug. Use niacinamide/tetracycline with caution in dogs with a seizure history.

Adverse Effects

Adverse effects of niacinamide in dogs are uncommon, but may include anorexia, vomiting, and lethargy. Occasionally, increases in liver enzymes may be noted. There have been some anecdotal reports of increased seizure frequencies in dogs.

Reproductive/Nursing Safety

While niacinamide alone should be safe to use in pregnant and lactating animals, its use in combination with tetracycline may not be safe.

Overdosage/Acute Toxicity

There is unlikely to be a problem with niacinamide overdoses other than acute GI distress.

Drug Interactions

Niacinamide and tetracycline treatment does not interfere with antibody production associated with routine vaccinations in dogs. Also see the tetracycline monograph for additional drug interactions if using combination therapy.

The following drug interactions have either been reported or are theoretical in humans or animals receiving niacinamide and may be of significance in veterinary patients:

- ■ **INSULIN/ORAL ANTIDIABETIC AGENTS:** In diabetic humans, dosage adjustments for insulin or oral antidiabetic agents have sometimes been necessary after initiating niacinamide therapy.

Doses

- ■ **DOGS:**

  For discoid lupus erythematosus:

  a) For dogs weighing 10 kg or more: 500 mg of niacinamide and 500 mg of tetracycline

PO q8h. For dogs weighing from 5–10 kg: 250 mg of each drug PO q8h. For dogs weighing less than 5 kg: 100 mg of each drug PO q8h. Improvement is usually noted within 6 weeks. (White 2000))

b) Dogs weighing more than 10 kg: 500 mg of niacinamide and 500 mg of tetracycline PO q8h. For dogs weighing less than 10 kg: 250 mg of each PO q8h. May use in combination with corticosteroids and Vitamin E. If adverse effects become a problem, reduce dose of niacinamide first. May also try this regimen for pemphigus foliaceous or pemphigus erythematous (approximately (Campbell 1999)

For various immune-mediated diseases (discoid lupus erythematosus, pemphigus erythematosus, pemphigus foliaceous, vasculitis, sterile pyelogranuloma, dermatomyositis, and lupoid onychodystrophy):

a) For dogs less than 10 kg: 250 mg each of niacinamide and tetracycline PO three times daily.

  For dogs larger than 10 kg: 500 mg each of niacinamide and tetracycline PO three times daily. May substitute doxycycline for tetracycline at 5 mg/kg PO once a day. (Tapp 2002)

b) For pemphigus foliaceous: Doses as above (with prednisone and azathioprine). Dogs that show improvement with this therapy do so within the first one or two months of therapy. Once remission has occurred the dose may be gradually tapered to once daily administration. (Marsella 2008)

c) For adjunctive therapy for pemphigus or discoid lupus erythematosus: 100 mg of each for dogs <5kg; 250 mg of each for dogs 5-10 kg; 500 mg of each for dogs >10 kg PO three times daily until resolve (90-120 days), then decrease by one dose per day per month (three times daily to two times daily to once daily and eventually to every other day for 30–60 days.) (Yu 2008)

Monitoring

- ■ Efficacy
- ■ Adverse effects (baseline and occasional monitoring of liver enzymes is suggested)

Client Information

- ■ Give as directed. Improvement may not be noted for 6–8 weeks.
- ■ If dog's condition deteriorates or if adverse effects are a problem, contact veterinarian.

Chemistry/Synonyms

Niacinamide, also commonly known as nicotinamide, occurs as a white crystalline powder. It is odorless or nearly odorless and has a bitter taste. It is freely soluble in water or alcohol.

Niacinamide may also be known as: nicotinamide, nicotinamidum, nicotinic acid amide, nicotylamide, Vitamin B(3), or Vitamin PP.

Storage/Stability

Store niacinamide tablets in tight containers at room temperature unless otherwise labeled. Niacinamide is **incompatible** with alkalis or strong acids.

Dosage Forms/Regulatory Status

VETERINARY-LABELED PRODUCTS: None

HUMAN-LABELED PRODUCTS:

Niacinamide (Nicotinamide) Tablets: 100 mg & 500 mg; generic; (OTC)

References

Bruner, S.R. (2006). Updates in therapeutics for veterinary dermatology. *Veterinary Clinics of North America-Small Animal Practice* **36**(1): 39–+.

Campbell, K. (1999). New Drugs in Veterinary Dermatology. Proceedings: Central Veterinary Conference, Kansas City.

Marsella, R. (2008). Autoimmune Skin Diseases: Diagnosis and Management. Proceedings: ACVC. Accessed via: Veterinary Information Network. http://goo.gl/xXhgN

Tapp, T. (2002). New drug therapy in dermatology. Proceedings: Atlantic Coast Veterinary Conference. Accessed via: Veterinary Information Network. http://goo.gl/Vjn2j

White, S. (2000). Veterinary Dermatology: New Treatments, 'New' Diseases. Proceedings: The North American Veterinary Conference, Orlando.

Yu, A. (2008). The autoimmune dermatoses. Proceedings: WVC. Accessed via: Veterinary Information Network. http://goo.gl/UFsvP

NITAZOXANIDE

(nye-tah-**zox**-ah-nide)   Navigator®

ANTIPARASITIC AGENT

Prescriber Highlights

▶ Drug that has activity against a variety of protozoa, nematodes, bacteria, & trematodes, including *Sarcocystis neurona*, giardia, cryptosporidia, & *Helicobacter pylori*

▶ Was approved for use in horses (EPM), but veterinary paste no longer marketed

▶ Interest in using in other companion animals (e.g., dogs, cats), but data is lacking to support use

▶ Adverse effects in dogs (GI, hypersalivation) may be therapy limiting; but very well tolerated in humans

Uses/Indications

Nitazoxanide may be useful as an alternative treatment for cryptosporidia in cats. In humans, nitazoxanide is FDA-approved for use in treating diarrhea caused by *Cryptosporidium parvum* and *Giardia lamblia* in pediatric patients from ages 1 to 11 years old. Because of the drug's spectrum of activity and apparent safety, there is considerable interest in using it in a variety of companion animal species, but data is lacking

for specific indications and dosages.

Nitazoxanide oral paste was approved for the treatment of horses with equine protozoal myeloencephalitis (EPM) caused by *Sarcocystis neurona*, but is no longer marketed in the USA.

Pharmacology

While the precise mechanism of action of nitazoxanide is unknown, its active metabolites tizoxanide and tizoxanide glucuronide, are thought to inhibit the pyruvate: ferredoxin oxidoreductase (PFOR) enzyme-dependent electron transfer reactions essential to anaerobic energy metabolism. Nitazoxanide has activity against a variety of protozoa, nematodes, bacteria, and trematodes, including *Sarcocystis neurona*, giardia, cryptosporidia, and *Helicobacter pylori*.

Pharmacokinetics

Following oral administration in horses, nitazoxanide is absorbed and rapidly converted to tizoxanide (desacetyl-nitazoxanide). Peak levels of tizoxanide are attained between 2–3 hours and are not detectable by 24 hours post dosing. In humans, nitazoxanide is not detectable in plasma, but peak levels of tizoxanide and tizoxanide glucuronide occur about 3–4 hours post dose. More than 99% of tizoxanide is bound to plasma proteins. Tizoxanide is excreted in the urine, bile, and feces; the glucuronide metabolite is secreted in the urine and bile.

Contraindications/Precautions/Warnings

In horses, the drug was labeled as contraindicated in horses less than one year of age and those that are sick or debilitated for reasons other than EPM. The drug should be used with caution in stallions and other horses predisposed to developing laminitis. Safety for use in animals with compromised renal or hepatic function has not been established; use with caution. The manufacturer has not evaluated nitazoxanide in horses weighing more than 545 kg (1200 lbs).

Adverse Effects

In horses, the following adverse effects are most commonly reported: fever, reduced appetite/anorexia, and lethargy/depression. Other adverse effects include decreased gut sounds, scant feces, loose/malodorous or discolored feces/diarrhea, colic, laminitis, increased water consumption, discolored urine, head and/or limb edema, or weight loss. The manufacturer states that stallions may be more prone to developing laminitis than either geldings or mares.

Nitazoxanide may disrupt normal flora in the horse leading to enterocolitis. If patient develops any of the following: a high fever (>103°F), scant or loose feces, diarrhea, colic, or signs of laminitis, nitazoxanide treatments should be stopped immediately and appropriate veterinary care be initiated.

A so-called "treatment crisis" may develop, particularly early in therapy (first two weeks) and is thought to be caused by CNS inflammation secondary to dead or dying protozoa. Common signs include neurological deficits, fever, lethargy, and decreasing appetite. Treatment with antiinflammatory agents may be indicated. Treatment may continue if horse is closely monitored for other adverse reactions (*e.g.*, anorexia, diarrhea, colic, laminitis).

In a study using nitazoxanide in dogs with naturally occurring *Giardia* spp. infections, 5 of 9 in the study developed excessive salivation, vomiting, or diarrhea that resulted in removal from the study (Lappin *et al.* 2008).

In humans, nitazoxanide appears to be well tolerated and adverse effect rates are similar to placebo. Rarely, sclera may turn yellow secondary to drug disposition, but return to normal after drug discontinuation.

Reproductive/Nursing Safety
The reproductive safety of nitazoxanide has not been determined in breeding stallions or in breeding or lactating mares. In pregnant humans, nitazoxanide is designated by the FDA as a category *B* drug (*Animal studies have not demonstrated risk to the fetus, but there are no adequate studies in pregnant women; or animal studies have shown an adverse effect, but adequate studies in pregnant women have not demonstrated a risk to the fetus during the first trimester of pregnancy, and there is no evidence of risk in later trimesters.*) Nitazoxanide did not affect male or female fertility in rats given approximately 66 times the human dose. It did not cause fetal harm in pregnant rats or rabbits given 48 times and 3 times the human dose, respectively. It is unknown if tizoxanide is excreted in milk.

Overdosage/Acute Toxicity
There is limited information available on the acute toxicity of nitazoxanide. It has been reported that overdoses of 2.5X in horses has been associated with fatalities. The oral LD_{50} for cats and dogs is greater than 10 grams/kg. Repeated doses of 450 mg/kg in rats caused intense salivation and increased liver and spleen weights. In horses given approximately 5 times the labeled dose, all developed anorexia, diarrhea, and lethargy, and testing was halted after 4 days of study. Human volunteers have taken doses of up to 4 grams without significant adverse effects occurring. In the event of an overdose, it is suggested to observe the patient closely and treat adverse effects in a supportive manner.

Drug Interactions
No specific drug interactions have been noted to date, but the veterinary and human manufacturers warn to use with caution if the patient is receiving other drugs that are highly protein bound and with a narrow therapeutic index.

Laboratory Considerations
■ No specific laboratory interactions or considerations noted.

Doses
■ **HORSES:**
For equine protozoal myeloencephalitis (EPM) caused by *Sarcocystis neurona*:
a) For a 28 day course of therapy: Days 1–5: 25 mg/kg (11.36 mg/lb) PO once daily; Days 6–28: 50 mg/kg (22.72 mg/lb) PO once daily. See directions for use in client information section that follows. (Package insert; *Navigator*®—Idexx). **Note:** Product has been withdrawn from the US market.
b) As a potentially effective therapy for relapsing EPM: Extend the treatment regimen from 28 to 56 days. (MacKay 2008)

■ **CATS:**
For cryptosporidia-associated diarrhea:
a) 25 mg/kg PO q12-24h. No drug is consistently effective. In cats, *Cryptosporidium* spp. associated diarrhea sometimes resolves after administration of tylosin, paromomycin, or nitazoxanide. (Lappin 2008)

Monitoring
■ Clinical efficacy
■ Weekly body weight
■ Adverse reactions; if adverse reactions occur, the manufacturer recommends performing a physical exam, CBC, serum albumin, total serum protein and body weight.

Client Information
■ For use in small animals, clients should understand that this drug has not been commonly used in dogs or cats and adverse effects may occur.

Chemistry/Synonyms
A nitrothiazolyl-salicylamide derivative antiparasitic agent, nitazoxanide occurs as a light yellow powder. It is slightly soluble in ethanol and practically insoluble in water.

Nitazoxanide may also be known as: PH-5776, *Alinia*®, *Daxon*®, *Heliton*®, and *Navigator*®.

Storage/Stability
The human-approved powder for oral suspension should be stored at 25°C (77°F); excursions permitted to 15–30°C (59–86°F). Once suspended with tap water, the oral suspension should be kept in tightly closed containers at room temperature and discarded after 7 days.

Dosage Forms/Regulatory Status
VETERINARY-LABELED PRODUCTS:
None. Nitazoxanide oral paste (32%); *Navigator*® was FDA-approved in the USA for horses, but the drug is no longer manufactured or marketed and approval has been withdrawn.

HUMAN-LABELED PRODUCTS:
Nitazoxanide Oral Tablets: 500 mg; *Alinia*® (Romark Laboratories); (Rx)

Nitazoxanide Powder for Oral Suspension: 20 mg/mL (100 mg/5 mL after reconstitution) in 60 mL; *Alinia*® (Romark Laboratories); (Rx)

References

Lappin, M.R. (2008). Giardia and Cryptosporidium Spp. Infections of Cats: Clinical and Zoonotic Aspects. Proceedings: ECVIM. Accessed via: Veterinary Information Network. http://goo.gl/ZyO3e

Lappin, M.R., M. Clark, et al. (2008). Treatment of Healthy Giardia Spp. Positive Dogs with Fenbendazole or Nitazoxanide. Accessed via: Veterinary Information Network. http://goo.gl/ZQYSU

MacKay, R. (2008). Equine Protozoal Myeloencephalitis: Managing Relapses. *Comp Equine*(Jan/Feb): 24–27.

NITENPYRAM

(nye-ten-*pye*-rum)   Capstar®, Program®

ORAL INSECTICIDE

Prescriber Highlights

▶ Oral insecticide used primarily as a flea adulticide in dogs & cats; may also have efficacy for other conditions (e.g., maggots)

▶ Very safe

▶ Not effective alone for flea eggs or other immature forms

▶ Over-the-counter

Uses/Indications

Nitenpyram is indicated as a flea adulticide in dogs and cats. It does not kill ticks, flea eggs, larvae or immature fleas. Nitenpyram may be effective for treating fly larvae (maggots) of various species. Fleas begin to fall from treated animals about 30 minutes after dosing and a single dose can protect animals for 1–2 days.

Pharmacology/Actions

Nitenpyram is in the class of neonicotinoid insecticides. It enters the systemic circulation of the adult flea after consuming blood from a treated animal. It binds to nicotinic acetylcholine receptors in the postsynaptic membranes and blocks acetylcholine-mediated neuronal transmission causing paralysis and death of the flea. Nitenpyram is 3500 times more selective for insect alpha-4beta-2 nicotinic receptors than in vertebrate receptors. It does not inhibit acetylcholinesterase. Efficacy appears to be greater than 99% (kill rate) in dogs or cats within 3-6 hours of treatment. When combined with an insect growth regulator (*e.g.*, lufenuron), immature stages of fleas may also be controlled.

Pharmacokinetics

Nitenpyram is rapidly and practically completely absorbed after oral administration. Peak levels occur about 80 minutes after dosing in dogs; about 40 minutes in cats. Elimination half-lives are about 3 hours for dogs; 8 hours for cats. Nitenpyram is excreted primarily unchanged in the urine. In dogs, about 3% of a dose is excreted in the feces; in cats about 5% is excreted in the feces.

Contraindications/Precautions/Warnings

Nitenpyram is not labeled to be used in animals under 2 pounds of body weight or under 4 weeks of age.

Adverse Effects

Nitenpyram is tolerated well. As fleas begin to die, animal may begin scratching. This effect is temporary and due to the fleas and not the medication.

Reproductive/Nursing Safety

Nitenpyram is probably safe to use in breeding, pregnant, or lactating animals.

Overdosage/Acute Toxicity

Nitenpyram is relatively safe in high dosages to mammals. The oral LD_{50} in rats is approximately 1.6 grams/kg. Cats or dogs given 10 times the usual dose for 14 days showed no untoward effects. In the circumstance of a massive overdose, contact an animal poison control center for additional guidance.

Drug Interactions

No specific drug interactions were located. Nitenpyram has reportedly been used safely with a variety of other medications and other flea products.

Laboratory Considerations

▪ No specific laboratory interactions or considerations noted.

Doses

▪ **DOGS:**

As a flea adulticide:

a) For dogs weighing 2–25 lb. (0.9–11.36 kg): Give one 11.4 mg tablet PO. May be given as often as once per day. For dogs weighing 25–125 lb. (11.36–56.8kg): Give one 57 mg tablet PO. May be given as often as once per day. May be given with or without food. (Label directions; *Capstar*®—Novartis)

▪ **CATS:**

As a flea adulticide:

a) For cats weighing 2–25 lb. (0.9–11.36 kg): Give one 11.4 mg tablet PO. May be given as often as once per day. May be given with or without food. (Label directions; *Capstar*®—Novartis)

▪ **REPTILES:**

a) For maggots: crush one 11.4 mg tablet into powder and give PO, as an enema, or on wound one time. (Klaphake 2005)

Monitoring

▪ Efficacy

Client Information

▪ All animals in household should be treated.

▪ Best dosed after a meal to increase absorption

▪ Because nitenpyram does not kill immature fleas, eggs, etc., it is usually used in combination with other products that will control those forms of fleas.

▪ Keep tablets out of reach of children.

Chemistry/Synonyms

A neonicotinoid insecticide, nitenpyram occurs as a pale yellow crystalline powder and is very soluble in water (840 mg/mL)

Nitenpyram may also be known as: TI-304, (E)-Nitenpyram, *Bestguard®*, and *Capstar®*.

Storage/Stability

Commercially available nitenpyram tablets should be stored at room temperature (15–30°C; 59–86°F). Shelf life is reported to be 3 years if stored below 25°C (76°F).

Dosage Forms/Regulatory Status

VETERINARY-LABELED PRODUCTS:

Nitenpyram Oral Tablets: 11.4 mg and 57 mg in boxes containing blister packs of 6 tablets; *Capstar®* (Novartis); (OTC); FDA-approved for use in dogs and cats.

Also available in combination packs with Lufenuron [*Program® Flavor Tabs* and *Capstar® Flea Management System for Dogs* and *Program® Flavor Tabs* (OTC); and *Capstar® Flea Management System for Cats* (OTC)] and in combination with milbemycin and lufenuron [*Sentinel® Flavor Tabs* and *Capstar® Flea Management System for Dogs* (Rx)].

HUMAN-LABELED PRODUCTS: None

References

Klaphake, E. (2005). Reptilian Parasites. Proceedings: Western Vet Conf. Accessed via: Veterinary Information Network. http://goo.gl/h07UP

NITROFURANTOIN

(nye-troe-fyoor-*an*-toyn)
Macrodantin®, Macrobid®

URINARY ANTIMICROBIAL

Prescriber Highlights

▶ Antibacterial used for susceptible UTI's

▶ Contraindications: Renal impairment; hypersensitivity to it

▶ Adverse Effects: Gastrointestinal disturbances & hepatopathy of most concern; may cause infertility in males or peripheral neuropathy

▶ Potentially teratogenic, may be toxic to neonates

Uses/Indications

Considered a urinary tract antiseptic, nitrofurantoin is used primarily in small animals, but also occasionally in horses in the treatment of lower urinary tract infections caused by susceptible bacteria. It is not effective in treating renal cortical or perinephric abscesses or other systemic infections.

Pharmacology/Actions

Nitrofurantoin usually acts as a bacteriostatic antimicrobial, but it may be bactericidal depending on the concentration of the drug and the susceptibility of the organism. The exact mechanism of action of nitrofurantoin has not been fully elucidated, but the drug apparently inhibits various bacterial enzyme systems, including acetyl coenzyme A. Nitrofurantoin has greater antibacterial activity in acidic environments.

Nitrofurantoin has activity against several gram-negative and some gram-positive organisms, including many strains of *E. coli*, Klebsiella, Enterobacter, Enterococci, *Staphylococcus aureus* and *epidermidis*, Enterobacter, Citrobacter, Salmonella, Shigella, and Corynebacterium. It has little or no activity against most strains of Proteus, Serratia, or Acinetobacter and has no activity against *Pseudomonas* spp.

Pharmacokinetics

Nitrofurantoin is rapidly absorbed from the GI tract and the presence of food may enhance the absorption of the drug. Macrocrystalline forms of the drug may be absorbed more slowly with less GI upset. Because of its slower absorption, urine levels of the drug may be prolonged.

Therapeutic levels in the systemic circulation are not maintained due to the rapid elimination of the drug after absorption. Approximately 20–60% of the drug is bound to serum proteins. Peak urine levels occur within 30 minutes of dosing. The drug crosses the placenta and only minimal quantities of the drug are found in milk.

Approximately 40–50% of the drug is eliminated into urine unchanged via both glomerular filtration and tubular secretion. Some of the drug is metabolized, primarily in the liver. Elimination half-lives in humans with normal renal function average 20 minutes.

Contraindications/Precautions/Warnings

Nitrofurantoin is contraindicated in patients with renal impairment as the drug is much less efficacious and the development of toxicity is much more likely. The drug is also contraindicated in patients hypersensitive to it.

Rats can develop neurotoxicity when given nitrofurantoin; avoid use.

Adverse Effects

In dogs and cats, gastrointestinal disturbances (primarily vomiting) and hepatopathy can occur with this drug. Rarely, reversible myasthenic-like effects have been seen in dogs. Neuropathies, chronic active hepatitis, hemolytic anemia, and pneumonitis have been described in humans, but are believed to occur very rarely in animals.

Reproductive/Nursing Safety

In humans, the drug is contraindicated in pregnant patients at term and neonates as hemolytic anemia can occur secondary to immature enzyme systems. Safe use of the drug during earlier stages of pregnancy has not been determined. Nitrofurantoin has been implicated in causing infertility in male dogs. Use only when the benefits of therapy outweigh the potential risks.

Nitrofurantoin is excreted into maternal milk in very low concentrations. Safety for use in the nursing mother or offspring has not been established.

Overdosage/Acute Toxicity

No specific information was located. Because the drug is rapidly absorbed and excreted, patients with normal renal function should require little therapy when mild overdoses occur. If the ingestion was relatively recent, massive overdoses should be handled by emptying the gut using standard protocols; patient should then be monitored for adverse effects (see above).

Drug Interactions

The following drug interactions have either been reported or are theoretical in humans or animals receiving nitrofurantoin and may be of significance in veterinary patients:

- ■ **FLUOROQUINOLONES (e.g., enrofloxacin, ciprofloxacin):** Nitrofurantoin may antagonize the antimicrobial activity of the fluoroquinolones and concomitant use is best avoided

- ■ **FOOD or ANTICHOLINERGIC DRUGS** may increase the oral bioavailability of nitrofurantoin

- ■ **MAGNESIUM TRISILICATE CONTAINING ANTACIDS:** May inhibit the oral absorption of nitrofurantoin

- ■ **PROBENECID:** May inhibit the renal excretion of nitrofurantoin potentially increasing its toxicity and reducing its effectiveness in urinary tract infections

Laboratory Considerations

- ■ Nitrofurantoin may cause false-positive **urine glucose** determinations if using cupric-sulfate solutions (Benedict's reagent, *Clinitest*®). Tests using glucose oxidase methods (*Tes-Tape*®, *Clinistix*®) are not affected by nitrofurantoin.

- ■ Nitrofurantoin may cause decreases in **blood glucose**, and increases in **serum creatinine, bilirubin** and **alkaline phosphatase.**

Doses

- ■ **DOGS:**

  For susceptible bacterial urinary tract infections:

  a) For prevention of re-infections with gram-negative organisms: nitrofurantoin 4 mg/kg PO once a day immediately before bedtime after the dog has urinated. May rarely cause drug-induced hepatopathy and liver enzymes should be evaluated if any adverse effects are suspected. Preventative therapy for repeated reinfection (> 2 per 6 months) should only be utilized after an extensive search for any underlying cause. This approach will not resolve existing UTI and should only be used after effective treatment using full therapeutic doses. (Adams 2009)

  b) For recurrent UTI: Conventional dose: 4 mg/kg, PO q8h; Prophylactic dose: 3–4 mg/kg, PO q24h (should be given at night after micturition and immediately before bedtime) (Polzin & Osborne 1985)

  c) 4 mg/kg PO q6–8h (Brovida 2003)

  d) 5 mg/kg PO q8h (Dowling 2007; Dowling 2009)

  e) 4.4 mg/kg PO three times daily (Senior 2005)

- ■ **CATS:**

  For susceptible bacterial urinary tract infections:

  a) 5 mg/kg PO q8h (Dowling 2007; Dowling 2009)

  b) For recurrent UTI: Conventional dose: 4 mg/kg, PO q8h; Prophylactic dose: 3–4 mg/kg, PO q24h (should be given at night after micturition and immediately before bedtime) (Polzin & Osborne 1985)

  c) 4 mg/kg PO q6–8h (Brovida 2003)

- ■ **HORSES:**

  For susceptible urinary tract infections:

  a) 2.5–4.5 mg/kg, PO three times daily (Robinson 1987)

  b) 10 mg/kg, PO daily (Huber 1988)

Monitoring

- ■ Clinical efficacy
- ■ Adverse effects
- ■ Periodic liver function tests should be considered with chronic therapy

Chemistry/Synonyms

A synthetic, nitrofuran antibacterial, nitrofurantoin occurs as a bitter tasting, lemon-yellow, crystalline powder with a pK_a of 7.2. It is very slightly soluble in water or alcohol.

Nitrofurantoin may also be known as: furadoninum or nitrofurantoinum, *Furadantin*®, *Macrobid*®, and *Macrodantin*®.

Storage/Stability

Nitrofurantoin preparations should be stored in tight containers at room temperature and protected from light. The oral suspension should not be frozen. Nitrofurantoin will decompose if it comes into contact with metals other than aluminum or stainless steel.

Dosage Forms/Regulatory Status

VETERINARY-LABELED PRODUCTS: None

HUMAN-LABELED PRODUCTS:

Nitrofurantoin Macrocrystals Oral Capsules: 25 mg, 50 mg & 100 mg (as macrocrystals) and 100 mg (as monohydrate/macrocrystals); *Macrodantin*® and *Macrobid*® (Procter & Gamble); generic; (Rx)

Nitrofurantoin Oral Suspension: 5 mg/mL (25 mg/5 mL) in 470 mL; *Furadantin*® (Sciele); (Rx)

References

Adams, L. (2009). Recurrent Urinary Tract Infections: Bad Bugs That Won't Go Away. Proceedings: WVC. Accessed via: Veterinary Information Network. http://goo.gl/eX3w6

Brovida, C. (2003). Urinary Tract Infection (UTI): How to diagnose correctly and treat. Proceedings: World Small Animal Veterinary Assoc World Congress. Accessed via: Veterinary Information Network. http://goo.gl/F2zcU

Dowling, P. (2007). Therapy of the "bad bugs" of UTI. Proceedings: Western Vet Conf. Accessed via: Veterinary Information Network. http://goo.gl/uHxBz

Dowling, P. (2009). Optimizing antimicrobial therapy of urinary tract infections. Proceedings: WVC. Accessed via: Veterinary Information Network. http://goo.gl/iXp5f

Huber, W.G. (1988). Aminoglycosides, Macrolides, Lincosamides, Polymyxins, Chloramphenicol, and other Antibacterial Drugs. *Veterinary Pharmacology and Therapeutics*. NH Booth and LE McDonald Eds. Ames, Iowa State University Press: 822–848.

Polzin, D.J. & C.A. Osborne (1985). Diseases of the Urinary Tract. *Handbook of Small Animal Therapeutics*. LE Davis Ed. New York, Churchill Livingstone: 333–395.

Robinson, N.E. (1987). Table of Common Drugs: Approximate Doses. *Current Therapy in Equine Medicine, 2*. NE Robinson Ed. Philadelphia, W.B. Saunders: 761.

Senior, D. (2005). Management of Urinary Tract Infection. Proceedings: WSAVA World Congress. Accessed via: Veterinary Information Network. http://goo.gl/gdfbm

NITROGLYCERIN, TOPICAL

(nye-troe-*gli*-ser-in)   NTG, Nitro-bid®, Minitran®

VENODILATOR

Prescriber Highlights

▶ Topical, oral, & injectable venodilator; occasionally used topically in veterinary medicine for CHF or hypertension

▶ Contraindications: anemia or hypersensitivity to nitrates. Caution: cerebral hemorrhage or head trauma, diuretic-induced hypovolemia, or other hypotensive conditions.

▶ Continuous use results in tolerance after 48–72 hours

▶ Adverse Effects: rashes at the application sites & orthostatic hypotension; transient headaches common in humans & may be a problem for some animals

▶ Rotate application sites

▶ Wear gloves when applying; avoid human skin contact

Uses/Indications

Topical nitroglycerin (NTG) in small animal medicine is used primarily as an adjunctive vasodilator in heart failure and cardiogenic edema. Because of questionable efficacy and rapid development of tolerance, nitroglycerine is not commonly used as an outpatient drug in vet-erinary medicine today. In humans, NTG is also used as an anti-anginal agent, antihypertensive (acute), and topically to treat Raynaud's disease.

Pharmacology/Actions

Nitroglycerin relaxes vascular smooth muscle primarily on the venous side, but a dose related effect on arterioles is possible. Preload (left end-diastolic pressure) is reduced from the peripheral pooling of blood and decreased venous return to the heart. Because of its arteriolar effects, depending on the dose, afterload may also be reduced. Myocardial oxygen demand and workload are reduced and coronary circulation can be improved.

Pharmacokinetics

Nitroglycerin topical ointment is absorbed through the skin, with an onset of action usually within 1 hour and duration of action of 2–12 hours. It is generally dosed in dogs and cats q6–8 hours (three to four times a day). The transdermal patches have a wide inter-patient bioavailability. Nitroglycerin has a very short half-life (1–4 minutes in humans) and is metabolized in the liver. At least two metabolites have some vasodilator activity and have longer half-lives than NTG.

Contraindications/Precautions/Warnings

Nitrates are contraindicated in patients with severe anemia or those hypersensitive to them. They should be used with caution (if at all) in patients with cerebral hemorrhage or head trauma, diuretic-induced hypovolemia or other hypotensive conditions.

Adverse Effects

Most common side effects seen are rashes at the application sites and orthostatic hypotension. If hypotension is a problem, reduce dosage. Transient headaches are a common side effect seen in humans and may be a problem for some animals.

Continuous use (48-72 hours) of nitroglycerin results in the rapid development of tolerance to the effects of the drug.

Reproductive/Nursing Safety

In humans, the FDA categorizes this drug as category *C* for use during pregnancy (*Animal studies have shown an adverse effect on the fetus, but there are no adequate studies in humans; or there are no animal reproduction studies and no adequate studies in humans.*) In a separate system evaluating the safety of drugs in canine and feline pregnancy (Papich 1989), this drug is categorized as class: *C* (*These drugs may have potential risks. Studies in people or laboratory animals have uncovered risks, and these drugs should be used cautiously as a last resort when the benefit of therapy clearly outweighs the risks.*)

It is not known whether nitrates are excreted in maternal milk; use with caution in nursing animals.

Overdosage/Acute Toxicity

If severe hypotension results after topical administration, wash the site of application to prevent any more absorption of ointment. Fluids may be administered if necessary. Epinephrine is contraindicated as it is ineffective and may complicate the animal's condition.

Drug Interactions

The following drug interactions have either been reported or are theoretical in humans or animals receiving nitroglycerin and may be of significance in veterinary patients:

■ **ANTIHYPERTENSIVE DRUGS, OTHER:** Use of nitroglycerin with other antihypertensive drugs may cause additive hypotensive effects

■ **PHENOTHIAZINES:** May increase hypotensive effects

■ **SILDENAFIL (and other PDE INHIBITORS):** May profoundly increase risk for hypotension

Doses

Note: For the treatment of heart failure, nitroglycerin is not generally used alone.

■ **DOGS:**

For adjunctive treatment of heart failure:

a) If nitroprusside not used, 2% NTG at ¼ to 1 inch q6–12h; apply to hairless area in the axilla or groin. (Macintire 2006)

b) Using the 2.5–10 mg/24hr transdermal patch: 12 hours on, 12 hours off (Fox 2003)

c) For adjunctive treatment of pulmonary edema: ¼–2 inches every 8 hours is applied cutaneously or directly to mucous membranes every 8 hours during the first 48 hours (all animals tolerate the paste given orally). (Lichtenberger 2009)

d) For any patient with cardiogenic pulmonary edema that is headed for oxygen: ¼ inch for small dogs up to 1 inch for large dogs on the inner ear pinnae, groin or axilla as needed q8h for the first 24 hours. Wear gloves to apply. (DeFrancesco 2006)

e) As a venodilator for the adjunctive treatment of systolic heart failure: ¼ inch per 5 kg of body weight of the 2% ointment applied topically three times daily for the first 24 hours. (Atkins 2007)

■ **CATS:**

For adjunctive treatment of heart failure:

a) Topical nitroglycerin might be beneficial in cats with severe pulmonary edema secondary to feline HCM; however, no studies have examined any effects of this drug in this species and its efficacy is suspect. But it is safe and some benefit may occur with its administration in some cats. ⅛th to ¼ inch of a 2% cream applied to a hairless area (e.g., inside the earflap) every 4–6 hours for the first 24 hours as long as furosemide is being administered concomitantly. Never rely on NTG to produce a beneficial effect and use is by no means mandatory. Tolerance develops rapidly in other species and probably does so in the cat, so prolonged administration is probably of even lesser benefit. Person applying should use gloves and avoid contact with the product. (Kittleson 2009).

b) To enhance resolution of pulmonary edema: ¼ to ½ inch topically q6h; to reduce nitrate tolerance, alternate 12 hrs with and 12 hrs without nitroglycerin therapy. (Fox 2007)

c) Using the 2.5–5 mg/24hr transdermal patch: 12 hours on, 12 hours off (Fox 2003)

d) For adjunctive treatment of pulmonary edema: ¼ inch every 8 hours is applied cutaneously or directly to mucous membranes every 8 hours during the first 48 hours (all animals tolerate the paste given orally). (Lichtenberger 2009)

e) For any patient with cardiogenic pulmonary edema that is headed for oxygen: ¼ inch on the inner ear pinnae, groin or axilla as needed q8h for the first 24 hours. Wear gloves to apply. (DeFrancesco 2006)

For adjunctive treatment of hypertension:

a) ¼ inch applied to pinna q6–8h (Norsworthy 2007)

■ **FERRETS:**

For adjunctive therapy for heart failure:

a) ⅛th inch strip applied to inside of pinna q12h for the first 24 hours of therapy (Hoeffer 2000)

b) For dilative cardiomyopathy: ⅛th of an inch applied to shaved skin once to twice daily. Apply to ear pinna or skin of thigh. May cause hypotension. (Williams 2000)

Monitoring

■ Clinical efficacy

■ Sites of application for signs of rash

■ Blood pressure, particularly if hypotensive effects are seen

Client Information

■ Dosage is measured in inches of ointment; use papers supplied with product to measure appropriate dose. Wear gloves (nonpermeable) when applying.

■ Do not pet animal where ointment has been applied

■ Rotate application sites. Recommended application sites include: groin, inside the ears, and thorax. Rub ointment into skin well. If rash develops, do not use that site again until cleared.

■ Contact veterinarian if rash persists or animal's condition deteriorates

■ There is no danger of explosion or fire with the use of this product

Chemistry/Synonyms

Famous as an explosive, nitroglycerin (NTG) occurs undiluted as a thick, volatile, white-pale yellow flammable, explosive liquid with a sweet, burning taste. The undiluted drug is soluble in alcohol and slightly soluble in water. Because of obvious safety reasons, nitroglycerin is diluted with lactose, dextrose, propylene glycol, alcohol, etc. when used for pharmaceutical purposes.

Nitroglycerin may also be known as: glyceryl trinitrate, glonoine, GTN; nitroglycerol, NTG, trinitrin, or trinitroglycerin, *Minitran®*, *Nitro-bid®*, *Nitrek®* and *Nitro-Dur®*.

Storage/Stability

The topical ointment should be stored at room temperature and the cap firmly attached. For storage/stability and compatibility for dosage forms other than the topical ointment, see specialized references or the package inserts for each product.

Dosage Forms/Regulatory Status

VETERINARY-LABELED PRODUCTS: None

The ARCI (Racing Commissioners International) has designated this drug as a class 3 substance. See the appendix for more information.

HUMAN-LABELED PRODUCTS:

Note: Many dosage forms of nitroglycerin are available for human use, including sublingual tablets, buccal tablets, lingual spray, extended-release oral capsules and tablets, and parenteral solutions for IV infusion. Because the use of nitroglycerin in small animal medicine is practically limited to the use of topical ointment or transdermal patches, those other dosage forms are not listed here.

Nitroglycerin Topical Ointment: 2% in a lanolin-white petrolatum base in 30 gram & 60 gram tubes and UD 1 gram; *Nitro-bid®* (Savage); generic; (Rx)

Nitroglycerin Transdermal Systems (patches): 0.1 mg/hr 0.2 mg/hr, 0.3 mg/hr, 0.4 mg/hr, 0.6 mg/hr & 0.8 mg/hr; *Minitran®* (3M); *Nitro-Dur®* (Key); *Nitrek®* (Bertek); generic; (Rx)

Note: Various products contain differing quantities of nitroglycerin and patch surface area size, but release rates of drug are identical for a given mg/hr.

References

Atkins, C. (2007). Canine Heart Failure—Current concepts. Proceedings: WSAVA World Congress. Accessed via: Veterinary Information Network. http://goo.gl/aWqPH

DeFrancesco, T. (2006). Refractory heart failure. Proceedings: IVECCS 2006. Accessed via: Veterinary Information Network. goo.gl/WObuJ

Fox, P. (2003). Congestive heart failure: Clinical approach and management. Proceedings: World Small Animal Veterinary Assoc World Congress. Accessed

via: Veterinary Information Network. http://goo.gl/xMFKn

Fox, P. (2007). Managing feline heart disease—an evidenced based approach. Proceedings: WSAVA World Congress. Accessed via: Veterinary Information Network. http://goo.gl/I4VeL

Hoeffer, H. (2000). Heart Disease in Ferrets. *Kirk's Current Veterinary Therapy: XIII Small Animal Practice*. J Bonagura Ed. Philadelphia, WB Saunders: 1144–1148.

Kittleson, M. (2009). Treatment of feline hypertrophic cardiomyopathy (HCM)—Lost Dreams. Proceedings: ACVIM. Accessed via: Veterinary Information Network. http://goo.gl/XvCZt

Lichtenberger, M. (2009). How I treat congestive heart failure I. Proceedings: WVC. Accessed via: Veterinary Information Network. http://goo.gl/UrCw8

Macintire, D. (2006). Cardiac Emergencies. Proceedings: ACVC 2006. Accessed via: Veterinary Information Network. http://goo.gl/KxqeK

Norsworthy, G. (2007). Complications of untreated hypertension. Proceedings: Western Vet Conf. Accessed via: Veterinary Information Network. http://goo.gl/kJikC

Papich, M. (1989). Effects of drugs on pregnancy. *Current Veterinary Therapy X: Small Animal Practice*. R Kirk Ed. Philadelphia, Saunders: 1291–1299.

Williams, B. (2000). Therapeutics in Ferrets. *Vet Clin NA: Exotic Anim Pract* **3:**1(Jan): 131–153.

NITROPRUSSIDE SODIUM

(nye-troe-***pruss***-ide)   Nitropress®, Sodium Nitroprusside

VASODILATOR

Prescriber Highlights

▶ Vascular, smooth muscle relaxant used for acute/severe hypertension; acute heart failure secondary to mitral regurgitation & in combination with dopamine for refractory CHF

▶ Contraindications: Compensatory hypertension, inadequate cerebral circulation, or during emergency surgery in patients near death. Caution: Geriatric patients, hepatic insufficiency, severe renal impairment, hyponatremia, or hypothyroidism.

▶ Adverse effects: Hypotensive effects; potentially: nausea, retching, restlessness, apprehension, muscle twitching, dizziness

▶ May be irritating at the infusion site; avoid extravasation.

▶ Continued use may lead to potential thiocyanate & cyanide toxicity

▶ Use only in an ICU setting; monitoring essential

Uses/Indications

In human medicine, nitroprusside is indicated for the management of hypertensive crises, acute heart failure secondary to mitral regurgitation, and severe refractory CHF (often in combination with dopamine or dobutamine). In patients with dilated cardiomyopathy, administering dobutamine first to improve contractility and increase cardiac output can offset the hypotensive effects of sodium nitroprusside (Erling & Mazzaferro 2008). Its use in veterinary medicine is generally reserved for the treatment of critically ill patients with those conditions only when constant blood pressure monitoring can be performed.

Pharmacology/Actions

Nitroprusside is an immediate acting intravenous hypotensive agent that directly causes peripheral vasodilation (arterial and venous) independent of autonomic innervation. It produces a lowering of blood pressure, an increase in heart rate, a mild decrease in cardiac output, and a significant reduction in total peripheral resistance. Preload, afterload and left ventricular end-diastolic pressures are reduced. Unlike the organic nitrates, tolerance does not develop to nitroprusside.

Pharmacokinetics

After starting an IV infusion of nitroprusside, reduction in blood pressure and other pharmacologic effects begin almost immediately. Blood pressure will return to pretreatment levels within 1–10 minutes following cessation of therapy.

Nitroprusside is metabolized non-enzymatically in the blood and tissues to cyanogen (cyanide radical). Cyanogen is converted in the liver to thiocyanate where it is eliminated in the urine, feces, and exhaled air. The half-life of cyanogen is 2.7–7 days if renal function is normal, but prolonged in patients with impaired renal function or with hyponatremia.

Contraindications/Precautions/Warnings

Nitroprusside is contraindicated in patients with compensatory hypertension (*e.g.*, AV shunts or coarctation of the aorta; Cushing's reflex), inadequate cerebral circulation, or during emergency surgery in patients near death.

Nitroprusside must be used with caution in patients with hepatic insufficiency, severe renal impairment, hyponatremia, or hypothyroidism. When nitroprusside is used for controlled hypotension during surgery, patients may have less tolerance to hypovolemia, anemia, or blood loss. Geriatric patients may be more sensitive to the hypotensive effects of nitroprusside.

Adverse Effects

Most adverse reactions from nitroprusside are associated with its hypotensive effects, particularly if blood pressure is reduced too rapidly. Clinical signs such as nausea, retching, restlessness, apprehension, muscle twitching, and dizziness have been reported in humans. These effects disappear when the infusion rate is reduced or stopped. Nitroprusside may be irritating at the infusion site; avoid extravasation.

Continued use may lead to potential thiocyanate and cyanide toxicity (see Overdosage section).

Reproductive/Nursing Safety

In humans, the FDA categorizes this drug as category *C* for use during pregnancy (*Animal studies have shown an adverse effect on the fetus, but there are no adequate studies in humans; or there are no animal reproduction studies and no adequate studies in humans.*) In a separate system evaluating the safety of drugs in canine and feline pregnancy (Papich 1989), this drug is categorized as class: *C* (*These drugs may have potential risks. Studies in people or laboratory animals have uncovered risks, and these drugs should be used cautiously as a last resort when the benefit of therapy clearly outweighs the risks.*)

It is not known whether nitroprusside and its metabolites are excreted in maternal milk.

Overdosage/Acute Toxicity

Acute overdosage is manifested by a profound hypotension. Treat by reducing or stopping the infusion and giving fluids. Monitor blood pressure constantly.

Excessive doses, prolonged therapy, a depleted hepatic thiosulfate (sulfur) supply, or severe hepatic or renal insufficiency may lead to profound hypotension, cyanogen, or thiocyanate toxicity. Acid/base status should be monitored to evaluate therapy and to detect metabolic acidosis (early sign of cyanogen toxicity). Tolerance to therapy is also an early sign of nitroprusside toxicity. Hydroxocobalamin (Vitamin B_{12a}) may prevent cyanogen toxicity. Thiocyanate toxicity may be exhibited as delirium in dogs. Serum thiocyanate levels may need to be monitored in patients on prolonged therapy, especially in those patients with concurrent renal dysfunction. Serum levels >100 micrograms/mL are considered toxic. It is suggested to refer to other references or contact an animal poison control center for further information should cyanogen or thiocyanate toxicity be suspected.

Drug Interactions

The following drug interactions have either been reported or are theoretical in humans or animals receiving nitroprusside and may be of significance in veterinary patients:

■ **ANESTHETICS, GENERAL:** The hypotensive effects of nitroprusside may be enhanced by concomitant administration of general anesthetics (*e.g.*, **halothane, enflurane**), or other circulatory depressants

■ **DOBUTAMINE:** Synergistic effects (increased cardiac output and reduced wedge pressure) may result if dobutamine is used with nitroprusside

■ **HYPOTENSIVE AGENTS, OTHER:** Patients receiving other hypotensive agents (*e.g.*, **beta-blockers, ACE inhibitors**, etc.) may be more sensitive to the hypotensive effects of nitroprusside

Doses

Directions for preparation of infusion: Add 2–3 mL D_5W to 50 mg vial to dissolve powder. Add dissolved solution to 1000 mL of D$_5$W and promptly protect solution from light (using aluminum foil or other opaque covering). Resultant solution contains 50 micrograms/mL of nitroprusside. Higher concentrations may be necessary in treating large animals. The administration set need not be protected from light. Solution may have a slight brownish tint, but discard solutions that turn to a blue, dark red or green color. Solution is stable for 24 hours after reconstitution. Do not add any other medications to IV running nitroprusside. Avoid extravasation at IV site. If using a Mini-Drip IV set (for small animals) (60 drops ≈ 1 mL; 1 drop contains approximately 0.83 micrograms of nitroprusside). Use an accurate flow control device (pump, controller, etc.) for administration.

■ **DOGS:**

For hypertensive crisis (systolic arterial BP >200 mm Hg):

a) Initiate dose at 1–2 micrograms/kg/minute; increase dosage incrementally every 3–5 minutes until a predetermined target BP is attained. Reduce BP 25% over 4-hour period to allow readaptation of cerebral blood vessels. (Proulx & Dhupa 2000)

For adjunctive treatment of heart failure (cardiogenic shock; fulminant pulmonary edema):

a) Goal is to decrease or maintain mean arterial pressure to support vital organ functions—approx. 70 mmHg): Dose as above (in "a"); concurrent use of dobutamine (5–10 micrograms/kg/min) often indicated. (Proulx & Dhupa 2000)

b) 0.5–10 micrograms/kg/min IV at a low fluid rate (≤2 mL/kg/hr) using D5W or other low sodium fluid. Usually start at 2 micrograms/kg/min and increase the base concentration by 1 microgram/kg every 20–30 minutes until there is an improvement in respiratory effort and thoracic auscultation. The patient is maintained on the effective dose for 48 hours. Monitor blood pressure; cyanide poisoning can occur if infusion lasts more than 3 days. After stabilized, drip is tapered as therapy with enalapril is initiated. (Macintire 2006)

c) For catastrophic pulmonary edema: As a CRI initiated at 1 microgram/kg/min and carefully titrated to effect by increasing by 1 microgram/kg/min increments every 15 minutes as long as BP remains stable and until perfusion and pulmonary function improves (usually requires between 2–5 micrograms/kg/min with the upper limit being 8–10 micrograms/kg/min). Maintain most effective

dose for 12–15 hours until respiratory distress resolves, lungs are clear, and the patient is stable with a normal blood pressure, pink mucous membranes, normal capillary refill time, and normal heart rate. Most animals at our clinic require 12 hours of treatment. The systolic blood pressure must remain greater than 90 mm Hg. If hypotension develops, the CRI should be stopped. Blood pressure will return to pretreatment levels within 1–10 minutes of discontinuing treatment and administration can be reinstituted at the previous lower dose. Administer with dobutamine to treat or prevent hypotension if severe myocardial failure is present based on an echocardiogram evaluation. Wean sodium nitroprusside over 6 hours first and then dobutamine over 6 hours. ACE inhibitor is added before tapering the infusions over 3–6 hours. (Lichtenberger 2006)

■ **CATS:**

For hypertensive crisis (systolic arterial BP >200 mm Hg):

a) Initiate dose at 0.5 micrograms/kg/minute; increase dosage incrementally every 3–5 minutes until a predetermined target BP is attained. Reduce BP 25% over 4-hour period to allow readaptation of cerebral blood vessels. (Proulx & Dhupa 2000)

For adjunctive treatment of heart failure (cardiogenic shock; fulminant pulmonary edema):

a) Goal to decrease or maintain mean arterial pressure to support vital organ functions—approx. 70 mmHg): Dose as above; concurrent use of dobutamine (1–5 micrograms/kg/min) often indicated. (Proulx & Dhupa 2000)

b) Initiate dose at 0.5 micrograms/kg/minute constant rate infusion and increase by 0.5–1 microgram/minute every 5 minutes to desired systolic pressure (90–100 mmHg). Cats are more sensitive to the oxidative damage that can be induced by nitroprusside and total dosages should be kept to a minimum. Use a dedicated line with an infusion pump; IV line and catheter should never be flushed. A nurse devoted for continuous monitoring should be in place during administration. Cover IV solution and IV line with opaque material and discard after 24 hours. (Proulx 2003)

c) For catastrophic pulmonary edema: As a CRI initiated at 1 microgram/kg/min and carefully titrated to effect by increasing by 1 microgram/kg/min increments every 15 minutes as long as BP remains stable and until perfusion and pulmonary function improves (cats usually requires between 1–2 micrograms/kg/min with the upper limit being 2 micrograms/kg/min). Maintain most effective dose for 12–15 hours until respiratory distress resolves, lungs are clear, and the patient is stable with a normal blood pressure, pink mucous membranes, normal capillary refill time and normal heart rate. Most animals at our clinic require 12 hours of treatment. The systolic blood pressure must remain greater than 90 mm Hg. If hypotension develops, the CRI should be discontinued. Blood pressure will return to pretreatment levels within 1–10 minutes of discontinuing treatment and administration can be reinstituted at the previous lower dose. Administer with dobutamine to treat or prevent hypotension if severe myocardial failure is present based on an echocardiogram evaluation. Wean sodium nitroprusside over 6 hours first and then dobutamine over 6 hours. ACE inhibitor is added before tapering the infusions over 3–6 hours. (Lichtenberger 2006)

Monitoring

■ Blood pressure must be constantly monitored

■ Acid/base balance

■ Electrolytes (especially Na^+)

Client Information

■ Must only be used by professionals in a setting where precise IV infusion and constant blood pressure monitoring can be performed.

Chemistry/Synonyms

A vascular smooth muscle relaxant, nitroprusside sodium occurs as practically odorless, reddish-brown crystals or powder. It is freely soluble in water and slightly soluble in alcohol. After reconstitution in D_5W, solution may have a brownish, straw, or light orange color and have a pH of 3.5–6.

Nitroprusside sodium may also be known as: disodium (OC-6-22)-pentakis(cyano-C)nitrosylferrate dihydrate, natrii nitroprussias, sodium nitroferricyanide dihydrate, sodium nitroprusside, or sodium nitroprussiate, and *Nitropress®*.

Storage/Stability

Nitroprusside sodium powder for injection should be stored protected from light and moisture and kept at room temperature (15–30°C). Nitroprusside solutions exposed to light will cause a reduction of the ferric ion to the ferrous ion with a resultant loss in potency and a change from a brownish-color to a blue color. Degradation is enhanced with nitroprusside solutions in *Viaflex®* (Baxter) plastic bags exposed to fluorescent light. After reconstitution, protect immediately by covering vial or infusion bag with aluminum foil or other opaque material. Discard solutions that turn to a blue, dark red, or green color. Solutions protected from light will remain stable for 24 hours after reconstitution. IV infusion tubing need not be protected from light while the infusion is running. It is not recommended to use IV infusion solutions other than D_5W or to add any other medications to the infusion solution.

Compatibility/Compounding Considerations

It is not recommended to use IV infusion solutions other than D_5W or to add any other medications to the infusion solution.

Dosage Forms/Regulatory Status

VETERINARY-LABELED PRODUCTS: None

HUMAN-LABELED PRODUCTS:

Nitroprusside Sodium Powder for Injection: 50 mg/vial in 2 mL Fliptop vials and 5 mL vials; *Nitropress®* (Hospira); generic; (Rx)

References

Erling, P. & E.M. Mazzaferro (2008). Left-sided congestive heart failure in dogs: Treatment and monitoring of emergency patients. *Compendium-Continuing Education for Veterinarians* 30(2): 94–+.

Lichtenberger, M. (2006). CHF in the ER: Keeping them alive. Proceedings: IVECCS. Accessed via: Veterinary Information Network. http://goo.gl/bXgF4

Macintire, D. (2006). Cardiac Emergencies. Proceedings: ACVC 2006. Accessed via: Veterinary Information Network. http://goo.gl/KxqeK

Papich, M. (1989). Effects of drugs on pregnancy. *Current Veterinary Therapy X: Small Animal Practice*. R Kirk Ed. Philadelphia, Saunders: 1291–1299.

Proulx, J. (2003). Intensive management of heart failure. Proceedings: Western Veterinary Conference. Accessed via: Veterinary Information Network. http://goo.gl/cii9Q

Proulx, J. & N. Dhupa (2000). Sodium Nitroprusside: Uses and precautions. *Kirk's Current Veterinary Therapy: XIII Small Animal Practice*. J Bonagura Ed. Philadelphia, WB Saunders: 194–197.

NIZATIDINE

(ni-*za*-ti-dine)   Axid®

H_2-RECEPTOR ANTAGONIST; PROKINETIC

Prescriber Highlights

▶ H_2 receptor antagonist similar to ranitidine; used primarily for its prokinetic activity; may be useful in preventing hemorrhagic necrosis in cats with pancreatitis. Not frequently used in veterinary medicine.

▶ Caution: Geriatric patients or those with hepatic or renal insufficiency

▶ Adverse Effects are rare

Uses/Indications

While nizatidine acts similarly to cimetidine and ranitidine as an H_2 blocker to reduce gastric acid secretion in the stomach, in small animal medicine its use has been primarily for its prokinetic effects. It may be useful to treat delayed gastric emptying, pseudo-obstruction of the intestine and constipation.

H_2 blockers may be useful in preventing hemorrhagic necrosis in feline pancreatitis.

Pharmacology/Actions

At the H_2 receptors of the parietal cells, nizatidine competitively inhibits histamine, thereby reducing gastric acid output both during basal conditions and when stimulated by food, amino acids, pentagastrin, histamine, or insulin.

While nizatidine may cause gastric emptying times to be delayed, it more likely will stimulate GI motility by inhibiting acetylcholinesterase (thereby increasing acetylcholine at muscarinic receptors). It may also have direct agonist effects on M_3 muscarinic receptors. Lower esophageal sphincter pressures may be increased by nizatidine. By decreasing the amount of gastric juice produced, nizatidine decreases the amount of pepsin secreted.

Pharmacokinetics

In the dog, oral absorption is rapid and nearly complete with minimal first pass effect. Food can enhance the absorption of nizatidine, but this is not considered clinically important. The drug is only marginally bound to plasma proteins. It is unknown if it enters the CNS. Nizatidine is metabolized in the liver to several metabolites, including at least one that has some activity. In animals with normal renal function over half the drug is excreted in the urine unchanged.

Contraindications/Precautions/Warnings

Nizatidine is contraindicated in patients who are hypersensitive to it. It should be used cautiously and, possibly, at reduced dosage in patients with diminished renal function. Nizatidine has caused increased serum ALT levels in humans receiving high IV doses for longer than 5 days. The manufacturer recommends that in high dose, chronic therapy, serum ALT values be monitored.

Adverse Effects

Nizatidine appears to be very well tolerated. Very rarely, anemia has been reported in humans taking the drug. CNS effects have been noted (headache, dizziness) but incidence is similar to those taking placebo. Rash and pruritus have also been reported in a few humans taking nizatidine.

Reproductive/Nursing Safety

Doses of up to 275 mg/kg per day in pregnant rabbits did not reveal any teratogenic or fetotoxic effects. Safety during pregnancy not firmly established, so use only when clearly warranted. In humans, the FDA categorizes this drug as category *B* for use during pregnancy (*Animal studies have not yet demonstrated risk to the fetus, but there are no adequate studies in pregnant women; or animal studies have shown an adverse effect, but adequate studies in pregnant women have not demonstrated a risk to the fetus in the first trimester of pregnancy, and there is no evidence of risk in later trimesters.*)

Nizatidine is excreted in maternal milk in a concentration of 0.1% of the oral dose in proportion to plasma concentrations and unlikely to cause significant effects in nursing offspring.

Overdosage/Acute Toxicity

Single oral doses of up to 800 mg/kg were not lethal in dogs. Adverse effects could include cholinergic effects (lacrimation, salivation, emesis, miosis and diarrhea); suggest treating supportively and symptomatically.

Drug Interactions

The following drug interactions have either been reported or are theoretical in humans or animals receiving nizatidine and may be of significance in veterinary patients:

■ **ANTICHOLINERGIC AGENTS (atropine, propantheline** etc.): May negate the prokinetic effects of nizatidine

■ **ASPIRIN:** Nizatidine may increase salicylate levels in patients receiving high doses of aspirin (or **other salicylates**)

Laboratory Considerations

■ False positive tests for **urobilinogen** may occur with patients receiving nizatidine

Doses

■ **DOGS:**

As a prokinetic agent:

a) 2.5–5 mg/kg PO once daily (Hall & Washabau 2000)

As an H_2 blocker to reduce gastric acid production:

a) 5 mg/kg PO once daily (dosage not well established). (Leib 2008)

■ **CATS:**

As a colonic prokinetic agent:

a) 2.5–5 mg/kg PO once daily (Washabau & Holt 2000)

b) In combination with cisapride: nizatidine 2.5–5 mg/kg PO q12h (Scherk 2003)

Monitoring

■ Clinical efficacy (dependent on reason for use); monitored by decrease in symptomatology, endoscopic examination, blood in feces, etc.

Client Information

■ To maximize the benefit of this medication, it must be administered as prescribed by the veterinarian; clinical signs may reoccur if dosages are missed.

Chemistry/Synonyms

Nizatidine occurs as an off-white to buff-colored crystalline powder. It has a bitter taste and a slight sulfur-like odor. Nizatidine is sparingly soluble in water.

Nizatidine may also be known as: LY-139037, nizatidinum, and *Axid*®.

Storage/Stability

Nizatidine oral tablets and capsules should be stored in tight, light-resistant containers at room temperature.

Dosage Forms/Regulatory Status

VETERINARY-LABELED PRODUCTS: None

The ARCI (Racing Commissioners International) has designated this drug as a class 5 substance. See the appendix for more information.

HUMAN-LABELED PRODUCTS:

Nizatidine Tablets: 75 mg; *Axid*® AR (Wyeth Consumer); (OTC)

Nizatidine Capsules: 150 mg & 300 mg; *Axid*® *Pulvules* (GlaxoSmithKline); generic; (Rx)

Nizatidine Oral Solution: 15 mg/mL in 480 mL; *Axid*® (Braintree); (Rx)

References

Hall, J. & R. Washabau (2000). Gastric Prokinetic Agents. *Kirk's Current Veterinary Therapy: XIII Small Animal Practice.* J Bonagura Ed. Philadelphia, WB Saunders: 609–617.

Leib, M.S. (2008). Drugs used to treat vomiting and upper GI diseases in dogs and cats. Proceedings: ACVC. Accessed via: Veterinary Information Network. http://goo.gl/R5KCS

Scherk, M. (2003). Feline megacolon. Proceedings: World Small Animal Veterinary Assoc World Congress. Accessed via: Veterinary Information Network. http://goo.gl/v69lu

Washabau, R. & D. Holt (2000). Feline Constipation and Idiopathic Megacolon. *Kirk's Current Veterinary Therapy: XIII Small Animal Practice.* J Bonagura Ed. Philadelphia, WB Saunders: 648–652.

NOVOBIOCIN SODIUM

(noe-ve-*bye*-oh-sin)   Albaplex®

Prescriber Highlights

▶ Antibiotic primarily effective against some gram-positive cocci

▶ Contraindications: hypersensitivity to it; Extreme caution: hepatic or hematopoietic dysfunction

▶ Adverse Effects: Systemic use: Fever, GI (nausea, vomiting, diarrhea), rashes, & blood dyscrasias

Uses/Indications

Novobiocin is FDA-approved in combination with penicillin G for use in dry dairy cattle as a mastitis tube. Novobiocin is available in combination with tetracycline and prednisolone for oral use in dogs.

Pharmacology/Actions

Novobiocin is believed to act in several ways in a bactericidal manner. It inhibits bacterial DNA gyrase, interfering with protein and nucleic acid synthesis and also interferes with bacterial cell wall synthesis. Activity of the drug is enhanced in an alkaline medium.

The spectrum of activity of novobiocin includes some gram-positive cocci (Staphs, Streptococcus pneumonia, and some group A streps). Activity is variable against other streptococci and weak against the Enterococci. Most gram-negative organisms are resistant to the drug, but some *Haemophilus* spp., *Neisseria* spp., and *Proteus* spp. may be susceptible.

Pharmacokinetics

After oral administration, novobiocin is well absorbed from the GI tract. Peak levels occur within 1–4 hours. The presence of food can decrease peak concentrations of the drug.

Novobiocin is only poorly distributed to body fluids with concentrations in synovial, pleural, and ascitic fluids less than those found in plasma. Only minimal quantities of the drug cross the blood-brain barrier, even when meninges are inflamed. Highest concentrations of novobiocin are found in the small intestine and liver. The drug is approximately 90% protein bound and is distributed into milk.

Novobiocin is primarily eliminated in the bile and feces. Approximately 3% is excreted into the urine; urine levels are usually less than those found in serum.

Contraindications/Precautions/Warnings

Novobiocin is contraindicated in patients hypersensitive to it. Additionally, the drug should be used with extreme caution in patients with preexisting hepatic or hematopoietic dysfunction.

Adverse Effects

Adverse effects reported with the systemic use of this drug include fever, GI disturbances (nausea, vomiting, diarrhea), rashes, and blood dyscrasias. In humans, occurrences of hypersensitivity reactions, hepatotoxicity, and blood dyscrasias have significantly limited the use of this drug.

Reproductive/Nursing Safety

Safety during pregnancy has not been established; use only when clearly indicated.

Overdosage/Acute Toxicity

Little information is available regarding overdoses of this drug. It is suggested that large oral overdoses be handled by emptying the gut following standard protocols; monitor and treat adverse effects symptomatically if necessary.

Drug Interactions

The following drug interactions have either been reported or are theoretical in humans or animals receiving novobiocin and may be of significance in veterinary patients:

■ **BETA-LACTAM ANTIBIOTICS:** Novobiocin reportedly acts similarly to probenecid by blocking the tubular transport of drugs. Although the clinical significance of this is unclear, the elimination rates of drugs excreted in this manner (*e.g.*, **penicillins, cephalosporins**) could be decreased and half-lives prolonged.

Laboratory Considerations

■ Novobiocin can be metabolized into a yellow-colored product that can interfere with **serum bilirubin** determinations.

■ Novobiocin may interfere with the determination **BSP** (bromosulfophthalein, sulfobromophthalein) uptake tests by altering BSP uptake or biliary excretion.

Doses

■ **DOGS:**

a) For susceptible infections using the combination product (with tetracycline and prednisolone): 22 mg/kg of each antibiotic and 0.55 mg prednisolone PO q12h for 48 hours (Package insert; *Delta Albaplex®*—Upjohn)

■ **CATTLE:**

a) For treatment of subclinical mastitis in dry cows: Infuse contents of one syringe into each quarter at the time of drying off; not later than 30 days prior to calving. Shake well before using. (Package directions; *Albadry Plus®*—Pharmacia & Upjohn)

Monitoring

■ Clinical efficacy

■ Adverse effects

■ Periodic liver function tests and CBC's are recommended if using long-term systemically.

Client Information

■ Shake mastitis tubes well before using

■ Do not exceed dosage recommendations or length of treatment

Chemistry/Synonyms

An antibiotic obtained from *Streptomyces niveus* or *spheroides*, novobiocin sodium occurs as white to light yellow, crystalline powder and is very soluble in water.

Novobiocin or novobiocin sodium may also be known as: crystallinic acid, PA-93, streptonivicin, U-6591, novobiocinum natricum, sodium novobiocin, *Albadry Plus®*, *Albamycin®*, *Biodry®* and *Delta Albaplex®*.

Storage/Stability

Novobiocin should be stored at room temperature in tight containers unless otherwise directed.

Dosage Forms/Regulatory Status

VETERINARY-LABELED PRODUCTS:

Novobiocin Combination Products:

Novobiocin (as the sodium salt): 400 mg and Penicillin G Procaine 200,000 Units per 10 mL *Plastet®* Syringe. *Albadry Plus®* (Pfizer); (OTC). FDA-approved for use in dry cows only. Do not use 30 days prior to calving. Milk must not be used for 72 hours after calving. Slaughter withdrawal (at labeled doses) = 30 days.

Novobiocin Sodium 60 mg, Tetracycline HCl 60 mg and Prednisolone 1.5 mg tablets; Novobiocin Sodium 180 mg, Tetracycline HCl 180 mg and Prednisolone 4.5 mg tablets; *Delta Albaplex®* and *Delta Albaplex® 3X* (Pfizer); (Rx). FDA-approved for use in dogs.

HUMAN-LABELED PRODUCTS: None

NYSTATIN (ORAL)

(nye-*stat*-in)   Nilstat®, Mycostatin®

ANTIFUNGAL (CANDIDA)

Prescriber Highlights

▶ Oral & topical antifungal (Candida); not absorbed systemically after PO

▶ Adverse Effects: GI effects possible at high dosages; hypersensitivity possible

Uses/Indications

Orally administered nystatin is used primarily for the treatment of oral or gastrointestinal tract Candida infections in dogs, cats, and birds; it has been used less commonly in other species for the same indications.

Pharmacology/Actions

Nystatin has a mechanism of action similar to that of amphotericin B. It binds to sterols in the membrane of the fungal cell altering the permeability of the membrane allowing intracellular potassium and other cellular constituents to "leak out." When given orally, the drug must come into contact with the organism to be effective.

Nystatin has activity against a variety of fungal organisms, but is clinically used against topical, oropharyngeal, and gastrointestinal Candida infections.

Pharmacokinetics

Nystatin is not measurably absorbed after oral administration and almost entirely excreted unchanged in the feces. The drug is not used parenterally because it is reportedly extremely toxic to internal tissues.

Contraindications/Precautions/Warnings

Nystatin is contraindicated in patients with known hypersensitivity to it.

Adverse Effects

Occasionally, high dosages of nystatin may cause GI upset (anorexia, vomiting, diarrhea). Rarely, hypersensitivity reactions have been reported in humans.

Reproductive/Nursing Safety

Although the safety of the drug during pregnancy has not been firmly established, the lack of appreciable absorption or case reports associating the drug with teratogenic effects appear to make it safe to use. In humans, the FDA categorizes this drug as category *B* for use during pregnancy (*Animal studies have not yet demonstrated risk to the fetus, but there are no adequate studies in pregnant women; or animal studies have shown an adverse effect, but adequate studies in pregnant women have not demonstrated a risk to the fetus in the first trimester of pregnancy, and there is no evidence of risk in later trimesters.*)

It is not known whether nystatin is excreted in maternal milk, but because the drug is not absorbed after oral administration it is unlikely to be of concern.

Overdosage/Acute Toxicity

Because the drug is not absorbed after oral administration, acute toxicity after an oral overdose is extremely unlikely, but transient GI distress may result.

Drug Interactions

■ No significant interactions reported for oral nystatin

Doses

■ **DOGS:**

For oral treatment of Candidal infections:

a) 100,000 Units PO q6h (Kirk 1989)

b) 50,000–150,000 Units PO q8h (Jenkins & Boothe 1987)

c) 22,000 Units/kg/day (Huber 1988)

■ **CATS:**

For oral treatment of Candidal infections:

a) 100,000 Units PO q6h (Kirk 1989)

■ **HORSES:**

For intrauterine infusion:

a) 250,000–1,000,000 IU; Mix with sterile water; precipitates in saline. Little science is available for recommending doses, volume infused, frequency, diluents, etc. Most intrauterine treatments are commonly performed every day or every other day for 3–7 days. (Perkins 1999)

■ **BIRDS:**

For crop mycosis and mycotic diarrhea (*Candida albicans*) in chickens and turkeys:

a) Feed at 50 grams per ton (*Mycostatin®-20*) or at 100 grams/ton for 7–10 days. (Label directions; *Mycostatin®-20*—Solvay)

For enteric yeast (Candidal) infections:

a) 200,000–300,000 Units/kg PO q8–12h. Relatively large volume must be administered (2–3 mL). May also be used prophylactically to prevent yeast infection in nestling birds treated with broad-spectrum antibiotics. Oral lesions may be missed if bird is tubed. (Flammer 2003)

b) For neonates on antibiotic therapy: Crush one fluconazole 100 mg tablet and mix with 20 mL of nystatin 100,000 Units/mL oral suspension. Dose at 0.5 mL/1000g of body weight PO twice daily for duration of antibiotic therapy. (Wissman 2003)

c) For treatment of candidiasis after antibiotic or in conjunction with antibiotics: One mL of the 100,000 Units/mL suspension per 300 grams body weight PO 1–3 times daily for 7–14 days. If treating mouth lesions do not give by gavage. Hand-fed babies should receive antifungal therapy if being treated with antibiotics. (Clubb 1986)

d) **Ratites:** 250,000–500,000 Units/kg PO twice daily (Jenson 1998)

■ **REPTILES:**

For susceptible infections:

a) For turtles with enteric yeast infections: 100,000 Units/kg PO once daily for 10 days (Gauvin 1993)

b) All species: 100,000 Units/kg PO once daily (Jacobson 1999)

Monitoring

■ Clinical efficacy

Client Information

■ Shake suspension well before administering

Chemistry/Synonyms

A polyene antifungal antibiotic produced by *Streptomyces noursei*, nystatin occurs as a yellow to light tan, hygroscopic powder having a cereal-like odor. It is very slightly soluble in water and slightly to sparingly soluble in alcohol. One mg of nystatin contains not less than 4400 Units of activity. According to the USP, nystatin used in the preparation of oral suspensions should not contain less than 5000 Units per mg.

Nystatin may also be known as: fungicidin, nistatina, or nystatinum, *Mycostatin®*, and *Nilstat®*.

Storage/Stability

Nystatin tablets and oral suspension should be stored at room temperature (15–30°C) in tight, light-resistant containers. Avoid freezing the oral suspension or exposing to temperatures greater than 40°C.

Nystatin deteriorates when exposed to heat, light, air or moisture.

Dosage Forms/Regulatory Status

VETERINARY-LABELED PRODUCTS:

None, for oral use. For topical use, see the topical dermatologic section in the appendix.

HUMAN-LABELED PRODUCTS:

Nystatin Oral Suspension: 100,000 Units/mL in 5 mL, 60 mL, 473 mL and 480 mL; *Nilstat®* (Lederle); generic; (Rx)

Nystatin Bulk powder: 50 million Units, 150 million Units, 500 million Units, 1 billion Units, 2 billion Units & 5 billion Units; generic; (Paddock); *Nilstat®* (Lederle); (Rx)

Nystatin Oral Tablets: 500,000 Units; *Mycostatin®* (Bristol-Myers Squibb), generic; (Rx)

Also available in oral troches, vaginal tablets, topical creams, powders and ointments.

References

Clubb, S.L. (1986). Therapeutics: Individual and Flock Treatment Regimens. *Clinical Avian Medicine and Surgery*. GJ Harrison and LR Harrison Eds. Philadelphia, W.B. Saunders: 327–355.

Flammer, K. (2003). Antifungal therapy in avian medicine. Proceedings: Western Veterinary Conference. Accessed via: Veterinary Information Network. http://goo.gl/rgOfo

Gauvin, J. (1993). Drug therapy in reptiles. *Seminars in Avian & Exotic Med* **2**(1): 48–59.

Huber, W.G. (1988). Antifungal and antiviral agents. *Veterinary Pharmacology and Therapeutics.* NH Booth and LE McDonald Eds. Ames, Iowa State University Press: 849–860.

Jacobson, E. (1999). Bacterial infections and antimicrobial treatment in reptiles. The North American Veterinary Conference, Orlando.

Jenkins, W.L. & D.M. Boothe (1987). Amphotericin B, Nystatin, Flucytosine, Imidazoles, Griseofulvin. *The Bristol Handbook of Antimicrobial Therapy.* DE Johnston Ed. Evansville, Veterinary Learning Systems: 270–271.

Jenson, J. (1998). Current ratite therapy. *The Veterinary Clinics of North America: Food Animal Practice* **16**:3(November).

Kirk, R.W., Ed. (1989). *Current Veterinary Therapy X, Small Animal Practice.* Philadelphia, W.B. Saunders.

Perkins, N. (1999). Equine reproductive pharmacology. *The Veterinary Clinics of North America: Equine Practice* **15**:3(December): 687–704.

Wissman, M. (2003). Avian pediatrics. Western Veterinary Conference.

OCTREOTIDE ACETATE

(ok-*trye*-oh-tide)   Sandostatin®

SOMATOSTATIN ANALOG

Prescriber Highlights

▶ Injectable long acting somatostatin analog that may be useful for adjunctive treatment of insulinomas & gastrinomas

▶ Limited experience, but appears safe

▶ Multiple daily SC injections are required

▶ No information for veterinary use of depot IM form

▶ Expensive (especially in large dogs)

▶ May affect GI fat absorption

Uses/Indications

Octreotide may be useful in the adjunctive treatment of hyperinsulinemia in patients with insulinomas (especially dogs, ferrets). Response is variable, presumably dependent on whether the tumor cells have receptors for somatostatin. Octreotide may also be useful in the diagnosis and symptomatic treatment of gastrinomas in dogs or cats. It may be of use in the treatment of acute pancreatitis, but more research is needed before it can be recommended for this use in veterinary patients. Octreotide has not been effective in reducing growth hormone levels or enhancing insulin sensitivity in cats with acromegaly.

Pharmacology/Actions

Octreotide is a synthetic long acting analog of somatostatin. It inhibits the secretion of insulin (in both normal and neoplastic beta cells), glucagon, secretin, gastrin and motilin. In humans, octreotide may bind to any one of 5 subtypes of somatostatin receptors found on neoplastic beta cells, but dogs only have one subtype. This, or octreotide's inhibition of glucagon and growth

hormone secretion, may explain the variable response dogs have to treatment.

Pharmacokinetics

Octreotide is absorbed and distributed rapidly from the injection site after SC administration. Half lives in humans average about 2 hours with duration of effect up to 12 hours. Treated dogs or ferrets generally require 2–3 injections per day to maintain blood glucose. About 32% of a dose is excreted unchanged in the urine and patients with severe renal dysfunction may need dosage adjustment.

Contraindications/Precautions/Warnings

Octreotide is contraindicated in patients hypersensitive to it. It should be used with caution in patients with biliary tract disorders.

Adverse Effects

Very limited experience in domestic animals, although it appears to be well tolerated thus far. GI effects (including biliary tract effects) are most commonly noted in human patients, particularly acromegalics.

Reproductive/Nursing Safety

In humans, the FDA categorizes this drug as category *B* for use during pregnancy (*Animal studies have not yet demonstrated risk to the fetus, but there are no adequate studies in pregnant women; or animal studies have shown an adverse effect, but adequate studies in pregnant women have not demonstrated a risk to the fetus in the first trimester of pregnancy, and there is no evidence of risk in later trimesters.*)

It is not known whether this drug is excreted in maternal milk.

Overdosage/Acute Toxicity

Serious adverse effects are unlikely. Human subjects have received up to 120 mg IV over 8 hours with no untoward effects.

Drug Interactions

The following drug interactions have either been reported or are theoretical in humans or animals receiving octreotide and may be of significance in veterinary patients:

■ **BETA-BLOCKERS:** Octreotide may cause additive bradycardic effects

■ **BROMOCRIPTINE:** Octreotide may increase oral bioavailability

■ **CALCIUM-CHANNEL BLOCKERS:** Octreotide may cause additive bradycardic effects

■ **CYCLOSPORINE:** Octreotide may reduce cyclosporine levels

■ **DIURETICS (and other agents that affect fluid/electrolyte balance):** Octreotide may enhance fluid/electrolyte imbalances

■ **FOOD:** Octreotide may reduce fat absorption

■ **INSULIN, ORAL HYPOGLYCEMICS:** Octreotide may can inhibit insulin

■ **QUINIDINE:** Octreotide may reduce the quinidine clearance

Doses

■ **DOGS:**

For medical treatment of insulinoma (beta cell tumor) particularly in patients refractory to or unable to tolerate other medical or surgical therapy:

a) 10–40 micrograms (total dose per dog) SC 2–3 times a day. Used in combination with dietary, glucocorticoid, and diazoxide treatment. (Nelson 2007)

b) Further studies needed to determine octreotide's efficacy and safety; has been administered at 2–4 micrograms/kg SC q8–12h (Hess 2005)

For adjunctive treatment of gastrinoma:

a) 2–20 micrograms/kg SC three times daily; with omeprazole. (Simpson 2005)

For adjunctive treatment of chylothorax:

a) 10–20 micrograms/kg SC three times a day for 2–3 weeks; prolonged treatment should be discouraged because people treated for longer than 4 weeks are at risk for gallstones. (Fossom 2006)

■ **CATS:**

For adjunctive treatment of chylothorax:

a) 10–20 micrograms/kg SC three times a day for 2–3 weeks; prolonged treatment should be discouraged because people treated for longer than 4 weeks are at risk for gallstones. (Fossom 2006)

■ **FERRETS:**

For medical treatment of insulinoma (particularly in patients refractory to or unable to tolerate other medical or surgical therapy):

a) 1–2 micrograms/kg SC 2–3 times a day (Meleo & Caplan 2000)

Monitoring

■ Blood glucose (for insulinoma treatment)

■ Clinical efficacy

Client Information

■ There is very limited experience with this medication in dogs and ferrets and therapy must be considered experimental.

■ Injections must be given 2–3 times a day per veterinarian instructions

■ The expense associated with this medication can be considerable.

Chemistry/Synonyms

Octreotide acetate is a synthetic polypeptide related to somatostatin. It is commercially available in injectable forms for subcutaneous or IV injection, and as an extended release suspension for IM administration.

Octreotide acetate may also be known as: SMS-201-995, *Longastatina®*, *Samilstin®*, *Sandostatin®*, *Sandostatina®*, or *Sandostatine®*.

Storage/Stability

When stored at room temperature and protected from light, octreotide acetate injection remains stable for 14 days. For long-term storage, keep refrigerated. If injecting solution that has been in the refrigerator, allow it to come to room temperature in the syringe before injecting. Do not use artificial warming techniques. It is recommended to use multidose vials within 14 days of initial use.

Dosage Forms/Regulatory Status

VETERINARY-LABELED PRODUCTS: None

HUMAN-LABELED PRODUCTS:

Octreotide Acetate for Injection: 0.05 mg/mL (50 micrograms/mL), 0.1 mg/mL (100 micrograms/mL), 0.2 mg/mL (200 micrograms/mL), 0.5 mg/mL (500 micrograms/mL) & 1 mg/mL (1,000 micrograms/mL) in 1 mg amps, single-dose vials and 5 mL multi-dose vials; *Sandostatin®* (Novartis); generic (Sicor); (Rx)

Octreotide Acetate Powder for Injectable Suspension: 10 mg/5 mL, 20 mg/5 mL & 30 mg/5mL in single-use kits; *Sandostatin® LAR Depot* (Novartis); (Rx)

References

Fossom, T. (2006). Chylothorax: Surgery is effective! Proceedings: WSAVA World Congress. Accessed via: Veterinary Information Network. http://goo.gl/0hWO1

Hess, R. (2005). Insulin-secreting islet cell neoplasia. *Textbook of Veterinary Internal Medicine, 6th Ed.* S Ettinger and E Feldman Eds., Elsevier: 1560–1563.

Meleo, K. & E. Caplan (2000). Treatment of insulinoma in the dogs, cat, and ferret. *Kirk's Current Veterinary Therapy: XIII Small Animal Practice.* J Bonagura Ed. Philadelphia, WB Saunders: 357–361.

Nelson, R. (2007). Hypoglycemia and Beta Cell Tumors, Proceedings: WSAVA. Accessed via: Veterinary Information Network. http://goo.gl/1V6xc

Simpson, K. (2005). Diseases of the stomach. *Textbook of Veterinary Internal Medicine, 6th Ed.* S Ettinger and E Feldman Eds., Elsevier: 1310–1331.

OLSALAZINE SODIUM

(ole-*sal*-a-zeen)   Dipentum®

ANTIINFLAMMATORY (LOCAL GI TRACT)

Prescriber Highlights

▶ Used for treatment of chronic colitis in dogs that either are unresponsive to or cannot tolerate sulfasalazine; limited experience

▶ Keratoconjunctivitis sicca (KCS) has been reported in some dogs

▶ Converted to 2 molecules of 5-ASA (mesalamine) in colon

▶ Expensive when compared to sulfasalazine

Uses/Indications

Olsalazine is used for treatment of dogs with chronic colitis that either cannot tolerate the adverse effects associated with sulfasalazine or the response to sulfasalazine has been ineffective.

Pharmacology/Actions

Olsalazine is cleaved in the intestine into 5-aminosalicylic acid (5-ASA, mesalamine) by bacteria in the gut. While its exact mechanism is unknown, mesalamine is thought to have efficacy for chronic colitis secondary to its antiinflammatory activity.

Pharmacokinetics

Olsalazine is poorly absorbed; approximately 98% of a dose reaches the colon intact and what drug is absorbed is rapidly eliminated. Serum half-life is about one hour.

Contraindications/Precautions/Warnings

Olsalazine is contraindicated in patients hypersensitive to it or to salicylates. Use with caution in animals with renal disease as renal toxicity has developed, though rarely, in human patients.

Adverse Effects

While keratoconjunctivitis sicca (KCS) is occasionally reported in dogs receiving olsalazine, it probably occurs less frequently than with sulfasalazine therapy. In humans, approximately 17% of patients developed more serious diarrhea (then they had prior to treatment) after receiving olsalazine.

Reproductive/Nursing Safety

In high dose rat studies, some fetal abnormalities were seen. Use during pregnancy only when benefits outweigh the risks. In humans, the FDA categorizes this drug as category *C* for use during pregnancy (*Animal studies have shown an adverse effect on the fetus, but there are no adequate studies in humans; or there are no animal reproduction studies and no adequate studies in humans.*)

Oral olsalazine given to lactating rats in doses 5–20 times the human dose produced growth retardation in their pups. Use with caution in nursing patients.

Overdosage/Acute Toxicity

Overdosage in dogs may cause vomiting, diarrhea and decreased motor activity; treat symptomatically and supportively. Dosages up to 2 grams/kg were not lethal in dogs.

Drug Interactions

The following drug interaction has either been reported or are theoretical in humans or animals receiving olsalazine and may be of significance in veterinary patients:

- ■ **WARFARIN:** Olsalazine may increase prothrombin times in patients receiving warfarin

Laboratory Considerations

- ■ Olsalazine may cause increases in **ALT** or **AST**

Doses

- ■ **DOGS:**

  a) For dogs who cannot tolerate sulfasalazine: 10–20 mg/kg PO three times daily (Leib 2000)

  b) 10–20 mg/kg PO q8h has had limited use

in dogs without causing apparent side effects. (Marks 2007)

  c) 10–15 mg/kg PO q8–12h (Hall 2004)

  d) Initially at 5–10 mg/kg PO three times daily, then reduce gradually. (Allensbach 2005; Allenspach 2009)

Monitoring

- ■ Clinical efficacy
- ■ Adverse effects

Client Information

- ■ Should be given with food in evenly spaced doses (if possible)
- ■ If diarrhea worsens or dogs eyes become dry, contact veterinarian

Chemistry/Synonyms

Olsalazine sodium occurs as a yellow crystalline powder that is soluble in water and stable under physiologic acidic and alkaline conditions. It is basically 2 molecules of mesalamine (5-ASA) connected at the azo bonding site.

Olsalazine sodium may also be known as: azodisal sodium, dimesalamine, CI mordant yellow 5, CI No. 14130, CJ-91B, olsalazinum natricum, sodium azodisalicylate, *Dipentum®* or *Rasal®*.

Storage/Stability

Store capsules at room temperature.

Dosage Forms/Regulatory Status

VETERINARY-LABELED PRODUCTS: None

The ARCI (Racing Commissioners International) has designated this drug as a class 4 substance. See the appendix for more information.

HUMAN-LABELED PRODUCTS:

Olsalazine Sodium Oral Capsules: 250 mg; *Dipentum®* (UCB Pharma); (Rx)

References

Allensbach, K. (2005). Innovative treatment options in dogs with chronic enteropathies. Proceedings: ECVIM.

Allenspach, K. (2009). Treatment of IBD. Proceediings: BSAVA. Accessed via: Veterinary Information Network. http://goo.gl/c5raP

Hall, E. (2004). Inflammatory Bowel Disease: Treatment. Proceedings: ACVIM Forum, Minneapolis. Accessed via: Veterinary Information Network. http://goo.gl/FzY5y

Leib, M. (2000). Chronic Colitis in Dogs. *Kirk's Current Veterinary Therapy: XIII Small Animal Practice.* J Bonagura Ed. Philadelphia, WB Saunders: 643–648.

Marks, S. (2007). Inflammatory Bowel Disease—More than a garbage can diagnosis. Proceedings: UCD Canine Medicine Symposium. Accessed via: Veterinary Information Network. http://goo.gl/ZGPg1

OMEPRAZOLE

(oh-*meh*-prah-zahl)   Gastrogard®, Prilosec®

PROTON PUMP INHIBITOR

Prescriber Highlights

▶ Proton pump inhibitor used for GI ulcers & erosions

▶ May need to adjust dosage with hepatic or renal disease

▶ Adverse Effects: Horses: Unlikely; potential hypersensitivity. Small Animals: Appears to be well tolerated. Potentially: GI distress (anorexia, colic, nausea, vomiting, flatulence, diarrhea), hematologic abnormalities, urinary tract infections, proteinuria, or CNS disturbances

Uses/Indications

Omeprazole is potentially useful in treating both gastroduodenal ulcer disease and to prevent or treat gastric erosions caused by ulcerogenic drugs (*e.g.*, aspirin). Omeprazole was superior to famotidine when used to prevent exercise-induced gastritis in racing Alaskan sled dogs (Williamson *et al.* 2010). An oral paste product is labeled for the treatment and prevention of recurrence of gastric ulcers in horses.

Pharmacology/Actions

Omeprazole is a substituted benzimidazole gastric acid (proton) pump inhibitor. In an acidic environment, omeprazole is activated to a sulphenamide derivative that binds irreversibly at the secretory surface of parietal cells to the enzyme, H^+/K^+ ATPase. There it inhibits the transport of hydrogen ions into the stomach. Omeprazole reduces acid secretion during both basal and stimulated conditions. There is a lag time between administration and efficacy. Omeprazole also inhibits the hepatic cytochrome P-450 mixed function oxidase system (see Drug Interactions below).

Pharmacokinetics

Omeprazole is rapidly absorbed from the gut; the human commercial product is in an enteric-coated granule form as the drug is rapidly degraded by acid. The equine paste is not enteric coated. In humans, peak serum levels occur within 0.5–3.5 hours and onset of action within 1 hour. Omeprazole is distributed widely, but primarily in gastric parietal cells. In humans, approximately 95% is bound to albumin and alpha$_1$-acid glycoprotein. It is unknown whether omeprazole enters maternal milk.

Omeprazole is extensively metabolized in the liver to at least six different metabolites. These are excreted principally in the urine, but also via the bile into feces. Significant hepatic dysfunction will reduce the first pass effect of the drug.

In humans and dogs with normal hepatic function, serum half-life averages about 1 hour, but the duration of therapeutic effect may persist for 24–72 hours or more. Effects on acid production in horses can last up to 27 hours, depending upon dose.

Contraindications/Precautions/Warnings

Omeprazole is contraindicated in patients hypersensitive to it. In patients with hepatic or renal disease, the drug's half–life may be prolonged and dosage adjustment may be necessary if the disease is severe.

Adverse Effects

The manufacturer does not note any adverse effects for use in horses at labeled dosages. There is an anecdotal case report of one horse developing urticaria after receiving omeprazole. The drug appears to be quite well tolerated in both dogs and cats at effective dosages. Potentially, GI distress (anorexia, colic, nausea, vomiting, flatulence, diarrhea) could occur, as well as hematologic abnormalities (rare in humans), urinary tract infections, proteinuria, or CNS disturbances. Chronic very high doses in rats caused enterochromaffin-like cell hyperplasia and gastric carcinoid tumors; effects occurred in dose related manner. The clinical significance of these findings for long-term low-dose clinical usage is not known, however, at the current time in humans, dosing for longer than 8 weeks is rarely recommended unless the benefits of therapy outweigh the potential risks. In dogs, omeprazole use is believed safe for at least 4 weeks of therapy. Treatment of horses for up to 90 days is believed safe.

Reproductive/Nursing Safety

Omeprazole's safety during pregnancy has not been established, but a study done in rats at doses of up to 345 times those recommended did not demonstrate any teratogenic effects; however, increased embryo–lethality has been noted in lab animals at very high dosages. In humans, the FDA categorizes this drug as category *C* for use during pregnancy (*Animal studies have shown an adverse effect on the fetus, but there are no adequate studies in humans; or there are no animal reproduction studies and no adequate studies in humans.*)

It is not known whether these agents are excreted in maternal milk. In rats, omeprazole administration during late gestation and lactation at doses of 35–345 times the human dose resulted in decreased weight gain in pups. In humans, because of the potential for serious adverse reactions in nursing infants, and the potential for tumorigenicity shown in rat carcinogenicity studies, nursing is discouraged if the drug is required.

Overdosage/Acute Toxicity

The LD$_{50}$ in rats after oral administration is reportedly >4 grams/kg. Humans have tolerated oral dosages of 360 mg/day without significant toxicity. Should a massive overdose occur, treat symptomatically and supportively.

Drug Interactions

The following drug interactions have either been reported or are theoretical in humans or animals receiving omeprazole and may be of significance in veterinary patients:

■ **BENZODIAZEPINES (e.g., diazepam):** Omeprazole may potentially alter benzodiazepine metabolism and prolong CNS effects

■ **CLARITHROMYCIN:** Increased levels of omeprazole, clarithromycin and 14-hydroxyclarithromycin are possible

■ **CYANOCOBALAMIN (oral):** Omeprazole may decrease oral absorption

■ **CYCLOSPORINE:** Omeprazole may reduce cyclosporine metabolism

■ **DRUGS REQUIRING DECREASED GASTRIC PH FOR OPTIMAL ABSORPTION (e.g., ketoconazole, itraconazole, iron, ampicillin esters):** Omeprazole may decrease drug absorption

■ **WARFARIN:** Omeprazole may increase anticoagulant effect

Laboratory Considerations

■ Omeprazole may cause increased **liver enzymes**

■ Omeprazole will increase **serum gastrin** levels early in therapy

Doses

Dose dependent on formulation, equine paste and human oral forms may not be interchangeable. Be wary of compounded formulations; bioequivalence is not assured.

■ **DOGS:**

For GI ulcer management/prevention:

a) 0.5−1 mg/kg PO once daily (Davenport 1992)(Haskins 2000)(Trepanier 2010)

b) For adjunctive treatment of uremic gastropathy: 0.5−1 mg/kg PO q24h; dosage may need to be modified in moderate or severe renal failure. (Vaden 2007)

c) To prevent exercise-induced gastritis in racing Alaskan sled dogs: In the study, dogs were dosed at approx. 0.85 mg/kg (one 20 mg tablet) once daily approximately 30 minutes before being fed. Dosing began approximately 48 hours before exercise. (Williamson *et al.* 2010)

d) For adjunctive treatment of esophagitis or gastric ulcers: 0.5−1 mg/kg PO q24h (Sellon 2007a; Sellon 2007b)

e) For some animals with gastrinomas or esophagitis (often H-2 receptor antagonists are adequate): 0.7−1.5 mg/kg PO q24h, but if severe esophagitis or gastrinomas may use up to 2 mg/kg PO q12h (Willard 2006)

f) 0.7 mg/kg PO q24h (20 mg/dog). (Marks 2008)

g) For esophagitis: 0.7 mg/kg PO twice daily. (Simpson 2008)

h) For adjunctive treatment of uremic vomiting: 0.7 mg/kg PO q12h. (Washabau 2009)

i) For Helicobacter infection/gastritis: Omeprazole 0.7 mg/kg PO once daily (or an H_2 blocker), amoxicillin 15 mg/kg PO twice daily, metronidazole 10 mg/kg PO twice daily, and Pepto Bismol ¼−2 tablets PO twice daily. All are given for 2 weeks. Other suggestions include omeprazole with either azithromycin 10−20 mg/kg PO once daily or clarithromycin 7.5 mg/kg PO twice daily. (Leib 2008)

■ **CATS:**

For GI ulcer management/prevention:

a) For adjunctive treatment of esophagitis or gastric ulcers: 0.5−1 mg/kg PO q24h (Sellon 2007a; Sellon 2007b; Trepanier 2010)

b) 0.7−1.5 mg/kg PO q12−24h (Willard 2003)

c) For adjunctive treatment of uremic gastropathy: 0.7 mg/kg PO q24h; dosage may need to be modified in moderate or severe renal failure. (Vaden 2007)

■ **FERRETS:**

a) For short-term treatment of gastroenteritis: 0.7 mg/kg PO q24h. (Johnson-Delaney 2009)

■ **HORSES: (Note:** ARCI UCGFS Class 5 Drug)

For gastric ulcers:

a) For treatment of gastric ulcers: 4 mg/kg PO once daily for 4 weeks; to prevent recurrence treat for at least another 4 weeks at 2 mg/kg PO once daily (Label Directions; *Gastrogard®*)

b) **Foals:** Preventative dose: 1 mg/kg PO q24h; Treatment dose: 4 mg/kg PO q24h. Will reduce gastric pH in a few hours. There has been a recent shift to not administering prophylactic antiulcer medication routinely to sick foals. (Stewart 2008)

c) For treatment or prophylaxis of gastric ulcers in foals: 4 mg/kg PO once daily for treatment, 1−2 mg/kg PO once daily for prophylaxis (Wilkins 2004)

d) **Foals:** 4 mg/kg PO q24h. Commonly foals will be started on ranitidine (1.5 mg/kg IV q8h; 6.6 mg/kg PO q8h) and omeprazole together. The ranitidine is quick acting histamine-2 antagonist and begins to alkalinize the gastric pH quickly. (Paradis 2008)

■ **SWINE:**

For ulcer management:

a) 40 mg of PO daily for two days; fasted for 48 hours (DeMint 1999)

Monitoring
■ Efficacy
■ Adverse effects

Client Information
■ Give before meals, preferably in the morning

Chemistry/Synonyms
A substituted benzimidazole proton pump inhibitor, omeprazole has a molecular weight of 345.4 and pK_a's of 4 and 8.8.

Omeprazole may also be known as: H-168/68, or omeprazolum, Gastrogard®, Prilosec®, Ulcergard® and Zegerid®.

Storage/Stability
Omeprazole oral paste should be stored below 86°F. Transient exposure to temperatures up to 104°F is permitted. Omeprazole tablets should be stored at room temperature in light-resistant, tight containers. Omeprazole pellets found in the capsules are fragile and should not be crushed. If needed to administer as a slurry, it has been suggested to mix the pellets carefully with fruit juices, not water, milk or saline.

Compatibility/Compounding Considerations
Use caution when using compounded omeprazole products; bioequivalence has been an issue with some compounded preparations. Omeprazole capsules or tablets should not be crushed or chewed. If reducing the dose of the commercially available capsules, the capsule contents should be re-inserted into a gelatin capsule so they cannot be chewed.

Compounded preparation stability: Omeprazole oral suspension compounded from the commercially available powder packets has been published (Johnson *et al.* 2007). Dissolving one (1) omeprazole 20 mg powder packet *qs ad* 10 ml in sterile water yields 2 mg/mL omeprazole oral suspension that retains >98% potency for 45 days when stored at 4°C; however, the resulting low concentration and strawberry flavoring may not be suitable for administration to veterinary patients. The efficacy of omeprazole 40 mg/mL oral suspension compounded by diluting commercially available equine paste 1:9 with sesame oil for use in dogs has been published (Tolbert *et al.* 2011). While the long term stability of this preparation has not yet been assayed, it meets the default beyond-use-date criteria of 180 days for non-aqueous oral suspensions.

Dosage Forms/Regulatory Status

VETERINARY-LABELED PRODUCTS:

Omeprazole Oral Paste, 2.28 g per syringe; Gastrogard® (Merial), (Rx); Ulcergard® (Merial), (OTC)

The ARCI (Racing Commissioners International) has designated this drug as a class 5 substance. See the appendix for more information.

HUMAN-LABELED PRODUCTS:

Omeprazole Oral Delayed-Release Capsules: 10 mg, 20 mg (tablets & capsules) & 40 mg; Prilosec® (AstraZeneca); Prilosec® OTC (Losec® in Canada; Procter & Gamble); generic; (Rx & OTC)

Omeprazole/Sodium Bicarbonate Oral Capsules (Immediate Release): 20 mg omeprazole/1,100 mg sodium bicarbonate; 40 mg omeprazole/1,100 mg sodium bicarbonate; Zegerid® (Santarus); (Rx)

Omeprazole/Sodium Bicarbonate Powder for Oral Suspension: 20 mg omeprazole/1,680 sodium bicarbonate; 40 mg omeprazole/1,680 sodium bicarbonate in 30 unit-dose packets; Zegerid® (Santarus); (Rx)

References

Davenport, D. (1992). Hematemesis: diagnosis and treatment. *Current Veterinary Therapy XI: Small Animal Practice*. R Kirk and J Bonagura Eds. Philadelphia, W.B. Saunders Company: 132–137.

DeMint, J. (1999). Gastric Ulcers. Proceedings: Central Veterinary Conference, Kansas City.

Haskins, S. (2000). Therapy for Shock. *Kirk's Current Veterinary Therapy: XIII Small Animal Practice*. J Bonagura Ed. Philadelphia, WB Saunders: 140–147.

Johnson, C.E., M.P. Cober, et al. (2007). Stability of partial doses of omeprazole-sodium bicarbonate oral suspension. *Ann Pharmacother* **41**(12): 1954–1961.

Johnson-Delaney, C. (2009). Gastrointestinal physiology and disease of carnivorous exotic companion animals. Proceedings: ABVP. Accessed via: Veterinary Information Network. http://goo.gl/iVI9w

Leib, M.S. (2008). Drugs used to treat vomiting and upper GI diseases in dogs and cats. Proceedings: ACVC. Accessed via: Veterinary Information Network. http://goo.gl/R5KCS

Marks, S. (2008). GI Therapeutics: Which Ones and When? Proceedings: IVECCS. Accessed via: Veterinary Information Network. http://goo.gl/rxwcs

Paradis, M. (2008). Gastrointestinal Problems in the Equine Neonate. Proceedings: World Veterinary Congress. Accessed via: Veterinary Information Network. http://goo.gl/pZkEx

Sellon, R. (2007a). Esophagitis. Proceedings: Western Vet Conf. Accessed via: Veterinary Information Network. http://goo.gl/6FdgL

Sellon, R. (2007b). Gastric Ulcers. Proceedings: Western Vet Conf. Accessed via: Veterinary Information Network. http://goo.gl/hW7b9

Simpson, K.W. (2008). How I Treat Esophagitis. Proceedings: WSAVA. Accessed via: Veterinary Information Network. http://goo.gl/nWWgW

Stewart, A. (2008). Equine Neonatal Sepsis. Proceedings: WVC. Accessed via: Veterinary Information Network. http://goo.gl/xT79V

Tolbert, K., S. Bissett, et al. (2011). Efficacy of Oral Famotidine and 2 Omeprazole Formulations for the Control of Intragastric pH in Dogs. *J Vet Intern Med* **25**(1): 47–54.

Trepanier, L. (2010). Acute Vomiting In Cats Rational treatment selection. *Journal of Feline Medicine and Surgery* **12**(3): 225–230.

Vaden, S. (2007). Management of chronic kidney disease. Proceedings: Western Vet Conf. Accessed via: Veterinary Information Network. http://goo.gl/CcxYX

Washabau, R. (2009). Difficult Vomiting Disorders: Therapy. Proceedings: WSAVA. http://goo.gl/aPwlv

Wilkins, P. (2004). Disorders of foals. *Equine Internal Medicine, 2nd Ed.* S Reed, W Bayly and D Sellon Eds. Philadelphia, Saunders: 1381–1431.

Willard, M. (2003). Diigestive system disorders. *Small Animal Internal Medicine, 3rd Ed.* R Nelson and C Couto Eds. St Louis, Mosby: 343–471.

Willard, M. (2006). Severe hematemesis and GI bleeding. Proceedings: IVECCS. Accessed via: Veterinary Information Network. http://goo.gl/fqsWD

Williamson, K.K., M.D. Willard, et al. (2010). Efficacy of Omeprazole versus High-Dose Famotidine for Prevention of Exercise-Induced Gastritis in Racing Alaskan Sled Dogs. *Journal of Veterinary Internal Medicine* 24(2): 285–288.

ONDANSETRON HCL

(on-*dan*-sah-tron)   Zofran®

5-HT$_3$ RECEPTOR ANTAGONIST

Prescriber Highlights

▶ 5-HT$_3$ receptor antagonist for severe vomiting

▶ Appears to be well tolerated in dogs

▶ Generic dosage forms now available, prices are much lower than previously

Uses/Indications

Used as an antiemetic when conventional antiemetics are ineffective, such as when administering cisplatin or for other causes of intractable vomiting. The use of ondansetron in cats is somewhat controversial and some state it should not be used in this species.

Pharmacology/Actions

Ondansetron is a 5-HT$_3$ (serotonin type 3) receptor antagonist. 5-HT$_3$ receptors are found peripherally on vagal nerve terminals and centrally in the chemoreceptor trigger zone (CTZ). It is not clear if ondansetron's effects are mediated centrally, peripherally or both.

Pharmacokinetics

No veterinary species data was located for ondansetron pharmacokinetics. In humans, ondansetron is well absorbed from the GI tract, but exhibits some first pass hepatic metabolism. Bioavailability is about 50–60%. Peak plasma levels occur about 2 hours after an oral dose. Ondansetron is extensively metabolized in the liver. Elimination half-lives are about 3–4 hours, but are prolonged in elderly patients.

Contraindications/Precautions/Warnings

Ondansetron is contraindicated in patients hypersensitive to it or other agents in this class. Ondansetron may mask ileus or gastric distention; it should not be used in place of nasogastric suction. Use with caution in patients with hepatic dysfunction as half-life may be prolonged.

In humans, ondansetron is reported to be pumped by P-glycoprotein (the protein encoded by the MDR1/*ABCB*1 gene), but there is currently no data stating whether they are or are not pumped by canine P-glycoprotein. It is suggested to use caution when administering ondansetron to dogs with the MDR1 mutation (WSU-VetClinPharmLab 2009)

Adverse Effects

Ondansetron appears to be well tolerated. Constipation, sedation, extrapyramidal clinical signs (head shaking), arrhythmias and hypotension are possible (incidence in humans <10%).

Reproductive/Nursing Safety

Safety in pregnancy not clearly established, but high dose studies in rodents did not demonstrate overt fetal toxicity or teratogenicity. In humans, the FDA categorizes this drug as category *B* for use during pregnancy (*Animal studies have not yet demonstrated risk to the fetus, but there are no adequate studies in pregnant women; or animal studies have shown an adverse effect, but adequate studies in pregnant women have not demonstrated a risk to the fetus in the first trimester of pregnancy, and there is no evidence of risk in later trimesters.*)

Ondansetron is excreted in the maternal milk of rats. Exercise caution when 5-HT$_3$ antagonists are administered to nursing patients.

Overdosage/Acute Toxicity

Overdoses of up to 10X did not cause significant morbidity in human subjects. If an overdose occurs, treat supportively.

Drug Interactions/Laboratory Considerations

■ **APOMORPHINE:** A human patient that received ondansetron and apomorphine developed severe hypotension. In humans, use together is contraindicated.

■ **DRUGS AFFECTING QTC INTERVAL** (*e.g.,* amiodarone, cisapride, halothane, isoflurane, sotalol): Theoretically, ondansetron may have additive effects on QTc interval; possible serious arrhythmias may result.

■ **TRAMADOL:** In humans, use together may reduce the efficacy of both drugs. Veterinary significance is not known.

Doses

■ **DOGS:**

a) 0.1–0.3 mg/kg IV given as a slow push every 8 to 12 hours (based on patient response). Has produced dramatic results in either controlling or at least significantly decreasing the frequency of vomiting in dogs with frequent or severe vomiting, including dogs with severe parvovirus enteritis or pancreatitis. (Tams 2007)

b) For chemotherapy–related vomiting: 0.5–1 mg/kg PO q8-12h; 0.1–0.5 mg/kg IV over 15 minutes q8h or 30 minutes before cisplatin infusion. (Kent 2009)

c) For adjunctive therapy of acute diarrhea: 0.5–1 mg/kg PO twice daily. Antagonizes neuronal 5-HT$_3$ receptors and inhibits Cl$^-$ and H$_2$O secretion from intestinal epithelial cells. (Washabau 2007)

d) As an antiemetic: 0.1–0.2 mg/kg IV

q6–12h or 0.1–1 mg/kg PO q12–24h (Otto 2005)

e) As an antiemetic for adjunctive treatment of uremia: 0.6–1 mg/kg PO or IV q12h; usually combined with metoclopramide. (Polzin 2005)

■ CATS:

a) Empiric dose: 0.5 mg/kg IV or PO twice daily. (Trepanier 2010)

b) As an anti-emetic for intractable vomiting: 0.1–0.15 mg/kg slow IV push q6–12h as needed (Scherk 2003)

c) As an antiemetic for adjunctive treatment of severe pancreatitis: 0.1–1 mg/kg PO or IV q12–24h (Armstrong 2007)

Monitoring
■ Clinical efficacy

Client Information
■ This medication is generally used in inpatient settings for treatment of serious vomiting.

Chemistry/Synonyms
A selective inhibitor of serotonin type 3 (5-HT₃), ondansetron HCl dihydrate occurs as a white to off-white powder that is soluble in water.

Ondansetron HCl may also be known as: GR-38032F or ondansetroni hydrochloridum, and *Zofran®*.

Storage/Stability
Unless otherwise labeled, store oral products in tight, light-resistant containers between 2–30°C. The injection should be stored between 2–30°C and protected from light.

Compatibility/Compounding Considerations
Drugs reported to be **compatible** with ondansetron when combined in a syringe and administered via a Y-site, include: alfentanil, atropine, fentanyl, glycopyrrolate, metoclopramide, midazolam, morphine, naloxone, neostigmine, and propofol.

Ondansetron is reported **compatible** with the following drugs when administered via a Y-site: amikacin, azithromycin, bleomycin, carboplatin, carmustine, cefotaxime, ceftazidime, cefuroxime, cisplatin, clindamycin, cyclophosphamide, cytarabine, dacarbazine, dactinomycin, daunorubicin, dexamethasone sodium phosphate, dexmedetomidine, diphenhydramine, dopamine, doxorubicin HCL (also liposome form), doxycycline, famotidine, filgrastim, fluconazole, gemcitabine, gentamicin, heparin, hydromorphone, hydroxyzine, ifosfamide, imipenem-cilastatin, mannitol, mesna, methotrexate, methylprednisolone sodium succinate, metoclopramide, mitoxantrone, morphine, piperacillin-tazobactam, potassium chloride, prochlorperazine, promethazine, ranitidine, vancomycin, vinblastine, vincristine, and zidovudine.

Compatibility is dependent upon factors such as pH, concentration, temperature, and diluent used; consult specialized references or a hospital pharmacist for more specific information.

Dosage Forms/Regulatory Status

VETERINARY-LABELED PRODUCTS: None

HUMAN-LABELED PRODUCTS:

Ondansetron HCl Tablets: 4 mg, 8 mg, 16 mg & 24 mg; *Zofran®* (GlaxoSmithKline), generic; (Rx)

Ondansetron Orally Disintegrating Tablets: 4 mg & 8 mg (as base); *Zofran® ODT* (GlaxoSmithKline), generic (Sandoz); (Rx)

Ondansetron HCl Oral Solution: 0.8 mg/ml (4 mg/5 mL) in 50 mL; *Zofran®* (GlaxoSmithKline), generic; (Rx)

Ondansetron HCl Injection: 2 mg/mL in 2 mL single-dose & 20 mL multi-dose vials; and 32 mg/50 mL (premixed; preservative free) in 50 mL single-dose containers; *Zofran®* (GlaxoSmithKline); generic; (Rx)

References

Armstrong, P. (2007). The clinical masquerade of feline pancreatitis. Proceedings: Western Vet Conference. Accessed via: Veterinary Information Network. http://goo.gl/4aH9I

Kent, M. (2009). Treating Chemotherapy Complications. Proceedings: BSAVA. Accessed via: Veterinary Information Network. http://goo.gl/c5DCW

Otto, C. (2005). Antiemetic update. Proceedings: IVECCS. Accessed via: Veterinary Information Network. http://goo.gl/oN4IJ

Polzin, D. (2005). Managing the acute uremic crisis. Proceedings: ACVC. Accessed via: Veterinary Information Network. http://goo.gl/iav1L

Scherk, M. (2003). Feline pancreatitis: underdiagnosed and overlooked. Proceedings: World Small Animal Veterinary Assoc World Congress. Accessed via: Veterinary Information Network. http://goo.gl/S8hdO

Tams, T. (2007). Update on Management of Vomiting in Dogs and Cats. Proceedings: ACVC. Accessed via: Veterinary Information Network. http://goo.gl/M1QEx

Trepanier, L. (2010). Acute Vomiting In Cats Rational treatment selection. *Journal of Feline Medicine and Surgery* 12(3): 225–230.

Washabau, R. (2007). Evidence-Based Medicine: GI Drugs in the ICU. Proceedings: IVECCS. Accessed via: Veterinary Information Network. http://goo.gl/IHZon

WSU-VetClinPharmLab (2009). "Problem Drugs." http://goo.gl/aIGlM.

o,p-DDD—see Mitotane

Opiate Antidiarrheals—See Separate Monographs for Diphenoxylate/Atropine, Loperamide, or Paregoric

ORBIFLOXACIN

(or-bi-*flox*-a-sin)   Orbax®

FLUOROQUINOLONE ANTIBIOTIC

Prescriber Highlights

▶ Fluoroquinolone antibiotic labeled for dogs & cats

▶ Contraindications: Immature dogs during the rapid growth phase; known hypersensitivity to this class of drugs. Caution: Known or suspected CNS disorders

▶ Adverse Effects: GI effects most likely

▶ Drug Interactions

Uses/Indications

Orbifloxacin is indicated for treatment in dogs and cats for bacterial infections susceptible to it. Orbifloxacin may also be of benefit in treating susceptible gram-negative infections in horses.

Pharmacology/Actions

Orbifloxacin is a concentration-dependent bactericidal agent. It acts by inhibiting bacterial DNA-gyrase (a type-II topoisomerase), thereby preventing DNA supercoiling and DNA synthesis. The net result is disruption of bacterial cell replication.

Orbifloxacin has good activity against many gram-negative and gram-positive bacilli and cocci, including most species and strains of *Klebsiella* spp., *Staphylococcus intermedius* or *aureus*, *E. coli*, Enterobacter, Campylobacter, Shigella, Proteus, Pasturella species. Some strains of *Pseudomonas aeruginosa* and *Pseudomonas* spp. are resistant to orbifloxacin and most *Enterococcus* spp. are resistant. Like other fluoroquinolones, orbifloxacin has weak activity against most anaerobes and is not a good choice when treating known or suspected anaerobic infections.

Pharmacokinetics

After oral administration in dogs or cats, orbifloxacin is apparently nearly completely absorbed. The drug is distributed well (V_d=1.5 L/kg in dogs and 1.4 L/kg in cats) and only bound slightly to plasma proteins (8% dogs; 15% cats). Orbifloxacin is eliminated primarily via the kidneys. Approximately 50% of the drug is excreted unchanged. Serum half-life is about 6 hours in both dogs and cats. Urine levels remain well above MIC's for susceptible organisms for at least 24 hours after dosing.

In horses, orbifloxacin is well absorbed after oral administration (bioavailability is about 70%) and distributes in many body fluids and endometrial tissue. Protein binding is relatively low (approx. 20%). Elimination half-life is approximately 6 hours.

Contraindications/Precautions/Warnings

Orbifloxacin, like other fluoroquinolones, can cause arthropathies in immature, growing animals. Because dogs appear to be more sensitive to this effect, the manufacturer states that the drug is contraindicated in immature dogs during the rapid growth phase (between 2–8 months in small and medium-sized breeds and up to 18 months in large and giant breeds). The drug is also contraindicated in dogs and cats known to be hypersensitive to orbifloxacin or other drugs in its class (quinolones).

The manufacturer states that orbifloxacin should be used with caution in animals with known or suspected CNS disorders (*e.g.*, seizure disorders) as, rarely, drugs in this class have been associated with CNS stimulation.

Adverse Effects

While the manufacturer reports that no adverse effects were reported during clinical studies (at 2.5. mg/kg dosing) in adult animals, higher doses or additional experience with use of the drug may demonstrate additional adverse effects. Gastrointestinal effects (anorexia, vomiting, diarrhea) would most likely be the first adverse effects noted.

Ophthalmic adverse effects are not likely in cats, but the FDA's Adverse Drug Reaction database received 10 reports (as of July 3, 2007) of blindness associated with orbifloxacin. Causal effect cannot be proven, but use higher dosages carefully.

Reproductive/Nursing Safety

Safety in breeding or pregnant dogs or cats has not been established. It is not known whether orbifloxacin enters maternal milk.

Overdosage/Acute Toxicity

Dogs and cats receiving up to 5X (37.5 mg/kg) for 30 days did not result in any significant adverse effects. Cats receiving the higher dosages exhibited soft feces and decreased body weight gains.

Drug Interactions

The following drug interactions have either been reported or are theoretical in humans or animals receiving orbifloxacin or related fluoroquinolones and may be of significance in veterinary patients:

■ **ANTACIDS/DAIRY PRODUCTS:** Containing cations (Mg^{++}, Al^{+++}, Ca^{++}) may bind to orbifloxacin and prevent its absorption; separate doses of these products by at least 2 hours

■ **ANTIBIOTICS, OTHER (aminoglycosides, 3rd-generation cephalosporins, penicillins—extended-spectrum):** Synergism may occur, but is not predictable, against some bacteria (particularly *Pseudomonas aeruginosa*) with these compounds. Although orbifloxacin has minimal activity against anaerobes, *in vitro* synergy has been reported when used with **clindamycin** against strains of Peptostreptococcus, Lactobacillus and *Bacteroides fragilis*.

■ **CYCLOSPORINE:** Fluoroquinolones may exacerbate the nephrotoxicity, and reduce the metabolism of, cyclosporine (used systemically)

■ **FLUNIXIN:** Has been shown in dogs to increase the AUC and elimination half-life of enrofloxacin and enrofloxacin increases the AUC and elimination half-life of flunixin; it is unknown if orbifloxacin also causes this effect or if other NSAIDs interact with orbifloxacin in dogs

■ **GLYBURIDE:** Severe hypoglycemia possible

■ **IRON, ZINC (oral):** Decreased orbifloxacin absorption; separate doses by at least two hours

■ **METHOTREXATE:** Increased MTX levels possible with resultant toxicity

■ **NITROFURANTOIN:** May antagonize the antimicrobial activity of the fluoroquinolones and their concomitant use is not recommended

■ **PHENYTOIN:** Orbifloxacin may alter phenytoin levels

■ **PROBENECID:** Blocks tubular secretion of ciprofloxacin and may also increase the blood level and half-life of orbifloxacin

■ **SUCRALFATE:** May inhibit absorption of orbifloxacin; separate doses of these drugs by at least 2 hours

■ **THEOPHYLLINE:** Orbifloxacin may increase theophylline blood levels

■ **WARFARIN:** Potential for increased warfarin effects

Doses

■ **DOGS/CATS:**

For susceptible infections:

Tablets:

Dogs and cats: 2.5 mg/kg–7.5 mg/kg, once daily PO. Higher end of the dosing range may be necessary in hospitalized patients, those with underlying disease (*e.g.*, malignancy) or structural alterations (*e.g.*, burns, complicated urinary tract infections, foreign body infections), infections associated with vascular compromise and infections caused by "problem" pathogens. (Package Insert; *Orbax®* —Schering)

Suspension:

Dogs: For the treatment of urinary tract infections (cystitis) in dogs caused by susceptible bacteria; and for the treatment of skin and soft tissue infections (wounds and abscesses) in dogs caused by susceptible bacteria (see package insert for actual species): 2.5–7.5 mg/kg PO once daily.

Cats: For the treatment of skin infections (wounds and abscesses) in cats caused by susceptible strains of *S. aureus*, *E. coli*,

and *P. multocida*: 7.5 mg/kg PO once daily. (Package insert; *Orbax® Suspension*—Intervet S-P)

■ **HORSES:**

For susceptible infections:

a) 5 mg/kg, once daily PO (Davis *et al.* 2006)

b) 7.5 mg/kg PO once daily (Haines *et al.* 2001)

Monitoring/Client Information

■ Efficacy is the most important monitoring parameter

■ Clients should be instructed on the importance of giving the medication as instructed and not to discontinue it on their own.

Chemistry/Synonyms

A 4-fluoroquinolone antibiotic, orbifloxacin is slightly soluble in water at neutral pH. Solubility increases in either an acidic or basic medium.

Orbifloxacin may also be known as marufloxacin or *Orbax®*.

Storage/Stability

The commercially available tablets should be stored between 2–30°C (36–86°F) and protected from excessive moisture.

The oral suspension should be stored between 2-25°C (36-77°F). It does not require refrigeration. Store upright. Shake well before use.

Compatibility/Compounding Considerations

An orbifloxacin 22.7 mg tablet crushed and mixed with mollases, dark corn syrup, water from canned tuna, Kame fish sauce, *Ora-Plus®*, *Syrplata®*, or simple syrup was relatively stable (>85% expected value) for up to 7 days when stored unrefrigerated, but protected from light. Mixing with oral supplements that contain calcium or magnesium (*e.g.*, *Lixotinic®*) showed significant inactivation of orbifloxacin by 4 days (Kukanich & Papich 2003).

Dosage Forms/Regulatory Status

VETERINARY-LABELED PRODUCTS:

Orbifloxacin Oral Tablets: 5.7 mg (yellow) in btls of 250; 22.7 mg (green; E-Z Break) in btls of 250; 68 mg (blue; E-Z Break) in btls of 100; *Orbax®* (Intervet Schering-Plough); (Rx). FDA-approved for use in dogs and cats. Federal law prohibits the use of the drug in food-producing animals.

Orbifloxacin Oral Suspension: 30mg/mL in 20 mL btls; *Orbax® Suspension* (Intervet Schering-Plough); (Rx). FDA-approved for use in dogs and cats. Federal law prohibits the use of the drug in food-producing animals.

HUMAN-LABELED PRODUCTS: None

References

Davis, J., M. Papich, et al. (2006). The pharmacokinetics of orbifloxacin in the horse following oral and intravenous administration. *J Vet Phamacol Ther* **29**(3): 191–197.

Haines, G., M. Brown, et al. (2001). Pharmacokinetics of orbifloxacin and its concentration in body fluids and in endometrial tissues of mares. *Can J Vet Res* **65**(3): 181–187.

Kukanich, B. & M. Papich (2003). Fluoroquinolone stability in vehicles for oral administration. Proceedings: ACVIM Forum. Accessed via: Veterinary Information Network. http://goo.gl/ecYeB

Ormetoprim–see

Sulfadimethoxine/Ormetoprim

OSELTAMIVIR PHOSPHATE

(oh-sell-*tam*-ih-vir)   Tamiflu®

NEURAMINIDASE INHIBITOR ANTIVIRAL

Prescriber Highlights

▶ Neuraminidase inhibitor antiviral for influenza A & B viruses; anecdotally, may be effective for parvovirus infections in dogs or other mixed bacterial/viral infections

▶ Very limited information on efficacy & safety in animals

▶ Due to public health issues, use in veterinary medicine is controversial

▶ Expense an issue, especially for treating horses

Uses/Indications

Oseltamivir has been suggested as a treatment for canine parvovirus infections. A recently published prospective, randomized, blinded, placebo-controlled clinical trial study, treated dogs showed statistically significant differences versus untreated dogs in weight gain and maintenance of white blood cell count (untreated dogs WBC's decreased). No major adverse effects were noted in the treated group. The authors concluded that while a clear advantage to oseltamivir treated dogs was not established, and the true role of oseltamivir for the treatment of parvoviral enteritis remains speculative, further investigation is warranted (Savigny & Macintire 2010). Oseltamivir may be of benefit for adjunctive treatment of other viral infections, particularly those with associated secondary bacterial components, but research or experience is lacking. A recent study performed in horses, experimentally infected with equine influenza A (H3N8), documented some efficacy in the attenuation of clinical signs (pyrexia), viral shedding, and secondary bacterial pneumonias (Yamanaka, T *et al.* 2006).

Because oseltamivir is the primary antiviral agent proposed for treatment or prophylaxis for an H5N1 influenza ("bird flu") pandemic in humans, its use in veterinary patients is controversial, particularly due to concerns of adequate drug supply for the human population and the potential for influenza virus resistance develop-

ment. In 2006, the FDA banned the extra-label use of oseltamivir and other influenza antivirals in chickens, turkeys and ducks.

Pharmacology/Actions

Oseltamivir phosphate is a prodrug that is converted after absorption into oseltamivir carboxylate, the active form of the drug. Oseltamivir carboxylate competitively inhibits influenza virus neuraminidase, an enzyme that is required for viral replication, release of virus from infected cells and the prevention of formation of viral aggregates after release from cells. Resistance to oseltamivir has been induced in the laboratory and from post-treatment isolates from infected humans. Oseltamivir or oseltamivir carboxylate do not act as substrates or inhibitors for any CYP-450 isoenzymes.

It has been postulated that oseltamivir may limit the ability of canine parvovirus to pass through intestinal mucosa and infect intestinal crypt cells. There is evidence that oseltamivir has this effect (increased mucous inactivation) on influenza viruses in the respiratory tract of humans. Additionally, it may reduce GI bacteria colonization, translocation and toxin production.

Pharmacokinetics

No information was located for the pharmacokinetic profiles of oseltamivir in dogs or cats.

In horses, oseltamivir and oseltamivir carboxylate (active metabolite) pharmacokinetics were evaluated after NG administration of 2 mg/kg. The drug was rapidly absorbed and peak levels were attained between 1-2 hours post-dose. Elimination half-lives were approximately 2 hours for oseltamivir and 2.5 hours of the carboxylate. When dosed at 2 mg/kg, the authors concluded that to maintain levels above the inhibitory concentrations against equine influenza A viruses administration intervals should be less than 10 hrs (Yamanaka, T. *et al.* 2007).

In humans, oseltamivir phosphate is readily absorbed and converted into the carboxylate (active) form predominantly via liver esterases. The bioavailability of oseltamivir carboxylate is about 75%; it is minimally bound to plasma proteins. Elimination of oseltamivir carboxylate is primarily via renal mechanisms, both glomerular filtration and tubular secretion. Elimination half-life is about 6–10 hours in patients with normal renal function. Up to 20% of a dose may be eliminated in the feces.

Contraindications/Precautions/Warnings

Oseltamivir should not be used in patients with documented hypersensitivity to it. For efficacy, treatment must begin as early as possible. Delay in treatment beyond 40 hours after the onset of clinical signs in humans with influenza is associated with minimal efficacy. Dosages may need adjustment in patients with severe renal insufficiency.

Studies where neonatal rats were administered 1 gram/kg levels of the prodrug in the brain were 1500X greater and the active metabolite was 3 times higher than those found in adult rats. Potentially, newborn puppies could exhibit similar findings; neurotoxicity is a possibility.

In 2006, the FDA banned the extra-label use of oseltamivir and other influenza antivirals in chickens, turkeys and ducks.

The UC-Davis Koret Shelter Medicine Program website (accessed October 2010) states: Oseltamivir is a drug developed for treatment of influenza in humans. This drug should not be used for treatment of canine influenza at this time. There are several reasons for this. We do not currently know the appropriate dose and duration for treatment of dogs. For best effect in humans, the drug needs to be started within 48 hours of infection. We rarely recognize canine flu this early. Most importantly, *Tamiflu®* represents a primary line of defense against a human influenza pandemic. Use of this drug may soon be restricted in order to best reserve its use for protection of human health.

Adverse Effects

Adverse effect profile in animals is not known. In the study mentioned above performed in horses, no adverse effects were noted. In humans, oseltamivir can cause gastrointestinal effects (nausea, vomiting), insomnia and vertigo. Bronchitis has been reported, but may be an artifact associated with influenza infection. Gastrointestinal effects are usually transient and may be alleviated by giving the medication with food.

Reproductive/Nursing Safety

Oseltamivir appears to be relatively safe during pregnancy. In rabbits, doses of 150 and 500 mg/kg (13X, 100X) caused dose-dependent increases of minor skeletal abnormalities. In humans, the FDA categorizes oseltamivir as category **C** for use during pregnancy (*Animal studies have shown an adverse effect on the fetus, but there are no adequate studies in humans; or there are no animal reproduction studies and no adequate studies in humans.*)

Oseltamivir and oseltamivir carboxylate have been detected in the milk of lactating rats. Safety during nursing cannot be guaranteed, but it is unlikely to pose significant risk in nursing veterinary patients.

Overdosage/Acute Toxicity

Oseltamivir has relatively low toxic potential. In humans, overdoses of up to 1000 mg have caused only nausea and vomiting.

Drug Interactions

The following drug interactions have either been reported or are theoretical in humans or animals receiving oseltamivir and may be of significance in veterinary patients:

■ **PROBENECID:** May increase 2-fold the exposure to oseltamivir carboxylate (active metabolite) by reducing tubular secretion. This could potentially be useful in reducing drug dosages or dosing frequency, or increasing serum concentrations at the usual dosage, however, supporting data is not readily available. Because of the implications associated with treating H5N1 influenza in humans, expect more information to be published on this interaction in the future. See the Probenecid monograph for more information.

■ **VACCINES, INFLUENZA (live):** Oseltamivir may potentially reduce the immune response to live influenza virus vaccines. There does not appear to be any effect on inactivated (killed) vaccines.

Laboratory Considerations
■ No concerns noted

Doses
■ **DOGS:**

For adjunctive treatment of canine parvovirus enteritis:

a) 2.2 mg/kg PO q12h. Should be administered as early as possible in the course of the disease. More data is needed to prove efficacy. (Macintire 2006)

b) 2.2 mg/kg PO twice daily for 5 days. To better insure that a vomiting patient will keep the drug down, recommend administering it 30 minutes after a chlorpromazine or other antiemetic injection. (Tams 2007)

■ **HORSES:**

For treatment of equine Influenza A:

a) 2 mg/kg PO twice daily for 5 days. Must be given early in the course of the disease to obtain satisfactory outcome. Dose used in this experimental study was based upon human pediatric dosage; not equine pharmacokinetic or pharmacodynamic data. This study also showed efficacy in reducing the clinical effects of influenza when used prophylactically. Dosage used was 2 mg/kg PO once daily for 5 days, but the authors concluded that this dosage may need to be given longer or changed for better prophylaxis. (Yamanaka, T *et al.* 2006)

Monitoring
■ Efficacy

Client Information
■ If used in veterinary patients, clients should understand the experimental nature of using this treatment

Chemistry/Synonyms

Oseltamivir phosphate occurs as a white crystalline solid. Molecular weights are 312.4 for the free base and 410.4 for the phosphate salt.

Oseltamivir phosphate may also be known as GS-4104/002, or Ro-64-0796/002 and *Tamiflu®*.

Storage/Stability

Oseltamivir capsules should be stored at 25°C, excursions are permitted to 15–30°C. The oral powder for reconstitution should be stored between 15–30°C. Once reconstituted with 23 mL of water, it should be stored at room temperature (15–30°C) or in the refrigerator (2–8°C) and protected from freezing. After reconstitution, it is stable for 10 days.

Compatibility/Compounding Considerations

A method of preparing an extemporaneously compounded oral suspension (15 mg/mL) has been published by the manufacturer of *Tamiflu®* at: http://goo.gl/pHCVk

Dosage Forms/Regulatory Status

VETERINARY-LABELED PRODUCTS: None

In 2006, the FDA banned the extra-label use of oseltamivir and other influenza antivirals in chickens, turkeys and ducks.

HUMAN-LABELED PRODUCTS:

Oseltamivir Phosphate Oral Capsules: 30 mg, 45 mg, & 75 mg (as base); *Tamiflu®* (Roche); (Rx)

Oseltamivir Phosphate Powder for Oral Suspension: 12 mg/mL (as base) after reconstitution in 25 mL bottles; *Tamiflu®* (Roche); (Rx)

References

Macintire, D. (2006). Treatment of parvoviral enteritis. Proceedings: Western Veterinary Conf 2006. Accessed via: Veterinary Information Network. http://goo.gl/0LWmI

Savigny, M.R. & D.K. Macintire (2010). Use of oseltamivir in the treatment of canine parvoviral enteritis. *Journal of Veterinary Emergency and Critical Care* 20(1): 132–142.

Tams, T. (2007). Update on management of parvoviral enteritis. Proceedings: ACVC. Accessed via: Veterinary Information Network. http://goo.gl/ZhLm8

Yamanaka, T., K. Tsujimura, et al. (2006). Efficacy of oseltamivir phosphate to horses inoculated with equine influenza A virus. *J Vet Med Sci* 68(9): 923–928.

Yamanaka, T., M. Yamada, et al. (2007). Clinical pharmacokinetics of oseltamivir and its active metabolite oseltamivir carboxylate after oral administration in horses. *Journal of Veterinary Medical Science* 69(3): 293–296.

OXACILLIN SODIUM

(ox-a-*sill*-in)

ANTI-STAPHYLOCOCCAL PENICILLIN

Prescriber Highlights

▶ Anti-staphylococcal penicillin; unavailability of appropriate dosage forms makes oral dosing impractical for animals

▶ Predominant adverse effects are GI in nature

▶ Must dose orally quite often (6–8h); owner compliance may be an issue

Uses/Indications

The veterinary use of these agents has been primarily in the treatment of bone, skin, and other soft tissue infections in small animals when penicillinase-producing Staphylococcus species have been isolated. Because of its rapid elimination with required frequent dosing, and the present unavailability of solid oral dosage forms, it is infrequently used.

Pharmacology/Actions

Cloxacillin, dicloxacillin and oxacillin have nearly identical spectrums of activity and can be considered therapeutically equivalent when comparing *in vitro* activity. These penicillinase-resistant penicillins have a narrower spectrum of activity than the natural penicillins. Their antimicrobial efficacy is aimed directly against penicillinase-producing strains of gram-positive cocci, particularly staphylococcal species. They are sometimes called anti-staphylococcal penicillins. There are documented strains of Staphylococcus that are resistant to these drugs (so-called methicillin-resistant or oxacillin-resistant Staph), but these strains have only begun to be a significant problem in veterinary species. While this class of penicillins does have activity against some other gram-positive and gram-negative aerobes and anaerobes, other antibiotics (penicillins and otherwise) are usually better choices. The penicillinase-resistant penicillins are inactive against Rickettsia, mycobacteria, fungi, Mycoplasma, and viruses.

Pharmacokinetics

Oxacillin sodium is resistant to acid inactivation in the gut, but is only partially absorbed after oral administration. The bioavailability after oral administration in humans has been reported to range from 30–35%, and, if given with food, both the rate and extent of absorption is decreased. After IM administration, oxacillin is rapidly absorbed and peak levels generally occur within 30 minutes.

The drug is distributed to the lungs, kidneys, bone, bile, pleural fluid, synovial fluid, and ascitic fluid. The volume of distribution is reportedly 0.4 L/kg in human adults and 0.3 L/kg in dogs. As with the other penicillins, only minimal amounts are distributed into the CSF, but levels are increased with meningeal inflammation. In humans, approximately 89–94% of the drug is bound to plasma proteins.

Oxacillin is partially metabolized to both active and inactive metabolites. These metabolites and the parent compound are rapidly excreted in the urine via both glomerular filtration and tubular secretion mechanisms. A small amount of the drug is also excreted in the feces via biliary elimination. The serum half-life in humans with normal renal function ranges from about 18–48 minutes. In dogs, the elimination half-life has been reported as 20–30 minutes.

Contraindications/Precautions/Warnings

Penicillins are contraindicated in patients with a history of hypersensitivity to them. Because there may be cross-reactivity, use penicillins cautiously in patients who are documented hypersensitive to other beta-lactam antibiotics (*e.g.*, cephalosporins, cefamycins, carbapenems).

Do not administer systemic antibiotics orally in patients with septicemia, shock, or other grave illnesses as absorption of the medication from the GI tract may be significantly delayed or diminished. Parenteral (preferably IV) routes should be used for these cases.

Adverse Effects
Adverse effects with the penicillins are usually not serious and have a relatively low frequency of occurrence.

Hypersensitivity reactions unrelated to dose can occur with these agents and can manifest as rashes, fever, eosinophilia, neutropenia, agranulocytosis, thrombocytopenia, leukopenia, anemias, lymphadenopathy, or full-blown anaphylaxis. In humans, it is estimated that 1-15% of patients hypersensitive to cephalosporins will also be hypersensitive to penicillins. The incidence of cross-reactivity in veterinary patients is unknown.

When given orally, penicillins may cause GI effects (anorexia, vomiting, diarrhea). Because the penicillins may also alter gut flora, antibiotic-associated diarrhea can occur and allow the proliferation of resistant bacteria in the colon (superinfections).

Neurotoxicity (*e.g.*, ataxia in dogs) has been associated with very high doses or very prolonged use. Although the penicillins are not considered hepatotoxic, elevated liver enzymes have been reported. Other effects reported in dogs include tachypnea, dyspnea, edema, and tachycardia.

Reproductive/Nursing Safety
Penicillins have been shown to cross the placenta and safe use of them during pregnancy has not been firmly established, but neither have there been any documented teratogenic problems associated with these drugs; however, use only when the potential benefits outweigh the risks. In humans, the FDA categorizes this drug as category *B* for use during pregnancy (*Animal studies have not yet demonstrated risk to the fetus, but there are no adequate studies in pregnant women; or animal studies have shown an adverse effect, but adequate studies in pregnant women have not demonstrated a risk to the fetus in the first trimester of pregnancy, and there is no evidence of risk in later trimesters.*) In a separate system evaluating the safety of drugs in canine and feline pregnancy (Papich 1989), this drug is categorized as class: *A* (*Probably safe. Although specific studies may not have proved he safety of all drugs in dogs and cats, there are no reports of adverse effects in laboratory animals or women.*)

Penicillins are excreted in maternal milk in low concentrations; use may cause diarrhea, candidiasis, or allergic response in nursing offspring.

Overdosage/Acute Toxicity
Acute oral penicillin overdoses are unlikely to cause significant problems other than GI distress, but other effects are possible (see Adverse effects). In humans, very high dosages of parenteral penicillins, especially in patients with renal disease, have induced CNS effects.

Drug Interactions
The following drug interactions have either been reported or are theoretical in humans or animals receiving oxacillin and may be of significance in veterinary patients:

- **AMINOGLYCOSIDES:** *In vitro* evidence of synergism with oxacillin against *S. aureus* strains

- **CYCLOSPORINE:** Oxacillin may reduce levels

- **PROBENECID:** Competitively blocks the tubular secretion of oxacillin, thereby increasing serum levels and serum half-lives

- **TETRACYCLINES:** Theoretical antagonism; use together usually not recommended

- **WARFARIN:** Oxacillin may cause decreased warfarin efficacy

Laboratory Considerations
- As penicillins and other beta-lactams can inactivate aminoglycosides *in vitro* (and *in vivo* in patients with renal failure), serum concentrations of **aminoglycosides** may be falsely decreased if the patient is also receiving beta-lactam antibiotics and the serum is stored prior to analysis. It is recommended that if the assay is delayed, samples be frozen and, if possible, drawn at times when the beta-lactam antibiotic is at a trough.

Doses
Note: Oxacillin is only available commercially in the USA for use as a parenteral injection and an oral suspension. For oral therapy, dicloxacillin capsules may be substituted for oxacillin.

- **DOGS/CATS:**
  For susceptible infections:
  a) 22-40 mg/kg PO, SC, IM, or IV q8h (Lappin 2003)

- **HORSES:**
  For susceptible infections:
  a) **Foals:** 20-30 mg/kg IV q6-8h (Dose extrapolated from adult horse data; use lower dose or longer interval in premature foals or those less than 7 days old.) (Brumbaugh 1999; Caprile & Short 1987)
  b) 25-50 mg/kg IM, IV twice daily (Robinson 1987)

Monitoring
- Because penicillins usually have minimal toxicity associated with their use, monitoring for efficacy is usually all that is required unless toxic signs develop. Serum levels and therapeutic drug monitoring are not routinely done with these agents.

Client Information

■ Unless otherwise instructed by the veterinarian, this drug should be given to an animal with an empty stomach, at least 1 hour before feeding or 2 hours after.

■ Keep oral solution in the refrigerator and discard any unused suspension after 14 days.

Chemistry/Synonyms

An isoxazolyl-penicillin, oxacillin sodium is a semi-synthetic penicillinase-resistant penicillin. It is available commercially as the monohydrate sodium salt, which occurs as a fine, white, crystalline powder that is odorless or has a slight odor. It is freely soluble in water and has a pK_a of about 2.8. One mg of oxacillin sodium contains not less than 815–950 micrograms of oxacillin. Each gram of the commercially available powder for injection contains 2.8 –3.1 mEq of sodium.

Oxacillin sodium may also be known as: sodium oxacillin, methylphenyl isoxazolyl penicillin (5-methyl-3-phenyl-4-isoxazolyl) penicillin sodium, oxacillinum natricum, oxacillinum natrium, P-12, or SQ-16423.

Storage/Stability

Oxacillin sodium powder for oral solution, and powder for injection should be stored at room temperature (15–30°C) in tight containers. After reconstituting with water, refrigerate and discard any remaining oral solution after 14 days. If kept at room temperature, the oral solution is stable for 3 days.

After reconstituting the sterile powder for injection with sterile water for injection or sterile sodium chloride 0.9%, the resultant solution with a concentration of 167 mg/mL is stable for 3 days at room temperature or 7 days if refrigerated. The manufacturer recommends using different quantities of diluent depending on whether the drug is to be administered IM, IV directly, or IV (piggyback). Refer to the package insert for specific instructions.

Compatibility/Compounding Considerations

Oxacillin sodium injection is reportedly physically **compatible** with the following fluids/drugs: dextrose 5% and 10% in water, dextrose 5% and 10% in sodium chloride 0.9%, lactated Ringer's injection, sodium chloride 0.9% amikacin sulfate, cephapirin sodium, chloramphenicol sodium succinate, dopamine HCl, potassium chloride, sodium bicarbonate, and verapamil.

Oxacillin sodium injection is reportedly physically **incompatible** with the following fluids/drugs: oxytetracycline HCl and tetracycline HCl. Compatibility is dependent upon factors such as pH, concentration, temperature, and diluent used; consult specialized references or a hospital pharmacist for more specific information.

Dosage Forms/Regulatory Status

VETERINARY-LABELED PRODUCTS: None

HUMAN-LABELED PRODUCTS:

Oxacillin Sodium Powder for Oral Solution: 250 mg/5 mL when reconstituted in 100 mL; generic; (Rx)

Oxacillin Sodium Powder for Injection: 500 mg, 1 gram & 2 grams in vials, *Add-Vantage* vials, and piggyback vials; 10 grams in bulk vials; generic; (Rx)

References

Brumbaugh, G. (1999). Clinical Pharmacology and the Pediatric Patient. 45th Annual AAEP Convention, Albuquerque.

Caprile, K.A. & C.R. Short (1987). Pharmacologic considerations in drug therapy in foals. *Vet Clin North Am (Equine Practice)* **3**(1): 123–144.

Lappin, M. (2003). Infectious disease. *Small Animal Internal Medicine, 3rd Ed.* R Nelson and C Couto Eds. St Louis, Mosby: 12229–11321.

Papich, M. (1989). Effects of drugs on pregnancy. *Current Veterinary Therapy X: Small Animal Practice.* R Kirk Ed. Philadelphia, Saunders: 1291–1299.

Robinson, N.E. (1987). Table of Common Drugs: Approximate Doses. *Current Therapy in Equine Medicine, 2.* NE Robinson Ed. Philadelphia, W.B. Saunders: 761.

OXAZEPAM

(ox-a-ze-pam)   Serax®

BENZODIAZEPINE

Prescriber Highlights

▶ Benzodiazepine used primarily as an appetite stimulant in cats, but may also be useful to treat behavior problems in dogs or cats

▶ Contraindications: Known benzodiazepine hypersensitivity, acute narrow angle glaucoma. Caution: Myasthenia gravis, hepatic dysfunction, seizure disorders.

▶ Adverse Effects: Primarily sedation & occasionally, ataxia.

▶ Possibly teratogenic

▶ C-IV Controlled substance

Uses/Indications

Oxazepam is used most frequently in small animal medicine as an appetite stimulant in cats and dogs. It may also be useful as an oral anxiolytic agent for adjunctive therapy of behavior-related disorders for both dogs and cats. Like lorazepam, it does not have any active metabolites so it may be a good choice for treating geriatric patients and those with liver dysfunction. Use in feline patients with liver dysfunction is somewhat controversial, as it has been anecdotally reported that oxazepam has been associated with fulminant hepatic failure in cats.

Pharmacology/Actions

The subcortical levels (primarily limbic, thalamic, and hypothalamic) of the CNS are depressed by oxazepam and other benzodiazepines thus producing the anxiolytic, sedative, skeletal muscle relaxant and anticonvulsant effects seen. The exact mechanism of action is unknown, but postulated mechanisms include: antagonism of serotonin, increased release of gamma-aminobutyric acid (GABA) and/or facilitation of GABA activity, and diminished release or turnover of acetylcholine in the CNS. Benzodiazepine specific receptors have been located in the mammalian brain, kidney, liver, lung, and heart. In all species studied, receptors are lacking in the white matter.

Pharmacokinetics

Oxazepam is absorbed from the GI tract, but it is one of the more slowly absorbed oral benzodiazepines. Oxazepam, like other benzodiazepines is widely distributed; it is highly bound to plasma proteins (97% in humans). While not confirmed, oxazepam may cross the placenta and enter maternal milk. Oxazepam is principally conjugated in the liver via glucuronidation to an inactive metabolite. Serum half-life in humans ranges from 3–21 hours.

Contraindications/Precautions/Warnings

Oxazepam is contraindicated in patients who are hypersensitive to it or other benzodiazepines or have acute narrow angle glaucoma. Benzodiazepines have been reported to exacerbate myasthenia gravis. While oxazepam is less susceptible to accumulation than many other benzodiazepines in patients with hepatic dysfunction, it should be used with caution nonetheless.

Use in feline patients with liver dysfunction is somewhat controversial, as it has been anecdotally reported that rarely, oxazepam has been associated with fulminant hepatic failure in cats.

Adverse Effects

The most prevalent adverse effects seen with oxazepam in small animals is sedation and occasionally, ataxia. These may be transient and dosage adjustment may be required to alleviate. Paradoxical effects such as excitability, vocalization or aggression are possible. When used to treat negative behaviors, a rebound effect can occur, particularly if the drug is not withdrawn slowly.

Rarely, oxazepam has reportedly precipitated tonic-clonic seizures; use with caution in susceptible patients. Potentially, oxazepam could cause hepatic toxicity in cats, but this occurs very rarely.

Reproductive/Nursing Safety

Safe use during pregnancy has not been established; teratogenic effects of similar benzodiazepines have been noted in rabbits and rats. In humans, the FDA categorizes this drug as category **D** for use during pregnancy (*There is evidence of human fetal risk, but the potential benefits from the use of the drug in pregnant women may be acceptable despite its potential risks.*)

Benzodiazepines are excreted in maternal milk. Since neonates metabolize benzodiazepines more slowly than adults do, accumulation of the drug and its metabolites to toxic levels is possible. Chronic diazepam use in nursing mothers reportedly caused human infants to be lethargic and lose weight; avoid the use of benzodiazepines in nursing patients.

Overdosage/Acute Toxicity

When used alone, oxazepam overdoses are generally limited to significant CNS depression (confusion, coma, decreased reflexes, etc.). Treatment of significant overdoses consists of standard protocols for removing and/or binding the drug (if taken orally) in the gut, and supportive systemic measures. The use of analeptic agents, (CNS stimulants such as caffeine, amphetamines, etc.) are generally not recommended. Flumazenil could potentially be used in life-threatening overdoses.

Drug Interactions

The following drug interactions have either been reported or are theoretical in humans or animals receiving oxazepam and may be of significance in veterinary patients:

- **CNS DEPRESSANT DRUGS:** If oxazepam administered with other CNS depressant agents (**barbiturates, narcotics, anesthetics,** etc.) additive effects may occur

- **PHENYTOIN:** May decrease oxazepam concentrations

- **PROBENECID:** May impair glucuronide conjugation (in dogs) and prolong effects

- **RIFAMPIN:** May induce hepatic microsomal enzymes and decrease the pharmacologic effects of benzodiazepines

- **ST. JOHN'S WORT:** May decrease oxazepam effectiveness

- **THEOPHYLLINES:** May decrease oxazepam effectiveness

Laboratory Considerations

- Benzodiazepines may decrease the thyroidal uptake of I^{123} or I^{131}.

Doses

- **DOGS:**

  For treating fears and phobias:

  a) 0.2–0.5 mg/kg PO q12–24h (Siebert 2003)

  b) 0.2–1 mg/kg PO q12–24h (Virga 2002; Virga 2007)

  c) 0.2–1 mg/kg one to two times a day (Landsberg 2005)

  d) 0.04–0.5 mg/kg PO q6h. The lowest dose and longest frequency between doses that alleviate the fear should be used. (Crowell-Davis 2008)

- **CATS:**

  As an appetite stimulant:

  a) 2 mg per cat (total dose) every 12 hours (Hartke *et al.* 1992)(Hodgkins & Franks 1991)

b) In cats with hepatic lipidosis, if cat has a small interest in eating: 0.1–0.3 mg/kg PO q12–24h (Twedt 2005)

c) 0.25–0.5 mg/kg PO one to two times daily. (Sparkes 2005)

For behavior-related conditions:

a) For treating fears and phobias: 1–2.5 mg per cat (total dose) PO every 12 hours (Siebert 2003)

b) For treating fears and phobias 0.2–0.5 mg/kg PO q12–24h (Virga 2002; Virga 2007)

c) For feline urine marking: 0.2–0.5 mg/kg PO once to twice a day. (Landsberg 2007)

d) For spraying or overgrooming: 0.2–0.5 mg/kg PO q12–24h (Seksel 2006)

e) For fears and phobias: 0.2–1 mg/kg PO q12h PO q6h. The lowest dose and longest frequency between doses that alleviate the fear should be used. (Crowell-Davis 2008)

Monitoring
■ Efficacy
■ Adverse effects

Client Information
■ Caution clients not to discontinue medication or adjust dosage without first checking with veterinarian.
■ Efficacy for anorexia may be improved if given just prior to feeding as effects are generally seen within 30 minutes.

Chemistry/Synonyms
A benzodiazepine, oxazepam occurs as a creamy white to pale yellow powder. It is practically insoluble in water.

Oxazepam may also be known as: oxazepamum, Wy-3498, and *Serax®*.

Storage/Stability
Store oxazepam capsules and tablets at room temperature in well-closed containers.

Dosage Forms/Regulatory Status
VETERINARY-LABELED PRODUCTS: None

The ARCI (Racing Commissioners International) has designated this drug as a class 2 substance. See the appendix for more information.

HUMAN-LABELED PRODUCTS:
Oxazepam Capsules: 10 mg, 15 mg & 30 mg; generic; (Rx; C-IV)

References
Crowell-Davis, S.L. (2008). Benzodiazepines: Pros and Cons for Fear and Anxiety. *Compendium-Continuing Education for Veterinarians* **30**(10): 526–+.
Hartke, J., J. Rojko, et al. (1992). Cachexia associated with cancer and immunodeficiency in cats. *Current Veterinary Therapy XI: Small Animal Practice.* R Kirk and J Bonagura Eds. Philadelphia, W.B. Saunders Company: 438–441.
Hodgkins, E. & P. Franks (1991). Nutritional requirements of the sick cat. *Consultations in Feline Internal Medicine.* J August Ed. Philadelphia, W.B. Saunders Company: 25–34.
Landsberg, G. (2005). Fear, anxiety and phobias—Diagnosis and treatment. Proceedings: ACVC 2005. Accessed via: Veterinary Information Network. http://goo.gl/HXM4j
Landsberg, G. (2007). Drug and natural alternatives for marking cats. Proceedings: Western Vet Conference. Accessed via: Veterinary Information Network. http://goo.gl/ro1SR
Seksel, K. (2006). Anxiety disorders in cats. Proceedings: Western Vet Conf. Accessed via: Veterinary Information Network. http://goo.gl/IyuKJ
Siebert, L. (2003). Psychoactive drugs in behavioral medicine. Western Veterinary Conference.
Sparkes, A. (2005). Assessing and tempting the 'finicky' cat. Proceedings: Western Vet Conf. Accessed via: Veterinary Information Network. http://goo.gl/43nyt
Twedt, D. (2005). The yellow cat: Updates on hepatic lipidosis. Proceediings: ACVC.
Virga, V. (2002). Which drug and why: An update on psychopharmacology. Proceedings: Atlantic Coast Veterinary Conference. Accessed via: Veterinary Information Network. http://goo.gl/m8qr4
Virga, V. (2007). Veterinary Psychopharmacology: Applications in Clinical Practice. Proceedings: ACVC. Accessed via: Veterinary Information Network. http://goo.gl/84nue

---

OXFENDAZOLE

(ox-*fen*-da-zole)   Synanthic®

ANTIPARASITIC AGENT (ANTHELMINTIC)

Prescriber Highlights

▶ Benzimidazole anthelmintic used primarily in cattle

▶ Contraindications: Not for use in female dairy cattle of breeding age

▶ Caution: Debilitated or sick horses; 7 day slaughter withdrawal in cattle

▶ Adverse Effects: Unlikely; hypersensitivity possible

Uses/Indications
Oxfendazole (*Synanthic®*) is indicated in cattle for the removal and control of lungworms, roundworms (including inhibited forms of *Ostertagia ostertagi*) and tapeworms.

Oxfendazole as *Benzelmin®* was indicated (no longer marketed in the USA) for the removal of the following parasites in horses: large roundworms (*Parascaris equorum*), large strongyles (*S. edentatus, S. equinus, S. vulgaris*), small strongyles, and pinworms (*Oxyuris equi*).

Oxfendazole has also been used extra-label in sheep, goats, and swine; see Dosage section for more information.

Pharmacology/Actions
Benzimidazole antiparasitic agents have a broad spectrum of activity against a variety of pathogenic internal parasites. In susceptible parasites, their mechanism of action is believed due to disrupting intracellular microtubular transport systems by binding selectively and damaging tubulin, preventing tubulin polymerization, and inhibiting microtubule formation. Benzimidazoles also act at higher concen-

trations to disrupt metabolic pathways within the helminth, and inhibit metabolic enzymes, including malate dehydrogenase and fumarate reductase.

Pharmacokinetics

Limited information is available regarding this compound's pharmacokinetics. Unlike most of the other benzimidazole compounds, oxfendazole is absorbed more readily from the GI tract. The elimination half-life has been reported to be about 7.5 hours in sheep and 5.25 hours in goats. Absorbed oxfendazole is metabolized (and vice-versa) to the active compound, fenbendazole (sulfoxide) and the sulfone.

After a single oral dose of 50 mg/kg to dogs, oxfendazole levels peaked at 8 hours. Elimination half-lives for the parent compound and the sulfoxide metabolite (active) were both about 5.5 hours. In dogs, oxfendazole plasma concentrations were significantly higher and resident times longer than that of either fenbendazole or albendazole following single oral administration at the same dose (50 mg/kg) (Gokbulut *et al.* 2007).

Contraindications/Precautions/Warnings

Not for use in female dairy cattle of breeding age. A 7 day slaughter withdrawal is required when using at labeled doses.

There are no contraindications to using this drug in horses, but it is recommended to use oxfendazole cautiously in debilitated or sick horses.

Adverse Effects

When used as labeled, it is unlikely any adverse effects will be noted. Hypersensitivity reactions secondary to antigen release by dying parasites are theoretically possible, particularly at high dosages.

Reproductive/Nursing Safety

Oxfendazole may be safely used in pregnant mares and foals.

Overdosage/Acute Toxicity

Doses of 10 times those recommended elicited no adverse reactions in horses tested. It is unlikely that this compound would cause serious toxicity when given alone.

Drug Interactions

The following drug interactions have either been reported or are theoretical in humans or animals receiving oxfendazole and may be of significance in veterinary patients:

■ **BROMSALAN FLUKICIDES (dibromsalan, tribromsalan):** Oxfendazole should not be given concurrently with these agents; abortions in cattle and death in sheep have been reported after using these compounds together

Doses

■ **DOGS:**
  a) For *Oslerus osleri*: 10 mg/kg PO once daily for 28 days. (Bowman 2006)

■ **HORSES:**
  a) For susceptible parasites: 10 mg/kg PO (Roberson 1988), (Package insert; *Benzelmin®*—Fort Dodge)

■ **CATTLE:**
  a) For susceptible parasites: 4.5 mg/kg either PO or via intraruminal injection (22.5% only). May repeat in 4–6 weeks. Dose of the 9.06% suspension is 2.5 mL per 100 lb (50 kg) of body weight PO. Dose of the 22.5% suspension is 1 mL per 100 lb (50 kg) of body weight either PO or intraruminal injection. See package label for specific directions if giving by intraruminal injection. (Package inserts; *Synanthic®* 9.06% and 22.5%—Fort Dodge)

■ **SWINE:**
  a) For susceptible parasites: 3–4.5 mg/kg PO (Roberson 1988)

■ **SHEEP:**
  a) For susceptible parasites: 5 mg/kg PO (Brander *et al.* 1982; Roberson 1988)

■ **GOATS:**
  a) For susceptible parasites: 7.5 mg/kg PO (Roberson 1988)

Monitoring

■ Efficacy

Client Information

■ Not to be used in horses intended for food purposes

■ Shake suspension well

■ Slaughter withdrawal in cattle is 7 days; not FDA-approved for lactating dairy cattle

Chemistry/Synonyms

A benzimidazole anthelmintic, oxfendazole occurs as white or almost white powder possessing a characteristic odor. It is practically insoluble in water. Oxfendazole is the sulfoxide metabolite of fenbendazole.

Oxfendazole may also be known as RS 8858; there are many international trade names.

Storage/Stability

Unless otherwise directed by the manufacturer, oxfendazole products should be stored at room temperature and protected from light. The manufacturer recommends discarding any unused suspension 24 hours after it has been reconstituted.

Dosage Forms/Preparations/Regulatory Status

VETERINARY-LABELED PRODUCTS:

Oxfendazole Oral Suspension: 9.06% in 1 liter and 4 liter; *Synanthic®* (BIVI); (OTC). FDA-approved for use in beef cattle and in female dairy cattle not of breeding age. Because a withdrawal time in milk has not been established, do not use in female dairy cattle of breeding age. At recommended dosages, slaughter withdrawal is 7 days.

Oxfendazole Oral Suspension: 22.5% in 500 mL and 1 liter; *Synanthic®* (BIVI); (Rx). FDA-approved for use in beef cattle and in female dairy cattle not of breeding age. Because a withdrawal time in milk has not been established, do not use in female dairy cattle of breeding age. At recommended dosages, slaughter withdrawal is 7 days.

HUMAN-LABELED PRODUCTS: None

References

Bowman, D. (2006). Canine respiratory parasites—a review. Proceedings: ACVC. Accessed via: Veterinary Information Network. http://goo.gl/g5qQR

Brander, C.G., D.M. Pugh, et al. (1982). *Veterinary Applied Pharmacology and Therapeutics*. London, Baillière Tindall.

Gokbulut, C., A. Bilgili, et al. (2007). Comparative plasma disposition of fenbendazole, oxfendazole and albendazole in dogs. *Veterinary Parasitology* **148**(3–4): 279–287.

Roberson, E.L. (1988). Antinematodal Agents. *Veterinary Pharmacology and Therapeutics*. NH Booth and LE McDonald Eds. Ames, Iowa State University Press: 882–927.

OXIBENDAZOLE

(ox-i-**ben**-da-zole)   Anthelcide EQ®

ANTIPARASITIC AGENT (ANTHELMINTIC)

Prescriber Highlights

▶ Benzimidazole anthelmintic used primarily in horses

▶ Resistance development an ongoing issue

▶ Contraindications: Severely debilitated horses or in horses suffering from colic, toxemia or infectious disease.

▶ Adverse Effects: Unlikely; hypersensitivity possible

Uses/Indications

Oxibendazole is indicated (labeled) for the removal of the following parasites in horses: large roundworms (*Parascaris equorum*), large strongyles (*S. edentatus, S. equinus, S. vulgaris*), small strongyles, threadworms, and pinworms (*Oxyuris equi*). Resistance to antiparasitic agents is an ongoing problem. It is recommended to perform fecal egg count reduction testing (FECRT) for strongyle nematodes. A value of less than 90% in 5-10 horses is the suggested cut-off for determining resistance on a given farm (Kaplan & Nielsen 2010).

Oxibendazole has also been used in cattle, sheep, and swine; see Dosage section for more information.

Pharmacology/Actions

Benzimidazole antiparasitic agents have a broad spectrum of activity against a variety of pathogenic internal parasites. In susceptible parasites, their mechanism of action is believed due to disrupting intracellular microtubular transport systems by binding selectively and damaging tubulin, preventing tubulin polymerization, and inhibiting microtubule formation. Benzimidazoles also act at higher concentrations to disrupt metabolic pathways within the helminth, and inhibit metabolic enzymes, including malate dehydrogenase and fumarate reductase.

Pharmacokinetics

No information was located.

Contraindications/Precautions/Warnings

Oxibendazole is stated by the manufacturer to be contraindicated in severely debilitated horses or in horses suffering from colic, toxemia, or infectious disease.

Adverse Effects

When used in horses at recommended doses, it is unlikely any adverse effects would be seen. Hypersensitivity reactions secondary to antigen release by dying parasites are theoretically possible, particularly at high dosages.

Oxibendazole in combination with diethylcarbamazine (*Filaribits Plus®*) was implicated in causing periportal hepatitis in dogs when it was marketed (1980s).

Reproductive/Nursing Safety

Oxibendazole is considered safe to use in pregnant mares.

Overdosage/Acute Toxicity

Doses of 60 times those recommended elicited no adverse reactions in horses tested. It is unlikely that this compound would cause serious toxicity when given alone to horses.

Drug Interactions

■ No significant interactions have been reported

Doses

■ **HORSES:**
For susceptible parasites:
a) 10 mg/kg PO; 15 mg/kg PO for strongyloides; horses maintained on premises where reinfection is likely to occur should be retreated in 6–8 weeks. (Package insert; *Anthelcide EQ®*—Pfizer)
b) 10 mg/kg, PO (Roberson 1988; Robinson 1987)

■ **CATTLE:**
For susceptible parasites:
a) 10–20 mg/kg PO (Brander *et al.* 1982)

■ **SWINE:**
For susceptible parasites:
a) 15 mg/kg, PO (Roberson 1988)

■ **SHEEP:**
For susceptible parasites:
a) 10–20 mg/kg PO (Brander *et al.* 1982)

Monitoring

■ Efficacy

Client Information

■ Protect suspension from freezing

■ Shake suspension well before using

■ Not for use in horses intended for food

Chemistry/Synonyms

A benzimidazole anthelmintic, oxibendazole occurs as a white powder that is practically insoluble in water.

Oxibendazole may also be known as SKF-30310 and *Anthelcide EQ®* and in the U.K. by the proprietary names: *Dio®* (Alan Hitchings), *Equidin®* (Univet), *Equitac®* (SKF) or *Loditac®* (SKF).

Storage/Stability

Unless otherwise directed by the manufacturer, oxibendazole products should be stored at room temperature; protect from freezing.

Dosage Forms/Regulatory Status

VETERINARY-LABELED PRODUCTS:

Oxibendazole Suspension: 100 mg/mL (10%) in gallons. *Anthelcide EQ® Suspension* (Pfizer); (Rx). FDA-approved for use in horses not used for food.

Oxibendazole Oral Paste: 227 mg/gram (22.7%) in 24-gram syringes. *Anthelcide EQ® Paste* (Pfizer); (OTC). FDA-approved for use in horses not used for food.

HUMAN-LABELED PRODUCTS: None

References

Brander, C.G., D.M. Pugh, et al. (1982). *Veterinary Applied Pharmacology and Therapeutics*. London, Baillière Tindall.

Kaplan, R.M. & M.K. Nielsen (2010). An evidence-based approach to equine parasite control: It ain't the 60s anymore. *Equine Veterinary Education* 22(6): 306–316.

Roberson, E.L. (1988). Antinematodal Agents. *Veterinary Pharmacology and Therapeutics*. NH Booth and LE McDonald Eds. Ames, Iowa State University Press: 882–927.

Robinson, N.E. (1987). Table of Common Drugs: Approximate Doses. *Current Therapy in Equine Medicine, 2*. NE Robinson Ed. Philadelphia, W.B. Saunders: 761.

OXYBUTYNIN CHLORIDE

(ox-i-*byoo*-tin-in)   Ditropan®, Oxytrol®

GENITOURINARY SMOOTH MUSCLE RELAXANT

Prescriber Highlights

▶ Urinary antispasmodic potentially useful in dogs or cats

▶ Cautions (risk vs. benefit): Obstructive GI tract disease or intestinal atony/paralytic ileus, angle closure glaucoma, hiatal hernia, cardiac disease (particularly associated with mitral stenosis, associated arrhythmias, tachycardia, CHF, etc.), myasthenia gravis, hyperthyroidism, prostatic hypertrophy, severe ulcerative colitis, urinary retention, or other obstructive uropathies

▶ Adverse Effects: Diarrhea, constipation, urinary retention, hypersalivation, & sedation

Uses/Indications

Oxybutynin may be useful for the adjunctive therapy of detrusor hyperreflexia in dogs and in cats with FeLV-associated detrusor instability.

Pharmacology/Actions

Considered a urinary antispasmodic, oxybutynin has direct antimuscarinic (atropine-like) and spasmolytic (papaverine-like) effects on smooth muscle. Spasmolytic effects appear to be most predominant on the detrusor muscle of the bladder and small and large intestine. It does not have appreciable effects on vascular smooth muscle. Studies done in patients with neurogenic bladders showed that oxybutynin increased bladder capacity, reduced the frequency of uninhibited contractions of the detrusor muscle and delayed initial desire to void. Effects were more pronounced in patients with uninhibited neurogenic bladders than in patients with reflex neurogenic bladders. Other effects noted in lab animal studies include moderate antihistaminic, local anesthetic, mild analgesic, very low mydriatic, and antisialagogue effects.

Pharmacokinetics

Oxybutynin is apparently rapidly and well absorbed from the GI tract. Studies done in rats show the drug distributed into the brain, lungs, kidneys, and liver. While elimination characteristics have not been well documented, oxybutynin apparently is metabolized in the liver and excreted in the urine. In humans, the duration of action is from 6–10 hours after a dose.

Contraindications/Precautions/Warnings

Because of the drug's pharmacologic actions, oxybutynin should be used when its benefits outweigh its risks if the following conditions are present: obstructive GI tract disease or intestinal atony/paralytic ileus, angle closure glaucoma, hiatal hernia, cardiac disease (particularly associated with mitral stenosis, associated arrhythmias, tachycardia, CHF, etc.), myasthenia gravis, hyperthyroidism, prostatic hypertrophy, severe ulcerative colitis, urinary retention or other obstructive uropathies.

Adverse Effects
While use in small animals is limited, diarrhea, constipation, urinary retention, hypersalivation, and sedation have been reported. Other adverse effects reported in humans, and potentially seen in animals, primarily result from the drug's pharmacologic effects, including: dry mouth or eyes, tachycardia, anorexia, vomiting, weakness, or mydriasis.

Reproductive/Nursing Safety
While safety during pregnancy has not been firmly established, studies in a variety of lab animals have demonstrated no teratogenic effect associated with the drug. In humans, the FDA categorizes this drug as category *B* for use during pregnancy (*Animal studies have not yet demonstrated risk to the fetus, but there are no adequate studies in pregnant women; or animal studies have shown an adverse effect, but adequate studies in pregnant women have not demonstrated a risk to the fetus in the first trimester of pregnancy, and there is no evidence of risk in later trimesters.*)

It is not known whether this drug is excreted in maternal milk. While oxybutynin may inhibit lactation, no documented problems associated with its use in nursing offspring have been noted.

Overdosage/Acute Toxicity
Overdosage may cause CNS effects (*e.g.*, restlessness, excitement, seizures), cardiovascular effects (*e.g.*, hyper- or hypotension, tachycardia, circulatory failure), fever, nausea or vomiting. Massive overdoses may lead to paralysis, coma, respiratory failure and death. Treatment of overdoses should consist of general techniques to limit absorption of the drug from the GI tract and supportive care as required; intravenous physostigmine may be useful. See the atropine monograph for more information on the use of physostigmine.

Drug Interactions
The following drug interactions have either been reported in humans or animals receiving oxybutynin and may be of significance in veterinary patients:

■ **ANTICHOLINERGIC AGENTS (e.g., atropine, propantheline, scopolamine, isopropamide, glycopyrrolate, hyoscyamine, tricyclic antidepressants, disopyramide, procainamide, antihistamines, etc.):** May intensify oxybutynin's anticholinergic effects

■ **AZOLE ANTIFUNGALS (ketoconazole, etc.):** May increase oxybutynin levels

■ **CNS DEPRESSANTS:** Other sedating drugs may exacerbate the sedating effects of oxybutynin

■ **MACROLIDE ANTIBIOTICS (erythromycin, clarithromycin):** May increase oxybutynin levels

Doses

■ **DOGS:**
To decrease bladder contractility (detrusor hyperreflexia):
a) 0.2 mg/kg PO q8–12h; most dogs are dosed at 1.25–3.75 mg (total dose) q12h. Juvenile animals may require a prolonged dosing interval. (Lane 2000)
b) 1.25–5 mg (total dose) PO q8–12h (Bartges 2003; Bartges 2009)
c) 2–5 mg (total dose) PO q8–12h (Vernau 2006)

■ **CATS:**
To decrease bladder contractility (detrusor hyperreflexia):
a) 0.5–1 mg (total dose) PO q8–12h. Juvenile animals may require a prolonged dosing interval. (Lane 2000)
b) 0.5–1.25 mg per cat PO q8–12h (Osborne *et al.* 2000)(Bartges 2003; Polzin 2005)

Monitoring
■ Efficacy
■ Adverse effects

Chemistry/Synonyms
A synthetic tertiary amine, oxybutynin chloride occurs as white to off-white crystals. It is freely soluble in water.

Oxybutynin chloride may also be known as: oxybutinyn HCl, 5058, MJ-4309-1, oxybutynini hydrochloridum, *Ditropan®* and *Oxytrol®*.

Storage/Stability
Tablets and oral solution should be stored at room temperature in tight containers. Protect oral solution from light. Tablets have an expiration date of 4 years after manufacture.

Dosage Forms/Regulatory Status
VETERINARY-LABELED PRODUCTS: None

HUMAN-LABELED PRODUCTS:

Oxybutynin Chloride Oral Tablets: 5 mg; generic; (Rx)

Oxybutynin Chloride Oral Extended release tablets: 5 mg, 10 mg & 15 mg; *Ditropan® XL* (Janssen); generic; (Rx)

Oxybutynin Chloride Oral Syrup: 1 mg/mL in 473 mL; generic; (Rx)

Oxybutynin Chloride Transdermal System, Topical: 36 mg of oxybutynin delivering 3.9 mg/day in 39 cm^2 system; *Oxytrol®* (Watson); (Rx)

Oxybutynin Topical Gel: 10% in 1 gram sachets; *Gelnique®* (Watson); (Rx)

References

Bartges, J. (2003). Canine lower urinary tract cases. Proceedings: ACVIM Forum. Accessed via: Veterinary Information Network. http://goo.gl/HH41u

Bartges, J. (2009). Pipes are leaking: Urinary Incontinence. Proceedings: WVC. Accessed via: Veterinary Information Network. http://goo.gl/X51gQ

Lane, I. (2000). Use of anticholinergic agents in lower urinary tract disease. *Kirk's Current Veterinary Therapy: XIII Small Animal Practice.* J Bonagura Ed. Philadelphia, WB Saunders: 899– 902.

Osborne, C., J. Kruger, et al. (2000). Feline Lower Urinary Tract Diseases. *Textbook of Veterinary Internal Medicine: Diseases of the Dog and Cat.* S Ettinger and E Feldman Eds. Philadelphia, WB Saunders. 2: 1710– 1747.

Polzin, D. (2005). Urinary Tract Therapeutics—What, When & How. Proceedings: ACVC. Accessed via: Veterinary Information Network. http://goo.gl/jRZ0n

Vernau, K. (2006). Dysuria: To pee or not to pee . . . Proceedings: UCD Veterinary Neurology Symposium. Accessed via: Veterinary Information Network. http://goo.gl/3KvT8

OXYMORPHONE HCL

(ox-ee-*mor*-fone)   Numorphan®

OPIATE AGONIST

Prescriber Highlights

▶ Injectable opiate sedative/restraining agent, analgesic, & preanesthetic

▶ Contraindications: Hypersensitivity to it, diarrhea caused by a toxic ingestion. Extreme Caution: Respiratory disease or acute respiratory dysfunction. Caution: Hypothyroidism, severe renal insufficiency (acute uremia), adrenocortical insufficiency, geriatric or severely debilitated patients, head injuries or increased intracranial pressure & acute abdominal conditions (e.g., colic).

▶ Adverse Effects: Respiratory depression & bradycardia. Decreased GI motility with resultant constipation possible. Cats (high dosages): ataxia, hyperesthesia, & behavioral changes (without concomitant tranquilization)

▶ Availability & expense are issues

▶ C-II controlled substance

Uses/Indications

Oxymorphone is used in dogs and cats as a sedative/restraining agent, analgesic, and preanesthetic; occasionally in horses as an analgesic and anesthesia induction agent. It may also be used in swine as an adjunctive analgesic with ketamine/xylazine anesthesia and small rodents as an analgesic/anesthetic for minor surgical procedures.

Oxymorphone is effective for moderate to severe pain and its effects on the cardiovascular system are usually not clinically significant. It causes less histamine release than morphine.

In a study done in dogs, oxymorphone was comparable to hydromorphone in potency and efficacy for pain control. Patients receiving hydromorphone vomited more than when oxymorphone was used, but hydromorphone was significantly less expensive (Bateman *et al.* 2008).

Pharmacology/Actions

Receptors for opiate analgesics are found in high concentrations in the limbic system, spinal cord, thalamus, hypothalamus, striatum, and midbrain. They are also found in tissues such as the gastrointestinal tract, urinary tract, and other smooth muscle.

The morphine-like agonists (morphine, meperidine, oxymorphone) have primary activity at the *mu* receptors, with some activity possible at the *delta* receptor. The primary pharmacologic effects of these agents include: analgesia, antitussive activity, respiratory depression, sedation, emesis, physical dependence, and intestinal effects (constipation/defecation). Secondary pharmacologic effects include: *CNS*: euphoria, sedation, and confusion. *Cardiovascular*: bradycardia due to central vagal stimulation, alpha-adrenergic receptors may be depressed resulting in peripheral vasodilation, decreased peripheral resistance, and baroreceptor inhibition. Orthostatic hypotension and syncope may occur. *Urinary*: Increased bladder sphincter tone can induce urinary retention.

Various species may exhibit contradictory effects from these agents. For example, horses, cattle, swine, and cats may develop excitement after morphine injections and dogs may defecate after morphine. These effects are in contrast to the expected effects of sedation and constipation. Dogs and humans may develop miosis, while other species (especially cats) may develop mydriasis. For more information, see the individual monographs for each agent.

Oxymorphone is approximately 10 times more potent an analgesic on a per weight basis when compared to morphine. It has less antitussive activity than morphine. In humans, it has more of a tendency to cause increased nausea and vomiting than does morphine, while in dogs the opposite appears to be true. At the usual doses employed, oxymorphone alone has good sedative qualities in the dog. Respiratory depression can occur especially in debilitated, neonatal or geriatric patients. Bradycardia, as well as a slight decrease in cardiac contractility and blood pressure, may also be seen. Like morphine, oxymorphone does initially increase the respiratory rate (panting in dogs) while actual oxygenation may be decreased and blood CO_2 levels may increase by 10 mmHg or more. Oxymorphone may cause more panting in dogs than morphine. Gut motility is decreased with resultant increases in stomach emptying times. Unlike either morphine or meperidine, oxymorphone does not appear to cause histamine release when administered IV and may cause less excitement than morphine.

Pharmacokinetics

Oxymorphone is absorbed when given by IV, IM, SC, and rectal routes. Although absorbed when given orally, bioavailability is reduced, probably from a high first-pass effect. After IV administration, analgesic efficacy usually occurs within 3–5 minutes. After 0.1 mg/kg IM administration to dogs, onset of action is about 15 minutes and duration of effect, 2-4 hours.

Like morphine, oxymorphone concentrates in the kidney, liver, and lungs; lower levels are found in the CNS. Oxymorphone crosses the placenta and narcotized newborns can result if mothers are given the drug before giving birth, but these effects can be rapidly reversed with naloxone.

The drug is metabolized in the liver; primarily by glucuronidation. Because cats are deficient in this metabolic pathway, half-lives in cats are probably prolonged. The kidneys excrete the glucuronidated metabolite.

Contraindications/Precautions/Warnings

All opiates should be used with caution in patients with hypothyroidism, severe renal insufficiency, adrenocortical insufficiency (Addison's), and in geriatric or severely debilitated patients. Oxymorphone is contraindicated in patients hypersensitive to narcotic analgesics, those receiving monamine oxidase inhibitors (MAOIs), or with diarrhea caused by a toxic ingestion until the toxin is eliminated from the GI tract.

Oxymorphone should be used with extreme caution in patients with head injuries, increased intracranial pressure or acute abdominal conditions (*e.g.*, colic) as it may obscure the diagnosis or clinical course of these conditions and suffering from respiratory disease or from acute respiratory dysfunction (*e.g.*, pulmonary edema secondary to smoke inhalation).

Oxymorphone can cause bradycardia and, therefore, should be used cautiously in patients with preexisting bradyarrhythmias.

In horses, opiates can mask the behavioral and cardiovascular clinical signs associated with mild colic.

Neonatal, debilitated, or geriatric patients may be more susceptible to the effects of oxymorphone and may require lower dosages. Patients with severe hepatic disease may have prolonged duration's of action of the drug. If used in cats at high dosages, it is recommended the drug be given along with a tranquilizing agent as oxymorphone can produce bizarre behavioral changes in this species. This also is true in cats for the other opiate agents, such as morphine.

Opiate analgesics are also contraindicated in patients who have been stung by the scorpion species *Centruroides sculpturatus* Ewing and *C. gertschi* Stahnke as it may potentiate these venoms.

Adverse Effects

Oxymorphone may cause respiratory depression and bradycardia (see above). Panting is commonly seen in dogs. When used in cats at high dosages, oxymorphone may cause ataxia, hyperesthesia, and behavioral changes such as hyperexcitability or aggression (without concomitant tranquilization). Decreased GI motility with resultant constipation has been described.

In horses, opiates may cause CNS excitement and pretreatment with drugs such as xylazine are usually administered to reduce the behavioral changes these drugs can cause.

Reproductive/Nursing Safety

In humans, the FDA categorizes this drug as category *C* for use during pregnancy (*Animal studies have shown an adverse effect on the fetus, but there are no adequate studies in humans; or there are no animal reproduction studies and no adequate studies in humans.*) In a separate system evaluating the safety of drugs in canine and feline pregnancy (Papich 1989), this drug is categorized as class: *B* (*Safe for use if used cautiously. Studies in laboratory animals may have uncovered some risk, but these drugs appear to be safe in dogs and cats or these drugs are safe if they are not administered when the animal is near term.*)

Most opioids appear in maternal milk, but effects on offspring may not be significant. Withdrawal symptoms have occurred in breastfeeding infants when maternal administration of an opioid-analgesic is stopped.

Overdosage/Acute Toxicity

Massive overdoses may produce profound respiratory and/or CNS depression in most species. Other effects may include cardiovascular collapse, hypothermia, and skeletal muscle hypotonia. Naloxone is the agent of choice in treating respiratory depression. In massive overdoses, naloxone doses may need to be repeated, and animals should be closely observed as naloxone's effects sometimes diminish before sub-toxic levels of oxymorphone are attained. Mechanical respiratory support should be considered in cases of severe respiratory depression.

Drug Interactions

The following drug interactions have either been reported or are theoretical in humans or animals receiving oxymorphone and may be of significance in veterinary patients:

- **BUTORPHANOL, BUPRENORPHINE, NALBUPHINE:** Potentially could antagonize opiate effects

- **CNS DEPRESSANTS, OTHER:** Additive CNS effects possible

- **DIURETICS:** Opiates may decrease efficacy in CHF patients

- **MONOAMINE OXIDASE INHIBITORS (e.g., amitraz, possibly selegiline):** Use MAOI's with oxymorphone with extreme caution as meperidine (a related opiate) is contraindicated in human patients receiving monamine oxidase (MAO) inhibitors for at least 14 days after receiving MAO inhibitors. Some human patients have exhibited signs of opiate overdose after receiving therapeutic doses of meperidine while taking MAOIs.

■ **MUSCLE RELAXANTS, SKELETAL:** Oxymorphone may enhance effects

■ **PHENOTHIAZINES:** Some phenothiazines may antagonize analgesic effects and increase risk for hypotension

■ **TRICYCLIC ANTIDEPRESSANTS (clomipramine, amitriptyline, etc.):** Oxymorphone may exacerbate the effects of tricyclic antidepressants

■ **WARFARIN:** Opiates may potentiate anticoagulant activity

Laboratory Considerations

■ As they may increase biliary tract pressure, opiates can increase plasma **amylase** and **lipase** values up to 24 hours following their administration.

Doses

■ **DOGS:**

For sedation for minor procedures:

a) Up to 0.2 mg/kg IM or IV; initially a maximum of 5 mg total dose (Combine with acepromazine 0.05–0.1 mg/kg IM or IV) (Shaw *et al.* 1986)

b) 0.05–0.1 mg/kg IV or 0.1–0.2 mg/kg IM, SC (Morgan 1988)

For analgesia (acute pain):

a) 0.1–0.2 mg/kg IM, IV, or SC q1–3h (Hendrix & Hansen 2000)

b) For animals with cardiovascular disease: 0.05–0.1 mg/kg IV, IM or SC q2–4h (Hansen 2003)

c) Epidural administration: 0.05 mg/kg. Recommend to dilute with sterile saline to a volume **not** to exceed 0.3 mL/kg to a maximum of 6 mL. Use of preservative-free opioids is best. (Matthews 2008)

d) 0.1–0.2 mg/kg IM or SC q3–4h for acute pain. (Gaynor 2007)

e) 0.05–0.4 mg/kg IV, IM, or SC q2–4h (Wagner 2002)

For premedication to anesthesia in healthy dogs:

a) 0.05–0.1 mg/kg IM, IV; 0.2 mg/kg for extra heavy sedation. Maximum initial dose: 5 mg. (Trim 2008)

■ **CATS:**

As a preanesthetic/analgesic:

a) 0.05–0.1 mg/kg IM; may cause dysphoria or excitement, add sedative. (Trim 2008)

As an analgesic (acute pain):

a) 0.05–0.1 mg/kg IM, SC or IV q1–3h; concomitant tranquilization recommended (Hendrix & Hansen 2000)

b) For animals with cardiovascular disease: 0.05–0.1 mg/kg IV, IM or SC q2–4h (Hansen 2003)

c) 0.025–0.1 mg/kg IV (IM or SC) q2–6h (Scherk 2003)

d) 0.02–0.1 mg/kg IV, IM, or SC q3–4h (Wagner 2002)

■ **FERRETS:**

a) 0.05–0.2 mg/kg IV or IM 2-4 times daily (Williams 2000)

b) 0.05–0.2 mg/kg SQ or IM q8-12 hrs (Hernandez-Divers 2008)

■ **RABBITS, RODENTS, SMALL MAMMALS:**

a) **Rabbits:** 0.2 mg/kg IM q2–4h (Ivey & Morrisey 2000)

b) Anesthetic/analgesic for minor surgical procedures: 0.15 mg/kg IM (for a hamster-sized animal) (Shaw *et al.* 1986)

c) **Hamsters, Gerbils, Mice, Rats, Guinea pigs:** 0.2–0.5 mg/kg SC, IM q6–12h for analgesia (Adamcak & Otten 2000)

d) **Rabbits, Rats, Mice, Gerbils, Guinea Pigs, Hamsters, Chinchillas:** 0.05–0.2 mg/kg SQ (or IM for rabbits only) q8-12 hrs (Hernandez-Divers 2008)

■ **HORSES:** (**Note:** ARCI UCGFS Class 1 Drug)

Note: Opiates (oxymorphone included) may cause CNS excitement in the horse. Some clinicians recommend pretreatment with acepromazine (0.02–0.04 mg/kg IV), or xylazine (0.3–0.5 mg/kg IV) to reduce the behavioral changes these drugs can cause.

Warning: Opiate analgesics can mask the behavioral and cardiovascular clinical signs associated with mild colic.

As an analgesic:

a) 0.01–0.02 mg/kg IV (Muir 1987)}

b) 0.01–0.022 mg/kg IV; up to 15 mg total (divide dose into 3–4 increments and give several minutes apart (Shaw *et al.* 1986)

c) 0.02–0.03 mg/kg IM (Robinson 1987)

d) 0.015–0.03 mg/kg IV (Thurmon & Benson 1987)

Anesthetic induction in severely compromised horses:

a) 0.01–0.022 mg/kg IV (after approx. 45 minutes, may be necessary to "top off" with another ⅓ of the original dose) (Shaw *et al.* 1986)

■ **SWINE:**

a) To increase analgesia when used with ketamine (2 mg/kg)/xylazine (2 mg/kg): 0.075 mg/kg IV (duration of anesthesia and recumbency: 20–30 minutes) (Shaw *et al.* 1986)

■ **ZOO, EXOTIC, WILDLIFE SPECIES:**

For use of oxymorphone in zoo, exotic and wildlife medicine refer to specific references, including:

a) *Zoo Animal and Wildlife Immobilization and Anesthesia.* West, G, Heard, D, Caulkett, N. (eds.). Blackwell Publishing, 2007.

b) *Handbook of Wildlife Chemical Immobilization, 3rd Ed.* Kreeger, T.J. and J.M. Arnemo. 2007.

c) *Restraint and Handling of Wild and Domestic Animals.* Fowler, M (ed.), Iowa State University Press, 1995

d) *Exotic Animal Formulary, 3rd Ed.* Carpenter, J.W., Saunders. 2005

e) The 2009 American Association of Zoo Veterinarian Proceedings by D. K. Fontenot also has several dosages listed for restraint, anesthesia, and analgesia for a variety of drugs for carnivores and primates. VIN members can access them at: http://goo.gl/BHRih or http://goo.gl/9UJse

Monitoring

- Respiratory rate/depth
- CNS level of depression/excitation
- Blood pressure (especially with IV use)
- Analgesic activity
- Cardiac rate

Client Information

- When given parenterally, this agent should be used in an inpatient setting or with direct professional supervision.

Chemistry/Synonyms

A semi-synthetic phenanthrene narcotic agonist, oxymorphone HCl occurs as odorless white crystals or white to off-white powder. It will darken in color with prolonged exposure to light. One gram of oxymorphone HCl is soluble in 4 mL of water; it is sparingly soluble in alcohol or ether. The commercially available injection has a pH of 2.7–4.5.

Oxymorphone HCl may also be known as: 7,8-Dihydro-14-hydroxymorphinone hydrochloride, or oximorphone hydrochloride, *Numorphan®* and *Opana®*.

Storage/Stability

The injection should be stored protected from light and at room temperature (15–30°C); avoid freezing. The commercially available suppositories should be stored at temperatures between 2–15°C.

Compatibility/Compounding Considerations

Oxymorphone has been reported to be physically **compatible** when mixed with acepromazine, atropine, glycopyrrolate, and ranitidine. It is physically **incompatible** when mixed with barbiturates or diazepam.

Dosage Forms/Regulatory Status

VETERINARY-LABELED PRODUCTS: None

The ARCI (Racing Commissioners International) has designated this drug as a class 1 substance. See the appendix for more information.

HUMAN-LABELED PRODUCTS:

Oxymorphone HCl Oral Tablets: 5 mg & 10 mg; *Opana®* (Endo); (Rx, C-II)

Oxymorphone HCl Extended-Release Oral Tablets: 5 mg, 7.5 mg, 10 mg, 15 mg, 20 mg, 30 mg & 40 mg; *Opana® ER* (Endo); (Rx, C-II)

Oxymorphone HCl for Injection: 1 mg/mL in 1 mL amps; *Opana®* (Endo); (Rx, C-II)

Note: Oxymorphone is a Class-II controlled substance. Very accurate record keeping is required as to use and disposition of stock.

References

Adamcak, A. & B. Otten (2000). Rodent Therapeutics. *Vet Clin NA: Exotic Anim Pract* **3:1**(Jan): 221–240.

Bateman, S.W., S. Haldane, et al. (2008). Comparison of the analgesic efficacy of hydromorphone and oxymorphone in dogs and cats: a randomized blinded study. *Veterinary Anaesthesia and Analgesia* **35**(4): 341–347.

Gaynor, J. (2007). Small Animal Acute Pain Control—NSAIDs and more. Proceedings: Western Vet Conference. Accessed via: Veterinary Information Network. http://goo.gl/9K2oy

Hansen, B. (2003). Opiate use in cardiovascular medicine. Proceedings: ACVIM Forum.

Hendrix, P. & B. Hansen (2000). Acute Pain Management. *Kirk's Current Veterinary Therapy: XIII Small Animal Practice.* J Bonagura Ed. Philadelphia, WB Saunders: 57–61.

Hernandez-Divers, S. (2008). Small Animal Anesthesia. Proceedings: AAZV. Accessed via: Veterinary Information Network. http://goo.gl/2Ta3J

Ivey, E. & J. Morrisey (2000). Therapeutics for Rabbits. *Vet Clin NA: Exotic Anim Pract* **3:1**(Jan): 183–216.

Matthews, N. (2008). Perioperative Analgesia: Part 1. Concepts and Drugs. Proceedings: ACVC. Accessed via: Veterinary Information Network. http://goo.gl/HgU4D

Morgan, R.V., Ed. (1988). *Handbook of Small Animal Practice.* New York, Churchill Livingstone.

Muir, W.W., III (1987). Analgesics in the treatment of colic. *Current Therapy in Equine Medicine.* NE Robinson Ed. Philadelphia, WB Saunders: 27–29.

Papich, M. (1989). Effects of drugs on pregnancy. *Current Veterinary Therapy X: Small Animal Practice.* R Kirk Ed. Philadelphia, Saunders: 1291–1299.

Robinson, N.E. (1987). Table of Common Drugs: Approximate Doses. *Current Therapy in Equine Medicine, 2.* NE Robinson Ed. Philadelphia, W.B. Saunders: 761.

Scherk, M. (2003). Feline analgesia in 2003. Proceedings: World Small Animal Veterinary Assoc World Congress. Accessed via: Veterinary Information Network. http://goo.gl/nXadm

Shaw, K., C.M. Trim, et al. (1986). The use of oxymorphone in veterinary medicine, University of Pennsylvania, Philadelphia.

Thurmon, J.C. & G.J. Benson (1987). Injectable anesthetics and anesthetic adjuncts. *Vet Clin North Am (Equine Practice)* **3**(1): 15–36.

Trim, C. (2008). Opioid Analgesia. Proceedings: WVC. Accessed via: Veterinary Information Network. http://goo.gl/VACG6

Wagner, A. (2002). Opioids. *Handbook of Veterinary Pain Management.* J Gaynor and W Muir Eds., Mosby: 164–183.

Williams, B. (2000). Therapeutics in Ferrets. *Vet Clin NA: Exotic Anim Pract* **3:1**(Jan): 131–153.

OXYTETRACYCLINE
OXYTETRACYCLINE HCL

(ox-it-tet-ra-sye-kleen)   Terramycin®

TETRACYCLINE ANTIBIOTIC

Prescriber Highlights

▶ Tetracycline antibiotic; while many bacteria are now resistant, it still may be very useful to treat mycoplasma, rickettsia, spirochetes, & Chlamydia

▶ Contraindications: Hypersensitivity to the tetracyclines. Extreme Caution: Pregnancy. Caution: Liver, renal insufficiency

▶ Adverse Effects: GI distress, staining of developing teeth & bones, superinfections, photosensitivity; long-term use may cause uroliths. *Cats* do not tolerate very well. *Horses:* if stressed may break with diarrheas (oral use). *Ruminants:* high oral doses can cause ruminal microflora depression & ruminoreticular stasis. Rapid IV of undiluted propylene glycol-based products can cause intravascular hemolysis & cardiodepressant effects. IM: local reactions, yellow staining & necrosis may be seen at the injection site.

Uses/Indications

Oxytetracycline products are FDA-approved for use in dogs and cats (no known products are being marketed, however), calves, non-lactating dairy cattle, beef cattle, swine, fish, and poultry. For more information, refer to the Doses section, below.

Pharmacology/Actions

Tetracyclines generally act as bacteriostatic antibiotics and inhibit protein synthesis by reversibly binding to 30S ribosomal subunits of susceptible organisms, preventing binding to those ribosomes of aminoacyl transfer-RNA. Tetracyclines also are believed to reversibly bind to 50S ribosomes and additionally alter cytoplasmic membrane permeability in susceptible organisms. In high concentrations, tetracyclines can also inhibit protein synthesis by mammalian cells.

As a class, the tetracyclines have activity against most mycoplasma, spirochetes (including the Lyme disease organism), Chlamydia, and Rickettsia. Against gram-positive bacteria, the tetracyclines have activity against some strains of staphylococci and streptococci, but resistance of these organisms is increasing. Gram-positive bacteria that are usually covered by tetracyclines, include *Actinomyces* spp., *Bacillus anthracis*, *Clostridium perfringens* and *tetani*, *Listeria*

monocytogenes, and Nocardia. Among gram-negative bacteria that tetracyclines usually have *in vitro* and *in vivo* activity include *Bordetella* spp., Brucella, Bartonella, *Haemophilus* spp., *Pasturella multocida*, Shigella, and *Yersinia pestis*. Many or most strains of *E. coli*, Klebsiella, Bacteroides, Enterobacter, Proteus and *Pseudomonas aeruginosa* are resistant to the tetracyclines. While most strains of *Pseudomonas aeruginosa* show *in vitro* resistance to tetracyclines, those compounds attaining high urine levels (*e.g.*, tetracycline, oxytetracycline) have been associated with clinical cures in dogs with UTI secondary to this organism.

Oxytetracycline and tetracycline share nearly identical spectrums of activity and patterns of cross-resistance. A tetracycline susceptibility disk is usually used for *in vitro* testing for oxytetracycline susceptibility.

In horses, oxytetracycline appears to be a potent inhibitor of matrix metalloproteinase-9 and a modest inhibitor of matrix metalloproteinase-2 (Fugler *et al.* 2009).

Pharmacokinetics

Both oxytetracycline and tetracycline are readily absorbed after oral administration to fasting animals. Bioavailabilities are approximately 60–80%. The presence of food or dairy products can significantly reduce the amount of tetracycline absorbed, with reductions of 50% or more possible. After IM administration of oxytetracycline (not long-acting), peak levels may occur in 30 minutes to several hours, depending on the volume and site of injection. The long-acting product (*LA-200*®) has significantly slower absorption after IM injection.

Tetracyclines as a class are widely distributed in the body, including to the heart, kidney, lungs, muscle, pleural fluid, bronchial secretions, sputum, bile, saliva, urine, synovial fluid, ascitic fluid, and aqueous and vitreous humor. Only small quantities of tetracycline and oxytetracycline are distributed to the CSF and therapeutic levels may not be attainable. While all tetracyclines distribute to the prostate and eye, doxycycline or minocycline penetrate better into these and most other tissues. Tetracyclines cross the placenta, enter fetal circulation and are distributed into milk. The volume of distribution of oxytetracycline is approximately 2.1 L/kg in small animals, 1.4 L/kg in horses, and 0.8 L/kg in cattle. The amount of plasma protein binding is about 10–40% for oxytetracycline. Oxytetracycline tissue concentrations are higher in diseased lung than in healthy lung and concentrations in milk are higher than serum when mammary glands are inflamed.

Both oxytetracycline and tetracycline are eliminated unchanged primarily via glomerular filtration. Patients with impaired renal function can have prolonged elimination half-lives and may accumulate the drug with repeated dosing.

These drugs apparently are not metabolized, but are excreted into the GI tract via both biliary and nonbiliary routes and may become inactive after chelation with fecal materials. The elimination half-life of oxytetracycline is approximately 4–6 hours in dogs and cats, 4.3–9.7 hours in cattle, 10.5 hours in horses, 6.7 hours in swine, and 3.6 hours in sheep.

Contraindications/Precautions/Warnings

Oxytetracycline is contraindicated in patients hypersensitive to it or other tetracyclines. Because tetracyclines can retard fetal skeletal development and discolor deciduous teeth, they should only be used in the last half of pregnancy when the benefits outweigh the fetal risks. Oxytetracycline and tetracycline are considered more likely to cause these abnormalities than either doxycycline or minocycline.

In patients with renal insufficiency or hepatic impairment, oxytetracycline and tetracycline must be used cautiously. Lower than normal dosages are recommended with enhanced monitoring of renal and hepatic function. Avoid concurrent administration of other nephrotoxic or hepatotoxic drugs with tetracyclines. Monitoring of serum levels should be considered if long-term therapy is required.

Adverse Effects

Oxytetracycline and tetracycline given to young animals can cause a yellow, brown, or gray discoloration of bones and teeth. High dosages or chronic administration may delay bone growth and healing. Tetracyclines in high levels can exert an antianabolic effect, which can cause an increase in BUN and/or hepatotoxicity, particularly in patients with preexisting renal dysfunction. As renal function deteriorates secondary to drug accumulation, this effect may be exacerbated.

In ruminants, high oral doses can cause ruminal microflora depression and ruminoreticular stasis. Rapid intravenous injection of undiluted propylene glycol-based products can cause intravascular hemolysis with resultant hemobinuria. Propylene glycol based products have also caused cardiodepressant effects when administered to calves. When administered IM, local reactions, yellow staining, and necrosis may be seen at the injection site.

In small animals, tetracyclines can cause nausea, vomiting, anorexia, and diarrhea. Cats do not tolerate oral tetracycline or oxytetracycline very well, and may present with clinical signs of colic, fever, hair loss, and depression. There are reports that long-term tetracycline use may cause urolith formation in dogs, but this is thought to occur very rarely.

Horses, who are stressed by surgery, anesthesia, trauma, etc., may break with severe diarrheas after receiving tetracyclines (especially with oral administration).

Tetracycline therapy (especially long-term)

may result in overgrowth (superinfections) of non-susceptible bacteria or fungi.

Tetracyclines have also been associated with photosensitivity reactions and, rarely, hepatotoxicity or blood dyscrasias.

Reproductive/Nursing Safety

In humans, the FDA categorizes this drug as category *D* for use during pregnancy (*There is evidence of human fetal risk, but the potential benefits from the use of the drug in pregnant women may be acceptable despite its potential risks.*) In a separate system evaluating the safety of drugs in canine and feline pregnancy (Papich 1989), this drug is categorized as class: *D* (*Contraindicated. These drugs have been shown to cause congenital malformations or embryotoxicity.*)

Tetracyclines are excreted in maternal milk. Milk to plasma ratios varies between 0.25 to 1.5. Because of the potential for serious adverse reactions, decide whether to discontinue nursing or discontinue the drug.

Overdosage/Acute Toxicity

Tetracyclines are generally well tolerated after acute overdoses. Dogs given more than 400 mg/kg/day orally or 100 mg/kg/day IM of oxytetracycline did not demonstrate any toxicity. Oral overdoses would most likely be associated with GI disturbances (vomiting, anorexia, and/or diarrhea). Should the patient develop severe emesis or diarrhea, fluids and electrolytes should be monitored and replaced if necessary. Chronic overdoses may lead to drug accumulation and nephrotoxicity.

High oral doses given to ruminants, can cause ruminal microflora depression and rumino-reticular stasis. Rapid intravenous injection of undiluted propylene glycol-based products can cause intravascular hemolysis with resultant hemoglobinuria.

Rapid intravenous injection of tetracyclines has induced transient collapse and cardiac arrhythmias in several species, presumably due to chelation with intravascular calcium ions. Overdose quantities of drug could exacerbate this effect if given too rapidly IV. If the drug must be given rapidly IV (less than 5 minutes), some clinicians recommend pre-treating the animal with intravenous calcium gluconate.

Drug Interactions

The following drug interactions have either been reported or are theoretical in humans or animals receiving oxytetracycline and may be of significance in veterinary patients:

- ■ **ATOVAQUONE:** Tetracyclines have caused decreased atovaquone levels

- ■ **BETA-LACTAM or AMINOGLYCOSIDE ANTIBIOTICS:** Bacteriostatic drugs, like the tetracyclines, may interfere with bactericidal activity of the penicillins, cephalosporins, and aminoglycosides; there is some controversy regarding the actual clinical significance of this interaction, however.

■ **DIGOXIN:** Tetracyclines may increase the bioavailability of digoxin in a small percentage of human patients and lead to digoxin toxicity. These effects may persist for months after discontinuation of the tetracycline.

■ **DIVALENT or TRIVALENT CATIONS (oral antacids, saline cathartics or other GI products containing aluminum, calcium, iron, magnesium, zinc, or bismuth cations):** When orally administered, tetracyclines can chelate divalent or trivalent cations that can decrease the absorption of the tetracycline or the other drug if it contains these cations; it is recommended that all oral tetracyclines be given at least 1–2 hours before or after the cation-containing products.

■ **METHOXYFLURANE:** Fatal nephrotoxicity has occurred in humans when used with tetracycline; concomitant use with oxytetracycline is not recommended

■ **WARFARIN:** Tetracyclines may depress plasma prothrombin activity and patients on anticoagulant) therapy may need dosage adjustment

Laboratory Considerations

■ Tetracyclines (not minocycline) may cause falsely elevated values of **urine catecholamines** when using fluorometric methods of determination.

■ Tetracyclines reportedly can cause false-positive **urine glucose** results if using the cupric sulfate method of determination (Benedict's reagent, *Clinitest®*), but this may be the result of ascorbic acid, which is found in some parenteral formulations of tetracyclines. Tetracyclines have also reportedly caused false-negative results in determining urine glucose when using the glucose oxidase method (*Clinistix®*, *Tes-Tape®*).

Doses

■ **DOGS:**

For susceptible infections:

a) For systemic infections: 22 mg/kg PO q8h for 7–14 days or 20 mg/kg IM (using repositol form) every 7 days as needed. (Greene *et al.* 2006)

b) 20 mg/kg PO q8–12h; (may give with food if GI upset occurs; avoid or reduce dose in animals with renal or severe liver failure; avoid in young, pregnant or breeding animals) (Vaden & Papich 1995)

c) For adjunctive treatment of Salmon poisoning (*Neorickettsia helmintheca*): 7 mg/kg IV every 8 h for 3–5 days. (Headley *et al.*)

d) As a chelating antibiotic for medial canthus syndrome (tear staining): 25–50 mg (total dose) PO once per day 2 weeks on and off and on. (Krohne 2008)

e) For diagnosis and treatment of idiopathic antibiotic-responsive diarrhea: 10–20 mg/kg PO q8h. (Allenspach 2009)

■ **CATS:**

For susceptible infections:

a) For hemotropic mycoplasmosis/feline hemoplasmosis: 10–25 mg/kg PO, IV q8h for 5–7 days (Greene *et al.* 2006). Oxytetracycline does not seem to clear the infection, as parasites may still be present three months after therapy. (Lobetti 2007)

b) 20 mg/kg PO q8–12h; (may give with food if GI upset occurs; avoid or reduce dose in animals with renal or severe liver failure; avoid in young, pregnant or breeding animals) (Vaden & Papich 1995)

c) As a trial for adjunctive treatment of inflammatory bowel disease: 10–20 mg/kg PO three times daily. (Simpson 2009)

■ **RABBITS, RODENTS, SMALL MAMMALS:**

a) **Rabbits:** 15 mg/kg SC, IM q8h; 15–50 mg/kg PO once daily; 1 mg/mL in drinking water (Ivey & Morrisey 2000)

b) For *E. cuniculi* infections in rabbits: 20 mg/kg SC once daily. (Bryan 2009)

c) **Chinchillas:** 50 mg/kg PO q12h (Hayes 2000); (Adamcak & Otten 2000)

d) **Gerbils:** 10 mg/kg PO q8h or 20 mg/kg SC q24h; **Guinea Pigs:** 50 mg/kg, PO q12h; **Hamsters:** 16 mg/kg, SC q24h; **Mice:** 10–20 mg/kg PO q8h; **Rats:** 10–20 mg/kg PO q8h or 6–10 mg/kg IM q12h (Adamcak & Otten 2000)

■ **CATTLE:**

For susceptible infections:

a) Using *Liquamycin LA-200®:* For bacterial pneumonia caused by *Pasteurella* spp. (shipping fever) in calves and yearlings, where retreatment is impractical due to husbandry conditions, such as cattle on range, or where their repeated restraint is inadvisable, or infectious bovine keratoconjunctivitis (pinkeye) caused by (M. bovis): 9 mg/lb (20 mg/kg) SC or IM once. Can also be given at 3–5 mg/lb (6.6–11 mg/kg) IM, SC, or IV once daily. In the treatment of severe footrot and advanced cases of other indicated diseases, a dosage level of 5 mg/lb (11 mg/kg) per day is recommended. Treatment should be continued 24–48 hours following remission of disease signs; however, treatment should not exceed a total of 4 consecutive days. (Label information; *Liquamycin LA-200®*—Pfizer)

b) Using *Tetradure-300®:* For the control of respiratory disease in cattle at high risk of developing BRD associated with *Mannheimia (Pasteurella) haemolytica:* 13.6 mg/lb (30 mg/kg) IM or SC once.

For bacterial pneumonia caused by *Pasteurella* spp (shipping fever) in calves and yearlings where retreatment is impractical due to husbandry conditions, such as cattle on range, or where their repeated restraint is inadvisable, or infectious bovine keratoconjunctivitis (pink eye) caused by *Moraxella bovis*: 9–13.6 mg/lb (20–30 mg/kg) IM or SC once.

For other indications (see label): 3–5 mg/lb (6.6–11 mg/kg) IM, SC or IV (IV slowly over a period of at least 5 minutes) once daily. In treatment of foot-rot and advanced cases of other indicated diseases, a dosage level of 5 mg/lb (11 mg/kg) per day is recommended. Treatment should be continued 24 to 48 hours following remission of disease signs, however, not to exceed a total of four consecutive days. If improvement is not noted within 24 to 48 hours of the beginning of treatment, diagnosis and therapy should be re-evaluated.

Do not administer intramuscularly in the neck of small calves due to lack of sufficient muscle mass. Use extreme care when administering this product by intravenous injection. Perivascular injection or leakage from an intravenous injection may cause severe swelling at the injection site. (Label information; *Tetradure-300®*—Merial)

c) For respiratory tract infections: Using 50 mg/mL product: 11 mg/kg IM or SC q24h or IV q12–24h;

Using 100 mg/mL, product: 20 mg/kg IM q24h;

Using 200 mg/mL, product (*LA-200®*): 20 mg/kg IM q3–4 days;

IM or SC doses should be injected into the neck and not more than 10 mL per site. IM route may lead to myositis and abscesses. Rapid IV injection may cause collapse. Phlebitis is possible with IV dosing. (Beech 1987)

d) For anthrax: 4.4 mg/kg IM or IV daily. Do not use in healthy animals recently vaccinated against anthrax as the protective effect of the vaccine may be negated. (Kaufmann 1986)

e) For bovine anaplasmosis:

For control: At start of vector season give 6.6–11 mg/kg (if using 50 mg/mL or 100 mg/mL product) or 20 mg/kg (if using depot form —*LA®-200*) every 21–28 days and extending 1–2 months after vector season ends.

To eliminate carrier state: If using 50 mg/mL or 100 mg/mL product: 22 mg/kg IM (not over 10 mL per injection site) or IV (diluted in saline) daily

for 5 days; or 11 mg/kg as above for 10 days. If using depot form (*LA®-200*): Give 20 mg/kg for 4 treatments deep IM in two separate injection sites at 3-day intervals.

For treatment of sick animals: Preferably using depot form (*LA®-200*): Give 20 mg/kg one time.

For temporary/prolonged protection for rest of herd: If using 50 mg/mL or 100 mg/mL product: 6.6–11 mg/kg IM (not over 10 mL per injection site) repeat at 21–28 day intervals throughout vector season for prolonged protection. If using depot form (*LA®-200*): Give 20 mg/kg IM as above and repeat at 28-day intervals for prolonged protection. (Richey 1986)

f) For pneumonia: If using 50 mg/mL or 100 mg/mL product: 11 mg/kg SC once daily. If using depot form (*LA®-200*): Give 20 mg/kg IM q48h (Hjerpe 1986)

g) For infectious bovine keratoconjunctivitis (*M. bovis*): 20 mg/kg once or twice followed by 2 grams/calf/day for 10 days. May give either PO or parenterally. (Angelos 2008)

h) For listeriosis (*L. monocytogenes*): Requires administration of very high doses to be effective; recommended oxytetracycline treatment scheme requires doses as high as 10 mg/kg per day for at least five days. (Wiedmann 2007)

■ **HORSES:**

For susceptible infections:

a) Foals: 5–10 mg/kg IV q12h diluted and given slowly, or 10–20 mg/kg IV q24h diluted and given slowly. Monitor creatinine and UA. (Bentz 2007)

b) Drug of choice for equine monocytic or granulocytic ehrlichiosis: 6.6 mg/kg IV q24h; to safeguard against adverse effects (muscle tremors, agitation or acute collapse) dilute at least in a 1:1 ratio and give IV slowly, or deliver it as an infusion in 500 mL or 1 liter of fluids. (Bentz 2007)

c) For Lyme disease: 5–6.6 mg/kg IV q12h for 3–4 weeks is typically regarded as the preferred treatment eliminating persistent *B. burgdorferi* infection. (Weese 2009)

d) For Potomac Horse Fever (*Neorickettsia risticii*) early in the clinical course of the disease: 6.6 mg/kg IV twice a day. Usually no more than 5 days treatment is necessary.

For Equine Granulocytic Ehrlichiosis: 7 mg/kg once daily for 5–7 days (Madigan & Pusterla 2000)

e) For proliferative enteropathy (*Lawsonia intracellularis*) in foals: Oxytetracycline 5–6.6 mg/kg IV q12h for 3–7 days followed by doxycycline (10 mg/kg PO q12h for 7–17 days). (Sampieri *et al.* 2006)

f) For proliferative enteropathy (*Lawsonia intracellularis*): Our recent clinical experiences suggest the use of metronidazole (10–15 mg/kg PO q8-12h) combined with either oxytetracycline (10–18 mg/kg slow IV infusion q24h) or chloramphenicol (44 mg/kg PO q6h). (Frazer 2007)

g) For intrauterine infusion: 1–5 grams; use povidone based products only. Little science is available for recommending doses, volume infused, frequency, diluents, etc. Most intrauterine treatments are commonly performed every day or every other day for 3–7 days. (Perkins 1999)

■ **SWINE:**

For susceptible infections:

a) Using *Tetradure-300®*: For bacterial pneumonia caused by *Pasteurella multocida* where retreatment is impractical due to husbandry conditions or where repeated restraint is inadvisable: 9 mg/lb (20 mg/kg) IM once. May also be used at 3–5 mg/lb (6.6–11 mg/kg) IM once per day. Treatment should be continued 24 to 48 hours following remission of disease signs; however, not to exceed a total of four (4) consecutive days. If improvement is not noted within 24 to 48 hours of the beginning of treatment, diagnosis and therapy should be re-evaluated.

For sows as an aid in the control of infectious enteritis in baby pigs: 3 mg/lb (6.6.mg/kg) IM once approximately eight (8) hours before farrowing or immediately after completion of farrowing.

For swine weighing 25 lbs (11.4 kg) or less, administer undiluted for treatment at 9 mg/lb (20 mg/kg), but should be administered diluted (see label for guidelines) for treatment at 3 or 5 mg/lb (6.6–11 mg/kg). (Label information; *Tetradure-300®*—Merial)

b) For anthrax: 4.4 mg/kg IM or IV daily. Do not use in healthy animals recently vaccinated against anthrax as the protective effect of the vaccine may be negated. (Kaufmann 1986)

c) 6–11 mg/kg IV or IM; 10–20 mg/kg PO q6h (Howard 1986)

d) If using 50 mg/mL or 100 mg/mL product: 10 mg/kg IM initially, then 7.5 mg/kg IM once daily (Baggot 1983)

■ **SHEEP & GOATS:**

For susceptible infections:

a) For anthrax: 4.4 mg/kg IM or IV daily. Do not use in healthy animals recently vaccinated against anthrax as the protective effect of the vaccine may be negated. (Kaufmann 1986)

b) For enteritis (*E. coli*) and pneumonia

(*P. multocida*): 22 mg/kg in water daily for 7 to 14 days. (Fajt 2008)

c) For campylobacteriosis in pregnant ewes: In the face of an outbreak, all pregnant ewes should be treated. Long acting oxytetracycline at 20 mg/kg can be used successfully. For large flocks when individual injections may be more difficult, tetracyclines may be added to the feed at a level of 250–300 mg/head/day until lambing is finished. (Menzies 2008)

■ **BIRDS:**

For chlamydiosis (Psittacosis):

a) Using 200 mg/mL product (*LA-200®*): 50 mg/kg IM once every 3–5 days in birds suspected or confirmed of having disease. Used in conjunction with other forms of tetracyclines. IM injections may cause severe local tissue reactions. (McDonald 1989)

b) Using 200 mg/mL, product (*LA-200®*): 200 mg/kg IM once daily for 3–5 days. Has worked well in treating breeding birds to control outbreak and while getting birds to eat oral forms doxycycline or chlortetracycline. (Clubb 1986)

■ **REPTILES:**

For susceptible infections:

a) For turtles and tortoises: 10 mg/kg PO once daily for 7 days (useful in ulcerative stomatitis caused by Vibrio) (Gauvin 1993)

Monitoring

■ Adverse effects

■ Clinical efficacy

■ Long-term use or in susceptible patients: periodic renal, hepatic, hematologic evaluations

Client Information

■ Avoid giving this drug orally within 1–2 hours of feeding, milk, or other dairy products

Chemistry/Synonyms

A tetracycline derivative obtained from *Streptomyces rimosus*, oxytetracycline base occurs as a pale yellow to tan, crystalline powder that is very slightly soluble in water and sparingly soluble in alcohol. Oxytetracycline HCl occurs as a bitter-tasting, hygroscopic, yellow, crystalline powder that is freely soluble in water and sparingly soluble in alcohol. Commercially available 50 mg/mL and 100 mg/mL oxytetracycline HCl injections are usually available in either propylene glycol or povidone-based products.

Oxytetracycline may also be known as: glomycin, hydroxytetracycline, oxytetracyclinum, riomitsin, terrafungine, *Biomycin®*, *Liquamycin®*, *Medamycin®*, *Oxyject®*, *Oxytet®*, and *Terramycin®*.

Storage/Stability

Unless otherwise directed by the manufacturer, oxytetracycline HCl and oxytetracycline products should be stored in tight, light-resistant containers at temperatures of less than 40°C (104°F) and preferably at room temperature (15–30°C); avoid freezing.

Compatibility/Compounding Considerations

The following information pertains to regular (not sustained–release) forms of oxytetracycline HCl. It is generally considered to be physically **compatible** with most commonly used IV infusion solutions, including D_5W, sodium chloride 0.9%, and lactated Ringer's, but can become relatively unstable in solutions with a pH >6, particularly in those containing calcium. This is apparently more of a problem with the veterinary injections that are propylene glycol based, rather than those that are povidone based. Other drugs that are reported to be physically **compatible** with oxytetracycline for injection include: colistimethate sodium, corticotropin, dimenhydrinate, insulin (regular), isoproterenol HCl, methyldopate HCl, norepinephrine bitartrate, polymyxin B sulfate, potassium chloride, tetracycline HCl, and vitamin B-complex with C.

Drugs that are reportedly physically **incompatible** with oxytetracycline, data conflicts, or compatibility is concentration/time dependent, include: amikacin sulfate, aminophylline, amphotericin B, calcium chloride/gluconate, carbenicillin disodium, cephalothin sodium, cephapirin sodium, chloramphenicol sodium succinate, erythromycin gluceptate, heparin sodium, hydrocortisone sodium succinate, iron dextran, methicillin sodium, methohexital sodium, oxacillin sodium, penicillin G potassium/sodium, pentobarbital sodium, phenobarbital sodium, and sodium bicarbonate. Compatibility is dependent upon factors such as pH, concentration, temperature, and diluent used; consult specialized references or a hospital pharmacist for more specific information.

Dosage Forms/Regulatory Status/Withdrawal Times

VETERINARY-LABELED PRODUCTS:

Oxytetracycline HCl 50 mg/mL, 100 mg/mL Injection: There are many FDA-approved oxytetracycline products marketed in these concentrations. Some trade names for these products include: *Terramycin®*, *Liquamycin®*, *Biomycin®* (Bio-Ceutic), *Medamycin®* (TechAmerica), *Biocyl®* (Anthony), *Oxyject®* (Fermenta), and *Oxytet®* (BIVI). Some are labeled for Rx (prescription) use only, while some are over-the-counter (OTC). Depending on the actual product, this drug may be FDA-approved for use in swine, cattle, beef cattle, chickens or turkeys. Products may also be labeled for IV, IM, or SC use. Withdrawal times vary with regard to individual products; when used as labeled, slaughter withdrawal times vary in cattle from 15–22 days, swine 20–26 days, and 5 days for chickens and turkeys. Refer to the actual labeled information for the product used for more information.

Oxytetracycline base 200 mg/mL Injection in 100, 250, and 500 mL bottles; *Liquamycin® LA-200* (Pfizer); (OTC or Rx). FDA-approved for use in swine and cattle. When used as labeled, slaughter withdrawal = 28 days for swine and cattle; Milk withdrawal = 96 hours

Oxytetracycline base 300 mg/mL Injection in 100 mL, 250 mL and 500 mL vials; *Tetradure®-300* (Merial); (Rx) FDA-approved for use in beef cattle, non-lactating dairy cattle, calves, including pre-ruminating (veal) calves, and swine. When used as labeled, slaughter withdrawal = 28 days

Oxytetracycline Oral Tablets (Boluses) 250 mg tablet; *Terramycin® Scours Tablets* (Pfizer); (OTC). FDA-approved for use in non-lactating dairy and beef cattle. Slaughter withdrawal (at labeled doses) = 7 days.

Oxytetracycline is also available in feed additive, premix, ophthalmic, and intramammary products.

Established residue tolerances: Uncooked edible tissues of swine, cattle, salmonids, catfish and lobsters: 0.10 ppm. Uncooked kidneys of chickens or turkeys: 3 ppm. Uncooked muscle, liver, fat or skin of chickens or turkeys: 1 ppm.

HUMAN-LABELED PRODUCTS: None

References

Adamcak, A. & B. Otten (2000). Rodent Therapeutics. *Vet Clin NA: Exotic Anim Pract* **3:**1(Jan): 221–240.

Allenspach, K. (2009). Treatment of IBD. Proceediings: BSAVA. Accessed via: Veterinary Information Network. http://goo.gl/c5raP

Angelos, D. (2008). Recent Discoveries About Infectious Bovine Keratoconjunctivitis. Procdings: ACVIM. Accessed via: Veterinary Information Network. http://goo.gl/5dSVs

Baggot, J.D. (1983). Systemic antimicrobial therapy in large animals. *Pharmacological Basis of Large Animal Medicine.* JA Bogan, P Lees and AT Yoxall Eds. Oxford, Blackwell Scientific Publications: 45–69.

Beech, J. (1987). Respiratory Tract—Horse, Cow. *The Bristol Handbook of Antimicrobial Therapy.* DE Johnston Ed. Evansville, Veterinary Learning Systems: 88–109.

Bentz, B. (2007). Antimicrobial selections for foals. Proceedings: Western Vet Conf. Accessed via: Veterinary Information Network. http://goo.gl/bA5Ny

Bryan, J. (2009). E. Cuniculi: Past, Present, and Future. Proceedings: Western Veterinary Conference. Accessed via: Veterinary Information Network. http://goo.gl/UEYVt

Clubb, S.L. (1986). Therapeutics: Individual and Flock Treatment Regimens. *Clinical Avian Medicine and Surgery.* GJ Harrison and LR Harrison Eds. Philadelphia, W.B. Saunders: 327–355.

Fajt, V.R. (2008). Small Ruminant Antimicrobial Decision-Making: Regimen Design. Proceedings: ACVIM. Accessed via: Veterinary Information Network. http://goo.gl/UWpmo

Frazer, M. (2007). A review of Lawsonia intracellularis: A significant equine pathogen. Proceedings: ACVIM. Accessed via: Veterinary Information Network. http://goo.gl/xyEwh

Fugler, L., S. Eades, et al. (2009). Evaluation of Various

Matrix Metalloproteinase Inhibitors (MMPIS) in the Horse. Proceedings: ACVIM. Accessed via: Veterinary Information Network. http://goo.gl/CgzCa

Gauvin, J. (1993). Drug therapy in reptiles. *Seminars in Avian & Exotic Med* 2(1): 48–59.

Greene, C., K. Hartmannn, et al. (2006). Appendix 8: Antimicrobial Drug Formulary. *Infectious Disease of the Dog and Cat.* C Greene Ed., Elsevier: 1186–1333.

Headley, S.A., D.G. Scorpio, et al. Neorickettsia helminthoeca and salmon poisoning disease: A review. *The Veterinary Journal* In Press, Corrected Proof.

Hjerpe, C.A. (1986). The bovine respiratory disease complex. *Current Veterinary Therapy: Food Animal Practice 2.* JL Howard Ed. Philadelphia, W.B. Saunders: 670–681.

Howard, J.L., Ed. (1986). *Current Veterinary Therapy 2, Food Animal Practice.* Philadelphia, W.B. Saunders.

Ivey, E. & J. Morrisey (2000). Therapeutics for Rabbits. *Vet Clin NA: Exotic Anim Pract* 3:1(Jan): 183–216.

Kaufmann, A.F. (1986). Anthrax. *Current Veterinary Therapy: Food Animal Practice 2.* JL Howard Ed. Philadelphia, W.B. Saunders: 566–567.

Krohne, S. (2008). Tear Staining & Pigment & Hairs—Oh My: Treating Medial Canthus Syndrome in Dogs. Proceedings: World Veterinary Conference. Accessed via: Veterinary Information Network. http://goo.gl/gjJG3

Lobetti, R. (2007). Feline Haemoplasmosis. Provceedings: Feline Haemoplasmosis. Accessed via: Veterinary Information Network. http://goo.gl/kketp

Madigan, J. & N. Pusterla (2000). Ehrlichial Diseases. *The Veterinary Clinics of North America: Equine Practice* 16:3(December).

McDonald, S.E. (1989). Summary of medications for use in psittacine birds. *JAAV* 3(3): 120–127.

Menzies, P. (2008). Control of Abortion in Sheep and Goats. Proceedings: World Veterinary Congress. Accessed via: Veterinary Information Network. http://goo.gl/6QIWc

Papich, M. (1989). Effects of drugs on pregnancy. *Current Veterinary Therapy X: Small Animal Practice.* R Kirk Ed. Philadelphia, Saunders: 1291–1299.

Perkins, N. (1999). Equine reproductive pharmacology. *The Veterinary Clinics of North America: Equine Practice* 15:3(December): 687–704.

Richey, E.J. (1986). Bovine anaplasmosis. *Current Veterinary Therapy: Food Animal Practice 2.* JL Howard Ed. Philadelphia, W.B. Saunders: 622–626.

Sampieri, F., K.W. Hinchcliff, et al. (2006). Tetracycline therapy of Lawsonia intracellularis enteropathy in foals. *Equine Veterinary Journal* 38(1): 89–92.

Simpson, K. (2009). Chronic diarrhea in the cat. Proceedings: WVC. Accessed via: Veterinary Information Network. http://goo.gl/WkGPw

Vaden, S. & M. Papich (1995). Empiric Antibiotic Therapy. *Kirk's Current Veterinary Therapy:XII.* J Bonagura Ed. Philadelphia, W.B. Saunders: 276–280.

Weese, J.S. (2009). Antimicrobial therapy for difficult to identify and atypical pathogens. *Equine Veterinary Education* 21(7): 388–392.

Wiedmann, M. (2007). Listeria Monocytogenes: Transmission and Disease in Ruminants. Proceedings: ACVIM. Accessed via: Veterinary Information Network. http://goo.gl/A6rTq

OXYTOCIN

(ox-i-*toe*-sin)   Pitocin®

HORMONAL AGENT

Prescriber Highlights

▶ Hypothalamic hormone used for induction or enhancement of uterine contractions at parturition, postpartum retained placenta & metritis, uterine involution after manual correction of prolapsed uterus in dogs, & agalactia.

▶ Contraindications: Known hypersensitivity, dystocia due to abnormal presentation of fetus(es) unless correction is made. When used prepartum, oxytocin should be used only when the cervix is relaxed naturally or by the prior administration of estrogens.

▶ Treat hypoglycemia or hypocalcemia before using

▶ Adverse Effects: Usually occur only when used in inappropriate patients or at too high a dosage.

▶ Drug Interactions

Uses/Indications

In veterinary medicine, oxytocin has been used for induction or enhancement of uterine contractions at parturition, treatment of postpartum retained placenta and metritis, uterine involution after manual correction of prolapsed uterus in dogs, and in treating agalactia.

Pharmacology/Actions

By increasing the sodium permeability of uterine myofibrils, oxytocin stimulates uterine contraction. The threshold for oxytocin-induced uterine contraction is reduced with pregnancy duration, in the presence of high estrogen levels and in patients already in labor.

Oxytocin can facilitate milk ejection, but does not have any galactopoietic properties. While oxytocin only has minimal antidiuretic properties, water intoxication can occur if it is administered at too rapid a rate and/or if excessively large volumes of electrolyte-free intravenous fluids are administered.

Pharmacokinetics

Oxytocin is destroyed in the GI tract and, therefore, must be administered parenterally. After IV administration, uterine response occurs almost immediately. Following IM administration, the uterus responds generally within 3–5 minutes. The duration of effect in dogs after IV or IM/SC administration has been reported to be 13 minutes and 20 minutes, respectively. While oxytocin can be administered intranasally, absorption can be erratic. Oxytocin is distributed throughout the extracellular fluid. It is believed that small quantities of the drug cross the placenta and enter the fetal circulation.

In humans, plasma half-life of oxytocin is about 3–5 minutes. In goats, this value has been reported to be about 22 minutes. Oxytocin is metabolized rapidly in the liver and kidneys and a circulating enzyme, oxytocinase can also destroy the hormone. Very small amounts of oxytocin are excreted in the urine unchanged.

Contraindications/Precautions/Warnings

Oxytocin is considered contraindicated in animals with dystocia due to abnormal presentation of fetus(es), unless correction is made. When used prepartum, oxytocin should be used only when the cervix is relaxed naturally or by the prior administration of estrogens (**Note:** Most clinicians avoid the use of estrogens, as natural relaxation is a better indicator for the proper time to induce contractions.) Oxytocin is also contraindicated in patients who are hypersensitive to it.

Before using oxytocin, treat hypoglycemia or hypocalcemia if present.

In humans, oxytocin is contraindicated in patients with significant cephalopelvic disproportion, unfavorable fetal positions, in obstetrical emergencies when surgical intervention is warranted, severe toxemia, or when vaginal delivery is contraindicated. Nasally administered oxytocin is contraindicated in pregnancy.

Adverse Effects

When used appropriately at reasonable dosages, oxytocin rarely causes significant adverse reactions. Most adverse effects are a result of using the drug in inappropriate individuals (adequate physical exam and monitoring of patient are essential) or at too high doses (see Overdosage below). Most of the older dosage recommendations for dogs or cats are obsolete as mini doses have been found to improve the frequency of uterine contractility, and are less hazardous to the bitch (uterine rupture) and to the fetuses (placental compromise). Hypersensitivity reactions are a possibility in non-synthetically produced products. Repeated bolus injections of oxytocin may cause uterine cramping and discomfort.

Overdosage/Acute Toxicity

Effects of overdosage on the uterus depend on the stage of the uterus and the position of the fetus(es). Hypertonic or tetanic contractions can occur leading to tumultuous labor, uterine rupture, fetal injury, or death.

Water intoxication can occur if large doses are infused for a long period, especially if large volumes of electrolyte-free intravenous fluids are concomitantly being administered. Early clinical signs can include listlessness or depression. More severe intoxication clinical signs can include coma, seizures and eventually death. Treatment for mild water intoxication is stopping oxytocin therapy and restricting water access until resolved. Severe intoxication may require the use of osmotic diuretics (mannitol, urea, dextrose) with or without furosemide.

Reproductive/Nursing Safety

In humans, oxytocin is contraindicated in patients with significant cephalopelvic disproportion, unfavorable fetal positions, in obstetrical emergencies when surgical intervention is warranted, severe toxemia, or when vaginal delivery is contraindicated. Nasally administered oxytocin is contraindicated in pregnancy.

No known indications for use in the first trimester exist other than in relation to spontaneous or induced abortion. Oxytocin is not expected to present a risk of fetal abnormalities when use as indicated.

Oxytocin may be found in small quantities in maternal milk but is unlikely to have significant effects.

Drug Interactions

The following drug interactions have either been reported or are theoretical in humans or animals receiving oxytocin and may be of significance in veterinary patients:

■ **THIOPENTAL:** One case in humans has been reported where thiopental anesthesia was delayed when oxytocin was being administered. The clinical significance of this interaction has not been firmly established.

■ **VASOCONSTRICTORS:** If sympathomimetic agents or other vasoconstrictors are used concurrently with oxytocin post-partum hypertension may result. Monitor and treat if necessary.

Doses

■ **DOGS:**

To augment uterine contractions during parturition:

a) 0.5–3 Units SC or IM every 30–60 minutes, best based upon the results of tokodynamometry. (Davidson 2004)

For uterine inertia:

a) For uterine inertia if no fetuses in birth canal, cervix is dilated, and fetal and maternal obstruction have been ruled out: Oxytocin at 5–20 Units (depending on size of animal) IM or as an IV drip (10 Units/liter) beginning as a slow drip and gradually increasing until effective contractions are observed. If no response to IM injection in 30 minutes, may repeat along with 10% dextrose IV slowly. If no response again in 30 minutes, repeat IM again. Some texts recommend giving calcium gluconate (2–10 mL slowly IV while monitoring ECG for bradycardia or arrhythmias). If no response to this medical management, perform Caesarian section. (Macintire 2006)

b) Use uterine and fetal monitors to guide oxytocin and calcium gluconate therapy. Generally, the administration of oxytocin increases the frequency of uterine contractions, while the administration of calcium increases their strength. Calcium is given before oxytocin in most cases, improving contraction strength before increasing frequency. Additionally, the action of oxytocin appears to be improved when given 15 minutes after calcium. Calcium gluconate 10% solution (0.465 mEq of calcium/mL) is given SC at 1 mL/5.5 kg of body weight BW as indicated by the strength of uterine contractions, generally no more frequently than every 4-6 hours. Oxytocin is effective at mini-doses, starting with 0.25 Units (total dose) SC or IM to a maximum dose of 4 Units per bitch or queen. Higher doses of oxytocin or intravenous boluses can cause tetanic, ineffective uterine contractions that can further compromise fetal oxygen supply by placental compression. The frequency of oxytocin administration is dictated by the labor pattern, and it is generally not given more frequently than hourly. (Davidson 2009a)

To induce milk let-down:

a) In bitches with adequate milk production and who tolerate nursing: Oxytocin nasal spray (*Syntocinon®*): 5–10 minutes prior to nursing three times daily (Loar 1989)

b) For secondary agalactia: oxytocin 0.25–1 Unit (total dose) SC q2h. Neonates are removed for 30 minutes post-injection, and then encouraged to suckle, or gentle stripping of the glands performed. Metoclopramide is given at 0.1–0.2 mg/kg SC q12h (dopamine antagonist) to promote milk production. Therapy is usually rewarding within 24 hours. (Davidson 2009b)

For adjunctive treatment of acute metritis:

a) Dam started on a broad-spectrum antibiotic with good tissue penetration into the reproductive tract, while waiting for the culture and sensitivity results. Institute fluid therapy if patient is dehydrated or in shock. Oxytocin at 0.5–5 Units (total dose) IM may be used if birth has occurred less than 24 hours prior or dinoprost (0.25 mg/kg SQ) may be used at any time to promote evacuation of the uterus. (Traas & O'Conner 2009)

To promote uterine involution after uterine prolapse manual reduction:

a) Digital manipulation can be attempted to replace the uterus using general and/or epidural anesthesia. If the tissue is very swollen, hyperosmotic fluids such as 50% dextrose or mannitol may assist in replacement. In some cases an episiotomy is required to successfully reduce the prolapse. Following reduction, oxytocin 0.5–5 Units IM will promote uterine involution. If the uterus cannot be reduced manually, laparotomy may be necessary. If tissue damage is significant, the potential for uterine vessel rupture and hemoabdomen is increased and ovariohysterectomy is indicated. (Traas & O'Conner 2009)

b) Anesthetize patient and apply sterile lubricant liberally to the exposed tissue. The uterine horn is flushed with sterile saline under pressure. Mannitol or hypertonic saline can be used to reduce edema if necessary before attempting reduction. Once the uterus is replaced, give 5–10 Units (total dose) of oxytocin IM to cause uterine involution. If the uterus stays in for 24 hours, further risk of prolapse is unlikely because the cervix should be closed. (Shaw 2007)

■ **CATS:**

To promote uterine involution after uterine prolapse manual reduction:

a) See the dog doses above.

To treat primary uterine inertia:

a) See the dog dose for uterine inertia "b" referenced to: (Davidson 2009a)

For adjunctive treatment of metritis:

a) Dam started on a broad-spectrum antibiotic with good tissue penetration into the reproductive tract, while waiting for the culture and sensitivity results. Institute fluid therapy if patient is dehydrated or in shock. Oxytocin at 0.5–5 Units IM may be used if birth has occurred less than 24 hours prior or dinoprost (0.25 mg/kg SQ) may be used at any time to promote evacuation of the uterus. (Traas & O'Conner 2009)

To induce milk let-down:

a) For secondary agalactia: oxytocin 0.25–1 Unit (total dose) SC q2h. Neonates are removed for 30 minutes post injection, and then encouraged to suckle, or gentle stripping of the glands performed. Metoclopramide is given at 0.1–0.2 mg/kg SC q12h (dopamine antagonist) to promote milk production. Therapy is usually rewarding within 24 hours. (Davidson 2009b)

■ **RABBITS, RODENTS, SMALL MAMMALS:**

a) Mice, Rats, Gerbils, Hamsters, Guinea pigs, Chinchillas: 0.2–3 Units/kg IV, IM or SC (Adamcak & Otten 2000)

■ **CATTLE:**

For retained placenta in patients

a) 40–60 Units oxytocin q2h (often used in conjunction with intravenous calcium therapy) as necessary. Of limited value after 48 hours postpartum as uterine sensitivity is reduced. (McClary 1986)

b) To reduce incidence of retained placenta: 20 Units IM immediately following calving and repeated 2–4 hours later (Hameida *et al.* 1986)

For mild to moderate cases of acute postpartum metritis:

a) 20 Units IM 3–4 times a day for 2–3 days (Hameida *et al.* 1986)

To augment uterine contractions during parturition:

a) 30 Units IM; repeat no sooner than 30 minutes if necessary (Wheaton 1989)

b) For obstetrical use in cows: 100 Units IV, IM or SC (Package Insert; Oxytocin Injection—Anthony Products)

For milk let-down in cows:

a) 10–20 Units IV (Package Insert; Oxytocin Injection—Anthony Products)

■ **HORSES:**

To augment or initiate uterine contractions during parturition in properly evaluated mares:

a) For induction: 2.5–5 Units IV, every 15–20 minutes until foal is born (McCue 2003)

To prevent luteolysis:

a) To prolong corpus luteum lifespan, oxytocin is given from day 7 to day 14 postovulation at a dose of 60 Units (3 ml) IM once daily. Mares have stayed out of heat for up to 45–60 days with this protocol. The negative aspect to using oxytocin in this manner is that ovulation must be documented (or estimated really closely). (Dascanio 2009)

For evacuation of uterine fluid:

a) 20 Units IV or IM one to three times a day (McCue 2003)

To aid in removal of retained fetal membranes:

a) Oxytocin: 30–100 Units in 1 liter of normal saline IV over 30–60 minutes *or* 10–120 Units IM *or* 10–40 Units by IV bolus (**Note:** large dose IV boluses are not recommended as they may cause uterine spasm and abdominal discomfort) (Perkins 1999)

b) Oxytocin: 20 Units IV or IM given every hour beginning 2–3 hours after foaling. Repeat as needed. (McCue 2003)

For mild to moderate cases of acute postpartum metritis:

a) 20 Units IM 3–4 times a day for 2–3 days (Hameida *et al.* 1986)

To treat esophageal obstruction ("choke"):

a) N-butylscopolammonium bromide (*Buscopan®*) at 0.3 mg/kg IV once and oxytocin 0.11–0.22 Units/kg IV once (oxytocin use should be avoided in mares, or dose significantly reduced. Do not use in pregnant mares.) (Beard 2008)

■ **SWINE:**

For adjunctive treatment of agalactia syndrome (MMA) in sows:

a) 30–40 Units per sow at 3–4 hours (Powe 1986)

b) 20–50 Units IM or 5–10 Units IV (Einarsson 1986)

For retained placenta in patients with uterine atony:

a) 20–30 Units oxytocin q2–3h as necessary (with broad-spectrum antibiotics) (McClary 1986)

To augment uterine contractions during parturition:

a) 10 Units IM; repeat no sooner than 30 minutes if necessary (Wheaton 1989)

b) For obstetrical use in sows: 30–50 Units IV, IM or SC (Package Insert; Oxytocin Injection—Anthony Products)

For mild to moderate cases of acute postpartum metritis:

a) 5–10 Units IM 3–4 times a day for 2–3 days (Hameida *et al.* 1986)

b) 5 Units IM; may need to be repeated as effect may be as short as 30 minutes (Meredith 1986)

For milk let-down in sows:

a) 5–20 Units IV (Package Insert; Oxytocin Injection—Anthony Products)

■ **SHEEP & GOATS:**

For retained placenta in patients with uterine atony:

a) 10–20 Units oxytocin. Of limited value after 48 hours postpartum as uterine sensitivity is reduced. If signs of metritis develop, treat with antibiotics. (McClary 1986)

For mild to moderate cases of acute postpartum metritis:

a) 5–10 Units IM 3–4 times a day for 2–3 days (Hameida *et al.* 1986)

To control post-extraction cervical and uterine bleeding after internal manipulations (*e.g.*, fetotomy, etc.):

a) Goats: 10–20 Units IV, may repeat SC in 2 hours (Franklin 1986)

■ **CAMELIDS (NW):**

For retained placenta:

a) 5–10 Units oxytocin may be given IM at 10-minute intervals with or without gentle traction. Strenuous traction may induce uterine prolapse. (Adams 2008)

■ **BIRDS:**

As a uterotonic agent:

a) 0.5 Units/kg IM; may repeat in 60 minutes (Pollock 2007)

For egg expulsion:

a) 0.01–0.1 mL once IM. Should be administered with Vitamin A and calcium (injectable) (Clubb 1986)

■ **REPTILES:**

For egg binding in combination with calcium (Calcium glubionate:

a) Calcium glubionate (10–50 mg/kg IM as needed until calcium levels back to normal or egg binding is resolved); oxytocin: 1–10 Units/kg IM. Use care when giving multiple injections. Not as effective in lizards as in other species. (Gauvin 1993)

To induce oviposition:

a) Doses range from 1–30 Units/kg. A dose of 10 Units/kg appears to be effective in many chelonians. May have to repeat in several hours, but there is a risk of oviduct rupture if cloaca is obstructed or eggs cannot pass for other reasons. (Lewbart 2001)

Monitoring

■ Uterine contractions, status of cervix

■ Fetal monitoring if available and indicated

Client Information

■ Oxytocin should only be used by individuals able to adequately monitor its effects.

Chemistry/Synonyms

A nonapeptide hypothalamic hormone stored in the posterior pituitary (in mammals), oxytocin occurs as a white powder that is soluble in water. The commercially available preparations are highly purified and have virtually no antidiuretic or vasopressor activity when administered at usual doses. Oxytocin potency is standardized according to its vasopressor activity in chickens and is expressed in USP Posterior Pituitary Units. One unit is equivalent of approximately 2–2.2 micrograms of pure hormone.

Commercial preparations of oxytocin injection have their pH adjusted with acetic acid to 2.5–4.5 and multi-dose vials generally contain chlorobutanol 0.5% as a preservative.

Oxytocin may also be known as: alpha-hypophamine, or oxytocinum and *Pitocin*®.

Storage/Stability

Oxytocin injection should be stored at temperatures of less than 25°C, but should not be frozen. Some manufacturers recommend storing the product under refrigeration (2–8°C), but some products have been demonstrated to be stable for up to 5 years if stored at less than 26°C.

Compatibility/Compounding Considerations

Oxytocin is reportedly physically **compatible** with most commonly used intravenous fluids and the following drugs: chloramphenicol sodium succinate, metaraminol bitartrate, netilmicin sulfate, sodium bicarbonate, tetracycline HCl, thiopental sodium, and verapamil HCl.

Oxytocin is reportedly physically **incompatible** with the following drugs: fibrinolysin, norepinephrine bitartrate, prochlorperazine edisylate, and warfarin sodium. Compatibility is dependent upon factors such as pH, concentration, temperature, and diluent used; consult specialized references or a hospital pharmacist for more specific information.

Dosage Forms/Regulatory Status

VETERINARY-LABELED PRODUCTS:

Oxytocin for Injection: 20 USP Units/mL in 10 mL, 30 mL, and 100 mL vials; available labeled generically from several manufacturers; (Rx). Oxytocin products are labeled for several species, including horses, dairy cattle, beef cattle, sheep, swine, cats, and dogs. There are no milk or meat withdrawal times specified for oxytocin.

HUMAN-LABELED PRODUCTS:

Oxytocin Solution for Injection: 10 Units/mL in 1 mL amps, 3 mL & 10 mL vials and 10 mL multiple-dose vials; *Pitocin*® (JHP Pharmaceuticals); generic; (Rx)

References

Adamcak, A. & B. Otten (2000). Rodent Therapeutics. *Vet Clin NA: Exotic Anim Pract* **3:1**(Jan): 221–240.

Adams, G. (2008). Eutocia, Dystocia and Post-Partum Care of the Dam and Neonatal Llama & Alpaca. Proceedings: WVC. http://goo.gl/Budm5

Beard, L. (2008). Respiratory disease in the geriatric patient. Proceedings: WVC. Accessed via: Veterinary Information Network. http://goo.gl/mNYAX

Clubb, S.L. (1986). Therapeutics: Individual and Flock Treatment Regimens. *Clinical Avian Medicine and Surgery*. GJ Harrison and LR Harrison Eds. Philadelphia, W.B. Saunders: 327–355.

Dascanio, J. (2009). Hormonal Control of Reproduction. Proceedings: ABVP. Accessed via: Veterinary Information Network. http://goo.gl/o2vHk

Davidson, A. (2004, Last Update). "Personal Communication."

Davidson, A. (2009a). Medical and Surgical Management of Dystocia. Proceedings: WVC. Accessed via: Veterinary Information Network. http://goo.gl/XINsz

Davidson, A. (2009b). Postpartum disorders in the bitch and queen. Proceedings: WVC. Accessed via: Veterinary Information Network. http://goo.gl/Z6o5F

Einarsson, S. (1986). Agalactia in Sows. *Current Therapy in Theriogenology 2: Diagnosis, Treatment and Prevention of Reproductive Diseases in Small and Large Animals*. DA Morrow Ed. Philadelphia, WB Saunders: 935–937.

Franklin, J.S. (1986). Dystocia and obstetrics in goats. *Current Therapy in Theriogenology 2: Diagnosis, Treatment and Prevention of Reproductive Diseases in Small and Large Animals*. DA Morrow Ed. Philadelphia, WB Saunders: 590–592.

Gauvin, J. (1993). Drug therapy in reptiles. *Seminars in Avian & Exotic Med* **2**(1): 48–59.

Hameida, N.A., B.K. Gustafsson, et al. (1986). Therapy of uterine infections: Alternatives to antibiotics. *Current Therapy in Theriogenology 2: Diagnosis, Treatment and Prevention of Reproductive Diseases in Small and Large Animals*. DA Morrow Ed. Philadelphia, WB Saunders: 45–47.

Lewbart (2001). Reptile Formulary. Proceedings: Atlantic Coast Veterinary Conference. Accessed via: Veterinary Information Network. http://goo.gl/EEQmM

Loar, A.S. (1989). Diseases of the mammary glands. *Handbook of Small Animal Practice*. RV Morgan Ed. New York, Churchill Livingstone: 707–717.

Macintire, D. (2006). Reproductive Emergencies. Proceedings: ACVC 2006. Accessed via: Veterinary Information Network. http://goo.gl/lotWY

McClary, D. (1986). Retained Placenta. *Current Veterinary Therapy: Food Animal Practice 2*. JL Howard Ed. Philadelphia, W.B. Saunders: 773–775.

McCue, P. (2003). Hormone therapy: new aspects. Proceedings: Western Veterinary Conference. Accessed via: Veterinary Information Network. http://goo.gl/RfyuN

Meredith, M.J. (1986). Bacterial endometritis. *Current Therapy in Theriogenology 2: Diagnosis, Treatment and Prevention of Reproductive Diseases in Small and Large Animals*. DA Morrow Ed. Philadelphia, WB Saunders: 953–956.

Perkins, N. (1999). Equine reproductive pharmacology. *The Veterinary Clinics of North America: Equine Practice* **15**:3(December): 687–704.

Pollock, C. (2007). Avian Reproductive Diseases. Proceedings: Western Vet Conf. Accessed via: Veterinary Information Network.

Powe, T.A. (1986). Lactation Failure: Dysglactia, Agalactia, Hypogalactia. *Current Veterinary Therapy: Food Animal Practice 2*. JL Howard Ed. Philadelphia, W.B. Saunders: 771–773.

Shaw, S. (2007). Dealing with Reproductive Emergencies. Proceedings: IVECCS. Accessed via: Veterinary Information Network. http://goo.gl/

Traas, A. & C. O'Conner (2009). Postpartum Emergencies. Peroceedings: IVECCS. Accessed via: Veterinary Information Network. http://goo.gl/CQmST

Wheaton, L.G. (1989). Drugs that affect uterine motility. *Current Veterinary Therapy X: Small Animal Practice*. RW Kirk Ed. Philadelphia, WB Saunders: 1299–1302.

PAMIDRONATE DISODIUM

(pah-*mih*-dro-nate)   Aredia®

BISPHOSPHONATE

Prescriber Highlights

▶ Bisphosphonate used IV for treating hypercalcemia associated with Vitamin D-analog toxicity or hypercalcemia of malignancy; being investigated for adjuvant treatment of osteosarcomas

▶ Must be given IV in saline over several hours

▶ Potentially can cause electrolyte abnormalities, anemias, or renal toxicity

▶ Expense may be an issue, but generic forms now available

Uses/Indications

Pamidronate may be useful in treating hypercalcemia associated with vitamin D-related toxicoses or hypercalcemia of malignancy. There is ongoing research on the use of this drug to determine if it has clinical usefulness in directly treating "micro-metastases" in osteosarcomas.

Pharmacology/Actions

Bisphosphonates at therapeutic levels inhibit bone resorption and do not inhibit bone mineralization via binding to hydroxyapatite crystals. They impede osteoclast activity, and induce osteoclast apoptosis. Pamidronate has approximately 100 times greater relative antiresorptive potency when compared to etidronate.

Bisphosphonates *in vitro* have direct cytotoxic or cytostatic effects on human osteosarcoma cell lines. They may also have antiangiogenic effects and inhibit cell migration in certain cancers.

Pharmacokinetics

After intravenous infusion in rats, 50–60% of the dose is rapidly absorbed by bone. Bone uptake is highest in areas of rapid bone turnover. The kidneys very slowly eliminate the drug. Terminal half-life is on the order of 300 days in rats.

Contraindications/Precautions/Warnings

Pamidronate is contraindicated in patients hypersensitive to it or any of the bisphosphonate drugs. It should be used with caution in patients with impaired renal function; the drug has been associated with renal toxicity. In humans, it has not been tested in patients with serum creatinine levels greater than 5 mg/dL.

Adverse Effects

Electrolyte abnormalities may occur with pamidronate therapy. One case of a dog developing hypomagnesemia and arrhythmias after pamidronate has been reported (Kadar *et al.* 2004). Pamidronate potentially can cause renal toxicity in dogs, but it is thought this can be minimized or avoided by infusing the drug over at least 2 hours. In humans, ophthalmic syndromes (*e.g.,* scleritis), transient bone pain, hypocalcemia, anemia, thrombocytopenia and granulocytosis have been reported.

Reproductive/Nursing Safety

In pregnant humans, the FDA lists pamidronate as a category **D** drug (*There is evidence of human fetal risk, but the potential benefits from the use of the drug in pregnant women may be acceptable despite its potential risks.*) Pamidronate has produced both maternal and embryo/fetal toxicity in laboratory animals when given at dosages therapeutically used in human patients. If it is used in pregnant veterinary patients, informed consent by the owner accepting the risks to both mother and offspring is recommended.

It is unknown if pamidronate is excreted into milk. Use with caution in nursing mothers.

Overdosage/Acute Toxicity

Overdosage of pamidronate may cause hypocalcemia, including tetany. Should this occur, treat with short-term, intravenous calcium.

Drug Interactions

The following drug interactions have either been reported or are theoretical in humans or animals receiving pamidronate and may be of significance in veterinary patients:

▪ **CALCIUM-AFFECTING DRUGS (*e.g.,* furosemide, corticosteroids):** Pamidronate must be used carefully (with monitoring) when used in conjunction with other drugs that can affect calcium

▪ **NEPHROTOXIC DRUGS (*e.g.,* cisplatin, aminoglycosides):** Use with caution, potential for increased risk for nephrotoxicity

Laboratory Considerations

▪ No specific laboratory interactions or considerations noted.

Doses

■ **DOGS:**

a) For refractory hypercalcemia: 1 mg/kg IV given over 2 hours in 250 mL of normal saline every 4 weeks. (Chun 2007)

b) For control of hypercalcemia: Treat each patient individually and if possible remove the underlying cause. If parenteral saline, furosemide and corticosteroids do not resolve the issue then bisphosphonates can be considered for more chronic control of hypercalcemia. Pamidronate 1.3–2 mg/kg in 150 mL of 0.9% saline with a 2 hour IV infusion; can repeat in 1–3 weeks. (Chew *et al.* 2003)

c) For treatment of cholecalciferol-induced toxicosis: 0.65–2 mg/kg in 0.9% NaCl on days 1 and 4 post-ingestion (Rumbeiha *et al.* 2000)

d) For attempting to reduce bone pain associated with osteosarcoma in combination with an NSAID: 1–2 mg/kg; diluted into 250 mL of 0.9% sodium chloride and administered as a CRI over 2 hours every 28 days. (Fan & de Lorimier 2003), (Fan *et al.* 2007)

e) For pain associated with skeletal neoplasias: 1–2 mg/kg IV over 2 hours every 21-28 days. Pamidronate has been shown to provide pain relief in ~50% of dogs with skeletal neoplasia. (Posner & papich 2009)

f) For calcitriene toxicosis: 1.3–2 mg/kg slow IV infusion. In most cases, a single dose will lower calcium levels back to normal levels. Recommended to monitor calcium levels daily for at least 10 days after they have returned to normal. (Gwaltney-Brant 2003)

g) For control of hypercalcemia: 1.05–2 mg/kg IV over 4 hours (from a retrospective study of 7 dogs). (Hostutler *et al.* 2005)

■ **CATS:**

a) For control of hypercalcemia: 1.5–2 mg/kg IV over 4 hours (from a retrospective study of 2 cats). (Hostutler *et al.* 2005)

Monitoring

■ Renal function (serum creatinine, etc.) and hydration status should be monitored before treating and prior to each dose

■ Serum calcium, phosphate, magnesium, potassium

■ CBC; baseline and continued if ongoing treatment

■ Urinalysis

Client Information

■ The medication must be given in an inpatient setting.

■ Clients should understand the costs for the medication, care, and monitoring associated with its use.

Chemistry/Synonyms

Pamidronate disodium a bisphosphonate inhibitor of bone resorption occurs as a white, crystalline powder that is soluble in water and practically insoluble in organic solvents.

Pamidronate may also be known as: ADP sodium, AHPrBP sodium, GCP-23339A, *Aminomux®, Aredia®, Aredronet®, Ostepam®,* or *Pamidran®.*

Storage/Stability

Do not store at temperatures greater than 30°C (86°F).

Once the lyophilized powder for injection is reconstituted (10 mL) with sterile water for injection, it may be stored in the refrigerator for 24 hours. Be sure drug is completely dissolved before withdrawing into syringe.

Compatibility/Compounding Considerations

Do not mix pamidronate with any intravenous fluid containing calcium (*e.g.,* Ringer's). It is recommended to use a dedicated IV solution (0.45% or 0.9% NaCl, or D_5W) and intravenous line.

Dosage Forms/Regulatory Status

VETERINARY-LABELED PRODUCTS: None

HUMAN-LABELED PRODUCTS:

Pamidronate Disodium Lyophilized Powder for Injection (IV infusion): 30 mg & 90 mg with 375 mg & 470 mg mannitol in vials; *Aredia®* (Novartis); generic (Sandoz); (Rx)

Pamidronate Disodium Injection: 3 mg/mL, 6 mg/mL & 9 mg/mL (may contain mannitol) in 10 mL vials; generic; (Rx)

References

Chew, D., P. Schenck, et al. (2003). Assessment and treatment of clinical cases with elusive disorders of hypercalcemia. Proceedings: ACVIM Forum. Accessed via: Veterinary Information Network. http://goo.gl/goje1

Chun, R. (2007). Paraneoplastic Syndromes: Hypercalcemia and beyond. Proceedings; Western Vet Conference. Accessed via: Veterinary Information Network. http://goo.gl/4fUKM

Fan, T. & L.-P. de Lorimier (2003). Bisphosphonates: molecular mechanisms and therapeutic uses in veterinary oncology. Proceedings: ACVIM Forum. Accessed via: Veterinary Information Network. http://goo.gl/UXMNf

Fan, T., L.-P. de Lorimier, et al. (2007). Single-agent pamidronate for palliative therapy of canine appendicular osteosarcoma bone pain. *J Vet Intern Med* 21(431–439).

Gwaltney-Brant, S. (2003). Terrible Toxicants. Proceedings: IVECC2003. Accessed via: Veterinary Information Network. http://goo.gl/6AZCf

Hostutler, R., D. Chew, et al. (2005). Uses and effectiveness of pamidronate disodium for treatment of dogs and cats with hypercalcemia. *J Vet Intern Med* **19**: 29–33.

Kadar, E., J. Rush, et al. (2004). Electrolyte disturbances and cardiac arrhythmias in a dog following pamidronate, calcitonin, and furosemide administration for hypercalcemia of malignancy. *J Am Anim Hosp Assoc* **40**(1): 75–81.

Posner, L.P. & M.G. papich (2009). Your patient is still in pain—Now what? "Rescue analgesia". Proceedings:

WVC. Accessed via: Veterinary Information Network. http://goo.gl/WMON9

Rumbeiha, W., S. Fitzgerald, et al. (2000). Use of pamidronate disodium to reduce cholecalciferol-induced toxicosis in dogs. *AM J Vet Res* 61(1): 9–13.

PANCRELIPASE

(pan-kree-*lih*-pase)

Viokase®, Pancreatic Enzymes, Lipase/Protease/Amylase

PANCREATIC ENZYMES

Prescriber Highlights

▶ Pancreatic enzymes used to treat exocrine pancreatic enzyme deficiency or to test for pancreatic insufficiency secondary to chronic pancreatitis

▶ Contraindications: Hypersensitivity to pork products

▶ Adverse Effects: High doses may cause GI distress

▶ Avoid inhalation of powder; may cause skin irritation; wash off if gets on hands

Uses/Indications

Pancrelipase is used to treat patients with exocrine pancreatic enzyme insufficiency (EPI).

The serum trypsin-like immunoreactivity (TLI) assay is used to establish the diagnosis in dogs. Dogs may have EPI and not respond to pancreatic enzyme replacement because: a) the enzyme product is poorly effective, b) the diet is too high in fat, and/or c) the dog has concurrent antibiotic responsive enteropathy. About 15% of dogs with EPI simply will not respond to therapy and have a bad prognosis (Willard 2009).

It may also be used in the attempt to test for pancreatic insufficiency secondary to chronic pancreatitis.

Pharmacology/Actions

The enzymes found in pancrelipase help to digest and absorb fats, proteins, and carbohydrates.

Contraindications/Precautions/Warnings

Pancrelipase products are contraindicated in animals that are hypersensitive to pork proteins.

Do not inhale the powder or bronchial/lung irritation can occur. Avoid contact with mucous membranes or skin.

Adverse Effects

High doses may cause GI distress (diarrhea, cramping, nausea). Concentrated pancreatic enzymes can cause oral or esophageal ulcers; follow dosing with food or water. Oral bleeding has been reported in dogs after receiving pancrelipase (Rutz *et al.* 2002). Dose reduction and moistening the food pancreatic/powder mix may also decrease the incidence of this adverse effect.

Reproductive/Nursing Safety

In humans, the FDA categorizes this drug as category *C* for use during pregnancy (*Animal studies have shown an adverse effect on the fetus, but there are no adequate studies in humans; or there are no animal reproduction studies and no adequate studies in humans.*)

These enzymes are unlikely to be excreted in maternal milk or pose risk to offspring.

Overdosage/Acute Toxicity

Overdosage may cause diarrhea or other intestinal upset. The effects should be temporary; treat by reducing dosage and supportively if diarrhea is severe.

Drug Interactions

The following drug interactions have either been reported or are theoretical in humans or animals receiving pancrelipase and may be of significance in veterinary patients:

▪ **ANTACIDS (magnesium hydroxide, calcium carbonate):** May diminish the effectiveness of pancrelipase

▪ **CIMETIDINE (or other H$_2$ antagonists):** May increase the amount of pancrelipase that reaches the duodenum

Doses

▪ **DOGS:**

For pancreatic exocrine insufficiency:

a) 1–1.5 teaspoonful with each meal mixed with food. Mix with food thoroughly and allow to stand for 15–20 minutes before feeding. Dosage should be adjusted as necessary. Best results are usually obtained by feeding small meals frequently (at least 3 times per day). (Package Insert; *Viokase®-V Powder*—Fort Dodge)

b) Initially, two teaspoons per 20 kg body weight per meal. Oral bleeding has recently been reported in 3 of 25 dogs with EPI treated with pancreatic enzyme supplements. The oral bleeding stopped in all 3 dogs after the dose of pancreatic enzymes was decreased. Moistening the food pancreatic/powder mix also appears to decrease the frequency of this side effect. When clinical signs have resolved, the amount of pancreatic enzymes given can be gradually decreased to the lowest effective dose, which may vary from patient to patient and from batch to batch of the pancreatic supplement. (Steiner 2008)

c) 1–2 teaspoonful of powder or finely crushed nonenteric-coated tablets to each of two meals of balanced canine ration. It is not necessary to incubate the enzyme preparation before feeding. Tailor regimen to maintain optimal body weight. (Bunch 2003)

d) Maintenance dose is usually 1 teaspoonful per meal. (Westermarck *et al.* 2005)

■ **CATS:**

Note: Cats reportedly "hate" the taste of the powder and may be more easily dosed using solid dosage forms (enteric-coated tablets or compounded capsules made from powder or crushed tablets). If using these products, be certain that the cat follows the tablets with water or food to reduce the risk for esophageal damage. It has also been reported that some cats will eat food mixed with one brand of veterinary powder and refuse another.

For pancreatic exocrine insufficiency:

a) 0.5–0.75 teaspoonful with each meal mixed with food. Mix with food thoroughly and allow it to stand for 15–20 minutes before feeding. Dosage should be adjusted as necessary. Best results are usually obtained by feeding small meals frequently (at least 3 times per day). (Package Insert; *Viokase®-V Powder—Fort* Dodge)

b) 1 teaspoonful of powder or finely crushed nonenteric-coated tablets to each of two meals of balanced feline ration. Cats that refuse to eat food treated with powder may be dosed with capsules filled with powder or crushed non-enteric coated tablets. It is not necessary to incubate the enzyme preparation before feeding. Tailor regimen to maintain optimal body weight. (Bunch 2003)

c) 0.5 teaspoonful of powder per meal. (Westermarck *et al.* 2005)

d) Initially, one teaspoon per cat per meal. When clinical signs have resolved, the amount of pancreatic enzymes given can be gradually decreased to the lowest effective dose, which may vary from patient to patient and from batch to batch of the pancreatic supplement. (Steiner 2008)

■ **RABBITS, RODENTS, SMALL MAMMALS:**

a) Rabbits: For gastric trichobezoars: 1 teaspoonful (5 mL) pancrelipase powder plus 3 teaspoonsful (15 mL) of yogurt; let stand for 15 minutes, then give 2–3 mL PO q12h. Questionable efficacy for removing "hairballs", but might help dissolve the protein matrix surrounding hair. (Ivey & Morrisey 2000)

■ **BIRDS:**

For pancreatic exocrine insufficiency (used in birds that are polyphagic "going light", passing whole seeds, and slow in emptying crops):

a) ⅛ tsp per kg. Mix with moistened feed or administer by gavage. Incubate with food for 15 minutes prior to gavage. (Clubb 1986)

Monitoring
■ Animal's weight

■ Stool consistency, frequency

Client Information
■ Powder spilled on hands should be washed off or skin irritation may develop; do not allow powder to contact eyes

■ Avoid inhaling powder; causes mucous membrane irritation and may trigger asthma attacks in susceptible individuals.

Chemistry/Synonyms
Pancrelipase contains pancreatic enzymes, primarily lipase but also amylase and protease, and is obtained from the pancreas of hogs. Each mg of pancrelipase contains not less than 24 USP Units of lipase activity, not less than 100 USP Units of protease activity, and not less than 100 USP Units of amylase activity. When compared on a per weight basis, pancrelipase has at least 4 times the trypsin and amylase content of pancreatin, and at least 12 times the lipolytic activity of pancreatin.

Pancrelipase may also be known as pancrelipasa, *Epizyme®*, *Panakare®*, *Pancrepowder Plus®*, *Pancreved®*, *Pancrezyme®*, and *Viokase®*.

Storage/Stability
Unless otherwise recommended by the manufacturer, store at room temperature in a dry place in tight containers. When present in quantities greater than trace amounts, acids will inactivate pancrelipase.

Dosage Forms/Regulatory Status
Note: There are several dosage forms (both human and veterinary-label) available containing pancrelipase, including oral capsules, oral delayed-release capsules, tablets, and delayed-released tablets. Most small animal practitioners feel that the oral powder is most effective in dogs.

VETERINARY-LABELED PRODUCTS:

Pancrelipase Powder containing (approximately) per teaspoonful (2.8 grams): 71,400 Units lipase; 388,000 Units protease; 460,000 Units amylase; in 8 oz bottle; *Viokase®-V Powder* (Fort Dodge), *Pancrezyme® Powder* (Virbac); *Pancrepowder Plus®* (Butler), *Pancreved® Powder* (Vedco), *Epizyme® Powder* (V.E.T.), *Panakare® Plus Powder* (Neogen); (Rx). Labeled for use in dogs and cats.

HUMAN-LABELED PRODUCTS:

There are capsules, tablets, and powders available containing lipase, protease, and amylase in varying units available for human consumption from many distributors.

References
Bunch, S. (2003). Hepatobiliary and exocrine pancreatic disorders. *Small Animal Internal Medicine, 3rd Ed.* R Nelson and C Couto Eds. St Louis, Mosby: 472–567.

Clubb, S.L. (1986). Therapeutics: Individual and Flock Treatment Regimens. *Clinical Avian Medicine and Surgery.* GJ Harrison and LR Harrison Eds. Philadelphia, W.B. Saunders: 327–355.

Ivey, E. & J. Morrisey (2000). Therapeutics for Rabbits. *Vet Clin NA: Exotic Anim Pract* **3:**1(Jan): 183–216.

Rutz, G.M., J.r.M. Steiner, et al. (2002). Oral bleeding associated with pancreatic enzyme supplementation in three dogs with exocrine pancreatic insufficiency. *Journal of the American Veterinary Medical Association* **221**(12): 1716–1718.

Steiner, J.M. (2008). How I Treat—Exocrine Pancreatic Insufficiency. Proceedings: WSAVA. Accessed via: Veterinary Information Network. http://goo.gl/aHIL4

Westermarck, E., M. Wiberg, et al. (2005). Exocrine pancreatic insufficiency in dogs and cats. *Textbook of Veterinary internal Medicine 6th Ed.* S Ettinger and E Feldman Eds., Elsevier: 1492–1495.

Willard, M. (2009). Canine Chronic Diarrheas: Diagnosis/Management of Non-Infiltrative Disorders. Proceedings: ACVIM. Accessed via: Veterinary Information Network. http://goo.gl/UMPrS

PANCURONIUM BROMIDE

(pan-kue-*roe*-nee-um)   Pavulon®

NON-DEPOLARIZING NEUROMUSCU-
LAR BLOCKER

Prescriber Highlights

▶ Non-depolarizing neuromuscular
   blocker used as an adjunct to general
   anesthesia

▶ Extreme Caution: Myasthenia gravis

▶ Caution: Renal dysfunction, hepatic or
   biliary disease; patients where tachycardias may be deleterious

▶ No analgesic or sedative/anesthetic
   actions

▶ Adverse Effects: Slight elevations in
   cardiac rate & blood pressure, hypersalivation (if not pretreated with
   an anticholinergic agent), prolonged
   or profound muscular weakness, &
   respiratory depression. Very Rarely:
   Histamine release with resultant hypersensitivity reaction

▶ Drug Interactions

Uses/Indications

Pancuronium is sometimes used as an adjunct to general anesthesia to produce muscle relaxation during surgical procedures or mechanical ventilation and to facilitate endotracheal intubation.

Pharmacology/Actions

Pancuronium is a nondepolarizing neuromuscular blocking agent and acts by competitively binding at cholinergic receptor sites at the motor endplate, inhibiting the effects of acetylcholine. It is considered 5 times as potent as d-tubocurarine and ⅓ as potent as vecuronium (some sources say that pancuronium is equipotent with vecuronium in animals). It has little effect on the cardiovascular system other than increasing heart rate slightly, and only rarely does it cause histamine release.

Pharmacokinetics

After intravenous administration, muscle relaxation sufficient for endotracheal intubation occurs generally within 2–3 minutes, but is dependent on the actual dose administered. Duration of action may persist 30–45 minutes, but this again is dependent on the dose. Additional doses may slightly increase the magnitude of the blockade and will significantly increase the duration of action.

In humans, pancuronium is approximately 87% bound to plasma proteins, but it may be used in hypoalbuminemic patients. Activity is non-affected substantially by either plasma pH or carbon dioxide levels.

The half-life in humans ranges from 90–161 minutes. Approximately 40% of the drug is excreted unchanged by the kidneys. The remainder is excreted in the bile (11%) or metabolized by the liver. In patients with renal failure, plasma half-lives are doubled; atracurium may be a better choice for these patients.

Contraindications/Precautions/Warnings

Pancuronium is contraindicated in patients hypersensitive to it. It should be used with caution in patients with renal dysfunction, or where tachycardias may be deleterious. Lower doses may be necessary in patients with hepatic or biliary disease. Pancuronium has no analgesic or sedative/anesthetic actions. In patients with myasthenia gravis, neuromuscular blocking agents should be used with extreme caution, if at all.

Adverse Effects

Adverse reactions seen with pancuronium include: slight elevations in cardiac rate and blood pressure, hypersalivation (if not pretreated with an anticholinergic agent), occasional rash (humans), and prolonged or profound muscular weakness and respiratory depression. Very rarely, pancuronium will cause substantial histamine release with resultant hypersensitivity reactions.

Reproductive/Nursing Safety

In humans, the FDA categorizes this drug as category *C* for use during pregnancy (*Animal studies have shown an adverse effect on the fetus, but there are no adequate studies in humans; or there are no animal reproduction studies and no adequate studies in humans.*) In a separate system evaluating the safety of drugs in canine and feline pregnancy (Papich 1989), this drug is categorized as class: *B* (*Safe for use if used cautiously. Studies in laboratory animals may have uncovered some risk, but these drugs appear to be safe in dogs and cats or these drugs are safe if they are not administered when the animal is near term.*)

It is not known whether these drugs are excreted in maternal milk.

Overdosage/Acute Toxicity

Monitoring muscle twitch response to peripheral nerve stimulation can minimize overdosage possibilities. Increased risks of hypotension and histamine release occur with overdoses, as well as prolonged duration of muscle blockade.

Besides treating conservatively (mechanical ventilation, O_2, fluids, etc.), reversal of blockade may be accomplished by administering an anticholinesterase agent (edrophonium, physostigmine, or neostigmine) with an anticholinergic (atropine or glycopyrrolate). A suggested dose for neostigmine is 0.06 mg/kg IV after atropine 0.02 mg/kg IV.

Drug Interactions
The following drug interactions have either been reported or are theoretical in humans or animals receiving pancuronium and may be of significance in veterinary patients:

■ **AZATHIOPRINE:** May reverse pancuronium's neuromuscular blocking effects

■ **AMINOGLYCOSIDES (gentamicin, etc.):** May enhance the neuromuscular blocking activity of pancuronium

■ **CALCIUM (IV):** May reverse the effects of nondepolarizing neuromuscular blocking agents

■ **LINCOSAMIDES: (clindamycin, etc.):** May enhance the neuromuscular blocking activity of pancuronium

■ **MAGNESIUM SULFATE or HCL:** May enhance the neuromuscular blocking activity of pancuronium

■ **QUINIDINE:** May enhance the neuromuscular blocking activity of pancuronium

■ **SUCCINYLCHOLINE:** Other muscle relaxant drugs may cause a synergistic or antagonistic effect. Succinylcholine may speed the onset of action and enhance the neuromuscular blocking actions of pancuronium. Do not give pancuronium until succinylcholine effects have subsided.

■ **THEOPHYLLINE:** May inhibit or reverse the neuromuscular blocking action of pancuronium and possibly induce arrhythmias

■ **TRICYCLIC ANTIDEPRESSANTS (e.g., clomipramine, amitriptyline):** Increased risk for cardiac arrhythmias when used with halothane anesthesia

Doses

■ **DOGS:**
  a) As a paralytic during mechanical ventilation: 0.05–0.1 mg/kg IV; lasts about an hour, must give sedation as well (Carr 2003)

  b) 0.044–0.11 mg/kg IV; higher dose used initially; lower doses required if repeated doses are necessary (Mandsager 1988)

  c) On occasions when anesthesia maintenance with IV or regional techniques are not adequate to prevent spontaneous movement and the addition of inhalational agents results in severe hypotension (not corrected with fluid therapy): 0.02–0.04 mg/kg IV provides 30–45 minutes of muscle relaxation. (Day 2005)

■ **CATS:**
  a) 0.044–0.11 mg/kg IV; higher dose used initially; lower dose required if repeated doses are necessary (Mandsager 1988)

■ **RABBITS, RODENTS, SMALL MAMMALS:**
  a) Rabbits: 0.1 mg/kg IV (Ivey & Morrisey 2000)

Monitoring
■ Level of neuromuscular blockade
■ Cardiac rate

Client Information
■ This drug should only be used by professionals familiar with using neuromuscular blocking agents in a supervised setting with adequate ventilatory support

Chemistry/Synonyms
A synthetic, non-depolarizing neuromuscular blocker, pancuronium bromide occurs as a white, odorless, bitter-tasting, hygroscopic, fine powder. It has a melting point of 215°C and one gram is soluble in 100 mL of water; it is very soluble in alcohol. Acetic acid is used to adjust the commercially available injection to a pH of approximately 4.

Pancuronium bromide may also be known as: NA-97, Org-NA-97, or pancuronii bromidum.

Storage/Stability
Pancuronium injection should be stored under refrigeration (2–8°C), but, according to the manufacturer, it is stable for 6 months at room temperature.

Do not store pancuronium in plastic syringes or containers as it may be adsorbed to plastic surfaces. It may be administered in plastic syringes, however.

Compatibility/Compounding Considerations
It is recommended that pancuronium NOT be mixed with barbiturates, as a precipitate may form, although data conflicts on this point. No precipitate was seen when pancuronium was mixed with succinylcholine, meperidine, neostigmine, gallamine, tubocurarine, or promethazine.

Dosage Forms/Regulatory Status
VETERINARY-LABELED PRODUCTS: None

The ARCI (Racing Commissioners International) has designated this drug as a class 2 substance. See the appendix for more information.

HUMAN-LABELED PRODUCTS:

Pancuronium Bromide for Injection: 1 mg/mL in 10 mL vials; 2 mg/mL in 2 mL & 5 mL vials & amps; generic; (Rx)

References
Carr, A. (2003). Short-term ventilator management: A practical discussion. Proceedings: IVECCS. Accessed via: Veterinary Information Network. http://goo.gl/TyFmj

Day, T. (2005). Anesthesia for the septic patient. Proceedings: IVECCS. Accessed via: Veterinary Information Network. http://goo.gl/NJZHH

Ivey, E. & J. Morrisey (2000). Therapeutics for Rabbits. *Vet Clin NA: Exotic Anim Pract* **3:1**(Jan): 183–216.

Mandsager, R.E. (1988, Last Update). "Personal Communication."

Papich, M. (1989). Effects of drugs on pregnancy. *Current Veterinary Therapy X: Small Animal Practice*. R Kirk Ed. Philadelphia, Saunders: 1291–1299.

PANTOPRAZOLE

(pan-*toe*-prah-zohl)   Protonix®, Pantoloc®

PROTON PUMP INHIBITOR

Prescriber Highlights

▶ Proton pump inhibitor similar to omeprazole; also available in IV dosage form

▶ May be useful in treating or preventing gastric acid-related pathologies in dogs, cats, foals & camelids

▶ Relatively limited research & experience in veterinary medicine, particularly when compared with omeprazole

▶ Appears well tolerated

Uses/Indications

Pantoprazole may be useful in treating or preventing gastric acid-related pathologies in dogs, cats, foals and camelids, particularly when the intravenous route is preferred. Pantoprazole is available in both intravenous and oral tablet (delayed-release) formulations. One study (Bersenas *et al.* 2005) performed in dogs, comparing the gastric pH effects of intravenous pantoprazole with oral omeprazole, intravenous ranitidine, and intravenous famotidine, found at the dosages used, that pantoprazole was more effective than ranitidine, but similar to famotidine, and that oral omeprazole was more effective in maintaining intragastric pH >3 for a longer period than pantoprazole.

Pantoprazole has been shown to directly reduce *in vitro* counts of *H. pylori* and is used in some *H. pylori* treatment protocols for humans.

Pharmacology/Actions

Pantoprazole is a substituted benzimidazole, similar to omeprazole and the other proton pump inhibitors (PPIs). At the secretory surface of gastric parietal cells, pantoprazole forms a covalent bond at two sites of the H^+/K^+ ATPase (proton pump) enzyme system. There it inhibits the transport of hydrogen ions into the stomach. Pantoprazole reduces acid secretion during both basal and stimulated conditions.

Pharmacokinetics

No specific information was located for pantoprazole pharmacokinetics in dogs or cats. In neonatal foals, intragastric (IG) administered pantoprazole bioavailability was 41% and drug was detected in plasma within 5 minutes of administration. Mean hourly gastric pH was increased for 2–24 hours versus untreated foals after either IV or IG administration, but IV administration increased pH significantly greater than IG administration, presumably due to low GI bioavailability (Ryan *et al.* 2005).In humans, it is rapidly absorbed after oral administration with an oral bioavailability of 77%. Food can reduce the rate of absorption, but does not appear to affect the extent of absorption. On average, 51% of gastric acid secretion is inhibited at 2.5 hours after a single dose and 85% is inhibited after the seventh day of daily administration. Protein binding is 98%, primarily to albumin. The drug is metabolized in the liver, primarily by CYP2C19 isoenzymes. CYP3A4, 2D6, 2C9, or 1A2 are minor components of pantoprazole biotransformation; pantoprazole does not appear to clinically affect (either induce or inhibit) the metabolism of other drugs using these isoenzymes for biotransformation. Metabolites of pantoprazole do not appear to have pharmacologic activity. Elimination half-life for both oral and IV administration is only about an hour, but the drug's pharmacologic action can persist for 24 hours or more, presumably due to irreversible binding at the receptor site. About 71% of a dose is excreted as metabolites in the urine, with the remainder in the feces as metabolites and unabsorbed drug.

Contraindications/Precautions/Warnings

Pantoprazole is contraindicated in patients known to be hypersensitive to it or other substituted benzimidazole PPIs.

Parenteral pantoprazole must be administered IV; **do not** give IM or SQ. Reconstituted injection (4 mg/mL) must be administered intravenously over not less than 2 minutes.

Adverse Effects

Use has been limited in small animals and an adverse effect profile is not well established; however, the drug appears to be tolerated well.

In humans, the most commonly reported adverse effects are diarrhea and headache. Hyperglycemia has been reported in about 1% of patients. Proton pump inhibitors have been associated with an increased risk of developing community-acquired pneumonia in humans. Injection site reactions (thrombophlebitis, abscess) have occurred with IV administration.

Reproductive/Nursing Safety

When pantoprazole was dosed in rats (98X human dose) and rabbits (16X), no affects on fertility or teratogenic effects were noted. In humans, the FDA categorizes pantoprazole as category *B* for use during pregnancy (*Animal studies have not yet demonstrated risk to the fetus, but there are no adequate studies in pregnant women; or animal studies have shown an adverse effect, but adequate studies in pregnant women have not demonstrated a risk to the fetus in the first trimester of pregnancy, and there is no evidence of risk in later trimesters.*)

Pantoprazole and its metabolites have been detected in milk, but it should be relatively safe to use in nursing veterinary patients.

Overdosage/Acute Toxicity

There is limited information available. A single oral dose of 887 mg/kg was lethal in dogs. Acute toxic signs included ataxia, hypo-activity, and tremor. In humans, single oral overdoses of up to 600 mg have been reported without adversity. In the event of a large overdose, it is recommended to contact an animal poison control center for guidance.

Drug Interactions

The following drug interactions have either been reported or are theoretical in humans or animals receiving pantoprazole and may be of significance in veterinary patients:

- ◼ **DRUGS REQUIRING DECREASED GASTRIC PH FOR OPTIMAL ABSORPTION (e.g., ketoconazole, itraconazole, iron, ampicillin esters):** Pantoprazole may decrease drug absorption
- ◼ **SUCRALFATE:** May decrease bioavailability of orally administered pantoprazole
- ◼ **WARFARIN:** Pantoprazole may increase anticoagulant effect

Laboratory Considerations

- ◼ Although not likely to be important for veterinary patients, pantoprazole may cause false-positive results for urine screening tests for THC (tetrahydrocannabinol)

Doses

- ◼ **DOGS/CATS:**
  a) Dogs: For intravenous treatment of stress-related mucosal disease: 0.7–1 mg/kg IV once daily. (Bateman 2003)
  b) Dogs, Cats: 0.5–1 mg/kg IV over 15 minutes q24h (once daily). (Marks 2008)
- ◼ **HORSES:**
  a) For gastric acid suppression in neonatal foals: 1.5 mg/kg IV once daily. **Note:** From an experimental study evaluating the pharmacokinetics and pharmacodynamics in normal neonatal foals. Further studies are required to investigate the use of this drug in critically ill patients. (Ryan *et al.* 2005)

Monitoring

- ◼ Efficacy
- ◼ Adverse effects (vomiting, diarrhea, injection site reactions if used IV)

Client Information

- ◼ Tablets must be given whole; do not split or crush
- ◼ If patient develops bloody diarrhea, tarry-black stools, or vomits blood, contact veterinarian immediately
- ◼ Contact veterinarian if vomiting or diarrhea persist or are severe

Chemistry/Synonyms

Pantoprazole sodium sesquihydrate occurs as a white to off-white crystalline powder and is racemic. It is freely soluble in water and very slightly soluble in phosphate buffer at a pH of 7.4. Stability of aqueous solutions is pH dependent. At room temperature, solutions of pH 5 are stable for about 3 hours; at a pH of 7.8, 220 hours.

Pantoprazole may also be known as BY-1023, or SKF-96022. International trade names include: *Controloc®, Pantoloc®, Zurcal, Pantozol®, Pantop®, Protonix®, Protium®, Somac-MA®*, and many others.

Storage/Stability

Delayed-release tablets should be stored between 15–30°C.

The powder for injection should be stored protected from light at 20–25°C; excursions are permitted to 15– 30°C. For a 2-minute IV infusion; reconstitute with 10 mL of 0.9% sodium chloride injection. To prepare the injection for a 15-minute IV infusion, reconstitute with 10 mL of 0.9% sodium chloride injection, then dilute further with 100 mL of D5W, 0.9% sodium chloride or lactated Ringer's injection to a final concentration of approximately 0.4 mg/mL. Reconstituted solutions (10 mL) are stable for up to 2 hours at room temperature. If further diluted (per 15 minute infusion), it is stable for up to 22 hours at room temperature. Reconstituted solutions do not need to be protected from light. Do not freeze. Do not use the IV solution if discoloration or precipitates are seen; should these be observed during the infusion, stop immediately.

Compatibility/Compounding Considerations

Pantoprazole injection is **not compatible** with midazolam and may not be compatible with solutions containing zinc.

Dosage Forms/Regulatory Status

VETERINARY-LABELED PRODUCTS: None

The ARCI (Racing Commissioners International) has designated this drug as a class 5 substance. See the appendix for more information.

HUMAN-LABELED PRODUCTS:

Pantoprazole Sodium Delayed-Release Tablets: 20 mg (as base) & 40 mg (as base); *Protonix®* (Wyeth-Ayerst); generic; (Rx)

Pantoprazole Lyophilized Powder for Injection Solution: 40 mg (as base) in vials; *Protonix I.V.®* (Wyeth-Ayerst); (Rx)

Pantoprazole Sodium Delayed-Release Granules for Suspension: 40 mg; *Protonix®* (Wyeth-Ayerst); (Rx)

References

Bateman, S. (2003). Gastroprotectants—which drug to use when? Proceedings: IVECCS 2003. Accessed via: Veterinary Information Network. http://goo.gl/atRuu

Bersenas, A., K. Mathews, et al. (2005). Effects of ranitidine, famotidine, pantoprazole, and omeprazole on intragastric pH in dogs. AJVR **66**(3): 425–431.

Marks, S. (2008). GI Therapeutics: Which Ones and When? Proceedings; IVECCS. Accessed via: Veterinary Information Network. http://goo.gl/rxwcs

Ryan, C., L. Sanchez, et al. (2005). Pharmacokinetics and pharmacodynamics of pantoprazole in clinically normal neonatal foals. Proceedings: ACVIM 2005. Accessed via: Veterinary Information Network. http://goo.gl/dW4cw

PARAPOX OVIS VIRUS IMMUNO-MODULATOR

(pair-ah-**poks oh**-vis)   Zylexis®

IMMUNOSTIMULANT

Prescriber Highlights

▶ Biologic immunostimulant labeled for use in healthy horses of 4 months of age & older as an aid in reducing upper respiratory disease caused by equine herpesvirus types 1 & 4

▶ Limited published information available on safety & efficacy

Uses/Indications

Parapox ovis virus immunomodulator is commercially available in the USA labeled for "use in healthy horses of 4 months of age and older as an aid in reducing upper respiratory disease caused by equine herpesvirus types 1 and 4."

A parapoxvirus product (*Baypamun®*) is reportedly available in some European countries for use in small animals.

Pharmacology/Actions

Parapox ovis is the virus responsible for "orf" in sheep, a contagious pustular dermatitis. The virus is inactivated in the commercial product. Parapoxvirus products are so-called "paramunity inducers" and are believed to prevent viral infection by pathogenic viruses via viral interference. By "infecting" host cells with a defective (non-replicating) virus, interference with infection with the pathogenic virus can occur. Postulated mechanisms of action include induction of interferons, cytokines and colony-stimulating factors, and activation of natural killer cells.

Pharmacokinetics

Effects on the immune system are reported to occur 4–6 hours after treating; effects persist for 1–2 weeks.

Contraindications/Precautions/Warnings

Do not be use in patients with prior hypersensitivity to the agent. The manufacturer warns that in the case of an anaphylactic reaction, administer epinephrine or equivalent.

Reproductive/Nursing Safety

No information was located.

Adverse Effects

No adverse effects are listed in the package insert, but anaphylaxis is possible.

Overdosage/Acute Toxicity

No information was located.

Drug Interactions

None noted

Laboratory Considerations

◾ None identified

Doses

◾ **HORSES:**

a) For an aid in reducing upper airway disease caused by herpesvirus types 1 and 4: After reconstituting with the sterile diluent provided, administer 2 mL IM. Repeat doses on days 2 and 9 following the initial dose. Retreatment is recommended during subsequent disease episodes or prior to stress inducing situations. (Label information; *Zylexis®*—Pfizer)

b) For hyper-responding or delayed uterine clearance (DUC) broodmares: A single IM dose of *Zylexis®* the day before breeding followed by 12 mg of dexamethasone sodium phosphate IV at the time of breeding and 1 mL (20 Units) oxytocin and 1 mL (250 micrograms) estradiol with or without uterine lavage 6 hours later. This protocol used with hyper-responders and DUC mares frequently eliminates most other treatment requirements other than a day or two of oxytocin treatments. (Foss 2009)

Monitoring

◾ Clinical Efficacy (respiratory infection improvement)

Chemistry/Synonyms

Zylexis® is provided commercially as a freeze-dried inactivated (killed) virus component with separate 2 mL vial of sterile diluent.

Parapox ovis virus immunomodulator may also be known as: PPOV, PIND-ORF, or *Baypamune®* and *Zylexis®*.

Storage/Stability

Zylexis® should be stored refrigerated (2–8°C), but not be frozen. After reconstituting, entire contents should be used.

Dosage Forms/Regulatory Status

VETERINARY-LABELED PRODUCTS:

Parapox Ovis Virus Immunomodulator Injection in boxes of 5-single dose vials for reconstitution with 5-2mL vials of sterile diluent; *Zylexis®* (Pfizer); Labeled for use in horses.

Note: This product is a USDA-licensed biologic and is not FDA-approved. The label for *Zylexis®* states that it should not be administered to horses within 21 days of slaughter.

HUMAN-LABELED PRODUCTS: None

References

Foss, R. (2009). Breeding the Problem Mare. Proceedings: WVC. Accessed via: Veterinary Information Network. http://goo.gl/FfGK8

PAREGORIC

(par-eh-*gore*-ik); Camphorated Tincture of Opium

OPIATE ANTIDIARRHEAL

Prescriber Highlights

▶ Opiate GI motility modifier for diarrhea

▶ Contraindications: Known hypersensitivity to narcotic analgesics, patients receiving monoamine oxidase inhibitors (MAOIs), diarrhea caused by a toxic ingestion until the toxin is eliminated from the GI tract

▶ Caution: Respiratory disease, hepatic encephalopathy, hypothyroidism, severe renal insufficiency, adrenocortical insufficiency (Addison's), head injuries, or increased intracranial pressure, acute abdominal conditions (e.g., colic), & in geriatric or severely debilitated patients

▶ Adverse Effects: *Dogs:* Constipation, bloat, & sedation. Potential for: paralytic ileus, toxic megacolon, pancreatitis, & CNS effects. *Cats:* Use is controversial, may exhibit excitatory behavior. *Horses:* With GI bacterial infection, may delay the disappearance of the microbe from the feces & prolong the febrile state

▶ Dose carefully in small animals; do not confuse with opium tincture

▶ Paregoric is a C-III controlled substance

Uses/Indications

Paregoric is occasionally used as a motility modifier for animals with diarrhea. Opiates as an antidiarrheal treatment in cats is controversial and many clinicians do not recommend their use in this species.

Pharmacology/Actions

Among their other actions, opiates inhibit GI motility and excessive GI propulsion. They also decrease intestinal secretion induced by cholera toxin, prostaglandin E_2 and diarrheas caused by factors in which calcium is the second messenger (non-cyclic AMP/GMP mediated). Opiates may also enhance mucosal absorption.

Pharmacokinetics

The morphine in paregoric is absorbed in a variable fashion from the GI tract. It is rapidly metabolized in the liver and serum morphine levels are considerably less than when morphine is administered parenterally.

Contraindications/Precautions/Warnings

All opiates should be used with caution in patients with hypothyroidism, severe renal insufficiency, adrenocortical insufficiency, (Addison's), in geriatric or those severely debilitated. Opiate antidiarrheals are contraindicated in cases where the patient is hypersensitive to narcotic analgesics, those receiving monoamine oxidase inhibitors (MAOIs), and with diarrhea caused by a toxic ingestion until the toxin is eliminated from the GI tract.

Opiate antidiarrheals should be used with caution in patients with head injuries or increased intracranial pressure and acute abdominal conditions (*e.g.*, colic), as it may obscure the diagnosis or clinical course of these conditions. It should be used with extreme caution in patients suffering from respiratory disease or acute respiratory dysfunction (*e.g.*, pulmonary edema secondary to smoke inhalation). Opiate antidiarrheals should be used with extreme caution in patients with hepatic disease with CNS clinical signs of hepatic encephalopathy; hepatic coma may result.

Adverse Effects

In dogs, constipation, bloat, and sedation are the most likely adverse reactions encountered when usual doses are used. Potentially, paralytic ileus, toxic megacolon, pancreatitis, and CNS effects could be seen.

Use of antidiarrheal opiates in cats is controversial; this species may react with excitatory behavior.

Opiates used in horses with acute diarrhea (or in any animal with a potentially bacterial-induced diarrhea) may have a detrimental effect. Opiates may enhance bacterial proliferation, delay the disappearance of the microbe from the feces, and prolong the febrile state.

Reproductive/Nursing Safety

Opium tincture is classified as category C for use during pregnancy (*Animal studies have shown an adverse effect on the fetus, but there are no adequate studies in humans; or there are no animal reproduction studies and no adequate studies in humans.*)

Safe use of paregoric during breastfeeding in women has not been established; use with caution in nursing animals.

Overdosage/Acute Toxicity

Acute overdosage of the opiate antidiarrheals could result in CNS, cardiovascular, GI, or respiratory toxicity. Because the opiates may significantly reduce GI motility, absorption from the GI may be delayed and prolonged. For more information, refer to the meperidine and morphine monographs found in the CNS section. Naloxone may be necessary to reverse the opiate effects.

Drug Interactions

The following drug interactions have either been reported or are theoretical in humans or animals

receiving opiate antidiarrheals and may be of significance in veterinary patients:

- **CNS DEPRESSANT DRUGS (e.g., anesthetic agents, antihistamines, phenothiazines, barbiturates, tranquilizers, alcohol, etc.):** May cause increased CNS or respiratory depression when used with opiate antidiarrheal agents

- **MONOAMINE OXIDASE INHIBITORS (including amitraz, and possibly selegiline):** Opiate antidiarrheal agents are contraindicated in human patients receiving monoamine oxidase (MAO) inhibitors for at least 14 days after receiving MAO inhibitors

Laboratory Considerations

- Plasma **amylase** and **lipase** values may be increased for up to 24 hours following administration of opiates.

Doses

- **DOGS:**
  a) For acute colitis: 0.06 mg/kg, PO three times daily (DeNovo 1988)
  b) For maldigestion; malabsorption; antidiarrheal: 0.05–0.06 mg/kg PO two to three times daily (Chiapella 1988), (Johnson 1984)
  c) As an antidiarrheal: 0.05–0.06 mg/kg PO q12h (Willard 2003)

- **CATS:**
  Note: Use of antidiarrheal opiates in cats is controversial; this species may react with excitatory behavior.
  For maldigestion, malabsorption, antidiarrheal:
  a) 0.05–0.06 mg/kg PO two to three times daily (Chiapella 1989), (Johnson 1984)

- **CATTLE:**
  a) Calves: 15–30 mL PO (Cornell 1985)

- **HORSES:**
  a) Foals: 15–30 mL PO; Adults: 15–60 mL PO (Cornell 1985)

Monitoring

- Clinical efficacy
- Fluid and electrolyte status in severe diarrhea
- CNS effects if using high dosages

Client Information

- If diarrhea persists or animal appears listless or develops a high fever, contact veterinarian.

Chemistry/Synonyms

Paregoric contains 2 mg of the equivalent of anhydrous morphine (usually as powdered opium or opium tincture) per 5 mL. Also included (per 5 mL) are 0.02 mL anise oil, 0.2 mL glycerin, 20 mg benzoic acid, 20 mg camphor, and a sufficient quantity of diluted alcohol to make a total of 5 mL. Paregoric should not be confused with opium tincture (tincture of opium), which con-

tains 50 mg of anhydrous morphine equivalent per 5 mL.

Paregoric is also known as camphorated tincture of opium.

Storage/Stability

Paregoric should be stored in tight, light-resistant containers. Avoid exposure to excessive heat or direct exposure to sunlight.

Dosage Forms/Regulatory Status

VETERINARY-LABELED PRODUCTS: None

HUMAN-LABELED PRODUCTS:

Paregoric (camphorated tincture of opium): 2 mg of morphine equiv. per 5 mL (45% alcohol) in 473 mL; generic; (Rx; C-III)

Note: Do not confuse with opium tincture, which contains 25 times more morphine per mL than paregoric.

References

Chiapella, A.M. (1989). Diseases of the Small Intestine. *Handbook of Small Animal Practice.* RV Morgan Ed. New York, Churchill Livingstone: 395–420.
Cornell, S. (1985). *Veterinary Drug Formulary: Cornell Research Foundation, Inc.* Baltimore, Williams & Wilkins.
Johnson, S.E. (1984). Clinical pharmacology of antiemetics and antidiarrheals. 8th Annual Kal Kan Symposium for the Treatment of Small Animal Diseases, Columbus, Kal Kan Foods, Inc.
Willard, M. (2003). Digestive system disorders. *Small Animal Internal Medicine, 3rd Ed.* R Nelson and C Couto Eds. St Louis, Mosby: 343–471.

PAROMOMYCIN SULFATE

(pair-oh-moe-*my*-sin)   Humatin®

ORAL AMINOGLYCOSIDE ANTIPARASITIC

Prescriber Highlights

- Aminoglycoside used primarily as an alternative for PO treatment of cryptosporidiosis in small animals
- Not appreciably absorbed when gut is intact when dosed orally in humans & dogs
- Some state that the drug is contraindicated in cats secondary to toxicity
- Adverse effects are usually limited to GI effects (N,V,D); cats may be susceptible to renal & ophthalmic toxicity
- Use with caution in patients with intestinal ulceration

Uses/Indications

Paromomycin may be useful as a secondary treatment for cryptosporidiosis in dogs and cats. It has also been used topically to treat cutaneous Leishmaniasis. In humans, it has been used as an alternative treatment for giardiasis, *Dientamoeba fragilis*, and hepatic coma.

Pharmacology/Actions

Paromomycin has an antimicrobial spectrum of activity similar to neomycin, but its primary therapeutic uses are for the treatment of protozoa, including *Leishmania* spp., *Entamoeba histolytica*, and *Cryptosporidium* spp. It also has activity against a variety of tapeworms, but there are better choices available for clinical use.

Pharmacokinetics

Like neomycin, paromomycin is very poorly absorbed when given orally. Potentially systemic toxicity (nephrotoxicity, ototoxicity, pancreatitis) could occur if used in patients with significant ulcerative intestinal lesions or for a prolonged period at high dosages.

Contraindications/Precautions/Warnings

Paromomycin is contraindicated in patients with known hypersensitivity to the drug, ileus or intestinal obstruction, and GI ulceration.

Use with caution in cats. Because of potential toxicity, some clinicians recommend not using the drug in this species.

Do not use in animals with blood in the stool as this may signal that the drug could be absorbed and cause nephrotoxicity.

Adverse Effects

Gastrointestinal effects (nausea, inappetence, vomiting, diarrhea) are the most likely adverse effects to be noted with therapy. Because paromomycin can affect gut flora, nonsusceptible bacterial or fungal overgrowths are a possibility. In patients with significant gut ulceration, paromomycin may be absorbed systemically with resultant nephrotoxicity, ototoxicity, or pancreatitis.

Use in cats has been associated with renal dysfunction, ototoxicity and blindness.

Reproductive/Nursing Safety

Because minimal amounts are absorbed when administered orally, paromomycin should be safe to use during pregnancy. It should not be used parenterally during pregnancy.

When used orally, paromomycin should be safe to use during lactation.

Overdosage/Acute Toxicity

Because paromomycin is not absorbed orally, acute overdose adverse effects should be limited to gastrointestinal distress in patients with an intact GI system. Chronic overdoses may lead to systemic toxicity.

Drug Interactions

The following drug interactions have either been reported or are theoretical in humans or animals receiving paromomycin and may be of significance in veterinary patients:

■ **DIGOXIN:** Paromomycin may reduce digoxin absorption

■ **METHOTREXATE:** Paromomycin may reduce methotrexate absorption

Laboratory Considerations

■ None were noted.

Doses

■ **DOGS:**
For treatment of cryptosporidiosis:
a) 125–165 mg/kg PO twice daily for 5 days (Blagburn 2003)
b) 150 mg/kg PO once a day for 5 days. **Caution:** nephrotoxicity. (Tams 2003)

■ **CATS:**
For treatment of cryptosporidiosis: **Note:** Higher dosages of paromomycin have caused renal or otic toxicity and/or blindness in some treated cats. Consider using an alternate treatment first (*e.g.*, azithromycin) or paromomycin at an initially reduced dosage level.
a) 125–165 mg/kg PO twice daily for 5 days. (Blagburn 2003)
b) 150 mg/kg PO once a day for 5 days. **Caution:** nephrotoxicity. (Tams 2003)
c) 150 mg/kg PO q12-24hr. Paromomycin can be nephrotoxic if absorbed. If the cat is responding to the first 7 days of therapy and toxicity has not been noted, continue treatment for 1 week past clinical resolution of diarrhea. (Lappin 2008)

■ **CAMELIDS (NWC):**
For treatment of cryptosporidiosis in crias: 50 mg/kg PO (*dosing interval not specified, assume once per day—Plumb*) for 5–10 days. (Walker 2009)

■ **REPTILES:**
For treatment of cryptosporidiosis: 300–800 mg/kg PO q24-48h for 7–14 days or as needed (de la Navarre 2003)

Monitoring

■ Efficacy

■ GI adverse effects

■ If used in cats, monitor renal function

Client Information

■ Unless otherwise instructed, give with food.

Chemistry/Synonyms

An aminoglycoside antibiotic, paromomycin sulfate occurs as an odorless, creamy white to light yellow, hygroscopic, amorphous powder having a saline taste. Paromomycin is very soluble in water (>1 gram/mL).

Paromomycin may also be known as: aminosidin sulphate, aminosidine sulphate, catenulin sulphate, crestomycin sulphate; estomycin sulphate, hydroxymycin sulphate, monomycin A sulphate, neomycin E sulphate, paucimycin sulphate, *Gabbromicina®, Gabbroral®, Gabroral®, Humagel®, Humatin®, Kaman®*, and *Sinosid®*.

Storage/Stability

Paromomycin capsules should be stored at room temperature (15–30°C; 59–86°F) in tight containers.

Dosage Forms/Regulatory Status

VETERINARY-LABELED PRODUCTS: None

HUMAN-LABELED PRODUCTS:

Paromomycin Sulfate Oral Capsules: 250 mg; *Humatin*® (Parke-Davis); generic; (Rx)

References

Blagburn, B. (2003). Current recognition, control and prevention of protozoan parasites affecting dogs and cats. Proceedings: Western Veterinary Conference. Accessed via: Veterinary Information Network. http://goo.gl/QsVOr

de la Navarre, B. (2003). Common parasitic diseases of reptiles and amphibians. Proceedings: Western Veterinary Conf. Accessed via: Veterinary Information Network. http://goo.gl/ZafJD

Lappin, M.R. (2008). Giardia and Cryptosporidium Spp. Infections of Cats: Clinical and Zoonotic Aspects. Proceedings: ECVIM. Accessed via: Veterinary Information Network. http://goo.gl/ZyO3e

Tams, T. (2003). Giardiasis, Clostridium perfringens enterotoxicosis, and Cryptosporidiosis. Proc: Atlantic Coast Veterinary Conf.

Walker, P. (2009). Differential Diagnosis of Diarrhea in Camelid Crias. Proceedings: ACVIM. Accessed via: Veterinary Information Network. http://goo.gl/0C6AM

PAROXETINE HCL

(pah-**rox**-a-teen)   Paxil®

SELECTIVE SEROTONIN REUPTAKE
INHIBITOR (SSRI) ANTIDEPRESSANT

Prescriber Highlights

▶ Selective serotonin reuptake inhibitor antidepressant related to fluoxetine used in dogs & cats for variety of behavior disorders

▶ Contraindications: Patients with known hypersensitivity or receiving monoamine oxidase inhibitors

▶ Caution: Patients with severe cardiac, renal or hepatic disease. Dosages may need to be reduced in patients with severe renal, or hepatic impairment. If patient is on the drug for an extended period, gradual withdrawal recommended.

▶ Adverse effect profile is not well established; potentially in *Dogs*: Anorexia, lethargy, GI effects, anxiety, irritability, insomnia/hyperactivity, or panting. Aggressive behavior in previously unaggressive dogs possible. *Cats*: May exhibit behavior changes (anxiety, irritability, sleep disturbances), anorexia, constipation & changes in elimination patterns

Uses/Indications

Paroxetine may be beneficial for the treatment of canine aggression, and stereotypic or other obsessive-compulsive behaviors. It has been used occasionally in cats as well.

Pharmacology/Actions

Paroxetine is a highly selective inhibitor of the reuptake of serotonin (SSRI) in the CNS, thus potentiating the pharmacologic activity of serotonin. Paroxetine apparently has little effect on other neurotransmitters (*e.g.*, dopamine or norepinephrine).

Pharmacokinetics

No veterinary data was located. In humans, paroxetine is slowly, but nearly completely, absorbed from the GI tract. Because of a relatively high first pass-effect, relatively small amounts reach the systemic circulation unchanged. Food does not impair absorption.

The drug is about 95% bound to plasma proteins. Paroxetine is extensively metabolized, probably in the liver. Half-life in humans ranges from 7–65 hours and averages about 24 hours.

Contraindications/Precautions/Warnings

Paroxetine is contraindicated in patients with known hypersensitivity to it or those receiving monoamine oxidase inhibitors (see Drug Interactions below). Use with caution in patients with seizure disorders, severe cardiac, hepatic, or renal disease. Dosages may need to be reduced in patients with severe hepatic or renal impairment.

If paroxetine is rapidly discontinued, withdrawal reactions can occur. If the patient has been receiving the drug for an extended period, a gradual withdrawal is recommended.

Adverse Effects

In dogs, paroxetine can cause lethargy, GI effects, anxiety, irritability, insomnia/hyperactivity, or panting. Anorexia is a common side effect in dogs (usually transient and may be negated by temporarily increasing the palatability of food and/or hand feeding). Some dogs have persistent anorexia that precludes further treatment. Aggressive behavior in previously unaggressive dogs has been reported. SSRIs may also cause changes in blood glucose levels and potentially, reduce seizure threshold.

Paroxetine in cats can cause behavior changes (anxiety, irritability, sleep disturbances), anorexia, constipation and changes in elimination patterns.

Reproductive/Nursing Safety

Paroxetine's safety during pregnancy has not been established. Preliminary studies done in rats demonstrated no overt teratogenic effects. In humans, the FDA categorizes this drug as category *C* for use during pregnancy (*Animal studies have shown an adverse effect on the fetus, but there are no adequate studies in humans; or there are no animal reproduction studies and no adequate studies in humans.*)

The drug is excreted into milk but at low levels; caution is advised in nursing patients.

Overdosage/Acute Toxicity

There is limited information available. Experience with overdoses in humans yields a mixed picture. While not as toxic as the tricyclic antidepressants, fatalities and significant morbidity have occurred after paroxetine overdoses.

There were 114 exposures to paroxetine reported to the ASPCA Animal Poison Control Center (APCC) during 2008-2009. In these cases 102 were dogs with 20 showing clinical signs, and 12 were cats with 4 showing clinical signs. Common findings in dogs recorded in decreasing frequency included hyperactivity, lethargy, mydriasis, and trembling. Common findings in cats included mydriasis.

In overdoses with small animals, it is recommended to err on the safe side and employ gut evacuation (if not contraindicated) and then treat supportively. Activated charcoal is very effective in binding paroxetine. Phenothiazine and cyproheptadine can be effective in controlling serotonin syndrome. Contact an animal poison control center for additional guidance.

Drug Interactions

The following drug interactions have either been reported or are theoretical in humans or animals receiving paroxetine and may be of significance in veterinary patients:

■ **BUSPIRONE:** Increased risk for serotonin syndrome

■ **CIMETIDINE:** May increase paroxetine levels

■ **CYPROHEPTADINE:** May decrease or reverse the effects of SSRIs

■ **DIGOXIN:** Paroxetine (in humans) can decrease digoxin AUC by 15%

■ **INSULIN:** May alter insulin requirements

■ **ISONIAZID:** Increased risk for serotonin syndrome

■ **MAO INHIBITORS (including amitraz and potentially, selegiline):** High risk for serotonin syndrome; use contraindicated; in humans, a 5 week washout period is required after discontinuing paroxetine and a 2 week washout period if first discontinuing the MAO inhibitor

■ **PENTAZOCINE:** Serotonin syndrome-like adverse effects possible

■ **PHENOBARBITAL:** May decrease paroxetine levels

■ **PHENYTOIN:** Increased plasma levels of phenytoin possible; may decrease paroxetine levels

■ **PROPRANOLOL, METOPROLOL:** Paroxetine may increase these beta-blockers' plasma levels and cause hypotension; atenolol may be safer to use if paroxetine required

■ **TRAMADOL:** SSRI's can inhibit the metabolism of tramadol to the active metabolites decreasing its efficacy and increasing the risk of toxicity (serotonin syndrome, seizures).

■ **TRICYCLIC ANTIDEPRESSANTS (e.g., clomipramine, amitriptyline):** Paroxetine may increase TCA blood levels and may increase the risk for serotonin syndrome

■ **THEOPHYLLINE:** Increased plasma levels of theophylline possible

■ **WARFARIN:** Paroxetine may increase the risk for bleeding

Doses

■ **DOGS:**

For SSRI responsive behavior problems:

a) For compulsive disorders: 1 mg/kg (up to 3 mg/kg) PO once daily (q24h) (Landsberg 2004)

b) For generalized anxiety disorder: 1–1.5 mg/kg q24h (Crowell-Davis 2009)

c) For adjunctive treatment of phobias, fears, and anxieties: 0.5–1 mg/kg PO once daily (Moffat 2007a)

■ **CATS:**

For SSRI responsive behavior problems:

a) 0.5–1 mg/kg q24h (2.5–5 mg per cat q24h) (Levine 2008)

b) For compulsive disorders: 0.5–1 mg/kg PO once daily (q24h) (Landsberg 2004)

c) For generalized anxiety disorder: 0.5–1.5 mg/kg q24h (Crowell-Davis 2009)

d) For marking: 0.5–1 mg/kg PO once daily (Landsberg 2007), (Neilson 2007)

e) For intercat aggression: 0.5–1 mg/kg PO once daily (Moffat 2007b)

f) 0.5–1.5 mg/kg PO q24-48h (Curtis 2008)

Monitoring

■ Efficacy

■ Adverse effects; including appetite (weight)

Client Information

■ Keep medication out of reach of children and pets

■ May cause GI effects (especially lack of appetite, constipation), behavior and sleep changes; if these become issues, contact veterinarian

Chemistry/Synonyms

A selective serotonin reuptake inhibitor (SSRI) antidepressant, paroxetine HCl occurs as an off-white, odorless powder. It has a solubility in water of 5.4 mg/mL and a pKa of 9.9.

Paroxetine may also be known as: BRL-29060, FG-7051, and *Paxil*®.

Storage/Stability

Paroxetine oral tablets should be stored at 15–30°C. The oral suspension should be stored below 25°C.

Dosage Forms/Regulatory Status

VETERINARY-LABELED PRODUCTS: None

The ARCI (Racing Commissioners International) has designated this drug as a class 2 substance. See the appendix for more information.

HUMAN-LABELED PRODUCTS:

Paroxetine Oral Tablets: 10 mg, 20 mg, 30 mg & 40 mg; *Paxil*® (GlaxoSmithKline); *Pexeva*® (Synthon); generic; (Rx)

Paroxetine Oral Tablets Controlled-release: 12.5 mg, 25 mg & 37.5 mg; *Paxil® CR* (Glaxo-SmithKline); generic; (Rx)

Paroxetine Oral Suspension: 2 mg/mL in 250 mL; *Paxil®* (GlaxoSmithKline); generic; (Rx)

References

Crowell-Davis, S.L. (2009). Generalized Anxiety Disorder. *Compendium-Continuing Education for Veterinarians* 31(9): 427–430.

Curtis, T. (2008). Human-directed aggression in the cat. *Vet Clin NA: Sm Anim Pract* **38**: 1131–1143.

Landsberg, G. (2004). A behaviorists approach to compulsive disorders. Proceedings: ACVIM Forum, Minneapolis. Accessed via: Veterinary Information Network. http://goo.gl/eRUh2

Landsberg, G. (2007). Drug and natural alternatives for marking cats. Proceedings: Western Vet Conference. Accessed via: Veterinary Information Network. http://goo.gl/ro1SR

Levine, E. (2008). Feline Fear and Anxiety. *Vet Clin NA: Sm Anim Pract* **38**: 1065–1079.

Moffat, K. (2007a). Fears, Anxieties & Phobias. Proceedings: Western Vet Conf. Accessed via: Veterinary Information Network. http://goo.gl/wM3GQ

Moffat, K. (2007b). Intercat aggression. Proceedings: Western Vet Conf. Accessed via: Veterinary Information Network. http://goo.gl/WXmv5

Neilson, J. (2007). Behavioral management of FLUTD: Thinking outside (& inside) the litterbox. Proceedings: Western Vet Conf. Accessed via: Veterinary Information Network. http://goo.gl/2DI7W

PEG 3550 Products—see Laxatives

PENICILLAMINE

(pen-i-*sill*-a-meen)   Depen®, Cuprimine®

ANTIDOTE; CHELATING AGENT

Prescriber Highlights

▶ Chelating agent used primarily for copper-storage hepatopathies (dogs). May be considered for lead poisoning or cystine urolithiasis

▶ Contraindications: History of penicillamine-related blood dyscrasias; lead present in GI tract

▶ Adverse Effects: Nausea, vomiting, & depression. Can reduce GI dietary mineral (zinc, iron, copper, and calcium) absorption and cause deficiencies; Rarely: Fever, lymphadenopathy, skin hypersensitivity reactions, or immune-complex glomerulonephropathy

▶ Potentially teratogenic

▶ Preferably given on an empty stomach

Uses/Indications

Penicillamine is used primarily for its chelating ability in veterinary medicine. It is the drug of choice for Copper storage-associated hepatopathies in dogs, but clinical improvement may require weeks to months of therapy. It can also be used for the long-term oral treatment of lead, or mercury poisoning or in cystine urolithiasis.

Because it has anti-fibrotic effects, penicillamine may be of benefit in chronic hepatitis, but doses necessary for effective treatment may be too high to be tolerated.

Pharmacology/Actions

Penicillamine chelates a variety of metals, including copper, lead, iron, and mercury, forming stable water soluble complexes that are excreted by the kidneys.

Penicillamine combines chemically with cystine to form a stable, soluble complex that can be readily excreted.

Penicillamine has antirheumatic activity. The exact mechanisms for this action are not understood, but the drug apparently improves lymphocyte function, decreases IgM rheumatoid factor and immune complexes in serum and synovial fluid.

Penicillamine possesses antifibrotic activity via inhibition of collagen crosslinking thereby causing collagen to be more susceptible to degradation.

Although penicillamine is a degradation product of penicillins, it has no antimicrobial activity.

Pharmacokinetics

In humans, penicillamine is well absorbed after oral administration and peak serum levels occur about one hour after dosing. The drug apparently crosses the placenta but, otherwise, little information is known about its distribution. Penicillamine that is not complexed with either a metal or cystine is thought metabolized by the liver and excreted in the urine and feces.

Contraindications/Precautions/Warnings

Penicillamine is contraindicated in patients with a history of penicillamine-related blood dyscrasias. Penicillamine potentially can cause enhanced absorption of lead from the gastrointestinal tract. If lead is still present in the gut, it should not be administered.

Adverse Effects

In dogs, the most prevalent adverse effects associated with penicillamine are nausea, vomiting, and depression. If vomiting is a problem, attempt to alleviate by giving smaller doses of the drug on a more frequent basis. Although food probably decreases the bioavailability of the drug, many clinicians recommend mixing the drug with food or giving at mealtimes if vomiting persists. Although thought infrequent or rare, fever, lymphadenopathy, skin hypersensitivity reactions, or immune-complex glomerulonephropathy may occur.

Penicillamine can reduce GI dietary mineral (zinc, iron, copper, and calcium) absorption and cause deficiencies with long-term use.

Reproductive/Nursing Safety

Penicillamine has been associated with the development of birth defects in offspring of rats given 10 times the recommended dose. There are also some reports of human teratogenicity. In humans, the FDA categorizes this drug as category *D* for use during pregnancy (*There is evidence of human fetal risk, but the potential benefits from the use of the drug in pregnant women may be acceptable despite its potential risks.*)

Lactation safety has not been established.

Overdosage/Acute Toxicity

No specific acute toxic dose has been established for penicillamine and toxic effects generally occur in patients taking the drug chronically. Any relationship of toxicity to dose is unclear; patients on small doses may develop toxicity.

Drug Interactions

The following drug interactions have either been reported or are theoretical in humans or animals receiving penicillamine and may be of significance in veterinary patients:

■ **4-AMINOQUINOLINE DRUGS (e.g., chloroquine, quinacrine):** Concomitant administration with these agents may increase the risks for severe dermatologic adverse effects

■ **CATIONS, ORAL including ZINC, IRON, CALCIUM, MAGNESIUM:** May decrease the effectiveness of penicillamine if given orally together

■ **FOOD, ANTACIDS:** The amount of penicillamine absorbed from the GI tract may be reduced by the concurrent administration of food or antacids

■ **GOLD COMPOUNDS:** May increase the risk of hematologic and/or renal adverse reactions

■ **IMMUNOSUPPRESSANT DRUGS (e.g., cyclophosphamide, azathioprine, but not corticosteroids):** May increase the risk of hematologic and/or renal adverse reactions

■ **PHENYLBUTAZONE:** May increase the risk of hematologic and/or renal adverse reactions

Laboratory Considerations

■ When using **technetium Tc 99m gluceptate** to visualize the kidneys, penicillamine may chelate this agent and form a compound that is excreted via the hepatobiliary system resulting in gallbladder visualization that could confuse the results.

Doses

■ **DOGS:**

For copper-associated hepatopathy:

a) 10–15 mg/kg PO q12h on an empty stomach. Do not give concurrently with any medication, including zinc or a vitamin-mineral supplement. (Jergens & Willard 2000)

b) Reduce copper intake (water, food), use chelation initially if liver copper >1,500 micrograms/gram dry wt, and thereafter may reduce enteric copper uptake with zinc. Chelation: penicillamine 15 mg/kg

PO twice daily 30 minutes before meals. Give supplemental pyridoxine. Chelate at least 6 months, and then use a second liver biopsy to determine efficacy and chronic treatment plan. If copper is critically lower, may be worth trying chronic zinc acetate, maintain dietary copper restriction, and watch ALT. If the patient is zinc intolerant, use chronic penicillamine at a dose restriction of 50%. Do not use chelation and zinc together; staggered dosing may still result in penicillamine-zinc chelation. (Center 2008)

c) 10–15 mg/kg PO two times a day 30 minutes prior to food. Start low and increase. (Webb 2007)

d) 15 mg/kg PO twice daily on an empty stomach. (Twedt 2009)

For cystine urolithiasis:

a) 15 mg/kg: PO twice daily. If nausea and vomiting occur, mix with food or give at mealtime. Some dogs may need to have the dosage slowly increased to full dose in order to tolerate the drug. (Osborne *et al.* 1989)

b) 15 mg/kg: PO twice daily with food (Lage *et al.* 1988)

For lead poisoning:

a) After initial therapy regimen with CaEDTA and if continued therapy is desired at home, may give penicillamine at 110 mg/kg/day, PO divided q6–8h for 1–2 weeks. If vomiting, depression, and anorexia occur, may reduce dose to 33–55 mg/kg/day divided q6–8h, which should be better tolerated. (Mount 1989)

b) As an alternate or adjunct to CaEDTA: 110 mg/kg/day divided q6–8h PO 30 minutes before feeding for 1–2 weeks. If vomiting a problem may premedicate with dimenhydrinate (2–4 mg/kg PO). Alternatively, may give 33–55 mg/kg/day divided as above. Dissolving medication in juice may facilitate administration. (Nicholson 2000)

■ **CATS:**

For lead poisoning:

a) After initial therapy with CaEDTA and if blood lead is greater than 0.2 ppm at 3–4 weeks post-treatment, may repeat CaEDTA or give penicillamine at 125 mg q12h PO for 5 days. (Reid & Oehme 1989)

■ **RUMINANTS:**

Note: When used in food animals, FARAD recommends a minimum milk withdrawal time of 3 days after the last treatment and a 21-day preslaughter withdrawal. (Haskell *et al.* 2005)

a) For copper toxicity in small ruminants: 52 mg/kg daily for 6 days is sometimes successful (Reilly 2004)

b) For copper toxicity in small ruminants: 26–52 mg/kg PO once daily for 6 days. (Boileau 2009)

c) For lead or mercury toxicity: 110 mg/kg PO for 1-3 weeks. To prevent continued metal absorption, must clear GI tract of toxic metal before therapy. (Osweiler 2007)

■ **BIRDS:**

For adjunctive treatment of lead poisoning:

a) 55 mg/kg PO q12h for 1–2 weeks. It has been suggested that combining CaEDTA and penicillamine for several days until symptoms dissipate followed by a 3–6 week treatment with penicillamine as the best regimen for lead toxicity. (Jones 2007)

Monitoring

■ Monitoring of penicillamine therapy is dependent upon the reason for its use; refer to the references in the Dose section above for further discussion on the diseases and associated monitoring of therapy.

Client Information

■ This drug should preferably be given on an empty stomach, at least 30 minutes before feeding. If the animal develops problems with vomiting or anorexia, three remedies have been suggested:

1) Give the same total daily dose, but divide into smaller individual doses and give more frequently

2) Temporarily reduce the daily dose and gradually increase to recommended dosage, or

3) Give with a small amount of food (*e.g.*, cheese or bread). Giving with full meals will probably reduce amount of drug absorbed, but may be necessary in some patients.

Chemistry/Synonyms

A monothiol chelating agent that is a degradation product of penicillins, penicillamine occurs as a white or practically white, crystalline powder with a characteristic odor. Penicillamine is freely soluble in water and slightly soluble in alcohol with pK_a values of 1.83, 8.03, and 10.83.

Penicillamine may also be known as: D-Penicillamine, beta,beta-Dimethylcysteine, D-3-Mercaptovaline, penicillaminum, *Depen*® and *Cuprimine*®.

Storage/Stability

Penicillamine should be stored at room temperature (15–30°C). The capsules should be stored in tight containers; tablets in well-closed containers.

Dosage Forms/Regulatory Status

VETERINARY-LABELED PRODUCTS: None

HUMAN-LABELED PRODUCTS:

Penicillamine Titratable Oral Tablets: 250 mg (scored); *Depen*® (Wallace); (Rx)

Penicillamine Oral Capsules: 125 mg & 250 mg; *Cuprimine*® (Aton Pharma); (Rx)

References

Boileau, M. (2009). Challenging cases in small ruminant medicine. Proceedings: ACVIM. Accessed via: Veterinary Information Network. http://goo.gl/ZEc1Z

Center, S. (2008). Update on Canine & Feline Liver Disease. Proceedings: ECVIM. Accessed via: Veterinary Information Network. http://goo.gl/jSTOR

Haskell, S., M. Payne, et al. (2005). Farad Digest: Antidotes in Food Animal Practice. *JAVMA* **226**(6): 884–887.

Jergens, A. & M. Willard (2000). Diseases of the large Intestine. *Textbook of Veterinary Internal Medicine: Diseases of the Dog and Cat*. S Ettinger and E Feldman Eds. Philadelphia, WB Saunders. **2**: 1238–1256.

Jones, M. (2007). Avian Toxicology. Proceedings: Western Vet Conf. Accessed via: Veterinary Information Network. http://goo.gl/YC7Vj

Lage, A.L., D. Polzin, et al. (1988). Diseases of the Bladder. *Handbook of Small Animal Practice*. RV Morgan Ed. New York, Churchill Livingstone: 605–620.

Mount, M.E. (1989). Toxicology. *Textbook of Veterinary Internal Medicine*. SJ Ettinger Ed. Philadelphia, WB Saunders. **1**: 456–483.

Nicholson, S. (2000). Toxicology. *Textbook of Veterinary Internal Medicine: Diseases of the Dog and Cat*. S Ettinger and E Feldman Eds. Philadelphia, WB Saunders. **1**: 357–363.

Osborne, C.A., A. Hoppe, et al. (1989). Medical Dissolution and Prevention of Cystine Urolithiasis. *Current Veterinary Therapy X: Small Animal Practice*. RW Kirk Ed. Philadelphia, WB Saunders: 1189–1193.

Osweiler, G. (2007). Detoxification and Antidotes for Ruminant Poisoning. Proceedings: ACVIM. Accessed via: Veterinary Information Network. http://goo.gl/h1YRI

Reid, F.M. & F.W. Oehme (1989). Toxicoses. *The Cat: Diseases and Clinical Management*. RG Sherding Ed. New York, Churchill Livingstone. **1**: 185–215.

Reilly, L. (2004). Anemia in small ruminants. Proceedings: ACVIM Forum, Mpls. Accessed via: Veterinary Information Network. http://goo.gl/0EJWv

Twedt, D. (2009). Treatment of liver disease. Proceedings: ACVC. Accessed via: Veterinary Information Network. http://goo.gl/7SUeb

Webb, C. (2007). Pushing the envelope in liver and pancreatic diseases. Proceedings: Western Vet Conference. Accessed via: Veterinary Information Network. http://goo.gl/bKTSb

PENICILLINS, GENERAL INFORMATION

(pen-i-*sill*-in)

Uses/Indications

Penicillins have been used for a wide range of infections in various species. FDA-approved indications/species, as well as non-FDA-approved uses, are listed in the Uses/Indications and Dosage section for each drug.

Pharmacology/Actions

Penicillins are usually bactericidal against susceptible bacteria and act by inhibiting mucopeptide synthesis in the cell wall resulting in a defective barrier and an osmotically unstable spheroplast. The exact mechanism for this effect has not been definitively determined, but beta-lactam antibiotics have been shown to bind to several enzymes (carboxypeptidases, transpeptidases, endopeptidases) within the bacterial cytoplasmic membrane that are involved with cell wall synthesis. The different affinities that various beta-lactam antibiotics have for these enzymes (also known as penicillin-binding proteins; PBPs) help explain the differences in spectrums of activity the drugs have that are not explained by the influence of beta-lactamases. Like other beta-lactam antibiotics, penicillins are generally considered more effective against actively growing bacteria.

The clinically available penicillins encompass several distinct classes of compounds with varying spectrums of activity: The so-called natural penicillins including penicillin G and V; the penicillinase-resistant penicillins including cloxacillin, dicloxacillin, oxacillin, nafcillin, and methicillin; the aminopenicillins including ampicillin, amoxicillin, cyclacillin, hetacillin, and bacampicillin; extended-spectrum penicillins including carbenicillin, ticarcillin, piperacillin, azlocillin, and mezlocillin; and the potentiated penicillins including amoxicillin-potassium clavulanate, ampicillin-sulbactam, piperacillin-tazobactam, and ticarcillin-potassium clavulanate.

The natural penicillins (G and K) have similar spectrums of activity, but penicillin G is slightly more active *in vitro* on a weight basis against many organisms. This class of penicillin has *in vitro* activity against most spirochetes and gram-positive and gram-negative aerobic cocci, but not penicillinase-producing strains. They have activity against some aerobic and anaerobic gram-positive bacilli such as *Bacillus anthracis*, *Clostridium* spp. (not *C. difficile*), Fusobacterium, and Actinomyces. The natural penicillins are customarily inactive against most gram-negative aerobic and anaerobic bacilli and all Rickettsia, mycobacteria, fungi, Mycoplasma, and viruses.

The penicillinase-resistant penicillins have a narrower spectrum of activity than the natural penicillins. Their antimicrobial efficacy is aimed directly against penicillinase-producing strains of gram-positive cocci, particularly staphylococcal species; these drugs are sometimes called anti-staphylococcal penicillins. There are documented strains of Staphylococcus that are resistant to these drugs (so-called methicillin-resistant or oxacillin-resistant Staph), but these strains have only begun to be a significant problem in veterinary species. While this class of penicillins does have activity against some other gram-positive and gram-negative aerobes and anaerobes, other antibiotics are usually better choices. The penicillinase-resistant penicillins are inactive against Rickettsia, mycobacteria, fungi, Mycoplasma, and viruses.

The aminopenicillins, also called the "broad-spectrum" or ampicillin penicillins, have increased activity against many strains of gram-negative aerobes not covered by either the natural penicillins or penicillinase-resistant penicillins, including some strains of *E. coli*, Klebsiella, and Haemophilus. Like the natural penicillins, they are susceptible to inactivation by beta-lactamase-producing bacteria (*e.g.*, Staph aureus). Although not as active as the natural penicillins, they do have activity against many anaerobic bacteria, including Clostridial organisms. Organisms that are generally not susceptible include *Pseudomonas aeruginosa*, Serratia, Indole-positive Proteus (*Proteus mirabilis* is susceptible), Enterobacter, Citrobacter, and Acinetobacter. The aminopenicillins also are inactive against Rickettsia, mycobacteria, fungi, Mycoplasma, and viruses.

The extended-spectrum penicillins, sometimes called anti-pseudomonal penicillins, include both alpha-carboxypenicillins (carbenicillin and ticarcillin) and acylaminopenicillins (piperacillin, azlocillin, and mezlocillin). These agents have similar spectrums of activity as the aminopenicillins but with additional activity against several gram-negative organisms of the family Enterobacteriaceae, including many strains of *Pseudomonas aeruginosa*. Like the aminopenicillins, these agents are susceptible to inactivation by beta-lactamases.

In order to reduce the inactivation of penicillins by beta-lactamases, potassium clavulanate and sulbactam have been developed to inactivate these enzymes and extend the spectrum of those penicillins. When used with penicillin, these combinations are often effective against many beta-lactamase-producing strains of otherwise resistant *E. coli*, *Pasturella* spp., *Staphylococcus* spp., Klebsiella, and Proteus. Type I beta-lactamases are often associated with *E. coli*, Enterobacter, and Pseudomonas, and not generally inhibited by clavulanic acid.

Pharmacokinetics (General)

The oral absorption characteristics of the penicillins are dependent upon its class. Penicillin G is the only available oral penicillin that is substantially affected by gastric pH and can be completely inactivated at a pH of less than 2. The other orally available penicillins are resistant to acid degradation but bioavailability can be decreased (not amoxicillin) by the presence of food. Of the orally administered penicillins, penicillin V and amoxicillin tend to have the greatest bioavailability in their respective classes.

Penicillins are generally distributed widely throughout the body. Most drugs attain therapeutic levels in the kidneys, liver, heart, skin, lungs, intestines, bile, bone, prostate, and peritoneal, pleural, and synovial fluids. Penetration into the CSF and eye only occur with inflammation and may not reach therapeutic levels. Penicillins are bound in varying degrees to plasma proteins and cross the placenta.

Most penicillin's are rapidly excreted largely unchanged by the kidneys into the urine via glomerular filtration and tubular secretion. Probenecid can prolong half-lives and increase serum levels by blocking the tubular secretion of penicillins. Except for nafcillin and oxacillin, hepatic inactivation and biliary secretion is a minor route of excretion.

Contraindications/Precautions/Warnings

Penicillins are contraindicated in patients with a history of hypersensitivity to them. Because there may be cross-reactivity, use penicillins cautiously in patients who are documented hypersensitive to other beta-lactam antibiotics (e.g., cephalosporins, cefamycins, carbapenems).

Do not administer systemic antibiotics orally in patients with septicemia, shock, or other grave illnesses, as absorption of the medication from the GI tract may be significantly delayed or diminished. Parenteral (preferably IV) routes should be used for these cases. Certain species (snakes, birds, turtles, Guinea pigs, and chinchillas) are reportedly sensitive to procaine penicillin G.

High doses of penicillin G sodium or potassium, particularly in small animals with a pre-existing electrolyte abnormality, renal disease, or congestive heart failure may cause electrolyte imbalances. Other injectable penicillins, such as ticarcillin, carbenicillin, and ampicillin, have significant quantities of sodium per gram and may cause electrolyte imbalances when used in large dosages in susceptible patients.

Adverse Effects

Adverse effects with the penicillins are usually not serious and have a relatively low frequency of occurrence.

Hypersensitivity reactions unrelated to dose can occur with these agents and can manifest as rashes, fever, eosinophilia, neutropenia, agranulocytosis, thrombocytopenia, leukopenia, anemias, lymphadenopathy, or full-blown anaphylaxis. In humans, it is estimated that up to 15% of patients hypersensitive to cephalosporins will also be hypersensitive to penicillins. The incidence of cross-reactivity in veterinary patients is unknown.

When given orally, penicillins may cause GI effects (anorexia, vomiting, diarrhea). Because the penicillins may also alter gut flora, antibiotic-associated diarrhea can occur and allow the proliferation of resistant bacteria in the colon (superinfections).

Neurotoxicity (e.g., ataxia in dogs) has been associated with very high doses or very prolonged use. Although the penicillins are not considered hepatotoxic, elevated liver enzymes have been reported. Other effects reported in dogs include tachypnea, dyspnea, edema, and tachycardia.

Some penicillins (ticarcillin, carbenicillin, azlocillin, mezlocillin, piperacillin and nafcillin) have been implicated in causing bleeding problems in humans. These drugs are infrequently used systemically in veterinary species and veterinary ramifications of this effect are unclear.

Reproductive/Nursing Safety

Penicillins have been shown to cross the placenta and safe use of them during pregnancy has not been firmly established, but neither have there been any documented teratogenic problems associated with these drugs. In humans, the FDA categorizes this drug as category *B* for use during pregnancy (*Animal studies have not yet demonstrated risk to the fetus, but there are no adequate studies in pregnant women; or animal studies have shown an adverse effect, but adequate studies in pregnant women have not demonstrated a risk to the fetus in the first trimester of pregnancy, and there is no evidence of risk in later trimesters.*) However, use only when the potential benefits outweigh the risks.

Penicillins are excreted in maternal milk in low concentrations; use potentially could cause diarrhea, candidiasis, or allergic response in the nursing offspring.

Overdosage/Acute Toxicity

Acute oral penicillin overdoses are unlikely to cause significant problems other than GI distress, but other effects are possible (see Adverse effects). In humans, very high dosages of parenteral penicillins, especially in patients with renal disease, have induced CNS effects.

Drug Interactions

The following drug interactions have either been reported or are theoretical in humans or animals receiving penicillins and may be of significance in veterinary patients:

- **AMINOGLYCOSIDES:** *In vitro* studies have demonstrated that penicillins can have synergistic or additive activity against certain bacteria when used with aminoglycosides or cephalosporins.

- **BACTERIOSTATIC ANTIBIOTICS (e.g., chloramphenicol, erythromycin, tetracyclines):** Use with penicillins is generally not recommended, particularly in acute infections where the organism is proliferating rapidly as penicillins tend to perform better on actively growing bacteria.

- **PROBENECID:** Competitively blocks the tubular secretion of most penicillins, thereby increasing serum levels and serum half-lives.

Laboratory Considerations

- Penicillins may cause false-positive **urine glucose** determinations when using cupric-sulfate solution (Benedict's Solution, *Clinitest®*). Tests utilizing glucose oxidase (*Tes-Tape®, Clinistix®*) are not affected by penicillin.

- In humans, clavulanic acid and high dosages of piperacillin have caused a false-positive direct **Combs' test.**

■ As penicillins and other beta-lactams can inactivate aminoglycosides *in vitro* (and *in vivo* in patients in renal failure), serum concentrations of **aminoglycosides** may be falsely decreased if the patient is also receiving beta-lactam antibiotics and the serum is stored prior to analysis. It is recommended that if the assay is delayed, samples be frozen and, if possible, drawn at times when the beta-lactam antibiotic is at a trough.

Monitoring

■ Because penicillins usually have minimal toxicity associated with their use, monitoring for efficacy is usually all that is required unless toxic signs develop.

■ Serum levels and therapeutic drug monitoring are not routinely done with these agents.

Client Information

■ Owners should be instructed to give oral penicillins on an empty stomach, unless using amoxicillin or GI effects (anorexia, vomiting) occur.

■ Compliance with the therapeutic regimen should be stressed.

■ Reconstituted oral suspensions should be kept refrigerated and discarded after 14 days, unless labeled otherwise.

PENICILLIN G

(pen-i-*sill*-in *jee*)

PENICILLIN ANTIBIOTIC

Prescriber Highlights

▶ Prototypical penicillin agent used for susceptible gram-positive aerobes & anaerobes; best used parenterally

▶ Contraindications: Known hypersensitivity (unless no other options)

▶ Adverse Effects: Hypersensitivity possible. Very high doses may cause CNS effects

▶ Benzathine penicillin only effective against extremely sensitive agents

▶ Certain species may be sensitive to procaine penicillin G

Uses/Indications

Natural penicillins remain the drugs of choice for a variety of infections, including group A beta-hemolytic streptococci, many gram-positive anaerobes, spirochetes, gram-negative aerobic cocci, and some gram-negative aerobic bacilli. Generally, if a bacteria remains susceptible to a natural penicillin, either penicillin G or V is preferred for treating that infection as long as adequate penetration of the drug to the site of the infection occurs and the patient is not hypersensitive to penicillins.

Pharmacology/Actions

Penicillins are usually bactericidal against susceptible bacteria and act by inhibiting mucopeptide synthesis in the cell wall resulting in a defective barrier and an osmotically unstable spheroplast. The exact mechanism for this effect has not been definitively determined, but beta-lactam antibiotics have been shown to bind to several enzymes (carboxypeptidases, transpeptidases, endopeptidases) within the bacterial cytoplasmic membrane that are involved in cell wall synthesis. The different affinities that various beta-lactam antibiotics have for these enzymes (also known as penicillin-binding proteins; PBPs) help explain the differences in spectrums of activity the drugs have that are not explained by the influence of beta-lactamases. Like other beta-lactam antibiotics, penicillins are generally considered more effective against actively growing bacteria. Penicillins are considered time dependent antibiotics as efficacy depends on the length of time that plasma (or tissue) concentrations exceed the MIC of pathogens.

The natural penicillins (G and K) have similar spectrums of activity, but penicillin G is slightly more active *in vitro* on a weight basis against many organisms. This class of penicillin has *in vitro* activity against most spirochetes and gram-positive and gram-negative aerobic cocci, but not penicillinase producing strains. They have activity against some aerobic and anaerobic gram-positive bacilli such as *Bacillus anthracis*, *Clostridium* spp. (not *C. difficile*), Fusobacterium, and Actinomyces. The natural penicillins are customarily inactive against most gram-negative aerobic and anaerobic bacilli, and all Rickettsia, mycobacteria, fungi, Mycoplasma, and viruses.

Pharmacokinetics

Penicillin G potassium is poorly absorbed orally because of rapid acid-catalyzed hydrolysis. When administered on an empty (fasted) stomach, oral bioavailability is only about 15–30%. If given with food, absorption rate and extent will be decreased.

Penicillin G potassium and sodium salts are rapidly absorbed after IM injections and yield high peak levels usually within 20 minutes of administration. In horses, equivalent doses given either IV or IM demonstrated that IM dosing will provide serum levels above 0.5 micrograms/mL for about twice as long as IV administration [approx. 3–4 hours (IV) vs. 6–7 hours (IM)].

Procaine penicillin G is slowly hydrolyzed to penicillin G after IM injection. Peak levels are much lower than with parenterally administered aqueous penicillin G sodium or potassium, but serum levels are more prolonged.

Benzathine penicillin G is also very slowly absorbed after IM injections after being hydrolyzed to the parent compound. Serum levels can be very prolonged, but levels attained generally only exceed MIC's for the most susceptible streptococci, and the use of benzathine penicillin G should be limited to these infections when other penicillin therapy is impractical.

After absorption, penicillin G is widely distributed throughout the body with the exception of the CSF, joints and milk. In lactating dairy cattle, the milk to plasma ratio is about 0.2. CSF levels are generally only 10% or less of those found in the serum when meninges are not inflamed. Levels in the CSF may be greater in patients with inflamed meninges or if probenecid is given concurrently. Binding to plasma proteins is approximately 50% in most species.

Penicillin G is principally excreted unchanged into the urine through renal mechanisms via both glomerular filtration and tubular secretion. Elimination half-lives are very rapid and are usually one hour or less in most species (if normal renal function exists).

Contraindications/Precautions/Warnings

Penicillins are contraindicated in patients with a history of hypersensitivity to them. Because there may be cross-reactivity, use penicillins cautiously in patients who are documented hypersensitive to other beta-lactam antibiotics (e.g., cephalosporins, cefamycins, carbapenems).

Do not administer systemic antibiotics orally in patients with septicemia, shock, or other grave illnesses as absorption of the medication from the GI tract may be significantly delayed or diminished; parenteral (preferably IV) routes should be used for these cases.

High doses of penicillin G sodium or potassium, particularly in small animals with a preexisting electrolyte abnormality, renal disease, or congestive heart failure may cause electrolyte imbalances. Other injectable penicillins, such as ticarcillin, carbenicillin, and ampicillin, have significant quantities of sodium per gram and may cause electrolyte imbalances when used in large dosages in susceptible patients.

Certain species (snakes, birds, turtles, Guinea pigs, and chinchillas) are reportedly sensitive to procaine penicillin G.

Adverse Effects

Adverse effects with the penicillins are usually not serious and have a relatively low frequency of occurrence.

Hypersensitivity reactions unrelated to dose can occur with these agents and can manifest as rashes, fever, eosinophilia, neutropenia, agranulocytosis, thrombocytopenia, leukopenia, anemias, lymphadenopathy, or full-blown anaphylaxis. In humans, it is estimated that up to 15% of patients hypersensitive to cephalosporins will also be hypersensitive to penicillins. The incidence of cross-reactivity in veterinary patients is unknown.

When given orally, penicillins may cause GI effects (anorexia, vomiting, diarrhea). Because the penicillins may also alter gut flora, antibiot-

ic-associated diarrhea can occur and allow the proliferation of resistant bacteria in the colon (superinfections).

Neurotoxicity (e.g., ataxia in dogs) has been associated with very high doses or very prolonged use. Although the penicillins are not considered hepatotoxic, elevated liver enzymes have been reported. Other effects reported in dogs include tachypnea, dyspnea, edema and tachycardia.

Reproductive/Nursing Safety

Penicillins have been shown to cross the placenta and safe use of them during pregnancy has not been firmly established, but neither has there been any documented teratogenic problems associated with these drugs; however, use only when the potential benefits outweigh the risks.

In humans, the FDA categorizes this drug as category **B** for use during pregnancy (*Animal studies have not yet demonstrated risk to the fetus, but there are no adequate studies in pregnant women; or animal studies have shown an adverse effect, but adequate studies in pregnant women have not demonstrated a risk to the fetus in the first trimester of pregnancy, and there is no evidence of risk in later trimesters.*) In a separate system evaluating the safety of drugs in canine and feline pregnancy (Papich 1989), this drug is categorized as class: **A** (*Probably safe. Although specific studies may not have proved he safety of all drugs in dogs and cats, there are no reports of adverse effects in laboratory animals or women.*)

Penicillins are excreted in maternal milk in low concentrations; use could potentially cause diarrhea, candidiasis, or allergic responses in nursing offspring.

Overdosage/Acute Toxicity

Acute oral penicillin overdoses are unlikely to cause significant problems other than GI distress, but other effects are possible (see Adverse Effects). In humans, very high dosages of parenteral penicillins, especially those with renal disease, have induced CNS effects.

Drug Interactions

The following drug interactions have either been reported or are theoretical in humans or animals receiving penicillin G and may be of significance in veterinary patients:

■ **AMINOGLYCOSIDES:** *In vitro* studies have demonstrated that penicillins can have synergistic or additive activity against certain bacteria when used with aminoglycosides or cephalosporins.

■ **BACTERIOSTATIC ANTIBIOTICS (e.g., chloramphenicol, erythromycin, tetracyclines):** Use with penicillins is generally not recommended, particularly in acute infections where the organism is proliferating rapidly as penicillins tend to perform better on actively growing bacteria.

■ **METHOTREXATE:** Penicillins may decrease renal elimination of MTX

■ **PROBENECID:** Competitively blocks the tubular secretion of most penicillins, thereby increasing serum levels and serum half-lives.

Laboratory Considerations

■ As penicillins and other beta-lactams can inactivate **aminoglycosides** *in vitro* (and *in vivo* in patients in renal failure), serum concentrations of aminoglycosides may be falsely decreased if the patient is also receiving beta-lactam antibiotics and the serum is stored prior to analysis. It is recommended that if the assay is delayed, samples be frozen and, if possible, drawn at times when the beta-lactam antibiotic is at a trough.

■ Penicillin G can cause falsely elevated **serum uric acid** values if the copper-chelate method is used; phosphotungstate and uricase methods are not affected

■ Penicillins may cause false-positive **urine glucose** determinations when using cupric-sulfate solution (Benedict's Solution, *Clinitest®*). Tests utilizing glucose oxidase (*Tes-Tape®*, *Clinistix®*) are not affected by penicillin.

Doses

■ **DOGS:**

For susceptible infections:

a) *Penicillin G potassium:*

For bacteremia, systemic infections: 20,000–40,000 Units/kg IV q4–6h for as long as necessary.

For orthopedic infections: 20,000–40,000 Units/kg IV q6h for as long as necessary.

Prophylaxis for orthopedic surgery: 40,000 Units/kg IV one hour prior to surgery, and if surgery lasts longer than 90 minutes a second dose is given.

For soft tissue infections: 40,000–60,000 Units/kg PO q8h for as long as necessary.

Penicillin G procaine: 20,000–40,000 Units/kg IM, SC q12–24h for as long as necessary.

Penicillin G benzathine: 40,000 Units/kg IM q5 days. (Greene *et al.* 2006)

b) For leptospiremia: 25,000–40,000 Units/kg IV or IM q12–24h for 14 days. For the renal carrier state of leptospirosis: Doxycycline 5–10 mg/kg PO twice daily of doxycycline for an additional 14 days after penicillin G therapy (Ross & Rentko 2000)

■ **CATS:**

For susceptible infections:

a) *Penicillin G potassium:*

For soft tissue, systemic infections: 40,000 Units/kg PO q6–8h for as long as necessary.

Penicillin G procaine:

For soft tissue infections: 20,000 Units/kg IM, SC q12h for as long as necessary.

For orthopedic infections: 20,000–40,000 Units/kg IM q8h for as long as necessary.

For resistant organisms (Actinomyces): 50,000–100,000 Units/kg IM, SC q12h for as long as necessary.

Penicillin G benzathine: 50,000 Units/kg IM q5 days. (Greene *et al.* 2006)

■ **FERRETS:**

For susceptible infections:

a) Procaine Pen G: 20,000–40,000 Units/kg IM once a day to twice daily;

Sodium or potassium Pen G: 20,000 Units/kg SC, IM or IV q4h or 40,000 Units/kg PO three times daily (Williams 2000)

■ **RABBITS, RODENTS, SMALL MAMMALS:**

a) **Rabbits:** Penicillin G Procaine 20,000–84,000 Units/kg SC, IM q24h for 5–7 days for venereal spirochetosis (Ivey & Morrisey 2000)

b) **Hedgehogs:** 40,000 Units/kg IM once daily (Smith 2000)

■ **CATTLE** (and other ruminants unless specified):

For susceptible infections:

a) *Penicillin G procaine:* 25,000 Units/kg (route not specified, assume IM or SC) once per day. For moderately susceptible bacteria give above dose twice daily. (Gunn 2008)

b) For clostridial abomasitis and enteritis in calves: Procaine Penicillin G 10,000–20,000 Units/kg PO q12-24 for 1–4 days. Oral penicillin is preferred over systemic as it is poorly absorbed from the GI tract and will provide activity in the intestinal lumen where the bacteria reside. (Callan & Rentko 2003)

c) For bovine respiratory disease complex: Procaine penicillin G 66,000 Units/kg IM or SC once daily. Recommend 20-day slaughter withdrawal at this dosage. (Hjerpe 1986)

d) *Procaine penicillin G:* 40,000 Units/kg IM once daily

Procaine penicillin G/benzathine penicillin G combination: 40,000 Units/kg IM once (Howard 1986)

e) *Procaine penicillin G:* 10,000–20,000 Units/kg IM q12–24h.

Benzathine penicillin G: 10,000–20,000 Units/kg, IM, SC q48h (Jenkins 1986)

■ **HORSES:**

For susceptible infections:

a) For gram-positive aerobes: Penicillin G potassium or sodium: 10,000–20,000 Units/kg IV or IM q6h.

For serious gram-positive infections (*e.g.*, tetanus, botulism, C. difficile enterocolitis in foals): Penicillin G sodium or potassium 22,000–44,000 Units/kg IV q6h

Susceptible bacterial infections: Penicillin G procaine: 22,000–44,000 Units/kg IM q12h (Whittem 1999)

b) Treatment of carriers with *S. equi* infections of the gutteral pouches: Administration of both systemic and topical penicillin G appears to improve treatment success rate. Before topical therapy, remove all visible inflammatory material removed from gutteral pouch. To make a gelatin/penicillin G mix of 50 mL for gutteral pouch instillation:

1) Weigh out 2 grams gelatin (Sigma G-6650 or household) and add 40 mL of sterile water.

2) Heat or microwave to dissolve. Cool to 45–50°C,

3) Add 10 mL sterile water to a 10 million Unit sodium penicillin G for injection vial and mix with the cooled gelatin to total volume of 50 mL.

4) Dispense into syringes and leave overnight in the refrigerator.

Instillation is easiest through a catheter inserted up the nose and endoscopically guided into the pouch opening with the last inch bent at an angle to aid entry under the pouch flap. Elevate horse's head for 20 minutes after infusion. (Verheyen *et al.* 2000)

c) For treatment of botulism: Penicillin G sodium or potassium 22,000–44,000 Units/kg IV four times daily (do not use oral penicillin therapy) (Johnston & Whitlock 1987)

d) For strangles: Early in infection when only fever and depression are present: procaine penicillin G 22,000 Units/kg IM or SC q12h, or aqueous salts (sodium or potassium) penicillin G 22,000 Units/kg IM, IV or SC q6h. If lymphadenopathy noted in otherwise healthy and alert horse do not treat. If lymphadenopathy present and horse is depressed, febrile, anorexic and especially if dyspneic, treat as above. (Foreman 1999)

e) For foals: Penicillin G Na or K: 20,000–50,000 Units/kg IV q6–8h; Procaine penicillin G 22,000–50,000 U/kg IM q12h (Brumbaugh *et al.* 1999)

f) For foals: Penicillin G sodium or potassium: 20,000–50,000 Units/kg IV q6h Penicillin G Procaine: 20,000–50,000 Units/kg IM q6h (Furr 1999)

g) Foals: Potassium penicillin G: 22,000 Units/kg q6h IV, IM (Excellent gram-positive coverage, expensive, high blood levels)

Procaine penicillin G: 22,000 Units/kg q12h IM (painful, lower blood levels) (Stewart 2008)

■ **SWINE:**

For susceptible infections:

a) Procaine penicillin G: 40,000 Units/kg IM once daily.

Procaine penicillin G/benzathine penicillin G combination: 40,000 Units/kg IM once (Howard 1986)

b) Procaine penicillin G: 6,600 Units/kg IM once daily for not more than 4 days

Procaine penicillin G/benzathine penicillin G combination: 11,000–22,000 Units/kg IM once (Wood 1986)

■ **BIRDS:**

For susceptible infections:

a) In turkeys: Procaine penicillin G/benzathine penicillin G combination: 100 mg/kg IM of each drug once a day or every 2 days. Use cautiously in small birds as it may cause procaine toxicity. (Clubb 1986)

Monitoring

■ Because penicillins usually have minimal toxicity associated with their use, monitoring for efficacy is usually all that is required unless toxic signs develop. Serum levels and therapeutic drug monitoring are not routinely done with these agents.

Client Information

■ Owners should be instructed to give oral penicillins to animals with an empty stomach, unless using amoxicillin or if GI effects (anorexia, vomiting) occur.

■ Compliance with the therapeutic regimen should be stressed.

Chemistry/Synonyms

Penicillin G is considered natural penicillin and is obtained from cultures *Penicillium chrysogenum* and is available in several different salt forms. Penicillin G potassium (also known as benzylpenicillin potassium, aqueous or crystalline penicillin) occurs as colorless or white crystals, or white crystalline powder. It is very soluble in water and sparingly soluble in alcohol. Potency of penicillin G potassium is usually expressed in terms of Units. One mg of penicillin G potassium is equivalent to 1440–1680 USP Units (1355–1595 USP Units for the powder for injection). After reconstitution, penicillin G potassium powder for injection has a pH of 6–8.5, and contains 1.7 mEq of potassium per 1 million Units.

Penicillin G sodium (also known as benzylpenicillin sodium, aqueous or crystalline penicillin) occurs as colorless or white crystals, or white to slightly yellow, crystalline powder. Approximately 25 mg are soluble in 1 mL of water. Potency of penicillin G sodium is usually expressed in terms of Units. One mg of penicillin G sodium is equivalent to 1500−1750 USP Units (1420−1667 USP Units for the powder for injection). After reconstitution, penicillin G sodium powder for injection has a pH of 6−7.5, and contains 2 mEq of sodium per 1 million Units.

Penicillin G procaine (also known as APPG, Aqueous Procaine Penicillin G, Benzylpenicillin Procaine, Procaine Penicillin G, Procaine Benzylpenicillin) is the procaine monohydrate salt of penicillin G. *In vivo* it is hydrolyzed to penicillin G and acts as a depot, or repository form, of penicillin G. It occurs as white crystals or very fine, white crystalline powder. Approximately 4−4.5 mg are soluble in 1 mL of water and 3.3 mg are soluble in 1 mL of alcohol. Potency of penicillin G procaine is usually expressed in terms of Units. One mg of penicillin G procaine is equivalent to 900−1050 USP Units. The commercially available suspension for injection is buffered with sodium citrate and has a pH of 5−7.5. It is preserved with methylparaben and propylparaben.

Penicillin G Benzathine (also known as Benzathine Benzylpenicillin, Benzathine Penicillin G, Benzylpenicillin Benzathine, Dibenzylethylenediamine Benzylpenicillin) is the benzathine tetrahydrate salt of penicillin G. It is hydrolyzed *in vivo* to penicillin G and acts as a long-acting form of penicillin G. It occurs as an odorless, white, crystalline powder. Solubilities are 0.2−0.3 mg/mL of water and 15 mg/mL of alcohol. One mg of penicillin G benzathine is equivalent to 1090−1272 USP Units. The commercially available suspension for injection is buffered with sodium citrate and has a pH of 5−7.5. It is preserved with methylparaben and propylparaben.

Penicillin G may also be known as: benzylpenicllin, crystalline penicillin G, penicillin, *Bicillin C-R®*, *Masti-Clear®*, *Permapen®*, and *Pfizerpen®*.

Storage/Stability
Penicillin G sodium and potassium should be protected from moisture to prevent hydrolysis of the compounds. Penicillin G potassium tablets and powder for oral solution should be stored at room temperature in tight containers; avoid exposure to excessive heat. After reconstituting, the oral powder for solution should be stored from 2−8°C (refrigerated) and discarded after 14 days.

Penicillin G sodium and potassium powder for injection can be stored at room temperature (15−30°C). After reconstituting, the injectable solution is stable for 7 days when kept refrigerated (2−8°C) and for 24 hours at room temperature.

Penicillin G procaine should be stored at 2−8°C; avoid freezing. Benzathine penicillin G should be stored at 2−8°C.

Compatibility/Compounding Considerations
All commonly used IV fluids (some Dextran products are physically **incompatible**) and the following drugs are reportedly physically **compatible** with penicillin G potassium: ascorbic acid injection, calcium chloride/gluconate, cephapirin sodium, chloramphenicol sodium succinate, cimetidine HCl, clindamycin phosphate, colistimethate sodium, corticotropin, dimenhydrinate, diphenhydramine HCl, ephedrine sulfate, erythromycin gluceptate/lactobionate, hydrocortisone sodium succinate, kanamycin sulfate, lidocaine HCl, methicillin sodium, methylprednisolone sodium succinate, metronidazole with sodium bicarbonate, nitrofurantoin sodium, polymyxin B sulfate, potassium chloride, prednisolone sodium phosphate, procaine HCl, prochlorperazine edisylate, sodium iodide, sulfisoxazole diolamine, and verapamil HCl.

The following drugs/solutions are either physically **incompatible** or **data conflicts** regarding compatibility with penicillin G potassium injection: amikacin sulfate, aminophylline, chlorpromazine HCl, dopamine HCl, heparin sodium, hydroxyzine HCl, lincomycin HCl, metoclopramide HCl, oxytetracycline HCl, pentobarbital sodium, prochlorperazine mesylate, promazine HCl, promethazine HCl, sodium bicarbonate, tetracycline HCl, and vitamin B-complex with C.

The following drugs/solutions are reportedly physically **compatible** with penicillin G sodium injection: Dextran 40 10%, dextrose 5% (some degradation may occur if stored for 24 hours), sodium chloride 0.9% (some degradation may occur if stored for 24 hours), calcium chloride/gluconate, chloramphenicol sodium succinate, cimetidine HCl, clindamycin phosphate, colistimethate sodium, diphenhydramine HCl, erythromycin lactobionate, gentamicin sulfate, hydrocortisone sodium succinate, kanamycin sulfate, methicillin sodium, nitrofurantoin sodium, polymyxin B sulfate, prednisolone sodium phosphate, procaine HCl, verapamil HCl, and vitamin B-complex with C.

The following drugs/solutions are either physically **incompatible** or **data conflicts** regarding compatibility with penicillin G sodium injection: amphotericin B, bleomycin sulfate, chlorpromazine HCl, heparin sodium, hydroxyzine HCl, lincomycin HCl, methylprednisolone sodium succinate, oxytetracycline HCl, potassium chloride, prochlorperazine mesylate, promethazine HCl and tetracycline HCl. Compatibility is dependent upon factors such as pH, concentration, temperature and diluent used; consult specialized references or a hospital pharmacist for more specific information.

Dosage Forms/Regulatory Status
VETERINARY-LABELED PRODUCTS:
Note: Withdrawal times are for labeled dosages only.

Penicillin G Procaine Injection 300,000 Units/mL in 100 mL and 250 mL vials: Variety of trade names available. Depending on product, FDA-approved for use in: cattle, sheep, horses, and swine. Not intended for use in horses used for food. Do not exceed 7 days of treatment in non-lactating dairy cattle, beef cattle, swine or sheep; 5 days in lactating dairy cattle. Treatment should not exceed 4 consecutive days.

Withdrawal times vary depending on the product are for the labeled dosage of 6,600 Units/kg once daily (rarely used clinically today). Actual withdrawal times may be longer. Milk withdrawal times (at labeled doses) = 48 hours. Slaughter withdrawal: Calves (non-ruminating) = 7 days; cattle = 4–10 days; sheep = 8–9 days; swine = 6–7 days; refer to label for more information.

Penicillin G Procaine Mastitis Syringes 100,000 Units/mL in 10 mL units: *Go-Dry®* (G.C. Hanford) (OTC) Milk withdrawal (at labeled doses) = 72 hours. Slaughter withdrawal (at labeled doses) = 14 days. For use in dry cows only. *Masti-Clear®* (G.C. Hanford) Milk withdrawal (at labeled doses) = 60 hours. Slaughter withdrawal (at labeled doses) = 3 days. Administer no more than 3 consecutive doses or withdrawal times must lengthen.

There are also mastitis syringes in combination with novobiocin (*Albadry Plus®*) or dihydro-streptomycin (*Quartermaster®*)

Penicillin G Benzathine 150,000 Units/mL with Penicillin G Procaine Injection 150,000 Units/mL for Injection in 100 mL and 250 mL vials: Variety of trade names available. FDA-approved (most products) in horses and beef cattle. Not FDA-approved for horses intended for food use. Slaughter withdrawal: cattle = 30 days (at labeled doses). Actual species approvals and withdrawal times may vary with the product; refer to the label of the product you are using.

HUMAN-LABELED PRODUCTS:

Penicillin G (Aqueous) Sodium Powder for Injection: 5,000,000 Units & 20,000,000 Units in vials; *Pfizerpen®* (Pfizer); generic (Sandoz); (Rx)

Penicillin G (Aqueous) Potassium Injection (Premixed, frozen): 1,000,000 Units, 2,000,000 Units & 3,000,000 Units in 50 mL Galaxy containers; generic (Baxter); (Rx)

Penicillin G Procaine Injection: 600,000 Units/vial in 1 mL *Tubex* & 1,200,000 Units/vial in 2 mL *Tubex*; generic; (Monarch); (Rx)

Penicillin G Benzathine Injection: 600,000 Units/dose in 1 mL *Tubex*; 1,200,000 Units/dose in 2 mL *Tubex* and 2 mL *Isoject*; 2,400,000 Units/dose in 4 mL pre-fillled syringes; *Bicillin L-A®* (Monarch); *Permapen®* (Roerig); (Rx)

Penicillin G Benzathine/Penicillin G Procaine IM Injection: 600,000 Units/dose (300,000 Units each penicillin G benzathine & penicillin G procaine) in 1 mL *Tubex*; 1,200,000 Units/dose (600,000 Units each penicillin G benzathine & penicillin G procaine) in 2 mL *Tubex*; 1,200,000 Units/dose (900,000 Units penicillin G benzathine & 300,000 Units penicillin G procaine) in 2 mL *Tubex*; *Bicillin C-R®* and *Bicillin C-R 900/300®* (Monarch); (Rx)

References

Brumbaugh, G., H. Lopez, et al. (1999). The pharmacologic basis for the treatment of laminitis. *The Veterinary Clinics of North America: Equine Practice* 15:2(August).

Callan, M.B. & V.T. Rentko (2003). Clinical application of a hemoglobin-based oxygen-carrying solution. *Veterinary Clinics of North America-Small Animal Practice* 33(6): 1277–+.

Clubb, S.L. (1986). Therapeutics: Individual and Flock Treatment Regimens. *Clinical Avian Medicine and Surgery*. GJ Harrison and LR Harrison Eds. Philadelphia, W.B. Saunders: 327–355.

Foreman, J. (1999). Equine respiratory pharmacology. *The Veterinary Clinics of North America: Equine Practice* 15:3(December): 665–686.

Furr, M. (1999). Antimicrobial treatments for the septic foal. Proceedings: The North American Veterinary Conference, Orlando.

Greene, C., K. Hartmannn, et al. (2006). Appendix 8: Antimicrobial Drug Formulary. *Infectious Disease of the Dog and Cat*. C Greene Ed., Elsevier: 1186–1333.

Gunn, A. (2008). Rational Use of Antimicrobial Therapy in Cattle. Proceedings: AVA. Accessed via: Veterinary Information Network. http://goo.gl/wghYb

Hjerpe, C.A. (1986). The bovine respiratory disease complex. *Current Veterinary Therapy: Food Animal Practice 2*. JL Howard Ed. Philadelphia, W.B. Saunders: 670–681.

Howard, J.L., Ed. (1986). *Current Veterinary Therapy 2, Food Animal Practice*. Philadelphia, W.B. Saunders.

Ivey, E. & J. Morrisey (2000). Therapeutics for Rabbits. *Vet Clin NA: Exotic Anim Pract* 3:1(Jan): 183–216.

Jenkins, W.L. (1986). Antimicrobial Therapy. *Current Veterinary Therapy: Food Animal Practice 2*. JL Howard Ed. Philadelphia, W.B. Saunders: 8–23.

Johnston, J. & R.H. Whitlock (1987). Botulism. *Current Therapy in Equine Medicine, 2*. NE Robinson Ed. Philadelphia, W.B. Saunders: 367–370.

Papich, M. (1989). Effects of drugs on pregnancy. *Current Veterinary Therapy X: Small Animal Practice*. R Kirk Ed. Philadelphia, Saunders: 1291–1299.

Ross, L. & V. Rentko (2000). Leptosirosis. *Kirk's Current Veterinary Therapy: XIII Small Animal Practice*. J Bonagura Ed. Philadelphia, WB Saunders: 298–300.

Smith, A. (2000). General husbandry and medical care of hedgehogs. *Kirk's Current Veterinary Therapy: XIII Small Animal Practice*. J Bonagura Ed. Philadelphia, WB Saunders: 1128–1133.

Stewart, A. (2008). Equine Neonatal Sepsis. Proceedings: WVC. Accessed via: Veterinary Information Network. http://goo.gl/xT79V

Verheyen, K., J. Newton, et al. (2000). Elimination of guttural pouch infection and inflammation in asymptomatic carriers of Streptococcus equi. *Equine Vet J* 32(6): 527–532.

Whittem, T. (1999). Appendix: Formulary of Common Equine Drugs. *The Veterinary Clinics of North America: Equine Practice* 15:3(December): 747–768.

Williams, B. (2000). Therapeutics in Ferrets. *Vet Clin NA: Exotic Anim Pract* 3:1(Jan): 131–153.

Wood, R.L. (1986). Swine Erysipelas. *Current Veterinary Therapy 2: Food Animal Practice*. JL Howard Ed. Philadelphia, WB Saunders: 561–562.

PENICILLIN V POTASSIUM

(pen-i-**sill**-in **Vee**)   Phenoxymethylpenicillin

ORAL PENICILLIN ANTIBIOTIC

Prescriber Highlights

▶ Oral natural penicillin

▶ Contraindications: Known hypersensitivity (unless no other options)

▶ Adverse Effects: GI effects or hypersensitivity possible

▶ Best to give on an empty stomach

Uses/Indications

Penicillins have been used for a wide range of infections in various species. See the dosage section for more information.

Pharmacology/Actions

The natural penicillins (G and K) have similar spectrums of activity, but penicillin G is slightly more active *in vitro* on a per weight basis against many organisms. This class of penicillin has *in vitro* activity against most spirochetes and gram-positive and gram-negative aerobic cocci, but not penicillinase producing strains. They have activity against some aerobic and anaerobic gram-positive bacilli such as *Bacillus anthracis*, *Clostridium* spp. (not *C. difficile*), Fusobacterium, and Actinomyces. The natural penicillins are customarily inactive against most gram-negative aerobic and anaerobic bacilli, and all Rickettsia, mycobacteria, fungi, Mycoplasma, and viruses. Although penicillin V may be slightly less active than penicillin G against organisms susceptible to the natural penicillins, its superior absorptive characteristics after oral administration make it a better choice against mild to moderately severe infections when oral administration is desired in monogastric animals.

Penicillins are usually bactericidal against susceptible bacteria and act by inhibiting mucopeptide synthesis in the cell wall resulting in a defective barrier and an osmotically unstable spheroplast. The exact mechanism for this effect has not been definitively determined, but beta-lactam antibiotics have been shown to bind to several enzymes (carboxypeptidases, transpeptidases, endopeptidases) within the bacterial cytoplasmic membrane that are involved with cell wall synthesis. The different affinities that various beta-lactam antibiotics have for these enzymes (also known as penicillin-binding proteins; PBPs) help explain the differences in spectrums of activity the drugs have that are not explained by the influence of beta-lactamases. Like other beta-lactam antibiotics, penicillins are generally considered more effective against actively growing bacteria.

Pharmacokinetics

The pharmacokinetics of penicillin V are very similar to penicillin G with the exception of oral bioavailability and the percent of the drug that is bound to plasma proteins. Penicillin V is significantly more resistant to acid-catalyzed inactivation in the gut and bioavailability after oral administration in humans is approximately 60–73%. In veterinary species, bioavailability in calves is only 30%, but studies performed in horses and dogs demonstrated that therapeutic serum levels can be achieved after oral administration. In dogs, food will decrease the rate and extent of absorption.

Distribution of penicillin V follows that of penicillin G but, at least in humans, the drug is bound to a larger extent to plasma proteins (approximately 80% with penicillin V vs. 50% with penicillin G).

Like penicillin G, penicillin V is excreted rapidly in the urine via the kidney. Elimination half-lives are generally less than 1 hour in animals with normal renal function; an elimination half-life of 3.65 hours has been reported after oral dosing in horses (Schwark et al. 1983).

Contraindications/Precautions/Warnings

Penicillins are contraindicated in patients with a history of hypersensitivity to them. Because there may be cross-reactivity, use penicillins cautiously in patients who are documented hypersensitive to other beta-lactam antibiotics (e.g., cephalosporins, cefamycins, carbapenems).

Do not administer systemic antibiotics orally in patients with septicemia, shock, or other grave illnesses as absorption of the medication from the GI tract may be significantly delayed or diminished. Parenteral (preferably IV) routes should be used for these cases.

Adverse Effects

Adverse effects with the penicillins are usually not serious and have a relatively low frequency of occurrence.

Hypersensitivity reactions unrelated to dose can occur with these agents and can manifest as rashes, fever, eosinophilia, neutropenia, agranulocytosis, thrombocytopenia, leukopenia, anemias, lymphadenopathy, or full-blown anaphylaxis. In humans, it is estimated that up to 15% of patients hypersensitive to cephalosporins will also be hypersensitive to penicillins. The incidence of cross-reactivity in veterinary patients is unknown.

When given orally, penicillins may cause GI effects (anorexia, vomiting, diarrhea). Because the penicillins may also alter gut flora, antibiotic-associated diarrhea can occur and allow the proliferation of resistant bacteria in the colon (superinfections).

Neurotoxicity (e.g., ataxia in dogs) has been associated with very high doses or very prolonged use. Although the penicillins are not considered hepatotoxic, elevated liver enzymes have been reported. Other effects reported in dogs include tachypnea, dyspnea, edema and tachycardia.

Reproductive/Nursing Safety

Penicillins have been shown to cross the placenta and safe use of them during pregnancy has not been firmly established, but neither has there been any documented teratogenic problems associated with these drugs; however, use only when the potential benefits outweigh the risks. Certain species (snakes, birds, turtles, Guinea pigs, and chinchillas) are reported to be sensitive to penicillins. High doses of penicillin G sodium or potassium, particularly in small animals with a preexisting electrolyte abnormality, renal disease, or congestive heart failure may cause electrolyte imbalances. Other injectable penicillins, such as ticarcillin, carbenicillin, and ampicillin, have significant quantities of sodium per gram and may cause electrolyte imbalances when used in large dosages in susceptible patients.

In humans, the FDA categorizes this drug as category *B* for use during pregnancy (*Animal studies have not yet demonstrated risk to the fetus, but there are no adequate studies in pregnant women; or animal studies have shown an adverse effect, but adequate studies in pregnant women have not demonstrated a risk to the fetus in the first trimester of pregnancy, and there is no evidence of risk in later trimesters*).

Penicillins are excreted in maternal milk in low concentrations; use could potentially cause diarrhea, candidiasis, or allergic response in nursing offspring.

Overdosage/Acute Toxicity

Acute oral penicillin overdoses are unlikely to cause significant problems other than GI distress, but other effects are possible (see Adverse effects). In humans, very high dosages of parenteral penicillins, especially in patients with renal disease, have induced CNS effects.

Drug Interactions

The following drug interactions have either been reported or are theoretical in humans or animals receiving penicillin V potassium and may be of significance in veterinary patients:

- **AMINOGLYCOSIDES:** *In vitro* studies have demonstrated that penicillins can have synergistic or additive activity against certain bacteria when used with aminoglycosides or cephalosporins.

- **BACTERIOSTATIC ANTIBIOTICS (e.g., chloramphenicol, erythromycin, tetracyclines):** Use with penicillins is generally not recommended, particularly in acute infections where the organism is proliferating rapidly as penicillins tend to perform better on actively growing bacteria.

- **METHOTREXATE:** Penicillins may decrease renal elimination of MTX

- **PROBENECID:** Competitively blocks the tubular secretion of most penicillins, thereby increasing serum levels and serum half-lives.

Laboratory Considerations

- As penicillins and other beta-lactams can inactivate **aminoglycosides** *in vitro* (and *in vivo* in patients in renal failure), serum concentrations of aminoglycosides may be falsely decreased if the patient is also receiving beta-lactam antibiotics and the serum is stored prior to analysis. It is recommended that if the assay is delayed, samples be frozen and, if possible, drawn at times when the beta-lactam antibiotic is at a trough.

- Penicillin V can cause falsely elevated **serum uric acid** values if the copper-chelate method is used; phosphotungstate and uricase methods are not affected

- Penicillins may cause false-positive **urine glucose** determinations when using cupric-sulfate solution (Benedict's Solution, *Clinitest®*). Tests utilizing glucose oxidase (*Tes-Tape®*, *Clinistix®*) are not affected by penicillin.

Doses

- **DOGS:**

  For susceptible infections:

  a) 5.5–11 mg/kg PO q6–8h (Aronson & Aucoin 1989)

  b) For soft tissue infections: 10 mg/kg PO q8h for 7 days. (Greene *et al.* 2006)

- **CATS:**

  For susceptible infections:

  a) 5.5–11 mg/kg PO q6–8h (Aronson & Aucoin 1989)

  b) For soft tissue infections: 10 mg/kg PO q8h for 7 days. (Greene *et al.* 2006)

- **HORSES:**

  For susceptible infections:

  a) 110,000 U/kg (68.75 mg/kg) PO q8h (may yield supra-optimal levels against uncomplicated infections by sensitive organisms) (Schwark *et al.* 1983)

  b) 110,000 U/kg PO q6–12h (Brumbaugh 1987)

Monitoring

- Because penicillins usually have minimal toxicity associated with their use, monitoring for efficacy is usually all that is required unless toxic signs develop. Serum levels and therapeutic drug monitoring are not routinely done with these agents.

Client Information

- Unless otherwise instructed by the veterinarian, this drug should be given on an empty stomach, at least 1 hour before feeding or 2 hours after feeding

- Keep oral suspension in the refrigerator and discard any unused suspension after 14 days

Chemistry/Synonyms

A natural-penicillin, penicillin V is produced from *Penicillium chrysogenum* and is usually commercially available as the potassium salt. Penicillin V potassium occurs as an odorless, white, crystalline powder that is very soluble in water and slightly soluble in alcohol. Potency of penicillin V potassium is usually expressed in terms of weight (in mg) of penicillin V, but penicillin V units may also be used. One mg of penicillin V potassium is equivalent to 1380–1610 USP Units of penicillin V. Manufacturers however generally state that 125 mg of penicillin V potassium is approximately equivalent to 200,000 USP units of penicillin V.

Penicillin V may also be known as: phenoxymethylpenicillin, fenoximetilpenicilina, penicillin, phenoxymethyl, phenomycilline, phenoxymethyl penicillin, phenoxymethylpenicillinum, and *Veetids*®.

Storage/Stability

Penicillin V potassium tablets and powder for oral solution should be stored in tight containers at room temperature (15–30°C). After reconstitution, the oral solution should be stored at 2–8°C (refrigerated) and any unused portion discarded after 14 days.

Dosage Forms/Regulatory Status

VETERINARY-LABELED PRODUCTS: None

HUMAN-LABELED PRODUCTS:

Penicillin V Potassium Tablets: 250 mg & 500 mg; *Veetids*® (Geneva); generic; (Rx)

Penicillin V Potassium Powder for Oral Solution: 25 mg/mL & 50 mg/mL in 100 mL & 200 mL; *Veetids*® (Geneva); generic; (Rx)

References

Aronson, A.L. & D.P. Aucoin (1989). Antimicrobial Drugs. *Textbook of Veterinary Internal Medicine.* SJ Ettinger Ed. Philadelphia, WB Saunders. **1:** 383–412.

Brumbaugh, G.W. (1987). Rational selection of antimicrobial drugs for treatment of infections in horses. *Vet Clin North Am (Equine Practice)* **3**(1): 191–220.

Greene, C., K. Hartmann, et al. (2006). Appendix 8: Antimicrobial Drug Formulary. *Infectious Disease of the Dog and Cat.* C Greene Ed., Elsevier: 1186–1333.

Schwark, W.S., N.G. Ducharme, et al. (1983). Absorption and distribution patterns of oral phenoxymethyl penicillin (penicillin V) in the horse. *Cornell Vet* **73**: 314–322.

PENTAZOCINE LACTATE PENTAZOCINE HCL

(pen-*taz*-oh-seen)   Talwin®

PARTIAL OPIATE AGONIST

Prescriber Highlights

▶ Partial opiate agonist analgesic used in a variety of species; usage and availability are decreasing

▶ Contraindications: Known hypersensitivity

▶ Caution: Head trauma, increased CSF pressure or other CNS dysfunction, hypothyroidism, severe renal insufficiency, adrenocortical insufficiency (Addison's), & geriatric or severely debilitated patients

▶ Not a replacement for surgery or medical treatment for horses with colic

▶ Adverse Effects: *Horses:* Transient ataxia, CNS excitement, increased pulse, & respiratory rate. *Dogs:* Salivation most prevalent; ataxia, fine tremors, seizures, emesis, & swelling at injection site possible

▶ Cats: Use is controversial; may cause dysphoric reactions

▶ C-IV controlled substance

Uses/Indications

Pentazocine is labeled for the symptomatic relief of pain of colic in horses and for the amelioration of pain accompanying postoperative recovery from fractures, trauma, and spinal disorders in dogs. It has also been used as an analgesic in cats (see Adverse Effects below) and swine.

Pharmacology/Actions

While considered a partial opiate agonist, pentazocine exhibits many of the same characteristics as the true opiate agonists. It is reported to have an analgesic potency of approximately one-half that of morphine and five times that of meperidine. It is a very weak antagonist at the *mu* opioid receptor when compared to naloxone. It will not antagonize the respiratory depression caused by drugs like morphine, but may induce symptoms of withdrawal in human patients physically dependent on narcotic agents. Pentazocine's mixed agonist/antagonist properties limit its maximal analgesic efficacy (ceiling effect).

Besides its analgesic properties, pentazocine can cause respiratory depression, decreased GI motility, sedation, and it possesses antitussive effects. Pentazocine tends to have less sedative qualities in animals than other opiates and is usually not used as a pre-operative medication.

In dogs, pentazocine can cause a transient decrease in blood pressure; in humans, increases in cardiac output, heart rate, and blood pressure can be seen.

Pharmacokinetics

Pentazocine is well absorbed following oral, IM, or SC administration. Because of a high first-pass effect, only about 20% of an oral dose will enter the systemic circulation in patients with normal hepatic function.

After absorption, the drug is distributed widely into tissues. In the equine, it has been shown to be 80% bound to plasma proteins. Pentazocine will cross the placenta and neonatal serum levels have been measured at 60–65% of maternal levels at delivery. It is not clearly known if or how much pentazocine crosses into milk.

The drug is primarily metabolized in the liver with resultant excretion by the kidneys of the metabolites. In the horse, approximately 30% of a given dose is excreted as the glucuronide. Pentazocine and its metabolites have been detected in equine urine for up to 5 days following an injection. Apparently, less than 15% of the drug is excreted by the kidneys in an unchanged form.

Plasma half-lives have been reported for various species: Humans = 2–3 hrs; Ponies = 97 min.; Dogs = 22 min.; Cats = 84 min.; Swine = 49 min. Volumes of distribution range from a high of 5.09 L/kg in ponies to 2.78 L/kg in cats. In horses, the onset of action has been reported to be 2–3 minutes following IV dosing with a peak effect at 5–10 minutes.

Contraindications/Precautions/Warnings

The drug is contraindicated in patients having known hypersensitivity to it. All opiates should be used with caution in patients with hypothyroidism, severe renal insufficiency, adrenocortical insufficiency (Addison's), and geriatric or severely debilitated patients.

Like other opiates, pentazocine must be used with extreme caution in patients with head trauma, increased CSF pressure or other CNS dysfunction (*e.g.*, coma). Pentazocine should not be used in place of appropriate therapy (medical &/or surgical) for equine colic, but only as adjunctive treatment for pain.

Adverse Effects

In dogs, the most predominant adverse reaction following parenteral administration is salivation. Other potential side effects at usual doses include fine tremors, emesis, and swelling at the injection site. At very high doses (6 mg/kg) dogs have been noted to develop ataxia, fine tremors, convulsions, and swelling at the injection site.

Horses may develop transient ataxia and clinical signs of CNS excitement. Pulse and respiratory rates may be mildly elevated.

The use of pentazocine in cats is controversial. Some clinicians claim that the drug causes dysphoric reactions that preclude its use in this species, while others disagree and state that drug may be safely used.

Reproductive/Nursing Safety

Because reproductive studies have not been done in dogs, the manufacturer does not recommend its use in pregnant bitches or bitches intended for breeding. Studies performed in laboratory animals have not demonstrated any indications of teratogenicity. In humans, the FDA categorizes this drug as category *C* for use during pregnancy (*Animal studies have shown an adverse effect on the fetus, but there are no adequate studies in humans; or there are no animal reproduction studies and no adequate studies in humans.*)

Safety for use during lactation has not been established.

Overdosage/Acute Toxicity

There is little information regarding acute overdose situations with pentazocine. For oral ingestions, the gut should be emptied if indicated and safe to do so. Clinical signs should be managed by supportive treatment (O_2, pressor agents, IV fluids, mechanical ventilation) and respiratory depression can be treated with naloxone. Repeated doses of naloxone may be necessary.

Drug Interactions

The following drug interactions have either been reported or are theoretical in humans or animals receiving pentazocine and may be of significance in veterinary patients:

- **CNS DEPRESSANTS, OTHER (*e.g.*, anesthetic agents, antihistamines, phenothiazines, barbiturates, tranquilizers, alcohol, etc.):** May cause increased CNS or respiratory depression; dosage may need to be decreased

- **FLUOXETINE (and OTHER SSRI'S):** May be at increased risk for serotonin syndrome

Laboratory Considerations

- Pentazocine may cause decreases for urinary **17-hydroxycorticosteroid** determinations

Doses

- **DOGS:**

  For analgesia:

  a) Initially 1.65 mg/kg; up to 3.3 mg/kg IM. Duration of effect generally lasts 3 hours. If dose is repeated, use different injection site. (Package Insert; *Talwin®-V—* Winthrop)

  b) 1–6 mg/kg IM or SC q1–3h (Hendrix & Hansen 2000)

  c) 1–4 mg/kg IM, IV q2–4h (Otero 2006)

- **CATS:**

  Note: Pentazocine can cause dysphoria in cats; alternative analgesics are recommended.

- **FERRETS:**

  a) 5–10 mg/kg SC or IM q4h (Williams 2000)

■ **RABBITS, RODENTS, SMALL MAMMALS:**
a) Rabbits: Post-operative analgesia: 5–20 mg/kg SC, IV, or IM q4h (Ivey & Morrisey 2000)

■ **HORSES:**
Studies have demonstrated that pentazocine is not as an effective analgesic as either butorphanol or flunixin in horses. Many clinicians no longer recommend its use. (**Note:** ARCI UCGFS Class 3 Drug)

For analgesia:
a) 0.33 mg/kg slowly in jugular vein. In cases of severe pain, a second dose (0.33 mg/kg) be given IM 15 minutes later (Package Insert; *Talwin®-V*—Winthrop)
b) 0.4–0.9 mg/kg IV. Duration of analgesia may last only 10–30 minutes following an IV dose. (Thurmon & Benson 1987)
c) For standing chemical restraint for castrations: Administer acepromazine at 0.088 mg/kg (or 40 mg/450 kg) IV after about 10 minutes when patient is obviously tranquilized, give pentazocine at 0.5 mg/kg (225 mg/450kg) IV and then administer local anesthetic to each cord and the incision sites on ventral surface of the scrotum. (Abrahamsen 2007)

Monitoring
■ Analgesic efficacy
■ Respiratory rate/depth
■ Appetite/bowel function
■ CNS effects

Client Information
■ Clients should report any significant changes in behavior, appetite, bowel, or urinary function in their animals.

Chemistry/Synonyms
A synthetic partial opiate agonist, pentazocine is commercially available as two separate salts. The hydrochloride salt, which is found in oral dosage forms, occurs as a white, crystalline powder. It is soluble in water and freely soluble in alcohol. The commercial injection is prepared from pentazocine base with the assistance of lactic acid. This allows the drug to be soluble in water. The pH of this product is adjusted to a range of 4–5. Pentazocine is a weak base with an approximate pK_a of 9.0.

Pentazocine may also be known as: NIH-7958, NSC-107430, pentazocinum, Win-20228, *Talacen®*, and *Talwin®*.

Storage/Stability
The tablet preparations should be stored at room temperature and in tight, light-resistant containers. The injectable product should be kept at room temperature; avoid freezing.

Compatibility/Compounding Considerations
The following agents have been reported to be physically **compatible** when mixed with pentazocine lactate: atropine sulfate, benzquinamide HCl, butorphanol tartrate, chlorpromazine HCl, dimenhydrinate, diphenhydramine HCl, droperidol, fentanyl citrate, hydromorphone, hydroxyzine HCl, meperidine HCl, metoclopramide, morphine sulfate, perphenazine, prochlorperazine edisylate, promazine HCl, promethazine HCl, and scopolamine HBr.

The following agents have been reported to be physically **incompatible** when mixed with pentazocine lactate: aminophylline, amobarbital sodium, flunixin meglumine, glycopyrrolate, pentobarbital sodium, phenobarbital sodium, secobarbital sodium, and sodium bicarbonate.

Dosage Forms/Regulatory Status

VETERINARY-LABELED PRODUCTS: None

The ARCI (Racing Commissioners International) has designated this drug as a class 3 substance. See the appendix for more information.

HUMAN-LABELED PRODUCTS:

Pentazocine Lactate Injection: 30 mg (as lactate)/mL in 10 mL vials, *Uni-Amps*; 1 mL *Uni-Amps*, 1 mL & 2 mL *Carpuject*; *Talwin®* (Abbott Hospital Products); (Rx, C-IV)

Pentazocine HCl and Naloxone HCl Tablets (Scored): 50 mg (as hydrochloride) & 0.5 mg naloxone; generic; (Royce); (Rx, C-IV)

Pentazocine HCl and Acetaminophen Tablets: 25 mg (as hydrochloride)/650 mg acetaminophen; *Talacen®* (Sanofi Winthrop); generic; (Rx, C-IV)

References
Abrahamsen, E. (2007). Standing chemical restraint techniques I. Proceedings: Western Vet Conference. Accessed via: Veterinary Information Network. http://goo.gl/o56co

Hendrix, P. & B. Hansen (2000). Acute Pain Management. *Kirk's Current Veterinary Therapy: XIII Small Animal Practice.* J Bonagura Ed. Philadelphia, WB Saunders: 57–61.

Ivey, E. & J. Morrisey (2000). Therapeutics for Rabbits. *Vet Clin NA: Exotic Anim Pract* **3:1**(Jan): 183–216.

Otero, P. (2006). Acute pain management in emergency. Proceedings: WSAVA World Congress. Accessed via: Veterinary Information Network. http://goo.gl/vB0lV

Thurmon, J.C. & G.J. Benson (1987). Injectable anesthetics and anesthetic adjuncts. *Vet Clin North Am (Equine Practice)* **3**(1): 15–36.

Williams, D. (2000). Exocrine Pancreatic Disease. *Textbook of Veterinary Internal Medicine: Diseases of the Dog and Cat.* S Ettinger and E Feldman Eds. Philadelphia, WB Saunders. **2**: 1345–1367.

PENTOBARBITAL SODIUM

(pen-toe-*bar*-bi-tal)   Nembutal®

BARBITURATE

Note: *Pentobarbital and combinations with pentobarbital (e.g., phenytoin) for euthanasia have a separate monograph listed under Euthanasia Agents*

Prescriber Highlights

▶ Barbiturate used therapeutically as a sedative/anesthetic, & treating intractable seizures; also used for euthanasia

▶ Contraindications: Known hypersensitivity, severe liver disease, nephritis, or severe respiratory depression (large doses). Caution: Hypovolemia, anemia, borderline hypoadrenal function, or cardiac or respiratory disease. Use with caution in cats (sensitive to respiratory depression).

▶ Adverse Effects: respiratory depression (if using for anesthesia have ventilatory support available), hypothermia, or excitement post-anesthesia (dogs)

▶ When giving IV, administer SLOWLY (unless for euthanasia); very irritating if given SC or perivascularly; do not give IA

▶ Numerous drug interactions

Uses/Indications

Once pentobarbital was the principal agent used for general anesthesia in small animals, but this has been largely supplanted by the use of inhalant anesthetic agents. It is still commonly used as an anesthetic in laboratory situations, for rodents and occasionally as a sedative agent in dogs and cats.

Pentobarbital can be used for treating intractable seizures secondary to convulsant agents (*e.g.*, strychnine) or secondary to CNS toxins (*e.g.*, tetanus). It should not be used to treat seizures caused by lidocaine intoxication. For refractory status epilepticus not controlled with diazepam and phenobarbital, pentobarbital can be used, but propofol is preferred by most today as it causes less cardiovascular depression and recoveries can be smoother.

Pentobarbital has been used as a sedative and anesthetic agent in horses, cattle, swine, sheep, and goats. Often the drug is given after a preanesthetic agent in order to reduce pentobarbital dosages and resultant side effects.

Pentobarbital is a major active ingredient in several euthanasia solutions. This indication is discussed in the monograph for Euthanasia Agents.

Pharmacology/Actions

While barbiturates are generally considered CNS depressants, they can invoke all levels of CNS mood alteration from paradoxical excitement to deep coma and death. While the exact mechanisms for the CNS effects caused by barbiturates are unknown, they have been shown to inhibit the release of acetylcholine, norepinephrine, and glutamate. The barbiturates also have effects on GABA and pentobarbital has been shown to be GABA-mimetic. At high anesthetic doses, barbiturates have been demonstrated to inhibit the uptake of calcium at nerve endings.

The degree of depression produced is dependent on the dosage, route of administration, pharmacokinetics of the drug, and species treated. Additionally, effects may be altered by patient age, physical condition, or concurrent use of other drugs. The barbiturates depress the sensory cortex, lessen motor activity, and produce sedation at low dosages. In humans, it has been shown that barbiturates reduce the rapid-eye movement (REM) stage of sleep. Barbiturates have no true intrinsic analgesic activity.

In most species, barbiturates cause a dose-dependent respiratory depression, but, in some species, they can cause slight respiratory stimulation. At sedative/hypnotic doses, respiratory depression is similar to that during normal physiologic sleep. As doses increase, the medullary respiratory center is progressively depressed with resultant decreases in rate, depth, and volume. Respiratory arrest may occur at doses four times lower than those will cause cardiac arrest. These drugs must be used very cautiously in cats; they are particularly sensitive to the respiratory depressant effects of barbiturates.

Besides the cardiac arresting effects of the barbiturates at euthanatizing dosages, the barbiturates have other cardiovascular effects. In the dog, pentobarbital has been demonstrated to cause tachycardia, decreased myocardial contractility and stroke volume, and decreased mean arterial pressure and total peripheral resistance.

The barbiturates cause reduced tone and motility of the intestinal musculature, probably secondary to its central depressant action. The thiobarbiturates (thiamylal, thiopental) may, after initial depression, cause an increase in both tone and motility of the intestinal musculature; however, these effects do not appear to have much clinical significance. Administration of barbiturates reduces the sensitivity of the motor end-plate to acetylcholine, thereby slightly relaxing skeletal muscle. Because the musculature is not completely relaxed, other skeletal muscle relaxants may be necessary for surgical procedures.

There is no direct effect on the kidney by the barbiturates, but severe renal impairment may occur secondary to hypotensive effects in overdose situations. Liver function is not directly affected when used acutely, but hepatic microsomal enzyme induction is well documented with extended barbiturate (especially phenobarbital) administration. Although barbiturates reduce oxygen consumption of all tissues, no change in metabolic rate is measurable when given at sedative dosages. Basal metabolic rates may be reduced with resultant decreases in body temperature when barbiturates are given at anesthetic doses.

Pharmacokinetics

Pentobarbital is absorbed quite rapidly from the gut after oral or rectal administration with peak plasma concentrations occurring between 30–60 minutes after oral dosing in humans. The onset of action usually occurs within 15–60 minutes after oral dosing and within 1 minute after IV administration.

Pentobarbital, like all barbiturates, distributes rapidly to all body tissues with highest concentrations found in the liver and brain. It is 35–45% bound to plasma proteins in humans. Although less lipophilic than the ultra-short acting barbiturates (e.g., thiopental), pentobarbital is highly lipid soluble and patient fat content may alter the distributive qualities of the drug. All barbiturates cross the placenta and enter milk (at concentrations far below those of plasma). In neonates, pentobarbital may cross into the CNS at levels up to 6 times those in adult animals.

Pentobarbital is metabolized in the liver principally by oxidation. Excretion of the drug is not appreciably enhanced by increased urine flow or alkalinizing the urine. Ruminants (especially sheep and goats) metabolize pentobarbital at a very rapid rate. The elimination half-life in the goat has been reported to be approximately 0.9 hrs. Conversely, the half-life in dogs is approximately 8 hours; in man, it ranges from 15–50 hours.

Contraindications/Precautions/Warnings

Use cautiously in patients who are hypovolemic, anemic, have borderline hypoadrenal function, or cardiac or respiratory disease. Large doses are contraindicated in patients with nephritis or severe respiratory dysfunction. Barbiturates are contraindicated in patients with severe liver disease or who have demonstrated previous hypersensitivity reactions to them. Use with caution in neonates, as pentobarbital levels in the CNS may be substantially higher than in adults.

When administering IV, give SLOWLY. Use for cesarean section is not recommended because of fetal respiratory depression. Cats tend to particularly sensitive to the respiratory depressant effects of barbiturates; use with caution in this species. Female cats appear to be more susceptible to the effects of pentobarbital than male cats.

Adverse Effects

Because of the respiratory depressant effects of pentobarbital, respiratory activity must be

closely monitored and respiratory assistance must be readily available when using anesthetic dosages. Pentobarbital may cause excitement in dogs during recovery from anesthetic doses. Hypothermia may develop in animals receiving pentobarbital if exposed to temperatures below 27°C (80.6°F). The barbiturates can be very irritating when administered SC or perivascularly; avoid these types of injections. Do not administer intra-arterially.

Reproductive/Nursing Safety

In humans, the FDA categorizes this drug as category *D* for use during pregnancy (*There is evidence of human fetal risk, but the potential benefits from the use of the drug in pregnant women may be acceptable despite its potential risks.*) In a separate system evaluating the safety of drugs in canine and feline pregnancy (Papich 1989), this drug is categorized as class: *D* (*Contraindicated. These drugs have been shown to cause congenital malformations or embryotoxicity.*)

Exercise caution when administering to the nursing mother, since small amounts are excreted in maternal milk. Drowsiness in nursing offspring has been reported.

Overdosage/Acute Toxicity

In dogs, the reported oral LD_{50} is 85 mg/kg and IV LD_{50} is 40–60 mg/kg. Fatalities from ingestion of meat from animals euthanized by pentobarbital have been reported in dogs. Treatment of pentobarbital overdose consists of removal of ingested product from the gut if appropriate and offering respiratory and cardiovascular support. Forced alkaline diuresis is of little benefit for this drug. Peritoneal or hemodialysis may be of benefit in severe intoxications.

Drug Interactions

Most clinically significant interactions have been documented in humans with phenobarbital; however, these interactions may also be of significance in animals receiving pentobarbital, especially with chronic therapy.

- ◼ **ACETAMINOPHEN:** Increased risk for hepatotoxicity, particularly when large or chronic doses of barbiturates are given.

- ◼ **LIDOCAINE:** Fatalities have been reported when dogs suffering from lidocaine-induced seizures were treated with pentobarbital. Until this interaction is further clarified, it is suggested that lidocaine-induced seizures in dogs be treated initially with diazepam.

- ◼ **PHENYTOIN:** Barbiturates may affect the metabolism of phenytoin, and phenytoin may alter barbiturate levels; monitoring of blood levels may be indicated.

- ◼ **RIFAMPIN:** May induce enzymes that increase the metabolism of barbiturates.

The following drugs may increase the effect of pentobarbital:
- ◼ **ANTIHISTAMINES**
- ◼ **CHLORAMPHENICOL**

- ◼ OPIATES
- ◼ PHENOTHIAZINES
- ◼ VALPROIC ACID

Pentobarbital (particularly after chronic therapy) may decrease the effect of the following drugs/drug classes by lowering their serum concentrations:

- ◼ ANTICOAGULANTS, ORAL (WARFARIN)
- ◼ BETA-BLOCKERS
- ◼ CHLORAMPHENICOL
- ◼ CLONAZEPAM
- ◼ CORTICOSTEROIDS
- ◼ CYCLOSPORINE
- ◼ DOXORUBICIN
- ◼ DOXYCYCLINE (may persist for weeks after barbiturate discontinued)
- ◼ ESTROGENS
- ◼ GRISEOFULVIN
- ◼ METHADONE
- ◼ METRONIDAZOLE
- ◼ QUINIDINE
- ◼ PAROXETINE
- ◼ PHENOTHIAZINES
- ◼ PROGESTINS
- ◼ THEOPHYLLINE
- ◼ TRICYCLIC ANTIDEPRESSANTS
- ◼ VERAPAMIL

Laboratory Considerations

- ◼ Barbiturates may cause increased retention of **bromosulfophthalein** (BSP; sulfobromophthalein) and give falsely elevated results. It is recommended that barbiturates not be administered within the 24 hours before BSP retention tests.

Doses

Note: In order to avoid possible confusion, doses used for euthanasia are listed separately under the monograph for euthanasia solutions.

- ◼ **DOGS:**

As a sedative:

a) 2–4 mg/kg IV (Kirk 1986)

b) 2–4 mg/kg PO q6h (Davis 1985b)

For anesthesia:

a) 30 mg/kg IV to effect (Kirk 1986)

b) 10–30 mg/kg IV to effect (Morgan 1988)

c) 24–33 mg/kg IV (Booth 1988)

For chemical restraint for ventilatory support:

a) For ventilator maintenance, pentobarbital is preferred and may be administered as a CRI from 1–3 mg/kg/hour IV; it is associated with relative cardiovascular stability, but may cause seizure-like movements during recovery from anesthesia. The author prefers to switch over to a shorter acting drug like propofol about 12 hours prior to weaning from the ventilator; this will allow the pentobarbital levels to decrease and will help attenuate any seizure-like activity. Adjunctive drugs include: Fentanyl 0.5–1 micrograms/kg/minute; Propofol 50–300 micrograms/kg/minute OR Midazolam 0.5 mg/kg/hour (Brainard 2008)

For status epilepticus:

a) Pentobarbital should be given to effect not as a specific dose (3–15 mg/kg body weight IV) as there is tremendous individual variation in response when used at standard safe doses. Pentobarbital is a general anesthetic with negligible anticonvulsant properties. Patients treated with "barbiturate coma" commonly require an extended period of mechanical ventilation in an intensive care setting. In general, the side effects of barbiturate coma include depression of myocardial metabolism, vasodilatation with a decrease in venous return, and decreased cardiac perfusion. These effects can be minimized by the use of saline infusion and small doses of dopamine. Patients can develop poikilothermia and decreased urinary output during myocardial depression and hypotension. Neurologic evaluation is difficult because spontaneous respiratory responses and spontaneous movements cease. (Platt 2009)

b) 2–15 mg/kg IV can effectively terminate the physical manifestations of seizure activity within several minutes, but it is not generally considered to be an effective anticonvulsant and is unlikely to stop seizure activity in the brain. (Fletcher 2009)

- ◼ **CATS:**

For chemical restraint for ventilatory support:

a) For ventilator maintenance, pentobarbital is preferred and may be administered as a CRI from 1–3 mg/kg/hour IV; it is associated with relative cardiovascular stability, but may cause seizure-like movements during recovery from anesthesia. The author prefers to switch over to a shorter acting drug like propofol about 12 hours prior to weaning from the ventilator; this will allow the pentobarbital levels to decrease and will help attenuate any seizure-like activity. Adjunctive drugs include: Midazolam 0.3–0.5 mg/kg/hour; Medetomidine 0.3–1 micrograms/kg/hour (**caution** with the use of medetomidine) (Brainard 2008)

As a sedative:

a) 2–4 mg/kg IV (Kirk 1986)

b) 2–4 mg/kg PO q6h (Davis 1985a)

For status epilepticus:

a) 5–15 mg/kg IV to effect (Morgan 1988)

b) 3–15 mg/kg IV SLOWLY to effect. Goal is heavy sedation, not surgical planes of anesthesia. May need to repeat in 4–8 hours. (Raffe 1986)

For anesthesia:

a) 25 mg/kg IV, an additional 10 mg/kg IV may be given if initial dose is inadequate (Booth 1988)

■ **SMALL MAMMALS/RODENTS:**
For chemical restraint:

Mice: 30–80 mg/kg IP

Rats: 40–60 mg/kg IP

Hamsters/Gerbils: 70–80 mg/kg IP

Guinea pig: 15–40 mg/kg IP; 30 mg/kg IV

Rabbits: 20–60 mg/kg IV (Burke 1999)

■ **CATTLE:**

a) 30 mg/kg IV to effect, repeat as needed for chlorinated hydrocarbon toxicity (Smith 1986)(

b) As an anesthetic in calves (over one month of age): 15–30 mg/kg IV (Thurmon & Benson 1986)

c) As a sedative: 1–2 grams IV in an adult cow (given until animal becomes unsteady and rear limb weakness occurs). 3 grams will usually induce recumbency. (Thurmon & Benson 1986)

■ **HORSES:**
Note: Pentobarbital is generally not considered an ideal agent for use in the adult horse due to possible development of excitement and injury when the animal is "knocked down." (**Note:** ARCI UCGFS Class 2 Drug)

a) 3–15 mg/kg IV (Robinson 1987)

b) 15–18 mg/kg IV for light anesthesia (Schultz 1986)

■ **SWINE:**

a) 30 mg/kg IV to effect (Howard 1986)

b) As an anesthetic: 15–30 mg/kg IV (Thurmon & Benson 1986)

■ **SHEEP:**
As an anesthetic:

a) 20–30 mg/kg IV (Thurmon & Benson 1986)

b) **Adult Sheep:** 11–54 mg/kg IV (average dose 24 mg/kg IV). Anesthesia required for longer than 15–30 minutes will require additional doses.

Lambs: 15–26 mg/kg IV (will induce anesthesia for 15 minutes). Additional 5.5 mg/kg IV will give another 30 minutes of effect. (Booth 1988)

■ **GOATS:**
As an anesthetic:

a) 20–30 mg/kg IV (Thurmon & Benson 1986)

b) 25 mg/kg IV slowly, duration of satisfactory anesthesia will last only 20 minutes or so. (Booth 1988)

Monitoring

■ Levels of consciousness and/or seizure control

■ Respiratory and cardiac signs

■ Body temperature

■ If using chronically, routine blood counts and liver function tests should be performed.

Client Information

■ This drug is best used in an inpatient setting or with close professional supervision.

■ If dosage forms are dispensed to clients, they must be in instructed to keep them away from children; dispense in child-resistant packaging.

Chemistry/Synonyms

Pentobarbital sodium occurs as odorless, slightly bitter tasting, white, crystalline powder or granules. It is very soluble in water and freely soluble in alcohol. The pK_a of the drug has been reported to range from 7.85–8.03 and the pH of the injection is from 9–10.5. Alcohol or propylene glycol may be added to enhance the stability of the injectable product.

Pentobarbital may also be known as: aethaminalum, mebubarbital, mebumal, pentobarbitalum, or pentobarbitone.

Storage/Stability

The injectable product should be stored at room temperature; the suppositories should be kept refrigerated. The aqueous solution is not very stable and should not be used if it contains a precipitate. Because precipitates may occur, pentobarbital sodium should not be added to acidic solutions.

Compatibility/Compounding Considerations

The following solutions and drugs have been reported to be physically **compatible** with pentobarbital sodium: dextrose IV solutions, Ringer's injection, lactated Ringer's injection, Saline IV solutions, dextrose-saline combinations, dextrose-Ringer's combinations, dextrose-Ringer's lactate combinations, amikacin sulfate, aminophylline, atropine sulfate (for at least 15 minutes, not 24 hours), calcium chloride, cephapirin sodium, chloramphenicol sodium succinate, hyaluronidase, hydromorphone HCl, lidocaine HCl, neostigmine methylsulfate, scopolamine HBr, sodium bicarbonate, sodium iodide, thiopental sodium, and verapamil HCl.

The following drugs have been reported to be physically **incompatible** with pentobarbital sodium: benzquinamide HCl, butorphanol tartrate, chlorpromazine HCl, cimetidine HCl, chlorpheniramine maleate, codeine phosphate, diphenhydramine HCl, droperidol, fentanyl citrate, glycopyrrolate, hydrocortisone sodium succinate, hydroxyzine HCl, insulin (regular), meperidine HCl, nalbuphine HCl, norepinephrine bitartrate, oxytetracycline HCl, penicillin G potassium, pentazocine lactate, phenytoin sodium, prochlorperazine edisylate, promazine HCl, promethazine HCl, and streptomycin sulfate. Compatibility is dependent upon factors such as pH, concentration, temperature, and diluent used; consult specialized references or a hospital pharmacist for more specific information.

Dosage Forms/Regulatory Status

VETERINARY-LABELED PRODUCTS: None

The ARCI (Racing Commissioners International) has designated this drug as a class 2 substance. See the appendix for more information.

HUMAN-LABELED PRODUCTS:

Pentobarbital Sodium Injection: 50 mg/mL in 2 mL *Tubex*; generic; (Wyeth-Ayerst); (Rx, C-II)

Pentobarbital is a Class-II controlled substance and detailed records must be maintained with regard to its use and disbursement.

References

Booth, N.H. (1988). Drugs Acting on the Central Nervous System. *Veterinary Pharmacology and Therapeutics - 6th Ed.* NH Booth and LE McDonald Eds. Ames, Iowa State University Press: 153–408.

Brainard, B. (2008). Long-term sedation for the ventilated patient. Proceedings: IVECCS. Accessed via: Veterinary Information Network. http://goo.gl/esktu

Burke, T. (1999). Husbandry and Medicine of Rodents and Lagomorphs. Proceedings: Central Veterinary Conference, Kansas City.

Davis, L.E. (1985a). General Care of the Patient. *Handbook of Small Animal Therapeutics.* LE Davis Ed. New York, Churchill Livingstone: 1–20.

Davis, L.E., Ed. (1985b). *Handbook of Small Animal Therapeutics.* New York, Churchill Livingstone.

Fletcher, D. (2009). Seizure Management and Anticonvulsant Therapy. Proceedings: ACVC. Accessed via: Veterinary Information Network. http://goo.gl/U6s6B

Howard, J.L., Ed. (1986). *Current Veterinary Therapy 2, Food Animal Practice.* Philadelphia, W.B. Saunders.

Kirk, R.W., Ed. (1986). *Current Veterinary Therapy IX, Small Animal Practice.* Philadelphia, W.B. Saunders.

Morgan, R.V., Ed. (1988). *Handbook of Small Animal Practice.* New York, Churchill Livingstone.

Papich, M. (1989). Effects of drugs on pregnancy. *Current Veterinary Therapy X: Small Animal Practice.* R Kirk Ed. Philadelphia, Saunders: 1291–1299.

Platt, S. (2009). Status Epilepticus. Proceedings: WVC. Accessed via: Veterinary Information Network. http://goo.gl/6cVWd

Raffe, M.R. (1986, Last Update). "Personal communication."

Robinson, N.E., Ed. (1987). *Current Therapy in Equine Medicine.* Philadelphia, W.B. Saunders.

Schultz, C.S. (1986). *Formulary, Veterinary Hospital Pharmacy, Washington State University.* Pullman, Washington, Washington State University Press.

Smith, J.A. (1986). Toxic encephalopathies in cattle. *Current Veterinary Therapy 2: Food Animal Practice.* JL Howard Ed. Philadelphia, WB Saunders: 855–863.

Thurmon, J.C. & G.J. Benson (1986). Anesthesia in ruminants and swine. *Current Veterinary Therapy 2: Food Animal Practice.* JL Howard Ed. Philadelphia, WB Saunders: 51–71.

PENTOSAN POLYSULFATE SODIUM

(*pen*-toe-san)
PPS, Cartrophen-Vet®, Elmiron®

ANTIINFLAMMATORY, OSTEOARTHRITIS DISEASE-MODIFIER

Prescriber Highlights

➤ May be useful in treating osteoarthritis in dogs, cats & horses; may be used as adjunctive treatment of feline interstitial cystitis (feline idiopathic lower urinary tract disease—FLUTD)

➤ Efficacy for FLUTD not well-documented

➤ Adverse effects uncommon, but can cause bleeding, GI effects

➤ Use with caution prior to surgery or with other drugs affecting coagulation

➤ In the USA, only human oral product available; may be expensive

Uses/Indications

Pentosan may be useful in treating osteoarthritis in dogs, cats, and horses. It has been used as an adjunctive treatment of feline interstitial cystitis (feline idiopathic lower urinary tract disease—FLUTD). Studies using pentosan for FLUTD have demonstrated that it is not effective for short-term, acute lower urinary tract disease.

Pharmacology/Actions

Pentosan has a mild analgesic effect when used for interstitial cystitis. The mechanism for its action in treating interstitial cystitis is not known, but it is postulated that it may adhere to bladder wall mucosal membranes and act as a "buffer" to prevent irritating compounds in urine from reaching bladder cells.

Pentosan has disease-modifying effects on osteoarthritic joints similar to polysulfated glycosoaminoglycans. It apparently modulates cytokine action, preserves preoteoglycan content and stimulates hyaluronic acid synthesis. Pentosan has antiinflammatory, hypolipidemic, anticoagulant (considerably weaker than heparin—1/15th), and fibrinolytic properties. These effects potentially could increase synovial blood flow and reduce joint inflammation.

Pharmacokinetics

In rats, 10–20% of the calcium derivative (pentosan polysulfate calcium) is absorbed after oral dosing. In humans, only about 3% of an oral dose of pentosan polysulfate sodium is absorbed. It distributes primarily to the uroepithelium of the genitourinary tract with smaller concentrations found in the liver, spleen, lung skin, bone marrow, and periosteum. About two-thirds of absorbed drug is desulfated in the liver and spleen within one hour; about 3.5% of the absorbed drug is excreted into the urine.

Contraindications/Precautions/Warnings

Pentosan is contraindicated in patients hypersensitive to it. Use this drug with caution in animals also receiving other medications that can affect coagulation, or having surgery in the near future.

Adverse Effects

Pentosan is usually well tolerated. Adverse effects of pentosan in veterinary species appear to be mild and transitory in nature. In dogs, vomiting, anorexia, lethargy, or mild depression are possible. When used orally in cats, pentosan seems to be tolerated well, but oral dosing twice daily can be stressful for both cat and owner. Because pentosan has some anticoagulant effects, bleeding is possible in any species and may be more likely in animals receiving other drugs that affect coagulation (*e.g.*, aspirin), or undergoing stressful exercise. In horses, pentosan causes dose-dependent increases in partial thromboplastin time (PTT) up to 24 hours post-dose. In a small percentage of humans (<2%) taking the medication, transient increases in liver enzymes have been reported.

Reproductive/Nursing Safety

In humans, pentosan is designated by the FDA as a category *B* drug (*Animal studies have not demonstrated risk to the fetus, but there are no adequate studies in pregnant women; or animal studies have shown an adverse effect, but adequate studies in pregnant women have not demonstrated a risk to the fetus during the first trimester of pregnancy, and there is no evidence of risk in later trimesters.*)

Pentosan is likely safe to use during nursing.

Overdosage/Acute Toxicity

Information regarding overdoses is not readily available. Potentially, overdoses could cause bleeding, thrombocytopenia, GI distress, and liver function abnormalities. At the present time, treatment recommendations are basically supportive in nature. If an oral overdose occurs, consider protocols for drug removal from the gut.

Drug Interactions

■ No specific drug interactions were located; use this drug cautiously with other **drugs that can affect coagulation (e.g., NSAIDs, aspirin, heparin, etc.).**

Laboratory Considerations

■ No laboratory interactions or considerations were noted

Doses

■ **DOGS:**

As a chondroprotective for osteoarthritis (OA):

a) High loading dose: 20 mg/kg PO twice weekly for 5 weeks (for treatment of OA

signs of pain, lameness and stiffness); Medium Loading dose: 10 mg/kg PO once weekly for 12 weeks (for management of OA after joint surgery); Maintenance dose: 10 mg/kg once weekly for 4 weeks as needed. Always give on an empty stomach. (Label information; *Cartrophen-Vet® Capsules*—Arthropharm)

b) 3 mg/kg IM or SC on four occasions with an interval of 5−7 days between injections (Label information; *Pentosan 100® Injection* —Nature Vet)

■ **CATS:**

For treatment of persistent or recurrent FLUTD (**Note:** Recent studies have not shown any statistical benefit):

a) 2−16 mg/kg PO q12h (Bartges 2002)

b) 8 mg/kg PO q12h (Lane 2002)

■ **HORSES:**

For treating osteoarthritis:

a) Intramuscular administration: 3 mg/kg IM on four occasions with an interval of 7 days between injections.

Intra-articular injection: Prepare site as for surgery. Avoid iodine based skin preps; use a neutral soapless skin cleanser. A 20 gauge non-cutting needle is preferred. Introduce into joint space with steady, even pressure. Allow approximately 1 mL of synovial fluid to escape. Attach syringe with pentosan into the syringe and withdraw more synovial fluid to enter syringe, if possible. Inject mixture back into joint; draw back once or twice to mix pentosan and joint fluid within the joint. Firmly bandage and confine for 3−4 hours, then remove bandage. Rest horse for 2 weeks and follow with another 2 weeks of graded walking exercise before returning to work. (Label information; *Pentosan Equine® Injection*—Nature Vet)

Monitoring

■ When used for veterinary indications clinical efficacy is the primary monitoring parameter.

■ When administered into joints, animals should be assessed for intra-articular bleeding.

Client Information

■ In cats, pentosan (human product) is usually dosed at ½ capsule (50 mg) twice daily. One half the contents of a commercially available capsule may be emptied into an empty gelatin capsule and administered.

■ Give oral medication on an empty stomach

Chemistry/Synonyms

A heparin-like compound, pentosan polysulfate sodium is a mixture of linear polymers of beta-1->4-linked xylose that are usually sulfated at the 2- and 3- positions. Average molecular weight is between 4000 and 6000. It is not derived from animal sources, but from Beechwood hemicellulose.

Pentosan may also be known as: pentosan polysulphate sodium; PZ-68; sodium pentosan polysulphate; sodium xylanpolysulphate; SP-54, *Cartrophen-Vet®*, *Fibrase®*, *Fibrezym®*, *Fibrocid®*, *Fibrocide®*, *Hemoclar®*, *Lelong Contusions®*, *Elmiron®*, *Pentosan®*, *Polyanion®*, *Tavan®-SP 54*, and *Thrombocid®*.

Storage/Stability

Unless otherwise labeled, store oral pentosan products at controlled room temperature (15–30°C; 59–86°F) and injectable pentosan products under refrigeration and protected from light.

Dosage Forms/Regulatory Status

VETERINARY-LABELED PRODUCTS:

No products currently available in USA.

In several other countries, *Cartrophen-Vet®* is available as oral 100 mg capsules (pentosan polysulfate calcium) labeled for use in dogs. Injectable pentosan polysulfate sodium 100 mg/mL (*Pentosan 100®* Injection, and *Cartrophen-Vet®* Injection) labeled for use in dogs and pentosan polysulfate sodium 250 mg/mL (*Pentosan Equine®* Injection) for horses are available in several countries.

HUMAN-LABELED PRODUCTS:

Pentosan Polysulfate Sodium Oral Capsules: 100 mg; *Elmiron®* (Ortho McNeil); (Rx)

References

Bartges, J. (2002). Idiopathic feline lower urinary tract disease. Proceedings: Western Veterinary Conference. Accessed via: Veterinary Information Network. http://goo.gl/IC0Ov

Lane, I. (2002). Feline urology update. Proceedings: Western Veterinary Conference. Accessed via: Veterinary Information Network. http://goo.gl/GNVpX

PENTOXIFYLLINE

(pen-tox-*ih*-fi-leen)   PTX, Trental®

HEMORRHEOLOGIC, IMMUNOMODULATORY AGENT

Prescriber Highlights

▶ Compound that increases erythrocyte flexibility & may decrease negative effects of endotoxemia

▶ Contraindications: Retinal or cerebral hemorrhage, intolerant or hypersensitive to it or other xanthines (*i.e.*, theophylline)

▶ Caution: Severe hepatic or renal impairment, or at risk for hemorrhage

▶ Adverse Effects: GI tract (vomiting/inappetence) most common. Potentially: Dizziness, other GI, CNS, or cardiovascular effects

Uses/Indications

In horses, pentoxifylline has been used as adjunctive therapy for cutaneous, vasculitis, endotoxemia and for the treatment of navicular disease.

Pentoxifylline has been used in dogs to treat immune-mediated dermatologic conditions, enhance healing, and reduce inflammation caused by ulcerative dermatosis in Shelties and Collies and for other conditions where improved microcirculation may be of benefit. There is some evidence for efficacy for pentoxifylline and misoprostol as antiallergic medications in dogs, but with their modest benefit, relatively high costs and adverse effects, these medications should probably not be used as first line medications to treat dogs with atopic dermatitis (Olivry *et al.* 2010). Pentoxifylline is being investigated for adjunctive therapy for dilated cardiomyopathy in Doberman pinschers and it has been tried in conjunction with prednisolone to decrease vasculitis associated with FIP in cats.

Pentoxifylline's major indications for humans include symptomatic treatment of peripheral vascular disease (*e.g.*, intermittent claudication, sickle cell disease, Raynaud's, etc.) and cerebrovascular diseases where blood flow may be impaired in the microvasculature.

Pharmacology/Actions

The mechanisms for pentoxifylline's actions are not fully understood. The drug increases erythrocyte flexibility probably by inhibiting erythrocyte phosphodiesterase and decreases blood viscosity by reducing plasma fibrinogen and increasing fibrinolytic activity. In horses, pentoxifylline appears to be a potent inhibitor of matrix metalloproteinase-9 and a modest inhibitor of matrix metalloproteinase-2 (Fugler *et al.* 2009).

Pentoxifylline is postulated to reduce negative

endotoxic effects of cytokine mediators via its phosphodiesterase inhibition.

Pharmacokinetics

In horses, after PO administration of crushed, sustained-release tablets, pentoxifylline is rapidly absorbed with a wide interpatient variation of bioavailability that averages around 68%. Bioavailability may decrease with continued administration over several days. The authors concluded that 10 mg/kg q12h PO yields serum levels equivalent to those observed after administration of therapeutic doses to humans and horses.

In dogs, pentoxifylline reportedly has a bioavailability of approximately 50% with peak levels occurring about 1–3 hours after dosing. Serum half-life is approximately 6–7 hours for the parent compound, 36 hours for active metabolite 1, and 8 hours for active metabolite 5.

In humans, pentoxifylline absorption from the gastrointestinal tract is rapid and almost complete, but a significant first-pass effect occurs. Food affects the rate, but not the extent, of absorption. While the distributive characteristics have not been fully described, it is known that the drug enters maternal milk. Pentoxifylline is metabolized both in the liver and erythrocytes; all identified metabolites appear to be active.

Contraindications/Precautions/Warnings

Pentoxifylline should be considered contraindicated in patients who have been intolerant to the drug or xanthines (e.g., theophylline, caffeine, theobromine) in the past and those with cerebral hemorrhage or retinal hemorrhage. It should be used cautiously in patients with severe hepatic or renal impairment and those at risk for hemorrhage.

Adverse Effects

Most commonly reported adverse effects involve the GI tract (vomiting, inappetence, loose stools) or CNS (excitement, nervousness). Erythema multiforme may occur rarely, secondary to pentoxifylline therapy in dogs.

In horses, IV administration may be associated with transient leukocytosis, muscle fasiculations, sweating on shoulders and flanks, and mild increases in heart rate. Oral dosing at 10 mg/kg or less appears to be well tolerated.

There are reports of dizziness and headache occurring in a small percentage of humans receiving the drug. Other adverse effects, primarily GI, CNS, and cardiovascular related, have been reported in people, but are considered to occur rarely. Veterinary experience is limited with pentoxifylline and animal adverse effects may differ.

Reproductive/Nursing Safety

In humans, the FDA categorizes this drug as category **C** for use during pregnancy (*Animal studies have shown an adverse effect on the fetus, but there are no adequate studies in humans; or there are no animal reproduction studies and no adequate studies in humans.*) Pentoxifylline may be teratogenic at high dosages.

Pentoxifylline and its metabolites are excreted in maternal milk. Because of the potential for tumorigenicity (seen in rats), use cautiously in nursing patients.

Overdosage/Acute Toxicity

Humans overdosed with pentoxifylline have demonstrated signs of flushing, seizures, hypotension, unconsciousness, agitation, fever, somnolence, GI distress and ECG changes. One patient who ingested 80 mg/kg recovered completely. Overdoses should be treated using the usual methods of appropriate gut emptying and supportive therapies.

Drug Interactions

The following drug interactions have either been reported or are theoretical in humans or animals receiving pentoxifylline and may be of significance in veterinary patients:

- ■ **ANTIHYPERTENSIVE DRUGS:** With pentoxifylline may increase hypotensive effect

- ■ **NSAIDS:** Use of non-steroidal antiinflammatory agents with pentoxifylline in horses is controversial. Some sources state that when used for endotoxemia in horses, pentoxifylline's beneficial effects are negated by NSAIDs, but one study showed superior efficacy when flunixin and pentoxifylline were used together, compared with either used alone.

- ■ **PLATELET-AGGREGATION INHIBITORS (e.g., aspirin, clopidogrel):** Increased risk for bleeding

- ■ **THEOPHYLLINE:** Serum levels may be increased when used concurrently with pentoxifylline

- ■ **WARFARIN:** When pentoxifylline is used with warfarin or other anticoagulants, increased risk of bleeding may result; use together with enhanced monitoring and caution

Doses

- ■ **DOGS:**

  a) For dermatologic conditions (e.g., dermatomyositis, ear margin seborrhea/necrosis, ulcerative dermatitis of collies/shelties, contact dermatitis, atopy and any disease with underlying vasculitis): 10 mg/kg PO q8h, if the disease does not respond, 15 mg/kg PO q8h may be effective (Merchant 2000)

  b) For atopic dermatitis: 10–25 mg/kg PO with food two to three times a day. Response may be improved by using with an antihistamine or a glucocorticoid. (Yu 2008)

  c) For dermatologic disorders including dermatomyositis, vasculitis, erythema multiforme, cutaneous and renal vasculitis of Greyhounds (Alabama rot), and allergic contact dermatitis: 10–30 mg/kg PO q 12 hours (Campbell 1999)

d) For familial canine dermatomyositis: 25 mg/kg PO q12h appears to be an effective beginning dose (Rees & Boothe 2003)

e) For atopic dermatitis: 10–15 mg/kg PO q8–12h. A 6–8 week course of therapy may be required to assess efficacy. (White 2003)

f) For vasculitis, dermatomyositis: 10 mg/kg PO q8h (Boord 2007)

g) For vasculitis: 15 mg/kg PO q8h (Hillier 2006)

h) In chronic pyoderma to help reverse chronic pathologic changes (scarring, fibrosis) and to aid in antibiotic tissue penetration: 20–30 mg/kg PO q12h. (Rosenkrantz 2009)

■ **HORSES: (Note:** ARCI UCGFS Class 4 Drug)

a) 10 mg/kg q12h PO yields serum levels equivalent to those observed after administration of therapeutic doses to humans and horses. OK to crush the sustained-release tablets and mix with molasses. If efficacy wanes with time, consider increasing the dose to 15 mg/kg PO twice daily or 10 mg/kg PO three times a day. In the experience of the authors, 10 mg/kg PO twice daily for 30 days results in clinical response in horses with cutaneous vasculitis. (Liska *et al.* 2006)

b) For adjunctive treatment to prevent GI thrombosis: 7.5 mg/kg IV q12 hours (can be easily filtered in a 0.5 micron filter for IV use); can make red blood cells more deformable, decrease blood viscosity, and inhibit some inflammatory cytokines. (Divers 2003)

To reduce cytokine effects in endotoxemia:

a) 7.5 mg/kg PO q12h, efficacy may be improved if used with flunixin (Smith 2003)

b) 8 mg/kg PO q8h (Barton 2003)

c) For adjunctive treatment (experimental) of sepsis in foals: 7.5 mg/kg IV bolus, followed by a CRI of 1.5 mg/kg/hour. Has been shown to increase regional blood flow and suppress coagulation. (McKenzie 2009)

For adjunctive treatment of equine pastern dermatitis:

a) If clinical signs do not resolve after 14 days of topical and other immunomodulating therapy, add pentoxifylline at 4–8 mg/kg PO q12h (Yu 2003)

To increase oxygenation of placenta in placentitis:

a) 7.5 mg/kg PO q12h (Troedsson 2003)

To increase the circulation to the podotrochlea:

a) 4.5–7 mg/kg PO three times daily (Turner 1999)

Monitoring
■ Efficacy
■ Adverse effects

Client Information
■ Give with food to reduce the GI effects of pentoxifylline
■ Clients should understand that veterinary experience with this medication is limited and that the risk versus benefit profile is not well-defined

Chemistry/Synonyms
A synthetic xanthine derivative structurally related to caffeine and theophylline, pentoxifylline occurs as a white, odorless, bitter-tasting, crystalline powder. At room temperature, approximately 77 mg are soluble in one mL of water and 63 mg in one mL of alcohol.

Pentoxifylline may also be known as: BL-191, oxpentifylline, or pentoxifyllinum and *Trental®*.

Storage/Stability
The commercially available tablets should be stored in well-closed containers, protected from light at 15–30°C.

Dosage Forms/Regulatory Status
VETERINARY-LABELED PRODUCTS: None

The ARCI (Racing Commissioners International) has designated this drug as a class 4 substance. See the appendix for more information.

HUMAN-LABELED PRODUCTS:

Pentoxifylline Controlled/Extended Release Tablets: 400 mg; *Trental®* (Hoechst Marion Roussel); generic; (Rx)

References
Barton, M. (2003). Endotoxemia. *Current Veterinary Therapy in Equine Medicine 5.* A Blikslager Ed. Philadelphia, Saunders: 104–108.
Boord, M. (2007). Treatment of pododermatitis. Proceedings: Western Vet Conf. Accessed via: Veterinary Information Network. http://goo.gl/1Qo9H
Campbell, K. (1999). New Drugs in Veterinary Dermatology. Proceedings: Central Veterinary Conference, Kansas City.
Divers, T.J. (2003). Prevention and treatment of thrombosis, phlebitis, and laminitis in horses with gastrointestinal diseases. *Veterinary Clinics of North America-Equine Practice* 19(3): 779–+.
Fugler, L., S. Eades, et al. (2009). Evaluation of Various Matrix Metalloproteinase Inhibitors (MMPIS) in the Horse. Proceedings: ACVIM. Accessed via: Veterinary Information Network. http://goo.gl/CgzCa
Hillier, A. (2006). Life threatening skin diseases. Proceedings: ACVC. Accessed via: Veterinary Information Network. http://goo.gl/GkQ1e
Liska, D., L. Akucewich, et al. (2006). Pharmacokinetics of pentoxifylline and its 5–hydroxyethyl metabolite after oral and intravenous administration to healthy adult horses. *AJVR* 67(9): 1621–1627.
McKenzie, E. (2009). Management of the Septic Foal. Proceedings: WVC. Accessed via: Veterinary Information Network. http://goo.gl/CXM0Q

Merchant, S. (2000). New Therapies in Veterinary Dermatology. Proceedings: American Animal Hospital Association 67th Annual Meeting, Toronto.

Olivry, T., D.J. DeBoer, et al. (2010). Treatment of canine atopic dermatitis: 2010 clinical practice guidelines from the International Task Force on Canine Atopic Dermatitis. *Veterinary Dermatology* 21(3): 233–248.

Rees, C. & D.M. Boothe (2003). Therapeutic response to pentoxifylline and its active metabolites in dogs with familial canine dermatomyositis. *Vet Therapeutics* 4(3): 234–241.

Rosenkrantz, W.S. (2009). Managing Challenging Pyoderma Cases. Proceedings: WVC. Accessed via: Veterinary Information Network. http://goo.gl/4Yupp

Smith, C. (2003). Critical care therapeutics for mature horses. *Current Veterinary Therapy in Equine Medicine 5*. C Kollias-Baker Ed. Philadelphia, Saunders: 19–23.

Troedsson, M. (2003). Placentitis. *Current Veterinary Therapy in Equine Medicine 5*. G Frazer Ed. Philadelphia, Saunders: 297–300.

Turner, T. (1999). Diagnosing lower limb lameness in the horse. Proceedings: Central Veterinary Conference, Kansas City.

White, S. (2003). Newly described diseases and treatments. Proceedings: World Animal Veterinary Assoc. World Congress. Accessed via: Veterinary Information Network. http://goo.gl/o5a92

Yu, A. (2003). Pastern dermatitis. *Current Veterinary Therapy in Equine Medicine 5*. S White Ed. Philadelphia, Saunders: 201–203.

Yu, A. (2008). Itchy, Chewy & Scratchy Dogs. What's in My Anti-Inflammatory Arsenal? Proceedings: WVC. Accessed via: Veterinary Information Network. http://goo.gl/6IXFP

PERGOLIDE MESYLATE

(*per*-go-lide)   Permax®

DOPAMINE AGONIST

Prescriber Highlights

▶ Dopamine agonist that can help control signs associated with pituitary pars intermedia dysfunction (PPID, equine Cushing's disease)

▶ Apparently, very well tolerated in horses; anorexia occurs in up to 10% of patients

▶ May be significant expense involved, since treatment is life-long

▶ Need to obtain via compounding pharmacies

Uses/Indications

The primary use for pergolide in veterinary medicine is in treatment of horses for pituitary pars intermedia dysfunction (PPID), commonly called equine Cushing's disease.

Pharmacology/Actions

Pergolide is a potent agonist at dopamine receptors D_1 and D_2 and is 10−1000 times more potent than bromocriptine. It is thought that pituitary pars intermedia dysfunction (PPID) in horses is a dopaminergic degenerative disease and pergolide (or dopamine) can reduce expression of proopiomelanocortin (POMC) peptides from the pars intermedia. These peptides are implicated in causing the signs associated with PPID.

Pharmacokinetics

In horses (6 in the study), pergolide was rapidly absorbed following oral administration (0.01 mg/kg), with plasma concentrations reaching maximum levels within 1 hour of dosing. Maximum plasma levels ranged from 1.07–3.38 nanograms/mL. Pergolide appears to be rapidly and widely distributed. Elimination half-life averaged 27 hours, but there was high interpatient variation (Gehring *et al.* 2010).

In humans, the drug is orally absorbed (estimated 60% bioavailable) and is 90% bound to plasma proteins. At least 10 different metabolites have been identified, some of which are active. The principle route of elimination is via the kidneys.

Contraindications/Precautions

Pergolide is contraindicated in patients hypersensitive to it or other ergot derivatives.

Adverse Effects

Pergolide appears to be very well tolerated in horses. Decreased appetite is seen during the first week of therapy in about 10% of horses treated; temporary dose reduction is often beneficial in alleviating this effect. Colic and diarrhea have been reported to occur more rarely.

Adverse effects reported in humans include: nervous system complaints (dyskinesia, hallucinations, somnolence and insomnia), gastrointestinal complaints (nausea, vomiting, diarrhea, constipation), transient hypotension, and rhinitis.

Reproductive/Nursing Safety

Safety of pergolide in pregnant horses has not been established. In humans, pergolide is designated by the FDA as a category **B** drug (*Animal studies have not demonstrated risk to the fetus, but there are no adequate studies in pregnant women; or animal studies have shown an adverse effect, but adequate studies in pregnant women have not demonstrated a risk to the fetus during the first trimester of pregnancy, and there is no evidence of risk in later trimesters.*)

It is not known if pergolide enters maternal milk; however, like other ergot-derivative dopamine agonists, it may interfere with lactation.

Overdosage/Acute Toxicity

There is limited information available on pergolide overdoses. Potential effects include GI disturbances, CNS effects, seizures, and hypotension.

There were 9 exposures to pergolide mesylate reported to the ASPCA Animal Poison Control Center (APCC) during 2008-2009. In these cases 8 were dogs with all 8 showing clinical signs, and the remaining 1 case was a horse showing no clinical signs. Common findings in dogs recorded in decreasing frequency included vomiting, lethargy, hypertension, and ptosis.

Treatment is supportive. Phenothiazines may decrease CNS stimulation effects.

Drug Interactions

The following drug interactions have either been reported or are theoretical in humans or animals receiving pergolide and may be of significance in veterinary patients:

- **DOPAMINE ANTAGONISTS (i.e., phenothiazines):** May decrease the effects of pergolide
- **METOCLOPRAMIDE:** May decrease the effects of pergolide

Laboratory Considerations

- No specific laboratory interactions or considerations were noted for this drug.

Doses

- **HORSES:**

  Note: The following doses each uses a different way of dosing (total dose, micrograms/kg, and mg/kg), do not be confused by them. For treatment of Equine "Cushing's-like" Disease [pituitary pars intermedia dysfunction (PPID)]:

  a) Initial dose of 1 mg (total dose) per day for horses and ponies with PPID. If the horse owner is willing to administer half the dose twice daily, this may be preferable on the basis of recent pharmacokinetic data. If anorexia or temporary dullness develop, treatment should be halted for 2 days or until appetite improves, and then restarted at 0.25 mg per day for 2 days, 0.5 mg per day for 2 days, and 0.75 mg per day for 2 days. (Frank 2010)

  b) 1.7–5.5 micrograms/kg; dose varies considerably. The higher doses are used in the more advanced cases or those refractory to treatment at a lower dose. (Messer 2009)

  c) Author's current opinion that initial medical treatment for equids with PPID should be pergolide at a dose of 0.002 mg/kg PO q24h. If no improvement is noted within 8-12 weeks (depending on season as hair coat changes will vary with the time of year that treatment is initiated), the daily dose can be increased by 0.002 mg/kg monthly up to a total dose of 0.006 mg/kg (3 mg/day for a 500 kg horse). If only a limited response is observed with the 0.006 mg/kg dose and endocrinologic test results remain abnormal, the author typically recommends addition of cyproheptadine (0.5 mg/kg PO q12h) to pergolide therapy. It is important to recognize that the rate of clinical improvement is higher than that for normalization of hyperglycemia and endocrinologic test results. Usually, only transient anorexia is recognized during the initial week of treatment and can be overcome in time or by cutting the dose in half for 2-4 days. (Schott II 2009)

Monitoring

- Dexamethasone suppression test (baseline and at 4–8 weeks post pergolide therapy initiation, repeat in 4–8 weeks if dosage is adjusted)
- Blood glucose (baseline, and if abnormal and repeat as per dexamethasone suppression test)
- Clinical signs (hair coat, weight, PU/PD, etc.)
- Periodic CBC and clinical chemistry panel

Client Information

- Clients should understand that pergolide does not cure the disease and it may take several weeks to months to see efficacy.
- Treatment is required for the life of the horse and the drug can be expensive.
- Proper nutrition and weight control can be very important to the successful treatment of this disease.

Chemistry/Synonyms

An ergot derivative, dopamine receptor agonist, pergolide occurs as white to off-white powder that is slightly soluble in water, dehydrated alcohol, or chloroform. It is very slightly soluble in acetone; practically insoluble in ether and sparingly soluble in methyl alcohol.

Pergolide mesylate may also be known as: LY-127809, pergolide mesilate, pergolidi mesilas, *Celance®, Nopar®, Parkotil®, Parlide®,* or *Pharken®.*

Storage/Stability

Store pergolide tablets in tight containers at room temperature (25°C; 77°F); excursions permitted to 15–30°C (59–86°F).

Compatibility/Compounding Considerations

As pergolide is no longer commercially available, compounding pharmacists must utilize the bulk powder pergolide mesylate to compound preparations of pergolide for horses. The compounder should account for the molecular weight of the mesylate salt by using a conversion factor of 1.3 when calculating the amount of pergolide mesylate to obtain an equivalent amount of pergolide base. Pergolide aqueous suspensions are unstable after compounding. Compounded pergolide formulations in aqueous vehicles should be stored in dark containers, protected from light, and refrigerated. Do not use more than 30 days after compounding. Formulations that have undergone a color change should be considered unstable and discarded (Davis *et al.* 2009).

Dosage Forms/Regulatory Status

VETERINARY-LABELED PRODUCTS: None

HUMAN-LABELED PRODUCTS: None

Due to an increased potential for heart valve damage associated with pergolide use in humans, all dosage forms were withdrawn from the US market in the spring of 2007. Pergolide may be available from compounding pharmacies for veterinary use.

References

Davis, J.L., L.M. Kirk, et al. (2009). Effects of compounding and storage conditions on stability of pergolide mesylate. *Javma-Journal of the American Veterinary Medical Association* 234(3): 385–389.

Frank, N. (2010). Which endocrine disorder are we dealing with? Pituitary pars intermedia dysfunction versus equine metabolic syndrome: treatment options. Proceedings: ACVIM. Accessed via: Veterinary Information Network. http://goo.gl/aFi5v

Gehring, R., L. Beard, et al. (2010). Single-Dose Oral Pharmacokinetics of Pergolide Mesylate in Healthy Adult Mares. *Vet Therapeutics* 11(1): E1–E8.

Messer, N.T. (2009). Diagnosis and Treatment of Pituitary Pars Intermedia. Proceedings: ABVP. Accessed via: Veterinary Information Network. http://goo.gl/U9gir

Schott II, H. (2009). Management of Pituitary Pars Intermedia Dysfunction. Proceedings: Western Vet Conf. Accessed via: Veterinary Information Network. http://goo.gl/2VC3p

PHENOBARBITAL SODIUM PHENOBARBITAL

(fee-noe-*bar*-bi-tal)   Phenobarbitone

BARBITURATE

Prescriber Highlights

▶ Barbiturate used primarily as an anti-seizure medication; also used as a sedative agent

▶ Contraindications: Known hypersensitivity, severe liver disease, nephritis, or severe respiratory depression (large doses)

▶ Caution: Hypovolemia, anemia, borderline hypoadrenal function, or cardiac or respiratory disease; use with caution in cats (sensitive to respiratory depression)

▶ Adverse Effects: *Dogs:* Anxiety/agitation or lethargy (when initiating treatment); profound depression, (even at low doses) is possible. Sedation, ataxia, polydipsia, polyuria, polyphagia can be seen at moderate to high serum levels. Increase in liver enzymes possible, but overt hepatotoxicity relatively uncommon. Rare: Anemia, thrombocytopenia or neutropenia.

▶ Adverse Effects: *Cats:* Ataxia, lethargy, polyphagia/weight gain & polydipsia/polyuria. Rare: Immune-mediated reactions & bone marrow hypoplasia

▶ When administering IV, give SLOWLY; do not give SC or perivascularly (very irritating)

▶ Drug Interactions; drug-lab interactions

▶ C-IV controlled substance

Uses/Indications

Although some believe that bromide salts are now the treatment of first choice for treating epilepsy in dogs (especially young dogs and those with liver disease), many still choose phenobarbital for dogs because of its favorable pharmacokinetic profile, relative safety, efficacy, low cost, and ability to treat epilepsy at subhypnotic doses. Phenobarbital is still widely considered the drug of first choice for treating epilepsy in cats. It is also occasionally used as an oral sedative agent in both species. Because it has a slightly longer onset of action, it is used principally in the treatment of status epilepticus in dogs, cats, and horses to prevent the recurrence of seizures after they have been halted with either a benzodiazepine or short-acting barbiturate. Phenobarbital may also useful in controlling excessive feline vocalization while riding in automobiles.

In cattle, the microsomal enzyme stimulating properties of phenobarbital has been suggested for its use in speeding the detoxification of organochlorine (chlorinated hydrocarbon) insecticide poisoning. Additionally, phenobarbital has been used in the treatment and prevention of neonatal hyperbilirubinemia in human infants. It is unknown if hyperbilirubinemia is effectively treated in veterinary patients with phenobarbital.

Pharmacology/Actions

While barbiturates are generally considered CNS depressants, they can invoke all levels of CNS mood alteration from paradoxical excitement to deep coma and death. While the exact mechanisms for the CNS effects caused by barbiturates are unknown, they have been shown to inhibit the release of acetylcholine, norepinephrine, and glutamate. The barbiturates also have effects on GABA and pentobarbital has been shown to be GABA-mimetic. At high anesthetic doses, barbiturates have been demonstrated to inhibit the uptake of calcium at nerve endings.

The degree of depression produced is dependent on the dosage, route of administration, pharmacokinetics of the drug, and species treated. Additionally, effects may be altered by patient age, physical condition, or concurrent use of other drugs. The barbiturates depress the sensory cortex, lessen motor activity, and produce sedation at low dosages. In humans, it has been shown that barbiturates reduce the rapid-eye movement (REM) stage of sleep. Barbiturates have no true intrinsic analgesic activity.

In most species, barbiturates cause a dose-dependent respiratory depression, but, in some species, they can cause slight respiratory stimulation. At sedative/hypnotic doses, respiratory depression is similar to that during normal physiologic sleep. As doses increase, the medullary respiratory center is progressively depressed with resultant decreases in rate, depth, and volume. Respiratory arrest may occur at doses four times lower than those will cause cardiac arrest. These drugs must be used very cautiously in cats; they are particularly sensitive to the respiratory depressant effects of barbiturates.

The barbiturates cause reduced tone and motility of the intestinal musculature, probably secondary to its central depressant action. Administration of barbiturates reduces the sensitivity of the motor endplate to acetylcholine, thereby slightly relaxing skeletal muscle. Because the musculature is not completely relaxed, other skeletal muscle relaxants may be necessary for surgical procedures.

There is no direct effect on the kidney by the barbiturates, but severe renal impairment may occur secondary to hypotensive effects in overdose situations. Liver function is not directly affected when used acutely, but hepatic microsomal enzyme induction is well documented with extended barbiturate (especially phenobarbital) administration. Although barbiturates reduce oxygen consumption of all tissues, no change in metabolic rate is measurable when given at sedative dosages. Basal metabolic rates may be reduced with resultant decreases in body temperature when barbiturates are given at anesthetic doses.

Pharmacokinetics

The pharmacokinetics of phenobarbital have been thoroughly studied in humans and in a more limited fashion in dogs, cats, and horses. Phenobarbital is slowly absorbed from the GI tract. Bioavailabilities range from 70–90% in humans, approximately 90% in dogs, and absorption is practically complete in adult horses. Peak levels occur in 4–8 hours after oral dosing in dogs, and in 8–12 hours in humans.

Phenobarbital is widely distributed throughout the body, but because of its lower lipid solubility, it does not distribute as rapidly as most other barbiturates into the CNS. The amount of phenobarbital bound to plasma proteins has been reported to be 40–60%. The reported apparent volumes of distribution are approximately: Horse ≈ 0.8 L/kg; Foals ≈ 0.86 L/kg; Dogs ≈ 0.75 L/kg.

The drug is metabolized in the liver primarily by hydroxylated oxidation to p-hydroxyphenobarbital; sulfate and glucuronide conjugates are also formed. The elimination half-lives reported in humans range from 2–6 days; in dogs from 12–125 hours with an average of approximately 2 days. Because of its ability to induce the hepatic enzymes used to metabolize itself (and other drugs), elimination half-lives may decrease with time along with concomitant reductions in serum levels. Some dogs may have half lives of less than 24 hours and may require 3 times daily dosing for maximal control. An elimination half-life of 34–43 hours has been reported in cats. Elimination half-lives in horses are considerably shorter with values reported of approximately 13 hours in foals and 18 hours in adult horses.

Phenobarbital will induce hepatic microsomal enzymes and it can be expected that elimination half-lives will decrease with time. Approximately 25% of a dose is excreted unchanged by the kidney. Alkalinizing the urine and/or substantially increasing urine flow will increase excretion rates. Anuric or oliguric patients may accumulate unmetabolized drug; dosage adjustments may need to be made.

Changes in diet, body weight, and body composition may alter the pharmacokinetics of phenobarbital in dogs and necessitate dosage adjustment.

Contraindications/Precautions/Warnings

Use cautiously in patients that are hypovolemic, anemic, have borderline hypoadrenal function, or cardiac or respiratory disease. Large doses are contraindicated in patients with nephritis or severe respiratory dysfunction. Barbiturates are contraindicated in patients with severe liver disease or who have demonstrated previous hypersensitivity reactions to them.

When administering IV, give slowly (not more than 60 mg/minute); too rapid IV administration may cause respiratory depression. Commercially available injectable preparations (excluding the sterile powder) must not be administered subcutaneously or perivascularly as significant tissue irritation and possible necrosis may result. Applications of moist heat and local infiltration of 0.5% procaine HCl solution have been recommended to treat these reactions.

Adverse Effects

Dogs may exhibit increased clinical signs of anxiety/agitation or lethargy when initiating therapy. These effects are generally transitory in nature. Occasionally dogs will exhibit profound depression at lower dosage ranges (and plasma levels). Polydipsia, polyuria, and polyphagia are also quite commonly displayed at moderate to high serum levels and may falsely infer a diagnosis of Cushing's disease; limiting intake of both food and water usually controls these signs. Sedation and/or ataxia often become significant concerns as serum levels reach the higher ends of the therapeutic range. Rarely, anemia, thrombocytopenia or neutropenia may occur which are reversible if detected early. Increases in liver enzymes are well described for phenobarbital in dogs and are not necessarily indicative of liver dysfunction, but if serum ALT or ALP are greater than 4–5 times the upper limit of normal, or if any elevation of AST and GGT are noted, it should raise concern. Phenobarbital should generally be discontinued if any increases in serum bilirubin, total serum bile acids or hypoalbumenemia are seen. Frank hepatic failure is uncommon and is usually associated with higher serum levels (>30–40 micrograms/mL).

Phenobarbital may rarely cause superficial necrolytic dermatitis (SND) in dogs associated with changes in hepatocytes (severe parenchymal collapse with glycogen-laden hepatocytes and moderate fibrosis sharply demarcated by nodules of normal hepatic parenchyma) distinct from that seen with phenobarbital hepatotoxicity.

Cats may develop ataxia, persistent sedation and lethargy, polyphagia/weight gain, and polydipsia/polyuria. Rarely, immune-mediated reactions and bone marrow hypoplasia (thrombocytopenia, neutropenia) may be seen. Cats, unlike dogs, apparently do not have the issues of increased liver enzymes. Very high dosages (10–40 mg/kg/day) have caused coagulopathies in cats.

As phenobarbital can potentially increase the metabolism of cortisol, it has been implicated in contributing to relative adrenal insufficiency.

Although there is much less information regarding its use in horses (and foals in particular), it would generally be expected that adverse effects would mirror those seen in other species.

Reproductive/Nursing Safety

Phenobarbital has been associated with rare congenital defects and bleeding problems in newborns, but may be safer than other anticonvulsants. In humans, the FDA categorizes this drug as category *D* for use during pregnancy (*There is evidence of human fetal risk, but the potential benefits from the use of the drug in pregnant women may be acceptable despite its potential risks.*) In a separate system evaluating the safety of drugs in canine and feline pregnancy (Papich 1989), this drug is categorized as class: *B* (*Safe for use if used cautiously. Studies in laboratory animals may have uncovered some risk, but these drugs appear to be safe in dogs and cats or these drugs are safe if they are not administered when the animal is near term.*)

Exercise caution when administering to a nursing mother since small amounts are excreted in maternal milk. Drowsiness in nursing offspring have been reported.

Overdosage/Acute Toxicity

There were 253 exposures to phenobarbital reported to the ASPCA Animal Poison Control Center (APCC) during 2008-2009. In these cases 228 were dogs with 99 showing clinical signs, 23 were cats with 10 showing clinical signs and the remaining 2 reported cases were a bird and a non human primate. The bird showed clinical signs while the non-human primate showed no clinical signs. Common findings in dogs recorded in decreasing frequency included ataxia, lethargy, sedation, recumbency, depression, hypothermia and coma. Common findings in cats recorded in decreasing frequency included ataxia, sedation, and recumbency.

Treatment of a phenobarbital overdose consists of removal of ingested product from the gut, if appropriate, and giving respiratory and cardiovascular support. Activated charcoal has been demonstrated to be of considerable benefit in enhancing the clearance of phenobarbital, even when the drug was administered parenterally. Charcoal acts as a "sink" for the drug to diffuse from the vasculature back into the gut. Forced alkaline diuresis can also be of substantial benefit in augmenting the elimination of phenobarbital in patients with normal renal function. Peritoneal dialysis or hemodialysis may be helpful in severe intoxications or in anuric patients.

Drug Interactions

The following drug interactions have either been reported or are theoretical in humans or animals receiving phenobarbital and may be of significance in veterinary patients:

- ■ **ACETAMINOPHEN:** Increased risk for hepatotoxicity, particularly when large or chronic doses of barbiturates are given
- ■ **CARPROFEN:** There may be an increased risk for hepatotoxicity secondary to carprofen metabolites. One source states: Patients should not receive phenobarbital or other hepatic drug metabolizing enzyme inducers when receiving this drug (Boothe 2005).
- ■ **MONAMINE OXIDASE (MAO) INHIBITORS (e.g., amitraz, possibly selegiline):** May prolong phenobarbital effects
- ■ **PHENYTOIN:** Barbiturates may affect the metabolism of phenytoin, and phenytoin may alter barbiturate levels; monitoring of blood levels may be indicated
- ■ **RIFAMPIN:** May induce enzymes that increase the metabolism of barbiturates

The following drugs may increase the effects of phenobarbital:

- ■ **ANTIHISTAMINES**
- ■ **CHLORAMPHENICOL**
- ■ **FELBAMATE**
- ■ **OPIATES**
- ■ **PHENOTHIAZINES**
- ■ **VALPROIC ACID**

Phenobarbital (particularly after chronic therapy) may decrease the effect of the following drugs/drug classes by lowering their serum concentrations:

- ■ **ANTICOAGULANTS, ORAL (WARFARIN)**
- ■ **BETA-BLOCKERS**
- ■ **CHLORAMPHENICOL**
- ■ **CLONAZEPAM**
- ■ **CORTICOSTEROIDS**
- ■ **CYCLOSPORINE**
- ■ **DOXORUBICIN**
- ■ **DOXYCYCLINE** (may persist for weeks after barbiturate discontinued)
- ■ **ESTROGENS**
- ■ **FELBAMATE:** Phenobarbital levels may increase and felbamate levels decrease
- ■ **GRISEOFULVIN**

- ■ ITRACONAZOLE
- ■ LAMOTRIGINE
- ■ LEVETIRACETAM (in dogs, 21 days of phenobarbital reduced levetiracetam elimination half-life by about 50%; 3.43 hrs to 1.73 hours) (Moore *et al.* 2009)
- ■ LEVOTHYROXINE
- ■ MEDROXYPROGESTERONE
- ■ METHADONE
- ■ METRONIDAZOLE
- ■ QUINIDINE
- ■ PAROXETINE
- ■ PHENOTHIAZINES
- ■ PRAZIQUANTEL
- ■ PROGESTINS
- ■ THEOPHYLLINE
- ■ TOPIRAMATE
- ■ TRICYCLIC ANTIDEPRESSANTS
- ■ VALPROIC ACID (may also increase risk for phenobarbital toxicity)
- ■ VERAPAMIL
- ■ WARFARIN

Laboratory Considerations

- ■ Barbiturates may cause increased retention of **bromosulfophthalein** (BSP; sulfobromophthalein) and give falsely elevated results. It is recommended that barbiturates not be administered within the 24 hours before BSP retention tests; or, if they must, (*e.g.*, for seizure control) the results be interpreted accordingly.

- ■ Phenobarbital can alter **thyroid** testing. Decreased total and free T4, normal T3, and either normal or increased TSH have been reported. It has been suggested to wait at least 4 weeks after discontinuing phenobarbital to perform thyroid testing.

- ■ In some dogs, phenobarbital may cause a false positive low dose **dexamethasone suppression test**, by increasing the clearance of dexamethasone. Phenobarbital apparently has no effect either on ACTH stimulation tests or on the hormonal equilibrium of the adrenal axis. As phenobarbital can potentially increase the metabolism of cortisol, it has been implicated in contributing to relative adrenal insufficiency.

Doses

- ■ **DOGS:**

    For treatment of idiopathic epilepsy:

    a) Initial oral dose is 2–2.5 mg/kg PO q12h. Serum phenobarbital concentrations should be monitored 2-3 weeks after initiating therapy and after any dosage adjustment. Therapeutic serum concentrations of 20-35 micrograms/mL are recommended in dogs, with the decrease in the high end of the range reflecting

suggested changes to minimize the potential for hepatotoxicity. (Munana 2010)

b) Initial maintenance dose: 2.5–3 mg/kg PO q12h. A CBC, serum biochemical evaluation and urinalysis should be performed before starting maintenance anticonvulsant therapy, both as part of the diagnostic evaluation and as a baseline before starting therapy. (Mariani 2010)

c) Initial oral dose: 2.5 mg/kg PO twice daily; to reach therapeutic levels faster may give an IV loading dose of 20 mg/kg. Adjust dosage based upon therapeutic levels, efficacy, and adverse effects. (Podell 2000)

d) Loading dose of 16–20 mg/kg once IV; maintenance dose of 2–5 mg/kg PO q12h. (Knipe 2006; Knipe 2009)

e) Begin at 3.5 mg/kg PO twice daily. Monitor at 2 to 4 weeks and 3 months later to detect induction. If response is insufficient, increase dose sufficiently to increase trough level by 3 to 5 micrograms/mL increments, rechecking at 2 to 4 weeks after each dose increase. Monitor at 3 to 12 month intervals once steady–state is achieved. As concentrations approach 30 micrograms/mL, begin monitoring hepatic function test (bile acids, albumin, BUN, chol). As concentrations approach 35 micrograms/mL, consider adding an additional drug. Avoid any other drug metabolized by the liver. Consider hepatoprotectant drugs if liver dysfunction is of concern. (Axlund 2004)

For treatment of status epilepticus:

a) If seizures persist after diazepam therapy (2 or more seizures recur; or gross motor activity persists) give phenobarbital bolus of 2–5 mg/kg (can be repeated at 20 minute intervals, up to two times). Add phenobarb to diazepam infusion at a rate of 2–10 mg/hour. If seizures are sustained or high frequency seizures recur, consider pentobarbital coma. (Quesnel 2000)

b) After using benzodiazepines (diazepam, midazolam), phenobarbital at 5–8 mg/kg IV; continue to administer every 4-6 hours until seizures are under control regardless of additional therapy. (Knipe 2009)

For sialadenosis:

a) From a case report of sialadenosis after removal of an esophageal body: 1 mg/kg PO q12h. After 3 months, dog was slowly weaned off phenobarbital. (Gilor *et al.* 2010)

For sedation:

a) 2.2–6.6 mg/kg PO twice daily (Walton 1986)

b) Treatment of irritable bowel syndrome: 2.2 mg/kg PO twice daily (Morgan 1988)

c) For adjunctive treatment of compulsive behaviors: 2–20 mg/kg q12–24h (Line 2000)

■ **CATS:**

Treatment of idiopathic epilepsy:

a) Initial oral dose is 2–2.5 mg/kg PO q12h. Serum phenobarbital concentrations should be monitored 2-3 weeks after initiating therapy and after any dosage adjustment. Optimum therapeutic levels of 23-30 micrograms/mL has been recommended in cats, in an attempt to maximize seizure control with the lowest potential for side effects. (Munana 2010)

b) For status epilepticus: If seizures persist after diazepam therapy (2 or more seizures recur; or gross motor activity persists) give phenobarbital bolus of 2–5 mg/kg (can be repeated at 20 minute intervals, up to two times). Add phenobarb to diazepam infusion at a rate of 2–10 mg/hour. If seizures are sustained or high frequency seizures recur, consider pentobarbital coma.

For oral maintenance therapy: 1–2 mg/kg PO every 12 hours; adjust dosages based upon serum levels (Shell 2000)

c) Loading dose of 16–20 mg/kg once IV; maintenance dose of 1–5 mg/kg PO q12h. (Knipe 2006), (Knipe 2009)

d) Starting dose is 1–2 mg/kg (usually 3.25–15 mg/cat) PO q12h. Measure trough serum levels 2–3 weeks after initiating therapy and after each dosage change. In the cat, therapeutic levels are likely 50–100 mcmol/L (lower than those in dogs). If seizure control is good, but levels are subtherapeutic, dose does not need to be increased. Measure phenobarbital levels, CBC and serum chemistries every 6 months. (Cochrane 2007)

e) Initial maintenance dose: 2.5–3 mg/kg PO q12h. A CBC, serum biochemical evaluation and urinalysis should be performed before starting maintenance anticonvulsant therapy, both as part of the diagnostic evaluation and as a baseline before starting therapy. (Mariani 2010)

f) Emergency seizure control involves intravenous diazepam (0.5 mg/kg up to three doses), along with phenobarbital 3 mg/kg IV. Phenobarbital may be repeated every 20 minutes up to 24 mg/kg in a 24-hour period, or it can be given as a "loading" of 10 mg/kg IV bolus. (Abramson 2009)

Sedation; for controlling excessive feline vocalization for situational distress (*e.g.*, riding in automobiles):

a) 2–3 mg/kg PO as needed (Overall 2000)

■ **FERRETS:**

a) 1–2 mg/kg PO 2–3 times daily (Williams 2000)

b) Loading dose of 16–20 mg/kg once IV; maintenance dose of 1–2 mg/kg PO q8–12h. (Knipe 2006), (Knipe 2009)

■ **CATTLE:**

For enzyme induction in organochlorine toxicity:

a) 5 grams PO for 3–4 weeks, off 3–4 weeks, then repeat for 3–4 more weeks (Smith 1986)

■ **HORSES: (Note:** ARCI UCGFS Class 2 Drug)

a) Loading dose of 12 mg/kg IV over 20 minutes, then 6.65 mg/kg IV over 20 minutes every 12 hours (Duran *et al.* 1987)

b) Adult horses: Loading dose of 16–20 mg/kg once IV; maintenance dose of 1–5 mg/kg PO twice daily.

Foals: Loading dose of 16–20 mg/kg once IV; maintenance dose of 100–500 mg (total dose) PO twice daily. (Knipe 2006), (Knipe 2009)

c) Foals for seizures: 20 mg/kg diluted with normal saline to a volume of 30–35 mL infused over 25–30 minutes IV, then 9 mg/kg diluted and infused as above q8h. Recommend monitoring serum levels if possible. (Spehar *et al.* 1984)

Monitoring

■ Anticonvulsant (or sedative) efficacy

■ Adverse effects (CNS related, PU/PD, weight gain)

■ Serum phenobarbital levels if lack of efficacy or adverse reactions noted. Some recommend that all dogs have their phenobarbital level monitored once or twice a year and cats monitored every 6 months. Although there is some disagreement among clinicians, therapeutic serum levels in dogs (15–45 micrograms/mL; 65-194 mcmol/L) are thought to be similar to those in humans. Optimum therapeutic levels of 23-30 micrograms/mL has been recommended in cats, in an attempt to maximize seizure control with the lowest potential for side effects. Similarly, serum levels of 20-35 micrograms/mL are recommended in the dog, with the decrease in the high end of the range reflecting suggested changes to minimize the potential for hepatotoxicity (Munana 2010). Animals on bromides and phenobarbital may require lower serum levels for seizure control. If phenobarbital was not "loaded", wait at least 5–6 half-lives (approximately 12–14 days in dogs and 9–10 days in cats) before measuring serum concentrations; time of sampling does not appear to be significant

■ If used chronically, routine CBC's, liver enzymes (especially ALT and AST), and bilirubin at least every 6 months.

Client Information

■ For successful epilepsy treatment compliance with prescribed therapy must be stressed. Encourage client to give doses at the same time each day.

■ Keep medications out of reach of children and stored in child-resistant packaging.

■ Veterinarian should be contacted if animal develops significant adverse reactions (including clinical signs of anemia and/or liver disease) or seizure control is unacceptable.

Chemistry/Synonyms

Phenobarbital, a barbiturate, occurs as white, glistening, odorless, small crystals or a white, crystalline powder with a melting point of 174°–178°C and a pK_a of 7.41. One gram is soluble in approximately 1000 mL of water; 10 mL of alcohol. Compared to other barbiturates it has a low-lipid solubility.

Phenobarbital sodium occurs as bitter-tasting, white, odorless, flaky crystals or crystalline granules or powder. It is very soluble in water, soluble in alcohol, and freely soluble in propylene glycol. The injectable product has a pH of 8.5–10.5.

SI units (mcmol/L) are multiplied by 0.232 to convert phenobarbital levels to conventional units (micrograms/mL).

Phenobarbital may also be known as fenobarbital, phenemalum, phenobarbitalum, phenobarbitone, phenylethylbarbituric acid, or phenylethylmalonylurea, *Luminal Sodium®* and *Solfoton®*.

Storage/Stability

Phenobarbital tablets should be stored in tight, light-resistant containers at room temperature (15–30°C); protect from moisture.

Phenobarbital elixir should be stored in tight containers at 20–20°C.

Phenobarbital sodium injection should be stored at room temperature (15–30°C).

Aqueous solutions of phenobarbital are not very stable. Propylene glycol is often used in injectable products to help stabilize the solution. Solutions of phenobarbital sodium should not be added to acidic solutions nor used if they contain a precipitate or are grossly discolored.

Compatibility/Compounding Considerations

The following solutions and drugs have been reported to be physically **compatible** with phenobarbital sodium: Dextrose IV solutions, Ringer's injection, lactated Ringer's injection, Saline IV solutions, dextrose-saline combinations, dextrose-Ringer's combinations, dextrose-Ringer's lactate combinations, amikacin sulfate, aminophylline, atropine sulfate (stable for at least 15 minutes, but not 24 hours), calcium chloride and gluconate, dimenhydrinate, polymyxin B sulfate, sodium bicarbonate, thiopental sodium, and verapamil HCl.

The following drugs have been reported to be physically **incompatible** with phenobarbital sodium: chlorpromazine HCl, codeine phosphate, ephedrine sulfate, fentanyl citrate, glycopyrrolate, hydralazine HCl, hydrocortisone sodium succinate, hydroxyzine HCl, insulin (regular), meperidine HCl, morphine sulfate, nalbuphine HCl, norepinephrine bitartrate, oxytetracycline HCl, pentazocine lactate, procaine HCl, prochlorperazine edisylate, promazine HCl, and promethazine HCl. Compatibility is dependent upon factors such as pH, concentration, temperature, and diluent used; consult specialized references or a hospital pharmacist for more specific information.

Dosage Forms/Regulatory Status

VETERINARY-LABELED PRODUCTS: None

The ARCI (Racing Commissioners International) has designated this drug as a class 2 substance. See the appendix for more information.

HUMAN-LABELED PRODUCTS:

Phenobarbital Tablets: 15 mg, 16 mg (tablets & capsules), 30 mg, 60 mg, 90 mg, & 100 mg; *Solfoton®* (ECR Pharm); generic; (Rx, C-IV)

Phenobarbital Elixir: 15 mg/5mL in pt & UD 5 mL, 10 mL & 20 mL; 20 mg/5mL in pt, gal, UD 5 mL & 7.5 mL; generic; (Rx, C-IV)

Phenobarbital Sodium Injection: 30 mg/mL, 60 mg/mL, 65 mg/mL, & 130 mg/mL in 1 mL *Tubex, Carpujects* & vials; *Luminal Sodium®* (Hospira); generic; (Rx; C-IV)

References

Abramson, C.J. (2009). Feline Neurology I. Proceedings: WVC. Accessed via: Veterinary Information Network. http://goo.gl/eWXb1

Axlund, T. (2004). Managing the seizuring dog: Phenobarbital and beyond. Proceedings: ACVC. Accessed via: Veterinary Information Network. http://goo.gl/H5D7K

Boothe, D.M. (2005). New information on nonsteroidal antiinflammatories: What every criticalist must know. Proceedings: IVECC. Accessed via: Veterinary Information Network. http://goo.gl/xUukK

Cochrane, S. (2007). Update on seizures in the dog and cat. Proceedings: WSAVA World Congress. Accessed via: Veterinary Information Network. http://goo.gl/9BB75

Duran, S.H., W.R. Ravis, et al. (1987). Pharmacokinetics of phenobarbital in the horse. *Am Jnl Vet Res* **48**(5): 807–810.

Gilor, C., S. Gilor, et al. (2010). Phenobarbital-Responsive Sialadenosis Associated With an Esophageal Foreign Body in a Dog. *Journal of the American Animal Hospital Association* **46**(2): 115–120.

Knipe, M. (2006). The essential guide to seizures. Proceedings: Vet Neuro Symposium. Accessed via: Veterinary Information Network. http://goo.gl/mhSI5

Knipe, M. (2009). The short and long of seizure management. Proceedings: UCD Veterinary Neurology Symposium. Accessed via: Veterinary Information Network. http://goo.gl/N66kW

Line, S. (2000). Sensory Mutilation and Related Behavior Syndromes. *Kirk's Current Veterinary Therapy: XIII Small Animal Practice*. J Bonagura Ed. Philadelphia, WB Saunders: 90–93.

Mariani, C. (2010). Maintenance therapy for the routine & difficult to control epileptic patient. Proceedings: ACVIM Forum. Accessed via: Veterinary Information Network. http://goo.gl/quX8P

Moore, S., K. Munana, et al. (2009). The Pharmacokinetics

of Levetiracetam in Dogs Concurrently Receiving Phenobarbital. Proceedings: ACVIM. Accessed via: Veterinary Information Network. http://goo.gl/McGT7

Morgan, R.V., Ed. (1988). *Handbook of Small Animal Practice.* New York, Churchill Livingstone.

Munana, K. (2010). Current Approaches to Seizure Management. Proceedings: ACVIM Forum. Accessed via: Veterinary Information Network. http://goo.gl/vl8Lp

Overall, K. (2000). Behavioral Pharmacology. Proceedings: American Animal Hospital Association 67th Annual Meeting, Toronto.

Papich, M. (1989). Effects of drugs on pregnancy. *Current Veterinary Therapy X: Small Animal Practice.* R Kirk Ed. Philadelphia, Saunders: 1291–1299.

Podell, M. (2000). Seizure management in dogs. *Kirk's Current Veterinary Therapy: XIII Small Animal Practice.* J Bonagura Ed. Philadelphia, WB Saunders: 959–963.

Quesnel, A. (2000). Seizures. *Textbook of Veterinary Internal Medicine: Diseases of the Dog and Cat.* S Ettinger and E Feldman Eds. Philadelphia, WB Saunders. **1:** 148–152.

Shell, L. (2000). Feline Seizure Disorders. *Kirk's Current Veterinary Therapy: XIII Small Animal Practice.* J Bonagura Ed. Philadelphia, WB Saunders: 963–966.

Smith, J.A. (1986). Toxic encephalopathies in cattle. *Current Veterinary Therapy 2: Food Animal Practice.* JL Howard Ed. Philadelphia, WB Saunders: 855–863.

Spehar, A.M., M.R. Hill, et al. (1984). Preliminary Study on the pharmacokinetics of phenobarbital in the neonatal foal. *Eq Vet Jnl* **16**(4): 368–371.

Williams, B. (2000). Therapeutics in Ferrets. *Vet Clin NA: Exotic Anim Pract* **3:1**(Jan): 131–153.

PHENOXYBENZAMINE HCL

(fen-ox-ee-*ben*-za-meen)   Dibenzyline®

ALPHA-ADRENERGIC BLOCKER

Prescriber Highlights

▶ Alpha-adrenergic blocker used in small animals: detrusor areflexia, pheochromocytoma (hypertension); horses: laminitis or diarrhea

▶ Contraindications: When hypotension would be deleterious; possibly glaucoma or diabetes mellitus, horses with clinical signs of colic. Caution: CHF or other heart disease, renal damage, or cerebral/coronary arteriosclerosis

▶ Adverse Effects: Hypotension, hypertension (rebound), miosis, increased intraocular pressure, tachycardia, inhibition of ejaculation, nasal congestion, weakness/dizziness, and GI effects (e.g., nausea, vomiting). Constipation may occur in horses.

▶ May need to be obtained from compounding pharmacy

▶ Drug Interactions

Uses/Indications

Phenoxybenzamine is used in small animals primarily for its effect in reducing internal urethral sphincter tone in dogs and cats when urethral sphincter hypertonus is present. It can also be used to treat the hypertension associated with pheochromocytoma prior to surgery or as adjunctive therapy in endotoxicosis.

Phenoxybenzamine has been reported to increase the effectiveness of acupuncture.

In horses, phenoxybenzamine has been used for preventing or treating laminitis in its early stages and to treat secretory diarrheas.

Pharmacology/Actions

Alpha-adrenergic response to circulating epinephrine or norepinephrine is noncompetitively blocked by phenoxybenzamine. The effect of phenoxybenzamine has been described as a "chemical sympathectomy." No effects on beta-adrenergic receptors or on the parasympathetic nervous system occur.

Phenoxybenzamine causes cutaneous blood flow to increase, but little effects are noted on skeletal or cerebral blood flow. Phenoxybenzamine can also block pupillary dilation, lid retraction, and nictitating membrane contraction. Both standing and supine blood pressures are decreased in humans.

Pharmacokinetics

No information was located on the pharmacokinetics of this agent in veterinary species. In humans, phenoxybenzamine is variably absorbed from the GI, with a bioavailability of 20–30%. Onset of action of the drug is slow (several hours) and increases over several days after regular dosing. Effects persist for 3–4 days after discontinuation of the drug.

Phenoxybenzamine is highly lipid soluble and may accumulate in body fat. It is unknown if it crosses the placenta or is excreted into milk. The serum half-life is approximately 24 hours in humans. It is metabolized (dealkylated) and excreted in both the urine and bile.

Contraindications/Precautions/Warnings

Phenoxybenzamine is contraindicated in horses with clinical signs of colic and in patients when hypotension would be undesirable (*e.g.*, shock, unless fluid replacement is adequate). One author (Labato 1988) lists glaucoma and diabetes mellitus as contraindications for the use of phenoxybenzamine in dogs.

Phenoxybenzamine should be used with caution in patients with CHF or other heart disease as drug-induced tachycardia can occur. It should be used cautiously in patients with renal damage or cerebral/coronary arteriosclerosis.

Adverse Effects

Adverse effects associated with alpha-adrenergic blockade include: hypotension, hypertension, miosis, increased intraocular pressure, tachycardia, sodium retention, inhibition of ejaculation, and nasal congestion. Additionally, it can cause weakness/dizziness and GI effects (*e.g.*, nausea, vomiting). Constipation may occur in horses.

Reproductive/Nursing Safety

Phenoxybenzamine has been shown to cause abnormalities in the closure of the patent ductus in guinea pigs. In humans, the FDA categorizes this drug as category *C* for use during pregnancy (*Animal studies have shown an adverse effect on the fetus, but there are no adequate studies in humans; or there are no animal reproduction studies and no adequate studies in humans.*)

It is unknown if phenoxybenzamine is excreted into milk.

Overdosage/Acute Toxicity

Overdosage of phenoxybenzamine may yield signs of postural hypotension (dizziness, syncope), tachycardia, vomiting, lethargy, or shock.

Treatment should consist of emptying the gut if the ingestion was recent and there are no contraindications to those procedures. Hypotension can be treated with fluid support. Epinephrine is contraindicated (see Drug Interactions) and most vasopressor drugs are ineffective in reversing the effects of alpha-blockade. Intravenous norepinephrine (levarterenol) may be beneficial, however, if clinical signs are severe.

Drug Interactions

The following drug interactions have either been reported or are theoretical in humans or animals receiving phenoxybenzamine and may be of significance in veterinary patients:

■ **EPINEPHRINE:** If used with drugs that have both alpha- and beta-adrenergic effects increased hypotension, vasodilatation or tachycardia may result

■ **PHENYLEPHRINE:** Phenoxybenzamine will antagonize the effects of alpha-adrenergic sympathomimetic agents

■ **RESERPINE:** Phenoxybenzamine can antagonize the hypothermic effects of reserpine

Doses

■ **DOGS:**

To treat functional urethral obstruction by decreasing sympathetic-mediated urethral tone:

a) 0.25 mg/kg PO q12-24h *or* 2.5-20 mg (total dose) PO q12-24h (Lane 2000)

b) 0.25 mg/kg PO q12h (Lulich 2004)

c) 0.25-0.5 mg/kg PO once or twice daily (Coates 2004)

d) 5-15 mg (total dose) PO q12h (Bartges 2003)

Treatment of hypertension associated with pheochromocytoma:

a) To minimize perioperative complications prior to surgical removal of tumor: Initially 0.5 mg/kg PO twice daily and gradually increase dosage every few days until clinical signs of hypotension (*e.g.*, lethargy, weakness, syncope), adverse drug reactions (*e.g.*, vomiting) or a maximum dosage of 2.5 mg/kg PO twice daily is attained. Surgery is recommended 1-2 weeks later. Continue phenoxybenzamine until the time of surgery. Close monitoring of the dog during the peri-

operative period is critical for a successful outcome. (Nelson 2008)

b) Initial dose is 0.25 mg/kg PO twice daily, dose is then gradually increased every few days until signs of hypotension or adverse drug reaction occur or a maximum dosage of 2.5 mg/kg twice a day is attained. In cases in where adrenalectomy is not an option, phenoxybenzamine should be used long-term to control blood pressure. Additional beta-blockers may be necessary in patients with severe tachycardia, but should not be given without prior alpha-blockade to avoid severe hypertension. (Reusch, C. 2006), (Reusch, C.E. *et al.* 2010)

For adjunctive treatment of endotoxicosis with appropriate antimicrobial agents, steroids (if indicated), and other supportive care:

a) 0.25-0.5 mg/kg PO q6h (Coppock & Mostrom 1986)

■ **CATS:**

To treat functional urethral obstruction by decreasing sympathetic-mediated urethral tone:

a) 2.5-7.5 mg/cat PO once to twice daily (Osborne *et al.* 2000)

b) 1.25-7.5 mg (total dose) PO q12-24h (Lane 2000)

c) 2.5-10 mg (total dose) PO q24h (Bartges 2003)

For short-term treatment of hypertension:

a) 0.5 mg/kg q12h (Sparkes 2003)

b) 2.5 mg (total dose) q12h increasing by 2.5 mg up to a maximum of 10 mg (total dose) q12h PO (Brovido 2002)

c) 2.5-7.5 mg per cat q8-12h (Waddell 2005)

■ **HORSES:** (**Note:** ARCI UCGFS Class 3 Drug)

a) To decrease urethral sphincter tone in horses with bladder paresis: 0.7 mg/kg PO 4 times a day (in combination with bethanechol at 0.25-0.75 mg/kg PO 2-4 times a day) (Schott II & Carr 2003)

b) For adjunctive treatment of laminitis (developmental phase): 1 mg/kg IV q12h for 2 doses (Brumbaugh *et al.* 1999)

c) For treatment of profuse, watery diarrhea: 200-600 mg q12h (Clark 1988)

Monitoring

■ Clinical efficacy (adequate urination, etc.)

■ Efficacy for urinary problems may take a week or longer and the drug should be given for several weeks before determining it is not effective

■ Blood pressure, if necessary/possible

Client Information

■ Contact veterinarian if animal has continuing problems with weakness, appears dizzy, collapses after standing, or has persistent vomiting. GI upset may be reduced if the drug is given with meals.

Chemistry/Synonyms

An alpha-adrenergic blocking agent, phenoxybenzamine HCl occurs as an odorless, white crystalline powder with a melting range of 136°–141° and a pK_a of 4.4. Approximately 40 mg are soluble in 1 mL of water and 167 mg are soluble in 1 mL of alcohol.

Phenoxybenzamine may also be known as: SKF-688A, *Dibenyline®, Dibenzyran®,* or *Fenoxene®.*

Storage/Stability

Phenoxybenzamine capsules should be stored at room temperature in well-closed containers.

Dosage Forms/Regulatory Status

VETERINARY-LABELED PRODUCTS: None

The ARCI (Racing Commissioners International) has designated this drug as a class 3 substance. See the appendix for more information.

HUMAN-LABELED PRODUCTS:

Phenoxybenzamine HCl Capsules: 10 mg; *Dibenzyline®* (Wellspring); (Rx)

References

Bartges, J. (2003). Canine lower urinary tract cases. Proceedings: ACVIM Forum. Accessed via: Veterinary Information Network. http://goo.gl/HH41u

Brovido, C. (2002). Hypertension in renal diseases and failure. The practical aspect. Proc: World Small Animal Association.

Brumbaugh, G., H. Lopez, et al. (1999). The pharmacologic basis for the treatment of laminitis. *The Veterinary Clinics of North America: Equine Practice* **15:**2(August).

Clark, D.R. (1988). Treatment of Circulatory Shock. *Veterinary Pharmacology and Therapeutics, 6th Ed.* NH Booth and LE McDonald Eds. Ames, Iowa State University Press: 563– 570.

Coates, J. (2004). Neurogenic micturition disorders. Proceedings: ACVIM Forum. Accessed via: Veterinary Information Network. http://goo.gl/260CO

Coppock, R.W. & M.S. Mostrom (1986). Intoxication Due to Contaminated Garbage, Food, and Water. *Current Veterinary Therapy IX: Small Animal Practice.* K R.W. Ed. Philadelphia, W.B. Saunders: 221–225.

Lane, I. (2000). Urinary Obstruction and Functional Urine Retention. *Textbook of Veterinary Internal Medicine: Diseases of the Dog and Cat.* S Ettinger and E Feldman Eds. Philadelphia, WB Saunders. **1:** 93–96.

Lulich, J. (2004). Managing functional urethral obstruction. Proceedings: ACVIM Forum. Accessed via: Veterinary Information Network. http://goo.gl/acf8d

Nelson, R. (2008). Unusual Endocrine Disorders. Proceedings: WVC. Accessed via: Veterinary Information Network. http://goo.gl/lII3J

Osborne, C., J. Kruger, et al. (2000). Feline Lower Urinary Tract Diseases. *Textbook of Veterinary Internal Medicine: Diseases of the Dog and Cat.* S Ettinger and E Feldman Eds. Philadelphia, WB Saunders. **2:** 1710–1747.

Reusch, C. (2006). Adrenal tumors in dogs. Proceedings: WSAVA World Congress. Accessed via: Veterinary Information Network. http://goo.gl/dY7Cm

Reusch, C.E., S. Schellenberg, et al. (2010). Endocrine Hypertension in Small Animals. *Veterinary Clinics of North America-Small Animal Practice* **40**(2): 335–+.

Schott II, H. & E. Carr (2003). Urinary incontinence in horses. Proceedings: ACVIM Forum. Accessed via: Veterinary Information Network. http://goo.gl/q7Uo2

Sparkes, A. (2003). Feline systemic hypertension-A hidden killer. Proceedings: World Small Animal Veterinary Assoc. Accessed via: Veterinary Information Network. http://goo.gl/QgVkr

Waddell, L. (2005). Feline Hypertension. Proceedings: IVECCS. Accessed via: Veterinary Information Network. http://goo.gl/BbBEi

PHENYLBUTAZONE

(fen-ill-*byoo*-ta-zone)   Butazolidin®, "Bute"

NON-STEROIDAL ANTIINFLAMMATORY AGENT

Prescriber Highlights

▶ NSAID used primarily in horses; little reason to use in dogs today

▶ Contraindications: Known hypersensitivity, history or preexisting hematologic or bone marrow abnormalities, preexisting GI ulcers, food producing animals

▶ Caution: Foals or ponies, preexisting renal disease, CHF, other drug allergies

▶ Adverse Effects: *Horses:* Oral & GI erosions & ulcers, hypoalbuminemia, diarrhea, anorexia, & renal effects. *Dogs:* GI ulceration, sodium & water retention, diminished renal blood flow, blood dyscrasias.

▶ Do not give IM or SC; IA injections may cause seizures

▶ Drug Interactions; lab interactions

Uses/Indications

One manufacturer lists the following as the indications for phenylbutazone: "For the relief of inflammatory conditions associated with the musculoskeletal system in dogs and horses." (Package Insert; *Butazolidin®*—Coopers). It has been used primarily for the treatment of lameness in horses and, occasionally, as an analgesic/ antiinflammatory, antipyretic in dogs, cattle, and swine.

Pharmacology/Actions

Phenylbutazone has analgesic, antiinflammatory, antipyretic, and mild uricosuric properties. The proposed mechanism of action is by the inhibition of cyclooxygenase, thereby reducing prostaglandin synthesis. Other pharmacologic actions phenylbutazone may induce include reduced renal blood flow and decreased glomerular filtration rate, decreased platelet aggregation, and gastric mucosal damage.

Pharmacokinetics

Following oral administration, phenylbutazone is absorbed from both the stomach and small intestine. The drug is distributed throughout the body with highest levels attained in the liver, heart, lungs, kidneys, and blood. Plasma protein binding in horses exceeds 99%. Both phenylbutazone and oxyphenbutazone cross the placenta and are excreted into milk.

The serum half-life in the horse ranges from 3.5–6 hours, and like aspirin is dose-dependent. Therapeutic efficacy, however, may last for more than 24 hours, probably due to the irreversible binding of phenylbutazone to cyclooxygenase. In horses and other species, phenylbutazone is nearly completely metabolized, primarily to oxphenbutazone (active) and gamma-hydroxyphenylbutazone. Oxyphenbutazone has been detected in horse urine up to 48 hours after a single dose. Phenylbutazone is more rapidly excreted into alkaline than acidic urine.

Other serum half-lives reported for animals are: Cattle ≈ 40–55 hrs; Dogs ≈ 2.5–6 hrs; Swine ≈ 2–6 hrs.; Rabbits ≈ 3 hrs.

Contraindications/Precautions/Warnings

Phenylbutazone is contraindicated in patients with a history of or preexisting hematologic or bone marrow abnormalities, preexisting GI ulcers, and in food producing animals or lactating dairy cattle. Cautious use in both foals and ponies is recommended because of increased incidences of hypoproteinemia and GI ulceration. Foals with a heavy parasite burden or that are undernourished may be more susceptible to developing adverse effects.

In horses with known or suspected EGUS, use should be avoided; single doses of phenylbutazone will probably not result in catastrophic consequences, but repeated doses can exacerbate gastric ulcers (Videla & Andrews 2009).

Phenylbutazone may cause decreased renal blood flow and sodium and water retention, and should be used cautiously in animals with preexisting renal disease or CHF.

Because phenylbutazone may mask clinical signs of lameness in horses for several days following therapy, unethical individuals may use it to disguise lameness for "soundness" exams. States may have different standards regarding the use of phenylbutazone in track animals. Complete elimination of phenylbutazone in horses may take 2 months and it can be detected in the urine for at least 7 days following administration. Phenylbutazone is contraindicated in patients demonstrating previous hypersensitivity reactions to it, and should be used very cautiously in patients with a history of allergies to other drugs.

Do not administer injectable preparation IM or SC as it is very irritating (swelling, to necrosis and sloughing). Intracarotid injections may cause CNS stimulation and seizures.

Adverse Effects

While phenylbutazone is apparently a safer drug to use in horses and dogs than in people, serious adverse reactions can still occur. Toxic effects that have been reported in horses include oral and GI erosions and ulcers, hypoalbuminemia, diarrhea, anorexia, and renal effects (azotemia, renal papillary necrosis). Unlike humans, it does not appear that phenylbutazone causes much

sodium and water retention in horses at usual doses, but edema has been reported. In dogs, however, phenylbutazone may cause sodium and water retention, and diminished renal blood flow. Phenylbutazone-induced blood dyscrasias and hepatotoxicity have also been reported in dogs.

Although gastric ulceration is frequently observed in adult horses and foals, evidence of an association between this disease and administration of NSAIDs such as phenylbutazone or flunixin at recommended dosages is lacking. On the basis of current evidence, prophylactic anti-ulcer medications for horses receiving therapeutic doses of NSAIDs is probably unnecessary in patients that are otherwise at low risk for gastric ulceration (Fennell & Franklin 2009).

The primary concerns with phenylbutazone therapy in humans include its bone marrow effects (agranulocytosis, aplastic anemia), renal and cardiovascular effects (fluid retention to acute renal failure), and GI effects (dyspepsia to perforated ulcers). Other serious concerns with phenylbutazone include hypersensitivity reactions, neurologic, dermatologic, and hepatic toxicities.

IM or SC injection can cause swelling, necrosis and sloughing. Intracarotid injections may cause CNS stimulation and seizures.

Therapy should be halted at first signs of any toxic reactions (e.g., anorexia, oral lesions, depression, reduced plasma proteins, increased serum creatinine or BUN, leukopenia, or anemias). The use of sucralfate or the H_2 blockers (cimetidine, ranitidine) have been suggested for use in treating the GI effects. Misoprostol, a prostaglandin E analog, may also be useful in reducing the gastrointestinal effects of phenylbutazone.

Reproductive/Nursing Safety

Although phenylbutazone has shown no direct teratogenic effects, rodent studies have demonstrated reduced litter sizes, increased neonatal mortality, and increased stillbirth rates. Phenylbutazone should, therefore, be used in pregnancy only when the potential benefits of therapy outweigh the risks associated with it.

In a system evaluating the safety of drugs in canine and feline pregnancy (Papich 1989), this drug is categorized as class: *C* (*These drugs may have potential risks. Studies in people or laboratory animals have uncovered risks, and these drugs should be used cautiously as a last resort when the benefit of therapy clearly outweighs the risks.*)

The safety of phenylbutazone during nursing has not been determined; use with caution.

Overdosage/Acute Toxicity

Manifestations (human) of acute overdosage with phenylbutazone include a prompt respiratory or metabolic acidosis with compensatory hyperventilation, seizures, coma, and acute hypotensive crisis. In an acute overdose, clinical signs of renal failure (oliguric, with proteinuria and hematuria), liver injury (hepatomegaly and jaundice), bone marrow depression, and ulceration (and perforation) of the GI tract may develop. Other symptoms reported in humans include: nausea, vomiting, abdominal pain, diaphoresis, neurologic and psychiatric symptoms, edema, hypertension, respiratory depression, and cyanosis.

There were 27 exposures to phenylbutazone reported to the ASPCA Animal Poison Control Center (APCC) during 2008-2009. In these cases 24 were dogs with 10 showing clinical signs, and 2 were equines with 1 showing clinical signs. The remaining reported case consisted of 1 cat that did not show any clinical signs. Common findings in dogs recorded in decreasing frequency included ataxia, seizures, tachycardia, trembling, and tremors.

Most common clinical signs in dogs (per unpublished APCC data) are tremors, seizures, ataxia, vomiting, and tachypnea. Oral LD50 in dogs is 332mg/kg (per RTECS 1988). Most common clinical signs in horses (per unpublished APCC data) are colic, anorexia, and ataxia.

Standard overdose procedures should be followed (empty gut following oral ingestion, etc.). Supportive treatment should be instituted as necessary and intravenous diazepam used to help control seizures. Monitor fluid therapy carefully, as phenylbutazone may cause fluid retention.

Drug Interactions

The following drug interactions have either been reported or are theoretical in humans or animals receiving phenylbutazone and may be of significance in veterinary patients:

■ **FUROSEMIDE:** Phenylbutazone may antagonize the increased renal blood flow effects caused by furosemide

■ **HEPATOTOXIC DRUGS:** Phenylbutazone administered concurrently with hepatotoxic drugs may increase the chances of hepatotoxicity developing

■ **NSAIDS:** Concurrent use with other NSAIDs may increase the potential for adverse reactions, however, some clinicians routinely use phenylbutazone concomitantly with flunixin in horses. One study did not show synergistic actions with flunixin, but did however, when phenylbutazone and ketoprofen were "stacked".

■ **PENICILLAMINE:** May increase the risk of hematologic and/or renal adverse reactions

■ **PENICILLIN G:** Phenylbutazone may increase plasma half-life of penicillin G

■ **SULFONAMIDES:** Phenylbutazone could potentially displace sulfonamides from plasma proteins; increasing the risk for adverse effects

■ **WARFARIN:** Phenylbutazone could potentially displace warfarin from plasma proteins; increasing the risk for bleeding

Laboratory Considerations

■ Phenylbutazone and oxyphenbutazone may interfere with **thyroid function tests** by competing with thyroxine at protein binding sites or by inhibiting thyroid iodine uptake. Interpretation of thyroid function tests may be complicated.

Doses

■ **DOGS:**

Note: With the release of safer and FDA-approved NSAIDs, it is this author's (Plumb) opinion that there is little reason to use this agent today in dogs.

a) 14 mg/kg PO three times daily initially (maximum of 800 mg/day regardless of weight), titrate dose to lowest effective dose (Package Insert; *Butazolidin®*—Coopers)

b) 15–22 mg/kg PO q12h (Posner & Papich 2009)

c) For analgesia: 1–5 mg/kg PO q8h (Taylor 2003)

■ **CATTLE:**

Note: The Food and Drug Administration (FDA) has issued an order prohibiting the extralabel use of phenylbutazone animal and human drugs in female dairy cattle 20 months of age or older. In addition, many believe that phenylbutazone use in any food animal should be banned.

a) 4–8 mg/kg PO or 2–5 mg/kg IV (Howard 1986)

b) 10–20 mg/kg PO, then 2.5–5 mg/kg q24h or 10 mg/kg every 48 hours PO (Jenkins 1987)

■ **HORSES:**

a) To reduced pain or pyrexia associated with pleuropneumonia: 2.2–4.4 mg/kg PO or IV q12h. NSAIDs are commonly used for the first week of treatment or longer. (Sprayberry 2009)

b) 1–2 grams IV per 454 kg (1000 lb.) horse. Injection should be made slowly and with care. Limit IV administration to no more than 5 successive days of therapy. Follow with oral forms if necessary; or 2–4 grams PO per 454 kg (1000 lb.) horse. Do not exceed 4 grams/day. Use high end of dosage range initially, then titrate to lowest effective dose. (Package Insert; *Butazolidin®*—Coopers)

c) For adjunctive treatment of colic (to reduce endotoxic effects): 2.2 mg/kg twice daily (Moore 1999)

d) For adjunctive treatment of laminitis: Phenylbutazone appears to be the most effective NSAID for the treatment of acute laminitis and is given at an initial dose of 4 grams (for an average adult-sized horse) and is immediately decreased to 1 to 1.5 grams twice daily. This lower dose is used to keep the horse comfortable, but not relieve pain to the extent the horse moves around excessively and won't lie down. (O'Grady 2008)

e) For osteoarthritis: Phenylbutazone remains widely used; minimal dose is 2.2 mg/kg PO twice daily to control pain. (Laverty 2008)

■ **SWINE:**

a) 4 mg/kg IV or orally q24h (Koritz 1986)

b) 4–8 mg/kg PO or 2–5 mg/kg IV (Howard 1986)

Monitoring

■ Analgesic/antiinflammatory/antipyretic effect

■ Regular complete blood counts with chronic therapy (especially in dogs). The manufacturer recommends weekly CBC's early in therapy, and biweekly with chronic therapy

■ Urinalysis &/or renal function parameters (serum creatinine/BUN) with chronic therapy

■ Plasma protein determinations, especially in ponies, foals, and debilitated animals.

Client Information

■ Do not administer injectable preparation IM or SC.

■ FDA-approved for use in dogs and horses not intended for food.

■ The Food and Drug Administration (FDA) has issued an order prohibiting the extralabel use of phenylbutazone animal and human drugs in female dairy cattle 20 months of age or older.

■ While phenylbutazone is not FDA-approved for use in beef cattle, and its use is discouraged, it is used. A general guideline for meat withdrawal times are: one dose = 30 days, 2 doses = 35 days, and 3 doses = 40 days. Contact FARAD for more information.

Chemistry/Synonyms

A synthetic pyrazolone derivative related chemically to aminopyrine, phenylbutazone occurs as a white to off-white, odorless crystalline powder that has a pK_a of 4.5. It is very slightly soluble in water and 1 gram will dissolve in 28 mL of alcohol. It is tasteless at first, but has a slightly bitter after-taste.

Phenylbutazone may also be known as: butadiene, fenilbutazona, bute, phenylbutazonum, or phenylbute.

Storage/Stability

Oral products should be stored in tight, child-resistant containers if possible. The injectable product should be stored in a cool place (46–56° F) or kept refrigerated.

Dosage Forms/Regulatory Status

VETERINARY-LABELED PRODUCTS:

Note: The Food and Drug Administration (FDA) has issued an order prohibiting the extralabel use of phenylbutazone animal and human drugs in female dairy cattle 20 months of age or older.

Phenylbutazone Tablets: 100 mg & 200 mg; many trade name and generic products available. FDA-approved for use in dogs. (Rx)

Phenylbutazone Tablets: 1 gram; many trade name and generic products available. FDA-approved for use in horses. Not to be used in animals used for food. (Rx)

Phenylbutazone Oral Powder: 1 gram in 10 grams of powder to be mixed into feed. *Phenylbute®* Powder (Phoenix); (Rx). Labeled for use in horses.

Phenylbutazone Paste Oral Syringes: containing 6 grams or 12 grams/syringe: Many trade name and generic products available. FDA-approved for use in horses not intended for food purposes. (Rx)

Phenylbutazone Injection: 200 mg/mL in 100 mL vials: Many trade name and generic products available. FDA-approved for use in horses. Not to be used in horses intended for food. (Rx)

HUMAN APPROVED PRODUCTS: None

References

Fennell, L.C. & R.P. Franklin (2009). Do nonsteroidal antiinflammatory drugs administered at therapeutic dosages induce gastric ulcers in horses? *Equine Veterinary Education* 21(12): 660–662.

Howard, J.L., Ed. (1986). *Current Veterinary Therapy 2, Food Animal Practice*. Philadelphia, W.B. Saunders.

Jenkins, W.L. (1987). Pharmacologic aspects of analgesic drugs in animals: An overview. *JAVMA* 191(10): 1231–1240.

Koritz, G.D. (1986). Therapeutic management of inflammation. *Current Veterinary Therapy 2: Food Animal Practice*. JL Howard Ed. Philaldelphia, WB Saunders: 23–27.

Laverty, S. (2008). Equine Osteoarthritis: Are We Moving Forward With Our Diagnosis and Therapy? Proceedings: World Veterinary Congress. Accessed via: Veterinary Information Network. http://goo.gl/fnOSK

Moore, R. (1999). Medical treatment of abdominal pain in the horse: Analgesics and IV fluids. Proceedings: The North American Veterinary Conference, Orlando.

O'Grady, S. (2008). A Realistic Approach to Treating Acute Laminitis. Proceedings: WVC. Accessed via: Veterinary Information Network. http://goo.gl/Co52f

Papich, M. (1989). Effects of drugs on pregnancy. *Current Veterinary Therapy X: Small Animal Practice*. R Kirk Ed. Philadelphia, Saunders: 1291–1299.

Posner, L.P. & M.G. Papich (2009). Your patient is still in pain—Now what? "Rescue analgesia". Proceedings: WVC. Accessed via: Veterinary Information Network. http://goo.gl/WMON9

Sprayberry, K. (2009). Pleuropneumonia. *Compendium Equine*(May): 166–175.

Taylor, S. (2003). Joint disorders. *Small Animal Internal Medicine, 3rd Ed.* R Nelson and C Couto Eds. St Louis, Mosby: 1079–1096.

Videla, R. & F.M. Andrews (2009). New Perspectives in Equine Gastric Ulcer Syndrome. *Veterinary Clinics of North America-Equine Practice* 25(2): 283–+.

PHENYLEPHRINE HCL

(fen-ill-ef-rin)   Neo-Synephrine®

ALPHA-ADRENERGIC AGONIST

Prescriber Highlights

▶ Alpha-adrenergic used parenterally to treat hypotension without overt cardio-stimulation

▶ Contraindications: Severe hypertension, ventricular tachycardia, or hypersensitive to it. Extreme Caution: Geriatric patients, patients with hyperthyroidism, bradycardia, partial heart block, or other heart disease

▶ Not a replacement for adequate volume therapy in patients with shock

▶ Adverse Effects: Reflex bradycardia, CNS effects (excitement, restlessness, headache), & rarely, arrhythmias

▶ Blood pressure must be monitored

▶ Extravasation injuries with phenylephrine can be very serious

Uses/Indications

Phenylephrine has been used to treat hypotension and shock (after adequate volume replacement), but many clinicians prefer to use an agent that also has cardiostimulatory properties. Phenylephrine is recommended for use to treat hypotension secondary to drug overdoses or idiosyncratic hypotensive reactions to drugs such as phenothiazines, adrenergic blocking agents, and ganglionic blockers. Its use to treat hypotension resulting from barbiturate or other CNS depressant agents is controversial. Phenylephrine has been used to increase blood pressure to terminate attacks of paroxysmal supraventricular tachycardia, particularly when the patient is also hypotensive. Phenylephrine has been used to both treat hypotension and prolong the effects of spinal anesthesia.

Ophthalmic uses of phenylephrine include use for some diagnostic eye examinations, reducing posterior synechiae formation, and relieving pain associated with complicated uveitis. It has been applied intranasally in an attempt to reduce nasal congestion.

Pharmacology/Actions

Phenylephrine has predominantly post-synaptic alpha-adrenergic effects at therapeutic doses. At usual doses, it has negligible beta effects, but these can occur at high doses.

Phenylephrine's primary effects, when given intravenously, include peripheral vasoconstriction with resultant increases in diastolic and systolic blood pressures, small decreases in cardiac output, and an increase in circulation time. A reflex bradycardia (blocked by atropine) can occur. Most vascular beds are constricted (renal splanchnic, pulmonary, cutaneous), but coronary blood flow is increased. Its alpha effects can cause contraction of the pregnant uterus and constriction of uterine blood vessels.

Pharmacokinetics

After oral administration, phenylephrine is rapidly metabolized in the GI tract and cardiovascular effects are generally unattainable via this route of administration. Following IV administration, pressor effects begin almost immediately and will persist for up to 20 minutes. The onset of pressor action after IM administration is usually within 10−15 minutes, and will last for approximately one hour.

It is unknown if phenylephrine is excreted into milk. It is metabolized by the liver, and the effects of the drug are also terminated by uptake into tissues.

Contraindications/Precautions/Warnings

Phenylephrine is contraindicated in patients with severe hypertension, ventricular tachycardia or those who are hypersensitive to it. It should be used with extreme caution in geriatric patients, patients with hyperthyroidism, bradycardia, and partial heart block or with other heart disease. Phenylephrine is not a replacement for adequate volume therapy in patients with shock.

Adverse Effects

At usual doses, a reflex bradycardia, CNS effects (excitement, restlessness, headache) and, rarely, arrhythmias are seen. Blood pressure must be monitored to prevent hypertension.

Extravasation injuries with phenylephrine can be very serious (necrosis and sloughing of surrounding tissue). Patient's IV sites should be routinely monitored. Should extravasation occur, infiltrate the site (ischemic areas) with a solution of 5−10 mg phentolamine (Regitine®) in 10−15 mL of normal saline. A syringe with a fine needle should be used to infiltrate the site with many injections.

Reproductive/Nursing Safety

In humans, the FDA categorizes this drug as category C for use during pregnancy (Animal studies have shown an adverse effect on the fetus, but there are no adequate studies in humans; or there are no animal reproduction studies and no adequate studies in humans.)

It is not known if these agents are excreted in maternal milk; exercise caution when administering to a nursing patient.

Overdosage/Acute Toxicity

There were 195 exposures to phenylephrine reported to the ASPCA Animal Poison Control Center (APCC) during 2008−2009. In these cases 189 were dogs with 51 showing clinical signs, 5 were cats with 1 showing clinic signs and 1 was a bird that did not show any clinical signs. Common findings in dogs recorded in decreasing frequency included vomiting, lethargy, depression, hyperactivity, and tachycardia.

Overdosage of phenylephrine can cause hypertension, seizures, vomiting, paresthesias, ventricular extrasystoles, and cerebral hemorrhage, but the margin of safety with phenylephrine overdose is fairly wide, especially after oral administration. Vomiting is commonly seen with overdoses. CNS stimulation (agitation, hyperactivity, and muscle tremors) or cardiovascular changes, most commonly tachycardia and hypertension are also seen. Cardiovascular changes often respond well to fluids. Beta-blockers or nitroprusside may be indicated when signs are refractory to fluids.

Drug Interactions

The following drug interactions have either been reported or are theoretical in humans or animals receiving phenylephrine (systemically) and may be of significance in veterinary patients:

- **ALPHA-ADRENERGIC BLOCKERS (phentolamine, phenothiazines, phenoxybenzamine):** Higher dosages of phenylephrine may be required to attain a pressor effect if these agents have been used prior to therapy

- **ANESTHETICS, GENERAL (halogenated):** Phenylephrine potentially may induce cardiac arrhythmias when used with halothane anesthesia

- **ATROPINE (and other anticholinergics):** Block the reflex bradycardia caused by phenylephrine

- **BETA-ADRENERGIC BLOCKERS:** The cardiostimulatory effects of phenylephrine can be blocked

- **DIGOXIN:** Use with phenylephrine may cause increased myocardium sensitization

- **MONAMINE OXIDASE (MAO) INHIBITORS (e.g., amitraz, possibly selegiline):** Monoamine oxidase (MAO) inhibitors should not be used with phenylephrine because of a pronounced pressor effect

- **OXYTOCIN:** When used concurrently with oxytocic agents, pressor effects may be enhanced

- **SYMPATHOMIMETIC AGENTS (epinephrine):** Tachycardia and serious arrhythmias are possible

Doses

- **DOGS:**
  a) As a CRI: Low dose is 1 microgram/kg/min; high dose is 3 micrograms/kg/min. Increases peripheral vascular resistance and mean arterial blood pressure. May see reflex bradycardia, and vasoconstriction can lead to excessive decreases in blood flow to liver, GI tract, and kidneys, although coronary blood flow is increased. (Quandt 2009)
  b) As a constant rate infusion: 2–10 micrograms/kg/minute. Can be useful when the patient suffers profound vasodilation due to septic shock. (Ko 2009)

  c) As a vasopressor in catastrophic stages of hypovolemic shock: 1–3 micrograms/kg/min (Rudloff 2002)

- **CATS:**
  a) When it is advantageous to increase blood pressure by vasoconstriction, phenylephrine may be useful in patients with pronounced systemic vasodilation (*e.g.,* visceral inflammation) or to increase blood pressure when increasing myocardial contractility may be disadvantageous (*e.g.,* hypertrophic cardiomyopathy): 1–2 micrograms/kg/minute as a CRI. In this study, infusions of 1 microgram/kg/min significantly increased mean arterial pressure without a change in cardiac output. At 2 micrograms/kg/min, cardiac index also was increased with an increase in stroke volume index. (Pascoe *et al.* 2006)
  b) As a constant rate infusion: 2–10 micrograms/kg/minute. Can be useful when the patient suffers profound vasodilation due to septic shock. (Ko 2009)
  c) As a vasopressor in catastrophic stages of hypovolemic shock: 1–3 micrograms/kg/min (Rudloff 2002)
  d) As a CRI: Low dose is 1 microgram/kg/min; high dose is 3 micrograms/kg/min. Increases peripheral vascular resistance and mean arterial blood pressure. May see reflex bradycardia, and vasoconstriction can lead to excessive decreases in blood flow to liver, GI tract, and kidneys, although coronary blood flow is increased. (Quandt 2009)

- **HORSES: (Note:** ARCI UCGFS Class 3 Drug)
  a) 5 mg IV (Enos & Keiser 1985)

Monitoring

- Cardiac rate/rhythm
- Blood pressure, and blood gases if possible

Client Information

- Parenteral phenylephrine should only be used by professionals in a setting where adequate monitoring is possible

Chemistry/Synonyms

An alpha-adrenergic sympathomimetic amine, phenylephrine HCl occurs as bitter-tasting, odorless, white to nearly white crystals with a melting point of 145–146°C. It is freely soluble in water and alcohol. The pH of the commercially available injection is 3–6.5.

Phenylephrine may also be known as: fenilefrina, phenylephrinum, or m-synephrine, *AH-chew D®*, *Little Colds Decongestant for Infants & Children®*, *Lusonal®*, *Nasop®*, *Neo-Synephrine®*, *Sudogest PE®*, and *Sudafed PE®*.

Storage/Stability

The injectable product should be stored protected from light. Do not use solutions if they are brown or contain a precipitate. Oxidation of the drug can occur without a color change. To protect against oxidation, the air in commercially available ampules for injection is replaced with nitrogen and a sulfite added.

Compatibility/Compounding Considerations

Phenylephrine is reported to be physically **compatible** with all commonly used IV solutions and the following drugs: chloramphenicol sodium succinate, dobutamine HCl, lidocaine HCl, potassium chloride, and sodium bicarbonate. While stated to be physically **incompatible** with alkalis, it is stable with sodium bicarbonate solutions. Phenylephrine is reported to be **incompatible** with ferric salts, oxidizing agents, and metals.

Dosage Forms/Regulatory Status

VETERINARY-LABELED PRODUCTS:

There are oral combination products marketed as "cough" syrups for veterinary use that contain phenylephrine, pyrilamine (antihistamine), guaifenesin, sodium citrate, and sometimes ammonium chloride.

The ARCI (Racing Commissioners International) has designated this drug as a class 3 substance. See the appendix for more information.

HUMAN-LABELED PRODUCTS:

Phenylephrine HCl Oral Tablets: 10 mg (regular & chewable); *AH-chew D*® (WE Pharm); *Sudafed PE*® (McNeil); *Sudogest PE*® (Major) (OTC or Rx)

Phenylephrine HCl Oral Solution/Liquid: 2.5 mg/mL (concentrate), 2.5 mg/5mL & 7.5 mg/5 mL; in 30 mL, 118 mL & 473 mL; *Little Colds Decongestant for Infants & Children*® (Vetco); *Lusonal*® (WraSer); *Pedia Care Children's Decongestant*® (Pfizer Cons Health); (OTC or Rx)

Phenylephrine HCl Oral Strips: 2.5 mg; *Triaminic Thin Strips Cold*® (Novartis Consumer Health); (OTC)

Phenylephrine HCl Injection: 1% (10 mg/mL) in 1 mL & 5 mL vials and 1 mL Uni-Nest amps; *Neo-Synephrine*® (Hospira); generic; (Rx)

Phenylephrine is also available in ophthalmic and intranasal dosage forms and in combination with antihistamines, analgesics, decongestants, etc., for oral administration in humans.

References

Enos, L.R. & K. Keiser (1985). Formulary: Veterinary Medical Teaching Hospital; University of California at Davis. Davis.

Ko, J. (2009). Anesthesia monitoring techniques and management. Proceedings: ACVC. Accessed via: Veterinary Information Network. http://goo.gl/ff1Ab

Pascoe, P.J., J.E. Ilkiw, et al. (2006). Effects of increasing infusion rates of dopamine, dobutamine, epinephrine, and phenylephrine in healthy anesthetized cats. American Journal of Veterinary Research 67(9): 1491–1499.

Quandt, J. (2009). The Use of Vasopressin & Positive Inotropes for the Treatment of Hypotension. Proceedings: ACVIM. Accessed via: Veterinary Information Network. http://goo.gl/6NqG0

Rudloff, E. (2002). Resuscitation from hypovolemic shock. World Small Animal Veterinary Assoc Proceedings. Accessed via: Veterinary Information Network. http://goo.gl/2qPib

PHENYL-PROPANOLAMINE HCL

(fen-ill-proe-pa-*nole*-a-meen)   PPA

SYMPATHOMIMETIC

Prescriber Highlights

▶ Sympathomimetic used primarily for urethral sphincter hypotonus

▶ Caution: Glaucoma, prostatic hypertrophy, hyperthyroidism, diabetes mellitus, cardiovascular disorders, or hypertension

▶ Adverse Effects: Restlessness, irritability, hypertension, & anorexia

Uses/Indications

Phenylpropanolamine is used chiefly for the treatment of urethral sphincter hypotonus and resulting incontinence in dogs and cats. It has also been used in an attempt to treat nasal congestion in small animals.

Pharmacology/Actions

While the exact mechanisms of phenylpropanolamine's actions are undetermined, it is believed that it indirectly stimulates both alpha- and beta-adrenergic receptors by causing the release of norepinephrine. Prolonged use or excessive dosing frequency can deplete norepinephrine from its storage sites, and tachyphylaxis (decreased response) may ensue. Tachyphylaxis has not been documented in dogs or cats when used for urethral sphincter hypotonus, however.

Pharmacologic effects of phenylpropanolamine include increased vasoconstriction, heart rate, coronary blood flow, blood pressure, mild CNS stimulation, and decreased nasal congestion and appetite. Phenylpropanolamine can also increase urethral sphincter tone and produce closure of the bladder neck; its principle veterinary indications are because of these effects.

Pharmacokinetics

No information was located on the pharmacokinetics of this agent in veterinary species. In humans, phenylpropanolamine is readily absorbed after oral administration and has an onset of action (nasal decongestion) of about 15–30 minutes with duration of effect lasting approximately 3 hours (regular capsules or tablets).

Phenylpropanolamine is reportedly distributed into various tissues and fluids, including the CNS. It is unknown if it crosses the placenta or enters milk. The drug is partially metabolized to an active metabolite, but 80–90% is excreted unchanged in the urine within 24 hours of dosing. The serum half-life is approximately 3–4 hours.

Contraindications/Precautions/Warnings
Phenylpropanolamine should be used with caution in patients with glaucoma, prostatic hypertrophy, hyperthyroidism, diabetes mellitus, cardiovascular disorders, or hypertension.

Adverse Effects
Most likely side effects include restlessness, anxiety, irritability, urine retention, tachycardia, and hypertension. Anorexia may be a problem in some animals. Rare reports of "stroke" have occurred in dogs given therapeutic dosages of phenylpropanolamine.

Reproductive/Nursing Safety
Phenylpropanolamine may cause decreased ovum implantation; uncontrolled clinical experience, however, has not demonstrated any untoward effects during pregnancy.

Overdosage/Acute Toxicity
Clinical signs of overdosage may consist of an exacerbation of the adverse effects listed above or, if a very large over-dose, severe cardiovascular (hypertension to rebound hypotension, bradycardias to tachycardias, and cardiovascular collapse) or CNS effects (stimulation to coma) can be seen.

A dog ingesting 48 mg/kg of PPA has been reported (Crandell and Ware 2005). Ventricular tachycardia and regions of myocardial necrosis were noted. All abnormalities resolved within 6 months.

There were 146 exposures to phenylpropanolamine reported to the ASPCA Animal Poison Control Center (APCC) during 2008-2009. In these cases 144 were dogs with 97 showing clinical signs. The remaining 2 cases were cats that showed no clinical signs. Common findings in dogs recorded in decreasing frequency included hypertension, vomiting, bradycardia, piloerection, mydriasis, and hyperthermia.

If the overdose was recent, empty the stomach using the usual precautions and administer charcoal and a cathartic. Treat clinical signs supportively as they occur. Do not use propranolol to treat hypertension in bradycardic patients and do not use atropine to treat bradycardia. Hypertension may be managed with a phenothiazine (*e.g.,* acepromazine—very low dose such as 0.02 mg/kg IV or IM). If phenothiazines do not normalize blood pressure, consider using a CRI of nitroprusside. Contact an animal poison control center for further guidance.

Drug Interactions
The following drug interactions have either been reported or are theoretical in humans or animals receiving phenylpropanolamine and may be of significance in veterinary patients:

■ **HALOTHANE:** An increased risk of arrhythmias developing can occur if phenylpropanolamine is administered to patients who have received cyclopropane or a halogenated hydrocarbon anesthetic agent. Propranolol may be administered should these occur.

■ **MONOAMINE OXIDASE (MAO) INHIBITORS (e.g., amitraz, possibly selegiline):** Phenylpropanolamine should not be given within two weeks of a patient receiving monoamine oxidase inhibitors

■ **NSAIDS:** An increased chance of hypertension if given concomitantly with NSAIDs, including aspirin

■ **RESERPINE:** An increased chance of hypertension if given concomitantly

■ **SYMPATHOMIMETIC AGENTS, OTHER:** Phenylpropanolamine should not be administered with other sympathomimetic agents (*e.g.,* ephedrine) as increased toxicity may result

■ **TRICYCLIC ANTIDEPRESSANTS (clomipramine, amitriptyline, etc.):** An increased chance of hypertension if given concomitantly

Doses
■ **DOGS:**
For urethral sphincter hypotonus:
a) 12.5–50 mg (total dose) or 1–2 mg/kg PO q8h (Bartges 2009)
b) Using the time-release 75 mg capsules: Dogs weighing less than 40 lbs: ½ capsule PO daily. Dogs 40–100 lbs: 1 capsule PO daily. Dogs weighing >100 lbs: 1.5 capsules PO per day. (Label information; *Cystolamine®* —VPL)
c) 1–1.5 mg/kg PO two to three times a day controls 74–92% of dogs with primary sphincter mechanism incontinence. Over half of dogs not responding to regular PPA will respond to sustained-release PPA. Incontinence control becomes less over time in some dogs. (Chew 2007)
d) 5–50 mg per dog PO q8h or 1.5 mg/kg PO q8h–12h (Vernau 2006)
For retrograde ejaculation:
a) 3–4 mg/kg PO twice daily may be tried. (Fontbonne 2007)
■ **CATS:**
For urethral sphincter hypotonus:
a) 12.5 mg PO q8h (Labato 1988)(Polzin & Osborne 1985)
b) 1–1.5 mg/kg PO q8h (Bartges 2009)
c) 1.1 –2.2 mg/kg PO two to three times daily (Lane 2003)

Monitoring
■ Clinical effectiveness
■ Adverse effects (see above)
■ Blood pressure

Client Information
■ In order for this drug to be effective, it must be administered as directed by the veterinar-

ian; missed doses will negate its effect. It may take several days for the full benefit of the drug to take place.

■ Contact veterinarian if the animal demonstrates ongoing changes in behavior (restlessness, irritability) or if incontinence persists or increases.

Chemistry/Synonyms

A sympathomimetic amine, phenylpropanolamine HCl occurs as a white crystalline powder with a slightly aromatic odor, a melting range between 191°–194°C, and a pK_a of 9.4. One gram is soluble in approximately 1.1 mL of water or 7 mL of alcohol.

Phenylpropanolamine may also be known as: (+/-)-norephedrine, dl-norephedrine or PPA, *Cystolamine®*, *Proin®*, *Propalin®*, *Uricon®*, and *Uriflex-PT®*.

Storage/Stability

Store phenylpropanolamine products at room temperature in light-resistant, tight containers.

Dosage Forms/Regulatory Status

VETERINARY-LABELED PRODUCTS:

Note: There are no phenylpropanolamine products (at the time of writing—February 2011) approved by the FDA for use in animals.

Phenylpropanolamine Chewable Tablets: 25 mg, 50 mg, & 75 mg; *Proin®* (PRN Pharmacal), *Propalin®* (Vetoquinol), *Uriflex-PT®* (Butler), *Uricon®* (Neogen); (Rx). Labeled for use in dogs.

Phenylpropanolamine Timed-Release Capsules: 75 mg; *Cystolamine®* (VPL); (Rx). Labeled for use in dogs.

Phenylpropanolamine oral solution: 25 mg/mL in 60 mL bottles; *Proin® Drops* (PRN Pharmacal) (Rx); 50 mg/mL in 30 mL and 100 mL bottles; (Rx). Labeled for use in dogs.

The ARCI (Racing Commissioners International) has designated this drug as a class 3 substance. See the appendix for more information.

In the USA, phenylpropanolamine is classified as a list 1 chemical (drugs that can be used as precursors to manufacture methamphetamine) and in some states it may be a controlled substance or have other restrictions placed upon its sale. Be alert to persons desiring to purchase this medication.

HUMAN-LABELED PRODUCTS:

Note: Because of potential adverse effects in humans, phenylpropanolamine has been removed from the US market for human use.

References

Bartges, J. (2009). Pipes are leaking: Urinary Incontinence. Proceedings: WVC. Accessed via: Veterinary Information Network. http://goo.gl/X51gQ

Chew, D. (2007). Urinary Incontinence in dogs—diagnosis and treatment. Proceedings: WSAVA World Congress. Accessed via: Veterinary Information Network. http://goo.gl/UryBh

Fontbonne, A. (2007). Approach to infertility in the bitch and the dog. Proceedings: WSAVA World Congress. Accessed via: Veterinary Information Network. http://goo.gl/OSre0

Lane, I. (2003). Incontinence and voiding disorders in cats. Proceedings: Western States Veterinary Conference. Accessed via: Veterinary Information Network. http://goo.gl/7jZKx

Polzin, D.J. & C.A. Osborne (1985). Diseases of the Urinary Tract. *Handbook of Small Animal Therapeutics*. LE Davis Ed. New York, Churchill Livingstone: 333–395.

Vernau, K. (2006). Dysuria: To pee or not to pee... Proceedings: UCD Veterinary Neurology Symposium. Accessed via: Veterinary Information Network. http://goo.gl/3KvT8

PHENYTOIN SODIUM

(fen-i-toe-in)   Dilantin®

ANTICONVULSANT, ANTIDYSRHYTHMIC

Prescriber Highlights

▶ Rarely used (in USA) for seizures in small animals; sustained release formulations may be useful (not available in USA)

▶ Potentially useful as a treatment for ventricular dysrhythmias in horses or digoxin-induced arrhythmias in dogs or horses; may be useful in cats with myokemia and neuromyotonia

▶ Contraindications: Hypersensitivity; IV use contraindicated for 2nd or 3rd degree heart block, sinoatrial block, Adams-Stokes syndrome, or sinus bradycardia.

▶ Adverse Effects: *Dogs:* Anorexia & vomiting, ataxia, sedation, gingival hyperplasia, hepatotoxicity. *Cats:* Ataxia, sedation, anorexia, dermal atrophy syndrome, thrombocytopenia

▶ Potentially teratogenic; many drug interactions possible

Uses/Indications

Because of its undesirable pharmacokinetic profiles in dogs and cats, the use of phenytoin as an anticonvulsant for long-term treatment of epilepsy has diminished over the years and few use it today for this purpose. It remains, however, of interest due to its efficacy in humans, and the potential for sustained-release products to be marketed for dogs. Until then, prerequisites for successful therapy in dogs include: a motivated client who will be compliant with multiple daily dosing and willing to assume the financial burden of high dose phenytoin therapy and therapeutic drug monitoring expenses.

Although not commonly used, phenytoin has been employed as an oral or IV antiarrhythmic agent in both dogs and cats. It has been described as the drug of choice for digitalis-induced ventricular arrhythmias in dogs. A cat with myokemia and neuromyotonia was treated with phenytoin in a recent case report (Galano *et al.* 2005).

Phenytoin has been studied as a treatment for ventricular dysrhythmias in horses and preliminary reports demonstrate efficacy (Wijnberg & Ververs 2004).

It has been suggested that phenytoin be used as adjunctive treatment of hypoglycemia secondary to hyperinsulinism, but apparently, little clinical benefit has resulted from this therapy.

Pharmacology/Actions
The anticonvulsant actions of phenytoin are thought to be caused by the promotion of sodium efflux from neurons, thereby inhibiting the spread of seizure activity in the motor cortex. It is believed that excessive stimulation or environmental changes can alter the sodium gradient, which may lower the threshold for seizure spread. Hydantoins tend to stabilize this threshold and limit seizure propagation from epileptogenic foci.

The cardiac electrophysiologic effects of phenytoin are similar (not identical) to that of lidocaine (Group 1B). It depresses phase O slightly and can shorten the action potential. Its principle cardiac use is in the treatment of digitalis-induced ventricular arrhythmias.

Phenytoin can inhibit insulin and vasopressin (ADH) secretion.

Pharmacokinetics
After oral administration, phenytoin is nearly completely absorbed in humans, but in dogs, bioavailabilities may only be about 40%. Phenytoin is well distributed throughout the body and about 78% bound to plasma proteins in dogs (vs. 95% in humans). Protein binding may be reduced in uremic patients. Small amounts of phenytoin may be excreted into the milk and it readily crosses the placenta.

The drug is metabolized in the liver with much of the drug conjugated to a glucuronide form and then excreted by the kidneys. Phenytoin will induce hepatic microsomal enzymes, which may enhance the metabolism of itself and other drugs. The serum half-life (elimination) differences between various species are striking. Phenytoin has reported half-lives of 2–8 hours in dogs, 8 hours in horses, 15–24 hours in humans, and 42–108 hours in cats. Because of the pronounced induction of hepatic enzymes in dogs, phenytoin metabolism is increased with shorter half-lives within 7–9 days after starting treatment. Puppies possess smaller volumes of distribution and shorter elimination half-lives (1.6 hours) than adult dogs.

Contraindications/Precautions/Warnings
Some data suggest that additive hepatotoxicity may result if phenytoin is used with either primidone or phenobarbital. Weigh the potential risks versus the benefits before adding phenytoin to either of these drugs in dogs.

Phenytoin is contraindicated in patients known to be hypersensitive to it or other hydantoins. Intravenous use of the drug is contraindicated in patients with 2nd or 3rd degree heart block, sinoatrial block, Adams-Stokes syndrome, or sinus bradycardia.

Adverse Effects
Adverse effects in dogs associated with high serum levels include anorexia and vomiting, ataxia, and sedation. Liver function tests should be monitored in patients on chronic therapy as hepatotoxicity (elevated serum ALT, decreased serum albumin, hepatocellular hypertrophy and necrosis, hepatic lipidosis, and extramedullary hematopoiesis) have been reported. Gingival hyperplasia has been reported in dogs receiving chronic therapy. Oral absorption may be enhanced and GI upset decreased if given with food.

Cats exhibit ataxia, sedation, and anorexia secondary to accumulation of phenytoin and high serum levels. Cats have also been reported to develop thrombocytopenia and a dermal atrophy syndrome secondary to phenytoin.

High plasma concentrations of phenytoin in horses can cause excitement and recumbency.

Reproductive/Nursing Safety
In humans, the FDA categorizes this drug as category **D** for use during pregnancy (*There is evidence of human fetal risk, but the potential benefits from the use of the drug in pregnant women may be acceptable despite its potential risks.*) In a separate system evaluating the safety of drugs in canine and feline pregnancy (Papich 1989), this drug is categorized as class: *C* (*These drugs may have potential risks. Studies in people or laboratory animals have uncovered risks, and these drugs should be used cautiously as a last resort when the benefit of therapy clearly outweighs the risks.*)

Phenytoin is excreted in maternal milk. Because of the potential for serious adverse reactions in nursing offspring, consider whether to accept the risks, discontinue nursing or to discontinue the drug.

Overdosage/Acute Toxicity
Clinical signs of overdosage may include sedation, anorexia, and ataxia at lower levels, and coma, hypotension, and respiratory depression at higher levels. Treatment of overdoses in dogs is dependent on the severity of the clinical signs demonstrated, since dogs rapidly clear the drug. Severe intoxications should be handled supportively.

Drug Interactions
■ **CHLORAMPHENICOL:** A case report of chloramphenicol increasing the serum half-life of phenytoin from 3 to 15 hours in a dog has been reported.

Note: The following interactions are from the human literature: because of the significant differences in pharmacokinetics in dogs and cats, their veterinary significance will be variable. This list includes only agents used in small animal medicine, in the human literature many more agents have been implicated.

■ **LITHIUM:** The toxicity of lithium may be enhanced.

■ **MEPERIDINE:** Phenytoin may decrease the analgesic properties meperidine, but enhance its toxic effects.

■ **PHENOBARBITAL/PRIMIDONE:** The pharmacologic effects of primidone may be altered. Some data suggest that additive hepatotoxicity may result if phenytoin is used with either primidone or phenobarbital. Weigh the potential risks versus the benefits before adding phenytoin to either of these drugs in dogs.

The following agents may **increase the effects of phenytoin:**

■ **ALLOPURINOL**
■ **CHLORAMPHENICOL**
■ **CHLORPHENIRAMINE**
■ **CIMETIDINE**
■ **DIAZEPAM**
■ **ETHANOL**
■ **ISONIAZID**
■ **PHENYLBUTAZONE**
■ **SALICYLATES**
■ **SULFONAMIDES**
■ **TRIMETHOPRIM**
■ **VALPROIC ACID**

The following agents may **decrease the pharmacologic activity of phenytoin:**

■ **ANTACIDS**
■ **ANTINEOPLASTICS**
■ **BARBITURATES**
■ **CALCIUM (DIETARY AND GLUCONATE)**
■ **DIAZOXIDE**
■ **ENTERAL FEEDINGS**
■ **FOLIC ACID**
■ **NITROFURANTOIN**
■ **PYRIDOXINE**
■ **THEOPHYLLINE**

Phenytoin may **decrease the pharmacologic activity of the following agents:**

■ **CORTICOSTEROIDS**
■ **DISOPYRAMIDE**
■ **DOPAMINE**
■ **DOXYCYCLINE**
■ **ESTROGENS**
■ **FUROSEMIDE**
■ **QUINIDINE**

Doses

■ **DOGS:**
For treatment of seizures:
a) 15–40 mg/kg PO three times daily (Morgan 1988)

b) 20–35 mg/kg three times daily (Bunch 1986)

c) Initially, 8.8–17.6 mg/kg PO in divided doses, then gradually increase or decrease dose to maintain control. May take several days for seizure control to be attained. (Package insert; *Dilantin® Veterinary*—Parke-Davis)

(**Plumb's Note**): Because of the extremely fast half-life of phenytoin in dogs, it is unlikely that this dosage regimen ("c") will attain serum levels of 10–20 micrograms/mL which are thought to be necessary for adequate seizure control.

For treatment of ventricular arrhythmias:
a) Up to 10 mg/kg IV in increments of 2–4 mg/kg or 20–35 mg/kg PO three times daily (Moses 1988)

b) 10 mg/kg slowly IV; 30–50 mg/kg PO q8h (Ware 2003)

For treatment (or prophylaxis) of digitalis intoxication:
a) 50 mg/kg PO q8h; long-term use may cause increases in serum alkaline phosphatase and increased hepatic cell size. (Kittleson 2006)

For treatment of hypoglycemia secondary to tumor:
a) 6 mg/kg PO two to three times daily (Morgan 1988)

■ **CATS:**
Note: Because cats can easily accumulate this drug and develop clinical signs of toxicity, the use of phenytoin is very controversial in this species. Diligent monitoring is required.
a) For treatment of ventricular arrhythmias: 2–3 mg/kg PO q24h (Wilcke 1985)

b) For treatment of seizures: 2–3 mg/kg daily PO; 20 mg/kg per week (Bunch 1986)

■ **HORSES:** (**Note:** ARCI UCGFS Class 4 Drug)
a) For seizures: 2.83–16.43 mg/kg PO q8h to obtain serum levels from 5–10 micrograms/mL. Suggest monitoring serum levels to adjust dosage. (Kowalczyk & Beech 1983)

b) For digoxin induced arrhythmias: 10–22 mg/kg PO q12h. Adverse effects are muscle fasciculations and sedation. (Mogg 1999)

c) For treatment of ventricular dysrhythmias: For persistent ventricular extra systoles or ventricular tachycardia where conventional treatment has failed: 20 mg/kg PO q12h initially for the first 3–4 doses, followed by a maintenance dose of 10–15 mg/kg PO q12h. Suggest monitoring plasma concentrations. (Wijnberg & Ververs 2004)

Monitoring
■ Level of seizure control; sedation/ataxia

- Body weight (anorexia)
- Liver enzymes (if chronic therapy) and serum albumin
- Serum drug levels if signs of toxicity or lack of seizure control

Client Information

- Notify veterinarian if patient becomes anorexic, lethargic, ataxic, or seizures are not adequately controlled.
- The importance of regular dosing is imperative for successful therapy.

Chemistry/Synonyms

A hydantoin-derivative, phenytoin sodium occurs as a white, hygroscopic powder which is freely soluble in water and warm propylene glycol, and soluble in alcohol.

Because phenytoin sodium slowly undergoes partial hydrolysis in aqueous solutions to phenytoin (base) with the resultant solution becoming turbid, the commercial injection contains 40% propylene glycol and 10% alcohol. The pH of the injectable solution is approximately 12.

Phenytoin sodium is used in the commercially available capsules (both extended and prompt) and the injectable preparations. Phenytoin (base) is used in the oral tablets and suspensions. Each 100 mg of phenytoin sodium contains 92 mg of the base.

Phenytoin may also be known as: diphenylhydantoin, DPH, fenitoina, phenantoinum, or phenytoinum, *Dilantin®*, and *Phenytek®*.

Storage/Stability

Store capsules at room temperature (below 86°F) and protect from light and moisture. Store phenytoin sodium injection at room temperature and protect from freezing. If injection is frozen or refrigerated, a precipitate may form which should resolubilize when warmed. A slight yellowish color will not affect either potency or efficacy, but do not use precipitated solutions. Injectable solutions at less than a pH of 11.5 will precipitate. No problems with adsorption to plastic have been detected thus far.

Compatibility/Compounding Considerations

Phenytoin sodium injection is generally physically **incompatible** with most IV solutions (upon standing) and drugs. It has been successfully mixed with sodium bicarbonate and verapamil HCl.

Because an infusion of phenytoin sodium is sometimes desirable, several studies have been performed to determine whether such a procedure can be safely done. The general conclusions and recommendations of these studies are: **1)** use either normal saline or lactated Ringer's; **2)** a concentration of 1 mg/mL phenytoin be used; **3)** start infusion immediately and complete in a relatively short time; **4)** use a 0.22 μm in-line IV filter; **5)** watch the admixture carefully.

Dosage Forms/Regulatory Status

VETERINARY-LABELED PRODUCTS: None

The ARCI (Racing Commissioners International) has designated this drug as a class 4 substance. See the appendix for more information.

HUMAN-LABELED PRODUCTS:

Phenytoin Sodium Extended-Release Capsules: 30 mg, 100 mg, 200 mg & 300 mg; *Dilantin Kapseals®* (Pfizer); *Phenytek®* (Bertek); generic (Rx)

Phenytoin Oral Suspension: 25 mg/mL in 240 mL; *Dilantin-125®* (Pfizer); generic; (Rx)

Phenytoin Tablets: 50 mg (chewable); *Dilantin® Infa-Tabs* (Pfizer); (Rx)

Phenytoin Sodium Injection: 50 mg/mL (46 mg/mL phenytoin) in 2 mL & 10 mL; generic; (Rx)

References

Bunch, S.E. (1986). Anticonvulsant drug therapy in companion animals. *Current Veterinary Therapy IX: Small Animal Practice*. RW Kirk Ed. Philadelphia, WB Saunders: 836–844.

Galano, H., N. Olby, et al. (2005). Myokymia and neuromyotonia in a cat. *JAVMA* 227(10): 1608–1612.

Kittleson, M. (2006). "Chapt 29: Drugs used in the treatment of cardiac arrhythmias." *Small Animal Cardiology, 2nd Ed.*

Kowalczyk, D.F. & J. Beech (1983). Pharmacokinetics of phenytoin in horses. *J Vet Pharmacol Ther* 6(2): 133–140.

Mogg, T. (1999). Equine Cardiac Disease: Clinical pharmacology and therapeutics. *The Veterinary Clinics of North America: Equine Practice* 15:3(December).

Morgan, R.V., Ed. (1988). *Handbook of Small Animal Practice*. New York, Churchill Livingstone.

Moses, B.L. (1988). Cardiac arrhythmias and cardiac arrest. *Handbook of Small Animal Practice*. RV Morgan Ed. New York, Churchill Livingstone: 71–90.

Papich, M. (1989). Effects of drugs on pregnancy. *Current Veterinary Therapy X: Small Animal Practice*. R Kirk Ed. Philadelphia, Saunders: 1291–1299.

Ware, W. (2003). Cardiovascular system disorders. *Small Animal Internal Medicine, 3rd Ed.* R Nelson and C Couto Eds. St Louis, Mosby: 1–209.

Wijnberg, I. & F. Ververs (2004). Phenytoin sodium as a treatment for ventricular dysrhythmia in horses. *J Vet Intern Med* 18(May/Jun): 350–353.

Wilcke, J.R. (1985). Cardiac Dysrhythmias. *Handbook of Small Animal Therapeutics*. LE Davis Ed. New York, Churchill Livingstone: 267–286.

PHEROMONES

(*fer*-i-mones)   Feliway®, D.A.P.®

PHEROMONE BEHAVIOR MODIFIER

Prescriber Highlights

▶ Commercially available pheromones may be useful in *Cats* for urine marking or spraying, vertical scratching, avoidance of social contact, loss of appetite, stressful situations, or inter-cat aggression; *Dogs:* Behaviors associated with fear or stress or for calming in new environments or situations; *Horses:* Alleviating stressful situations

▶ May need adjunctive therapy (behavior modification, drug therapy) for negative behaviors

▶ Dog/Cat products are administered via the environment; Equine product administered intranasally

▶ Appears to be safe

Uses/Indications

Pheromones may be useful adjuncts to reduce anxiety and stress. In cats, FFP may be useful in treating urine marking or spraying, vertical scratching, avoidance of social contact, loss of appetite, stressful situations, or inter-cat aggression. Behavioral modification and/or concomitant drug therapy may be required.

In dogs, DAP may be useful in treating behaviors associated with fear or stress (*e.g.*, separation anxiety, destruction, excessive barking, house soiling, licking, phobias) or calming animals in new environments or situations.

In horses, EAP may be useful in alleviating stressful situations (*e.g.*, transport, shoeing, clipping, new environments, training).

Pharmacology/Actions

Appeasing pheromones produced during nursing are thought to exist with all mammals. They are detected by the Jacobson's organ or vomeronasal organ (VNO). The VNO is more sensitive in young animals, but is believed to continue to function in older animals as well. It is not well understood what neurotransmitters or neurochemical processes are involved for pheromones to exhibit their effects. In most animals, pheromones have a general calming effect. In cats, the F3 facial pheromone is thought to inhibit urine marking, encourage feeding, and enhance exploratory behaviors in unfamiliar situations. The F4 pheromone is a so-called allomarking pheromone that calms and familiarizes the cat with its surroundings.

Pharmacokinetics

No information located.

Contraindications/Precautions/Reproductive Safety

No information located.

Adverse Effects

No significant adverse effects were located for these products and are unlikely to occur.

Overdosage/Acute Toxicity

No specific animal toxicity data was located. Although the ingredients in these products are not thought toxic, the manufacturer recommends that humans accidentally exposed resulting in an adverse reaction should report to a physician or poison control center.

Drug Interactions

■ None were located. Effects may be reduced or negated by concurrent use of drugs that cause CNS stimulation.

Laboratory Considerations

■ No information was located.

Doses

■ CATS:

a) Diffusers: Diffuser vial lasts approximately 4 weeks and covers 500–650 sq. ft. Plug diffuser into electric outlet in the room most often used by the animal. Do not cover diffuser or place behind or under furniture. When plugged in, do not touch diffuser with wet hands or metal objects. Do not touch diffuser with uncovered hands during, or immediately after use. May require up to 72 hours to saturate area, so effects may not be immediate. (Label Information; *Feliway® Diffuser*—VPL)

b) Spray: Do not spray directly on cats. Pump spray approximately 4 inches from site, 8 inches from the floor. One spray per application site. Clean urine marks with clear water only. Urine marks and prominent objects (furniture, window or doorframes) should be sprayed 1–2 times daily for 30 days. If cat is observed rubbing its own facial pheromones onto a spot, treatment is no longer necessary at that location. Maintenance sprays every 2–3 days may be required. Inter-cat aggression problems may require behavior modification and concomitant drug therapy. (Label Information; *Feliway® Spray*—VPL)

■ DOGS:

a) Diffusers: Diffuser vial lasts approximately 4 weeks and covers 500–650 sq. ft. Plug diffuser into electric outlet in the room most often used by the animal. Do not cover diffuser or place behind or under furniture. When plugged in, do not touch diffuser with wet hands or metal objects. Do not touch diffuser with uncovered hands during, or immediately after use. May require up to 72 hours to saturate area, so effects may not be immediate. (Label Information; *D.A.P.® Diffuser—VPL*)

b) Spray: Do not spray directly on dogs. May spray in car, kennels, crates, carriers, or on neck bandanas. Spray approximately 20 minutes prior to travel, etc. When entering unfamiliar places/rooms, spray twice day in the area. (Label Information; *D.A.P.® Spray—VPL*)

■ **HORSES:**

a) Administer 2 sprays into each nostril ½ hour before anticipated stress or event. After administration, keep horse in a non-stressful environment for ½ hour to achieve best results. (Label Information; *Modipher EQ® Spray—VPL*)

Monitoring
■ Clinical efficacy

Chemistry
Mammalian pheromones are fatty acids. Dog appeasing pheromone (DAP) is a synthetic derivative of bitch intermammary pheromone. Feline pheromone is a synthetic analog of feline cheek gland secretions (feline facial pheromone; FFP). The commercially available product available in the USA is an analog of the F3 fraction of the pheromone. Equine appeasing pheromone (EAP) is derived from maternal pheromones found in the "wax area" close to the mammae of nursing mares.

Storage/Stability
Unless otherwise labeled, store at room temperature and do not mix with other ingredients or substances. Keep products out of reach of children.

Dosage Forms/Regulatory Status
VETERINARY-LABELED PRODUCTS:

Feline Facial Pheromone (FFP-F3 fraction) Diffuser (electric diffuser plus a 2% FFP vial) 48 mL vial; *Feliway® Diffuser* (Farnam); *Comfort Zone® Feline* (Farnam); (OTC)

Feline Facial Pheromone (FFP-F3 fraction) Spray 10% 75 mL bottle; *Feliway® Spray* (VPL); *Comfort Zone® Spray for Cats* (Farnam); (OTC)

Dog Appeasing Pheromone (DAP) Diffuser (electric diffuser plus a 2% DAP vial) 48 mL vial; *D.A.P.® Diffuser* (VPL); (OTC)

Dog Appeasing Pheromone 2% (DAP) Spray 60 mL bottle; *D.A.P.® Spray* (VPL); *Comfort Zone® Spray for Dogs* (Farnam); (OTC)

Dog Appeasing Pheromone (DAP) 48 mL with or without plug in adapter; *Comfort Zone® Canine* (Farnam); (OTC)

Dog Appeasing Pheromone Collar; *D.A.P.® Collar* (VPL); (OTC)

Equine Appeasing Pheromone (EAP) 0.1% Spray 7.5 mL bottle, *Modipher EQ® Mist with E.A.P.* (VPL); (OTC)

A product (not currently available in the USA) called *FeliFriend®* contains a synthetic F4 fraction of FFP.

HUMAN-LABELED PRODUCTS: None

PHOSPHATE, PARENTERAL POTASSIUM PHOSPHATE SODIUM PHOSPHATE

ELECTROLYTE

Prescriber Highlights

▶ For treatment or prevention of hypophosphatemia

▶ Contraindications: Hyperphosphatemia, hypocalcemia, oliguric renal failure, or if tissue necrosis is present; Potassium phosphate contraindicated if hyperkalemia present; sodium phosphate if hypernatremia present

▶ Caution: Cardiac (esp. if receiving digoxin) or renal disease

▶ Adverse Effects: Hyperphosphatemia, resulting in hypocalcemia, hypotension, renal failure or soft tissue mineralization; hyperkalemia or hypernatremia are possible

▶ Dilute before giving IV

Uses/Indications
Phosphate is useful in large volume parenteral fluids to correct or prevent hypophosphatemia when adequate oral phosphorous intake is not possible. Hypophosphatemia may cause hemolytic anemia, thrombocytopenia, neuromuscular and CNS disorders, bone and joint pain, and decompensation in patients with cirrhotic liver disease. There is some controversy whether "a low phos" indicates that treatment is necessary.

Pharmacology/Actions
Phosphate is involved in several functions in the body, including calcium metabolism, acid-base buffering, B-vitamin utilization, bone deposition, and several enzyme systems.

Pharmacokinetics
Intravenously administered phosphate is eliminated via the kidneys. It is glomerularly filtered, but up to 80% is reabsorbed by the tubules.

Contraindications/Precautions/Warnings
Both potassium and sodium phosphate are contraindicated in patients with hyperphosphatemia, hypocalcemia, oliguric renal failure, or if tissue necrosis is present. Potassium phosphate is contraindicated in patients with hyperkalemia. It should be used with caution in patients

with cardiac or renal disease. Particular caution should be used in using this drug in patients receiving digitalis therapy.

Sodium phosphate is also contraindicated in patients with hypernatremia.

Adverse Effects

Overuse of parenteral phosphate can result in hyperphosphatemia, resulting in hypocalcemia (refer to the Overdose section for more information). Phosphate therapy can also result in hypotension, renal failure or soft tissue mineralization. Either hyperkalemia or hypernatremia may result in susceptible patients.

Reproductive/Nursing Safety

In humans, the FDA categorizes this drug as category *C* for use during pregnancy (*Animal studies have shown an adverse effect on the fetus, but there are no adequate studies in humans; or there are no animal reproduction studies and no adequate studies in humans.*)

It is not known whether this drug is excreted in maternal milk. It is unlikely to be of concern.

Overdosage/Acute Toxicity

Patients developing hyperphosphatemia secondary to intravenous therapy with potassium phosphate should have the infusion stopped and be given appropriate parenteral calcium therapy to restore serum calcium levels. Serum potassium should be monitored and treated if required.

Drug Interactions

The following drug interactions have either been reported or are theoretical in humans or animals receiving phosphates and may be of significance in veterinary patients:

- **ALUMINUM and CALCIUM SALTS (oral) and SEVELAMER:** May reduce phosphorus levels
- **ANGIOTENSIN CONVERTING ENZYME INHIBITORS (ACE Inhibitors):** May cause potassium retention. When used with potassium products such as potassium phosphate, hyperkalemia can result.
- **DIGOXIN:** Potassium salts (potassium phosphate) must be used very cautiously in patients on digitalis therapy and should not be used in digitalized patients with heart block
- **POTASSIUM SPARING DIURETICS (e.g., spironolactone):** May cause potassium retention. When used with potassium products such as potassium phosphate, hyperkalemia can result.

Doses

Both sodium and potassium phosphate injections must be diluted before intravenous administration.

- **DOGS/CATS:**

  For hypophosphatemia:

  a) The goal in treatment of hypophosphatemia is to maintain serum levels above 2 mg/dL. For mild to moderate hypophosphatemia, oral supplementation in

the form of sodium phosphate or potassium phosphate can be administered. Treatment with intravenous supplementation should begin when levels are less than 1-1.5 mg/dL or if clinical symptoms are present. Intravenous administration of potassium phosphate is recommended at 0.01–0.06 mMol/kg/hr IV mixed in saline or dextrose. Serum phosphate levels should be monitored every 4–6 hours. Once levels exceed 2–2.5 mg/dL, the patient may be maintained on oral phosphorus supplementation. (Schropp & Kovacic 2007)

b) For hypophosphatemia associated with diabetic ketoacidosis: Phosphorus can be added to IV fluids in the form of potassium phosphate. Dosing ranges from 0.03–0.12 mMol/kg/hour are added to the IV fluids. Alternatively, ⅓–½ of the calculated dose of potassium supplementation can be added as potassium phosphate, with KCl used for the remainder. (O'Brien 2010)

c) Correct underlying cause if possible. If serum phosphorus concentration is >1.5 mg/dL and unlikely to decrease further, no treatment is usually necessary. If <1.5 mg/dL, clinical signs or hemolysis present, treat. Also, consider treating during the first 24 hours of therapy for DKA. Goal of therapy is to maintain serum phosphorus >2 mg/dL without causing hyperphosphatemia. Oral phosphate supplementation is preferred; either a buffered phosphate laxative (*e.g.*, Phospho-Soda), balanced commercial diet or milk. Severe hypophosphatemia is treated with intravenous therapy: Using either potassium phosphate (3 mMol phosphate/mL and 4.4 mEq potassium/mL) or sodium phosphate (if potassium supplementation is contraindicated; 3 mMol phosphate/mL and 4 mEq sodium/mL), give 0.01–0.03 mMol/kg/hr preferably by CRI. Avoid hyperphosphatemia. Monitor serum phosphorus every 6–8 hours and adjust dose. (Nelson & Elliott 2003)

d) In treating diabetic ketoacidosis, ⅓ of the IV potassium should be administered as potassium phosphate, particularly in small dogs and cats who are most susceptible to hemolysis caused by hypophosphatemia. Use caution as over supplementation of phosphorus can result in metastatic calcification and hypocalcemia. (Greco 2007)

e) Cats with DKA and a serum phosphorus of < 2 mg/dL: CRI of potassium phosphate at 0.03–0.06 mMol/kg/hr; severe cases of hypophosphatemia (< 1 mg/dL) may require doses as high as

0.12−0.2 mMol/kg/hr. Recheck phosphorus after 6−12 hours. Alternatively may provide half the potassium requirements as KCl and half as K Phos. (Waddell 2007)

■ **RUMINANTS:**

For hypophosphatemia:

a) Oral phosphate is the preferred method of administration in ruminants with rumen motility. Recommended dose is: 200 grams of feed grade monosodium phosphate (contains 50 grams of phosphate) administered in gelatin boluses, drench, or by ororuminal intubation. Almost all commercially available intravenous solutions use phosphite or hypophosphite salts as the source of phosphorus because these salts are very soluble, even in the presence of calcium and magnesium, but the phosphorous in phosphite and hypophosphite is unavailable to ruminants, meaning that the vast majority of "phosphate" containing solutions have no efficacy in treating hypophosphatemia. Instead, the monobasic monophosphate form of sodium phosphate (NaH_2PO_4) should be administered. The pH of the solution should be mildly acidic (pH=5.8) to maintain phosphate solubility in cold weather, but is not needed in warm ambient temperatures. A recommended treatment to adult cattle with severe hypophosphatemia is 300 mL of 10% NaH_2PO_4 (monohydrate) solution by slow IV injection, this provides 7 grams of phosphate and increases plasma phosphate concentrations for at least 6 hours (the calculated phosphorus deficit in adult cattle is approximately 5 grams phosphate). A major drawback with IV administration of phosphate solutions is that they should not be administered within 2 hours of intravenous calcium administration because of concerns that calcium-phosphate precipitates may be formed in the plasma of cattle with treatment-induced hypercalcemia and hyperphosphatemia. (Constable 2008)

Monitoring

■ Serum inorganic phosphate (phosphorous)

■ Other electrolytes, including calcium

Chemistry

Potassium phosphate injection is a combination of 224 mg monobasic potassium phosphate and 236 mg dibasic potassium phosphate. The pH of the injection is 6.5 and has an osmolarity of 7357 mOsm/L.

Sodium phosphate injection is a combination of 276 mg monobasic sodium phosphate and 142 mg dibasic sodium phosphate. The pH of the injection is 5.7 and has an osmolarity of about 7000 mOsm/L.

Because commercial preparations are a combination of monobasic and dibasic forms, prescribe and dispense in terms of mMoles of phosphate.

Storage/Stability

Unless otherwise instructed by the manufacturer, store potassium or sodium phosphate injection at room temperature; protect from freezing.

Compatibility/Compounding Considerations

Phosphates may be physically **incompatible** with metals such as calcium and magnesium.

Potassium phosphate injection is reportedly physically **compatible** with the following intravenous solutions and drugs: amino acids 4%/dextrose 25%, D_{10}LRS, D_{10}Ringer's, Dextrose 2.5%−10% injection, sodium chloride 0.45%−0.9%, magnesium sulfate, metoclopramide HCl, and verapamil HCl.

Potassium phosphate injection is reportedly physically **incompatible** with the following solutions or drugs: $D_{2.5}$ in half normal Ringer's or LRS, D_5 in Ringer's, D_{10}/sodium chloride 0.9%, Ringer's injection, LRS, and dobutamine HCl. Compatibility is dependent upon factors such as pH, concentration, temperature and diluent used; consult specialized references or a hospital pharmacist for more specific information.

Dosage Forms/Regulatory Status

VETERINARY-LABELED PRODUCTS: None

There are no parenteral phosphate-only products FDA-approved for veterinary medicine. There are several proprietary phosphate-containing products available that may also include calcium, magnesium, potassium, and/or dextrose; refer to the individual product's labeling for specific dosage information. Trade names for these products include: *Magnadex®*—Osborn, *Norcalciphos®*—SKB, *Cal-Dextro® Special*, and *#2*, (Fort Dodge), and *CMPK®*, and *Cal-Phos® #2* (TechAmerica). They are legend (Rx) drugs.

HUMAN-LABELED PRODUCTS:

Potassium Phosphate Injection; each mL provides 3 mM of phosphate (99.1 mg/dL of phosphorous) and 4.4 mEq of potassium per mL in 5, 10, 15, 30, and 50 mL vials; generic; (Rx)

Sodium Phosphate Injection; each mL provides 3 mM of phosphate (93 mg/dL of phosphorous) and 4 mEq of sodium per mL in 10, 15, 30, and 50 mL vials; generic; (Rx)

References

Constable, P.D. (2008). Metabolic Disease of Beef Cattle: Diagnosis, Treatment, & Prevention. Western Veterinary Conference. Accessed via: Veterinary Information Network. http://goo.gl/vmVKl

Greco, D. (2007). Ketoacidosis, hypoglycemia, & hyperosmolar emergencies. Proceedings Western Vet Conf. Accessed via: Veterinary Information Network. http://goo.gl/Cq3AG

Nelson, R. & D. Elliott (2003). Metabolic and electrolyte disorders. *Small Animal Internal Medicine, 3rd Ed.* R Nelson and C Couto Eds. St Louis, Mosby: 816–846.

O'Brien, M.A. (2010). Diabetic Emergencies in Small Animals. *Veterinary Clinics of North America-Small Animal Practice* **40**(2): 317–+.

Schropp, D. & J. Kovacic (2007). Phosphorus and phosphate metabolism in veterinary patients. *J Vet Emerg Crit Care* **17**((2)): 127–134.

Waddell, L. (2007). Diabetic ketoacidosis in cats. Proceedings: Western Vet Conference. Accessed via: Veterinary Information Network. http://goo.gl/YKWAL

PHYSOSTIGMINE SALICYLATE

(fye-zoh-*stig*-meen sah-*lis*-ah-layt)
Antilirium®

CHOLINESTERASE INHIBITOR

Prescriber Highlights

▶ Cholinesterase inhibitor that may be used for the adjunctive treatment of ivermectin toxicity in dogs, as a provocative agent for the diagnosis of narcolepsy in dogs & horses, or as a treatment for anticholinergic toxicity

▶ Crosses into the CNS, so it is effective for treating central anticholinergic toxicity, but also increases the risks for central physostigmine toxic effects (e.g., seizures)

▶ Must be administered with direct patient supervision; toxic effects from this drug can be serious

Uses/Indications

Physostigmine has been used for the adjunctive treatment of ivermectin toxicity in dogs, as a provocative agent for the diagnosis of narcolepsy in dogs and horses, and as a treatment for anticholinergic toxicity. Because of the potential for serious adverse effects, use of physostigmine as an antidote is generally reserved for very serious toxicity affecting the CNS. Otherwise, safer alternatives such as neostigmine or pyridostigmine are preferred.

While physostigmine has been used to antagonize the CNS depressant effects of benzodiazepines in humans, it should not be used for this purpose because of the potential toxicity and non-specific action of physostigmine.

Pharmacology/Actions

Physostigmine reversibly inhibits the destruction of acetylcholine by acetylcholinesterase, thereby increasing acetylcholine at receptor sites. Because physostigmine is a tertiary amine, unlike the quaternary amine cholinesterase inhibitors neostigmine and pyridostigmine, it crosses the blood-brain barrier and inhibits acetylcholinesterase both centrally and peripherally. Pharmacologic effects include miosis, bronchial constriction, hypersalivation, muscle weakness, and sweating (in species with sweat

glands). At higher dosages, cholinergic crisis can occur; seizures, bradycardia, tachycardia, asystole, nausea, vomiting, diarrhea, depolarizing neuromuscular block, pulmonary edema, and respiratory paralysis are possible.

Pharmacokinetics

Physostigmine is rapidly absorbed from the GI tract (no oral dosage form available), subcutaneous tissue or mucous membranes. After parenteral administration, physostigmine readily crosses the blood-brain barrier into the CNS. Peak effects occur within 5 minutes after IV administration; about 25 minutes after IM dosing. The majority of administered drug is rapidly destroyed via hydrolysis by cholinesterases. Very small amounts can be eliminated unchanged into the urine. Duration of pharmacologic effects can be from 30 minutes to 5 hours; average duration is 30–60 minutes.

Contraindications/Precautions/Warnings

Contraindications for humans and, presumably, animal patients include: prior hypersensitivity reactions to physostigmine or sulfites, bronchoconstrictive disease (asthma), gangrene, diabetes mellitus, cardiovascular disease, mechanical obstruction of the GI or urinary tract, any vagotonic state, or the concurrent use of choline esters (*e.g.*, bethanechol, methacholine) or neuromuscular blocking agents (*e.g.*, succinylcholine)—see Drug Interactions.

When physostigmine is used in the absence of anticholinergic toxicity or to treat tricyclic or tetracyclic antidepressant overdoses, there is an increased risk for cholinergic crisis.

Rapid IV administration increases the potential for bradycardia, hypersalivation, or seizures. In humans, it should be given intravenously at a slow, controlled rate not exceeding 1 mg/minute (adults) and 0.5 mg/min (children).

Because of the risks for toxicity, atropine should be readily available (see Overdosage).

Physostigmine injection contains benzyl alcohol that may be toxic in neonatal animals.

Adverse Effects

Adverse effects are a result of the drug's pharmacologic actions and, except for hypersensitivity reactions, are dose related depending upon concurrent anticholinergic effects secondary to anticholinergics on board. Pharmacologic effects include miosis, bronchial constriction, hypersalivation, muscle weakness, and sweating (in species with sweat glands). At higher dosages, cholinergic crisis can occur; seizures, bradycardia, tachycardia, asystole, nausea, vomiting, diarrhea, depolarizing neuromuscular block, pulmonary edema, and respiratory paralysis are possible.

Reproductive/Nursing Safety

Little information is available, but it would be expected that physostigmine would cross the placenta. Teratogenic effects (behavioral, biochemical and metabolic) have reportedly been observed in mice studies. Weigh the potential risks of using physostigmine during pregnancy versus its potential benefits. In humans, the FDA categorizes alendronate as category **C** for use during pregnancy (*Animal studies have shown an adverse effect on the fetus, but there are no adequate studies in humans; or there are no animal reproduction studies and no adequate studies in humans.*)

It is not known if physostigmine enters milk, but it would unlikely pose much risk to nursing offspring.

Overdosage/Acute Toxicity

Overdoses or acute toxicity can be life-threatening (see Adverse Reactions), however, because of the short duration of effect, supportive care may be all that is required. Treatment of serious acute toxicity includes mechanical ventilation, repeated bronchial aspiration, and administration of IV atropine. Refer to the Atropine monograph for dosages for cholinergic toxicity. Readministration of atropine may be required. Pralidoxime (2-PAM) may be useful in reversing the ganglionic and skeletal muscle effects of physostigmine. Refer to the Pralidoxime monograph for more information. An animal poison control center may be helpful in assisting with case management.

Drug Interactions

The following drug interactions have either been reported or are theoretical in humans or animals receiving physostigmine and may be of significance in veterinary patients:

- ■ **CHOLINE ESTERS (bethanechol, carbachol, methacholine) or ORGANOPHOSPHATES:** Physostigmine may cause additive adverse effects
- ■ **SUCCINYLCHOLINE:** Physostigmine (high doses) may cause muscle fasiculations or depolarization block (very high doses), which may be additive to the effects of succinylcholine-like neuromuscular blockers

Laboratory Considerations

- ■ None were noted

Doses

- ■ **DOGS:**
  a) To temporarily reverse the CNS effects of ivermectin toxicosis in support of the diagnosis: 1 mg (total dose) IV (Mealey 2006)
  b) To temporarily reverse the CNS effects of ivermectin toxicosis in support of the diagnosis: 1 mg (total dose)/12 hours IV. May reverse ivermectin-induced coma for 30–90 minutes. In comatose patients, it does not appear to induce seizures, but seizure-like activity can be observed in patients with only minor ataxia and confusion. (Estrada 2002)
  c) Provocative test for narcolepsy/cataplexy if feeding test (*10 pieces of highly tasty food that the dog loves to eat in a row 12–*

24 inches apart; affected dogs will usually take 2 minutes or longer to eat the food and will have several attacks) is not successful: Physostigmine at 0.025 mg/kg IV, wait 9–15 minutes and observe response to stimulus (food test or similar). If clinical signs do not appear, may try a higher dose of 0.05 mg/kg as above. Subsequent testing can be done at doses of 0.075 mg/kg and 1 mg/kg as above. Increased severity of signs that may persist for 15–45 minutes in response to stimulus is indicative of cataplexy/narcolepsy. (Shell 2003)

- ■ **HORSES: (Note:** RCI Class 3 drug)
  a) Provocative test in diagnosing cataplexy or narcolepsy: 0.05–0.1 mg/kg slow IV will precipitate a cataplectic attack within 3–10 minutes after administration in affected horses. Untoward effects may include colic or cholinergic stimulation. (Andrews & Matthews 2004).
  b) Provocative test in diagnosing cataplexy or narcolepsy: 0.06–0.08 mg/kg IV. Lack of positive response does not rule out diagnosis of narcolepsy. Diarrhea can occur and caution is advised as horse can cause colic. (Mayhew 2005)

- ■ **CATTLE:**
  a) For reversal of tall larkspur (*Delphinium barbeya*) poisoning: 0.04–0.08 mg/kg IV rapidly; serial injections may be necessary. (Pfister *et al.* 1994)

Monitoring

- ■ Direct patient supervision required for monitoring adverse effects
- ■ Heart rate, blood pressure; monitor heart rhythm if heart rate is abnormal

Client Information

- ■ This medication must be administered in a setting where direct veterinary supervision is available

Chemistry/Synonyms

Physostigmine salicylate is made from an extract of *Physostigma venenosum* (Calabar Bean) seeds. It occurs as white, shining, odorless, crystals or crystalline powder. Upon exposure to heat, light, air, or exposure to traces of metals for a long period, it develops a red tint. One gram is soluble in 75 mL of water and 16 mL of alcohol. The injection has a pH of 3.5–5.

Physostigmine salicylate may also be known as eserine salicylate, physostigmine monosalicylate and *Anticholium*®.

Storage/Stability

The injection (ampules) should be stored below 40°C and preferably between 15–30°C. Protect from light and freezing.

Compatibility/Compounding Considerations

Physostigmine is labeled for human use to be administered IV undiluted. It may be given via a Y-site or stopcock port on IV set, but it should **not** be added to IV solutions. IM dosing (although not FDA-approved) is not uncommon in humans.

Dosage Forms/Regulatory Status

VETERINARY-LABELED PRODUCTS: None

The ARCI (Racing Commissioners International) has designated this drug as a class 3 substance. See the appendix for more information.

HUMAN-LABELED PRODUCTS:

Physostigmine Salicylate Injection: 1mg/mL (contains benzyl alcohol 2% and 0.1% sodium metabisulfite) in 2 mL ampules; generic; (Rx)

References

Andrews, F. & H. Matthews (2004). Seizures, narcoplexy, and cataplexy. *Equine Internal Medicine, 2nd Ed.* S Reed, W Bayly and D Sellon Eds. Philadelphia, Saunders: 560–579.

Estrada, K. (2002). Ivermectin Toxicity. Proceedings: ACVIM 2002. Accessed via: Veterinary Information Network. http://goo.gl/1NWyI

Mayhew, J. (2005). Sleep disorders, seizures and epilepsy in horses. Proceedings: ACVIM2005. Accessed via: Veterinary Information Network. http://goo.gl/cTGQ1

Mealey, K. (2006). Ivermectin: Macrolide Antiparasitic Agents. *Small Animal Toxicology, 2nd Ed.* M Peterson and P Talcott Eds., Elsevier: 785–794.

Pfister, J., K. Panter, et al. (1994). Reversal of tall larkspur (Delphinium barbeyi) poisoning in cattle with physostigmine. *Vet Hum Toxicol* **36**(6): 511–514.

Shell, L. (2003). "Narcolepsy/Cataplexy."

PHYTONADIONE
VITAMIN K1

(fye-toe-na-*dye*-ohne)
Vitamin K1, Mephyton®

ANTIDOTE, FAT SOLUBLE VITAMIN

Prescriber Highlights

▶ Used for the treatment of anticoagulant rodenticide toxicity, dicumarol toxicity associated with sweet clover ingestion in ruminants, sulfaquinoxaline toxicity, & in bleeding disorders associated with faulty formation of vitamin K-dependent coagulation factors

▶ Contraindications: Hypersensitivity; does not correct hypoprothrombinemia due to hepatocellular damage.

▶ Adverse Effects: Anaphylactoid reactions after IV administration, IM use may result in acute bleeding from the site of injection during the early stages of treatment. SC injections or oral dosages may be slowly or poorly absorbed in hypovolemic animals.

▶ May require 6–12 hours for effect

▶ Small gauge needles are recommended for use when injecting SC or IM

Uses/Indications

The principal use of exogenously administered phytonadione is in the treatment of anticoagulant rodenticide toxicity. It is also used for treating dicumarol toxicity associated with sweet clover ingestion in ruminants, sulfaquinoxaline toxicity, and in bleeding disorders associated with faulty formation of vitamin K-dependent coagulation factors.

Pharmacology/Actions

Vitamin K_1 is necessary for the synthesis of blood coagulation factors II, VII, IX, and X in the liver. It is believed that Vitamin K_1 is involved in the carboxylation of the inactive precursors of these factors to form active compounds.

Pharmacokinetics

Phytonadione is absorbed from the GI tract in monogastric animals via the intestinal lymphatics, but only in the presence of bile salts. Oral absorption of phytonadione may be significantly enhanced by administration with fatty foods. The relative bioavailability of the drug is increased 4–5 times in dogs given canned dog food with the dose. After oral administration, increases in clotting factors may not occur until 6–12 hours later.

In humans, oral administration may be more rapidly absorbed than with SC administration.

Phytonadione may concentrate in the liver for a short period of time, but is not appreciably stored in the liver or other tissues. Only small amounts are distributed across the placenta in pregnant animals. Exogenously administered phytonadione enters milk. The elimination of Vitamin K_1 is not well understood.

Contraindications/Precautions/Warnings

Many veterinary clinicians state that the intravenous use of phytonadione is contraindicated because of increased risk of anaphylaxis development, and while intravenous phytonadione is used in human medicine and several intravenous dosage regimens are outlined below in the Dosage section, the FDA-CVM has warned to avoid administering the drug IV. However, in human medicine, intravenous phytonadione is recommended (with caution) for severe bleeding associated with very high INR. Phytonadione is contraindicated in patients hypersensitive to it or any component of its formulation.

Vitamin K does not correct hypoprothrombinemia due to hepatocellular damage.

Adverse Effects

Anaphylactoid reactions have been reported following IV administration of Vitamin K_1; use with extreme caution (See Contraindications above). Intramuscular administration may result in acute bleeding from the site of injection during the early stages of treatment. Small gauge needles are recommended for use when injecting SC or IM. Subcutaneous injections or oral dosages may be slowly or poorly absorbed in animals that are hypovolemic.

Because 6–12 hours may be required for new clotting factors to be synthesized after phytonadione administration, emergency needs for clotting factors must be provided by giving blood products.

Reproductive/Nursing Safety

Phytonadione crosses the placenta only in small amounts, but its safety has not been documented in pregnant animals. In humans, the FDA categorizes this drug as category *C* for use during pregnancy (*Animal studies have shown an adverse effect on the fetus, but there are no adequate studies in humans; or there are no animal reproduction studies and no adequate studies in humans.*)

Vitamin K is excreted in maternal milk, but is unlikely to have negative effects in nursing offspring.

Overdosage/Acute Toxicity

Phytonadione is relatively non-toxic, and it would be unlikely that toxic clinical signs would result after a single overdosage. However, refer to the Adverse Effects section for more information.

Drug Interactions

The following drug interactions have either been reported or are theoretical in humans or animals receiving phytonadione and may be of significance in veterinary patients:

■ **ANTIBIOTICS, ORAL:** Although chronic antibiotic therapy should have no significant effect on the absorption of phytonadione, these drugs may decrease the numbers of vitamin K producing bacteria in the gut

■ **MINERAL OIL:** Concomitant administration of oral mineral oil may reduce the absorption of oral vitamin K.

■ **WARFARIN:** As would be expected, phytonadione antagonizes the anticoagulant effects of coumarin (and indanedione agents. There are many drugs that may prolong or enhance the effects of anticoagulants and antagonize some of the therapeutic effects of phytonadione, including: **phenylbutazone, aspirin, chloramphenicol, sulfonamides diazoxide, allopurinol, cimetidine, metronidazole, anabolic steroids, erythromycin, ketoconazole, propranolol,** and **thyroid** drugs.

Doses

■ **DOGS/CATS:**

For adjunctive therapy of acute liver failure:
a) 1–5 mg/kg PO or SC q24h (Rosanski 2002)

For anticoagulant rodenticide toxicity:
a) For the exposed but non-bleeding patient, inducing emesis along with repeated doses of activated charcoal and cathartic will help reduce further absorption of the rodenticide. If the exposure dose is high enough, phytonadione at

1.25–2.5 mg/kg PO twice daily with a fatty meal for 2-4 weeks. Only give SC with starting dose if patient is vomiting or activated charcoal was administered.

In the bleeding patient, decontamination procedures are generally not worthwhile due to time delay between ingestion and onset of bleeding. When clotting times are prolonged, plasma transfusions are a necessity. Blood transfusions may be necessary if the patient is severely anemic. Phytonadione at 2.5 mg/kg PO twice daily with a fatty meal should be administered for a minimum of 4 weeks. Other supportive measures may include broad-spectrum antibiotics, oxygen therapy and exercise restriction. Removing free blood from the thoracic cavity should only be performed when respiratory function is severely compromised. It is recommended that clotting times be re-examined 2–3 days following cessation of phytonadione therapy. (Talcott 2008)

b) In symptomatic patients, give a loading dose of 2.5–5 mg/kg PO. In cases of large ingestions, begin phytonadione therapy at 3–5 mg/kg PO divided twice daily. Treat pocket pets at the high end of this dosage range. SC dosing may be required in vomiting or anorectic patients or pocket pets, but PO is preferred. For first-generation anticoagulants, treatment with phytonadione for 14 days is usually sufficient. For a second-generation anticoagulant or if the anticoagulant is unknown, treatment should be instituted for at least 30 days. Absorption is enhanced when a fatty meal is fed at the same time the dose is given. In all patients, check the PT or PIVKA 48 hours after stopping phytonadione therapy, and if the test result is prolonged, continue treatment for another week. Again, a patient must be tested for adequate clotting 48 hours after phytonadione has been discontinued. (Merola 2002)

■ **RABBITS, RODENTS, SMALL MAMMALS:**

a) Stabilize the animal if clinical signs are evident. Transfusions with whole blood or plasma may be necessary to replace clotting factors. Decontamination is only effective early; do **not** attempt to induce emesis in rodents, rabbits, or birds. 3% hydrogen peroxide is an effective emetic for ferrets. Following its use, the mouth could be gently rinsed with water to dilute the remaining peroxide. (An option would be apomorphine 5 mg/kg SC, however, adverse effects include sedation or hyperexcitability.) Activated charcoal (1–3 grams/kg body weight) effectively adsorbs anticoagulants and can facilitate excretion via the feces. Injectable forms of phytonadione can be given PO at 5 mg/kg/day divided q8-12h. Give with a fatty meal, such as peanut butter, to enhance absorption. Phytonadione should not be given IV; SC administration can cause anaphylaxis. (Richardson & Gwaltney-Brant 2002)

b) In symptomatic patients, give a loading dose of 2.5–5 mg/kg PO. In cases of large ingestions, begin phytonadione therapy at 3–5 mg/kg PO divided twice daily. Treat pocket pets at the high end of this dosage range. SC dosing may be required in vomiting or anorectic patients or pocket pets, but PO is preferred. For first-generation anticoagulants, treatment with phytonadione for 14 days is usually sufficient. For a second-generation anticoagulant or if the anticoagulant is unknown, treatment should be instituted for at least 30 days. Absorption is enhanced when a fatty meal is fed at the same time the dose is given. In all patients, check the PT or PIVKA 48 hours after stopping phytonadione therapy, and if the test result is prolonged, continue treatment for another week. Again, a patient must be tested for adequate clotting 48 hours after phytonadione has been discontinued. (Merola 2002)

■ **CATTLE:**

For anticoagulant rodenticide toxicity:

a) Initially 0.5–2.5 mg/kg IV in D_5W at a rate of 10 mg/minute. Subsequent doses may be given IM or SC. Second generation agents may require 3–4 weeks of treatment. (Bailey 1986)

b) 0.5–2.5 mg/kg IM, if IV use is necessary (avoid if possible), dilute in saline or D_5W/saline and give very slowly (not to exceed 5 mg/minute). (Upson 1988)

c) For acute hypoprothrombinemia with hemorrhage: 0.5–2.5 mg/kg IV, not to exceed 10 mg/minute in mature animals and 5 mg/minute in newborn and very young animals.

For non-acute hypoprothrombinemia: 0.5–2.5 mg/kg IM or SC (Label directions; *Veda-K₁®*—Vedco)

For sweet clover (*Melilotus* spp.) or lespedeza (*Lespedeza* sp.) toxicity:

a) 1–1.5 mg/kg SC for several days, remove from source, avoid stress/injury. (Oehme 2009)

■ **HORSES:**

For warfarin (or related compounds) toxicity:

a) 500 mg SC q4–6h until one-stage prothrombin time (OSPT) returns to normal control values. Whole blood or fresh

plasma may also be necessary early in the course of treatment. (Byars 1987)

b) 0.5–2.5 mg/kg IM, if IV use is necessary (avoid if possible), dilute in saline or D_5W/saline and give very slowly (not to exceed 5 mg/minute). (Upson 1988)

■ **SWINE:**

For warfarin (or related compounds) toxicity:

a) 0.5–2.5 mg/kg IM, if IV use is necessary (avoid if possible), dilute in saline or D_5W/saline and give very slowly (not to exceed 5 mg/minute). (Upson 1988)

■ **SHEEP & GOATS:**

For warfarin (or related compounds) toxicity:

a) 0.5–2.5 mg/kg IM, if IV use is necessary (avoid if possible), dilute in saline or D_5W/saline and give very slowly (not to exceed 5 mg/minute). (Upson 1988)

■ **BIRDS:**

For hemorrhagic disorders:

a) 0.25–0.5 mL/kg IM of the 10 mg/mL injectable product. Commonly used before surgery where hemorrhage is anticipated. (McDonald 1989)

b) 0.2–2.5 mg/kg IM as needed; usually only 1–2 injections are required. May also be used prophylactically when amprolium and sulfas are administered. (Clubb 1986)

Monitoring

■ Clinical efficacy (lack of hemorrhage)

■ One-stage prothrombin time (OSPT); INR

Client Information

■ Because it may take several weeks to eliminate some of the anticoagulant rodenticides from the body, clients must be counseled on the importance of continuing to administer the drug (phytonadione) for as long as instructed or renewed bleeding may occur.

■ Unless otherwise instructed, oral phytonadione should be administered with food, preferably foods high in fat content.

■ During therapy, animals should be kept quiet whether at home or hospitalized.

Chemistry/Synonyms

A naphthoquinone derivative identical to naturally occurring vitamin K_1, phytonadione occurs as a clear, yellow to amber, viscous liquid. It is insoluble in water, slightly soluble in alcohol and soluble in lipids.

Phytonadione may also be known as: methylphytylnaphthochinonum, phylloquinone, phytomenadionum, phytomenadione, vitamin K_1, *AmTech®, Glakay®, Aqua-Mephyton®, K1®, K-Caps®, K-Chews®, K-Ject®, KP®, Kanakion®, Kanavit®, Kavit®, Kaytwo®, Kaywan®, Kenadion®, Konakion®, Konakion Novum®,*

Mephyton®, Pertix-Solo®, Veda-K1, Vikatron®, Vita-Jec®, or *Vitamon K®.*

Storage/Stability

Phytonadione should be protected from light at all times, as it is quite sensitive to light. If used as an intravenous infusion, the container should be wrapped with an opaque material. Tablets and capsules should be stored in well-closed, light-resistant containers.

Compatibility/Compounding Considerations

Because most veterinary clinicians state that phytonadione is contraindicated for intravenous use; consult specialized references or a hospital pharmacist for more specific information on compatibility of phytonadione with other agents.

Dosage Forms/Regulatory Status

VETERINARY-LABELED PRODUCTS:

Phytonadione Oral Capsules: 25 mg; *K-Caps®* (Butler), *Veda-K1® Capsules* (Vedco), *Veta-K₁®* (Bimeda), *Vitamin K₁* (Phoenix Pharmaceutical, RXV); (Rx) Labeled for use in dogs and cats.

Phytonadione Oral Capsules: 50 mg; *Vitamin K₁ Double Strength®* (Phoenix); (Rx) Labeled for use in dogs.

Phytonadione Oral Tablets, Chewable: 25 mg, 50 mg; *Vitamin K₁ Chewable®* (V.E.T.), *Vitamin K1 Chewablet®* (Pala-Tech), *K-Chews®* (Butler); (Rx). Products may be labeled for use in dogs and cats.

Phytonadione Aqueous Colloidal Solution for Injection: 10 mg/mL in 30 mL and 100 mL vials; *K-Ject®* (Butler), *Veda-K₁® Injection* (Vedco), *Vita-Jec®* (RXV), *Vitamin K₁* (Vet Tek, Bimeda, Neogen, Phoenix Pharmaceutical); (Rx) Labeled for use dogs, cats, cattle, calves, horses, swine, sheep, and goats. No withdrawal times listed.

HUMAN-LABELED PRODUCTS:

Phytonadione Oral Tablets: 5 mg; *Mephyton®* (Aton); (Rx)

Phytonadione Injection, Emulsion: 2 mg/mL & 10 mg/mL in 0.5 mL & 1 mL amps; generic (Hospira); (Rx)

References

Bailey, E.M. (1986). Management and treatment of toxicosis in cattle. *Current Veterinary Therapy 2: Food Animal Practice.* JL Howard Ed. Philadelphia, WB Saunders: 341–354.

Byars, T.D. (1987). Disseminated Intravascular Coagulation. *Current Therapy in Equine Medicine 2.* NE Robinson Ed. Phialdelphia, WB Saunders: 306–309.

Clubb, S.L. (1986). Therapeutics: Individual and Flock Treatment Regimens. *Clinical Avian Medicine and Surgery.* GJ Harrison and LR Harrison Eds. Philadelphia, W.B. Saunders: 327–355.

McDonald, S.E. (1989). Summary of medications for use in psittacine birds. *JAAV* 3(3): 120–127.

Merola, V. (2002). Anticoagulant rodenticides: Deadly for pets, dangerous for pets. *Vet Med*(October): 716–722.

Oehme, F. (2009). The 10 Most Common Poisonings in Production Animals I. Proceedings: WVC. Accessed via: Veterinary Information Network. http://goo.gl/alNR5

Richardson, J.A. & S. Gwaltney-Brant (2002). Tips for treating anticoagulant rodenticide toxicity in small mammals. *Exotic DVM* 4(1): 5.

Rosanski, E. (2002). Acute liver failure. Proceedings: Tufts Animal Expo. Accessed via: Veterinary Information Network. http://goo.gl/BiTmT

Talcott, P. (2008). Common and Uncommon Toxins for "Roaming Around" Pets. Proceedings: WVC. http://goo.gl/o5xPu

Upson, D.W. (1988). *Handbook of Clinical Veterinary Pharmacology.* Manhattan, Dan Upson Enterprises.

PIMOBENDAN

(pi-moe-*ben*-den)   Vetmedin®

INODILATOR

Prescriber Highlights

▶ Oral drug that may be useful in treatment of congestive heart failure in dogs

▶ Give on an empty stomach

▶ May increase risks for arrhythmias

Uses/Indications

Pimobendan is used to treat dogs with congestive heart failure (CHF) secondary to dilated cardiomyopathy (DCM) or chronic mitral valve insufficiency (CMVI), myxomatous/degenerative mitral valve disease (MMVD, DMVD). Two recent studies (Häggström *et al.* 2008; Lombard, C.W. *et al.* 2006) have shown that in dogs with MMVD and heart failure pimobendan can improve survival times and quality of life when compared with standard treatment consisting of an ACE inhibitor and furosemide. A study done in Doberman Pinschers concluded that pimobendan should be used as first-line therapy in Doberman Pinschers for the treatment of CHF caused by DCM (O'Grady, M. *et al.* 2008). Pimobendan has been shown that it may be–viable as a first line or adjunctive treatment option for dogs with PHT secondary to mitral valve disease (Atkinson *et al.* 2009). In the 2009 ACVIM Consensus Statement: Guidelines for the Diagnosis and Treatment of Canine Chronic Valvular Heart Disease (Atkins *et al.* 2009) the panel recommended to incorporate pimobendan (0.25–0.3 mg/kg PO q12h) in the acute and chronic treatment of stage C heart failure (Patients have a structural abnormality and current or previous clinical signs of heart failure caused by CVHD).

Ongoing studies may help determine if pimobendan should be used in the occult or preclinical stage of heart failure, or if additional significant benefit occurs when used concurrently with an ACE inhibitor.

While pimobendan is not FDA-approved for use in cats, there is some anecdotal evidence for use in restrictive and dilated cardiomyopathy. One small (11 cats) case series has been reported. However, since cats with heart failure predominantly have hypertrophic cardiomyopathy and positive inotropic therapy is generally contraindicated, it probably has a limited role in cats (Cote 2008).

Pharmacology/Actions

Pimobendan is a so-called inodilator; it has both inotropic and vasodilator effects. Pimobendan usually decreases heart rate (negative chronotrope) in animals with CHF. Its inotropic effects occur via inhibition of phosphodiesterase III (PDE-III) and by increasing intracellular calcium sensitivity in the cardiac contractility apparatus. Cardiac contractility is enhanced without an increase in myocardial oxygen consumption, as pimobendan does not increase intracellular calcium levels. Commercially available pimobendan is a 50:50 mixture of *l*- and *d*-isomers. In dogs, the *l*-isomer of pimobendan has about 1.5X greater inotropic activity than the *d*-isomer. Pimobendan's vasodilator effects are via vascular PDE-III inhibition and both arterial and venous dilation occur. Pimobendan also possesses antithrombotic activity.

Pharmacokinetics

In dogs, following a single oral administration of 0.25 mg/kg pimobendan peak levels of the parent compound and the active metabolite were observed 1–4 hours post-dose (mean: 2 and 3 hours, respectively). Food decreased the bioavailability of an aqueous solution of pimobendan, but the effect of food on the absorption of pimobendan from chewable tablets is unknown. The steady-state volume of distribution of pimobendan is 2.6 L/kg. Protein binding of pimobendan and the active metabolite in dog plasma is >90%. Pimobendan is oxidatively demethylated to a pharmacologically active metabolite that is then conjugated with sulfate or glucuronic acid and excreted mainly via feces. Clearance of pimobendan is approximately 90 mL/min/kg, and the terminal elimination half-lives of pimobendan and the active metabolite are approximately 0.5 hours and 2 hours, respectively. Plasma levels of pimobendan and the active metabolite were below quantifiable levels by 4 and 8 hours respectively after oral administration.

In humans with heart failure, pimobendan is rapidly absorbed with peak levels occurring in less than one hour after dosing. The volume of distribution was about 3.2 L/kg; clearance about 25 mL/min/kg. Terminal half-life is slightly less than 3 hours.

Contraindications/Precautions/Warnings

Pimobendan is contraindicated in animals hypersensitive to it, with hypertrophic cardiomyopathy, aortic stenosis, or any other condition where an augmentation of cardiac output is inappropriate for functional or anatomic reasons. It should be used with caution in patients with uncontrolled cardiac arrhythmias.

The label states the drug has not been evaluated in dogs younger than 6 months of age, dogs with congenital heart defects, diabetes mellitus or other serious metabolic diseases, dogs used for breeding, or pregnant or lactating bitches.

Adverse Effects

The primary adverse effects that have been noted in dogs are gastrointestinal effects. There is some evidence that pimobendan may increase the development of arrhythmias. Atrial fibrillation or increased ventricular ectopic beats have been reported in dogs on pimobendan, but because cardiomyopathy can cause arrhythmias, a causative effect has not been fully established. A trial of pimobendan in humans with heart failure demonstrated an increased mortality rate while on the drug, but this result has not been duplicated in canine studies. In a US field trial (56 day) done in dogs, the adverse effect incidence (at least one occurrence reported per dog) was: poor appetite (38%), lethargy (33%), diarrhea (30%), dyspnea (29%), azotemia (14%), weakness and ataxia (13%), pleural effusion (10%), syncope (9%), cough (7%), sudden death (6%), ascites (6%), and heart murmur (3%). As experience with the drug continues, a more detailed adverse effect profile will be developed.

In a study comparing cardiac adverse effects of pimobendan with benazepril (Chetboul *et al.* 2007), dogs with mitral valve regurgitation had increases in systolic function but also developed worsening mitral valve disease and specific mitral valve lesions (acute hemorrhages, endocardial papilloform hyperplasia on the dorsal surfaces of the leaflets, and infiltration of *chordae tendinae* by glycosaminoglycans) not seen in the benazepril group. The authors recommend that patients with mitral valve disease that are treated chronically with pimobendan be regularly and cautiously examined for any worsening mitral valvular lesions and regurgitation.

Reproductive/Nursing Safety

The label states the drug has not been evaluated in dogs used for breeding, or pregnant or lactating bitches. When pimobendan was given in high dosages (300 mg/kg) to pregnant laboratory animals, increased resorptions occurred. Rabbits given 100 mg/kg showed no adverse fetal effects.

No information on the safety of pimobendan during nursing was located.

Overdosage/Acute Toxicity

There were 20 exposures to pimobendan reported to the ASPCA Animal Poison Control Center (APCC) during 2008-2009. In these cases, 19 were dogs with 4 showing clinical signs, and 1 was a ferret that showed no clinical signs. Common findings in dogs included tachycardia.

Dose dependent increases in heart rate were seen at 2 and 8 mg/kg IV in a 4-week study in dogs. In a six-month toxicity study in dogs, mild heart murmurs developed in 1 dog at 3x (1.5 mg/kg) and in 2 dogs at 5x (2.5 mg/kg). The murmurs were non-clinical. Treatment:

Decontamination (induce emesis and give activated charcoal early), monitor heart rate, blood pressure, and EKG if needed. Control hypotension with IV fluids and dopamine.

Drug Interactions

The drug is labeled as being used safely with furosemide, digoxin, enalapril, atenolol, nitroglycerin, hydralazine, diltiazem, antiparasitic products (including heartworm preventative), antibiotics, famotidine, theophylline, levothyroxin, diphenhydramine, hydrocodone, metoclopramide and butorphanol.

The U.K. label states that "pimobendan-induced increases in contractility of the heart are attenuated in the presence of the calcium antagonist **verapamil** and the beta-antagonist **propranolol**." It is assumed that other drugs in these categories (*e.g.*, diltiazem, atenolol) may also have effect.

Milrinone, a human drug that also inhibits phosphodiesterase, has been used with a variety of other drugs (*e.g.*, cardiac glycosides, lidocaine, hydralazine, prazosin, quinidine, nitroglycerin, furosemide, warfarin, spironolactone, heparin, potassium) without apparent problems, but because pimobendan also increases calcium sensitivity, comparing the two drugs may not be fully informative.

Laboratory Considerations

■ No laboratory interactions or special considerations were located.

Doses

■ **DOGS:**

a) For management of the signs of mild, moderate or severe congestive heart failure due to AV valve insufficiency or dilated cardiomyopathy: 0.5 mg/kg total daily dose. Divide daily dose into two portions that are not necessarily equal (using whole and half tablets) and administer approximately 12 hours apart. (Label directions; *Vetmedin*®—B-I)

b) For treatment of congestive heart failure secondary to myxomatous mitral valve disease (MMVD): 0.4–0.6 mg/kg PO divided twice daily (Lombard, C. 2004)

c) For treatment of heart failure secondary to dilated cardiomyopathy or chronic mitral valve insufficiency: 0.25 mg/kg PO twice daily (O'Grady, MR *et al.* 2004)

d) 0.2–0.6 mg/kg PO divided q12h (U.K. Label directions; *Vetmedin*®—BI; 2003)

e) As an adjunctive drug for the emergency treatment of CHF (if the case is not overtly critical and a strong positive oral inotrope is needed): 0.1–0.3 mg/kg PO q12h. (Erling & Mazzaferro 2008)

f) For adjunctive treatment of acute or chronic stage D heart failure [patients have clinical signs of failure refractory to standard treatment for Stage C heart failure

from CVHD (chronic valvular heart disease)]: No consensus was reached by the panel regarding the following, but some panelists increase the pimobendan dose to 0.3 mg/kg PO to three times daily. Because this dosage recommendation is outside of the FDA-approved labeling for pimobendan, this use of the drug should be explained to, and approved by the client. (Atkins *et al.* 2009)

■ **CATS:**

a) For management of myocardial failure (DCM), especially if the DCM is not associated with taurine deficiency: However, because this is a relatively rare condition in cats, there is little information about clinical efficacy. Additionally, the manufacturers have not conducted any trials in cats to determine efficacy or safety, but there do not appear to be any obvious safety concerns. The dose of pimobendan in cats is 1.25–1.5 mg/cat PO q12hrs. (Rishniw 2005)

Monitoring

■ Cardiovascular parameters used to monitor heart function, including ECG (rate/rhythm), blood pressure, echo studies, clinical signs, etc.

Client Information

■ Give medication approximately one hour before feeding.

■ Pimobendan is a treatment and not a cure for heart failure.

■ Compliance with the veterinarian's instructions is essential.

■ Keep out of reach of children.

Chemistry/Synonyms

A benzimidazole-derivative phosphodiesterase inhibitor, pimobendan occurs as a white or slightly yellowish, hygroscopic powder. It is practically insoluble in water and slightly soluble in acetone or methyl alcohol. Pimobendans's chemical name is: 4,5-Dihydro-6-[2-(p-methyoxyphenyl)-5-benzimidazolyl]-5-methyl-3(2H)pyridazinone. It has a molecular weight of 334.4.

Pimobendan may also be known as: UDCG-115, *Acardi*®, and *Vetmedin*®.

Storage/Stability

Unless otherwise labeled, pimobendan chewable tablets or capsules should be stored at room temperature below 25°C (77°F) in a dry place.

Dosage Forms/Regulatory Status

VETERINARY-LABELED PRODUCTS:

Pimobendan Chewable Tablets: 1.25 mg, 2.5 mg and 5 mg: *Vetmedin*® (B-I); (Rx). FDA-approved for use in dogs.

HUMAN-LABELED PRODUCTS: None

References

Atkins, C., J. Bonagura, et al. (2009). Guidelines for the Diagnosis and Treatment of Canine Chronic Valvular Heart Disease. *Journal of Veterinary Internal Medicine* 23(6): 1142–1150.

Atkinson, K., D. Fine, et al. (2009). Evaluation of Pimobendan and N-Terminal Probrain Natriuretic Peptide in the Treatment of Pulmonary Hypertension Secondary to Degenerative Mitral Valve Disease in Dogs. *Journal of Veterinary Internal Medicine* 23(6): 1190–1196.

Chetboul, V., H. Lefebvre, et al. (2007). Comparative adverse cardiac effects of pimobendan and benazepril monotherapy in dogs with mild degenerative mitral valve disease: a prospective, controlled, blinded, and randomized study. *J Vet Intern Med* 21(4): 742–753.

Cote, E. (2008). Positive Inotropes: Digoxin, Pimobendan, and Others. Proceedings: WORLDVC. Accessed via: Veterinary Information Network. http://goo.gl/9iNIC

Erling, P. & E.M. Mazzaferro (2008). Left-sided congestive heart failure in dogs: Treatment and monitoring of emergency patients. *Compendium-Continuing Education for Veterinarians* 30(2): 94–+.

Häggström, J., A. Boswood, et al. (2008). Effect of Pimobendan or Benazepril Hydrochloride on Survival Times in Dogs with Congestive Heart Failure Caused by Naturally Occurring Myxomatous Mitral Valve Disease: The QUEST Study. *Journal of Veterinary Internal Medicine* 22(5): 1124–1135.

Lombard, C. (2004). Pimobendan in mitral regurgitation vs dilated cardiomyopathy. Proceedings: ACVIM Forum, Minneapolis. Accessed via: Veterinary Information Network. http://goo.gl/Gkd0Y

Lombard, C.W., O. Jons, et al. (2006). Clinical efficacy of pimobendan versus benazepril for the treatment of acquired atrioventricular valvular disease in dogs. *Journal of the American Animal Hospital Association* 42(4): 249–261.

O'Grady, M., S. Minors, et al. (2008). Effect of Pimobendan on Case Fatality Rate in Doberman Pinschers with Congestive Heart Failure Caused by Dilated Cardiomyopathy. *Journal of Veterinary Internal Medicine* 22(4): 897–904.

O'Grady, M., S. Minors, et al. (2004). The assessment and ability of pimobendan to increase the frequency of ventricular ectopy in dogs with CHF due to DCM and chronic mitral valve insufficiency. Proceedings: ACVIM Forum, Minneapolis. Accessed via: Veterinary Information Network. http://goo.gl/fEil9

Rishniw, M. (2005). "Pimobendan: Medical FAQs." 2010, http://goo.gl/7xxAa.

PIPERACILLIN SODIUM

(**pype**-er-ah-sill-in)   Pipracil®

EXTENDED SPECTRUM PENICILLIN

Prescriber Highlights

▶ Extended-action penicillin, with good gram-negative spectrum, including many strains of Pseudomonas

▶ Limited experience in veterinary medicine, but appears quite safe

▶ Also available with a beta-lactamase inhibitor (tazobactam); see the next monograph

Uses/Indications

Although veterinary experience is limited with piperacillin or piperacillin/tazobactam, these drugs have expanded coverage against many bacteria and may be suitable for empiric use until culture and susceptibility data are available, or for surgical prophylaxis when gram-negative or mixed aerobic/anaerobic infections are concerns.

Pharmacology/Actions

Piperacillin is a bactericidal, extended action acylaminopenicillin that inhibits septum formation and cell wall synthesis in susceptible bacteria. It has a wide spectrum of activity against many aerobic and anaerobic gram-positive (including many enterococci) and gram-negative bacteria. It has a similar spectrum of activity as the aminopenicillins, but with additional activity against several gram-negative organisms of the family Enterobacteriaceae, including many strains of *Pseudomonas aeruginosa*. Like the aminopenicillins, it is susceptible to inactivation by beta-lactamases. The addition of a beta-lactamase inhibitor (tazobactam) in the product *Zosyn*® (see next monograph), increases piperacillin's spectrum of activity against many beta lactamase producing strains of bacteria.

Pharmacokinetics

Limited information is available for veterinary species. In mares, piperacillin has an elimination half-life of about 7 hours. IM bioavailability is 86% and protein binding about 19%.

In humans, piperacillin is not appreciably absorbed from the gut so it must be administered parenterally. After IM administration peak levels occur in about 30 minutes. The drug exhibits low protein binding and has a volume of distribution of 0.1L/kg. It is widely distributed into many tissues and fluids including lung, gallbladder, intestinal mucosa, uterus, bile, and interstitial fluid. With inflamed meninges, piperacillin levels in the CSF are approximately 30% those in serum. If meninges are normal, CSF concentrations are only about 6% of serum levels. Piperacillin crosses the placenta and is distributed into milk in low concentrations. Piperacillin is metabolized somewhat in the liver to a desethyl metabolite that has only minimal antibacterial activity. Piperacillin is primarily (68%) eliminated unchanged in the urine via active tubular secretion and glomerular filtration; it is also excreted in the bile. Elimination half-life in humans is approximately one hour.

Contraindications/Precautions/Warnings

Piperacillin should not be used in patients with documented hypersensitive reactions to a beta-lactam.

Because of sodium content, high dosages of piperacillin may adversely affect patients with cardiac failure or hypernatremic conditions.

Dosage adjustment may be required in patients with significantly decreased renal function (CrCl <40 mL/min).

Adverse Effects

Piperacillin is generally well tolerated. Hypersensitivity reactions are possible. Local effects (thrombophlebitis, etc.) associated with intravenous injection or pain after IM injection may occur. Alterations in gut flora may lead to antibiotic-associated diarrhea.

In humans, piperacillin has caused coagulation abnormalities on occasion, particularly in patients with renal failure. Very high doses may cause neurotoxicity (seizures); again, these are more likely in patients with diminished renal function. Superinfections with *Clostridium difficile* have been reported rarely.

Reproductive/Nursing Safety

Piperacillin is thought relatively safe to use during pregnancy. No teratogenic effects have been attributed to it in either humans or laboratory animals. In humans, the FDA categorizes piperacillin as category *B* for use during pregnancy (*Animal studies have not yet demonstrated risk to the fetus, but there are no adequate studies in pregnant women; or animal studies have shown an adverse effect, but adequate studies in pregnant women have not demonstrated a risk to the fetus in the first trimester of pregnancy, and there is no evidence of risk in later trimesters.*)

Piperacillin is distributed in milk in low concentrations; it is likely safe to use during nursing.

Overdosage/Acute Toxicity

Single overdoses are unlikely to pose much risk although very large overdoses may cause vomiting, diarrhea, or neurotoxicity. Dogs receiving up to 800 mg/kg/day of piperacillin/tazobactam for 6 months demonstrated no serious toxic effects. Doses at 400 mg/kg/day or greater caused some transient effects to the liver (glycogen granules in the cytoplasm and increases in smooth endoplasmic reticulum in hepatocytes) that were mostly reversed after one month.

Treatment for overdoses, if required, is supportive.

Drug Interactions

The following drug interactions have either been reported or are theoretical in humans or animals receiving piperacillin and may be of significance in veterinary patients:

■ **AMINOGLYCOSIDES (amikacin, gentamicin, tobramycin):** *In vitro* studies have demonstrated that penicillins can have synergistic or additive activity against certain bacteria when used with aminoglycosides. Beta-lactam antibiotics, however, can inactivate aminoglycosides *in vitro* and *in vivo* in patients in renal failure or when penicillins are used in massive dosages. Amikacin is considered the most resistant aminoglycoside to this inactivation.

■ **ANTICOAGULANTS:** Because piperacillin may rarely affect platelets, increased monitoring of coagulation parameters is suggested for patients on heparin or warfarin

■ **METHOTREXATE:** Piperacillin may increase MTX serum levels

■ **PROBENECID:** Can reduce the renal tubular secretion of piperacillin thereby maintain-

ing higher systemic levels for longer periods; this potential "beneficial" interaction requires further investigation before dosing recommendations can be made for veterinary patients

■ **VECURONIUM:** Piperacillin may prolong neuromuscular blockade

Laboratory Considerations

■ **Urine glucose determinations** when using cupric sulfate solution (Benedict's Solution, *Clinitest®*): Piperacillin may cause false-positive results; tests utilizing glucose oxidase (*Tes-Tape®, Clinistix®*) are not affected by piperacillin

■ **Aminoglycoside serum quantitative analysis:** As penicillins and other beta-lactams can inactivate aminoglycosides *in vitro* (and *in vivo* in patients in renal failure or when penicillins are used in massive dosages), serum concentrations of aminoglycosides may be falsely decreased if the patient is also receiving beta-lactam antibiotics and the serum is stored prior to analysis. It is recommended that if the aminoglycoside assay is delayed, samples be frozen and, if possible, drawn at times when the beta-lactam antibiotic is at a trough.

■ **Direct antiglobulin (Coombs') tests:** False-positive results may occur

■ **Urine protein:** May produce false-positive urine protein results with the sulfosalicylic acid and boiling test, nitric acid test, or the acetic acid test. Strips using bromophenol blue reagent (*e.g., Multi-Stix®*) do not appear to be affected by high levels of penicillins in the urine.

Doses

■ **DOGS/CATS:**

a) For bacteremia with or without endocarditis: 30 mg/kg IV q6h for 7–14 days. (Calvert & Wall 2006)

b) For respiratory infections: 25–50 mg/kg IV q8h. (Greene & Reinero 2006)

c) Dogs: For systemic treatment of otitis media or proliferative otitis externa complicated by gram-negative (especially Pseudomonas) bacteria: 20 mg/kg SC three times daily. (Bloom 2006)

■ **BIRDS:**

a) For *Bordetella avium* infections: 150 mg/kg IM q8–12h; minimum treatment period is two weeks. (Flammer, K 2006)

b) For susceptible infections: 100 mg/kg IM two to three times daily. (Antinoff 2004)

c) For empirical treatment in Psittacines of gram-negative bacterial infections: 100 mg/kg IM 3-4 times a day if immunocompetent; 4 times a day if immunocompromised. (Flammer, K. 2006)

■ **HORSES:**
a) For susceptible infections: 15–50 mg/kg IV or IM q6–12h. (Bertone & Horspool 2004)

■ **REPTILES:**
a) For susceptible infections: 100 mg/kg route not specified q48h. (Antinoff 2004)

b) Snakes: 100 mg/kg IM q24h (Mader 2004)

Monitoring
Efficacy for the infection treated (WBC, clinical signs, etc.)

Client Information
■ Limited experience in veterinary medicine
■ Best suited for inpatient use

Chemistry/Synonyms
Piperacillin sodium occurs as a white or almost white, hygroscopic powder. It is freely soluble in water or alcohol. A 40% solution has a pH of 5–7.

Piperacillin sodium for injection contains 42.5 mg (1.85 mEq) sodium per gram.

Piperacillin may also be known as: piperacillinum, BL-P 1908, Cl 867, CL 227 193, T 12220, TA 058, *Pipracil®*, and *Pipril®*.

Storage/Stability
Piperacillin powder for injection vials should be stored at controlled room temperature (20–25°C).

Conventional vials should be reconstituted with 5 mL of diluent per gram of piperacillin. Suitable diluents include 0.9% sodium chloride, sterile water for injection, D5W, and bacteriostatic saline or water for injection. Once reconstituted, further dilute for intravenous infusion with 50–150 mL of 0.9% sodium chloride, LRS (must be given within 2 hours) or D5W. IV infusion of diluted products should be over at least 30 minutes. IV infusion from the contents of the reconstituted vials should be administered over at least 3–5 minutes to reduce the chance of vein irritation.

Once reconstituted, vials should be used within 4 hours of initial puncture. The manufacturer recommends not freezing reconstituted vials. IV bags (50–150 mL) containing further diluted product are stable for up to 24 hours at room temperature and one week if refrigerated. As no preservatives are used, sterility is not assured in stored reconstituted products.

Compatibility/Compounding Considerations
For IM use, 5 mL of 0.5% or 1% lidocaine injection (without epinephrine) may be added to a 2 gram vial and used immediately.

Do not mix with aminoglycosides. Intravenous admixture solutions containing potassium, clindamycin, or hydrocortisone sodium succinate are reportedly **compatible** with piperacillin.

Dosage Forms/Regulatory Status
VETERINARY-LABELED PRODUCTS: None

HUMAN-LABELED PRODUCTS:
Piperacillin Sodium Injection (powder for reconstitution): 2 gram, 3 gram, & 4 gram (as base) vials, 40 gram bulk vials; generic (American Pharmaceutical Partners); (Rx)

References

Antinoff, N. (2004). Traumatic injuries in exotic pets. Proceedings: IVECC Symposium. Accessed via: Veterinary Information Network. http://goo.gl/4JjDs

Bertone, J. & L. Horspool (2004). Appendix: Drug and Dosages for use in Equines. *Equine Clinical Pharmacology*, Saunders: 365–380.

Bloom, P. (2006). Practical approach to otitis externa in the dog. Proceedings: Western Vet Conf 2006. Accessed via: Veterinary Information Network. http://goo.gl/a9ogZ

Calvert, C. & M. Wall (2006). Cardiovascular Infections. *Infectious Diseases of the Dog and Cat, 3rd Ed.* C Greene Ed., Elsevier: 841–865.

Flammer, K. (2006). Antibiotic drug selection in companion birds. *Journal of Exotic Pet Medicine* 15(3): 166–176.

Flammer, K. (2006). Managing Avian Bacterial Diseases II. Proceedings: WVC2006. Accessed via: Veterinary Information Network. http://goo.gl/wPvdh

Greene, C. & C. Reinero (2006). Bacterial Respiratory Infections. *Infectious Diseases of the Dog and Cat, 3rd Ed.* C Greene Ed., Elsevier: 866–882.

Mader, D. (2004). Antibiotic therapy in reptiles. Proceedings: WVC2004. Accessed via: Veterinary Information Network. http://goo.gl/G77UM

PIPERACILLIN SODIUM + TAZOBACTAM

(*pype*-er-ah-sill-in; tay-zoh-*bak*-tam)
Zosyn®

EXTENDED SPECTRUM PENICILLIN + BETA-LACTAMASE INHIBITOR

Prescriber Highlights

▶ Extended action parenteral penicillin with a beta lactamase inhibitor; has increased spectrum of activity when compared with piperacillin alone, but is more expensive

▶ Limited experience or research in veterinary medicine, but appears quite safe

Uses/Indications
Although veterinary experience is limited with piperacillin or piperacillin/tazobactam, these drugs have expanded coverage against many bacteria and may be suitable for empiric use until culture and susceptibility data are available, or for surgical prophylaxis when gram-negative or mixed aerobic/anaerobic infections are concerns.

Pharmacology/Actions
For information on piperacillin, refer to the preceding monograph. Tazobactam irreversibly binds to beta-lactamases thereby "protecting" the beta-lactam ring of piperacillin from hydrolysis. When tazobactam is combined with piperacillin, it extends piperacillin's spectrum of activity to those bacteria that produce beta-

lactamases of Richmond-Sykes types II-V that would otherwise render it ineffective. It has slightly more activity than either clavulanate or sulbactam against some Type I beta-lactamases.

Tazobactam has minimal antibacterial activity when used alone, but in combination with piperacillin, synergistic effects may result. It is more potent than sulbactam and, unlike clavulanic acid, does not induce chromosomal beta-lactamases at serum concentrations achieved.

Pharmacokinetics

For information on the pharmacokinetics of piperacillin, refer to the previous monograph; tazobactam's pharmacokinetics generally mirrors that of piperacillin. In dogs, piperacillin reduced the renal clearance of tazobactam, presumably due to competition for tubular secretion.

Contraindications/Precautions/Warnings

Piperacillin/tazobactam should not be used in patients with documented hypersensitive reactions to a beta-lactam or beta-lactamase inhibitor.

Because of sodium content, high dosages of piperacillin/tazobactam may adversely affect patients with cardiac failure or hypernatremic conditions.

Dosage adjustment may be required in patients with significantly decreased renal function (CrCl <40 mL/min).

Adverse Effects

Piperacillin/tazobactam is generally well tolerated. Hypersensitivity reactions are possible. Local effects (thrombophlebitis, etc.) associated with intravenous injection may occur. Alterations in gut flora may lead to antibiotic-associated diarrhea.

In humans, piperacillin has caused coagulation abnormalities on occasion, particularly in patients with renal failure. Very high doses may cause neurotoxicity (seizures); again, this is more likely in patients with diminished renal function. Superinfections with *Clostridium difficile* have been rarely reported.

Reproductive/Nursing Safety

Piperacillin/tazobactam is thought relatively safe to use during pregnancy. No teratogenic effects have been attributed to either drug in either humans or laboratory animals. In humans, the FDA categorizes piperacillin/tazobactam as category *B* for use during pregnancy (*Animal studies have not yet demonstrated risk to the fetus, but there are no adequate studies in pregnant women; or animal studies have shown an adverse effect, but adequate studies in pregnant women have not demonstrated a risk to the fetus in the first trimester of pregnancy, and there is no evidence of risk in later trimesters.*)

Piperacillin is distributed in milk in low concentrations. It is not known if tazobactam enters milk. This drug combination is likely safe to use during nursing.

Overdosage/Acute Toxicity

Single overdoses are unlikely to pose much risk although very large overdoses may cause vomiting, diarrhea, or neurotoxicity. Dogs receiving up to 800 mg/kg/day of piperacillin/tazobactam for 6 months demonstrated no serious toxic effects. Doses at 400 mg/kg/day or greater caused some transient effects to the liver (glycogen granules in the cytoplasm and increases in smooth endoplasmic reticulum in hepatocytes) that were mostly reversed after one month.

Treatment for overdoses, if required, is supportive.

Drug Interactions

The following drug interactions have either been reported or are theoretical in humans or animals receiving piperacillin/tazobactam and may be of significance in veterinary patients:

- ■ **AMINOGLYCOSIDES (amikacin, gentamicin, tobramycin):** *In vitro* studies have demonstrated that penicillins can have synergistic or additive activity against certain bacteria when used with aminoglycosides. Beta-lactam antibiotics however, can inactivate aminoglycosides *in vitro* and *in vivo* in patients in renal failure or when penicillins are used in massive dosages. Amikacin is considered the most resistant aminoglycoside to this inactivation.

- ■ **ANTICOAGULANTS:** Because piperacillin may rarely affect platelets, increased monitoring of coagulation parameters is suggested for patients on heparin or warfarin.

- ■ **METHOTREXATE:** Piperacillin may increase MTX serum levels

- ■ **PROBENECID:** Can reduce the renal tubular secretion of both piperacillin and tazobactam, thereby maintaining higher systemic levels for a longer period of time; this potential "beneficial" interaction requires further investigation before dosing recommendations can be made for veterinary patients.

- ■ **VECURONIUM:** Piperacillin may prolong neuromuscular blockade

Laboratory Considerations

- ■ **Urine glucose determinations** when using cupric sulfate solution (Benedict's Solution, *Clinitest®*): Piperacillin may cause false-positive results. Tests utilizing glucose oxidase (*Tes-Tape®, Clinistix®*) are not affected by piperacillin.

- ■ **Aminoglycoside serum quantitative analysis:** As penicillins and other beta-lactams can inactivate aminoglycosides *in vitro* (and *in vivo* in patients in renal failure or when penicillins are used in massive dosages), serum concentrations of aminoglycosides may be falsely decreased if the patient is also receiving beta-lactam antibiotics and the serum is stored prior to analysis. It is recommended that if the aminoglycoside assay is delayed, samples be frozen and, if possible, drawn at times when the beta-lactam antibiotic is at a trough.

■ **Direct antiglobulin (Coombs') tests:** False-positive results may occur

■ **Urine protein:** Piperacillin may produce false-positive urine protein results with the sulfosalicylic acid and boiling test, nitric acid test, or the acetic acid test. Strips using bromophenol blue reagent (*e.g.*, *Multi-Stix®*) do not appear to be affected by high levels of penicillins in the urine.

Doses

■ **DOGS/CATS:**

a) For single-agent therapy of intra-abdominal sepsis: 50 mg/kg IV or IM q4–6h for 5–7 days; dose extrapolated from human dosage with limited studies in dogs or cats. (Greene 2006)

b) For bacterial sepsis in dogs: 3.375 grams (total dose per dog) IV q6h or 4.5 grams (total dose per dog) IV q8h for 7 days. (Greene *et al.* 2006)

■ **BIRDS:**

a) For susceptible infections: Reconstitute to 200 mg/mL and administer at 100 mg/kg IM q8–12h; for severe polymicrobic bacteremia give 100 mg/kg IV q6h; for preoperative orthopedic or coelomic surgery: 100 mg/kg IM q12h. (Nemetz & Lennox 2006)

Monitoring

■ Efficacy for the infection treated (CBC, clinical signs, etc.)

Client Information

■ Limited experience in veterinary medicine

■ Best suited for inpatient use

Chemistry/Synonyms

Piperacillin sodium/tazobactam sodium occurs as a white or almost white, cryodessicated powder. Tazobactam is structurally related to sulbactam and a penicillanic acid sulfone derivative. The commercially available piperacillin/tazobactam injection contains 2.79 mEq of sodium and 0.25 mg of EDTA per gram of piperacillin.

Tazobactam may also be known as: CL 298741, or YTR 830H. Piperacillin may also be known as piperacillinum, BL-P 1908, Cl 867, CL 227193, T 12220, and TA 058. International trade names for piperacillin/tazobactam include: *Tazobac®*, *Tazocin®*, *Zosyn®* and others.

Storage/Stability

Piperacillin/tazobactam injection vials and *ADD-Vantage* vials should be stored at controlled room temperature (20–25°C).

Conventional vials should be reconstituted with 5 mL of diluent per gram of piperacillin. Suitable diluents include 0.9% sodium chloride, sterile water for injection, and bacteriostatic saline or water for injection. Once reconstituted,

further dilute for intravenous infusion with 50–150 mL of 0.9% sodium chloride, LRS (reformulated product only—see below) or D5W. IV infusion should be over at least 30 minutes.

Once reconstituted, vials should be used immediately. It is recommended to discard after 24 hours if kept at room temperature or 48 hours if stored in the refrigerator. The manufacturer recommends not freezing reconstituted vials. IV bags (50–150 mL) containing further diluted product are stable for up to 24 hours at room temperature and one week if refrigerated. As no preservatives are used, sterility is not assured in stored reconstituted products.

Compatibility/Compounding Considerations

Zosyn® (piperacillin/tazobactam) injection underwent a formulation change in 2006. Sodium citrate (buffer) and EDTA (metal chelator) were added that made it **compatible** with lactated Ringer's injection and via simultaneous Y-site administration at specific concentrations of gentamicin and amikacin (but not tobramycin). This reformulated product has a yellow background behind the *Zosyn®* name on the label. Refer to the package insert for specific information on diluent and concentration compatibility.

Dosage Forms/Regulatory Status

VETERINARY-LABELED PRODUCTS: None

HUMAN-LABELED PRODUCTS:

Piperacillin Sodium & Tazobactam Injection (powder for solution); *Zosyn®* (Wyeth); (Rx):

2.25 grams, concentrate (piperacillin 2 grams/tazobactam 0.25 g), preservative free, in vials and *ADD-Vantage®* vials

3.375 grams (piperacillin 3 grams/tazobactam 0.375 grams) preservative free, in vials and *ADD-Vantage®* vials

4.5 grams (piperacillin 4 grams/tazobactam 0.5 grams) preservative free, in vials and *ADD-Vantage®* vials

40.5 grams (piperacillin 36 grams/ tazobactam 4.5 grams) preservative free; in bulk vials

Also available in 3.375 grams/50 mL (piperacillin 3 grams/tazobactam 0.375 grams) and 4.5 grams/100 mL (piperacillin 4 grams/tazobactam 0.5 grams) premixed, frozen *Galaxy* containers.

References

Greene, C. (2006). Gastrointestinal and Intraabdominal Infections. *Infectious Diseases of the Dog and Cat, 3rd Ed.* C Greene Ed., Elsevier: 883–912.

Greene, C., K. Hartmannn, et al. (2006). Appendix 8: Antimicrobial Drug Formulary. *Infectious Disease of the Dog and Cat.* C Greene Ed., Elsevier: 1186–1333.

Nemetz, L. & A. Lennox (2006). Zosyn: A replacement for Pipracil in the avian patient. Proceedings: AAV 2004. Accessed via: Veterinary Information Network. http://goo.gl/2Ay44

PIPERAZINE

(pi-per-a-*zeen*)   Pipa-Tabs®

ANTIPARASITIC (ASCARIDS)

Prescriber Highlights

▶ Anthelmintic for ascarids in a variety of species

▶ Contraindications: Chronic liver, kidney disease, & gastrointestinal hypomotility.

▶ Caution: Seizure disorders, horses with heavy infestations of P. equorum

▶ Adverse Effects: Unlikely, but diarrhea, emesis, or ataxia possible

Uses/Indications

Piperazine is used for the treatment of ascarids in dogs, cats, horses, swine and poultry. Piperazine is considered safe to use in animals with concurrent gastroenteritis and during pregnancy.

Pharmacology/Actions

Piperazine is thought to exert "curare-like" effects on susceptible nematodes, thereby paralyzing or narcotizing the worm and allowing it to be passed out with the feces. The neuromuscular blocking effect is believed to be caused by blocking acetylcholine at the myoneural junction. In ascarids, succinic acid production is also inhibited.

Pharmacokinetics

Piperazine and its salts are reportedly readily absorbed from the proximal sections of the GI tract and the drug is metabolized and excreted by the kidneys. Absorptive, distribution, and elimination kinetics on individual species were not located.

Contraindications/Precautions/Warnings

Piperazine should be considered contraindicated in patients with chronic liver or kidney disease, and those with gastrointestinal hypomotility. There is some evidence in humans that high-dose piperazine may provoke seizures in patients with a history of seizures, or with renal disease.

If used in horses with heavy infestations of *P. equorum*, rupture or blockage of intestines is possible due to the rapid death and detachment of the worm.

Adverse Effects

Adverse effects are uncommon at recommended doses, but diarrhea, emesis, and ataxia may be noted in dogs or cats. Horses and foals generally tolerate the drug quite well, even at high dosage rates, but a transient softening of the feces may be seen. Other adverse effects have been seen at toxic dosages; refer to the Overdosage section below for more information.

Reproductive/Nursing Safety

In a system evaluating the safety of drugs in canine and feline pregnancy (Papich 1989), this drug is categorized as class: *A (Probably safe. Although specific studies may not have proved he safety of all drugs in dogs and cats, there are no reports of adverse effects in laboratory animals or women.)*

No information was located on use during nursing, but it probably is safe to use.

Overdosage/Acute Toxicity

Acute massive overdosage can lead to paralysis and death, but the drug is generally considered to have a wide margin of safety. The oral LD_{50} of piperazine adipate in mice is 11.4 grams/kg.

In cats, adverse effects occur within 24 hours after a toxic dose is ingested. Emesis, weakness, dyspnea, muscular fasciculations of ears, whiskers, tail and eyes, rear limb ataxia, hypersalivation, depression, dehydration, head-pressing, positional nystagmus and slowed pupillary responses have all been described after toxic ingestions. Many of these effects may also be seen in dogs after toxic piperazine ingestions.

Treatment is symptomatic and supportive. If ingestion was recent, use of activated charcoal and a cathartic has been suggested. Intravenous fluid therapy and keeping the animal in a quiet, dark place is recommended. Recovery generally takes place within 3–4 days.

Drug Interactions

The following drug interactions have either been reported or are theoretical in humans or animals receiving piperazine and may be of significance in veterinary patients:

■ **CHLORPROMAZINE:** Although data conflicts, piperazine and chlorpromazine may precipitate seizures if used concomitantly

■ **LAXATIVES:** The use of purgatives (laxatives) with piperazine is not recommended as the drug may be eliminated before its full efficacy is established

■ **PYRANTEL/MORANTEL:** Piperazine and pyrantel/morantel have antagonistic modes of action and should generally not be used together

Laboratory Considerations

■ Piperazine can have an effect on **uric acid** blood levels, but references conflict with regard to the effect. Both falsely high and low values have been reported; interpret results cautiously.

Doses

Caution: Piperazine is available in several salts that contain varying amounts of piperazine base (see Chemistry below). Many of the doses listed below do not specify what salt (if any) is used in the dosage calculations. If the dose is in question, refer to the actual product information for the product you are using.

■ **DOGS:**

For treatment of ascarids (**Note:** Because larval stages in the host's tissues may not be affected by the drug, many clinicians recommend retreating about 2–3 weeks after the first dose):

a) 45–65 mg of base/kg PO; for pups less than 2.5 kg: 150 mg maximum. (Cornelius & Roberson 1986)

b) 110 mg/kg PO (Chiapella 1989)

c) 100 mg/kg PO; repeat in 3 weeks (Morgan 1988)

d) 20–30 mg/kg PO once (Davis 1985)

e) 110 mg/kg PO; repeat in 21 days (Kirk 1989)

f) 45–65 mg/kg (as base) PO (Roberson 1988)

■ **CATS:**

For treatment of ascarids (**Note:** Because larval stages in the host's tissues may not be affected by the drug, many clinicians recommend retreating about 2–3 weeks after the first dose):

a) 45–65 mg of base/kg PO; 150 mg maximum (Cornelius & Roberson 1986)

b) 110 mg/kg PO (Chiapella 1989)

c) 100 mg/kg PO; repeat in 3 weeks (Morgan 1988)

d) 20–30 mg/kg PO once (Davis 1985)

e) 110 mg/kg PO; repeat in 21 days (Kirk 1989)

f) 45–65 mg/kg (as base) PO (Roberson 1988)

■ **RABBITS, RODENTS, SMALL MAMMALS:**

a) **Mice, rats, hamsters, gerbils, and rabbits:** For pinworms: Piperazine citrate in drinking water at 3 grams/liter for 2 weeks. (Burke 1999)

b) **Rabbits:** For Pinworms: Piperazine citrate 100 mg/kg PO q24h for 2 days. Piperazine adipate: Adults: 200–500 mg/kg PO q24h for 2 days. Young rabbits: 750 mg/kg, PO once daily for 2 days. Wash the perianal area. (Ivey & Morrisey 2000)

c) **Mice, Rats, Gerbils, Hamsters, Guinea pigs, Chinchillas:** For pinworms/tapeworms using piperazine citrate: 2–5 mg/mL drinking water for 7 days, off 7 days and repeat (Adamcak & Otten 2000)

■ **HORSES:**

There are combination products available for use in horses (see Dosage Forms/Preparations section) that contain piperazine with increased efficacy against nematodes and other helminths. Refer to the individual products' package insert for more information.

a) 110 mg/kg (base) PO; repeat in 3–4 weeks. Retreating at 10-week intervals for

P. equorum infections in young animals is recommended. (Roberson 1988)

b) 200 mg/kg, PO. Maximum of 80 grams in adults, 60 grams in yearlings, and 30 grams in foals. (Brander *et al.* 1982)

■ **CATTLE, SHEEP & GOATS:**

Because of high resistance of many nematode species to piperazine, it is rarely used alone in these species.

■ **SWINE:**

For *Ascaris suum* and *Oesophagostomum*:

a) 0.2–0.4% in the feed, or 0.1–0.2% in the drinking water. All medicated water or feed must be consumed within 12 hours, so fasting or withholding water overnight may be beneficial to ensure adequate dosing; retreat in 2 months. Safe in young animals, and during pregnancy. Drug withdrawal times not determined for swine. (Paul 1986)

b) 110 mg/kg (as base). Citrate salt usually used in feed as a one-day treatment, and hexahydrate in drinking water. Dose must be consumed in 8–12 hours. Withholding water or feed the previous night may be beneficial. (Roberson 1988)

■ **BIRDS:**

a) For ascarids in poultry (not effective in psittacines): 100–500 mg/kg PO once; repeat in 10–14 days (Clubb 1986)

b) For nematodes: Piperazine citrate: 45–100 mg/kg single dose or 6–10 grams/gallon for 1–4 days. In raptors: 100 mg/kg. In parakeets and canaries: 0.5 mg/gram (Stunkard 1984)

c) For *Ascaridia galli* in poultry: 32 mg/kg (as base) (approximately 0.3 grams for each adult) given in each of 2 successive feedings or for 2 days in drinking water. Citrate or adipate salts are usually used in feed and the hexahydrate in drinking water. (Roberson 1988)

■ **REPTILES:**

a) For nematodes: 40–60 mg/kg PO. Repeat in two weeks, followed by a fecal examination 14 days after the second dose. If positive for parasites, a third dose is given and the cycle continued until the parasites are cleared from the animal. (de la Navarre 2008)

Monitoring

■ Clinical and/or laboratory efficacy

■ Adverse effects

Client Information

■ Clients should be instructed to administer only the amount prescribed and to relate any serious adverse effects to the veterinarian.

Chemistry/Synonyms

Piperazine occurs as a white, crystalline powder that may have a slight odor. It is soluble in water and alcohol. Piperazine is available commercially in a variety of salts, including citrate, adipate, phosphate, hexahydrate, and dihydrochloride. Each salt contains a variable amount of piperazine (base): adipate (37%), chloride (48%), citrate (35%), dihydrochloride (50–53%), hexahydrate (44%), phosphate (42%), and sulfate (46%).

Piperazine may also be known as diethylendiamin, dispermin, hexahydropropyrazin, piperazinum, and *Pipa-Tabs®*.

Storage/Stability
Unless otherwise specified by the manufacturer, piperazine products should be stored at room temperature (15–30°C).

Dosage Forms/Regulatory Status

VETERINARY-LABELED PRODUCTS:

Piperazine Dihydrochloride tablets equivalent to 50 mg or 250 mg base. *Pipa-Tabs®* (Vet-A-Mix); (Rx). FDA-approved for use in dogs and cats.

Additional OTC products and combination products may be available for a variety of species. Products and/or trade names include: *Alfalfa Pellet Horse Wormer, Tasty Paste® Dog & Puppy Wormer, Wonder Wormer™ for Horses, D-Worm™ Liquid Wormer for Cats and Dogs, Wazine®-17, Wazine®-34, Hartz® Advanced Care™ Liquid Wormer, Hartz® Advanced Care™ Once-a-Month® Wormer for Kittens and Cats, Hartz® Advanced Care™ Once-a-Month® Wormer for Dogs, Sergeant's® Vetscription® Worm-Away® for Cats, Sergeant's® Vetscription® Sure Shot® Liquid Wormer for Cats & Kittens, Piperazine-17 Medicated, WormEze™ Canine Anthelmintic, WormEze™ Feline Anthelmintic Paste, WormEze™ Canine & Feline Anthelmintic Liquid.*

HUMAN-LABELED PRODUCTS: None

References

Adamcak, A. & B. Otten (2000). Rodent Therapeutics. *Vet Clin NA: Exotic Anim Pract* **3:**1(Jan): 221–240.

Brander, C.G., D.M. Pugh, et al. (1982). *Veterinary Applied Pharmacology and Therapeutics*. London, Baillière Tindall.

Burke, T. (1999). Husbandry and Medicine of Rodents and Lagomorphs. Proceedings: Central Veterinary Conference, Kansas City.

Chiapella, A.M. (1989). Diseases of the Small Intestine. *Handbook of Small Animal Practice*. RV Morgan Ed. New York, Churchill Livingstone: 395–420.

Clubb, S.L. (1986). Therapeutics: Individual and Flock Treatment Regimens. *Clinical Avian Medicine and Surgery*. GJ Harrison and LR Harrison Eds. Philadelphia, W.B. Saunders: 327–355.

Cornelius, L.M. & E.L. Roberson (1986). Treatment of gastrointestinal parasitism. *Current Veterinary Therapy IX: Small Animal Practice*. K R.W. Ed. Philadelphia, W.B. Saunders: 921–924.

Davis, L.E. (1985). General Care of the Patient. *Handbook of Small Animal Therapeutics*. LE Davis Ed. New York, Churchill Livingstone: 1–20.

de la Navarre, B. (2008). Identification & treatment of common parasitic diseases of reptiles and amphibians. Proceedings: Western Veterinary Conf. Accessed via: Veterinary Information Network. http://goo.gl/lSN3C

Ivey, E. & J. Morrisey (2000). Therapeutics for Rabbits. *Vet Clin NA: Exotic Anim Pract* **3:**1(Jan): 183–216.

Kirk, R.W., Ed. (1989). *Current Veterinary Therapy X, Small Animal Practice*. Philadelphia, W.B. Saunders.

Morgan, R.V., Ed. (1988). *Handbook of Small Animal Practice*. New York, Churchill Livingstone.

Papich, M. (1989). Effects of drugs on pregnancy. *Current Veterinary Therapy X: Small Animal Practice*. R Kirk Ed. Philadelphia, Saunders: 1291–1299.

Paul, J.W. (1986). Anthelmintic Therapy. *Current Veterinary Therapy: Food Animal Practice 2*. JL Howard Ed. Philadelphia, W.B. Saunders: 39–44.

Roberson, E.L. (1988). Antinematodal Agents. *Veterinary Pharmacology and Therapeutics*. NH Booth and LE McDonald Eds. Ames, Iowa State University Press: 882–927.

Stunkard, J.M. (1984). *Diagnosis, Treatment and Husbandry of Pet Birds*. Edgewater, MD, Stunkard Publishing.

PIRLIMYCIN HCL

(per-li-*mye*-sin)   Pirsue®

INTRAMAMMARY LINCOSAMIDE ANTIBIOTIC

Prescriber Highlights

▶ Lincosamide antibiotic for intramammary use in dairy cattle

▶ Milk withdrawal (at labeled doses) = 36 hours after last treatment; Meat withdrawal (at labeled doses) = 9 days

Uses/Indications

Pirlimycin mastitis tubes are indicated for the treatment of clinical and subclinical mastitis caused by susceptible organisms in lactating dairy cattle.

Pharmacology/Actions

Like other lincosamides, pirlimycin acts by binding to the 50S ribosomal subunit of susceptible bacterial RNA, thus interfering with bacterial protein synthesis. It is primarily active against gram-positive bacteria, including a variety of species of staphylococcus (*S. aureus, S. epidermidis, S. chromogenes, S. hyicus, S. xylosus*), streptococcus (*S. agalactiae, S. dysgalactiae, S. uberis, S. bovis*) and *Enterococcus faecalis*.

Organisms with a MIC of ≤2 micrograms/mL are considered susceptible, and organisms with a MIC value of 4 micrograms/mL are considered resistant. If using a 2 microgram disk for Kirby-Bauer plate testing, a zone diameter of ≤12mm indicates resistance and a diameter of ≥13mm indicates susceptibility.

Pharmacokinetics

Little information is available; the manufacturer states that the drug penetrates the udder well and is absorbed systemically from the udder and then secreted into the milk of all four quarters. Tissue levels in treated quarters of pirlimycin are approximately 2–3 times those found in the extracellular fluid.

Contraindications/Precautions/Warnings

No information was noted.

Adverse Effects

No adverse affects, including udder irritation have been reported thus far.

Milk from untreated quarters must be disposed of during withdrawal time as residues may be detected from untreated quarters.

Reproductive/Nursing Safety

No information was noted.

Overdosage/Acute Toxicity

No data was located.

Drug Interactions

■ Because **erythromycin** and clindamycin have shown antagonism *in vitro*, this could also occur with pirlimycin.

Laboratory Considerations

■ The established tolerance of pirlimycin in milk is 0.4 ppm.

Doses

■ **CATTLE:**

a) Lactating Dairy Cattle: Infuse contents of one syringe into each affected quarter. Use proper teat end preparation, sanitation and intramammary infusion technique. Repeat treatment after 24 hours. Daily treatment may be repeated at 24-hour intervals for up to 8 consecutive days. (Package Insert; *Pirsue®*—Pfizer)

Monitoring

■ Efficacy

■ Withdrawal periods

Client Information

■ Be sure clients understand dosage recommendations and withdrawal periods.

■ Milk from untreated quarters must be disposed of during withdrawal time as residues may be detected from untreated quarters.

Chemistry/Synonyms

Pirlimycin HCl is a lincosamide antibiotic. It has a molecular weight of 465.4.

Pirlimycin HCl may also be known as U-57930E and *Pirsue®*.

Storage/Stability

Store syringes at or below 25°C (77°F); protect from freezing.

Dosage Forms/Regulatory Status

VETERINARY-LABELED PRODUCTS:

Pirlimycin HCl Sterile Solution 50 mg (equiv. to free base) in a 10 mL disposable teat syringe; *Pirsue® Aqueous Gel* (Pfizer); (Rx). FDA-approved for use in lactating dairy cattle. Milk withdrawal (at labeled doses) = 36 hours after last treatment. Meat withdrawal if two infusions 24 hours apart are used = 9 days; following any extended duration of therapy (more than two infusions at a 24-hour interval, up to 8 consecutive days), animals must not be slaughtered for 21 days.

HUMAN-LABELED PRODUCTS: None

PIROXICAM

(peer-ox-i-kam)   Feldene®

NON-STEROIDAL ANTIINFLAMMATORY, ANTI-TUMOR

Prescriber Highlights

▶ NSAID with antiinflammatory & antitumor (indirect) activity

▶ Low dose metronomic (continuous) therapy with cyclophosphamide shows promise for preventing sarcoma recurrence in dogs with fewer adverse effects then high dose treatment.

▶ Contraindications: Hypersensitivity or severely allergic to aspirin or other NSAIDs. Extreme Caution: Active, or a history of GI ulcer disease or bleeding disorders. Caution: Severely compromised cardiac function

▶ Use in cats is controversial; use with caution

▶ Adverse Effects: GI ulceration & bleeding, renal papillary necrosis, & peritonitis

▶ Probably safer NSAIDs available for pain/inflammation for dogs & cats

Uses/Indications

In dogs, piroxicam may be beneficial in reducing the pain and inflammation associated with degenerative joint disease, but there are safer alternatives available. Its primary use is in dogs as adjunctive treatment of bladder transitional cell carcinoma. It may also be of benefit in squamous cell carcinoma, mammary adenocarcinoma, and transmissible venereal tumor (TVT). There is some use of it in cats for its anti-tumor effects, but there presently are no studies published documenting its safety or efficacy in cats and it should be used with caution in this species.

Pharmacology/Actions

Like other non-steroidal antiinflammatory agents, piroxicam has antiinflammatory, analgesic, and antipyretic activity. The drug's antiinflammatory activity is thought to be primarily due to its inhibition of prostaglandin synthesis, but additional mechanisms (*e.g.*, superoxide formation inhibition) may be important. As with other NSAIDs, piroxicam can affect renal function, cause GI mucosal damage, and inhibit platelet aggregation.

Piroxicam's antitumor effects are believed to be due to its action on the immune system and not because of direct effects on tumor cells.

Pharmacokinetics

After oral administration, piroxicam is well absorbed from the gut. While the presence of food will decrease the rate of absorption, it will not decrease the amount absorbed. It is not believed that antacids significantly affect absorption.

In dogs, piroxicam has high oral bioavailability (100%) with peak plasma levels reached around 3 hours after dosing. Volume of distribution is about 0.3 L/kg; total body clearance is 0.066 L/hour and elimination half-life is about 40 hours (Galbraith & McKellar 1991).

After single oral doses in cats, piroxicam is well absorbed with an oral bioavailability of about 80%. Peak levels occur in approximately 3 hours. Elimination half-life after intravenous or oral dosing is about 12-13 hours.

Piroxicam is highly bound to plasma proteins. In humans, synovial levels are about 40% of those found in plasma. Maternal milk concentrations are only about 1% of plasma levels.

In humans, piroxicam has a very long plasma half-life (about 50 hours). The drug is principally excreted as metabolites in the urine after hepatic biotransformation.

Contraindications/Precautions/Warnings

Piroxicam is contraindicated in patients hypersensitive to it or who are severely allergic to aspirin or other NSAIDs. It should be used only when its potential benefits outweigh the risks in patients with active or history of GI ulcer disease or bleeding disorders. Because peripheral edema has been noted in some human patients, it should be used with caution in patients with severely compromised cardiac function.

Piroxicam has not been evaluated for use in cats. It must be used with extreme caution, if at all, in this species.

Adverse Effects

Like other NSAIDs used in dogs, piroxicam has the potential for causing significant GI ulceration and bleeding. The therapeutic window for the drug is very narrow in dogs, as doses as low as 1 mg/kg given daily have caused significant GI ulceration, renal papillary necrosis, and peritonitis. Other adverse effects reported in humans and potentially possible in dogs include: CNS effects (headache, dizziness, etc.), otic effects (tinnitus), elevations in hepatic function tests, pruritus and rash, and peripheral edema. Renal papillary necrosis has been seen in dogs at postmortem but, apparently, clinical effects have not been noted with these occurrences.

In cats, GI effects (vomiting, anorexia, diarrhea) may be seen, particularly early in therapy. There are anecdotal reports of piroxicam decreasing hematocrits in cats when dosed daily for 7-14 days. Renal toxicity is possible if used for prolonged periods.

Reproductive/Nursing Safety

Animal studies have not demonstrated any teratogenic effects associated with piroxicam. The drug is excreted into milk in very low concentrations (about 1% found in maternal plasma). In humans, the FDA categorizes this drug as category *C* for use during pregnancy (*Animal studies have shown an adverse effect on the fetus, but there are no adequate studies in humans; or there are no animal reproduction studies and no adequate studies in humans.*) If using in the third trimester or near delivery in humans, the FDA categorizes all NSAIDs as category *D* for use during pregnancy (*There is evidence of human fetal risk, but the potential benefits from the use of the drug in pregnant women may be acceptable despite its potential risks.*)

Most NSAIDs are excreted in maternal milk; use with caution in nursing patients.

Overdosage/Acute Toxicity

There is limited information available, but dogs may be more sensitive to the drugs ulcerative effects than are humans.

There were 63 exposures to piroxicam reported to the ASPCA Animal Poison Control Center (APCC) during 2008-2009. In these cases 58 were dogs with 12 showing clinical signs and 5 were cats with 1 showing clinical signs. Common findings in dogs recorded in decreasing frequency included vomiting, and bloody vomitus.

As with any NSAID, overdosage can lead to gastrointestinal and renal effects. Decontamination with emetics and/or activated charcoal is appropriate. For doses where GI effects are expected, the use of gastrointestinal protectants is warranted. If renal effects are also expected, fluid diuresis is should be considered. Patients ingesting significant overdoses should be monitored carefully and treated supportively.

Drug Interactions

The following drug interactions have either been reported or are theoretical in humans or animals receiving piroxicam and may be of significance in veterinary patients:

- ◼ **AMINOGLYCOSIDES (gentamicin, amikacin, etc.):** Increased risk for nephrotoxicity
- ◼ **ANTICOAGULANTS (heparin, LMWH, warfarin):** Increased risk for bleeding possible
- ◼ **ASPIRIN:** When aspirin is used concurrently with piroxicam, plasma levels of piroxicam could decrease and an increased likelihood of GI adverse effects (blood loss) could occur. Concomitant administration of aspirin with piroxicam cannot be recommended.
- ◼ **BISPHOSPHONATES (alendronate, etc.):** May increase risk for GI ulceration
- ◼ **CISPLATIN:** Piroxicam may potentiate the renal toxicity of cisplatin when used in combination
- ◼ **CORTICOSTEROIDS:** Concomitant administration with NSAIDs may significantly increase the risks for GI adverse effects
- ◼ **FUROSEMIDE:** Piroxicam may reduce the saluretic and diuretic effects of furosemide
- ◼ **HIGHLY PROTEIN BOUND DRUGS (e.g., phenytoin, valproic acid, oral anticoagulants, other antiinflammatory agents, salicylates,**

sulfonamides, and the sulfonylurea antidiabetic agents): Because piroxicam is highly bound to plasma proteins (99%), it potentially could displace other highly bound drugs; increased serum levels and duration of actions may occur. Although these interactions are usually of little concern clinically, use together with caution.

■ **METHOTREXATE:** Serious toxicity has occurred when NSAIDs have been used concomitantly with methotrexate; use together with extreme caution

Laboratory Considerations

■ Piroxicam may cause falsely elevated **blood glucose** values when using the glucose oxidase and peroxidase method using ABTS as a chromogen.

Doses

■ **DOGS:**

As an adjunctive therapy of transitional cell carcinomas, squamous cell carcinomas, and palliative therapy for other neoplastic diseases:

a) 0.3 mg/kg PO once a day (Frimberger & London 2003)

b) 0.3 mg/kg PO once a day. Give with food. Consider adding misoprostol at 3 micrograms/kg, PO q8h for dogs who tolerate NSAIDs poorly. Discontinue if severe irritation or ulceration occurs. Treat ulcers and if signs abate, may resume piroxicam with misoprostol. (Frimberger 2000)

c) For adjuvant therapy for splenic hemangiosarcoma (stage II): Etoposide 50 mg/m^2 PO once daily for 3 weeks, alternating 3 week cycles with cyclophosphamide at 12.5–25 mg/m^2 PO once daily. Piroxicam is given at 0.3 mg/kg PO every day. Continue until disease recurrence and progression is noted. (Lana et al. 2007)

d) For transitional cell carcinoma after laser ablation of the primary tumor: Mitoxantrone at IV 5 mg/m^2 every 3 weeks for 4 treatments. Piroxicam was given at a dosage of 0.3 mg/kg PO once daily for the remaining life of the dog. (Upton et al. 2006)

e) To inhibit local recurrence in dogs with incompletely resected soft tissue sarcomas: piroxicam at 0.3 mg/kg PO once daily with cyclophosphamide at 10 mg/m^2 (NOT mg/kg) PO once daily. If dog develops unacceptable adverse effects dosing interval increased to every other day. (Elmslie et al. 2008)

As an antiinflammatory/analgesic:

a) 0.3 mg/kg PO every other day (q48h) (Boothe 1992)(Hansen 2003)

b) For cancer pain: 0.3 mg/kg PO q24-48h. (Gaynor 2008)

c) For adjunctive treatment of Idiopathic lymphoplasmacytic rhinitis (LPR): Long-term administration of antibiotics having immunomodulatory effects (doxycycline 3–5 mg/kg PO q12h; or azithromycin 5 mg/kg PO q24h) combined with NSAIDs can be helpful in some dogs. Piroxicam 0.3 mg/kg PO q24h is recommended. If clinical improvement is observed within 2 weeks, daily piroxicam therapy is continued but the frequency of administration of doxycycline is reduced to once daily or azithromycin reduced to twice weekly. Therapy will likely be required for a minimum of 6 months, if not indefinitely. (Kuehn 2007b)

■ **CATS:**

As adjunctive therapy for neoplasia:

a) For adjunctive therapy of transitional cell carcinomas: 0.3 mg/kg PO q24–72h. Gastric protectants (misoprostol, H$_2$ blockers sucralfate, omeprazole) may be useful to prevent/treat GU ulceration. Use with caution in patients with pre-existing renal disease and avoid use with other nephrotoxic drugs. Fluid supplementation may be warranted. (Smith 2003)

b) For an adjunctive therapy of transitional cell carcinomas, but may be of limited utility in squamous cell carcinoma: Doses of 0.3 mg/kg PO every 24–48 hours have been used for neoplastic diseases; it is unknown if this dose provides anti-inflammatory or analgesic effects. (Lascelles et al. 2007)

As an antiinflammatory/analgesic:

a) For cancer pain: 0.3 mg/kg PO q24-48h or 1 mg (total dose) per cat PO q24h for a maximum of 7 days. (Gaynor 2008)

b) 1 mg per cat (total dose) PO once daily for a maximum of 7 days. (Note: After compounding, drug is stable for 10 days). (Rochette 2007)

c) Idiopathic chronic rhinosinusitis: Some cats' clinical signs can be reduced with piroxicam at 0.3 mg/kg PO once daily or every other day. (Kuehn 2007a)

■ **HORSES:**

For neoplastic diseases:

a) From a case report treating mucocutaneous squamous cell carcinoma: 80 mg (total dose) PO once daily; lip lesion resolved completely over 3 months, but patient developed colic signs twice. Dose was eventually reduced to every other day or every third day. (Moore et al. 2003)

b) From a case report treating a squamous cell carcinoma of the third eyelid after surgical excision: 80 mg (total dose) PO once daily. (Iwabe et al. 2009)

■ **RABBITS, RODENTS, SMALL MAMMALS:**
For fracture associated limb swelling:

a) **Rabbits:** 0.1–0.2 mg/kg PO q8h for 3 weeks (Ivey & Morrisey 2000)

Monitoring

■ Adverse Effects (particularly GI bleeding)

■ Liver function and renal function tests should be monitored occasionally with chronic use

Client Information

■ Have clients monitor for GI ulceration/bleeding (anorexia, tarry stools, etc.).

■ Do not exceed dosage recommendations without veterinarian's approval. It has been suggested to give the drug with food to reduce GI upset potential.

Chemistry/Synonyms

An oxicam derivative non-steroidal antiinflammatory agent, piroxicam occurs as a white, crystalline solid. It is sparingly soluble in water. Piroxicam is structurally not related to other non-steroidal antiinflammatory agents.

Piroxicam may also be known as: CP-16171, piroxicamum or PIRO; many trade names are available.

Storage/Stability

Capsules should be stored at temperatures less than 30°C in tight, light-resistant containers. When stored as recommended, capsules have an expiration date of 36 months after manufacture.

Dosage Forms/Regulatory Status

VETERINARY-LABELED PRODUCTS: None

The ARCI (Racing Commissioners International) has designated this drug as a class 4 substance. See the appendix for more information.

HUMAN-LABELED PRODUCTS:

Piroxicam Oral Capsules: 10 mg & 20 mg; *Feldene®* (Pfizer); generic; (Rx)

References

Boothe, D. (1992). Control of pain in small animals. Proceedings of the Tenth Annual Veterinary Medical Forum, San Diego, American College of Veterinary Internal Medicine.

Elmslie, R.E., P. Glawe, et al. (2008). Metronomic Therapy with Cyclophosphamide and Piroxicam Effectively Delays Tumor Recurrence in Dogs with Incompletely Resected Soft Tissue Sarcomas. *Journal of Veterinary Internal Medicine* 22(6): 1373–1379.

Frimberger, A. (2000). Anticancer Drugs: New Drugs or Applications for Veterinary Medicines. *Kirk's Current Veterinary Therapy: XIII Small Animal Practice.* J Bonagura Ed. Philadelphia, WB Saunders: 474–478.

Frimberger, A. & C. London (2003). Principles of oncology. *Handbook of Small Animal Practice, 4th Ed.* R Morgan, R Bright and M Swartout Eds. Philadelphia, Saunders: 719–734.

Galbraith, E.A. & Q.A. McKellar (1991). Pharmacokinetics and pharmacodynamics of piroxicam in dogs. *Veterinary Record* 128(24): 561–565.

Gaynor, J.S. (2008). Control of Cancer Pain in Veterinary Patients. *Veterinary Clinics of North America-Small Animal Practice* 38(6): 1429–+.

Hansen, B. (2003). Updated opinions on analgesic techniques. Proceedings: ACVIM Forum.

Ivey, E. & J. Morrisey (2000). Therapeutics for Rabbits. *Vet Clin NA: Exotic Anim Pract* 3:1(Jan): 183–216.

Iwabe, S., L. Ramirez-Lopez, et al. (2009). The use of piroxicam as an adjunctive treatment for squamous cell carcinoma in the third eyelid of a horse. *Veterinaria Mexico* 40(4): 389–395.

Kuehn, N. (2007a). Chronic rhinitis in cats. Proceedings: ACVIM. Accessed via: Veterinary Information Network. http://goo.gl/wPcsU

Kuehn, N. (2007b). Chronic rhinitis in dogs. Proceedings; ACVIM. Accessed via: Veterinary Information Network. http://goo.gl/YSuy2

Lana, S., L. U'ren, et al. (2007). Continuous low-dose oral chemotherapy for adjuvant therapy of splenic hemangiosarcoma in dogs. *J Vet Intern Med* 21: 764–769.

Lascelles, D., M.H. Court, et al. (2007). Nonsteroidal anti-inflammatory drugs in cats: a review. *Veterinary Anaesthesia and Analgesia* 34(4): 228–250.

Moore, A.S., S.L. Beam, et al. (2003). Long-term control of mucocutaneous squamous cell carcinoma and metastases in a horse using piroxicam. *Equine Veterinary Journal* 35(7): 715–718.

Rochette, J. (2007). Nerve Blocks and Management of Oral Pain. Proceedings: AAFP. Accessed via: Veterinary Information Network. http://goo.gl/vwn6n

Smith, A. (2003). Special concerns in cat chemotherapy. Proceedings: ACVIM Forum. Accessed via: Veterinary Information Network. http://goo.gl/dnmJ3

Upton, M., C. Tanger, et al. (2006). Evaluation of carbon dioxide laser ablation combined with mitoxantrone and piroxicam treatment in dogs with transitional cell carcinoma. *JAVMA* 228(4): 549–552.

Plasma-Lyte—see the section on intravenous fluids in the Appendix

POLYSULFATED GLYCOSAMINO-GLYCAN (PSGAG)

(*pol*-ee-*sulf*-ayte-ed glye-*kose*-a-meen-ohe-glye-kan)   Adequan®, Chondroprotec®

PROTEOLYTIC ENZYME INHIBITOR; CHONDROPROTECTANT

Prescriber Highlights

▶ Proteolytic enzyme inhibitor used IM or intra-articularly for non-infectious &/or traumatic joint dysfunction & associated lameness of the carpal joints in horses & non-infectious degenerative &/or traumatic arthritis in dogs

▶ Contraindications: Intra-articular injection if patient hypersensitive to PSGAG. Should not be used in place of other treatments when infection suspected or present, or when surgery or joint immobilization required

▶ Adverse Effects: IM use: Unlikely. Intra-articular: Post-injection inflammation possible. *Dogs:* Dose-related inhibition of coagulation/hemostasis possible.

Uses/Indications

PSGAG administered either IM or IA is indicated for the treatment of non-infectious and/or traumatic joint dysfunction and associated lameness of the carpal joints in horses. Some studies have indicated that PSGAG is much less effective in joints where there has been acute trauma but no degradative enzymes present.

It is also FDA-approved for the control of signs associated with non-infectious degenerative and/or traumatic arthritis in dogs.

Pharmacology/Actions

In joint tissue, PSGAG inhibits proteolytic enzymes that can degrade proteoglycans (including naturally occurring glycosaminoglycans), thereby preventing or reducing decreased connective tissue flexibility, resistance to compression, and resiliency. By acting as a precursor, PSGAG increases the synthesis of proteoglycans, reduces inflammation by reducing concentrations of prostaglandin E_2 (released in response to joint injury) and increases hyaluronate concentrations in the joint, thereby restoring synovial fluid viscosity.

Pharmacokinetics

PSGAG is deposited in all layers of articular cartilage and preferentially taken up by osteoarthritic cartilage. When administered IM, articular levels will with time exceed those found in the serum. After IM injection, peak joint levels are reached in 48 hours and persist up to 96 hours.

Contraindications/Precautions/Warnings

PSGAG is contraindicated for intra-articular administration in patients hypersensitive to it. While the manufacturer states there are no contraindications for IM use of the drug, the drug should not be used in place of other therapies in cases where infection is present or suspected, or in place of surgery or joint immobilization where indicated.

Some clinicians feel that PSGAG should not be used within one week of arthrotomy in dogs, because it may cause increased bleeding. This effect apparently has not been confirmed in the literature, however.

Adverse Effects

Adverse effects are unlikely when using the IM route. Intra-articular administration may cause a post-injection inflammation (joint pain, effusion, swelling, and associated lameness) secondary to sensitivity reactions, traumatic injection technique, overdosage, or the number or frequency of the injections. Treatment consisting of antiinflammatory drugs, cold hydrotherapy, and rest is recommended. Although uncommon, joint sepsis secondary to intraarticular injection is possible; strict aseptic technique should be employed to minimize this occurrence. Several sources recommend adding 125 mg of amikacin if PSGAG is to be injected in joints of horses.

In dogs, a dose-related inhibition of coagulation/hemostasis has been described.

Reproductive/Nursing Safety

Reproductive studies have apparently not been performed; use with caution during pregnancy or in breeding animals (the manufacturer does not recommend use in breeding animals).

In humans, the FDA categorizes glycosaminoglycans as category **B** for use during pregnancy (*Animal studies have not yet demonstrated risk to the fetus, but there are no adequate studies in pregnant women; or animal studies have shown an adverse effect, but adequate studies in pregnant women have not demonstrated a risk to the fetus in the first trimester of pregnancy, and there is no evidence of risk in later trimesters.*)

It is not known whether glycosaminoglycans are excreted in maternal milk, but is unlikely to be of significant concern.

Overdosage/Acute Toxicity

Doses five times those recommended (2.5 grams) given IM to horses twice weekly for 6 weeks revealed no untoward effects. Approximately 2% of horses receiving overdoses (up to 1250 mg) IA showed transient clinical signs associated with joint inflammation.

Drug Interactions

The following drug interactions have either been reported or are theoretical in humans or animals receiving PSGAG and may be of significance in veterinary patients:

While specific drug interactions have not been detailed to date, using this product in conjunction with either steroids or non-steroidal antiinflammatory agents could mask the signs and clinical signs associated with septic joints.

There is some concern that since PSGAG is a heparin analog that it should not be used in conjunction with other NSAIDs or other anticoagulants. Clinical significance remains unclear, but use together with caution.

Doses

■ **HORSES:**

a) For IM administration: 500 mg IM (of IM product) every 4 days for 28 days. Thoroughly cleanse injection site before injecting. Do not mix with other drugs or chemicals. (Package Insert; *Adequan® I.M.*)

For intra-articular administration: 250 mg (of IA product) IA once a week for 5 weeks. Joint area should be shaved, and cleansed as if a surgical procedure, prior to injecting. Do not mix with other drugs or chemicals. (Package Insert; *Adequan® I.A.*)

b) For IM injection: 500 mg IM every 3–4 days for a minimum of 4 and preferably, 7 treatments.

For intra-articular injection: As above; author recommends adding 125 mg of amikacin for injection into the IA injection to reduce potential for infection. (Nixon 1992)

■ **DOGS:**

For the treatment of non-infectious degenerative and/or traumatic arthritis:

a) 4.4 mg/kg IM twice weekly for up to 4 weeks. (Label information; *Adequan® Canine*—Luitpold)

b) 1.1–4.8 mg/kg IM every 4 days for six doses and then as needed (Kelly 1995)

c) Osteoarthritis: 5 mg/kg IM twice a week (McLaughlin 2000)

d) Osteoarthritis: 5 mg/kg IM once weekly (Hardie & Grauer 2007)

■ **CATS:**

As a chondroprotective drug:

a) 1.1–4.8 mg/kg IM every 4 days for six doses and then as needed (Kelly 1995)

b) 2 mg/kg IM every 3–5 days for 4 treatments; only anecdotal experience in cats. (Kerwin 2007)

■ **RABBITS, RODENTS, SMALL MAMMALS:**

a) **Rabbits:** For arthritis: 2.2 mg/kg SC or IM every 3 days for 21–28 days, then once every 2 weeks (Ivey & Morrisey 2000)

Monitoring

■ Efficacy

■ Joint inflammation/infection if administered IA.

Client Information

■ The IA product must be administered by veterinary professionals; the IM product could, with proper instruction, be administered by the owner.

Chemistry/Synonyms

Polysulfated glycosaminoglycan (PSGAG) is chemically similar to natural mucopolysaccharides found in cartilaginous tissues. PSGAG is reportedly an analog of heparin.

Polysulfated glycosaminoglycan is also known as PSGAG, *Adequan®* and *Chondroprotec®*.

Storage/Stability

Commercial products should be stored in a cool place 8–15°C (46–59°F). The manufacturer recommends discarding any unused portion from the vial or ampule and, also does not recommend mixing with any other drug or chemical.

Dosage Forms/Regulatory Status

VETERINARY-LABELED PRODUCTS:

Polysulfated Glycosaminoglycan for Intra-Articular Injection: 250 mg/mL in 1 mL single use vials, boxes of 6; *Adequan® I.A.* (Luitpold); (Rx). FDA-approved for use in horses, (not in those intended for food).

Polysulfated Glycosaminoglycan for Intra-Muscular Injection: 100 mg/mL in 5 mL glass ampules or vials and 20 mL, 30 mL, and 50 mL multi-dose vials; *Adequan® I.M.* (Luitpold); (Rx). FDA-approved for use in horses, (not in those intended for food).

Polysulfated Glycosaminoglycan for IM Injection: 100 mg/mL; *Adequan® Canine* (Luitpold); (Rx). FDA-approved for use in dogs.

Polysulfated Glycosaminoglycan Topical Solution: sterile solution of 1000 mg in 10 mL vials. FDA-approved for use on horses. No reported side effects. *Chondroprotec®* (Neogen) (Rx)

HUMAN-LABELED PRODUCTS: None

References

Hardie, E. & G. Grauer (2007). Treating the dog with osteoarthritis and chronic kidney disease. Proceedings: Western Vet Conf. Accessed via: Veterinary Information Network. http://goo.gl/572Rl

Ivey, E. & J. Morrisey (2000). Therapeutics for Rabbits. *Vet Clin NA: Exotic Anim Pract* **3:**1(Jan): 183–216.

Kelly, M. (1995). Pain. *Textbook of Veterinary Internal Medicine: Diseases of the Dog and Cat.* S Ettinger and E Feldman Eds. Philadelphia, WB Saunders: 21–25.

Kerwin, S. (2007). Feline Osteoarthritis. Proceedings: Western Vet Conf. Accessed via: Veterinary Information Network. http://goo.gl/2clD0

McLaughlin, R. (2000). Management of Osteoarthritic Pain. *Vet ClinNA: Small Anim Pract* **30:**4(July): 933–947.

Nixon, A. (1992). Intra-articular medication. *Current Therapy in Equine Medicine 3.* N Robinson Ed. Philadelphia, W.B. Saunders Co.: 127–131.

PONAZURIL

(poe-*naz*-yoor-ill)   Marquis®

ANTIPROTOZOAL

Prescriber Highlights

▶ Equine FDA-approved triazine for treating EPM

▶ Adverse Effect profile not well established; in field trials: rashes, hives, blisters, or GI signs noted

▶ Treatment is relatively expensive

Uses/Indications

Ponazuril is indicated for the treatment of equine protozoal myeloencephalitis (EPM) caused by *Sarcocystis neurona*.

Ponazuril could potentially be useful in treating *Neospora caninum* and Toxoplasma or other protozoal infections in other species (*e.g.*, dogs, cats, birds, reptiles, ruminants).

Pharmacology/Actions

The triazine class of antiprotozoals is believed to target the "plastid" body, an organelle found in the members of the Apicomplexa phylum, including *Sarcocystis neurona. In vitro* levels required to kill *Sarcocystis neurona* range from 0.1–1 micrograms/mL.

Pharmacokinetics

When administered orally to horses in water, ponazuril has an approximate bioavailability of 30% and elimination half-life of 80 hours. After daily (5 mg/kg) oral administration to horses, ponazuril reaches its peak serum levels in about 18 days and peak CSF levels in about 15 days. Peak CSF levels are about $^{1}/_{20}$ th (0.21 micrograms/mL) those found in the serum. Elimination half-life from serum averages about 4.5 days. If ponazuril is given orally (2.2 mg/kg) dissolved in DMSO, bioavailability is significantly enhanced (Dirikolu, Karpiesiuk *et al.* 2009).

In cattle, 5 mg/kg oral doses of ponazuril are relatively well absorbed and have an approximate elimination half-life of 58 hours (Dirikolu, Yohn *et al.* 2009).

Contraindications/Precautions/Warnings

None were noted. Before treating, other conditions that can cause ataxia should be ruled out.

Adverse Effects

Field trials showed some animals developing blisters on nose and mouth or a rash/hives. Single animals developed diarrhea, mild colic or seizures.

Successful treatment may not negate all the clinical signs associated with EPM.

Keratoconjunctivitis sicca (KCS) has been reported in some dogs, especially those breeds with a predilection towards developing KCS or when the drug was given in overdose quantities.

Reproductive/Nursing Safety

Safety during pregnancy or in lactating mares has not been evaluated.

Overdosage/Acute Toxicity

Daily doses of up to 30 mg/kg (6X) primarily caused loose feces. Moderate edema of the uterine epithelium was noted on histopathology for female horses receiving the 6X dose.

Drug Interactions/Laboratory Considerations

■ None noted

Doses

■ **DOGS/CATS:**

a) For Neosporosis or Toxoplasmosis: 7.5–15 mg/kg PO once daily for 28 days. Dose extrapolated between doses for horses and mice. (Greene *et al.* 2006)

b) For coccidiosis: Anecdotally, 15–30 mg/kg PO once or repeated after 7–10 days. (Hurley 2007)

c) **Cats:** For coccidiosis: 20 mg/kg PO daily for 3 days; must be compounded for administration in kittens or cats. Has been well tolerated and been associated with rapid resolution of diarrhea and eradication of coccidia in infected kittens. (Marks, S. 2007), (Marks, S.L. 2009)

■ **SMALL MAMMALS:**

a) **Rabbits:** For adjunctive treatment of Eimeria species: 20 mg/kg PO q24h for 7 days. (Kelleher 2008)

■ **HORSES:**

a) For EPM: 5 mg/kg, PO once daily for 28 days. See the package insert for specific dosing instructions. (Package insert; *Marquis®*—Bayer)

■ **CAMELIDS (NW):**

a) For *Eimeria macusaniensis* in Crias: 20 mg/kg, PO once daily for 3 days. Because *E. mac* can cause clinical disease or even death before oocysts are present in feces, prophylactic treatment should be considered in camelids that have unexplained weight loss with concurrent hypoproteinemia and without severe anemia. The commercially available paste (*Marquis®*) is too concentrated to be given to camelids and should be diluted before being administered. Recommend diluting the paste to 100 mg/mL by taking 40 grams of paste, q.s. with distilled water to 60 grams total and mixing well. It is very water-soluble and can be easily syringed into the animal. (Walker 2009)

■ **BIRDS:**

a) **Falcons:** For Cryptosporidium respiratory disease: Case report of two patients: 20 mg/kg PO (as a compounded suspension) once daily for 7 days. (Van Sant & Stewart 2009)

■ **REPTILES:**

a) **Bearded dragons:** For coccidians 30 mg/kg PO twice 48 hours apart. (Mitchell 2008)

Monitoring

■ Clinical efficacy

Client Information

■ For this drug to be effective it must be given as prescribed.

■ Contact veterinarian if rashes, hives, blisters, or GI signs develop.

■ Clients should be forewarned of the considerable expense associated with this drug and that clinical improvement may be marginal or not occur at all in some horses treated.

Chemistry/Synonyms

Related to other antiprotozoals such as toltrazuril, ponazuril is a triazine antiprotozoal (anticoccidial) agent. The commercially available oral paste is white to off-white in color and odorless; pH is 5.7–6. Solubility of ponazuril in DMSO is 250 mg/mL.

Ponazuril may also be known as: toltrazolone sulfone, ICI-128436, *Marquis®*, and *Ponalrestat®*.

Storage/Stability

Store the paste at room temperature (15–30°C).

Dosage Forms/Regulatory Status

VETERINARY-LABELED PRODUCTS:

Ponazuril Oral Paste (15% w/w): 127-gram tubes; each gram of paste contains 150 mg of ponazuril; each syringe is enough to treat a 1200 lb. horse for 7 days. *Marquis®* (Bayer); (Rx). Not for use in horses intended for food.

HUMAN-LABELED PRODUCTS: None

References

Dirikolu, L., W. Karpiesiuk, et al. (2009). Synthesis and detection of toltrazuril sulfone and its pharmacokinetics in horses following administration in dimethylsulfoxide. *Journal of Veterinary Pharmacology and Therapeutics* 32(4): 368–378.

Dirikolu, L., R. Yohn, et al. (2009). Detection, quantifications and pharmacokinetics of toltrazuril sulfone (Ponazuril((R))) in cattle. *Journal of Veterinary Pharmacology and Therapeutics* 32(3): 280–288.

Greene, C., K. Hartmannn, et al. (2006). Appendix 8: Antimicrobial Drug Formulary. *Infectious Disease of the Dog and Cat.* C Greene Ed., Elsevier: 1186–1333.

Hurley, K. (2007). Identification & management of diarrhea outbreaks in animal shelter. Proceedings: Western Vet Conference. Accessed via: Veterinary Information Network. http://goo.gl/ksvJG

Kelleher, S. (2008). Rabbit GI Disease. Proceedings: WVC. Accessed via: Veterinary Information Network. http://goo.gl/Iaajp

Marks, S. (2007). What's the latest on parasitic causes of diarrhea in dogs and cats? Proceedings: ACVIM 2007. Accessed via: Veterinary Information Network. http://goo.gl/fw8Kw

Marks, S.L. (2009). Frustrating Kitten Diarrhea. Proceedings: WVC. Accessed via: Veterinary Information Network. http://goo.gl/4fwQa

Mitchell, M.A. (2008). Gastroenterology of Reptiles. Proceedings: ACVC. Accessed via: Veterinary Information Network. http://goo.gl/xo98I

Van Sant, F. & G. Stewart (2009). Ponazuril Used as a Treatment for Suspected Cryptosporidium Infection in 2 Hybrid Falcons. Proceedings: AAV. Accessed via: Veterinary Information Network. http://goo.gl/c1zIG

Walker, P. (2009). Differential Diagnosis of Diarrhea in Camelid Crias. Proceedings: ACVIM. Accessed via: Veterinary Information Network. http://goo.gl/0C6AM

Potassium Bromide—see Bromides
Potassium Iodide—see Iodide, Potassium

POTASSIUM CHLORIDE POTASSIUM GLUCONATE

(po-*tass*-ee-um)   Cal-Dextro® K, Tumil-K®

ELECTROLYTE

Prescriber Highlights

▶ Used for treatment or prevention of hypokalemia

▶ Contraindications: Hyperkalemia, renal failure or severe renal impairment, severe hemolytic reactions, untreated Addison's disease, acute dehydration, GI motility impairment (solid oral dosage forms)

▶ Caution: Patients on digoxin

▶ Adverse Effects: Hyperkalemia. Oral therapy: GI distress; IV therapy may be irritating to veins

▶ Intravenous potassium salts must be diluted before administering & drug must be given slowly

▶ Acid/base, hydration status important

▶ Drug Interactions

Uses/Indications

Potassium supplementation is used to prevent or treat potassium deficits. When feasible and appropriate, because it is generally safer, oral or nutritional therapy is generally preferred over parenteral potassium administration.

Pharmacology/Actions

Potassium is the principal intracellular cation in the body. It is essential in maintaining cellular tonicity; nerve impulse transmission; smooth, skeletal and cardiac muscle contraction; and maintenance of normal renal function. Potassium is also used in carbohydrate utilization and protein synthesis.

Potassium requirements in mature dogs are approximately 3.7 mEq/kg/day, and in mature cats approximately 1.5 mEq/kg/day. Puppies and kittens require higher dietary potassium than do mature animals.

Pharmacokinetics

Approximately 98% of total body potassium is found in the intracellular fluid space while only 2% is in the extracellular fluid space. Plasma pH can alter distribution. Acidosis can shift potassium out of the intracellular space and conversely, alkalosis shifts potassium into the intracellular space. Potassium is primarily (80–90%) excreted via the kidneys with the majority of the remainder excreted in the feces. Very small amounts may be excreted in perspiration (animals with sweat glands).

Contraindications/Precautions/Warnings

Potassium salts are contraindicated in patients with hyperkalemia, renal failure or severe renal impairment, severe hemolytic reactions, untreated Addison's disease, and acute dehydration. Solid oral dosage forms should not be used in patients where GI motility is impaired. Use cautiously in digitalized patients (see Drug Interactions).

Because potassium is primarily an intracellular electrolyte, serum levels may not adequately reflect the total body stores of potassium. Acid-base balance may also mask the actual potassium picture. Patients with systemic acidosis conditions may appear to have hyperkalemia when, in fact, they may be significantly low in total body potassium. Conversely, alkalosis may cause a falsely low serum potassium value. Assess renal and cardiac function prior to therapy and closely monitor serum potassium levels. Supplementation should generally occur over 3–5 days to allow equilibration to occur between extracellular and intracellular fluids. Some clinicians feel that if acidosis is present or a concern, use potassium acetate, citrate or bicarbonate; if alkalosis is present, use potassium chloride.

Adverse Effects

The major problem associated with potassium supplementation is the development of hyperkalemia which is usually much more serious than hypokalemia. Clinical signs associated with hyperkalemia can range from muscular weakness and/or GI disturbances to cardiac conduction disturbances. Clinical signs can be exacerbated by concomitant hypocalcemia, hyponatremia, or acidosis. Intravenous potassium salts must be diluted before administering and given slowly (see Doses).

Oral therapy can cause GI distress and IV therapy may be irritating to veins.

Reproductive/Nursing Safety

Monitored potassium supplementation is unlikely to have negative effects during pregnancy or lactation.

Overdosage/Acute Toxicity

Fatal hyperkalemia may develop if potassium salts are administered too rapidly IV or if potassium renal excretory mechanisms are impaired. Clinical signs associated with hyperkalemia are noted in the Adverse Effects section above. Treatment of hyperkalemia is dependent upon the cause and/or severity of the condition and can consist of: discontinuation of the drug with ECG, acid/base and electrolyte monitoring, glucose/insulin infusions, sodium bicarbonate, calcium therapy, and polystyrene sulfonate resin. It is suggested to refer to other references appropriate for the species being treated for specific protocols for the treatment of hyperkalemia.

Drug Interactions

The following drug interactions have either been reported or are theoretical in humans or animals receiving potassium and may be of significance in veterinary patients:

- **ACE INHIBITORS (e.g., enalapril):** Potassium retention may occur; increased risk for hyperkalemia

- **DIGOXIN:** In patients with severe or complete heart block who are receiving digitalis therapy, it is often recommended not to use potassium salts

- **NSAIDS:** Oral potassium given with nonsteroidal antiinflammatory agents may increase the risk of gastrointestinal adverse effects

- **POTASSIUM-SPARING DIURETICS (e.g., spironolactone):** Potassium retention may occur; increased risk for hyperkalemia

Doses

- **DOGS/CATS:**

  For hypokalemia:

  a) Treatment of chronic mild hypokalemia (3.0-3.5 mEq/L) can be accomplished with dietary measures or commercially available oral potassium supplement tablets and elixirs (diluted in water) at 0.5–1 mEq/kg mixed in food once or twice daily. If using the commercially available *Tumil-K®* powder, it is dosed at ¼ teaspoonful (2 mEq) per 4.5 kg body weight PO in food twice daily; adjust as necessary.

  For moderate to severe (<3.0 mEq/L) or acute hypokalemia with or without metabolic alkalosis requiring the administration of IV potassium; no accurate formulas available for calculating the exact amount of KCL needed to restore normokalemia. The *rate* of administration of intravenous KCL is more critical than the total amount administered. Under most circumstances the rate should not exceed 0.5 mEq/kg/hour. But, under the most dire circumstances (serum potassium < 2.0 mEq/L), rate can be increased to 1.5 mEq/kg/hour along with close EKG monitoring. Amounts exceeding more than 10 mEq/hour to a small animal (<10 kg body weight) can be potentially life-threatening because of the effects of a more concentrated solution on the wall of the right ventricle, if the solution is given through a central intravenous line.

  KCL supplemented fluids can also be safely given in patients weighing less than 10 kg. Isotonic fluids such as lactated Ringers or 0.9% saline containing 30–35 mEq/L KCl per Liter and administered at a dose of 150 mL SC every 12 hours. (Schaer 2009)

  b) Oral using *Tumil-K®* (Virbac): ¼ teaspoonful (2 mEq) per 4.5 kg body weight PO in food twice daily. Adjust dose as necessary. (Package insert; *Tumil-K®*—Virbac).

c) Intravenous replacement: potassium chloride IV at a rate not to exceed 0.5 mEq/hour. Concentration of replacement fluid should exceed 60 mEq/L. Begin oral supplementation as soon as possible using potassium gluconate for dogs at a dose of 2–44 mEq/day depending on body size; cats get 2–4 mEq/day. (Peres 2000)

d) Potassium administration should be considered on the basis of how much potassium to administer to the patient, not how much to add to a bag of fluid. Dosages usually range from maintenance (0.05–0.1 mEq/kg/hour) to 0.5 mEq/kg/hour. (Hansen 2007)

e) There are no exact formulas for calculating the total body potassium depletion, nor the requirement for supplementation. Guidelines should always be modified based on patient response. Patients with hypokalemia and an osmotic diuresis will have a much higher requirement for potassium than ones with normal urine output. Guidelines are: Serum K+ <2 mEq/L = 60 mEq/1000 mL IV fluid; Serum K+ 2-2.5 mEq/L = 40 mEq/1000 mL IV fluid; Serum K+ 2.5-3 mEq/L = 30 mEq/1000 mL IV fluid; Serum K+ 3–3.5 mEq/L = 20 mEq/1000 mL IV fluid. Infusion rates should generally not exceed 0.5 mEq/kg/hour; however, higher rates may be required in some patients. Rates as high as 1.5 mEq/kg/hour can be used as long as the patient's heart rate and electrocardiogram are monitored continuously. Hypomagnesemia should be ruled out in patients with refractory hypokalemia. (Devey 2009)

■ **HORSES:**

For hypokalemia:

a) To counteract potassium depletion in a completely anorectic horse, IV fluids should be supplemented with KCl (at least 50 mEq/hour). Hypertonic oral KCL pastes can be administered to horses with diarrhea. (Schott II 2009)

■ **RUMINANTS:**

For hypokalemia:

a) In "downer" cows: 80 grams sodium chloride and 20 grams potassium chloride in 10 liters of water PO via stomach tube. Provide a bucket containing similar solution for cow to drink and another containing fresh water. (Caple 1986)

b) 50 grams PO daily; 1 mEq/kg/hour IV drip (Howard 1986)

c) For severe hypokalemia (<2.3 mEq/L) with severe muscle weakness or recumbency: Isotonic potassium chloride (11.5 grams of potassium chloride per 1 liter of sterile water) at a rate of 4 mL/kg/hour. Combined with large doses of oral potassium salts (*i.e.*, 200 grams of KCl per day). (Smith 2006)

Monitoring

Level and frequency of monitoring associated with potassium therapy is dependent upon the cause and/or severity of hypokalemia, acid/base abnormalities, renal function, concomitant drugs administered, or disease states and can include:

■ Serum potassium
■ Other electrolytes
■ Acid/base status
■ Glucose
■ ECG
■ CBC
■ Urinalyses

Chemistry/Synonyms

Potassium chloride occurs as either white, granular powder or as colorless, elongated, prismatic, or cubical crystals. It is odorless and has a saline taste. One gram is soluble in about 3 mL of water and is insoluble in alcohol. The pH of the injection ranges from 4–8. One gram of potassium chloride contains 13.4 mEq of potassium. A 2 mEq/mL solution has an osmolarity of 4000 mOsm/L. Potassium chloride may also be known as KCl.

Potassium gluconate occurs as white to yellowish white, crystalline powder or granules. It is odorless, has a slightly bitter taste, and is freely soluble in water. One gram of potassium gluconate contains 4.3 mEq of potassium.

Potassium Chloride may also be known as: KCl, cloreto de potassio, E508, kalii chloridum, or kalium chloratum.

Potassium Gluconate may also be known as: E577, *K-G Elixir®*, *Kaon®*, *Kaylixir®*, *Potasoral®*, *Potassiject®*, *Potassium-Rougier®*, *Renakare®*, *Sopa-K®*, *Tumil-K®*, and *Ultra-K®*.

Storage/Stability

Potassium gluconate oral products should be stored in tight, light resistant containers at room temperature (15–30°C), unless otherwise instructed by the manufacturer.

Unless otherwise directed by the manufacturer, potassium chloride products should be stored in tight, containers at room temperature (15–30°C); protect from freezing.

Compatibility/Compounding Considerations

Potassium chloride for injection is reportedly physically **compatible** with the following intravenous solutions and drugs (as an additive): all commonly used intravenous replacement fluids (not 10% fat emulsion), aminophylline, amiodarone HCl, bretylium tosylate, calcium gluconate, chloramphenicol sodium succinate, cimetidine HCl, clindamycin phosphate, corticotropin (ACTH), cytarabine, dimenhydrinate, dopamine HCl, erythromycin gluceptate/lactobionate, heparin sodium, hydrocortisone sodium succinate, isoproterenol HCl, lidocaine HCl, metaraminol bitartrate, methicillin sodium, methyldopate HCl, metoclopramide HCl, nafcillin sodium, norepinephrine bitartrate, oxacillin sodium, oxytetracycline HCl, penicillin G potassium, phenylephrine HCl, piperacillin sodium, sodium bicarbonate, tetracycline HCl, thiopental sodium, vancomycin HCl, verapamil HCl, and vitamin B-complex with C.

Potassium chloride for injection **compatibility information conflicts** or is dependent on diluent or concentration factors with the following drugs or solutions: fat emulsion 10%, amikacin sulfate, dobutamine HCl, methylprednisolone sodium succinate (at Y-site), penicillin G sodium, and promethazine HCl (at Y-site). Compatibility is dependent upon factors such as pH, concentration, temperature, and diluent used; consult specialized references or a hospital pharmacist for more specific information.

Potassium chloride for injection is reportedly physically **incompatible** with the following solutions or drugs: amphotericin B, diazepam (at Y-site), and phenytoin sodium (at Y-site).

Dosage Forms/Regulatory Status

VETERINARY-LABELED PRODUCTS:

There are several products for parenteral use that contain potassium; refer to the tables in the appendix or individual proprietary veterinary products for additional information.

Potassium Chloride IV Solution: 2 mEq (149 mg) in 10 mL vials; *Potassiject®* (Butler-Schein); generic; (Rx)

Oral Products:

Potassium Gluconate Tablets: 2 mEq (468 mg). Labeled for use in cats and dogs; *Tumil-K®* (Virbac), *Renakare®* (Neogen); (Rx)

Potassium Gluconate Oral Powder: Each 0.65 gram (¼ teaspoonful) contains 2 mEq of potassium in 4 oz. Containers; *Renakare®* (Neogen); *Tumil-K®* (Virbac) (Rx). Labeled for use in dogs and cats.

Potassium Gluconate Gel: Each 2.34 grams (½ teaspoonful) contains 2 mEq of potassium in 5 oz tubes; *Tumil-K® Gel* (Virbac), *Renakare®* (Neogen) (Rx). Labeled for use in dogs and cats.

HUMAN-LABELED PRODUCTS: Not a complete list.

Parenteral Products:

Potassium Chloride for Injection Concentrate **(Must be diluted before administering):** 2 mEq/mL in 250 mL & 500 mL bulk pkgs; 10 mEq in 5 mL & 10 mL single-dose vials and 50 mL & 100 mL containers; 20 mEq in 10 mL single-dose vials, and 50 & 100 mL containers; 30 mEq in 15 mL single-dose vials and 100 mL containers; 40 mEq in 20 mL & 30 mL single-dose vials and 100 mL containers; 60 mEq in 30 mL multiple-use vials; generic; (Rx)

Potassium acetate for injection and potassium phosphate for injection (see Phosphate monograph) are also available. There are a multitude of human-labeled potassium salts for oral use available in several dosage forms; refer to human drug references for more information on these products. Tablets, controlled/sustained release tablets and capsules, effervescent tablets, liquids, and powder in varying strengths available; (OTC and Rx)

References

Caple, I., W. (1986). Downer Cow Syndrome. *Current Veterinary Therapy: Food Animal Practice 2*. JL Howard Ed. Philadelphia, W.B. Saunders: 327–328.

Devey, J. (2009). What's All the Salt About? Understanding Sodium, Chloride and Potassium. Proceedings: ABVP. Accessed via: Veterinary Information Network. http://goo.gl/bVCaG

Hansen, B. (2007). Tips and tricks for fluid therapy. Proceedings: Western Vet Conf. Accessed via: Veterinary Information Network. http://goo.gl/U4vTe

Howard, J.L., Ed. (1986). *Current Veterinary Therapy 2, Food Animal Practice*. Philadelphia, W.B. Saunders.

Peres, Y. (2000). Hyponatremia and hypokalemia. *Textbook of Veterinary Internal Medicine: Diseases of the Dog and Cat*. S Ettinger and E Feldman Eds. Philadelphia, WB Saunders. **1:** 222–227.

Schaer, M. (2009). Hypokalemia—A Problem to Be Reckoned With. Proceedings: IVECCS. Accessed via: Veterinary Information Network. http://goo.gl/tInSS

Schott II, H. (2009). Disorders of Sodium & Potassium Balance in the Foal & Adult Horse. Proceedings: ACVIM. Accessed via: Veterinary Information Network. http://goo.gl/lTsJj

Smith, G. (2006). Fluid therapy in adult ruminants. Proceedings: Western Vet Conference. http://goo.gl/aeRIE

Potassium Citrate—see Citrate Salts

PRALIDOXIME CHLORIDE
2-PAM CHLORIDE

(pra-li-*dox*-eem)   Protopam Chloride®

ANTIDOTE; CHOLINESTERASE REACTIVATOR

Prescriber Highlights

▶ Cholinesterase reactivator used for adjunctive treatment of organophosphate poisoning

▶ Contraindications: Hypersensitivity; generally not recommended for carbamate poisoning

▶ Caution: Renal impairment, patients receiving anticholinesterase agents for the treatment of myasthenia gravis

▶ Adverse Effects: Rapid IV injection may cause tachycardia, muscle rigidity, transient neuromuscular blockade, or laryngospasm

▶ Most-effective if given within 24 hours of exposure

Uses/Indications

Pralidoxime is used in the treatment of organophosphate poisoning, often in conjunction with atropine and supportive therapy.

Pharmacology/Actions

Pralidoxime reactivates cholinesterase that has been inactivated by phosphorylation secondary to certain organophosphates. Via nucleophilic attack, the drug removes and binds the offending phosphoryl group attached to the enzyme, which is then excreted.

Pharmacokinetics

Pralidoxime is only marginally absorbed after oral dosing; oral dosage forms are no longer available in the United States. It is distributed primarily throughout the extracellular water. Because of its quaternary ammonium structure, it is not believed to enter the CNS in significant quantities, but recent studies and clinical responses have led some to question this belief.

Pralidoxime is thought to be metabolized by the liver and excreted as both metabolite(s) and unchanged drug in the urine.

Contraindications/Precautions/Warnings

Pralidoxime is contraindicated in patients hypersensitive to it. Pralidoxime is generally not recommended for use in instances of carbamate poisoning because inhibition is rapidly reversible, but there is some controversy regarding this issue.

Pralidoxime should be used with caution in patients receiving anticholinesterase agents for the treatment of myasthenia gravis as it may precipitate a myasthenic crisis. It should also be used cautiously and at a reduced dosage rate in patients with renal impairment.

Adverse Effects

At usual doses, pralidoxime generally is safe and free of significant adverse effects. Rapid IV injection may cause tachycardia, muscle rigidity, transient neuromuscular blockade, and laryngospasm.

Pralidoxime must generally be given within 24 hours of exposure to be effective, but some benefits may occur, particularly in large exposures, if given within 36–48 hours.

Reproductive/Nursing Safety

In humans, the FDA categorizes this drug as category *C* for use during pregnancy (*Animal studies have shown an adverse effect on the fetus, but there are no adequate studies in humans; or there are no animal reproduction studies and no adequate studies in humans.*)

It is not known whether this drug is excreted in maternal milk; exercise caution.

Overdosage/Acute Toxicity

The acute LD_{50} of pralidoxime in dogs is 190 mg/kg and, at high dosages, causes signs associated with its own anticholinesterase activity. Clinical signs of toxicity in dogs may be exhibited as muscle weakness, ataxia, vomiting, hyperventilation, seizures, respiratory arrest, and death.

Drug Interactions

The following drug interactions have either been reported or are theoretical in humans or animals receiving pralidoxime and may be of significance in veterinary patients:

- ▆ **BARBITURATES:** Anticholinesterases can potentiate the action of barbiturates; use with caution.

- ▆ **CIMETIDINE, SUCCINYLCHOLINE, THEOPHYLLINE, RESERPINE, and RESPIRATORY DEPRESSANT DRUGS (e.g., narcotics, phenothiazines):** Use should be avoided in patients with organophosphate toxicity.

Doses

Note: Often used in conjunction with atropine; refer to that monograph and/or the references below for more information.

- ▆ **DOGS/CATS:**
  For organophosphate poisoning:
  a) Pralidoxime works best when combined with atropine. Pralidoxime at 20 mg/kg, 2–3 times a day. Initial dose may be given either IM or slow IV. Subsequent doses may be given IM or SC. (Refer to reference for more specific guidelines regarding adjunctive therapy) (Fikes 1990)

  b) 10–15 mg/kg IM or SC q8–12h; 36 hour minimum (Firth 2000)

  c) Give atropine first at 0.1 mg/kg IV, followed by an additional 0.3 mg/kg IM. Then pralidoxime at 50 mg/kg diluted in 10% glucose and administered via slow IV. If a severe poisoning and muscle weakness has not been relieved, may give another dose in one hour. For small dogs or cats, pralidoxime may be administered IM or IP. Reduce dose in presence of renal failure. Recovery should occur gradually over 48 hours. (El Bahri 2002)

  d) Dogs: 50 mg/kg; Cats 20 mg/kg. Give IV slowly or with fluids over a 30-minute period. Repeat in one hour if clinical signs persist and then q8h for 24–48 hours. Author recommends using pralidoxime in animals that are severely depressed, weak, and anorectic one or more days after exposure if not previously treated with pralidoxime. In animals that have clinical signs intensified (e.g., respiratory depression), reduce dose and give as repeated one-hour infusions every 4–8 hours in combination with atropine (0.04–0.4 mg/kg) once or as needed (Mount 1989)

  e) Cats: 20 mg/kg IM or IV within first 24 hours of exposure. May repeat q6–8h and combine with atropine or give separately. Do not use in carbamate toxicity. (Reid & Oehme 1989)

■ **RUMINANTS:**

Note: When used in food animals, FARAD recommends a 28-day meat and a 6-day milk withdrawal time. (Haskell *et al.* 2005)

For organophosphate poisoning:

a) Cattle: 30 mg/kg IM q8h. (Osweiler 2007)

b) Cattle: 25–50 mg/kg as a 20% solution IV over 6 minutes; or as a maximum of 100 mg/kg/day as an IV drip (Smith 1986)

■ **HORSES:**

For organophosphate poisoning:

a) 20 mg/kg (may require up to 35 mg/kg) IV and repeat q4–6h (Oehme 1987)

■ **BIRDS:**

For organophosphate poisoning:

a) 10–20 mg/kg q8–12h (route not specified) with atropine (0.2–0.5 mg/kg IM q3–4h). (Jones 2007)

b) 10–100 mg/kg IM q24-48h or repeat once in 6 hours. (Johnson-Delaney & Reavill 2009)

Monitoring

■ Pralidoxime therapy is monitored via the clinical signs associated with organophosphate poisoning. For more information, refer to one of the references outlined in the dosage section.

Client Information

■ This agent should only be used with close professional supervision.

Chemistry/Synonyms

A quaternary ammonium oxime cholinesterase reactivator, pralidoxime chloride occurs as a white to pale yellow, crystalline powder with a pK_a of 7.8–8. It is freely soluble in water. The commercially available injection has a pH of 3.5–4.5 after reconstitution.

Pralidoxime Chloride may also be known as: 2-Formyl-1-methylpyridinium chloride oxime, 2-PAM, 2-PAM chloride, 2-PAMCl, 2-pyridine aldoxime methochloride and *Protopam*®.

Storage/Stability

Unless otherwise instructed by the manufacturer, pralidoxime chloride powder for injection should be stored at room temperature. After reconstituting with sterile water for injection, the solution should be used within a few hours. Do not use sterile water with preservatives added.

Dosage Forms/Regulatory Status

VETERINARY-LABELED PRODUCTS: None

HUMAN-LABELED PRODUCTS:

Pralidoxime Chloride Powder for Injection: 1 gram in 20 mL single-use vials; *Protopam*® *Chloride* (Wyeth-Ayerst); (Rx)

References

El Bahri, L. (2002). Pralidoxime. *Comp Contin Educ Pract Vet* **24**(11): 884–886.

Fikes, J.D. (1990). Organophosphorous and Carbamate Insecticides. *Vet Clinics of North Amer: Small Anim Pract* **20**(2): 353–367.

Firth, A. (2000). Treatments used in small animal toxicoses. *Kirk's Current Veterinary Therapy: XIII Small Animal Practice.* J Bonagura Ed. Philadelphia, WB Saunders: 207–211.

Haskell, S., M. Payne, et al. (2005). Farad Digest: Antidotes in Food Animal Practice. *JAVMA* **226**(6): 884–887.

Johnson-Delaney, C. & D. Reavill (2009). Toxicoses in Birds: Ante- and Postmortem Findings for Practitioners. Proceedings: AAV. Accessed via: Veterinary Information Network. http://goo.gl/LVYYE

Jones, M. (2007). Avian Toxicology. Proceedings: Western Vet Conf. Accessed via: Veterinary Information Network. http://goo.gl/YC7Vj

Mount, M.E. (1989). Toxicology. *Textbook of Veterinary Internal Medicine.* SJ Ettinger Ed. Philadelphia, WB Saunders. **1:** 456–483.

Oehme, F.W. (1987). Insecticides. *Current Therapy in Equine Medicine.* NE Robinson Ed. Philadelphia, WB Saunders: 658–660.

Osweiler, G. (2007). Detoxification and Antidotes for Ruminant Poisoning. Proceedings: ACVIM. Accessed via: Veterinary Information Network. http://goo.gl/h1YRI

Reid, F.M. & F.W. Oehme (1989). Toxicoses. *The Cat: Diseases and Clinical Management.* RG Sherding Ed. New York, Churchill Livingstone. **1:** 185–215.

Smith, J.A. (1986). Toxic encephalopathies in cattle. *Current Veterinary Therapy 2: Food Animal Practice.* JL Howard Ed. Philadelphia, WB Saunders: 855–863.

PRAZIQUANTEL

(pra-zi-*kwon*-tel)   Droncit®

ANTICESTODAL ANTIPARASITIC

Prescriber Highlights

▶ Anticestodal anthelmintic also may be useful for some other parasites

▶ Contraindications: Puppies less than 4 weeks old or kittens less than 6 weeks old; hypersensitivity to the drug

▶ Adverse Effects: Uncommon after oral use; pain at injection site, anorexia, salivation, vomiting, lethargy, weakness, or diarrhea possible after using injectable

For information on the spot-on combination product containing praziquantel and emodepside (Profender®), see the Emodepside monograph.

For information on the combination product containing praziquantel and moxidectin (Quest Plus®), see the Moxidectin monograph.

Uses/Indications

Praziquantel is indicated for (FDA-approved labeling) for the treatment of *Dipylidium caninum*, *Taenia pisiformis*, and *Echinococcus granulosis* in dogs, and *Dipylidium caninum* and *Taenia taeniaeformis* in cats. Fasting is not required nor recommended before dosing. A single dose is usually effective, but measures should be taken to prevent reinfection, particularly against *D. caninum*. Praziquantel can also be used for treating *Alaria* spp. in dogs and cats and *Spirometra mansonoides* infections in cats.

Praziquantel has been used in birds and other animals, but it is usually not economically feasible to use in large animals. In humans, praziquantel is used for schistosomiasis, other trematodes (lung, liver, intestinal flukes) and tapeworms. It is not routinely effective in treating *F. hepatica* infections in humans.

Combination products can give a wide spectrum of internal parasite control in a variety of species.

Pharmacology/Actions

Praziquantel's exact mechanism of action against cestodes has not been determined, but it may be the result of interacting with phospholipids in the integument causing ion fluxes of sodium, potassium and calcium. At low concentrations *in vitro*, the drug appears to impair the function of their suckers and stimulates the worm's motility. At higher concentrations *in vitro*, praziquantel increases the contraction (irreversibly at very high concentrations) of the worm's strobilla (chain of proglottids). In addition, praziquantel causes irreversible focal vacuolization with subsequent cestodal disintegration at specific sites of the cestodal integument.

In schistosomes and trematodes, praziquantel directly kills the parasite, possibly by increasing calcium ion flux into the worm. Focal vacuolization of the integument follows and the parasite is phagocytized.

Pharmacokinetics

Praziquantel is rapidly and nearly completely absorbed after oral administration, but there is a significant first-pass effect. Peak serum levels are achieved between 30–120 minutes in dogs.

Praziquantel is distributed throughout the body. It crosses the intestinal wall and across the blood-brain barrier into the CNS.

Praziquantel is metabolized in the liver via CYP3A enzymes to metabolites of unknown activity. It is excreted primarily in the urine; elimination half-life is approximately 3 hours in the dog. In dogs, orally administered grapefruit juice can increase the area under the curve by 150–200%.

Contraindications/Precautions/Warnings

The manufacturer recommends not using praziquantel in puppies less than 4 weeks old or in kittens less than 6 weeks old. However, a combination product containing praziquantel and febantel from the same manufacturer is FDA-approved for use in puppies and kittens of all ages. No other contraindications are listed for this compound from the manufacturer. In humans, praziquantel is contraindicated in patients hypersensitive to the drug.

Adverse Effects

When used orally, praziquantel can cause anorexia, vomiting, lethargy, or diarrhea in dogs, but the incidence of these effects is less than 5%. In cats, adverse effects were quite rare (<2%) in

field trials using oral praziquantel, with salivation and diarrhea being reported.

A greater incidence of adverse effects has been reported after using the injectable product. In dogs, pain at the injection site, vomiting, drowsiness, and/or a staggering gait were reported from field trials with the drug. Some cats (9.4%) showed clinical signs of diarrhea, weakness, vomiting, salivation, sleepiness, transient anorexia, and/or pain at the injection site.

Reproductive/Nursing Safety

Praziquantel is considered safe to use in pregnant dogs or cats. In humans, the FDA categorizes this drug as category *B* for use during pregnancy (*Animal studies have not yet demonstrated risk to the fetus, but there are no adequate studies in pregnant women; or animal studies have shown an adverse effect, but adequate studies in pregnant women have not demonstrated a risk to the fetus in the first trimester of pregnancy, and there is no evidence of risk in later trimesters.*) In a separate system evaluating the safety of drugs in canine and feline pregnancy (Papich 1989), this drug is categorized as class: *A* (*Probably safe. Although specific studies may not have proved he safety of all drugs in dogs and cats, there are no reports of adverse effects in laboratory animals or women.*)

Praziquantel appears in maternal milk at a concentration of approximately 25% of that in maternal serum, but is unlikely to pose harm to nursing offspring.

Overdosage/Acute Toxicity

Praziquantel has a wide margin of safety. In rats and mice, the oral LD50 is at least 2 g/kg. An oral LD50 could not be determined in dogs, as at doses greater than 200 mg/kg, the drug induced vomiting. Parenteral doses of 50–100 mg/kg in cats caused transient ataxia and depression; injected doses at 200 mg/kg were lethal in cats.

There were 22 exposures to praziquantel reported to the ASPCA Animal Poison Control Center (APCC) during 2001-2009. In these cases 12 were cats with 4 showing clinical signs. The remaining 10 were dogs that showed no clinical signs.

Drug Interactions

Reportedly in humans, synergistic activity occurs with praziquantel and oxamniquine in the treatment of schistosomiasis. The clinical implications of this synergism in veterinary patients are not clear.

Doses

- ■ DOGS:
  a) For susceptible cestodes:
     IM or SC using the 56.8 mg/mL injectable product:
     Body weight: Dose
     ≤5 lbs: 17 mg (0.3 mL)
     6–10 lbs: 28.4 mg (0.5 mL)
     11–25 lbs: 56.8 mg (1 mL)

≥25 lbs: 0.2 mL/5 lb body weight; maximum 3 mL

Oral: Using the 34 mg canine tablet:

Body weight: Dose

≤5 lbs: 17 mg (½ tab)

6–10 lbs: 34 mg (1 tab)

11–15 lbs: 51 mg (1.5 tabs)

16–30 lbs: 68 mg (2 tabs)

31–45 lbs: 102 mg (3 tabs)

46–60 lbs: 136 mg (4 tabs)

≥60 lbs: 170 mg (5 tabs maximum); (Package insert; *Droncit® Injectable and Tablets*—Bayer)

b) For *Taenia, Echinococcus, Dipylidium caninum, Mesocestoides* (adult): 5 mg/kg PO or SC.

For *Diphyllobothrium*: 7.5 mg/kg PO either once or for 2 days.

For *Sparganum proliferum (adult)*: 7.5 mg/kg or 25 mg/kg PO or SC daily for 2 days. (Conboy 2009)

c) For *Echinococcus granulosis*: 10 mg/kg (Sherding 1989)

d) For *Spirometra mansonoides* or *Diphyllobothrium erinacei*: 7.5 mg/kg, PO once daily for 2 days (Roberson 1988)

e) For treatment of Paragonimiasis (*Paragonimus kellicotti*): 23–25 mg/kg PO q8h for 3 days (Reinemeyer 1995), (Hawkins 2000)

f) For treatment of liver flukes (Platynosum or Opisthorchiidae families): 20–40 mg/kg PO once daily for 3–10 days (Taboada 1999)

g) For *Alaria* spp.: 20 mg/kg PO (Ballweber 2004)

h) For giardia using *Drontal Plus®*: Use label dose once daily PO for 3 days. (Lappin 2006)

i) For adjunctive treatment of the flukes (*Nanophyetus salmincola*) associated with Salmon poisoning: Single dose of 10–30 mg/kg PO or SC. (Headley *et al.*)

■ **CATS:**

a) For susceptible cestodes:

IM or SC using the 56.8 mg/mL injectable product:

Body weight: Dose

<5 lbs: 11.4 mg (0.2 mL)

5–10 lbs: 22.7 mg (0.4 mL)

≥10 lbs: 34.1 mg (0.6 mL maximum)

Oral: Using the 23 mg feline tab

Body weight: Dose

<4 lbs:11.5 mg (½ tab)

5–11 lbs: 23 mg (1 tab)

>11 lbs: 34.5 mg (1.5 tabs)

(Package insert; *Droncit® Injectable and Tablets*—Bayer)

b) For susceptible parasites using combination product with pyrantel pamoate (*Drontal®*): Administer a minimum dose of 2.27 mg praziquantel and 9.2 mg pyrantel pamoate per pound of body weight according to the dosing tables on labeling. May be given directly by mouth or in a small amount of food. Do not withhold food prior to or after treatment. If reinfection occurs, treatment may be repeated. (Package insert; *Drontal®*—Bayer)

c) For treatment of Paragonimiasis (*Paragonimus kellicotti*): 23–25 mg/kg PO q8h for 3 days (Reinemeyer 1995)(Hawkins 2000)

d) For treatment of Giardia infections: Give two small dog tablets of *Drontal Plus®* (febantel 113.4 mg; pyrantel 22.7 mg; praziquantel 22.7 mg) once daily PO for 5 days. (Scorza *et al.* 2004)

e) For *Alaria* spp.: 20 mg/kg PO (Ballweber 2004)

f) For *Spirometra mansonoides*: 30–35 mg/kg PO. (Bowman 2006)

g) For *Taenia, Echinococcus, Dipylidium caninum, Mesocestoides* (adult): 5 mg/kg PO or SC.

For *Diphyllobothrium (adult)*: 35 mg/kg PO once has been recommended.

For *Sparganum proliferum (adult)*: 7.5 mg/kg or 25 mg/kg PO or SC daily for 2 days. (Conboy 2009)

■ **RABBITS, RODENTS, SMALL MAMMALS:**

a) **Chinchillas:** 6–10 mg/kg PO (Hayes 2000)

b) **Mice, Rats, Hamsters and Gerbils:** For tapeworms: 30 mg/kg, PO once (note the high dosage required) (Burke 1999)

c) **Mice, Rats, Gerbils, Hamsters, Guinea pigs, Chinchillas:** For tapeworms: 6–10 mg/kg PO (Adamcak & Otten 2000)

d) **Rabbits:** For cestodes and trematodes: 5–10 mg/kg PO once. (Bryan 2009)

■ **SHEEP & GOATS:**

a) For all species of Moniezia, Stilesia, or Avitellina: 10–15 mg/kg (Roberson 1988)

■ **HORSES:**

For labeled parasites using the oral gel combination of moxidectin/praziquantel:

a) Dial in the weight of the animal on the syringe. Administer gel by inserting the syringe applicator into the animal's mouth through the interdental space and depositing the gel in the back of the mouth near the base of the tongue. Once the syringe is removed, the animal's head should be raised to insure proper swallowing of the gel. Horses weighing more than 1250 lb require additional gel from a second syringe. (Label Directions; *Quest® Plus*—Fort Dodge)

■ **LLAMAS:**

For susceptible parasites:

a) 5 mg/kg, PO (Fowler 1989)

■ **BIRDS:**

For susceptible parasites (tapeworms):

a) ¼ of one 23 mg tablet/kg PO; repeat in 10–14 days. Add to feed or give by gavage. Injectable form is toxic to finches. (Clubb 1986)

b) For common tapeworms in chickens: 10 mg/kg (Roberson 1988)

c) For cestodes and some trematodes: Direct dose: 5–10 mg/kg PO or IM as a single dose -or- 12 mg of crushed tablets baked into a 9"x9"x2" cake. Finches should have their regular food withheld and be pre-exposed to a non-medicated cake. (Marshall 1993)

■ **REPTILES/AMPHIBIANS**

a) Reptiles: For cestodes and some trematodes in most species: 7.5 mg/kg PO once; repeat in 2 weeks PO (Gauvin 1993)

b) For removal of common tapeworms in snakes: 3.5–7 mg/kg (Roberson 1988)

c) For cestodes and trematodes in reptiles and amphibians: 7–8 mg/kg PO, IM, SC. (de la Navarre 2003)

Monitoring

■ Clinical efficacy

Client Information

■ Fasting is neither required nor recommended before dosing. A single dose is usually effective, but measures should be taken to prevent reinfection, particularly against *D. caninum*.

■ Tablets may be crushed or mixed with food.

■ Because tapeworms are often digested, worm fragments may not be seen in the feces after using.

Chemistry/Synonyms

A prazinoisoquinoline derivative anthelmintic, praziquantel occurs as a white to practically white, hygroscopic, bitter tasting, crystalline powder, either odorless or having a faint odor. It is very slightly soluble in water and freely soluble in alcohol.

Praziquantel may also be known as: EMBAY-8440, praziquantelum, *Biltricide®*, *Bio-Cest®*, *Cercon®*, *Cesol®*, *Cestox®*, *Cisticid®*, *ComboCare®*, *Cysticide®*, *Droncit®*, *Drontal®*, *Ehliten®*, *Equimax®*, *Extiser Q®*, *Mycotricide®*, *Opticide®*, *Quest® Plus*, *Praquantel®*, *Prasikon®*, *Prazite®*, *Prozitel®*, *Sincerck®*, *Teniken®*, *Virbantel®*, *Waycital®*, or *Zifartel®* and *Zimecterin Gold Paste®*.

Storage/Stability

Unless otherwise instructed by the manufacturer, praziquantel tablets should be stored in tight containers at room temperature. Protect from light.

Dosage Forms/Regulatory Status

VETERINARY-LABELED PRODUCTS:

Praziquantel Tablets: 23 mg (feline); 34 mg (canine); *Droncit® Tablets* (Bayer); generic; (Rx; OTC). FDA-approved for use in cats and dogs.

Praziquantel Injection: 56.8 mg/mL in 10 mL and 50 mL vials; *Droncit® Injection* (Bayer); generic; (Rx). FDA-approved for use in cats and dogs.

Combination Products:

Tablets: Praziquantel 13.6 mg/pyrantel pamoate 54.3 mg (as base) for 2–5.9 lb cats and kittens; Praziquantel 18.2 mg/pyrantel pamoate 72.6 mg (as base); Praziquantel 27.2 mg/pyrantel pamoate 108.6 mg (as base) for 6-24 lb. cats; *Drontal® Tablets* (Bayer); (OTC); some sizes may be available as generics or under various trade names (OTC). FDA-approved for use in cats and kittens that are 2 months of age or older and weigh 2 lb. or greater.

Chewable Tablets: Praziquantel 30 mg/pyrantel pamoate 30 mg; & Praziquantel 114 mg/pyrantel pamoate 114 mg chewable tablets; *Virbantel Flavored Chewables®* (Virbac); (OTC). FDA-approved for use in dogs.

Chewable Tablets: Fenbendazole 454 mg, Ivermectin 27 micrograms, & Praziquantel 23 mg (2.16 grams small chews) Chewable Tablets; *Panacur Plus® Soft Chews* (Intervet); (Rx). FDA-approved for use in adult dogs.

Chewable Tablets: Fenbendazole 1.134 grams, Ivermectin 68 micrograms, & Praziquantel 57 mg (5.4 grams large chews) Chewable Tablet; *Panacur Plus® Soft Chews* (Intervet); (Rx). FDA-approved for use in adult dogs. Tablets: Praziquantel/pyrantel pamoate plus febantel; *Drontal® Plus Tablets* (Bayer); (Rx); small, medium and large dog sizes. FDA-approved for dogs and puppies 3 weeks of age or older and weighing 2 lb. or greater.

Oral Gel: containing 20 mg/mL moxidectin and 125 mg/mL of praziquantel in 11.6 grams syringes (sufficient to treat one 1150 lb horse); *Quest® Plus* (Fort Dodge); *ComboCare® Equine Oral Gel* (Farnam); (OTC). FDA-approved for use in horse or ponies not intended for food purposes.

Oral Paste: containing 1.87% ivermectin and 14.03% of praziquantel in oral syringes (sufficient to treat one 1320 lb horse); *Equimax®* (Pfizer); (OTC). FDA-approved for use in horse or ponies not intended for food purposes.

Oral Paste: containing 1.55% ivermectin and 7.75% of praziquantel in oral syringes (sufficient to treat one 1250 lb horse); *Zimecterin Gold Paste®* (Merial); (OTC). FDA-approved for use in horse or ponies not intended for food purposes.

HUMAN-LABELED PRODUCTS:

Praziquantel Oral Tablets (Film-coated): 600 mg; *Biltricide®* (Schering); (Rx)

References

Adamcak, A. & B. Otten (2000). Rodent Therapeutics. *Vet Clin NA: Exotic Anim Pract* **3**:1(Jan): 221–240.

Ballweber, L. (2004). Internal parasites in dogs and cats. Proceedings; Western Vet Conf. Accessed via: Veterinary Information Network. http://goo.gl/YMwbR

Bowman, D. (2006). Feline gastrointestinal parasites. Proceedings: ACVC. Accessed via: Veterinary Information Network. http://goo.gl/DMPMV

Bryan, J. (2009). Rabbit GI Physiology: What do I do now? Proceedings: WVC. Accessed via: Veterinary Information Network. http://goo.gl/cAD9L

Burke, T. (1999). Husbandry and Medicine of Rodents and Lagomorphs. Proceedings: Central Veterinary Conference, Kansas City.

Clubb, S.L. (1986). Therapeutics: Individual and Flock Treatment Regimens. *Clinical Avian Medicine and Surgery*. GJ Harrison and LR Harrison Eds. Philadelphia, W.B. Saunders: 327–355.

Conboy, G. (2009). Cestodes of Dogs and Cats in North America. *Veterinary Clinics of North America-Small Animal Practice* **39**(6): 1075–+.

de la Navarre, B. (2003). Common parasitic diseases of reptiles and amphibians. Proceedings: Western Veterinary Conf. Accessed via: Veterinary Information Network. http://goo.gl/ZafJD

Fowler, M.E. (1989). *Medicine and Surgery of South American Camelids*. Ames, Iowa State University Press.

Gauvin, J. (1993). Drug therapy in reptiles. *Seminars in Avian & Exotic Med* 2(1): 48–59.

Hawkins, E. (2000). Pulmonary Parenchymal Diseases. *Textbook of Veterinary Internal Medicine: Diseases of the Dog and Cat*. S Ettinger and E Feldman Eds. Philadelphia, WB Saunders. 2: 1061–1091.

Hayes, P. (2000). Diseases of Chinchillas. *Kirk's Current Veterinary Therapy: XIII Small Animal Practice*. J Bonagura Ed. Philadelphia, WB Saunders: 1152–1157.

Headley, S.A., D.G. Scorpio, et al. Neorickettsia helminthoeca and salmon poisoning disease: A review. *The Veterinary Journal* **In Press, Corrected Proof.**

Lappin, M. (2006). Giardia infections. Proceedings: WSAVA World Congress. Accessed via: Veterinary Information Network. http://goo.gl/aywXP

Marshall, R. (1993). Avian anthelmintics and antiprotozoals. *Seminars in Avian & Exotic Med* 2(1): 33–41.

Papich, M. (1989). Effects of drugs on pregnancy. *Current Veterinary Therapy X: Small Animal Practice*. R Kirk Ed. Philadelphia, Saunders: 1291–1299.

Reinemeyer, C. (1995). Parasites of the respiratory system. *Kirk's Current Veterinary Therapy:XII*. J Bonagura Ed. Philadelphia, W.B. Saunders: 895–898.

Roberson, E.L. (1988). Anticestodal and antitrematodal drugs. *Veterinary Pharmacology and Therapeutics*. NH Booth and LE McDonald Eds. Ames, Iowa State University Press: 928–949.

Scorza, A., S. Radecki, et al. (2004). Efficacy of febantel/pyrantel/praziquantel for the treatment of giardia infection in cats. Proceedings: ACVIM Forum. Accessed via: Veterinary Information Network. http://goo.gl/Hp31u

Sherding, R.G. (1989). Diseases of the small bowel. *Textbook of Veterinary Internal Medicine*. SJ Ettinger Ed. Philadelphia, WB Saunders. **2:** 1323–1396.

Taboada, J. (1999). How I treat gastrointestinal pythiosis. Proceedings: The North American Veterinary Conference, Orlando.

PRAZOSIN HCL

(pra-zoe-*sin*)   Minipress®

ALPHA-1 ADRENERGIC BLOCKER

Prescriber Highlights

▶ Alpha1-blocker that may be useful for adjunctive treatment of CHF, systemic hypertension, or pulmonary hypertension in dogs

▶ Also used to reduce sympathetic tone to treat functional urethral obstruction in dogs & cats

▶ Caution: Chronic renal failure or preexisting hypotensive conditions

▶ Adverse Effects: Potentially hypotension, CNS effects (lethargy, dizziness, etc.), & GI effects

Uses/Indications

Prazosin is less well studied in dogs than hydralazine, and its capsule dosage form makes it less convenient for dosing. Prazosin, however, appears to have fewer problems with causing tachycardia, and its venous dilation effects may be an advantage over hydralazine when preload reduction is desired. It could be considered for therapy for the adjunctive treatment of CHF, particularly when secondary to mitral or aortic valve insufficiency when hydralazine is ineffective or not tolerated. Prazosin may also be used for the treatment of systemic hypertension or pulmonary hypertension in dogs.

Pharmacology/Actions

Prazosin's effects are a result of its selective, competitive inhibition of alpha$_1$-adrenergic receptors. It reduces blood pressure and peripheral vascular resistance and, unlike hydralazine, has dilatory effects on both the arterial and venous side.

Prazosin significantly reduces systemic arterial and venous blood pressures, and right atrial pressure; cardiac output is increased in patients with CHF. Moderate reductions in blood pressure, pulmonary vascular resistance, and systemic vascular resistance are seen in these patients. Heart rates can be moderately decreased or unchanged. Unlike hydralazine, prazosin does not seem to increase renin release so diuretic therapy is not mandatory with this agent (but is usually beneficial in CHF).

Pharmacokinetics

The pharmacokinetic parameters for this agent were not located for veterinary species. In humans, prazosin is variably absorbed after oral administration. Peak levels occur in 2–3 hours.

Prazosin is widely distributed throughout the body and is approximately 97% bound to plasma proteins. Prazosin is minimally distributed into milk. It is unknown if it crosses the placenta.

Prazosin is metabolized in the liver and some metabolites have activity. Metabolites and some unchanged drug (5–10%) are primarily eliminated in feces via the bile.

Contraindications/Precautions/Warnings

Prazosin should be used with caution in patients with chronic renal failure or preexisting hypotensive conditions.

There are some anecdotal reports that dogs with the *ABCB*1 mutation (MDR1) may be overly sensitive to the effects of prazosin; use with caution in breeds known to be susceptible to this mutation. Alternate drugs should be considered for dogs tested positive for this mutation until more information becomes available; if this is not possible, consider reducing the dosage and increase monitoring (particularly blood pressure).

Adverse Effects

An experimental study done in dogs using IV prazosin at 0.025 mg/kg caused significant decreases in systolic, diastolic and mean arterial blood pressures (Fischer *et al.* 2003). Whether this is a clinical concern when using prazosin orally to decrease urethral resistance is unclear.

Syncope secondary to orthostatic hypotension has been reported in people after the first dose of the drug. This effect may persist if the dosage is too high for the patient. CNS effects (lethargy, dizziness, etc.) may occur, but are usually transient in nature. GI effects (nausea, vomiting, diarrhea, constipation, etc.) have been reported. Tachyphylaxis (drug tolerance) has been reported in humans, but dosage adjustment, temporarily withdrawing the drug, &/or adding an aldosterone antagonist (*e.g.*, spironolactone) usually corrects this.

Reproductive/Nursing Safety

In humans, the FDA categorizes this drug as category *C* for use during pregnancy (*Animal studies have shown an adverse effect on the fetus, but there are no adequate studies in humans; or there are no animal reproduction studies and no adequate studies in humans.*)

Prazosin is excreted in small amounts in maternal milk and unlikely to pose much risk to nursing offspring.

Overdosage/Acute Toxicity

There were 12 exposures to prazosin reported to the ASPCA Animal Poison Control Center (APCC) during 2008-2009. In these cases 6 were dogs with none showing clinical signs and 6 were cats with 1 showing clinical signs. Common findings in dogs recorded in decreasing frequency included hyperactivity, tachycardia, hyperthermia, panting and agitation. Common findings in cats in decreasing frequency included tachycardia.

Evacuate gastric contents and administer activated charcoal using standard precautionary measures if the ingestion was recent and if cardiovascular status has been stabilized. Monitor heart rate and blood pressure. Treat shock using volume expanders and pressor agents if necessary. Monitor and support renal function.

Drug Interactions

The following drug interactions have either been reported or are theoretical in humans or animals receiving prazosin and may be of significance in veterinary patients:

■ **BETA-BLOCKING AGENTS (e.g., propranolol):** May enhance the postural hypotensive effects seen after the first dose of prazosin

■ **CLONIDINE:** May decrease prazosin antihypertensive effects

■ **SILDENAFIL (and other PDE INHIBITORS):** May increase risk for hypotension

■ **VERAPAMIL or NIFEDIPINE:** May cause synergistic hypotensive effects when used concomitantly with prazosin

Doses

■ **DOGS:**

a) For adjunctive treatment of heart failure: 1 mg PO three times daily for dogs weighing less than 15 kg; 2 mg three times daily PO for dogs weighing more than 15 kg (Atkins 2007; Kittleson 1985)

b) For hypertension: 1–4 mg (total dose) PO q12–24 hours (Brown & Henik 2000)

c) For hypertension in a large dog: 1 mg (total dose) PO q8–12h (Ware 2003)

d) To decrease urethral resistance: 1 mg per 15 kg of body weight PO q8h (Lane 2000)

e) For functional urethral obstruction: 1 mg/15 kg of body weight PO q8–24h (Lulich 2004)

f) To decrease urethral resistance: 1 mg per 15 kg of body weight PO q12–24h (Bartges 2006; Vernau 2006)

g) To reduce urethral tone: 1 mg/15 kg body weight PO two to three times a day. (Dickinson 2010)

■ **CATS:**

To decrease urethral resistance:

a) 0.5 mg (total dose) PO q8h or 0.03 mg/kg IV (Lane 2000)

b) 0.03 mg/kg IV (Osborne *et al.* 2000)

c) For functional urethral obstruction: 0.25–0.5 mg/cat (total dose) PO q12–24h (Coates 2004; Lulich 2004), (Vernau 2006)

d) For urethral spasm: 0.25–1 mg/cat (total dose) PO q8-12h; initially give for 5–7 days then wean off if possible. (Gunn-Moore & Casey 2009)

e) To reduce urethral tone: 0.5 mg/cat (total dose) PO once to two times a day. (Dickinson 2010)

Monitoring

■ Baseline thoracic radiographs

■ Mucous membrane color; CRT

■ If possible, arterial blood pressure and venous PO$_2$

Client Information

■ Compliance with directions is necessary to maximize the benefits from this drug. If possible, give medication with food.

■ Notify veterinarian if patient's condition deteriorates or if the animal becomes lethargic or depressed.

Chemistry/Synonyms

A quinazoline-derivative postsynaptic alpha$_1$-adrenergic blocker, prazosin HCl occurs as a white to tan powder. It is slightly soluble in water and very slightly soluble in alcohol.

Prazosin may also be known as: CP-12299-1, furazosin hydrochloride, prazosini hydrochloridum; many trade names are available.

Storage/Stability

Prazosin capsules should be stored in well-closed containers at room temperature.

Dosage Forms/Regulatory Status

VETERINARY-LABELED PRODUCTS: None

The ARCI (Racing Commissioners International) has designated this drug as a class 3 substance. See the appendix for more information.

HUMAN-LABELED PRODUCTS:

Prazosin Capsules: 1 mg, 2 mg & 5 mg (as base); *Minipress®* (Pfizer); generic; (Rx)

References

Atkins, C. (2007). Canine Heart Failure—Current concepts. Proceedings: WSAVA World Congress. Accessed via: Veterinary Information Network. http://goo.gl/aWqPH

Bartges, J. (2006). Broken plumbing: urinary incontinence. Proceedings: ACVC 2006. Accessed via: Veterinary Information Network. http://goo.gl/XgEUd

Brown, S. & R. Henik (2000). Therapy for Systemic Hypertension in Dogs and Cats. *Kirk's Current Veterinary Therapy: XIII Small Animal Practice.* J Bonagura Ed. Philadelphia, WB Saunders: 838–841.

Coates, J. (2004). Neurogenic micturition disorders. Proceedings: ACVIM Forum. Accessed via: Veterinary Information Network. http://goo.gl/260CO

Dickinson, P. (2010). Disorders of micturition and continence. Proceedings: UCD Veterinary Neurology Symposium. Accessed via: Veterinary Information Network. http://goo.gl/wo3hl

Fischer, J.R., I.F. Lane, et al. (2003). Urethral pressure profile and hemodynamic effects of phenoxybenzamine and prazosin in non-sedated male beagle dogs. *Canadian Journal of Veterinary Research-Revue Canadienne De Recherche Veterinaire* 67(1): 30–38.

Gunn-Moore, D. & R. Casey (2009). Feline Lower Urinary Tract Disease. Proceedings: BSAVA. Accessed via: Veterinary Information Network. http://goo.gl/IUYv5

Kittleson, M.D. (1985). Pathophysiology and treatment of heart failure. *Manual of Small Animal Cardiology.* LP Tilley and JM Owens Eds. New York, Churchill Livingstone: 308–332.

Lane, I. (2000). Urinary Obstruction and Functional Urine Retention. *Textbook of Veterinary Internal Medicine: Diseases of the Dog and Cat.* S Ettinger and E Feldman Eds. Philadelphia, WB Saunders. 1: 93–96.

Lulich, J. (2004). Managing functional urethral obstruction. Proceedings: ACVIM Forum. Accessed via: Veterinary Information Network. http://goo.gl/acf8d

Osborne, C., J. Kruger, et al. (2000). Feline Lower Urinary Tract Diseases. *Textbook of Veterinary Internal Medicine: Diseases of the Dog and Cat.* S Ettinger and E Feldman Eds. Philadelphia, WB Saunders. 2: 1710–1747.

Vernau, K. (2006). Dysuria: To pee or not to pee . . . Proceedings: UCD Veterinary Neurology Symposium. Accessed via: Veterinary Information Network. http://goo.gl/3KvT8

Ware, W. (2003). Cardiovascular system disorders. *Small Animal Internal Medicine, 3rd Ed.* R Nelson and C Couto Eds. St Louis, Mosby: 1–209.

PREDNISOLONE
PREDNISOLONE SODIUM SUCCINATE
PREDNISOLONE ACETATE
PREDNISONE

(pred-*niss*-oh-lone); (*pred*-ni-zone)

For more information refer to the monograph: Glucocorticoids, General Information or to the manufacturer's product information for veterinary labeled products.

Note: Although separate entities, prednisone and prednisolone are often considered bioequivalent; most species rapidly convert prednisone to prednisolone in the liver. *Horses, cats* and *patients in frank hepatic failure* do not appear to either absorb or convert prednisone to prednisolone efficiently. Use either prednisolone or an alternative glucocorticoid in these patients when possible.

Prescriber Highlights

▶ Classic glucocorticoids used for many conditions in many species. Antiinflammatory activity is 4X more potent than hydrocortisone; has some mineralocorticoid activity

▶ Contraindications (relative): Systemic fungal infections

▶ Caution: Active bacterial infections, corneal ulcer, Cushingoid syndrome, diabetes, osteoporosis, chronic psychotic reactions, predisposition to thrombophlebitis, hypertension, CHF, renal insufficiency

▶ Goal of therapy is to use as much as is required & as little as possible for as short an amount of time as possible

▶ Prednisone poorly absorbed after oral use in horses; prednisone may not be readily converted to prednisolone in cats. Prednisolone is preferred in these two species.

▶ Primary adverse effects are "Cushingoid" in nature with sustained use

▶ Many potential drug & lab interactions

Uses/Indications

Glucocorticoids have been used in an attempt to treat practically every malady that afflicts man or animal, but for prednisolone/prednisone, there are there are four primary uses and dose ranges: **1)** replacement or supplementation (*e.g.*, relative adrenal insufficiency associated with septic shock) of glucocorticoid effects secondary to hypoadrenocorticism, **2)** as an antiinflammatory, **3)** as an immunosuppressive, and, **4)** as an antineoplastic agent. Current evidence does not support high dose use for hemorrhagic or hypovolemic shock, head trauma, spinal cord injury, or sepsis. In general, in using glucocorticoids, the following principles should be followed:

1. Glucocorticoids can mask disease! Try not to use them until you have a diagnosis.
2. Make a specific diagnosis!
3. Determine course from outset.
4. Determine endpoint before you starting treating.
5. Use the least potent form for the minimal time.
6. Know where glucocorticoids inappropriate. (Behrend 2007)

Pharmacology/Actions

Prednisolone and prednisone are intermediate acting corticosteroids with a biologic "half-life" of 12–36 hours. Glucocorticoids have effects on virtually every cell type and system in mammals. For more information, refer to the Glucocorticoid Agents, General Information monograph.

Pharmacokinetics

In cats, prednisolone is much better absorbed when administered orally than prednisone. Reported bioavailabilities (of active prednisolone) are 100% and 21%, respectively.

Plasma half-life is not meaningful from a therapy standpoint when evaluating systemic corticosteroids. Prednisolone and prednisone are intermediate acting corticosteroids with a biologic "half-life" of 12–36 hours.

Contraindications/Precautions/Warnings

Systemic use of glucocorticoids is generally considered contraindicated in systemic fungal infections (unless used for replacement therapy in Addison's), when administered IM in patients with idiopathic thrombocytopenia, and those hypersensitive to a particular compound. Sustained-released injectable glucocorticoids are considered contraindicated for chronic corticosteroid therapy of systemic diseases.

Animals that have received glucocorticoids systemically, other than with "burst" therapy, should be tapered off the drugs. Patients who have received the drugs chronically should be tapered off slowly as endogenous ACTH and corticosteroid function may return slowly. Should the animal undergo a "stressor" (*e.g.*, surgery, trauma, illness, etc.) during the tapering process

or until normal adrenal and pituitary function resume, additional glucocorticoids should be administered.

Animals, particularly cats, at risk for diabetes mellitus or with concurrent cardiovascular disease should receive glucocorticoids with caution due to these agents' potent hyperglycemic effect.

Adverse Effects

Adverse effects are generally associated with long-term administration of these drugs, especially if given at high dosages or not on an alternate day regimen. Effects generally are manifested as clinical signs of hyperadrenocorticism. When administered to young, growing animals, glucocorticoids can retard growth. Many of the potential effects, adverse and otherwise, are outlined above in the Pharmacology section.

In dogs, polydipsia (PD), polyphagia (PP), and polyuria (PU) may all be seen with short-term "burst" therapy as well as with alternate-day maintenance therapy on days when giving the drug. Adverse effects in dogs can include: dull, dry haircoat, weight gain, panting, vomiting, diarrhea, elevated liver enzymes, pancreatitis, GI ulceration, lipidemias, activation or worsening of diabetes mellitus, muscle wasting, and behavioral changes (depression, lethargy, viciousness). Discontinuation of the drug may be necessary; changing to an alternate steroid may also alleviate the problem. With the exception of PU/PD/PP, adverse effects associated with antiinflammatory therapy are relatively uncommon. Adverse effects associated with immunosuppressive doses are more common and potentially more severe.

Cats generally require higher dosages than dogs for clinical effect, but tend to develop fewer adverse effects. Glucocorticoids appear to have a greater hyperglycemic effect in cats than other species. Occasionally, polydipsia, polyuria, polyphagia with weight gain, diarrhea, or depression can be seen. Long-term, high dose therapy can lead to "Cushingoid" effects, however.

Reproductive/Nursing Safety

Corticosteroid therapy may induce parturition in large animal species during the latter stages of pregnancy. In humans, the FDA categorizes this drug as category **C** for use during pregnancy (*Animal studies have shown an adverse effect on the fetus, but there are no adequate studies in humans; or there are no animal reproduction studies and no adequate studies in humans.*) In a separate system evaluating the safety of drugs in canine and feline pregnancy (Papich 1989), this drug is categorized as class: **C** (*These drugs may have potential risks. Studies in people or laboratory animals have uncovered risks, and these drugs should be used cautiously as a last resort when the benefit of therapy clearly outweighs the risks.*)

Use with caution in nursing dams. Glucocorticoids unbound to plasma proteins will enter milk. High dosages or prolonged administration to mothers may potentially inhibit growth, interfere with endogenous corticosteroid production or cause other unwanted effects in nursing offspring. In humans, however, several studies suggest that amounts excreted in breast milk are negligible when prednisone or prednisolone doses in the mother are less than or equal to 20 mg/day or methylprednisolone doses are less than or equal to 8 mg/day. Larger doses for short periods may not harm the infant.

Overdosage/Acute Toxicity

Overdoses of glucocorticoids used alone are unlikely to cause harmful effects, but gastrointestinal signs can be seen in dogs. Should clinical signs occur, use supportive treatment if required. Chronic usage of glucocorticoids can lead to serious adverse effects. Refer to Adverse Effects above for more information.

There were 175 exposures to prednisone reported to the ASPCA Animal Poison Control Center (APCC) during 2008-2009. In these cases, 164 were dogs with 16 showing clinical signs, and 10 were cats with 2 showing clinical signs. The remaining 1 case was a bird that showed no clinical signs. Common findings in dogs included polydipsia and polyuria.

Drug Interactions

The following drug interactions have either been reported or are theoretical in humans or animals receiving oral prednisolone/prednisone and may be of significance in veterinary patients:

- **AMPHOTERICIN B:** When administered concomitantly with glucocorticoids may cause hypokalemia
- **ANTICHOLINESTERASE AGENTS (e.g., pyridostigmine, neostigmine, etc.):** In patients with myasthenia gravis, concomitant glucocorticoid with these agents may lead to profound muscle weakness. If possible, discontinue anticholinesterase medication at least 24 hours prior to corticosteroid administration.
- **ASPIRIN (salicylates):** Glucocorticoids may reduce salicylate blood levels. In dogs, prednisone with ultra low-dose (0.5 mg/kg) aspirin does not increase the severity of GI lesions when compared with prednisone alone, but may increase incidence of diarrhea (Graham & Leib 2009).
- **CYCLOPHOSPHAMIDE:** Glucocorticoids may also inhibit the hepatic metabolism of cyclophosphamide; dosage adjustments may be required.
- **CYCLOSPORINE:** Concomitant administration of may increase the blood levels of each, by mutually inhibiting the hepatic metabolism of each other; clinical significance of this interaction is not clear
- **DIGOXIN:** Secondary to hypokalemia, increased risk for arrhythmias

- **DIURETICS, POTASSIUM-DEPLETING (furosemide, thiazides):** When administered concomitantly with glucocorticoids may cause hypokalemia
- **EPHEDRINE:** May increase metabolism of glucocorticoids
- **ESTROGENS:** The effects of hydrocortisone, and possibly other glucocorticoids, may be potentiated by concomitant administration with estrogens
- **INSULIN:** Requirements may increase in patients receiving glucocorticoids
- **KETOCONAZOLE:** May decrease metabolism of glucocorticoids
- **MITOTANE:** May alter the metabolism of steroids; higher than usual doses of steroids may be necessary to treat mitotane-induced adrenal insufficiency
- **NSAIDS:** Administration of other ulcerogenic drugs with glucocorticoids may increase risk
- **PHENOBARBITAL:** May increase the metabolism of glucocorticoids
- **PHENYTOIN:** May increase the metabolism of glucocorticoids
- **RIFAMPIN:** May increase the metabolism of glucocorticoids
- **VACCINES:** Patients receiving corticosteroids at immunosuppressive dosages should generally not receive live attenuated-virus vaccines as virus replication may be augmented; a diminished immune response may occur after vaccine, toxoid, or bacterin administration in patients receiving glucocorticoids

Laboratory Considerations

- Glucocorticoids may increase serum **cholesterol** and **urine glucose** levels.
- Glucocorticoids may decrease serum **potassium**.
- Glucocorticoids can suppress the release of thyroid stimulating hormone (TSH) and reduce T_3 & T_4 values. Thyroid gland atrophy has been reported after chronic glucocorticoid administration. Uptake of I^{131} by the thyroid may be decreased by glucocorticoids.
- Reactions to **skin tests** may be suppressed by glucocorticoids.
- False-negative results of the **nitroblue tetrazolium test for systemic bacterial infections** may be induced by glucocorticoids.

Doses

There are a plethora of doses and protocols associated with many specific indications for systemic administration of glucocorticoids, but there are four primary uses and dose ranges: **1)** replacement or supplementation (e.g., relative adrenal insufficiency associated with septic shock) of glucocorticoid effects secondary to hypoadrenocorticism, **2)** as an antiinflammatory, **3)** as an immunosuppressive, and, **4)** as an antineoplastic agent. Current evidence does not support high dose use for hemorrhagic or hypovolemic shock, head trauma, spinal cord trauma, or sepsis.

■ **DOGS/CATS:**

Use PO prednisolone in place of prednisone in cats whenever possible as they do not absorb or convert prednisone to prednisolone as well as dogs. If PO prednisone must be used in cats, consider increasing the dose.

Note: If given daily, therapy for longer than one-two weeks will suppress the HPA axis and recovery will take longer than one week. Therefore, if corticosteroids are used for longer than a few days, dosage must be tapered off using alternate day therapy. Many glucocorticoid responsive diseases can be managed with chronic alternate day therapy; avoid if possible, doses greater than 1 mg/kg (prednisolone equivalent) every other day. Larger doses saturate the dog's ability to fully metabolize the last dose before the next dose is given and can negate the benefits of alternate day therapy. However, to induce remission of clinical signs or manage their recurrence requires institution of daily therapy at an appropriate dose to control clinical signs, then tapering to reach a minimum daily dose that will control signs followed by alternate day therapy to manage the disease. Individuals vary greatly in their response to the therapeutic and adverse effects of glucocorticoids and there may be qualitative differences between the effects of different glucocorticoids in the same patient. (Maddison 2009)

As an antiinflammatory agent:

a) **Dogs:** 0.5–1 mg/kg PO per day. See above note for additional information. (Maddison 2009)

b) **Dogs or Cats:** 0.55–1.1 mg/kg PO per day, either once per day or divided twice per day. (Lowe *et al.* 2008)

As an immunosuppressive:

a) **Dogs:** Doses up to 2.2 mg/kg PO per day. Doses above 2.2 mg/kg/day do not give more immunosuppression, but do cause more adverse effects. If further immunosuppression is required, an additional immunosuppressive drug is needed. Many internists believe that prednisone doses should not exceed 80 mg per day, regardless of dog's weight. A sample prednisone immunosuppressive protocol for dogs follows but doses and dosage schedule must be tailored to the ongoing requirements of the individual patient: 2.2 mg/kg/day (not to exceed 80 mg total dose per day) for 3 weeks, then 1 mg/kg/day for 3 weeks, then 0.5 mg/kg/day for 3 weeks, then 0.5 mg/kg every other day.

Cats: Often require up to 4.4 mg/kg/day PO for immunosuppression. If further immunosuppression is required, an additional immunosuppressive drug is needed. A sample prednisolone immunosuppressive protocol for cats follows but doses and dosage schedule must be tailored to the ongoing requirements of the individual patient: 4.4 mg/kg/day for 3 weeks, then 2.2 mg/kg/day for 3 weeks, then 1 mg/kg/day for 3 weeks, then 1 mg/kg every other day. (Wilson 2010; Wilson 2011)

b) **Dogs:** >1.5 mg/kg, up to 4 mg/kg PO per day; no clinical advantage in using a higher dose and risk of side effects increase. See above note for additional information. (Maddison 2009)

c) **Cats** (prednisolone): 2.2–8.8 mg/kg per day. Some authors believe that dividing the daily dose is indicated to decrease GI irritation. (Lowe *et al.* 2008)

As an antineoplastic/cytotoxic:

When prednis(ol)one is used as an antineoplastic agent, whether alone or in a multi-drug chemotherapy protocol, the following dosages should be used only as a general guide. Consultation with a veterinary oncologist and referral to current veterinary oncology references [*e.g.*, (Henry & Higginbotham 2009); (Argyle *et al.* 2008); (Withrow & Vail 2007); (Villalobos 2007); (Ogilvie & Moore 2006); (Ogilvie & Moore 2001)] is *strongly recommended.*

a) **Dogs:** 2 mg/kg per day. Cats are relatively steroid resistant and require higher doses than dogs. Doses can usually be safely doubled compared to dogs. See above note for additional information. (Maddison 2009) (Note: When used with other cytotoxic agents in chemo protocols, prednis(ol)one doses may be reduced.)

b) When prednis(ol)one is used as a single agent, the dose must be kept fairly high. When using it as part of a multi-drug protocol, the dose will be tapered. (Wilson 2010; Wilson 2011)

As adjunctive treatment for hypoadrenocorticism:

a) Acute treatment: After second blood draw for cortisol measurement (ACTH stimulation test), prednisolone sodium succinate 2–20 mg/kg IV. If animal is in shock, give steroids at shock doses instead of trying to get an immediate diagnosis, then give dexamethasone (0.05–0.1 mg/kg IV q12h) in IV fluids until able to switch to PO steroids.

For oral glucocorticoid replacement (ongoing, with a mineralocorticoid): Prednisone initially at 0.1–0.22 mg/kg, then taper to lowest dose to control clinical signs. (Scott-Moncrieff 2010)

b) For physiologic replacement, it is common for dogs to require no more than 0.1 mg/kg once per day of prednis(ol)one, and often less will be sufficient to prevent recurrence of signs of glucocorticoid insufficiency. When on fludrocortisone (*Florinef*®), approximately half of the cases do not require any additional prednisone as there is enough glucocorticoid activity in fludrocortisone for those dogs. However, if on desoxycorticosterone pivalate (*Percorten*®), all cases require additional prednisone as it only has mineralocorticoid activity. (Wilson 2010; Wilson 2011)

■ **CATTLE:**

For adjunctive therapy of cerebral edema secondary to polioencephalomalacia:

a) Prednisolone 1–4 mg/kg intravenously (Dill 1986)

For adjunctive therapy of aseptic laminitis:

a) Prednisolone (assuming sodium succinate salt) 100–200 mg IM or IV; continue therapy for 2–3 days (Berg 1986)

For glucocorticoid activity:

a) Prednisolone sodium succinate: 0.2–1 mg/kg IV or IM. (Howard 1986)

■ **RABBITS, RODENTS, SMALL MAMMALS:**

a) **Rabbits:** Rarely indicated. Use with caution; concurrent gastroprotectant is recommended. For spinal trauma: 0.25–0.5 mg/kg PO q12h for 3 days, then once daily for 3 days, then once every other day for 3 doses.

As an antiinflammatory: 0.5–2 mg/kg PO (Ivey & Morrisey 2000)

b) **Mice, Rats, Gerbils, Hamsters, Guinea pigs, Chinchillas:** 0.5–2.2 mg/kg IM or SC (Adamcak & Otten 2000)

■ **FERRETS:**

As an antiinflammatory or for insulinoma (postsurgical or nonsurgical cases):

a) 0.5–2 mg/kg PO or IM (frequency not specified) (Williams 2000)

■ **HORSES:** (**Note:** ARCI UCGFS Class 4 Drug) **Note:** Prednisone does not appear to be absorbed very well after oral dosing; use prednisolone or another oral steroid.

For adjunctive therapy of Recurrent Airway Obstruction (RAO; Heaves):

a) For short term treatment with environmental control: In the study, dexamethasone sodium phosphate was given (0.1 mg/kg IM once daily for 4 days, 0.075 mg/kg IM once daily for 4 days, and 0.05 mg/kg IM for 4 days) or oral prednisolone (1 mg/kg PO for 4 days, 0.75 mg/kg for 4 days, 0.5 mg/kg PO for

4 days). Except for bronchoalveolar lavage cytology, prednisolone was as effective as IM dexamethasone. (Courouce-Malblanc *et al.* 2008)

b) In this study, horses were under continuous antigen exposure: Dexamethasone was given (0.05 mg/kg PO once daily for 7 days) or prednisolone (2 mg/kg PO once daily for 7 days). Both were effective, but dexamethasone more so. (Leclere *et al.* 2010)

For adjunctive therapy of neoplasias:

a) Prednisolone: Typical dose is 1 mg/kg PO every other day. (Mair & Couto 2006)

For glucocorticoid effects:

a) Prednisolone sodium succinate: 0.25–1 mg/kg IV, Predniso(lo)ne tablets 0.25–1 mg/kg PO; Prednisolone acetate: 0.25–1 mg/kg IM or 10–25 mg subconjunctivally (Robinson 1987)

■ **LLAMAS:**

For steroid-responsive pruritic dermatoses secondary to allergic origins:

a) Prednisone: 0.5–1 mg/kg PO initially, gradually reduce dosage to lowest effective dose given every other day (Rosychuk 1989)

■ **SWINE:**

For glucocorticoid activity:

a) Prednisolone sodium succinate: 0.2–1 mg/kg IV or IM (Howard 1986)

■ **BIRDS:**

As an antiinflammatory:

a) Prednisolone: 0.2 mg/30 gram body weight, or dissolve one 5 mg tablet in 2.5 mL of water and administer 2 drops orally. Give twice daily. Decrease dosage schedule if using long-term. (Clubb 1986)

For treatment of shock:

a) Prednisolone sodium succinate (10 mg/mL): 0.1–0.2 mL/100 grams body weight. Repeat every 15 minutes to effect. In large birds, dosage may be decreased by ½. (Clubb 1986)

■ **REPTILES:**

For shock in most species using prednisolone sodium succinate:

a) 5–10 mg/kg IV as needed (Gauvin 1993)

Monitoring

Monitoring of glucocorticoid therapy is dependent on its reason for use, dosage, agent used (amount of mineralocorticoid activity), dosage schedule (daily versus alternate day therapy), duration of therapy, and the animal's age and condition. The following list may not be appropriate or complete for all animals; use clinical assessment and judgment should adverse effects be noted:

■ Weight, appetite, signs of edema

- Serum and/or urine electrolytes
- Total plasma proteins, albumin
- Blood glucose
- Growth and development in young animals
- ACTH stimulation test if necessary

Client Information

- Clients should carefully follow the dosage instructions and not discontinue the drug abruptly without consulting with veterinarian beforehand.
- Clients should be briefed on the potential adverse effects that can be seen with these drugs and instructed to contact the veterinarian should these effects become severe or progress.

Chemistry/Synonyms

Prednisolone and prednisone are synthetic glucocorticoids. Prednisolone and prednisone acetate occur as odorless, white to practically white, crystalline powders. Prednisolone is very slightly soluble in water and slightly soluble in alcohol. The acetate ester is practically insoluble in water and slightly soluble in alcohol. The sodium succinate ester is highly water-soluble.

Prednisone occurs as an odorless, white to practically white, crystalline powder. Prednisone is very slightly soluble in water and slightly soluble in alcohol.

Prednisolone is also known as deltahydrocortisone or metacortandralone.

Prednisone may also be known as: delta(1)-cortisone, 1,2-dehydrocortisone, deltacortisone, deltadehydrocortisone, metacortandracin, NSC-10023, prednisonum; many trade names are available.

Storage/Stability

Prednisolone and prednisone tablets should be stored in well-closed containers. All prednisone and prednisolone products should be stored at temperatures less than 40°, and preferably between 15–30°C; avoid freezing liquid products. Do not autoclave. Oral liquid preparations of prednisone should be stored in tight containers. Do not refrigerate prednisolone syrup.

Prednisolone sodium succinate should be stored at room temperature and protected from light (store in carton). After reconstitution, the product is recommended for immediate use and not to be stored for later use.

Compatibility/Compounding Considerations

Little data appears to be available regarding the compatibility of prednisolone sodium succinate injection (*Solu-Delta Cortef®*—Pfizer) with other products. A related compound, prednisolone sodium phosphate is reportedly physically **compatible** with the following drugs/solutions: ascorbic acid injection, cytarabine, erythromycin lactobionate, fluorouracil, heparin sodium, methicillin sodium, penicillin G potassium/sodium, tetracycline HCl, and vitamin B-Complex

with C. It is reportedly physically **incompatible** with: calcium gluconate/gluceptate, dimenhydrinate, metaraminol bitartrate, methotrexate sodium, prochlorperazine edisylate, polymyxin B sulfate, promazine HCl, and promethazine. Compatibility is dependent upon factors such as pH, concentration, temperature, and diluent used; consult specialized references or a hospital pharmacist for more specific information.

Dosage Forms/Regulatory Status

VETERINARY-LABELED PRODUCTS:

A zero tolerance of residues in milk for these compounds have been established for dairy cattle. All these agents require a prescription (Rx). Known FDA-approved-veterinary products for systemic use are indicated below.

The ARCI (Racing Commissioners International) has designated this drug as a class 4 substance. See the appendix for more information.

Prednisolone Sodium Succinate for Injection *act-o-vial®* System 100 mg (equivalent to 10 mg prednisolone) & 500 mg (equivalent to 50 mg prednisolone) per 10 mL vial; *Solu-Delta-Cortef®* (Pfizer); (Rx). FDA-approved for use in dogs, cats, and horses.

Prednisolone Tablets: 5 mg, 20 mg: *Prednis-Tab®* (various); generic; (Rx). FDA-approved for use in dogs.

Prednisolone, Tetracycline, Novobiocin Tablets: each tablet contains 60 mg tetracycline, 60 mg novobiocin, 1.5 mg prednisolone. *Delta Albaplex®*; each tablet contains 180 mg tetracycline, 180 mg novobiocin, and 4.5 mg prednisolone *Delta Albaplex® 3X* (Pfizer); (Rx). FDA-approved for use in dogs.

Prednisolone & Trimeprazine Tartrate Tablets: each tablet contains trimeprazine 5 mg and prednisolone 2 mg. *Temaril-P®* (Pfizer Animal Health); (Rx). FDA-approved for use in dogs.

HUMAN-LABELED PRODUCTS:

Prednisolone Oral Tablets: 5 mg; generic; (Rx)

Prednisolone Sodium Phosphate Orally Disintegrating Tablets: 10 mg, 15 mg & 30 mg (as base); *Orapred ODT®* (Sciele); (Rx)

Prednisolone Syrup/Oral Liquid or Solution: 1 mg/mL, 2 mg/mL, 3 mg/mL, 4 mg/mL; *Pediapred®* (Celltech Pharmaceuticals); *Millipred®* (Laser); *Orapred®* (Sciele); *Veripred 20* (Hawthorn); *Flo-Pred®* (Taro); generic; (Rx)

Prednisone Tablets: 1 mg, 2.5 mg, 5 mg, 10 mg, 20 mg & 50 mg; generic; (Rx)

Prednisone Oral Solution/Syrup: 1 mg/mL; *Prednisone* and *Prednisone Intensol® Concentrate* (Roxane); (Rx)

Ophthalmic solutions/suspensions are available.

References

Adamcak, A. & B. Otten (2000). Rodent Therapeutics. *Vet Clin NA: Exotic Anim Pract* **3:1**(Jan): 221–240.

Argyle, D., M. Brearly, et al. (2008). *Decision Making in Small Animal Oncology*, Wiley-Blackwell.

Behrend, E. (2007). Approach to glucocorticoid therapy. Proceedings: Western Vet Conference. Accessed via: Veterinary Information Network. http://goo.gl/XSDaM

Berg, J.N. (1986). Aseptic laminitis in cattle. *Current Veterinary Therapy: Food Animal Practice 2*. JL Howard Ed. Philadelphia, W.B. Saunders: 896–898.

Clubb, S.L. (1986). Therapeutics: Individual and Flock Treatment Regimens. *Clinical Avian Medicine and Surgery*. GJ Harrison and LR Harrison Eds. Philadelphia, W.B. Saunders: 327–355.

Courouce-Malblanc, A., G. Fortier, et al. (2008). Comparison of prednisolone and dexamethasone effects in the presence of environmental control in heaves-affected horses. *Veterinary Journal* **175**(2): 227–233.

Dill, S.G. (1986). Polioencephalomalacia in Ruminants. *Current Veterinary Therapy: Food Animal Practice 2*. JL Howard Ed. Philadelphia, W.B. Saunders: 868–869.

Gauvin, J. (1993). Drug therapy in reptiles. *Seminars in Avian & Exotic Med* **2**(1): 48–59.

Graham, A.H. & M.S. Leib (2009). Effects of Prednisone Alone or Prednisone with Ultralow-Dose Aspirin on the Gastroduodenal Mucosa of Healthy Dogs. *Journal of Veterinary Internal Medicine* **23**(3): 482–487.

Henry, C. & M. Higginbotham (2009). *Cancer Management in Small Animal Practice*, Saunders.

Howard, J.L., Ed. (1986). *Current Veterinary Therapy 2, Food Animal Practice*. Philadelphia, W.B. Saunders.

Ivey, E. & J. Morrisey (2000). Therapeutics for Rabbits. *Vet Clin NA: Exotic Anim Pract* **3:1**(Jan): 183–216.

Leclere, M., J. Lefebvre-Lavoie, et al. (2010). Efficacy of oral prednisolone and dexamethasone in horses with recurrent airway obstruction in the presence of continuous antigen exposure. *Equine Veterinary Journal* **42**(4): 316–321.

Lowe, A.D., K.L. Campbell, et al. (2008). Glucocorticoids in the cat. *Veterinary Dermatology* **19**(6): 340–347.

Maddison, J. (2009). Cortocosteroids—Friend or Foe? Proceedings: WSAVA. Accessed via: Veterinary Information Network. http://goo.gl/CUecU

Mair, T.S. & C.G. Couto (2006). The use of cytotoxic drugs in equine practice. *Equine Veterinary Education* **18**(3): 149–156.

Ogilvie, G. & A. Moore (2001). *Feline Oncology: A Comprehensive Guide to Compassionate Care*, Veterinary Learning Systems.

Ogilvie, G. & A. Moore (2006). *Managing the Canine Cancer Patient: A Practical Guide to Compassionate Care*, Veterinary Learning Systems.

Papich, M. (1989). Effects of drugs on pregnancy. *Current Veterinary Therapy X: Small Animal Practice*. R Kirk Ed. Philadelphia, Saunders: 1291–1299.

Robinson, N.E. (1987). Table of Common Drugs: Approximate Doses. *Current Therapy in Equine Medicine, 2*. NE Robinson Ed. Philadelphia, W.B. Saunders: 761.

Rosychuk, R.A.W. (1989). Llama Dermatology. *Vet Clin of North Amer: Food Anim Prac* **5**(1): 203–215.

Scott-Moncrieff, J.C. (2010). Hypoadrenocorticism in dogs and cats: Update on diagnosis & treatment. Proceedings: ACVIM Forum. Accessed via: Veterinary Information Network. http://goo.gl/DV3Xh

Villalobos, A. (2007). *Canine and Feline Geriatric Oncology*. Ames, Blackwell.

Williams, B. (2000). Therapeutics in Ferrets. *Vet Clin NA: Exotic Anim Pract* **3:1**(Jan): 131–153.

Wilson, S. (2010, Last Update). "VIN BOARDS: Diabetic with post lysodren treatment for Cushings."

Wilson, S. (2011, Last Update). "Personal Communication."

Withrow, S. & D. Vail (2007). *Withrow and MacEwen's Small Animal Clinical Oncology 4th Ed*. Philadelphia, Elsevier.

PREGABALIN

(pre-**gab**-ah-lin)   Lyrica®

ANTICONVULSANT; NEUROPATHIC PAIN AGENT

Prescriber Highlights

▶ Similar to gabapentin; may be useful as an anticonvulsant or to treat neuropathic pain

▶ Little information available on safety and efficacy in dogs or cats

▶ Most common adverse effects are sedation and ataxia

▶ Currently very expensive

Uses/Indications

Like gabapentin, pregabalin may be useful as adjunctive therapy for refractory or complex partial seizures and in treating chronic pain, particularly neuropathic pain in small animals.

In an open label, non-comparative study in dogs that were not controlled with phenobarbital and/or bromides, in 7/9 dogs pregabalin reduced seizures by about 60%. Two dogs were considered non-responders to pregabalin (Dewey *et al.* 2009).

Pharmacology/Actions

Pregabalin has antiepileptic, analgesic, and anxiolytic activity. Like gabapentin, pregabalin is a structural analog of the inhibitory neurotransmitter gamma-aminobutyric acid (GABA). The mechanism of action of pregabalin, for either its anticonvulsant or analgesic actions is not fully understood, but it appears to bind to CaVa2-d (alpha2-delta subunit of the voltage-gated calcium channels). By decreasing calcium influx, release of excitatory neurotransmitters (*e.g.*, substance P, glutamate, norepinephrine) is inhibited. It is 3-10 times as potent as gabapentin.

Pharmacokinetics

After single oral doses in six dogs, pregabalin median parameters were: T max = 1.5 hours; Cmax = 7.15 micrograms/mL; elimination half-life = 6.9 hours (Salazar *et al.* 2009).

After single oral doses in six cats, pregabalin median parameters were: T max = 2.9 hours; Cmax = 8.3 micrograms/mL; elimination half-life = 10.4 hours (Cautela *et al.* 2009).

In humans, oral bioavailability is about 90%. Presence of food can delay the rate, but not the amount absorbed and it can be administered regardless of feeding status. Pregabalin is not bound to plasma proteins and it has an apparent volume of distribution of about 500 mL/kg. Hepatic metabolism is negligible and it does not appear to affect hepatic enzymes. The drug is almost exclusively cleared unchanged by renal routes with a renal clearance of 67-81 mL/minute in young, healthy subjects. Elimination half-life is approximately 6 hours. Dosage adjustment may be required in patients with diminished renal function.

Contraindications/Precautions/Warnings

Pregabalin is contraindicated in patients hypersensitive to it. Use with caution in patients with renal insufficiency; if required, dosage adjustment should be considered. In humans, pregabalin doses are adjusted based on creatinine clearance. Pregabalin is used with caution in human patients with heart failure.

In humans, abrupt discontinuation may lead to increased seizure frequency, diarrhea, headache, insomnia, or nausea.

Adverse Effects

Most common adverse effects reported include sedation and ataxia. Because use to date is limited in animals, adverse effect profile may evolve with additional clinical experience.

In humans, the most common adverse effects reported are: somnolence, dizziness, ataxia, difficulty with concentration/attention/memory, blurred vision, dry mouth, peripheral edema, constipation and weight gain. Syncope and congestive heart failure have been reported less frequently. Rarely, renal failure (reversible) and rhabdolmyolysis have been reported. Hypersensitivity reactions have included angioedema, rash, blisters, and wheezing. Pregabalin therapy has been associated with decreased platelet production or increased creatine kinase levels in some human patients.

Reproductive/Nursing Safety

In humans, the FDA categorizes this drug as category **C** for use during pregnancy *(Animal studies have shown an adverse effect on the fetus, but there are no adequate studies in humans; or there are no animal reproduction studies and no adequate studies in humans.)* Very high dosages of pregabalin have caused skeletal malformations in offspring when given to pregnant rats and rabbits. Pregabalin is excreted into milk, and safety has not been established. Weigh the potential risks of treating versus the benefits when using this drug in pregnant or nursing animals.

Overdosage/Acute Toxicity

There is limited experience with overdoses of pregabalin. One human ingested 8 grams without significant effect. There is no specific antidote for overdose with pregabalin. Standard decontamination protocols can be employed if indicated. Contact an animal poison center for more information.

Drug Interactions

The following drug interactions have either been reported or are theoretical in humans or animals receiving pregabalin and may be of significance in veterinary patients:

- ■ **ACE INHIBITORS (e.g., benazepril, enalapril):** In humans, co-administration with pregabalin may increase risks edema and hives

- ■ **CNS DEPRESSANTS:** Pregabalin may cause additive CNS depression

- ■ **NSAIDS:** In humans, ketorolac and naproxen have been cited as possibly reducing anticonvulsant effectiveness. Substantive evidence is weak, however.

Laboratory Considerations

- ■ None noted.

Doses

- ■ **DOGS:**
  a) In a small single-dose pharmacokinetic study, the authors concluded that 4 mg/kg PO twice daily would produce plasma levels within the extrapolated (from humans) therapeutic range; further studies evaluating its safety and efficacy for the treatment of neuropathic pain and seizures in dogs is warranted. (Salazar *et al.* 2009)

  b) For seizure disorders: 3−4 mg/kg PO every 8 hours; to minimize side effects, it is suggested that dogs initially be started on 2 mg/kg and the dose increased by 1 mg/kg each week until the target dose is reached. (Munana 2010),

  c) The major side effect noted in dogs is sedation and the dose must be gradually increased from 2 mg/kg PO to 3−4 mg/kg q8−12h as needed for effectiveness. (Bailey & Dewey 2009)

  d) If seizure control cannot be obtained with a combination of phenobarbital and bromides, then a third anticonvulsant medication may be added (*e.g.,* zonisamide, levetiracetam, felbamate, gabapentin or pregabalin). If trying pregabalin: 2 mg/kg q8-12h, increasing 1 mg/kg/dose each week to a total of 3−4 mg/kg. (Mariani 2010)

- ■ **CATS:**
  a) For seizure disorders: There are anecdotal reports of pregabalin use in cats; 1−2 mg/kg PO q12h is most commonly mentioned. (Munana 2010)

  b) Based on their single-dose pharmacokinetic study in 6 cats, the authors theorize that a dose of 1−2 mg/kg PO twice daily would be a reasonable starting dose in cats. Further clinical trials are warranted based on a favorable pharmacokinetic profile. (Cautela *et al.* 2009)

Monitoring

- ■ Efficacy/Adverse effects
- ■ At present, pregabalin plasma levels are not routinely monitored in human medicine

Client Information

- ■ Most common adverse effects seen in animals are sleepiness and sometimes difficulty walking; if these are severe or persist contact veterinarian
- ■ Advise clients that there is little clinical experience with this medication at present,

and to report any adverse effects (other than those noted above) that are seen. If allergic effects are noted (rash, hives, wheezing, or collapse) they should contact veterinarian immediately.

■ Do not stop this medication abruptly without veterinarian's approval. Stopping the medication abruptly may cause increased adverse effects and increase seizures in patients with epilepsy.

Chemistry/Synonyms

Pregabalin is (S)-3-(Aminomethyl)-5-methylhexanoic acid). It is freely soluble in water and in both basic and acidic aqueous solutions.

Pregabalin may also be known as CI-1008, PD-144723, pregabalina, prégabaline or pregabalinum. A common trade name is *Lyrica®*.

Storage/Stability

Store capsules and oral solution at room temperature, 25°C (77°F); excursions permitted between 15-30°C (59-86°F).

Use the oral solution within the first 45 days after opening the bottle.

Dosage Forms/Regulatory Status

VETERINARY-LABELED PRODUCTS: None

HUMAN-LABELED PRODUCTS:

Pregabalin Oral Capsules: 25 mg, 50 mg, 75 mg, 100 mg, 150 mg, 200 mg, 225 mg, & 300 mg; *Lyrica®* (Pfizer); (Rx; C-V controlled substance)

Pregabalin Oral Solution: 20 mg/mL; *Lyrica®* (Pfizer); (Rx; C-V controlled substance)

References

Bailey, K.S. & C.W. Dewey (2009). THE SEIZURING CAT Diagnostic work-up and therapy. *Journal of Feline Medicine and Surgery* 11(5): 385–394.

Cautela, M., C.W. Dewey et al. (2009). Pharmacokinetics of oral pregabalin in catsa after single dose administration. Proceedings: ACVIM. Accessed via: Veterinary Information Network. http://goo.gl/a5fLW

Dewey, C.W., S. Cerda-Gonzalez, et al. (2009). Pregabalin as an adjunct to phenobarbital, potassium bromide, or a combination of phenobarbital and potassium bromide for treatment of dogs with suspected idiopathic epilepsy. *Javma-Journal of the American Veterinary Medical Association* 235(12): 1442–1449.

Mariani, C. (2010). Maintenance therapy for the routine & difficult to control epileptic patient. Proceedings: ACVIM Forum. Accessed via: Veterinary Information Network. http://goo.gl/quX8P

Munana, K. (2010). Current Approaches to Seizure Management. Proceedings: ACVIM Forum. Accessed via: Veterinary Information Network. http://goo.gl/vl8Lp

Salazar, V., C.W. Dewey, et al. (2009). Pharmacokinetics of single-dose oral pregabalin administration in normal dogs. *Veterinary Anaesthesia and Analgesia* 36(6): 574–580.

PRIMAQUINE PHOSPHATE

(*prim*-ah-kwin)

ANTIPROTOZOAL

Prescriber Highlights

▶ Antiprotozoal agent considered the drug of choice for treating *Babesia felis* in cats; does not apparently "cure" the infection; repeated courses of therapy may be necessary

▶ May also be useful in treating *Hepatazoon canis* in dogs or *Plasmodium* spp. in birds

▶ Most common adverse effect in cats is nausea; giving with food may help

▶ Very narrow therapeutic index (safety margin); must be careful in determining dosages

▶ Monitoring CBC mandatory

Uses/Indications

Primaquine is considered the drug of choice for treating *Babesia felis* in cats. Primaquine does not apparently "cure" the infection; repeated courses of therapy may be necessary. It may be useful in treating *Hepatazoon canis* in dogs or *Plasmodium* spp. in birds. In humans, primaquine is used for treatment and prophylaxis for malaria and treating *Pneumocystis* pneumonia.

Pharmacology/Actions

Primaquine's antiprotozoal mechanism of action is not well understood, but it may be related to it binding and altering protozoal DNA.

Pharmacokinetics

No pharmacokinetic information was located for small animals. In humans, primaquine is rapidly absorbed with high (96%) systemic bioavailability. It is extensively distributed and rapidly metabolized in the liver to carboxyprimaquine. It is not known if this metabolite has any antiprotozoal activity. Elimination half-life is around 6 hours for primaquine; 24 hours for carboxyprimaquine.

Contraindications/Precautions/Warnings

Primaquine is contraindicated in patients with known hypersensitivity to it. In humans, it is contraindicated in patients receiving other bone marrow suppressant medications or patients susceptible to granulocytopenia (*e.g.*, lupus, rheumatoid arthritis). The CDC states the drug is contraindicated in individuals with G-6-PD deficiency, and during pregnancy or lactation (unless nursing infant determined not to be G-6-PD deficient).

Adverse Effects

Vomiting is the most common adverse effect in cats associated with primaquine; dosing with food may help alleviate this problem. Other concerns include myelosuppression, methemoglobinemia and hemolysis. Safety margin is particularly narrow with this drug in cats (see Overdoses).

Reproductive/Nursing Safety

The CDC recommends using chloroquine or mefloquine for humans during pregnancy and to defer using primaquine until after delivery primarily because primaquine can cause hemolytic anemia in G-6-PD deficient fetuses. It is also contraindicated during lactation in nursing infants unless they are determined not to be G-6-PD deficient. While significance for veterinary patients is not clear, primaquine should be avoided during pregnancy and lactation.

Overdosage/Acute Toxicity

In cats, it has been reported that dosages greater than 1 mg/kg can be lethal. Overdoses should initially be handled aggressively using standardized protocols for removal of drug from the gut and to prevent absorption. Because of the potential seriousness of overdoses, it is recommended to contact an animal poison control center for guidance.

Drug Interactions

The following drug interactions have either been reported or are theoretical in humans or animals receiving primaquine and may be of significance in veterinary patients:

- **QUINACRINE:** May potentiate the toxicity of one another; use of primaquine within 3 months of quinacrine is not recommended

- **BONE MARROW DEPRESSANT DRUGS (e.g., amphotericin B, azathioprine, chloramphenicol, many antineoplastic drugs) or HEMOLYTIC DRUGS (e.g., acetohydroxamic acid, sulfonylureas, quinidine, sulfonamides):** Use with primaquine may cause increased risk for toxicity

Laboratory Considerations

- No specific concerns noted

Doses

- **CATS:**

  Note: Dosing for humans for primaquine is usually described in terms of primaquine base, but dosages for cats may not directly specify whether primaquine is being dosed as the phosphate or as the base. Because primaquine has an extremely narrow therapeutic index in cats, this is problematic as a 26.3 mg primaquine phosphate tablet contains only 15 mg of primaquine base. Additionally, commercially available tablets are usually too concentrated to be accurately dosed in domestic cats; a specialized compounding pharmacy should be employed to prepare a suitable dosage form. Be clear as to the amount of primaquine *base or phosphate* wanted per dose.

  a) For *Babesia felis:* 0.5 mg (as base)/kg PO once daily for 1–3 days. (Greene *et al.* 2006)

  b) For *Babesia felis:* 1 mg (total dose per cat) primaquine phosphate PO every 36 hours for 4 treatments, then 1 mg (total dose) per cat every 7 days for 4 treatments. The drug does not sterilize the infection. (Lobetti 2005)

  c) For *Babesia felis:* Primaquine phosphate 1 mg/kg IM one time. (Birkinheuer 2005) **Note:** IM dosage form must be compounded.

Monitoring

- CBC; weekly while treating

- Improved clinical signs (increased appetite and body weight, improvement in anemia)

Client Information

- This drug has a very low safety margin when used in cats; exact adherence with the prescribed dosage is very important; do not double-up the next dose if a dose was previously missed

- Give dose with food to reduce chance for GI problems (vomiting)

Chemistry/Synonyms

Primaquine phosphate is an 8-amino-quinoline compound that occurs as an orange-red, odorless, bitter-tasting, crystalline powder. It is soluble (1 gram in 15 mL) in water and practically insoluble in alcohol. 1 mg of primaquine phosphate contains 0.57 mg of primaquine base.

Primaquine may also be known as primachina, primachinum, primaquina or SN 13272.

Storage/Stability

Primaquine phosphate tablets should be stored in a tight, light resistant container below 40°C, preferably between 15–30°C.

Dosage Forms/Regulatory Status

VETERINARY-LABELED PRODUCTS: None

HUMAN-LABELED PRODUCTS:

Primaquine Phosphate Oral Tablets: 26.3 mg (equiv. to 15 mg primaquine base); generic (Sanofi Winthrop); (Rx)

References

Birkenheuer, A. (2005). Babesiosis. *The 5–minute Veterinary Consult: Canine and Feline 3rd Ed.* L Tilley and F Smith Eds., Lippincott Williams & Wilkins.

Greene, C., K. Hartmannn, et al. (2006). Appendix 8: Antimicrobial Drug Formulary. *Infectious Disease of the Dog and Cat.* C Greene Ed., Elsevier: 1186–1333.

Lobetti, R. (2005). Tropical Diseases. *Textbook of Veterinary Internal Medicine 6th Ed.* S Ettinger and E Feldman Eds., Elsevier: 699–702.

PRIMIDONE

(*pri*-mi-done)   Mysoline®, Neurosyn®
ANTICONVULSANT

Prescriber Highlights

> ▶ Phenobarbital precursor that may be useful for treating seizures in dogs; most recommend using phenobarbital instead
>
> ▶ Contraindications: Severe liver disease or patients with demonstrated previous hypersensitivity. Large Doses Contraindicated: Nephritis or severe respiratory dysfunction
>
> ▶ Extreme Caution: Cats
>
> ▶ Caution: Hypovolemic, anemic, have borderline hypoadrenal function, or cardiac or respiratory disease
>
> ▶ Adverse Effects: *Dogs:* anxiety & agitation when initiating therapy, increases in liver enzymes, hepatic lipidosis, hepatocellular hypertrophy/necrosis, extramedullary hematopoiesis, depression, polydipsia, polyuria, & polyphagia, anorexia, tachycardia, dermatitis, episodic hyperventilation, urolith formation; rarely megaloblastic anemia
>
> ▶ Possibly more hepatotoxic than phenobarbital to dogs
>
> ▶ Most of the anticonvulsant activity comes from the phenobarbital metabolite of primidone
>
> ▶ Drug Interactions, lab interactions

Uses/Indications

Primidone is indicated for seizure control (idiopathic epilepsy, epileptiform convulsions) in the dog. Because it is rapidly converted into phenobarbital in this species (see Pharmacokinetics below), and has a greater incidence of hepatotoxicity and behavioral effects, most neurologists do not recommend its use. However, some clinicians feel that some animals not responding to phenobarbital do benefit from primidone therapy, perhaps as a result that PEMA has been demonstrated to potentiate the anticonvulsant activity of phenobarbital in animals. When compared with phenobarbital, increased incidence of hepatotoxicity associated with primidone is considered the major limitation to long-term therapy with this agent. Primidone is considered more toxic in rabbits and cats than in humans or dogs.

Pharmacology/Actions

Primidone and its active metabolites, phenylethamalonamide (PEMA) and phenobarbital have similar anticonvulsant actions. While the exact mechanism for this activity is unknown, these agents raise seizure thresholds or alter seizure patterns.

Pharmacokinetics

Primidone is slowly absorbed after oral administration in the dog, with peak levels occurring 2–4 hours after dosing. The bioavailability of primidone in humans has been reported as 60–80%.

Primidone is rapidly converted to PEMA and phenobarbital in the dog. Serum half-lives of primidone, PEMA, and phenobarbital have been reported to be 1.85 hrs, 7.1 hrs, and 41 hours, respectively (Yeary 1980). In dogs, the conversion rate of primidone to phenobarbital is approximately 4 to 1; a 250 mg dose of primidone is approximately equivalent to 60 mg of phenobarbital (Platt 2005).

Primidone, like phenobarbital (possibly due to the phenobarbital?), can induce hepatic microsomal enzymes that can increase the rate of metabolism of itself and other drugs.

For more information on the pharmacokinetics of phenobarbital, refer to its monograph.

Contraindications/Precautions/Warnings

Many clinicians and the veterinary manufacturers of primidone feel that primidone is contraindicated in cats, other clinicians dispute this, but it is recommended that primidone be used in cats only with extreme caution. Use cautiously in patients who are hypovolemic, anemic, have borderline hypoadrenal function, or cardiac or respiratory disease. Large doses are contraindicated in patients with nephritis or severe respiratory dysfunction. Primidone is contraindicated in patients with severe liver disease or have had hypersensitivity reactions.

When converting dogs from primidone to phenobarbital, it has been suggested do this slowly (¼ of the dose each month) (Platt 2005).

Adverse Effects

Adverse effects in dogs are similar for both primidone and phenobarbital. Dogs may exhibit increased clinical signs of anxiety and agitation when initiating therapy. These effects may be transitory in nature and often will resolve with small dosage increases. Occasionally, dogs will exhibit profound depression at lower dosage ranges (and plasma levels). Polydipsia, polyuria, and polyphagia are quite commonly displayed at moderate to high serum levels; these are best controlled by limiting intake of both food and water. Sedation and/or ataxia often become significant concerns as serum levels reach the higher ends of the therapeutic range.

Increases in liver enzymes (ALT, ALP, glutamate dehydrogenase) and decreased serum albumin with chronic therapy are common (up to 70% of dogs treated), and more prevalent than with phenobarbital. Hepatic lipidosis, hepatocellular hypertrophy and necrosis, and extramedullary hematopoiesis can be seen after 6 months of therapy. Serious hepatic injury probably occurs in approximately 6–14% of dogs treated.

In dogs, anorexia, tachycardia, dermatitis, episodic hyperventilation, urolith formation and, rarely, megaloblastic anemia have also been reported with primidone therapy.

A urolith consisting of primidone has been reported in one cat (Osborne *et al.* 1999).

Reproductive/Nursing Safety

The effects of primidone in pregnancy are unknown. In pregnant humans, primidone is designated by the FDA as a category **D** drug (*There is evidence of human fetal risk, but the potential benefits from the use of the drug in pregnant women may be acceptable despite its potential risks.*) In a separate system evaluating the safety of drugs in canine and feline pregnancy (Papich 1989), this drug is categorized as class: **C** (*These drugs may have potential risks. Studies in people or laboratory animals have uncovered risks, and these drugs should be used cautiously as a last resort when the benefit of therapy clearly outweighs the risks.*)

Primidone appears in maternal milk in substantial quantities. It is suggested that if somnolence occurs in nursing newborns to consider discontinue nursing.

Overdosage/Acute Toxicity

Because primidone is rapidly metabolized to phenobarbital in dogs, similar clinical signs (sedation to coma, anorexia, vomiting, nystagmus) are seen and corresponding procedures should be used for the treatment of acute primidone overdose. This includes the removal of ingested product from the gut if appropriate, and offering respiratory and cardiovascular support. Activated charcoal has been demonstrated to be of considerable benefit in enhancing the clearance of phenobarbital, even when the drug was administered parenterally. Charcoal acts as a "sink" for the drug to diffuse from the vasculature back into the gut. Forced alkaline diuresis can be of considerable benefit in augmenting the elimination of phenobarbital in patients with normal renal function. Peritoneal or hemodialysis may also be helpful in severe intoxications or in anuric patients.

Drug Interactions

The following drug interactions have either been reported or are theoretical in humans or animals receiving primidone or phenobarbital (primidone's active metabolite) and may be of significance in veterinary patients:

- **ACETAMINOPHEN:** Increased risk for hepatotoxicity, particularly when large or chronic doses of barbiturates are given
- **CARBONIC ANHYDRASE INHIBITORS (e.g., acetazolamide):** Oral administration may decrease the GI absorption of primidone.
- **MONAMINE OXIDASE (MAO) INHIBITORS (e.g., amitraz, possibly selegiline):** May prolong phenobarbital effects
- **PHENYTOIN:** Barbiturates may affect the metabolism of phenytoin, and phenytoin may

alter barbiturate levels; monitoring of blood levels may be indicated

- **RIFAMPIN:** May induce enzymes that increase the metabolism of barbiturates

The following drugs may increase the effects of phenobarbital:

- **ANTIHISTAMINES**
- **CHLORAMPHENICOL**
- **OPIATES**
- **PHENOTHIAZINES**
- **VALPROIC ACID**
- **PHENOBARBITAL** (particularly after chronic therapy) may decrease the effect of the following drugs/drug classes by lowering their serum concentrations:
- **ANTICOAGULANTS, ORAL (WARFARIN)**
- **BETA-BLOCKERS**
- **CHLORAMPHENICOL**
- **CLONAZEPAM**
- **CORTICOSTEROIDS**
- **CYCLOSPORINE**
- **DOXORUBICIN**
- **DOXYCYCLINE** (may persist for weeks after barbiturate discontinued)
- **ESTROGENS**
- **GRISEOFULVIN**
- **METHADONE**
- **METRONIDAZOLE**
- **QUINIDINE**
- **PAROXETINE**
- **PHENOTHIAZINES**
- **PROGESTINS**
- **THEOPHYLLINE**
- **TRICYCLIC ANTIDEPRESSANTS**
- **VERAPAMIL**

Laboratory Considerations

- Barbiturates may cause increased retention of **bromosulfophthalein** (BSP; sulfobromophthalein) and give falsely elevated results. It is recommended that barbiturates not be administered within the 24 hours before BSP retention tests; or if they must, (*e.g.*, for seizure control) the results be interpreted accordingly.

- Primidone/phenobarbital can alter **thyroid** testing. Decreased total and free T4, normal T3, and either normal or increased TSH have been reported. It has been suggested to wait at least 4 weeks after discontinuing phenobarbital to perform thyroid testing.

- In some dogs, primidone/phenobarbital may cause a false positive low dose **dexamethasone suppression test,** by increasing the clearance of dexamethasone. Phenobarbital apparently has no effect either on ACTH stimulation tests or on the hormonal equilibrium of the adrenal axis.

Doses

- **DOGS:**
  a) Initially, 10–30 mg/kg per day divided into 2–3 doses (LeCouteur 1999)

  b) 10 mg/kg PO q8h; not recommended as first choice (Taylor 2003)

- **CATS:**
  a) 20 mg/kg, PO q12h (Neff-Davis 1985)

Monitoring

- Anticonvulsant efficacy
- Adverse effects (CNS related, PU/PD, weight gain)
- Serum phenobarbital levels if lack of efficacy or adverse reactions noted. Although there is some disagreement, therapeutic serum levels in dogs are thought to mirror those in people at 15–40 micrograms/mL. See the phenobarbital monograph for more information.
- If used chronically, routine CBCs and liver enzymes at least every 6 months

Client Information

- Compliance with therapy must be stressed to clients for successful epilepsy treatment. Encourage giving daily doses at same time each day.
- Veterinarian should be contacted if animal develops significant adverse reactions (including clinical signs of anemia and/or liver disease) or if seizure control is unacceptable.

Chemistry/Synonyms

An analog of phenobarbital, primidone occurs as a white, odorless, slightly bitter-tasting, crystalline powder with a melting point of 279°–284°C. One gram is soluble in approximately 2000 mL of water or 200 mL of alcohol.

Primidone may also be known as: hexamidinum, primaclone, primidonum, *Cyral®*, *Epidona®*, *Liskantin®*, *Mylepsinum®*, *Mysoline®*, *Neurosyn®*, *Prysoline®*, *Resimatil®*, or *Sertan®*.

Storage/Stability

Tablets should be stored in well-closed containers preferably at room temperature. The oral suspension should be stored in tight, light-resistant containers preferably at room temperature; avoid freezing. Commercially available suspension and tablets generally have expiration dates of 5 years after manufacture.

Dosage Forms/Regulatory Status

VETERINARY-LABELED PRODUCTS:

Primidone Tablets: 50 mg and 250 mg; *Neurosyn®* (BI-Vetmedica); (Rx). FDA-approved for use in dogs.

The ARCI (Racing Commissioners International) has designated this drug as a class 3 substance. See the appendix for more information.

HUMAN-LABELED PRODUCTS:

Primidone Tablets: 50 mg & 250 mg; *Mysoline®* (Xcel Pharm); generic; (Rx)

References

LeCouteur, R. (1999). Seizures in Dogs and Cats. American Animal Hospital Association: Proceedings from the 1999 Annual Meeting, St Louis.

Neff-Davis, C.A. (1985). Clinical monitoring of drug concentrations. Handbook of Small Animal Therapeutics. LE Davis Ed. New York, Churchill Livingstone: 633–655.

Osborne, C.A., J.P. Lulich, et al. (1999). Drug induced urolithiasis. Vet Clin NA: Sm Anim Pract 28(1): 251–266.

Papich, M. (1989). Effects of drugs on pregnancy. Current Veterinary Therapy X: Small Animal Practice. R Kirk Ed. Philadelphia, Saunders: 1291–1299.

Platt, S. (2005). Anticonvulsant use for epileptics. Proceedings: WSAVA World Congress. Accessed via: Veterinary Information Network. http://goo.gl/HgN0z

Taylor, S. (2003). Neuromuscular disorders. Small Animal Internal Medicine, 3rd Ed. R Nelson and C Couto Eds. St Louis, Mosby: 946–1070.

Yeary, R.A. (1980). Serum concentrations of primidone and its metabolites, phenylethylmalonamide and phenobarbital in the dog. Am J Vet Res 41(10): 1643–1645.

PROBENECID

(proh-*ben*-eh-sid)   Benemid®, Benuryl®

URICOSURIC; RENAL TUBULAR SECRETION INHIBITOR

Prescriber Highlights

- ▶ Uricosuric & renal tubular secretion inhibitor that may be useful for treating gout (particularly in reptiles)
- ▶ Probenecid is associated with many drug interactions as it inhibits the renal tubular secretion of numerous drugs, including several beta-lactam antibiotics; some interactions may be beneficial, others may increase potential for toxicity
- ▶ Little experience using this drug in mammals other than humans

Uses/Indications

Although there has been very limited clinical use or research on probenecid in veterinary medicine, it can be useful in treating gout (hyperuricemia), particularly in reptiles.

Probenecid's effect in inhibiting renal tubular secretion of certain beta-lactam antibiotics and other weak organic acids is of interest for increasing serum concentrations, or reducing doses and dosing frequency of these drugs. This may allow greater efficacy (but also toxic effects) and reduce the cost or dosing frequency of expensive human drugs. Probenecid has a significantly long elimination half-life in dogs (about 18 hours), which may make it particularly useful in this species; however, at present there is little research supporting this use of probenecid in veterinary patients.

Pharmacology/Actions

Probenecid reduces serum uric acid concentrations by enhancing uric acid excretion into the urine by competitively inhibiting urate reabsorption at the proximal renal tubules.

Probenecid competitively inhibits tubular secretion of weak organic acids including the penicillins, some cephalosporins (not ceftriaxone, ceftazidime, or cefoperazone), sulbactam and tazobactam (not clavulanic acid), oseltamivir, etc.

Pharmacokinetics

There is limited information available for veterinary species. In dogs, information on oral bioavailability was not located, but after intravenous administration the distribution half-life was 2.3 hours and apparent volume of distribution at steady state was 0.46 L/kg. Probenecid exhibits biphasic concentration dependent plasma protein binding characteristics in the dog and appears to bind less to plasma proteins than in humans. Plasma clearance was 0.343 mL/min/kg and elimination half-life was 17.7 hours, which is considerably longer than in humans (6.5 hrs) or sheep (1.55 hrs) (Kakizaki *et al.* 2005).

After administration to mares, probenecid had an oral bioavailability of approximately 90%. The drug is highly bound (99.9%) to equine plasma proteins. Elimination half-life is approximately 90–120 minutes.

In humans, absorption after oral administration is rapid and complete. The drug is converted in the liver to glucuronidated, carboxylated, and hydroxylated compounds that have uricosuric and renal tubular secretion inhibition activity. Elimination half-life is dosage dependent and large dosages (above 500 mg) have longer half-lives.

Contraindications/Precautions/Warnings

Probenecid should not be used in patients with, or susceptible to, uric acid renal or bladder calculus formation or urate nephropathy (*e.g.*, cancer chemotherapy with rapidly cytolytic agents). Probenecid requires sufficient renal function to be effective; efficacy decreases with increasing renal function impairment. The drug has no efficacy in human patients with a creatine clearance of less than 30 mL/min.

Probenecid is not usually recommended for treating gout in birds as it can exacerbate the condition.

Adverse Effects

An accurate adverse effect profile for probenecid has not been determined for animal patients. In humans, probenecid occasionally causes headache, gastrointestinal effects (inappetence, nausea, mild vomiting), or rashes. When used for gout, it can initially cause an increased rate of gouty attacks unless prophylaxis with colchicine is used concurrently. Rarely, hypersensitivity, bone marrow suppression, hepatotoxicity, or nephrotic syndrome have been reported in humans.

Reproductive/Nursing Safety

Probenecid apparently crosses the placenta, but adverse effects to fetuses have not been reported.

In humans, the FDA categorizes probenecid as category *B* for use during pregnancy (*Animal studies have not yet demonstrated risk to the fetus, but there are no adequate studies in pregnant women; or animal studies have shown an adverse effect, but adequate studies in pregnant women have not demonstrated a risk to the fetus in the first trimester of pregnancy, and there is no evidence of risk in later trimesters.*)

It is unknown if probenecid enters milk, but it is unlikely to pose much risk to nursing offspring.

Overdosage/Acute Toxicity

Limited information is available. One massive (>45 g) overdose in a human patient caused CNS stimulation, seizures, protracted vomiting and respiratory failure.

Consider contacting an animal poison control center for guidance with large overdoses. Generally, probenecid overdoses should initially be handled using standardized protocols for removal of drug from the gut and preventing absorption. Treat supportively, but use caution co-administrating drugs that may compete with probenecid for tubular secretion.

Drug Interactions

The following drug interactions have either been reported or are theoretical in humans or animals receiving probenecid and may be of significance in veterinary patients:

- **ACYCLOVIR:** Increased acyclovir serum concentrations; probenecid can decrease renal excretion

- **ANTINEOPLASTICS (rapidly cytolytic):** Increased chance of uric acid nephropathy

- **ASPIRIN (and other salicylates):** Salicylates antagonize the uricosuric effects of probenecid

- **BENZODIAZEPINES (lorazepam, oxazepam):** Probenecid may prolong action or reduce time for onset of action

- **BETA-LACTAM ANTIBIOTICS (including penicillins and some cephalosporins):** Probenecid may increase serum concentrations by reducing renal excretion

- **BETA-LACTAMASE INHIBITORS (including sulbactam and tazobactam, but not clavulanic acid):** Probenecid may increase serum concentrations by reducing renal excretion

- **CHLORPROPAMIDE (and potentially other sulfonylureas):** Probenecid decreases elimination; hypoglycemia is possible

- **CIPROFLOXACIN/ENROFLOXACIN:** Probenecid reduces renal tubular secretion of ciprofloxacin by about 50%. In goats, probenecid significantly reduced renal excretion of enrofloxacin (Narayan *et al.* 2009).

- **DAPSONE:** Possible accumulation of dapsone or its active metabolites

- **FUROSEMIDE:** Increased serum furosemide levels

■ **HEPARIN:** Probenecid may increase and pro-long heparin's effects

■ **METHOTREXATE:** Probenecid may increase levels; increased risks for toxicity

■ **NSAIDS (including carprofen, ketoprofen & potentially others):** Probenecid may in-crease plasma levels and increase risks for toxicity

■ **NITROFURANTOIN:** Reduced urine levels; in-creased chance for systemic toxicity

■ **OSELTAMIVIR:** Probenecid may increase serum concentrations by reducing renal excretion

■ **RIFAMPIN:** Probenecid may reduce hepatic uptake of rifampin and serum levels can be increased; use together is not recommend-ed as effect is inconsistent and can lead to toxicity

■ **SULFONAMIDES:** Probenecid decreases renal elimination of sulfonamides, but as free se-rum concentrations of sulfonamides are not increased this interaction is not therapeuti-cally beneficial and may increase risks for sulfonamide toxicity

■ **THIOPENTAL:** Anesthesia may be extended or dose required for anesthesia decreased

Laboratory Considerations

The following laboratory alterations have been reported in humans with probenecid and may be of significance in veterinary patients:

■ **Urine glucose determinations:** When using cupric sulfate solution (Benedict's Solution, *Clinitest®*): Probenecid may cause false-pos-itive results. Tests utilizing glucose oxidase (*Tes-Tape®, Clinistix®*) are not affected.

■ **Theophylline levels:** Serum theophylline levels may be falsely elevated (Schack and Waxtler technique)

■ **17-ketosteroid concentrations in urine:** May be decreased

■ **Phosphorus:** Probenecid may increase phos-phorus reabsorption in hypoparathyroid patients

■ **Aminohippuric acid (PAH) or Phenolsulphon-phthalein (PSP) clearance studies:** Proben-ecid decreases renal clearance

■ **Renal function studies using iodohippurate sodium I 123 or I 131, or technetium TC 99:** Decreased kidney uptake

■ **Homovanillic acid (HVA) or 5-Hydroxyindole-acetic acid (5-HIAA):** Probenecid inhibits transport from CSF into blood

Doses

■ **REPTILES:**
For gout:
a) 250 mg PO q12h; can be increased as needed. Suggested dosage based upon human data as dose is not established for reptiles. (Johnson-Delaney 2005)

b) 40 mg/kg PO q12h (Coke 2004)

c) 250 mg (total dose) PO twice daily; may increase as needed. (de la Navarre 2003)

Monitoring

■ Depending on purpose for use: serum and urine uric acid, if concomitant urine alka-linization is used, consider monitoring acid-base balance

Client Information

■ In small animals, there is little scientific data supporting using probenecid for increas-ing blood levels of drugs that compete with probenecid for renal excretion; probenecid's adverse effects are not well known in these patients

Chemistry/Synonyms

Probenecid is a sulfonamide derivative that oc-curs as a white, to practically white, practically odorless, fine, crystalline powder. It is practically insoluble in water and soluble in alcohol.

Probenecid may also be known as: proben-ecidas, probenecidum, *Benemid®* and *Benuryl®*.

Storage/Stability

Probenecid tablets should be stored at room temperature in well-closed containers. Expiration dates are generally 3−5 years after manufacture.

Dosage Forms/Regulatory Status

VETERINARY-LABELED PRODUCTS: None

HUMAN-LABELED PRODUCTS:

Probenecid Tablets: 500 mg; generic; (Rx)

Also available as fixed-dose tablets containing probenecid 500 mg and colchicine 0.5 mg, but this dosage form is unlikely to be useful in vet-erinary patients.

References

Coke, R. (2004). Practical reptile nutrition. Proceedings: Western Veterinary Conference. Accessed via: Veterinary Information Network. http://goo.gl/kK1ar

de la Navarre, B. (2003). Acute and chronic renal disease (specifically in lizard species). Proceedings: Western Veterinary Conference. Accessed via: Veterinary Information Network. http://goo.gl/coWpS

Johnson-Delaney, C. (2005). Osteodystrophy and renal dis-ease in reptiles. Proceedings: Atlantic Coast Veterinary Conference. Accessed via: Veterinary Information Network. http://goo.gl/iuvuG

Kakizaki, T., Y. Yokoyama, et al. (2005). Probenecid: Its chromatographic determination, plasma protein bind-ing, and in vivo pharmacokinetics in dogs. *J Vet Med Sci* 68(4): 361−365.

Narayan, J., N. Kumar, et al. (2009). Effect of probenecid on kinetics of enrofloxacin in lactating goats after subcu-taneous administration. *Indian J Exp Biol* 47(1): 53−56.

PROCAINAMIDE HCL

(proe-kane-*a*-mide)   Pronestyl®

ANTIARRHYTHMIC

Prescriber Highlights

▶ Antiarrhythmic used primarily for treatment of atrial fibrillation, ventricular premature complexes (VPC's), ventricular tachycardia

▶ Contraindications: Myasthenia gravis; hypersensitive to drug, procaine or other chemically related drugs; torsade de pointes; or 2nd or 3rd degree heart block (unless artificially paced)

▶ Extreme Caution: Cardiac glycoside intoxication, systemic lupus; Caution: Significant hepatic, renal disease or CHF

▶ Adverse Effects: *Dogs:* Blood level related: GI effects, weakness, hypotension, negative inotropism, widened QRS complex & QT intervals, AV block, multiform ventricular tachycardias. Possible: fevers & leukopenias

▶ Profound hypotension can occur if injected too rapidly IV

▶ Consider dosage reduction in patients with renal failure, CHF, or critically ill

▶ Drug Interactions

Uses/Indications

Procainamide potentially may be useful for the treatment of ventricular premature complexes (VPC's), ventricular tachycardia, or supraventricular tachycardias associated with wide QRS complexes. When a tachycardia with a wide QRS is seen that that cannot be definitively identified as supraventricular or ventricular in origin, procainamide is an ideal first-line IV therapeutic agent because of its broad spectrum of activity for atrial and ventricular arrhythmias (Saunders *et al.* 2009).

Pharmacology/Actions

A class 1A antiarrhythmic agent, procainamide exhibits cardiac action similar to that of quinidine. It is considered both a supraventricular and ventricular antidysrhythmic. Procainamide prolongs the refractory times in both the atria and ventricles, decreases myocardial excitability, and depresses automaticity and conduction velocity. It has anticholinergic properties that may contribute to its effects. Procainamide's effects on heart rate are unpredictable, but it usually causes only slight increases or no change. It may exhibit negative inotropic actions on the heart, although cardiac outputs are generally not affected.

On ECG, QRS widening, and prolonged PR and QT intervals can be seen. The QRS complex and T wave may occasionally show some slight decreases in voltage.

Pharmacokinetics

After IM or IV administration, the onset of action is practically immediate. After oral administration in humans, approximately 75–95% of a dose is absorbed in the intestine, but some patients absorb less than 50% of a dose. Food, delayed gastric emptying, or decreased stomach pH may delay oral absorption. In dogs, it has been reported that the oral bioavailability is approximately 85% and the absorption half-life is 0.5 hours; however, there is an apparent large degree of variability in both bioavailability and half-life of absorption.

Distribution of procainamide is highest into the CSF, liver, spleen, kidneys, lungs, heart and muscles. The volume of distribution in dogs is approximately 1.4–3 L/kg. It is only approximately 20% protein bound in humans and 15% in dogs. Procainamide can cross the placenta and is excreted into milk.

The elimination half-life in dogs has been reported to be variable; most studies report values between 2–3 hours. In humans, procainamide is metabolized to N-acetyl-procainamide (NAPA), an active metabolite. It appears, however, that dogs do not form appreciable amounts of NAPA from procainamide as they are unable to appreciably acetylate aromatic and hydrazine amino groups. In the dog, approximately 90% (50–70% unchanged) of an intravenous dose is excreted in the urine as procainamide and metabolites within 24 hours after dosing.

Contraindications/Precautions/Warnings

Procainamide may be contraindicated in patients with myasthenia gravis (see Drug Interactions). Procainamide is contraindicated in patients hypersensitive to it, procaine or other chemically related drugs. In humans, procainamide is contraindicated in patients with systemic lupus erythematosus (SLE), but it is unknown if it adversely affects dogs with this condition. Procainamide should not be used in patients with torsade de pointes, or with 2nd or 3rd degree heart block (unless artificially paced).

Procainamide should be used with extreme caution, if at all, in patients with cardiac glycoside intoxication. It should be used with caution in patients with significant hepatic or renal disease or with congestive heart failure.

It has been recommended to not use procainamide in Doberman pinschers and boxers with dilated cardiomyopathy or dogs with subaortic stenosis; the drug may be proarrhythmic in certain patients susceptible to tachyarrhythmic-induced sudden death. (Kittleson 2006)

Adverse Effects

Adverse effects are generally dosage (blood level) related in the dog. Gastrointestinal effects may include anorexia, vomiting, or diarrhea. Effects related to the cardiovascular system can include weakness, hypotension, negative inotropism, widened QRS complex and QT intervals, AV block, multiform ventricular tachycardias. Fevers and leukopenias are a possibility. Profound hypotension can occur if injected too rapidly IV. In humans an SLE syndrome can occur, but its incidence has not been established in the dog.

Dosages should usually be reduced in patients with renal failure, congestive heart failure, or those who are critically ill.

Reproductive/Nursing Safety

In humans, the FDA categorizes this drug as category *C* for use during pregnancy (*Animal studies have shown an adverse effect on the fetus, but there are no adequate studies in humans; or there are no animal reproduction studies and no adequate studies in humans.*) In a separate system evaluating the safety of drugs in canine and feline pregnancy (Papich 1989), this drug is categorized as class: *B* (*Safe for use if used cautiously. Studies in laboratory animals may have uncovered some risk, but these drugs appear to be safe in dogs and cats or these drugs are safe if they are not administered when the animal is near term.*)

Both procainamide and NAPA are excreted in maternal milk and absorbed in nursing offspring. It should be used with caution in nursing patients; consider using milk replacer if the drug is to be continued.

Overdosage/Acute Toxicity

Clinical signs of overdosage can include hypotension, lethargy, confusion, nausea, vomiting, and oliguria. Cardiac signs may include widening of the QRS complex, junctional tachycardia, ventricular fibrillation, or intraventricular conduction delays.

If an oral ingestion, emptying of the gut and charcoal administration may be beneficial to remove any unabsorbed drug. IV fluids, plus dopamine, phenylephrine, or norepinephrine could be considered to treat hypotensive effects. A 1/6 molar intravenous infusion of sodium lactate may be used in an attempt to reduce the cardiotoxic effects of procainamide. Forced diuresis using fluids and diuretics along with reduction of urinary pH can enhance the renal excretion of the drug. Temporary cardiac pacing may be necessary should severe AV block occur.

Drug Interactions

The following drug interactions have either been reported or are theoretical in humans or animals receiving procainamide and may be of significance in veterinary patients:

Use with caution with other antidysrhythmic agents, as additive cardiotoxic or other toxic effects may result.

■ **AMIODARONE:** May increase procainamide levels, procainamide dose may need to be reduced

■ **ANTICHOLINESTERASE AGENTS** (*e.g.*, pyridostigmine, neostigmine): Procainamide may antagonize effects in patients with myasthenia gravis

■ **CIMETIDINE:** May increase procainamide levels

■ **HYPOTENSIVE DRUGS:** Procainamide may enhance effect

■ **LIDOCAINE:** Toxic effects may be additive, and cardiac effects unpredictable

■ **NEUROMUSCULAR BLOCKING AGENTS:** Procainamide may potentiate or prolong the neuromuscular blocking activity

■ **QUINIDINE:** Toxic effects may be additive, and cardiac effects unpredictable

■ **PHENYTOIN:** Toxic effects may be additive, and cardiac effects unpredictable

■ **PROPRANOLOL:** Toxic effects may be additive, and cardiac effects unpredictable

■ **RANITIDINE:** May increase procainamide levels

■ **TRIMETHOPRIM:** May increase procainamide levels

Doses

■ **DOGS:**

a) For ventricular tachyarrhythmias: When used IV: intermittent boluses of 2–4 mg/kg IV slowly (over two minutes) up to a total dose of 12–20 mg/kg until arrhythmia controlled and then a CRI may be started at 10–40 micrograms/kg/minute. PO use at: 20–30 mg/kg PO q6–8h (could be too low—previous recommendations of 8–20 mg/kg PO q6–8h are almost certainly too low). (Kittleson 2006)

b) For acute management of SVT's: After drugs have been used to slow AV nodal conduction (*i.e.*, diltiazem), procainamide at 6–8 mg/kg IV over 3 minutes or 6–20 mg/kg IM may terminate atrial tachyarrhythmias.

For chronic management: 10–20 mg/kg PO q6–8h; higher dosages of up to 40 mg/kg q6h have been necessary to treat junctional SVT's in some dogs (Wright 2000)

c) For ventricular tachycardia: For acute treatment of VT: 10–15 mg/kg IV bolus over 1–2 minutes; if continued parenteral administration required may use a constant rate IV infusion at 25–50 micrograms/kg/minute. For chronic treatment: 10–20 mg/kg PO q6h (Moise 2000)

d) For ventricular tachycardia: 6.6–8.8 mg/kg slowly IV over 5 minutes, then give as a CRI at 40–100 micrograms/kg/minute. (Fine 2006)

e) For chronic treatment of ventricular arrhythmias: 20–23 mg/kg PO q8h (Meurs 2002)

f) Using sustained-release tablets:

20 mg/kg PO q8h; For intravenous therapy: 6−8 mg/kg IV bolus, 20−40 micrograms/kg/min CRI (Hogan 2004)

g) For acute treatment of atrial fibrillation: 5−15 mg/kg IV slowly to effect. (Saunders *et al.* 2009)

h) If lidocaine ineffective for ventricular tachycardia: 20−50 micrograms/kg/min IV or 6−15 mg/kg IM q4-6h. (Rush 2006)

■ **CATS:**

For chronic management of SVT's:

a) 3−8 mg/kg PO q6−8h. (Wright 2000)

b) 1−2 mg/kg slowly IV; 10−20 micrograms/kg/minute constant rate IV infusion. Oral dose: 7.5−20 mg/kg q 6−8h (Ware 2000)

■ **HORSES:** (**Note:** ARCI UCGFS Class 4 Drug)

a) For atrial fibrillation (not as effective as quinidine); also has been used for ventricular tachycardia: IV at 1 mg/kg/min, not too exceed 20 mg/kg (20 minutes) total dose. Alternatively administer 25−35 mg/kg PO q8h. (Kimberly & McGurrin 2006)

b) For V-Tach: 1 mg/kg/minute IV up to a total dose of 20 mg/kg; or 25−35 mg/kg PO q8h (Mogg 1999)

Monitoring

■ ECG; continuously with IV dosing

■ Blood pressure, during IV administration

■ Clinical signs of toxicity (see Adverse Effects/Overdosage)

■ Serum levels

Because of the variability in pharmacokinetics reported in the dog, it is recommended to monitor therapy using serum drug levels. Because dogs apparently do not form the active metabolite NAPA in appreciable quantities, the therapeutic range for procainamide is controversial. Therapeutic ranges from 3−8 micrograms/mL to 8−20 micrograms/mL have been suggested. This author would suggest using the lower range as a guideline to initiate therapy, but not to hesitate increasing doses to attain the higher values if efficacy is not achieved and toxicity is not a problem. Digitalis-induced ventricular arrhythmias may require substantially higher blood levels for control. Trough levels are usually specified when monitoring oral therapy. Because NAPA is routinely monitored with procainamide in human medicine, it may be necessary to request to the laboratory that NAPA values need not be automatically run for canine patients.

In horses, therapeutic levels have been suggested as 4−10 micrograms/mL for procainamide and 10−30 micrograms/dL as procainamide and NAPA together. (Kimberly & McGurrin 2006)

Client Information

■ Oral products should be administered at evenly spaced intervals throughout the day/ night. Unless otherwise directed, give the medication at least 1 hour before feeding to animal with an empty stomach.

■ Notify veterinarian if animal's condition deteriorates or clinical signs of toxicity (*e.g.*, vomiting, diarrhea, weakness, etc.) occur.

Chemistry/Synonyms

Structurally related to procaine, procainamide is used as an antiarrhythmic agent. Procainamide HCl differs from procaine by the substitution of an amide group for the ester group found on procaine. It occurs as an odorless, white to tan, hygroscopic, crystalline powder with a pK_a of 9.23 and a melting range from 165°−169°C. It is very soluble in water and soluble in alcohol. The pH of the injectable product ranges from 4−6.

Procainamide may also be known as: novocainamidum. procainamidi chloridum, procainamidi hydrochloridum, *Biocoryl®*, *Procan®*, *Procanbid®*, or *Pronestyl®*.

Storage/Stability

The solution may be used if the color is no darker than a light amber. Refrigeration may retard the development of oxidation, but the solution may be stored at room temperature.

The injectable product is reportedly physically **compatible** with sodium chloride 0.9% injection, and water for injection. Procainamide is also physically **compatible** with dobutamine HCl, lidocaine HCl, and verapamil HCl. Compatibility is dependent upon factors such as pH, concentration, temperature, and diluent used; consult specialized references or a hospital pharmacist for more specific information.

Compatibility/Compounding Considerations

The injectable product is reportedly physically **compatible** with sodium chloride 0.9% injection, and water for injection. Procainamide is also physically **compatible** with dobutamine HCl, lidocaine HCl, and verapamil HCl. Compatibility is dependent upon factors such as pH, concentration, temperature, and diluent used; consult specialized references or a hospital pharmacist for more specific information.

Dosage Forms/Regulatory Status

VETERINARY-LABELED PRODUCTS: None

The ARCI (Racing Commissioners International) has designated this drug as a class 4 substance. See the appendix for more information.

HUMAN-LABELED PRODUCTS:

Procainamide HCl Injection Solution: 100 mg/mL in 10 mL multi-dose vials and 500 mg/mL in 2 mL vials; generic; (Rx)

Procainamide HCl Oral Capsules: 250 mg & 375 mg; generic; (Rx)

Procainamide HCl Extended-Release Oral Tablets: 250 mg, 500 mg, & 1000 mg (**Note:** These products are not recommended for initial therapy and have not been extensively used in veterinary medicine.); *Procanbid®* (Monarch); generic; (Rx)

References

Fine, D. (2006). Emergency management of cardiac arrhythmias. Proceedings: ACVIM. Accessed via: Veterinary Information Network. http://goo.gl/ieCZL

Hogan, D. (2004). Arrhythmias: diagnosis and treatment. Proceedings: ACVIM Forum. Accessed via: Veterinary Information Network. http://goo.gl/voENn

Kimberly, M. & K. McGurrin (2006). Update on antiarrhythmic therapy in horses. Proceedings; ACVIM. Accessed via: Veterinary Information Network. http://goo.gl/kSS8b

Kittleson, M. (2006). "Chapt 29: Drugs used in the treatment of cardiac arrhythmias." *Small Animal Cardiology, 2nd Ed.*

Meurs, K. (2002). Ventricular arrhythmias: When to treat and which drugs. Proceedings: Western Veterinary Conf. Accessed via: Veterinary Information Network. http://goo.gl/51j7h

Mogg, T. (1999). Equine Cardiac Disease: Clinical pharmacology and therapeutics. *The Veterinary Clinics of North America: Equine Practice* **15:3**(December).

Moise, N. (2000). CVT Update: Ventricular Arrhythmias. *Kirk's Current Veterinary Therapy: XIII Small Animal Practice.* J Bonagura Ed. Philadelphia, WB Saunders: 733–737.

Papich, M. (1989). Effects of drugs on pregnancy. *Current Veterinary Therapy X: Small Animal Practice.* R Kirk Ed. Philadelphia, Saunders: 1291–1299.

Rush, B. (2006). Use of inhalation therapy in management of recurrent airway obstruction. Proceedings: ACVIM. Accessed via: Veterinary Information Network. http://goo.gl/LhZJ8

Saunders, A., S. Gordon, et al. (2009). Canine Atrial Fibrillation. *Comp CE*(November): E1–E!).

Ware, W. (2000). Therapy for Critical Arrythmias: New Advances. Proceedings: The North American Veterinary Conference, Orlando.

Wright, K. (2000). Assessment and treatment of supraventricular tachyarrhythmias. *Kirk's Current Veterinary Therapy: XIII Small Animal Practice.* J Bonagura Ed. Philadelphia, WB Saunders: 726–730.

PROCARBAZINE HCL

(proe-**kar**-ba-zeen)   Matulane®

ANTINEOPLASTIC

Prescriber Highlights

▶ Atypical alkylating agent that is used in MOPP lymphoma protocols for dogs/cats & for GME in dogs; enters CNS

▶ Contraindications: Hypersensitivity to drug, inadequate bone marrow reserve

▶ Caution: Hepatic/renal impairment, use with other CNS depressant drugs

▶ Adverse Effects: GI, myelosuppression, central & peripheral nervous system, hepatic

▶ Teratogen

▶ Drug interactions

▶ May need to be reformulated in an oil-based solution to dose appropriately; commercial preparation may be very expensive

Uses/Indications

In veterinary medicine, procarbazine is used as part of MOPP protocols (mechlorethamine, vincristine, procarbazine, prednisone) to treat lymphoma in dogs and cats. It may be of benefit in treating granulomatous meningoencephalitis (GME) in dogs.

Pharmacology/Actions

Procarbazine's precise mode of action is not well understood, but it is considered by most to be an alkylating agent, as it appears to inhibit protein, RNA, and DNA synthesis. Procarbazine is autooxidized into hydrogen peroxide, which may also directly damage DNA.

Pharmacokinetics

No data specific for dogs or cats was located. In humans, procarbazine is well absorbed after oral administration and rapidly equilibrates between the CSF and plasma. Peak levels in plasma occur in about one hour; in the CSF, about 30–90 minutes after dosing. Procarbazine is almost entirely metabolized in the liver and kidney. Metabolic products are cytotoxic and excreted in the urine.

Contraindications/Precautions/Warnings

Procarbazine is contraindicated in patients known to be hypersensitive to it or with inadequate bone marrow reserve as determined by bone marrow aspirate.

Because procarbazine can cause CNS depression, use with extreme caution with other CNS depressant drugs.

Use with caution in patients with impaired renal or hepatic function.

Adverse Effects

When dosed as recommended for dogs and cats, procarbazine is relatively well tolerated. In dogs, procarbazine toxicity appears to mirror that seen in humans. Gastrointestinal effects (nausea, vomiting, hepatotoxicity) and myelosuppression (thrombocytopenia, leukopenia) can be seen. Thrombocytopenia nadirs usually occur at about 4 weeks. Because it is often used in combination with other chemotherapy agents (MOPP), myelosuppression and GI effects (hemorrhagic gastritis) may be enhanced. CNS effects may be noted and include sedation or agitation. Peripheral neuropathy can occur and includes loss of tendon reflexes, paresthesias and myalgia.

In humans, it is recommended to discontinue therapy if any of the following occur: CNS signs, leukopenia (WBC <4000 mm³), thrombocytopenia (platelets <100,000 mm³), hypersensitivity, stomatitis (at sign of first ulceration), diarrhea, and hemorrhage or bleeding. Resume therapy at a lower dosage only when effects clear.

Reproductive/Nursing Safety

Procarbazine is potential teratogen. In pregnant humans, procarbazine is designated by the FDA as a category *D* drug (*There is evidence of human fetal risk, but the potential benefits from the use of the drug in pregnant women may be acceptable despite its potential risks.*)

It is unknown if procarbazine enters milk. It is recommended to use milk replacer if the dam requires procarbazine.

Overdosage/Acute Toxicity

The LD_{50} for laboratory animals range from 150 mg/kg (rabbits) to 1.3 grams/kg (mice). Treat overdoses aggressively to remove drug from the gut if overdose was within an hour or two. Anticipated adverse effects would be extensions of the drug's adverse effect profile (GI, bone marrow suppression, CNS effects). Monitor and support as necessary. Contact an animal poison control center for further guidance.

Drug Interactions

The following drug interactions have either been reported or are theoretical in humans or animals receiving procarbazine and may be of significance in veterinary patients:

■ **ALCOHOL/ETHANOL:** May cause severe nausea and vomiting

■ **CNS DEPRESSANT DRUGS (e.g., barbiturates, opiates, antihistamines, phenothiazines, etc.):** Because procarbazine can cause CNS depression, use with extreme caution with other CNS depressant drugs. Coma and death have been reported when procarbazine has been used with opiates.

■ **FOODS WITH HIGH TYRAMINE CONTENT (aged cheese, yogurt):** Procarbazine exhibits some monoamine oxidase inhibitory (MAOI) activity; serious hypertension may result

■ **SYMPATHOMIMETICS (phenylpropanolamine, etc.):** Procarbazine exhibits some monoamine oxidase inhibitory (MAOI) activity; serious hypertension may result

■ **TRICYCLIC ANTIDEPRESSANTS (e.g., clomipramine, amitriptyline, etc.):** Procarbazine exhibits some monoamine oxidase inhibitory (MAOI) activity. Do not use concurrently with tricyclic antidepressant drugs.

Laboratory Considerations

■ None were noted

Doses

Note: Because of the potential toxicity of this drug to patients, veterinary personnel and clients, and since chemotherapy indications, treatment protocols, monitoring and safety guidelines often change, the following dosages should be used only as a general guide. Consultation with a veterinary oncologist and referral to current veterinary oncology references [e.g., (Henry & Higginbotham 2009); (Argyle et al. 2008); (Withrow & Vail 2007); (Villalobos 2007); (Ogilvie & Moore 2006); (Ogilvie & Moore 2001)] is strongly recommended.

■ **DOGS:**

For lymphoma rescue: When procarbazine is used, it is part of a protocol in combination with other antineoplastic agents and usually given for the first 14 days of the treatment cycle. Usual doses for dogs are: 50 mg/m² PO.

For treatment of granulomatous meningoencephalitis (GME):

a) 25–50 mg/m² PO once daily, initially with prednisone treatment. After the first month of therapy, we attempt to reduce procarbazine dose to every other day. Monitor CBC weekly for first month, and then monthly thereafter. Wear gloves when handling. To prepare a 10 mg/mL oil-based solution: Five 50 mg capsules, oil-based flavor (chicken, liver, fish) drops, 0.25 teaspoonful of silica gel (to keep in suspension), and gradually add sesame oil to a total of 25 mL. Assigned expiration date of 30 days. (Cuddon & Coates 2002)

■ **CATS:**

For MOPP lymphoma rescue: When procarbazine is used, it is part of a protocol in combination with other antineoplastic agents and usually given for the first 14 days of the treatment cycle. Usual doses for cats are: 50 mg/m² PO or 10 mg (total dose per cat).

Monitoring

■ Baseline: CBC, hepatic and renal function, urinalysis

■ Repeat CBC at least once weekly for the first month of treatment and then monthly

■ In humans, it is recommended to repeat urinalysis, transaminases/alkaline phosphatase, and BUN at least weekly

Client Information

■ Avoid skin contact with the medication. Wear gloves or wash hands thoroughly after dosing. Avoid contact with patient's saliva or urine.

■ Contact veterinarian immediately if any signs associated with toxicity occur. These could include vomiting, lack of appetite, diarrhea, bleeding, depression or agitation, bleeding, sores in mouth, lameness, etc.

Chemistry/Synonyms

A derivative of hydrazine, procarbazine HCl occurs as a white to pale yellow crystalline powder having a slight odor. It is soluble, but unstable in water or aqueous solutions.

Procarbazine may also be known as: Ibenzemethyzin, NSC-77213, Ro-4-6467/1, MIH, N-Methylhydrazine, *Matulane®*, *Natulan®*, and *Natulanar®*.

Storage/Stability

Procarbazine capsules should be stored in airtight containers, protected from light at temperatures less than 40°C (preferably between 15–30°C, (59–86°F). An expiration date of 4 years is assigned after the date of manufacture.

Dosage Forms/Regulatory Status

VETERINARY-LABELED PRODUCTS: None

HUMAN-LABELED PRODUCTS:

Procarbazine HCl Capsules: 50 mg; *Matulane®* (Sigma-Tau); (Rx)

References

Argyle, D., M. Brearly, et al. (2008). *Decision Making in Small Animal Oncology*, Wiley-Blackwell.

Cuddon, P. & J. Coates (2002). New treatments for granulomatous meningoencephalitis. Proceedings: ACVIM Forum. Accessed via: Veterinary Information Network. http://goo.gl/CaD7L

Henry, C. & M. Higginbotham (2009). *Cancer Management in Small Animal Practice*, Saunders.

Ogilvie, G. & A. Moore (2001). *Feline Oncology: A Comprehensive Guide to Compassionate Care*, Veterinary Learning Systems.

Ogilvie, G. & A. Moore (2006). *Managing the Canine Cancer Patient: A Practical Guide to Compassionate Care*, Veterinary Learning Systems.

Villalobos, A. (2007). *Canine and Feline Geriatric Oncology*. Ames, Blackwell.

Withrow, S. & D. Vail (2007). *Withrow and MacEwen's Small Animal Clinical Oncology 4th Ed.* Philadelphia, Elsevier.

PROCHLORPERAZINE

(proe-klor-*per*-a-zeen)

Compazine®, Compro®

PHENOTHIAZINE ANTIEMETIC

Prescriber Highlights

▶ Phenothiazine used alone as an antiemetic; formerly in combination with an anticholinergic for other GI effects (*e.g.*, diarrhea)

▶ Relative Contraindications: Hypovolemia/dehydration or shock & in patients with tetanus or strychnine intoxication

▶ Caution: Hepatic dysfunction, cardiac disease, general debilitation, or very young animals

▶ Adverse Effects: Sedation or hypotension

Uses/Indications

Prochlorperazine as a single agent is used in dogs and cats as an antiemetic. The only FDA-approved products for animals were combination products containing prochlorperazine, isopropamide, with or without neomycin (*Darbazine®, Neo-Darbazine®*—SKB Labs). These products are no longer marketed in the USA. The FDA-approved indications for these products were: vomiting, non-specific gastroenteritis, drug induced diarrhea, infectious diarrhea, spastic colitis, and motion sickness in dogs and cats (injectable product only).

Pharmacology/Actions

The basic pharmacology of prochlorperazine is similar to that of the other phenothiazines (refer to the acepromazine monograph for more information). Prochlorperazine has weak anticholinergic effects, strong extrapyramidal effects, and moderate sedative effects. Antiemetic activity of prochlorperazine is due to its effects primarily in the brain's emetic center and chemoreceptor trigger zone, but it also has some peripheral activity. Alpha-adrenergic, dopaminergic, histaminergic, and cholinergic receptor antagonism all contribute to its antiemetic action.

Pharmacokinetics

Little information is available regarding the pharmacokinetics of prochlorperazine in animals, although it probably follows the general patterns of other phenothiazine agents in absorption, distribution, and elimination.

Contraindications/Precautions/Warnings

Animals may require lower dosages of general anesthetics following phenothiazines. Cautious use and smaller doses of phenothiazines should be given to animals with hepatic dysfunction, cardiac disease, or general debilitation. Because of their hypotensive effects, phenothiazines are relatively contraindicated in patients with hypovolemia/dehydration or shock. Phenothiazines may exacerbate depression in patients with CNS depression. It should not be used for tetanus or strychnine intoxication due to effects on the extrapyramidal system. Use cautiously in very young or debilitated animals.

Adverse Effects

Alone, prochlorperazine is most likely to cause sedation or hypotension. Muscle fasciculations/tremors, and prolactin release have been reported in small animals

Reproductive/Nursing Safety

In humans, the FDA categorizes this drug as category *C* for use during pregnancy (*Animal studies have shown an adverse effect on the fetus, but there are no adequate studies in humans; or there are no animal reproduction studies and no adequate studies in humans.*) In a separate system evaluating the safety of drugs in canine and feline pregnancy (Papich 1989), this drug is categorized as class: *B* (*Safe for use if used cautiously. Studies in laboratory animals may have uncovered some risk, but these drugs appear to be safe in dogs and cats or these drugs are safe if they are not administered when the animal is near term.*)

A related compound, chlorpromazine has been detected in maternal milk. Although few cases are documented, a milk to plasma ratio of 0.5–0.7 or less is reported. Prochlorperazine is unlikely to pose significant risk to nursing animals.

Overdosage/Acute Toxicity

Refer to the information listed in the acepromazine monograph. Acute extrapyramidal clinical signs (torticollis, tremor, salivation) have been successfully treated with injectable diphenhydramine in humans.

Drug Interactions

The following drug interactions have either been reported or are theoretical in humans or animals receiving prochlorperazine or other phenothiazines and may be of significance in veterinary patients:

- **ANTACIDS:** May cause reduced GI absorption of oral phenothiazines

- **ANTIDIARRHEAL MIXTURES (e.g., Kaolin/pectin, bismuth subsalicylate mixtures):** May cause reduced GI absorption of oral phenothiazines

- **CNS DEPRESSANT AGENTS (barbiturates, narcotics, anesthetics, etc.):** May cause additive CNS depression if used with phenothiazines

- **DOPAMINE:** Phenothiazines may decrease pressor effects

- **EPINEPHRINE:** Phenothiazines block alpha-adrenergic receptors and concomitant epinephrine can lead to unopposed beta-activity causing vasodilation and increased cardiac rate

- **METOCLOPRAMIDE:** Phenothiazines may potentiate the extrapyramidal effects of metoclopramide

- **OPIATES:** May enhance the hypotensive effects of the phenothiazines; dosages of prochlorperazine may need to be reduced when used with an opiate

- **ORGANOPHOSPHATE AGENTS:** Phenothiazines should not be given within one month of worming with these agents as their effects may be potentiated

- **PARAQUAT:** Toxicity of the herbicide paraquat may be increased by prochlorperazine

- **PHENYTOIN:** Metabolism may be decreased if given concurrently with phenothiazines

- **PHYSOSTIGMINE:** Toxicity may be enhanced by prochlorperazine

- **PROCAINE:** Activity may be enhanced by phenothiazines

- **PROPRANOLOL:** Increased blood levels of both drugs may result if administered with phenothiazines

- **WARFARIN:** Prochlorperazine may decrease anticoagulant effect

Doses

- **DOGS:**

  As an antiemetic:

  a) 0.5 mg/kg IM or SC q8h; ensure adequate hydration (Washabau and Elie 1995) (Marks 2006; Simpson 2003)

  b) 0.1 mg/kg IM q6–8h; use with extreme caution in dehydrated or hypotensive animals. (Silverstein 2003)

  c) 0.1–0.5 mg/kg IM or SC q6–8h (Otto 2005)

- **CATS:**

  As an antiemetic:

  a) 0.5 mg/kg SC or IM three times a day; ensure adequate hydration (Simpson 2003)

  b) 0.5 mg/kg IM or SC q8h (Washabau and Elie 1995)(Marks 2006)

  c) 0.1–0.5 mg/kg IM or SC q6–8h (Otto 2005)

Monitoring

- Cardiac rate/rhythm/blood pressure if indicated and possible to measure

- Anti-emetic/anti-spasmodic efficacy; hydration and electrolyte status

- Body temperature (especially if ambient temperature is very hot or cold)

Client Information

- Observe animal for at least one hour following dosing. Dry mouth may be relieved by applying small amounts of water to animal's tongue for 10–15 minutes.

- May discolor the urine to a pink or red-brown color; this is not abnormal.

- Protracted vomiting and diarrhea can be serious; contact veterinarian if clinical signs are not alleviated. Contact veterinarian if animal exhibits abnormal behavior, becomes rigid or displays other abnormal body movements.

Chemistry/Synonyms

Prochlorperazine, a piperazine phenothiazine derivative, is available commercially as the base in rectal formulations, the edisylate salt in injectable and oral solutions, and as the maleate salt in oral tablets and capsules. Each 8 mg of the maleate salt and 7.5 mg of the edisylate salt are approximately equivalent to 5 mg of prochlorperazine base.

The base occurs as a clear, to pale yellow, viscous liquid that is very slightly soluble in water and freely soluble in alcohol. The edisylate salt occurs as white to very light yellow, odorless, crystalline powder. 500 mg are soluble in 1 mL of water and 750 mL of alcohol. The maleate salt occurs as a white or pale yellow, practically odorless, crystalline powder. It is practically insoluble in water or alcohol.

The commercial injection is a solution of the edisylate salt in sterile water. It has a pH of 4.2–6.2.

Prochlorperazine may also be known as: chlormeprazine, prochlorpemazine, *Compazine®, Compro®, Prochlor®, Prorazin®, Stemetil®,* or *Tementil®.*

Storage/Stability

Store in tight, light resistant containers at room temperature. Avoid temperatures above 40°C and below freezing. A slight yellowing of the oral or injectable solution has no effects on potency or efficacy, but do not use if a precipitate forms or the solution is substantially discolored.

Compatibility/Compounding Considerations

The following products have been reported to be physically **compatible** when mixed with prochlorperazine edisylate injection: all usual IV fluids, ascorbic acid injection, atropine sulfate, butorphanol tartrate, chlorpromazine HCl, dexamethasone sodium phosphate, droperidol, fentanyl citrate, glycopyrrolate, hydroxyzine HCl, lidocaine HCl, meperidine HCl, metoclopramide, morphine sulfate, nafcillin sodium, nalbuphine HCl, pentazocine lactate, perphenazine, promazine HCl, promethazine, scopolamine HBr, sodium bicarbonate, and vitamin B complex with C.

The following drugs have been reported to be physically **incompatible** when mixed with prochlorperazine edisylate: aminophylline, amphotericin B, ampicillin sodium, calcium gluceptate, chloramphenicol sodium succinate, chlorothiazide sodium, dimenhydrinate, hydrocortisone sodium succinate, methohexital sodium, penicillin G sodium, phenobarbital sodium, pentobarbital sodium, and thiopental sodium. Do not mix with other drugs/diluents having parabens as preservatives. Compatibility is dependent upon factors such as pH, concentration, temperature, and diluent used; consult specialized references or a hospital pharmacist for more specific information.

Dosage Forms/Regulatory Status

VETERINARY-LABELED PRODUCTS:

None; *Darbazine®* is no longer available.

The ARCI (Racing Commissioners International) has designated this drug as a class 2 substance. See the appendix for more information.

HUMAN-LABELED PRODUCTS:

Prochlorperazine for Injection: 5 mg/mL in 2 mL vials; generic; (Rx)

Prochlorperazine Tablets: 5 mg & 10 mg (as maleate); generic; (Rx)

Prochlorperazine (base) Suppositories: 25 mg; *Compro®* (Paddock); generic; (Rx)

References

Marks, S. (2006). Diagnostic and therapeutic approach to the chronically vomiting dog and cat. Proceedings: Western Vet Conf. Accessed via: Veterinary Information Network. http://goo.gl/nsCGW

Otto, C. (2005). Antiemetic update. Proceedings: IVECCS. Accessed via: Veterinary Information Network. http://goo.gl/oN4lJ

Papich, M. (1989). Effects of drugs on pregnancy. *Current Veterinary Therapy X: Small Animal Practice*. R Kirk Ed. Philadelphia, Saunders: 1291–1299.

Silverstein, D. (2003). Intensive care treatment of severe Parvovirus enteritis. Proceedings: IVECCS. Accessed via: Veterinary Information Network. http://goo.gl/S5gKe

Simpson, K. (2003). Managing persistent vomiting. Proceedings: ACVIM Forum. Accessed via: Veterinary Information Network. http://goo.gl/nRqvI

PROMETHAZINE HCL

(proe-*meth*-a-zeen)   Phenergan®

PHENOTHIAZINE

Prescriber Highlights

▶ Phenothiazine used as an antihistamine & antiemetic in small animals
▶ Relatively little experience with this drug in veterinary medicine; not frequently recommended for use
▶ Adverse Effects: sedation or anticholinergic effects

Uses/Indications

Promethazine may be useful in dogs and cats as an antiemetic. Because of its antihistamine actions, it has been tried for treating pruritus in atopic dogs, but its efficacy has been poor.

Pharmacology/Actions

The basic pharmacology of promethazine is similar to that of the other phenothiazines (refer to the acepromazine monograph for more information). It exhibits antiemetic, antihistaminic, anticholinergic, sedative, and local anesthetic actions.

Pharmacokinetics

Little information is available regarding the pharmacokinetics of promethazine in animals, although it probably follows the general patterns of other phenothiazine agents in absorption, distribution, and elimination.

In humans, the drug is well absorbed following oral or rectal administration, and via IM injection. Sedative effects occur within minutes of IV administration and persist for several hours. The drug is metabolized in the liver and these metabolites are eliminated primarily in the urine. Elimination half-life in humans is about 10 hours.

Contraindications/Precautions/Warnings

Animals may require lower dosages of general anesthetics following phenothiazines. Cautious use and smaller doses of phenothiazines should be given to animals with hepatic dysfunction, cardiac disease, or general debilitation. Because of their hypotensive effects, phenothiazines are relatively contraindicated in patients with hypovolemia or shock. Do not use in patients with tetanus or strychnine intoxication due to effects on the extrapyramidal system. Use cautiously in very young or debilitated animals.

In humans, promethazine has a "black box warning" to not use the medication in children less than 2 years old; fatal respiratory depression has occurred in that patient group.

Adverse Effects

Little experience has been reported with this drug in animals, but prochlorperazine would most likely cause sedation or anticholinergic effects (dry mouth, etc.).

Reproductive/Nursing Safety

In humans, the FDA categorizes this drug as category *C* for use during pregnancy (*Animal studies have shown an adverse effect on the fetus, but there are no adequate studies in humans; or there are no animal reproduction studies and no adequate studies in humans.*)

It is not known whether promethazine is distributed into milk; a related compound, chlorpromazine has been detected in maternal milk. Although few cases are documented, a milk to plasma ratio of 0.5–0.7 or less is reported. Promethazine is unlikely to pose significant risk to nursing animals.

Overdosage/Acute Toxicity

Refer to the information listed in the acepromazine monograph. Acute extrapyramidal clinical signs (torticollis, tremor, salivation) have been successfully treated with injectable diphenhydramine in humans.

Drug Interactions

The following drug interactions have either been reported or are theoretical in humans or animals receiving promethazine or other phenothiazines and may be of significance in veterinary patients:

- **ANTACIDS:** May cause reduced GI absorption of oral phenothiazines
- **ANTIDIARRHEAL MIXTURES (e.g., Kaolin/ pectin, bismuth subsalicylate mixtures):** May cause reduced GI absorption of oral phenothiazines
- **ATROPINE & OTHER ANTICHOLINERGICS:** May have additive effects when used with promethazine
- **CNS DEPRESSANT AGENTS (barbiturates, narcotics, anesthetics, etc.):** May cause additive CNS depression if used with phenothiazines
- **EPINEPHRINE:** Phenothiazines block alpha-adrenergic receptors and concomitant epinephrine can lead to unopposed beta-activity causing vasodilation and increased cardiac rate
- **METOCLOPRAMIDE:** Phenothiazines may potentiate the extrapyramidal effects of metoclopramide
- **MONOAMINE OXIDASE INHIBITORS:** May potentiate extrapyramidal effects
- **OPIATES:** May enhance the hypotensive effects of the phenothiazines; dosages of prochlorperazine may need to be reduced when used with an opiate
- **ORGANOPHOSPHATE AGENTS:** Phenothiazines should not be given within one month of worming with these agents as their effects may be potentiated

Laboratory Considerations

- Promethazine can cause false positive results for **salicylates** in urine
- Promethazine can cause false positive or false negative results for **chorionic gonadotropin** in urine

Doses

- **DOGS/CATS:**

  As an antiemetic:

  a) 2 mg/kg PO or IM once daily (Dowling 2003)

  As an antihistamine:

  a) 0.2–0.4 mg/kg PO three to four times a day. (Morgan 2003)

  b) 1–2 mg/kg PO q12h. (Mueller 2000)

Monitoring

- Efficacy

Client Information

- Dry mouth may be relieved by applying small amounts of water to animal's tongue for 10–15 minutes
- May cause sedation or behavior changes; contact veterinarian if these are a concern
- Protracted vomiting or diarrhea can be serious; contact veterinarian if clinical signs are not alleviated
- Contact veterinarian if animal exhibits abnormal movements or becomes rigid

Chemistry/Synonyms

Promethazine HCl occurs as a white to faint yellow, practically odorless, crystalline powder. It slowly oxidizes and acquires a blue color on prolonged exposure to air. Promethazine HCl is freely soluble in water, in hot dehydrated alcohol, and in chloroform, but practically insoluble in acetone, ether, or ethyl acetate. The pH of a 5% solution in water is between 4–5.

Promethazine may also be known as: Lilly 01516, PM 284, RP 3277, prometazina or *Phenergan®*. There are many other trade names available.

Storage/Stability

Store tablets at room temperature (20–25°C) in tight, light resistant containers. The syrup should be stored from 15–25°C and protected from light.

The injection should be stored at room temperature 20–25°C and protected from light. Keep in covered carton until time of use. Do not use if a precipitate forms or the solution is discolored. Promethazine can be adsorbed to plastic IV bags and tubing.

Promethazine suppositories should be stored in the refrigerator (2–8°C)

Compatibility/Compounding Considerations

The following products have been reported to be physically **compatible** when promethazine injection is mixed with them: all usual IV fluids, amikacin, ascorbic acid, buprenorphine, butorphanol, cimetidine, diphenhydramine, fentanyl, fluconazole, glycopyrrolate, hydromorphone, hydroxyzine, meperidine, metoclopramide, midazolam, ondansetron, pancuronium, pentazocine, procainamide, and ranitidine.

Solutions of promethazine hydrochloride are **incompatible** with alkaline substances, which can precipitate promethazine base.

The following drugs have been reported to be physically **incompatible** when mixed with promethazine HCl: aminophylline, barbiturates, benzylpenicillin salts, carbenicillin sodium, chloramphenicol sodium succinate, chlorothiazide sodium, cefoperazone, dimenhydrinate, doxorubicin (in a liposomal formulation), furosemide, heparin sodium, hydrocortisone sodium succinate, morphine sulfate, and nalbuphine HCl. Compatibility is dependent upon factors such as pH, concentration, temperature, and diluent used; consult specialized references or a hospital pharmacist for more specific information.

Dosage Forms/Regulatory Status
VETERINARY-LABELED PRODUCTS: None

The ARCI (Racing Commissioners International) has designated this drug as a class 3 substance. See the appendix for more information.

HUMAN-LABELED PRODUCTS:

Promethazine HCl for Injection: 25 mg/mL in 1 mL amps & 50 mg/mL in 1 mL amps; *Phenergan*® (Wyeth); generic; (Rx)

Promethazine HCl Oral syrup: 1.25 mg/mL in 473 mL; generic; (Rx)

Promethazine HCl Oral Tablets: 12.5 mg, 25 mg & 50 mg; *Phenergan*® (Wyeth); generic; (Rx)

Promethazine HCl Rectal Suppositories: 12.5 mg, 25 mg, & 50 mg; *Phenergan*® (Wyeth), *Phenadoz*® (Paddock), *Promethegan*® (G & W Labs); generic; (Rx)

References
Dowling, P. (2003). GI Therapy: When what goes in won't stay down. Proceedings: Western Veterinary Conference. Accessed via: Veterinary Information Network. http://goo.gl/co8V8

Morgan, R. (2003). Appendix IV: Recommended Drug Dosages. *Handbook of Small Animal Practice 4th Ed.* R Morgan, R Bright and M Swartout Eds. Philadelphia, Saunders: 1279–1308.

Mueller, R. (2000). *Dermatology for the Small Animal Practitioner*, Teton New Media.

PROPANTHELINE BROMIDE

(proe-*pan*-the-leen)   Pro-Banthine®

QUATERNARY ANTIMUSCARINIC

Prescriber Highlights

▶ Quaternary antimuscarinic agent used for its antispasmodic/antisecretory for treatment of diarrhea, hyperreflexic detrusor or urge incontinence & anticholinergic responsive bradycardias. In horses, IV to reduce colonic peristalsis & relax rectum to allow easier examination & surgery.

▶ Contraindications: Hypersensitivity to anticholinergics, tachycardias secondary to thyrotoxicosis or cardiac insufficiency, myocardial ischemia, unstable cardiac status during acute hemorrhage, GI obstructive disease, paralytic ileus, severe ulcerative colitis, obstructive uropathy, or myasthenia gravis (unless used to reverse adverse muscarinic effects secondary to therapy).

▶ Extreme Caution: Known or suspected GI infections, autonomic neuropathy. Caution: hepatic or renal disease, hyperthyroidism, hypertension, CHF, tachyarrhythmias, prostatic hypertrophy, esophageal reflux, & geriatric or pediatric patients.

▶ Adverse Effects: Similar to atropine (dry mouth, dry eyes, urinary hesitancy, tachycardia, constipation, etc.), but less effects on eye or CNS. Cats may exhibit vomiting & hypersalivation. High doses may cause ileus.

Uses/Indications
In small animal medicine propantheline bromide has been used for its antispasmodic/antisecretory effects in the treatment of diarrhea. It is also employed in the treatment of hyperreflexic detrusor or urge incontinence and as oral treatment in anticholinergic responsive bradycardias. In horses, propantheline has been used intravenously to reduce colonic peristalsis and for relaxing the rectum to allow easier rectal examination and surgery.

Pharmacology/Actions
An antimuscarinic with similar actions as atropine, propantheline is a quaternary ammonium compound and does not cross appreciably into the CNS. It should not exhibit the same extent of CNS adverse effects that atropine possesses. For further information, refer to the atropine monograph.

Pharmacokinetics
Quaternary anticholinergic agents are not completely absorbed after oral administra-

tion because they are completely ionized. In humans, peak levels occur about 2 hours after oral administration. Food apparently decreases the amount of drug absorbed. Propantheline is reportedly variably absorbed in dogs; dosages should be adjusted for each patient.

The distribution of propantheline has not been extensively studied, but like other quaternary antimuscarinics, propantheline is poorly lipid soluble and does not extensively penetrate into the CNS or eye.

Propantheline is believed to be prevalently metabolized in the GI and/or liver; less than 5% of an oral dose is excreted unchanged in the urine.

Contraindications/Precautions/Warnings

Use of propantheline should be considered contraindicated if the patient has a history of hypersensitivity to anticholinergic drugs, tachycardias secondary to thyrotoxicosis or cardiac insufficiency, myocardial ischemia, unstable cardiac status during acute hemorrhage, GI obstructive disease, paralytic ileus, severe ulcerative colitis, obstructive uropathy, or myasthenia gravis (unless used to reverse adverse muscarinic effects secondary to therapy).

Antimuscarinic agents should be used with extreme caution in patients with known or suspected GI infections. Propantheline or other antimuscarinic agents can decrease GI motility and prolong retention of the causative agent(s) or toxin(s) resulting in prolonged clinical signs. Antimuscarinic agents must also be used with extreme caution in patients with autonomic neuropathy.

Antimuscarinic agents should be used with caution in patients with hepatic disease, renal disease, hyperthyroidism, hypertension, CHF, tachyarrhythmias, prostatic hypertrophy, esophageal reflux, and in geriatric or pediatric patients.

Adverse Effects

With the exception of fewer effects on the eye and the CNS, propantheline can be expected to have a similar adverse reaction profile as atropine (dry mouth, dry eyes, urinary hesitancy, tachycardia, constipation, etc.). Vomiting and hypersalivation have also been reported in cats. High doses may lead to the development of ileus with resultant bacterial overgrowth in susceptible animals. For more information, refer to the atropine monograph.

Reproductive/Nursing Safety

In humans, the FDA categorizes this drug as category **B** for use during pregnancy (*Animal studies have not yet demonstrated risk to the fetus, but there are no adequate studies in pregnant women; or animal studies have shown an adverse effect, but adequate studies in pregnant women have not demonstrated a risk to the fetus in the first trimester of pregnancy, and there is no evidence of risk in later trimesters.*)

Although anticholinergics (especially atropine) may be excreted in milk and can cause toxicity and reduce milk production, it is unknown if propantheline enters maternal milk. Use with caution in nursing patients.

Overdosage/Acute Toxicity

Because of its quaternary structure, it would be expected that minimal CNS effects would occur after an overdose of propantheline when compared to atropine. See the information listed in the atropine monograph for more information on the clinical signs that may be seen following an overdose.

If a recent oral ingestion, emptying gut contents and administration of activated charcoal and saline cathartics may be warranted. Treat clinical signs supportively and symptomatically. Do not use phenothiazines as they may contribute to anticholinergic effects. Fluid therapy and standard treatments for shock may be instituted.

The use of physostigmine is controversial and should probably be reserved for cases where the patient exhibits either extreme agitation and is at risk for injuring themselves or others, or where supraventricular tachycardias and sinus tachycardias are severe or life threatening. The usual dose for physostigmine (human) is 2 mg IV slowly (for average sized adult); if no response may repeat every 20 minutes until reversal of toxic antimuscarinic effects or cholinergic effects takes place. The human pediatric dose is 0.02 mg/kg slow IV (repeat q10 minutes as above) and may be a reasonable choice for treatment of small animals. Physostigmine adverse effects (bronchoconstriction, bradycardia, seizures) may be treated with small doses of IV atropine.

Drug Interactions

The following drug interactions have either been reported or are theoretical in humans or animals receiving propantheline and may be of significance in veterinary patients:

- **ANTIHISTAMINES:** May enhance the activity of propantheline

- **BENZODIAZEPINES:** May enhance the activity of propantheline

- **CIMETIDINE:** Propantheline may decrease the absorption of cimetidine

- **CORTICOSTEROIDS (long-term use):** May increase intraocular pressure

- **MEPERIDINE:** May enhance the activity of propantheline

- **NITRATES:** May potentiate the adverse effects of propantheline

- **NITROFURANTOIN:** Propantheline may enhance actions

- **PHENOTHIAZINES:** May enhance the activity of propantheline

- **SYMPATHOMIMETICS:** Propantheline may enhance actions

- **RANITIDINE:** Propantheline delays the absorption, but increases the peak serum level of ranitidine; the relative bioavailability of ranitidine may be increased by 23% when propantheline is administered concomitantly with ranitidine

■ **THIAZIDE DIURETICS:** Propantheline may enhance actions

Doses

■ **DOGS:**

For detrusor hyperreflexia, urge incontinence:

a) 0.2 mg/kg PO q6−8h; increase dose if necessary to the lowest dose that will control clinical signs (Polzin & Osborne 1985)

b) 7.5−30 mg (total dose) PO once a day to q8h (Bartges 2003)

c) 7.5−15 mg (total dose) PO q12h; occasionally dosages of 30 mg q8h are required (Lane 2000)

For sinus bradycardia, incomplete AV block, etc.

a) 0.25−0.5 mg/kg PO q8−12h (Hogan 2004)

b) 7.5−30 mg PO q8−12h; usually well tolerated, but improvement is usually partial and often temporary. (Rishniw & Thomas 2000)

For colitis, irritable bowel syndrome, etc.

a) 0.25 mg/kg PO three times a day; do not use longer than 48−72 hours (48 hours for acute colitis) (DeNovo, R.C. 1988)

b) 0.5 mg/kg two to three times daily (Chiapella 1986)

As an antiemetic/antidiarrheal:

a) 0.25 mg/kg PO q8h (DeNovo, R.C., Jr. 1986)

■ **CATS:**

For detrusor hyperreflexia, urge incontinence:

a) 0.25−0.5 mg/kg PO q12−24h. Empirical dosage. Further studies required to substantiate beneficial effect. (Osborne *et al.* 2003)

b) 5−7.5 mg (total dose) PO once a day to once every 3 days (Lane 2000)

c) 5−7.5 mg (total dose) PO q8h; 7.5 mg PO q72h (Bartges 2003)

For sinus bradycardia, incomplete AV block, etc.:

a) Although generally ineffective, a trial may be attempted using: 0.8−1.6 mg/kg three times daily (Harpster 1986)

b) 7.5 mg PO q8−12h; usually well tolerated, but improvement is usually partial and often temporary (Rishniw & Thomas 2000)

For chronic colitis:

a) 0.5 mg/kg two to three times daily (Chiapella 1986)

As an antiemetic/antidiarrheal:

a) 0.25 mg/kg PO q8h (DeNovo, R.C., Jr. 1986)

■ **HORSES:**

To reduce rectal contractions:

a) During oocyte collection: 0.04 mg/kg IV (Carnevale & Coutinho da Silva 2003)

b) 30 mg IV to inhibit peristalsis for 2 hours during rectal surgery (Merkt *et al.* 1979)

Note: There is no commercially available injectable product available in the U.S.A. Should a preparation be made from oral tablets, it should be freshly prepared and filtered through a 0.22 micron-filter before administering. Use with caution.

Monitoring

Dependent on reason for use:

■ Clinical efficacy

■ Heart rate and rhythm if indicated

■ Adverse effects

Client Information

■ Dry mouth may be relieved by applying small amounts of water to animal's tongue for 10−15 minutes.

■ Protracted vomiting and diarrhea can be serious; contact veterinarian if symptoms are not alleviated.

Chemistry/Synonyms

A quaternary ammonium antimuscarinic agent, propantheline bromide occurs as bitter-tasting, odorless, white or practically white crystals, with a melting range of 156−162° (with decomposition). It is very soluble in both water and alcohol.

Propantheline bromide may also be known as: bromuro de propantelina, propanthelini bromidum, *Banthine®*, *Bropantil®*, *Corrigast®*, *Ercorax Roll-on®*, *Ercoril®*, *Ercotina®*, *Pantheline®*, *Probamide®*, *Propantel®*, or *Propanthel®*.

Storage/Stability

Propantheline bromide tablets should be stored at room temperature in tight containers.

Dosage Forms/Regulatory Status

VETERINARY-LABELED PRODUCTS: None

HUMAN-LABELED PRODUCTS:

Propantheline Bromide Tablets: 7.5 mg & 15 mg; *Pro-Banthine®* (Schiapparelli Searle); generic; (Rx)

References

Bartges, J. (2003). Canine lower urinary tract cases. Proceedings: ACVIM Forum. Accessed via: Veterinary Information Network. http://goo.gl/HH41u

Carnevale, E. & M. Coutinho da Silva (2003). Assisted reproduction techniques. *Equine Internal Medicine, 2nd Ed.* S Reed, W Bayly and D Sellon Eds. Philadelphia, Saunders: 1130−1135.

Chiapella, A. (1986). Diagnosis and management of chronic colitis in the dog and cat. *Current Veterinary Therapy IX: Small Aniaml Practice*. RW Kirk Ed. Philadelphia, WB Saunders: 896–903.

DeNovo, R.C. (1988). Diseases of the Large Bowel. *Handbook of Small Animal Practice*. RV Morgan Ed. New York, Churchill Livingstone: 421–439.

DeNovo, R.C., Jr. (1986). Therapeutics of gastrointestinal diseases. *Current Veterinary Therapy (CVT) IX Small Animal Practice*. RW Kirk Ed. Philadelphia, W.B. Saunders: 862–871.

Harpster, N.K. (1986). Feline myocardial diseases. *Current Veterinary Therapy IX: Small Animal Practice*. RW Kirk Ed. Philadelphia, WB Saunders: 380–398.

Hogan, D. (2004). Arrhythmias: diagnosis and treatment. Proceedings: ACVIM Forum. Accessed via: Veterinary Information Network. http://goo.gl/voENn

Lane, I. (2000). Use of anticholinergic agents in lower urinary tract disease. *Kirk's Current Veterinary Therapy: XIII Small Animal Practice*. J Bonagura Ed. Philadelphia, WB Saunders: 899– 902.

Merkt, H., A. Graser, et al. (1979). [Perforation of the rectum in the horse. Trials on temporary inhibition of peristalsis by drugs.] Mastdarmperforation beim pferd. Versuche zur temporaren medikamentosen Peristalikhemmung. Abstract. *Praktische Tierarzt* **60**(3): 189–190.

Osborne, C., J. Lulich, et al. (2003). Idiopathic feline lower urinary tract disease: Therapeutic rights and wrongs. Proceedings: World Small Animal Veterinary Association World Congress. Accessed via: Veterinary Information Network. http://goo.gl/knB2k

Polzin, D.J. & C.A. Osborne (1985). Diseases of the Urinary Tract. *Handbook of Small Animal Therapeutics*. LE Davis Ed. New York, Churchill Livingstone: 333–395.

Rishniw, M. & W. Thomas (2000). Bradyarrhythmias. *Kirk's Current Veterinary Therapy: XIII Small Animal Practice*. J Bonagura Ed. Philadelphia, WB Saunders: 719–725.

PROPIONIBACTERIUM ACNES INJECTION

(*proe*-pee-ohe-bak-*ter*-ee-um *ak*-nees)
Immunoregulin®, Eqstim®

IMMUNOSTIMULANT

Prescriber Highlights

▶ Immunostimulant for Staph pyoderma, FeLV, feline herpes, equine respiratory infections

▶ Contraindications: Hypersensitivity to compound, canine lymphoma, or leukemias with CNS involvement. Caution: Cardiac dysfunction

▶ Adverse Effects: Lethargy, hyperthermia, chills, & anorexia. Anaphylactic reactions are possible

▶ Extravasation may cause local tissue inflammation

Uses/Indications

The manufacturer's label notes the product (*Immunoregulin®*) ". . . indicated in the dog as adjunct to antibiotic therapy in the treatment of chronic recurring canine pyoderma to decrease the severity and extent of lesions and increase the percentage of dogs free of lesions after the appropriate therapeutic period." The equine product (*EqStim®*) is labeled as an immunostimulant for adjunctive therapy of primary or secondary viral or bacterial respiratory tract infections.

Additionally, it has been used as an immunostimulant for the adjunctive treatment of feline rhinotracheitis and feline leukemia virus-induced disease. In dogs, it may be of use in the adjunctive treatment of oral melanoma and mastocytoma. Unfortunately, controlled studies documenting efficacy were not located for these potential indications.

Pharmacology/Actions

A non-specific immunostimulant, Propionibacterium acnes injection may induce macrophage activation, lymphokine production, increase natural killer cell activity, and enhance cell-mediated immunity.

Pharmacokinetics

No information was noted.

Contraindications/Precautions/Warnings

Propionibacterium acnes injection is contraindicated in patients hypersensitive to it. It should also be considered contraindicated in canine lymphoma or leukemias with CNS involvement. Use with caution in patients with cardiac dysfunction. One source states that its use is contraindicated in cats with FIV or FIP (Hartmann 2009).

Adverse Effects

Occasionally within hours after injection, lethargy, increased body temperature, chills, and anorexia may be noted. Anaphylactic reactions have also been reported. Extravasation may cause local tissue inflammation. Long-term toxicity studies have demonstrated vomiting, anorexia, malaise, fever, acidosis, increased water consumption, and hepatitis.

Reproductive/Nursing Safety

Safe use during pregnancy has not been established.

Overdosage/Acute Toxicity

No overdosage information was noted; the manufacturer states that the antidote is epinephrine, presumably for the treatment of anaphylactic reactions.

Drug Interactions

The manufacturer states that the immunostimulant effects may be compromised if given concomitantly with **glucocorticoids** or **other immune suppressing drugs**; manufacturer recommends discontinuing steroids at least 7 days prior to initiating therapy.

Doses

■ **DOGS:**

For labeled indications (as adjunct to antibiotic therapy in the treatment of chronic recurring canine pyoderma):
a) Shake well. Give via intravenous route at the following dosages: For animals weighing up to 15 lbs = 0.25–0.5 mL;

15–45 lbs = 0.25–1 mL; 45–75 lbs = 1–1.5 mL; >75 lbs = 1.5–2 mL. During the first two weeks, give 4 times at 3–4 day intervals, then once weekly until symptoms abate or stabilize. Maintenance doses once per month are recommended. (Package Insert; *Immunoregulin®*)

b) For adjunctive therapy of chronic recurrent canine pyoderma: 0.03–0.07 mL/kg twice weekly for 10 weeks (combined with antibiotic therapy) (Barta 1992)

■ **CATS:**

For adjunctive therapy of feline retrovirus infections:

a) 0.5 mL IV twice weekly for 2 weeks, then one injection weekly for 20 weeks or until cat is seronegative. (McCaw 1994)

b) 0.25–0.5 mL IV twice weekly then every other week for 16 weeks (Levy 2004)

c) As an antiviral immunostimulant in cats to increase hematopoiesis in FeLV-positive cats: 5 lb cats: 0.25 mL IV, IP twice weekly for 2 weeks, then once weekly until remission and once monthly after that to maintain clinical improvement. For 10 lb cats: 0.5 mL IV, IP twice weekly for 2 weeks, then once weekly for 3 weeks and once monthly for 2 months for a total of nine injections after that to maintain clinical improvement. Some protocols suggest follow-up with injections once weekly for 20 weeks or longer as needed. Others suggest follow-up with once weekly until clinical remission, and then once per month. (Greene *et al.* 2006)

■ **HORSES:**

As an immunostimulant for adjunctive therapy of primary or secondary viral or bacterial respiratory tract infections:

a) Using *EqStim®*: 1 mL per 114kg (250 lb) body weight IV q48-72h (Flamino 2003)

b) Using *EqStim®*: 1 mL per 114kg (250 lb) body weight IV. Repeat dosage on day 3 (or day 4), at day 7, and weekly as needed (Label information; *Eqstim®*—Neogen)

c) As an adjunctive treatment to improve fertility in mares with endometritis: Using *EqStim®*: 1 mL per 114 kg (250 lb) body weight IV. Given days 0, 2, and 6. Best results in mares bred 2 days before to 8 days after initial administration. (Dascanio 2009; Rohrbach *et al.* 2007)

Monitoring
■ Efficacy
■ Adverse effects (see above)

Chemistry/Synonyms
Propionibacterium acnes injection is an immunostimulant agent, containing nonviable *Propionibacterium acnes* suspended in 12.5% ethanol in saline.

Propionibacterium acnes may also be known as: *Corynebacterium parvum*; NSC-220537, *Arthrokehlan A®*, *Coparvax®*, *Corymunun®*, *Eqstim®*, *Imunoparvum®*, and *Immunoregulin®*.

Storage/Stability
Store refrigerated; do not freeze. Shake well before using.

Dosage Forms/Regulatory Status
VETERINARY-LABELED PRODUCTS:

Propionibacterium acnes (non-viable) IV: 0.4 mg/mL in 5 mL and 50 mL vials; *Immunoregulin®* (Neogen); (OTC-biologic; manufacturer states that use is restricted to use by, or under the supervision of a veterinarian). Labeled for use in dogs. *Eqstim®* (Neogen). For use in horses and restricted to use by or under the supervision of a veterinarian.

HUMAN-LABELED PRODUCTS: None

References

Barta, O. (1992). Immunoadjuvant therapy. *Current Veterinary Therapy XI: Small Animal Practice*. R Kirk and J Bonagura Eds. Philadelphia, W.B. Saunders Company: 217–223.

Dascanio, J. (2009). Hormonal Control of Reproduction. Proceedings: ABVP. Accessed via: Veterinary Information Network. http://goo.gl/o2vHk

Flamino, M.J.B.F. (2003). Immunomodulators in respiratory disease treatment. *Current Therapy in Equine Medicine 5*. A Hoffman Ed. Philadelphia, Saunders: 6–11.

Greene, C., K. Hartmannn, et al. (2006). Appendix 8: Antimicrobial Drug Formulary. *Infectious Disease of the Dog and Cat*. C Greene Ed., Elsevier: 1186–1333.

Hartmann, K. (2009). Immunomodulators in Veterinary Medicine—Is There Evidence of Efficacy? Proceedings: ACVIM. Accessed via: Veterinary Information Network. http://goo.gl/WplyC

Levy, J. (2004). FELV: Afraid of a positive? Proceedings: ACVIM Forum. Accessed via: Veterinary Information Network. http://goo.gl/gGs7t

McCaw, D. (1994). Advances in therapy for retroviral infections. *Consultations in Feline Internal Medicine: 2*. J August Ed. Philadelphia, W.B. Saunders Company: 21–25.

Rohrbach, B.W., P.C. Sheerin, et al. (2007). Effect of adjunctive treatment with intravenously administered Propionibacterium acnes on reproductive performance in mares with persistent endometritis. *Javma-Journal of the American Veterinary Medical Association* **231**(1): 107–113.

PROPOFOL

(*proe*-po-fole)
Rapinovet®, PropoFlo®, Diprivan®

INJECTABLE ANESTHETIC

Prescriber Highlights

▶ Short-acting injectable hypnotic agent

▶ Contraindications: Hypersensitivity to it or any component of the product

▶ Caution: Severe stress or having undergone trauma, hypoproteinemia, hyperlipidemia, seizures, or anaphylaxis history

▶ Adverse Effects: Transient respiratory depression is common but usually clinically tolerable. Apnea possible, especially if given too rapidly. May cause histamine release; anaphylactoid reactions possible. Hypotension, seizure-like clinical signs (paddling, opisthotonus, myoclonic twitching) during induction. Repeated doses in Cats: Increased Heinz body production, slowed recoveries, anorexia, lethargy, malaise, & diarrhea

▶ Little, if any, analgesia is provided

▶ Consider dose reduction if using other CNS depressant

▶ Sufficient monitoring & patient-support capabilities are mandatory

▶ Cats with preexisting liver disease may be susceptible to longer recovery times

Uses/Indications

In appropriate patients, propofol may be useful as an induction agent (especially before endotracheal intubation or an inhalant anesthetic), and as an anesthetic for outpatient diagnostic or minor procedures (*e.g.*, laceration repair, radiologic procedures, minor dentistry, minor biopsies, endoscopy, etc.).

Propofol is used as a treatment for refractory status epilepticus, as it tends to cause less cardiovascular depression and recoveries can be smoother than with pentobarbital. Propofol may be of particular usefulness for use in Greyhounds and in patients with preexisting cardiac dysrhythmias. At low dosages, propofol is being investigated as an appetite stimulant in dogs.

Propofol may be safely used in animals with liver or renal disease and mild to moderate cardiac disease.

In dogs, propofol's labeled indications are: 1) for induction of anesthesia; 2) for maintenance of anesthesia for up to 20 minutes; 3) for induction of general anesthesia where maintenance is provided by inhalant anesthetics.

Pharmacology/Actions

Propofol is a short acting hypnotic unrelated to other general anesthetic agents. Its mechanism of action is not well understood.

In dogs, propofol produces rapid yet smooth and excitement-free anesthesia induction (in 30–60 seconds) when given slowly IV. Subanesthetic dosages will produce sedation, restraint and an unawareness of surroundings. Anesthetic dosages produce unconsciousness and good muscle relaxation.

Propofol's cardiovascular effects include arterial hypotension, bradycardia, (especially in combination with opiate premedicants) and negative inotropism. It causes significant respiratory depression, particularly with rapid administration or very high dosages. Propofol also decreases intraocular pressure, increases appetite and has antiemetic properties. It does not appear to precipitate malignant hyperthermia and has little or no analgesic properties.

Pharmacokinetics

After IV administration, propofol rapidly crosses the blood brain barrier and has an onset of action usually within one minute. Duration of action after a single bolus lasts about 2–5 minutes. It is highly bound to plasma proteins (95–99%), crosses the placenta, is highly lipophilic, and reportedly enters maternal milk.

Propofol's short duration of action is principally due to its rapid redistribution from the CNS to other tissues. It is rapidly biotransformed in the liver via glucuronide conjugation to inactive metabolites, which are then excreted primarily by the kidneys. Because cats do not glucuronidate as well as dogs or humans, this may help explain their problems with consecutive day administration (see Adverse Effects below).

There is limited data available on propofol's pharmacokinetic parameters in dogs. The steady state volume of distribution is >3L/kg, elimination half-life about 1.4 hours, and clearance about 50 mL/kg/min.

Contraindications/Precautions/Warnings

Propofol is contraindicated in patients hypersensitive to it or any component of the product. It should not be used in patients where general anesthesia or sedation is contraindicated.

Propofol should only be used in facilities where sufficient monitoring and patient-support (intubation/ventilation) capabilities are available. Because patients that are in shock, under severe stress, or have undergone trauma may be overly sensitive to the cardiovascular and respiratory depressant effects of propofol, it should be used with caution in these patients. Adequate perfusion should be maintained before and during propofol anesthesia; dosage adjustments may be necessary.

As propofol is so highly bound to plasma proteins, patients with hypoproteinemia may be susceptible to untoward effects; general anesthetic agents may be a safer choice in these patients.

Propofol does not provide analgesia and perioperative analgesics should be considered. The benefits of propofol should be weighed against its risks in patients with a history of hyperlipidemia, seizures or anaphylactic reactions. Cats with preexisting liver disease may be susceptible to longer recovery times.

Adverse Effects

Transient respiratory depression is common but is usually clinically tolerable. However, there is a relatively high incidence of apnea with resultant cyanosis if propofol is given too rapidly; it should be given slowly (25% of the calculated dose every 30 seconds until desired effect). Treat with assisted ventilation until spontaneous ventilation resumes.

Propofol has been documented to cause histamine release in some patients and anaphylactoid reactions (rare) have been noted in humans. Propofol has direct myocardial depressant properties and resultant arterial hypotension has been reported.

Occasionally, dogs may exhibit seizure-like clinical signs (paddling, opisthotonus, myoclonic twitching) during induction, that, if persist, may be treated with intravenous diazepam. Propofol may have both anticonvulsant and seizure-causing properties. It should be used with caution in patients with a history of, or active seizure disorders, but some clinicians believe however, that propofol is actually more appropriate to use in seizure patients or in high seizure-risk procedures (e.g., myelography) than is thiopental.

While propofol is not inexpensive, it should ideally be used in a single-use fashion, as it is a good growth medium (contains no preservative) for bacteria.

When used in combination with other CNS depressant premedicants (e.g., acepromazine, narcotics, diazepam, etc.), a decrease in dosage of about 25% (from the single agent dose) should be considered. In very thin animals, consider dosage reduction as well.

When used repeatedly (once daily) or as a prolonged CRI in cats, increased Heinz body production, slowed recoveries, anorexia, lethargy, malaise, and diarrhea have been noted. Heinz body formation is due to oxidative injury to RBCs and has been documented in cats with other phenolic compounds as well. Consecutive use in dogs appears to be safe.

Pain upon injection has been reported in humans, but does not appear to be a clinically significant problem for dogs or cats. Extravasation of injection is not irritating nor does it cause tissue sloughing.

Propofol does not provide good analgesia, so appropriate analgesic agents should be used before and after painful procedures.

Reproductive/Nursing Safety

Propofol crosses the placenta and its safe use during pregnancy has not been established. High dosages (6X) in laboratory animals caused increased maternal death and decreased offspring survival rates after birth. In humans, the FDA categorizes this drug as category **B** for use during pregnancy (*Animal studies have not yet demonstrated risk to the fetus, but there are no adequate studies in pregnant women; or animal studies have shown an adverse effect, but adequate studies in pregnant women have not demonstrated a risk to the fetus in the first trimester of pregnancy, and there is no evidence of risk in later trimesters.*)

In humans, propofol is not recommended for use in nursing mothers because propofol is excreted in maternal milk and the effects of oral absorption of small amounts of propofol are not known. Use with caution in nursing veterinary patients.

Overdosage/Acute Toxicity

Overdosages are likely to cause significant respiratory depression and, potentially, cardiovascular depression. Treatment should consist of propofol discontinuation, artificial ventilation with oxygen, and if necessary, symptomatic and supportive treatment for cardiovascular depression (*e.g.*, intravenous fluids, pressors, anticholinergics, etc.).

Drug Interactions

The following drug interactions have either been reported or are theoretical in humans or animals receiving propofol and may be of significance in veterinary patients:

- **ANESTHETICS, INHALATION (halothane, isoflurane):** Propofol serum concentrations may be increased

- **ANESTHETICS, LOCAL:** Propofol dosage requirements for sedation or hypnosis reduced

- **ANTICHOLINERGICS:** Propofol-induced bradycardia may be exacerbated in animals, particularly when opiate premedicants are used

- **CHLORAMPHENICOL:** May decrease clearance of propofol and increase recovery times.

- **CLONIDINE:** When used as a premed, may reduce propofol dosage requirements

- **CNS DEPRESSANTS:** Increased sedative, anesthetic, and cardiorespiratory depression possible

- **DRUGS THAT INHIBIT THE HEPATIC P-450 ENZYME SYSTEM (e.g., chloramphenicol, cimetidine, ketoconazole, etc.):** May potentially increase the recovery times associated with propofol; clinical significance is unclear, but it may be of significance in cats

- **FENTANYL:** In pediatric (human) patients increased risk for bradycardia

- **MEDETOMIDINE:** When propofol is used after medetomidine, hypoxemia may occur;

dosage adjustments may be required along with adequate monitoring

■ **METOCLOPRAMIDE:** In humans, metoclopramide reduced the propofol dose required for induction by 20–25%

■ **MIDAZOLAM:** May have synergistic effects with propofol, midazolam plasma concentrations may be increased up to 20%

■ **OPIATES:** May increase the serum concentrations of both the opiate and propofol if used together

Doses

■ **DOGS/CATS:**

Dogs: For induction of general anesthesia using *PropoFlo®*

Dose should be titrated against the response of the patient over 30-60 seconds or until clinical signs show the onset of anesthesia. Rapid injection of propofol (<5 seconds) may be associated with an increased incidence of apnea. The average propofol induction dose rates for healthy dogs given propofol alone, or when propofol is preceded by a premedicant, are indicated in the table below. This table is for guidance only. The dose and rate should be based upon patient response.

Induction Dosage Guidelines: Dogs

Preanesthetic	Propofol Induction Dose: Dogs (mg/kg)	Propofol Rate of Administration		
		Seconds	mg/kg/min	mL/kg/min
None	5.5	40-60	5.5–8.3	0.55–0.83
Acepromazine	3.7	30-50	4.4–7.4	0.44–0.74
Acepromazine / Oxymorphone	2.6	30-50	3.1–5.2	0.31–0.52

Propofol doses and rates for the above premedicants were based upon the following average dosages which may be lower than the label directions for their use as a single medication: Acepromazine 0.06 mg/kg IM, SC, IV; Oxymorphone 0.09 mg/kg IM, SC, IV; Xylazine 0.33 IM, SC, The use of these drugs as preanesthetics markedly reduces propofol requirements. As with other sedative hypnotic agents, the amount of opioid and/or alpha2 agonist premedication will influence the response of the patient to an induction dose of propofol. In the presence of premedication, the dose of propofol may be reduced with increasing age of the animal. The dose of propofol should always be titrated against the response of the patient. During induction, additional low doses of propofol, similar to those used for maintenance with propofol, may be administered to facilitate intubation or the transition to inhalant maintenance anesthesia.

DOGS: Maintenance Of General Anesthesia Using *PropoFlo®*

A. Intermittent Propofol Injections: Anesthesia can be maintained by administering propofol in intermittent IV injections. Clinical response will be determined by the amount and the frequency of maintenance injections. The following table is provided for guidance:

Preanesthetic	Propofol Maintenance Dose: Dogs mg/kg	Propofol Rate of Administration		
		Seconds	mg/kg/min	mL/kg/min
None	2.2	10-30	4.4–13.2	0.44–1.32
Acepromazine	1.6	10-30	3.2–9.6	0.32–0.96
Acepromazine / Oxymorphone	1.8	10-30	3.6–10.8	0.36–1.08

Repeated maintenance doses of propofol do not result in increased recovery times or dosing intervals, indicating that the anesthetic effects of propofol are not cumulative.

B. Maintenance by Inhalant Anesthetics: Due to the rapid metabolism of propofol, additional low doses of propofol, similar to those used for maintenance with propofol, may be required to complete the transition to inhalant maintenance anesthesia. Clinical trials using propofol have shown that it may be necessary to use a higher initial concentration of the inhalant anesthetic halothane than is usually required following induction using barbiturate anesthetics, due to rapid recovery from propofol. (Label Information; *PropoFlo®*—Abbott)

CATS: Induction of General Anesthesia Using *PropoClear®*

Induction dose guidelines are 4.1−8 mg/kg for cats that do not receive a preanesthetic, and 2.7−8 mg/kg for cats that receive a preanesthetic. The induction dose is reduced by 16-24% for cats that receive a preanesthetic (dose sparing effect). Anesthesia is usually observed within 60 seconds after the end of the induction dose administration. Duration of anesthesia following the recommended induction dose is approximately 3 minutes without a preanesthetic and 3-6 minutes with a preanesthetic. Full standing recovery occurs within approximately 30 minutes in cats. Individual anesthesia times vary. Induction doses for cats given propofol alone, or when it is preceded by a preanesthetic, are indicated in the following table. The table is for guidance only. The actual induction dose should be based on patient response.

Propofol (*PropoClear®*) 10 mg/mL Induction Dose Guidelines: Cat			
Preanesthetic	**Mean Induction Dose (mg/kg)**	**Induction Dose Range (mg/kg)**	**Induction Dose Sparing (%)**
None	7.4	4.1–8	0%
Phenothiazine + Opioid	6.2	2.7–8	16%
Alpha2-Adrenergic Agonist	5.6	3.3–8	24%
Benzodiazepine + Opioid	6.2	3.1–8	16%

CATS: Maintenance of General Anesthesia Using *PropoClear®*

Anesthesia can be maintained by administration of propofol using intermittent IV injections. For cats, the duration of anesthesia following each propofol maintenance dose is approximately 3-5 minutes. Clinical response may vary, and is determined by the dose, rate of administration and frequency of maintenance injections. Propofol maintenance dose sparing is greater in cats that receive a preanesthetic. The maintenance dose and frequency should be based on the patient's response. The following table is provided for guidance.

Propofol 10 mg/mL (*PropoClear®*) Maintenance Dose Guidelines: Cat		
Preanesthetic	**Mean Maintenance Dose (mg/kg)**	**Maintenance Dose Range (mg/kg)**
None	1.9	0.6–3.3.
Phenothiazine + Opioid	2.3	0.8–5
Alpha2-Adrenergic Agonist	2.2	1–3.4
Benzodiazepine + Opioid	2.3	1.1–3.6

Inhalant Anesthetic Maintenance of General Anesthesia in Cats: Additional low doses of propofol, similar to a maintenance dose, may be necessary to facilitate the transition to inhalant maintenance anesthesia. (Label Information; *PropoClear®*—Pfizer)

Note: The following dosages are for propofol macroemulsion unless otherwise noted.

As an anesthetic:

a) As a single injection (25% of the calculated dose every 30 seconds until desired effect):

For healthy, unpremedicated animal: 6 mg/kg IV;

For healthy, premedicated animal: After tranquilizer (*e.g.*, acepromazine) = 4 mg/kg IV; after sedative (*e.g.*, xylazine, opioids) = 3 mg/kg IV.

As a constant infusion:

For sedation only: 0.1 mg/kg/minute;

For minor surgery: 0.6 mg/kg/min, or 1 mL (10 mg) per minute per 12–25 kg of body weight (Robinson *et al.* 1993)

b) Dogs: For induction without premedication: 5–6 mg/kg IV;

With acepromazine (0.05 mg/kg IM, IV, or SC), propofol given at 3–4 mg/kg IV;

With acepromazine and oxymorphone (0.09 mg/kg IM, IV or SC), propofol given at 2.3 mg/kg IV. Xylazine or medetomidine premeds may reduce propofol dose further.

Cats: Premed with acepromazine (0.05–1 mg/kg IM) with or with-

out an analgesic such as butorphanol (0.2–0.4 mg/kg IM) and induce with propofol at 4–6 mg/kg IV. Doses of propofol at 8–13 mg/kg IV will allow intubation without topical anesthesia, lower propofol dose if topical anesthesia is used. (Mathews 1999)

c) 6 mg/kg IV; in healthy animals 25% of the calculated dose is administered every 30 seconds until intubation is possible. After induction, duration of anesthesia is only 2.5–9.4 minutes. Maintenance anesthesia obtained using either inhalational agents or a continuous infusion of propofol at approximately 0.4 mg/kg/minute. If anesthesia appears inadequate, a small bolus of 1 mg/kg followed by an increase in the infusion rate by 25%. If infusion is too deep, discontinue infusion until suitable anesthesia level is achieved. An infusion dose of 0.1 mg/kg/min appears to be suitable dose for sedation in the dog. (Ilkiw 1992)

d) As an induction agent for halothane or isoflurane anesthesia: 6.6 mg/kg IV given over 60 seconds to unpremedicated dogs. Best achieved by early intubation and administration of the inhalant following propofol induction. (Bufalari *et al.* 1998)

For refractory status epilepticus:

a) Propofol may be used as a substitute for pentobarbital if general anesthesia is required to control seizure activity. Because of its short duration of action, it must be given as a CRI: 6 mg/kg IV initial bolus followed by 0.1−0.6 mg/kg/min CRI. Substantial respiratory depression can occur and anesthesia must be closely monitored. Also, propofol can have pro-convulsant effects in some patients. Some consider this to be the treatment of choice for patients in status epilepticus secondary to hepatic encephalopathy (typically after surgical repair of a portosystemic shunting vessel). (Mariani 2010)

b) If seizures persist after diazepam and phenobarbital therapy: 3−6 mg/kg IV followed by an infusion of 8−12 mg/kg/hour. Must closely monitor for hypoventilation and may require mechanical ventilatory support. (Munana 2004)

c) If seizures persist after diazepam and phenobarbital therapy in dogs: Propofol IV bolus at 1−3.5 mg/kg up to 6 mg/kg followed by a CRI using a syringe pump of 0.1−0.25 mg/kg/minute (up to 0.6 mg/kg/minute) for 6−12 hours and then gradually decreased; maximum duration of propofol CRI is approximately 48 hours. If used in cats, carefully monitor PVC and CBC (Heinz body anemia, hemolytic anemia) and propofol dose should be kept as low, and duration of treatment as short, as possible. (Knipe 2006)

■ **RABBITS, RODENTS, SMALL MAMMALS:**
a) Rabbits: 5−14 mg/kg slow IV (20 mg/kg/minute) to effect; not recommended as the sole agent for maintenance (Ivey & Morrisey 2000)

b) Mice: 26 mg/kg IV. Rats: 10 mg/kg IV (Adamcak & Otten 2000)

■ **REPTILES:**
a) Iguanas: 3 mg/kg IV via either intraosseous catheter or into the coccygeal or ventral abdominal vein. Wait 3−5 minutes before giving additional increments. May also be used in tortoises. (Heard 1999)

b) 5−15 mg/kg IV or IO; in snakes intracardiac route is usually used (Innis 2003)

■ **ZOO, EXOTIC, WILDLIFE SPECIES:**
For use of propofol in zoo, exotic and wildlife medicine refer to specific references, including:
a) *Zoo Animal and Wildlife Immobilization and Anesthesia.* West, G, Heard, D, Caulkett, N. (eds.). Blackwell Publishing, 2007.

b) *Handbook of Wildlife Chemical Immobilization, 3rd Ed.* Kreeger, T.J. and J.M. Arnemo. 2007.

c) *Restraint and Handling of Wild and Domestic Animals.* Fowler, M (ed.), Iowa State University Press, 1995

d) *Exotic Animal Formulary, 3rd Ed.* Carpenter, J.W., Saunders. 2005

e) The 2009 American Association of Zoo Veterinarian Proceedings by D. K. Fontenot also has several dosages listed for restraint, anesthesia, and analgesia for a variety of drugs for carnivores and primates. VIN members can access them at: http://goo.gl/BHRih or http://goo.gl/9UJse

Monitoring
■ Level of anesthesia/CNS effects
■ Respiratory depression
■ Cardiovascular status (cardiac rate/rhythm; blood pressure)

Chemistry/Synonyms
Propofol is an alkylphenol derivative (2,6-diisopropylphenol). The commercially available injections are either a milky-white macroemulsion containing 100 mg/mL of soybean oil, 22.5 mg/mL of glycerol, and 12 mg/mL of egg lecithin with a pH of 7-8.5 or a clear (at room temperature) lipid-free microemulsion that contains methylparaben and propylparaben as preservatives

Propofol may also be known as: disoprofol, ICI-35868, propofolum, *Ansiven®, Bioprofol®, Cryotol®, Diprofol®, Diprivan®, Disoprivan®, Fresofol®, Ivofol®, Klimofol®, Oleo-Lax®, Pofol®, Profolen®, Pronest®, Propoabbott®, Propocam®, PropoClear®, PropoFlo®' Propovan®, Provive®, Rapinovet®, Recofol®,* or *Recofol®.*

Storage/Stability
Macroemulsion: Store propofol (macroemulsion) injection below 22°C (72°F), but not below 4°C (40°F.); do not refrigerate or freeze. Protect from light. Shake well before using. Do not use if the emulsion has separated. The manufacturer recommends discarding any unused portion at the end of the anesthetic procedure or after 6 hours, whichever occurs sooner.

Microemulsion: Store propofol (microemulsion) injection protected from light at controlled room temperature. Do not store above 30°C and do not refrigerate. Exposure for an extended period to temperatures below 20°C may result in a cloudy appearance. A clear appearance will return upon allowing the product to warm to 20−30°C. Gentle agitation will speed the process. Do not administer if opaque or precipitates are noted. Discard unused portions 28 days after first use.

Compatibility/Compounding Considerations
Propofol (macroemulsion) is physically **compatible** with the commonly used IV solutions (*e.g.*, LRS, D$_5$W) when injected into a running IV line. Drugs that are reported to be **compatible** with propofol (macroemulsion) at Y-site administration include (partial listing): ampicillin, butorphanol, calcium gluconate, cefazolin, cefoxitin, clindamycin, dexamethasone sodium phosphate, dexmetomidine, diphenhydramine, dobutamine, dopamine, epinephrine, fentanyl,

furosemide, heparin sodium, insulin, ketamine, lorazepam, magnesium sulfate, mannitol, naloxone, pentobarbital, phenobarbital, potassium chloride, propranolol, sodium bicarbonate, succinylcholine, thiopental, and vecuronium. It is **incompatible** with atracurium and vecuronium. Refer to specialized references or a hospital pharmacist for more information.

Dosage Forms/Regulatory Status

VETERINARY-LABELED PRODUCTS:

Propofol Injectable (macroemulsion): 10 mg/mL in 5 mL and 20 mL (single use) vials; *Rapinovet*® (Schering Plough); *PropoFlo*® (Abbott); (Rx). FDA-approved for use in dogs and cats.

Propofol Injectable (microemulsion): 10 mg/mL in 20 mL, 50 mL and 100 mL multi-dose vials; *PropoClear*® (Pfizer); (Rx). FDA-approved for use in dogs and cats.

The ARCI (Racing Commissioners International) has designated this drug as a class 2 substance. See the appendix for more information.

HUMAN-LABELED PRODUCTS:

Propofol Injectable Emulsion: 10 mg/mL in 20 mL amps & vials, 50 mL & 100 mL vials; 50 mL & 100 mL infusion vials and 50 mL prefilled single-use syringes; *Diprivan*® (AstraZeneca); Propofol (Baxter); *Fresenius Propoven*® (APP Pharmaceutical); (Rx)

References

Adamcak, A. & B. Otten (2000). Rodent Therapeutics. *Vet Clin NA: Exotic Anim Pract* **3:**1(Jan): 221–240.

Bufalari, A., S. Miller, et al. (1998). The use of propofol as an induction agent for halothane and isoflurane anesthesia in dogs. *AAHA* **34:** 83–91.

Heard, D. (1999). Advances in Reptile Anesthesia. The North American Veterinary Conference, Orlando.

Ilkiw, J. (1992). Other potentially useful new injectable anesthetic agents. *The Veterinary Clinics of North America; Small Animal Practice* **22**(2: March): 281–293.

Innis, C. (2003). Advances in anesthesia and analgesia in reptiles. Proceedings: Western Veterinary Conference. Accessed via: Veterinary Information Network. http://goo.gl/yOsua

Ivey, E. & J. Morrisey (2000). Therapeutics for Rabbits. *Vet Clin NA: Exotic Anim Pract* **3:**1(Jan): 183–216.

Knipe, M. (2006). Make it stop! Managing status epilepticus. Proceedings; Vet Neuro Symposium. Accessed via: Veterinary Information Network. http://goo.gl/sDYLA

Mariani, C. (2010). Treatment of cluster seizures and stauts epilepticus. Proceedings: ACVIM Forum. Accessed via: Veterinary Information Network. http://goo.gl/QhJST

Mathews, N. (1999). Propofol - How to use it. Proceedings: Central Veterinary Conference, Kansas City.

Munana, K. (2004). Managing the Refractory Epileptic. Proceedings: ACVIM Forum, Minneapolis. Accessed via: Veterinary Information Network. http://goo.gl/nQ9ba

Robinson, E., S. Sanderson, et al. (1993, Last Update). "Personal Communication."

PROPRANOLOL HCL

(proe-*pran*-oh-lole)   Inderal®
BETA-ADRENERGIC BLOCKER

Prescriber Highlights

▶ Non specific beta blocker primarily used in veterinary medicine as an antiarrhythmic agent

▶ Contraindications: Heart failure, hypersensitivity to this class of agents, greater than 1st degree heart block, or sinus bradycardia; generally contraindicated in patients with CHF unless secondary to a tachyarrhythmia responsive to beta-blockers or with bronchospastic lung disease

▶ Caution: Significant renal or hepatic insufficiency, sinus node dysfunction, labile diabetic patients, digitalized or digitalis intoxicated patients

▶ Adverse Effects: Bradycardia, lethargy, & depression, impaired AV conduction, CHF or worsening of heart failure, hypotension, syncope, diarrhea, hypoglycemia, & bronchoconstriction

▶ May mask (treat) clinical signs of thyrotoxicosis

▶ If discontinuing drug, consider gradual withdrawal

▶ Drug Interactions

Uses/Indications

While propranolol is used for hypertension, migraine headache prophylaxis, and angina in human patients, it is used primarily in veterinary medicine for its antiarrhythmic effects. Dysrhythmias treated with propranolol include: atrial premature complexes, ventricular premature complexes, supraventricular premature complexes and tachyarrhythmias, ventricular or atrial tachyarrhythmias secondary to digitalis, atrial tachycardia secondary to Wolff-Parkinson-White (WPW) with normal QRS complexes, and atrial fibrillation (generally in combination with digoxin). Propranolol reportedly improves cardiac performance in animals with hypertrophic cardiomyopathy. It has been used to treat systemic hypertension and clinical signs associated with thyrotoxicosis and pheochromocytoma.

Pharmacology/Actions

Propranolol blocks both beta$_1$- and beta$_2$-adrenergic receptors in the myocardium, bronchi, and vascular smooth muscle. Propranolol does not have any intrinsic sympathomimetic activity (ISA). Additionally, propranolol possesses membrane-stabilizing effects (quinidine-like) affecting the cardiac action potential and direct myocardial depressant effects. Cardiovascular effects secondary to propranolol include: decreased sinus heart rate, depressed AV conduction, diminished cardiac output at rest and during exercise, decreased myocardial oxygen demand, decreased hepatic and renal blood flow, reduced blood pressure, and inhibition of isoproterenol-induced tachycardia. Electrophysiologic effects on the heart include decreased automaticity, increased or no effect on effective refractory period, and no effect on conduction velocity.

Additional pharmacologic effects of propranolol, include increased airway resistance (especially in patients with bronchoconstrictive disease), prevention of migraine headaches, increased uterine activity (more so in the non-pregnant uterus), decreased platelet aggregability, inhibited glycogenolysis in cardiac and skeletal muscle, and increased numbers of circulating eosinophils.

Pharmacokinetics

Propranolol is well absorbed after oral administration, but a rapid first-pass effect through the liver reduces systemic bioavailability to approximately 2–27% in dogs, thereby explaining the significant difference between oral and intravenous dosages. These values reportedly increase with chronic dosing. Hyperthyroid cats may have increased bioavailability of propranolol when compared with normal cats.

Propranolol is highly lipid soluble and readily crosses the blood-brain barrier. The apparent volume of distribution has been reported to 3.3–11 L/kg in the dog. Propranolol crosses the placenta and enters milk (at very low levels). In humans, propranolol is approximately 90% bound to plasma proteins.

Propranolol metabolization occurs principally by the liver. An active metabolite, 4-hydroxypropranolol, has been identified after oral administration in humans. Less than 1% of a dose is excreted unchanged into the urine. The half-life in dogs has been reported to range from 0.77–2 hours, and in horses, less than 2 hours. It has been reported that hyperthyroid cats have a decreased clearance of propranolol when compared with normal cats.

Contraindications/Precautions/Warnings

Propranolol is contraindicated in patients with overt heart failure, hypersensitivity to this class of agents, greater than 1st degree heart block, or sinus bradycardia. Non-specific beta-blockers are generally contraindicated in patients with CHF unless secondary to a tachyarrhythmia responsive to beta-blocker therapy. They are also relatively contraindicated in patients with bronchospastic lung disease.

Propranolol should be used cautiously in patients with significant renal or hepatic insufficiency, or with sinus node dysfunction.

Propranolol can mask the clinical signs associated with hypoglycemia. It can also cause hypoglycemia or hyperglycemia and, therefore, should be used cautiously in labile diabetic patients.

Propranolol can mask the clinical signs associated with thyrotoxicosis, but it has been used clinically to treat the clinical signs associated with this condition.

Use propranolol cautiously with digitalis or in digitalis intoxicated patients; severe bradycardias may result.

Adverse Effects

It is reported that adverse effects most commonly occur in geriatric animals or those that have acute decompensating heart disease. Clinically relevant adverse effects include: bradycardia, lethargy and depression, impaired AV conduction, CHF or worsening of heart failure, hypotension, hypoglycemia, and bronchoconstriction. Syncope and diarrhea have also been reported in canine patients.

Exacerbations of clinical signs have been reported following abrupt cessation of beta-blockers in humans. It is recommended to withdraw therapy gradually in patients who have been receiving the drug chronically.

Reproductive/Nursing Safety

In humans, the FDA categorizes this drug as category *C* for use during pregnancy (*Animal studies have shown an adverse effect on the fetus, but there are no adequate studies in humans; or there are no animal reproduction studies and no adequate studies in humans.*) In a separate system evaluating the safety of drugs in canine and feline pregnancy (Papich 1989), this drug is categorized as class: *C* (*These drugs may have potential risks. Studies in people or laboratory animals have uncovered risks, and these drugs should be used cautiously as a last resort when the benefit of therapy clearly outweighs the risks.*)

Propranolol is excreted in maternal milk. Use with caution in nursing patients.

Overdosage/Acute Toxicity

The most predominant clinical signs expected would be hypotension and bradycardia. Other possible effects could include: CNS (depressed consciousness to seizures), bronchospasm, hypoglycemia, hyperkalemia, respiratory depression, pulmonary edema, other arrhythmias (especially AV block), or asystole.

There were 115 exposures to propranolol reported to the ASPCA Animal Poison Control Center (APCC) during 2008-2009. In these cases 96 were dogs with 6 showing clinical signs, 18 were cats with 3 showing clinical signs, and 1 was a ferret that showed clinical signs. Common findings in dogs recorded in decreasing frequency included bradycardia and lethargy.

If overdose is secondary to a recent oral ingestion, emptying the gut and charcoal administration may be considered. Seizures are reported in people, but in a review of the APCC database, seizures were not reported in animals. Monitor patient's ECG, blood glucose, potassium and, if possible, blood pressure; treatment of the cardiovascular and CNS effects are symptomatic. Use fluids and pressor agents to treat hypotension. Bradycardia may be treated with atropine. If atropine fails, isoproterenol given cautiously has been recommended. Use of a transvenous pacemaker may be necessary. Cardiac failure can be treated with digoxin, diuretics, oxygen and, if necessary, IV aminophylline. Glucagon (5–10 mg IV; human dose) may increase heart rate and blood pressure and reduce the cardiodepressant effects of propranolol. Seizures generally will respond to IV diazepam.

Drug Interactions

The following drug interactions have either been reported or are theoretical in humans or animals receiving propranolol and may be of significance in veterinary patients:

- **ANTACIDS:** May reduce oral propranolol absorption; separate doses by at least one hour
- **ANESTHETICS, GENERAL:** Additive myocardial depression may occur with the concurrent use of propranolol and myocardial depressant anesthetic agents
- **ANTICHOLINERGICS:** May negate cardiac effects of beta-blockers
- **CALCIUM CHANNEL BLOCKERS:** Concurrent use of beta-blockers with calcium channel blockers (or other negative inotropes) should be done with caution, particularly in patients with preexisting cardiomyopathy or CHF
- **CIMETIDINE:** May decrease the metabolism of propranolol and increase blood levels
- **DIURETICS:** May increase risk for hypotension
- **EPINEPHRINE:** Unopposed alpha effects of epinephrine may lead to rapid increases in blood pressure and decrease in heart rate
- **FLUOXETINE:** May decrease propranolol metabolism; complete heart block reported in one human
- **INSULIN and other ANTIDIABETIC DRUGS:** Propranolol may prolong the hypoglycemic effects of insulin therapy
- **LIDOCAINE:** Clearance may be impaired by propranolol
- **METHIMAZOLE, PROPYLTHIOURACIL:** Propranolol doses may need to be decreased when initiating therapy
- **PHENOBARBITAL:** May increase the metabolism of propranolol
- **PHENOTHIAZINES:** May increase risk for hypotension
- **RESERPINE:** May have additive effects with propranolol
- **SUCCINYLCHOLINE, TUBOCURARINE:** Effects may be enhanced with propranolol therapy
- **SYMPATHOMIMETICS (metaproterenol, terbutaline, beta effects of epinephrine, phenyl-**

propanolamine, etc.): May have their actions blocked by propranolol
- **THEOPHYLLINE:** Effects of theophylline (bronchodilation) may be blocked by propranolol
- **THYROID HORMONES:** May decrease the effects of beta blocking agents

Doses

- **DOGS:**
  a) For susceptible cardiac arrhythmias: 0.02 mg/kg IV slowly (up to a maximum of 1 mg/kg). Oral dose: 0.1–0.2 mg/kg initially PO q8h, up to a maximum of 1.5 mg/kg q8h (Ware 2000)

  b) As a beta-blocker for adjunctive therapy in heart failure: 0.1–0.2 mg/kg PO q8h (start low and titrate) (Fox 2003)

  c) For loud-noise phobias: 5–40 mg/dog q8h (Crowell-Davis 1999)

  d) For treatment of tachycardia associated with serotonin syndrome: 0.02 mg/kg slowly IV; titrate up as needed. (Wismer 2000)

- **CATS:**
  a) For susceptible cardiac arrhythmias: 0.02 mg/kg IV slowly (up to a maximum of 1 mg/kg). Oral dose: 2.5 mg (up to 10 mg) total dose per cat q 8–12h. (Ware 2000)

  b) For susceptible cardiac arrhythmias: 0.02 mg/kg IV over one minute; can repeat up to a maximum of four times as needed based upon response (Cote 2004)

  c) As a beta-blocker for adjunctive therapy in heart failure: 2.5–10 mg (total dose) PO q8h (start low and titrate) (Fox 2003)

  d) For adjunctive therapy of hypertension: 2.5–5 mg (total dose) PO q8–12h (Sparkes 2003)

  e) For adjunctive therapy (to control neuromuscular and cardiovascular effects) in feline hyperthyroidism: 2 mg/kg (6.25 mg per cat) once daily (Behrend 1999)

- **FERRETS:**
  For hypertrophic cardiomyopathy:
  a) 0.5–2 mg/kg PO or SC once a day to twice a day (Williams 2000)

  b) 0.2–2 mg/kg PO q8-12h. (Heatley 2009)

- **HORSES: (NOTE:** ARCI UCGFS Class 3 Drug)
  a) For V-Tach: 0.05–0.16 mg/kg IV. **Note:** negative inotropic and chronotropic effects may be undesirable. (Mogg 1999)

  b) For V-Tach: 0.03–0.15 mg/kg IV or 0.3–0.7 mg/kg PO q8h. Considered not as effective as lidocaine; decreases ventricular rate even if it does not restore sinus rhythm. Toxic effects include bradycardia, AV block, proarrhythmic, negative inotrope and hypotension. Use with caution in animals with airway disease (bronchoconstriction). (Kimberly & Mc-Gurrin 2006)

c) Oral: Days 1 and 2: 175 mg three times a day; Days 3 and 4: 275 mg three times a day; Days 5 and 6: 350 mg three times daily.

Intravenous: Days 1 and 2: 25 mg two times a day; Days 3 and 4: 50 mg two times a day; Days 5 and 6: 75 mg twice daily (Hilwig 1987)

Monitoring
- ECG
- Toxicity (see Adverse Effects/Overdosage)
- Blood pressure if administering IV

Client Information
- To be effective, the animal must receive all doses as prescribed.
- Notify veterinarian if animal becomes lethargic or becomes exercise intolerant, begins wheezing, develops shortness of breath or cough, or presents a change in behavior or attitude.

Chemistry/Synonyms
A non-specific beta-adrenergic blocking agent, propranolol HCl occurs as a bitter tasting, odorless, white to almost white powder with a pK_a of 9.45 and a melting point of about 161°C. One gram of propranolol is soluble in about 20 mL of water or alcohol. At a pH from 4-5, solutions of propranolol will fluoresce. The commercially available injectable solutions are adjusted with citric acid to a pH 2.8–3.5.

Propranolol may also be known as: AY-64043, ICI-45520, NSC-91523, propranololi hydrochloridum; many trade names are available.

Storage/Stability
All propranolol preparations should be stored at room temperature (15–30°C) and protected from light. Propranolol solutions will decompose rapidly at alkaline pH.

Compatibility/Compounding Considerations
Propranolol injection is reported to be physically **compatible** with D_5W, 0.9% sodium chloride, or lactated Ringer's injection. It is also physically **compatible** with dobutamine HCl, verapamil HCl, and benzquinamide HCl.

Dosage Forms/Regulatory Status
VETERINARY-LABELED PRODUCTS: None

HUMAN-LABELED PRODUCTS:

Propranolol HCl Oral Tablets: 10 mg, 20 mg, 40 mg, 60 mg & 80 mg; generic; (Rx)

Propranolol HCl Extended/Sustained-Release Capsules: 60 mg, 80 mg, 120 mg & 160 mg; *Inderal® LA* (Akrimax); *InnoPran® XL* (Reliant); generic; (Rx)

Propranolol for Injection: 1 mg/mL in 1 mL amps or vials; *Inderal®* (Wyeth-Ayerst); generic; (Rx)

Propranolol Oral Solution: 4 mg/mL & 8 mg/mL in 500 mL; generic; (Rx)

In addition, fixed dose combination products containing propranolol and hydrochlorothiazide are available to treat hypertension in humans.

References
Behrend, E. (1999). Update on the diagnosis and treatment of feline hyperthyroidism. American College of Veterinary Internal Medicine: 17th Annual Veterinary Medical Forum, Chicago.

Cote, E. (2004). Feline arrhythmias. Proceedings: ACVIM Forum. Accessed via: Veterinary Information Network. http://goo.gl/jigyx

Crowell-Davis, S. (1999). Behavior Psychopharmacology Part 2: Anxiolytics, hormones, narcotic antagonists and Miscellaneous. Proceedings: Central Veterinary Conference, Kansas City.

Fox, P. (2003). Congestive heart failure: Clinical approach and management. Proceedings: World Small Animal Veterinary Assoc World Congress. Accessed via: Veterinary Information Network. http://goo.gl/xMFKn

Heatley, J. (2009). Small Exotic Mammal Cardiovascular Disease. Proceedings: ABVP. Accessed via: Veterinary Information Network. http://goo.gl/rzlia

Hilwig, R.W. (1987). Cardiac arrhythmias. *Current Therapy in Equine Medicine*. NE Robinson Ed. Philadelphia, WB Saunders: 154–164.

Kimberly, M. & K. McGurrin (2006). Update on antiarrhythmic therapy in horses. Proceedings; ACVIM. Accessed via: Veterinary Information Network. http://goo.gl/kSS8b

Mogg, T. (1999). Equine Cardiac Disease: Clinical pharmacology and therapeutics. *The Veterinary Clinics of North America: Equine Practice* **15:3**(December).

Papich, M. (1989). Effects of drugs on pregnancy. *Current Veterinary Therapy X: Small Animal Practice*. R Kirk Ed. Philadelphia, Saunders: 1291–1299.

Sparkes, A. (2003). Feline systemic hypertension-A hidden killer. Proceedings: World Small Animal Veterinary Assoc. Accessed via: Veterinary Information Network. http://goo.gl/QgVkr

Ware, W. (2000). Therapy for Critical Arrythmias: New Advances. Proceedings: The North American Veterinary Conference, Orlando.

Williams, B. (2000). Therapeutics in Ferrets. *Vet Clin NA: Exotic Anim Pract* **3:1**(Jan): 131–153.

Wismer, T. (2000). Toxicology Brief: Antidepressant Overdoses. *Vet Med*(July).

Prostaglandin F2 alpha—see Dinoprost Tromethamine

PROTAMINE SULFATE
(proe-ta-meen)

ANTIDOTE (HEPARIN)

Prescriber Highlights
- Protein that complexes with heparin (treatment of overdoses); may also be useful for Bracken Fern poisoning
- Contraindications: Hypersensitivity to protamine
- Adverse Effects: If injected IV too rapidly: Acute hypotension, bradycardia, pulmonary hypertension, & dyspnea; hypersensitivity possible
- Monitor for heparin "rebound effect"

Uses/Indications

Protamine is used in all species for the treatment of heparin overdosage when significant bleeding occurs. While protamine will neutralize the anti-thrombin effects of low molecular weight heparins (*e.g.*, dalteparin or enoxaparin), it does not completely inhibit their anti-Xa activity. Laboratory animal studies however, shows it does improve microvascular bleeding associated with LMWH overdoses. Protamine has been suggested for use for Bracken Fern toxicity in ruminants (see Doses).

Pharmacology/Actions

Protamine is strongly basic and heparin, strongly acidic; protamine complexes with heparin to form an inactive stable salt. Protamine has intrinsic anticoagulant activity, but its effects are weak and rarely cause problems.

Pharmacokinetics

After IV injection, protamine binds to heparin within 5 minutes. The exact metabolic fate of the heparin-protamine complex is not known, but there is evidence that the complex is partially metabolized and/or degraded by fibrinolysin thus freeing heparin.

Contraindications/Precautions/Warnings

Protamine is contraindicated in patients who have demonstrated hypersensitivity or intolerance to the drug in the past.

Adverse Effects

If protamine sulfate is injected IV too rapidly, acute hypotension, bradycardia, pulmonary hypertension, and dyspnea can occur. These effects are usually absent or minimized when the drug is administered slowly (over 1–3 minutes). Hypersensitivity reactions have also been reported.

A heparin "rebound" effect has been reported where anticoagulation and bleeding occur several hours after heparin has apparently been neutralized. This may be due to either a release of heparin from extravascular compartments or the release of heparin from the protamine-heparin complex.

Reproductive/Nursing Safety

In humans, the FDA categorizes this drug as category **C** for use during pregnancy (*Animal studies have shown an adverse effect on the fetus, but there are no adequate studies in humans; or there are no animal reproduction studies and no adequate studies in humans.*)

It is not known whether this drug is excreted in milk.

Overdosage/Acute Toxicity

Because protamine has inherent anticoagulant activity, overdoses of protamine may, theoretically, result in hemorrhage; however, in one human study, overdoses of 600–800 mg resulted only in mild, transient effects on coagulation. The LD_{50} of protamine in mice is 100 mg/kg.

Drug Interactions; Laboratory Considerations

■ None were located.

Doses

■ **DOGS/CATS** (and presumably other species): For heparin overdosage:

a) Give 1–1.5 mg protamine sulfate to antagonize each mg (≈100 units) of heparin via slow IV injection. Reduce dose as time increases between heparin dose and start of treatment (after 30 minutes give only 0.5 mg). (Bailey 1986)

b) Administer 1 mg protamine for each 100 Units of heparin to be inactivated. Decrease protamine dose by ½ for every 30 minutes that have lapsed since heparin was administered (*Plumb's Note*: This may be ineffective if heparin has been administered by deep SC injection). Give dose slowly IV, do not give at a rate faster than 50 mg over a 10-minute period. (Adams 1988)

■ **CATTLE:**
For Bracken Fern (*Pteridium* spp.) poisoning:

a) In combination with whole blood (2.25–4.5 L), 1 injection of 10 mL of 1% protamine sulfate IV (Osweiler & Ruhr 1986)

Monitoring

■ See the Heparin monograph

Client Information

■ Should only be used in a setting where adequate monitoring facilities are available.

Chemistry/Synonyms

Simple, low molecular weight, cationic proteins, protamines occur naturally in the sperm of fish. Commercially available protamine sulfate is produced from protamine obtained from the sperm or mature testes of salmon (or related species). It occurs as a fine, white to off-white crystalline or amorphous powder that is sparingly soluble in water and very slightly soluble in alcohol. The injection is available as either a prepared solution with a pH of 6–7 or a lyophilized powder that has a pH of 6.5–7.5 after reconstituting.

Protamine Sulfate may also be known as: protamine sulphate, protamini sulfas, sulfato de protamina, *Prosulf®*, or *Prota®*.

Storage/Stability

The powder for injection should be stored at room temperature (15–30°C), and the injection (liquid) in the refrigerator (2–8°C); avoid freezing. The injection is stable at room temperature for at least 2 weeks, however. The powder for injection should be used immediately if reconstituted with Sterile Water for Injection and within 72 hours if reconstituted with Bacteriostatic Water for Injection.

It is recommended to use either D_5W or normal saline for protamine sulfate infusions. Cimetidine and verapamil are reported to be physically **compatible** with protamine sulfate for injection.

Dosage Forms/Regulatory Status

VETERINARY-LABELED PRODUCTS: None

HUMAN-LABELED PRODUCTS:

Protamine Sulfate Injection: 10 mg/mL preservative-free in 5 mL and 25 mL vials; generic; (Rx)

References

Adams, H.R. (1988). Hemostatic and Anticoagulant Drugs. *Veterinary Pharmacology and Therapeutics.* NH Booth and LE McDonald Eds. Ames, Iowa State University Press: 481–494.

Bailey, E.M. (1986). Emergency and general treatment of poisonings. *Current Veterinary Therapy (CVT) IX Small Animal Practice.* RW Kirk Ed. Philadelphia, W.B. Saunders: 135–144.

Osweiler, G.D. & L.P. Ruhr (1986). Plants affecting blood coagulation. *Current Veterinary Therapy: Food Animal Practice 2.* JL Howard Ed. Philadelphia, W.B. Saunders: 404–406.

PSEUDOEPHEDRINE HCL

(soo-doe-e-*fed*-rin)   Equiphed®, Sudafed®

SYMPATHOMIMETIC

Prescriber Highlights

▶ Oral sympathomimetic used primarily for urethral sphincter hypotonus when phenylpropanolamine unavailable; may be used as an oral decongestant or for retrograde ejaculation.

▶ Caution: Glaucoma, prostatic hypertrophy, hyperthyroidism, diabetes mellitus, cardiovascular disorders, or hypertension

▶ Adverse Effects: Restlessness, irritability, hypertension, & anorexia

▶ Restricted drug in USA; can be used as a precursor to manufacture methamphetamine

Uses/Indications

Pseudoephedrine is used primarily as a substitute for phenylpropanolamine for the treatment of urinary incontinence (dribbling) in dogs. One study showed that it was not as effective and had more adverse effects then phenylpropanolamine in dogs with urinary incontinence (Byron *et al.* 2007). It may also be used as an oral decongestant or for treating retrograde ejaculation.

Pharmacology/Actions

While the exact mechanisms of pseudoephedrine's actions are undetermined, it is believed that it indirectly stimulates both alpha- and beta- (to a lesser degree) adrenergic receptors by causing the release of norepinephrine.

Pharmacologic effects of pseudoephedrine include increased vasoconstriction, heart rate, coronary blood flow, blood pressure, mild CNS stimulation, and decreased nasal congestion and appetite. Pseudoephedrine can also increase urethral sphincter tone and produce closure of the bladder neck.

Pharmacokinetics

Pseudoephedrine is rapidly and nearly completely absorbed from the GI tract. Food may delay the absorption somewhat, but not the extent. In children, the apparent volume of distribution is about 2.5 L/kg. Pseudoephedrine is only partially metabolized and the bulk is excreted unchanged in the urine. Urine pH can affect excretion rates. Alkaline urine (pH 8) can prolong half-life while acidic urine (pH 5) can decrease it.

Contraindications/Precautions/Warnings

Pseudoephedrine should be used with caution in patients with glaucoma, prostatic hypertrophy, hyperthyroidism, diabetes mellitus, cardiovascular disorders or hypertension.

Adverse Effects

Adverse effects are dose related and adrenergic in nature with panting, decreased appetite, lethargy, and rapid heart rate the most likely to be seen at usual doses; CNS excitement/restlessness/insomnia are possible. Increases in blood pressure and arrhythmias can occur in susceptible individuals, particularly at high doses.

Because pseudoephedrine may be used to manufacture methamphetamine, be alert for clients wanting to purchase very large amounts of the drug.

Reproductive/Nursing Safety

Safe use has not been established during pregnancy; use with care. In humans, the FDA categorizes this drug as category **C** for use during pregnancy (*Animal studies have shown an adverse effect on the fetus, but there are no adequate studies in humans; or there are no animal reproduction studies and no adequate studies in humans.*)

In humans, it is not recommended to use systemic pseudoephedrine during breastfeeding as the drug enters maternal milk and infants may be very susceptible to the drug's effects. Use with caution in veterinary patients.

Overdosage/Acute Toxicity

Overdoses of pseudoephedrine can cause hyperthermia, mydriasis, tachycardia, hypertension, vomiting, disorientation, and seizures. In small animals, adverse reactions may develop at doses of 5–6 mg/kg. Deaths have occurred at doses >10–12 mg/kg.

There were 221 exposures to pseudoephedrine reported to the ASPCA Animal Poison Control Center (APCC) during 2008-2009. In these cases 213 were dogs with 64 showing clinical signs and 8 were cats with 3 showing clinical signs. Common findings in dogs recorded in decreasing frequency included hyperactivity, tachycardia, agitation, mydriasis, restlessness, head bobbing, and panting. Common findings in cats included tachycardia.

Large overdoses should be treated with gastric evacuation (if not contraindicated); otherwise, treat supportively and symptomatically (*e.g.,* propranolol for tachycardia). Phenothiazines are preferred to treat hyperactivity, agitation, and tremors as diazepam may worsen dysphoria. It is recommended to contact an animal poison control center for further guidance in the case of a large pseudoephedrine overdose.

Drug Interactions

The following drug interactions have either been reported or are theoretical in humans or animals receiving pseudoephedrine and may be of significance in veterinary patients:

- **◼ MONAMINE OXIDASE (MAO) INHIBITORS (e.g., amitraz, possibly selegiline):** Pseudoephedrine should not be given within two weeks of a patient receiving monoamine oxidase inhibitors

- **◼ RESERPINE:** An increased chance of hypertension if given concomitantly

- **◼ SYMPATHOMIMETIC AGENTS, OTHER:** Phenylpropanolamine should not be administered with other sympathomimetic agents (*e.g.,* **ephedrine**) as increased toxicity may result

- **◼ TRICYCLIC ANTIDEPRESSANTS (clomipramine, amitriptyline, etc.):** An increased chance of hypertension if given concomitantly

Doses

- **◼ DOGS:**
  a) For urinary incontinence, or as a decongestant: 0.2–0.4 mg/kg [or practically, 15–60 mg (total dose) per dog] PO q8–12h (Tilley & Smith 2000)
  b) To increase urethral tone: 1.5 mg/kg PO two to three times a day. (Dickinson 2010)
  c) For retrograde ejaculation: 4–5 mg/kg PO three times daily or 1 to 3 hours before semen collection or attempted breeding may be tried. (Fontbonne 2007)

- **◼ CATS:**
  a) As a decongestant: 1 mg/kg PO q8h (Scherk 2010)

- **◼ HORSES: (NOTE: ARCI UCGFS CLASS 3 DRUG)**
  a) For use when an antihistamine/decongestant may be useful using the pyrilamine/pseudoephedrine oral granules: ½ ounce (1 tablespoonful) per 1,000 lb body weight. May mix with feed and repeated at 12 our intervals if needed. Do not use at least 72 hours before sporting events. (Label information—veterinary products listed below)

Monitoring

- ◼ Efficacy
- ◼ Adverse effects (heart rate, CNS stimulation, appetite)

Client Information

- ◼ For this drug to be effective, it must be administered as directed by the veterinarian; missed doses will negate its effect. It may take several days for the full benefit of the drug to take place.

- ◼ Contact veterinarian if the animal demonstrates ongoing changes in behavior (restlessness, irritability) or if incontinence persists or increases.

Chemistry/Synonyms

A sympathomimetic, pseudoephedrine HCl is the stereoisomer of ephedrine. It occurs as a fine, white to off-white powder or crystals. Approximately 2 grams are soluble in one mL of water.

Pseudoephedrine may also be known as: pseudoephedrini, pseudoephedrina, *Equi-Phar Equi-Hist 1200 Granules®, Drixoral®, Equiphed®, Histgranules®, Sudafed®,* and *Tri-Hist®.*

Storage/Stability

Oral pseudoephedrine products should be stored at room temperature in tight containers. Oral liquid preparations should be protected from light and freezing.

Dosage Forms/Regulatory Status

In the USA, pseudoephedrine is classified as a list 1 chemical (drugs that can be used as precursors to manufacture methamphetamine) and in some states it may be a controlled substance or have other restrictions placed upon its sale. Be alert to persons desiring to purchase this medication.

VETERINARY-LABELED PRODUCTS:

Pseudoephedrine HCl 600 mg/oz and Pyrilamine maleate 600 mg/oz Granules in 20 oz, 5 lb and 10 lb containers; *Equiphed®* (AHC), *Equi-Phar Equi-Hist 1200 Granules®* (Vedco); *Tri-Hist® Granules* (Neogen); *Histgranules®* (Butler); (Rx). FDA-approved for use in horses not intended for food. Do not use at least 72 hours before sporting events.

The ARCI (Racing Commissioners International) has designated this drug as a class 3 substance. See the appendix for more information.

HUMAN-LABELED PRODUCTS:

Pseudoephedrine HCl Tablets and Capsules: 30 mg & 60 mg; Extended/Controlled Release: 120 mg and 240 mg (immediate-release 60 mg, controlled-release 180 mg). A common trade name is *Sudafed®,* but there are many others and generically labeled pseudoephedrine is available. All are OTC, but sales are now restricted to "behind-the-counter" status.

Pseudoephedrine Liquid: 3 mg/mL and

6 mg/mL in 118 mL, 120 mL, 237 mL, 480 mL and 3.8 L. A common trade name is *Sudafed®*, but there are many others, including generically labeled pseudoephedrine available. All are OTC, restricted.

Pseudoephedrine Oral Drops: 7.5 mg/0.8 mL in 15 mL & 30 mL; *Kid Kare®* (Rugby); Nasal Decongestant Oral (various); (OTC, restricted)

References

Byron, J.K., P.A. March, et al. (2007). Effect of phenylpropanolamine and pseudoephedrine on the urethral pressure profile and continence scores of incontinent female dogs. *Journal of Veterinary Internal Medicine* **21**(1): 47–53.

Dickinson, P. (2010). Disorders of micturition and continence. Proceedings: UCD Veterinary Neurology Symposium. Accessed via: Veterinary Information Network. http://goo.gl/wo3hl

Fontbonne, A. (2007). Approach to infertility in the bitch and the dog. Proceedings: WSAVA World Congress. Accessed via: Veterinary Information Network. http://goo.gl/OSre0

Scherk, M. (2010). Snots and Snuffles Rational approach to chronic feline upper respiratory syndromes. *Journal of Feline Medicine and Surgery* **12**(7): 548–557.

Tilley, L. & F. Smith (2000). *The 5–Minute Veterinary Consult: Canine and Feline.*

PSYLLIUM HYDROPHILIC MUCILLOID

(**sill**-i-yum hye-droe-**fill**-ik **myoo**-sill-oid)
Metamucil®, Equi-Psyllium®

BULK FORMING GI LAXATIVE/ ANTIDIARRHEAL

Prescriber Highlights

▶ Bulk-forming agent used for treatment & prevention of sand colic in horses, as a laxative, & to increase stool consistency in patients with chronic, watery diarrhea

▶ Contraindications: Rabbits. Where prompt intestinal evacuation is required, & when fecal impaction or intestinal obstruction is present.

▶ Adverse Effects: Flatulence; if insufficient liquid is given, increased possibility of esophageal or bowel obstruction

Uses/Indications

Bulk forming laxatives are used in patients where constipation is a result a too little fiber in their diets or when straining to defecate may be deleterious. Psyllium is considered the laxative of choice in the treatment and prevention of sand colic in horses.

Psyllium has also been used to increase stool consistency in patients with chronic, watery diarrhea. The total amount of water in the stool remains unchanged.

Pharmacology/Actions

By swelling after absorbing water, psyllium increases bulk in the intestine and is believed to induce peristalsis and decrease intestinal transit time. In the treatment of sand colic in horses, psyllium is thought to help collect sand and to help lubricate its passage through the GI tract.

Pharmacokinetics

Psyllium is not absorbed when administered orally. Laxative action may take up to 72 hours to occur.

Contraindications/Precautions/Warnings

Bulk-forming laxatives should not be used in cases where prompt intestinal evacuation is required, or when fecal impaction (no feces being passed) or intestinal obstruction is present. Psyllium products are not recommended for use in rabbits as they may damage intestinal mucosa and cause blockage.

Adverse Effects

With the exception of increased flatulence, psyllium very rarely produces any adverse reactions if adequate water is given or is available to the patient. If insufficient liquid is given, there is an increased possibility of esophageal or bowel obstruction occurring.

Reproductive/Nursing Safety

Because there is no appreciable absorption of psyllium from the gut, it should be safe to use in pregnant animals. In humans, the FDA categorizes this drug as category *B* for use during pregnancy (*Animal studies have not yet demonstrated risk to the fetus, but there are no adequate studies in pregnant women; or animal studies have shown an adverse effect, but adequate studies in pregnant women have not demonstrated a risk to the fetus in the first trimester of pregnancy, and there is no evidence of risk in later trimesters.*)

Psyllium should be safe to administer to lactating animals.

Overdosage/Acute Toxicity

If administered with sufficient liquid, psyllium overdose should cause only an increased amount of soft or loose stools.

Drug Interactions

The following drug interactions have either been reported or are theoretical in humans or animals receiving psyllium and may be of significance in veterinary patients:

▪ **ASPIRIN (and other SALICYLATES):** Potential exists for psyllium to bind and reduce absorption if given at the same time; if possible, separate doses by 3 hours or more

▪ **DIGOXIN:** Potential exists for psyllium to bind and reduce absorption if given at the same time; if possible, separate doses by 3 hours or more

▪ **NITROFURANTOIN:** Potential exists for psyllium to bind and reduce absorption if given at the same time; if possible, separate doses by 3 hours or more

Doses

■ **DOGS:**

a) For a trial to treat chronic idiopathic large bowel diarrhea using *Metamucil®*: Median dose is 2 tablespoonsful (1.33 grams/kg/day; range: 0.32–4.9 grams/kg/day) per day added to a highly digestible diet such as Hill's *i/d®* (Leib 2004; Leib 2005)

b) To increase fiber in dogs with chronic colitis: Add 1–2 tablespoonful (15–30 mL) per 25 kg body weight to animal's regular diet. (Jergens 2007)

c) In cases of predominantly large bowel diarrhea (colitis with typical clinical presentation) if parasiticide treatment and elimination diet fail, a therapeutic trial can be made: metronidazole 20–25 mg/kg PO twice daily for 5-10 days with the addition of fiber to the diet (*e.g.,* psyllium at 0.5 tablespoon for toy breeds, 1 tablespoon for small dogs, 2 tablespoons for medium dogs, and 3 tablespoons for large dogs). However, sampling of mucosal biopsies prior to further treatment may be the best course of action. (Gaschen 2008)

d) In dogs prone to constipation, 2% psyllium was added as part of diet. 80% of studied dogs had easier defecation process. (Tortola *et al.* 2009)

e) As an adjunct (source of soluble fiber) for treatment of hepatic encephalopathy: 1–3 teaspoons per day as a dietary supplement. (Twedt 2009)

■ **CATS:**

a) For chronic constipation: 1–4 teaspoonsful per meal added to canned cat food. Be sure cat is properly hydrated. (Washabau 2001)

b) For adjunctive treatment of feline megacolon: 1–4 teaspoonsful mixed with food PO q12–24h (Scherk 2003)

■ **HORSES:**

a) For sand colic: 1 gram/kg twice daily. Administration of psyllium, approximately 1 lb, in powdered form can be given via nasogastric tube once the powder has been mixed with water; mix and administer immediately via NG tube or mixture will thicken. If giving orally to foals, esophageal obstruction can occur. Give small amounts of the mixture at a time and confirm that the foal swallows after each bolus. A liquid-like versus paste-like mixtures can help also. Pelleted psyllium is also available and most horses find this form more palatable than if the powdered form is mixed with dry or moistened feed. If horse refuses the pelleted form, experimentation with different flavors and smells produced by different suppliers of psyllium pellets may be helpful. Another option is to try mixing the psyllium pellets with the horse's favorite treat or grain source to improve intake. (Tillotson & Traub-Dargatz 2003)

b) For sand colic: In this experimental study, 0.5 kg psyllium was mixed with 1 liter of mash and given twice daily and 2 liters of mineral oil via NG tube were administered once daily. This combination was more effective (measured ash content of feces) than giving mineral oil alone. (Hotwagner & Iben 2008)

c) For sand impactions: 8 ounces in water via NG tube q24h. (Blikslager 2006)

Monitoring

■ Stool consistency, frequency

Client Information

■ Contact veterinarian if patient begins vomiting

■ Be sure animal has free access to water

Chemistry/Synonyms

Psyllium is obtained from the ripe seeds of varieties of Plantago species. The seed coating is high in content of hemicellulose mucilage that absorbs and swells in the presence of water.

Psyllium may also be known as *Metamucil®*; many other trade names are available.

Storage/Stability

Store psyllium products in tightly closed containers; protect from excess moisture or humidity.

Dosage Forms/Regulatory Status

VETERINARY-LABELED PRODUCTS:

Equine Enteric Colloid® (Techmix); *Equi-Phar® Sweet Psyllium* (Vedco); (not for horses intended for food); *Sandclear®* (Farnam), *Anipsyll® Powder* (AHC), *Purepsyll® Powder* (AHC), *Vita-Flex Sand Relief®* (Vita-lex), *Equa Aid Psyllium®* (Equi Aid); (OTC). Products may be available in 28 oz, 56 oz, 1 lb, 10 lb and 30 lb pails and are labeled for use in horses.

Vetasyl Fiber Tablets for Cats® 500 mg, & 1000 mg tablets in bottles of 60 or 180; (Virbac) (OTC); Labeled for use in cats. Also contains barley malt extract powder, acacia and thiamine.

HUMAN-LABELED PRODUCTS:

There are many human-approved products containing psyllium, most products contain approximately 3.4 grams of psyllium per rounded teaspoonful. Dosages of sugar-free products may be different from those containing sugar.

References

Blikslager, A. (2006). Differential diagnosis or impaction colic in horses. Proceedings: Western Vet Conf. Accessed via: Veterinary Information Network. http://goo.gl/bdOC4

Gaschen, F. (2008). How I Treat Chronic Canine Enteropathies. Peroceedings: WSAVA. Accessed via: Veterinary Information Network. http://goo.gl/cGz2Y

Hotwagner, K. & C. Iben (2008). Evacuation of sand from the equine intestine with mineral oil, with and without psyllium. *Journal of Animal Physiology and Animal Nutrition* **92**(1): 86–91.

Jergens, A. (2007). Chronic Large Bowel Diarrheas. Proceedings: Western Vet Conf. Accessed via: Veterinary Information Network. http://goo.gl/Mn735

Leib, M. (2004). Chronic idiopathic large bowel diarrhea in dogs. Proceedings: ACVIM Forum. Accessed via: Veterinary Information Network. http://goo.gl/Nwoz8

Leib, M. (2005). Idiopathic large intestinal diarrhea in dogs. Proceedings: Western Veterinary Conference 2005, Accessed via the Veterinary Information Network Jan 2007. Accessed via: Veterinary Information Network. http://goo.gl/rYA0d

Scherk, M. (2003). Feline megacolon. Proceedings: World Small Animal Veterinary Assoc World Congress. Accessed via: Veterinary Information Network. http://goo.gl/v69lu

Tillotson, K. & J. Traub-Dargatz (2003). Gastrointestinal protectants and cathartics. *Vet Clin Equine* **19**: 599–615.

Tortola, L., L. Zaine, et al. (2009). Psyllium (Plantago psyllium) Uses In The Management Of Constipation In Dogs. Proceedings: WSAVA. Accessed via: Veterinary Information Network. http://goo.gl/pejpb

Twedt, D. (2009). Treatment of liver disease. Proceedings: ACVC. Accessed via: Veterinary Information Network. http://goo.gl/7SUeb

Washabau, R. (2001). Feline constipation, obstipation and megacolon: Prevention, diagnosis and treatment. Proceedings: World Small Animal Assoc. World Congress. Accessed via: Veterinary Information Network. http://goo.gl/bpU1s

PYRANTEL PAMOATE

(pi-*ran*-tel *pam*-oh-ate)
Strongid T®, Nemex®

ANTIPARASITIC

Prescriber Highlights

▶ Pyrimidine anthelmintic used primarily for ascarids in a variety of species

▶ Contraindications: Severely debilitated animals

▶ Adverse Effects: Unlikely, emesis possible in small animals

Uses/Indications

Pyrantel has been used for the removal of the following parasites in dogs: ascarids (*Toxocara canis, T. leonina*), hookworms (*Ancylostoma caninum, Uncinaria stenocephala*), and stomach worm (Physaloptera). *A. caninum* resistance has been reported. Although not FDA-approved for use in cats, it is useful for similar parasites and is considered safe to use.

Pyrantel is indicated (labeled) for the removal of the following parasites in horses: *Strongylus vulgaris* and *equinus, Parasacaris equorum*, and *Probstymayria vivapara*. It has variable activity against *Oxyuris equi, S. edentatus*, and small strongyles. Pyrantel is active against ileocecal tapeworm (*A. perfoliata*) when used at twice the recommended dose, although resistance has been reported. Resistance to antiparasitic agents is an ongoing problem. It is recommended to perform fecal egg count reduction testing

(FECRT) for strongyle nematodes. A value of less than 90% in 5-10 horses is the suggested cut-off for determining resistance on a given farm (Nielsen & Kaplan 2009).

Although there are apparently no pyrantel products FDA-approved for use in cattle, sheep, or goats, the drug is effective (as the tartrate) for the removal of the following parasites: *Haemonchus* spp., *Ostertagia* spp., *Trichostrongylus* spp., *Nematodirus* spp., *Chabertia* spp., *Cooperia* spp. and *Oesophagostomum* spp.

Pyrantel tartrate is indicated (labeled) for the removal or prevention of the following parasites in swine: large roundworms (*Ascaris suum*) and *Oesophagostomum* spp. The drug has activity against the swine stomach worm (*Hyostrongylus rubidus*).

Although not FDA-approved, pyrantel has been used in pet birds and llamas. See the Dosage section for more information.

Pharmacology/Actions

Pyrantel acts as a depolarizing, neuromuscular-blocking agent in susceptible parasites, which paralyzes the organism. The drug possesses nicotine-like properties and acts similarly to acetylcholine. It also inhibits cholinesterase.

Pharmacokinetics

Pyrantel pamoate is poorly absorbed from the GI tract, thus allowing it to reach the lower GI in dogs, cats and equines. Pyrantel tartrate is absorbed more readily than the pamoate salt. Pigs and dogs absorb pyrantel tartrate more so than do ruminants, with peak plasma levels occurring 2–3 hours after administration. Peak plasma levels occur at highly variable times in ruminants.

Absorbed drug is rapidly metabolized and excreted into the urine and feces.

Contraindications/Precautions/Warnings

Use with caution in severely debilitated animals. The manufacturers usually recommend not administering the drug to severely debilitated animals.

Adverse Effects

When administered at recommended doses, adverse effects are unlikely. Emesis may possibly occur in small animals receiving pyrantel pamoate.

Reproductive/Nursing Safety

In humans, the FDA categorizes this drug as category *C* for use during pregnancy (*Animal studies have shown an adverse effect on the fetus, but there are no adequate studies in humans; or there are no animal reproduction studies and no adequate studies in humans.*) In a separate system evaluating the safety of drugs in canine and feline pregnancy (Papich 1989), this drug is categorized as class: *A* (*Probably safe. Although specific studies may not have proved he safety of all drugs in dogs and cats, there are no reports of adverse effects in laboratory animals or women.*)

Pyrantel is considered safe to use in nursing veterinary patients.

Overdosage/Acute Toxicity

Pyrantel has a moderate margin of safety. Dosages up to approximately 7 times recommended generally result in no toxic reactions. In horses, doses of 20X yielded no adverse effects. The LD$_{50}$ in mice and rats for pyrantel tartrate is 170 mg/kg; >690 mg/kg for pyrantel pamoate in dogs.

Chronic dosing of pyrantel pamoate in dogs resulted in clinical signs when given at 50 mg/kg/day, but not at 20 mg/kg/day over 3 months. Clinical signs of toxicity that may be seen include increased respiratory rates, profuse sweating (in species with sweat glands), ataxia or other cholinergic effects.

Drug Interactions

■ **DIETHYLCARBAMAZINE:** Increased risk for adverse effects

■ **LEVAMISOLE:** Because of similar mechanisms of action (and toxicity), do not use concurrently with pyrantel

■ **MORANTEL:** Because of similar mechanisms of action (and toxicity), do not use concurrently with pyrantel

■ **ORGANOPHOSPHATES:** Increased risk for adverse effects

■ **PIPERAZINE:** Pyrantel and piperazine have antagonistic mechanisms of action; do not use together

Doses

All doses are for pyrantel pamoate unless otherwise noted. **Caution:** Listed dosages are often not specified as to whether using the salt or base.

For additional information using this drug in dogs in cats, see: Companion Animal Parasite Council recommendations: http://goo.gl/wJBq1

■ **DOGS:**

For susceptible parasites:

a) For dogs weighing <5 lb: 10 mg/kg (as base) PO; for dogs weighing >5 lbs: 5 mg/kg (as base) PO. Treat puppies at 2, 3, 4, 6, 8, and 10 weeks of age. Treat lactating bitches 2–3 weeks after whelping. Do follow-up fecal 2–4 weeks after treating to determine need for retreatment. (Label directions; *Nemex® Tabs*—Pfizer)

b) For hookworms, or roundworms: 5 mg/kg PO after meals; repeat in 7–10 days (Willard 2003)

c) Puppies: Can be treated as early as 2–3 weeks of age at 5–10 mg/kg PO; can be repeated every 2–3 weeks until at least 12 weeks of age. (Hoskins 2005)

d) 20 mg/kg PO; be sure that liquid is well mixed before using; tablets may be broken for accurate dosing. Not FDA-approved for cats but very safe and effective. (Blagburn 2005)

■ **CATS:**

For susceptible parasites:

a) For susceptible parasites using combination product with praziquantel (*Drontal®*): Administer a minimum dose of 2.27 mg praziquantel and 9.2 mg pyrantel pamoate per pound of body weight according to the dosing tables on labeling. May be given directly by mouth or in a small amount of food. Do not withhold food prior to or after treatment. If reinfection occurs, treatment may be repeated. (Package insert; *Drontal®*—Bayer)

b) Ascarids, Hookworms, Physaloptera: 5 mg/kg, PO; repeat in 2 weeks (one time only for Physaloptera) (Dimski 1989)

c) 10 mg/kg PO, repeat in 3 weeks (Kirk 1989)

d) Kittens: Can be treated as early as 2–3 weeks of age at 5–10 mg/kg PO; can be repeated every 2–3 weeks until at least 12 weeks of age. (Hoskins 2005)

■ **RABBITS, RODENTS, SMALL MAMMALS:**

a) Rabbits: 15–10 mg/kg PO, repeat in 2–3 weeks (Ivey & Morrisey 2000)

■ **HORSES:**

For susceptible parasites:

a) 6.6 mg/kg PO every 6-8 weeks for ascarid control in foals and every 4 weeks for ascarid control on some farms. For tapeworm control, double the dose (13.2 mg/kg PO) and use once to twice yearly. (Taylor 2010)

b) 6.6 mg (as base)/kg PO; 13.2 mg (as base)/kg for cestodes (Roberson 1988; Robinson 1987)

■ **SWINE:**

For susceptible parasites:

a) To remove *Ascaris suum* or *Oesophagostomum* spp.: Pyrantel tartrate: 22 mg/kg PO (or in feed at a rate of 800 grams/ton) as a single treatment. For *Ascaris suum* only: in feed at a rate of 96 grams/ton (2.6 mg/kg) for 3 days. (Paul 1986) (Label instructions from several pyrantel tartrate premix products)

b) For ascarids and nodular worms in pot-bellied pigs: 6.6 mg/kg PO (Braun 1995)

■ **CATTLE, SHEEP & GOATS:**

For susceptible parasites:

a) Pyrantel tartrate: 25 mg/kg, PO (Roberson 1988)

■ **LLAMAS:**

a) 18 mg/kg, PO for one day (Cheney & Allen 1989; Fowler 1989)

■ **BIRDS:**

For intestinal nematodes:

a) Psittacines: In endemic areas, outdoor breeding birds and their offspring should be routinely dewormed for ascarids: 25 mg/kg PO q2 weeks. (Lightfoot 2008)

b) 100 mg/kg, PO as a single dose in psittacines and passerines (Marshall 1993)

Client Information

■ Shake suspensions well before administering.

Chemistry/Synonyms

A pyrimidine-derivative anthelmintic, pyrantel pamoate occurs as yellow to tan solid and is practically insoluble in water and alcohol. Each gram of pyrantel pamoate is approximately equivalent to 347 mg (34.7%) of the base.

Pyrantel may also be known as: CP-10423-16, pyrantel embonate, pirantel pamoate, *Anthel®, Antiminth®, Ascarical®, Aut®, Bantel®, Cobantril®, Combantrin®, Combantrin®, Early Bird®, Helmex®, Helmintox®, Jaa Pyral®, Lombriareu®, Nemex®, Nemocid®, Pin-X®, Pirantrim®, Pyrantin®, Pyrantrin®, Pyrapam®, Reese's® Pinworm, Strongid®, Trilombrin®,* or *Vertel®.*

Storage/Stability

Pyrantel pamoate products should be stored in tight, light-resistant containers at room temperature (15–30°C) unless otherwise directed by the manufacturer.

Dosage Forms/Regulatory Status

VETERINARY-LABELED PRODUCTS:

Note: Many products available; a partial listing of products follows:

Pyrantel Pamoate Tablets: 22.7 mg (of base), 113.5 mg (of base); (OTC). FDA-approved for use in dogs. A commonly known product is *Nemex® Tabs* (Pfizer).

Pyrantel Pamoate Oral Suspension: 4.54 mg/mL (as base) (for dogs only); in 60 mL, 120 mL 280 mL and 473 mL bottles. Many products are available; a commonly known trade name is *Nemex-2®* (Pfizer).

Pyrantel Pamoate Oral Suspension: 50 mg/mL (of base); Many products are available; a commonly known trade name is *Strongid® T* (Pfizer); (OTC). FDA-approved for use in horses not intended for food.

Pyrantel Pamoate Oral Paste: 43.9% w/w pyrantel base in 23.6 grams (20 mL) paste (180 mg pyrantel base/mL); several products are available. A commonly known trade name is *Strongid® Paste* (Pfizer); (OTC). FDA-approved for use in horses not intended for food.

Pyrantel Tartrate 1.06% (4.8 grams/lb) Top Dress: in 25 lb pails: *Strongid C®* (Pfizer); (OTC). Labeled for use in horses (not intended for food).

Combination Products:

Tablets: Praziquantel 13.6 mg/pyrantel pamoate 54.3 mg (as base) for 2–5.9 lb cats and kittens; Praziquantel 18.2 mg/pyrantel pamoate 72.6 mg (as base); Praziquantel

27.2 mg/pyrantel pamoate 108.6 mg (as base) for 6-24 lb. cats; *Drontal® Tablets* (Bayer); (OTC). *Drontal® Tablets* (Bayer); some sizes may be available as generics or under various trade names (OTC). FDA-approved for use in cats and kittens that are 2 months of age or older and weigh 2 lb. or more.

Praziquantel 30 mg/pyrantel pamoate 30 mg; & Praziquantel 114 mg/pyrantel pamoate 114 mg Chewable Tablets: *Virbantel Flavored Chewables®* (Virbac), generic; (OTC). FDA-approved for use in dogs.

Praziquantel/pyrantel pamoate plus febantel Tablets: Small, medium and large dog sizes. *Drontal® Plus Tablets* (Bayer); (Rx); FDA-approved for dogs and puppies 3 weeks of age or older and weighing 2 lb. or greater.

Ivermectin/Pyrantel Oral Chewable Tablets: 68 micrograms/57 mg, 136 micrograms/114mg, 272 micrograms/228 mg; *Heartgard® Plus Chewables* (Merial); *Tri-Heart® Plus Chewable Tablets* (Schering); (Rx). FDA-approved for use in dogs.

HUMAN-LABELED PRODUCTS:

Pyrantel Pamoate Oral Suspension: 50 mg/mL & 144 mg/mL (equiv to 50 mg/mL pyrantel base) in 30 mL; *Reese's® Pinworm* (Reese); *Pin-X®* (Penn); (OTC)

Pyrantel Soft-gel Oral Capsules: 180 mg (equivalent to 62.5 mg pyrantel base); *Pin-Rid®* (Apothecary); *Reese's® Pinworm* (Reese); (OTC)

Pyrantel Pamoate Oral Tablets: 180 mg & 720.5 mg (chewable); *Reese's Pinworm®* (Reese); *Pin-X®* (Penn); (OTC)

References

Blagburn, B. (2005). Update on treatment and control of parasites and parasitic diseases of companion animals. Proceedings: ACVC2005. Accessed via: Veterinary Information Network. http://goo.gl/CdZGi

Braun, W. (1995). Potbellied pigs: General medical care. *Kirk's Current Veterinary Therapy:XII.* J Bonagura Ed. Philadelphia, W.B. Saunders: 1388–1389.

Cheney, J.M. & G.T. Allen (1989). Parasitism in Llamas. *Vet Clin North America: Food Animal Practice* 5(1): 217–232.

Dimski, D.S. (1989). Helminth and noncoccidial protozoan parasites of the gastrointestinal tract. *The Cat: Diseases and Clinical Management.* RG Sherding Ed. New York, Churchill Livingstone. 1: 459–477.

Fowler, M.E. (1989). *Medicine and Surgery of South American Camelids.* Ames, Iowa State University Press.

Hoskins, J. (2005). Veterinary pediatrics of the puppy and kitten. Proceedings: ACVC 2006. Accessed via: Veterinary Information Network. http://goo.gl/otqkb

Ivey, E. & J. Morrisey (2000). Therapeutics for Rabbits. *Vet Clin NA: Exotic Anim Pract* 3:1(Jan): 183–216.

Kirk, R.W., Ed. (1989). *Current Veterinary Therapy X, Small Animal Practice.* Philadelphia, W.B. Saunders.

Lightfoot, T. (2008). Pediatric Psittacine Diseases. Proceedings: WVC. Accessed via: Veterinary Information Network. http://goo.gl/L46Is

Marshall, R. (1993). Avian anthelmintics and antiprotozoals. *Seminars in Avian & Exotic Med* 2(1): 33–41.

Nielsen, M. & R.M. Kaplan (2009). Diagnosis & Management of Anthelmintic Resistance in Equid

Parasites. Proceedings: ACVIM. Accessed via: Veterinary Information Network. http://goo.gl/oIqSj

Papich, M. (1989). Effects of drugs on pregnancy. *Current Veterinary Therapy X: Small Animal Practice.* R Kirk Ed. Philadelphia, Saunders: 1291–1299.

Paul, J.W. (1986). Anthelmintic Therapy. *Current Veterinary Therapy: Food Animal Practice 2.* JL Howard Ed. Philadelphia, W.B. Saunders: 39–44.

Roberson, E.L. (1988). Antinematodal Agents. *Veterinary Pharmacology and Therapeutics.* NH Booth and LE McDonald Eds. Ames, Iowa State University Press: 882–927.

Robinson, N.E. (1987). Table of Common Drugs: Approximate Doses. *Current Therapy in Equine Medicine, 2.* NE Robinson Ed. Philadelphia, W.B. Saunders: 761.

Taylor, D. (2010). Equine Parasite Control in the New Century. Proceedings: WVC. Accessed via: Veterinary Information Network. http://goo.gl/CsjXG

Willard, M. (2003). Digestive system disorders. *Small Animal Internal Medicine, 3rd Ed.* R Nelson and C Couto Eds. St Louis, Mosby: 343–471.

PYRIDOSTIGMINE BROMIDE

(peer-i-oh-*stig*-meen)   Mestinon®

ANTICHOLINESTERASE AGENT

Prescriber Highlights

▶ Anticholinesterase used for treatment of myasthenia gravis

▶ Contraindications: hypersensitivity to this class of compounds or bromides, patients with mechanical or physical obstructions of the urinary or GI tract

▶ Caution: bronchospastic disease, epilepsy, hyperthyroidism, bradycardia or other arrhythmias, vagotonia, or GI ulcer diseases

▶ Adverse Effects: Usually dose related cholinergic effects GI (nausea, vomiting, diarrhea), salivation, sweating, respiratory (increased bronchial secretions, bronchospasm, pulmonary edema, respiratory paralysis), ophthalmic (miosis, blurred vision, lacrimation), cardiovascular (bradycardia or tachycardia, cardiospasm, hypotension, cardiac arrest), muscle cramps, & weakness

Uses/Indications

Pyridostigmine is used in the treatment of myasthenia gravis (MG) in dogs (and rarely in cats). It is considered to be much more effective in acquired MG, than in congenital MG.

Pharmacology/Actions

Pyridostigmine inhibits the hydrolysis of acetylcholine by directly competing with acetylcholine for attachment to acetylcholinesterase. Because the pyridostigmine-acetylcholinesterase complex is hydrolyzed at a much slower rate than the acetylcholine-acetylcholinesterase complex, acetylcholine tends to accumulate at cholinergic synapses with resultant cholinergic activity.

At usual doses, pyridostigmine does not cross into the CNS (quaternary ammonium structure), but overdoses can cause CNS effects.

Pharmacokinetics

Pyridostigmine is only marginally absorbed from the GI tract and absorption may be more erratic with the sustained-release tablets than the regular tablets. The onset of action after oral dosing is generally within one hour.

At usual doses, pyridostigmine is apparently distributed to most tissues, but not to the brain, intestinal wall, fat or thymus. The drug crosses the placenta.

Pyridostigmine is metabolized by both the liver and hydrolyzed by cholinesterases.

Contraindications/Precautions/Warnings

Pyridostigmine is contraindicated in patients hypersensitive to this class of compounds or bromides, or in those who have mechanical or physical obstructions of the urinary or GI tract.

The drug should be used with caution in patients with bronchospastic disease, epilepsy, hyperthyroidism, bradycardia or other arrhythmias, vagotonia, or GI ulcer diseases.

Adverse Effects

Adverse effects associated with pyridostigmine are generally dose related and cholinergic in nature. Although usually mild and easily treatable with dosage reduction, severe adverse effects are possible (see Overdosage below).

Reproductive/Nursing Safety

In humans, the FDA categorizes this drug as category *C* for use during pregnancy (*Animal studies have shown an adverse effect on the fetus, but there are no adequate studies in humans; or there are no animal reproduction studies and no adequate studies in humans.*)

Pyridostigmine is excreted in maternal milk; use with caution in nursing patients.

Overdosage/Acute Toxicity

Overdosage of pyridostigmine may induce a cholinergic crisis. Clinical signs of cholinergic toxicity can include: GI effects (nausea, vomiting, diarrhea), salivation, sweating (species with sweat glands), respiratory effects (increased bronchial secretions, bronchospasm, pulmonary edema, respiratory paralysis), ophthalmic effects (miosis, blurred vision, lacrimation), cardiovascular effects (bradycardia or tachycardia, cardiospasm, hypotension, cardiac arrest), muscle cramps, and weakness.

Overdoses in myasthenic patients can be very difficult to distinguish from the effects associated with a myasthenic crisis. The time of onset of clinical signs or an edrophonium challenge may help to distinguish between the two.

Treatment of pyridostigmine overdosage consists of both respiratory and cardiac supportive therapy and atropine if necessary. Refer to the atropine monograph for more information on its use for cholinergic toxicity.

Drug Interactions

The following drug interactions have either been reported or are theoretical in humans or animals receiving pyridostigmine and may be of significance in veterinary patients:

■ **ATROPINE:** Atropine will antagonize the muscarinic effects of pyridostigmine but concurrent use should be used cautiously as atropine can mask the early clinical signs of cholinergic crisis

■ **CORTICOSTEROIDS:** May decrease the anticholinesterase activity of pyridostigmine. After stopping corticosteroid therapy, drugs like pyridostigmine may cause increased anticholinesterase activity

■ **DEXPANTHENOL:** Theoretically, dexpanthenol may have additive effects when used with pyridostigmine

■ **DRUGS WITH NEUROMUSCULAR BLOCKING ABILITY (e.g., aminoglycoside antibiotics):** May necessitate increased dosages of pyridostigmine in treating or diagnosing myasthenic patients

■ **MAGNESIUM:** Anticholinesterase therapy may be antagonized by administration of parenteral magnesium therapy, as it can have a direct depressant effect on skeletal muscle

■ **MUSCLE RELAXANTS:** Pyridostigmine may prolong the Phase I block of depolarizing muscle relaxants (e.g., **succinylcholine, decamethonium**) and edrophonium antagonizes the actions of non-depolarizing neuromuscular blocking agents (e.g., **pancuronium, tubocurarine, gallamine, vecuronium, atracurium,** etc.)

Doses

■ **DOGS:**

For myasthenia gravis (MG):

a) 1–3 mg/kg PO q8-12h. The dosage is titrated to effect to minimize adverse effects and maximize muscle strength. For animals that cannot tolerate oral medications, it may be used as an IV constant rate infusion at 0.01–0.03 mg/kg/hour. (Vernau 2009)

b) 0.5–3 mg/kg PO q8-12 hours with food. With high doses, weakness may occur as a result of a cholinergic crisis and therefore a low dose of pyridostigmine is initially given then slowly increased until weakness is resolved. A liquid formulation of pyridostigmine is recommended so dose can be easily adjusted to control clinical signs. An H2 antagonist (e.g., famotidine at 5 mg/kg/day) may reduce nausea and GI irritation associated with pyridostigmine. (Platt 2009)

c) For acquired MG: After oral regurgitation is abolished with parenteral therapy (neostigmine), may begin oral therapy with pyridostigmine at 7.5–30 mg PO two times a day. Once patient is stable and infections have resolved, begin corticosteroid therapy (antiinflammatory doses of prednisone) and continue concurrently with anticholinesterase drugs for 2 weeks, then pyridostigmine may be gradually reduced. (Pedroia 1989)

d) 0.5–3 mg/kg PO two to three times a day. If no response, add prednisone (0.5–1 mg/kg day; increase to 1–2 mg/kg after a few days). (Kornegay 2006)

e) 0.5–1 mg/kg PO two to three times a day with or without prednisone (2 mg/kg PO twice daily). Not uncommon for dogs to fully recover without treatment (spontaneous remission). (LeCouteur 2005)

■ **CATS:**

For myasthenia gravis (MG):

a) 0.5–3 mg/kg daily PO in divided doses, dose depending on response. (Jones 2009)

b) 1–3 mg/kg PO q8–12h. (Inzana 2000)

c) 0.5–3 mg/kg PO per day with corticosteroids (Wheeler 2006)

Monitoring

■ Animals should be routinely monitored for clinical signs of cholinergic toxicity (see Overdosage section above) and efficacy of the therapy

Client Information

■ Clients should be instructed to report to the veterinarian clinical signs of excessive salivation, GI disturbances, weakness, or difficulty breathing

Chemistry/Synonyms

An anticholinesterase agent, pyridostigmine bromide is a synthetic quaternary ammonium compound that occurs as an agreeable smelling, bitter tasting, hydroscopic, white or practically white, crystalline powder. It is freely soluble in water and in alcohol. The pH of the commercially available injection is approximately 5.

Pyridostigmine Bromide may also be known as: pyridostigmini bromidum, *Distinon®*, *Kalymin®, Mestinon®,* or *Regonol®*.

Storage/Stability

Unless otherwise instructed by the manufacturer, store pyridostigmine products at room temperature. The oral solution and injection should be protected from light and freezing. Pyridostigmine tablets should be kept in tight containers.

The extended-release tablets may become mottled with time, but this does not affect their potency.

Pyridostigmine injection is unstable in alkaline solutions.

Compatibility/Compounding Considerations

Pyridostigmine injection is reportedly physically **compatible** with glycopyrrolate, heparin sodium, hydrocortisone sodium succinate, potassium chloride, and vitamin B-complex with C. Compatibility is dependent upon factors such as pH, concentration, temperature and diluent used; consult specialized references or a hospital pharmacist for more specific information.

Dosage Forms/Regulatory Status

VETERINARY-LABELED PRODUCTS: None

The ARCI (Racing Commissioners International) has designated this drug as a class 3 substance. See the appendix for more information.

HUMAN-LABELED PRODUCTS:

Pyridostigmine Bromide Tablets: 60 mg; *Mestinon®* (ICN); generic, (Rx)

Pyridostigmine Bromide Extended-Release Tablets: 180 mg; *Mestinon®* (ICN); (Rx)

Pyridostigmine Bromide Syrup: 12 mg/mL in 480 mL; *Mestinon®* (ICN); (Rx)

Pyridostigmine Bromide Injection: 5 mg/mL in 2 mL amps; *Mestinon®* (ICN); (Rx)

References

Inzana, K. (2000). Peripheral Nerve Disorders. *Textbook of Veterinary Internal Medicine: Diseases of the Dog and Cat.* S Ettinger and E Feldman Eds. Philadelphia, WB Saunders. **1:** 662–684.

Jones, B. (2009). Feline Neuromuscular Disease. Proceedings: ECVIM-CA Congress. Accessed via: Veterinary Information Network. http://goo.gl/fIe7J

Kornegay, J. (2006). Neuromuscular disease I & II. Proceedings: Western Vet Conf. Accessed via: Veterinary Information Network. http://goo.gl/mH597

LeCouteur, R. (2005). Neuropathies, junctionopathies & myopathies of dogs and cats: 1–5. Proceedings: Veterinary Neurology Seminar. Accessed via: Veterinary Information Network. http://goo.gl/jUyAu

Pedroia, V. (1989). Disorders of the Skeletal Muscles. *Textbook of Veterinary Internal Medicine.* SJ Ettinger Ed. Philadelphia, WB Saunders. **1:** 733–744.

Platt, S. (2009). Neuromuscular Causes of Weakness and Collapse. Proceedings: WSAVA. Accessed via: Veterinary Information Network. http://goo.gl/9iuiF

Vernau, K. (2009). Beyond Tensilon and Titers: Myasthenia Gravis. Veterinary Neurology Symposium; Univ. of Calif.-Davis. Accessed via: Veterinary Information Network. http://goo.gl/UHXuc

Wheeler, S. (2006). The paralyzed cat. Proceedings: WSAVA World Congress. Accessed via: Veterinary Information Network. http://goo.gl/St3pJ

PYRIDOXINE HCL (VITAMIN B-6)

(peer-ih-*dox*-een)

NUTRITIONAL B VITAMIN, ANTIDOTE

Prescriber Highlights

▶ Pyridoxine may be beneficial in the treatment of isoniazid or crimidine toxicity, or delaying cutaneous toxicity of *Doxil®* (liposomal doxorubicin)

▶ Overdoses may cause peripheral neuropathy

Uses/Indications

Pyridoxine use in veterinary medicine is relatively infrequent. It may be of benefit in the treatment of isoniazid (INH) or crimidine (an older rodenticide) toxicity. Pyridoxine deficiency is apparently extremely rare in dogs or cats able to ingest food. Cats with severe intestinal disease may have a greater requirement for pyridoxine in their diet. Experimentally, pyridoxine has been successfully used in dogs to reduce the cutaneous toxicity associated with doxorubicin containing pegylated liposomes (*Doxil®*). Pyridoxine has been demonstrated to suppress the growth of feline mammary tumors (cell line FRM) *in vitro*.

In humans, labeled uses for pyridoxine include pyridoxine deficiency and intractable neonatal seizures secondary to pyridoxine dependency syndrome. Unlabeled uses include premenstrual syndrome (PMS), carpal tunnel syndrome, tardive dyskinesia secondary to antipsychotic drugs, nausea and vomiting in pregnancy, hyperoxaluria type 1 and oxalate kidney stones, and for the treatment of isoniazid (INH), cycloserine, hydrazine or Gyometra mushroom poisonings.

Pharmacology/Actions

In erythrocytes, pyridoxine is converted to pyridoxal phosphate and, to a lesser extent, pyridoxamine, which serve as coenzymes for metabolic functions affecting protein, lipid and carbohydrate utilization. Pyridoxine is necessary for tryptophan conversion to serotonin or niacin, glycogen breakdown, heme synthesis, synthesis of GABA in the CNS, and oxalate conversion to glycine. Pyridoxine can act as an antidote by enhancing the excretion of cycloserine or isoniazid.

Pyridoxine requirements increase as protein ingestion increases.

Pharmacokinetics

Pyridoxine is absorbed from the GI tract primarily in the jejunum. Malabsorption syndromes can significantly impair pyridoxine absorption. Pyridoxine is not bound to plasma proteins, but pyridoxal phosphate is completely bound to plasma proteins. Pyridoxine is stored primarily in the liver with smaller amounts stored in the brain and muscle. It is biotransformed in the liver and various tissues, and excreted almost entirely as metabolites into the urine. Elimination half-life in humans is approximately 15–20 days.

Contraindications/Precautions/Warnings

Weigh potential risks versus benefits in patients with documented sensitivity to pyridoxine.

Adverse Effects

Pyridoxine is generally well tolerated unless doses are large (see Overdosage). In humans, paresthesias and somnolence have been reported. Reduced serum folic acid levels have occurred.

Reproductive/Nursing Safety

While pyridoxine is a nutritional agent and very safe at recommended doses during pregnancy, very large doses during pregnancy can cause a pyridoxine dependency syndrome in neonates.

Pyridoxine administration at low dosages should be safe during nursing. Pyridoxine requirements of the dam may be increased during nursing.

Overdosage/Acute Toxicity

Single overdoses are not considered overly problematic, unless they are massive. Laboratory animals given 3–4 grams/kg developed seizures and died. Dogs (Beagles) repeatedly given 3 gram oral daily doses developed uncoordinated gait and neurologic signs. Neuronal lesions were noted in sensory, dorsal root ganglia, and trigeminal ganglia. Signs generally resolved over a 2-month drug free period.

Drug Interactions

The following drug interactions have either been reported or are theoretical in humans or animals receiving pyridoxine and may be of significance in veterinary patients:

- **CHLORAMPHENICOL:** May cause increased pyridoxine requirements
- **ESTROGENS:** May cause increased pyridoxine requirements
- **HYDRALAZINE:** May cause increased pyridoxine requirements
- **IMMUNOSUPPRESSANTS (e.g., azathioprine, chlorambucil, cyclophosphamide, corticosteroids):** May cause increased pyridoxine requirements
- **ISONIAZID:** May cause increased pyridoxine requirements
- **PENICILLAMINE:** May cause increased pyridoxine requirements
- **LEVODOPA:** Pyridoxine may reduce levodopa efficacy (no interaction when levodopa is used with carbidopa)
- **PHENOBARBITAL:** High dose pyridoxine may decrease phenobarbital serum levels
- **PHENYTOIN:** High dose pyridoxine may decrease phenytoin serum concentration

Laboratory Considerations

The following laboratory alterations have been reported in humans with pyridoxine and may be of significance in veterinary patients:

- **Urobilinogen in the spot test using Ehrlich's reagent:** Pyridoxine may cause false-positive results
- **AST:** Excessive dosages of pyridoxine may elevate AST

Doses

- **DOGS/CATS:**
  a) Dogs: For isoniazid (INH) toxicity: If quantity of INH ingested is known, give pyridoxine on a mg for mg (1:1) basis. If it is not known, give pyridoxine initially at 71 mg/kg as a 5–10% IV infusion over 30–60 minutes (some sources say it can be given as an IV bolus). Pyridoxine injection can usually be obtained from human hospital pharmacies. Do not use injectable B-complex vitamins. (Gwaltney-Brant 2003)
  b) To replace pyridoxine antagonized by crimidine ingestion: 20 mg/kg IV (Dalefield & Oehme 2006)
  c) Dogs: To delay the development of cutaneous toxicity (PPES; palmer-plantar-dyerythrodysesthesia) associated with doxorubicin containing pegylated liposomes (*Doxil®*): 50 mg PO three times daily during chemotherapy protocol period. (Vail et al. 1998)

Monitoring

- Other than evaluating efficacy for its intended use, no significant monitoring is required

Client Information

- Do not give more than prescribed by the veterinarian
- Contact veterinarian if animal develops any abnormal signs such as difficulty walking, using stairs, etc.

Chemistry/Synonyms

Pyridoxine (vitamin B6) is a water-soluble vitamin present in many foods (liver, meat, eggs, cereals, legumes, and vegetables). The commercially available form (pyridoxine HCl) found in medications is obtained synthetically. Pyridoxine HCl occurs as white or practically white, crystals or crystalline powder with a slightly bitter, salty taste. It is freely soluble in water and slightly soluble in alcohol.

Pyridoxine or Vitamin B6 may also be known by the following synonyms or analogs: adermine, pyridoxal, pyridoxal-5-phosphate, pyridoxamine, pirodoxamina, piridossima, piridoxolum, piridossina, *Aminoxin®*, and *Vitelle Nestrex®*.

Storage/Stability

Unless otherwise specified by the manufacturer, pyridoxine tablets should be stored below 40°C (104°F), preferably between 15–30°C (59–86°F), in well-closed containers protected from light.

Pyridoxine HCl injection should be stored below 40°C (104°F), preferably between 15–30°C (59–86°F), protected from light and freezing.

Pyridoxine HCl injection can be administered undiluted or added to commonly used IV solutions. It is reportedly **compatible** with doxapram when mixed in a syringe and with fat emulsion 10%. It is reportedly **incompatible** with alkaline or oxidizing solutions, and iron salts.

Dosage Forms/Regulatory Status

VETERINARY-LABELED PRODUCTS:

No single ingredient pyridoxine products were located. There are a multitude of various veterinary-labeled products that contain pyridoxine as one of several ingredients.

HUMAN-LABELED PRODUCTS:

Pyridoxine Tablets 50 mg, 100 mg, 250 mg, & 500 mg; Vitamin B6; generic (various); (OTC)

Pyridoxine (as pyridoxal-5'-phosphate) Tablets (enteric-coated): 20 mg; *Aminoxin®* (Tyson); (OTC)

Pyridoxine HCl Injection: 100 mg/mL in 1 mL vials; generic; (Rx)

Pyridoxine is also an ingredient in many combination products (*e.g.*, B-Complex, multivitamins).

References

Dalefield, R. & F. Oehme (2006). Antidotes for specific poisons. *Small Animal Toxicology*. M Peterson and P Talcott Eds., Elsevier: 459–474.

Gwaltney-Brant, S. (2003). Terrible Toxicants. Proceedings: IVECC2003. Accessed via: Veterinary Information Network. http://goo.gl/6AZCf

Vail, D., R. Chun, et al. (1998). Efficacy of pyridoxine to ameliorate the cutaneous toxicity associated with doxorubicin containing pegylated (stealth) liposomes: A randomized, double-blind clinical trial using a canine model. *Clinical Cancer Res* 4(June): 1567–1571.

PYRILAMINE MALEATE

(pye-*ril*-a-meen)   Histall®, Equiphed®

ANTIHISTAMINE

Prescriber Highlights

▶ Injectable antihistamine

▶ Contraindications: None noted

▶ Adverse Effects: Horses: CNS stimulation (nervousness, insomnia, convulsions, tremors, ataxia), palpitation, GI disturbances, CNS depression (sedation), muscular weakness, anorexia, lassitude & incoordination

▶ Drug Interactions

Uses/Indications

Antihistamines are used in veterinary medicine to reduce or help prevent histamine mediated adverse effects; predominantly used in horses.

Pharmacology/Actions

Antihistamines (H_1-receptor antagonists) competitively inhibit histamine at H_1 receptor sites. They do not inactivate, nor prevent the release of histamine, but can prevent histamine's action on the cell. Besides their antihistaminic activity, these agents also have varying degrees of anticholinergic and CNS activity (sedation). Pyrilamine is considered to be less sedating and have fewer anticholinergic effects when compared to most other antihistamines.

Pharmacokinetics

The pharmacokinetics of this agent have apparently not been extensively studied in cattle, dogs or cats. In horses, pyrilamine is poorly bio-

available (18%) after oral administration. After IV administration, elimination half-life was about 1.7 hours. After a single dose, pyrilamines principle metabolite, *O*-desmethylpyrilamine (O-DMP), can be detected in urine for at least two days, and possibly up to one week after dosing. (Dirikolu *et al.* 2009)

Contraindications/Precautions/Warnings

The manufacturer indicates that the use of this product ". . . should not supersede the use of other emergency drugs and procedures."

Adverse Effects

Adverse effects in horses can include CNS stimulation (nervousness, insomnia, convulsions, tremors, ataxia), palpitation, GI disturbances, CNS depression (sedation), muscular weakness, anorexia, lassitude and incoordination.

Reproductive/Nursing Safety

At usual doses, pyrilamine is probably safe to use during pregnancy. Rats and mice treated with 10–20 times the human dose had an increased frequency of embryonic, fetal or perinatal death, but a study in pregnant women, showed no increase in teratogenic or fetocidal rates.

It is unknown if pyrilamine enters milk.

Overdosage/Acute Toxicity

Treatment of overdosage is supportive and symptomatic. One manufacturer (*Histavet-P®*—Schering) suggests using "careful titration" of barbiturates to treat convulsions, and analeptics (caffeine, ephedrine, or amphetamines) to treat CNS depression. Most toxicologists however, recommend avoiding the use of CNS stimulants in the treatment of CNS depressant overdoses. Phenytoin (IV) is recommended in the treatment of seizures caused by antihistamine overdose in humans; barbiturates and diazepam are to be avoided.

Drug Interactions

The following drug interactions have either been reported or are theoretical in humans or animals receiving pyrilamine and may be of significance in veterinary patients:

■ **ANTICOAGULANTS (heparin, warfarin):** Antihistamines may partially counteract the anticoagulation effects of heparin or warfarin

■ **CNS DEPRESSANT DRUGS:** Increased sedation can occur if pyrilamine is combined with other CNS depressant drugs

■ **EPINEPHRINE:** Pyrilamine may enhance the effects of epinephrine

Laboratory Considerations

■ Antihistamines can decrease the wheal and flare response to antigen **skin testing**. In humans, it is suggested that antihistamines be discontinued at least 4 days before testing.

Doses

■ **DOGS:**
a) 12.5–25 mg PO four times a day; 25–125 mg IM (Swinyard 1975)

■ **CATTLE:**

a) 0.5–1.5 grams IM (Swinyard 1975)

b) For adjunctive treatment of aseptic laminitis: 55–110 mg/100 kg IV or IM (Berg 1986)

■ **HORSES: (NOTE: ARCI UCGFS CLASS 3 DRUG)**

a) 0.88–1.32 mg/kg (2–3 mL of 20 mg/mL solution per 100 lbs body weight) IV (slowly), IM or SC; may repeat in 6–12 hours if necessary. Foals: 0.44 mg/kg (1 mL of 20 mg/mL solution per 100 lbs. body weight) IV (slowly), IM or SC; may repeat in 6–12 hours if necessary. (Package Insert; *Histavet-P*®—Schering)

b) 1 mg/kg IV, IM or SC (Robinson 1987)

c) 0.5–1.5 grams IM) (Swinyard 1975)

■ **SHEEP, SWINE:**

a) 0.25–0.5 gram IM (Swinyard 1975)

Monitoring

■ Clinical efficacy

■ Adverse effects

Chemistry/Synonyms

An ethylenediamine antihistamine, pyrilamine maleate occurs as a white, crystalline powder with a melting range of 99–103°. One gram is soluble in approximately 0.5 mL of water or 3 mL alcohol.

Pyrilamine Maleate may also be known as: pyranisamine hydrochloride, pyrilamine hydrochloride, mepyramine hydrochloride, mepyramini maleas, myranisamine maleate, myrilamine maleate, mepyramine maleate, *Anihist*®, *Alergitanil*®, *Antemesyl*®, *Anthisan*®, *Anthisan*®, *Equi-Phar*® *Equi-Hist*®, *Equiphed*®, *Fluidasa*®, *Histall*®, *Histagranules*®, *Histamed*®, *Mepyraderm*®, *Mepyrimal*®, *Pyramine*®, *Pyriped*®, *Relaxa-Tabs*®, and *Tri-Hist*®.

Storage/Stability

Avoid freezing the injectable product.

Dosage Forms/Regulatory Status

VETERINARY-LABELED PRODUCTS:

Pyrilamine Granules: 600 mg/oz in 20 oz containers; *Histall*® (AHC); (OTC). Labeled for use in horses. Do not use at least 72 hours before sporting events.

The following products contain pseudoephedrine. In the USA, pseudoephedrine is classified as a list 1 chemical (drugs that can be used as precursors to manufacture methamphetamine) and in some states it may be a controlled substance or have other restrictions placed upon its sale. Be alert to persons desiring to purchase this medication.

Pseudoephedrine HCl 600 mg/oz and Pyrilamine maleate 600 mg/oz Granules: in 20 oz, 5 lb and 10 lb containers; *Equiphed*® (AHC), *Equi-Phar Equi-Hist 1200 Granules*® (Vedco), *Tri-Hist Granules*® (Neogen), *Histagranules*® (Butler); (Rx). Labeled for use in horses. Do not use at least 72 hours before sporting events.

Pyrilamine 600 mg/oz and Guaifenesin 2400 mg/oz Granules: in 20 oz, 5 lb and 25 lb containers; *Anihist*® (AHC), *Hist-EQ*® (Butler); (OTC). Labeled for use in horses. Do not use at least 72 hours before sporting events.

There are also combination cough syrups containing pyrilamine labeled for use in small animals.

The ARCI (Racing Commissioners International) has designated this drug as a class 3 substance. See the appendix for more information.

HUMAN-LABELED PRODUCTS: None

References

Berg, J.N. (1986). Aseptic laminitis in cattle. *Current Veterinary Therapy: Food Animal Practice 2.* JL Howard Ed. Philadelphia, W.B. Saunders: 896–898.

Dirikolu, L., A.F. Lehner, et al. (2009). Pyrilamine in the horse: detection and pharmacokinetics of pyrilamine and its major urinary metabolite O-desmethylpyrilamine. *Journal of Veterinary Pharmacology and Therapeutics* 32(1): 66–78.

Robinson, N.E. (1987). Table of Common Drugs: Approximate Doses. *Current Therapy in Equine Medicine, 2.* NE Robinson Ed. Philadelphia, W.B. Saunders: 761.

Swinyard, E.A. (1975). Histamine and Antihistamines. *Remington's Pharmaceutical Sciences.* A Osol Ed. Easton, Mack Publishing Co.: 1055–1066.

PYRIMETHAMINE

(pye-ri-*meth*-a-meen)   Daraprim®

ANTIPROTOZOAL

Note: *Also see the Pyrimethamine/Sulfadiazine, and Sulfadiazine/Trimethoprim monographs*

Prescriber Highlights

▶ Folic acid inhibitor used primarily (in combination) for toxoplasmosis, *H. americanum*, neosporosis, & equine protozoal myeloencephalitis

▶ Caution: Hematologic disorders; cats

▶ Adverse Effects: *Small animals:* Anorexia, malaise, vomiting, depression, & bone marrow depression (anemia, thrombocytopenia, leukopenia). Cats may be more likely to develop adverse reactions. *Horses:* Leukopenias, thrombocytopenia, & anemias; Baker's yeast or folinic acid may treat/prevent.

▶ Potentially teratogenic; avoid use in pregnancy

▶ Dosage form (25 mg tab only) may be inconvenient; unpalatable to cats

Uses/Indications

In veterinary medicine, pyrimethamine is used to treat *Hepatozoon americanum* infections, and toxoplasmosis in small animals (often in combination with sulfonamides). In horses, it is used to treat equine protozoal myeloencephalitis, sometimes called equine toxoplasmosis.

In humans, pyrimethamine is used for the treatment of toxoplasmosis and as a prophylactic agent for malaria.

Pharmacology/Actions

Pyrimethamine is a folic acid antagonist similar to trimethoprim. It acts by inhibiting the enzyme, dihydrofolate reductase that catalyzes the conversion of dihydrofolic acid to tetrahydrofolic acid.

Pharmacokinetics

No pharmacokinetic data was located for veterinary species. In humans, pyrimethamine is well absorbed from the gut after oral administration. It is distributed primarily to the kidneys, liver, spleen, and lungs, but does cross the blood-brain barrier. It has a volume of distribution of about 3 L/kg and is 80% bound to plasma proteins. Pyrimethamine enters milk in levels greater than those found in serum and can be detected in milk up to 48 hours after dosing.

In humans, plasma half-life is approximately 3–5 days. It is unknown how or where the drug is metabolized, but metabolites are found in the urine.

Contraindications/Precautions/Warnings

Pyrimethamine is contraindicated in patients hypersensitive to it and should be used cautiously in patients with preexisting hematologic disorders. Some clinicians recommend avoiding its use in cats because of its adverse effect profile.

Adverse Effects

In small animals, anorexia, malaise, vomiting, depression, and bone marrow depression (anemia, thrombocytopenia, leukopenia) have been seen. Adverse effects may be more prominent in cats and noted 4–6 days after starting combination therapy. Some clinicians recommend avoiding its use in this species. Hematologic effects can develop rapidly and frequent monitoring is recommended, particularly if therapy persists longer than 2 weeks. Oral administration of folinic acid at 1 mg/kg PO, folic acid 5 mg/day, or Brewer's yeast 100 mg/kg/day have been suggested to alleviate adverse effects.

The drug is unpalatable to cats when mixed with food and the 25 mg tablet dosage size makes successful dosing a challenge.

In horses, pyrimethamine has caused leukopenias, thrombocytopenia and anemias when used in combination with sulfonamides. Baker's yeast and folinic acid have been suggested to antagonize these adverse effects. Alternatively, folic acid supplement may be used (an example is Folic Acid and Vitamin E Pak from Buckeye Feed Mills in Dalton, Ohio).

Reproductive/Nursing Safety

Pyrimethamine has been demonstrated to be teratogenic in rats. Fetal abnormalities have been seen in foals after mares have been treated, however, it has been used in treating women with toxoplasmosis during pregnancy.

Clearly, the risks associated with therapy must be weighed against the potential for toxicity, the severity of the disease, and any alternative therapies available (*e.g.*, clindamycin in small animals). Concomitant administration of folinic acid has been recommended if the drug is to be used during pregnancy by some, but others state that pregnant mares should not receive folic acid during therapy as it may exacerbate fetal abnormalities or mortality. In humans, the FDA categorizes this drug as category *C* for use during pregnancy (*Animal studies have shown an adverse effect on the fetus, but there are no adequate studies in humans; or there are no animal reproduction studies and no adequate studies in humans.*)

Pyrimethamine is excreted in maternal milk; consider using milk replacer.

Overdosage/Acute Toxicity

Reports of acute overdosage of pyrimethamine in animals were not located. In humans, vomiting, nausea, anorexia, CNS stimulation (including seizures), and hematologic effects can be seen. Recommendations for treatment include: standard procedures in emptying the gut or preventing absorption, parenteral barbiturates for seizures, folinic acid for hematologic effects, and long-term monitoring (at least 1 month) of renal and hematopoietic systems.

Drug Interactions

The following drug interactions have either been reported or are theoretical in humans or animals receiving pyrimethamine and may be of significance in veterinary patients:

- **p-AMINOBENZOIC ACID (PABA):** PABA is reportedly antagonistic towards the activity of pyrimethamine; clinical significance is unclear
- **SULFONAMIDES:** Pyrimethamine is synergistic with sulfonamides in activity against toxoplasmosis (and malaria)
- **TRIMETHOPRIM:** Use with pyrimethamine/sulfa is not recommended in humans as adverse effects may be additive, however, this combination has been used clinically in horses

Doses

- **DOGS:**

    For protozoal diseases:

    a) For toxoplasmosis: 0.5–1 mg/kg PO once daily for 2 days, then 0.25 mg/kg PO once daily for 2 weeks. Given with sulfadiazine at 30–50 mg/kg PO divided two to four times a day for 1–2 weeks (Murtaugh & Ross 1988)

    b) For Toxoplasmosis: 0.25–0.5 mg/kg once daily for 28 days; For Neospora (with trimethoprim sulfa): 1 mg/kg once daily for 28 days; For *Hepatazoon canis* (with trimethoprim sulfa and clindamycin): 0.25–0.5 mg/kg once daily for 2–4 weeks (Lappin, M. 2000)

c) For *Hepatazoon americanum*: Trimethoprim/sulfa (15 mg/kg PO q12h), pyrimethamine (0.25 mg/kg PO q24h), and clindamycin (10 mg/kg q8h). Once remission attained, decoquinate (see monograph) can maintain. (Baneth 2007)

d) For *Hepatazoon americanum*: Trimethoprim/sulfa (15 mg/kg PO q12h for 14 days), pyrimethamine (0.25 mg/kg PO q24h for 14 days), and clindamycin (10 mg/kg q8h for 14 days). Once remission attained, decoquinate (see monograph) can maintain.

For neosporosis: pyrimethamine (1 mg/kg PO daily) with trimethoprim/sulfa (15–30 mg/kg PO twice daily). (Blagburn 2005)

■ **CATS: SEE WARNINGS ABOVE.**

For toxoplasmosis:

a) 0.5–1 mg/kg PO once daily for 2 days, then 0.25 mg/kg PO once daily for 2 weeks. Given with sulfadiazine at 30–50 mg/kg PO divided two to four times a day for 1–2 weeks (Murtaugh & Ross 1988)

b) For enteroepithelial cycle: 2 mg/kg, PO once daily. For extraintestinal cycle: 0.5–1 mg/kg PO divided two to three times daily combined with sulfonamides (*e.g.*, triple sulfa, sulfadiazine) at 60 mg/kg PO or IM divided two to three times daily (Lappin, M.R. 1989)

c) For protozoal myocarditis: Pyrimethamine 1 mg/kg PO once daily for 3 days, then decrease dose to 0.5 mg/kg PO once a day, with sulfadimethoxine 25 mg/kg PO, IV, or IM once a day (Ogburn 1988)

d) Pyrimethamine: 0.5 mg/kg PO per day with sulfadiazine at 30 mg/kg, PO q12h for 7–10 days. Do not use continuously for longer than 2 weeks. Supplementation with folic acid 5 mg/day or folinic acid 1 mg/kg/day may alleviate toxicity. (Swango *et al.* 1989)

■ **HORSES:**

See also the next monograph (Pyrimethamine + Sulfadiazine)

For equine protozoal myeloencephalitis:

a) Pyrimethamine 1 mg/kg PO once a day for 90–120 days (or longer). Given with a sulfa or potentiated sulfa (sulfadiazine 20 mg/kg PO once or twice a day). Monitor CBC's. (MacKay *et al.* 2000)

■ **BIRDS:**

For Coccidian organisms in raptors:

a) 0.5 mg/kg PO twice daily for 14–28 days (especially effective against Toxoplasmosis, Atoxoplasmosis and Sarcocystis). (Jones 2007)

Monitoring

■ See adverse effects; CBC with platelet count

■ Clinical efficacy

Client Information

■ Clients should he instructed to monitor for clinical signs of abnormal bleeding, lassitude, etc. that may signal development of hematologic disorders.

■ Accurate dosing of the tablets in cats may be very difficult as only 25 mg tablets are commercially available. Preferably, custom prepared capsules containing the accurate dosage should be prepared.

Chemistry/Synonyms

An aminopyrimidine agent structurally related to trimethoprim, pyrimethamine occurs as an odorless, white, or almost white, crystalline powder or crystals. It is practically insoluble in water and slightly soluble in alcohol.

Pyrimethamine may also be known as: BW-50-63, pirimetamina, pyrimethaminum, RP-4753, *Daraprim®*, *Malocide®*, or *Pirimecidan®*.

Storage/Stability

Pyrimethamine tablets should be stored in tight, light-resistant containers.

Pyrimethamine tablets may be crushed to make oral suspensions of the drug. Although stable in an aqueous solution, sugars tend to adversely affect the stability of pyrimethamine. If cherry syrup, corn syrup, or sucrose-containing liquids are used in the preparation of the suspension, it is recommended to store the suspension at room temperature and discard after 7 days.

Dosage Forms/Regulatory Status

VETERINARY-LABELED PRODUCTS: None

HUMAN-LABELED PRODUCTS:

Pyrimethamine Tablets: 25 mg; *Daraprim®* (GlaxoSmithKline); (Rx)

References

Baneth, G. (2007). Canine and Feline Hepatozoonosis—More than one disease. Proceedings: WSAVA World Congress. Accessed via: Veterinary Information Network. http://goo.gl/naPZN

Blagburn, B. (2005). Treatment and control of tick borne diseases and other important parasites of companion animals. Proceedings: ACVC2005. Accessed via: Veterinary Information Network. http://goo.gl/Pexfa

Jones, M. (2007). Falconry and raptor medicine. Proceedings: Western Vet Conf. Accessed via: Veterinary Information Network. http://goo.gl/40QbS

Lappin, M. (2000). Protozoal and Miscellaneous Infections. *Textbook of Veterinary Internal Medicine: Diseases of the Dog and Cat.* S Ettinger and E Feldman Eds. Philadelphia, WB Saunders. **1:** 408–417.

Lappin, M.R. (1989). Feline Toxoplasmosis. *Current Veterinary Therapy X: Small Animal Practice.* RW Kirk Ed. Philadelphia, WB Saunders: 1112–1115.

MacKay, R., D. Granstrom, et al. (2000). Equine protozoal myeloencephalitis. *The Veterinary Clinics of North America: Equine Practice* **16:3**(December).

Murtaugh, R.J. & J.N. Ross (1988). Cardiac Arrhythmias: Pathogenesis and Treatment in the Trauma Patient, 10:3, 1988, p.). *Comp CE* **10**(2): 332–339.

Ogburn, P.N. (1988). Myocardial Diseases. *Handbook of Small Animal Practice.* RV Morgan Ed. New York, Churchill Livingstone: 109–128.

Swango, L.J., K.W. Bankemper, et al. (1989). Bacterial, Rickettsial, Protozoal, and Miscellaneous Infections. *Textbook of Veterinary Internal Medicine.* SJ Ettinger Ed. Philadelphia, WB Saunders. **1:** 265–297.

PYRIMETHAMINE + SULFADIAZINE

(pye-ri-*meth*-a-meen + sul-fa-*dye*-a-zeen)
ReBalance®

ANTIPROTOZOAL

Note: *Also see the Pyrimethamine, and Sulfadiazine/Trimethoprim monographs*

Prescriber Highlights

▶ Tetrahydrofolic acid inhibitor suspension labeled for the treatment of horses with equine protozoal myeloencephalitis (EPM) caused by *Sarcocystis neurona*

▶ May cause bone marrow suppression, GI effects, & "treatment crisis" (patient's signs worsen after beginning therapy)

▶ Daily treatment may be required for 3–9 months

Uses/Indications

ReBalance® (pyrimethamine/sulfadiazine suspension in a 1:20 concentration) is labeled for the treatment of horses with equine protozoal myeloencephalitis (EPM) caused by *Sarcocystis neurona.* Some combine pyrimethamine and sulfadiazine with ponazuril or diclazuril in treating relapsing EPM.

Although not labeled for use in small animals it potentially could be useful for treating protozoal infections such as Toxoplasmosis in cats or Neosporosis in dogs.

Pharmacology/Actions

Sulfonamides inhibit the conversion of para-aminobenzoic acid (PABA) to dihydrofolic acid (DFA) by competing with PABA for dihydropteroate synthase. Pyrimethamine blocks the conversion of DFA to tetrahydrofolic acid by inhibiting dihydrofolate reductase. When sulfas and dihydrofolate reductase inhibitors (*e.g.*, trimethoprim, pyrimethamine) are used together, synergistic effects can occur. When comparing pyrimethamine and trimethoprim, pyrimethamine is more active against protozoal dihydrofolate reductase and trimethoprim is more active against bacterial dihydrofolate reductase.

Pharmacokinetics

No specific information was located for the pharmacokinetics of this drug combination and dosage form (oral suspension) in horses. Previous reports in horses using other dosage forms reported pyrimethamine oral bioavailability of approximately 56% and elimination half-life of about 12 hours. CNS levels are approximately 25–50% of those found in plasma. Sulfadiazine is apparently well absorbed after oral administration to horses and enters the CSF. Volume of distribution is approximately 0.58 L/kg; elimination half-life is about 3–4 hours.

Contraindications/Precautions/Warnings

This drug combination is contraindicated in horses hypersensitive to either pyrimethamine or sulfadiazine. It should not be used in horses intended for human consumption. Because it may cause bone marrow suppression, use with caution in horses with preexisting hematologic abnormalities or those receiving other drugs that may cause bone marrow suppression.

Adverse Effects

Adverse effects in horses reported during field trials for pyrimethamine/sulfadiazine suspension include bone marrow suppression (anemia, leukopenia, neutropenia, thrombocytopenia), reduced appetite/anorexia, loose stools/diarrhea, and urticaria. CNS effects may be noted (seizures, depression), but are probably a result of the disease (EPM).

Baker's yeast or folinic acid have been suggested to antagonize the drug combination's bone marrow depressive effects, but efficacy has not been proven.

During the initial period (first few days) of treatment, neurologic signs may worsen—so-called treatment crisis—and may persist up to 5 weeks. It is thought this may be the result of an inflammatory reaction secondary to dying parasites in the central nervous system.

Reproductive/Nursing Safety

The label for *ReBalance®* (pyrimethamine/sulfadiazine suspension) states that the safe use of this product in horses for breeding purposes, during pregnancy, or in lactating mares has not been evaluated. Pyrimethamine has been demonstrated to be teratogenic in rats. Fetal abnormalities have been seen in foals after mares have been treated; however, it has been used in treating women with toxoplasmosis during pregnancy. Risks associated with therapy must be weighed against the potential for toxicity, the severity of the disease, and any alternative therapies available. Some have recommended concomitant administration of folinic acid if the drug is to be used during pregnancy, but others state that pregnant mares should not receive folic acid during therapy as it may exacerbate fetal abnormalities or mortality. In humans, the FDA categorizes pyrimethamine as category *C* for use during pregnancy (*Animal studies have shown an adverse effect on the fetus, but there are no adequate studies in humans; or there are no animal reproduction studies and no adequate studies in humans.*)

Sulfas cross the placenta and fetal serum levels may be up to 50% of that found in maternal serum. Teratogenicity has been reported in some laboratory animals when given at very high doses. Sulfas should be used in pregnant animals only when the benefits clearly outweigh the risks of therapy.

Sulfonamides are distributed into milk. Pyrimethamine is excreted in maternal milk and safety for nursing offspring has not been established; consider using milk replacer.

Overdosage/Acute Toxicity

Acute overdosage information for pyrimethamine/sulfadiazine in horses (greater than 2X) was not located. *ReBalance®* (pyrimethamine/ sulfadiazine suspension) was administered at 2X the labeled dose for 92 days to 49 horses. Signs noted included loose stools, slight increases in ALP in some horses, declines in RBC, HCT, Hgb, and PCV, and depressed appetite.

Drug Interactions

The label for *ReBalance®* (pyrimethamine/sulfadiazine suspension) states that the safety of this product with concomitant therapies in horses has not been evaluated.

In humans, the following drug interactions with sulfas and/or pyrimethamine have been reported or are theoretical and may be of significance in veterinary patients:

■ **ANTACIDS:** May decrease the bioavailability of sulfonamides if administered concurrently

■ **HIGHLY PROTEIN-BOUND DRUGS (e.g., methotrexate, phenylbutazone, thiazide diuretics, salicylates, probenecid, phenytoin, warfarin):** Sulfonamides may displace other highly bound drugs

■ **p-AMINOBENZOIC ACID (PABA):** PABA is reportedly antagonistic towards the activity of pyrimethamine; clinical significance is unclear

■ **TRIMETHOPRIM:** Use with pyrimethamine/ sulfa is not recommended in humans as adverse effects may be additive, however, this combination has been used clinically in horses

Laboratory Considerations

The following laboratory alterations have been reported in humans taking sulfonamides and may be of significance in veterinary patients:

■ **Urine glucose:** Sulfonamides may give false-positive results when using the Benedict's method

Doses

■ **HORSES:**

For treatment of EPM:

a) 20 mg/kg sulfadiazine with 1 mg/kg pyrimethamine; equivalent to 4 mL of *ReBalance®* suspension per 50 kg (110 lb) body weight PO once daily at least 1 hour before feeding with hay or grain. Administer using a suitable oral dosing syringe; insert nozzle through the interdental space and deposit the dose on the back of the tongue by depressing the plunger.

Treatment duration is based upon clinical response, but usually ranges from 90–270 days. (Label information; *ReBalance®*— Phoenix)

b) For horses that have had two relapses, intermittent sulfa-pyrimethamine may be effective in maintaining clinical remission. After completing regular therapy for EPM, give pyrimethamine/sulfadiazine twice weekly (first and fourth day of each week). (MacKay 2008)

Monitoring

■ CBC (including platelets): baseline and at least monthly during therapy

■ GI adverse effects

■ Clinical Efficacy: Improvement in neuro signs, CSF Western Blot test negative

Client Information

■ Shake well before using and store at room temperature; see dosage information for instructions on proper administration

■ Horse may develop worsening signs after beginning treatment, probably due to local inflammation from dying parasites

■ Watch for signs that may indicate toxicity including depression, bleeding, bruising, bloody diarrhea, etc.; contact veterinarian if these occur

Chemistry/Synonyms

Pyrimethamine is an aminopyrimidine agent structurally related to trimethoprim. It occurs as an odorless, white, or almost white, crystalline powder or crystals. It is practically insoluble in water and slightly soluble in alcohol.

Sulfadiazine occurs as an odorless or nearly odorless, white to slightly yellow powder. It is practically insoluble in water and sparingly soluble in alcohol.

Sulfadoxine and Pyrimethamine may also be known as *Fansidar®* and *ReBalance®*.

Storage/Stability

ReBalance® suspension should be stored at controlled room temperature (15–30°C) and protected from freezing.

Dosage Forms/Regulatory Status

VETERINARY-LABELED PRODUCTS:

Sulfadiazine (as the sodium salt) 250 mg/mL and Pyrimethamine 12.5 mg/mL Oral Suspension in quart (946.4 mL) bottles; *ReBalance® Antiprotozoal Oral Suspension* (Phoenix); (Rx) FDA-approved for use in horses; not for use in horses intended for human consumption.

HUMAN-LABELED PRODUCTS:

A related compound for humans that contained Sulfadoxine & Pyrimethamine *Fansidar®*, has been discontinued in the US market.

References

MacKay, R. (2008). Equine Protozoal Myeloencephalitis: Managing Relapses. *Comp Equine*(Jan/Feb): 24–27.

QUINACRINE HCL

(*qwin*-a-krin)

ANTIPROTOZOAL

Prescriber Highlights

▶ Antiprotozoal that may be useful for treatment of Giardia, Leishmania, & coccidia. May improve clinical signs associated with giardial infection, but not eliminate infection

▶ Contraindications: Potentially, if hepatic dysfunction or pregnancy

▶ Adverse Effects: Yellowing of skin & urine color, (not of clinical importance); GI (anorexia, nausea, vomiting, diarrhea), abnormal behaviors ("fly biting", agitation), pruritus, & fever. Potentially: Hypersensitivity, hepatopathy, aplastic anemia, corneal edema, & retinopathy.

▶ Availability an issue

▶ Potential teratogen

▶ Give with meals; have liquid available

Uses/Indications

While quinacrine has activity against a variety of protozoans and helminths, its use against all but Giardia and Trichomonas has been superseded by safer or more effective agents. In humans, quinacrine may be used for treatment of mild to moderate discoid lupus erythromatosis, transcervically as a sterilizing agent, or in powder form as an intrapleural sclerosing agent.

Pharmacology/Actions

Quinacrine's mechanism of action for its antiprotozoal activity against Giardia is not understood, however, it does bind to DNA by intercalation to adjacent base pairs thereby inhibiting RNA transcription and translocation. Additionally, quinacrine interferes with electron transport and inhibits succinate oxidation and cholinesterase. Quinacrine binds to nucleoproteins that (in humans at least) can suppress lupus erythromatosis (LE) cell factor.

Pharmacokinetics

Quinacrine is absorbed well from the GI tract or after intrapleural administration. It is distributed throughout the body, but CSF levels are only 1–5% of those found in plasma. Drug is concentrated in the liver, spleen, lungs, and adrenals. It is relatively highly bound to plasma proteins in humans (80–90%). Quinacrine crosses the placenta, but only small amounts enter maternal milk.

Quinacrine is eliminated very slowly (half life in humans: 5–14 days). Quinacrine is slowly metabolized, but primarily eliminated by the kidneys; acidifying the urine will increase renal excretion somewhat. Significant amounts may be detected in urine up to 2 months after drug discontinuation.

Contraindications/Precautions/Warnings

In humans, quinacrine is relatively contraindicated in patients with psychotic disorders, psoriasis, or porphyria as it may exacerbate these conditions. Veterinary relevance is unknown. The drug should be used with extreme caution in patients with hepatic dysfunction.

Adverse Effects

In small animals, a yellowing of skin and urine color can occur, but is not of clinical importance (does not indicate jaundice). Additionally, gastrointestinal disturbances (anorexia, nausea, vomiting, diarrhea), abnormal behaviors ("fly biting", agitation), lethargy, pruritus, and fever have been noted.

Potentially hypersensitivity reactions, hepatopathy, aplastic anemia, corneal edema, and retinopathy could occur (all reported rarely in humans, primarily with high dose long-term use).

Reproductive/Nursing Safety

Quinacrine crosses the placenta and has been implicated in causing a case of renal agenesis and hydrocephalus in a human infant. In high doses, it has caused increased fetal death rates in rats. Weigh the potential benefits with the risks when considering use in pregnant animals.

In humans, the FDA categorizes this drug as category **C** for use during pregnancy (*Animal studies have shown an adverse effect on the fetus, but there are no adequate studies in humans; or there are no animal reproduction studies and no adequate studies in humans.*)

Overdosage/Acute Toxicity

Overdosage may be serious depending on the dose. In humans, a dose as low as 6.8 grams (administered intraduodenally) caused death. Clinical signs associated with acute toxicity include CNS excitation (including seizures), GI disturbances, vascular collapse, and cardiac arrhythmias. Treatment consists of gut emptying protocols, and supportive and symptomatic therapies. Urinary acidification with ammonium chloride and forced diuresis (with adequate fluid therapy) may be beneficial in enhancing urinary excretion of the drug.

Drug Interactions

The following drug interactions have either been reported or are theoretical in humans or animals receiving quinacrine HCl and may be of significance in veterinary patients:

◼ **ALCOHOL:** Quinacrine may cause a "disulfiram-reaction" if used with alcohol.

◼ **HEPATOTOXIC DRUGS:** Quinacrine concentrates in the liver and should be used with caution with hepatotoxic drugs (clinical significance unknown).

◼ **PRIMAQUINE:** Quinacrine increases the toxicity of primaquine (generally not used in veterinary medicine), and the two should not be used simultaneously.

Laboratory Considerations

■ When urine is acidic, quinacrine can cause it to turn a deep yellow color. By causing an interfering fluorescence, quinacrine can cause falsely elevated values of **plasma and urine cortisol** values.

Doses

■ **DOGS:**

As a drug of second-choice in the treatment of Giardia or other susceptible protozoa:
a) 6.6 mg/kg PO q12h for 5 days (Papich 1992), (Sherding & Johnson 1994), (Blagburn 2003; Blagburn 2005)
b) 9 mg/kg PO q24h for 6 days. (Lappin 2006)

■ **CATS:**

a) Giardia: 9 mg/kg PO once daily for 6 days; Coccidiosis: 10 mg/kg PO once daily for 5 days (Blagburn 2003), (Blagburn 2005)
b) Giardia: 11 mg/kg PO q24h for 12 days (Lappin 2006)
c) Coccidiosis: 10 mg/kg PO once daily for 5 days (Greene & Watson 1998)

■ **REPTILES:**

a) For hemoprotozoal infections: 19−100 mg/kg PO q48h (every other day) for 2−3 weeks (de la Navarre 2003)

Monitoring

■ Efficacy (fecal exams, reduction in diarrhea)

■ Adverse effects

Client Information

■ Quinacrine should preferably be given after meals with plenty of liquids available.

■ Make sure clients understand the importance of compliance with directions and to watch for signs of adverse effects.

Chemistry/Synonyms

A synthetic acridine derivative anthelmintic, quinacrine HCl occurs as a bright yellow, odorless, crystalline powder having a bitter taste. It is sparingly soluble in water.

Quinacrine HCl may also be known as mepacrine HCl.

Storage/Stability

Tablets should be stored in tight, light-resistant containers at room temperature. Quinacrine is not stable in solution for any length of time; however, it may be crushed and mixed with foods to mask its very bitter taste.

Dosage Forms/Regulatory Status

VETERINARY-LABELED PRODUCTS: None

HUMAN-LABELED PRODUCTS: None

There currently are no quinacrine products being marketed in the USA. It may be available from compounding pharmacies.

References

Blagburn, B. (2003). Giardiasis and coccidiosis updates. Proceedings: Western Veterinary Conference. Accessed via: Veterinary Information Network. http://goo.gl/EZqfI

Blagburn, B. (2005). Treatment and control of tick borne diseases and other important parasites of companion animals. Proceedings: ACVC2005. Accessed via: Veterinary Information Network. http://goo.gl/Pexfa

de la Navarre, B. (2003). Common parasitic diseases of reptiles and amphibians. Proceedings: Western Veterinary Conf. Accessed via: Veterinary Information Network. http://goo.gl/ZafJD

Greene, C. & A. Watson (1998). Antimicrobial Drug Formulary. Infectious Diseases of the Dog and Cat. C Greene Ed. Philadelphia, WB Saunders: 790–919.

Lappin, M. (2006). Giardia infections. Proceedings: WSAVA World Congress. Accessed via: Veterinary Information Network. http://goo.gl/aywXP

Papich, M. (1992). Table of Common Drugs: Approximate Dosages. Current Veterinary Therapy XI: Small Animal Practice. R Kirk and J Bonagura Eds. Philadelphia, W.B. Saunders Company: 1233–1249.

Sherding, R. & S. Johnson (1994). Diseases of the intestines. Saunders Manual of Small Animal Practice. S Birchard and R Sherding Eds. Philadelphia, W.B. Saunders Company: 687–714.

QUINIDINE GLUCONATE QUINIDINE POLY-GALACTURONATE QUINIDINE SULFATE

(**qwin**-i-deen)   Quinidex®

ANTIARRHYTHMIC

Prescriber Highlights

▶ Antiarrhythmic agent used in small animals & horses

▶ Contraindications: Hypersensitivity, myasthenia gravis; complete AV block with an AV junctional or idioventricular pacemaker; intraventricular conduction defects; digitalis intoxication with associated arrhythmias or AV conduction disorders; aberrant ectopic impulses; or abnormal rhythms secondary to escape mechanisms

▶ Extreme Caution: Any form of AV block or if any clinical signs of digoxin toxicity are exhibited

▶ Caution: Uncorrected hypokalemia, hypoxia, & disorders or acid-base balance; hepatic or renal insufficiency

▶ Adverse Effects: *Dogs:* GI effects, weakness, hypotension (especially with too rapid IV administration), negative inotropism, widened QRS complex & QT intervals, AV block, & multiform ventricular tachycardias hypotension. *Horses:* inappetence, depression, swelling of the nasal mucosa, ataxia, diarrhea, colic, hypotension & rarely, laminitis, paraphimosis & the development of urticarial wheals; cardiac arrhythmias including AV block, circulatory collapse & sudden death

▶ Consider monitoring blood levels

▶ Administer at evenly spaced intervals throughout the day/night

▶ GI upset may be decreased if administered with food

▶ Do not allow animal to chew or crush sustained-release oral dosage forms

▶ Many drug interactions

Uses/Indications

Quinidine is used in small animal or equine medicine for the treatment of ventricular arrhythmias (VPCs, ventricular tachycardia), refractory supraventricular tachycardias, and supraventricular arrhythmias associated with anomalous conduction in Wolff-Parkinson-White (WPW) syndrome. Chronic use of quinidine for controlling ventricular arrhythmias and supraventricular tachycardia in dogs has diminished over the years as other drugs appear to be more effective. It is still used in dogs and horses to convert atrial fibrillation to sinus rhythm. Oral therapy is generally not used in cats.

Pharmacology/Actions

A class IA antiarrhythmic, quinidine has effects similar to that of procainamide. It depresses myocardial excitability, conduction velocity, and contractility. Quinidine will prolong the effective refractory period, which prevents the reentry phenomenon and increases conduction times. Quinidine also possesses anticholinergic activity, which decreases vagal tone and may facilitate AV conduction.

Pharmacokinetics

After oral administration, quinidine salts are nearly completely absorbed from the GI, however, the actual amount that reaches the systemic circulation will be reduced due to the hepatic first-pass effect. The extended-release formulations of quinidine sulfate and gluconate, as well as the polygalacturonate tablets, are more slowly absorbed than the conventional tablets or capsules.

Quinidine is distributed rapidly to all body tissues except the brain. Protein binding varies from 82–92%. The reported volumes of distribution in various species are: horses ≈ 15.1 L/kg; cattle ≈ 3.8 L/kg; dogs ≈ 2.9 L/kg; cats ≈ 2.2 L/kg. Quinidine is distributed into milk and crosses the placenta.

Quinidine is metabolized in the liver, primarily by hydroxylation. Approximately 20% of a dose may be excreted unchanged in the urine within 24 hours after dosing. Serum half-lives reported in various species are: horses ≈ 8.1 hours; cattle ≈ 2.3 hours; dogs ≈ 5.6 hours; cats ≈ 1.9 hours; swine≈ 5.5 hours; goats ≈ 0.9 hours. Acidic urine (pH <6) can increase renal excretion of quinidine and decrease its serum half-life.

Contraindications/Precautions/Warnings

Quinidine is generally contraindicated in patients who have demonstrated previous hypersensitivity reactions to it; myasthenia gravis; complete AV block with an AV junctional or idioventricular pacemaker; intraventricular conduction defects (especially with pronounced QRS widening); digitalis intoxication with associated arrhythmias or AV conduction disorders; aberrant ectopic impulses; or abnormal rhythms secondary to escape mechanisms. It should be used with extreme caution, if at all, in any form of AV block or if any clinical signs of digitalis toxicity are exhibited.

Quinidine should be used with caution in patients with uncorrected hypokalemia, hypoxia, and disorders or acid-base balance. Use cautiously in patients with hepatic or renal insufficiency as accumulation of the drug may result.

When using to cardiovert horses with atrial fibrillation, monitor the ECG throughout treatment. Heart rates above 80 bpm, a widening of QRS beyond 125% of baseline, and abnormal complexes are all indicators to discontinue medication (McGurrin 2010).

Adverse Effects

In dogs, gastrointestinal effects may include anorexia, vomiting, or diarrhea. Effects related to the cardiovascular system can include weakness, hypotension (especially with too rapid IV administration), negative inotropism, widened QRS complex and QT intervals, AV block, and multiform ventricular tachycardias.

Horses may exhibit inappetence and depression commonly after quinidine therapy but this does not necessarily indicate toxicity. Signs of toxicity include swelling of the nasal mucosa, ataxia, diarrhea, colic, hypotension and, rarely, laminitis, paraphimosis and the development of urticarial wheals. Urticaria or upper respiratory tract obstruction can be treated by discontinuing the drug and administering corticosteroids if necessary. If obstruction persists, nasotracheal tube placement or tracheostomy may be required. Horses may develop cardiac arrhythmias including AV block, circulatory collapse, and sudden death.

Patients exhibiting signs of toxicity or lack of response may be candidates for therapeutic serum monitoring. The therapeutic range is thought to be 2.5–5 micrograms/mL in dogs. Toxic effects usually are not seen unless levels are >10 micrograms/mL.

Reproductive/Nursing Safety

In humans, the FDA categorizes this drug as category *C* for use during pregnancy (*Animal studies have shown an adverse effect on the fetus, but there are no adequate studies in humans; or there are no animal reproduction studies and no adequate studies in humans.*) In a separate system evaluating the safety of drugs in canine and feline pregnancy (Papich 1989), this drug is categorized as class: *B* (*Safe for use if used cautiously. Studies in laboratory animals may have uncovered some risk, but these drugs appear to be safe in dogs and cats or these drugs are safe if they are not administered when the animal is near term.*)

Quinidine is excreted into maternal milk with a milk:serum ratio of approximately 0.71. Use caution when quinidine is administered to nursing patients. The American Academy of Pediatrics considers quinidine compatible with breastfeeding.

Overdosage/Acute Toxicity

Clinical signs of overdosage can include depression, hypotension, lethargy, confusion, seizures, vomiting, diarrhea, and oliguria. Cardiac signs may include depressed automaticity and conduction, or tachyarrhythmias. The CNS effects are often delayed after the onset of cardiovascular effects but may persist after the cardiovascular effects have begun to resolve.

If a recent oral ingestion, emptying of the gut and charcoal administration may be beneficial to remove any unabsorbed drug. IV fluids, plus metaraminol or norepinephrine, can be considered to treat hypotensive effects. A 1/6 molar intravenous infusion of sodium lactate may be used in an attempt to reduce the cardiotoxic effects of quinidine. Forced diuresis using fluids and diuretics along with reduction of urinary pH may enhance the renal excretion of the drug. Temporary cardiac pacing may be necessary should severe AV block occur. Hemodialysis will effectively remove quinidine, but peritoneal dialysis will not.

Drug Interactions

The following drug interactions have either been reported or are theoretical in humans or animals receiving quinidine and may be of significance in veterinary patients:

- **ACETAZOLAMIDE:** May reduce quinidine clearance
- **AMIODARONE:** May increase quinidine levels (significantly)
- **ANTACIDS:** May delay oral absorption; separate dosages
- **ANTIARRHYTHMIC AGENTS:** Use with caution with other antidysrhythmic agents, as additive cardiotoxic or other toxic effects may result
- **ANTICHOLINESTERASES (e.g., pyridostigmine, neostigmine):** Quinidine may antagonize the effects of anticholinesterases in patients with myasthenia gravis
- **AUROTHIOGLUCOSE:** Increased risk for blood dyscrasias
- **CIMETIDINE:** Cimetidine may increase the levels of quinidine by inhibiting hepatic microsomal enzymes
- **CISAPRIDE:** Increased risk for QTc interval prolongation
- **COLCHICINE:** Quinidine may increase colchicine levels
- **CLARITHROMYCIN:** Increased risk for torsade de pointes
- **DEXAMETHASONE:** In dogs, dexamethasone increased quinidine volume of distribution (49-78%) and elimination half-life (1.5-2.3X). (Zhang *et al.* 2006)
- **DIGOXIN:** Digoxin levels may increase considerably in patients stabilized on digoxin who receive quinidine. Some cardiologists recommend decreasing the digoxin dosage

by ½ when adding quinidine. Therapeutic drug monitoring of both quinidine and digoxin may be warranted in these cases.

- **DILTIAZEM:** Possible decreased clearance; increased elimination half-life of quinidine
- **HYPOTENSIVE AGENTS:** Quinidine may potentiate the effects of other drugs having hypotensive effects
- **FLUCONAZOLE:** Increased risk for cardiotoxicity
- **FLUOROQUINOLONE ANTIBIOTICS (e.g., ciprofloxacin, enrofloxacin, etc):** Increased risk for cardiotoxicity
- **ITRACONAZOLE:** Increased risk for quinidine toxicity
- **KETOCONAZOLE:** May reduce the metabolism of quinidine
- **NEUROMUSCULAR BLOCKING AGENTS:** Quinidine may increase the neuromuscular blocking effects of drugs like succinylcholine, tubocurarine, or atracurium
- **PHENOBARBITAL, PHENYTOIN:** May induce hepatic enzymes that metabolize quinidine thus reducing quinidine serum half-life by 50%
- **PHENOTHIAZINES:** Additive cardiac depressant effects may be seen
- **RESERPINE:** Additive cardiac depressant effects may be seen
- **RIFAMPIN:** May induce hepatic enzymes that metabolize quinidine thus reducing quinidine serum half-life by 50%
- **TRICYCLIC ANTIDEPRESSANTS (e.g., amitriptyline, clomipramine, doxepin, imipramine):** Increased risk for QTc interval prolongation and tricyclic adverse effects
- **URINARY ACIDIFIERS (e.g., methionine, ammonium chloride):** Drugs that acidify the urine (may increase the excretion of quinidine and decrease serum level)
- **URINARY ALKALINIZERS (carbonic anhydrase inhibitors, thiazide diuretics, sodium bicarbonate, antacids, etc.):** Drugs that alkalinize the urine may decrease the excretion of quinidine, prolonging its half-life
- **VERAPAMIL:** Possible decreased clearance; increased elimination half-life of quinidine; increased risk for hypotension
- **WARFARIN:** Coumarin anticoagulants with quinidine may increase the likelihood of bleeding problems

Doses

- **DOGS:**
  a) For VPC's or ventricular tachycardia:
    Quinidine gluconate: 6.6−22 mg/kg IM q2−4h or q8−12h PO (delayed dosage forms).

    Quinidine Sulfate: 6.6−22 mg/kg PO q6−8h; may be given initially q2h as a loading dose until arrhythmia is controlled or toxicity is induced (Ettinger 1989)

b) 6–20 mg/kg IM q6h (loading dose 14–20 mg/kg); 6–16 mg/kg PO q6h; Sustained action oral preparations: 8–20 mg/kg PO q8h (Ware 2000)

c) 6–16 mg/kg PO or IM q6h (q8h with sustained release products) (Fox 2003)

d) For conversion of atrial fib to sinus rhythm in dogs without underlying heart disease: Initially attempted with quinidine gluconate at 6–11 mg/kg IM q6h. Some dogs will convert in the first 24 hours of therapy. If rapid ventricular response occurs, may give either digoxin or a beta-blocker to slow rate of conduction across AV node. (Russell & Rush 1995), (Smith 2009)

■ **CATS:**

a) 6–16 mg/kg IM or PO q8h (Ware 2000)

■ **HORSES: (Note:** ARCI UCGFS Class 4 Drug)

a) For atrial fib without signs of heart failure: Keep horse quiet during dosing stage. Monitor ECG either continuously or before each dose. Horses with recent onset (<7 days) or whom develop atrial fib during anesthesia: Quinidine gluconate 1.1–2.2 mg/kg IV every 10 minutes to a total dose of 8.8–11 mg/kg (or until conversion or toxicity develop).

For horses who have had atrial fib for >7 days: Give quinidine sulfate 22 mg/kg via NG tube every 2 hours for a total dose of 88–132 mg/kg (or until conversion or toxicity develop). If this fails to convert and no signs of toxicity are evident may continue at 22 mg/kg, PO q6h for an additional 2–4 or more days. Discontinue if QRS duration is >125% of baseline. Rapid SVT's (>100 BPM) or ventricular arrhythmias may necessitate specific antiarrhythmic therapy.

For V-Tach: Quinidine gluconate 0.5–2.2 mg/kg IV boluses every 10 minutes up to a total of 8.8–11 mg/kg (Mogg 1999)

b) For atrial fibrillation in a horse without heart failure:

Oral (via NG tube) Dosing: give quinidine sulfate 22 mg/kg PO via nasogastric tube every two hours until cardioversion, toxic effects, or six doses have been given. If AF remains continue administration every 6 hours until cardioversion or adverse effects.

Alternate *IV dosing* method: 0.5–2.2 mg/kg IV bolus every 5–10 minutes to effect or until adverse effects seen. Maximum IV dose is 12mg/kg. Conversion of ventricular tachycardia has occurred with a single 0.5 mg/kg dose.

Monitor ECG throughout treatment. Heart rate in excess of 80 bpm, widening QRS complex >125% of baseline, or abnormal complexes are indicators to discontinue treatment.

Toxic effects are variable. Mild signs include nasal edema, and mild depression. More severe signs include marked ataxia, hypotension, colic, diarrhea, seizures, sustained tachycardia, syncope and sudden death. Adverse effects not necessarily dose dependent. Hypokalemia increases risk for torsades de pointes. Therapeutic levels 3–5 micrograms/mL. (Kimberly & McGurrin 2006)

c) For atrial fibrillation:

Oral (via NG tube) Dosing: give quinidine sulfate 22 mg/kg PO via nasogastric tube every two hours for 4–6 doses, followed by dosing q6h if needed for conversion. Withhold food for 12 hours prior to starting treatment to ensure maximum oral absorption. Quinidine dissolves poorly so 1–2 liters of water may be needed per dose. Oral ulcers can occur if attempting to administer by mouth. If nasal edema or urticaria occurs, discontinue immediately. Heart rate in excess of 100 bpm, widening QRS complex >125% of baseline, ventricular arrhythmias or abnormal complexes are indicators to discontinue treatment or prolong dosing interval. Suggest monitoring levels. (Risberg 2005)

Monitoring

■ ECG, continuous if possible

■ Blood pressure, during IV administration

■ Clinical signs of toxicity (see Adverse Reactions/Overdosage)

■ Serum levels. Therapeutic serum levels are believed to range from 2–7 micrograms/mL (2–5 micrograms/mL in horses). Levels >10 micrograms/mL are considered toxic.

Client Information

■ Oral products should be administered at evenly spaced intervals throughout the day/night. GI upset may be decreased if administered with food.

■ Do not allow animal to chew or crush sustained-release oral dosage forms.

■ Notify veterinarian if animal's condition deteriorates or signs of toxicity (*e.g.*, vomiting, diarrhea, weakness, etc.) occur.

Chemistry/Synonyms

Used as an antiarrhythmic agent, quinidine is an alkaloid obtained from cinchona or related plants, or is prepared from quinine. It is available commercially in three separate salts: gluconate, polygalacturonate, or sulfate.

Quinidine gluconate occurs as a very bitter

tasting, odorless, white powder. It is freely soluble in water and slightly soluble in alcohol. The injectable form has a pH of 5.5–7.

Quinidine polygalacturonate occurs as a bitter tasting, creamy white, amorphous powder. It is sparingly soluble in water and freely soluble in hot 40% alcohol.

Quinidine sulfate occurs as very bitter tasting, odorless, fine, needle-like, white crystals that may cohere in masses. One gram is soluble in approximately 100 mL of water or 10 mL of alcohol.

Quinidine Gluconate may also be known as: quinidinium gluconate, *Duraquin®*, *Quinaglute®*, *Quinalan®*, and *Quinate®*.

Quinidine Sulfate may also be known as: chinidini sulfas, chinidinsulfate, chinidinum sulfuricum, or quinidini sulfas; many trade names are available.

Quinidine Polygalacturonate may also be known as: *Cardioquin®*, *Cardioquin®*, *Cardioquine®*, *Galactoquin®*, *Naticardina®*, or *Neochinidin Ritmocor®*.

Storage/Stability

All quinidine salts darken upon exposure to light (acquire a brownish tint) and should be stored in light-resistant, well-closed containers. Use only colorless, clear solutions of quinidine gluconate for injection.

Quinidine gluconate injection is usually administered intramuscularly, but may be given very slowly (1 mL/minute) intravenously. It may be diluted by adding 10 to 40 mL of D_5W.

Compatibility/Compounding Considerations

Quinidine gluconate is reported to be physically **compatible** with bretylium tosylate, cimetidine HCl, and verapamil HCl. It is reportedly physically **incompatible** with alkalies and iodides.

Dosage Forms/Regulatory Status

VETERINARY-LABELED PRODUCTS: None

The ARCI (Racing Commissioners International) has designated this drug as a class 4 substance. See the appendix for more information.

HUMAN-LABELED PRODUCTS:

Quinidine Sulfate (contains 83% anhydrous quinidine alkaloid) Tablets: 100 mg, 200 mg & 300 mg; generic; (Rx)

Quinidine Sulfate (contains 83% anhydrous quinidine alkaloid) Sustained-Release Tablets: 300 mg; generic; (Rx)

Quinidine Gluconate Sustained-Release Tablets: 324 mg; generic; (Rx)

Quinidine Gluconate Injection: 80 mg/mL (50 mg/mL of quinidine base) in 10 mL multidose vials; generic (Lilly); (Rx)

References

Ettinger, S.J. (1989). Cardiac Arrythmias. *Textbook of Veterinary Internal Medicine.* SJ Ettinger Ed. Philadelphia, WB Saunders. 1: 1051–1096.

Fox, P. (2003). Congestive heart failure: Clinical approach and management. Proceedings: World Small Animal Veterinary Assoc World Congress. Accessed via: Veterinary Information Network. http://goo.gl/xMFKn

Kimberly, M. & K. McGurrin (2006). Update on antiarrhythmic therapy in horses. Proceedings; ACVIM. Accessed via: Veterinary Information Network. http://goo.gl/kSS8b

McGurrin, M. (2010). Therapeutic Options in Atrial Fibrillation. Proceedings: ACVIM. Accessed via: Veterinary Information Network. http://goo.gl/pFM13

Mogg, T. (1999). Equine Cardiac Disease: Clinical pharmacology and therapeutics. *The Veterinary Clinics of North America: Equine Practice* **15:3**(December).

Papich, M. (1989). Effects of drugs on pregnancy. *Current Veterinary Therapy X: Small Animal Practice.* R Kirk Ed. Philadelphia, Saunders: 1291–1299.

Risberg, A. (2005). Equine atrial fibrillation; new treatment options. Proceedings: ACVIM. Accessed via: Veterinary Information Network. http://goo.gl/Fo5hI

Russell, L. & J. Rush (1995). Cardiac Arrhythmias in Systemic Disease. *Kirk's Current Veterinary Therapy:XII.* J Bonagura Ed. Philadelphia, W.B. Saunders: 161–166.

Smith, F. (2009). Update on Antiarrhythmic Therapy. Proceedings: Western Veterinary Conference. Accessed via: Veterinary Information Network. http://goo.gl/aiVDJ

Ware, W. (2000). Therapy for Critical Arrythmias: New Advances. Proceedings: The North American Veterinary Conference, Orlando.

Zhang, K.W., S. Kohno, et al. (2006). Clinical oral doses of dexamethasone decreases intrinsic clearance of quinidine, a cytochrome P450 3A substrate in dogs. *Journal of Veterinary Medical Science* **68**(9): 903–907.

RAMIPRIL

(***ram**-ih-prill*)   Altace®, Vasotop®

ANGIOTENSIN CONVERTING ENZYME (ACE) INHIBITOR

Prescriber Highlights

▶ ACE inhibitor used primarily as a vasodilator in the treatment of heart failure or hypertension; may be of benefit in the treatment of chronic renal failure or protein losing nephropathies

▶ Not as much information or experience available as some other ACE inhibitors (e.g., enalapril) in dogs or cats

▶ Contraindications: Hypersensitivity to ACE inhibitors

▶ Caution: Pregnancy, patients with hyponatremia, coronary or cerebrovascular insufficiency, preexisting hematologic abnormalities, or a collagen vascular disease (e.g., SLE)

▶ Adverse Effects: Appears well tolerated in both dogs & cats. GI effects (anorexia, vomiting, diarrhea) possible; potentially: weakness, hypotension, & hyperkalemia

Uses/Indications

Ramipril is a long-acting angiotensin converting enzyme (ACE) inhibitor that may be useful in treating heart failure or hypertension in dogs or cats. It is an approved product in the UK for treating heart failure in dogs. In cats, ramipril has been used for treating arterial hypertension. A recent study (MacDonald *et al.* 2006) did not show any significant benefit using ramipril in treating Maine Coon cats with hypertrophic cardiomyopathy without heart failure.

Like other ACE inhibitors, it may potentially be useful as adjunctive treatment in chronic renal failure and protein losing nephropathies. In dogs with moderate renal impairment (such as might be found with CHF), there is apparently no need to adjust ramipril dosage.

Pharmacology/Actions

Ramipril is a pro-drug that has little pharmacologic activity until converted into ramiprilat. Ramiprilat prevents the formation of angiotensin-II (a potent vasoconstrictor) by competing with angiotensin-I for the enzyme angiotensin-converting enzyme (ACE). ACE has a much higher affinity for ramiprilat than for angiotensin-I. Because angiotensin-II concentrations are decreased, aldosterone secretion is reduced and plasma renin activity is increased.

The cardiovascular effects of ramiprilat in patients with CHF include decreased total peripheral resistance, pulmonary vascular resistance, mean arterial and right atrial pressures, and pulmonary capillary wedge pressure with no change or decrease in heart rate. Increased cardiac index and output, stroke volume, and exercise tolerance also occur. Renal blood flow can be increased with little change in hepatic blood flow. In animals with glomerular disease, ACE inhibitors probably decrease proteinuria and help to preserve renal function.

Pharmacokinetics

After oral administration to dogs, ramipril is rapidly converted via de-esterification into ramiprilat. Bioavailability of ramiprilat after a dose of 0.25 mg/kg per day of ramipril is about 6.7%. At this dose, ACE activity never exceeded 60% in either healthy dogs or those with experimentally induced renal dysfunction (GFR reduced 58%) (Lefebvre *et al.* 2006).

After oral administration to cats with ramipril doses ranging from 0.125 mg/kg to 1 mg/kg once daily for 9 days, ramipril peak concentrations occurred in about 0.5 hours. Ramipril is rapidly converted into its active metabolite ramiprilat, which peaks at 1 hour post-administration. Repeated doses of 0.125 mg/kg inhibited serum ACE activity by 94% at maximum to 55% 24 hours post-dose. At a dose of 1 mg/kg, ACE activity was 97% inhibited at maximum, and 83% inhibited 24 hours post-dose (Coulet & Burgaud 2002).

When cats were administered radio-labeled ramipril orally, 85–89% of the radioactivity was recovered in the feces. It is unclear how much of this represents unabsorbed drug or absorbed parent compound/metabolites eliminated in the feces. Approximately 10% of administered drug was recovered in the urine. Excretion of radio-labeled compounds was complete by 168 hours after dosing.

Contraindications/Precautions/Warnings

The labeling for the UK product approved for dogs (*Vasotop®*) states that it should not be used in clinical cases of vascular stenosis (*e.g.*, aortic stenosis), obstructive hypertrophic cardiomyopathy, or with potassium-sparing diuretics (see Drug Interactions).

Adverse Effects

While information is limited, ramipril appears to be well tolerated in dogs and cats. Gastrointestinal effects are probably the most likely adverse effects to be noted. Weakness, hypotension, or hyperkalemia are possible.

Reproductive/Nursing Safety

The labeling for the product approved in the UK (*Vasotop®*) suggests not using in bitches during pregnancy or lactation. Weigh the potential risks associated with using this medication (see human data below) in veterinary patients with the potential benefits of therapy. Dosages of up to 500 mg/kg/day did not impair fertility in rats. While no teratogenic effects have been detected with ramipril in studies performed in mice, rats, rabbits, and cynomolgus monkeys, fetal risk is increased in humans.

If used in humans during the 2nd and 3rd trimesters increased rates of fetal death, neonatal hypotension, skull hypoplasia, anuria, renal failure, oligohydramnios leading to fetal limb contractures, craniofacial deformation, and hypoplastic lung development were noted. In humans, ramipril has a "black box" warning regarding its use in pregnancy that states "When used in pregnancy during the second and third trimesters, angiotensin-converting enzyme (ACE) inhibitors can cause injury and even death to the developing fetus. When pregnancy is detected, ramipril should be discontinued as soon as possible." For humans, the FDA categorizes ramipril as category *D* for use during the 2nd and 3rd trimesters of pregnancy *(There is evidence of human fetal risk, but the potential benefits from the use of the drug in pregnant women may be acceptable despite its potential risks)* and as category *C* for use during the first trimester of pregnancy *(Animal studies have shown an adverse effect on the fetus, but there are no adequate studies in humans; or there are no animal reproduction studies and no adequate studies in humans.)*

It is unknown whether ramipril (or ramiprilat) enters milk. Both the veterinary label (UK) and human label recommended not using the drug during nursing.

Overdosage/Acute Toxicity

In dogs, ramipril appears quite safe; dosages as high as 1 gram/kg induced only mild GI distress. Lethal doses in rats and mice were noted at 10–11 grams/kg. No information was located on overdoses in cats. In overdose situations, the primary concern is hypotension; supportive treatment with volume expansion with normal saline is recommended to correct blood pressure. Because of the drug's long duration of action, prolonged monitoring and treatment may be required.

Drug Interactions

The following drug interactions have either been reported or are theoretical in humans or animals receiving ramipril and may be of significance in veterinary patients:

■ **ASPIRIN:** Aspirin may potentially negate the decrease in systemic vascular resistance induced by ACE inhibitors. However, in one study in dogs using low-dose aspirin, hemodynamic effects of enalaprilat (active metabolite of enalapril, a related drug) were not affected.

■ **ANTIDIABETIC AGENTS (insulin, oral agents):** Possible increased risk for hypoglycemia; enhanced monitoring recommended

■ **DIURETICS (e.g., furosemide, hydrochlorothiazide):** Potential for increased hypotensive effects

■ **DIURETICS, POTASSIUM SPARING (e.g., spironolactone, triamterene):** Increased hyperkalemic effects, enhanced monitoring of serum potassium

■ **NSAIDS:** Potential for increased risk of renal dysfunction or hyperkalemia

■ **POTASSIUM SUPPLEMENTS:** Increased risk for hyperkalemia

Laboratory Considerations

■ ACE inhibitors may cause a reversible decrease in localization and excretion of **iodohippurate sodium I^{123}/I^{134}, or Technetium Tc^{99} pententate** renal imaging in the affected kidney in patients with renal artery stenosis, which could lead to confusion in test interpretation

Doses

■ **DOGS:**

a) For treatment of heart failure: Initially, 0.125 mg/kg PO once daily; depending on the severity of pulmonary congestion, dose may be increased to 0.25 mg/kg PO once daily (Label information; *Vasotop®*—Intervet UK)

■ **CATS:**

a) For treatment of arterial hypertension: 0.125 mg/kg PO once daily (Graff & Herve 2003)

■ **HORSES:**

a) For CHF: There is anecdotal evidence that ACE inhibitors may be beneficial in horses and ramipril at 0.2 mg/kg PO once daily has been used, but pharmacokinetic studies are lacking. (Giguere 2008)

Monitoring

■ Clinical signs of CHF

■ Serum electrolytes, creatinine, BUN, urine protein

■ CBC with differential, periodic

■ Blood pressure (if treating hypertension or clinical signs associated with hypotension arise)

Client Information

■ For this drug to be maximally effective it must be given once daily at about the same time each day

■ Do not abruptly stop or reduce therapy without veterinarian's approval

■ Contact veterinarian if vomiting or diarrhea persist, are severe, or if animal's condition deteriorates

Chemistry/Synonyms

Ramipril occurs as a white to almost white, crystalline powder that is sparingly soluble in water and freely soluble in methyl alcohol.

Ramipril may also be known as Hoe-498, ramiprilis, or ramiprilium. There are many international trade names, including: *Altace®*, *Cardase®*, *Delix®*, *Ramase®*, *Triatec®*, and *Tritace®*.

Storage/Stability

Capsules should be stored at room temperature (15–30°C) protected from light in tight containers.

Dosage Forms/Regulatory Status

VETERINARY-LABELED PRODUCTS:

None in the USA; in the UK and in other European countries: Ramipril Tablets: 0.625 mg, 1.25 mg, 2.5 mg, & 5 mg; *Vasotop®* (Intervet); (Rx). Approved for use in dogs.

HUMAN-LABELED PRODUCTS:

Ramipril Oral Tablets/Capsules: 1.25 mg, 2.5 mg, 5 mg, & 10 mg; *Altace®* (Monarch); generic; (Rx)

References

Coulet, M. & S. Burgaud (2002). Pharmacokinetics of ramipril and ramiprilat and angiotensin converting enzyme (ACE) activity after single and repeated oral administration of ramipril to cats. Proceedings: 12th ECVIM-CA Congress. Accessed via: Veterinary Information Network. http://goo.gl/jkrfB

Giguere, S. (2008). Diagnostic Approach to the Equine Patient with Cardiac Disease: A Proceedingts; Case Series. Proceedings: IVECCS. Accessed via: Veterinary Information Network. http://goo.gl/Qk01s

Graff, J. & C. Herve (2003). Efficacy of ramipril in the treatment of arterial hypertension in cats. Proceedings: 13th ECVIM-CA Congress. Accessed via: Veterinary Information Network. http://goo.gl/EKA0e

Lefebvre, H., E. Jeunesse, et al. (2006). Pharmacokinetic and pharmacodynamic parameters of ramipril and ramiprilat in healthy dogs and dogs with reduced glomerular filtration rate. *J Vet Intern Med* **20:** 499–507.

MacDonald, K., M. Kittleson, et al. (2006). The effect of ramipril on left ventricular mass, myocardial fibrosis, diastolic function, and plasma neurohormones in Maine Coon cats with familial hypertrophic cardiomyopathy without heart failure. *J Vet Intern Med* **20**(5): 1093–1105.

RANITIDINE HCL

(rah-*nit*-a-deen)   Zantac®

H₂ RECEPTOR ANTAGONIST;
PROKINETIC

Prescriber Highlights

▶ H₂ receptor antagonist similar to cimetidine, but fewer drug interactions; used to reduce acid output in stomach; also has prokinetic activity

▶ Contraindications: Hypersensitivity. Caution: Geriatric patients, hepatic or renal insufficiency

▶ Adverse Effects: Rare. IV boluses may cause vomiting. Potentially: Mental confusion, agranulocytosis, & transient cardiac arrhythmias (too rapid IV injection). Pain at the injection site after IM administration.

Uses/Indications

In veterinary medicine, ranitidine has been used for the treatment and/or prophylaxis of gastric, abomasal, and duodenal ulcers, uremic gastritis, stress-related or drug-induced erosive gastritis, esophagitis, duodenal gastric reflux and esophageal reflux. It has also been employed to treat hypersecretory conditions associated with gastrinomas and systemic mastocytosis. Because of its effects on gastric motility, ranitidine may be useful in increasing gastric emptying, particularly when delayed gastric emptying is associated with gastric ulcer disease. Ranitidine may also be useful to stimulate colonic activity in cats via its prokinetic effects.

Pharmacology/Actions

At the H₂ receptors of the parietal cells, ranitidine competitively inhibits histamine, thereby reducing gastric acid output both during basal conditions and when stimulated by food, amino acids, pentagastrin, histamine, or insulin. Ranitidine is between 3–13 times more potent (on a molar basis) as cimetidine.

While ranitidine may cause gastric emptying times to be delayed, it more likely will stimulate GI motility by inhibiting acetylcholinesterase (thereby increasing acetylcholine at muscarinic receptors). Lower esophageal sphincter pressures may be increased by ranitidine. By decreasing the amount of gastric juice produced, ranitidine decreases the amount of pepsin secreted.

Ranitidine, unlike cimetidine, does not appear to have any appreciable effect on serum prolactin levels, although it may inhibit the release of vasopressin.

Pharmacokinetics

In dogs, the oral bioavailability is approximately 81%, serum half-life is 2.2 hours and volume of distribution 2.6 L/kg.

In horses, oral ranitidine has a bioavailability of about 27% in adults and 38% in foals. Peak levels after oral dosing occur in about 100 minutes in adults and 60 minutes in foals. Apparent volume of distribution is approximately 1.1 L/kg and 1.5 L/kg in adults and foals, respectively. Clearance in adults is approximately 10 mL/min/kg and 13.3 mL/min/kg in foals.

In humans, ranitidine is absorbed rapidly after oral administration, but undergoes extensive first-pass metabolism with a net systemic bioavailability of approximately 50%. Peak levels occur at about 2–3 hours after oral dosing. Food does not appreciably alter the extent of absorption or the peak serum levels attained.

Ranitidine is distributed widely throughout the body and is only 10–19% bound to plasma proteins. Ranitidine is distributed into human milk at levels 25–100% of those found in plasma.

Ranitidine is both excreted in the urine by the kidneys (via glomerular filtration and tubular secretion) and metabolized in the liver to inactive metabolites; accumulation of the drug can occur in patients with renal insufficiency. The serum half-life of ranitidine in humans averages 2–3 hours. The duration of action at usual doses is from 8–12 hours.

Contraindications/Precautions/Warnings

Ranitidine is contraindicated in patients who are hypersensitive to it. It should be used cautiously and possibly at reduced dosage in patients with diminished renal function. Ranitidine has caused increased serum ALT levels in humans receiving high, IV doses for longer than 5 days. The manufacturer recommends that with high dose, chronic therapy, serum ALT values be considered for monitoring.

Adverse Effects

Adverse effects appear to be very rare in animals at the dosages generally used. Potential adverse effects (documented in humans) that might be seen include mental confusion and headache. Rarely, agranulocytosis may develop and, if given rapidly IV, transient cardiac arrhythmias may be seen. Pain at the injection site may be noted after IM administration. IV boluses have been associated with vomiting in small animals.

Reproductive/Nursing Safety

In humans, the FDA categorizes this drug as category **B** for use during pregnancy (*Animal studies have not yet demonstrated risk to the fetus, but there are no adequate studies in pregnant women; or animal studies have shown an adverse effect, but adequate studies in pregnant women have not demonstrated a risk to the fetus in the first trimester of pregnancy, and there is no evidence of risk in later trimesters.*) In a separate system evaluating the safety of drugs in canine and feline pregnancy (Papich 1989), this drug is categorized as class: **B** (*Safe for use if used cautiously. Studies in laboratory animals may have uncovered some risk, but these drugs appear to be safe in dogs and cats* *or these drugs are safe if they are not administered when the animal is near term.*)

Ranitidine is excreted in human breast milk with milk:plasma ratios of approximately 5:1 to 12:1. The drug is not recommended to be used in nursing humans; use with caution in nursing veterinary patients.

Overdosage/Acute Toxicity

Clinical experience with ranitidine overdosage is limited. In laboratory animals, very high dosages (225 mg/kg/day) have been associated with muscular tremors, vomiting and rapid respirations. Single doses of 1 gram/kg in rodents did not cause death.

Treatment of overdoses in animals should be handled using standard protocols for oral ingestions of drugs; clinical signs may be treated symptomatically and supportively if necessary. Hemodialysis and peritoneal dialysis have been noted to remove ranitidine from the body.

Drug Interactions

Unlike cimetidine, ranitidine appears to have much less effect on the hepatic metabolism of drugs and is unlikely to cause clinically relevant drug interactions via this mechanism. The following drug interactions have either been reported or are theoretical in humans or animals receiving ranitidine and may be of significance in veterinary patients:

- ■ **ACETAMINOPHEN:** Ranitidine (dose-dependent) may inhibit acetaminophen metabolism
- ■ **ANTACIDS (high doses):** May decrease the absorption of ranitidine; give at separate times (2 hours apart) if used concurrently
- ■ **KETOCONAZOLE, ITRACONAZOLE:** Absorption may be reduced secondary to increased gastric pH
- ■ **METOPROLOL:** Ranitidine may increase metoprolol half-life, and peak levels
- ■ **NIFEDIPINE:** Ranitidine may increase nifedipine AUC by 30%
- ■ **PROPANTHELINE:** Delays the absorption but increases the peak serum level of ranitidine; relative bioavailability of ranitidine may be increased by 23% when propantheline is administered concomitantly with ranitidine
- ■ **VITAMIN B-12:** Long-term ranitidine use may reduce oral absorption of B-12

Laboratory Considerations

- ■ Ranitidine may cause a false-positive **urine protein** reading when using *Multistix®*. The sulfosalicylic acid reagent is recommended for determining urine protein when the patient is concomitantly receiving ranitidine.

Doses

■ **DOGS:**

For esophagitis:

a) 1–2 mg/kg PO twice daily (Watrous 1989)

For chronic gastritis:

a) 0.5 mg/kg PO twice daily (Hall, J.A. & Twedt 1989)

For ulcer disease:

a) 0.5–2 mg/kg PO, IV or IM q8–12h (Haskins 2000)

b) 2 mg/kg PO, IV q8h (Matz 1995)

c) 1–2 mg/kg PO, IV, SC q12h (also used for esophagitis) (Sellon 2007)

d) 2 mg/kg PO, IV q12h (Waddell 2007)

For gastrinoma:

a) 1–2 mg/kg PO, SC, IV q8–12h (Zerbe & Washabau 2000)

b) 0.5 mg/kg PO, IV or SC twice daily (Kay & Richter 1988)

To treat hypergastrinemia secondary to chronic renal failure:

a) 1–2 mg/kg PO twice daily (Morgan 1988)

To treat hyperhistaminemia secondary to mast cell tumors:

a) 2 mg/kg q12h (Fox 1995)

As a prokinetic agent to stimulate gastric contractions:

a) 1–2 mg/kg PO q12h (Hall, J. & Washabau 2000)

■ **CATS:**

For ulcer disease/esophagitis:

a) 2.5 mg/kg IV q12h or 3.5 mg/kg PO q12h (Matz 1995), (Johnson 1996)

b) 1–2 mg/kg PO, IV, SC q12h (Sellon 2007)

c) 2 mg/kg PO, IV q12h (Waddell 2007)

As a prokinetic agent to stimulate colonic motility:

a) 1–2 mg/kg PO q8–12h (Washabau & Holt 2000)

b) 1–2 mg/kg PO q12h (Scherk 2003)

■ **FERRETS:**

a) For *Helicobacter mustelae*: Ranitidine bismuth citrate (**Note:** Not available commercially in USA; must be compounded) at 24 mg/kg PO q8-12h and clarithromycin (12.5 mg/kg PO q8-12h). Treat with both for 14 days. (Johnson-Delaney 2008)

■ **HORSES: (Note:** ARCI UCGFS Class 5 Drug)

a) Foals: 1.5 mg/kg IV q8h or 6.6 mg/kg PO q8h often used with omeprazole (4 mg/kg PO q24h). (Paradis 2008)b)

Foals: 6.6 mg/kg IV q4h *or* 0.8–2.2 mg/kg IV four times a day; 5–10 mg/kg PO two to four times a day. (Wilkins 2004)

c) 1.5–2 mg/kg IV or IM q6–8h; 6.6 mg/kg PO q8h (Sanchez 2004)

■ **SMALL MAMMALS:**

a) As a prokinetic in rabbits: 0.5 mg/kg IV q24 with cisapride (0.5 mg/kg PO q8h). (Lichtenberger 2008)

b) For suspected gastric ulceration in rabbits: 2–5 mg/kg PO twice daily. (Bryan 2009)

Monitoring
■ Clinical efficacy (dependent on reason for use); monitored by decrease in clinical signs, endoscopic examination, blood in feces, etc.

Client Information
■ To maximize the benefit of this medication, it must be administered as prescribed by the veterinarian; symptoms may reoccur if dosages are missed.

Chemistry/Synonyms
An H_2 receptor antagonist, ranitidine HCl occurs as a white to pale-yellow granular substance with a bitter taste and a sulfur-like odor. The drug has pK_as of 8.2 and 2.7. One gram is approximately soluble in 1.5 mL of water or 6 mL of alcohol. The commercially available injection has a pH of 6.7–7.3.

Ranitidine HCl may also be known as: AH-19065, ranitidini hydrochloridum; many trade names are available.

Storage/Stability
Ranitidine tablets should be stored in tight, light-resistant containers at room temperature. The injectable product should be stored protected from light and at a temperature less than 30°C. A slight darkening of the injectable solution does not affect the potency of the drug.

Compatibility/Compounding Considerations
Ranitidine injection is reportedly stable up to 48 hours when mixed with the commonly used IV solutions (including 5% sodium bicarbonate).

Dosage Forms/Regulatory Status
VETERINARY-LABELED PRODUCTS: None

The ARCI (Racing Commissioners International) has designated this drug as a class 5 substance. See the appendix for more information.

HUMAN-LABELED PRODUCTS:

Ranitidine HCl Oral Tablets: 75 mg, 150 mg & 300 mg; *Zantac*® (GlaxoSmithKline); *Zantac*® *75* (Boehringer Ingelheim); generic; (Rx or OTC)

Ranitidine HCl Effervescent Oral Tablets: 25 mg & 150 mg; *Zantac*® *EFFERdose* (GlaxoSmithKline); (Rx)

Ranitidine HCl Solution: 15 mg/mL in 473 mL & 480 mL; *Zantac*® (GlaxoSmithKline); generic; (Rx)

Ranitidine HCl Injection: 1 mg/mL (premixed) & 25 mg/mL in 2 mL single-dose and 6 mL multi-dose vials; *Zantac*® (GlaxoSmithKline); generic (Bedford); (Rx)

References
Bryan, J. (2009). Rabbit GI Physiology: What do I do now? Proceedings: WVC. Accessed via: Veterinary Information Network. http://goo.gl/cAD9L

Fox, L. (1995). The paraneoplastic disorders. Kirk's Current Veterinary Therapy:XII. J Bonagura Ed. Philadelphia, W.B. Saunders: 530–542.

Hall, J. & R. Washabau (2000). Gastric Prokinetic Agents. Kirk's Current Veterinary Therapy: XIII Small Animal Practice. J Bonagura Ed. Philadelphia, WB Saunders: 609–617.

Hall, J.A. & D.C. Twedt (1989). Diseases of the Stomach. Handbook of Small Animal Practice. RV Morgan Ed. New York, Churchill LIvingstone: 371–384.

Haskins, S. (2000). Therapy for Shock. Kirk's Current Veterinary Therapy: XIII Small Animal Practice. J Bonagura Ed. Philadelphia, WB Saunders: 140–147.

Johnson, S. (1996). Nonsteroidal antiinflammatory analgesics to manage acute pain in dogs and cats. Comp CE(October 1996): 1117–1123.

Johnson-Delaney, C. (2008). Gastrointestinal Diseases in Ferrets. Proceedings: WVC. Accessed via: Veterinary Information Network. http://goo.gl/UC3zs

Kay, A.D. & K.P. Richter (1988). Diseases of the parathyroid glands. Handbook of Small Animal Practice. RV Morgan Ed. New York, Churchill Livingstone: 521–526.

Lichtenberger, M. (2008). What's new in small mammal critical care. Proceedings: AAV. http://goo.gl/f4wXv

Matz, M. (1995). Gastrointestinal ulcer therapy. Kirk's Current Veterinary Therapy:XII. J Bonagura Ed. Philadelphia, W.B. Saunders: 706–710.

Morgan, R.V., Ed. (1988). Handbook of Small Animal Practice. New York, Churchill Livingstone.

Papich, M. (1989). Effects of drugs on pregnancy. Current Veterinary Therapy X: Small Animal Practice. R Kirk Ed. Philadelphia, Saunders: 1291–1299.

Paradis, M. (2008). Gastrointestinal Problems in the Equine Neonate. Proceedings: World Veterinary Congress. Accessed via: Veterinary Information Network. http://goo.gl/pZkEx

Sanchez, C. (2004). Disorders of the stomach. Equine Internal Medicine, 2nd Ed. S Reed, W Bayly and D Sellon Eds. Philadelphia, Saunders: 863–872.

Scherk, M. (2003). Feline megacolon. Proceedings: World Small Animal Veterinary Assoc World Congress. Accessed via: Veterinary Information Network. http://goo.gl/v69lu

Sellon, R. (2007). Gastric Ulcers. Proceedings: Western Vet Conf. Accessed via: Veterinary Information Network. http://goo.gl/hW7b9

Waddell, L. (2007). Acute renal failure. Proceedings: Western Vet Conference. Accessed via: Veterinary Information Network. http://goo.gl/RlcNc

Washabau, R. & D. Holt (2000). Feline Constipation and Idiopathic Megacolon. Kirk's Current Veterinary Therapy: XIII Small Animal Practice. J Bonagura Ed. Philadelphia, WB Saunders: 648–652.

Watrous, B.J. (1989). Diseases of the esophagus. Handbook of Small Animal Practice. RV Morgan Ed. New York, Churchill LIvingstone: 357–370.

Wilkins, P. (2004). Disorders of foals. Equine Internal Medicine, 2nd Ed. S Reed, W Bayly and D Sellon Eds. Philadelphia, Saunders: 1381–1431.

Zerbe, C. & R. Washabau (2000). Gastrointestinal endocrine disease. Textbook of Veterinary Internal Medicine: Diseases of the Dog and Cat. S Ettinger and E Feldman Eds. Philadelphia, WB Saunders. 2: 1500–1508.

1206   REMIFENTANIL HCL

REMIFENTANIL HCL

(rem-i-*fen*-ta-nil)   Ultiva®

ULTRA-SHORT ACTING OPIOID ANALGESIC

Prescriber Highlights

▶ Opioid similar to fentanyl; used primarily as an anesthesia adjunct

▶ Degraded by esterases in plasma, red cells, and tissues; can be used for prolonged procedures in patients with renal or hepatic dysfunction

▶ Because of its short duration of action, may reduce recovery times

▶ Little veterinary clinical experience at present

▶ Currently much more expensive than fentanyl

Uses/Indications

Remifentanil is a *mu*-opioid structurally related to fentanyl. Because remifentanil is primarily metabolized by tissue and red cell esterases, it can safely be used in patients with either hepatic or renal impairment. Its very short duration of action also is beneficial, because if adverse effects occur (*e.g.*, respiratory depression, bradycardia), reversal with naloxone should rarely be required. A possible advantage of using remifentanil versus fentanyl as an anesthesia adjunct is that recovery times may be faster with remifentanil. There is some remifentanil research on dogs and cats published, but there is little clinical experience in veterinary medicine with this agent.

Pharmacology/Actions

Remifentanil hydrochloride is a *mu*-opioid agonist with rapid onset of analgesic action and peak effect, and short duration of action. *Mu*-receptors are found primarily in the pain regulating areas of the brain. They are thought to contribute to the analgesia, euphoria, respiratory depression, physical dependence, miosis, and hypothermic actions of opiates. Receptors for opiate analgesics are found in high concentrations in the limbic system, spinal cord, thalamus, hypothalamus, striatum, and midbrain. They are also found in tissues such as the gastrointestinal tract, urinary tract, and in other smooth muscles. The pharmacology of the opiate agonists is discussed in more detail in the monograph, Narcotic (opiate) Agonist Analgesics.

Unlike other opioids, remifentanil is rapidly metabolized by hydrolysis of the propanoic acid-methyl ester linkage by nonspecific blood and tissue esterases. Remifentanil is not appreciably metabolized by the liver or metabolized by plasma cholinesterase (pseudocholinesterase). Adverse effects (bradycardia, respiratory depression, hypotension) are dose dependent and similar to other *mu*-opioids. When used as an anesthesia adjunct, remifentanil, like other

opioids, has a ceiling effect (increased doses do not enhance analgesia).

Opioid activity of remifentanil is antagonized by antagonists such as naloxone.

In dogs, remifentanil is equally efficacious, but about half as potent, as fentanyl but recovery from remifentanil anesthesia is much more rapid, especially after continuous infusions maintained for 6+ hours (Michelsen *et al.* 1996). Remifentanil reduced sevoflurane MAC similarly to fentanyl in dogs, but allowed shorter recovery times (Martinez & Lepiz 2008). In another dog study, remifentanil given as a CRI reduced the dosage requirements of propofol for maintaining target-controlled infusion system−based anesthesia. (Beier *et al.* 2009) The principle carboxylic acid metabolite of remifentanil (GR90291) has been shown to be at least 4000 times less potent in dogs as the parent drug (Hoke *et al.* 1997).

In cats, remifentanil reduced isoflurane MAC similarly (about 25% reduction) at the three doses studied (Ferreira *et al.* 2009). However in another cat study, remifentanil did not alter the MAC thresholds for isoflurane, but did produce analgesia, reflected by increased thermal thresholds. The authors state that the extent or existence of an analgesic-MAC relationship cannot be assumed for all analgesics in all species. They concluded that measures of anesthetic immobility need not bear any relation to measures of analgesic efficacy. Consequently, MAC-sparing effects should not be used to infer analgesic effects without prior validation of the nature of such a relationship for a specific agent and species (Brosnan *et al.* 2009).

Pharmacokinetics

In dogs, remifentanil is rapidly distributed into the CNS with a blood-brain equilibration half-life of 2.3−5.2 minutes. It has an terminal elimination half-life of 6 minutes (Hoke *et al.* 1997).

In cats, remifentanil has a moderately high volume of distribution (7.6 L/kg) and a high clearance (766 mL/min/kg) and a short terminal elimination half-life (17.4 minutes). In anesthetized (isoflurane) cats, volume of distribution of remifentanil is decreased (1.65 L/kg), but elimination half-life is not significantly altered (Pypendop *et al.* 2008).

In humans after IV doses, remifentanil is rapidly distributed into the CNS and has a peak effect 1-3 minutes after administration. Remifentanil is approximately 70% bound to plasma proteins with the majority bound to alpha-1-acid-glycoprotein. Remifentanil has an effective biological half-life of 3-10 minutes in human patients. The pharmacokinetics of remifentanil are not appreciably altered in patients with renal or hepatic failure.

Contraindications/Precautions/Warnings

Remifentanil is contraindicated in patients hypersensitive to it or other fentanyl analogs. As the injection contains glycine, it is contraindicated for epidural or intrathecal administration.

Because of the possibility of significant respiratory depression or bradycardia, it should be administered only in a monitored anesthesia care setting. Continuous infusions should only be administered by an infusion device.

In morbidly obese patients, the drug dose should be based upon ideal body weight.

Adverse Effects

Remifentanil has an adverse effect profile similar to other *mu*-opioids. Respiratory depression, including apnea, bradyarrhythmias and hypotension are possible. Increased body temperatures in cats may be noted. Anaphylaxis is very rare, but possible.

Reproductive/Nursing Safety

Remifentanil appears to be relatively safe to use during pregnancy. No teratogenic effects were observed after administration of remifentanil at doses up to 5 mg/kg in rats and 0.8 mg/kg in rabbits. For humans, the FDA categorizes this drug as category C for use during pregnancy *(Animal studies have shown an adverse effect on the fetus, but there are no adequate studies in humans; or there are no animal reproduction studies and no adequate studies in humans.)* It is unknown if remifentanil is excreted into milk, but clinical effect in offspring seems unlikely. However, weigh the potential risks of using this medication versus the benefits in pregnant or nursing animals.

Overdosage/Acute Toxicity

As with all potent opioid analgesics, overdosage should manifest as enhancement of the drug's non-analgesic pharmacological effects. Clinical signs may include: apnea, chest-wall rigidity, seizures, hypoxemia, hypotension, and bradycardia.

Discontinue drug administration and give supportive therapy including mechanical ventilation and oxygen administration. Oftentimes, this is all that is required since the drug is cleared so rapidly. Additional supportive therapy can include IV fluids, glycopyrrolate or atropine for bradycardia or hypotension. Naloxone may also be used to reverse the drug's *mu*-activity, but can lead to acute pain and sympathetic hyperactivity.

Drug Interactions

Remifentanil clearance is not altered by concomitant administration of thiopental, isoflurane, or propofol.

The following drug interactions have either been reported or are theoretical in humans or animals receiving fentanyl and may apply to remifentanil and be of significance in veterinary patients:

- ■ **CNS DEPRESSANTS, OTHER:** Additive CNS effects possible

- ■ **DIURETICS:** Opiates may decrease efficacy in CHF patients

- ■ **MONOAMINE OXIDASE INHIBITORS (e.g., amitraz, and possibly selegiline):** Severe and unpredictable opiate potentiation may be seen; fentanyl not recommended (in humans) if MAO inhibitor has been used within 14 days

- ■ **MUSCLE RELAXANTS, SKELETAL:** Remifentanil may enhance neuromuscular blockade

- ■ **NITROUS OXIDE:** High remifentanil doses may cause cardiovascular depression

- ■ **TRICYCLIC ANTIDEPRESSANTS (clomipramine, amitriptyline, etc.):** Fentanyl may exacerbate the effects of tricyclic antidepressants

- ■ **WARFARIN:** Opiates may potentiate anticoagulant activity

Laboratory Considerations

- ■ As they may increase biliary tract pressure, opiates can increase plasma amylase and lipase values up to 24 hours following their administration.

Doses

Note: Do not confuse microgram/kg/HOUR and microgram/kg/MINUTE CRI rates

- ■ **DOGS:**
  As an analgesic adjunct to general anesthesia:

  a) 4 micrograms/kg bolus IV, followed by 6–20 micrograms/kg/hr CRI. (Spelts 2009)

  b) 1 microgram/kg IV loading dose slowly over 2–3 minutes, followed by a 0.1–0.2 microgram/kg/minute CRI. (Grint 2008)

- ■ **CATS:**
  As an analgesic adjunct to general anesthesia:

  a) In the study, in propofol-anesthetized (0.3 micrograms/kg/minute) cats an infusion rate of remifentanil at 0.2 micrograms/kg/minute allowed ovariohysterectomies to be performed; an infusion rate of 0.3 micrograms/kg/minute was required to reduce the incidence of stimulus-induced movement after electrical noxious stimulation. (Correa *et al.* 2007)

Monitoring

- ■ Cardiac and respiratory rate

- ■ Pulse oximetry or other methods to measure blood oxygenation when used for anesthesia

- ■ Blood pressure

Chemistry/Synonyms

Remifentanil hydrochloride has a pKa of 7.07 and partition coefficient n-octanol:water of 17.9 at pH 7.3. The commercially available injection has a pH of 2.5–3.5.

Remifentanil may also be known as: GI-87084B, remifentanilo, rémifentanil, or remifentanili. Trade names include: *Ultiva*® and *Remicit*®.

Storage/Stability

Prior to reconstitution, store lyophilized powder for solution between 2°-25°C (36°-77° F). It is stable for 24 hours at room temperature after reconstitution and further dilution to concentrations of 20–250 micrograms/mL with the following IV fluids: sterile water for injection; D_5W; D_5NS, 0.9% sodium chloride, 0.45% sodium chloride; D_5LR; it is stable for 4 hours at room temperature after reconstitution and further dilution to concentrations of 20–250 micrograms/mL with lactated Ringer's injection. The UK licensed product information states that it should NOT be mixed with lactated Ringer's injection with or without 5% glucose.

Compatibility/Compounding Considerations

To reconstitute solution, add 1 mL of diluent per mg of remifentanil. Shake well to dissolve. When reconstituted as directed, the solution contains approximately 1 mg of remifentanil activity per mL. It should then be further diluted to a final concentration of 20, 25, 50, or 250 micrograms per mL prior to administration. Do not administer remifentanil without dilution.

Dosage Forms/Regulatory Status

VETERINARY-LABELED PRODUCTS: None

HUMAN-LABELED PRODUCTS:

Remifentanil HCl Powder for reconstitution (IV use only): 1 mg (3 mL vial), 2 mg (5 mL vial), 5 mg (10 mL vial); *Ultiva®* (Bioniche); (Rx, C-II controlled substance)

References

Beier, S.L., A.J.D. Aguiar, et al. (2009). Effect of remifentanil on requirements for propofol administered by use of a target-controlled infusion system for maintaining anesthesia in dogs. *American Journal of Veterinary Research* 70(6): 703–709.

Brosnan, R.J., B.H. Pypendop, et al. (2009). Effects of remifentanil on measures of anesthetic immobility and analgesia in cats. *American Journal of Veterinary Research* 70(9): 1065–1071.

Correa, M.D., A.J.D. Aguiar, et al. (2007). Effects of remifentanil infusion regimens on cardiovascular function and responses to noxious stimulation in propofol-anesthetized cats. *American Journal of Veterinary Research* 68(9): 932–940.

Ferreira, T.H., A.J.A. Aguiar, et al. (2009). Effect of remifentanil hydrochloride administered via constant rate infusion on the minimum alveolar concentration of isoflurane in cats. *American Journal of Veterinary Research* 70(5): 581–588.

Grint, N. (2008). Constant Rate Infusions (CRIS) in Pain Management. Proceedings: BSAVA. Accessed via: Veterinary Information Network. http://goo.gl/CIXUX

Hoke, J.F., F. Cunningham, et al. (1997). Comparative pharmacokinetics and pharmacodynamics of remifentanil, its principle metabolite (GR90291) and alfentanil in dogs. *Journal of Pharmacology and Experimental Therapeutics* 281(1): 226–232.

Martinez, E. & M. Lepiz (2008). Effect of Remifentanil and Fentanyl on Minimum Alveolar Concentration and Recovery in Sevoflurane-Anesthetized Dogs. Proceedings: IVECCS. Accessed via: Veterinary Information Network. http://goo.gl/8kdv7

Michelsen, L.G., M. Salmenpera, et al. (1996). Anesthetic potency of remifentanil in dogs. *Anesthesiology* 84(4): 865–872.

Pypendop, B.H., R.J. Brosnan, et al. (2008). Pharmacokinetics of remifentanil in conscious cats and cats anesthetized with isoflurane. *American Journal of Veterinary Research* 69(4): 531–536.

Spelts, K. (2009). Anesthesia for the critically ill patient. Proceedings: WVC. Accessed via: Veterinary Information Network. http://goo.gl/fzgwp

RIFAMPIN

(*rif*-am-pin)   Rifadin®, Rimactane®

ANTIMICROBIAL

Prescriber Highlights

▶ Antimicrobial with activity against a variety of microbes (Rhodococcus, mycobacteria, staphylococci; has some antifungal & antiviral activity as well.

▶ Contraindications: Hypersensitivity to it or other rifamycins

▶ Caution: Preexisting hepatic dysfunction (may need to reduce dosage)

▶ Adverse Effects: Uncommon; potentially rashes, GI distress, & increases in liver enzymes.

▶ Should not be used alone as resistance develops rapidly

▶ Preferably, give on an empty stomach

▶ May cause red/orange urine, tears, & sweat (harmless)

▶ Drug Interactions, lab interactions

Uses/Indications

The principle use of rifampin in veterinary medicine is in the treatment of *Rhodococcus equi* (*Corynebacterium equi*) infections (usually with erythromycin estolate) in young horses. It may also be useful to treat proliferative enteropathy caused by *Lawsonia intracellularis* in foals.

In small animals, the drug is sometimes used in combination with other antifungal agents (amphotericin B and 5-FC) in the treatment of histoplasmosis or aspergillosis with CNS involvement.

Pharmacology/Actions

Rifampin may act as either a bactericidal or bacteriostatic antimicrobial dependent upon the susceptibility of the organism and the concentration of the drug. Rifampin acts by inhibiting DNA-dependent RNA polymerase in susceptible organisms, thereby suppressing the initiation of chain formation for RNA synthesis. It does not inhibit the mammalian enzyme.

Rifampin is active against a variety of mycobacterium species and *Staphylococcus aureus*, Neisseria, Haemophilus, and *Rhodococcus equi* (*C. equi*). At very high levels, rifampin has activity against poxviruses, adenoviruses, and *Chlamydia trachomatis*. Rifampin has antifungal activity when combined with other antifungal agents.

Pharmacokinetics

After oral administration, rifampin is relatively well absorbed from the GI tract. Oral bioavailability is reportedly about 40−70% in horses and 37% in adult sheep. If food is given concurrently, peak plasma levels may be delayed and slightly reduced.

Rifampin is very lipophilic and readily penetrates most body tissues (including bone and prostate), cells and fluids (including CSF). It also penetrates abscesses and caseous material. Rifampin is 70−90% bound to serum proteins, is distributed into milk and crosses the placenta. Mean volume of distribution is approximately 0.9 L/kg in horses, and 1.3 L/kg in sheep.

Rifampin is metabolized in the liver to a deacetylated form that also has antibacterial activity. Both this metabolite and unchanged drug are excreted primarily in the bile, but up to 30% may be excreted in the urine. The parent drug is substantially reabsorbed in the gut, but the metabolite is not. Reported elimination half-lives for various species are: 6−8 hours (horses), 8 hours (dogs), 3−5 hour's (sheep). Because rifampin can induce hepatic microsomal enzymes, elimination rates may increase with time.

Contraindications/Precautions/Warnings

Rifampin is contraindicated in patients hypersensitive to it or to other rifamycins. It should be used with caution in patients with preexisting hepatic dysfunction.

Adverse Effects

Rifampin can cause red-orange colored urine, tears, sweat, and saliva. There are no harmful consequences from this effect. In some species (*e.g.*, humans) rashes, GI distress, and increases in liver enzymes may occur, particularly with long-term use.

Because resistance develops rapidly when rifampin is used alone, it should be used in combination with other effective antibiotics.

Adverse effects in horses are apparently rare, but when combined with erythromycin, mild diarrhea (self-limiting) to severe enterocolitis in foals and mares, hyperthermia, and acute respiratory distress can occur. Although not commercially available, intravenous rifampin has caused CNS depression, sweating, hemolysis, and anorexia in horses.

Reproductive/Nursing Safety

Rodents given high doses of rifampin 150−250 mg/kg/day resulted in some congenital malformations in offspring, but the drug has been used in pregnant women with no reported increases in teratogenicity. In humans, the FDA categorizes this drug as category *C* for use during pregnancy (*Animal studies have shown an adverse effect on the fetus, but there are no adequate studies in humans; or there are no animal reproduction studies and no adequate studies in humans.*)

Rifampin is excreted in maternal milk; use with caution in nursing veterinary patients.

Overdosage/Acute Toxicity

Clinical signs associated with overdosage of oral rifampin generally are extensions of the adverse effects outlined above (GI, orange-red coloring of fluids, and skin), but massive overdoses may cause hepatotoxicity.

There were 8 exposures to rifampin reported to the ASPCA Animal Poison Control Center (APCC) during 2008-2009. In these cases 4 were dogs with 2 showing clinical signs and 3 were cats with all 3 showing clinical signs. Common findings in dogs included central nervous system depression. Common findings in cats included erythema.

Should a massive oral overdosage occur, the gut should be emptied following standard protocols. Liver enzymes should be monitored and supportive treatment initiated if necessary.

Drug Interactions

The following drug interactions have either been reported or are theoretical in humans or animals receiving rifampin and may be of significance in veterinary patients:

- ■ **FLUOROQUINOLONES:** *In vitro* antagonism has been reported when rifampin is used concurrently with fluoroquinolone antibiotics and concurrent use should be avoided

Because rifampin has been documented to induce hepatic microsomal enzymes, drugs that are metabolized by these enzymes may have their elimination half-lives shortened and serum levels decreased; drugs/classes that may be affected by this process include:

- ■ **BARBITURATES**
- ■ **BENZODIAZEPINES (*e.g.*, diazepam)**
- ■ **CHLORAMPHENICOL**
- ■ **CORTICOSTEROIDS**
- ■ **DAPSONE**
- ■ **KETOCONAZOLE**
- ■ **PROPRANOLOL**
- ■ **QUINIDINE**
- ■ **WARFARIN**

Laboratory Considerations

- ■ Microbiologic methods of assaying serum **folate** and **vitamin B$_{12}$** are interfered with by rifampin.
- ■ Rifampin can cause false-positive **BSP** (bromosulfophthalein, sulfobromophthalein) test results by inhibiting the hepatic uptake of the drug

Doses

Note: Because resistance develops rapidly when rifampin is used alone, it should be used in combination with other effective antibiotics.

- ■ **DOGS:**
  a) For combination therapy of atypical Mycobacteria infections; treatment of resistant Staph endocarditis (in combination with amoxicillin/clavulanate or trimethoprim/sulfa): 10−20 mg/kg PO q8−12h (Trepanier 1999)

b) As an alternate treatment for scarred pyo-granulomatous pyoderma: 5–10 mg/kg PO q24h. Must be used with another antibiotic to reduce risk for resistance development. Author generally uses cephalexin or a potentiated sulfonamide. To monitor for potential toxicity, CBC's, liver screens, and a urinalysis should be performed every 2 to 3 weeks. Rifampin is generally used for 4-8 weeks. (Rosenkrantz 2009)

c) For actinomycosis: 10–20 mg/kg PO q12h PO (Hardie 1984)

■ **HORSES:**

For treatment of *Rhodococcus equi* (*C. equi*) infections in foals:

a) Rifampin 5 mg/kg PO two times daily with erythromycin 15–25 mg/kg, PO q12–24h. Conventional treatment, but erythromycin has numerous side effects including enterocolitis in foals and mares, hyperthermia, and acute respiratory distress. Clarithromycin may be superior. (Chaffin 2006)

b) Rifampin 5 mg/kg PO two times daily or 10 mg/kg PO once daily with erythromycin 25 mg/kg, PO q6–8h. Duration of therapy usually takes 4–9 weeks. (Giguere 2003)

For susceptible infections in foals:

a) For treatment of proliferative enteropathy caused by *Lawsonia intracellularis* in foals: Erythromycin estolate (25 mg/kg PO q6–8h) alone or in combination with rifampin: 10 mg/kg PO once daily for a minimum of 21 days (Lavoie & Drolet 2003)

■ **BIRDS:**

For treatment of mycobacteriosis:

a) Rifampin (45 mg/kg PO once daily) in combination with ethambutol (30 mg/kg PO once daily) and one of the following: clofazimine (6 mg/kg PO once daily) or isoniazid (30 mg/kg PO once daily). (Pollock 2007)

Monitoring

■ Clinical efficacy

■ For monitoring *C. equi* infections in foals and response to rifampin/erythromycin: Chest radiographs and plasma fibrinogen levels have been suggested as prognostic indicators when done after 1 week of therapy. (Hillidge and Zertuche 1987)

■ Adverse effects: may consider liver function monitoring with long-term therapy.

Client Information

■ Rifampin may cause urine and other secretions (tears, saliva, etc.) to turn red-orange in color; this is not abnormal

■ Preferably give on an empty stomach

■ May cause softening of stools in horses/foals

Chemistry/Synonyms

A semi-synthetic zwitterion derivative of rifamycin B, rifampin occurs as a red-brown, crystalline powder with a pK_a of 7.9. It is very slightly soluble in water and slightly soluble in alcohol.

Rifampin may also be known as: Ba-41166/E, L-5103, NSC-113926, rifaldazine, rifampicinum, rifamycin AMP; many trade names are available.

Storage/Stability

Rifampin capsules should be stored in tight, light-resistant containers, preferably at room temperature (15–30°C).

Dosage Forms/Regulatory Status

VETERINARY-LABELED PRODUCTS: None

HUMAN-LABELED PRODUCTS:

Rifampin Oral Capsules: 150 mg & 300 mg; *Rifadin*® (Aventis); *Rimactane*® (Novartis); generic; (Rx)

Rifampin Lyophilized Powder for Injection Solution: 600 mg; *Rifadin*® (Aventis); generic; (Rx)

References

Chaffin, M. (2006). Treatment and chemoprophylaxis of Rhodococcus equi pneumonia in foals. Proceedings: ACVIM. Accessed via: Veterinary Information Network. http://goo.gl/wuP4O

Giguere, S. (2003). Rhodococcus equi infections. *Current Therapy in Equine Medicine 5*. C Kollias-Baker Ed. Philadelphia, Saunders: 60–63.

Hardie, E.M. (1984). Actinomycosis and Nocardiosis. *Clinical Microbiology and Infectious Diseases of the Dog and Cat*. CE Greene Ed. Philadelphia, WB Saunders: 663–674.

Lavoie, J.-P. & R. Drolet (2003). Proliferative enteropathy in foals. Proceedings: ACVIM Forum. Accessed via: Veterinary Information Network. http://goo.gl/Q17MH

Pollock, C. (2007). Avian Mycobacteriosis. Proceedings: Western Vet Conf. Accessed via: Veterinary Information Network. http://goo.gl/FsF5P

Rosenkrantz, W. (2009). Pyoderma: Topical and Systemic Treatment. Proceedings: Western Veterinary Conference. Accessed via: Veterinary Information Network. http://goo.gl/Y2VCi

Trepanier, L. (1999). Treating resistant infections in small animals. Proceedings: 17th Annual American College of Veterinary Internal Medicine Meeting, Chicago.

ROBENACOXIB

(roe-ben-ah-*cox*-ib)   Onsior®
NSAID

Prescriber Highlights

▶ Coxib-class NSAID licensed (not FDA-approved in USA at time of writing) for dogs and cats

▶ Appears to be relatively COX-2 specific in both species

▶ Limited clinical experience, but GI effects are the most likely adverse effect seen

Uses/Indications

Robenacoxib is a coxib class non-steroidal anti-inflammatory drug (NSAID) that is available for use in dogs and cats in some countries. Robenacoxib appears to be a selective inhibitor for COX-2 in cats (Giraudel *et al.* 2009; Schmid, Seewald *et al.* 2010) and dogs (King *et al.* 2010). In the UK, the oral tablets are labeled as recommended for the treatment of pain and inflammation associated with chronic osteoarthritis in dogs and for the treatment of acute pain and inflammation associated with musculoskeletal disorders in cats. The injection is labeled for the treatment of pain and inflammation associated with orthopedic or soft tissue surgery in dogs and for the treatment of pain and inflammation associated with soft tissue surgery in cats (*Onsior*®; UK label information).

In an acute synovitis model in dogs, robenacoxib had equivalent analgesic and antiinflammatory efficacy as meloxicam (Schmid, Spreng *et al.* 2010). In a non-inferiority field trial in cats that compared robenacoxib flavored tablets with ketoprofen, robenacoxib had equivalent (non-inferior) efficacy and tolerability, and better palatability. The primary adverse effects in both groups were GI-related and included diarrhea and vomiting (Giraudel *et al.* 2010).

Pharmacology/Actions

Like other NSAIDs in its class, robenacoxib is a selective inhibitor of the cyclooxygenase-2 enzyme (COX-2). COX-2 is the inducible form of the enzyme and is primarily responsible for the production of mediators such as prostaglandin E that can induce pain, inflammation or fever.

In dogs and cats, robenacoxib is approximately 140X (dogs) and 500X (cats) selective for COX-2 as compared to COX-1 when using an *in vitro* whole blood assays for each species.

Creatinine clearance in cats was not altered when determined immediately after a single dose (2 mg/kg SC) of robenacoxib or ketoprofen (Pelligand *et al.* 2010).

Pharmacokinetics

In dogs, peak blood concentrations occur approximately 30 minutes after dosing; food decreases peak levels somewhat. It is highly bound to plasma proteins (>99%). Robenacoxib is metabolized by the liver in dogs and terminal half-life in blood is about 1.2-1.7 hours. Robenacoxib persists longer and at higher concentrations at sites of inflammation than in blood. In dogs, robenacoxib resides longer at inflamed joints compared to blood in both healthy and dogs with osteoarthritis (Silber *et al.* 2010). Excretion is primarily via the biliary route (~65%); remainder is excreted renally. Robenacoxib does not appear to induce hepatic enzymes in dogs.

In cats, after oral administration peak blood concentrations of robenacoxib occur at about 30 minutes and the presence of small amount of food does not impact absorption. As in dogs,

robenacoxib is highly bound to plasma proteins (>99%) and extensively metabolized by the liver. Terminal elimination half-life is about 1.7 hours. Elimination is 70% biliary and 30% renal.

Contraindications/Precautions/Warnings

Robenacoxib is contraindicated in patients with GI ulcers or that are hypersensitive to it (or any of its excipients). It is also contraindicated in dogs with hepatic disease.

Use with caution in dogs or cats with impaired cardiac or renal function or that are dehydrated, hypovolemic or hypotensive and in cats with hepatic dysfunction. If use cannot be avoided in these cases, careful monitoring is required.

Robenacoxib should not be used concurrently with corticosteroids or other NSAIDs. The manufacturer states that: Pre-treatment with other anti-inflammatory medicines may result in additional or increased adverse effects and accordingly a treatment-free period with such substances should be observed for at least 24 hours before the commencement of treatment with robenacoxib. The treatment-free period, however, should take into account the pharmacokinetic properties of the products used previously.

The UK label states: Use this product under strict veterinary monitoring in dogs or cats with a risk of gastrointestinal ulcers, or if the animal previously displayed intolerance to other NSAIDs.

The manufacturer recommends that robenacoxib be used cautiously with other drugs that may affect renal blood flow (*e.g.*, diuretics, ACE inhibitors); additional clinical monitoring is recommended. They also recommend avoiding use with other potentially nephrotoxic drugs as there is a possibility for an increased risk for renal toxicity.

Adverse Effects

In pre-marketing field studies in dogs, GI effects (decreased appetite, vomiting, soft feces, diarrhea) were commonly reported, but were usually mild and self-limiting. Blood in the feces was seen in some patients.

In pre-marketing field studies in cats, transient, mild diarrhea, soft feces or vomiting were commonly reported.

As there is limited clinical experience with this drug, the adverse effect profile will likely change with time.

Reproductive/Nursing Safety

Because the safety of robenacoxib has not been established during pregnancy and lactation in dogs or cats used for breeding, the manufacturer does not recommended its use in pregnant or lactating dogs or cats.

Overdosage/Acute Toxicity

No acute toxicity data was located. Acute overdoses may potentially cause GI, kidney, or liver toxicity. In chronic toxicity studies in healthy young dogs (doses of up to 10 mg/kg/day for 6 months) of robenacoxib did not produce any signs of toxicity. In healthy young cats aged 10 months, once daily doses of 4 mg/kg (2X) SC for 2 days and 10 mg/kg (5X) SC for 3 consecutive days did not produce any signs of toxicity.

Symptomatic, supportive therapy including administration of gastrointestinal protective agents and forced diuresis may be appropriate. Contact an animal poison center for more information.

Drug Interactions

See the Contraindications section above for the manufacturer's warnings on use of robenacoxib with other medications. In addition, the following drug interactions have either been reported or are theoretical in humans or animals receiving NSAIDs and may be of significance in veterinary patients receiving robenacoxib:

- ■ **ACE INHIBITORS (e.g., enalapril, benazepril):** Some NSAIDs can reduce effects on blood pressure
- ■ **ASPIRIN:** May increase the risk of gastrointestinal toxicity (e.g., ulceration, bleeding, vomiting, diarrhea)
- ■ **CORTICOSTEROIDS (e.g., prednisone):** May increase the risk of gastrointestinal toxicity (e.g., ulceration, bleeding, vomiting, diarrhea)
- ■ **DIGOXIN:** NSAIDS may increase serum levels
- ■ **FLUCONAZOLE:** Administration has increased plasma levels of celecoxib in humans and potentially could also affect robenacoxib levels in dogs
- ■ **FUROSEMIDE:** NSAIDs may reduce the saluretic and diuretic effects
- ■ **HIGHLY PROTEIN BOUND DRUGS (phenytoin, valproic acid, oral anticoagulants, other antiinflammatory agents, salicylates, sulfonamides, sulfonylurea antidiabetic agents):** As robenacoxib is highly bound to plasma proteins (>99%) in dogs and cats, it may displace other highly bound drugs or those agents could displace robenacoxib. Increased serum levels, duration of actions and toxicity could occur.
- ■ **METHOTREXATE:** Serious toxicity has occurred when NSAIDs have been used concomitantly with **methotrexate**; use together with extreme caution
- ■ **NEPHROTOXIC DRUGS (e.g., furosemide, aminoglycosides, amphotericin B, etc.):** May enhance the risk of nephrotoxicity development

Laboratory Considerations
- ■ None noted

Doses

- ■ **DOGS:**
  For pain and inflammation associated with chronic osteoarthritis:
  a) 1 mg/kg with a range of 1–2 mg/kg PO

once daily (at the same time every day). A clinical response is normally seen within a week; discontinue after 10 days if no clinical improvement seen. For long term treatment, can adjust to lowest effective dose for the patient. (Adapted from label information; *Onsior*—Novartis. U.K.)

For treatment of pain and inflammation associated with orthopedic or soft tissue surgery:
a) 2 mg/kg SC *once* approximately 30 minutes before the start of surgery. (Adapted from label information; *Onsior Injection*®—Novartis. U.K.)

- ■ **CATS:**
  For the treatment of acute pain and inflammation associated with musculoskeletal disorders:
  a) 1 mg/kg; with a range of 1–2.4 mg/kg PO once daily (at the same time each day) for up to 6 days. Equates to 1 tablet for cats weighing 2.5–<6 kg and 2 tablets for cats weighing 6 kg–<12 kg. Give either without food or with a small amount of food; tablets should not be divided or broken. (Adapted from label information; *Onsior*®—Novartis. U.K.)

For pain and inflammation associated with chronic osteoarthritis:
a) 2 mg/kg SC *once* approximately 30 minutes before the start of surgery. (Adapted from label information; *Onsior Injection*®—Novartis. U.K.)

Monitoring
- ■ Baseline and periodic physical exam including clinical efficacy and adverse effect queries
- ■ Baseline and periodic: CBC, liver function, renal function, and electrolytes; urinalysis. For long term therapy in dogs, the manufacturer recommends that liver enzymes be monitored at the start of therapy, and after 2, 4 and 8 weeks; thereafter it is recommended to continue regular monitoring (every 3–6 months). Therapy should be discontinued if liver enzyme activities increase markedly or the dog shows clinical signs such as anorexia, apathy or vomiting in combination with elevated liver enzymes.

Client Information
- ■ Do not give with food to dogs; give at least 30 minutes before or after food
- ■ Give without or with a small amount of food to cats; do not divide, break or crush tablets
- ■ The manufacturer recommends washing hands after contact with tablets; pregnant women who are near term should wear gloves when handling the drug
- ■ If your animal shows signs of drug toxicity (collapse, listlessness, yellowing of the whites of the eyes) or if vomiting or diarrhea

persist, are severe, or bloody, contact veterinarian immediately

Chemistry/Synonyms

A coxib-class NSAID, robenacoxib's chemical name is 5-ethyl-2-[(2,3,5,6-tetrafluorophenyl)amino]phenyl acetic acid. The commercially available injection is a clear, colorless to slightly pink solution.

Robenacoxib may also be known as robenacoxibum or robénacoxib. Its trade name is *Onsior®*.

Storage/Stability

Store the flavored canine tablets at 25°C (77°F) or less and the feline flavored tablets at no more than 30°C (86°F). The injection should be stored in the refrigerator (2°-8°C) in its original outer carton.

Compatibility/Compounding Considerations

The manufacturer states: In the absence of compatibility studies, this veterinary medicinal product must not be mixed with other veterinary medicinal products.

Dosage Forms/Regulatory Status

VETERINARY-LABELED PRODUCTS: None in USA

In the UK and elsewhere:

Robenacoxib Flavored (yeast, artificial beef) Oral Tablets (not scored): 5 mg, 10 mg, 20 mg, 40 mg; *Onsior®* (Novartis); (Rx). Licensed (in UK) for use in dogs.

Robenacoxib Flavored (yeast) Tablets (not scored): 6 mg; *Onsior®* (Novartis); (Rx). Licensed (in UK) for use in cats.

Robenacoxib Solution for Injection: 20 mg/mL in 20 mL multi-dose vials; *Onsior®* (Novartis); (Rx). Licensed (in UK) for use in dogs and cats.

HUMAN-LABELED PRODUCTS: None

References

Giraudel, J.M., P. Gruet, et al. (2010). Evaluation of orally administered robenacoxib versus ketoprofen for treatment of acute pain and inflammation associated with musculoskeletal disorders in cats. *American Journal of Veterinary Research* 71(7): 710–719.

Giraudel, J.M., P.L. Toutain, et al. (2009). Differential inhibition of cyclooxygenase isoenzymes in the cat by the NSAID robenacoxib. *Journal of Veterinary Pharmacology and Therapeutics* 32(1): 31–40.

King, J.N., C. Rudaz, et al. (2010). In vitro and ex vivo inhibition of canine cyclooxygenase isoforms by robenacoxib: A comparative study. *Research in Veterinary Science* 88(3): 497–506.

Pelligand, L., J.N. King, et al. (2010). Effect of Robenacoxib and Ketoprofen on Exogenous Serum Creatinine Clearance in Conscious Healthy Cats. Proceedings: ECVIM. Accessed via: Veterinary Information Network. http://goo.gl/ylB5I

Schmid, V.B., W. Seewald, et al. (2010). In vitro and ex vivo inhibition of COX isoforms by robenacoxib in the cat: a comparative study. *Journal of Veterinary Pharmacology and Therapeutics* 33(5): 444–452.

Schmid, V.B., D.E. Spreng, et al. (2010). Analgesic and anti-inflammatory actions of robenacoxib in acute joint inflammation in dog. *Journal of Veterinary Pharmacology and Therapeutics* 33(2): 118–131.

Silber, H.E., C. Burgener, et al. (2010). Population Pharmacokinetic Analysis of Blood and Joint Synovial Fluid Concentrations of Robenacoxib from Healthy Dogs and Dogs with Osteoarthritis. *Pharmaceutical Research* 27(12): 2633–2645.

ROCURONIUM BROMIDE

(roe-kyoo-*roe*-nee-um)

Zemuron®, Esmeron®

NON-DEPOLARIZING NEUROMUSCULAR BLOCKER

Prescriber Highlights

▶ Nondepolarizing neuromuscular blocking agent with a rapid to intermediate onset depending on dose and an intermediate duration of action (Alderson et al. 2007)

▶ Faster onset of action than vecuronium or atracurium and fewer adverse effects than succinylcholine

▶ Limited information and clinical experience in dogs, cats, or horses

Uses/Indications

Rocuronium bromide is an aminosteroidal competitive, nondepolarizing neuromuscular blocking agent with a rapid to intermediate onset depending on dose and an intermediate duration of action. Rocuronium has minimal cardiovascular and histamine-releasing effects. It has a similar duration of action as vecuronium and atracurium but a faster onset of action (2–3 times faster than vecuronium). Unlike both vecuronium and atracurium, it is stable in aqueous solutions. Rocuronium's onset of action is nearly as rapid as succinylcholine but it has fewer adverse effects. Clinical experience with rocuronium in veterinary patients is limited but it potentially can be used for rapid endotracheal intubation and to provide muscle relaxation during surgery.

Pharmacology/Actions

Rocuronium is a nondepolarizing neuromuscular blocking agent structurally similar to vecuronium, with a dose-dependent rapid to intermediate onset of action and an intermediate duration. Its mechanism of action is to compete for cholinergic receptors at the motor end plate. Effects are antagonized by acetylcholinesterase inhibitors (*e.g.*, edrophonium or neostigmine). Rocuronium does not appear to induce malignant hyperthermia (MH) as it did not cause hyperthermia in (MH)-susceptible swine. Rocuronium is mildly vagolytic and a slight, transient tachycardia is occasionally seen in human patients.

In dogs, a dose of 0.4 mg/kg IV produces complete neuromuscular blockade in about 2–3 minutes (Dugdale *et al.* 2002). Cats administered 0.6 mg/kg IV caused complete neuromuscular blockade in 90% of cats in the study within

30–60 seconds and did not significantly affect HR in any of the animals. At doses of 0.6 mg/kg, rocuronium appears to have a longer duration of action in dogs (20 minutes) and horses (55 minutes) than in cats (13 minutes) (Auer & Mosing 2006; Auer *et al.* 2007).

Pharmacokinetics

Specific pharmacokinetic parameters for dogs, cats, or horses were not located. Onset of effect and duration of action are noted above. It has been reported that rocuronium is eliminated primarily by the liver in dogs and cats. The principle metabolite, 17-desacetyl-rocuronium has approximately $^1/_{20}$th the neuromuscular-blocking potency of rocuronium in cats.

Contraindications/Precautions/Warnings

Rocuronium is contraindicated in patients hypersensitive to it or other neuromuscular blocking agents. It should only be used in settings where patients can be fully monitored and intubation, mechanical ventilation, oxygen therapy, and antagonist drugs are immediately available.

Rocuronium use should only be undertaken in patients that are adequately anesthetized or sedated.

There are conflicting reports whether rocuronium should be used in patients with hepatic or renal impairment and some have stated that atracurium is preferred in these patients.

Adverse Effects

Other than the effects associated with pharmacologic neuromuscular blockade, rocuronium appears to be well tolerated in the limited number of animals studied. Changes in heart rate and blood pressure may be noted. A more accurate picture of the drug's true adverse effect profile in veterinary patients may be forthcoming if it is more widely used.

In humans, the most common adverse reactions noted are effects on blood pressure (hypo- or hypertension). These are transient and usually mild and have been reported in only about 2% of patients. Severe anaphylaxis has been reported in humans. While rocuronium is thought to possess little histamine releasing effects, histaminoid reactions have been reported. Because the drug reportedly can cause a severe burning pain at the injection site, it is recommended that rocuronium be given only when a deep stage of anesthesia has been achieved.

Reproductive/Nursing Safety

When administered to pregnant laboratory animals, rocuronium did not demonstrate teratogenic effects and it is likely safe to use as long as the patient does not become hypoxic during use. For humans, the FDA categorizes this drug as category *C* for use during pregnancy *(Animal studies have shown an adverse effect on the fetus, but there are no adequate studies in humans; or there are no animal reproduction studies and no adequate studies in humans.)*

The molecular weight of rocuronium is low enough for excretion into milk, but because the drug is ionized at physiologic pH, any clinical effect in offspring seems unlikely. However, weigh the potential risks of using this medication versus the benefits in pregnant or nursing animals.

Overdosage/Acute Toxicity

Overdosage with neuromuscular blocking agents may result in prolonged neuromuscular blockade. The primary treatment is maintenance of the patient's airway, mechanical ventilation and oxygenation, and adequate sedation until recovery function is assured. Only after evidence of recovery is seen should administration of an anticholinesterase drug with an anticholinergic agent be considered. Blood pressure and heart rate should be monitored during an overdose with any necessary supportive treatment considered.

Rocuronium's effects can be reversed by the drug, sugammadex, a binding agent that is specific for rocuronium (and to a lesser extent vecuronium and pancuronium). However in 2008, the FDA (USA) rejected the new drug application based upon concerns that it could cause anaphylaxis.

Drug Interactions

The following drug interactions have either been reported or are theoretical in humans or animals receiving rocuronium and may be of significance in veterinary patients:

- **NON-DEPOLARIZING MUSCLE RELAXANT DRUGS, OTHER:** May have a synergistic effect if used with rocuronium
- **SUCCINYLCHOLINE:** May speed the onset of action and enhance the neuromuscular blocking actions of rocuronium; do not give rocuronium until succinylcholine effects have subsided

The following agents may enhance or prolong the neuromuscular blocking activity of rocuronium:

- **AMINOGLYCOSIDES** (e.g., gentamicin, amikacin)
- **ANESTHETICS** (halothane, isoflurane, sevoflurane)
- **CLINDAMYCIN, LINCOMYCIN**
- **DANTROLENE**
- **MAGNESIUM SALTS**
- **PIPERACILLIN, MEZLOCILLIN**
- **QUINIDINE**
- **TETRACYCLINES**
- **VERAPAMIL**

Laboratory Considerations

- No special consideration noted.

Doses

- **DOGS:**

  As a neuromuscular blocker:

  a) In the study, rocuronium was given as a bolus dose of 0.5 mg/kg and then a CRI was started immediately at

0.2 mg/kg/hour. The authors concluded that rocuronium administered this way was effective in dogs and easily applicable to clinical practice, but that further work is required on infusion titration. (Alderson *et al.* 2007)

■ **CATS:**

As a neuromuscular blocker:

a) In the study, the dose used was 0.6 mg/kg IV. The authors concluded that rocuronium appears to be an effective nondepolarizing muscle relaxant in cats; has a rapid onset and a short duration of action and does not cause significant changes in heart rate. (Auer & Mosing 2006)

■ **HORSES:**

As a neuromuscular blocker:

a) In the study, the dose used was 0.6 mg/kg IV. The authors concluded that rocuronium provided predictable neuromuscular blockade, without hemodynamic changes in isoflurane-anesthetized horses, but there was large variation between the individuals in response to a given dose; monitoring of the neuromuscular block is essential. (Auer *et al.* 2007)

Monitoring

■ Degree of neuromuscular blockade; the manufacturer recommends use of a peripheral nerve stimulator to determine drug response, need for additional doses, and to evaluate recovery

Chemistry/Synonyms

Rocuronium bromide is an aminosteroidal competitive, nondepolarizing neuromuscular blocking agent. It occurs as an almost white or pale yellow, slightly hygroscopic powder. It is freely soluble in water and in dehydrated alcohol. A 1% solution (in water) has a pH 8.9-9.5. The commercially available injection is a sterile, non-pyrogenic, isotonic solution that is clear, colorless to yellow/orange. Each mL contains 10 mg rocuronium bromide and 2 mg sodium acetate and is adjusted to isotonicity with sodium chloride. The pH is adjusted to 4 with acetic acid and/or sodium hydroxide.

Rocuronium may also be known as: ORG-9426, rocuronii, rocuronio, rokuroniowy, or rokuronyum. Rocuronium may also be known by the trade names: *Zemuron®* or *Esmeron®*.

Storage/Stability

Store at 2°-8°C (36°-46°F). Do not freeze. When removed from refrigeration to room temperature storage conditions (25°C; 77°F), use within 60 days. Use opened vials of rocuronium within 30 days. Infusion solutions should be used within 24 hours of mixing. Unused portions of infusion solutions should be discarded.

Compatibility/Compounding Considerations

Rocuronium for injection is **compatible** in solution with: 0.9% NaCl, sterile water for injection, D_5W, D_5NS, and LRS. Rocuronium concentrations up to 5 mg/mL in these solutions are stable for 24 hours at room temperature in plastic bags, glass bottles, and plastic syringe pumps.

Rocuronium is physically **incompatible** when mixed with the following drugs: Amphotericin B, hydrocortisone sodium succinate, amoxicillin, insulin, azathioprine, lipid emulsion (Intralipid), cefazolin, ketorolac, cloxacillin, lorazepam, dexamethasone, methohexital, diazepam, methylprednisolone, erythromycin, thiopental, famotidine, trimethoprim, furosemide, and vancomycin.

Dosage Forms/Regulatory Status

VETERINARY-LABELED PRODUCTS: None

HUMAN-LABELED PRODUCTS:

Rocuronium Bromide for Injection 10 mg/mL in 5 mL & 10 mL multi-dose vials; *Zemuron®* (Schering-Plough), generic; (Rx)

References

Alderson, B., J.M. Senior, et al. (2007). Use of rocuronium administered by continuous infusion in dogs. *Veterinary Anaesthesia and Analgesia* **34**(4): 251–256.

Auer, U. & M. Mosing (2006). A clinical study of the effects of rocuronium in isoflurane-anaesthetized cats. *Veterinary Anaesthesia and Analgesia* **33**(4): 224–228.

Auer, U., C. Uray, et al. (2007). Observations on the muscle relaxant rocuronium bromide in the horse - a dose-response study. *Veterinary Anaesthesia and Analgesia* **34**(2): 75–81.

Dugdale, A.H.A., W.A. Adams, et al. (2002). The clinical use of the neuromuscular blocking agent rocuronium in dogs. *Veterinary Anaesthesia and Analgesia* **29**(1): 49–53.

ROMIFIDINE HCL

(roe-*mif*-ih-deen)   Sedivet®

ALPHA-2 AGONIST SEDATIVE
ANALGESIC

Prescriber Highlights

▶ Alpha-2 agonist with sedative, muscle relaxant & analgesic effects

▶ Indicated in USA for adult horses as a sedative & analgesic to facilitate handling, clinical examinations & procedures, minor surgical procedures, & as preanesthetic prior to the induction of general anesthesia

▶ Labeled in some European countries for use in dogs & cats; has been used extra-label in foals & cattle

▶ Adverse effects in *horses* include bradycardia (possibly profound), first- & second-degree atrioventricular heart block, sinus arrhythmias (dose dependent), initial hypertension followed by hypotension, ataxia, sweating, piloerection, salivation, muscle tremors, penile-relaxation, urination, swelling of face, lips & upper airways, stridor, decreased GI motility, flatulence & mild colic; anaphylaxis possible

▶ In dogs & cats, romifidine may cause bradycardia, cardiac arrhythmias, hypotension, transient hyperglycemia, & alterations in thermoregulation. Dogs may pant, salivate, vomit (less likely than in cats), & develop muscle twitching. Vomiting in cats may be a problem

▶ Adjust dosage if used with other CNS depressant drugs

Uses/Indications

Romifidine is an alpha-2 agonist with sedative, muscle relaxant and analgesic effects. It is indicated (in the USA) for use in adult horses as a sedative and analgesic to facilitate handling, clinical examinations and procedures, minor surgical procedures, and as a preanesthetic prior to the induction of general anesthesia.

In certain European countries, it is approved for use in dogs and cats as a sedative/preanesthetic.

Although not approved, romifidine has been used in cattle and foals.

Pharmacology/Actions

A potent alpha$_2$-adrenergic agonist, romifidine is classified as a sedative/analgesic with muscle relaxant properties. Alpha-2 receptors are found in the CNS and several tissues peripherally; both presynaptically and postsynaptically. In the CNS, the primary action is a feedback inhibition of norepinephrine release. Opioids and alpha-2 agonists may have synergistic analgesic effects.

Pharmacologic effects of romifidine include sedation, analgesia, and reduced catecholamine release from the CNS. Thermoregulatory mechanisms may be altered. Peripherally, an initial vasoconstrictive response occurs with increases in blood pressure. Within minutes a hypotensive phase occurs. Heart rate can significantly decrease secondary to a vagal response to hypertension. A second-degree atrioventricular block may also occur. Antimuscarinic agents can prevent bradycardia, but their use is controversial as they can potentially cause hypertension, increased myocardial oxygen demand, and reduced GI motility. Alpha-2 agonists can transiently slow duodenal motility and increase micturition in horses and can inhibit insulin release from pancreatic islet cells resulting in hyperglycemia. Other effects seen in horses include sweating, mydriasis, decreases in hematocrit, and increased uterine pressure in non-pregnant mares.

In horses, when compared with other alpha-2 agonists (xylazine, detomidine, medetomidine), romifidine does not appear to cause as much ataxia at sedative dosages and has the longest duration of sedation. Duration of analgesia is shorter than the duration of sedation.

Pharmacokinetics

In horses, romifidine has a volume of distribution of approximately 2–3 L/kg, a clearance of about 100 mL/min/kg and an elimination half-life around 135 minutes (Wojtsiak-Wypart *et al.* 2008).

In dogs and cats, bioavailability after IM administration is 86% and 95%, respectively. Bioavailability after subcutaneous injection in dogs is 92%. Peak levels after IM injection occur in approximately 50 minutes in dogs and 25 minutes in cats. After IV injection, volumes of distribution are about 3 L/kg in dogs, and 6 L/kg in cats. Romifidine is biotransformed in the liver. In dogs, about 80% of an administered dose is eliminated in the urine; 20% in the feces. Elimination half-lives are approximately 2 hours for dogs, 6 hours for cats.

Contraindications/Precautions/Warnings

Romifidine should not be used in animals hypersensitive to it or in combination with intravenous potentiated sulfonamides. The label states that this medication should not be used in horses with respiratory disease, hepatic or renal disease, or other systemic conditions of compromised health. It also states that the effects of this medication have not been evaluated in horses with colic, or in foals. Because of its effects on heart rhythm and blood pressure, use very cautiously in horses with preexisting cardiac conditions.

The manufacturer cautions that using with other sedatives, tranquilizers, or opioids may potentiate the adverse effects of romifidine and to avoid using epinephrine as it may potentiate the effects of alpha-2 agonists.

Although animals may appear to be deeply sedated, some may respond (kick, etc.) to external stimuli; use appropriate caution.

When used in dogs and cats, the label for *Romydis®* (Virbac—Ireland) states: "Animals should be restrained to prevent injury, ensure that animals have sufficient fluid intake, and if undergoing prolonged sedation, animals should be prevented from becoming hypothermic. Additionally, care should be taken when used in animals in poor health, suffering from respiratory distress, or in cases of cardiovascular, renal, hepatic or pancreatic disease." Cats with pancreatitis should be closely monitored. Because dogs and, particularly, cats may vomit after receiving romifidine, the manufacturer recommends not feeding for at least 12 hours prior to use.

When used epidurally in dogs, romifidine causes cardiovascular effects similar to when it is administered IV and equivalent monitoring must be performed (Martin-Bouyer *et al.* 2010).

This medication can be absorbed through the skin and via oral routes. Persons administering the medication should handle it carefully and avoid self-exposure.

Adverse Effects

In horses, romifidine may cause bradycardia (possibly profound), first- and second-degree atrioventricular heart block, and sinus arrhythmias (dose dependent). Initially, hypertension may occur followed by hypotension. Other adverse effects can include: ataxia, sweating, piloerection, salivation, muscle tremors, penile-relaxation, urination (occurs about one hour after dose), swelling of face, lips and upper airways, stridor, decreased GI motility, flatulence and mild colic. There is a possibility that horses may react paradoxically (excitation) to romifidine. Rarely, anaphylactic reactions to alpha-2 agonists have been reported in horses.

In dogs and cats romifidine may cause bradycardia, cardiac arrhythmias, hypotension, transient hyperglycemia, and alterations in thermoregulation (body temperature may increase or decrease depending on ambient temperature). Dogs may pant, salivate, vomit (less likely than in cats), and develop muscle twitching.

In cats, vomiting associated with romifidine use can be seen and persist up to 24 hours after dosing. Pancreatitis has been noted in some cats receiving the drug repeatedly every 2 days for 6 days; dose related increases in BUN have been observed. Localized injection site reactions have occurred in cats receiving the medication intramuscularly.

Reproductive/Nursing Safety

The label for the US product states that the effects of this medication have not been evaluated in pregnant mares, horses intended for breeding, or foals.

The labeling for the equine and small animal products approved in Europe states that the drug is contraindicated in pregnant horses during the last month of pregnancy and during pregnancy in dogs and cats.

Overdosage/Acute Toxicity

Horses have received up to 600 micrograms/kg (5X) in experimental studies. Signs exhibited included sinus bradycardia, 2nd degree heart block, occasional apnea and mild respiratory stridor, deep sedation, frequent urination, and sweating. No clinically significant alterations in blood gases, acid-base, hematological or chemical parameters were noted. If necessary, a reversal agent such as atipamezole (at a dose of 30−80 micrograms/kg) or yohimbine may be used to reduce the duration and extent of adverse effects associated with acute toxicity.

Dogs have been administered doses of up to 1 mg/kg (approx. 8−10X) IV daily for up to 4 weeks with no serious adverse effects reported.

Drug Interactions

- ■ **INTRAVENOUS POTENTIATED SULFON-AMIDES (e.g., trimethoprim/sulfa):** The manufacturer warns against using this agent with intravenous potentiated sulfonamides as fatal dysrhythmias may occur

- ■ **OTHER ALPHA-2 AGONISTS (e.g., xylazine, medetomidine, detomidine, clonidine and including epinephrine):** Not recommended to be used together with romifidine as effects may be additive

- ■ **PHENOTHIAZINES (e.g., acepromazine):** Severe hypotension can result

The following drug interactions have either been reported or are theoretical in humans receiving a similar alpha-2 agonist, dexmetomidine and may be of significance in veterinary patients:

- ■ **ANESTHETICS, OPIATES, SEDATIVE/HYPNOTICS:** Effects may be additive; dosage reduction of one or both agents may be required; potential for increased risk for arrhythmias when used in combination with thiopental, ketamine or halothane

Laboratory Considerations

- ■ **ADP-induced platelet aggregation:** Can be inhibited in cats by medetomidine (a related alpha-2 agonist); not known if romifidine can have this effect

Doses

- ■ **HORSES (ADULTS):**
    - a) **For sedation and analgesia:** 40−120 micrograms/kg IV slowly one time. This dose is equivalent to 0.4−1.2 mL per 100 kg (220 lb) body weight using the 1% (10 mg/mL) injection. Degree of sedation and analgesia is dose and time dependent. Onset of action occurs between 30 seconds to 5 minutes and gradually subsides during the next 2−4 hours. Duration of analgesia is shorter than the du-

ration of sedation. See the package insert for expected onset and duration times for sedation and analgesia based upon dose.

As a preanesthetic: 100 micrograms/kg as slow, single IV injection. Induce anesthesia after maximal sedation is achieved. Mild to moderate sedation occurs in 2−4 minutes. Anesthetic doses may need to be decreased to prevent an overdose as romifidine has anesthesia-sparing effects. (Label information; *Sedavet®*—B-I Vetmedica)

■ **DOGS:**

a) **For sedation:** 40−120 micrograms/kg IV, IM or SQ. IV administration causes sedation within approximately 5 minutes. With SC or IM injection sedation is delayed until about 30 minutes post-injection. Sedation depth is also lower than with IV injection. Atipamezole may be used to hasten recovery. A dose of 200 micrograms/kg atipamezole IM will reverse a dose of 120 micrograms/kg of romifidine.

As a preanesthetic: 40−120 micrograms/kg IV, IM or SQ. Induce anesthesia (with propofol or thiopental) approximately 10 minutes after IV injection and 10−15 minutes after IM or SC injection. Label states to maintain anesthesia with halothane. (Label information; *Romydis®*—Virbac-Ireland)

b) **As an analgesic adjunct:** 10−20 micrograms/kg IM, SQ. May combine with an anticholinergic agent in exercise-tolerant patients free from heart disease. (Lamont & Tranquilli 2002)

■ **CATS:**

a) **For sedation:** 200−400 micrograms/kg IV or IM. An IM injection of 200 micrograms/kg gives sedation in about 10 minutes and persists for about 60 minutes. IV administration gives a more rapid onset of action (5 minutes) and the duration is similar to IM. Atipamezole IM 30 minutes after IM romifidine injection may be used to hasten recovery. A dose of 400 micrograms/kg atipamezole IM will reverse a dose of 400 micrograms/kg of romifidine.

As a preanesthetic: 200 micrograms/kg IM 10−15 minutes prior to giving ketamine at 10 mg/kg IM will provide surgical anesthesia for up to 30 minutes. Increasing the dose of romifidine to 400 micrograms/kg will extend period of surgical anesthesia. A "top-up dose" of 50% of the initial doses of romifidine and ketamine can be used to prolong anesthesia. (Label information; *Romydis®*—Virbac-Ireland)

b) **As an analgesic adjunct:** 20−40 micrograms/kg IM, IV. May combine with an anticholinergic agent in exercise-tolerant patients free from heart disease. (Lamont & Tranquilli 2002)

■ **CATTLE:**

Note: Romifidine is not FDA-approved for use in cattle or other food-producing animals in the USA. For guidance with determining withdrawal times, contact FARAD (see Phone Numbers & Websites in the appendix for contact information).

a) **For epidural anesthesia for paralumbar analgesia or laparotomy:** Romifidine 50 micrograms/kg plus morphine 0.1 mg/kg. Duration of analgesia is 12 hours maximum. (Anderson 2006)

Monitoring

■ Level of sedation/analgesia

■ Respiratory rate

■ Heart rate/rhythm; blood pressure (during general anesthesia)

■ Body temperature for longer procedures using higher dosages

Client Information

■ This medication should only be administered by veterinary professionals

■ If clients are involved with handling horses after they are dosed with romifidine, they should be warned that although the horse looks fully sedated it may respond defensively (*e.g.,* kick) when stimulated

Chemistry/Synonyms

Romifidine HCl is an alpha-2 adrenoreceptor agonist that is structurally related to clonidine. It has a molecular weight of 258.1 and occurs as a crystalline, white, odorless substance that is soluble in water. Its chemical name is 2-(2-Bromo-7-fluoroanilino-)-2-imidazoline or 2-Bromo-6-fluoro-N-(1-imidazolin-2yl)analine.

Romifidine may also be known as: STH-2130, romifidiini, romifidin, romifidina, romifidinum, *Romidys®*, *Sedivet®*, and *Sedivan®*.

Storage/Stability

Romifidine HCl injection should be stored at controlled room temperature (15−30°C).

Dosage Forms/Regulatory Status

VETERINARY-LABELED PRODUCTS:

Romifidine HCl 1% (10 mg/mL) Injection; *Sedivet®* (B-I Vetmedica); (Rx). In the USA: FDA-approved for use in horses not intended for human consumption. In the UK, slaughter withdrawal is 6 days for horses.

A small animal product, *Romidys®* (Virbac) containing 1 mg/mL is approved for use in dogs and cats in some European countries.

HUMAN-LABELED PRODUCTS: None

References

Anderson, D. (2006). Urogenital surgery in cows. Proceedings: ACVIM 2006. Accessed via: Veterinary Information Network. http://goo.gl/lu6YB

Lamont, L. & W. Tranquilli (2002). Alpha2–Agonists. *Handbook of Veterinary Pain Management.* J Gaynor and W Muir Eds., Mosby: 199–220.

Martin-Bouyer, V., S. Schauvliege, et al. (2010). Cardiovascular effects following epidural injection of romifidine in isoflurane-anaesthetized dogs. *Veterinary Anaesthesia and Analgesia* 37(2): 87–96.

Wojtsiak-Wypart, M., L. Soma, et al. (2008). Pharmacokinetics and Pharmacodynamics of Romifidine Hydrochloride in the Horse. Peroceedings: IVECCS. Accessed via: Veterinary Information Network. http://goo.gl/pJDHg

RONIDAZOLE

(roe-*nid*-ah-zole)

ANTIPROTOZOAL

Prescriber Highlights

▶ Nitroimidazole antibiotic/antiparasitic drug that appears to be useful in treating *Tritrichomonas foetus* infections in cats; also used for treating trichomonas infections in non-food birds

▶ Potentially carcinogenic; avoid human exposure

▶ Neurotoxicity (reversible): more likely at higher doses (50 mg/kg twice daily), but can occur at lower dosages as well; GI effects possible

▶ Many potential drug interactions

▶ Must be compounded from bulk powder (100%) & ideally, put in gelatin capsules

Uses/Indications

Ronidazole is a nitroimidazole antibiotic/antiparasitic drug that appears to be useful in treating *Tritrichomonas foetus* infections in cats. The drug is not commercially available in the USA and must be compounded from bulk powder by a compounding pharmacy. The drug is also used for treating Trichomonas infections in non-food animal birds.

Pharmacology/Actions

Ronidazole, like other 5-nitroimidazoles such as metronidazole is converted by hydrogenosomes (an organelle found in trichomonads) into polar autotoxic anion radicals. *T. foetus* infections in cats have been resistant to treatment by metronidazole, and ronidazole appears to have greater activity against the organism, but ronidazole resistance has been documented (Gookin *et al.* 2010).

Pharmacokinetics

In cats, ronidazole is completely absorbed and bioavailable after oral dosing. Volume of distribution (steady state) is about 0.7 L/kg and clearance approximately 0.8 mL/kg/min. Elimination half-life is long at around 10 hours (LeVine *et al.* 2008).

Contraindications/Precautions/Warnings

Ronidazole should not be used in patients hypersensitive to it or other 5-nitroimidazoles (*e.g.*, metronidazole).

The compound has been demonstrated to be carcinogenic in mice but not rats. While humans should avoid contact with this compound or with animal waste from treated patients, it can be safely compounded using a biological safety cabinet.

The FDA prohibits this drug for use in food animals.

Adverse Effects

Reversible neurotoxicity similar to that reported with metronidazole, has been reported in cats with ronidazole. Initial signs may include lethargy, anorexia, ataxia, nystagmus, seizures or behavior changes. Should neurotoxicity be diagnosed, discontinue ronidazole, treat supportively, and if necessary, consider administering a benzodiazepine such as diazepam to competitively inhibit GABA receptors in the CNS. Incidence of neurotoxicity appears to be higher when using the 50 mg/kg twice daily dosage, but may occur at lower dosages as well. Potentially, gastrointestinal effects can occur (anorexia, vomiting). Ronidazole is very bitter and should be administered to cats in capsule form.

Ronidazole has been shown to increase the rate of benign mammary tumors in rats and increase the rates of benign and malignant pulmonary tumors in mice at dosages at or above 20 mg/kg/day.

Dogs given 30 mg/kg per day for two years (40 mg/kg/day the first month) showed some testicular toxicity (type not specified), but no tumors.

Reproductive/Nursing Safety

Safety of this compound during pregnancy is not established. Teratology studies have been performed in mice, rats, and rabbits. In rabbits given 30 mg/kg/day, no embryotoxicity occurred, but fetal weights were significantly decreased. Mice demonstrated no teratogenic effects at dosages of up to 200 mg/kg/day. Rats given up to 150 mg/kg/day demonstrated no embryotoxic effects, but at dosages of 200 mg/kg/day both maternal and fetal weights were decreased.

If this compound is to be used in pregnant cats, weigh the potential benefits of treating with the potential for adverse effects in the offspring and queen.

It is not known if ronidazole is distributed into milk and safety cannot be assured. Consider using milk replacer if treating nursing queens.

Overdosage/Acute Toxicity

No specific information was located. Cats receiving doses of 50 mg/kg twice daily appear to have greater incidences of neurotoxicity (see Adverse Reactions). A case report of an overdose causing neurotoxicity, hemorrhage and death in society finches after consuming ronidazole in drinking water has been published (Woods *et al.* 2010). If overdoses cause neurotoxicity, discontinue further therapy and treat supportively.

Consider administering a GABA inhibitor such as diazepam, to competitively inhibit GABA receptors in the CNS.

Drug Interactions

In humans, the following drug interactions with metronidazole, a compound similar to ronidazole, have been reported or are theoretical and may be of significance in veterinary patients in patients receiving ronidazole:

- **ALCOHOL:** May induce a disulfiram-like (nausea, vomiting, cramps, etc.) reaction
- **CIMETIDINE, KETOCONAZOLE:** May decrease the metabolism of ronidazole and increase the likelihood of dose-related side effects occurring
- **CYCLOSPORINE, TACROLIMUS (systemic):** Ronidazole may increase the serum levels of cyclosporine or tacrolimus
- **FLUOROURACIL (systemic):** Ronidazole may increase the serum levels of fluorouracil and increase risk for toxicity
- **LITHIUM:** Ronidazole may increase lithium serum levels and increase risk for lithium toxicity
- **OXYTETRACYCLINE:** Reportedly may antagonize the therapeutic effects of metronidazole (and presumably ronidazole)
- **PHENOBARBITAL, RIFAMPIN or PHENYTOIN:** May increase the metabolism of ronidazole thereby decreasing blood levels
- **WARFARIN:** Metronidazole (and potentially ronidazole), may prolong INR/PT in patients taking coumarin anticoagulants; avoid concurrent use if possible; otherwise intensify monitoring

Laboratory Considerations

- **AST, ALT, LDH (lactic dehydrogenase), Triglycerides, Hexokinase glucose:** A related compound, metronidazole can cause falsely decreased readings when determined using methods measuring decreases in ultraviolet absorbance when NADH is reduced to NAD. It is not known if ronidazole can also cause falsely decreased values.

Doses

- **CATS:**
  a) For treatment of *T. foetus* infections: Recent studies investigating the pharmacokinetics of ronidazole in cats suggest that 30 mg/kg PO q24h for 14 days is likely to be most effective in resolving diarrhea and eradicating *T. foetus* infection. (Tolbert & Gookin 2009)

Monitoring

- Clinical efficacy (diarrhea improvement)
- Adverse effects (neurotoxicity, vomiting, anorexia)
- PCR testing (can be used to confirm infection, but negative results after treatment do not conclusively prove that infection has been eradicated)

Client Information

- Ronidazole must be given by mouth twice daily (approximately 12 hours apart) for 14 days for it to be effective. Do not skip doses.
- Store capsules in the freezer.
- This drug is considered a carcinogen. Do not open or crush capsules; give whole. It is recommended to wear disposable gloves when administering this medication.
- When cleaning litter box, wear disposable gloves; double bag feces and dispose in trash.
- Contact veterinarian immediately if cat shows signs of behavior changes, eyes moving back and forth (nystagmus), or has difficulty walking, climbing stairs, etc. (ataxia). These could be signs that drug toxicity is occurring.

Chemistry/Synonyms

Ronidazole is a 5-nitroimidazole compound that occurs as a white to yellowish-brown, odorless or almost odorless, bitter-tasting, powder. It is very slightly soluble in water or alcohol.

Ronidazole may also be known as ronidazol, ronidazolum, *Belga®, Ridsol-S®, Ronida®, Ronivet®, Ronizol®, Turbosol®, Tricho Plus®, Trichocure®,* or *Trichorex®.*

Storage/Stability

Compounded capsules should be stored in child-resistant, tight containers protected from light. Until further stability studies can be performed, capsules should be stored in the freezer.

Aqueous solutions are reportedly not very stable. It is recommended that fresh solutions using the 10% powder for addition to drinking water (used for pigeons) be freshly prepared every day.

Dosage Forms/Regulatory Status

VETERINARY-LABELED PRODUCTS:

None in the USA; a 10% ronidazole powder to be added to drinking water for treating Trichomonas infections in pigeons is available in some countries, but these products are unsuitable for use in cats due to the dosage required and the unpalatability (very bitter) of the powder and solution. Capsules prepared from 100% bulk powder for an individual feline patient should be obtained from a compounding pharmacy that can prepare the capsules in a bio-safety hood that will protect the compounder from drug exposure.

The FDA prohibits this drug for use in food animals.

HUMAN-LABELED PRODUCTS: None

References

Gookin, J.L., S.H. Stauffer, et al. (2010). Documentation of In Vivo and In Vitro Aerobic Resistance of Feline Tritrichomonas foetus Isolates to Ronidazole. *Journal of Veterinary Internal Medicine* 24(4): 1003–1007.

LeVine, D., M. Papich, et al. (2008). Ronidazole Pharmacokinetics in Cats After IV Administration and Oral Administration of an Immediate Release Capsule and a Colon-Targeted Delayed Release Tablet. Procedings: ACVIM. Accessed via: Veterinary Information Network. http://goo.gl/gCeAN

Tolbert, M.K. & J.L. Gookin (2009). Tritrichomonas foetus: A New Agent of Feline Diarrhea. *Compendium-Continuing Education for Veterinarians* 31(8): 374–+.

Woods, L.W., R.J. Higgins, et al. (2010). Ronidazole Toxicosis in 3 Society Finches (Lonchura striata). *Veterinary Pathology* 47(2): 231–235.

S-ADENOSYL-METHIONINE (SAMe) ADEMETIONINE

(ess-ah-*den*-oh-seel meth-*ie*-oh-neen)

HEPATOPROTECTANT

Prescriber Highlights

▶ "Nutraceutical" that can be used as an adjunctive treatment for liver disease (chronic hepatitis), osteoarthritis, or treatment of acetaminophen toxicity in small animals

▶ Well tolerated

▶ Not a regulated drug; choose products carefully

Uses/Indications

In small animal medicine, SAMe is most commonly used as an adjunctive treatment for liver disease (chronic hepatitis, hepatic lipidosis, cholangiohepatitis, feline triad disease, etc.). It may also be of benefit in osteoarthritis, age-related cognitive dysfunction, treatment of acute hepatotoxin-induced liver toxicity (*e.g.*, acetaminophen, xylitol toxicity), and at-risk patients on long-term therapy using drugs with hepatotoxic potential.

In humans, SAMe is being used as a treatment for depression, osteoarthritis, AIDS-related myopathy, intrahepatic cholestasis, liver disease, alcoholic liver cirrhosis, fibromyalgia, adult ADHD, Alzheimer's, migraines, etc.

Pharmacology/Actions

S-adenosyl-methionine (SAMe) is an endogenous molecule synthesized by cells throughout the body. SAMe is formed from the amino acid methionine and ATP, in conjunction with SAMe synthetase enzyme (an enzyme manufactured in the liver, a rate-limiting step in the presence of liver compromise). SAMe is an essential part of three major biochemical pathways: transmethylation, transsulfuration, and aminopropylation. Normal function of these pathways is especially vital to the liver as many metabolic reactions occur there. In the transmethylation pathway, SAMe serves as a methyl donor (necessary for many substances and drugs to be activated and/or eliminated). Transmethylation is essential in phospholipid synthesis important

to cell membrane structure, fluidity, and function. In aminopropylation, SAMe donates aminopropyl groups and is a source of polyamines. Aminopropylation is important in producing substances that have antiinflammatory effects, protein and DNA synthesis, and promoting cell replication and liver mass regeneration. In transulfuration, SAMe generates sulfur containing compounds important for conjugation reactions used in detoxification and as a precursor to glutathione (GSH). Glutathione is important in many metabolic processes and cell detoxification. The conversion of SAMe to glutathione requires the presence of folate, cyanocobalamin (B_{12}), and pyridoxine (B_6). Normally, the liver produces ample SAMe, but in liver disease or in the presence of hepatotoxic substances, endogenous conversion to glutathione may be deficient. Exogenous SAMe has been shown to increase liver and red cell glutathione levels and/or prevent its depletion. SAMe inhibits apoptosis secondary to alcohol or bile acids in hepatocytes.

In humans, the mechanism for its antidepressant effects are not well understood, but it apparently increases serotonin turnover and increases dopamine and norepinephrine levels. Neuro-imaging studies in humans show that SAMe affects the brain similarly to other antidepressant medications.

Pharmacokinetics

Oral bioavailability is dependent on the salt used to stabilize SAMe. Oral bioavailability of the tosylate salt is reportedly 1% whereas the 1,4-butanedisulfonate form has a bioavailability of 5%. Regardless of oral dosage form administered, presence of food in the gut can substantially reduce the amount of drug absorbed. Peak levels occur in 1–6 hours after oral dosing with the enteric coated tablets. Once absorbed, SAMe enters the portal circulation and is primarily metabolized in the liver. In humans, 17% of a dose of radio-labeled SAMe was recovered in the urine within 48 hours of dosing; 27% in the feces.

In dogs, a chewable non-hygroscopic formulation of SAMe (*Denosyl® Chewable*) yielded similar areas under-the-curve when compared with the enteric-coated tablets (*Denosyl®*), but peak levels occurred sooner with the chewable tablets (Griffin *et al.* 2009).

Contraindications/Precautions/Warnings

There are no apparent contraindications to the use of SAMe.

Adverse Effects

Adverse effects appear to be minimal or nonexistent in treated animals. Most studies in humans have shown adverse effects similar to that of placebo. There have been reports of immediate post-dose vomiting, anorexia, and anxiety. Oral SAMe in humans may cause anorexia, nausea, vomiting, diarrhea, flatulence, constipation, dry mouth, insomnia/nervousness, headache, sweating, and dizziness.

Reproductive/Nursing Safety

The safety of exogenous SAMe has not been proven in pregnancy; use with caution. Limited studies in laboratory animals and in pregnant women with liver disease have not demonstrated any ill effects to mother or fetus.

It is unknown if SAMe enters maternal milk.

Overdosage/Acute Toxicity

SAMe appears to be quite safe. LD_{50} in rodents exceeds 4.65 grams/kg, and toxicity studies in dogs and cats at the usual prescribed dosages demonstrated no deleterious effects. In the case of an overdose, gastrointestinal effects may be observed, but unlikely to require treatment.

Drug Interactions

No interactions have been documented, but theoretically, concurrent use of SAMe with **tramadol, meperidine, dextromethorphan, pentazocine**, monoamine oxidase inhibitors (**MAOIs**) including **selegiline**, selective serotonin reuptake inhibitors (**SSRIs**) such as **fluoxetine**, or other antidepressants (*e.g.*, **amitriptyline, clomipramine**) could cause additive serotonergic effects.

Laboratory Considerations

■ No specific laboratory interactions or considerations noted.

Doses

■ **DOGS/CATS:**

Daily dose for animals with body weights of:

up to 12 pounds (5.5 kg): one 90 mg tablet;

12−25 pounds (5.5−11 kg): two 90 mg tablets (or one 225 mg tablet, if more convenient);

25−35 pounds (11−16 kg): one 225 mg tablet;

35−65 pounds (16−29.5 kg): two 225 mg tablets;

65−90 pounds (29.5 kg−41 kg): three 225 mg tablets;

over 90 pounds (41 kg+): four 225 mg tablets.

Daily dosage may also be calculated based on 18 mg/kg of body weight and rounded to the closest tablet size or combination of sizes. Product should be given on an empty stomach, at least one hour before feeding. If giving more than one tablet, may divide total daily dosage and give twice daily. The number of tablets can be gradually reduced or may be increased at any time depending on the pet's needs. (Package information; *Denosyl®* —Nutramax)

For Liver Disease:

a) For adjunctive treatment of necro-inflammatory/cholestatic liver disease, vacuolar hepatopathy, feline hepatic lipidosis: 20 mg/kg PO once daily on an empty stomach; use a proven bioavailable product. (Center 2008)

b) 20 mg/kg once daily (Willard 2006)

Monitoring

■ Clinical signs (appetite, activity, attitude)

■ Liver enzymes, bilirubin, bile acids

■ Liver biopsies

■ Hepatic and erythrocyte glutathione levels (available at research institutions only at this time); may require 1−4 months before any changes in lab values are noted

Client Information

■ Administer tablets to animal with an empty stomach, preferably at least one hour before feeding

■ Keep tablets in original packaging until administration. Do not crush or split enteric-coated tablets.

Chemistry/Synonyms

S-adenosyl-methionine (SAMe) is a naturally occurring molecule found throughout the body. Because pure SAMe is highly reactive and unstable, commercially available forms of SAMe are salt forms; sulfate, sulfate-p-toluenesulfonate (also known as tosylate), and butanedisulfonate salts can all be procured.

SAMe may also be known as: S-adenosyl-L-methionine, S-adenosylmethionine, SAM, SAM-e, adenosylmethionine, Sammy, methioninyl adenylate, *Donamet®, Gumbaral®, Isimet®, MoodLift®, S Amet®, Samyr®, Transmetil®,* and *Tunik®.*

Storage/Stability

Unless otherwise labeled, SAMe tablets should be stored at room temperature. Avoid conditions of high temperature or humidity. SAMe is inherently unstable in acidic or aqueous environments; store in tightly sealed, moisture-resistant containers.

Dosage Forms/Regulatory Status

VETERINARY-LABELED PRODUCTS:

None as a pharmaceutical. SAMe is considered a nutritional supplement by the FDA. No standards have been accepted for potency, purity, safety, or efficacy by regulatory bodies. Supplements are available from a wide variety of sources and dosage forms include tablets in a variety of concentrations.

There are specific products marketed for use in animals, including:

Denosyl® (Nutramax) which is a 1, 4 −butanediolsulfonate salt in 90 mg, 225 mg, & 425 mg enteric-coated, blister-packed tablets and 225 mg chewable tablets.

Zentonil® (Vetoquinol) which is a tosylate salt in 100 mg, 200 mg and 400 mg tablets. Bioequivalence between SAMe products is not assured.

A combination product *Denamarin®* (Nutramax), containing SAMe and silybin (silymarin) is also labeled for use in dogs and cats.

HUMAN-LABELED PRODUCTS:

None as a pharmaceutical.

References

Center, S. (2008). Update on Canine & Feline Liver Disease. Proceedings: ECVIM. Accessed via: Veterinary Information Network. http://goo.gl/jSTOR

Griffin, D., M. Whalen, et al. (2009). Bioavailability of a Novel Formulation of S-Adenosylmethioine in Beagle Dogs. Preoceedings: ACVIM. Accessed via: Veterinary Information Network. http://goo.gl/wq06l

Willard, M. (2006). General considerations in hepatic disease: part 2. Proceedings: ACVC. Accessed via: Veterinary Information Network. http://goo.gl/BITIz

SELAMECTIN

(sell-a-*mek*-tin)   Revolution®

AVERMECTIN (TOPICAL) ANTIPARASITIC

Prescriber Highlights

▶ Topical avermectin antiparasiticide FDA-approved for multiple indications in dogs & cats

▶ Applied monthly (usually; some indications one time dosing)

▶ Adverse effect profile appears minimal

Uses/Indications

Topical selamectin (*Revolution®*—Pfizer) is indicated for flea infestations (*Ctenocephalides felis*), prevention of heartworm disease (*Dirofilaria immitis*), and for ear mites (*Otodectes cynotis*) in both dogs and cats. Additionally in dogs, it is indicated for sarcoptic mange (*Sarcoptes scabeii*), and tick infestations (*Dermacentor variabilis*). In cats it is indicated for hookworms (*Ancylostoma tubaeforme*) and roundworms (*Toxocara cati*).

The product (*Revolution®*) is labeled as not effective against either adult heartworms or clearing circulating microfilaria, but it possibly may have some efficacy with prolonged, continuous administration (Atkins 2007).

Topical selamectin has been used off-label successfully to treat a variety of ectoparasites in small animals, including notoedric mange (*Notoedres cati*), nasal mites in dogs (*Pneumonyssoides caninum*), cheyletiellosis in dogs, cats and rabbits, and cordylobiolosis (cutaneous myiasis, *Cordylobia anthropophaga*) in dogs.

Selamectin has not been successful for treating generalized demodicosis.

Pharmacology/Actions

Like other compounds in its class, selamectin is believed to act by enhancing chloride permeability or enhancing the release of gamma amino butyric acid (GABA) at presynaptic neurons. GABA acts as an inhibitory neurotransmitter and blocks the post-synaptic stimulation of the adjacent neuron in nematodes or the muscle

fiber in arthropods. By stimulating the release of GABA, it causes paralysis of the parasite and eventual death. As liver flukes and tapeworms do not use GABA as a peripheral nerve transmitter, selamectin would probably be ineffective against these parasites.

Pharmacokinetics

After topical administration to dogs, about 5% of the drug is bioavailable and peak plasma levels occur about 3 days later. Selamectin bioavailability may be higher in female dogs. Elimination half-life after topical administration is about 11 days.

After topical administration to cats, about 75% of the drug is bioavailable and peak plasma levels occur about 15 hours later. Elimination half-life after topical administration is about 8 days. In cats, bioavailability is about 75% and peak levels may be 64 times those in dogs.

The persistence of the drug in the body is believed to be due to the drug forming reservoirs in skin sebaceous glands. It is secreted into the intestine to kill susceptible endoparasites in cats.

Contraindications/Precautions/Warnings

The manufacturer recommends caution when using in sick, underweight, or debilitated dogs or cats. It is not recommended for use in dogs under 6 weeks of age and in cats under 8 weeks of age.

At labeled doses of selamectin, dogs at risk for MDR1-allele mutation (Collies, Australian Shepherds, Shelties, Long-haired Whippet, etc.) should tolerate the medication, but use cautiously. Higher doses may cause neurological toxicity in these dogs.

Adverse Effects

In field trials (limited numbers of animals) adverse effects were rare. Approximately 1% of cats showed a transient, localized alopecia at the area of administration. Other effects reported (< or = 0.5% incidence) include diarrhea, vomiting, muscle tremors, anorexia, pruritus/urticaria, erythema, lethargy, salivation and tachypnea. Very rarely, seizures and ataxia have been reported in dogs.

Reproductive/Nursing Safety

Selamectin appears to be safe to use in pregnant or lactating dogs or cats.

Overdosage/Acute Toxicity

Dogs: Oral overdoses of up to 15 mg/kg did not cause adverse effects (except for ataxia in one avermectin sensitive collie). Topical overdoses (10x) to puppies caused no adverse effects; topical overdoses to avermectin-sensitive Collies caused salivation.

Cats: Oral ingestion may cause salivation and vomiting. Topical overdoses of up to 10x caused no observable adverse effects.

There were 97 exposures to selamectin reported to the ASPCA Animal Poison Control Center (APCC) during 2008-2009. In these cases 48 were dogs with 12 showing clinical signs and 53 cases were cats with 28 showing clinical signs. The remaining 3 cases consisted of 2 lagomorphs and 1 ferret none of which had clinical signs. Common findings in dogs recorded in decreasing frequency included hypersalivation and polydipsia. Common findings in cats recorded in decreasing frequency included hypersalivation, licking lips, vomiting, anorexia, depression, and lethargy.

Drug Interactions

None documented, but caution is advised if using other drugs that can inhibit **p-glycoprotein**. Those dogs at risk for MDR1-allele mutation (Collies, Australian Shepherds, Shelties, Long-haired Whippet, etc "white feet") should probably not receive selamectin with the following drugs, unless tested "normal": Drugs and drug classes involved include:

- **AMIODARONE**
- **CARVEDILOL**
- **CLARITHROMYCIN**
- **CYCLOSPORINE**
- **DILTIAZEM**
- **ERYTHROMYCIN**
- **ITRACONAZOLE**
- **KETOCONAZOLE**
- **QUINIDINE**
- **SPIRONOLACTONE**
- **TAMOXIFEN**
- **VERAPAMIL**

Laboratory Considerations

- None reported.

Doses

- **DOGS:**

  a) For prophylaxis and treatment of dirofilariasis, it is suggested to review the guidelines published by the American Heartworm Society at www.heartwormsociety.org for more information: The recommended topical dose is 6 mg/kg. Dosing frequency: Heartworm prevention, flea control = monthly; Ticks = monthly (if heavy infestations, may repeat 2 weeks after the first dose); Ear Mites, Sarcoptes = once, repeat in one month if necessary. See the package for specific instructions on administration technique. (Label information; *Revolution®*—Pfizer)

  b) For nasal mites in dogs (*Pneumonyssoides caninum*): In the study, dogs were dosed at 6−24 mg/kg for three times at 2-week intervals. (Gunnarsson *et al.* 2004)

  c) For cheyletiellosis: 6−12 mg/kg topically every other week for a total of four treatments. (Mueller & Bettenay 2002)

  d) For biting lice: 6 mg/kg topically once. (Shanks *et al.* 2003)

- **CATS:**

  a) The recommended topical dose is 6 mg/kg. Dosing frequency: Heartworm prevention, flea control = monthly; Ear Mites = once, repeat in one month if necessary. Hookworms, Roundworms = once. See the package for specific instructions on administration technique. (Label information; *Revolution®*—Pfizer)

  b) For notoedric (face/head) mange (*Notoedres cati*): 6 mg/kg topically once. (Arther 2009)

  c) For biting lice: 6 mg/kg topically once. (Shanks *et al.* 2003)

- **FERRETS:**

  a) For heartworm prevention: 18 mg/kg topically every 30 days. (Johnson 2006)

- **RABBITS:**

  a) For ear mites (*P. cunuculi*): 6−18 mg/kg topically (McTier *et al.* 2003)

Monitoring

- Clinical efficacy
- Owner compliance with treatment regimen

Client Information

- Follow label directions for administration technique; do not massage into skin, and do not apply if hair coat is wet. Because the product contains alcohol, do not apply to broken skin.

- Avoid contact with animal while the application site is wet.

- Wait two hours or more after applying to bathe the animal (or allow to go swimming).

- Avoid getting the product on human skin; if contact occurs, wash off immediately. Dispose of tubes in regular household refuse.

- Do not expose to flame as the product is flammable.

Chemistry/Synonyms

A semi-synthetic avermectin, selamectin is commercially available as a colorless to yellow solution (flammable).

Selamectin may also be known as UK-124114, or *Revolution®*.

Storage/Stability

The commercially available solution should be stored below 30°C (86°F). Keep away from flame or other igniters.

Dosage Forms/Regulatory Status

VETERINARY-LABELED PRODUCTS:

Selamectin Topical Solution for Cats; Revolution® (Pfizer); (Rx):

Up to 5 lbs in wt, Pkg. Color: mauve. 15 mg/tube. Tube volume: 0.25 mL

5.1−15 lbs in wt, Pkg. Color: blue. 45 mg/tube. Tube volume: 0.75 mL

Selamectin Topical Solution for Dogs; Revolution® (Pfizer); (Rx)

Up to 5 lbs in wt, Pkg. Color: mauve. 15 mg/tube. Tube volume: 0.25 mL

5.1–10 lbs in wt, Pkg. Color: purple. 30 mg/tube. Tube volume: 0.25 mL

10.1–20 lbs in wt, Pkg. Color: brown. 60 mg/tube. Tube volume: 0.5 mL

20.1–40 lbs in wt, Pkg. Color: red. 120 mg/tube. Tube volume: 1 mL

40.1–85 lbs in wt, Pkg. Color: teal. 240 mg/tube. Tube volume: 2 mL

85.1–130 lbs in wt, Pkg. Color: plum. One 120 mg tube and one 240 mg tube. Total volume: 3 mL

HUMAN-LABELED PRODUCTS: None

References

Arther, R. (2009). Mites and Lice: Biology and Control. *Vet Clin Small Anim* **39**: 1159–1171.

Atkins, C. (2007). What's new in heartworms. Proceedings: WVC. Accessed via: Veterinary Information Network. http://goo.gl/5EDFH

Gunnarsson, L., G. Zakrisson, et al. (2004). Efficacy of selamectin in the treatment of nasal mite (Pneumonyssoides caninum) infection in dogs. *Journal of the American Animal Hospital Association* **40**(5): 400–404.

Johnson, D. (2006). Ferrets: the other companion animal. Proceedings: ACVC. Accessed via: Veterinary Information Network. http://goo.gl/bSeol

McTier, T., J. Hair, et al. (2003). Efficacy and safety of topical administration of selamectin for treatment of ear mite infestation in rabbits. *J Am Vet Med Assoc* **223**(3): 322–324.

Mueller, R.S. & S.V. Bettenay (2002). Efficacy of selamectin in the treatment of canine cheyletiellosis. *Veterinary Record* **151**(25): 773–773.

Shanks, D.J., R. Gautier, et al. (2003). Efficacy of selamectin against biting lice on dogs and cats. *Veterinary Record* **152**(8): 234–+.

SELEGILINE HCL
L-DEPRENYL

(se-*le*-ji-leen)   Anipryl®, Eldepryl®

MONAMINE OXIDASE INHIBITOR

Prescriber Highlights

▶ MAO-B inhibitor that may be useful for cognitive dysfunction syndrome in dogs or cats or canine Cushing's (efficacy in doubt for Cushing's)

▶ Contraindications: Potentially in patients receiving opiates (see Drug Interactions)

▶ Adverse Effects: Vomiting & diarrhea; CNS effects manifested by restlessness, repetitive movements, or lethargy; salivation & anorexia. Diminished hearing/deafness, pruritus, licking, shivers/trembles/shakes possible

▶ Drug Interactions

Uses/Indications

Selegiline is FDA-approved for use in dogs for the treatment of Cushing's disease and for Canine Cognitive Dysfunction (so-called "old dog dementia"). Its use for Cushing's disease is somewhat controversial as clinical studies evaluating its efficacy have shown disappointing results. In humans, selegiline's primary indication is for the adjunctive treatment of Parkinson's disease. Selegiline may have a role in treating dogs with chronic anxiety, particularly those that have high prolactin levels (Pageat *et al.* 2007). Combined with a benzodiazepine and a beta-blocker such as propranolol, selegiline may be particularly useful in treating social or noise phobias.

Selegiline may be of use in feline cognitive dysfunction syndrome.

Pharmacology/Actions

Selegiline's mechanism of action for treatment of Cushing's disease (pituitary dependent hyperadrenocorticism—PDH) is complex; a somewhat simplified explanation follows: In the hypothalamus, corticotropin-releasing hormone (CRH) acts to stimulate the production of ACTH in the pituitary and dopamine acts to inhibit the release of ACTH. As dogs age, there is a tendency for a decrease in dopamine production that can contribute to the development of PDH.

As dopamine is metabolized by monamine oxidase-B (MAO-B) and selegiline inhibits MAO-B, dopamine levels can be increased at receptor sites after selegiline administration. In theory, this allows the levels of dopamine and CRH to be in balance in the hypothalamus, thereby reducing the amount of ACTH produced and ultimately, cortisol.

While selegiline is labeled as a MAO-B inhibitor, at higher than labeled dosages, the drug loses its MAO-B specificity and also inhibits MAO-A. Two of three metabolites of selegiline are amphetamine and methamphetamine that may contribute to both the efficacy and the adverse effects of the drug.

Pharmacokinetics

There is only limited information on the pharmacokinetics of selegiline in dogs. A study done in 4 dogs showed that selegiline was absorbed rapidly and had an absolute bioavailability of about 10%. The volume of distribution of the central compartment was measured at approximately 7 L/kg. Terminal half-life was about one hour.

In humans, selegiline pharmacokinetics have wide interpatient variability. The drug has a high first pass effect where extensive metabolism to L-desmethylselegiline, methylamphetamine, and L-amphetamine occur. Each of these metabolites is active. While L-desmethylselegiline does inhibit MAO-B, the others do not, but thye are CNS stimulants. The drug is excreted in the urine, primarily as conjugated and unconjugated metabolites.

Contraindications/Precautions/Warnings

Selegiline is contraindicated in patients known to be hypersensitive to it. In human patients, it is contraindicated in patients receiving meperidine and possibly with other opioids as well.

The manufacturer cautions to perform appropriate diagnostic tests to confirm the diagnosis before starting therapy and not to attempt to treat hyperadrenocorticism not of pituitary origin.

Adverse Effects

Adverse reports reported thus far in dogs include, vomiting, diarrhea, CNS effects manifested by restlessness, repetitive movements or lethargy, salivation, and anorexia. Should GI effects be a problem, discontinue the drug for a few days and restart at a lower dose. Diminished hearing/deafness, pruritus, licking, shivers/trembles/shakes have also been reported. The manufacturer advises to observe animals carefully for atypical responses.

Adverse effects that have been reported in human patients include nausea (10%), hallucinations, confusion, depression, loss of balance, insomnia, and hypersexuality. These effects are noted because of their "subjective" nature and they could help explain untoward behavioral changes in canine patients should they occur.

Because selegiline could potentially be abused by humans, veterinarians should be alert for drug "shoppers." Selegiline is classified by the Association of Racing Commissioners International (ARCI) as a class 2 agent (high abuse potential in racing horses).

Reproductive/Nursing Safety

Safety of selegiline in pregnant, breeding or lactating animals has not been established. Rat studies have not demonstrated overt teratogenicity. In humans, the FDA categorizes this drug as category **C** for use during pregnancy (*Animal studies have shown an adverse effect on the fetus, but there are no adequate studies in humans; or there are no animal reproduction studies and no adequate studies in humans.*)

It is not known whether selegiline is excreted in maternal milk.

Overdosage/Acute Toxicity

Oral LD_{50} in laboratory animals was approximately 200–445 mg/kg. In limited data, dogs receiving 3x dosages showed signs of decreased weight, salivation, decreased pupillary response, panting, stereotypic behaviors and decreased skin elasticity (dehydration). Overdoses, if severe, should be treated with appropriate gut emptying and supportive treatments.

Drug Interactions

Evaluating the potential for drug interactions for selegiline in dogs is problematic. There are a plethora of significant interactions with monamine oxidase inhibitors in humans for selegiline, but because there are significant species differences in quantities and locations of MOA-A and B and selegiline's effects at various dosages on these enzymes, they may not apply to dogs. However, the following drug interactions are some of the more significant interactions reported or are theoretical in humans or animals

receiving selegiline and potentially could be of significance in veterinary patients; caution is advised particularly if using selegiline at higher than labeled dosages:

- ◾ **AMITRAZ:** The manufacturer recommends not using selegiline concurrently with amitraz (*Mitaban®*) in dogs
- ◾ **BUPROPION:** Potential for serotonin syndrome
- ◾ **EPHEDRINE:** The manufacturer recommends not using selegiline concurrently with ephedrine in dogs
- ◾ **MEPERIDINE/OPIOIDS:** In humans, severe agitation, hallucinations and death have occurred in some patients receiving meperidine and an MAO inhibitor. Until the data can be clarified, it is recommended not to use selegiline and meperidine together. A separation of two weeks has been recommended. Other opioids (*e.g.*, morphine) should be safer, but use with extreme caution, if at all.
- ◾ **PHENYLPROPANOLAMINE, PSEUDOEPHEDRINE:** Possibility for increased risk for hypertension, hyperpyrexia
- ◾ **SSRI'S (e.g., fluoxetine):** Potentially, the so-called serotonin syndrome could occur if selegiline is used concurrently with selective serotonin reuptake inhibitors (SSRIs); several sources recommend a 5-week washout before administering selegiline in dogs after fluoxetine is discontinued and to wait 2 weeks if switching from selegiline to an SSRI.
- ◾ **TRAMADOL:** Use contraindicated in humans; serotonin syndrome, nausea, vomiting, cardiovascular collapse
- ◾ **TRICYCLIC & TETRACYCLIC ANTIDEPRESSANTS (clomipramine, amitriptyline, etc.):** Potentially, the so-called serotonin syndrome could occur if selegiline is used concurrently with these agents and use together is not advised at this time; a 2-week separation between these compounds and selegiline is recommended.

Doses

- ◾ **DOGS:**

  For Cushing's disease:

  a) 1 mg/kg PO in the AM (with food as needed); Reevaluate clinically over next 2 mos.; if no improvement, may increase to 2 mg/kg once daily; if no improvement or signs increase, reevaluate diagnosis or consider alternate treatment (Package Insert; *Anipryl®*—Pfizer).

  For Canine Cognitive Dysfunction:

  a) 0.5–1 mg/kg, PO once daily, preferably in the AM. Initially, dose to the nearest whole tablet; adjustments should then be made based upon response and tolerance to the drug (Package Insert; *Anipryl®*—Pfizer).

b) 0.5 mg/kg PO q24h; if no response after 4 weeks give 1 mg/kg PO q24h. Also useful in some anxiety problems and sleep disorders. (Seksel 2008)

■ **CATS:**

For Cognitive Dysfunction Syndrome:

a) 0.25–1 mg/kg PO once daily. There are no drugs licensed for the treatment of CDS in cats. However, a small open trial using selegiline showed a positive effect and the American Association of Feline Practitioners supports the use of this drug for the treatment of CDS. (Gunn-Moore 2008)

b) For anxiety, disturbed sleep wake cycles and excessive vocalization associated with aging: 0.5–1 mg/kg PO once daily. (Seksel 2008)

Monitoring

■ Clinical efficacy

■ Adverse effects. No correlation between low dose dexamethasone suppression test results and clinical efficacy of the drug. The manufacturer recommends physical exam and history as the primary methods to measure response to therapy.

Client Information

■ Keep this and all medications out of reach of children

■ Have clients monitor closely for adverse effects

■ Clients should be advised on the importance of complying with the dosing recommendations to adequately evaluate therapeutic response to the drug

■ When used for cognitive dysfunction, drug may take several weeks to show any benefit

Chemistry/Synonyms

Selegiline HCl, also commonly called l-deprenyl, occurs as a white to off-white crystalline powder that is freely soluble in water. It has a pKa of 7.5.

Selegiline HCl may also be known as: deprenyl, L-deprenyl, selegilini hydrochloridum; many trade names are available.

Storage/Stability

Commercially available veterinary tablets should be stored at controlled room temperature 20–25°C (68–77°F). The commercially available human-labeled tablets and capsules are recommended to be stored from 15–30°C.

Dosage Forms/Regulatory Status

VETERINARY-LABELED PRODUCTS:

Selegiline HCl Oral Tablets: 2 mg, 5 mg, 10 mg, 15 mg, 30 mg in blister-packs of 30 tablets; *Anipryl®* (Pfizer); (Rx). FDA-approved for use in dogs.

The ARCI (Racing Commissioners International) has designated this drug as a class 2 substance. See the appendix for more information.

HUMAN-LABELED PRODUCTS:

Selegiline HCl Tablets and Capsules: 1.25 mg (orally disintegrating) & 5 mg; *Eldepryl®* (Somerset); *Zelapar®* (Valeant Pharmaceuticals); generic; (Rx)

Selegiline HCl Transdermal Patch: 6 mg/24 h (20 mg/20 cm^2); 9 mg/24 h (30 mg/30 cm^2) & 12 mg/24 hours (40 mg/40 cm^2); *Emsam®* (Dey); (Rx)

References

Gunn-Moore, D. (2008). Geriatric Cats and Cognitive Dysfunction Syndrome. Procedings: WSAVA. Accessed via: Veterinary Information Network. http://goo.gl/cubmX

Pageat, P., C. Lafont, et al. (2007). An evaluation of serum prolactin in anxious dogs and response to treatment with selegiline or fluoxetine. *Applied Animal Behaviour Science* 105(4): 342–350.

Seksel, K. (2008). To medicate or not to medicate—That is the question! What to use, when and why. Proceedings: World Veterinary Congress. Accessed via: Veterinary Information Network. http://goo.gl/KjRxj

SERTRALINE HCL

(*sir*-trah-leen)   Zoloft®

SELECTIVE SEROTONIN REUPTAKE INHIBITOR (SSRI)

Prescriber Highlights

▶ A selective serotonin reuptake inhibitor that may be useful in treating a variety of behavior-related diagnoses in dogs & cats, including aggression, anxiety-related behaviors & other obsessive-compulsive behaviors

▶ Caution: geriatric patients or those with severe hepatic disease; dosages may need to be adjusted

▶ Adverse effect profile not well established. Potentially, *Dogs:* Anorexia, lethargy, GI effects, anxiety, irritability, insomnia/hyperactivity, or panting. Aggressive behavior in previously non-aggressive dogs possible. *Cats:* Sedation, decreased appetite/anorexia, vomiting, diarrhea, behavior changes (anxiety, irritability, sleep disturbances), & changes in elimination patterns

▶ Drug-drug interactions

▶ Relatively inexpensive generic products now available

Uses/Indications

Sertraline may be considered for use in treating a variety of behavior-related diagnoses in dogs and cats, including aggression, and anxiety-related or other obsessive-compulsive behaviors.

Pharmacology/Actions

Sertraline is a highly selective inhibitor of the reuptake of serotonin (5-hydroxytryptamine)

in the CNS thus potentiating its pharmacologic activity. Sertraline apparently has little effect on dopamine or norepinephrine, and apparently no effect on other neurotransmitters.

Pharmacokinetics

In dogs, sertraline's volume of distribution is 25 L/kg and is 97% bound to plasma proteins. High first-pass metabolism occurs; clearance is greater than 35 mL/min/kg. Bile is the major route of excretion in the dog.

In humans, sertraline peak levels occur 30–45 minutes after oral dosing. It is 98% bound to plasma proteins. Sertraline appears to be highly metabolized primarily to N-desmethylsertraline, which is active. Elimination half-lives for sertraline and desmethylsertraline average 26 and 80 hours respectively.

Contraindications/Precautions/Warnings

Sertraline is contraindicated in patients hypersensitive to it or any SSRI, or receiving a monoamine oxidase inhibitor (MAOI) or cisapride. Use with caution in geriatric patients and those with hepatic impairment; dosages may need to be decreased or dosing interval increased.

Adverse Effects

Limited use of sertraline in dogs or cats makes it difficult to compare its adverse effect profile with other SSRIs (e.g., fluoxetine, paroxetine, fluvoxamine). In dogs, SSRIs can cause lethargy, GI effects, anxiety, irritability, insomnia/hyperactivity, or panting. Anorexia is a common side effect in dogs (usually transient and may be negated by temporarily increasing the palatability of food and/or hand feeding). Some dogs have persistent anorexia that precludes further treatment. Aggressive behavior in previously nonaggressive dogs has been reported. SSRI's in cats can cause sedation, decreased appetite/anorexia, vomiting, diarrhea, behavior changes (anxiety, irritability, sleep disturbances), and changes in elimination patterns.

Reproductive/Nursing Safety

In humans, the FDA categorizes sertraline as a category *C* drug for use during pregnancy (*Animal studies have shown an adverse effect on the fetus, but there are no adequate studies in humans; or there are no animal reproduction studies and no adequate studies in humans.*) In rats and rabbits, sertraline was implicated in causing delayed ossification. Sertraline decreased pup survival in rats exposed in utero.

It is unknown if sertraline enters maternal milk.

Overdosage/Acute Toxicity

With overdoses, the SSRI's can cause vomiting, diarrhea, hypersalivation, and lethargy. Serotonin syndrome may occur with signs that include muscle tremors, rigidity, agitation, hyperthermia, vocalization, hypertension or hypotension, tachycardia, seizures, coma, and death. Most dog exposures below 20 mg/kg are not se-

rious. Human overdoses of as little as 2.5 grams have caused death, but one patient survived after taking 13.5 grams.

There were 345 exposures to sertraline reported to the ASPCA Animal Poison Control Center (APCC) during 2008-2009. In these cases 316 were dogs with 65 showing clinical signs and 27 were cats with 5 showing clinical signs. The remaining 2 cases were birds that showed no clinical signs. Common findings in dogs recorded in decreasing frequency included lethargy, tachycardia, somnolence, vomiting, and vocalization. Common findings in cats included hypersalivation.

Management of sertraline overdoses should be handled aggressively with supportive and symptomatic treatment. Veterinarians are encouraged to contact an animal poison control center for further guidance.

Drug Interactions

The following drug interactions have either been reported or are theoretical in humans or animals receiving sertraline and may be of significance in veterinary patients:

- **BUSPIRONE:** Increased risk for serotonin syndrome
- **CIMETIDINE:** May increase sertraline levels
- **CYPROHEPTADINE:** May decrease or reverse the effects of SSRIs
- **DIAZEPAM:** Sertraline may decrease diazepam clearance
- **ISONIAZID:** Increased risk for serotonin syndrome
- **MAO INHIBITORS (including amitraz and potentially, selegiline):** High risk for serotonin syndrome; use contraindicated; in humans, a 5 week washout period is required after discontinuing sertraline and a 2 week washout period is required if first discontinuing the MAO inhibitor
- **PENTAZOCINE:** Serotonin syndrome-like adverse effects possible
- **TRAMADOL:** SSRI's can inhibit the metabolism of tramadol to the active metabolites decreasing its efficacy and increasing the risk of toxicity (serotonin syndrome, seizures)
- **TRICYCLIC ANTIDEPRESSANTS (e.g., clomipramine, amitriptyline):** Sertraline may increase TCA blood levels and may increase the risk for serotonin syndrome
- **WARFARIN:** Sertraline may increase the risk for bleeding

Laboratory Considerations

- No significant laboratory interactions or considerations were located.

Doses

- **DOGS:**
  a) For treatment of compulsive disorders: 2–4 mg/kg PO once daily or divided twice daily (Landsberg 2004)

b) 1−2 mg/kg PO q24h (once daily) (allow 6−8 weeks for initial trial) (Virga 2005)

c) 1−3 mg/kg PO once daily. Plan is to use the drug for a limited time (3−6 months) during which time behavioral modification is also employed. The animal should learn appropriate behavior in previously problematic situations. Then the animal should be weaned off the medication over a 2 to 4 week period by halving the dose weekly (Neilson 2002)

d) For treatment of behavioral diagnoses: 0.25−0.5 mg/kg PO q24h (once a day). **Note:** must treat for 3−5 weeks minimum to assess effects; then treat until "well" until either has no signs associated with diagnosis or some low, consistent level (a minimum of another 1−2 months). Then treat for another 1−2 months (minimum), so that reliability of assessment is reasonably assured. If weaning off the drug do so over 3−5 weeks (or longer). Treatment should last for a minimum 4−6 months once initiating therapy. (Overall 2001)

e) For compulsive disorder, anxiety: 1−4 mg/kg PO q24h (once daily) (Seibert 2003)

f) 0.5−4 mg/kg PO once daily. (Haug 2008)

g) For generalized anxiety disorder: 0.5−4 mg/kg PO once daily. (Crowell-Davis, S.L. 2009)

■ **CATS:**

a) For treatment of compulsive disorders: 0.5 mg/kg PO once daily (Landsberg 2004)

b) For urine marking (spraying), aggression, anxiety—including anxiogenic house soiling, phobias, fears: 0.5−1 mg/kg PO q24h (once daily) (Virga 2002)

c) For treatment of behavioral diagnoses: 1 mg/kg PO q24h (once a day). **Note:** must treat for 3−5 weeks minimum to assess effects; then treat until "well" until either has no signs associated with diagnosis or some low, consistent level (a minimum of another 1−2 months). Then treat for another 1−2 months (minimum), so that reliability of assessment is reasonably assured. If weaning off the drug do so over 3−5 weeks (or longer). Treatment should last for a minimum 4−6 months once initiating therapy. (Overall 2001)

d) For treatment of fear, affective or dominance aggression: 0.5−1 mg/kg PO once daily (Crowell-Davis, S. 2003b), (Crowell-Davis, S. 2003a). For generalized anxiety disorder: 0.5−1.5 mg/kg PO q24h. (Crowell-Davis, S.L. 2009)

e) For treatment of compulsive disorder, anxiety: 0.5−1 mg/kg PO q24h (once daily) (Seibert 2003)

f) 0.25−1.3 mg/kg PO q24h. (Curtis 2008)

Monitoring
■ Efficacy
■ Adverse Effects; including appetite (weight)
■ Consider doing baseline liver function tests and ECG; re-test as needed

Client Information
■ Because there has not as yet been widespread use of sertraline in dogs or cats, its adverse effect and efficacy profiles have not been yet fully determined; clients should report any significant abnormal findings to the veterinarian.

■ Clients should understand that this drug is unlikely to have an immediate effect (or even in the short-term) and must commit to using the drug for months to determine efficacy

Chemistry/Synonyms
A selective serotonin reuptake inhibitor, sertraline hydrochloride is a white crystalline powder that is slightly soluble in water and isopropyl alcohol; sparingly soluble in ethanol. The commercially available oral solution contains 12% ethanol and has a menthol scent.

Sertraline may also be known as: CP-51974-01; *Altruline®, Anilar®, Aremis®, Atenix®, Besitran®, Bicromil®, Gladem®, Insertec®, Irradial®, Lustral®, Novativ®, Sealdin®, Serad®, Sercerin®, Serlain®, Serta®, Tatig®, Tolrest®, Tresleen®* or *Zoloft®.*

Storage/Stability
Store commercially available sertraline tablets and oral solution at controlled room temperature (25°C; 77°F); excursions permitted to 15−30°C (59−86°F). The manufacturer states to dilute the oral solution only in the following liquids: water, orange juice, ginger ale, lemonade or lemon/lime soda; use immediately after dilution.

Dosage Forms/Regulatory Status
VETERINARY-LABELED PRODUCTS: None

The ARCI (Racing Commissioners International) has designated this drug as a class 2 substance. See the appendix for more information.

HUMAN-LABELED PRODUCTS:

Sertraline HCl Tablets: 25 mg, 50 mg & 100 mg (as base); *Zoloft®* (Pfizer); generic; (Rx)

Sertraline HCl Oral Solution Concentrate: 20 mg/mL in 60 mL; *Zoloft®* (Pfizer); generic; (Rx)

References
Crowell-Davis, S. (2003a). Human-directed aggression in cats. Proceedings: Western Veterinary Conference. Accessed via: Veterinary Information Network. http://goo.gl/kRXNT

Crowell-Davis, S. (2003b). Intraspecies aggression in cats. Proceedings: Western Veterinary Conference. Accessed via: Veterinary Information Network. http://goo.gl/ZnhsI

1230   SEVELAMER HCL

Crowell-Davis, S.L. (2009). Generalized Anxiety Disorder. *Compendium-Continuing Education for Veterinarians* **31**(9): 427–430.

Curtis, T. (2008). Human-directed aggression in the cat. *Vet Clin NA: Sm Anim Pract* **38**: 1131–1143.

Haug, L. (2008). Canine aggression toward unfamiliar people and dogs. *Vet Clin NA: Sm Anim Pract* **38**: 1023–1041.

Landsberg, G. (2004). A behaviorists approach to compulsive disorders. Proceedings: ACVIM Forum, Minneapolis. Accessed via: Veterinary Information Network. http://goo.gl/eRUh2

Neilson, J. (2002). Serotonergic Drug Therapy. Proceedings: Western Veterinary Conference. Accessed via: Veterinary Information Network. http://goo.gl/LgRfY

Overall, K. (2001). Pharmacology and Behavior: Practical Applications. Proceedings: Atlantic Coast Veterinary Conference. Accessed via: Veterinary Information Network. http://goo.gl/7RRam

Seibert, L. (2003). Antidepressants in behavioral medicine. Proceedings: Western Veterinary Conference. Accessed via: Veterinary Information Network. http://goo.gl/LyQ8m

Virga, V. (2002). Which drug and why: An update on psychopharmacology. Proceedings: Atlantic Coast Veterinary Conference. Accessed via: Veterinary Information Network. http://goo.gl/m8qr4

Virga, V. (2005). Psychopharmacology for anxiety disorders. Proceedings: Western Vet Cong 2005. Accessed via: Veterinary Information Network. http://goo.gl/4uZW3

SEVELAMER HCL

(se-*vel*-a-mer)   Renagel®

PHOSPHORUS BINDING AGENT

Prescriber Highlights

▶ Phosphorus binding agent (in the gut) for hyperphosphatemia associated with chronic renal failure

▶ May be useful if patient cannot tolerate aluminum salts or aluminum salts are commercially unavailable

▶ Expensive when compared to aluminum hydroxide or calcium carbonate products

▶ Drug-drug interactions including nutrients

Uses/Indications

Sevalamer may be useful for treating hyperphosphatemia associated with chronic renal failure, particularly when oral aluminum salts are not tolerated.

Pharmacology/Actions

Sevelamer binds phosphorus in the gut; when combined with decreased phosphorus in the diet it can substantially reduce serum phosphorus levels. It also reduces serum low-density lipoproteins and total cholesterol.

Pharmacokinetics

Sevelamer is administered orally, but is not absorbed systemically.

Contraindications/Precautions/Warnings

Sevelamer is contraindicated in patients with hypophosphatemia, or bowel obstruction and in patients hypersensitive to it.

Adverse Effects

Adverse effects in humans are reported to be the same as placebo. Potentially some GI effects occur.

As oral vitamin absorption may be reduced by sevelamer, consider the addition of vitamin supplementation during therapy.

Reproductive/Nursing Safety

Safety during pregnancy is not established; because of the potential for binding vitamins, additional vitamins (both fat and water soluble) may be necessary. In humans, the FDA categorizes this drug as category *C* for use during pregnancy (*Animal studies have shown an adverse effect on the fetus, but there are no adequate studies in humans; or there are no animal reproduction studies and no adequate studies in humans.*)

There are no adequate and well-controlled studies in nursing mothers.

Overdosage/Acute Toxicity

As sevelamer is not absorbed, acute toxicity potential appears to be negligible.

Drug Interactions

The following drug interactions have either been reported or are theoretical in humans or animals receiving sevelamer and may be of significance in veterinary patients:

■ **ANTICONVULSANTS (oral):** Sevelamer may reduce oral absorption; give at least one hour before or three hours after sevelamer capsules

■ **ANTIARRHYTHMICS (oral):** Sevelamer may reduce oral absorption; give at least one hour before or three hours after sevelamer capsules

■ **CIPROFLOXACIN:** Concurrent administration with sevelamer may decrease absorption by 50%; administer ciprofloxacin and other oral fluoroquinolones at least one hour before or 3 hours after sevelamer

■ **ORAL MEDICATIONS:** There are only a few medications having documented reductions in oral administration when administered with sevelamer; consider dosing other oral drugs separately, particularly for drugs with narrow therapeutic indexes

■ **VITAMINS:** Sevelamer may reduce vitamin absorption from food; consider administering vitamin supplements separately from sevelamer dose

Doses

■ **DOGS:**
a) For medium to large sized dog: 400 mg PO with meals (Vaden 2007)

■ **CATS:**
a) Has been used at 200 mg 2–3 times daily. Anecdotally appears to be safe and effective. (Sparkes 2006)

Monitoring

■ Serum phosphorus (and other electrolytes calcium, bicarbonate, chloride)

■ Consider a baseline coagulation screening test before and after sevalamer therapy implementation as vitamin K absorption may be impacted by the drug

Chemistry/Synonyms

A phosphorus binding agent, sevalamer HCl is a complex chemical that is hydrophilic, but insoluble in water.

Sevelamer may also be known as GT16-026A and *Renagel®*.

Storage/Stability

Sevelamer capsules should be stored at room temperature and protected from moisture.

Dosage Forms/Regulatory Status

VETERINARY-LABELED PRODUCTS: None

HUMAN-LABELED PRODUCTS:

Sevalamer HCl Oral Tablets: 400 mg & 800 mg; *Renagel®* (Genzyme); *Renvela®* (Genzyme); (Rx)

Sevalamer Powder for Oral Suspension: 0.8 grams/packet & 2.4 grams/packet; *Renvela®* (Genzyme); (Rx)

References

Sparkes, A. (2006). Chronic renal failure in the cat. Proceedings: WSAVA Congress. Accessed via: Veterinary Information Network. http://goo.gl/xrddI
Vaden, S. (2007). Management of chronic kidney disease. Proceedings: Western Vet Conf. Accessed via: Veterinary Information Network. http://goo.gl/CcxYX

SEVOFLURANE

(see-voe-*floo*-rane)   SevoFlo®, Ultane®

INHALATIONAL ANESTHETIC

Prescriber Highlights

▶ Inhalational anesthetic similar to isoflurane, but with more rapid induction & recovery

▶ Currently much more expensive than isoflurane

Uses/Indications

Sevoflurane may be useful in a variety of species when rapid induction and/or rapid recoveries are desired with an inhalational anesthetic. The advantages of sevoflurane include rapid inductions and recoveries and the ability to change depth of anesthesia faster than with isoflurane. When mask inductions are necessary, sevoflurane is preferred over isoflurane or desflurane as it is better accepted and inductions are faster and smoother than with isoflurane. Sevoflurane may be of particular usefulness in debilitated or geriatric cats as it tends to cause less hypotension than isoflurane.

Pharmacology/Actions

While the precise mechanism that inhalant anesthetics exert their general anesthetic effects is not precisely known, they may interfere with functioning of nerve cells in the brain by acting at the lipid matrix of the membrane. Sevoflurane has a very low blood:gas partition coefficient (0.6) allowing very rapid anesthesia induction and recovery. Rapid mask induction is possible.

Pharmacologic effects of sevoflurane are similar to isoflurane and include: CNS depression, depression of body temperature regulating centers, increased cerebral blood flow, respiratory depression, hypotension, vasodilatation, myocardial depression (less so than with halothane), and muscular relaxation.

Minimal Alveolar Concentration (MAC; %) in oxygen reported for sevoflurane in various species: Dog = 2.09–2.4; Cat = 2.58; Horse = 2.31; Sheep = 3.3; Swine = 1.97–2.66; Human (adult) = 1.71–2.05. Several factors may alter MAC (acid/base status, temperature, other CNS depressants on board, age, ongoing acute disease, etc.).

Pharmacokinetics

Because of its low solubility in blood, only small concentrations of sevoflurane in the blood are required to be dissolved in blood before alveolar partial pressures are in equilibrium with arterial partial pressures. This low solubility means that sevoflurane is rapidly removed from the lungs. It is unknown what percent sevoflurane is bound to plasma proteins. The majority of sevoflurane is excreted via the lungs, but about 3% is metabolized in the liver via the cytochrome P450 2E1 isoenzyme system.

Contraindications/Precautions/Warnings

Sevoflurane is contraindicated in patients with a history or predilection towards malignant hyperthermia. It should be used with caution (benefits vs. risks) in patients with increased CSF or head injury, or renal insufficiency.

Because of its rapid action, use caution not to overdose during the induction phase. Because of the rapid recovery associated with sevoflurane use caution (and appropriate sedation during the recovery phase), particularly with large animals.

Geriatric animals may require less inhalation anesthetic.

In rabbits, sevoflurane (and isoflurane) can cause breath holding and struggling; premedication and close observation are required. Sevoflurane may have a low margin of safety in guinea pigs.

Sevoflurane can react with carbon dioxide absorbents to produce "compound A", a nephrotoxin. After extensive clinical use in humans and dogs nephrotoxicity has not been demonstrated to be of clinical concern. However sevoflurane should be used with good maintenance

1232   SEVOFLURANE

of the carbon dioxide absorbent (*i.e.*, should be changed regularly to prevent exhaustion or excessive drying) and should not be used with extremely low oxygen flows (*i.e.*, less than 500 mL/min) (Mathews 2008).

Adverse Effects

Sevoflurane seems to be well tolerated. Hypotension may occur and is considered dose related. Dose-dependent respiratory depression and GI effects (nausea, vomiting, ileus) have been reported. While cardiodepression generally is minimal at doses causing surgical planes of anesthesia, it may occur; bradycardia is possible.

Malignant hyperthermia may be triggered by this agent (like other inhalational anesthetics).

Sevoflurane should be used in precision, agent-specific, out of circuit vaporizers.

In ferrets, sevoflurane (and isoflurane) can cause temporary decreases in erythrocyte and white cell counts and total protein. Within 45 minutes after discontinuation of sevoflurane, this effect begins to revert to normal and is reversed within 2 hours.

Reproductive/Nursing Safety

No overt fetotoxicity or teratogenicity has been demonstrated in lab animal studies, but definite safety has not been established for use during pregnancy.

Overdosage/Acute Toxicity

In the event of an overdosage, discontinue sevoflurane; maintain airway and support respiratory and cardiac function as necessary.

Drug Interactions

The following drug interactions have either been reported or are theoretical in humans or animals receiving sevoflurane and may be of significance in veterinary patients:

■ **AMINOGLYCOSIDES, LINCOSAMIDES:** May enhance neuromuscular blockade

■ **BARBITURATES (phenobarbital, pentobarbital, etc.):** May increase concentrations of inorganic fluoride

■ **ISONIAZID:** May increase concentrations of inorganic fluoride

■ **MIDAZOLAM:** May potentiate sevoflurane effects; decrease MAC

■ **NON-DEPOLARIZING NEUROMUSCULAR BLOCKING AGENTS (atracurium, pancuronium, vecuronium):** Additive neuromuscular blockade may occur

■ **OPIATES:** May potentiate sevoflurane effects; decrease MAC

■ **ST. JOHNS WORT:** Increased risk for anesthetic complications; recommend discontinuing St. John's Wort 5 days in advance of surgery

■ **SUCCINYLCHOLINE:** Sevoflurane may enhance effects

■ **SYMPATHOMIMETICS (dopamine, epinephrine, norepinephrine, ephedrine, metarami-** nol, etc.): While sevoflurane sensitizes the myocardium to the effects of sympathomimetics less so than halothane, arrhythmias may still result; caution and monitoring is advised

■ **TRAMADOL:** May decrease MAC requirements

■ **VERAPAMIL:** May cause cardiodepression

Laboratory Considerations

■ Inhalational anesthetics may cause transient increases in **liver function tests, WBCs,** and **glucose**

Doses

Minimal Alveolar Concentration (MAC; %) in oxygen reported for sevoflurane in various species: Dog = 2.09–2.4; Cat = 2.58; Horse = 2.31; Sheep = 3.3; Swine = 1.97–2.66; Human (adult) = 1.71–2.05. Several factors may alter MAC (acid/base status, temperature, other CNS depressants on board, age, ongoing acute disease, etc.)

■ **DOGS/CATS:**

a) Dogs: Inspired Concentration: The delivered concentration of *SevoFlo®* (sevoflurane) should be known. Since the depth of anesthesia may be altered easily and rapidly, only vaporizers producing predictable percentage concentrations of sevoflurane should be used. Sevoflurane should be vaporized using a precision vaporizer specifically calibrated for sevoflurane. Sevoflurane contains no stabilizer. Nothing in the drug product alters calibration or operation of these vaporizers. The administration of general anesthesia must be individualized based on the patient's response. When using sevoflurane, patients should be continuously monitored and facilities for maintenance of patient airway, artificial ventilation, and oxygen supplementation must be immediately available.

Replacement of Desiccated CO2 Absorbents: When a clinician suspects that the CO2 absorbent may be desiccated, it should be replaced. An exothermic reaction occurs when sevoflurane is exposed to CO2 absorbents. This reaction is increased when the CO2 absorbent becomes desiccated.

Premedication: No specific premedication is either indicated or contraindicated with sevoflurane. The necessity for and choice of premedication is left to the discretion of the veterinarian. Preanesthetic doses for premedicants may be lower than the label directions for their use as a single medication.

Induction: For mask induction using sevoflurane, inspired concentrations up to 7% sevoflurane with oxygen are employed to induce surgical anesthesia in the healthy dog. These concentrations can be expected to produce surgical anesthesia in 3 to 14 minutes. **Due to the rapid and dose dependent changes in anesthetic depth, care should be taken to prevent overdosing. Respiration must be monitored closely in the dog and supported when necessary with supplemental oxygen and/or assisted ventilation.**

Maintenance: *SevoFlo®* may be used for maintenance anesthesia following mask induction using sevoflurane or following injectable induction agents. The concentration of vapor necessary to maintain anesthesia is much less than that required to induce it. Surgical levels of anesthesia in the healthy dog may be maintained with inhaled concentrations of 3.7–4% sevoflurane in oxygen in the absence of premedication and 3.3–3.6% in the presence of premedication. The use of injectable induction agents without premedication has little effect on the concentrations of sevoflurane required for maintenance. Anesthetic regimens that include opioid, alpha2-agonist benzodiazepine or phenothiazine premedication will allow the use of lower sevoflurane maintenance concentrations. (Label directions; *SevoFlo®*—Abbott Animal Health)

b) Dogs/Cats: Where required, mask induction (particularly of cats) is achieved easily via a non-rebreathing system, usually starting at a concentration of around 4–4.5%. Maximum concentration (8%) is possible using the vaporizer and can be used for fresh gas flow for 'chamber' inductions as the concentrations in the box take time to reach high levels. However, concentrations administered must be reduced as soon as the animal loses consciousness (*i.e.*, take animal out of the box). For maintenance, vaporizer settings with non-rebreathing systems depend on the fresh gas flow rates as well as the residual effects of injectable drugs; a vaporizer setting of 3% for a circle system is a reasonable initial concentration. (Clarke 2008)

Monitoring
- Respiratory and ventilatory status
- Cardiac rate/rhythm; blood pressure (particularly with "at risk" patients)
- Level of anesthesia

Chemistry/Synonyms
Sevoflurane is an isopropyl ether inhalational anesthetic with a molecular wt. of 200, saturate vapor pressure at 20°C of 160 mmHg and a boiling pt. of 58.5°C. It is reported to have a pleasant odor and is not irritating to airways. It is non-

flammable and non-explosive. Sevoflurane is a clear, colorless liquid that is miscible with ethanol or ether and slightly soluble in water. It does not possess an objectionable odor.

Sevoflurane may also be known as: BAX-3084, MR-654, *Sevocris®*, *SevoFlo®*, *Sevorane®*, or *Ultane®*.

Storage/Stability
Sevoflurane should be stored at room temperature. Sevoflurane does not react with metal.

Dosage Forms/Regulatory Status

VETERINARY-LABELED PRODUCTS:
Sevoflurane in 250 mL btls; *SevoFlo®* (Halocarbon Prod.); *Petrem®* (Minrad); (Rx). FDA-approved for use in dogs.

HUMAN-LABELED PRODUCTS:
Sevoflurane in 250 mL btls; *Ultane®* (Abbott); *Sojourn®* (Minrad); (Rx)

References
Clarke, K.W. (2008). Options for inhalation anaesthesia. *In Practice* **30**(9): 513–518.
Mathews, N.S. (2008). Newer Anesthetics: 2. Proceedings: ACVC. Accessed via: Veterinary Information Network. http://goo.gl/Yxy45

SILDENAFIL CITRATE

(sil-*den*-ah-fil)   Viagra®, Revatio®

VASODILATOR; PHOSPHODIESTERASE TYPE 5 INHIBITOR

Prescriber Highlights

▶ Used in veterinary medicine for treating pulmonary hypertension

▶ Contraindicated if patients receiving organic nitrates

▶ Adverse effects not well-known; inguinal flushing, possible GI effects reported

▶ Treatment may be very expensive

Uses/Indications
Sildenafil may be of benefit in the adjunctive treatment of pulmonary hypertension in small animals.

In humans, sildenafil is indicated for erectile dysfunction or pulmonary hypertension.

Pharmacology/Actions
Sildenafil inhibits cyclic guanosine monophosphate (cGMP) specific phosphodiesterase type-5 (PDE5) found in the smooth muscle of the pulmonary vasculature, corpus cavernosum and elsewhere, where PDE5 is responsible for degradation of cGMP. Sildenafil increases cGMP thereby resulting in nitric oxide mediated vasodilatation within pulmonary vascular smooth muscle cells.

Pharmacokinetics
The pharmacokinetics of sildenafil has been reported in dogs (Walker *et al.* 1999). Oral

bioavailability is approximately 50% (higher than humans); volume of distribution is about 5.2 L/kg (versus 1.2 L/kg in humans); elimination half-life approximately 6 hours (significant interpatient variability; average human half life is about 4 hours).

Contraindications/Precautions/Warnings

Sildenafil should not be used concurrently with nitrates (see drug interactions) or in patients documented hypersensitive to it.

Pulmonary vasodilators may significantly worsen the cardiovascular status of patients with pulmonary veno-occlusive disease (PVOD).

Use with extreme caution in patients with resting hypotension, fluid depletion, severe left ventricular outflow obstruction, or autonomic dysfunction.

Adverse Effects

Because of limited use in dogs, the adverse effect profile is not fully known. Cutaneous flushing of the inguinal region has been reported and GI effects are possible. In humans, headache, visual disturbances, dyspepsia, nasal congestion, myalgia, priapism, dizziness, and back pain have been reported.

Reproductive/Nursing Safety

No evidence of teratogenicity, embryotoxicity or fetotoxicity was observed in pregnant rats or rabbits, dosed at 200 mg/kg/day during organogenesis. In a rat pre- and postnatal development study, the no-observed-adverse-effect dose was 30 mg/kg/day. In humans, the FDA categorizes this drug as category **B** for use during pregnancy (*Animal studies have not yet demonstrated risk to the fetus, but there are no adequate studies in pregnant women; or animal studies have shown an adverse effect, but adequate studies in pregnant women have not demonstrated a risk to the fetus in the first trimester of pregnancy, and there is no evidence of risk in later trimesters.*)

It is not known if sildenafil or its metabolites are excreted in milk.

Overdosage/Acute Toxicity

Little information is available. An adult woman ingested 2000 mg and survived but developed tachycardia, nonspecific ST-T changes on ECG, headache, dizziness, and flushing.

It is expected that overdoses in animals would mirror the drugs adverse effect profile; treat supportively.

Drug Interactions

The following drug interactions have either been reported or are theoretical in humans or animals receiving sildenafil and may be of significance in veterinary patients:

- **ALPHA-ADRENERGIC BLOCKERS (e.g., phentolamine, phenothiazines, phenoxybenzamine):** May increase hypotensive effects
- **AMLODIPINE:** Potential to increase hypotensive effects

- **ANTIHYPERTENSIVE, HYPOTENSIVE DRUGS:** Potentially could increase hypotensive effects
- **AZOLE ANTIFUNGALS (ketoconazole, itraconazole):** May reduce sildenafil metabolism and increase AUC
- **CIMETIDINE:** May reduce sildenafil metabolism and increase AUC
- **ERYTHROMYCIN, CLARITHROMYCIN:** May reduce sildenafil metabolism and increase AUC
- **HEPARIN:** May increase bleeding risks
- **NITRATES (e.g., NTG, Isosorbide):** Significant potentiation of vasodilatory effects; life-threatening hypotension possible
- **NITROPRUSSIDE SODIUM:** Significant potentiation of vasodilatory effects; life-threatening hypotension possible
- **PHENOBARBITAL:** May decrease sildenafil concentrations
- **RIFAMPIN:** May decrease sildenafil concentrations

Laboratory Considerations

- None were noted.

Doses

- **DOGS/CATS:**

  For pulmonary hypertension:

  a) Dogs: From a retrospective study: median dose was 1.9 mg/kg (range from 0.5–2.7 mg/kg) q8–24h. Dogs may have been also treated with oxygen, ACE inhibitors, furosemide, amlodipine, diltiazem, theophylline, phenobarbital and/or antibiotics. (Bach et al. 2006)

  b) For pulmonary hypertension documented by Doppler, chronic pulmonary disease, right-sided heart failure (HW disease; congenital): 0.5–1 mg/kg PO two times daily (higher dose of 2 –3 mg/kg three times a day may be tolerated and needed) (Tilley 2007)

  c) In dogs and cats with moderate to severe PH secondary to either left heart disease or primary lung disease: 1 mg/kg PO q8h. (Henik 2007)

  d) Dogs: 1–2 mg/kg PO three times daily. (Oyama 2009)

Monitoring

- Clinical efficacy (improved syncope, cough, respiratory effort)
- Pulmonary artery pressure, systemic blood pressure
- Adverse effects

Client Information

- Brief clients on the experimental nature of using this medication in small animals and the costs of therapy
- Report any adverse effects to the veterinarian

Chemistry/Synonyms

Sildenafil citrate occurs as a white to off-white crystalline powder with a solubility of 3.5 mg/mL in water and a molecular weight of 666.7.

Sildenafil may also be known as UK 92480, UK 92480-10, *Aphrodil®*, *Revatio®*, or *Viagra®*.

Storage/Stability

Sildenafil tablets should be stored at room temperature (25°C; 77°F); excursions permitted to 15–30°C (59–86°F).

Dosage Forms/Regulatory Status

VETERINARY-LABELED PRODUCTS: None

HUMAN-LABELED PRODUCTS:

Sildenafil Citrate Oral Tablets: 20 mg *Revatio®* (Pfizer); (Rx) and 25 mg, 50 mg & 100 mg (of sildenafil); *Viagra®* (Pfizer); (Rx)

Sildenafil Injection Solution: 10 mg/12.5 mL (dextrose 50.5 mg/mL) in 12.5 mL single-use vials; *Revatio®* (Pfizer); (Rx)

References

Bach, J., E. Rozanski, et al. (2006). Retrospective evaluation of sildenafil citrate as a therapy for pulmonary hypertension in dogs. *J Vet Intern Med* **20**: 1132–1135.

Henik, R. (2007). Pulmonary Hypertension: More than Viagra. Proceedings: IVECCS. Accessed via: Veterinary Information Network. http://goo.gl/MYyCw

Oyama, M. (2009). Pulmonary Hypertension: What you can't see can kill you. Proceedings: ACVC. Accessed via: Veterinary Information Network. http://goo.gl/0jNQb

Tilley, L. (2007). A cardiac drug formulary. Proceedings: WVC. Accessed via: Veterinary Information Network. http://goo.gl/HEgQe

Walker, D., M. Ackland, et al. (1999). Pharmacokinetics and metabolism of sildenafil in mouse, rat, rabbit, dog and man. *Xenobiotica* **29**(3): 297–310.

SILYMARIN
MILK THISTLE

(sill-e-*mar*-in)   Marin®

NUTRACEUTICAL HEPATO-PROTECTANT

Prescriber Highlights

▶ Nutraceutical that may be useful for treatment of chronic & acute liver disease, cirrhosis; as a hepato-protective agent when hepatotoxins (*e.g., Aminita phalloide*) ingested

▶ Appears well-tolerated; potentially could cause GI effects

▶ Do not confuse Milk Thistle with Blessed Thistle

▶ Potential drug interactions

Uses/Indications

While controlled studies demonstrating efficacy and a standardized form and concentration of silymarin are lacking, it is being used to treat a variety of liver diseases in humans and domestic companion animals (birds, dogs, cats, horses, rabbits). It is mostly of interest in treating chronic and acute liver disease, cirrhosis, and as a hepato-protective agent when hepatotoxic agents are ingested (*e.g., Aminita phalloide*; "Death Cap Mushrooms"). There is laboratory data that silymarin may be beneficial in preventing certain cancers and in improving the efficacy and reducing the negative effects of chemotherapy for certain tumors.

Pharmacology/Actions

Silymarin has a variety of pharmacologic actions that may contribute to its apparent effects in treating liver disease. It inhibits lipid peroxidase and beta-glucuronidase and acts as an anti-oxidant and free radical scavenger. Silymarin also inhibits the cytotoxic, inflammatory, and apoptotic effects of tumor necrosis factor (TFN). It apparently can alter outer hepatocyte cell membranes that can prevent toxin penetration. Silymarin is thought to reduce hepatic collagen formation and increase hepatic glutathione content.

Pharmacokinetics

In humans, silymarin has an oral bioavailability of less than 50% and peak levels occur 2–4 hours post-dose. When silibinin (silybin, sylibin) is complexed with phosphatidylcholine, oral absorption can be increased. The drug undergoes extensive enterohepatic circulation and has significantly higher concentrations in liver cells and bile than in plasma. Elimination half-life in humans averages 6 hours. The majority of the drug is eliminated unchanged in the feces, but 20–40% is converted into glucuronide and sulfate conjugates which are eliminated in the feces; only about 8% is excreted in the urine.

Contraindications/Precautions/Warnings

There are no reported absolute contraindications to silymarin in animals. Extracts from the plant parts of Milk Thistle (not the seeds which are used to make the extract silymarin), may possess estrogen-like activity and should not be used in patients where exogenous estrogens would be contraindicated.

Adverse Effects

Silymarin is apparently well tolerated when administered orally. In humans, GI disturbances have been reported on occasion (nausea to diarrhea). Patients who have allergies to other members of the Asteraceae/Compositae plant family (includes ragweed, marigolds, daisies, etc.) may exhibit allergic reactions to Milk Thistle derivatives. Do not confuse Milk Thistle with Blessed Thistle.

Reproductive/Nursing Safety

Data on the safety of silymarin use during pregnancy or nursing is not available; its potential benefit must be weighed against the uncertainty of its safety.

Overdosage/Acute Toxicity

Overdoses are unlikely to cause significant morbidity. Gastrointestinal effects may be seen and treated in a supportive manner.

Drug Interactions

While no specific drug interactions have been reported, silymarin may inhibit cytochrome P450 isoenzyme 2C9 (CYP2C9). Drugs with narrow therapeutic indexes that are metabolized by this isoenzyme should be used with caution when using silymarin. Drugs that could be affected include: **warfarin, amitriptyline, verapamil,** etc.

Silymarin also may inhibit CYP3A4, but thus far this interaction does not appear to be clinically significant. Silymarin may increase the clearance of drugs that undergo hepatic glucuronidation (not cats), including: **acetaminophen, diazepam, morphine, and lamotrigine.** Clinical significance has not been determined for this interaction and the usefulness of silymarin for treating acetaminophen toxicity has not been determined.

Laboratory Considerations

■ No interactions with laboratory tests are reported.

Doses

■ **DOGS/CATS:**

a) Therapeutic dosage is unknown, but suggested doses range from 50–250 mg/day (Twedt 2004)

b) For adjunctive therapy for chronic liver disease: 20–50 mg/kg per day (extrapolated from human, monkey, rodent and dog research) (Center 2002)

c) For chronic liver disease and ameliorating the effects of anticonvulsants: Dosages vary from 50–200 mg given every 12–24 hours (Tams 2001)

d) For hepatotoxicity, hepatic recovery/regeneration, hepatic fibrosis: 20–50 mg/kg/day. (Webb 2007)

e) Cats: 4–8 mg/kg/day (Zoran 2006)

Monitoring

■ Clinical efficacy

Client Information

■ May cause diarrhea or vomiting. If these persists or are severe, contact veterinarian.

■ These products are not evaluated or approved by the FDA

Chemistry/Synonyms

Milk Thistle, the common name for *Silybum marianum*, has been used as a medicinal agent for at least two thousand years. The medicinal extract from the seeds of the plant is silymarin that contains the four flavolignans: silichristin (sylichristin), isosilibinin, silydianin (silidianin), and the most biological active component, silibinin (sylibin, silybin, silibide). Milk Thistle extract contains approximately 70% silymarin of which about 70% is silibinin. Silymarin is reportedly fairly insoluble in water.

Silymarin or Milk thistle may also be known as *Carduus marianus*, Holy Thistle, Legalon,

or Marian Thistle. Blessed Thistle is a different compound.

Storage/Stability

Unless otherwise labeled, commercially available products containing silymarin should be stored at room temperature in tight containers. Avoid storing the products in areas of high humidity.

Dosage Forms/Regulatory Status

VETERINARY-LABELED PRODUCTS:

Milk Thistle or silymarin is considered a nutritional supplement by the FDA. No standards have been accepted for potency, etc. by regulatory bodies. Supplements are available from a wide variety of sources and dosage forms include tablets and capsules in a variety of concentrations (150–1000 mg). When choosing a product it is recommended to purchase ones that state the concentration (usually 70–80%) of silymarin contained in the product.

Silybin A+B 9 mg (in a phosphatidylcholine complex) & Vitamin E 50 Units Tablets: *Marin®* *for Cats* (Nutramax); Not considered a drug by the FDA.

Silybin A+B 24 mg (in a phosphatidylcholine complex), Vitamin E 105 Units, & Zinc 17 mg Chewable Tablets: *Marin® for Dogs* (Nutramax); Not considered a drug by the FDA. Labeled for use in small to medium dogs.

Silybin A+B 70 mg (in a phosphatidylcholine complex), Vitamin E 300 Units, & Zinc 45 mg Chewable Tablets: *Marin® for Dogs* (Nutramax); not considered a drug by the FDA. Labeled for use in large dogs.

A combination product (*Denamarin®*, Nutramax) containing SAMe and silybin (silymarin) is also labeled for use in dogs and cats.

HUMAN-LABELED PRODUCTS: None as pharmaceuticals

References

Center, S. (2002). Chronic hepatitis. Proceedings: Western Veterinary Conference. Accessed via: Veterinary Information Network. http://goo.gl/pvWQX

Tams, T. (2001). Management of chronic liver disease. Proceedings: Atlantic Coast Veterinary Conference. Accessed via: Veterinary Information Network. http://goo.gl/Vsos8

Twedt, D. (2004). Nutraceuticals in liver disease. Proceedings: ACVIM Forum. Accessed via: Veterinary Information Network. http://goo.gl/6LVwJ

Webb, C. (2007). Pushing the envelope in liver and pancreatic diseases. Proceedings: Western Vet Conference. Accessed via: Veterinary Information Network. http://goo.gl/bKTSb

Zoran, D. (2006). Inflammatory liver disease in cats. Proceedings: ABVP 2006. Accessed via: Veterinary Information Network. http://goo.gl/IFyUT

SODIUM BICARBONATE

(soe-*dee*-um bye-*kar*-boe-nate)   Neut®

ALKALINIZER

Prescriber Highlights

▶ Alkalinizing agent used to treat metabolic acidosis & alkalinize urine; may be used adjunctively for hypercalcemic or hyperkalemic crises

▶ Contraindications: Parenteral bicarbonate is generally contraindicated in patients with metabolic or respiratory alkalosis, excessive chloride loss secondary to vomiting or GI suction, at risk for development of diuretic-induced hypochloremic alkalosis, or with hypocalcemia where alkalosis may induce tetany

▶ Extreme Caution: Hypocalcemia Caution: CHF, nephrotic syndrome, hypertension, oliguria or volume overload

▶ Adverse Effects: Especially with parenteral (high dose): metabolic alkalosis, hypokalemia, hypocalcemia, "overshoot" alkalosis, hypernatremia, volume overload, congestive heart failure, shifts in the oxygen dissociation curve causing decreased tissue oxygenation, & paradoxical CNS acidosis leading to respiratory arrest. If used during CPR: hypercapnia, if the patient is not well ventilated; patients may be predisposed to ventricular fibrillation.

▶ Drug Interactions

Uses/Indications

Sodium bicarbonate is indicated to treat metabolic acidosis and alkalinize the urine. It is also used as adjunctive therapy in treating hypercalcemic or hyperkalemia crises.

Pharmacology/Actions

Bicarbonate ion is the conjugate base component of bicarbonate: carbonic acid buffer, the principal extracellular buffer in the body.

Contraindications/Precautions/Warnings

Parenterally administered sodium bicarbonate is considered generally contraindicated in patients with metabolic or respiratory alkalosis, excessive chloride loss secondary to vomiting or GI suction, at risk for development of diuretic-induced hypochloremic alkalosis, or with hypocalcemia where alkalosis may induce tetany.

Use with extreme caution and give very slowly in patients with hypocalcemia. Because of the potential sodium load, use with caution in patients with CHF, nephrotic syndrome, hypertension, oliguria, or volume overload.

Adverse Effects

Sodium bicarbonate therapy (particularly high-dose parenteral use) can lead to metabolic alkalosis, hypokalemia, hypocalcemia, "overshoot" alkalosis, hypernatremia, volume overload, congestive heart failure, shifts in the oxygen dissociation curve causing decreased tissue oxygenation, and paradoxical CNS acidosis leading to respiratory arrest.

When sodium bicarbonate is used during cardiopulmonary resuscitation, hypercapnia may result if the patient is not well ventilated; patients may be predisposed to ventricular fibrillation.

Oral and parenteral bicarbonate (especially at higher doses) may contribute significant amounts of sodium and result in hypernatremia and volume overload; use with caution in patients with CHF, or acute renal failure.

Reproductive/Nursing Safety

Reproductive safety studies have not been performed. Assess risk versus benefit before using.

Overdosage/Acute Toxicity

Sodium bicarbonate can cause severe alkalosis, with irritability or tetany if overdosed or given too rapidly. Dosages should be thoroughly checked and frequent monitoring of electrolyte and acid/base status performed.

Treatment may consist of simply discontinuing bicarbonate if alkalosis is mild or by using a rebreathing mask. Severe alkalosis may require intravenous calcium therapy. Sodium chloride or potassium chloride may be necessary if hypokalemia is present.

Drug Interactions

The following drug interactions have either been reported or are theoretical in humans or animals receiving sodium bicarbonate and may be of significance in veterinary patients:

■ **ANTICHOLINERGIC AGENTS:** Concomitant oral sodium bicarbonate may reduce absorption; administer separately

■ **AZOLE ANTIFUNGALS (ketoconazole, itraconazole):** Concomitant oral sodium bicarbonate may reduce absorption; administer separately

■ **CIPROFLOXACIN; ENROFLOXACIN:** The solubility of ciprofloxacin and enrofloxacin is decreased in an alkaline environment; patients with alkaline urine should be monitored for signs of crystalluria

■ **CORTICOSTEROIDS:** Patients receiving high dosages of sodium bicarbonate and ACTH or glucocorticoids may develop hypernatremia

■ **DIURETICS (e.g., thiazides, furosemide):** Concurrent use of sodium bicarbonate in patients receiving potassium-wasting diuretics may cause hypochloremic alkalosis

■ **EPHEDRINE:** When urine is alkalinized by sodium bicarbonate, excretion may be decreased

■ **HISTAMINE$_2$ BLOCKING AGENTS (e.g., ci-metidine, ranitidine):** Concomitant oral sodium bicarbonate may reduce absorption; administer separately

■ **IRON PRODUCTS:** Concomitant oral sodium bicarbonate may reduce absorption; administer separately

■ **ORAL MEDICATIONS:** Because oral sodium bicarbonate can either increase or reduce the rate and/or extent of absorption of many orally administered drugs, it is recommended to avoid giving other drugs within 1–2 hours of sodium bicarbonate

■ **QUINIDINE:** When urine is alkalinized by sodium bicarbonate, excretion may be decreased

■ **SALICYLATES:** When urine is alkalinized by sodium bicarbonate, excretion of weakly acidic drugs may be increased

■ **SUCRALFATE:** Oral sodium bicarbonate may reduce the efficacy of sucralfate if administered concurrently

■ **TETRACYCLINES:** Concomitant oral sodium bicarbonate may reduce absorption; administer separately

Doses

■ **DOGS/CATS:**

For severe metabolic acidosis:

a) Main therapeutic goal should be to eliminate the underlying cause of acidosis. If causes are not readily reversible, arterial pH is <7.2 (7.1 if diabetic ketoacidosis), and ventilatory procedures have not reduced acidemia, bicarbonate therapy should be considered. mEq of bicarbonate required = 0.5 x body weight in kg x(desired total CO_2 mEq/L minus measured total CO_2 mEq/L). Give ½ of the calculated dose slowly over 3–4 hours IV. Recheck blood gases and assess the clinical status of the patient. Avoid over-alkalinization. (Schaer 2006)

b) For metabolic acidosis secondary to uremia: In the majority of patients, definitive treatment of the urinary tract disorder and fluid diuresis is usually all that is required. In the unstable dog or cat with a pH <7.0 due to metabolic acidosis, sodium bicarb administration should be considered. The formula often recommended is 0.3 x body weight (kilograms) x the base deficit. This gives an approximation for the total bicarbonate deficit. Administration of one third of this dose slowly IV and the rest placed in the intravenous fluids will correct the metabolic acidosis over several hours. If measurement of blood gas is not possible and it is believed that the animal is severely acidemic, 1–2 mEq/kg of bicarbonate can be given as a slow IV bolus. Rapid intravenous

boluses of sodium bicarbonate should be avoided because of the production of carbon dioxide and its diffusion into the central nervous system making CSF acidosis even worse. Other disadvantages of sodium bicarbonate administration include shifting of the oxygen/hemoglobin dissociation curve to the left and increasing osmolality. When monitoring the response to bicarbonate through the measurement of blood gases, remember that bicarbonate will increase initially in the intravascular space but then will be buffered by intracellular buffers. Immediate measurement of blood gases after bicarbonate administration may over-estimate the effect of the therapy. Diffusion and buffering of administered bicarbonate by intracellular buffers takes approximately 2-4 hours and a blood gas analysis should be performed after this time period as well. (Drobatz 2009)

c) For metabolic acidosis in acutely critical situations (cardiac arrest): Sodium bicarbonate is generally not necessary unless a metabolic acidosis was present before the arrest or the CPR is extending beyond 10-20 minutes. It is definitely not given in those animals not being ventilated well. Both venous and arterial blood gas analysis is recommended to accurately determine if or how much bicarbonate is required. In most cases of CPR, hyperventilation alone is enough to circumvent the acidosis that occurs during CPR. (Crowe 2008)

For adjunctive therapy of diabetic ketoacidosis:

Note: Use of bicarb for this indication is somewhat controversial and its use is falling out of favor. Bicarb therapy can be dangerous in DKA for several reasons. Like insulin, bicarbonate drives potassium intracellularly, potentially worsening hypokalemia. Bicarbonate shifts the oxyhemoglobin curve to the left decreasing oxygen release at the tissue level and can lead to paradoxic central nervous system acidosis, fluid overload, lactic acidosis, persistent ketosis, and cerebral edema (O'Brien 2010).

a) If plasma bicarbonate is ≤11 mEq/L give bicarbonate therapy. Dose (in mEq) = body weight in kgs. x 0.4 x (12–patient's bicarbonate) x 0.5. Give above dose over 6 hours in IV fluids and then recheck plasma bicarbonate or total venous CO_2. If still ≤11 mEq/L, recalculate dose and repeat therapy. (Nelson & Feldman 1988)

For adjunctive treatment of hypercalcemic crisis:

a) The mEq of bicarbonate required = 0.3 x body weight in kg x (desired plasma bicarbonate mEq/L — measured plasma bicarbonate mEq/L); or 1 mEq/kg IV every 10–15 minutes; maximum total dose: 4 mEq/L (Kruger *et al.* 1986)

For adjunctive therapy for hyperkalemic crises:

a) If serum bicarbonate or total CO_2 is unavailable: 2–3 mEq/kg IV over 30 minutes if patient has decreased tissue perfusion or renal failure and does not have diabetic ketoacidosis. Must be used judiciously. (Willard 1986)

b) 1–2 mEq/kg IV slowly (Macintire 2006)

To alkalinize the urine:

a) Dosage must be individualized to the patient. Initially give 10–90 grains (650 mg–5.85 grams) PO per day, depending on the size of the patient and the pretreatment urine pH value. Goal of therapy is to maintain a urine pH of about 7; avoid pH >7.5.) (Osborne *et al.* 1989)

b) For adjunctive therapy in dissolution and/or prevention of urate urolithiasis in dogs: 0.5–1 gram (⅛–¼ tsp.) per 5 kg of body weight three times daily PO. Goal of therapy is to attain a urine pH of from 7–7.5. (Senior 1989)

■ **HORSES:**

For metabolic acidosis:

a) Associated with colic; if pH is <7.3 and base deficit is >10 mEq/L estimate bicarbonate requirement using the formula: bicarbonate deficit (HCO^{-3} mEq) = base deficit (mEq/L) x 0.4 x body weight (kg). May administer as a 5% sodium bicarbonate solution. Each L of solution contains 600 mEq of bicarbonate (hypertonic) and should not be administered any faster than 1–2 L/hr. Because acidotic horses with colic tend also to be dehydrated, may be preferable to give as isotonic sodium bicarbonate (150 mEq/L). (Stover 1987)

■ **RUMINANTS:**

For acidosis:

a) 2–5 mEq/kg IV for a 4–8 hour period (Howard 1986)

b) For severely dehydrated (10–16% dehydrated) acidotic calves (usually comatose): Use isotonic sodium bicarbonate (156 mEq/L). Most calves require about 2 liters of this solution given over 1–2 hours, then change to isotonic saline and sodium bicarbonate or a balanced electrolyte solution. Isotonic sodium bicarbonate may be made by dissolving 13 grams of sodium bicarbonate in 1 L of sterile water. Isotonic saline and sodium bicarbonate may be made by: mixing 1 L of isotonic saline with 1 L of isotonic sodium bicarbonate. (Radostits 1986)

■ **BIRDS:**

For metabolic acidosis:

a) 1 mEq/kg initially IV (then SC) for 15–30 minutes to a maximum of 4 mEq/kg (Clubb 1986)

Monitoring

■ Acid/base status

■ Serum electrolytes

■ Urine pH (if being used to alkalinize urine)

Chemistry/Synonyms

An alkalinizing agent, sodium bicarbonate occurs as a white, crystalline powder having a slightly saline or alkaline taste. It is soluble in water and insoluble in alcohol. One gram of sodium bicarbonate contains about 12 mEq (mMol) each of sodium and bicarbonate; 84 mg of sodium bicarbonate contains 1 mEq each of sodium and bicarbonate. A 1.5% solution of sodium bicarbonate is approximately isotonic. An 8.4% solution of sodium bicarbonate can be made isotonic by diluting each mL with 4.6 mL of sterile water for injection.

Because converting volume measurements into weights is not very accurate for powders, it is recommended to actually weigh powders when using them for pharmaceutical purposes. However, if this is not possible, one (1) level teaspoon (5 mL) of commercially-available baking soda contains approximately 4.8–5.9 grams of sodium bicarbonate.

Sodium Bicarbonate may also be known as: baking soda, E500, monosodium carbonate, natrii bicarbonas, natrii hydrogenocarbonas, sal de vichy, sodium acid carbonate, $NaHCO_3$, sodium hydrogen carbonate; many trade names are available.

Storage/Stability

Sodium bicarbonate tablets should be stored in tight containers, preferably at room temperature (15–30°C). Sodium bicarbonate injection should be stored at temperatures less than 40°C and preferably at room temperature; avoid freezing.

Sodium bicarbonate powder is stable in dry air, but will slowly decompose upon exposure to moist air.

Compatibility/Compounding Considerations

Sodium bicarbonate for injection is reportedly physically **compatible** with the following intravenous solutions and drugs: Dextrose in water, dextrose/saline combinations, dextrose-Ringer's combinations, sodium chloride injections, amikacin sulfate, aminophylline, amphotericin B, atropine sulfate, bretylium tosylate, cefoxitin sodium, chloramphenicol sodium succinate, chlorothiazide sodium, cimetidine HCl, clindamycin phosphate, ergonovine maleate, erythromycin gluceptate/lactobionate, heparin sodium, hyaluronidase, hydrocortisone sodium succinate, kanamycin sulfate, lidocaine HCl, metaraminol bitartrate, methotrexate sodium, oxytocin, phenobarbital sodium, phenylephrine HCl, phenytoin sodium, phytonadione, potassium chloride, prochlorperazine edisylate, and sodium iodide.

Sodium bicarbonate for injection **compatibility information conflicts** or is dependent on diluent or concentration factors with the following drugs or solutions: lactated Ringer's injection, Ringer's injection, sodium lactate 1/6 M, ampicillin sodium, calcium chloride/gluconate, penicillin G potassium, pentobarbital sodium, promazine HCl, thiopental sodium, vancomycin HCl, verapamil HCl, and vitamin B-complex with C. Consult specialized references or a hospital pharmacist for more specific information.

Sodium bicarbonate for injection is reportedly physically **incompatible** with the following solutions or drugs: alcohol 5%/dextrose 5%, D$_5$ lactated Ringer's, amrinone lactate, ascorbic acid injection, carmustine, cisplatin, codeine phosphate, corticotropin, dobutamine HCl, epinephrine HCl, glycopyrrolate, hydromorphone HCl, imipenem-cilastatin, regular insulin, isoproterenol HCl, labetolol HCl, levorphanol bitartrate, magnesium sulfate, meperidine HCl, methadone HCl, metoclopramide HCl, norepinephrine bitartrate, oxytetracycline HCl, pentazocine lactate, and succinylcholine chloride.

Because converting volume measurements into weights is not very accurate for powders, it is recommended to actually weigh powders when using them for pharmaceutical purposes. However, if this is not possible, one (1) level teaspoon (5 mL) of commercially-available baking soda contains approximately 4.8–5.9 grams of sodium bicarbonate.

Dosage Forms/Regulatory Status

VETERINARY-LABELED PRODUCTS:

Sodium Bicarbonate Injection: 8.4% (1 mEq/mL) in 50 mL (50 mEq/vial), 100 mL (100 mEq/vial) and 500 mL (500 mEq/vial) vials; available generically labeled; (Rx)

HUMAN-LABELED PRODUCTS:

Injectable Products:

Sodium Bicarbonate Neutralizing Additive Solution: 4% (0.48 mEq/mL) in 5 mL (2.4 mEq) vials; 4.2% (0.5 mEq/mL) in 5 mL fill in 6 mL vials (2.5 mEq); *Neut*® (Abbott); generic (American Pharmaceutical Partners); (Rx)

Sodium Bicarbonate Injection: 4.2% (0.5 mEq/mL) in 10 mL (5 mEq) syringes, 10 mL (5 mEq) *Bristoject* syringes; generic; (Rx)

Sodium Bicarbonate Injection: 5% (0.6 mEq/mL) in 500 mL vials (297.5 mEq); generic; (Rx)

Sodium Bicarbonate Injection: 7.5% (0.9 mEq/mL) in 50 mL (44.6 mEq) amps, syringes, vials, *Bristoject* syringes and 200 mL (179 mEq) *MaxiVials*; generic; (Rx)

Sodium Bicarbonate Injection: 8.4% (1 mEq/mL) in 10 mL (10 mEq) and 50 mL (50 mEq) syringes and 50 mL vials (50 mEq/vial); generic; (Rx)

Oral Products:

Sodium Bicarbonate Tablets: 325 mg & 650 mg; generic; (OTC)

Powder: 120 grams, 300 grams & 1 lb; generic; (OTC)

Omeprazole/Sodium Bicarbonate Capsules (immediate release): 20 mg omeprazole/1,100 mg sodium bicarbonate & 40 mg omeprazole/1,100 mg sodium bicarbonate; *Zegerid*® (Santarus); (Rx)

Omeprazole/Sodium Bicarbonate Powder for Oral Suspension: 20 mg omeprazole/1,680 mg sodium bicarbonate & 40 mg omeprazole/1,680 mg sodium bicarbonate in unit-dose packets; *Zegerid*® (Santarus); (Rx)

References

Clubb, S.L. (1986). Therapeutics: Individual and Flock Treatment Regimens. *Clinical Avian Medicine and Surgery*. GJ Harrison and LR Harrison Eds. Philadelphia, W.B. Saunders: 327–355.

Crowe, D. (2008). Cardiac Arrest Prevention and Management: New Paradigm Shifts That Must Be Taken. Proceedings: ACVC. Accessed via: Veterinary Information Network. http://goo.gl/aQNgL

Drobatz, K.J. (2009). Emergencies of the urogenital tract. Proceedings: IVECCS. Accessed via: Veterinary Information Network. http://goo.gl/n6v1j

Kruger, J.M., C.A. Osborne, et al. (1986). Treatment of hypercalcemia. *Current Veterinary Therapy (CVT) IX Small Animal Practice*. RW Kirk Ed. Philadelphia, W.B. Saunders: 75–90.

Macintire, D. (2006). Cardiac Emergencies. Proceedings: ACVC 2006. Accessed via: Veterinary Information Network. http://goo.gl/KxqeK

Nelson, R.W. & E.C. Feldman (1988). Diseases of the Endocrine Pancreas. *Handbook of Small Animal Practice*. RV Morgan Ed. New York, Churchill Livingstone: 527–535.

O'Brien, M.A. (2010). Diabetic Emergencies in Small Animals. *Veterinary Clinics of North America-Small Animal Practice* 40(2): 317–+.

Osborne, C.A., D.J. Polzin, et al. (1989). Canine Urolithiasis. *Textbook of Veterinary Internal Medicine*. SJ Ettinger Ed. Philadelphia, WB Saunders. 2: 2083–2107.

Radostits, O.M. (1986). Neonatal diarrhea in ruminants (calves, lambs and kids). *Current Veterinary Therapy 2: Food Animal Practice*. JL Howard Ed. Philadelphia, WB Saunders: 105–113.

Schaer, M. (2006). Acute adrenocortical insufficiency. Proceedings: WSAVA World Congress. Accessed via: Veterinary Information Network. http://goo.gl/QpFSa

Senior, D.F. (1989). Medical Management of Urate Uroliths. *Current Veterinary Therapy X: Small Animal Practice*. RW Kirk Ed. Philadelphia, WB Saunders: 1178–1181.

Stover, S.M. (1987). Pre- and postoperative management of the colic patient. *Current Therapy in Equine Medicine: 2*. NE Robinson Ed. Philadelphia, WB Saunders: 33–38.

Willard, M.D. (1986). Treatment of hyperkalemia. *Current Veterinary Therapy IX: Small Animal Practice*. RW Kirk Ed. Phialdelphai, W.B. Saunders: 94–101.

Sodium Bromide—see Bromides

Sodium Chloride Injections—see the Intravenous Fluids section in the appendix

Sodium Citrate—see Citrate Salts

Sodium Hyaluronate—see
Hyaluronate Sodium

Sodium Iodide—see Iodide,
Sodium

Sodium Nitroprusside—see
Nitroprusside Sodium

Sodium Phosphate—see
Phosphate, Parenteral

SODIUM POLYSTYRENE SULFONATE

(soe-**dee**-um pol-ee-**stye**-reen **sulf**-foe-nate)
Kayexalate®, SPS

CATIONIC EXCHANGE RESIN (HYPER-
KALEMIA)

Prescriber Highlights

▶ Cation exchange resin used to treat
hyperkalemia

▶ Contraindications: Patients who cannot
tolerate a large sodium load

▶ Cause of hyperkalemia must be addressed

▶ Adverse Effects: Constipation, anorexia,
vomiting, or nausea. Overdosage/over-
use may lead to hypokalemia, hypocalcemia & hypomagnesemia.

▶ If given PO, often mixed with sorbitol to expedite removal of resin (&
potassium)

▶ Drug Interactions

Uses/Indications

SPS is indicated as adjunctive treatment of
hyperkalemia. The cause of the hyperkalemia
should be elucidated and corrected if possible.

Pharmacology/Actions

SPS is a resin that exchanges sodium for other
cations. After being given orally, hydrogen ions
will be exchanged for sodium (in an acidic environment). As the resin travels through the intestinal tract, the hydrogen ions will be exchanged
with other more concentrated cations. Primary
exchange with potassium occurs predominantly
in the large intestine. When given as a retention enema, SPS generally exchanges sodium
for potassium directly in the colorectum. While
theoretically, up to 3.1 mEq of potassium could
be exchanged per gram of SPS, it is unlikely that
more than one mEq will be exchanged per gram
of resin administered.

Pharmacokinetics

SPS is not absorbed from the GI tract. Its onset
of action may be from hours to days; so severe

hyperkalemia may require other treatments
(*e.g.*, dialysis) in the interim.

Contraindications/Precautions/Warnings

Because large quantities of sodium may be
released and absorbed, patients on severely
restricted sodium diets (severe CHF, hypertension, oliguria) may benefit from alternative
methods of treatment. Overdosage/overuse
may lead to hypokalemia, hypocalcemia and
hypomagnesemia.

Adverse Effects

Large doses may cause constipation (fecal impactions have been reported rarely), anorexia,
vomiting or nausea. Dose related hypocalcemia,
hypokalemia and sodium retention have also
been noted. To hasten the drug's action and prevent constipation, SPS is generally mixed with
70% sorbitol (3–4 mL per one gram of resin)
when dosed orally.

Reproductive/Nursing Safety

While reproductive studies have apparently not
been performed, it is unlikely the drug carries
much teratogenic potential. In humans, the FDA
categorizes this drug as category *C* for use during pregnancy (*Animal studies have shown an
adverse effect on the fetus, but there are no adequate studies in humans; or there are no animal
reproduction studies and no adequate studies in
humans.*)

As SPS is not absorbed, it should be safe to use
during nursing.

Overdosage/Acute Toxicity

Overdosage may cause the adverse effects noted
(above); treat symptomatically.

Drug Interactions

The following drug interactions have either been
reported or are theoretical in humans or animals
receiving SPS and may be of significance in veterinary patients:

▪ **ANTACIDS, LAXATIVES (calcium- or magnesium-containing):** SPS may bind with magnesium or calcium found in laxatives (milk
of magnesia, magnesium sulfate, etc.) or
antacids which can prevent bicarbonate ion
neutralization and lead to metabolic alkalosis. Concurrent use is not recommended
during SPS therapy.

Doses

If dosed orally, to hasten the drug's action and to
prevent constipation SPS is generally mixed with
70% sorbitol (3–4 mL per one gram of resin);
shake well before using.

▪ **DOGS:**
   a) For hyperkalemia: 2 grams of resin/kg
   of body weight (each gram should be
   suspended in 3–4 mL of water; or use
   commercially prepared suspension products) divided into 3 daily doses. If given
   orally, give with a cathartic. Do not use
   a cathartic if using as a retention enema
   as it must be in the colon for at least 30

minutes. To prepare a retention enema from the powder: add 15 grams per 100 mL of a 1% methylcellulose solution or 10% dextrose. If hyperkalemia is severe: 3–4 times the normal amount of resin may be given. (Willard 1986)

b) For mild hyperkalemia (<6 mEq/L): 2 grams/kg PO in 3–4 divided doses with 20% sorbitol; may also be give as an enema without sorbitol. (Cowgill & Francey 2005)

■ **HORSES:**

a) For life-threatening hyperkalemia in neonatal foals: 15 grams of resin in 100 mL of 10% dextrose via enema. Monitor serum potassium and sodium closely. (Madigan 2002)

Monitoring

■ Serum electrolytes (sodium potassium (at least once a day), calcium, magnesium

■ Acid/base status, ECG, if warranted

Chemistry/Synonyms

A sulfonated cation exchange resin, sodium polystyrene sulfonate (SPS) occurs as a golden brown, fine powder. It is odorless and tasteless. Each gram contains 4.1 mEq of sodium and has an *in vitro* exchange capacity of about 3.1 mEq of potassium (in actuality a maximum of 1 mEq is usually exchanged).

Sodium Polystyrene Sulfonate may also be known as: natrii polystyrenesulfonas, sodium polystyrene sulphonate, *Elutit-Natrium®*, *K-Exit®*, *Kayexalate®*, *Kexelate®*, *Kionex®*, *Resinsodio®*, *Resonium®*, *Resonium A®*, or *SPS®*.

Storage/Stability

Store products in well-closed containers at room temperature; do not heat. Suspensions made from powder should be freshly prepared and used within 24 hours.

Dosage Forms/Regulatory Status

VETERINARY-LABELED PRODUCTS: None

HUMAN-LABELED PRODUCTS:

Sodium Polystyrene Sulfonate Powder: Sodium content is approximately 100 mg (4.1 mEq) per g; in 1 lb. jars & 454 g; *Kayexalate®* (Sanofi Winthrop); *Kionex®* (Paddock); (Rx)

Sodium Polystyrene Sulfonate Suspension: 15 grams/60 mL (sodium 1.5 grams, 65 mEq) in 60 mL, 120 mL, 200 mL, 480 mL, 500 mL and UD 60 mL; *SPS®* (Carolina Medical Products Co); generic (Roxane); (Rx)

References

Cowgill, L. & T. Francey (2005). Acute uremia. *Textbook of Veterinary Internal Medicine, 6th Ed.* S Ettinger and E Feldman Eds., Elsevier: 1731–1751.

Madigan, J. (2002). Renal and urinary disorders in equine neonates. Proceedings: Western Veterinary Conference. Accessed via: Veterinary Information Network. http://goo.gl/i5uXP

Willard, M.D. (1986). Treatment of hyperkalemia. *Current Veterinary Therapy IX: Small Animal Practice*. RW Kirk Ed. Phialdelphai, W.B. Saunders: 94–101.

SODIUM STIBOGLUCONATE SODIUM ANTIMONY GLUCONATE

(sti-boe-*gloo*-koe-nate; an-ti-*moe*-nee *gloo*-koe-nate)   Pentostam®

ANTILEISHMANIAL

Prescriber Highlights

▶ Antimony compound for treatment of leishmaniasis in humans & dogs

▶ Not commercially available in USA (CDC distributes)

▶ Contraindicated in renal failure, preexisting arrhythmias

▶ Many potential adverse effects, including some very serious

Uses/Indications

Sodium stibogluconate is used for the treatment of leishmaniasis in dogs.

Pharmacology/Actions

Sodium stibogluconate's exact mode of action is unknown. It is believed that it may reduce ATP and GTP synthesis in susceptible amistigotes.

Pharmacokinetics

In dogs, stibogluconate's volume of distribution (steady-state) was 0.25 L/kg, clearance 1.71 L/kg/hr, and terminal half-life ranged from 0.6–1.5 hours. The main route of excretion is via the kidneys; glomerular filtration rate determines excretion rate.

Contraindications/Precautions/Warnings

Stibogluconate is contraindicated in patients with pre-existing cardiac arrhythmias, or significantly impaired renal function. It should not be used in those that have had a serious adverse reaction to a previous dose.

Adverse Effects

Dogs given 40 mg/kg of stibogluconate developed increased AST levels. Other reported adverse effects (incidence unknown) include pain on injection, musculoskeletal pain, hemolytic anemia, leukopenia, vomiting, diarrhea, pancreatitis, myocardial injury and arrhythmias, renal toxicity, shock and sudden death. Intravenous administration can cause thrombophlebitis. Reportedly, the incidence of adverse effects increases if the drug is administered for longer than 2 months.

Reproductive/Nursing Safety

Sodium stibogluconate has not been shown to cause fetal harm, but the manufacturer states that the drug should be withheld during pregnancy unless the benefits outweigh the risks.

The use of this drug during nursing is controversial. Some (*e.g.*, The American Academy of

Pediatrics) say that it is usually compatible with breast-feeding, but the manufacturer states that it should not be used in nursing mothers.

Overdosage/Acute Toxicity
In the unlikely event of a parenterally administered overdose, it is suggested to contact an animal poison control center. Potentially, antimony can be chelated with dimercaptosuccinic acid (DMSA) or d-penicillamine.

Drug Interactions
■ No specific drug interactions were noted. Stibogluconate has reportedly been used with allopurinol, paromomycin, or pentamidine without problems.

Laboratory Considerations
No specific laboratory interactions or considerations noted.

Doses

■ **DOGS:**
  a) For treatment of cutaneous leishmaniasis: 30–50 mg/kg IV or SC daily for 3–4 weeks (Anon 2004; Brosey 2005)
  b) For visceral leishmaniasis: 30–50 mg/kg IV or SC q24h for one month. Has severe side effects and may not be obtainable in the USA; allopurinol alone is usually used initially. (Petersen & Barr 2009)

Monitoring
■ Laboratory and clinical signs associated with adverse effects (CBC, liver enzymes, renal function tests, ECG, etc.)
■ Bone marrow cultures for Leishmania
■ Clinical efficacy

Client Information
■ Clients should understand the potential public health implications of this disease (dependent on country) in dogs, the guarded prognosis (even with treatment), risks of treatment and associated expenses.

Chemistry/Synonyms
Sodium stibogluconate is a pentavalent antimony compound that contains between 30–34% antimony and is a colorless, odorless or almost odorless, amorphous powder. Sodium stibogluconate is very soluble in water and practically insoluble in alcohol or ether. The commercially available (not in the USA) injection has a pH between 5–5.6.

Sodium stibogluconate may also be known as: sodium antimony gluconate, *stiboglucat-natrium*, natriumstibogluconat-9-wasser, solusurmin, stibogluconat, *sodio stibogluconato*, and *natrii stibogluconas*.

Storage/Stability
The commercially available injection (*Pentostam®*) should be stored at temperatures below 25°C (76°F) and protected from freezing and exposure to light. After removing the first dose, the vial should not be used after one month.

Dosage Forms/Regulatory Status
VETERINARY-LABELED PRODUCTS: None
HUMAN-LABELED PRODUCTS: None in the USA.

Sodium Stibogluconate (sodium antimony gluconate) 100 mg (of antimony)/mL for injection in 6 mL and 100 mL (*Pentostam®*—Wellcome Foundation) is available from the Centers for Disease Control (CDC). It may or may not be released for use in domestic animals. Contact the CDC at 404-639-3670 from 8 AM–4:30 PM Eastern Time, Monday-Friday for more information or go to their website: www.cdc.gov/ncidod/srp/drugs/drug-service.html

Pentostam® is available commercially in several countries.

References
Anon (2004). "Cutaneous Leishmaniasis." *Associate Library*. Veterinary Information Network
Brosey, B. (2005). Leishmaniasis. Proceedings: ACVIM 2005. Accessed via: Veterinary Information Network. http://goo.gl/qQ0Yr
Petersen, C.A. & S.C. Barr (2009). Canine Leishmaniasis in North America: Emerging or Newly Recognized? *Veterinary Clinics of North America-Small Animal Practice* 39(6): 1065–+.

SODIUM THIOSULFATE

(soe-*dee*-um thye-oh-*sul*-fayte)
Sodium Hyposulfite
ANTIDOTE (ARSENIC, CYANIDE)

Prescriber Highlights

▶ Used for cyanide or arsenic poisoning
▶ Contraindications: None
▶ Adverse Effects: Large doses by mouth may cause profuse diarrhea
▶ Injectable forms should be given slowly IV

Uses/Indications
Sodium thiosulfate (alone or in combination with sodium nitrite) is useful in the treatment of cyanide toxicity. It has been touted for use in treating arsenic or other heavy metal poisonings, but its efficacy is in question for these purposes. However, because sodium thiosulfate is relatively non-toxic and inexpensive, it may be tried to treat arsenic poisoning. When used in combination with sodium molybdate, sodium thiosulfate may be useful for the treatment of copper poisoning.

Sodium thiosulfate may be useful for the topical treatment for some fungal infections (Tinea). In humans, sodium thiosulfate has been used to reduce the nephrotoxicity of cisplatin therapy. A 3 or 4% solution has been used to infiltrate the site of extravasations of cisplatin, carboplatin, or dactinomycin. In combination with steroids, sodium thiosulfate may reduce the healing time associated with doxorubicin extravasation.

Pharmacology/Actions

By administering thiosulfate, an exogenous source of sulfur is available to the body, thereby hastening the detoxification of cyanide using the enzyme rhodanese. Rhodanese (*thiosulfate cyanide sulfurtransferase*) converts cyanide to the relatively nontoxic thiocyanate ion; thiocyanate is then excreted in the urine.

Sodium thiosulfate has been used in humans to treat extravasation injuries secondary to carboplatin or cisplatin, for prophylaxis to prevent nephrotoxicity after cisplatin overdoses and ototoxicity with carboplatin overdoses.

Sodium thiosulfate's topical antifungal activity is probably due to its slow release of colloidal sulfur.

While sodium thiosulfate has been recommended for treating arsenic (and some other heavy metal) poisoning, the proposed mechanism of action is not known and its efficacy is in question. Presumably, the sulfate moiety may react with and chelate the metal allowing its removal.

Pharmacokinetics

Sodium thiosulfate is relatively poorly absorbed from the GI tract. When substantial doses are given PO, it acts a saline cathartic. When administered intravenously, it is distributed in the extracellular fluid and then rapidly excreted via the urine.

Contraindications/Precautions/Warnings

There are no absolute contraindications to the use of the drug.

Adverse Effects

The drug is relatively non-toxic. Large doses by mouth may cause profuse diarrhea. Injectable forms should be given slowly IV.

Reproductive/Nursing Safety

Safe use during pregnancy has not been established; use when benefits outweigh the potential risks. In humans, the FDA categorizes this drug as category *C* for use during pregnancy (*Animal studies have shown an adverse effect on the fetus, but there are no adequate studies in humans; or there are no animal reproduction studies and no adequate studies in humans.*)

No lactation information was found.

Drug Interactions/Laboratory Considerations

■ No specific drug or laboratory interactions or considerations were noted.

Doses

■ **DOGS/CATS:**

a) For cyanide toxicity: Contact an animal poison control center for guidance.

b) For treating extravasation injuries secondary to doxorubicin, carboplatin, cisplatin infusions: **Note:** These are recommendations for human patients.

Doxorubicin: Subcutaneous sodium thiosulfate 2% added to therapy with subcutaneous hydrocortisone and topical betamethasone decreased the healing time by half for cytotoxic drug extravasation (including doxorubicin and epirubicin) when compared to therapy without sodium thiosulfate.

Carboplatin: Prepare a 0.17 moles/L solution by mixing 4 mL sodium thiosulfate 10% w/v with 6 mL sterile water for injection. Inject 5 mL into extravasation site.

Cisplatin: For extravasation of large amounts (greater than 20 mL) of highly concentrated (greater than 0.5 mg/mL) solutions: Prepare a 0.17 moles/L solution by mixing 4 mL sodium thiosulfate 10% w/v with 6 mL sterile water for injection. Inject into extravasation site. (*Drugdex*® Evaluations. Micromedex Healthcare Series; Thompson, 2007)

■ **HORSES:**

a) For cyanide toxicity: First give sodium nitrite at a dose of 16 mg/kg IV followed with a 20% solution of sodium thiosulfate given at a dose of 30–40 mg/kg IV. If repeating treatment, use sodium thiosulfate only. (Bailey & Garland 1992)

b) For cyanide toxicity: First give sodium nitrite in a 20% solution at a dose of 10–20 mg/kg IV followed with a 20% solution of sodium thiosulfate given at a dose of 30–40 mg/kg IV (Osweiler 2003)

c) For arsenic toxicity: Sodium thiosulfate at 20–30 grams in 300 mL of water orally with dimercaprol (BAL) 3 mg/kg IM q4h (Jones 2004)

■ **RUMINANTS:**

Note: When used in food animals, FARAD states that this salt is rapidly excreted in and is not considered a residue concern in animal tissues; therefore, a 24 hour preslaughter withdrawal interval (WDI) would be sufficient. (Haskell *et al.* 2005)

a) In combination with sodium molybdate for the treatment of copper poisoning: In conjunction with fluid replacement therapy, 500 mg sodium thiosulfate in combination with 200 mg ammonium or sodium molybdate PO daily for up to 3 weeks will help decrease total body burden of copper (Thompson & Buck 1993)

b) For treatment of cyanide toxicity secondary to cyanogenic plants: 660 mg/kg IV sodium thiosulfate in a 30% solution given rapidly using a 12 or 14 gauge needle. (Post & Keller 2000)

c) For treatment of arsenic poisoning: 30–60 grams PO every 6 hours for 3–4 days and 30–60 grams as a 10–20% solution IV may be potentially useful in binding arsenic. Adjunctive fluid and electrolyte replacement is necessary. (Galey 1993)

Chemistry/Synonyms

Sodium thiosulfate occurs as large, colorless crystals or coarse, crystalline powder. It is very soluble in water, deliquescent in moist air and effloresces in dry air at temperatures >33°C.

Sodium thiosulfate may also be known as: natrii thiosulfas, natrium thiosulfuricum, sodium hyposulphite or sodium thiosulphate.

Storage/Stability

Unless otherwise stated by the manufacturer, store at room temperature. Crystals should be stored in tight containers.

Sodium thiosulfate is **not compatible** mixed with cyanocobalamin.

Dosage Forms/Regulatory Status

VETERINARY-LABELED PRODUCTS: None

HUMAN-LABELED PRODUCTS:

Sodium Thiosulfate for Injection: 10% (100 mg/mL, as pentahydrate) & 25% (250 mg/mL as pentahydrate) preservative-free in 10 mL & 50 mL single-use vials; generic; (Rx)

References

Bailey, E. & T. Garland (1992). Management of Toxicoses. *Current Therapy in Equine Medicine 3*. N Robinson Ed. Philadelphia, W.B. Saunders Co.: 346–353.

Galey, F. (1993). Arsenic toxicosis. *Current Veterinary Therapy 3: Food Animal Practice*. J Howard Ed. Philadelphia, W.B. Saunders Co.: 394–396.

Haskell, S., M. Payne, et al. (2005). Farad Digest: Antidotes in Food Animal Practice. *JAVMA* **226**(6): 884–887.

Jones, S. (2004). Inflammatory diseases of the gastrointestinal tract causing diarrhea. *Equine Internal Medicine 2nd Ed*. S Reed, W Bayly and D Sellon Eds. Philadelphia, Saunders: 884–912.

Osweiler, G. (2003). Toxicity of natural products in horses. Proceedings: Western Veterinary Conference. Accessed via: Veterinary Information Network. http://goo.gl/ttKbu

Post, L. & W. Keller (2000). Current status of food animal antidotes. *The Veterinary Clinics of North America: Food Animal Practice* 16:3(November).

Thompson, J.R. & W.B. Buck (1993). Copper-Molybdenum Toxicosis. *Current Veterinary Therapy 3: Food Animal Practice*. JL Howard Ed. Philadelphia, W.B. Saunders: 396–398.

SOMATOTROPIN (GROWTH HORMONE)

(soe-ma-toe-*troe*-pin)

HORMONE

Prescriber Highlights

▶ Used for canine hypopituitary dwarfism or growth hormone-responsive dermatosis (in adult dogs).

▶ May cause diabetes mellitus

▶ Availability & expense issues

Uses/Indications

Somatotropin may be useful in treating hypopituitary dwarfism or growth hormone-responsive dermatosis (in adult dogs).

Pharmacology/Actions

Growth hormone (somatotropin) is responsible for, or contributes to, linear and skeletal growth, organ growth, and cell growth. It also is a factor in protein, carbohydrate, lipid, connective tissue, and mineral metabolism.

Pharmacokinetics

No canine information was located. Both the liver and kidney are major elimination organs for somatotropin.

Contraindications/Precautions/Warnings

Growth hormone derived from other species is contraindicated in patients hypersensitive to it.

Adverse Effects

Growth hormone may cause diabetes mellitus in dogs. This may be transient or permanent even after discontinuing treatment. Blood and urine glucose should be routinely monitored. If blood glucose exceeds 150 mg/dL, therapy should be stopped. Hypersensitivity reactions are possible, but less so if using porcine origin product. Long-term treatment at high doses may cause acromegaly. Acromegaly in dogs can cause increased size of paws and head, increased skin folds around head and neck area, prognathism, and inspiratory stridor.

Reproductive/Nursing Safety

In humans, the FDA categorizes this drug as category *C* for use during pregnancy (*Animal studies have shown an adverse effect on the fetus, but there are no adequate studies in humans; or there are no animal reproduction studies and no adequate studies in humans.*)

Overdosage/Acute Toxicity

Acute overdosage could cause hypoglycemia initially and then hyperglycemia. Blood glucose should be monitored and supportive treatment (glucose/insulin) performed.

Drug Interactions

The following drug interactions have either been reported or are theoretical in humans or animals receiving somatotropin and may be of significance in veterinary patients:

■ **GLUCOCORTICOIDS:** May inhibit the growth promoting effect of somatotropin. When concurrent adrenal insufficiency is diagnosed, adjust glucocorticoid dose carefully to avoid negative effects on growth.

Doses

■ **DOGS:**

a) For treatment of hypopituitary dwarfism: 0.1 Unit (0.05 mg)/kg SC three times per week for 4–6 weeks. **Note:** May also require life-long thyroid hormone supplementation and if secondary adrenal insufficiency present, glucocorticoid treatment. If after successful treatment, dermatologic signs recur, may dose as above (0.1 Unit/kg three times weekly for one week). Repeat these weekly regimens at intervals determined by the time lapse between treatments and relapse. (Feldman & Nelson 1996)

b) For treatment of growth hormone-responsive dermatosis in adult dogs: Dose as above (a), but thyroid and steroid supplementation not required (Feldman & Nelson 1996)

c) For Alopecia X: 0.15 Units/kg of porcine growth hormone SC 2 times weekly for 6 weeks. (Hillier 2006)

Monitoring

■ Clinical efficacy

■ Blood glucose (weekly)

■ Urine glucose (daily)

■ Thyroid function, adrenal function initially and then periodically (pituitary dwarfism pts.)

Client Information

■ Clients should be instructed on the methods for SC injection and testing urine glucose

■ May be expensive to treat and diabetes (permanent) can occur

Synonyms

Somatotropin may also be known as: CB-311, HGH, human growth hormone, LY-137998, somatropinum; many trade names are available.

Dosage Forms/Regulatory Status

There are several manufacturers of human recombinant DNA origin somatotropin products, but these are expensive, can cause immunogenicity reactions in dogs, and not sold for veterinary use.

The bovine recombinant growth hormone product (*Posilac®*—Monsanto) is not suitable for canine use as it is a sustained release formulation and not easily diluted down to the smaller doses required for dogs.

Porcine growth hormone appears to have little immunogenicity in dogs and reportedly can be obtained via: Dr A. F. Partlow at: 310-222-3537 E-Mail: Partlow@HUMC.edu WEBSITE: www.humc.edu/hormones

The ARCI (Racing Commissioners International) has designated this drug as a class 2 substance. See the appendix for more information.

References

Feldman, E. & R. Nelson (1996). *Canine and Feline Endocrinology and Reproduction*. Philadelphia, Saunders.

Hillier, A. (2006). Alopecia: is an endocrine disorder responsible? Proceedings: ACVC. Accessed via: Veterinary Information Network. http://goo.gl/6xjBy

SOTALOL HCL

(**soh**-ta-lole)   Betapace®

BETA-ADRENERGIC BLOCKER

Prescriber Highlights

▶ Non-selective beta blocker/Class III antiarrhythmic for ventricular tachycardia

▶ Adverse Effects: Most serious: negative inotropism & pro-arrhythmic but dyspnea/bronchospasm, fatigue/dizziness, & nausea/vomiting possible

▶ Generic forms available, so cost is less of an issue than in the past

Uses/Indications

Sotalol may be useful in the treatment of ventricular tachycardias and, possibly, supraventricular tachycardias in dogs and cats. It is most often used in Boxers or in cases with ventricular tachycardia that are refractory to lidocaine.

Pharmacology/Actions

Sotalol is a non-selective beta-blocker and Class III antiarrhythmic agent. The beta blocking activity of sotalol is about 30% that of propranolol. Its primary usage in veterinary medicine is associated with its antiarrhythmic activity. Like other Class III drugs, it prolongs repolarization and refractoriness without affecting conduction. The pharmacologic action is believed caused by selectively inhibiting potassium channels.

Pharmacokinetics

Unlike propranolol, sotalol does not have any appreciable first pass effect after oral administration. Food may reduce the bioavailability of sotalol by approximately 20% (human data) and, if given on an empty stomach, bioavailability is 90–100%. The drug has relatively low lipid solubility and virtually no protein binding. Elimination is almost all via the kidney and most of the drug is excreted unchanged. In dogs, sotalol's elimination half-life is 5 hours; in humans about 12 hours.

Contraindications/Precautions/Warnings

Sotalol is considered contraindicated in patients with asthma, sinus bradycardia, 2nd or 3rd degree heart block (unless artificially paced), long Q-T syndromes, cardiogenic shock or uncontrolled CHF. Because of the potential for negative inotropic effects, use with caution in CHF. Also, use with caution in patients with diabetes mellitus, or hyperthyroidism (may mask signs). Use with caution in patients with renal dysfunction; dosage intervals may need to be extended.

Adverse Effects

Primary concerns with sotalol in dogs are the potential for negative inotropic and proarrhythmic effects. These generally are not clinically important if dosage is not excessive. Other potential adverse effects include dyspnea/bronchospasm, fatigue/dizziness, and nausea/vomiting. Sotalol's beta blocking effects can worsen syncope or cause lethargy, particularly if the ventricular tachyarrhythmia coexists with intermittent bradycardia (*e.g.*, AV block).

Reproductive/Nursing Safety

Sotalol did not cause any fetotoxicity or teratogenicity when given to pregnant lab animals at high dosages, but clear safety in pregnancy has not been established. Sotalol enters maternal milk in concentrations up to 5X found in the serum; consider using milk replacer in nursing animals.

In humans, the FDA categorizes this drug as category *B* for use during pregnancy (*Animal studies have not yet demonstrated risk to the fetus, but there are no adequate studies in pregnant women; or animal studies have shown an adverse effect, but adequate studies in pregnant women have not demonstrated a risk to the fetus in the first trimester of pregnancy, and there is no evidence of risk in later trimesters.*)

Sotalol is excreted in milk; use with caution in nursing patients. It is not recommended for use in nursing humans.

Overdosage/Acute Toxicity

Overdoses may result in bradycardia, hypotension, CHF, bronchospasm, and hypoglycemia. Use gut evacuation (if not contraindicated) when significant risk of morbidity is possible. Treat adverse effects symptomatically and supportively.

Drug Interactions

The following drug interactions have either been reported or are theoretical in humans or animals receiving sotalol and may be of significance in veterinary patients:

- ■ **AMIODARONE:** May prolong refractory periods; concurrent use not recommended in human patients
- ■ **ANESTHETICS, GENERAL:** Additive myocardial depression may occur with the concurrent use of sotalol and myocardial depressant anesthetic agents
- ■ **ANTACIDS:** May reduce oral sotalol absorption; separate doses by at least 2 hours
- ■ **ANTIARRHYTHMICS, CLASS IA (quinidine, procainamide, disopyramide):** May prolong refractory periods; concurrent use not recommended in human patients; may also prolong QT interval
- ■ **ANTIARRHYTHMICS, CLASS IB, 1C (lidocaine, mexiletine, phenytoin, flecainide etc.):** May prolong QT interval
- ■ **CALCIUM CHANNEL BLOCKERS (verapamil, diltiazem, etc.):** Potential to increase hypotensive effects; may have additive effects on AV conduction or ventricular function; use with caution, particularly in patients with preexisting cardiomyopathy or CHF

- ■ **CISAPRIDE:** May prolong QT interval
- ■ **CLONIDINE:** If clonidine is discontinued after concomitant therapy with sotalol, there is an increased risk for rebound hypertension
- ■ **DIGOXIN:** Potential for increased risks for proarrhythmic events
- ■ **ERYTHROMYCIN; CLARITHROMYCIN:** May prolong QT interval
- ■ **LIDOCAINE:** Clearance may be impaired by sotalol
- ■ **PHENOTHIAZINES:** May prolong QT interval
- ■ **RESERPINE:** May have additive effects (hypotension, bradycardia) with sotalol
- ■ **SYMPATHOMIMETICS, BETA 2 AGONISTS (e.g., metaproterenol, terbutaline, albuterol):** May have their actions blocked by sotalol
- ■ **TRICYCLIC ANTIDEPRESSANTS:** May prolong QT interval

Laboratory Considerations

- ■ Beta-blockers may produce hypoglycemia and interfere with **glucose** or insulin tolerance tests
- ■ Sotalol may falsely elevate urine **metanephrine** levels (pheochromocytoma screen) if using a fluorometric or photometric assay

Doses

- ■ **DOGS:**
  - a) 1–2 mg/kg PO q12h (Fox 2003), (Moise 2002), (Marks 2009; Smith 2007)
  - b) 1–3 mg/kg PO twice daily. (Henik 2007)
  - c) For ventricular tachycardia: 1–2 mg/kg PO twice daily (Atkins 2007)
  - d) For ventricular tachyarrhythmias in Boxers in combination with mexiletine: Sotalol 1.5–3 mg/kg PO twice daily with mexiletine (5–7.5 mg/kg PO three times daily). (Prosek *et al.* 2006)
  - e) In Boxers: 40–80 mg (total dose) PO q12h. (Mucha 2009)
- ■ **CATS:**
  - a) 2 mg/kg PO twice daily (Atkins 2003)
  - b) For ventricular tachyarrhythmias: 2 mg/kg PO q12h (Cote 2010)
  - c) 1–2 mg/kg PO q12h. (Marks 2009)
  - d) ⅛th of an 80 mg tablet PO twice daily, or approximately 2 mg/kg PO twice daily. (Henik 2007)

Monitoring

- ■ Efficacy (ECG)
- ■ Adverse effects

Client Information

- ■ Relatively limited clinical experience; but appears safe
- ■ Must be given as prescribed; do not stop drug suddenly or alter dosing without veterinarian guidance
- ■ Report adverse effects to veterinarian immediately

Chemistry/Synonyms

A non-selective beta-blocker and Class III antiarrhythmic agent, sotalol HCl is a racemic mixture of the d- and l- forms. Both isomers exhibit antiarrhythmic (Class II) activity, but only the Levo- form has beta blocking activity. Sotalol HCl occurs as white, crystalline solid that is soluble in water.

Sotalol may also be known as: MJ-1999, d,l-sotalol hydrochloride, or sotaloli hydrochloridum; many trade names are available.

Storage/Stability

Store tablets at room temperature.

Dosage Forms/Approval

VETERINARY-LABELED PRODUCTS: None

The ARCI (Racing Commissioners International) has designated this drug as a class 3 substance. See the appendix for more information.

HUMAN-LABELED PRODUCTS:

Sotalol HCl Tablets: 80 mg, 120 mg, 160 mg & 240 mg; *Betapace*® (Bayer); generic; (Rx)

Sotalol Injection Solution Concentrate: 15 mg/mL in 10 mL vials; generic (Academic Pharmaceutical); (Rx)

References

Atkins, C. (2003). Therapeutic strategies in feline heart disease. Proceedings: ACVIM Forum. Accessed via: Veterinary Information Network. http://goo.gl/NSJtl

Atkins, C. (2007). Canine Heart Failure—Current concepts. Proceedings: WSAVA World Congress. Accessed via: Veterinary Information Network. http://goo.gl/aWqPH

Cote, E. (2010). Feline Arrhythmias: An Update. *Veterinary Clinics of North America-Small Animal Practice* **40**(4): 643–+.

Fox, P. (2003). Congestive heart failure: Clinical approach and management. Proceedings: World Small Animal Veterinary Assoc World Congress. Accessed via: Veterinary Information Network. http://goo.gl/xMFKn

Henik, R. (2007). New Information on Cardiac Drugs. Proceedings: IVECCS. Accessed via: Veterinary Information Network. http://goo.gl/QGlS2

Marks, S.L. (2009). A review of drugs for the ER. Proceedings: IVECCS. Accessed via: Veterinary Information Network. http://goo.gl/XI8qP

Moise, N. (2002). Chronic management of tachyarrhythmias in the dog. Proceedings: Waltham/OSU Symposium. Accessed via: Veterinary Information Network. http://goo.gl/1hgYI

Mucha, C. (2009). Therapeutics in Heart Disease. Proceedings: WSAVA. Accessed via: Veterinary Information Network. http://goo.gl/ca6mX

Prosek, R., A. Estrada, et al. (2006). Comparison of sotalol and mexiletine versus stand alone sotalol in treatment of Boxer dogs with ventricular arrhythmias. Proceedings: ACVIM. Accessed via: Veterinary Information Network. http://goo.gl/wnpJV

Smith, F. (2007). Updates on arrhythmic therapies. Proceedings: Western Vet Conf. Accessed via: Veterinary Information Network. http://goo.gl/NJQmQ

SPECTINOMYCIN HCL
SPECTINOMYCIN SULFATE

(spek-ti-noe-*mye*-sin)   Adspec®, Spectam®

AMINOCYCLITOL ANTIBIOTIC

Prescriber Highlights

▶ Aminocyclitol antibiotic used primarily in food producing animals; relatively broad spectrum but minimal activity against anaerobes & most strains of Pseudomonas

▶ Contraindications: Hypersensitive to it

▶ Adverse Effects: Appears to have minimal adverse effects at labeled dosages; probably less nephrotoxicity/ototoxicity than other aminocyclitols. Can cause neuromuscular blockade. May cause swelling at SC injection sites.

Uses/Indications

Although occasionally used in dogs, cats, and horses for susceptible infections, Spectinomycin only has FDA-approved dosage forms for cattle, chickens, turkeys, and swine. Refer to the Dosage section below for more information on FDA-approved uses.

Pharmacology/Actions

Spectinomycin is primarily a bacteriostatic antibiotic that inhibits protein synthesis in susceptible bacteria by binding to the 30S ribosomal subunit.

Spectinomycin has activity against a wide variety of gram-positive and gram-negative bacteria, including *E. coli*, Klebsiella, Proteus, Enterobacter, Salmonella, Streptococci, Staphylococcus, and Mycoplasma. It has minimal activity against anaerobes, most strains of Pseudomonas, Chlamydia, or Treponema.

In human medicine, spectinomycin is used principally for its activity against *Neisseria gonorrhoeae*.

Pharmacokinetics

After oral administration only about 7% of the dose is absorbed, but the drug that remains in the GI tract is active. When injected SC or IM, the drug is reportedly absorbed well with peak levels occurring in about 1 hour.

Tissue levels of absorbed drug are lower than those found in the serum. Spectinomycin does not appreciably enter the CSF or the eye and is not bound significantly to plasma proteins. It is unknown whether spectinomycin crosses the placenta or enters milk.

Absorbed drug is excreted via glomerular filtration into the urine mostly unchanged. In cattle, terminal half-life is about 2 hours.

Contraindications/Precautions/Warnings

Spectinomycin is contraindicated in patients hypersensitive to it.

Adverse Effects

When used as labeled, adverse effects are unlikely with this drug. It is reported that parenteral use of this drug is much safer than with other aminocyclitol antibiotics, but little is known regarding its prolonged use. It is probably safe to say that spectinomycin is significantly less ototoxic and nephrotoxic than other commonly used aminocyclitol antibiotics, but can cause neuromuscular blockade. Parenteral calcium administration will generally reverse the blockade.

Adverse effects that have been reported in human patients receiving the drug in single or multidose studies include soreness at injection site, increases in BUN, alkaline phosphatase and SGPT, and decreases in hemoglobin, hematocrit, and creatinine clearance. Although increases in BUN and decreases in creatinine clearance and urine output have been noted, overt renal toxicity has not been demonstrated with this drug.

Cattle receiving the sulfate form subcutaneously have developed swelling at the injection site.

Reproductive/Nursing Safety

In humans, the FDA categorizes this drug as category *B* for use during pregnancy (*Animal studies have not yet demonstrated risk to the fetus, but there are no adequate studies in pregnant women; or animal studies have shown an adverse effect, but adequate studies in pregnant women have not demonstrated a risk to the fetus in the first trimester of pregnancy, and there is no evidence of risk in later trimesters.*)

It is not known whether spectinomycin is excreted in milk; use caution when administering to nursing patients.

Overdosage/Acute Toxicity

No specific information was located on oral overdoses, but because the drug is negligibly absorbed after oral administration, significant toxicity is unlikely via this route.

Injected doses of 90 mg produced transient ataxia in turkey poults.

Drug Interactions

■ Antagonism has been reported when spectinomycin is used with **chloramphenicol** or **tetracycline**.

Doses

■ **DOGS:**

For susceptible infections:

a) 5.5–11 mg/kg q12h IM or 22 mg/kg PO q12h (for enteric infections; not absorbed) (Kintzer & Peterson 1989)

b) 5–10 mg/kg IM q12h (Davis 1985)

c) For acute infectious gastroenteritis: 5–12 mg/kg IM q12h (DeNovo 1986)

■ **CATS:**

For susceptible infections:

a) For acute infectious gastroenteritis: 5–12 mg/kg IM q12h (DeNovo 1986)

■ **CATTLE:**

For susceptible infections:

a) For bronchopneumonia and fibrinous pneumonia: 33 mg/kg SC q8h. Suggested withdrawal time is 60 days. (Hjerpe 1986)

b) 22–39.6 mg/kg/day IM divided three times daily (Upson 1988)

c) For bovine respiratory disease: 10–15 mg/kg SC (in the neck; not more than 50 mL per site) once daily (q24h) for 3–5 consecutive days (Label directions; *Adspec®*)

■ **HORSES:**

For susceptible infections:

a) 20 mg/kg, IM three times daily (Robinson 1987)

b) For pneumonia: 20 mg/kg IM q8h; may cause local myositis. Insufficient data to comment on use. (Beech 1987)

■ **SWINE:**

For susceptible enteric infections:

a) 10 mg/kg, PO q12h (Howard 1986)

b) For bacterial enteritis (white scours) in baby pigs associated with E. coli susceptible to spectinomycin: 50 mg/10 lbs of body weight PO twice daily for 3–5 days (Label directions; *Spectam Scour-Halt®*—Ceva)

c) 10 mg/kg, IM q12h (Baggot 1983)

■ **BIRDS:**

a) For airsacculitis associated with *M. meleagridis* or chronic respiratory disease associated with *E. coli* in turkey poults (1–3 days old): Inject 0.1 mL (10 mg) SC in the base of the neck.

For control and to lessen mortality due to infections from *M. synoviae, S. typhimurium, S. infantis,* and *E. coli* in newly hatched chicks: Dilute injection with normal saline to a concentration of 2.5–5 mg/0.2 mL and inject SC. (Label directions; *Spectam® Injectable*—Ceva)

b) For prevention and control of chronic respiratory disease associated with *Mycoplasma gallisepticum* in broilers: Add sufficient amount to drinking water to attain a final concentration of 2 grams/gallon.

For infectious synovitis associated with *Mycoplasma synoviae* in broilers: Add sufficient amount to drinking water to attain a final concentration of 1 gram/gallon.

For improved weight gain/feed efficiency in floor-raised broilers: Add sufficient amount to drinking water to attain a final concentration of 0.5 grams/gallon. (Label directions; *Spectam® Water-Soluble*—Ceva)

Monitoring

■ Clinical efficacy

Chemistry/Synonyms

An aminocyclitol antibiotic obtained from *Streptomyces spectabilis*, spectinomycin is available as the dihydrochloride pentahydrate and hexahydrate sulfate salts. It occurs as a white to pale buff, crystalline powder with pK$_a$s of 7 and 8.7. It is freely soluble in water and practically insoluble in alcohol.

Spectinomycin may also be known as: M-141, actinospectacin, spectinomycini, U-18409AE, *Adspec®*, *Amtech Spectam®*, *Kempi®*, *Kirin®*, *Spectoguard Scour-Chek®*, *Stanilo®*, *Togamycin®*, *Trobicin®*, *Trobicine®*, or *Vabicin®*.

Storage/Stability

Unless otherwise instructed by the manufacturer, spectinomycin products should be stored at room temperature (15−30°C). Protect from freezing.

Dosage Forms/Regulatory Status

VETERINARY-LABELED PRODUCTS:

Spectinomycin Sulfate Injection: 100 mg/mL in 500 mL vials; *Adspec®*; (Pharmacia & Upjohn); (Rx). When used as labeled, slaughter withdrawal in cattle = 11 days; not to be used in veal calves or in dairy cattle 20 months of age or older.

Spectinomycin Injection: 100 mg/mL in 500 mL vials; *Spectam® Injectable* (Teva); (OTC). FDA-approved for use in 1–3 days old turkey poults and newly hatched chicks.

Spectinomycin Water Soluble Concentrate: 0.5 gram of spectinomycin per gram *Spectam® Water Soluble* (Bimeda); (OTC). FDA-approved for use in chickens (not layers). Slaughter withdrawal (at labeled doses) = 5 days.

Spectinomycin Oral Solution: 50 mg/mL in 240 mL pump bottle and 500 and 1000 mL without pump; *Spectam Scour-Halt®*, (Teva), *Spectoguard Scour-Chek®* (Bimeda), *Spectam Scour-Halt®*, (AgriPharm); (OTC). FDA-approved for use in swine (Weighing less than 15 lbs and not older than 4 weeks of age). Slaughter withdrawal (at labeled doses) = 21 days.

Spectinomycin/Lincomycin in a 2:1 ratio

LS 50 Water Soluble Powder® (Pharmacia & Upjohn); Sepclinx-50® (Bimeda); generic; in 2.65 oz packets. Each packet contains lincomycin 16.7 grams and spectinomycin 33.3 grams. FDA-approved for use in chickens up to 7 days of age.

Lincomycin 50 mg/Spectinomycin 100 mg per mL in 20 mL vials; *Linco-Spectin® Sterile Solution* (Pharmacia & Upjohn); (OTC). FDA-approved for use in semen extenders only.

HUMAN-LABELED PRODUCTS: None

References

Baggot, J.D. (1983). Systemic antimicrobial therapy in large animals. *Pharmacological Basis of Large Animal Medicine*. JA Bogan, P Lees and AT Yoxall Eds. Oxford, Blackwell Scientific Publications: 45–69.

Beech, J. (1987). Respiratory Tract—Horse, Cow. *The Bristol Handbook of Antimicrobial Therapy*. DE Johnston Ed. Evansville, Veterinary Learning Systems: 88–109.

Davis, L.E., Ed. (1985). *Handbook of Small Animal Therapeutics*. New York, Churchill Livingston.

DeNovo, R.C., Jr. (1986). Therapeutics of gastrointestinal diseases. *Current Veterinary Therapy (CVT) IX Small Animal Practice*. RW Kirk Ed. Philadelphia, W.B. Saunders: 862–871.

Hjerpe, C.A. (1986). The bovine respiratory disease complex. *Current Veterinary Therapy: Food Animal Practice 2*. JL Howard Ed. Philadelphia, W.B. Saunders: 670–681.

Howard, J.L., Ed. (1986). *Current Veterinary Therapy 2, Food Animal Practice*. Philadelphia, W.B. Saunders.

Kintzer, P.P. & M.E. Peterson (1989). Mitotane (o,p'-DDD) treatment of cortisol-secreting adrenocortical neoplasia. *Current Veterinary Therapy X: Small Animal Practice*. RW Kirk Ed. Philadelphia, WB Saunders: 1034–1037.

Robinson, N.E. (1987). Table of Common Drugs: Approximate Doses. *Current Therapy in Equine Medicine, 2*. NE Robinson Ed. Philadelphia, W.B. Saunders: 761.

Upson, D.W. (1988). *Handbook of Clinical Veterinary Pharmacology*. Manhattan, Dan Upson Enterprises.

SPINOSAD

(***spin***-oh-sad)   Comfortis®

ORAL FLEA ADULTICIDE

Prescriber Highlights

▶ Oral flea adulticide for dogs; labeled for one month prevention/treatment

▶ Rapid action

▶ Appears very safe and well tolerated in dogs

▶ Give with food

Uses/Indications

Spinosad is indicated for the prevention and treatment of flea (*Ctenocephalides felis*) infestations for one month in dogs 14 weeks of age and older (Label Information; *Comfortis®*). Advantages of this drug include: rapid response for a systemic once monthly product, killing adult fleas before egg laying is initiated, efficacy is not affected by bathing or swimming, and FDA-approved (not EPA-approved as are many topical flea products) (Ihrke 2009).

While the drug is not labeled for use against ticks and it has been stated that it is not effective for this use, a pilot study evaluating the efficacy of spinosad dosed at 50 mg/kg (1.7X minimum flea dose) and 100 mg/kg (3.3X minimum flea dose) against adult brown dog tick (*R. sanguineus*) infestations in dogs, demonstrated high efficacy in killing ticks within 24 hours of dosing. The results suggested that some post-treatment residual tick control persisted up to 1 month.

The authors concluded that the role of spinosad as a useful adjunct to currently marketed acaricidal products needs to be explored (Snyder *et al.* 2009).

In humans, spinosad as a topical suspension has been used to treat pediculosis capitis (head lice).

Pharmacology/Actions

Spinosad is a macrocyclic lactone containing two natural occurring macrocyclic lactones (spinosyn A and spinosyn D). Its primary mode of action in insects is as a nicotinic acetylcholine D-alpha receptor agonist causing involuntary muscle contractions and tremors secondary to motor neuron activation. Prolonged exposure causes paralysis and flea death. Flea death begins within 30 minutes of dosing and is complete in 4 hours. In insects, spinosad also opens chloride channels similarly to other macrocyclic lactones.

Pharmacokinetics

After oral administration of spinosad (with food) to dogs, peak plasma levels for spinosyn A and spinosyn D occur in about 2 and 3 hours, respectively. Spinosyn D levels are about 5 times greater than those of spinosyn A. Spinosyn A & B are extensively bound to canine plasma proteins with a resultant plasma elimination half-life of about 10 days.

Contraindications/Precautions/Warnings

No labeled contraindications; not approved for use in cats. It has been recommended not to use spinosad with the high extra-label doses of ivermectin (Jazic 2010; Kuhl 2009).

The product label cautions use in breeding females and dogs with pre-existing epilepsy at higher than labeled dosages may decrease seizure threshold.

The chewable tablets are beef flavored and while they do not contain beef proteins, pork proteins and hydrolyzed soy are used. Dogs with pork or soy allergies may react (Rosenkrantz 2010).

A study evaluating the safety of spinosad (doses up to 5X) with or without milbemycin (doses up to 10X) in Collies homozygous and heterozygous for the *ABCB1* (MDR1) mutation did not cause signs of neuro-toxicosis (Sherman *et al.* 2010).

Adverse Effects

Spinosad appears to be very well tolerated in dogs and most animals will not show any adverse effects after dosing. The following adverse reactions are possible and based on post-approval adverse drug event reporting; listed in decreasing order of frequency: vomiting, depression/lethargy, anorexia, ataxia, diarrhea, pruritus, trembling, hypersalivation and seizures.

Reproductive/Nursing Safety

The manufacturer states to use with caution in breeding females, but the drug appears to be relatively safe to use during pregnancy or lactation. In female Beagles dosed at 1.3X and 4.4X every 28 days prior to mating, during gestation, and during a six-week lactation period, no changes in dam conception rates or mortality, body temperature, necropsy, or histopathology were seen in dams or puppies. Treated dams experienced more vomiting, especially at one hour post-dose, than control dams. Puppies from dams treated at 1.3X had lower body weights and those from the 4.4X group experienced more lethargy, dehydration, weakness and felt cold. Safe use in breeding males has not been evaluated.

In a pilot study in 3 dogs, spinosyns were excreted in milk at levels about 2.5X of that found in the plasma. Puppy mortality and morbidity was highest in puppies from the dam with the highest spinosyn milk levels, but causal effect cannot be inferred due to the small sample size of the study.

Overdosage/Acute Toxicity

Spinosad appears to be very safe in mammals with the oral LD50 in mice >5000 mg/kg. Acute overdoses in dogs appear relatively innocuous. In a dose tolerance study, in adult Beagles dosed orally up to 100 mg/kg (16.7X) PO once daily for 10 consecutive days, vomiting was routinely seen after the dose was administered. No significant changes in hematology, blood coagulation or urinalysis parameters were noted, but phospholipidosis (vacuolation) of the lymphoid tissue and mild elevations in ALT occurred in all dogs.

Drug Interactions

The following drug interactions have either been reported or are theoretical in humans or animals receiving spinosad and may be of significance in veterinary patients:

■ **IVERMECTIN:** It has been recommended not to use with the high extra-label doses of ivermectin (Kuhl 2009). When used with heartworm preventatives at their labeled doses, spinosad appears safe to use. No signs of signs of neuro-toxicosis were seen in Collies homozygous and heterozygous in the *ABCB1* (MDR1) mutation in a study evaluating the safety of spinosad (doses up to 5X) with or without milbemycin (doses up to 10X) (Sherman *et al.* 2010).

Laboratory Considerations

■ No specific concerns noted

Doses

■ **DOGS:**

For prevention or treatment of fleas infestations:

a) 30–60 mg/kg (minimum dosage of 30 mg/kg) PO once monthly with food. (Adapted from label information; *Comfortis®*—Lilly)

Monitoring

■ Efficacy

Client Information

■ Give with food

■ If vomiting occurs within an hour of administration, redose with another full dose.

■ If a dose is missed, administer with food and resume a monthly dosing schedule.

Chemistry/Synonyms

Spinosad is a spinosyn class insecticide and contains two major factors, spinosyn A and spinosyn D that are derived from the naturally occurring bacterium, *Saccharopolyspora spinosa*. Spinosad may also be known as spinosyn A & B, DE-105, or XDE-105. Trade names include *Comfortis*® and *Natroba*® (human topical), or *Extinosad*®.

Storage/Stability

Chewable tablets should be stored at 20-25°C (68-77°F), excursions permitted between 15–30°C (59-86°F).

Dosage Forms/Regulatory Status

VETERINARY-LABELED PRODUCTS:

Spinosad Chewable Tablets: 140 mg, 270 mg, 560 mg, 810 mg, 1620 mg; *Comfortis*® (Lilly); (Rx). FDA-approved for use in dogs.

HUMAN-LABELED PRODUCTS:

None for systemic use. There is a topical product (for head lice) Spinosad 0.9% topical suspension in 120 mL: *Natroba*® (ParaPro; Pernix); (Rx)

References

Ihrke, P. (2009). Managing flea allergy- Where are we in 2009? Proceedings: WVC. Accessed via: Veterinary Information Network. http://goo.gl/7zZ05

Jazic, E. (2010). Out With the Old, In With the New: New Approaches to the Management of Canine and Feline Demodicosis. Proceedings: WVC. Accessed via: Veterinary Information Network. http://goo.gl/13495

Kuhl, K. (2009). Integrated Parasite Control in Dogs. Proceedings: WVC. Accessed via: Veterinary Information Network. http://goo.gl/7yKXe

Rosenkrantz, W.S. (2010). Flea Control Update. Proceedings: WVC. Accessed via: Veterinary Information Network. http://goo.gl/RNehD

Sherman, J.G., A.J. Paul, et al. (2010). Evaluation of the safety of spinosad and milbemycin 5–oxime orally administered to Collies with the MDR1 gene mutation. *American Journal of Veterinary Research* 71(1): 115–119.

Snyder, D.E., L.R. Cruthers, et al. (2009). Preliminary study on the acaricidal efficacy of spinosad administered orally to dogs infested with the brown dog tick, Rhipicephalus sanguineus (Latreille, 1806) (Acari: Ixodidae). *Veterinary Parasitology* 166(1–2): 131–135.

SPIRONOLACTONE

(speer-on-oh-*lak*-tone)   Aldactone®

ALDOSTERONE ANTAGONIST

Prescriber Highlights

▶ Aldosterone antagonist used as a potassium sparing diuretic or for adjunctive treatment for heart failure (use is somewhat controversial for CHF in dogs); should not be substituted for furosemide in CHF

▶ Contraindications: Hyperkalemia, Addison's disease, anuria, acute renal failure or significant renal impairment

▶ Caution: Any renal impairment or hepatic disease

▶ Adverse Effects: Facial dermatitis in cats. Hyperkalemia, hyponatremia, & dehydration possible; increased BUN & mild acidosis in patients with renal impairment. GI distress (vomiting, anorexia, etc.), CNS effects (lethargy, ataxia, etc.), & endocrine changes possible

Uses/Indications

Spironolactone may be used in patients with congestive heart failure who do not adequately respond to furosemide and ACE inhibitors, who develop hypokalemia on other diuretics, and are unwilling or unable to supplement with exogenous potassium sources. It may also be effective in treating ascites as it has less potential to increase ammonia levels than other diuretics. Spironolactone may find a role in treating renal disease. In rats, it has been shown to decrease proteinuria and glomerulosclerosis in experimental models of renal disease.

Pharmacology/Actions

Aldosterone is competitively inhibited by spironolactone in the distal renal tubules with resultant increased excretion of sodium, chloride, and water, and decreased excretion of potassium, ammonium, phosphate, and titratable acid. Spironolactone has no effect on carbonic anhydrase or renal transport mechanisms and has its greatest effect in patients with hyperaldosteronism. When used alone in healthy dogs, spironolactone does not appear to cause significant diuresis (Jeunesse *et al.* 2004).

Spironolactone is not commonly used alone as most sodium is reabsorbed at the proximal tubules. Combining it with a thiazide or loop diuretic will yield maximum diuretic effect.

After cats received 2.7 mg/kg spironolactone twice daily for 7–9 days, the following serum values increased (on average) significantly: potassium 0.39 mEq/L, calcium 0.48 mg/dL, creatinine 0.22 mg/dL, phosphorus 0.63 mg/dL and total protein 0.51 mg/dL. (Abbott & Saker 2006)

In humans, spironolactone can have antifibrotic effects on cardiac muscle. Whether this occurs in veterinary patients with heart failure is controversial. One study in Maine Coon cats with hypertrophic cardiomyopathy, but not in heart failure showed that spironolactone did not yield significant changes in diastolic function or left ventricular mass after 4 months of treatment (MacDonald *et al.* 2008). A study published in dogs with moderate to severe mitral regurgitation, concluded that spironolactone added to conventional therapy, decreased the risk for death, euthanasia or severe worsening of signs (Bernay *et al.* 2010). This study has met with skepticism by some who are unconvinced that the data supports this conclusion.

Pharmacokinetics

Because spironolactone is unstable if frozen and thawed, pharmacokinetic studies in animals are not readily performed. In fasted dogs, oral bioavailability of spironolactone (measured via its main metabolites) is approximately 50%, but increases up to 90% when given with food. About 70% of a dose is found in the feces and 18% in the urine. In a recent pharmacodynamic study done in 15 Beagles, the dose required to inhibit the action of aldosterone by 50% was estimated to be about 1.1 mg/kg and the authors suggest that the dose for spironolactone would be about 2 mg/kg PO once daily to obtain concentrations effective at inhibiting the aldosterone levels associated with CHF in dogs (Guyonnet *et al.* 2010).

In humans, spironolactone is >90% bioavailable and peak levels are reached within 1–2 hours. The diuretic action of spironolactone (when used alone) is gradually attained and generally reaches its maximal effect on the third day of therapy.

Spironolactone and its active metabolite, canrenone, are both about 98% bound to plasma proteins. Both spironolactone and its metabolites may cross the placenta. Canrenone has been detected in breast milk. Spironolactone is rapidly metabolized (half-life of 1–2 hours) to several metabolites, including canrenone, which has diuretic activity. Canrenone is more slowly eliminated, with an average half-life of around 20 hours.

Contraindications/Precautions/Warnings

Spironolactone is contraindicated in patients with hyperkalemia, Addison's disease, anuria, acute renal failure or significant renal impairment. It should be used cautiously in patients with hepatic disease, but is often used to treat ascites.

Adverse Effects

Adverse effects are usually considered mild and reversible upon discontinuation of the drug. Electrolyte (hyperkalemia, hyponatremia) and water balance (dehydration) abnormalities are the most likely effects with spironolactone therapy, but electrolytes in dogs do not appear to be significantly affected.

In a study in Maine Coon cats, approximately ⅓ of treated subjects developed severe facial dermatitis.

Transient increases in BUN and mild acidosis may occur in patients with renal impairment. GI distress (vomiting, anorexia, etc.), CNS effects (lethargy, ataxia, headaches in humans, etc.), and endocrine changes (gynecomastia in human males) are all possible.

Use of spironolactone in patients with renal impairment may lead to hyperkalemia. Spironolactone reportedly inhibits the synthesis of testosterone and may increase the peripheral conversion of testosterone to estradiol. Long-term toxicity studies in rats have demonstrated that spironolactone is tumorigenic in that species.

Reproductive/Nursing Safety

Spironolactone or its metabolites may cross the placental barrier. Feminization occurs in male rat fetuses. In humans, the FDA categorizes this drug as category *D* for use during pregnancy (*There is evidence of human fetal risk, but the potential benefits from the use of the drug in pregnant women may be acceptable despite its potential risks.*)

Canrenone, a metabolite of spironolactone, appears in maternal milk. In humans, the estimated maximum dose to the infant is approximately 0.2% of the mother's daily dose. Use with caution in nursing patients, but it is unlikely of clinical significance in veterinary patients.

Overdosage/Acute Toxicity

Information on overdosage of spironolactone is apparently unavailable. Should an acute overdose occur, it is suggested to follow the guidelines outlined in the chlorothiazide and furosemide monographs. Contact an animal poison control center for further guidance.

Drug Interactions

The following drug interactions have either been reported or are theoretical in humans or animals receiving spironolactone and may be of significance in veterinary patients:

- ■ **DIGOXIN:** Spironolactone may increase the half-life of digoxin; enhanced monitoring of digoxin serum levels and effects are warranted when spironolactone is used with these agents

- ■ **MITOTANE:** Spironolactone may mute the effects of mitotane if given concurrently, but very limited information is available on this potential interaction; monitor carefully.

- ■ **NEUROMUSCULAR BLOCKERS, NON-DEPOLARIZING:** Increase in neuromuscular blockade effects possible

- ■ **POTASSIUM-SPARING DIURETICS, OTHER (e.g., triamterene):** Hyperkalemia possible

- ■ **POTASSIUM SUPPLEMENTS:** Hyperkalemia possible

■ **SALICYLATES:** Spironolactone's diuretic effects may be decreased if **aspirin** or other salicylates are administered concomitantly

Laboratory Considerations

■ Spironolactone may give falsely elevated **digoxin** values, if using a radioimmune assay (RIA) method.

■ Fluorometric methods of determining plasma and urinary **17-hydroxycorticosteroids** (cortisol) may be interfered with by spironolactone.

Doses

■ **DOGS:**

As a diuretic in CHF:

a) When furosemide and ACE inhibitors alone do not control fluid accumulation in refractory CHF: 1–2 mg/kg PO q12h (Ware & Keene 2000)

b) With other diuretics when hypokalemia is an issue: 2–4 mg/kg PO once daily (Kittleson, 2000)

c) To allow further reduction of furosemide dose (target dose for furosemide during maintenance phase: 1–2 mg/kg PO q24–48h): Spironolactone dose varies between 0.5 mg/kg PO once daily (aldosterone blockage, weak diuretic effect) to 2 mg/kg twice daily (stronger diuretic effect). (de Madron 2004)

For treating ascites:

a) Using the fixed dose combination with hydrochlorothiazide (*Aldactazide®*): The empirical dosage, based on the spironolactone component, is 0.5–1 mg/kg PO twice daily. (Trepanier 2008)

b) Attempt at treating underlying abnormality. When ascites is caused by right-sided heart failure: Be sure owner is administering medication properly and the prescription is correct. Increase furosemide to 4–6 mg/kg PO q8h (generally speaking dose should be increased until all the abnormal accumulated fluid is eliminated or unacceptable azotemia develops). Optimize ACE inhibitor dose. Restrict dietary sodium. Add spironolactone at 1–2 mg/kg PO q12h. Initially (3 times weekly) substitute one of the oral furosemide doses with a SC dose. Consider adding hydrochlorothiazide initially at 2 mg/kg PO every other day. (Connolly 2006)

For adjunctive treatment of hypertension:

a) 1–2 mg/kg PO q12h (Stepian 2006)

b) As a fourth step drug for systolic hypertension >160 mmHg, diastolic >120 mmHg; after **1)** enalapril/benazepril (0.5 mg/kg q12h); **2)** amlodipine (0.1 mg/kg q24h); **3)** amlodipine (0.2 mg/kg q24h); **4)** spironolactone (1–2 mg/kg twice daily);

5) hydralazine 0.5 mg/kg PO twice daily. Each step added (except when increasing amlodipine dose) if after 1–2 weeks systolic BP > 160 mmHg. (Henik 2007)

■ **CATS:**

As a diuretic in CHF:

a) When furosemide and ACE inhibitors alone do not control fluid accumulation in refractory CHF: 1–2 mg/kg PO q12h (Ware & Keene 2000)

b) 1 mg/kg q12h PO when serum potassium is low (Bonagura 1989)

For adjunctive treatment of hypertension:

a) 1–2 mg/kg PO q12h (Stepian 2006)

b) As a 3rd step drug when systolic BP >160 mmHg, diastolic >120 mmHg: **1)** amlodipine (0.625 mg per cat q24h; if cat greater then 6 kg, 1.25 mg/cat q24h), add ACE inhibitor if proteinuric; **2)** ACE inhibitor (benazepril/enalapril 0.5 mg/kg q12h); **3)** spironolactone (1–2 mg/kg twice daily); **4)** hydralazine 0.5 mg/kg PO twice daily. Each step added (except when increasing amlodipine dose) if after 1-2 weeks systolic BP > 160 mmHg. (Henik 2007)

For adjunctive treatment of primary hyperaldosteronism:

a) If potassium supplementation alone does not control clinical signs: 1–2 mg/kg PO twice daily. (Caney 2009)

Monitoring

Serum electrolytes, BUN, creatinine

Hydration status

Blood pressure, if indicated

Clinical signs of edema/ascites; patient weight, if indicated

Client Information

■ Notify veterinarian if GI symptoms (*e.g.*, vomiting, diarrhea, anorexia), lethargy, or other CNS effects are severe or persist

Chemistry/Synonyms

A synthetically produced aldosterone antagonist, spironolactone occurs as a cream-colored to light tan, crystalline powder with a faint mercaptan-like odor. It has a melting range of 198°–207°, with decomposition. Spironolactone is practically insoluble in water and soluble in alcohol.

Spironolactone may also be known as: espironolactona, SC-9420, spirolactone, spironolactonum; many trade names are available.

Storage/Stability

Spironolactone tablets should be stored at room temperature in tight, light-resistant containers.

Compatibility/Compounding Considerations

An extemporaneously prepared oral suspension can be prepared by pulverizing commercially available tablets and adding cherry syrup. This preparation is reportedly stable for at least one month when refrigerated.

Dosage Forms/Regulatory Status

VETERINARY-LABELED PRODUCTS: None

The ARCI (Racing Commissioners International) has designated this drug as a class 4 substance. See the appendix for more information.

HUMAN-LABELED PRODUCTS:

Spironolactone Oral Tablets: 25 mg, 50 mg & 100 mg; *Aldactone®* (Searle); generic; (Rx)

Spironolactone/Hydrochlorothiazide Oral Tablets: 25 mg/25 mg & 50 mg/50 mg; *Aldactazide®* (Searle); generic; (Rx)

References

Abbott, J. & K. Saker (2006). Serum chemistry variables of healthy cats receiving spironolactone, Proceedings: ACVIM. Accessed via: Veterinary Information Network. http://goo.gl/q7Q1n

Bernay, F., J.M. Bland, et al. (2010). Efficacy of Spironolactone on Survival in Dogs with Naturally Occurring Mitral Regurgitation Caused by Myxomatous Mitral Valve Disease. Journal of Veterinary Internal Medicine 24(2): 331–341.

Bonagura, J.D. (1989). Cardiovascular Diseases. The Cat: Diseases and Clinical Management. RG Sherding Ed. New York, Churchill Livingstone. 2: 649–686.

Caney, S. (2009). Feline adrenal disease: Diagnosis and management. Proceedings: BSAVA. Accessed via: Veterinary Information Network. http://goo.gl/iY5jX

Connolly, D. (2006). The ascitic dog. Proceedings: BSAVA Congress. Accessed via: Veterinary Information Network. http://goo.gl/BB9AX

de Madron, E. (2004). Diuretics in CHF: New strategies. Proceedings: ACVIM Forum. Accessed via: Veterinary Information Network. http://goo.gl/lPzdM

Guyonnet, J., J. Elliott, et al. (2010). A preclinical pharmacokinetic and pharmacodynamic approach to determine a dose of spironolactone for treatment of congestive heart failure in dog. Journal of Veterinary Pharmacology and Therapeutics 33(3): 260–267.

Henik, R. (2007). Stepwise therapy of systemic hypertension. Proceedings: IVECCS. Accessed via: Veterinary Information Network. http://goo.gl/nofKU

Jeunesse, E., F. Wohrle, et al. (2004). Spironolactone as a diuretic agent in the dog: Is the water becoming muddy? Proceedings: ACVIM Forum. Accessed via: Veterinary Information Network. http://goo.gl/yr8Nr

Kittleson, M. (2000). Therapy of Heart Failure. Textbook of Veterinary Internal Medicine: Diseases of the Dog and Cat. S Ettinger and E Feldman Eds. Philadelphia, WB Saunders. 1: 713-737.

MacDonald, K.A., M.D. Kittleson, et al. (2008). Effect of spironolactone on diastolic function and left ventricular mass in maine coon cats with familial hypertrophic cardiomyopathy. Journal of Veterinary Internal Medicine 22(2): 335–341.

Stepian, R. (2006). Therapeutic management of systemic hypertension. Proceedings: ACVIM Forum.

Trepanier, L. (2008). Choosing therapy for chronic liver disease. Proceedings: WSAVA. Accessed via: Veterinary Information Network. http://goo.gl/NLh4X

Ware, W. & B. Keene (2000). Outpatient management of chronic heart failure. Kirk's Current Veterinary Therapy: XIII Small Animal Practice. J Bonagura Ed. Philadelphia, WB Saunders: 748–752.

STANOZOLOL

(stah-*no*-zo-lahl)   Winstrol®-V

ANABOLIC STEROID

Prescriber Highlights

▶ Anabolic steroid; FDA-approved products no longer marketed in USA

▶ Contraindications: Pregnant animals, breeding stallions, food animals. Extreme Caution: Cats, hepatic dysfunction, hypercalcemia, history of myocardial infarction, pituitary insufficiency, prostate carcinoma, mammary carcinoma, benign prostatic hypertrophy, & during the nephrotic stage of nephritis. Caution: Cardiac & renal dysfunction with enhanced fluid & electrolyte monitoring.

▶ Adverse Effects: Potentially high incidence of hepatotoxicity in cats. Other possible effects: sodium, calcium, potassium, water, chloride, & phosphate retention; hepatotoxicity, behavioral (androgenic) changes, & reproductive abnormalities (oligospermia, estrus suppression)

▶ Category "X" for pregnancy; teratogenicity outweighs any possible benefit

▶ Controlled substance in the USA

▶ Drug Interactions; lab interactions

Uses/Indications

Labeled indications for the previously marketed veterinary stanozolol product *Winstrol®-V* (Winthrop/Upjohn) included ". . . to improve appetite, promote weight gain, and increase strength and vitality . . ." in dogs, cats and horses. The manufacturer also stated that: "Anabolic therapy is intended primarily as an adjunct to other specific and supportive therapy, including nutritional therapy." In a review of the evidence supporting anabolic steroid use in horses, the authors conclude: "Level 1 evidence for the efficacy of anabolic steroids in horses for therapeutic uses is not found in the biomedical literature. Evidence in other species exists for the efficacy of anabolic steroids in treating anemia and increasing muscle mass after illness or injury, but that evidence is not unequivocal, and the applicability to horses has not been demonstrated. There is little evidence in other species for the efficacy of anabolic steroids for increasing appetite." (Fajt & McCook 2008)

Like nandrolone, stanozolol has been used to treat anemia of chronic disease. Because stanozolol has been demonstrated to enhance fibrinolysis after parenteral injection, it may be efficacious in the treatment of feline aortic thromboembolism or thrombosis in nephrotic syndrome; however, clinical studies and/or experience are apparently lacking for this indication at present.

Pharmacology/Actions

Stanozolol possesses the actions of other anabolic agents but it may be less androgenic than other anabolics that are used in veterinary medicine. Refer to the discussion in the boldenone monograph for more information.

Pharmacokinetics

No specific information was located for this agent. It is generally recommended that the injectable suspension be dosed on a weekly basis in both small animals and horses.

Contraindications/Precautions/Warnings

Stanozolol is contraindicated in pregnant animals and in breeding stallions and should not be administered to horses intended for food purposes. Because of reported hepatotoxicity associated with this drug in cats, it should only be used in this species with extreme caution.

The manufacturer recommends using stanozolol cautiously in patients with cardiac and renal dysfunction with enhanced fluid and electrolyte monitoring.

In humans, anabolic agents are contraindicated in patients with hepatic dysfunction, hypercalcemia, patients with a history of myocardial infarction (can cause hypercholesterolemia), pituitary insufficiency, prostate carcinoma, benign prostatic hypertrophy, during the nephrotic stage of nephritis, and in selected patients with breast carcinoma.

Adverse Effects

The manufacturer (Winthrop/Upjohn) lists as adverse effects in dogs, cats, and horses only "mild androgenic effects" and then only when used with excessively high doses for a prolonged period of time.

One study in cats, demonstrated a very high incidence of hepatotoxicity associated with stanozolol use and the authors recommended that this drug not be used in cats until further toxicological studies are performed.

Potentially (from human data), adverse reactions of the anabolic agents in dogs and cats could include: sodium, calcium, potassium, water, chloride, and phosphate retention, hepatotoxicity, behavioral (androgenic) changes, and reproductive abnormalities (oligospermia, estrus suppression).

Reproductive/Nursing Safety

In humans, the FDA categorizes this drug as category *X* for use during pregnancy (*Studies in animals or humans demonstrate fetal abnormalities or adverse reaction; reports indicate evidence of fetal risk. The risk of use in pregnant women clearly outweighs any possible benefit.*) In a separate system evaluating the safety of drugs in canine and feline pregnancy (Papich 1989), this drug is categorized as in class: *D* (*Contraindicated. These drugs have been shown to cause congenital malformations or embryotoxicity.*)

It is not known whether anabolic steroids are excreted in maternal milk. Because of the potential for serious adverse reactions in nursing offspring, use in nursing patients with extreme caution.

Overdosage/Acute Toxicity

No information was located for this specific agent. In humans, sodium and water retention can occur after overdosage of anabolic steroids. It is suggested to treat supportively and monitor liver function should an inadvertent overdose be administered.

Drug Interactions

The following drug interactions have either been reported or are theoretical in humans or animals receiving stanozolol and may be of significance in veterinary patients:

■ **ANTICOAGULANTS (heparin, warfarin):** Anabolic agents as a class may potentiate the effects of anticoagulants; monitoring of INR/PT's and dosage adjustment, if necessary, of the anticoagulant are recommended

■ **CORTICOSTEROIDS:** Anabolics may enhance the edema that can be associated with ACTH or adrenal steroid therapy

■ **INSULIN:** Diabetic patients receiving insulin may need dosage adjustments if anabolic therapy is added or discontinued; anabolics may decrease blood glucose and decrease insulin requirements

Laboratory Considerations

■ Concentrations of protein bound iodine (PBI) can be decreased in patients receiving androgen/anabolic therapy, but the clinical significance of this is probably not important. Androgen/anabolic agents can decrease amounts of thyroxine-binding globulin and decrease **total T_4** concentrations and increase resin uptake of T_3 **and** T_4. Free thyroid hormones are unaltered and there is no evidence of dysfunction.

■ Both **creatinine** and **creatine** excretion can be decreased by anabolic steroids.

■ Anabolic steroids can increase the urinary excretion of **17-ketosteroids.**

■ Androgenic/anabolic steroids may alter **blood glucose** levels.

■ Androgenic/anabolic steroids may suppress **clotting factors** II, V, VII, and X.

■ Anabolic agents can affect **liver function tests** (BSP retention, SGOT, SGPT, bilirubin, and alkaline phosphatase).

Doses

■ **DOGS:**

As an anabolic agent per labeled indications:

a) Small Breeds: 1–2 mg PO twice daily; or 25 mg deep IM, may repeat weekly.

Large Breeds: 2–4 mg PO twice daily; or 50 mg deep IM, may repeat weekly.

Treatment should continue for several weeks, depending on response and condition of animal. (Package Insert; *Winstrol®-V* —Winthrop/Upjohn)

For anemia secondary to chronic renal failure:

a) 1–4 mg PO once daily (Ross *et al.* 1989)

b) For anemias secondary to uremia: 2–10 mg PO twice daily (Maggio-Price 1988)

As an anabolic/appetite stimulant:

a) 1–4 mg PO twice daily (Weller 1988)

b) 1–2 mg PO twice daily or 25–50 mg IM weekly (Bartges 2003; Macy & Ralston 1989)

For canine cognitive dysfunction:

a) 2 mg/kg IM for 4–6 weeks with 1–2 mg (total dose) PO once daily for dogs less than 23 kg and 4 mg (total dose) PO once daily for dogs greater than 23 kg. If drug has some positive effect, maintain oral dosing and gradually reduce injections to every 3–4 weeks. (Hoskins 1999)

■ **CATS: NOTE: SEE WARNINGS ABOVE**

As an anabolic agent per labeled indications:

a) 1–2 mg PO twice daily; or 25 mg deep IM, may repeat weekly. Treatment should continue for several weeks, depending on response and condition of animal. (Package Insert; *Winstrol®-V* —Winthrop/Upjohn)

■ **FERRETS:**

a) 0.5 mg/kg PO or SC twice daily; use with caution in hepatic disease (Williams 2000)

■ **RABBITS, RODENTS, SMALL MAMMALS:**

a) Rabbits: As an appetite stimulant: 0.5–2 mg PO once (Ivey & Morrisey 2000)

■ **HORSES:** (**Note:** ARCI UCGFS Class 4 Drug) As an anabolic agent per labeled indications:

a) 0.55 mg/kg (25 mg per 100 pounds of body weight) IM deeply. May repeat weekly for up to and including 4 weeks. (Package Insert; *Winstrol®-V*—Winthrop/Upjohn)

■ **SHEEP & GOATS:**

For acute or subacute aflatoxicosis in ruminants:

a) Stanozolol 2 mg/kg IM (plus activated charcoal 6.7 mg/kg as a 30% w/v slurry in M/15, pH 7 phosphate buffer). Do not combine with oxytetracycline therapy. (Hatch 1988)

■ **BIRDS:**

As an anabolic agent to promote weight gain and recovery from disease:

a) 0.5–1 mL/kg (25–50 mg/kg) IM once or twice weekly. Use with caution in birds with renal disease. (Clubb 1986)

■ **REPTILES:**

For most species post-surgically and in very debilitated animals:

a) 5 mg/kg IM once a week as needed (Gauvin 1993)

Monitoring

■ Androgenic side effects
■ Fluid and electrolyte status, if indicated
■ Liver function tests if indicated
■ RBC count, indices, if indicated
■ Weight, appetite

Client Information

■ Tablets may be crushed and administered with food
■ Because of the potential for abuse of anabolic steroids this agent is a controlled drug; it should be kept in a secure area and out of the reach of children

Chemistry/Synonyms

An anabolic steroid, stanozolol occurs as an odorless, nearly colorless, crystalline powder that can exist in two forms: prisms that melt at approximately 235°C, and needles that melt at about 155°C. It is sparingly soluble in alcohol and insoluble in water.

Stanozolol may also be known as: androstanazole, estanozolol, methylstanazole, NSC-43193, stanozololum, win-14833, *Menabol®*, *Neurabol®*, *Stanol®*, *Stromba®*, *Strombaject®* and *Winstrol®*.

Storage/Stability

Stanozolol tablets should be stored in tight, light-resistant packaging, preferably at room temperature.

Dosage Forms/Regulatory Status

VETERINARY-LABELED PRODUCTS: None

Winstrol®-V (Pfizer) tablets and injection were previously available. Stanozolol may be available from compounding pharmacies.

The ARCI (Racing Commissioners International) has designated this drug as a class 4 substance. See the appendix for more information.

HUMAN-LABELED PRODUCTS: None

References

Bartges, J. (2003). Enteral Nutrition. Proceedings: World Small Animal Veterinary Assoc. World Congress. Accessed via: Veterinary Information Network. http://goo.gl/IZLCY

Clubb, S.L. (1986). Therapeutics: Individual and Flock Treatment Regimens. *Clinical Avian Medicine and Surgery*. GJ Harrison and LR Harrison Eds. Philadelphia, W.B. Saunders: 327–355.

Fajt, V.R. & C. McCook (2008). An evidence-based analysis of anabolic steroids as therapeutic agents in horses. *Equine Veterinary Education* 20(10): 542–544.

Gauvin, J. (1993). Drug therapy in reptiles. *Seminars in Avian & Exotic Med* 2(1): 48–59.

Hatch, R.C. (1988). Poisons causing abdominal distress or liver or kidney damage. *Veterinary Pharmacology and Therapeutics*. NH Booth and LE McDonald Eds. Ames, Iowa State Univ. Press: 1102–1125.

Hoskins, J. (1999). Old dog mental deterioration. Proceedings: American College of Veterinary Internal Medicine: 17th Annual Veterinary Medical Forum, Chicago.

Ivey, E. & J. Morrisey (2000). Therapeutics for Rabbits. *Vet Clin NA: Exotic Anim Pract* **3:**1(Jan): 183–216.

Macy, D.W. & S.L. Ralston (1989). Cause and control of decreased appetite. *Current Veterinary Therapy X: Small Animal Practice.* RW Kirk Ed. Philadelphia, WB Saunders: 18–24.

Maggio-Price, L. (1988). Disorders of Red Blood Cells. *Handbook of Small Animal Practice.* RV Morgan Ed. New York, Churchill Livingstone: 725–748.

Papich, M. (1989). Effects of drugs on pregnancy. *Current Veterinary Therapy X: Small Animal Practice.* R Kirk Ed. Philadelphia, Saunders: 1291–1299.

Ross, L.A., E.B. Breitschwerdt, et al. (1989). Diseases of the Kidney. *Handbook of Small Animal Practice.* RV Morgan Ed. New York, Churchill Livingstone: 567–593.

Weller, R.E. (1988). Paraneoplastic Syndromes. *Handbook of Small Animal Practice.* RV Morgan Ed. New York, Churchill Livingstone: 819–827.

Williams, B. (2000). Therapeutics in Ferrets. *Vet Clin NA: Exotic Anim Pract* **3:**1(Jan): 131–153.

STAPHYLOCOCCAL PHAGE LYSATE

(*staf-loe-kok-*al *faje* lye-*sate*)   Staphage Lysate (SP)®, SPL

IMMUNE STIMULANT

Prescriber Highlights

▶ Injectable immune stimulant used to treat dogs with recurrent, idiopathic, staphylococcal pyodermas

▶ May cause hypersensitivity (local or systemic)

Uses/Indications

Staphylococcal phage lysate (SPL) is labeled for treatment of canine pyoderma and related staphylococcal hypersensitivity, or polymicrobial skin infections with a staphylococcal component. Veterinary dermatologists use SPL most commonly to treat recurrent, idiopathic, staphylococcal pyodermas in combination (at least initially) with an appropriate antibiotic.

Pharmacology/Actions

SPL apparently enhances cell-mediated immunity. It stimulates the production of tumor necrosis factor, interleukin-6, interleukin-γ, and γ-interferon.

Pharmacokinetics

No information was located.

Contraindications/Precautions/Warnings

The label states that "there are no known contraindications to the use of *SPL®* except that in highly allergic patients, reduced desensitizing doses may be indicated." However, use with extreme caution, if at all, in patients with prior systemic hypersensitivity reactions to it or documented hypersensitivity reactions to beef products (contains unfiltered beef heart infusion broth).

Avoid administering subsequent doses at the same injection site.

The product contains no preservative so it must be handled aseptically. It is recommended to use the entire contents when the vial is opened.

Adverse Effects

Adverse effects reported for SPL include post vaccine-type reactions (fever, malaise, etc.) and injection site reactions (redness, itching, swelling) that may occur in 2–3 hours after injection and persisting up to 3 days. If these effects are excessive, the manufacturer recommends dosage reduction.

Systemic hypersensitivity reactions are thought to occur rarely. Signs could include weakness, vomiting, diarrhea, severe itching, rapid breathing, and/or fatigue/lassitude. Should an anaphylactic-type reaction occur, treat supportively; the manufacturer recommends epinephrine and atropine as antidotes.

Reproductive/Nursing Safety

Studies performed in rats and rabbits demonstrated no impaired fertility or fetal harm.

No information was located on safety during nursing, but it is unlikely to be of concern.

Overdosage/Acute Toxicity

No specific information was located. Other than an increased risk for local or systemic hypersensitivity reactions, significant morbidity appears unlikely.

Drug Interactions

◼ **CELL-MEDIATED   IMMUNOSUPPRESSIVE DRUGS (*e.g.*, corticosteroids, cyclosporine):** These drugs may reduce the efficacy of SPL

Laboratory Considerations

◼ No significant concerns noted.

Doses

◼ **DOGS:**

a) For labeled indications: Highly allergic patients: Skin test with 0.05–0.1 mL intradermally. Therapy: Initially, 0.2 mL SC, then incremental increases of 0.2 mL once a week to 1 mL (a total of 5 injections). Then continue at 1 mL SC weekly for approximately 10–12 weeks.

For non-allergic patients: 0.5 mL SC twice weekly for 10–12 weeks, then 0.5–1 mL every 1–2 weeks.

Concomitant antibiotic therapy is recommended for an initial 4–6 week period.

Maximum dose should be decreased in small dogs and can be increased cautiously, if necessary, in large dogs to 1.5 mL. This dose is continued until improvement is demonstrated then the interval may be lengthened gradually to the longest interval that maintains adequate clinical control. (Label information; *Staphage Lysate (SPL)®*—Delmont Labs)

b) For idiopathic, recurrent pyoderma: Typically given 0.5 mL SC twice weekly for 10–12 weeks, then tapered to effect. This agent is rarely needed, because in most cases, an underlying cause can be identified and treated. (Gram 2005)

c) For chronic recurrent idiopathic pyoderma: Pyoderma needs to be under control as this product is not a substitute for antibiotics. Injections are administered twice weekly (0.5 mL) and slowly reduced to 0.5 mL every 2 weeks. (Waisglass 2009)

Monitoring

■ Clinical efficacy

■ Local and systemic reactions (see adverse effects)

Client Information

■ This medication should ideally be administered at a veterinary practice where suitable treatment can be instituted should a serious adverse effect (*e.g.*, anaphylaxis) occur

■ Report to veterinarian any adverse effects noted (*e.g.*, local effects at injection site, itching, change in behavior or activity level, difficulty or unexplained rapid breathing, vomiting, diarrhea)

Chemistry/Synonyms

SPL is prepared by lysing cultures of *Staphylococcal aureas* (Cowan serologic types I & III; human strains) by a staphylococcal bacteriophage. Pre-lysed cell counts (120–180 CFU/mL) are used to standardize the product; ultrafiltration achieves bacteriologic sterility. The prepared solution contains *Staphylococcal aureas* components (protein A extracts), bacteriophage, and unfiltered beef heart infusion.

Storage/Stability

SPL should be stored in the refrigerator (2–7°C); do not freeze.

Unopened, properly stored vials and ampules have an average expiration date of one year past the shipment date. The product contains no preservative and must be handled aseptically. It is recommended using the entire contents of the vial after opening. Do not use if contents are cloudy.

Compatibility/Compounding Considerations

Do not mix with other drugs or solutions prior to administration.

Dosage Forms/Regulatory Status

VETERINARY-LABELED PRODUCTS:

Staphylococcal Phage Lysate (serotypes I & III): in 1 mL ampules (box of 10) and 10 mL multidose vials (no preservative added and manufacturer recommends using entire contents when opened); *Staphage Lysate (SPL)®* (Delmont Labs); (Biologic OTC)

Note: This product is a USDA-licensed biologic and is not an FDA-approved product.

HUMAN-LABELED PRODUCTS: None

References

Gram, D. (2005). Chronic recurrent pyoderma. Proceedings: Western Veterinary Conference 2005. Accessed via: Veterinary Information Network. http://goo.gl/2q9xz

Waisglass, S. (2009). New Perspectives on Pyoderma—Something Old and Something New. Proceedings: WVC. Accessed via: Veterinary Information Network. http://goo.gl/ZNgzx

STREPTOZOCIN

(strep-toe-**zoe**-sin)   Zanosar®

ANTINEOPLASTIC

Prescriber Highlights

▶ Antineoplastic used primarily for treating recurrent insulinoma in dogs

▶ May be nephrotoxic, myelotoxic, hepatotoxic

▶ Vomiting after treatment may occur

▶ To reduce nephrotoxicity, must give saline diuresis during administration

Uses/Indications

At present the primary purpose for streptozocin use in veterinary medicine is as a treatment for insulinomas in dogs, particularly those with refractory hypoglycemia and when tumors are non-resectable or have metastasized. Streptozocin potentially could be used for other oncologic conditions as well.

Pharmacology/Actions

While streptozocin has activity against gram-positive and gram-negative bacteria, its cytotoxicity prevents it from clinical usefulness for this purpose. While its antineoplastic activity is not well understood, streptozocin is considered an alkylating agent and it inhibits DNA synthesis, probably by inhibiting precursor incorporation into DNA.

Streptozocin also exhibits a species-specific (in dogs, not humans) diabetogenic effect via reducing nicotinamide adenine dinucleotide (NAD) concentration in pancreatic beta cells. This effect is usually irreversible in animals with preexisting normal beta cell function.

Pharmacokinetics

Streptozocin must be administered IV. Its distribution characteristics are not well known, but the drug does distribute to most tissues; concentrations in the pancreas are higher than those found in plasma. Streptozocin is metabolized, probably in the liver. Both unchanged and metabolized drug are excreted in the urine.

Contraindications/Precautions/Warnings

Should be used for recurrent insulinoma only in dogs that have undergone previous surgery in which all of the tumor could not be resected. Confirmed histologic diagnosis is mandatory.

Streptozocin must be used with extreme caution in patients with decreased renal, bone marrow, or hepatic function.

Adverse Effects

The primary concern when used for treating insulinomas in dogs is the potential for the development of serious, permanent renal toxicity. Aggressive saline diuresis during drug administration appears to reduce this concern. Additionally, GI effects (vomiting/nausea) often occur and can be severe or protracted. Less commonly, hematologic changes (mild myelosuppression) and increases in liver enzymes can occur. Injection site reactions (including severe necrosis) may occur if the drug extravasates.

Reproductive/Nursing Safety

Streptozocin has been shown to be teratogenic in rats; use during pregnancy when the benefits outweigh the risks. In humans, the FDA categorizes this drug as category *C* for use during pregnancy (*Animal studies have shown an adverse effect on the fetus, but there are no adequate studies in humans; or there are no animal reproduction studies and no adequate studies in humans.*)

It is not known whether streptozocin is excreted in milk. Because of the potential for serious adverse reactions in nursing offspring, consider using milk replacer if used in nursing patients.

Overdosage/Acute Toxicity

Severe toxicity may result if acutely overdosed (see Adverse Effects); calculate dosages carefully.

Drug Interactions

The following drug interactions have either been reported or are theoretical in humans or animals receiving streptozocin and may be of significance in veterinary patients:

- **DOXORUBICIN:** Streptozocin may prolong the half-life of doxorubicin; dosage adjustment may be required
- **MYELOSUPPRESSIVE DRUGS, OTHER:** When streptozocin is used with other myelosuppressive drugs (*e.g.,* **carmustine**) additive or synergistic myelosuppression may occur
- **NEPHROTOXIC DRUGS, OTHER (aminoglycosides, amphotericin B, cisplatin, etc.):** May cause additive nephrotoxicity when used with streptozocin
- **NIACINAMIDE (nicotinamide):** Can block the diabetogenic effects of streptozocin without altering its antineoplastic activity; this may be beneficial or detrimental depending on the reason for use

Doses

- **DOGS:**
  a) For "investigational" treatment of recurrent insulinoma after surgery: Begin saline diuresis: Give normal saline at 18–20 mL/kg/hour for 7–8 hours. Over the 4th–5th hour, give streptozocin in the saline solution at a dose of 500 mg/m^2 IV. Give an antiemetic (*e.g.,* butorphanol) at the end of the 7-hour period. (Meleo & Caplan 2000)
  b) Normal saline is given IV at 18.3 mL/kg/hr for 3 hours, then streptozocin is administered at 500 mg/m^2 over two hours with the saline diuresis continuing. After streptozocin infusion completed, continue saline diuresis for another 2 hours. Butorphanol is administered as an antiemetic immediately after streptozocin. May repeat at 3 week intervals until evidence of tumor progression, recurrence of hypoglycemia, or drug toxicity. Monitor for myelosuppression and nephrotoxicity. (Moore *et al.* 2002)

Monitoring

- Blood glucose (efficacy)
- Baseline renal function tests (including urinalyses) and after treatment
- CBC
- Baseline liver function tests and before retreatment
- Hydration status (especially for the first few days after treatment or if vomiting a problem).

Client Information

- Clients should understand the "experimental" nature of this treatment and the potential risks for serious adverse effects; follow-up monitoring is essential.

Chemistry/Synonyms

Streptozocin is an antineoplastic antibiotic produced by *Streptomyces achromogenes*, although the commercial product is prepared synthetically. It occurs as an ivory colored, crystalline powder. It is very soluble in water and has a pKa of 1.35.

Streptozocin may also be known as: NSC-85998, streptozotocin, U-9889 and *Zanosar®*.

Storage/Stability

The lyophilized powder for injection should be stored in the refrigerator and protected from light. It is stable for at least 3 years after manufacture. If stored at room temperature, it is stable for at least one year after manufacture.

After reconstitution, the lyophilized powder for injection has a pH of 3.5–4.5. Dextrose 5% or 0.9% sodium chloride are used to reconstitute the solution. Citric acid is added to buffer the solution at a concentration of 22 mg/mL. The solution is stable for 48 hours at room temperature and 96 hours if refrigerated, but as no preservative is added the manufacturer recommends using the drug within 12 hours of mixing.

Dosage Forms/Regulatory Status

VETERINARY-LABELED PRODUCTS: None

HUMAN-LABELED PRODUCTS:

Streptozocin Powder for Injection: 1 gram (100 mg/mL) in vials; *Zanosar®* (Genesia Sicor); (Rx)

References

Meleo, K. & E. Caplan (2000). Treatment of insulinoma in the dogs, cat, and ferret. *Kirk's Current Veterinary Therapy: XIII Small Animal Practice.* J Bonagura Ed. Philadelphia, WB Saunders: 357–361.

Moore, A., D. Nelson, et al. (2002). Streptozocin for treatment of pancreatic islet cell tumors in dogs: 17 cases. *JAVMA* 221: 811–818.

SUCCIMER

(*sux*-i-mer)   Chemet®, DMSA, Dimercaptosuccinic acid

ANTIDOTE; CHELATOR

Prescriber Highlights

▶ Oral heavy metal chelator

▶ Appears to be safe & effective despite limited experience

▶ Most likely adverse effects noted are GI in nature; may also cause increased liver enzymes, rash

▶ High doses may be fatal in birds

▶ Unpleasant odor of capsules; may give feces, urine, saliva, etc. a very unpleasant smell

▶ Cost is an issue

Uses/Indications

In veterinary medicine, succimer may be useful for the oral treatment of lead poisoning in small animals (including birds). Potentially, it also may be of benefit for the treatment of other toxic heavy metals such as arsenic or mercury, but more research must be done before this can be recommended.

Pharmacology/Actions

Succimer physically chelates heavy metals such as lead, mercury, and arsenic. These water-soluble chelates are then excreted via the kidneys.

Pharmacokinetics

No veterinary information was located. In humans, the drug is rapidly absorbed after oral ingestion, but only incompletely. Absorbed drug is excreted primarily through the kidneys into the urine. Half-life in humans is about 2 days.

Contraindications/Precautions/Warnings

Succimer is contraindicated in patients hypersensitive to it. Chelation therapy should only be attempted if the source of lead is removed to prevent further exposure.

Adverse Effects

Most common adverse reactions reported in humans are GI related effects (vomiting, diarrhea, etc.) or "flu-like" symptoms (body aches, fatigue, etc.). Increases in liver enzymes and rashes have also been reported.

Reproductive/Nursing Safety

It is unknown if succimer is safe to use during pregnancy. At high doses it was fetotoxic and teratogenic in mice. Mothers are discouraged from nursing when taking succimer. In humans, the FDA categorizes this drug as category *C* for use during pregnancy (*Animal studies have shown an adverse effect on the fetus, but there are no adequate studies in humans; or there are no animal reproduction studies and no adequate studies in humans.*)

It is not known whether this drug is excreted in breast milk. Discourage mothers requiring therapy from nursing their infants.

Overdosage/Acute Toxicity

In toxicology studies, doses of up to 200 mg/kg per day in dogs did not cause overt toxicity. Doses of 300 mg/day did cause fatalities in dogs; primarily kidney and GI tract lesions were seen. Doses of 80 mg/kg, PO q12h did cause a significant number of fatalities in Cockatiels (but 40 mg/kg q12h did not). If an overdose situation is encountered, standardized gut evacuation with subsequent activated charcoal protocols are recommended.

Drug Interactions

The following drug interactions have either been reported or are theoretical in humans or animals receiving succimer and may be of significance in veterinary patients:

■ **CHELATING AGENTS, OTHER (CaEDTA, dimercaprol, trientine, penicillamine, etc.):** Concomitant use with other chelating agents is not recommended in humans

Laboratory Considerations

■ False positive **urine ketones** can be reported when using nitroprusside reagents (*e.g.*, as in *Ketostix®*)

■ Falsely low measurements of **CPK** or serum **uric acid** can be caused by succimer

Doses

■ **DOGS:**

For lead poisoning:

a) 10 mg/kg PO q8h for 10 days. Succimer has a good therapeutic index, few side effects, spares most other elements from being chelated and does not cause enhanced lead uptake from the gut. Blood lead levels should be rechecked a few days following the last dose of succimer; a second round of chelation therapy may be necessary to reduce the lead load. (Talcott 2008)

b) 10 mg/kg PO three times daily for 5 days, followed by 10 mg/kg PO twice daily for 2 weeks (Poppenga 2002)

■ **CATS:**

For lead poisoning:

a) 10 mg/kg PO three times daily for 5 days, followed by 10 mg/kg PO twice daily for 2 weeks (Poppenga 2002)

b) See the dog dose referenced to Talcott above.

■ BIRDS:

For lead poisoning:

a) 15–35 mg/kg PO twice daily for 5 days (Calvert & Mieurs 2000)

b) 30 mg/kg PO twice daily for a minimum of 7 days. If severe neurologic signs, may supplement with one dose of CaEDTA (edetate calcium disodium; <50 mg/kg of body weight IM) (Hoogesteijn *et al.* 2003)

Monitoring

■ Blood lead

■ GI adverse effects

■ Liver enzymes (AST, ALT)

Client Information

■ Capsules may have an unpleasant odor; this is no problem with the drug, but unpleasant odor may be transferred to saliva, urine, feces

■ Contents of capsules may be sprinkled on soft food

■ Animals must be adequately hydrated as the lead chelates are excreted in the urine

Chemistry/Synonyms

A heavy metal chelating agent also known as meso-2,3 dimercaptosuccinic acid (DMSA), succimer is an analog of dimercaprol. It has an unpleasant odor.

Succimer may also be known as: meso-2,3 dimercaptosuccinic acid, dimercaptosuccinic acid, DIM-SA, DMSA, *Chemet*® or *Succicaptal*®.

Storage/Stability

Unless otherwise labeled, store succimer capsules in tight containers at room temperature. Protect from light.

Dosage Forms/Regulatory Status

VETERINARY-LABELED PRODUCTS: None

HUMAN-LABELED PRODUCTS:

Succimer Capsules: 100 mg; *Chemet*® (Ovation); (Rx)

References

Calvert, C. & K. Mieurs (2000). CVT Update: Doberman Pinscher Occult Cardiomyopathy. *Kirk's Current Veterinary Therapy: XIII Small Animal Practice.* J Bonagura Ed. Philadelphia, WB Saunders: 756–760.

Hoogesteijn, A., B. Raphael, et al. (2003). Oral treatment of avian lead intoxication with meso-2,3,dimercaptosuccinic acid. *J Zoo Wildli Med* **34**(1): 82–87.

Poppenga, R. (2002). Decontaminating and detoxifying the poisoned patient. Proceedings: Western Veterinary Conf. Accessed via: Veterinary Information Network. http://goo.gl/Hq3dC

Talcott, P. (2008). New and Used Topics in Toxicology. Proceedings: Western Veterinary Conference. Accessed via: Veterinary Information Network. http://goo.gl/g6SuY

SUCCINYLCHOLINE CHLORIDE

(**suks**-sin-i-nil-**koe**-leen)   Anectine®

NEUROMUSCULAR BLOCKING AGENT

Prescriber Highlights

▶ Depolarizing neuromuscular blocking agent

▶ Contraindications: Severe liver disease, chronic anemias, malnourishment, glaucoma or penetrating eye injuries, predisposition to malignant hyperthermia, & increased CPK values with resultant myopathies

▶ Extreme Caution: Traumatic wounds or burns, receiving quinidine or digoxin therapy, hyperkalemia or electrolyte imbalances

▶ Caution: Pulmonary, renal, cardiovascular, metabolic or hepatic dysfunction

▶ Adverse Effects: Muscle soreness, histamine release, malignant hyperthermia, excessive salivation, hyperkalemia, rash, & myoglobinemia/myoglobinuria. Cardiovascular effects, (bradycardia, tachycardia, hypertension, hypotension, or arrhythmias)

▶ Specific recommendations for use in horses (see Contraindications below)

▶ No analgesic or anesthetic effects

Uses/Indications

Succinylcholine chloride is indicated for short-term muscle relaxation needed for surgical or diagnostic procedures, to facilitate endotracheal intubation in some species, and reducing the intensity of muscle contractions associated with electro- or pharmacological-induced convulsions. Dogs, cats, and horses are the primary veterinary species where succinylcholine chloride has been used. Its use has been largely supplanted by newer agents (*e.g.*, atracurium) with fewer adverse effects.

Pharmacology/Actions

An ultrashort-acting depolarizing skeletal muscle relaxant, succinylcholine bonds with motor endplate cholinergic receptors to produce depolarization (perceived as fasciculations). The neuromuscular block remains as long as sufficient quantities of succinylcholine remain, and is characterized by a flaccid paralysis. Other pharmacologic effects are discussed in the precautions and adverse effects sections.

Pharmacokinetics

The onset of action, with complete muscle relaxation, after IV administration is usually within 30-60 seconds. In humans, this effect lasts for 2–3 minutes and then gradually diminishes within 10 minutes. The very short duration of action after a single IV dose is thought to occur because the drug diffuses away from the motor end plate. If multiple injections or a continuous infusion is performed, the brief activity is a result of rapid hydrolysis by pseudocholinesterases at the site of action. After IM injection, the onset of action is generally within 2–3 minutes and may persist for 10–30 minutes. Dogs exhibit a prolonged duration of action ($\approx$ 20 minutes); this species appears unique in this idiosyncratic response.

Succinylcholine is metabolized by plasma pseudocholinesterases to succinylmonocholine and choline; 10% is excreted unchanged in the urine. Succinylmonocholine is partially excreted in the urine and may accumulate in patients with impaired renal function. Succinylmonocholine has approximately $^1/_{20}$ th the neuromuscular blocking activity of succinylcholine, but if it accumulates, prolonged periods of apnea may result.

Contraindications/Precautions/Warnings

Succinylcholine is contraindicated in patients with severe liver disease, chronic anemias, malnourishment (chronic), glaucoma or penetrating eye injuries, predisposition to malignant hyperthermia, and increased CPK values with resultant myopathies. As succinylcholine can exacerbate the effects of hyperkalemia, it should be used with extreme caution in patients who have suffered traumatic wounds or burns, are receiving quinidine or digoxin therapy, or have preexisting hyperkalemia or electrolyte imbalances as arrhythmias or cardiac arrest may occur. It should be used with caution in patients with pulmonary, renal, cardiovascular, metabolic, or hepatic dysfunction.

Succinylcholine should not be used if organophosphate agents have been given or applied recently.

Succinylcholine chloride does not have analgesic effects; and should be used with appropriate analgesic, sedative, and anesthetic agents.

In horses, The American Association of Equine Practitioners have made the following additional recommendations:

1) Inform the owner that succinylcholine chloride is to be used as a restraining agent, not as an anesthetic.

2) Obtain history before use; do not use in horses if within 30 days they have received, an antibiotic ending in "mycin", organophosphate insecticides or anthelmintics, any other cholinesterase inhibitor, or procaine.

3) Do not use in debilitated, excited, or exhausted horses.

4) If possible, withhold food for 4–6 hours before use.

5) Dosage of 0.088 mg/kg IV may be used to paralyze skeletal muscles without causing respiratory depression. Higher doses may cause apnea and death without respiratory support. Lower doses may be possible if used with a preanesthetic agent.

6) After administration, have someone hold the horse that is familiar with the actions of succinylcholine chloride so that the animal does not fall forward on its nose. Be prepared to administer oxygen and artificial respiration.

7) If death occurs, a necropsy should be performed.

Adverse Effects

Succinylcholine chloride can cause muscle soreness, histamine release, malignant hyperthermia, excessive salivation, hyperkalemia, rash, and myoglobinemia/myoglobinuria. Cardiovascular effects can include bradycardia, tachycardia, hypertension, hypotension, or arrhythmias.

Reproductive/Nursing Safety

It is unknown if succinylcholine can cause fetal harm. The drug does cross the placenta in low concentrations and a newly delivered neonate may show signs of neuromuscular blockade if the mother received high doses or prolonged administration of the drug prior to delivery. In humans, the FDA categorizes this drug as category *C* for use during pregnancy (*Animal studies have shown an adverse effect on the fetus, but there are no adequate studies in humans; or there are no animal reproduction studies and no adequate studies in humans.*) In a separate system evaluating the safety of drugs in canine and feline pregnancy (Papich 1989), this drug is categorized as in class: *B* (*Safe for use if used cautiously. Studies in laboratory animals may have uncovered some risk, but these drugs appear to be safe in dogs and cats or these drugs are safe if they are not administered when the animal is near term.*)

It is not known whether this drug is excreted into milk; exercise caution when succinylcholine is administered to a nursing patient.

Overdosage/Acute Toxicity

Inadvertent overdoses, or standard doses in patients deficient in pseudocholinesterase may result in prolonged apnea. Mechanical ventilation with O_2 should be used until recovery.

Repeated or prolonged high dosages may cause patients to convert from a phase I to a phase II block.

Drug Interactions

The following drug interactions have either been reported or are theoretical in humans or animals receiving succinylcholine and may be of significance in veterinary patients:

- ■ **AMPHOTERICIN B:** May increase succinylcholine's effects by causing electrolyte imbalances

- ■ **DIGOXIN:** Succinylcholine may cause a sudden outflux of potassium from muscle cells, thus causing arrhythmias in digitalized patients

■ **OPIATES:** Potential for increased incidences of bradycardia and sinus arrest

■ **THIAZIDE DIURETICS:** May increase succinylcholine's effects by causing electrolyte imbalances

The following drugs/drug classes may increase or prolong neuromuscular blockade if used concurrently with succinylcholine:

■ **AMINOGLYCOSIDES**

■ **ANESTHETICS, INHALATION (ISOFLURANE, DESFLURANE)**

■ **ANTIARRHYTHMICS (QUINIDINE, LIDOCAINE, PROCAINAMIDE)**

■ **BETA-ADRENERGIC BLOCKERS**

■ **CHLOROQUINE**

■ **CLINDAMYCIN**

■ **CORTICOSTEROIDS**

■ **CYCLOPHOSPHAMIDE**

■ **MAGNESIUM SALTS**

■ **MAO INHIBITORS**

■ **METOCLOPRAMIDE**

■ **NEOSTIGMINE**

■ **ORGANOPHOSPHATES**

■ **OXYTOCIN**

■ **PANCURONIUM**

■ **PHENOTHIAZINES**

■ **PROCAINE (IV)**

■ **TERBUTALINE**

■ **THIOTEPA**

Doses

■ **DOGS:**
  a) 0.07 mg/kg IV (Morgan 1988)
  b) 0.22 mg/kg IV (Mandsager 1988)

■ **CATS:**
  a) 0.06 mg/kg IV (Morgan 1988)
  b) 0.11 mg/kg IV (Mandsager 1988)

■ **HORSES:**
  See Precautions above. (**Note:** ARCI UCGFS Class 2 Drug)
  a) 0.088–0.11 mg/kg IV, IM (Mandsager 1988)

■ **REPTILES:**
  a) To relax an animal to allow intubation: 0.5–1 mg/kg IM. Especially helpful with turtles and crocodilians. (Lewbart 2001)

Monitoring

■ Level of muscle relaxation

■ Cardiac rate/rhythm

■ Respiratory depressant effect

Client Information

■ This drug should only be used by professionals familiar with its use

Chemistry/Synonyms

A depolarizing neuromuscular blocking agent, succinylcholine chloride occurs as an odorless, white, crystalline powder. The dihydrate

form melts at 190°C and the anhydrous form at 160°C. Aqueous solutions are acidic with a pH of approximately 4. One gram is soluble in about 1 mL of water and about 350 mL of alcohol. Commercially available injections have a pH from 3–4.5.

Succinylcholine chloride may also be known as: choline chloride succinate, succicurarium chloride, succinylcholine chloride, suxamethonii chloridum, suxametonklorid, suxamethonium chloride; many trade names are available.

Storage/Stability

Commercial injectable solutions should be stored refrigerated (2°–8°C). One manufacturer (*Anectine®*—Glaxo Wellcome) states that multiple dose vials are stable up to 2 weeks at room temperature with no significant loss of potency.

The powder forms of the drug are stable indefinitely when stored unopened at room temperature. After reconstitution with either D_5W or normal saline, they are stable for 4 weeks at 5°C or 1 week at room temperature, but because they contain no preservative, it is recommended they be used within 24 hours.

Compatibility/Compounding Considerations

Succinylcholine chloride is physically **compatible** with all commonly used IV solutions, amikacin sulfate, isoproterenol HCl, meperidine HCl, norepinephrine bitartrate, and scopolamine HBr. It **may not be compatible** with pentobarbital sodium and is physically **incompatible** with sodium bicarbonate and thiopental sodium.

Dosage Forms/Regulatory Status

VETERINARY-LABELED PRODUCTS: None

The ARCI (Racing Commissioners International) has designated this drug as a class 2 substance. See the appendix for more information.

HUMAN-LABELED PRODUCTS:

Succinylcholine Chloride Injection: 20 mg/mL in 10 mL vials and 5 mL *Abboject* syringes; *Anectine®* (GlaxoWellcome); *Quelicin®* (Hospira); (Rx)

Succinylcholine Chloride Injection, Solution: 100 mg/mL in 5 mL & 10 mL single-use, preservative free vials & 20 mL multidose vials; *Quelicin-1000®* (Hospira); (Rx)

Succinylcholine Chloride Powder for Infusion: 500 mg & 1 gram in vials; *Anectine® Flo-Pak* (GlaxoWellcome); (Rx)

References

Lewbart (2001). Reptile Formulary. Proceedings: Atlantic Coast Veterinary Conference. Accessed via: Veterinary Information Network. http://goo.gl/EEQmM

Mandsager, R.E. (1988, Last Update). "Personal Communication."

Morgan, R.V., Ed. (1988). *Handbook of Small Animal Practice*. New York, Churchill Livingstone.

Papich, M. (1989). Effects of drugs on pregnancy. *Current Veterinary Therapy X: Small Animal Practice*. R Kirk Ed. Philadelphia, Saunders: 1291–1299.

SUCRALFATE

(soo-**kral**-fate)   Carafate®

GASTROPROTECTANT

Prescriber Highlights

▶ Locally-acting treatment for GI ulcers; may also protect somewhat against GI ulceration. Potentially could be useful for lowering serum phosphorus in renal patients.

▶ Contraindications: None, use with caution where decreased GI transit times may be harmful

▶ Adverse Effects: Unlikely; constipation possible. Vomiting reported in cats.

▶ Give on empty stomach if possible

▶ Drug Interactions

Uses/Indications

Sucralfate has been used in the treatment of oral, esophageal, gastric, and duodenal ulcers. It has also been employed to prevent drug-induced (e.g., aspirin) gastric erosions, but efficacy for this is somewhat sporadic.

Sucralfate has been used in human patients with hyperphosphatemia secondary to renal failure and potentially could be useful for this in animals as well. In a study done in six healthy cats, sucralfate did not significantly change serum or urine phosphorus levels (Quimby & Lappin 2008).

Pharmacology/Actions

While the exact mechanism of action of sucralfate as an antiulcer agent is not known, the drug has a local effect rather than a systemic one. After oral administration, sucralfate reacts with hydrochloric acid in the stomach to form a paste-like complex that will bind to the proteinaceous exudates that generally are found at ulcer sites. This insoluble complex forms a barrier at the site and protects the ulcer from further damage caused by pepsin, acid, or bile. Sucralfate can inactivate pepsin and bind bile acids.

Sucralfate may have some cytoprotective effects, possibly by stimulation of prostaglandin E_2 and I_2. Sucralfate also has some antacid activity, but it is believed that this is not of clinical importance.

Sucralfate does not significantly affect gastric acid output, or trypsin or pancreatic amylase activity. It may decrease the rate of gastric emptying.

As an aluminum salt, sucralfate can bind to gastrointestinal phosphorus.

Pharmacokinetics

Animal studies have indicated that only 3–5% of an oral dose is absorbed which is excreted in the urine unchanged within 48 hours. By reacting with hydrochloric acid in the gut, the remainder

of the drug is converted to sucrose sulfate, which is excreted in the feces within 48 hours. The duration of action (binding to ulcer site) may persist up to 6 hours after oral dosing.

Contraindications/Precautions/Warnings

There are no known contraindications to the use of sucralfate. Because it may cause constipation, it should be used with caution in animals where decreased intestinal transit times might be deleterious.

Adverse Effects

Adverse effects are uncommon with sucralfate therapy. Constipation is the most prominent adverse effect reported in humans (2%) and dogs receiving the drug. Vomiting has been reported in cats.

Reproductive/Nursing Safety

It is unknown if sucralfate crosses the placenta and whether it may definitively be used safely during pregnancy. In rats, dosages up to 38 times those used in humans caused no impaired fertility and doses up to 50 times normal caused no symptoms of teratogenicity. In humans, the FDA categorizes this drug as category **B** for use during pregnancy (*Animal studies have not yet demonstrated risk to the fetus, but there are no adequate studies in pregnant women; or animal studies have shown an adverse effect, but adequate studies in pregnant women have not demonstrated a risk to the fetus in the first trimester of pregnancy, and there is no evidence of risk in later trimesters.*) In a separate system evaluating the safety of drugs in canine and feline pregnancy (Papich 1989), this drug is categorized as in class: **A** (*Probably safe. Although specific studies may not have proved he safety of all drugs in dogs and cats, there are no reports of adverse effects in laboratory animals or women.*)

It is not known whether this drug is excreted in milk, but it is unlikely to be of concern.

Overdosage/Acute Toxicity

Overdosage is unlikely to cause any significant problems. Laboratory animals receiving up to 12 grams/kg orally demonstrated no incidence of mortality.

Drug Interactions

The following drug interactions have either been reported or are theoretical in humans or animals receiving sucralfate and may be of significance in veterinary patients:

Sucralfate may impair the oral absorption of the following medications; separate dosing by at least 2 hours to minimize this effect:

■ AZITHROMYCIN

■ CIPROFLOXACIN/ENROFLOXACIN (assume other **oral fluoroquinolones** as well)

■ DICLOFENAC

■ DIGOXIN

■ DOXYCYCLINE

■ ERYTHROMYCIN

■ **KETOCONAZOLE**

■ **LEVOTHYROXINE**

■ **PENICILLAMINE**

■ **TETRACYCLINE**

■ **THEOPHYLLINE**

■ **VITAMINS (fat soluble)**

■ **WARFARIN**

Doses

■ **DOGS:**

a) For esophagitis: 0.5–1 gram PO three times a day. Suspensions are more therapeutic than intact tablets. (Washabau 2000)

b) For large dogs: 1 gram PO q8; for smaller dogs: 0.5 gram PO q8h (Zerbe & Washabau 2000)

c) 0.5–1 gram PO 2–4 times a day; patients with severe GI blood loss give an initial loading dose of 3–6 grams and then resume lower dose. If also using an H2 blocker, administer sucralfate 30–60 minutes later. (Hall 2000)

d) For eliminating Helicobacter gastritis infections: Using triple therapy: Metronidazole 33 mg/kg once daily, amoxicillin 11 mg/kg q12h and either sucralfate (0.25–0.5 grams q8h) or omeprazole 0.66 mg/kg once daily (Hall 2000)

e) In patients with severe hematemesis and anemia we sometimes give a loading dose of 3–6 grams initially and then decrease to 1 gram PO three to four times a day. May not always work in vomiting dogs. Suspensions may have less tendency to be vomited up in these patients. (Willard 2006)

f) For gastric ulcers, esophagitis: 0.5–1 gram PO per dog q8–12h (Sellon 2007)

g) For GI ulcers/esophagitis associated with acute renal failure: 1 gram per 30 kg body weight PO q6h (Waddell 2007)

■ **CATS:**

a) 0.25–0.5 grams PO q8–12h (Zerbe & Washabau 2000)

b) Empirical dosage of sucralfate is ¼ of a 1 gram tablet per cat PO three to four times a day. (Trepanier 2010)c)

For gastric ulcers, esophagitis: 0.25–0.5 grams PO per cat PO q8–12h (Sellon 2007)

■ **FERRETS:**

a) 75 mg/kg PO q4–6h; give 10 minutes prior to feeding (Williams 2000)

■ **HORSES:**

a) For adjunctive treatment (used with acid suppressive drugs) for preventing stress-induced ulcers in foals: 10–20 mg/kg PO q6–8h (Sanchez 2004)

b) For treating equine gastric ulcer syndrome: 20–40 mg/kg PO q8h (Sanchez 2004), (Nadeau & Andrews 2003)

c) Sucralfate alone may not be beneficial in treatment of equine gastric ulcer syndrome, but can be used in conjunction with acid-suppressive therapy and may be more suited for treatment of right dorsal colitis (colonic ulcers) at a dose of 22 mg/kg PO q6-8h. (Videla & Andrews 2009)

■ **REPTILES:**

a) For GI irritation in most species: 500–1,000 mg/kg PO q6–8h (Gauvin 1993)

Monitoring

■ Clinical efficacy (dependent on reason for use); monitored by decrease in symptomatology, endoscopic examination, blood in feces, etc.

Client Information

■ To maximize the benefit of this medication, it must be administered as prescribed by the veterinarian; clinical signs may reoccur if dosages are missed

■ Unless otherwise instructed, give this medication to animal having an empty stomach (1 hour before feeding or 2 hours after) and at bedtime

Chemistry/Synonyms

A basic, aluminum complex of sucrose sulfate, sucralfate occurs as a white, amorphous powder. It is practically insoluble in alcohol or water.

Sucralfate is structurally related to heparin, but does not possess any appreciable anticoagulant activity. It is also structurally related to sucrose, but is not utilized as a sugar by the body.

Sucralfate is also known as aluminum sucrose sulfate, basic and *Carafate®*.

Storage/Stability

Store sucralfate tablets in tight containers at room temperature.

Compatibility/Compounding Considerations

A sucralfate 200 mg/mL suspension can be extemporaneously prepared. To make 100 mL: crush twenty (20) sucralfate 1 gram tablets and add sufficient quantity of distilled water to bring the volume to 100 mL. Suspending agents such as acacia or tragacanth should not be used, as they can bind to sucralfate and make it inactive. Label "shake well" and "refrigerate." When refrigerated it is stable for 14 days.

Dosage Forms/Regulatory Status

VETERINARY-LABELED PRODUCTS: None

HUMAN-LABELED PRODUCTS:

Sucralfate Tablets: 1 gram; *Carafate®* (Axcan Sandipharm); generic; (Rx)

Sucralfate Suspension: 1 gram/10 mL in 10 mL unit dose cups & 415 mL; *Carafate®* (Axcan Scandipharm); generic (Precision Dose); (Rx)

References

Gauvin, J. (1993). Drug therapy in reptiles. *Seminars in Avian & Exotic Med* 2(1): 48–59.

Hall, J. (2000). Diseases of the Stomach. *Textbook of Veterinary Internal Medicine: Diseases of the Dog and Cat.* S Ettinger and E Feldman Eds. Philadelphia, WB Saunders. 2: 1154–1182.

Nadeau, J. & F. Andrews (2003). Gastric Ulcer Syndrome. *Current Therapy in Equine Medicine 5.* A Blikslager Ed. Philadelphia, Saunders: 94–99.

Papich, M. (1989). Effects of drugs on pregnancy. *Current Veterinary Therapy X: Small Animal Practice.* R Kirk Ed. Philadelphia, Saunders: 1291–1299.

Quimby, J. & M.R. Lappin (2008). Effects of Sucralfate on the Serum Phosphorus Concentration and Urinary Fractional Excretion of Phosphorus in Healthy Cats. Proceedings: ACVIM. Accessed via: Veterinary Information Network. http://goo.gl/cO4BV

Sanchez, L. (2004). Diseases of the stomach. *Equine Internal Medicine 2nd Ed.* S Reed, W Bayly and D Sellon Eds. Philadelphia, Saunders: 863–872.

Sellon, R. (2007). Gastric Ulcers. Proceedings: Western Vet Conf. Accessed via: Veterinary Information Network. http://goo.gl/hW7b9

Trepanier, L. (2010). Acute Vomiting in Cats: Rational treatment selection. *Journal of Feline Medicine and Surgery* 12(3): 225–230.

Videla, R. & F.M. Andrews (2009). New Perspectives in Equine Gastric Ulcer Disease. *Veterinary Clinics of North America-Equine Practice* 25(2): 283–+.

Waddell, L. (2007). Acute renal failure. Proceedings: Western Vet Conference. Accessed via: Veterinary Information Network. http://goo.gl/RlcNc

Washabau, R. (2000). Diseases of the Esophagus. *Textbook of Veterinary Internal Medicine: Diseases of the Dog and Cat.* S Ettinger and E Feldman Eds. Philadelphia, WB Saunders. 2: 1142–1154.

Willard, M. (2006). Severe hematemesis and GI bleeding. Proceedings: IVECCS. Accessed via: Veterinary Information Network. http://goo.gl/fqsWD

Williams, B. (2000). Therapeutics in Ferrets. *Vet Clin NA: Exotic Anim Pract* 3:1(Jan): 131–153.

Zerbe, C. & R. Washabau (2000). Gastrointestinal endocrine disease. *Textbook of Veterinary Internal Medicine: Diseases of the Dog and Cat.* S Ettinger and E Feldman Eds. Philadelphia, WB Saunders. 2: 1500–1508.

SUFENTANIL CITRATE

(soo-**fen**-ta-nil)   Sufenta®

OPIATE AGONIST

Prescriber Highlights

▶ Injectable, extremely potent opiate that may be useful for adjunctive anesthesia or epidural analgesia

▶ Marginal veterinary experience & little published data available to draw conclusions on appropriate usage in veterinary species

▶ Dose-related respiratory & CNS depression most likely adverse effects

▶ Class-II controlled substance; expensive when compared to fentanyl

Uses/Indications

An opioid analgesic, sufentanil may be useful as an anesthesia adjunct or as an epidural analgesic. In humans, it has been used as the primary anesthetic in intubated patients with assisted ventilation, and as a post-operative analgesic.

Pharmacology/Actions

Sufentanil is a potent *mu* opioid with the expected sedative, analgesic, and anesthetic properties. When comparing analgesic potencies, 0.01–0.04 mg of sufentanil is equivalent to 0.4–0.8 mg of alfentanil, 0.1–0.2 mg of fentanyl, and approximately 10 mg of morphine, when all are injected IM. Like fentanyl, sufentanil appears to have less circulatory effects than does morphine. Sufentanil has a rapid onset of action (1–3 minutes) and a faster recovery time than fentanyl.

Pharmacokinetics

No information on the pharmacokinetics of sufentanil in domestic animals was located. In humans, the drug has rapid onset of action (1–3 minutes) after intravenous injection. The drug is highly lipid soluble and has volume of distribution in the central compartment of 0.1 L/kg. Approximately 93% is bound to plasma proteins; plasma concentrations rapidly decline due to redistribution. Terminal elimination half-life is about 2.5 hours. Plasma clearance has been reported to be 11.8 mL/min/kg. Sufentanil is metabolized primarily in the liver and small intestine via O-demethylation and N-dealkylation. The parent drug and these metabolites are excreted primarily in the urine. While the manufacturer states to use with caution in patients with impaired renal of hepatic function, limited pharmacokinetic studies in these patients, rarely showed any drug accumulation.

Contraindications/Precautions/Warnings

Sufentanil is contraindicated in patients hypersensitive to it or other opioids. It should be used with caution in debilitated or geriatric patients and those with severely diminished renal or hepatic function.

Because of the drug's potency and potential for significant adverse effects, it should only be used in situations where patient vital signs can be continuously monitored. Initial dosage reduction may be required in geriatric or debilitated patients, particularly those with diminished cardiopulmonary function.

Adverse Effects

Adverse effects are generally dose related and consistent with other opiate agonists. Respiratory depression and/or CNS depression are most likely to be encountered.

In humans, bradycardia that is usually responsive to anticholinergic agents can occur. Dose-related skeletal muscle rigidity is not uncommon, and neuromuscular blockers are routinely used. Sufentanil has rarely been associated with asystole, hypercarbia and hypersensitivity reactions.

Respiratory or CNS depression may be exacerbated if sufentanil is given with other drugs that can cause those effects.

Reproductive/Nursing Safety

In humans, the FDA categorizes sufentanil as a category **C** drug for use during pregnancy (*Animal studies have shown an adverse effect on the fetus, but there are no adequate studies in humans; or there are no animal reproduction studies and no adequate studies in humans.*) While sufentanil is indicated for epidural use (mixed with bupivacaine ± epinephrine) in women for labor/delivery, it should not be administered systemically to a mother close to giving birth as offspring may show behavioral alterations (hypotonia, depression) associated with opioids.

The effects of sufentanil on lactation or its safety for nursing offspring is not well-defined, but sufentanil milk levels approximate those found in serum. This coupled with its low oral bioavailability, make it unlikely to cause significant effects in nursing offspring.

Overdosage/Acute Toxicity

In dogs, the LD_{50} of intravenous sufentanil is 10.1–19.5 mg/kg. Intravenous severe overdoses may cause apnea, circulatory collapse, pulmonary edema, seizures, cardiac arrest and death. Treatment is a combination of supportive therapy and administration of an opiate antagonist such as naloxone. Although sufentanil has a fairly rapid half-life, multiple doses of naloxone may be necessary. Because of the drug's potency, the use of a tuberculin syringe to measure dosages less than 1 mL, with a dosage calculation and measurement double-check system is recommended.

Drug Interactions

The following drug interactions have either been reported or are theoretical in humans or animals receiving sufentanil and may be of significance in veterinary patients:

- **BETA-ADRENERGIC BLOCKERS:** May increase bradycardia and hypotension
- **CALCIUM-CHANNEL BLOCKERS:** May increase bradycardia and hypotension
- **CNS DEPRESSANTS, OTHER:** Additive effects can occur if sufentanil is used concurrently with other drugs that can depress CNS or respiratory function (*e.g.*, **barbiturates**, etc.)
- **NITROUS OXIDE:** Can cause cardiovascular depression if used with high dose sufentanil

Laboratory Considerations

- Because opiates can increase biliary tract pressure and raise serum **amylase** and **lipase** values, these values may be unreliable for 24 hours after sufentanil is administered.

Doses

Note: In very obese patients, figure dosages based upon lean body weight.

- **DOGS:**
  a) As a pre-med: 3 micrograms/kg IV. As a combination for induction: Sufentanil

  3 micrograms/kg IV first, then diazepam or midazolam 0.2–0.5 mg IV. (Banyard 2004)
  b) For epidural analgesia: 0.7–1 micrograms/kg diluted to a volume of 0.26 mL/kg with sterile saline. Onset of action in 10–15 minutes; duration 1–4 hours. (Otero 2006b)
  c) Acute pain relief in an emergency: 0.75–2 micrograms/kg IV; constant rate infusion of 1–2 micrograms/kg/hour. (Otero 2006a)
  d) For surgical pain: 5 micrograms/kg IV prior to a CRI. Duration of effect: 2–6 hours. CRI (post-operative) of 0.1 micrograms/kg/hour. (Ogilvie 2004)

- **CATS:**
  a) Acute pain relief in an emergency: 0.1–0.5 micrograms/kg IV; constant rate infusion of 0.5–1 micrograms/kg/hour. (Otero 2006a)

Monitoring

- Anesthetic and/or analgesic efficacy
- Cardiac and respiratory rate
- Pulse oximetry or other methods to measure blood oxygenation when used for anesthesia

Client Information

- Sufentanil is a very potent opiate that should only be used by professionals in a setting where adequate patient monitoring is available.

Chemistry/Synonyms

A phenylpiperidine derivative opioid related to fentanyl, sufentanil citrate occurs as a white or almost white powder that is soluble in water, sparingly soluble in alcohol, acetone, or chloroform. The commercially available injection has a pH (adjusted with citric acid) of 3.5–6.

Sufentanil citrate may also be known as: R-33800, sufentanili citras, fentathienel citrate, sufentanyl citrate, sulfentanil citrate, *Fastfen®*, *Fentaientel®* and *Sufenta®*.

Storage/Stability

Unless otherwise labeled, sufentanil injection should be stored protected from light at room temperature. Sufentanil citrate is hydrolyzed in acidic solutions.

Compatibility/Compounding Considerations

Sufentanil citrate is reportedly **compatible** with D5W and bupivacaine. For Y-site injection it is **compatible** with solutions containing: atropine, dexamethasone sodium phosphate, diazepam, diphenhydramine, etomidate, metoclopramide, midazolam, phenobarbital, and propofol. It is **incompatible** with lorazepam, phenytoin and thiopental.

Dosage Forms/Regulatory Status

VETERINARY-LABELED PRODUCTS: None

The ARCI (Racing Commissioners International) has designated this drug as a class 1 substance. See the appendix for more information.

HUMAN-LABELED PRODUCTS:

Sufentanil Citrate Injection: 50 micrograms/mL (as base) in 1 mL, 2 mL & 5 mL amps; *Sufenta*® (preservative free) (Taylor); generic; (Rx, C-II).

References

Banyard, J. (2004). Drugs commonly used in anesthesia., Accessed from Forms Library; Veterinary Information Network 2004. http://goo.gl/mRb4n

Ogilvie, G. (2004). Fulfilling the first commandment: providing analgesia and compassionate care. Proceedings: WSAVA. Accessed via: Veterinary Information Network. http://goo.gl/MkWjI

Otero, P. (2006a). Acute pain management in emergency. Proceedings: WSAVA World Congress. Accessed via: Veterinary Information Network. http://goo.gl/vB0IV

Otero, P. (2006b). Epidural anesthesia and analgesia. Proceedings: WSAVA World Congress. Accessed via: Veterinary Information Network. http://goo.gl/GUkw8

SULFACHLORPYRIDA-ZINE SODIUM

(sul-fa-klor-pye-*rid*-a-zeen)   Vetisulid®

SULFONAMIDE ANTIMICROBIAL AGENT

Prescriber Highlights

▶ Contraindications: Hypersensitivity to sulfas, thiazides, or sulfonylurea agents; severe renal or hepatic impairment

▶ Caution: Diminished renal or hepatic function, or urinary obstruction

▶ Adverse Effects: Can precipitate in the urine (especially with high dosages for prolonged periods, acidic urine if highly concentrated urine); Dogs: Keratoconjunctivitis sicca, bone marrow depression, hypersensitivity reactions (rashes, dermatitis), focal retinitis, fever, vomiting, & nonseptic polyarthritis possible

▶ Potentially teratogenic; weigh risk vs. benefit

▶ Too-rapid IV injection may cause muscle weakness, blindness, ataxia, & collapse; SC or IM injection may cause tissue irritation

Uses/Indications

Sulfachlorpyridazine is indicated for the treatment of diarrhea caused or complicated by *E. coli* in calves less than one month of age or colibacillosis in swine. It is also used parenterally as a general-purpose sulfonamide in adult cattle and other species.

Pharmacology/Actions

Sulfonamides are usually bacteriostatic agents when used alone. They are thought to prevent bacterial replication by competing with para-aminobenzoic acid (PABA) in the biosynthesis of tetrahydrofolic acid in the pathway to form folic acid. Only microorganisms that synthesize their own folic acid are affected by sulfas.

Microorganisms that are usually affected by sulfonamides include some gram-positive bacteria, including some strains of streptococci, staphylococcus, *Bacillus anthracis*, *Clostridium tetani*, *C. perfringens*, and many strains of Nocardia. Sulfas have *in vitro* activity against some gram-negative species, including some strains of Shigella, Salmonella, *E. coli*, Klebsiella, Enterobacter, Pasturella, and Proteus. Sulfas also have activity against some rickettsia and protozoa (Toxoplasma, Coccidia). Unfortunately, resistance to sulfas is a progressing phenomenon and many strains of bacteria that were once susceptible to this class of antibacterial are now resistant. The sulfas are less efficacious in pus, necrotic tissue, or in areas with extensive cellular debris.

Pharmacokinetics

Very limited information is available on the specific pharmacokinetics for this agent. In general, sulfonamides are readily absorbed from the GI tract of non-ruminants, but absorption can vary depending on the drug, species, disease process, etc. Food delays the rate, but usually not the extent of absorption. Peak levels occur within 1–2 hours in non-ruminant (and young pre-ruminant) animals. Adult ruminants may have significant delays before the drug is absorbed orally.

Sulfas are well distributed throughout the body and some reach significant levels in the CSF. Levels of the drugs tend to be highest in liver, kidney, and lung, and lower in muscle and bone. The sulfas can be highly bound to serum proteins, but the extent of binding is species and drug dependent. When bound to proteins the sulfa is not active.

Sulfonamides are both renally excreted and metabolized. Renal excretion of unchanged drug occurs via both tubular secretion and glomerular filtration. Protein bound drug is not filtered by the glomeruli. Metabolism is performed principally in the liver, but extra-hepatic metabolism is also involved. Mechanisms of metabolism are usually acetylation and glucuronidation. The acetylated metabolites may be less soluble and crystallization in the urine can occur with some sulfonamides, particularly at lower pH. The serum half-life of sulfachlorpyridazine is approximately 1.2 hours in cattle.

Contraindications/Precautions/Warnings

Sulfonamides are contraindicated in patients hypersensitive to them, thiazides, or sulfonylurea agents. They are also considered contraindicated in patients with severe renal or hepatic impairment and should be used with caution in patients with diminished renal or hepatic function, or urinary obstruction.

Oral sulfonamides can depress the normal cellulytic function of the ruminoreticulum, but this effect is generally temporary and the animal adapts.

Adverse Effects

Sulfonamides (or their metabolites) can precipitate in the urine, particularly when given at high dosages for prolonged periods. Acidic or highly concentrated urine may also contribute to increased risk of crystalluria, hematuria, and renal tubule obstruction. Different sulfonamides have different solubilities at various pH's. Alkalinization of the urine using sodium bicarbonate may prevent crystalluria, but it also decreases the amount available for tubular reabsorption. Crystalluria can usually be avoided with most of the commercially available sulfonamides by maintaining an adequate urine flow. Normal urine pH in herbivores is usually 8 or more, so crystalluria is not frequently a problem. Sulfonamides can also cause various hypersensitivity reactions or diarrhea by altering the normal gut flora.

Too rapid intravenous injection of the sulfas can cause muscle weakness, blindness, ataxia, and collapse.

In dogs, keratoconjunctivitis sicca has been reported with sulfonamide therapy. In addition, bone marrow depression, hypersensitivity reactions (rashes, dermatitis), focal retinitis, fever, vomiting and nonseptic polyarthritis have been reported in dogs.

Oral sulfonamides can depress the normal cellulytic function of the ruminoreticulum, but this effect is generally temporary and the animal adapts.

Because solutions of sulfonamides are usually alkaline, they can cause tissue irritation and necrosis if injected intramuscularly or subcutaneously.

Reproductive/Nursing Safety

Sulfas cross the placenta and may reach fetal levels of 50% or greater those found in maternal serum; teratogenicity has been reported in some laboratory animals when given at very high doses. They should be used in pregnant animals only when the benefits clearly outweigh the risks of therapy.

Sulfonamides are distributed into milk. Safe use during lactation cannot be assumed; use with caution.

Overdosage/Acute Toxicity

Acute toxicity secondary to overdoses apparently occurs only rarely in veterinary species. In addition to the adverse effects listed above, CNS stimulation and myelin degeneration have been noted after very high dosages.

Drug Interactions

The following drug interactions have either been reported or are theoretical in humans or animals receiving sulfachlorpyridazine and may be of significance in veterinary patients:

■ **ANTACIDS:** May decrease the oral bioavailability of sulfonamides if administered concurrently

Laboratory Considerations

■ Sulfonamides may give false-positive results for **urine glucose** determinations when using the Benedict's method.

Doses

■ **CATTLE:**
In calves for labeled indications: 33–49.5 mg/kg PO, or IV twice daily for 1–5 days; suggest initiating therapy with intravenous preparation and then changing to oral if possible (Package insert; *Vetisulid*®—Fort Dodge)

■ **SWINE:**
For labeled indications: 44–77 mg/kg PO per day (divide dose and give twice daily if treating individual animals) for 1–5 days (Package insert; *Vetisulid*®—Fort Dodge)

■ **BIRDS:**
For enteric bacterial infections:

a) Using the oral powder: Mix ¼ teaspoonful per liter of water and use as only supply of drinking water for 5–10 days. May be effective for many *E. coli* enteric infections. (Clubb 1986)

b) Using the oral powder: Mix ¾ teaspoonful per 2 quarts of water. Fairly effective for enteric infections, particularly *E. coli*. Reserved for clients who are unable to give other medications by mouth or parenterally. (McDonald 1989)

c) For pigeons: 1200 mg per gallon of drinking water. Very effective for *E. coli* and it is a good coccidiostat. (Harlin 2006)

Monitoring

■ Clinical efficacy
■ Adverse effects

Client Information

■ To help reduce the possibility of crystalluria occurring, animals should have free access to water; avoid dehydration.

Chemistry/Synonyms

Sulfachlorpyridazine sodium is listed as a short to intermediate-acting, low lipid soluble sulfonamide antibacterial. It is reportedly very soluble in urine at usual pH's.

Sulfachlorpyridazine may also be known as cluricol, sulphachlorpyridazine, or *Vetisulid®*.

Storage/Stability

The injection should be stored at room temperature and protected from light; avoid freezing. The oral suspension should be stored at room temperature; avoid freezing. The oral boluses and powder should be stored at room temperature; avoid excessive heat (above 40°; 104°F).

Dosage Forms/Regulatory Status

VETERINARY-LABELED PRODUCTS:

Sulfachlorpyridazine Sodium Oral powder: 54 grams per bottle; *Vetisulid®* Powder (BIVI); (OTC) FDA-approved for use in calves under one month of age and swine. Slaughter withdrawal (at labeled doses) = 4 days for swine. When used orally in the milk or milk replacer for ruminating calves, treated calves must not be slaughtered for food during treatment and for 7 days after the last treatment.

Sulfachlorpyridazine Sodium Oral Suspension: 50 mg/mL in 180 mL bottles; *Vetisulid®* Oral Suspension (BIVI); (OTC). FDA-approved for use in swine. Slaughter withdrawal (at labeled doses) = 4 days for swine.

HUMAN-LABELED PRODUCTS: None

References

Clubb, S.L. (1986). Therapeutics: Individual and Flock Treatment Regimens. *Clinical Avian Medicine and Surgery*. GJ Harrison and LR Harrison Eds. Philadelphia, W.B. Saunders: 327–355.

Harlin, R. (2006). Practical pigeon medicine. Proceedings: AAV 2006. Accessed via: Veterinary Information Network. http://goo.gl/EW76N

McDonald, S.E. (1989). Summary of medications for use in psittacine birds. *JAAV* 3(3): 120–127.

Sulfadiazine/Pyrimethamine—See Pyrimethamine/Sulfadiazine

SULFADIAZINE/ TRIMETHOPRIM

SULFA-METHOXAZOLE/ TRIMETHOPRIM

(sul-fa-*dye*-a-zeen; sul-fa-meth-*ox*-a-zole/trye-*meth*-ohe-prim)   Co-trimoxazole, Tribrissen®, Bactrim®, Septra®

POTENTIATED SULFONAMIDE ANTIMICROBIAL

Note: *In the USA, two separate combinations with trimethoprim are used clinically. There are trimethoprim/sulfadiazine products FDA-approved for use in dogs, cats, and horses in both parenteral and oral dosage forms. Many veterinarians also use the human FDA-approved, trimethoprim/sulfamethoxazole oral products. In Canada, sulfadoxine is available in combination with trimethoprim for veterinary use.*

Prescriber Highlights

▶ Potentiated sulfonamide antimicrobial agent

▶ Contraindications: Hypersensitivity to sulfas, thiazides, or sulfonylurea agents; severe renal or hepatic impairment; Doberman pinschers

▶ Caution: Diminished renal or hepatic function, or urinary obstruction or urolithiasis

▶ Adverse Effects: *Dogs:* Keratoconjunctivitis sicca, hypersensitivity (type 1 or type 3), acute neutrophilic hepatitis with icterus, vomiting, anorexia, diarrhea, fever, hemolytic anemia, urticaria, polyarthritis, facial swelling, polydipsia, crystalluria, hematuria, polyuria, cholestasis, hypothyroidism, anemias, agranulocytosis, idiosyncratic hepatic necrosis in dogs. *Cats:* Anorexia, crystalluria, hematuria, leukopenias & anemias. *Horses:* Transient pruritic (after IV injection). Oral: diarrhea, hypersensitivity reactions & hematologic effects (anemias, thrombocytopenia, or leukopenias

▶ Local injection effects possible (check label for product recommendation for injection technique)

▶ Potentially teratogenic, weigh risk vs. benefit

Uses/Indications

Although only FDA-approved for use in dogs and horses, trimethoprim/sulfadiazine etc. is used in many species to treat infections caused by susceptible organisms. See Dosage section for more information.

Trimethoprim/sulfa can be effective for prostate infections and for infections caused by many strains of methicillin-resistant staphylococci.

Pharmacology/Actions

Alone, sulfonamides are bacteriostatic agents and trimethoprim is bactericidal, but when used in combination, the potentiated sulfas are bactericidal. Potentiated sulfas sequentially inhibit enzymes in the folic acid pathway, inhibiting bacterial thymidine synthesis. The sulfonamide blocks the conversion of para-aminobenzoic acid (PABA) to dihydrofolic acid (DFA), and trimethoprim blocks the conversion of DFA to tetrahydrofolic acid by inhibiting dihydrofolate reductase. Infected tissue and cellular debris can inhibit the activity of trimethoprim/sulfa by secreting PABA and thymidine.

The *in vitro* optimal ratio for most susceptible bacteria is approximately 1:20 (trimethoprim:sulfa), but synergistic activity can reportedly occur with ratios of 1:1–1:40. The serum concentration of the trimethoprim component is considered more important than the sulfa concentration. For most susceptible bacteria, the MIC's for TMP are generally above 0.5 micrograms/mL.

The potentiated sulfas have a fairly broad spectrum of activity. Gram-positive bacteria that are generally susceptible include most streptococci, many strains of staphylococcus (including many strains of MRSA and MRSI), and Nocardia. In horses, approximately 30% of strains tested of *Streptococcus zooepidemicus* are resistant to TMP/Sulfa. Many gram-negative organisms of the family Enterobacteriaceae are susceptible to the potentiated sulfas, but not *Pseudomonas aeruginosa*. Some protozoa (*Pneumocystis carinii*, Coccidia, and Toxoplasma) are also inhibited by the combination. Potentiated sulfas reportedly have little activity against most anaerobes, but opinions vary.

Resistance will develop more slowly to the combination of drugs than to either one alone. In gram-negative organisms, resistance is usually plasmid-mediated.

Pharmacokinetics

Trimethoprim/sulfa is well absorbed after oral administration, with peak levels occurring about 1–4 hours after dosing; the drug is more slowly absorbed after subcutaneous absorption, however. In ruminants greater than 8 weeks old, trimethoprim is apparently trapped in the ruminoreticulum after oral administration and undergoes some degradation limiting its usefulness.

Trimethoprim/sulfa is well distributed in the body. When meninges are inflamed, the drugs enter the CSF in levels of about 50% those found in the serum. Both drugs cross the placenta and are distributed into milk. Trimethoprim/sulfa is relatively well distributed into the prostate.

The volume of distribution for trimethoprim in various species are: 1.49 L/kg (dogs); 0.59–1.51 L/kg (horses). The volume of distribution for sulfadiazine in dogs is 1.02 L/kg.

Trimethoprim/sulfa is both renally excreted unchanged via glomerular filtration and tubular secretion and metabolized by the liver. The sulfas are primarily acetylated and conjugated with glucuronic acid and trimethoprim is metabolized to oxide and hydroxylated metabolites. Trimethoprim may be more extensively metabolized in the liver in adult ruminants, than in other species. The serum elimination half-lives for trimethoprim in various species is: 2.5 hours (dogs), 1.91–3 hours (horses), 1.5 hours (cattle). The serum elimination half-lives for sulfadiazine in various species is: 9.84 hours (dogs), 2.71 hours (horses), and 2.5 hours (cattle). While trimethoprim is rapidly eliminated from the serum, the drug may persist for a longer period of time in tissues.

Because of the number of variables involved, it is extremely difficult to apply pharmacokinetic values in making dosage recommendations with these combinations. Each drug (trimethoprim and the sulfa) has different pharmacokinetic parameters (absorption, distribution, elimination) in each species. Since different organisms have different MIC values and the optimal ratio of trimethoprim to sulfa differs from organism to organism, this problem is exacerbated.

There is considerable controversy regarding the frequency of administration of these combinations. The veterinary product, trimethoprim/sulfadiazine is labeled for once daily administration in dogs and horses, but many clinicians believe that the drug is more efficacious if given twice daily, regardless of which sulfa is used.

Contraindications/Precautions/Warnings

The manufacturer states that trimethoprim/sulfadiazine should not be used in dogs or horses showing marked liver parenchymal damage, blood dyscrasias, or those with a history of sulfonamide sensitivity. It is not for use in horses (or FDA-approved for other animals) intended for food.

Doberman pinschers appear to be very susceptible to sulfonamide-induced poly-systemic immune complex disease and most believe that these drugs are contraindicated in them.

This combination should be used with caution in patients with pre-existing hepatic or renal disease.

Because of its potential for crystallization in the urine, it may be wise to avoid the use of sulfadiazine in dogs known to have uroliths, at increased risk for developing uroliths or known to have highly concentrated (dehydration) or acidic urine.

Adverse Effects

Adverse effects noted in dogs include: keratoconjunctivitis sicca (which may be irreversible), acute neutrophilic hepatitis with icterus, vomiting, anorexia, diarrhea, fever, hemolytic anemia, urticaria, polyarthritis, facial swelling, polydipsia, polyuria and cholestasis. Potentiated sulfonamides may cause hypothyroidism in dogs, particularly with extended therapy. Acute hypersensitivity reactions manifesting as Type I (anaphylaxis) or Type III reaction (serum sickness) can be seen. Hypersensitivity reactions appear to be more common in large breed dogs; Doberman Pinschers may possibly be more susceptible to this effect than other breeds. Other hematologic effects (anemias, agranulocytosis) are possible, but fairly rare. TMP/Sulfa has rarely been noted to cause an idiosyncratic, moderate to massive hepatic necrosis. TMP/Sulfa may be a risk factor for developing acute pancreatitis, but cause and effect have not been definitively shown.

Adverse effects noted in cats may include anorexia, leukopenias and anemias.

In horses, transient pruritus has been noted after intravenous injection. Oral therapy has resulted in diarrhea in some horses, but incidence is relatively low. Previous administration of potentiated sulfas has been implicated in increasing the mortality rate of associated with severe diarrhea. If the 48% injectable product is injected IM, SC, or extravasates after IV administration, swelling, pain and minor tissue damage may result. Hypersensitivity reactions and hematologic effects (anemias, thrombocytopenia, or leukopenias) may also be seen; long-term therapy should include periodic hematologic monitoring.

Sulfonamides (or their metabolites) can precipitate in the urine, particularly when given at high dosages for prolonged periods. Acidic urine or highly concentrated urine may also contribute to increased risk of crystalluria, hematuria, and renal tubule obstruction.

Reproductive/Nursing Safety

Safety of trimethoprim/sulfa has not been clearly established in pregnant animals. Reports of teratogenicity (cleft palate) have been reported. Studies thus far in male animals have not demonstrated any decreases in reproductive performance. In humans, the FDA categorizes this drug as category *C* for use during pregnancy (*Animal studies have shown an adverse effect on the fetus, but there are no adequate studies in humans; or there are no animal reproduction studies and no adequate studies in humans.*) In a separate system evaluating the safety of drugs in canine and feline pregnancy (Papich 1989), this drug is categorized as in class: *B* (*Safe for use if used cautiously. Studies in laboratory animals may have uncovered some risk, but these drugs appear to be safe in dogs and cats or these drugs are safe if they are not administered when the animal is near term.*)

Use TMP/sulfa products in nursing animals with caution. TMP-SMZ is not recommended for human use in the nursing period as sul-fonamides are excreted in milk and may cause kernicterus. Premature infants and infants with hyperbilirubinemia or G-6-PD deficiency are also at risk for adverse effects.

Overdosage/Acute Toxicity

Manifestations of an acute overdosage can include clinical signs of GI distress (nausea, vomiting, diarrhea), CNS toxicity (depression, headache, and confusion), facial swelling, bone marrow depression and increases in serum aminotransferases. Oral overdoses can be treated by emptying the stomach, (following usual protocols), and initiating symptomatic and supportive therapy. Acidification of the urine may increase the renal elimination of trimethoprim, but could also cause sulfonamide crystalluria, particularly with sulfadiazine containing products. Complete blood counts (and other laboratory parameters) should be monitored as necessary. Bone marrow suppression associated with chronic overdoses may be treated with folinic acid (leucovorin) if severe. Peritoneal dialysis is not effective in removing TMP or sulfas from the circulation.

Drug Interactions

The following drug interactions have either been reported or are theoretical in humans or animals receiving trimethoprim/sulfa and may be of significance in veterinary patients:

- ◼ **AMANTADINE:** A human patient developed toxic delirium when receiving amantadine with TMP/sulfa

- ◼ **ANTACIDS:** May decrease the bioavailability of sulfonamides if administered concurrently

- ◼ **CYCLOSPORINE:** TMP/sulfa may increase the risk of nephrotoxicity

- ◼ **DIGOXIN:** TMP/sulfa may increase digoxin levels

- ◼ **DIURETICS, THIAZIDE:** May increase risk for thrombocytopenia

- ◼ **HYPOGLYCEMIC AGENTS, ORAL:** TMP/sulfa may potentiate effects

- ◼ **METHOTREXATE:** TMP/sulfa may displace from plasma proteins and increase risk for toxic effects; it can also interfere with MTX assays (competitive protein binding technique)

- ◼ **PHENYTOIN:** TMP/sulfa may increase half-life

- ◼ **TRICYCLIC ANTIDEPRESSANTS:** TMP/sulfa may decrease efficacy

- ◼ **WARFARIN:** TMP/sulfa may prolong INR/PT

Laboratory Considerations

- ◼ When using the Jaffe alkaline picrate reaction assay for **creatinine** determination, trimethoprim/sulfa may cause an overestimation of approximately 10%.

- ◼ Sulfonamides may give false-positive results for **urine glucose** determinations when using the Benedict's method.

Doses

Note: There is significant controversy regarding the frequency of dosing these drugs. See the pharmacokinetic section above for more information. Unless otherwise noted, doses are for combined amounts of trimethoprim/sulfa.

■ **DOGS:**

For susceptible infections:

a) For UTI, pyoderma, soft tissue infections: 30 mg/kg PO q24h (not soft tissue infections) or 15 mg/kg PO q12h for 14 days.

For chronic pyoderma, acanthamebiasis: 30 mg/kg PO q12h for 21–42 days.

For systemic infections; bacteremia: 30–45 mg/kg PO q12h for 3–5 days. (Greene *et al.* 2006)

b) For bacterial UTI: 30 mg/kg q12h PO (Bartges 2007)

c) For protozoal diseases:

For toxoplasmosis: 15 mg/kg, PO q12h for 28 days.

For Neospora: 15 mg/kg, PO q12h for 4 weeks. Used concurrently with clindamycin (10 mg/kg q12h for 4 weeks) *or* pyrimethamine (1 mg/kg PO once daily for 4 weeks).

For *Hepatazoon canis*: 15 mg/kg, PO q12h for 2–4 weeks. Used concurrently with clindamycin (10 mg/kg PO q8h for 2–4 weeks) *and* pyrimethamine (0.25 mg/kg PO once daily for 2–4 weeks) (Lappin 2000b)

d) For coccidiosis: 30 mg/kg PO once daily for 10 days (Matz 1995)

e) For pneumocystosis (*Pneumocystis carinii*): 15 mg/kg PO q8h or 30 mg/kg PO q12h, both for 3 weeks. May be given with cimetidine and levamisole as potential immune stimulants. (Hawkins 2000)

f) For *Hepatazoon americanum*: TMP/sulfa (15 mg/kg PO q12h), pyrimethamine (0.25 mg/kg PO q24h), and clindamycin (10 mg/kg q8h). Once remission attained decoquinate (see monograph) can maintain. (Baneth 2007)

g) For *Hepatazoon americanum*: TMP/sulfa (15 mg/kg PO q12h for 14 days), pyrimethamine (0.25 mg/kg PO q24h for 14 days), and clindamycin (10 mg/kg PO q8h for 14 days). Once remission attained decoquinate (see monograph) can maintain.

For neosporosis: pyrimethamine (1 mg/kg PO daily) with TMP/sulfa (15–30 mg/kg PO twice daily. (Blagburn 2005)

■ **CATS:**

For susceptible infections:

a) For UTI: 30 mg/kg PO q24h for 7–14 days.

For UTI, soft tissue infections: 15 mg/kg PO q12h for 7–14 days. (Greene *et al.* 2006)

b) 30 mg/kg q12h (if treating Nocardia, double dose) (Ford & Aronson 1985)

c) For toxoplasmosis: 15 mg/kg PO q12h for 28 days (Lappin 2000a)

d) For bacterial UTI: 30 mg/kg q12h PO (Bartges 2007)

■ **FERRETS:**

For susceptible infections:

a) 30 mg/kg PO twice daily (Williams 2000)

b) For coccidiosis: 30 mg/kg PO once daily for 14 days. (Johnson 2006)

■ **RABBITS, RODENTS, SMALL MAMMALS:**

a) **Rabbits:** 15–30 mg/kg, PO q12–24h; 30–48 mg/kg SC q12h. Sulfadiazine has a very short half-life (approx. 1 hour) in rabbits. (Ivey & Morrisey 2000)

b) **Chinchillas, Gerbils, Guinea Pigs, Hamsters, Mice, Rats:** 15–30 mg/kg PO q12h; or 30 mg/kg IM q12h (Adamcak & Otten 2000)

c) **Chinchillas:** 30 mg/kg PO, SC or IM q12h (Hayes 2000)

■ **CATTLE:**

For susceptible infections:

a) 44 mg/kg once daily IM or IV using 48% suspension (Upson 1988)

b) 25 mg/kg, IV or IM q24h (Burrows 1980)

c) **Calves:** 48 mg/kg IV or IM q24h (Baggot 1983)

■ **HORSES:**

For susceptible infections:

a) For respiratory tract infections: 15–30 mg/kg PO q12h. Give 30 minutes prior to feeding hay (grain is OK) (Foreman 1999)

b) **Foals:** 15 mg/kg IV q12h; 30 mg/kg PO q12h (Brumbaugh 1999)

c) 22 mg/kg IV q24h or 30 mg/kg, PO q24h (Upson 1988)

d) 30 mg/kg PO once daily or 21.3 mg/kg IV once daily (Package inserts; *Tribrissen®*—Coopers)

e) **Foals:** 15 mg/kg PO or IV twice daily (Furr 1999)

■ **SWINE:**

For susceptible infections:

a) 48 mg/kg, IM q24h (Baggot 1983)

■ **BIRDS:**

For susceptible infections:

a) Using TMP/SMX oral suspension (240 mg/5 mL): 2 mL/kg PO twice daily. Good for many gram-positive and negative enteric and respiratory infections, particularly in hand-fed babies. May cause emesis in Macaws. (McDonald 1989)

b) For respiratory and enteric infections in psittacines using the 24% injectable suspension: 0.22 mL/kg IM once to twice daily.

For coccidiosis in toucans and my-nahs using TMP/SMX oral suspension (240 mg/5 mL): 2.2 mL/kg once daily for 5 days. May be added to feed.

For respiratory and enteric infections in hand-fed baby psittacines using TMP/SMX oral suspension (240 mg/5 mL): 0.22 mL/30 grams twice daily to three times daily for 5–7 days. (Clubb 1986)

c) Using oral suspension: 50–100 mg/kg (of combined product) PO q12h (Hoeffer 1995)

d) Ratites: For Toxoplasma gondii: 30–50 mg/kg IM twice daily (Jenson 1998)

■ **REPTILES:**
For susceptible infections:

a) For most species: 30 mg/kg IM (upper part of body) once daily for 2 treatments, then every other day for 5–12 treatments. May be useful for enteric infections. (Gauvin 1993)

b) For all species: 30 mg/kg IM, first two doses 24 hours apart and then every other day (Jacobson 1999)

c) 15–25 mg/kg/day IM for 7–14 days (Lewbart 2001)

Monitoring
■ Clinical efficacy

■ Adverse effects; with chronic therapy, peri-odic complete blood counts should be considered

■ In dogs, monitor tear production (one suggestion is in 5 days and every 2–3 weeks)

■ Thyroid function tests should be considered (baseline and ongoing) particularly in dogs receiving long-term treatment. Some do not feel this is necessary.

Client Information
■ If using oral suspension, shake well before using; does not need to be refrigerated

■ Animals must be allowed free access to water and must not become dehydrated while on therapy

■ If dogs eyes are dry or become irritated contact veterinarian

Chemistry/Synonyms
Trimethoprim occurs as odorless, bitter-tasting, white to cream-colored crystals or crystalline powder. It is very slightly soluble in water and slightly soluble in alcohol.

Sulfadiazine occurs as an odorless or nearly odorless, white to slightly yellow powder. It is practically insoluble in water and sparingly soluble in alcohol.

Sulfamethoxazole occurs as a practically odorless, white to off-white, crystalline powder. Approximately 0.29 mg are soluble in 1 mL of water and 20 mg are soluble in 1 mL of alcohol.

In combination, these products may be known as: Co-trimoxazole, SMX-TMP, TMP-SMX, trimethoprim-sulfamethoxazole, sul-famethoxazole-trimethoprim, sulfadiazine-trimethoprim, trimethoprim-sulfadiazine, TMP-SDZ, SDZ-TMP, Co-trimazine or by their various trade names.

Storage/Stability
Unless otherwise instructed by the manufac-turer, trimethoprim/sulfadiazine and co-tri-moxazole products should be stored at room temperature (15–30°C) in tight containers.

Dosage Forms/Regulatory Status/Withdrawal Times

VETERINARY-LABELED PRODUCTS:

Trimethoprim (TMP)/Sulfadiazine (SDZ) Oral Paste: Each gram contains 67 mg trimethoprim and 333 mg sulfadiazine. Available in 37.5 gram (total weight) syringes; *Tribrissen® 400 Oral Paste* (Schering-Plough); (Rx). FDA-approved for use in horses not intended for food.

Trimethoprim/Sulfadiazine Sterile Injection: 48% in 100 mL vials: *Di-Biotic® 48%* (Phoenix Pharmaceutical), *Tribrissen® 48% Injection* (Schering-Plough); (Rx) FDA-approved for use in horses not intended for food.

Trimethoprim/Sulfadiazine Powder: 67 mg tri-methoprim and 333 mg sulfadiazine per gram: *Tucoprim® Powder* (Pharmacia & Upjohn) in 200 grams & 400 grams bottles and 2000 grams pails, *Uniprim® Powder* (Macleod) in 37.5 grams and 1,125 grams packets, 200 grams jar, and 12 kg box; (Rx). FDA-approved for use in hors-es not intended for food.

In Canada, trimethoprim and sulfadoxine are available for use in cattle and swine (*Trive-trin®*—Wellcome; *Borgal®*—Hoechst). Slaugh-ter withdrawal = 10 days; milk withdrawal = 96 hours.

HUMAN-LABELED PRODUCTS:

Trimethoprim (alone) Tablets: 100 mg and 200 mg; *Proloprim®* (Glaxo Wellcome); *Trimpex®* (Roche); generic; (Rx)

Trimethoprim & Sulfamethoxazole (Co-Tri-moxazole; TMP-SMZ) Oral Tablets: 80 mg trimethoprim & 400 mg sulfamethoxazole; Double Strength Tablets: 160 mg trimethoprim & 800 mg sulfamethoxazole; *Bactrim® & Bac-trim® DS* (AR Scientific); *Septra® & Septra® DS* (Monarch); generic; (Rx)

Trimethoprim 8 mg/mL and Sulfamethoxa-zole 40 mg/mL oral suspension in 100 mL, 150 mL, 200 mL, 473 mL, and 480 mL; *Septra®* (GlaxoWellcome); *Cotrim® Pediatric* (Lem-mon), *Sulfatrim®*, (various); generic; (Rx)

Trimethoprim & Sulfamethoxazole Injection: 80 mg sulfamethoxazole, 16 mg trimethoprim per mL in 5 mL single-use vials, 10 mL, or 30 mL multiple-dose vials; generic; (Rx)

References

Adamcak, A. & B. Otten (2000). Rodent Therapeutics. *Vet Clin NA: Exotic Anim Pract* **3:1**(Jan): 221–240.

Baggot, J.D. (1983). Systemic antimicrobial therapy in large animals. *Pharmacological Basis of Large Animal Medicine*. JA Bogan, P Lees and AT Yoxall Eds. Oxford, Blackwell Scientific Publications: 45–69.

Baneth, G. (2007). Canine and Feline Hepatozoonosis—More than one disease. Proceedings: WSAVA World Congress. Accessed via: Veterinary Information Network. http://goo.gl/naPZN

Bartges, J. (2007). Urinary tract infections: Which antimicrobials work best? Proceedings: Western Vet Conf. Accessed via: Veterinary Information Network. http://goo.gl/vZZDm

Blagburn, B. (2005). Treatment and control of tick borne diseases and other important parasites of companion animals. Proceedings: ACVC2005. Accessed via: Veterinary Information Network. http://goo.gl/Pexfa

Burrows, G.E. (1980). Systemic antibacterial drug selection and dosage. *Bovine Practioner* **15**: 103–110.

Clubb, S.L. (1986). Therapeutics: Individual and Flock Treatment Regimens. *Clinical Avian Medicine and Surgery*. GJ Harrison and LR Harrison Eds. Philadelphia, W.B. Saunders: 327–355.

Ford, R.B. & A.L. Aronson (1985). Antimicrobial Drugs and Infectious Diseases. *Handbook of Small Animal Therapeutics*. LE Davis Ed. New York, Churchill Livingstone: 45–88.

Foreman, J. (1999). Equine respiratory pharmacology. *The Veterinary Clinics of North America: Equine Practice* **15:3**(December): 665–686.

Furr, M. (1999). Antimicrobial treatments for the septic foal. Proceedings: The North American Veterinary Conference, Orlando.

Gauvin, J. (1993). Drug therapy in reptiles. *Seminars in Avian & Exotic Med* **2**(1): 48–59.

Greene, C., K. Hartmannn, et al. (2006). Appendix 8: Antimicrobial Drug Formulary. *Infectious Disease of the Dog and Cat*. C Greene Ed., Elsevier: 1186–1333.

Hawkins, E. (2000). Pulmonary Parenchymal Diseases. *Textbook of Veterinary Internal Medicine: Diseases of the Dog and Cat*. S Ettinger and E Feldman Eds. Philadelphia, WB Saunders. **2**: 1061–1091.

Hayes, P. (2000). Diseases of Chinchillas. *Kirk's Current Veterinary Therapy: XIII Small Animal Practice*. J Bonagura Ed. Philadelphia, WB Saunders: 1152–1157.

Hoeffer, H. (1995). Antimicrobials in pet birds. *Kirk's Current Veterinary Therapy:XII*. J Bonagura Ed. Philadelphia, W.B. Saunders: 1278–1283.

Ivey, E. & J. Morrisey (2000). Therapeutics for Rabbits. *Vet Clin NA: Exotic Anim Pract* **3:1**(Jan): 183–216.

Jacobson, E. (1999). Bacterial infections and antimicrobial treatment in reptiles. The North American Veterinary Conference, Orlando.

Jenson, J. (1998). Current ratite therapy. *The Veterinary Clinics of North America: Food Animal Practice* **16:3**(November).

Johnson, D. (2006). Ferrets: the other companion animal. Proceedings: ACVC. Accessed via: Veterinary Information Network. http://goo.gl/bSeol

Lappin, M. (2000a). Infectious causes of feline diarrhea. The North American Veterinary Conference, Orlando.

Lappin, M. (2000b). Protozoal and Miscellaneous Infections. *Textbook of Veterinary Internal Medicine: Diseases of the Dog and Cat*. S Ettinger and E Feldman Eds. Philadelphia, WB Saunders. **1**: 408–417.

Lewbart (2001). Reptile Formulary. Proceedings: Atlantic Coast Veterinary Conference. Accessed via: Veterinary Information Network. http://goo.gl/EEQmM

Matz, M. (1995). Gastrointestinal ulcer therapy. *Kirk's Current Veterinary Therapy:XII*. J Bonagura Ed. Philadelphia, W.B. Saunders: 706–710.

McDonald, S.E. (1989). Summary of medications for use in psittacine birds. *JAAV* **3**(3): 120–127.

Papich, M. (1989). Effects of drugs on pregnancy. *Current Veterinary Therapy X: Small Animal Practice*. R Kirk Ed. Philadelphia, Saunders: 1291–1299.

Upson, D.W. (1988). *Handbook of Clinical Veterinary Pharmacology*. Manhattan, Dan Upson Enterprises.

Williams, B. (2000). Therapeutics in Ferrets. *Vet Clin NA: Exotic Anim Pract* **3:1**(Jan): 131–153.

SULFADIMETHOXINE

(sul-fa-*dye*-meth-ox-een)   Albon®

SULFONAMIDE ANTIMICROBIAL

Prescriber Highlights

➤ Sulfonamide antimicrobial agent

➤ Contraindications: Hypersensitivity to sulfas, thiazides, or sulfonylurea agents; severe renal or hepatic impairment; Dobermans

➤ Caution: Diminished renal or hepatic function, or urinary obstruction.

➤ Adverse Effects: Can precipitate in the urine (esp. with high dosages for prolonged periods, acidic urine or highly concentrated urine). Dogs: Keratoconjunctivitis sicca, bone marrow depression, hypersensitivity reactions (rashes, dermatitis), focal retinitis, fever, vomiting & nonseptic polyarthritis possible

➤ Potentially teratogenic; weigh risk vs. benefit

Uses/Indications

Sulfadimethoxine injection and tablets are FDA-approved for use in dogs and cats for respiratory, genitourinary, enteric and soft tissue infections caused by susceptible organisms. Sulfadimethoxine is used in the treatment of coccidiosis in dogs although not FDA-approved for this indication.

In horses, sulfadimethoxine injection is FDA-approved for the treatment of respiratory infections caused by *Streptococcus equi*.

In cattle, the drug is FDA-approved for treating shipping fever complex, calf diphtheria, bacterial pneumonia and foot rot caused by susceptible organisms.

In poultry, sulfadimethoxine is added to drinking water to treat coccidiosis, fowl cholera, and infectious coryza.

Pharmacology/Actions

Sulfonamides are usually bacteriostatic agents when used alone. They are thought to prevent bacterial replication by competing with para-aminobenzoic acid (PABA) in the biosynthesis of tetrahydrofolic acid in the pathway to form folic acid. Only microorganisms that synthesize their own folic acid are affected by sulfas.

Microorganisms that are usually affected by sulfonamides include some gram-positive bacteria, including some strains of streptococci, staphylococcus, *Bacillus anthracis*, *Clostridium tetani*, *C. perfringens*, and many strains of Nocardia. Sulfas also have *in vitro* activity against some gram-negative species, including some strains of Shigella, Salmonella, *E. coli*, Klebsiella, Enterobacter, Pasturella, and

Proteus. Sulfas have activity against some rickettsia and protozoa (Toxoplasma, Coccidia). Unfortunately, resistance to sulfas is a progressing phenomenon and many strains of bacteria that were once susceptible to this class of antibacterial are now resistant. The sulfas are less efficacious in pus, necrotic tissue, or in areas with extensive cellular debris.

Pharmacokinetics

In dogs, cats, swine, and sheep, sulfadimethoxine is reportedly readily absorbed and well distributed. Relative volumes of distribution range from 0.17 L/kg in sheep to 0.35 L/kg in cattle and horses. The drug is highly protein bound.

In most species, sulfadimethoxine is acetylated in the liver to acetylsulfadimethoxine and excreted unchanged in the liver. In dogs, the drug is not appreciably hepatically metabolized and renal excretion is the basis for the majority of elimination of the drug. Sulfadimethoxine's long elimination half-lives are a result of its appreciable reabsorption in the renal tubules. Serum half-lives reported in various species are: swine 14 hours; sheep 15 hours; horses 11.3 hours.

Contraindications/Precautions/Warnings

Sulfonamides are contraindicated in patients hypersensitive to them, thiazides, or sulfonylurea agents. They are also considered contraindicated in patients with severe renal or hepatic impairment and should be used with caution in patients with diminished renal or hepatic function, or urinary obstruction.

Doberman pinschers appear to be very susceptible to sulfonamide-induced poly-systemic immune complex disease and most believe that these drugs are contraindicated in them.

Oral sulfonamides can depress the normal cellulytic function of the ruminoreticulum, but this effect is generally temporary and the animal adapts.

Adverse Effects

Sulfonamides (or their metabolites) can precipitate in the urine, particularly when given at high dosages for prolonged periods. Acidic urine or highly concentrated urine may also contribute to increased risk of crystalluria, hematuria, and renal tubule obstruction. Different sulfonamides have different solubilities at various pH's. Alkalinization of the urine using sodium bicarbonate may prevent crystalluria, but it also decreases the amount available for tubular reabsorption. Crystalluria can usually be avoided with most of the commercially available sulfonamides by maintaining an adequate urine flow. Normal urine pH in herbivores is usually 8 or more, so crystalluria is not frequently a problem. Sulfonamides can also cause various hypersensitivity reactions or diarrhea by altering the normal gut flora.

Too rapid intravenous injection of the sulfas can cause muscle weakness, blindness, ataxia, and collapse.

In dogs, keratoconjunctivitis sicca, bone mar-row depression, hypersensitivity reactions (rashes, dermatitis), focal retinitis, fever, vomiting and nonseptic polyarthritis have been reported with sulfonamides.

Oral sulfonamides can depress the normal cellulytic function of the ruminoreticulum, but this effect is generally temporary and the animal adapts.

Because solutions of sulfonamides are usually alkaline, they can cause tissue irritation and necrosis if injected intramuscularly or subcutaneously.

Reproductive/Nursing Safety

Sulfas cross the placenta and may reach fetal levels of 50% or greater of those found in maternal serum; teratogenicity has been reported in some laboratory animals when given at very high doses. They should be used in pregnant animals only when the benefits clearly outweigh the risks of therapy.

Sulfonamides are distributed into milk.

Overdosage/Acute Toxicity

Acute toxicity secondary to overdoses apparently occurs only rarely in veterinary species. In addition to the adverse effects listed above, CNS stimulation and myelin degeneration have been noted after very high dosages.

Drug Interactions

The following drug interactions have either been reported or are theoretical in humans or animals receiving sulfonamides and may be of significance in veterinary patients:

■ **ANTACIDS:** May decrease the oral bioavailability of sulfonamides if administered concurrently

Laboratory Considerations

■ Sulfonamides may give false-positive results for **urine glucose** determinations when using the Benedict's method.

Doses

■ **DOGS:**

For susceptible infections:

a) 25 mg/kg PO, IV, or IM once daily (Davis 1985), (Kirk 1989)

b) 100 mg/kg PO, IV or IM once daily (Upson 1988)

c) 55 mg/kg PO, or IV, or SC initially, then 27.5 mg/kg once daily thereafter (Package insert; *Albon*®—Roche)

For coccidiosis:

a) 55 mg/kg PO initially on the first day of therapy, then 27.5 mg/kg PO once daily for 9 days (Matz 1995)

b) 50 mg/kg once daily for 10–14 days will eliminate oocyst excretion in most dogs and cats. (Marks 2007)

c) During the infant period (2–6 weeks): 50 mg/kg PO on the first day followed by a daily dose of 25 mg/kg PO until symptoms regress (Macintire 2004)

■ **CATS:**

For susceptible infections:

a) 25 mg/kg PO, IV, or IM once daily (Davis 1985), (Kirk 1989)

b) 100 mg/kg PO, IV or IM once daily (Upson 1988)

c) 55 mg/kg PO, or IV, or SC initially, then 27.5 mg/kg once daily thereafter (Package insert; *Albon*®—Roche)

For coccidiosis:

a) 50 mg/kg once daily for 10–14 days will eliminate oocyst excretion in most dogs and cats. (Marks 2007)

■ **FERRETS:**

For susceptible infections:

a) 25 mg/kg PO, SC or IM once daily (Williams 2000)

b) For coccidiosis: 25 mg/kg PO once daily for 14 days. (Johnson 2006)

■ **RABBITS, RODENTS, SMALL MAMMALS:**

a) **Rabbits:** 10–15 mg/kg PO q12h (Ivey & Morrisey 2000)

b) **Rabbits:** For coccidiosis: 25 mg/kg PO once daily (Burke 1999)

c) **Hedgehogs:** 2–20 mg/kg/day IM, SC or PO (Smith 2000)

d) **Mice, Rats, Gerbils, Hamsters, Guinea pigs, Chinchillas:** As a coccidiostat: 50 mg/kg PO once, then 25 mg/kg PO once daily for 10–20 days *or* 75 mg/kg PO for 7–14 days (Adamcak & Otten 2000)

■ **CATTLE:**

For susceptible infections:

a) 110 mg/kg PO or IV once daily (Upson 1988)

b) 55 mg/kg IV initially, then 27.5 mg/kg IV once daily (Baggot 1983)

c) 110 mg/kg, PO q24h (Burrows 1980)

d) 55 mg/kg PO or IV initially, then 27.5 mg/kg q24h (Jenkins 1986)

e) 55 mg/kg IV or PO initially, then 27.5 mg/kg q24h IV or PO for up to 5 days. If using sustained release boluses: 137.5 mg/kg PO every 4 days (Package insert; *Albon*®—Roche)

■ **HORSES:**

For susceptible infections:

a) 55 mg/kg, PO or IV q12h (Upson 1988)

b) 55 mg/kg IV or PO initially, then 27.5 mg/kg q24h IV (Package insert; *Albon*®—Roche)

■ **CAMELIDS (NWC):**

a) For coccidiosis ("regular" coccidia: *E. alpacae, E. lamae, E. punoensis, E. peruviana*): 15 mg/kg PO twice daily for 5 days; monitor for signs of polioencephalomalacia. (Walker 2009)

b) Treatment of Eimeria infection is generally directed at clinically affected animals using sulfadimethoxine at 110 mg/kg

PO q24h (or amprolium). Treatments are effective only against the immature stages and therefore may not have a significant impact on fecal oocyst count initially. Given the long prepatent period, it is prudent to treat *E. macusaniensis* infections for 10-15 days. Treatment should be directly administered to the animal rather than by medicating water supplies. (McKenzie 2008)

■ **REPTILES:**

For susceptible infections:

a) For coccidia: 90 mg/kg PO on day one and then 45 mg/kg PO on 5 successive days; may also be given IM or IV. Maintain adequate hydration. (Lewbart 2001)

Chemistry/Synonyms

A long-acting sulfonamide, sulfadimethoxine occurs as an odorless or almost odorless, creamy white powder. It is very slightly soluble in water and slightly soluble in alcohol.

Sulfadimethoxine may also be known as: solfadimetossina, solfadimetossipirimidina, sulphadimethoxine, *Albon*®, *Amtech*®, *Chemiosalfa*®, *Deltin*®, *Di-Methox*®, *Risulpir*®, *Ritarsulfa*®, *SDM*®, *Sulfadren*®, *Sulfastop*®, or *Sulfasol*®, and *Sulfathox*®.

Storage/Stability

Unless otherwise instructed by the manufacturer, store sulfadimethoxine products at room temperature and protect from light. If crystals form due to exposure to cold temperatures, either warm the vial or store at room temperature for several days to resolubilize the drug; efficacy is not impaired by this process.

Dosage Forms/Regulatory Status

VETERINARY-LABELED PRODUCTS:

Sulfadimethoxine Injection: 400 mg/mL (40%) in 100 mL vials; *Albon*® *Injection 40%* (Pfizer); *Di-Methox*® *Injection 40%* (AgriLabs), generic; (Rx) FDA-approved for use in dogs, cats, horses, swine and cattle. Not to be used in horses intended for food or calves to be processed for veal. Slaughter withdrawal (at labeled doses) = 5 days (cattle); milk withdrawal (at labeled doses) = 60 hours.

Sulfadimethoxine Oral Tablets: 125 mg, 250 mg, and 500 mg; *Albon*® *Tablets* (Pfizer); (Rx). FDA-approved for use in dogs and cats.

Sulfadimethoxine Oral Suspension: 50 mg/mL in 2 oz. and 16 oz. Bottles; *Albon*® (Pfizer); (Rx). FDA-approved for use in dogs and cats.

Sulfadimethoxine Oral Boluses: 5 grams, and 15 grams; *Albon*® (Pfizer); (OTC). FDA-approved for use in cattle. Not to be used in calves to be processed for veal. No withdrawal period has been established for this in preruminating calves. Slaughter withdrawal (at labeled doses) = 7 days (cattle); milk withdrawal (at labeled doses) = 60 hours.

Sulfadimethoxine Oral Boluses Sustained-Release: 12.5 g; *Albon® SR* (Pfizer); (Rx) FDA-approved for use in non-lactating cattle. Slaughter withdrawal (at labeled doses) = 21 days (cattle), a withdrawal period has not been established for pre-ruminating calves. Not for use in calves intended to be processed for veal.

Sulfadimethoxine Soluble Powder: 94.6 grams/packet (for addition to drinking water); *Albon®* (Pfizer), generic; FDA-approved for use in dairy calves, dairy heifers, beef cattle, broiler and replacement chickens only, and meat-producing turkeys. Slaughter withdrawal (at labeled doses) = 7 days (cattle); 5 days (poultry—do not use in chickens over 16 weeks old or in turkeys over 24 weeks old).

Sulfadimethoxine 12.5% Concentrated Solution (for addition to drinking water): *Albon®* (Pfizer), generic; (OTC). FDA-approved for use in chickens, turkeys and cattle. Slaughter withdrawal (at labeled doses) = 7 days (for dairy calves, dairy heifers and beef cattle only. Withdrawal for pre-ruminating calves has not been established. Not to be used in calves to be processed for veal; 5 days (poultry—do not use in chickens over 16 weeks old or in turkeys over 24 weeks old).

HUMAN-LABELED PRODUCTS: None

References

Adamcak, A. & B. Otten (2000). Rodent Therapeutics. *Vet Clin NA: Exotic Anim Pract* **3:1**(Jan): 221–240.

Baggot, J.D. (1983). Systemic antimicrobial therapy in large animals. *Pharmacological Basis of Large Animal Medicine*. JA Bogan, P Lees and AT Yoxall Eds. Oxford, Blackwell Scientific Publications: 45–69.

Burke, T. (1999). Husbandry and Medicine of Rodents and Lagomorphs. Proceedings: Central Veterinary Conference, Kansas City.

Burrows, G.E. (1980). Systemic antibacterial drug selection and dosage. *Bovine Practioner* **15:** 103–110.

Davis, L.E., Ed. (1985). *Handbook of Small Animal Therapeutics*. New York, Churchill Livingston.

Ivey, E. & J. Morrisey (2000). Therapeutics for Rabbits. *Vet Clin NA: Exotic Anim Pract* **3:1**(Jan): 183–216.

Jenkins, W.L. (1986). Antimicrobial therapy. *Current Veterinary Therapy: Food Animal Practice 2*. JL Howard Ed. Philadelphia, W.B. Saunders: 8–23.

Johnson, D. (2006). Ferrets: the other companion animal. Proceedings: ACVC. Accessed via: Veterinary Information Network. http://goo.gl/bSeol

Kirk, R.W., Ed. (1989). *Current Veterinary Therapy X, Small Animal Practice*. Philadelphia, W.B. Saunders.

Lewbart (2001). Reptile Formulary. Proceedings: Atlantic Coast Veterinary Conference. Accessed via: Veterinary Information Network. http://goo.gl/EEQmM

Macintire, D. (2004). Pediatric Emergencies. Proceedings: ACVIM Forum. Accessed via: Veterinary Information Network. http://goo.gl/hIEyv

Marks, S. (2007). What's the latest on parasitic causes of diarrhea in dogs and cats? Proceedings: ACVIM 2007. Accessed via Veterinary Information Network. http://goo.gl/fw8Kw

Matz, M. (1995). Gastrointestinal ulcer therapy. *Kirk's Current Veterinary Therapy:XII*. J Bonagura Ed. Philadelphia, W.B. Saunders: 706–710.

McKenzie, E. (2008). Diagnosis & Management of Diseases of Neonatal & Juvenile Camelids. Proceedings: ACVIM. Accessed via: Veterinary Information Network. http://goo.gl/yIfEV

Smith, A. (2000). General husbandry and medical care of hedgehogs. *Kirk's Current Veterinary Therapy: XIII*

Small Animal Practice. J Bonagura Ed. Philadelphia, WB Saunders: 1128–1133.

Upson, D.W. (1988). *Handbook of Clinical Veterinary Pharmacology*. Manhattan, Dan Upson Enterprises.

Walker, P. (2009). Differential Diagnosis of Diarrhea in Camelid Crias. Proceedings: ACVIM. Accessed via: Veterinary Information Network. http://goo.gl/0C6AM

Williams, B. (2000). Therapeutics in Ferrets. *Vet Clin NA: Exotic Anim Pract* **3:1**(Jan): 131–153.

SULFADIMETHOXINE/ ORMETOPRIM

(or-me-*toe*-prim)   Primor®

POTENTIATED SULFONAMIDE ANTIMICROBIAL

Prescriber Highlights

▶ Potentiated sulfa similar to trimethoprim/sulfa, but may have fewer adverse effects and is labeled for once daily dosing.

▶ Does not appear to be effective for prostate infections and is more expensive then generic trimethoprim/sulfa.

▶ The following apply to TMP/Sulfa & may apply to this agent as well:

▶ Contraindications: Hypersensitive to sulfas, thiazides, or sulfonylurea agents; severe renal or hepatic impairment; Dobermans

▶ Caution: Diminished renal or hepatic function, or urinary obstruction or urolithiasis

▶ Adverse Effects: *Dogs:* Keratoconjunctivitis sicca, hypersensitivity (type 1 or type 3) acute neutrophilic hepatitis with icterus, vomiting, anorexia, diarrhea, fever, hemolytic anemia, urticaria, polyarthritis, facial swelling, polydipsia, crystalluria, hematuria, polyuria, cholestasis, hypothyroidism, anemias, agranulocytosis, idiosyncratic hepatic necrosis in dogs. *Cats:* Anorexia, crystalluria, hematuria, leukopenias & anemias

▶ Potentially teratogenic, weigh risk vs. benefit

Uses/Indications

Sulfadimethoxine/ormetoprim is FDA-approved for the treatment of skin and soft tissue infections in dogs caused by susceptible strains of *Staphylococcus aureus* and *E. coli*. Some fell that it has fewer adverse effects in dogs than trimethoprim/sulfa and can be dosed once daily. It is more expensive than trimethoprim/sulfa and does not appear to penetrate into the prostate as well.

Pharmacology/Actions

Sulfadimethoxine/ormetoprim shares mechanisms of action and probably the bacterial spectrum of activity with trimethoprim/sulfa. Alone, sulfonamides are bacteriostatic agents, but in combination with either ormetoprim or trimethoprim, the potentiated sulfas are bactericidal. Potentiated sulfas sequentially inhibit enzymes in the folic acid pathway, thereby inhibiting bacterial thymidine synthesis. The sulfonamide blocks the conversion of para-aminobenzoic acid (PABA) to dihydrofolic acid (DFA) and ormetoprim blocks the conversion of DFA to tetrahydrofolic acid by inhibiting dihydrofolate reductase.

The potentiated sulfas have a fairly broad spectrum of activity. Gram-positive bacteria that are generally susceptible include most streptococci, many strains of staphylococcus, and Nocardia. Many gram-negative organisms of the family Enterobacteriaceae are susceptible to the potentiated sulfas, but not *Pseudomonas aeruginosa*. Some protozoa (*Pneumocystis carinii*, Coccidia and Toxoplasma) are also inhibited by the combination. Potentiated sulfas reportedly have little activity against most anaerobes, but opinions on this vary.

Resistance will develop more slowly to the combination of drugs, than to either one alone. In gram-negative organisms, resistance is usually plasmid-mediated.

Pharmacokinetics

The pharmacokinetics of sulfadimethoxine are outlined in the previous monograph. Pharmacokinetic data for ormetoprim is not available at the time of this writing, but the manufacturer states that therapeutic levels are maintained over 24 hours at recommended doses. Unlike trimethoprim/sulfa, ormetoprim does not apparently attain clinically effective levels in the prostate for treating bacterial prostatic infections.

Contraindications/Precautions/Warnings

The manufacturer states that ormetoprim/sulfadimethoxine should not be used in dogs showing marked liver parenchymal damage, blood dyscrasias, or in those with a history of sulfonamide sensitivity.

Doberman pinschers appear to be very susceptible to sulfonamide-induced poly-systemic immune complex disease and most believe that these drugs are contraindicated in them.

This combination should be used with caution in patients with pre-existing hepatic or thyroid disease.

Adverse Effects

This combination would be expected to exhibit an adverse reaction profile in dogs similar to that seen with trimethoprim/sulfa, including: keratoconjunctivitis sicca (which may be irreversible), acute neutrophilic hepatitis with icterus, vomiting, anorexia, diarrhea, fever, hemolytic anemia, urticaria, polyarthritis, facial swelling, polydipsia, polyuria, and cholestasis. Acute hypersensitivity reactions manifesting as Type I,

(anaphylaxis) or Type III reaction (serum sickness) can also be seen. Hypersensitivity reactions appear to be more common in large breed dogs; Doberman Pinschers may possibly be more susceptible to this effect than other breeds. Other hematologic effects (anemias, agranulocytosis) are possible, but fairly rare.

Long-term (8 weeks) therapy at recommended doses with ormetoprim/sulfadimethoxine (27.5 mg/kg once daily) resulted in elevated serum cholesterol, thyroid and liver weights, mild follicular thyroid hyperplasia, and enlarged basophilic cells in the pituitary. The manufacturer states that the principal treatment-related effect of extended or excessive usage is hypothyroidism.

Reproductive/Nursing Safety

Safety of ormetoprim/sulfadimethoxine has not been established in pregnant animals. Reports of teratogenicity (cleft palate) have been reported in some lab animals with trimethoprim/sulfa.

Overdosage/Acute Toxicity

In experimental studies in dogs, doses greater than 80 mg/kg resulted in slight tremors and increased motor activity in some dogs. Higher doses may result in depression, anorexia, or seizures.

It is suggested that very high oral overdoses be handled by emptying the gut using standard precautions and protocols and by treating clinical signs supportively and symptomatically.

Drug Interactions; Laboratory Considerations

■ None have been noted for this combination, but it would be expected that the potential interactions outlined for the trimethoprim/sulfa monograph would also apply to this combination; refer to that monograph for more information.

Doses

■ **DOGS:**

For susceptible infections:

a) Initially 55 mg/kg (combined drug) PO on the first day of therapy, then 27.5 mg/kg PO once daily for at least 2 days after remission of clinical signs. Not approved for treatment longer than 21 days. (Package insert; *Primor®*—Pfizer)

Monitoring

■ Clinical efficacy

■ Adverse effects

■ In dogs, monitor tear production (one suggestion is in 5 days after starting treatment and then every 2-3 weeks)

Client Information

■ Animals must be allowed free access to water and must not become dehydrated while on therapy.

Chemistry/Synonyms

A diaminopyrimidine structurally related to trimethoprim, ormetoprim occurs as a white, almost tasteless powder. The chemistry of sulfadimethoxine is described in the previous monograph.

Sulfadimethoxine may also be known as: solfadimetossina, solfadimetossipirimidina, sulphadimethoxine, *Chemiosalfa®*, *Deltin®*, *Risulpir®*, *Ritarsulfa®*, *Sulfadren®*, *Sulfastop®*, or *Sulfathox®*.

Ormetoprim may also be known as NSC-95072, ormetoprima, ormétoprime, ormetoprimum, or Ro-5-9754.

Storage/Stability

Unless otherwise instructed by the manufacturer, store tablets in tight, light resistant containers at room temperature.

Dosage Forms/Regulatory Status

VETERINARY-LABELED PRODUCTS:

Sulfadimethoxine/Ormetoprim Tablets (scored)

120's: 100 mg Sulfadimethoxine, 20 mg Ormetoprim

240's: 200 mg Sulfadimethoxine, 40 mg Ormetoprim

600's: 500 mg Sulfadimethoxine, 100 mg Ormetoprim

1200's: 1000 mg Sulfadimethoxine, 200 mg Ormetoprim; *Primor®* (Pfizer); (Rx) FDA-approved for use in dogs.

Sulfadimethoxine/Ormetoprim medicated premix: 113.5 grams sulfadimethoxine and 68.1 grams ormetoprim per pound in 50 lb bags. FDA-approved for use in chickens [broilers, replacements (breeders and layers)], turkeys, ducks, & Chukar partridges. Slaughter withdrawal (at labeled doses) = 5 days. Do not feed to chickens over 16 weeks or age, turkeys or ducks producing eggs for food. *Rofenaid® 40* (Alpharma), *Romet® 30* (Alpharma)—FDA-approved for use in salmonids (trout and salmon) and catfish. Slaughter or release as stocker fish = 42 days. (OTC)

HUMAN-LABELED PRODUCTS: None

SULFASALAZINE

(sul-fa-*sal*-a-zeen)   Azulfidine®

SULFONAMIDE/SALICYLATE ANTI-BACTERIAL/IMMUNOSUPPRESSIVE

Prescriber Highlights

▶ Sulfa-analog that has GI antibacterial & antiinflammatory activity used for inflammatory bowel disease; has also been used for vasculitis

▶ Contraindications: Hypersensitivity to it, sulfas or salicylates; intestinal or urinary obstructions; Dobermans

▶ Caution: Liver, renal or hematologic diseases; cats

▶ Adverse Effects: *Dogs:* Keratoconjunctivitis sicca, anorexia, vomiting, cholestatic jaundice, hemolytic anemia, leukopenia, vomiting, decreased sperm counts & an allergic dermatitis. *Cats:* Anorexia, vomiting, anemias

Uses/Indications

Sulfasalazine is used for the treatment of inflammatory large bowel (colonic) disease in dogs and cats. It has also been suggested for adjunctive use in treating vasculitis in dogs. It is not effective for small intestinal inflammation as colonic bacteria are required to cleave the drug into mesalamine (5-ASA) and sulfapyridine.

Pharmacology/Actions

While the exact mechanism of action for its therapeutic effects in treating colitis in small animals has not been determined, it is believed that after sulfasalazine is cleaved into sulfapyridine and 5-aminosalicylic acid (5-ASA, mesalamine) by bacteria in the gut the antibacterial (sulfapyridine) and/or antiinflammatory (mesalamine) activity alters the clinical signs/course of the disease. Levels of both drugs in the colon are higher then by giving them orally as separate agents.

Pharmacokinetics

Only about 10–33% of an orally administered dose of sulfasalazine is absorbed. Apparently, some of this absorbed drug is then excreted unchanged in the bile. Unabsorbed and biliary excreted drug is cleaved into 5-ASA and sulfapyridine in the colon by bacterial flora. The sulfapyridine component is rapidly absorbed, but only a small percentage of the 5-ASA is absorbed.

Absorbed sulfapyridine and 5-ASA are hepatically metabolized and then renally excreted.

Contraindications/Precautions/Warnings

Sulfasalazine is contraindicated in animals hypersensitive to it, sulfonamides or salicylates. It is also contraindicated in patients with intestinal or urinary obstructions. Doberman pinschers appear to be very susceptible to sulfonamide-induced polysystemic immune complex disease and most believe that these drugs are contraindicated in them.

It should be used with caution in animals with preexisting liver, renal or hematologic diseases. Because cats can be sensitive to salicylates (see the aspirin monograph), use caution when using this drug in this species.

Adverse Effects

Although adverse effects do occur in dogs, with keratoconjunctivitis sicca (KCS) reported most frequently, they are considered to occur relatively uncommonly. Other potential adverse effects include anorexia, vomiting, cholestatic jaundice, hemolytic anemia, leukopenia, vomiting, decreased sperm counts and an allergic dermatitis. Should decreased tear production be noted early, either reducing the dose or discontinuing the drug may prevent progression of KCS or increase tear production.

Cats can occasionally develop anorexia and vomiting which may be alleviated by use of the enteric-coated tablets. Anemias secondary to sulfasalazine are also potentially possible in cats.

Reproductive/Nursing Safety

Although sulfasalazine has not been proven harmful to use during pregnancy and incidences of neonatal kernicterus in infants born to women taking sulfasalazine are low, it should only be used when clearly indicated. In laboratory animal studies (rats, rabbits), doses of six times normal (human) caused impairment of fertility in male animals; this effect is thought to be caused by the sulfapyridine component and was reversible upon discontinuation of the drug.

In humans, the FDA categorizes this drug as category **B** for use during pregnancy (*Animal studies have not yet demonstrated risk to the fetus, but there are no adequate studies in pregnant women; or animal studies have shown an adverse effect, but adequate studies in pregnant women have not demonstrated a risk to the fetus in the first trimester of pregnancy, and there is no evidence of risk in later trimesters.*) In a separate system evaluating the safety of drugs in canine and feline pregnancy (Papich 1989), this drug is categorized as in class: **B** (*Safe for use if used cautiously. Studies in laboratory animals may have uncovered some risk, but these drugs appear to be safe in dogs and cats or these drugs are safe if they are not administered when the animal is near term.*)

Sulfonamides are excreted in milk. In human newborns, they compete with bilirubin for binding sites on plasma proteins and may cause kernicterus. Use with caution in nursing patients.

Overdosage/Acute Toxicity

Little specific information is available regarding overdoses with this agent, but because massive overdoses could cause significant salicylate and/or sulfonamide toxicity, standard protocols (empty stomach, cathartics, etc.) should be considered. Urine alkalinization and forced diuresis may also be beneficial in selected cases.

Drug Interactions

The following drug interactions have either been reported or are theoretical in humans or animals receiving sulfasalazine and may be of significance in veterinary patients:

- ◼ **CHLORPROPAMIDE:** Hypoglycemic effects could be potentiated

- ◼ **DIGOXIN:** Sulfasalazine may reduce absorption

- ◼ **FERROUS SULFATE or other iron salts:** May decrease the blood levels of sulfasalazine if administered concurrently; clinical significance is unknown

- ◼ **FOLIC ACID:** Oral absorption may be inhibited

- ◼ **WARFARIN:** Potentially sulfasalazine could potentiate warfarin

Doses

◼ **DOGS:**

For inflammatory large bowel disease:

a) Usual initial dose: 20–40 mg/kg q8h for 3 weeks, followed by 20–40 mg/kg q12h for 3 weeks, and 10–20 mg/kg q12h for 3 weeks. (Marks 2009)

b) 20–48.4 mg/kg (maximum total dose of one gram in refractory patients) PO q8h. May consider an initial dose of 12.5 mg/kg, q8h. Continue initial dose for a minimum of 4 weeks before modifying dosage. After signs of disease resolve, reduce dosage by 25% at 2 week intervals and eventually discontinue while maintaining dietary management. (Jergens & Willard 2000)

c) For chronic colitis: If hypoallergenic diet does not control signs, sulfasalazine 20–50 mg/kg (up to a maximum of 1 gram) three times daily. Initial dosage usually 20–30 mg/kg three times daily. Dose may be reduced at 2–4 week intervals if stool remains normal using the following protocol: Initially same dose given twice daily, then 50% of initial dose twice daily, then 50% of that dose once daily, then discontinue. Some dogs may require chronic therapy. (Leib 2000)

d) 10–25 mg/kg PO three times a day for 4–6 weeks. With resolution of clinical signs, reduce dose by 25 percent at 2 week intervals and eventually discontinue while maintaining dietary management. (Washabau 2005)

For adjunctive treatment of vasculitis:

a) 20–40 mg/kg PO q8h (Hillier 2006), (Griffin 2006)

b) 25 mg/kg PO three times a day. (Bloom 2006)

✕ CATS:

For inflammatory large bowel disease:

a) 10–20 mg/kg PO once daily. Use cautiously in cats because of their sensitivity to salicylates (Jergens & Willard 2000)

b) 10–20 mg/kg PO q24 hours (once daily) tapered to the lowest effective dose (Moore 2004), (Marks 2007)

c) 10–20 mg/kg PO q8–12h (maximum of 10 days) (Dimski 1995)

d) 10–20 mg/kg PO q8–24h; up to a maximum of 10 days treatment (Krecic 2002)

✕ FERRETS:

a) 10–20 mg/kg PO 2–3 times a day (Williams 2000)

b) 25 mg (total dose) PO twice daily (Weiss 2002)

Monitoring

■ Efficacy

■ Adverse effects, particularly KCS; Schirmer tear tests should be performed prior to therapy (and on rechecks), especially in middle-aged to older dogs

■ Occasional CBC, liver function tests are warranted with chronic therapy

Client Information

■ Clients should monitor for clinical signs of KCS (dry cornea, blepharospasm, bilateral mucopurulent discharge) and report them to the veterinarian immediately.

Chemistry/Synonyms

Sulfasalazine is basically a molecule of sulfapyridine linked by a diazo bond to the diazonium salt of salicylic acid. It occurs as an odorless, bright yellow to brownish-yellow fine powder. Less than 0.1 mg is soluble in 1 mL of water and about 0.34 mg is soluble in 1 mL of alcohol.

Sulfasalazine may also be known as: salazosulfapyridine, salicylazosulfapyridine, sulfasalazinum, sulphasalazine, *Azulfidine®*, *Aculfin®*, *Azulfin®*, *Colo-Pleon®*, *Pleon RA®*, *Pyralin®*, *SAS®*, *Salazine®*, *Salazopirina®*, *Salazoprin®*, *Salazopyrin®*, *Salazopyrina®*, *Salazopyrine®*, *Salisulf Gastroprotetto®*, *Salopyrine®*, *Saridine®*, *Sazo®*, *Sulazine®*, or *Ulco®*.

Storage/Stability

Sulfasalazine tablets (either plain or enteric-coated) should be stored at temperatures less than 40°C and preferably at room temperature (15–30°C, 59–86°F) in well-closed containers. The oral suspension should be stored at room temperature (15–30°C, 59–86°F); avoid freezing.

Dosage Forms/Regulatory Status

VETERINARY-LABELED PRODUCTS: None

HUMAN-LABELED PRODUCTS:

Sulfasalazine Tablets: 500 mg; *Azulfidine®* (Pfizer); generic; (Rx)

Sulfasalazine Delayed-Release Tablets: 500 mg

(enteric coated); *Azulfidine® EN-tabs®* (Pfizer); generic; (Rx)

References

Bloom, P. (2006). Diagnosis and treatment of vasculitis. Proceedings: Western Vet Conf 2006. Accessed via: Veterinary Information Network. http://goo.gl/dLi6e

Dimski, D. (1995). Therapy of inflammatory bowel disease. *Kirk's Current Veterinary Therapy:XII.* J Bonagura Ed. Philadelphia, W.B. Saunders: 723–728.

Griffin, C. (2006). Dermatologic diseases of the auricle. Proceedings: WSAVA Congress. Accessed via: Veterinary Information Network. http://goo.gl/Qllpg

Hillier, A. (2006). Life threatening skin diseases. Proceedings: ACVC. Accessed via: Veterinary Information Network. http://goo.gl/GkQ1e

Jergens, A. & M. Willard (2000). Diseases of the large Intestine. *Textbook of Veterinary Internal Medicine: Diseases of the Dog and Cat.* S Ettinger and E Feldman Eds. Philadelphia, WB Saunders. **2:** 1238–1256.

Krecic, M. (2002). Feline IBD: Diagnostic challenges, treatment, and monitoring. Proceedings: ACVIM Forum. Accessed via: Veterinary Information Network. http://goo.gl/oxEm2

Leib, M. (2000). Chronic Colitis in Dogs. *Kirk's Current Veterinary Therapy: XIII Small Animal Practice.* J Bonagura Ed. Philadelphia, WB Saunders: 643–648.

Marks, S. (2007). Inflammatory Bowel Disease—More than a garbage can diagnosis. Proceedings: UCD Canine Medicine Symposium. Accessed via: Veterinary Information Network. http://goo.gl/ZGPg1

Marks, S. (2009). How I treat inflammatory bowel disease in dogs. Proceedings: WSAVA. Accessed via: Veterinary Information Network. http://goo.gl/IpRpO

Moore, L. (2004). Beyond corticosteroids for therapy of inflammatory bowel disease in dogs and cats. Proceedings: ACVIM Forum. Accessed via: Veterinary Information Network. http://goo.gl/MOJ1B

Papich, M. (1989). Effects of drugs on pregnancy. *Current Veterinary Therapy X: Small Animal Practice.* R Kirk Ed. Philadelphia, Saunders: 1291–1299.

Washabau, R. (2005). The Colon: Dietary & medical management of colonic disease. Proceedings: ACVIM. Accessed via: Veterinary Information Network. http://goo.gl/s27tF

Weiss, C. (2002). Newly recognized diseases of ferrets. Proceedings: Atlantic Coast Veterinary Conference. Accessed via: Veterinary Information Network. http://goo.gl/5RFXi

Williams, B. (2000). Therapeutics in Ferrets. *Vet Clin NA: Exotic Anim Pract* **3:**1(Jan): 131–153.

TADALAFIL

(ta-*dal*-a-fil)   Cialis®

PHOSPHODIESTERASE TYPE 5 INHIBITOR

Prescriber Highlights

▶ PDP5 inhibitor that may be useful for treating pulmonary arterial hypertension in dogs

▶ Very limited clinical experience or published data for use in dogs

▶ Appears to have a longer duration action than sildenafil

▶ Contraindicated if patients receiving organic nitrates

▶ Adverse effects not well-known for dogs; inguinal flushing, GI effects reported with sildenafil

▶ Currently, very expensive

Uses/Indications

Tadalafil is a phosphodiesterase-5 inhibitor similar to sildenafil and may be useful for treating pulmonary arterial hypertension (PAH) in dogs. A pilot study done in dogs with PAH, showed that tadalafil (1 mg/kg PO) caused modest, but significant decreases in diastolic pulmonary arterial pressure (PAP), mean PAP and tricuspid regurgitation suggesting that oral tadalafil, when added to conventional heart failure therapy, decreases PAP in dogs with PAH. Because of its longer duration of action, tadalafil has some advantages over sildenafil but it is currently very expensive.

In humans, tadalafil is approved for use in treating pulmonary artery hypertension (*Adcirca®*) and erectile dysfunction (*Cialis®*). Off-label uses include treating Raynaud's phenomenon.

Pharmacology/Actions

Tadalafil is a selective inhibitor of cyclic guanosine monophosphate (cGMP)–specific phosphodiesterase type 5 (PDE5). PDE5 is the enzyme responsible for the degradation of cGMP and is found (in humans) in the corpus cavernosum smooth muscle, pulmonary vascular and visceral smooth muscle, skeletal muscle, platelets, kidney, lung, cerebellum, and pancreas. In patients with PAH, vascular endothelium nitric oxide release is impaired with associated reduction of cGMP. PDE5 is the primary phosphodiesterase in pulmonary vasculature and tadalafil's PDE5 inhibition increases cGMP thereby relaxing pulmonary vascular smooth muscle with resultant vasodilation.

Pharmacokinetics

No pharmacokinetic data for tadalafil for dogs was located.

In humans, after oral administration maximum plasma concentrations occur at around 4 hours in patients with PAH. Food does not alter the rate or extent of absorption. Tadalafil is 94% bound to human plasma proteins. Tadalafil is metabolized by CYP3A4 to a catechol metabolite that then undergoes methylation and glucuronidation. These metabolites are not thought to be active. In PAH patients, mean terminal half-life is 35 hours. Excretion is primarily of the drug's metabolites via fecal routes (61%) with the majority of the remainder in the urine (approximately 36%).

Contraindications/Precautions/Warnings

Tadalafil is contraindicated in human patients using (either regularly or intermittently) any form of organic nitrate, and in those with serious hypersensitivity to tadalafil. Dosage reductions may be required in patients with severe hepatic or renal impairment.

Adverse Effects

An adverse effect profile for dogs at suggested doses for PAH has not been determined. Cutaneous flushing of the inguinal region has been reported with sildenafil in dogs. GI effects are possible. In a 12-month tadalafil chronic toxicity study done in dogs, no disseminated arteritis was observed as was seen in rodent studies, but 2 dogs exhibited marked decreases in neutrophils and moderate decreases in platelets with inflammatory signs when dosed at approximately 4X to 18X the equivalent human dose. These effects were reversible within 2 weeks after discontinuing the drug.

Most common adverse effects of tadalafil reported in humans with PAH, include: dyspepsia, nausea, back pain, myalgia, nasal congestion, flushing and headache. Rare, but serious adverse effects include hypersensitivity, optic neuropathy, seizures, Stevens-Johnson syndrome and exfoliative dermatitis, and deafness.

Reproductive/Nursing Safety

Tadalafil animal reproduction studies in rats and mice demonstrated no evidence of teratogenicity, embryotoxicity, or fetotoxicity when tadalafil was given to pregnant rats or mice at exposures of up to 11X (human equivalent dose). The FDA categorizes tadalafil as category *B* for use during pregnancy (*Animal studies have not yet demonstrated risk to the fetus, but there are no adequate studies in pregnant women; or animal studies have shown an adverse effect, but adequate studies in pregnant women have not demonstrated a risk to the fetus in the first trimester of pregnancy, and there is no evidence of risk in later trimesters.*)

Tadalafil and/or its metabolites are secreted into the milk in lactating rats at concentrations approximately 2.4-fold found in the plasma. It is unlikely to pose much risk to nursing offspring.

Overdosage/Acute Toxicity

Little information is available. Single doses of up to 500 mg have been given to healthy men, and multiple daily doses of up to 100 mg have been given to men with erectile dysfunction; adverse reactions were similar to those seen at lower doses.

It is expected that overdoses in animals would mirror the drugs adverse effect profile; treat supportively. Contact an animal poison control center for guidance, if necessary.

Drug Interactions

The following drug interactions have either been reported or are theoretical in humans or animals receiving tadalafil and may be of significance in veterinary patients:

- **ALPHA-ADRENERGIC BLOCKERS (*e.g.*, phentolamine, phenothiazines, phenoxybenzamine):** May increase hypotensive effects

- **AMLODIPINE:** Potential to increase hypotensive effects

- **ANTIHYPERTENSIVE, HYPOTENSIVE DRUGS:** Potentially could increase hypotensive effects

- **AZOLE ANTIFUNGALS (ketoconazole, itraconazole):** May reduce tadalafil metabolism and increase AUC

■ **CIMETIDINE:** May reduce tadalafil metabolism and increase AUC

■ **ERYTHROMYCIN, CLARITHROMYCIN:** May reduce tadalafil metabolism and increase AUC

■ **NITRATES (e.g., NTG, Isosorbide):** Significant potentiation of vasodilatory effects; life-threatening hypotension possible

■ **NITROPRUSSIDE SODIUM:** Significant potentiation of vasodilatory effects; life-threatening hypotension possible

■ **PHENOBARBITAL:** May decrease tadalafil concentrations

■ **RIFAMPIN:** May decrease tadalafil concentrations

Laboratory Considerations
■ None noted

Doses
■ **DOGS:**
For pulmonary arterial hypertension:

a) From a case report in a Yorkshire terrier: 1 mg/kg PO q48h (every other day) was added to the background treatment (furosemide, spironolactone, benazepril, dexamethasone and oxygen). Dog's condition rapidly (<24 hours) improved and 7-day follow-up showed a decrease (up to 26 mmHg) in systolic pulmonary arterial pressure and disappearance of all respiratory and cardiac signs of PAH (cyanosis, syncope and tachypnea). Authors' recommend long-term studies in more animals. (Serres *et al.* 2006)

b) 1 mg/kg PO once daily. (Oyama 2009)

Monitoring
■ Clinical efficacy (improved syncope, cough, respiratory effort)

■ Pulmonary artery pressure, systemic blood pressure

■ Adverse effects

Client Information
■ Brief clients on the experimental nature of using this medication in small animals and the costs of therapy

■ Report any adverse effects to the veterinarian

Chemistry/Synonyms
Tadalafil has a molecular weight of 389.41. It is insoluble in water and slightly soluble in ethanol.

Tadalafil may also be known as: GF-196960, IC-351, tadalafiili, tadalafilo, or tadalafilum. *Cialis®* and *Adcirca®* are trade names for tadalafil.

Storage/Stability
Tadalafil tablets should be stored at room temperature between 59°-86°F (15° and 30°C).

Dosage Forms/Regulatory Status
VETERINARY-LABELED PRODUCTS: None

HUMAN-LABELED PRODUCTS:
Tadalafil Oral Tablets: 2.5 mg, 5 mg, 10 mg, 20 mg: *Cialis®*, *Adcirca®* (Lilly); (Rx)

References
Oyama, M. (2009). Pulmonary Hypertension: What you can't see can kill you. Proceedings: ACVC. Accessed via: Veterinary Information Network. http://goo.gl/0jNQb

Serres, F., A. Nicole, et al. (2006). Efficacy of Oral Tadalafil, a New Long-acting Phosphodiesterase-5 Inhibitor, for the Short-term Treatment of Pulmonary Arterial Hypertension in a Dog. *J Vet Med A* **53**: 129–133.

TAURINE
(*tor*-een)

AMINO ACID NUTRITIONAL

Prescriber Highlights

▶ Amino acid used primarily for the treatment of taurine deficiency cardiomyopathies in cats & dogs

▶ May also be useful for many other conditions (*e.g.*, seizures, hepatic lipidosis), but little supporting data available

▶ Very low toxic potential

▶ Laboratory considerations

Uses/Indications
Taurine has proven beneficial in preventing retinal degeneration and the prevention and treatment of taurine-deficiency dilated cardiomyopathy in cats. Although modern commercial feline diets have added taurine, some cats still develop taurine-deficiency associated dilated cardiomyopathy. It may also be of benefit in taurine (±carnitine) deficient cardiomyopathy in American Cocker Spaniels and certain other breeds such as, Golden Retrievers, Labrador Retrievers, Newfoundlands, Dalmations, Portuguese Water Dogs, and English Bulldogs. Preliminary studies have shown evidence that it may be useful as adjunctive treatment for cardiac disease in animals even if taurine deficiency is not present. Because of its low toxicity, some have suggested it be tried for a multitude of conditions in humans and animals; unfortunately, little scientific evidence exists for these uses.

Pharmacology/Actions
While classically considered a "non-essential" nutrient, taurine has been found to play several "essential" roles in various mammalian species. Taurine is important for bile acid conjugation, especially in cats and dogs. *In vivo*, taurine is synthesized from methionine. Cysteinesulfinic acid decarboxylase (CSAD) and vitamin B_6 are involved with this synthesis. Deficiencies of either will depress taurine synthesis. Cats are particularly susceptible to taurine deficiency as they have low CSAD activity and use taurine almost exclusively for bile acid conjugation.

Additionally taurine is important in the

modulation of calcium flux, thereby reducing platelet aggregation, stabilizing neuronal membranes, and affecting cardiac function. Taurine's effects on cardiac function include positive inotropic activity without affecting resting potential and modulating ionic currents across the cell membrane. Taurine is important for normal development of the CNS and it has a GABA-like effect that may make it useful for treating some seizure disorders.

Pharmacokinetics

No specific information was located. Excess taurine is rapidly excreted in the kidneys, but if a deficiency exists, urinary excretion is reduced via reabsorption.

Contraindications/Precautions/Warnings

While taurine is safe, it should not be used as a substitute for adequate diagnosis.

Adverse Effects

Taurine appears to be very well tolerated. Minor GI distress potentially could occur after oral dosing.

Overdosage/Acute Toxicity

No specific information was located, but toxic potential appears to be very low.

Drug Interactions

■ None noted

Laboratory Considerations

■ Because plasma levels may reflect the acute changes associated with dosing, whole blood levels are preferred to measure actual status of taurine in the body. Because intracellular levels of taurine are much higher than in plasma, hemolysis or collection of the buffy coat will negate the results.

Doses

■ **DOGS:**

a) For taurine-deficiency related cardiomyopathy: In American Cocker Spaniels: Give 500 mg taurine PO q12h (with 1 gram of carnitine PO q12h). (Kittleson 2000)

b) Complementary therapy for seizures: 400 mg/40 lbs of body weight PO twice daily. "May" help decrease seizure activity (Neer 2000)

c) For taurine-related cardiomyopathy: 500–1500 mg (total dose) PO per day. (Reynolds 2009)

d) Recommendations for taurine supplementation in dilated cardiomyopathy are: **1)** All American Cocker spaniels; **2)** Consider in animals with dilated cardiomyopathy and cysteine or urate urolithiasis (*e.g.,* English Bulldogs and Dalmatians); **3)** Consider in golden retrievers, Newfoundland dogs, Portuguese water dogs and any atypical breeds for dilated cardiomyopathy

The suggested taurine dose for dogs with

dilated cardiomyopathy is 500–1000 mg PO q8-12h for dogs weighing under 25 kg and 1–2 grams PO q8-12h for dogs weighing > 25 kg. (Smith 2009)

■ **CATS:**

a) For taurine-deficiency related cardiomyopathy: 250 mg (per cat) PO q12-24h. Because taurine is safe and inexpensive, recommend using for any case of myocardial failure. (Fox 2000)

b) Complementary therapy for seizures: 500 mg per cat PO twice daily. "May" help decrease seizure activity (Neer 2000)

c) For adjunctive treatment of hepatic lipidosis: 250–500 mg/day is valuable. Taurine may be hepatoprotective and is required for bile conjugation. It plays a role in membrane stability and function. Cats with hepatic lipidosis waste taurine in their urine and anorexia causes a decrease in serum taurine levels. (Scherk 2007)

Monitoring

■ Clinical efficacy

■ Taurine levels (if possible and affordable; whole blood levels preferable to plasma/serum levels)

Chemistry/Synonyms

Taurine, an amino acid also known as 2-aminosulphonic acid, has a molecular wt. of 125. Solubility in 100 mL of water at 20°C is 8.8 grams.

Storage/Stability

Unless otherwise labeled, store taurine tablets or capsules at room temperature. Protect from light and moisture.

Dosage Forms/Regulatory Status

VETERINARY-LABELED PRODUCTS:

The following products are labeled (not FDA-approved drugs) for use in animals:

Taurine Tablets: 250 mg: *Formula V® Taurine Tablets* (PetAg); Labeled for use in cats.

Taurine Liquid: 375 mg/4 mL (one pump); *Dyna-Taurine®* (Harlmen); Labeled for use in dogs and cats.

HUMAN-LABELED PRODUCTS:

There are several oral dosage form products available for taurine. Technically considered a "nutrient" they are all OTC and may need to be obtained from health food stores. Most dosage forms available range from 125 mg to 500 mg.

References

Fox, P. (2000). Feline Cardiomyopathies. *Textbook of Veterinary Internal Medicine: Diseases of the Dog and Cat.* S Ettinger and E Feldman Eds. Philadelphia, WB Saunders. **1:** 896–923.

Kittleson, M. (2000). Taurine- and Carnitine-responsive dilated cardiomyopathy in American Cocker spaniels. *Kirk's Current Veterinary Therapy: XIII Small Animal Practice.* J Bonagura Ed. Philadelphia, WB Saunders: 761–762.

Neer, T. (2000). The refractory seizure patient: What

should be my diagnostic and therapeutic approach? American Animal Hospital Assoc, Toronto.

Reynolds, C. (2009). Non-conventional Drugs for Heart Disease: Off the Beaten Path. Proceedings: ACVC. Accessed via: Veterinary Information Network. http://goo.gl/GVHmw

Scherk, M. (2007). Mellow Yellow: Winning with Hepatic Lipidosis. Proceedings: ACVC. Accessed via: Veterinary Information Network. http://goo.gl/GuQCT

Smith, F. (2009). Feline Cardiomyopathies: Diagnosis and treatment. Proceedings: WVC. Accessed via: Veterinary Information Network. http://goo.gl/w4AMz

Telazol®—See Tiletamine/ Zolazepam

TEPOXALIN

(te-**pox**-a-lin)   Zubrin®

NONSTEROIDAL ANTIINFLAMMATORY AGENT

Prescriber Highlights

▶ NSAID dual inhibitor of COX & LOX indicated for the treatment of pain & inflammation associated with osteoarthritis in dogs

▶ Adverse effect profile still being determined, but may cause more vomiting & diarrhea than some other FDA-approved NSAIDs

▶ Rapidly disintegrating tablet dosage form may be useful in difficult to pill dogs

Uses/Indications

Tepoxalin is indicated for the treatment of pain and inflammation associated with osteoarthritis in dogs. Because of the drug's inhibitory effects on leukotrienes, there is interest in seeing if it would be beneficial in the adjunctive treatment of allergic conditions in dogs.

Pharmacology/Actions

Tepoxalin is a dual inhibitor of both cyclooxygenase (COX) and 5-lipoxygenase (LOX). It inhibits both COX-1 and COX-2 enzymes, but it is not clear if it is COX-2 preferential in the dog (it is not COX-2 preferential in sheep uterine cells) or if its LOX inhibition reduces the adverse effects associated with COX-1 inhibition. COX inhibition in dogs persists for only about 6 hours after dosing. By inhibiting COX-2 enzymes, tepoxalin reduces the production of prostaglandins associated with pain, hyperpyrexia and inflammation. Its inhibition of LOX potentially reduces the production of leukotrienes, including leukotriene B_4. As leukotriene B_4 may contribute to increased GI tract inflammation by increasing cytokine production, neutrophil longevity and release of proteinases, inhibition may reduce the GI effects routinely seen in dogs with COX-1 inhibitors. Leukotrienes may also contribute to inflammatory responses seen in osteo-

arthritic conditions and their inhibition could reduce clinical signs seen with the condition.

Pharmacokinetics

After oral administration to dogs, tepoxalin is readily absorbed and peak levels occur between 2–3 hours post-dose. The presence of food in the gut increases bioavailability. Tepoxalin is rapidly metabolized to several metabolites, including one that it active (tepoxalin pyrazole acid). Tepoxalin and tepoxalin pyrazole acid are highly bound to plasma proteins (98–99%). Elimination half-lives for tepoxalin and tepoxalin pyrazole acid are about 2 hours and 13 hours, respectively. Metabolites are eliminated in the feces; only 1% of the drug is eliminated in the urine.

In cats, tepoxalin elimination half-life is about 5 hours; the active metabolite half-life is approximately 4 hours.

Contraindications/Precautions/Warnings

Tepoxalin is contraindicated in dogs demonstrating prior hypersensitivity reactions to tepoxalin. It should be used with caution in patients with impaired hepatic, cardiovascular or renal function, or at risk for developing nephrotoxic affects associated with NSAIDs (*i.e.*, dehydrated or on concomitant diuretic therapy). Patients with active gastrointestinal ulcers should probably not receive this drug.

Dogs weighing less than 3 kg cannot be accurately dosed with available dosage forms. Safety in dogs less than 6 months old has not been established.

Adverse Effects

Adverse effects most likely seen in dogs include diarrhea, vomiting, anorexia/inappetence, enteritis, and lethargy. In one study where dogs received labeled doses for 4 weeks, 22% of dogs developed diarrhea and 20% vomited. It is unknown if giving the drug with food will decrease vomiting incidence. Other adverse effects reported (incidences <1%) include incoordination, incontinence, increased appetite, eating grass, flatulence, hair loss, and trembling. While all NSAIDs can potentially cause renal dysfunction, a study done in healthy dogs did not show that tepoxalin altered renal blood flow or renal function when used alone or with benazepril (for 7 days) or with enalapril (for 28 days) (Fusellier *et al.* 2005).

The manufacturer warns to discontinue the drug if signs such as inappetence, vomiting, fecal abnormalities, anemia, icterus, or lethargy are observed. Safety studies in dogs less than 6 months of age have not been completed.

Reproductive/Nursing Safety

Safety of this drug has not been determined in pregnant, breeding, or lactating dogs; use with caution and with informed consent of client.

Overdosage/Acute Toxicity

Information on acute overdosage of tepoxalin was not located. Dogs receiving 300 mg/kg/day for 6 months showed decreases in total protein, albumin and calcium concentrations. At necropsy, all dogs showed gastric lesions. An acute overdose may cause significant GI distress and ulceration with GI bleeding. It is suggested to treat supportively and monitor CBC, hydration, renal function, and for evidence of GI bleeding. Contact an animal poison control center for more information.

Drug Interactions

A study in normal dogs showed no significant changes in renal function when **enalapril** was used with tepoxalin.

The following drug interactions have either been reported or are theoretical in humans or animals receiving tepoxalin and may be of significance in veterinary patients:

- **ASPIRIN:** May increase the risk of gastrointestinal toxicity (*e.g.*, ulceration, bleeding, vomiting, diarrhea)

- **CORTICOSTEROIDS:** As concomitant corticosteroid therapy may increase the occurrence of gastric ulceration, avoid the use of these drugs when also using tepoxalin

- **DIGOXIN:** NSAIDS may increase serum levels

- **FLUCONAZOLE:** Administration has increased plasma levels of celecoxib in humans, it is unknown if fluconazole affects tepoxalin levels in dogs

- **FUROSEMIDE:** NSAIDs may reduce saluretic and diuretic effects

- **METHOTREXATE:** Serious toxicity has occurred when NSAIDs have been used concomitantly with methotrexate; use together with extreme caution

- **NEPHROTOXIC DRUGS (e.g., furosemide, aminoglycosides, amphotericin B, etc.):** May enhance the risk of nephrotoxicity

- **NSAIDS, OTHER:** May increase the risk of gastrointestinal toxicity (*e.g.*, ulceration, bleeding, vomiting, diarrhea)

- **WARFARIN:** The manufacturer cautions to closely monitor patients also receiving drugs that are highly bound to plasma proteins (*e.g.*, warfarin), as tepoxalin and its active metabolite are 98–99% protein bound in the dog

Laboratory Considerations

- No specific laboratory interactions or considerations noted

Doses

- **DOGS:**

  For pain and inflammation associated with osteoarthritis:

  a) On first day of treatment give 20 mg/kg PO (or 10 mg/kg PO); subsequently give 10 mg/kg PO once daily. Duration of treatment should be based on clinical response and patient tolerance to therapy. (Package insert; *Zubrin*®—Schering-Plough)

Monitoring

- Clinical efficacy

- Baseline and periodic CBC, chemistry panel (including bilirubin and serum creatinine)

- Signs associated with adverse effects (GI effects, appetite, vomiting, diarrhea, etc.)

Client Information

- When dosing, the person administering the tablet should place it in dog's mouth and hold mouth closed for approximately 4 seconds to assure tablet disintegration

- Absorption may be enhanced (and vomiting reduced?) if given with food

- Owners should be instructed to discontinue the drug and contact their veterinarian if diarrhea is severe or persists, or signs such as inappetence, vomiting, fecal abnormalities, anemia, icterus or lethargy are observed

- Dogs should have access to water; dehydration should be avoided

- The manufacturer provides a client information sheet and states to "Always provide client information sheet . . ."

Chemistry/Synonyms

A non-steroidal antiinflammatory agent (NSAID), tepoxalin occurs as a white, tasteless, crystalline material that is insoluble in water and soluble in alcohol and most organic solvents. The commercially available tablets contain a micronized form of the drug in a highly porous matrix that rapidly disintegrates in the mouth. Drug particles are released into the saliva and swallowed by the dog where it is absorbed in the intestines.

Tepoxalin may also be known as ORF-20485, RWJ-20485 and *Zubrin*®.

Storage/Stability

Tablets should be kept in their foil blister packs until used and stored at temperatures between 2–30°C (36–86°F).

Dosage Forms/Regulatory Status

VETERINARY-LABELED PRODUCTS:

Tepoxalin Oral (rapidly-disintegrating) Tablets: 30 mg, 50 mg, 100 mg, 200 mg in foil blisters containing 10 tablets in boxes of 10 foil blisters; *Zubrin*® (Schering-Plough); (Rx). FDA-approved for use in dogs.

HUMAN-LABELED PRODUCTS: None

References

Fusellier, M., J.C. Desfontis, et al. (2005). Effect of tepoxalin on renal function in healthy dogs receiving an angiotensin-converting enzyme inhibitor. *Journal of Veterinary Pharmacology and Therapeutics* **28**(6): 581–586.

TERBINAFINE HCL

(ter-*bin*-ah-fin)   Lamisil®

ANTIFUNGAL

Prescriber Highlights

▶ Oral & topical antifungal; used primarily for dermatophytic infections, but may be useful for other fungi (e.g., aspergillus), especially in birds

▶ Comparatively (with azole antifungals) few drug interactions

▶ Appears to be very well tolerated, but limited experience; vomiting most likely adverse effect

▶ Caution if liver or renal disease

▶ Treatment is relatively expensive, but generics are now available

Uses/Indications

Terbinafine may be useful for treating dermatophytic and other fungal infections in dogs and cats.

Terbinafine may also be useful for treating birds for systemic mycotic (*e.g.*, aspergillosis) infections.

Pharmacology/Actions

Terbinafine is an inhibitor of the synthesis of ergosterol, a component of fungal cell membranes. By blocking the enzyme squalene monooxygenase (squalene 2,3-epoxidase), terbinafine inhibits the conversion of squalene to sterols (especially ergosterol) and causes accumulation of squalene. Both these effects are thought to contribute to its antifungal action. Terbinafine's mechanism for inhibiting ergosterol is different from the azole antifungals.

Unlike the azole agents, terbinafine's actions are not mediated via the cytochrome P-450 enzyme system, and, therefore, do not have the concerns of drug interactions or altering testosterone or cortisol.

Terbinafine primarily has clinical activity (fungicidal) against dermatophytic organisms (*Microsporum* spp., *Trichophyton* spp., etc.). It may only be fungistatic against the yeasts (*Candida* spp.). Terbinafine has activity against Aspergillus, Blastomyces, and Histoplasma but is usually not used clinically for infections caused by these organisms.

Pharmacokinetics

Little small animal specific information is available. In cats dosed at 34–46 mg/kg PO once daily for 14 days, terbinafine persisted in hair above MIC for several weeks. (Foust *et al.* 2007)

In six horses, orally administered terbinafine pharmacokinetic values have been reported. The maximum plasma concentration was 0.31 (range: 0.21-0.61) micrograms/mL and occurred at 1.7 (range: 0.75-4) hours after dosing.

Mean half-life was about 8 hours, but ranged widely (range: 3.9-11.6 hours); volume of distribution (Vd/F) was about 131 L/kg (range: 50-266 L/kg); clearance was 187 mL/min/kg (range: 132–282 mL/min/kg). As intravenous terbinafine was not administered, volume of distribution, and clearance are reported per fraction of drug available (KuKanich *et al.* 2009).

In humans, terbinafine given orally is greater than 70% absorbed; after first pass, metabolism bioavailability is about 40%. Food may enhance absorption somewhat. Terbinafine is distributed to skin and into the sebum. Over 99% of drug in plasma is bound to plasma proteins. Drug in the circulation is metabolized in the liver and the effective elimination half-life is about 36 hours. The drug may persist in adipose tissue and skin for very long periods.

Contraindications/Precautions/Warnings

Terbinafine is contraindicated in patients hypersensitive to it. The manufacturer does not recommend its use in patients with active or chronic liver disease or with significantly impaired renal function. If terbinafine is to be used in veterinary patents with markedly impaired liver or renal function, do so with extreme caution; dosage adjustments should be considered.

Adverse Effects

Because of limited usage in veterinary patients the adverse effect profile is not well defined, but thus far, the drug appears to be well tolerated. GI effects (vomiting, inappetence, diarrhea) are possible. In case report in two cats, one cat developed lethargy (Nuttall *et al.* 2008).

Very rarely in humans, liver failure, neutropenia or serious skin reactions (*e.g.*, TEN, Stevens-Johnson syndrome) have occurred after terbinafine use.

Reproductive/Nursing Safety

High dose studies in pregnant rabbits and rats have not demonstrated overt fetotoxicity or teratogenicity, but definitive safety in pregnancy has not been determined. Use with caution (manufacturer recommends NOT using in pregnant women). In humans, the FDA categorizes this drug as category *B* for use during pregnancy (*Animal studies have not yet demonstrated risk to the fetus, but there are no adequate studies in pregnant women; or animal studies have shown an adverse effect, but adequate studies in pregnant women have not demonstrated a risk to the fetus in the first trimester of pregnancy, and there is no evidence of risk in later trimesters.*)

The drug enters maternal milk at levels 7 times that found in plasma; the manufacturer recommends that mothers not nurse while taking this drug. Use with caution in nursing veterinary patients.

Overdosage/Acute Toxicity

Limited information; humans have taken doses of up to 5 grams without serious effects.

Drug Interactions

The following drug interactions have either been reported or are theoretical in humans or animals receiving terbinafine and may be of significance in veterinary patients:

■ **CYCLOSPORINE:** Terbinafine may increase the elimination of cyclosporine

■ **RIFAMPIN:** May increase terbinafine clearance

As it shares the same metabolic pathway (CYP2D6), terbinafine could affect the metabolism of:

■ **BETA-BLOCKERS**

■ **MAO INHIBITORS (amitraz, selegiline)**

■ **SSRI'S (fluoxetine, etc.)**

■ **TRICYCLIC ANTIDEPRESSANTS**

Laboratory Considerations

■ No apparent issues

Doses

■ **DOGS/CATS:**

For dermatophytic infections:

a) Using pulse therapy in cats: In the study, cats given 20 mg/kg PO once daily for 7 days and then 21 days off had clinical and mycological cures and terbinafine concentrations in hair were maintained above therapeutic concentrations. Cats given higher doses (40 mg/kg) or continuous administration accumulated higher concentrations, but some developed emesis in the first week of therapy, and higher hepatic enzyme serum activities. There were no alterations in the values of ALT and FA in the pulse therapy group. (Balda & Larsson 2009)

b) 10–20 mg/kg PO once daily; appears to be better tolerated than either ketoconazole or itraconazole. (MacDonald 2008)

c) In cases where other drugs are not tolerated: 25 mg/kg PO q24h. (Rosenkrantz 2006)

d) For dermatophyte (*M. canis*) mycetomas in cats (from a case report in two cats): Both cats achieved clinical and mycological cure after 12–14 weeks therapy with 26–31 mg/kg PO q24h. (Nuttall *et al.* 2008)

For adjunctive treatment (with topical therapy) of nasal Aspergillus infections if the cribriform pate is penetrated:

a) 5–10 mg/kg PO q12h for 3–6 months (Kuehn 2007)

For pythiosis where advanced disease precludes complete surgical excision:

a) 10 mg/kg PO q24h with itraconazole (10 mg/kg PO twice daily) (Marks 2007)

For lagendiosis where disease precludes complete surgical excision:

a) 5–10 mg/kg PO q24h with itraconazole (10 mg/kg PO q24h) with repeated aggressive surgical resection was effective in one dog with multifocal cutaneous lesions, but no systemic lesions. (Grooters 2007)

For cryptococcal infections in cats that have become resistant to the azoles:

a) 10 mg/kg PO per day can rectify the clinical signs though cats with CNS cryptococcus usually require treatment for life. (Legendre 2010)

■ **BIRDS:**

For avian mycotic infections:

a) For Aspergillus: 10–15 mg/kg PO every 12-24 hours and appears to be well tolerated by a number of avian species. It can also be administered by nebulization as a 1 mg/mL aqueous solution. (Black 2008)

b) 10–15 mg/kg PO q12–24h (suspend a 250 mg tablet in 25 mL water); Nebulization: 1 mg/mL (500 mg terbinafine plus 1 mL *Mucomyst*® plus 500 mL of distilled water). Terbinafine can be used in combination with itraconazole. (Flammer 2003)

c) Aspergillosis: Birds suspected of aspergillosis (leukocytosis and pulmonary nodules) should be treated with terbinafine at 10–15 mg/kg PO q12h for 4 weeks. (Lichtenberger & Orosz 2007)

Monitoring

■ Clinical efficacy

■ Baseline liver enzymes and then as needed (especially if treating long-term)

Client Information

■ Costs of treating can be considerable

■ Give with food, particularly if vomiting is a problem

Chemistry/Synonyms

A synthetic allylamine antifungal, terbinafine HCl occurs as a white to off-white, fine, crystalline powder. It is slightly soluble in water and soluble in ethanol.

Terbinafine HCl may also be known as: *Alamil*®, *Daskil*®, *Daskyl*®, *DesenexMax*®, *Finex*®, *Lamisil*®, *Maditez*®, *Micosil*®, or *Terekol*®.

Storage/Stability

Terbinafine tablets should be stored at room temperature, in tight containers; protect from light.

Dosage Forms/Regulatory Status

VETERINARY-LABELED PRODUCTS: None

HUMAN-LABELED PRODUCTS:

Terbinafine HCl Oral Tablets: 250 mg; *Lamisil*® (Novartis); *Terbinex*® (JSJ); generic; (Rx)

Terbinafine HCl Oral Granules (film-coated): 125 mg/packet & 187.5 mg/packet (as base); *Lamisil*® (Novartis); (Rx)

A topical cream and spray (1%) are also available (Rx).

References

Balda, A. & C. Larsson (2009). Evaluation of Terbinafine Hair Concentration in Persian Cats with Dermatophytosis and Healthy Carriers of Microsporum canis Treated with Pulse or Continuous Therapy. Proceedings; WSAVA. Accessed via: Veterinary Information Network. http://goo.gl/v5oxW

Black, D. (2008). Avian Aspergillosis. Proceedings: UEP. Accessed via: Veterinary Information Network. http://goo.gl/XK2xx

Flammer, K. (2003). Antifungal therapy in avian medicine. Proceedings: Western Veterinary Conference. Accessed via: Veterinary Information Network. http://goo.gl/rgOfo

Foust, A., R. Marsella, et al. (2007). Evaluation of persistence of terbinafine in the hair of normal cats after 14 days of daily therapy. Vet Derm 18(4): 246–251.

Grooters, A. (2007). Lagendium infection in dogs. Proceedings: ACVIM. Accessed via: Veterinary Information Network. http://goo.gl/wVUm8

Kuehn, N. (2007). Chronic rhinitis in dogs. Proceedings; ACVIM. Accessed via: Veterinary Information Network. http://goo.gl/YSuy2

KuKanich, B., M. Montgomery, et al. (2009). Pharmacokinetics of Orally Administered Terbinafine in Horses. Proceedings: ACVIM. Accessed via: Veterinary Information Network. http://goo.gl/8kVYI

Legendre, A.M. (2010). Novel Antifungal Drug Therapies for Deep Mycoses. Proceedings: ACVIM. Accessed via: Veterinary Information Network. http://goo.gl/mPeBb

Lichtenberger, M. & S.E. Orosz (2007). Acute Respiratory Distress (ARD) - From Anatomy through Treatment, Proceedings: AAV.

MacDonald, J. (2008). Yeastie Beasties & Ohter Mycotic issues. Proceedings: WVC. Accessed via: Veterinary Information Network. http://goo.gl/RulYJ

Marks, S. (2007). Fungal and viral enteropathies in dogs and cats: What have we learned? Proceedings: ACVIM. Accessed via: Veterinary Information Network. http://goo.gl/GHMZW

Nuttall, T.J., A.J. German, et al. (2008). Successful resolution of dermatophyte mycetoma following terbinafine treatment in two cats. Veterinary Dermatology 19(6): 405–410.

Rosenkrantz, W. (2006). Appropriate therapy for Malassezia dermatitis. Proceedings: Western Vet Conf. Accessed via: Veterinary Information Network. http://goo.gl/ri2z1

TERBUTALINE SULFATE

(ter-*byoo*-ta-leen)   Brethine®

BETA-ADRENERGIC AGONIST

Prescriber Highlights

▶ Beta agonist used as a bronchodilator & sometimes to treat bradyarrhythmias or as a tocolytic

▶ Looks promising as a test to quantitate anhidrosis in horses

▶ Caution: Diabetes, hyperthyroidism, hypertension, seizure disorders, or cardiac disease (especially with concurrent arrhythmias)

▶ Adverse Effects: Increased heart rate, tremors, CNS excitement (nervousness) & dizziness; after parenteral injection in horses, sweating & CNS excitation are possible

Uses/Indications

Terbutaline is used as a bronchodilating agent in the adjunctive treatment of cardiopulmonary diseases (including tracheobronchitis, collapsing trachea, pulmonary edema, and allergic bronchitis) in small animals. It may be of some benefit in treating bradyarrhythmias in dogs and cats.

Terbutaline has been used occasionally in horses for its bronchodilating effects, but adverse effects, short duration of activity after IV administration and poor oral absorption have limited its use. It has been shown to be useful as a diagnostic agent to diagnose anhidrosis in horses after intradermal injection.

Oral and intravenous terbutaline has been used successfully in humans for the inhibition of premature labor clinical signs.

Pharmacology/Actions

Terbutaline stimulates beta-adrenergic receptors found principally in bronchial, vascular, and uterine smooth muscles ($beta_2$); bronchial and vascular smooth muscle relaxation occurs with resultant reduced airway resistance. At usual doses it has little effect on cardiac ($beta_1$) receptors and usually does not cause direct cardiostimulatory effects. Occasionally, a tachycardia develops which may be a result of either direct beta stimulation or a reflex response secondary to peripheral vasodilation. Terbutaline has virtually no alpha-adrenergic activity.

Pharmacokinetics

The pharmacokinetics of this agent have apparently not been thoroughly studied in domestic animals. In humans, only about 33–50% of an oral dose is absorbed; peak bronchial effects occur within 2–3 hours and activity persists up to 8 hours. Terbutaline is well-absorbed following SC administration with an onset of action occurring within 15 minutes, peak effects at 30–60 minutes, and duration of activity up to 4 hours.

In horses, terbutaline is very poorly absorbed after oral administration with a bioavailability <1%. When given IV, mean residence time is about 30 minutes in horses and the drug probably needs to be given as a constant rate infusion if used therapeutically.

Terbutaline is distributed into milk at levels approximately 1% of the oral dose given to the mother. Terbutaline is principally excreted unchanged in the urine (60%), but is also metabolized in the liver to an inactive sulfate conjugate.

Contraindications/Precautions/Warnings

Terbutaline is contraindicated in patients hypersensitive to it. One veterinary school formulary (Schultz 1986) states that terbutaline is contraindicated in dogs and cats with heart disease, especially with CHF or cardiomyopathy. It should be used with caution in patients with diabetes, hyperthyroidism, hypertension, seizure disorders, or cardiac disease (especially with concurrent arrhythmias).

Adverse Effects

Most adverse effects are dose-related and those that would be expected with sympathomimetic agents, including increased heart rate, tremors, CNS excitement (nervousness) and dizziness. These effects are generally transient, mild and do not require discontinuation of therapy. After parenteral injection in horses, sweating and CNS excitation have been reported.

Transient hypokalemia has been reported in humans receiving beta-adrenergic agents. If an animal is susceptible to developing hypokalemia, it is suggested that additional serum potassium monitoring be done early in therapy.

Reproductive/Nursing Safety

In humans, the FDA categorizes this drug as category *B* for use during pregnancy (*Animal studies have not yet demonstrated risk to the fetus, but there are no adequate studies in pregnant women; or animal studies have shown an adverse effect, but adequate studies in pregnant women have not demonstrated a risk to the fetus in the first trimester of pregnancy, and there is no evidence of risk in later trimesters.*)

Terbutaline is excreted in milk. In humans, nursing is not recommended with systemic terbutaline therapy.

Overdosage/Acute Toxicity

Clinical signs of significant overdose after systemic administration may include arrhythmias (bradycardia, tachycardia, heart block, extrasystoles), hypertension, fever, vomiting, mydriasis, and CNS stimulation. If a recent oral ingestion, it should be handled like other overdoses (empty gut, give activated charcoal and a cathartic) if the animal does not have significant cardiac or CNS effects. If cardiac arrhythmias require treatment, a beta-blocking agent (*e.g.*, propranolol) can be used, but may precipitate bronchoconstriction.

Drug Interactions

The following drug interactions have either been reported or are theoretical in humans or animals receiving terbutaline and may be of significance in veterinary patients:

- ■ **ANESTHETICS, INHALATION (e.g., halothane, isoflurane, methoxyflurane):** Use with inhalation anesthetics may predispose the patient to ventricular arrhythmias, particularly in patients with preexisting cardiac disease—use cautiously

- ■ **BETA-ADRENERGIC BLOCKING AGENTS (e.g., propranolol):** May antagonize the actions of terbutaline

- ■ **DIGOXIN:** Use with digitalis glycosides may increase the risk of cardiac arrhythmias

- ■ **MONOAMINE OXIDASE INHIBITORS:** May potentiate the vascular effects of terbutaline

- ■ **SYMPATHOMIMETICS, OTHER:** Use of terbutaline with other sympathomimetic amines may increase the risk of developing adverse cardiovascular effects

- ■ **TRICYCLIC ANTIDEPRESSANTS:** May potentiate the vascular effects of terbutaline

Doses

■ **DOGS:**

a) For a trial to treat intrathoracic tracheal collapse, expiratory cough or dyspnea and marked exercise intolerance: 1.25–5 mg (total dose) PO two to three times daily (Johnson, LR 2004)

b) As a bronchodilator in chronic bronchitis: Small dogs: 0.625–1.25 mg (total dose) PO q12h; medium-sized dogs: 1.25–2.5 mg (total dose) PO q12h; large dogs: 2.5–5 mg PO q12h (Johnson, L 2000)

c) For bradyarrhythmias: 0.2 mg/kg PO q8–12h; improvement usually partial and often temporary (Rishniw & Thomas 2000)

d) For treatment of premature labor: The initial dose is 0.03 mg/kg PO or SC q8h. The drug should be discontinued 48 hours prior to the calculated delivery date to permit normal labor and delivery to occur. Exogenous progesterone can be added if myometrial contractility cannot be controlled with tocolytics. (Davidson 2008)

e) For tracheal collapse: Small dogs: 0.625–1.25 mg (total dose) PO q12h; medium-sized dogs: 1.25–2.5 mg (total dose) PO q12h; large dogs: 2.5–5 mg PO q12h; 0.01 mg/kg IV, IM or SC (Ettinger & Kantrowitz 2005)

■ **CATS:**

a) For acute exacerbations of feline asthma treated at home: 0.01 mg/kg SC or IM; Beneficial response (decrease of respiratory rate or effort by 50%) occurs in 15–30 minutes. A heart rate that approaches 240 BPM indicates that the drug has been absorbed. (Padrid 2000))

b) For feline asthma: 0.312–0.625 mg (total dose) per cat PO two to three times daily; may adjust dose up to 1.25 mg in larger cats if needed (Noone 1999)

c) For bradyarrhythmias: 0.625 mg PO q8–12h; improvement usually partial and often temporary (Rishniw & Thomas 2000)

d) For acute bronchoconstriction (initial crisis): 0.01 mg/kg IV, SC, IM (Cohn 2007)

■ **HORSES:** (**Note:** ARCI UCGFS Class 3 Drug)

a) For use as a quantitative intradermal terbutaline sweat test (QITST) to identify anhidrosis (preliminary study): In the study a 6 cm wide strip of skin was clipped parallel with and 3 cm below the dorsal margin of the neck on the left side. Beginning at the caudal aspect of this strip, eight 0.1 mL intradermal injections of serial 10-fold dilutions of terbutaline sulfate in 0.9% saline were made through a 25 gauge needle at approximately 5 cm intervals as follows: 0 (control), 0.001,

0.01, 0.1, 1, 10, 100 and 1000 mg/L. Individual sections of absorbent pad (3 x 3 cm; *Stayfree® Ultrathin* regular pads) were preweighed within plastic bags. Pads were then taped over each injection site. Thirty minutes later, they were removed, replaced in plastic bags and reweighed. Sweat weights at saline control sites were, in all cases, ≤8 mg. Sweat weights increased significantly at each successive terbutaline concentration up to a mean weight of 491 mg at the 1000 mg/L dose. The lower one-sided 95% confidence limits for sweat weights were 19, 57, 96, 195 and 267 mg for terbutaline concentrations of 0.1, 1, 10, 100 and 1000 mg/L, respectively. (MacKay 2008)

b) 0.0033 mg/kg IV (Robinson 1987)

Monitoring
- Clinical symptom improvement; auscultation
- Cardiac rate, rhythm (if indicated)
- Serum potassium, early in therapy if animal susceptible to hypokalemia

Client Information
- Contact veterinarian if animal's condition deteriorates or if it becomes acutely ill

Chemistry/Synonyms
A synthetic sympathomimetic amine, terbutaline sulfate occurs as a slightly bitter-tasting, white to gray-white, crystalline powder that may have a faint odor of acetic acid. One gram is soluble in 1.5 mL of water or 250 mL of alcohol. The commercially available injection has its pH adjusted to 3–5 with hydrochloric acid.

Terbutaline Sulfate may also be known as: KWD-2019, terbutaline sulphate, terbutalini sulfas; many trade names are available.

Storage/Stability
Terbutaline tablets should be stored in tight containers at room temperature (15–30°C). Tablets have an expiration date of 3 years beyond the date of manufacture. Terbutaline injection should be stored at room temperature (15–30°C) and protected from light. The injection has an expiration date of 2 years after the date of manufacture.

Terbutaline injection is stable over a pH range of 1–7. Discolored solutions should not be used.

Compatibility/Compounding Considerations
Terbutaline injection is physically **compatible** with D_5W and aminophylline.

Dosage Forms/Regulatory Status
VETERINARY-LABELED PRODUCTS: None

The ARCI (Racing Commissioners International) has designated this drug as a class 3 substance. See the appendix for more information.
HUMAN-LABELED PRODUCTS:

Terbutaline Sulfate Tablets: 2.5 mg & 5 mg; *Brethine®* (aaiPharma); generic; (Global) (Rx)

Terbutaline Injection: 1 mg/mL in 1 mL vials & 2 mL amps with 1 mL fill; *Brethine®* (aaiPharma); generic; (Rx)

References

Cohn, L. (2007). Breathing easy: How to help cats with asthma. Proceedings: Western Vet Conf. Accessed via: Veterinary Information Network. http://goo.gl/9gP2F

Davidson, A. (2008). Breeder Myths and the Veterinarian. Proceedings: WVC. Accessed via: Veterinary Information Network. http://goo.gl/OqjwC

Ettinger, S. & B. Kantrowitz (2005). Diseases of the trachea. *Textbook of Veterinary Internal Medicine, 6th Ed.* SJ Ettinger and E Feldman Eds. Philadelphia, Elsevier: 1217–1232.

Johnson, L. (2000). CVT Update: Canine Chronic Bronchitis. *Kirk's Current Veterinary Therapy: XIII Small Animal Practice.* J Bonagura Ed. Philadelphia, WB Saunders: 801–805.

Johnson, L. (2004). Canine airway collapse. Proceedings: ACVIM Forum. Accessed via: Veterinary Information Network. http://goo.gl/yKRzG

MacKay, R.J. (2008). Quantitative intradermal terbutaline sweat test in horses. *Equine Veterinary Journal* 40(5): 518–520.

Noone, K. (1999). Feline Bronchial asthma. Proceedings: American College of Veterinary interanl Medicine: 17th Annual Veterinary Medical Forum, Chicago.

Padrid, P. (2000). Feline bronchial disease: Therapeutic recommendations for the 21st Century. Proceedings: The North American Veterinary Conference, Orlando.

Rishniw, M. & W. Thomas (2000). Bradyarrhythmias. *Kirk's Current Veterinary Therapy: XIII Small Animal Practice.* J Bonagura Ed. Philadelphia, WB Saunders: 719–725.

Robinson, N.E. (1987). Table of Common Drugs: Approximate Doses. *Current Therapy in Equine Medicine, 2.* NE Robinson Ed. Philadelphia, W.B. Saunders: 761.

TESTOSTERONE CYPIONATE TESTOSTERONE ENANTHATE TESTOSTERONE PROPIONATE

(tess-**toss**-ter-ohn)
ANDROGENIC HORMONE

Prescriber Highlights

- Principle endogenous androgen used primarily for the treatment of testosterone-responsive urinary incontinence in neutered male dogs/cats; in bovine medicine to produce an estrus-detector animal
- Contraindications: Known hypersensitivity to the drug; prostate carcinoma. Caution: Renal, cardiac, or hepatic dysfunction
- Adverse Effects: Uncommon, but perianal adenomas, perineal hernias, prostatic disorders, & behavior changes possible
- Testosterone products are controlled substances (C-III)

Uses/Indications

The use of injectable esters of testosterone in veterinary medicine is limited primarily to its use in dogs (and perhaps cats) for the treatment of testosterone-responsive urinary incontinence in neutered males. Testosterone has been used to treat a rare form of dermatitis (exhibited by bilateral alopecia) in neutered male dogs. These drugs are also used in bovine medicine to produce an estrus-detector (teaser) animal in cull cows, heifers, and steers.

The effectiveness of testosterone to increase libido, treat hypogonadism, aspermia, and infertility in domestic animals has been disappointing.

Pharmacology/Actions

The principle endogenous androgenic steroid, testosterone is responsible for many secondary sex characteristic of the male as well as the maturation and growth of the male reproductive organs and increasing libido.

Testosterone has anabolic activity with resultant increased protein anabolism and decreased protein catabolism. Testosterone causes nitrogen, sodium, potassium and phosphorus retention and decreases the urinary excretion of calcium. Nitrogen balance is improved only when an adequate intake of both calories and protein occurs.

By stimulating erythropoietic stimulating factor, testosterone can stimulate the production of red blood cells. Large doses of exogenous testosterone can inhibit spermatogenesis through a negative feedback mechanism inhibiting luteinizing hormone (LH).

Testosterone may help maintain the normal urethral muscle tone and integrity of the urethral mucosa in male dogs. It may also be necessary to prevent some types of dermatoses.

Pharmacokinetics

Orally administered testosterone is rapidly metabolized by the GI mucosa and the liver (first-pass effect); very little reaches the systemic circulation. The esterified compounds, testosterone enanthate and cypionate are less polar than testosterone and more slowly absorbed from lipid tissue after IM injection. The duration of action of these compounds may persist for 2–4 weeks after IM injection. Testosterone propionate reportedly has a much shorter duration of action than the enanthate or cypionate esters. Because absorption is dependent upon several factors (volume injected, perfusion, etc.), duration of action may be variable.

Testosterone is highly bound to a specific testosterone-estradiol globulin (98% in humans). The quantity of this globulin determines the amount of drug that is in the free or bound form. The free form concentration determines the plasma half-life of the hormone.

Testosterone is metabolized in the liver and is, with its metabolites, excreted in the urine

($\approx$90%) and the feces ($\approx$6%). The plasma half-life of testosterone has been reported to be between 10–100 minutes in humans. The plasma half-life of testosterone cypionate has been reported to be 8 days.

Contraindications/Precautions/Warnings

Testosterone therapy is contraindicated in patients with known hypersensitivity to the drug or prostate carcinoma. It should be used with caution in patients with renal, cardiac or hepatic dysfunction.

Adverse Effects

Adverse effects are reportedly uncommon when injectable testosterone products are used in male dogs to treat hormone-responsive incontinence. Perianal adenomas, perineal hernias, prostatic disorders, and behavior changes (aggression) are all possible, however. Behavioral changes have been reported in cats. Polycythemia has been reported in humans receiving high dosages of testosterone. High dosages or chronic usage may result in oligospermia or infertility in intact males.

Reproductive/Nursing Safety

In humans, the FDA categorizes this drug as category X for use during pregnancy (*Studies in animals or humans demonstrate fetal abnormalities or adverse reaction; reports indicate evidence of fetal risk. The risk of use in pregnant women clearly outweighs any possible benefit.*) In a separate system evaluating the safety of drugs in canine and feline pregnancy (Papich 1989), this drug is categorized as in class: *D* (*Contraindicated. These drugs have been shown to cause congenital malformations or embryotoxicity.*)

It is not known whether androgens are excreted in milk; consider using milk replacer if using testosterone in nursing patients.

Overdosage/Acute Toxicity

No specific information was located; refer to the Adverse Effects section for further information.

Drug Interactions

The following drug interactions have either been reported or are theoretical in humans or animals receiving testosterone and may be of significance in veterinary patients:

- ■ **CORTICOSTEROIDS:** Androgens may enhance the edema that can be associated with ACTH or adrenal steroid therapy

- ■ **INSULIN; ORAL ANTIDIABETIC AGENTS:** Testosterone may decrease serum glucose levels

- ■ **PROPRANOLOL:** Testosterone cypionate may increase propranolol clearance

- ■ **WARFARIN:** Testosterone may increase anticoagulant effects

Laboratory Considerations

- ■ Concentrations of protein bound iodine (PBI) can be decreased in patients receiving testosterone therapy, but the clinical significance of this is probably not important. Androgen agents can decrease amounts of thyroxine-binding globulin and decrease **total T₄** concentrations and increase resin uptake of T_3 and T_4. Free thyroid hormones are unaltered and clinically, there is no evidence of dysfunction.

■ Both **creatinine** and **creatine** excretion can be decreased by testosterone

■ Testosterone can increase the urinary excretion of **17-ketosteroids**

■ Androgenic/anabolic steroids may alter **blood glucose** levels

■ Androgenic/anabolic steroids may suppress **clotting factors II, V, VII, and X**

Doses

■ **DOGS:**

For testosterone-responsive urinary incontinence (may be used with phenylpropanolamine) in males:

a) Testosterone propionate: approximately 2 mg/kg IM or SC 3 times per week. Testosterone cypionate: 200 mg IM once per month (Labato 1989; Polzin & Osborne 1985)

b) Testosterone propionate: 2.2 mg/kg IM q2-3 days. Testosterone cypionate: 2.2 mg/kg IM once per month (Chew *et al.* 1986; Moreau & Lappin 1989)

c) Testosterone cypionate: 2.2 mg/kg IM q4-8 weeks (Lane 2002)

d) Testosterone propionate: 2.2 mg/kg IM or SC every 2-3 days. Testosterone cypionate: 2.2 mg/kg every 30 days or 200 mg IM every 30 days. (Bartges 2006)

For estrus control:

a) Testosterone enanthate or cypionate 0.5 mg/kg IM once every 5 days or methyltestosterone tablets 25 mg PO twice a week; this dose is for Greyhound-sized dogs. (Purswell 1999)

To reduce mammary gland enlargement seen in pseudopregnancy:

a) Testosterone enanthate or cypionate 0.5-1 mg/kg IM once (Purswell 1999)

■ **CATS:**

For infertility or reduced libido: Using either testosterone cypionate or propionate:

a) 0.1-1 mg every other day or every third day for 3-5 injections IM or SC. Not indicated for testis descent. (Verstegen 2000)

For testosterone-responsive urinary incontinence (may be used with phenylpropanolamine) in males:

a) Testosterone propionate 5-10 mg IM as needed. (Barsanti & Finco 1986; Osborne *et al.* 2000), (Bartges 2006)

■ **CATTLE:**

To produce an estrus-detector (teaser) animal (cull cows, heifers, steers):

a) Testosterone propionate 200 mg IM on day 1 and on days 4-9. On day 10, give 1 gram IM and attach a chinball marker and put with the breeding herd. To maintain the teaser give 1 gram booster every 10-14 days.

Alternatively, initially give testosterone enanthate 0.5 gram IM and 1.5 gram SC (divided in two separate locations). After 4 days attach chinball marker and put in with breeding herd. To maintain, give 0.5-0.75 gram SC every 10-14 days. (Wolfe 1986)

Monitoring

■ Efficacy
■ Adverse effects

Chemistry/Synonyms

The esterified compounds, testosterone cypionate, enanthate, and propionate are available commercially as injectable products. Testosterone cypionate occurs as an odorless to having a faint odor, creamy white or white, crystalline powder. It is insoluble in water, soluble in vegetable oils, and freely soluble in alcohol. Testosterone cypionate has a melting range of 98°-104°C. It may also be known as testosterone cyclopentylpropionate.

Testosterone enanthate occurs as an odorless to having a faint odor, creamy white or white, crystalline powder. It is soluble in vegetable oils, insoluble in water and melts between 34-39°C.

Testosterone propionate occurs as odorless, creamy white to white, crystals or crystalline powder. It is insoluble in water, freely soluble in alcohol and soluble in vegetable oils. Testosterone propionate melts between 118-123°C.

Testosterone Cypionate may also be known as: testosterone cyclopentylpropionate, testosterone cypionate, *Deposteron®*, *Depotrone®*, *Depo-Testosterone®*, *Duratest®*, *Scheinpharm Testone-Cyp®*, *T-Cypionate®*, *Testex®*, *Testiormina®*, *Testred®*, *Virilon®*, or *depAndro®*.

Testosterone Propionate may also be known as: NSC-9166, testosteroni propionas, *Malogen in Oil®*, *Sostenon®*, *Sustanon®*, *Testanon 25®*, *Testex®*, *Testoviron®*, *Testoviron Depot®*, *Testovis®*, *Tesurene®*, or *Virormone®*.

Storage/Stability

The commercially available injectable preparations of testosterone cypionate, enanthate and propionate should be stored at room temperature; avoid freezing or exposing to temperatures greater than 40°C. If exposed to low temperature a precipitate may form, but should redissolve with shaking and rewarming. If a wet needle or syringe is used to draw up the parenteral solutions, cloudy solutions may result, but will not affect the drug's potency.

Dosage Forms/Regulatory Status

VETERINARY-LABELED PRODUCTS:

No known testosterone products (with the exception of combinations with estradiol as growth promotant implants) FDA-approved for use in veterinary species were located. Testosterone propionate (200 mg) is available in combination with estradiol benzoate (20 mg) as a growth promotant. Trade names include *Component E-H®* (VetLife); (OTC) and *Synovex-H®* (Fort Dodge); (OTC). For use in heifers weighing 400 or more pounds.

Testosterone propionate (200 mg) with estradiol benzoate (28 mg); *Synovex-Plus®* (Fort Dodge); (OTC); for steers.

The ARCI (Racing Commissioners International) has designated this drug as a class 4 substance. See the appendix for more information.

HUMAN-LABELED PRODUCTS:

Testosterone Cypionate (in oil) Injection: 100 mg/mL & 200 mg/mL in 1 mL & 10 mL vials; *Depo-Testosterone®* (Pfizer); generic; (Rx, C-III)

Testosterone Enanthate (in oil) Injection: 200 mg/mL in 5 mL multi-dose vials; *Delatestyl®* (Indevus); generic (Paddock); (Rx, C-III)

Testosterone Pellets Implant for subcutaneous implantation: 75 mg in 1 pellet/vials; *Testopel®* (Bartor Pharmacal); (Rx, C-III)

Testosterone Transdermal System: Release Rates: 5 & 2.5 mg/24 hour, total testosterone contents: 24.3 mg & 12.2 mg (respectively): *Androderm®* (Watson Pharma); (Rx, C-III)

Testosterone Gel: 1% (50 mg testosterone) in unit-dose packets and tubes or 75 gram metered multiple dose pumps; *AndroGel® 1%* (Solvay); *Testim®* (Auxilium); (Rx, C-III)

Testosterone, Buccal System: 30 mg testosterone in blister packs; *Striant®* (Columbia); (Rx, C-III)

References

Barsanti, J.A. & D.R. Finco (1986). Feline Urinary Incontinence. *Current Veterinary Therap IX: Small Animal Practice.* RW Kirk Ed. Philadelphia, W.B. Saunders: 1159–1163.

Bartges, J. (2006). Broken plumbing: urinary incontinence. Proceedings: ACVC 2006. Accessed via: Veterinary Information Network. http://goo.gl/XgEUd

Chew, D.J., S.P. DiBartola, et al. (1986). Pharmacologic Manipulation of Urination. *Current Veterinary Therapy IX: Small Animal Practice.* RW Kirk Ed. Philadelphia, W.B. Saunders: 1207–1212.

Labato, M.A. (1989). Disorders of Micturation. *Handbook of Small Animal Practice.* RV Morgan Ed. New York, Churchill Livingstone: 621–628.

Lane, I. (2002). Micturition disorders. Proceedings: Western Veterinary Conf. Accessed via: Veterinary Information Network. http://goo.gl/wT1Ro

Moreau, P.M. & M.R. Lappin (1989). Pharmacologic management of urinary incontinence. *Current Veterinary Therapy X: Small Animal Practice.* RW Kirk Ed. Philadelphia, Saunders: 1214–1222.

Osborne, C., J. Kruger, et al. (2000). Feline Lower Urinary Tract Diseases. *Textbook of Veterinary Internal Medicine: Diseases of the Dog and Cat.* S Ettinger and E Feldman Eds. Philadelphia, WB Saunders. **2:** 1710–1747.

Papich, M. (1989). Effects of drugs on pregnancy. *Current Veterinary Therapy X: Small Animal Practice.* R Kirk Ed. Philadelphia, Saunders: 1291–1299.

Polzin, D.J. & C.A. Osborne (1985). Diseases of the Urinary Tract. *Handbook of Small Animal Therapeutics.* LE Davis Ed. New York, Churchill Livingstone: 333–395.

Purswell, B. (1999). Pharmaceuticals used in canine theriogenology - Part 1 & 2. Proceedings: Central Veterinary Conference, Kansas City.

Verstegen, J. (2000). Feline Reproduction. *Textbook of Veterinary Internal Medicine: Diseases of the Dog and Cat.* S Ettinger and E Feldman Eds. Philadelphia, WB Saunders. **2:** 1585–1598.

Wolfe, D.F. (1986). Surgical procedures of the reproductive system of the bull. *Current Therapy in Theriogenology 2: Diagnosis, treatment and prevention of reproductive diseases in small and large animals.* DA Morrow Ed. Philadelphia, WB Saunders: 353–379.

TETRACYCLINE HCL

(tet-ra-sye-kleen)   Aquadrops®, Panmycin®

TETRACYCLINE ANTIBIOTIC

Prescriber Highlights

▶ Prototype tetracycline antibiotic; many bacteria are now resistant, but still may be very useful to treat mycoplasma, rickettsia, spirochetes, & Chlamydia

▶ Dosing frequency may be an issue for small animals

▶ Extreme Caution: Pregnancy

▶ Caution: Liver or renal insufficiency

▶ Adverse Effects: GI distress, staining of developing teeth & bones, superinfections, photosensitivity; long-term use may cause uroliths. *Cats:* Do not tolerate very well. *Horses:* If stressed may break with diarrheas (oral use). *Ruminants:* High oral doses can cause ruminal microflora depression & ruminoreticular stasis; rapid IV of undiluted propylene glycol-based products can cause intravascular hemolysis & cardiodepressant effects; *IM:* local reactions, yellow staining & necrosis may be seen at the injection site

Uses/Indications

While tetracycline still is used as an antimicrobial, most small animal clinicians prefer doxycycline and large animal clinicians prefer oxytetracycline when a tetracycline is indicated to treat susceptible infections. The most common use of tetracycline HCl today is in combination with niacinamide for the treatment of certain immune-mediated skin conditions in dogs, such as pemphigus.

Pharmacology/Actions

Tetracyclines generally act as time-dependent antibiotics and inhibit protein synthesis by reversibly binding to 30S ribosomal subunits of susceptible organisms, thereby preventing binding to those ribosomes of aminoacyl transfer-RNA. Tetracyclines have been deemed bacteriostatic antibiotics, but this nomenclature is more of historical importance than descriptive of their antibacterial actions. Tetracyclines are believed to reversibly bind to 50S ribosomes and additionally alter cytoplasmic membrane permeability in susceptible organisms. In high concentrations, tetracyclines can inhibit protein synthesis by mammalian cells.

As a class, the tetracyclines have activity against most mycoplasma, spirochetes (including the Lyme disease organism), Chlamydia, and Rickettsia. Against gram-positive bacteria, the tetracyclines have activity against some strains of staphylococcus and streptococci, but resistance of these organisms is increasing. Gram-positive bacteria that are usually covered by tetracyclines include *Actinomyces* spp., *Bacillus anthracis*, *Clostridium perfringens* and tetani, *Listeria monocytogenes*, and Nocardia. Among gram-negative bacteria that tetracyclines usually have *in vitro* and *in vivo* activity include *Bordetella* spp., Brucella, Bartonella, *Haemophilus* spp., *Pasturella multocida*, Shigella, and Yersinia pestis. Many or most strains of *E. coli*, Klebsiella, Bacteroides, Enterobacter, Proteus and *Pseudomonas aeruginosa* are resistant to the tetracyclines. While most strains of Pseudomonas aeruginosa show *in vitro* resistance to tetracyclines, those compounds attaining high urine levels (*e.g.*, tetracycline, oxytetracycline) have been associated with clinical cures in dogs with UTI secondary to this organism. Hemoglobin at the site of the infection can reduce the antimicrobial activity of tetracycline.

Oxytetracycline and tetracycline share nearly identical spectrums of activity and patterns of cross-resistance and a tetracycline susceptibility disk is usually used for *in vitro* testing for oxytetracycline susceptibility.

Tetracyclines have antiinflammatory and immunomodulating effects. They can suppress antibody production and chemotaxis of neutrophils; inhibit lipases, collagenases, prostaglandin synthesis, and activation of complement component 3.

Pharmacokinetics

Both oxytetracycline and tetracycline are readily absorbed after oral administration to fasting animals. Bioavailabilities are approximately 60–80%. The presence of food or dairy products can significantly reduce the amount of tetracycline absorbed, with reductions of 50% or more possible. After IM administration, tetracycline is erratically and poorly absorbed with serum levels usually lower than those attainable with oral therapy.

Tetracyclines as a class, are widely distributed to heart, kidney, lungs, muscle, pleural fluid, bronchial secretions, sputum, bile, saliva, urine, synovial fluid, ascitic fluid, and aqueous and vitreous humor. Only small quantities of tetracycline and oxytetracycline are distributed to the CSF, and therapeutic levels may not be achievable. While all tetracyclines distribute to the prostate and eye, doxycycline or minocycline penetrate better into these and most other tissues. Tetracyclines cross the placenta, enter fetal circulation and are distributed into milk. The volume of distribution of tetracycline is approximately 1.2–1.3 L/kg in small animals. The amount of plasma protein binding is about 20–67% for tetracycline. In cattle, the volume of distribution for oxytetracycline is between 1 and 2.5 L/kg. Milk to plasma ratios for oxytetracycline and tetracycline are 0.75 and 1.2–1.9, respectively.

Both oxytetracycline and tetracycline are eliminated unchanged primarily via glomerular filtration. Patients with impaired renal function can have prolonged elimination half-lives and accumulate the drug with repeated dosing. These drugs apparently are not metabolized, but are excreted into the GI tract via both biliary and nonbiliary routes and may become inactive after chelation with fecal materials. The elimination half-life of tetracycline is approximately 5–6 hours in dogs and cats.

Contraindications/Precautions/Warnings

Tetracycline is contraindicated in patients hypersensitive to it or other tetracyclines. Because tetracyclines can retard fetal skeletal development and discolor deciduous teeth, they should only be used in the last half of pregnancy when the benefits outweigh the fetal risks. Oxytetracycline and tetracycline are considered more likely to cause these abnormalities than either doxycycline or minocycline.

In patients with renal insufficiency or hepatic impairment, tetracycline must be used cautiously; lower than normal dosages are recommended with enhanced monitoring of renal and hepatic function. Avoid concurrent administration of other nephrotoxic or hepatotoxic drugs if tetracyclines are administered to these patients. Monitoring of serum levels should be considered if long-term therapy is required.

Adverse Effects

Oxytetracycline and tetracycline given to young animals can cause discoloration of bones and teeth to a yellow, brown, or gray color. High dosages or chronic administration may delay bone growth and healing.

Tetracyclines in high levels can exert an antianabolic effect that can cause an increase in BUN and/or hepatotoxicity, particularly in patients with preexisting renal dysfunction. As renal function deteriorates secondary to drug accumulation, this effect may be exacerbated.

In ruminants, high oral doses can cause ruminal microflora depression and ruminoreticular stasis. Rapid intravenous injection of undiluted propylene glycol-based products can cause intravascular hemolysis with resultant hemoglobinuria. Propylene glycol based products have also caused cardiodepressant effects when administered to calves. When administered IM, local reactions, yellow staining, and necrosis may be seen at the injection site.

In small animals, tetracyclines can cause nausea, vomiting, anorexia, and diarrhea. Cats do not tolerate oral tetracycline or oxytetracycline very well, and may present with clinical signs of colic, fever, hair loss, and depression. There are reports that long-term tetracycline use may cause urolith formation in dogs.

Horses that are stressed by surgery, anesthesia, trauma, etc., may break with severe diarrheas after receiving tetracyclines (especially with oral administration).

Tetracycline therapy (especially long-term) may result in overgrowth of non-susceptible bacteria or fungi (superinfections).

Tetracyclines have also been associated with photosensitivity reactions and, rarely, hepatotoxicity, formation of anti-nuclear antibodies, or blood dyscrasias.

Reproductive/Nursing Safety

In humans, the FDA categorizes this drug as category **D** for use during pregnancy (*There is evidence of human fetal risk, but the potential benefits from the use of the drug in pregnant women may be acceptable despite its potential risks.*) In a separate system evaluating the safety of drugs in canine and feline pregnancy (Papich 1989), this drug is categorized as in class: **D** (*Contraindicated. These drugs have been shown to cause congenital malformations or embryotoxicity.*)

Tetracyclines are excreted in milk, but because much of the drug will be bound to calcium in milk, it is unlikely to be of significant risk to nursing animals.

Overdosage/Acute Toxicity

Tetracyclines are generally well tolerated after acute overdoses. Dogs given more than 400 mg/kg/day orally or 100 mg/kg/day IM of oxytetracycline did not demonstrate any toxicity. Oral overdoses would most likely be associated with GI disturbances (vomiting, anorexia, and/or diarrhea). Should the patient develop severe emesis or diarrhea, fluids and electrolytes should be monitored and replaced if necessary. Chronic overdoses may lead to drug accumulation and nephrotoxicity.

High oral doses given to ruminants, can cause ruminal microflora depression and ruminoreticular stasis. Rapid intravenous injection of undiluted propylene glycol-based products can cause intravascular hemolysis with resultant hemoglobinuria.

Rapid intravenous injection of tetracyclines has induced transient collapse and cardiac arrhythmias in several species, presumably due to chelation with intravascular calcium ions. Overdose quantities of drug could exacerbate this effect if given too rapidly IV. If the drug must be given rapidly IV (less than 5 minutes), some clinicians recommend pre-treating the animal with intravenous calcium gluconate.

Drug Interactions

The following drug interactions have either been reported or are theoretical in humans or animals receiving tetracyclines and may be of significance in veterinary patients:

- **ATOVAQUONE:** Tetracyclines have caused decreased atovaquone levels

- **BETA-LACTAM OR AMINOGLYCOSIDE ANTIBIOTICS:** Bacteriostatic drugs, like the tetracyclines, have been historically thought to interfere with bactericidal activity of the penicillins, cephalosporins, and aminoglycosides but the actual clinical significance of this interaction is doubtful.

- **DIGOXIN:** Tetracyclines have increased the bioavailability of digoxin in a small percentage of human patients and caused digoxin toxicity. These effects may persist for months after discontinuation of the tetracycline.

- **DIVALENT OR TRIVALENT CATIONS (oral antacids, saline cathartics or other GI products containing aluminum, calcium, iron, magnesium, zinc, or bismuth cations):** When orally administered, tetracyclines can chelate divalent or trivalent cations that can decrease the absorption of the tetracycline or the other drug if it contains these cations; it is recommended that all oral tetracyclines be given at least 1–2 hours before or after the cation-containing products.

- **METHOXYFLURANE:** Fatal nephrotoxicity has occurred in humans when used with tetracycline; concomitant use with oxytetracycline not recommended

- **SUCRALFATE:** Sucralfate may impair the oral absorption of tetracycline; separate dosing by at least 2 hours to minimize this effect

- **WARFARIN:** Tetracyclines may depress plasma prothrombin activity and patients on anticoagulant therapy may need dosage adjustment

Laboratory Considerations

- Tetracyclines (not minocycline) may cause falsely elevated values of **urine catecholamines** when using fluorometric methods of determination.

- Tetracyclines reportedly can cause false-positive **urine glucose results** if using the cupric sulfate method of determination (Benedict's reagent, *Clinitest®*), but this may be the result of ascorbic acid that is found in some parenteral formulations of tetracyclines. Tetracyclines have also reportedly caused false-negative results in determining urine glucose when using the glucose oxidase method (*Clinistix®*, *Tes-Tape®*).

Doses

■ **DOGS:**

For discoid lupus erythematosus:

a) For dogs weighing 10 kg or more: 500 mg of niacinamide and 500 mg of tetracycline PO q8h. For dogs weighing from 5−10 kg: 250 mg of each PO q8h. For dogs weighing <5 kg: 100 mg of each PO q8h. Improvement is usually noted within 6 weeks. (White 2000)

b) Dogs weighing more than 10 kg: 500 mg of niacinamide and 500 mg of tetracycline PO q8h. For dogs weighing less than 10 kg: 250 mg of each PO q8h. May use in combination with corticosteroids and Vitamin E. If adverse effects become a problem, reduce dose of niacinamide first. May also try this regimen for pemphigus foliaceous or pemphigus erythematous. (Campbell 1999)

c) For various immune-mediated diseases (discoid lupus erythematosus, pemphigus erythematosus, pemphigus foliaceous, vasculitis, sterile pyelogranuloma, dermatomyositis and lupoid onychodystrophy: For dogs less than 10 kg: 250 mg each of niacinamide and tetracycline PO three times daily. For dogs larger than 10 kg: 500 mg each of niacinamide and tetracycline PO three times daily. May substitute doxycycline for tetracycline at 5 mg/kg PO once a day. (Tapp 2002)

For susceptible infections:

a) For UTI: 16 mg/kg PO q8h for 7−14 days; For Rickettsiosis, Borreliosis: 22 mg/kg PO q8h for 14 days;

For systemic bacteremia, brucellosis: 22−50 mg/kg PO q8h for 28 days. (Greene *et al.* 2006)

b) For Rocky Mountain Spotted Fever: 22 mg/kg q8h for 14−21 days (Sellon & Breitschwerdt 1995)

c) 20 mg/kg PO q8−12h; (may give with food if GI upset occurs; avoid or reduce dose in animals with renal or severe liver failure; avoid in young, pregnant or breeding animals) (Vaden & Papich 1995)

d) For susceptible UTI's: 18 mg/kg PO q8h (Dowling 2009)

e) For Lyme disease: 22 mg/kg PO q8h for 14 days (Breitschwerdt 2000)

f) For small intestinal bacterial overgrowth: 5−10 mg/kg PO q8h for 28 days; has been effective for uncomplicated cases (Ludlow & Davenport 2000)

g) For Ehrlichiosis: 22 mg/kg PO q8h for 28 days. (Ford 2009)

For facial tear staining:

a) 5−10 mg/kg/day or 50 mg per dog per day. Results are variable. (Kern 1986)

For pleurodesis:

a) Using capsules or aqueous solution; mix 20 mg/kg in 4 mL per kg of saline and infuse into pleural space (Morgan 1988)

■ **CATS:**

For susceptible infections:

a) For soft tissue infections: 20 mg/kg PO q8h for 21 days;

For Hemotropic mycoplasmosis: 10−25 mg/kg PO q8−12h for 21 days;

For bacteremia, systemic infections: 7 mg/kg IV, IM q12h as long as necessary. (Greene *et al.* 2006)

b) For rickettsial diseases: 16 mg/kg, PO three times daily for 21 days (Morgan 1988)

c) 20 mg/kg PO q8−12h; (may give with food if GI upset occurs; avoid or reduce dose in animals with renal or severe liver failure; avoid in young, pregnant or breeding animals) (Vaden & Papich 1995)

d) 22−33 mg/kg PO q8h (Aronson & Aucoin 1989)

■ **FERRETS:**

For susceptible infections:

a) 25 mg/kg PO 2−3 times daily (Williams 2000)

■ **RABBITS, RODENTS, SMALL MAMMALS:**

a) **Rabbits:** 50−100 mg/kg PO q8−12h (Ivey & Morrisey 2000)

b) **Chinchillas:** 50 mg/kg PO q8−12h (Hayes 2000)

c) **Chinchillas, Guinea Pigs, Rats:** 20 mg/kg, PO q12h. **Mice:** 20 mg/kg, PO q12h or 50−60 mg/liter of drinking water **Hamsters:** 30 mg/kg, PO q6h or 400 mg/liter, drinking water. **Gerbils:** 20 mg/kg, PO or IM q24h (Adamcak & Otten 2000)

■ **CATTLE:**

For susceptible infections in calves:

a) 11 mg/kg orally (Howard 1986)

b) 11 mg/kg, PO twice daily for up to 5 days (Label directions; *Polyotic®*—American Cyanamid)

■ **SHEEP:**

For susceptible infections:

a) 11 mg/kg, PO twice daily for up to 5 days (Label directions; *Polyotic®*—American Cyanamid)

■ **HORSES:**

For susceptible infections:

a) 5−7.5 mg/kg IV q12h (Brumbaugh 1987)

■ **SWINE:**

For susceptible infections:

a) 22 mg/kg, PO for 3 to 5 days in drinking water (Label directions; *Polyotic®*— American Cyanamid)

■ **BIRDS:**

For susceptible infections:

a) For treatment of psittacosis in conjunction with *LA-200®* (see oxytetracycline doses) and/or medicated pellets and/or *Keet Life*: Using 25 mg/mL oral suspension, mix 2 teaspoonsful to 1 cup of soft food.

For mild respiratory disease (especially flock treatment): Mix 1 teaspoonful of 10 grams/6.4 oz. soluble powder per gallon of drinking water. Used as an adjunct for psittacosis with other tetracycline forms. Will not reach therapeutic levels by itself. Prepare fresh solution twice daily, as potency is rapidly lost. (McDonald 1989)

b) Mix 1 teaspoonful of 10 grams/6.4 oz. soluble powder per gallon of drinking water and administer for 5–10 days. Prepare fresh solution 2–3 times daily, as potency is rapidly lost.

For converting regimen to pelleted feeds administer oral suspension by gavage at 200–250 mg/kg once or twice daily until feeds are accepted. Is not an adequate therapy for long-term treatment of chlamydiosis (psittacosis) (Clubb 1986)

Monitoring

■ Adverse effects

■ Clinical efficacy

■ Long-term use or in susceptible patients: periodic renal, hepatic, hematologic evaluations

Client Information

■ Avoid giving this drug orally within 1–2 hours of feeding, giving milk or other dairy products

■ If gastrointestinal upset occurs, giving with a small amount of food may help, but this may also reduce the amount of drug absorbed

Chemistry/Synonyms

An antibiotic obtained from *Streptomyces aureofaciens* or derived semisynthetically from oxytetracycline, tetracycline HCl occurs as a moderately hygroscopic, yellow, crystalline powder. About 100 mg/mL is soluble in water and 10 mg/mL soluble in alcohol. Tetracycline base has a solubility of about 0.4 mg per mL of water and 20 mg per mL of alcohol. Commercially available tetracycline HCl for IM injection also contains magnesium chloride, procaine HCl and ascorbic acid.

Tetracycline may also be known as: tetracyclini hydrochloridum; many trade names are available.

Storage/Stability

Unless otherwise instructed by the manufacturer, tetracycline oral tablets and capsules should be stored in tight, light resistant containers at room temperature (15–30°C). The oral suspension and powder for injection should be stored at room temperature; avoid freezing the oral suspension.

Dosage Forms/Regulatory Status

VETERINARY-LABELED PRODUCTS:

There are a variety of Tetracycline HCl Soluble Powder (as a water additive) products that are available in various concentrations and sizes. Usual concentrations are either 25 grams/lb or 324 grams/lb and these products may be available in several sizes; may be FDA-approved for use in swine, cattle, or poultry. Withdrawal time may vary depending on age of animal and product.

An oral combination product containing tetracycline, novobiocin and prednisone (*Delta Albaplex®*) is also available; see the novobiocin monograph for more information.

HUMAN-LABELED PRODUCTS:

Tetracycline HCl Capsules: 250 mg & 500 mg; *Sumycin® -250 & -500* (Par); generic; (Rx)

Tetracycline HCl Oral Suspension: 25 mg/mL in 473 mL; *Sumycin® Syrup* (Par); (Rx)

References

Adamcak, A. & B. Otten (2000). Rodent Therapeutics. *Vet Clin NA: Exotic Anim Pract* **3:**1(Jan): 221–240.

Aronson, A.L. & D.P. Aucoin (1989). Antimicrobial Drugs. *Textbook of Veterinary Internal Medicine.* SJ Ettinger Ed. Philadelphia, WB Saunders. **1:** 383–412.

Breitschwerdt, E. (2000). Rocky Mountain Spotted Fever. Proceedings: American Animal Hospital Association 67th Annual Meeting, Toronto.

Brumbaugh, G.W. (1987). Rational selection of antimicrobial drugs for treatment of infections in horses. *Vet Clin North Am (Equine Practice)* **3**(1): 191–227.

Campbell, K. (1999). New Drugs in Veterinary Dermatology. Proceedings: Central Veterinary Conference, Kansas City.

Clubb, S.L. (1986). Therapeutics: Individual and Flock Treatment Regimens. *Clinical Avian Medicine and Surgery.* GJ Harrison and LR Harrison Eds. Philadelphia, W.B. Saunders: 327–355.

Dowling, P. (2009). Optimizing antimicrobial therapy of urinary tract infections. Proceedings: WVC. Accessed via: Veterinary Information Network. http://goo.gl/iXp5f

Ford, R. (2009). Tick-Borne Disease Diagnosis: Moving from 3Dx to 4Dx. Proceedings: ACVC. Accessed via: Veterinary Information Network. http://goo.gl/0Pb6s

Greene, C., K. Hartmannn, et al. (2006). Appendix 8: Antimicrobial Drug Formulary. *Infectious Disease of the Dog and Cat.* C Greene Ed., Elsevier: 1186–1333.

Hayes, D. (2000). Diseases of Chinchillas. *Kirk's Current Veterinary Therapy: XIII Small Animal Practice.* J Bonagura Ed. Philadelphia, WB Saunders: 1152–1157.

Howard, J.L., Ed. (1986). *Current Veterinary Therapy 2, Food Animal Practice.* Philadelphia, W.B. Saunders.

Ivey, E. & J. Morrisey (2000). Therapeutics for Rabbits. *Vet Clin NA: Exotic Anim Pract* **3:**1(Jan): 183–216.

Kern, T.J. (1986). Disorders of the Lacrimal System. *Current Veterinary Therapy IX: Small Animal Practice.* RW Kirk Ed. Philadelphia, W.B. Saunders: 634–641.

Ludlow, C. & D. Davenport (2000). Small Intestinal Bacterial Overgrowth. *Kirk's Current Veterinary*

Therapy: XIII Small Animal Practice. J Bonagura Ed. Philadelphia, WB Saunders: 637–641.

McDonald, S.E. (1989). Summary of medications for use in psittacine birds. *JAAV* 3(3): 120–127.

Morgan, R.V., Ed. (1988). *Handbook of Small Animal Practice.* New York, Churchill Livingstone.

Papich, M. (1989). Effects of drugs on pregnancy. *Current Veterinary Therapy X: Small Animal Practice.* R Kirk Ed. Philadelphia, Saunders: 1291–1299.

Sellon, R. & E. Breitschwerdt (1995). CVT Update: Rocky Mountain Spotted Fever. *Kirk's Current Veterinary Therapy:XII.* J Bonagura Ed. Philadelphia, W.B. Saunders: 293–297.

Tapp, T. (2002). New drug therapy in dermatology. Proceedings: Atlantic Coast Veterinary Conference. Accessed via: Veterinary Information Network. http://goo.gl/Vjn2j

Vaden, S. & M. Papich (1995). Empiric Antibiotic Therapy. *Kirk's Current Veterinary Therapy:XII.* J Bonagura Ed. Philadelphia, W.B. Saunders: 276–280.

White, S. (2000). Veterinary Dermatology: New Treatments, 'New' Diseases. Proceedings: The North American Veterinary Conference, Orlando.

Williams, B. (2000). Therapeutics in Ferrets. *Vet Clin NA: Exotic Anim Pract* 3:1(Jan): 131–153.

Theophylline—see Aminophylline

Thiacetarsamide (no longer available)—See Melarsomine

THIAMINE HCL
VITAMIN B1

(thye-a-min)

NUTRITIONAL; B VITAMIN

Prescriber Highlights

▶ A "B" vitamin used for treatment or prevention of thiamine deficiency. May be useful for adjunctive treatment of lead poisoning & ethylene glycol toxicity

▶ Adverse Effects: hypersensitivity/ana-phylactic reactions (rarely); tenderness, or muscle soreness after IM injection

▶ Drug Interactions; lab interactions

Uses/Indications

Thiamine is indicated in the treatment or prevention of thiamine deficiency states. Clinical signs of thiamine deficiency may be manifested as gastrointestinal (anorexia, salivation), neuromuscular/CNS signs (ataxia, seizures, loss of reflexes), or cardiac effects (brady- or tachyar-rhythmias). Deficiency states may be secondary to either a lack of thiamine in the diet or the presence of thiamine destroying compounds in the diet (e.g., bracken fern, raw fish, amprolium, thiaminase-producing bacteria in ruminants). Thiamine may be supplemented in camelids and other species when long-term amprolium is used.

Thiamine has also been used in the adjunctive treatment of lead poisoning and ethylene glycol toxicity (to facilitate the conversion of glyoxylate to nontoxic metabolites).

Pharmacology/Actions

Thiamine combines with adenosine triphosphate (ATP) to form a compound (thiamine diphosphate/thiamine pyrophosphate) that is employed for carbohydrate metabolism, but does not effect blood glucose concentrations.

Absence of thiamine results in decreased transketolase activity in red blood cells and increased pyruvic acid blood concentrations. Without thiamine triphosphate, pyruvic acid is not converted into acetyl-CoA; diminished NADH results with anaerobic glycolysis producing lactic acid. Lactic acid production is further increased secondary to pyruvic acid conversion; lactic acidosis may occur.

Pharmacokinetics

Thiamine is absorbed from the GI tract and is metabolized by the liver. Elimination is renal, the majority of the drug is eliminated as metabolites.

Contraindications/Precautions/Warnings

Thiamine injection is contraindicated in animals hypersensitive to it or to any component of it.

Adverse Effects

Hypersensitivity reactions have occurred after injecting this agent. Rarely, a vasovagal anaphylactic response (cardiac arrest or severe bradycardia, cardiac arrhythmias, apnea, hypotension, collapse, seizure, and protracted neuromuscular weakness), has been observed in a small number of cats when thiamine hydrochloride was administered subcutaneously. Some tenderness or muscle soreness may result after IM injection.

Reproductive/Nursing Safety

In humans, the FDA categorizes this drug as category **A** for use during pregnancy (*Adequate studies in pregnant women have not demonstrated a risk to the fetus in the first trimester of pregnancy, and there is no evidence of risk in later trimesters.*) If used in doses greater than the RDA, the FDA categorizes this drug as category **C** for use during pregnancy (*Animal studies have shown an adverse effect on the fetus, but there are no adequate studies in humans; or there are no animal reproduction studies and no adequate studies in humans.*)

It is not known whether this drug is excreted in milk, but it should not be of clinical concern.

Overdosage/Acute Toxicity

Very large doses of thiamine in laboratory animals have been associated with neuromuscular or ganglionic blockade, but the clinical significance is unknown. Hypotension and respiratory depression may also occur with massive doses. A lethal dose of 350 mg/kg has been reported. Generally, no treatment should be required with most overdoses.

Drug Interactions

The following drug interactions have either been reported or are theoretical in humans or animals

receiving thiamine and may be of significance in veterinary patients:

■ **NEUROMUSCULAR BLOCKING AGENTS:** Thiamine may enhance the activity of neuromuscular blocking agents; clinical significance is unknown

Laboratory Considerations

■ Thiamine may cause false-positive **serum uric acid** results when using the phosphotungstate method of determination or urobilinogen urine spot tests using Ehrlich's reagent

■ The Schack and Wexler method of determining **theophylline concentrations** may be interfered with by large doses of thiamine

Doses

■ **DOGS:**

For thiamine deficiency:

a) 5–50 mg IM, SC, or IV (depending on formulation) (Phillips 1988)

b) 1–2 mg IM (Greene & Braund 1989)

c) 2 mg/kg, PO once daily (Davis 1985)

d) 100–250 mg SC twice daily for several days until regression of symptoms with complete recovery (Hoskins 1988)

For adjunctive treatment for ethylene glycol toxicity:

a) 100 mg/day PO (Morgan 1988)

■ **CATS:**

For thiamine deficiency:

a) 100–250 mg parenterally twice a day (experimentally, as little as 1 mg is effective) (Armstrong & Hand 1989)

b) 10–20 mg/kg IM for several days. (Abramson 2009)

c) For adjunctive treatment of hepatic lipidosis: If neck ventroflexion is present, consider electrolyte or thiamine insufficiency; check electrolytes (potassium, phosphate, and magnesium); provide supplements as appropriate. Give 100 mg of thiamine in one liter of crystalloid fluids with additional soluble B vitamins (riboflavin, niacinamide, D-panthenol, pyridoxine, and cyanocobalamin). (Center 2005)

d) 100–250 mg SC twice daily for several days until regression of symptoms with complete recovery (Hoskins 1988)

e) 10–20 mg/kg IM or SC two to three times daily until signs abate, then 10 mg/kg PO once daily for 21 days (Morgan 1988)

■ **CATTLE:**

For thiamine deficiency:

a) For polioencephalomalacia: Initially, 10 mg/kg IV; then, 10 mg/kg IM twice daily for 2–3 days. If no improvement within 4 days, may be advisable to recommend slaughter. (Dill 1986)

b) 10–20 mg/kg IM or SC 3 times daily; if giving IV dilute in isotonic saline or isotonic dextrose. (Walz 2006)

c) 10 mg/kg up to 4 times a day; first dose may be given via slow IV and subsequent doses IM. Less severely affected animals may respond to lower or less frequent dosing. Severely affected animals may benefit from corticosteroids (dexamethasone 1–2 mg/kg) and mannitol (1 gram/kg in a 20% solution IV through a filtered IV set). (Cebra, C. 2005)

For adjunctive therapy of lead poisoning:

a) 2 mg/kg IM (at same time as CaEDTA therapy); total daily dose 8 mg/kg (Brattan & Kowalczyk 1989)

■ **HORSES:**

For thiamine deficiency:

a) 0.5–5 mg/kg IV, IM or PO (Robinson 1987)

b) 100–1000 mg IM, SC, or IV (depending on formulation) (Phillips 1988)

For adjunctive treatment of perinatal asphyxia syndrome (hypoxic ischemic encephalopathy):

a) Foals: 1 gram in one liter of fluids IV once a day (Slovis 2003)

As part of a parenteral nutrition (PN) formula:

a) B complex vitamins (thiamine 12.5 mg/mL; niacinamide 12.5 mg/mL; pyridoxine 5 mg/mL; d-panthenol 5 mg/mL; riboflavin 2 mg/mL; cyanocobalamin 5 mg/mL) should be supplied at a rate of 1–2 mL/45 kg daily, diluted in fluids or PN. Vitamin C should be supplied at a rate of 20 mg/kg/day enterally whenever possible. (Magdesian 2010)

■ **SWINE:**

For thiamine deficiency:

a) 5–100 mg IM, SC, or IV (depending on formulation) (Phillips 1988)

■ **SHEEP & GOATS:**

For thiamine deficiency:

a) For polioencephalomalacia: Initially, 10 mg/kg IV; then, 10 mg/kg IM twice daily for 2–3 days. If no improvement within 4 days, may be advisable to recommend slaughter. (Dill 1986)

b) Sheep: 20–200 mg IM, SC, or IV (depending on formulation) (Phillips 1988)

■ **CAMELIDS (NWC):**

a) For prophylaxis when animals with *E. macusaniensis* treated with amprolium for >5 days (from a retrospective study): 10 mg/kg SC q24h after the 5th day of amprolium. (Cebra, C.K. *et al.* 2007)

Monitoring

■ Efficacy

Client Information

■ Epidemiologic investigation as to the cause of thiamine deficiency (diet, plants, raw fish, etc.) should be performed with necessary changes made to prevent recurrence

Chemistry/Synonyms

A water-soluble "B" vitamin, thiamine HCl occurs as bitter-tasting, white, small hygroscopic crystals, or crystalline powder that has a characteristic yeast-like odor. Thiamine HCl is freely soluble in water, slightly soluble in alcohol and has pK$_a$s of 4.8 and 9.0. The commercially available injection has a pH of 2.5–4.5.

Thiamine HCl may also be known as: aneurine hydrochloride, thiamin hydrochloride, thiamine chloride, thiamini hydrochloridum, thiaminii chloridum, vitamin B-1; many trade names available.

Storage/Stability

Thiamine HCl for injection should be protected from light and stored at temperatures less than 40°C and preferably between 15–30°C; avoid freezing.

Thiamine HCl is unstable in alkaline or neutral solutions or with oxidizing or reducing agents. It is most stable at a pH of 2.

Compatibility/Compounding Considerations

Thiamine HCl is reportedly physically **compatible** with all commonly used intravenous replacement fluids.

Do **not** mix thiamine with alkaline drugs or alkalinizing agents (barbiturates, citrates, carbonates, acetates, copper ions) or oxidizing/reducing agents (*e.g.*, sulfites).

Compatibility is dependent upon factors such as pH, concentration, temperature, and diluent used; consult specialized references or a hospital pharmacist for more specific information.

Dosage Forms/Regulatory Status

VETERINARY-LABELED PRODUCTS:

Thiamine HCl for Injection: 200 mg/mL in 100 mL and 250 mL vials & Thiamine HCl for Injection: 500 mg/mL in 100 mL vials; generic; (Rx). Labeled for use in horses, dogs and cats.

Thiamine HCl Dietary Supplement: 8,200 mg per lb.; *Horse Care Durvit B-1 Crumbles®* (Durvet); (OTC), Labeled for use in horses.

Thiamine HCl Supplement: 500 mg/oz in 1.5 lb, 4 lb and 20 lb containers; *Thia-Dex®* (Neogen), *Vitamin B-1 Powder®* (AHC); (OTC). Labeled for use in dogs & horses.

There are several B-complex vitamin preparations available that may also have thiamine included.

HUMAN-LABELED PRODUCTS:

Thiamine Tablets: 50 mg, 100 mg& 250 mg; generic; (OTC)

Thiamine Enteric Coated Tablets: 20 mg; *Thiamilate®* (Tyson); (OTC)

Thiamine HCl Injection: 100 mg/mL in 1 mL in 2 mL *Tubex*, 2 mL multi-dose vials; generic; (Rx)

References

Abramson, C.J. (2009). Feline Neurology I. Proceedings: WVC. Accessed via: Veterinary Information Network. http://goo.gl/eWXb1

Armstrong, P.J. & M.S. Hand (1989). Nutritional Disorders. *The Cat: Diseases and Clinical Management.* RG Sherding Ed. New York, Churchill Livingstone. **1**: 141–161.

Brattan, G.R. & D.F. Kowalczyk (1989). Lead Poisoning. *Current Veterinary Therapy (CVT) X Small Animal Practice.* RW Kirk Ed. Philadelphia, W.B. Saunders: 152–159.

Cebra, C. (2005). Polioencephalomalacia. Proceedings: ACVIM. Accessed via: Veterinary Information Network. http://goo.gl/1h9LH

Cebra, C.K., B.A. Valentine, et al. (2007). Eimeria macusaniensis infection in 15 llamas and 34 alpacas. *Javma-Journal of the American Veterinary Medical Association* **230**(1): 94–100.

Center, S.A. (2005). Feline hepatic lipidosis. *Veterinary Clinics of North America-Small Animal Practice* **35**(1): 225–+.

Davis, L.E., Ed. (1985). *Handbook of Small Animal Therapeutics.* New York, Churchill Livingston.

Dill, S.G. (1986). Polioencephalomalacia in Ruminants. *Current Veterinary Therapy: Food Animal Practice 2.* JL Howard Ed. Philadelphia, W.B. Saunders: 868–869.

Greene, C.E. & K.G. Braund (1989). Diseases of the Brain. *Textbook of Veterinary Internal Medicine.* SJ Ettinger Ed. Philadelphia, WB Saunders. **1**: 578–623.

Hoskins, J.D. (1988). Juvenile Nutritional Disorders. *Handbook of Small Animal Practice.* RV Morgan Ed. New York, Churchill Livingstone: 1061–1066.

Magdesian, K.G. (2010). Parenteral nutrition in the mature horse. *Equine Veterinary Education* **22**(7): 364–371.

Morgan, R.V., Ed. (1988). *Handbook of Small Animal Practice.* New York, Churchill Livingstone.

Phillips, R.W. (1988). Water-soluble Vitamins. *Veterinary Pharmacology and Therapeutics - 6th Ed.* NH Booth and LE McDonald Eds. Ames, Iowa State University Press: 698–702.

Robinson, N.E. (1987). Table of Common Drugs: Approximate Doses. *Current Therapy in Equine Medicine, 2.* NE Robinson Ed. Philadelphia, W.B. Saunders: 761.

Slovis, N. (2003). Perinatal asphyxia syndrome (Hypoxic ischemic encephalopathy). Proceedings: ACVIM Forum. Accessed via: Veterinary Information Network. http://goo.gl/I6TgF

Walz, P. (2006). Neurologic diseases of cattle. Proceedings: ABVP. Accessed via: Veterinary Information Network. http://goo.gl/vQeWD

THIOGUANINE

(thye-oh-**gwah**-neen)

ANTINEOPLASTIC

Prescriber Highlights

▶ Oral purine analog antineoplastic that may be useful as adjunctive treatment for acute lymphocytic or granulocytic leukemia in dogs or cats

▶ **Contraindications:** Hypersensitivity to thioguanine

▶ **Caution:** Hepatic dysfunction, bone marrow depression, infection, renal function impairment (adjust dosage), or history of urate urinary stones

▶ Potentially mutagenic & teratogenic; use milk replacer if nursing

▶ **Adverse Effects:** GI effects, bone marrow suppression, hepatotoxicity, pancreatitis, GI (including oral) ulceration, & dermatologic reactions

▶ Cats may be more susceptible than dogs to adverse effects

▶ Low therapeutic index; monitoring mandatory

Uses/Indications

Thioguanine may be useful as adjunctive therapy for acute lymphocytic or granulocytic leukemia in dogs or cats.

Pharmacology/Actions

Intracellularly, thioguanine is converted to ribonucleotides that cause the synthesis and utilization of purine nucleotides to be blocked. The drug's cytotoxic effects are believed to occur when these substituted nucleotides are inserted into RNA and DNA. Thioguanine has limited immunosuppressive activity. Extensive cross-resistance usually occurs between thioguanine and mercaptopurine.

Pharmacokinetics

Thioguanine is administered orally, but absorption is variable. In humans, only about 30% of a dose is absorbed. Thioguanine is distributed into the DNA and RNA of bone marrow, but several doses may be necessary for this to occur. It does not apparently enter the CNS, but does cross the placenta. It is unknown whether it enters maternal milk.

Thioguanine is rapidly metabolized primarily in the liver to a methylate derivative that is less active (and toxic) than the parent compound. This and other metabolites are eliminated in the urine.

Contraindications/Precautions/Warnings

Thioguanine is contraindicated in patients hypersensitive to it. The drug should be used cautiously (risk versus benefit) in patients with hepatic dysfunction, bone marrow depression, infection, renal function impairment (adjust dosage) or with a history of urate urinary stones. Thioguanine has a very low therapeutic index and should only be used by clinicians with experience in the use of cytotoxic agents and able to monitor therapy appropriately.

Adverse Effects

At usual doses, GI effects (nausea, anorexia, vomiting, diarrhea) may occur in small animals. However, bone marrow suppression, hepatotoxicity, pancreatitis, GI (including oral) ulceration, and dermatologic reactions are potentially possible. Cats may be particularly susceptible to the hematologic effects of thioguanine.

Reproductive/Nursing Safety

Thioguanine is potentially mutagenic and teratogenic and not recommended for use during pregnancy. In humans, the FDA categorizes this drug as category **D** for use during pregnancy (*There is evidence of human fetal risk, but the potential benefits from the use of the drug in pregnant women may be acceptable despite its potential risks.*)

Although it is unknown whether thioguanine enters milk, use of milk replacer is recommended for nursing bitches or queens.

Overdosage/Acute Toxicity

Toxicity may be acute (GI effects) or delayed (bone marrow depression, hepatotoxicity, gastroenteritis). It is suggested to use standard protocols to empty the GI tract if ingestion was recent and treat supportively.

Drug Interactions

The following drug interactions have either been reported or are theoretical in humans or animals receiving thioguanine and may be of significance in veterinary patients:

◼ **HEPATOTOXIC DRUGS (e.g., halothane, ketoconazole, valproic acid, phenobarbital, primidone, etc.):** Thioguanine should be used cautiously with other drugs that can cause hepatotoxicity

◼ **IMMUNOSUPPRESSIVE DRUGS (e.g., azathioprine, cyclophosphamide, corticosteroids):** Use with other immunosuppressant drugs may increase the risk of infection

◼ **MYELOSUPPRESSIVE DRUGS (e.g., chloramphenicol, flucytosine, amphotericin B, or colchicine):** Use extreme caution when used concurrently with other drugs that are also myelosuppressive, including many of the other antineoplastics and other bone marrow depressant drugs; bone marrow depression may be additive

◼ **VACCINES, LIVE:** Live virus vaccines should be used with caution during therapy, if at all

Laboratory Considerations

◼ Thioguanine may increase serum **uric acid** levels in some patients

Doses

■ **DOGS:**

Note: Because of the potential toxicity of this drug to patients, veterinary personnel and clients, and since chemotherapy indications, treatment protocols, monitoring and safety guidelines often change, the following dosages should be used only as a general guide. Consultation with a veterinary oncologist and referral to current veterinary oncology references [*e.g.,* (Henry & Higginbotham 2009); (Argyle *et al.* 2008); (Withrow & Vail 2007); (Villalobos 2007); (Ogilvie & Moore 2006); (Ogilvie & Moore 2001)] are *strongly recommended.*

a) For acute lymphocytic and granulocytic leukemia: 40 mg/m^2 PO once daily (q24 hours) for 4–5 days, then every 3rd day thereafter (Jacobs *et al.* 1992)

b) As part of protocols for treatment of acute myelogenous leukemias: Protocol 1: Cytarabine 100 mg/m^2 SC daily for 2–6 days; Thioguanine 50 mg/m^2 PO q24–48h. Protocol 2: Cytarabine 100 mg/m^2 SC daily for 2–6 days; Thioguanine 50 mg/m^2 PO q24–48h; Doxorubicin 10 mg/m^2 IV once a week (Couto 2003)

■ **CATS:**

a) For acute lymphocytic and granulocytic leukemia: 25 mg/m^2 PO once daily (q24 hours) for 1–5 days, then every 30 days thereafter as necessary (Jacobs *et al.* 1992)

Monitoring

■ Hemograms (including platelets) should be monitored closely; initially every 1-2 weeks and every 1–2 months once on maintenance therapy. It is recommended by some clinicians that if the WBC count drops to between 5,000–7,000 cells/mm^3 the dose be reduced by 25%. If WBC count drops below 5,000 cells/mm^3 treatment should be discontinued until leukopenia resolves

■ Liver function tests; serum amylase, if indicated

■ Efficacy

Client Information

■ Clients must be briefed on the possibilities of severe toxicity developing from this drug, including drug-related neoplasms or mortality.

■ Clients should contact veterinarian if the animal exhibits clinical signs of abnormal bleeding, bruising, anorexia, vomiting, jaundice, or infection.

■ Although, no special precautions are necessary with handling intact tablets, it is recommended to wash hands after administering the drug.

Chemistry/Synonyms

A purine analog antineoplastic agent, thioguanine occurs as a pale yellow, odorless or practically odorless, crystalline powder. It is insoluble in water or alcohol.

Thioguanine may also be known as: NSC-752, 6- thioguanine, TG, 6-TG, 2-Amino-6-mercaptopurine, WR-1141, *Lanvis®, Tabloid®,* or *Tioguanina®.*

Storage/Stability

Store tablets in tight containers at room temperature.

Dosage Forms/Regulatory Status

VETERINARY-LABELED PRODUCTS: None

HUMAN-LABELED PRODUCTS:

Thioguanine Tablets: 40 mg; *Tabloid®* (GlaxoSmithKline); (Rx)

References

Argyle, D., M. Brearly, et al. (2008). *Decision Making in Small Animal Oncology,* Wiley-Blackwell.

Couto, C. (2003). Oncology. *Small Animal Internal Medicine, 3rd Ed.* R Nelson and C Couto Eds. St Louis, Mosby: 1093–1155.

Henry, C. & M. Higginbotham (2009). *Cancer Management in Small Animal Practice,* Saunders.

Jacobs, R., J. Lumsden, et al. (1992). Canine and Feline Reference Values. *Current Veterinary Therapy XI: Small Animal Practice.* R Kirk and J Bonagura Eds. Philadelphia, W.B. Saunders Company: 1250–1277.

Ogilvie, G. & A. Moore (2001). *Feline Oncology: A Comprehensive Guide to Compassionate Care,* Veterinary Learning Systems.

Ogilvie, G. & A. Moore (2006). *Managing the Canine Cancer Patient: A Practical Guide to Compassionate Care,* Veterinary Learning Systems.

Villalobos, A. (2007). *Canine and Feline Geriatric Oncology.* Ames, Blackwell.

Withrow, S. & D. Vail (2007). *Withrow and MacEwen's Small Animal Clinical Oncology 4th Ed.* Philadelphia, Elsevier.

THIOPENTAL SODIUM

(thye-oh-*pen*-tal)   Pentothal®

ULTRA-SHORT ACTING
  THIOBARBITURATE

Prescriber Highlights

▶ Ultra-short acting thiobarbiturate used for anesthesia induction or anesthesia for very short procedures

▶ Contraindications: Absolute contraindications: absence of suitable veins for IV administration, history of hypersensitivity reactions to barbiturates, status asthmaticus. Relative contraindications: severe cardiovascular disease or preexisting ventricular arrhythmias, shock, increased intracranial pressure, myasthenia gravis, asthma, & conditions where hypnotic effects may be prolonged (*e.g.*, severe hepatic disease, myxedema, severe anemia, excessive premedication, etc.). Greyhounds (& other sight hounds) metabolize thiobarbiturates much more slowly than other breeds; consider using methohexital instead. *Horses:* preexisting leukopenia; thiopental alone may cause excessive ataxia & excitement

▶ Avoid: Extravasation, intra-carotid or intra-arterial injections, & use of concentrations of less than 2% in sterile water. Too rapid IV administration can cause significant vascular dilatation & hypoglycemia

▶ Adverse Effects: *Dogs:* Ventricular bigeminy *Cats:* Apnea after injection, mild arterial hypotension. *Horses:* Excitement & severe ataxia (if used alone); transient leukopenias, hyperglycemia, apnea, moderate tachycardia, mild respiratory acidosis

▶ Severe CNS toxicity & tissue damage has occurred in horses receiving intra-carotid injections of thiobarbiturates

▶ C-III controlled substance

Uses/Indications

Because of its rapid action and short duration, in young, healthy animals, thiopental is excellent induction agent (rapid IV bolus) for general anesthesia with other anesthetics or as the sole anesthetic agent for very short procedures. In sick or debilitated animals, thiopental may be used in a more cautious manner (IV, slowly to effect).

Pharmacology/Actions

Because of their high lipid solubility, thiobarbiturates rapidly enter the CNS and produce profound hypnosis and anesthesia. They are also known as ultrashort-acting barbiturates. See the monograph: Barbiturates, Pharmacology of, for additional information.

Pharmacokinetics

Following IV injection of therapeutic doses, hypnosis and anesthesia occur within one minute and usually within 15-30 seconds. The drug rapidly enters the CNS and then redistributes to muscle and adipose tissue in the body. The short duration of action (10−30 minutes) after intravenous dosing of thiopental is due less to rapid metabolism than to this redistribution out of the CNS and into muscle and fat stores. Greyhounds and other sight hounds may exhibit longer recovery times than other breeds. This may be due to these breeds low body fat levels or differences in the metabolic handling of the thiobarbiturates. Although anesthesia is short, recovery periods may require several hours.

Thiopental is metabolized by the hepatic microsomal system and several metabolites have been isolated. The elimination half-life in dogs has been reported as being approximately 7 hours and in sheep, 3−4 hours. Very little of the drug is excreted unchanged in the urine (0.3% in humans), so dosage adjustments are not necessary in patients with chronic renal failure.

Contraindications/Precautions/Warnings

The following are considered **absolute contraindications** to the use of thiopental: absence of suitable veins for IV administration, history of hypersensitivity reactions to the barbiturates, and status asthmaticus. **Relative contraindications** include: severe cardiovascular disease or preexisting ventricular arrhythmias, shock, increased intracranial pressure, myasthenia gravis, asthma, and conditions where hypnotic effects may be prolonged (*e.g.*, severe hepatic disease, myxedema, severe anemia, excessive premedication, etc.). These relative contraindications do not preclude the use of thiopental, but dosage adjustments must be considered and the drug must be given slowly and cautiously.

Patients with renal dysfunction or acidemia may show increased sensitivity to thiopental.

Because greyhounds (and other sight hounds) metabolize thiobarbiturates much more slowly than methohexital, many clinicians recommend using methohexital instead. In horses, thiopental should not be used if the patient has preexisting leukopenia. Some clinicians feel that thiopental should not be used alone in the horse as it may cause excessive ataxia and excitement.

Concentrations of less than 2% in sterile water should not be used as they may cause hemolysis. Extravasation and intra-arterial injections should be avoided because of the high alkalinity of the solution. Severe CNS toxicity and tissue damage has occurred in horses receiving intra-carotid injections of thiobarbiturates.

Adverse Effects

In dogs, thiopental has an approximate arrhythmogenic incidence of 40%. Ventricular bigeminy is the most common arrhythmia seen; it is usually transient and generally responds to additional oxygen. Administration of catecholamines may augment the arrhythmogenic effects of the thiobarbiturates, while lidocaine may inhibit it. Cardiac output may also be reduced, but is probably only clinically significant in patients experiencing heart failure. Dose-related apnea and hypotension may be noted.

Cats are susceptible to developing apnea after injection and may develop a mild arterial hypotension.

Horses can exhibit clinical signs of excitement and severe ataxia during the recovery period if the drug is used alone. Horses can develop transient leukopenias and hyperglycemia after administration. A period of apnea and moderate tachycardia and a mild respiratory acidosis may also develop after dosing.

Too rapid IV administration can cause significant vascular dilatation and hypoglycemia. Repeated administration of thiopental is not advised as recovery times can become significantly prolonged. Parasympathetic side effects (*e.g.*, salivation, bradycardia) may be managed with the use of anticholinergic agents (atropine, glycopyrrolate).

Prolonged recoveries may occur when repeated dosages of thiopental are administered.

Thiopental's high pH (10–11) can cause significant tissue irritation and necrosis if administered perivascularly; administration through an IV catheter is advised.

Reproductive/Nursing Safety

Thiopental readily crosses the placental barrier and should be used with caution during pregnancy. In humans, the FDA categorizes this drug as category *C* for use during pregnancy (*Animal studies have shown an adverse effect on the fetus, but there are no adequate studies in humans; or there are no animal reproduction studies and no adequate studies in humans.*) In a separate system evaluating the safety of drugs in canine and feline pregnancy (Papich 1989), this drug is categorized as in class: *C* (*These drugs may have potential risks. Studies in people or laboratory animals have uncovered risks, and these drugs should be used cautiously as a last resort when the benefit of therapy clearly outweighs the risks.*)

Small amounts of thiopental may appear in milk following administration of large doses, but is unlikely to be of clinical significance in nursing animals.

Overdosage/Acute Toxicity

Treatment of thiobarbiturate overdosage consists of supporting respirations (O_2, mechanical ventilation) and giving cardiovascular support (do not use catecholamines, *e.g.*, epinephrine, etc.).

Drug Interactions

A fatal interaction has been reported in a dog receiving the proprietary product, *Diathal®* (no longer marketed; contained procaine penicillin G, dihydrostreptomycin sulfate, diphemanil methylsulfate, and chlorpheniramine) and the related compound thiamylal.

The following drug interactions have either been reported or are theoretical in humans or animals receiving thiopental and may be of significance in veterinary patients:

- ◼ **CLONIDINE:** IV clonidine prior to induction may reduce thiopental dosage requirements by up to 37%
- ◼ **CNS DEPRESSANTS, OTHER:** May enhance respiratory and CNS depressant effects
- ◼ **DIAZOXIDE:** Potential for hypotension
- ◼ **EPINEPHRINE, NOREPINEPHRINE:** The ventricular fibrillatory effects of epinephrine and norepinephrine may be potentiated when used with thiobarbiturates and halothane
- ◼ **METOCLOPRAMIDE:** Given prior to induction may reduce thiopental dosage requirements
- ◼ **MIDAZOLAM:** May potentiate hypnotic effects
- ◼ **OPIATES:** Given prior to induction may reduce thiopental dosage requirements
- ◼ **PHENOTHIAZINES:** May potentiate thiopental effects; hypotension possible
- ◼ **PROBENECID:** May displace thiopental from plasma proteins
- ◼ **SULFONAMIDES:** Thiopental and sulfas may displace one another from plasma proteins

Doses

Note: Atropine sulfate (or glycopyrrolate) is often administered prior to thiobarbiturate anesthesia to prevent parasympathetic side effects; however, some clinicians question whether routine-administration of anticholinergic agents is necessary.

Thiobarbiturates are administered strictly to effect; *doses are guidelines only.*

- ◼ **DOGS:**
    a) 13.2–26.4 mg/kg IV depending on duration of anesthesia required (Package insert; *Pentothal®*—Ceva Laboratories)
    b) 15–17 mg/kg IV for brief (7–10 minutes) anesthesia; 18–22 mg/kg IV for moderate (10–15 minutes) duration; 22–29 mg/kg IV for longer (15–25 minutes) duration (Booth 1988)
    c) 22 mg/kg IV; or 15.4 mg/kg IV after tranquilization; or 11 mg/kg IV after narcotic premedication (Mandsager 1988)
    d) Usually dosed at 12–15 mg/kg, with one-third of the drug administered rapidly and any additional amount administered to effect. Repeated doses will accumulate resulting in prolonged recoveries; residual effect may last several hours. (Hellyer 2005)

■ **CATS:**

a) 13.2−26.4 mg/kg IV depending on duration of anesthesia required (Package insert; *Pentothal®*—Ceva Laboratories)

b) 22 mg/kg IV; or 15.4 mg/kg IV after tranquilization; or 11 mg/kg IV after narcotic premedication (Mandsager 1988)

c) Usually dosed at 12−15 mg/kg, with one-third of the drug administered rapidly and any additional amount administered to effect. Repeated doses will accumulate resulting in prolonged recoveries; residual effect may last several hours. (Hellyer 2005)

■ **RABBITS, RODENTS, SMALL MAMMALS:**

a) **Rabbits:** 15−30 mg/kg IV to effect (Ivey & Morrisey 2000)

b) For chemical restraint: **Mice:** 50 mg/kg IP; **Rats:** 40 mg/kg IP; **Hamsters/ Gerbils:** 30−40 mg/kg IP; **Guinea pig:** 15−30 mg/kg IV; **Rabbits:** 15−30 mg/kg IV (Burke 1999)

c) For anesthesia in rabbits: 10−12 mg/kg IV to effect. (Kaiser-Klingler 2009)

■ **CATTLE:**

a) 8.14−15.4 mg/kg IV; for unweaned calves from which food has been withheld for 6−12 hours: no more than 6.6 mg/kg IV for deep surgical anesthesia (*Pentothal®* package insert; Ceva Laboratories)

b) For calves under 2 weeks of age: 15−22 mg/kg IV slowly until complete muscular relaxation takes place, duration of anesthesia usually lasts 10−12 minutes (Booth 1988)

c) 5.5 mg/kg IV after sedation and administration with guaifenesin; or 8.8−11 mg/kg IV after tranquilization (Mandsager 1988)

■ **HORSES: (Note:** ARCI UCGFS Class 2 Drug)

a) With preanesthetic tranquilization: 6−12 mg/kg IV (an average of 8.25 mg/kg is recommended); Without preanesthetic tranquilization: 8.8−15.4 mg/kg IV (an average horse: 9.9−11 mg/kg IV) (Package insert; *Pentothal®*—Ceva Laboratories)

b) One gram of thiopental per 90 kg body weight as a 10% solution given evenly over 20 seconds 15 minutes after premedication with either 0.22 mg/kg IV xylazine or 0.05 mg/kg IV acepromazine (Booth 1988)

c) 5.5 mg/kg IV after sedation and administration with guaifenesin; or 8.8−11 mg/kg IV after tranquilization (Mandsager 1988)

■ **SWINE:**

a) 5.5−11 mg/kg IV (Package insert; *Pentothal®*—Ceva Laboratories)

b) For swine weighing 5−50 kg: 10−11 mg/kg IV (Booth 1988)

■ **SHEEP:**

a) 9.9−15 mg/kg IV depending on depth of anesthesia required (Package insert; *Pentothal®*—Ceva Laboratories)

■ **GOATS:**

a) 20−22 mg/kg IV after atropine (0.7 mg/kg) IM (Booth 1988)

Monitoring

■ Level of hypnosis/anesthesia

■ Respiratory status; cardiac status (rate/ rhythm/blood pressure)

Client Information

This drug should only be used by professionals familiar with its effects in a setting where adequate respiratory support can be performed.

Chemistry/Synonyms

A thiobarbiturate, thiopental occurs as a bitter tasting, white to off-white, crystalline powder or a yellow-white hygroscopic powder. It is soluble in water (1 gram in 1.5 mL) and alcohol. Thiopental has a pK_a of 7.6 and is a weak organic acid. Thiopental solutions are very alkaline (pH>10).

Thiopental sodium may also be known as: thiopentone sodium, natrium isopentylaethylthiobarbituricum, penthiobarbital sodique, thiomebumalnatrium cum natrii carbonate, thiopentalum natricum, thiopentobarbitalum solubile, tiopentol sodico, *Anesthal®*, *Bensulf®*, *Farmotal®*, *Hipnopento®*, *Inductal®*, *Intraval®*, *Nesdonal®*, *Pensodital®*, *Pentothal®*, *Sandothal®*, *Sodipental®*, *Thionembutal®*, *Thiopentax®*, *Tiobarbital®*, or *Trapanal®*.

Storage/Stability

When stored in the dry form, thiopental sodium is stable indefinitely. Thiopental should be diluted with only sterile water for injection, sodium chloride injection, or D$_5$W. Concentrations of less than 2% in sterile water should not be used as they may cause hemolysis. After reconstitution, solutions are stable for 3 days at room temperature and 7 days if refrigerated; however, as no preservative is present, it is recommended it be used within 24 hours after reconstitution. After 48 hours, the solution has been reported to attack the glass bottle in which it is stored. Thiopental may also adsorb to plastic IV tubing and bags. Do not administer any solution that has a visible precipitate.

Compatibility/Compounding Considerations

Preparation of Solution for Administration: Use only sterile water for injection, normal saline, or D$_5$W to dilute. A 5 gram vial diluted with 100 mL will yield a 5% solution and diluted with 200 mL will yield a 2.5% solution. Discard reconstituted solutions after 24 hours

The following agents have been reported to be physically **compatible** when mixed with thiopental: aminophylline, chloramphenicol sodium succinate, hyaluronidase, hydrocortisone sodium succinate, neostigmine methylsulfate, oxytocin, pentobarbital sodium, phenobarbital sodium, potassium chloride, propofol (1:1 mixture), scopolamine HBr, sodium iodide, and tubocurarine chloride (recommendations **conflict** with regard to tubocurarine; some clinicians recommend not mixing with thiopental).

The following agents have been reported to be physically **incompatible** when mixed with thiopental: Ringer's injection, Ringer's injection lactate, amikacin sulfate, atropine sulfate, chlorpromazine, codeine phosphate, dimenhydrinate, diphenhydramine, ephedrine sulfate, glycopyrrolate, hydromorphone, insulin (regular), levorphanol bitartrate, meperidine, metaraminol, morphine sulfate, norepinephrine bitartrate, penicillin G potassium, prochlorperazine edisylate, promazine HCl, promethazine HCl, succinylcholine chloride, and tetracycline HCl. Compatibility is dependent upon factors such as pH, concentration, temperature, and diluent used; consult specialized references or a hospital pharmacist for more specific information.

Dosage Forms/Regulatory Status

VETERINARY-LABELED PRODUCTS:

None presently being marketed in USA.

The ARCI (Racing Commissioners International) has designated this drug as a class 2 substance. See the appendix for more information.

HUMAN-LABELED PRODUCTS:

At the time of writing (February 2011), thiopental is not available for the US market.

Thiopental Sodium Powder for Injection: 2% (20 mg/mL) in 1 gram, 2.5 grams and 5 grams kits; 400 mg *Min-I-Mix* vials with *Min-I-Mix* injector, *Ready-to-Mix* and *Ready-to-MixLifeShield* syringes; 2.5% (25 mg/mL) in 250 mg & 500 mg *Min-I-Mix* vials, 500 mg, 1 gram, 2.5 grams, 5 grams & 10 grams kits, 250 mg and 500 mg *Ready-to-Mix* syringes and *Ready-to-Mix LifeShield* syringes; *Pentothal®* (Abbott); generic; (Rx, C-III)

References

Booth, N.H. (1988). Drugs Acting on the Central Nervous System. *Veterinary Pharmacology and Therapeutics - 6th Ed.* NH Booth and LE McDonald Eds. Ames, Iowa State University Press: 153–408.

Burke, T. (1999). Husbandry and Medicine of Rodents and Lagomorphs. Proceedings: Central Veterinary Conference, Kansas City.

Hellyer, P. (2005). Anesthetic induction drugs. Proceedings: Western Vet Conf. Accessed via: Veterinary Information Network. http://goo.gl/3fD0w

Ivey, E. & J. Morrisey (2000). Therapeutics for Rabbits. *Vet Clin NA: Exotic Anim Pract* **3:1**(Jan): 183–216.

Kaiser-Klingler, S. (2009). Exotic animal anesthesia for the small animal practice. Proceedings: World Veterinary Congress. Accessed via: Veterinary Information Network. http://goo.gl/SdnQy

Mandsager, R.E. (1988, Last Update). "Personal Communication."

Papich, M. (1989). Effects of drugs on pregnancy. *Current Veterinary Therapy X: Small Animal Practice.* R Kirk Ed. Philadelphia, Saunders: 1291–1299.

THIOTEPA

(thye-oh-*tep*-ah)

ANTINEOPLASTIC

Prescriber Highlights

▶ Rarely used antineoplastic for carcinomas (systemic administration), intracavitary for neoplastic effusions, & intravesical for transitional carcinomas

▶ Contraindications: Hypersensitivity to thiotepa; Caution: Hepatic dysfunction, bone marrow depression, infection, tumor cell infiltration of bone marrow, renal dysfunction, or history of urate urinary stones

▶ Adverse Effects: Leukopenia most likely adverse effect; other hematopoietic toxicity (thrombocytopenia, anemia, pancytopenia), GI toxicity possible. Intracavitary or intravesical instillation can also cause hematologic toxicity.

▶ Potentially teratogenic; use milk replacer if patient nursing

▶ Monitor diligently

Uses/Indications

Veterinary indications for thiotepa include: systemic use for adjunctive therapy against carcinomas, and intracavitary use for neoplastic effusions. In dogs with transitional cell bladder carcinoma, intravesical instillation of thiotepa had significantly less efficacy (mean survival time = 57 days) when compared to a systemic doxorubicin/cyclophosphamide protocol (mean survival time = 259 days).

Pharmacology/Actions

Thiotepa is an alkylating agent, thereby interfering with DNA replication and RNA transcription. It is cell cycle non-specific. Thiotepa has some immunosuppressive activity. When given via the intracavitary route, thiotepa is thought to control malignant effusions by a direct antineoplastic effect.

Pharmacokinetics

Thiotepa is poorly absorbed from the GI tract. Systemic absorption is variable from the pleural cavity, bladder, and after IM injection. Some studies in humans have shown that absorption from bladder mucosa ranges from 10–100% of an administered dose. Distribution characteristics are not well described; it is unknown if the drug enters maternal milk. Thiotepa is extensively metabolized and then excreted in the urine.

Contraindications/Precautions/Warnings

Thiotepa is contraindicated in patients hypersensitive to it. The drug should be used cautiously (weigh risk versus benefit) in patients with hepatic dysfunction, bone marrow depression, infection, tumor cell infiltration of bone marrow, renal function impairment (adjust dosage) or with a history of urate urinary stones. Thiotepa has a very low therapeutic index and should only be used by clinicians with experience in the use of cytotoxic agents and able to monitor therapy appropriately.

Adverse Effects

When used systemically, leukopenia is the most likely adverse effect seen in small animals. Other hematopoietic toxicity (thrombocytopenia, anemia, pancytopenia) may be noted. Intracavitary or intravesical instillation of thiotepa may cause hematologic toxicity. GI toxicity (vomiting, diarrhea, stomatitis, intestinal ulceration) may be noted and human patients have reported dizziness and headache as well.

Reproductive/Nursing Safety

Thiotepa is potentially mutagenic and teratogenic and is not recommended for use during pregnancy. In humans, the FDA categorizes this drug as category *D* for use during pregnancy (*There is evidence of human fetal risk, but the potential benefits from the use of the drug in pregnant women may be acceptable despite its potential risks.*)

Although it is unknown whether thiotepa enters milk, use of milk replacer is recommended for nursing bitches or queens.

Overdosage/Acute Toxicity

There is no specific antidote for thiotepa overdose. Supportive therapy, including transfusions of appropriate blood products, may be beneficial for treatment of hematologic toxicity.

Drug Interactions

The following drug interactions have either been reported or are theoretical in humans or animals receiving thiotepa and may be of significance in veterinary patients:

- ◾ **IMMUNOSUPPRESSIVE DRUGS (e.g., azathioprine, cyclophosphamide, corticosteroids):** Use with other immunosuppressant drugs may increase the risk of infection

- ◾ **MYELOSUPPRESSIVE DRUGS (e.g., chloramphenicol, flucytosine, amphotericin B, or colchicine):** Use extreme caution when used concurrently with other drugs that are also myelosuppressive, including many of the other antineoplastics and other bone marrow depressant drugs; bone marrow depression may be additive

- ◾ **VACCINES, LIVE:** Live virus vaccines should be used with caution during therapy, if at all

Laboratory Considerations

- ◾ Thiotepa may increase serum **uric acid** levels in some patients

Doses

- ◾ **DOGS:**

    Note: Because of the potential toxicity of this drug to patients, veterinary personnel and clients, and since chemotherapy indications,

treatment protocols, monitoring and safety guidelines often change, the following dosages should be used only as a general guide. Consultation with a veterinary oncologist and referral to current veterinary oncology references [*e.g.,* (Henry & Higginbotham 2009); (Argyle *et al.* 2008); (Withrow & Vail 2007); (Villalobos 2007); (Ogilvie & Moore 2006); (Ogilvie & Moore 2001)] are *strongly recommended.*

a) For intracavitary use neoplastic effusions or systemically for adjunctive therapy of carcinomas: $0.2–0.5$ mg/m^2 intracavitary; IV. (Jacobs *et al.* 1992)

Monitoring

- ◾ Efficacy
- ◾ CBC with platelets

Client Information

- ◾ Clients must be briefed on the possibilities of severe toxicity developing from this drug, including drug-related neoplasms or mortality
- ◾ Clients should contact veterinarian should the animal exhibit clinical signs of abnormal bleeding, bruising, anorexia, vomiting, jaundice, or infection

Chemistry/Synonyms

An ethylene derivative alkylating agent antineoplastic, thiotepa occurs as fine, white crystalline flakes. The drug has a faint odor and is freely soluble in water or alcohol.

Thiotepa may also be known as: NSC-6396, TESPA, thiophosphamide, triethylenethiophosphoramide, TSPA, WR-45312, *Ledertepa®, Onco Tiotepa®, Tespamin®,* or *Thioplex®.*

Storage/Stability

Store both the powder and the reconstituted solution refrigerated (2–8°C) and protected from light. Do not use solution that is grossly opaque (slightly opaque is OK) or if a precipitate is present. If refrigerated, reconstituted solutions are stable for up to 5 days.

Dosage Forms/Regulatory Status

VETERINARY-LABELED PRODUCTS: None

HUMAN-LABELED PRODUCTS:

Thiotepa Lyophilized Powder for Injection: 15 mg & 30 mg in vials; *Thioplex®* (Amgen); generic, (Sicor); (Rx)

References

Argyle, D., M. Brearly, et al. (2008). *Decision Making in Small Animal Oncology,* Wiley-Blackwell.
Henry, C. & M. Higginbotham (2009). *Cancer Management in Small Animal Practice,* Saunders.
Jacobs, R., J. Lumsden, et al. (1992). Canine and Feline Reference Values. *Current Veterinary Therapy XI: Small Animal Practice.* R Kirk and J Bonagura Eds. Philadelphia, W.B. Saunders Company: 1250–1277.
Ogilvie, G. & A. Moore (2001). *Feline Oncology: A Comprehensive Guide to Compassionate Care,* Veterinary Learning Systems.
Ogilvie, G. & A. Moore (2006). *Managing the Canine Cancer Patient: A Practical Guide to Compassionate Care,* Veterinary Learning Systems.

Villalobos, A. (2007). *Canine and Feline Geriatric Oncology*. Ames, Blackwell.

Withrow, S. & D. Vail (2007). *Withrow and MacEwen's Small Animal Clinical Oncology 4th Ed.* Philadelphia, Elsevier.

THYROTROPIN
THYROTROPIN ALFA
(rhTSH)

(thye-roe-*troe*-pin)
Thyroid Stimulating Hormone, TSH

HORMONE

Prescriber Highlights

▶ Hormone used for thyroid stimulating hormone (TSH) test for thyroid function

▶ Contraindications: Adrenocortical insufficiency, hyperthyroidism, coronary thrombosis, hypersensitivity to bovine thyrotropin

▶ Adverse Effects: Hypersensitivity (especially with repeated injections)

▶ Expense (human product) may be an issue

Uses/Indications

The labeled indications for the formerly available bovine-source veterinary product *Dermathycin®* (Mallinckrodt) was for "the treatment of acanthosis nigricans and for temporary supportive therapy in hypothyroidism in dogs." In actuality however, TSH is used in veterinary medicine principally as a diagnostic agent in the TSH stimulation test to diagnose primary hypothyroidism.

Pharmacology/Actions

Thyrotropin increases iodine uptake by the thyroid gland and increases the production and secretion of thyroid hormones. With prolonged use, hyperplasia of thyroid cells may occur.

Pharmacokinetics

No specific information was located; exogenously administered TSH apparently exerts maximal increases in circulating T_4 approximately 4–8 hours after IM or IV administration.

Contraindications/Precautions/Warnings

A previous veterinary manufacturer (Coopers), listed adrenocortical insufficiency and hyperthyroidism as contraindications to TSH use for treatment purposes in dogs. In humans, TSH is contraindicated in patients with coronary thrombosis, untreated Addison's disease, or hypersensitive to bovine thyrotropin.

Adverse Effects

Because the commercially available product is derived from human sources, hypersensitivity reactions may occur in patients sensitive to human proteins, particularly with repeated use.

Reproductive/Nursing Safety

In humans, the FDA categorizes this drug as category **C** for use during pregnancy (*Animal studies have shown an adverse effect on the fetus, but there are no adequate studies in humans; or there are no animal reproduction studies and no adequate studies in humans.*)

It is not known whether the drug is excreted in milk, but is unlikely to be clinically significant when used for diagnostic purposes.

Overdosage/Acute Toxicity

Chronic administration at high dosages can produce clinical signs of hyperthyroidism. Massive overdoses can cause clinical signs resembling thyroid storm. Refer to the levothyroxine monograph for more information on treatment.

Drug Interactions; Laboratory

Considerations

▪ Refer to the information listed in the Levothyroxine monograph for more information.

Doses

▪ **DOGS:**

For TSH stimulation test:

a) Using the human recombinant product. From a study where dogs received 75 micrograms (total dose) IV. Blood samples were taken before and 6 hours after rhTSH administration for determination of total serum thyroxine (T4) concentration. The authors concluded: The TSH-stimulation test with rhTSH is a valuable diagnostic tool to assess thyroid function in selected dogs in which a diagnosis of hypothyroidism cannot be based on basal T4 and canine TSH concentrations alone. (Boretti *et al.* 2006)

b) Using the human recombinant product: 50–100 micrograms (0.05–0.1 mg) IV; Measure serum T_4 at 0 hours (pre-sample) and 4 hours post. Product may be frozen for at least 8 weeks with no loss of potency. (Scott-Moncrieff 2006)

▪ **BIRDS:**

For TSH stimulation test:

a) Draw pre-dose baseline sample. Administer 1 Unit/kg IM. Collect sample for T_4 6 hours after dose. (Greenacre 2009)

Chemistry/Synonyms

Commercially available thyrotropin (human; rhTSH) is now available only as a lyophilized powder for reconstitution obtained via DNA recombinant technology. Originally obtained from bovine anterior pituitary glands, thyrotropin is a highly purified preparation of thyroid-stimulating hormone (TSH). Thyrotropin is a glycoprotein and has a molecular weight of approximately 28,000–30,000. Thyrotropin is measured in International Units (IU), which is abbreviated as Units in this reference. 7.5 micrograms of thyrotropin are approximately equivalent to 0.037 Units.

Thyrotropin may also be known as: thyroid-stimulating hormone, thyrotrophic hormone, thyrotropin, TSH, *Ambinon®, Thyreostimulin®, Thyrogen®,* or *Thytropar®.*

Storage/Stability

Thyrotropin alfa (unreconstituted) should be stored between 2–8°C (36–46°F). If necessary, the reconstituted solution can be stored up to 24 hours between 2–8°C (36–46°F), while avoiding microbial contamination. However, it is reportedly stable if kept refrigerated (2–8°C) up to 4 weeks and up to 8 weeks if frozen (-20°C).

After reconstitution visually inspect each vial for particulate matter or discoloration before use. Do not use any vial exhibiting particulate matter or discoloration. Do not use after the expiration date on the vial. Protect from light.

Dosage Forms/Regulatory Status

VETERINARY-LABELED PRODUCTS: None

HUMAN-LABELED PRODUCTS:

Recombinant (human) Thyrotropin (Thyroid Stimulating Hormone) Powder for Injection, Lyophilized: 1.1 mg per vial; *Thyrogen®* (Genzyme); (Rx)

References

Boretti, F.S., N.S. Sieber-Ruckstuhl, et al. (2006). Evaluation of recombinant human thyroid-stimulating hormone to test thyroid function in dogs suspected of having hypothyroidism. *American Journal of Veterinary Research* 67(12): 2012–2016.

Greenacre, C. (2009). Diagnostic Testing in the Field: The Researcher's Prospective on Thyroid Testing in Psittacine Birds. Proceedings: AAV. Accessed via: Veterinary Information Network. http://goo.gl/du7Wc

Scott-Moncrieff, J. (2006). Diagnosis and Treatment of Canine Hypothyroidism and Thyroiditis. Proceedings: ACVC. Accessed via: Veterinary Information Network. http://goo.gl/goI9N

Thyroxine Sodium See Levothyroxine Sodium

TIAMULIN

(tye-*am*-myoo-lin)   Denagard®

DITERPINE PLEUROMUTILIN ANTIBIOTIC

Prescriber Highlights

▶ Antibiotic used primarily in swine

▶ Contraindications: Access to feeds containing polyether ionophores (*e.g.,* monensin, lasalocid, narasin, or salinomycin); swine over 250 pounds

▶ Adverse Effects are unlikely

▶ Variable withdrawal times depending on dosage

Uses/Indications

Tiamulin is FDA-approved for use in swine to treat pneumonia caused by susceptible strains of *Haemophilus pleuropneumoniae* and swine dysentery caused by *Treponema hyodysenteriae.* As a feed additive, it is used to cause increased weight gain in swine.

Pharmacology/Actions

Tiamulin is a pleuromutilin antibiotic that is usually bacteriostatic, but can be bactericidal in very high concentrations against susceptible organisms. The drug acts by binding to the 50S ribosomal subunit, thereby inhibiting bacterial protein synthesis.

Tiamulin has good activity against many gram-positive cocci, including most Staphylococci and Streptococci (not group D streps). It also has good activity against Mycoplasma and spirochetes. With the exception of *Haemophilus* spp. and some *E. coli* and Klebsiella strains, the drug's activity is quite poor against gram-negative organisms.

Pharmacokinetics

Tiamulin is well absorbed orally by swine. Approximately 85% of a dose is absorbed and peak levels occur between 2–4 hours after a single oral dose. Tiamulin is apparently well distributed, with highest levels found in the lungs.

Tiamulin is extensively metabolized to over 20 metabolites, some having antibacterial activity. Approximately 30% of these metabolites are excreted in the urine with the remainder excreted in the feces.

Contraindications/Precautions/Warnings

Tiamulin should not be administered to animals having access to feeds containing polyether ionophores (*e.g.,* monensin, lasalocid, narasin, or salinomycin) as adverse reactions may occur. Not for use in swine over 250 pounds.

Reproductive/Nursing Safety

Teratogenicity studies done in rodents demonstrated no teratogenic effects at doses up to 300 mg/kg. The manufacturer has concluded that the drug is not tumorigenic, carcinogenic, teratogenic, or mutagenic.

Adverse Effects

Adverse effects occurring with this drug at usual doses are considered unlikely. Rarely, redness of the skin, primarily over the ham and underline, has been observed. It is recommended to discontinue the medication, provide clean drinking water, and hose down the area or move affected animals to clean pens.

Overdosage/Acute Toxicity

Oral overdoses in pigs may cause transient salivation, vomiting, and CNS depression (calming effect). Discontinue drug and treat symptomatically and supportively if necessary.

Drug Interactions

◼ **POLYETHER IONOPHORES (*e.g.,* monensin, lasalocid, narasin, or salinomycin):** Tiamulin should not be administered to animals having access to feeds containing polyether ionophores as adverse reactions may occur

■ **LINCOSAMIDES, MACROLIDES (e.g., clindamycin, lincomycin, erythromycin, tylosin):** Although not confirmed with this drug, concomitant use with other antibiotics that bind to the 50S ribosome could lead to decreased efficacy secondary to competition at the site of action

Doses

■ **SWINE:**

a) For swine dysentery: 7.7 mg/kg PO daily in drinking water for 5 days. See package directions for dilution instructions. (Package insert; *Denagard® Liquid Concentrate*)

b) For swine pneumonia: 23.1 mg/kg PO daily in drinking water for 5 days. See package directions for dilution instructions. (Package insert; *Denagard® Liquid Concentrate*)

c) For use as a medicated premix: See the label for the product.

Monitoring

■ Clinical efficacy

Client Information

■ Prepare fresh medicated water daily

■ Avoid contact with skin or mucous membranes as irritation may occur

Chemistry/Synonyms

A semisynthetic diterpene-class antibiotic derived from pleuromulin, tiamulin is available commercially for oral use as the hydrogen fumarate salt. It occurs as white to yellow, crystalline powder with a faint but characteristic odor. Approximately 60 mg of the drug are soluble in 1 mL of water.

Tiamulin may also be known as: 81723-hfu, SQ-14055, SQ-22947 (tiamulin fumarate), and *Denagard®*.

Storage/Stability

Protect from moisture; store in a dry place. In unopened packets, the powder is stable up to 5 years. Fresh solutions should be prepared daily when using clinically.

Dosage Forms/Regulatory Status

VETERINARY APPROVED PRODUCTS:

Tiamulin Medicated Premix: 10 grams/1 lb in 35 lb bags. FDA-approved for use in swine not weighing over 250 lbs. Slaughter withdrawal period at the 35 grams/ton use is 2 days and at the 200 grams/ton dose is 7 days. *Denagard® 10* (Novartis); (OTC).

Tiamulin Solution: 12.3% tiamulin hydrogen fumarate in an aqueous base in 32 oz bottles. FDA-approved for use in swine. Slaughter withdrawal: treatment at 3.5 mg/lb = 3 days, at 10.5 mg/lb = 7 days. *Denagard® Liquid Concentrate* (Boehringer Ingelheim); *TiaGard®* (Teva); (OTC)

Tiamulin Soluble Powder: 45% in 2.28 oz packets (29.1 gram tiamulin per packet). FDA-approved for use in swine. Slaughter withdrawal: treatment at 3.5 mg/lb = 3 days, at 10.5 mg/lb = 7 days. *Denagard® Liquid Concentrate* (Boehringer Ingelheim); *TiaGard®* (Teva); (OTC)

There is also a chlortetracycline/tiamulin premix approved by the FDA.

HUMAN APPROVED PRODUCTS: None

TICARCILLIN DISODIUM + CLAVULANATE POTASSIUM

(tye-kar-*sill*-in; klav-yoo-*lan*-ate)
Timentin®

PARENTERAL EXTENDED SPECTRUM
PENICILLIN + BETA-LACTAMASE
INHIBITOR

Prescriber Highlights

▶ Parenteral, extended action penicillin with a beta lactamase inhibitor; has increased spectrum of activity when compared with ticarcillin alone, but is more expensive

▶ Used for serious systemic infections & as a compounded otic prep for Pseudomonas otitis

▶ Limited experience or research in veterinary medicine, but appears quite safe

▶ Patients with significantly impaired renal function or those receiving very high dosages may be more prone to develop platelet function abnormalities (bleeding) or CNS effects

Uses/Indications

Ticarcillin/clavulanate is used systemically to treat serious infections such as sepsis or nosocomial pneumonias in dogs, cats and horses. By adding clavulanate, enhanced spectrum of activity against beta-lactamase producing bacteria can be obtained. This drug combination is sometimes used to treat Pseudomonas otitis in dogs.

Pharmacology/Actions

Penicillins are usually bactericidal against susceptible bacteria and act by inhibiting mucopeptide synthesis in the cell wall resulting in a defective barrier and an osmotically unstable spheroplast. The exact mechanism for this effect has not been definitively determined, but beta-lactam antibiotics have been shown to bind to several enzymes (carboxypeptidases, transpeptidases, endopeptidases) within the bacterial cytoplasmic membrane that are involved with cell wall synthesis. The different affinities that various beta-lactam antibiotics have for these enzymes (also known as penicillin-binding proteins; PBPs) help explain the differences in spectrums of activity the drugs have that are not explained by the influence of beta-lactamases. Like other beta-lactam antibiotics, penicillins are generally considered more effective against actively growing bacteria.

The extended-spectrum penicillins, sometimes called anti-pseudomonal penicillins, include both alpha-carboxypenicillins (carbenicillin and ticarcillin) and acylaminopenicillins (piperacillin, azlocillin, and mezlocillin). These agents have similar spectrums of activity as the aminopenicillins but with additional activity against several gram-negative organisms of the family Enterobacteriaceae, including many strains of *Pseudomonas aeruginosa*. Like the aminopenicillins, these agents are susceptible to inactivation by beta-lactamases.

By adding clavulanate, ticarcillin's efficacy can be extended against beta-lactamase-producing strains of otherwise resistant *E. coli*, *Pasturella* spp., *Staphylococcus* spp., Klebsiella, and Proteus. Clavulanic acid acts by competitively and irreversibly binding to beta-lactamases, including types II, III, IV, and V, and penicillinases produced by Staphylococcus. Type I beta-lactamases that are often associated with *E. coli*, Enterobacter, and Pseudomonas are not generally inhibited by clavulanic acid.

Clavulanic acid has only weak antibacterial activity when used alone and at present is only available in fixed-dose combinations with either amoxicillin (oral) or ticarcillin (parenteral). Unlike sulbactam or tazobactam, clavulanic acid (clavulanate) can induce chromosomal beta-lactamases.

Synergy against *Pseudomonas aeruginosa* can occur when used with an aminoglycoside, but the drugs cannot be mixed together (see Drug Interactions).

Pharmacokinetics

Ticarcillin is not appreciably absorbed after oral administration and must be given parenterally to achieve therapeutic serum levels. When given IM to humans, the drug is readily absorbed with peak levels occurring about 30–60 minutes after dosing. The reported bioavailability in the horse after IM administration is about 65%.

After parenteral injection, ticarcillin is distributed into pleural fluid, interstitial fluid, bile, sputum, and bone. Like other penicillins, CSF levels are low in patients with normal meninges (about 6% of serum levels), but increased (39% of serum levels) if meninges are inflamed. The volume of distribution is reportedly 0.34 L/kg in dogs and 0.22–0.25 L/kg in the horse. The drug is 45–65% bound to serum proteins (human). Ticarcillin is thought to cross the placenta and found in small quantities in milk. In cattle, mastitic milk levels of ticarcillin are approximately twice those found in normal milk, but are too low to treat most causal organisms.

Ticarcillin is eliminated primarily by the kidneys, via both tubular secretion and glomerular filtration. Concurrent probenecid administration can slow elimination and increase blood levels. In humans, about 10–15% of the drug is metabolized by hydrolysis to inactive compounds. The half-life in dogs and cats is reportedly 45–80 minutes; about 54 minutes in the horse. Clearance is 4.3 mL/kg/min in the dog and 2.8–3.2 mL/kg/min in the horse.

There is no evidence to suggest that the addition of clavulanic acid alters ticarcillin pharmacokinetics.

Clavulanic acid has an apparent volume of distribution of 0.32 L/kg in dogs and is distributed (with ticarcillin) into the lungs, pleural fluid and peritoneal fluid. Low concentrations of both drugs are found in the saliva, sputum and CSF (uninflamed meninges). Higher concentrations in the CSF are expected when meninges are inflamed, but it is questionable whether therapeutic levels are attainable. Clavulanic acid is 13% bound to proteins in dog serum.

Clavulanic acid is extensively metabolized in the dog (and rat) primarily to 1-amino-4-hydroxybutan-2-one. It is not known if this compound possesses any beta-lactamase inhibiting activity. Clavulanic acid is also excreted unchanged in the urine via glomerular filtration. In dogs, 34–52% of a dose is excreted in the urine as unchanged drug and metabolites, 25–27% in the feces, and 16–33% into respired air. The elimination half-life for clavulanic acid in dogs is faster than is ticarcillin.

Contraindications/Precautions/Warnings

Do not use this medication in patients with documented hypersensitivity reactions to penicillins or other beta-lactams.

Dosage adjustments should be made in patients with significantly impaired renal function.

Adverse Effects

Although clinical experience with this medication in veterinary patients is limited, it appears to be well tolerated; potentially, hypersensitivity reactions can occur. In humans, high dosages (particularly in patients with renal insufficiency) have caused platelet dysfunction and bleeding, and CNS effects (headache, giddiness, hallucinations, seizures). Intramuscular administration can cause pain, but reconstituting with 1% lidocaine (see Storage/Stability) can alleviate this effect. Local irritation to veins after IV administration is possible and best avoided by using dilute concentrations administered over not less than 30 minutes.

Antibiotic-associated diarrhea or colitis may occur.

Reproductive/Nursing Safety

Penicillins have been shown to cross the placenta and safe use during pregnancy has not been firmly established, but neither have there been any documented teratogenic problems associated with these drugs; however, use only when the potential benefits outweigh the risks. In humans, the FDA categorizes ticarcillin/clavulanate as category *B* for use during pregnancy (*Animal studies have not yet demonstrated risk to the fetus, but there are no adequate studies in pregnant women; or animal studies have shown an adverse effect, but adequate studies in pregnant women have not demonstrated a risk to the fetus in the first trimester of pregnancy, and there is no evidence of risk in later trimesters.*)

Although penicillins can be distributed into milk, it is unlikely that ticarcillin/clavulanate would be of significant clinical concern for nursing veterinary patients.

Overdosage/Acute Toxicity
A single inadvertent overdose is unlikely to cause significant morbidity. In humans, very high dosages of parenteral penicillins such as ticarcillin, especially in patients with renal disease, have induced CNS effects (hallucinations, headaches, seizures) and alterations in platelet function (bleeding).

Drug Interactions
The following drug interactions have either been reported or are theoretical in humans or animals receiving ticarcillin/clavulanate and may be of significance in veterinary patients:

- **AMINOGLYCOSIDES (e.g., amikacin, gentamicin, tobramycin):** *In vitro* studies have demonstrated that penicillins can have synergistic or additive activity against certain bacteria when used with aminoglycosides. However, beta-lactam antibiotics can inactivate aminoglycosides *in vitro* and *in vivo* in patients in renal failure or when penicillins are used in massive dosages. Amikacin is considered the most resistant aminoglycoside to this inactivation.

- **PROBENECID:** Can reduce the renal tubular secretion of ticarcillin, thereby maintaining higher systemic levels for a longer period of time; it does not affect the elimination of clavulanate

- **WARFARIN; HEPARIN:** As ticarcillin has been implicated in rarely causing bleeding, use with caution in patients receiving anticoagulant therapy

Laboratory Considerations
- **Aminoglycoside serum quantitative analysis:** As penicillins and other beta-lactams can inactivate aminoglycosides *in vitro* (and *in vivo* in patients in renal failure or when penicillins are used in massive dosages), serum concentrations of aminoglycosides may be falsely decreased if the patient is also receiving beta-lactam antibiotics and the serum is stored prior to analysis. It is recommended that if the aminoglycoside assay is delayed, samples be frozen and, if possible, drawn at times when the beta-lactam antibiotic is at a trough.

- **Direct antiglobulin (Coombs') tests:** False-positive results may occur

- **Urine protein:** May produce false-positive protein results with the sulfosalicylic acid and boiling test, nitric acid test, and the acetic acid test. Strips using bromophenol blue reagent (*e.g., Multi-Stix®*) do not appear to be affected by high levels of penicillins in the urine

Doses
Note: Unless otherwise indicated, this drug combination is dosed on the basis of ticarcillin content.

- **DOGS:**
  - a) For sepsis: 40–50 mg/kg q6–8h IV (Hardie 2000)
  - b) 15–50 mg/kg q6–8h IV, IM or SC (Lappin 2003)

    For *Pseudomonas* sepsis/bacteremia: 20–50 mg/kg IV q6–8h (Greene *et al.* 2006)
  - c) As an otic solution for adjunctive treatment of Pseudomonas otitis using the ticarcillin/clavulanic acid product—*Timentin®*): Dilute according to manufacturer's directions, then draw into 2 mL aliquots and freeze. Thaw and use each aliquot as 0.5 mL in each ear, twice daily. (White 2003)

- **CATS:**
  - a) For sepsis: 40–50 mg/kg q6–8h IV (Hardie 2000)
  - b) For *Pseudomonas* sepsis/bacteremia: 40 mg/kg IV q6h (Greene *et al.* 2006)
  - c) 50 mg/kg IV or IM 4 times daily; may need more frequent dosing or constant rate infusion for resistant Pseudomonas infections (Trepanier 1999)
  - d) 15–50 mg/kg q6–8h IV, IM or SC (Lappin 2003)

- **HORSES:**
  For susceptible infections:
  - a) 50 mg/kg IV q6h (Bertone 2003)
  - b) Foals (neonatal septicemia): 40–60 mg/kg IV or IM q8h (Paradis 2003)
  - c) Foals: 50 mg/kg IV or IM q6–8h (Brumbaugh 1999)
  - d) For intrauterine infusion: 3–6 grams with a minimum of 200 mL of saline. Mares need to be treated frequently (every 4–6 h) in order to maintain drug concentrations above MIC. (LeBlanc 2009)

Monitoring
- Efficacy for the infection treated (WBC, clinical signs, etc.)

- Serum levels and therapeutic drug monitoring are not routinely performed with this drug

Client Information

■ Limited experience in veterinary medicine when used systemically

■ Best suited for inpatient use

Chemistry/Synonyms

An alpha-carboxypenicillin, ticarcillin disodium occurs as a white to pale yellow, hygroscopic powder or lyophilized cake with pK_as of 2.55 and 3.42. More than 600 mg is soluble in 1 mL of water. Potency of ticarcillin disodium is expressed in terms of ticarcillin and one gram of the disodium contains not less than 800 mg of ticarcillin anhydrous. One gram of the commercially available injection contains 5.2–6.5 mEq of sodium.

A beta-lactamase inhibitor, clavulanate potassium occurs as an off-white, crystalline powder that has a pK_a of 2.7 (as the acid) and is very soluble in water and slightly soluble in alcohol at room temperatures. Although available commercially as the potassium salt, potency is expressed in terms of clavulanic acid.

Ticarcillin Disodium may also be known as: BRL-2288, or ticarcillinum natricum. Clavulanate potassium may also be known by the following synonyms: clavulanic acid, BRL-14151K, or kalii clavulanas. International trade names for ticarcillin/clavulanate include *Timentin®* and *Claventin®*.

Storage/Stability

Unused vials should be stored at room temperature (below 24°C, 75°F).

A darkening of the sterile powder or solution indicates degradation and loss of potency of clavulanate.

For IM use, reconstitute vial with 2 mL of sterile water for injection, sodium chloride for injection, or 1% lidocaine (without epinephrine) per gram of ticarcillin. Each mL of the resulting solution will contain approximately 385 mg/mL (1 gram per 2.6 mL) ticarcillin. For humans, IM injections are recommended to be made into a relatively large muscle and not to administer more than one gram (2.6 mL) IM per injection site.

For IV use, initially reconstitute 3.1 gram vials with 13 mL of sodium chloride injection, dextrose 5% or LRS. Resulting solution will contain approximately 200 mg of ticarcillin per mL. If administered IV at this concentration, give as slowly as possible. Ideally, dilute further to a concentration of 10–100 mg (ticarcillin)/mL with a suitable diluent (*e.g.*, NS, LRS, D5W). Concentrations of 50 mg/mL or less will cause less vein irritation; the solution should be administered as slowly as possible (over at least 30 minutes).

When vials are reconstituted (as above) to 200 mg/mL, the resulting solution is stable for 6 hours at room temperature and 72 hours when refrigerated. Stability for solutions diluted for IV infusion (10–100 mg/mL):

Diluent	Room Temp	Refrigerated	Frozen
NS	24 hrs	7 days	30 days
D5W	24 hrs	3 days	7 days
LRS	24 hrs	7 days	30 days

All thawed solutions should be used within 8 hours and not refrozen.

Compatibility/Compounding Considerations

Ticarcillin/clavulanate should **not** be mixed with aminoglycosides (*e.g.*, gentamicin, amikacin) and **may not be compatible** when infused at a Y-site with solutions containing amphotericin B cholesteryl sulfate complex, azithromycin, or vancomycin. Y-site **compatible** drugs include (partial listing): propofol, dexmetomidine, cefepime, diltiazem, doxorubicin HCl liposomes, etoposide, famotidine, fluconazole, heparin sodium, hetastarch, regular insulin, meperidine, morphine sulfate, and ondansetron.

Dosage Forms/Regulatory Status

VETERINARY-LABELED PRODUCTS: None

HUMAN-LABELED PRODUCTS:

Ticarcillin Disodium Powder for Injection (contains 4.75 mEq sodium/g) and Clavulanate Potassium (contains 0.15 mEq potassium/g): 3 grams ticarcillin and 0.1 gram clavulanic acid in 3.1 gram vials, piggyback bottles, ADD-Vantage vials, 100 mL premixed, frozen Galaxy plastic containers, and 31 gram pharmacy bulk packages; *Timentin®* (GlaxoSmithKline); (Rx)

Ticarcillin Powder for Injection (contains 18.7 mEq sodium/100 mL) and Clavulanate Potassium (contains 0.5 mEq potassium/100 mL): 3 grams ticarcillin and 0.1 gram clavulanic acid/100 mL in; *Timentin®* (GlaxoSmithKline); (Rx)

Ticarcillin (alone) has now been discontinued.

References

Bertone, J. (2003). Rational antibiotic choices. Proceedings: Western Veterinary Conf. Accessed via: Veterinary Information Network. http://goo.gl/MxKfS

Brumbaugh, G. (1999). Clinical Pharmacology and the Pediatric Patient. 45th Annual AAEP Convention, Albuquerque.

Greene, C., K. Hartmannn, et al. (2006). Appendix 8: Antimicrobial Drug Formulary. *Infectious Disease of the Dog and Cat*. C Greene Ed., Elsevier: 1186–1333.

Hardie, E. (2000). Therapeutic Mangement of Sepsis. *Kirk's Current Veterinary Therapy: XIII Small Animal Practice*. J Bonagura Ed. Philadelphia, WB Saunders: 272–275.

Lappin, M. (2003). Practical Antimicrobial Chemotherapy. *Small Animal Internal Medicine, 3rd Ed*. R Nelson and C Couto Eds. St Louis, Mosby: 1240–1249.

LeBlanc, M.M. (2009). The current status of antibiotic use in equine reproduction. *Equine Veterinary Education* 21(3): 156–167.

Paradis, M. (2003). Neonatal Septicemia. *Current Therapy in Equine Medicine 5*. N Robinson Ed., Elsevier: 656–665.

Trepanier, L. (1999). Treating resistant infections in small animals. Proceedings: 17th Annual American College of Veterinary Internal Medicine Meeting, Chicago.

White, S. (2003). Medical treatment of otitis externa. Proceedings: World Small Animal Vet Assoc World Congress. Accessed via: Veterinary Information Network. http://goo.gl/hE5TM

TILETAMINE HCL/ ZOLAZEPAM HCL

(tye-*let*-a-meen and zoe-*laze*-a-pam)
Telazol®

INJECTABLE ANESTHETIC/
TRANQUILIZER

Prescriber Highlights

▶ Injectable anesthetic/tranquilizer combination similar to ketamine/diazepam

▶ Contraindications: Pancreatic disease, rabbits, severe cardiac disease, use in cesarean section, or pulmonary disease

▶ Caution: Renal disease, large exotic cats, especially tigers (use avoided)

▶ Protect patient's eyes after using

▶ Dosages may need to be reduced in geriatric, debilitated, or animals with renal dysfunction

▶ Adverse Effects: Respiratory depression, pain after IM injection, athetoid movements, tachycardia (esp. dogs), emesis during emergence, excessive salivation & bronchial/tracheal secretions, transient apnea, vocalization, erratic &/or prolonged recovery, involuntary muscular twitching, hypertonia, cyanosis, cardiac arrest, pulmonary edema, muscle rigidity, & either hypertension or hypotension

▶ Monitor body temperature (may cause hypothermia)

▶ Class-III controlled substance

▶ Cost and shelf-life may be issues

Uses/Indications

Telazol® is indicated for restraint or anesthesia combined with muscle relaxation in cats, and for restraint and minor procedures of short duration ($\approx$30 minutes) which require mild to moderate analgesia in dogs. Although not officially FDA-approved, it has been used also in horses and many exotic and wild species.

Pharmacology/Actions

In cats, tiletamine decreases cardiac rate and blood pressure after IM injections. Its effect on respiratory activity is controversial, and until these effects have been clarified, respiratory function should be closely monitored. The pharmacology of this drug combination is similar to that of ketamine and diazepam; for more information, refer to their monographs.

Pharmacokinetics

Little pharmacokinetic information is available for these agents. The onset of action may be variable and be very rapid; animals should be observed carefully after injection.

In cats, the onset of action is reported to be within 1–7 minutes after IM injection. Duration of anesthesia is dependent on dosage, but is usually about 0.33–1 hour at peak effect. This is reported to be approximately 3 times the duration of ketamine anesthesia. The duration of effect of the zolazepam component is longer than that of the tiletamine, so there is a greater degree of tranquilization than anesthesia during the recovery period. The recovery times vary in length from approximately 1–5.5 hours. Reported elimination half-life for tiletamine is 2.5 hours and 4.5 hours for zolazepam.

In dogs, the onset of action following IM injection averages 7.5 minutes. The mean duration of surgical anesthesia is about 27 minutes, with recovery times averaging approximately 4 hours. The duration of the tiletamine effect is longer than that of zolazepam, so there is a shorter duration of tranquilization than there is anesthesia. Less than 4% of the drugs are reported excreted unchanged in the urine in the dog. Reported elimination half-life for tiletamine is 2.5 hours and 1.5 hours for zolazepam.

Contraindications/Precautions/Warnings

Telazol® is contraindicated in animals with pancreatic disease, or severe cardiac or pulmonary disease. Animals with renal disease may have prolonged duration of anesthetic action or recovery times.

Because *Telazol*® may cause hypothermia, susceptible animals (small body surface area, low ambient temperatures) should be monitored carefully and supplemental heat applied if needed. Like ketamine, *Telazol*® does not abolish pinnal, palpebral, pedal, laryngeal, and pharyngeal reflexes and its use (alone) may not be adequate if surgery is to be performed on these areas.

It has been reported that this drug is contraindicated in rabbits due to renal toxicity.

Telazol® is generally avoided for use in large, exotic cats (contraindicated in tigers) as it may cause seizures, permanent neurologic abnormalities, or death.

Cats' eyes remain open after receiving *Telazol*®, and they should be protected from injury and an ophthalmic lubricant (*e.g.,* *Lacrilube*®) should be applied to prevent excessive drying of the cornea. Cats reportedly do not tolerate endotracheal tubes well with this agent.

Dosages may need to be reduced in geriatric, debilitated, or animals with renal dysfunction.

Adverse Effects

Respiratory depression is a definite possibility, especially with higher dosages of this product. Apnea may occur; observe animal carefully. Pain after IM injection (especially in cats) has been noted which may be a result of the low pH of the solution. Athetoid movements (constant succession of slow, writhing, involuntary movements of flexion, extension, pronation, etc.) may occur;

do not give additional *Telazol®* in the attempt to diminish these actions. Large doses given SC or IM, versus small doses given IV, may result in longer, rougher recoveries.

In dogs, tachycardia may be a common effect and last for 30 minutes. Insufficient anesthesia after recommended doses has been reported in dogs.

Telazol® has been implicated in causing nephrosis in lagamorphs (rabbits/hares) and is usually not recommended for use in these species.

Other adverse effects listed by the manufacturer include: emesis during emergence, excessive salivation and bronchial/tracheal secretions (if atropine not administered beforehand), transient apnea, vocalization, erratic and/or prolonged recovery, involuntary muscular twitching, hypertonia, cyanosis, cardiac arrest, pulmonary edema, muscle rigidity, and either hypertension or hypotension.

Reproductive/Nursing Safety

Telazol® crosses the placenta and may cause respiratory depression in newborns; the manufacturer lists its use in cesarean section as being contraindicated. The teratogenic potential of the drug is unknown, and it is not recommended for use during any stage of pregnancy.

Overdosage/Acute Toxicity

The manufacturer claims a 2X margin of safety in dogs, and a 4.5X margin of safety in cats. A preliminary study in dogs (Hatch et al. 1988) suggests that doxapram at 5.5 mg/kg will enhance respirations and arousal after *Telazol®*. In massive overdoses, it is suggested that mechanically assisted ventilation be performed if necessary and other clinical signs treated symptomatically and supportively.

High doses of tiletamine have caused acute tubular necrosis in New Zealand white rabbits.

Drug Interactions

Little specific information is available presently on drug interactions with this product.

- **ANESTHETICS, INHALATIONAL:** Dosage may need to be reduced when used concomitantly with *Telazol®*
- **BARBITURATES:** Dosage may need to be reduced when used concomitantly with *Telazol®*
- **CHLORAMPHENICOL:** In dogs, chloramphenicol apparently has no effect on recovery times with *Telazol®*, but in cats, anesthesia is prolonged on average of 30 minutes by chloramphenicol.
- **PHENOTHIAZINES:** Can cause increased respiratory and cardiac depression

For potential additional interactions from the related compounds, ketamine and midazolam:

Ketamine:

- **NEUROMUSCULAR BLOCKERS (e.g., succinylcholine and tubocurarine):** May cause enhanced or prolonged respiratory depression

- **THYROID HORMONES:** When given concomitantly with ketamine, thyroid hormones have induced hypertension and tachycardia in humans; beta-blockers (*e.g.*, **propranolol**) may be of benefit in treating these effects

Midazolam:

- **ANESTHETICS, INHALATIONAL:** Midazolam may decrease the dosages required
- **AZOLE ANTIFUNGALS (ketoconazole, itraconazole, fluconazole):** May increase midazolam levels
- **CALCIUM CHANNEL BLOCKERS (diltiazem, verapamil):** May increase midazolam levels
- **CIMETIDINE:** May increase midazolam levels
- **CNS DEPRESSANTS, OTHER:** May increase the risk of respiratory depression
- **MACROLIDES (erythromycin, clarithromycin):** May increase midazolam levels
- **OPIATES:** May increase the hypnotic effects of midazolam and hypotension has been reported when used with meperidine.
- **PHENOBARBITAL:** May decrease peak levels and AUC of midazolam
- **RIFAMPIN:** May decrease peak levels and AUC of midazolam
- **THIOPENTAL:** Midazolam may decrease the dosages required

Doses

- **DOGS:**
  a) For diagnostic purposes: 6.6–9.9 mg/kg IM

     For minor procedures of short duration: 9.9–13.2 mg/kg IM;

     If supplemental doses are necessary, give doses less than the initial dose and total dosage should not exceed 26.4 mg/kg. Atropine 0.04 mg/kg should be used concurrently to control hypersalivation. (Package Insert; *Telazol®*—Robins)

  b) Based upon the combination of drugs: 3–10 mg/kg IM or SC or 2–5 mg/kg IV (Mama 2002)

  c) For aggressive (difficult to handle) dogs that require more sedation and only if insufficient sedation from opioid, higher dose medetomidine, and midazolam: 1–2 mg/kg IM. (Moffat 2008)

- **CATS:**
  a) 9.7–11.9 mg/kg IM for procedures such as dentistry, abscess treatment, foreign body removal, etc. For procedures that require mild to moderate levels of analgesia (lacerations, castration, etc.) use 10.6–12.5 mg/kg IM.

     For ovariohysterectomy and onychectomy use 14.3–15.8 mg/kg IM.

     If supplemental doses are necessary, give doses less than the initial dose and the total dosage should not exceed 72 mg/kg.

Atropine 0.04 mg/kg should be used concurrently to control hypersalivation. (Package Insert; *Telazol®*—Robins)

b) Based upon the combination of drugs: 3–10 mg/kg IM or SC or 2–5 mg/kg IV (Mama 2002)

■ **RUMINANTS:**
As an induction agent for cattle, llamas/alpacas, goats, sheep:

a) Xylazine at 0.05–0.1 mg/kg IV, IM, then *Telazol®* at 2–4 mg/kg IV (IM). Caution: xylazine can cause severe hypoxemia and pulmonary edema in sheep. (Haskell 2005)

b) **Llamas:** 4.7–6 mg/kg IM. (Wolff 2009)

■ **RABBITS, RODENTS, SMALL MAMMALS:**
For chemical restraint:

a) **Gerbils:** 20 mg/kg IP (in combination with xylazine 10 mg/kg) (Huerkamp 1995)

b) **Mice:** 80–100 mg/kg IM.
Rats: 20–60 mg/kg IM.
Hamsters/Gerbils: 20–80 mg/kg IM.
Guinea pig: 10–80 mg/kg IM.
Rabbits: Not recommended (Burke 1999)

c) **Chinchillas:** 20–40 mg/kg IM.
Hamsters: 50–80 mg/kg IP for immobilization/anesthesia.
Gerbils: 10–30 mg/kg IP.
Mice: 80 mg/kg IP for immobilization
Rats: 40 mg/kg IP for light anesthesia.
Guinea pigs: 40–60 mg/kg IM for immobilization (Adamcak & Otten 2000)

d) **Small rodents:** 6–10 mg/kg IM is adequate prior to inhalation anesthesia. Advantages over ketamine include better muscle relaxation, small volume of injection, rapid induction time and a wide margin of safety. Disadvantages of this drug combination are increased respiratory secretions, variability in recovery times, and short self-life after reconstitution. (Bennett 2009)

■ **FERRETS:**
As a sedative/analgesic:

a) 22 mg/kg IM combined with glycopyrrolate (0.01 mg/kg IM). Rapid onset, but slow and rough recovery (3–4 hours) (Finkler 1999)

b) *Telazol®* alone: 22 mg/kg IM;
Telazol® (1.5 mg/kg) plus xylazine (1.5 mg/kg) IM; may reverse xylazine with yohimbine (0.05 mg/kg IM)
Telazol® (1.5 mg/kg) plus butorphanol (1.5 mg/kg) plus xylazine (0.2 mg/kg) IM; may reverse xylazine with yohimbine (0.05 mg/kg IM) (Williams 2000)

c) 22 mg/kg IM. (Kaiser-Klingler 2009)

■ **HORSES:** (**Note:** ARCI UCGFS Class 2 Drug)

a) Xylazine 1.1 mg/kg IV, 5 minutes prior to *Telazol®* at 1.65–2.2 mg/kg IV (Hubbell *et al.* 1989)

■ **REPTILES:**

a) Large Snakes: 3 mg/kg IM to facilitate handling and anesthesia. Administer 30–45 minutes prior to handling. Sedation may persist for up to 48 hours. May also be used in Crocodilians at 4–8 mg/kg. (Heard 1999)

b) 3–10 mg/kg IM. Lizards and snakes can generally be treated with lower end of dosage range and chelonians may require high end. If sedation is inadequate, may give incrementally up to the maximum dose. Monitor closely for apnea and ventilate if required. (Innis 2003)

c) Significant interspecies and interpatient differences in effectiveness. At lower doses of 4–10 mg/kg sedation may be sufficient for some procedures (venipuncture, gastric lavage, intubation for inhalation anesthesia). At higher doses (15–40 mg/kg), recovery may be greatly prolonged. Suggest starting out at 7–15 mg/kg the first few times this is used on reptiles in your practice (and to use on your own "in house" pets first!), and then use increasing dosages as needed. (Funk 2002)

d) Best used for sedation and tranquillization or to facilitate intubation, especially in large boids, crocodilians and venomous species. Author starts with a dose of 5 mg/kg IM and repeats if needed. Higher doses (6 mg/kg) are associated with very long recovery times, especially in chelonians (72 hours). (Mehler 2009)

■ **BIRDS:**

a) Ratites: 5 mg/kg IM or IV (Jenson 1998)

■ **ZOO, EXOTIC, WILDLIFE SPECIES:**
For use of *Telazol®* in zoo, exotic and wildlife medicine refer to specific references, including:

a) *Zoo Animal and Wildlife Immobilization and Anesthesia.* West, G, Heard, D, Caulkett, N. (eds.). Blackwell Publishing, 2007.

b) *Handbook of Wildlife Chemical Immobilization, 3rd Ed.* Kreeger, T.J. and J.M. Arnemo. 2007.

c) *Restraint and Handling of Wild and Domestic Animals.* Fowler, M (ed.), Iowa State University Press, 1995

d) *Exotic Animal Formulary, 3rd Ed.* Carpenter, J.W., Saunders. 2005

e) The 2009 American Association of Zoo Veterinarian Proceedings by D. K. Fontenot also has several dosages listed for restraint, anesthesia, and analgesia for a variety of drugs for carnivores and primates. VIN members can access them at: http://goo.gl/BHRih or http://goo.gl/9UJse

Monitoring

■ Level of anesthesia/analgesia

■ Respiratory function; cardiovascular status (rate, rhythm, BP if possible)

■ Monitor eyes to prevent drying or injury

■ Body temperature

Client Information

Should only be administered by individuals familiar with its use.

Chemistry/Synonyms

Tiletamine is an injectable anesthetic agent chemically related to ketamine. Zolazepam is a diazepinone minor tranquilizer. The pH of the injectable product, after reconstitution, is 2.2–2.8.

Tiletamine HCl may also be known as: CI-634, CL-399, CN-54521-2, or *Telazol®*.

Zolazepam HCl may also be known as: CI-716.

Storage/Stability

After reconstitution, solutions may be stored for 4 days at room temperature and 14 days if refrigerated. Do not use solutions that contain a precipitate or are discolored.

Dosage Forms/Regulatory Status

VETERINARY-LABELED PRODUCTS:

Tiletamine HCl (equivalent to 250 mg free base) and Zolazepam HCl (equivalent to 250 mg free base) as lyophilized powder/vial in 5 mL vials. When 5 mL of sterile diluent (sterile water) is added a concentration of 50 mg/mL of each drug (100 mg/mL combined) is produced; *Telazol®* (Pfizer); (Rx, C-III). FDA-approved for use in cats and dogs. *Telazol®* is a Class-III controlled substance.

HUMAN-LABELED PRODUCTS: None

References

Adamcak, A. & B. Otten (2000). Rodent Therapeutics. *Vet Clin NA: Exotic Anim Pract* **3:**1(Jan): 221–240.

Bennett, R. (2009). Small Mammal Anesthesia—Rabbits and Rodents. Proceedings: ACVC. Accessed via: Veterinary Information Network. http://goo.gl/hRqTS

Burke, T. (1999). Husbandry and Medicine of Rodents and Lagomorphs. Proceedings: Central Veterinary Conference, Kansas City.

Finkler, M. (1999). Anesthesia in Ferrets. Proceedings: Central Veterinary Conference, Kansas City.

Funk, R. (2002). Anesthesia in reptiles. Proceedings: Western Veterinary Conf. Accessed via: Veterinary Information Network. http://goo.gl/9l98U

Haskell, R. (2005). Caprine surgery and anesthesia. Proceedings: WVC. Accessed via: Veterinary Information Network. http://goo.gl/1diCH

Heard, D. (1999). Advances in Reptile Anesthesia. The North American Veterinary Conference, Orlando.

Hubbell, J.A.E., R.M. Bednarski, et al. (1989). Xylazine and tiletamine-zolazepam anesthesia in horses. *Am J Vet Res* **50**(5): 737–742.

Huerkamp, M. (1995). Anesthesia and postoperative management of rabbits and pocket pets. *Kirk's Current Veterinary Therapy:XII.* J Bonagura Ed. Philadelphia, W.B. Saunders: 1322–1327.

Innis, C. (2003). Advances in anesthesia and analgesia in reptiles. Proceedings: Western Veterinary Conference. Accessed via: Veterinary Information Network. http://goo.gl/yOsua

Jenson, J. (1998). Current ratite therapy. *The Veterinary Clinics of North America: Food Animal Practice* **16:**3(November).

Kaiser-Klinger, S. (2009). Exotic animal anesthesia for the small animal practice. Proceedings: World Veterinary Congress. Accessed via: Veterinary Information Network. http://goo.gl/SdnQy

Mama, K. (2002). Injectable anesthesia: Pharmacology and clinical use of contemporary agents. Proceedings: World Small Animal Veterinary Association. Accessed via: Veterinary Information Network. http://goo.gl/1Z7Iy

Mehler, S. (2009). Anaesthesia and care of the reptile. Proceedings: BSAVA. Accessed via: Veterinary Information Network. http://goo.gl/2QYZU

Moffat, K. (2008). Addressing canine and feline aggression in the veterinary clinic. *Vet Clin NA: Sm Anim Pract* **38:** 983–1003.

Williams, B. (2000). Therapeutics in Ferrets. *Vet Clin NA: Exotic Anim Pract* **3:**1(Jan): 131–153.

Wolff, P. (2009). Camelid Medicine. Proceedings: AAZV. Accessed via: Veterinary Information Network. http://goo.gl/4TEAy

TILMICOSIN

(til-mi-**coe**-sin)   Micotil®, Pulmotil®

MACROLIDE ANTIBIOTIC

Prescriber Highlights

▶ Macrolide antibiotic used in cattle, sheep, & sometimes rabbits; used in swine as a medicated feed article

▶ Contraindications: Not to be used in automatically powered syringes or to be given IV, camelids(?)

▶ May be fatal in swine (when injected) & non-human primates; potentially in horses

▶ Adverse Effects: IM injections may cause a local tissue reaction resulting in trim loss; edema is possible at SC injection site

▶ Avoid contact with eyes

▶ In case of human injection, contact physician immediately

Uses/Indications

Tilmicosin is indicated for the treatment of bovine or ovine respiratory diseases (BRD) caused by *Mannheimia* (*Pasturella*) *haemolytica*.

Pharmacology/Actions

Like other macrolides, tilmicosin has activity primarily against gram-positive bacteria, although some gram-negative bacteria are affected and the drug reportedly has some activity against mycoplasma. Preliminary studies have shown that 95% of studied isolates of *Pasturella haemolytica* are sensitive. Bacterial isolates susceptible to tilmicosin at concentrations of 8 micrograms/mL or less are reported as susceptible to tilmicosin. The MIC_{90} value reported for *M. haemolytica* and *P. multocida* in cattle with BRD is 32 micrograms/mL.

Pharmacokinetics

Tilmicosin apparently concentrates in lung tissue. At 3 days post injection, the lung:serum ratio is about 60:1. MIC_{95} concentrations (3.12 micrograms/mL) for *P. Haemolytica* persist for a minimum of 3 days after a single injection.

Contraindications/Precautions/Warnings

Not to be used in automatically powered syringes or to be given intravenously as fatalities may result. Tilmicosin has been shown to be fatal in swine (when injected), non-human primates and potentially, in horses. Avoid contact with eyes.

There have been anecdotal reports of severe reactions in some camelids.

Adverse Effects

If administered IM, a local tissue reaction may occur resulting in trim loss. Edema may be noted at the site of subcutaneous injection.

Accidental self-injection can be fatal in humans. Do not use in automatically powered syringes. Emergency treatment includes applying ice to injection site and contacting a physician immediately. Emergency medical telephone numbers are 1-800-722-0987 or 1-317-276-2000.

Reproductive/Nursing Safety

Safe use in pregnant animals or animals to be used for breeding purposes has not been demonstrated.

Overdosage/Acute Toxicity

The cardiovascular system is apparently the target of toxicity in animals. In cattle, doses up to 50 mg/kg IM did not cause death, but SC doses of 150 mg/kg did cause fatalities, as well as IV doses of 5 mg/kg. Doses as low as 10 mg/kg in swine caused increased respiration, emesis and seizures; 20 mg/kg IM caused deaths in most animals tested. In monkeys, 10 mg/kg administered once caused no signs of toxicity, but 20 mg/kg caused vomiting; 30 mg/kg caused death.

In cases of human injection, contact physician immediately. The manufacturer has emergency telephone numbers to assist in dealing with exposure: 1-800-722-0987 or 1-317-276-2000.

Drug Interactions

In swine, **epinephrine** increased the mortality associated with tilmicosin. No other specific information was noted; refer to the erythromycin monograph for possible interactions.

Doses

■ **CATTLE:**

For susceptible infections (subcutaneous injection under the skin in the neck, or if not accessible, behind the shoulders and over the ribs is suggested).

a) For treatment of pneumonic pasteurellosis: 10 mg/kg SC every 72 hours (Shewen & Bateman 1993)

b) 10 mg/kg SC (not more than 15 mL per injection site. (Package insert; *Micotil® 300*—Elanco)

■ **SHEEP:**

For susceptible infections:

a) 10 mg/kg SC (not more than 15 mL per injection site). Subcutaneous injection under the skin in the neck, or if not accessible, behind the shoulders and over the ribs is suggested. Do not use in lambs less than 15 kg of body weight. (Package insert; *Micotil® 300*—Elanco)

■ **RABBITS, RODENTS, SMALL MAMMALS:**

a) **Rabbits:** Two regimens:

1) 25 mg/kg SC once; repeat in 3 days if necessary.

2) 5 mg/kg SC on day 0, if no reaction, give 10 mg/kg SC on days 7 and 14. Can cause weakness, pallor, tachypnea and sudden death. May cause acute death if given IV. SC injections can cause local swelling and necrosis. (Ivey & Morrisey 2000)

Monitoring

■ Efficacy
■ Withdrawal times

Client Information

■ If clients are administering the drug, they should be warned about the potential toxicity to humans, swine, and horses if accidentally injected

■ Carefully instruct in proper injection techniques

■ Avoid contact with eyes

Chemistry/Synonyms

A semi-synthetic macrolide antibiotic, tilmicosin phosphate is commercially available in a 300 mg/mL (of tilmicosin base) injection with 25% propylene glycol.

Tilmicosin may also be known as EL-870, LY-177370, *Micotil®* or *Pulmotil®*.

Storage/Stability

Store the injection at or below room temperature. Avoid exposure to direct sunlight.

Dosage Forms/Regulatory Status

VETERINARY-LABELED PRODUCTS:

Tilmicosin for Subcutaneous Injection: 300 mg/mL in 50 mL, 100 mL and 250 mL multi-dose vials; *Micotil® 300 Injection* (Elanco); (Rx). FDA-approved for use in cattle and sheep. Not FDA-approved for use in female dairy cattle 20 months or older. Do not use in lactating ewes if milk is to be used for human consumption. Do not use in veal calves. Slaughter withdrawal (at labeled doses) = 28 days.

Tilmicosin Feed Medication: 90.7 grams/lb. *Pulmotil® 90* (Elanco); (OTC). FDA-approved for veterinary use in swine only. Slaughter withdrawal (at labeled doses) = 7 days.

HUMAN-LABELED PRODUCTS: None

References

Ivey, E. & J. Morrisey (2000). Therapeutics for Rabbits. *Vet Clin NA: Exotic Anim Pract* **3:1**(Jan): 183–216.
Shewen, P. & K. Bateman (1993). Pasteurellosis in Cattle. *Current Veterinary Therapy 3: Food Animal Practice.* J Howard Ed. Philadelphia, W.B. Saunders Co.: 555–559.

TILUDRONATE DISODIUM TILUDRONIC ACID

(til-yoo-*droe*-nate)   Tildren®, Skelid®

BISPHOSPHONATE BONE RESORPTION INHIBITOR

Prescriber Highlights

▶ Bisphosphonate bone resorption inhibitor available in some countries for the intravenous treatment of navicular disease in horses

▶ Adverse effects: Signs of colic, muscle tremor (hypocalcemia), fatigue/lassitude, sweating, injection site effects, salivation, tail hypertonia

▶ Must be legally imported into the USA

Uses/Indications

Tiludronate disodium (tiludronic acid) is a bisphosphonate bone resorption inhibitor that is available in some countries for the intravenous treatment of navicular disease in horses. It may be beneficial in managing lameness isolated to the navicular bone and distal tarsal osteoarthritis by decreasing bone resorption and inflammation (Kamm *et al.* 2008). Treatment earlier in the course of the disease apparently results in greater efficacy.

For humans, there is an orally administered FDA-approved product for treating Paget's disease (osteitis deformans).

Pharmacology/Actions

Tiludronate, like other bisphosphonates, inhibit osteoclastic bone resorption by inhibiting osteoclast function after binding to bone hydroxyapatite thereby helping to regulate bone remodeling.

Pharmacokinetics

After intravenous injection in horses the drug is rapidly distributed to bone. Binding is greater to cancellous bone than cortical bone. Plasma protein binding is reported to be approximately 85% and elimination half-life is approximately 4.5 hours. Repeated daily doses do not result in accumulation in plasma. Unbound drug is eliminated unchanged in the urine. Approximately 25–50% of a single IV dose is eliminated in the urine over 96 hours.

Contraindications/Precautions/Warnings

The labeling for *Tildren®* states that the drug should not be used in horses with renal dysfunction or those producing milk for human consumption. Because there is an absence of data on the effects the drug may have on the skeleton of young animals, the manufacturer states to not administer to horses less than 3 years old.

Since the safety of tiludronate has not been studied in pregnant or lactating mares, the manufacturer recommends not using it during pregnancy or lactation.

Use with caution in horses with hypocalcemia or cardiac dysfunction. If used in these patients, slow the rate of injection and watch these patients carefully for the first few hours post-injection.

Adverse Effects

Acute adverse effects reported in horses include colic (reduced appetite, abdominal discomfort, pawing/scratching at ground, restlessness), muscle tremor, fatigue/lassitude and sweating. The incidences of these effects are reported at 5% or less and are postulated to be due to a mild hypoglycemic effect. The onset of colic signs appear within a few hours of treatment and generally resolve without treatment. Should they persist, conventional colic treatments are recommended. Muscle tremors may be treated with intravenous calcium if required.

Up to 9% of patients develop local reactions at the injection site (*e.g.,* phlebitis), particularly after the 4th injection.

Other adverse effects reported include salivation and tail hypertonia.

Reproductive/Nursing Safety

Studies performed in male and female rats at dosages as high as 75 mg/kg/day demonstrated no effects on fertility.

Studies in pregnant rabbits given 2X–5X human dosages showed no skeletal abnormalities. Pregnant mice given 7X human dosages showed some adverse effects (decreased litter size, malformed paws in 6 fetuses from one litter). Rat studies have shown decreased litter sizes, but no teratogenic effects. In humans, the FDA categorizes tiludronate as category *C* for use during pregnancy (*Animal studies have shown an adverse effect on the fetus, but there are no adequate studies in humans; or there are no animal reproduction studies and no adequate studies in humans.*)

As the safety of tiludronate has not been studied in pregnant or lactating mares, the manufacturer recommends not using it during pregnancy or lactation.

Overdosage/Acute Toxicity

Limited information is available. The manufacturer reports that doses of 3X in horses caused an increased frequency of adverse effects, particularly signs of colic and muscle tremor. Intravenous calcium administration may be considered for signs associated with hypocalcemia.

Drug Interactions

■ **CALCIUM- or MAGNESIUM-CONTAINING INTRAVENOUS FLUIDS:** May complex with tiludronate and reduce its availability; do not mix with fluids or administer with fluids such as *Lactated Ringer's, Ringer's, Plasma-Lyte®, Normasol®,* etc.

Laboratory Considerations

No specific concerns were noted.

Doses

■ **HORSES:**
For navicular disease:

a) 0.1 mg/kg tiludronic acid slow IV (over 20–30 seconds per 10 mL given) once daily for 10 days. Alternate injection sites from day to day. (Label information; *Tildren®*—Ceva/ Sanofi)

Monitoring

■ Clinical Efficacy

■ Serum Calcium

■ Adverse Effects (particularly within first 4 hours after dosing)

Client Information

■ This medication should be administered by a veterinary professional

■ Patient should be observed for up to 4 hours post-administration for signs of hypocalcemia (muscle tremors, etc.) or colic

Chemistry/Synonyms

Tiludronate disodium is a bisphosphonate that occurs as a white powder having a molecular weight of 380.6. Commercially available products contain the disodium salt of tiludronic acid. 120 mg of tiludronate disodium is equivalent to 100 mg of tiludronic acid.

Tiludronate disodium or tiludronic acid may also be known as ME-3737, SR-41319, acidum tiludronicum, *Tildren®* or *Skelid®*.

Storage/Stability

Unless otherwise indicated, store the unreconstituted powder and diluent at room temperature (15–30°C) in the outer carton.

Shelf life of properly stored unreconstituted product is generally 3 years. Reconstitute the powder by aseptically adding 10 mL of the provided diluent and mix gently. The resulting solution contains 5 mg/mL of tiludronic acid.

After reconstitution, use immediately. Any remaining product should be discarded.

Do not mix or administer with intravenous fluids containing calcium or magnesium (*e.g.*, LRS, Ringer's, etc.).

Dosage Forms/Regulatory Status

VETERINARY-LABELED PRODUCTS:

None in the USA; it is available in France, Spain, The Netherlands, and Italy as:

Tiludronic Acid: 50 mg (as tiludronate disodium) per vial, with one 10 mL vial of sterile water for reconstitution; *Tildren®* (Sanofi/Ceva). Labeled for use in horses.

Not permitted for use in lactating animals producing milk for human consumption. Labeled meat and offal withdrawal = 0 days. Refer to individual product labels for more information.

The FDA may allow legal importation of this medication for compassionate use in animals; for more information, see the *Instructions for Legally Importing Drugs for Compassionate Use in the USA* found in the appendix.

One source recommended for obtaining *Tildren®* via this process is: manorveterinaryexports.com

HUMAN-LABELED PRODUCTS:

Tiludronate Disodium Oral Tablets: 240 mg (equiv. to 200 mg tiludronic acid); *Skelid®* (Sanofi-Aventis); (Rx)

Note: The information presented in this monograph pertains to the veterinary-labeled intravenous product only.

References

Kamm, L., W. McLlwraith, et al. (2008). A review of the efficacy of tiludronate in the horse. *Journal of Equine Veterinary Science* 28(4): 209–214.

TINIDAZOLE

(tye-*ni*-dah-zole)   Tindamax®

NITROIMIDAZOLE ANTIPROTOZOAL/ ANTIBIOTIC

Prescriber Highlights

▶ Drug similar to metronidazole, potentially useful for treating anaerobic infections (especially in the mouth), trichomoniasis, amebiasis and balantidiasis

▶ Little experience in veterinary medicine

▶ Adverse effects most likely GI-related; like metronidazole and ronidazole, tinidazole could cause neurotoxicity

▶ Many potential drug interactions

Uses/Indications

Little information is presently available on the use of tinidazole in dogs, cats, or horses. It potentially could be useful for treating anaerobic infections, particularly associated with dental infections in small animals. Because of its antiprotozoal effects, it has been used as an alternative for treating giardiasis in small animals, and it could have efficacy against amebiasis, trichomoniasis or balantidiasis in veterinary species, but documentation of efficacy is not available. Tinidazole has a longer duration of action in dogs and cats than does metronidazole. In a small study done in cats experimentally infected with *T. foetus*, tinidazole doses at 30 mg/kg PO once daily for 14 days, decreased fecal shedding of *T. foetus* but failed to eradicate the infection from 2 of 4 cats (Gookin *et al.* 2007).

In humans, oral tinidazole is FDA-approved for treating extraintestinal and intestinal amebiasis, (*Entamoeba histolytica*), giardiasis (*Giardia duodenalis/lamblia*), and trichomoniasis (*T. vaginalis*).

Pharmacology/Actions

Tinidazole is a 5-nitroimidazole similar to metronidazole. It is bactericidal against susceptible bacteria. Its exact mechanism of action is not completely understood, but it is taken-up by anaerobic organisms where it is reduced to an unidentified polar compound. It is believed that this compound is responsible for the drug's antimicrobial activity by disrupting DNA and nucleic acid synthesis in the bacteria.

Tinidazole has activity against many obligate anaerobes and *H. pylori*. It has excellent activity against *Porphyromonas* spp. found in canine gingiva.

Tinidazole is also trichomonacidal and amebicidal. Its mechanism of action for its antiprotozoal activity is not well understood. It has therapeutic activity against *Entamoeba histolytica*, Trichomonas, and Giardia.

Pharmacokinetics

In dogs and cats, tinidazole is practically completely absorbed after oral administration. Apparent volumes of distribution are 0.66 L/kg in dogs and 0.54 L/kg in cats. Dogs clear the drug about twice as fast as cats; elimination half-lives are about 4.4 hours in dogs, 8.4 hours in cats.

In horses, tinidazole is practically completely absorbed after oral administration. Apparent volume of distribution is 0.66 L/kg an elimination half-life of about 5.2 hours.

Contraindications/Precautions/Warnings

Tinidazole should not be used in patients documented to be hypersensitive to it or other 5-nitroimidazoles (*e.g.*, metronidazole).

Tinidazole is metabolized by the liver; use with caution in patients with hepatic dysfunction.

As other 5-nitroimidazoles (metronidazole, ronidazole) have been associated with neurotoxic signs in dogs and cats and seizures have been reported rarely with tinidazole use in humans, use with caution in animals susceptible to seizures.

The human labeling for tinidazole carries a "black box warning" stating: "Carcinogenicity has been seen in mice and rats treated chronically with another agent in the nitroimidazole class (metronidazole). Although such data have not been reported for tinidazole, avoid unnecessary use of tinidazole. Reserve its use for the conditions for which it is indicated."

Adverse Effects

The adverse effect profiles for dogs, cats or horses are not well described since clinical use of this medication has been limited. Gastrointestinal effects including vomiting, inappetence, and diarrhea are most likely. Giving the medication with food may help alleviate these effects. Other 5-nitroimidazoles (metronidazole, ronidazole) have been associated with neurotoxic signs in dogs and cats; seizures have been reported rarely with tinidazole use in humans.

Tinidazole reportedly is very bitter tasting. If using compounded products, consider using capsules or having a flavored suspension prepared.

Reproductive/Nursing Safety

In studies performed on male rats tinidazole decreased fertility and caused testicular histopathology.

Tinidazole crosses the placenta. While studies in mice and rats have not demonstrated significant fetal effects, because of its mutagenic potential, it is stated that it should not be used in women during the first trimester of pregnancy. In humans, the FDA categorizes tinidazole as category *C* for use during pregnancy (*Animal studies have shown an adverse effect on the fetus, but there are no adequate studies in humans; or there are no animal reproduction studies and no adequate studies in humans.*) If considering use of this product in a pregnant animal, weigh the potential benefits of treatment versus the risks.

Tinidazole is distributed into maternal milk at levels approximating those found in serum. It is suggested that milk replacer be used if tinidazole is necessary for treating a nursing dam.

Overdosage/Acute Toxicity

Very limited information is available. In studies done in rats and mice, the oral LD50 was >3.6 grams/kg for mice and >2 grams/kg for rats. Treatment of acute overdoses of tinidazole is symptomatic and supportive. Gastric lavage or induction of emesis may be helpful. Hemodialysis can remove approximately 43% of the amount in the body (human) in a 6 hour session.

Drug Interactions

In humans, the following drug interactions with metronidazole have been reported or are theoretical and may be of significance in veterinary patients receiving tinidazole:

- ■ **ALCOHOL:** May induce a disulfiram-like (nausea, vomiting, cramps, etc.) reaction
- ■ **CIMETIDINE, KETOCONAZOLE:** May decrease the metabolism of tinidazole and increase the likelihood of dose-related side effects occurring

■ **CYCLOSPORINE, TACROLIMUS (systemic):** Tinidazole may increase the serum levels of cyclosporine or tacrolimus

■ **FLUOROURACIL (systemic):** Tinidazole may increase the serum levels of fluorouracil and increase the risk of toxicity

■ **LITHIUM:** Tinidazole may increase lithium serum levels and increase the risk for lithium toxicity

■ **OXYTETRACYCLINE:** Reportedly, may antagonize the therapeutic effects of metronidazole (and presumably tinidazole)

■ **PHENOBARBITAL, RIFAMPIN OR PHENYTOIN:** May increase the metabolism of tinidazole thereby decreasing blood levels

■ **WARFARIN:** Metronidazole (and potentially tinidazole) may prolong the prothrombin time (PT) in patients taking warfarin or other coumarin anticoagulants. Avoid concurrent use if possible; otherwise, intensify monitoring.

Laboratory Considerations

■ **AST, ALT, LDH, Triglycerides, Hexokinase glucose:** Tinidazole, like metronidazole may interfere with enzymatic coupling of the assay to oxidation-reduction of nicotinamide adenine. Falsely low values, including zero, may result.

Doses

■ **DOGS:**
a) For stomatitis, anaerobic infections: 15–25 mg/kg PO q12h for 7 days. (Greene *et al.* 2006)

b) For giardiasis: 44 mg/kg PO q24h for 6 days. Potentially may be useful for treating trichomoniasis, amebiasis and balantidiasis, but efficacy data lacking for animals. (Barr 2006)

■ **CATS:**
a) For stomatitis, anaerobic infections: 15 mg/kg PO q24h for 7 days. (Greene *et al.* 2006)

■ **HORSES:**
a) For susceptible anaerobic infections: 10–15 mg/kg PO q12h (Pvorala *et al.* 1990)

Monitoring

■ Clinical efficacy in treating the infection

Client Information

■ Give this medication with food
■ Animals should not have access to alcohol when receiving this medication
■ If gastrointestinal signs (vomiting, lack of appetite, diarrhea) are severe or persist, contact veterinarian
■ Contact veterinarian immediately if animal shows signs of behavior changes, eyes moving back and forth (nystagmus), convulsions, or if patient has difficulty walking, climbing stairs, etc. (ataxia); these could be signs that drug toxicity is occurring

Chemistry/Synonyms

Tinidazole occurs as an almost white or pale yellow, crystalline powder. It is practically insoluble in water, soluble in acetone, and sparingly soluble in methyl alcohol.

Tinidazole may also be known as CP-12574 or tinidazolum. International trade names include: *Estovyn-T®*, *Fasigyn®*, *Tindamax®*, *Tiniba®*, *Tiniameb®*, or *Tinidazol®*.

Storage/Stability

Store tinidazole tablets at controlled room temperature (20–25°C) protected from light.

Dosage Forms/Regulatory Status

VETERINARY-LABELED PRODUCTS: None

As tinidazole is a nitroimidazole, its use is prohibited in animals to be used for food.

HUMAN-LABELED PRODUCTS:

Tinidazole Tablets (scored): 250 mg & 500 mg; *Tindamax®* (Mission Pharmacal); generic; (Rx)

References

Barr, S. (2006). Giardiasis. *Infectious Diseases of the Dog and Cat*. C Greene Ed., Elsevier: 736–742.

Gookin, J.L., S.H. Stauffer, et al. (2007). Efficacy of tinidazole for treatment of cats experimentally infected with Tritrichomonas foetus. *American Journal of Veterinary Research* **68**(10): 1085–1088.

Greene, C., K. Hartmannn, et al. (2006). Appendix 8: Antimicrobial Drug Formulary. *Infectious Disease of the Dog and Cat*. C Greene Ed., Elsevier: 1186–1333.

Pvorala, S., T. Kotilainen, et al. (1990). Pharmacokinetics of tinidazole in the horse. *J Vet Pharmacol Ther* **13**(1): 76–80.

TIOPRONIN

(tye-oh-*proe*-nin)   Thiola®, 2-MPG

ANTIUROLITHIC (CYSTINE) AGENT

Prescriber Highlights

▶ Drug for prevention (& treatment) of cystine urolithiasis

▶ Cautions: Agranulocytosis, aplastic anemia, thrombocytopenia or other significant hematologic abnormality, impaired renal or hepatic function, or sensitivity to either tiopronin or penicillamine

▶ Adverse Effects: Coombs'-positive regenerative spherocyte anemia, aggressiveness, proteinuria, thrombocytopenia, elevations in liver enzymes, dermatologic effects, & myopathy

▶ Relatively expensive

Uses/Indications

Tiopronin is indicated for the prevention of cystine urolithiasis in patients where dietary therapy combined with urinary alkalinization is not completely effective. It may also be useful in combination with urine alkalinization and dietary (ultra-low protein diet) modification to dissolve stones.

Pharmacology/Actions

Tiopronin is considered an antiurolithic agent. It undergoes thiol-disulfide exchange with cystine (cysteine-cysteine disulfide) to form tiopronin-cystine disulfide. This complex is more water-soluble and is readily excreted thereby preventing cystine calculi from forming.

Pharmacokinetics

Tiopronin has a rapid onset of action and in humans, up to 48% of a dose is found in the urine within 4 hours of dosing. Tiopronin has a relatively short duration of action and its effect in humans disappears in about 10 hours. Elimination is primarily via renal routes.

Contraindications/Precautions/Warnings

Tiopronin's risks versus its benefits should be considered before using in patients with agranulocytosis, aplastic anemia, thrombocytopenia or other significant hematologic abnormality, impaired renal or hepatic function, or sensitivity to either tiopronin or penicillamine.

Adverse Effects

There is limited information available on the adverse effect profile of tiopronin in dogs. In a retrospective study evaluating tiopronin treatment for cystinuria in about 16% of treated dogs, proteinuria, thrombocytopenia, anemia, increased liver enzymes and bile acids, lethargy, dermatologic effects (small pustules of the skin, dry crusty nose) aggressiveness, sulfur odor of the urine, or myopathy (noted as staggering and difficulty chewing) were noted (Hoppe & Denneberg 2001). Tiopronin has been associated with Coombs'-positive regenerative spherocyte anemia in dogs. Should this effect occur, the drug should be discontinued and appropriate treatment started (corticosteroids, blood component therapy) as needed.

While tiopronin is thought to have fewer adverse effects than penicillamine in humans, adverse effects that occur more frequently include dermatologic effects (ecchymosis, itching, rashes, mouth ulcers, jaundice) and GI distress; less frequently allergic reactions (specifically adenopathy), arthralgias, dyspnea, fever, hematologic abnormalities, edema, and nephrotic syndrome.

Reproductive/Nursing Safety

There is limited information on the reproductive safety of tiopronin. Skeletal defects, cleft palates and increased resorptions were noted when rats were given 10 times the human dose of penicillamine and, therefore, may also be of concern with tiopronin. Other animal studies have suggested that tiopronin may affect fetus viability at high doses. In humans, the FDA categorizes this drug as category *C* for use during pregnancy (*Animal studies have shown an adverse effect on the fetus, but there are no adequate studies in hu-*

mans; or there are no animal reproduction studies and no adequate studies in humans.)

Because tiopronin may be excreted in milk, at present it is not recommended for use in nursing animals.

Overdosage/Acute Toxicity

There is little information available. It is suggested to contact an animal poison control center for further information in the event of an overdose situation.

Drug Interactions

Potentially use of tiopronin with **other drugs causing nephrotoxicity, hepatotoxicity, or bone marrow depression** could cause additive toxic effects. Clinical significance is not clear.

Doses

■ DOGS:

For treatment or prevention of recurrence of cystine urinary calculi:

a) Prophylactic treatment: 30 mg/kg PO q12h. Increase water intake and urine diuresis. Alkalinize urine (pH 6.5–7.0) using potassium citrate. In cases with low cystine excretion and low urolith recurrence rate, tiopronin dose may be individually decreased (<30 mg/kg) or stopped.

Dissolution of uroliths: Approximately 40 mg/kg PO q12h. Reevaluation of uroliths with ultrasound or radiography every 4th week. After urolith dissolution, give prophylactic dose of tiopronin. If urolith dissolution is not achieved after 2–3 months, surgery is recommended. Reexamination recommended 1, 3, 6, & 12 months after start of treatment and thereafter twice a year, including: physical examination, ultrasonography/radiography of the urinary tract, urinalyses (specific gravity, protein, pH, sediment, and cyanide nitroprusside reaction) using AM samples of urine, CBC (with platelets), liver enzymes (alkaline phos, ALT). Quantitative measurements of urinary cystine excretion related to the urinary creatinine excretion, AM urine samples, before start of treatment and once a year during treatment. If adverse reactions occur, stop treatment for 4 weeks. Blood and urine analysis every 1-2 weeks until remission of signs. When the adverse reactions disappear, start tiopronin again, gradually increasing the dose from 10–15 mg/kg q12h. If the adverse reactions reappear despite a lowered dose, tiopronin treatment has to be abandoned. (Hoppe & Denneberg 2001)

b) In conjunction with an alkalinizing, protein and sodium restricted diet (*e.g.*, *u/d*®), 30–40 mg/kg PO divided into two daily doses. (Cowan 1994)

c) Treatment: 20 mg/kg PO twice daily for 1–3 months; relatively high incidence of adverse effects; Prevention: 15 mg/kg PO twice daily. (Adams & Syme 2005)

Monitoring
■ See the recommendations for monitoring in the dose section (Hoppe and Denneberg reference)

Client Information
■ Clients should be counseled on the importance of adequate compliance with this drug to maximize efficacy and detailed on the clinical signs to watch for regarding adverse effects.

Chemistry/Synonyms
A sulfhydryl compound related to penicillamine, tiopronin has a molecular weight of 163.2. It occurs as a white crystalline powder that is freely soluble in water.

Tiopronin may also be known as: SF 522, N-(2-Mercaptopropionyl)-glycine (MPG), 2-MPG, thiopronine, *Acadione®*, *Captimer®*, *Epatiol®*, *Mucolysin®*, *Mucosyt®*, *Sutilan®*, *Thiola®*, *Thiosol®*, or *Tioglis®*.

Storage/Stability
Store tablets at room temperature in tight containers.

Dosage Forms/Regulatory Status
VETERINARY-LABELED PRODUCTS: None

HUMAN-LABELED PRODUCTS:

Tiopronin Tablets: 100 mg; *Thiola®* (Mission); (Rx)

References
Adams, L. & H. Syme (2005). Canine lower urinary tract diseases. *Textbook of Veterinary Internal Medicine, 6th Ed.* S Ettinger and E Feldman Eds., Elsevier: 1850–1874.

Cowan, L. (1994). Diseases of the urinary bladder. *Saunders Manual of Small Animal Practice.* S Birchard and R Sherding Eds. Philadelphia, W.B. Saunders Company: 826–836.

Hoppe, A. & T. Denneberg (2001). Cystinuria in the dog: Clinical studies during 14 years of medical treatment. *Journal of Veterinary Internal Medicine* 15(4): 361–367.

TOBRAMYCIN SULFATE

(toe-bra-*mye*-sin)   Nebcin®, TOBI®

AMINOGLYCOSIDE ANTIBIOTIC

Prescriber Highlights

▶ Parenteral aminoglycoside antibiotic that has "good" activity against a variety of bacteria, predominantly gram-negative aerobic bacilli, also in ophthalmic preps

▶ Because of potential adverse effects usually reserved for serious infections when given systemically, may be less nephrotoxic than gentamicin

▶ Adverse Effects: Nephrotoxicity, ototoxicity, neuromuscular blockade

▶ Cats may be more sensitive to toxic effects

▶ Risk factors for nephrotoxicity: Pre-existing renal disease, age (both neonatal & geriatric), fever, sepsis, & dehydration

Uses/Indications
While most veterinarians use gentamicin or amikacin and there are no FDA-approved veterinary tobramycin products in the U.S., tobramycin can be useful clinically to treat serious gram-negative infections in most species. It is often used in settings where gentamicin-resistant bacteria are a clinical problem. The inherent toxicity of the aminoglycosides limit their systemic use to serious infections when there is either a documented lack of susceptibility to other less toxic antibiotics or when the clinical situation dictates immediate treatment of a presumed gram-negative infection before culture and susceptibility results are reported.

Whether tobramycin is less nephrotoxic than either gentamicin or amikacin when used clinically is controversial. Laboratory studies indicate that in a controlled setting in laboratory animals, it may indeed be so.

Pharmacology/Actions
Tobramycin, like the other aminoglycoside antibiotics, act on susceptible bacteria presumably by irreversibly binding to the 30S ribosomal subunit thereby inhibiting protein synthesis. It is considered a bactericidal antibiotic.

Tobramycin's spectrum of activity includes coverage against many aerobic gram-negative and some aerobic gram-positive bacteria, including most species of *E. coli*, Klebsiella, Proteus, *Pseudomonas*, *Salmonella*, Enterobacter, Serratia, Shigella, Mycoplasma, and Staphylococcus.

Antimicrobial activity of the aminoglycosides is enhanced in an alkaline environment.

The aminoglycoside antibiotics are inactive against fungi, viruses and most anaerobic bacteria.

Pharmacokinetics

Tobramycin, like the other aminoglycosides, is not appreciably absorbed after oral or intra-uterine administration, but it is absorbed from topical administration (not skin or urinary bladder) when used in irrigations during surgical procedures. Patients receiving oral aminoglycosides with hemorrhagic or necrotic enteritises may absorb appreciable quantities of the drug. Subcutaneous injection results in slightly delayed peak levels and more variability than after IM injection. Bioavailability from extravascular injection (IM or SC) is greater than 90%.

The pharmacokinetics of tobramycin in horses has been reported (Hubenov *et al.* 2007). Approximate values are (**Note:** First value is calculated value from a microbiologic assay and second from an HPLC assay): volume of distribution (steady-state): 0.24-0.55 L/kg; clearance: 101–130 mL/kg/hr; elimination half-life: 2.5–4 hours.

After absorption, aminoglycosides are distributed primarily in the extracellular fluid. They are found in ascitic, pleural, pericardial, peritoneal, synovial and abscess fluids, and high levels are found in sputum, bronchial secretions and bile. Aminoglycosides (other than streptomycin) are minimally protein bound (<20%) to plasma proteins. Aminoglycosides do not readily cross the blood-brain barrier nor penetrate ocular tissue. CSF levels are unpredictable and range from 0-50% those found in the serum. Therapeutic levels are found in bone, heart, gallbladder and lung tissues after parenteral dosing. Aminoglycosides tend to accumulate in certain tissues such as the inner ear and kidneys, which may help explain their toxicity. Aminoglycosides cross the placenta and fetal concentrations range from 15–50% those found in maternal serum.

Elimination of aminoglycosides after parenteral administration occurs almost entirely by glomerular filtration. Patients with decreased renal function can have significantly prolonged half-lives. In humans with normal renal function, elimination rates can be highly variable with the aminoglycoside antibiotics.

Contraindications/Precautions/Warnings

Aminoglycosides are contraindicated in patients who are hypersensitive to them. Because these drugs are often the only effective agents in severe gram-negative infections, there are no other absolute contraindications to their use; however, they should be used with extreme caution in patients with preexisting renal disease with concomitant monitoring and dosage interval adjustments made. Other risk factors for the development of toxicity include age (both neonatal and geriatric patients), fever, sepsis, and dehydration.

Because aminoglycosides can cause irreversible ototoxicity, they should be used with caution in "working" dogs (*e.g.*, "seeing-eye", herding, dogs for the hearing impaired, etc.).

Aminoglycosides should be used with caution in patients with neuromuscular disorders (*e.g.*, myasthenia gravis) due to their neuromuscular blocking activity.

Because aminoglycosides are eliminated primarily through renal mechanisms, they should be used cautiously, preferably with serum monitoring and dosage adjustment in neonatal or geriatric animals.

Aminoglycosides are generally considered contraindicated in rabbits/hares as they adversely affect the GI flora balance in these animals.

Adverse Effects

The aminoglycosides are infamous for their nephrotoxic and ototoxic effects. The nephrotoxic (tubular necrosis) mechanisms of these drugs are not completely understood, but are probably related to interference with phospholipid metabolism in the lysosomes of proximal renal tubular cells, resulting in leakage of proteolytic enzymes into the cytoplasm. Nephrotoxicity normally manifests by increases in BUN, creatinine, nonprotein nitrogen in the serum and decreases in urine specific gravity and creatinine clearance. Proteinuria and cells or casts may also be seen in the urine. Nephrotoxicity is usually reversible once the drug is discontinued. While gentamicin may be more nephrotoxic than the other aminoglycosides, the incidences of nephrotoxicity with all of these agents require equal caution and monitoring.

Ototoxicity (8th cranial nerve toxicity) of the aminoglycosides can manifest with either auditory and/or vestibular clinical signs and may be irreversible. Vestibular clinical signs are more frequent with streptomycin, gentamicin, or tobramycin. Auditory clinical signs are more frequent with amikacin, neomycin, or kanamycin, but either form can occur with any of the drugs. Cats are apparently very sensitive to the vestibular effects of the aminoglycosides.

The aminoglycosides can also cause neuromuscular blockade, facial edema, pain or inflammation at the injection site, peripheral neuropathy, and hypersensitivity reactions. Rarely, GI clinical signs, hematologic, and hepatic effects have been reported.

Reproductive/Nursing Safety

Tobramycin can cross the placenta and concentrate in fetal kidneys and while rare, cause 8th cranial nerve toxicity or nephrotoxicity in fetuses. Total irreversible deafness has been reported in some human babies whose mothers received tobramycin during pregnancy. Because the drug should only be used in serious infections, the benefits of therapy may exceed the potential risks. In humans, the FDA categorizes this drug as category *D* for use during pregnancy (*There is evidence of human fetal risk, but the potential benefits from the use of the drug in pregnant women may be acceptable despite its potential risks.*) In a separate system evaluating the safety of drugs in canine and feline pregnancy (Papich 1989), this drug is categorized as in class: **C** (*These drugs may have potential risks. Studies in people or laboratory animals have uncovered risks, and these drugs should be used cautiously as a last resort when the benefit of therapy clearly outweighs the risks.*)

Small amounts of aminoglycoside antibiotics are excreted in milk, but are unlikely to cause clinically significant effects in nursing offspring.

Overdosage/Acute Toxicity
Should an inadvertent overdosage be administered, three treatments have been recommended: 1) Hemodialysis is very effective in reducing serum levels of the drug, but is not a viable option for most veterinary patients; 2) Peritoneal dialysis also will reduce serum levels, but is much less efficacious; 3) Complexation of drug with either carbenicillin or ticarcillin (12–20 grams/day in humans) is reportedly nearly as effective as hemodialysis.

Drug Interactions
The following drug interactions have either been reported or are theoretical in humans or animals receiving tobramycin and may be of significance in veterinary patients:

■ **BETA-LACTAM ANTIBIOTICS (penicillins, cephalosporins):** May have synergistic effects against some bacteria; some potential for inactivation of aminoglycosides *in vitro* (do not mix together) and *in vivo* (patients in renal failure)

■ **CEPHALOSPORINS:** The concurrent use of aminoglycosides with cephalosporins is somewhat controversial. Potentially, cephalosporins could cause additive nephrotoxicity when used with aminoglycosides, but this interaction has only been well documented with cephaloridine and cephalothin (both no longer marketed).

■ **DIURETICS, LOOP (e.g., furosemide, torsemide) or OSMOTIC (e.g., mannitol):** Concurrent use with loop or osmotic diuretics may increase the nephrotoxic or ototoxic potential of the aminoglycosides

■ **NEPHROTOXIC DRUGS, OTHER (e.g., cisplatin, amphotericin B, polymyxin B, or vancomycin):** Potential for increased risk for nephrotoxicity

■ **NEUROMUSCULAR BLOCKING AGENTS & ANESTHETICS, GENERAL:** Concomitant use with general anesthetics or neuromuscular blocking agents could potentiate neuromuscular blockade

Laboratory Considerations
■ Tobramycin serum concentrations may be falsely decreased if the patient is also receiving **beta-lactam antibiotics** and the serum is stored prior analysis. It is recommended that if assay is delayed, samples be frozen and, if possible, drawn at times when the beta-lactam antibiotic is at a trough level.

Doses
Note: There is significant inter-patient variability with aminoglycoside pharmacokinetic parameters. To insure therapeutic levels and to minimize the risks for toxicity development, consider monitoring serum levels for this drug. Like other aminoglycosides, most now recommend dosing mammals once daily; consider giving the total daily dose as a single dose (*e.g.*, if dose listed is 2 mg/kg q8h, give 6 mg/kg once daily).

■ **DOGS/CATS:**
For small animals, one pair of authors (Aronson and Aucoin 1989) make the following recommendations with regard to minimizing risks of toxicity, yet maximizing efficacy:

1. Dose according to animal size. The larger the animal, the smaller the dose (on a mg/kg basis).

2. The more risk factors (age, fever, sepsis, renal disease, dehydration) the smaller the dose.

3. In old patients or those suspected of renal disease, increase dosing interval from q8h to q16–24h.

4. Determine serum creatinine prior to therapy and adjust by changes in level even if it remains in "normal range."

5. Monitor urine for changes in sediment (*e.g.*, casts) or concentrating ability. Not very useful in patients with UTI.

6. Therapeutic drug monitoring is recommended when possible.

a) 2 mg/kg IV, IM, or SC q8h (avoid use or reduce dosage in patients with renal failure; recommend therapeutic drug monitoring, particularly in young animals) (Vaden & Papich 1995)

b) For susceptible UTI: 1–2 mg/kg SC q8h (Brovida 2003)

c) For sepsis: 2–4 mg/kg IV three times daily (q8h) (Tello 2003)

d) Dogs:
For soft tissue, systemic infections: 1–1.7 mg/kg IV q8h or 3–5.1 mg/kg IV q24h for less than 7 days;
For systemic infections: 2 mg/kg SC q8–12h or 4–6 mg/kg SC q24h for less than 7 days;
For persistent bacteremia: 3–5 mg/kg IV, IM, SC q8h or 9–15 mg/kg IV, IM or SC q24h for 7 days or less. (Greene *et al.* 2006)

e) Cats:
For soft tissue, systemic infections:

2 mg/kg IV, IM or SC q12h or 4 mg/kg IV, IM, SC q24h for 5 days or less;

For persistent bacteremia: 2 mg/kg IV, IM, SC q8h or 6 mg/kg IV, IM or SC q24h for 5 days or less.

(Greene *et al.* 2006)

■ **HORSES:**

For susceptible infections:

a) Based upon a limited pharmacokinetic study (6 horses): The repeated dosing of 4 mg/kg q24h will result in the same concentration profile every day as no accumulation takes place, with the exception of a possible trapping in proximal tubule cells. These data suggest that the this dose will allow achievement of Cmax/MIC ratio higher than 10 for pathogen strains with a MIC of 1 microgram/mL. Further studies are required to define the real breakpoint values for Cmax/MIC ratio for tobramycin not only in healthy horses, but also in diseased animals. (Hubenov *et al.* 2007)

■ **LLAMAS:**

For susceptible infections:

a) 4 mg/kg IV q24h; 0.75 mg/kg IV q8h (Baird 2003)

■ **BIRDS:**

For susceptible infections:

a) 5 mg/kg IM every 12 hours (Bauck & Hoefer 1993)

b) 2.5–5 mg/kg/day; must be given parenterally (Flammer 2003)

■ **REPTILES:**

For susceptible infections:

a) 2.5 mg/kg once daily IM (Gauvin 1993)

Monitoring

■ Efficacy (cultures, clinical signs associated with infection)

■ Renal toxicity; baseline urinalysis, and serum creatinine/BUN. Casts in the urine are often the initial sign of impending nephrotoxicity. Frequency of monitoring during therapy is controversial, but daily urinalysis and serum creatinine may not be too frequent.

■ Gross monitoring of vestibular or auditory toxicity is recommended

■ Serum levels if possible

Client Information

■ With appropriate training, owners may give subcutaneous injections at home, but routine monitoring of therapy for efficacy and toxicity must still be done

■ Clients should understand that the potential exists for severe toxicity (nephrotoxicity, ototoxicity) developing from this medication

Chemistry/Synonyms

An aminoglycoside derived from Streptomyces tenebrarius, tobramycin occurs as a white to off-white, hygroscopic powder that is freely soluble in water and very slightly soluble in alcohol. The sulfate salt is formed during the manufacturing process. The commercial injection is a clear, colorless solution and the pH is adjusted to 6–8 with sulfuric acid and/or sodium hydroxide.

Tobramycin Sulfate may also be known as: tobramycin sulphate, *Brulamycin®*, *Gernebcin®*, *Mytobrin®*, *Nebcina®*, *Nebcine®*, *Nebicina®*, *Obracin®*, *Tobra®*, *Tobra Gobens®*, *TOBI®*, *Tobra Laf®*, *Tobra-cell®*, *Tobracil®*, *Tobradistin®*, *Tobramina®*, *Tobraneg®*, *Tobrasix®*, *Tobrex®*, *Tomycin®*, or *Trazil®*.

Storage/Stability

Tobramycin sulfate for injection should be stored at room temperature (15–30°C); avoid freezing and temperatures above 40°C. Do not use the product if discolored.

Compatibility/Compounding Considerations

While the manufacturers state that tobramycin should not be mixed with other drugs, it is reportedly physically **compatible** and stable in most commonly used intravenous solutions (**not** compatible with dextrose and alcohol solutions, Polysal, Polysal M, or Isolyte E, M or P) and **compatible** with the following drugs: aztreonam, bleomycin sulfate, calcium gluconate, cefoxitin sodium, ciprofloxacin lactate, clindamycin phosphate (not in syringes), floxacillin sodium, metronidazole (with or without sodium bicarbonate), ranitidine HCl, and verapamil HCl.

The following drugs or solutions are reportedly physically **incompatible** or only compatible in specific situations with tobramycin: cefamandole naftate, furosemide and heparin sodium. Compatibility is dependent upon factors such as pH, concentration, temperature, and diluent used; consult specialized references or a hospital pharmacist for more specific information.

In vitro inactivation of aminoglycoside antibiotics by beta-lactam antibiotics is well documented; see the information in the Drug Interaction and Laboratory Consideration sections.

Dosage Forms/Regulatory Status

VETERINARY-LABELED PRODUCTS: None

HUMAN-LABELED PRODUCTS:

Tobramycin Sulfate Injection: 0.8 mg/mL and 1.2 mg/mL (as sulfate) in 100 mL & 50 mL (respectively) single-dose containers; Solution for Injection: 10 mg/mL in 2 mL vials and 40 mg/mL in 1.5 mL & 2 mL syringes, & 2 mL and 30 mL vials; generic; (Rx)

Tobramycin Sulfate Powder for Injection: 1.2 grams (40 mg/mL after reconstitution), preservative free in 50 mL bulk package vial; generic; (Rx)

Tobramycin Solution for inhalation: 60 mg/mL in 5 mL amps; *TOBI®* (Novartis); (Rx)

Also available in ophthalmic preparations.

References

Baird, N. (2003). Antibiotic use in camelids. Proceedings: Western Veterinary Conference. Accessed via: Veterinary Information Network. http://goo.gl/6JhBQ

Bauck, L. & H. Hoefer (1993). Avian antimicrobial therapy. *Seminars in Avian & Exotic Med* 2(1): 17–22.

Brovida, C. (2003). Urinary Tract Infection (UTI): How to diagnose correctly and treat. Proceedings: World Small Animal Veterinary Assoc World Congress. Accessed via: Veterinary Information Network. http://goo.gl/F2zcU

Flammer, K. (2003). Antimicrobic selection criteria in avian medicine. Proceedings: Western Veterinary Conf. Accessed via: Veterinary Information Network. http://goo.gl/l8kX7

Gauvin, J. (1993). Drug therapy in reptiles. *Seminars in Avian & Exotic Med* 2(1): 48–59.

Greene, C., K. Hartmannn, et al. (2006). Appendix 8: Antimicrobial Drug Formulary. *Infectious Disease of the Dog and Cat.* C Greene Ed., Elsevier: 1186–1333.

Hubenov, H., D. Bakalov, et al. (2007). Pharmacokinetic studies on tobramycin in horses. *Journal of Veterinary Pharmacology and Therapeutics* 30(4): 353–357.

Papich, M. (1989). Effects of drugs on pregnancy. *Current Veterinary Therapy X: Small Animal Practice.* R Kirk Ed. Philadelphia, Saunders: 1291–1299.

Tello, L. (2003). Septic patient: Approach and medical management. Proceedings: World Small Animal Veterinary Assoc World Congress. Accessed via: Veterinary Information Network. http://goo.gl/Tt7BL

Vaden, S. & M. Papich (1995). Empiric Antibiotic Therapy. *Kirk's Current Veterinary Therapy:XII.* J Bonagura Ed. Philadelphia, W.B. Saunders: 276–280.

TOCERANIB PHOSPHATE

(toe-**ser**-a-nib)   Palladia®

TYROSINE KINASE INHIBITOR
ANTINEOPLASTIC

Prescriber Highlights

▶ Tyrosine kinase inhibitor FDA-approved for grades II or III canine mast cell tumors

▶ Most common adverse effects are: diarrhea, decreased/loss of appetite, lameness, weight loss and blood in the stool

▶ Adverse effects can be serious and require treatment pause or dose reduction

▶ Monitoring essential

Uses/Indications

Toceranib is indicated for the treatment of Patnaik grade II or III, recurrent, cutaneous mast cell tumors with or without regional lymph node involvement in dogs.

Toceranib may prove useful for treating a variety of tumors in dogs, including sarcomas, carcinomas, melanomas, and myeloma. Toceranib as part of metronomic protocol (using low doses of chemotherapy and/or other anti-cancer agents to inhibit tumor angiogenesis and growth) is being investigated.

Pharmacology/Actions

Toceranib is a small molecule tyrosine kinase inhibitor (TKIs) that selectively inhibits the tyrosine kinase activity of several split kinase receptor tyrosine kinases (RTK), including VEGFR-2 (vascular endothelial growth factor receptor-2), PDGFR-Beta (platelet-derived growth factor receptor-Beta), Kit (stem cell growth factor receptor), among others. These kinases are believed to be involved in growth, pathologic angiogenesis, and metastatic processes of certain tumors. By inhibiting TKIs, toceranib competitively inhibits ATP, preventing receptor phosphorylation and subsequent downstream signal transduction. Toceranib exerts an antiproliferative effect on endothelial cells (*in vitro*) and can induce cell cycle arrest and subsequent apoptosis in tumor cell lines expressing activating mutations in Kit. As canine mast cell tumor growth can be enhanced by activating mutations in Kit, toceranib inhibition can reduce angiogenesis and subsequent growth of these cells.

Calcitriol may enhance the antiproliferative activity of toceranib in dogs with mast cell tumors and investigations exploring this potential are ongoing (Malone *et al.* 2010).

Pharmacokinetics

Oral bioavailability of toceranib phosphate in dogs is about 77%. The presence of food does not significantly impact absorption. Binding to canine plasma proteins is around 94% and the volume of distribution is very large (>20 L/kg). Terminal elimination half-life is about 17 hours (after IV) and 31 hours (oral). While the metabolic fate of toceranib has not been completely determined, it appears that the drug is metabolized via cytochrome P450 and/or flavin monooxygenase to an N-oxide metabolite.

Contraindications/Precautions/Warnings

The label lists toceranib contraindications as breeding, pregnant or lactating bitches. Safe use has not been evaluated in dogs less than 24 months of age or weighing less than 5 kg. Because toceranib can cause vascular dysfunction leading to edema and thromboembolism (including pulmonary emboli), wait at least 3 days after stopping drug before performing surgery.

Use caution when handling this medication. See drug company's Client Information Sheet for more details.

When toceranib is used in the presence of systemic mast cell tumors significant mast cell degranulation with resultant adverse effects may result. The manufacturer states that attempt should be made to rule out systemic mastocytosis prior to starting toceranib.

Toceranib can cause clinical signs similar to those seen with aggressive mast cell tumors, when these occur, the drug should be stopped and the patient re-evaluated (Johannes 2010). The package insert has specific monitoring requirements with dosage adjustment or therapy pause guidelines when certain adverse effects (severe diarrhea, GI bleeding) occur or when laboratory monitoring indicates toxicity. Refer to the Monitoring section below, or the package insert for more information.

Adverse Effects

Most common adverse effects seen with toceranib in dogs include: diarrhea, decreased/loss of appetite, lameness, weight loss and blood in the stool. Severe diarrhea or GI bleeding require immediate treatment and dictate dose interruption or dose reduction (see monitoring below). Other potential adverse effects include muscle cramping, neutropenia, hypoalbuminemia, thromboembolic disease, vasculitis, pancreatitis, nasal depigmentation, change in coat or skin color, epistaxis, seizures and pruritus.

One author (London 2010) suggests starting certain drugs 4-7 days prior to staring toceranib to reduce the likelihood of toxicity. These include antacids (famotidine, omeprazole), an antihistamine (diphenhydramine) and prednisone (to reduce tumor inflammation and possibly decrease mast cell tumor mediators' effects) and sucralfate (if dog has a positive stool hemoccult). Additionally, dogs that experience inappetence or vomiting after therapy has begun, either metoclopramide, ondansetron, or maropitant may be effective. Loperamide can be given on toceranib dosing days help prevent or lessen diarrhea. Others have found metronidazole useful. Another author states that prednisone can be continued after treatment has begun, but should only given on days when toceranib is not given and that NSAIDs and prednisone should never be used together (Garrett 2010).

Reproductive/Nursing Safety

Toceranib is a likely teratogen and should not be used in pregnant females. It is labeled as contraindicated in breeding, pregnant, or lactating bitches.

Overdosage/Acute Toxicity

No acute toxicity data was located, but toceranib has a narrow margin of safety. In the event of an acute overdose, consider immediate gut decontamination; contact an animal poison center for further guidance.

Drug Interactions

The following drug interactions have either been reported or are theoretical in humans or animals receiving toceranib and may be of significance in veterinary patients:

■ **NSAIDS:** The package insert states: to use NSAIDs with caution in conjunction with toceranib due to an increased risk of gastrointestinal ulceration or perforation. However, NSAIDs (e.g., piroxicam) are often sometimes used with toceranib as part of metronomic drug protocols, they should be used with extreme caution in dogs receiving toceranib; and should never be given on the same day as GI toxicity can be exacerbated (London 2010).

■ **CYP3A4 INHIBITORS** (e.g., ketoconazole, fluconazole, itraconazole, grapefruit juice, clarithromycin, verapamil): May increase toceranib concentrations. This interaction with toceranib has not been documented in dogs to date and presently is speculative. However, use caution.

Laboratory Considerations

■ None noted.

Doses

■ **DOGS:**

For Patnaik grade II or III, recurrent, cutaneous mast cell tumors with or without regional lymph node involvement:

a) Initial dose 3.25 mg/kg PO every other day (q48h). Dose reductions of 0.5 mg/kg (to a minimum dose of 2.2 mg/kg every other day and dose interruptions (cessation of treatment) for up to two weeks may be utilized, if needed, to manage adverse reactions. May be administered with or without food. Do not split tablets. The package insert has a dosage table to determine the appropriate strength and number of tablets to use for a given dog's weight. (Adapted from label information; *Palladia®*—Pfizer)

b) Recent clinical experience with toceranib in dogs suggests that dosing at 2.5–2.75 mg/kg every other day is better tolerated than the higher dose, resulting in less toxicity, better owner compliance, and fewer drug holidays. Some dogs do not tolerate this dosing regimen even at the 2.5 mg/kg dose rate. The author and some other medical oncologists have found that a Monday/Wednesday/Friday schedule of dosing may be better tolerated by some dogs. This may be particularly useful when toceranib is combined with other drugs, such as cyclophosphamide or NSAIDs as part of a metronomic treatment protocol. When a dog cannot tolerate the M/W/F schedule, every third day dosing may be attempted, but this is not ideal and may result in sub-therapeutic drug exposure. (London 2010)

Monitoring

■ CBC, Hematocrit, Serum Albumin, Creatinine, Serum Phosphate. Manufacturer recommends weekly (approximately) veterinary assessment for the first 6 weeks of therapy and every 6 weeks (approximately) thereafter.

■ The package insert states: Temporarily discontinue drug if anemia, azotemia, hypoalbuminemia, and hyperphosphatemia occur simultaneously. Resume treatment at a dose reduction of 0.5 mg/kg after 1 to 2 weeks when values have improved and albumin is >2.5 g/dL. Temporary treatment interruptions may be needed if any one of these occurs alone: hematocrit <26%, creatinine ≥2 mg/dL or albumin <1.5 g/dL. Then resume treatment at a dose reduction of 0.5 mg/kg once the hematocrit is >30%, the creatinine is <2.0 mg/dL, and the albumin is >2.5 g/dL. Temporarily discontinue the use of toceranib if neutrophil count is ≤1000/microL. Resume treatment after 1 to 2 weeks at a dose reduction of 0.5 mg/kg, when neutrophil count has returned to >1000/microL. Further dose reductions may be needed if severe neutropenia reoccurs.

■ Other laboratory tests that have been suggested for monitoring early (first 6 weeks) include urinalysis, and full chemistry panels

■ Adverse Effects (Diarrhea): If ≥4 watery stools/day or ≥ 2 days stop drug until formed stools and institute supportive care. When dosing is resumed, decrease dose by 0.5 mg/kg.

■ Adverse Effects (GI-Bleeding): If fresh blood in stool or black tarry stool for > 2 days or frank hemorrhage or blood clots in stool. Stop drug and institute supportive care until resolution of all clinical signs of blood in stool, then decrease dose by 0.5 mg/kg.

■ Tumor Size

Client Information

■ In the package insert, the manufacturer states to: "Always provide Client Information Sheet with prescription." In addition, it is highly recommended to verbally reiterate some of the key points found on the client information sheet, including the sections: "How do I give *Palladia* to my dog?"; "Stop *Palladia* immediately and contact your veterinarian if you notice any of the following changes in your dog"; and "Handling Instructions".

■ May be given with or without food; do not split or crush tablets

Chemistry/Synonyms

Toceranib phosphate is an idolinone with a molecular weight of 494.46. Toceranib may also be known as: PHA-291639, SU-11654, UNII-59L7Y0530C, toceranibum, or tocéranib.

Storage/Stability

Toceranib phosphate tablets should be stored at controlled room temperature 20–25°C (68–77° F).

Dosage Forms/Regulatory Status

VETERINARY-LABELED PRODUCTS:

Toceranib Phosphate Oral Tablets: 10 mg, 15 mg, 50 mg; *Palladia®* (Pfizer); (Rx)

HUMAN-LABELED PRODUCTS: None

References

Garrett, L. (2010). New Therapies for Cancer: The Role of Tyrosine Kinase Inhibitors in Practice. Proceedings: WVC. Accessed via: Veterinary Information Network. http://goo.gl/MHJRY

Johannes, C. (2010). Toceranib Phosphate (PalladiaTM): A New Treatment Option for Canine MCT. Proceedings: ACVIM. Accessed via: Veterinary Information Network. http://goo.gl/PtGuk

London, C.A. (2010). Tyrosine Kinase Inhibitor (TKI) Therapy in Companion Animals: Year One. Proceedings: ACVIM. Accessed via: Veterinary Information Network. http://goo.gl/v01GA

Malone, E.K., K.M. Rassnick, et al. (2010). Calcitriol (1,25–dihydroxycholecalciferol) enhances mast cell tumour chemotherapy and receptor tyrosine kinase inhibitor activity in vitro and has single-agent activity against spontaneously occurring canine mast cell tumours. *Veterinary and Comparative Oncology* 8(3): 209–220.

TOLAZOLINE HCL

(toe-*laz*-oh-leen)   Tolazine®

ALPHA-ADRENERGIC BLOCKER

Prescriber Highlights

▶ Alpha-adrenergic blocker used primarily as a reversal agent for xylazine

▶ Contraindications: Horses exhibiting signs of stress, debilitation, cardiac disease, sympathetic blockage, hypovolemia or shock, hypersensitivity, or with coronary artery or cerebrovascular disease

▶ Adverse Effects: *Horses:* Transient tachycardia; peripheral vasodilatation presenting as sweating & injected mucous membranes of the gingiva & conjunctiva; hyperalgesia of the lips (licking, flipping of lips); piloerection; clear lacrimal & nasal discharge; muscle fasciculations; apprehensiveness

Uses/Indications

Tolazoline is FDA-approved and indicated for the reversal of effects associated with xylazine in horses. It has also been used for this purpose in a variety of other species as well, but less safety and efficacy data is available.

In humans, the primary uses for tolazoline are: treatment of persistent pulmonary hypertension in newborns, adjunctive treatment and diagnosis of peripheral vasospastic disorders, and as a provocative test for glaucoma after subconjunctival injection.

Pharmacology/Actions

By directly relaxing vascular smooth muscle, tolazoline has peripheral vasodilating effects and decreases total peripheral resistance. Tolazoline also is a competitive alpha$_1$ and alpha$_2$-adrenergic blocking agent, explaining its mechanism for reversing the effects of xylazine. Tolazoline is rapid acting (usually within 5 minutes of IV administration), but has a short duration of action and repeat doses may be required.

Pharmacokinetics

After IV injection in horses, tolazoline is widely distributed. Animal studies have demonstrated that tolazoline is concentrated in the liver and kidneys. Half-life in horses at recommended doses is approximately 1 hour.

Contraindications/Precautions/Warnings

The manufacturer does not recommend use in horses exhibiting signs of stress, debilitation, cardiac disease, sympathetic blockage, hypovolemia, or shock. Safe use for foals has not been established and some believe it should not be used in foals. as adverse reactions and fatalities have been reported.

Tolazoline should be considered contraindicated in patients known to be hypersensitive to it, or with coronary artery or cerebrovascular disease. Humans having any of the above-contraindicated conditions should use extra caution when handling the agent.

Adverse Effects

In horses adverse effects that may occur include: transient tachycardia; peripheral vasodilatation presenting as sweating and injected mucous membranes of the gingiva and conjunctiva; hyperalgesia of the lips (licking, flipping of lips); piloerection; clear lacrimal and nasal discharge; muscle fasciculations; apprehensiveness. Adverse effects should diminish with time and generally disappear within 2 hours of dosing. The potential for adverse effects increases if tolazoline is given at higher than recommended dosages or if xylazine has not be previously administered.

Reproductive/Nursing Safety

Safety during pregnancy, in breeding or lactating animals has not been established. It is unknown if the drug enters maternal milk.

Overdosage/Acute Toxicity

In horses given tolazoline alone (no previous xylazine), doses of 5X recommended resulted in gastrointestinal hypermotility with resultant flatulence and defecation or attempt to defecate. Some horses exhibited mild colic and transient diarrhea. Intraventricular conduction may be slowed when horses are overdosed, with a prolongation of the QRS-complex noted. Ventricular arrhythmias may occur resulting in death with higher overdoses (5X). In humans, ephedrine (NOT epinephrine or norepinephrine) has been recommended to treat serious tolazoline-induced hypotension.

A llama that received 4.3 mg/kg IV and again 45 minutes later (approximately a 5X overdose) developed signs of anxiety, hyperesthesia, profuse salivation, GI tract hypermotility, diarrhea, convulsions, hypotension, and tachypnea. Treatment including IV diazepam, phenylephrine, IV fluids, and oxygen was successful. (Reed *et al.* 2000).

Drug Interactions

The following drug interactions have either been reported or are theoretical in humans or animals receiving tolazoline and may be of significance in veterinary patients:

■ **ALCOHOL:** Accumulation of acetaldehyde can occur if tolazoline and alcohol are given simultaneously

■ **EPINEPHRINE, NOREPINEPHRINE:** If large doses of tolazoline are given with either norepinephrine or epinephrine, a paradoxical drop in blood pressure can occur followed by a precipitous increase in blood pressure

Doses

■ **DOGS/CATS:**

For reversal of xylazine effects:

a) 4 mg/kg slow IV (4 mL/220 lb. of body weight); administration rate should approximate 1 mL/second (Package Insert; *Tolazine®*—Lloyd Laboratories; New Zealand)

Note: If reversal is warranted, the high concentration (100 mg/mL) of the veterinary drug may make accurate dosing difficult; yohimbine or the human-labeled tolazoline product (25 mg/mL) may be safer alternatives than *Tolazine®* (100 mg/mL). **Note:** Tolazoline is not FDA-approved for use in dogs and cats in the USA and the US manufacturer does not recommend its use.

■ **HORSES:**

For reversal of xylazine effects:

a) 4 mg/kg slow IV (4 mL/220 lb. of body weight); administration rate should approximate 1 mL/second (Package Insert; *Tolazine®*—Lloyd Laboratories)

■ **LLAMAS/ALPACAS:**

For reversal of xylazine effects:

a) 1–2 mg/kg IM or give 50% of initial dose slowly IV or IM and then determine if more is needed. Use with caution IV in camelids. (Wolff 2009)

b) 1–2 mg/kg IV or IM; Caution: acute death has been reported after rapid IV administration of tolazoline at high dosages. (Anderson 2005)

■ **BIRDS:**

As a reversal agent for alpha2-adrenergic agonists (*e.g.*, xylazine, detomidine, etc.):

a) 15 mg/kg IV (Clyde & Paul-Murphy 2000)

■ **DEER:**

Note: Not FDA-approved in the USA for use in food animals

For reversal of xylazine effects:

a) 2–4 mg/kg slow IV; titrate to effect; Slaughter withdrawal: 30 days (Label Directions; *Tolazine®*—Lloyd Laboratories; New Zealand)

■ **CATTLE:**

Note: Not FDA-approved in the USA for use in food animals

For reversal of xylazine effects:

a) 2–4 mg/kg slow IV; titrate to effect; Slaughter withdrawal: 30 days (Label Directions; *Tolazine®*—Lloyd Laboratories; New Zealand)

b) The amount of reversal agent used depends on the dose and time elapsed after administering xylazine. Emergency doses of yohimbine (0.1 mg/kg IV) or tolazoline at 2 mg/kg IM can be administered, but tolazoline should not be administered IV rapidly as this can result in cardiac asystole. When dosed properly the effects of reversal should start to become evident about 10 minutes following IM administration. (Anderson & Abrahamsen 2008)

■ **SHEEP & GOATS:**

Note: Not FDA-approved in the USA for use in food animals

For reversal of xylazine effects:

a) 2–4 mg/kg slow IV; titrate to effect; Slaughter withdrawal: 30 days (Label Directions; *Tolazine®*—Lloyd Laboratories; New Zealand)

b) Small Ruminants: 1–2 mg /kg IM. Give 50% of initial dose slow IV or IM and then determine if more is needed. (Snyder 2009)

Monitoring/Client Information
■ Reversal effects (efficacy)
■ Adverse effects (see above). Because of the risks associated with the use of xylazine and reversal by tolazoline, these drugs should be administered and monitored by veterinary professionals only.

Chemistry/Synonyms
An alpha-adrenergic blocking agent, tolazoline HCl is structurally related to phentolamine. It occurs as a white to off-white, crystalline powder possessing a bitter taste and a slight aromatic odor. Tolazoline is freely soluble in ethanol or water. The commercially available (human) injection has pH between 3–4.

Tolazoline HCl may also be known as: benzazoline hydrochloride, tolazolinium chloratum, *Priscol®*, *Priscoline®*, *Tolazine®* or *Vaso-Dilatan®*.

Storage/Stability
Commercially available injection products should be stored between 15–30°C and protected from light.

Compatibility/Compounding Considerations
The drug is reportedly physically **compatible** with the commonly used IV solutions.

Dosage Forms/Regulatory Status
VETERINARY-LABELED PRODUCTS:

Tolazoline HCl Injection: 100 mg/mL in 100 mL multi-dose vials; *Tolazine®* (Lloyd); (Rx). FDA-approved for use in horses; not to be used in food-producing animals.

HUMAN-LABELED PRODUCTS: None

References
Anderson, D. (2005). Camelid anesthesia and surgery. Proceedings: Western Vet Conf. Accessed via: Veterinary Information Network. http://goo.gl/93zbj

Anderson, D. & E. Abrahamsen (2008). Chemical Restraint in the Field—New Uses For Old Drugs. Proceedings: World Vet Congress. Accessed via: Veterinary Information Network. http://goo.gl/G6BXN

Clyde, V. & J. Paul-Murphy (2000). Avian Analgesia. *Kirk's Current Veterinary Therapy: XIII Small Animal Practice.* J Bonagura Ed. Philadelphia, WB Saunders: 1126–1128.

Reed, M., T. Duke, et al. (2000). Suspected tolazoline toxicosis in a llama. *J Am Vet Med Assoc* **216**: 227–229.

Snyder, J. (2009). Small Ruminant Medicine & Surgery for Equine and Small Animal Practitioners I & II. Proceedings: WVC. Accessed via: Veterinary Information Network. http://goo.gl/hkoer

Wolff, P. (2009). Camelid Medicine. Proceedings: AAZV. Accessed via: Veterinary Information Network. http://goo.gl/4TEAy

TOLFENAMIC ACID

(tole-fen-a-mik)   Tolfedine®

NONSTEROIDAL ANTIINFLAMMATORY AGENT

Prescriber Highlights

▶ NSAID approved for dogs & cats in Canada, Europe

▶ Available (not in USA) in both oral & injectable dosage forms

▶ Relatively safe for short-term use

Uses/Indications
Tolfenamic acid may be useful for the treatment of acute or chronic pain and/or inflammation in dogs and acute pain/inflammation in cats. In Europe, it is also approved for use in cattle.

Pharmacology/Actions
Tolfenamic acid exhibits pharmacologic actions similar to those of aspirin. It is a potent inhibitor of cyclooxygenase, thereby inhibiting the release of prostaglandins. It also has direct inhibition of prostaglandin receptors. Tolfenamic acid has significant anti-thromboxane activity and is not recommended for use pre-surgically because of its effects on platelet function.

Pharmacokinetics
Tolfenamic acid is absorbed after oral administration. In dogs, peak levels occur from 2–4 hours after dosing. Enterohepatic recirculation is increased if given with food. This can increase the bioavailability, but also creates more variability in bioavailability than when given to fasted dogs. The vol-

ume of distribution in dogs is reported to be 1.2 L/kg and it has an elimination half-life of about 6.5 hours. Duration of antiinflammatory effect is 24–36 hours. Dogs with experimentally induced renal failure had significantly increased clearances of the drug presumably via increasing hepatic metabolism or enterohepatic recycling of tolfenamic acid (Lefebvre *et al.* 1997).

Contraindications/Precautions/Warnings

Tolfenamic acid is contraindicated in animals hypersensitive to it or to other drugs in its class (*i.e.*, meclofenamic acid). Like other NSAIDs, it should not be used in animals with active GI bleeding or ulceration. Use with caution in patients with decreased renal or hepatic function.

Adverse Effects

Tolfenamic acid is relatively safe when given as recommended in dogs and cats. Vomiting and diarrhea have been reported after oral use. Experimental studies did not demonstrate significant renal or GI toxicity until doses were more than 10 times labeled.

Because of its anti-thromboxane activity and resultant effects on platelet function, tolfenamic acid is not recommended for use pre-surgically.

Reproductive/Nursing Safety

No specific information was located; like other NSAIDs, tolfenamic acid should be used with caution in pregnancy.

Overdosage/Acute Toxicity

No specific information was located. It is suggested that if an acute, overdose occurs treatment follows standard overdose procedures (empty gut following oral ingestion, etc.). Supportive treatment should be instituted as necessary and IV diazepam used to help control seizures. Monitor for GI bleeding. Because tolfenamic acid may cause renal effects, monitor electrolyte and fluid balance carefully and manage renal failure using established guidelines.

Drug Interactions

The following drug interactions have either been reported or are theoretical in humans or animals receiving tolfenamic acid or other NSAIDs and may be of significance in veterinary patients:

- **ASPIRIN:** May increase the risk of gastrointestinal toxicity (*e.g.*, ulceration, bleeding, vomiting, diarrhea)
- **CORTICOSTEROIDS:** As concomitant corticosteroid therapy may increase the occurrence of gastric ulceration, avoid the use of these drugs when also using tolfenamic acid
- **DIGOXIN:** NSAIDS may increase serum levels
- **FLUCONAZOLE:** Administration has increased plasma levels of celecoxib in humans and potentially could also affect tolfenamic acid levels in dogs
- **FUROSEMIDE:** NSAIDs may reduce saluretic and diuretic effects
- **METHOTREXATE:** Serious toxicity has occurred when NSAIDs have been used con-

comitantly with methotrexate; use together with extreme caution

- **NEPHROTOXIC DRUGS (*e.g.*, furosemide, aminoglycosides, amphotericin B, etc.):** May enhance the risk of nephrotoxicity
- **NSAIDS, OTHER:** May increase the risk of gastrointestinal toxicity (*e.g.*, ulceration, bleeding, vomiting, diarrhea)
- **WARFARIN:** Closely monitor patients also receiving drugs that are highly bound to plasma proteins (*e.g.*, warfarin), as tolfenamic acid and its active metabolite are 98–99% protein bound in the dog

Doses

- **DOGS:**
  a) For acute pain: 4 mg/kg once daily SC, IM or PO for 3–5 days.

  For chronic pain: 4 mg/kg, PO once daily for 3–5 consecutive days per week. The injectable is suggested for the first dose only. (Dowling 2000)

  b) First dose: 4 mg/kg SC or IM; follow with tablets at 4 mg/kg PO once daily for 2–4 days. The treatment may be repeated once a week as required, or as recommended by the veterinarian, PO once daily for 3–5 days. (Label information; *Tolfedine®*—Vetoquinol Canada)

- **CATS:**
  a) For acute pain: 4 mg/kg once daily SC, IM or PO for 3–5 days. The injectable is suggested for the first dose only. (Dowling 2000)

  b) 4 mg/kg PO once daily for 3–5 days or as recommended by the veterinarian. (Label information; *Tolfedine®*—Vetoquinol Canada)

- **CATTLE:**
  a) As registered for use in Australia: As an aid in the treatment of pneumonia and acute mastitis in cattle: Pneumonia: 2 mg/kg by IM injection high in the neck. Treatment may be repeated once only after 48 hours. Mastitis: 4 mg/kg as a single intravenous injection. DO NOT inject cattle other than into muscle tissues high on the side of the neck. Meat withdrawal = 10 days (IM), 4 days (IV); Milk withdrawal = 12 hours (1 milking). (Label Information; *Tolfejec®*—Troy Labs, Australia)

- **SWINE:**
  a) As registered for use in Australia: As an aid in the treatment of metritis-mastitis-agalactia in pigs: 2 mg/kg IM once. Meat withdrawal = 6 days. (Label Information; *Tolfejec®*—Troy Labs, Australia)

Monitoring

- Clinical efficacy
- Adverse effects

Client Information

■ The weekly dosing regimen (3–5 consecutive days per week for dogs) is important to follow to minimize risks of adverse effects

■ Report any changes in appetite, water consumption, or GI distress to veterinarian

Chemistry/Synonyms

A non-steroidal antiinflammatory agent in the anthranilic acid (fenamate) category, tolfenamic acid is related chemically to meclofenamic acid.

Tolfenamic Acid may also be known as: acidum tolfenamicum, *Bifenac®, Clotam®, Clotan®, Fenamic®, Flocur®, Gantil®, Migea®, Polmonin®, Purfalox®, Rociclyn®, Tolfamic®, Tolfedine®, Tolfejec®* or *Turbaund®*.

Storage/Stability

Unless otherwise labeled, store tolfenamic acid tablets and solution at room temperature.

Dosage Forms/Regulatory Status

VETERINARY-LABELED PRODUCTS: None in the USA.

In Canada, New Zealand, Australia and Europe: Tolfenamic Acid Tablets: 6 mg, 30 mg, 60 mg and Tolfenamic Acid Injection 40 mg/mL are available. Common trade name is *Tolfedine®* (Vetoquinol).

HUMAN-LABELED PRODUCTS: None in the USA

References

Dowling, P. (2000). Non-steroidal anti-inflammatory drugs for small animal practitioners. District of Columbia Academy of Veterinary Medicine, Fairfax VA.

Lefebvre, H.P., V. Laroute, et al. (1997). The effect of experimental renal failure on tolfenamic acid disposition in the dog. *Biopharmaceutics & Drug Disposition* 18(1): 79–91.

TOLTRAZURIL

(tole-*traz*-yoo-ril)   Baycox®

ANTIPROTOZOAL/ANTICOCCIDIAL

Prescriber Highlights

▶ Antiprotozoal labeled for treating coccidia in poultry (in Europe)

▶ May be considered as an alternative for treating coccidiosis in dogs & cats, oocyst shedding stage of toxoplasmosis in cats, etc.

▶ Not commercially available in the USA, must be legally imported

▶ Adverse effect profile not well described

Uses/Indications

Toltrazuril is an antiprotozoal agent that may be considered as an alternative treatment for coccidiosis in dogs and cats, Isospora or Hepatazoon infections, or for treating the oocyst shedding stage of toxoplasmosis in cats. It has also been used as a treatment for overwhelming parasitic loads in lizards (Bearded Dragons).

Toltrazuril has activity against parasites of the genus *Hepatozoon*, but other drugs (*e.g.*, imidocarb, primaquine, doxycycline) are generally used. Toltrazuril can induce initial excellent clinical responses in dogs with American canine hepatozoonosis (ACH), but cannot completely eliminate the parasites, and remission is transient in most dogs.

While toltrazuril has been used to treat equine protozoal myeloencephalitis (EPM) caused by *Sarcocystis neurona*, use of FDA-approved products now available (*e.g.*, ponazuril, pyrimethamine/sulfadiazine) is preferred.

Toltrazuril has been used in some countries to treat *Isospora suis* in piglets.

Pharmacology/Actions

Toltrazuril is the parent compound to ponazuril (toltrazuril sulfone). Its mechanism of action is not well understood, but it appears to inhibit protozoal enzyme systems.

Toltrazuril has activity against *Hepatozoon*, *Isospora*, *Sarcocystis*, *Toxoplasma*, and all intracellular stages of coccidia.

Pharmacokinetics

Little information is available. Toltrazuril is about 50% absorbed after oral consumption in poultry. Highest concentrations are found in the liver; it is rapidly metabolized into the sulfone derivative (ponazuril).

Contraindications/Precautions/Warnings

Toltrazuril should not be used in patients who have had prior hypersensitivity reactions to it or other triazinone (triazine) antiprotozoals (*e.g.*, ponazuril, diclazuril).

The principle metabolite of toltrazuril reportedly persists in the environment and can contaminate groundwater, however there appears to be little risk for significant environmental contamination when toltrazuril is used in dogs, cats, horses, or other companion animals (pet birds, reptiles).

Adverse Effects

Toltrazuril appears to be well tolerated in birds. An adverse effect profile in mammals is not well described. Potentially, GI signs could occur. Some horses receiving the related drug ponazuril, developed blisters on their nose and mouth, and some, a rash or hives during field trials.

Reproductive/Nursing Safety

No reproductive or nursing safety information was located; weigh potential risks versus benefits of use during pregnancy or lactation.

Overdosage/Acute Toxicity

Very limited information is available. Doses of up to 10X in horses were tolerated without significant adverse effects. 5X overdoses in poultry have been tolerated without clinical signs noted. Decreased water intake has been seen if overdoses are greater than 5X.

Drug Interactions

■ None reported

Laboratory Considerations

■ No issues were noted.

Doses

■ **DOGS:**

a) For coccidiosis (Cystoisosporosis): 10–20 mg/kg PO one time to all puppies at 3–4 weeks of age will help prevent problems associated with intestinal coccidiosis (Daugschies *et al.* 2000)

b) For coccidiosis: 15 mg/kg PO once daily for 3–6 days (Dubey, J. & Greene 2006)

c) For *Isospora* spp. infections: 10–30 mg/kg PO once daily for 1–3 days. (Dubey, J.P. *et al.* 2009)

d) For coccidiosis: 20 mg/kg PO once daily for 3 days. (Marks 2007)

■ **CATS:**

a) For enteroepithelial cycle of toxoplasmosis (oocyst shedding): 5–10 mg/kg PO once daily for 2 days (Dubey, J. & Lappin 2006)

b) For coccidiosis: 30 mg/kg PO once daily for 2–3 days (Greene *et al.* 2006)

c) For coccidiosis: 20 mg/kg PO once daily for 3 days. (Marks 2007)

■ **SHEEP:**

a) For ovine coccidiosis (*Eimeria ovinoidalis*): Controlled study comparing efficacy against diclazuril: 20 mg/kg PO once. (Mundt *et al.* 2009)

■ **BIRDS:**

a) For coccidiosis in raptors: 7 mg/kg PO once daily for 2–3 days (Jones 2004)

■ **REPTILES:**

a) For parasitism in Bearded Dragons: 5–15 mg/kg PO once daily for 3 days (Kramer 2006)

Monitoring

■ Clinical efficacy

Client Information

■ Avoid direct contact with this medication; the manufacturer recommends wearing synthetic rubber gloves when handling the 2.5% solution. Wash exposed skin after use.

Chemistry/Synonyms

Related to other antiprotozoals such as ponazuril, toltrazuril is a triazinone (triazine) antiprotozoal (anticoccidial) agent. The commercially available (in Europe) 2.5% oral solution is an alkaline, clear, colorless to yellow brown solution that also contains triethanolamine 30 mg/mL and polyethylene glycol 80.7 mg/mL. Toltrazuril has a molecular weight of 425.4

Toltrazuril may also be known as Bay-Vi-9142, toltrazurilo, toltrazurilum and *Baycox®*.

Storage/Stability

The 2.5% solution should be stored at temperatures at 25°C or below.

Dilutions in drinking water more concentrated than 1:1000 (1 mL of the 2.5% solution to 1 liter of water) may precipitate. After dilution, the resulting solution is stable for 24 hours. It is recommended that medicated drinking water not consumed after 24 hours be discarded.

Dosage Forms/Regulatory Status

VETERINARY-LABELED PRODUCTS: None in the USA

In some European countries: Toltrazuril 2.5% (25 mg/ml) solution for dilution in drinking water in 1 liter bottles; *Baycox® 2.5% Solution* (Bayer); (Rx). FDA-approved for treatment of coccidiosis in poultry. In the UK, slaughter withdrawal is 18 days for poultry. Not for use in birds producing eggs for human consumption.

The FDA may allow legal importation of this medication for compassionate use in animals; for more information, see the *Instructions for Legally Importing Drugs for Compassionate Use in the USA* found in the appendix.

HUMAN-LABELED PRODUCTS: None

References

Daugschies, A., H. Mundt, et al. (2000). Toltrazuril treatment of cystoisosporosis in dogs under experimental and field conditions. *Parisol Res* **86**: 797–799.

Dubey, J. & C. Greene (2006). Enteric coccidiosis. *Infectious Diseases of the Dogs and Cat, 3rd Ed.* C Greene Ed., Elsevier: 775–784.

Dubey, J. & M. Lappin (2006). Toxoplasmosis and Neosporosis. *Infectious Diseases of the Dogs and Cat, 3rd Ed.* C Greene Ed., Elsevier: 754–775.

Dubey, J.P., D.S. Lindsay, et al. (2009). Toxoplasmosis and Other Intestinal Coccidial Infections in Cats and Dogs. *Veterinary Clinics of North America-Small Animal Practice* **39**(6): 1009–+.

Greene, C., K. Hartmannn, et al. (2006). Appendix 8: Antimicrobial Drug Formulary. *Infectious Disease of the Dog and Cat.* C Greene Ed., Elsevier: 1186–1333.

Jones, M. (2004). Update on infectious diseases of birds of prey. Proceedings: Western Veterinary Conference. Accessed via: Veterinary Information Network. http://goo.gl/DHagK

Kramer, M. (2006). Bearded Dragon Medicine. Proceedings: Western Veterinary Confernce. Accessed via: Veterinary Information Network. http://goo.gl/GAfJR

Marks, S. (2007). What's the latest on parasitic causes of diarrhea in dogs and cats? Proceedings: ACVIM 2007. Accessed via: Veterinary Information Network. http://goo.gl/fw8Kw

Mundt, H.C., K. Dittmar, et al. (2009). Study of the Comparative Efficacy of Toltrazuril and Diclazuril against Ovine Coccidiosis in Housed Lambs. *Parasitology Research* **105**: S141–S150.

TOPIRAMATE

(toe-*pie*-rah-mate) Topamax®

ANTICONVULSANT

Prescriber Highlights

▶ Antiseizure medication that may be useful for seizure disorders in dogs, particularly partial seizure activity; may be of benefit in treating cats, but little information available

▶ Very short half-life in dogs (2–4 hours), but therapeutic activity may persist secondary to high affinity for receptors in brain

▶ Adverse effect profile may include GI distress, inappetence, & irritability in dogs; in cats, sedation & inappetence have been noted

▶ Expense may be an issue; generics now available

Uses/Indications

Topiramate may be useful for treating seizures in dogs, particularly partial seizure activity. It may also be of benefit in treating cats, but little information is available.

Pharmacology/Actions

While the exact mechanism for its antiseizure action is not known, topiramate possesses three properties that probably play a role in its activity: Topiramate blocks in a time-dependent manner action potentials elicited repetitively by a sustained depolarization of neurons; it increases the frequency that GABA activates $GABA_A$ receptors; and it antagonizes the kainite/AMPA receptors without affecting the NMDA receptor subtype. Topiramate's actions are concentration-dependent; effects can first be seen at 1microMole and maximize at 200 microMoles. Topiramate is a weak inhibitor of carbonic anhydrase isoenzymes CA-II and CA-IV, but it is believed that this effect does not contribute significantly to its antiepileptic actions.

Pharmacokinetics

In dogs, topiramate is rapidly absorbed after oral administration, but absolute bioavailability varies between 30–60%. Half-life ranges from 2–4 hours after multiple doses (Streeter *et al.* 1995). Comparatively, the half-life in humans is about 21 hours in adults, but shorter in children. In humans, the drug is not extensively metabolized and about 70% is excreted unchanged in the urine.

Contraindications/Precautions/Warnings

Topiramate is contraindicated in patients hypersensitive to it. It should be used with caution (in humans) with impaired hepatic or renal function.

Adverse Effects

Because this drug rarely has been used in veterinary patients, an accurate adverse effect profile is not known. In dogs, most prevalent adverse effects reported include GI distress, inappetence, and irritability. In cats, sedation and inappetence have been noted.

In humans, the most likely adverse effects include somnolence, dizziness, nervousness, confusion, and ataxia. Very rarely, acute myopia with secondary angle closure glaucoma has been reported. Incidence of kidney stones is about 2–4 times higher in patients taking topiramate than in the general population. Topiramate can cause a hyperchloremic metabolic acidosis and reduce citrate excretion in the urine thus increasing urine pH leading to calcium phosphate renal calculi.

Reproductive/Nursing Safety

In humans, the FDA categorizes topiramate as a category *C* drug for use during pregnancy (*Animal studies have shown an adverse effect on the fetus, but there are no adequate studies in humans; or there are no animal reproduction studies and no adequate studies in humans.*) Teratogenic effects were noted in mice and rats given topiramate at dosages equivalent to those used in humans.

Topiramate enters maternal milk; use with caution in nursing patients.

Overdosage/Acute Toxicity

Overdoses in humans have cause convulsions, drowsiness/lethargy, slurred speech, blurred and double vision, impaired mentation/ stupor, ataxia, metabolic acidosis, hypotension, agitation, and abdominal pain.

There were 140 exposures to topiramate reported to the ASPCA Animal Poison Control Center (APCC) during 2008-2009. In these cases 129 were dogs with 16 showing clinical signs and 11 were cats with 5 showing clinical signs. Common findings in dogs recorded in decreasing frequency included ataxia and lethargy.

Treatment consists of gut emptying protocols if the ingestion was recent, and supportive therapy. Hemodialysis is effective in enhancing the elimination of topiramate from the body.

Drug Interactions

The following drug interactions have either been reported or are theoretical in humans or animals receiving topiramate and may be of significance in veterinary patients:

▪ **AMITRIPTYLINE:** Topiramate may increase levels

▪ **CARBONIC ANHYDRASE INHIBITORS (acetazolamide, dichlorphenamide, etc.):** Used concomitantly with topiramate, may increase the risk of renal stone formation

▪ **CNS DEPRESSANT DRUGS, OTHER:** Other CNS depressant drugs may exacerbate the adverse effects of topiramate

■ **LAMOTRIGINE:** May increase topiramate levels

■ **PHENYTOIN:** May decrease topiramate levels; phenytoin levels may increase

■ **VALPROIC ACID:** May decrease topiramate and VPA levels

Laboratory Considerations

■ No specific laboratory interactions or considerations were noted. Plasma concentrations of topiramate are usually not monitored in human patients, but therapeutic levels are thought to range from 2–25 mg/L.

Doses

■ **DOGS:**

a) As an alternative second line anticonvulsant: 5–10 mg/kg PO q12h (Shell 2003)

b) As an alternative treatment for refractory generalized and focal seizures: 5–10 mg/kg PO twice daily (Smith 2002)

c) Initial dose of 2–10 mg/kg PO q12h. (Podell 2006)

d) 5–10 mg/kg PO twice daily; start at the lower dosage to reduce adverse effects. (Kortz 2005)

e) For refractory epilepsy: Presently, the author is using this drug at 2.5–5 mg/kg PO three times daily, but at this stage there is not enough data to know how effective this treatment will be. (Platt 2008)

■ **CATS:**

a) 12.5–25 mg PO (total dose) q8–12h. In author's experience, topiramate has been most useful to treat automatisms (especially running fits) and focal seizure activity. Gradual adaptation in dosing is recommended. Inappetence is a major adverse effect with higher doses. (Podell 2006; Podell 2008)

Monitoring

■ Efficacy
■ Adverse effects

Client Information

■ Clients must understand that the clinical use of this agent is relatively "investigational" in veterinary patients, that it must be dosed often in dogs, and the potential costs

■ Caution clients not to stop therapy abruptly or "rebound" seizures may occur

■ Have clients maintain a seizure diary to help determine efficacy

Chemistry/Synonyms

A sulfamate-substituted derivative of D-fructose antiepileptic, topiramate occurs as a white crystalline powder with a bitter taste. Its solubility in water is 9.8 mg/mL; it is freely soluble in alcohol.

Topiramate may also be known as: McN-4853, RWJ-17021, *Epitomax®*, *Topamac®*, *Topamax®*, or *Topimax®*.

Storage/Stability

Topiramate tablets should be stored in tight containers at room temperature (15–30°C; 59–86°F); protect from moisture. Topiramate sprinkle capsules should be stored in tight containers at temperatures below 25°C (76°F); protect from moisture.

Dosage Forms/Regulatory Status

VETERINARY-LABELED PRODUCTS: None

The ARCI (Racing Commissioners International) has designated this drug as a class 2 substance. See the appendix for more information.

HUMAN-LABELED PRODUCTS:

Topiramate Tablets: 25 mg, 50 mg & 100 mg; Sprinkle Capsules: 15 mg & 25 mg; *Topamax®* (Janssen); *Topiragen®* (Upsher-Smith); generic; (Rx)

References

Kortz, G. (2005). From gold beads to Keppra: Update on anticonvulsant therapy. Proceedings: UCD Veterinary Neurology Symposium. Accessed via: Veterinary Information Network. http://goo.gl/v1l8m

Platt, S.R. (2008). Options for Refractory Epilepsy. Proceedings: WSAVA. Accessed via: Veterinary Information Network. http://goo.gl/BNDiH

Podell, M. (2006). New Horizons in the treatment of epilepsy. Proceedings: ACVIM. Accessed via: Veterinary Information Network. http://goo.gl/PlHdG

Podell, M. (2008). Novel approaches to feline epilepsy. Proceedings: ACVIM. Accessed via: Veterinary Information Network. http://goo.gl/cZuVg

Shell, L. (2003). "Primary Epilepsy."

Smith, M. (2002). Managing refractory seizure disorders. Proceedings: Western Veterinary Conference. Accessed via: Veterinary Information Network. http://goo.gl/ZjyAv

Streeter, A.J., P.L. Stahle, et al. (1995). Pharmacokinetics and bioavailability of topiramate in the beagle dog. *Drug Metabolism and Disposition* 23(1): 90–93.

TORSEMIDE

(**tor**-she-myde)   Demadex®, Torasemide

LOOP DIURETIC

Prescriber Highlights

▶ Potent loop diuretic potentially useful for adjunctive treatment of CHF in dogs & cats; very little information available on clinical use in veterinary medicine

▶ Approximately 10X more potent, longer diuretic action, & more potassium-sparing (in dogs) than furosemide

▶ May be more expensive than furosemide, but tablets are now available generically

Uses/Indications

Torsemide is a loop diuretic similar to furosemide, but it is more potent, its diuretic effects persist for a longer period, and it does not cause as much potassium excretion (in dogs). While clinical use in dogs and cats thus far has been minimal, it potentially may be a useful adjunctive treatment for congestive heart failure in dogs and cats, particularly in patients that have become refractory to furosemide.

Torsemide could be considered for use as an alternative to furosemide particularly in those patients that have become refractory to furosemide therapy. Torsemide is approximately 10 times more potent than furosemide, so a starting dose of 10% of the furosemide dose could be considered. As torsemide has a more persistent diuretic effect (approximately 12 hours), dosing frequency may also be reduced. A study comparing furosemide (2 mg/kg PO twice daily) with torsemide (0.2 mg/kg PO twice daily) demonstrated that diuretic resistance developed after 14 days of furosemide, but not torsemide. But both drugs were associated with increased BUN and plasma creatinine concentrations, compared with values before treatment (Hori *et al.* 2007).

Pharmacology/Actions

Torsemide, like furosemide inhibits sodium and chloride reabsorption in the ascending loop of Henle via interference with the chloride-binding site of the $1Na^+$, $1K^+$, $2Cl^-$ cotransport system.

Torsemide increases renal excretion of water, sodium, potassium, chloride, calcium, magnesium, hydrogen, ammonium, and bicarbonate. In dogs, excretion of potassium is affected much less so than is sodium (20:1); this is approximately twice the ratio of Na:K excreted than with furosemide. In cats, torsemide's effects on potassium excretion appear to be similar to that of furosemide. In dogs, torsemide appears to have differing effects on aldosterone than furosemide. When compared to furosemide, torsemide increases plasma aldosterone levels and inhibits the amount of receptor-bound aldosterone, however, additional research must be performed to determine the clinical significance of these effects.

Pharmacokinetics/Pharmacodynamics

Limited information is available. Oral bioavailability has been reported to be between 80–100% in dogs and cats. Elimination half-life in dogs is about 8 hours which is longer than furosemide. In dogs, diuretic activity begins within one hour of dosing, peaks at about 2 hours and persists for approximately 12 hours.

In cats, peak diuresis occurs about 4 hours post-dose and persists for 12 hours.

Contraindications/Precautions/Warnings

Torsemide should not be used in patients with known hypersensitivity to it or other sulfonylureas, or in anuric patients.

Use torsemide cautiously in patients with significant hepatic dysfunction, hyperuricemia (may increase serum uric acid), or diabetes mellitus (may increase serum glucose).

The ARCI (Racing Commissioners International) has designated this drug as a class 3 substance when used in horses.

The injection should be administered IV slowly over a period of 2 minutes. Ototoxicity has occurred in human patients receiving rapid IV administration of other loop diuretics.

Adverse Effects

Adverse effect profiles for dogs and cats have not been established due to the limited use of this drug in veterinary medicine. Furosemide, a related drug, can induce fluid and electrolyte abnormalities. Patients should be monitored for hydration status and electrolyte imbalances (especially potassium, calcium, magnesium and sodium). Prerenal azotemia may result if moderate to severe dehydration occurs. Hyponatremia is probably the greatest concern, but hypocalcemia, hypokalemia, and hypomagnesemia may all occur. Animals with normal food and water intake are much less likely to develop water and electrolyte imbalances than those that do not.

Other potential adverse effects include gastrointestinal disturbances, hematologic effects (anemia, leukopenia), weakness, and restlessness. Torsemide, unlike furosemide, apparently only rarely causes significant ototoxic effects in humans; very high doses in laboratory animals have induced ototoxicity.

Reproductive/Nursing Safety

No effects on fertility were noted when female and male rats were administered up to 25 mg/kg/day.

No adverse teratogenic effects were seen when pregnant rats and rabbits were administered up to 15X (human dose) and 5X (human dose), respectively. Larger doses did increase fetal resorptions, decreased average body weight, and delayed fetal ossification. In humans, the FDA categorizes torsemide as category *B* for use during pregnancy (*Animal studies have not yet demonstrated a risk to the fetus, but there are no adequate studies in pregnant women; or animal studies have shown an adverse effect, but adequate studies in pregnant women have not demonstrated a risk to the fetus in the first trimester of pregnancy, and there is no evidence of risk in later trimesters.*)

It is unknown if torsemide enters milk, but furosemide is distributed in milk. Clinical significance for nursing offspring is unknown.

Overdosage/Acute Toxicity

In dogs, the oral LD50 is >2 grams/kg. Fluid and electrolyte imbalance is the most likely risk associated with an overdose. Consider gut emptying protocols for very large or quantity unknown ingestions. Acute overdoses should generally be managed by observation with fluid, electrolyte and acid-base monitoring; supportive treatment should be initiated if required.

Drug Interactions

The following drug interactions have either been reported or are theoretical in humans or animals

receiving torsemide and may be of significance in veterinary patients:

■ **ACE INHIBITORS (e.g., enalapril, benazepril):** Increased risks for hypotension, particularly in patients who are volume or sodium depleted secondary to diuretics

■ **AMINOGLYCOSIDES (gentamicin, amikacin, etc.):** Other diuretics have been associated with increasing the ototoxic or nephrotoxic risks of aminoglycosides. It is unknown if torsemide can also have these effects and if so, what the clinical significance may be.

■ **AMPHOTERICIN B:** Loop diuretics may increase the risk for nephrotoxicity development

■ **DIGOXIN:** Can increase the area under the curve of torsemide by 50%, but is unlikely to be of significance clinically; torsemide-induced hypokalemia may increase the potential for digoxin toxicity

■ **LITHIUM:** Torsemide may reduce lithium clearance

■ **NSAIDS:** Some NSAIDs may reduce the natriuretic effects of torsemide

■ **PROBENECID:** Can reduce the diuretic efficacy of torsemide

■ **SALICYLATES:** Torsemide can reduce the excretion of salicylates

Laboratory Considerations

Torsemide can affect **serum electrolytes, glucose, uric acid,** and **BUN** concentrations.

Doses

■ **DOGS/CATS:**

a) For adjunctive treatment of refractory congestive heart failure: Injectable furosemide can restore a diuresis in some animals, and torsemide (*now only available PO in the USA*) can also be tried at approximately 0.2–0.3 mg/kg q12-24 hours when other diuretics have become ineffective. (Rush 2008)

b) 0.2 mg/kg PO once a day to three times a day. (Atkins 2008)

Monitoring

■ Serum electrolytes, BUN, creatinine, glucose (if diabetic)

■ Hydration status

■ Blood pressure, if indicated

■ Clinical signs of edema, patient weight, if indicated

Client Information

■ Contact veterinarian if clinical signs of water or electrolyte imbalance occur. Signs such as excessive thirst, lethargy, restlessness, increased urination, GI distress or rapid heart rate may indicate electrolyte or water balance problems.

Chemistry/Synonyms

Torsemide is a pyridyl sulfonylurea loop diuretic that occurs as white to off-white, crystalline powder. It is practically insoluble in water and slightly soluble in alcohol. The injection (no longer marketed in USA) has a pH >8.3.

Torsemide may also be known as torasemide, AC-3525, AC 4464, BM-02.015, JDL-464, and *Demadex®*. International trade names include *Torem®* and *Unat®*.

Storage/Stability

Torsemide tablets should be stored below 40°C; preferably between 15–30°C (59–86°F).

Dosage Forms/Regulatory Status

VETERINARY-LABELED PRODUCTS: None

The ARCI (Racing Commissioners International) has designated this drug as a class 3 substance.

HUMAN-LABELED PRODUCTS:

Torsemide Oral Tablets: 5 mg, 10 mg, 20 mg, & 100 mg; *Demadex®* (Meda); generic; (Rx)

References

Atkins, C. (2008). Therapeutic advances in the management of heart disease: An overview. Proceedings: World Veterinary Congress. Accessed via: Veterinary Information Network. http://goo.gl/qVJsN

Hori, Y., F. Takusagawa, et al. (2007). Effects of oral administration of furosemide and torsemide in healthy dogs. *American Journal of Veterinary Research* **68**(10): 1058–1063.

Rush, J. (2008). Heart failure in dogs and cats. Proceedings: IVECCS. Accessed via: Veterinary Information Network. http://goo.gl/cFKka

TRAMADOL HCL

(*tram*-ah-doll)   Ultram®

OPIATE-LIKE (*MU*-RECEPTOR) AGONIST

Prescriber Highlights

▶ Synthetic *mu*-receptor opiate-like agonist that also inhibits reuptake of serotonin & norepinephrine

▶ May be useful as an analgesic or antitussive. May take up to two weeks for full analgesic activity in chronic pain states.

▶ Not a controlled drug in USA, but has some potential for human abuse

▶ Appears well tolerated in dogs; sedation most likely adverse effect

▶ Avoid use with SSRIs (*e.g.,* fluoxetine) or MAOIs (*e.g.,* selegiline)

▶ Relatively inexpensive

Uses/Indications

Tramadol may be a useful alternative or adjunct for the treatment of post-operative or chronic pain or cough in dogs and potentially, other species. When used in combination with NSAIDs, or other analgesic drugs (*e.g.,* amantadine, gabapentin, alpha-2 agonists) it may be particularly useful for chronic pain conditions. Epidurally administered tramadol may also be useful as an analgesic in horses, but no appropriate commercial dosage forms are presently available in the USA.

Pharmacology/Actions

Tramadol is a centrally acting opiate-like agonist that has primarily *mu*-receptor activity, but also inhibits reuptake of serotonin and norepinephrine. These pharmacologic actions all contribute to its analgesic properties. At least one metabolite (O-desmethyltramadol; ODT; M1) has activity. When compared to tramadol in lab animal studies, M1 is 6 times more potent an analgesic and has 20 times more potency in binding to *mu*-receptors. Naloxone only partially antagonizes the analgesic effects of tramadol.

Pharmacokinetics

In dogs after oral administration of immediate-release tablets, bioavailability is about 65%, but there is significant interpatient variability. Rectal bioavailability is only about 10%. Volume of distribution is approximately 3.8 L/kg. Total body clearance and half-life are about 55 mL/kg/min and 1.7 hours, respectively. Tramadol is extensively metabolized via several metabolic pathways. At least one metabolite (M1) has agonist activity, but is a minor metabolite in dogs; M1 has a half-life of about 2 hours after oral tramadol administration in dogs.

One study in 8 cats using the immediate release oral tablet, showed high interpatient variability in absorption (with two cats there was not enough data to analyze). The elimination half-life for the parent compound was about 2.5 hours; for the M1 metabolite, 4.5 hours. Neurologic effects (mydriasis, dysphoria) were seen in 25% of cats (2 of 4 females) in the study group and the drug was observed to be unpalatable to cats (Papich & Bledsoe 2007). Another study in 6 cats demonstrated approximate values of: oral bioavailability—60%, volume of distribution (steady-state)—2 L/kg, clearance—12 mL/min/kg, and terminal half-life—191 minutes. Terminal half-life for ODT after oral administration was about 290 minutes (Pypendop & Ilkiw 2007).

In neonatal and weaned foals, tramadol has different pharmacokinetics. After oral administration, higher bioavailability (53% vs. 20%), shorter time to peak concentration (1 hr. vs. 1.25 hr.), and peak levels occurred with neonatal (2 week old) versus weaned foals (4 months old). Elimination half-life did not significantly differ (approx. 2 hours). The active metabolite (M1; ODT) remained above the reported therapeutic concentration for humans for 3 hours in neonatal foals and 8 hours in weaned foals (Stewart *et al.* 2006). In adult horses, tramadol has relatively poor oral absorption (approx. 14%) and an elimination half-life has been reported to be

approximately 2–10 hours, depending on the study. The active metabolite, (m1; ODT) is reported as 4 hours (Cox *et al.* 2010).

Contraindications/Precautions/Warnings

Tramadol is contraindicated in patients hypersensitive to it or other opioids. The combination product containing acetaminophen is contraindicated in cats.

Use with caution in conjunction with other drugs that can cause CNS or respiratory depression. Because tramadol has caused seizures in humans, it should be used with caution in animals with preexisting seizure disorders or receiving other drugs that may reduce the seizure threshold. Like other opiate-like compounds, tramadol should be used with caution in geriatric or severely debilitated animals. Patients with impaired renal or hepatic function may need dosage adjustments.

While the risk of physical dependence occurring is less than that of several other opiates, it has been reported in humans. The drug should be withdrawn gradually in animals that have received it chronically. While not a controlled substance in the USA, humans can potentially abuse tramadol and significant diversion of the drug reportedly occurs. Veterinarians should be alert to "clients" seeking tramadol for their animals.

Extended-release tablets (generally not currently recommended or used in veterinary patients) must not be broken, crushed or chewed or toxicity could occur.

Adverse Effects

Tramadol appears to be well tolerated in dogs. Potentially, it could cause a variety of adverse effects associated with its pharmacologic actions, including: CNS effects (excessive sedation, agitation, anxiety, tremor, dizziness), or GI (inappetence, vomiting, constipation to diarrhea).

Very limited information is available on the adverse effects in cats. Dysphoria, mydriasis, and dose avoidance (unpalatability) have been reported.

Approximately 10% of humans receiving the drug develop pruritus. Injectable tramadol may cause respiratory and cardiac depression.

Reproductive/Nursing Safety

In humans, the FDA categorizes tramadol as a category *C* drug for use during pregnancy (*Animal studies have shown an adverse effect on the fetus, but there are no adequate studies in humans; or there are no animal reproduction studies and no adequate studies in humans.*) At dosages 3–15 times usual, tramadol was embryotoxic and fetotoxic in laboratory animals. Tramadol and its active metabolite enter maternal milk in very low levels, but the drug's safety in neonates has not been established.

Overdosage/Acute Toxicity

Acute oral overdoses may cause either CNS depressive signs or serotonin syndrome. Lethargy, mydriasis, ataxia and vomiting are most common, but stimulatory signs (tachycardia, tremors, vocalization) may also be seen.

There were 308 exposures to tramadol reported to the ASPCA Animal Poison Control Center (APCC) during 2008-2009. In these cases 246 were dogs with 46 showing clinical signs, 60 were cats with 33 showing clinical signs, 1 case involved a bird that showed clinical signs and the remaining 1 case involved a lagomorph that showed no clinic signs. Common findings in dogs recorded in decreasing frequency included sedate, ataxia, agitation, somnolence, and seizures. Common findings in cats recorded in decreasing frequency included mydriasis, hypersalivation, tachycardia, agitation, lethargy, and ataxia.

Treatment is primarily supportive (maintaining respiration, treating seizures with benzodiazepines or barbiturates, etc.). Naloxone may NOT be useful in tramadol overdoses as it may only partially reverse some of the effects of the drug and may, in fact, increase the risk of seizures. Naloxone did not decrease the drug's lethality in tramadol overdoses given to mice. Cyproheptadine and phenothiazines can be used to treat the stimulatory signs.

Drug Interactions

The following drug interactions have either been reported or are theoretical in humans or animals receiving tramadol and may be of significance in veterinary patients:

■ **DIGOXIN:** In humans, tramadol has been rarely linked to digoxin toxicity

■ **MAO INHIBITORS (including amitraz and possibly, selegiline):** Potential for serotonin syndrome; use together should be avoided

■ **ONDANSETRON:** In humans, use together may reduce the effectiveness of both drugs

■ **QUINIDINE:** May increase tramadol concentrations and decrease M1 (active metabolite) concentrations

■ **SAMe:** Theoretically, concurrent use of SAMe with tramadol could cause additive serotonergic effects

■ **SEVOFLURANE:** Pretreatment with tramadol reduced MAC values by approximately 30% in dogs (Seddighi *et al.* 2009), and 40% in cats (Dirikolu *et al.* 2009).

■ **SSRI ANTIDEPRESSANTS (fluoxetine, sertraline, paroxetine, etc.):** Can inhibit the metabolism of tramadol to its active metabolites thereby decreasing its efficacy and increasing the risk of toxicity (serotonin syndrome, seizures).

■ **TRICYCLIC ANTIDEPRESSANTS (clomipramine, amitriptyline, etc.):** Increased risk for seizures; amitriptyline may inhibit tramadol metabolism

■ **WARFARIN:** In humans, increased PT and INR in patients taking tramadol has been reported (relatively rare)

Laboratory Considerations

■ No specific laboratory interactions or considerations were noted.

Doses

■ **DOGS:**

a) Current dosing recommendations for dogs are 5 mg/kg PO q6-8h and up to 10 mg/kg PO q6-8h in non-responsive dogs. The efficacy of these dosages has not been evaluated. It is important to remember that maximum analgesic effects may not occur immediately and may be delayed up to 14 days for chronic pain conditions such as cancer and degenerative joint disease. (KuKanich 2010)

b) As an analgesic: Recent investigations and clinical use suggest a starting dose of 2–5 mg/kg four times daily. (Hellyer 2006)

c) For chronic pain: 2–5 mg/kg PO 2-3 times a day is reasonable for mild pain, although both dose and dosing interval may need to be adjusted for more severe pain. The pharmacokinetics in the dog are somewhat erratic, so the drug is best used as multimodal therapy with NSAIDs or other analgesic drugs. (Grubb 2010)

■ **CATS:**

a) Based upon the pharmacokinetics of tramadol and O-desmethyltramadol (ODT) in cats, a dose of 2 mg/kg twice daily is a reasonable starting dose. (Boothe 2010)

b) Current dosing recommendations for cats is 1–2 mg/kg PO q12h. The efficacy of these dosages has not been evaluated. It is important to remember that maximum analgesic effects may not occur immediately and may be delayed up to 14 days for chronic pain conditions such as cancer and degenerative joint disease. (KuKanich 2010)

c) For chronic pain: 1–4 mg/kg PO 2–3 times a day is reasonable for mild pain, although both dose and dosing interval may need to be adjusted for more severe pain. (Grubb 2010)

■ **HORSES:**

a) In a study of 10 horses with chronic laminitis pain: tramadol at 5 mg/kg PO twice daily for seven days, alone or with ketamine at 0.6 mg/kg/hr IV during six hours each day for the first 3 days of treatment, pain relief was enhanced. (Guedes *et al.* 2009)

■ **ZOO, EXOTIC, WILDLIFE SPECIES:**

For use of tramadol in zoo, exotic and wildlife medicine refer to specific references, including:

a) *Exotic Animal Formulary, 3rd Ed.* Carpenter, J.W., Saunders. 2005

b) The 2009 American Association of Zoo

Veterinarian Proceedings by D. K. Fontenot also has several dosages listed for restraint, anesthesia, and analgesia for a variety of drugs for carnivores and primates. VIN members can access them at: http://goo.gl/BHRih or http://goo.gl/9UJse

Monitoring

■ Clinical efficacy
■ Adverse effects

Client Information

■ May be given with or without food
■ Keep out of reach of children
■ May cause changes in alertness or behavior
■ Clients should understand that the clinical experience with this drug in animals is limited and to report adverse effects to the veterinarian

Chemistry/Synonyms

A *mu*-receptor opiate agonist, tramadol HCl occurs as a white crystalline powder that is freely soluble in water or alcohol, and very slightly soluble in acetone. Tramadol is not derived from opium nor is it a semi-synthetic opioid, but is entirely synthetically produced.

Tramadol HCl may also be known as: CG-315; CG-315E; tramadoli hydrochloridum; U-26225A; many trade names are available.

Storage/Stability

Unless otherwise labeled, tramadol tablets should be stored at room temperature 25°C (77°F); excursions permitted to 15–30°C (59–86°F). Dispense in tight, light-resistant containers.

Compatibility/Compounding Considerations

Tramadol HCl injection 50 mg/mL (not available commercially in the USA) is reportedly **not compatible** when mixed in the same syringe with injectable diazepam, diclofenac sodium, indomethacin, midazolam, piroxicam, phenylbutazone, or lysine aspirin.

Dosage Forms/Regulatory Status

VETERINARY-LABELED PRODUCTS: None

The ARCI (Racing Commissioners International) has designated this drug as a class 2 substance. See the appendix for more information.

HUMAN-LABELED PRODUCTS:

Tramadol HCl Oral Tablets (film-coated) 50 mg; *Ultram®* (Janssen); generic; (Rx)

Tramadol HCl Extended-Release Tablets 100 mg, 200 mg & 300 mg; *Ultram ER®* (Ortho-McNeil); *Ryzolt®* (Purdue Pharma); generic; (Rx). **Note:** Dogs apparently do not absorb this product as well as humans, and potentially could "overdose" if the tablet is chewed.

Tramadol HCl Oral Disintegrating Tablets: 50 mg in UD 30s; *Rybix ODT®* (Victory Pharma); (Rx)

Tramadol is also available in a fixed dose combination of tramadol HCl 37.5 mg and acetaminophen 325 mg tablets. USA trade name is *Ultracet®* (Ortho-McNeil); (Rx). **Warning:** Be certain this combination product is not dispensed for cats.

In several countries (but not the USA), tramadol injection is available commercially.

References

Boothe, D.M. (2010). Chronic Pain Management in Cats: What Are the Options? Proceedings: ACVIM. Accessed via: Veterinary Information Network. http://goo.gl/QkzhB

Cox, S., N. Villarino, et al. (2010). Determination of oral tramadol pharmacokinetics in horses. *Research in Veterinary Science* 89(2): 236–241.

Dirikolu, L., A.F. Lehner, et al. (2009). Pyrilamine in the horse: detection and pharmacokinetics of pyrilamine and its major urinary metabolite O-desmethylpyrilamine. *Journal of Veterinary Pharmacology and Therapeutics* 32(1): 66–78.

Grubb, T. (2010). What Do We Really Know About the Drugs We Use to Treat Chronic Pain? *Topics in Companion Animal Medicine* 25(1): 10–19.

Guedes, A., N.S. Matthews, et al. (2009). Analgesic Role of Tramadol and Ketamine in Horses with Laminitis-Associated Pain. Proceedings: IVECCS. Accessed via: Veterinary Information Network. http://goo.gl/fw3GG

Hellyer, P. (2006). Pain assessment and multimodal analgesic therapy in dogs and cats. Proceedings: ABVP. Accessed via: Veterinary Information Network. http://goo.gl/LMXcX

KuKanich, B. (2010). Managing Severe Chronic Pain: Maintaining Quality of Life in Dogs. Proceedings ACVIM. Accessed via: Veterinary Information Network. http://goo.gl/X6AAd

Papich, M. & D. Bledsoe (2007). Tramadol pharmacokinetics in cats after oral administration of an immediate release product. Proceedings: ACVIM. Accessed via: Veterinary Information Network. http://goo.gl/fNpsk

Pypendop, B.H. & J.E. Ilkiw (2007). Pharmacokinetics of Tramadol and O-Desmethyltramadol in Cats. Proceedings: IVECCS. Accessed via: Veterinary Information Network. http://goo.gl/vUVqC

Seddighi, M.R., C.M. Egger, et al. (2009). Effects of tramadol on the minimum alveolar concentration of sevoflurane in dogs. *Veterinary Anaesthesia and Analgesia* 36(4): 334–340.

Stewart, A., D.M. Boothe, et al. (2006). Pharmacokinetics of tramadol in 2–week and 4–month-old foals. Proceedings: IVECC. Accessed via: Veterinary Information Network. http://goo.gl/B8iRi

TRAZODONE HCL

(*traz*-oh-done)   Desyrel®

SEROTONIN 2A ANTAGONIST/REUPTAKE INHIBITOR

Prescriber Highlights

▶ Antidepressant that may be useful for adjunctive treatment of behavioral disorders (esp. anxiety- or phobia-related) in dogs

▶ Little research or clinical experience available regarding veterinary use

▶ Relatively inexpensive

Uses/Indications

Trazodone may be useful in treating behavioral disorders in small animals, particularly as an adjunctive treatment in those patients that do not adequately respond to conventional therapies.

In a retrospective study of 56 dogs (Gruen & Sherman 2008), evaluating trazodone as an adjunctive treatment for anxiety disorders in dogs, it was found to be well tolerated over a wide dose range and enhanced behavioral calming. The authors concluded that further controlled studies are needed to more fully evaluate the pharmacokinetics, safety profile, and efficacy of this drug in dogs.

In humans, trazodone is used for treating depression, aggressive behavior, alcohol or cocaine withdrawal, migraine prevention, and insomnia. It has fewer anticholinergic effects than the tricyclic antidepressants and is among the antidepressants with the lowest seizure risk.

Pharmacology/Actions

Trazodone is classified as a serotonin 2A antagonist/reuptake inhibitor (SARI) that primarily potentiates serotonin activity in the CNS. In laboratory animals, trazodone selectively inhibits serotonin uptake by brain synaptosomes and potentiates the behavioral changes induced by the serotonin precursor, 5-hydroxytryptophan. In dogs, trazodone exerts qualitatively different and less pronounced cardiac conduction effects than do the tricyclic antidepressants. Trazodone can antagonize alpha-1 adrenergic receptors and reduce blood pressure. As trazodone can antagonize 5-HT2 receptors and cause their downregulation, it can augment the efficacy of SSRIs (Virga 2010).

Pharmacokinetics

No information was located regarding the pharmacokinetics of trazodone in dogs. In humans, oral bioavailability of trazodone (immediate-release tablets) is about 65%; presence of food increases absorption (AUC is increased), but decreases Cmax (peak plasma level) and delays Tmax (time of peak level). It is approximately 90–95% bound to plasma proteins. Volume of distribution ranges from 0.47–0.84 L/kg. Metabolism is extensive and occurs primarily in the liver. An active metabolite, m-chlorophenyl-piperazine (mCCP) is formed via oxidative cleavage by CYP3A4 that is further metabolized to inactive compounds via CYP2D6. Excretion is mostly (70–75%) via renal mechanisms with only a very small amount (0.13%) excreted unchanged in the urine. About 21% of a dose is excreted in the feces. Elimination half-life of the parent compound is around 7 hours (immediate-release tablets) and 10 hours (sustained-release tablets).

Contraindications/Precautions/Warnings

Trazodone is contraindicated in patients hypersensitive to it or those receiving MAO inhibitors (including amitraz and possibly, selegiline). It should be used with caution in patients with severe cardiac disease or hepatic or renal impairment.

Adverse Effects

The adverse effect profile for trazodone in dogs is not well documented. Potential adverse effects include sedation, lethargy, ataxia, cardiac conduction disturbances, increased anxiety, and aggression. In a retrospective study in 56 dogs (Gruen & Sherman 2008), trazodone adverse effects were in general mild, and only 3 dogs had to have the drug discontinued. Approximately 80% of the dogs in the study had no reported adverse effects. Adverse effects that were reported included: vomiting/gagging (2), behavioral changes (within hours of a dose) such as getting onto counters (1), or into trash (1), increased excitement (2), sedation (2), increased appetite (2) and colitis (1). Should trazodone be used more extensively in dogs, a more defined adverse effect profile may be discerned.

Trazodone alone is unlikely to cause serotonin syndrome at clinically used dosages, but when used with other serotonergic drugs, it is possible. The most common clinical signs seen with serotonin syndrome in dogs include (in descending order): vomiting, diarrhea, seizures, hyperthermia, hyperesthesia, depression, mydriasis, vocalization, death, blindness, hypersalivation, dyspnea, ataxia/paresis, disorientation, hyperreflexia, and coma (Wismer 2006).

In humans, the most common adverse effects include blurred vision; confusion, dizziness, dry mouth, orthostatic hypotension, sweating, lethargy or somnolence. QT prolongation can occur, but is much less common in humans with trazodone than with the tricyclic antidepressants. Priapism has been reported rarely in men taking trazodone.

Reproductive/Nursing Safety

Trazodone appears to be relatively safe to use during pregnancy. At very high dosages (15–50X) in rats and rabbits, some increase in fetal death/resorption rates and congenital abnormalities were noted. For humans, the FDA categorizes trazodone as category *C* for use during pregnancy *(Animal studies have shown an adverse effect on the fetus, but there are no adequate studies in humans; or there are no animal reproduction studies and no adequate studies in humans.)* Tramadol is excreted into milk at very low levels and clinical effects in offspring seem unlikely. However, weigh the potential risks of using this medication versus the benefits in pregnant or nursing animals.

Overdosage/Acute Toxicity

No specific information was located regarding trazodone overdoses in veterinary patients. In humans, incidence of serious toxicity from trazodone overdose (alone) was low compared with tricyclic antidepressant overdoses. However, in the event of substantial overdose of trazodone, it is recommended to contact an animal poison control center for further guidance.

Drug Interactions

The following drug interactions have either been reported or are theoretical in humans or animals receiving trazodone and may be of significance in veterinary patients:

- **ANTIHYPERTENSIVE DRUGS:** Trazodone may increase reductions in blood pressure and cause hypotension
- **ASPIRIN:** Increase risk for GI bleeding; monitor
- **AZOLE ANTIFUNGALS (e.g., ketoconazole, fluconazole):** May increase trazodone blood levels
- **CNS DEPRESSANTS:** Use with trazodone may cause additive CNS depressant effects
- **DIGOXIN:** Trazodone may increase digoxin levels
- **MACROLIDE ANTIBIOTCS (e.g., erythromycin, clarithromycin):** May increase trazodone blood levels
- **METOCLOPRAMIDE:** Increased risk for serotonin syndrome
- **NSAIDS:** Increased risk for GI bleeding; monitor
- **PHENOTHIAZINES:** May increase trazodone blood levels; cause additive CNS effects
- **SSRI ANTIDEPRESSANTS (e.g., fluoxetine):** Increased risk for serotonin syndrome. Trazodone is commonly used together with SSRI's, but be alert for signs associated with serotonin syndrome (see adverse effects above).

Laboratory Considerations

- None noted

Doses

- **DOGS:**

    As an adjunctive treatment of anxiety-related disorders:

    a) From a retrospective study of 56 dogs. To allow dogs to become tolerant to the drug and avoid potential gastrointestinal adverse effects, trazodone was begun at an initial dose that was half of the target dose and administered for 3 days. Then the target dose was established as the lowest effective dose needed for behavioral calming. Additional dose increments were made empirically over time.

Weight (kg)	Initial Dosage (total; NOT mg/kg) Range	Target Dosage (total; NOT mg/kg) Range
<10 kg	≤ 25 mg q8-24h	≤ 50 mg q8-24h
≥10-20 kg	50 mg q12-24h	100 mg q8-24h
≥20-40 kg	100 mg q12-24h	200 mg q8-24h
>40 kg	100 mg q12-24h	200–300 mg q8-24h

In the study, the following minimum, maximum and mean daily dosages and dosing frequencies were used:

Daily medication only: 1.9 mg/kg/day–16.2 mg/kg/day (mean = 7.3 mg/kg/day)

As needed only: 2.2 mg/kg/day–14 mg/kg/day (mean 7.7 mg/kg/day)

Daily medication and as needed: 1.7 mg/kg/day–19.5 mg/kg/day (mean 7.25 mg/kg/day) (Gruen & Sherman 2008)

b) 1 mg/kg PO q12h for 7 days, then up to 3 mg/kg PO q12h. (Frank 2010)

c) 1–4.8 mg/kg PO twice daily; (titrate to effect in 1 mg increments every 7 days). (Virga 2010)

d) In addition to the daily serotonin enhancing medication, trazodone can be used as an adjunctive drug to increase clinical control of anxiety related conditions. It is given about an hour prior to the onset of anxiety and with a typical starting dose between 2–5 mg/kg and adjusting upwards as necessary to get control (maximum dose 14 mg/kg/day). (Neilson 2010)

Monitoring

- Clinical efficacy and adverse effects

Client Information

- Preferably give with food
- Clients should understand that trazodone has not been used extensively in dogs and to report any unforeseen adverse effects to the veterinarian

Chemistry/Synonyms

Trazodone is a triazolopyridine antidepressant agent. It occurs as a white to off-white crystalline powder and is sparingly soluble in water, alcohol, or chloroform.

Trazodone may also be known as AF-1161, trazodona, trazodon, or "sleepeasy." A common trade name is *Desyrel®*.

Storage/Stability

Store between 20-25°C (68-77°F); excursions are permitted to 15-30°C (59-86°F). Keep in an airtight container and protect from light.

Dosage Forms/Regulatory Status

VETERINARY-LABELED PRODUCTS: None

HUMAN-LABELED PRODUCTS:

Trazodone Oral Tablets: 50 mg, 100 mg, 150 mg, & 300 mg; generic; (Rx)

Trazodone Extended-Release (24-hour) Oral Tablets: 150 mg & 300 mg; *Oleptro®* (Labopharm); (Rx)

References

Frank, D. (2010). Selection of Patients for Treatment with Psychotropic Medication. Proceedings: CVMA. Accessed via: Veterinary information Network. http://goo.gl/FcMQ0

Gruen, M.E. & B.L. Sherman (2008). Use of trazodone as an adjunctive agent in the treatment of canine anxiety disorders: 56 cases (1995–2007). *Javma-Journal of the American Veterinary Medical Association* **233**(12): 1902–1907.

Neilson, J. (2010). Drug Therapy for Behavioral Problems. Proceedings: Western Veterinary Conference. Accessed via: Veterinary Information Network. http://goo.gl/Auokc

Virga, V. (2010). Case Files in Anxiety: Practical Management from the Trenches III, IV. Proceedings: WVC. Accessed via: Veterinary Information Network. http://goo.gl/ND2yn

Wismer, T. (2006). Serotonin Syndrome. Proceedings: IVECC Symposium. Accessed via: Veterinary Information Network. http://goo.gl/ua96I

TRIAMCINOLONE ACETONIDE

(trye-am-**sin**-oh-lone)   Vetalog®

GLUCOCORTICOID

Prescriber Highlights

▶ Oral, parenteral, topical & inhaled glucocorticoid that is 4–10X (some say up to 40X) more potent than hydrocortisone; no appreciable mineralocorticoid activity

▶ Contraindications (relatively): Systemic fungal infections, manufacturer lists: "in viral infections, . . . animals with arrested tuberculosis, peptic ulcer, acute psychoses, corneal ulcer, & Cushingoid syndrome. The presence of diabetes, osteoporosis, chronic psychotic reactions, predisposition to thrombophlebitis, hypertension, CHF, renal insufficiency, & active tuberculosis necessitates carefully controlled use."

▶ If using systemically for therapy, goal is to use as much as is required & as little as possible for as short an amount of time as possible

▶ Primary adverse effects are "Cushingoid" in nature with sustained use

▶ Many potential drug & lab interactions

Uses/Indications

The systemic veterinary labeled product (*Vetalog® Injection*) is labeled as "indicated for the treatment of inflammation and related disorders in dogs, cats, and horses. It is also indicated for use in dogs and cats for the management and treatment of acute arthritis, allergic and dermatologic disorders."

In horses, intra-articular (IA) injection of triamcinolone acetonide (TA), particularly in high motion joints is often recommended as studies have demonstrated that IA injection can improve clinical lameness and reduce articular protein, inflammatory cell infiltration, intimal hyperplasia and subintimal fibrosis, and synovial levels of hyaluronan and glycosaminoglycan can be increased. Combining TA with a local anesthetic (*e.g.*, mepivacaine) has been shown not to alter the potency or duration of action of

TA and may be useful to both confirm the joint causing lameness and to reduce synovitis (Kay *et al.* 2008). There is some evidence supporting the IA use of TA with hyaluronic acid. In clinically normal horses, IA triamcinolone acetonide diffused directly from the distal interphalangeal joint with or without hyaluronic acid and, after additional studies, may prove to be useful in treating navicular syndrome (Boyce *et al.* 2010).

Intralesional injection of triamcinolone into esophageal strictures has been done in dogs and cats prior to dilation (Richter 2009).

Glucocorticoids have been used in an attempt to treat practically every malady that afflicts man or animal, but there are three broad uses and dosage ranges for use of these agents. 1) Replacement of glucocorticoid activity in patients with adrenal insufficiency, 2) as an antiinflammatory agent, and 3) as an immunosuppressive. Among some of the uses for glucocorticoids include treatment of: endocrine conditions (*e.g.*, adrenal insufficiency), rheumatic diseases (*e.g.*, rheumatoid arthritis), collagen diseases (*e.g.*, systemic lupus), allergic states, respiratory diseases (*e.g.*, asthma), dermatologic diseases (*e.g.*, pemphigus, allergic dermatoses), hematologic disorders (*e.g.*, thrombocytopenias, autoimmune hemolytic anemias), neoplasias, nervous system disorders (increased CSF pressure), GI diseases (*e.g.*, ulcerative colitis exacerbations), and renal diseases (*e.g.*, nephrotic syndrome). Some glucocorticoids are used topically in the eye and skin for various conditions or are injected intra-articularly or intra-lesionally. The above listing is certainly not complete.

Pharmacology/Actions

Triamcinolone acetonide is considered an intermediate acting (metabolic activity of 24-48 hours when given orally) glucocorticoid that is approximately 4-10 times more potent than hydrocortisone. When injected IM, duration of activity may persist for 4-6 (and sometimes up to 8) weeks.

Glucocorticoids have effects on virtually every cell type and system in mammals. For more information, refer to the Glucocorticoid Agents, General Information monograph.

Contraindications/Precautions/Warnings

Systemic use of glucocorticoids is generally considered contraindicated in systemic fungal infections (unless used for replacement therapy in Addison's), when administered IM in patients with idiopathic thrombocytopenia or hypersensitive to a particular compound. Sustained-release injectable glucocorticoids use is considered contraindicated for chronic corticosteroid therapy of systemic diseases.

Animals that have received glucocorticoids systemically, other than with "burst" therapy, should be tapered off the drugs. Patients who have received the drugs chronically should be tapered off slowly as endogenous ACTH and corticosteroid function may return slowly. Should the animal undergo a "stressor" (*e.g.*, surgery, trauma, illness, etc.) during the tapering process or until normal adrenal and pituitary function resume, additional glucocorticoids should be administered.

Corticosteroid therapy may induce parturition in large animal species during the latter stages of pregnancy.

Adverse Effects

Adverse effects are generally associated with long-term administration of these drugs, especially if given at high dosages or not on an alternate day regimen. Effects generally are manifested as clinical signs of hyperadrenocorticism. When administered to young, growing animals, glucocorticoids can retard growth. Many of the potential effects, adverse and otherwise, are outlined above in the Pharmacology section.

In dogs, polydipsia (PD), polyphagia (PP) and polyuria (PU), may all be seen with short-term "burst" therapy as well as with alternate-day maintenance therapy on days when giving the drug. Adverse effects in dogs can include dull, dry haircoat, weight gain, panting, vomiting, diarrhea, elevated liver enzymes, pancreatitis, GI ulceration, lipidemias, activation or worsening of diabetes mellitus, muscle wasting and behavioral changes (depression, lethargy, viciousness). Discontinuation of the drug may be necessary; changing to an alternate steroid may also alleviate the problem. With the exception of PU/PD/PP, adverse effects associated with antiinflammatory therapy are relatively uncommon. Adverse effects associated with immunosuppressive doses are more common and potentially, more severe.

Cats generally require higher dosages than dogs for clinical effect, but tend to develop fewer adverse effects. Occasionally polydipsia, polyuria, polyphagia with weight gain, diarrhea, or depression can be seen. Long-term, high dose therapy can lead to "Cushingoid" effects, however.

Administration of dexamethasone or triamcinolone may play a role in the development of laminitis in horses.

Reproductive/Nursing Safety

Glucocorticoids are probably necessary for normal fetal development. They may be required for adequate surfactant production, myelin, retinal, pancreas and mammary development.

Excessive dosages early in pregnancy may lead to teratogenic effects. In horses and ruminants, exogenous steroid administration may induce parturition when administered in the latter stages of pregnancy. In humans, the FDA categorizes this drug as category *C* for use during pregnancy (*Animal studies have shown an adverse effect on the fetus, but there are no adequate studies in humans; or there are no animal reproduction studies and no adequate studies in humans.*)

Glucocorticoids unbound to plasma proteins will enter milk. High dosages or prolonged administration to mothers may potentially inhibit the growth of nursing newborns.

Overdosage/Acute Toxicity

Glucocorticoids when given short-term are unlikely to cause harmful effects, even in massive dosages. One incidence of a dog developing acute CNS effects after accidental ingestion of glucocorticoids has been reported. Should clinical signs occur, use supportive treatment if required.

Chronic usage of glucocorticoids can lead to serious adverse effects. Refer to Adverse Effects above for more information.

Drug Interactions

The following drug interactions have either been reported or are theoretical in humans or animals receiving triamcinolone and may be of significance in veterinary patients:

■ **AMPHOTERICIN B:** Administered concomitantly with glucocorticoids may cause hypokalemia

■ **ANALGESICS, OPIATE and/or ANESTHETICS, LOCAL (epidural injections):** Combination with glucocorticoids in epidurals has caused serious CNS injuries and death; do not use more volume than very small intrathecal test doses of these agents with glucocorticoids

■ **ANTICHOLINESTERASE AGENTS (e.g., pyridostigmine, neostigmine, etc.):** In patients with myasthenia gravis, concomitant glucocorticoid and anticholinesterase agent administration may lead to profound muscle weakness. If possible, discontinue anticholinesterase medication at least 24 hours prior to corticosteroid administration

■ **ASPIRIN:** Glucocorticoids may reduce salicylate blood levels

■ **BARBITURATES:** May increase the metabolism of glucocorticoids and decrease blood levels

■ **CYCLOPHOSPHAMIDE:** Glucocorticoids may also inhibit the hepatic metabolism of cyclophosphamide; dosage adjustments may be required

■ **CYCLOSPORINE:** Concomitant administration of glucocorticoids and cyclosporine may increase the blood levels of each, by mutually inhibiting the hepatic metabolism of each other; the clinical significance of this interaction is not clear

■ **DIURETICS, POTASSIUM-DEPLETING (e.g., spironolactone, triamterene):** Administered concomitantly with glucocorticoids may cause hypokalemia

■ **ERYTHROMYCIN, CLARITHROMYCIN:** May increase TMC levels

■ **ESTROGENS:** The effects of TMC, and possibly other glucocorticoids, may be potentiated by concomitant administration with estrogens

■ **INSULIN:** Insulin requirements may increase in patients receiving glucocorticoids

■ **ISONIAZID:** TMC may decrease isoniazid levels

■ **KETOCONAZOLE and other AZOLE ANTI-FUNGALS:** May decrease the metabolism of glucocorticoids and increase TMC blood levels; ketoconazole may induce adrenal insufficiency when glucocorticoids are withdrawn by inhibiting adrenal corticosteroid synthesis

■ **MITOTANE:** May alter the metabolism of steroids; higher than usual doses of steroids may be necessary to treat mitotane-induced adrenal insufficiency

■ **NSAIDS:** Administration of ulcerogenic drugs with glucocorticoids may increase the risk of gastrointestinal ulceration

■ **PHENOBARBITAL:** May increase the metabolism of glucocorticoids and decrease TMC blood levels

■ **RIFAMPIN:** May increase the metabolism of glucocorticoids and decrease TMC blood levels

■ **VACCINES:** Patients receiving corticosteroids at immunosuppressive dosages should generally not receive live attenuated-virus vaccines as virus replication may be augmented; a diminished immune response may occur after vaccine, toxoid, or bacterin administration in patients receiving glucocorticoid

■ **WARFARIN:** TMC may affect INR's; monitor

Laboratory Considerations

■ Glucocorticoids may increase **serum cholesterol**

■ Glucocorticoids may increase **serum and urine glucose** levels

■ Glucocorticoids may decrease **serum potassium**

■ Glucocorticoids can suppress the release of thyroid stimulating hormone (TSH) and reduce T_3 & T_4 values. Thyroid gland atrophy has been reported after chronic glucocorticoid administration. Uptake of I^{131} by the thyroid may be decreased by glucocorticoids.

■ Reactions to **skin tests** may be suppressed by glucocorticoids

■ False-negative results of the **nitroblue tetrazolium** test for systemic bacterial infections may be induced by glucocorticoids

■ Glucocorticoids may cause **neutrophilia** within 4–8 hours after dosing and return to baseline within 24–48 hours after drug discontinuation

■ Glucocorticoids can cause **lymphopenia** which can persist for weeks after drug discontinuation in dogs

Doses

■ **DOGS:**

For glucocorticoid effects:

a) 2 mg PO once daily for 7 days; 0.11–0.22 mg/kg IM or SC (Kirk 1989)

b) For antiinflammatory effects: 0.05 mg/kg PO two to three times daily (Williamson 2003)

c) For tablets: 0.11 mg/kg PO initially once a day, may increase to 0.22 mg/kg PO once daily if initial response is unsatisfactory. As soon as possible, but not later than 2 weeks, reduce dose gradually to 0.028–0.055 mg/kg/day. (Package insert; *Vetalog® Tablets*—Solvay)

d) For injectable product: 0.11–0.22 mg/kg for inflammatory or allergic disorders, and 0.22 mg/kg for dermatological disorders. Effects generally persist for 7–15 days; if symptoms recur, may repeat or institute oral therapy.

For intralesional injection: Usual dose is 1.2–1.8 mg; inject around lesion at 0.5–2.5 cm intervals. Do not exceed 0.6 mg at any one site or 6 mg total dose. May repeat as necessary. (Package insert; *Vetalog® Injection*—Solvay)

e) To prevent re-stricture after esophageal dilation: Using an endoscopically directed needle, inject 0.5–1 mL of *Vetalog®* (2 mg/mL) submucosally at time of dilation procedure. Infiltration is done circumferentially at four points around the site. (Marks 2004)

■ **CATS:**

a) 0.25–0.5 mg PO once daily for 7 days (Kirk 1989)

b) For pododermatitis, feline plasmacytic pharyngitis: 2–4 mg (total dose) PO once a day or every other day 0.4–0.6 mg/kg PO once daily, then taper. For pemphigus complex: 0.4–0.8 mg/kg/day PO (Williamson 2003)

c) For tablets: 0.11 mg/kg PO initially once a day, may increase to 0.22 mg/kg PO once daily if initial response is unsatisfactory. As soon as possible, but not later than 2 weeks, reduce dose gradually to 0.028–0.055 mg/kg/day (Booth 1988), (Package insert; *Vetalog® Tablets*—Solvay)

d) For injectable product: 0.11–0.22 mg/kg for inflammatory or allergic disorders, and 0.22 mg/kg for dermatological disorders. Effects generally persist for 7–15 days; if symptoms recur, may repeat or institute oral therapy.

For intralesional injection: Usual dose is 1.2–1.8 mg; inject around lesion at 0.5–2.5 cm intervals. Do not exceed 0.6 mg at any one site or 6 mg total dose.

May repeat as necessary. (Package insert; *Vetalog® Injection*—Solvay)

e) To prevent re-stricture after esophageal dilation: Using an endoscopically directed needle, inject 0.5−1 mL of *Vetalog®* (2 mg/mL) submucosally at time of dilation procedure. Infiltration is done circumferentially at four points around the site. (Marks 2004)

f) For adjunctive treatment of miliary dermatitis: 0.2−0.6 mg/kg PO once daily for 10-14 days, then tapered. (Beale 2008)

■ **CATTLE:**

For glucocorticoid effects:

a) 0.02−0.04 mg/kg IM; 6−18 mg intra-articularly. (Howard 1986)

■ **HORSES:** (**Note:** ARCI UCGFS Class 4 Drug) For glucocorticoid effects:

a) 0.011−0.022 mg/kg PO twice daily; 0.011−0.022 mg/kg IM or SC;

6−18 mg intra-articularly or intrasynovially, may repeat after 3−4 days (Package inserts; *Vetalog® Powder* and *Injection*—Solvay)

b) For intra-articular injection: 12 mg IA on days 0, 13, 27 (McClure 2002)

Monitoring

Monitoring of glucocorticoid therapy is dependent on its reason for use, dosage, agent used (amount of mineralocorticoid activity), dosage schedule (daily versus alternate day therapy), duration of therapy, and the animal's age and condition. The following list may not be appropriate or complete for all animals; use clinical assessment and judgment should adverse effects be noted:

■ Weight, appetite, signs of edema

■ Serum and/or urine electrolytes

■ Total plasma proteins, albumin

■ Blood glucose

■ Growth and development in young animals

■ ACTH stimulation test if necessary

Chemistry/Synonyms

Triamcinolone acetonide, a synthetic glucocorticoid, occurs as slightly odorous, white to cream-colored, crystalline powder with a melting point between 290−294°C. It is practically insoluble in water, very soluble in dehydrated alcohol and slightly soluble in alcohol. The commercially available sterile suspensions have a pH range of 5−7.5.

Triamcinolone acetonide may also be known as: triamcinoloni acetonidum; many trade names are available.

Storage/Stability

Triamcinolone acetonide products should be stored at room temperature (15−30°C); the injection should be protected from light.

Dosage Forms/Regulatory Status

VETERINARY-LABELED PRODUCTS:

Triamcinolone Acetonide Tablets: 0.5 mg, 1.5 mg; *Vetalog®* (BIVI), generic; (Rx). FDA-approved for use in dogs and cats.

Triamcinolone acetonide Suspension for Injection: 2 mg/mL; 6 mg/mL; *Vetalog® Parenteral* (BIVI); (Rx). FDA-approved for use in dogs, cats, and horses not intended for food.

The ARCI (Racing Commissioners International) has designated this drug as a class 4 substance. See the appendix for more information.

HUMAN-LABELED PRODUCTS:

Triamcinolone Acetonide Injection: 10 mg/mL suspension & 40 mg/mL suspension in 1 mL, 5 mL and 10 mL vials; *Kenalog-10* & *-40* (Bristol-Myers Squibb); (Rx)

Triamcinolone Hexacetonide Injection: 5 mg/mL & 20 mg/mL suspension in 1 mL & 5 mL vials; *Aristospan Intralesional®* & *Intra-articular®* (Sandoz); (Rx)

Many topical preparations are available, alone and in combination with other agents. Oral mucosal paste & Inhaled products are also FDA-approved. All are Rx.

References

Beale, K. (2008). Dealing with Miliary Dermatitis. Proceedings: WVC. Accessed via: Veterinary Information Network. http://goo.gl/oBh6l

Boyce, M., E.D. Malone, et al. (2010). Evaluation of diffusion of triamcinolone acetonide from the distal interphalangeal joint into the navicular bursa in horses. *American Journal of Veterinary Research* 71(2): 169–175.

Howard, J.L., Ed. (1986). *Current Veterinary Therapy 2, Food Animal Practice.* Philadelphia, W.B. Saunders.

Kay, A.T., D.M. Bolt, et al. (2008). Anti-inflammatory and analgesic effects of intra-articular injection of triamcinolone acetonide, mepivacaine hydrochloride, or both on lipopolysaccharide-induced lameness in horses. *American Journal of Veterinary Research* 69(12): 1646–1654.

Kirk, R.W., Ed. (1989). *Current Veterinary Therapy X, Small Animal Practice.* Philadelphia, W.B. Saunders.

Marks, S. (2004). What's new in veterinary endoscopy? Proceedings: ACVIM Forum. Accessed via: Veterinary Information Network. http://goo.gl/aMVlh

McClure, S. (2002). An opinion on joint therapy. Proceedings: Western Veterinary Conf. Accessed via: Veterinary Information Network. http://goo.gl/wVJwW

Richter, K. (2009). Esophageal Strictures—Update on Therapeutic Options. Proceedings: ACVIM. Accessed via: Veterinary Information Network. http://goo.gl/a5psU

Williamson, N. (2003). Immune-mediated skin diseases. P Ashley Ed. Handbook of Small Animal Practice, 4th Ed, Saunders: 894–908.

TRIAMTERENE

(trye-*am*-the-reen)   Dyrenium®

POTASSIUM-SPARING DIURETIC

Prescriber Highlights

▶ Potassium-sparing diuretic that may be considered as an alternative to spironolactone for treating CHF in dogs; limited clinical experience with this drug in dogs/cats

▶ Contraindications: Anuria, severe or progressive renal disease, severe hepatic disease, hypersensitivity to triamterene, preexisting hyperkalemia, concurrent therapy with another potassium-sparing agent (spironolactone, amiloride) or potassium supplementation

▶ Hyperkalemia possible; must monitor serum K+

Uses/Indications

Triamterene is a potassium-sparing diuretic that potentially could be used as an alternative to spironolactone for the adjunctive treatment of congestive heart failure in dogs, however, there is little experience associated with its use in dogs or cats.

Pharmacology/Actions

By exerting a direct effect on the distal renal tubule, triamterene inhibits the reabsorption of sodium in exchange for hydrogen and potassium ions. Unlike spironolactone, it does not competitively inhibit aldosterone. Triamterene increases excretion of sodium, calcium, magnesium and bicarbonate; urinary pH may be slightly increased. Serum concentrations of potassium and chloride may be increased. When used alone, triamterene has little effect on blood pressure. Triamterene can reduce GFR slightly, probably by affecting renal blood flow. This effect is reversible when the medication is discontinued.

Pharmacokinetics

Pharmacokinetic data for dogs or cats was not located. In humans, triamterene is rapidly absorbed after oral administration and oral bioavailability is about 85%. Onset of diuresis occurs in 2–4 hours and diminishes after about 8 hours. Triamterene is metabolized in the liver to 6-p-hydroxytriamterine and its sulfate conjugate. These metabolites are eliminated in the bile/feces and urine; elimination half-life is about 2 hours.

Contraindications/Precautions/Warnings

Triamterene is contraindicated for human patients (and presumably dogs and cats) with anuria, severe or progressive renal disease, severe hepatic disease, hypersensitivity to triamterene, preexisting hyperkalemia, history of triamterene-induced hyperkalemia, concurrent therapy with another potassium-sparing agent (spironolactone, amiloride) or potassium supplementation.

Adverse Effects

Because triamterene has been infrequently used in veterinary medicine, an accurate adverse effect profile for small animals is not known, however, hyperkalemia is a definite possibility and monitoring of electrolytes and renal function are necessary. In humans, hyperkalemia rarely occurs in patients with normal urine output and potassium intake.

Less common adverse effects reported in humans include headache/dizziness, GI effects, hyponatremia, and an increased sensitivity to sunlight. Rarely, hypersensitivity reactions have occurred in human patients taking triamterene. Other rare adverse effects include triamterene-nephrolithiasis, agranulocytosis, thrombocytopenia, or megaloblastosis.

Reproductive/Nursing Safety

Studies to determine triamterene's effects on fertility have not been performed.

Studies in pregnant rats given triamterene at 6–20X (human dose) did not show adverse effects to the fetuses. Triamterene crosses the placental barrier. For humans, triamterene is either in FDA category *B* or category *C*, depending on the reference. Category *C* for use during pregnancy states: *Animal studies have shown an adverse effect on the fetus, but there are no adequate studies in humans; or there are no animal reproduction studies and no adequate studies in humans.* If considering use of this product in a pregnant animal, weigh the potential benefits of treatment versus the risks.

Triamterene is distributed into milk. Although unlikely to pose much risk to nursing animals, safety during nursing cannot be assured.

Overdosage/Acute Toxicity

The oral LD50 for triamterene in mice is 380 mg/kg. Fluid and electrolyte imbalance is the most likely risk associated with an overdose. GI effects or hypotension are also possible. Consider gut emptying protocols for very large or quantity unknown ingestions. Acute overdoses should generally be managed by observation, with fluid, electrolyte (especially serum potassium) and acid-base monitoring. Supportive treatment should be initiated if required.

Drug Interactions

The following drug interactions have either been reported or are theoretical in humans or animals receiving triamterene and may be of significance in veterinary patients:

◾ **ACE INHIBITORS (e.g., enalapril, benazepril):** Increased risks for hyperkalemia

◾ **ANTIDIABETIC AGENTS (insulin, oral hypoglycemic agents):** Triamterene may increase blood glucose

■ **ANTIHYPERTENSIVE AGENTS:** Possible potentiation of hypotensive effects

■ **DIURETICS, POTASSIUM-SPARING (spironolactone, amiloride):** Increase risk of hyperkalemia; use of these drugs with triamterene in humans is contraindicated

■ **LITHIUM:** Triamterene may reduce lithium clearance

■ **NSAIDS:** Triamterene with NSAIDs (esp. **indomethacin**) may increase the risks of nephrotoxicity

■ **POTASSIUM SUPPLEMENTS or HIGH POTASSIUM FOODS:** Increased risk for hyperkalemia

Laboratory Considerations

■ **Quinidine:** Triamterene may interfere with fluorescent assay of quinidine

Doses

■ **DOGS:**
   a) For adjunctive treatment of recurrent heart failure associated with chronic mitral valve insufficiency: 1–2 mg/kg PO q12h. Documentation of use is limited; spironolactone is drug of choice. (Haggstrom *et al.* 2005)

   b) As a diuretic for adjunctive treatment of CHF: 2–(4) mg/kg/day PO (Ware 2003)

Monitoring

■ Serum electrolytes (especially potassium), BUN, creatinine

■ Hydration status

■ Blood pressure, if indicated

■ Signs of edema; patient weight, if indicated

Client Information

■ Give this medication with food to help prevent stomach upset

■ Urine may develop a bluish hue, this is normal

■ Because this medication has not been used very much in dogs or cats; report any unusual effects to the veterinarian

Chemistry/Synonyms

Triamterene is structurally related to folic acid and occurs as a yellow, odorless, crystalline powder. It is practically insoluble in water and very slightly soluble in alcohol. At 50°C, it is slightly soluble in water. In acidified solutions, triamterene gives off a blue fluorescence.

Triamterene may also be known as NSC-77625, KF-8542, FI-6143, triamteren, trimaterenum, triamtereen, or *Dyrenium®*. International trade names include *Dytac®*, *Dyazide®*, *Maxzide-25®* and *Triteren®*. There are many international trade names for combination products with hydrochlorothiazide.

Storage/Stability

Triamterene capsules should be stored between 15–30°C (59–86°F) in tight, light-resistant containers.

Dosage Forms/Regulatory Status

VETERINARY-LABELED PRODUCTS: None

The ARCI (Racing Commissioners International) has designated this drug as a class 4 substance.

HUMAN-LABELED PRODUCTS:

Triamterene Capsules: 50 mg & 100 mg; *Dyrenium®* (SmithKline Beecham); (Rx)

In humans, triamterene is often prescribed as a fixed-dose combination with hydrochlorothiazide. Products include:

Triamterene 37.5 mg/Hydrochlorothiazide 25 mg Tablets and Capsules; generic, *Dyazide®*, *Maxzide-25MG®*; generic; (Rx)

Triamterene 50 mg/Hydrochlorothiazide 25 mg Capsules; generic; (Rx)

Triamterene 75 mg/Hydrochlorothiazide 50 mg Tablets; *Maxzide®*; generic; (Rx)

References

Haggstrom, J., C. Kvart, et al. (2005). Acquired Valvular Heart Disease. *Textbook of Veterinary Internal Medicine, 6th Ed.* S Ettinger and E Feldman Eds., Elsevier: 1022–1039.

Ware, W. (2003). Cardiovascular system disorders. *Small Animal Internal Medicine, 3rd Ed.* R Nelson and C Couto Eds. St Louis, Mosby: 1–209.

TRIENTINE HCL

(trye-en-*teen*)   Syprine®

CHELATING AGENT

Prescriber Highlights

▶ Oral copper chelating agent for copper hepatopathy

▶ Probably fewer adverse effects then penicillamine, but acute renal failure possible

▶ Very limited experience with this drug

▶ More expensive than penicillamine; may need to be compounded into smaller dosages

▶ Give on an empty stomach

Uses/Indications

Trientine may be useful for the treatment of copper-associated hepatopathy in dogs, particularly when dogs cannot tolerate the adverse effects (*e.g.*, vomiting) associated with penicillamine.

Pharmacology/Actions

Trientine is an effective chelator of copper and increases its elimination via urinary excretion. It apparently has a greater affinity for copper in plasma than penicillamine, but penicillamine has a greater affinity for tissue copper.

Pharmacokinetics

No data was located.

Contraindications/Precautions/Warnings

Trientine is contraindicated in patients hypersensitive to it. It is not indicated for cystinuria, rheumatoid arthritis, or biliary cirrhosis.

Adverse Effects

Albeit with limited veterinary experience, trientine has had relatively minimal adverse effects in dogs treated for copper hepatotoxicity, but acute renal failure has been reported. Human patients have developed iron deficiency anemia after taking trientine long-term. There is a chance for topical dermatitis developing if trientine gets on skin; wash off immediately. The drug should be given in a capsule (may need to be compounded) and not sprinkled on food.

Reproductive/Nursing Safety

Trientine is a potential teratogen. It was teratogenic in rats given doses similar to those for humans and should only be used in pregnancy when the benefits to the mother outweigh the risks to offspring. In humans, the FDA categorizes this drug as category *C* for use during pregnancy (*Animal studies have shown an adverse effect on the fetus, but there are no adequate studies in humans; or there are no animal reproduction studies and no adequate studies in humans.*)

It is not known whether this drug is excreted in breast milk. Exercise caution when administering to nursing patients.

Overdosage/Acute Toxicity

Little information is available; a case of a human ingesting 30 grams of trientine without significant morbidity has been reported.

Drug Interactions

The following drug interactions have either been reported or are theoretical in humans or animals receiving trientine and may be of significance in veterinary patients:

- ▉ **IRON:** Iron and trientine inhibit the absorption of one another; if iron therapy is needed, give doses at least 2 hours apart from one another

- ▉ **ZINC:** Because trientine may also chelate zinc or other minerals, separate doses as above

Doses

- ▉ **DOGS:**

As a chelator for copper hepatotoxicity:

a) 10–15 mg/kg PO twice daily; 1–2 hours before a meal (Twedt 1999)

b) 10–15 mg/kg PO q12h; give one hour before meals (Johnson 2000)

c) 15–30 mg/kg PO twice daily (q12h). Give prior to meals (Richter 2002)

Monitoring

- ▉ Periodic quantitative hepatic copper levels

Client Information

- ▉ While it is preferable to give on an empty stomach, if the drug causes vomiting or lack of appetite give with a small amount of food

Chemistry/Synonyms

An oral copper chelator, trientine HCl occurs as a white to pale yellow crystalline powder. It is hygroscopic and freely soluble in water.

Trientine HCl may also be known as: MK-0681, 2,2,2-tetramine, trien hydrochloride, triethylenetetramine dihydrochloride, trientine hydrochloride or *Syprine®*.

Storage/Stability

Store trientine capsules in the refrigerator (2–8°C) in tightly closed containers.

Dosage Forms/Regulatory Status

VETERINARY-LABELED PRODUCTS: None

HUMAN-LABELED PRODUCTS:

Trientine HCl Oral Capsules: 250 mg; *Syprine®* (Aton); (Rx)

References

Johnson, S. (2000). Chronic Hepatic Disorders. *Textbook of Veterinary Internal Medicine: Diseases of the Dog and Cat.* S Ettinger and E Feldman Eds. Philadelphia, WB Saunders. **2:** 1298–1325.

Richter, K. (2002). Common canine hepatopathies. Proceedings: ACVIM Forum. Accessed via: Veterinary Information Network. http://goo.gl/pqRDc

Twedt, D. (1999). Treatment of chronic hepatitis: Scientific research examines traditional therapies. Proceedings: American College of Veterinary Internal Medicine: 17th Annual Veterinary Medical Forum, Chicago.

TRILOSTANE

(***trye***-low-stane)   Vetoryl®

ADRENAL STEROID SYNTHESIS INHIBITOR

Prescriber Highlights

- ▶ Competitive inhibitor of 3-beta hydroxysteroid dehydrogenase thereby reducing synthesis of cortisol, aldosterone, & adrenal androgens

- ▶ May be useful in dogs for treatment of pituitary-dependent hyperadrenocorticism, adrenal dependent hyperadrenocorticism, Alopecia X in Pomeranians & Alaskan malamutes; in cats for treatment of feline pituitary dependent hyperadrenocorticism, & in horses for equine hyperadrenocorticism (HAC)

- ▶ Potential adverse effects in dogs include lethargy, inappetence, vomiting, electrolyte abnormalities, & diarrhea

- ▶ Rare case reports of hypoadrenocorticism & death

- ▶ Expense of treatment may be an issue

Uses/Indications

Trilostane may be useful for treating pituitary-dependent hyperadrenocorticism or adrenal dependent hyperadrenocorticism in dogs, feline pituitary-dependent hyperadrenocorticism, and equine hyperadrenocorticism (HAC). It may also be useful in treating Pomeranians with

Alopecia X and Alaskan malamutes with adult-onset alopecia.

Pharmacology/Actions

Trilostane is a competitive inhibitor of 3-beta hydroxysteroid dehydrogenase thereby reducing synthesis of cortisol, aldosterone, and adrenal androgens. Inhibition is reversible and apparently dose dependent.

Pharmacokinetics

In dogs, orally administered trilostane is rapidly, but erratically absorbed with peak levels occurring between 1.5–2 hours post dose. It is unknown whether the presence of food in the gut significantly alters absorption characteristics. After 18 hours, the drug reportedly returns to baseline levels. Effects on cortisol production apparently last for no more than 20 hours, and more likely wane within 10 hours of dosing. Trilostane is metabolized in the liver to several metabolites including ketotrilostane, which is active.

Contraindications/Precautions/Warnings

Trilostane is contraindicated in animals hypersensitive to it. It should be used with caution in patients with renal or hepatic impairment. Do not use in pregnant dogs.

When used for controlling clinical signs of Cushing's in dogs with adrenal tumors, trilostane will not shrink the tumor and adrenal glands may actually increase in size during treatment.

Adverse Effects

Trilostane appears to be relatively well tolerated in dogs, but up to 63% of treated dogs can develop lethargy, mild electrolyte abnormalities (hyponatremia, hyperkalemia), vomiting, diarrhea and inappetence are commonly noted during the first few days of therapy secondary to steroid withdrawal. These effects are usually relatively mild and self-limiting. Withholding the drug for a few days and then giving it every other day for a week may alleviate lethargy and vomiting. Although adrenal suppression caused by trilostane is reversible in most cases, rarely adrenal necrosis and death have occurred in dogs.

In one study of trilostane given to 20 horses with equine Cushing's (McGowan & Neiger 2003), no adverse effects were noted.

Reproductive/Nursing Safety

Because trilostane can significantly reduce the synthesis of progesterone *in vivo*, it should not be used in pregnancy. Trilostane reportedly (not confirmed) is classified by the FDA as a category X drug (*Contraindicated in pregnancy*).

Information on trilostane levels in maternal milk were not located; use with caution in lactating animals.

Overdosage/Acute Toxicity

Specific information on trilostane acute toxicity was not located. One source states that trilostane overdoses would be unlikely to threaten life and no clinical signs would be expected. However, blood pressure, hydration status, and electrolyte balance should be monitored. If the animal is stressed, consider giving exogenous corticosteroids short-term. Because the drug's effects are relatively short lived, monitoring of patients without complications should only be required for a few days post ingestion.

Drug Interactions

The following drug interactions have either been reported or are theoretical in humans or animals receiving trilostane and may be of significance in veterinary patients:

- ■ **ACE INHIBITORS (e.g., benazepril, enalapril):** Could increase risk for hyperkalemia
- ■ **AMINOGLUTETHIMIDE:** May potentiate the effects of trilostane and lead to hypoadrenocorticism
- ■ **KETOCONAZOLE:** May potentiate the effects of trilostane and lead to hypoadrenocorticism
- ■ **MITOTANE:** May potentiate the effects of trilostane and lead to hypoadrenocorticism
- ■ **POTASSIUM-SPARING DIURETICS (e.g., spironolactone):** Could increase risk for hyperkalemia
- ■ **POTASSIUM-SUPPLEMENTS; HIGH POTASSIUM FOODS:** Could increase risk for hyperkalemia

Laboratory Considerations

- ■ No specific laboratory interactions or considerations were located.

Doses

- ■ **DOGS:**

   For treatment of canine hyperadrenocorticism (HAC):

   a) The starting dose for the treatment of hyperadrenocorticism in dogs is 2.2–6.7 mg/kg PO once a day with food based on body weight and capsule size. The package insert has a dosing table (Table 1) to help determine the appropriate size and number of capsules to administer.

   After approximately 10-14 days at this dose, re-examine the dog and conduct a 4-6 hour post-dosing ACTH stimulation test. If physical examination is acceptable adjust dose according to Table 2 (found in the package insert). Individual dose adjustments and close monitoring are essential. Re-examine and conduct an ACTH stimulation test 10-14 days after every dose alteration. Care must be taken during dose increases to monitor the dog's clinical signs and serum electrolyte concentrations. Once daily administration is recommended. However, if clinical signs are not controlled for the full day, twice daily dosing may be needed. To switch from a once daily dose to a twice daily dose, increase the total daily dose by

⅓ to ½ and divide the total amount into two doses given 12 hours apart. (Label Information; *Vetoryl®*—Dechra)

b) For treatment of canine hyperadreno-corticism (HAC) whether due to adrenal tumor or PDH: Initial therapy at 2–10 mg/kg PO once daily. Adjust dosage per monitoring parameters below. Doses of up to 50 mg/kg/day divided twice daily have been given without untoward side effects. Give with food. Some dogs require twice daily administration.

ACTH stimulation test done at 10–14 days, 30 days and 90 days after starting therapy. ACTH stimulation tests should be performed 4–6 hours post-trilostane dose. Interpret ACTH test in light of physical exam. If ACTH Stim results are <20 nMol/L (0.72 micro-grams/dL), then the drug is discontinued for 48–72 hours and then restarted at a lower dosage. If ACTH Stim results are >200 nMol/L (7.2 micro-grams/dL), then the dose is increased. If the ACTH Stim results are between these two values and the dog is clinically well-controlled, then no change. If between these two results and the patient appears not to be clinically well-controlled, then the drug may need to be given twice daily. Once the dog is stable, repeat ACTH Stim test every 3–6 months. (Neiger 2004)

c) Author's (Feldman) experience is that trilostane is not more effective or safer than mitotane and that trilostane is less predictable (under dose, over dose, resolution of signs, or the need for dosing more than once per day) than mitotane.

If using trilostane current recommendation is: Initiate at 1 mg/kg PO once daily and continue for about one week until a veterinary recheck can occur. Have owners collect a small urine sample from their dog before leaving home the morning of the scheduled recheck prior to trilostane administration. Trilostane should then be given and the dog should be seen by veterinarian 2-3 hours later. The goal of therapy is an owner who is completely pleased with the response. The urine should be checked, at a minimum, for specific gravity, glucose and urine cortisol:creatinine ratio (UCCR). An ACTH stimulation test should be started at the time that the dog is seen (about 2-3 hours after trilostane dose). The UCCR result should be within the reference interval and the post-ACTH serum cortisol concentration should be between 1.5 and 5.5 micrograms/dL. If the serum cortisol concentration is within that goal and the UCCR is abnormal, the medica-

tion should be given twice daily. If the serum cortisol concentration is too high, the trilostane dose should be increased and if the serum cortisol concentration is too low, the dose should be decreased. This approach should be utilized at each recheck until the dog is doing well. (Feldman 2007)

For treatment of Alopecia X:

a) In Alaskan Malamutes: 3–3.6 mg/kg PO twice a day for 4–6 months. Three dogs treated; no adverse effects reported. (Leone *et al.* 2005)

b) In Miniature poodles and Pomeranians: Average dose was 10.85 mg/kg per day given either once a day or divided twice a day for 4–8 weeks. (Cerundolo *et al.* 2004)

■ **CATS:**

a) For treatment of feline hyperadrenocorticism: 7 mg/kg/day divided and given twice daily. Doses of up to 60 mg per cat per day have been used in a small number of cats with PDH. (Greco 2007)

b) Treatment with trilostane may improve clinical signs, but cats typically remain diabetic. Effective doses range from 15 mg (total dose) PO once daily to 60 mg (total dose) PO q12h. ACTH stimulation tests should be used to titrate the dose, similar to the protocol for dogs. (Scott-Moncrieff 2010)

■ **HORSES:**

a) For treatment of equine Cushing's syndrome: 0.4–1 mg/kg (total dose 120–240 mg) PO once daily. (McGowan & Neiger 2003)

Monitoring

■ Clinical effects
■ Adverse effects
■ Serum electrolytes
■ Urinalysis including specific gravity, glucose and urine cortisol:creatinine ratio (UCCR)
■ ACTH stimulation tests (see doses for recommendations). For long-term monitoring, the manufacturer recommends: Once an optimum dose has been reached, re-examine the dog at 30 days, 90 days and every 3 months thereafter. At a minimum, this monitoring should include a thorough history and physical examination, ACTH stimulation test (conducted 4-6 hours after trilostane administration), and serum biochemical tests (with particular attention to electrolytes, renal and hepatic function). A post-ACTH stimulation test resulting in a cortisol of <1.45 micrograms/dL (<40 nMol/L), with or without electrolyte abnormalities, may precede the development of clinical signs of hypoadrenocorticism. Good control is indicated by favor-

able clinical signs as well as post-ACTH serum cortisol of 1.45-9.1 micrograms/dL (40-250 nMol/L). If the ACTH stimulation test is <1.45 micrograms/dL (<40 nMol/L) and/or if electrolyte imbalances characteristic of hypoadrenocorticism (hyperkalemia and hyponatremia) are found, trilostane should be temporarily discontinued until recurrence of clinical signs consistent with hyperadrenocorticism and test results return to normal (1.45-9.1 micrograms/dL or 40-250 nMol/L). Trilostane may then be reintroduced at a lower dose.

Client Information
- Keep out of reach of children and pets
- Trilostane capsules do not require any special safety handling precautions. The manufacturer states: Wash hands after use. Do not empty capsule contents and do not attempt to divide the capsules. Do not handle the capsules if pregnant or if trying to conceive. Clients should report any adverse effects to the veterinarian
- Give the drug with food, unless otherwise directed by veterinarian
- Clients should understand that trilostane is a treatment for the condition and not a cure

Chemistry/Synonyms
A synthetic steroid analog, trilostane has a molecular weight of 329.4 and its chemical name is 4-alpha, 5-alpha-Epoxy-17-beta-hydroxy-3-oxoandrostane-2-alpha-carbonitrile. It reportedly is relatively insoluble in water.

Trilostane may also be known as: WIN 24540, *Vetoryl®*, *Desopan®*, *Modrastane®* or *Modrenal®*.

Storage/Stability
Commercially available trilostane capsules should be stored at room temperature in tight, light-resistant containers.

Dosage Forms/Regulatory Status
VETERINARY-LABELED PRODUCTS: None in the USA.

Trilostane Oral Capsules: 10 mg, 30 mg, & 60 mg packaged in aluminum foil blister cards of 10 capsules; *Vetoryl®* (Dechra); (Rx).

HUMAN-LABELED PRODUCTS:

Modrastane® is reportedly still an FDA-approved human drug, but was withdrawn from the market in the USA in 1994.

References
Cerundolo, R., D. Lloyd, et al. (2004). Treatment of Alopecia X with trilostane. *Vet Derm* 15: 285–293.
Feldman, E. (2007). Medical management of canine hyperadrenocorticism: A comparison of trilostane to mitotane. Proceedings: UCD Canine Medicine Symposium. Accessed via: Veterinary Information Network. http://goo.gl/WbO8k
Greco, D. (2007). Feline adrenal gland disorders. Proceedings Western Vet Conf. Accessed via: Veterinary Information Network. http://goo.gl/pz6kw
Leone, F., A. Vercelli, et al. (2005). The use of trilostane for the treatment of Alopecia X in Alaskan Malamutes. *J Am Anim Hosp Assoc* 41: 336–342.

McGowan, C. & R. Neiger (2003). Efficacy of trilostane in the treatment of equine Cushing's syndrome. *Equine Vet Jnl* 35: 414–418.
Neiger, R. (2004). Hyperadrenocorticism: The animal perspective-Comparative efficacy and safety of trilostane. Proceedings: ACVIM Forum, Minneapolis. Accessed via: Veterinary Information Network. http://goo.gl/ocgpy
Scott-Moncrieff, J.C. (2010). Update on treatment of hyperadrenocorticism: What is the current recommendation? Proceedings: ACVIM Forum. Accessed via: Veterinary Information Network. http://goo.gl/OsV6A

TRIMEPRAZINE TARTRATE WITH PREDNISOLONE

(trye-*mep*-ra-zeen)   Temaril-P®

PHENOTHIAZINE ANTIHISTAMINE & CORTICOSTEROID

Prescriber Highlights

▶ Combination phenothiazine antihistamine & corticosteroid used for pruritus & potentially as an antitussive

▶ Relatively Contraindicated: Systemic fungal infections, hypovolemia, or shock & in patients with tetanus or strychnine intoxication. Caution: Hepatic dysfunction, cardiac disease, active bacterial or viral infections, peptic ulcer, acute psychoses, corneal ulcer, Cushingoid syndrome, diabetes, osteoporosis, chronic psychotic reactions, predisposition to thrombophlebitis, hypertension, CHF, renal insufficiency, general debilitation, very young animals

▶ Primary adverse effects: Sedation, may cause significant hypotension, cardiac rate abnormalities, hypo- or hyperthermia, "Cushingoid" effects with sustained use

▶ Many potential drug & lab interactions

Uses/Indications
Trimeprazine with prednisolone is used for the treatment of pruritic conditions, especially if induced by allergic conditions. Many dermatologists believe, and there is reasonable evidence to support, that when prednisolone is combined with trimeprazine (*Temaril-P®*), less prednisolone is required to control pruritus. The manufacturer suggests the drug is for use in dogs either for pruritic conditions or as an antitussive.

Pharmacology/Actions
Trimeprazine has antihistaminic, sedative, antitussive, and antipruritic qualities. The veterinary FDA-approved product also has prednisolone in its formulation that provides additional antiinflammatory effects.

Pharmacokinetics

The pharmacokinetics of trimeprazine have apparently not been studied.

Contraindications/Precautions/Warnings

The contraindications and precautions of this product follow those of the other phenothiazines and antihistaminic agents. For more information, it is suggested to review the acepromazine and chlorpheniramine monographs.

Adverse Effects

For trimeprazine, possible adverse reactions include: sedation, depression, hypotension and extrapyramidal reactions (rigidity, tremors, weakness, restlessness, etc.).

Additional adverse effects, if using the product containing steroids include: elevated liver enzymes, weight loss, polyuria/polydipsia, vomiting, and diarrhea. If used chronically, therapy must be withdrawn gradually and Cushing's syndrome may develop.

The manufacturer of the veterinary combination product (*Temaril®-P*) includes the following adverse effects in its package insert: sodium retention and potassium loss, negative nitrogen balance, suppressed adrenocortical function, delayed wound healing, osteoporosis, possible increased susceptibility to and/or exacerbation of bacterial infections, sedation, protruding nictitating membrane, blood dyscrasias. In addition, intensification and prolongation of the action of sedatives, analgesics or anesthetics can be noted and potentiation of organophosphate toxicity and of procaine HCl activity.

Reproductive/Nursing Safety

The manufacturer of the veterinary combination product (*Temaril®-P*) warns that corticosteroids can induce the first stages of parturition if administered during the last trimester of pregnancy.

Overdosage/Acute Toxicity

Acute overdosage should be handled as per the acepromazine monograph found at the beginning of the book.

Drug Interactions

The following drug interactions have either been reported or are theoretical in humans or animals receiving promethazine (a related phenothiazine antihistamine) or prednisolone and may be of significance in veterinary patients:

- **ACE INHIBITORS:** Phenothiazines may increase effects

- **AMPHOTERICIN B:** When administered concomitantly with glucocorticoids may cause hypokalemia

- **ANTACIDS:** May cause reduced GI absorption of oral phenothiazines

- **ANTIDIARRHEAL MIXTURES (e.g., Kaolin/pectin, bismuth subsalicylate mixtures):** May cause reduced GI absorption of oral phenothiazines

- **ANTICHOLINESTERASE AGENTS (e.g., pyridostigmine, neostigmine, etc.):** In patients with myasthenia gravis, concomitant glucocorticoid with these agents may lead to profound muscle weakness. If possible, discontinue anticholinesterase medication at least 24 hours prior to corticosteroid administration.

- **ASPIRIN (salicylates):** Glucocorticoids may reduce salicylate blood levels

- **CISAPRIDE:** Increased risk for cardiac arrhythmias when used with phenothiazines

- **CNS DEPRESSANT AGENTS (barbiturates, narcotics, anesthetics, etc.):** May cause additive CNS depression if used with phenothiazines

- **CYCLOPHOSPHAMIDE:** Glucocorticoids may also inhibit the hepatic metabolism of cyclophosphamide; dosage adjustments may be required.

- **CYCLOSPORINE:** Concomitant administration of may increase the blood levels of each, by mutually inhibiting the hepatic metabolism of each other; clinical significance of this interaction is not clear

- **DIGOXIN:** Secondary to hypokalemia, increased risk for arrhythmias

- **DIURETICS, POTASSIUM-DEPLETING (furosemide, thiazides):** When administered concomitantly with glucocorticoids may cause hypokalemia

- **EPHEDRINE:** May increase metabolism

- **ESTROGENS:** The effects of hydrocortisone, and possibly other glucocorticoids, may be potentiated by concomitant administration with estrogens

- **INSULIN:** Requirements may increase in patients receiving glucocorticoids

- **KETOCONAZOLE:** May decrease metabolism

- **MITOTANE:** May alter the metabolism of steroids; higher than usual doses of steroids may be necessary to treat mitotane-induced adrenal insufficiency

- **NSAIDS:** Administration of other ulcerogenic drugs with glucocorticoids may increase risk

- **PAROXETINE:** May increase phenothiazine plasma levels

- **PHENOBARBITAL:** May increase the metabolism of glucocorticoids

- **PHENYTOIN:** May increase the metabolism of glucocorticoids

- **RIFAMPIN:** May increase the metabolism of glucocorticoids

- **VACCINES:** Patients receiving corticosteroids at immunosuppressive dosages should generally not receive live attenuated-virus vaccines as virus replication may be augmented; a diminished immune response may occur after vaccine, toxoid, or bacterin administration in patients receiving glucocorticoids

Laboratory Considerations

■ Glucocorticoids may increase serum **cholesterol** and **urine glucose** levels.

■ Glucocorticoids may decrease serum **potassium**.

■ Glucocorticoids can suppress the release of thyroid stimulating hormone (TSH) and reduce T_3 & T_4 values. Thyroid gland atrophy has been reported after chronic glucocorticoid administration. Uptake of I^{131} by the thyroid may be decreased by glucocorticoids.

■ Reactions to **skin tests** may be suppressed by glucocorticoids or trimeprazine.

■ False-negative results of the **nitroblue tetrazolium test for systemic bacterial infections** may be induced by glucocorticoids.

Doses

■ **DOGS:**

a) For antipruritic and antitussive therapy: Weight up to 10 lb = ½ tab PO twice daily; 11–20 lb = 1 tablet twice daily; 21–40 lb = 2 tablets twice daily; over 40 lb = 3 tablets twice daily. After 4 days reduce dose to ½ of initial dose or to an amount just sufficient to maintain remission of symptoms; adjust as necessary. (Package Insert; *Temaril®-P*—Pfizer)

b) For treatment of pruritus: 1 tablet per 10 kg of body weight once daily for 3–5 days, then every other day. Giving with an EFA (essential fatty acid) may reduce the dose and frequency, if not the need for, glucocorticoids. (White 2003)

c) For atopic dermatitis: 1 tablet of *Temaril®-P* per 5 kg body weight q12h for one week, then once daily for one week, then q48h (every other day). (Hillier 2006)

Monitoring

■ Efficacy

■ Degree of sedation, and anticholinergic effects

■ Adverse effects associated with corticosteroids

Client Information

■ Follow veterinarians dosage recommendations carefully

■ Dog's appetite and water consumption may increase

■ If side effects are worrisome, contact veterinarian

Chemistry/Synonyms

A phenothiazine antihistamine related to promethazine, trimeprazine tartrate occurs as an odorless, white, to off-white crystalline powder with a melting range of 160–164°C. Approximately 0.5 gm is soluble in 1 mL water, and 0.05 gram is soluble in 1 mL of alcohol.

Trimeprazine Tartrate may also be known as: trimeprazine tartrate, alimemazine tartrate, *Chemists Own Peetalix®, Nedeltran®, Panectyl®, Repeltin®, Temaril®, Theralen®, Theralene®, Theralene®, Vallergan®,* or *Variargil®*.

Storage/Stability

Store trimeprazine products at room temperature (15–30°C); protect tablets from light.

Dosage Forms/Regulatory Status

VETERINARY-LABELED PRODUCTS:

No single agent trimeprazine products are FDA-approved for veterinary medicine.

Trimeprazine Tartrate 5 mg; Prednisolone 2 mg Tablets; *Temaril-P® Tablets* (Pfizer); (Rx). FDA-approved for use in dogs. Trade name in Canada is *Vanectyl-P®*.

The ARCI (Racing Commissioners International) has designated this drug as a class 4 substance. See the appendix for more information.

HUMAN-LABELED PRODUCTS: None

References

Hillier, A. (2006). Therapeutic options for atopic dermatitis. Proceedings: ACVC. Accessed via: Veterinary Information Network. http://goo.gl/dtZEv

White, P. (2003). Medical management of canine pruritus. Proceedings: Western Veterinary Conf. Accessed via: Veterinary Information Network. http://goo.gl/2P8ET

Trimethoprim/Sulfa—See Sulfadiazine/Trimethoprim

TRIPELENNAMINE HCL

(tri-pel-*ehn*-a-meen)   Re-Covr®

ANTIHISTAMINE

Prescriber Highlights

▶ Injectable antihistamine

▶ Contraindications: Do not give IV to horses

▶ Adverse Effects: CNS stimulation (if given IV to horses), sedation, depression, ataxia, GI effects (oral use)

Uses/Indications

Antihistamines are used in veterinary medicine to reduce or help prevent histamine mediated adverse effects. Tripelennamine has been used as a CNS stimulant in "Downer cows" when administered slow IV.

Pharmacology/Actions

Antihistamines (H_1-receptor antagonists) competitively inhibit histamine at H_1 receptor sites. They do not inactivate or prevent the release of histamine, but can prevent histamine's action on the cell. Besides their antihistaminic activity, these agents also have varying degrees of anticholinergic and CNS activity (sedation). Tripelennamine is considered to have moderate sedative activity and minimal anticholinergic activity when compared to other antihistamines.

Pharmacokinetics

The pharmacokinetics of tripelennamine have apparently not been thoroughly studied in domestic animals or humans. One study performed in horses and camels (Wasfi *et al.* 2000), showed that after IV administration similar pharmacokinetic profiles were obtained for both species. Terminal elimination half-lives were around 2+ hours; volumes of distribution steady-state approximately 1.5–3 L/kg; protein binding was 80% and total body clearance approximately 1 L/hour/kg.

Contraindications/Precautions/Warnings

Do not administer Tripelennamine IV in horses (see Adverse Effects).

Adverse Effects

CNS stimulation (hyperexcitability, nervousness, and muscle tremors) lasting up to 20 minutes, has been noted in horses after receiving tripelennamine intravenously. Other effects seen (in all species) include CNS depression, incoordination, and GI disturbances.

Overdosage/Acute Toxicity

Overdosage of tripelennamine reportedly can cause CNS excitation, seizures and ataxia. Treat symptomatically and supportively if clinical signs are severe. Phenytoin (IV) is recommended in the treatment of seizures caused by antihistamine overdose in humans; barbiturates and diazepam are generally avoided.

Drug Interactions

The following drug interactions have either been reported or are theoretical in humans or animals receiving tripelennamine and may be of significance in veterinary patients:

- ◼ **CNS DEPRESSANTS, OTHER:** Increased sedation can occur if chlorpheniramine is combined with other CNS depressant drugs

- ◼ **HEPARIN, WARFARIN:** Antihistamines may partially counteract the anti-coagulation effects of heparin or warfarin.

Laboratory Considerations

- ◼ Antihistamines can decrease the wheal and flare response to **antigen skin testing.** In humans, it is suggested that antihistamines be discontinued at least 4 days prior to testing.

Doses

It is recommended to warm the solution to near body temperature before injecting; give IM injections into large muscle areas. **Note:** Oral dosage forms may no longer be obtainable.

- ◼ **DOGS:**
  a) 1mg/kg PO q12h; 1 mg/kg IM (Kirk 1986)

- ◼ **CATS:**
  a) 1 mg/kg PO q12h; 1 mg/kg IM (Kirk 1986)

- ◼ **CATTLE:**
  a) 1.1 mg/kg (2.5 mL per 100 lbs body weight) IV (for more immediate effect)

or IM q6–12h as needed (Package Insert; *Re-Covr®*—Solvay)

  b) As adjunctive treatment in "Downer Cow Syndrome" as a CNS stimulant: 0.5 mg/kg slow IV in conjunction with parenteral mineral treatment (Caple 1986)

  c) 1 mg/kg IV or IM (Howard 1986)

- ◼ **HORSES: (Note:** ARCI UCGFS Class 3 Drug)
  a) 1.1 mg/kg (2.5 mL per 100 lbs body weight) IM q6–12h as needed (Package Insert; *Re-Covr®*—Solvay)

  b) 1 mg/kg IM (Robinson 1987)

- ◼ **SWINE:**
  a) 1 mg/kg IV or IM (Howard 1986)

Monitoring

- ◼ Clinical efficacy
- ◼ Adverse effects

Chemistry/Synonyms

An ethylenediamine-derivative antihistamine, tripelennamine HCl occurs as a white, crystalline powder that will slowly darken upon exposure to light. It has a melting range of 188–192°C and pK$_a$s of 3.9 and 9.0. One gram is soluble in 1 mL of water or 6 mL of alcohol.

Tripelennamine HCl may also be known as: tripelennaminium chloride, *Azaron®*, *Etono®*, *Fenistil®*, *PBZ®*, *Pelamine®*, *Pyribenzamine®*, *Re-Covr®* or *Vaginex®*.

Storage/Stability

Store the injection at room temperature and protect from light; avoid freezing or excessive heat.

Dosage Forms/Regulatory Status

VETERINARY-LABELED PRODUCTS:

Tripelennamine HCl for Injection: 20 mg/mL in 20 mL, 100 mL, and 250 mL vials; *Re-Covr®* (Fort Dodge) Note: This product is still listed as FDA-approved, but may not be available commercially; generic (various manufacturers and trade names); (Rx). Tripelennamine HCl injection is FDA-approved for use in cattle and horses. Treated cattle must not be slaughtered for food purposes for 4 days following the last treatment. Milk must not be used for food for 24 hours (2 milkings) after treatment. No specific tolerance for residues has been published.

The ARCI (Racing Commissioners International) has designated this drug as a class 3 substance. See the appendix for more information.

HUMAN-LABELED PRODUCTS: None

References

Caple, I., W. (1986). Downer Cow Syndrome. Current Veterinary Therapy: Food Animal Practice 2. JL Howard Ed. Philadelphia, W.B. Saunders: 327–328.

Howard, J.L., Ed. (1986). Current Veterinary Therapy 2, Food Animal Practice. Philadelphia, W.B. Saunders.

Kirk, R.W., Ed. (1986). Current Veterinary Therapy IX, Small Animal Practice. Philadelphia, W.B. Saunders.

Robinson, N.E. (1987). Table of Common Drugs: Approximate Doses. Current Therapy in Equine Medicine, 2. NE Robinson Ed. Philadelphia, W.B. Saunders: 761.

Wasfi, I.A., A.A.A. Hadi, et al. (2000). Comparative disposition of tripelennamine and camels after intravenous administration. Journal of Veterinary Pharmacology and Therapeutics 23(3): 145–152.

TRYPAN BLUE

(*trip*-ann *bloo*)

ANTI-BABESIAL AGENT; OPTHO SURGERY DYE

Prescriber Highlights

➤ Uncommonly used alternative treatment for babesia (*B. canis*) in dogs that can rapidly alleviate clinical signs, but does not eliminate parasite

➤ Must follow-up treatment with other antibabesial drugs (e.g., diminazene, imidocarb)

➤ Must be given IV

➤ Will stain all body tissues and secretions for several weeks

➤ Likely teratogen when used systemically

Uses/Indications

Trypan blue was among the first agents used to treat Babesia. It may be useful as an adjunctive treatment for dogs with mild, to moderate signs of infection with babesiosis (*B. canis*). Some have recommended its use in dogs with severe infections as it does not possess imidocarb's anticholinergic effects or the CNS toxic effects of some of the other diamidine drugs (*e.g.*, diminazene, pentamidine). Trypan blue suppresses parasitemia and can alleviate clinical signs, but it does not eliminate the infection and results can be variable. Other treatments (*e.g.*, imidocarb, diminazene) must be used within a month of trypan blue to be curative (Greene & Ewing 2006; Taboada & Lobetti 2006). In a study comparing the effects of trypan blue and diminazene on hematocrit and parasitemia in dogs with clinically mild to moderate, uncomplicated babesiosis, there were no significant differences between diminazene and trypan blue on hematocrit or parasite clearance (Jacobson *et al.* 1996).

Trypan blue is also used as a dye in eye surgery to stain the anterior capsule of the lens and the epiretinal membranes.

Pharmacology/Actions

Trypan blue blocks the C3b receptor on both the erythrocyte membrane and the Babesia organism and likely prevents the parasite from entering the erythrocyte.

Pharmacokinetics

No information was located.

Contraindications/Precautions/Warnings

As trypan blue is a known teratogen it should be used during pregnancy in dogs only when the benefits to the dam outweigh the potential effects on puppies.

Adverse Effects

Trypan blue is well tolerated in dogs. The bluish-color change of secretions, urine, eyes and mucous membranes is most often the only adverse effect seen. This effect can persist for several weeks after treatment.

Reproductive/Nursing Safety

Trypan blue is teratogenic when used systemically in rats, mice, rabbits, hamsters, dogs, guinea pigs, and pigs. Systemically administered trypan blue to rats was teratogenic at 50 mg/kg (single dose) and 25 mg/kg/day (multiple doses). The FDA categorizes trypan blue used as a ophthalmologic dye as category *C* for use during pregnancy (*Animal studies have shown an adverse effect on the fetus, but there are no adequate studies in humans; or there are no animal reproduction studies and no adequate studies in humans.*)

Trypan blue can distribute into milk and cause it to have a bluish-tint. Safety in nursing offspring has not been established.

Overdosage/Acute Toxicity

No information located; figure dosages carefully.

Drug Interactions

■ None noted

Laboratory Considerations

■ Trypan blue can tint plasma to a bluish color it may affect photometric-based test results or affect erythrocyte monitoring.

Doses

■ **DOGS:**

For *B. canis*:

a) 10 mg/kg IV (only) once. (Schoeman 2008)

b) 10 mg/kg IV as a 1% solution once. (Taboada & Lobetti 2006)

Monitoring

■ Efficacy against babesia organism's effects on patient (bluish color change in plasma may make blood smear evaluation more difficult and affect erythrocyte counts and hematocrit determination)

Client Information

■ This medication may cause a bluish color change in the dog's mucous membranes, eyes, urine, or secretions. This should diminish in a few weeks, but secretions may stain fabrics.

■ Trypan blue does not completely eradicate the organism and additional treatments are required using other drugs

Chemistry/Synonyms

Trypan blue is an azo-naphthalene dye derived from toluidine.

Trypan blue may also be known as azidione blue 3B, benzamine blue 3B, Niagara blue, Congo blue, diamine blue, CI Direct Blue 14, or trypanum caeruleum. Trade names include VisionBlue® and MembranBlue®.

Storage/Stability

Trypan blue powder or solutions should be stored at 15-25°C (59-77°F). Protect from direct sunlight.

Compatibility/Compounding Considerations

A 1% solution (10 mg/mL) is usually given intravenously. Trypan blue for injection that is compounded from powder should be administered through an in-line filter during intravenous administration.

Dosage Forms/Regulatory Status

VETERINARY-LABELED PRODUCTS: None in the USA

HUMAN-LABELED PRODUCTS:

Trypan blue powder is available and it is also available as an ophthalmic stain in 0.06% and 0.15% solutions; VisionBlue®, MembraneBlue® (Dutch Ophthalmic); (Rx)

References

Greene, C. & S. Ewing (2006). Antiprotozoal Chemotherapy. *Infectious Diseases of the Dog and Cat*, 3rd Ed. C Greene Ed., Elsevier: 672–676.

Jacobson, L.S., F. Reyers, et al. (1996). Changes in haematocrit after treatment of uncomplicated canine babesiosis: A comparison between diminazene and trypan blue, and an evaluation of the influence of parasitaemia. *Journal of the South African Veterinary Association-Tydskrif Van Die Suid-Afrikaanse Veterinere Vereniging* 67(2): 77–82.

Schoeman, J. (2008). Canine Babesiosis: An Update. Proceedings: WSAVA. Accessed via: Veterinary Information Network. http://goo.gl/cF5PQ

Taboada, J. & R. Lobetti (2006). Babesia. *Infectious Diseases of the Dog and Cat, 3rd Ed.* C Greene Ed., Elsevier: 722–736.

TSH—See Thyrotropin

TULATHROMYCIN

(too-*la*-throe-*mye*-sin)   Draxxin®

INJECTABLE MACROLIDE ANTIBIOTIC

Prescriber Highlights

▶ Injectable macrolide antibiotic for cattle & swine

▶ Very long tissue half-lives; one dose treatment

▶ Not for lactating dairy cattle or veal calves

▶ Local injection site reactions most likely adverse effect

Uses/Indications

In beef and non-lactating dairy cattle, tulathromycin is indicated for the treatment of bovine respiratory disease (BRD) associated with *Mannheimia haemolytica*, *Pasteurella multocida*,

Histophilus somni (*Haemophilus somnus*) and *Mycoplasma bovis*; and for the control of respiratory disease in cattle at high risk of developing BRD, associated with *Mannheimia haemolytica*, *Pasteurella multocida* and *Histophilus somni* (*Haemophilus somnus*). It is also FDA-approved for the treatment of bovine foot rot (interdigital necrobacillosis) associated with *Fusobacterium necrophorum* and *Porphyromonas levii* and for the treatment of infectious bovine keratoconjunctivitis (IBK) associated With *Moraxella bovis*.

In swine, tulathromycin is indicated for the treatment of swine respiratory disease (SRD) associated with *Actinobacillus pleuropneumoniae*, *Pasteurella multocida*, *Bordetella bronchiseptica*, *Haemophilus parasuis*, and *Mycoplasma hyopneumoniae*.

Tulathromycin may prove useful as a treatment of *Rhodococcus equi* infections in foals and in treating various infections in small ruminants.

Pharmacology/Actions

While tulathromycin is a macrolide antibiotic such as erythromycin or azithromycin, it is structurally unique in that it has three amine groups (tribasic), while erythromycin and azithromycin have one (monobasic) and two (dibasic) groups, respectively. The tribasic group of compounds are called triamilide macrolides.

It is believed that tulathromycin's tribasic structure allows it to better penetrate gram-negative pathogenic bacteria and its low affinity for bacterial efflux pumps may allow the drug to remain and accumulate within the bacteria.

The mechanism of action of tulathromycin is similar to other macrolides in that it inhibits protein synthesis by penetrating the cell wall and binding to the 50S ribosomal subunits in susceptible bacteria. It is considered a bacteriostatic antibiotic, but it possesses some bactericidal activity as well, particularly for *Mannheimia haemolytica* and *Pasteurella multocida*.

Tulathromycin's efficacy is probably enhanced by its ability to accumulate and be released by host phagocytic cells. Neither time-dependent nor concentration-dependent models may accurately predict or describe the drug's efficacy. Some modern macrolides (*e.g.*, azithromycin) efficacy may be more predictive by assessing the total drug exposure to the pathogen; the AUC:MIC ratio may be helpful.

Bacterial isolates susceptible to tulathromycin at concentrations of 16 micrograms/mL or less are reported as susceptible to tulathromycin. The MIC_{90} values reported for *M. haemolytica* and *P. multocida* in cattle with BRD are 2 micrograms/mL and 1 microgram/mL, respectively. To date, resistance development to tulathromycin has not been a major problem.

Pharmacokinetics

In feeder calves given 2.5 mg/kg SC (in the neck), tulathromycin is rapidly and nearly completely absorbed (bioavailability >90%). Peak plasma concentrations generally occur within 15 minutes after dosing. Volume of distribution is very large (approximately 11 L/kg) and total systemic clearance is approximately 170 mL/hr/kg. This extensive volume of distribution is largely responsible for the long elimination half-life of this compound. In plasma, elimination half life is approximately 2.75 days, but in lung tissue it is about 8.75 days. Tulathromycin is eliminated from the body primarily unchanged via biliary excretion.

Following intramuscular administration to feeder pigs at a dosage of 2.5 mg/kg, tulathromycin is readily and rapidly absorbed (bioavailability 88%) with peak levels occurring in about 15 minutes. Tulathromycin rapidly distributes into body tissues, and the volume of distribution is 13–15 L/kg. Plasma half-life is approximately 60–90 hours, but lung tissue half life is about 5.9 days. Tulathromycin is eliminated from the body primarily unchanged via the feces and urine.

Contraindications/Precautions/Warnings

Tulathromycin is contraindicated in animals with a prior hypersensitivity reaction to the drug.

Cattle intended for human consumption must not be slaughtered within 18 days from the last treatment. Do not use in female dairy cattle 20 months of age or older. A withdrawal period has not been established for this product in pre-ruminating calves. Do not use in calves to be processed for veal.

Swine intended for human consumption must not be slaughtered within 5 days from the last treatment.

Adverse Effects

At labeled doses, adverse effects appear to be minimal in cattle and swine. Transient hypersalivation has been reported and one feeder calf in field studies developed transient dyspnea. Injection site reactions are most commonly reported and there have been some reports to the FDA's Adverse Drug Reporting database of anorexia in cattle.

Hypersensitivity reactions are possible, but no reports were located.

Subcutaneous or intramuscular injection can cause a transient local tissue reaction that may result in trim loss at slaughter.

Reproductive/Nursing Safety

Reproductive safety is not known, the product is labeled: "The effects of *Draxxin*® on bovine (and porcine) reproductive performance, pregnancy and lactation have not been determined.

Overdosage/Acute Toxicity

In cattle (feeder calves), single subcutaneous doses of up to 25 mg/kg caused transient indications of pain at the injection, including head shaking and pawing at the ground. Injection site swelling, discoloration of the subcutaneous tissues at the injection site and corresponding histopathologic changes were seen in animals in all dosage groups.

In swine, single IM doses of up to 25 mg/kg caused transient indications of pain at the injection site, restlessness, and excessive vocalization. Tremors occurred briefly in one animal receiving 7.5 mg/kg BW.

No systemic treatment for single overdoses should be necessary, localized treatment at the injection site (*e.g.*, ice pack) to reduce swelling and pain as well as FDA-approved analgesic medications can be considered.

Drug Interactions

■ No drug interactions are noted in the manufacturer's label and none could be found in other references for tulathromycin.

Laboratory Considerations

■ No concerns were noted

Doses

■ **CATTLE:**

For labeled indications:

a) Inject subcutaneously as a single dose in the neck at a dosage of 2.5 mg/kg (1.1 mL/100 lb) body weight (BW). Do not inject more than 10 mL per injection site. (Label directions; *Draxxin*®—Pfizer)

■ **SWINE:**

For labeled indications:

a) Inject intramuscularly as a single dose in the neck at a dosage of 2.5 mg/kg (0.25 mL/22 lb) BW. Do not inject more than 2.5 mL per injection site. (Label directions; *Draxxin*®—Pfizer)

■ **HORSES:**

a) For foals with *R. equi*: Anecdotally, 2.5 mg/kg IM every 5–7 days has been used successfully in milder clinical cases. (Divers 2009)

Monitoring

■ Clinical efficacy

Client Information

■ Follow dosing guidelines exactly; adhere to withdrawal times

■ Not for female dairy cattle (20 months or older) or veal calves

■ Cattle are dosed subcutaneously in the neck, not more than 10 mL per injection site

■ Swine are dosed intramuscularly in the neck, not more than 2.5 mL per injection site

Chemistry/Synonyms

Tulathromycin is a semi-synthetic macrolide antibiotic of the subclass triamilide. It occurs as white to of-white-crystalline powder that is readily soluble in water at pH<8. At a pH of 7.4 (physiological pH), tulathromycin (a weak base) is approximately 50 times more soluble in hydrophilic than hydrophobic media.

The commercially available injection contains 100 mg/mL of tulathromycin in an equilibrated mixture of the two isomeric forms of tulathromycin in a 9:1 ratio. The injectable vehicle consists of 50% propylene glycol, monothioglycerol (5 mg/mL); citric and hydrochloric acids are added to adjust pH. It has a relatively low viscosity.

Tulathromycin may also be known as tulathromycine, tulathromycinum, CP-472295 (component A), CP-547272 (component B), or *Draxxin®*.

Storage/Stability

Tulathromycin injection should be stored at, or below 25°C (77°F). The product is stable at room temperature for up to 36 months.

Dosage Forms/Regulatory Status

VETERINARY-LABELED PRODUCTS:

Tulathromycin Injection 100 mg/mL in 50, 100, 250, & 500 mL vials: *Draxxin®* (Pfizer); FDA-approved for use in cattle and swine. Cattle intended for human consumption must not be slaughtered within 18 days from the last treatment. Do not use in female dairy cattle 20 months of age or older. A withdrawal period has not been established for this product in pre-ruminating calves. Do not use in calves to be processed for veal.

Swine intended for human consumption must not be slaughtered within 5 days from the last treatment.

HUMAN-LABELED PRODUCTS: None

References

Divers, T.J. (2009). Diagnosing, treating and preventing Rhodococcus equi. Proceedings: WVC. Accessed via: Veterinary Information Network. http://goo.gl/rGGeM

TYLOSIN

(**tye**-loe-sin)   Tylan®

MACROLIDE ANTIBIOTIC

Prescriber Highlights

▶ Macrolide antibiotic related to erythromycin, used primarily in cattle & swine; sometimes used orally in cats/dogs for chronic colitis; has been used anecdotally in cats as an immunomodulating agent for treating FIP

▶ Contraindications: hypersensitivity to it or other macrolide antibiotics; probably contraindicated in horses

▶ Adverse Effects: Pain & local reactions after IM injection, GI upset (anorexia, & diarrhea). May cause severe diarrheas if administered PO to ruminants or by any route to horses. *Swine:* edema of rectal mucosa & mild anal protrusion with pruritus, erythema, & diarrhea

Uses/Indications

Although the injectable form of tylosin is FDA-approved for use in dogs and cats, it is rarely used parenterally in those species. Oral tylosin is sometimes recommended for the treatment of chronic colitis in small animals (see Doses). A double-blinded prospective study, comparing tylosin to placebo in dogs with a history of chronic diarrhea that was thought to be responsive to tylosin in the past, showed that 85% dogs receiving tylosin had perceived normal fecal consistency versus 29% of those receiving placebo (Kilpienn *et al.* 2009). Tylosin has been used has been used anecdotally in cats as an immunomodulating agent for treating FIP. In dogs, tylosin has been used orally to treat tear staining (epiphora).

Tylosin is also used clinically in cattle and swine for infections caused by susceptible organisms.

Pharmacology/Actions

Tylosin is thought to have the same mechanism of action as erythromycin (binds to 50S ribosome and inhibits protein synthesis) and exhibits a similar spectrum of activity. It is a bacteriostatic antibiotic. Tylosin may also have immunomodulatory effects on cell-mediated immunity. In dogs, tylosin increases concentrations of enterococci (*Enterococcus fecalis*) in the jejunum. Enterococci are thought to have probiotic effects.

For more specific information on organisms where tylosin is usually active, refer to the erythromycin monograph; cross-resistance with erythromycin occurs.

Pharmacokinetics

Tylosin tartrate is well absorbed from the GI tract, primarily from the intestine. The phosphate salt is less well absorbed after oral administration. Tylosin base injected SC or IM is reportedly rapidly absorbed.

Like erythromycin, tylosin is well distributed in the body after systemic absorption, with the exception of penetration into the CSF. The volume of distribution of tylosin is reportedly 1.7 L/kg in small animals and 1–2.3 L/kg in cattle. In lactating dairy cattle, the milk to plasma ratio is reported to be between 1–5.4.

Tylosin is eliminated in the urine and bile apparently as unchanged drug. The elimination half-life of tylosin is reportedly 54 minutes in small animals, 139 minutes in newborn calves, and 64 minutes in calves 2 months of age or older.

Contraindications/Precautions/Warnings

Tylosin is contraindicated in patients hypersensitive to it or other macrolide antibiotics (*e.g.*, erythromycin). Most clinicians feel that tylosin is contraindicated in horses, as severe and sometimes fatal diarrheas may result from its use in that species.

Adverse Effects

Most likely adverse effects with tylosin are pain and local reactions at intramuscular injection sites, and mild GI upset (anorexia and diarrhea). Tylosin may induce severe diarrheas if administered orally to ruminants or by any route to horses. In swine, adverse effects reported include edema of rectal mucosa and mild anal protrusion with pruritus, erythema, and diarrhea.

Reproductive/Nursing Safety

In a system evaluating the safety of drugs in canine and feline pregnancy (Papich 1989), this drug is categorized as in class: *B (Safe for use if used cautiously. Studies in laboratory animals may have uncovered some risk, but these drugs appear to be safe in dogs and cats or these drugs are safe if they are not administered when the animal is near term.)*

Overdosage/Acute Toxicity

Tylosin is relatively safe in most overdose situations. The LD_{50} in pigs is greater than 5 grams/kg orally, and approximately 1 gram/kg IM. Dogs are reported to tolerate oral doses of 800 mg/kg. Long-term (2 year) oral administration of up to 400 mg/kg produced no organ toxicity in dogs. Shock and death have been reported in baby pigs overdosed with tylosin, however.

Drug Interactions

Drug interactions with tylosin have not been well documented. It has been suggested that tylosin may increase **digoxin** blood levels with resultant toxicity. It is suggested to refer to the erythromycin monograph for more information on potential interactions.

Laboratory Considerations

■ Macrolide antibiotics may cause falsely elevated values of **AST** (SGOT), and **ALT** (SGPT) when using colorimetric assays.

■ Fluorometric determinations of **urinary catecholamines** can be altered by concomitant macrolide administration.

Doses

■ **DOGS:**

When using *Tylan® Soluble* (100 grams per bottle) powder: Using volumetric containers to measure powders is not necessarily accurate, but 1 level teaspoonful (5 mL) of powder contains approximately 2.5–2.7 grams of tylosin; ⅛th of a teaspoonful contains approximately 325 mg tylosin.

a) For small intestinal bacterial overgrowth: 10–20 mg/kg PO q12h; recommended for chronic cases, may require therapy for as long as 6 weeks. (Ludlow & Davenport 2000)

b) For adjunctive treatment of IBD: 10 mg/kg PO three times daily. Therapeutic trial for 21 days to evaluate efficacy. (Simpson 2003)

c) For clostridial colitis: 10–40 mg/kg PO twice daily. Practically (using the wettable powder): 1/16th of teaspoon 2–3 times daily for dogs (<7kg); ⅛th of a teaspoon 2–3 times a day for medium dogs (7–15 kg); and ¼ teaspoon 2–3 times a day for larger dogs (>15 kg). Mix with food to hide unpleasant taste or put into capsules. Animals with chronic clostridial colitis can often be controlled with one treatment every 2–3 days. (Willard 2006)

d) For IBD and antibiotic responsive diarrhea: 20–40 mg/kg PO q12h (Marks 2007)

e) 25 mg/kg PO once daily (in the study dogs were treated for 7 days, but the authors state that in dogs with tylosin-responsive diarrhea the stool remains normal as long as treatment continues, but diarrhea reappears within weeks after discontinuation). (Kilpienn *et al.* 2009)

■ **CATS:**

When using *Tylan® Soluble* (100 grams per bottle) powder: Using volumetric containers to measure powders is not necessarily accurate, but 1 level teaspoonful (5 mL) of powder contains approximately 2.5–2.7 grams of tylosin; ⅛th of a teaspoonful contains approximately 325 mg tylosin.

a) For adjunctive treatment of IBD: 10 mg/kg PO three times daily. Therapeutic trial for 21 days to evaluate efficacy. (Simpson 2003)

b) For treatment of IBD or diarrheas caused by *C. perfringens*: 20–40 mg/kg PO twice daily (Marks 2002)

c) For IBD: 40 mg/kg PO q12h (Zoran 2007)

d) For clostridial colitis: 10–40 mg/kg PO twice daily. Practically (using the wettable powder): 1/16th of teaspoon 2–3 times daily. Mix with food to hide unpleasant taste or put into capsules. Animals with chronic clostridial colitis can often be controlled with one treatment every 2–3 days. (Willard 2006)

■ **FERRETS:**

For susceptible infections:

a) 10 mg/kg PO once to twice daily (Williams 2000)

■ **RABBITS, RODENTS, SMALL MAMMALS:**

a) **Rabbits:** 10 mg/kg PO, SC, IM q12–24h (Ivey & Morrisey 2000)

b) **Gerbils, Hamsters, Rats:** 10 mg/kg SC q24h (Adamcak & Otten 2000)(

■ **CATTLE:**

For susceptible infections:

a) 17.6 mg/kg IM once daily. Continue treatment for 24 hours after symptoms have stopped, not to exceed 5 days. Do not inject more than 10 mL per site. Use the 50 mg/mL formulation in calves weighing less than 200 pounds. (Package insert; *Tylosin® Injection*—TechAmerica)

b) For bronchopneumonia and fibrinous pneumonia in cattle associated with penicillin G-refractory *C. pyogenes* infections or other bacteria sensitive to tylosin and resistant to sulfas, penicillin G and tetracyclines: using Tylosin 200 mg/mL: 44 mg/kg IM q24h. Recommend a 21-day slaughter withdrawal at this dosage. (Hjerpe 1986)

c) 5–10 mg/kg IM or slow IV once daily; not to exceed 5 days (Huber 1988)

d) Tylosin base injectable: 10 mg/kg IM initially, then 6 mg/kg IM q8h (q8–12h in calves) (Baggot 1983)

■ **SWINE:**

For susceptible infections:

a) 8.8 mg/kg IM twice daily. Continue treatment for 24 hours after symptoms have stopped, not to exceed 3 days. Do not inject more than 5 mL per site. (Package insert; *Tylosin® Injection*—TechAmerica)

b) 5–10 mg/kg until 24 hours after remission of disease signs; not to exceed 3 days therapy (Huber 1988)

c) Tylosin base injectable: 12.5 mg/kg IM q12h (Baggot 1983)

■ **SHEEP & GOATS:**

For susceptible infections:

a) 10 mg/kg, treatment not to exceed 5 days (Huber 1988)

■ **BIRDS:**

For susceptible infections:

a) For initial therapy in caged birds for upper respiratory infections (especially if mycoplasma suspected).

Using 200 mg/mL injectable: 40 mg/kg IM. Used in combination with aminoglycosides. (McDonald 1989)

b) For initial therapy of upper respiratory infections and air sacculitis. Using 50 mg/mL or 200 mg/mL injectable: 10–40 mg/kg IM twice daily or three times daily (Clubb 1986)

c) 30 mg/kg IM q12h (Hoeffer 1995)

■ **REPTILES:**

For susceptible infections:

a) For tortoises: 5 mg/kg IM once daily for at least 10 days. Used primarily for chronic respiratory infections or when Mycoplasma is suspected (Gauvin 1993)

b) All species: 5 mg/kg IM once daily (Jacobson 1999)

Monitoring

■ Clinical efficacy

■ Adverse effects

Client Information

■ Follow veterinarians dosage recommendations carefully

■ Tylosin powder in food can be very unpalatable. Placing the proper dose in a gelatin capsule and dosing may be preferable to mixing in food. Another suggestion for dogs or cats that absolutely won't eat food that has tylosin in it is to: Melt approximately ¼ teaspoon of butter and place in one of the compartments in a mini-ice tray. Add the proper dose of tylosin powder, mix well and freeze. (**Note:** Stability information for this procedure has not been performed).

■ When administered orally to small animals, tylosin is usually very well tolerated, but contact veterinarian if adverse effects are seen.

Chemistry/Synonyms

A macrolide antibiotic related structurally to erythromycin, tylosin is produced from *Streptomyces fradiae*. It occurs as an almost white to buff-colored powder with a pK_a of 7.1. It is slightly soluble in water and soluble in alcohol. Tylosin is considered highly lipid soluble. The tartrate salt is soluble in water. The injectable form of the drug (as the base) is in a 50% propylene glycol solution.

Tylosin may also be known as Desmycosin, tilosina, tylozin, tylosiini, tylosinum, tylozyna or *Tylan®*.

Storage/Stability

Unless otherwise instructed by the manufacturer, injectable tylosin should be stored in well-closed containers at room temperature. Tylosin, like erythromycin, is unstable in acidic (pH <4) media. It is not recommended to mix the parenteral injection with other drugs.

Compatibility/Compounding Considerations

Because converting volume measurements into weights is not very accurate for powders, it is recommended to actually weigh powders when using them for pharmaceutical purposes. However, if this is not possible, one (1) level teaspoon (5 mL) of commercially-available tylosin tartrate (*Tylan® Soluble*) contains approximately 2.5–2.7 grams of tylosin; ⅛th of a teaspoonful contains approximately 325 mg tylosin.

Tylan tartrate powder added to food can be very unpalatable for dogs or cats. Placing the proper dose in a gelatin capsule and dosing may be preferable to mixing in food. Another suggestion for dogs or cats that absolutely won't eat food that has tylosin in it is to: Melt approximately ¼ teaspoon of butter and place in one of the compartments in a mini-ice tray. Add the proper dose of tylosin powder, mix well and freeze. (**Note:** Stability information for this procedure has not been performed).

Dosage Forms/Regulatory Status

VETERINARY-LABELED PRODUCTS:

Note: The product *Tylan® Plus Vitamins* was used extensively orally in companion animals, but has been withdrawn from the market.

Tylan® Soluble may be substituted, but is significantly more concentrated than *Tylan® Plus Vitamins* and dosage sizes (teaspoons are not equivalent) will be different.

Tylosin Injection: 50 mg/mL, 200 mg/mL; *Tylan®* (Elanco); generic; (OTC). FDA-approved for use in nonlactating dairy cattle, beef cattle, swine, dogs, and cats. Slaughter withdrawal (at labeled doses): cattle = 21 days; swine = 14 days. **Note:** Although this author (Plumb) was unable to locate parenteral products FDA-approved for use in lactating dairy animals, one source (Huber 1988a) states that tylosin has a 72 hour milk withdrawal for dairy cattle, and 48 hour milk withdrawal in dairy goats and sheep. Contact FARAD for more information before using in lactating dairy animals.

Tylosin Tartrate Powder: (approximately 2.5–2.7 grams/level teaspoonful) in 100 gram bottles; *Tylan® Soluble* (Elanco); (OTC). FDA-approved for use in turkeys (not layers), chickens (not layers) and swine. Slaughter withdrawal swine = 2 days; chickens = 1 day; turkeys = 5 days.

There are many FDA-approved tylosin products for addition to feed or water for use in beef cattle, swine, and poultry. Many of these products have other active ingredients included in their formulations.

HUMAN-LABELED PRODUCTS: None.

References

Adamcak, A. & B. Otten (2000). Rodent Therapeutics. *Vet Clin NA: Exotic Anim Pract* **3:**1(Jan): 221–240.

Baggot, J.D. (1983). Systemic antimicrobial therapy in large animals. *Pharmacological Basis of Large Animal Medicine*. JA Bogan, P Lees and AT Yoxall Eds. Oxford, Blackwell Scientific Publications: 45–69.

Clubb, S.L. (1986). Therapeutics: Individual and Flock Treatment Regimens. *Clinical Avian Medicine and Surgery*. GJ Harrison and LR Harrison Eds. Philadelphia, W.B. Saunders: 327–355.

Gauvin, J. (1993). Drug therapy in reptiles. *Seminars in Avian & Exotic Med* 2(1): 48–59.

Hjerpe, C.A. (1986). The bovine respiratory disease complex. *Current Veterinary Therapy: Food Animal Practice 2*. JL Howard Ed. Philadelphia, W.B. Saunders: 670–681.

Hoeffer, H. (1995). Antimicrobials in pet birds. *Kirk's Current Veterinary Therapy:XII*. J Bonagura Ed. Philadelphia, W.B. Saunders: 1278–1283.

Huber, W.G. (1988). Aminoglycosides, Macrolides, Lincosamides, Polymyxins, Chloramphenicol, and other Antibacterial Drugs. *Veterinary Pharmacology and Therapeutics*. NH Booth and LE McDonald Eds. Ames, Iowa State University Press: 822–849.

Ivey, E. & J. Morrisey (2000). Therapeutics for Rabbits. *Vet Clin NA: Exotic Anim Pract* **3:**1(Jan): 183–216.

Jacobson, E. (1999). Bacterial infections and antimicrobial treatment in reptiles. The North American Veterinary Conference, Orlando.

Kilpienn, S., T. Spillman, et al. (2009). Effect of Tylosin on Dogs with Diarrhea: A Placebo-Controlled, Randomized, Double-Blinded, Prospective Clinical Trial. Proceedings: ECVIM. Accessed via: Veterinary Information Network. http://goo.gl/aawdt

Ludlow, C. & D. Davenport (2000). Small Intestinal Bacterial Overgrowth. *Kirk's Current Veterinary Therapy: XIII Small Animal Practice*. J Bonagura Ed. Philadelphia, WB Saunders: 637–641.

Marks, S. (2002). Diagnostic and therapeutic approach to the cat with chronic diarrhea. Proceedings: World Small Anim Assoc World Congress. Accessed via: Veterinary Information Network. http://goo.gl/X48gF

Marks, S. (2007). Inflammatory Bowel Disease—More than a garbage can diagnosis. Proceedings: UCD Canine Medicine Symposium. Accessed via: Veterinary Information Network. http://goo.gl/ZGPg1

McDonald, S.E. (1989). Summary of medications for use in psittacine birds. *JAAV* **3**(3): 120–127.

Papich, M. (1989). Effects of drugs on pregnancy. *Current Veterinary Therapy X: Small Animal Practice*. R Kirk Ed. Philadelphia, Saunders: 1291–1299.

Simpson, K. (2003). Chronic enteropathies: How should I treat them. Proceedings: ACVIM Forum. Accessed via: Veterinary Information Network. http://goo.gl/nicNM

Willard, M. (2006). Chronic Diarrhea: Part 2. Proceedings: ACVC. Accessed via: Veterinary Information Network. http://goo.gl/LXXZ0

Williams, B. (2000). Therapeutics in Ferrets. *Vet Clin NA: Exotic Anim Pract* **3:**1(Jan): 131–153.

Zoran, D. (2007). Diarrhea in kittens and cats: What can you do? Proceedings; Western Vet Conf. Accessed via: Veterinary Information Network. http://goo.gl/oC0Qg

URSODIOL

(ur-soe-*dye*-ole)
Actigall®, Ursodeoxycholic acid

BILE ACID

Prescriber Highlights

▶ Bile acid that may be useful for adjunctive treatment of hepatobiliary disease in dogs/cats. May also be used for cholesterol containing gallstones

▶ Contraindications: Rabbits & other hindgut fermenters. Caution: Complications associated with gallstones (e.g., biliary obstruction, biliary fistulas, cholecystitis, pancreatitis, cholangitis)

▶ Adverse Effects: Appears to be well tolerated in dogs/cats

Uses/Indications

In small animals, ursodiol may be useful as adjunctive therapy for the medical management of cholesterol-containing gallstones and/or in patients with chronic liver disease, particularly where cholestasis (bile toxicity) plays an important role. Ursodiol's benefit in treating canine or feline hepatobiliary disease is unknown at the time of writing (studies are ongoing), but it may be of help in slowing the progression of inflammatory hepatic disorders, particularly autoimmune hepatitis and acute hepatotoxicity.

Pharmacology/Actions

After oral administration, ursodiol suppresses hepatic synthesis and secretion of cholesterol. Ursodiol also decreases intestinal absorption of cholesterol. By reducing cholesterol saturation in the bile, it is thought that ursodiol allows solubilization of cholesterol-containing gallstones. Ursodiol also increases bile flow and in patients with chronic liver disease, it apparently reduces the hepatocyte toxic effects of bile salts by decreasing their detergent action, and may protect hepatic cells from toxic bile acids (*e.g.*, lithocholate, deoxycholate, and chenodeoxycholate).

Pharmacokinetics

Ursodiol is well absorbed from the small intestine after oral administration. In humans, up to 90% of dose is absorbed. After absorption, it enters the portal circulation. In the liver, it is extracted and combined (conjugated) with either taurine or glycine and secreted into the bile. Only very small quantities enter the systemic circulation and very little is detected in the urine. After each entero-hepatic cycle, some quantity of conjugated and free drug undergoes bacterial degradation; eventually most of the drug is eliminated in the feces after being oxidized or reduced to less soluble compounds. Ursodiol detected in the systemic circulation is highly bound to plasma proteins.

Contraindications/Precautions/Warnings

Ursodiol is contraindicated in rabbits and other hindgut fermenters as it is converted into lithocholic acid (toxic). Patients sensitive to other bile acid products may also be sensitive to ursodiol. The benefits of using ursodiol should be weighed against its risks in patients with complications associated with gallstones (*e.g.*, biliary obstruction, biliary fistulas, cholecystitis, pancreatitis, cholangitis). While ursodiol may be useful in treating patients with chronic liver disease, some patients may experience further impairment of bile acid metabolism.

Adverse Effects

While ursodiol use in animals has been limited, it appears to be well tolerated in dogs and cats. Although hepatotoxicity has not been associated with ursodiol therapy, some human patients have an inability to sulfate lithocholic acid (a naturally occurring bile acid and also a metabolite of ursodiol). Lithocholic acid is a known hepatotoxin; veterinary significance is unclear. Diarrhea and other GI effects have rarely been noted in humans taking ursodiol. Ursodiol will not dissolve calcified radiopaque stones or radiolucent bile pigment stones.

Reproductive/Nursing Safety

In humans, the FDA categorizes this drug as category ***B*** for use during pregnancy (*Animal studies have not yet demonstrated risk to the fetus, but there are no adequate studies in pregnant women; or animal studies have shown an adverse effect, but adequate studies in pregnant women have not demonstrated a risk to the fetus in the first trimester of pregnancy, and there is no evidence of risk in later trimesters.*)

It is not known whether ursodiol is excreted in breast milk.

Overdosage/Acute Toxicity

Overdosage of ursodiol would most likely cause diarrhea. Treatment, if required, could include supportive therapy; oral administration of an aluminum-containing antacid (*e.g.*, aluminum hydroxide suspension); gastric emptying (if large overdose) with concurrent administration of activated charcoal or cholestyramine suspension.

Drug Interactions

The following drug interactions have either been reported or are theoretical in humans or animals receiving ursodiol and may be of significance in veterinary patients:

- ■ **ALUMINUM-CONTAINING ANTACIDS:** May bind to ursodiol, thereby reducing its efficacy

- ■ **CHOLESTYRAMINE RESIN:** May bind to ursodiol, thereby reducing its efficacy

- ■ **TAURINE:** Although not documented, concern has been raised that chronic administration of ursodiol in cats may lead to taurine deficiency.

Laboratory Considerations

- ■ As ursodiol is detected by many **serum bile acid** tests, bile acids may remain falsely elevated. One study in normal dogs did not show any effects. However if possible, stop ursodiol for 2-3 days before running test.

Doses

■ **DOGS:**

For adjunctive treatment of chronic hepatitis:

a) 5–15 mg/kg PO divided q12h, with immunosuppressive therapy. (**Note:** Use of this drug at this dose is preliminary, but promising) (Johnson & Sherding 1994)

b) 10–15 mg/kg PO once daily. Little work has yet been done in dogs and cats, but at 10 mg/kg it is safe and potentially beneficial in cases of cholestatic liver disease, cholangitis/cholangiohepatitis, chronic hepatitis, and copper-associated hepatopathy. (Webb & Twedt 2008)

c) For use in chronic active hepatitis, fibrosis and cirrhosis. May use as primary or adjunctive therapy. Dose: 11–15.4 mg/kg PO either once daily or divided twice daily (Tams 2000)

■ **CATS:**

For adjunctive treatment of chronic hepatitis:

a) 10–15 mg/kg PO once daily. Little work has yet been done in dogs and cats, but at 10 mg/kg it is safe and potentially beneficial in cases of cholestatic liver disease, cholangitis/cholangiohepatitis, chronic hepatitis, and copper-associated hepatopathy. (Webb & Twedt 2008)

b) For use in chronic active hepatitis, fibrosis, and cirrhosis. May use as primary or adjunctive therapy. Dose: 11–15.4 mg/kg PO either once daily or divided twice daily. Cats usually get 1/6th of a capsule mixed with a small amount of food. Cats may still eat their food even if drug is sprinkled on top. (Tams 2000)

c) 10 mg/kg/day PO (Zoran 2006)

■ **BIRDS:**

For adjunctive treatment of liver disease:

a) 10–15 mg/kg PO once daily. (Oglesbee 2009)

Monitoring

■ Efficacy (ultrasonography for gallstones; improved liver function tests for chronic hepatic disease)

■ Monitoring of SGPT/SGOT (AST/ALT) on a routine basis (in humans these tests are recommended to be performed at the initiation of therapy and at 1 and 3 months after starting therapy; then every 6 months).

Client Information

■ Because ursodiol dissolves more rapidly in the presence of bile or pancreatic juice, it should be given with food.

Chemistry/Synonyms

A naturally occurring bile acid, ursodiol, also known as ursodeoxycholic acid has a molecular weight of 392.6.

Ursodiol may also be known as: acidum ursodeoxycholicum, UDCA, ursodesoxycholic acid; many trade names are available, including *Actigall*®.

Storage/Stability

Unless otherwise specified by the manufacturer, ursodiol capsules should be stored at room temperature (15–30°C) in tight containers.

Dosage Forms/Regulatory Status

VETERINARY-LABELED PRODUCTS: None

HUMAN-LABELED PRODUCTS:

Ursodiol Oral Capsules: 300 mg; *Actigall*® & generic (Watson); (Rx)

Ursodiol Oral Tablets: 250 mg & 500 mg; *URSO® 250* & *-Forte* (Axcan Scandipharm); generic; (Rx)

References

Johnson, S. & R. Sherding (1994). Diseases of the liver and biliary tract. *Saunders Manual of Small Animal Practice*. S Birchard and R Sherding Eds. Philadelphia, W.B. Saunders Company: 722–760.

Oglesbee, B. (2009). Liver disease in pet birds. Proceedings: WVC. Accessed via: Veterinary Information Network. http://goo.gl/6wL9s

Tams, T. (2000). Diagnosis and Management of Liver Disease in Dogs. Proceedings: American Animal Hospital Association 67th Annual Meeting, Toronto.

Webb, C. & D. Twedt (2008). Oxidative Stress and Liver Disease. *Vet Clin Small Anim* **38**: 125–135.

Zoran, D. (2006). Inflammatory liver disease in cats. Proceedings: ABVP 2006. Accessed via: Veterinary Information Network. http://goo.gl/lFyUT

VALPROIC ACID
VALPROATE SODIUM
DIVALPROEX SODIUM

(*val*-proe-*ik*; val-*proe*-ayte; die-*val*-proe-ex)

Depakene®, Depakote®, Depacon®

Prescriber Highlights

▶ 2nd to 4th line anticonvulsant that may be useful as adjunctive treatment in some dogs; most do not recommend its use in veterinary patients

▶ Contraindications: Significant hepatic disease or dysfunction, previous hypersensitivity

▶ Caution: Thrombocytopenia or altered platelet aggregation function

▶ Adverse Effects: GI effects (may be diminished by giving with food) most likely; hepatotoxicity, CNS (sedation, ataxia, behavioral changes, etc.), dermatologic reactions, (alopecia, rash, etc.), hematologic reactions, (thrombocytopenia, reduced platelet aggregation, leukopenias, anemias, etc.), pancreatitis, & edema are possible

▶ May be teratogenic

Uses/Indications

Because of its cost, apparent unfavorable pharmacokinetic profile, and potential hepatotoxicity, valproic acid must be considered at best, a third or fourth line drug in the treatment of seizures in the dog. Some clinicians feel it is of benefit when added to phenobarbital in patients not adequately controlled with that drug alone. Additionally, it is less protein bound in dogs than in humans, so the human serum therapeutic range of the drug (40–100 micrograms/mL) may be too high in dogs. The drug (free form) actually may concentrate in the CSF, and anticonvulsant effects may persist even after valproate levels are non-detectable in CSF, lending to the idea that serum levels do not accurately reflect clinical efficacy. Clearly, additional studies are needed to determine the clinical role, if any, for this drug.

Pharmacology/Actions

The mechanism of the anticonvulsant activity of valproic acid is not understood. Animal studies have demonstrated that valproic acid inhibits GABA transferase and succinic aldehyde dehydrogenase causing increased CNS levels of GABA. Additionally, one study has demonstrated that valproic acid inhibits neuronal activity by increasing potassium conductance.

Pharmacokinetics

Sodium valproate is rapidly converted to valproic acid in the acidic environment of the stomach where it is rapidly absorbed from the GI tract. The bioavailability reported in dogs following oral administration is approximately 80%; peak levels occur in approximately 1-hour. Food may delay absorption, but does not alter the extent of it. Divalproex in its enteric-coated form has an approximately 1-hour delay in its oral absorption. Patients' who exhibit GI (nausea, vomiting) adverse effects may benefit from this dosage form.

Valproic acid is rapidly distributed throughout the extracellular water spaces and plasma. It is approximately 80–95% plasma protein bound in humans, and 78–80% plasma protein bound in dogs. CSF levels are approximately 10% those found in plasma. Milk levels are 1–10% those found in plasma; it readily crosses the placenta.

Valproic acid is metabolized in the liver and is conjugated with glucuronide. These metabolic conjugates are excreted in the urine; only very small amounts of unchanged drug are excreted in the urine. The elimination half-life in humans ranges from 5–20 hours; in dogs from 1.5–2.8 hours.

Contraindications/Precautions/Warnings

Valproic acid is contraindicated in patients with significant hepatic disease or dysfunction, or exhibiting previous hypersensitivity to the drug. It should be used with caution in patients with thrombocytopenia or altered platelet aggregation function.

Adverse Effects

Because of the limited experience with this agent, the following adverse effects may not be complete nor valid for dogs: Gastrointestinal effects consisting of nausea, vomiting, anorexia, and diarrhea are the most common adverse effects seen in people and also apparently,, in dogs. GI effects may be diminished by administration with food. Hepatotoxicity is the most serious potential adverse (human) reaction reported and must be considered for canine patients also. Dose related increases in liver enzymes may be seen and, rarely, hepatic failure and death may occur. In humans, incidences of hepatotoxicity are greater in very young (<2 yr. old) patients, those on other anticonvulsants, or with multiple congenital abnormalities.

Other potential adverse effects include: CNS (sedation, ataxia, behavioral changes, etc.), dermatologic (alopecia, rash, etc.), hematologic (thrombocytopenia, reduced platelet aggregation, leukopenias, anemias, etc.), pancreatitis, and edema.

Reproductive/Nursing Safety

A 1–2% incidence of neural tube defects in children born of mothers taking valproic acid during the first trimester of pregnancy has been reported. Use in pregnant dogs only when the benefits outweigh the risks of therapy. In humans, the FDA categorizes this drug as category **D** for use during pregnancy (*There is evidence of human fetal risk, but the potential benefits from the use of the drug in pregnant women may be acceptable despite its potential risks.*) In a separate system evaluating the safety of drugs in canine and feline pregnancy (Papich 1989), this drug is categorized as in class: **C** (*These drugs may have potential risks. Studies in people or laboratory animals have uncovered risks, and these drugs should be used cautiously as a last resort when the benefit of therapy clearly outweighs the risks.*)

Concentrations of valproic acid in maternal milk are 1–10% serum concentrations. It is unknown if this would have any detrimental effect on nursing offspring.

Overdosage/Acute Toxicity

There were 14 exposures to valproic acid/valproate reported to the ASPCA Animal Poison Control Center (APCC) during 2008–2009. In these cases 11 were dogs with 1 showing clinical signs and the remaining 3 reported cases were cats that showed no clinical signs. Common findings in dogs recorded in decreasing frequency included sedation.

Severe overdoses can cause profound CNS depression, asterixis, motor restlessness, hallucinations, and death. One human patient recovered after a serum level of 2000 micrograms/mL (20 times over therapeutic) was measured. Treatment consists of supportive measures and maintenance of adequate urine output is considered mandatory. Because the drug is rapidly absorbed, emesis or gastric lavage may be of limited value. Because of its delayed absorptive characteristics, the divalproex form may be removed by lavage or emesis if ingestion occurred recently. Naloxone is reported to be of benefit in reversing some of the CNS effects of valproic acid, but may also reverse the anticonvulsant properties of the drug.

Drug Interactions

The following drug interactions have either been reported or are theoretical in humans or animals receiving valproic acid and may be of significance in veterinary patients:

- ■ **ANTICOAGULANTS:** Valproic acid may have effects on platelet aggregation; use with caution with other drugs that affect coagulation status

- ■ **ASPIRIN:** Salicylates may displace valproic acid from plasma protein sites, thus increasing valproic acid levels

- ■ **CLONAZEPAM:** The sedative effects of clonazepam may be enhanced by valproic acid and the anticonvulsant efficacy of both may be diminished

- ■ **CNS DEPRESSANTS, OTHER:** VPA may enhance the CNS depressant effects of other CNS active drugs

- ■ **PHENOBARBITAL, PRIMIDONE:** Valproic acid may increase serum levels of phenobarbital and primidone

Laboratory Considerations

■ A keto-metabolite of valproic acid is excreted into the urine and may yield false positive **urine ketone** tests.

■ Altered **thyroid function tests** have been reported in humans with unknown clinical significance.

Doses

Note: Because of its very short half-life in dogs, most neurologists do not recommend using VPA in dogs.

■ **DOGS:**
    a) Add on therapy with phenobarbital or bromide: 60 mg/kg PO q8h (Thomas 2000)

Monitoring

■ Anticonvulsant efficacy

■ If used chronically, routine CBC's and liver enzymes at least every 6 months

Client Information

■ Compliance with therapy must be stressed to clients for successful epilepsy treatment. Encourage administering daily doses at same time each day, preferably with food.

■ Veterinarian should be contacted if animal develops significant adverse reactions (including clinical signs of anemia and/or liver disease) or if seizure control is unacceptable.

Chemistry/Synonyms

Structurally unrelated to other anticonvulsant agents; valproic acid, valproate sodium, divalproex sodium are derivatives of carboxylic acid. Valproic acid occurs as a colorless to pale yellow clear liquid. It is slightly viscous; has a characteristic odor, a pK$_a$ of 4.8, is slightly soluble in water and freely soluble in alcohol. It is also known as Dipropylacetic acid, DPA, 2-propylpentanoic acid, and 2-propylvaleric acid.

Valproate sodium occurs as a white, crystalline, saline tasting, very hygroscopic powder. It is very soluble in water or alcohol. The commercially available oral solution has a pH of 7–8.

Divalproex sodium is a stable compound in a 1:1 molar ratio of valproic acid and valproate sodium. It occurs as a white powder with a characteristic odor. It is insoluble in water and very soluble in alcohol.

Valproate sodium may also be known as: Abbott-44090, natrii valproas; many trade names are available.

Valproic acid may also be known as: Abbott-44089, acidum valproicum; many trade names are available.

Storage/Stability

Valproic acid capsules should be stored at room temperature (15–30°C) and in tight containers; avoid freezing. Valproate sodium oral solution should be stored at room temperature and in tight containers; avoid freezing. Divalproex sodium enteric-coated tablets should be stored at room temperature in tight, light resistant containers.

Dosage Forms/Regulatory Status

VETERINARY-LABELED PRODUCTS: None

HUMAN-LABELED PRODUCTS:

Valproic Acid Oral Capsules: 250 mg; *Depakene®* (Abbott); generic; (Rx)

Valproate Sodium Syrup: 250 mg/5 mL in 473 mL; *Depakene®* (Abbott); generic; (Rx)

Divalproex Sodium Delayed/Extended Release Tablets/Capsules: 125 mg, 250 mg, 500 mg; *Depakote®* & *Depakote ER®* (Abbott); *Stavzor®* (Noven); generic; (Rx)

Divalproex Sodium Oral Capsules (Sprinkle): 125 mg; *Depakote®* (Abbott); generic; (Rx)

Valproate Sodium Injection Concentrate: 100 mg/mL in 5 mL single-dose vials (may be preservative free); *Depacon®* (Abbott); generic; (Rx)

References

Papich, M. (1989). Effects of drugs on pregnancy. *Current Veterinary Therapy X: Small Animal Practice.* R Kirk Ed. Philadelphia, Saunders: 1291–1299.

Thomas, W. (2000). Idiopathic epilepsy in dogs. *Vet Clin NA: Small Anim Pract* **30:1**(Jan): 183–206.

VANADIUM
VANADYL SULFATE

(van-*aye*-dee-um; van-ah-*dil*)
Vanadyl Fuel®

TRACE METAL

Prescriber Highlights

▶ Trace metal "nutraceutical" that may be useful as an adjunctive treatment for diabetes mellitus in cats

▶ Efficacy questionable, but probably safe

Uses/Indications

Vanadium supplementation may be useful in the adjunctive treatment of diabetes mellitus, particularly in cats. There is controversy whether or not this treatment is beneficial.

Pharmacology/Actions

In humans with non-insulin dependent diabetes mellitus (NIDDM), vanadium can reduce fasting blood glucose and glycosylated hemoglobin levels, reduces hepatic glucose release, and increases peripheral glucose disposal and uptake into skeletal muscle mediated by insulin. Vanadium does not influence blood glucose levels in normal patients. While the exact mechanism of action of vanadium is unknown, it apparently inhibits protein tyrosine phosphatase (PTP). PTP is important in signal transduction and allows vanadium to act via both insulin-dependent and insulin-independent pathways.

Pharmacokinetics

Little information on the pharmacokinetics of vanadium was located. Only about 5% is absorbed from foodstuffs. *In vivo* it is converted to the vanadyl cation and forms complexes with ferritin and transferrin. Highest vanadium concentrations are found in the liver, bone and kidney. Vanadium is eliminated via renal routes. Effects on glucose in NIDDM humans may persist for weeks after discontinuation of therapy.

Contraindications/Precautions/Warnings

Vanadium supplements could potentially exacerbate renal insufficiency; use with caution in these patients.

Adverse Effects

Gastrointestinal effects have been reported in some cats receiving vanadium supplements; anorexia and vomiting is most commonly reported. It has been reported that cats initially unable to tolerate vanadium, can have therapy re-instituted without ill effect. Vanadium in high dosages may have renal toxic effects.

Reproductive/Nursing Safety

It is unknown if supplemental vanadium is safe in pregnancy.

Vanadium is unlikely to have negative effects in nursing kittens.

Overdosage/Acute Toxicity

Vanadyl sulfate may be mildly toxic. The oral LD_{50} in rats is 450 mg/kg. Consider gut removal protocols if an acute overdose occurs. Contact an animal poison control center for further guidance. Chronic overdoses may cause kidney damage.

Drug Interactions

■ No specific interactions of note were located. When used with other agents for diabetes management, effects may be additive.

Laboratory Considerations

■ No specific laboratory interactions or considerations were noted

Doses

Note: Because vanadium is given as a salt, do not confuse dosages for vanadium with vanadyl sulfate. Vanadyl sulfate reportedly contains 31% elemental vanadium, but labeled amounts of vanadium vary considerably.

■ **CATS:**

a) Using *Super Vanadyl Fuel*® (Twin Labs; also contains chromium): ½ capsule PO once daily with food. (Dowling 2000)

b) For adjunctive use in treating feline type 2 diabetes: Vanadium (**Note:** salt not specified, assume elemental vanadium) 0.2 mg/kg PO once daily in food or water. (Greco 2002)

c) For diabetes mellitus: Vanadyl sulfate 1 mg/kg PO once daily or vanadium 0.2 mg/kg PO once daily. (Wynn 2002)

d) For early NIDDM using *Vanadyl Fuel*® (Twin Labs; also contains chromium): One capsule PO once daily (q24h) (Melendez & Lorenz 2002)

Monitoring

■ As there is no reliable way to measure vanadium in the body, a clinical trial is the only way to determine whether vanadium is effective in helping to control blood glucose. Standard methods for monitoring efficacy of diabetes treatment should be followed (*e.g.*, fasting blood glucose, appetite, attitude, body condition, PU/PD resolution and, perhaps, serum fructosamine and/or glycosylated hemoglobin levels).

Client Information

■ Clients should give the medication only as prescribed and not change brands without their veterinarian's guidance

■ Give with food

Chemistry/Synonyms

A trace element, vanadium (V, atomic number 23) is usually given in the form of the inorganic salt, vanadyl sulfate. Vanadyl sulfate occurs as blue crystals and is very soluble in water. Vanadyl sulfate reportedly contains 31% elemental vanadium.

Vanadyl sulfate may also be known as: vanadium (IV) sulfate oxide; vanadium oxysulfate, oxo[sulfato(2-)-O]-vanadium, oxysulfato vanadium (IV); vanadyl (IV) sulfate, or vanadyl (IV)-sulfate hydrate.

Storage/Stability

While vanadyl sulfate is stable under ordinary conditions, refer to the label for each product used.

Dosage Forms/Regulatory Status

VETERINARY-LABELED PRODUCTS: None

HUMAN-LABELED PRODUCTS:

No oral products are FDA-approved as pharmaceuticals.

Oral vanadyl sulfate products are considered nutritional supplements by the FDA. No standards have been accepted for potency, purity, safety or efficacy by regulatory bodies.

Supplements are available from a wide variety of sources. Common products include 7.5 mg, and 10 mg tablets or 15 mg capsules. One proprietary product that has been used in cats is *Super Vanadyl Fuel*® (Twin Labs). This is a combination product that contains per capsule (among many other ingredients): 150 micrograms chromium (from chromium nicotinate and picolinate) and 1.25 mg of elemental vanadium (from BMOV [bi (maltolato) oxovanadium] and vanadyl sulfate). Bioequivalence between products cannot be assumed.

References

Dowling, P. (2000). Two transition metals show promise in treating diabetic cats. *Vet Med*(March): 190–192.

Greco, D. (2002). Feline Diabetes Mellitus II. Proceedings

Western Vet Conf. Accessed via: Veterinary Information Network. http://goo.gl/jCEFQ

Melendez, L. & M. Lorenz (2002). Feline Insulin Resistance and Diabetes Mellitus. Proceedings: Western Veterinary Conference. Accessed via: Veterinary Information Network. http://goo.gl/PrwTk

Wynn, S. (2002). Nutraceutical options in veterinary medicine. Proceedings Western Veterinary Conference. Accessed via: Veterinary Information Network. http://goo.gl/JdSbp

VANCOMYCIN HCL

(van-koe-*mye*-sin)   Vancocin®

GLYCOPEPTIDE ANTIBIOTIC

Prescriber Highlights

▶ Glycopeptide antibiotic reserved for IV use for multi-drug resistant Staph or Enterococcus infections; can also be used PO to treat *Clostridium difficile* diarrhea

▶ Oral vancomycin is not absorbed systemically and is only useful for treating GI *C. difficile* overgrowth

▶ When used systemically, must be given IV; severe pain & tissue injury occurs with SC or IM injection

▶ May be synergistic with aminoglycoside therapy, but increased risk of nephrotoxicity, ototoxicity & neutropenia also possible

▶ If decreased renal dysfunction, adjust dosage

Uses/Indications

Vancomycin should only be used to treat infections that are documented resistant to other antibiotics and susceptible to vancomycin, usually methicillin-resistant *Staphylococcus* spp. (MRSA) or multidrug-resistant *Enterococcus* spp. It potentially is useful for oral treatment of pseudomembranous colitis caused by *Clostridia difficile*.

Pharmacology/Actions

Vancomycin inhibits cell-wall synthesis and bacterial cell-membrane permeability. It also affects bacterial RNA synthesis. It is only effective against gram-positive bacteria, including many strains of streptococci, staphylococci, and enterococci. Vancomycin is generally a bactericidal antibiotic, but is bacteriostatic against enterococci. Vancomycin also has activity against *Clostridium difficile*, *Listeria monocytogenes*, Corynebacterium, and *Actinomyces* spp.. Vancomycin and aminoglycosides can have synergistic action against susceptible bacteria. Pus and cellular debris may bind to vancomycin and reduce its efficacy.

Resistance to vancomycin by certain strains of enterococci and staphylococci is an increasing concern in human medicine and potentially, for veterinary patients.

Pharmacokinetics

When given orally, vancomycin is not appreciably absorbed. After intravenous administration, vancomycin is widely distributed. Therapeutic levels can be found in pleural, ascitic, pericardial, and synovial fluids. At usual serum levels, it does not readily distribute into the CSF.

The elimination half-life of vancomycin in patients with normal renal function is approximately 4–6 hours. Prolonged dosing can allow the drug to accumulate. The drug is eliminated primarily via glomerular filtration; small amounts are excreted into the bile.

Contraindications/Precautions/Warnings

Vancomycin is an important antibiotic for treating multi-drug resistant infections in humans. It should not be used in veterinary patients when other antibiotics can be used to successfully treat the infection; some believe that the drug should never be used in veterinary patients.

Patients with decreased renal function that require vancomycin should have dosages reduced or dosing interval increased. Serum levels should be monitored.

Adverse Effects

When given parenterally, nephrotoxicity and ototoxicity are the most serious potential adverse effects of vancomycin. Unlike aminoglycosides, these effects are believed to be uncommon. In humans, dermatologic reactions and hypersensitivity can occur; it is unknown if these effects are issues for veterinary patients. Reversible neutropenia has been reported in humans, particularly when dosage is high and prolonged.

Do not administer IV rapidly or as a bolus; thrombophlebitis, severe hypotension or cardiac arrest (rare) have been reported. Vancomycin must be given over at least 30 minutes as a dilute solution.

Do not give IM, SC, or IP. Severe tissue damage and pain may occur.

Oral therapy may cause GI effects (nausea, inappetence).

Reproductive/Nursing Safety

When used orally, vancomycin is relatively safe to use during pregnancy (FDA category *B*). When used IV, it is not known whether vancomycin can cause fetal harm. A limited study performed in humans did not detect fetal harm, but the numbers studied were small. In humans, the FDA categorizes IV vancomycin as a category *C* drug for use during pregnancy (*Animal studies have shown an adverse effect on the fetus, but there are no adequate studies in humans; or there are no animal reproduction studies and no adequate studies in humans.*) Because in veterinary patients, vancomycin should only be used for serious infections, the potential benefits of therapy will probably outweigh the risks in most circumstances.

Vancomycin is excreted into milk. Because the drug is not appreciably absorbed, it is unlikely to pose significant harm to nursing animals, although diarrhea could occur.

Overdosage/Acute Toxicity

Patients with colitis associated with *Clostridia difficile* taking an oral overdose, could potentially absorb enough drug to cause adverse effects. The IV LD_{50} for vancomycin in mice and rats is 400 mg/kg and 319 mg/kg, respectively. Intravenous overdoses of vancomycin may cause an increased risk of adverse effects, particularly ototoxicity and nephrotoxicity. Supportive care is advised. Hemodialysis does not appear to remove the drug in significant amounts.

Drug Interactions

The following drug interactions have either been reported or are theoretical in humans or animals receiving vancomycin and may be of significance in veterinary patients:

- **AMINOGLYCOSIDES:** Vancomycin may increase the risk of aminoglycoside-related ototoxicity or nephrotoxicity. Because this combination of drugs may be medically required (there is evidence of synergy against staphylococci and enterococci), only enhanced monitoring is suggested.

- **ANESTHETIC AGENTS:** In children, vancomycin used with anesthetic agents has caused erythema and a histamine-like flushing

- **NEPHROTOXIC DRUGS, OTHER (e.g., amphotericin B, cisplatin):** Use with caution with other nephrotoxic drugs

Laboratory Considerations

- No specific concerns were noted

Doses

To prepare parenteral solution using vancomycin 500 mg or 1 gram powder for injection: Reconstitute the 500 mg for injection vial by adding 10 mL of sterile water for injection. Add 20 mL to the 1 gram vial. Before administering to patient, further dilute reconstituted solutions with (at least 100 mL for 500 mg; 200 mL for 1 gram vial) a compatible diluent (*e.g.*, D_5W, lactated Ringer's, 0.9% NaCl).

- **DOGS:**

  For susceptible infections:

  Note: *Oral vancomycin is not appreciably absorbed and is only effective for susceptible enteric infections.*

  a) For confirmed bacteremia/septicemia for enterococci or staphylococci resistant to other commonly used antibiotics: 15 mg/kg IV over 30–60 minutes q6–8h. (Ford 2005)

  b) 15 mg/kg IV over 30–60 minutes q6h. For successful therapy of serious infections, an aminoglycoside such as gentamicin or amikacin should also be administered. (Papich 2003)

  c) For oral use to treat *C. difficile* enterocolitis: 10–20 mg/kg PO q6h for 5–7 days;

For IV use to treat skin, urinary, soft tissue infections: 10–20 mg/kg IV q12h for 7–10 days;

For IV use to treat systemic infections, bacteremia: 15 mg/kg IV q6h for 10 days. (Greene *et al.* 2006)

- **CATS:**

  For susceptible infections:

  a) For confirmed bacteremia/septicemia for enterococci or staphylococci resistant to other commonly used antibiotics: 15 mg/kg IV over 30–60 minutes q6–8h. (Ford 2005)

  b) 15 mg/kg IV over 30–60 minutes q6h. For successful therapy of serious infections, an aminoglycoside such as gentamicin or amikacin should also be administered. (Papich 2003)

Monitoring

When used parenterally:

- Renal function, baseline and periodic

- Vancomycin levels, maintain trough level above 5 micrograms/mL (some say troughs between 10–15 micrograms/mL)

- Periodic CBC if therapy is prolonged

Client Information

- Parenteral vancomycin is used in an inpatient setting

- Oral vancomycin may be used for outpatient therapy; clients should be counseled to give as prescribed

- May give oral dosage forms with a small amount of food

Chemistry/Synonyms

A glycopeptide antibiotic, vancomycin HCl occurs as an odorless, tan to brown free-flowing powder. It is freely soluble in water. A 5% aqueous solution has a pH of 2.5–4.5.

Vancomycin may also be known as: vanco, vancomycini, or *Vancocin®*; there are many registered international trade names available.

Storage/Stability

Vancomycin should be stored at room temperature in tight containers that are protected from light. Once reconstituted (see directions in package insert or in the Doses section), the injectable or oral solutions are stable for 14 days if refrigerated. If diluted further with D_5W or sodium chloride 0.9% for parenteral administration, solutions are stable for 24 hours at room temperature and 2 months if refrigerated.

Compatibility/Compounding Considerations

Vancomycin is **compatible** with D_5W, 0.9% NaCl, and lactated Ringer's injection.

Dosage Forms/Regulatory Status

VETERINARY-LABELED PRODUCTS: None

HUMAN-LABELED PRODUCTS:

Vancomycin HCl Oral Capsules: 125 mg & 250 mg; *Vancocin®* (ViroPharma); (Rx)

Vancomycin HCl Powder for Injection Solution: 500 mg, 750 mg, 1 gram, 5 grams, & 10 grams (some preservative free) in single-dose vials, 100 mL pharmacy bulk packagers and premixed 100 mL & 200 mL *Galaxy* containers; generic; (Rx)

References

Ford, R. (2005). Resistant Infections: The cruelest reality show. Proceedings IVECCS. Accessed via: Veterinary Information Network. http://goo.gl/LvXNe

Greene, C., K. Hartmannn, et al. (2006). Appendix 8: Antimicrobial Drug Formulary. *Infectious Disease of the Dog and Cat*. C Greene Ed., Elsevier: 1186–1333.

Papich, M. (2003). Multi-resistant bacterial pathogens. Proceedings: ACVIM Forum.

VASOPRESSIN

(vay-soe-*press*-in)   Pitressin®

HORMONE

Prescriber Highlights

▶ Hormone used primarily as a diagnostic agent & sometimes for treatment of diabetes insipidus; it may be useful for the adjunctive treatment of shock syndromes and cardio-pulmonary cerebral resuscitation (CPCR)

▶ Contraindications: Chronic nephritis until nitrogen retention is resolved to reasonable levels, or patients hypersensitive to it; Caution: Vascular disease, seizure disorders, heart failure, or asthma

▶ Adverse Effects: Local irritation at the injection site (including sterile abscesses), skin reactions, abdominal pain, hematuria, &, rarely, a hypersensitivity (urticarial) reaction

▶ Overdosage can lead to water intoxication

Uses/Indications

Vasopressin is used in veterinary medicine as a diagnostic agent and in the treatment of diabetes insipidus in small animals. In recent years, there has been significant interest in using vasopressin for treating shock syndromes and for cardiopulmonary cerebral (CPCR) in humans and animals. In ventricular asystole or pulseless electrical activity, vasopressin has some advantages over epinephrine. Vasopressin can act as a vasoconstricting agent even when acidosis is present and may cause less vasoconstriction of coronary and renal vasculature, thereby increasing myocardial perfusion and does not have the arrhythmogenic or chronotropic effects that are associated with epinephrine. Ongoing research is being conducted.

In human medicine, vasopressin has been used to treat acute GI hemorrhage and to stimulate GI peristalsis. Vasopressin CRI is also being used for treatment of hypotensive septic patients unresponsive to conventional vasopressor. Prior to radiographic procedures, it has been used to dispel interfering gas shadows or help concentrate contrast media.

Pharmacology

Vasopressin or antidiuretic hormone (ADH) acts through at least 5 different receptors (three subtypes, V1, V2, V3, the oxytocin receptor, and the purinergic P2 receptor). It promotes the renal reabsorption of solute-free water in the distal convoluted tubules and collecting duct. ADH increases cyclic adenosine monophosphate (cAMP) at the tubule which increases water permeability at the luminal surface resulting in increased urine osmolality and decreased urine flow. Without vasopressin, urine flow can be increased up to 90% greater than normal.

At doses above those necessary for antidiuretic activity, vasopressin can cause smooth muscle contraction. Capillaries and small arterioles are most affected, with resultant decreased blood flow to several systems. Hepatic flow may actually be increased, however.

Vasopressin can cause contraction of smooth muscle of the bladder and gall bladder and increase intestinal peristalsis, particularly of the colon. Vasopressin may decrease gastric secretions and increase GI sphincter pressure; gastric acid concentration remains unchanged.

Vasopressin possesses minimal oxytocic effects, but at large doses may stimulate uterine contraction. Vasopressin also causes the release of corticotropin, growth hormone, and follicle-stimulating hormone (FSH).

Pharmacokinetics

Vasopressin is destroyed in the GI prior to being absorbed and therefore must be administered either intranasally or parenterally. After IM or SC administration in dogs, aqueous vasopressin has antidiuretic activity for 2–8 hours.

Vasopressin is distributed throughout the extracellular fluid. The hormone apparently is not bound to plasma proteins.

Vasopressin is rapidly destroyed in the liver and kidneys. The plasma half-life has been reported to be only 10–20 minutes in humans.

Contraindications/Precautions/Warnings

In humans, vasopressin is contraindicated in patients hypersensitive to it or with chronic nephritis until nitrogen retention is resolved to reasonable levels.

Because of its effects on other systems, particularly at high doses, vasopressin should be used with caution in patients with vascular disease, seizure disorders, heart failure, or asthma.

Adverse Effects

Adverse effects that can be seen include local irritation at the injection site (including sterile abscesses), skin reactions, platelet aggregation, bilirubinemia, abdominal pain, hematuria, and, rarely, a hypersensitivity (urticarial) reaction.

Overdosage can lead to water intoxication (see below).

Reproductive/Nursing Safety

Although the drug has minimal effects on uterine contractions at usual doses, it should be used with caution in pregnant animals. In humans, the FDA categorizes this drug as category *C* for use during pregnancy (*Animal studies have shown an adverse effect on the fetus, but there are no adequate studies in humans; or there are no animal reproduction studies and no adequate studies in humans.*)

Overdosage/Acute Toxicity

Early clinical signs of overdose-induced water intoxication can include listlessness or depression. More severe intoxication clinical signs can include coma, seizures, and eventually death. Treatment for mild intoxication is stopping vasopressin therapy and restricting water access until resolved. Severe intoxication may require the use of osmotic diuretics (mannitol, urea, or dextrose) with or without furosemide.

Drug Interactions

The following drugs may **inhibit** the antidiuretic activity of vasopressin:

- **ALCOHOL**
- **DEMECLOCYCLINE**
- **EPINEPHRINE (large doses)**
- **HEPARIN**
- **NOREPINEPHRINE (large doses)**

The following drugs may **potentiate** the antidiuretic effects of vasopressin:

- **ANTIDEPRESSANTS, TRICYCLIC**
- **CARBAMAZEPINE**
- **CHLORPROPAMIDE**
- **CLOFIBRATE**
- **FLUDROCORTISONE**
- **PHENFORMIN**
- **UREA**

Doses

- **DOGS:**

  As a diagnostic agent after the water deprivation test (WDT); monitor carefully. The WDT is considered contraindicated in animals that are dehydrated or have known renal disease and is used to characterize whether DI is central or nephrogenic in origin. Refer to a current small animal internal medicine text for further information.

  a) Exogenous vasopressin test: After WDT, empty bladder and start IV catheter and slowly reintroduce water. Give aqueous vasopressin in D_5W IV at a dose of 2.5 mU/kg over one hour. To make one liter of a 5 mU/mL solution add 5 Units of vasopressin to one liter of D_5W. Empty bladder and collect urine at 30 minutes, 60 minutes, and 90 minutes. If urine specific gravity >1.1015 = ADH-responsive DI; if <1.015 = either nephrogenic DI or medullary washout effect. (Nichols & Miller 1989)

For adjunctive treatment of shock/CPCR:

a) In patients with vasodilatory shock that is unresponsive to fluid resuscitation and catecholamine (dobutamine, dopamine, and norepinephrine) administration: 0.01–0.04 Units/minute IV (*Note*: This dose is not dependent upon patient weight). DO NOT exceed 0.04 Units/minute. Risk of myocardial ischemia. DO NOT use in patients with cardiogenic shock.

  For CPCR with pulseless electrical activity or ventricular asystole, vasopressin may be beneficial for myocardial and cerebral blood flow: 0.2–0.8 Units/kg, IV once. (**Note:** *This reference has a stepwise guidance flowchart for treating vasodilatory shock and CPCR with pulseless electrical activity or ventricular asystole that veterinary practices are encouraged to have on hand—Plumb*) (Scroggin & Quandt 2009)

For treatment of central diabetes insipidus: [**Note:** Because vasopressin tannate in oil is no longer commercially available; most clinicians are using desmopressin (DDAVP) for treating central DI. Refer to that monograph for more information.]

- **CATS:**

  As a diagnostic agent after the water deprivation test (WDT): The WDT is generally considered contraindicated in animals that are dehydrated or have known renal disease and is used to characterize whether DI is central or nephrogenic in origin.

  a) Immediately after the end-point of the WDT, give aqueous vasopressin 0.5 U/kg IM; continue to withhold food and water. At 30, 60, and 120 minutes after vasopressin, empty bladder and determine specific gravity (osmolality). Upon completion, the cat is gradually allowed access to water. Inability to concentrate urine during the water deprivation test followed by a rise in urine specific gravity above 1.025 after vasopressin is indicative of central DI. (Peterson & Randolph 1989)

For adjunctive treatment of shock/CPCR:

a) In patients with vasodilatory shock that is unresponsive to fluid resuscitation and catecholamine (dobutamine, dopamine, and norepinephrine) administration: 0.01–0.04 Units/minute IV.

  For CPCR with pulseless electrical activity or ventricular asystole, vasopressin may be beneficial for myocardial and cerebral blood flow: 0.2–0.8 Units/kg, IV once. (**Note:** *This reference has a stepwise guidance flowchart for treating vasodila-*

tory shock and CPCR with pulseless electrical activity or ventricular asystole that veterinary practices are encouraged to have on hand—Plumb) (Scroggin & Quandt 2009)

For treatment of central diabetes insipidus: [**Note:** Because vasopressin tannate in oil is no longer commercially available; most clinicians are using desmopressin (DDAVP) for treating central DI. Refer to that monograph for more information.]

Monitoring

■ Urine output/frequency

■ Water consumption

■ Urine specific gravity &/or osmolality

Chemistry/Synonyms

A hypothalamic hormone stored in the posterior pituitary, vasopressin is a 9-amino acid polypeptide with a disulfide bond. In most mammals (including dogs and humans), the natural hormone is arginine vasopressin, while in swine the arginine is replaced with lysine. Lysine vasopressin has only about ½ the antidiuretic activity of arginine vasopressin. The commercially available vasopressin products may be a combination of arginine or lysine vasopressin derived from natural sources or synthetically prepared. The products are standardized by their pressor activity in rats [USP posterior Pituitary (pressor) Units]; their antidiuretic activity can be variable. Commercially available vasopressin has little, if any, oxytocic activity at usual doses.

Vasopressin injection occurs as a clear, colorless or practically colorless liquid with a faint, characteristic odor. Vasopressin is soluble in water.

Vasopressin may also be known as: ADH, antidiuretic hormone, 8-arginine vasopressin, beta-hypophamine, *Neo-Lidocaton®*, *Pitressin®* or *Pressyn®*.

Storage/Stability

Vasopressin (aqueous) injection should be stored at room temperature; avoid freezing.

Compatibility/Compounding Considerations

If the aqueous injection is to be administered as an intravenous or intra-arterial infusion, it may be diluted in either D_5W or normal saline. For infusion use in humans, it is usually diluted to a concentration of 0.1–1 Unit/mL.

Dosage Forms/Regulatory Status

VETERINARY-LABELED PRODUCTS: None

HUMAN-LABELED PRODUCTS:

Vasopressin Injection: 20 pressor Units/mL in 0.5 mL, 1 mL & 10 mL vials; *Pitressin® Synthetic* (JHP Pharm); generic; (Rx)

Vasopressin Tannate Sterile Suspension in oil is no longer commercially available.

References

Nichols, C.E. & J.B. Miller (1989). Diseases of the Pituitary Gland. *Handbook of Small Animal Practice.* RV Morgan Ed. New York, Churchill Livingstone: 501–506.

Peterson, M.E. & J.F. Randolph (1989). Endocrine Diseases. *The Cat: Diseases and Clinical Management.* RG Sherding Ed. New York, Churchill Livingstone. **2:** 1095–1161.

Scroggin, R.D. & J. Quandt (2009). The use of vasopressin for treating vasodilatory shock and cardiopulmonary arrest. *Journal of Veterinary Emergency and Critical Care* **19**(2): 145–157.

VECURONIUM BROMIDE

(vek-yew-*roe*-nee-um)   Norcuron®

NONDEPOLARIZING NEUROMUSCULAR BLOCKER

Prescriber Highlights

▶ Nondepolarizing neuromuscular blocking agent

▶ Caution: Severe renal dysfunction, hepatic, or biliary disease; extreme caution: myasthenia gravis

▶ Adverse Effects: None, other than pharmacologic actions

▶ No analgesia or anesthetic effects

Uses/Indications

Vecuronium is indicated as an adjunct to general anesthesia to produce muscle relaxation during surgical procedures or mechanical ventilation and to facilitate endotracheal intubation. It causes very minimal cardiac effects and generally does not cause the release of histamine. Vecuronium has been used topically to cause mydriasis in birds.

Pharmacology/Actions

Vecuronium is a nondepolarizing neuromuscular blocking agent and acts by competitively binding at cholinergic receptor sites at the motor endplate, thereby inhibiting the effects of acetylcholine. The potency of vecuronium when compared to pancuronium (on a weight basis) has been described as being equipotent to up to 3 times as potent.

Pharmacokinetics

The onset of neuromuscular blockade after IV injection is dependent upon the dose administered. In dogs administered 0.1 mg/kg IV, full neuromuscular block occurs within 2 minutes and the duration of action at this dose is approximately 25 minutes (also receiving halothane anesthesia). Vecuronium has a shorter duration of action than pancuronium (approx. ⅓–½ as long), but is very similar to that of atracurium.

A study done in rats showed that vecuronium was absorbed after intratracheal administration with an onset of action that was slower than intravenous administration, but faster than intramuscular. Intratracheal administration resulted in a longer duration of action then intravenous dosing (Sunaga *et al.* 2006).

1378 VECURONIUM BROMIDE

Vecuronium is partially metabolized; it and its metabolites are excreted into the bile and urine. Prolonged recovery times may result in patients with significant renal or hepatic disease.

Contraindications/Precautions/Warnings

Vecuronium is contraindicated in patients hypersensitive to it. It should be used with caution in patients with severe renal dysfunction. Lower doses may be necessary in patients with hepatic or biliary disease. Vecuronium has no analgesic or sedative/anesthetic actions. In patients with myasthenia gravis, neuromuscular blocking agents should be used with extreme caution, if at all. One case of successful use in a dog with myasthenia gravis has been reported.

Adverse Effects

In human studies and one limited dog study, adverse effects other than what would be seen pharmacologically (skeletal muscle weakness to profound, prolonged musculoskeletal paralysis) have not been reported.

Reproductive/Nursing Safety

In humans, the FDA categorizes this drug as category C for use during pregnancy (*Animal studies have shown an adverse effect on the fetus, but there are no adequate studies in humans; or there are no animal reproduction studies and no adequate studies in humans.*)

Overdosage/Acute Toxicity

No cases of vecuronium overdosage have yet been reported (human or veterinary). Should an inadvertent overdose occur, treat conservatively (mechanical ventilation, O_2, fluids, etc.). Reversal of blockade might be accomplished by administering an anticholinesterase agent (edrophonium, physostigmine, or neostigmine) with an anticholinergic (atropine or glycopyrrolate). A suggested dose for neostigmine is 0.06 mg/kg IV after atropine 0.02 mg/kg IV.

Drug Interactions

The following drug interactions have either been reported or are theoretical in humans or animals receiving vecuronium and may be of significance in veterinary patients:

- **NON-DEPOLARIZING MUSCLE RELAXANT DRUGS, OTHER:** May have a synergistic effect if used with vecuronium
- **SUCCINYLCHOLINE:** May speed the onset of action and enhance the neuromuscular blocking actions of vecuronium; do not give vecuronium until succinylcholine effects have subsided

The following agents may enhance or prolong the neuromuscular blocking activity of vecuronium:

- **AMINOGLYCOSIDES**
- **ANESTHETICS (HALOTHANE, ISOFLURANE, SEVOFLURANE)**
- **CLINDAMYCIN, LINCOMYCIN**
- **DANTROLENE**
- **MAGNESIUM SALTS**
- **PIPERACILLIN, MEZLOCILLIN**
- **QUINIDINE**
- **TETRACYCLINES**
- **VERAPAMIL**

Doses

- **DOGS:**
  a) 0.1 mg/kg IV initially (after meperidine and/or acepromazine pre-op 30 minutes before); may give subsequent incremental doses of 0.04 mg/kg IV. Duration of action after initial dose averages 25 minutes. (Jones & Seymour 1985)
  b) 10–20 micrograms/kg IV (Morgan 2003)
  c) If using CRI propofol-fentanyl anesthesia: CRI maintenance infusion rate of vecuronium at 0.2 mg/kg/hr;
  If using CRI fentanyl-isoflurane or fentanyl-sevoflurane anesthesia: CRI maintenance infusion rate of vecuronium at 0.1 mg/kg/hr. (Nagahama *et al.* 2006)
- **CATS:**
  a) 20–40 micrograms/kg (0.02–0.04 mg/kg) IV (Morgan 2003)

Monitoring
- Level of neuromuscular relaxation

Client Information
- This drug should only be used by professionals familiar with its use

Chemistry/Synonyms

Structurally similar to pancuronium, vecuronium bromide is a synthetic, nondepolarizing neuromuscular blocking agent. It contains the steroid (androstane) nucleus, but is devoid of steroid activity. It occurs as white to off-white, or slightly pink crystals or crystalline powder. In aqueous solution, it has a pK_a of 8.97, and the commercial injection has a pH of 4 after reconstitution. 9 mg are soluble in 1 mL of water; 23 mg are soluble in 1 mL of alcohol.

Vecuronium Bromide may also be known as: Org-NC-45, *Curlem®*, *Norcuron®*, *Rivecrum®*, *Vecural®*, or *Vecuron®*.

Storage/Stability

The commercially available powder for injection should be stored at room temperature and protected from light. After reconstitution with sterile water for injection, vecuronium bromide is stable for 24 hours at either 2–8°C or at room temperature (less than 30°C) if stored in the original container. As it contains no preservative, unused portions should be discarded after reconstitution. The drug is stable for 48 hours at room temperature or refrigerated when stored in plastic or glass syringes, but the manufacturer recommends that it be used within 24 hours.

Compatibility/Compounding Considerations

Vecuronium bromide has been shown to be physically **compatible** with D_5W, normal saline, D_5 in normal saline, and lactated Ringer's.

It should **not** be mixed with alkaline solutions (*e.g.*, thiobarbiturates).

Dosage Forms/Regulatory Status

VETERINARY-LABELED PRODUCTS: None

HUMAN-LABELED PRODUCTS:

Vecuronium Bromide Powder for Injection: 10 mg & 20 mg; in 10 mL & 20 mL vials, with and without diluent; *Norcuron®* (Organon); generic; (Rx)

References

Jones, R.S. & C.J. Seymour (1985). Clinical observations on the use of vecuronium as a muscle relaxant in the dog. *J Small Anim Pract* **26**(4): 213–218.

Morgan, R. (2003). Appendix IV: Recommended Drug Dosages. *Handbook of Small Animal Practice 4th Ed*. R Morgan, R Bright and M Swartout Eds. Philadelphia, Saunders: 1279–1308.

Nagahama, S., R. Nishimura, et al. (2006). The effects of propofol, isoflurane and sevoflurane on vecuronium infusion rates for surgical muscle relaxation in dogs. *Vet Anaesth Analg* **33**(3): 169–174.

Sunaga, H., M. Kaneko, et al. (2006). The Efficacy of Intratracheal Administration of Vecuronium in Rats, Compared with Intravenous and Intramuscular Administration. *Anesth Analg* **103**: 601–607.

VERAPAMIL HCL

(ver-*ap*-a-mill)   Calan®, Isoptin®, Verelan®

CALCIUM-CHANNEL BLOCKER

Prescriber Highlights

▶ Calcium channel blocking agent used for supraventricular tachycardias in dogs & cats

▶ Contraindications: Cardiogenic shock or severe CHF (unless secondary to a supraventricular tachycardia), hypotension, sick sinus syndrome, 2nd or 3rd degree AV block, digoxin intoxication, or hypersensitive to verapamil. IV is contraindicated within a few hours of IV beta-adrenergic blockers.

▶ Caution: Heart failure, hypertrophic cardiomyopathy, & hepatic or renal impairment. Use very cautiously in patients with atrial fibrillation & Wolff-Parkinson-White (WPW) syndrome.

▶ Adverse Effects: Hypotension, bradycardia, tachycardia, exacerbation of CHF, peripheral edema, AV block, pulmonary edema, nausea, constipation, dizziness, headache, or fatigue

▶ Drug Interactions

Uses/Indications

Veterinary experience with this agent is somewhat limited, but in dogs and cats verapamil may be useful for supraventricular tachycardias and, possibly, treatment of atrial flutter or fibrillation. Verapamil is being studied as an adjunctive treatment for pharmaco-resistant epilepsy.

Pharmacology/Actions

A slow-channel calcium blocking agent, verapamil is classified as a class IV antiarrhythmic drug. Verapamil exerts its actions by blocking the transmembrane influx of extracellular calcium ions across membranes of vascular smooth muscle cells and myocardial cells. The result of this blocking is to inhibit the contractile mechanisms of vascular and cardiac smooth muscle. Verapamil has inhibitory effects on the cardiac conduction system and these effects produce its antiarrhythmic properties. Electrophysiologic effects include increased effective refractory period of the AV node, decreased automaticity and substantially decreased AV node conduction. On ECG, heart rate and RR intervals can be increased or decreased; PR and A-H intervals are increased. Verapamil has negative effects on myocardial contractility and decreases peripheral vascular resistance.

Verapamil is an inhibitor of P-glycoprotein which is the mechanism proposed for its potential to treat pharmaco-resistant epilepsy.

Pharmacokinetics

In humans, about 90% of a dose of verapamil is rapidly absorbed after oral administration, but because of a high first-pass effect, only about 20–30% is available to the systemic circulation. Patients with significant hepatic dysfunction may have considerably higher percentages of the drug systemically bioavailable. Food will decrease the rate and extent of absorption of the sustained-release tablets, but less so with the conventional tablets.

Verapamil's volume of distribution is between 4.5–7 L/kg in humans and has been reported to be approximately 4.5 L/kg in dogs. In humans, approximately 90% of the drug in the serum is bound to plasma proteins. Verapamil crosses the placenta and milk levels may approach those in the plasma.

Verapamil is metabolized in the liver to at least 12 separate metabolites, with norverapamil being the most predominant. The majority of the amounts of these metabolites are excreted into the urine. Only 3–4% is excreted unchanged in the urine. In humans, the half-life of the drug is 2–8 hours after a single IV dose, but it can increase after 1–2 days of oral therapy (presumably due to a saturable process of the hepatic enzymes). Serum half-lives of 0.8 hours and 2.5 hours have been reported in the dog.

Contraindications/Precautions/Warnings

Verapamil is contraindicated in patients with cardiogenic shock or severe CHF (unless secondary to a supraventricular tachycardia amenable to verapamil therapy), hypotension (<90 mmHg systolic), sick sinus syndrome, 2nd or 3rd degree AV block, digoxin intoxication, or hypersensitive to verapamil.

IV verapamil is contraindicated within a few hours of IV beta-adrenergic blocking agents (*e.g.*, propranolol) as they both can depress myocardial contractility and AV node conduction. Use of this combination in patients with wide complex ventricular tachycardia (QRS >0.11 seconds) can cause rapid hemodynamic deterioration and ventricular fibrillation.

Verapamil should be used with caution in patients with heart failure, hypertrophic cardiomyopathy, and hepatic or renal impairment. Toxicity may be potentiated in patients with hepatic dysfunction. It should be used very cautiously in patients with atrial fibrillation and Wolff-Parkinson-White (WPW) syndrome as fatal arrhythmias may result.

Because verapamil may increase blood glucose in dogs, it should be used with caution in diabetic animals.

Verapamil is potentially a neurotoxic substrate of P-glycoprotein; use with caution in those herding breeds (*e.g.*, Collies) that may have the gene mutation that causes a nonfunctional protein.

Adverse Effects

The following adverse reactions may occur: hypotension, bradycardia, tachycardia, exacerbation of CHF, peripheral edema, AV block, pulmonary edema, nausea, constipation, dizziness, headache or fatigue.

Reproductive/Nursing Safety

Oral verapamil in rats with doses 1.5−6 times the human dose was embryocidal and retarded fetal growth and development, probably due to reduced weight gains in dams. Verapamil crosses the placenta and can be detected in umbilical vein blood at delivery. In humans, the FDA categorizes this drug as category *C* for use during pregnancy (*Animal studies have shown an adverse effect on the fetus, but there are no adequate studies in humans; or there are no animal reproduction studies and no adequate studies in humans.*)

Verapamil is excreted in milk. Consider discontinuing nursing if the dam requires verapamil therapy.

Overdosage/Acute Toxicity

Clinical signs of overdosage may include bradycardia, hypotension, hyperglycemia, junctional rhythms, and 2nd or 3rd degree AV block.

If overdose is secondary to a recent oral ingestion, emptying the gut and charcoal administration may be considered. Treatment is generally supportive in nature; vigorously monitor cardiac and respiratory function. Intravenous calcium salts (1 mL of 10% solution per 10 kgs of body weight) have been suggested to treat the negative inotropic clinical signs, but may not adequately treat clinical signs of heart block. Use of fluids and pressor agents (*e.g.*, dopamine, norepinephrine, etc.) may be utilized to treat hypotensive clinical signs. The AV block and/or bradycardia can be treated with isoproterenol, norepinephrine, atropine, or cardiac pacing. Patients that develop a rapid ventricular rate after verapamil due to antegrade conduction in flutter/fibrillation with WPW syndrome, have been treated with D.C. cardioversion, lidocaine, or procainamide.

Drug Interactions

The following drug interactions have either been reported or are theoretical in humans or animals receiving verapamil and may be of significance in veterinary patients:

■ **ACE INHIBITORS:** May cause additive hypotensive effects

■ **ALPHA-ADRENERGIC BLOCKERS (e.g., prazosin):** May cause additive hypotensive effects

■ **BETA-ADRENERGIC BLOCKERS (e.g., propranolol):** May cause additive negative cardiac inotrope and chronotrope effects

■ **DOXORUBICIN:** Verapamil may increase concentrations

■ **COPP CHEMOTHERAPY (cyclophosphamide, vincristine, procarbazine, prednisone):** May decrease oral absorption of verapamil

■ **CYCLOSPORINE:** Verapamil may increase levels

■ **DANTROLENE:** Cardiovascular collapse reported in animals when used with verapamil

■ **DIGOXIN:** Verapamil may increase the blood levels of digoxin; monitoring of digoxin levels recommended

■ **DISOPYRAMIDE:** May cause additive effects; impair left ventricular function; use together within 24−48 hours not recommended

■ **DIURETICS:** May cause additive hypotensive effects

■ **ERYTHROMYCIN, CLARITHROMYCIN:** May increase verapamil levels

■ **FLECAINIDE:** Possible additive effects; use is together with verapamil is to be avoided in humans

■ **NEUROMUSCULAR BLOCKERS:** Neuromuscular blocking effects of nondepolarizing muscle relaxants may be enhanced by verapamil

■ **PHENOBARBITAL:** May reduce verapamil levels

■ **QUINIDINE:** Additive alpha-adrenergic blocking activity; increased hypotensive effect; verapamil can block quinidine's AV conductive effects and increase quinidine levels

■ **RIFAMPIN:** May reduce verapamil levels

■ **THEOPHYLLINE:** Verapamil may increase serum levels of theophylline and lead to toxicity

■ **VINCRISTINE:** Calcium channel blockers may increase intracellular vincristine by inhibiting the drug's outflow from the cell

Laboratory Considerations

■ Verapamil may elevate blood glucose in dogs and confuse **blood glucose** determinations

Doses

■ **DOGS:**
a) Initial dose of 0.05 mg/kg IV slowly, can repeat every 5 minutes up to a total dose of 0.15−0.2 mg/kg; Oral Dose: 0.5−2 mg/kg PO q8h (Ware 2000)

b) For treatment of hypertension: 1–5 mg/kg PO q8h (Brovida 2002)

c) For emergency treatment for hemodynamically unstable and sustained (continuous) supraventricular tachycardia: As an alternative to diltiazem, verapamil can be given IV in a series of 0.05 mg/kg boluses IV (slowly) up to a total dose of 0.15 mg/kg. (Smith 2009)

d) 1–5 mg/kg PO three times daily; 0.05–0.25 mg/kg IV slowly (Kramer 2003)

e) For the acute termination of supraventricular tachycardia: Initial dose of 0.05 mg/kg should be administered over 1–2 minutes while ECG is monitored; if not effective, may repeat in 5–10 minutes. If arrhythmia still not terminated, may give one last dose of 0.05 mg/kg (total = 0.15 mg/kg). Effect may persist for 30 minutes or less. For longer control, may give as a CRI at 2–10 micrograms/kg/minute. (Kittleson 2006)

■ **CATS:**

a) Initial dose of 0.025 mg/kg IV slowly, can repeat every 5 minutes up to a total dose of 0.15–0.2 mg/kg; Oral Dose: 0.5–1 mg/kg PO q8h (Ware 2000)

■ **HORSES: (NOTE: ARCI UCGFS CLASS 4 DRUG)**

a) To control ventricular rate in atrial fibrillation: 0.025–0.05 mg/kg IV q 30 minutes; give less than 0.2 mg/kg total dose (Reimer 2002)

■ **SMALL MAMMALS:**

a) **Hamsters:** 0.25–0.5 mg (total dose per hamster) SC;

Rabbits: 8–16 mg/kg PO + 0.5–2 mg/kg SC once daily (q24h). (Heatley 2009)

Monitoring

■ ECG

■ Clinical signs of toxicity (see Adverse Effects);

■ Blood pressure, during acute IV therapy

■ Serum concentration, if efficacy or toxicity warrant (100–300 ng/mL is considered therapeutic)

Client Information

■ To be effective, the animal must receive all doses as prescribed

■ If animal becomes lethargic or becomes exercise intolerant, begins wheezing, has shortness of breath or cough, or develops a change in behavior or attitude, notify veterinarian.

Chemistry/Synonyms

A calcium channel blocking agent, verapamil HCl occurs as a bitter-tasting, nearly white, crystalline powder. It is soluble in water and the injectable product has a pH of 4–6.5.

Verapamil HCl tablets should be stored at room temperature (15–30°C); the injectable product should be stored at room temperature (15–30°C) and protected from light and freezing.

Verapamil may also be known as: CP-16533-1, D-365, iproveratril hydrochloride, verapamili hydrochloridum; many trade names are available.

Compatibility/Compounding Considerations

Verapamil HCl for injection is physically **compatible** when mixed with all commonly used intravenous solutions. However, a crystalline precipitate may form if verapamil is added to an infusion line with 0.45% sodium chloride with sodium bicarbonate running. Verapamil is reported to be physically **compatible** with the following drugs: amikacin sulfate, aminophylline, ampicillin sodium, ascorbic acid, atropine sulfate, bretylium tosylate, calcium chloride/gluconate, cefazolin sodium, cefotaxime sodium, cefoxitin sodium, chloramphenicol sodium succinate, cimetidine HCl, clindamycin phosphate, dexamethasone sodium phosphate, diazepam, digoxin, dobutamine HCl (slight discoloration due to dobutamine oxidation), dopamine HCl, epinephrine HCl, furosemide, gentamicin sulfate, heparin sodium, hydrocortisone sodium phosphate, hydromorphone HCl, insulin, isoproterenol, lidocaine HCl, magnesium sulfate, mannitol, meperidine HCl, metaraminol bitartrate, methylprednisolone sodium succinate, metoclopramide HCl, morphine sulfate, multivitamin infusion, nitroglycerin, norepinephrine bitartrate, oxytocin, pancuronium Br, penicillin G potassium/sodium, pentobarbital sodium, phenobarbital sodium, phentolamine mesylate, phenytoin sodium, potassium chloride/phosphate, procainamide HCl, propranolol HCl, protamine sulfate, quinidine gluconate, sodium bicarbonate, sodium nitroprusside, tobramycin sulfate, vasopressin, and vitamin B complex with C.

The following drugs have been reported to be physically **incompatible** with verapamil: albumin injection, amphotericin B, hydralazine HCl, and trimethoprim/sulfamethoxazole. Compatibility is dependent upon factors such as pH, concentration, temperature, and diluent used; consult specialized references or a hospital pharmacist for more specific information.

Dosage Forms/Regulatory Status

VETERINARY-LABELED PRODUCTS: None

The ARCI (Racing Commissioners International) has designated this drug as a class 4 substance. See the appendix for more information.

HUMAN-LABELED PRODUCTS:

Verapamil HCl Tablets: 40 mg, 80 mg & 120 mg; *Calan®* (Pfizer); generic; (Rx)

Verapamil HCl Sustained/Extended-Release Tablets/Capsules: 100 mg, 120 mg, 180 mg, 200 mg, 240 mg, 300 mg & 360 mg; *Calan® SR*

& *Covera-HS®* (Pfizer); *Isoptin® SR* (FSC Laboratories); *Verelan®* & *Verelan® PM* (Schwarz Pharma); generic; (Rx)

Verapamil HCl for Injection: 2.5 mg/mL in 2 mL & 4 mL vials, amps and syringes, 2 mL fill in single-use 2 mL *Carpuject* & *Carpuject Interlink* syringes; generic; (Rx)

References

Brovida, C. (2002). Hypertension in renal diseases and failure. The practical aspect. Proceedings: World Small Animal Association. Accessed via: Veterinary Information Network. http://goo.gl/5iMw3

Heatley, J. (2009). Small Exotic Mammal Cardiovascular Disease. Proceedings: ABVP. Accessed via: Veterinary Information Network. http://goo.gl/rzlia

Kittleson, M. (2006). "Chapt 29: Drugs used in the treatment of cardiac arrhythmias." *Small Animal Cardiology, 2nd Ed.*

Kramer, G. (2003). Treatment of arrhythmias: Case-based presentation. Proceedings: Atlantic Coast Veterinary Conf. Accessed via: Veterinary Information Network. http://goo.gl/U6WTk

Reimer, J. (2002). Treating life-threatening cardiac arrhythmias in the horse. Proceedings: ACVIM Forum. Accessed via: Veterinary Information Network. http://goo.gl/Fxb6n

Smith, F. (2009). Update on Antiarrhythmic Therapy. Proceedings: Western Veterinary Conference. Accessed via: Veterinary Information Network. http://goo.gl/aiVDJ

Ware, W. (2000). Therapy for Critical Arrythmias: New Advances. Proceedings: The North American Veterinary Conference, Orlando.

VINBLASTINE SULFATE

(vin-*blas*-teen)   Velban®

ANTINEOPLASTIC

Prescriber Highlights

▶ A Vinca alkaloid antineoplastic used for a variety of tumors in dogs (& sometimes cats)

▶ Contraindications: Preexisting leukopenia or granulocytopenia (unless a result of the disease being treated) or active bacterial infection; reduce dose if hepatic disease

▶ Adverse Effects: Gastroenterocolitis (nausea/vomiting), myelosuppression (more so than with vincristine; may also cause constipation, alopecia, stomatitis, ileus, inappropriate ADH secretion, jaw & muscle pain, & loss of deep tendon reflexes

▶ Cats can develop neurotoxicity causing constipation or paralytic ileus & aggravating anorexia; can also develop reversible axon swelling & paranodal demyelination

▶ Potentially teratogenic

▶ Avoid extravasation; wear gloves & protective clothing when preparing or administering

▶ Drug Interactions

Uses/Indications

Vinblastine may be employed in the treatment of lymphomas, carcinomas, mastocytomas, and splenic tumors in small animals. It is more effective than vincristine in the treatment of canine mast cell tumors.

Pharmacology/Actions

Vinblastine apparently binds to microtubular proteins (tubulin) in the mitotic spindle, thereby preventing cell division during metaphase. It also interferes with amino acid metabolism by inhibiting glutamic acid utilization and preventing purine synthesis, citric acid cycle, and urea formation.

Pharmacokinetics

Vinblastine is administered IV. After injection, it is rapidly distributed to tissues. In humans, approximately 75% is bound to tissue proteins and the drug does not appreciably enter the CNS.

Vinblastine is extensively metabolized by the liver and is primarily excreted in the bile/feces; lesser amounts are eliminated in the urine.

Contraindications/Precautions/Warnings

Vinblastine is contraindicated in patients with preexisting leukopenia or granulocytopenia (unless a result of the disease being treated), or active bacterial infection.

Doses of vinblastine should be reduced in patients with hepatic disease. A 50% reduction in dose should be considered if serum bilirubin levels are greater than 2 mg/dL.

Because vinblastine is potentially a neurotoxic substrate of P-glycoprotein, it should be used with caution in those herding breeds (*e.g.*, Collies) that may have the gene mutation (MDR1; *ABCB1*) that causes a nonfunctional protein. Bone marrow suppression (decreased blood cell counts, particularly neutrophils) and GI toxicity (anorexia, vomiting, diarrhea) are more likely to occur at normal doses in dogs with the *ABCB1* mutation. To reduce the likelihood of severe toxicity in these dogs (mutant/normal or mutant/mutant), the Veterinary Clinical Pharmacology Laboratory at Washington State University recommends reducing the dose by 25-30% and carefully monitoring these patients (WSU-VetClinPharmLab 2009).

As vinblastine may be a skin irritant, gloves and protective clothing should be worn when preparing or administering the medication. If skin/mucous membrane exposure occurs, thoroughly wash area with soap and water.

Adverse Effects

Vinblastine can cause gastroenterocolitis (nausea/vomiting), which generally lasts less than 24-hours. It can be myelosuppressive at usual dosages (nadir at 4–9 days after treatment; recovery at 7–14 days). Vinblastine is considered more myelosuppressive than is vincristine.

Vinblastine may not possess the degree of peripheral neurotoxic effects seen with vincristine, but at high doses, these effects may be seen.

Additionally, vinblastine may cause constipation, alopecia, stomatitis, ileus, inappropriate ADH secretion, jaw and muscle pain, and loss of deep tendon reflexes.

Cats can develop neurotoxicity that can be associated with constipation or paralytic ileus thereby aggravating anorexia. They may develop reversible axon swelling and paranodal demyelination.

Extravasation of vinblastine may cause significant tissue irritation and cellulitis. Because of the vesicant action of this drug, it is recommended to use a different needle for injecting the drug than the one used to withdraw the drug from the vial. Should clinical signs of extravasation be noted, discontinue infusion immediately at that site and apply moderate heat to the area to help disperse the drug. Injections of hyaluronidase have also been suggested to help diffuse the drug.

Reproductive/Nursing Safety

Little is known about the effects of vinblastine on developing fetuses, but it is believed that the drug possesses some teratogenic and embryotoxic properties. It may also cause aspermia in males. In humans, the FDA categorizes this drug as category *D* for use during pregnancy (*There is evidence of human fetal risk, but the potential benefits from the use of the drug in pregnant women may be acceptable despite its potential risks.*)

It is not known whether vinblastine is excreted in milk. Because of the potential for serious adverse reactions in nursing offspring, consider using milk replacer if dams are being given this drug.

Overdosage/Acute Toxicity

In dogs, the lethal dose for vinblastine has been reported as 0.2 mg/kg. Effects of an overdosage of vinblastine are exacerbations of the adverse effects outlined above. Additionally, neurotoxic effects similar to those associated with vincristine may also be noted.

A case report of a cat receiving a 4X IV overdose has been published (Grant *et al.* 2010). The following were noted with this patient after the overdose: Within hours the cat developed depression and was unable to jump; days 1-11 anorexia; days 2-6 neutropenia with a fever on day 4; days 2-10 thrombocytopenia and anemia; days 4-10 vomiting and diarrhea, and on days 3-10 syndrome of inappropriate ADH (SIADH). Aggressive therapeutic interventions supporting the patient resulted in a positive outcome.

In humans, cardiovascular and hematologic monitoring are performed after an overdose. Treatment can include anticonvulsants, and prevention of ileus. Additionally, an attempt is made to prevent the effects associated with the syndrome of inappropriate antidiuretic hormone (SIADH) with fluid restriction and loop diuretics to maintain serum osmolality.

Drug Interactions

The following drug interactions have either been reported or are theoretical in humans or animals receiving vinblastine and may be of significance in veterinary patients:

■ **OTOTOXIC DRUGS (e.g., cisplatin, carboplatin):** May cause additive risk for ototoxicity

Caution is advised if using other drugs that can inhibit **p-glycoprotein** particularly in those dogs at risk for MDR1-allele mutation (Collies, Australian Shepherds, Shelties, Long-haired Whippet, etc. "white feet"), unless tested "normal". Drugs and drug classes involved include:

■ **AMIODARONE**

■ **AZOLE ANTIFUNGALS (e.g., ketoconazole)**

■ **CARVEDILOL**

■ **CYCLOSPORINE**

■ **DILTIAZEM**

■ **ERYTHROMYCIN; CLARITHROMYCIN**

■ **QUINIDINE**

■ **SPIRONOLACTONE**

■ **TAMOXIFEN**

■ **VERAPAMIL**

Laboratory Considerations

■ Vinblastine may significantly increase both blood and urine concentrations of **uric acid**

Doses

Note: Because of the potential toxicity of this drug to patients, veterinary personnel and clients, and since chemotherapy indications, treatment protocols, monitoring and safety guidelines often change, the following dosages should be used only as a general guide. Consultation with a veterinary oncologist and referral to current veterinary oncology references [*e.g.,* (Henry & Higginbotham 2009); (Argyle *et al.* 2008); (Withrow & Vail 2007); (Villalobos 2007); (Ogilvie & Moore 2006); (Ogilvie & Moore 2001)] are *strongly recommended.*

■ **DOGS/CATS:**
The following are doses are general guidelines (see above). Depending on the protocol and the disease treated, vinblastine doses are usually 2–2.2 mg/m^2 IV every 1-2 weeks often in combination with other chemo drugs (*e.g.,* in dogs, cyclophosphamide and prednisolone). There is one protocol for dogs (Woods 2010), where it is given on four subsequent days every 3 weeks.

Monitoring

■ Efficacy

■ Toxicity (complete blood counts with platelets; liver function tests prior to therapy and repeated as necessary; serum uric acid)

Client Information

■ Clients must be briefed on the possibilities of severe toxicity developing from this drug, including drug-related mortality

■ Contact the veterinarian if the patient exhibits any symptoms of profound depression, abnormal bleeding (including bloody diarrhea) and/or bruising

Chemistry/Synonyms

Commonly referred to as a Vinca alkaloid, vinblastine sulfate is isolated from the plant Cantharanthus roseus (*Vinca rosea Linn*) and occurs as a white or slightly yellow, hygroscopic, amorphous or crystalline powder that is freely soluble in water. The commercially available injection has a pH of 3–5.5.

Vinblastine may also be known as: 29060-LE, NSC-49842, sulfato de vimblastina, vinblastini sulfas, vincaleukoblastine sulphate, VBL, *Alkaban®, Blastovin®, Cellblastin®, Cytoblastin®, Ifabla®, Lemblastine®, Periblastine®, Serovin®, Solblastin®, Velban®, Velbe®, Velsar®,* or *Xintoprost®*.

Storage/Stability

The sterile powder for injection, solution for injection and reconstituted powder for injection should all be protected from light. The powder for injection and injection should be stored in the refrigerator (2–8°C). The intact powder for injection is stable at room temperature for at least one month. After reconstituting with bacteriostatic saline, the powder for injection is stable for 30 days if refrigerated.

Compatibility/Compounding Considerations

Vinblastine sulfate is reportedly physically **compatible** with the following intravenous solutions and drugs: D_5W and bleomycin sulfate. In syringes or at Y-sites with: bleomycin sulfate, cisplatin, cyclophosphamide, droperidol, fluorouracil, leucovorin calcium, methotrexate sodium, metoclopramide HCl, mitomycin, and vincristine sulfate.

Vinblastine sulfate **compatibility information** conflicts or is dependent on diluent or concentration factors with the following drugs or solutions: doxorubicin HCl and heparin sodium (in syringes).

Vinblastine sulfate is reportedly physically **incompatible** with furosemide.

Compatibility is dependent upon factors such as pH, concentration, temperature and diluent used; consult specialized references or a hospital pharmacist for more specific information.

Dosage Forms/Regulatory Status

VETERINARY-LABELED PRODUCTS: None

HUMAN-LABELED PRODUCTS:

Vinblastine Sulfate Injection: 1 mg/mL in 10 mL & 25 mL vials; generic; (Rx)

Vinblastine Powder for Injection: 10 mg in vials; *Velban®* (Lilly); generic; (Rx)

References

Argyle, D., M. Brearly, et al. (2008). *Decision Making in Small Animal Oncology*, Wiley-Blackwell.

Grant, I.A., K. Karnik, et al. (2010). Toxicities and salvage therapy following overdose of vinblastine in a cat. *Journal of Small Animal Practice* 51(2): 127–131.

Henry, C. & M. Higginbotham (2009). *Cancer Management in Small Animal Practice*, Saunders.

Ogilvie, G. & A. Moore (2001). *Feline Oncology: A Comprehensive Guide to Compassionate Care*, Veterinary Learning Systems.

Ogilvie, G. & A. Moore (2006). *Managing the Canine Cancer Patient: A Practical Guide to Compassionate Care*, Veterinary Learning Systems.

Villalobos, A. (2007). *Canine and Feline Geriatric Oncology*. Ames, Blackwell.

Withrow, S. & D. Vail (2007). *Withrow and MacEwen's Small Animal Clinical Oncology 4th Ed*. Philadelphia, Elsevier.

Woods, J. (2010). Medical & Surgical Oncology: Diagnosis & Management of Mast Cell Tumors in Dogs & Cats. Proceedings: ACVIM. Accessed via: Veterinary Information Network. http://goo.gl/DDcFd

WSU-VetClinPharmLab (2009). "Problem Drugs." http://goo.gl/aIGlM.

VINCRISTINE SULFATE

(vin-**kris**-teen)   Oncovin®

ANTINEOPLASTIC

Prescriber Highlights

▶ A Vinca alkaloid antineoplastic used for a variety of tumors in dogs & cats (primarily lymphoid & hematopoietic neoplasms); also used for the treatment of immune-mediated thrombocytopenia

▶ Caution: Hepatic disease, leukopenia, infection, or preexisting neuromuscular disease; reduce dose if hepatic disease

▶ Adverse Effects: Much less myelosuppressive than vinblastine, but may cause more peripheral neurotoxic effects; neuropathic clinical signs can include proprioceptive deficits, spinal hyporeflexia, or paralytic ileus with resulting constipation; Cats can develop neurotoxicity causing constipation or paralytic ileus & aggravating anorexia; can also develop reversible axon swelling & paranodal demyelination

▶ Potentially teratogenic

▶ Avoid extravasation; wear gloves & protective clothing when preparing or administering

▶ Drug Interactions

Uses/Indications

Vincristine is used as an antineoplastic primarily in combination drug protocols in dogs and cats in the treatment of lymphoid and hematopoietic neoplasms. In dogs, it may be used alone in the therapy of transmissible venereal neoplasms.

Because vincristine can induce thrombocytosis (at low doses) and has some immunosuppressant activity, it may also be employed in the treatment of immune-mediated thrombocytopenia, but efficacy is questionable.

Pharmacology/Actions

Vincristine apparently binds to microtubular proteins (tubulin) in the mitotic spindle, thereby preventing cell division during metaphase. It also interferes with amino acid metabolism by inhibiting glutamic acid utilization and preventing purine synthesis, citric acid cycle and urea formation. Tumor resistance to one Vinca alkaloid does not imply resistance to another..

Vincristine can induce thrombocytosis (mechanism unknown) and has some immunosuppressant activity.

Pharmacokinetics

Vincristine is administered IV as it is unpredictably absorbed from the GI tract. After injection it is rapidly distributed to tissues. In humans, approximately 75% is bound to tissue proteins and the drug does not appreciably enter the CNS.

Vincristine is extensively metabolized, presumably by the liver and primarily excreted in the bile/feces; lesser amounts are eliminated in the urine. The elimination half-life in dogs is reportedly biphasic with an alpha half-life of 13 minutes and a beta half-life of 75 minutes.

Contraindications/Precautions/Warnings

Vincristine should be used with caution in patients with hepatic disease, leukopenia, infection, or preexisting neuromuscular disease.

Doses of vincristine should be reduced in patients with hepatic disease. A 50% reduction in dose should be considered if serum bilirubin levels are greater than 2 mg/dL.

Because vincristine is potentially a neurotoxic substrate of P-glycoprotein, it should be used with caution in those herding breeds (e.g., Collies) that may have the gene mutation that causes a nonfunctional protein. Bone marrow suppression (decreased blood cell counts, particularly neutrophils) and GI toxicity (anorexia, vomiting, diarrhea) are more likely to occur at normal doses in dogs with the ABCB1 mutation. To reduce the likelihood of severe toxicity in these dogs (mutant/normal or mutant/mutant), the Veterinary Clinical Pharmacology Laboratory at Washington State University recommends reducing the dose by 25-30% and carefully monitoring these patients (WSU-VetClinPharmLab 2009).

As vincristine may be a skin irritant, gloves and protective clothing should be worn when preparing or administering the medication. If skin/mucous membrane exposure occurs, thoroughly wash area with soap and water.

Adverse Effects

Although structurally related to and having a similar mechanism of action as vinblastine, vincristine has a different adverse reaction profile. Vincristine is much less myelosuppressive (mild leukopenia) at usual doses than is vinblastine, but may cause more peripheral neurotoxic effects. Neuropathic clinical signs may include proprioceptive deficits, spinal hyporeflexia, or paralytic ileus with resulting constipation. In humans, vincristine commonly causes mild sensory impairment and peripheral paresthesias. These may also occur in animals, but are not usually noted due to difficulty in detection. Cats, however, can develop neurotoxicity that can be associated with constipation or paralytic ileus thereby aggravating anorexia. They can develop reversible axon swelling and paranodal demyelination.

Additionally, in small animals, vincristine may cause impaired platelet aggregation, increased liver enzymes, inappropriate ADH secretion, jaw pain, alopecia, stomatitis, or seizures.

A case report of cat developing pulmonary edema attributed to vincristine administration has been published (Polton & Elwood 2008).

Extravasation injuries associated with perivascular injection of vincristine can range from irritation to necrosis and tissue sloughing. Because of the vesicant action of this drug, it is recommended to use a different needle for injecting the drug than the one used to withdraw it from the vial. Recommendations of therapy for extravasation include discontinuing the infusion immediately at that site and applying moderate heat to the area to help disperse the drug. Injections of hyaluronidase have been suggested to help diffuse the drug. Others have suggested applying ice to the area to limit the drug's diffusion and minimize the area affected. Topical dimethyl sulfoxide (DMSO) has also been recommended by some to treat the area involved.

Reproductive/Nursing Safety

Little is known about the effects of vincristine on developing fetuses, but it is believed that the drug possesses some teratogenic and embryotoxic properties. It may also cause aspermia in males. In humans, the FDA categorizes this drug as category *D* for use during pregnancy (*There is evidence of human fetal risk, but the potential benefits from the use of the drug in pregnant women may be acceptable despite its potential risks.*) In a separate system evaluating the safety of drugs in canine and feline pregnancy (Papich 1989), this drug is categorized as in class: *C* (*These drugs may have potential risks. Studies in people or laboratory animals have uncovered risks, and these drugs should be used cautiously as a last resort when the benefit of therapy clearly outweighs the risks.*)

It is not known whether this drug is excreted in milk. Because of the potential for serious adverse reactions in nursing offspring, consider using milk replacer if dams are being given this drug.

Overdosage/Acute Toxicity

In dogs, it is reported that the maximally tolerated dose of vincristine is 0.06 mg/kg every 7 days for 6 weeks. Animals receiving this dose showed signs of slight anemia, leukopenia, increased liver enzymes, and neuronal shrinkage in the peripheral and central nervous systems.

In cats, the lethal dose of vincristine is reportedly 0.1 mg/kg. Cats receiving toxic doses showed clinical signs of weight loss, seizures, leukopenia, and general debilitation. A case report of cat receiving a 10X overdose (5 mg/m2) has been published (Hughes *et al.* 2009). Despite intensive treatment including using calcium folinate, the cat died 72 hours after the overdose.

In humans, cardiovascular and hematologic monitoring are performed after an overdose. Treatment can include anticonvulsants, and prevention of ileus. Additionally, an attempt is made to prevent the effects associated with the syndrome of inappropriate antidiuretic hormone (SIADH) with fluid restriction and loop diuretics to maintain serum osmolality. There have been some reports of leucovorin calcium being used to treat vincristine overdoses in humans, but efficacy of this treatment has not yet been confirmed.

Drug Interactions

The following drug interactions have either been reported or are theoretical in humans or animals receiving vincristine and may be of significance in veterinary patients:

■ **ASPARAGINASE:** Additive neurotoxicity may occur; is apparently less common when asparaginase is administered after vincristine

■ **MITOMYCIN:** In humans who have previously or simultaneously received mitomycin-C with Vinca alkaloids, severe bronchospasm has occurred

Caution is advised if using other drugs that can inhibit **p-glycoprotein** particularly in those dogs at risk for MDR1-allele mutation (Collies, Australian Shepherds, Shelties, Long-haired Whippet, etc. "white feet"), unless tested "normal". Drugs and drug classes involved include:

■ **AMIODARONE**

■ **AZOLE ANTIFUNGALS (e.g., ketoconazole)**

■ **CARVEDILOL**

■ **CYCLOSPORINE**

■ **DILTIAZEM**

■ **ERYTHROMYCIN; CLARITHROMYCIN**

■ **QUINIDINE**

■ **SPIRONOLACTONE**

■ **TAMOXIFEN**

■ **VERAPAMIL**

Laboratory Considerations

■ Vincristine may significantly increase both blood and urine concentrations of **uric acid**

Doses

Note: Because of the potential toxicity of this drug to patients, veterinary personnel and clients, and since chemotherapy indications, treatment protocols, monitoring and safety guidelines often change, the following dosages should be used only as a general guide. Consultation

with a veterinary oncologist and referral to current veterinary oncology references [*e.g.,* (Henry & Higginbotham 2009); (Argyle *et al.* 2008); (Withrow & Vail 2007); (Villalobos 2007); (Ogilvie & Moore 2006); (Ogilvie & Moore 2001)] are *strongly recommended*.

■ **DOGS:**

For neoplastic diseases (usually used in combination protocols with other drugs; consultation with a veterinary oncologist is encouraged before use; see above): Vincristine is usually dosed in dogs at 0.5–0.75 mg/m^2 (*NOT* mg/kg) IV and administered every 1–2 weeks. When used for transmissible venereal tumor, vincristine is used as sole therapy usually at 0.5 mg/m^2 (maximum dose 1 mg) IV once weekly for 4-6 weeks of therapy.

For adjunctive treatment of immune-mediated thrombocytopenia:

a) 0.5 mg/m^2 IV if platelet count <10-20,000 cells/mcL or bleeding; consider bone marrow aspiration to document presence of megakaryocytes. (Saxon 2008)

b) If refractory to prednisone (3–5 days), give vincristine at 0.5–0.7 mg/m^2 IV bolus or as an infusion over 4–6 hours. (Trepanier 1999)

c) 0.02 mg/kg IV once; generally single use (Cohn 2004)

■ **CATS:**

For neoplastic diseases; (consultation with a veterinary oncologist is encouraged before use; see above): Vincristine is usually dosed in cats at 0.5–0.75 mg/m^2 (*NOT* mg/kg) IV and administered every 1-3 weeks.

■ **HORSES:**

For neoplastic diseases; consultation with a veterinary oncologist is encouraged before use:

a) Usual doses used in horses are: 0.5 mg/m^2 (usually 2.5–3 mg total dose per horse) IV weekly. For generalized lymphoma the CAP protocol was used at the time of publication by one of the authors: cytarabine (cytosine arabinoside) at an average dose of 1–1.2 grams (total dose), SC or IM once every 1–2 weeks; cyclophosphamide at a dose of 1 gram (total dose) IV every 2 weeks (alternating with cytarabine); and prednisolone at a dose of 1 mg/kg PO every other day. Vincristine at 2.5 mg (total dose) IV is added on the weeks when the cytarabine is administered if there is no response. These are starting doses; the total doses can be increased by 20–30% without expecting complications. With remission, the starting doses are maintained for 2–3 months and then the horse is switched onto a maintenance protocol. The first cycle of maintenance therapy increases the treatment interval for each drug by one week (except prednisolone which is kept at the same frequency but with a reducing dose). If horse is still in remission after 2–3 months of the first cycle, the second cycle is begun by adding a further week to the treatment intervals of each drug. (Mair & Couto 2006)

Monitoring

■ Efficacy (tumor burden reduction or platelet count)

■ Toxicity (peripheral neuropathic clinical signs; complete blood counts with platelets; liver function tests prior to therapy and repeated as necessary; serum uric acid)

Client Information

■ Clients must be briefed on the possibilities of severe toxicity developing from this drug, including drug-related mortality

■ Clients should contact the veterinarian if the patient exhibits any signs of profound depression, abnormal bleeding (including bloody diarrhea) and/or bruising, severe constipation, or severe peripheral neuropathic signs

■ Avoid contact with treated patient's urine, saliva or feces after treatment. Vincristine or metabolites have been detected in dogs' urine up to 7 days after treatment.

Chemistry/Synonyms

Commonly referred to as a Vinca alkaloid, vincristine sulfate is isolated from the plant *Cantharanthus roseus* (*Vinca rosea Linn*) and occurs as a white or slightly yellow, hygroscopic, amorphous or crystalline powder that is freely soluble in water and slightly soluble in alcohol. The commercially available injection has a pH of 3–5.5. Vincristine sulfate has pK$_a$s of 5 and 7.4

Vincristine Sulfate may also be known as: leurocristine sulfate, VCR, LCR compound 37231, leurocristine sulphate, NSC-67574, 22-oxovincaleukoblastine sulphate, sulfato de vincristina, vincristini sulfas and *Oncovin®*; many other trade names are available.

Storage/Stability

Vincristine sulfate injection should be protected from light and stored in the refrigerator (2–8°C).

Compatibility/Compounding Considerations

Vincristine sulfate is reportedly physically **compatible** with the following intravenous solutions and drugs: D$_5$W, bleomycin sulfate, cytarabine, fluorouracil, and methotrexate sodium. In syringes or at Y-sites with: bleomycin sulfate, cisplatin, cyclophosphamide, doxorubicin HCl, droperidol, fluorouracil, heparin sodium, leucovorin calcium, methotrexate sodium, metoclopramide HCl, mitomycin, and vinblastine sulfate.

Vincristine sulfate is reportedly physically **incompatible** with furosemide. Compatibility is dependent upon factors such as pH, concentration, temperature, and diluent used; consult specialized references or a hospital pharmacist for more specific information.

Dosage Forms/Regulatory Status

VETERINARY-LABELED PRODUCTS: None

HUMAN-LABELED PRODUCTS:

Vincristine Sulfate Injection: 1 mg/mL in 1 mL, 2 mL & 5 mL vials and flip-top vials; *Vincasar® PFS* (Sicor); generic; (Rx)

References

Argyle, D., M. Brearly, et al. (2008). *Decision Making in Small Animal Oncology*, Wiley-Blackwell.

Cohn, L. (2004). Immune mediated blood dyscrasias: Therapeutic options. Proceedings: ACVIM Forum. Accessed via: Veterinary Information Network. http://goo.gl/iGm0U

Henry, C. & M. Higginbotham (2009). *Cancer Management in Small Animal Practice*, Saunders.

Hughes, K., T.J. Scase, et al. (2009). Vincristine overdose in a cat: clinical management, use of calcium folinate, and pathological lesions. *Journal of Feline Medicine and Surgery* 11(4): 322–325.

Mair, T.S. & C.G. Couto (2006). The use of cytotoxic drugs in equine practice. *Equine Veterinary Education* 18(3): 149–156.

Ogilvie, G. & A. Moore (2001). *Feline Oncology: A Comprehensive Guide to Compassionate Care*, Veterinary Learning Systems.

Ogilvie, G. & A. Moore (2006). *Managing the Canine Cancer Patient: A Practical Guide to Compassionate Care*, Veterinary Learning Systems.

Papich, M. (1989). Effects of drugs on pregnancy. *Current Veterinary Therapy X: Small Animal Practice*. R Kirk Ed. Philadelphia, Saunders: 1291–1299.

Polton, G.A. & C.M. Elwood (2008). Pulmonary oedema as a suspected adverse drug reaction following vincristine administration to a cat: A case report. *Veterinary Journal* 177(1): 130–133.

Saxon, W. (2008). Thrombocytopenia & Other Platelet Disorders. Proceedings: WVC. Accessed via: Veterinary Information Network. http://goo.gl/ZNM0g

Trepanier, L. (1999). Practical tips in immunosuppressive therapy. American Animal Hospital Association: Proceedings from the 1999 Annual Meeting, Denver.

Villalobos, A. (2007). *Canine and Feline Geriatric Oncology*. Ames, Blackwell.

Withrow, S. & D. Vail (2007). *Withrow and MacEwen's Small Animal Clinical Oncology 4th Ed*. Philadelphia, Elsevier.

WSU-VetClinPharmLab (2009). "Problem Drugs." http://goo.gl/aIGlM.

VITAMIN E/SELENIUM
VITAMIN E

(se-*lee*-nee-um)

NUTRITIONAL; FAT SOLUBLE VITAMIN

Prescriber Highlights

► Lipid-soluble vitamin (E) with or without selenium used alone for discoid lupus erythematosus, canine demodicosis, acanthosis nigricans, hepatic fibrosis, or adjunctive therapy of exocrine pancreatic deficiency or hepatopathy in dogs & cats; used in combination for selenium-tocopherol deficiency (white muscle disease)

► Contraindications: Vitamin E/selenium products should only be used in the species for which they are FDA-approved

► Selenium overdoses can be extremely toxic

► Adverse Effects: Anaphylactoid reactions; IM injections may cause transient muscle soreness. Selenium ODs can cause depression, ataxia, dyspnea, blindness, diarrhea, muscle weakness, & a "garlic" odor on the breath

Uses/Indications

Depending on the actual product and species, vitamin E/selenium is indicated for the treatment or prophylaxis of selenium-tocopherol deficiency (STD) syndromes in ewes and lambs (white muscle disease), sows, weanling and baby pigs (hepatic necrosis, mulberry heart disease, white muscle disease), calves and breeding cows (white muscle disease), and horses (myositis associated with STD).

Vitamin E may be useful as adjunctive treatment of discoid lupus erythematosus, canine demodicosis, and acanthosis nigricans in dogs. It may also be of benefit in the adjunctive treatment of hepatic fibrosis or adjunctive therapy of copper-associated hepatopathy in dogs. There is some evidence that vitamin E and silymarin have synergistic effects on hepatocytes. Some dogs and cats with dilated cardiomyopathy have low vitamin E levels, but it is unknown if vitamin E supplementation has any clinical effect.

Pharmacology/Actions

Both vitamin E and selenium are involved with cellular metabolism of sulfur. Vitamin E has antioxidant properties and, with selenium, protects against red blood cell hemolysis and prevents the action of peroxidase on unsaturated bonds in cell membranes.

Pharmacokinetics

After absorption, vitamin E is transported in the circulatory system via beta-lipoproteins. It is distributed to all tissues and stored in adipose tissue. Vitamin E is only marginally transported across the placenta. Vitamin E is metabolized in the liver and excreted primarily into the bile. Absorption of vitamin E may be impaired in patients with severe cholestatic liver disease or in animals with fat malabsorption syndromes.

Pharmacokinetic parameters for selenium were not located.

Contraindications/Precautions/Warnings

Vitamin E/selenium products should only be used in the species for which they are FDA-approved. Because selenium can be extremely toxic, the promiscuous use of these products cannot be condoned.

Give slowly when administering intravenously to horses.

Adverse Effects

Anaphylactoid reactions have been reported. Intramuscular injections may be associated with transient muscle soreness. Other adverse effects are generally associated with overdoses of selenium (see below).

Overdosage/Acute Toxicity

Selenium is quite toxic in overdose quantities, but has a fairly wide safety margin. Cattle have tolerated chronic doses of 0.6 mg/kg/day with no adverse effects (approximate therapeutic dose is 0.06 mg/kg). Clinical signs of selenium toxicity include depression, ataxia, dyspnea, blindness, diarrhea, muscle weakness, and a "garlic" odor on the breath. Horses suffering from selenium toxicity may become blind, paralyzed, slough their hooves, and lose hair from the tail and mane. Dogs may exhibit clinical signs of anorexia, vomiting, and diarrhea at high dosages.

Large overdoses of vitamin E can cause coagulopathies.

Drug Interactions

The following drug interactions have either been reported or are theoretical in humans or animals receiving vitamin E/selenium and may be of significance in veterinary patients:

■ **IRON:** Large doses of vitamin E may delay the hematologic response to iron therapy in patients with iron deficiency anemia.

■ **MINERAL OIL:** May reduce the absorption of orally administered vitamin E

■ **VITAMIN A:** Absorption, utilization and storage may be enhanced by vitamin E

■ **WARFARIN:** Vitamin E may increase the effects of warfarin

Doses (Vitamin E alone):

For doses of vitamin E/selenium products see the Dosage Form section

■ **DOGS:**

For adjunctive treatment of discoid lupus erythematosus, canine demodicosis or acanthosis nigricans:

a) 200–400 Units PO three times daily; variable efficacy, but relatively innocuous at these dosages (White 2000)

For adjunctive treatment of cholestatic hepatopathies; necro-inflammatory hepatopathies:

a) 10−15 Units/kg per day PO as alpha-tocopherol acetate. (Webster & Cooper 2009)

For adjunctive treatment of copper-associated hepatopathy:

a) 400−600 Units PO per day (Johnson, S. 2000)

For treatment of tocopherol deficiency associated with exocrine pancreatic disease:

a) 100−400 Units PO once daily for one month then every 1−2 weeks as needed (Williams 2000)

■ **CATS:**

For treatment of tocopherol deficiency associated with exocrine pancreatic disease:

a) 30 Units PO once daily for one month then every 1−2 weeks as needed (Williams 2000)

For adjunctive treatment of hepatic lipidosis:

a) 10 Units/kg once PO once daily. (Scherk & Center 2005)

■ **HORSES:**

For adjunctive treatment of ionophore (monensin) toxicity:

a) 4−12 Units/kg PO once daily (Mogg 1999)

For adjunctive therapy for EPM:

a) 8000−9000 Units PO per day (Dowling 1999)

For adjunctive therapy for metabolic syndrome:

a) 10,000 Units PO once daily (Johnson, P. 2003)

For adjunctive treatment of perinatal asphyxia syndrome (hypoxic ischemic encephalopathy):

a) Foals: 4,000 Units PO once daily; Mares: 10,000 Units PO once daily (Slovis 2003)

Monitoring

■ Clinical efficacy

■ Blood selenium levels (when using the combination product). Normal values for selenium have been reported as: >1.14 micromol/L in calves, >0.63 micromol/L in cattle, >1.26 micromol/L in sheep, and >0.6 micromol/L in pigs. Values indicating deficiency are: <0.40 micromol/L in cattle, <0.60 micromol/L in sheep, and <0.20 micromol/L in pigs. Intermediate values may result in suboptimal production

■ Optionally, glutathione peroxidase activity may be monitored

Chemistry/Synonyms

Vitamin E is a lipid soluble vitamin that can be found in either liquid or solid forms. The liquid forms occur as clear, yellow to brownish red, viscous oils that are insoluble in water, soluble in alcohol and miscible with vegetable oils. Solid forms occur as white to tan-white granular powders that disperse in water to form cloudy suspensions. Vitamin E may also be known as alpha tocopherol.

Selenium in commercially available veterinary injections is found as sodium selenite. Each mg of sodium selenite contains approximately 460 micrograms (46%) of selenium.

Storage/Stability

Vitamin E/Selenium for injection should be stored at temperatures less than 25°C (77°F).

Dosage Forms/Regulatory Status

VETERINARY-LABELED PRODUCTS:

Vitamin E (Alone) Injection

Vitamin E Injection: 300 mg/mL in 250 mL vials; *Emulsivit® E-300* (Vedco); *Vital E®-300* (Schering-Plough); (OTC or Rx)

Vitamin E/Selenium Oral

Equ-SeE® (Vet-A-Mix) (one teaspoonful contains 1 mg selenium and 220 Units vitamin E) and *Equ-Se5E®* (one teaspoonful contains 1 mg selenium and approximately 1100 Units vitamin E); (Vet-a-Mix); (OTC) FDA-approved for oral use in horses.

Other top dress equine products containing Vitamin E and Selenium include: Vitamin E and Selenium Powder (Farnam, Horse Health), *Vitamin E and Selenium Crumbles®* (Horse Health)

Vitamin E/Selenium Injection

Mu-Se® (Schering); (Rx): Each mL contains: selenium 5 mg (as sodium selenite); Vitamin E 68 Units; 100 mL vial for injection. FDA-approved for use in non-lactating dairy cattle and beef cattle. Slaughter withdrawal (at labeled doses) = 30 days. Dose: For weanling calves: 1 mL per 200 lbs. body weight IM or SC. For breeding beef cows: 1 mL per 200 lbs. body weight during middle third of pregnancy and 30 days before calving IM or SC.

Bo-Se® (Schering); (Rx): Each mL contains selenium 1 mg (as sodium selenite) and Vitamin E 68 Units; 100 mL vial for injection. FDA-approved for use in calves, swine and sheep. Slaughter withdrawal (at labeled doses) = 30 days (calves); 14 days (lambs, ewes, sows, and pigs). Dose: Calves: 2.5–3.75 mL/100 lbs body weight (depending on severity of condition and geographical area) IM or SC. Lambs (2 weeks of age or older): 1 mL per 40 lbs. body weight IM or SC (1 mL minimum). Ewes: 2.5 mL/100 lbs. body weight IM or SC. Sows and weanling pigs: 1mL/40 lbs. body weight IM or SC (1 mL minimum). Do not use on newborn pigs.

L-Se® (Schering); (Rx): Each mL contains: selenium 0.25 mg (as sodium selenite) and Vitamin E 68 Units in 30 mL vials. FDA-approved for use in lambs and baby pigs. Slaughter withdrawal (at labeled doses) = 14 days. Dose: Lambs: 1 mL SC or IM in newborns and 4 mL SC or IM in lambs 2 weeks of age or older; Baby Pigs: 1 mL SC or IM.

E-Se® (Schering); (Rx): Each mL contains selenium 2.5 mg (as sodium selenite) and Vitamin E 68 Units in 100 mL vials. FDA-approved for use in horses. Dose: Equine: 1 mL/100 lbs. body weight slow IV or deep IM (in 2 or more sites; gluteal or cervical muscles). May be repeated at 5–10 day intervals.

Seletoc® (Schering); (Rx): Each mL contains selenium 1 mg (as sodium selenite) and Vitamin E 68 Units in 10 mL vials. FDA-approved for use in dogs. Dose: Dogs: Initially, 1 mL per 20 pounds of body weight (minimum 0.25 mL; maximum 5 mL) SC, or IM in divided doses in 2 or more sites. Repeat dose at 3 day intervals until satisfactory results then switch to maintenance dose. If no response in 14 days reevaluate. Maintenance dose: 1 mL per 40 lbs body weight (minimum 0.25 mL) repeat at 3–7 day intervals (or longer) to maintain.

HUMAN-LABELED PRODUCTS:

Vitamin E Tablets: 100 Units, 200 Units, 400 Units, 500 Units & 800 Units; generic (various; OTC)

Vitamin E Capsules: 100 Units, 200 Units, 400 Units & 1000 Units; *Mixed E 400 Softgels®* & *d'ALPHA E 1000 Softgels®* (Naturally); *Vita-Plus E®* (Scot-Tussin); generic; (OTC)

Vitamin E Drops: 15 Units/0.3 mL in 12 mL & 30 mL; *Aquasol E®* (Mayne Pharma); *Aquavit-E®* (Cypress); (OTC)

Vitamin E Liquid: 15 Units/30 mL in 30 mL, 60 mL & 120 mL; 798 Units/30 mL in 473 mL; Vitamin E (Freeda); *Nutr-E-Sol®* (Advanced Nutritional Technology); (OTC)

Topicals are available. There are no FDA-approved vitamin E/selenium products, but there are many products that contain either vitamin E (alone, or in combination with other vitamins ± minerals) or selenium (as an injection alone or in combination with other trace elements) available.

References

Dowling, P. (1999). Clinical pharmacology of nervous system diseases. *The Veterinary Clinics of North America: Equine Practice* **15**:3(December): 575–588.

Johnson, P. (2003). Metabolic syndrome in horses. Proceedings: ACVIM Forum. Accessed via: Veterinary Information Network. http://goo.gl/KRXvm

Johnson, S. (2000). Chronic Hepatic Disorders. *Textbook of Veterinary Internal Medicine: Diseases of the Dog and Cat.* S Ettinger and E Feldman Eds. Philadelphia, WB Saunders. **2**: 1298–1325.

Mogg, T. (1999). Equine Cardiac Disease: Clinical pharmacology and therapeutics. *The Veterinary Clinics of North America: Equine Practice* **15**:3(December).

Scherk, M. & S. Center (2005). Toxic, metabolic, infections, and neoplastic liver diseases. *Textbook of Veterinary Internal Medicine, 6th Ed.* S Ettinger and E Feldman Eds., Elsevier: 1464–1478.

Slovis, N. (2003). Perinatal asphyxia syndrome (Hypoxic ischemic encephalopathy). Proceedings: ACVIM Forum. Accessed via: Veterinary Information Network. http://goo.gl/l6TgF

Webster, C.R.L. & J. Cooper (2009). Therapeutic Use of Cytoprotective Agents in Canine and Feline Hepatobiliary Disease. *Veterinary Clinics of North America-Small Animal Practice* **39**(3): 631–+.

White, S. (2000). Veterinary Dermatology: New Treatments, 'New' Diseases. Proceedings: The North American Veterinary Conference, Orlando.

Williams, D. (2000). Exocrine Pancreatic Disease. *Textbook of Veterinary Internal Medicine: Diseases of the Dog and Cat.* S Ettinger and E Feldman Eds. Philadelphia, WB Saunders. **2**: 1345–1367.

VORICONAZOLE

(vor-ih-*koh*-nah-zohl)   Vfend®

SECOND GENERATION TRIAZOLE ANTIFUNGAL

Prescriber Highlights

▶ Broad-spectrum oral/parenteral triazole antifungal

▶ Very little clinical experience thus far in veterinary medicine; extremely expensive

▶ Cats appear to be susceptible to adverse effects. Until further pharmacokinetic and safety studies can be done, it should only used in cats as a last resort.

▶ Like other compounds in this class, there are many potential drug interactions

Uses/Indications

Voriconazole may be a useful treatment for a variety of fungal infections in veterinary patients, particularly against *Blastomyces, Cryptococcus,* and *Aspergillus.* It has high oral bioavailability in a variety of species and can cross into the CNS. Currently available human dosage forms are extremely expensive, however, and little clinical experience has occurred using voriconazole in veterinary patients. There is considerable interest in using voriconazole for treating aspergillosis in pet birds as their relative small size may allow the drug to be affordable; additional research must be performed before dosing regimens are available.

Pharmacology/Actions

Voriconazole a synthetic derivative of fluconazole, has broad-spectrum antifungal activity against a variety of organisms, including *Candida, Aspergillus, Trichosporon, Histoplasma, Cryptococcus, Blastomyces,* and *Fusarium* species. Like the other azole/triazole antifungals it inhibits cytochrome P-450-dependent 14-alpha-sterol demethylase that is required for ergosterol biosynthesis in fungal cell walls. Unlike fluconazole, voriconazole also inhibits 24-methylene dehydrolanosterol demethylation in molds such as *Aspergillus* giving it more activity against these fungi.

Pharmacokinetics

In dogs, voriconazole is rapidly and essentially completely absorbed after oral administration. Peak levels occur about 3 hours after oral dosing. Voriconazole is only moderately (51%) bound to canine plasma proteins and volume of distribution is about 1.3 L/kg. It is metabolized in the liver to a variety of metabolites with the N-oxide metabolite being the primary circulating metabolite. This metabolite has only weak (<100X as active as the parent) antifungal activity. The elimination pharmacokinetics of voriconazole in dogs is very complex. Both dose-dependent non-linear elimination and auto-induced metabolism after multiple dosages are seen complicating any dosage regimen scenarios; dosages may need to be increased over time. Auto-induction of metabolism apparently does not occur in humans, rabbits or guinea pigs.

In horses, voriconazole is well absorbed after oral administration with peak levels occurring at approximately 1-3 hours post-dose. Voriconazole has low protein binding (31%); volume of distribution is about 1.35-1.6 L/kg. The drug is distributed into the CSF, tears and synovial fluid. Elimination half-life is quite long—approximately 13 hours after oral dosing. It is not known if voriconazole self-induces hepatic metabolism after multiple doses in the horse.

After single oral doses to alpacas, voriconazole had a low bioavailability (approx. 24%), but IV doses of 4 mg/kg yielded plasma levels above 0.1 micrograms/mL for at least 24 hours. Elimination half-life is about 8 hours (Chan *et al.* 2009).

In Hispaniolan Amazon parrots, oral voriconazole had a short half-life (about one hour). The authors concluded that the drug could be safely administered to this species at a dose of 18 mg/kg PO q8h for 11 days, but that further studies were necessary to determine safety and efficacy of long-term treatment (Guzman *et al.* 2010).

Contraindications/Precautions/Warnings

Voriconazole is contraindicated in patients hypersensitive to it other azole antifungals. It should be given with caution to patients with hepatic dysfunction, or proarrhythmic conditions.

The intravenous product contains 3200 mg of sulfobutyl ether beta-cyclodextrin sodium (SBECD) per vial. This compound can accumulate in patients with decreased renal function.

Adverse Effects

Accurate adverse effect profiles are unknown for veterinary species. Liver enlargement and up to a 2–3 fold increase in cytochrome P450 hepatic microsomal enzyme concentrations were noted in dogs orally dosed for 30 days. This may significantly impact the metabolism of other drugs that are hepatically metabolized (See Drug Interactions).

Two cats initially treated with 10 mg/kg PO once daily developed significant adverse reactions, including azotemia, inappetence, lethargy, and weight loss. One developed a presumed cutaneous drug reaction which resolved when voriconazole was discontinued and the other cat developed ataxia and hind limb paresis (Smith & Hoffman 2010). In another published case report (Quimby *et al.* 2010), three cats receiving voriconazole at doses from 10–13 mg/kg PO once daily developed neurologic signs that included: ataxia in all subjects; 2 of the 3 cats developed paraplegia of hind limbs, 2 of the 3 cats had visual signs (mydriasis, decreased or absent pupillary light responses, and reduced menace response). One cat developed an arrhythmia and in one cat, hypokalemia was noted.

In humans, commonly encountered adverse effects include visual disturbances (blurring, spots, wavy lines) usually within 30 minutes of dosing or if higher drug concentrations are attained, and rashes (usually mild to moderate in severity). Less frequent adverse effects include gastrointestinal effects (nausea, vomiting, diarrhea), hepatotoxicity (jaundice, abnormal liver function tests), hypertension/hypotension, tachycardia, peripheral edema, hypokalemia, and hypomagnesemia. Rarely, eye hemorrhage, anemia, leukopenia, thrombocytopenia, pancytopenia, QT prolongation, torsade de pointes, and nephrotoxicity have been reported.

Reproductive/Nursing Safety

Voriconazole was teratogenic in rats at low dosages (10 mg/kg) and embryotoxic in rabbits at higher dosages (100 mg/kg). In humans, the FDA categorizes voriconazole as category *D* for use during pregnancy *(There is evidence of human fetal risk, but the potential benefits from the use of the drug in pregnant women may be acceptable despite its potential risks.)* Weigh the risks of treatment versus the benefits when considering use in pregnant patients.

It is unknown if voriconazole enters milk.

Overdosage/Acute Toxicity

The minimum lethal dose in rats and mice was 300 mg/kg (4–7X maintenance dose). Toxic effects included increased salivation, mydriasis, ataxia, depression, dyspnea, and seizures. Accidental single overdoses of up to 5X in human pediatric patients caused only brief photophobia. No antidote is known for voriconazole overdoses. Gut emptying should be considered for very large oral overdoses, followed by close observation and supportive treatment if required.

Drug Interactions

There are many potential drug interactions involving voriconazole. The following partial listing includes reported or theoretical interactions in humans receiving voriconazole that may also be of significance in veterinary patients. Because, in dogs, voriconazole induces hepatic microsomal enzymes (in humans it does not) additional interactions and further clarification may be reported as clinical use increases in veterinary patients.

■ **ANTIDIABETIC AGENTS (sulfonylureas):** Voriconazole may increase serum concentrations of these drugs and increase risk for hypoglycemia

■ **BARBITURATES (phenobarbital):** Decreased voriconazole concentrations; use together contraindicated

■ **BENZODIAZEPINES:** Voriconazole may increase benzodiazepine concentrations

■ **CALCIUM-CHANNEL BLOCKERS (amlodipine, diltiazem, verapamil):** Voriconazole may increase serum concentrations, dosage adjustment may be required

■ **CARBAMAZEPINE:** Decreased voriconazole concentrations; use together contraindicated

■ **CISAPRIDE:** Potential for serious cardiac arrhythmias; use is contraindicated

■ **CORTICOSTEROIDS (prednisolone):** Potentially increased AUC for prednisolone

■ **IMMUNOSUPPRESSIVE AGENTS (systemic: cyclosporine, tacrolimus):** Increased cyclosporine and tacrolimus concentrations; decrease cyclosporine dosage by 50% when starting voriconazole; decrease tacrolimus dosage by 33% when starting voriconazole

■ **METHADONE:** Voriconazole may increase plasma concentrations of R-methadone; monitor for methadone toxicity and adjust dosage if necessary

■ **PHENYTOIN:** Can decrease voriconazole concentrations and voriconazole can increase phenytoin concentrations; monitoring and dosage adjustment may be required

■ **PIMOZIDE:** Potential for serious cardiac arrhythmias; use is contraindicated

■ **PROTON-PUMP INHIBITORS (omeprazole):** Voriconazole may increase omeprazole (and potentially other PPI's) concentrations

■ **QUINIDINE:** Potential for serious cardiac arrhythmias; use is contraindicated

■ **RIFAMPIN, RIFABUTIN:** Decreased voriconazole concentrations; use together contraindicated

■ **VINCA ALKALOIDS (vincristine, vinblastine):** Possible increased Vinca alkaloid concentrations; monitor for toxicity

■ **WARFARIN:** Voriconazole may potentiate warfarin's effects

Laboratory Considerations

■ No specific concerns were noted; see Monitoring for additional information.

Doses

■ **DOGS:**
a) For coccidioidomycosis: 4 mg/kg PO q12h. (Graupmann-Kuzma et al. 2008)

■ **CATS:**
a) From a published case report in 3 cats: Two of the cats were treated with oral voriconazole for orbital aspergillosis initially at 10 mg/kg PO once daily. Both responded to treatment, but significant systemic reactions were noted. Authors concluded that based on their experience, voriconazole should be used with caution as adverse side effects may be common. (Smith & Hoffman 2010)

■ **HORSES:**
a) Based upon pharmacokinetic studies, doses of 3 mg/kg PO q24h should be sufficient to treat aspergillosis, but higher doses (4–5 mg/kg) are probably necessary to treat infections with *Fusarium* spp. However, clinical experience is lacking, and the drug is currently too expensive for practical use. (Davis 2008)

■ **BIRDS:**
a) Based upon this pharmacokinetic study in Hispaniolan Amazon parrots the authors concluded that the drug could be safely administered to this species at a dose of 18 mg/kg PO q8h for 11 days, but that further studies were necessary to determine safety and efficacy of long-term treatment (Guzman *et al.* 2010).

b) For avian aspergillosis: 12.5 mg/kg PO twice daily for 60-90 days or by nebulization as a 1 mg/mL solution for 60 minutes once daily. (Black 2008)

Monitoring

■ Efficacy

■ Liver function tests, serum electrolytes

Client Information

■ Inform clients of the investigational nature of using this drug in veterinary species and the associated expense

■ Give at least one hour before or one hour after feeding

■ Because experience with this medication has been limited, report any possible adverse effects to the veterinarian immediately, including itching/rash, yellowing of whites of the eyes, reduced appetite, difficulty walking, vision problems, etc.

Chemistry/Synonyms

A triazole antifungal, voriconazole occurs as a white to light colored powder with a molecular weight of 349.3. Aqueous solubility is 0.7 mg/mL.

Voriconazole may also be known as UK-109496, voriconazol, voraconazolum, or *Vfend®*.

Storage/Stability

Voriconazole tablets should be stored at 15–30°C.

The unreconstituted powder for oral suspension should be stored in the refrigerator

(2–8°C); it has a shelf-life of approximately 18 months. Once reconstituted, it should be stored in tightly closed containers at room temperature (15–30°C); do not refrigerate or freeze. After reconstitution, the suspension is stable for 14 days. The suspension should be shaken well for 10 seconds prior to each administered dose.

The powder for injection should be stored at room temperature (15–30°C). After reconstituting with 19 mL of sterile water for injection, the manufacturer recommends using immediately; however, chemical and physical stability remain for up to 24 hours if stored in the refrigerator (2–8°C). Discard solution if it is not clear or particles are visible.

Compatibility/Compounding Considerations
The injectable solution must be further diluted to a concentration of 5mg/mL or less for administration over 1–2 hours. Suitable diluents for IV infusion include (partial list): NS, LRS, D5LRS, and D5W. Voriconazole is **not compatible** with simultaneous infusion with blood products.

Voriconazole tablets can be crushed and made into a 2.5 mg/mL oral suspension by mixing a crushed tablet with 25:75 *v/v* water:*OraPlus®* (Paddock Labs). This suspension will pass through a 10-French feeding needle. To prepare, mix a crushed 200-mg tablet with 20 mL water and then add 60 mL *OraPlus®*. The suspension should be thoroughly vortex-mixed or shaken until no particles are visible (usually takes 2-3 minutes) and then for ~30-60 seconds before each use. The suspension is stable under refrigeration for 14 days. (Guzman *et al.* 2010), (Flammer 2008)

Dosage Forms/Regulatory Status
VETERINARY-LABELED PRODUCTS: None

HUMAN-LABELED PRODUCTS:

Voriconazole Tablets: 50 mg & 200 mg; *Vfend®* (Roerig); (Rx)

Voriconazole Powder for Oral Suspension: 45 grams (40 mg/mL after reconstitution); in 100 mL bottles; *Vfend®* (Roerig); (Rx)

Voriconazole Powder for Injection, Lyophilized: 200 mg in single-use vials; *Vfend I.V.®* (Roerig); (Rx). Also contains 3200 mg of sulfobutyl ether beta-cyclodextrin sodium (SBECD) per vial (See Warnings) to solubolize the drug for IV administration.

References
Black, D. (2008). Avian Aspergillosis. Proceedings: UEP. Accessed via: Veterinary Information Network. http://goo.gl/XK2xx

Chan, H.M., S.H. Duran, et al. (2009). Pharmacokinetics of voriconazole after single dose intravenous and oral administration to alpacas. *Journal of Veterinary Pharmacology and Therapeutics* 32(3): 235–240.

Davis, J. (2008). The use of antifungals. *Comp Equine*(April): 128–133.

Flammer, K. (2008). Avian Mycoses: Managing those difficult cases. Proceedings: AAV. Accessed via: Veterinary Information Network. http://goo.gl/iDsnR

Graupmann-Kuzma, A., B.A. Valentine, et al. (2008).

Coccidioidomycosis in dogs and cats: A review. *Journal of the American Animal Hospital Association* 44(5): 226–235.

Guzman, D.S.M., K. Flammer, et al. (2010). Pharmacokinetics of voriconazole after oral administration of single and multiple doses in Hispaniolan Amazon parrots (Amazona ventralis). *American Journal of Veterinary Research* 71(4): 460–467.

Quimby, J.M., S.B. Hoffman, et al. (2010). Adverse Neurologic Events Associated with Voriconazole Use in 3 Cats. *Journal of Veterinary Internal Medicine* 24(3): 647–649.

Smith, L.N. & S.B. Hoffman (2010). A case series of unilateral orbital aspergillosis in three cats and treatment with voriconazole. *Veterinary Ophthalmology* 13(3): 190–203.

WARFARIN SODIUM

(*war*-far-in)   Coumadin®

ANTICOAGULANT

Prescriber Highlights

▶ Coumarin derivative anticoagulant used primarily for long-term treatment (or prevention of recurrence) of thrombotic conditions, primarily in cats, dogs, or horses

▶ Contraindications: Preexistent hemorrhage, pregnancy, those undergoing or contemplating eye or CNS surgery, major regional lumbar block anesthesia, surgery of large, open surfaces, active bleeding from the GI, respiratory, or GU tract; aneurysm, acute nephritis, cerebrovascular hemorrhage, blood dyscrasias, uncontrolled or malignant hypertension, hepatic insufficiency, pericardial effusion, & visceral carcinomas

▶ Adverse Effects: Dose-related hemorrhage

▶ Teratogenic; contraindicated in pregnancy

▶ Must actively monitor coagulation status

▶ Many potentially significant drug interactions

Uses/Indications
In veterinary medicine, warfarin is used primarily for the oral, long-term treatment (or prevention of recurrence) of thrombotic conditions, primarily in cats, dogs, or horses. Use of warfarin in veterinary species is somewhat controversial and due to unproven benefit in reducing mortality, increased expense associated with monitoring, and potential for serious effects (bleeding), many do not recommend its use.

Pharmacology/Actions
Warfarin acts indirectly as an anticoagulant (it has no direct anticoagulant effect) by interfering with the action of vitamin K_1 in the synthesis of the coagulation factors II, VII, IX, and X.

Sufficient amounts of vitamin K_1 can override this effect. Warfarin is administered as a racemic mixture of S (+) and R (-) warfarin. The S enantiomer is a significantly more potent vitamin K antagonist than the R enantiomer in species studied.

Pharmacokinetics

Warfarin is administered as a racemic mixture of S (+) and R (-) warfarin. Warfarin is rapidly and completely absorbed in humans after oral administration. In cats, warfarin is also rapidly absorbed after oral administration.

After absorption, warfarin is highly bound to plasma proteins in humans, with approximately 99% of the drug bound. In cats, more than 96% of the drug is protein bound. It is reported that there are wide species variations with regard to protein binding; horses have a higher free (unbound) fraction of the drug than do rats, sheep or swine. Only free (unbound) warfarin is active. While other coumarin and indanedione anticoagulants are distributed in milk, warfarin does not enter milk in humans.

Warfarin is principally metabolized in the liver to inactive metabolites that are excreted in urine and bile (and then reabsorbed and excreted in the urine). The plasma half-life of warfarin may be several hours to several days, depending on the patient (and species?). In cats, the terminal half-life of the S enantiomer is approximately 23–28 hours and the R enantiomer approximately 11–18 hours.

Contraindications/Precautions/Warnings

Warfarin is contraindicated in patients with preexistent hemorrhagic tendencies or diseases, those undergoing or contemplating eye or CNS surgery, major regional lumbar block anesthesia, or surgery of large, open surfaces. It should not be used in patients with active bleeding from the GI, respiratory, or GU tract. Other contraindications include: aneurysm, acute nephritis, cerebrovascular hemorrhage, blood dyscrasias, uncontrolled or malignant hypertension, hepatic insufficiency, pericardial effusion, pregnancy, and visceral carcinomas.

Adverse Effects

The principal adverse effect of warfarin use is dose-related hemorrhage, which may manifest with clinical signs of anemia, thrombocytopenia, weakness, hematomas and ecchymoses, epistaxis, hematemesis, hematuria, melena, hematochezia, hemathrosis, hemothorax, intracranial and/or pericardial hemorrhage, and death.

Reproductive/Nursing Safety

Warfarin is embryotoxic, can cause congenital malformations and considered contraindicated during pregnancy. If anticoagulant therapy is required during pregnancy, most clinicians recommend using low-dose heparin. In humans, the FDA categorizes this drug as category *X* for use during pregnancy (*Studies in animals or humans demonstrate fetal abnormalities or adverse reaction; reports indicate evidence of fetal risk. The risk of use in pregnant women clearly outweighs any possible benefit.*) In a separate system evaluating the safety of drugs in canine and feline pregnancy (Papich 1989), this drug is categorized as in class: *D* (*Contraindicated. These drugs have been shown to cause congenital malformations or embryotoxicity.*)

Based on very limited published data, warfarin has not been detected in the breast milk of humans treated, but there are reports of some breast-fed infants whose mothers were treated having prolonged prothrombin times. Use with caution in nursing patients.

Overdosage/Acute Toxicity

Acute overdosages of warfarin may result in life-threatening hemorrhage. In dogs and cats, single doses of 5–50 mg/kg have been associated with toxicity. It must be remembered that a lag time of 2–5 days may occur before signs of toxicity occur, and animals must be monitored and treated accordingly.

Cumulative toxic doses of warfarin have been reported as 1–5 mg/kg for 5–15 days in dogs and 1 mg/kg for 7 days in cats.

If overdosage is detected early, prevent absorption from the gut using standard protocols. If clinical signs are noted, they should be treated with blood products and vitamin K_1 (phytonadione). Refer to the phytonadione monograph for more information.

Drug Interactions

Drug interactions with warfarin are perhaps the most important in human medicine. The following drug interactions have either been reported or are theoretical in humans or animals receiving warfarin and may be of significance in veterinary patients:

A multitude of drugs have been documented or theorized to interact with warfarin. The following drugs or drug classes may **increase** the **anticoagulant response** of warfarin (not necessarily complete):

- **ACETAMINOPHEN**
- **ALLOPURINOL**
- **AMIODARONE**
- **ANABOLIC STEROIDS**
- **AZITHROMYCIN**
- **CHLORAMPHENICOL**
- **CIMETIDINE**
- **CISAPRIDE**
- **CO-TRIMOXAZOLE (trimethoprim/sulfa)**
- **DANAZOL**
- **DIAZOXIDE**
- **ERYTHROMYCIN**
- **ETHACRYNIC ACID**
- **FLUOROQUINOLONES**
- **FLUOXETINE**
- **HEPARIN**
- **METRONIDAZOLE**

- ✖ NSAIDS
- ✖ PENTOXIFYLLINE
- ✖ PROPYLTHIOURACIL
- ✖ QUINIDINE
- ✖ SALICYLATES
- ✖ SERTRALINE
- ✖ SULFONAMIDES
- ✖ THYROID MEDICATIONS
- ✖ ZAFIRLUKAST

The following drugs or drug classes may **decrease** the **anticoagulant response** of warfarin (not necessarily complete):

- ✖ **BARBITURATES (phenobarbital, etc.)**
- ✖ **CORTICOSTEROIDS**
- ✖ **ESTROGENS**
- ✖ **GRISEOFULVIN**
- ✖ **MERCAPTOPURINE**
- ✖ **RIFAMPIN**
- ✖ **SPIRONOLACTONE**
- ✖ **SUCRALFATE**
- ✖ **VITAMIN K**

Should concurrent use of any of the above drugs with warfarin be necessary, enhanced monitoring is required. Refer to other references on drug interactions for more specific information.

Laboratory Considerations

- ✖ Warfarin may cause falsely decreased **theophylline** values if using the Schack and Waxler ultraviolet method of assay

Doses

- ✖ **DOGS:**

  For adjunctive therapy of thromboemboli:

  a) For adjunctive maintenance therapy for venous thrombosis with or without pulmonary thromboembolism (PTE): warfarin may be considered at a dose of 0.22 mg/kg PO q12h initially and then adjusted to achieve a PT prolongation of 1.25 to 1.5 times the pretreatment value. (Lunsford & Mackin 2007)

  b) 0.22 mg/kg PO q12h; target dosage to prolong PT by 1.25–1.5 times the pretreatment value. (Brooks 2000)

  c) For prophylactic use in patients with glomerular disease and severe proteinuria: Initially, 0.22 mg/kg, PO once daily. Monitor PT and adjust dose so that PT is maintained at 1.5 times normal. (Grauer & DiBartola 2000)

- ✖ **CATS:**

  For adjunctive therapy of thromboembolism:

  a) For adjunctive maintenance therapy for venous thrombosis with or without pulmonary thromboembolism (PTE): warfarin may be considered at a dose of 0.5 mg (total dose per cat) PO once daily and then adjusted to achieve a PT prolongation of 1.25 to 1.5 times the pretreatment value.

For maintenance therapy for feline arterial thromboembolism: Aspirin (ultra-low dose 5 mg) is often preferred over warfarin as it is difficult to dose accurately (active enantiomers not evenly distributed in tablets and they must be finely crushed and carefully compounded for precise dosing), and frequent and costly monitoring is required. Pharmacokinetic and pharmacodynamic studies in cats have demonstrated that a warfarin dose of 0.06 to 0.09 mg/kg/day is appropriate. Heparinization is recommended during the first 5 to 7 days that warfarin is administered. (Lunsford & Mackin 2007)

b) For long-term thromboprophylaxis: Initially warfarin at 0.06–0.09 mg/kg per day PO. Due to unequal drug distribution, tablets should be crushed and mixed well. PT, adjusted to international normalized ratio (INR) is used to monitor therapy, but may not be applicable to cats. Overlap heparin and warfarin therapy by at least 4–5 days. Reevaluate anticoagulation status with any change in concurrent drug therapy. (Smith 2004)

c) Initially, 0.25–0.5 mg (total dose) per cat PO once daily. Adjust dosage to prolong PT to twice normal value, or INR to be between 2–3. Overlap therapy with heparin. (Fox 2007)

d) For cardiogenic arterial thromboembolism: 0.25–0.5 mg total dose per cat PO q24h (once daily). If using 1 mg tablets = ¼–½ tab. Heparin (150–250 Units/kg SC q8h should be administered concurrently during the first 4-6 days of warfarin therapy. Cats on warfarin should generally be kept indoors to prevent traumatic events, but these can occur indoors as well. Monitoring is done by evaluating prothrombin time (PT) or INR. Baseline values should be obtained prior to initiating therapy and repeated daily during the first week of therapy then twice weekly for 2-4 weeks. If stable, the PT is repeated weekly for 1-2 months followed by once every 1-3 months. The target range is 1.3-1.6 times baseline value. If using INR, target INR range is typically 2.0-3.0 and monitoring times are the same as for PT. (Hogan 2007)

- ✖ **HORSES:** (**Note:** ARCI UCGFS Class 5 Drug) As an anticoagulant:

  a) For adjunctive treatment of laminitis: 0.0198 mg/kg PO once daily; monitor OSPT (one-step prothrombin time) until prolonged 2–4 seconds beyond baseline (Brumbaugh *et al.* 1999)

  b) Initially, 0.018 mg/kg PO once daily and increase dose by 20% every day until baseline PT is doubled. Final dose rates may be from 0.012 mg/kg to 0.57 mg/kg daily. (Vrins *et al.* 1983)

Monitoring

Note: The frequency of monitoring is controversial, and is dependent on several factors including dose, patient's condition, concomitant problems, etc. See the Dosage section above for more information.

■ While Prothrombin Times (PT) or International Normalized Ratio (INR; not validated for veterinary patients) are most commonly used to monitor warfarin, PIVKA (proteins induced by vitamin K antagonists) has been suggested as being more sensitive. PT's are usually recommended to be 1.5–2X normal and INR's to be between 2–3.

■ Platelet counts and hematocrit (PCV) should be done periodically

■ Occult blood in stool and urine; other observations for bleeding

■ Clinical efficacy

Client Information

■ Clients must be counseled on both the importance of administering the drug as directed

■ Immediately report any signs or symptoms of bleeding

Chemistry/Synonyms

A coumarin derivative, warfarin sodium occurs as a slightly bitter tasting, white, amorphous or crystalline powder. It is very soluble in water and freely soluble in alcohol. The commercially available products contain a racemic mixture of the two optical isomers.

Warfarin Sodium may also be known as: sodium warfarin, warfarinum natricum, *Coumadin®*, *Jantoven®*, or *Panwarfin®*; there are many other trade names internationally.

Storage/Stability

Warfarin sodium tablets should be stored in tight, light-resistant containers at temperatures less than 40°C, preferably at room temperature. Warfarin sodium powder for injection should be protected from light and used immediately after reconstituting.

Compatibility/Compounding Considerations

A method of suspending warfarin tablets in an oral suspension has been described (Enos 1989). To make 30 mL of a 0.25 mg/mL suspension: Crush three 2.5 mg tablets with a mortar and pestle. Add 10 mL glycerin to form a paste; then 10 mL of water; add sufficient amount of dark corn syrup (*Karo®*) to obtain a final volume of 30 mL. Warm gently; shake well and use within 30 days.

Dosage Forms/Regulatory Status

VETERINARY-LABELED PRODUCTS: None

The ARCI (Racing Commissioners International) has designated this drug as a class 5 substance. See the appendix for more information.

HUMAN-LABELED PRODUCTS:

Warfarin Sodium Oral Tablets (scored): 1 mg, 2 mg, 2.5 mg, 3 mg, 4 mg, 5 mg, 6 mg, 7.5 mg & 10 mg; *Coumadin®* (Bristol-Myers Squibb), *Jantoven®* (Upsher-Smith), generic; (Rx)

Warfarin Sodium Powder for Injection, lyophilized: 5.4 mg (2 mg/mL when reconstituted) preservative-free in 5 mg vials; *Coumadin®* (Bristol-Myers Squibb); (Rx)

References

Brooks, M. (2000). Coagulopathies and thrombosis. *Textbook of Veterinary Internal Medicine: Diseases of the Dog and Cat.* S Ettinger and E Feldman Eds. Philadelphia, WB Saunders. **2:** 1829–1841.

Brumbaugh, G., H. Lopez, et al. (1999). The pharmacologic basis for the treatment of laminitis. *The Veterinary Clinics of North America: Equine Practice* **15:**2(August).

Enos, L.R. (1989, Last Update). "Personal Communication."

Fox, P. (2007). Feline thromboembolism—New clinical perspectives. Proceedings: WSAVA World Congress. Accessed via: Veterinary Information Network. http://goo.gl/i0wsm

Grauer, G. & S. DiBartola (2000). Glomerular Disease. *Textbook of Veterinary Internal Medicine: Diseases of the Dog and Cat.* S Ettinger and E Feldman Eds. Philadelphia, WB Saunders. **2:** 1662–1678.

Hogan, D. (2007). Big Hearts and Big Clots in Cats: What's New? Proceedings: ACVIM. Accessed via: Veterinary Information Network. http://goo.gl/OSDnV

Lunsford, K.V. & A.J. Mackin (2007). Thromboembolic therapies in dogs and cats: An evidence-based approach. *Veterinary Clinics of North America-Small Animal Practice* **37**(3): 579–+.

Papich, M. (1989). Effects of drugs on pregnancy. *Current Veterinary Therapy X: Small Animal Practice.* R Kirk Ed. Philadelphia, Saunders: 1291–1299.

Smith, S. (2004). Feline arterial thromboembolism: An update. Proceedings: ACVIM Forum. Accessed via: Veterinary Information Network. http://goo.gl/fJeSR

Vrins, A., G. Carlson, et al. (1983). Warfarin: A review with emphasis on its use in the horse. *Can Vet Jnl* **24:** 211–213.

XYLAZINE HCL

(**zye**-la-zeen)   Rompun®

ALPHA2-ADRENERGIC AGONIST

Prescriber Highlights

▶ Alpha$_2$-adrenergic agonist used for its sedative & analgesic in a variety of species; sometimes used as an emetic in cats

▶ Contraindications: Animals receiving epinephrine or having active ventricular arrhythmias. Extreme caution: preexisting cardiac dysfunction, hypotension or shock, respiratory dysfunction, severe hepatic or renal insufficiency, preexisting seizure disorders, or if severely debilitated. Should generally not be used in the last trimester of pregnancy, particularly in cattle. Do not give to ruminants that are debilitated, dehydrated, or with urinary tract obstruction. Horses may kick after a stimulatory event (usually auditory); use caution. Avoid intra-arterial injection; may cause severe seizures & collapse. Caution in patients treated for intestinal impactions. Use cautiously in horses during the vasoconstrictive development phase of laminitis.

▶ Adverse Effects: *Cats:* emesis, muscle tremors, bradycardia with partial A-V block, reduced respiratory rate, movement in response to sharp auditory stimuli, & increased urination.

▶ Adverse Effects: *Dogs:* Muscle tremors, bradycardia with partial A-V block, reduced respiratory rate, movement in response to sharp auditory stimuli, emesis, bloat from aerophagia which may require decompression.

▶ Adverse Effects: *Horses:* Muscle tremors, bradycardia with partial A-V block, reduced respiratory rate, movement in response to sharp auditory stimuli, sweating, increased intracranial pressure, or decreased mucociliary clearance.

▶ Adverse Effects: *Cattle:* Salivation, ruminal atony, bloating, regurgitation, hypothermia, diarrhea, bradycardia, premature parturition, & ataxia.

▶ Yohimbine, atipamezole, & tolazoline may be used alone or in combination to reverse effects or speed recovery times

▶ Dosages between species can be very different; be certain of product concentration when drawing up into syringe, especially if treating ruminants

▶ Drug Interactions

Uses/Indications

Xylazine is FDA-approved for use in dogs, cats, horses, deer, and elk. It is indicated in dogs, cats, and horses to produce a state of sedation with a shorter period of analgesia, and as a preanesthetic before local or general anesthesia.

Xylazine use in small animals is somewhat controversial and because it can cause arrhythmias, reduce cardiac output, and increase risk for general anesthesia-related death, it is usually reserved for "healthy animals."

Because of the emetic action of xylazine in cats, it is occasionally used to induce vomiting after ingesting toxins.

Pharmacology/Actions

A potent alpha$_2$-adrenergic agonist, xylazine is classified as a sedative/analgesic with muscle relaxant properties. Although xylazine possesses several of the same pharmacologic actions as morphine, it does not cause CNS excitation in cats, horses or cattle, but causes sedation and CNS depression. In horses, the visceral analgesia produced has been demonstrated to be superior to that produced by meperidine, butorphanol or pentazocine.

Xylazine can also have alpha$_1$-agonist activity and is less selective for alpha$_2$-receptors then detomidine, dexmedetomidine or romifidine.

Xylazine causes skeletal muscle relaxation through central mediated pathways. Emesis is often seen in cats, and occasionally in dogs receiving xylazine. While thought to be centrally mediated, neither dopaminergic blockers (*e.g.*, phenothiazines) nor alpha-blockers (yohimbine, tolazoline) block the emetic effect. Xylazine does not cause emesis in horses, cattle, sheep or goats. Xylazine depresses thermoregulatory mechanisms and either hypothermia or hyperthermia is a possibility depending on ambient air temperatures.

Effects on the cardiovascular system include an initial increase in total peripheral resistance with increased blood pressure followed by a longer period of lowered blood pressures (below baseline). A bradycardic effect can be seen with some animals developing a second-degree heart block or other arrhythmias. An overall decrease in cardiac output of up to 30% may be seen. Xylazine has been demonstrated to enhance the arrhythmogenic effects of epinephrine in dogs with or without concurrent halothane.

Xylazine's effects on respiratory function are usually clinically insignificant, but at high dosages it can cause respiratory depression with decreased tidal volumes and respiratory rates, and an overall decreased minute volume. Brachycephalic dogs and horses with upper airway disease may develop dyspnea.

Xylazine can increase blood glucose secondary to decreased serum levels of insulin; in non-diabetic animals, there appears to be little clinical significance associated with this effect.

In horses, sedatory signs include a lowering of

the head with relaxed facial muscles and drooping of the lower lip. The retractor muscle is relaxed in male horses, but unlike acepromazine, no reports of permanent penile paralysis have been reported. Although, the animal may appear to be thoroughly sedated, auditory stimuli may provoke arousal with kicking and avoidance responses.

With regard to the sensitivity of species to xylazine, definite differences are seen. Ruminants are extremely sensitive to xylazine when compared with horses, dogs, or cats. Ruminants generally require approximately $1/10^{th}$ the dosage that is required for horses to exhibit the same effect. In cattle (and occasionally cats and horses), polyuria is seen following xylazine administration, probably because of decreased production of vasopressin (anti-diuretic hormone, ADH). Bradycardia and hypersalivation are also seen in cattle and diminished by pretreating with atropine. Because swine require 20−30 times the ruminant dose, it is not routinely used.

Pharmacokinetics

Absorption is rapid following IM injection, but bioavailabilities are incomplete and variable. Bioavailabilities of 40−48% in horses, 17−73% in sheep, and 52−90% in dogs have been reported after IM administration.

In horses, the onset of action following IV dosage occurs within 1−2 minutes with a maximum effect 3−10 minutes after injection. The duration of effect is dose dependent but may last for approximately 1.5 hours. The serum half-life after a single dose of xylazine is approximately 50 minutes in the horse; recovery times generally take from 2−3 hours.

In dogs and cats, the onset of action following an IM or SC dose is approximately 10−15 minutes, and 3−5 minutes following an IV dose. The analgesic effects may persist for only 15−30 minutes, but the sedative actions may last for 1−2 hours depending on the dose given. The serum half-live of xylazine in dogs has been reported as averaging 30 minutes. Complete recovery after dosing may take 2−4 hours in dogs and cats.

Xylazine is not detected in milk of lactating dairy cattle at 5 and 21 hours post-dose, but the FDA has not approved its use in dairy cattle and no meat or milk withdrawal times have been specified.

Contraindications/Precautions/Warnings

Xylazine is contraindicated in animals receiving epinephrine or having active ventricular arrhythmias. It should be used with extreme caution in animals with preexisting cardiac dysfunction, hypotension or shock, respiratory dysfunction, severe hepatic or renal insufficiency, preexisting seizure disorders, or if severely debilitated. Because it may induce premature parturition, it should generally not be used in the last trimester of pregnancy, particularly in cattle.

Be certain of product concentration when drawing up into syringe, especially if treating ruminants. Do not give to ruminants that are dehydrated, debilitated, or with urinary tract obstruction. It is not FDA-approved for any species to be consumed for food purposes.

Horses have been known to kick after a stimulatory event (usually auditory); use caution. The addition of opioids (e.g., butorphanol) may help temper this effect, but may cause increased risks for hypotension or ileus development. Avoid intra-arterial injection; may cause severe seizures and collapse. The manufacturers warn against using xylazine in conjunction with other tranquilizers. Because this drug may inhibit gastrointestinal motility, use with caution in patients treated for intestinal impactions. Use cautiously in horses during the vasoconstrictive development phase of laminitis as xylazine has been shown to reduce digital flow of blood for about 8 hours after administration.

Adverse Effects

Emesis is generally seen within 3−5 minutes after xylazine administration in cats and occasionally in dogs. To prevent aspiration, do not induce further anesthesia until this time has lapsed. Other adverse effects listed in the package insert (*Gemini*®, Butler) for dogs and cats include: muscle tremors, bradycardia with partial A-V block, reduced respiratory rate, movement in response to sharp auditory stimuli, and increased urination in cats.

Xylazine can reduce tear production in cats and cause diuresis in dogs.

Dogs may develop bloat from aerophagia that may require decompression. Because of gaseous distention of the stomach, xylazine's use before radiography can make test interpretation difficult.

Adverse effects listed in the package insert (*AnaSed*®, Lloyd) for horses include: muscle tremors, bradycardia with partial A-V block, reduced respiratory rate, movement in response to sharp auditory stimuli, and sweating (rarely profuse). Additionally, horses receiving xylazine may develop transient hypertension, or decreased mucociliary clearance rates.

Adverse reactions reported in cattle include: salivation, ruminal atony, bloating and regurgitation, hypothermia, diarrhea, and bradycardia. Hypersalivation and bradycardia may be alleviated by pretreating with atropine.

Large animals may become ataxic following dosing and caution should be observed.

Reproductive/Nursing Safety

Limited information was located on the safety of xylazine in pregnancy; apparently, there are no reports of teratogenicity in animals. Xylazine may induce premature parturition in cattle.

Xylazine does not appear to be excreted in detectable quantities in cows' milk.

Overdosage/Acute Toxicity

In the event of an accidental overdosage, cardiac arrhythmias, hypotension, and profound CNS and respiratory depression may occur. Seizures have also been reported after overdoses. There has been much interest in using alpha-blocking agents as antidotes or reversal agents to xylazine. Yohimbine, atipamezole, and tolazoline have been suggested for use alone and in combination to reverse the effects of xylazine or speed recovery times. Separate monographs for yohimbine and atipamezole are available with suggested doses.

To treat the respiratory depressant effects of xylazine toxicity, mechanical respiratory support with respiratory stimulants (*e.g.*, doxapram) have been recommended for use.

Drug Interactions

The manufacturers warn against using xylazine in conjunction with **other tranquilizers.**

■ **ACEPROMAZINE:** The combination use of acepromazine with xylazine is generally considered safe, but there is potential for additive hypotensive effects and this combination should be used cautiously in animals susceptible to hemodynamic complications.

■ **CHLORAMPHENICOL:** Prolonged sedation and gastrointestinal stasis possible (Davis 2007)

■ **CNS DEPRESSANT AGENTS, OTHER (barbiturates, narcotics, anesthetics, phenothiazines, etc.):** May cause additive CNS depression if used with xylazine. Dosages of these agents may need to be reduced.

■ **EPINEPHRINE:** The use of epinephrine with or without the concurrent use of halothane with xylazine may induce the development of ventricular arrhythmias.

■ **RESERPINE:** A case of a horse developing colic-like clinical signs after reserpine and xylazine has been reported. Until more is known about this potential interaction, use of these two agents together should be avoided.

Doses

■ **DOGS:**

a) 1.1 mg/kg IV, 1.1−2.2 mg/kg IM or SC (Package Insert; *Rompun®*—Miles) **Note:** Many believe the labeled dosage is too high.

b) As a preanesthetic: Dosage range for xylazine 0.2−1 mg/kg IV, IM or SC is very broad, and dosages on the label are relatively high. Xylazine has depressant, sedative, analgesic, and muscle relaxing effects. It is very effective for restraint and analgesia, but does not produce immobilization and sedated animals can respond to noxious stimuli and noise. Xylazine is associated with significant cardiac rhythm disturbances when dosed according to the recommendations on the label, especially in dogs. In low doses, the benefits of xylazine can be realized while

eliminating some of its detrimental side effects. (Hartsfield 2007)

c) Alpha-2 agonists can be used in low doses with opioids to provide dependable and profound restraint in healthy animals. Healthy animals can be given xylazine at a dose of 0.05−0.2 mg/kg (route not listed). (Dyson 2008)

d) For epidural injection: 0.02−0.25 mg/kg; dilute with sufficient quantity of sterile saline to a volume of 0.26 mL/kg. Onset of action 20−30 minutes; 2−5 hour duration.

Xylazine 0.02 mg/kg with morphine 0.1 mg/kg; dilute with sufficient quantity of sterile saline to a volume of 0.26 mL/kg. Onset of action 30−60 minutes; 10−20 hour duration.

As an analgesic: 0.1−1 mg/kg IV, IM or SC. For post-operative anxiety: 0.1−0.5 mg/kg IV, IM or SC (Carroll 1999)

■ **CATS:**

a) 1.1 mg/kg IV, 1.1−2.2 mg/kg IM or SC (Package Insert; *Rompun®*—Miles) **Note:** Many believe the labeled dosage is too high.

b) As a preanesthetic: Dosage range for xylazine 0.2−1 mg/kg IV, IM or SC is very broad, and dosages on the label are relatively high. Xylazine has depressant, sedative, analgesic, and muscle relaxing effects. It is very effective for restraint and analgesia, but does not produce immobilization and sedated animals can respond to noxious stimuli and noise. Xylazine is associated with significant cardiac rhythm disturbances when dosed according to the recommendations on the label, especially in dogs. In low doses, the benefits of xylazine can be realized while eliminating some of its detrimental side effects. (Hartsfield 2007)

b) As an emetic: 0.44 mg/kg IM (Morgan 1988; Riviere 1985)

c) As an analgesic: 0.1−1 mg/kg IV, IM or SC. For post-operative anxiety: 0.1−0.5 mg/kg IV, IM or SC (Carroll 1999)

■ **RABBITS, RODENTS, SMALL MAMMALS:**

a) **Rabbits:** For minimally invasive procedures lasting less than 30−45 minutes: 5 mg/kg once SC or IM in combination with ketamine (35 mg/kg). **Mice/Rats:** General anesthesia 13 mg/kg once IP in combination with ketamine (87 mg/kg). **Hamsters/Guinea pigs:** General anesthesia 8−10 mg/kg once IP in combination with ketamine (200 mg/kg for hamsters and 60 mg/kg for Guinea pigs) (Huerkamp 1995)

b) **Rabbits: 1)** Ketamine 35 mg/kg + xylazine 5 mg/kg IM; surgical anesthesia for 20-30 min, good relaxation, sleep time is 60–120 min, some effects reversible with atipamezole. **2)** Ketamine 25 mg/kg + xylazine 5 mg/kg + butorphanol 0.1 mg/kg IM; surgical anesthesia for 60-90 min, good relaxation, sleep time is 120–180 min. **3)** Ketamine 25 mg/kg + xylazine 5 mg/kg + acepromazine 1 mg/kg IM; surgical anesthesia for 45-75 min, good relaxation, sleep time is 100-150 min. **Gerbils:** Ketamine 50 mg/kg + xylazine 2 mg/kg IP; **Guinea Pigs:** Ketamine 40 mg/kg + xylazine 5 mg/kg IP; **Hamsters:** Ketamine 200 mg/kg + xylazine 10 mg/kg IP; **Mice:** Ketamine 80 mg/kg + xylazine 10 mg/kg IP; **Rats:** Ketamine 75 mg/kg + xylazine 10 mg/kg IP; Atipamezole 1 mg/kg SC, IM, IO or IV can be used to reverse xylazine. (Flecknell 2008)

c) **Rodents:** Xylazine (5 mg/kg) + ketamine (50 mg/kg) + atropine (0.05 mg/kg) IP. (Bennett 2009)

■ **FERRETS:**

a) As a sedative/analgesic: Xylazine: 0.5–2 mg/kg IM or SC. Usually combined with atropine (0.05 mg/kg) or glycopyrrolate (0.01 mg/kg IM) or Butorphanol/Xylazine: Butorphanol 0.2 mg/kg plus Xylazine (2 mg/kg) IM (Finkler 1999)

b) Xylazine (2 mg/kg) plus butorphanol (0.2 mg/kg) IM;

Telazol (1.5 mg/kg) plus xylazine (1.5 mg/kg) IM; may reverse xylazine with yohimbine (0.05 mg/kg IM)

Telazol (1.5 mg/kg) plus xylazine (1.5 mg/kg) plus butorphanol (0.2 mg/kg) IM; may reverse xylazine with yohimbine (0.05 mg/kg IM) (Williams 2000)

■ **BIRDS:**

a) As a sedative/analgesic: 1–4 mg/kg IM, provides sedation for ketamine anesthesia. Has been used at dosages of up to 10 mg/kg in small psittacines (Clyde & Paul-Murphy 2000)

b) In combination with ketamine: Ketamine 10–30 mg/kg IM; Xylazine 2–6 mg/kg IM; birds less than 250 grams require a higher dosage (per kg) than birds weighing greater than 250 g. Xylazine is not recommended for use in debilitated birds because of its cardiodepressant effects. (Wheler 1993)

■ **CATTLE:**

Caution: Cattle are extremely sensitive to xylazine's effects; be certain of dose and dosage form. Pretreatment with atropine can decrease bradycardia and hypersalivation.

a) For analgesia and restraint for standing procedures in cattle: A protocol for use of IM butorphanol/xylazine/ketamine

(BXK) has been reported (Miesner 2009). It consists of butorphanol (0.01–0.025 mg/kg) + xylazine (0.02–0.05 mg/kg) + ketamine (0.04–0.1 mg/kg). For a 450 kg animal, 5 mg butorphanol, 10 mg xylazine, and 20 mg ketamine would constitute the low end of the dosing range. Up to an hour of cooperation was accomplished using this protocol, but more fractious patients may require increased doses. Suggested to give no more than 10 mg butorphanol or 20 mg of xylazine for the initial dose to an animal greater than 450 kg. (Coetzee 2010)

b) 0.1–0.3 mg/kg IM; 0.05–0.15 mg/kg IV; 0.05–0.07 mg/kg epidurally. When used IV/IM, analgesia can be very short-lived (½ hour). (Walz 2006)

■ **HORSES: (Note:** ARCI UCGFS Class 3 Drug)

a) 1.1 mg/kg IV; 2.2 mg/kg IM. Allow animal to rest quietly until full effect is reached. (Package Insert; *Rompun®*—Bayer)

b) Sedative/analgesic for colic: 0.2–0.5 mg/kg IV (will provide analgesia for 20–30 minutes); or 0.6–1 mg/kg IM (effects for 1–2 hours). Evaluate heart rate prior to therapy. (Moore 1999)

c) For sedation analgesia: 0.2–1.1 mg/kg IV, or IM; higher doses IM are required to achieve same effect as IV.

As a caudal epidural for analgesia:

Alone in first coccygeal space: 0.03–0.35 mg/kg; perineal sweating common; 3–5 hour duration of effect.

In combination in first coccygeal space: xylazine 0.17 mg/kg with lidocaine (0.22 mg/kg); can cause ataxia or recumbency, perineal sweating; duration of effect 5-6 hours.

For lumbosacral analgesia (via catheter): 0.2 mg/kg (Sellon 2007)

d) As a short-acting, potent analgesic for mild, to moderate colic that will control pain but allow an estimate of the severity of the colic episode: 0.3–0.5 mg/kg IV; may be combined with butorphanol (0.01 mg/kg) and dosed at 0.3 mg/kg IV.

If the signs of colic are so violent as to prevent safe IV administration, an increased dose of xylazine (1.1 mg/kg) or detomidine (0.02 mg/kg) may be administered IM. The general rule is to double the IV dose. Expect a longer duration of effect with the IM route. (Blikslager 2008)

e) For field anesthesia: Sedate with xylazine (1 mg/kg IV; 2 mg/kg IM) given 5–10 minutes (longer for IM route) before induction of anesthesia with ketamine (2 mg/kg IV). Horse must be adequately sedated (head to the knees) before giving the ketamine (ketamine can cause muscle rigidity and seizures). If adequate sedation does not occur, either: **1)** Redose xylazine: up to half the original dose, **2)** Add butorphanol (0.02–0.04 mg/kg IV). Butorphanol can be given with the original xylazine if you suspect that the horse will be difficult to tranquilize (*e.g.*, high-strung Thoroughbreds) or added before the ketamine. This combination will improve induction, increase analgesia and increase recumbency time by about 5–10 minutes. **3)** Diazepam (0.03 mg/kg IV). Mix the diazepam with the ketamine. This combination will improve induction when sedation is marginal, improve muscle relaxation during anesthesia and prolong anesthesia by about 5–10 minutes. **4)** Guaifenesin (5% solution administered IV to effect) can also be used to increase sedation and muscle relaxation. (Mathews 1999)

f) As part of a balanced anesthesia protocol: 0.5–1 mg/kg IV given over ½–1 minute. (MAC sparing effect approximately 20-34%). (Driessen 2008)

■ **SHEEP & GOATS:**
Note: Use xylazine with extreme caution in these species. Use only the 20 mg/mL solution.

a) 0.01 mg/kg IV for light standing sedation to 0.2 mg/kg IM for recumbency of an hour's duration. Goats are bit more sensitive than sheep. When beginning to use these drugs, it is advisable to start with a conservative dose until one develops a feel for level of sedation provided. A reversal agent should always be on hand; reversal of sedative effects also reverses analgesic effects. (Snyder 2009)

■ **CAMELIDS:**
Note: Use xylazine with extreme caution in these species. Use only the 20 mg/mL solution.

a) For procedural pain (*e.g.*, castrations) when recumbency (up to 30 minutes) is desired: Alpacas: butorphanol 0.046 mg/kg; xylazine 0.46 mg/kg; ketamine 4.6 mg/kg. Llamas: butorphanol 0.037 mg/kg; xylazine 0.37 mg/kg; ketamine 3.7 mg/kg. All drugs are combined in one syringe and given IM. May administer 50% of original dose of ketamine and xylazine during anesthesia to prolong effect up to 15 minutes.

If doing mass castrations on 3 or more animals, can make up bottle of the "cocktail." Add 10 mg (1 mL) of butorphanol and 100 mg (1 mL) xylazine to a 1 gram (10 mL) vial) of ketamine. This mixture is dosed at 1 mL/40 lbs. (18 kg) for alpacas, and 1 mL/50 lbs. (22 kg) for

llamas. Handle quietly and allow plenty of time before starting procedure. Expect 20 minutes of surgical time; patient should stand 45 minutes to 1 hour after injection. (Miesner 2009)

■ **ZOO, EXOTIC, WILDLIFE SPECIES:**
For use of xylazine in zoo, exotic and wildlife medicine refer to specific references, including:

a) *Zoo Animal and Wildlife Immobilization and Anesthesia.* West, G, Heard, D, Caulkett, N. (eds.). Blackwell Publishing, 2007.

b) *Handbook of Wildlife Chemical Immobilization, 3rd Ed.* Kreeger, T.J. and J.M. Arnemo. 2007.

c) *Restraint and Handling of Wild and Domestic Animals.* Fowler, M (ed.), Iowa State University Press, 1995

d) *Exotic Animal Formulary, 3rd Ed.* Carpenter, J.W., Saunders. 2005

e) The 2009 American Association of Zoo Veterinarian Proceedings by D. K. Fontenot also has several dosages listed for restraint, anesthesia, and analgesia for a variety of drugs for carnivores and primates. VIN members can access them at: http://goo.gl/BHRih or http://goo.gl/9UJse

Monitoring
■ Level of anesthesia/analgesia
■ Respiratory function; cardiovascular status (rate, rhythm, BP if possible)
■ Hydration status if polyuria present

Client Information
■ Xylazine should only be used by individuals familiar with its use

Chemistry/Synonyms
Xylazine HCl is an alpha$_2$-adrenergic agonist structurally related to clonidine. The pH of the commercially prepared injections is approximately 5.5. Dosages and bottle concentrations are expressed in terms of the base.

Xylazine HCl may also be known as Bay-Va-1470, *Rompun®*, *AnaSed®*, *Sedazine®*, *X-Ject®*, or *Xyla-Ject®*.

Storage/Stability
Do not store above 30°C (86°F).

Compatibility/Compounding Considerations
Xylazine is reportedly physically **compatible** in the same syringe with several compounds, including: acepromazine, buprenorphine, butorphanol, chloral hydrate, and meperidine.

A study (Taylor *et al.* 2009) evaluating the stability, sterility, pH, particulate formation and efficacy in laboratory rodents of compounded ketamine, acepromazine and xylazine ("KAX") supported the finding that the drugs are stable and efficacious for at least 180 days after mixing if stored at room temperature in the dark.

Dosage Forms/Regulatory Status

VETERINARY-LABELED PRODUCTS:

Xylazine Injection: 20 mg/mL in 20 mL vials or 100 mg/mL in 50 mL vials: *Rompun®* (Bayer), *AnaSed®*, *Cervizine®* (300 mg/mL; for deer and elk) (Lloyd); *Sedazine®* (BIVI); *Chanazine®* (Teva); generic; (Rx); FDA-approved for use (depending on strength and product) in dogs, cats, horses, deer, and elk.

While xylazine is not FDA-approved for use in cattle in the USA, at labeled doses in Canada it reportedly has been assigned withdrawal times of 3 days for meat and 48 hours for milk. FARAD has reportedly suggested a withdrawal of 7 days for meat and 72 hours for milk for extra-label use.

The ARCI (Racing Commissioners International) has designated this drug as a class 3 substance. See the appendix for more information.

HUMAN-LABELED PRODUCTS: None

References

Bennett, R. (2009). Small Mammal Anesthesia—Rabbits and Rodents. Proceedings: ACVC. Accessed via: Veterinary Information Network. http://goo.gl/hRqTS

Blikslager, A.T. (2008). Managing Pain Associated with Colic. *Comp Equine* **294**–307(July/August).

Carroll, G. (1999). Analgesics and pain. *Vet Clin of NA: Small Animal Pract* **29**:3(May): 701–717.

Clyde, V. & J. Paul-Murphy (2000). Avian Analgesia. *Kirk's Current Veterinary Therapy: XIII Small Animal Practice*. J Bonagura Ed. Philadelphia, WB Saunders: 1126–1128.

Coetzee, H. (2010). How Do We Manage Pain in Cattle Effectively? Proceedings: WVC. Accessed via: Veterinary Information Network. http://goo.gl/ybT9N

Davis, J. (2007). Potential Drug Interactions: What Every Technician Should Know. Proceedings: IVECCS. Accessed via: Veterinary Information Network. http://goo.gl/rBCo2

Driessen, B. (2008). Balanced Anesthesia in the Equine: Techniques That Work in Practice. Proceedings: IVECCS. Accessed via: Veterinary Information Network. http://goo.gl/9ykAr

Dyson, D.H. (2008). Analgesia and Chemical Restraint for the Emergent Veterinary Patient. *Veterinary Clinics of North America-Small Animal Practice* **38**(6): 1329–+.

Finkler, M. (1999). Anesthesia in Ferrets. Proceedings: Central Veterinary Conference, Kansas City.

Flecknell, P. (2008). Anaesthesia of Rodents, Rabbits and Ferrets. Proceedings: WVC. Accessed via: Veterinary Information Network. http://goo.gl/SpAC7

Hartsfield, S. (2007). Preanesthetic Drugs in Small Animal Anesthesia. Proceedings: ACVC. Accessed via: Veterinary Information Network. http://goo.gl/ZSiXS

Huerkamp, M. (1995). Anesthesia and postoperative management of rabbits and pocket pets. *Kirk's Current Veterinary Therapy:XII*. J Bonagura Ed. Philadelphia, W.B. Saunders: 1322–1327.

Mathews, N. (1999). Anesthesia in large animals—Injectable (field) anesthesia: How to make it better. Proceedings: Central Veterinary Conference, Kansas City.

Miesner, M. (2009). Field anesthesia techniques in camelids. Proceedings: WVC. Accessed via: Veterinary Information Network. http://goo.gl/aYHQB

Moore, R. (1999). Medical treatment of abdominal pain in the horse: Analgesics and IV fluids. Proceedings: The North American Veterinary Conference, Orlando.

Morgan, R.V., Ed. (1988). *Handbook of Small Animal Practice*. New York, Churchill Livingstone.

Riviere, J.E. (1985). Clinical management of of toxico-

ses and adverse drug reactions. *Handbook of Small Animal Therapeutics*. LE Davis Ed. New York, Churchill Livingstone: 657–683.

Sellon, D. (2007). New Alternatives for Pain Management in Horses. Proceedings: New Alternatives for Pain Management in Horses. Accessed via: Veterinary Information Network. http://goo.gl/gXMfb

Snyder, J. (2009). Anesthesia and pain management: Minor surgeries. Proceedings: WVC. Accessed via: Veterinary Information Network. http://goo.gl/ljAl5

Taylor, B.J., S.A. Orr, et al. (2009). Beyond-Use Dating of Extemporaneously Compounded Ketamine, Acepromazine, and Xylazine: Safety, Stability, and Efficacy over Time. *Journal of the American Association for Laboratory Animal Science* **48**(6): 718–726.

Walz, P. (2006). Practical management of pain in cattle. Proceedings: ABVP. Accessed via: Veterinary Information Network. http://goo.gl/hScVv

Wheler, C. (1993). Avian anesthetics, analgesics, and tranquilizers. *Seminars in Avian & Exotic Med* **2**(1): 7–12.

Williams, B. (2000). Therapeutics in Ferrets. *Vet Clin NA: Exotic Anim Pract* **3**:1(Jan): 131–153.

YOHIMBINE HCL

(yo-***him***-been)   Yobine®, Antagonil®

ALPHA$_2$-ADRENERGIC ANTAGONIST

Prescriber Highlights

▶ Alpha$_2$-adrenergic antagonist used to reverse xylazine, other alpha$_2$ agonists & potentially amitraz; may be used prophylactically before amitraz dips

▶ Caution: Renal disease, seizure disorders

▶ Adverse Effects: Transient apprehension or CNS excitement, muscle tremors, salivation, increased respiratory rates, & hyperemic mucous membranes; more likely in small animals and horses

▶ Drug interactions

Uses/Indications

Yohimbine is indicated to reverse the effects of xylazine in dogs, but it is being used clinically for other alpha$_2$ agonists and in several other species as well.

Yohimbine may be efficacious in reversing some of the toxic effects associated with other agents (*e.g.*, amitraz) and can be used prophylactically before amitraz dips.

Pharmacology/Actions

Yohimbine is an alpha$_2$-adrenergic antagonist that can antagonize the effects of xylazine. Alone, yohimbine increases heart rate, blood pressure, causes CNS stimulation and antidiuresis, and has hyperinsulinemic effects.

By blocking central alpha$_2$-receptors, yohimbine causes sympathetic outflow (norepinephrine) to be enhanced. Peripheral alpha$_2$-receptors are also found in the cardiovascular system, genitourinary system, GI tract, platelets, and adipose tissue.

Pharmacokinetics

The pharmacokinetics of this drug have been reported in steers, dogs, and horses (Jernigan et al. 1988). The apparent volume of distribution (steady-state) is approximately 5 L/kg in steers, 2–5 L/kg in horses, and 4.5 L/kg in dogs. The total body clearance is approximately 70 mL/min/kg in steers, 35 mL/min/kg in horses, and 30 mL/min/kg in dogs. The half-life of the drug is approximately 0.5–1 hours in steers, 0.5–1.5 hours in horses, and 1.5–2 hours in dogs.

Yohimbine is believed to penetrate the CNS quite readily and, when used to reverse the effects of xylazine, onset of action generally occurs within 3 minutes. The metabolic fate of the drug is not known.

Contraindications/Precautions/Warnings

Yohimbine is contraindicated in patients hypersensitive to it. In humans, yohimbine is contraindicated in patients with renal disease.

Yohimbine should be used cautiously in patients with seizure disorders. When used to reverse the effects xylazine, normal pain perception may result.

Adverse Effects

Yohimbine may cause transient apprehension or CNS excitement, muscle tremors, salivation, increased respiratory rates, and hyperemic mucous membranes. Adverse effects appear to be more probable in small animals and horses.

Reproductive/Nursing Safety

Safe use of yohimbine in pregnant animals has not been established. No information on safety during lactation was located.

Overdosage/Acute Toxicity

Dogs receiving 0.55 mg/kg (5 times recommended dose) exhibited clinical signs of transient seizures and muscle tremors.

There were 5 exposures to yohimbine reported to the ASPCA Animal Poison Control Center (APCC) during 2008-2009. In these cases, all 5 were dogs with 2 showing clinical signs. Reported findings in dogs included diarrhea, disorientation, hyperactivity, panting, tachycardia, and hypersalivation.

For more information on clinical effects and treatment for yohimbine toxicity see: (Volmer et al. 1994)

Drug Interactions

Little information is available, use with caution with **other alpha₂-adrenergic antagonists** or **other drugs that can cause CNS stimulation.**

The following drug interaction has been reported in humans receiving yohimbine and may be of significance in veterinary patients:

■ **TRICYCLIC ANTIDEPRESSANTS:** In humans, yohimbine is not recommended for use with antidepressants or other mood-altering agents; hypertension has been reported with tricyclics

Doses

■ **DOGS:**

For alpha₂ agonist reversal:
a) For xylazine: 0.11 mg/kg IV slowly (Package insert; *Yobine®*—Lloyd)
b) For xylazine: 0.1 mg/kg IV (Gross & Tranquilli 1989)
c) For medetomidine: 0.11 mg/kg IV. (Park *et al.* 2009)

For reversal or prevention of amitraz effects:
a) To reverse centrally mediated bradycardia and hypotension associated with amitraz ingestion: 0.1 mg/kg IV; repeat as necessary (Manning 2000)
b) In cases of toxicity or to prevent a dog from having an acute episode of toxicity associated with demodicosis treatment: Yohimbine at 0.11 mg/kg IV or 0.25 mg/kg IM with atipamezole (50 micrograms/kg IM). (Torres 2007)
c) For treatment or prevention of side effects associated with amitraz dips: 0.1 mg/kg IV; may give prior to, or after bathing to prevent effects. (Hillier 2006)

As an antiemetic:
a) 0.25–0.5 mg/kg SC or IM q12h. (Washabau & Elie 1995), (Encarnacion *et al.* 2009), (Neiger 2007)

■ **RABBITS, RODENTS, SMALL MAMMALS:**

To reverse the effects of xylazine and to partially antagonize the effects of ketamine and acepromazine:
a) **Rabbits:** 0.2 mg/kg IV as needed
b) **Mice/Rats:** 0.2 mg/kg IP as needed (Huerkamp 1995)

■ **BIRDS:**

As a reversal agent for alpha2-adrenergic agonists (*e.g.*, xylazine):
a) 0.1 mg/kg IV (Clyde & Paul-Murphy 2000)

■ **CATTLE:**

For xylazine reversal:
a) 0.125 mg/kg IV (Gross & Tranquilli 1989)
b) Yohimbine (or tolazoline) may be used to reverse the effects of xylazine to facilitate a quicker recovery at the end of a procedure and minimize the risks of gastrointestinal complications. IM administration of the reversal agent is preferred in all but emergency situations as it decreases the risk of CNS excitement or cardiovascular complications. The amount of reversal agent used depends on the dose and time elapsed after administrating xylazine. Reversal of xylazine should not be attempted until sufficient time has elapsed to allow any ketamine or *Telazol®* used to resolve (30–45 min. post IM and 15–30 min. post-IV administration) to reduce the chances of a rough recovery.

When dosed properly the effects of reversal should start to become evident about 10 minutes following IM administration. Emergency doses of yohimbine at 0.1 mg/kg can be administered IV, but the shorter duration of action when given IV can result in the return of the effects of IM administered xylazine. (Anderson & Abrahamsen 2008)

■ **HORSES:** (**Note:** ARCI UCGFS Class 2 Drug)
For xylazine reversal:

a) 0.075 mg/kg IV (Gross & Tranquilli 1989)

■ **LLAMAS:**
For xylazine reversal:

a) 0.25 mg/kg IV or IM (Fowler 1989)

■ **ZOO, EXOTIC, WILDLIFE SPECIES:**
For use of yohimbine in zoo, exotic and wildlife medicine refer to specific references, including:

a) *Zoo Animal and Wildlife Immobilization and Anesthesia*. West, G, Heard, D, Caulkett, N. (eds.). Blackwell Publishing, 2007.

b) *Handbook of Wildlife Chemical Immobilization, 3rd Ed.* Kreeger, T.J. and J.M. Arnemo. 2007.

c) *Restraint and Handling of Wild and Domestic Animals.* Fowler, M (ed.), Iowa State University Press, 1995

d) *Exotic Animal Formulary, 3rd Ed.* Carpenter, J.W., Saunders. 2005

e) The 2009 American Association of Zoo Veterinarian Proceedings by D. K. Fontenot also has several dosages listed for restraint, anesthesia, and analgesia for a variety of drugs for carnivores and primates. VIN members can access them at: http://goo.gl/BHRih or http://goo.gl/9UJse

Monitoring

■ CNS status (arousal level, etc.)

■ Cardiac rate; rhythm (if indicated), blood pressure (if indicated and practical)

■ Respiratory rate

Client Information

■ This agent should be used with direct professional supervision only

Chemistry/Synonyms

A Rauwolfia or indolealkylamine alkaloid, yohimbine HCl has a molecular weight of 390.9. It is chemically related to reserpine.

Yohimbine may also be known as: aprhodine hydrochloride, chlorhydrate de quebrachine, corynine hydrochloride, *Aphrodyne®, Dayto Himbin®, Pluriviron mono®, Prowess Plain®, Urobine®, Virigen®, Yobine®, Yocon®, Yocoral®, Yohimex®, Yohydrol, Yomax®,* or *Zumba®.*

Storage/Stability

Yohimbine injection should be stored at room temperature (15–30°C) and protected from light and heat.

Dosage Forms/Regulatory Status

VETERINARY-LABELED PRODUCTS:

Yohimbine Sterile Solution for Injection: 2 mg/mL in 20 mL vials; *Yobine®* (Lloyd); (Rx). FDA-approved for use in dogs.

HUMAN-LABELED PRODUCTS:

Oral 5.4 mg tablets are available, but would unlikely to be of veterinary benefit.

References

Anderson, D. & E. Abrahamsen (2008). Chemical Restraint in the Field—New Uses For Old Drugs. Proceedings: World Vet Congress. Accessed via: Veterinary Information Network. http://goo.gl/G6BXN

Clyde, V. & J. Paul-Murphy (2000). Avian Analgesia. *Kirk's Current Veterinary Therapy: XIII Small Animal Practice.* J Bonagura Ed. Philadelphia, WB Saunders: 1126–1128.

Encarnacion, H.J., J. Parra, et al. (2009). Vomiting. *Compendium-Continuing Education for Veterinarians* 31(3): 122–+.

Fowler, M.E. (1989). *Medicine and Surgery of South American Camelids.* Ames, Iowa State University Press.

Gross, M.E. & W.J. Tranquilli (1989). Use of Alpha 2-Adrenergic Receptor Atagonists. *JAVMA* 195(3): 378–381.

Hillier, A. (2006). Update on canine demodicosis. Proceedings: ACVC. Accessed via: Veterinary Information Network. http://goo.gl/O2tAz

Huerkamp, M. (1995). Anesthesia and postoperative management of rabbits and pocket pets. *Kirk's Current Veterinary Therapy:XII.* J Bonagura Ed. Philadelphia, W.B. Saunders: 1322–1327.

Manning, A. (2000). Alpha- and Beta-Agonist Intoxications. *Kirk's Current Veterinary Therapy: XIII Small Animal Practice.* J Bonagura Ed. Philadelphia, WB Saunders: 153–157.

Neiger, R. (2007). What's New in Antiemetic Therapy. Proceedings: ECVIM. Accessed via: Veterinary Information Network. http://goo.gl/UuS6T

Park, C., K. Heo, et al. (2009). Antagonism of medetomidine sedation in dogs by yohimbine. Peroceedings: WSAVA. Accessed via: Veterinary Information Network. http://goo.gl/g2uFu

Torres, S. (2007). Diagnosis and treatment of canine and feline demodicosis. Proceedings: Western Vet Conf. Accessed via: Veterinary Information Network. http://goo.gl/Yt1sh

Volmer, P.A., W.J. Tranquilli, et al. (1994). Acute Oral Yohimbine Toxicosis in a Dog. *Canine Practice* 19(2): 18–19.

Washabau, R. & M. Elie (1995). Antiemetic therapy. *Kirk's Current Veterinary Therapy:XII.* J Bonagura Ed. Philadelphia, W.B. Saunders: 679–684.

ZAFIRLUKAST

(zah-*fur*-luh-kast)   Accolate®

LEUKOTRIENE-RECEPTOR ANTAGONIST

Prescriber Highlights

▶ Leukotriene-receptor antagonist; potentially useful for canine atopic dermatitis, feline asthma, or inflammatory bowel disease, but efficacy has either been disappointing or not well studied in veterinary patients

▶ Not for treatment of acute bronchospasm

▶ Well tolerated

▶ Dose on an empty stomach

Uses/Indications

While zafirlukast potentially could be useful for treating a variety of conditions (*e.g.,* feline asthma, atopic dermatitis, inflammatory bowel disease) where leukotrienes are thought to contribute to morbidity, to date, efficacy has been shown to be disappointing, limited, or not fully studied. A study using zafirlukast to evaluate effects on pruritus (owner subjective evaluation) in dogs with atopic dermatitis, showed that only 11% of treated dogs had at least 50% reductions in pruritus (Senter *et al.* 2002).

Pharmacology/Actions

Zafirlukast selectively and competitively inhibits leukotriene receptors, specifically receptors for leukotriene D_4 and E_4 (LTD$_4$ and LTE$_4$). Additionally, it competes for receptors with some components of slow-reacting substance of anaphylaxis (SRS-A). These substances have all been implicated in the inflammatory and bronchoconstrictive aspects of bronchial asthma.

Pharmacokinetics

No specific veterinary data was located. In humans, zafirlukast is rapidly absorbed after oral administration. Food may impair the absorption of the drug, therefore, give on an empty stomach. Peak plasma levels occur about 3 hours after dosing. Zafirlukast is highly bound to plasma proteins (>99%). The drug is extensively metabolized; less than 10% of a dose is excreted in the urine, the rest in the feces. Half lives in humans average about 10 hours.

Contraindications/Precautions/Warnings

Zafirlukast is contraindicated in patients hypersensitive to it.

Zafirlukast is not indicated for, and is ineffective for treating bronchospasm associated with acute asthma attacks.

Patients with significantly decreased hepatic function may have reduced clearances (and increased plasma levels) of zafirlukast.

Adverse Effects

Veterinary experience is very limited, but some dogs reportedly have vomited after oral dosing. In humans, the adverse effect profile seems to be minimal; headache was noted most often, but incidence is not much different than placebo.

Reproductive/Nursing Safety

In humans, the FDA categorizes this drug as category *B* for use during pregnancy *(Animal studies have not yet demonstrated risk to the fetus, but there are no adequate studies in pregnant women; or animal studies have shown an adverse effect, but adequate studies in pregnant women have not demonstrated a risk to the fetus in the first trimester of pregnancy, and there is no evidence of risk in later trimesters.)*

Zafirlukast is excreted in milk, but it is probably safe to administer to nursing veterinary patients.

Overdosage/Acute Toxicity

In dogs, doses of up to 500 mg/kg were tolerated without mortality.

Drug Interactions

The following drug interactions have either been reported or are theoretical in humans or animals receiving zafirlukast and may be of significance in veterinary patients:

■ **ASPIRIN:** May significantly increase zafirlukast plasma levels

■ **ERYTHROMYCIN:** May decrease the bioavailability of zafirlukast

■ **THEOPHYLLINE:** May decrease plasma levels of zafirlukast

■ **WARFARIN:** Zafirlukast may significantly increase the prothrombin time of patients taking warfarin.

Laboratory Considerations

■ None were noted

Doses

■ **DOGS:**

For adjunctive treatment of atopic dermatitis:

a) 20 mg (total dose) PO twice daily; only moderate success (Foil 2003)

b) In the study dogs received: 5 mg PO q12h, if the dog weighed less than 11.4 kg (25 lb); 10 mg PO q12h, if 11.4–22.3 kg (25–49 lb); 20 mg PO q12h, if 22.7–34.1 kg (50–75 lb); and 30 mg PO q12h, if greater than 34.1 kg (75 lb). Given on an empty stomach, 1 hour before, or 2 hours after meals. (Senter *et al.* 2002)

■ **CATS:**

For adjunctive treatment of feline bronchial "asthma."

a) 1–2 mg/kg PO once to twice daily (Noone 1999)

b) 0.5–1 mg/kg q12–24h. (Scherk 2010)

c) 5 mg (total dose) per cat PO q12h. (Lappin 2008)

For adjunctive treatment of mild inflammatory bowel disease:

a) 0.15–0.2 mg/kg PO once daily. Author has used a combination of zafirlukast (3 months), famotidine (4 weeks), and sucralfate (2 weeks) (along with a low-allergen diet) to successfully treat a case. (Boothe 2009)

Monitoring

■ Clinical efficacy

Client Information

■ Preferably give on an empty stomach.

■ Give this medication even if animal appears well; do not use to treat acute asthma clinical signs.

■ Because experience in veterinary medicine is limited, report any untoward effects to the veterinarian.

Chemistry/Synonyms

A leukotriene-receptor antagonist, zafirlukast occurs as a white to pale yellow, fine amorphous powder. It is practically insoluble in water.

Zafirlukast may also be known as: ICI-204219, *Accolate®, Accoleit®, Aeronix®, Azimax®, Olmoran®, Resma®, Vanticon®, Zafarismal®, Zafirst®,* or *Zuvair®.*

Storage/Stability

Zafirlukast tablets should be stored at room temperature and protected from light and moisture. The manufacturer states that the tablets should be dispensed only in the original, unopened container.

Dosage Forms/Regulatory Status

VETERINARY-LABELED PRODUCTS: None

The ARCI (Racing Commissioners International) has designated this drug as a class 4 substance. See the appendix for more information.

HUMAN-LABELED PRODUCTS:

Zafirlukast Tablets (film-coated): 10 mg & 20 mg; *Accolate®* (AstraZeneca); (Rx)

References

Boothe, D.M. (2009). Control of Inflammatory Allergic Disease in Cats II. Proceedings; WVC. http://goo.gl/q6uOz

Foil, C. (2003). New drugs in dermatology. Proceedings: Western Veterinary Conf. Accessed via: Veterinary Information Network. http://goo.gl/iEYic

Lappin, M.R. (2008). Update on the Diagnosis, Treatment, and Prevention of Feline Lower Respiratory Diseases. Proceedings: ACVIM. Accessed via: Veterinary Information Network. http://goo.gl/eYyOC

Noone, K. (1999). Feline Bronchial asthma. Proceedings: American College of Veterinary interanl Medicine: 17th Annual Veterinary Medical Forum, Chicago.

Scherk, M. (2010). SNOTS AND SNUFFLES Rational approach to chronic feline upper respiratory syndromes. *Journal of Feline Medicine and Surgery* 12(7): 548–557.

Senter, D.A., D.W. Scott, et al. (2002). Treatment of canine atopic dermatitis with zafirlukast, a leukotriene-receptor antagonist: a single-blinded, placebo-controlled study. *Canadian Veterinary Journal-Revue Veterinaire Canadienne* 43(3): 203–206.

ZIDOVUDINE (AZT)

(zid-o-vew-den)   Retrovir®

ANTIRETROVIRAL

Prescriber Highlights

▶ Antiretroviral agent that may be useful for adjunctive treatment of FeLV or FIV in cats

▶ Use with caution if renal, hepatic, or bone marrow dysfunction present

▶ Anemia (non-regenerative) most common adverse effect in cats

Uses/Indications

In veterinary medicine, zidovudine may be useful for treating feline immunodeficiency virus (FIV) or feline leukemia virus (FeLV). While zidovudine can reduce the viral load in infected cats and improve clinical signs, it may not alter the natural course of the disease to a great extent.

Pharmacology/Actions

Zidovudine is considered an antiretroviral agent. While its exact mechanism of action is not fully understood, zidovudine is converted *in vivo* to an active metabolite (triphosphate) that interferes with viral RNA-directed DNA polymerase (reverse transcriptase). This causes a virustatic effect in retroviruses.

Zidovudine has some activity against gram-negative bacteria and can be cytotoxic as well.

Pharmacokinetics

Zidovudine is well absorbed after oral administration. In cats, oral bioavailability is approximately 95%. When administered with food, peak levels may be decreased, but total area under the curve may not be affected; peak levels occur about one hour post-dosing in cats. The drug is widely distributed, including into the CSF. It is only marginally bound to plasma proteins. Zidovudine is rapidly metabolized and excreted in the urine. Half-life in cats is about 1.5 hours.

Contraindications/Precautions/Warnings

Zidovudine is considered contraindicated in patients who have developed life threatening hypersensitivity reactions to it in the past.

Use zidovudine with caution in patients with bone marrow, renal or hepatic dysfunction. The European Advisory Board on Cat Diseases (ABCD) guidelines on prevention and management of feline immunodeficiency state that: Cats with bone marrow suppression should not be treated (with zidovudine; see monitoring guidelines, below). Dosage adjustment may be necessary in cats with renal or hepatic dysfunction.

Adverse Effects

In cats, reductions in RBC's, PCV and hemoglobin are the most common adverse effects reported. Anemia may be non-regenerative and is most commonly seen with the higher end of the dosage range (10–15 mg/kg). Diarrhea and weakness have also been reported. While there are many adverse effects reported in humans, granulocytopenia and GI effects appear to be the most likely to occur.

Reproductive/Nursing Safety

In humans, the FDA categorizes this drug as category C for use during pregnancy (*Animal studies have shown an adverse effect on the fetus, but there are no adequate studies in humans; or there are no animal reproduction studies and no adequate studies in humans.*)

Zidovudine is excreted in milk. Clinical significance is not clear for nursing offspring.

Overdosage/Acute Toxicity

Human adults and children have survived oral overdoses of up to 50 grams without permanent sequelae. Vomiting and transient hematologic effects are the most consistent adverse effects reported with overdoses.

Drug Interactions

The following drug interactions have either been reported or are theoretical in humans or animals receiving zidovudine and may be of significance in veterinary patients:

■ **ANTIFUNGALS, AZOLE (ketoconazole, etc.):** May increase zidovudine levels

■ **ATOVAQUONE:** May increase zidovudine levels

■ **DOXORUBICIN:** May antagonize each other's effects; avoid use together

■ **INTERFERON ALFA:** Increased risk for hematologic and hepato-toxicity

■ **PROBENECID:** May increase zidovudine levels

■ **MYELO-/CYTOTOXIC DRUGS (e.g., chloramphenicol, doxorubicin, flucytosine, vincristine, vinblastine):** Administered with zidovudine may increase the risk of hematologic toxicity

■ **RIFAMPIN:** May decrease blood levels (AUC) of zidovudine

Laboratory Considerations

■ None were noted.

Doses

■ **CATS:**

For adjunctive therapy of FeLV and FIV:

a) 5–10 mg/kg q12h PO or SC. The higher dose should be used carefully as side effects can develop. For SC injection, the lyophilized product should be diluted in isotonic sodium chloride solution to prevent local irritation. For PO dosing, syrup or gelatin capsules (dosage/weight calculated individually for each cat) can be given. See the ABCB monitoring guidelines below. (Hosie *et al.* 2009)

b) 5–10 mg PO or SC q12h. The higher dose should be carefully used in FeLV-infected

cats because side effects, particularly non-regenerative anemia, can develop. (Levy *et al.* 2008)

c) For FELV: 5 mg/kg PO or SC q12h. If giving SC dilute in sterile normal saline to prevent local irritation. Check CBC weekly the first month as anemia (non-regenerative) can be seen. If values are stable; may monitor monthly. Some cats develop mild decreases in hematocrit that resolves even if treatment is continued. (Hartmannn 2007)

d) For FIV encephalopathy: 20 mg/kg PO q12h (Taylor 2003)

Monitoring

■ The European Advisory Board on Cat Diseases (ABCD) guidelines on prevention and management of feline immunodeficiency (Hosie *et al.* 2009) recommends: During treatment, a CBC should be performed weekly for the first month, because non-regenerative anemia is common, especially at higher doses. If the values are stable, monthly checks are sufficient. If hematocrit drops below 20%, treatment should be discontinued, and anemia then usually resolves within a few days.

■ CD4/CD8 rates, if possible

■ Clinical efficacy

Client Information

■ Must be considered "experimental" therapy for cats

■ Must be administered as prescribed for efficacy

■ Regular blood tests required

Chemistry/Synonyms

A thymidine analog, zidovudine is synthetically produced and occurs as a white to beige-colored, odorless, crystalline solid. Approximately 20 mg are soluble in one mL of water.

Zidovudine may also be known as: ZDV, azidodeoxythymidine, 3'-azido-2',3'-dideoxythymidine, azidothymidine, AZT, BW-A509U, BW-509U, compound-S, zidovudinum or *Retrovir®*; many other trade names are available.

Storage/Stability

Zidovudine oral tablets or capsules should be stored at room temperature. Protect from heat, light and moisture. The oral solution should be stored at room temperature. Zidovudine injection (for IV infusion) should be store at room temperature and protected from light.

Dosage Forms/Regulatory Status

VETERINARY-LABELED PRODUCTS: None

HUMAN-LABELED PRODUCTS:

Zidovudine Oral Tablets: 300 mg; *Retrovir®* (GlaxoSmithKline); generic; (Rx)

Zidovudine Oral Capsules: 100 mg; *Retrovir®* (GlaxoSmithKline); generic; (Rx)

Zidovudine Oral Syrup: 50 mg/5 mL in 240 mL; *Retrovir*® (GlaxoSmithKline); generic; (Rx)

Zidovudine Injection Solution: 10 mg/mL in 20 mL single-use vials; *Retrovir*® (GlaxoSmith-Kline); (Rx)

References

Hartmannn, K. (2007). Update on management and treatment of feline leukemia virus-infected cats. Proceedings: ACVIM. Accessed via: Veterinary Information Network. http://goo.gl/5PphR

Hosie, M.J., D. Addie, et al. (2009). Feline Immunodeficiency ABCD guidelines on prevention and management. *Journal of Feline Medicine and Surgery* 11(7): 575–584.

Levy, J., C. Crawford, et al. (2008). 2008 American Association of Feline Practitioners' feline retrovirus management guidelines. *Journal of Feline Medicine and Surgery* 10(3): 300–316.

Taylor, S. (2003). Neuromuscular disorders. *Small Animal Internal Medicine, 3rd Ed.* R Nelson and C Couto Eds. St Louis, Mosby: 946–1070.

ZINC ACETATE
ZINC SULFATE
ZINC GLUCONATE

(*zink*)

NUTRITIONAL; TRACE ELEMENT

Prescriber Highlights

▶ Metal nutritional agent that may be used for zinc deficiency, to reduce copper toxicity in susceptible dog breeds (Bedlington Terriers, West Highland White Terriers) with hepatic copper toxicosis, & treat hepatic fibrosis in dogs. Has astringent & antiseptic activity topically.

▶ Contraindications: None; consider obtaining zinc & copper levels before treating.

▶ Adverse Effects: Large doses may cause GI disturbances or hematologic abnormalities (usually hemolysis), particularly if a coexistent copper deficiency exists

▶ Zinc overdoses (e.g., U.S. pennies) can be serious

Uses/Indications

Zinc sulfate is used systemically as a nutritional supplement in a variety of species. Oral zinc acetate has been shown to reduce copper toxicity in susceptible dog breeds (Bedlington Terriers, West Highland White Terriers) with hepatic copper toxicosis. Zinc therapy may also be of benefit in the treatment of hepatic fibrosis in the dog. Zinc sulfate is used topically as an astringent and as a weak antiseptic both for dermatologic and ophthalmic conditions.

For more information, the reader is encouraged to refer to a thorough review of zinc physi-

ology, pathophysiology, toxicity and deficiency in veterinary patients (Cummings & Kovacic 2009).

Pharmacology/Actions

Zinc is a necessary nutritional supplement; it is required by over 200 metalloenzymes for proper function. Enzyme systems that require zinc include alkaline phosphatase, alcohol dehydrogenase, carbonic anhydrase, and RNA polymerase. Zinc is also necessary to maintain structural integrity of cell membranes and nucleic acids. Zinc dependent physiological processes include sexual maturation and reproduction, cell growth and division, vision, night vision, wound healing, immune response, and taste acuity.

When administered orally, large doses of zinc can inhibit the absorption of copper.

Pharmacokinetics

About 20–30% of dietary zinc is absorbed, principally from the duodenum and ileum. Bioavailability is dependent upon the food in which it is present. Phytates can chelate zinc and form insoluble complexes in an alkaline pH. Zinc is stored mostly in red and white blood cells, but is also found in the muscle, skin, bone, retina, pancreas, liver, kidney, and prostate. Elimination is primarily via the feces, but some is also excreted by the kidneys and in sweat. Zinc found in feces may be reabsorbed from the colon.

Contraindications/Precautions/Warnings

Zinc supplementation should be carefully considered before administering to patients with copper deficiency.

When dosing, do not confuse the concentrations of zinc salts with elemental zinc.

Adverse Effects

Large doses may cause GI disturbances. Hematologic abnormalities (usually hemolysis) may occur with large doses or serum levels greater than 1000 micrograms/dL (1 mg/dL), particularly if a coexistent copper deficiency exists. Zinc acetate or methionine may be less irritating to the stomach. Mixing the contents of the capsule with a small amount of tuna or hamburger may minimize vomiting.

Reproductive/Nursing Safety

Although zinc deficiency during pregnancy has been associated with adverse perinatal outcomes, other studies report no such occurrences. In humans, since zinc deficiency is very rare, the routine use of zinc supplementation during pregnancy is not recommended. In humans, the FDA categorizes this drug as category *C* for use during pregnancy (*Animal studies have shown an adverse effect on the fetus, but there are no adequate studies in humans; or there are no animal reproduction studies and no adequate studies in humans.*)

Overdosage/Acute Toxicity

Signs associated with overdoses of zinc in mammals include hemolytic anemia, hypotension, jaundice, vomiting, and pulmonary edema. Suggestions for treatment of overdoses of oral zinc include removing the source, dilution with milk or water, and chelation therapy using edetate calcium disodium (Calcium EDTA). Refer to that monograph for possible doses and usage information.

Zinc intoxication in birds is relatively common, but clinical signs of intoxication in birds are varied and nonspecific. They include lethargy, anorexia, regurgitation, polyuria, polydipsia, hematuria, hematochezia, pallor, dark or bright green diarrhea, foul-smelling feces, paresis, seizures, and sudden death (Puschner & Poppenga 2009). Treatment involves removing the source of zinc, chelation therapy (edetate calcium disodium or succimer), and supportive care.

Drug Interactions

The following drug interactions have either been reported or are theoretical in humans or animals receiving zinc and may be of significance in veterinary patients:

- ◼ **COPPER:** Large doses of zinc can inhibit copper absorption in the intestine; if this interaction is not desired, separate copper and zinc supplements by at least two hours

- ◼ **FLUOROQUINOLONES (e.g., enrofloxacin, ciprofloxacin):** Zinc salts may reduce the oral absorption of some fluoroquinolones

- ◼ **PENICILLAMINE:** May potentially inhibit zinc absorption; clinical significance is not clear

- ◼ **TETRACYCLINES:** Zinc salts may chelate oral tetracycline and reduce its absorption; separate doses by at least two hours

- ◼ **URSODIOL:** May potentially inhibit zinc absorption; clinical significance is not clear

Doses

- ◼ **DOGS:**

  For adjunctive treatment and prophylaxis of hepatic copper toxicosis:

  a) Initially, give a loading dose of 100 mg *elemental* zinc (zinc acetate used in this study) twice daily (separate doses by at least 8 hours) for about 3 months; then reduce dose to 50 mg (elemental zinc) twice daily. If animal vomits, give doses with a small piece of meat. Do not give within one hour of a meal. Monitoring of zinc levels every 2–3 months initially is recommended. Target zinc levels are 200–500 micrograms/dL. Do not allow levels to increase higher than 1000 micrograms/dL. May require 3–6 months of therapy before significant efficacy is noted. (Brewer *et al.* 1992)

  b) 5–10 mg/kg *elemental* zinc q12h; use high end of dosage range initially for 3 months, then 50 mg PO q12h for maintenance. Separate dosage from meals by 1–2 hours. Zinc acetate or methionine may be less irritating to the GI than other

salts. Mixing the contents of the capsule with a small amount of tuna or hamburger may also minimize vomiting. In dogs with active copper-induced hepatitis, do not use zinc alone, but in combination with a chelator (*e.g.,* D-penicillamine, trientine). Target zinc plasma levels >200 micrograms/dL but <400 micrograms/dL. Monitor levels every 2–3 months and adjust dosage as necessary. (Johnson 2000)

  c) 10 mg/kg *elemental* zinc (given as zinc acetate or zinc gluconate) PO twice daily. Give one hour before each meal. (Rothuizen 2003)

  d) 1.5–2.5 mg/kg zinc gluconate PO three times daily; 0.67 mg/kg zinc sulfate PO three times daily; or 100 mg (total dose) *elemental* zinc (as zinc acetate) PO twice daily. Goal is to achieve zinc plasma concentrations of 200–600 micrograms/dL. After a 3–6 month loading period, dose is decreased to approximately half the original dose. Serum zinc concentrations are measured every 4–6 months. If serum level drops below 150 micrograms/dL, increase dose to original level. If vomiting is a problem, may mix dosage with a tablespoonful of tuna fish (in oil). (Richter 2002)

  For hepatic fibrosis:

  a) 200 mg of *elemental* zinc PO once daily for a 10–25 kg dog. Keep zinc plasma levels between 200–300 micrograms/dL. (Rutgers 2000)

  b) Empirical dosage is 15 mg/kg of *elemental* zinc per day, (or 200 mg elemental zinc per medium sized dog per day, tapered to 50–100 mg per dog per day based on serum zinc levels). The goal is for serum zinc levels of 200–500 micrograms/dL (2–5 micrograms/mL). Zinc should ideally be given on an empty stomach (1 hour before or after a meal); mix with tuna oil if nausea noted. Author prefers to add zinc in as a single drug after stabilization of the patient with hepatoprotective agents and glucocorticoids (if indicated). (Trepanier 2008)

  For zinc-related dermatoses:

  a) Rapidly growing dogs: 10 mg/kg, day PO of zinc sulfate (Willemse 1992)

  b) For zinc-responsive dermatoses found in Siberian huskies, Alaskan malamutes, Great Danes, and Doberman pinschers: Zinc sulfate: 10 mg/kg PO with food either once daily or divided q12h. Alternatively, zinc methionine: 2 mg/kg PO once daily. Correct any dietary imbalances (high calcium and phytate). Lifetime therapy usually required. If vomiting occurs, lower dose or give with food.

For syndrome seen in puppies: Dietary corrections alone usually resolve the syndrome, but zinc supplementation as above, can expedite process. Some puppies require supplementation until maturity. (Kwochka 1994)

As an appetite stimulant:

a) 1 mg/kg of *elemental* zinc PO once a day (Bartges 2003)

■ **CATS:**

For adjunctive therapy of severe hepatic lipidosis:

a) 7–10 mg/kg PO once daily, in B-Complex mixture if possible (Center 1994)

As an appetite stimulant:

a) 1 mg/kg of *elemental* zinc PO once a day (Bartges 2003)

Monitoring; Client Information

■ See information in individual doses above

■ There is poor correlation between serum zinc levels and zinc-deficient states in dogs, and zinc levels may have more value in detection of potentially toxic intake or corroboration of a clinical diagnosis of toxicity or deficiency (Cummings & Kovacic 2009).

Client Information

■ Although it is best to give oral zinc acetate on an empty stomach, if vomiting occurs mix with hamburger or tuna fish to decrease this side effect

Chemistry/Synonyms

Zinc acetate occurs as white crystals or granules. It has a faint acetous odor and effloresces slightly. One gram is soluble in 2.5 mL of water or 30 mL of alcohol. Zinc acetate contains 30% elemental zinc (100 mg zinc acetate = 30 mg elemental zinc).

Zinc sulfate occurs as a colorless granular powder, small needles, or transparent prisms. It is odorless but has an astringent metallic taste. 1.67 grams are soluble in one mL of water. Zinc sulfate is insoluble in alcohol and contains 23% zinc by weight (100 mg zinc sulfate = 23 mg elemental zinc).

Zinc gluconate occurs as white or practically white powder or granules. It is soluble in water; very slightly soluble in alcohol. Zinc gluconate contains 14.3% zinc (100 mg zinc gluconate = 14.3 mg elemental zinc).

Zinc methionine contains 18-21% elemental zinc. For very 5 mg of zinc methionine there is approximately 1 mg of elemental zinc.

Zinc acetate may also be known as: E650, or zinci acetas dihydricus.

Zinc sulfate may also be known as: zinc sulphate; zinci sulfas, zincum sulfuricum; many trade names are available.

Storage/Stability

Store zinc acetate crystals in tight containers. Unless otherwise recommended by the manufacturer, store zinc sulfate products in tight containers at room temperature.

Dosage Forms/Regulatory Status

VETERINARY-LABELED PRODUCTS:

None as single-ingredient products for systemic use; several vitamin/mineral supplements contain zinc, however.

HUMAN-LABELED PRODUCTS:

Zinc Acetate is available from chemical supply houses.

Zinc Acetate Capsules: 25 mg & 50 mg as zinc acetate; *Galzin*® (Gate Pharmaceuticals); (Rx)

Zinc Injection: 1 mg/mL (as sulfate; as 4.39 mg heptahydrate or 2.46 mg anhydrous) in 10 mL & 30 mL vials; 5 mg/mL (as 21.95 mg sulfate) in 5 mL & 10 mL vials; 1 mg/mL (as 2.09 mg chloride) in 10 mL vials; *Zinca-Pak*® (Smith & Nephew SoloPak); generic; (Rx)

Zinc Gluconate Tablets: 10 mg (1.4 mg zinc), 15 mg (2 mg zinc) & 50 mg (7 mg zinc); generic; (OTC)

Zinc sulfate is also available in topical ophthalmic preparations.

References
Bartges, J. (2003). Enteral Nutrition. Proceedings: World Small Animal Veterinary Assoc. World Congress. Accessed via: Veterinary Information Network. http://goo.gl/IZLCY

Brewer, G.J., R.D. Dick, et al. (1992). Use of zinc acetate to treat copper toxicosis in dogs. *JAVMA* **201**(August 15, 1992): 564–568.

Center, S. (1994). Hepatic lipidosis. *Consultations in Feline Internal Medicine: 2.* J August Ed. Philadelphia, W.B. Saunders Company: 87–101.

Cummings, J.E. & J.P. Kovacic (2009). The ubiquitous role of zinc in health and disease. *Journal of Veterinary Emergency and Critical Care* **19**(3): 215–240.

Johnson, S. (2000). Chronic Hepatic Disorders. *Textbook of Veterinary Internal Medicine: Diseases of the Dog and Cat.* S Ettinger and E Feldman Eds. Philadelphia, WB Saunders. 2: 1298–1325.

Kwochka, K. (1994). Keratinization Defects. *Saunders Manual of Small Animal Practice.* S Birchard and R Sherding Eds. Philadelphia, W.B. Saunders Company: 318–325.

Puschner, B. & A. Poppenga (2009). Lead and Zinc Intoxication in Companion Birds. *Comp CE*(January): E1–E12.

Richter, K. (2002). Common canine hepatopathies. Proceedings: ACVIM Forum. Accessed via: Veterinary Information Network. http://goo.gl/pqRDc

Rothuizen, J. (2003). Copper-associated liver diseases in dogs. Proceedings: World Small Animal Veterinary Assoc World Congress. Accessed via: Veterinary Information Network. http://goo.gl/c7fL0

Rutgers, H. (2000). Hepatic Fibrosis in the Dog. *Kirk's Current Veterinary Therapy: XIII Small Animal Practice.* J Bonagura Ed. Philadelphia, WB Saunders.

Trepanier, L. (2008). Choosing therapy for chronic liver disease. Proceedings: WSAVA. Accessed via: Veterinary Information Network. http://goo.gl/NLh4X

Willemse, T. (1992). Zinc-related cutaneous disorders of dogs. *Current Veterinary Therapy XI: Small Animal Practice.* R Kirk and J Bonagura Eds. Philadelphia, W.B. Saunders Company: 532–534.

Zolazepam—see Tiletamine HCl/ Zolazepam HCl

ZONISAMIDE

(zoh-*niss*-a-mide)   Zonegran®

ANTICONVULSANT

Prescriber Highlights

▶ Antiseizure medication that may be useful as an "add-on" drug for refractory epilepsy. May be considered for initial treatment as monotherapy in dogs.

▶ Half-life of 15 hours makes twice daily dosing possible in dogs; 33 hour half-life in cats may allow once daily dosing.

▶ Adverse effect profile not fully elucidated for dogs; sedation, ataxia, & inappetence have been reported

▶ Known teratogen in dogs

▶ Contraindicated in patients hypersensitive to sulfonamides

▶ Generics now available

Uses/Indications

Zonisamide may be useful as an "add-on" drug for refractory epilepsy in dogs. It has been suggested that it could be useful as monotherapy as the initial choice for dogs, particularly when the client wishes to avoid adverse effects associated with phenobarbital or bromides (Thomas 2010).

Pharmacology/Actions

The exact mechanism of action for zonisamide is not known. It may produce its antiseizure activity by blocking sodium channels and reducing transient inward currents, thereby stabilizing neuronal membranes and suppressing neuronal hypersynchronization. It does not appear to potentiate GABA. Zonisamide has weak carbonic anhydrase inhibitory activity.

Pharmacokinetics

In dogs, zonisamide is well absorbed (bioavailability about 70%) after oral administration and has low protein binding. Zonisamide has been demonstrated to be absorbed rectally in dogs. The elimination half-life in dogs is about 15 hours. Most of the drug is excreted via the kidneys into the urine, but about 20% is metabolized, primarily in the liver. Unlike in humans, zonisamide exhibits linear pharmacokinetics (dose to plasma trough concentrations) in dogs (at doses between 5–30 mg/kg PO twice daily) (Fukunaga *et al.* 2010).

Zonisamide has a long half-life in cats of approximately 33 hours (Hasegawa *et al.* 2008).

Contraindications/Precautions/Warnings

Zonisamide is contraindicated in patients hypersensitive to it or to any of the sulfonamide drugs.

Adverse Effects

Because there has been limited use of this drug in veterinary patients the adverse effect profile is not fully known. Adverse effects that have been reported in dogs include sedation (usually transient), ataxia, and inappetence. Because it is a sulfonamide, there is concern (yet no reports as of writing) that zonisamide may cause KCS or other sulfonamide-related adverse effects in dogs or cats.

In a combined pharmacokinetic and toxicity study in cats, half of cats receiving 20 mg/kg per day developed adverse effects that included inappetence, diarrhea, vomiting, ataxia and somnolence (Hasegawa *et al.* 2008). Tolerance to therapy is possible.

In humans, the most common adverse effects associated with zonisamide include anorexia, nausea, dizziness, somnolence, agitation and headache. Rarely, serious dermatologic reactions (Stevens-Johnson syndrome, TEN), blood dyscrasias, oligohidrosis, and hyperthermia have been reported in humans.

Reproductive/Nursing Safety

When zonisamide was administered to pregnant dogs at 10 or 30 mg/kg/day (approximate therapeutic dosages in dogs), ventricular septal defects, cardiomegaly and various valvular and arterial anomalies were seen at the higher dose. A plasma level of 25 micrograms/mL was the threshold level for malformation. If this drug is to be used in pregnant dogs, the owner must accept the significant risks associated with its use.

It is not known if zonisamide enters maternal milk; use with caution in nursing animals.

Overdosage/Acute Toxicity

The LD_{50} of zonisamide in dogs is reportedly 1 gram/kg. In human overdoses, effects reported include coma, bradycardia, hypotension, and respiratory depression. Treatment recommendations include GI evacuation, if ingestion was recent, and supportive therapy. Because of the drug's long half-life, support may be required for several days.

Drug Interactions

The following drug interactions have either been reported or are theoretical in humans or animals receiving zonisamide and may be of significance in veterinary patients:

■ **PHENOBARBITAL:** In dogs, phenobarbital may increase the clearance of zonisamide as repeated phenobarbital dosing decreased the bioavailability, peak concentrations, half-life, and area under the curve of zonisamide, but it did not affect the time to peak level or the volume of distribution of zonisamide. This effect persisted up to 10 weeks after phenobarbital discontinuation (Orito *et al.* 2008). See the dose section for suggestions on altering zonisamide doses for dogs on phenobarbital.

Laboratory Considerations

■ No specific laboratory interactions or considerations were noted

■ While plasma concentrations of zonisamide are not routinely monitored in human patients, in dogs, the therapeutic range has been suggested to be from 10–40 micrograms/mL

Doses

■ **DOGS:**

a) 5–10 mg/kg PO q12h. The high end of the dose range is needed when used in combination with phenobarbital, probably as a result of phenobarbital-induced microsomal enzyme induction. (Munana 2010)

b) As monotherapy: Initially at 5 mg/kg PO twice daily (q12h). When used in combination with phenobarbital: 10 mg/kg PO q12h. (Thomas 2010), (Martin-Jimenez 2010)

c) As initial monotherapy: 3–5 mg/kg PO q12h. As an add-on agent: 10 mg/kg PO q12h. (Mariani 2010)

d) Initial dose: 5–10 mg/kg PO q12h; gradual adaptation in dosing is recommended. Reduce phenobarbital doses by 25% at the time of starting zonisamide. (Podell 2006)

■ **CATS:**

a) There are anecdotal reports of the use of zonisamide in cats, with oral doses of 5 mg/kg every 12-24 hours most commonly utilized. (Munana 2010)

b) Because of its long half-life, doses of 5–10 mg/kg PO once daily are likely to be appropriate in cats, although additional studies are needed to determine this. The authors report using the drug in 2 cats that were refractory to phenobarbital therapy; one developed anorexia and the drug had to be discontinued, but the other responded well. (Bailey & Dewey 2009)

c) 10–20 mg/kg PO once daily. (Martin-Jimenez 2010)

Monitoring

■ Efficacy

■ Monitoring zonisamide blood levels may be useful in veterinary patients, but this has not been confirmed nor have veterinary therapeutic blood concentrations been identified. Therapeutic levels for humans are thought to be: 10–40 micrograms/mL.

■ Adverse effects

Client Information

■ Caution clients not to stop therapy abruptly or "rebound" seizures may occur

■ Have clients maintain a seizure diary to help determine efficacy

Chemistry/Synonyms

A sulfonamide unrelated to other antiseizure drugs, zonisamide occurs as a white powder with a pKa of 10.2. It is moderately soluble in water (0.8 mg/mL).

Zonisamide may also be known as: AD-810, CI-912, PD-110843, *Excegran®*, or *Zonegran®*.

Storage/Stability

Zonisamide capsules should be stored at 25°C (76°F); excursions permitted to 15–30°C (59–86°F). Store in a dry place and protected from light.

Dosage Forms/Regulatory Status

VETERINARY-LABELED PRODUCTS: None

HUMAN-LABELED PRODUCTS:

Zonisamide Capsules: 25 mg, 50 mg & 100 mg; *Zonegran®* (Eisai); generic; (Rx)

References

Bailey, K.S. & C.W. Dewey (2009). The Seizuring Cat: Diagnostic work-up and therapy. *Journal of Feline Medicine and Surgery* 11(5): 385–394.

Fukunaga, K., M. Saito, et al. (2010). Steady-state pharmacokinetics of zonisamide in plasma, whole blood, and erythrocytes in dogs. *Journal of Veterinary Pharmacology and Therapeutics* 33(1): 103–106.

Hasegawa, D., M. Kobayashi, et al. (2008). Pharmacokinetics and toxicity of zonisamide in cats. *Journal of Feline Medicine and Surgery* 10(4): 418–421.

Mariani, C. (2010). Maintenance therapy for the routine & difficult to control epileptic patient. Proceedings: ACVIM Forum. Accessed via: Veterinary Information Network. http://goo.gl/quX8P

Martin-Jimenez, T. (2010). Newer agents for the treatment of epileptic disorders. Proceedings: WVC. Accessed via: Veterinary Information Network. http://goo.gl/L5HIt

Munana, K. (2010). Current Approaches to Seizure Management. Proceedings: ACVIM Forum. Accessed via: Veterinary Information Network. http://goo.gl/vI8Lp

Orito, K., M. Saito, et al. (2008). Pharmacokinetics of zonisamide and drug interaction with phenobarbital in dogs. *Journal of Veterinary Pharmacology and Therapeutics* 31(3): 259–264.

Podell, M. (2006). New Horizons in the treatment of epilepsy. Proceedings: ACVIM. Accessed via: Veterinary Information Network. http://goo.gl/PlHdG

Thomas, W.B. (2010). Idiopathic Epilepsy in Dogs and Cats. *Veterinary Clinics of North America-Small Animal Practice* 40(1): 161–+.

Appendix

Ophthalmic Products, Topical

The following section lists the majority of veterinary-labeled ophthalmic topical products and some of the more commonly used human-labeled products in veterinary medicine; written by Gigi Davidson, DICVP with input from Michael Davidson, DVM, DACVO. Drugs are listed by therapeutic class.

For additional information, an excellent review on veterinary ophthalmic pharmacology and therapeutics can be found in both of the following textbooks: Slatter's Fundamentals of Veterinary Ophthalmology, 4th Edition. David Maggs, Paul Miller, Ron Ofri, Editors, Elsevier,

2007, 496 pages, and Veterinary Ophthalmology, 4th Edition; Kirk N Gelatt, Editor; Lippincott Williams & Wilkins, Media, Pennsylvania, 2007. 1568 pp.

Routes of Administration For Ophthalmic Drugs

The route of administration selected to deliver therapy for an ocular condition is critical to successful therapy. The following table lists advantages and disadvantages of each route of administration for ocular medications.

Route	Tissues Reached	Dosage Forms	Advantages	Disadvantages	Comments
Topical	Conjunctiva; Cornea; Anterior uvea; Lids	Solutions Suspensions	Easier administration for small animals; minimal interference with vision; lower incidence of contact dermatitis; less toxic to interior of eye if penetrating wound	More difficult to administer to horses; less contact time with eye; requires more frequent application than ointment; diluted by tearing; generally more expensive than ointment; more systemic absorption	Doses >1 drop rarely indicated in small animals (maximum tear capacity is 10−20 ml, volume of a drop is 25−50 ml); allow 5 minutes between drops; instill in order of least viscous to most; instill in order of aqueous prior to oil base
		Ointments	Longer contact time; less frequent administration; protect cornea from drying; not diluted by tearing; generally less expensive than solutions/ suspensions	Contribute to volume of ocular discharge; temporary blurring of vision; more difficult for client administration; more contact dermatitis; should not be applied to penetrating corneal wounds as oils will cause a granulomatous uveitis; difficult to determine exact dose; metal tubes often fatigue and split before all medication is used	Owners should be counseled to avoid contact of application tube with eye; observe patient for short while after application due to temporarily blurred vision
Subconjunctival injection	Cornea; Anterior uvea	Sterile solutions and suspensions	Longer duration of action; higher anterior chamber concentrations than topical;	Limited number of injections can be performed; may create scar tissue; cannot be removed once applied; temporary pain; drug vehicle residues	Indicated for poorly compliant owners, uncooperative patients; indicated for drugs with poor corneal penetration
Retrobulbar injection	Posterior segment; Optic nerve	Sterile solutions and suspensions			Primarily used for local anesthetic prior to enucleation of the eye
Intracameral injection	Anterior chamber; Posterior segment	Sterile solutions and suspensions	Allows very high drug concentrations for intraocular infections	Risk of hemorrhage, retinal detachment, cataract formation, and retinal degeneration	Rarely used except for severe intraocular infections or for administration of tPA to dissolve fibrin clots in the anterior chamber
Systemic Drugs	Lids; Posterior segment; Optic nerve; Anterior uvea (occasionally)	Oral Intramuscular Subcutaneous Intravenous	Allows drug penetration to areas where topical therapy will not reach	Systemic toxicity; Does not reach cornea; expense directly proportional to body weight in most cases	See monographs for use of systemic agents.

Diagnostic Agents

Note: A logical sequence of diagnostic tests must be used to perform ocular examination based on the special needs of each diagnostic agent and test. For example, evaluation of the tear film is performed with the Schirmer Tear Test and must be done before the eye is manipulated or any drug agents are instilled in order to provide a true picture of tear production. Likewise, cultures of the external ocular structures must be done prior to extensive cleaning or administration of any drugs that may alter bacterial culture. The use of mydriatics is essential to examination of the interior elements of the eye, but must not be given prior to measuring intraocular pressure as these agents will likely affect aqueous humor outflow. Intraocular pressure determination requires topical anesthetic, but must quickly be recorded prior to excessive manipulation of the eye or before the patient becomes anxious and uncooperative.

FLUORESCEIN SODIUM
(flure-e-seen)

Indications/Pharmacology

Fluorescein sodium is a yellow water-soluble dye that fluoresces under a Wood's Lamp, but is plainly visible after binding to corneal stroma through an ophthalmic examination light source. It is used most commonly to delineate full thickness loss of corneal epithelium indicating the presence of a corneal ulceration. In this instance, it will stain the corneal stroma. The epithelium is not stained because its outer lipid cell membrane repels the stain. Descemet's membrane will not stain with fluorescein stain and this is used to indicate descemetocele formation, an ocular emergency.

Fluorescein stain is applied to the precorneal tear film in dogs and cats and the break-up of this stain with time, as observed through a slit lamp biomicroscope using a cobalt blue light source, is used to determine the tear film break-up time (normal 19 seconds), an indicator of tear film quality.

Fluorescein stain is applied to the tear film of dogs to determine patency of the nasolacrimal outflow system. The normal wait time is 2–5 minutes in dogs and up to 10 minutes in cats. A positive test indicates patency of the system. A negative test is not indicative of disease, as the test is negative in a large percentage of normal animals. Fluorescein stain, then, can be added to irrigating solution to flush the nasolacrimal system, making detecting the irrigation solution at the nose more obvious during flushing of the system.

Suggested Dosages/Precautions/Adverse Effects

Fluorescein stain is applied by dropping a drop of irrigating solution onto the sterile strip and then allowing the drop to fall on the eye. The strip should not contact the cornea or it will cause false positive stain retention at the site of contact with the epithelial cells. Fluorescein impregnated paper strips are preferred to fluorescein solution to insure sterility. After a few seconds, the excess fluorescein is irrigated from the eye, staining areas of full thickness epithelial loss.

For procedures requiring topical anesthesia as well as a disclosing agent, benoxinate is added to fluorescein solutions in a ratio of 0.25% fluorescein to 0.4% benoxinate. These solutions are useful for removal of foreign bodies or sutures, but are not commonly used in veterinary medicine.

Conjunctival or corneal epithelial cells for fluorescent antibody testing should be collected prior to application of fluorescein stain, which can cause a false positive test for several days after application of the stain.

Fluorescein may rarely cause hypersensitivity reactions. Temporary staining of fur and skin may result. Do not use during intraocular surgery.

Dosage Forms/Regulatory Status

VETERINARY-LABELED PRODUCTS: None

HUMAN-LABELED PRODUCTS:

Sterile strips of paper impregnated with fluorescein sodium are the most commonly used form in veterinary medicine. Solutions (2%) of fluorescein are available, however they are not popular following one study indicating that Pseudomonas is readily grown in such solutions. Injectable products are also available (for ophthalmic angiography), but are not routinely used in veterinary medicine.

Fluorescein Sodium Strips: 0.6 mg, *Ful-Glo®* (Barnes Hind); 1 mg, *Fluor-I-Strip®-A.T.* (W-A); 9 mg, *Fluor-I-Strip®* (W-A); (all Rx); 1 mg *Bio-Glo®*, 100 ct or 300 ct (Wilson Ophthalmic,) *AK Flor 10% Injection* (Akorn) 5 mL ampules

Fluorescein Sodium:Benoxinate: *Fluress®* (Akorn) 0.25:0.4% Drops in 5 mL, *Flurox®* (Hub) 0.25:0.4% Drops in 5 mL, *Flurate®* (Bausch and Lomb) 0.25:0.4% Drops in 5 mL.

LISSAMINE GREEN
(lis-ah-meen)

Indications/Pharmacology

Lissamine green is used for diagnosis of corneal damage and to quantify tear production. These strips work by staining the cornea blue upon instillation, resulting in a "speckling" of the cornea. This speckling marks any corneal ulcerations as well as dry patches from any muco-deficient or damaged corneal cells. A white or blue light may be used on the slit lamp during detection. Lissamine green possesses a therapeutic advantage in that it does not sting the eye like Rose Bengal; however, as interpretation of lissamine green results requires broader experience than that of Rose Bengal and fluorescein, fluorescein staining is considered a more reliable indicator of corneal damage.

Suggested Dosages/Precautions/Adverse Effects

Lissamine Green impregnated strips are placed in the conjunctival sac and staining is scored based on 6 areas of staining.

Dosage Forms/Regulatory Status

VETERINARY-LABELED PRODUCTS: None

HUMAN-LABELED PRODUCTS:

Lissamine Green Ophthalmic Strips (Imperial Chemical Industries—available through distributors such as Wilson Ophthalmic) 1.5 mg, 100 individually wrapped strips per box.

PHENOL RED THREAD
(*fee*-nol)

Indications/Pharmacology

Measurement of tear production is an important diagnostic test when deficiency of the lacrimal system is suspected. Tear production is evaluated qualitatively by assessment of the corneal surface for moistness and luster. Tear production is measured quantitatively with either the Schirmer Tear Test or the Phenol Red Thread Test. The Phenol Red Thread (PRT) test is a new, fast and equally accurate method to test tear production as compared to the Schirmer Tear Test. The PRT test has a 75mm long yellow-colored thread that is impregnated with phenol red, a pH sensitive indicator.

Suggested Dosages/Precautions/Adverse Effects

The 3mm indentation at the end of the thread is inserted into the inferior conjunctival sac for 15 seconds. As tears travel up the thread, the alkaline pH of the tears turns the thread red. The PRT requires only 15 seconds for diagnostic results as opposed to 1 minute for the Schirmer Tear Test in dogs. Normal tear production via PRT in cats at 15 seconds is 18.4 to 27.7 mm/15 seconds and, in dogs, 29.7 to 38.6 mm/15 seconds.

Dosage Forms/Regulatory Status

VETERINARY-APPROVED PRODUCTS: None

HUMAN-LABELED PRODUCTS:

Phenol Red Thread Test: *Zone-QuickDiagnostic Threads®*, 100 per box, (Menicon—available through distributors such as Wilson Ophthalmic)

ROSE BENGAL
(*rose ben*-gall)

Indications/Pharmacology

Rose bengal is a vital stain and stains dead epithelial cells and mucus. Full thickness loss of the corneal epithelium is not necessary (only dead cells need be present) to obtain rose bengal stain uptake. It does not stain epithelial defects and does not pass into intercellular spaces.

Rose bengal stain is most commonly employed in the detection of the presence of viral keratitis in the cat. Because feline herpes virus tends to infect one cell, moving then to an adjacent cell (causing the so called dendritic tracts in the cornea) without full thickness loss of corneal epithelium initially, rose bengal is an ideal diagnostic agent for this infection. Rose Bengal can also be used to detect damaged corneal epithelium on the dorsal cornea in early cases of keratoconjunctivitis sicca. Rose bengal stain is virucidal although no information is available relative to its use as a therapeutic agent.

Suggested Dosages/Precautions/Adverse Effects

Rose Bengal is applied as a solution (1–2 drops in conjunctival sac before examination) or from an impregnated strip (saturate tip of strip with sterile irrigating solution; touch bulbar conjunctiva or lower fornix with moistened strip; cause patient to blink several times to distribute the stain).

Rose bengal is apparently toxic to the cornea and conjunctiva and should be thoroughly flushed from the eye after use to prevent irritation. Hypersensitivity reactions are possible. May stain clothing.

Dosage Forms/Regulatory Status

VETERINARY-LABELED PRODUCTS: None

HUMAN-LABELED PRODUCTS:

Rose Bengal Solution: 1% in 5 mL dropper bottles (Spectrum); (Rx)

Rose Bengal Strips: 1.3 mg per strip; *Rosets®* (Akorn); generic (Barnes-Hind); (Rx)

SCHIRMER TEAR TEST
(*shir*-mer)

Indications/Dosages/Precautions

Measurement of tear production is an important diagnostic test when deficiency of the lacrimal system is suspected. Tear production is evaluated qualitatively by assessment of the corneal surface for moistness and luster. Tear production is measured quantitatively by the Schirmer Tear Test or the Phenol Red Thread Test. The Schirmer Tear Test measures the aqueous aspect of tears and is the most commonly used test for measuring tear production.

Suggested Dosages/Precautions/Adverse Effects

Because of the risk of false readings, the following should be avoided prior to conducting a Schirmer Tear Test: excessive manipulation of the eyelids, topical anesthesia, and topical or systemic drugs (*e.g.,* tranquilizers and atropine). The round end of the test paper is bent while still in the envelope and positioned to avoid contamination. The bent end should be positioned in the lacrimal lake at the junction of the lateral and middle thirds of the lower eyelid. Most animals will close the eye during the test but this does not affect results. The Schirmer Tear Test should be left in position for one minute as results are not linear and cannot be extrapolated from shorter test times. Schirmer tear test values are as follows for the following species: Dogs: 21.9 ± 4.0 mm wetting per minute, Rabbits: 5.3 ± 2.9 mm wetting per minute, Cats: 20.2 ± 4.5 mm wetting per minute.

Dosage Forms/Regulatory Status

VETERINARY-LABELED PRODUCTS:

Schirmer Tear Test®: 300 individually wrapped strips, (Schering Plough/Intervet)

HUMAN-LABELED PRODUCTS:

Clemente Clarke® *Schirmer Tear Test Strips*: 50 pair/box, *Schirmer Tear Test Strips*® (Alcon)

Ocular Anesthetics

Local anesthetic effect is dependent upon chemical structure and concentration. Local anesthetic agents structurally consist of a hydrophobic aromatic ring (benzoic acid derivatives), a linkage site between the aromatic ring and an intermediate chain, and a hydrophilic amine. The hydrophobic portion is essential for activity, as it is the portion that enables diffusion through the lipid membrane of nerves increasing hydrophobicity increases access of the anesthetic to its site of action and decreases its metabolism, thereby increasing potency and duration. Greater hydrophobicity is also associated with increased toxicity. The hydrophilic amine portion may exist in an uncharged, poorly water-soluble form, or as the positively charged ammonium ion.

Topical anesthetics adversely affect the epithelial surface and delay wound healing. Adverse effects range from superficial punctate keratitis, decreased tearing, and decreased blinking, to corneal edema, pain, and diffuse necrotizing keratitis. Long-term administration inhibits cell migration and mitosis leading to retarded wound healing and infection. For this reason, topical anesthetics are never administered therapeutically.

Contraindications to topical anesthetics include liver disease (decreased clearance), concurrent anticholinergic therapy (prevents metabolism of esters), perforating ocular injury, and for collection of ocular surface cultures (due to inhibition of microbial growth.)

PROPARACAINE HCL
(proe-*par*-a-kane)

Indications/Pharmacology

Proparacaine is a rapid acting topical anesthetic useful for a variety of ophthalmic procedures including tonometry (intraocular pressure measurement), relief of corneal pain to facilitate examination, biopsy/sample collection, and to distinguish between corneal and uveal pain. Proparacaine primarily anesthetizes the cornea; with limited penetration into conjunctiva. Anesthesia is of short duration (5–10 minutes).

Suggested Doses/Precautions/Adverse Effects

Usual dose is 1–2 drops prior to examination or procedure. For prolonged procedures only requiring local anesthesia; may repeat 1 drop doses every 5–10 minutes for 5–7 doses.

Dosage Forms/Regulatory Status

VETERINARY-LABELED PRODUCTS:

Proparacaine HCl Solution: 0.5% in 15 mL bottles; *Ophthaine*® (Solvay); (Rx). Protect from light. Refrigerate.

HUMAN-LABELED PRODUCTS:

Proparacaine HCl Solution: 0.5% in 2 & 15 mL bottles; *Ophthetic*® (Allergan), *Alcaine*® (Alcon), *Ophthaine*® (Squibb), *AK-Taine*® (Akorn), Generic; (Rx). Protect from light. Some products should be refrigerated; check label.

TETRACAINE HCL
(*teh*-trah-kane)

Indications/Pharmacology

Tetracaine is more irritating than proparacaine but is sometimes used in veterinary medicine. It is indicated to produce local anesthesia of short duration for ophthalmic procedures including measurement of intraocular pressure (tonometry), removal of foreign bodies and sutures, and conjunctival and corneal scraping in diagnosis and gonioscopy. Tetracaine is also indicated to produce local anesthesia prior to surgical procedures in humans such as cataract extraction and pterygium excision, usually as an adjunct to locally injected anesthetics. Ophthalmic solutions used for intraocular procedures should be preservative-free. Preservatives may cause damage to the corneal epithelium if a significant quantity of solution enters the eye through the incision.

Suggested Dosages/Precautions/Adverse Effects

Usual dose is 1–2 drops prior to examination or procedure. The onset of action is about 15 seconds. The duration of action usually extends with repeated applications.

Topical anesthetics should not be used to treat painful eye disease. Prolonged use may retard wound healing and cause corneal epithelial ulcers. Because the blink reflex may be suppressed, the eye should be protected from external injury during use. Repeated use may lead to rapid development of tolerance. Local allergic-type reactions have been rarely reported in humans.

Dosage Forms/Regulatory Status

VETERINARY-LABELED PRODUCTS: None

HUMAN-LABELED PRODUCTS:

Tetracaine Solution 0.5%: 15 mL; *Ak-Taine®* (Akorn), *Alcaine®* (Alcon), *Ocu-Caine®*, *Ophthaine®*, *Ophthetic®*, *Spectro-Caine®*; (Rx)

Tetracaine Solution 2%; 15 mL and 30 mL bottles; *Pontocaine®* (Hospira); (Rx)

Tetracaine Injection 10 mg/mL; 2 mL ampules; *Pontocaine®* (Hospira); (Rx)

BENOXINATE
(bin-*ak*-sin-ate)

Indications/Pharmacology

Benoxinate is only available in combination with vital dyes, either sodium fluorescein 0.25% or disodium fluorexon 0.35% (a high-molecular-weight fluorescein that does not stain hydrogel contact lenses, allowing contacts to be worn sooner following administration, without concern of staining). It has a similar onset, intensity, and duration of action to that of tetracaine 0.5% and proparacaine 0.5%. Benoxinate has not been evaluated in veterinary ophthalmology.

Dosage Forms/Regulatory Status

VETERINARY-LABELED PRODUCTS: None

HUMAN-LABELED PRODUCTS:

Fluorescein Sodium:Benoxinate: *Fluress®* (Akorn) 0.25:0.4% Drops in 5 mL, *Flurox®* (Hub) 0.25:0.4% Drops in 5 mL, *Flurate®* (Bausch and Lomb) 0.25:0.4% Drops in 5 mL.

Ocular Hypotensive Agents, Topical

Note: It is important to review the basic pathophysiology of glaucoma in order to understand drug therapy of this disease. Aqueous humor production results from ciliary body secretion and ultrafiltration of plasma. Carbonic anhydrase is a vital enzyme in the production of aqueous humor. Outflow of aqueous humor flows from the posterior chamber into the anterior chamber and exits at the iridocorneal angle, or exits through the iris, ciliary body, choroids, and sclera. The balance of generation and outflow of aqueous humor maintains the intraocular pressure at between 15 and 25 mmHg. By definition, glaucoma is an increase in intraocular pressure with resulting visual deficits. Delayed

inadequate or inappropriate therapy can result in severe pain and irreversible blindness as well as a cosmetically unappealing eye. Generally, once acute congestive primary glaucoma (generally breed-related and hereditary) is noted in one eye in the dog, it is treated as an emergency using a topical prostaglandin such as latanoprost. Surgery may be considered for lasting control of intraocular pressure. The following topical drugs are used "in general" as a preventative measure to prevent the occurrence of primary glaucoma in the unaffected eye in canine patients. Topical ocular antihypertensive medications are sometimes employed for pressure control with secondary glaucomas also. Because primary glaucoma in dogs is a progressive disorder, many patients are initially treated with single agents but combinations of drugs are often ultimately necessary to maintain pressure control.

Primary glaucoma in the feline species is increasingly being recognized in several forms. Although breed-related glaucoma in Siamese and Persian cat breeds has been noted, many veterinary ophthalmologists feel that domestic shorthaired cats are most likely affected. One form involving misdirected flow of aqueous humor into the vitreous, secondarily resulting in a forward displacement of the lens-iris diaphragm, has been described in the literature. The forward displacement of the iris has resulted in an average intraocular pressure of 30 mmHg in most patients. Topical medications have been successful in preventing progressive vision loss in most of these cats. Other forms of feline glaucomas that are presumably genetic are being noted sporadically in clinical practice and most of these cases, in complete contrast with primary glaucoma in the canine, are managed successfully with medications. Pharmacologic agents utilized for medical treatment of glaucoma are noted below categorized by therapeutic class but not by therapeutic priority.

Parasympathomimetics (Miotics)

The parasympathomimetic nervous system utilizes acetylcholine as the pre- and post-synaptic neurotransmitter. Parasympathomimetic drugs act either directly by mimicking acetylcholine, or indirectly by preventing its breakdown by acetylcholinesterase. Parasympathomimetics are useful ocular therapeutic agents by virtue of inducing contraction of the intraocular smooth muscle (miosis), which reduces intraocular pressure.

CARBACHOL
(*kar*-beh-call)

Indications/Pharmacology

Carbachol is a direct-acting parasympathomimetic but also has some indirect action through inhibition of acetylcholinesterase. It cannot penetrate intact epithelium and when used topically (rarely), its use must be accompanied with a surfactant (benzalkonium chloride) to enhance penetration.

Carbachol has been used to induce miosis in treatment of glaucoma, but more commonly, is used by veterinary ophthalmologists as an intracameral 0.01% injection at the conclusion of phacoemulsification surgery (cataract removal) to protect against postoperative increases in intraocular pressure (Crasta *et al.* 2010; Stuhr *et al.* 1998).

Suggested Dosages/Precautions/Adverse Effects

Carbachol 0.75% has been used topically, although rarely, to reduce intraocular pressures in dogs at a dose of 1 drop every 4-8 hours. Carbachol is administered intraoperatively at a dose of 0.5 mL of a 0.01% solution. Carbachol shares the potential for the same adverse effects of all other miotic agents, and in humans has been noted to cause severe headaches and accommodative muscle spasms. Corneal clouding, persistent bullous keratopathy, retinal detachment and postoperative iritis have been reported in humans following intracameral injection of carbachol following cataract extraction.

Dosage Forms/Regulatory Status

VETERINARY-LABELED PRODUCTS: NONE

HUMAN-LABELED PRODUCTS:

Carbachol 0.01% Injection, for intraocular use only, 10 x 1 mL ampules, *Carbastat®* (Novartis), *Miostat®* Intraocular (Alcon); (Rx)

Carbachol Ophthalmic Solution: 0.75%, 1.5%, 2.25%, and 3%, in 15 mL plastic dropper bottles; *Isopto Carbachol®* (Alcon), *Carboptic®* (Optopics); (Rx)

References

Crasta, M., A.B. Clode, et al. (2010). Effect of three treatment protocols on acute ocular hypertension after phacoemulsification and aspiration of cataracts in dogs. Veterinary Ophthalmology 13(1): 14-19.

Stuhr, C.M., P. Miller, et al. (1998). Effect of intracameral administration of carbachol on the post-operative increase in intraocular pressure in dogs undergoing cataract extraction. JAVMA 212: 18885-11888.

PILOCARPINE HCL

(pye-loe-*kar*-peen)

Indications/Pharmacology

Pilocarpine is a cholinergic agonist (miotic) that is rarely used in the treatment of canine primary glaucoma. Pilocarpine causes the ciliary body muscle to constrict placing posteriorly directed tension on the base of the iris to mechanically pull open the iridocorneal angle structures. By causing miosis, it may prevent closure of the iridocorneal angle by preventing excess iris tissue from peripherally compromising the outflow of aqueous humor. It should be noted however, that cholinergic agonists reduce uveoscleral outflow, making them less useful in species that are more dependent on uveoscleral outflow for maintenance of intraocular pressure (*e.g.*, horses). Evaluation of pilocarpine 2% to normal mares did not reduce intraocular pressure although it did induce miosis (van der Woerdt *et al.* 1998).

Pilocarpine has also been used for diagnostic localization of parasympathetic denervation of the iris sphincter caused by lesions or trauma to Cranial Nerve III. The popularity of treatment of KCS with ophthalmic cyclosporine and tacrolimus has been associated with a decline in the use of pilocarpine for this disease; however, pilocarpine is still used orally as the primary treatment of neurogenic keratoconjunctivitis sicca in dogs as this condition does not respond to cyclosporine or tacrolimus.

Pilocarpine is available in various solutions and gels with a low and potentially irritating pH of 4.5-5.5 in order to maintain drug stability. A buffered-tip formulation of pilocarpine enables administration of a pH 7.0 solution, which may decrease ocular side effects without compromising efficacy.

Suggested Dosages/Precautions/Adverse Effects

One drop in affected eye(s) 3 times daily. Usually 1% or 2% is most commonly used in veterinary medicine.

Pilocarpine can cause local irritation initially accompanied by a profound miosis that significantly decreases visual acuity, in humans. This irritation reportedly diminishes after 3 days of therapy. It may also cause inflammation of the uveal tract, especially with repeated applications and can cause hyphema. Chronic use may result in an irreversible miosis due to dilator muscle atrophy and sphincter muscle fibrosis. Pilocarpine should not be used in secondary glaucoma cases. With repeated use, pilocarpine may cause systemic effects (vomiting, diarrhea, increased salivation, bronchiolar spasm, and pulmonary edema). Pilocarpine should be avoided in dogs with glaucoma secondary to uveitis as well as in dogs with lens luxation or subluxation due to potential for papillary block.

For diagnosis of parasympathetic denervation or other conditions caused by cranial nerve III lesions, a 0.2% solution of pilocarpine is applied topically. For neurogenic keratoconjunctivitis sicca, a 2% solution of pilocarpine is given orally (in food) at a dose of 2 drops per 20 lbs of body weight twice daily. The dose is increased weekly until signs of toxicity or until control of symptoms is achieved.

Dosage Forms/Regulatory Status

VETERINARY-LABELED PRODUCTS: None

HUMAN-LABELED PRODUCTS:

Pilocarpine HCl Ophthalmic Solution: 0.25%, 0.5%, 1%, 2%, 3%, 4%, and 6% (in addition there are 8% and 10% solutions and a 4% gel is available from Alcon) in 15 mL and 30 mL containers; *Isopto Carpine*® (Alcon); *Ocu-Carpine*® (Iomed); *Piloptic*® (Optopics); *Pilostat*® (Bausch and Lomb), generic; (Rx)

See also the epinephrine monograph for information on epinephrine/pilocarpine fixed dose combination products.

References
van der Woerdt, A., B.C. Gilger, et al. (1998). Normal variation in, and effect of 2% pilocarpine on, intraocular pressure and pupil size in female horses. *American Journal of Veterinary Research* 59(11): 1459-1462.

DEMECARIUM BROMIDE
(deh-meh-*kar*-ee-um)

Indications/Pharmacology
Demecarium is a potent, long-acting carbamate inhibitor that may reduce intraocular pressures for up to 48 hours in canines. Demecarium reversibly inhibits anticholinesterase thereby causing miosis. Demecarium is generally used in preventive management of the contralateral eye in canine patients after the diagnosis of an acute congestive crisis of primary glaucoma in the other eye. It is not used in secondary glaucoma. Demecarium has the advantage of once or twice daily dosing.

Suggested Dosages/Precautions/Adverse Effects
One drop once or twice daily. Demecarium is contraindicated during pregnancy. Because of additive effects, demecarium should be used with caution with other cholinesterase inhibitors (*e.g.*, carbamate/organophosphate antiparasiticides), or succinylcholine. Demecarium can cause ciliary body muscle spasm, producing a headache and blurred vision, as well as local inflammation (alleviated by addition of topical corticosteroids) and systemic adverse effects (vomiting, diarrhea, increased salivation, cardiac effects), particularly with high dosages or in very small dogs.

Dosage Forms/Regulatory Status
VETERINARY-LABELED PRODUCTS: None

HUMAN-LABELED PRODUCTS:

Formerly available as: Demecarium 0.125% or 0.25% in 5 mL dropper bottles; *Humorsol*® (Merck); (Rx). Do not freeze and protect from heat. Demecarium must be obtained from an appropriately qualified compounding pharmacy.

ECHOTHIOPHATE IODIDE
(ek-oh-*thye*-oh-fate *eye*-oh-dide)

Indications/Pharmacology
Echothiophate iodide for ophthalmic solution is a long-acting, irreversible cholinesterase inhibitor for topical use that enhances the effect of endogenously liberated acetylcholine in iris, ciliary muscle, and other parasympathetically innervated structures of the eye. It thereby causes miosis, increase in facility of outflow of aqueous humor, fall in intraocular pressure, and potentiation of accommodation. Echothiophate iodide for ophthalmic solution will depress both plasma and erythrocyte cholinesterase levels in most patients after a few weeks of eye drop therapy.

Suggested Doses/Precautions/Adverse Effects
One drop twice daily. Echothiophate is contraindicated in the presence of active uveal inflammation, and in most cases of angle-closure glaucoma, due to the possibility of increasing angle block. Temporary or permanent discontinuation of the drug may be required if cardiac irregularities, urinary incontinence, diarrhea, muscle weakness, nausea, abdominal cramps, fatigue, weakness or respiratory difficulties occur. Echothiophate should be avoided in patients with asthma, gastric ulcers, bradycardia, hypotension, epilepsy or other disorders that may respond adversely to vagotonic effects. Carbamate and organophosphate pesticides should not be used on patients receiving echothiophate.

Dosage Forms/Regulatory Status
VETERINARY-LABELED PRODUCTS: None

HUMAN-LABELED PRODUCTS:

Echothiophate Iodide Solution: 0.125% in 5 mL; *Phospholine Iodide*® (Wyeth); (Rx). Store under refrigeration. Once reconstituted, may be stored at room temperature for up to 4 weeks.

Sympathomimetics (Alpha₂-Agonists)
Alpha-agonists reduce intraocular pressure by activation of presynaptic alpha-receptors, inhibiting release of norepinephrine, blocking adrenergic stimulation of the ciliary body and decreasing production of aqueous humor. Chronic use of these agents also results in increased uveoscleral outflow.

APRACLONIDINE
(a-pra-*kloe*-ni-deen)

Indications/Pharmacology
Apraclonidine is an alpha2 adrenergic agonist used to reduce aqueous humor formation. Apraclonidine is a relatively selective, alpha-adrenergic agonist and does not have significant membrane stabilizing (local anesthetic) activity. The primary ocular side effects noted following use of apraclonidine include conjunctival

blanching, eyelid elevation, and mydriasis. While its systemic side effects are relatively mild compared to those of the beta-blockers, apraclonidine can cause dry eye or dry mouth, as well as mild elevations in resting heart rate, blood pressure, and respiration. Chronic use of apraclonidine can lead to decrease in therapeutic response. The onset of action is within 3–5 hours of a single dose. It apparently is less effective than brimonidine in dogs and is very potent, causing vomiting and diarrhea in dogs and cats (Miller & Rhaesa 1996). Severe side effects such as bradycardia, salivation and vomiting preclude use of apraclonidine in cats. Apraclonidine will reduce aqueous production, but it must be combined with other agents for adequate control. Neither the beta-blockers nor alpha-agonists are as effective as the carbonic anhydrase inhibitors in decreasing aqueous production.

Suggested Dosage/Precautions/Adverse Effects

1% solution applied as 1 drop 2–3 times daily. Apraclonidine should be used with caution in the face of hepatic and renal function impairment (since a structurally related medication, clonidine, is partly metabolized in the liver and undergoes a significant increase in half life in humans with renal impairment). Apraclonidine should not be used in cats due to severe adverse effects including vomiting, diarrhea, bradycardia and salivation. Ironically, in humans the 0.5% concentration is more likely to cause cardiovascular adverse effects than the 1% solution. In humans the following side effects have been noted: For 0.5% ophthalmic apraclonidine: Allergic reaction, abnormal coordination, arrhythmia, asthma, blepharitis, blepharoconjunctivitis, conjunctivitis, blurred vision or change in vision, chest pain, contact dermatitis, corneal erosion, corneal infiltrate, foreign body sensation, keratitis, keratopathy, depression, dizziness, dyspnea, edema of eye, eyelid, or conjunctiva, eye discharge, facial edema, lid retraction, paresthesia, or peripheral edema. For 1% ophthalmic apraclonidine: allergic reaction, arrhythmia, or ocular inflammation or injection.

Dosage Forms/Regulatory Status

VETERINARY-LABELED PRODUCTS: None

HUMAN-LABELED PRODUCTS:

Apraclonidine 0.5% Solution: 5 mL & 10 mL; 1% *Iopidine®* (Alcon); (Rx). Supplied as follows: 0.1 mL in plastic ophthalmic dispensers, packaged two per pouch. These dispensers are enclosed in a foil overwrap as an added barrier to evaporation.

References

Miller, P.E. & S.L. Rhaesa (1996). Effects of topical administration of 0.5% apraclonidine on intraocular pressure, pupil size, and heart rate in clinically normal cats. *American Journal of Veterinary Research* 57(1): 83–86.

BRIMONIDINE
(bri-*moe*-ni-deen)

Indications/Pharmacology

Brimonidine tartrate is an alpha-adrenergic receptor agonist with a greater affinity for alpha$_2$ receptors than apraclonidine. Brimonidine has a longer duration of action than apraclonidine as it binds to melanin, which acts as a reservoir to slowly release brimonidine. When used as a monotherapy, it is recommended that brimonidine be administered every 8 hours. Every 12-hour administration is acceptable when brimonidine is used in combination with timolol, latanoprost or dorzolamide. Brimonidine may also provide a protective effect to the retina and optic nerve (Karakucuk *et al.* 2009). However, this effect has not been clinically explored nor utilized in animals. Fluorophotometric studies in animals and humans suggest that brimonidine tartrate has a dual mechanism of action by reducing aqueous humor production and by and increasing uveoscleral outflow. After ocular administration of either a 0.1% or 0.2% solution, plasma concentrations peaked within 0.5 to 2.5 hours and declined with a systemic half-life of approximately 2 hours. In humans, systemic metabolism of brimonidine is extensive. It is metabolized primarily by the liver. Urinary excretion is the major route of elimination of the drug and its metabolites. Approximately 87% of an orally administered radioactive dose was eliminated within 120 hours, with 74% found in the urine.

Suggested Dosages/Precautions/Adverse Effects

The usual dosage is 1 drop in the affected eye twice daily. Adverse events in humans include: allergic conjunctivitis, conjunctival hyperemia, and eye pruritus, burning sensation, conjunctival folliculosis, hypertension, oral dryness, and visual disturbance. Brimonidine also causes an increase in eyelash growth in humans and it is used in the cosmetic industry for this purpose. Brimonidine appears to be better tolerated in animals than apraclonidine.

Dosage Forms/Regulatory Status

VETERINARY-LABELED PRODUCTS: None

HUMAN-LABELED PRODUCTS:

Brimonidine 0.15% solution: 5 mL, 10 mL, & 15 mL; *Alphagan P®* (Allergan); various generics as 0.1% and 0.2% solutions; (Rx)

Brimonidine 0.2%/Timolol maleate: 0.5% in 5 mL & 10 mL; *Combigan®* (Allergan); (Rx)

References

Karakucuk, S., Y. Yuce, et al. (2009). The effects of antiglaucomatous topical medications on retinal ganglion cell apoptosis. *Erciyes Medical Journal* 31: 310-317.

DIPIVEFRIN, TOPICAL
(dye-*pi*-ve-frin)

Indications/Pharmacology
Dipivefrin is a lipophilic prodrug to epinephrine allowing penetration through the corneal epithelium into the stroma where it is converted to epinephrine by esterases. Once converted to epinephrine, aqueous humor production is decreased primarily through vasoconstriction of ciliary body vessels and increases outflow through the trabecular meshwork. A study in beagles demonstrated that epinephrine at 1% and 2% and dipivefrin at 0.5% were effective in decreasing intraocular pressure (Gwin *et al.* 1978). While the drug has reasonable efficacy in humans, the associated local adverse effects of burning, hyperemia, hyperpigmentation, and cardiovascular stimulation have caused both epinephrine and dipivefrin to be replaced by the other alpha$_2$ agonists, apraclonidine and brimonidine.

Suggested Dosage/Precautions/Adverse Effects
Dipivefrin is not recommended for use due to significant local adverse effects including burning, hyperemia, hyperpigmentation, and cardiovascular stimulation.

Dosage Forms/Regulatory Status
VETERINARY-LABELED PRODUCTS: None

HUMAN-LABELED PRODUCTS:

Dipivefrin 1% solution in 5 mL, 10 mL or 15 mL vials; *Propine®* (Allergan); (Rx)

References
Gwin, R.M., K.N. Gelatt, et al. (1978). Effects of topical 1-epinephrine and dipivalyl epinephrine on intraocular pressure and pupil size in normotensive and glaucomatous beagles. *American Journal of Veterinary Research* 39(1): 83–86.

EPINEPHRINE, TOPICAL
(ep-i-*nef*-rin)

Indications/Pharmacology
Epinephrine is a direct-acting alpha- and beta-agonist. Its primary use in veterinary ophthalmology is for intracameral injection to facilitate mydriasis and prevent bleeding during intraocular procedures. Epinephrine (usually in combination with pilocarpine due to epinephrine's mydriatic effects) is usually used as a preventative measure to prevent glaucoma in the unaffected eye. Epinephrine acts on both alpha and beta adrenergic receptors, thereby causing conjunctival decongestion, transient mydriasis (less so in cats) and decreased IOP (intraocular pressure). Decreased IOP is probably due primarily to increased aqueous humor outflow, but decreased aqueous humor production may occur

secondary to vasoconstriction. Epinephrine is ineffective as a sole mydriatic in cats.

Suggested Dosages/Precautions/Adverse Effects
One drop 2–3 times daily in the unaffected eye. Epinephrine may cause ocular discomfort upon instillation. When injected intracamerally, it may be injected as a 1:10,000 dilution or added to ophthalmic irrigating solutions at a 1:100,000,000 dilution. If used intracamerally, epinephrine solutions should be preservative-free and bisulfate-free to avoid endothelial toxicity.

Dosage Forms/Regulatory Status
VETERINARY-LABELED PRODUCTS: None

HUMAN-LABELED PRODUCTS:

Epinephrine (HCl) Solution: 0.25%, 0.5%, 1% & 2%: 10 or 15 mL btls; *Epifrin®* (Allergan), *Glaucon®* (Alcon); (Rx)

Epinephrine (Borate) Solution: 0.5%, 1% & 2%: 7.5 mL btls; *Eppy/N®* (Pilkington/Barnes-Hind), *Epinal®* (Alcon); (Rx)

Epinephrine Bitartrate 1% in combination with Pilocarpine HCl Solution: 1%, 2%, 3%, 4% or 6%; *E-Pilo-1® -2, -3, -4, -6* (Iolab); *P1 E1®* (Alcon); (Rx)

Beta-Adrenergic Antagonists

This class of ocular hypotensive drugs currently consists of both non-selective and beta$_1$-selective agents. At the time of writing, it is not known how blockade of the ciliary body epithelium beta-receptors reduces intraocular pressure. Several mechanisms have been postulated including: beta-blockade of norepinephrine-induced tonic sympathetic stimulation, decreased activation of cAMP in the ciliary body leading to decreased aqueous humor production, inhibition of Na^+K^+ATPase activity, or action through a vasoactive mechanism. Because beta-blockers significantly affect function of the cardiovascular and pulmonary systems, patients with heart block, bradycardia, heart failure, asthma, chronic bronchitis or other cardiopulmonary conditions are poor candidates for use of topical beta-blockers to reduce intraocular pressure. Topical use of beta-blockers also can affect membrane stabilizing ability and induce local anesthesia. While this property is of no clinical value, adverse effects such as punctuate keratitis and epitheliopathies have been reported with chronic use in humans.

BETAXOLOL
(be-*tax*-oh-lol)

Indications/Pharmacology
Betaxolol HCl is a specific beta$_1$-adrenergic blocking agent that theoretically reduces the potential for beta$_2$-induced adverse pulmonary effects; however, its cardiac effects are the

same as non-selective beta-antagonists. Either levobunolol HCl or betaxolol HCl would be the first choice beta-blocking agent in a feline patient with glaucoma and asthma, although a topical carbonic anhydrates inhibitor should be considered before a beta-blocking agent in this situation. Betaxolol and the other beta-blockers should be used with caution in patients with cardiac disease. Betaxolol also inhibits glutamine-induced increases in intracellular calcium thereby providing a potential protective effect against ischemic insult to the retina (Bartlett *et al.* 2008).

Suggested Dosages/Precautions/Adverse Effects

Like timolol maleate, betaxolol HCl is supplied in a 0.5% and 0.25% solution. Because in animal patients, minimal pressure reduction is noted with concentrations below 0.5% with timolol maleate, many veterinary ophthalmologists only consider use of the 0.5% betaxolol HCl product. One drop of the 0.5% betaxolol HCl solution is instilled twice daily alone or in combination with other glaucoma medications. A study (Miller *et al.* 2000) utilizing 0.5% betaxolol as prophylaxis in the normal eye of dogs with unilateral glaucoma demonstrated a delay in onset of glaucoma in the normal eye relative to dogs who received no prophylaxis (31 months versus 8 months respectively). While problems have rarely been noted in veterinary medicine, ophthalmic beta-blockers should be used with caution in patients with bronchoconstrictive disease or congestive heart failure, although the selective beta$_1$-blocking properties of this particular drug would tend to minimize these risks for patients with pulmonary disease.

Dosage Forms/Regulatory Status

VETERINARY-LABELED PRODUCTS: None

HUMAN-LABELED PRODUCTS:

Betaxolol HCl 0.5% and 0.25% Solution: 2.5, 5, 10, & 15 mL bottles; *Betoptic®* & *Betoptic-S®* (Alcon); (Rx)

References

Bartlett, J., R. Fiscella, et al. (2008). Ocular Hypotensive Drugs. *Clinical Ocular Pharmacology 5th ed.* J Bartlett and S Jaanus Eds. St Louis, Butterworth-Heinenmann: 139-174.

Miller, P.E., G.M. Schmidt, et al. (2000). The efficacy of topical prophylactic antiglaucoma therapy in primary closed angle glaucoma in dogs: A multicenter clinical trial. *Journal of the American Animal Hospital Association* 36(5): 431-438.

CARTEOLOL
(*kar*-tee-oh-loll)

Indications/Pharmacology

Carteolol HCl is a nonspecific beta-adrenergic blocking agent. In addition to the typical therapeutic profile for non-specific beta-blockers, carteolol also possesses intrinsic sympathomimetic activity. This partial agonism of beta-receptors may be advantageous in patients experiencing bradycardia from other non-selective beta-blockade. Carteolol is a suitable substitute for timolol maleate or any of the other beta-blocking agents although it is rarely used in veterinary medicine, and no studies evaluating veterinary use of carteolol have been published. In humans, similar IOP reducing effects have been shown for all members of this class. Substitutes are necessary when one particular product induces topical irritation upon application or when potential beta agonism may be desirable.

Suggested Dosages/Precautions/Adverse Effects

One drop twice daily of the 1% solution. While problems have rarely been noted in veterinary medicine, ophthalmic beta-blockers should be used with caution in patients with bronchoconstrictive disease or congestive heart failure.

Dosage Forms/Regulatory Status

VETERINARY-LABELED PRODUCTS: None

HUMAN-LABELED PRODUCTS:

Carteolol HCl 1% Solution: 5, 10 & 15 mL bottles; *Ocupress®* (Otsuka America); (Rx)

LEVOBUNOLOL HCL
(lee-voe-*byoo*-noe-lole)

Indications/Pharmacology

Levobunolol HCl is a non-selective beta-blocking agent but without the potential for myocardial depression or airway constriction noted rarely in veterinary medicine and occasionally in human patients. Levobunolol is used in humans with glaucoma responsive to beta adrenergic blocking agents but who suffer cardiac and respiratory side effects associated with timolol. A study (Pugliese *et al.* 2009) comparing 0.5% levobunolol with 0.5% timolol-2% dorzolamide in normal dogs found levobunolol to be less effective than the combination therapy when used twice daily. Levobunolol HCl and then carteolol HCl would be suitable beta-blocking agents for feline patients with glaucoma and asthma, although carbonic anhydrase inhibitors should be used in such cases prior to adding a beta-blocking agent.

Suggested Dosages/Precautions/Adverse Effects

One drop twice daily of the 0.5% concentration. Miosis may develop in veterinary patients after application of topical beta-blocking antiglaucoma medications.

Dosage Forms/Regulatory Status

VETERINARY-LABELED PRODUCTS: None

HUMAN-LABELED PRODUCTS:

Levobunolol HCl 0.25% or 0.5% solution: 5, 10, & 15 mL. *Betagan®* (Allergan); (Rx)

References

Pugliese, M., A. Scardillo, et al. (2009). Comparison of effects of topical levobunolol to a combination of timolol-dorzolamide on intraocular pressure and pulse rate of healthy dogs. *Veterinary Research Communications* 33: S205-S207.

METIPRANOLOL

(meti-*pran*-oh-lol)

Indications/Pharmacology

Metipranolol is a nonselective beta-blocking agent and can be used as a substitute for timolol maleate. Pilot studies have suggested that metipranolol is as effective as timolol maleate and is significantly less expensive then trade name timolol preparations, but not the generically labeled products. Metipranolol has been useful for the management of primary open angle glaucoma in cats, however, no studies evaluating veterinary use of metipranolol have been performed.

Suggested Dosages/Precautions/Adverse Effects

One drop twice daily of the 0.3% solution. While problems have rarely been noted in veterinary medicine, ophthalmic beta-blockers should be used with caution in patients with bronchoconstrictive disease or congestive heart failure.

Dosage Forms/Regulatory Status

VETERINARY-LABELED PRODUCTS: None

HUMAN-LABELED PRODUCTS:

Metipranolol Solution 0.3%: 2, 5, & 10 mL; *OptiPranolol®* (Bausch & Lomb); (Rx)

TIMOLOL

(tye-moe-lole), (teh-moe-loll)

Indications/Pharmacology

Timolol is a non-selective beta-blocker supplied as 0.25% or 0.5% maleate salts, 0.25% or 0.5% hemihydrates salts, 0.47% potassium sorbate, or 0.25% or 0.5% gel-forming solutions. The 0.25% and 0.5% solutions have comparable efficacy in humans, while the potassium sorbate formulation has increased lipophilicity, resulting in greater anterior chamber relative to plasma concentrations (and therefore potentially fewer systemic side effects). Evaluation of 0.25 and 0.5% timolol in normotensive and glaucomatous eyes of Beagles with open-angle glaucoma, caused a reduction of 4-5 mmHg in glaucomatous eyes only (Gum *et al.* 1991). The 0.5% gel-forming solution, applied once daily for seven days, reduced IOP in normotensive dogs by a mean of 5.3 mmHg (Takiyama *et al.* 2006). Timolol has been evaluated in normotensive cats. In a comparison utilizing q12h and q8h administration of 2% dorzolamide with dorzolamide q8h in combination with 0.5% timolol q12h, no greater decrease was found with the addition of timolol compared to the q8h dorzolamide alone (Dietrich *et al.* 2007). Timolol has also been evaluated in horses utilizing a 0.5% solution alone or in combination with 2% dorzolamide and both studies indicate that every 12 hour dosing is preferred utilizing either regimen to effectively reduce intraocular pressure (van der Woerdt *et al.* 2000; Willis *et al.* 2001).

Timolol maleate is used primarily to prevent the development of primary glaucoma in the contralateral eye of a dog that has developed primary glaucoma in one eye. It only reduces intraocular pressure 3–10 mmHg and, therefore is of minimal usefulness in patients requiring treatment of primary acute congestive glaucoma. Timolol may cause slight miosis in dogs and cats. It is rarely used alone, but is combined with dorzolamide solution (*Cosopt®*). Caution is advised with use of beta-blocking agents in cats with concurrent asthma. As timolol maleate is now available in generic form, it is the primary beta-blocker agent now used.

Suggested Dosages/Precautions/Adverse Effects

One drop twice daily of the 0.5% solution. The 0.25% concentration has minimal efficacy in animals. While problems have rarely been noted in veterinary medicine, ophthalmic beta-blockers should be used with caution in patients with bronchoconstrictive disease or congestive heart failure.

Dosage Forms/Regulatory Status

VETERINARY-LABELED PRODUCTS: None

HUMAN-LABELED PRODUCTS:

Timolol Maleate 0.25% (see dosage above) or 0.5% Solution: 2.5, 5, 10, & 15 mL *Ocumeter®* bottles; *Timoptic®* (MSD); Istalol® (ISTA Pharmaceuticals); generic; (Rx)

Timolol Maleate 0.5% and Dorzolamide 2% Solution: 5 mL & 10 mL *Ocumeter®* bottles, *Cosopt®* (MSD); (Rx)

References

Dietrich, U.M., M.J. Chandler, et al. (2007). Effects of topical 2% dorzolamide hydrochloride alone and in combination with 0.5% timolol maleate on intraocular pressure in normal feline eyes. *Veterinary Ophthalmology* 10: 95-100.

Gum, G., R. Larocca, et al. (1991). The effect of topical timolol maleate on intraocular pressure in normal beagles and beagles with inherited glaucoma. *Progress in Veterinary Ophthalmology* 1: 141-150.

Takiyama, N., S. Shoji, et al. (2006). The effects of a timolol maleate gel-forming solution on normotensive beagle dogs. *Journal of Veterinary Medical Science* 68(6): 631-633.

van der Woerdt, A., D.A. Wilkie, et al. (2000). Effect of single- and multiple-dose 0.5% timolol maleate on intraocular pressure and pupil size in female horses. *Veterinary Ophthalmology* 3: 165-168.

Willis, A.M., T.E. Robbin, et al. (2001). Effect of topical administration of 2% dorzolamide hydrochloride or 2% dorzolamide hydrochloride-0.5% timolol maleate on intraocular pressure in clinically normal horses. *American Journal of Veterinary Research* 62(5): 709-713.

Carbonic Anhydrase Inhibitors

Carbonic anhydrase is found within the cytosol, mitochondria and salivary glands and catalyzes the conversion of carbon dioxide and water to carbonic acid and free hydrogen molecules. In the eye, bicarbonate ions are then transported into the posterior chamber where water follows the concentration gradient. Inhibition of carbonic anhydrase leads to decreased production of aqueous humor. Carbonic anhydrase inhibitors are most useful in treating primary open-angle glaucoma and secondary glaucomas in humans. Systemic use of these agents has generally been replaced by use of topical carbonic anhydrase inhibitors. For information on systemic carbonic anhydrase inhibitors, see individual monographs for Acetazolamide, Dichlorphenamide, and Methazolamide in the systemic drug monograph section of this reference.

BRINZOLAMIDE HCL
(brin-*zoh*-la-mide)

Indications/Pharmacology

Brinzolamide is chemically similar to dorzolamide and reduces aqueous humor production by altering H+/Na+ active transport mechanisms associated with aqueous humor production in the ciliary epithelial cells. It can be used as a substitute for dorzolamide and some patients that exhibit excessive topical irritation following application of dorzolamide drops, tolerate brinzolamide better or vice versa. Cats seem to be particularly sensitive to irritation from topical dorzolamide and often brinzolamide can be used in these patients. Comparative data is available suggesting that brinzolamide and dorzolamide are equally effective in animal patients, although brinzolamide has a higher affinity for the carbonic anhydrase enzyme allowing it to be dosed twice daily as compared to 3 times daily for dorzolamide in humans. While there have not been any compelling studies conducted with brinzolamide for dogs and cats, an evaluation of brinzolamide in horses indicated that once daily dosing was equally effective to twice daily dosing with no evidence of ocular or systemic effects (Germann *et al.* 2008).

Suggested Dosages/Precautions/Adverse Effects

One drop three times daily is the standard treatment frequency, adjusted based on clinical response. Like dorzolamide, may also cause stinging upon application.

Dosage Forms/Regulatory Status

VETERINARY-LABELED PRODUCTS: None

HUMAN-LABELED PRODUCTS:

Brinzolamide HCl 1% solution: 2.5, 5, 10 & 15 mL containers; *Azopt®* (Alcon); (Rx)

References

Germann, S.E., F.L. Matheis, et al. (2008). Effects of topical administration of 1% brinzolamide on intraocular pressure in clinically normal horses. *Equine Veterinary Journal* 40(7): 662-665.

DORZOLAMIDE HCL
(dor-*zole*-a-mide)

Indications/Pharmacology

Dorzolamide was the first topical carbonic anhydrase inhibitor marketed. Its chemical structure allows it to be both lipophilic and hydrophilic, thereby enabling penetration of the cornea and sclera. It is often used in the contralateral eye of a dog with primary glaucoma to prevent development of bilateral disease. It is also an excellent agent to consider for most secondary glaucomas in dogs and cats because it has no effect on pupil size. Like the related oral carbonic anhydrase inhibitors (dichlorphenamide or *Daranide®*, methazolamide or *Neptazane®*), dorzolamide decreases aqueous humor production by the ciliary body epithelium by altering pH and affecting the H^+/Na^+ active transport exchange mechanism. Oral carbonic anhydrase inhibitors cause numerous systemic side effects such as metabolic acidosis and panting, diarrhea, vomiting, anorexia and others, all of which can be avoided with topical carbonic anhydrase inhibitors. Investigations of dorzolamide have been conducted to establish efficacy in dogs and cats (McLean *et al.* 2008; Rainbow & Dziezyc 2003). Studies in horses indicate that dorzolamide is an effective monotherapy however, twice daily dosing is required (Willis *et al.* 2001).

Suggested Dosages/Precautions/Adverse Effects

One drop two to three times daily is the standard treatment frequency, adjusted based on clinical response. Dorzolamide may cause stinging (related to the low pH of the solution) upon topical application, particularly in cats. Superficial punctuate keratitis or local hypersensitivity may occur. Approximately 5-10% of humans will experience irritation with use of topical dorzolamide. Systemic effects are not usually associated with topical administration.

Dosage Forms/Regulatory Status

VETERINARY-LABELED PRODUCTS: None

HUMAN-LABELED PRODUCTS:

Dorzolamide HCl 2% Solution: 5, 10 & 15 mL; *Trusopt®* (Merck); (Rx)

Timolol Maleate 0.5% and Dorzolamide 2% Solution: 5 & 10 mL *Ocumeter®* bottles, *Cosopt®* (Merck); (Rx)

References

McLean, N.S.J., D.A. Ward, et al. (2008). The effect of a single dose of topical 0.005% latanoprost and 2% dorzolamide/0.5% timolol combination on the blood-aqueous barrier in dogs: a pilot study. *Veterinary Ophthalmology* 11(3): 158-161.

Rainbow, M.E. & J. Dziezyc (2003). Effects of twice daily application of 2% dorzolamide on intraocular pressure in normal cats. *Veterinary Ophthalmology* 6(2): 147-150.

Willis, A.M., T.E. Robbin, et al. (2001). Effect of topical administration of 2% dorzolamide hydrochloride or 2% dorzolamide hydrochloride-0.5% timolol maleate on intraocular pressure in clinically normal horses. *American Journal of Veterinary Research* 62(5): 709-713.

Prostaglandins

Ophthalmic prostaglandin analogues are chemically modified versions of PGF2-alpha, an endogenous inflammatory mediator, that have ocular hypotensive effects. Chemical modification of these agents improves lipid solubility and allows them to pass through the epithelium where corneal esterases activate them to the active metabolite, 17-phenyl-PGF2-alpha that acts on prostanoid receptors to lower intraocular pressure by effecting extensive uveoscleral matrix remodeling, reducing resistance to outflow. This remodeling is believed to be due to increased levels of metalloproteinases that degrade collagen within the extracellular matrix.

LATANOPROST
(la-*ta*-noe-prost)

Indications/Pharmacology

Latanoprost was the first drug marketed in this class; it is labeled for once daily use in humans. Clinical studies show reduced effectiveness when once daily treatment is exceeded in humans. Although latanoprost is initially dosed once daily in the evening for canine glaucoma, a study (Gelatt & MacKay 2001) was performed evaluating once versus twice daily administration of latanoprost in dogs that demonstrated that twice daily administration of latanoprost produced greater and more significant control of intraocular pressure. The canine uveal tract apparently metabolizes latanoprost at a rate higher than in humans as IOP reduction is profound, but it persists only for 12–15 hours in most dogs. Latanoprost will provide the greatest amount of pressure reduction in canine primary glaucoma cases compared with any other single oral or topical agent and efficacy is even greater when combined with carbonic anhydrase inhibitors. Latanoprost has not been found to be useful in the management of glaucoma in cats (Studer *et al.* 2000). Equine glaucoma is usually secondary to uveitis and latanoprost treatment for glaucoma in horses is not considered effective and is associated with a high incidence of side effects, including ocular discomfort. (Davidson *et al.* 2002; van der Woerdt *et al.* 2000).

Suggested Dosages/Precautions/Adverse Effects

One drop of latanoprost is applied in the PM initially, but with progression of the glaucoma, twice daily treatment schedules will provide additional reduction in intraocular pressure. Latanoprost may cause topical irritation. Conjunctival hyperemia is commonly noted in patients using this medication. A direct stimulation of iris melanocytes results in excess melanin production in the iris of people using this medication, causing an irreversible dark brown color change to the iris, and reversible hyperpigmentation of the eyelid. Hypertrichosis, conjunctival hyperemia, allergy, cystoid macular edema, anterior uveitis, and punctuate corneal erosions have also been reported. Profound miosis is noted with the use of latanoprost in dogs. It is not recommended for use in cats and horses due to adverse effects.

Dosage Forms/Regulatory Status

VETERINARY-LABELED PRODUCTS: None

HUMAN-LABELED PRODUCTS:

Latanoprost 0.005% Solution: 2.5 mL; *Xalatan®* (Pharmacia & Upjohn); (Rx). Store under refrigeration until use; may be stored at room temperature for 6 weeks after opened.

References

Davidson, H., C. Martin, et al. (2002). Effect of topical ophthalmic latanoprost on intraocular pressure in normal horses. *Vet Therapeutics* 3: 1220-1224.

Gelatt, K.N. & E.O. MacKay (2001). Effect of different dose schedules of latanoprost on intraocular pressure and pupil size in the glaucomatous Beagle. *Veterinary Ophthalmology* 4(4): 283-288.

Studer, M.E., C.L. Martin, et al. (2000). Effects of 0.005% latanoprost solution on intraocular pressure in healthy dogs and cats. *American Journal of Veterinary Research* 61(10): 1220-1224.

van der Woerdt, A., D.A. Wilkie, et al. (2000). Effect of single- and multiple-dose 0.5% timolol maleate on intraocular pressure and pupil size in female horses. *Veterinary Ophthalmology* 3: 165-168.

BIMATOPROST
(bi-*ma*-toe-prost)

Indications/Pharmacology

While bimatoprost is grouped in the prostaglandin-analog class, it is considered a synthetic prostamide. It is derived from anandamide, a fatty acid precursor. Prostamides interact only weakly with prostaglandin receptors, and the mechanism of action in reducing intraocular pressure remains unknown. Bimatoprost is available in solutions containing minimal concentrations of benzalkonium chloride and causes less ocular discomfort than latanoprost or travoprost. Bimatoprost also is initially administered once daily in the evening, but an evaluation in dogs (Gelatt & MacKay 2002) demonstrated that twice daily dosing provided for less fluctuation in intraocular pressure. Since latanoprost does not seem to be effective for most forms of feline glaucoma, it is unlikely bimatoprost will prove effective in these cases either.

Suggested Dosages/Precautions/Adverse Effects
Bimatoprost is dosed 1–2 drops once daily in the evening and increased to twice daily as glaucoma progresses. Bimatoprost shares the same adverse effects profile as latanoprost.

Dosage Forms/Regulatory Status
VETERINARY-LABELED PRODUCTS: None

HUMAN-LABELED PRODUCTS:
Bimatoprost 0.03% Solution 2.5 mL, 5 mL, 7.5 mL bottles; *Lumigan*® (Allergan); (Rx), *Latisse*® (Allergan); (Rx)

References
Gelatt, K.N. & E.O. MacKay (2002). Effect of different dose schedules of bimatoprost on intraocular pressure and pupil size in the glaucomatous Beagle. *Journal of Ocular Pharmacology and Therapeutics* 18(6): 525-534.

TRAVOPROST
(tra-vo-*prost*)

Indications/Pharmacology
Travoprost is a PGF2-alpha analog that is available preserved with benzalkonium chloride as well as in a benzalkonium chloride-free product that avoids the toxic epithelial effects commonly noted with this preservative in humans. As with latanoprost, travoprost is dosed once daily in the evening and produces mean intraocular pressure reductions of 7-8 mmHg. It shares the same adverse effect profile as latanoprost. Since latanoprost does not seem to be effective for most forms of feline glaucoma, it is not likely travoprost will prove effective in these cases either.

Suggested Dosages/Precautions/Adverse Effects
Travoprost is dosed 1-2 drops in the evening and increased to twice daily dosing with progression of glaucoma.

Dosage Forms/Regulatory Status
VETERINARY-LABELED PRODUCTS: None

HUMAN-LABELED PRODUCTS:
Travoprost 0.004% Solution; 2.5 mL, 5 mL bottles, *Travatan*® (Alcon); (Rx)

UNOPROSTONE ISOPROPYL
(ooh-no-*prah*-stone i-so-*proe*-pel)

Indications/Pharmacology
Unoprostone is a prostaglandin analog that is no longer commercially available in the United States. It is converted by ocular esterases to the active free acid form of isopropyl unoprostone instead of PGF2-alpha like other ocular prostaglandin prodrugs. Evaluations of unoprostone in dogs (Ofri *et al.* 2000) demonstrated that once daily evening dosing or twice daily dosing produced the best intraocular pressure control as well as the fewest adverse effects. Like latanoprost, unoprostone did not demonstrate any effects in lowering intraocular pressure in cats (Bartoe *et al.* 2005).

Suggested Dosages/Precautions/Adverse Effects
Unoprostone is dosed 1–2 drops in the evening and increased to twice daily dosing with progression of glaucoma.

Dosage Forms/Regulatory Status
VETERINARY-LABELED PRODUCTS: None

HUMAN-LABELED PRODUCTS:
None currently available in the United States, but may be obtained through importation or through the services of appropriately qualified pharmacy.

References
Bartoe, J.T., H.J. Davidson, et al. (2005). The effects of bimatoprost and unoprostone isopropyl on the intraocular pressure of normal cats. *Veterinary Ophthalmology* 8(4): 247-252.
Ofri, R., D. Raz, et al. (2000). The effect of 0.12% unoprostone isopropyl (Rescula) on intraocular pressure in normotensive dogs. *Journal of Veterinary Medical Science* 62(12): 1313-1315.

Osmotic Agents For Treatment of Glaucoma
Osmotic agents increase the osmotic pressure of plasma and create a concentration gradient that will draw fluid out of the intraocular environment. Effective osmotic agents should be non-toxic, small in molecular weight, and have poor intraocular penetration (else intraocular pressure may increase). These agents are systemically administered with concurrent water deprivation (4–6 hrs) and are indicated only for acute episodes of glaucoma, not maintenance. For further information, see systemic monographs for Mannitol, Glycerin, and Isosorbide.

Mydriatic-Cycloplegic-Vasoconstrictors

CYCLOPENTOLATE
(sye-kloe-*pen*-toe-late)

Indications/Pharmacology
Cyclopentolate is an anticholinergic agent that induces relaxation of the sphincter of the iris and the ciliary muscles. When applied topically to the eyes, it causes a rapid, intense cycloplegic and mydriatic effect that is maximal in 15–60 minutes; recovery usually occurs within 24

hours. The cycloplegic and mydriatic effects are slower in onset and longer in duration in animal patients who have darkly pigmented irises. Cyclopentolate is used mainly to produce mydriasis and cycloplegia for diagnostic purposes.

Suggested Dosages/Precautions/Adverse Effects

1 drop instilled in the eye(s), followed by a second drop 5 minutes later, if necessary. Drops should be administered 40–50 minutes prior to diagnostic procedure. Cyclopentolate increases intraocular pressure and should not be used in animals with glaucoma. Slight stinging is noted with the higher (1%) concentration of the drug.

Dosage Forms/Regulatory Status

VETERINARY-LABELED PRODUCTS: None

HUMAN-LABELED PRODUCTS:

Cyclopentolate Solution 0.5%, 1%, & 2%: in 2, 5 & 15 mL bottles: *AK-Pentolate®* (Akorn); *Cyclogyl®* (Alcon); generic; (Rx)

PHENYLEPHRINE HCL
(fen-il-*ef*-rin)

Indications/Pharmacology

Phenylephrine is a direct-acting alpha1 agonist vasoconstrictor that is most commonly used in veterinary medicine as an adjunct preoperative medication to induce mydriasis prior to phacoemulsification for cataract removal. Phenylephrine is also used prior to minor surface (*e.g.*, conjunctival) procedures to limit bleeding. Phenylephrine can be used to confirm the diagnosis of Horner's syndrome. Dilution of 2.5% phenylephrine solution with saline (1:10) produces a 0.25% solution. Normal eyes will not demonstrate mydriasis in response to this low concentration of phenylephrine. Third order Horner's syndrome of greater than two weeks duration is associated with receptor up regulation and therefore a response to 0.25% phenylephrine is noted. In this way, the diagnosis of Horner's is confirmed and a suggestion as to whether or not the condition is 2nd or 3rd order in nature.

In dogs, maximum mydriasis persists for about 2 hours and effects may last for up to 18 hours. Phenylephrine has significant alpha-adrenergic effects (vasoconstriction and pupillary dilation) and minimal effects on beta-receptors. When used alone, phenylephrine is reportedly not efficacious in the cat unless used with other mydriatics.

Suggested Dosages/Precautions/Adverse Effects

For diagnosis and characterization of Horner's syndrome: Apply 0.25% solution (see above) in both eyes. If there is a response in the miotic eye, it is 3rd order. If no response in 20–30 minutes, apply 2.5% solution; if there is a response in both

eyes it confirms Horner's and probably is 2nd order.

For treatment of Horner's syndrome: Treatment is indicated only if patient experiences visual difficulty because third eyelid is elevated over pupil; then given on an as needed basis with an average duration of effect of 3–6 hours.

Prior to cataract or intraocular surgery: 2.5% or 10% given every 15 minutes for two hours. Smaller animals (*e.g.*, cats and dogs weighing <5kg) are more susceptible to life-threatening systemic effects on blood pressure and cardiac rhythm and preoperative use of phenylephrine in these animals is generally not recommended. In larger animals, repeated dosing is also associated with cardiovascular adverse effects. Phenylephrine is ineffective as a sole mydriatic in cats or horses and it should be combined with atropine to achieve adequate mydriasis.

Local discomfort may occur after instillation and chronic use may lead to inflammation. In some species (cats, rabbits, humans), transient stromal clouding may occur if used when corneal epithelium is damaged.

Dosage Forms/Regulatory Status

VETERINARY-LABELED PRODUCTS: None

HUMAN-LABELED PRODUCTS:

Phenylephrine HCl 0.12% Solution: 15 mL or 20 mL bottles; generic; (OTC)

Phenylephrine HCl 2.5% Solution: 2, 5 or 15 mL bottles; generic; (Rx)

Phenylephrine HCl 10% Solution: 1, 2, 5 or 15 mL bottles; *Neo-Synephrine®* (Sanofi Winthrop), generic; (Rx)

ATROPINE SULFATE
(*a*-troe-peen)

Indications/Pharmacology

Atropine is a potent mydriatic-cycloplegic utilized for therapeutic (not diagnostic) purposes. When used topically on the eye, atropine acts by blocking the cholinergic receptors of the sphincter muscle of the iris and the ciliary body to cause mydriasis (pupillary dilation) and accommodation paralysis (cycloplegia). Atropine is significantly ionized at physiological pH and it has limited corneal penetration. Atropine controls pain secondary to corneal and uveal disease; to maximally dilate the pupil prior to intraocular surgery; to dilate the pupil and prevent pupillary block in glaucoma and uveitis. In the dog, atropine causes maximal mydriasis in about 1 hour and it may persist for up to 120 hours. Cats also show a delayed onset of action and mydriasis may persist for up to 144 hours (dose dependent). Atropine is particularly long acting in horses and may last days to weeks.

Atropine may be used in combination with 10% phenylephrine to achieve mydriasis and cycloplegia in cases of anterior uveitis. Atropine may also be used in uveitis to break up synechiae.

Suggested Dosages/Precautions/Adverse Effects

Ointments or drops are routinely used in dogs. One percent is commonly used, but 2% solutions may be required in severe cases of uveitis. Ointments are generally used in cats to prevent hypersalivation associated with the bitter taste of this medication. Dosage frequencies are variable depending on the condition and its severity. Commonly, atropine is given as one drop 2–3 times a day or every other day until pupillary dilation is achieved and once daily thereafter to maintain this response.

Atropine may precipitate acute, congestive primary glaucoma in dogs predisposed to primary glaucoma; do not use in primary glaucoma. Repeated topical application prior to surgery can result in systemic atropine toxicosis (mania, hyperthermia, etc.). Salivation may result in dogs as well as cats (see above) secondary to the bitter taste. Atropine may also decrease tear production in small animals.

Reportedly, very frequent treatment with atropine may induce colic in horses secondary to systemic absorption and atropine's vagal parasympathetic effects. However, clinically this effect is only rarely noted.

Dosage Forms/Regulatory Status

VETERINARY-LABELED PRODUCTS:

Atropine Sulfate Ophthalmic Ointment: 10 mg/gm (1%) in 3.5 gm tubes; *Atrophate®* (Schering-Plough); (Rx)

HUMAN-LABELED PRODUCTS:

Atropine Sulfate Ophthalmic Ointment: 5 mg/gm (0.5%), & 10 mg/gm (1%) in 3.5 gm tubes; various trade names & generic; (Rx)

Atropine Sulfate Ophthalmic Solution: 0.5%, 1%, and 2% in unit dose droppers, 2, 5, & 15 mL bottles; various trade names & generic; (Rx)

TROPICAMIDE
(troe-*pik*-a-mide)

Indications/Pharmacology

Tropicamide, like atropine, causes mydriasis and cycloplegia, but has more mydriatic than cycloplegic activity. It has excellent corneal penetration because it is minimally ionized at physiological pH. The action of tropicamide is also less affected by intraocular pigment than are other mydriatics. Tropicamide has a more rapid onset (maximum mydriasis in 15–30 minutes) of action and a shorter duration of action (pupil returns to normal in 6–12 hours in most animals) than does atropine, thereby making it more useful for funduscopic examinations. In dogs, intraocular pressure is apparently not af-

fected by tropicamide. Tropicamide is also indicated following cataract removal to prevent synechiae formation that is associated with post-cataract atropine administration. As the half-life of tropicamide is shorter than that of atropine, this allows iris contraction preventing synechial adhesions.

Suggested   Dosages/Precautions/Adverse Effects

Once or twice application to eye, prior to exam. Following cataract surgery: apply 2–3 times daily to keep pupil constantly changing in size and reduce formation of synechiae associated with prolonged pupillary dilation (atropine).

Tropicamide is less effective in pain control (cycloplegia) than atropine.

Tropicamide may cause salivation, particularly in cats. It may also sting when applied. Tropicamide may precipitate acute congestive glaucoma in predisposed patients. Tropicamide has been reported to decrease Schirmer Tear Test values for several hours following application in cats and horses.

Dosage Forms/Regulatory Status

VETERINARY-LABELED PRODUCTS: None

HUMAN-LABELED PRODUCTS:

Tropicamide Solution 0.5% and 1%: 2 mL & 15 mL bottles; *Mydriacyl®* (Alcon), *Opticyl®* (Optopics), *Tropicacyl®* (Akorn), generic; (Rx)

Anti-inflammatory/ Analgesic Ophthalmic Agents

Mast Cell Stabilizers, Antihistamines, Decongestants

CROMOLYN SODIUM
(*kroe*-moe-lin)

Indications/Pharmacology

Cromolyn sodium is a mast cell stabilizing agent that blocks release of histamine and slow-reacting substance of anaphylaxis from mast cells following antigen recognition. Similar to lodoxamine tromethamine, cromolyn sodium has no intrinsic vasoconstrictor, antihistaminic, cyclooxygenase inhibition or other anti-inflammatory properties. Mast cell stabilizing agents are most useful in animal patients suffering from allergic conjunctivitis.

Suggested Dosages/Precautions/Adverse Effects

For relief of seasonal allergy, one drop 2–6 times daily. A stinging sensation is noted in a low percentage of people using this medication.

Dosage Forms/Regulatory Status

VETERINARY-LABELED PRODUCTS: None

HUMAN-LABELED PRODUCTS:

Cromolyn Sodium 4% Solution: 2.5, & 10 mL; *Crolom®* (Bausch & Lomb); (Rx)

LODOXAMINE TROMETHAMINE
(loe-*dox*-a-mide)

Indications/Pharmacology

Lodoxamine tromethamine is a mast cell stabilizer that inhibits Type-I hypersensitivity responses by preventing antigen mediated histamine release. Lodoxamine stabilizes mast cells by blocking calcium influx into the cell upon antigen recognition, thereby blocking histamine release. Lodoxamine has no intrinsic vasoconstrictor, antihistaminic, cyclooxygenase inhibition or other anti-inflammatory properties. Lodoxamine is used in people for management of conjunctivitis associated with seasonal allergy and other histamine mediated disorders. In veterinary medicine, lodoxamine tromethamine has been used in horses and small animal patients with presumed allergic conjunctivitis.

Suggested Dosages/Precautions/Adverse Effects

Prior to surgery: One drop 2–4 times daily. A stinging sensation is noted in a low percentage of people using this medication.

Dosage Forms/Regulatory Status

VETERINARY-LABELED PRODUCTS: None

HUMAN-LABELED PRODUCTS:

Lodoxamine Tromethamine 0.1%: 10 mL; *Alomide®* (Alcon); (Rx)

OLOPATADINE HCL
(oh-loe-pa-*ta*-deen)

Indications/Pharmacology

Olopatadine HCl is a selective H$_1$ receptor antagonist and inhibitor of histamine release from mast cells. It is marketed for topical use to alleviate symptoms of allergic conjunctivitis in humans and is thought to be safe for use in children three years of age and older. Olopatadine, upon topical application in humans, was shown to have very limited systemic absorption. It was detectable in the milk of nursing rats, after topical application, and like most medications should be avoided in pregnant or nursing animals.

Suggested Doses/Precautions/Adverse Effects

Olopatadine eye drops are applied as needed in people for temporary relief of itchiness associated with seasonal allergy. They can be used in dogs two to three times daily for allergic conjunctivitis.

Dosage Forms/Regulatory Status

VETERINARY-LABELED PRODUCTS: None

HUMAN-LABELED PRODUCTS:

Olopatadine HCl ophthalmic solution 0.1%; *Patanol®* (Alcon); (Rx)

Non-Steroidal Antiinflammatory Agents

Non-steroidal anti-inflammatory drugs (NSAIDs), administered topically or systemically, are used in ophthalmology to control inflammation and provide analgesia. However, corticosteroids remain the standard for topical anti-inflammatory effect. NSAIDs are administered perioperatively to induce mydriasis and reduce inflammatory-mediated breakdown of the blood-aqueous barrier during cataract extraction, and postoperatively to reduce inflammation and facilitate corneal healing. NSAIDs are also used in allergic conjunctivitis.

NSAIDs safe for topical ophthalmic use include indole acetic acid, aryl acetic acid, and aryl propionic acid derivatives that are readily formulated as solutions due to their water-soluble nature. Salicylates, fenamates, and pyrazolones are too toxic for topical ocular use. As most NSAIDs are weakly acidic, they exist in their ionized form in the tear film pH and thus only weakly penetrate the cornea. Reducing the pH of topical formulations increases the unionized fractions and intraocular penetration, however it also increases the local irritant effects following administration. Additionally, the anionic nature of NSAIDs favors formation of insoluble complexes with cationic quaternary ammonium preservatives such as benzalkonium chloride.

Adverse effects from topical NSAIDs include local reactions such as hyperemia and contact dermatitis, punctuate keratitis (chronic use, especially diclofenac), keratomalacia, corneal toxicity (through disruption of corneal epithelial arachidonic acid metabolism and through disruption of matrix metalloproteinase), and impaired wound healing (particularly products containing thimerosal). Systemic adverse effects may also occur and are associated with an increased risk for gastrointestinal ulceration, altered platelet function, renal damage, bronchospasm, and bone marrow suppression in cats (Giuliano 2004).

References

Giuliano, E.A. (2004). Nonsteroidal anti-inflammatory drugs in veterinary ophthalmology. *Veterinary Clinics of North America-Small Animal Practice* 34(3): 707-+.

BROMFENAC
(brome-fen-ak)

Indications/Pharmacology
Bromfenac is a nonsteroidal anti-inflammatory drug (NSAID) by virtue of its ability to block prostaglandin synthesis by inhibiting cyclooxygenase 1 and 2. Bromfenac is indicated for treatment of postoperative inflammation in patients who have undergone cataract extraction.

Suggested Doses/Precautions/Adverse Effects
One drop twice daily.

Bromfenac is contraindicated in patients with known hypersensitivity to any ingredient in the formulation. Bromfenac ophthalmic solution contains sodium sulfite, a sulfite known to cause allergic reactions especially in asthmatic patients. Caution should be exercised when utilizing bromfenac in patients who have previously exhibited sensitivity to other NSAID drugs as there is potential for cross-sensitivity. There have been reports that ocularly applied NSAIDs may cause increased belled of ocular tissues (including hyphema) in conjunction with ocular surgery due to interference with platelet aggregation. All topical NSAIDs may slow or delay healing. Concomitant use with topical steroidal agents may increase the potential for delayed healing. Use of topical NSAIDs may result in keratitis due to epithelial breakdown, corneal thinning, corneal erosion, corneal ulceration or corneal perforation. Use of bromfenac should be discontinued immediately in patients exhibiting evidence of corneal epithelial breakdown. Post marketing experience with topical NSAIDs suggests that use more than 24 hours prior to surgery or use beyond 14 days after surgery may increase patient risk for the occurrence of corneal adverse events. Bromfenac should be used with caution in patients with known bleeding tendencies or who are receiving other medications, which may prolong bleeding time. The most commonly reported adverse experiences reported following use of bromfenac include: abnormal sensations in the eye, conjunctival hyperemia, eye irritation (including burning/stinging), eye pain, eye pruritus, eye redness, headache, and iritis. These events were reported in 2–7% of human patients.

Dosage Forms/Regulatory Status
VETERINARY-LABELED PRODUCTS: None
HUMAN-LABELED PRODUCTS:

Bromfenac 0.09% solution: 7.5 mL & 10 mL; *Xibrom*® (ISTA) (Rx). Store at room temperature.

DICLOFENAC SODIUM
(dye-*kloe*-fen-ak)

Indications/Pharmacology
Diclofenac sodium is a phenylacetic acid that inhibits cyclooxygenase, inhibiting prostaglandin synthesis. Diclofenac sodium topical solution reduces inflammation following cataract extraction in people and counteracts photophobia in humans having refractive corneal surgery. In veterinary medicine, diclofenac sodium is used for treatment of uveitis following surgery on the eye or other causes of uveitis especially when corneal infection is suspected or in diabetic patients whose insulin regulation could be altered by the systemic uptake of topical corticosteroids. Diclofenac can be combined with topical corticosteroids for better control of uveitis in animals when the condition is severe.

Suggested Dosages/Precautions/Adverse Effects
Prior to surgery: One drop 4 times at 20-minute intervals. One drop four times daily following cataract surgery or for the treatment of uveitis. Caution should be used when applying any anti-inflammatory agent on the cornea in the face of corneal stromal infection because of the positive role inflammation plays in the immune response to microbial invasion of tissue. A stinging sensation is noted in 15% of people using this medication.

Dosage Forms/Regulatory Status
VETERINARY-LABELED PRODUCTS: None
HUMAN-LABELED PRODUCTS:

Diclofenac Sodium 0.1% Solution: 2.5 & 5 mL; *Voltaren*® (Novartis); (Rx)

FLURBIPROFEN SODIUM
(flure-*bi*-proe-fen)

Indications/Pharmacology
Flurbiprofen is a non-steroidal anti-inflammatory agent that probably acts by inhibiting the cyclo-oxygenase enzyme system, thereby reducing the biosynthesis of prostaglandins. Prostaglandins may mediate certain kinds of ocular inflammation. They may disrupt the blood-aqueous humor barrier, cause vasodilation, increase intraocular pressure and leukocytosis, and increase vascular permeability. Prostaglandins may also cause iris sphincter constriction (miosis) independent of cholinergic mechanisms. Flurbiprofen can inhibit this intraocular miosis and it may be useful in the management of uveal inflammation (usually in addition to topical steroids).

Suggested Dosages/Precautions/Adverse Effects

Prior to surgery: One drop 4 times at 20-minute intervals.

Because flurbiprofen may be as immunosuppressive as topical corticosteroids, it should not be used in patients with infected corneal ulcers. By blocking prostaglandin synthesis, arachidonic acid metabolites may be shunted into leukotriene pathways and this effect may result in a transient increase in intraocular pressure commonly noted after intraocular surgery. Postoperative pressure spikes following cataract surgery have been the subject of much study in recent years and a general trend away from the use of flurbiprofen prior to cataract surgery has resulted from these studies.

Dosage Forms/Regulatory Status

VETERINARY-LABELED PRODUCTS: None

HUMAN-LABELED PRODUCTS:

Flurbiprofen Sodium 0.03% Solution: 2.5 mL, 5 mL & 10 mL btls; *Ocufen*® (Allergan); generic; (Rx)

KETOROLAC TROMETHAMINE
(kee-toe-*role*-ak)

Indications/Pharmacology

Ketorolac tromethamine is a pyrrolol-pyrrole nonsteroidal anti-inflammatory agent that inhibits prostaglandin formation. Ketorolac tromethamine is marketed for use before cataract extraction in human patients (to prevent miosis during surgery) and for control of post surgical inflammation, especially following cataract surgery. Ketorolac is also effective in treating postoperative cystoid macular edema and ocular surface inflammation. It is also approved for management of conjunctivitis associated with seasonal allergy in people. In veterinary medicine, ketorolac tromethamine is primarily used to control surgical or nonsurgical uveitis particularly in cases with concurrent corneal bacterial infection or ulceration when topical corticosteroids are contraindicated. It is also used in diabetic patients, especially smaller patients, adversely affected by systemic uptake of topically applied corticosteroids. Nonsteroidal agents like ketorolac tromethamine can be combined with topical steroids in patients with severe uveal inflammation.

Suggested Dosages/Precautions/Adverse Effects

Prior to surgery: One drop 4 times at 20-minute intervals. One drop four times daily; following cataract surgery, treatment of uveitis, or management of allergic conjunctivitis.

The manufacturer indicates that ketorolac tromethamine does not enhance the spread of pre-existing corneal fungal, viral or bacterial infections in animal models. Ketorolac tromethamine does not induce postoperative pressure elevation beyond which that frequently follows cataract extraction in people and animals.

Dosage Forms/Regulatory Status

VETERINARY-LABELED PRODUCTS: None

HUMAN-LABELED PRODUCTS:

Ketorolac Tromethamine Solution 0.5%: 3, 5, & 10 mL; *Acular*® (Allergan); (Rx)

NEPAFENAC
(ne-pa-*fen*-ak)

Indications/Pharmacology

Nepafenac is a nonsteroidal anti-inflammatory and analgesic prodrug. After topical ocular dosing, nepafenac penetrates the cornea where it is converted by ocular tissue hydrolases to amfenac, a nonsteroidal anti-inflammatory drug. Amfenac is thought to inhibit the action of prostaglandin H synthase (cyclooxygenase), an enzyme required for prostaglandin production. Nepafenac is indicated for the treatment of pain and inflammation associated with cataract surgery.

Suggested Dosages/Precautions/Adverse Effects

One drop three times daily. Shake well before use.

Nepafenac is contraindicated in patients who have demonstrated hypersensitivity to any of the ingredients in the formulation or to other NSAIDs. Caution should be exercised when utilizing nepafenac in patients who have previously exhibited sensitivity to other NSAID drugs as there is potential for cross-sensitivity.

There have been reports that ocularly applied NSAIDs may cause increased bleeding of ocular tissues (including hyphema) in conjunction with ocular surgery due to interference with platelet aggregation. All topical NSAIDs may slow or delay healing. Concomitant use with topical steroidal agents may increase the potential for delayed healing. Use of topical NSAIDs may result in keratitis due to epithelial breakdown, corneal thinning, corneal erosion, corneal ulceration or corneal perforation. Use of nepafenac should be discontinued immediately in patients exhibiting evidence of corneal epithelial breakdown. Post marketing experience with topical NSAIDs suggests that use more than 24 hours prior to surgery or use beyond 14 days after surgery may increase patient risk for the occurrence of corneal adverse events. Nepafenac should be used with caution in patients with known bleeding tendencies or who are receiving other medications, which may prolong bleeding time. In controlled clinical studies, the most frequently reported ocular adverse events following cataract surgery were capsular opacity, decreased visual acuity, foreign body sensation, increased intraocular pressure, and sticky sensation. These events occurred in approximately 5–10% of patients. Other ocular adverse events occurring at an incidence of approximately 1–5% included conjunctival edema, corneal edema, dry eye, lid margin crusting, ocular discomfort, ocular hyperemia, ocular pain, ocular pruritus, photophobia, tearing and vitreous detachment. Some of these events may be the consequence of the cataract surgical procedure. Non-ocular adverse events reported at an incidence of 1–4% included headache, hypertension, nausea/vomiting, and sinusitis. Nepafenac ophthalmic suspension may be administered in conjunction with other topical ophthalmic medications such as beta-blockers, carbonic anhydrase inhibitors, alpha-agonists, cycloplegics, and mydriatics.

Dosage Forms/Regulatory Status

VETERINARY-LABELED PRODUCTS: None

HUMAN-LABELED PRODUCTS:

Nepafenac Ophthalmic Suspension: 0.1% in 3 mL; *Nevanac®* (Alcon); (Rx). Shake well and store at room temperature.

SUPROFEN
(su-*pro*-phen)

Indications/Pharmacology

Suprofen is a non-steroidal anti-inflammatory agent similar to flurbiprofen. Suprofen and flurbiprofen are phenylalkanoic acids that inhibit the cyclo-oxygenase enzymes responsible for conversion of arachadonic acid from cell membranes into various prostaglandins. These prostaglandins mediate certain aspects of ocular inflammation including disruption of the blood-aqueous barrier, uveal vasodilation, increases in intraocular pressure, and leakage of white blood cells and protein from uveal vessels into the aqueous humor. Prostaglandins cause iris sphincter constriction (miosis) independent of cholinergic mechanisms. Suprofen can inhibit this intraocular miosis and may be useful in the management of uveal inflammation (usually in addition to topical steroids).

Suggested Dosages/Precautions/Adverse Effects

Prior to surgery: One drop 4 times at 20-minute intervals.

Because suprofen may be as immunosuppressive as topical corticosteroids, it should not be used in patients with bacterial corneal ulcers. By blocking prostaglandin synthesis, arachidonic acid metabolites may be shunted into leukotriene pathways and this effect may result in a transient increase in intraocular pressure commonly noted after intraocular surgery. Postoperative pressure spikes following cataract surgery have been the subject of much study in recent years

and a general trend away from the use of suprofen or flurbiprofen prior to cataract surgery has resulted from these studies.

Dosage Forms/Regulatory Status

VETERINARY-LABELED PRODUCTS: None

HUMAN-LABELED PRODUCTS:

Suprofen Sodium 1% Solution in 2.5 mL btls; *Profenal®* (Alcon); (Rx)

Steroidal Anti-inflammatory Agents

Topical corticosteroids are used to treat diseases of the eye involving the conjunctiva, sclera, cornea, and anterior chamber. Efficacy of corticosteroids applied topically to the eye is dependent on many patient-related and drug-related factors. Patient factors include frequency and route of administration as well as conditions influencing penetration such as corneal ulceration or ocular inflammation. Topically delivered corticosteroids are best able to penetrate the cornea if they are both hydrophilic and lipophilic. The solubility can be improved by utilizing salts that are more lipophilic in nature (*e.g.* acetates), hydrophilic in nature (*e.g.* sodium phosphate or hydrochloride) or biphasic (*e.g.* alcohol derivatives). Hydrophilic ocular preparations are usually supplied as solutions while lipophilic agents are usually supplied as ointments or suspensions. In order to increase efficacy of topically administered corticosteroids, frequency of administration is increased instead of drug concentration (*e.g.*, prednisolone acetate 1% suspension is equally efficacious as 1.5% and 3% suspensions when used at the same frequency.) Penetration of topically applied corticosteroids into the eyelids is poor as is penetration to the posterior segment of the eye. Corticosteroid-responsive conditions affecting these areas are usually managed with systemically administered agents (with or without adjunctive topically applied medications).

Ocular side effects of ophthalmic corticosteroids can be numerous, including the development of cataracts, increased IOP, infection, decreased would healing, mydriasis, and calcific keratopathy. While these side effects may be frequent in humans, some are less common in animals. With the exceptions of mydriasis and calcific keratopathy, these side effects may occur in association with systemically administered corticosteroids as well. Systemic side effects of topical ophthalmic corticosteroids include glucocorticoid-induced hepatopathy, suppression of endogenous glucocorticoid production, or local alopecia. It is important to note that such side effects occur more readily with systemic administration of corticosteroids, but occur in a dose and duration-dependent manner following topical ophthalmic administration.

Conjunctivitis in animals is often treated symptomatically, particularly during the first occurrence of the condition for any particular patient. Antibiotic agents with hydrocortisone or dexamethasone, or antibiotic agents alone initially, are used for conjunctivitis in the dog and the horse. Allergic and eosinophilic conjunctivitis are rare diagnoses in the cat. Topically applied corticosteroids should not be used to treat conjunctivitis in cats. Herpes virus is the most common feline conjunctival pathogen and topically applied steroids can induce prolonged disease, steroid dependency and corneal complications including ulcerative keratitis and/or corneal sequestrum formation.

Inflammatory conditions of the canine sclera and episclera include episcleritis, scleritis, nodular granulomatous episclerokeratitis, Collie granuloma and others. Potency and penetration of corticosteroid agents is important in the management of these conditions. Dexamethasone sodium phosphate ointment is often employed and the relatively reduced penetration of the fibrous ocular tunics of this medication compared with that of 1% prednisolone acetate ophthalmic suspension is made up for by increased contact time of the ointment form of this drug and by the increased potency of dexamethasone (30X cortisone) relative to prednisolone (4–5X cortisone). Dexamethasone products alone (without antibiotics) are becoming increasingly scarce in the marketplace and because of this, dexamethasone is often used in combination with an antibiotic for availability reasons only. Four times daily treatment is often the initial frequency with tapering paralleled to clinical response. Topical treatment is often used following subconjunctival injection of corticosteroid agents into or adjacent to the lesion (if focal). Systemic steroid treatment is usually not necessary.

Non-ulcerative inflammatory conditions of the cornea of animals include chronic superficial keratitis (pannus) of the German Shepherd and other breeds, eosinophilic keratitis of the cat and certain, often poorly understood, keratopathies of the equine, including Onchocerca related keratitis. German Shepherd pannus may be better managed using cyclosporine ophthalmic solution or ointment with or without concurrent topical steroids initially followed by long term management with cyclosporine ophthalmic solution (see cyclosporine ophthalmic). Eosinophilic keratitis is often treated with subconjunctival corticosteroids in addition to topical 0.1% dexamethasone ophthalmic ointment or solution or 1% prednisolone acetate ophthalmic suspension 4 times daily, tapering the dosage frequency based on clinical response. Recent research reveals that eosinophilic keratitis may be an unusual immune response to latent feline herpes virus in the corneal stroma, calling into question the value of topical steroids in the management of a disease with an infectious etiology. Despite new information pertaining to possible causes of eosinophilic keratitis in the cat, the condition continues to be well managed in most cases with infrequent topical corticosteroid treatment. Non-ulcerative, immune mediated and/or parasitic equine keratitis are treated with 0.1% dexamethasone ointment 4 times daily with tapering of the treatment frequency based on the clinical response.

Corticosteroids are also used to manage anterior uveal inflammatory disease of companion animals. In small animals, 1% prednisolone acetate ophthalmic suspension is generally used for this purpose because of superior penetration into the anterior segment of the eye in comparison with dexamethasone products. The frequency of treatment depends on the severity of the condition. Severe anterior uveitis can be treated with subconjunctival corticosteroids given in combination with hourly topical corticosteroids with reevaluation performed again 24 hours after beginning treatment. Moderate to mild uveitis and that found following surgery of the anterior segment is often treated initially at the QID level with tapering based on clinical response. Anterior uveitis in animals can often be associated with an underlying systemic infectious or neoplastic condition in animals. Clinicians are advised to evaluate the patient for generalized infectious or neoplastic conditions prior to or concurrent with a course of corticosteroid antiinflammatory therapy, particularly if the condition dictates systemic treatment with these agents in combination with subconjunctival and topical treatment. Uveitis has also been successfully treated utilizing subconjunctival injections of triamcinolone acetonide. As commercially available triamcinolone injections are preserved with benzyl alcohol, veterinary ophthalmologists centrifuge triamcinolone injections and remove the alcohol-containing supernatant vehicle. An equal volume of non-preserved sodium chloride injection is then utilized to reconstitute the remaining triamcinolone to provide for an acceptable subconjunctival injection. Uveitis in the equine species is often treated with either 1% prednisolone acetate ophthalmic suspension or with 0.1% dexamethasone ointment. Many clinicians prefer to use the ointment because of increased contact time and potency and the logistics of frequent treatment of this species. 1% prednisolone acetate can be passed through a subpalpebral lavage catheter very frequently to treat equine patients with anterior uveitis when necessary.

Inflammatory conditions of the posterior segment require systemic treatment because of poor penetration of topically applied agents.

PREDNISOLONE
(pred-*nis*-oh-lone)

Indications/Pharmacology
Prednisolone is an intermediate-acting synthetic corticosteroid available as acetate or phosphate salts. The acetate derivative has superior anti-inflammatory activity in comparison to the phosphate derivative, and it is considered the most effective drug for anterior uveitis. Prednisolone acetate ophthalmic suspension is generally used for anterior uveitis because of superior penetration into the anterior segment of the eye in comparison with dexamethasone products. The frequency of treatment depends on the severity of the condition. Severe anterior uveitis can be treated with subconjunctival corticosteroids given in combination with hourly topical corticosteroids with reevaluation performed again 24 hours after beginning treatment. Moderate to mild uveitis and that found following surgery of the anterior segment is often treated initially at four times daily with tapering based on clinical response.

Other routes of administration: Systemically administered corticosteroids (usually orally) may be indicated for non-infectious inflammatory ocular conditions and following intraocular surgery. Subconjunctival steroids are useful in anterior segment inflammatory disease and following cataract surgery and intraocular glaucoma surgery. Subconjunctival steroids may be absorbed systemically and should be used with caution in patients with endocrinopathies (*e.g.*, diabetes mellitus) or infectious diseases. Even frequent topical steroid application in small animal patients under 20 kg can cause difficulties with diabetes mellitus regulation and after the peak inflammatory response has been suppressed, nonsteroidal antiinflammatory drugs should be considered for ongoing maintenance treatment.

Dosage Forms/Regulatory Status
VETERINARY-LABELED PRODUCTS: None

HUMAN-LABELED PRODUCTS:

Prednisolone Acetate Drops: 0.12% Suspension: *Pred Mild®* (Allergan); 0.125% Suspension: *Econopred®* (Alcon); 1% Suspension: *Econopred Plus®* (Alcon); *Pred Forte®* (Allergan), generic; (Rx)

Prednisolone Sodium Phosphate Drops: 0.125 & 1% Solution; (various); (Rx)

Prednisolone (0.25%) and Atropine (1%) Drops in 5 mL btls; *Mydrapred®* (Alcon); (Rx)

DEXAMETHASONE
(dex-a-*meth*-a-sone)

Indications/Pharmacology
Dexamethasone is a long-acting synthetic corticosteroid, available as alcohol or phosphate derivative suspensions or solutions, or as a phosphate derivative ointment. The anti-inflammatory efficacy of the alcohol is superior to that of the phosphate derivative.

Dosage Forms/Regulatory Status
VETERINARY-LABELED PRODUCTS: None

HUMAN-LABELED PRODUCTS:

Dexamethasone Sodium Phosphate 0.1% Solution, 5 mL bottles, generic; (Rx)

Dexamethasone Phosphate 0.05% Ointment, 3.5 gram tubes, generic; (Rx)

BETAMETHASONE
(bay-ta-*meth*-a-sone)

Indications/Pharmacology
Betamethasone is a long-acting corticosteroid was formerly available as a veterinary-approved antimicrobial-steroid combination (*Gentocin Durafilm®*—Schering).

Dosage Forms/Regulatory Status
VETERINARY-LABELED PRODUCTS: None

HUMAN-LABELED PRODUCTS: None

Note: Compounding pharmacists can still provide the combination of gentamicin and betamethasone, but this preparation should never be utilized if corneal abrasion or ulceration are suspected, and should not be used to treat herpes keratitis in cats.

FLUOROMETHOLONE
(flor-o-*meth*-a-lone)

Indications/Pharmacology
Fluorometholone is actually an analog of progesterone instead of cortisol, available in alcohol or acetate salt formulations. Fluorometholone alcohol formulations have less anti-inflammatory effect than prednisolone acetate, but acetate salts have activity comparable to prednisolone acetate suspensions. Higher concentrations of fluorometholone (0.25%) have been noted to raise intraocular pressure (Sendrowski *et al.* 2008).

Dosage Forms/Regulatory Status
VETERINARY-LABELED PRODUCTS: None

HUMAN-LABELED PRODUCTS:

Fluorometholone 0.1% ointment, 3.5 gram tube: *FML S.O.P.®* (Allergan); (Rx)

Fluorometholone 0.25% alcohol suspension, 5 mL, 10 mL bottles, *FML Forte®* (Allergan); (Rx)

Fluorometholone acetate 0.1% suspension, 5 mL, 10 mL, 15 mL bottles, *FML®* (Allergan); *Flarex®* (Alcon), generic; (Rx)

References
Sendrowski, D., S. Jaanus, et al. (2008). Anti-Inflammatory Drugs. *Clinical Ocular Pharmacology 5th ed.* J Bartlett and S Jaanus Eds. St Louis, Butterworth-Heinenmann: 221-244.

LOTEPREDNOL
(lo-teh-*pred*-nal)

Indications/Pharmacology
Loteprednol etabonate is synthesized from an inactive metabolite of the parent drug (*i.e.* a "soft drug") that is briefly activated to the active metabolite *in vivo*, exerts its pharmacological effects, and then is transformed back to the inactive metabolite. Loteprednol antiinflammatory effect is comparable to other topical corticosteroids and it has a lower risk of raising intraocular pressure.

Dosage Forms/Regulatory Status
VETERINARY-LABELED PRODUCTS: None

HUMAN-LABELED PRODUCTS:

Loteprednol 0.5% suspension: 2.5 mL, 5 mL, 10 mL, 15 mL bottles; *Lotemax®* (Bausch & Lomb); (Rx)

Loteprednol 0.2% suspension: 5 mL, 10 mL; *Alrex®* (Bausch & Lomb); (Rx)

RIMELOXOLONE
(rem-eh-*lox*-a-lone)

Indications/Pharmacology
Rimeloxolone is a topical corticosteroid agent that has comparable anti-inflammatory activity to prednisolone acetate. It is used for treatment of uveitis and is administered in aggressive pulse doses to patients with mild to moderate inflammation.

Dosage Forms/Regulatory Status
VETERINARY-LABELED PRODUCTS: None

HUMAN-LABELED PRODUCTS:

Rimeloxolone 1% suspension, 5 mL and 10 mL bottles; *Vexol®* (Alcon); (Rx)

Ophthalmic Analgesics

MORPHINE SULFATE
(*mor*-feen)

Indications/Pharmacology
A recent study showed that topical use of 1% morphine sulfate solution in dogs with corneal ulcers provided analgesia and did not interfere with normal wound healing. Both *mu* and *delta* opioid receptors were identified in normal corneas of dogs, although the *mu* receptors were present only in small numbers. Dogs treated with morphine sulfate 1% topical solution had significantly less blepharospasm and lower esthesiometer readings than did control dogs. Morphine sulfate is a Schedule II controlled substance.

Suggested Dosages/Precautions/Adverse Effects
1 drop of 1% morphine sulfate solution in the affected eye(s) three times daily. Preserved solutions of morphine should not be used.

Dosage Forms/Regulatory Status
VETERINARY-LABELED PRODUCTS: None

HUMAN-LABELED PRODUCTS: None

A 1% morphine sulfate ophthalmic solution may be compounded by utilizing the preservative-free morphine 2.5% injectable solution diluted with sterile saline observing appropriate aseptic technique.

NALBUPHINE
(*nal*-byoo-feen)

Indications/Pharmacology
A review of the literature reveals that solutions of topical nalbuphine were used clinically to provide analgesia and reduce ophthalmic pain in humans as early as 1983. Nalbuphine hydrochloride is a potent analgesic. Its analgesic potency is essentially equivalent to that of morphine on a milligram basis. Receptor studies show that nalbuphine hydrochloride binds to *mu, kappa,* and *delta* receptors, but not to *sigma* receptors. Nalbuphine hydrochloride is primarily a *kappa* agonist/partial *mu* antagonist analgesic. Nalbuphine hydrochloride by itself has potent opioid antagonist activity at doses equal to or lower than its analgesic dose. When administered following or concurrent with *mu* agonist opioid analgesics (*e.g.,* morphine, oxymorphone, fentanyl), nalbuphine hydrochloride may partially reverse or block opioid-induced activity from the *mu* agonist analgesic. Nalbuphine hydrochloride may precipitate withdrawal in patients dependent on opioid drugs. Nalbuphine hydrochloride should be used with caution in patients who have been receiving *mu* opioid analgesics on a regu-

lar basis. Nalbuphine is not commercially available for ophthalmic use, but may be obtained through appropriately qualified compounding pharmacies.

Suggested Dosages/Precautions/Adverse Effects

One drop two to six times daily as needed for corneal pain. Do not use in conjunction with topical morphine as nalbuphine will reverse the effects of morphine at the *mu* receptor.

Dosage Forms/Regulatory Status

VETERINARY-LABELED PRODUCTS: None

HUMAN-LABELED PRODUCTS: None

The 10 mg/mL (1%) nalbuphine injection may be applied as an ophthalmic solution. A 1% nalbuphine ophthalmic solution may also be compounded by utilizing nalbuphine 20 mg/mL injectable solution diluted with 1:1 with sterile saline observing appropriate aseptic technique.

Antimicrobial Ophthalmic Therapy

Antibiotics, Single & Combination Products

Antimicrobials are critical to the management of ocular disease, however several considerations determine appropriate use. For prophylactic use, drugs effective against pathogens likely at the site should be selected as well as potential for microbial resistance or adverse reactions. For therapeutic use, the causative agent should be determined and an appropriate antimicrobial applied again monitoring for development of resistance or adverse effects.

Aminoglycosides, Ocular

Aminoglycosides inhibit bacterial protein synthesis via inhibition of the 30S bacterial ribosome and are therefore primarily effective against gram-negative organisms such as Pseudomonas, Proteus, and Enterobacter (with the exception of neomycin which is considered ineffective against *Pseudomonas aeruginosa*). Gram-positive activity is restricted to *Staphylococcus aureus*. Aminoglycosides are not effective against anaerobes. Aminoglycosides are poorly absorbed after oral administration, and use is limited to parenteral or topical administration.

Penicillins and cephalosporins can inactivate aminoglycosides and administration must be separated by a time lapse if concurrently administered.

Aminoglycosides induce ototoxicity (auditory and vestibular) and nephrotoxicity when administered systemically. Topical ophthalmic adverse effects include corneal epithelial damage, conjunctival damage, and hypersensitivity reactions. Intravitreal injection of gentamicin is toxic to the retina and the ciliary body and has been used therapeutically to treat end-stage glaucoma (chemical enucleation). Aminoglycosides should be used carefully and monitored in patients with renal disease.

AMIKACIN SULFATE
(am-eh-*kaye*-sin *suhl*-fate)

Indications/Pharmacology

Although amikacin is not commercially available as a topical preparation, it has been compounded for use in corneal infections caused by gram-negative bacilli that have become resistant to gentamicin or tobramycin. Subconjunctival injection does raise ocular concentrations of amikacin; however, parenteral administration does not demonstrate benefit in treating ocular infections. Of the aminoglycosides, amikacin demonstrates the least retinal toxicity, making it useful in treating endophthalmitis.

Suggested Dosages/Precautions/Adverse Effects

Amikacin may be compounded to a concentration of 8mg/ml as a sterile, fortified ophthalmic antibiotic solution.

Dosage Forms/Regulatory Status

VETERINARY-LABELED PRODUCTS: None

HUMAN-LABELED PRODUCTS: None

Fortified solutions of amikacin sulfate may be compounded in concentrations of 8 mg/mL.

NEOMYCIN SULFATE
(nee-o-*mye*-sin *suhl*-fate)

Indications/Pharmacology

Neomycin is commonly included in triple antibiotic formulations. It has minimal corneal penetration in the presence of intact corneal epithelium, but is useful for treatment of superficial corneal ulceration or surface ocular infections.

Suggested Dosages/Precautions/Adverse Effects

Neomycin may cause contact sensitivity and it is contraindicated in patients with a history of such.

Dosage Forms/Regulatory Status

VETERINARY-LABELED PRODUCTS:

Bacitracin zinc 400 units/Neomycin 3.5 mg/Polymyxin B Sulfate 10,000 Units per gram Ophthalmic Ointment: 3.5 gm tubes; *Mycitracin®* (Upjohn); (**Note:** contains 500 mg bacitracin/gm); *Neobacimyx®* (Schering); *Trioptic-P®* (Pfizer); *Vetropolycin®* (Dechra); generic; (Rx). Approved for dogs and cats.

Neomycin 3.5 mg/Polymyxin B Sulfate 10,000 Units per mL Ophthalmic Solution: *Optiprime®* (Syntex); (Rx). Approved for use in dogs.

HUMAN-LABELED PRODUCTS:

There is a wide variety of human-labeled ophthalmic combination products available. Most are a combination of bacitracin/neomycin/polymyxin B. However, there are variations of this theme (*e.g.*, gramicidin in place of bacitracin in topical solutions-*Neosporin® Ophthalmic Solution*). All of these products require a prescription.

GENTAMICIN SULFATE
(jen-ta-*mye*-sin *suhl*-fate)

Indications/Pharmacology

Gentamicin may be administered topically or subconjunctivally and is primarily used for keratitis caused by *Pseudomonas aeruginosa*. The commercially available 0.3% solution is generally too dilute to achieve topical efficacy, and solutions with concentrations greater than 13.6 mg/ml may be compounded for use in ocular infections. The primary antimicrobial spectrum for gentamicin is gram-negative organisms making it less useful for prophylaxis, as agents of concern on the ocular surface tend to be gram-positive organisms. Gentamicin has minimal penetration of intact corneal epithelium but does penetrate in the presence of infection. Subconjunctival injection may increase ocular drug levels, but systemic absorption is a possibility after this route of administration, particularly in smaller patients. Gentamicin is toxic to the intraocular structures (retina and ciliary body) and is used therapeutically for chemical enucleation in end-stage glaucoma.

Suggested Dosages/Precautions/Adverse Effects

Three to four times daily as an ointment or solution. For chemical enucleation in end-stage glaucoma: 0.25 mL of gentamicin 100 mg/ml injection.

Dosage Forms/Regulatory Status
VETERINARY-LABELED PRODUCTS:

Gentamicin Ophthalmic Ointment: 3 mg/gram in 3.5 gm tubes; *Gentocin®* (Schering); (Rx). FDA-approved for use in dogs and cats.

Gentamicin Ophthalmic Drops: 3 mg/mL in 5 mL btls; *Gentocin®* (Schering); (Rx). FDA-approved for use in dogs and cats.

HUMAN-LABELED PRODUCTS:

Gentamicin Ophthalmic Ointment: 3 mg/gram in 3.5 gm tubes; *Garamycin®* (Schering); *Genoptic®* (Allergan); generic; (Rx)

Gentamicin Ophthalmic Drops: 3 mg/mL in 5 mL btls *Garamycin®* (Schering); *Genoptic®* (Allergan); generic; (Rx)

TOBRAMYCIN SULFATE
(toe-*bra*-mye-sin *suhl*-fate)

Indications/Pharmacology

Tobramycin possesses a similar spectrum of activity to that of gentamicin. The commercially available solutions and ointments are sometimes not concentrated enough to achieve therapeutic effect and fortified concentrations of greater than 14.5 mg/mL are compounded for use. Ocular drug levels of tobramycin can be increased with use of subconjunctival injections, however, systemic use of tobramycin does not demonstrate benefit in ocular infections.

Suggested Dosages/Precautions/Adverse Effects

Solution: One drop three to four times daily. Ointment: ½ inch strip three to four times daily.

Dosage Forms/Regulatory Status
VETERINARY-LABELED PRODUCTS: None

HUMAN-LABELED PRODUCTS:

Tobramycin Ophthalmic Ointment: 3 mg/gram in 3.5 gm tubes; *Tobrex®* (Alcon); (Rx)

Tobramycin Ophthalmic Drops: 3 mg/mL in 5 mL btls; *Tobrex®* (Alcon); (Rx)

Fluoroquinolones, Ocular

Fluoroquinolones (FQNs) are bactericidal through inhibition of bacterial DNA gyrase thereby disrupting bacterial DNA replication. Nalidixic acid is considered the first fluoroquinolone with a spectrum of activity limited to gram-negative organisms and weak activity against *Pseudomonas aeruginosa*. Second generation FQNs (lomefloxacin, norfloxacin, enoxacin, enrofloxacin, ciprofloxacin and ofloxacin) also demonstrate weak activity against *Pseudomonas aeruginosa*, and *Streptococcus* spp are also increasing in resistance to second generation FQN. Third generation FQNs (sparfloxacin, gemifloxacin and levofloxacin) are rarely used in ophthalmology. Fourth generation FQNs (gatifloxacin, moxifloxacin and besifloxacin) have a greater efficacy against gram-positive organisms compared to earlier generation FQNs, but are still relatively ineffective against *Pseudomonas* spp. Moxifloxacin has consistently demonstrated superior ocular penetration when compared to other FQNs (Solomon *et al.* 2005; Yagci *et al.* 2007).

References

Solomon, R., E.D. Donnenfeld, et al. (2005). Penetration of topically applied gatifloxacin 0.3%, moxifloxacin 0.5%, and ciprofloxacin 0.3% into the aqueous humor. *Ophthalmology* 112(3): 466-469.

Yagci, R., Y. Oflu, et al. (2007). Penetration of second-, third-, and fourth-generation topical fluoroquinolone into aqueous and vitreous humour in a rabbit endophthalmitis model. Eye 21(7): 990-994.

CIPROFLOXACIN
GATIFLOXACIN
LEVOFLOXACIN
MOXIFLOXACIN
NORFLOXACIN
OFLOXACIN

Indications/Pharmacology

These fluroquinolone ophthalmic antibiotics are primarily useful for established gram-negative corneal infections. They are not recommended for prophylactic use prior to or after surgery. See the main enrofloxacin/ciprofloxacin monograph for additional pharmacologic information.

Clinicians are strongly cautioned regarding the development of retinal neurotoxicity at or above the formerly recommended *systemic* enrofloxacin dosage in cats. There are no reports at the time of writing of retinal toxicity in cats administered topical fluroquinolone ophthalmic products.

Precautions/Adverse Effects

Ciprofloxacin may cause crusting or crystalline precipitates in the superficial portion of corneal defects. Other potential adverse effects with quinolones include: conjunctival hyperemia, bad taste in mouth, itching foreign body sensation, photophobia, lid edema, tearing keratitis and nausea. Allergic reactions have been reported with quinolone eye preps.

Dosage Forms/Regulatory Status

VETERINARY-LABELED PRODUCTS: None

HUMAN-LABELED PRODUCTS:

Ciprofloxacin 3 mg/mL drops in 2.5 & 5 mL btls; *Ciloxan®* (Alcon); (Rx)

Ciprofloxacin:Dexamethasone 0.3%:0.1% drops in 7.5 mL btls; *Ciprodex®* (Alcon); (Rx)

Gatifloxacin 0.3% drops in 5 mL btls; *Zymar®* (Allergan); (Rx)

Levofloxacin 0.5% drops in 5 mL btls, *Quixin®* (JOM); 1.5% drops, 5 mL btls; *Iquix®* (JOM); (Rx)

Moxifloxacin 5 mg/mL drops: 3 mL & 6 mL btls; *Vigamox®* (Alcon); (Rx)

Norfloxacin 3 mg/mL drops in 5 mL btls; *Chibroxin®* (Merck); (Rx)

Ofloxacin 3 mg/mL drops in 5 mL btls; *Ocuflox®* (Allergan); (Rx)

Macrolides, Ocular

Macrolides inhibit bacterial growth through binding the bacterial 50S ribosomal subunit preventing protein synthesis. Bacterial resistance to macrolides occurs when bacteria alter ribosomal RNA preventing binding of macrolides to the resulting subunit. Bacterial typically resistant to macrolides include *Staphylococcus aureus*, coagulase-negative Staph spp, and *Streptococcus* spp. While systemic macrolide therapy (azithromycin and clarithromycin) has been used to treat animals with systemic diseases that have ocular manifestations, topical ocular therapy is limited to erythromycin.

ERYTHROMYCIN
(ee-*rith*-rowe-*mye*-sin)

Indications/Pharmacology

Erythromycin has a spectrum against gram-positive organisms except for enterococci. Use of erythromycin in ophthalmology is targeted towards infections caused by *Mycoplasma* spp, *Chlamydia* spp, and *Borrelia burgdorferi*. Resistance to erythromycin is still limited enough that it remains a potentially useful therapeutic option for diseases caused by these organisms.

Suggested Dosages/Precautions/Adverse Effects

½ inch strip three to four times daily.

Dosage Forms/Regulatory Status

VETERINARY-LABELED PRODUCTS: None

HUMAN-LABELED PRODUCTS:

Erythromycin 0.5% ophthalmic ointment, 3.5 gram tube, generic (Rx)

Tetracyclines, Ocular

Tetracyclines exert an antimicrobial effect through inhibition of bacterial protein synthesis at the 30S ribosomal subunit. While tetracyclines have a broad spectrum of antimicrobial coverage, their clinical usefulness is limited by efflux mechanisms in bacteria that actively pump tetracyclines out of cells to create resistant strains. *Pseudomonas* spp are considered resistant to tetracyclines.

Tetracyclines are also useful as anti-inflammatory agents by virtue of their ability to inhibit matrix metalloproteinases (MMP). The role of MMP in destroying corneal collagen can be blocked by tetracyclines administered orally to patients with melting corneal ulcers. Oral administration of doxycycline at doses of 20 mg/kg PO twice daily have resulted in detectable levels of doxycycline in aqueous humor (Davis *et al.* 2006).

References

Davis, J.L., J.H. Salmon, et al. (2006). Pharmacokinetics and tissue distribution of doxycycline after oral administration of single and multiple doses in horses. *American Journal of Veterinary Research* **67**(2): 310-316.

OXYTETRACYCLINE
(ox-ee-tet-ra-**sye**-kleen)

Indications/Pharmacology
The tetracyclines are most useful in cats for the treatment of Chlamydial and Mycoplasma conjunctivitis as well as nonspecific or symptomatic therapy for undiagnosed (causative organism not determined) conjunctivitis in cats.

Suggested Dosages/Precautions/Adverse Effects
For Chlamydial/Mycoplasma keratoconjunctivitis: Apply 4 times daily. Dramatic improvement should be noted in 3–4 days, but treatment should continue for 3–4 weeks for Chlamydia to break the reproductive cycle of this organism. Expect potential recurrence after discontinuation of topical treatment from organisms dormant in the nasal passage. As oral doxycycline has been documented to eliminate the carrier state of Chlamydia in cats, better treatment is oral doxycycline 25 mg PO twice daily for three weeks.

Dosage Forms/Regulatory Status
VETERINARY-LABELED PRODUCTS:
Oxytetracycline HCl 5 mg/Polymyxin B Sulfate 10,000 Units/gm: 3.5 gram tubes; *Terramycin®* *Ophthalmic Ointment* (Pfizer); (Rx)

HUMAN-LABELED PRODUCTS: None

TETRACYCLINE
(tet-ra-**sye**-kleen)

Indications/Pharmacology
The tetracyclines are most useful in cats for the treatment of Chlamydial and Mycoplasma conjunctivitis as well as nonspecific or symptomatic therapy for undiagnosed (causative organism not determined) conjunctivitis in cats.

At the time of writing, there are no commercially available ophthalmic dosage forms of tetracycline.

Suggested Dosages/Precautions/Adverse Effects
For Chlamydial/Mycoplasma keratoconjunctivitis: Apply 4 times daily. Dramatic improvement should be noted in 3–4 days, but treatment should continue for 3–4 weeks for Chlamydia to break the reproductive cycle of this organism. Expect potential recurrence after discontinuation of topical treatment from organisms dormant in the nasal passage. As oral doxycycline has been documented to eliminate the carrier state of Chlamydia in cats, better treatment is oral doxycycline 25 mg PO twice daily for three weeks.

Dosage Forms/Regulatory Status
VETERINARY-LABELED PRODUCTS: None

HUMAN-LABELED PRODUCTS: None

Formerly available as Tetracycline HCl Ophthalmic Ointment: 10 mg/gram in 3.75 gram tubes; *Achromycin®* (Storz/Lederle); (Rx)

Formerly available as Tetracycline HCl Ophthalmic Suspension: 10 mg/mL in 4 mL btls; *Achromycin®* (Storz/Lederle); (Rx)

Miscellaneous Antibiotics, Ocular

BACITRACIN
(bah-si-**trey**-sun)

Indications/Pharmacology
Bacitracin inhibits bacterial cell wall synthesis through inhibition of a peptidoglycan precursor, and exhibits a spectrum of action primarily against gram-positive organisms. Bacitracin is unstable in solution, however, it is a common component of combination antibiotic ointments. It is usually combined with polymyxin B and neomycin due to their greater gram-negative activity. This broad spectrum of activity makes triple antibiotic products useful in prophylaxis and therapy for corneal and ocular surface infections. Bacitracin poorly penetrates the cornea and is of limited value in deep corneal or intraocular infections.

Suggested Dosages/Precautions/Adverse Effects
The primary adverse effect associated with bacitracin is local hypersensitivity.

Dosage Forms/Regulatory Status
VETERINARY-LABELED PRODUCTS:
Bacitracin zinc 400 units/Neomycin 3.5 mg/Polymyxin B Sulfate 10,000 Units per gram Ophthalmic Ointment: 3.5 gm tubes; *Mycitracin®* (Upjohn) (**Note:** contains 500 mg bacitracin/gram); *Neobacimyx®* (Schering); *Trioptic-P®* (Pfizer); *Vetropolycin®* (Dechra); generic; (Rx). Approved for dogs and cats.

HUMAN-LABELED PRODUCTS:
There is a wide variety of human-labeled ophthalmic combination products available. Most are a combination of bacitracin/neomycin/polymyxin B. However, there are variations of this theme (*e.g.*, gramicidin in place of bacitracin in topical solutions-*Neosporin® Ophthalmic Solution*). All these products require a prescription.

CHLORAMPHENICOL
(klor-am-*fen*-i-call)

Indications/Pharmacology

A broad spectrum antibiotic, chloramphenicol has the ability to cross the corneal barrier and enter the anterior chamber. However, very few infections occur in the anterior chamber and if bacteria are actually present, the blood ocular barrier is lost and systemically administered antibiotics can achieve therapeutic levels. Typically, Staph spp. and Strep spp. are susceptible to chloramphenicol while Pseudomonas spp. are resistant.

Because of the potential toxicity associated with chloramphenicol to humans, chloramphenicol's use in veterinary ophthalmology is becoming less widespread. It may be useful, however, in treating cats with suspected Mycoplasma or chlamydial conjunctivitis, and at the time of printing is one of the few commercially available ophthalmic antibiotics available in an ointment form.

Suggested Dosages/Precautions/Adverse Effects

For prophylaxis following surgery or for cats with Mycoplasma or chlamydial conjunctivitis: One drop (or 1/4 inch strip if using ointment) four times daily. For established corneal infection: Application may be very frequent (up to hourly).

Chloramphenicol exposure in humans has resulted in fatal aplastic anemia. For this reason, this drug should be used with caution in veterinary patients and some ophthalmologists avoid its use entirely. Clients should be cautioned to use appropriate safeguards when applying the drug and avoiding contact with drops or solutions after application.

Labels state to not use longer than 7 days in cats, although three times daily application of ointment for 21 days to cats did not cause toxicity. Must not be used in any food producing animal.

Dosage Forms/Regulatory Status

VETERINARY-LABELED PRODUCTS: None

HUMAN-LABELED PRODUCTS:

Chloramphenicol 1% Ophthalmic Ointment in 3.5 gm tubes; *Chloromycetin*® (Parke Davis); *Chloroptic*® (Allergan); generic (Rx)

Chloramphenicol 0.5% Ophthalmic Drops in 7.5 mL; *Chloroptic*® (Allergan); generic; (Rx). Refrigerate until dispensed. These products are sporadically available commercially and may need to be compounded by an appropriately qualified compounding pharmacy.

POLYMYXIN B
(pahl-ee-*mix*-in bee)

Indications/Pharmacology

Polymyxin B is a cationic surfactant (detergent) that disrupts cell membrane integrity through interaction with cell phospholipids. The antimicrobial spectrum is against gram-negative organisms and it is therefore frequently combined with antimicrobials possessing gram-positive activity (*e.g.* bacitracin).

Suggested Dosages/Precautions/Adverse Effects

Local reactions can be noted in hypersensitive patients.

Dosage Forms/Regulatory Status

VETERINARY-LABELED PRODUCTS:

Oxytetracycline HCl 5 mg/Polymyxin B Sulfate 10,000 U/gm: 3.5 gm tubes; *Terramycin*® *Ophthalmic Ointment* (Pfizer); (Rx)

HUMAN-LABELED PRODUCTS:

There is a wide variety of human-labeled ophthalmic combination products available. Most are a combination of bacitracin/neomycin/polymyxin B. However, there are variations of this theme (*e.g.*, gramicidin in place of bacitracin in topical solutions-*Neosporin*® *Ophthalmic Solution*). All are Rx.

SULFACETAMIDE
(sul-fa-*see*-ta-mide)

Indications/Pharmacology

For the treatment of conjunctivitis and other superficial ocular infections due to susceptible microorganisms, and as an adjunctive in systemic sulfonamide therapy of trachoma, *Escherichia coli*, *Staphylococcus aureus*, *Streptococcus pneumoniae*, Streptococcus (viridans group), *Haemophilus Muenzae*, Klebsiella species and Enterobacter species. Topically applied sulfonamides do not provide adequate coverage against Neisseria species, *Serratia marcescens* and *Pseudomonas aeruginosa*. A significant percentage of staphylococcal isolates are completely resistant to sulfa drugs.

Precautions/Adverse Effects

For conjunctivitis and other superficial ocular infections: Instill one or two drops into the conjunctival sac(s) of the affected eye(s) every two to three hours initially. Dosages may be tapered by increasing the time interval between doses as the patient responds. The usual duration of treatment is seven to ten days. Owners with sulfa allergies should be cautioned to avoid all contact with this medication. Adverse effects seen in animals include gastrointestinal disturbances, allergic skin reactions, renal damage and blood dyscrasias. In dogs, sulfonamides are known to cause keratoconjunctivitis sicca associated with direct toxic effect to the lacrimal acinar cells. This effect is caused by the nitrogen-containing pyridine and pyrimidine rings in sulfonamides and is dose-related. The estimated incidence is 15%-25% in dogs treated with sulfonamides and may occur long after treatment. Dogs demonstrating squinting or excess ocular mucous discharge should be evaluated for this adverse effect, which may be reversible if sulfonamides are discontinued in time.

Sulfonamides are contraindicated in patients with known hypersensitivity or with blood dyscrasias.

Dosage Forms/Regulatory Status

VETERINARY-LABELED PRODUCTS: None

HUMAN-LABELED PRODUCTS:

Sulfacetamide Ophthalmic Solution 10%: 15 mL btls; *Sulf-10*®, *AK-10*® (Akorn); *Bleph-10*® (Allergan); (Rx)

Sulfacetamide Ophthalmic Ointment 10%: *Bleph-10*® (Allergan); (Rx)

VANCOMYCIN
(**vank**-o-**mye**-sin)

Indications/Pharmacology
Vancomycin inhibits bacterial cell wall synthesis through inhibition of peptidoglycan development. Vancomycin has strong activity against gram-positive organisms, particularly Staphylococcus and Streptococcus species. Vancomycin is generally reserved for those gram-positive species that have been classified as methicillin-resistant. Vancomycin is used for topical administration in infectious keratitis or bacterial endophthalmitis. An evaluation of vancomycin to treat methicillin-resistant Staph keratitis in rabbits, demonstrated that concentrations of 0.3%-1% vancomycin are effective (Eguchi *et al.* 2009). Injection of vancomycin nanoparticles into the anterior chamber of rabbits demonstrated good prophylactic activity against MRSA with minimal adverse effects (Kodjikian *et al.* 2010).

Suggested Dosages/Precautions/Adverse Effects
Systemic vancomycin therapy can be associated with ototoxicity, potentially leading to permanent deafness, and nephrotoxicity with resultant fatal uremia.

Dosage Forms/Regulatory Status
VETERINARY-LABELED PRODUCTS: None
HUMAN-LABELED PRODUCTS: None

Vancomycin topical solutions intended for ocular use may be prepared by appropriately qualified compounding pharmacists in concentrations from 0.3%-1%.

References

Eguchi, H., H. Shiota, et al. (2009). The inhibitory effect of vancomycin ointment on the manifestation of MRSA keratitis in rabbits. *Journal of Infection and Chemotherapy* 15(5): 279-283.
Kodjikian, L., J. Couprie, et al. (2010). Experimental Intracameral Injection of Vancomycin Microparticles in Rabbits. *Investigative Ophthalmology & Visual Science* 51(8): 4125-4132.

ANTIBIOTIC COMBINATIONS

Indications/Pharmacology
These combination products exhibit a broad-spectrum of activity and are considered the first choice for symptomatic treatment of conjunctivitis in dogs and for prophylactic treatment of small animals prior to or after eye surgery. These agents are also used prophylactically for corneal injuries/wounds.

Suggested Dosages/Precautions/Adverse Effects
Usually applied 4 times daily to prevent infection and up to every 30 minutes in established corneal infections. See individual product label information and the information noted previously.

Neomycin has been reported to cause allergic reactions in dogs and cats, particularly after prolonged usage. As noted above, avoid neomycin treatment in cats unless absolutely necessary. Interestingly, anaphylactic reactions in cats have only been associated with neomycin products in ointment form in the absence of cortisone, but not with antibiotic-steroid combination preparations.

Dosage Forms/Regulatory Status
VETERINARY-LABELED PRODUCTS:

Bacitracin zinc 400 Units/Neomycin 3.5 mg/Polymyxin B Sulfate 10,000 Units/gram Ophthalmic Ointment: 3.5 gram tubes; *Mycitracin*® (Upjohn) (**Note:** contains 500 mg bacitracin/gm); *Neobacimyx*® (Schering); *Trioptic-P*® (Pfizer); *Vetropolycin*® (Dechra); generic; (Rx). FDA-approved for dogs and cats.

Oxytetracycline HCl 5 mg/Polymyxin B Sulfate 10,000 Units/gram Ophthalmic Ointment: 3.5 gm tubes; *Terramycin*® *Ophthalmic Ointment* (Pfizer); (OTC). FDA-approved for use in dogs, cats, sheep, cattle, and horses.

Neomycin 3.5 mg/Polymyxin B Sulfate 10,000 Units per mL Ophthalmic Solution: *Optiprime*® (Syntex); (Rx). FDA-approved for use in dogs.

HUMAN-LABELED PRODUCTS:

There is a wide variety of human-labeled ophthalmic combination products available. Most are a combination of bacitracin/neomycin/polymyxin B. However, there are variations of this theme (*e.g.*, gramicidin in place of bacitracin in topical solutions-*Neosporin*® *Ophthalmic Solution*). All these products require a prescription.

ANTIBIOTIC AND CORTICOSTEROID COMBINATIONS

Indications/Pharmacology

There are three basic categories of these products that are routinely used in veterinary medicine; antibiotic combinations with hydrocortisone, antibiotic combinations with dexamethasone, and individual antibiotics (*e.g.*, gentamicin or chloramphenicol) with a steroid.

Antibiotic combinations with hydrocortisone (ointment or solution) are used in dogs and horses for conjunctivitis as nonspecific therapy after ruling out other causes for red painful eyes, including glaucoma and anterior uveitis. They generally are applied 4 times daily and then on a tapering schedule based on the response to therapy. The hydrocortisone is relatively weak as an antiinflammatory agent and is not effective for intraocular inflammatory disease such as anterior uveitis. The relative penetration and potency of hydrocortisone in these preparations makes them relatively ineffective for immune mediated extraocular disease including scleritis, episcleritis and or nodular granulomatous episclerokeratitis. Anterior uveitis is statistically more common in horses than simple conjunctivitis and the steroid in these agents would not be helpful in improving the clinical signs of immune mediated uveitis.

Antibiotic combinations with dexamethasone are valuable for use in cases of more severe canine or equine conjunctivitis, nonulcerative keratitis and for immune-mediated scleral or corneal conditions such as chronic superficial keratitis (German shepherd pannus), feline eosinophilic keratitis, scleritis, episcleritis and nodular granulomatous episclerokeratitis. For these conditions, the antibiotic agent is not necessary but dexamethasone-only products are not always available. These medications are also used in the equine species with equine uveitis because the ointment forms persist on the cornea longer than drops.

Single agent antibiotic (gentamicin) and potent steroid (betamethasone) combination products (*e.g.*, *Gentocin Durafilm®*) are commonly used in veterinary medicine. However, there are few instances in veterinary ophthalmology in which a very potent corticosteroid agent and an aminoglycoside antibiotic are necessary in combination. Simple conjunctivitis in dogs and horses is adequately treated with antibiotic combinations with hydrocortisone. Avoid use of this agent in cats with conjunctivitis for the reasons noted below.

Suggested Dosages/Precautions/Adverse Effects

See individual product label information and the information noted above.

Avoid use of antibiotic/steroid combination agents in cats with conjunctivitis as the most common cause of conjunctivitis in the cat is primary or recurring infection with exposure to, or reactivation of, latent feline herpes virus. Recent research indicates that topical steroids increase the length of the typical course of feline herpes virus related conjunctivitis and/or keratitis and can induce corneal involvement in cases that might otherwise have remained confined to conjunctiva. Corneal sequestration has been noted to occur in cats with herpes virus conjunctivitis after treatment with topical steroids. Recommended treatment for feline herpes virus conjunctivitis is tetracycline ointment *QID* during active disease, as this drug is effective against Mycoplasma and Chlamydia (**Note:** concurrent systemic treatment with doxycycline will likely be necessary to clear Chlamydia organisms from the nasal and/or GI passages in cats as discussed above).

Dosage Forms/Regulatory Status

VETERINARY-LABELED PRODUCTS:

Triple Antibiotic Ointments with Hydrocortisone:

Bacitracin zinc 400 units/Neomycin 3.5 mg/Polymyxin B Sulfate 10,000 Units & Hydrocortisone acetate 1% per gram in 3.5 gm tubes; *Neobacimyx H®* (Schering); *Trioptic-S®* (Pfizer); *Vetropolycin HC®* (Dechra); generic; (Rx). Approved for dogs and cats.

Other Antibiotic/Steroid Ointments:

Neomycin Sulfate 5 mg & Prednisolone 2 mg (0.2%) per gram in 3.5 gram tubes; *Optisone®* (Evsco); (Rx). Approved for use in dogs and cats.

Neomycin Sulfate 5 mg & Isoflupredone acetate 1 mg (0.1%) per gram in 3.5 & 5 gram tubes; *Neo-Predef®* *Sterile Ointment* (Upjohn); (Rx). Approved for use in horses, cattle, dogs and cats.

Chloramphenicol 1% and Prednisolone acetate 2.5 mg (0.25%) in 3.5 gm tubes; *Chlorasone®* (Evsco) (Rx). Approved for use dogs and cats.

Drops:

Gentamicin Ophthalmic Drops 3 mg/mL & Betamethasone acetate 1 m/mL in 5 mL btls; *Gentocin Durafilm®* (Schering); (Rx). Approved for use in dogs.

HUMAN-LABELED PRODUCTS:

There is a wide variety of human-labeled ophthalmic antibiotic/steroid combination products available. Some of the more commonly used combinations include:

Ointments:

Bacitracin/Neomycin/Polymyxin B and Hydrocortisone; *Cortisporin®* (BW); (Rx)

Neomycin/Polymyxin B & Dexamethasone; *Maxitrol®* (Alcon); (Rx)

Neomycin and Dexamethasone; *NeoDecadron®* (Merck); (Rx)

Drops:

Neomycin/Polymyxin B and Hydrocortisone; *Cortisporin®* (BW, etc.); (Rx)

Neomycin/Polymyxin B & Dexamethasone; *Maxitrol®* (Alcon); (Rx)

Neomycin and Dexamethasone; *NeoDecadron®* (Merck); (Rx)

Antifungals, Ocular

Antifungal agents act primarily by inhibition of fungal cell wall and fall into four classes: polyenes, pyrimidines, azoles, or echinocandins. Polyenes (amphotericin, nystatin and natamycin) bind ergosterol in a dose-related effect causing fungal cell wall leakage and cell death. Fungal keratitis is a serious corneal disease, most commonly reported in the horse. The species selectivity of this disease is related to the environment of this animal, which is often contaminated with fungal elements. An increased incidence of fungal keratitis in people was directly related to the development of multiple topical steroid agents for treatment of eye diseases. In the horse, many cases of fungal keratitis are noted in association with prior treatment of conjunctival and/or corneal diseases with topical steroid agents. Aspergillus is the most common cause of fungal keratitis in the horse, although there is a great deal of variation in fungal isolates from the cornea depending upon geographical location. Studies in people and anecdotal reports from veterinarians suggest that fungal keratitis due to fusarium organisms are more resistant to therapy than are those caused by aspergillus. Most studies in the equine suggest that about 50% of cases of fungal keratitis in the horse result in perforation of the corneal and enucleation of the eye. Medical and surgical therapy (keratectomy, corneal debridement, and conjunctival grafting) are used to treat such cases with the goals of therapy including arresting infection, mechanical removal of organisms from the cornea, and support of the cornea. All antifungal agents available for use in the equine suffer from poor penetration into the corneal stroma. Conjunctival grafting may further hinder drug penetration as a trade off to improving vascular availability to the cornea and mechanical support. Pathologic specimens from horses with fungal keratitis indicate that fungal organisms, unlike bacterial organisms, have a propensity to multiply deep in the stroma, directly adjacent to Descemet's membrane, making corneal penetration an important issue. Because the prognosis for return of vision and saving the globe in cases of fungal keratitis cases is guarded and because treatment is labor intensive, referral to teaching or other hospitals for 24 hour care and observation is recommended.

AMPHOTERICIN B

(am-foe-*ter*-i-sin **B**)

Indications/Pharmacology

Amphotericin B is a broad spectrum antifungal drug derived from *Streptomyces nodosus*. Originally formulated as a colloidal suspension to overcome poor water solubility, amphotericin frequently caused significant systemic toxicity to kidneys, liver and blood. Amphotericin is now provided in a variety of dosage forms to reduce the risk for systemic toxicity including liposomal injection, lipid complex injection, and colloidal dispersion. No ocular topical dosage form of amphotericin is commercially available, however, the colloidal suspension has been used topically and subconjunctivally to treat cases of equine fungal keratitis. When reconstituting amphotericin, sterile water should be utilized as saline decreases the stability of amphotericin. Resulting dilutions should be refrigerated and protected from light. Amphotericin B is fungistatic or fungicidal depending on the concentration obtained in body fluids and the susceptibility of the fungus. Amphotericin B has been shown to be effective against the following fungi: *Histoplasma capsulatum*, *Coccidioides immitis*, Candida species, *Blastomyces dermatitidis*, Rhodotorula, *Cryptococcus neoformans*, *Sporothrix schenckii*, *Mucor mucedo*, and *Aspergillus fumigatus*. While *Candida albicans* is generally quite susceptible to amphotericin B, non-albicans species may be less susceptible. *Pseudallescheria boydii* and *Fusarium* spp. are often resistant to amphotericin B.

Suggested Dosages/Precautions/Adverse Effects

Instill 0.2 mL of a 0.15% solution in the eye or the palpebral lavage catheter every 2–6 hours, or 0.25 mL of a 0.5 mg/mL solution subconjunctivally every 48 hours. There are no commercially available amphotericin B ophthalmic products, but the non-liposomal injectable formulation can be reconstituted with sterile water to make sterile solutions suitable for topical or subconjunctival administration. Amphotericin B should not be reconstituted with sodium chloride containing solutions as this encourages degradation of the drug.

Dosage Forms/Regulatory Status

VETERINARY-LABELED PRODUCTS: None

HUMAN-LABELED PRODUCTS: None

Sterile solutions for topical ophthalmic administration or subconjunctival injection may be prepared by reconstituting commercially available amphotericin B injection lyophilized powder and diluting to appropriate concentrations with sterile water for injection. Chemical stability is concentration dependent, but most resulting solutions may be stored for at least 7 days under refrigeration and protected from light.

NATAMYCIN

(na-ta-*mye*-sin)

Indications/Pharmacology

Natamycin (pimaricin) is a semisynthetic polyene antibiotic and has an improved antimycotic spectrum compared to amphotericin B. It is well-tolerated and induces fewer ocular toxicities compared to amphotericin B. However, natamycin is poorly water-soluble and will not penetrate the intact corneal epithelium. Natamycin is the only antifungal agent approved for use on the eye and the only commercially available eye drug for treatment of fungal keratitis.

Suggested Dosages/Precautions/Adverse Effects

The product comes as a thick white suspension that complicates the use of subpalpebral lavage apparatus for frequent treatment of the cornea of the horse. This drug will obstruct catheter systems used for medication. It will cause dramatic swelling and pain in the upper eyelid if it leaks out of the tubing into the subcutaneous tissues of the eyelid. Corneal penetration is poor and the medication is very expensive. Fungal keratitis cases are treated aggressively with hourly or bi-hourly treatment the first 1–3 days and gradual reduction in treatment frequency with signs of clinical improvement. Cytology and repeated cultures of the cornea are used to indicate treatment effectiveness. Worsening of the corneal edema and cellular infiltration can be a sign of treatment response. This is thought to be due to antigenic release associated with killing of fungal organisms (like the pulmonary response noted in dogs with institution of antifungal therapy for blastomycosis, etc.). Four to six weeks of treatment is not uncommon for fungal keratitis cases.

Dosage Forms/Regulatory Status

VETERINARY-LABELED PRODUCTS: None

HUMAN-LABELED PRODUCTS:

Natamycin Ophthalmic Suspension 5%: 15 mL btls; *Natacyn*® (Alcon); (Rx)

MICONAZOLE

(mi-*kon*-a-zole)

Indications/Pharmacology

Miconazole is a broad spectrum imidazole antifungal agent with some antibacterial activity. Miconazole will penetrate the intact corneal epithelium. Topical miconazole therapy has been a favorite first choice agent for treatment of fungal keratitis in the horse by veterinary ophthalmologists for several years. Miconazole may be delivered by subconjunctival route, but with some local irritation, and topical use is the most commonly employed treatment method.

Suggested Dosages/Precautions/Adverse Effects

Miconazole was formerly available as a 10 mg/mL injectable solution for IV use in humans. It can now only be obtained through s. It is a clear solution readily delivered through subpalpebral lavage apparatus systems. The medication is significantly less expensive compared with natamycin and its corneal penetration is more favorable, although still less than optimal. Treatment is generally delivered hourly or bi-hourly during the first several days of treatment. Once clinical improvement is noted and cytology specimens and repeated cultures indicate eradication of fungal organisms, the treatment frequency is gradually reduced. Most fungal keratitis cases are treated 4–6 weeks.

Dosage Forms/Regulatory Status

VETERINARY-LABELED PRODUCTS: None

HUMAN-LABELED PRODUCTS: None suitable for the eye.

All commercially available miconazole topical preparations contain alcohols or other agents that cause corneal damage. It is imperative that a 1% miconazole solution be compounded without alcohols for use on the cornea.

POVIDONE IODINE

Indications/Pharmacology

Dilute solutions of povidone iodine (1%–5%) have been utilized for chemical debridement of loose epithelium in canine indolent ulcers. 5% povidone iodine has also been used as an antifungal for fungal keratitis, but must be lavaged from the eye within 5 minutes to prevent damage to corneal epithelium. Generally, povidone iodine is only used once daily and then rinsed off when used in the eye as an anti-fungal. There has also been a renewed interest in utilizing povidone iodine in treating feline herpes keratitis. Solutions of commercially available 10% povidone iodine are diluted in physiologic saline to concentrations of 0.5–1% and applied 1 drop twice to four times daily for treatment of chronic feline herpes keratitis and may also be used prophylactically for feline herpes-virus (FHV) cats with a history of recurring ulcer.

Suggested Dosages/Precautions/Adverse Effects

Solutions of 1% are applied twice to four times daily for treatment and prophylaxis of feline herpes-virus (FHV) keratitis and for chemical debridement of epithelium for canine indolent ulcers. Solutions of concentration greater than 1% should be lavaged from the eye after no more than 5 minutes to prevent corneal epithelial damage.

Dosage Forms/Regulatory Status

VETERINARY-LABELED PRODUCTS: None

HUMAN-LABELED PRODUCTS: None

Products must be compounded and diluted from the commercially available povidone iodine 10% solutions and diluted to final concentrations of 0.5–1% for antiviral indications and no more than 5% for use as an ophthalmic irrigant.

SILVER SULFADIAZINE

(*sil*-ver sul-fa-*dye*-a-zeen)

Indications/Pharmacology

Silver sulfadiazine cream is a broad spectrum agent that covers bacteria (gram-positive and -negative) and fungal agents. It has been used extensively in people suffering from skin burns. It is nontoxic to the skin, conjunctiva and cornea and has been used in the last several years for cases of fungal keratitis. Particularly good results have been noted in cases of superficial keratitis prior to development of advanced disease. Clinical response is better when used early in the course of the disease. Treatment with silver sulfadiazine is considered non-conventional in people. It is gaining in popularity in the treatment of equine fungal keratitis by veterinary ophthalmologists. For medico-legal reasons, in very expensive horses in which litigation may be an issue, treatment with more conventional therapy (natamycin) may be indicated first, or consideration can be given to signed consent regarding treatment with silver sulfadiazine. The initial response to this drug has been promising, however.

Suggested Dosages/Precautions/Adverse Effects

The commercially available product is a cream, but can be delivered into the conjunctival sac using a tuberculin syringe, without the needle. A typical treatment dose is 0.2 mL drawn into a syringe. It will not pass through standard sized subpalpebral lavage catheters, although it may be administered through large medication administration systems using red rubber feeding tubes passed through the lid, with variable results getting the medication to pass through the tube. It is probably best applied manually. The cream sticks well to the cornea that probably improves effectiveness, similar to natamycin, as compared to miconazole. Treatment regimes are similar to the other antifungal agents with very frequent applications necessary during the early phases of the treatment and reduction in therapy based upon clinical response. Daily debridement of the necrotic corneal stroma and epithelium will improve penetration of the drug and the clinical response.

The medication is inexpensive and is available from any pharmacy, but it is not labeled for use in eyes. The label (package insert) specifically states "not to be used in eyes" so liability for use in eyes rests solely with the prescribing veterinarian and some pharmacists may be unwilling to dispense this medication for ophthalmic use. Argyrism has been reported in patients receiving topical silver sulfadiazine on a chronic basis.

Dosage Forms/Regulatory Status

VETERINARY-LABELED PRODUCTS: None

HUMAN-LABELED PRODUCTS:

Silver Sulfadiazine Topical (*not an ophthalmic product*): 10 mg per gram in a water miscible cream base; 20, 50, 400, and 1000 g containers; *Silvadene®* (Marion); *Flint SSD®* (Flint); (Rx). Preferably dispensed aseptically in single use sterile tuberculin syringes for application to the conjunctival sac.

ITRACONAZOLE

(i-tra-*koe*-na-zole)

Indications/Pharmacology

Itraconazole is a broad spectrum synthetic antifungal agent effective against a wide range of filamentous fungi, dimorphic fungi, and yeasts. It is the most popular systemic antifungal agent for treatment of blastomycosis related and other systemic fungal infections in dogs and people. Itraconazole specifically targets oxidative enzymes of fungal organisms thereby increasing efficacy while lowering toxicity. Itraconazole prepared as a 1% ointment in 30% dimethylsulfoxide (DMSO) is well tolerated in horses with keratomycosis with reported good results. Itraconazole is relatively insoluble in water and must be diluted in DMSO to achieve solution. Itraconazole 1% suspensions in a vehicle of 30% DMSO and 70% artificial tears have also been used successfully to treat fungal keratitis in horses. It is important to note that the DMSO may be topically irritating to many horses. The fungal species most commonly isolated from cases of equine keratomycosis and their particular sensitivity to specific antifungal agents varies greatly by geography in the United States. In vitro sensitivity testing can be done at select laboratories on fungal isolates from the equine eye but this information generally takes several weeks to become available. Because of these considerations, the selection of a particular antifungal drug for an individual case is largely based on local clinical experience and impressions.

Suggested Doses/Precautions/Adverse Effects

Compounded itraconazole/DMSO preparation is applied to the cornea frequently in horses with confirmed keratomycosis. Initially, treatment every 2–3 hours is not uncommon; tapering of the treatment based on clinical response. Individuals treating horses need to use routine precautions (gloves) while handling this medication to minimize any skin uptake enhanced by the DMSO solvent.

Dosage Forms/Regulatory Status

VETERINARY-LABELED PRODUCTS: None

HUMAN-LABELED PRODUCTS:

Compounded product. Must be obtained from an appropriately qualified compounding pharmacy as a 1% suspension or ointment in a DMSO 30% base.

VORICONAZOLE
(vor-i-*kon*-a-zole)

Indications/Pharmacology

Voriconazole is derived from fluconazole and is considerably more efficacious than amphotericin B for filamentous organisms. Following oral (4 mg/kg) or IV (1 mg/kg) doses to horses, voriconazole demonstrated excellent absorption, bioavailability and tolerance (Davis *et al.* 2006). Although there are currently no approved ocular formulations of voriconazole, compounded solutions of 1% voriconazole have been shown to achieve acceptable ocular concentrations in the aqueous humor (Clode *et al.* 2006).

Voriconazole has been used clinically for the treatment of equine fungal keratitis. Voriconazole is a triazole antifungal agent. The primary mode of action of voriconazole is the inhibition of fungal cytochrome P-450-mediated 14 alpha-lanosterol demethylation, an essential step in fungal ergosterol biosynthesis. The accumulation of 14 alpha-methyl sterols correlates with the subsequent loss of ergosterol in the fungal cell wall and may be responsible for the antifungal activity of voriconazole. Voriconazole has been shown to be more selective for fungal cytochrome P-450 enzymes than for various mammalian cytochrome P-450 enzyme systems. Voriconazole has demonstrated *in vitro* activity against *Aspergillus* (*A. fumigatus, A. flavus, A. niger* and *A. terreus*), *Candida* (*C. albicans, C. glabrata, C. krusei, C. parapsilosis* and *C. tropicalis*), *Scedosporium apiospermum* and *Fusarium* spp., including *Fusarium solani*. Voriconazole drug resistance development has not been adequately studied *in vitro* against *Candida, Aspergillus, Scedosporium* and *Fusarium* species. The frequency of drug resistance development for the various fungi for which this drug is indicated is not known. Fungal isolates exhibiting reduced susceptibility to fluconazole or itraconazole may also show reduced susceptibility to voriconazole, suggesting cross-resistance can occur among these azoles. The relevance of cross-resistance and clinical outcome has not been fully characterized. Clinical cases where azole cross-resistance is demonstrated may require alternative antifungal therapy. There are no approved ophthalmic formulations of voriconazole, however, a suitable solution for ophthalmic administration can be prepared by utilizing the approved voriconazole injectable product.

Suggested Dosages/Precautions/Adverse Effects

0.2 mL in the eye or palpebral lavage catheter every 2–4 hours. Voriconazole is contraindicated in patients with known hypersensitivity to voriconazole or its excipients. There is no information regarding cross-sensitivity between voriconazole and other azole antifungal agents. Caution should be used when prescribing voriconazole to patients with hypersensitivity to other azoles. Voriconazole treatment-related visual disturbances are common in humans. In therapeutic trials, approximately 21% of patients experienced abnormal vision, color vision change and/or photophobia. The visual disturbances were generally mild and rarely resulted in discontinuation. Visual disturbances may be associated with higher plasma concentrations and/or doses. Since topical administration of voriconazole has not been evaluated in humans, it is not known if this adverse event occurs with topical administration. The mechanism of action of the visual disturbance is unknown, although the site of action is most likely to be within the retina. In a study in healthy volunteers investigating the effect of 28-day treatment with voriconazole on retinal function, voriconazole caused a decrease in the electroretinogram (ERG) waveform amplitude, a decrease in the visual field, and an alteration in color perception. The ERG measures electrical currents in the retina. The effects were noted early in administration of voriconazole and continued through the course of study drug dosing. Fourteen days after end of dosing, ERG, visual fields and color perception returned to normal. Dermatological reactions are also common in human patients treated with voriconazole. The mechanism underlying these dermatologic adverse events remains unknown. In clinical trials, rashes considered related to therapy were reported by 7% (110/1655) of voriconazole-treated patients. The majority of rashes were of mild to moderate severity. Cases of photosensitivity reactions appear to be more likely to occur with long-term treatment. Human patients have rarely developed serious cutaneous reactions, including Stevens-Johnson syndrome, toxic epidermal necrolysis and erythema multiforme during treatment with VFEND. If patients develop a rash, they should be monitored closely and consideration given to discontinuation of VFEND. It is recommended that patients avoid strong, direct sunlight during VFEND therapy. The extent of these adverse drug reactions in animals is unknown at this time.

Dosage Forms/Regulatory Status

VETERINARY-LABELED PRODUCTS: None

HUMAN-LABELED PRODUCTS: None

There are no commercially available ophthalmic dosage forms of voriconazole. A suitable solution for ophthalmic administration may be prepared by aseptically adding 19 mL of sterile water for injection to a 200 mg vial of *VFend®* injection to result in a sterile 1% solution. Resulting solution should be stored under refrigeration and discarded 28 days after reconstitution.

References

Clode, A.B., J.L. Davis, et al. (2006). Evaluation of concentration of voriconazole in aqueous humor after topical and oral administration in horses. *American Journal of Veterinary Research* 67(2): 296-301.

Davis, J., J. Salmon, et al. (2006). Pharmacokinetics of voriconazole after oral and intravenous administration to horses. *AJVR* 67(6): 1070-1075.

Antivirals, Ocular

Antiviral drugs are used most commonly in clinical practice for the treatment of feline ocular herpes virus infections. Simple acute conjunctivitis is best managed with symptomatic antibiotic therapy alone (*i.e.*, tetracycline treatment or systemic doxycycline treatment). The development of concurrent corneal disease, however, indicates that consideration should be given to the use of antiviral drugs. Persistent cases of conjunctivitis in the cat due to feline herpes virus infection may also benefit from treatment with topical antiviral drugs. Although *in vitro* studies indicate that trifluridine is the most effective agent against feline herpes virus, idoxuridine is a less irritating, more economical alternative. In general, all antivirals are virustatic (not cidal) and require application every 2 hours for the first 24 hours followed by 5–6 times daily treatment thereafter. While this appendix focuses mostly on topical ophthalmic therapies, it is important to note that studies support use of l-lysine at 500 mg orally twice daily in cats to prevent or reduce the severity of feline herpes virus ocular infections through disruption of viral replication.

TRIFLURIDINE (TRIFLUORO-THYMIDINE)

(trye-*flure*-i-deen)

Indications/Pharmacology

Trifluridine (trifluorothymidine; *Viroptic®*) is a pyrimidine nucleoside analog. It is structurally related to 2-deoxythymidine, the natural precursor of DNA synthesis and exerts its effects via inhibition of thymidylate synthetase. An *in vitro* study in which several strains of feline herpes virus were collected from the United States and were used to infect kidney epithelial cells showed that trifluridine was more effective at lower concentrations compared with several other agents. For this reason, trifluridine was the first choice drug employed in the treatment of feline herpes virus ocular disease for many years. Because of the topical toxicity associated with use of trifluridine in cats, its popularity has diminished greatly. In many milder cases, the irritation associated with topical trifluridine is more intense than the inflammation induced by viral infection. Antiviral agents have also been used in the treatment of superficial punctate keratitis in the horse, thought to be associated with equine herpes virus-2 (EHV-2) infection of the cornea.

Suggested Dosages/Precautions/Adverse Effects

Trifluridine must be applied very frequently. Many veterinary ophthalmologists recommend treatment every 2 hours (waking hours) during the first 2 days of therapy to establish effective corneal drug levels. After this time, treatment 4–6 times daily is indicated. Because trifluridine is virostatic and not viricidal, treatment 1 week beyond the resolution of clinical signs is recommended, to prevent a rebound effect associated with poor surface immunity in combination with residual active viral agents. However, a maximum supply of 3 weeks medication should initially be dispensed as trifluridine is a corneal toxin and can retard corneal epithelial healing. Additionally, if cats do not respond favorably to trifluridine therapy within three weeks, they are not likely to respond with longer durations of therapy. If no improvement is noted in three weeks, trifluridine (or any antiviral) should be discontinued for a rest period and then a different antiviral initiated.

Anecdotally, improvement with antiviral agents is noted in about 50% of cats in which the treatment is employed. In some cats, the ocular disease persists despite treatment with antiviral agents. It is not certain if these are truly cases of feline herpes virus infection or other disease. Except in acute cases with respiratory and ocular involvement, the confirmation of feline herpes virus infection is exceedingly difficult in private practice, primarily due to the logistics of performing specific viral isolation tests. Chronic conjunctivitis in the cat seems to be the most resistant to treatment with antiviral agents. Conjunctival and lid margin irritation are commonly reported with trifluridine use.

Dosage Forms/Regulatory Status

VETERINARY-LABELED PRODUCTS: None

HUMAN-LABELED PRODUCTS:

Trifluridine Ophthalmic Solution: 1% in 7.5 mL btls; *Viroptic®* (Monarch); (Rx)

IDOXURIDINE
(eye-dox-*yoor*-i-deen)

Indications/Pharmacology
Idoxuridine (IDU) is chemically similar to thymidine and its substitution into viral DNA causes misreading of the viral genetic code thereby inhibiting viral replication. Because IDU is a non-specific inhibitor of DNA synthesis, it affects any cellular function requiring thymidine and is not suitable for systemic use. Even with topical therapy, corneal toxicity can occur. Like trifluridine, IDU is considered virostatic rather than viricidal. IDU was found to be second to trifluridine in efficacy *in vitro* against common strains of feline herpes virus growing in kidney epithelial cells. IDU is extremely well tolerated in cats and this feature alone makes it the most popular antiviral currently available for use in cats with presumed or established feline herpes virus infection. Although trifluridine was shown to be more effective *in vitro*, the topical irritation it induces in cats frequently negates any beneficial effect that might be noted clinically. Stinging upon application is a rare feature with IDU/artificial tear preparations.

Suggested Doses/Precautions/Adverse Effects
IDU, like trifluridine, penetrates poorly into the cornea (except in instances of ulceration) and conjunctiva and therefore must initially be applied frequently. Most treatment protocols involve application every two to three hours during waking hours the first two days of acute infection, followed by four to five times daily treatment continued a week beyond resolution of clinical signs.

Dosage Forms/Regulatory Status
VETERINARY-LABELED PRODUCTS: None

HUMAN-LABELED PRODUCTS: None.

Formerly approved as *Stoxil*® and *Herplex*®; must be obtained from appropriately qualified compounding pharmacies as a 0.1% ophthalmic solution or a 0.5% ophthalmic ointment.

INTERFERON ALPHA
(in-ter-*feer*-on *al*-fa)

Indications/Pharmacology
Interferon alpha-2B is thought to stimulate local immunity against viral infection and has been advocated as an adjunct therapy for treatment of feline herpes viral keratitis. Few peer-reviewed, placebo controlled, prospective clinical trials evaluating interferon administration to FHV cats exist at the time of writing, and until further studies are conducted, the dosage, frequency and efficacy of interferon in FHV cannot be stated.

Furthermore, the stability of interferon for long term administration has not been scientifically evaluated. The gastric degradation of interferon by peptidases precludes likely systemic absorption of this drug; however, absorption across the oropharyngeal mucosa may occur and low concentrations of interferon may be amplified via a cascade effect (Weigent *et al.* 1984).

Suggested Dosages/Precautions/Adverse Effects
It has been used both systemically (30 Units PO q24h) and/or topically (30–50 Units/mL in artificial tears in both eyes 3–5 times daily) for refractory cases of feline herpes keratitis although these doses, routes and frequencies have not been scientifically evaluated.

Dosage Forms/Regulatory Status
VETERINARY-LABELED PRODUCTS: None

HUMAN-LABELED PRODUCTS: None.

The human interferon alpha-2B injection (*Intron-A*®—Schering) is diluted to a final concentration of 30–50 Units/mL in saline or artificial tears and administered orally or topically respectively.

References
Weigent, D.A., M.P. Langford, et al. (1984). Interferon-induced transfer of viral resistance by human lymphocyte-B and lymphocyte-T. *Cellular Immunology* 87(2): 678-683.

ACYCLOVIR
VALACYCLOVIR
FAMCICLOVIR
GANCICLOVIR
CIDOFOVIR
PENCICLOVIR

Indications/Pharmacology
These antiviral drugs represent the acyclic nucleoside analogs and require three phosphorylation steps for activation: catalyzation by thymidine kinase, followed by phosphorylation by host enzymes. Because the Feline Herpes virus (FHV) thymidine kinase enzyme is less active than the human Herpes simplex virus (HSV), these agents are not as effective against FHV as they are against HSV.

A 0.5% acyclovir ophthalmic ointment administered 5 times daily demonstrated a mean time of 10 days to resolution of clinical signs (Williams *et al.* 2005). Ophthalmic ganciclovir is available as a 0.15% topical gel for human use, but at the time of writing has not been studied in cats. Systemic anti-retroviral agents have been tried in cats with persistent herpes keratitis, but myelosuppression and nephrotoxicity following systemic use is a serious risk with acyclovir and valacyclovir. Acyclovir should only be used systemically as a last resort and CBC should be monitored weekly in cats receiving this drug. Valacyclovir apparently has no effect on feline herpes replication and should **never** be used in cats due to fatal myeloid dysplasia. The pharmacokinetics of systemic famciclovir in cats are extremely complex and this drug should be used with caution in this species. However, a study of famciclovir administered at 90 mg/kg orally three times daily in experimentally infected FHV cats demonstrated significantly reduced clinical signs, serum globulin concentrations, histologic evidence of conjunctivitis, viral shedding, and serum FHV titers with no evidence of adverse clinical, hematologic or biochemical effects (Thomasy et al. 2010). As other agents in this drug class are myelosuppressive, extreme caution is recommended regarding famciclovir therapy in cats. Topically administered cidofovir 0.5% solutions have recently been shown to reduce the severity and duration of FHV-1 infections. The in vitro efficacy of commonly available antiviral agents for FHV-1 has been studied and is as follows: trifluridine > ganciclovir = idoxuridine = cidofovir = penciclovir = vidarabine > acyclovir >> foscarnet.

Suggested Doses/Precautions/Adverse Effects

Acyclovir 0.5% ointment applied 5-6 times daily. Cidofovir 0.5% topical solution, 1 drop in each eye twice daily. Until further data is available, systemic use of these agents is not recommended in cats. Topical use of these agents should be conducted with caution in cats as they are likely to groom off medication and experience systemic adverse effects.

Dosage Forms/Regulatory Status

VETERINARY-LABELED PRODUCTS: None

HUMAN-LABELED PRODUCTS: None

Sterile solutions of cidofovir suitable for ophthalmic administration may be prepared by diluting the commercially available injection to a final concentration of 5 mg/mL using 1% carboxymethylcellulose solutions (Fontenelle et al. 2008). Acyclovir 0.5% ophthalmic ointment may be obtained from appropriately qualified compounding pharmacies.

References

Fontenelle, J.R., C.C. Powell, et al. (2008). Effect of topical ophthalmic application of cidofovir on experimentally induced primary ocular feline herpesvirus-1 infection in cats. American Journal of Veterinary Research 69(2): 289-293.

Thomasy, S., C. Lim, et al. (2010). Safety and efficacy of orally administered famciclovir in cats experimentally infected with feline herpesvirus-1-. AJVR IN PRESS.

Williams, D.L., J.C. Robinson, et al. (2005). Efficacy of topical aciclovir for the treatment of feline herpetic keratitis: results of a prospective clinical trial and data from in vitro investigations. Veterinary Record 157(9): 254-257.

Keratoconjunctivitis Sicca

Keratoconjunctivitis sicca (KCS) is a common ocular disorder in dogs. Recent research efforts indicate that KCS in dogs is an immune mediated disease. It is similar to Sjogren's Syndrome in humans except we do not recognize a connective tissue disorder in the dog compared to this disease in people (man-dry eye, dry mouth, and connective tissue disorder like rheumatoid arthritis; dogs just dry eye). Immune mediated lacrimal adenitis can result in complete destruction of tear producing glands in dogs. Glandular fibrosis produces absolute sicca and these cases may be better managed with a parotid duct transposition surgery because there may be little remaining gland tissue to treat.

CYCLOSPORINE
(sye-kloe-spor-een)

Indications/Pharmacology

Cyclosporine is a polypeptide agent first isolated from a fungus. The agent interferes with interleukin synthesis by T-lymphocytes and in so doing, has been employed extensively in people following major organ transplantation to prevent immune rejection. Cyclosporine is extremely hydrophobic and was originally compounded by pharmacists in virgin olive oil or purified corn oil for the topical application to dogs with keratoconjunctivitis sicca. Topical cyclosporine is now commercially available as a 0.2% ointment (Optimmune®; Schering). The mechanism of action of cyclosporine in the treatment of keratoconjunctivitis sicca is still not fully understood, although it has been employed in the treatment of KCS in dogs for several years. It stimulates increased tear production in normal dogs and for this reason it is thought to have a direct stimulatory effect on the tear gland. It may do this acting as a prolactin analog, fitting onto lacrimal prolactin receptors. Its interleukin blocking effects likely are the major mechanism of action. Halting local inflammatory mediator production appears to arrest self perpetuating lacrimal adenitis resulting in resumption of normal or improved tear production after several weeks of therapy, however, cessation of therapy results in return of symptoms in a matter of days. Cyclosporine in the cornea appears to have the ability to lessen granulation and pigment development. This property appears to be unrelated to its tear producing effect.

The reported success rate of alleviating the signs of KCS in dogs with treatment with cyclosporine is 75−85%. Some studies indicate that the higher the Schirmer value prior to starting therapy, the more likely that the dog will be well managed with cyclosporine alone. Absolute sicca may be associated with extensive fibrosis of the tear glands, leaving little tissue for stimulation or repair.

Cyclosporine is effective in the management of German Shepherd Pannus or chronic superficial keratitis in the dog. This condition is an immune disease of the cornea and likely is interleukin mediated. Cyclosporine may be preferred for the treatment of pannus because of the lack of systemic side effects noted in dogs with chronic topical administration of cyclosporine. Chronic topical corticosteroid treatment is associated with biochemical changes in the blood of large and small dogs.

Cyclosporine has been tried in the management of the rare case of keratoconjunctivitis sicca in the cat. Dry eye in cats is usually associated with herpes virus destruction of lacrimal epithelial cells and or stenosis of the ductules or openings of the ductules due to chronic viral conjunctivitis. Preliminary results have not been promising. Topical cyclosporine often aggravates ophthalmic herpes virus infections in people. Cyclosporine has not shown promising effects in the management of feline eosinophilic keratitis, a condition now thought to be related to chronic stromal herpes virus infection in cats.

Suggested Dosages/Precautions/Adverse Effects

Cyclosporine is an immunosuppressive agent used to facilitate tear production in canine keratoconjunctivitis sicca (KCS). Multiple mechanisms of action have been attributed to cyclosporine. Cyclosporine suppresses T-cell mediated destruction of the lacrimal gland and conjunctival epithelium. Conjunctival mucin stores are also increased leading to improved quality of the tear film and a direct lacrimomimetic effect contributes to the mechanism of action of treating KCS. Cyclosporine is initiated generally as the first course of therapy for confirmed dry eye cases in the dog. The topical half-life of cyclosporine is about 8 hours and most canine cases of KCS are managed with twice daily therapy with 0.2% ointment (*Optimmune®*). Three times a day therapy has been employed during the initial phases of treatment in more difficult or slow responding cases. For unknown reasons (reversal of lacrimal adenitis > reorganization of lacrimal epithelial cell function > formation of secretory granules > tear production) 3–8 weeks of therapy are necessary before a dramatic increase in the Schirmer tear test becomes evident. Patients are generally maintained for life on cyclosporine ophthalmic once or twice daily depending on the response. Discontinuation of therapy is usually associated with the return of clinical signs of KCS within a few days. Reinstitution of therapy, at this time, is usually associated with an almost immediate return of tear production (versus the initial lag phase noted). This likely is related to the degree of inflammatory disease noted with short discontinuation of therapy versus that present initially, prior to the diagnosis of KCS.

If tear production is very low, cyclosporine is often used in combination with artificial tears during the initial phases of therapy. Once tear production is improved, artificial tears can generally be removed completely or their frequency reduced in the treatment plan. After treatment is initiated, reevaluation of tear production in one month is recommended. If ulcerative keratitis complicates keratoconjunctivitis sicca in the dog, more frequent evaluation is necessary. Cyclosporine, although an immunomodulating agent, is considered safe in the face of ulcerative keratitis, with concurrent antibiotic therapy. Caution is advised, however.

When cyclosporine is delivered topically, no systemic toxicity has been noted in dogs given this drug chronically. This is probably associated with the poor absorption of this drug across the GI tract and because it is delivered to the eye at very low concentrations which even if 100% absorbed, when divided over the body weight of the dog is well below even the therapeutic dose. Advanced detection methods have made it possible to measure trace levels of cyclosporine in the blood of dogs being topically treated for dry eye. The clinical implication of this finding is uncertain at this time.

Dosage Forms/Regulatory Status

Optimmune® ointment is the approved formulation of topical cyclosporine for the management of dry eye in dogs. Compounding of topical cyclosporine drops was popular before the introduction, approval, and marketing of *Optimmune®* ointment. Clinicians persistently using compounded formulations of cyclosporine eye drops may be outside of expected ethical and legal standards of practice except under very specific situations. The use of commercially available ophthalmic products instead of compounded medications is highly recommended. *Optimmune®* is first applied 2 or 3 times daily and frequency of daily application is adjusted based on clinical response.

VETERINARY-LABELED PRODUCTS:

Cyclosporine Ophthalmic Ointment 0.2%; *Optimmune®* (Schering-Plough); (Rx)

HUMAN-LABELED PRODUCTS:

Cyclosporine 0.05% Ophthalmic Emulsion; *Restasis®* (Allergan). **Note:** the concentration of this product has not been shown to increase tear production in dogs. Patients failing to respond to the veterinary approved ophthalmic ointment may respond to compounded cyclosporine 1% ophthalmic solution or tacrolimus 0.03% ophthalmic solution.

TACROLIMUS

(ta-*kroe*-li-mus)

Indications/Pharmacology

Tacrolimus was originally studied at the University of Tennessee College of Veterinary Medicine where investigators found it equally effective as cyclosporine and effective for cyclosporine-resistant cases of KCS. Tacrolimus is a macrolide antibiotic that exerts it effects in KCS through mechanisms similar to that of cyclosporine, however exact mechanisms of action in causing tear production are still being determined.

Dosage Forms/Regulatory Status

VETERINARY-LABELED PRODUCTS: None

HUMAN-LABELED PRODUCTS:

None appropriate for the eye. At the time of publication, Fujisawa, Inc. has granted exclusive rights to Sucampo, Inc. to study, develop, and market an ophthalmic tacrolimus formulation for use in KCS. **Note:** *Protopic®* topical ointment is a topical tacrolimus formulated with propylene carbonate that is known to deplete cholinesterase and to be an ophthalmic irritant and should not be used in the eye. Tacrolimus 0.01–0.03% solutions and ointments should be prescribed through an appropriately qualified compounding pharmacy until a suitable commercially available product is available.

PIMECROLIMUS

(pee-*mek*-rowe-*li*-mus)

Indications/Pharmacology

Pimecrolimus is similar in mechanism of action to tacrolimus, with a greater sensitivity. An evaluation of pimecrolimus 1% solution given three times daily to KCS patients demonstrated a favorable response (Nell *et al.* 2005). A comparison of pimecrolimus 1% solution to cyclosporine 0.2% ointment in dogs with KCS demonstrated comparable improvement from both drugs over the 8-week study period (Ofri *et al.* 2009).

Suggested Dosages/Precautions/Adverse Effects

Pimecrolimus should be administered as a 1% ophthalmic solution twice daily.

Dosage Forms/Regulatory Status

VETERINARY-LABELED PRODUCTS: None

HUMAN-LABELED PRODUCTS: None

Compounding pharmacists may prepare a pimecrolimus 1% solution for use in dogs with KCS that are unresponsive to *Optimmune®* 0.2% Ophthalmic Ointment.

References

Nell, B., I. Walde, et al. (2005). The effect of topical pimecrolimus on keratoconjunctivitis sicca and chronic superficial keratitis in dogs: results from an exploratory study. *Veterinary Ophthalmology* 8(1): 39-46.

Ofri, R., G.N. Lambrou, et al. (2009). Clinical evaluation of pimecrolimus eye drops for treatment of canine keratoconjunctivitis sicca: A comparison with cyclosporine A. *Veterinary Journal* 179(1): 70-77.

Artificial Tear Products/ Ocular Lubricants

ARTIFICIAL TEARS/ OCULAR LUBRICANTS

Indications/Pharmacology

Various solutions and ointments have been designed to replace (in quality or quantity) the precorneal tear film with the goal of restoring ocular comfort and corneal protection. Artificial tear solutions are aqueous, isotonic, pH buffered viscous solutions with appropriate surface tension that serve as a lubricant for dry eyes and associated eye irritation due to dry eye syndromes. They are often useful adjuncts in keratoconjunctivitis sicca in dogs early in cyclosporine therapy. Most are water-based preparations that may also include polymers (methylcellulose, polyvinyl alcohol, povidone, dextran and propylene glycol) and other agents (gelatin, glycerin, polyethylene glycol, pluronic gel and polysorbate 80) to increase viscosity, lubrication and retention time. Tonicity and pH are achieved through use of sodium chloride, potassium chloride and boric acid. Preservatives may be present or absent, however, preservatives may add to disease through toxicity to the corneal epithelium.

Ocular lubricant ointments are white petrolatum-based products that serve to lubricate and protect eyes. They are particularly useful during anesthetic procedures where animals' eyes may remain open and during which time tear production is dramatically reduced.

Dosage Forms/Regulatory Status

VETERINARY-LABELED PRODUCTS: None

HUMAN-LABELED PRODUCTS:

There is a plethora of products available with a variety of formulations and trade names. All are OTC. Some commonly known products include:

Artificial Tear Products (Methylcellulose-based): *Adsorbotear®* (Alcon); *Comfort Tears®* (Pilkington Barnes Hind); *GenTeal®* (Ciba Vision); *Isopto-Tears®* (Alcon); *Tears Naturale®* (Alcon); *Lacril®* (Allergan)

Artificial Tear Products (Polyvinyl Alcohol-based): *Hypotears®* (Iolab); *Liquifilm Tears®* (Allergan); *Tears Plus®* (Allergan)

Artificial Tear Products (Glycerin-based): *Dry Eye Therapy®* (Bausch & Lomb); *Eye Lube A®* (Optopics)

Ocular Lubricants (Petrolatum-based): *Lacri-Lube® S.O.P.* (Allergan); *Akwa Tears®* (Akorn)

OPHTHALMIC IRRIGANTS

Indications/Pharmacology

The primary use of ocular irrigation solutions is during intraocular surgery (cataract removal). Ocular irrigating solutions maintain the shape of the anterior chamber during surgery, cool phacoemulsification handpieces, and lavage emulsified lens and surgical byproducts from the eye. The ideal ocular irrigation solution mimics the composition of the aqueous humor in terms of physiologic pH, osmolality and ion composition. Sterile isotonic solutions are also used for flushing the nasolacrimal system and for removing debris from the eye. They are also used to remove excess stain after diagnostic staining of the cornea. Sterile lactated Ringer's solution (LRS) is well tolerated by the surface of the eye as is a balanced salt solution (BSS). Extraocular irrigating solutions may contain preservatives. Intraocular irrigating solutions (used during surgical procedures) do not contain preservatives and contain electrolytes that are required for normal cell function. Intraocular irrigating solutions may also have added glutathione, which is responsible for stabilizing endothelial cell junctions and intraocular pumping functions. Other additives include heparin, epinephrine, antibiotics and local anesthetics to exert desired pharmacological effects. A study evaluating cooled versus room temperature irrigating solutions have demonstrated no significant adverse effects between the two temperatures (Praveen *et al.* 2009).

Suggested Dosages/Precautions/Adverse Effects

Extraocular: Use to flush eye as necessary; control rate of flow by exerting pressure on bottle. Intraocular: Refer to both established practices for each surgical procedure as well as the specific manufacturers' recommendations.

Dosage Forms/Regulatory Status

VETERINARY-LABELED PRODUCTS:

Eye Rinse® (Butler); (OTC): Contains: water, boric acid, zinc sulfate, glycerin, camphor. Note: This product is not labeled for use as an irrigant per se, but as an aid in cleaning the eye and removing eye stains.

HUMAN-LABELED PRODUCTS:

Common trade name products for extraocular irrigation: *AK-Rinse®* (Akorn), *Blinx®* (Pilkington Barnes Hind), *Collyrium for Fresh Eyes Eye Wash®* (Wyeth-Ayerst), *Dacriose®* (Iolab), *Eye Irrigating Solution®* (Rugby), *Eye-Stream®* (Alcon), *Eye Wash®* (several manufacturers), *Eye Irrigating Wash®* (Roberts Hauck), *Irrigate Eye Wash®* (Optopics), *Optigene®* (Pfeiffer), *Star-Optic Eye Wash®* (Stellar), *Visual-Eyes®* (Optopics). All are OTC.

Common trade name products for intraocular irrigation: **Note:** Most of these products contain Balanced Salt Solution (BSS) = NaCl 0.64%, KCl 0.075%, $CaCl_2 \cdot 2H_2O$ 0.048%, $MgCl_2 \cdot 6H_2O$ 0.03%, Na acetate trihydrate 0.39%, sodium citrate dihydrate 0.17%, sodium hydroxide and/or hydrochloric acid to adjust pH, and water: Balanced Salt Solution (various manufacturers), *BSS®* (Alcon), *Iocare Balanced Salt Solution®* (Iolab); All are Rx.

BSS + solutions that also contain dextrose, glutathione, bicarbonate, phosphate are also available as: *BSS Plus®* (Alcon) and *AMO Endosol Extra®* (Allergan); All are Rx.

References

Praveen, M.R., A.R. Vasavada, et al. (2009). Effect of room temperature and cooled intraocular irrigating solution on the cornea and anterior segment inflammation after phacoemulsification: a randomized clinical trial. *Eye* 23(5): 1158-1163.

Topical Hyperosmotic Agents

POLYSULFATED GLYCOSAMINO-GLYCAN

Indications/Pharmacology

Polysulfated glycosaminoglycan (PSGAG) *Adequan®* (Luitpold) inhibits a number of enzymes (lysozyme, hyaluronidase, and serine proteases), decreases prostaglandin E_2 synthesis, reduces production of toxic superoxide radicals, and increases synthesis of collagen proteoglycans and hyaluronic acid. Thus polysulfated glycosaminoglycan, originally developed for use in degenerative osteoarthritis cases, has intriguing properties suggesting usefulness in corneal ulcer management. It has anecdotally been effective in promoting healing of indolent corneal ulcers in dogs but no studies in dogs have been published to date. A Brazilian study reported that when using a 5% PSGAG formulation was applied to indolent ulcers of horses, that 86% of eyes treated were considered healed within 3 weeks of initiation of therapy.

Fibronectin and epidermal growth factors have also been applied in treating indolent ulcers but scientific studies remain to be published regarding efficacy. At the time of publication, surgical keratectomy remains the most reliable treatment for indolent ulcers.

Suggested Dosages/Precautions/Adverse Effects

1 drop of a 5% PSGAG solution in artificial tears applied to the affected eye(s) three times daily.

Dosage Forms/Regulatory Status

VETERINARY-LABELED PRODUCTS:

None, however the veterinary approved *Adequan*® injection may be diluted 1:1 with sterile artificial tears to produce a 5% PSGAG solution.

HUMAN-LABELED PRODUCTS: None

HYPERTONIC SODIUM CHLORIDE

Indications/Pharmacology

The stroma of the cornea is the middle layer located between the outer epithelial layer on the surface of the eye and the inner single epithelial layer lining the cornea, called the corneal endothelium. The stroma consists of highly organized collagen bundles and a few keratocytes (fibroblasts). The spacing of the collagen bundles is critical to absolute clarity of the cornea. The spacing of these bundles is disturbed when fluid enters the stroma. Surrounded by water to the exterior (tears) and on the interior (aqueous humor) the relative dehydration of the stroma is maintained by an active ATP-dependent pump mechanism in the corneal endothelial cells. Degeneration of the corneal endothelium is a relatively common eye problem in older dogs and is a known genetic condition in Boston Terrier and Chihuahua dogs. Fluid continuously seeps into the corneal stroma via the tear film and through aqueous humor passing between corneal endothelial cells. When the endothelial pumping capacity deteriorates, fluid retention in the stroma causes two problems. Visual impairment can eventually develop. The other common complication is the development of corneal ulcers. Edema fluid retained in the cornea pools into pockets called bullae which progressively migrate to the surface of the cornea, eventually draining through and disrupting the surface epithelium. This results in very slow healing and painful corneal erosions in dogs (type II refractory ulcers). Hyperosmotic agents applied 2–3 times daily help to prevent recurrence of bullae and subsequent corneal ulcers <u>after</u> the erosions have healed. Because osmotic agents require an intact epithelial barrier in which to induce a pressure gradient (5% NaCl commercial preparation versus 0.9% NaCl body fluids), they are not effective with respect to healing of stubborn corneal ulcers when present. They simply help to prevent re-ulceration once an intact epithelial barrier has been established. It may be said that these agents simply aggravate irritation already present when used in the face of ulcerative keratitis.

Suggested Dosages/Precautions/Adverse Effects

5% NaCl (*Muro 128*® or equivalent) eye drops or ointment are applied two to three times daily on an indefinite basis to the surface of eyes with corneal endothelial degeneration to prevent corneal ulceration. In the event of corneal ulceration, treatment is discontinued and substituted for antibiotic and mydriatic treatment in addition to procedures to promote healing of refractory type corneal ulcers. NaCl eye drops are available at a 2% and 5% concentration and ointment is available at a 5% concentration. Because of limited contact time with eye drops, the 2% solution would not be considered for use in animals. Because of prolonged contact time associated with ointments, the 5% ointment is probably the best of the available products for use in animals.

Dosage Forms/Regulatory Status

VETERINARY-LABELED PRODUCTS: None

HUMAN-LABELED PRODUCTS:

Sodium Chloride 2% Ophthalmic Solution in 15 mL btls; *Adsorbonac*® (Alcon), *Muro 128*® (Bausch & Lomb); (OTC)

Sodium Chloride 5% Ophthalmic Solution in 15 mL btls; *Adsorbonac*® (Alcon), *Muro 128*® (Bausch & Lomb), *AK-NaCl*® (Akorn), *Muroptic-5*® (Optopics); (OTC)

Sodium Chloride 5% Ophthalmic Ointment in 15 mL btls; *Muro 128*® (Bausch & Lomb), *AK-NaCl*® (Akorn); (OTC)

Viscoelastic Substances

Viscoelastic substances are vital to ocular surgery, minimizing loss of fluid from the anterior chamber while maintaining intraocular space during surgical procedures. The purity and integrity of viscoelastics ensure tissue protection during and after surgery. Viscoelastics generally fall into two categories: cohesives, that tend to stick together, and dispersives, that are more likely to diffuse out into the anterior chamber. Cohesives, in general, create and maintain space very well in the anterior chamber and help stabilize tissue. Such viscoelastics are easily washed away at the end of the case, but are also, unfortunately, all too easily removed during phacoemulsification. Dispersives, that have lower viscosity, remain in the eye more readily, making them well-suited for difficult cases. They are also excellent for various maneuvers, such as retrieving a lost lens fragment, attempting to viscoelevate cortex, or partitioning away a small piece that continues to get caught on the phacoemulsifier tip. Ophthalmic surgeons should be familiar with the advantages and disadvantages of several viscoelastics and realize the limitations encountered if the surgeon chooses to rely on a single viscoelastic. Veterinary ophthalmologist loyalty to brands of viscoelastics is well-earned as newcomer products to this field have frequently resulted in surgical disasters.

Viscoelastics are also vital to tear replacement.

HYALURONIC ACID
(hye-a-loo-*ron*-ik *as*-id)

Indications/Pharmacology

Hyaluronic acid is a natural complex sugar of the glycosaminoglycan family and is a long-chain polymer containing repeating disaccharide units of Na-glucuronate-N-acetylglucosamine. Hyaluronic acid is indicated for use as a surgical aid in cataract extraction (intra-and extracapsular), IOL implantation, corneal transplant, glaucoma filtration and retinal attachment surgery. Hyaluronic acid is a naturally occurring polymer and has wound healing properties. In surgical procedures in the anterior segment of the eye, instillation of hyaluronic acid serves to maintain a deep anterior chamber within corneal endothelium and other surrounding tissues. Furthermore, its viscoelasticity helps to push back the vitreous face and prevent formation of a postoperative flat chamber. In posterior segment surgery, hyaluronic acid serves as a surgical aid to gently separate, maneuver and hold tissues. Hyaluronic acid creates a clear field of vision thereby facilitating intra- and post-operative inspection of the retina and photocoagulation.

Suggested Dosages/Precautions/Adverse Effects

A sufficient amount of hyaluronic acid (generally 10% concentration) is slowly, and carefully introduced (using a cannula or needle into the anterior chamber. Injection of hyaluronic acid can be performed either before or after delivery of the lens. Injection prior to lens delivery will, however, have the additional advantage of protecting the corneal endothelium from possible damage arising from the removal of the cataractous lens. Hyaluronic acid may also be used to coat surgical instruments and the IOL prior to insertion. Additional hyaluronic acid can be injected during surgery to replace any hyaluronic acid lost during surgical manipulation. Topical solutions of hyaluronic acid are also used to provide a viscoelastic shield to the cornea and provide prolonged relief from ocular surface discomfort.

Dosage Forms/Regulatory Status

VETERINARY-LABELED PRODUCTS:

Hyaluronic acid 10% Solution: 2 mL pre-filled syringe; *Hylartin-V*® (Pfizer Pharmacia); *I-Drop Med*® 0.3% solution, 20 x 1 mL preservative-free unit dose containers; (Rx)

HUMAN-LABELED PRODUCTS:

Hyaluronic acid 10%–23%: *Healon*® products (Pfizer); (Rx)

Cytotoxic Ophthalmic Agents

CISPLATIN BEADS
(sis-*pla*-tin)

Indications/Pharmacology

Cisplatin 1.6 mg biodegradable beads are used for intralesional chemotherapy in various cutaneous neoplasia including squamous cell carcinoma and sarcoids in equine patients. A recent retrospective case series study demonstrated that implantation of cisplatin beads into cutaneous neoplasia was an effective method of treatment for these tumors. Implantation of commercially available beads is less time consuming and safer than intralesional injection of cytotoxic agents suspended in fixed oils.

Dosage Forms/Regulatory Status

VETERINARY-LABELED PRODUCTS: Matrix III Cisplatin Beads: 1.6 mg per 3 mm bead; 3 beads per packet; (Royer Biomedical, Inc.), (Rx) At the time of writing was being considered for approval by FDA.

HUMAN-LABELED PRODUCTS: None

5-FLUOROURACIL
(flure-oh-*yoor*-a-sil)

Indications/Pharmacology/Suggested Dosage

5-fluorouracil is a potent cytotoxic chemo-therapeutic agent used for the topical therapy of equine limbal and eyelid squamous cell carcinoma. It is also used as an antimetabolite to limit fibrosis over the body of gonioimplant devices used to artificially shunt aqueous humor out of the eye in glaucoma as well as improve long-term filtering performance of the implant.

1% solution applied to the affected eye three times daily. **Note:** Ingestion of fluorouracil products by dogs has resulted in significant toxicity and a high rate of mortality. All fluorouracil products should be kept well out of the reach of dogs.

Dosage Forms/Regulatory Status

VETERINARY-LABELED PRODUCTS: None

HUMAN-LABELED PRODUCTS: None.

Must be compounded from the injectable product by an appropriately qualified compounding pharmacist in a biological safety cabinet approved for preparation of cytotoxic agents

MITOMYCIN-C
(mye-toe-*mye*-sin)

Indications/Pharmacology
Mitomycin C is a potent cytotoxic chemotherapeutic agent used for topical therapy of equine limbal and eyelid squamous cell carcinoma. It is also used as an antimetabolite to limit fibrosis over the body of gonioimplant devices used to artificially shunt aqueous humor out of the eye in glaucoma as well as improve long-term filtering performance of the implant.

Suggested Doses/Precautions
0.4% solution applied initially followed by 0.04% solution applied topically three times daily for 21 days in a cycle of 7 days on followed by 7 days off. Caregivers should be counseled in proper handling of cytotoxic drugs and contact with biological waste from treated patients.

Dosage Forms/Regulatory Status
VETERINARY-LABELED PRODUCTS: None
HUMAN-LABELED PRODUCTS: None

Must be compounded from the injectable product by an appropriately trained compounding pharmacist in a biological safety cabinet approved for preparation of cytotoxic agents.

Sympathomimetics

HYDROXY-AMPHETAMINE
(hye-*drox*-ee-am-*fe*-ta-meen)

Indications/Pharmacology
Hydroxyamphetamine is an indirectly acting alpha-agonist that is used to diagnose Cranial Nerve III denervation syndromes such as Horner's Syndrome. Hydroxyamphetamine stimulates release of norepinephrine from postganglionic neurons and therefore amplifies pupil dilation response in hypersensitive, denerved neurons.

Dosage Forms/Regulatory Status
VETERINARY-LABELED PRODUCTS: None
HUMAN-LABELED PRODUCTS: None

Must be compounded by an appropriately qualified compounding pharmacist.

COCAINE
(koe-*kane*)

Indications/Pharmacology
Cocaine is an indirectly acting sympathomimetic which is used to diagnose Cranial Nerve III denervation syndromes such as Horner's Syndrome. Cocaine prevents reuptake of norepinephrine into postganglionic neurons and therefore amplifies pupil dilation response in hypersensitive, denerved neurons. Adrenergic agonist activity of cocaine prevents norepinephrine reuptake allowing maintenance of sympathetic stimulation, so it does not localize lesions but confirms diagnosis of sympathetic denervation syndromes.

Dosage Forms/Regulatory Status
VETERINARY-LABELED PRODUCTS: None
HUMAN-LABELED PRODUCTS: None

Must be compounded by an appropriately qualified compounding pharmacist.

Anticollagenase Agents

ACETYLCYSTEINE
(a-se-teel-*sis*-teen)

Indications/Pharmacology
Acetylcysteine is a mucolytic agent that is also used to stop the melting effect of collagenases and proteases on the cornea. Acetylcysteine is useful in halting melting through inhibition of metalloproteinases, but is not felt to be useful for melting caused by infectious agents.

Suggested Dosages/Precautions/Adverse Effects
Acetylcysteine 5% solution is dosed 1 drop in the affected eye every 1–2 hours for the first 24 hours and then 3–4 times daily for the next 7–10 days. Acetylcysteine solutions are diluted with artificial tears to a final concentration of 5% prior to administration as commercially available solutions of 10% and 20% are topically irritating. Acetylcysteine possesses a foul, sulfur-like smell and owners should be informed that this foul odor does not indicate drug deterioration. Acetylcysteine is unstable at room temperature and solutions should be refrigerated.

Dosage Forms/Regulatory Status
VETERINARY-LABELED PRODUCTS: None
HUMAN-LABELED PRODUCTS:

None; *Mucomyst*® 10% and 20% solution for inhalation may be used to compound a 5% solution in artificial tears.

EDETATE DISODIUM
(*ed*-a-tayt)

Indications/Pharmacology
Edetate Disodium (Sodium EDTA) is a chelating agent that is also used to stop the melting effect of collagenases and proteases on the cornea.

EDTA is useful in halting melting through inhibition of matrix metalloproteinases, but is not felt to be useful for melting caused by infectious agents. As the effect of EDTA on metalloproteinases is reversible, it must be administered several times daily to be effective.

Suggested Dosages/Precautions/Adverse Effects

0.05%-1% solution applied as 1 drop in the affected eye several times daily.

Dosage Forms/Regulatory Status

VETERINARY-LABELED PRODUCTS: None

HUMAN-LABELED PRODUCTS: None

EDTA solutions must be compounded by an appropriately qualified compounding pharmacist.

Fibrinolytics/Antifibrinolytic Agents, Ocular

Fibrin clot formation results from activation of the clotting cascade in an effort to control hemorrhage. Intraocular fibrin formation can result in complications (synechia formation, pupillary seclusion, occlusion of gonioimplants, formation of traction bands) that compromise ocular integrity and vision, so lysis of the clot before these complications occur is essential. Agents developed for fibrinolysis in humans include urokinase, streptokinase and tissue plasminogen activator (tPA). At the time of writing, tPA is the only fibrinolytic commercially available for intraocular use.

Antifibrinolytic agents can be useful to inhibit the breakdown of fibrin clots when control of intraocular bleeding is desired. These agents are used particularly as antidotes following overdosage of fibrinolytics.

Fibrinolytic Agents

TISSUE PLASMINOGEN ACTIVATOR (tPA)

(**tiss**-u plaz-**men**-o-jen **ak**-tiv-ate-or)

Indications/Pharmacology

Recombinant human tPA is a fibrinolytic agent that is injected by the intracameral route to achieve lysis of intraocular clots. Intracameral injection of tPA in humans following cataract removal in doses of 10 micrograms dissolved fibrin clots, reduced posterior synechiae, and did not result in any re-bleeding (Heiligenhaus et al. 1998). Topical application of tPA to dogs does not result in therapeutic aqueous humor concentrations (Gerding et al. 1994). Intracameral injection of 25 micrograms of tPA caused fibrinolysis without corneal toxicity in dogs and cats, while doses of 50 micrograms have lead to

corneal endothelial toxicity (Gerding et al. 1992; Hrach et al. 2000).

Suggested Dosages/Precautions/Adverse Effects

Tissue Plasminogen Activator, reconstituted to 250 micrograms/mL is injected intracamerally at 0.1 mL per dose. Adverse effects include repeat bleeding and profound hypotonia and corneal epithelium toxicity at doses equal to or greater than 50 micrograms.

Dosage Forms/Regulatory Status

VETERINARY-LABELED PRODUCTS: None

HUMAN-LABELED PRODUCTS:

Tissue Plasminogen Activator Lyophilized Powder for Injection: 2 mg, 50 mg, 100 mg, *Activase®* (Genentech); (Rx)

References

Gerding, P.A., D. Essexsorlie, et al. (1992). Use of tissue plasminogen-activator for intraocular fibrinolysis in dogs. *American Journal of Veterinary Research* 53(6): 894–896.

Gerding, P.A., R.E. Hamor, et al. (1994). Evaluation of topically administered tissue-plasminogen activator for intraocular fibrinolysis in dogs. *American Journal of Veterinary Research* 55(10): 1368–1370.

Heiligenhaus, A., B. Steinmetz, et al. (1998). Recombinant tissue plasminogen activator in cases with fibrin formation after cataract surgery: a prospective randomised multicentre study. *British Journal of Ophthalmology* 82(7): 810–815.

Hrach, C.J., M.W. Johnson, et al. (2000). Retinal toxicity of commercial intravitreal tissue plasminogen activator solution in cat eyes. *Archives of Ophthalmology* 118(5): 659–663.

Antifibrinolytic Agents

AMINOCAPROIC ACID

(a-**mee**-no-ka-**pro**-ik **ass**-id)

Indications/Pharmacology

Aminocaproic acid may be administered systemically or topically. Systemic administration significantly decreases intraocular re-bleeding episodes, but side effects can be severe and include nausea, dizziness, hypotension, and thrombosis of retinal vessels. Topical administration achieves therapeutic concentrations in aqueous humor in rabbits and humans, but clinical antifibrinolytic efficacy by this route is variable. Aminocaproic acid has also been used in patients with persistent corneal ulceration in order to maintain Fibronectin in the wound promoting re-epithelialization (Regnier et al. 2005).

Suggested Dosages/Precautions/Adverse Effects

If administered topically, aminocaproic acid is compounded in a concentration of 30% in 2% carboxypolymethylene gel.

Dosage Forms/Regulatory Status

VETERINARY-LABELED PRODUCTS: None

HUMAN-LABELED PRODUCTS: None

Aminocaproic acid 30% solution in 2% carboxypolymethylene gel may be compounded by an appropriately qualified compounding pharmacist.

References

Regnier, A., G. Cazalot, et al. (2005). Topical treatment of non-healing corneal epithelial ulcers in dogs with aminocaproic acid. Veterinary Record 157(17): 510-513.

Principles of Compounding Ophthalmic Products

GIGI DAVIDSON, DICVP

Physiochemical Considerations for Compounding Ophthalmic Preparations

The availability of suitable commercially available products for every veterinary ophthalmic indication is highly unlikely. Many agents used in veterinary ophthalmology are no longer or never were commercially available. Examples of agents that are commonly used by veterinarians but are no longer commercially available currently include oxytetracycline ophthalmic ointment, idoxuridine ophthalmic solution and ointment, miconazole solution, vidarabine ophthalmic solution, trifluridine ophthalmic solution, tetracycline ophthalmic solution, rose bengal solution, and chloramphenicol ophthalmic ointment. Even if commercially available, products may be of inappropriate concentration to achieve a therapeutic effect in a given patient (e.g., cyclosporine A) or may have agents and excipients that have adverse effects in animal patients (e.g., neomycin sulfate in cats). In other cases, no product is commercially available and must be compounded from other non-ophthalmic drugs or from bulk chemicals (e.g., acetylcysteine ophthalmic solution and disodium edetate ophthalmic solution). For these reasons, pharmacists are frequently called upon to compound products to be used in the animal eye. These products may be administered topically in the form of solutions, suspensions or ointments, by periocular or intraocular injection, by drug-implanted collagen shields, or by drug-impregnated disposable contact lens delivery systems. The quality and sterility of these products is critical. To ensure adequate stability, uniformity, and sterility, both the American Society of Health-Systems Pharmacists and the United States Pharmacopoeial (USP) Convention have published guidelines for pharmacy-prepared ophthalmic products. These guidelines address the following areas of concern.

Validation of Formulation:

Before compounding any product for ophthalmic use, the pharmacist should obtain documentation that substantiates the stability, safety and benefit of the requested formulation. Pharmacists may call the manufacturer of the drug, refer to primary literature, call regional eye centers, or call professional compounding organizations to obtain such information. If no such documentation is available, the pharmacist must employ professional judgment in determining a suitable formulation for ophthalmic administration. Factors to consider when making this judgment include: sterility, tonicity, pH and buffering, toxicity of the drug, need for preservatives, solubility, stability in the chosen vehicle, viscosity, packaging, and any precautions necessary to keep drug residues from occurring in any food-producing animals.

Documentation:

A written procedure for each ophthalmic product compounded should be recorded and kept in a readily retrievable place. This master formulation sheet should indicate the name of the product, the dosage form, the specifications and source of each ingredient used, the weights and measures of each ingredient used, the equipment required, a complete description of each step in the compounding process with special notation of aseptic techniques utilized and which method of terminal sterilization is appropriate, beyond-use dating, storage requirements, specific packaging requirements, sample label and auxiliary labeling, quality control testing performed, and references for formula. Production records for each batch should include the date of compounding, lot or batch number assigned, the manufacturer and lot number and expiration date of each ingredient used, a sign-off provision for compounder and checker, the amount compounded, and the projected beyond-use date for the batch compounded.

Sterility:

Ophthalmic dosage forms must be compounded in aseptic conditions. Sterile Compounding Guidelines should be consulted in the United States Pharmacopeia General Chapter <797>. Sterility is the most important consideration for ophthalmic products. Contaminated ophthalmic products can result in eye infections leading to blindness or even loss of the eye, especially if pathogens such as Pseudomonas are present. Eye infections from contamination can also lead to systemic infections requiring hospitalization and may even result in death. All ophthalmics should be compounded in a laminar flow hood that has undergone annual checkups and certification of acceptable performance. It is also important to note that the laminar flow hood does not guarantee sterility. The compounding pharmacist must also use impeccable aseptic technique when handling products intended for use in the eye. All products must be rendered sterile after formulation in the laminar flow hood. Sterilization of the final product is most easily achieved through filtration through 0.2μ filters, which also remove particulate matter. This method is obviously only suitable for ophthalmic solutions. Ophthalmic suspensions and ointments must be sterilized by other means to avoid filtering out active drug. Other methods of sterilization available to the pharmacist include dry heat, autoclaving, and ethylene oxide gas sterilization. Gamma radiation is also commercially available for bulk sterilization, but is very expensive. Preservatives may also be added to prevent bacterial growth, especially if the container is intended for multiple use. The preservative selected must be compatible with the active drug and excipients as well as non-toxic to the eye or to the patient. A description of commonly used ophthalmic preservatives and maximal concentrations in provided in Table 1.

Table 1. Agents used for preserving ophthalmic products.

Agent	Maximum concentration (%)*
Benzalkonium chloride	*0.01*
Benzethonium chloride	0.01
Phenylmercuric acetate	0.004
Phenylmercuric nitrate	0.004
Methylparaben	0.2
Propylparaben	0.04
Thimerosal	0.01
Chlorobutanol	0.5

*As recommended by FDA Advisory Review Panel on OTC Ophthalmic Drug Products

Clarity:
Drugs prepared as ophthalmic solutions should be free from foreign particles. This can be accomplished through filtration with a 0.45μ filter needle attached to a sterile syringe, or through the use of clarifying agents such as polysorbate 20 (maximum of 1%) and polysorbate 80 (maximum of 1%). Drugs prepared as ophthalmic suspensions, obviously cannot be filtered, but must be of a particle size that does not irritate or scratch the cornea. A micronized form of the drug is required. The use of an ointment mill is highly recommended to decrease particle size for ophthalmic ointments.

Tonicity:
Ophthalmic products do not need to be isotonic if the contact time with the cornea is only for a few minutes. The eye can tolerate a range of 200–600 mOsm/L for short periods of time. For ointments, irrigations and products that will remain in contact with the eye longer than a few minutes, isotonic products should be used. Hypotonic agents may cause corneal edema and hypertonic agents may dehydrate the cornea and cause pain. Tear fluid and normal saline have identical osmotic pressures making 0.9% sodium chloride an excellent vehicle for ophthalmic products. For products that are hypotonic,

sodium chloride equivalencies can be used to determine how much sodium chloride to render the product isotonic.

Buffering and pH:
Ophthalmic preparations are generally buffered in a range from 4.5–11.5. Buffering is necessary to provide maximal stability of the drug or for comfort and safety of the patient. Alkaloids such as atropine and pilocarpine are usually buffered. If the activity and stability of the drug are not pH dependent, and the pH of the product is not irritating, then buffers may be omitted from the formulation. Commonly used buffers for ophthalmic preparations include Palitzsch buffer, boric acid buffer, boric acid/sodium borate buffer, sodium acetate/boric acid buffer, Sorensen's modified phosphate buffer, Atkins and Pantin buffer solution, Feldman buffer, and Gilford ophthalmic buffer. Formulations for these solutions and ratios required to achieve a desired pH are referenced in the International Journal of Pharmaceutical Compounding, Vol. 2, No. 3 May/June 1998.

Viscosity Enhancers:
Because tears and blinking reflexes reduce the total amount of drug available for penetration, an increase in residence time in the eye will increase drug absorption. Increasing the viscosity of the drug is the most common way to prolong contact time. Methylcellulose is the most commonly used agent and is generally formulated at a concentration of 0.25%. Hydroxypropylmethylcellulose is used in concentrations of 0.5–1%. Polyvinyl alcohol has also been used in concentrations of 0.5–1% w/v. Agents used to increase the viscosity of ophthalmic products are shown in Table 2.

Table 2. Agents used to increase viscosity of ophthalmic solutions and suspensions.

Agent	Maximum Concentration (%)
Hydroxyethylcellulose	0.8
Hydroxypropylmethylcellulose	1.0
Methylcellulose	2.0
Polyvinyl alcohol	1.5
Polyvinylpyrrolidone	1.7

Quality Control:
Finished products should be thoroughly inspected visually for clarity and uniformity of suspension. The pH of the final product should always be checked and the value recorded on the master formula record for that batch. Most compounded products should have a pH of 5–7 unless otherwise indicated for stability or penetration of ocular tissue. Practitioners compounding large volumes of ophthalmic products should periodically perform testing to ensure sterility. Various agencies provide this service. The nearest college of pharmacy can be consulted for a list of providers of this service.

Packaging:

Ophthalmic preparations should be packaged in sterile dropper bottles (glass or plastic), or individual doses can be placed in sterile syringes with sterile tip caps. Ointments should be packaged in sterile ointment tubes and heat-sealed.

Beyond Use Dating:

The USP/NF standards for preparation of ophthalmic medications indicate that, unless otherwise documented, the beyond-use date for water containing formulations is 14 days. For non-aqueous liquids, the recommendation is not more than 25% of the time remaining until the expiration date of the starting product or six months, whichever is earlier. For all other products, the expiration dating should be the duration of therapy or 30 days whichever is shorter. These beyond-use recommendations can be extended in the face of supporting, valid, scientifically conducted stability information.

Considerations for use of ophthalmics in veterinary patients:

Veterinary patients experience many of the same ophthalmic diseases and conditions as humans, and treatments are often based on human therapy. Animals, however, have a variety of species-related characteristics that might cause human-designed therapies to fail or be toxic. Behavioral characteristics such as grooming may significantly reduce the contact time of ophthalmic agents with the eye, and increase systemic exposure through ingestion. Anatomical differences such as size must be considered. Horses and other large animals may simply elevate their eyes out of a caregiver's reach if ophthalmic treatments are objectionable. Specialized delivery devices have been created to treat these patients. Subcutaneous palpebral lavage systems are tunneled under the skin over the animal's brow and allow for passage of medication through long catheters that are easily reachable by caregivers. Food-producing animals require special consideration. Systemic absorption of ophthalmic agents in food-producing animals could result in violative drug residues in food intended for human consumption.

General Principles of Ocular Penetration

Corneal penetration:

Drugs must generally be administered topically to treat corneal and intraocular conditions. While the eye would appear to be an easy target for topical administration, the eye has several anatomical barriers to prevent penetration by foreign substances. Instantaneous tear production, strong blinking reflexes, and alternating layers of lipophilic and hydrophilic tissue all work in conjunction to prevent entry of foreign substances. The clear tissue known as the cornea covers the visible outer surface of the eye between the lids. The cornea must be clear in order to allow for vision, and nature has accomplished this by omitting blood vessels in the cornea. Because of this lack of vascular tissue, systemically administered drugs do not penetrate into the cornea. The cornea is composed of several layers of lipophilic (outer layers) and hydrophilic (inner layer) tissue. For a topically administered drug to fully penetrate the cornea, the drug must be able to exist in ready equilibrium between both ionized and non-ionized forms (e.g., chloramphenicol, atropine, and pilocarpine). Most antibiotics are water-soluble and will not penetrate the lipophilic outer layer of the cornea unless ulcers are present. Small molecular weight (<350) and high local concentration of drugs will also increase penetration even if the drugs are ionized and hydrophilic. Topical administration is ideal as it allows for very high local concentrations of drug on the cornea. For a topically administered drug to reach the anterior chamber and bind to intraocular structures (e.g., ciliary body, iris, aqueous humor), the drug must pass through the cornea. Drugs may also reach the anterior chamber to some extent by passive absorption through the conjunctiva.

Key points for corneal penetration of drugs:
- lipophilic
- equilibrium between ionized and non-ionized forms
- small molecular weight (<350)
- high local concentrations

Intravitreal Penetration:

Topically administered drugs reach the vitreous only in very small concentrations. To treat severe conditions of the anterior chamber (uveitis) as well as intravitreal conditions, drugs must be administered by periocular or intraocular injection. The periocular routes include subconjunctival injection and sub-Tenon's membrane injection while the intraocular routes are intracameral injection (directly into the aqueous humor) or intravitreal injection (directly into the vitreous humor). Periocular injections can be administered under sedation and topical anesthesia. Intraocular injections are usually only performed in the operating room while the patient is completely anesthetized. These routes bypass the outermost chemical and physical ocular defenses and allow for better concentration of drug in the vitreous. The volume of administration for these routes is relatively small. Periocular injections should not exceed 0.5–1.0 mL in small animals and 2 mL in large animals. Intraocular injections should not exceed 0.1 mL in small animals and 0.25 mL in large animals due to the risk in increasing intraocular pressure. Drugs injected into the eye should be free of preservatives and buffers.

Route of Therapy for Given Ocular Target:

Tissue	Routes of Administration
Eyelids	Topical, systemic
Corneal surface	Topical
Anterior segment	Topical if good penetration or mild disease
	Systemic if poor penetration or severe disease
Posterior segment	Systemic or intraocular injection (rarely)
Any site where multiple dosing is impractical	Subconjunctival depot injection

Questions to Ponder Prior to Compounding Ophthalmic Products:

1. Where is the target of therapy? (eyelids, corneal surface, cornea, anterior segment, posterior segment)
2. What is the character of the drug?
   - Lipophilic? Hydrophilic?
   - What is the molecular weight?
   - What is the inherent toxicity of the drug to the eye (gentamicin)? To the caregiver (chloramphenicol); to the patient (neomycin sulfate in cats)?
   - Is there data to support what concentration is necessary for corneal penetration?
   - Is the drug soluble in a vehicle that is not toxic to the eye?
   - If not soluble, will the particle size of the suspension or the ointment scratch the corneal or conjunctiva?
   - What is the pH of the final product? Is this in an acceptable range to avoid irritation (4.5–11.5)?
   - What is the tonicity of the final product? Hypertonic? Hypotonic? How long will the product be in contact with the cornea if not isotonic?
   - Will the viscosity need to be enhanced in order to prolong contact with the eye? Which agent is compatible?
   - What is the duration of therapy? Will the product require preservation if long term multiple use? Which preservative is compatible?

Dermatological Agents, Topical

The following section lists many of the active ingredients and corresponding preparations used topically for their local action in veterinary medicine. It includes both veterinary-labeled dermatological products and some potentially useful human-labeled products. Active ingredients are listed by therapeutic class. The drug sponsor, availability and formulation of these products tend to change rapidly in the marketplace so this listing should be used as a basic guide.

Products that are applied topically, but are absorbed systemically and used primarily for their systemic effects are found in the general monograph section. For veterinary products, refer to the complete label for additional information.

Portions of this section are adapted from: Koch, Torres, & Plumb. (2011). *Canine and Feline Dermatology Drug Handbook*. IN PRESS. Wiley-Blackwell. This reference provides additional detail on these, and other compounds and products.

Note: While many of these products do not legally require a prescription (OTC), they are often marketed as "Sold only through licensed veterinarians" or "Sold by professionals only."

Antipruritics/Antiinflammatories, Topical
Non-Corticosteroids

ALUMINUM ACETATE SOLUTION (BUROW'S SOLUTION OR MODIFIED BUROW'S SOLUTION)
(ah-*loo*-mi-num *ass*-ih-tate)
For otic use, refer to the Otics section

Indications/Actions
An astringent antipruritic agent, aluminum acetate solution (Burow's solution, modified Burow's solution) can be useful for adjunctive treatment of minor skin irritations such as insect bites, and localized inflamed and exudative skin conditions, including acute moist dermatitis, fold dermatitis (intertrigo) and contact dermatitis. It can also be used for the treatment of otitis externa (see Otics section).

In addition to Burow's solution's astringent and antipruritic actions, it also has acidifying effects and it mildly antiseptic. The exact mechanisms of action for these effects are not fully understood.

Suggested Dosages/Use

Topical use of Burow's solution (alone) is usually as a wet compress, dressing or soak. Application for 15–30 minutes is generally recommended and the affected area is air-dried between applications. Use can be as often as necessary, but every 4–6 hours is often employed. The veterinary-labeled products containing hydrocortisone may be directly applied. As Burow's solution products come in various dosage forms (powder or tablets for dissolving, liquid); refer to package directions for proper dilutions. Dilutions of 1:40, 1:20, or 1:10 are commonly used.

Precautions/Adverse Effects

Do not use plastic or any occlusive dressing material to prevent evaporation. Use room temperature water for dissolving and application. Avoid contact with eyes. Clients should wash hands after application or wear gloves when applying.

Burow's solution may cause dry skin or skin irritation on some patients.

Veterinary-Labeled Aluminum Acetate Solution Products

Product (Company)	Form: Concentration All contain: Hydrocortisone 1%; Aluminum Acetate 2%	Label Status	Other Ingredients; Comments; Size(s)
Cort/Astrin Solution® (Vedco)	Solution	OTC	1 oz. dropper btl, 16 oz.
Corti-Derm Solution® (First Priority)	Solution	OTC	1 oz.
Hydro-Plus® (Phoenix)	Solution	OTC	1, 2, 16 oz.
Bur-O-Cort 2:1® (Q.A. Labs)	Solution	OTC	1, 16 oz.
Hydro-B 1020® (Butler)	Solution	OTC	1, 2, 16 oz.

Human-Labeled Aluminum Acetate Solution Products

Product (Company)	Form: Concentration	Label Status	Other Ingredients; Size(s)
Domeboro Powder® (Bayer)	Powder Packets: Aluminum sulfate and Calcium acetate	OTC (Human)	Packets of 12 or 100/box. One packet dissolved in 16 oz (480 mL) of water makes a 1:40 (2.5%) modified Burow's sol.
Pedi-Boro Soak Paks® (Pedinol)	Powder Packets: Aluminum sulfate and Calcium acetate 2.7 g	OTC (Human)	Packets of 12 or 100/box. One packet dissolved in 16 oz (480 mL) of water makes a 1:40 (2.5%) modified Burow's sol.
Domeboro Tablets® (Bayer)	Effervescent Tablets: Aluminum sulfate and Calcium acetate	OTC (Human)	Tablets of 12 or 100/box. One tablet dissolved in 16 oz (480 mL) of water makes a 1:40 (2.5%) modified Burow's sol.
Burow's Solution (various)	Solution: Aluminum acetate (Burow's)	OTC (Human)	480 mL bottles

COLLOIDAL OATMEAL

(ko-*loyd*-al *ote*-meel)

Indications/Actions

Colloidal oatmeal is used topically as an antiinflammatory and antipruritic, but an exact mechanism for this effect is not known. It is thought that as the concentration of oatmeal increases, both its drying and antipruritic effects increase; it has been suggested that it may inhibit prostaglandin synthesis.

Suggested Dosages/Use

Spray can be used 2–3 times per day as needed for itching or pain. Shampoo or conditioner is usually used once a day to once a week. Shampoo should be in contact with skin for at least 10 minutes and then rinsed well. Refer to each product's label for further details.

Precautions/Adverse Effects

Other than the potential for increased drying of already dry skin, colloidal oatmeal is very safe. In humans, there are some reports of contact dermatitis associated with its use.

Veterinary-Labeled Colloidal Oatmeal Products

Note: Products listed are those containing only colloidal oatmeal as the principle active ingredient. For other products that contain colloidal oatmeal, see Diphenhydramine, Pramoxine, Hydrocortisone, Permethrin, or Pyrethrins listings.

Product (Company)	Form: Concentration	Label Status	Other Ingredients; Comments; Size(s)
Dermallay® Oatmeal Spray (Dechra)	Leave-On Spray: 0.75%	OTC	12 oz; 1 gal
Dermallay® Conditioner (Dechra)	Conditioner: 0.75%	OTC	8 oz; 1 gal
Epi-Soothe® Cream Rinse (Virbac)	Cream Rinse: 1%	OTC	Lactic acid. 8, 16 oz; 1 gal
ResiSoothe® Leave-On Lotion (Virbac)	Lotion: % not listed	OTC	Sunflower oil (omega 6 FA's), vitamin E. 8 oz. Shake well.
Aloe & Oatmeal Skin and Coat Conditioner® (Vet Solutions, Vetoquinol)	Conditioner: % not listed	OTC	Aloe vera gel, vitamins A, D & E, chamomile. 16 oz; 1 gal.
Dermallay® Oatmeal Shampoo (Dechra)	Shampoo: 2%	OTC	12 oz; 1 gal
Epi-Soothe® Shampoo (Virbac)	Shampoo: 2%	OTC	Chitosanide, glycerin. Ingredients in free form and in Spherulites®. 8, 16 oz; 1 gal
Cortisoothe Shampoo® (Virbac)	Shampoo: Colloidal Oatmeal % not listed; Hydrocortisone 1%	Rx	8, 16 oz Labeled for dogs and cats.
Hartz Soothing Botanicals Skin Moisturizing Shampoo® (Hartz Mountain)	Shampoo: % not listed	OTC	Aloe vera. 15 oz
Hartz Groomer's Best Oatmeal Shampoo® (Hartz Mountain)	Shampoo: % not listed	Rx	18 oz
Aloe & Oatmeal Shampoo® (Sogeval, Vet Solutions, Vetoquinol)	Shampoo: % not listed	Rx	Aloe vera. 16 oz; 1 gal.
Foaming Silk Bath® (AAH)	Shampoo: % not listed	Rx	Aloe vera, vitamins A & E. 16 oz

Human-Labeled Colloidal Oatmeal Products
Note: There are several human products available containing colloidal oatmeal, including creams, lotions and products to be added to the bath. Common trade names include: *Aveeno®, Geri SS®,* and *Actibath®.*

ESSENTIAL FATTY ACIDS, TOPICAL

For systemic use of essential fatty acids, refer to the Fatty Acids, Essential monograph found in the main section.

Indications/Actions
Essential fatty acids are indicated primarily for pruritic and inflammatory conditions such as atopic dermatitis and sebaceous adenitis, and keratinization disorders such as seborrhea. They may also be used to improve coat quality and ameliorate dry skin. Some of these products may contain other active ingredients, including other natural oils, which may have other adjunctive indications.

The exact mechanism of action of essential fatty acids is not well understood. However, essential fatty acids affect the arachadonic acid levels in plasma lipids and platelet membranes. They affect production of inflammatory prostaglandins in the body, thereby reducing inflammation and pruritus. Essential oils may also play a role in restoring the skin barrier.

Suggested Uses/Dosages
If using spray: up to 2–3 times applications a day or as needed. If spot-on: treatment may vary from weekly to every 2 weeks or monthly. If shampoo or conditioner: daily to weekly baths/after baths; leave shampoo in contact with the skin for at least 10 minutes prior to rinsing well. Refer to product label for details on individual use.

Precautions/Adverse Effects
No specific precautions or adverse effects are described for these products.

Veterinary-Labeled Topical Essential Fatty Acids Products

Product (Company)	Form: Concentration	Label Status	Ingredients; Comments; Size(s)
Dermoscent® Atop7 (Animal Dermo-Care)	Spray	OTC	Capparis spinosa extract, essential fatty acids from hamp and neen, essential oils of cajputi and melaleuca. Indicated for itchy or allergy prone skin. Labeled for dogs. 75 mL
Dermoscent® Cicafolia (Animal Dermo-Care)	Spray	OTC	Cajputi essential oil and Amazonian Croton lechleri sap extract, peptids, Margosa's essential fatty acids, gamma oryzanol and silicon. Labeled for dogs and cats. 30 mL
HyLyt® EFA Bath Oil (DVM)	Spray	OTC	Omega 6 fatty acids. Labeled for dogs and cats. 8 oz
Dermoscent® Essential 6 Spot-On (Animal Dermo-Care)	Spot on	OTC	Essential oils of rosemary, lavender, melaleuca, cedar, oregano, essential fatty acids from hemp grain and neem, vitamin E. Labeled for dogs and cats. Pipettes of 0.4, 0.6, 1.2, & 2.4 mL depending package labeling.
Dermoscent® Essential Mousse (Animal Dermo-Care)	Mousse	OTC	Oils and polyunsatured fatty acids as well as soothing *Cucurbitine®*. Soap free. Labeled for dogs and cats. 150 ml.
HyLyt® EFA Shampoo (DVM)	Shampoo	OTC	Omega 6 fatty acids. Soap free. Labeled for dogs and cats. 8, 12 (spray) oz; 1 gal.
Dermoscent® EFA Treatment Shampoo (Animal Dermo-Care)	Shampoo	OTC	Essential fatty acids from hamp grain, Cucurbitine (lichen plant extract), Niaouli essential oil. Soap free. Labeled for dogs and cats. 200 mL
DermaLyte® Shampoo (Dechra)	Shampoo	OTC	Omega 6 fatty acids, Vitamin E, Coconut oil. Soap free. 1 oz pouch, 12 oz; 1 gal.
Hyliderm® Shampoo (Sogeval)	Shampoo	OTC	Omega 6 fatty acids. Soap free. Labeled for dogs and cats. 2, 8, 16 oz; 1 gal.
Allermyl® Shampoo (Virbac)	Shampoo	OTC	Omega 6 fatty acids (linoleic acid), Ceramides 1, 3 and 6, Cholesterol, L-rhamnose, D-mannose, D-galactose; polysaccharide: alkyl polyglucoside. Fragrance free. Indicated for control of pruritus, specifically labeled for management of allergic skin conditions in dogs and cats. Also has skin barrier restoring properties. 8, 16 oz
Allerderm Spot-on® (Virbac)	Spot-on	OTC	Free fatty acids, Ceramides 1, 3 and 6, Cholesterol Indicated specifically for allergic dermatitis, contact allergies, keratinization disorders and chronic microbial infections. May also be used for the treatment of sebaceous adenitis. 2 mL, 4 mL.
HyLyt® EFA Crème Rinse (DVM)	Creme Rinse	OTC	Labeled for dogs and cats. 8 oz; 1 gal.

Human-Labeled Topical Essential Fatty Acids Products

Note: Several human over-the-counter products are available in the USA but may contain other ingredients. They are generally not used in dogs and cats.

DIPHENHYDRAMINE HCL, TOPICAL

(dye-fen-**hye**-dra-meen)   Benadryl®

For systemic use, see the monograph found in the main section

Indications/Actions

A first generation antihistamine, diphenhydramine has some local anesthetic activity that probably is its main antipruritic mechanism of action. Diphenhydramine may be absorbed in small amounts transdermally, but should not cause systemic side effects.

Suggested Dosages/Use

Topical creams, gels, lotion or sprays are usually applied 2–3 times a day. The shampoos and conditioners are generally used once a day to once a week after bathing. Shampoos should remain in contact with skin for at least 10 minutes prior to rinsing.

Precautions/Adverse Effects

Avoid contact with eyes or mucous membranes. Do not apply to blistered or oozing areas of skin. Clients should wash hands after application or wear gloves when applying.

Prolonged use could potentially cause local irritation and/or hypersensitization. Residual activity may affect intradermal or allergy serum tests; it has been suggested to stop use 2 weeks prior to allergy testing.

Veterinary-Labeled Topical Diphenhydramine Products

Product (Company)	Form: Concentration	Label Status	Other Ingredients; Comments; Size(s)
ResiHist® Leave-On Lotion (Virbac)	Lotion: 2%	Rx	Water, cetyl alcohol base. 8 oz Labeled for use on dogs and cats

Human-Labeled Topical Diphenhydramine Products

Product (Company)	Forms: Concentration	Label Status	Other Ingredients; Comments; Size(s)
Products include: Benadryl®, Dermamycin®, Dermarest®, Ziradryl® (various manufacturers and additional trade name modifiers such as Maximum Strength, etc may be found)	Spray: 1%, 2% Lotion: 0.5%, 1% Gel: 1%, 2% Cream 1%, 2%, 4%	OTC (Human)	These products may also contain astringents (calamine, zinc oxide or acetate), other antihistamines (pyrilamine, tripelennamine), and/or counter irritants (menthol, camphor)

LIDOCAINE, TOPICAL
LIDOCAINE/PRILOCAINE (EMLA CREAM)
(*lye*-doe-kane; *prye*-loe-kane)

For systemic use of lidocaine, see the monograph found in the main section

Indications/Actions

Lidocaine is used topically as a dermal anesthetic or antipruritic and is included in several products used for acute moist dermatitis, pruritic lesions, or painful skin conditions. When combined with prilocaine (commonly called EMLA cream), it may be useful for dermal anesthesia prior to painful or invasive procedures (*e.g.*, catheter placement, etc).

Lidocaine exerts its anesthetic properties via alteration of cell membrane ion permeability, thereby inhibiting conduction from sensory nerves.

Suggested Dosages/Use

Thin layers can be applied every 3-4 hours as needed.

Precautions/Adverse Effects

Topical lidocaine may be absorbed systemically, but systemic toxicity is unlikely to occur unless used on a significant percentage of body area, for prolonged times or at high concentrations. Be extra vigilant in patients also receiving Class-I antiarrhythmics (*e.g.*, lidocaine, mexiletine). Avoid contact with eyes and do not use in ears, unless specifically labeled for such. Clients should wash hands after application or wear gloves when applying.

Hypersensitivity reactions or skin irritation (burning, tenderness, etc.) are possible, but apparently do not occur commonly. Products containing prilocaine (EMLA) may be more likely to cause methemoglobinemia or systemic toxicity, but these occur rarely.

Veterinary-Labeled Topical Lidocaine Products

Product (Company)	Form: Concentration	Label Status	Other Ingredients; Comments; Size(s)
Allercaine® (Tomlyn)	Spray: 2.4%	OTC	Denatonium benzoate (bittering agent), Benzalkonium Chloride 0.1%. Do not apply to entire body or to large areas of broken skin. 4, 12 oz.
Allerspray® (Vetoquinol)	Spray: 2.4%	OTC	Denatonium benzoate (bittering agent), Benzalkonium Chloride 0.1%, aloe vera gel, allantoin, PEG-75 lanolin. 4 oz.
Dermacool w/ Lidocaine Spray® (Virbac)	Spray: 1.5%	OTC	Hamamelis extract, lactic acid, colloidal oatmeal, PCMX. 4 oz
Hexa-Caine® (PRN Pharmacal)	Spray: 2.4%	OTC	Denatonium benzoate (bittering agent), Benzalkonium Chloride 0.1%, aloe vera gel, allantoin, lanolin. 4, 8, 16 oz.
Biocain® (Tomlyn)	Lotion: 2%	OTC	*Bittran*® II (bittering agent), Benzalkonium Chloride 0.1%. 2, 4 oz.

Human-Labeled Topical Lidocaine Products

There are also several topical OTC products listed for human use, including sprays (2–2.5%), liquids (2–4%), creams (0.5–2%), gels (0.5–2.5%) and topical patches.

Product (Company)	Form: Concentration	Label Status	Other Ingredients; Size(s)
EMLA® (Astra) Lidocaine/Prilocaine Cream (Generic various)	Cream: Lidocaine 2.5%; Prilocaine 2.5%	Rx (Human)	Depending on manufacturer: 5, 15, 30 g.

PHYTOSPHINGOSINE

(fye-tos-*fin*-joe-seen)   DOUXO®

Indications/Actions

The *Douxo® Calm* products containing phytosphingosine are labeled as indicated for localized and generalized inflammatory conditions that may be associated with pruritus including allergic diseases such as atopic dermatitis. *Douxo Gel®* is also indicated as a liquid wound dressing for localized inflammation and after surgery (can be sprayed on sutures). There are also products marketed for seborrheic conditions and an otic cleanser.

Phytosphingosine is a modified pro-ceramide with salicylic acid and a key molecule in the natural defense mechanism of the skin. Ceramides comprise 40-50% of the main lipids responsible for maintaining the cohesion of the stratum corneum, therefore; restoring the skin lipid barrier, controlling local flora (antibacterial and antifungal effects), and maintaining the correct moisture balance. It is also anti-inflammatory as it has anti-IL-1 activity, impairing the production of PGE2 and inhibits kinase protein C.

Suggested Dosages/Use

If using spray or gel: up to 2–3 times a day as needed for itching/pain relief. If shampoo or conditioner: daily to weekly baths/after baths; leave shampoo in contact with the skin for at least 10 minutes prior to rinsing well. Refer to product label for details on individual use.

Precautions/Adverse Effects

Skin redness or irritation may occur.

Veterinary-Labeled Phytosphingosine Products

Product (Company)	Form: Concentration	Label Status	Other Ingredients; Comments; Size(s)
DOUXO® Calm Gel (Sogeval)	Gel: 0.1%	OTC	Hinokitiol 0.2%, Raspberry seed oil, natural tocopherol, extract of creosote bush. 2 oz.
DOUXO® Calm Micro-emulsion Spray (Sogeval)	Spray: 0.05%	OTC	Hinokitiol 0.1%, Raspberry seed oil. 6.8 oz.
DOUXO® Calm Shampoo (Sogeval)	Shampoo: 0.05%	OTC	Hinokitiol 0.1%, Raspberry seed oil, allantoin, lipidure C. 6.8, 16.9 oz, 3L.
DOUXO® Seborrhea Shampoo (Sogeval)	Shampoo: 0.1%	OTC	Fomblin (stabilizer), cationic conditioners; 6.8 oz
DOUXO® Chlorhexidine PS (Sogeval)	Shampoo: Chlorhexidine 3% Phytosphigosine 0.05%	OTC	*Lipicid®* C8G; 6.8 oz
DOUXO® Seborrhea MicroEmulsion Spray (Sogeval)	Spray: 0.2%	OTC	Boswellia serrata extract, glycerin; 6.8 oz
DOUXO® Seborrhea Spot-on (Sogeval)	Spot-on Solution: 1%	OTC	Transcutol (surface diffuser)

Human-Labeled Phytosphingosine Products

Note: There are several over-the-counter human cosmetic products containing phytosphingosine in the USA. These products target mostly lipid barrier restoration and are generally not used in dogs and cats.

PRAMOXINE HCL
(pra-**moks**-een)

Indications/Actions
Pramoxine is a surface and local anesthetic affecting peripheral nerves. It is not related structurally to procaine-type anesthetics. Pramoxine is often combined with other topical medications to reduce pain and/or itching. Precise mechanism of action is not known.

Suggested Dosages/Use
Depending on the product labeling, pramoxine 1% may be applied every 3–4 hours. Peak local anesthetic effects occur within 3–5 minutes of application. It provides only temporary effects. Shampoos are used once daily to once weekly and should remain in contact with the skin for at least 10 minutes prior to rinsing well.

Precautions/Adverse Effects
Avoid contact with eyes; pramoxine is too irritating for ophthalmic use. Depending on product labeling, clients should wash hands after application or wear gloves when applying. Adverse effects are unlikely, but localized dermatitis is possible.

Veterinary-Labeled Pramoxine Products

Product (Company)	Form: Concentration	Label Status	Other Ingredients; Comments; Size(s)
Micro-Pearls Advantage Dermal-Soothe® Anti-Itch Spray (Vetoquinol)	Spray: 1%	OTC	Lactamide monoethanolamine and *Novasome®* microvesicles. 12 oz. Shake well and repeat as necessary.
Relief® Spray (DVM)	Spray: 1%	OTC	Colloidal oatmeal. 8 oz. For dogs or cats.
Relief® HC Spray (DVM)	Spray: Hydrocortisone 1% Pramoxine 1%	Rx	Colloidal oatmeal. 8 oz.
Pramoxine Anti-Itch® Spray (Davis)	Spray: 1%	OTC	8 oz. For dogs or cats. Labeled for daily use or as directed by DVM
Pramosoothe® HC Spray (Sogeval)	Spray: Hydrocortisone 1% Pramoxine1%	Rx	Colloidal oatmeal, essential fatty acids. 8 oz.
Resiprox® Leave-On Lotion (Virbac)	Lotion: 1.5%	Rx	Water, cetyl alcohol, stearyl alcohol base. 8 oz. Shake well. Use daily or as directed by DVM
Micro-Pearls Advantage Dermal-Soothe® Anti-Itch Shampoo (Vetoquinol)	Shampoo: 1%	OTC	Colloidal Oatmeal, *Novasome®* microvesicles, Skin respiratory factor. 12 oz, 1 gal. Labeled for dogs, cats, horses.
Pramoxine Anti-Itch® Shampoo (Davis)	Shampoo: 1%	OTC	Colloidal oatmeal, emollients. 12 oz, 1 gal. Labeled for dogs, cats, puppies, kittens
Relief® Shampoo (DVM)	Shampoo: 1%	OTC	Colloidal oatmeal, Omega-6 FA's. 8, 12 oz, 1 gal.
Micro-Pearls Advantage Dermal-Soothe® Anti-Itch Cream Rinse (Vetoquinol)	Rinse: 1%	OTC	Colloidal Oatmeal, *Novasome®* microvesicles, Skin respiratory factor. 12 oz, 1 gal. Labeled for dogs, cats, & horses.
Pramoxine Anti-Itch® Creme Rinse (Davis)	Rinse: 1%	OTC	Colloidal oatmeal, emollients, Omega-6 FA's. 12 oz, 1 gal. Labeled for dogs, cats, puppies, kittens
Relief® Creme Rinse (DVM)	Rinse: 1%	OTC	Colloidal oatmeal, emollients, Omega-6 FA's. 8, 12 oz, 1 gal.

Human-Labeled Pramoxine Products

Product (Company)	Form: Concentration	Label Status	Other Ingredients; Comments; Size(s)
AmLactin® AP (UpsherSmith)	Cream: 1%	OTC (Human)	Usually used for extremely dry, painful or itchy skin in humans.
Prax® (Ferndale)	Lotion: 1%	OTC (Human)	Usually used for extremely dry, painful or itchy skin in humans.
Tronothane® (Abbott)	Lotion: 1%	OTC (Human)	Usually used for extremely dry, painful or itchy skin in humans.
Itch-X® (Ascher)	Spray: 1%	OTC (Human)	Benzyl alcohol 10%, aloe vera gel. 60 mL
Itch-X® (Ascher)	Gel: 1%	OTC (Human)	Benzyl alcohol 10%, aloe vera gel. 35.4 g.
PrameGel® (GenDerm)	Gel: 1%	OTC (Human)	0.5% menthol, emollient base, benzyl alcohol. 118 g.

PHENOL/MENTHOL/CAMPHOR
(*fee*-nol; *men*-thol; *kam*-for)

Indications/Actions
When used in low concentrations, these agents can be used as counterirritants and may be added to proprietary or compounded products primarily as antipruritics. Camphor and phenol may also have some antiseptic properties.

Precautions/Adverse Effects
These compounds may cause local irritation and should not be used around, or in eyes. Products containing phenol should not be used on cats.

Veterinary-Labeled Phenol, Menthol, or Camphor Products
Note: There are also several over the counter products not listed containing menthol, phenol or camphor used primarily on equine patients for overexertion, soreness, or stiffness. These include a variety of liniments (*e.g.*, white liniment, Choate's liniment) or gels (*e.g.*, *Cool Gel®*, *Ice-O-Gel®*, *Shin-O-Gel®*, etc.).

Product (Company)	Form/Concentration	Label Status	Other Ingredients; Size(s)
Scarlet Oil Pump Spray (Dominion)	Spray: Menthol, Phenol, Oil of Camphor, Oil of Eucalyptus & Oil of Pine each at 7.5mg/mL; Oil of Thyme 2.8mg/mL; Peru Balsam 1.5mg/mL; Biebrich Scarlet Red 100 ppm.	OTC	Labeled for superficial cuts, wounds, burns, etc. for horses and mules. Shake well. 500 mL

ZINC GLUCONATE (NEUTRALIZED), TOPICAL
For otic use, refer to the Otics section.

Indications/Actions
Can be used alone for mild itching or as an adjunctive treatment for more pruritic conditions, mild bacterial infections, or dry skin. It can be used for minor skin irritations such as insect bite reactions, acute moist dermatitis, acral lick dermatitis, fold dermatitis (intertrigo), feline acne and post surgery wounds.

Exact mechanism of action is unknown. Zinc plays a role in extra-cellular matrix remodeling, wound healing, connective tissue repair, inflammation, and cell proliferation. Zinc also has antiseptic and astringent properties.

Suggested Dosages/Use
May be applied to affected areas 2 times a day or as needed to relief itching and soothe the skin. Refer to product label for details on individual use.

Precautions/Adverse Effects
Avoid contact with eyes.

Veterinary-Labeled Topical Neutralized Zinc Products

Product (Company)	Form: Concentration	Label Status	Other Ingredients; Comments; Size(s);
Maxi/Guard® ZN7 Derm (Addison)	Solution and Spray: Zinc gluconate 0.9–1.1%	OTC	Taurine, L-lysine, glycerin. 2 oz btl.

Human-Labeled Topical Neutralized Zinc Products
There are several OTC zinc gluconate or zinc oxide products available for use in humans, and many of the products contain other ingredients. A common trade name is *Calamine lotion*, which contains zinc oxide and 0.5% iron(III) oxide.

Corticosteroids, Topical

Note: There are at least 20 chemical entities (plus a variety of salts) used in humans for topical corticosteroid therapy. The following section includes many veterinary topical products and some human products that may be of use in veterinary medicine. Also, see the *Otics section* for more products.

> ## BETAMETHASONE, TOPICAL
> (bet-ah-*meth*-ah-zone)
>
> *For systemic use, see the monograph found in the main section*

Indications/Actions

Considered a high potency topical corticosteroid, betamethasone may useful for adjunctive treatment of localized pruritic or inflammatory conditions. Because risks associated with betamethasone (HPA axis suppression, systemic corticosteroid effects, skin atrophy) are greater than with hydrocortisone, betamethasone products are generally reserved for more serious localized pruritic conditions or when hydrocortisone is not effective. All veterinary-labeled products are in combination with gentamicin and labeled indications are for treatment of infected superficial lesions caused by bacteria sensitive to gentamicin. Additional otic products are available that contain gentamicin and clotrimazole, but these can be used in an extra-label manner for treating mixed bacterial and yeast infections when strong antiinflammatory activity is desired. Sole ingredient betamethasone topical forms are available with human labeling.

Corticosteroids are non-specific anti-inflammatory agents. They probably act by inducing phospholipase A2 inhibitory proteins (lipocortins) in cells, thereby reducing the formation, activity, and release of endogenous inflammatory mediators (*e.g.*, histamine, prostaglandins, kinins, etc.). Corticosteroids also reduce DNA synthesis via an anti-mitotic effect on epidermal cells. Topically applied corticosteroids also inhibit the migration of leukocytes and macrophages to the area reducing erythema, pruritus and edema.

Suggested Dosages/Use

Betamethasone formulations are best suited for focal (*e.g.*, pedal) or multifocal lesions for relatively short durations (*e.g.*, less than 2 months). Initially, topical corticosteroids are usually used sparingly 1–4 times per day and then frequency is tapered when control is achieved. Long term, frequent use can cause HPA axis suppression and risk can be reduced by treating for only as long as necessary on as small an area as possible. Refer to individual product labeling for actual dosing recommendations for veterinary products.

Precautions/Adverse Effects

Several veterinary topical products list tuberculosis of the skin or pregnancy as a contraindication. Systemic corticosteroids can be teratogenic or induce parturition during the third trimester of pregnancy in animals. If considering use during pregnancy, weigh the respective risks with treating versus potential benefits. Clients should wash hands after application or wear gloves when applying. Avoid contact with eyes. Do not allow animal to lick or chew at affected sites for at least 20–30 minutes after application.

Residual activity may affect intradermal or allergy serum tests; it has been suggested to stop use 2 weeks prior to allergy testing.

Use care when treating large areas, or when used on smaller patients. Risks can be reduced by treating for only as long as necessary on as small an area as possible. Increased risks of HPA axis suppression, systemic corticosteroid effects (polydipsia/polyuria, Cushing's, gastrointestinal effects) and skin atrophy (skin fragility, alopecia, localized pyoderma and comedones are other possible complications) occur as product concentration and duration of use increases. Betamethasone may delay wound healing particularly if used longer than 7 days in duration. Vomiting and diarrhea have been reported with use of the products containing betamethasone. Local skin reactions (burning, itching, redness) are possible, but unlikely to occur.

Veterinary-Labeled Topical Betamethasone Products

Note: At time of writing there are no veterinary-labeled sole active ingredient betamethasone products in the USA.

Product (Company)	Form: Concentration	Label Status	Other Ingredients; Comments; Size(s)
Gentocin Topical Spray® (Intervet/Schering) **Gentaspray®** (Butler) **Betagen Topical Spray®** (Med-Pharmex) **Gentamicin Topical Spray®** (RXV) **Gentaved Topical Spray®** (Vedco)	Spray (all products listed): Gentamicin 0.57 mg/mL; Betamethasone (as valerate) 0.284 mg/mL	All are Rx	Depending on product: 15 & 30 g, 60, 72, 120, 240 mL
Otomax® Ointment (Intervet/Schering) **DVMAX® Ointment** (DVM) **Vetromax® Ointment** (Dechra) **MalOtic® Ointment** (Vedco)	Ointment (otic): All Products contain: Gentamicin 3 mg/g; Betamethasone (as valerate) 1 mg/g; Clotrimazole 10 mg/g	Rx	Mineral oil base. Approved for otic use in dogs; used in extra-label manner for bacterial skin lesions or Malassezia dermatitis; 7.5, 10, 15, 20 and 215 g bottles or tubes
Fuciderm Gel® (Dechra)	Gel: Betamethasone valerate 0.1% Fusidic acid 0.5%	Rx (not in USA); available in EU and Canada	Labeled for dogs. Can be used extra-label in cats. 15, 30 g tubes.

Human-Labeled Topical Betamethasone Products

Note: Partial listing; there are also topical branded products (two common trade names are *Diprosone®* and *Maxivate®*) available with betamethasone dipropionate. Do not confuse products containing *augmented* betamethasone dipropionate (*Diprolene®*, etc.) with betamethasone dipropionate. Augmented betamethasone dipropionate is not equivalent with betamethasone dipropionate as it is more potent. For more information on human-labeled betamethasone products, refer to a comprehensive human drug reference (*e.g.*, *Facts and Comparisons*) or contact a pharmacist.

Product (Company)	Form: Concentration	Label Status	Size(s); Comments
Betamethasone Dipropionate Ointment	Ointment: 0.05%	Rx (Human)	15, 45 g.
Betamethasone Dipropionate Cream	Cream: 0.05%	Rx (Human)	15, 45 g.
Betamethasone Dipropionate Lotion	Lotion: 0.05%	Rx (Human)	20, 30, 60 mL
Diprosone® (Westwood Squibb)	Aerosol Spray: 0.1%	Rx (Human)	85 g. 10% isopropyl alcohol, mineral oil
Clotrimazole & Betamethasone Diprop. (Fougera) **Lotrisone®** (Schering)	Lotion: Clotrimazole 1% Betamethasone dip. 0.05%	Rx (Human)	30 mL
Clotrimazole & Betamethasone Diprop. (Fougera) **Lotrisone®** (Schering)	Cream: Clotrimazole 1% Betamethasone dip. 0.05%	Rx (Human)	15, 45 g.

HYDROCORTISONE, TOPICAL

(hye-droe-**kor**-ti-zone)

Indications/Actions

Considered a low potency topical corticosteroid, hydrocortisone may useful for adjunctive treatment of localized pruritic and/or inflammatory conditions. Because risks associated with hydrocortisone are significantly less when compared to higher potency corticosteroids, hydrocortisone is a reasonable first choice, particularly when treating large areas, or when used on smaller patients. Some products also contain the astringent Burow's solution, which may have additional antipruritic effects.

Corticosteroids are non-specific anti-inflammatory agents. They probably act by inducing phospholipase A2 inhibitory proteins (lipocortins) in cells, thereby reducing the formation, activity, and release of endogenous inflammatory mediators (*e.g.*, histamine, prostaglandins, kinins, etc.). Corticosteroids also reduce DNA synthesis via an anti-mitotic effect on epidermal cells. Topically applied corticosteroids also inhibit the migration of leukocytes and macrophages to the area reducing erythema, pruritus and edema.

Suggested Dosages/Use

Hydrocortisone formulations are best suited for focal (*e.g.*, pedal) or multifocal lesions for relatively short durations (*e.g.*, less than 2 months). Initially, topical corticosteroids are usually used sparingly 1-4 times per day and then frequency is tapered when control is achieved. In contrast to some of the more potent topical corticosteroids, hydrocortisone can be applied more frequently and over a greater surface area without undue risk for local or systemic adverse effects. Long term, frequent use can cause HPA axis suppression and risk can be reduced by treating for only as long as necessary on as small an area as possible.

Shampoos containing hydrocortisone are generally used once a day to once a week. They should remain in contact with skin for at least 10 minutes prior to rinsing. Refer to individual product labeling for actual dosing recommendations for veterinary products.

Precautions/Adverse Effects

Several veterinary topical products list tuberculosis of the skin or pregnancy as contraindications. Clients should wash hands after application or wear gloves when applying. Avoid contact with eyes. Do not allow animal to lick or chew at affected sites for at least 20-30 minutes after application.

Local skin reactions are possible, but unlikely to occur. Atrophy associated with skin fragility, superficial follicular cysts (milia) and comedones may be seen with long term, frequent use, but this occurs more commonly when using more potent, topical corticosteroids. Although systemic absorption is rare with hydrocortisone, long term use may lead to HPA axis suppression.

Residual activity may affect intradermal or allergy serum tests; it has been suggested to stop use 2 weeks prior to allergy testing.

Veterinary-Labeled Topical Hydrocortisone Products

Product (Company)	Form: Concentration	Label Status	Other Ingredients; Comments; Size(s)
Corticalm Lotion® (DVM)	Lotion: 1%	Rx	3, 6 oz.
Sulfodene HC Anti-Itch Lotion® (Farnam)	Lotion: 0.5%	OTC	1.5 oz.
Zymox Topical Cream® (PKB)	Cream: 1%	Rx	Lactoperoxidase, lysozyme, lactoferrin. 1 oz.
Zymox Topical Wipes® (PKB)	Wipes: 1%	Rx	Lactoperoxidase, lysozyme, lactoferrin. 30 count jar.
Malacetic HC Wipes® (Dechra)	Wipes: Hydrocortisone 1% Acetic Acid 1% Boric Acid 1%	Rx	25 count jar.
Relief® HC Spray (DVM)	Spray: Hydrocortisone 1% Pramoxine 1%	Rx	Colloidal oatmeal. 8 oz.
Pramosoothe® HC Spray (Sogeval)	Spray: Hydrocortisone 1% Pramoxine1%,	Rx	Colloidal oatmeal, essential fatty acids. 8 oz.
Cortispray® (DVM)	Spray: 1%	Rx	Labeled for use on dogs, cats, and horses. 60 mL
Dermacool HC Spray® (Virbac)	Spray: 1%	Rx	Colloidal oatmeal, hamamelis extract, lactic acid, menthol, propylene glycol. 2, 4 oz.
Hartz Advanced Care Hydrocortisone Spray w/Aloe® (Hartz Mountain)	Spray: 0.5%	OTC	Aloe. 5 oz.
Zymox Topical Spray® (PKB)	Spray: Hydrocortisone 1%	Rx	Lactoperoxidase, lysozyme, lactoferrin. 2 oz.
Malacetic Ultra Spray® (Dechra)	Spray: Hydrocortisone 1% Ketoconazole 0.15%	Rx	Acetic Acid 1%, Boric Acid 2%; 8 oz.
Cort/Astrin Solution® (Vedco) **Corti-Derm Solution®** (First Priority) **Hydro-Plus®** (Phoenix) **Bur-O-Cort 2:1®** (Q.A. Labs) **Hydro-B 1020®** (Butler)	Solution: Hydrocortisone 1% Burow's Solution 2%	OTC	Depending on product: 1, 2, 16 oz btl
Cortisoothe Shampoo® (Virbac)	Shampoo: Hydrocortisone1% Colloidal oatmeal 1%	Rx	Labeled for dogs and cats. 8, 16 oz.
Chlorhexidine 4% HC Shampoo (Sogeval)	Chlorhexidine 4% Hydrocortisone 1%	Rx	Labeled for dogs and cats. 8, 16 oz.
Malacetic Ultra Shampoo® (Dechra)	Hydrocortisone 1% Ketoconazole 0.15% Acetic Acid 1% Boric Acid 2%	Rx	Labeled for dogs and cats. 8 oz.
Resicort Leave-On Lotion® (Virbac)	Lotion: 1%	Rx	8, 16 oz.

Human-Labeled Topical Hydrocortisone Products

Note: Partial listing; there are many branded products available with hydrocortisone. For more information on human-labeled hydrocortisone products, refer to a comprehensive human drug reference (*e.g.*, *Facts and Comparisons*) or contact a pharmacist.

Product (Company)	*Form: Concentration*	*Label Status*	*Size(s)*
Hydrocortisone Ointment	Ointment: 0.5, 1%	OTC/Rx (Human). Status determined by labeling	15, 20, 28.4, 30 60, 120, 454 g.
Hydrocortisone Ointment	Ointment: 2.5%	Rx (Human)	20, 30 g
Hydrocortisone Cream	Cream: 0.5, 1%	OTC/Rx (Human). Status determined by labeling	1 g pkts, 15, 20, 28.4, 30, 60, 120, 454 g.
Hydrocortisone Cream	Cream: 2.5%	Rx (Human)	15, 20, 30, 60, 240, 454 g
Hydrocortisone Lotion	Lotion: 0.5, 1%	OTC/Rx (Human). Status determined by labeling	30, 60, 120 mL
Hydrocortisone Lotion	Lotion: 2.5%	Rx (Human)	60, 120mL
Hydrocortisone Gel (various))	Gel: 1%	OTC (Human)	15, 30 g
Hydrocortisone Gel	Gel: 2%	Rx (Human)	43 g
Hydrocortisone Solution; Liquid	Solution: 1%, 2.5%	Rx (Human)	30, 45, 60, 75, 120, 600 mL
Hydrocortisone Spray	Spray: 1%	OTC (Human)	45 mL

ISOFLUPREDONE ACETATE, TOPICAL

(eye-soe-*flue*-pre-done *ass*-i-tate)

Indications/Actions

Considered a high potency topical corticosteroid, isoflupredone in combination with neomycin and tetracaine may be useful for adjunctive treatment of otic or topical localized pruritic or inflammatory conditions that may be associated with a bacterial skin infection and pain. Because risks associated with isoflupredone (HPA axis suppression, systemic corticosteroid effects, skin atrophy) are greater than with hydrocortisone, these products are generally reserved for more serious localized pruritic conditions or when hydrocortisone is not effective. All veterinary-labeled products (*Tritop® Ointment* and *Neo-Predef w/Tetracaine Powder®*) have labeled indications for conditions associated with neomycin-susceptible organisms and/or allergy with anesthetic properties due to tetracaine, or as a superficial dressing applied to minor cuts, wounds, lacerations, and abrasions, and for post-surgical pain application where reduction in pain and inflammatory response is deemed desirable. In addition, *Tritop® Ointment* is also labeled for acute (and possibly chronic) otitis externa, acute moist dermatitis and anal sac inflammation/infection, and *Neo-Predef w/Tetracaine Powder®* for acute otitis externa, acute moist dermatitis and interdigital dermatitis in dogs and cats.

Corticosteroids are non-specific anti-inflammatory agents. They probably act by inducing phospholipase A2 inhibitory proteins (lipocortins) in cells, thereby reducing the formation, activity, and release of endogenous inflammatory mediators (*e.g.*, histamine, prostaglandins, kinins, etc.). Corticosteroids also reduce DNA synthesis via an anti-mitotic effect on epidermal cells. Topically applied corticosteroids also inhibit the migration of leukocytes and macrophages to the area reducing erythema, pruritus and edema.

Suggested Dosages/Use

Labeled dose for *Tritop®* when used on skin or mucous membranes: Cleanse area, apply a small amount and spread and rub in gently. Involved area may be treated 1–3 times daily and continued in accordance with clinical response.

Labeled dose for *Neo-Predef w/Tetracaine Powder®*: Cleanse area, apply by compressing bottle with short, sharp squeezes; once daily application usually sufficient, but may use 1–3 times as required.

Precautions/Adverse Effects

Several veterinary topical products containing corticosteroids list tuberculosis of the skin or pregnancy as a contraindication. Systemic corticosteroids can be teratogenic or induce parturition during the third trimester of pregnancy in animals. If considering use during pregnancy, weigh the respective risks with treating versus potential benefits. Residual activity may affect intradermal or allergy serum tests; it has been suggested to stop use 2 weeks prior to allergy testing.

Clients should wash hands after application or wear gloves when applying. Avoid contact with eyes. Do not allow the animal to lick or chew at affected sites for at least 20-30 minutes after application. Isoflupredone may delay wound healing particularly if used longer than 7 days in duration.

Use care when treating large areas, or when used on smaller patients. Treat for only as long as necessary on as small an area as possible. Risk for HPA axis suppression, systemic corticosteroid effects (polydipsia/polyuria, Cushing's, gastrointestinal effects) and skin atrophy increase with prolonged duration of use. Local skin reactions (burning, itching, redness) are possible, but unlikely to occur. Hypersensitivity reactions to neomycin and/or tetracaine are possible.

Veterinary-Labeled Topical Isoflupredone Products

Note: At time of writing there are no veterinary-labeled sole active ingredient isoflupredone products in the USA.

Product (Company)	Form: Concentration	Label Status	Other Ingredients; Comments; Size(s)
Tritop® (Pfizer)	Ointment: Isoflupredone acetate 0.1%; Neomycin sulfate 0.5%; Tetracaine HCl 0.5%	Rx	10 g. tube. Labeled for dogs and cats.
Neo-Predef w/ Tetracaine Powder® (Pfizer)	Powder: Isoflupredone acetate 1mg/g; Neomycin Sulf. 5 mg/g; Tetracaine HCl 5 mg/g	Rx	Myristyl-gamma-picolinium Cl (germicidal surfactant) 0.2 mg/g. 15 g. insufflator bottle. Store in dry place, do not allow tip of bottle to contact moisture. Labeled for use on dogs and cats.

Human-Labeled Topical Isoflupredone Products

None

MOMETASONE FUROATE

(moe-**met**-a-zone **fyur**-oh-ate))

For otic use, refer to the Otics section.

Indications

Considered a highly potent topical corticosteroid, mometasone furoate may be useful for adjunctive treatment of pruritic and/or inflammatory conditions that may be associated with bacterial and/or yeast skin infections. Because risks associated with mometasone (HPA axis suppression, skin atrophy) are greater than with hydrocortisone, mometasone products are generally reserved for more serious pruritic conditions or when hydrocortisone is not effective. Mometasone is found in a veterinary-labeled suspension (*MoMetaMax®*) in combination with gentamicin and clotrimazole indicated for otic use. It can also be used extra-label for yeast and/or bacterial skin infections sensitive to clotrimazole and gentamicin, when a strong anti-inflammatory effect is also needed.

Corticosteroids are non-specific anti-inflammatory agents. They probably act by inducing phospholipase A2 inhibitory proteins (lipocortins) in cells, thereby reducing the formation, activity, and release of endogenous inflammatory mediators (*e.g.*, histamine, prostaglandins, kinins, etc.). Corticosteroids also reduce DNA synthesis via an anti-mitotic effect on epidermal cells. Topically applied corticosteroids also inhibit the migration of leukocytes and macrophages to the area reducing erythema, pruritus and edema.

Suggested Dosages/Use

Initially, topical corticosteroids are usually used sparingly 1–2 times per day, then tapered to less frequent use. Mometasone formulations are best suited for focal (*e.g.* pedal) or multifocal lesions and for relatively short durations (*e.g.*, less than 2 months). However, clinicians must tailor the frequency and duration of application to the severity of clinical signs. Refer to the actual product labeling for additional usage information.

Precautions/Adverse Effects

Several veterinary topical products list tuberculosis of the skin or pregnancy as a contraindication. Use care when treating large areas, or when used on smaller patients. Risks can be reduced by treating for only as long as necessary on as small an area as possible. Increased risks of HPA axis suppression, systemic corticosteroid effects (polydipsia/polyuria, Cushing's, gastrointestinal effects) and cutaneous atrophy associated with skin fragility, alopecia, localized pyoderma, superficial follicular cysts (milia) and comedones occur as product concentration and duration of use increases. Local skin reactions (burning, itching, redness) are possible, but unlikely to occur. Mometasone may delay wound healing particularly if used longer than 7 days in duration.

Residual activity may affect intradermal or allergy serum tests; it has been suggested to stop use 2 weeks prior to allergy testing.

Clients should wash hands after application or wear gloves when applying. Avoid contact with eyes. Do no let animal lick or chew at affected areas for at least 20-30 minutes after application.

Veterinary-Labeled Mometasone Products

Product (Company)	Form: Concentration	Label Status	Other Ingredients; Comments; Size(s)
MoMetaMax Otic Suspension® (Intervet/Schering-Plough)	Suspension (otic): Per gram: Mometasone 1 mg; Gentamicin 3 mg; Clotrimazole 10 mg	Rx	Mineral-oil base. Approved for otic use in dogs, but used extra-label (see above). In 7.5, 15, 30, 215 g tubes

Human-Labeled Topical Mometasone Products

Note: Partial listing; for more information on human-labeled mometasone products (nasal, etc), refer to a comprehensive human drug reference (*e.g.*, *Facts and Comparisons*) or contact a pharmacist.

Product (Company)	Form: Concentration	Label Status	Other Ingredients; Comments; Size(s)
Elocon® (Schering- Plough); generic	Cream, Ointment, Lotion: 0.1%	Rx	Cream: stearyl alcohol. 15, 45 g. Ointment: 15, 45 g. Lotion: Propylene glycol, isopropyl alcohol. 30, 60 mL

TRIAMCINOLONE ACETONIDE, TOPICAL

(trye-am-*sin*-ohe-lone ass-si-*toe*-nide)

For systemic use, see the monograph found in the main section.

Indications/Actions

Considered a medium potency topical corticosteroid when used at concentrations less than 0.5% (high potency), triamcinolone acetonide may useful for adjunctive treatment of pruritic conditions. Because risks associated with triamcinolone (HPA axis suppression, skin atrophy) are greater than with hydrocortisone, triamcinolone acetonide products are generally reserved for more serious pruritic conditions or when hydrocortisone is not effective. Triamcinolone can be found in a veterinary-labeled sole agent cream (*Medalone®*) or spray (*Genesis®*). It is also an ingredient in combination with antibiotics and anti-yeast ingredients in several veterinary products (*e.g.*, *Panalog®*) that are labeled for otic use. However, these products can be used in an extra-label manner to treat bacterial and yeast skin infections sensitive to gentamicin and nystatin, including pododermatitis and anal sac disease, when a strong anti-inflammatory effect is needed.

Corticosteroids are non-specific anti-inflammatory agents. They probably act by inducing phospholipase A2 inhibitory proteins (lipocortins) in cells, thereby reducing the formation, activity, and release of endogenous inflammatory mediators (*e.g.*, histamine, prostaglandins, kinins, etc). Corticosteroids also reduce DNA synthesis via an anti-mitotic effect on epidermal cells. Topically applied corticosteroids also inhibit the migration of leukocytes and macrophages to the area reducing erythema, pruritus and edema.

Suggested Dosages/Use

Triamcinolone formulations are best suited for focal (*e.g.*, pedal) or multifocal lesions for relatively short durations (*e.g.*, less than 2 months). Initially, topical corticosteroids are usually used sparingly 1-4 times per day and then frequency is tapered when control is achieved. Long term, frequent use can cause HPA axis suppression and risk can be reduced by treating for only as long as necessary on as small an area as possible. Refer to individual product labeling for actual dosing recommendations for veterinary products.

Precautions/Adverse Effects

Several veterinary topical products list tuberculosis of the skin or pregnancy as a contraindication. Systemic corticosteroids can be teratogenic or induce parturition during the third trimester of pregnancy in animals. If considering use during pregnancy, weigh the respective risks with treating versus potential benefits. Clients should wash hands after application or wear gloves when applying. Avoid contact with eyes. Do not allow animal to lick or chew at affected sites for at least 20-30 minutes after application.

Residual activity may affect intradermal or allergy serum tests; it has been suggested to stop use 2 weeks prior to allergy testing.

Use care when treating large areas, or when used on smaller patients. Risks can be reduced by treating for only as long as necessary on as small an area as possible. Increased risks of HPA axis suppression, systemic corticosteroid effects (polydipsia/polyuria, Cushing's, gastrointestinal effects) and skin atrophy (skin fragility, alopecia, localized pyoderma and comedones are other possible complications) occur as product concentration and duration of use increases. Local skin reactions (burning, itching, redness) are possible, but unlikely to occur.

Veterinary-Labeled Topical Triamcinolone Acetonide Products

Product (Company)	Form: Concentration	Label Status	Other Ingredients; Comments; Size(s)
Medalone Cream® (Med-Pharmex) **Cortalone Cream®** (Vedco)	Cream: 0.1%	Rx	7.5, 15 g. Approved for dogs. Indications include allergic dermatitis and summer eczema.
Genesis Spray® (Virbac)	Spray: 0.015%	Rx	16 oz spray bottle. Approved for dogs. Indication is for control of pruritus associated with allergic dermatitis. Bacterial skin infection needs to be resolved prior to use. Strongly recommend referring to the package insert information for maximum allowable dosages, treatment durations, etc.
Derma-Vet Cream® (Med-Pharmex)	Cream: Nystatin 100,000 units/g Triamcinolone Acet. 1 mg Neomycin Sulf. 2.5 mg Thiostrepton 2,500 units	Rx	Aqueous vanishing cream. 7.5, 15 g. Panalog and Derma-Vet labeled for use in dogs or cats. Cortalone labeled for dogs only.
Panalog Ointment® (Pfizer) **Animax Ointment®** (Pharmaderm) **Quadratop Ointment®** (Butler) **Derma-Vet Ointment®** (Med-Pharmex) **Dermalog Ointment®** (RXV) **Dermalone Ointment®** (Vedco)	Ointment: Nystatin 100,000 units/g Triamcinolone Acet. 1 mg Neomycin Sulf. 2.5 mg Thiostrepton 2,500 units	Rx	Labeled for use in dogs or cats. 7.5, 15, 30, 240 mL

Human-Labeled Topical Triamcinolone Acetonide Products

Note: Partial listing; there are several topical branded products (two common trade names are *Aristocort®* and *Kenalog®*) available with triamcinolone. For more information on human-labeled triamcinolone products, refer to a comprehensive human drug reference (*e.g.*, *Facts and Comparisons*) or contact a pharmacist.

Product (Company)	Form: Concentration	Label Status	Size(s); Comments
Triamcinolone Acetonide Ointment	Ointment: 0.025, 0.1, 0.5%	Rx (Human)	15, 20, 28.4, 30, 60, 120, 454 g.
Triamcinolone Acetonide Cream	Cream: 0.025, 0.1, 0.5%	Rx (Human)	15, 20, 30, 60, 120, 240 454 g.
Triamcinolone Acetonide Lotion	Lotion: 0.025, 0.1%	Rx (Human)	15, 60 mL
Kenalog® (Westwood Squibb)	Aerosol Spray: 0.1%	Rx (Human)	23, 63 g. 10.3% alcohol
Nystatin-Triamcinolone Acetonide (various)	Cream: Nystatin 100,000 units/g Triamcinolone Acet. 0.1%	Rx (Human)	Depending on product: 1.5 g. pkts, 15, 30, 60, 120 g.

Antimicrobials, Topical

Antibacterial Agents

*See also the **Sulfur** listing the keratolytic section*

BACITRACIN AND BACITRACIN COMBINATIONS, TOPICAL

(bass-ih-*trase*-in)

Indications/Actions

Bacitracin is used topically to prevent infection after dermal lacerations, scrapes or minor burns. Bacitracin acts by inhibiting cell wall synthesis of susceptible bacteria and is either bactericidal or bacteriostatic depending on drug concentration and bacterial susceptibility. Bacitracin is primarily active against gram-positive bacteria, but *Staphylococci* spp. are becoming increasingly resistant. Bacitracin activity is not impaired by blood, pus, necrotic tissue or large inocula. Bacitracin is not recommended in the treatment of ulcerated and chronic canine dermatoses (sensitization may occur).

Suggested Dosages/Use

May be applied up to 3 times daily and be covered by a suitable dressing. Use is usually not recommended to continue more than one week.

Precautions/Adverse Effects

Bacitracin topical ointment should not be used in or around eyes, for the treatment of ulcerated lesions, or in patients known to be hypersensitive to it. There have been anecdotal reports of cats developing fatal anaphylactic reactions after administered ophthalmic "triple" antibiotic ointment. Deep puncture wounds, animal bites or deep cutaneous infections may require systemic antibiotic therapy. While topical administration generally results in negligible systemic levels, if used over large areas of the body or on serious burns or puncture wounds, measurable absorption and potential toxicity may occur. Do no let animal lick or chew at affected areas for at least 20-30 minutes after application. Clients should wash hands after application or wear gloves when applying.

Veterinary-Labeled Bacitracin Topical Products

Veterinary-labeled bacitracin formulations for topical use are not available. However, ophthalmic preparations containing bacitracin in combination with other antibiotics w/ or w/o hydrocortisone could be used in an extra-label manner.

Human-Labeled Topical Bacitracin Products

Bacitracin ointment is available alone as 500 Units/g in various tube sizes. There are many OTC human products available with formulas equivalent to the formally available veterinary-labeled triple antibiotic preparations that contained neomycin, polymyxin B, and bacitracin. A well-known trade name is *Neosporin®* or it is available generically as Triple Antibiotic Ointment. When combined with only polymyxin B, a common trade name is *Polysporin®*.

Product (Company)	Form: Concentration	Label Status	Other Ingredients; Size(s)
Bacitracin (various generic)	Ointment: 500 Units/gram	OTC (Human)	Depending of manufacturer: white petrolatum, mineral oil. 14, 28, 120 g. tubes, 1 lb. jars

BENZOYL PEROXIDE
(ben-*zoyl* per-*oks*-ide)

Indications/Actions

Benzoyl peroxide products are used topically either as gels or in shampoos. Shampoos are generally used for oily and scaly skin (seborrhea oleosa), superficial and deep pyodermas, crusty pyodermas (such as seborrheic dermatitis/pyoderma commonly seen in Cocker Spaniels), furunculosis, and as adjunctive therapy for generalized demodicosis and Schnauzer comedo syndrome. Gels may be useful for treating localized superficial and deep pyodermas, chin acne, fold pyodermas, and localized Demodex lesions.

Benzoyl peroxide possesses antimicrobial (especially antibacterial), comedolytic ("follicular flushing"), keratolytic and antiseborrheic actions. It also is It has some mild antipruritic activity and wound healing effects, and is thought to increase follicular flushing. Benzoyl peroxide's antimicrobial activity is due to the oxidative benzoyl peroxy radicals formed that disrupt cell membranes.

Suggested Dosages/Use

Gels are usually recommended for use once to twice daily and shampoos up to once daily. Shampoos should remain in contact with skin for at least 10 minutes before rinsing. For veterinary products, refer to product label for details on use.

Precautions/Adverse Effects

Avoid contact with eyes or mucous membranes. Clients should wash hands after application or wear gloves when applying. Benzoyl peroxide will bleach colored fabrics, jewelry, clothing or carpets and may bleach the patient's fur. Clients should be advised to keep treated animals away from fabrics during treatment. Do no let animal lick or chew at affected areas for a few minutes after application.

Benzoyl peroxide can be drying or irritating (erythema, pruritus, pain) in some patients particularly at higher (>5%) concentrations. Reducing frequency of use, application of emollients after bathing, or using shampoos with moisturizing microvesicles may alleviate or prevent this problem. Benzoyl peroxide shampoos do not lather well.

Veterinary-Labeled Topical Benzoyl Peroxide Products

Product (Company)	Form: Active Ingredients; Concentration	Label Status	Other Ingredients; Comments; Size(s)
Pyoben Gel® (Virbac)	Gel: 5%	Rx	Labeled for dogs and cats and for use once or twice daily after cleaning. 30 g
Oxydex Gel® (DVM)	Gel: 5%	Rx	Labeled for dogs and cats and for use once or twice daily after cleaning. Rub in well so that no residue remains. Prevent pet from licking area until dries (1−2 minutes). 30 g
Micro-Pearls Advantage Benzoyl-Plus® (Vetoquinol)	Shampoo: 2.5%	Rx	*Novasome®* microvesicles. Labeled for dogs & cats. Shake well; wear gloves. May be used up to once daily as directed. 12 oz, 1 gal
Benzoyl Peroxide Shampoo® (Davis)	Shampoo: 2.5%	OTC	Labeled for OTC use. 12 oz, 1 gal
OxyDex Shampoo® (DVM)	Shampoo: 2.5%	OTC	Labeled for OTC use. 8, 12 oz, 1 gal.
Pyoben Shampoo® (Virbac)	Shampoo: 3%	Rx	*Spherulites®* microcapsules, chitosanide. Labeled for dogs and cats. Use initially 2−3 times/week, then once a week or as directed by DVM. 8, 16 oz.
Vet Solutions BPO-3® Shampoo (Vetoquinol)	Shampoo: 3%	Rx	Labeled for dogs and cats. 16 oz; 1 gal.
Sulf OxyDex Shampoo® (DVM)	Shampoo: Benzoyl Peroxide 2.5% Sulfur (micronized) 2%	OTC	Shake well. May be used prn or as directed by DVM. 8, 12 oz, 1 gal
Oxyderm® Shampoo (Sogeval)	Shampoo: Benzoyl peroxide 3% Sulfur 2% Salicylic acid 2% Phytosphingosine	OTC	Labeled for dogs and cats. 8, 16 oz.
Dermabenss® Shampoo® (DermaPet)	Shampoo: Benzoyl peroxide 2.5%, Sulfur 1%, Salicylic Acid 1%	OTC	Moisturizing factors, Vitamin E. 8 oz, 1 gal

Human-Labeled Topical Benzoyl Peroxide Products

There are many human products available containing benzoyl peroxide (2.5%-10%), but with the possible exception of the 5% gel products, the veterinary formulations would be more suitable for use on dogs or cats. Benzoyl peroxide 5% gel can be labeled as either Rx or OTC depending on product and are available as generics or with the following trade names: *Benzac®, Desquam-X®,* or *PanOxyl®.*

CLINDAMYCIN, TOPICAL

(klin-da-*mye*-sin)   Cleocin®, ClinzGard®

For systemic use, see the monograph found in the main section

Indications/Actions

Topical clindamycin may be used for the treatment of feline acne or other localized skin infections caused by bacteria susceptible to it. The veterinary product (*ClinzGard®*) is labeled as indicated for the treatment of anal sac and tissue abscesses, puncture wounds and surgical incisions. It has been recommended by some veterinary dermatologists that topical clindamycin only be used when other topical antibiotics such as gentamicin have failed. Ideally, treatment should be based on culture and susceptibility results.

Clindamycin inhibits bacterial protein synthesis by binding to the 50S ribosome; primary activity is against anaerobic and gram-positive aerobic bacteria. For more information on the pharmacology of clindamycin, refer to the monograph for systemic use found in the main section.

Suggested Dosages/Use

When used for feline acne, topical clindamycin is generally applied in a thin film once to twice daily. *ClinzGard®* is used as a single application that has sustained-release over 7-10 days. It must be applied to cleaned and, if necessary, debrided surfaces.

Precautions/Adverse Effects

Topical clindamycin should not be used in patients with a history of hypersensitivity to clindamycin or lincomycin. Avoid contact with eyes. Clients should wash hands after application or wear gloves when applying.

Contact reactions (pain, burning erythema, itching, drying, peeling) are possible. Clindamycin lotions and gels may cause less burning than the topical solutions or foams. As clindamycin can be absorbed through the skin, systemic adverse effects are possible. Antibiotic associated diarrheas are potentially possible, but severe, life-threatening diarrheas (so-called Pseudomembranous colitis) are thought to occur very rarely in animal patients when clindamycin is used systemically.

Veterinary-Labeled Topical Clindamycin Products

Product (Company)	Form: Concentration	Label Status	Other Ingredients; Comments; Size(s)
ClinzGard® (TriLogic)	Gel: 1%	Rx	Labeled for dogs and cats. Sterile single-dose syringes (box with 4 units).

Human-Labeled Topical Clindamycin Products

Product (Company)	Form: Concentration	Label Status	Other Ingredients; Comments; Size(s)
Clindamycin Phosphate (various generic)	Lotion: 1%	Rx (Human)	30, 60 g.
Cleocin T® (Pharmacia Upjohn)	Lotion: 1%	Rx (Human)	Cystostearyl alcohol, glycerin, methylparaben. 60 mL
Clindamax® (PharmaDerm)	Lotion: 1%	Rx (Human)	Cystostearyl alcohol, glycerin, methylparaben. 60 mL
Clindamycin Phosphate (various generic)	Gel: 1%	Rx (Human)	30, 60 g.
Cleocin T® (Pharmacia Upjohn)	Gel: 1%	Rx (Human)	Methylparaben. 30, 60 g.
Clindagel® (Galderma)	Gel: 1%	Rx (Human)	Methylparaben. 7.5, 42 & 77 g.
Clindamax® (PharmaDerm)	Gel: 1%	Rx (Human)	Methylparaben. 30, 60 g.
Clindamycin Phosphate (various generic)	Solution: 1%	Rx (Human)	30, 60 mL
Cleocin T® (Pharmacia Upjohn)	Solution: 1%	Rx (Human)	Isopropyl alcohol 50%. Single-use pledgets 30 & 60 mL
Clindets® (Stiefel)	Pledgets: 1%	Rx (Human)	Isopropyl alcohol 52%. 1 mL pledgets
Evoclin® (Connetics)	Aerosol Foam: 1%	Rx (Human)	Cetyl alcohol, ethanol 58%, stearyl alcohol, propylene glycol. 50 g.

GENTAMICIN SULFATE, TOPICAL

(jen-ta-*mye*-sin *sul*-fate)   Gentocin®

For systemic use, see the monograph found in the main section.

Indications/Actions

Topical gentamicin can be useful for treating both primary and secondary superficial bacterial skin infections caused by bacteria susceptible to it. It can also be used prophylactically after lacerations/abrasions or after minor surgery. In small animal medicine, topical gentamicin is usually used in combination with the corticosteroid betamethasone to treat superficial lesions, including "hot spots" (acute moist dermatitis, pruritic lesions).

The products containing betamethasone or mometasone and clotrimazole are labeled for otic use, but can also be used in an extra-label manner for yeast and/or bacterial skin infections sensitive to gentamicin and clotrimazole, when an anti-inflammatory effect is also desired. Formulations containing betamethasone ore mometasone are best suited for focal (*e.g.*, pedal) or multifocal lesions for relatively short durations (*e.g.*, less than 2 months). Initially, topical corticosteroids are usually used sparingly 1-4 times per day and then frequency is tapered when control is achieved. Sole ingredient gentamicin sulfate topical forms are available with human labeling.

Gentamicin has activity against many Streptococci, Staphylococci (coagulase negative/positive and some penicillinase-producing strains) and gram-negative bacteria including many Klebsiella, *E. coli*, and some strains of Pseudomonas. Gentamicin-resistant strains of Pseudomonas are an ongoing issue.

Suggested Dosages/Use

Topical gentamicin/betamethasone sprays are labeled for use 2–4 times day for up to 7 days. Topical gentamicin creams and ointments are generally applied to affected areas up to four times daily. Creams are generally used for secondary or greasy infections; ointments on dry skin infections.

Precautions/Adverse Effects

Topical gentamicin may be absorbed systemically if used on ulcers, burned or denuded skin. Creams are more likely to be absorbed than are ointments. Systemic toxicity is unlikely to occur unless used on a significant percentage of body area or for prolonged times. Do not let animal lick or chew at affected areas for at least 20-30 minutes after application.

With products containing betamethasone or mometasone, long-term or frequent use can cause HPA axis suppression. Risk can be reduced by treating for only as long as necessary on as small an area as possible. Residual activity may affect intradermal or allergy serum tests; it has been suggested to stop use 2 weeks prior to allergy testing.

Avoid contact with eyes. Clients should wash hands after application or wear gloves when applying.

Refer to individual product labeling for actual dosing recommendations for veterinary products.

Veterinary-Labeled Topical Gentamicin Products

Product (Company)	Form: Concentration	Label Status	Other Ingredients; Size(s)
Gentocin Topical Spray® (Intervet Schering-Plough) **Gentaspray®** (Butler) **Betagen Topical Spray®** (Med-Pharmex) **Gentamicin Topical Spray®** (RXV; Priority Care 1) **Gentaved Topical Spray®** (Vedco) **GenOne Spray®** (VetOne)	Spray (all products listed): Gentamicin 0.57 mg/mL; Betamethasone (as valerate) 0.284 mg/mL	Rx	All products listed are labeled for dogs and contain isopropyl alcohol, propylene glycol and parabens. Sizes range from 60 mL to 240 mL
Otomax® Ointment (Schering) **DVMAX® Ointment** (DVM) **Vetromax® Ointment** (Dechra)	Ointment (otic): Gentamicin 3 mg/g; Betamethasone 1 mg/g; Clotrimazole 10 mg/g	Rx	Approved for otic use in dogs; used in extra-label manner for bacterial skin lesions or Malassezia dermatitis; Depending on product: 7.5, 15, 20 g tubes & 215 g bottles
MoMetaMax Otic Suspension® (Intervet Schering-Plough)	Suspension (otic): Gentamicin 3 mg/g Mometasone 1 mg/g Clotrimazole 10 mg/g	Rx	Mineral oil based. Approved for otic use in dogs. Extra label use in dogs and cats with localized inflamed or infected cutaneous lesions (e.g., bacterial skin lesions or Malassezia dermatitis.) 7.5, 15, 30, 215 g tubes.

Human-Labeled Topical Gentamicin Products

Product (Company)	Form: Concentration	Label Status	Other Ingredients; Comments; Size(s)
Gentamicin (various generic)	Cream: 0.1% (as base) Ointment: 0.1% (as base)	Rx (Human)	Cream may contain propylene glycol and parabens. 15 g tubes Ointment may contain white petrolatum and parabens. 15 g. tubes

MUPIROCIN (PSEUDOMONIC ACID A)

(myoo-*pye*-roe-sin)   Bactroban®, Bactoderm®

Indications/Actions

Mupirocin is FDA-approved for treating infections in dogs (*e.g.*, superficial pyoderma, fold pyoderma, interdigital cysts/draining tracts, acne, pressure point pyodermas, etc) caused by susceptible strains of *Staphylococcus aureus* or *Staphylococcus (pseudo)intermedius*, including beta-lactamase producing and methicillin-resistant strains. It may also be of use in other species and conditions (*e.g.*, feline acne, equine pyoderma, superficial pyoderma, interdigital abscesses, pressure point pyodermas, etc). It may also be of use in feline acne. It also shows activity against other gram-positive pathogens, including strains of Corynebacterium, Clostridium, Proteus and Actinomyces.

Mupirocin is not related structurally to other commercially available antibiotics and acts by inhibiting bacterial protein synthesis by binding to bacterial isoleucyl transfer-RNA sythetase. While bacterial resistance is rare, resistant strains of *Staphylococcal aureus* have been identified and resistance transference is thought to be plasmid-mediated. It is thought that resistance occurs more frequently when mupirocin is used over a prolonged period and over larger areas of skin, therefore; it may be best to use mupirocin for short-term treatment and on small, localized areas. Cross-resistance with other antimicrobials has not been identified. Mupirocin also has activity against some gram-negative bacteria, but it is not used clinically for gram-negative infections. Pseudomonas is particularly resistant to mupirocin.

Mupirocin is not significantly absorbed through the skin into the systemic circulation, but does penetrate well into granulomatous deep pyoderma lesions. It is not suitable for application to burns.

Suggested Dosages/Use

Mupirocin is labeled for twice daily application on dogs. It requires 10 minutes of contact time to be active. In cats with feline acne, once a course of once to twice daily mupirocin therapy has been completed (control attained), some cats can be maintained with 1–2 applications per week.

Precautions/Adverse Effects

Mupirocin is contraindicated in patients with a history of hypersensitive reactions it or other ointments containing polyethylene glycol. Because the ointment has a polyethylene glycol base, the manufacturer warns that nephrotoxicity may potentially develop if used on extensive deep lesions. Avoid contact with eyes.

Mupirocin appears to be very well tolerated; contact reactions (pain, erythema, itching) are possible, but thought to occur rarely. Overgrowth of non-susceptible organisms (superinfection) is also possible with prolonged use. Anecdotally, very rare renal toxicity has been reported.

Veterinary-Labeled Topical Mupirocin Products

Product (Company)	Form: Concentration	Label Status	Other Ingredients; Size(s)
Muricin® (Dechra)	Ointment: 2%	Rx	Labeled for use on dogs; Polyethylene glycol base. 15 g.

Human-Labeled Topical Mupirocin Products

Product (Company)	Form: Concentration	Label Status	Other Ingredients; Size(s)
Mupirocin (various generic)	Ointment: 2%	Rx (Human)	Polyethylene glycol base. 22 g.
Bactroban® Ointment (GlaxoSmithKline)	Ointment: 2%	Rx (Human)	Polyethylene glycol base. 22 g.
Centany® (Medimetriks)	Ointment: 2%	Rx (Human)	Castor oil, hard fat base. 30 g
Bactroban® Cream (GlaxoSmithKline)	Cream: 2%	Rx (Human)	Oil/water base. 15 & 30 g

NITROFURAZONE, TOPICAL

(nye-troe-*fur*-ah-zone)   Furazone®

Indications/Actions

Nitrofurazone is a nitrofuran antibacterial that can be used topically as an antibacterial for treating or preventing superficial infections. It is bactericidal for many bacteria, including *E. coli, S. aureus,* etc. Clinical efficacy demonstrating efficacy for the treatment of minor burns or surface bacterial infections is apparently unavailable.

Nitrofurazone's mechanism of action is thought to be associated with inhibiting bacterial enzymes that primarily degrade glucose and pyruvate.

Suggested Dosages/Use

Apply once daily until lesions resolve or as directed by the veterinarian. For veterinary products, refer to product label for details on individual use.

Precautions/Adverse Effects

As nitrofurazone has been shown to cause mammary tumors when fed in high doses to rats and ovarian tumors in mice, **U.S.A. federal law prohibits the use of nitrofurazone products in (or on) food animals, including horses to be used for food.**

The soluble dressing contains polyethylene glycols and if used on large areas of denuded skin significant amounts of polyethylene glycol could be absorbed and cause nephrotoxicity.

Avoid ointment contact with eyes or mucous membranes. Clients should wash hands after application or wear gloves when applying. Do not allow animal to lick or chew treated area for at least 30 minutes. Avoid exposure to sunlight, strong fluorescent lighting, excessive heat, or alkaline materials.

Topical nitrofurazone appears to be well tolerated; hypersensitivity or skin reactions (pain, erythema, itching) are possible, but thought to occur rarely. Overgrowth of non-susceptible organisms (superinfection) is also possible with prolonged use.

Veterinary-Labeled Topical Nitrofurazone Products

Product (Company)	Form: Concentration	Label Status	Other Ingredients; Comments; Size(s)
Nitrofurazone Soluble Dressing (Generic; Med-Pharmex, AgriLabs, Vedco, etc.) Also available under a variety of trade names.	Ointment (soluble): 0.2%	OTC	Water-soluble or polyethylene glycol base. 1 lb. jars.
NFZ® Puffer (AgriLabs, Durvet, Aspen, etc)	Soluble Powder: 0.2%	OTC	Labeled for eye and ear infections, surface wounds, cuts and abrasions in dogs and cats. Shake or rotate to loosen powder. Restricted drug in California. 45 g.

Human-Labeled Topical Nitrofurazone Products
None. Nitrofurazone products are apparently no longer available with human labeling in the USA.

SILVER SULFADIAZINE (SSD)
(*sil*-ver sul-fa-*dye*-ah-zeen)   Silvadene®

Indications/Actions
Topical silver sulfadiazine (SSD) is labeled (human) for topical prophylaxis and treatment of 2nd and 3rd degree burns. In veterinary medicine, it is can be useful in treating localized bacterial skin infections, particularly those caused by *Pseudomonas* spp.

SSD has extensive antimicrobial activity and is bactericidal for yeasts and many gram-negative and gram-positive bacteria. SSD acts by disrupting microbial cell membranes and cell walls; this differs from the antibacterial actions of silver nitrate or sodium sulfadiazine. It can enhance epithelization, but can retard granulation.

Suggested Dosages/Use
When used for burns SSD is applied once to twice daily at a thickness of approx. 1/16th of an inch (1–2 mm). Dressings may be applied over the cream. When used for localized bacterial infections once to twice daily treatment with the cream rubbed in is suggested.

Precautions/Adverse Effects
Patients hypersensitive to sulfonamides may also react to SSD. Risks of continued treatment must be weighed against the risks of not treating with SSD. Patients with significant hepatic or renal dysfunction may accumulate drug, particularly when used over large areas. Because SSD can retard granulation, avoid use in non-granulated wounds. Avoid contact with eyes. Clients should wash hands after application or wear gloves when applying.

Adverse effects associated with sulfonamides (*e.g.*, KCS in dogs, blood dyscrasias in dogs/cats, etc.) are possible particularly when used over large areas or for extended periods. Refer to the Sulfadiazine/Trimethoprim monograph in the main section of the reference for more information.

Veterinary-Labeled Silver Sulfadiazine Products
There are no topical products labeled for veterinary patients. An otic preparation (*Baytril Otic*®) contains SSD. See the Otics section for more information.

Human-Labeled Silver Sulfadiazine Products

Product (Company)	Form: Concentration	Label Status	Other Ingredients; Size(s)
Silvadene® (Hoechst MR)	Cream: 1% (10 mg/gm)	Rx (Human)	Water-miscible base containing white petrolatum, stearyl alcohol, methylparaben. 20, 50, 85, 400 & 1000 g.
SSD AF Cream® (Boots)	Cream: 1% (10 mg/gm)	Rx (Human)	Water-miscible base containing white petrolatum, stearyl alcohol, methylparaben. 50, 400 & 1000 g.
Thermazene® (Sherwood)	Cream: 1% (10 mg/gm)	Rx (Human)	Water-miscible base containing white petrolatum, stearyl alcohol, methylparaben. 50, 400 & 1000 g.
SSD Cream® (Boots)	Cream: 1% (10 mg/gm)	Rx (Human)	Water-miscible base containing cetyl alcohol, white petrolatum, stearyl alcohol, methylparaben. 25, 50, 85, 400 & 1000 g.

Antiseptics

ACETIC ACID/BORIC ACID
(ah-*see*-tik *ass*-id; *Bor*-ik *ass*-id)

Indications/Actions
Indicated for the treatment of skin infections caused by bacteria including *Staphylococcus* spp., *Pseudomonas* spp. and yeast such as *Malassezia* spp. Also indicated for fold dermatitis, acute moist dermatitis, pododermatitis, and seborrhea oleosa. Some products contain other antimicrobials such as chlorhexidine and ketoconazole or antiinflammatory agents such as hydrocortisone for anti-pruritic effects.

Acetic and boric acids are potent antibacterial and antifungal agents with a rapid killing effect. They also possess ceruminolytic, keratolytic, keratoplastic, and astringent activities.

Suggested Uses/Dosages
If using spray or wipes: up to 2–3 times a day. If shampoo or conditioner: daily to weekly baths/after baths according to the veterinarian's recommendations. Leave shampoos in contact with the skin for at least 10 minutes prior to rinsing. Refer to the product for individual label directions.

Precautions/Adverse Effects
Skin redness and irritation may occur. Do no let animal lick or chew at affected areas for at least 20-30 minutes after application.

Veterinary-Labeled Topical Acetic and Boric Acid Products

Product (Company)	Form: Active Ingredients; Concentration	Label Status	Other Ingredients; Comments; Size(s);
Malacetic Ultra Spray® (Dechra)	Spray: Acetic Acid 1% Boric Acid 2% Ketoconazole 0.15% Hydrocortisone 1%	OTC	Labeled for dogs and cats. 8 oz.
Mal-A-Ket Wipes® (Dechra)	Wipes: Acetic Acid 2% Chlorhexidine 2% Ketoconazole 1%	OTC	Labeled for dogs and cats. 50 count jar.
Malacetic HC Wipes® (Dechra)	Wipes: Acetic Acid 1% Boric Acid 2% Hydrocortisone 1%	OTC	Labeled for dogs and cats. 25 count jar.
Malacetic Wet Wipes® (Dechra)	Wipes: Acetic Acid 1% Boric Acid 1%	OTC	Labeled for dogs and cats. Indicated for anal sac expression, skin folds and cleaning of ears. 25 and 100 count jars and 25-count brick pack.
Malacetic Spray® (Dechra)	Leave-on Spray: Acetic Acid 2% Boric Acid 2%	OTC	Labeled for dogs and cats. 8, 16 oz.
Malacetic Shampoo® (Dechra)	Shampoo: Acetic Acid 2% Boric Acid 2%	OTC	Labeled for dogs and cats. 12, 16 oz; 1 gal.
Malacetic Ultra Shampoo® (Dechra)	Shampoo: Ketoconazole 0.15% Hydrocortisone 1% Acetic Acid 1% Boric Acid 2%.	Rx	Labeled for dogs and cats. 8 oz.
Mal-A-Ket® Shampoo (Dechra)	Shampoo: Ketoconazole 2% Acetic Acid 2% Chlorhexidine 2%	Rx	Labeled for dogs and cats. 1 oz pouch, 8 oz; 1 gal.

Human-Labeled Topical Acetic and Boric Acid Products
There are several OTC human products available containing acetic acid or boric acid (alone or containing other ingredients). For more information on human-labeled acetic acid or boric acid products, refer to a comprehensive human drug reference (*e.g., Facts and Comparisons*) or contact a pharmacist.

CHLORHEXIDINE
(klor-*heks*-ih-deen)   Nolvasan®

Indications/Actions
A topical antiseptic, chlorhexidine has activity against many bacteria, but apparently, it is not predictably active against *Pseudomonas* or *Serratia* spp. It is available with veterinary labels in many different forms (solutions, shampoos, scrubs, ointments, sprays, etc.).

Because it causes less drying and is usually less irritating than benzoyl peroxide, it is sometimes used in patients that cannot tolerate benzoyl peroxide. However, it does not have the keratolytic, comedolytic or degreasing effects of benzoyl peroxide. Chlorhexidine possesses some residual effects and can remain active on skin after rinsing. Chlorhexidine products may also contain other ingredients such as antifungals (ketoconazole and miconazole), salicylic acid, phytosphingosine, etc.

At usual concentrations, chlorhexidine acts by damaging bacterial cytoplasmic membranes. Antifungal activity can be obtained with 2% or higher concentrations.

Suggested Dosages/Use

For wound irrigation or foot soaking, 0.05–0.1% dilution in water is recommended. If using spray or wipes/pads: 1-2 times a day. If using shampoo or conditioner: daily to weekly baths/after baths; leave shampoo in contact with the skin for at least 10 minutes prior to rinsing. For veterinary products, refer to product label for details on individual use.

Precautions/Adverse Effects

Keep away from eyes as chlorhexidine products can damage eyes. Clients should wash hands after application or wear gloves when applying. Chlorhexidine is safe used on cats, although irritation and corneal ulcers have been reported.

Hypersensitivity and local skin irritant reactions are possible. Likelihood of irritation increases with increased concentrations. Chlorhexidine may retard wound healing; not recommended for long-term use particularly on granulating lesions.

Veterinary-Labeled Topical Chlorhexidine Products

There are also a several teat dip and udder wash products, a lubricant, and oral rinses are available. There are several trade names used for chlorhexidine products, including *Nolvasan®, Chlorhexiderm®, Dermachlor®, Chlorasan®, Chloradine®, Privasan®,* and *Chlorhex®.*

Product (Company)	Form: Concentration	Label Status	Other Ingredients; Comments; Size(s)
Chlorhexidine Spray (various manufacturers and trade names)	Spray: 4%	OTC	Aloe. 8 oz. Shake well. Labeled for dogs, cats, & horses
Malaseb® Spray (DVM)	Spray: Miconazole 2% Chlorhexidine 2%	Rx	Alcohol 30%. 8 oz. Labeled for use in dogs, cats, & horses.
DOUXO® Chlorhexidine PS Micro-emulsion Spray (Sogeval)	Spray: Chlorhexidine 3% Phytosphingosine 0.05%	OTC	Labeled for dogs and cats. 6.8 oz.
Chlorhex 2X 4%® Spray (Vedco)	Spray: 4%	OTC	4% Isopropyl alcohol. Labeled for dogs and cats. 8 oz.
ChlorhexiDerm Spray® (DVM)	Spray: 4%	OTC	Labeled for dogs and cats. 8 oz.
Ketoseb-D® Spray (Sogeval)	Spray: Chlorhexidine 2% Ketoconazole 1%	Rx	Labeled for dogs and cats. 8 oz.
Mal-A-Ket Plus TrizEDTA Spray® (Dechra)	Leave-on Spray: Chlorhexidine 2% Ketoconazole 1% TrizEDTA	Rx	Labeled for dogs and cats. 8 oz.
TrizChlor 4® Spray (Dechra)	Leave-on Spray: Chlorhexidine 4% TrizEDTA	OTC	Labeled for dogs and cats. 8 oz, 1 gal.
Chlorhexidine Solution (various manufacturers and trade names)	Solution: 2%	OTC	As the gluconate. 16 oz, 1 gal. May be labeled for use on dogs, horses, cattle and swine.
Chlorhexidine Concentrate (Davis)	Solution for dilution: 20%	OTC	For 1%: Dilute 6 oz into 1 gal water or shampoo. For 2%: 12 oz into one gal.
DOUXO®Chlorhexidine 3% PS pads (Sogeval)	Medicated pads: Chlorhexidine 3% Climbazole 0.5% Phytosphingosine 0.05%	Rx	Alcohol free. Labeled for dogs and cats. 30 count jar.
Ketoseb-D® Wipes (Sogeval)	Wipes: Chlorhexidine 2% Ketoconazole 1%	Rx	Labeled for dogs and cats. 50 count jar.
Mal-A-Ket® Wipes (Dechra)	Wipes: Chlorhexidine 2% Ketoconazole 1% Acetic Acid 2%	Rx	Labeled for dogs and cats. 50 count jar.
TrizChlor® 4 Wipes (Dechra)	Wipes: Chlorhexidine 4% TrizEDTA	OTC	Labeled for dogs and cats. 50 count jar.

Product (Company)	Form: Concentration	Label Status	Other Ingredients; Comments; Size(s)
Malaseb Pledgets® (DVM)	Pledget (medicated pad): 20 mg Chlorhexidine, 17.4 Miconazole	Rx	Alcohol 30%. 60 per container. Labeled for use in dogs, cats, & horses.
Malaseb Towelettes® (DVM)	Towelette (medicated pad 6X6 inches): 72 mg Chlorhexidine, 63 mg Miconazole	Rx	Polypropylene 60%, alcohol 30%. 60 per container. Labeled for use in dogs, cats, & horses.
Chlorhexidine Flush (various manufacturers and trade names)	Flush: Depending on product concentration may not be not listed	OTC	4, 12 oz
TrizChlor® Flush (Dechra)	Flush: Chlorhexidine 0.15% TrizEDTA	OTC	Labeled for dogs and cats. 4 oz.
Mal-A-Ket Plus TrizEDTA® Flush (Dechra)	Flush: Chlorhexidine 0.15% Ketoconazole 0.15% TrizEDTA	Rx	A multicleanse flush to aid in the treatment of bacterial and fungal (dermatophytosis and malassezia) infections. pH 8. Labeled for dogs and cats. 4, 12 oz.
Dermachlor Flush Plus® (Butler)	Flush: Lidocaine 0.5% Chlorhexidine 0.2%	OTC	Propylene glycol, malic acid, benzoic acid, salicylic acid, glycerin. 4 oz.
Hexadene Flush® (Virbac)	Flush: Chlorhexidine 0.25% Triclosan	OTC	Spherulites® Microcapsules. Labeled for dogs and cats. 12 oz.
Malaseb® Flush (DVM)	Flush: Chlorhexidine 2% Miconazole nitrate 2%	OTC	Labeled for dogs and cats. 4, 12 oz.
ChlorhexiDerm® Flush (DVM)	Flush: 2%	OTC	Labeled for dogs and cats. 4, 12 oz.
Chlorhexidine 0.2% Solution® (Sogeval)	Flush: Chlorhexidine 2%	OTC	Isopropyl alcohol, glycerin, castor oil. Labeled for dogs and cats. 4, 8, 16 oz.
Ketoseb-D® Flush (Sogeval)	Flush: Chlorhexidine 2% Ketoconazole 1%	OTC	Labeled for dogs and cats. 4, 16 oz.
Chlorhexidine Ointment (various manufacturers and trade names)	Ointment: 1%	OTC	1 & 7 oz, 1 lb.
Nolvasan Shampoo® (Pfizer)	Shampoo: 0.5%	OTC	8 oz, 1 gal.
Chlorhexidine Shampoo 2% (various manufacturers and trade names)	Shampoo: 2%	OTC	8, 16 oz, 1 gal
Chlorhexidine Shampoo 4% (various manufacturers and trade names)	Shampoo: 4%	OTC	Depending manufacturer: 8,12, 16 oz., 1 gal.
Ketochlor Shampoo® (Virbac)	Shampoo: Chlorhexidine 2.3% Ketoconazole 1%	Rx	Spherulites® Microcapsules. Glycotechnology (monosaccharides: L-rhamnose, D-mannose, D-galactose; polysaccharide: alkyl polyglucoside), chitosanide. Labeled for dogs and cats. 8, 16 oz, 1 gal.
Malaseb Shampoo® (DVM)	Shampoo: Miconazole nitrate 2% Chlorhexidine 2%	OTC	8, 12 oz, 1 gal.
Malaseb® Concentrate Rinse (DVM)	Rinse: Miconazole nitrate 5.2% Chlorhexidine 5.9%	OTC	Labeled for use on dogs, cats, & horses. Must be diluted before use. Do not allow animal to lick the treated areas until dry. 8, 32 oz.
TrizChlor 4® Shampoo (Dechra)	Shampoo: Chlorhexidine 4% TrizEDTA	OTC	Labeled for dogs and cats. 8 oz, 1 gal.
ResiKetoChlor Leave-On Conditioner® (Virbac)	Conditioner: Chlorhexidine 4% Ketoconazole 1%	OTC	Spherulites® Microcapsules. Glycotechnology (monosaccharides: L-rhamnose, D-mannose, D-galactose; polysaccharide: alkyl polyglucoside), chitosanide. Labeled for dogs and cats. 8 oz.
Chlorhexidine Scrub (various)	Scrub: 2%, 4%	OTC	1 gal.
ChlorhexiDerm® Plus Scrub (DVM)	Scrub: 2%	OTC	Labeled for dogs and cats. 1 gal.

Human-Labeled Topical Chlorhexidine Products
There are several topical skin cleansers available in the 2–4% range. Trade names include: *Hibiclens®*, *Hibistat®*, *Betasept®*, *Exidine®*, *Dyna-Hex®* and *BactoShield®*.

CHLOROXYLENOL (PCMX)
(Kloro-zye-len-ol)

For otic use, refer to the Otics section

Indications/Actions
Chloroxylenol is an antimicrobial disinfectant with demonstrated efficacy against gram-negative and gram-positive bacteria, in addition to a wide variety of fungal organisms, and against RNA and DNA viruses. It can be used in pre-surgical preparation of skin, cleaning wounds and in the treatment of bacterial, fungal and yeast skin infections.

Chloroxylenol, also known as PCMX, is a chlorinated phenolytic antiseptic. Its antibacterial action is due to disruption of bacterial cytoplasmic membranes by blocking production of adenosine triphosphate.

Suggested Uses/Dosages
If using shampoo, leave shampoo in contact with the skin for at least 10 minutes prior to rinsing. Refer to product label for details on individual use.

Precautions/Adverse Effects
May cause skin irritation.

Veterinary-Labeled Topical Chloroxylenol Products
This list contains only products where chloroxylenol is one of the main active ingredients. For more products containing chloroxylenol (PCMX), see other topical compounds in this section.

Product (Company)	Form: Concentration	Label Status	Other Ingredients; Comments; Size(s)
Chloroxylenol Scrub® (Vedco)	Scrub: 2%	OTC	Propylene glycol, citric acid. Used for surgical scrub and preoperative skin preparation. Use full strength. Do not dilute. Labeled for dogs and cats. 1 gal.
Medicated Shampoo® (Sogeval)	Shampoo: Chloroxylenol 2% Salicylic acid 2% Sodium thiosulfate 2%	OTC	Propylene glycol, citric acid. Also has antiseborrheic effect. Labeled for dogs and cats. 16 oz; 1 gal.
Vet Solutions Sebozole Shampoo® (Vetoquinol)	Solution: Chloroxylenol 1% Miconazole nitrate 1%	OTC	Also has antimycotic effect. Labeled for dogs and cats. 8, 16 oz; 1 gal.
Vet Solutions Universal Medicated Shampoo® (Vetoquinol)	Solution: Chloroxylenol 2% Salicylic acid 2% Sodium thiosulfate 2%	OTC	Propylene glycol, citric acid. Also has antiseborrheic effect. Labeled for dogs and cats. 16 oz.
VPS Medicated Shampoo® (Jeffers)	Solution: Chloroxylenol 2% Salicylic acid 2% Sodium thiosulfate 2%	OTC	Also has antiseborrheic effect. Labeled for dogs and cats. 16 oz; 1 gal.

Human-Labeled Topical Chloroxylenol Products
There are several topical products available containing chloroxylenol usually combined with other ingredients such as hydrocortisone, menthol, pramoxine, and benzocaine. They are presented in different forms (creams, ointments, lotions and shampoos), but are not commonly used in dogs and cats. Trade names include: *Aurinol®*, *Calamycin®*, *Cortamox®*, *Cortane-B®*, *Dermacoat®* and *Foille®*

ENZYMES, TOPICAL (LACTOPEROXIDASE, LYSOZYME, LACTOFERRIN)
For otic use, refer to the Otics section

Indications/Actions
These products may be useful for bacterial and fungal skin infections and are reported to be effective against *Staphylococcus* spp., *Pseudomonas* spp., *Malassezia* spp., *Candida albicans*, *Microsporum* spp.

The can be used alone, or especially with products containing hydrocortisone, for mild itching or as an adjunctive treatment for more pruritic conditions such as atopic dermatitis.

The veterinary products contain the milk-derived enzymes lactoperoxidase, lysozyme and lactoferrin. These enzymes are reported to be effective against bacterial, fungal and viral microorganisms. Lactoperoxidase combined with hydrogen peroxide, thiocyanate, and/or iodide produce hypothiocyanate or hypoiodite ions that are bactericidal by oxidizing components of bacterial cell walls. Hypoiodite also is fungicidal. Lactoferrin acts as a bacteriostatic agent against many bacteria by depriving them of iron.

Suggested Uses/Dosages
If using spray, cream or wipes: 1–2 times a day applications. If shampoo or rinse: daily to weekly baths/after baths; leave shampoo in contact with the skin for at least 10 minutes prior to rinsing well. May be applied to affected areas 2 times a day or as needed to relief itching and soothe the skin. Refer to product label for details on individual use.

Precautions/Adverse Effects
Overall appears to be safe. No reported side effects, but skin irritation is possible.

Veterinary-Labeled Topical Products

Product (Company)	Form: Concentration	Label Status	Ingredients; Comments; Size(s)
Zymox Topical Spray® (PKB)	Spray	OTC	Lactoperoxidase, lysozyme, lactoferrin. Available with and without Hydrocortisone 1%. 2 oz.
Zymox Topical Cream® (PKB)	Cream	OTC	Lactoperoxidase, lysozyme, lactoferrin. Available with and without Hydrocortisone 1%. 1 oz.
Zymox Topical Wipes® (PKB)	Wipes	OTC	Lactoperoxidase, lysozyme, lactoferrin. Available with and without hydrocortisone 1%. 30 wipes.
Zymox Enzymatic Shampoo® (PKB)	Shampoo	OTC	Lactoperoxidase, lysozyme, lactoferrin. 12 oz.
Zymox Enzymatic Rinse® (PKB)	Rinse	OTC	Lactoperoxidase, lysozyme, lactoferrin. 12 oz.

Human-Labeled Topical Products
None

ETHYL LACTATE
(*eth*-il *lak*-tate) Etiderm®

Indications/Actions
Ethyl lactate shampoos can be used for bacterial skin infections, including surface and superficial pyodermas. It also has a keratoplastic effect, which provides anti-seborrheic activity.

A lipid soluble compound, ethyl lactate rapidly penetrates hair follicles and sebaceous glands where bacterial lipases convert it into lactic acid and ethanol, which are responsible for its antibacterial action. Ethanol helps solubolize fats and reduces sebaceous secretions. It is not as active as benzoyl peroxide against staphylococcal organisms, but it is less irritating and drying.

Suggested Dosages/Use
Daily to 2–3 weekly baths. Shampoo should remain in contact with the skin for at least 10 minutes prior to rinsing well. Refer to product label for details on individual use.

Precautions/Adverse Effects
Ethyl lactate shampoos are often used in conjunction with oral antibiotics and are usually used 2–3 times per week initially; frequency of use may be reduced when pyoderma is under control.

Avoid contact with eyes. Clients should wash hands after application or wear gloves when applying.

Adverse effects are unlikely, but local effects (erythema, pain, itching) are possible.

Veterinary-Labeled Topical Ethyl Lactate Products

Product (Company)	Form: Concentration	Label Status	Other Ingredients; Comments; Size(s)
Etiderm Shampoo® (Virbac)	Shampoo: 10% (in Spherulite® and free form)	OTC	Chitosanide (in Spherulite® and free form), benzalkonium chloride (in encapsulated form), lactic acid, propylene glycol in a shampoo base. Labeled for dogs & cats. Shake well. 8, 16 oz, 1 gal.

Human-Labeled Topical Ethyl Lactate Products
None

HYPOCHLOROUS ACID
SODIUM HYPOCHLORITE
(hye-poe-*klor*-us *ass*-id)

Indications/Actions

The proprietary products, *Vetericyn®* and *Microcyn®* contain hypochlorous acid and sodium hypochlorite and are labeled for the management of wounds, abscesses, cuts, abrasions, skin irritations, ulcers, post surgical incision sites, burns and wound odors and to accelerate healing. It may be used for prevention of bacterial skin infections or as an adjunctive topical therapy for bacterial skin infections, including Methicillin-Resistant *Staphylococcus* spp. and *Pseudomonas* spp. Hypochlorous acid also has anti-fungal and antiviral properties and is reported to reduce inflammation, pain and itching.

These products are a proprietary formulation and have broad-spectrum antimicrobial activity and act rapidly against gram-positive and gram-negative bacteria and fungal/yeast organisms. They may also be effective against viruses. The products *Vetericyn®* and *Microcyn®* contain oxychlorine (bleach-like) compounds and have a neutral pH. Mode of action is to disrupt the cellular membrane of single cell organisms. Because mode of action is primarily chemical in nature, resistance does not appear to be an issue.

Suggested Dosages/Use

Clip hair if necessary and apply spray or gel to affected areas up to 3 times a day; may be used with dressing applications on wounds. Refer to product label for details on individual use. No rinsing is required. Labeled as safe to use around eyes, nose and mouth.

Precautions/Adverse Effects

No precautions or adverse effects reported. Reported as non-toxic; does not sting or irritate the skin, however treated area may become reddened secondary to increased blood flow.

Veterinary-Labeled Topical Hypochlorous Acid Products

Product (Company)	Form: Concentration	Label Status	Other Ingredients; Comments; Size(s)
Vetericyn® VF (Innovacyn)	Spray/liquid: Hypochlorous Acid <0.1% Sodium hypochlorite 0.001%	OTC	Labeled for dogs and cats, including puppies and kittens. 4, 8, 16 oz.
Vetericyn® VF Hydrogel (Innovacyn)	Spray/gel: Hypochlorous Acid <0.1% Sodium Hypochlorite 0.001% Boric Acid 0.5%	OTC	Labeled for dogs and cats, including puppies and kittens. 4, 8, 16 oz.
Vetericyn® Wound and Infection Treatment (Innovacyn) **Vetericyn® Hot Spot Spray** (Innovacyn) **Vetericyn® Wound and Infection Treatment** (Innovacyn)	Spray/liquid: (all products contain the same formula): Hypochlorous Acid <0.01% Sodium Hypochlorite 0.001%	OTC	Depending on product, labeled for dogs, cats, horses, or all animals. 4, 8, 16 oz.

Human-Labeled Topical Hypochlorous Acid Products

Product (Company)	Form: Concentration	Label Status	Other Ingredients; Comments; Size(s)
Microcyn® Skin & Wound HydroGel **Microcyn® Dermatology HydroGel** **Microcyn® Dermatology Spray** **Microcyn® Solution with Preservatives** **Microcyn® Skin and Wound Care** **Microcyn® Negative -Pressure Wound Therapy Solution** **Puracyn® Wound and Skin Care** All products are by: Oculus Innovative	All products contain: Hypochlorous Acid 0.008% Sodium Hypochlorite 0.002%	Depending on label-ing either OTC or Rx	Product sizes range from 1.5 oz to 990 mL
Myclyns® Spray (Union Spring)	Spray: Hypochlorous Acid 0.00025% Sodium Hypochlorite 0.0036%	OTC	pH: 6.2-7.8. 2 oz.

POVIDONE IODINE

(*poe*-vi-done *eye*-oh-dine) Betadine®

Indications/Actions

Povidone iodine can be used as a topical pre-surgical skin cleanser/antiseptic and may be used for superficial pyoderma and *Malassezia* dermatitis, however; it is infrequently used in small animal dermatology due to its drying, irritating and staining effects.

An iodophore antiseptic, povidone iodine is rapidly bactericidal (against gram-positive and –negative bacteria) at low concentration. It is also fungicidal and sporicidal (as a 1% aqueous solution). Povidone acts by slowly releasing iodine to tissues. It has prolonged activity (4–6 hours), but not as long as chlorhexidine. Povidone iodine also has mild degreasing and debriding activity.

Suggested Dosages/Use

For veterinary products, refer to product label for details on individual use

Precautions/Adverse Effects

Povidone may be drying, irritating and staining to skin, hair and fabrics. Can be extremely irritating to the scrotal skin and external ears. Use with emollients may alleviate the drying effects. Avoid contact with eyes. Clients should wash hands after application or wear gloves when applying. Systemic absorption can result in renal and thyroid dysfunction.

Veterinary-Labeled Topical Povidone Iodine Products

There are several trade names used for povidone iodine products, including *Poviderm®*, *Prodine®*, *Vetadine®*, *Betadine®*, *Lanodine®*, *Viodine®* and *Povidine®*. There are also (not listed) hoof dressings, teat dips, and udder washes available that contain povidone iodine.

Note: 10% povidone iodine yields 1% titratable iodine and so forth. Labels may be confusing.

Product (Company)	Form: Concentration	Label Status	Other Ingredients; Comments; Size(s)
Poviderm Medicated Shampoo® (Butler)	Shampoo: 5%	OTC	8 oz, 1 gal.
Viodine Medicated Shampoo® (Farnam)	Shampoo: 5%	OTC	1 pt.
Povidone Iodine Solution (various manufacturers and trade names)	Solution: 10%	OTC	1 qt, 1 gal
Povidone Iodine Ointment (various manufacturers and trade names)	Ointment: 10%	OTC	1 lb.
Povidone Iodine Surgical Scrub (various manufacturers and trade names)	Scrub: 7.5%	OTC	1 gal

Human-Labeled Topical Povidone Iodine Products

There are several trade names used for povidone iodine products, including *Betadine®*, *Betagen®*, *Biodine®*, *Etodine®*, *Mallisol®*, *Minidyne®*, *Polydine®* and *Povidine®*. There are also (not listed) vaginal gels, swabs, and foaming skin cleansers available.

Product (Company)	Form: Concentration	Label Status	Other Ingredients; Size(s)
Povidone Iodine Solution (various manufacturers and trade names)	Solution: 10%	OTC (Human)	15, 30, 120 mL, 1 pt, 1 qt, 1 gal
Povidone Iodine Spray (various manufacturers and trade names)	Spray: 10%	OTC (Human)	30, 60 mL, 1 pt, 1 gal
	Aerosol: 5%	OTC (Human)	89 mL
Povidone Iodine Surgical Scrub (various manufacturers and trade names)	Scrub: 5.5 − 7.5%	OTC (Human)	15 mL, 1 pt, 1 gal
Povidone Iodine Ointment (various manufacturers and trade names)	Ointment: 10%	OTC (Human)	1 g pkts, 30, 120 g, 1 lb.

TRICLOSAN (IRGASAN)

(trye-*klose*-san)

Indications/Actions

Found in several products, often with other active ingredients, triclosan's antibacterial effects may be useful in treating superficial pyodermas. Veterinary products labeled for small animals containing triclosan as the sole active ingredient are all shampoos.

Triclosan is a bis-phenol disinfectant/antiseptic. It has activity against a wide range of organisms, including both gram-positive and gram-negative bacteria and acts via inhibiting bacterial fatty acid synthesis leading to disruption of cell membrane integrity. Triclosan reportedly is not effective against *Pseudomonas* spp. and may be less effective against staphylococci than either chlorhexidine or ethyl lactate.

Suggested Dosages/Use

Daily to weekly baths; leave shampoo in contact with the skin for at least 10 minutes prior to rinsing. For veterinary products, refer to product label for details on individual use

Precautions/Adverse Effects

Triclosan should not be used on burned or denuded skin, or mucous membranes. Avoid contact with eyes.

Triclosan is not recommended as a surgical scrub. Clients should wash hands after application or wear gloves when applying. Allergic contact reactions may occur.

Veterinary-Labeled Triclosan Products

There are also triclosan products labeled for use as teat sealants (*Uddergold Dry*®) in cattle.

Product (Company)	Form: Concentration	Label Status	Other Ingredients; Comments; Size(s)
Sebalyt Shampoo® (DVM)	Shampoo: Triclosan 0.5% Sulfur 2% Salicylic acid 2%	OTC	Labeled for dogs and cats. 8, 12 oz, 1 gal.
Triclosan Shampoo (Davis)	Shampoo: % not listed	OTC	12 oz, 1 gal.

Human-Labeled Triclosan Products

There are several human triclosan products labeled as hand, face or body washes for acne treatment. Trade names include *Septisoft*®, *Clearasil Antibacterial*®, *Clearasil Daily Face Wash*®, *Stri-Dex*®, *Oxy Medicated Soap*®, and *ASC*®.

Antifungals

CLOTRIMAZOLE, TOPICAL
(kloe-*trye*-ma-zole)   Lotrimin®

Indications/Actions

Topical clotrimazole has activity against dermatophytes and yeasts; it may be useful for localized lesions associated with *Malassezia*. It is not very effective in treating dermatophytosis in cats. Most veterinary products contain gentamicin and either, betamethasone or mometasone, and are labeled for otic use. However, these products may be used in an extra-label manner for bacterial and yeast skin infections with concurrent inflamed/pruritic skin.

Clotrimazole inhibits the biosynthesis of ergosterol, a component of fungal cell membranes leading to increased membrane permeability and probable disruption of membrane enzyme systems.

Suggested Dosages/Use

If sprays, twice daily applications are usually recommended. Ointments are generally applied to affected areas up to four times daily. For veterinary products, refer to product label for details on individual use.

Precautions/Adverse Effects

Products with clotrimazole alone:

Avoid contact with eyes and mucous membranes. Clients should wash hands after application or wear gloves when applying. Skin irritation is possible, but unlikely to occur with products containing only clotrimazole.

If using products containing betamethasone or mometasone:

Several veterinary topical products list tuberculosis of the skin or pregnancy as a contraindication. Systemic corticosteroids can be teratogenic or induce parturition during the third trimester of pregnancy in animals. If considering use during pregnancy, weigh the respective risks with treating versus potential benefits. Clients should wash hands after application or wear gloves when applying. Avoid contact with eyes. Do not allow animal to lick or chew at affected sites for at least 20–30 minutes after application. Residual activity may affect intradermal or allergy serum tests; it has been suggested to stop use 2 weeks prior to allergy testing.

Use care when treating large areas, or when used on smaller patients. Risks can be reduced by treating for only as long as necessary on as small an area as possible. Increased risks of HPA axis suppression, systemic corticosteroid effects (polydipsia/polyuria, Cushing's, gastrointestinal effects) and skin atrophy (skin fragility, alopecia, localized pyoderma and comedones are other possible complications) occur as product concentration and duration of use increases. Betamethasone may delay wound healing particularly if used longer than 7 days in duration. Vomiting and diarrhea have been reported with use of the products containing betamethasone. Local skin reactions (burning, itching, redness) are possible, but unlikely to occur.

Veterinary-Labeled Topical Clotrimazole Products
Note: There are several products containing clotrimazole for otic use; refer to that section for more information.

Product (Company)	Form: Concentration	Label Status	Other Ingredients; Size(s)
Clotrimazole Solution (Vet Solutions, Butler, Vedco)	Spray or Solution: 1%	Rx	30 mL
Otomax® Ointment (Intervet/Schering) **DVMAX® Ointment** (DVM) **Vetromax® Ointment** (Dechra) **MalOtic® Ointment** (Vedco)	Ointment (otic): All Products contain: Gentamicin 3 mg/g; Betamethasone (as valerate) 1 mg/g; Clotrimazole 10 mg/g	Rx	Mineral oil base. Approved for otic use in dogs; used in extra-label manner for bacterial skin lesions or Malassezia dermatitis; 7.5, 10, 15, 20 and 215 g bottles or tubes
MoMetaMax Otic Suspension® (Intervet/Schering-Plough)	Suspension (otic): Per gram: Mometasone 1 mg; Gentamicin 3 mg; Clotrimazole 10 mg	Rx	Mineral-oil base. Approved for otic use in dogs, but used extra-label (see above). In 7.5, 15, 30, 215 g tubes.

Human-Labeled Topical Clotrimazole Products
In addition to the products listed below, there vaginal creams and suppositories, and oral 10 mg troches.

Product (Company)	Form: Concentration	Label Status	Other Ingredients; Size(s)
Clotrimazole (various); **Cruex®** (Novartis); **Lotrimin AF®** (Schering-P); **Desenex®** (Novartis)	Solution: 1%	OTC/Rx (Human). Status determined by labeling	Depending on product: 105–113 mL
Lotrimin AF® (Schering-P);	Lotion: 1%	OTC (Human)	20 mL
Clotrimazole & Betamethasone Diprop. (Fougera) **Lotrisone®** (Schering	Lotion: Clotrimazole 1% Betamethasone dip. 0.05%	Rx (Human)	30 mL
Clotrimazole (various); **Lotrimin AF®** (Schering)	Cream: 1%	OTC/Rx (Human). Status determined by labeling	Depending on product: 10, 30 mL
Clotrimazole & Betamethasone Diprop. (generic) **Lotrisone®** (Schering)	Cream: Clotrimazole 1% Betamethasone dip. 0.05%	Rx (Human)	15, 45 g.

ENILCONAZOLE
(ee-nil-**kon**-a-zole)

Indications/Actions
Although no dosage forms are currently commercially available for topical use in the USA, enilconazole is used topically for treating dermatophytosis in small animals and horses using compounded products. A commercially available topical rinse *Imaverol®* (Janssen) 10% is available with canine, bovine and equine use labeling in many countries. Intranasal instillation of enilconazole after plaque debridement has also been shown useful in treating nasal aspergillosis in small animals.

Use of topical enilconazole on cats with dermatophytosis is somewhat controversial as there are apparently no products with feline labeling available in Europe or Canada. There are reports of safely and successfully using enilconazole on dermatophytic cats alone, or in combination with oral itraconazole.

A topical product and a poultry environmental disinfectant product (*Clinafarm EC®*) are available in the USA. This formulation has been used off-label to treat dermatophytosis at a dilution of 55.6 ml per gallon water as a topical antifungal. However, it is technically illegal to use this product other than it is labeled, as it is an EPA-licensed product in the USA.

Suggested Dosages/Use
Using *Imaverol®*: dilute as directed and wash or dip 4 times, at 3-day intervals or as directed by veterinarian. Refer to product label for details on individual use.

Precautions/Adverse Effects
Avoid contact with eyes. Clients should wear gloves when applying and use eye protection.

When used topically in cats, hypersalivation, vomiting, anorexia/weight loss, muscle weakness, and a slight increase in serum ALT levels have been reported.

Veterinary-Labeled Topical Enilconazole Products

Product (Company)	Form: Concentration	Label Status	Other Ingredients; Comments; Size(s)
Imaverol® (Janssen)	Concentrate: 10%	Not available in USA	Concentrate is diluted to 0.2% (1 part concentrate to 50 parts water). For Dogs: Dilute as directed and wash 4 times, at 3–day intervals. May also use as a dip. Not labeled for use on cats. 100 mL
Clinafarm EC® (Schering Plough)	Emulsifiable Concentrate: 13.8%	OTC-EPA Pesticide	Labeled for the control of Aspergillus fumigates contamination in poultry hatchery equipment. It is a violation of US Federal Law to use this product in a manner inconsistent with its labeling. Corrosive; may cause irreversible eye damage. Labeling includes several warnings on ingestion or exposure. 750 mL

Human-Labeled Topical Enilconazole Products
None

KETOCONAZOLE, TOPICAL

(kee-toe-*kah*-na-zole)   Nizoral®, Ketochlor®

For systemic use, see the monograph found in the main section
For otic use, see the Otics section

Indications/Actions
Topical ketoconazole has activity against dermatophytes and yeasts and ketoconazole shampoos can be effective treatment for *Malassezia* dermatitis. Patients with severe, generalized infections may require additional systemic therapy. Topical ketoconazole shampoos are generally ineffective (or minimally effective) when used alone for dermatophytosis.

Suggested Dosages/Use
If using spray or wipes/pads: 1–2 times a day. If shampoo or conditioner: daily to weekly baths/after baths; leave shampoo in contact with skin for at least 10 minutes prior to rinsing. For veterinary products, refer to product label for details on individual use.

Precautions/Adverse Effects
Avoid contact with eyes. Clients should wash hands after application or wear gloves when applying. Skin irritation is possible.

Veterinary-Labeled Topical Ketoconazole Products

Product (Company)	Form: Concentration	Label Status	Other Ingredients; Comments; Size(s)
Ketoseb-D® Spray (Sogeval)	Spray: Chlorhexidine 2% Ketoconazole 1%	Rx	Labeled for dogs and cats. 8 oz.
Mal-A-Ket Plus TrizEDTA Spray® (Dechra)	Leave-on Spray: Chlorhexidine 2% Ketoconazole 1% TrizEDTA	Rx	Labeled for dogs and cats. 8 oz.
Malacetic Ultra Spray® (Dechra)	Spray: Ketoconazole 0.15% Hydrocortisone 1% Acetic Acid 1% Boric Acid 2%	Rx	Labeled for dogs and cats. 8 oz.
Ketoseb-D® Wipes (Sogeval)	Wipes: Chlorhexidine 2% Ketoconazole 1%	Rx	Labeled for dogs and cats. 50 count jar.
Mal-A-Ket® Wipes (Dechra)	Wipes: Chlorhexidine 2% Ketoconazole 1% Acetic Acid 2%	Rx	Labeled for dogs and cats. 50 count jar.
Mal-A-Ket Plus TrizEDTA® Flush (Dechra)	Flush: Chlorhexidine 0.15% Ketoconazole 0.15% TrizEDTA	Rx	A multicleanse flush to aid in the treatment of bacterial and fungal (dermatophytosis and malassezia) infections. pH 8. Labeled for dogs and cats. 4, 12 oz.
Ketoseb-D® Flush (Sogeval)	Flush: Chlorhexidine 2% Ketoconazole 1%	OTC	Labeled for dogs and cats. 4, 16 oz.

Product (Company)	Form: Concentration	Label Status	Other Ingredients; Comments; Size(s)
Mal-A-Ket® Shampoo (Dechra)	Shampoo: Ketoconazole 2% Acetic Acid 2% Chlorhexidine 2%	Rx	Labeled for dogs and cats. 1 oz pouch, 8 oz; 1 gal.
Ketochlor Shampoo® (Virbac)	Shampoo: Chlorhexidine 2.3% Ketoconazole 1%	Rx	Spherulites® Microcapsules. Glycotechnology (monosaccharides: L-rhamnose, D-mannose, D-galactose; polysaccharide: alkyl polyglucoside), chitosanide. Labeled for dogs and cats. 8, 16 oz, 1 gal.
ResiKetoChlor Leave-On Conditioner® (Virbac)	Conditioner: Chlorhexidine 4% Ketoconazole 1%	OTC	Spherulites® Microcapsules. Glycotechnology (monosaccharides: L-rhamnose, D-mannose, D-galactose; polysaccharide: alkyl polyglucoside), chitosanide. Labeled for dogs and cats. 8 oz.

Human-Labeled Topical Ketoconazole Products

Product (Company)	Form: Concentration	Label Status	Other Ingredients; Size(s)
Nizoral A-D® (McNeil)	Shampoo: 1%	OTC (Human)	207 mL
Nizoral® (McNeil)	Shampoo: 2%	Rx (Human)	Aqueous suspension. 120 mL
Ketoconazole (Clay-Park)	Shampoo: 2%	Rx (Human)	118 mL
Ketoconazole (Teva)	Cream: 2%	Rx (Human)	Aqueous vehicle containing cetyl alcohol, stearyl alcohol, sodium sulfite. 15, 30 60 g.
Nizoral® (McNeil)	Cream: 2%	Rx (Human)	15, 30, 60 g.

LIME SULFUR (SULFURATED LIME SOLUTION)

(lyme sul-fur)   Lymdyp®

Indications/Actions

Lime sulfur applications are very effective and relatively inexpensive as a generalized topical treatment for dermatophytosis. Both lime sulfur and enilconazole are thought to have the most topical activity against *M. canis* of commercially available compounds. In addition, it is the most efficacious treatment of surface demodicosis (*Demodex gatoi*) in cats. Lime sulfur can also be useful in the adjunctive treatment of Malassezia dermatitis, Cheyletiellosis, Chiggers, Sarcoptic and Notoedric mange, fur mites, lice, canine demodicosis and sarcoptic mange.

Lime sulfur has antibacterial and antifungal (and some anti-yeast) properties secondary to the formation of pentathionic acid and hydrogen sulfide after application. Both lime sulfur and enilconazole are thought to have the most topical activity against *M. canis*. Lime sulfur may also have keratolytic, keratoplastic, antiparasitic, and antipruritic effects.

Suggested Dosages/Use

Labeled dose for *LymDyp®* and *Vet Solutions Lime Sulfur Dip®*: Shake well; dilute 4 oz. of concentrate in one gal of water. Mix well. Apply as a rinse or dip at 5–7 day intervals. Do not rinse. For more chronic or resistant cases, may be used at 8 oz per gal.

Labeled dose for *LimePlus Dip®* and *Lime Sulfur Dip®*: Pour 4 oz. of concentrate in one gal of water. Mix well. Bathe animal prior to application. Rinse off shampoo. Pour entire contents of diluted *LimePlus Dip®* onto pet and work into skin. Apply as a rinse, spray or dip at 5–7 day intervals. Allow to dry on the animal. Do not rinse. When used for dermatophytosis, once to twice weekly treatments have been recommended, if patients can tolerate the treatment's irritating effects, until 2 consecutive negative cultures are obtained. When used for confirmed cases of feline surface demodicosis, applications are recommended every 5–7 days for a total of 6 treatments. If using lime sulfur as a treatment trial for surface demodicosis, 3 applications should be performed and if there is significant improvement in clinical signs, 3 more applications should be performed to complete treatment. If no significant improvement is seen after 3 applications, demodicosis should be ruled out and other diagnosis should be considered.

Precautions/Adverse Effects

Avoid contact with eyes and mucous membranes. Can stain porous surface (*e.g.*, concrete, porcelain) or permanently discolor jewelry. Clients should wear gloves and protect skin and eyes from solution. Because of its very unpleasant odor, application should be performed in a well-ventilated area or clients should wear a protective (respirator-type) mask.

While reasonably non-toxic, lime sulfur may cause skin irritation or drying. Adding mineral oil to the solution may reduce its drying effects. Lime sulfur can stain (temporarily) light colored fur and rarely cause hair loss on the pinnae in cats. Lime sulfur's odor may persist on treated animals, but generally is tolerable once the patient dries. Oral ingestion can rarely cause nausea and oral ulcers, mainly in cats; an Elizabethan collar may help prevent this from occurring.

Veterinary-Labeled Lime Sulfur Products

Product (Company)	Form: Concentration	Label Status	Other Ingredients; Comments; Size(s)
LymDyp® (DVM)	Concentrate: 76.9%	OTC	Labeled for dogs, puppies, kittens and cats. Shake well and dilute before use (see dosages above). 16 oz, 1 gal.
LimePlus Dip® (Dechra)	Concentrate: 97.8%	OTC	Labeled for dogs, puppies, kittens and cats. Shake well and dilute before use (see dosages above). 4, 16 oz., 1 gal.
Vet Solutions Lime Sulfur Dip® (Vetoquinol)	Concentrate: 97.8%	OTC	Labeled for dogs, puppies, kittens and cats. Shake well and dilute before use (see dosages above). 4, 16 oz.
Lime Sulfur Dip® (Davis)	Concentrate: 97.8%	OTC	Labeled for dogs, puppies, kittens and cats. Shake well and dilute before use (see dosages above). 16 oz.
LymDyp® Spray (DVM)	Solution: 76.9%	Rx	Labeled for dogs, puppies, kittens and cats. Scented (less strong odor compared to concentrated solutions). Already diluted and ready to use. 16 oz.

Human-Labeled Lime Sulfur Products
None

MICONAZOLE, TOPICAL
(mye-**kah**-nah-zole)

For otic use, refer to the Otics section

Indications/Actions
Topical miconazole has activity against dermatophytes and yeast. It is especially effective for the treatment of *Malassezia* dermatitis. Patients with severe, generalized infections may require systemic therapy. Lotions, sprays and creams are generally used for localized lesions associated with *Malassezia* sp. or dermatophytes. Topical miconazole products are generally ineffective (or minimally effective) when used alone for dermatophytosis; adjunctive systemic treatment is usually required.

Miconazole's actions are a result of altering permeability of fungal cellular membranes and interfering with peroxisomal and mitochondrial enzymes, leading to intracellular necrosis. Miconazole products are fungicidal with repeated application.

Suggested Dosages/Use
If using spray, creams, lotions or wipes/pads: 1–2 times a day applications. If using a shampoo or conditioner: daily to weekly baths; leave in contact with skin for at least 10 minutes prior to rinsing. For veterinary products, refer to product label for details on individual use.

Precautions/Adverse Effects
Avoid contact with eyes. Clients should wash hands after application or wear gloves when applying. Do not allow animal lick or chew at affected areas for at least 20-30 minutes after application.

Skin irritation is possible, but unlikely to occur, but in very inflamed, eroded to ulcerated skin, the pledgets, wipes, towelettes, and spray containing alcohol (*Malaseb®*) can be severely irritating.

Veterinary-Labeled Topical Miconazole Products
Note: Miconazole nitrate is the salt generally used in pharmaceutical products. While technically, a 1% concentration of miconazole nitrate contains less than 1% miconazole, the following products are rounded to the closest full percent regardless of how much miconazole base is actually in each product.

Product (Company)	Form: Concentration	Label Status	Other Ingredients; Comments; Size(s)
Micro-Pearls Advantage Miconazole 1% Spray® (Vetoquinol)	Spray: 1%	Rx	Labeled for dogs, cats, & horses. 4 oz.
Conofite Spray® 1% (Intervet/Schering-Plough)	Spray: 1%	Rx	Labeled for dogs and cats. 60 mL
Micaved Spray® 1% (Vedco)	Spray: 1%	Rx	Labeled for use on dogs and cats. 60 mL
Malaseb® Spray (DVM)	Spray: Miconazole nitrate 2% Chlorhexidine 2%	OTC	Alcohol 30%. Labeled for use in dogs, cats, & horses. 8 oz.

Product (Company)	Form: Concentration	Label Status	Other Ingredients; Comments; Size(s)
Micazole Spray® (Butler)	Spray: 1%	Rx	Labeled for use on dogs and cats. 120, 240 mL
Malaseb® Flush (DVM)	Flush: Miconazole nitrate 2% Chlorhexidine 2%	OTC	Labeled for use on dogs and cats. 4, 12 oz.
Malaseb® Concentrate Rinse (DVM)	Rinse: Miconazole nitrate 5.2% Chlorhexidine 5.9%	Rx	Labeled for use on dogs, cats, and horses. Must be diluted before use. 8, 32 oz.
Malaseb® Pledgets (DVM)	Pledget (medicated pad): 17.4 Miconazole 20 mg Chlorhexidine	OTC	Alcohol 30%. Labeled for use in dogs, cats, & horses. 60 per container.
Malaseb® Towelettes (DVM)	Towelettes: Miconazole 20 mg Chlorhexidine 20 mg	OTC	Alcohol 30%. Labeled for dogs, and cats. 12 and 60 count jars.
Conofite Cream® 2% (Intervet/Schering-Plough)	Cream: 2%	Rx	Labeled for use on dogs and cats. 15 g
Resizole Leave-On Lotion® (Virbac)	Lotion: 2%	Rx	Labeled for use on dogs and cats. 8 oz.
Priconazole Lotion® 1% (First Priority)	Lotion: 1%	Rx	Polyethylene glycol, ethyl alcohol. Labeled for dogs and cats. 60 mL
Miconosol Lotion 1%® (Med-Pharmex)	Lotion: 1%	Rx	Labeled for use on dogs and cats. 60 mL
Conofite Lotion® 1% (Intervet/Schering-Plough)	Lotion: 1%	Rx	Labeled for use on dogs and cats. 30 mL
Micaved Lotion® 1% (Vedco)	Lotion: 1%	Rx	Labeled for use on dogs and cats. 60 mL
Micazole Lotion® 1% (Butler)	Lotion: 1%	Rx	Labeled for use on dogs and cats. 60 mL
Sebazole® Shampoo (Vet Solutions)	Shampoo: Miconazole 2%, Chlorxylenol 1%	Rx	Salicylic acid, sodium thiosulfate. Labeled for dogs, cats, and horses. 8, 12 oz, 1 gal.
Dermazole Shampoo® (Virbac)	Shampoo: Miconazole 2%, Salicylic Acid 2%	Rx	Labeled for use on dogs and cats. 6, 16 oz.
Malaseb Shampoo® (DVM)	Shampoo: Miconazole 2%, Chlorhexidine 2%	OTC	Labeled for dogs, cats, and horses. 8, 12 oz, 1 gal.

Human-Labeled Topical Miconazole Products

In addition to the products listed below, there are 2% topical vaginal creams, vaginal suppositories, 2% powders and spray powders available. Most human-labeled products are OTC.

Product (Company)	Form: Concentration	Label Status	Other Ingredients; Size(s)
Micatin® (Ortho); **Neosporin AF®** (Pfizer); **Lotrimin AF®** (Schering); **Prescription Strength Desenex®** (Ciba)	Spray (liquid): 2%	OTC (Human)	Depending on product: 90-115 mL
Tetterine® (SSS Co.)	Ointment: 2%	OTC (Human)	30 g.
Zeosorb-AF® (Stiefel)	Gel: 2%	OTC (Human)	24 g.
Miconazole Nitrate (Taro); **Micatin®** (Ortho); **Monistat-Derm®** (Ortho); **Neosporin AF®** (Pfizer)	Cream: 2%	OTC (Human)	Depending on product: 15, 30, 90 g

NYSTATIN

(nye-**sta**-tin)

For oral use, see the monograph found in the main section.

Indications/Actions

Because of limited dosage forms and other alternative antiyeast medications readily available, nystatin is not usually used alone in small animal medicine. The combination products (*e.g.*, *Panalog®*, etc.) can be useful for topical lesions caused by yeasts or yeast-like organisms; they have been used for mixed otitis infections for many years.

Nystatin has efficacy against many yeasts and yeast-like organisms (*Malassezia*). Its mechanism of action is believed secondary to binding to sterols in the fungal cell membranes thereby increasing membrane permeability with leakage of intracellular components. Nystatin does not have activity against bacteria and is ineffective against other fungi.

Suggested Dosages/Use

Nystatin (topical) is rarely used alone in veterinary medicine. In humans, the cream is usually used instead of the ointment in treating candidal-infections involving intertriginous areas; nystatin topical powder is best used for very moist lesions.

Nystatin products that contain triamcinolone are best suited for focal (*e.g.*, pedal) or multifocal lesions for relatively short durations (*e.g.*, less than 2 months). Initially, topical corticosteroids are usually used sparingly 1–4 times per day and then frequency is tapered when control is achieved.

Precautions/Adverse Effects

Avoid contact with eyes. Clients should wash hands after application or wear gloves when applying

Nystatin alone is very safe, although hypersensitivity reactions are possible. The combination veterinary products are usually well tolerated when used on skin. Neomycin can cause localized sensitivity and those containing glucocorticoids can potentially cause cutaneous atrophy HPA-axis suppression.

Veterinary-Labeled Nystatin-Containing Topical Products

Product (Company)	Form: Concentration	Label Status	Other Ingredients; Comments; Size(s)
Derma-Vet Cream® (Med-Pharmex)	Cream: Nystatin 100,000 units/g Triamcinolone Acet. 1 mg Neomycin Sulf. 2.5 mg Thiostrepton 2,500 units	Rx	Aqueous vanishing cream. Labeled for use in dogs or cats. 7.5, 15 g.
Panalog Ointment® (Pfizer) **Animax Ointment®** (Dechra) **Quadratop Ointment®** (Butler) **Derma-Vet Ointment®** (Med-Pharmex) **Dermalog Ointment®** (RXV)	Ointment: Nystatin 100,000 units/g Triamcinolone Acet. 1 mg Neomycin Sulf. 2.5 mg Thiostrepton 2,500 units	Rx	Labeled for use in dogs or cats. 7.5, 15, 30, 240 mL

Human-Labeled Topical Nystatin Products

In addition to the products listed below, there are vaginal tablets and oral products. Oral products are found in the main section.

Product (Company)	Form: Concentration	Label Status	Other Ingredients; Size(s)
Nystatin (various)	Powder: 100,000 units/g	Rx (Human)	Depending on product: 15, 30, 60 g.
Nystatin (various)	Ointment: 100,000 units/g	Rx (Human)	Depending on product: 15, 30 g.
Nystatin (various)	Cream: 100,000 units/g	Rx (Human)	Depending on product: 15, 30, 240 g.
Nystatin-Triamcinolone Acetonide (various) **Mycogen II®** (Goldline) **Mycolog-II®** (Bristol Meyers Squibb) **Myco-Triacet II®** (Lemmon)	Ointment: Nystatin 100,000 units/g Triamcinolone Acet. 0.1%	Rx (Human)	Depending on product: 15, 30, 60, 120 g.
Nystatin-Triamcinolone Acetonide (various) **Mycogen II®** (Goldline) **Mycolog-II®** (Bristol Meyers Squibb) **Myco-Triacet II®** (Lemmon) **Myconel®** (Marnel)	Cream: Nystatin 100,000 units/g Triamcinolone Acet. 0.1%	Rx (Human)	Depending on product: 1.5 g. pkts, 15, 30, 60, 120 g.

SELENIUM SULFIDE

(si-*leen*-ee-um *sul*-fide)

Indications/Actions

Selenium sulfide may be useful in seborrheic disorders (mainly for seborrhea oleosa) and for adjunctive treatment of *Malassezia* dermatitis, particularly in dogs exhibiting signs of waxy, greasy or scaly (seborrheic) dermatitis. There may be some residual activity on the skin.

Selenium sulfide possesses antifungal (including sporicidal activity), keratolytic, keratoplastic and degreasing properties. It affects cells of the epidermis and follicular epithelium (alters the epidermal turnover) and interferes with hydrogen bond formation of keratin thereby reducing corneocyte production. Selenium sulfide's antifungal mechanism of action is not well understood.

Suggested Dosages/Use

Frequency of shampooing will vary according to the patient's needs. When using a medicated shampoo allow 10 minutes contact time. Another acceptable regimen is to allow the shampoo act for 3–5 minutes, rinse it thoroughly and thereafter repeat the procedure. Completely rinse to prevent skin irritation and/or excessive drying.

Precautions/Adverse Effects
Selenium sulfide products should **not be used on cats.** Avoid contact with eyes. Selenium sulfide can discolor jewelry. Clients should wear gloves when using these products.

Selenium sulfide can be irritating, cause excessive drying and hair-coat staining. Mucous membranes and scrotal areas may be particularly sensitive to the irritating effects of the drug.

After discontinuation, a rebound seborrhea can occur where signs could be worse than prior to treatment. Gastrointestinal effects (nausea, vomiting, diarrhea) may occur selenium sulfide is ingested orally. Neurologic signs are possible if large quantities are ingested. Contact an animal poison center if a substantial oral ingestion occurs.

Veterinary-Labeled Topical Selenium Sulfide Products
There apparently are no labeled veterinary products containing selenium sulfide currently available in the USA; *Seleen*® may be available in other countries.

Human-Labeled Topical Selenium Sulfide Products

Product (Company)	Form: Concentration	Label Status	Other Ingredients; Size(s)
Selenium Sulfide (various)	Shampoo/Lotion: 1%	OTC (Human)	210 mL
Selsun Blue Medicated Treatment® (Chattem)	Shampoo/Lotion: 1%	OTC (Human)	Menthol. 325 mL
Head & Shoulders Intensive Treatment® (P&G)	Shampoo/Lotion: 1%	OTC (Human)	400 mL
Selenium Sulfide (various)	Lotion: 2.5%	Rx (Human)	120 mL
Selsun® (Abbott)	Lotion: 2.5%	Rx (Human)	120 mL

TERBINAFINE HCL, TOPICAL

(ter-**bin**-a-feen)   Lamisil®

For systemic use, see the monograph found in the main section

Indications/Actions
An allylamine antifungal agent, terbinafine may be useful for localized lesions associated with *Malassezia*. With its current topical dosage forms, it does not appear to be very useful for treating dermatophytosis in cats.

Terbinafine inhibits the biosynthesis of ergosterol, but its mechanism for inhibiting ergosterol is different from the azole antifungals. Terbinafine inhibits the fungal squalene epoxidase enzyme. The resultant depletion of ergosterol within the fungal cell membrane and the intracellular accumulation of squalene are believed to be responsible for the fungicidal effect of terbinafine. It is fungicidal against dermatophytes, but may only be fungistatic against yeasts.

Suggested Dosages/Use
Topical terbinafine is not commonly used in veterinary medicine at present, but it could be used topically to affected areas once to twice a day.

Precautions/Adverse Effects
Avoid contact with eyes and mucous membranes. Clients should wash hands after application or wear gloves when applying. Skin irritation is possible, but unlikely to occur.

Veterinary-Labeled Topical Terbinafine Products
None

Human-Labeled Topical Terbinafine Products

Product (Company)	Form: Concentration	Label Status	Other Ingredients; Size(s)
Lamisil AT® (Ciba-Geigy); generic	Cream: 1%	OTC (Human)	15, 30 g
Lamisil® (Ciba-Geigy)	Solution: 1%	Rx (Human)	Alcohol. 30 mL
Lamisil AT®	Spray: 1%	OTC (Human)	Ethanol, benzyl alcohol. 30 mL
Lamisil Advanced® (Ciba-Geigy)	Gel: 1%	OTC (Human)	Ethanol, propylene glycol. 6 & 12 g

Keratolytic Agents

Also see the:
- ■ **BENZOYL PEROXIDE** monograph in the Antibacterials section
- ■ **PHYTOSPHINGOSINE** monograph in the Non-Corticosteroid Antipruritic/Antiinflammatories section
- ■ **SELENIUM SULFIDE** monograph in the Antifungals section

SALICYLIC ACID
(sal-i-*sil*-ic *ass*-id)

Indications/Actions
Often combined with sulfur, salicylic acid shampoos are employed to treat patients with seborrheic disorders (seborrhea sicca and oleosa) exhibiting mild to moderate scaling, with mild waxy and keratinous debris. When combined with benzoyl peroxide, salicylic acid and sulfur containing shampoos can also be used to manage seborrhea oleosa. In higher concentrations, topicals such as *Kerasolv® Gel* (6.6% salicylic acid) can be used to remove localized excessive tissues associated with hyperkeratotic disorders, such as calluses and idiopathic thickening of the planum nasale and footpads.

Salicylic acid has mildly antipruritic, antibacterial (bacteriostatic), keratoplastic and keratolytic actions. Lower concentrations are primarily keratoplastic and higher concentrations, keratolytic. Salicylic acid lowers skin pH, increases corneocyte hydration and dissolves the intercellular binder between corneocytes. Salicylic acid and sulfur are thought to be synergistic in their keratolytic actions.

Suggested Dosages/Use
Frequency of shampooing will vary according to the patient's needs. When using a medicated shampoo allow 10 minutes contact time. Another acceptable regimen is to allow the shampoo act for 3-5 minutes, rinse it thoroughly and thereafter repeat the procedure. Completely rinse to prevent skin irritation and/or excessive drying.

Precautions/Adverse Effects
Avoid contact with eyes, mucous membranes and open sores/cuts. Clients should wash hands after application or wear gloves when applying.

Skin irritation is possible. Burning, itching, pain, erythema, swelling can occur from salicylic acid, particularly when used in higher concentrations (> 2%). A rebound seborrheic effect can occur.

Veterinary-Labeled Topical Salicylic Acid Products

Product (Company)	Form: Concentration	Label Status	Other Ingredients; Size(s)
Kerasolv Gel® (DVM)	Gel: 6.6%	OTC	Labeled for use on dogs, cats, & horses. Other ingredients (humectants): sodium lactate and urea, propylene glycol. Rub in well. Usually used once daily initially, may reduced to 2−3 times per week once remission occurs. Often requires life-long treatment. 30 mL
Derma-Clens® Cream (Pfizer)	Cream: Salicylic acid, Benzoic acid, Malic acid. Concentrations not listed (proprietary).	OTC	Labeled as an acidic cleansing cream for use on wounds, abrasions, burns, and other dermatological conditions. 1oz, 14 oz.
Dermazole Shampoo® (Virbac)	Shampoo: Miconazole 2% Salicylic Acid 2%	Rx/OTC	6, 16 oz.
Sebalyt Shampoo® (DVM)	Shampoo: Triclosan 0.5% Sulfur 2% Salicylic acid 2%	OTC	8, 12 oz, 1 gal.
Nova Pearls Medicated Dandruff Shampoo® (Tomlyn)	Shampoo: Salicylic Acid 2% Sulfur 2%	OTC	Novasome® moisturizers. 12 oz, 1 gal.
Keratolux Shampoo® (Virbac)	Shampoo: Salicylic Acid 1% Zinc Gluconate 0.5% Pyridoxine 0.5%	OTC	Spherulites®, fatty acids, tea tree leaf oil. Shake well; wear gloves. 8, 16 oz; 1 gal
Sebolux Shampoo® (Virbac)	Shampoo: Salicylic Acid 2% Sulfur 2%	OTC	Chitosanide, urea, glycerin. Ingredients in free form and in Spherulites®. Shake well; wear gloves. 8, 16 oz; 1 gal
Oxiderm® Shampoo (Sogeval)	Shampoo: Salicylic acid 2% Benzoyl peroxide 3% Sulfur 2%	OTC	8, 16 oz,

Product (Company)	Form: Concentration	Label Status	Other Ingredients; Size(s)
Oxiderm® Shampoo + PS (Sogeval)	Shampoo: Salicylic acid 2% Benzoyl peroxide 3% Microsized sulfur 2% Phytosphingosine HCl 0.05%	OTC	8, 16 oz, 1 gal
Micro Pearls Advantage Seba-Moist Shampoo® (Vetoquinol)	Shampoo: Salicylic Acid 2% Sulfur 2%	Rx	Novasome® microvesicles. Labeled for dogs and cats. Shake well; wear gloves. 12 oz, 1 gal.
Micro Pearls Advantage Seba-Hex Shampoo® (Vetoquinol)	Shampoo: Chlorhexidine 2% Salicylic Acid 2% Sulfur 2%	Rx	Novasome® microvesicles. Labeled for dogs, cats and horses. Shake well; wear gloves. 12 oz, 1 gal.
Vet Solutions Universal Medicated Shampoo® (Vetoquinol)	Solution: Chloroxylenol 2% Salicylic acid 2% Sodium thiosulfate 2%	OTC	Propylene glycol, citric acid. Also has antiseborrheic effect. Labeled for dogs and cats. 16 oz.
NuSal-T® (DVM)	Shampoo: Salicylic acid 3%, Coal Tar 2%, menthol 1%	OTC	Labeled for dogs; in 237 mL, 355 mL & 3.78 L

Human-Labeled Topical Salicylic Acid Products
Note: There are many topical salicylic acid products labeled for human use, including topical creams, ointments, transdermal patches, liquids and gels that are principally labeled for wart removal. Except for one product (*Salex®*; 6% cream), they are available OTC. There are also many OTC skin cleansers and shampoos containing salicylic acid and usually sulfur (sometimes coal tar or menthol). As there are several similar products formulated and labeled for animal use, human products will not be listed. For more information on these products, refer to a comprehensive human drug reference or contact a pharmacist.

SULFUR, PRECIPITATED
(**sul**-fer)

Indications/Actions
Often combined with salicylic acid, sulfur-containing shampoos are often employed to treat patients with seborrheic disorders exhibiting mild to moderate scaling, with mild waxiness and keratinous debris.

Sulfur has keratoplastic and keratolytic actions. Lower concentrations of sulfur are primarily keratoplastic secondary to assisting conversion of cysteine to cystine, thought an important factor in the maturation of corneocytes. Like salicylic acid, sulfur's keratolytic effects increase with concentration. Salicylic acid and sulfur are believed synergistic in their keratolytic actions. Sulfur also has mild degreasing effects and can be mildly antipruritic.

Sulfur also has antibacterial, antifungal, and antiparasitic effects secondary to sulfur conversion to hydrogen sulfide and pentathionic acid by bacteria and keratocytes.

Suggested Dosages/Use
Frequency of shampooing will vary according to the patient's needs. When using a medicated shampoo allow 10 minutes contact time. Another acceptable regimen is to allow the shampoo act for 3-5 minutes, rinse it thoroughly and thereafter repeat the procedure. Completely rinse to prevent skin irritation and/or excessive drying.

Precautions/Adverse Effects
Avoid contact with eyes, mucous membranes and open sores/cuts. Clients should wash hands after application or wear gloves when applying.

Skin irritation is possible. Sulfur can be drying, cause pruritus and be irritating. Residual odor is often bothersome to clients. Sulfur may stain fabrics and hair. A rebound seborrheic effect can occur when using shampoo products containing sulfur.

Veterinary-Labeled Topical Sulfur Products

Product (Company)	Form: Concentration	Label Status	Other Ingredients; Size(s)
Sebalyt Shampoo® (DVM)	Shampoo: Triclosan 0.5% Sulfur 2% Salicylic acid 2%	OTC	8, 12 oz, 1 gal.
Micro Pearls Advantage Seba-Hex Shampoo® (Vetoquinol)	Shampoo: Chlorhexidine 2% Salicylic Acid 2% Sulfur 2%	Rx	*Novasome®* microvesicles. Labeled for dogs, cats and horses. Shake well; wear gloves. 12 oz, 1 gal.
Micro Pearls Advantage Seba-Moist Shampoo® (Vetoquinol)	Shampoo: Salicylic Acid 2% Sulfur 2%	Rx	*Novasome®* microvesicles. Labeled for dogs and cats. Shake well; wear gloves. 12 oz, 1 gal.
Sebolux Shampoo® (Virbac)	Shampoo: Salicylic Acid 2% Sulfur 2%	OTC	Chitosanide, urea, glycerin. Ingredients in free form and in *Spherulites®*. Shake well; wear gloves. 8, 16 oz; 1 gal
Oxiderm® Shampoo (Sogeval)	Shampoo: Sulfur 2% Salicylic acid 2% Benzoyl peroxide 3%	OTC	8, 16 oz
Oxiderm Shampoo + PS (Sogeval)	Shampoo: Microsized sulfur 2% Salicylic acid 2% Benzoyl peroxide 3% Phytosphingosine HCl 0.05%	OTC	8, 16 oz, 1 gal
Keratolux Shampoo® (Virbac)	Shampoo: Salicylic Acid 1% Zinc Gluconate 0.5% Pyridoxine 0.5%	OTC	*Spherulites®*, fatty acids, tea tree leaf oil. Shake well; wear gloves. 8, 16 oz, 1 gal
Dermapet Dermasebs Shampoo® (Dermapet)	Shampoo: Salicylic Acid 2% Sulfur 2%	OTC	8 oz, 1 gal
Nova Pearls Medicated Dandruff Shampoo® (Tomlyn)	Shampoo: Salicylic Acid 2% Sulfur 2%	OTC	*Novasome®* moisturizers. 12 oz, 1 gal.
Paraguard Shampoo® (First Priority)	Shampoo: Captan 2% Sulfur 1%	OTC	Labeled as an anti-ringworm, antifungal, antibacterial shampoo for dogs, cats & horses. 32 oz.
Sulf OxyDex Shampoo® (DVM)	Shampoo: Benzoyl peroxide 2.5% Sulfur (micronized) 2%	Rx	8, 12 oz, 1 gal.
Medicated Shampoo (Vet Solutions, Sogeval)	Shampoo: Sodium Thiosulfate 2% (source of soluble sulfur) Salicylic Acid 2% Chloroxylenol 2%	OTC	16 oz, 1 gal

Human-Labeled Topical Sulfur Products

Note: There are several topical products containing sulfur labeled for human use, including topical creams, lotions, shampoos, soaps and masks that are principally labeled for acne or dandruff. For more information on these products, refer to a comprehensive human drug reference (*e.g., Facts and Comparisons*) or contact a pharmacist.

COAL TAR
(kole tar)

Indications/Actions
Use of coal tar containing shampoos in veterinary medicine is somewhat controversial, particularly since almost all veterinary-labeled products have been withdrawn from the market. However, coal tar shampoos have been used in dogs for treating greasy dermatoses (seborrhea oleosa) for many years.

Coal tar possesses keratoplastic, keratolytic, vasoconstrictive, antipruritic, and degreasing actions. Coal tar's mechanism of keratoplastic (keratoregulating) action is probably secondary to decreasing mitosis and DNA synthesis of basal epidermal cells.

Suggested Dosages/Use

Frequency of shampooing will vary according to the patient's needs. When using a medicated shampoo allow 10 minutes contact time. Another acceptable regimen is to allow the shampoo act for 3–5 minutes, rinse it thoroughly and thereafter repeat the procedure. Completely rinse to prevent skin irritation and/or excessive drying.

Precautions/Adverse Effects

The carcinogenic risks associated with coal tar products are hotly debated. At present, most (including the FDA) believe that coal tar products with concentrations of 5% or less are safe for human use. However, should they be used on animals, clients should wear gloves when applying and wash off any product that contacts their skin. Carcinogenic risk assessment for dogs using coal tar products was not located.

Coal tar products should **not be used on cats**, patients who have prior sensitivity reactions to tar products or have dry scaling dermatoses.

Be careful in comparing coal tar concentrations on labels. Coal tar solution contains approximately 20% coal tar extract or refined tar. For example, a 10% coal tar solution contains approximately 2% coal tar (refined).

Photosensitization, skin drying and skin irritation are possible with tar therapy. Adverse effects are more likely with tar concentrations greater than 3%. Residual odor is often bothersome to clients. Tar may stain fabrics or haircoats and discolor jewelry.

Veterinary-Labeled Coal Tar-Containing Products

Product (Company)	Form: Concentration (Concentrations listed as refined tar or extract)	Label Status	Other Ingredients; Size(s)
NuSal-T® (IVX)	Shampoo: Coal Tar 2%, Salicylic acid 3%, menthol 1%	OTC (Human)	Labeled for dogs; in 237 mL, 355 mL & 3.78 L

Human-Labeled Coal Tar-Containing Products

There several products labeled for human use that contain coal tar, including ointments, lotions, creams, and shampoos available in concentrations ranging from 0.5%-5% coal tar (not coal tar extract).

Antiseborrheic Products

See the:

■ **BENZOYL PEROXIDE** monograph in the Antibacterials section

■ **ESSENTIAL FATTY ACIDS, TOPICAL** monograph in the Non-Corticosteroid Antipruritic/Antiinflammatories section

■ **PHYTOSPHINGOSINE** monograph in the Non-Corticosteroid Antipruritic/Antiinflammatories section

■ **SELENIUM SULFIDE** monograph in the Antifungals section

■ **SALICYLIC ACID, SULFUR and COAL TAR** monographs in the Keratolytics section

Immunomodulators, Topical

IMIQUIMOD, TOPICAL

(imi-i-*kwi*-mod)   Aldara®

Indications/Actions

An immune response modifier, imiquimod may be useful in the treatment of a variety of topical conditions in animals. It is labeled for use on humans as a treatment for genital or perianal warts, superficial basal cell carcinomas and actinic keratoses of the face and scalp. In dogs and cats, imiquimod potentially may be of benefit in treating feline herpes virus dermatitis, actinic keratosis, squamous cell carcinoma and Bowen's disease, papillomas virus lesions, and localized solar dermatitis or solar carcinoma *in situ*. Many of these indications are based upon anecdotal evidence, as there are very few studies published for veterinary use. In horses, imiquimod has been anecdotally used with success in treating sarcoids.

Imiquimod stimulates the patient's own immune system to release a variety of cytokines including interferon-alpha and interleukin-12. This locally generated cytokine milieu induces a Th1-immune response with the generation of cytotoxic effectors Imiquimod itself does not have in vitro activity against wart viruses, but stimulates monocytes and macrophages to release cytokines that induce a regression in viral protein production.

Suggested Dosages/Use

Use in animals is still rather limited and ongoing research on this agent is being performed. Doses and treatment regimens will vary depending on the disease treated and tolerance to the drug. At present, dosing ranges from applying a thin film once daily to 2–3 times weekly or every-other-week. Treatment duration and frequency may need to be adjusted depending on patient response and adverse reactions.

Precautions/Adverse Effects

Clients administering the drug should wear gloves when handling or applying the cream. It is advised to avoid getting in eyes or on mucous membranes; but dogs with oral mucosal papillomas have been treated without significant problems. While there are low chances the drug would be absorbed systemically, do not allow animal to groom/lick the applied site; occlusive dressings should not be used over the treatment site. Application site should not be touched after application. Avoid exposure of the site to sunlight; there is concern that there may be an increased risk for sunburn after use (not proven).

Local skin reactions are common with imiquimod therapy and include application site reactions: erythema, burning, tenderness, pain, irritation, oozing/exudate and erosion. Treatment duration and frequency may need to be adjusted depending on response and irritant reactions. Depigmentation and hair loss may occur at application sites as post-treatment sequelae.

Veterinary-Labeled Imiquimod Products
None

Human-Labeled Imiquimod Products

Product (Company)	Form: Concentration	Label Status	Other Ingredients; Size(s)
Aldara® (Graceway)	Cream: 5%	Rx (Human)	Cetyl alcohol, stearyl alcohol, white petrolatum, benzyl alcohol, parabens. Single use 250 mg packets in boxes of 12.
Zyclara® (Graceway)	Cream: 3.75%	Rx (Human)	Single use 250 mg packets in boxes of 28.

PIMECROLIMUS, TOPICAL
(pim-e-*kroe*-li-mus)   Elidel®

Indications/Actions

A relatively new addition to the human topical armamentarium, pimecrolimus cream may be of benefit in veterinary patients in the adjunctive treatment of atopic dermatitis, discoid lupus erythematosus, pemphigus erythematosus or foliaceous, pinnal vascular disease or other cutaneous vasculopathies, alopecia areata, vitiligo, perianal fistulas (terminal phase or maintenance treatment after cyclosporine therapy), and for feline proliferative and necrotizing otitis externa. Unlike topical corticosteroids, pimecrolimus does not have atrophogenic or metabolic effects associated with long-term or large area treatment.

Pimecrolimus acts similarly as cyclosporine and tacrolimus, namely inhibiting T-lymphocyte activation primarily by inhibiting the phosphatase activity of calcineurin. It also inhibits the release of inflammatory cytokines and mediators from mast cells and basophils. Pimecrolimus may not have identical mechanisms of action as tacrolimus, as it did not impair the primary immune response (as did tacrolimus) in mice after a contact sensitizer was applied. Both drugs did impair the secondary response however. Any clinical significance associated with this difference is not yet clear.

Suggested Dosages/Use

Only limited experience has occurred with this drug in veterinary patients. Most dosing recommendations are to use the product twice daily until signs are controlled, then reduce application frequency to the fewest times that allow control of the disease.

Precautions/Adverse Effects

Both tacrolimus and pimecrolimus have FDA-mandated "black box" warnings that use may increase risks for skin cancer and lymphomas in humans, although a causal relationship has not been established. Because of the rarity of these occurrences in humans, these drugs are probably relatively safe to use in veterinary patients. However, clients should be informed and instructed to wear gloves or use an applicator (*e.g.*, a Q-tip) when applying the cream. The long-term adverse effects of topical pimecrolimus are currently unknown; therefore, it is prudent to avoid using this medication on a continuous maintenance basis. When long-term treatment is required, the ultimate goal should be to achieve the lowest possible dose that keeps the disease under control.

Topical pimecrolimus appears well tolerated in dogs, but localized irritation and pruritus have been reported in humans and dogs using the drug. Early anecdotal reports state that pimecrolimus may be less irritating than tacrolimus in dogs, but that it also may not be as effective. The cost of the medication may be prohibitive for some clients.

Veterinary-Labeled Topical Pimecrolimus Products
None

Human-Labeled Topical Pimecrolimus Products

Product (Company)	Form: Concentration	Label Status	Other Ingredients; Size(s)
Elidel® (Novartis)	Cream: 1%	Rx (Human)	30, 60, 100 g.

TACROLIMUS, TOPICAL
(ta-*kroe*-li-mus)   Protopic®

Indications/Actions
Tacrolimus ointment may be of benefit in veterinary patients in the adjunctive treatment of atopic dermatitis, discoid lupus erythematosus, pemphigus erythematosus or foliaceous, pinnal vascular disease, alopecia areata, vitiligo and for perianal fistulas (terminal phase or maintenance treatment after cyclosporine therapy). Unlike topical corticosteroids, tacrolimus or pimecrolimus do not have atrophogenic or metabolic effects associated with long-term or large area treatment.

Tacrolimus acts similarly as cyclosporine, namely inhibiting T-lymphocyte activation primarily by inhibiting the phosphatase activity of calcineurin. It also inhibits the release of inflammatory cytokines and mediators from mast cells and basophils.

Suggested Dosages/Use
Only limited experience has occurred with this drug in veterinary patients. Most dosing recommendations are to use the product twice daily until signs are controlled, then reduce application frequency to the fewest times that allow control of the disease.

Precautions/Adverse Effects
Both tacrolimus and pimecrolimus have FDA-mandated "black box" warnings that use may increase risks for skin cancer and lymphomas in humans, although a causal relationship has not been established. Because of the rarity of these occurrences in humans, these drugs are probably relatively safe to use in veterinary patients. However, clients should be informed and instructed to wear gloves or use an applicator (*e.g.*, a Q-tip) when applying the ointment. The long-term adverse effects of topical tacrolimus are currently unknown; therefore, it is prudent to avoid using this medication on a continuous maintenance basis. When long-term treatment is required, the ultimate goal should be to achieve the lowest possible dose that keeps the disease under control.

The commercially available ointment should not be used as, or compounded into an ophthalmic preparation for treating KCS in dogs as it contains propylene carbonate, a known ocular toxin.

Thus far, topical tacrolimus is appears to be well tolerated in dogs, but localized irritation and pruritus have been reported in humans and dogs using the drug. Early anecdotal reports state that pimecrolimus may be less irritating than tacrolimus in dogs, but that it may also not be as effective. The cost of the medication may be cost prohibitive for some clients.

Veterinary-Labeled Topical Tacrolimus Products
None

Human-Labeled Topical Tacrolimus Products

Product (Company)	Form: Concentration	Label Status	Other Ingredients; Size(s)
Protopic® (Astellas Pharma)	Ointment: 0.03, 0.1%	Rx (Human)	30, 60, 100 g.

Retinoids, Topical

TRETINOIN (TRANS-RETINOIC ACID; VITAMIN A ACID)
(*tret*-in-oyn)   Retin-A®

Indications/Actions
Topical tretinoin may be useful in treating localized follicular or hyperkeratotic disorders such as acanthosis nigrans, idiopathic nasal and footpad hyperkeratosis, callous pyodermas, or chin acne.

Tretinoin's exact mechanism of action is not well understood, but it stimulates cellular mitotic activity, increases cell turnover, and decreases the cohesiveness of follicular epithelial cells.

Suggested Dosages/Use
In small animals, topical tretinoin gel is usually used initially at a concentration of 0.05% and is applied once daily. Treatment continues as long as the animal tolerates the treatment or until controlled. Once controlled, usage is then reduced to as needed. In animals unable to tolerate therapy, concentration may be reduced to 0.025–0.01% in an attempt to balance efficacy with adverse effects.

Precautions/Adverse Effects
Avoid sun exposure during treatment with tretinoin. Avoid contact with eyes, nostrils, inner ears, or mouth. Clients should wear gloves when applying the product.

Adverse effects can include hypersensitivity reactions or local irritation (erythema, dryness, peeling, pruritus).

Veterinary-Labeled Topical Tretinoin Products
None

Human-Labeled Topical Tretinoin Products

Product (Company)	Form: Concentration	Label Status	Other Ingredients; Size(s)
Renova® (OrthoDerm)	Cream: 0.02%	Rx (Human)	40 g.
Retin-A® (Ortho), **Avita®** (Bertek), **Altinac®** (Upsher-Smith); generic	Cream: 0.025%	Rx (Human)	20, 40 g.
Retin-A® (Ortho), **Altinac®** (Upsher-Smith), **Renova®** (OrthoDerm); generic	Cream: 0.05%	Rx (Human)	20, 45, 60 g.
Retin-A® (Ortho); generic	Cream: 0.1%	Rx (Human)	20, 45 g.
Retin-A® (Ortho); generic	Gel: 0.01%	Rx (Human)	15, 45 g.
Retin-A® (Ortho), **Avita®** (Bertek); generic	Gel: 0.025%	Rx (Human)	15, 20, 45 g.
Retin-A Micro® (Ortho)	Gel: 0.04%	Rx (Human)	Microspheres. 20, 45 g.
Retin-A Micro® (Ortho)	Gel: 0.05%	Rx (Human)	Microspheres. 20, 45 g.

Antiparasitic Agents, Topical

For agents such as **eprinomectin, ivermectin, levamisole, moxidectin** and **selamectin** that may be administered topically, but absorbed through the skin to treat internal parasites as well as external parasites, refer to the monographs in the main (systemic drugs) section of the Handbook. Also see monographs in the main section for those products administered orally for their external parasitic actions, including **lufenuron, nitenpyram, milbemycin,** and **spinosad.**

AMITRAZ
(a-mi-*traz*)   Mitaban®, Taktic® EC, Preventic®, ProMeris® for Dogs

Indications/Actions
In dogs, amitraz solution is used topically primarily in the treatment of generalized demodicosis. A topical spot-on solution (*ProMeris® for Dogs*) and a collar (*Preventic®*) are available for treatment and prevention of flea and tick infestation. It is also used as a general insecticidal/miticidal agent in several other species (see label information). The pharmacologic action of amitraz is not well understood, but it is a monoamine oxidase (MAO) inhibitor (in mites) and may have effects on the CNS of susceptible organisms. It apparently also possesses alpha-2 adrenergic activity and inhibits prostaglandin synthesis. Amitraz can cause a significant increase in plasma glucose levels, presumably by inhibiting insulin release via its alpha2-adrenergic activity. Yohimbine (alpha$_2$ blocker) or atipamezole can antagonize this effect.

Suggested Dosages/Use

◼ DOGS:

For treatment of generalized demodicosis:
Note: The general rule of thumb for therapy duration independent of the protocol chosen involves treating for 30 days past two consecutive negative skin scrapings.

Labeled Dose Protocol

Long and medium haired dogs should be clipped closely and given a shampoo with mild soap and water prior to first treatment. Topically treat at a concentration of 250 ppm (one 10.6 mL bottle of *Mitaban®* in 2 gallons of warm water), by applying to entire animal and allowing to air dry. DO NOT rinse or towel dry. Use a freshly prepared dilution for additional dogs or additional treatments. Repeat every 14 days for 3–6 treatments (continue until six treatments done or two successive skin scrapings demonstrate no live mites). Chronic cases may require additional courses of therapy. (Package Insert; *Mitaban®*—Upjohn)

Extra-label Protocols:

1) For dogs whose owners accept the risk of using the drug in an "unlicensed" manner with the goal of increasing efficacy, first try the 250 ppm solution (as above) *once weekly* for 4 weeks. If positive response is seen, continue treatment for an additional 30 days after obtaining two consecutive negative skin scrapings (rule of thumb). If weekly 250 ppm application fails, a 500 ppm solution may be tried (1 bottle in 1 gallon of water) weekly as above. In dogs failing 500 ppm, 1000 ppm may also be attempted, but likelihood of toxicity increases and the authors have no experience using this high concentration. If these methods fail, the dog is unlikely to be cured using amitraz.

2) Prepare a 0.125% solution by diluting 1 mL of the 12.5% commercially available large animal product (*Taktic®*) in 100 mL of water. Using a sponge rub the diluted solution (0.125%) *daily onto one-half of the dog's body and alternate sides on a daily basis.* Air dry. During the first week of therapy, keep dog hospitalized and observe for adverse effects. Follow rule of thumb above for duration of therapy.

Dogs with severe pododemodicosis should be also treated with daily foot soaks of the 0.125% solution. Dogs with otic demodicosis can be treated with a diluted solution of amitraz (1 mL of Tactic in 8.5 mL of mineral oil) every 3–7 days unless irritation develops. Owners accepting the extra-label therapy, must be carefully screened and trained to carefully handle the amitraz solutions.

◼ CATS:

For follicular demodicosis (*Demodex cati*) (**Note:** extra-label; not labeled for use on cats): Dilute amitraz to 0.0125% (125 ppm) and apply every 7–14 days. Monitor cats very closely for potential side effects. Place an Elizabethan-collar until the solution is completely dry.

For surface demodicosis (*Demodex gatoi*) (**Note:** extra-label; not labeled for use on cats): Dilute amitraz to 0.0125% (125 ppm) and apply every 7 days for 12 weeks. Monitor cats very closely for potential side effects. Place an Elizabethan-collar until the solution is completely dry. (Saari S. AM. et al. Acta Veterinaria Scandinavica; 51:40, 2009).

Mice, Rats, Gerbils, Hamsters, Guinea pigs, Chinchillas:

1.4 mL per liter topically every 2 weeks (q14 days) for 3–6 treatments. **Caution:** Not recommended in young animals or *rabbits.* (Adamcak, A. & B. Otten (2000). Rodent Therapeutics. Vet Clin NA: Exotic Anim Pract 3:1(Jan): 221-240)

Precautions/Adverse Effects/Drug Interactions

Amitraz liquid concentrates are flammable until diluted with water. Do not stress animals for at least 24 hours after application of *Mitaban®.* When mixing with water, protect exposed skin with rubber gloves, etc. After application to anima, wash hands and arms well. Dispose of unused diluted solution by flushing down the drain. Rinse *Mitaban®* container with water and dispose; do not re-use. Do not re-use collar or container; wrap in newspaper and throw in trash. Avoid inhalation of vapors. Animals treated may exhibit signs of sedation; if animal is un-arousable or sedation persists for longer than 72 hours, contact your veterinarian.

Safety has not been demonstrated in dogs less than 4 months of age. The manufacturer of *Mitaban®* does not recommend use in these animals. Toy breeds may be more susceptible to CNS effects (transient sedation); lower dose rates (½ of recommended) have been recommended in these breeds. Because of the drug's effects on plasma glucose, use with caution in brittle diabetic patients. Reproductive safety has not been established. Use only when benefits outweigh potential risks of therapy

The most commonly reported adverse effect after amitraz topical administration is transient sedation that may persist for up to 72 hours (24 hours is usual). If treating around eyes, use an ophthalmic protectant (*e.g.*, petrolatum ophthalmic ointment) before treating. Do not use if dog has deep pyodermas with drainage tracts; postpone application until lesions improve after treating with antibiotic and shampoo therapy. Other adverse effects include: ataxia, bradycardia, vomiting, diarrhea, hypothermia and a transient hyperglycemia. Rarely, seizures have been reported. Topical effects can include edema, erythema and pruritus. Adverse effects are more likely to be seen in debilitated, geriatric, or very small breed dogs.

Amitraz can be toxic to cats and rabbits and it is probably best to avoid its use in these species, although amitraz has been used safely in cats in diluted form for the treatment of demodicosis.

Amitraz may be toxic if swallowed (by either animals or humans). Beagles receiving 4 mg/kg PO daily for 90 days, demonstrated transient ataxia, CNS depression, hyperglycemia, decreased pulse rates and lowered body temperature. No animals died.

Amitraz toxicity can be significant if amitraz-containing insecticide collars are ingested. Treatment should consist of emesis, retrieval of the collar using endoscopy if possible and administration of activated charcoal and a cathartic to remove any remaining collar fragments. Because of the risk of an increased chance of gastric dilatation, gastrotomy may not be a viable option. Yohimbine at a dose of 0.11– 0.2 mg/kg IV (start with low dosage) may be of benefit for overdose effects. Because yohimbine has a short half-life it may need to be repeated, particularly if the animal has ingested an amitraz-containing collar that has not been retrieved from the GI tract. Atipamezole has also been used to treat amitraz toxicity; refer to that monograph for more information. Contact a poison center for more information, if necessary.

Because of their immunosuppressive effects, **corticosteroids** and **other immunosuppressant drugs** (*e.g.*, azathioprine, cyclophosphamide, etc) should not be used in animals with demodicosis.

Amitraz may interact with other MAO inhibitors (including **selegiline**) or tricyclic antidepressants (**amitriptyline, clomipramine**). Concomitant use is not recommended.

Clients should wear gloves when applying and wash off any product that contacts their skin.

Veterinary-Labeled Amitraz Products

Product (Company)	Form: Concentration	Label Status	Other Ingredients; Comments; Size(s)
Mitaban® (Pfizer) **Note:** This product's availability has been undependable in past years; may not be available	Solution for Dilution: 19.9%	Rx	10.6 mL btls. FDA labeled and approved for use on dogs. **Note:** Liquid is flammable until diluted.
Taktic®EC (Intervet)	Solution (emulsifiable concentrate) for Dilution: 12.5%	OTC-EPA	760 mL cans. EPA labeled for use on swine, dairy or beef cattle. Label states not to use on dogs or horses.
ProMeris® for Dogs (BIVI)	Spot-On Solution: amitraz 150 mg/mL; metaflumizone 150 mg/mL	OTC-EPA	For dogs and puppies 8 weeks of age or older. Must not be used on cats. See the product label for more information. Packaged in 5 different sizes according to dog's weight.
Preventic® (Virbac)	Collar: 9% amitraz; 25 inch	OTC-EPA	25 in. adjustable (cut off excess). EPA labeled for dogs 12 weeks and older only. Effective for 3 months.

Human-Labeled Amitraz Products
None

CROTAMITON

(**kroe**-ta-mye-ton)   Eurax®

Indications/Actions

Crotamiton is a topical miticide/scabicide and has been used primarily for adjunctive treatment (with ivermectin) for treating mite infections (*e.g.*, Knemidopkoptes) in birds. Crotamiton has both miticidal and antipruritic actions, but the mechanism for each is not known.

Suggested Dosages/Use

Once to twice daily applications are usually recommended.

Precautions/Adverse Effects

Do not apply around eyes or mouth. Little is known of the compound's safety profile; irritation or hypersensitivity reactions are possible.

Veterinary-Labeled Crotamiton Products

None

Human-Labeled Topical Crotamiton Products

Product (Company)	Form: Concentration	Label Status	Other Ingredients; Size(s)
Eurax® (Ranbaxy)	Cream: 10%	Rx (Human)	Cetyl alcohol, vanishing base. 60 g.
Eurax® (Ranbaxy)	Lotion: 10%	Rx (Human)	Cetyl alcohol, emollient base. 60, 454 g.

DELTAMETHRIN

(del-ta-*meeth*-rin)

Indications/Actions

In the United States, deltamethrin-impregnated collars are labeled for killing fleas and ticks on dogs. In countries where leishmaniasis is a problem, deltamethrin-impregnated collars are also indicated for repelling and killing the phlebotomine sandfly vectors.

Deltamethrin is a synthetic pyrethroid and acts by disrupting the sodium channel current in arthropod nerve cell membranes, resulting in paralysis and death.

Suggested Dosages/Use

The manufacturer recommends applying a new collar every 6 months and claims that maximum effect may not occur before 2 to 3 weeks after collar placement. Follow label for specific use instructions.

Precautions/Adverse Effects

Collars containing deltamethrin should not be used in dogs younger than 12 weeks of age. Avoid contact with eyes, skin or clothing. Consult a veterinarian before using on debilitated, pregnant, nursing, old or medicated animals. Skin reactions at the application site may occur. Mammalian exposure to deltamethrin is classified as safe; however, it should be used very carefully around water because deltamethrin is highly toxic to aquatic animals, especially fish

Veterinary-Labeled Deltamethrin Products

Product (Company)	Form: Concentration	Label Status	Other Ingredients; Size(s)
Scalibor® Protector Band for Dogs (Intervet/Schering-Plough)	Deltamethrin 4%	OTC-EPA	One size fits all. 0.9 oz

Human-Labeled Deltamethrin Products
None

DINOTEFURAN + PYRIPROXYFEN (± PERMETHRIN)

Indications/Actions

The product containing dinotefuran and pyriproxyfen (*Vectra*®) labeled for dogs and cats is used for control of adult and all immature flea stages including eggs, larvae and pupae. The exclusive dog product contains in addition to dinotefuran and pyriproxyfen, permethrin (*Vectra 3D*®), which kills and repels adult and immature fleas, ticks and mosquitoes.

Dinotefuran is a nitroguanidine, neonicotinoid insecticide with a structure similar to acetylcholine. It permanently binds to the same insect receptor sites as acetylcholine and activates the nerve impulse at the synapse causing stimulation, which results in tremors, incoordination and insect death. Dinotefuran does not bind to mammalian acetylcholine receptor sites.

The commercially available products also contain pyriproxyfen (a second-generation insect growth regulator) and, in the case of *Vectra 3D* (for dogs only), permethrin.

Suggested Dosages/Use

Refer to the package information for specific instructions on application and dosages of dinotefuran-containing products. Monthly applications are recommended for dogs and cats. It is labeled for cats and kittens 8 weeks of age or older and dogs or puppies 7 weeks of age or older. Apparently bathing or swimming does not interfere with efficacy; however, the authors do not recommend bathing the pet until two days after application.

Precautions/Adverse Effects

The dog product containing permethrin (*Vectra 3D*®) **must not be used on cats or on dogs that cohabit with a cat**. The manufacturer recommends not using *Vectra 3D*® or *Vectra*® on debilitated, aged, medicated, pregnant or nursing animals and animals known to be sensitive to pesticide products. Mild transitory skin erythema may occur at the application site. Avoid eye and oral contact since Dinotefuran can cause substantial, but temporary eye irritation.

Veterinary-Labeled Topical Dinotefuran Products

Product (Company)	Form: Concentration	Label Status	Comments; Size(s)
Vectra® for Cats and Kittens (Summit VetPharm)	Topical Solution: Dinotefuran 22% Pyriproxyfen 3%	EPA-OTC	For cats and kittens under 9 lbs and over 8 weeks of age: dose size = 0.8 mL
Vectra® for Cats (Summit VetPharm)	Topical Solution: Dinotefuran 22% Pyriproxyfen 3%	EPA-OTC	For cats weighting 9 lbs or over: dose size— 1.2 mL
Vectra for Dogs & Puppies® (Summit VetPharm)	Topical Solution: Dinotefuran 4.95% Pyriproxyfen 0.44%	EPA-OTC	Can be used on dogs and puppies 8 weeks of age or older.

For dogs and puppies 2.5 to 10 lbs— dose volume 1.3 mL

For dogs and puppies 11 to 20 lbs— dose volume 2 mL

For dogs 21 to 55 lbs—dose volume 4 mL

For dogs 56-100 lbs—dose volume 6 mL |
| Vectra 3D® (Summit VetPharm) | Topical Solution: Dinotefuran 4.95% Pyriproxyfen 0.44% Permethrin 36.08% | EPA-OTC | Must not be used on cats or on dogs that co-habit with a cat. For dogs and puppies 2.5 to 20 lbs, 7 weeks of age or over—dose volume 1.6 mL

For dogs and puppies 21 to 55 lbs, 7 weeks of age or over— dose volume 3.6 mL

For dogs 56 to 95 lbs—dose volume 4.7 mL

For dogs over 95 lbs—dose volume 8 mL |

Human-Labeled Dinotefuran Products
None

FIPRONIL ± (S)-METHOPRENE±
(**fip**-roe-nil; meth-oh-preen)   Frontline®, Frontline® Plus

Indications/Actions
In the USA, Fipronil is indicated for the treatment of fleas, ticks and chewing lice infestations in dogs and cats. It has also been used successfully for *Trombicula autumnalis* (chigger) infestation, sarcoptic mange, cheyletiellosis, chewing lice and otoacariosis.

Fipronil is a phenylpyrazole antiparasitic agent that in invertebrates interferes with the passage of chloride ions in GABA regulated chloride channels, thereby disrupting CNS activity causing death of the flea or tick. The manufacturer states that fipronil collects in the oils of the skin and hair follicles and continues to be released over a period a time resulting in long residual activity. Topically applied, the drug apparently spreads over the body in approximately 24 hours via translocation.

When fipronil is combined with the insect growth regulator (S)-methoprene (*Frontline® Plus*), additionally flea eggs and flea larvae are killed. (S)-methoprene mimics flea juvenile growth hormone, halting development during metamorphosis and larval development. It also concentrates in female flea ovaries, causing non-viable eggs to be produced.

Suggested Dosages/Use
For fleas, ticks or chewing lice:
Monthly treatments are usually recommended when used for fleas, ticks or chewing lice. See product labels for specific directions on administration and recommendations on bathing/swimming, etc after administration.

For Trombicula autumnalis infestation:
Fipronil *spray* (0.25%) is recommended Monthly applications throughout the trombiculid season at the dose of 3 to 6 mL/kg. It is important to thoroughly wet the coat with special emphasis on the areas typically affected (feet, ears, face, perineum and tail). In some cases, the interval between applications needs to be shortened to every 14 days.

For otoacariosis:
Apply 0.05 mL of fipronil solution inside each ear canal and 0.4 mL between the shoulder blades. Resolution of clinical signs can be seen as early as seven days post-treatment. Additional applications may be needed. Fipronil needs to be applied in the ear canals to be effective.

Precautions/Adverse Effects
Do not use on puppies or kittens less than 8 weeks of age. This product is reportedly contraindicated in rabbits as deaths have occurred with the spray. Do not apply or spray in eyes. While temporary irrita-

tion may occur at the site of administration, animals that have demonstrated sensitivity reactions to fipronil or any of the ingredients in the product should probably not be retreated.

The manufacturer recommends consulting a veterinarian before using on debilitated, aged, or medicated patients.

Do not contaminate food or water and dispose of container properly. Avoid human contact with skin, eyes or clothing and wear gloves when applying/spraying. If using spray, do so in a well ventilated area. Avoid contact with animal until dry. Wash well with soap and water if contact occurs.

Product is labeled as remaining effective after bathing (but do not shampoo within 48 hours of application), water immersion, or exposure to sunlight. Spotted areas may appear wet or oily for up to 24 hours after application.

Temporary irritation may occur at the site of administration. Rarely, hypersensitivity has been reported.

Veterinary-Labeled Fipronil w/ & w/o (s)-Methoprene Products

Product (Company)	Form: Concentration	Label Status	Other Ingredients; Comments; Size(s)
Frontline® Spray Treatment (Merial)	Spray: 0.29% fipronil	OTC-EPA	Labeled for use on dogs, cats, puppies, kittens 8 weeks of age or older. 8.5, 17 oz.
Frontline® Top Spot for Cats and Kittens (Merial)	Solution: 9.7% fipronil	OTC-EPA	Labeled for use on cats or kittens 8 weeks of age or older. Single dose applicators 50 mL in 3's & 6's.
Frontline® Plus for Cats and Kittens (Merial)	Solution: 9.8% fipronil, (s)-methoprene 11.8%	OTC-EPA	Labeled for use on cats or kittens 8 weeks of age or older. Single dose applicators 50 mL in 3's & 6's.
Frontline® Top Spot for Dogs and Puppies (Merial)	Solution: 9.7% fipronil	OTC-EPA	Labeled for use on dogs or puppies 8 weeks of age or older. Single dose applicators 50 mL in 3's & 6's.
Frontline® Plus for Dogs & Puppies (Merial)	Solution: 9.8% fipronil, (s)-methoprene 8.8%	OTC-EPA	Single dose applicators in 3's and 6's; Labeled for dogs or puppies 8 weeks of age or older. For dogs weighing 11−22 lb.: 0.67 mL For dogs weighing 23−44 lb.: 1.34 mL For dogs weighing 45−88 lb.: 2.68 mL For dogs weighing 89−132 lb.: 4.02 mL

Human-Labeled Fipronil Products
None

IMIDACLOPRID
IMIDACLOPRID WITH PERMETHRIN
IMIDACLOPRID WITH MOXIDECTIN

(eye-mi-da-*kloe*-prid, per-*meth*-rin, *mox*-ih-dek-tin)   Advantage®, K9 Advantix®, Advantage®, Advocate®

Indications/Actions

Imidacloprid topical solution (*Advantage®*) is indicated for the treatment of adult and larval stage fleas in dogs and cats. The combination product with permethrin (*K9 Advantix®*) is indicated for adulticide/larvicide for fleas, to repel and kill ticks, and mosquitoes in dogs only. The canine combination product with moxidectin (*Advantage® Multi for Dogs* in USA and *Advocate®* in Europe) is indicated for the prevention of heartworm disease, adult fleas, adult and immature hookworms, adult roundworms, and adult whipworms. It has been also used successfully for the treatment of sarcoptic mange, cheyletiellosis and mild cases of demodicosis.

The feline combination product (*Advantage® Multi for Cats*) is indicated for the prevention of heartworm disease, adult fleas, ear mites, adult and immature hookworms, and adult roundworms.

Imidacloprid's mechanism of action as an insecticide is to act on nicotinic acetylcholine receptors on the postsynaptic membrane causing CNS impairment and death. Certain insect species are more sensitive to these agents than are mammalian receptors. This is a different mechanism of action than other insecticidal agents (organophosphates, pyrethrins, carbamates, insect growth regulators (IGR's) and insect development inhibitors (IDI's). The manufacturer states that imidacloprid is non-teratogenic, non-hypersensitizing, non-mutagenic, non-allergenic, non-carcinogenic, and non-photosensitizing. The manufacturer states that when applied topically the compound is not absorbed into the bloodstream or internal organs. One combination product for dogs (*K9 Advantix®*) also contains permethrin, a pyrethroid (synthetic pyrethrin) that will kill and repel ticks and mosquitoes. Permethrin's insecticidal activity is as a neurotoxin in susceptible species by slowing sodium ions through sodium channels in neuron membranes. Moxidectin is found in combination products (*Advantage® Multi for Dogs* and *Cats*) with imidacloprid. Moxidectin is a macrocyclic lactone that binds to the glutamate-gated ion channels specific to parasites thereby increasing the influx of chloride ions resulting in hyperpolarization of neuronal cells causing paralysis and death.

Suggested Dosages/Use
Refer to the package information for specific instructions on application of imidacloprid products. They are generally administered once monthly. While swimming, bathing, and rain do not apparently significantly affect the duration of action, repeated shampooing may require additional treatment(s) before the monthly dosing interval is completed. Do not reapply more often than once weekly for these animals.

Precautions/Adverse Effects
The manufacturer lists the following contraindications for imidacloprid (alone): Do not use in puppies younger than 7 weeks old or kittens younger than 8 weeks old. The manufacturer recommends consulting a veterinarian before using on debilitated, aged, pregnant, or nursing animals or those on medication.

The combination product with permethrin (*K9 Advantix®*) **must not be used on cats**. Use with caution in households with both dogs and cats, particularly if cats are in close contact or will groom dogs in the household.

When used as directed, adverse effects are unlikely. Because the drug is bitter tasting, oral contact may cause excessive salivation. Do not get product in eyes. If eye contact occurs (human or animal), flush well with ophthalmic irrigation solution or water. While gloving is not mandated it should be encouraged, as contact with skin should be avoided. Wash hands with soap and water after handling. Keep out of reach of children and do not contaminate feed or food. Dispose of product carefully (in the trash); the permethrin-containing product is extremely toxic to fish.

Imidacloprid topical solutions are usually very well tolerated. Dermal irritation has been reported at the site of application. Hypersalivation, tremors, vomiting and reduced appetite may occur in cats after oral exposure to *Advantage Multi®*. Uncommon to rare adverse reactions reported in dogs treated with *Advantage Multi®* in a field study included pruritus, lethargy, reduced appetite and hyperactivity.

Overdoses/Acute Toxicity
Most problems are seen following oral dosing of topical products. Signs include hypersalivation and vomiting, oral ulcers have been rarely reported in cats. There were 119 exposures to imidacloprid reported to the ASPCA Animal Poison Control Center (APCC) during 2008-2009. In these cases 57 were dogs with 25 showing clinical signs, 60 cases were cats in which 42 showed clinical signs, 1 case was a turtle that showed clinical signs and the remaining case was a lagomorph that showed no clinical signs. Common findings in dogs recorded in decreasing frequency included vomiting, hypersalivation, and trembling. Common findings in cats recorded in decreasing frequency included hypersalivation, vomiting, lethargy, and hiding.

Veterinary-Labeled Imidacloprid Topical Products

Product (Company)	Form: Concentration	Label Status	Other Ingredients; Comments; Size(s)
Advantage® For Dogs (Bayer)	Topical Solution: imidacloprid 9.1%	OTC-EPA	Flea adulticide/larvicide for use on dogs and puppies 7 weeks of age and older. In cards of 4 or 6 tubes: Under 10 lb. = 0.4 mL (green) 11−20 lb. = 1 mL (teal) 21−55 lb. = 2.5 mL (red) Over 55 lb. = 4 mL (blue)
Advantage® for Cats (Bayer)	Topical Solution: imidacloprid 9.1%	OTC-EPA	Flea adulticide/larvicide for use on cats and kittens 8 weeks of age and older. In cards of 4 or 6 tubes: 9 lb and under = 0.4 mL (orange) Over 9 lb. = 0.8 mL (purple)
K9 Advantix® (Bayer)	Topical Solution: imidacloprid 8.8%, permethrin 44%	OTC-EPA	Flea adulticide/larvicide, tick and mosquito repellant and treatment. For use on dogs and puppies 7 weeks of age and older. In cards of 4 or 6 tubes: Under 10 lb. = 0.4 mL (green) 11−20 lb. = 1 mL (teal) 21−55 lb. = 2.5 mL (red) Over 55 lb. = 4 mL (blue)
Advantage Multi® for Dogs (Bayer)	Topical Solution: imidacloprid 10%, moxidectin 2.5%	Rx	Approved for use on dogs 7 weeks of age or greater, and more than 3 lb body weight
Advantage Multi® for Cats (Bayer)	Topical Solution: imidacloprid 10%, moxidectin 1%	Rx	Approved for use on cats 9 weeks of age or greater, and more than 2 lb body weight.

Human-Labeled Imidacloprid Products
None

METAFLUMIZONE
(met-ah-*floo*-mih-zone)   ProMeris®

Indications/Actions
The canine product (*ProMeris® For Dogs*) contains metaflumizone and amitraz (see amitraz monograph for more information) and is labeled for control of fleas (*Ctenocephalides* spp.), ticks, chewing lice and Demodectic mange mites on dogs and puppies 8 weeks of age and older. The feline product (*ProMeris® For Cats*) is labeled for control of fleas (*Ctenocephalides* sp.) on cats and kittens 8 weeks of age and older.

Metaflumizone blocks the influx of sodium required to propagate a nerve impulse along the axon and dendrite of the neuron causing a reduction in feeding, loss of coordination, paralysis and death of the parasite. Amitraz is a formamidine compound that acts by inhibiting mixed function oxidases in addition to monoamine oxidase. It apparently also has alpha$_2$ adrenergic activity and inhibits prostaglandin synthesis.

Suggested Dosages/Use
Refer to the package information for specific instructions on recommended dosages and application of metaflumizone products. For cats, the label states that a single dose is effective for up to 7 weeks in controlling fleas. Apply a single dose prior to exposure. Reapplication at monthly intervals may be appropriate depending upon the level of flea challenge and animal sensitivities (*i.e.* flea allergy dermatitis). Do not apply more than once monthly.

For dogs, the product's label states: A single dose is effective for up to 6 weeks in controlling fleas and up to 4 weeks for ticks. Apply a single dose prior to exposure. Monthly application is recommended for effective control of fleas, ticks, chewing lice and Demodectic mange mites and to prevent re-infestation of fleas, ticks and chewing lice. Do not apply more than once monthly.

Precautions/Adverse Effects
The manufacturer does not recommend using in lactating/nursing dogs or cats until at least 5 days post delivery. However, it can be used in breeding dogs (males and females) as well as in pregnant dogs and cats. **The canine formulation must not be used in cats** because it contains amitraz. The manufacturer recommends consulting a veterinarian before applying these products in aged or debilitated animals or animals on medications. The manufacturer also advises contacting a veterinarian if skin irritation, behavior changes, vomiting or diarrhea occurs and persists after application of these products.

Adverse application site events such as focal inflammation, pruritus or alopecia are uncommon. A subset of dogs treated with the combined product may experience clinical signs similar to pemphigus foliaceus (pemphigus-like disease) after one or multiple applications of the product. Lesions may be limited to the application site and surrounding skin or be present at distant sites such as face and feet.

Accidental oral exposure of the combined product containing amitraz (*ProMeris® For Dogs*) may result in decreased activity.

Veterinary-Labeled Topical Metaflumizone Products

Product (Company)	*Form: Concentration*	*Label Status*	*Other Ingredients; Comments; Size(s)*
ProMeris® for Cats (Pfizer)	Topical Solution: Metaflumizone 9.1%	OTC-EPA	For use on cats and kittens 8 weeks of age and older. Product comes in two sizes: for cats less than 9 lbs, and for those over 9 lbs.
ProMeris® for Dogs (Pfizer)	Spot-On Solution: amitraz 14.34%; metaflumizone 14.34% mg/mL	OTC-EPA	For dogs and puppies 8 weeks of age or older. Must not be used on cats. See the product label for more information. Packaged in 5 different sizes according to dog's weight.

Human-Labeled Metaflumizone Products
None

(S)-METHOPRENE COMBINATIONS

(meth-oh-*preen*)

Also see the Fipronil ± (s)-Methoprene listing

Indications/Actions

Methoprene is added to premise sprays and topical products to eliminate insects (usually fleas) via its ability prevent maturation of eggs or larva.

(s)-methoprene mimics insect juvenile growth hormone, halting development during metamorphosis and larval development. It also concentrates in female flea ovaries, causing non-viable eggs to be produced. When combined with an adulticide (*e.g.*, permethrin, fipronil, phenothrin) all stages of the parasite are killed and re-infestation is less likely.

Suggested Dosages/Use

For specific use and dosage recommendations, refer to the actual product's label.

Precautions/Adverse Effects

Methoprene may be found in products also containing **permethrin or phenothrin, which can be toxic to cats,** particularly small kittens. **Only use in cats those products containing permethrin or other pyrethroids labeled specifically for use on cats.** Hypersensitivity can occur to these compounds. Do not use in eyes or on mucous membranes.

Methoprene (used alone) has low toxicity in mammals. Potentially, skin irritation or hypersensitivity reactions could occur. As methoprene is broken down by UV light, protect unused product from light.

Veterinary-Labeled (s)-Methoprene Topical Products

Product (Company)	Form: Concentration	Label Status	Other Ingredients; Comments; Size(s)
Adams Spot On® Flea & Tick Control (Farnam)	Topical Solution: (s)-Methoprene: 3% Permethrin: 45%	OTC-EPA	Kills and repels adult fleas, ticks and mosquitoes. It also prevents flea eggs from developing into adult fleas. For dogs 6 months of age or older. Must not be used on cats or on dogs that cohabit with a cat. Packaged and labeled by the dog's weight in tubes of 3: <15-30 lbs = 0.034 oz; 31-60 lbs = 0.068 oz; > 60 lbs = 0.101 oz
Bio Spot On® Flea & Tick Control For Dogs (Farnam)	Topical Solution: (s)-Methoprene: 3% Permethrin: 45%	OTC-EPA	Kills and repels adult fleas, ticks and mosquitoes. It also prevents flea eggs from developing into adult fleas. For dogs 6 months of age or older Must not be used on cats or on dogs that cohabit with a cat. Packaged and labeled by the dog's weight in tubes of 3: <15-30 lbs = 0.034 oz; 31-60 lbs = 0.068 oz; > 60 lbs = 0.101 oz
Frontline® Plus for Cats and Kittens (Merial)	Topical Solution: (s)-Methoprene: 11.8%, Fipronil: 9.7%	OTC-EPA	Labeled for use on cats or kittens 8 weeks of age or older. Single dose applicators 50 mL in 3's & 6's.
Frontline® Plus for Dogs & Puppies (Merial)	Topical Solution: (s)-Methoprene: 8.8%, Fipronil: 9.7%	OTC-EPA	Single dose applicators in 3's and 6's; Labeled for dogs or puppies 8 weeks of age or older. For dogs weighing 11−22 lb.: 0.67 mL For dogs weighing 23−44 lb.: 1.34 mL For dogs weighing 45−88 lb.: 2.68 mL For dogs weighing 89−132 lb.: 4.02 mL
Hartz UltraGuard Plus® Flea & Tick Drops for Dogs and Puppies®; Hartz UltraGuard Pro® (Hartz Mountain)	Topical Solution: (s)-Methoprene: 2.3% Phenothrin: 85.7%	OTC-EPA	**Note:** Phenothrin is a pyrethroid similar to permethrin; refer to the permethrin monograph for more information. For dogs 12 weeks of age and older or weighting more than 4 pounds. Kills fleas, ticks, mosquitoes and flea eggs for 30 days; repels fleas and ticks. Must not be used on cats or on dogs that cohabit with a cat. Packaged and labeled by dogs weight in tubes of 3: 4−15 lb. = 1.1 mL; 16−30 lb. = 1.3 mL; 31−60 lb. = 4.1 mL; > 60 lb. = 5.9 mL
Hartz UltraGuard One Spot® Treatment for Cats and Kittens® (Hartz Mountain)	Topical Solution: (s)-Methoprene: 2.9%	OTC-EPA	For kittens 12 weeks of age and older. Kills and prevents flea eggs and larvae for up to 30 days. 1 mL

Product (Company)	Form: Concentration	Label Status	Other Ingredients; Comments; Size(s)
Hartz UltraGuard Plus® **Drops for Cats; Hartz** **UltraGuard Pro®** (Hartz Mountain)	Topical Solution: (s)-Methoprene: 3.6% Etofenprox: 40%	OTC-EPA	For kittens 12 weeks of age and older. Kills fleas, flea eggs and deer ticks; kills and repels mosquitoes. 1.8 mL applicators.
Bio-Spot® Flea & Tick **Spray for Dogs and Puppies** (Farnam)	Topical Spray: (s)-Methoprene: 0.27% Pyrethrins: 0.2% Piperonyl Butoxide: 0.37%	OTC-EPA	Kills and repels fleas, ticks and mosquitoes. Prevents flea eggs from hatching. For dogs 12 weeks of age or older. 24 oz.

Human-Labeled (s)-Methoprene Products
None

PERMETHRIN

(per-*meth*-rin)

Also see the Imidacloprid $\pm$ Permethrin listing

Indications/Actions
Permethrin is synthetic pyrethroid that acts as an adulticide insecticide/miticide. It has knockdown activity against fleas, lice, ticks, and certain mites (*e.g.*, Cheyletiella, *Sarcoptes scabiei*). Permethrin also has repellant activity. In small animal medicine, it is used primarily for fleas and ticks on dogs. In large animal and food animal medicine, there are many products (not listed below) available for pour-on, dusting, and spray use for flies, lice, mites, mosquitoes, ticks and keds.

Permethrin acts by disrupting the sodium channel current in arthropod nerve cell membranes, resulting in paralysis and death.

Suggested Dosages/Use
For specific dosage recommendations, refer to the actual product's label.

Precautions/Adverse Effects
Permethrin and other synthetic pyrethroids can be toxic to cats, particularly small kittens. **Only use products containing pyrethroids labeled for use on cats on this species.** Hypersensitivity can occur to these compounds. Do not use in eyes or on mucous membranes. Clients should wear gloves when applying and wash off any product that contacts their skin.

Pruritus or mild skin irritation can occur at application site, but occur uncommonly.

Veterinary-Labeled Topical Permethrin Products
Not inclusive; many shampoos, pour-ons, sprays, dusts are available.

Product (Company)	Form: Concentration	Label Status	Other Ingredients; Comments; Size(s)
Adams Spot On® **Flea & Tick Control** (Farnam)	Topical Solution: Permethrin: 45% (s)-Methoprene: 3%	OTC-EPA	Kills and repels adult fleas, ticks and mosquitoes. It also prevents flea eggs from developing into adult fleas. For dogs 6 months of age or older. Must not be used on cats or on dogs that cohabit with a cat. Packaged and labeled by the dog's weight in tubes of 3: <15-30 lbs = 0.034 oz 31-60 lbs = 0.068 oz > 60 lbs = 0.101 oz
Bansect® Squeeze-On **Flea & Tick Control** **for Dogs®** (Sergeant's)	Topical Solution: Permethrin 45%	OTC-EPA	Kills and repels fleas and ticks. For dogs, older than 6 months old. Must not be used on cats or on dogs that cohabit with a cat. Individual packaging for dog's weighing: < 33 lb. = 1.5 mL >33 lb. = 3 mL 3 per package.
Bio Spot On® Flea & **Tick Control For Dogs** (Farnam)	Topical Solution: Permethrin: 45% (s)-Methoprene: 3%	OTC-EPA	Kills and repels adult fleas, ticks and mosquitoes. It also prevents flea eggs from developing into adult fleas. For dogs 6 months of age or older. Must not be used on cats or on dogs that cohabit with a cat. Packaged and labeled by the dog's weight in tubes of 3: <15-30 lbs = 0.034 oz 31-60 lbs = 0.068 oz > 60 lbs = 0.101 oz

Product (Company)	Form: Concentration	Label Status	Other Ingredients; Comments; Size(s)
Flea Halt® Flea and Tick Spray for Dogs (Farnam)	Topical Spray: Permethrin 0.1% Pyrethrins 0.05% Piperonyl Butoxide 0.5%	OTC-EPA	Kills and repels fleas, ticks, flies, mosquitoes, gnats, chiggers and lice. For dogs older than 3 months of age. Must not be used on cats or on dogs that cohabit with a cat. 32 oz bottle.
Freedom® 45 Spot-On for Dogs (Star Horse)	Topical Solution Permethrin 45%	OTC-EPA	Kills fleas, ticks, mosquitoes, lice and mites. For dogs 12 weeks of age or older. It cannot be used on cats or on dogs that cohabit with a cat. In cards of 2 to 3 tubes 33 lbs and under = 1.5 cc applicators 33 to 66 lbs = 3 cc applicators Over 66 lbs = 6 cc applicators
K9 Advantix® (Bayer)	Topical Solution: Permethrin 44% Imidacloprid 8.8%,	OTC-EPA; Manufacturer restricts sales to licensed veterinarians	Flea adulticide/larvicide, tick and mosquito repellant. For use on dogs and puppies 7 weeks of age and older. It cannot be used on cats or on dogs that cohabit with a cat. In cards of 4 or 6 tubes: Under 10 lb. = 0.4 mL (green) 11−20 lb. = 1 mL (teal) 21−55 lb. = 2.5 mL (red) Over 55 lb. = 4 mL (blue)
Liberty 50 Plus IGR Spot-On® (Star Horse)	Topical Solution: Permethrin 50% Pyriproxyfen 1.2%	OTC-EPA	Kills and repels fleas, ticks, mosquitoes, lice and mites. Kills flea larvae and prevents eggs from hatching. For use on dogs over 12 weeks of age. Must not be used on cats or on dogs that cohabit with a cat. Available for extra small, small, large and extra large dogs.
ProTICall® Insecticide for Dogs (Intervet-Schering-Plough)	Spot-On Liquid: Permethrin 65%	EPA	Kills and repels fleas, ticks and mosquitoes. Dosing amounts vary with dog weight; refer to directions. Labeled for use on puppies over 4 weeks of age. Must not be used on cats or on dogs that cohabit with a cat. 6 X 1 mL applicators.
Scratchex® Flea & Tick Spray For Dogs and Cats (Farnam)	Topical Spray: Permethrin 0.05% Pyrethrins 0.056% Related compounds 0.004%	OTC-EPA	Kills and ticks. For dogs and cats 12 weeks of age or older. 7 oz bottle.
Vectra 3D® (Summit VetPharm)	Topical Solution: Permethrin 36.08%, Pyripoxyfen 0.44%, Dinotefuran, 4.95%	OTC-EPA	For use on dogs over 7 weeks old only. Must not be used on cats or on dogs that cohabit with a cat. In 4 different package sizes for dogs weighing >2.5. lb.
Virbac Long Acting Knockout® (Virbac)	Topical Spray: Permethrin 2 % Pyriproxyfen 0.05%	OTC-EPA	Kills adult and immature fleas and ticks. Use only on dogs 12 weeks of age or older. Re-apply every 2 months. It cannot be used on cats or on dogs that cohabit with a cat. 16 oz.

Human-Labeled Topical Permethrin Products

Product (Company)	Form: Concentration	Label Status	Other Ingredients; Comments; Size(s)
Generic (various), Elimite® (Allergan), Acticin® (Bertek)	Cream: Permethrin 5%	Rx (Human)	Used for treating scabies in humans. 60 g.
Generic (various)	Lotion/Cream Rinse: Permethrin 1%	OTC (Human)	Used for treating head lice in humans. 60 mL

PYRETHRINS AND PYRETHRIN COMBINATIONS, TOPICAL

(pye-*ree*-thrins)

For otic use, refer to the Otics section

Indications/Actions

Pyrethrins are naturally derived insecticides that act as adulticide insecticides/miticides. They have knockdown activity against fleas, lice, ticks, and Cheyletiella. In small animal medicine, pyrethrins are used primarily for fleas and ticks on dogs and cats. In large animal and food animal medicine, there are many products (not listed below) available for pour-on, dusting, and spray use.

Pyrethrins act by disrupting the sodium channel current in arthropod nerve cell membranes, resulting in paralysis and death. Pyrethrins are often found in combination with the insect growth regulators, methoprene or pyriproxyfen and with the synergist piperonyl butoxide. Piperonyl butoxide inhibits insect metabolic enzymes (P450 system) allowing a lower dose of primary insecticide to be used.

Suggested Dosages/Use
For specific dosage recommendations, refer to the actual product's label.

Precautions/Adverse Effects
Pyrethrins are among the safest insecticidal products available, but cats should not be allowed to groom wet product after using dips or sprays. Hypersensitivity can occur to these compounds. Do not use in eyes or on mucous membranes. Avoid hypothermia when using liquid products (sprays, dips, etc), particularly in small animals and when ambient temperatures are low.

Pruritus or mild skin irritation can occur at application site, but occur uncommonly.

Clients should wear gloves when applying and wash off any product that contacts their skin.

Veterinary-Labeled Pyrethrin Products
Not an inclusive list, but representative of the types of products available; many shampoos, pour-ons, sprays, dusts, ointments are available.

Product (Company)	Form: Concentration	Label Status	Other Ingredients; Comments; Size(s)
Adams Flea & Tick Dust II® (VPL)	Dust: Pyrethrins 0.1% Carbaryl 12.5% Piperonyl butoxide 1%	OTC-EPA	Silica gel 10%. Odorless. Labeled for dogs, cats, puppies, & kittens over 12 weeks old. 3 oz.
Adams Flea & Tick Mist with IGR® (Farnam) **Adams Flea & Tick Mist for Cats®** (Farnam)	Topical Spray: Pyrethrins 0.18% Pyriproxyfen 0.125%	OTC-EPA	N-octyl bicyclohepane dicarboxamide 1% (insecticide synergist). For dogs and cats. 16, 32 oz.
Vet-Kem Ovitrol Plus Flea, Tick & Bot Spray® (Wellmark)	Topical Spray: (s)-Methoprene: 0.27% Pyrethrins: 0.2% Piperonyl Butoxide 0.37%	OTC-EPA	N-octyl bicycloheptene dicarboximide: 0.62%. 16 oz., 1 gal. Labeled for use on dogs, cats, puppies, kittens, horses, and ponies. Not for puppies or kittens less than 12 weeks old.
Bio-Spot® Flea & Tick Spray for Dogs and Puppies (Farnam)	Topical Spray: Pyrethrins: 0.2% Piperonyl Butoxide: 0.37% (s)-Methoprene: 0.27%	OTC-EPA	Kills and repels fleas, ticks and mosquitoes. Prevents flea eggs from hatching. For dogs 12 weeks of age or older. 24 oz.
Bio-Spot® Flea & Tick Repellent for Puppies (Farnam)	Topical Spray: Pyrethrins: 0.2% Piperonyl Butoxide: 0.37% (s)-Methoprene: 0.1%	OTC-EPA	Kills fleas and ticks and prevents flea eggs from hatching. For puppies 12 weeks of age or older. 16 oz.
Flea Halt® Flea and Tick Spray for Dogs (Farnam)	Topical Spray: Pyrethrins 0.05% Permethrin 0.1% Piperonyl Butoxide 0.5%	OTC-EPA	Kills and repels fleas, ticks, flies, mosquitoes, gnats, chiggers and lice. For dogs older than 3 months of age. Must not be used on cats or on dogs that cohabit with a cat. 32 oz bottle.
Scratchex® Flea & Tick Spray For Dogs and Cats (Farnam)	Topical Spray: Pyrethrins 0.056% Permethrin 0.05%	OTC-EPA	Kills fleas and ticks. For dogs and cats 12 weeks of age and older. 7 oz bottle.
Bio Spot Shampoo® for Dogs and Puppies (Farnam)	Shampoo: Pyrethrins 0.15% (s)-methoprene 0.1% Piperonyl butoxide 1.5%	OTC-EPA	For dogs and cats 12 weeks of age or older. 12 oz.
Adams® Plus Flea & Tick Shampoo with Insect Growth Regulator (IGR) (Farnam)	Shampoo: Pyrethrins 0.075% Pyriproxyfen 0.086% Piperonyl butoxide 0.75%	OTC-EPA	Kills fleas, ticks and lice. Prevent flea eggs from hatching. For dogs and cats. 12 oz.
Vet-Kem Ovitrol Plus Flea & Tick Shampoo® (Wellmark)	Shampoo: (s)-Methoprene: 1.1% Pyrethrins: 0.15% Piperonyl butoxide:1.05%	OTC-EPA	12 oz. Not for puppies or kittens less than 12 weeks old.
Ectokyl 3X Flea & Tick Shampoo® (DVM)	Shampoo: Pyrethrins: 0.15% Piperonyl butoxide:1% N-octyl bicycloheptene dicarboxamide 0.5% Di-n-propyl isocinchomerate 0.5%	OTC-EPA	Oatmeal, aloe. Not for puppies or kittens less than 12 weeks old. 8 oz, 1 gal.

Product (Company)	Form: Concentration	Label Status	Other Ingredients; Comments; Size(s)
Ecto-Soothe® 3X Shampoo (Virbac)	Shampoo: Pyrethrins 0.15% Piperonyl butoxide 1.5% Spherulite® microcapsules	OTC-EPA	N-octyl bicycloheptane dicarboxamide (MGK 264) 0.5%. Kills ticks, fleas, and lice. For dogs and cats 12 weeks of age or older. 8 oz, 16 oz, 1 gal.
Vet-Kem Ovitrol Plus Flea & Tick Shampoo® (Wellmark)	Shampoo: Pyrethrins: 0.15% Piperonyl butoxide:1.05% (s)-Methoprene: 1.1%	OTC-EPA	Kills adult fleas, ticks and lice and prevents flea larvae from hatching. Not for puppies or kittens less than 12 weeks old. 12 oz.
Adams Pyrethrin Dip® (Farnam)	Dip: Pyrethrins: 0.97% Piperonyl butoxide: 3.74%	OTC-EPA	N-octyl bicycloheptene dicarboxamide 5.7% Di-n-propyl isocinchomerate 1.94%. Kills and repels fleas, ticks, lice, gnats, mosquitoes and flies. Not for puppies or kittens less than 12 weeks old. Must be diluted before use. 4 oz.
Bio Spot® Pyrethrin Dip (Farnam)	Dip: Pyrethrin 0.97% Piperonyl butoxide 3.74%	OTC-EPA	N-octyl bicycloheptene dicarboxamide 5.7% Di-n-propyl isocinchomeronate 1.94%. Kills and repels fleas, ticks, lice, gnats, mosquitoes and flies. For dogs and cats over 12 weeks of age. 4 oz.
Pyrethrins Dip and Spray® (Davis)	Dip & Spray: Pyrethrins 3% Piperonyl butoxide 30%	OTC-EPA	Petroleum distillate 12%. Kills fleas, ticks and lice. For puppies or kittens over 6 weeks old. Must be diluted before use. Keep away from open flame. 16 oz, 1 gal.

Human-Labeled Pyrethrin Products
None

PYRIPROXYFEN & PYRIPROXYFEN COMBINATIONS, TOPICAL

(pye-ri-**proks**-i-fen)   Nylar®

Also see to the Dinotefuran listing

Indications/Actions

Pyriproxyfen is a second-generation insect growth regulator and is added to premise sprays and topical products to eliminate insects (usually fleas) via its ability to prevent maturation of eggs or larva.

Pyriproxyfen mimics insect juvenile growth hormone, halting development during metamorphosis and larval development. It also concentrates in female flea ovaries, causing non-viable eggs to be produced. When combined with an adulticide (*e.g.*, permethrin, fipronil) all stages of the parasite are killed and re-infestation is less likely. It is more resistant to UV light than is methoprene.

Suggested Dosages/Use

For specific dosage recommendations, refer to the actual product's label.

Precautions/Adverse Effects

Pyriproxyfen may be found in products also containing **permethrin, which can be toxic to cats**, particularly small kittens. **Only use in cats those products containing permethrin or other pyrethroids labeled specifically for use on cats.**

Pyriproxyfen (used alone) has low toxicity in mammals. Potentially, skin irritation or hypersensitivity reactions could occur.

Clients should wear gloves when applying products containing permethrin or other insecticides and wash off any product that contacts their skin.

Veterinary-Labeled Topical Pyriproxyfen Products

Not necessarily inclusive, there are premise sprays and other topical products containing pyriproxyfen.

Product (Company)	Form: Concentration	Label Status	Other Ingredients; Comments; Size(s)
Adams® Plus Flea & Tick Mist with Insect Growth Regulator (IGR) (Farnam)	Topical Spray: Pyriproxyfen 0.125% Pyrethrins 0.18%	OTC-EPA	Kills and repels fleas, ticks and mosquitoes. Also kills flea eggs and larvae. For dogs and cats. N-octyl bicycloheptane dicarboxamide 1% (insecticide synergist). 16 and 32 oz.

Product (Company)	Form: Concentration	Label Status	Other Ingredients; Comments; Size(s)
Adams® Flea & Tick Mist for Cats (Farnam)	Topical Spray: Pyriproxyfen 0.125% Pyrethrins 0.18%	OTC-EPA	Kills and repels fleas, ticks and mosquitoes. Also kills flea eggs and larvae. For cats. N-octyl bicycloheptane dicarboxamide 1% (insecticide synergist). 16 oz.
Adams® Plus Flea & Tick Shampoo with Insect Growth Regulator (IGR) (Farnam)	Shampoo: Pyriproxyfen 0.086% Pyrethrins 0.075% Piperonyl butoxide 0.75%	OTC-EPA	Kills fleas, ticks and lice. Prevent flea eggs from hatching. For dogs and cats. 12 oz.
Bio Spot® Shampoo (Farnam)	Shampoo: Pyriproxyfen 0.01% Pyrethrins 0.1% Piperonyl butoxide 0.5%	OTC-EPA	Kills adult and larval fleas, and ticks. For dogs only. 12 oz.
Liberty® 50 Plus IGR Spot-On (Star Horse)	Topical Solution: Pyriproxyfen 1.2% Permethrin 50%	OTC-EPA	Kills and repels fleas, ticks, mosquitoes, lice and mites. Kills flea larvae and prevents eggs from hatching. For use on dogs over 12 weeks of age. It must not be used on cats or on dogs that cohabit with a cat. Available for extra small, small, large and extra large dogs. Available in three dosage sizes: < 33 lbs; 33-66 lbs.; >66 lbs
TriForce® Canine Squeeze-On (Tradewinds)	Topical Solution: Pyriproxyfen 2% Cyphenothrin 40%	OTC-EPA	Kills and repels fleas, ticks and mosquitoes. Kills flea larvae and prevents eggs from hatching. For use on dogs 12 weeks of age or older. Must not be used on cats or on dogs that cohabit with a cat. Available in four dosage sizes: 9-20 lbs; 21-39 lbs; 40-60 lbs; 61 lbs and over

Human-Labeled Pyriproxyfen Topical Products
None

SPINETORAM

Indications/Actions
Topical spinetoram is labeled for the prevention and treatment of flea infestations in cats and kittens 8 weeks of age or older.

Spinetoram is a spinosyn compound related to spinosad. It activates the nicotinic acetylcholine receptors (nAChRs) causing the death of fleas.

Suggested Dosages/Use
One low-volume dose treats cats of all sizes/body weights. The manufacturer recommends applying the tube content topically to the skin at the base of the cat's neck once monthly. The manufacturer claims that the product starts working within 30 minutes and kills 98%–100% of fleas within 12 hours.

Precautions/Adverse Effects
None reported by the manufacturer.

Veterinary-Labeled Spinetoram Products

Product (Company)	Ingredients	Label Status	Size
Assurity® (Elanco)	Spinetoram 39.6%	OTC-EPA	Do not use on kittens less than eight (8) weeks of age. One applicator tube contains 0.019 oz (0.57 mL). Single-dose and six-dose dispensing packs.

Human-Labeled Spinetoram Products
None

Otic Preparations

While not a complete list, the following examples are representative of the types of topical otic preparations available to veterinarians. Included are both veterinary-labeled and human-labeled products that may be of use in veterinary medicine. Much of this section is adapted from: Koch, Torres, & Plumb. (2011). *Canine and Feline Dermatology Drug Handbook* IN PRESS. Wiley-Blackwell. This reference provides additional detail on these, and other related compounds and products.

Ceruminolytic Agents

Ceruminolytic products emulsify and remove ceruminous and purulent exudate by providing a surfactant, detergent and bubbling activity. They work best if applied 10-15 minutes prior to cleaning. Ceruminolytic agents should not be used with ruptured tympanic membrane because of potential for ototoxicity (be especially careful in cats with ruptured tympanum). If they are needed during in-hospital ear flushing procedures, their use should be followed by multiple flushes with warm sterile isotonic saline. Docusate sodium (DSS), calcium sulfosuccinate, and urea (carbamide) peroxide are considered potent ceruminolytic agents. Squalene, triethanolamine polypeptide elite condensate and hexamethyltetracosane are less potent agents. Propylene glycol, glycerin and oil are considered very mild ceruminolytic agents. Urea peroxide containing products will release oxygen when activated and produce a foaming action that helps breakdown down cerumen. This product however, can be irritating to already inflamed ears. If mild ceruminolytic products will be used at home by the client (intact tympanic membrane), it is important to demonstrate the cleaning technique in the examination room. Advise the client to discontinue product application and contact the veterinarian if the ears become redder or more inflamed at any time during the course of cleaning. The frequency of cleaning varies according to the needs of the individual patient.

Trade Name (Manufacturer)	Ingredients	Sizes
ADL Foaming Ear Cleanser® (ADL)	Cocamidopropyl betaine, isosteramidopropyl morpholine lactate, salicylic acid, eucalyptol	4 oz, 8 oz
Cerumene® (Vetoquinol)	25% squalene in isopropyl myristate liquid, petrolatum base	4 oz
ClearX Ear Cleaning Solution® (DVM)	Docusate (DSS) 6.5%; urea (carbamide) peroxide 6%	4 oz
Corium-20® (Virbac)	Purified water, SDA-40B 23%, glycerol	8 oz
KlearOtic® Ear Cleanser (Dechra)	Squalene 22%	4 oz
Douxo® Micellar Solution (Sogeval)	Phytosphingosine, polysorbate, propylene glycol, poloxamer 184, imidazolidin urea, polidocanol, polysaccharides, alcohol, light fragrance	4.2, 8.4 oz
Ear Cleansing Solution® (Vet Solutions)	De-ionized water, aloe vera gel, SD alcohol 40-2, propylene glycol, lactic acid, glycerin, docusate (DSS), salicylic acid, fragrance, benzoic acid and benzyl acid	8, 16 oz
Earoxide Ear Cleanser® (Tomlyn)	Carbamide peroxide 6.5% in a glycerin base	2, 4 oz
OtiFoam® (DVM)	Water, cocamidopropyl betaine, PEG-60 almond glycerides, mackalene 426, salicylic acid and oil of eucalyptus.	8 oz
OtiRinse® Solution (DVM)	Salicylic acid, benzoic acid, docusate sodium (DSS), aloe vera	8 oz
Vet Solutions Ear Cleansing Solution for Dogs and Cats® (Vetoquinol)	Docusate sodium (DSS), ethanol, aloe vera	4, 8, 16 oz, 1 gal

Cleaning/Drying Agents

Cleaning and drying agents are typically used after debris or exudate has been removed from the ear canals with a ceruminolytic agent. Their ingredients are usually an acid or isopropyl alcohol. Cleaning and drying ear solutions can be used on a maintenance regimen to help prevent ear infections and after bathing or swimming to keep the external ear canals water free. It is important to demonstrate the cleaning technique in the examination room. Advise the client to discontinue application and contact the veterinarian if the ears become more red or more inflamed at any time during the course of cleaning. The frequency of cleaning varies according to the needs of the individual patient.

Trade Name (Manufacturer)	Ingredients	Sizes
ADL Ear Flushing Drying Lotion® (ADL)	Isopropyl alcohol, salicylic acid, eucalyptol, acetamine MEA, propylene glycol, acetic acid, aluminum acetate, hydrolyzed oat protein, wheat amino acids	8 oz
Alocetic Ear Rinse® (DVM)	Water, acetic acid, nonoxynol-12, fragrance, methylparaben, DMDM hydantoin, aloe vera gel	4, 12 oz
Clearx Ear Drying Solution® (DVM)	Acetic acid, colloidal sulfur, hydrocortisone	4 oz
Corium-20® (Virbac)	SDA-40B 23%, glycerol	8 oz

Trade Name (Manufacturer)	Ingredients	Sizes
Domeboro® Otic (Miles) Note: human product	Acetic acid 2%, aluminum acetate	2 oz
Ear Cleaning Solution® (Vetoquinol)	Aloe vera gel, SD alcohol 40-2, propylene glycol, lactic acid, glycerin, docusate sodium (DSS), salicylic acid, fragrance, benzoic acid and benzyl acid	8, 16 oz
Epi-Otic® Cleanser with Spherulites (Virbac)	Lactic acid 2.5%, salicylic acid 0.1%, Spherulites® microcapsules, encapsulated chitosanide, docusate sodium, propylene glycol, PCMX	4, 8, 16 oz
Epi-Otic Advanced® (Virbac)	Salicylic acid 0.2%, disodium EDTA, docusate sodium, PCMX, a monosaccharide complex, odor neutralizer	4, 8 oz
Euclens Otic Cleanser® (Butler Schein)	Propylene glycol, malic acid, benzoic acid, eucalyptus oil	4, 16 oz
Gent-L-Clens® (Intervet/Schering-Plough)	Lactic acid, salicylic acid in propylene glycol	4 oz
MalAcetic Otic®, MalAcetic Otic® AP (contains apple fragrance) (Dechra)	Acetic acid 2%, boric acid 2%	4, 8, 16 oz
Oti-Calm® (DVM)	Benzoic acid, malic acid, salicylic acids; oil of eucalyptus	4 oz, 12 oz
Oti-Clens® (Pfizer)	Propylene glycol, malic acid, benzoic acid, salicylic acid	4 oz
Oti-Soothe®+ PS with Aloe Vera (Sogeval) Oti-Soothe® + PS with Cucumber Melon (Sogeval)	Aloe vera gel, lactic acid, salicylic acid, benzoic acid, propylene glycol, SD alcohol 40, glycerin, docusate (DSS), fragrance, benzyl alcohol; phytosphingosine: 0.01%	4, 8, 16 oz & 1 gallon
Oti-Soothe® with Aloe Vera (Sogeval) Oti-Soothe® with Cucumber Melon (Sogeval)	Aloe vera gel, lactic acid, salicylic acid, benzoic acid, propylene glycol, SD alcohol 40, glycerin, docusate sodium (DSS), fragrance, benzyl Alcohol	4, 8, 16 oz & 1 gallon
OtiRinse® Solution (DVM)	Salicylic acid, benzoic acid, docusate (DSS), aloe vera	8 oz
Otocetic Solution® (Vedco)	Acetic acid 2%, hamamelis, anodyne with surfactants	4, 16 oz

Antiseptic Agents

Topical antiseptic ear flushes include acetic acid, chlorhexidine and ketoconazole containing products. These products are typically used as adjunctive therapy for ear infections (e.g., bacterial and/or yeast) but can also be used as sole treatment in mild, first time infections. Acetic acid works as an acidifying and antimicrobial agent. Chlorhexidine has activity against gram-positive and gram-negative bacteria and fungi. Chlorhexidine containing products should be used cautiously in ear canals with ruptured tympanic membranes because of potential for ototoxicity. Ketoconazole is a fungistatic antifungal. When recommending ear flushing as part of the treatment regimen, it is important to demonstrate the cleaning technique in the examination room and advise the client to discontinue application and contact the veterinarian if the ears become more red or more inflamed at any time during the course of cleaning. The frequency of cleaning varies according to the needs of the individual patient.

Trade Name (Manufacturer)	Active Ingredients	Sizes
Bausch & Lomb Acetic Acid 2% in Aqueous Aluminum (B&L)	Acetic acid, aluminum acetate	60 mL
MalAcetic Otic® MalAcetic Otic® AP (Dechra)	Acetic acid 2%, boric acid 2%; MalAcetic® Otic AP contains apple fragrance	4, 8, 16 oz
MalAcetic® Ultra Otic (Dechra)	Acetic acid 1%, boric acid 1%, ketoconazole 0.15%, Hydrocortisone 1%	2, 8 oz
Mal-A-Ket Plus TrizEDTA Flush® (Dechra)	Ketoconazole (0.15%), chlorhexidine 0.15%, tris-EDTA	4, 12 oz
Otocetic Solution® (Vedco)	Acetic acid 2%, hamamelis	4, 16 oz

Antibiotic Potentiating Agents

Tromethamine-ethylenediaminetetraacetic acid (tris-EDTA) has antimicrobial and antibiotic potentiating activity. It is alkalinizing (pH8), blocks the Pseudomonas efflux pump, potentiates antibiotics such as enrofloxacin and aminoglycosides, disrupts the bacterial cell wall by chelating metal ions and making it more porous, inhibits the effects of ulcerating bacterial enzymes. Tris-EDTA is non-ototoxic and safe to use in the middle ear. Tris-EDTA containing products are most effective when applied 15-30 minutes before the topical antibiotic.

Products containing tris-EDTA are available as a sole ingredient or combined with chlorhexidine or ketoconazole. When recommending ear flushing as part of the treatment regimen, it is important to demonstrate the cleaning technique in the examination room and advise the client to discontinue application and contact the veterinarian if the ears become redder or more inflamed at any time during the course of cleaning. The frequency of cleaning varies according to the needs of the individual patient.

Trade Name (Manufacturer)	Active Ingredients	Sizes
KetoTris Flush + PS® (Sogeval)	Ketoconazole 0.1%, EDTA, phytosphingosine 0.01%	4, 16 oz
KetoTris Flush® (Sogeval)	Ketoconazole 0.1%, EDTA	4, 16 oz
Mal-A-Ket Plus TrizEDTA Flush® (Dechra)	Ketoconazole 0.15%, chlorhexidine 0.15%, tris-EDTA	4, 12 oz
TrizEDTA®, Aqueous or Crystals (Dechra)	tris-EDTA	4, 16 oz
TrizULTRA + Keto® (Dechra)	tris-EDTA, ketoconazole 0.15%	4, 12 oz
TrizCHLOR® (Dechra)	tris-EDTA, chlorhexidine 0.15%	4 oz
T8 Keto® Flush (DVM)	tris-EDTA, ketoconazole 0.1%	4, 12 oz
T8 Solution® Ear Rinse (DVM)	tris-EDTA, benzyl alcohol, nonoxynol 12, lanolin	4, 12 oz

Corticosteroid Preparations

Corticosteroid-containing ear medications are used in cases of acute or chronic otitis with the goal of reducing inflammation, edema, tissue hyperplasia, pain and pruritus. In addition, they are helpful in decreasing secretions from sebaceous and apocrine glands thereby reducing the build up of debris in ear canals. Ear cleaning solutions that contain glucocorticoids without an antibiotic can be used as maintenance therapy in cases of allergic otitis, but use the least potent glucocorticoid at the lowest possible frequency to balance efficacy and prevent undesirable side effects.

Trade Name (manufacturer)	Active Ingredients	Sizes
Clearx Drying Solution® (DVM)	Hydrocortisone 1%, acetic acid, colloidal sulfur.	1 oz
Cort/Astrin Solution® (Vedco)	Hydrocortisone 1%, Burow's solution	1, 16 oz
MalAcetic ® Ultra Otic (Dechra)	Hydrocortisone 1%, boric acid 2%, acetic acid 1%, ketoconazole 0.15%	2, 8 oz
Synotic Otic Solution® (Pfizer)	Fluocinolone 0.01%; DMSO 60%	8 & 60 mL

Antibacterials

Refer also to Corticosteroid Preparations and Injectable Antimicrobial (Antibacterial) Preparations

Antibacterial ear preparations are commonly used to treat infections caused by *Staphylococcus* spp. or *Pseudomonas* spp. Very few otic products containing solely an antibiotic are commercially available to treat bacterial otitis; therefore, the clinician often must use ophthalmic products or injectable antibiotics directly into the ear canals to treat these infections. When using acidifying ear cleansers and with an aminoglycoside- or fluoroquinolone-containing agent, it is recommended to use these products about one hour apart since low pH can decrease the activity of aminoglycosides and fluoroquinolones. When treating a Pseudomonas ear infection, culture and susceptibility should be performed to select the appropriate antibiotic as resistance is a major concern.

These products should be used two to three times daily in adequate amounts to coat the entire ear canal. Advise the client to discontinue the medication and contact the veterinarian if the ears become more red or more inflamed at any time during treatment. Patients should be rechecked before discontinuing treatment.

Trade Name (Manufacturer)	Active Ingredients	Sizes
Baytril Otic® (Bayer)	Enrofloxacin 0.5%, Silver sulfadiazine (SSD) 1%.	15 mL, 30 mL
Gentocin® Ophthalmic Solution (Schering-Plough) generic	Gentamicin sulfate 0.3%	5 mL
Tobrex® Ophthalmic Solution (Alcon Ophthalmic)	Tobramycin 0.3%,	5 mL

Antifungals

Refer also to the Corticosteroid + Antimicrobial section

Antifungal ear preparations are used to treat *Malassezia* otitis and rarely otic candidiasis. Most of the commercially available products also contain an antibiotic and/or a glucocorticoid. Listed here are exclusively the products without an antibiotic agent.

These products should be used two to three times daily in adequate amounts to coat the entire ear canal. Advise the client to discontinue the medication and contact the veterinarian if the ears become more red or more inflamed at any time during treatment. Patients should be rechecked before discontinuing treatment.

Trade Name (Manufacturer)	Active Ingredients	Sizes
Clotrimatop® Solution (Butler)	Clotrimazole 1%	30 mL
Clotrimazole Solution (VET Solutions)	Clotrimazole 1%	30 mL
Lotrimin® Solution (Schering-Plough); Generics	Clotrimazole 1%	10 mL, 30 mL
MicaVed® Lotion (Vedco)	Miconazole 1%	120 mL

Trade Name (Manufacturer)	Active Ingredients	Sizes
Micazole® Lotion (Butler)	Miconazole 1%	60 mL
Miconosol® Lotion (Med Pharmex)	Miconazole 1%	60 mL
Priconazole® Lotion 1% (Priority Care)	Miconazole 1%	30 mL, 60 mL

Corticosteroid + Antimicrobial Preparations

Most otic antimicrobial preparations commercially available combine an antifungal, an antibiotic and a glucocorticoid agent

These products should be used two to three times daily in adequate amounts to coat the entire ear canal. Advise the client to discontinue the medication and contact the veterinarian if the ears become more red or more inflamed at any time during treatment. Patients should be rechecked before discontinuing treatment.

Trade Name (Manufacturer)	Active Ingredients	*Size(s)*
Antibiotic Ear Solution® (Rugby) **Cortisporin® Otic Suspension** (Monarch) **Cortomycin®** (Major) **Oti-Sone® Otic Suspension** (Ocumed) **Pediotic® Otic Suspension** (GlaxoSmithKline) **Generics**	Neomycin sulfate 3.5 mg/mL, Polymyxin B 10,000 Units/mL, Hydrocortisone 10 mg/mL	7.5 mL or 10 mL depending on brand
Betagen® Otic Solution (Med-Pharmex) **GenOne Otic Solution®** (VetOne) **Gentaotic®** (Butler) **GentaVed Otic Solution®** (Vedco) **Topagen® Ointment** (Intervet/Schering-Plough)	Gentamicin sulfate 3 mg/mL, Betamethasone valerate 1 mg/mL	Depending on brand: 7.5, 15, & 240 mL
Animax® Ointment (Dechra) **Derma Vet® Ointment** (Med-Pharmex) **Dermalog Ointment®** (RXV) **Dermalone Ointment®** (Vedco) **Quadritop® Ointment** (Butler) **Panolog® Ointment** (Pfizer)	Nystatin 100,000 Units/mL, Neomycin sulfate 0.25%, Thiostrepton 2,500 Units, Triamcinolone acetonide 0.1%	Depending on brand: 7.5, 15, 30 & 240 mL
MoMetaMax® Otic Suspension (Schering-Plough)	Gentamicin 3 mg/gram, Mometasone 1 mg/gram, Clotrimazole 10 mg/gram	15, 30 g
DVMax® Ointment (DVM) **Gentizol® Ointment** (VetOne) **Malotic® Ointment** (Vedco) **Otibiotic® Ointment** (Butler) **Otomax® Ointment** (Intervet/Schering-Plough); **Tri-Otic®** (Med-Pharmex) **Vetromax®** (Dechra)	Clotrimazole 1%, Gentamicin sulfate 0.3%, Betamethasone valerate 0.1%	Depending on brand: 7.5, 10, 15, 20, 25, 30 & 215 g
Posatex® Otic Suspension (Intervet)	Posaconazole 0.1%, Orbifloxacin 1%, Mometasone furoate monohydrate 0.1%	7.5, 15 & 30 g
Quadritop® Ointment (Vetus)	Nystatin 100,000 units/mL, Neomycin sulfate 2.5 mg/mL, Thiostrepton 2,500 units/mL, Triamcinolone acetonide 1.0 mg/mL	240 mL
Surolan® Otic Suspension (Vetoquinol)	Miconazole 23 mg/mL, Polymyxin B 0.5293 mg/mL, Prednisolone acetate 5 mg/mL	15 & 30 mL
Tresaderm® (Merck)	Neomycin 0.25%, Dexamethasone 0.1%, Thiabendazole 4%	7.5 mL, 15
Tritop® Ointment (Pfizer)	Neomycin sulfate 0.5%, Isoflupredone acetate 0.1%, Tetracaine hydrochloride 0.5%	10 g
TobraDex® Ophthalmic Solution (Alcon); Generics	Tobramycin 0.3%, Dexamethasone 0.1%	2.5
Zymox® Otic (Three Point Enzyme System)	Lysozyme, Lactoferrin, Lactoperoxidase, Hydrocortisone 1%	3

Antiparasitic Preparations

Refer also to the Selamectin and Fipronil monographs

Included are only preparations labeled to be applied directly into the ear ca... eatment of otoacariosis. However, parasiticides with systemic or more generalized eff... lamectin or fipronil are preferred because *Otodectes cynotis* mites are known to also live nals and can re-infest the ears.

Trade Name (manufacturer)	Active Ingredients	Dose/Use	Comments; Size(s)
Acarexx® Otic Suspension (Idexx)	0.01% Ivermectin	Clean ear and apply 0.5 ml in each ear; repeat one time if necessary	For ear mite infestation in cats or kittens four weeks of age or older. 12 foil pouches with 2 ampules per foil pouch containing 0.5 mL.
Adams Pene-Mite® (Farnam)	Pyrethrins 0.05% Piperonyl butoxide 0.5%	Clean ear and apply every-other-day for 12 days	Recommended for dogs and cats 12 weeks of age or older. 0.5 oz
Cerumite 3x® (Vetoquinol)	Pyrethrins 0.15% Piperonyl butoxide 1.5%	Clean ear and apply a sufficient amount to coat the ear canals not more frequent than twice a week	N-octyl bicycloheptene dicarboximide. For ear mite infestation in dogs and cats. 0.5 oz
Cooper's Best Ear Mite Lotion® (Aspen)	Oil of pennyroyal, Oil of lemongrass, Oil of lavender	Clean ear and apply daily for 7 to 10 days. Repeat the procedure in two weeks if needed.	Aloe. For ear mite infestation on dogs and cats. 6 oz
Ear Mite Solution® (Durvet)	Rotenone 0.12%	Clean ear and apply twice allowing one day interval.	Associated resins 0.16%. For ear mite infestation on dogs and cats 12 weeks of age or older. 4 oz
Ear Miticide® (Phoenix)	Rotenone 0.12%	Clean ear and apply twice allowing one day interval.	Associated resins 0.16%. For ear mite infestation on dogs and cats 12 weeks of age or older. 2 oz
EarMed Mite Lotion® (Davis)	Oil of pennyroyal, Oil of lemongrass, Oil of lavender	Clean ear and apply once daily for 7-10 days. Repeat in two weeks if needed.	Aloe. For ear mite infestation on dogs and cats. 2 oz
Eradimite® (Pfizer)	Pyrethrins 0.15%, Piperonyl butoxide 1.5%	Clean ear and apply once daily every 2 days until resolution of infestation	For ear mite and spinose ear tick infestation on dogs and cats. 1 oz
Happy Jack Mitex® (Happy Jack)	Pyrethrins 0.05% Piperonyl butoxide 0.5%	Clean ear and apply once daily for 7-10 days. Repeat in two weeks if needed.	For ear mite infestation on dogs and cats. 0.5, 1 oz
Hartz Advanced Care® Ear Mite Treatment (Hartz)	Pyrethrins 0.05% Piperonyl butoxide 0.5%	Clean ear and apply once daily for 7-10 days. Repeat in two weeks if needed.	Aloe. For ear mite infestation on cats 12 weeks of age or older. 3 mL
MilbeMite® Otic (Novartis)	Milbemycin oxime 0.1%	Clean ear and apply entire contents of tube in external ear canal; one tube per ear. Repeat in 30 days if recommended by the veterinarian.	For ear mite infestation on cats or kittens four weeks of age or older. Box of 10 pouches of 2 tubes of 0.25 mL each
Mita-Clear® Lotion (Pfizer)	Pyrethrins 0.15%, Technical piperonyl butoxide 1.5%,	Clean ear; instill enough to wet ear canal and massage. Retreat in 7 days.	N-octyl bicycloheptene dicarboximide 0.5%, di-n-propyl isocinchomeronate 1%. For ear mite infestation on dogs and cats. 22 mL
Otomite Plus® (Virbac)	Pyrethrins 0.15%, Technical piperonyl butoxide 1.5%,	Clean ear and instill enough to wet ear canal and massage. Retreat in 7 days.	N-octyl bicycloheptene dicarboximide 0.5%, di-n-propyl isocinchomeronate 1%. For ear mite infestation on dogs and cats. 15 mL
ormer Ear Mite r® (Agrilabs)	Pyrethrins 0.15%, Piperonyl butoxide 1%	Apply daily for 7 to 10 days.	N-Octyl bicycloheptene dicarboximide 0.5%, di-n-propyl isocinchomeronate 1%. For ear mite infestation on dogs and cats 12 weeks of age or older. 6 oz
Clear® Ear Drops®	Pyrethrin 0.61 mg/mL, Sesquiterpenoid 25 mg/mL, Salicin 0.61 mg/mL, Property blend of carvacrol 58 mg/mL	Clean ears and apply twice daily for 7-10 days.	1-8 cineol,thymol, menthol, cinnamic aldehyde. For ear mite infestation on dogs and cats. Other manufacturer's recommendations include: bacterial and yeast ear infections. 1 oz
RMITEfree (Sor Dogs®	Pyrethrins 0.06%, Piperonyl butoxide 0.6%	Clean ears and apply twice daily until the infestation is resolved.	For mite and tick ear infestation on dogs 12 weeks of age or older. 1 oz
EaMITEfree (SeCats®	Pyrethrins 0.06%, Piperonyl butoxide 0.6%	Clean ears and apply twice daily until the infestation is resolved.	For mite and tick ear infestation on cats 12 weeks of age or older. 1 oz
Ear otion Trea	Pyrethrins 0.06%, Piperonyl butoxide 0.6%	Clean ears and apply twice daily until the infestation is resolved.	For use on cats 12 weeks of age or older. 3 oz

Overdose and Toxin Exposure Decontamination Guidelines

CAMILLE DECLEMENTI, VMD, DABT
ASPCA Animal Poison Control Center

All patients should be stabilized prior to attempts at decontamination. Once stabilization has been accomplished, decontamination should be considered to prevent systemic absorption of the toxicant. The specific method of decontamination chosen in each case must be guided by the species exposed and the exposure circumstances. When a patient has ingested a potentially toxic dose of a substance, the clinician has many options for decontamination including dilution, induction of emesis, gastric lavage, the use of adsorbents, cathartics, and administration of enemas. In many cases, the best treatment plan will include more than one of these methods.

Dilution using a small amount of milk or water is recommended in cases where irritant or corrosive materials have been ingested. A dose of 2-6 ml/kg is suggested (Mathews, 2006), which for an average-sized cat, would be approximately only 1−2 teaspoons. Using only a small amount is important since using excessive amounts could lead to vomiting and re-exposure of the esophagus to the damaging material (Rosendale, 2002). Juicy fruits and vegetables can be fed to accomplish dilution in some patients, especially birds and reptiles. Dilution is not appropriate in patients who are at an increased risk for aspiration, including those who are actively seizing or obtunded (Rosendale, 2002). Dilution with milk, yogurt and cottage cheese has been useful in cases of oral irritation following ingestion of plants containing insoluble calcium oxalate crystals (Philodendron species, for example) (Means, 2004).

Emetics are usually most effective if used within 2−3 hours after the ingestion (Rosendale, 2002) but in some cases, emesis may be effective even after that time frame. If the substance ingested could coalesce to form a bezoar in the stomach or a timed-released medication was ingested, emesis may be effective later than 3 hours after the ingestion. Chocolate (Albretsen, 2004) and chewable medications are examples of products, which may form bezoars. Emetics generally empty 40−60% of the stomach contents (Beasley and Dorman, 1990). Feeding a small moist meal before inducing vomiting can increase the chances of an adequate emesis.

Animals that are able to vomit safely include dogs, cats, ferrets, and potbelly pigs. Emetics should not be used in birds, rodents, rabbits, horses or ruminants. Rodents are unable to vomit. Rabbits have a thin-walled stomach putting them at risk for gastric rupture if they vomit (Donnelly, 2004).

Induction of emesis is *contraindicated* with ingestion of corrosive agents including alkalis and acids. The protective epithelial lining of the esophagus may be damaged initially when one of these products is swallowed. The muscular layer of the esophagus may be exposed and at risk for ulceration, perforation and scarring if vomiting does occur (Beasley and Dorman, 1990). Emesis is also not recommended after petroleum distillate ingestion due to the risk of aspiration. The clinician must also take into account when deciding whether to induce emesis, any pre-existing conditions of the patient that can cause vomiting to be hazardous including severe cardiac disease or seizure disorder. In all instances the attending veterinarian must carefully weigh the benefits of emesis against the risks. Emesis may not be needed if the animal has already vomited and is not appropriate if the animal is already exhibiting clinical signs such as coma, seizures or recumbency, which make emesis hazardous. Additionally, if the patient has ingested a CNS stimulant and is already agitated, the additional stimulation of vomiting could lead to seizures (Rosendale, 2002).

Hydrogen peroxide, apomorphine hydrochloride and xylazine hydrochloride are commonly used emetics in the veterinary clinical setting. Preliminary data obtained from the ASPCA Animal Poison Control's toxicology database indicate that hydrogen peroxide and apomorphine are effective emetics in dogs. Emesis was successful in ninety-two percent of dogs when administered either 3% hydrogen peroxide or apomorphine. No significant adverse effects were reported in dogs after emetic use. Apomorphine was poorly effective as an emetic in cats and using it in cats is controversial. Xylazine was an effective emetic in only fifty-seven percent of cats. When emesis was successfully induced, sixty-eight percent of patients vomited some portion of the ingested toxicant (Khan, 2009). Please see the monographs in the text for additional information on using these as emetics.

Several other agents have been suggested by various sources as emetics. These include table salt, liquid dishwashing liquid, syrup of ipecac and powdered mustard. They are not as effective as those mentioned, and salt and syrup of ipecac may cause significant adverse effects. Table salt (sodium chloride) has been associated with hypernatremia and CNS dysfunction (Beasley and Dorman, 1990) and there are concerns that syrup of ipecac can be cardiotoxic (Rosendale, 2002). Human pediatricians no longer routinely recommend syrup of ipecac for home use and The American Association of Poison Control Centers reported in 2001 that the use of ipecac in human exposures has fallen by more than 95% over a 15-year period (Shannon, 2003).

An October 12, 2010 bulletin by the American Society of Health-System Pharmacists indicates that syrup of ipecac has been discontinued (http://goo.gl/dwbY2).

Gastric lavage can be considered in cases where emesis is contraindicated, not possible or has been unsuccessful. For example, lavage is an option if the patient is agitated, seizing or recumbent or has other health concerns, such as recent abdominal surgery, that increase the risks associated with induction of emesis. Gastric lavage should be considered in rabbits and rodents, which are unable to vomit safely. Lavage is unlikely to be as effective as emesis (Beasley and Dorman, 1990) and is associated with significant potential risks (Rosendale, 2002). For these reasons, it should not be chosen routinely as a decontamination method over emesis. Lavage should also not be used to remove caustic materials or volatile hydrocarbons for the same reasons emesis is contraindicated in such cases (Rosendale, 2002).

The patient should be under general anesthesia when performing gastric lavage unless the patient is comatose. In all instances, a cuffed endotracheal tube should be in place to prevent aspiration. If the patient is a species with cheek pouches, the cheek pouches should be emptied gently with a finger or swab prior to the lavage. Risks associated with gastric lavage include esophageal or stomach damage or perforation, electrolyte abnormalities, hypothermia and the accidental placement of the tube in the trachea and the instillation of fluid into the patient's lungs (Rosendale, 2002).

Adsorbents may be utilized instead of or in addition to using an emetic or performing gastric lavage to prevent further systemic absorption of a toxicant. These agents act by adsorbing to a chemical or toxicant in the gastrointestinal tract and facilitating its excretion in the feces. Activated charcoal is the most commonly used adsorbent.

Activated charcoal is composed of large porous particles that adsorb to and therefore trap a wide range of organic compounds within the gastrointestinal tract. It is created from materials such as coal, wood, rye starch and coconut shells through a process using acid and steam treatments. The surface binding area of activated charcoal is large, in the range of 900–1500 m^2/g (Rosendale, 2002). Charcoal tablets and capsules available over the counter, which are used to control flatulence, and bloating are not likely to be as effective adsorbents as the commercially prepared products (Buck and Bratich, 1986). The concentration of charcoal in the capsules is often low and the binding area much smaller.

Repeated doses of activated charcoal should be considered in some instances where toxicants are known to undergo enterohepatic recircula-

tion. In enterohepatic recirculation, the toxicant is first carried to the liver by either the portal vein after absorption from the gastrointestinal tract or via the systemic circulation. Once in the liver, the toxicant enters the bile and is excreted into the gastrointestinal tract where it is again available for absorption. Examples of toxicants known to undergo this type of recycling include most NSAIDs, marijuana and digoxin.

Another instance where multiple doses of activated charcoal are appropriate is in the treatment of ivermectin toxicosis. Ivermectin is a substrate for the P-glycoprotein pump that transports drugs across cell membranes. This pump is found in various cells including intestinal epithelial cells and brain capillary endothelial cells. In the intestine, ivermectin is absorbed into the enterocyte. However, once in the cell, the P-glycoprotein pump acts to move the ivermectin back into the gastrointestinal lumen. This cycling allows the ivermectin molecules to have multiple opportunities to bind with the repeated doses of activated charcoal (DeClementi, 2007). Other P-glycoprotein substrates include loperamide, diltiazem and doxorubicin (Mealey, 2006).

When repeated doses are indicated, half the original dose should be given at 4 to 8 hour intervals (Peterson, 2006). It is important to mention that if medications are excreted in the bile, activated charcoal can be beneficial regardless of the route the medication was administered. Thus if a patient received an overdose of injectable ivermectin subcutaneously, use of activated charcoal will still be a very useful (DeClementi, 2007).

Administration of activated charcoal does carry some risks and it does not bind all compounds equally. Some chemicals that are not bound effectively include: ethanol, methanol, fertilizer, fluoride, petroleum distillates, most heavy metals, iodides, nitrates, nitrites, sodium chloride, and chlorate. Activated charcoal should not be given to animals that have ingested caustic materials. It is unlikely to bind them, can be additionally irritating to the mucosal surfaces, and make visualization of oral and esophageal burns difficult (Buck and Bratich, 1986). Activated charcoal can cause a false positive on an ethylene glycol test since propylene glycol is found in many formulations. Additionally, the timing of the activated charcoal administration should be taken into account when deciding on dosing of other oral medications since the charcoal can also bind them.

Activated charcoal administration carries a significant risk of aspiration. If a patient does aspirate the charcoal, the prognosis is poor, hence proper placement of the stomach tube and a protected airway are required in symptomatic patients. Constipation and black bowel movements are possible making it difficult to determine if melena is present. If the activated charcoal resides within the gastrointestinal tract for a significant period, it may release the compound it has adsorbed. It is for this reason that activated charcoal is frequently administered with a cathartic. Many commercially available preparations do contain a cathartic such as sorbitol.

Hypernatremia is another possible adverse effect of activated charcoal administration. In humans, hypernatremia has been reported primarily in children when multiple doses of a charcoal-sorbitol mixture were administered. The mechanism for hypernatremia is attributed to a water shift from the intracellular and extracellular spaces into the gastrointestinal tract as a result of the osmotic pull of the sorbitol cathartic (Allerton and Strom, 1991). The ASPCA Animal Poison Control Center (APCC) has also received reports of elevated serum sodium following activated charcoal administration in dogs. Hypernatremia appears to be reported more often in small dogs receiving multiple doses of activated charcoal, but it has also been reported in large dogs and in cases receiving only a single dose. Furthermore, unlike the human reports, elevated serum sodium has also been noted in cases where no cathartic was present in the charcoal (APCC unpublished data). In hypernatremia cases, the APCC has found that administration of a warm water enema is effective at lowering the serum sodium and controlling the resultant central nervous system effects (DeClementi, 2007).

Cathartics enhance elimination of substances, including administered activated charcoal, by promoting their movement through the gastrointestinal tract. Activated charcoal only binds to toxicants by weak chemical forces, so without cathartics the bound toxicant can eventually be released and reabsorbed (Rosendale, 2002). When used with activated charcoal, the cathartic is given immediately following or mixed with the charcoal. Cathartics are *contraindicated* if the animal is dehydrated, has diarrhea, if ileus is present, or if intestinal obstruction or perforation are possible (Peterson, 2006).

There are bulk, osmotic, and lubricant cathartics. The most commonly used bulk cathartic is psyllium hydrophilic mucilloid (*e.g.*, *Metamucil®*). Another bulking cathartic that can be used in dogs and cats is unspiced canned pumpkin. In birds and reptiles, dilute peanut butter, fruit or vegetables can be used as bulking agents. Timothy hay can be utilized in rabbits. Osmotic cathartics have limited absorption from the gastrointestinal tract so they are able to pull water into the gastrointestinal tract, thereby increasing the fluid volume and stimulating motility to hasten expulsion in the feces.

There are saline and saccharide osmotic cathartics. Sorbitol is the most commonly used saccharide osmotic cathartic; it is the cathartic of choice and is frequently combined with activated charcoal in commercially prepared charcoal products. The saline cathartics include sodium sulfate (Glauber's salts) and magnesium sulfate (Epsom salts). Saline cathartics *should not* be used in patients with renal insufficiency or in birds or reptiles.

Of the lubricant cathartics, mineral oil is the most often used. Mineral oil is *not recommended following activated charcoal administration* as the mineral oil may render the charcoal less effective (Buck and Bratich, 1986; Galey, 1992). Since all cathartics alter the water balance in the gastrointestinal tract, electrolyte abnormalities, especially hypernatremia, are a potential risk to their use. Hydration status should be monitored frequently and fluids administered, intravenously or via an enema as needed.

Enemas may be indicated when elimination of toxicants from the lower gastrointestinal tract is desired (Beasley and Dorman, 1990). Medications formulated as extended-release or controlled-release are absorbed from the entire gastrointestinal tract, including the colon (Buckley et al., 1995). An enema can be used to move those medications through the colon quickly and lessen additional systemic effects. The general technique is to use plain warm water or warm soapy water. Phosphate enema solutions should be avoided due to the risk of electrolyte and acid-base disturbances (Beasley and Dorman, 1990). In reptiles, enemas may be useful since ingested materials often lag for prolonged periods in the colon. Enemas are *not recommended for birds* since they already have a rapid gastrointestinal transit time.

References

Albretsen, J.C. (2004). Methylxanthines. In "Clinical Veterinary Toxicology" (K.H. Plumlee, Ed.), pp. 322–326. Mosby, St. Louis.

Allerton, J.P., and Strom, J.A. (1991). Hypernatremia due to repeated doses of charcoal-sorbitol. Am J Kidney Dis 17, 581-584.

Beasley, V.R., and Dorman, D.C. (1990). Management of Toxicoses. Vet Clin North Am Small Anim Pract 20, 307-337.

Buck, W.B., and Bratich, P.M. (1986). Activated charcoal: preventing unnecessary death by poisoning. Vet Med 81, 73-77.

Buckley, N.A., Dawson, A.H., and Reith, D.A. (1995). Controlled release drugs in overdose Clinical considerations. Drug Safety 12, 73-84.

DeClementi, C. (2007). Prevention and treatment of poisoning. In "Veterinary Toxicology Basic and Clinical Principles" (R.C. Gupta, Ed.), pp. 1143–1147. Elsevier, Amsterdam.

Donnelly, T.M. (2004). Rabbits. Basic Anatomy, Physiology, and Husbandry. In "Ferrets, Rabbits, and Rodents Clinical Medicine and Surgery" (K.E. Quesenberry and J.W. Carpenter, Eds.), 2nd Ed, pp. 136-139. Saunders, St. Louis.

Galey, F.D. (1992). Diagnostic Toxicology. In "Current Therapy in Equine Medicine 3" (N.E. Robinson, Ed.), pp. 337-340. W.B. Saunders Company, Philadelphia.

Khan, S., McLean, M.K., Hansen, S., Luchinski, D., and Zawistowski, S. (2009) ASPCA Animal Poison Control Center uses its databases to study the efficacy and safety of three different emetics in dogs and cats utilizing 3R principles. Poster presented at 7th World Congress on Alternatives and Animal Use in the Life Sciences. Rome, Italy.

Mathews, K.A. (2006). "Veterinary Emergency and Critical Care Manual." Lifelearn Inc., Guelph. Pp. 4-8, 12-17, 85, 630-640, 655-659.

Mealey, K.L. (2006). Adverse drug reactions in herding-breed dogs: the role of P-glycoprotein. Compend Contin Educ Pract Vet 28, 23-33.

Means, C. (2004). Insoluble Calcium Oxalates. In "Clinical Veterinary Toxicology" (K.H. Plumlee, Ed.), pp. 340-341. Mosby, St. Louis.

Peterson, M.E. (2006). Toxicological Decontamination. In "Small Animal Toxicology" (M.E. Peterson and P.A. Talcott, Eds.), 2nd Ed, pp. 127-141. Elsevier Inc., St. Louis.

Rosendale, M.E. (2002). Decontamination strategies. Vet Clin North Am Small Anm Prac 32, 311-321.

Shannon, M. (2003). The demise of ipecac. J Pediatr Vol. 112, 1180-1181.

Importation of Unapproved New Animal Drugs into the USA

As of October 2009, the Food and Drug Administration's Center for Veterinary Medicine is no longer accepting requests nor issuing "no-objection" letters facilitating veterinarians' personal importation of foreign animal drugs that are not approved for use in the United States. FDA previously allowed licensed veterinarians to apply for permission to import small amounts of unapproved animal drugs under the Medically Necessary Personal Import Policy (a 13 step letter detailing the intended use for a specific patient under specific circumstances, such as when the drug posed no threat to human or animal health and there were no adequate drug substitutes available.) The burden of importation now appears to rest upon the exporter in completing necessary Customs and Border Patrol (CBP) documents that will allow the drugs to clear US Customs upon entry into the United States. It is important to note that drug shipments may still be seized by US Customs and returned to the exporter in spite of efforts to provide necessary documentation.

Veterinarians seeking to import these types of foreign animal drugs are now directed to FDA's guidance on the Coverage of Personal Importation, which is available at: http://goo.gl/GiWys

This supplier from the U.K. has been recommended to the author and may be able to assist U.S. veterinarians in obtaining medically necessary products from abroad:

Manor Veterinary Exports
Telephone (from USA): 01144-1993-830-278
Email: johngrippervet@compuserve.com
www.manorveterinaryexports.com

Conversion Tables for Weight in Kilograms to Body Surface Area (m²)

The following tables are derived from the equation:

Approximate surface area in $m^2 =$

$$\frac{10.1 \ (10.0 \ for \ cats) \ x \ (weight \ in \ grams)^{2/3}}{10000}$$

Dogs

Weight in Kg	m²
0.5	0.06
1	0.1
2	0.15
3	0.2
4	0.25
5	0.29
6	0.33
7	0.36
8	0.4
9	0.43
10	0.46
11	0.49
12	0.52
13	0.55
14	0.58
15	0.6
16	0.63
17	0.66
18	0.69
19	0.71
20	0.74
21	0.76
22	0.78
23	0.81
24	0.83
25	0.85
26	0.88
27	0.9
28	0.92
29	0.94
30	0.96
32	1.01
34	1.05
36	1.09
38	1.13
40	1.17
42	1.21
44	1.25
46	1.28
50	1.36
54	1.44
58	1.51
62	1.58
66	1.65
70	1.72
74	1.78
80	1.88

Cats

Weight in Kg	m²
2	0.159
2.5	0.184
3	0.208
3.5	0.231
4	0.252
4.5	0.273
5	0.292
5.5	0.311
6	0.33
6.5	0.348
7	0.366
7.5	0.383
8	0.4
8.5	0.416
9	0.432
9.5	0.449
10	0.464

Tables of Parenteral Fluids

(Not a complete listing; includes both human- and veterinary-approved products)

Sodium Chloride Solutions	Sodium (mEq/L)	Chloride (mEq/L)	Osmolality (mOsm/L)	Available as:
Sodium Chloride 0.2%	34	34	69	3 mL
Sodium Chloride 0.45% (Half-Normal Saline)	77	77	155	3, 5, 500, and 1000 mL
Sodium Chloride 0.9% (Normal Saline)	154	154	310	1, 2, 2.5. 3, 4, 5, 10, 20, 25, 30, 50, 100, 130, 150, 250, 500, & 1000 mL
Sodium Chloride 3%	513	513	1030	500 mL
Sodium Chloride 5%	855	855	1710	500 mL

Dextrose Solutions	Dextrose (g/L)	Calories (kCal/L)	Osmolality (mOsm/L)	Available as:
Dextrose 2.5%	25	85	126	250, 500, & 1000 mL
Dextrose 5%	50	170	253	10, 25, 50, 100, 130, 150, 250, 400, 500, 1000 mL
Dextrose 10%	100	340	505	250, 500, & 1000 mL
Dextrose 20%	200	680	1010	500 & 1000 mL
Dextrose 25%	250	850	1330	in 10 mL syringes
Dextrose 30%	300	1020	1515	500 & 1000 mL
Dextrose 38.5%	385	1310	1945	1000 mL
Dextrose 40%	400	1360	2020	500 & 1000 mL
Dextrose 50%	500	1700	2525	50, 250, 500, & 1000 mL
Dextrose 60%	600	2040	3030	500 & 1000 mL
Dextrose 70%	700	2380	3535	250, 500, & 1000 mL

Dextrose & Saline Solutions	Sodium (mEq/L)	Chloride (mEq/L)	Dextrose (g/L)	Calories (kCal/L)	Osmolality (mOsm/L)	Available as:
D$_{2.5}$ & 0.45% NaCl	77	77	25	85	280	250, 500, & 1000 mL
D$_5$ & 0.11% NaCl	19	19	50	170	290	500 & 1000 mL
D$_5$ & 0.2% NaCl	34	34	50	170	320	250, 500, & 1000 mL
D$_5$ & 0.33% NaCl	56	56	50	170	365	250, 500, & 1000 mL
D$_5$ & 0.45% NaCl	77	77	50	170	405	250, 500, & 1000 mL
D$_5$ & 0.9% NaCl	154	154	100	170	560	250, 500, & 1000 mL
D$_{10}$ & 0.45% NaCl	77	77	100	340	660	1000 mL
D$_{10}$ & 0.9% NaCl	154	154	100	340	815	500 & 1000 mL

Electrolyte Solutions	Na+ (mEq/L)	K+ (mEq/L)	Ca++ (mEq/L)	Mg++ (mEq/L)	Cl- (mEq/L)	Gluconate (mEq/L).4;	Lactate (mEq/L)	Acetate (mEq/L)	Osmolarity (mOsm/L)	Available as:
Ringer's Injection	147	4	4		156				310	250, 500, 1000 mL
Lactated Ringer's Injection (LRS)	130	4	4		109		28		272	250, 500, 1000, 5000 mL
Plasma-Lyte® 56	40	13		3	40			16	111	500 & 1000 mL
Plasma-Lyte® R	140	10	5	3	103		8	47	312	1000 mL
Plasma-Lyte A; Normosol®-R pH 7.4	140	5		3	98	23		27	294	500, 1000, & 5000 mL
Isolyte® S pH 7.4	141	5		3	98	23		29	295	500 & 1000 mL

Dextrose & Electrolyte Solutions	D5 In Ringer's	D2.5 In Half-strength lactated Ringer's	D5 In lactated Ringer's	Normosol®-M w/D5; Plasma-Lyte 56 w/D5	Plasma-Lyte® 148 and D5	Normosol®-R and D5
Dextrose (g/L)	50	25	50	50	50	50
Calories (kCal/L)	170	89	179	170	190	185
Na+ (mEq/L)	147	65.5	130	40	140	140
K+ (mEq/L)	4	2	4	13	5	5
Ca++ (mEq/L)	4.5	1.4	2.7			
Mg++ (mEq/L)				3	3	3
Cl- (mEq/L)	156	54	109	40	98	98
Gluconate (mEq/L)					23	23
Lactate (mEq/L)		14	28			
Acetate (mEq/L)				16	27	27
Osmolarity (mOsm/L)	562	263	527	368 (363)	547	552
Available as:	500 & 1000 mL	250, 500 & 1000 mL	250, 500 & 1000 mL	500 & 1000 mL	500 & 1000 mL	500 & 1000 mL

Abbreviations Used in Prescription Writing

A warning and the strange case of S.I.D.: Although prescription abbreviations are used throughout many references and they are generally fairly well recognized, they do increase the potential for mistakes to occur. When writing a prescription, this author recommends writing out the directions in plain English and avoiding the use of abbreviations entirely. If abbreviations are to be used, definitely avoid q.d., q.o.d., q.i.d. and s.i.d. because they can be easily confused with other abbreviations.

S.I.D. is an abbreviation virtually unknown to health professionals outside of veterinary medicine and the vast majority of pharmacists have never seen it. **S.I.D. should be eliminated from all veterinary usage and replaced with "once a day."** The additional time to write out "once a day" versus "SID" is approximately 3 seconds, but by doing so, a potentially serious, avoidable error could be prevented.

a.c.	before meals
a.d.	right ear
a.s.	left ear
a.u.	both ears
amp.	ampule
b.i.d.	twice a day
c.	with
cap.	capsule
cc	cubic centimeter
disp.	dispense
g or gm	gram
gtt(s).	drop(s)
h.	hour
h.s.	at bedtime
IM	intramuscular
IO	intraosseous
IP	intraperitoneal
IV	intravenous
lb.	pound
m2	meter squared
mg.	milligram
ml. or mL	milliliter

o.d.	right eye
o.s.	left eye
o.u	both eyes
p.c.	after meals
p.o	by mouth
p.r.n.	as needed
q.	every
q4h, etc	every 4 hours
q.i.d.	four times a day
q.o.d.	every other day
q.s.	a sufficient quantity
q4h	every 4 hours, etc.
s.i.d.	once a day
Sig:	directions to pt.
stat	immediately
SubQ, SQ, SC, Subcut	subcutaneous
susp.	suspension
t.i.d.	three times a day
tab	tablet
Tbsp., T	tablespoon (15 mL)
tsp., t	teaspoon (5 mL)
Ut dict	as directed

Solubility Definitions

The following definitions are used throughout the book in the chemistry section for each agent:

Descriptive Term	Parts of Solvent for 1 Part of Solute
Very Soluble	Less than 1
Freely Soluble	From 1 to 10
Soluble	From 10 to 30
Sparingly Soluble	From 30 to 100
Slightly Soluble	From 100 to 1000
Very Slightly Soluble	From 1000 to 10,000
Practically Insoluble, or Insoluble	More than 10,000

Conversion: Weights; Temperature; Liquids

1 pound (lb) = 0.454 kg = 454 grams = 16 ounces
1 kilogram (kg) = 2.2 pounds = 1000 grams
1 grain (gr.) = 64.8 mg (often rounded to 60 or 65 mg)
1 gram = 15.43 grains = 1000 mg
1 ounce = 28.4 grams
1 gram = 1000 mg
1 milligram (mg) = 1000 mcg (μg)
1 microgram (mcg or μg) = 1000 nanograms (ng)

TEMPERATURE CONVERSION:
9 x (°C) = (5 x °F) − 160
°C to °F = (°C x 1.8) + 32 = °F
°F to °C = (°F − 32) x 0.555 = °C

LIQUID MEASURE:
1 gallon (gal.) = 4 qts. = 8 pts. = 128 fl. oz. = 3.785 liters = 3785 mL
1 quart (qt) = 2 pints = 32 fl. oz. = 946 mL
1 pint = 2 cups = 16 fl. oz. = 473 mL
1 cup = 8 fl. oz = 237 mL = 16 tablespoons
1 tablespoon = 15 mL = 3 teaspoons
1 teaspoon = 5 mL
4 liters = 1.057 gals.
1 liter = 1000 mL = 10 deciliters
1 deciliter (dl) = 100 mL
1 milliliter (mL) = 1 cubic centimeter (cc) = 1000 microliters (μl; mcl)

Milliequivalents & Molecular Weights

Milliequivalents: The term milliequivalents (mEq) is usually used to express the quantities of electrolytes administered to patients. A mEq is 1/1000 of an equivalent (Eq). For pharmaceutical purposes an equivalent may be thought of as equal to the equivalent weight of a given substance. This, in practical terms, is the molecular weight of the substance divided by the valence or the radical. For example:

How many milligrams are equivalent to 1 mEq of potassium chloride (KCl)?

1. Determine the equivalent weight = gram atomic weight ÷ valence; Molecular weight of KCl = 74.5; Valence = 1 (K^+; Cl^-); Equivalent weight = 74.5 ÷ 1 = 74.5 grams
2. Determine the mEq weight: Equivalent weight ÷ 1000; 74.5 ÷ 1000 = 74.5 mg = 1 mEq of KCl = 1 mEq of K^+ & 1 mEq of Cl^-

If the substance would have been $CaCl_2$, the process would be identical using the gram molecular weight of $CaCl_2$ (MW 111 if anhydrous; 147 if dihydrate) and a valence of 2.

Listed below are several commonly used electrolytes with their molecular weights and valences in parentheses:

Electrolyte	Molecular Weight (valence)
Sodium Chloride	58.44 (1)
Sodium Bicarbonate	84 (1)
Sodium Acetate, anhydrous	82 (1)
Sodium Acetate, trihydrate	136 (1)
Sodium Lactate	112 (1)
Potassium Chloride	74.55 (1)
Potassium Gluconate	234.25 (1)
Calcium Gluconate	430.4 (2)
Calcium Lactate, anhydrous	218.22 (2)
Calcium Chloride, anhydrous	111 (2)
Calcium Chloride, dihydrate	147 (2)
Magnesium Sulfate, heptahydrate	246.5 (2)
Magnesium Sulfate, anhydrous	120.4 (2)
Magnesium Chloride, anhydrous	95.21 (2)
Magnesium Chloride, hexahydrate	203.3 (2)

"Normal" Vital Signs

Temperature	Celsius (°C)	Fahrenheit (°F)
Dog	37.5–39.2	99.5–102.5
Cat	37.8–39.5	100–102.5
Ferret	37.8–39.2	100–102.5
Cattle, up to one year old	38.6–39.4	101.5–103.5
Cattle, over one year old	37.8–39.2	100–102.5
Horse, adult	37.2–38.5	99–101.3
Horse, foal	37.5–39.3	99.5–102.7
Goat	38.5–40.2	101.3–104.5
Sheep	38.5–40	101.3–104
Swine, piglet	38.9–40	102–104
Swine, adult	37.8–38.9	100–102
Rabbit	38.5–39.3	100.4–105

Temperature (Rectal): Temperatures will normally fluctuate over the course of the day. The following may increase body temperature: Time of day (evening), food intake, muscular activity, approaching estrus, during gestation, high external temperatures. The following may decrease body temperature: intake of large quantities of cool fluids, time of day (morning), and low atmospheric temperature. Small breed dogs tend to have higher normal tempertures than large breeds.

Pulse Rates	BPM
Cattle, calves	100−120
Cattle, adults	55−80
Cat, young	130−140
Cat, old	100−120
Dog, young	110−120
Dog, adult large breed	80−120
Ferret	300
Goat	70−120
Horse, adult	28−40
Horse, 3 months−2 years	40−80
Horse, foals−3 months	64−128
Rabbit	120−150
Sheep	66−115
Swine, young	100−130
Swine, adult	60−90

Pulse Rates (resting and healthy) in beats per minute (BPM). Pulse rates for very young animals are usually in the higher ranges and older animals in the lower ranges of those values listed.

Respiratory Rates	RPM
Cattle, young	15−40
Cattle, adults	10−30
Cats	20−30
Dog	15−30
Ferret	33−36
Horse	10−14
Swine	8−18
Rabbit	50−60
Sheep, Goat	10−30

Respiratory Rates (resting & healthy) respirations per minute

Estrus and Gestation Periods for Dogs & Cats

	Dog	Cat
Appearance of first estrus at the age of:	7−9 months	4−12 months
Estrous cycle in animals not served:	Mean = 7 months Range = every 5−8 months	Every 4−30 days (14−19 day model) if constant photoperiod
Duration of estrus period:	7−42 days (proestrus plus estrus)	2−19 days
First occurrences after parturition:	Pregnancy does not alter interval	7−9 days
Gestation Period	Mean = 63 days; Range 58−71 days	Mean = 63 days; Range 58−70 days
Number of Young	8−12 Large Breeds 6−10 Medium Breeds 2−4 Small Breeds	4−6
Suckling Period	3−6 weeks	3−6 weeks

Conversion of Conventional Chemistry Units to SI Units

The Système Internationale d'Unites (SI), or the International System of Units was recommended for use in the health professions by the World Health Assembly in 1977. It is slowly being adopted in the United States and many journals now require its use. The following is an abbreviated table of conversion values for some of the more commonly encountered tests that may now be reported in SI Units.

	Chemistry Units to SI Units
Albumin	g/dl x 10 = g/L
Ammonia	mg/dl x 0.5872 = mmol/L
Bilirubin	mg/dl x 17.10 = mmol/L
Calcium	mg/dl x 0.2495 = mmol/L
Cholesterol	mg/dl x 0.02586 = mmol/L
CO2 pressure, pCO2	mmHg x 0.1333 = kPa
Creatinine	mg/dl x 88.4 = mmol/L
Glucose	mg/dl x 0.05551 = mmol/L
Lactate	mg/dl x 0.111 = mmol/L
Magnesium	mg/dl x 0.4114 = mmol/L
O2 pressure, pO2	mmHg x 0.1333 = kPa
Phosphorus	mg/dl x 0.3229 = mmol/L
Protein	g/dl x 10 = g/L
Urea Nitrogen	mg/dl x 0.7140 = mmol/L
Amylase	IU/L = U/L
AST (SGOT)	IU/L = U/L
ALT (SGPT)	IU/L = U/L
Lipase	IU/L = U/L
ALP	IU/L = U/L
SDH (Sorbitol)	IU/L = U/L

Bicarbonate, Chloride, CO_2 (total), Potassium, & Sodium do not require conversion from conventional to SI units.

Reference Laboratory Ranges

Note: The following reference ranges are as a general reference only; refer to the "normals" for the laboratory you are using

Chemistry: Canine, Feline, Bovine, Equine

Values are from: Marshfield Clinic Laboratories, Veterinary Diagnostic Service; http://www.marshfieldlabs.org/veterinary/ Data accessed: 2011

Test	Units	Canine	Feline	Bovine	Equine
Glucose	mg/dl	74−145	56−153	50−79	52−121
AST (SGOT)	Units/L	13−81	14−54	57−108	156−597
ALT (SGPT)	Units/L	14−151	26−128	11−47	3−60
Alkaline phosphatase	Units/L	13−289	14−102	26−78	86−262
Total bilirubin	mg/dL	0.1−0.5	0.0−0.2	0.1−0.4	0.4−3.3
Cholesterol	mg/dL	98−300	71−218	112−331	59−125
Total protein	gm/dL	5.0−8.3	5.9−8.4	6.3−8.5	5.2−8.2
Albumin	gm/dL	2.6−4.0	2.3−3.9	3.2−4.3	2.8−3.8
Urea nitrogen	mg/dL	8−30	18−36	8−22	9−27
Creatinine	mg/dL	0.5−2.0	0.6−2.0	0.6−1.4	0.4−1.9
Phosphorus	mg/dL	2.5−7.9	2.7−7.5	4.4−9.2	1.7−5.8
Calcium	mg/dL	8.7−12.0	8.7−11.7	7.9−10.5	10.2−13.4
Sodium	mmol/L	141−159	146−160	140−151	130−144
Potassium	mmol/L	3.4−5.6	3.3−5.4	3.7−5.6	2.9−5.6
Chloride	mmol/L	100−118	110−123	100−109	92−107

Test	Units	Canine	Feline	Bovine	Equine
Bicarbonate	mmol/L	16−31	15−24	22−29	21−33
CK	Units/L	50−554	55−688	50−271	96−620
GGT	Units/L	3−19	0−5	12−30	5−51
Magnesium	mg/dL	1.5−3.4	2.0−2.8	1.8−2.9	1.6−2.3
Amylase	Units/L	268−1653	422−1328	*	1−10
Lipase	Units/L	81−696	8−289	*	14−50
SDH	Units/L	0.7−20.0	0.0−10.9	12.2−46.0	2.7−8.3
LDH	Units/L	19−396	52−331	806−1250	151−776
Triglycerides	mg/dL	18−248	17−133	*	10−61
T4	μg/dL	0.8−4.0	1.9−4.8	2.8−7.0	2.5−4.8
Bile acid, fasting	μmol/L	0.0−12.0	0 0−5.0	0.0−12.0	4.6−13.3
Bile acid, postprandial	μmol/L	0.0−25.0	5.0−15.0	0.0−12.0	*
Fructosamine	μmol/L	181−400	172−370	*	232−365
Iron	μg/dL	46−214	50−141	*	89−262
BHBA	mg/dL	0.7−3.2	0.1−4.6	0.4−8.8	*
Uric acid	mg/dL	0.1−1.4	0.0−0.5	0.6−1.7	0.1−0.6
Direct bilirubin	mg/dL	0.0−0.2	0.0−0.2	0.0−0.2	0.0−0.2

*no normal range established in this laboratory

Hematology: Canine, Feline, Bovine, Equine

Values are from: Marshfield Clinic Laboratories, Veterinary Diagnostic Service; http://www.marshfieldlabs.org/veterinary/ Accessed: 2011

Test	Units	Canine	Feline	Bovine	Equine
Red Blood Count (RBC)	x 106/μL	4.48−8.53	5.8−11.0	5.0−10.0	5.63−12.09
Hemoglobin	g/dL	10.5−20.1	8.6−16.0	8.0−15.0	9.8−17.1
Hematocrit	%	33.6−58.7	28.0−47.0	24.0−46.0	27.0−47.5
Mean corp. vol. (MCV)	fL	63.0−78.3	37.7−50.0	40.0−60.0	33.5−55.8
Mean corp. Hgb (MCH)	pg	15.3−39.2	12.3−17.2	11.0−17.0	12.2−19.3
Mean corp. Hgb conc. (MCHC)	g/dL	30.8−35.9	31.1−36.0	30.0−36.0	32.4−37.4
Red cell dis. width (RDW)	%	13.4−18.1	17.0−24.0	26.0−30.0	20.6−29.0
Platelet count	x 103/μL	110−460	160−660	230−690	95−385
White blood count (WBC)	x 103/μL	4.0−17.6	3.7−20.5	4.0−12.0	4.1−14.3
Segmented neutrophil absolute no.	x 103/μL	2.5−14.3	1.3−15.7	0.6−4.0	1.7−10.4
Banded neutrophil absolute no.	x 103/μL	0.0−0.2	0.0−0.5	0.0−0.12	0.0−0.1
Lymphocyte absolute no.	x 103/μL	0.3−3.9	1.0−7.9	2.5−7.5	0.6−6.7
Monocyte absolute no.	x 103/μL	0.0-1.4	0.0-1.0	0.03-0.84	0.0-0.9
Eosinophil absolute no.	x 103/μL	0.0−1.3	0.1−2.0	0.0−2.4	0.0−0.5
Basophil absolute no.	x 103/μL	0.0−0.1	0.0−0.1	0.0−0.2	0.0−0.2

Coagulation: Canine, Feline, Bovine, Equine

Values are from: Marshfield Clinic Laboratories, Veterinary Diagnostic Service; http://www.marshfieldlabs.org/veterinary/ Accessed: 2011

Test	Units	Canine	Feline	Bovine	Equine
Antithrombin III	%	84.0−128.0	87.0−143.0	*	*
APTT (Activated Partial Thromboplastin Time	seconds	9.1−15.6	9.9−23.4	21.3−35.8	33.0−55.0
D-Dimer	μg/mL	0.0−0.4	0.0−0.4	*	*
Fibrin split products	μg/mL	0.0−4.0	0.0−4.0	*	*
Fibrinogen, Semi-quantitative	mg/dL	*	*	300−700	100−400
PIVKA	seconds	12.0−18.0	19.0−33.0	*	17.0−23.0
PT (Prothrombin time)	seconds	5.4−8.8	7.2−12.5	16.8−20.7	9.1−12.6

*no normal range established in this laboratory

Urinalysis: Canine, Feline

Test	Units	Canine	Feline
Specific Gravity		1.001−1.070	1.001−1.080
pH		5.5−7.5	5.5−7.5
Volume	mL/kg/day	24−41	22−30
Osmolality		500−1200 50 min; 2400 max.	50 min; 3000 max.
Sediment: erythrocytes (per HPF)		0−5	0−5
Sediment: leukocytes (per HPF)		0−5	0−5
Sediment: casts (per HPF)		0	0
Glucose/Ketones		0	0
Bilirubin		0−trace	0
Calcium	mEq/L	2−10	
Creatinine	mg/dL	100−300	110−280
Chloride	mEq/L	0−400	
Magnesium	mg/kg/24h	1.7−3.0	3
Phosphorus	mEq/L	50−180	
Potassium	mEq/L	20−120	
Sodium	mEq/L	20−165	
Urea Nitrogen	mg/kg/24h	140−2302	374−1872

Cerebral Spinal Fluid: Canine, Feline

Test	Units	Canine	Feline
Pressure	mm of Water	<170	<100
Specific gravity		1.005−1.007	1.005−1.007
Lymphocytes	per mcl	<5	<5
Pandy's		neg.−trace	neg.
Protein	mg/dL	<25	<25
CK	Units/L	9−28	

Ferret: Male Albino

Values are from: Marshfield Clinic Laboratories, Veterinary Diagnostic Service; http://www.marshfieldlabs.org/veterinary/ Accessed: 2011. Adapted from *Biology and Disease of the Ferret* by James G. Fox

Test	Units	Range
WBC	103/μL	4.4−19.1
RBC	x 106/μL	7.3−12.18
HGB	gm/dL	16.3−18.2
HCT	%	44−61
PLT	103/μL	297−730
Seg	%	11−82
Lymph	%	12−54
Mono	%	0−9
EOS	%	0−7
Baso	%	0−2
Glu	mg/dL	94−207
AST	Units/L	28−120
Alk Phos	Units/L	9−84
T Bili	mg/dL	<1.0
Chol	mg/dL	64−296
TP	gm/dL	5.1−7.4
ALB	gm/dL	2.6−3.8
BUN	mg/dL	10−45

Test	Units	Range
Creat	mg/dL	0.4−0.9
Phos	mg/dL	4.0−9.1
CA	mg/dL	8.0−11.8
NA	mEq/L	137−162
K	mEq/L	4.5−7.7
CL	mEq/L	106−125

Rabbit: Female New Zealand White

Values are from: Marshfield Clinic Laboratories, Veterinary Diagnostic Service; http://www.marshfieldlabs.org/veterinary/ Accessed: 2011. Adapted from *Animal Models in Toxicology* by GAD and Chengelis

Test	Units	Range
WBC	103/µL	4.0−13.0
RBC	x 106/µL	5.0−7.2
HGB	gm/dL	10.5−15.0
HCT	%	32−45
MCV	fL	55−70
MCH	pg	19−23
MCHC	%	30−35
PLT	x 103/uL	300−750
Neutrophil	x 103/uL	1.0−6.0
Lymph	x 103/uL	2.0−9.0
Mono	x 103/uL	0−0.5
EOS	x 103/uL	0−0.4
Baso	x 103/uL	0−1.0
GLU	mg/dL	100−190
AST	Units/L	15−45
ALKP	Units/L	40−140
ALT	Units/L	15−50
T bili	mg/dL	0.1−0.5
Chol	mg/dL	30−100
TP	gm/dL	5.2−7.5
ALB	gm/dl	3.5−5.5
BUN	MG/dL	11−25
Creat	mg/dL	0.9−1.7
Phos	mg/dL	2.0−9.0
CA	mg/dL	12.5−15.5
NA	mEq/L	133−150
K	mEq/L	3.5−6.0
CL	mEq/L	96−106
Trig	mg/dL	30−180
GGT	Units/L	0−10

Avian: Macaws

Values are from: Marshfield Clinic Laboratories, Veterinary Diagnostic Service; http://www.marsh-fieldlabs.org/veterinary/ Accessed: 2011

Test	Units	Range
GLU	mg/dL	136–464
AST	Units/L	70–316
GGT	Units/L	2–21
Alk phos	Units/L	22–233
LDH	Units/L	19–178
Chol	mg/dL	102–386
TP	g/dL	3.3–4.9
Phos	mg/dL	2.1–11.2
CA	mg/dL	8.9–11.7
NA	mmol/L	144–163
K	mmol/L	2.1–5.0
CL	mmol/L	113–120
Bicarb	mmol/L	23–27
Uric acid	mg/dL	2.9–10.4
Anion gap	mmol/L	12.7–19.6

Avian: Parrots, African Grey

Values are from: Marshfield Clinic Laboratories, Veterinary Diagnostic Service; http://www.marsh-fieldlabs.org/veterinary/ Accessed: 2011

Test	Units	Range
GLU	mg/dL	185–294
AST	Units/L	78–149
Chol	mg/dL	179–417
TP	gm/dL	3.1–4.4
Phos	mg/dL	3.2–5.4
CA	mg/dL	8.4–10.4
NA	mmol/L	156–164
K	mmol/L	2.9–4.6
CL	mmol/L	118–127
Bicarb	mmol/L	8–14
Uric acid	mg/dL	3.4–10.8
Anion gap	mmol/L	24.2–37

Hematology: Sheep, Goats, Swine

Test	Units	Sheep	Goats	Swine
PCV	%	27–45	22–38	32–50
HGB	g/dL	9–15	8–12	10–16
RBC	x 106/µL	9–15	8–18	5–8
WBC	x 103/µL	4–12	4–13	11–22
Total Protein (TPP)	g/dL	6.0–7.5	6–7.5	6–8
MCV	fL	28–40	16–25	50–68
MCH	pg	8–12	5.2–8	17–21
MCHC	g/dL	31–34	30–36	30–34
Reticulocytes	%	0	0	0–1.0
RBC diameter	microns	3.2–6	2.5–3.9	4–8
RBC life	days	140–150	125	75–98
M:E ratio		0.77–1.68:10	0.69:10	1.77–0.52:10
Platelets	x 103/µL	250–750	300–600	325–715
Icterus Index			<5 Units	2–5
Fibrinogen	mg/dL	100–500	100–400	1–500
WBC Diff.	Absolute count/ µL (% of total)			
stabs		rare	rare	0–900 (0–4)
segs		400–6000 (10–50)	1200–6250 (30–48)	3100–10350 (28–47)
lymphs		1600–9000 (40–75)	2000–9100 (50–70)	1550–13650 (39–62)
monos		0–750 (0–6)	0–550 (0–4)	200–2200 (2–10)
eos		0–1200 (0–10)	50–1050 (1–8)	50–2400 (0.5–11)
basos		0–350 (0–3)	0–150 (0–1)	0–450 (0–2)
Coagulation		seconds		
PT		13.5–15.9		
PTT		27.9–40.7		
TT		4.8–8.0		

Chemistry: Sheep, Goats, Swine

Test	Units	Sheep	Goats	Swine
Blood Urea Nitro.	mg/dL	8–20	13–28	8–24
Sodium (Na+)	mEq/L	139–152	135–154	135–150
Potassium (K+)	mEq/L	3.9–5.4	4.6–9.8	7.8–10.9
Chloride (Cl-)	mEq/L	95–103	105–120	94–106
Glucose	g/dL	42–76	60–100	65–95
Calcium, Total	mg/dL	11.5–12.8	8.6–10.6	10.2–11.9
Creatinine	mg/dL	1–2.7	0.9–1.8	1–3
Phosphorus	mg/dL	5–7.3	4.2–9.8	7.8–10.9
Alk. Phosphatase	Units/L	68–387	9–131	9–20
Bilirubin Total	mg/dL	0.14–0.32	0–0.9	0–0.7
Creatine Kinase	Units/L	42–62	<38	
Gamma GT	Units/L	25–59	24–39	
Total Protein (TP)	g/dL	6–7.9	6.4–7.8	7.4
Albumin	g/dL	2.4–3	2–4.4	3.4
SDH	Units/L	5.8–27.9	14–23.6	

Phone Numbers & Websites

Governmental Veterinary Drug-Related Websites

Food and Drug Administration Center for Veterinary Medicine (FDA-CVM)
Call to report an adverse effect for a pharmaceutical, etc. 888-463-6332 (888-INFO-FDA); Emergency: 866-300-4374. After hours call and leave a recorded message. May also file a report on-line www.fda.gov/cvm/

U.S. Department of Agriculture (USDA)
For adverse effect reporting on biologics: 800-752-6255. May also file a report on-line at: http://goo.gl/5hoCO

U.S. Environmental Protection Agency (EPA)
Most of the products used topically for the control of ectoparasites and insects on animals are regulated by the Environmental Protection Agency (EPA) under the Federal Insecticide Fungicide and Rodenticide Act. The EPA may be reached at 800-858-7378.

The National Pesticide Information Center has a hotline and an online site for veterinarians or their staff to report adverse effects of topical pesticides: 800-858-7378; http://pi.ace.orst.edu/vetrep/

Food Animal Residue Avoidance & Depletion Program (FARAD)
1-888-USFARAD (1-888-873-2723)
http://www.farad.org/

Drug Enforcement Administration (DEA)
800-882-9539 Toll-free number for registration information. www.deadiversion.usdoj.gov/

OUTSIDE OF USA:
Australia: APVMA Website: http://www.apvma.gov.au/
Canada: Health Canada website with many veterinary links: http://goo.gl/cGDua_
New Zealand: NZFSA Ag Compounds and Vet Medicines website: http://goo.gl/UvHLa
United Kingdom: Veterinary Medicines Directorate website: http://www.vmd.gov.uk/

Drug Shortage Websites
The Food and Drug Administration (FDA) maintains a drug shortage web page. E-mail notification service is available: http://goo.gl/16ICZ

The American Society of Health-System Pharmacists (ASHP) has a website for drug shortages (human drugs): http://www.ashp.org/shortages

Animal Poison Centers

ASPCA Animal Poison Control Center
1-888-426-4435
www.apcc.aspca.org
A consultation fee may be applied to a credit card.

Pet Poison HELPLINE
1- 800-213-6680
www.petpoisonhelpline.com
A consultation fee may be applied to a credit card.

Angell Poison Control Hotline
1-877-2ANGELL
http://goo.gl/oJ8jX
A consultation fee may be applied to a credit card.

There are many regional poison centers that may be of assistance with animal poisonings; refer to your local poison center for more information.

Animal Blood Banks

Animal Blood Resources
Michigan: 517-851-8244
California: 800-243-5759
http://www.abrint.net/index.html

Canadian Animal Blood Bank Inc.
Tel: 204-632-2856
FAX: 204-632-4859
http://www.rrc.mb.ca/abb/

Eastern Veterinary Blood Bank
(410) 384-9441 - Customer line
(800) 949-EVBB (3822) - Customer & Donor lines
(410) 224-BANK (2265) - Donor line
www.evbb.com

Hemopet
Phone: (714) 891-2022
FAX: (714) 891-2123
www.hemopet.com

LifeStream Animal Blood Bank Inc. (Canada)
Tel: 1-866-696-0099
FAX: 613-531-0732
www.animalbloodbank.ca

Penn Animal Blood Bank (PABB)
Tel: 215-573-PABB
http://goo.gl/5ub6F

Sun States Animal Blood Bank
Phone: 954-630-2231
FAX: 954-630-3120
www.sunstates.org/

The Animal Blood Bank at The Ohio State University
614-292-5551
http://vet.osu.edu/vmc/animal-blood-bank

The Pet Blood Bank
Tel: 800-906-7059
FAX: 512-267-8860
www.pettransfusion.com

The Veterinarians' Blood Bank
Phone: 1-877-838-8533
Fax: 812-358-0083
www.vetbloodbank.com

Companion Animal Diet Websites

The Nutrition Support Service at The Ohio State University Veterinary Hospital maintains a website at:

http://vet.osu.edu/vmc/nutrition-support-service

This site has a variety of useful information for the veterinary professional, including a: Body Condition Scoring Chart, Diet Manual, Food and Feeding Management Guide and information on Home-Made Diets. The diet search function on this site is particularly useful. It can be found at: http://goo.gl/xVaMJ

Dog and Cat Food Company Websites

The following are links to some of the major canine and feline dog food companies in the USA.

Del Monte
www.delmonte.com/brands/

Eukanuba/Iams
www.iams.com
www.eukanuba.com

Hill's/Science Diet
www.hillspet.com

Nutro
www.thenutrocompany.com

PetAg
www.petag.com

Purina
www.purina.com

Royal Canin/IVD
www.royalcanin.us/

Veterinary Pharmaceutical Manufacturers/ Suppliers

The following lists customer service phone numbers and website URLs for several companies that provide veterinary drug-related products for the USA market.

3M Animal Care Products
800-848-0829
www.3M.com/animalcare

Abbott Laboratories
888-299-7416
www.abbottanimalhealth.com

Agri Laboratories LTD
800-542-8916
www.agrilabs.com

Alpharma Inc. Animal Health Division
800-834-6470
www.alpharma.com

Aspen Veterinary Resources Ltd.
816-415-4324
www.aspenveterinaryresources.com

B.E.T. Labs
859-273-3036
http://www.betlabs.com/

Bayer HealthCare LLC, Animal Health Division
General Inquiries: 800-255-6517
www.bayer-ah.com

Bimeda, Inc., Div. Cross Vetpharm Group, Ltd.
888-524-6332
www.bimeda.com

Bioniche Animal Health USA, Inc.
800-265-5464
www.bioniche.com

Boehringer Ingelheim Vetmedica, Inc.
800-325-9167
www.bi-vetmedica.com

Butler Schein Animal Health
800-456-0400
www.butlerschein.com

Colorado Serum Company
800-525-2065
www.colorado-serum.com

Davis Mfg.
800-292-2424
www.davismfg.com

Dechra Veterinary Products
913-327-0015
www.pharmadermah.com

Delmont Laboratories, Inc.
800-562-5541
www.delmont.com

Dermapet
301-983-8387
www.dermapet.com

Durvet, Inc.
800-821-5570
www.durvet.com

Elanco Animal Health
A Division of Eli Lilly & Co.
800-428-4441
www.elanco.com
www.elancopet.co

Farnam
800-234-2269
www.farnam.com

Figuerola Laboratories
800-219-1147
http://www.figuerola-labs.com/

First Priority, Inc.
800-650-4899
www.prioritycare.com

Ford Dodge Labs
—See Pfizer

Greer Laboratories, Inc.
877-777-1080
www.greerlabs.com

Halocarbon Products Corporation
201-262-8899
www.halocarbon.com

Hanford Pharmaceuticals
800-234-4263
www.hanford.com

Happy Jack, Incorporated
800-326-5225
www.happyjackinc.com

The Hartz Mountain Corporation
800-275-1414
www.hartz.com

Heska Corporation
800-464-3752 (800-GO HESKA)
www.heska.com

IDEXX Laboratories, Inc.
800-548-6733
www.idexx.com

Innovacyn, Inc
866-318-3116
www.vetericyn.com

Intervet Schering-Plough Animal Health Corporation
800-224-5318 Companion Animals
800-211-3573 Livestock
800-219-9286 Poultry
www.intervetusa.com

Janssen Animal Health
+32(0)14 60 2017 (Belgium)
www.janssenanimalhealth.com

Lloyd Laboratories
800-831-0004
www.lloydinc.com

Luitpold Pharmaceuticals, Inc.
800-458-0163
www.luitpoldanimalhealth.com/

MVP Laboratories, Inc
800-856-4648
www.mvplabs.com

Macleod Pharmaceuticals, Inc.
800-850-5432
www.macleodpharma.com

Med-Pharmex, Inc.
www.med-pharmex.com

Merial Ltd.
678-638-3000
www.merial.com

Modern Veterinary Therapeutics, LLC
305-669-4150
www.modernveterinarytherapeutics.com

Neogen Corporation
800-525-2022
www.neogen.com

Novartis Animal Health USA, Inc.
800-637-0281
www.ah.novartis.com

Nutramax Laboratories, Inc.
888-886-6442
www.nutramaxlabs.com

OPK Biotech
866-933-2472
www.opkbiotech.com

Pala-Tech Laboratories, Inc.
888-337-2446
www.palatech.com

PetAg, Inc.
800-323-6878
www.petag.com

Pfizer Animal Health
Customer Service: 800-733-5500
Veterinary Medical Information & Product
Support: 800-366-5288
www.pfizerah.com

Pharmacia & Upjohn Company
—see Pfizer

Phibro Animal Health
888-403-0074
www.phibroah.com

PRN Pharmacal
800-874-9764
www.prnpharmacal.com

Purica
866-334-2463
www.purica.com/

Schering
—see Intervet Schering-Plough

Sergeant's Pet Care Products, Inc.
800-224-7387 (800-224-PETS)
www.sergeants.com

Sogeval Laboratories, Inc.
866-866-8896
www.sogevalus.com

Sparhawk Laboratories, Inc.
800-255-6368
www.sparhawklabs.com

Star Horse Products
www.starhorseproducts.com

Summit VetPharm
800-999-0297
www.summitvetpharm.com

The Hartz Mountain Corporation
800-275-1414
www.hartz.com

Tomlyn Products
877-580-7729
www.tomlyn.com

Tradewinds Inc.
877-734-7565
www.tradewindsforpets.com

TriLogic Pharma
866-562-8042
www.trilogicpharma.com

Van Beek Natural Science
800-346-5311
www.vanbeeknaturalscience.com/

Vedco, Inc.
816-238-8840
www.vedco.com

Vet One
www.vetone.net

Vet Solutions
A Division of Vetoquinol USA
800-267-5707
http://goo.gl/Iilzs

Vet-A-Mix, A Division of Lloyd, Inc.
800-831-0004
www.lloydinc.com

Veterinary Products Laboratories
www.vpl.com

Vetoquinol USA, Inc.
800-267-5707
www.vetoquinolusa.com

Virbac Corporation
817-831-5030 (US)
www.virbac.com

Vortech Pharmaceuticals, Ltd.
800-521-4686
www.vortechpharm.com

Wellmark
800-877-6374; 800-263-2740 (Canada)
www.wellmarkinternational.com

Wildlife Pharmaceuticals, Inc.
866-823-9314
www.wildpharm.com

Zinpro Corporation
952-983-4000
www.zinpro.com

Systemic Drugs Sorted by Therapeutic Class or Major Indication

The following lists systemic drugs by their therapeutic class or major indication, followed by species where dosages are listed, and the page number for the monograph. The following species codes are used in parentheses after the drug name:

A = Avian; Pet Bird
B = Bovine, Cattle
C = Cat, Feline
D = Dog, Canine
Fer = Ferret
Fi = Fish
H = Horse, Equine
L = Llama, Alpacas, Camelids
Po = Pocket Pets, Rabbits, Small Lab Animals
O = Ostrich, Ratite
R = Reptiles/Amphibians
Sh = Sheep/Goats; Ovine/Caprine
Sw = Swine, Pigs
Z = Wildlife/Zoo Animals

Note: As some drugs have multiple indications, there may not be a specific dosage listed for that indication for every species noted.

Antihistamines

Cetirizine (D, C, H) 258
Chlorpheniramine (D, C, Fer, A) 276
Clemastine Fumarate (D, C) 305
Cyproheptadine (D, C, H) 357
Diphenhydramine (D, C, Fer, Po, A, H, B) 454
Doxepin (D, C, A) 481
Hydroxyzine (D, C, Fer, H, A) 691
Meclizine (D, C, Po) 845
Promethazine (D, C) 1161
Pyrilamine (D, B, H, Sh, Sw) 1189
Trimeprazine (D) 1357
Tripelennamine (D, C, B, H, Sw) 1359

Central Nervous System Drugs

(including antiinflammatories, analgesics, muscle relaxants)

CNS/RESPIRATORY STIMULANTS
Doxapram (D, C, Po, B, Sw, H, A, R) 478

ANALGESICS, OPIOID AGONISTS
Alfentanil (D) 38
Codeine Phosphate (D, C, Po) 333
Fentanyl (D, C, Fer, Po, H, Sh, Sw) 560
Hydromorphone (D, C, Fer, Po) 682
Meperidine (D, C, Fer, Po, Sh, Sw, B, H) 869
Methadone (D, C, H) 880
Morphine (D, C, Po, H, Sw, Sh, L, Z) 955
Oxymorphone (D, C, Fer, H, Sw, Po, Z) 1025
Sufentanil (D, C) 1267
Tramadol (D, C, H, Z) 1342

ANALGESICS, OPIOID AGONIST/ANTAGONISTS
Buprenorphine (D, C, Po, Fer, H, Z) 169
Butorphanol (D, C, Fer, Po, B, H, A, L, R, Z) 177
Pentazocine (D, C, Po, Fer, H) 1067

ANALGESICS, OTHER
Amantadine (D, C, H) 50
Clonidine (B) 321
Gabapentin (D, C) 613
Ketamine (D, C, Po, Fer, B, H, Sw, Sh, L, R, A, Z) 762
Pregabalin (D, C) 1145

NONSTEROIDAL ANTIINFLAMMATORY/ ANALGESIC AGENTS
Acetaminophen (D, Po) 8
Aspirin (D, C, Po, Fer, B, H, Sw, A) 112
Carprofen (D, C, Po, H, B, A, R, Z) 207
Colchicine (D, A) 335
Deracoxib (D) 381
Diclofenac (H) 421
Dimethyl Sulfoxide (D, H) 445
Etodolac (D) 538
Firocoxib (D, C, H) 571
Flunixin (D, Fer, Po, B, H, Sh, Sw, A, Z) 588
Ketoprofen (D, C, Fer, Po, H, A, Z) 775
Ketorolac Tromethamine (D, C, Sh, Po) 779
Mavacoxib (D) 841
Meloxicam (D, C, H, B, Sw, Fer, A, Z) 864
Naproxen (D, Po, H) 977
Phenylbutazone (D, B, H, Sw) 1089
Piroxicam (D, C, H, Po) 1121
Robenacoxib (D, C) 1210
Tepoxalin (D) 1287
Tolfenamic Acid (D, C, B, Sw) 1335

BEHAVIOR-MODIFYING AGENTS
Amitriptyline (D, C, A) 68
Buspirone (D, C) 172
Clomipramine HCl (D, C, A) 316
Clorazepate (D, C) 328
Diazepam (D, C, Fer, Po, B, H, Sw, Sh, A, Z) 408
Fluoxetine (D, C) 594
Fluvoxamine (D, C) 600
Imipramine (D, C, H) 704
Lorazepam (D, C) 820
Methylphenidate (D) 901
Paroxetine HCl (D, C) 1052
Pheromones (D, C, H) 1101
SAMe (D, C) 1221
Sertraline (D, C) 1227
Trazodone (D) 1345

TRANQUILIZERS/SEDATIVES
Acepromazine (D, C, Fe, P, B, H, Sw, Sh, Z) 4
Alprazolam (D, C) 44
Azaperone (Sw) 133
Chlordiazepoxide (D, C) 269
Detomidine (H, B, Sh, L, A) 391
Dexmedetomidine (D, C) 400
Diazepam (D, C, Po, Fer, A, B, H, Sw, Sh, Z) 408
Doxepin (D, C, A) 481
Lorazepam (D, C) 820
Medetomidine (D, C, Po, Fer, A, R, Z) 846
Midazolam (D, C, Po, A, H, Z) 927
Romifidine (D, C, H, B) 1216
Tiletamine/Zolazepam (D, C, Po, B, Sh, Fer, H, R, A, Z) 1317
Xylazine (D, C, Fer, Po, A, B, H, Sh, L, Z) 1397

ANESTHETIC AGENTS, BARBITURATES
Methohexital Sodium (D, C) 893
Pentobarbital (D, C, Po, B, H, Sw, Sh) 1081
Thiopental (D, C, Po, B, H, Sw, Sh) 1306

ANESTHETIC AGENTS, INHALANTS
Desflurane 383
Halothane (D, C, Po, H) 656
Isoflurane (D, C, Po, R, A) 735
Sevoflurane (D, C) 1231

ANESTHETIC AGENTS, MISCELLANEOUS
Alfaxalone (D, C, Po) 36
Alfentanil (D) 38
Etomidate (D, C, Fe, Po) 541
Fentanyl (D, C, Fer, Po, H, Sh, Sw) 560
Ketamine (D, C, Po, Fer, B, H, Sw, Sh, L, R, A, Z) 762
Propofol (D, C, Po, R, Z) 1168
Remifentanil (D, C) 1206
Sufentanil (D, C) 1267
Tiletamine/Zolazepam (D, C, Po, B, Sh, Fer, H, A, R, Z) 1317
Xylazine (D, C, Po, Fer, A, B, H, Sh, L, Z) 1397

REVERSAL AGENTS
Atipamezole (D, C, Po, B, Sh, A, R, Z) 120
Flumazenil (D, C, Z) 584
Naloxone (D, C, Po, H) 970
Naltrexone (D, C, Z) 972
Neostigmine (D, C, B, H, Sw, Sh) 985
Tolazoline (D, C, H, L, A, Sh, B, Z) 1333
Yohimbine (D, Po, A, B, H, L, Z) 1402

ANTICONVULSANTS
Bromides (D, C) 161
Carbamazepine (D, H) 198
Clonazepam (D, C) 319
Clorazepate (D, C) 328
Diazepam (D, C, Po, Fer, A, B, H, Sw, Sh, Z) 408
Felbamate (D) 554
Gabapentin (D, C) 613
Levetiracetam (D, C) 798
Lorazepam (D, C) 820
Phenobarbital (D, C, Fer, B, H) 1081
Phenytoin (D, C, H) 1097
Pregabalin (D, C) 1145
Primidone (D, C) 1149
Topiramate (D, C) 1339
Valproic Acid (D) 1369
Zonisamide (D, C) 1411

MUSCLE RELAXANTS, SKELETAL
Atracurium (D, C, Po, H) 124
Baclofen (D) 143
Dantrolene (D, C, H, Sw) 371
Guaifenesin (D, B, H, L, Sh) 653
Methocarbamol (D, C, B, H) 891
Pancuronium (D, C, Po) 1044
Rocuronium (D, C, H) 1213
Succinylcholine (D, C, H, R) 1262
Vecuronium (D, C) 1377

Euthanasia Agents
Pentobarbital/Phenytoin (D, C) 1081

Cardiovascular Agents
INOTROPIC AGENTS
Digoxin (D, C, Fer, Po, B, H, A) 431
Dobutamine (D, C, H) 465
Inamrinone Lactate (D, C) 708
Pimobendan (D, C) 1110

ANTIARRHYTHMIC DRUGS
Amiodarone (D, H) 65
Disopyramide (D) 463
Lidocaine (D, C, H) 805

Mexiletine (D) 923
Procainamide (D, C, H) 1154
Quinidine (D, C, H) 1196
Verapamil (D, C, H, Po) 1379

ANTICHOLINERGICS
Atropine (D, C, B, H, Po, Fer, Sw, Sh, A, R) 126
Glycopyrrolate (D, C, Fer, Po, H, R) 641
Hyoscyamine (D) 693

ACE INHIBITORS
Benazepril (D, C) 145
Captopril (D, C) 196
Enalapril (D, C, Fer, A) 499
Lisinopril (D, C) 814
Ramipril (D, C, H) 1200

CALCIUM CHANNEL BLOCKING AGENTS
Amlodipine (D, C) 70
Diltiazem (D, C, Fer) 438
Verapamil (D, C, H, Po) 1379

VASODILATING AGENTS
Hydralazine (D, C, H) 667
Isosorbide (D, C) 742
Isoxsuprine (H, D) 746
Nitroglycerine (D, C, Fer) 994
Nitroprusside (D, C) 996
Sildenafil (D, C) 1233
Tadalafil (D) 1283

AGENTS USED IN TREATMENT OF SHOCK
Dobutamine (D, C, H) 465
Dopamine 473
Epinephrine (D, C, A, H, B, Sh, Sw) 512
Isoproterenol HCl (D, C, H) 740
Phenylephrine (D, C, H) 1093

ALPHA-ADRENERGIC BLOCKING AGENTS
Phenoxybenzamine (D, C, H) 1087
Prazosin (D, C) 1137

BETA-ADRENERGIC BLOCKING AGENTS
Atenolol (D, C, Fer) 117
Carvedilol (D) 210
Esmolol (D, C) 528
Metoprolol (D, C) 913
Propranolol (D, C, Fer, H) 1173
Sotalol HCl (D, C) 1246

ANTIHYPERTENSIVE AGENTS
Irbesartan (D) 730
Nitroprusside (D, C) 996

OTHER CARDIOVASCULAR AGENTS
Carnitine (D, C) 205
Taurine (D, C) 1285

Respiratory Drugs
SYMPATHOMIMETICS
Albuterol (D, C, H) 31
Clenbuterol (H) 307
Ephedrine (D, C) 510
Epinephrine (D, C, A, H, B, Sh, Sw) 512
Isoproterenol HCl (D, C, H) 740
Pseudoephedrine HCl (D, C, H) 1178
Terbutaline (D, C, H) 1291

XANTHINES
Aminophylline/Theophylline (D, C, Fer, H) 60

ANTITUSSIVES
Butorphanol (D, C, Fer, Po, B, H, A, L, R, Z) 177
Codeine (D, C, Po) 333
Hydrocodone (D, C) 674

MUCOLYTICS
Acetylcysteine (D, C, H) 15

OTHER RESPIRATORY AGENTS
Cromolyn Sodium (H) 344
Ipratropium Br (H, Po) 728
Montelukast (C) 952
Zafirlukast (D, C) 1405

Renal & Urinary Tract Agents
DIURETICS, CARBONIC ANHYDRASE INHIBITORS
Acetazolamide (D, C, B, H, Sh, Sw) 10
Dichlorphenamide (D, C) 416
Methazolamide (D, C) 882

DIURETICS, THIAZIDES
Chlorothiazide (D, C, B) 273
Hydrochlorothiazide (D, C, H) 670

DIURETICS, LOOP
Furosemide (D, C, Fer, Po, B, H, A, R) 609
Torsemide (D, C) 1340

DIURETICS, POTASSIUM SPARING
Spironolactone (D, C) 1252
Triamterene (D) 1352

DIURETICS, OSMOTIC
Glycerine, Oral (D, C) 640
Mannitol (D, C, B, Sw, Sh, H) 832

**AGENTS FOR URINARY INCONTINENCE/
    RETENTION**
Baclofen (D) 143
Bethanechol (D, C, H, B) 151
Ephedrine (D, C) 510
Flavoxate (D) 574
Imipramine (D, C, H) 704
Oxybutynin (D, C) 1023
Phenoxybenzamine (D, C, H) 1087
Phenylpropanolamine (D, C) 1095
Pseudoephedrine HCl (D, C, H) 1178

URINARY ALKALINIZERS
Sodium Bicarbonate (D, C, H, B, Sh, A) 1237

URINARY ACIDIFIERS
Ammonium Chloride (D, C, H, B, Sh) 73
Methionine (D, C, B, H) 889

AGENTS FOR UROLITHIASIS
Acetohydroxamic Acid (D) 14
Allopurinol (D, A, R) 40
Ammonium Chloride (D, C, H, B, Sh) 73
Citrate Salts (D, C) 300
Methionine (D, C, B, H) 889
Tiopronin (D) 1325

MISCELLANEOUS RENAL/URINARY AGENTS
Amitriptyline (D, C, A) 68
Pentosan (D, C, H) 1074
Probenecid (R) 1151

Gastrointestinal Agents
ANTIEMETIC AGENTS
Chlorpromazine (D, C, B, H, Sw, Sh) 278
Dimenhydrinate (D, C) 441
Diphenhydramine (D, C, Fer, Po, A, H, B) 454
Dolasetron (D, C) 469
Granisetron (D, C) 649
Maropitant (D, C) 838
Meclizine (D, C, Po) 845
Metoclopramide (D, C, Po, H) 909
Mirtazapine (D, C) 940
Ondansetron (D, C) 1010
Prochlorperazine (D, C) 1159
Promethazine (D, C) 1161

ANTACIDS
Aluminum Hydroxide (D, C, Po, B, H) 48
Calcium Salts, Oral (D, C, B, H, Sh, Sw, A, R) 191
Sodium Bicarbonate (D, C, H, B, Sh, A) 1237

H-2 ANTAGONISTS
Cimetidine (D, C, Fer, Po, H, Sw, R) 288
Famotidine (D, C, Fer, Po H) 545
Nizatidine (D, C) 999
Ranitidine (D, C, Fer, H, Po) 1203

GASTROMUCOSAL PROTECTANTS
Sucralfate (D, C, Fer, H, R) 1265

PROSTAGLANDIN E ANALOGS
Misoprostol (D, H) 942

PROTON PUMP INHIBITORS
Omeprazole (D, C, Fer, H, Sw) 1007
Pantoprazole (D, C, H) 1046

APPETITE STIMULANTS
Cyproheptadine (D, C, H) 357
Diazepam (D, C, Fer, Po, A, B, H, Sw, Sh, Z) 408
Mirtazapine (D, C) 940
Oxazepam (D, C) 1018

GI ANTISPASMODICS-ANTICHOLINERGICS
Aminopentamide (D, C) 59
Hyoscyamine (D, C) 693
N-Butylscopolammonium Br (H) 980
Propantheline (D, C, H) 1163

GI STIMULANTS
Cisapride (D, C, Po, H) 294
Dexpanthenol (D, C, H) 404
Domperidone (D, C, H) 471
Metoclopramide (D, C, Po, H) 909
Neostigmine (D, C, B, H, Sw, Sh) 985

DIGESTIVE ENZYMES
Pancrelipase (D, C, Po, A) 1042

LAXATIVES
Bisacodyl (D, C) 154
Docusate (D, C, H) 467
Lactulose (D, C, A, R) 781
Laxatives, Hyperosmotic (D, C, H, B, Sh, Sw, A) 784
Magnesium Hydroxide (D, C, B, H, Sh) 826
Mineral Oil (D, C, Po, B, H, Sw, Sh, A) 935
Psyllium (D, C, H) 1180

ANTIDIARRHEALS
Bismuth Subsalicylate (D, C, B, H, Fer, Sw) 155
Clonidine (D, C) 321
Diphenoxylate/Atropine (D, C) 458
Kaolin/Pectin (D, C, Fer, Po, B, H, Sw, Sh, A) 760
Loperamide (D, C, Po) 818
Paregoric (D, C H, B) 1049

EMETICS
Apomorphine (D, C) 104
Hydrogen Peroxide % (D, C, Fer, Sw) 680
Xylazine (D, C, Po, Fer, A, B, H, Sh, L, Z) 1397

MISCELLANEOUS GI DRUGS
Bismuth Subsalicylate (D, C, Fer, B, H, Sw) 155
Budesonide (D, C) 167
Dirlotapide (D) 460
Glutamine (D, C) 637
Olsalazine Sodium (D) 1005
SAMe (D, C) 1221
Silymarin (D, C) 1235
Sulfasalazine (D, C, Fer) 1281
Ursodiol (D, C, A) 1367

Hormones/Endocrine/Reproductive Agents
SEX HORMONES, ESTROGENS
Diethylstilbestrol (DES) (D, C) 426
Estradiol (D, C, B, H) 530

SEX HORMONES, PROGESTINS
Altrenogest (D, H, Sw) 46
Medroxyprogesterone (D, C, H, A) 850
Megestrol Acetate (D, C) 853

SEX HORMONES, ANDROGENS
Danazol (D, C) 368
Methyltestosterone (D, C) 907
Mibolerone (D, C) 925
Testosterone (D, C, B) 1293

ANABOLIC STEROIDS
Boldenone (H, C) 160
Nandrolone (D, C, R) 974
Stanozolol (D, C, Fer, Po, H, Sh, A, R) 1255

POSTERIOR PITUITARY HORMONES
Desmopressin (D, C, H) 386
Vasopressin (D, C) 1375

OXYTOCICS
Oxytocin (D, C, Po, B, H, Sw, Sh, A, L, R) 1035

ADRENAL CORTICAL STEROIDS
Corticotropin-ACTH (D, C, B, H, A) 338
Cortisone Acetate (D) 340
Cosyntropin (D, C, H) 342

MINERALOCORTICOIDS
Desoxycorticosterone Piv. (D, C) 389
Fludrocortisone (D, C, Fer) 582

GLUCOCORTICOIDS
Betamethasone (D, H) 148
Dexamethasone (D, C, Po, B, H, Sw, L, A, R) 393
Flumethasone (D, C, H) 585
Fluticasone (D, C, H) 597
Hydrocortisone (D, C, B, H) 676
Isoflupredone (B, H, Sw) 733
Methylprednisolone (D, C, H) 903
Prednisolone (D, C, Po, Fer, B, H, L, Sw, A, R) 1139
Prednisone (D, C, Po, Fer, B, H, L, Sw, A, R) 1139
Triamcinolone (D, C, B, H) 1348

ADRENAL STEROID INHIBITORS
Ketoconazole (D, C, H, Po, A, R) 769
Metyrapone (C) 921
Mitotane (D, Fer) 945
Selegiline (D, C) 1225
Trilostane (D, C, H) 1354

ANTIDIABETIC AGENTS
Acarbose (D, C) 1
Chlorpropamide (D, C) 280
Chromium (C) 287
Glimepiride (C) 625
Glipizide (C) 626
Glyburide (C) 638
Insulin (D, C, Fer, B, H, A) 710
Metformin (C, A) 878
Vanadium (C) 1371

GLUCOSE ELEVATING AGENTS
Diazoxide, Oral (D, C, Fer) 414
Glucagon (D, C, B) 629
Octreotide Acetate (D, C, Fer) 1004

THYROID HORMONES
Levothyroxine (D, C, H, A, R) 801
Liothyronine (D, C) 812
Thyrotropin (D, A) 1311

ANTITHYROID DRUGS
Carbimazole (C) 201
Ipodate Sodium (C) 727
Methimazole (D, C) 886

PROSTAGLANDINS
Cloprostenol (D, B, H, Sw, Sh, L) 325
Dinoprost (D, C, B, H, Sw, Sh) 450

MISC. ENDOCRINE/REPRODUCTIVE DRUGS
Aglepristone (D, C) 22
Bromocriptine (D, C, H) 165
Cabergoline (D, C, A) 183
Chorionic Gonadotropin-HCG (D, C, Fer, Po, A, B, H) 284
Deslorelin (D, H) 385
Finasteride (D, Fer) 570
Gonadorelin (D, C, Fer, B, Sh) 647
Leuprolide (Fer, A) 792
Melatonin (D, C, Fer) 861
Metergoline (D, C) 876
Mibolerone (D, C) 925
Octreotide Acetate (D, C, Fer) 1004
Pergolide (H) 1079
Somatotropin (D) 1245

Anti-infective Drugs

ANTIPARASITICS

Albendazole (D, C, Po, B, Sw, Sh, A) 25
Atovaquone (D, C) 122
Clorsulon (B, Sh, L) 329
Dichlorvos (Po, Sw) 418
Diclazuril (D, C, H, B, Sh) 419
Diethylcarbamazine (D, C, Fer, B) 424
Diminazene (D, C, H, B, Sh) 448
Doramectin (D, C, B, Sw, Po) 476
Emodepside + Praziquantel (C, R) 497
Eprinomectin (C, H) 519
Epsiprantel (D, C) 520
Fenbendazole (D, C, Po, B, H, Sw, Sh, L, A, R, Z) 555
Furazolidone (D, C, H) 607
Imidocarb (D, C, Sh, H) 699
Ivermectin (D, C, B, Fer, Po, H, Sw, Sh, L, A, R) 753
Levamisole (D, C, Po, H, B, L, Sw, Sh, A, R) 794
Lufenuron (D, C, Po) 822
Meglumine Antimoniate (D) 857
Melarsomine (D) 859
Metronidazole (D, C, Fer, Po, H, A, R) 916
Milbemycin Oxime (D, C, R) 931
Miltefosine (D) 933
Morantel (B, Sh) 953
Moxidectin (D, C, Sh, L, H, B) 961
Nitazoxanide (D, C, H) 989
Nitenpyram (D, C, R) 991
Oxfendazole (D. H, B, Sw, Sh) 1020
Oxibendazole (H, B, Sw, Sh) 1022
Paromomycin (D, C, L, R) 1050
Piperazine (D, C, Po, H, B, Sh, Sw, A, R) 1118
Ponazuril (D, C, Po, H, L, A, R) 1126
Praziquantel (D, C, Po, Sh, L, A, R) 1133
Primaquine (C) 1147
Pyrantel (D, C, Po, H, Sw, B, L, A, Sh) 1182
Pyrimethamine (D, C, H, A) 1190
Pyrimethamine + Sulfadiazine (H) 1193
Quinacrine (D, C, R) 1195
Ronidazole (C) 1219
Selamectin (D, C, Fer, Po) 1223
Sodium Stibogluconate (D) 1242
Spinosad (D) 1250
Tinidazole (D, C, H) 1323
Trypan Blue (D) 1361

ANTICOCCIDIAL AGENTS

Amprolium (D, C, Fer, Po, B, Sw, Sh, L, A) 97
Decoquinate (D, B, Sh, L) 378
Diclazuril (D, C, B, Sh) 419
Toltrazuril (D, C, Sh, A, R) 1337

ANTIBIOTICS, AMINOCYCLITOLS

Amikacin (D, C, B, Fer, Fi, Po, H, A, R) 52
Apramycin (B, Sw, A) 106
Gentamicin (D, C, Fer, Po, H, Sw, A, R) 619
Neomycin (D, C, Po, Fer, B, H, Sw, Sh, A, R) 981
Spectinomycin (D, C, B, H, Sw, A) 1248
Tobramycin (D, C, H, L, A, R) 1327

ANTIBIOTICS, CARBAPENEMS

Ertapenem (D, C) 522
Imipenem-Cilastatin (D, C, H) 701
Meropenem (D, C) 874

ANTIBIOTICS, CEPHALOSPORINS

Cefaclor (D, C) 214
Cefadroxil (D, C, Fer) 216
Cefazolin (D, C, H, R) 218
Cefepime (D, H) 221
Cefixime (D, C) 223

Cefotaxime (D, C, H, A, R) 225
Cefotetan Disodium (D, C) 228
Cefovecin (D, C) 230
Cefoxitin (D, C, H) 232
Cefpodoxime Proxetil (D, C, H) 234
Ceftazidime (D, C, R) 236
Ceftiofur (D, C, A, B, Sw, Sh, H, R, Z) 239, 242, 245
Ceftriaxone (D, C, H) 249
Cefuroxime (D) 251
Cephalexin (D, C, Po, Fer, H, A) 253
Cephapirin (B) 256

ANTIBIOTICS, MACROLIDES

Azithromycin (D, C, H, Po, A) 138
Clarithromycin (D, C, Fer, H) 303
Erythromycin (D, C, Fer, A, B, H, Sw, Sh) 524
Tulathromycin (B, Sw, H) 1362
Tylosin (D, C, Fer, Po, B, Sw, Sh, A, R) 1364

ANTIBIOTICS, PENICILLINS

Amoxicillin (D, C, Po, Fer, B, H, A, R) 77
Amoxicillin/Clavulanate (D, C, Fer, A) 81
Ampicillin (D, C, B, H, Fer, Sw, Po, A, R) 90
Ampicillin/Sulbactam (D, C) 95
Cloxacillin (D, C, B) 331
Dicloxacillin (D, C) 422
Oxacillin (D, C, H) 1016
Penicillin G (D, C, Fer, Po, B, H, Sw, A) 1059
Penicillin V (D, C, H) 1065
Piperacillin (D, C, H, A, R) 1113
Piperacillin/Tazobactam (D, C, A) 1115
Ticarcillin/Clavulanate (D, C, H) 1313

ANTIBIOTICS, TETRACYCLINES

Chlortetracycline (D, C, Po, A, B, Sw) 282
Doxycycline (D, C, Po, H, A, R) 486
Minocycline HCl (D, C) 937
Oxytetracycline (D, C, B, Po, Sw, Sh, H, A, R) 1029
Tetracycline (D, C, Fer, Po, B, Sh, H, Sw, A) 1296

ANTIBIOTICS, LINCOSAMIDES

Clindamycin (D, C, Fer, A, R) 309
Lincomycin (D, C, Fer, Sw) 809
Pirlimycin (B) 1120
Tilmicosin (B, Sh, Po) 1320

ANTIBIOTICS, QUINOLONES

Ciprofloxacin (D, C, Fer, Po, A) 291
Danofloxacin (B) 369
Difloxacin (D, H) 429
Enrofloxacin (D, C, H, B, Fer, Po, R, A, L) 504
Ibafloxacin (D, C) 695
Marbofloxacin (D, C, R) 836
Orbifloxacin (D, C, H) 1012

ANTIBIOTICS, SULFONAMIDES

Sulfachlorpyridazine (B, Sw, A) 1269
Sulfadiazine/Trimethoprim (D, C, Fer, Po, B, H, Sw, A, R) 1271
Sulfamethoxazole/Trimethoprim (D, C, Fer, Po, B, H, Sw, A, R) 1271
Sulfadimethoxine (D, C, Fer, Po, B, H, L, R) 1276
Sulfadimethoxine/Ormetoprim (D) 1279

MISCELLANEOUS ANTIBIOTICS, ANTIBACTERIALS

Aztreonam (D, Fi) 141
Chloramphenicol (D, C, Po, Fer, H, A, R) 266
Clofazimine (D, C, A) 313
Dapsone (D, C, H) 374
Ethambutol (D, C, A) 533
Florfenicol (D, C, B, Sh, Sw) 575
Fosfomycin (D, H) 606
Isoniazid (D, C) 737
Methenamine (D, C) 884
Metronidazole (D, C, Po, Fer, H, A, R) 916
Nitrofurantoin (D, C, H) 992
Novobiocin (D, B) 1001
Rifampin (D, H, A) 1208
Sodium Iodide (D, C, B, Sh, H) 722
Tiamulin (Sw) 1312
Tinidazole (D, C, H) 1323
Vancomycin (D, C) 1373

ANTIFUNGAL AGENTS

Amphotericin B (D, C, H, Po, L, A, R) 84
Caspofungin (D, C) 213
Fluconazole (D, C, H, Po, A) 577
Flucytosine (D, C, A) 580
Griseofulvin (D, C, Po, B, Sh, H, Sw, A) 650
Itraconazole (D, C, Po, A, H) 748
Ketoconazole (D, C, Po, H, A, R) 769
Nystatin (D, C, H, A, R) 1002
Terbinafine HCl (D, C, A) 1289
Voriconazole (D, C, H, A) 1390

ANTIVIRAL AGENTS

Acyclovir (A, C, H) 20
Amantadine (D, C, H) 50
Famciclovir (C) 544
Interferon Alfa (D, C) 718
Interferon Omega (D, C) 721
Lysine (C) 824
Oseltamivir (D, H) 1004
Zidovudine (AZT) (C) 1406

Blood Modifying Agents

ANTICOAGULANTS/ANTITHROMBOTICS

Aspirin (D, C, Fer, Po, B, H, Sw, A) 112
Clopidogrel (D, C) 323
Dalteparin (D, C, H) 366
Enoxaparin (D, C, H) 502
Heparin (D, C, H) 661
Warfarin (D, C, H) 1393

ERYTHROPOIETIC AGENTS

Cyanocobalamin (D, C, H, Sw, B, Sh) 345
Darbepoetin (D, C) 376
Epoetin Alfa (Erythropoietin) (D, C, Fer, Po) 516
Ferrous Sulfate (D, C, B, H, Sw, Sh) 565
Folic Acid (D, C, H) 602
Iron Dextran (D, C, Fer, Sw, A) 731

MISC. BLOOD MODIFYING AGENTS

Aminocaproic Acid (D) 57
Filgrastim (D, C) 568
Gemfibrozil (D, C) 618
Hemoglobin Glutamer (D, C) 658
Pentoxifylline (D, H) 1076
Phytonadione (D, C, Po, H, B, Sw, Sh, A) 1107
Protamine Sulfate (D, C, B) 1176

FLUID & ELECTROLYTE MODIFIERS

Albumin (D, C) 28
Aluminum Hydroxide (D, C) 48
Butaphosphan (H, B, Sw, A) 176
Calcitonin (D, R) 185
Calcitriol (D, C) 187
Calcium Acetate (D, C) 189
Calcium Salts (D, C, B, H, Sh, Sw, A, R) 191
Dextran (D, C, B) 406
Dihydrotachysterol (D, C) 436
Ergocalciferol (D, C) 520
Etidronate (D, C) 537
Glycerine, Oral (D, C) 640
Hydroxyethyl Starch (D, C, H, A, L) 686
Lanthanum Carbonate (C) 783
Magnesium (D, C, B, H, Sh, Sw) 828
Mannitol (D, C, B, Sw, Sh, H) 832
Pamidronate (D, C) 1040
Phosphate (D, C, B, Sh) 1102
Potassium (D, C, H, B, Sh) 1128
Sevelamer HCl (D, C) 1230
Sodium Polystyrene Sulfonate (D) 1241

Antineoplastics

ANTINEOPLASTICS, ALKYLATING AGENTS

Busulfan (D, C) 174
Carboplatin (D, C, Po) 203
Chlorambucil (D, C, H) 263
Cisplatin (D, C) 297
Cyclophosphamide (D, C, H, Po) 348
Dacarbazine (D) 362
Ifosfamide (D, C) 697
Lomustine (D, C) 816
Mechlorethamine (D, C) 843
Melphalan (D, C) 867
Procarbazine (D, C) 1157
Thiotepa (D) 1309

ANTINEOPLASTICS, ANTIMETABOLITES

Cytarabine (D, C, H) 360
Fluorouracil (5-FU) (D, C, H) 592
Mercaptopurine (D) 873
Methotrexate (D, C) 895
Thioguanine (D, C) 1304

ANTINEOPLASTICS, ANTIBIOTICS

Bleomycin (D, C) 158
Dactinomycin (D) 364
Doxorubicin (D, C, Fer) 483
Streptozocin (D) 1259

ANTINEOPLASTICS, MITOTIC INHIBITORS

Vinblastine (D, C) 1382
Vincristine (D, C, H) 1384

ANTINEOPLASTICS, MISCELLANEOUS

Asparaginase (D, C) 110
Gemcitabine (D, C) 616
Hydroxyurea (D, C) 689
Mitoxantrone (D, C) 950
Piroxicam (D, C, H, Po) 1121
Toceranib (D) 1340

Immunomodulators

IMMUNOSUPPRESSIVE DRUGS

Azathioprine (D, C, Fer, H) 134
Cyclophosphamide (D, C, H, Po) 348
Cyclosporine (D, C) 352
Dexamethasone (D, C, Po, B, H, Sw, L, A, R) 393
Flumethasone (D, C, H) 585
Immune Globulin (Human), Intravenous (D) 706
Leflunomide (D, C) 788
Mercaptopurine (D) 873
Methotrexate (D, C) 895
Methylprednisolone (D, C, H) 903
Mycophenolate (D, C) 967
Prednisolone (D, C, Po, Fer, B, H, L, Sw, A, R) 1139
Prednisone (D, C, Po, Fer, B, H, L, Sw, A, R) 1139
Triamcinolone (D, C, B, H) 1348

GOLD COMPOUNDS

Aurothioglucose (D, C, H) 644
Auranofin (D, C) 131
Gold Sodium Thiomalate (D, C, H) 644

IMMUNOSTIMULANTS

Acemannan (D, C) 2
Mycobacterial Cell Wall Fraction Immunomodulator (D, H) 965
Parapox Ovis Virus Immunomodulator (H) 1048
Propionibacterium acnes Inj. (D, C, H) 1166
Staphylococcal Phage Lysate (D) 1258

Antidotes

Acetylcysteine (D, C, H) 15
Ammonium Molybdate (Sh) 76
Ammonium Tetrathiomolybdate (Sh) 76
Antivenin Black Widow Spider (D, C) 103
Antivenin Coral Snake (D, C, H) 101
Antivenin Crotalidae (D, C, H) 99
Atipamezole (D, C, Po, B, Sh, A, R, Z) 120
Charcoal, Activated (D, C, H, B, Sh) 260
Deferoxamine (D, C) 379
Dexrazoxane (D) 405
Dimercaprol (D, C, H, B, Sh, Sw) 443
Edetate Calcium Disodium (D, C, Po, H, A, B, Sw, Sh) 492
Ethanol (D, C) 535
Fat Emulsion, Intravenous 549
Fomepizole (D, C) 604
Leucovorin Calcium (D, C, H) 790
Methylene Blue (D, C, B, Sh, H) 899
Naloxone (D, C, Po, H) 970
Penicillamine (D, C, B, Sh, A) 1054
Physostigmine (D, H, B) 1105
Phytonadione (D, C, Po, B, H, Sw, Sh, A) 1107
Pralidoxime (D, C, B, Sh, H, A) 1131
Protamine Sulfate (D, C, B) 1176
Pyridoxine (D, C) 1187
SAMe (D, C) 1221
Silymarin (D, C) 1235
Sodium Polystyrene Sulfonate (D) 1241
Sodium Sulfate (B, Sh, Sw) 785
Sodium Thiosulfate (D, C, H, B, Sh) 1243
Succimer (D, C, A) 1261
Thiamine (D, C, B, H, Sw, Sh, L) 1301
Trientine HCl (D) 1353
Zinc Acetate/Sulfate (D, C) 1408

Bone/Joint Agents

Alendronate Sodium (D, C) 34
Allopurinol (D, A, R) 40
Glucosamine±Chondroitin (D, C, H) 634
Hyaluronate (D, H) 665
Etidronate (D, C) 537
Pentosan (D, C, H) 1074
Polysulfated Glycosaminoglycan (H, D, C, Po) 1124
Tiludronate Disodium (H) 1322

Dermatologic Agents (Systemic)

Acitretin (D, C) 18
Fatty Acids, Essential (D, C) 552
Isotretinoin (D, C) 744
Pentoxifylline (D, H) 1076

Vitamins & Minerals/Nutrients

Ascorbic Acid (C, Po, H, B) 108
Carnitine (D, C) 205
Cyanocobalamin (D, C, H, Sw, B, Sh) 345
Fat Emulsion, Intravenous 549
Fatty Acids, Essential (D, C) 552
Folic Acid (D, C, H) 602
Medium Chain Triglycerides (D) 849
Niacinamide (D) 987
Pyridoxine (D, C) 1187
Thiamine (D, C, B, H, Sw, Sh, L) 1301
Vitamin E/Selenium (D, C, H) 1388
Zinc (D, C) 1408

Cholinergic Muscle Stimulants

Edrophonium Chloride (D, C) 495
Pyridostigmine (D, C) 1185

Systemic Acidifiers

Acetazolamide (D, C, B, H, Sh, Sw) 10
Acetic Acid (B, Sh, H) 13

Systemic Alkalinizers

Sodium Bicarbonate (D, C, H, B, Sh, A) 1237

Unclassified

Aminocaproic Acid (D) 57
Colchicine (D, A) 335
Iohexol (D, C, A) 724

Index

NOW IN A FULLY UPDATED SEVENTH EDITION, Plumb's *Veterinary Drug Handbook* remains the most complete source of drug information relevant for animals available. Providing referenced dosing recommendations in each monograph, this book offers doses for a wide range of species, including dogs, cats, exotic animals, and farm animals, in a single resource. The book also includes detail on key aspects for appropriate use of each drug, including pharmacology, pharmacokinetics, contraindications, adverse effects, safety during pregnancy or nursing, overdoses, drug interactions, monitoring, chemistry and stability, storage, compatibility, and available products.

The seventh edition adds 22 new drug monographs, as well as updated dosages and information for existing drugs. A noteworthy feature is the Prescriber Highlights section found at the beginning of each monograph that allows readers a quick method of finding important information for that drug.

This is the 5 x 8-inch pocket size, offering convenience and ease of use; Plumb's Veterinary Drug Handbook is also available in the convenient 8½ x 11-inch desk size and as a mobile version. Plumb's exhaustive one-volume coverage of drugs approved for veterinary species and non-approved (human) drugs that are used in veterinary practices today make this book an essential reference for veterinarians, veterinary technicians, veterinary pharmacologists, pharmacists with veterinary patients, animal research or zoological facilities, and libraries that serve these groups.

Key Features

- Fully updated edition of the classic Veterinary Drug Handbook
- Features 22 new drugs, as well as updated dosages and information for existing monographs.
- Lists references after each monograph for easier access
- Offers current information on compounding stability for key drugs
- Provides detail on monitoring, chemistry, storage, and dosages
- A must-have reference for veterinarians and veterinary students

The Author

Donald Plumb was formerly Director of Pharmacy Services and Hospital Director at the University of Minnesota's Veterinary Medical Center. Now retired from the University of Minnesota, he focuses full-time on providing veterinary drug information to veterinarians, other health professionals, and animal caretakers.